THE METABOLIC BASIS OF INHERITED DISEASE

THE METABOLIC BASIS OF INHERITED DISEASE

EDITORS

John B. Stanbury, M.D.
Professor, Unit of Experimental Medicine
Department of Nutrition and Food Science
Massachusetts Institute of Technology
Faculty Member, Harvard-M.I.T.
School of Health Sciences and Technology

James B. Wyngaarden, M.D.
Frederic M. Hanes Professor of Medicine
Chairman, Department of Medicine
Duke University Medical Center

Donald S. Fredrickson, M.D.
Director of Intramural Research, and
Chief, Molecular Disease Branch
National Heart and Lung Institute
National Institutes of Health

Third Edition

McGraw-Hill Book Company
A Blakiston Publication

New York St. Louis San Francisco Düsseldorf Johannesburg Kuala Lumpur London
Mexico Montreal New Delhi Panama Rio de Janeiro Singapore Sydney Toronto

NOTICE

Medicine is an ever-changing science. As new research and clinical experience broaden our knowledge, changes in treatment and drug therapy are required. The editors and the publisher of this work have made every effort to ensure that the drug dosage schedules herein are accurate and in accord with the standards accepted at the time of publication. The reader is advised, however, to check the product information sheet included in the package of each drug he plans to administer to be certain that changes have not been made in the recommended dose or in the contraindications for administration. This recommendation is of particular importance in regard to new or infrequently used drugs.

THE METABOLIC BASIS OF INHERITED DISEASE

Library of Congress Catalog Card Number 76-163304

07-060724-9

5 6 7 8 9 0 DODO 7 9 8 7 6 5 4

This book was set in Times Roman by York Graphic Services, Inc., and printed and bound by R. R. Donnelley & Sons Company. The designer was Richard Paul Kluga; the drawings were done by John Cordes, J. & R. Technical Services, Inc. The editors were Paul K. Schneider and Stuart D. Boynton. Robert R. Laffler supervised production.

CONTENTS

LIST OF CONTRIBUTORS

HUGO AEBI, M.D.
Professor of Biochemistry, and Director, Medizinisch-Chemisches Institut, Bern University, Bern, Switzerland

K. FRANK AUSTEN, M.D.
Professor, Department of Medicine, Harvard Medical School; Physician-in-Chief, Robert B. Brigham Hospital; Physician, Peter Bent Brigham Hospital, Boston, Massachusetts

JAMES A. BAIN, Ph.D.
Professor, Department of Pharmacology, and Director, Division of Basic Health Sciences, and Associate Dean, School of Medicine, Emory University, Atlanta, Georgia

FREDERIC C. BARTTER, M.D.
Chief, Endocrinology Branch, National Heart and Lung Institute, National Institutes of Health, Bethesda, Maryland

ALEXANDER G. BEARN, M.D.
Professor and Chairman, Department of Medicine, Cornell University Medical College; and Physician-in-Chief, The New York Hospital, New York, New York

ERNEST BEUTLER, M.D.
Chairman, Division of Medicine, City of Hope Medical Center, Duarte, California; Clinical Professor of Medicine, University of Southern California, Los Angeles, California

ALFRED M. BONGIOVANNI, M.D.
William H. Bennett Professor and Chairman, Department of Pediatrics, University of Pennsylvania School of Medicine; and Physician-in-Chief, The Children's Hospital of Philadelphia, Philadelphia, Pennsylvania

MAURICE B. BURG, M.D.
Head, Unit on Renal Transport, Laboratory of Kidney and Electrolyte Metabolism, National Heart and Lung Institute, National Institutes of Health, Bethesda, Maryland

GEORGE F. CAHILL, Jr., M.D.
Professor, Department of Medicine, Harvard Medical School; Director, Elliot P. Joslin Research Laboratory; and Physician, Peter Bent Brigham Hospital, Boston, Massachusetts

HARTWIG CLEVE, M.D.
Associate Professor, Division of Human Genetics, Department of Medicine, Cornell University Medical College; and Associate Attending Physician, The New York Hospital, New York, New York

ALAN S. COHEN, M.D.
Professor, Department of Medicine, Boston University School of Medicine; and Head, Arthritis and Connective Tissue Disease Section, University Hospital, Boston, Massachusetts

RICHARD A. COOPER, M.D.
Assistant Professor, Department of Medicine, Harvard Medical School; and Chief, Hematology Division, Harvard Medical Unit, Boston City Hospital, Boston, Massachusetts

JOSEPH DANCIS, M.D.
Professor, Department of Pediatrics, New York University School of Medicine, New York, New York

ROBERT J. DESNICK, Ph.D.
The Dight Institute of Genetics, University of Minnesota School of Medicine, Minneapolis, Minnesota

ALBERT DORFMAN, M.D., Ph.D.
Richard T. Crane Distinguished Service Professor, and Chairman, Department of Pediatrics, Pritzker School of Medicine, University of Chicago, Chicago, Illinois

MARY L. EFRON, M.D.
Late Assistant in Neurology and Assistant Biochemist, Neurology Service, Massachusetts General Hospital, Boston, Massachusetts

ERIC ENGEL, M.D.
Professor, Department of Medicine, Vanderbilt University School of Medicine, Nashville, Tennessee

THOMAS B. FITZPATRICK, M.D., Ph.D.
Edward Wigglesworth Professor of Dermatology; Head, Department of Dermatology, Harvard Medical School; and Chief, Dermatology Service, Massachusetts General Hospital, Boston, Massachusetts

DONALD S. FREDRICKSON, M.D.
Director of Intramural Research, and Chief, Molecular Disease Branch, National Heart and Lung Institute, National Institutes of Health, Bethesda, Maryland

GEORGE W. FRIMPTER, M.D.
Professor, Department of Physiology and Medicine, and Head, Section of Genetics, University of Texas School of Medicine, San Antonio, Texas

E. RUDOLF FROESCH, M.D.
Associate Professor, Metabolic Unit, Department of Medicine, University of Zurich, Zurich, Switzerland

THEO GERRITSEN, D.Sc.
Associate Professor, Department of Pediatrics and Physiological Chemistry, University of Wisconsin School of Medicine, Madison, Wisconsin

H. GHADIMI, M.D.
Professor of Pediatrics, Downstate Medical Center, State University of New York, New York, New York; and Director, Department of Pediatrics, Methodist Hospital of Brooklyn, Brooklyn, New York

EGIL GJONE, M.D.
Professor of Medicine, Medical Department A, University Hospital, Rikshospitalet, Oslo, Norway

JOHN A. GLOMSET, M.D.
Research Associate Professor, Department of Medicine, and Regional Primate Research Center, University of Washington School of Medicine, Seattle, Washington

LEIV R. GJESSING, M.D.
Chief, Central Laboratory, Dikemark Hospital, Asker, Norway

ANTONIO M. GOTTO, Jr., M.D., Ph.D.
Head, Section on Molecular Structure, Molecular Disease Branch, National Heart and Lung Institute, National Institutes of Health, Bethesda, Maryland

GARY M. GRAY, M.D.
Associate Professor of Medicine, Division of Gastroenterology, Stanford University School of Medicine, Stanford, California

HOWARD H. HIATT, M.D.
Professor, Department of Medicine, Harvard Medical School; and Physician-in-Chief, Beth Israel Hospital, Boston, Massachusetts

MAHLON B. HOAGLAND, M.D.
Director, Worcester Foundation for Experimental Biology, Shrewsbury, Massachusetts

R. RODNEY HOWELL, M.D.
Associate Professor, Department of Pediatrics, The Johns Hopkins University School of Medicine, Baltimore, Maryland

CHARLES M. HUGULEY, Jr., M.D.
Professor, Department of Medicine (Hematology), Emory University School of Medicine, Atlanta, Georgia

R. G. HUNTSMAN, M.D., M.R.C.P., M.R.C.Path.
Reader in Haematology, University of London; and Honorary Consultant Haematologist, Lambeth and St. Thomas' Hospitals, London, England

JAMES H. JANDL, M.D.
George Richards Minot Professor of Medicine, Harvard Medical School, Boston, Massachusetts

JOHN B. JEPSON, M.A., B.Sc., D.Phil., F.R.I.C., F.I.Biol.
Professor, Courtauld Institute of Biochemistry, The Middlesex Hospital Medical School, London, England

KRISHNA KALYANARAMAN, M.D.
Research Fellow in Medicine, University of California School of Medicine, Los Angeles, California

ALAN S. KEITT, M.D.
Assistant Professor, Department of Medicine, University of Florida College of Medicine, Gainesville, Florida

WILLIAM N. KELLEY, M.D.
Associate Professor of Medicine, and Chief, Division of Rheumatic and Genetic Diseases, Department of Medicine, Duke University Medical Center, Durham, North Carolina

BERNARD KLIONSKY, M.D.
Professor of Pathology, University of Pittsburgh School of Medicine; and Director of Laboratories, Magee-Womens Hospital, Pittsburgh, Pennsylvania

W. EUGENE KNOX, M.D.
Professor, Department of Biological Chemistry, Harvard Medical School; and New England Deaconess Hospital, Boston, Massachusetts

STEPHEN M. KRANE, M.D.
Professor, Department of Medicine, Harvard Medical School; and The Arthritis Unit, Massachusetts General Hospital, Boston, Massachusetts

WILLIAM KRIVIT, M.D.
Department of Pediatrics, University of Minnesota School of Medicine, Minneapolis, Minnesota

BERT N. LA DU, M.D., Ph.D.
Professor and Chairman, Department of Pharmacology, New York University School of Medicine, New York, New York

HERMANN LEHMANN, M.D., Sc.D., F.R.C.P., F.R.I.C., F.R.C.Path.
Professor of Clinical Biochemistry and Honorary Director, Medical Research Council Abnormal Haemoglobin Unit, University of Cambridge, Cambridge, England

MORTIMER LEVITZ, Ph.D.
Professor, Department of Obstetrics and Gynecology, New York University School of Medicine, New York, New York

ROBERT I. LEVY, M.D.
Head, Section of Lipoproteins Molecular Disease Branch, National Heart and Lung Institute, National Institutes of Health, Bethesda, Maryland

JAMES LIDDELL, M.D., M.R.C.Path.
Consultant Chemical Pathologist, Guy's Hospital, London, England

CHARLES C. LOBECK, M.D.
Professor and Chairman, Department of Pediatrics, University of Wisconsin School of Medicine, Madison, Wisconsin

HARVEY S. MARVER, M.D.
Late Associate Professor of Medicine, Department of Internal Medicine, University of Texas Southwestern Medical School of Dallas, Dallas, Texas

REUBEN MATALON, M.D.
Assistant Professor and Joseph P. Kennedy, Jr. Scholar, Department of Pediatrics, Pritzker School of Medicine, University of Chicago, Chicago, Illinois

EZIO MERLER, M.D.
Department of Bacteriology and Immunology, Harvard Medical School; and The Children's Hospital, Boston, Massachusetts

HUGO W. MOSER, M.D.
Associate Professor, Department of Neurology, Harvard Medical School; and Neurologist, Massachusetts General Hospital, Boston, Massachusetts; and Assistant Superintendent, Walter E. Fernald State School, Waverley, Massachusetts

KAARE R. NORUM, M.D.
Associate Professor, Institute of Nutrition Research Medical School, University of Oslo, Oslo, Norway

WILLIAM L. NYHAN, M.D., Ph.D.
Professor and Chairman, Department of Pediatrics, University of California School of Medicine, San Diego, La Jolla, California

JOHN S. O'BRIEN, M.D.
Professor and Chairman, Department of Neurosciences, University of California School of Medicine, San Diego, La Jolla, California

JACK ORLOFF, M.D.
Chief, Laboratory of Kidney and Electrolyte Metabolism, National Heart and Lung Institute, National Institutes of Health, Bethesda, Maryland

CARL M. PEARSON, M.D.
Professor, Department of Medicine, University of California School of Medicine, Los Angeles, California

THOMAS L. PERRY, M.D.
Professor, Department of Pharmacology, Faculty of Medicine, University of British Columbia School of Medicine, Vancouver, Canada

MYRON POLLYCOVE, M.D.
Professor and Vice-Chairman, Department of Clinical Pathology and Laboratory Medicine, University of California School of Medicine, San Francisco; and Director, Clinical Laboratories, San Francisco General Hospital, San Francisco, California

JOHN T. POTTS, Jr., M.D.
Chief, Endocrine Unit, Massachusetts General Hospital, Boston, Massachusetts

WALTER C. QUEVEDO, Jr., Ph.D.
Professor, Department of Biology, Division of Biological and Medical Sciences, Brown University, Providence, Rhode Island

OSCAR D. RATNOFF, M.D.
Professor of Medicine and Career Investigator of the American Heart Association, Case Western Reserve University School of Medicine; and University Hospitals of Cleveland, Cleveland, Ohio

ALBERT E. RENOLD, M.D.
Professor of Clinical Biochemistry, and Director, Institut de Biochimie Clinique, Faculty of Medicine, University of Geneva, Geneva, Switzerland

FRED S. ROSEN, M.D.
Department of Pediatrics, Harvard Medical School; and The Children's Hospital, Boston, Massachusetts

LEON E. ROSENBERG, M.D.
Associate Professor, Department of Medicine and Pediatrics, Yale University School of Medicine, New Haven, Connecticut

SHAUN RUDDY, M.D.
Assistant Professor, Department of Medicine, Harvard Medical School; Associate Physician, Robert B. Brigham Hospital; and Investigator, Howard Hughes Medical Institute, Boston, Massachusetts

RUDI SCHMID, M.D., Ph.D.
Professor, Department of Medicine, University of California School of Medicine, San Francisco, San Francisco, California

JERRY A. SCHNEIDER, M.D.
Assistant Professor, Department of Pediatrics, University of California School of Medicine, San Diego, La Jolla, California; and Established Investigator of the American Heart Association

CHARLES R. SCRIVER, M.D.
Professor, Department of Pediatrics; and Associate Professor of Genetics (Human Sector), McGill University School of Medicine, Montreal, Canada

J. EDWIN SEEGMILLER, M.D.
Professor, Department of Medicine, University of California School of Medicine, San Diego, La Jolla, California

STANTON SEGAL, M.D.
Professor, Department of Pediatrics and Medicine, University of Pennsylvania School of Medicine; Senior Physician, Children's Hospital of Philadelphia; and Attending Physician, Medical Services, Hospital of the University of Pennsylvania, Philadelphia, Pennsylvania

DONALD W. SELDIN, M.D.
William Buchanan Professor of Medicine and Chairman, Department of Medicine, University of Texas Southwestern Medical School at Dallas, Dallas, Texas

VIVIAN E. SHIH, M.D.
Assistant Professor, Department of Neurology, Harvard Medical School; and Assistant in Neurology, Massachusetts General Hospital, Boston, Massachusetts

HOWARD R. SLOAN, M.D., Ph.D.
Head, Section on Genetics and Lipid Biochemistry, Molecular Disease Branch, National Heart and Lung Institute, National Institutes of Health, Bethesda, Maryland

LLOYD H. SMITH, Jr., M.D.
Professor and Chairman, Department of Medicine, University of California School of Medicine, San Francisco, California

JOHN B. STANBURY, M.D.
Professor, Unit of Experimental Medicine, Department of Nutrition and Food Science, Massachusetts Institute of Technology, Cambridge, Massachusetts; Faculty Member, Harvard-M.I.T. School of Health Sciences and Technology

WERNER STAUFFACHER, M.D.
Research Associate, and Associate Director, Institut de Biochimie Clinique, Faculty of Medicine University of Geneva, Geneva, Switzerland

DANIEL STEINBERG, M.D.
Professor, Department of Medicine; and Head, Division of Metabolic Disease, University of California School of Medicine, San Diego, La Jolla, California

HEDI SUTER
Associate, Medizinisch-Chemisches Institut, Bern University, Bern, Switzerland

KUNIHIKO SUZUKI, M.D.
Associate Professor, Department of Neurology, University of Pennsylvania School of Medicine, Philadelphia, Pennsylvania

YOSHIYUKI SUZUKI, M.D.
Instructor, Department of Neurology, University of Pennsylvania School of Medicine, Philadelphia, Pennsylvania
Present address: Department of Pediatrics, University of Tokyo, Faculty of Medicine, Tokyo, Japan

CHARLES C. SWEELEY, Ph.D.
Professor, Department of Biochemistry, Michigan State University, East Lansing, Michigan

KOUICHI R. TANAKA, M.D.
Professor, Department of Medicine, University of California School of Medicine, Los Angeles, California; and Chief, Division of Hematology, Harbor General Hospital, Torrance, California

SAMUEL O. THIER, M.D.
Associate Professor, Department of Medicine, University of Pennsylvania School of Medicine; and Associate Director, Medical Services, Hospital of the University of Pennsylvania, Philadelphia, Pennsylvania

FRANK H. TYLER, M.D.
Division of Metabolism, Department of Internal Medicine, University of Utah College of Medicine, Salt Lake City, Utah

WILLIAM N. VALENTINE, M.D.
Professor and Chairman, Department of Medicine, University of California School of Medicine, Los Angeles, California

HARRY A. WAISMAN, M.D., Ph.D.
Late Professor, Department of Pediatrics; and Director, Joseph P. Kennedy, Jr. Laboratories, University of Wisconsin School of Medicine, Madison, Wisconsin

D. J. WEATHERALL, M.D., F.R.C.P., M.R.C.Path.
Reader in Hematology, Department of Medicine, University of Liverpool School of Medicine; and Honorary Consultant Physician (Hematology), United Liverpool Hospitals and Liverpool Royal Infirmary, Liverpool, England

HIBBARD E. WILLIAMS, M.D.
Professor, Department of Medicine, University of California School of Medicine, San Francisco, California; Chief, Medical Service, San Francisco General Hospital, San Francisco, California

T. FRANKLIN WILLIAMS, M.D.
Professor, Department of Medicine, University of Rochester School of Medicine and Dentistry; Medical Director, Monroe Community Hospital; and Attending Physician, Strong Memorial Hospital, Rochester, New York

JEAN D. WILSON, M.D.
Professor, Department of Medicine, University of Texas Southwestern Medical School at Dallas, Dallas, Texas

ROBERT W. WINTERS, M.D.
Professor, Department of Pediatrics, College of Physicians and Surgeons, Columbia University, New York, New York

JAMES B. WYNGAARDEN, M.D.
Frederic M. Hanes Professor of Medicine, and Chairman, Department of Medicine, Duke University Medical Center, Durham, North Carolina

PREFACE

Twelve eventful years have passed since the first edition of *The Metabolic Basis of Inherited Disease* was published. The present edition has become necessary not only because of much new knowledge about the diseases described in the previous editions, but also because new discoveries have placed several other disorders among those due to inherited metabolic errors. Furthermore, many fundamental concepts in this field have undergone substantial transformation and development.

Perhaps the most significant emerging point of view is that inherited diseases of metabolism do not necessarily arise from unique errors in the genotype, but that a spectrum of clinical expression occurs because of multiple alleles for a given gene. The molecular base for this concept has been beautifully developed, for example, by Perutz and Lehmann in studies on the hemoglobin molecule. They have examined the structure and function of hemoglobin from samples of blood of patients with various hemoglobinopathies and have clearly demonstrated that the degree of functional impairment of the hemoglobin molecule is dependent upon the strategic location of a particular amino acid substitution or deletion, each by inference arising from a different mutational change in the corresponding DNA. The large number of variants of the glucose-6-phosphate dehydrogenase molecule offers another example. Thus, variability in clinical expression and severity of an inherited disease may arise in part from the existence of a series of slightly different but allelic genes, each of which is responsible for an altered enzyme (or structural protein), or in some cases for no gene product at all. Clearly, many patients previously classed as homozygotes for a given abnormality may in fact be heterozygous for two abnormal genes. Indeed it is now quite certain that similar minor and well-tolerated alterations in molecular structure provide for the normal inherited variations among individuals. Identification of the variations in molecular structure of the proteins which are involved in the inherited diseases is a formidable but realizable goal for the future.

Every chapter from the previous edition has been extensively revised and most have been completely rewritten. Rapid evolution in understanding of the nature of genetic control and expression has required a thorough rewriting of the introductory chapter on the variability of human inheritance. Progress in this field is so rapid that some of the tables may already be incomplete. Similarly, developments achieved in molecular biology have required extensive revision of the chapter on genetic information processing, and prodigious progress in the field of human chromosomal accidents has necessitated a completely new chapter on these congenital disorders.

A proliferation of diseases has required subdivision of old and addition of new chapters. In some instances what was thought to be a single disease now appears to be due to two or more different genetic defects, but with common or overlapping clinical expression. Examples are primary hyperoxaluria and galactosemia, each earlier thought to be a single disease entity but now subdivided into nonallelic forms arising from different enzyme defects with similar or identical phenotypic expression. New diseases closely related metabolically to those described in the previous edition have been defined. To the section on branched-chain amino aciduria in the earlier edition is now added hypervalinemia and isovaleric aciduria. New metabolic entities have been added to the syndrome of familial adrenal hyperplasia, and an extraordinary disorder of purine metabolism closely related to classic gout, the Lesch-Nyhan syndrome, has been identified and given status as a separate chapter. The nonspherocytic hereditary hemolytic anemias have now become a well-defined group of diseases which arise from a series of different defects in glycolysis in the erythrocyte. There has continued an awesome proliferation in the hemoglobin variants and in the glucose-6-phosphate dehydrogenase deficiency syndromes.

In addition to many new disorders which fall within the scope of the chapters of the previous edition, the present one includes 12 additional chapters on new diseases. Within the section on disorders related to amino acid metabolism there is now a chapter on the errors of propionate, methylmalonate, and vitamin B_{12} metabolism; one on hypersarcosinemia; and another on disorders of beta-alanine and carnosine metabolism. Disturbances in glycine metabolism are now treated in two chapters, one on nonketotic hyperglycinemia and another on familial iminoglycinuria. The section on abnormal lipid metabolism has been extensively reorganized, and chapters have been added on Krabbe's disease, lecithin:cholesterol acyl transferase deficiency, G_{M1} gangliosidoses, Wolman's disease, hepatic cholesteryl ester storage disease, normolipidemic xanthomatosis, and phytanic acid storage disease. Chapters on intestinal disaccharidase deficiencies and glucose-galactose malabsorption, and on the inherited abnormalities of the complement system have also been added.

The inevitability of continuing growth in the area covered by this volume is exhilarating, but has created problems for us as editors. We have again had to make arbitrary decisions concerning the choice of new subject matter. In general we have included those disorders for which there has been both good evidence for inheritance and sufficient information to localize the metabolic error within a biochemical area. Had time for preparation permitted, we should like to have included xeroderma pigmentosa, that extraordinary skin disease which reveals the intricate mechanism by which DNA is constantly monitored and repaired, as well as coverage of myeloperoxidase deficiency, lysosomal acid phosphatase deficiency, and several other diseases which have been the subjects of signal advances in recent times.

It is an unhappy task to record the deaths of six contributors to the first two editions of this book: Dr. Charles Burnett, Dr. Mary Efron, Dr. Harry Heller, Dr. Harvey Marver, Dr. Milton Shy, and Dr. Harry Waisman. Their influence continues in their fields of endeavor and in this book.

The value that resides in this book is directly traceable to the authority and competence of our contributors and their cooperation in seeking a uniformity of presentation, sophistication, and style. Without exception they have tolerated our questions and our suggestions and have sought with us to achieve clarity and to avoid ambiguity. Their willingness to take leave of busy schedules in order to write their chapters is an indication of their belief in the validity and importance of the study of the abnormal metabolism of inherited human disease.

It is a privilege to thank our secretaries, Mrs. Shirley Stratton and Mrs. Harriet Gordon, who have devoted countless hours to the production of this volume and have immeasurably lightened the burden of our task.

John B. Stanbury
James B. Wyngaarden
Donald S. Fredrickson

PART ONE

INTRODUCTION

CHAPTER ONE

INHERITED VARIATION AND METABOLIC ABNORMALITY

The Editors

This volume is concerned with the inherited variations of man which can be described in biochemical terms. Most of the variations included are diseases, in that they produce unpleasant symptoms, or unwelcome structural abnormalities, which impair the fitness of the individual. The etiologic agent of these disorders is the mutant gene. Attention is focused chiefly upon the mechanism by which the mutant gene produces clinical manifestations, and upon methods for interrupting that mechanism or compensating for it.

Some of the heritable diseases presented in this book are common; many are rare. The latter are important out of proportion to their numerical incidence, for they teach us much about the nature of normal metabolic events and their genetic controls. The details of many metabolic sequences and systems, of ganglioside catabolism or the clotting of blood, for example, first became visible through experiments of nature in which a specific biochemical reaction was faulty because of an inborn metabolic error. Studies of hereditary disorders continue to offer tantalizing clues to the understanding of metabolic regulation, growth, differentiation, cellular and humoral defenses, neoplastic transformation, and other fundamental biologic mechanisms.

GENETIC AND BIOCHEMICAL INDIVIDUALITY

The correct chromosome number of man was established as 46 by Tjio and Levan in 1956 [1]. The inheritance of man is determined by the information carried on these 23 pairs of chromosomes, which are estimated to contain 20,000 to 40,000 different gene pairs, or loci [2]. The structure of each gene is subject to variation. Variant genes of a given locus are called *alleles.* The cause of genetic heterogeneity, i.e., of differences among homologous gene pairs, is *mutation* of gene structure. Variations of chromosome content are introduced by *recombination,* a process in which genetic material is exchanged between homologous chromosomes during the pairing that takes place in meiosis, and perhaps on rare occasions by *translocation,* a process in which chromosomal breakage and reunion result in the insertion of whole segments of chromosomes in new positions within the same or another chromosome (intra- or interchromosomal translocation). Additional variation of the genetic constitution, or genotype, results from the *random distribution* ("independent assortment") of one member of each paired chromosome into daughter cells during reductive division of the germ cells. The interplay of all these forces provides each human being, except monovular twins, with a unique inheritance.

Certain genes specify the sequence of amino acids in proteins, others control the rates or times of protein synthesis. The immediate consequence of gene mutation is a change in quality or quantity of a specific protein. In recent years examination of the structure and properties of many proteins has disclosed an abundant degree of both qualitative and quantitative variation among healthy individuals. Many variations are trivial, lead to no recognizable biologic advantage or disadvantage, and are probably neutral from the evolutionary point of view. Others lead to some slight advantage in fitness or reproductive capacity in the heterozygous state, and produce a positive selection pressure in the population. The best-known example is the relative resistance to malignant tertian malaria of the person heterozygous for the sickle-cell hemoglobin trait. These observations provide a basis for an understanding of the structural and biochemical individuality of man. Structural individuality is everywhere visible. Biochemical individuality is exhibited in variations of protein composition, of constituents of tissues and body fluids, of quantitative needs for specific nutrients, pharmacologic responses to specific drugs, and numerous other ways.

In certain instances a mutation proves to be harmful to its bearer because the change in quality or quantity of protein results in a structural or functional change which reduces the fitness or reproductive capacity of the individual. Some mutations are deleterious in single dose, e.g., that causing acute intermittent hepatic porphyria. Others require a double dose, i.e., either the homozygous state (characterized by two *identical* mutant alleles at one locus) or the "compound heterozygous" state (characterized by two *different* mutant alleles at one locus), in order to produce deleterious effects. Harris [3] estimates that normal individuals may be heterozygous at perhaps as many as 16 percent of loci. It has also been estimated that the average healthy individual is a heterozygous carrier of at least three to five harmful mutations, of the type responsible in homozygous state for disorders described in this book. The majority of mutations responsible for genetic disorders are probably not fundamentally different in kind or mechanism from those that account for the subtle or even gross variation considered to fall within the range of normal for the species. Possible exceptions are those involving gross chromosomal damage, including certain translocations or deletions.

McKusick [4] has published a catalogue of Mendelian characteristics of man in which he lists 1,545 genetically determined variations reported until 1967. Most of these are diseases, usually rare and often involving many organ systems. In most of these disorders it is not yet possible to identify the product of the mutant gene, whose presence is suggested by the Mendelian distribution of the phenotype.

In only about 20 percent has a relation between a given gene and a particular metabolic function been recognized; in only about 10 percent is information sufficient to indicate that either the quality or the availability of a specific protein has been altered [5]. This volume treats chiefly this last subgroup of genetically determined disorders of man. In a limited number of these the precise structural modification of a protein is known, and from this information the specific modification of DNA structure can be deduced.

Few if any diseases are either wholly genetic or wholly environmental in their pathogenesis. Even such disorders as phenylketonuria and galactosemia are not exclusively genetic, for control of diet can induce important modifications in phenotype. The controversy of an earlier day between genetics and environment, nature and nurture, has been resolved: it is now widely appreciated that both factors are important and are coordinated.

HISTORICAL CONSIDERATIONS

Concept of Inborn Errors of Metabolism (Garrod)

Shortly before the turn of the present century Sir Archibald Garrod began his studies on alcaptonuria which were to culminate in his classic Croonian Lectures in 1908 [6] and in his monograph, *Inborn Errors of Metabolism,* which appeared in 1909 and again in 1923 [7].

Garrod had observed that patients with alcaptonuria [8] excreted large, rather constant quantities of homogentisic acid throughout their lifetimes, whereas other persons excreted none at all. He observed that this condition had a familial distribution and that while frequently one or more sibs were involved, parents and more distant relatives were always normal. He was particularly impressed by the fact that there was a high incidence of consanguine marriages in the parents of his patients, as well as in the parents of similar patients studied elsewhere. On conferring with Bateson, one of the earliest of the great school of British geneticists, Garrod learned that the situation could readily be explained as a recessive condition in terms of the recently rediscovered laws of Mendel [9, 10].

From his observations on alcaptonuria, albinism, cystinuria, and pentosuria, Garrod developed the concept that certain diseases of lifelong duration arise because an enzyme governing a single metabolic step is reduced in activity or missing altogether. Garrod viewed the accumulation of homogentisic acid in alcaptonuria as evidence that this substance is a normal metabolite in the dissimilation of tyrosine, and he correctly attributed its accumulation to a failure of oxidation of homogentisic acid. A half-century later Garrod's hypothesis was proved by the demonstration of unmeasurable activity of homogentisic acid oxidase in the liver of a patient with alcaptonuria [11].

Similarly, the failure of pigment formation in the skin in albinism, the excretion of large amounts of cystine in the urine in cystinuria, and the appearance of pentose in the urine in essential pentosuria were viewed by Garrod as the results of blocks in normal metabolic pathways. He attributed the first instance to failure of melanin formation and the other two to excretion of metabolites accumulating proximal to a metabolic block. His interpretation of the defect in cystinuria has required modification, but the prescience of his remaining hypotheses has been supported by subsequent studies.

Garrod's work was almost ignored by geneticists for a generation, but time has corrected this oversight; the importance of the contributions of Garrod in the history of genetics and inherited diseases is now acknowledged by all.

Genetic Information and Chemical Function

Studies on the inheritance of flower colors, initiated by a contemporary of Garrod, probably were the first to demonstrate genetic influence at the molecular level. These investigations, begun by Wheldale [12–14] and extended by Scott-Moncrieff [15], Lawrence [16], and others, mark the beginnings of biochemical genetics. The differences in color of the principal water-soluble plant pigments, the anthocyanins, were found to depend on methylation or hydroxylation at specific molecular locations. These pigment differences were recognized as inheritable characteristics attributable to variations of anthocyanin structures.

It is now known that a gene governing a given chemical step in the production of plant pigments exerts its influence by controlling the synthesis of the enzyme which catalyzes that step [17, 18]. The early intuition of Wheldale that inheritable differences in flower color correspond to specific differences in pigment molecules was clearly a forerunner of the concept that a single chemical reaction may be under the control of a specific genetic locus.

One Gene—One Enzyme Concept

The term *gene* was first applied to the hereditary determinant of a unit characteristic by Johannsen in 1911 [19]. The relationship between gene and enzyme attained clear definition in the one gene–one enzyme principle, first succinctly stated by Beadle in 1945 [20]. This formulation, now a biologic precept, emerged gradually from studies of eye color in the fruit fly, *Drosophila,* by Beadle and Tatum [21, 22] and Ephrussi [23]. It received extensive support from the classic studies of Beadle and Tatum on induced mutants of *Neurospora crassa,* in which the acquisitions of requirements for specific metabolites in the culture medium were traced to losses of single chemical transformations, each dependent on a different enzyme [22, 24].

The one gene–one enzyme concept which developed from these experiments has been well expressed by Tatum [25] as follows:

1. All biochemical processes in all organisms are under genic control.
2. These biochemical processes are resolvable into series of individual stepwise reactions.
3. Each biochemical reaction is under the ultimate control of a different single gene.
4. Mutation of a single gene results only in an alteration in the ability of the cell to carry out a single primary chemical reaction.

In recent years the one gene–one enzyme hypothesis has been made more precise [26], and extended to cover proteins that are not enzymes, as well as complex proteins composed of nonidentical polypeptide chains, linked in various ways. The functional unit of DNA which controls the structure of a single polypeptide chain is frequently called a *cistron* [27]. The one gene–one enzyme principle has been redefined as the *one cistron–one polypeptide* concept (see Chap. 2).

With the growth of knowledge of gene types and of control of gene action, exceptions to Tatum's last statement have emerged. Certain genes control the function of other genes, or specify the structure of RNA molecules concerned with general processes, rather than the synthesis of a particular protein. A proposed modification of the fourth item of Tatum's statement is given here; its justification follows in succeeding sections of this chapter, and in Chap. 2.

4. Mutation of a *structural* gene causes a change in structure of a specific protein and may affect the quantity of a limited number of other proteins. Mutation of a *control* gene alters the extent of function of one or more structural genes and therefore alters the amount of one or more proteins without changing their structure. Mutations of other types of genes may have a variety of complex effects, difficult to classify at present.

GENETIC CONTROL OF PROTEIN SYNTHESIS

Genetic Information

The gene is deoxyribonucleic acid, DNA. Its information is determined by the sequence of purine (adenine and guanine) and pyrimidine (cytosine and thymine) bases in the gene. DNA forms a template on which other nucleic acid molecules of precise structure are synthesized. The exposed surfaces of the purine of the DNA chain will pair only with pyrimidine bases, and the exposed surfaces of pyrimidine pair only with purine bases. These obligatory pairings are shown in Table 1-1. The constraints of pairing allow genes to specify the sequences of bases of complementary molecules of DNA or RNA. Gene replication depends on synthesis of complementary molecules of DNA. Growth, differentiation, and cell function depend on synthesis of complementary molecules of RNA.

Table 1-1. BASE PAIRINGS OF NUCLEIC ACID BIOSYNTHESIS

DNA → DNA	DNA → RNA
A-T	A-U
G-C	G-C
C-G	C-G
T-A	T-A

There are several types of RNA that serve different roles in the cell. A gene which specifies the sequence of amino acids in a protein is called a *structural gene.* Such a gene first transfers its information to a molecule of "messenger RNA," which carries the message to the ribosome where protein synthesis takes place. The insertion of a particular amino acid into a growing peptide chain is determined by a specific sequence of three nucleotides in the messenger RNA, which in turn reflects the genetic code for that amino acid in the DNA. The DNA and RNA triplet codes [28] for each of 20 amino acids are shown in Table 1-2. The ribosome on which protein synthesis occurs is composed of one-half protein and one-half "ribosomal RNA." Each ribosome contains over 50 types of proteins [29] which vary only slightly from species to species. Each ribosome contains two types of RNA, of about 16S and 23S respectively. The assemblage of amino acids into polypeptide chains involves one or more specific carrier molecules of "soluble" or "transfer RNA" for each amino acid. At least one specific transfer RNA exists for each RNA code word. Some have more than one [30], and mutant tRNAs are also known [31]. The base sequences of ribosomal and transfer RNAs are determined by specific genes with multiple representation in the genome. Among the recent triumphs of science are the isolation of a structural gene in 1969 [32] and the chemical synthesis in vitro of complete proteins (ribonucleases A and S) in 1969 [33] and of the gene for $tRNA_{alanine}$ in 1970 [34].

The transfer of information from DNA to RNA involves no change of language (nucleotide → nucleotide) and is called *transcription;* the transfer of information from RNA to polypeptide involves a new language (nucleotide → amino acid) and is called *translation.* Insofar as is presently known, this is the exclusive route of information flow in man. There is now evidence that certain RNAs may code for DNA, but this exception is presently limited to the action of some (not all) RNA viruses upon infection of mammalian cells. Those RNA viruses capable of this function are associated with induction of tumors in animals. This observation, first made by Temin in 1964 [35], and recently confirmed [36, 37], has exceedingly important implications.

Regulation of Gene Action in Bacteria

A central theme of modern biology involves regulation of transcription and of translation. The normal process of de-

Table 1-2. THE GENETIC CODE

First nucleotide	*Second Nucleotide*				*Third nucleotide*
	A or *U*	G or *C*	T or *A*	C or *G*	
A	**AAA** *UUU* Phe	**AGA** *UCU*	**ATA** *UAU* Tyr	**ACA** *UGU* Cys	A or *U*
or	**AAG** *UUC*	**AGG** *UCC* Ser	**ATG** *UAC*	**ACG** *UGC*	G or *C*
U	**AAT** *UUA* Leu	**AGT** *UCA*	**ATT** *UAA* Stop	**ACT** *UGA* Stop	T or *A*
	AAC *UUG*	**AGC** *UCG*	**ATC** *UAG*	**ACC** *UGG* Trp	C or *G*
G	**GAA** *CUU*	**GGA** *CCU*	**GTA** *CAU* His	**GCA** *CGU*	A or *U*
or	**GAG** *CUC* Leu	**GGG** *CCC* Pro	**GTG** *CAC*	**GCG** *CGC* Arg	G or *C*
C	**GAT** *CUA*	**GGT** *CCA*	**GTT** *CAA* Gln	**GCT** *CGA*	T or *A*
	GAC *CUG*	**GGC** *CCG*	**GTC** *CAG*	**GCC** *CGG*	C or *G*
T	**TAA** *AUU*	**TGA** *ACU*	**TTA** *AAU* Asn	**TCA** *AGU* Ser	A or *U*
or	**TAG** *AUC* Ile	**TGG** *ACC* Thr	**TTG** *AAC*	**TCG** *AGC*	G or *C*
A	**TAT** *AUA*	**TGT** *ACA*	**TTT** *AAA* Lys	**TCT** *AGA* Arg	T or *A*
	TAC *AUG* Met	**TGC** *ACG*	**TTC** *AAG*	**TCC** *AGG*	C or *G*
C	**CAA** *GUU*	**CGA** *GCU*	**CTA** *GAU* Asp	**CCA** *GGU*	A or *U*
or	**CAG** *GUC* Val	**CGG** *GCC* Ala	**CTG** *GAC*	**CCG** *GGC* Gly	G or *C*
G	**CAT** *GUA*	**CGT** *GCA*	**CTT** *GAA* Glu	**CCT** *GGA*	T or *A*
	CAC *GUG*	**CGC** *GCG*	**CTC** *GAG*	**CCC** *GGG*	C or *G*

Note: The DNA codons appear in boldface type; the complementary RNA codons are in italics. A = adenine, C = cytosine, G = guanine, T = thymine, U = uridine (replaces thymine in RNA). In RNA, adenine is complementary to thymine of DNA; uridine is complementary to adenine of DNA; cytosine is complementary to guanine, and vice versa. "Stop" = punctuation. The amino acids are abbreviated as follows:

Ala = alanine	Leu = leucine
Arg = arginine	Lys = lysine
Asn = asparagine	Met = methionine
Asp = aspartic acid	Phe = phenylalanine
Cys = cysteine	Pro = proline
Gln = glutamine	Ser = serine
Glu = glutamic acid	Thr = threonine
Gly = glycine	Trp = tryptophan
His = histidine	Tyr = tyrosine
Ile = isoleucine	Val = valine

velopment occurs by differential gene action, i.e., by activity of certain genes but not of others in particular tissues at particular times. The mechanisms controlling the switching of one gene on and another off at particular stages are unknown. Some insights are provided from studies of enzyme induction in bacteria, which show that certain genes have the function not of specifying the primary structure of a protein but of controlling the rate of synthesis of one or more proteins through regulation of the rate of production of specific messenger RNAs.

The conceptual base of the genetic regulation of protein synthesis was first clearly formulated by Jacob and Monod in 1961 [38]. They proposed a model for the control of structural gene activity, based chiefly on studies of the induction of enzymes concerned with metabolism of β-galactosides in an extensive series of mutants of *Escherichia coli.* In their model, messenger RNA synthesis by the structural gene is regulated by two types of control genes, called *operator* and *regulator* genes.

The operator gene, located adjacent to the structural gene, or perhaps constituting the first portion of it, controls the initiation of synthesis of messenger RNA. A single operator may control the transcription of one or of several contiguous structural genes. A group of contiguous genes regulated by a single operator is called an *operon.* An essential feature of the operator gene is that it affects only the adjacent structural gene or genes on the same strand of DNA, and has no effect on the homologous structural gene in diploid organisms.

The activity of the operator gene (or locus) is controlled by the regulator gene, which may be located some distance from the operator gene by genetic mapping techniques. The regulator gene determines the production of a specific substance called a *repressor.* The repressor can associate reversibly with the operator locus. Association blocks the initiation of transcription of the whole operon and thereby prevents synthesis of proteins governed by the structural genes comprising the operon. The repressor is capable of affecting both members of homologous operator genes of diploid organisms. In this model, regulation of transcription is negative; the structural gene is active in synthesis of messenger RNA unless inhibited by repressor [39].

Enzyme induction is brought about when an inducer, a low-molecular-weight compound, interacts with repressor, a protein, to cause a conformational change which results in its release from the operator locus. Conversely, *enzyme repression* occurs when an inactive product of a regulator gene, an aporepressor, is activated by combination with a small molecule (e.g., the end product of the metabolic sequence controlled by the genetic system in question) and rendered capable of blocking the synthesis of specific messenger RNA and specific protein.

The basic features of this model have now been confirmed by experimental observation. The repressor of the *lac* operon of *E. coli* [40] and that of the λ-phage [41] have been isolated and shown to be proteins capable of binding to the DNA of the operator locus and, in the case of *lac* repressor, of responding to inducer [42].

This model does not explain all bacterial regulation. There is evidence that certain inducible operons are controlled by positive regulators rather than by repressors [43]. The positive regulators are also thought to be protein products of specific regulatory genes, which in the presence of externally added inducer stimulate rather than inhibit the expression of the operon.

The synthesis of all types of cellular RNA is mediated by an enzyme, DNA-dependent RNA polymerase, of which mammalian cells possess more than one variety. A second protein component, called *sigma factor,* stimulates transcription, and determines which regions of DNA are transcribed [44–46]. Evidence suggests that sigma factor acts at the level of initiation of synthesis of RNA chains, and that there may be several, perhaps many, different sigma factors, each capable of selectively promoting transcription of specific genetic regions [47, 48]. Additionally a specific protein component, called *rho factor,* controls release of messenger RNA from its structural gene [49]. Sigma and rho factors thus become positive control elements of genomic transcription.

In addition, several factors have been identified which are required for initiating, elongating, and terminating new polypeptide chains in microbial systems [50]. These may be viewed as positive control elements of messenger translation.

Regulation of Protein Levels in Higher Organisms

In bacteria, protein synthesis occurs on a complex of DNA with messenger RNA, ribosomes, enzymes, and other substances involved in peptide bond formation. Regulation of transcription indirectly also regulates translation, because the half-life of messenger RNA is very short. In eukaryotic cells, the bulk of DNA is enclosed within the nuclear membrane, whereas the bulk of protein synthesis takes place in the cytoplasm. (Mitochondrial DNA and nuclear ribosomal protein synthesis are important but quantitatively minor exceptions.) Thus the site of transcription of the genetic message is separated from the site of translation of messenger RNA into protein.

Control of protein synthesis in eukaryotic cells is probably a very complex process, operating at many levels through coordinated mechanisms [50–53]. These may be viewed as consisting of pretranscriptional, transcriptional, posttranscriptional, translational, and posttranslational controls. This arbitrary scheme provides a convenient approach to discussion of this field.

Pretranscriptional Controls

One current hypothesis proposes that nuclear histones play a governing role in transcription in mammalian cells [54]. Histones are basic proteins of two types, arginine-rich and lysine-rich, which are complexed to the acidic phosphate residues of DNA. Expression of genetic information may require the uncovering of specific genes by removal of histones. There is a body of observation that associates acetylation [55] or phosphorylation [56] of histones with gene activation, perhaps in determining availability of DNA templates rather than their immediate function in RNA synthesis. The histones themselves do not possess enough structural diversity for serving as specific information carriers in nuclear function. Moreover, they do not appear to occupy the narrow groove of the DNA helix which is the site of reading by RNA polymerase [57].

Transcriptional Controls

In bacterial enzyme induction, the rate of synthesis of induced protein may be increased quite suddenly by more than a thousandfold, and in a fully induced organism the quantity of new enzyme may amount to 5 to 7 percent of the dry weight [58]. Nothing quite so startling takes place in higher cells; yet there is abundant evidence that regulation of gene activity underlies certain important adaptations and responses of cells of complex organisms. Enzyme induction or repression, operating by control of transcription, may result in changes of five- to twentyfold, rarely 100-fold, in activity of specific enzymes in response to dietary changes, hormone action, or drug administration [52, 53]. Examples include the decline in activity of a number of hepatic enzymes in the rat subjected to protein restriction. Refeeding of a diet rich in protein results in return of enzyme levels toward normal. In several instances it has been demonstrated that recovery is dependent on synthesis of new RNA and enzyme, and is not merely attributable to reduction of enzyme turnover [53].

A number of enzymes are induced by hormones. For example, hydrocortisone increases levels of tryptophan pyrrolase and tyrosine α-ketoglutarate aminotransferase in rat liver [59, 60] and in hepatoma cells in tissue culture [61–63]. Experiments with inhibitors suggest that the increase in rate of enzyme synthesis in cell and tissue cultures brought about by corticosteroids is proportional to the accumulation of new specific messenger RNA [64, 65]. Actions of other steroid hormones such as aldosterone, testosterone, and estrogens, and of polypeptide hormones, such as gonadotropins, follicle-stimulating hormone, and luteinizing hormone, also depend on alterations of gene activity for their effects in target tissues.

The mechanism of control of transcription in eukaryotic cells in unknown. Although there is much interest in applying the Monod-Jacob model of regulation of transcription in bacteria to the regulation of enzyme induction in mammalian cells, there is no experimental basis to justify this extension. Current postulates of structural, regulator, temporal, and organizational genes [66] or of sensor genes, integrator genes (i.e., regulator), receptor (i.e., operator), and producer (i.e., structural) genes operating as single or as overlapping batteries [67], are additional examples of attempts to construct models for the regulation of genetic events of complex organisms, on the basis of concepts developed in simple cells.

Cells of higher organisms probably possess very complex regulatory mechanisms for switching off large portions of the genome for long periods of time or indeed permanently. These mechanisms play critical roles in cell differentiation, which is almost certainly based on regulation of gene activity, so that for each state of differentiation a certain set of genes is active in transcription and other genes are inactive. The differentiation of sporulating cells, in which sigma factors determine which families of genes are transcribed [68], offers an interesting model of potential relevance to differentiation of eukaryotic cells.

Each mammalian cell contains approximately 1,000 times as many DNA nucleotide pairs as a bacterium—sufficient to code for 5 million cistrons per haploid genome [62]. The added complement of genes is presumably involved in specifying the primary structure of a larger array of proteins, and in guiding the complex problems of tissue and organ differentiation and architectural specification.

Posttranscriptional Controls

In analysis of the regulation of gene expression in higher organisms, it is also necessary to consider the role of giant DNA-like RNA (D-RNA) strands in the nucleus [69], the role of the 30S particles which contain most if not all of the nuclear D-RNA [70], and the recently postulated regulation of transport of messenger RNA across the nuclear membrane which involves selection of D-RNAs to be destroyed in the cell nucleus or transferred to the cytoplasm in packages called *informasomes* [71].

An additional pretranslational control concerns the stability of messenger RNA in the mammalian cell, in which the half-life of certain messengers is much longer than in bacteria. For example, hepatic [72] and brain [73] messenger RNAs have half-lives of 10 to 15 hr, and reticulocytes are capable of synthesizing hemoglobin for 72 to 96 hr after nuclear material has been extruded and messenger synthesis has ceased [74]. By contrast, when synthesis of new messenger RNA is inhibited in bacteria, the capacity to synthesize bacterial protein disappears in a few minutes [75].

Translational Controls

Translational control of protein synthesis is a new concept which rests on a developing body of evidence [50, 51]. Two examples will be given.

In rats depleted of protein and then refed, with concomitant administration of glucose, synthesis of serine dehydratase is blocked for 6 to 10 hr. During this time messenger RNA specific for the enzyme accumulates: glucose feeding blocks translation but not transcription [76]. The glucose effect is antagonized by glucagon, and cyclic AMP administration to intact rats increases synthesis of serine dehydratase [77]. This is a type of "catabolite repression" in a mammalian system, a process in which cAMP has been implicated in bacteria [78].

In the hepatoma tissue culture system, tyrosine amino transferase messenger RNA is stable, yet enzyme synthesis stops when steroid inducer is removed. This suggests that inducer is required for translation of amino transferase messenger. In addition, both in vivo and in vitro, large doses of inhibitors of RNA synthesis, such as actinomycin D or 5-fluorouracil, administered after enzyme induction is underway, further *increase* the synthesis of induced tyrosine amino transferase. Tomkins et al. [79] propose that the rate of translation of amino transferase messenger is normally limited by a labile "cytoplasmic repressor." They suggest that both the mRNA for the repressor and the repressor itself turn over much more rapidly than the mRNA for tyrosine amino transferase. Stimulation of enzyme synthesis in preinduced cells by inhibitors of RNA synthesis may result from inhibition of repressor mRNA formation, followed by rapid decrease in the total repressor messenger available. The requirement for continued presence of inducer in the stimulation of amino transferase synthesis suggests that inducer antagonizes the action of cytoplasmic repressor in this system.

In addition, specific factors are required for initiation of synthesis of new and complete proteins in mammalian systems as in bacteria. At least three factors, M_1, M_2, and M_3, are required for initiating new hemoglobin α and β chains [79*a*].

Posttranslational Controls: Regulation of Protein Turnover

The capacity of microorganisms to adjust rapidly to environmental change is largely dependent on regulation of synthesis of labile specific messenger RNAs for control of production of stable proteins. The capability for lowering enzyme content when the stimulus for high enzyme level is no longer present is met by simple dilution in rapidly dividing organisms. Specific messenger RNA is rapidly degraded when inducer is withdrawn, and the concentration of its protein product is progressively reduced throughout succeeding generations of daughter cells.

In cells of higher organisms the biologic half-lives of enzymes are relatively short compared with the longevity of the cell. The level of an enzyme is determined by the steady state, and changes of an enzyme level can be achieved by alteration of its rate of degradation as well as of its rate of synthesis. For example, a shift of rats from a high-protein diet to one of modest restriction results in a decline in arginase activity attributable to acceleration of the rate of degradation of the enzyme. When rats are then shifted to a starvation regimen, arginase activity increases because of total cessation of arginase turnover [80].

Mutations leading to increased enzyme lability are common, as for example in various types of human glucose-6-phosphate dehydrogenase deficiency. Mutations to increased stability are also known, though less common. One example is the Panay variant of G6PD [81]. Another is one variant of hypoxanthine-guanine phosphoribosyl transferase (HGPRT) deficiency [82]. A mutation that changes the rate of turnover of an enzyme may operate (1) by altering the properties of the protein as a substrate for degradation, (2) through an effect on concentrations of stabilizer molecules, or (3) by altering the activity of the degradative system itself. Knowledge of the mechanisms of control of enzyme turnover is limited at present.

Regulation of Enzyme Activity in Higher Organisms

The cell has intricate regulatory mechanisms for governing the activities of biosynthetic pathways. In 1954 Novick and Szilard [83] observed that a tryptophan auxotroph failed to accumulate a tryptophan precursor when the medium contained tryptophan. This suggested that tryptophan inhibits an early enzyme of its own biosynthetic pathway. In the first study of this type of metabolic control at the enzyme level, Umbarger [84] demonstrated that isoleucine specifically inhibits threonine deaminase, an enzyme which catalyzes an early reaction in isoleucine biosynthesis. He proposed a general mechanism of regulation in which the end product inhibits the first specific and essentially irreversible reaction of its own biosynthetic pathway. Almost simultaneously, Yates and Pardee [85] observed that pyrimidine ribonucleotides inhibit the initial reaction of pyrimidine biosynthesis. Numerous other examples have been described in higher organisms as well as in bacteria, and the Umbarger postulate has become a biologic precept. The terms *Novick-Szilard-Umbarger effect, feedback inhibition,* and *end-product inhibition* have been proposed for this phenomenon; end-product inhibition has become the favored term.

The fundamental characteristic of regulatory enzymes is their susceptibility to activation and inhibition by metabolites or cofactors that are not involved in the primary reaction. The kinetics of many regulatory enzymes are "abnormal," in that a plot of reaction velocity against substrate concentration is sigmoidal in shape. Regulatory enzymes are composed of subunits which interact with substrates or with inhibitors (negative effectors) or activators (positive effectors). There is often no structural similarity between effector and substrate molecules, and many regulatory enzymes can be made insensitive to end-product inhibitors by laboratory procedures which cause no loss of catalytic activity. This proves that substrate- and effector-binding sites are independent of one another. In aspartate transcarbamylase, the catalytic site and the regulator site are located on different subunits [86]. There is evidence for different conformational states of aspartate transcarbamylase in the presence and absence of specific ligands [87].

In 1963 Monod, Changeux, and Jacob [88] proposed that regulatory enzymes which undergo a conformational change when binding an inhibitor or activator be called *allosteric proteins.* The site at which such an inhibitor or activator was bound was called an *allosteric site,* and the conformational change which occurred in the protein was an *allosteric transition.*

There are two major models for enzyme regulation by allosteric transition. In one it is proposed that the change in enzyme conformation on binding of effector at the allosteric site alters the affinity of the enzyme for its substrate at the active site [89]. This model is an extension of Koshland's induced-fit hypothesis of substrate-enzyme interaction [90].

In the other, two conformational states of the enzyme are assumed to exist in equilibrium. One of these forms is catalytically active, the other is not. When allosteric inhibitor is present, it combines with the inactive form and thus traps the enzyme in a noncatalytic conformation [91]. This formulation assumes no interaction between binding sites. Changes of conformation are considered to be the result of tautomerism within the protein, rather than of catalyzed transformation.

Metabolic controls involving modulation of enzyme activity include many examples of activation as well as of inhibition. In some instances, the rationality of activation is understood easily, as in the activation of aspartate transcarbamylase (the first enzyme of pyrimidine biosynthesis) by adenosine-5′-triphosphate, which antagonizes the inhibition by cytidine-5′-triphosphate [92]. In others, such as the activation of acetyl–coenzyme A carboxylase by isocitrate [93], the role in the economy of metabolic regulation is still obscure.

There are a number of examples of mutations which have altered the susceptibility of regulatory enzymes to effector molecules in bacteria [94, 95], or Ehrlich's ascites cells [96]. Studies in fibroblasts have provisionally identified two patients with gout and purine overproduction in which end-product inhibition of purine biosynthesis appears to be reduced in effectiveness [97].

INHERITED DISORDERS AS ERRORS IN PROTEIN SYNTHESIS

Mutation

Point Mutation

Point mutations derive from changes affecting a single nucleotide. When the term *mutation* is used without further specification it usually refers to a *replacement,* a change in which one base has been substituted for another in DNA. Copy errors occur approximately once in 10^5 replications. A purine-purine or pyrimidine-pyrimidine substitution is called a *transition;* a purine-pyrimidine or pyrimidine-purine substitution is called a *transversion*. A variety of replacement mutagens and mechanisms of action are known, and are discussed in Chap. 2.

A second type of point mutation involves *insertion* or *loss* of a single base in DNA. Such mutations can be produced in bacteria or bacteriophage with acridine or proflavin [98]; they result in "frame-shift mutants." These polycyclic mutagens appear to intercalate covalently between the planar rings of successive nucleotide bases of DNA. As a consequence, during replication an extra, uncoded nucleotide may be incorporated to match the acridine in the template; or an intercalation in the growing replica may cause it to skip a nucleotide. For example, in a DNA segment of triplets -AAA-AGT-TCT-CTA-CCA-, corresponding to -Phe-Ser-Arg-Asp-Gly-, loss of "C" from the third triplet produces a new code segment, -AAA-AGT-TTC-TAC-CAX-, corresponding to -Phe-Ser-Lys-Met-Val-. Frame-shift mutations result in synthesis of a new amino acid sequence beyond the mutation. Unless the mutation is corrected by a second mutation within the same gene, for example, a loss followed by an insertion, with production of only a short altered polypeptide segment in a noncritical portion of the molecule, the new protein is apt to be nonfunctional.

From the viewpoint of the gene product, point mutations may, therefore, be of two varieties, *mis-sense* and *no-sense.* In mis-sense mutations a different amino acid is substituted at a given site in a particular protein. In no-sense mutations the change of base sequence in DNA is such that no protein is formed. A replacement mutation which changes CTT to CAT, or CTC to CAC, will cause a substitution of valine for glutamic acid in the protein product. This change is the one which occurs in the 6 position of the β chain of sickle-cell hemoglobin. Replacement mutations may alter the properties of the protein so drastically that it may be inactive as enzyme, may function with limited efficiency, may be unusually labile, or less soluble, or, if the substitution is in a noncritical region of the protein, perhaps cause little or no functional or physical change. The effects of replacement mutations are perhaps most explicitly understood with hemoglobin, the precise three-dimensional structure of which has been established. Perutz and Lehmann [99] have pointed out how known substitutions at specific loci might affect the structure and function of the molecule, and have correlated these changes with the clinical findings in patients homozygous for the mutant hemoglobin.

A no-sense mutation may result from any of several changes in the gene. The simplest change is perhaps a replacement mutation to a *non-sense DNA codon,* ATT, ATC, or ACT. For example, a mutation from ATA to ATT changes the information from "tyrosine" to "stop." Such a mutation results in premature termination of the polypeptide chain during its synthesis, with release of an incomplete protein, probably unrecognizable as enzyme by tests of functional activity. A no-sense mutation could also result from a frame-shift mutation which generates a non-sense codon through insertion or loss of a nucleotide. Finally, no-sense mutations may also result from *deletions,* mutations which consist of loss of more than one nucleotide—often hundreds or thousands of them. Deletions may involve a portion of one gene or all of several contiguous genes.

In general, mis-sense mutations are CRM-positive (pronounced "krim"), and no-sense mutations are CRM-negative. CRM means *cross-reactive material* and refers to protein which reacts immunologically with specific antibody developed against normal enzyme, whether or not it is functionally effective. The test is widely applied in bacterial genetics and is being used increasingly in the study of human mutations. For example, there are two types of hereditary angioneurotic edema due to deficiency of a normal serum inhibitor of C′l-esterase. In some families C′l-esterase inhibitor activity is greatly diminished and immunologic assays show a markedly reduced concentration of inhibitor (CRM-negative). Other families have no detectable inhibitor activity although normal levels of the protein can be demonstrated immunochemically (CRM-positive) [100]. Most patients with isolated growth hormone deficiency have no hormone detectable by immunoassay; these are CRM-negative cases. A few have immunologically detectable substance which is apparently nonfunctional as growth hormone; these are CRM-positive cases [101]. Both hemophilias A and B occur as CRM-negative and -positive varieties [102, 103].

The Structural-rate Hypothesis

A replacement point mutation may change a DNA codon without resulting in an amino acid substitution. For example, both GCA and GCC code for arginine. In terms of the primary structure of the protein, the mutation GCA → GCC is *silent.* If, however, *CGG* (the complementary messenger RNA codon) codes for a $tRNA_{Arg}$ present in very limited quantities, the limited availability of the latter tRNA could introduce a marked reduction in the rate of translation of the mutant (*CGU → CGG*) messenger RNA. This has been offered as one possible explanation of the observation that in patients heterozygous for the sickle-cell trait, sickle-cell hemoglobin always amounts to less than half the total [104]. In the homozygous state, such a mutation could in theory result in a severe deficiency or virtual absence of protein.

One human variant of glucose-6-phosphate dehydrogenase, G6PD Hektoen, which differs from normal G6PD in a single amino acid substitution, His → Tyr [105], is associated with a fourfold increase in rate of enzyme synthesis. This G6PD variant shows normal heat stability, pH optima, and K_m values for G6P and NADP [106]. This example indicates that a single-step base substitution in a structural gene may also result in an increase in synthesis of a variant protein. One potential mechanism is that discussed above, operating in the reverse of the direction cited in the example of sickle-cell hemoglobin.

Polarity Mutations

Genes are transcribed in one direction only, i.e., they have *polarity*. RNA-polymerase can initiate RNA synthesis only at certain segments, or starter points, of DNA, called *promoter regions* [107]. In the case of an operon, the synthesis of a long polycistronic messenger RNA molecule begins only at one promoter region adjacent to the operator locus, which may be the first portion of the most proximal structural gene of that operon.

Certain mutations within the operator locus will abolish synthesis of proteins of the entire operon. Similarly, certain mutations within a structural gene will reduce synthesis of all protein coded beyond the mutation. Most "polarity mutations" are caused by a mutation to a non-sense DNA codon [107] resulting from a single base replacement, insertion, or loss, or from a frame-shift mutation [108] resulting in a new "gibberish" code throughout the remainder of the polycistronic messenger RNA. However, some polarity mutations have proved to be due to chromosomal aberrations such as gross insertions or deletions [107].

Reversions

In a point mutation there is always a finite chance that a second mutation may occur at the site of the original mutation. If such a mutation corrects the genetic change, it is called a *reversion*. In fact, in bacterial systems point mutations are recognized by their ability to undergo true reversion, deletions by their failure to give rise to reversions.

Suppressor Mutations

The phenotypic expression of one mutation may be modified toward the normal by a second mutation. If a second mutation corrects the genetic change at a site different from the original mutation, it is called a *suppressor mutation*. Examples of suppressor mutations in human genetics include hemoglobin Harlem [109], in which a second mis-sense mutation has occurred in the β chain of hemoglobin S (Hb Harlem $\beta^{6\text{ Glu}\rightarrow\text{Val}}$, $\beta^{73\text{ Asp}\rightarrow\text{Asn}}$), and hemoglobin Memphis/S [110], in which mis-sense mutations are present in both the α and β chains ($\alpha^{23\text{ Glu}\rightarrow\text{Gln}}$, $\beta^{6\text{ Glu}\rightarrow\text{Val}}$). In both instances the deleterious effects of the sickle-cell gene have been ameliorated. Suppressor mutations may also operate by a variety of other mechanisms involving control of protein synthesis.

Nonhomologous Pairing and Unequal Crossing-over

During the meiotic process of gametogenesis, homologous chromosomes pair and exchange genetic material by a process called *crossing-over*. If the pairing is not precise, unequal crossing-over occurs and results in either deletion or duplication of genetic material. Certain mutant hemoglobins appear to have arisen by a process of deletion of a part of a gene or of two contiguous genes rather than from point mutations. In hemoglobin Gun Hill, amino acids 93 through 97 are missing from the β chain, so that this hemoglobin has only 141 residues, rather than 146 [111]. Hemoglobin Freiburg is missing residue 23 (valine) from its β chain [112]. Hemoglobin Lepore appears to be composed of the N-terminal portion of the δ chain and the C-terminal portion of the β chain. No normal δ or β chains are formed in homozygous individuals. The genes for the β chains of hemoglobin A and the δ chain of hemoglobin A_2 are probably contiguous. A fusion gene specifying a hybrid polypeptide of this type could have arisen by unequal crossing-over [113]. Two families with Lepore hemoglobin are known. The δ fraction of one Lepore hemoglobin is longer than the other [114].

Chromosomal Abnormalities

This class of mutations includes abnormalities of chromosome number (resulting from errors in chromosome segregation during cell division) and of chromosome structure (resulting from chromosome breakage). These may be associated with mild or severe abnormalities of somatic structure or development, but they have not been identified with disorders that can be assigned to an error of a single biochemical transformation. Many are known to be transmissible to the next generation, e.g., the D/G translocation associated with Down's syndrome. About one-fifth of spontaneous abortions show a detectable chromosomal abnormality. This group is discussed fully in Chap. 3.

Gene Duplication

Complete gene duplication may result from nonhomologous pairing and unequal crossing-over during recombination. A variety of other kinds of chromosomal rearrangement due to breaks and aberrant reunions and resulting in gene duplication may also be envisaged [115]. Complete gene duplication, however it comes about, is potentially of considerable evolutionary significance, for it is a process by which the organism can experiment in the evolution of new proteins, through mutation in one copy while retaining the essential function of the original gene. The gene products resulting from duplicate genes differ from one another according to the antiquity of the duplication. The concept can be illustrated effectively by considering the structurally similar polypeptide chains, α, β, γ, and δ, which occur in the A, A_2, and F forms of normal hemoglobin. There are extensive homologies in the amino acid sequences of these four polypeptides, which also show some degree of homology with myoglobin. These findings can be most simply accounted for by assuming that the genes which determine these proteins were originally derived from a common ancestral gene [116].

Gene duplication of more recent evolutionary occurrence may be envisaged in the case of the haptoglobins of man, in which the multiple polymers characteristic of types 2-2 and 2-1, attributed to sequentially aligned gene duplicates in the same chromosome, have not been found in comparative studies on a number of primate haptoglobins [117]. Or perhaps even more interestingly, a Melanesian population appears to have only a single Hb-α locus, whereas in populations of European origin, two Hb-α loci are believed to be present. Melanesians heterozygous for Hb $J_{Tongariki}$ ($\alpha^{115\ Ala \rightarrow Asp}$) have 45 to 50 percent of the Hb J component, and two subjects homozygous for Hb J have no Hb A[118]. By contrast, in Europeans and Americans heterozygous for α-chain variants, one usually finds only 20 to 30 percent of the abnormal component [114]. This suggests the presence of four Hb-α genes, only one of which has undergone mutation. The concept of duplicated α-chain loci receives strong support in a Hungarian family in which two distinct α-chain mutants were found together with normal Hb A in the same individual [119].

An estimate of the extent of gene duplication of structural genes of common proteins may be made from the study of nonallelic isozymes of erythrocytes conducted by Brewer and Sing [120]. They found evidence for two or more loci in 10 of 16 enzymes from human erythrocytes, and in 9 of 16 from sheep erythrocytes.

A rather special circumstance is proposed to explain the unique structural relationships of the γ-globulins. Both light and heavy chains have variable and constant sequence regions. The variable regions of the two chain types have a moderate degree of homology. The constant region of the heavy chain is divisible into three repeating homology regions, each of which has extensive homology with the others and with the constant region of the light chain. It is likely that a primitive C gene (C for constant segment) doubled and tripled, thereby forming a larger heavy-chain C gene whose segments then became somewhat different, as reflected in the amino acid sequences. By a similar process the two kinds of chains, heavy and light, appear to have had a common ancestor [121, 122]. The light chain is then coded by the V-C gene (V for variable segment), the heavy chains by a V′-C′-C″-C′″ gene. Each individual is capable of making several different immunoglobulins, composed of four types of heavy chains, (γ, α, μ, and δ) and two types of light chains (κ and λ). The variable regions of all types of light and heavy chains fall into a limited number of classes, which nevertheless may differ extensively one from another in different specific antibodies in any one individual. It is widely suspected that the number of different sets of molecules in the total immunoglobulin population of any one person is vast, numbering in the thousands or more. Three theories have been proposed to explain the diversity of variable regions [123]. (1) A large number of genes, one for each variable region, could have arisen in the course of evolution. (2) There could be one V gene which mutates in an individual's body cells during development to produce the required variety. (3) Several V genes could evolve by mutation, be selected during evolution, and then be recombined with C genes in many ways in the animal. The latter hypothesis is currently favored, and it is proposed that the required diversity of antibodies can be achieved by somatic recombination within a relatively small set of V genes, coupled with translocation and integration of a V gene into the C gene [123].

The discussion thus far has concerned gene duplications giving rise to gene multiples that are transmitted from one generation to the next and are subject to independent mutation. Another type of gene duplication has been proposed to account for the cytologic evidence from disparate sources that each unit of information encoded as a DNA base sequence is serially repeated. There is also chemical evidence in support of this concept. For example, RNA-DNA hybridization studies indicate that the genes for both 16- and 23S ribosomal RNA may be represented 100 times in the genome of the animal cell [124]. Callan [125] and Whitehouse [126] have proposed a master-slave gene model, in which the master gene is subject to mutation, recombination, replication, and transmission to progeny cells, and also subject to amplification to form a potentially large number of slave genes, not subject to recombination but made congruent to the master sequence once per life cycle. The formation of lateral lampbrush loops in meiotic prophase, after synapsis, is claimed to represent the outcome of the master-slave gene-matching process [125]. Maintenance of the identity of slave genes with the master gene of the family through the rectification process permits one to envisage numerous copies of any one gene within the cell, without postulating more "loci" than the number of master genes, for only master genes are in the chromatin and subject to recombination, whereas slave genes are removed from the chromatin at the time of crossing-over. Such removal could be brought about by a crossover between the first and last members of the linear series of identical genes. All except one would thereby be detached in the form of closed circles [126]. The postulate of multiple slave genes, all identical to the master gene, does not therefore lead to conceptual difficulty in explaining the heterozygous state, for all gene copies of the mutant allele would contain the same mutation, and a transmissible mutation could occur only within the master copy. This postulate could explain the very large number of presumably identical genes for ribosomal RNAs. If the process is general, it provides an explanation for the function of the bulk of the DNA of mammalian cells, which is fiftyfold in excess of the amount required to accommodate the postulated number of structural loci.

Isozymes

Isozymes are different molecular forms of an enzyme serving the same or a closely related function. The term is general and connotes no specific type of structural relationship between the protein species which may be observed to have similar enzyme activities. Isozymes may be generated in a number of different ways, which may conveniently be classified in three distinct categories [127].

1 *Multiple gene loci coding structurally distinct polypeptide chains of a protein.* In some cases the several polypeptides may be associated in various members of the set of isozymes, so that the individual isozymes vary in the particular combinations of polypeptides they possess. An example is the case of the five standard lactic dehydrogenase isozymes in which the A and B polypeptides form a tetramer series A_4, A_3B, A_2B_2, AB_3, and B_4 [128]. In other cases the polypeptide products of different loci may separately form the various members of the set of isozymes. This is probably the case with phosphoglucomutase, for which there are three distinct loci, at each of which multiple alleles occur, giving rise to a series of isozymes and extensive heterogeneity of the protein in the population [129, 130]. Individuals homozygous at all three loci show at least eight phosphoglucomutase isozymes. There is no evidence of hybrid isozyme formation between products of different loci. In an individual heterozygous at one of more loci—PGM_1, PGM_2, and PGM_3—the isozyme patterns are more complex.

2 *Multiple alleles at a single locus.* Heterozygotes, since they carry two different alleles, may be expected to show a more complex pattern of isozymes than homozygotes. The example already cited for any one PGM locus may be recalled. Heterozygosity at the PGM_1 locus gives rise to more than eight isozymes in one individual. Multiple alleles at this locus give rise to an array of isozymes in the population. At least eight alleles of PGM_1, five of PGM_2, and two of PGM_3 have been recognized [3].

3 *Secondary modifications of protein structure.* The complexity of isozymes of either category discussed above is further increased by the wide variety of structural changes which may modify the assembled protein. These may involve, for example, deamination of glutamine or asparagine residues, phosphorylation of serine residues, addition of carbohydrate groupings, removal of components of the polypeptide chain by proteolytic enzymes, and so on. Characteristic sets of isozymes, the several members of which all appear to be products of a single allele, have been observed in studies of allelic variants of phosphoglucomutase [3], adenylate kinase [131], adenosine deaminase [130], and peptidase B [132]. It is probable that the minor components of lactic dehydrogenase that are often found in addition to the five major tetrameric forms are attributable to secondary modifications of the primary protein products formed.

Qualitative Heterogeneity of Proteins

Understanding of genetic variation in a population will ultimately require disclosure of differences in sequences of nucleotides in the DNA of the cells of different persons, or if that is impossible, disclosure of sequence differences in messenger RNAs. At present these demonstrations are lacking, and inferences about gene differences must be drawn from observations of differences in qualities or quantities of proteins whose composition these nucleic acids determine. These inferences would be valid only if the distribution of the protein difference in families should be found to conform to genetic principles.

Table 1-3 lists human proteins of which more than one genetically determined variety is known [5, 133–135]. Most are associated with no discernible abnormality of phenotype. Most of these variants are demonstrated by electrophoresis, some by immunologic methods, at least one (hypoxanthine-guanine phosphoribosyl transferase) by heat stability, and

Table 1-3. PROTEINS IN WHICH GENETICALLY DETERMINED STRUCTURAL VARIATION HAS BEEN DEMONSTRATED IN MAN

Acetyl transferase	Hemoglobin, δ chain
Adenine phosphoribosyl transferase	Hypoxanthine-guanine phosphoribosyl transferase
Adenosine deaminase	Immunoglobulins, IgA (Am-1)
Adenylate kinase	Immunoglobulins, IgA (Am-2)
Albumin	Immunoglobulins, IgG, heavy chains (Gm)
Amylase	Immunoglobulins, IgG, light chains (InV)
Antihemophilic globulin	Lactate dehydrogenase, A chain
α_1-Antitrypsin	Lactate dehydrogenase, B chain
Carbonic anhydrase	β-Lipoprotein (Ag types)
Catalase	β-Lipoprotein (Ld types)
Ceruloplasmin	β-Lipoprotein (Lp types)
Cholinesterase (E_1 locus)	β-Lipoprotein (Lt types)
Cholinesterase (E_2 locus)	α_2-Macroglobulin (Xm)
Complement component C'1 esterase-inhibitor	Malate dehydrogenase, mitochondrial
Complement component C'3	Malate dehydrogenase, cytoplasmic
Complement component C'4	Methemoglobin reductase
Esterase (acetyl esterase)	Myoglobin
Factor VIII	Peptidase A
Factor IX	Peptidase B
Fibrinogen	Peptidase C
Galactose-1-phosphate uridyl transferase	Peptidase D
α_2-Globulin (PA types)	Peptidase E
α_1-Acid glycoprotein	Phosphate, acid
Glucose-6-phosphate dehydrogenase	Phosphatase, alkaline
Glutamic oxaloacetic transaminase, mitochondrial	Phosphoglucomutase-1 (PGM-1)
Glutathione reductase	Phosphoglucomutase-2 (PGM-2)
Glycoprotein, α_1-acid	Phosphoglucomutase-3 (PGM-3)
Group-specific component (GC)	6-Phosphogluconate dehydrogenase
Growth hormone	Phosphohexose isomerase
Haptoglobin, α chain	Prealbumin
Haptoglobin, β chain	Prothrombin
Hemoglobin, α chain	Pyruvate kinase
Hemoglobin, β chain	Tetrazolium oxidase
Hemoglobin, γ chain	Transferrin

Source: From McKusick [133], with additions.

Table 1-4. DISORDERS IN WHICH A DEFICIENT ACTIVITY OF A SPECIFIC ENZYME HAS BEEN DEMONSTRATED IN MAN

Condition	Enzyme with deficient activity
Acatalasia	Catalase
Acid phosphatase deficiency	Acid phosphatase
Adrenal hyperplasia I	21-Hydroxylase*
Adrenal hyperplasia II	11-β-Hydroxylase*
Adrenal hyperplasia III	3-β-Hydroxysteroid dehydrog.*
Adrenal hyperplasia V	17-Hydroxylase*
Albinism	Tyrosinase
Aldosterone synthesis, defect in	18-Hydroxylase*
Alcaptonuria	Homogentisic acid oxidase
Angiokeratoma, diffuse (Fabry)	Ceramide-trihexosidase
Apnea, drug-induced	Pseudocholinesterase
Argininemia	Arginase
Argininosuccinic aciduria	Argininosuccinase
Aspartylglycosaminuria	Specific hydrolase (AADG-ase)
Carnosinemia	Carnosinase
Cholesterol ester deficiency (Norum-Gjone disease)	Lecithin cholesterol acetyl transferase (LCAT)
Citrullinemia	Arginosuccinic acid synthetase
Crigler-Najjar syndrome	Glucuronyl transferase
Cystathioninuria	Cystathionase
Disaccharide intolerance I	Invertase
Disaccharide intolerance II	Invertase, maltase
Disaccharide intolerance III	Lactase
Formimino transferase deficiency	Formimino transferase
Fructose intolerance	Fructose-1-phosphate aldolase
Fructosuria	Hepatic fructokinase
Fucosidosis	Fucosidase
Galactokinase deficiency	Galactokinase
Galactosemia	Galactose-1-phosphate uridyl transferase
Gangliosidosis, generalized	β-Galactosidase
Gaucher's disease	Glucocerebrosidase
G6PD deficiency (favism, primaquine sensitivity, etc.)	Glucose-6-phosphate dehydrogenase
Glycogen storage disease I	Glucose-6-phosphatase
Glycogen storage disease II	α-1,4-Glucosidase
Glycogen storage disease III	Amylo-1,6-glucosidase
Glycogen storage disease IV	Amylo-(1,4 to 1,6)-transglucosidase
Glycogen storage disease V	Muscle phosphorylase
Glycogen storage disease VI	Liver phosphorylase*
Glycogen storage disease VII	Muscle phosphofructokinase
Glycogen storage disease VIII	Liver phosphorylase kinase
Gout, primary (one form)	Hypoxanthine-guanine phosphoribosyl transferase
Hemolytic anemia I	Adenosine triphosphatase
Hemolytic anemia II	Diphosphoglycerate mutase
Hemolytic anemia III	Glucose-6-phosphate dehydrogenase
Hemolytic anemia V	Glutathione reductase
Hemolytic anemia VI	Hexokinase
Hemolytic anemia VII	Pyruvate kinase
Hemolytic anemia VIII	Triosephosphate isomerase
Hemolytic anemia IX	Hexosephosphate isomerase
Hemolytic anemia X	Phosphoglycerate kinase
Histidinemia	Histidinase
Homocystinuria	Cystathionine synthetase
Hydroxyprolinemia	Hydroxyproline oxidase
Hyperammonemia I	Ornithine transcarbamylase
Hyperammonemia II	Carbamyl phosphate synthetase
Hyperglycinemia, ketotic form	Propionate carboxylase*
Hyperlysinemia	Lysine-ketoglutarate reductase
Hyperoxaluria, with I Glycolic aciduria	2-Oxo-glutarate-glyoxylate carboligase
II Glyceric aciduria	D-Glyceric dehydrogenase
Hyperprolinemia I	Proline oxidase
Hyperprolinemia II	δ-1-Pyrroline-5-carboxylate dehydrogenase*
Hypophosphatasia	Alkaline phosphatase
Intestinal lactase deficiency (adult)	Lactase
Isovaleric acidemia	Isovaleric acid CoA dehydrogenase
Leigh's necrotizing encephalomyelopathy	Pyruvate carboxylase
Lesch-Nyhan syndrome	Hypoxanthine-guanine phosphoribosyl transferase
Lipase deficiency, congenital	Lipase (pancreatic)
Lysine intolerance	L-lysine:NAD-oxido-reductase
Mannosidosis	α-Mannosidase
Maple sugar urine disease	Keto acid decarboxylase
Metachromatic leukodystrophy	Arylsulfatase A (sulfatide sulfatase)
Methemoglobinemia	NAD-methemoglobin reductase
Methylmalonic aciduria I	Methylmalonic CoA carboxymutase
Methylmalonic aciduria II	5′ Deoxyadenosylcobalamin synthetase*
Myeloperoxidase deficiency with disseminated candidiasis	Myeloperoxidase
Neonatal jaundice	Glutathione peroxidase
Niemann-Pick disease	Sphingomyelinase
Orotic aciduria	Orotidylic pyrophosphorylase and orotidylic decarboxylase
Pentosuria	L-Xylulose reductase
Phenylketonuria	Phenylalanine hydroxylase
Porphyria, acute intermittent	Uroporphyrinogen I synth.*
Porphyria, congenital erythropoietic	Uroporphyrinogen III cosynthetase
Pulmonary emphysema (one type)	α-1-Antitrypsin
Pyridoxine-dependent infantile convulsions	Glutamic acid decarboxylase*
Pyridoxine-responsive anemia	δ-Aminolevulinic acid synthetase*
Refsum's disease	Phytanic acid α-oxidase
Sulfite oxidase deficiency	Sulfite oxidase
Tay-Sachs disease	Hexosaminidase A
Testicular feminization	Δ^4-5α-Reductase
Thyroid hormonogenesis, defect in	Iodotyrosine dehalogenase (deiodinase)
Trypsinogen deficiency disease	Trypsinogen
Tyrosinemia I	Para-hydroxyphenylpyruvate oxidase
Tyrosinemia II	Tyrosine transaminase
Valinemia	Valine transaminase
Vitamin D–resistant rickets	Cholecalciferase*
Wolman's disease	Acid lipase
Xanthinuria	Xanthine oxidase
Xanthurenic aciduria	Kynureninase
Xeroderma pigmentosum	DNA-specific endonuclease

* Inferred from functional deficit. Specific assays not performed.

Source: From McKusick [133], with additions.

one (pseudocholinesterase) by difference of response to inhibitors. The tissue from which the protein was derived was most often serum (or plasma), and next most often, red blood cells. White blood cells, liver, placenta, and saliva have been the source of material in some instances. Multiple alleles have been demonstrated for many of these proteins [134, 135].

This list can be only a beginning, since these variants have been detected primarily in the more accessible tissues. Furthermore, the list is a product of the methods employed. The test of amino acid sequence has been most widely applied in the case of the variant hemoglobins. At least 22 amino acid substitutions are known for the α chain, 42 for the β chain, 3 for the γ chain, and 3 for the δ chain [114]. The array of variations of primary structure of immunoglobulins has already been cited. Though not inborn errors of metabolism of the type comprising this volume, the myeloma proteins constitute a special example of qualitative heterogeneity of proteins, since in all likelihood no two patients will produce precisely the same molecular species.

Sequence data on human mutant enzymes are limited, but two variants of glucose-6-phosphate dehydrogenase are known in which a single amino acid substitution occurs (GGPD-A variant, Asn $\rightarrow$ Asp [136]; GGPD-Hektoen, His $\rightarrow$ Tyr) [105]. Similarly, a mutant human erythrocyte carbonic anhydrase, Ic_{Guam}, differs from the normal enzyme by a single amino acid substitution, Gly $\rightarrow$ Arg [137]. A much larger body of information exists on the structure of mutant bacterial enzymes, in which genetic mapping and sequence data have provided a striking documentation of the principle of collinearity of gene and polypeptide structures [138].

Table 1-5. SOME BLOOD PROTEINS IN WHICH QUANTITATIVE ABNORMALITY HAS BEEN DEMONSTRATED

Protein	Phenotype
Albumin*	Analbuminemia
α_1-Antitrypsin*	α_1-Antitrypsin deficiency (degenerative lung disease)
C′1 esterase inhibitor*	Angioneurotic edema
C′2 complement component	C′2 complement component deficiency
Ceruloplasmin*	Wilson's disease
Growth hormone	Ateliotic dwarfism
Immunoglobulins	Immunoglobulin-deficiency disorders
Insulin	Childhood diabetes
α-Lipoprotein	Tangier disease (analphalipoproteinemia; high-density lipoprotein deficiency)
β-Lipoprotein*	Abetalipoproteinemia
Thyroxine-binding globulin (TBG)	*a.* Increased TBG *b.* Decreased TBG *c.* Absent TBG
Transferrin*	Atransferrinemia
Vitamin B_{12}–binding α-globulin	No phenotypic abnormality

*Also listed in Table 1-3.
Source: From McKusick [133], with additions.

Quantitative Heterogeneity of Proteins

Table 1-4 lists disorders in which a deficient activity of a specific enzyme has been demonstrated in man [133]. Tables 1-5 and 1-6 list blood proteins and clotting factors for which quantitative abnormalities have been observed [133].

Table 1-6. QUANTITATIVE VARIATION IN CLOTTING FACTORS IN PLASMA

Clotting factor	Other name(s) of clotting factor	Clinical name of deficiency state
Factor I	Fibrinogen	Afibrinogenemia
Factor II	Prothrombin	Hypoprothrombinemia
Factor V	Labile factor	Factor V deficiency (labile factor deficiency; Owren's parahemophilia)
Factor VII	Proconvertin	Factor VII deficiency (hypoproconvertinemia)
Factor VIII	Antihemophilic factor, or globulin (AHF, AHG)	*a.* Hemophilia A (classic hemophilia) *b.* von Willebrand's disease
Factor IX	Plasma thromboplastin component (PTC)	Hemophilia B (Christmas disease; PTC deficiency)
Factor X	Stuart-Prower factor	Factor X deficiency
Factor XI	Plasma thromboplastin antecedent (PTA)	Factor XI deficiency
Factor XII	Hageman factor	Hageman factor deficiency
Factor XIII	Fibrin-stabilizing factor; fibrinase	Factor XIII deficiency
Pechet's factor	....	Pechet's factor deficiency

Source: From McKusick [133].

The activity or availability of a protein may be reduced or increased for any of several reasons. The enzyme may be inhibited, activated, or stabilized in some way; the degradative system may be altered; or synthesis may be decreased or increased. It may be difficult to distinguish among these alternatives, especially when data on primary structure are not obtainable, and the distinction between allelism and genes at different loci may be impossible to make [5].

When the Jacob-Monod model of regulation of gene activity in the *lac* system of *E. coli* was first proposed in 1961, there followed immediately several applications of the concepts of structural and control genes to anomalies of human hemoglobins [139, 140] and the "missing-enzyme" diseases [141]. Zuckerkandl [142] even proposed the division of inborn errors into two large categories, called molecular diseases [143] and controller-gene diseases, to accommodate disorders in which protein structure was altered and disorders in which the protein was either missing or present in much reduced amount but presumably of normal structure.

This distinction has hueristic appeal, but the lesson of recent years is that it may be an untrustworthy distinction when casually made, for usually when steps have been taken to test the possibility, structural variations of the molecules have been found [5]. For example, certain of the catalase-deficiency variants with minimal residual activity have enzymes of abnormal electrophoretic mobility [144]. This is also true for many of the variants of G6PD with reduced activity [145] (see Chap. 55). In the Lesch-Nyhan syndrome, what was initially interpreted as a total absence of hypoxanthine-guanine phosphoribosyl transferase activity has now been shown to reflect the extreme instability of a mutant enzyme, which also shows no stabilization by substrate nor inhibition by nucleotides such as are found with normal enzyme [146, 147]. In xanthurenic aciduria and in cystathioninuria, the enzyme deficiency now appears to be a consequence of a structural change manifested as a marked decrease in affinity for a specific coenzyme, in these instances pyridoxal phosphate [148]. The occurrence of CRM-positive variants of "missing-protein" diseases of man has already been cited.

Even in those instances in which no protein is detected, either by assay or by immunologic search, one is not justified a priori in assuming a control-gene mutation. There are several types of structural-gene mutations which could order synthesis of a nonfunctioning protein or abolish specific protein synthesis altogether. A point mutation introducing an amino acid substitution having a critically deleterious effect on substrate binding, or causing the protein to assume an altered secondary, tertiary, or quaternary conformation, could appear to be a missing-enzyme disease by enzyme assay alone. A point mutation or a frame-shift mutation to a non-sense ("stop"—Table 1-2) RNA codon might lead to premature chain termination. Deletions or insertions arising from unequal crossing-over might shorten or lengthen polypeptide chains. Frame-shift mutations to a new triplet sequence might lead to synthesis of a novel polypeptide beyond the mutation. There are other possibilities whereby mutations could exert their effects on cell organization and activity. In spite of these precautionary statements, one may anticipate that in time a number of disorders of man will be firmly established as disorders of control genes, which must surely exist in higher organisms, even if they are as yet poorly defined.

The Operon Concept in Higher Organisms

The first attempts to apply the concept of regulatory genes to man were made by Ingram and Streeton [149], who suggested that the thalassemias might represent "tap" defects in which a mutation at a control gene somehow resulted in a reduced rate of synthesis of a hemoglobin chain of normal structure. The next efforts involved application of the concepts of Jacob and Monod [38] to the normal postnatal switching-off of synthesis of fetal hemoglobin ($\alpha_2\gamma_2$) and the switching-on of synthesis of adult hemoglobins $A(\alpha_2\beta_2)$ and $A_2(\alpha_2\delta_2)$ [150]. It was suggested that the closely linked β and δ genes were controlled by an adjacent operator gene. During fetal development the operator gene activates expression of β and δ chains, and as a secondary effect, it suppresses synthesis of γ chains in a reciprocal relationship. The gene for persistent fetal hemoglobin synthesis is considered to be allelic or closely linked to the β gene, and to involve a mutation of the operator gene, causing failure of normal activation of synthesis of β and δ chains [150]. In the homozygous state of persistent high fetal hemoglobin, no β or δ chains are synthesized [139]. The mutation proposed [150] was considered an analogue of the 0^- mutation of the lac operator of *E. coli* in which no lac operon proteins are synthesized [38, 39]. The persistent high-fetal-hemoglobin state could, however, be equally well explained by a structural gene mutation of the linked β/δ-gene loci, e.g., an extensive deletion. Currently the latter explanation is favored [150*a*].

The operon concept has also been invoked in hereditary orotic aciduria to explain the total deficiency of activity of two enzymes which catalyze successive steps in pyrimidine biosynthesis. The structural genes for these enzymes, orotidylic pyrophosphorylase and decarboxylase, are located within an operon in *E. coli* [151]. Both enzymes are decreased in activity to 20 or 25 percent of normal in human heterozygous carriers of the defect. It has been suggested that a mutation of a repressor or operator locus could explain these findings [152]. In tissue culture, fibroblasts of affected homozygotes also show markedly depressed activity values of both enzymes. However, when incubated with azauridine or barbituric acid they will develop normal activities of both enzymes with no change of the normal activity values of dihydro-orotic dehydrogenase, which catalyzes the preceding step of pyrimidine biosynthesis [153]. These results suggest that two structural genes are switched off in patients with orotic aciduria, and that they may be switched on in vitro by these pyrimidine analogues. It is not yet known whether the enzymes thus induced are structurally and functionally normal. Several alternative mechanisms not involving the operon concept also need to be considered, such as enzyme stabilization, induction of sigma factors stimulating mRNA synthesis at nonlinked loci, and stabilization of a polypeptide chain which is a component of two discrete enzymes. Nevertheless, at present the orotic aciduria syndrome represents one of the better candidates in human genetics for eventual explanation by the operon concept. The normal pyrophosphorylase activity with absence of only the decarboxylation function in one patient with orotic aciduria presumably represents a different mutation [154].

Evidence for polycistronic transcription in higher organisms is circumstantial [155]. In animal cells and in the cells of certain eukaryotic microorganisms, clusters of genes controlling either metabolic or morphologic units are known. Long stretches of DNA-like RNA are found in the nucleus [69, 70]. Against the concept in higher organisms are recent studies of Samarina et al. [70, 71], which suggest that only single cistron lengths of messenger RNA traverse the nuclear membrane. In addition, the average length of polyribosomes in animal cells suggests that single cistrons are the usual units of transcription.

Consequences of Metabolic Defects

The consequences of a genetic alteration in quality or quantity of a protein will depend on the role normally served by that protein. Disabilities based solely on defects of structural proteins will not be considered in this volume, even though a number of genetically determined disorders of this type are known. Certain disturbances of circulating transport proteins will be considered in detail. Included in this group are the disorders of hemoglobin (Chaps. 57 and 58), lipoproteins (Chap. 26), and other plasma proteins (Chap. 69). Also, a number of disorders to be considered fall into a category suggestive of defects of membrane transport. These may involve malfunctions of carrier substances serving quasi-enzymatic roles. The majority of the disorders included in this volume may be considered consequences of derangements of enzymatic function, or of defects of control of rates of reaction sequences. A brief inquiry into the potential consequences of enzymatic defects will provide an orientation for the chapters to follow.

Failure of Formation of a Specific Product

In the presence of a metabolic block, the product of the defective reaction will be reduced in quantity, or perhaps be absent altogether. Metabolites derived uniquely from this product will also be wanting. In a few circumstances failure of formation of a specific product explains the clinical manifestations of the disease and may be the most prominent diagnostic feature of the disorder. In von Gierke's disease, absence of glucose-6-phosphatase activity leads to hypoglycemia on fasting. Failure of specific steps in thyroxine or hydrocortisone synthesis leads to goitrous cretinism or the adrenogenital syndrome. In one type of albinism a defect in tyrosinase activity accounts for the failure of melanin formation.

Accumulation of Precursors of the Blocked Reaction

A metabolic block also results in accumulation of precursors of the defective reaction, or in excessive production of substances derived from these precursors through alternative pathways. If the accumulated metabolites are soluble, their concentrations in body fluids may be raised and their excretion in urine increased. In some instances, such as alcaptonuria, it is the immediate precursor of the blocked reaction, homogentisic acid, which accumulates and is excreted. In other circumstances where the reactions preceding the block are reversible, steady state factors may lead to accumulation of a more distant metabolite, such as lactate in von Gierke's disease. The precursors of the blocked reaction may undergo metabolic transformations to give increased production of products which are normally of minor quantitative significance. In phenylketonuria the block in phenylalanine hydroxylase activity results both in accumulation of phenylalanine and in gross overproduction of phenylketone products. In Type I hyperoxaluria a block in metabolism of glyoxylate leads to its excessive conversion to oxalate. A precursor of the blocked reaction may be stored if it is poorly soluble. The so-called thesauroses, or storage diseases, fall largely into this category. Among these are the disorders of lipid storage, the Hunter-Hurler group, and the glycogen deposition diseases. The "lysosomal diseases" may represent a special class, in which, for example, glycogen may accumulate because of a deficiency of a lysosomal enzyme (Type II, Chap. 7), or cystine may accumulate because of a postulated membrane transport defect (Cystinosis, Chap. 62).

Overproduction Diseases

There are no unequivocal examples of overproduction diseases attributable to excess activity of a regulatory enzyme as a direct effect of mutation. The marked increase in activity of ALA (δ-aminolevulinic acid) synthetase in acute intermittent hepatic porphyria, initially attributed to a possible operator-gene mutation [156], is now more plausibly assigned to enzyme induction by 5β-steroid metabolites [157], or to derepression secondary to a defect in heme synthesis (Chap. 45). If either of the latter mechanisms is correct, the reduced activity of the steroid Δ^4-5α-reductase [157] or of uroporphyrinogen I synthetase (Chap. 45) must be critical even in the heterozygous state, for the disease behaves as a dominant trait.

In the Lesch-Nyhan syndrome, and in one heterogeneous subtype of gout, a block in a purine-salvage pathway leads to enhanced purine biosynthesis because of increased availability of a precursor of the initial reaction of the chain, decreased end-product control of this reaction, or both [158]. These two diseases represent examples of disorders of enzyme synthesis on the one hand and enzyme control on the other, but in both instances these are epiphenomena, not direct consequences of the mutation.

EXPRESSION OF THE INHERITED METABOLIC DISORDERS

There is great variability in expression of different inherited metabolic defects and in the manifestations of the same defect in different individuals. Perhaps the simplest point of reference from which such variability may be considered is the degree of incapacitation of the affected individual.

Severity

Asymptomatic and without Consequence

Many disorders that are discovered accidentally may be classified simply as metabolic "variants." Examples of such trivial but informative conditions are pentosuria, most cases of fructosuria, β-aminoisobutyric aciduria [159], albumin B anomaly, and the curious inherited differences in ability to taste the thiourea derivatives [160].

Asymptomatic Except for Accidental Circumstances

Some of the inherited diseases become symptomatic only occasionally and then quite often because some accidental environmental circumstance has intervened. Trauma is required for expression of many of the inherited deficiencies in blood clotting factors. Several other diseases, such as hemolytic anemia associated with glucose-6-phosphate dehydrogenase deficiency or acute intermittent hepatic porphyria, may be revealed only by exposure to certain drugs. This category includes many of the inborn errors often referred to as "pharmacogenetic disorders."

Mild to Moderate

The inherited diseases are sometimes troublesome and symptomatic but compatible with long life and productivity. Patients with familial bilirubinemia are relatively asymptomatic unless they develop biliary stones. Acatalasia seems benign in the absence of nasopharyngeal infections. Alcaptonuria, gout, and even Gaucher's disease may pose little threat to a reasonably normal existence.

Severe to Lethal

Many of these conditions have severe consequences to the patient and may be lethal. Branched-chain amino aciduria and untreated phenylketonuria may be associated with irreversible changes in the central nervous system. The same is true of several of the lipid storage diseases, which are often fatal in infancy. The retarded development of congenital mutant cretinism may be irreversible. Severe hepatic and neurologic disturbances accompany Wilson's disease, and many of the organ systems of the body are severely damaged in hemochromatosis. The number of inherited metabolic disorders which are manifested only as abortion, miscarriage, or stillbirth is, of course, unknown.

For some mutations both the heterozygous and homozygous state cause sufficient disability to be considered disease. The homozygous state may be more severe but still compatible with life. An example is type II hyperlipoproteinemia.

Age of Onset

Though the fundamental defects in these disorders must be congenitally present, they do not necessarily become clinically evident at an early age. Failure to thrive and retardation in development may be apparent almost from the day of birth in patients with branched-chain amino aciduria, phenylketonuria, galactosemia, or metabolic cretinism. On the other hand, many of the hereditary metabolic diseases become fully manifest only in the adult. Several, such as gout, hemochromatosis, familial periodic paralysis, or some of the hyperlipoproteinemic states, rarely appear before the third decade.

The age of onset of the clinical manifestations of some of the heritable diseases bears a strong relationship to severity of the disease and to survival. In several of the lipid storage diseases, such as Niemann-Pick disease and Gaucher's disease, the expression of the defect during the infantile period when the brain is being actively myelinated results in much more serious disability and limitation of life. These storage disorders, of which Tangier disease is a particularly pertinent example, continue relentlessly throughout life, and their clinical effects tend to be cumulative, steadily worsening with time.

Conversely, some inborn metabolic diseases appear to improve as the patients become older. Galactosemic patients who survive their early years with the help of lactose-free diets may become more tolerant of milk as adults, although their uridine diphospho (UDP)-galactose transferase activity remains permanently missing. For unknown reasons, patients with adynamia episodica hereditaria and periodic paralysis also may cease having attacks in their later years.

Effects of Sex

Some of the inherited metabolic disorders are sex-linked. Hemophilia A, childhood muscular dystrophy, Fabry's disease, and the Lesch-Nyhan syndrome, for example, appear exclusively in hemizygous males and are transmitted by female carriers. The female heterozygote may display some features of the disease, presumably because of the inability of the normal X chromosome to compensate fully for the expression of those mutant X chromosomes not randomly inactivated during "lyonization." Thus, carriers of a gene defective for HGPRT whose fibroblasts are mosaics of cells able and unable to utilize hypoxanthine, being either normal or deficient in activity of hypoxanthine-guanine phosphoribosyl transferase [161], are frequently hyperuricemic [162]. Carriers of Fabry's disease may show corneal clouding, and perhaps minimal renal disease attributable to accumulation of small quantities of ceramide-trihexoside. Other disorders are sex-limited for reasons not always understood. For example, there is at present no good explanation for why hyperuricemia (other than X-linked varieties) occurs so predominantly in males. On the other hand, hemochromatosis is undoubtedly far more common in males because females have in the menstrual cycle a means of decreasing the iron available for tissue storage.

THE DIAGNOSIS OF METABOLIC DEFECTS

Identification of Accumulated or Missing Metabolite

The earliest recognized inborn errors of metabolism came to Garrod's attention because of the absence of melanin in albinism or the presence of an abnormal quantity of an unusual metabolite in pentosuria, cystinuria, and alcaptonuria. Identification of the specific metabolite depended on qualitative chemical tests and on preparation of derivatives which could be characterized by chemical or physical methods.

With the scientific and technologic advances of recent decades it is now possible to apply a sophisticated battery of laboratory procedures to the identification and elucidation of a suspected metabolic disorder.

Screening of Body Fluids for Abnormal Metabolites

Among the simple screening tests which exist for the presumptive identification of metabolic diseases are the ferric chloride test for phenylketonuria, the cyanide-nitroprusside test for disulfides such as cystine, and the phenylhydrazine test for keto acids.

More definitive tests involve application of paper, anion- or cation-exchange, or gas-liquid chromatographic procedures, coupled with appropriate staining, chemical, or optical methods for identification of the substances separated. The widespread use of chromatography has permitted delineation of a number of new amino acidurias, several of which were found by systematic screening of patients, particularly children, in mental institutions. The recent development of high-resolution column chromatographic analyzers of ultraviolet-absorbing materials [163] or carbohydrate-containing compounds [164] may well disclose a succession of new disorders.

Direct Enzyme Assay

Chemical identification of the accumulated metabolite has frequently led rather promptly to recognition of the site of the metabolic derangement and to confirmation by direct assay for activity of the suspect enzyme in appropriate tissue. Often full disclosure of the biochemical abnormality has had to await the elucidation of the normal pathways of synthesis and degradation of the compound. Indeed, metabolic errors have served as a stimulus for biochemists to define the related pathways of normal metabolism, as in the case of gangliosidoses. Only then has it been possible to demonstrate conclusively the site of the specific enzymatic deficiency.

Diagnosis by direct enzyme assay may be made on blood or on tissue obtained by biopsy. Samples of intestinal mucosa may be readily obtained at negligible risk, and biopsies of liver and thyroid have provided critical information in some instances in which it would have been unobtainable in any other way. A particularly useful technique is that of assay on white blood cells. These may be selectively concentrated and used to demonstrate a variety of disorders, such as the defect in maple syrup urine disease, methylmalonic aciduria, some of the glycogen storage diseases, orotic aciduria, and others. At least 35 disorders produce enzymatic or phenotypic abnormalities of the leukocyte [165]. An equally large number of inborn errors can be demonstrated in the red blood cells. Among these are deficiencies in 10 of 25 enzymes involving the glycolytic and oxidative pathways of glucose metabolism, acatalasia, other enzymatic disorders, and of course the hemoglobinopathies [114].

Identification of Protein Variants

Polymorphism of proteins has largely been detected on the basis of abnormal electrophoretic mobility, attributable to a change in net charge of the molecule. However, it has been estimated that only one-third of amino acid substitutions result in a charge difference and altered mobility of protein on electrophoresis [166].

In enzyme deficiency states in which some residual activity is detected, certain observations may suggest an enzyme variant rather than a reduction in number of normal enzyme molecules. Among these are changed electrophoretic behavior, abnormal kinetics disclosed by different Michaelis constants, altered response to substrates or cofactors, altered sensitivity to inhibitors, increased or decreased heat lability, or different pH optima. Immunologic procedures may disclose the presence of cross-reactive material, presumably representing a protein variant, in the absence of enzymatic activity. Combinations of these methods have revealed approximately 40 variants of erythrocyte glucose-6-phosphate dehydrogenase, each of which presumably represents a different amino acid substitution in a single polypeptide chain [145].

Sequence data disclosing differences, the ultimate demonstration of protein polymorphism, are available in an increasing number of variant proteins, including a limited number of enzymes. New techniques for isolating pure proteins in quantity based on the principle of affinity chromatography [166*a*] greatly increase the likelihood that the structural abnormalities in many more mutant proteins will be uncovered in the next few years.

Cell Culture Studies

The technology of cell culture has now progressed to the point where it is relatively easy to grow somatic cells in vitro. In recent years this technique has been widely exploited in the study of genetics of human disorders [167, 168]. Single cells can be isolated and cloned. Cultures can be synchronized for study of events of the cell cycle. Biochemical studies of varying levels of complexity can be performed on the cells. The full potential of cell culture in the study of hereditary disease is just being realized.

All lines of cultured mammalian cells perform a constellation of biosynthetic activities, including synthesis of purine and pyrimidine nucleotides, of 7 of the 20 structural amino acids, and of DNA, RNA, and protein. Many enzymes can be assayed, and their kinetic properties, inhibition characteristics, and thermal stabilities studied. The enzymatic defect of at least 25 inborn errors has been demonstrated in fibroblast cultures. In at least 15 others the morphologic appearance of the cultured cells is abnormal, and in some instances diagnostic for a specific disorder [165]. A particularly interesting observation is that of Fratantoni, Hall, and Neufeld [169], who found that the medium in which fibroblasts from a patient with Hurler's disease had grown was able to correct the defect in the cells from a patient with Hunter's disease, and conversely that the medium from Hunter's cells was able to correct the defect of Hurler's cells (cf. Chap. 49). In each case the metachromatic inclusion bodies which had accumulated during the first incubation disappeared during the second. These observations were the first to indicate the nature of the biochemical defects, viz., a deficiency of a different catabolic enzyme involved in mucopolysaccharide metabolism in each case. They furthermore provide a glimmering hope for a new approach to therapy, if a diffusible substance can correct the defect [170]. The fibroblast culture technique, unfortunately, is not applicable to the study of all inborn errors, since the metabolic activity at fault may not be a property native to the fibroblast. For example, phenylalanine hydroxylase activity is confined to the hepatic parenchymal cell; accordingly phenylketonuria cannot be diagnosed with fibroblast cultures.

A particularly interesting property of fibroblasts in culture has come to light recently. Normal skin fibroblasts can repair ultraviolet irradiation damage to DNA if the damaged segment is excised and new bases are inserted in the form of small patches [171]. Cells from patients with xeroderma pigmentosum carry a mutation that causes repair of DNA to be greatly reduced in comparison with normal fibroblasts. One of the enzymes involved in repair of DNA damage, viz., an endonuclease, is deficient in this autosomal recessive disease [172]. The relationship of failure of DNA repair in the skin to carcinogenesis, which occurs in sun-exposed areas of the skin of these patients, is not yet clear [173].

Cells in culture offer unique opportunities for testing genetic mechanisms. Five X-limited mutations have been used in cell cultures to test the single active X hypothesis of Lyon, and in every case random inactivation of either the paternal or maternal X chromosome in each cell of heterozygous females occurred. Similar inactivation does not occur in autosomal loci [168]. Nor does it appear that inactivation of one X is necessarily complete at all loci: present evidence suggests that both Xg(a) alleles are expressed in cells of heterozygous females [174].

Somatic cell hybrids whose nuclei contain genomes from different species, including serially propagatable hybrids of mouse and human fibroblast cells, have now been prepared in a number of laboratories [167, 168]. Following hybridization there is a gradual noncoordinate reduction in chromosome number in which human chromosomes are preferentially eliminated. This has made possible the identification of a chromosome of the E group (No. 17 or possibly No. 18) as that bearing the human gene for thymidine kinase [175], and of the C group as that bearing the gene for the A polypeptide of LDH (lactic dehydrogenase) [176], and for phosphoglucomutase (PGM_1) [177]. This technology opens the possibility of genetic mapping of the autosomes of man, a chore done painstakingly and only to a limited degree for the sex chromosomes heretofore. Patients with inborn errors of metabolism will furnish the cells which will contribute most to the exploitation of cell hybridization in the biocartography of the future.

This approach will then supplement pedigree data for assignment, and linkage studies for mapping, of the X chromosome; and cytogenic studies for associating abnormalities of specific metabolic functions with particular structural anomalies, such as linkage of the gene for the Duffy blood group to the region of secondary constriction of chromosome 1 [172]. Known chromosomal assignments of specific genes in man are summarized in Table 1-7.

Successful DNA-mediated transformation of a subline of human heteronuclear cells has been reported by Szybalska and Szybalski [187]. The recipient cells lacked hypoxanthine phosphoribosyl transferase activity, but after exposure to DNA from donor cells having catalytic activity for this enzyme, a fraction of them acquired ability to utilize hypoxanthine. The implications of this kind of experiment in the genetic engineering of the future are great indeed.

Prenatal Detection of Hereditary Defects

Certain inherited disorders can be detected with cells from amniotic fluid, which may be obtained safely as early as

Table 1-7. CHROMOSOMAL ASSIGNMENT OF SPECIFIC GENES IN MAN

Chromosome No.	Gene product, or phenotype	Ref.
1	Duffy blood group	[178]
	Congenital cataract	[179]
2/4	MN blood group	[180]
5	Triose-phosphate isomerase	[181]
6	Hageman factor	[182]
C-group (6–12)	LDH-A	[176]
	Phosphoglucomutase (PGM_1)	[177]
16	Haptoglobin	[183]
	HL-A	[184]
17 or 18	Thymidine kinase	[175]
18	IgA	[185]
X	A total of at least 68 phenotypes and specific gene products, including:	[4]
	Ceramide trihexosidase	
	Factor VIII	
	Factor IX	
	Glucose-6-phosphate dehydrogenase	
	Hypoxanthine-guanine phosphoribosyl transferase	[161]
	Phosphorylase kinase	[186]

the fifteenth week [188]. The primary cells obtained by centrifugation of fluid have limited value. Their chief use has been in sex determination by noting the presence or absence of a Barr body, the "resting" female chromosome. Far more information has been obtained by culture of the amniotic cells, which also eliminates any contamination from maternal cells. Culturing, by fostering cell division, permits karyotyping, and furthermore often allows the latent characteristics of the cell to emerge. A number of cases are on record of prenatal diagnosis of Down's syndrome on the basis of D/G translocation [189].

The most promising area of prenatal diagnosis involves biochemical studies of cultured cells. Accumulation of metachromatic granules in cells may indicate one of several hereditary storage diseases, such as a mucopolysaccharidosis, or cystic fibrosis [190]. Since metachromatic granules may appear in cultured cells rather nonspecifically [191, 192], one must at present interpret such a finding with great caution. Failure of detection of specific enzyme activity in cultured amniotic cells must also be interpreted conservatively and with full knowledge of the variability in maturation which is displayed by the enzyme in question at the stage in embryogenesis when the fluid was obtained. Prenatal diagnoses of the Lesch-Nyhan syndrome [193], galactosemia, Hurler's and Hunter's syndromes, cystic fibrosis of the pancreas, acid phosphatase deficiency, and Pompe's disease have already been made [158].

Amniocentesis involves minimal risk to the fetus. If a diagnostic tap is done at the fifteenth week of gestation, the 6-week delay required for culture of an adequate number of cells for biochemical study brings one only to the twenty-first week, when pregnancy may still be interrupted safely [188]. Karyotyping can be done earlier [217].

The development of appropriate standards for determining deficiencies in activity of various enzymes in cells derived prenatally is a paramount problem in the application of this important technique.

TREATMENT AND PREVENTION

Some of these diseases lend themselves unusually well to the ingenious employment of therapeutic maneuvers, and often the results are especially gratifying. In many conditions, however, there is as yet no specific therapy. The type of approach varies with the nature of the defect and the means available to overcome it.

Supplying the Missing Metabolite

When the metabolic block prevents formation of sufficient end product, the disease can sometimes be alleviated by supplying the needed metabolite. The macrocytic anemia of orotic aciduria is relieved by feeding cytidine and uridine. Much can be done to ameliorate metabolic cretinism if thyroxine is given sufficiently early. Administration of cortisone inhibits the stimulated pituitary of the adrenogenital syndrome, with gratifying relief of signs and symptoms.

Supplying the Vitamin Cofactor

A limited number of inherited abnormalities are manifested by responsiveness to pharmacologic doses of specific vitamins [148]. In some the nature of the defect is unknown, in at least two there appears to be a defect in conversion of vitamin precursor into its active form, and in several a defective enzyme with reduced affinity for its vitamin cofactor is suspected. Although in all cases the biochemical abnormality is correctable, clinical improvement does not necessarily ensue. For example, in homocystinuria the excessive quantities of homocystine respond to treatment with pyridoxine, but the structural abnormalities of this condition remain.

Limiting the Intake of a Precursor Which May Undergo Toxic Accumulation

It may be possible to withhold from the diet a substance which gives rise to toxic products because its metabolism is blocked [194]. Considerable success has attended the treatment of phenylketonuric children with diets low in phenylalanine. Phenylalanine itself is essential in only minute amounts, provided tyrosine is in adequate supply. Galactosemic children improve remarkably on lactose-free diets, and the toxic form of fructosuria can be prevented by avoiding fructose. Reducing the branched-chain amino acids is beneficial in branched-chain amino aciduria, as is reduction of the phytol precursor of phytanic acid in the diet of patients with Refsum's disease.

Use of Metabolic Inhibitors

In instances in which a metabolite accumulates as a consequence of a metabolic error it may be possible to control production by use of an appropriate metabolic inhibitor. Allopurinol is an effective inhibitor of xanthine oxidase and a successful agent for regulating production of uric acid in gout. Sodium hydroxymethane sulfonate, an inhibitor of an enzyme involved in conversion of glyoxylate to oxalate, is a possible prototype of a therapeutic agent in oxalosis [195]. Clofibrate, which inhibits synthesis or release of glyceride from the liver, is effective in reducing blood lipids to normal levels in type III hyperlipoproteinemia.

Depletion of Stored Substances

It is sometimes possible to deplete the body of a storage substance with toxic properties. Thus with British antilewisite (BAL) or with penicillamine, copper can be partially removed from the body, with benefit to the patient with Wilson's disease. Much can be done for hemochromatosis by frequent phlebotomy, and for gout with uricosuric substances such as probenecid and sulfinpyrazone which increase the elimination of uric acid. Urinary tract stones in cystinuria may be reduced with penicillamine by formation of the soluble mixed disulfide. Cholestyramine, capable of binding bile acids and of upsetting the balance between synthesis and catabolism of cholesterol, can reduce plasma cholesterol by 50 percent or more in heterozygotes with type II hyperlipoproteinemia.

Environmental Manipulation

The therapeutic resource in the group of patients with metabolic idiosyncrasy is obvious once the diagnosis has been made. The avoidance of drugs known to induce hemolytic anemia in sensitive patients is effective and readily achieved. Likewise, the avoidance of cholinesterase inhibitors in patients with pseudocholinesterase deficiency and of barbiturates in patients with porphyria is to be strongly recommended.

Induction of Metabolizing Enzymes

Phenobarbital and certain other drugs have the interesting property of stimulating production of increased amounts of smooth endoplasmic reticulum. One result is an increase in the rate of oxidation or conjugation of a variety of drugs and steroids. The stimulation of synthesis of enzymes of the endoplasmic reticulum is selective. For example, the activities of NADPH-cytochrome *c* reductase, cytochrome (s) P-450, and several drug-hydroxylating enzymes are increased four- to fivefold, whereas the synthesis of cytochrome b_5 is essentially unchanged, and that of certain membrane proteins is decreased [53]. Therapy of patients with unconjugated hyperbilirubinemia in a variant of the Crigler-Najjar syndrome [196], or with Gilbert's syndrome [197], may result in a fall in plasma bilirubin levels. Present evidence supports the view that phenobarbital administration has led to induction of hepatic glucuronyl transferase, although enzyme stabilization has not been excluded.

Supplying the Missing Protein

A limited number of inborn errors can be treated by administration of a missing enzyme or protein. Examples include treatment of agammaglobulinemia with γ-globulin, analbuminemia with albumin, hemophilia with antihemophilic globulin, and Fabry's disease with normal plasma [197*a*]. Treatment of Wilson's disease with ceruloplasmin has not been of value [198]. The mouth lesions of acatalasia could perhaps be treated by local application of catalase [199] or by transfusion of catalase-containing normal erythrocytes. Injection of protein as replacement therapy may result in antibody formation, as has been seen in some patients given parathormone or insulin.

Organ Transplantation

A potentially more permanent means of supplying the missing enzyme is transplantation of an appropriate organ from a normal individual. This approach will require further progress in breaking the immunologic barriers. Success may be anticipated chiefly in instances where the new organ can manufacture a critical circulating protein for export, e.g., antihemophilic globulin or γ-globulin; or in instances where the concentration of some diffusible metabolite, present in excess, can be brought down by its repeated transit in the blood through a competent organ.

Attempts at treatment of quite different inborn conditions by means of organ transplantation have been made. These include transplantation of the spleen in canine hemophilia [200] and classic human [201] hemophilia, of kidney in gout [202], oxalosis [203], and cystinosis [204], and of the thymus in di George's syndrome [205, 206]. Temporary successes have been reported.

The most daring experiments have involved transplantation of allogeneic marrow into patients with immunologic deficiency states, including lymphopenic hypogammaglobulinemia (Swiss type) and bone marrow aplasia [207] and Wiscott-Aldrich syndrome [208]. A limited number of successes has been achieved; graft-versus-host disease remains a serious problem, often precluding a permanently successful outcome.

Other Therapeutic Possibilities

Introduction of missing genetic material into cells through "genetic engineering" is currently much discussed, particularly in the lay press. The isolation [32] and chemical synthesis [34] of a gene have evoked both wonder and horror at the potentialities disclosed by these accomplishments. The feasibility of transformation of human cells has been disclosed by the experiments of Szybalska and Szybalski [187] already discussed. The demonstration of the capacity of certain RNA viruses to code for DNA synthesis [35–37], presently correlated with oncogenic potentiality, may also have opened avenues for genetic therapy. Rogers [209] has suggested that the apparently benign lifelong infection of laboratory workers with the Shope rabbit papilloma (DNA) virus which is associated in animals with elevated activity levels of arginase in epithelial cells [201], and, in animals and man with reduced blood arginine levels [211], might be considered as therapy in patients with argininemia who lack arginase activity.

A second major area of potential endeavor is the stabilization of mutant enzymes having increased turnover, either through use of pharmacologic agents designed for this task, or through inhibition of enzymes responsible for their degradation. It is possible that the responsiveness of certain disorders to administration of massive doses of cofactor vitamins may be brought about through enzyme stabilization.

Limiting the Frequency of Undesirable Genes

Since inherited metabolic diseases cannot yet be cured in a true sense, the reduction of incidence becomes mainly an exercise in eugenics. Perhaps ultimately the prevention of harmful mutations will become a clearly defined public health discipline.

Most of the diseases in this volume have an autosomal recessive pattern of inheritance. Care to exclude consanguine marriages in tainted families will cause these diseases, especially those with low gene frequency, such as phenylketonuria, to become increasingly rare, until the disease incidence is governed by the statistical risk of homozygosity in random matings and the equilibrium achieved between spontaneous mutations and gene loss. A lesser effect will be noted, of course, on the incidence of diseases with greater gene frequency, such as drug-induced hemolytic anemia.

Diseases with an autosomal dominant mode of inheritance generally are limited in incidence only by any decline in fecundity of patients with the disease. Here, too, the frequency of the disease in offspring and possibly a greater degree of severity in the presence of a double dose of the offending dominant gene are factors which may be influenced by the avoidance of doubly tainted matings.

The necessities of family counseling [212, 213] highlight the need for methods of identifying the heterozygous carrier of recessive traits. Considerable success has already been achieved. In some instances measurements of a specific metabolite or an enzyme activity in the presumed heterozygote have improved to the point where they can be clearly distinguished from the distribution of normal values. In the presumed heterozygote for cystathioninuria the excretion of cystathionine in the urine is elevated, but not so much as in the patient with the homozygous disease. In acatalasia type I, erythrocyte catalase activity values are approximately one-half normal in the heterozygous carrier. Ceramide trihexosidase activity in heterozygotes for Fabry's disease is low in plasma, as is the activity of hexosaminidase A in leukocytes in carriers of Tay-Sachs disease.

Additional tests for the heterozygous state depend mainly on detection of a failure to handle an abnormal load of substrate. Thus, in presumed heterozygotes for phenylketonuria, there is reduced tolerance to an administered load of phenylalanine, which is a better discriminant than the slight elevation of phenylalanine levels in the blood. Such tolerance tests detect heterozygotes only in instances in which the intermediate activity value of the enzyme being tested can be made limiting. This is often not possible. For example, in alcaptonuria one cannot detect heterozygotes this way. Even if the activity of homogentisic oxidase is presumed to be half-normal in liver of the heterozygote (this has not been studied), such a liver would be able to metabolize more than 500 gm homogentisic acid per day. The homozygote excretes only 2 to 10 gm per day. Detection of the heterozygote for accessible proteins which can be studied by physical methods has been highly successful. Thus the heterozygotes for the abnormal hemoglobins and for the diseases characterized by abnormalities of circulating plasma proteins are now routinely identified.

Heterozygous female sibs or daughters of mothers who have given birth to male children with the Lesch-Nyhan syndrome may be identified by study of fibroblasts in culture. The detection of cells lacking HGPRT (hypoxanthine-guanine phosphoribosyl transferase) activity may require preliminary incubation in a medium containing a toxic purine antimetabolite, such as thioguanine [214] or azaguanine [215], which will be destructive only to the normal cell capable of converting the analogue to its active ribonucleotide derivative.

It must be emphasized that the presence of a single gene for a recessive disease is not demonstrated conclusively by an abnormal result of a tolerance test or by a finding of depressed enzyme activity values alone. Such results must be correlated with pedigree data and, in addition, must be interpreted with care to exclude both nongenetic causes for the test abnormality and the homozygous state of a milder form of the disorder, as in the Duarte variant of galactosemia [216].

BIBLIOGRAPHY

1. Tjio, J. H., and Levan, A.: The chromosome number of man. Hereditas, **42,** 1, 1956.
2. Neel, J. V., and Schull, W. J.: *Human Heredity.* The University of Chicago Press, Chicago, 1954.
3. Harris, H.: *The Principles of Human Biochemical Genetics.* American Elsevier, New York, 1970.
4. McKusick, V. A.: *Mendelian Inheritance in Man: Catalogs of Autosomal Dominant, Recessive, and X-linked Phenotypes,* 2d ed., 521 pp. Johns Hopkins, Baltimore, 1968.
5. Childs, B., and Der Kaloustian, V. M.: Genetic heterogeneity. New Engl. J. Med., **279,** 1205–1212; 1267–1274, 1968.
6. Garrod, A. E.: Inborn errors of metabolism (Croonian Lectures). Lancet, **2,** 1, 73, 142, 214, 1908.
7. Garrod, A. E.: *Inborn Errors of Metabolism.* Oxford, London, 1923.
8. Garrod, A. E.: A contribution to the study of alkaptonuria. Proc. Roy. Med. Chir. Soc., n.s., **2,** 130, 1899.
9. Garrod, A. E.: The incidence of alkaptonuria: a study in chemical individuality. Lancet, **2,** 1616, 1902.
10. Mendel, G.: *Versuche über Pflanzenhybriden.* Engelmann, Leipzig, 1901.
11. La Du, B. N., Zannoni, V. A., Laster, L., and Seegmiller, J. E.: The nature of the defect in tyrosine metabolism in alcaptonuria. J. Biol. Chem., **230,** 251, 1958.
12. Wheldale, M.: On the nature of anthocyanin. Proc. Cambridge Phil. Soc., **15,** 137, 1909.
13. Wheldale, M.: Our present knowledge of the chemistry of the Mendelian factors for flower colour. Part I. J. Genet., **4,** 109, 1914.
14. Wheldale, M.: Our present knowledge of the chemistry of the Mendelian factors for flower colour. Part II. J. Genet., **4,** 369, 1915.
15. Scott-Moncrieff, R.: The genetics and biochemistry of flower color variation. Ergebn. Enzymforsch., **8,** 277, 1939.
16. Lawrence, W. J. C., and Price, J. R.: The genetics and chemistry of flower color variation. Biol. Rev., **14,** 35, 1940.
17. Jorgensen, E. C., and Geissman, T. A.: The chemistry of flower pigments in *Antirrhinum majus* color genotypes. III. Relative anthocyanin and aurone concentrations. Arch. Biochem. Biophys., **55,** 389, 1955.
18. Jorgensen, E. C., and Geissman, T. A.: The chemistry of flower pigmentation in *Antirrhinum majus.* II. Glycosides of PPmmYY, PPMMYY, ppmmYY, and ppMMYY color genotypes. Arch. Biochem. Biophys., **54,** 72, 1955.
19. Johannsen, W.: The genotype conception of heredity. Amer. Naturalist, **45,** 129, 1911.
20. Beadle, G. W.: Biochemical genetics. Chem. Rev., **37,** 15, 1945.
21. Beadle, G. W., and Tatum, E. L.: Experimental control of developmental reactions. Amer. Naturalist, **75,** 107, 1941.
22. Beadle, G. W., and Tatum, E. L.: Genetic control of biochemical reactions in *Neurospora.* Proc. Nat. Acad. Sci. U.S.A., **27,** 499, 1941.
23. Ephrussi, B.: Chemistry of "eye color hormones" of *Drosophila.* Quart. Rev. Biol., **17,** 327, 1942.
24. Beadle, G. W.: Genes and chemical reactions in *Neurospora.* Science, **129,** 1715, 1959.
25. Tatum, E. L.: A case history in biological research. Science, **129,** 1711, 1959.
26. Horowitz, N. H., and Leupold, U.: Some recent studies bearing on the one gene one enzyme hypothesis. Sympos. Quant. Biol., **16,** 65, 1951.
27. Benzer, S.: The elementary units of heredity, in *The Chemical Basis of Heredity,* edited by W. D. McElroy and B. Glass, p. 70. Johns Hopkins, Baltimore, 1957.
28. Frisch, L. (editor): The genetic code. Sympos. Quant. Biol., **31,** 762 pp., 1966.
29. Trout, R. R., Delius, H., Ahmed-Zadeh, C., Bickle, T. A., Pearson, P., and Tissières, A.: Ribosomal proteins of *E. coli:* stoichiometry and implications for ribosome structure. Sympos. Quant. Biol., **34,** 25, 1969.
30. Bergquist, P. L.: Degenerate transfer RNAs from brewer's yeast. Sympos. Quant. Biol., **31,** 435, 1966.
31. Carbon, J., Berg, P., and Yanofsky, C.: Missense suppression due to a genetically altered tRNA. Sympos. Quant. Biol., **31,** 487, 1966.
32. Shapiro, J., Machattie, L., Eron, L., Ihler, G., Ippen, K., and Beckwith, J.: Isolation of pure lac operon DNA. Nature (London), **224,** 768, 1969.
33. Marglin, A., and Merrifield, R. B.: Chemical synthesis of peptides and proteins. Ann. Rev. Biochem., **39,** 841, 1970.
34. Agarwal, K. L., Buchi, H., Caruthers, M. H., Gupta, N., Khorana, H. G., Kleppe, K., Kumar, A., Ohtsuka, E., Rajbhandary, U. L., Van de Saude, J. H., Sgaramella, V., Weber, H., and Yamada, Y.: Total synthesis of the gene for an alanine transfer ribonucleic acid from yeast. Nature (London), **227,** 27, 1970.
35. Temin, H. M.: The participation of DNA in Rous sarcoma virus reproduction. Virology, **23,** 486, 1964.
36. Baltimore, D.: RNA-dependent DNA polymerase in virions of RNA tumour viruses. Nature (London), **226,** 1209, 1970.
37. Temin, H. M., and Mizutani, S.: RNA-dependent DNA polymerase in virions of Rous sarcoma virus. Nature (London), **226,** 1211, 1970.
38. Jacob, F., and Monod, J.: Genetic regulatory mechanisms in the synthesis of proteins. J. Molec. Biol., **3,** 318, 1961.
39. Jacob, F., and Monod, J.: On the regulation of gene activity. Sympos. Quant. Biol., **38,** 193, 1963.
40. Gilbert, W., and Müller-Hill, B.: Isolation of the *lac* repressor. Proc. Nat. Acad. Sci. U.S.A., **56,** 1891, 1966.
41. Ptashne, M.: Isolation of the λ-phage repressor. Proc. Nat. Acad. Sci. U.S.A., **57,** 306, 1967.
42. Gilbert, W., and Müller-Hill, B.: The *lac* operator is DNA. Proc. Nat. Acad. Sci. U.S.A., **58,** 2415, 1967.
43. Sheppard, D., and Englesberg, E.: Positive control in the L-arabinose gene-enzyme complex of *Escherichia coli* B/r as exhibited with stable merodiploids. Sympos. Quant. Biol., **31,** 345, 1966.
44. Burgess, R. R., Travers, A. A., Dunn, J. J., and Bautz, E. K. F.: Factor stimulating transcription by RNA polymerase. Nature (London), **221,** 43, 1969.
45. Bautz, E. K. F., Bautz, F. A., and Dunn, J. J.: *E. coli* σ factor: A positive control element in phage T4 development. Nature (London), **223,** 1022, 1969.
46. Travers, A. A.: Bacteriophage sigma factor for RNA polymerase. Nature (London), **223,** 1107, 1969.
47. Travers, A. A., and Burgess, R. R.: Cyclic re-use of the RNA polymerase sigma factor. Nature (London), **222,** 537, 1969.
48. Sugiura, M., Okamoto, T., and Takanami, M.: RNA polymerase σ-factor and the selection of initiation site. Nature (London), **225,** 598, 1970.
49. Roberts, J. W.: Termination factor for RNA synthesis. Nature (London), **224,** 1168, 1969.
50. Lengyel, P.: The process of translation as seen in 1969. Sympos. Quant. Biol., **34,** 828, 1969.
51. Boyer, S. H.: An appraisal of genetic regulation of protein synthesis in higher organisms: 1969, in *Modern Trends in Human Genetics,* edited by A. E. H. Emery. Butterworth, London, 1970.
52. Wyngaarden, J. B.: Genetic control of enzyme activity in higher organisms. Biochem. Genet., **4,** 105, 1970.
53. Schimke, R. T., and Doyle, D.: Control of enzyme levels in animal tissues. Ann. Rev. Biochem., **39,** 929, 1970.
54. Georgiev, G. P.: Histones and the control of gene action. Ann. Rev. Genet., **3,** 155, 1969.
55. Allfrey, V. G.: Some observations on histone acetylation and its temporal relationship to gene activation, in *Regulatory Mechanisms for Protein Synthesis in Mammalian Cells,* edited by A. San Pietro, M. R. Lamborg, and F. T. Kenney, pp. 65–100. Academic, New York, 1968.
56. Langan, T. A.: Histone phosphorylation: stimulation by adenosine 3′,5′-monophosphate. Science, **162,** 579, 1968.
57. Simpson, R. T.: Interaction of a reporter molecule with chromatin: evidence suggesting that the histones do not occupy the minor groove of deoxyribonucleic acid. Biochemistry **9,** 4815, 1970.
58. Jacob, F., and Wollman, E. L.: *Sexuality and the Genetics of Bacteria.* Academic, New York, 1961.
59. Lin, E. C. C., and Knox, W. E.: Adaptation of the rat liver tyrosine-α-ketoglutarate transaminase. Biochim. Biophys. Acta, **26,** 85, 1957.

60. Knox, W. E., and Auerbach, V. H.: The hormonal control of tryptophan peroxidase in the rat. J. Biol. Chem., **214**, 307, 1955.
61. Thompson, E. B., Tomkins, G. M., and Curran, J. E.: Induction of tyrosine α-ketoglutarate transaminase by steroid hormones in a newly established tissue culture cell line. Proc. Nat. Acad. Sci. U.S.A., **56**, 296, 1966.
62. Tomkins, G. M.: Enzyme induction in tissue culture, in *Regulatory Mechanisms for Protein Synthesis in Mammalian Cells,* edited by A. San Pietro, M. R. Lamborg, and F. T. Kenney, pp. 269–282. Academic, New York, 1968.
63. Kenney, F. T., Reel, J. R., Hager, C. B., and Wittliff, J. L.: Hormonal induction and repression, in *Regulatory Mechanisms for Protein Synthesis in Mammalian Cells,* edited by A. San Pietro, M. R. Lamborg, and F. T. Kenney, pp. 119–142. Academic, New York, 1968.
64. Peterkofsky, B., and Tomkins, G. M.: Effect of inhibitors of nucleic acid synthesis on steroid-mediated induction of tyrosine aminotransferase in hepatoma cell cultures. J. Molec. Biol., **30**, 49, 1967.
65. Peterkofsky, B., and Tomkins, G. M.: Evidence for the steroid-induced accumulation of tyrosine-aminotransferase messenger RNA in the absence of protein synthesis. Proc. Nat. Acad. Sci. U.S.A., **60**, 222, 1967.
66. Paigen, K.: The genetic control of enzyme realization, in *Second International Conference on Congenital Malformations,* edited by M. Fishbein, pp. 181–190. International Medical Congress, Ltd., New York, 1964.
67. Britten, R. J., and Davidson, E. H.: Gene regulation for higher cells: a theory. Science, **165**, 349, 1969.
68. Losick, R., and Sonenshein, A. L.: Change in the template specificity of RNA polymerase during sporulation of *Bacillus subtilis.* Nature (London), **224**, 35, 1969.
69. Attardi, G., Parnas, H., Hwang, M., and Attardi, M.: Giant size rapidly labeled nuclear RNA and cytoplasmic messenger RNA in immature duck erythrocytes. J. Molec. Biol., **20**, 145, 1966.
70. Samarina, O. P., Lukanidin, E. M., Molnar, J., and Georgiev, G. P.: Structural organization of nuclear complex containing DNA-like RNA. J. Molec. Biol., **33**, 251, 1968.
71. Georgiev, G. P.: The regulation of the biosynthesis and transport of messenger RNA in animal cells, in *Regulatory Mechanisms for Protein Synthesis in Mammalian Cells,* edited by A. San Pietro, M. R. Lamborg, and F. T. Kenney, pp. 25–48. Academic, New York, 1968.
72. Revel, M., and Hiatt, H. H.: The stability of liver messenger RNA. Proc. Nat. Acad. Sci. U.S.A., **51**, 810, 1964.
73. Appel, S. H.: The turnover of brain messenger RNA. Nature (London), **213**, 1253, 1967.
74. Marks, P. A., Burka, E. R., and Schlessinger, D.: Protein synthesis in erythroid cells. I. Reticulocyte ribosomes active in stimulating amino acid incorporation. Proc. Nat. Acad. Sci. U.S.A., **48**, 2163, 1962.
75. Rouvière, J., Wyngaarden, J. B., Cantoni, J., Gros, F., and Kepes, A.: Effect of T_4 infection on messenger RNA synthesis in *Escherichia coli.* Biochim. Biophys. Acta, **166**, 94, 1968.
76. Jost, J. P., Khairallah, E., and Pitot, H. C.: Studies on the induction and repression of enzymes in rat liver. V. Regulation of the rate of synthesis and degradation of serine dehydratase by dietary amino acids and glucose. J. Biol. Chem., **243**, 3057, 1968.
77. Jost, J. P., Hsie, A., Hughes, S. D., and Ryan, L.: Role of cyclic adenosine 3′,5′-monophosphate in the induction of hepatic enzymes. I. Kinetics of the induction of rat liver serine dehydratase by cyclic adenosine 3′,5′-monophosphate. J. Biol. Chem., **245**, 351, 1970.
78. Perlman, R. L., De Chrombrugghe, B., and Pasten, I.: Cyclic AMP regulates catabolite and transient repression in *E. coli.* Nature (London), **223**, 810, 1969.
79. Tomkins, G. M., Gelehrter, T. D., Granner, D., Martin, D., Jr., Samuels, H. H., and Thompson, E. B.: Control of specific gene expression in higher organisms. Science, **166**, 1474, 1969.
79*a*. Prichard, P. M., Gilbert, J. M., Shafritz, D. A., and Anderson, W. F.: Factors for the initiation of haemoglobin synthesis by rabbit reticulocyte ribosomes. Nature (London), **226**, 511, 1970.
80. Schimke, R. T.: The importance of both synthesis and degradation in the control of arginase levels in rat liver. J. Biol. Chem., **239**, 3803, 1964.
81. Fernandez, M. N., and Fairbanks, V. F.: A new glucose-6-phosphate dehydrogenase (G6PD) variant in the Philippines (G6PD Panay). Clin. Res., **16**, 297, 1968.
82. Kelley, W. N., Greene, M. L., Rosenbloom, F. M., Henderson, J. F., and Seegmiller, J. E.: Hypoxanthine-guanine phosphoribosyltransferase deficiency in gout. Ann. Intern. Med., **70**, 155, 1969.
83. Novick, A., and Szilard, L.: Experiments with the chemostat on the rates of amino acid synthesis in bacteria, in *Dynamics of Growth Processes,* p. 21. Princeton, Princeton, N.J., 1954.
84. Umbarger, H. E.: Evidence for a negative-feedback mechanism in the biosynthesis of isoleucine. Science, **123**, 848, 1956.
85. Yates, R. A., and Pardee, A. B.: Control of pyrimidine biosynthesis in *Escherichia coli* by a feed-back mechanism. J. Biol. Chem., **221**, 757, 1956.
86. Gerhart, J. C., and Schachman, H. K.: Distinct subunits for the regulation and catalytic activity of aspartate transcarbamylase. Biochemistry, **4**, 1054, 1965.
87. Gerhart, J. C., and Schachman, H. K.: Allosteric interactions in aspartate transcarbamylase. II. Evidence for different conformational states of the protein in the presence and absence of specific ligands. Biochemistry, **7**, 538, 1968.
88. Monod, J., Changeux, J. P., and Jacob, F.: Allosteric proteins and cellular control systems. J. Molec. Biol., **6**, 306, 1963.
89. Koshland, D. E., Jr., Némethy, G., and Filmer, D.: Comparison of experimental binding data and theoretical models in proteins containing subunits. Biochemistry, **5**, 365, 1966.
90. Koshland, D. E., Jr.: The role of flexibility in enzyme action. Sympos. Quant. Biol., **28**, 473, 1963.
91. Monod, J., Wyman, J., and Changeux, J.-P.: On the nature of allosteric transitions: a plausible model. J. Molec. Biol., **12**, 88, 1965.
92. Gerhart, J. C., and Pardee, A. B.: Aspartate transcarbamylase, an enzyme designed for feedback inhibition. Fed. Proc., **23**, 727, 1964.
93. Ryder, E., Gregolin, C., Chang, H.-C., and Lane, M. D.: Liver acetyl CoA carboxylase: insight into the mechanism of activation by tricarboxylic acids and acetyl CoA. Proc. Nat. Acad. Sci. U.S.A., **57**, 1455, 1967.
94. Moyed, H. S.: Interference with feedback control of enzyme activity. Sympos. Quant. Biol., **26**, 323, 1961.
95. Ames, B. N., and Hartman, P. E.: The histidine operon. Sympos. Quant. Biol., **28**, 389, 1963.
96. Henderson, J. F., Caldwell, I. C., and Paterson, A. R. P.: Decreased feedback inhibition in a 6-methylmercaptopurine ribonucleoside resistant tumor. Cancer Res., **27**, 1773, 1967.
97. Henderson, J. F., Rosenbloom, F. M., Kelley, W. N., and Seegmiller, J. E.: Variations in purine metabolism of cultured skin fibroblasts from patients with gout. J. Clin. Invest., **47**, 1511, 1968.
98. Crick, F. H. C., Barnett, L., Brewer, S., and Watts-Tobin, R. J.: General nature of the genetic codes for protein. Nature (London), **192**, 1227, 1961.
99. Perutz, M. F., and Lehmann, H.: Molecular pathology of human haemoglobin. Nature (London), **219**, 902, 1968.
100. Ruddy, S., and Austen, K. F.: Inherited abnormalities of the complement system in man. Progr. Med. Genet., **7**, 69, 1970.
101. Daughaday, W. H., Laron, Z., Pertzelan, A., and Heins, J. N.: Defective sulfation factor generation: a possible etiological link in dwarfism. Trans. Ass. Amer. Physicians, **82**, 129, 1969.
102. Hoyer, L. W., and Breckenridge, R. T.: Immunologic studies of antihemophilic factor (AHF, Factor VIII). II. Properties of cross-reacting material. Blood, **35**, 809, 1970.
103. Brown, P. E., Hougie, C., and Roberts, H. R.: The genetic heterogeneity of hemophilia B. New Eng. J. Med., **283**, 61, 1970.
104. Itano, H. A.: The human hemoglobins: their properties and genetic control. Advances Protein Chem., **12**, 215, 1957.
105. Yoshida, A.: An amino acid substitution (histidine to tyrosine) in a human glucose-6-phosphate dehydrogenase variant associated with increased enzyme synthesis. Program abstracts, p. 49, American Society on Human Genetics, San Francisco, Oct. 1–4, 1969.
106. Dern, R. J.: A new hereditary quantitative variant of glucose-

6-phosphate dehydrogenase characterized by a marked increase in enzyme activity. J. Lab. Clin. Med., **68**, 560, 1966.
107. Martin, R. G.: Control of gene expression. Ann. Rev. Genet., **3**, 181, 1969.
108. Malamy, M. H.: Frameshift mutations in the lactose operon of *E. coli.* Sympos. Quant. Biol., **31**, 189, 1966.
109. Bookchin, R. M., Nagel, R. L., and Ranney, H. M.: Structure and properties of hemoglobin C_{Harlem}, a human hemoglobin variant with amino acid substitutions in two residues of the β-polypeptide chain. J. Biol. Chem., **242**, 248, 1967.
110. Kraus, L. M., Miyaji, T., Iuchi, I., and Kraus, A. P.: Characterization of $\alpha^{23gluNH_2}$ in hemoglobin Memphis. Hemoglobin Memphis/S, a new variant of molecular disease. Biochemistry, **5**, 3701, 1966.
111. Bradley, T. B., Wohl, R. C., and Reider, R. F.: Hemoglobin Gun Hill: deletion of five amino acid residues and impaired heme-globin binding. Science, **157**, 1581, 1967.
112. Jones, R. T., Brimhall, B., Huisman, T. H., Kleihauer, E., and Betke, K.: Hemoglobin Freiburg: abnormal hemoglobin due to deletion of a single amino acid residue. Science, **154**, 1024, 1966.
113. Baglioni, C.: The fusion of two peptide chains in hemoglobin Lepore and its interpretation as a genetic deletion. Proc. Nat. Acad. Sci. U.S.A., **48**, 1880, 1962.
114. Huisman, T. H. J.: Human hemoglobin, in *Biochemical Methods in Red Cell Genetics,* edited by J. J. Yunis, p. 391. Academic, New York, 1969.
115. Watts, R. L., and Watts, D. C.: The implications for molecular evolution of possible mechanisms of primary gene duplication. J. Theor. Biol., **20**, 277, 1968.
116. Ingram, V. M.: Gene evolution and the haemoglobins. Nature (London), **189**, 704, 1961.
117. Parker, W. C., and Bearn, A. G.: Haptoglobin and transferrin variations in humans and primates: two new transferrins in Chinese and Japanese populations. Ann. Hum. Genet., **25**, 227, 1961.
118. Abramson, R. K., Rucknagel, D. L., Shreffler, D. C., and Saave, J. J.: Homozygous Hb J Tongariki: evidence for only one alpha chain structural locus in Melanesians. Science, **169**, 194, 1970.
119. Brimhall, B., Hollan, S., Jones, R. T., Kohlen, R. D., Stocklen, Z., and Szelenyi, J. G.: Multiple alpha-chain loci for human hemoglobin. Clin. Res., **18**, 184, 1970.
120. Brewer, G. J., and Sing, C. F.: Survey of isozymes of human erythrocytes, in *Biochemical Methods in Red Cell Genetics,* edited by J. J. Yunis, p. 377. Academic, New York, 1969.
121. Hill, R. L., Delaney, R., Fellows, R. E., Jr., and Lebovitz, H. E.: The evolutionary origins of the immunoglobulins. Proc. Nat. Acad. Sci. U.S.A., **56**, 1762, 1966.
122. Singer, S. J., and Doolittle, R. F.: Antibody active sites and immunoglobulin molecules. Science, **153**, 13, 1966.
123. Gally, J. A., and Edelman, G. M.: Somatic translocation of antibody genes. Nature (London), **227**, 341, 1970.
124. Attardi, G., and Amaldi, F.: Structure and synthesis of ribosomal RNA. Ann. Rev. Biochem., **39**, 183, 1970.
125. Callan, H. G.: The organization of genetic units in chromosomes. J. Cell. Sci., **2**, 1, 1967.
126. Whitehouse, H. L. K.: A cycloid model for the chromosome. J. Cell. Sci., **2**, 9, 1967.
127. Harris, H.: Genes and isozymes. Proc. Roy. Soc. Biol., **174**, 1, 1969.
128. Markert, C. L.: The molecular basis of isozymes. Ann. N.Y. Acad. Sci., **151**, 14, 1968.
129. Hopkinson, A. H., and Harris, H.: Evidence for a second "structural" locus determining human phosphoglucomutase. Nature (London), **208**, 410, 1965.
130. Hopkinson, A. H., and Harris, H.: A third phosphoglucomutase locus in man. Ann. Hum. Genet., **31**, 359, 1968.
131. Fields, R. A., and Harris, H.: Genetically determined variation of adenylate kinase in man. Nature (London), **209**, 261, 1966.
132. Lewis, W. H. P., and Harris, H.: Human red cell peptidases. Nature (London), **215**, 351, 1967.
133. McKusick, V. A.: Human genetics. Ann. Rev. Genet., **4**, 1–46, 1970.
134. Sutton, H. E.: Human genetics. Ann. Rev. Genet., **1**, 1, 1967.
135. Knudson, A. G., Jr.: Inborn errors of metabolism. Ann. Rev. Genet., **3**, 1, 1969.
136. Yoshida, A.: A single amino acid substitution (asparagine to aspartic acid) between normal (B+) and the common Negro variant (A+) of human glucose-6-phosphate dehydrogenase. Proc. Nat. Acad. Sci. U.S.A., **57**, 835, 1967.
137. Tashian, R. E., Riggs, S. K., and Yu, Y.-S. L.: Characterization of a mutant human erythrocyte carbonic anhydrase: carbonic anhydrase Ic_{Guam}. Arch. Biochem. Biophys., **117**, 320, 1966.
138. Yanofsky, C.: Amino acid replacements associated with mutation and recombination in the A gene and their relationship to in vitro coding data. Sympos. Quant. Biol., **28**, 581, 1963.
139. Wheeler, J. T., and Krevans, J. R.: The homozygous state of persistent fetal hemoglobin and the interaction of persistent fetal hemoglobin with thalassemia. Bull. Johns Hopkins Hosp., **109**, 217, 1961.
140. Neel, J. V.: The hemoglobin genes: a remarkable example of the clustering of related genetic functions on a single mammalian chromosome. Blood, **18**, 769, 1961.
141. Parker, W. C., and Bearn, A. G.: Application of genetic regulatory mechanisms to human genetics. Amer. J. Med., **34**, 680, 1963.
142. Zuckerkandl, E.: Controller-gene diseases: the operon model as applied to β-thalassemia, familial fetal hemoglobinemia and the normal switch from the production of fetal hemoglobin to that of adult hemoglobin. J. Molec. Biol., **8**, 128, 1964.
143. Pauling, L., Itano, H. A., Singer, S. J., and Wells, I. C.: Sickle cell anemia, a molecular disease. Science, **110**, 543, 1949.
144. Aebi, H.: Inborn errors of metabolism. Ann. Rev. Biochem., **36**, 271, 1967.
145. Motulsky, A. G., and Yoshida, A.: Methods for the study of red cell glucose-6-phosphate dehydrogenase, in *Biochemical Methods in Red Cell Genetics,* edited by J. J. Yunis, p. 51. Academic, New York, 1969.
146. Kelley, W. N.: Studies on hypoxanthine-guanine phosphoribosyl transferase in fibroblasts from patients with the Lesch-Nyhan syndrome. Submitted for publication.
147. Fukimoto, W. Y., and Seegmiller, J. E.: Hypoxanthine-guanine phosphoribosyltransferase deficiency: activity in normal, mutant, and heterozygote-cultured human skin fibroblasts. Proc. Nat. Acad. Sci. U.S.A., **65**, 577, 1970.
148. Rosenberg, L. E.: Vitamin-dependent genetic disease. Hosp. Pract., **5**, 59, 1970.
149. Ingram, V. M., and Streeton, A. O. W.: Genetic basis of the thalassemia diseases. Nature (London), **184**, 1903, 1959.
150. Motulsky, A.: Controller genes in synthesis of human haemoglobin. Nature (London), **194**, 607, 1962.
150*a*. Huisman, T. H. J., Schroeder, W. A., Adams, H. R., Shelton, J. B., and Apell, G.: A possible subclass of the hereditary persistence of fetal hemoglobin. Blood, **36**, 1, 1970.
151. Beckwith, J. R., Pardee, A. B., Austrian, R., and Jacob, F.: Coordination of the synthesis of the enzymes in the pyrimidine pathway of *E. coli.* J. Molec. Biol., **5**, 618, 1962.
152. Smith, L. H., Jr.: Hereditary orotic aciduria: pyrimidine auxotrophism in man. Amer. J. Med., **38**, 1, 1965.
153. Pinsky, L., and Krooth, R. S.: Studies on the control of pyrimidine biosynthesis in human diploid cell strains. II. Effects of 5-azoorotic acid, barbituric acid, and pyrimidine precursors on cellular phenotype. Proc. Nat. Acad. Sci. U.S.A., **57**, 1267, 1967.
154. Fox, R. M., O'Sullivan, W. J., and Firkin, B. G.: Orotic aciduria. Differing enzyme patterns. Amer. J. Med., **47**, 332, 1969.
155. Tomkins, G. M., and Ames, B. N.: The operon concept in bacteria and in higher organisms. Nat. Cancer Inst. Monograph No. 27, pp. 221, 1967.
156. Granick, S.: The induction in vitro of the synthesis of δ-aminolevulinic acid synthetase in chemical porphyria: a response to certain drugs, sex hormones, and foreign chemicals. J. Biol. Chem., **241**, 1359, 1966.
157. Strand, L. J., Felsher, B. F., Redeker, A. G., and Marver, H. S.: Heme biosynthesis in intermittent acute porphyria: decreased hepatic conversion of porphobilinogen to porphyrins and increased delta-aminolevulinic acid synthetase activity. Proc. Nat. Acad. Sci. U.S.A., **67**, 1315, 1970.

158. Rosenbloom, F. M., Henderson, J. F., Caldwell, I. C., Kelley, W. N., and Seegmiller, J. E.: Biochemical bases of accelerated purine biosynthesis de novo in human fibroblasts lacking hypoxanthine-guanine phosphoribosyl transferase. J. Biol. Chem., **243,** 1166, 1968.
159. Sutton, H. E.: Beta-aminoisobutyricaciduria, in *The Metabolic Basis of Inherited Disease,* edited by J. B. Stanbury, J. B. Wyngaarden, and D. S. Fredrickson, 1st ed., p. 792. McGraw-Hill, New York, 1960.
160. Harris, H.: *An Introduction to Human Biochemical Genetics,* p. 69. Cambridge, New York, 1953.
161. Rosenbloom, F. M., Kelley, W. N., Henderson, J. F., and Seegmiller, J. E.: Lyon hypothesis and X-linked disease. Lancet, **2,** 305, 1967.
162. Emmerson, B. T., and Wyngaarden, J. B.: Purine metabolism in heterozygous carriers of hypoxanthine-guanine phosphoribosyltransferase deficiency. Science, **166,** 1533, 1969.
163. Scott, C. D.: Analysis of urine for its ultraviolet-absorbing constituents by high-pressure anion-exchange chromatography. Clin. Chem., **14,** 521, 1968.
164. Jolley, R. L., and Freeman, M. L.: Automated carbohydrate analysis of physiological fluids. Clin. Chem., **14,** 538, 1968.
165. Hsia, D. Y.-Y.: Study of hereditary metabolic diseases using in vitro techniques. Metabolism, **19,** 309, 1970.
166. Shaw, C. R.: Electrophoretic variation in enzymes. Science, **149,** 936, 1965.
166*a*. Cuatrecasas, P.: Topography of the active site of staphylococcal nuclease. Affinity labeling with diazonium substrate analogues. J. Biol. Chem., **245,** 574, 1970.
167. Migeon, B. R., and Childs, B.: Hybridization of mammalian somatic cells. Progr. Med. Genet., **7,** 1, 1970.
168. Krooth, R. S., Darlington, G. A., and Velazquez, A. A.: The genetics of cultured mammalian cells. Ann. Rev. Genet., **2,** 141, 1968.
169. Fratantoni, J. C., Hall, C. W., and Neufeld, E. F.: The defect in Hurler's and Hunter's syndromes: faulty degradation of mucopolysaccharide. Proc. Nat. Acad. Sci. U.S.A., **60,** 699, 1968.
170. Neufeld, E. F., and Fratantoni, J. C.: Inborn errors of mucopolysaccharide metabolism. Science, **169,** 141, 1970.
171. Witkin, E. M.: Ultraviolet-induced mutation and DNA repair. Ann. Rev. Genet., **3,** 525, 1969.
172. Cleaver, J. E.: Xeroderma pigmentosum: a human disease in which an initial stage of DNA repair is defective. Proc. Nat. Acad. Sci. U.S.A., **63,** 428, 1969.
173. Reed, W. B., Landing, B., Sugarman, G., Cleaver, J. E., and Melnyk, J.: Xeroderma pigmentosum. Clinical and laboratory investigation of its basic defect. J.A.M.A., **207,** 2073, 1969.
174. Fialkow, P. J., Lisker, R., Giblett, E. R., and Zavala, C.: Xg locus: failure to detect inactivation in females with chronic myelocytic leukaemia. Nature (London), **226,** 367, 1970.
175. Matsuya, Y., Green, H., and Basilico, C.: Properties and uses of human-mouse hybrid cell lines. Nature (London), **220,** 1199, 1968.
176. Ruddle, F. H., Chapman, V. M., Chen, T. R., and Klebe, R. J.: Linkage between human lactate dehydrogenase A and B and peptidase B. Nature (London), **227,** 251, 1970.
177. Conover, J. H., and Hirschhorn, K.: A system for the localization of autosomal traits via somatic cell hybridization. Program abstracts, p. 23, American Society of Human Genetics, San Francisco, Oct. 1–4, 1969.
178. Donahue, R. P., Bias, W. B., Renwick, J. H., and McKusick, V. A.: Probable assignment of the Duffy blood group locus to chromosome 1 in man. Proc. Nat. Acad. Sci. U.S.A., **61,** 949, 1968.
179. Renwick, J. H., and Lawler, S. D.: Probable linkage between a congenital cataract locus and the Duffy blood group locus. Ann. Hum. Genet., **27,** 67, 1963.
180. German, J. L., Walker, M. E., Stiefel, F. H., and Allen, F. H., Jr.: Autoradiographic studies of human chromosomes. II. Data concerning the position of the MN locus. Vox Sang., **16,** 130, 1969.
181. Sparkes, R. S., Carrel, R. E., and Paglia, D. E.: Probable localization of a triosephosphate isomerase gene to the short arm of a number 5 human chromosome. Nature (London), **224,** 367, 1969.
182. De Grouchy, J., Veslot, J., Bonnette, J., and Roidot, M.: A case of ?6p-chromosomal aberration. Amer. J. Dis. Child., **115,** 93, 1968.
183. Robson, E. B., Polani, P. E., Dart, S. J., Jacobs, P. A., and Renwick, J. H.: Probable assignment of the alpha locus of haptoglobin to chromosome 16 in man. Nature (London), **223,** 1163, 1969.
184. Dr. Wilma Bias: Personal communication, 1970.
185. Hecht, F.: IgA and partial deletions of chromosome 18. Lancet, **1,** 100, 1969.
186. Lyon, J. B.: The X-chromosome and the enzymes controlling muscle glycogen: Phosphorylase kinase. Biochem. Genet., **4,** 169, 1970.
187. Szybalska, E. H., and Szybalski, W.: Genetics of human cell lines. IV. DNA-mediated heritable transformation of a biochemical trait. Proc. Nat. Acad. Sci. U.S.A., **48,** 2026, 1962.
188. Nadler, H. L., and Gerbie, A. B.: Role of amniocentesis in the intrauterine detection of genetic disorders. New Eng. J. Med., **282,** 596, 1970.
189. Valenti, C., Schutta, E. J., and Kehaty, T: Cytogenetic in utero diagnosis of mongolism. J.A.M.A., **207,** 1513, 1969.
190. Danes, B. S.: Cell cultures and genetic disease. Hosp. Pract., **4,** 88, 1969.
191. Taysi, K., Kistenmacher, M. L., Punnett, H. H., and Mellman, W. J.: Limitations of metachromasia as a diagnostic aid in pediatrics. New Eng. J. Med., **281,** 1108, 1969.
192. Milunsky, A., and Littlefield, J. W.: Diagnostic limitations of metachromasia. New Eng. J. Med., **281,** 1128, 1969.
193. Boyle, J. A., Raivio, K. O., Astrin, K. H., Schulman, J. D., Graf, M. L., Seegmiller, J. E., and Jacobsen, C. B.: Lesch-Nyhan syndrome: preventive control by prenatal diagnosis. Science, **169,** 688, 1970.
194. Holtzman, N. A.: Dietary treatment of inborn errors of metabolism. Ann. Rev. Med., **21,** 335, 1970.
195. Frederick, E. W., Rabkin, M. T., and Smith, L. H., Jr.: Primary hyperoxaluria: a defect in glyoxylate metabolism. J. Clin. Invest., **41,** 1358, 1962.
196. Arias, I. M., Gartner, L. M., Cohen, M., Benn-Ezzer, J., and Levi, A. J.: Chronic nonhemolytic unconjugated hyperbilirubinemia with hepatic glucuronyl transferase deficiency: evidence for genetic heterogeneity. Trans. Ass. Amer. Physicians, **81,** 66, 1968.
197. Kreek, M. J., and Sleisenger, M. H.: Reduction of serum unconjugated bilirubin with phenobarbitone in adult congenital non-haemolytic unconjugated hyperbilirubinaemia. Lancet, **1,** 73, 1968.
197*a*. Mapes, C. A., Anderson, R. L., and Sweeley, C. G., Enzyme replacement in Fabry's disease, an inborn error of metabolism. Science, **169,** 981, 1970.
198. Bickel, H., Schultze, H. E., Grüter, W., and Göllner, I.: Versuche zur Coeruloplasmin-substitution bei der hepatocerebralen Degeneration (Wilsonsche Krankheit). Klin. Wschr., **15,** 961, 1956.
199. Editorial: Blood catalase and oral ulceration. Lancet, **2,** 1121, 1952.
200. McKee, P. A., Coussons, R. T., Buckner, G. R., Williams, G. R., and Hampton, J. W.: Effects of the spleen on canine factor VIII levels. J. Lab. Clin. Med., **75,** 391, 1970.
201. Hathaway, W. E., Mull, M. M., Githens, J. H., Groth, C. G., Marchioro, T. L., and Starzl, T. E.: Attempted spleen transplant in classical hemophilia. Transplantation, **7,** 73, 1969.
202. Sorensen, L. B.: Suppression of the shunt pathway in primary gout by azathioprine. Proc. Nat. Acad. Sci. U.S.A., **55,** 571, 1966.
203. Deodhar, S. D., Tung, K. S. K., Zühlke, V., and Nakamoto, S.: Renal transplantation in a patient with primary familial oxalosis. Arch. Path. (Chicago), **87,** 118, 1969.
204. Mahoney, C. P., Striker, G. E., Hickman, R. O., Manning, G. B., and Marchioro, T. L.: Renal transplantation for childhood cystinosis. New Eng. J. Med., **283,** 397, 1970.
205. August, C. S., Rosen, F. S., Filler, R. M., Janeway, C. A., Markowski, B., and Kay, H. E. M.: Implantation of a foetal thymus, restoring immunological competence in a patient with thymic aplasia (DiGeorge's syndrome). Lancet, **2,** 1210, 1968.
206. Cleveland, W. W., Fogel, B. J., Brown, W. T., and Kay, H. E. M.: Foetal thymic transplant in a case of DiGeorge's syndrome. Lancet, **2,** 1211, 1968.
207. Meuwissen, H. J., Gatti, R. A., Terasaki, P. I., Hong, R., and Good, R. A.: Treatment of lymphopenic hypogammaglobulinemia and bone-marrow aplasia by transplantation of allogeneic marrow. New Eng. J. Med., **281,** 691, 1969.

208. Bach, F. H., Albertini, R. J., Joo, P., Anderson, J. L., and Bortin, M. M.: Bone-marrow transplantation in a patient with the Wiskott-Aldrich syndrome. Lancet, **2,** 1364, 1968.

209. Rogers, S.: Skills for genetic engineers. New Scientist, pp. 194–196, Jan. 29, 1970.

210. Rogers, S., and Moore, M.: Studies of the mechanism of action of the Shope rabbit papilloma virus. I. Concerning the nature of the induction of arginase in the infected cells. J. Exp. Med., **117,** 521, 1963.

211. Rogers, S.: Shope papilloma virus: a passenger in man and its significance to the potential control of the host genome. Nature (London), **212,** 1220, 1966.

212. Edwards, J. H.: Familial predisposition in man. Brit. Med. Bull., **25,** 58, 1969.

213. Edwards, J. H.: Analysis of pedigree data, in *Advances in Human Genetics,* edited by H. Harris and K. Hirschhorn, vol. 1, p. 1. Plenum, New York, 1970.

214. Migeon, B. R.: X-linked hypoxanthine-guanine phosphoribosyl transferase deficiency: detection of heterozygotes by selective medium. Biochem. Genet., **4,** 377, 1970.

215. Felix, J. S., and DeMars, R.: Detection of females heterozygous for the Lesch-Nyhan mutation by 8-azaguanine resistant growth of cultured fibroblasts. In press, 1970.

216. Beutler, E., Saluda, M. C., Sturgeon, P., and Day, R. W.: Genetics of galactose-1-phosphate uridyl transferase deficiency. J. Lab. Clin. Med., **68,** 646, 1966.

217. Milunsky, A., Littlefield, J. W., Kanfer, J. N., Kolodny, E. H., Shih, V. E., and Atkins, L.: Prenatal genetic diagnosis. New Eng. J. Med., **283,** 1370, 1441, 1489, 1970.

CHAPTER TWO

CODING, INFORMATION TRANSFER, AND PROTEIN SYNTHESIS*

Mahlon B. Hoagland

This chapter is designed to furnish a molecular background for the problems in human genetics and metabolic disease to be discussed in chapters to follow. In particular, it will review current knowledge of the structure and mode of replication of the genetic material—deoxyribonucleic acid (DNA), the mechanism of transcription of its message, and the chemistry of the process by which cells translate this message into protein molecules. This biosynthetic conversion of genotype to phenotype appears in principle to be quite simple: genetic information is written in a language of four letters (the nucleotide bases of DNA) and its ultimate expression, protein, in a language of 20 letters (the amino acids). The common mechanism used by all living systems to carry out the process is now understood in considerable detail.

Experimentally, there have been two broad approaches to our present knowledge. The first alters the genetic material by mutation and asks how such alteration affects the structure of the final product, protein. By the use of increasingly fine genetic analysis to localize the mutational defect on the one hand and rigorous chemical dissection of protein on the other, it becomes possible to deduce structural relationships between gene and gene product. This approach asks no questions about *intermediate* processes. The second approach is a direct assault on mechanism: the cell is disrupted in such a way as to preserve its biosynthetic activity in cell-free systems, and the components of the machinery are scrutinized in fine detail. The union of these two approaches in recent years has been remarkably fruitful.

The reader will note frequent reference to results obtained with bacteria and viruses as experimental material. The reason for this is that the rapidity of their growth in simple, well-defined media and the ease with which their genetics may be manipulated make them ideal subjects. But it becomes increasingly apparent that at the underlying molecular level bacteria and men use the same tools. And, in such a volume as this, it is worth recalling that the clinical observation of the patient with sickle-cell anemia led a physician, William Castle, to suggest to a chemist, Linus Pauling, that the genetic defect might be an alteration of the structure of the hemoglobin molecule [1]. The proof of this by Itano and Pauling, and Ingram's subsequent demonstration that the chemical alteration involved a single amino acid substitution [2] gave strong impetus to the search for simple systems amenable to detailed genetic analysis. As William Hayes, an outstanding microbial geneticist, has said: "Arrogant microbial geneticists should note that this is not the first time that the biochemical and genetic study of man has helped to illuminate their problems."

In this chapter I do not aim at completeness so much as at contributing some insight into the accomplishments and problems of molecular biologists. At the end of this chapter I have supplied some general references (*A*–*G*) where the subject is discussed in full detail and with thorough documentation. References to original papers are sprinkled sparsely throughout the chapter according to whim.

*The preparation of this chapter has been aided by a research grant from the Public Health Service.

THE GENETIC MATERIAL—DNA

There are two kinds of nucleic acid: deoxyribonucleic acid (DNA) and ribonucleic acid (RNA). They are chemically similar but functionally quite different. DNA, residing in the nucleus, is the substance of the gene. The evidence for this statement will be examined after we have considered its structure.

It is now clear that at least in viruses and in bacteria the total genome, which behaves genetically as a single linkage group, is a single molecule. It is possible now to isolate single intact molecules of DNA of some 10^9 molecular weight units. It may be that in higher organisms the total genetic information in a single chromosome may also reside in a single molecule (of which there may be more than one copy), but this is still undetermined.

Molecular Structure

When a molecule of DNA is hydrolyzed by appropriate chemical and enzymatic means, it is found to consist of three kinds of molecular subunits: phosphoric acid, a sugar deoxyribose,[1] and a group of aromatic ring structures—*purine* and *pyrimidine bases.* There are four of these bases in DNA—thymine (T), adenine (A), guanine (G), and cytosine (C), and their chemical structure is illustrated in Fig. 2-1. The next level of complexity is the *nucleoside,* a purine or pyrimidine base linked to the sugar deoxyribose: thymidine,[2] deoxyadenosine, deoxyguanosine, and deoxycytidine (Fig. 2-2). Next is the *nucleotide* (also shown in Fig. 2-2), a phosphoric acid ester of a nucleoside: thymidylic acid, deoxyadenylic acid, deoxyguanylic acid, and deoxycytidylic acid—also referred to as thymidine (3′- or 5′-) monophos-

[1] The "deoxy-" prefix denotes the absence of a hydroxyl group in the 2′ position of ribose (the sugar present in ribonucleic acid).
[2] Note that since thymine with rare exception occurs only in DNA and is thus always associated with deoxyribose, its derivatives are customarily not prefixed with "deoxy-."

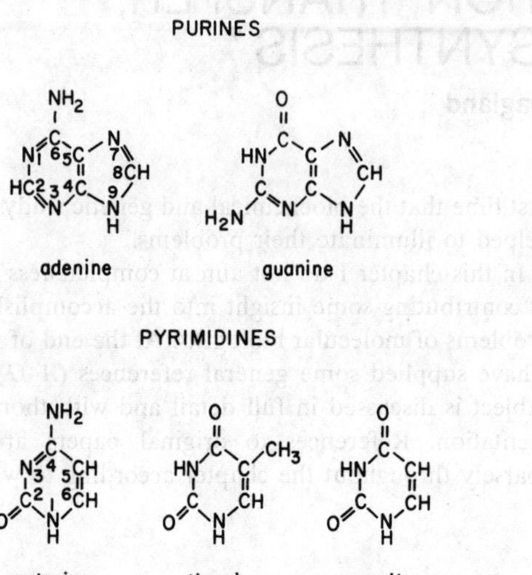

Figure 2-1. The five purine and pyrimidine bases naturally occurring in DNA and RNA.

phate, deoxyadenosine (3′- or 5′-) monophosphate, etc. (We shall see in a subsequent section that the nucleotides exist in cells with either one or two more phosphate groups linked to the first: nucleoside 5′-diphosphates and -triphosphates. The latter are used by the cell to build DNA.) These singly phosphorylated nucleotides are the basic repeating subunits of the DNA molecule and are linked in DNA as shown in Fig. 2-3. Each nucleotide is linked through its phosphate group to the deoxyribose 3′-hydroxyl of the adjacent nucleotide. A polynucleotide of 10^8 molecular weight units (such as the DNA of a bacterial virus) would thus contain a string of as many as 300,000 nucleotide bases.

The Double Helix

Physicochemical studies of native DNA early revealed that it is a rigid rodlike structure and strongly acidic (because of the ionizable phosphate groups). Studies, notably by Chargaff and his associates at Columbia University, of its relative content of the four bases revealed some interesting

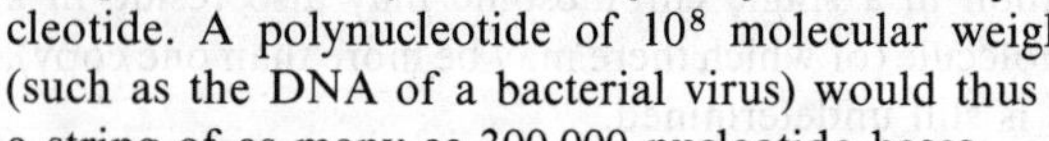

purine base (adenine)
nucleoside (deoxy-adenosine)
sugar (deoxyribose)
nucleotide (deoxy-adenylic acid)
phosphate

Figure 2-2. Organization of phosphate, sugar, and adenine in deoxyadenylic acid, one of the four mononucleotide subunits of DNA.

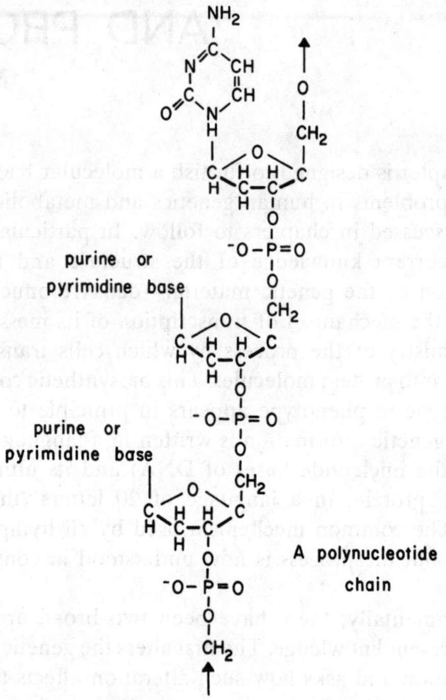

purine or pyrimidine base
purine or pyrimidine base
A polynucleotide chain

Figure 2-3. The structure of a polydeoxy-nucleotide.

relationships. First, the content of thymine always equaled the content of adenine, and the content of guanine equaled that of cytosine. Second, although the ratio of G + C to A + T varied widely from species to species, the total number of pyrimidine bases always equaled the total number of purine bases: that is, A + G = T + C.

X-ray diffraction has been an invaluable tool for elucidating macromolecular structure. It involves an analysis of the refractions of x-ray beams by a regularly repeating crystalline or semicrystalline structure. By 1952 Wilkins and his associates [3, 4] had added, from an extensive study of x-ray diffraction photographs of DNA fibers, several more valuable pieces of information about the structure: (1) the DNA chain consists of more than one helix winding around a central axis, and each full turn is 34 Å from the next along the axis; (2) the flat purine and pyrimidine bases are stacked parallel to each other, 3.4 Å apart and perpendicular to the long axis of the helix.

These various facts were available to Crick and Watson as they pondered the structure of DNA. Using models of hypothetical DNA structures and aided by brilliant intuition they arrived at the remarkable structure shown in Fig. 2-4 [5].[3] This consists of a double helix in which the phosphate-sugar groups form backbones, while the purine and pyrimidine bases face inward, the plane of their rings at right angles

[3] Dr. Watson has written a popular, highly personal, and controversial account of the evolution of this important discovery, which makes delightful reading (J. D. Watson, *The Double Helix*. New York: Atheneum, 1968).

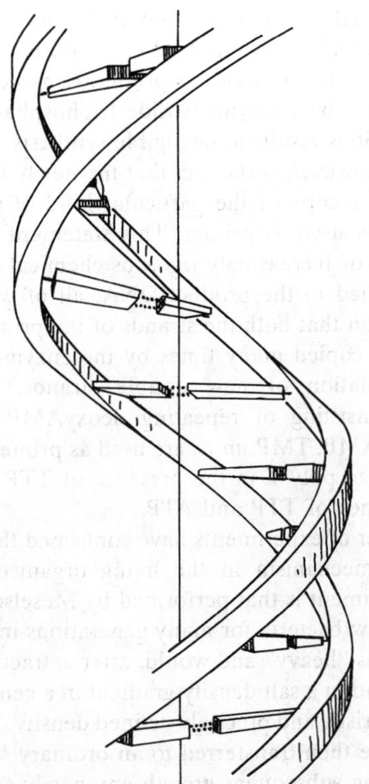

Figure 2-4. A diagrammatic portion of the DNA double helix. The phosphate-sugar backbone forms the framework ascending around a central axis. The bases are pictured as plates opposite one another, perpendicular to the helix axis, interacting through hydrogen bonds (dots).

to the axis of the helix. The bases thus form, as it were, the steps of a "spiral" staircase, and the phosphate-sugar backbone forms the supporting framework. The 34-Å repeat in the x-ray photographs was thus one full turn of the helix. Figure 2-5 shows the details of the interaction of the four bases: each "step" consists of a purine attached to one chain and a pyrimidine attached to the other. The neatness of fit is provided by the exact complementary configuration of the two kinds of bases; this permits the sharing of hydrogen atoms (hydrogen bonds) and consequent stabilization of the configuration. It can be seen that the physical repeat distance between turns of the helix accommodates 10 nucleotide units, and, because of the complementary relationship of the purines and pyrimidines, there are always as many thymine as adenine residues and as many cytosine as guanine residues. The structure also requires that the sum of the pyrimidines equals the sum of the purines.

Structure of RNA

RNA is very similar in structure to DNA, although, as we shall see, RNA, unlike DNA, exists in several distinct forms with quite different functions and is not generally as regular in secondary structure. Instead of deoxyribose the backbone sugar is ribose (an extra hydroxyl group at the 2′ position), and replacing thymine is uracil (Fig. 2-1). The hydrogen-bonding properties of uracil are identical to those in thymine, so that under certain conditions RNA can form stable double helixes as well as "hybrid" helixes composed of one RNA strand and one complementary DNA strand. This is possible, of course, only if the RNA has extensive structural homology with the DNA.

One of the more significant generalizations that has come from these studies of nucleic acid—and, indeed, of protein structure—is the great importance in biology of *weak* chemical linkages, notably hydrogen bonds. Indeed, such low-energy links between nucleotides not only determine the high fidelity of DNA replication and RNA synthesis but also are critical as we shall see, to specification of amino acid sequence in the process of protein synthesis.

Replication of DNA

It was immediately apparent to Watson and Crick that implicit in this structure was a clear indication of its mode

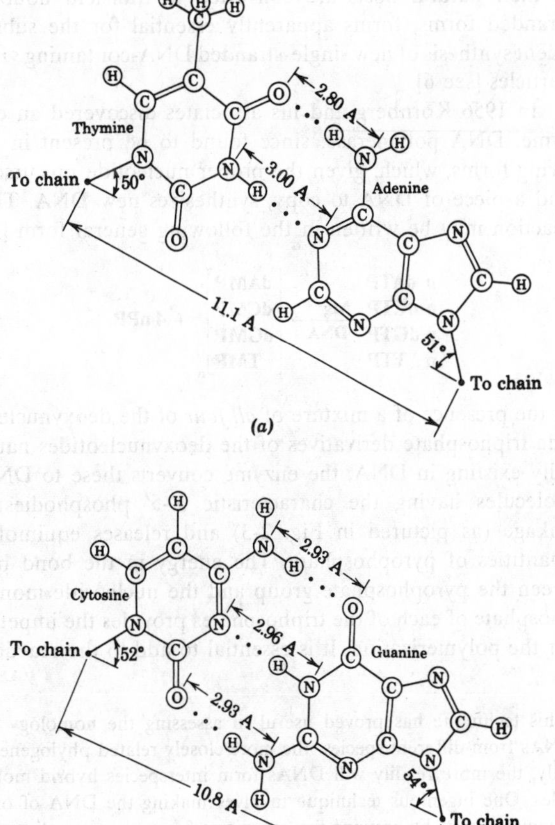

Figure 2-5. The geometry of base interaction through hydrogen bonding. (*From Pauling and Corey, Arch. Biochem.*, **65**, 164, 1956.)

of replication. Simply by uncoiling the two strands and laying down new bases (A opposite T and C opposite G) a pair of new double strands could be formed, each a perfect copy of the original. We shall see how thoroughly experiment has borne out this prediction.

In the years since the proposal of this remarkable model a variety of ingenious experiments have established beyond any reasonable doubt the validity both of the structure of DNA and of the proposed general mechanism of its replication. A number of these pieces of evidence may be examined briefly:

1 By heating solutions of DNA to temperatures of 80 to 90°C and then rapidly cooling the solution it is possible to separate the two strands of the native DNA, i.e., to "denature" it. The once-rigid double-stranded rods are converted to limp coils of single-stranded DNA. If such heated solutions are cooled very *slowly,* the single strands have time to find and reunite with their complementary sisters to re-form partially the original rigid duplex molecules.[4]

2 Naturally occurring single-stranded DNAs and RNAs have been discovered in viruses, which before replication in their natural hosts are converted to transient double-stranded forms, forms apparently essential for the subsequent synthesis of new single-stranded DNA-containing viral particles [see 6].

3 In 1956 Kornberg and his associates discovered an enzyme, DNA polymerase, since found to be present in all living forms, which, given the proper nucleotide precursors and a piece of DNA to copy, synthesizes new DNA. This reaction may be written in the following general form [7]:

$$\begin{matrix}\text{n dATP}\\ \text{n dCTP}\\ \text{n dGTP}\\ \text{n TTP}\end{matrix} \xrightarrow[\text{DNA}]{\text{Mg}^{++}} \begin{bmatrix}\text{dAMP}\\ \text{dCMP}\\ \text{dGMP}\\ \text{TMP}\end{bmatrix}_n + 4\ \text{nPP}$$

In the presence of a mixture of *all four* of the deoxynucleoside triphosphate derivatives of the deoxynucleotides naturally existing in DNA, the enzyme converts these to DNA molecules having the characteristic 3′-5′ phosphodiester linkage (as pictured in Fig. 2-3) and releases equimolar quantities of pyrophosphate. The energy in the bond between the pyrophosphate group and the nucleoside monophosphate of each of the triphosphates provides the impetus for the polymerization. It is essential to add to the reaction mixture a small amount of DNA to "prime" the reaction. The product DNA is synthesized in quantities far exceeding the amount of DNA added as primer. Omission of primer, of any one of the deoxynucleoside triphosphate substrates, or of Mg^{++} ions results in negligible synthesis. Most important of all, however, is the fact that the newly formed DNA is an accurate copy of the particular kind of naturally occurring DNA used as primer. This statement is supported by a variety of increasingly rigorous chemical and physical criteria applied to the product DNA, all of which lead to the conclusion that both the strands of the primer DNA are sequentially copied many times by the enzyme, leading to the accumulation of new double strands.[5] If artificial "DNAs" consisting of repeating deoxyAMP units or of alternating AMP, TMP units, are used as primer, the system will synthesize poly-T in the presence of TTP, or poly-AT in the presence of TTP and ATP.

4 A number of experiments have confirmed the postulated replication mechanism in the living organism. The now classic experiment is that performed by Meselson and Stahl [8]. They grew bacteria for many generations in ^{15}N, so that the DNA was "heavy" and would, after extraction from the bacteria, band in a salt density gradient in a centrifugal field at a characteristic and precisely defined density. The "heavy" bacteria were then transferred to an ordinary ^{14}N medium, so that during subsequent growth any newly formed DNA would be "light." The replication mechanism implicit in the Watson-Crick model would predict the following outcome (where the full line is "heavy" DNA and the dotted line is "light" DNA):

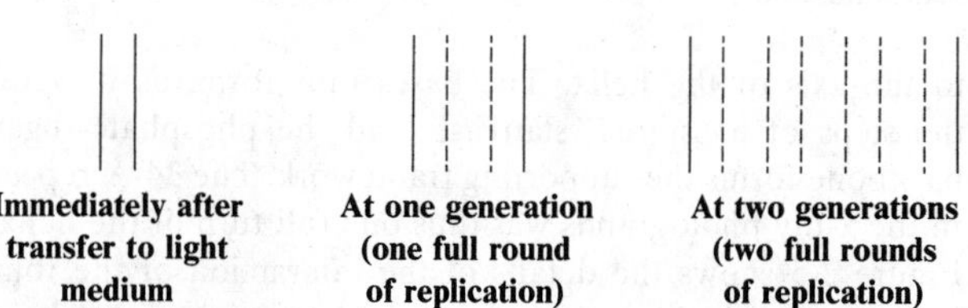

[4]This technique has proved useful in assessing the homology of DNAs from different species: the more closely related phylogenetically, the more readily will DNAs form interspecies hybrid molecules. One ingenious technique involves making the DNA of one organism heavy by growing the organisms for many generations in ^{15}N, which gives it a greater density when centrifuged through a salt gradient. The heavy DNA of one organism is mixed with the light DNA of another, heated, and slow-cooled, and a hybrid molecule is found to have a characteristic density intermediate between the two parental molecules.

[5]A polynucleotide chain has an unambiguous direction, or polarity, as indicated by the arrows in Fig. 2-3: reading up we pass along a series of $3' \rightarrow 5'$ phosphodiester linkages. The Watson-Crick model clearly predicted that in order to obtain base pairing of the kind suggested, the two strands of the double helix would have to be of *opposite* polarity: if one strand read $3' \rightarrow 5'$, the other must read $5' \rightarrow 3'$. Using DNA polymerase and an ingenious technique called *nearest-neighbor frequency analysis,* it has been possible to show that, in fact, the two strands are of opposite polarity. The enzyme is permitted to synthesize DNA-containing radioactive phosphate groups. The DNA is then hydrolyzed by an enzyme that leaves the phosphate, originally introduced in one nucleotide, attached to its nearest neighbor! The statistical frequency with which each of the four nucleotides is found next to itself and the other three may thus be determined. The opposite polarity model puts definite restrictions on nearest-neighbor frequencies, which are borne out by the analysis. (The technique, incidentally, also shows that these frequencies in DNA are *not* random—a finding to be expected for a molecule bearing genetic information.)

After one full round of replication, all the molecules of DNA would be expected to be half light and half heavy; i.e., they would have a density intermediate between fully heavy and fully light DNA. After a second round of replication, each of the half-heavy, half-light molecules of DNA would have replicated again, this time generating two all-light double-stranded chains and again two mixed chains. This was indeed exactly what was found: at one generation of bacterial growth the DNA produced a single band of intermediate density, and at the second generation two bands were evident, one at intermediate density and another corresponding to the known density of all-light DNA. Similar techniques have subsequently been used to show that the phenomenon of genetic recombination—by which, in the sexual reproductive process, genetic traits are mixed—probably involves actual breakage and reunion of DNA strands; i.e., segments of the DNA of one parent actually become covalently linked to segments of the DNA of the other parent [9].

Perhaps the most graphic picture of DNA replication has been given us by Cairns [10]. He has been able to obtain from *Escherichia coli* radioautographs of complete extended chromosomes (tritium-labeled) which have the dimensions of a double-stranded molecule of DNA. (Genetically the chromosome of this bacterium behaves as a single linkage group as mentioned before.) The structure is continuous (i.e., a circle), as had been predicted from certain genetic data. Such chromosomes taken from bacteria in progressive stages of replicating their DNA in a tritiated medium can be seen on radioautography to become labeled progressively from one end to the other, starting from a single point. This clearly indicates that replication proceeds along both strands in parallel, resulting in the final duplication of the whole molecule.

Furthermore, the labeling pattern is such that between the first and second generations of growth in labeled medium one replicating arm of the splitting circle is exactly twice as dense as the other, precisely according to the prediction of the Watson-Crick model: the first round of replication would have produced a double strand, one labeled and the other not, and the second round would produce two strands, one doubly labeled and one laying down labeled DNA on an unlabeled DNA. This interpretation is diagrammed in Fig. 2-6.

There have been two puzzling features about DNA replication that made it difficult to reconcile in vitro results with in vivo observations. The first is that DNA polymerase synthesizes new DNA unidirectionally, from the 5′ end to the 3′ end [11]. However, the double-stranded molecule is composed of two chains of opposite polarity (see footnote 5), i.e., one chain reads 5′ → 3′ while the other reads 3′ → 5′. The Cairns model suggested that in vivo replication proceeds unidirectionally. This implied that the enzyme moved along the DNA synthesizing the two chains in opposite directions! The paradox can be resolved as follows: suppose the polymerase copied one DNA strand (*A*) in the conventional way (5′ → 3′) and the other (*B*) *dis*continuously, in short segments 5′ → 3′. Thus:

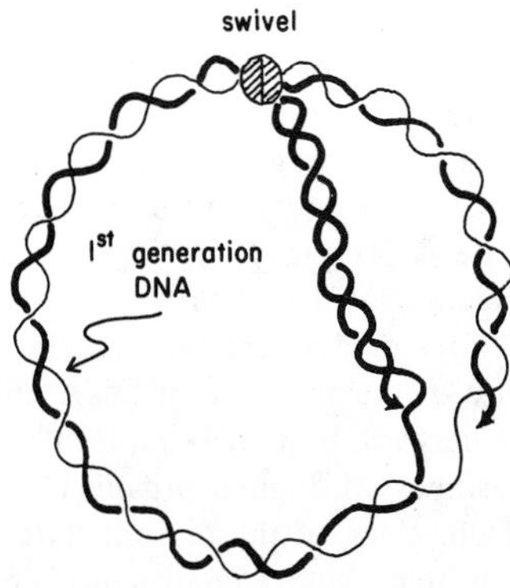

Figure 2-6. A diagrammatic interpretation of the experiment of Cairns [10]. DNA made during the first generation in tritiated medium would contain one tritiated strand (dark line) and one unlabeled strand (light line). The latter would therefore not show up on the radioautograph. During the second generation of replication, which is pictured as having proceeded a bit less than halfway, new tritiated DNA would be laid down on the separating strands, making a Y-shaped molecule in radioautographs, one arm of which is twice as radioactive as the other arm and as the base. A hypothetical swivel is provided to allow the DNA to unwind.

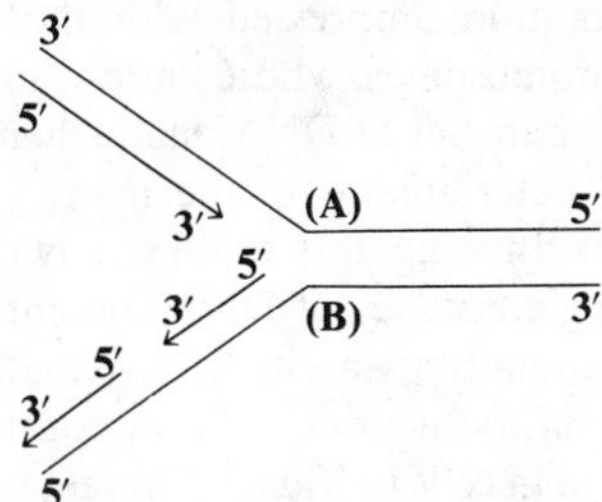

If these short strands could then be joined by another enzyme, it would account for the overall picture seen in vivo. Recent experiments strongly support this mechanism. (1) Newly synthesized DNA in vivo is released as short segments when the molecules are denatured; and (2) an enzyme, DNA ligase, has been discovered which can join gaps between segments of DNA [see *G*, vol. XXXIII, p. 129].

The other puzzling feature was that DNA polymerase until recently was never able to synthesize a biologically active DNA. This has now been accomplished [12]. Success in this endeavor depended on having a continuous (i.e., circular) DNA template and the ligase enzyme to join the two ends of the newly made DNA strands.

Very recently, a rapidly increasing body of evidence indicates that the Kornberg DNA polymerase may not in fact be the true DNA replicase in living cells. Mutants of bacteria have been isolated which appear to lack this enzyme [42].

Also, membrane-bound replicating complexes have been isolated from cells which contain the growing point of newly forming DNA. These complexes can autonomously synthesize DNA and lack Kornberg DNA polymerase activity (for example see Ref. 43). It may prove to be that the "classical" DNA polymerase is primarily an enzyme used by the cell to repair damaged DNA (see below).

Such varied lines of evidence all contribute to a rather definitive picture of the structure of DNA and its mode of replication. We may ask how these molecules are organized in the chromosomes of higher organisms. Although the picture is far from clear, at the present state of knowledge the consensus is that the basic structural and replicative processes are probably the same, and that it may well be that a single genetic linkage group in higher organisms is a single DNA molecule arranged in some kind of package representing the morphologic entity, the chromosome itself. Models for such a structure have been suggested [see *C*, part I, p. 65], but will not be discussed here, since they do not contribute to our understanding of the molecular aspects of information-transfer processes.

DNA as Genetic Arbiter

The evidence that DNA is in fact the substance of the gene is now very impressive. First isolated and studied just about one hundred years ago by Miescher and known for many years to be localized in the chromosomes, DNA was not early a favorite candidate for the genetic material. Workers were somewhat more impressed with the proteins to be found in the chromosomes, whose variety, in contrast to the rather uniform character of DNA, made them more appealing as possible determinants of the many genetic traits of living organisms. Investigators could not avoid noting, however, the striking constancy of DNA content of the somatic cells of a given organism, and its relative metabolic stability, unlike the variability of other cellular constituents such as RNA and protein in cells in widely different metabolic states. The fact, furthermore, that the haploid germ cells of organisms contained exactly one-half the quantity of DNA found in its somatic cells did not go without serious notice.

DNA was enthroned by the painstaking studies of Avery and his associates at the Rockefeller Institute, published in 1944 [13]. These showed that bacterial *transformation,* the process by which extracts of bacteria of one genotype could permanently alter the heredity of bacteria of another genotype, was caused by DNA. Earlier work by Griffiths had shown that a mixture of living nonvirulent pneumococci and a heat-killed suspension of virulent organisms, when injected into mice, produced virulent organisms which were lethal to the host.[6] Virulence is a genetically determined trait, depending on the ability of these organisms to produce a characteristic polysaccharide capsule. The virulence acquired by this exposure to dead organisms was stably inherited indefinitely thereafter. The vague interpretation of this remarkable finding at that time was that in some manner the few nonvirulent organisms had picked up from the products of the dead virulent forms some "antigens" somehow conferring the property of virulence. In the intervening years other investigators refined the study of genetic transformation chiefly by making it possible for the work to be carried out in vitro using crude extracts of cells. In their now classic paper, Avery, MacLeod, and McCarty described their systematic chemical attack on such extracts and their final conclusion that the transforming principle was, indeed, DNA. An important part of their evidence was that an enzyme specific for hydrolysis of DNA also destroyed transforming ability. Although some doubts lingered, particularly because of small amounts of protein associated with the DNA, from that date onward DNA was considered for practical experimental purposes the basic material of the gene.

Transformation studies have since been extended to other genetic markers (such as drug resistance and metabolic enzymes), have given us some insight into the mechanisms of the process, and have extended the phenomenon to include animal cells as well. There are several separate aspects of the process of transformation. (1) Cells must be *competent:* they must be able to take up DNA and be transformed by it. Not all cells are competent, and those that are may be so only under certain conditions of growth, nutritional environment, stage of division cycle, etc. Very little is known about the factors underlying competence. (2) There is the actual uptake of the DNA by the cells, a rather nonspecific process independent of, but essential to, subsequent events. (3) There follows a stage in which the DNA becomes integrated in some way with the DNA of the host cell, an event that must precede the formation of a recombinant progeny chromosome containing genetic markers introduced by the transforming DNA. Transforming DNA preparations now contain less than 0.02 percent of protein, but we cannot yet be certain that this protein is not an essential element in transformation.

Study of the chemical events occurring during infection of a bacterium by a virus pioneered by Hershey and associates have also supplied important evidence on the role of DNA as genetic arbiter. The virulent bacteriophages T2, T4, and T6 infect their natural host *E. coli* by attaching to the surface of the cell and injecting their DNA into the host cytoplasm. The protein coat of the virus remains outside the bacterium and may be sheared off mechanically without altering the subsequent course of events. Very shortly after this event, the bacterium ceases to synthesize its own RNA and protein. During a latent period lasting several minutes the biosynthetic machinery of the host synthesizes, *under viral direction,* a series of enzymes necessary for the synthesis of viral DNA and protein. Soon new viral DNA appears and becomes enclosed in new viral coat protein, and shortly

[6] Here is another instance in which studies motivated primarily by medical considerations led to one of the most important discoveries in the history of biology.

thereafter the bacterial cells burst (as a result of the action of a newly synthesized viral lysozyme), and 100 to 200 new viruses are liberated.

This total transformation of the host's metabolic machinery to one whose sole function is to produce viral components is the dramatic outcome of the injection of a foreign DNA. The mechanism by which this is accomplished will be discussed later. Basically similar phenomena seem to occur upon infection of animal cells by animal viruses.

During the course of studies of various chemical mutagenic agents it has become clear that analogues of the bases of DNA are highly effective mutagens. They are incorporated into DNA in place of the analogous natural base and during subsequent copying of the DNA allow errors to be introduced by mechanisms to be discussed in the next section. This fact in itself—that chemical analogues of the subunits of DNA are mutagenic—constitutes important support for the proof of the role of DNA as genetic arbiter.

Finally, perhaps the most telling evidence equating DNA and the gene comes from the proof of *collinearity:* mutational alterations of single bases in DNA result in collinear alterations of amino acids in proteins. This evidence will be examined in a later section.

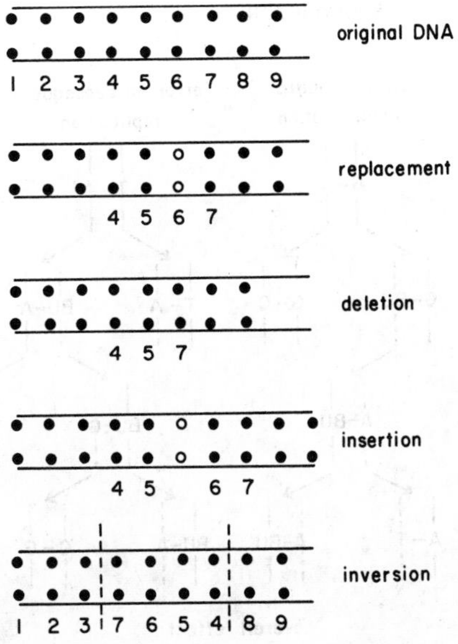

Figure 2-7. Some kinds of mutations. *(From D. Freese.)*

MOLECULAR MECHANISMS OF MUTATION

Before proceeding to the evidence supporting the concept of collinearity it is fitting to discuss briefly the chemical mechanism of mutation. We shall equate the chromosome with DNA with some confidence now, keeping in mind, however, that the DNA may be arranged in some complex way involving protein and other factors. Chromosomal variations may be divided into large changes detectable cytologically, such as increase or decrease in chromosome number, and changes in information content observable only by genetic analysis. This chapter is concerned exclusively with the latter. Changes in information content in DNA may be brought about by transformation, by transduction (virus-mediated transfer of genetic material from one bacterium to another), or by the sexual process. All these cases involve a recombination of information derived from two separate pieces of DNA. Information changes may also be brought about by mutation.

In Fig. 2-7 some kinds of mutational base alterations in DNA are shown. Replacements of one base pair by another are usefully subdivided into *transitions,* i.e., pyrimidine-pyrimidine or purine-purine interchange (C ↔ T, A ↔ G), or *transversions,* i.e., purine-pyrimidine interchanges (A ↔ C, A ↔ T, G ↔ C, G ↔ T). Genetically, a base-pair change is observed as a *point* mutation. A point mutation, since it involves an alteration of a single base pair, has a finite chance to revert to the original wild genotype, unlike a deletion mutation or an inversion, in which one or more bases are actually removed from the DNA or transposed.

Chemical Mutagens

A wide variety of chemical and physical mutagenic agents is now known, a few examples of which will be given to illustrate general principles.

5-Bromouracil (BU), an analogue of thymine in which a bromine atom replaces the methyl group, has been one of the most thoroughly studied chemical mutagens. The nucleoside derivative of BU, bromodeoxyuridine, is readily phosphorylated by cells and thence incorporated into DNA in place of thymidine. Indeed, in cells starved of thymine most of this base can be replaced in DNA by BU. This analogue apparently induces base-pair transitions by either of two mechanisms: (1) during DNA synthesis it may enter the newly forming strand opposite G—i.e., a mistake in *incorporation* is made; or (2) it may, after having entered DNA by pairing normally with A, pair with G during a subsequent round of replication—a mistake in *replication.* In the former case the G of a GC pair in DNA would generate a G-BU pair, which on further replication would generate a BU-A pair, since A is the "normal" companion of BU (or T). In the next replication, A would pair normally with T. Thus the intervention of BU would convert, by an initial mistake in incorporation, a GC pair into an AT pair. This series of events is illustrated in Fig. 2-8. In the second case, the mistake in replication, BU pairs "normally" with A on incorporation into DNA (generating an A-BU pair) but, on further replication, pairs with G (generating G-BU). The G of this pair would then normally pair in the next round with C. Thus, an original AT pair has been converted to a GC pair (see Fig. 2-8).

Another highly mutagenic agent is 2-aminopurine (AP), an analogue of adenine, which apparently can pair on occa-

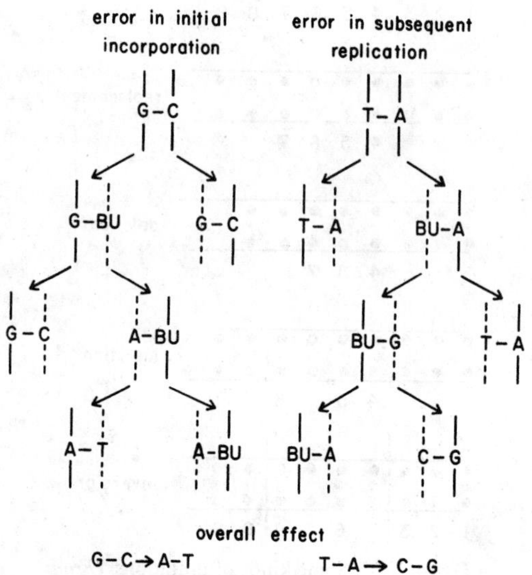

Figure 2-8. The probable molecular mechanism of mutagenesis by bromouracil. (The dotted line at each generation is the newly formed strand.)

sion with T and more rarely with C. The former pairing would not be expected to be mutagenic (since proper pairing would not be altered), but the latter would, by the same arguments used above (i.e., a normal GC pair is converted to AP-C, which next generates AP-T and finally AT, as the T pairs normally with A). On chemical grounds the frequency of pairing of AP with C should be higher than that of BU with G, and this is probably why AP is highly mutagenic even though it is incorporated into DNA only to a small extent.

The effects of both AP and BU are to produce transitions. Other mutagens, notably the sulfur and nitrogen mustards and ethylene oxides and ethylethane sulfonate, the so-called *alkylating agents,* also produce base transitions. The main effect of alkylating agents is upon guanine, the alkylated form of which tends to pair erroneously with thymine. The resulting G-T pair generates a T-A pair at the next round of replication.

Acridine dyes such as proflavin and acridine orange constitute another class of effective mutagens and appear to act by becoming sandwiched between two layers of base pairs in the DNA duplex, thus causing distortions in the regularity of the base spacing. Such distortions then lead to errors in replication by inducing deletions or additions of single bases or small groups of bases. Since, as we shall see in a later section, the genetic information in DNA is read out, base by base, in a unidirectional process, deletions or additions of bases can have a devastating effect on the translation process.

For a more detailed discussion on chemical mutagens see reference [14].

Physical Agents

The important physical mutagenic agents are, of course, x-rays and ultraviolet light. The actions of the two are quite different: x-rays act indirectly, damage to the DNA being produced by free radicals induced transiently in the vicinity of the DNA molecule. The effect of ultraviolet light is direct, the nucleic acid molecule preferentially absorbing light of a particular wavelength, with resulting damage. In both cases, a variety of effects is induced, from breaks in chain continuity to alterations of a single or several bases.

One of the striking findings that has emerged from the study of chemical and physical mutagens is that each agent causes mutation in particular sites in the DNA, or "hot spots" [15]. These favored sites of mutation are different for each mutagen and are in turn different from those for "spontaneous" mutations.

Repair of Mutationally Altered DNA

Recent experimental work has revealed that living systems are remarkably agile in carrying out repair of DNA. It now appears that enzymes are constantly monitoring DNA and repairing any damage they detect. Indeed, this continuous repair process requires that we modify our concept of DNA as an inert macromolecule, uninvolved in the dynamic turnover characteristic of all other macromolecular species. Our newer knowledge comes from studies of molecular events occurring during the course of repair of damage to the genetic material produced in bacteria by ultraviolet irradiation [see *G*, vol. XXXIII]. One of the effects of this physical mutagenic agent is the production of thymine dimers—chemical bonds between neighboring thymines on a DNA strand. Repair of such damage is an elaborate process. It involves four distinct steps, each requiring a specific enzyme activity: (1) *opening* of the chain by breaking a phosphodiester linkage near the site of damage; (2) *removal* of the offending section; (3) *restoration* of the section by normal DNA polymerase action; and (4) *closure* of the final phosphodiester link by DNA ligase. This fascinating healing process is another dramatic illustration of the importance of DNA's double-strandedness: the "memory" preserved in the intact strand serves to ensure the fidelity of repair of the damaged strand.

A Brief Digression into Protein Structure

It is now clear that proteins, as enzymes, carry out the functions of the living organisms and define the specificity of species. That is, just as DNA is the molecular substratum of genotype, protein is the molecular basis of phenotype. This is the important concept behind our attempt to link DNA and protein synthesis.

Proteins are linear unbranched polymers with complex

secondary, tertiary, and quaternary structures. They are composed of 20 basic building blocks, the amino acids, arranged in a specific order in peptide linkage, and they may be several hundred amino acids in length. The order of amino acids in these chains is referred to as the *primary* structure (Fig. 2-9). It seems highly probable that the genetically defined specificity of a protein molecule depends entirely upon the *kind* of amino acids it contains and their *sequence,* and that subsequent folding is generally a spontaneous process. For it has been observed now with a number of quite different proteins that they may be fully denatured, i.e., unfolded into their one-dimensional structure, and when the denaturing conditions are removed, they return spontaneously to their former native configuration. It is a reasonable working hypothesis that a newly forming polypeptide chain in the cell also folds spontaneously as it grows in length into its most comfortable form energetically. Substantial segments of these polypeptide chains form helixes through hydrogen bonding (*secondary* structure), while the helixes and nonhelical stretches in turn are folded into complex stabilized *tertiary* structures, through a variety of covalent and noncovalent linkages. A number of proteins (many enzymes, hemoglobin, antibodies, etc.) are composed of more than one of these folded polypeptide chains (*quaternary* structure). The ingenious techniques pioneered by Sanger [16] have made it possible to work out complete amino acid sequences of a number of pure proteins. Refinements in the techniques of x-ray diffraction have permitted the visualization of primary, secondary, and tertiary structure of several proteins; indeed, the now-attained resolution of 2 Å permits one to locate and identify individual amino acids [17].

Specificity of Protein Structure

A striking and important fact about protein structure is the specificity of its amino acid content and sequence; i.e., in general these parameters vary only slightly for a given protein species from a variety of organisms. Thus insulins,

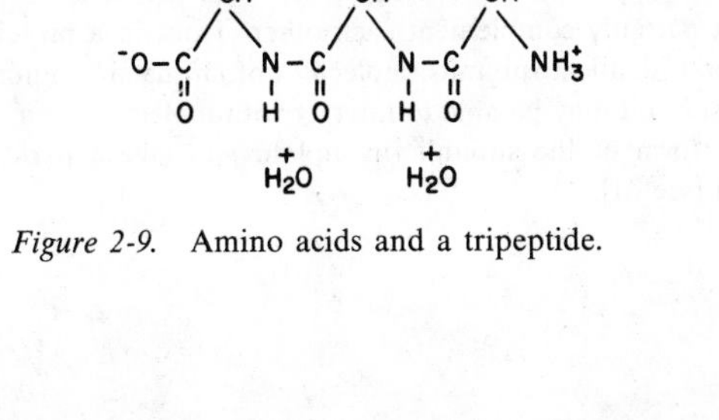

Figure 2-9. Amino acids and a tripeptide.

hemoglobins, and ribonucleases from different sources are remarkably similar in amino acid content and sequence. Clearly the synthetic mechanism must be one that selects and orders amino acids with a high degree of precision. As far as selection is concerned, experiment has shown that amino acid analogues, closely resembling their natural counterparts, are excluded from protein in vivo with remarkable accuracy by the living cell.

Having emphasized the specificity of protein structure we may also note that it is by no means inflexible. Mutational amino acid substitutions in proteins occur which produce no detectable alteration in their physicochemical or enzymatic properties. A substitution which replaces a charged residue with an uncharged one, as in sickle-cell hemoglobin, will have a much more drastic effect than the replacement of, say, a glycine by an alanine residue. The replacement of an amino acid like proline, for example, which seems to be involved in making key corners in protein chains, would be highly destructive. Again, a substitution in or near the active site of an enzyme is likely to be more damaging than a substitution elsewhere in the molecule. Thus, both specificity of structure and some flexibility in construction serve the needs of the living organism.

As the complete amino acid sequence of an increasingly large number of proteins is worked out it has become clear that, for a given protein species, evolution has preserved long sequences of amino acids as essential to function. But it is equally obvious that extensive changes (sometimes involving as many as half of the total number of amino acids) can occur without altering the critical function. This kind of study sheds light not only upon biochemical evolution, but also upon the extent to which certain portions of a protein molecule are essential to their particular job in the cell [18] [see also *F*].

FINE-STRUCTURE GENETICS AND PROTEIN ALTERATION

The concept of the gene has undergone considerable modification in recent years. Through the pioneering work of Mendel, Morgan, and Muller it came to be visualized as a heritable unit that somehow determined a phenotypic trait or function. It soon became clear, of course, that gross genetic characteristics such as eye color were the result of the complex interaction of a number of proteins, enzymes, and structural elements, the alteration of any one of which by mutation could result in a gross change.

Beadle and Tatum [19, 20], as a result of their studies of x-ray-induced nutritional mutants of the mold *Neurospora,* introduced the modern era with the notion that a gene is a heritable unit governing the synthesis of a single enzyme—the so-called one-gene–one-enzyme hypothesis. This definition is generally accepted today, modified by a greater sophistication about the complexity of enzyme structure. For it is now known that many enzymes are not single proteins but complexes of more than one polypeptide chain, linked in various ways. Such protein subunits of enzymes may be identical or nonidentical polypeptides. In the latter case a gene governing the synthesis of such an enzyme is a *complex gene,* containing as many different subunits as there are different subunit proteins in the enzyme.

Complementation Analysis

Exquisitely fine genetic analysis has been made possible by the use of bacteria and their viruses. The keys to their usefulness are (1) they grow very rapidly, permitting the analysis of large populations in short times; (2) they are largely haploid so that any induced genetic alteration is immediately expressed in phenotype; (3) applicable procedures for the selection of *rare* mutant forms are extremely sensitive. In practice, for fine-structure genetic analysis, the gene is delineated by *complementation,* just as in classical genetics. Given two mutants of a given organism with identical phenotypes, the critical question is whether they are defective in the same gene or in different genes. For example, one may irradiate a culture of bacteria which ordinarily are able to synthesize the amino acid leucine. The irradiated culture may then be plated on a medium lacking leucine but containing an agent such as penicillin which will kill all the organisms able to grow without leucine (the parental types). Mutant forms, incapable of making leucine, will survive because they do not grow. The latter organisms may then be isolated on plates containing leucine. These surviving organisms will have mutational alterations in any one of several enzymes involved in leucine biosynthesis.

Now there are means by which these normally haploid organisms may be made diploid for particular genetic characters one wishes to study ("abortive" transduction, "sex duction" in bacterial mating, etc.). One thus establishes stable diploid organisms by combining the relevant genes from each of the mutants in question. If the function which was lacking in each of the mutants separately—ability to synthesize leucine in our example—is restored in the diploid, one concludes that each of the mutants is defective in *different* genes; if the function is not restored, the mutants are defective in the *same* gene. In molecular terms, failure to restore function in a diploid composed of two mutant DNAs means that the same enzyme of the leucine biosynthetic pathway is defective. Restoration of function means that each mutant has a different defective enzyme, and therefore each also has one normal enzyme. This restoration of function is called *complementation*—i.e., two wild-type (nonmutated) genes complementing each other in the diploid. R. D. Hotchkiss has offered the following analogy: A man "wants to go somewhere and has two defective motor cars. If one of the cars has a flat tire and the other a faulty carburetor, the man can fulfill his engagement by replacing either the flat tire or the faulty carburetor with a good one from the other car; but if both cars have useless carburetors he can do nothing" [*D*, p. 94].

The *complex genes,* of course, introduce an added subtlety, for in this case one might have mutations in two separate subunits of the *same* gene which could complement each other in diploids. The minimal noncomplementing genetic element has generally been defined as that which governs the synthesis of a *single polypeptide chain.*[7]

Definition of the Gene

Now we may return to chemistry. Evidence that DNA is the genetic material has been presented. All genetic mapping data are consistent with the hypothesis that the genome is a linear unbranched structure. All chemical evidence finds DNA to be a linear unbranched polymer. This suggests a molecular definition of the gene: a *linear sequence of bases in DNA of determinate length that defines a collinear sequence of amino acids in a single functional protein unit.*

Genetic Mapping

As mentioned at the beginning of this chapter, the dramatic demonstration that sickle-cell hemoglobin differs from normal hemoglobin by the substitution of a single amino acid residue spurred the search for systems more amenable to fine genetic analysis. This search can be said to have been abundantly successful—the microbial systems have permitted genetic analysis to probe to the level of the individual nucleotide. We have seen how the complementation test permits the geneticist to define the gene precisely in operational terms. He may then obtain a wide variety of mutants *defective in the same gene* and map—by genetic recombi-

[7] This minimal noncomplementing genetic element is now usually called a *cistron,* after Benzer. This name is confusing but pervades the literature. It derives from the following considerations: two mutations in different locations on two different pieces of DNA are said to be in position *trans* to each other, thus: A——— / ———B. If they are both within a noncomplementing unit, as we have said, there will be no function. If, however, in what might be considered a never-performed control experiment, both mutations were in the *same* piece of DNA: A——— / B———, i.e., in position *cis,* function would be restored, because one whole gene (B), or cistron, is present. In some current usage the terms "gene" and "cistron" are given identical meaning: both are the minimal unit of complementation.

It is becoming increasingly clear, however, that the phenomenon of intracistronic complementation can occur, thus placing restrictions on the usefulness of complementation tests in defining the cistron. That is, it appears that certain mutations in the *same* cistron may at least partially complement each other. Thus, in a protein made of several identical subunits, molecules of an inactive mutant form of the subunit may be able to interact with molecules of a different mutant form of the subunit (in diploids) to give a partial active protein [see 21].

nation—the actual linear order of the defects within the gene. This is accomplished by determining the frequency with which haploid, wild-type recombinant progeny appear after a genetic cross between any two parent organisms having defects in the gene in question. (In bacteria this is done by sexual conjugation or transduction; in bacteriophage, by mixed infection of a single bacterial host with two mutant phages.) Recombinant frequency is a direct measure of the linear distance separating two defects; the closer the defects are to each other, the rarer will be the recombinants. (Of course, if the defects are at exactly the same site, there will be no recombinants.) For example, suppose we have three mutants—A, B, and C—defective in the same gene by complementation tests. By crossing mutant A first with mutant B and then with mutant C, and B and C with each other, we obtain the following recombination frequencies (the percentage of progeny having the wild phenotype): $A \times B = 0.08$, $A \times C = 0.03$, and $B \times C = 0.05$. We may then locate the mutations with respect to one another along the gene as

$$\mathbf{A \leftarrow 0.03 \rightarrow C \leftarrow 0.05 \rightarrow B}$$
$$\longleftarrow \mathbf{0.08} \longrightarrow$$

The detection of wild-type recombinant progeny is so sensitive that it is possible, by equating recombinant frequency with total amount of DNA in an organism, to map mutations separated in the DNA by only one or two nucleotides! It is important to emphasize that the initial assumption of linearity of genetic information is borne out by such genetic analysis.

Collinearity of DNA and Protein

The question one next asks, therefore, is: Is the linearity of genetic information in DNA correlated directly with linear information in the protein made from this DNA? Here one not only requires a delicate genetic test for restoration of function; one also must have in hand the pure enzyme whose amino acid sequence is determined by the gene in question. The most thoroughly studied case to date, the tryptophan-synthetase system of *E. coli*, so brilliantly exploited by Yanofsky, may be used as an example [22]. The genes mediating the synthesis of the enzymes involved in tryptophan biosynthesis have been accurately mapped on the *E. coli* chromosome. The enzymes themselves have been purified, and the amino acid sequence of one of the proteins has been largely worked out. It is important here to point out that while many mutations result in synthesis of no protein at all, many others result in synthesis of immunologically related but inactive or poorly active protein, or active protein with detectably altered physical properties. Thus it is possible to obtain protein products of *mutated genes* upon which amino acid analysis may be performed. When the mutational alterations in the genetic map are correlated with the amino acid analysis of the altered proteins, there is indeed found to be a collinear relationship between the two; i.e., in our example above, where mutants A, B, and C are found to be linearly related to one another as $A \leftarrow 0.03 \rightarrow C \leftarrow 0.05 \rightarrow B$, the protein of mutant A is found to have a single amino acid change at a given point, mutant C an altered amino acid to the right of it, and mutant B an alteration still farther to the right.

A most elegant demonstration of collinearity has been offered by Sarabhai et al. [23]. They have studied a special group of bacteriophage mutants that are defective in synthesis of head protein. This particular set of mutants contain "nonsense," i.e., nontranslatable, mutations. The different mutants thus make head proteins of varying lengths. When the lengths of the proteins made by a series of mutants are correlated with the location of the mutation in the controlling gene (as determined by genetic mapping), they are found to be collinear; i.e., the longer the protein the farther the mutation is from one end of the gene. The synthetic machinery vigorously completes the proteins up to "nonsense" mutations and can proceed no further.

TRANSCRIPTION OF THE MESSAGE AND ITS CONTROL AT THE GENETIC LEVEL

We have thus far looked at the beginning and the end of the information transfer system without asking questions about mechanism. It remains now to examine the actual chemical mechanism of transcription of the genetic message. The assembly of amino acids into polypeptide chains occurs on ribosomes in the cytoplasm, while the DNA, particularly in higher forms, is sequestered in the nucleus. Thus the message of DNA must be transcribed into a utilizable cytoplasmic form before it can be secondarily translated into the language of protein.[8]

Messenger RNA

Figure 2-10 is a schematic outline of the present picture of the transcription process and the mechanisms by which its expression is controlled. It will be useful to refer to it in this and the following sections. At the level of DNA, segments are designated "structural loci." These are the sequences of nucleotides collinear with the sequences of amino acids in protein—the genes—as defined in the previous section. Thus they determine the primary structure of protein. Presumably a large fraction of the total DNA of a cell is made up of these structural genes. (A bacterial cell such as *E. coli* can make some one to two thousand different

[8]The term *transcription* is used to denote the process by which the cell reads out the information in DNA (the production of a message); *translation* refers to the final conversion of this information into protein (the reading of the message).

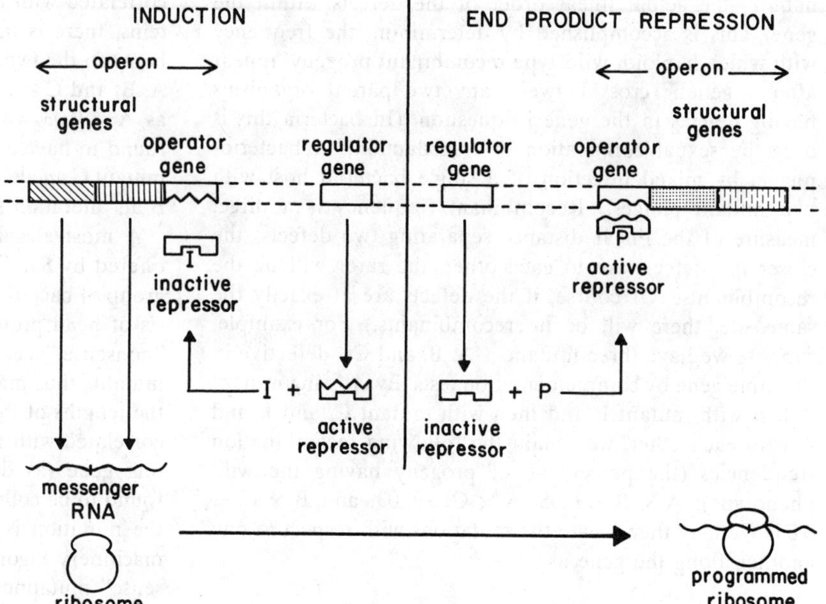

Figure 2-10. A scheme for the repressive control of messenger output at the gene level. I is the small molecular inducer, P the small molecule end product. The systems are shown as they would be functioning in the presence of I and P. In their absence the exact opposite effect would be observed: the left-hand system would be repressed, the right-hand system active. The affinity of repressors for operators is indicated by their complementary shapes.

species of protein molecules; an animal cell, many times this number.) An enzyme, RNA polymerase, copies from one strand of the DNA a replica RNA—messenger RNA (mRNA). Messenger RNA passes to the cytoplasm and is bound to the ribosomes, where it is used by the protein synthetic machinery to make protein. This is a dynamic process in which the messenger serves a limited number of times as template and is then destroyed. The lifetime of a messenger RNA molecule is probably much longer in animal cells.

Some of the lines of evidence supporting this scheme may be briefly recounted:

1 In bacteria, the synthesis of a newly needed enzyme occurs with remarkable rapidity. This phenomenon led Pardee, Jacob, and Monod [24] early to wonder whether the cell might possess some mechanism for the rapid transmission of genetic information to the site of protein synthesis. The then-known mechanism of protein synthesis did not indicate such a mechanism, but the following observation, made earlier but not originally accorded its present significance, suggested a possible mechanism.

2 When a bacteriophage introduces its DNA into a bacterial cell, all synthesis of bacterial RNA and protein ceases, and a new RNA fraction appears which rapidly turns over (as judged by a rapid rate of incorporation of labeled RNA precursors); i.e., it is synthesized and destroyed very rapidly, never amounting to more than a few percent of the total RNA of the cell [25]. The base composition of this RNA is an accurate reflection of the base composition of the viral DNA and differs from that of the bulk RNA of the bacterial cell. Concomitant with the appearance of this RNA new protein begins to appear, all of it involved in the production of new virus. This observation was originally very puzzling: why should phage DNA induce the synthesis of a mimic RNA when it did not itself contain RNA? It was later shown, after the possible significance of this finding was aired, that this RNA can attach reversibly (depending chiefly on the Mg^{++} concentration) to ribosomes already present in the bacterium [26]. This RNA was named *messenger RNA* because of the clear implication that it carried a message from DNA to the protein synthetic machinery. The molecular weight of messenger RNA fraction is generally high and heterogeneous, in keeping with its role as mediator of the synthesis of proteins of large and varied size.

Similar rapidly turning over RNA fractions have since been identified in normal uninfected bacterial, plant, and animal cells.

3 An enzyme, RNA polymerase, which has been isolated from numerous bacterial and animal sources, synthesizes RNA when supplied with all four of the *ribo*nucleoside triphosphates, Mg^{++}, *and* DNA [see *C*]. (The reader will note the similarity in requirements of this enzyme to DNA polymerase.) The product made is an RNA whose base composition and other characteristics are an accurate reflection of the DNA used as "primer." The RNA product will reversibly associate with ribosomes in vitro and can be used for protein synthesis. Actinomycin D, a potent inhibitor of RNA synthesis in the cell, also stops protein synthesis. Using this antibiotic to inhibit further messenger synthesis, it is possible to measure the rate of decay of the remaining messenger molecules. This measurement, together with a determination of the residual protein synthesis, gives the number of protein molecules made per messenger molecule: this comes out to be of the order of 10 to 20 in bacteria.

4 A *synthetic* messenger RNA, produced by the enzyme

polynucleotide phosphorylase,[9] will reversibly associate with ribosomes in vitro and can be used by the natural protein synthetic machinery to make a synthetic protein whose amino acid content is dictated by the bases incorporated into the messenger. This remarkable synthesis has been found to occur in both bacterial and animal systems.

Control of Gene Action

We may now consider how the transcription process may be regulated at the genetic level. Our information here is derived entirely from microbial systems. In the scheme in Fig. 2-10 note that there are other genes designated *regulator genes,* which are pictured as producing *repressors.* The repressor substance interacts with a DNA locus adjacent to a structural locus, thereby shutting off the synthesis of messenger RNA by that structural gene. The locus with which the repressor interacts is called an *operator* locus, or operator gene. The operator locus and the contiguous structural gene or genes[10] are referred to as an *operon* [27].

Regulation by Repression

Bacteria respond dramatically to the introduction of a new energy source, such as a sugar, by synthesizing the appropriate enzyme to utilize it. The synthesis of the enzyme is said to be *induced* by the sugar. This response ensures the ready adaptation of the cells to new nutrients in their environment. Cells lacking the structural gene for the enzyme or containing a damaged gene, of course, cannot so respond. But genetic analysis reveals that the ability to respond to inducer is based not only on an intact *structural* gene but also on another genetic site, the *regulator* locus, frequently mapping at a distance from the structural gene. This regulator locus synthesizes a product (the repressor) which shuts off enzyme synthesis; the action of the repressor is reversed by the inducing agent. The evidence for this is, first, that a mutation in this locus causes the organism to make the enzyme constitutively, i.e., in the *absence* of inducer, suggesting that the cell's capacity to make enzyme is normally restricted, or repressed. Second, when this gene is present on a chromosome in a stable diploid state, it can repress the synthesis of the enzyme mediated by an intact structural gene on *another* chromosome. This means that the influence of the regulator gene can be exerted over a distance; i.e., the wild-type gene must make something that can diffuse to a gene on another piece of DNA and shut off its expression. The third piece of evidence comes from an ingenious experiment of Pardee, Jacob, and Monod [24], illustrated in Fig. 2-11. In a sexual cross in *E. coli,* the regulator gene together with the structural gene for an enzyme (β-

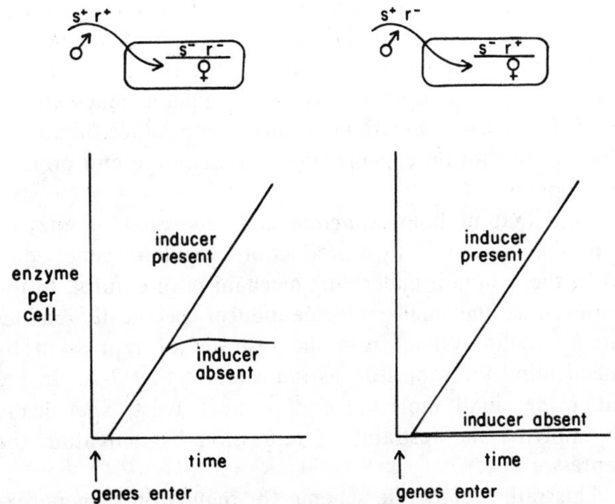

Figure 2-11. The experiment of Pardee, Jacob, and Monod [24]. Above the experimental curves are the genetic experiments. In the left-hand experiment the intact, or wild-type (+), structural gene (s) and regulator gene (r) are injected by a male into a female having defective (−) s and r genes. The events occurring immediately (~ about 2 min) after gene entry are shown below. In the right-hand experiment a competent structural gene (and functionless regulator gene) is injected into a female with an intact regulator gene, and the ensuing events are pictured below. The immediate constitutive synthesis of enzyme in the first case but not in the second is taken to mean that the presence of the intact regulator gene in the female established a milieu incompatible with the expression of the structural gene. The shutoff of synthesis in the first case suggests that it takes time to establish this milieu (i.e., to accumulate repressor).

galactosidase) was introduced into a female whose genome contained inoperative (mutant) alleles of both these genes. It was noted that immediately upon entry of the two genes, enzyme began to be synthesized at a rapid rate in the *absence* of inducer. After a while synthesis ceased; it resumed only if inducer was added. If, on the other hand, the female contained a functional regulator gene, synthesis occurred only if inducer was present. This was interpreted to mean that a female with a defective regulator gene could not synthesize repressor, and therefore synthesis of enzyme proceeded until enough repressor was made by the newly introduced regulator gene to shut off synthesis. The inducer was needed to counteract the effect of repressor.

Another area of study contributing to the general scheme of control by repression is that of the biosynthetic enzymes—those enzymes in bacteria which synthesize the essential building blocks of protoplasm, amino acid, nucleotides, etc. It is striking that bacteria genetically capable of synthesizing these enzymes do not do so when the amino acid or nucleotide is presented to them in the medium. Thus it appears that such metabolites shut off, or *repress,* their own synthesis when they are available to the cell. If one limits their supply, the bacterium overcompensates by synthesizing enormous quantities of the enzymes that make them—sometimes more

[9]This enzyme is discussed more fully on p. 48.

[10]Often several genes, governing the synthesis of a series of enzymes carrying out sequential biosynthetic operations, are located sequentially in space on the chromosome.

than 10 percent of their total cell protein! This overcompensation is in itself a dramatic demonstration of the normal capacity of the bacterial cell to regulate enzyme synthesis. Again, genetic analysis reveals that regulator genes are involved here also: mutations in such loci produce organisms that *fail* to shut off enzyme synthesis when the end product is supplied.

Note that in both *induction* and *repression* of enzyme synthesis, repression by a product of a regulator gene seems to be the common underlying mechanism of control. In the former case the small molecule inducer specifically *releases* the synthetic system from the restraint of repression by inactivating the repressor, as indicated in Fig. 2-10. In the latter the small molecule end product assists specifically in applying the restraint of repression by activating the repressor.

This rather elaborate scheme for regulation of gene expression by repression was deduced almost entirely from genetic evidence. Until about 4 years ago, direct evidence for the existence of repressor substances was wholly lacking. Evidence has now been brought forward that repressors actually do exist, that they are proteins that bind specifically with inducers, and that they are in extremely low concentrations in bacterial cells [28, 29].

Repression by Control of Transcription

Most of the evidence now available supports the idea that repressors act upon DNA directly by interfering with the production of mRNA. It has recently been demonstrated that bacterial cells "derepressed" for synthesis of a particular enzyme contain a messenger RNA specific for that enzyme, while cells that have not been derepressed lack such a messenger RNA. Specific messenger RNA may be demonstrated by showing that the rapidly labeled RNA fraction of derepressed cells will form a hybrid with the DNA from cells possessing the structural gene for that enzyme, under appropriate conditions. No hybrid is formed with the RNA from the repressed cells or with DNA from an organism lacking the gene in question.

The Operon

The evidence for *operator loci* (O) comes from the discovery of mutations (O^c) that occur very close to, but not within, a sequence of structural genes and result in constitutive synthesis of the enzymes involved; i.e., the series of enzymes is made whether or not inducer is present. Further genetic analysis shows that in order to express itself this type of gene must be contiguous with the structural genes it controls. This is in contrast to the regulator gene, which can express itself even when on another piece of DNA, as we have seen. The reasonable interpretation of these experiments is that the operator locus is the site with which the repressor interacts to block transcription of the adjacent structural gene: somehow the mutation causes the gene to lose its sensitivity to repressor.

The concept of the operon derives from the observation, in such inducible and repressible systems as we have discussed, that frequently regulator genes govern the expression of more than one structural gene. When the operator locus and the related structural genes are clustered together on the chromosome, they are referred to as an *operon.* Regulator mutations affect the expression of these genes in parallel.

The reader will not fail to note that most of the experimental evidence presented is derived from studies on bacteria and viruses. Such organisms require biosynthetic machinery that can respond rapidly to changes in environment. Differentiated cells, on the other hand, must maintain a stable intracellular biosynthetic establishment, which is accomplished in part by a stable extracellular environment. One might then not be surprised to find that the *regulation* of biosynthetic pathways might be quite different in bacterial and animal cells, even though the pathways themselves are very similar. Animal cells are much more difficult to study, both genetically and biochemically, at this level, and our information is consequently more fragmentary. Nonetheless, it is impressive to see that bacteria and higher animals use identical building blocks for DNA, RNA, and protein and identical pathways for their synthesis, and that, to date, the similarities even at the level of regulation—induction, repression, messenger RNA—are more impressive than the differences. It would appear that the evolutionary process may have fixed upon certain optimal building blocks, synthetic pathways, and control circuits that have been useful to all living forms. However, the price we have paid in the last 15 years for the rapid advances in our understanding of microbial systems is neglect of experimental interest in animal systems. Medical science has its fads like other fields of endeavor. At this writing one can begin to detect the rebirth of interest in the serious study of regulatory mechanisms in mammalian systems, and the next decade should produce many new insights. In addition to the obvious difference between bacteria and animals with respect to the problems of gene expression alluded to above, there are two additional broad areas of interest that are becoming the focus of biochemical concern. One is the nature of memory storage—a process by which specialized animal cells are able to convert environmental information into molecular structure. The other is the mechanism of growth control. Neither phenomenon seems to have any counterpart in the simple life of the bacterium. Our first glimpse of mechanistic detail in growth regulation, for example, reveals that animal cells maintain a high rate of synthesis and breakdown of all their macromolecular constituents in remarkable balance over long periods of time, and that mechanisms exist by which the cell may *directly* control the rate of functioning of the protein synthetic machinery in the cytoplasm [30].

THE MECHANISM OF PROTEIN SYNTHESIS

Although the early studies of Caspersson in Sweden and Brachet in Belgium pointed to the importance of RNA in protein synthesis, the real beginnings of our understanding came in the late 1940s when ^{14}C-labeled amino acids became available. This permitted the detection of traces of synthetic activity in tissue preparations. The development of improved methods for tissue fractionation by centrifugal means paralleled the use of isotopes and further contributed to the exponential growth of our knowledge. With these two techniques it became possible to inject animals with ^{14}C-labeled amino acids and, by subsequently isolating the various intracellular particulate and soluble components of the tissues, to follow the flow of amino acids into new protein molecules. It is interesting in the light of our heavy emphasis thus far on microbial systems that the early important advances in protein synthesis were made using animal cells [31].

The Ribosome

It soon became abundantly clear that the site of formation of the first new peptide bonds following injection of an animal with a labeled amino acid were the ribosomes, small cytoplasmic particles rich in RNA and protein, which line the endoplasmic reticular membrane within most adult animal cells (see Fig. 2-12). Only after radioactivity had appeared in the nascent protein of these ribosomes did it appear in other fractions of the cell cytoplasm such as mitochondrial and soluble protein.

Ribosomes are found in all living forms. In bacteria and in rapidly proliferating animal cells they are found free in the cytoplasm. In differentiated animal cells, most of them are found in intimate association with membranes of the endoplasmic reticulum. This reticulum appears in electron micrographs to be arranged in an elaborate system of canals, or tubes, along the walls of which the ribosomes are distributed in regular rows. The number of ribosomes per cell is a rather direct function of the rate at which the cells grow, particularly in bacteria.

Ribosomes are composed of three kinds of RNA, defined on the basis of their sedimentation constants in the ultracentrifuge—28S, 18S, and 5S for animal cells and 23S, 16S, and 5S in bacterial cells. They also contain a very large number of proteins—about fifty—many of which have special functions. The arrangement of these RNAs and proteins in the particle is not presently known but is the subject of intensive current investigation [see *G*, chap. XXXIV]. The particles are approximately 250 Å in diameter, and their molecular weight is approximately 5×10^6 for animal ribosomes and 4×10^6 for bacterial ribosomes.

Ribosomes are rich in Mg^{++} ions, there being one Mg^{++} for every three phosphate residues of their RNA. When isolated ribosomes are exposed to conditions which chelate the Mg^{++}, they dissociate reversibly into two subunits (the cap and nut of the acorn). The larger particle contains the 28S RNA, the 5S RNA, and some thirty proteins; the smaller particle contains the 18S RNA and some twenty proteins. (Since ribosomes cannot be separated into different functional units, it is not yet known whether there may be classes of ribosomes containing a few proteins, as opposed to a situation in which all ribosomes contain all the proteins.) The functional significance of ribosomal dissociation will be discussed later.

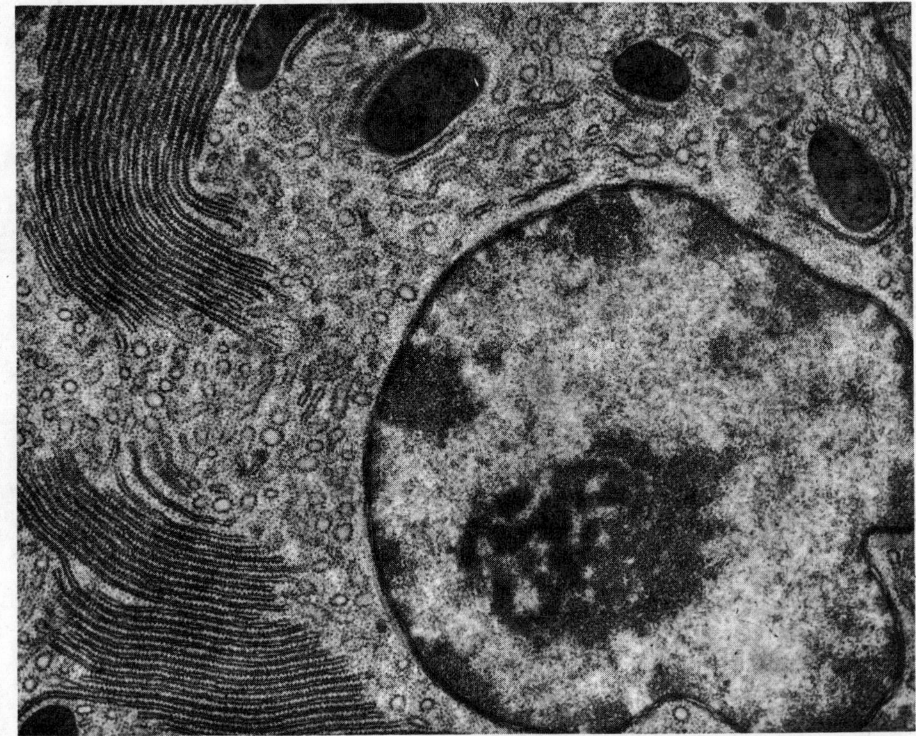

Figure 2-12. An electron micrograph of a mammalian cell (bat pancreas) with a profusion of endoplasmic reticulum seen as fine channels, some cut longitudinally and some in cross section, lined with dense ribosomes. A nucleus and a number of mitochondria may also be seen. Magnification is about ×11,000. (*Photograph generously supplied by Dr. D. W. Fawcett.*)

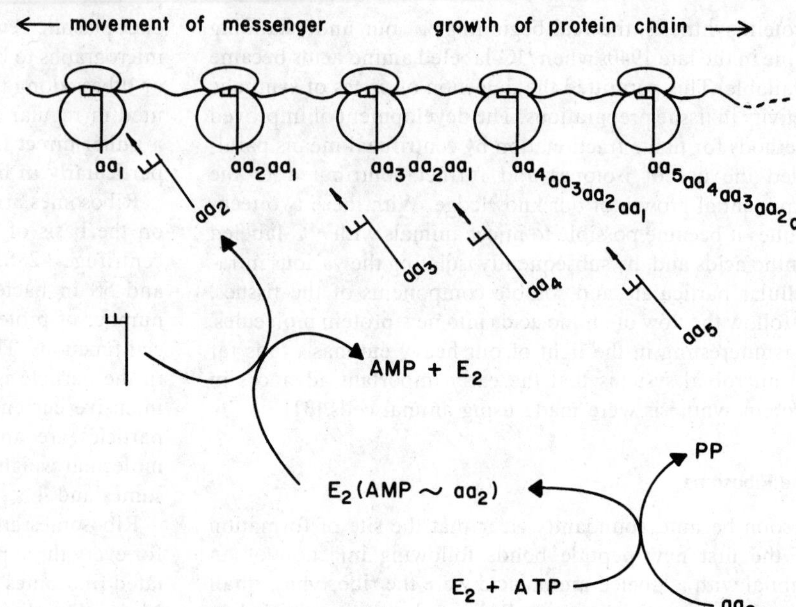

Figure 2-13. Scheme of protein synthesis including amino acid activation, attachment of amino acid to tRNA, and transfer of amino acids to protein in ribosomes. Five ribosomes are shown threaded with their messenger. Transfer RNA molecules are three-pronged at one end to represent three nucleotides which recognize the codon on the messenger.

In order to obtain more information on the role of ribosomes in protein synthesis, it was necessary to obtain a system capable of synthesizing protein in vitro. This was accomplished in the early 1950s and permitted a rapid advance in our knowledge of mechanism. We now know that in order to obtain an active cell-free protein-synthesizing system of bacterial, plant, or animal cell origin, we require in addition to ribosomes and messenger RNA the following components: (1) amino acids, activating enzymes and ATP; (2) transfer RNA (tRNA); and (3) GTP (guanosine-triphosphate) and several transfer factors (see Fig. 2-13 for an overall scheme).

Amino Acid Activation

The condensation of an amino acid carboxyl group with the amino group of an adjacent amino acid to form a peptide bond requires an external source of energy. ATP is the energy donor, as it is for many other biosyntheses. The reaction in which ATP supplies this energy is called *amino acid activation* and is catalyzed by *amino acid–activating enzymes* in the manner pictured in Fig. 2-14. An amino acid–specific enzyme, ATP, and one of the 20 amino acids interact to produce an amino acyl–adenylate compound, which remains firmly bound to the enzyme. Inorganic pyrophosphate is ejected as product. The energy of the pyrophosphoryl-AMP bond of ATP (a "high-energy" bond) is *preserved* in an amino acid carboxyl–phosphoanhydride bond (amino acyl–AMP bond). The reaction is thus reversible, and the carboxyl group of the amino acid is now in an "activated" form. Indeed, these compounds are highly reactive and would readily form indiscriminate peptide linkages with other amino acids had not the cell arranged to keep the compound firmly bound to the enzyme. This reaction may thus be considered the initial step in protein synthesis. Presumably each of the 20 amino acids is activated by its own specific enzyme. These enzymes are found in all cells among the soluble proteins of cytoplasm.

An important feature of this reaction points up a generalization about DNA, RNA, and protein synthesis. In all three processes, pyrophosphate (PP) is eliminated as a reaction product. This would appear to be wasteful, since the bond between these two phosphates is "energy-rich." However, all cells possess an enzyme, pyrophosphatase, which rapidly hydrolyzes PP to two molecules of orthophosphate. This hydrolysis eliminates PP as a reaction product, thereby for-

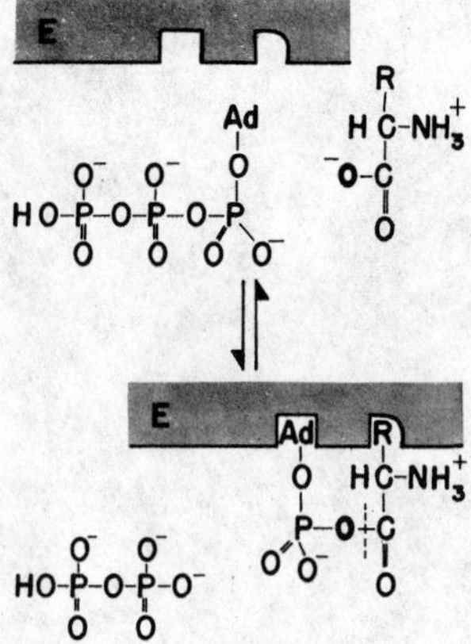

Figure 2-14. Detail of amino acid activation. One activating enzyme (E) is shown with sites specific for the adenosine portion of adenosine triphosphate and for the specific amino acid side chain (R). Activation involves an attack by the amino acid carboxyl group upon the innermost phosphate of ATP to form an amino acyl-adenylate compound, firmly bound to the enzyme, as shown. (*From M. B. Hoagland et al., J. Biol. Chem.,* **218**, 345, 1956.)

cing the reaction equilibrium in the direction of further synthesis. If PP were allowed to accumulate in the cell it would gradually bring synthesis to a halt through a mass-action effect on these macromolecular syntheses.

Amino Acid Linkage to Transfer RNA

The next step in protein synthesis proved to be a puzzling reaction at first but is a most essential step preparatory to the arrangement of amino acids in a specific order in the finished protein. The activating enzymes each attach their specific activated amino acid to the end of an RNA molecule called *transfer* RNA (tRNA). This reaction is schematized in Fig. 2-13. A special type of ester bond is formed between the carboxyl group of the amino acid and the hydroxyl group on the ribose of the last nucleotide of a transfer RNA chain, thus liberating the enzyme and the AMP portion of the amino acyl–adenylate compound. Again the reaction is reversible, indicating that the carboxyl group is still activated, though now forming a new compound. These transfer RNA molecules are ubiquitous and are found in the soluble portion of the cytoplasm. They are of approximately 25,000 molecular weight units (some seventy nucleotides), and there is at least one for each of the 20 amino acids:[11] each amino acid is attached to its own specific tRNA molecule. It has been possible to fractionate some of the specific tRNA species and directly demonstrate their specificity for single amino acids. A peculiar feature of the tRNA story is the following: all tRNAs have the same terminal three nucleotides at the amino acid acceptor end. These three nucleotides are attached by a specific series of reactions unrelated to the synthesis of the rest of the molecule.

The first two steps of protein synthesis not only activate amino acids and attach them to tRNA but also function as a screening device. Certain amino acid analogues (fluorophenylalanine is an example) are known to be incorporated to a small extent into protein. These are found to be activated and transferred to tRNA to some extent. Others, which have been found never to get into protein, are probably not activated or, if activated, are not transferred to tRNA. It seems highly probable that in vivo these first two steps in protein synthesis protect the cell from unwanted amino acid substitutes.

The Adapter Hypothesis

The discovery that amino acids attached to RNA molecules *before* they even arrived at the ribosome, which is clearly the initial site of protein synthesis, suggested the "adapter hypothesis" [32, 33], which has since received substantial experimental support. The ribosome must supply to the synthetic machinery a template for protein synthesis—a

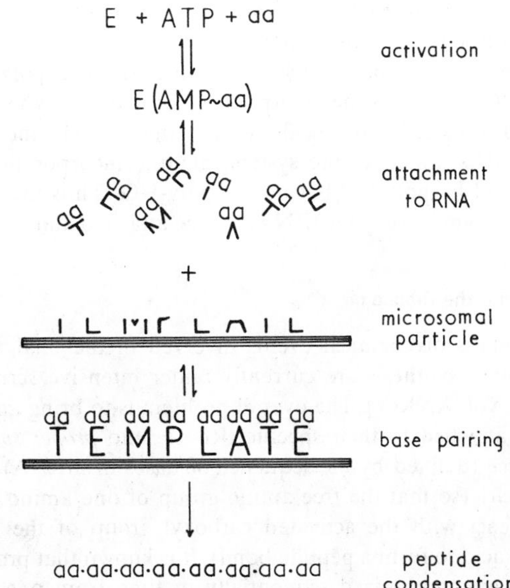

Figure 2-15. The adapter hypothesis. (*From M. B. Hoagland, in Structure and Function of Genetic Elements. Brookhaven Symposia in Biology, no.* 12, 1959.)

linear sequence of bases accurately reflecting a sequence in DNA—presumably messenger RNA.[12] We have already reviewed the evidence that messenger RNA is synthesized on DNA and may associate with ribosomes. Since base pairing by hydrogen bonding is a characteristic and specific feature of RNA-RNA interaction (as it is in DNA), would it not be useful to attach each amino acid first to tRNA molecules with characteristic base sequences complementary to specific sequences on the template? This would serve to locate the amino acid on a particular base sequence on the template with a high degree of precision. Once the amino acid is affixed to such an "adapter" it would have no further role in finding its proper location. This idea is rather whimsically pictured in Fig. 2-15.

One may isolate these ^{14}C-amino acyl–tRNA compounds free of other cellular components and incubate them with ribosomes, and the attached labeled amino acids will all be converted to peptide linkage in protein [34]. This reaction requires two other kinds of components of the synthetic system: GTP and certain soluble transfer factors.

That the site of peptide bond formation recognizes the tRNA and not the amino acid, in confirmation of the adapter hypothesis, was demonstrated by an ingenious experiment [35]. Using cysteine and its activating enzyme, one makes cysteine-tRNA and treats it with Raney nickel, which converts the cysteine to alanine without damaging the tRNA. A synthetic messenger, poly-UC (see "The Genetic Code,"

[11] We now know that there are several tRNAs per amino acid, an indication of degeneracy in the amino acid code (see "The Genetic Code," further on in this chapter).

[12] At the time the adapter hypothesis was suggested, messenger RNA was unknown, but it was simply assumed that the *ribosomal* RNA contained this message, earlier obtained from DNA, in the form of *its own* RNA.

further on in this chapter), vigorously promotes the incorporation of cysteine on its proper transfer RNA into a synthetic protein in the ribosome system while another polymer, poly-UG, promotes the incorporation of alanine. When the treated transfer RNA specific for cysteine with alanine now attached is added to the system, alanine incorporation is promoted by poly-UC but not by poly-UG. Thus the template recognizes only the tRNA, not the attached amino acid.

Events on the Ribosome

The details of chemical events involved in the final steps of protein synthesis are currently under intensive scrutiny [see *G*, vol. XXXIV]. The overall problem is to bring amino acids, attached to their specific tRNAs, into *proper spatial sequence* (defined by the sequence of bases in mRNA) and *proximity* (so that the free amino group of one amino acid may react with the activated carboxyl group of the next amino acid to form a peptide bond). It is known that protein chains are synthesized sequentially in time from one end (amino end) to the other (carboxyl end), not randomly or simultaneously [36]. Another requirement is that the growing peptide chain must remain attached to the site of synthesis until it is completed; and when it is completed it must be removed. Finally, the underlying mechanism for the ordering of amino acids must involve the recognition of a short sequence of bases in the mRNA (the codon) by a short sequence of bases in the tRNA (the anticodon); this is depicted in Fig. 2-16.

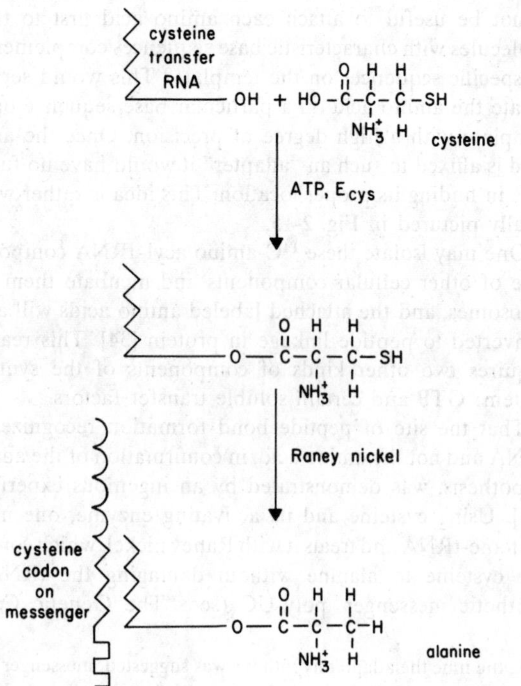

Figure 2-16. Base pairing interaction of amino acyl–tRNA and -mRNA.

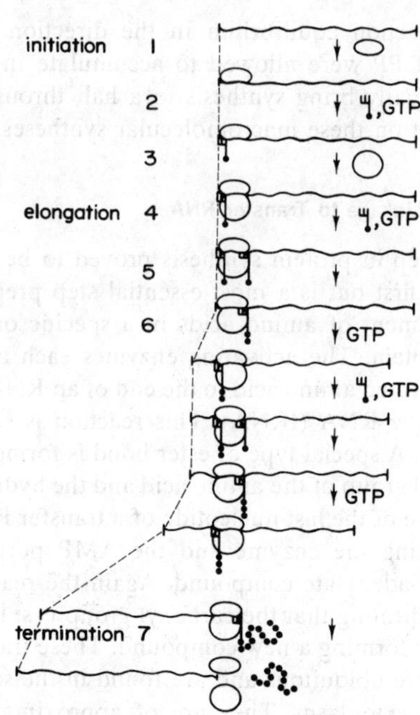

Figure 2-17. Initiation, elongation, and termination reactions in protein synthesis. Reaction 1: binding of the smaller of the ribosomal subunits to mRNA. Reaction 2: binding of special initiating amino acyl–tRNA to subunit–mRNA complex. Reaction 3: attachment of larger ribosomal subunit to the complex. Reaction 4: binding of the second amino acyl–tRNA. Reaction 5: peptide bond formation between first two amino acids. Reaction 6: translocation of mRNA–peptidyl-tRNA unit one codon further on. This elongation reaction sequence is repeated until the last (terminator) codon is reached. Reaction 7: release of finished polypeptide from the terminal tRNA and dissociation of the complex. All the above reactions require protein factors (not shown). The scale depicted is much reduced in length, and only one ribosome is depicted where in reality many ribosomes would be simultaneously carrying out the identical reaction sequence on this mRNA.

The present picture of the sequence of reactions on the ribosome which accomplishes these objectives is shown in Fig. 2-17 [see *G*, vol. XXXIV]; it may be summarized as follows (all reactions require one or more special protein factors):

Initiation

REACTION 1: The smaller ribosomal subunit binds to the mRNA, at an initiator codon (AUG).

REACTION 2: The first amino acyl–tRNA compound is bound to the 30S subunit-mRNA complex.

In bacteria and in certain other systems which utilize 70S ribosomes, the initiating event involves a unique tRNA species: it is acylated by the amino acid methionine, and its anticodon recognizes the only codon for methionine, AUG. In addition, however, the amino group of the methionine attached to this special tRNA is formylated by an enzyme catalyzing the transfer of a formyl group on N^{10}-tetrahydrofolate to the methionyl-tRNA. Thus the amino group of methionine on the initiator tRNA is effectively blocked, giving the amino acid the "appearance" of a peptide. Since all subsequent reactions in the scheme of polymerization involve adding amino acids to a growing peptide chain, this first step provides a simulated peptide to which the next amino acid may be added. (It might be expected that such a mechanism of initiation would result in all the proteins of an organism having N-formyl methionine as the amino-terminal residue. In *E. coli,* where this mechanism has been studied most thoroughly, many protein sequences do indeed start with methionine. However, others do not, and it appears that enzymes exist in these cells which remove the formyl group from methionine and *also* remove one or more of the amino-terminal amino acids as well.)

REACTION 3: The larger ribosomal subunit now binds to the complex.

Elongation

REACTION 4: The second amino acyl–tRNA compound binds to the complex by codon-anticodon pairing.

REACTION 5: The activated carboxyl group of amino acid 1 reacts with the contiguous amino group of amino acid 2 to form a *peptide bond.* The dipeptide remains attached, through the carboxyl group of amino acid 2, to the second tRNA. The first tRNA is ejected from the ribosome.

REACTION 6: The dipeptidyl-tRNA-ribosome unit is translocated one codon further along the mRNA in preparation for a repeat of the elongation cycle (i.e., Reactions 4 and 5). This cycle is repeated as many times as there are amino acids in the protein undergoing synthesis. (It should be noted that the translocation step involves movement of the mRNA relative to the ribosome, a process which requires the expenditure of energy. The energy is supplied by GTP, by a mechanism unknown.)

Termination

REACTION 7: Evidence is now available that one or more of the codons UAA, UAG, and UGA, which code for none of the 20 naturally occurring amino acids, are natural chain-terminating codons: i.e., when they are encountered by the tRNA reading machinery, synthesis ceases. Furthermore, enzymes have recently been isolated which appear to recognize the polypeptide-terminal tRNA-terminator codon complex, and catalyze hydrolysis of the carboxyl-ribose linkage binding the finished polypeptide to the synthetic complex. This effectively releases the polypeptide and completes the synthetic cycle.

It is awesome to realize that the total sequence of reactions of protein synthesis can polymerize amino acids at a rate of some ten amino acids per second per ribosome! Further amplification is facilitated by an ingenious device: a single messenger is read *simultaneously* by many ribosomes. Such multiribosome–messenger RNA complexes may be seen in electron micrographs and can be isolated by appropriate techniques. They are called *polyribosomes,* or *polysomes.*

THE GENETIC CODE

One of the more diverting pastimes of the theoretical biologist in the last decade has been consideration of the coding problem: how to discover the sequences of bases in the DNA that determine each of the amino acids in protein. *Collinearity* has been a basic assumption, and we have seen how it has been proved by experiment. The obvious direct experimental approach to the code would be the chemical determination of base sequence in DNA or in specific messenger RNAs and its correlation with the sequence of amino acids in protein. The problems associated with determination of sequences in polymers composed of only four units and of molecular weight in the millions—as opposed to polymers of 20 units and of molecular weight of tens of thousands—are formidable, though they have been solved in recent years.

The discovery of tRNA and the realization that there was one (or more) of these molecules specific for each of the 20 amino acids ignited much excitement and intensive effort to isolate pure tRNAs and determine their structure. According to the adapter hypothesis they should contain somewhere among their 70-odd bases a few which code for their specific amino acid (the anticodon). Progress in fractionation of tRNAs and elucidation of total base sequence has gone forward very rapidly, but without other information identification of the anticodon would be extremely difficult if not hopeless. No one in the field anticipated the astonishing discovery of Nirenberg and Matthaei which led in a few short years to the "cracking" of the code: supplying ribosomes with *artificial* messengers of known base composition resulted in synthesis of artificial proteins whose amino acid composition was defined by the composition of the message. This development will be discussed below, but before proceeding to it we will take a brief look at the theoretical background of coding.

The Problems of Coding

If one has an encoded tape written in a four-letter language, an important question is: How many of these letters code for each amino acid? In other words, what is the size of the *codon?* This may be approximated by determining the *coding ratio:* given the total length of the DNA of an organism, the length of one protein made by the organism, and the fraction of the total genetic map occupied by the *gene* for that protein, one may estimate the average number of nucleotides per amino acid residue. From the examples studied in viruses and bacteria this number turns out to be substantially less than 10. The work of Yanofsky on the tryptophan-synthetase system quoted earlier gives a more precise figure: the protein produced by the A structural gene of the tryptophan locus has 280 amino acids in it. Assuming a coding ratio of 3 or 4, the gene must be 840 to 1,120 nucleotides long—say, about 1,000. Two mutations (A-23 and A-46) of this A gene have been found which map one one-thousandth of the total gene map distance apart. These two mutations must then be *in the same codon.* Analysis of the amino acid alteration in the A proteins of these two mutants showed that the *same* amino acid position was in fact affected: a position in the wild type occupied by glycine contained glutamic acid in mutant A-46 and arginine in A-23! This confirmed the assumption that the coding ratio was 3 or 4. Since there are 20 amino acids to be taken care of, a codon of 3 is a convenient minimum: there are only 16 (4^2) possible combinations of 4 letters taken 2 at a time, while there are 64 (4^3) possible combinations of the 4 taken in groups of 3. We shall therefore in subsequent discussion assume a coding ratio of 3.

Another important question is: How is the code read—randomly or from one end to the other? If a code is read randomly, a serious problem arises: How does the machinery recognize the correct codons? If, on the other hand, the code is read sequentially, this problem is obviated. There is now direct evidence that amino acids are assembled sequentially [36]. We may therefore dispense with much of the highly ingenious theorizing in this field designed to devise systems for unambiguous random reading.

Genetic Evidence for the Reading Mechanism

A number of remarkably clever genetic experiments, notably those of Crick and associates [37], have supported the concept of unidirectional reading, and a coding ratio of 3. Briefly, these experiments involve the use of acridine-induced mutations, alluded to in an earlier section, which appear to be insertions or deletions of single-base pairs in the DNA. If the mRNA is read in codons of three from one end, addition or deletion of a single base should shift the "frame" of reading such that the protein product is totally altered in amino acid sequence distal to the mutation. By the same argument, genetic combination of two mutants, one with a deletion and another with an addition, should produce a protein with amino acids altered between the two mutational sites. Finally, a similar combination of mutations involving three deletions, or three additions, should give correct reading distal to the altered bases. All these predictions have been borne out by experiment.

Assignment of Codons

Now we may examine the system that permits us to make actual code-letter assignments to each of the amino acids. The enzyme polynucleotide phosphorylase supplies the artificial messenger RNA molecules. It catalyzes the reaction

$$\text{n NDP} \underset{}{\overset{\text{Mg}}{\rightleftharpoons}} [\text{NMP}]_n + \text{n P}_i$$

Using *ribo*nucleoside *di*phosphates as substrates, the enzyme catalyzes their polymerization to high-molecular-weight material, releasing inorganic phosphate (P_i) as product. The nature of the linkage between subunits is the same as that in natural RNA-3′-,5′-phosphodiester linkages. However, the composition of the polymer is determined by the concentration and kind of diphosphate added to the reaction mixture. Thus, supplying UDP results in the synthesis of poly-U, ADP results in poly-A, etc. Mixtures of diphosphates give mixed polymers, or heteropolymers, in which the relative quantity of bases in the polymer is proportional to the relative proportions of diphosphates in the incubation mixture. As far as is known, the distribution of bases in such copolymers is *random.* Thus a 5:1 molar ratio of UDP to CDP will be polymerized to a polymer having a 5:1 molar ratio of U to C, distributed in a statistically random order.[13]

The initial discovery of Nirenberg and Matthaei [38] arose from an attempt to determine the capacity of various RNAs, including these synthetic polymers, to stimulate the incorporation of amino acids into protein in the bacterial cell-free amino acid incorporation system (ribosomes, tRNA, transfer factors, and GTP). When ^{14}C-phenylalanine was used as amino acid and poly-U as messenger, there was a surprisingly large incorporation of the amino acid into an acid-insoluble product identified as polyphenylalanine. Clearly, the normal biologic system was able to use a synthetic messenger to make a synthetic protein! The implications of this observation for solving the code were immediately apparent and were exploited by the Nirenberg group at the National Institutes of Health and by Ochoa and his associates at New York University. The basic approach is as follows: *assuming that the code is based on triplets,* one assigns the triplet UUU to phenylalanine (i.e., UUU is the *codon* for phenylalanine). One then synthesizes a series of polymers containing a certain proportion of U and various proportions of the other bases. Since the polymer is random, the probability of occurrence of triplets containing one, two, or three of the other bases may then be calculated. For example, in poly-UC (5:1), i.e., containing five times as much U as C, if the relative frequency of occurrence of UUU is set at 1, the chance of occurrence of the triplet UUC would be $1 \times 1 \times \frac{1}{5} = 0.2$; of UCC, $1 \times \frac{1}{5} \times \frac{1}{5} = 0.04$; and of CCC, $\frac{1}{5} \times \frac{1}{5} \times \frac{1}{5} = 0.008$. Next, one sets up a series of identical incubations of the cell-free system, to which the polymer is added in optimal concentration. All tubes contain a complete mixture of amino acids, and each tube has a different one labeled. At the end of the incubation, the

[13] Note that the action of this enzyme is in striking contrast to DNA polymerase and RNA polymerase: the character of the polymer made is determined not by a macromolecule used as primer but by the concentration and kind of substrate used.

acid-insoluble protein formed in each tube is isolated and counted. Since the polymer contains considerable U, the polypeptides formed will contain phenylalanine, whose relative incorporation is set at 1. The extent of incorporation of each of the other amino acids is then noted in relation to that of phenylalanine. These figures are compared to the probability of occurrence of a particular triplet, and where good matching is obtained, a tentative triplet assignment is made.

To take an example: poly-UC containing 39 percent U and 61 percent C was used. Relative frequency of occurrence of UUU = 1; UUC = 1.57 ($1 \times 1 \times {}^{61}/_{39}$); UCC = 2.44 ($1 \times {}^{61}/_{39} \times {}^{61}/_{39}$); CCC = 3.82 (${}^{61}/_{39} \times {}^{61}/_{39} \times {}^{61}/_{39}$). Amino acids were incorporated as follows: phenylalanine 1, arginine 0, alanine 0, serine 1.60, proline 2,85, tyrosine 0, valine 0, etc. (Figures are moles of amino acid incorporated per mole of phenylalanine incorporated × 100.) Thus the triplet UUC is assigned to serine and UCC to proline. Of course the order of the nucleotides in the codon is not known. Using this technique, it is possible to assign codons to most of the amino acids.

A second technique, also developed by Nirenberg and his associates [39], depends on the fact that nucleotide triplets of known base sequence will bind readily to ribosomes and, in turn, will promote the binding of specific amino acyl–tRNA compound. Such experiments not only strongly support a triplet code but also permit assignment of the order of bases in the triplet. A third approach pioneered by Khorana [40], that of chemically synthesizing mRNAs of considerable length and known sequence, which are then used in cell-free systems, further confirms ordered code-letter assignments. Finally, the codon assignments obtained from cell-free systems can be validated by using them to predict the kinds of amino acid substitutions that would occur as a result of exposure to known mutagenic agents. All the above experiments give remarkable agreement and have produced the definitive code shown in Table 2-1.

Table 2-1. THE GENETIC CODE

First nucleotide	Second nucleotide				Third nucleotide
	U	C	A	G	
U	phe	ser	tyr	cys	U
	phe	ser	tyr	cys	C
	leu	ser	C.T.	C.T.	A
	leu	ser	C.T.	trp	G
C	leu	pro	his	arg	U
	leu	pro	his	arg	C
	leu	pro	gln	arg	A
	leu	pro	gln	arg	G
A	ile	thr	asn	ser	U
	ile	thr	asn	ser	C
	ile	thr	lys	arg	A
	met (C.I.)	thr	lys	arg	G
G	val	ala	asp	gly	U
	val	ala	asp	gly	C
	val	ala	glu	gly	A
	val (C.I.)	ala	glu	gly	G

Note: C.T., chain terminator; C.I., chain initiator.

An examination of the code reveals some interesting features. The most striking finding is the high level of *degeneracy:* almost all the amino acids are represented by more than one codon. Thus three amino acids have six codons; five have four; one has three; nine have two; and only two have a single codon. Degeneracy implies evolutionary survival value. Had there been only one codon for each amino acid, the code would be highly vulnerable to mutations. In the existing code, mutations will often have no effect on the protein product (if they occur in position 3) or will be "mis-sense"—the replacement of one amino acid by another in the gene product. Many of these latter mutations may be "silent," harmless, and indeed provide a possibility for improvement of the protein structure. Degeneracy also invokes the possibility of rate regulation by *scarcity.* For example, the existence of six codons for leucine requires six specific tRNAs for leucine. If certain of these tRNAs are relatively rarer than others, then a codon specifying a rare tRNA will become rate-limiting during reading. That this phenomenon does in fact occur has recently been demonstrated in a cell-free system [41].

It is also of interest that the code has "wobble" in the third position: all codons assigned to a given amino acid differ in the third base only, with one exception (serine). Note that position 3 for a given amino acid is generally either a purine or pyrimidine. This suggests the possibility that early in evolution the code may have been a two-letter code specifying 15 "primordial" amino acids. As five more amino acids became necessary in the progression of evolutionary complexity, a third letter was required in the code to specify them unambiguously (asparagine, glutamine, methionine, tyrosine, and tryptophan).

Three codons are provided as chain terminator codons: i.e., they are codons recognized by none of the tRNAs, as noted earlier. We have also noted that the codon for methionine has been implicated in chain initiation (C.I.). There is also evidence that one of the codons for valine is a chain initiator. Thus the code provides all the required information for beginning and ending polypeptide chains.

There is a striking negative feature of the code which is to be expected from the adapter hypothesis. There is no clear-cut stereochemical relationship between the codons themselves and the amino acids specified by them.

Finally, a variety of studies on mutagenesis and in cell-free systems have established that the genetic code is *universal.* Just as all living forms today use the same 20 amino acids, so too they use the same code for specifying the sequence of the amino acids. Bacteria probably existed as long as 3 billion years ago and the code's universality suggests that the code may be equally ancient, having arisen but once in life's history.

It is aesthetically satisfying to end on a note of universality.

Unfortunately, the curiosity of the biologist is not satiated by this comforting conclusion. There is a long way yet to go in the understanding of cellular mechanism; indeed we have only defined a base from which to operate. Having triumphed in understanding universal biosynthetic mechanism, we now have the task of getting at the biochemical basis of *diversity*. What we really want to know is the fundamental qualities underlying the *differences* between bacterial and animal cells. The coming years will surely witness an increasingly zestful focus on the unique properties of specialized animal cells, and are likely to lead us to even more provocative insights, much more nearly applicable to human affairs and the problems of genetic disease.

BIBLIOGRAPHY

1. Pauling, L.: *Abnormality of Hemoglobin Molecules in Hereditary Hemolytic Anemias.* Harvey Lectures, Academic, New York, 1954.
2. Ingram, V. M.: *Hemoglobin and Its Abnormalities.* Charles C Thomas, Springfield, Ill., 1961.
3. Wilkins, M. F. H., Stokes, A. R., and Wilson, H. R.: Molecular structure of deoxypentose nucleic acids. Nature (London), **171,** 738, 1953.
4. Franklin, R. E., and Gosling, R. G.: Molecular configuration of sodium thymonucleate. Nature (London), **171,** 740, 1953.
5. Watson, J. D., and Crick, F. H. C.: Molecular structure of nucleic acids (737); genetic implications of the structure of deoxyribonucleic acid (964). Nature (London), **171,** 737, 964, 1953.
6. Sinsheimer, R. L., Starman, B., Nagler, C., and Guthrie, S.: The process of infection with bacteriophage øX174. I. Evidence for a "replicative form." J. Molec. Biol., **4,** 142, 1962.
7. Kornberg, A.: *Enzymatic Synthesis of DNA.* Ciba Lectures in Microbial Biochemistry, Wiley, New York, 1961.
8. Meselson, M., and Stahl, F. W.: The replication of DNA in *Escherichia coli.* Proc. Nat. Acad. Sci. U.S.A., **44,** 671, 1958.
9. Meselson, M.: On the mechanism of genetic recombination between DNA molecules. J. Molec. Biol., **9,** 734, 1964.
10. Cairns, J.: The bacterial chromosome and its manner of replication as seen by autoradiography. J. Molec. Biol., **6,** 208, 1963.
11. Mitra, S., and Kornberg, A.: Enzymatic mechanisms of DNA replication. J. Gen. Physiol., **49,** 59, 1966.
12. Goulian, M., Kornberg, A., and Sinsheimer, R. L.: Enzymatic synthesis of DNA, XXIV. Synthesis of infectious phage øX174 DNA. J. Molec. Biol., **24,** 429, 1967.
13. Avery, O. T., MacLeod, C. M., and McCarty, M.: Studies on the chemical nature of the substance inducing transformation of pneumococcal types. J. Exp. Med., **79,** 137, 1944.
14. Auerbach, C.: The chemical production of mutations. Science, **158,** 1141, 1967.
15. Benzer, S.: *Genetic Fine Structure.* Harvey Lectures, Academic, New York, 1960–1961.
16. Sanger, F.: in *Currents in Biochemical Research,* edited by D. E. Green. Interscience, New York, 1956.
17. Kendrew, J. C.: in *Biological Structure and Function,* edited by T. W. Goodwin and O. Lindberg, vol. I, p. 5. Academic, New York, 1960.
18. Smith, E. L.: *The Evolution of Proteins.* Harvey Lectures, ser. 62, p. 231, Academic, New York, 1968.
19. Beadle, G. W., and Tatum, E. L.: Genetic control of biochemical reactions in *Neurospora.* Proc. Nat. Acad. Sci. U.S.A., **27,** 499, 1941.
20. Beadle, G. W.: Biochemical genetics. Chem. Rev., **37,** 15, 1945.
21. Schlesinger, M. J., and Levinthal, C.: Hybrid protein formation of *E. coli* alkaline phosphatase leading to *in vitro* complementation. J. Molec. Biol., **7,** 1, 1963.
22. Henning, U., and Yanofsky, C.: An alteration in the primary structure of a protein predicted on the basis of genetic recombination data. Proc. Nat. Acad. Sci. U.S.A., **48,** 183, 1962.
23. Sarabhai, A. S., Stretton, A. O. W., Brenner, S., and Bolle, A.: Colinearity of the gene with the polypeptide chain. Nature (London), **201,** 13, 1964.
24. Pardee, A. B., Jacob, F., and Monod, J.: The genetic control and cytoplasmic expression of "inducibility" in the synthesis of β-galactosidase by *E. coli.* J. Molec. Biol., **1,** 165, 1959.
25. Volkin, E., and Astrachan, L.: in *The Chemical Basis of Heredity,* edited by W. D. McElroy and B. Glass, p. 686. Johns Hopkins, Baltimore, 1957.
26. Brenner, S., Jacob, F., and Meselson, M.: An unstable intermediate carrying information from genes to ribosomes for protein synthesis. Nature (London), **190,** 576, 1961.
27. Jacob, F., and Monod, J.: Genetic regulatory mechanisms in the synthesis of proteins. J. Molec. Biol., **3,** 318, 1961.
28. Gilbert, W., and Muller-Hill, B.: Isolation of the "lac" repressor. Proc. Nat. Acad. Sci. U.S.A., **56,** 1891, 1966.
29. Ptashe, M.: Specific binding of the α phage repressor to α DNA. Nature, **214,** 232, 1967.
30. Scornik, O. A.: *In vivo* rate of translation by ribosomes of normal and regenerating liver. J. Molec. Biol. (in press).
31. Zamecnik, P. C.: *Historical and Current Aspects of the Problems of Protein Synthesis.* Harvey Lectures, Academic, New York, 1958–1959.
32. Crick, F. H. C.: On protein synthesis. Sympos. Soc. Exp. Biol., **12,** 138, 1958.
33. Hoagland, M. B.: in *A Symposium of Molecular Biology,* edited by R. E. Zirkle. The University of Chicago Press, Chicago, 1959.
34. Hoagland, M. B., Stephenson, M. L., Scott, J. F., Hecht, L. I., and Zamecnik, P. C.: A soluble ribonucleic acid intermediate in protein synthesis. J. Biol. Chem., **231,** 241, 1958.
35. Chapeville, F., Lipmann, F., von Ehrenstein, G., Weisblum, B., Ray, W. J., and Benzer, S.: On the role of soluble ribonucleic acid in coding for amino acids. Proc. Nat. Acad. Sci. U.S.A., **48,** 1086, 1962.
36. Dintzis, H. M.: Assembly of peptide chains of hemoglobin. Proc. Nat. Acad. Sci. U.S.A., **47,** 247, 1961.
37. Crick, F. H. C., Barnett, L., Brenner, S., and Watts-Toben, R. J.: General nature of the genetic code for proteins. Nature (London), **192,** 1227, 1961.
38. Nirenberg, M. W., and Matthaei, J. H.: The dependence of cell-free protein synthesis in *E. coli* upon naturally occurring or synthetic polyribonucleotides. Proc. Nat. Acad. Sci. U.S.A., **47,** 1588, 1961.
39. Nirenberg, M. W., and Leder, P.: RNA codewords and protein synthesis. Science, **145,** 1399, 1964.
40. Khorana, G.: *Polynucleotide Synthesis and the Genetic Code.* Harvey Lectures, ser. 62, o. 79, Academic, New York, 1968.
41. Anderson, W. F., and Gilbert, J. M.: tRNA-Dependent translational control of *in vitro* hemoglobin synthesis. Biochem. Biophys. Res. Commun., **36,** 456, 1969.
42. DeLucia, P., and Cairnes, J.: Isolation of *E. coli* strain with a mutation affecting DNA polymerase. Nature, **224,** 1164, 1969.
43. Fuchs, E., and Hanawalt, P.: Isolation and characterization of the DNA replication complex from *E. coli.* J. Molec. Biol., **52,** 301, 1970.

GENERAL REFERENCES

A. Watson, J. D.: *The Molecular Biology of the Gene.* Benjamin, New York, 1970. An extremely lucid, imaginatively written and illustrated text on bioenergetics, gene structure and function, nucleic acid and protein synthesis, coding and regulation.

B. Chargaff, E., and Davidson, J. N., editors: *The Nucleic Acids,* vols. I (1955), II (1955), and III (1960). Academic, New York. A definitive work on the chemistry and physical chemistry of nucleic acids, written by experts in the various fields of specialization. (See also succeeding volumes of *Progress in Nucleic Acid Research,* edited by J. N. Davidson and W. E. Cohn, vol. I. Academic, New York.)

C. Taylor, J. H., editor: *Molecular Genetics,* part I, 1963; part II, 1967.

Academic, New York. Contains able articles by specialists on DNA and RNA synthesis, chromosome organization and mutation mechanisms, regulation and coding.

D. Hayes, W.: *Genetics of Bacteria and Their Viruses.* Wiley, New York, 1964. A clearly written and excellently illustrated textbook, for graduate students, covering classical and modern genetics, including aspects at the molecular level.

E. Davis, B. D., Dulbecco, R., Eisen, H. N., Ginsberg, H. S., and Wood, W. B.: *Principles of Microbiology and Immunology.* Harper & Row, New York, 1968. A comprehensive and up-to-date microbiology text covering all aspects of the material discussed in this chapter.

F. Jukes, T. H.: *Molecules and Evolution.* Columbia, New York, 1966. An easily read account of protein and nucleic acid structure from the point of view of evolutionary determinants.

G. Cold Spring Harbor Symposia on Quantitative Biology, vol. XXVI, 1961: Cellular Regulatory Mechanisms; vol. XXVIII, 1963: Synthesis and Structure of Macromolecules; vol. XXXI, 1966: The Genetic Code; vol. XXXIII, 1968: Replication of DNA in Micro-organisms; vol. XXXIV, 1970: The Mechanism of Protein Synthesis. These volumes contain thorough experimental documentation for the subjects discussed in this chapter. The articles are generally highly technical and are recommended only for the serious student of molecular biology. Each volume also contains a summary chapter, covering the symposium's deliberations, written by a distinguished investigator in the field.

CHAPTER THREE

THE CHROMOSOME BASIS OF HUMAN HEREDITY

Eric Engel

Although chromosome aberrations, which are responsible for congenital anomalies in man, were unrecognized only 15 years ago, their frequency and diversity are now well established. This new knowledge has been possible because of various technical achievements, especially improvements in cell culture methods.

A review of the progress in genetics of the last 100 years discloses that the cellular basis of Mendel's laws was not understood until the key phenomenon of meiosis was discovered. Observation of the segregation and assortment of the chromosomes in the germ cells provided a mechanism mirroring as well as explaining the patterns of transmission of the Mendelian factors at the cellular level. Light microscopy was the instrument of this achievement. Mendel died before this technical advance gave the human eye the power to visualize what his mind had foreseen 35 years earlier. But the new eye, after much masterly searching which revealed many new cellular structures, needed new kinds of objects to obtain new answers. Thus, for all its refinements, microscopy had been unable even to elucidate man's karyotype: in his tissues dividing cells were too few, sections were too thick, or chromosome bodies were too entangled to permit an accurate count of their number and shape. Nowadays, the direct observation of dividing cells is routine. It requires cell cultivation for an ample yield of cells in mitoses, arrest at metaphase for further accumulation of metaphase plates at a propitious stage, some clear water to swell the space which chromosomes can occupy in the cell, and fast drying to flatten them on the plane of a slide.

It could be anticipated that meiosis, by occasionally failing to meet the precision essential for its purpose, would create a series of errors which would prove deleterious to a proportion of human zygotes and individuals. It took over half a century until this toll, already documented for years in domestic flies, could be assessed in man. The toll is staggering: it now appears that close to 5 percent of all conceptuses carry the consequences, often lethal, of a chromosome error, usually due to faulty division. This may indeed be more than all genetic defects due to point mutations.

It has been a long time since the methods of the cell gardener have replaced those of the plant grower of Brunn; but, as the scene has moved from the sanctuary of the monastery to the commonplace of the laboratory, it may be hoped that the causes and mechanisms of chromosome anomalies will be elucidated, anticipated, and ultimately avoided.

This chapter is aimed at presenting some of the facts as human cytogeneticists know them at this moment.

MEIOSIS

For all their complexity the two meioses which result in the formation of the gametes can be described in simple terms. In man the primordial germ cells contain two sets of 23 chromosomes (i.e., 46 chromosomes), each set inherited from one of the two parents. Except for the XY sex pair in males, each member of a set has its homologue in the other set. At the first meiotic division, homologues which have initially replicated their DNA material recognize each other and synapse lengthwise to form pairs (bivalents) and exchange corresponding strands of genetic material (crossing-over). The X and Y chromosomes form only a loose, terminal association. By the end of the first meiosis the two members of each pair, while clearly double-stranded as a result of earlier DNA replication, have migrated to opposite poles of the spindle, and each pair is represented in each of the two resulting daughter cells by one of its two members. Thus, as a result of the first meiotic division, a cell with two sets of double-stranded chromosomes has formed two daughter cells, each with one set of still double-stranded chromosomes (reductional division). The second meiotic division achieves the formation of cells each containing one single set of single-stranded chromosomes. This is done by the longitudinal splitting of the centromeres and migration to opposite poles of the two chromatids of each replicated chromosome present in the set (equational division). At fertilization two cells each with one set of single-stranded chromosomes fuse to form a zygote in which the diploid number of chromosomes of the species is restored.

NORMAL HUMAN KARYOTYPES

Morphologic Pattern

A normal diploid set in man consists of 23 pairs of chromosomes, including one pair of sex chromosomes and 22 pairs of nonsex chromosomes, or autosomes. One member of every pair, a so-called haploid set, is derived from each parent. A pictorial display in which an attempt is made to pair homologous chromosomes and to arrange them according to size is known as a *karyotype,* or *idiogram* (Fig. 3-1). Human chromosomes are usually studied during mitosis, typically at metaphase, because they become greatly contracted and condensed during cell division and individually distinguishable. Deoxyribonucleic acid replication occurs during late interphase, so that each metaphase chromosome consists of a pair of chromatids held together at the centromere. Chromosomes are described as metacentric, submetacentric, acrocentric, or telocentric, depending on whether the centromere is at the exact center of the chromosome (dividing it into arms of equal length), near the center, near one end, or at one end of the chromosome. Another identifying feature is the possession by certain chromosomes of small terminal projections known as satellite bodies.

There is general agreement that every chromosome in a normal set can be assigned reliably to one of seven groups, labeled A to G in order of decreasing size. A major limitation of human chromosome studies is that it is still not possible to distinguish individually all members of every group, although considerable progress has been made in this direction. Each of the three pairs of large chromosomes in the A groups (pairs 1 to 3) can be identified with relative certainty. The first and third are metacentric but differ slightly in size, whereas the second is intermediate in size but submetacentric. The B group (pairs 4 and 5) consists of two pairs of large submetacentric chromosomes. The C group contains pairs 6 to 12 in addition to the X chromosome(s). This large group is made up of submetacentric chromosomes, which decrease in size so gradually that, in general, individual identification is not possible. The D group (pairs 13 to 15) includes three pairs of large acrocentric

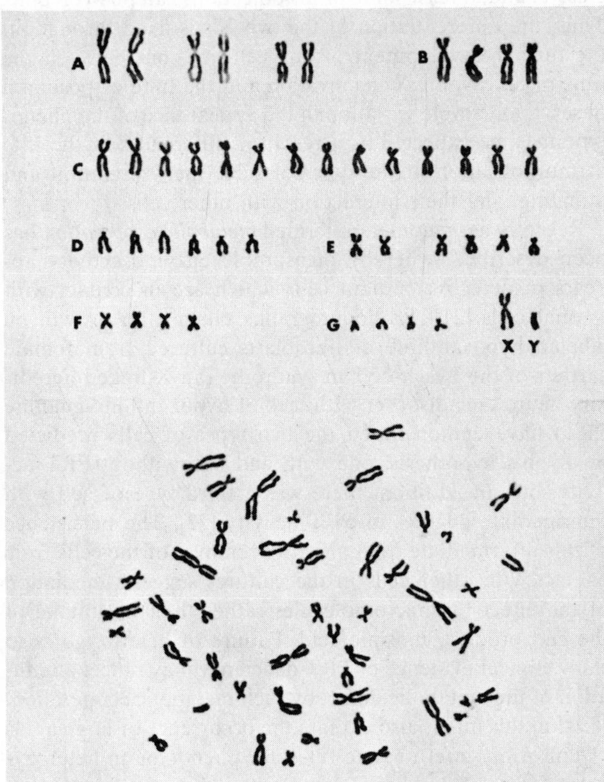

Figure 3-1. 46,XY, normal male karyotype showing typical XY complement (*lower right*). In females, a second X replaces the Y chromosome.

chromosomes. These sometimes have satellite bodies. The E group (pairs 16 to 18) is composed of three pairs of small submetacentric chromosomes. Pair 16 is somewhat larger and more nearly metacentric than the other members of the group. The two small metacentric pairs of the F group (pairs 19 and 20) are indistinguishable. There is no general agreement that the two pairs of satellited, short acrocentric chromosomes in the G group (pairs 21 and 22) can be distinguished reliably by morphologic criteria alone. In addition to the autosomes, the female carries two X chromosomes, which are members of the C group. The male has a single X in the C group and a much smaller Y chromosome in the G group. The Y chromosome can usually be distinguished from the other G-group members by its dark staining and the typically close proximity of its two long arms.

An abbreviated scheme for describing the karyotype was agreed upon at a conference in Chicago in 1966. The total number of chromosomes is listed, then the sex chromosome complement, and finally a description of any anomaly. Normal female and male karyotypes are respectively written 46,XX and 46,XY. A male with one more Y chromosome and a girl with only one X are written respectively 47,XYY and 45,X; a girl with an extra autosome in the G group is written 47,XX,G+; a girl lacking the short arm of a pair-18 chromosome (one of the three E chromosome pairs) is referred to as 46,XX,18p− or 46,XX,E_{18p-} (as *p* is the symbol for the chromosome short arm). The symbol for the long arm is *q*; a girl lacking part (or all) of an E_{18} long arm will be described by the formula 46,XX,E_{18q-}. A translocation with centric fusion of two large acrocentric chromosomes of the D group will reduce the complement to 45 discrete chromosomes, since two D members have become attached into one single larger member, including both chromosome long arms and one of the two centromeres. This defect will be read (in a girl) 45,XX, D−,D−,t (Dq Dq)+, where *t* stands for translocation.

Autoradiographic Patterns

Assessment of the pattern of DNA replication by radioautography after the addition of tritiated thymidine to growing cells has proved to be a useful procedure for differentiating the members of several chromosome groups. Pair five can be distinguished from pair four by early replication of the long arm [2]. The three pairs in the D group also have distinctive labeling patterns. D_1, the member involved in the D-trisomy syndrome (discussed later), shows late replication of the long arm; in a second pair, D_2, replication of the centromere region is delayed, whereas the third pair, D_3, replicates early [3]. The E_{17} and E_{18} pairs are almost similar morphologically, but the E_{18} pair is late in replicating [4]. The chromosome present in triplicate in Down's syndrome (mongolism, discussed later) usually replicates later than the other G-group pair [5]. One of the two X chromosomes in normal females characteristically shows a delayed pattern of DNA replication.

Normal Variants

According to Court Brown [6], between 2 and 3 percent of the members of the adult population show a normal variant affecting an autosome, and variation in the length of the Y chromosome is seen in between 2 and 3 percent of males. The autosomes commonly involved are those known to have secondary constrictions, particularly the large and small acrocentric autosomes and those of pair 16. When an acrocentric autosome is affected, there is an increase in the length of its short arm which can be noted in all suitable cells. These changes may represent localized anomalies of coiling which are genetically determined. On present evidence they appear to be harmless to their carriers, and they are classed as normal variants in order to distinguish them as a group from changes which are the outcome of structural rearrangements following chromosome breakage.

There is evidence that in adults the frequency of aneuploid cells increases with age [7–9]. This increase is more obvious in women and is first detectable in the fifth decade, about ten years before it is detectable in men. In both sexes the change is due to an increase in the frequency of cells with an XO sex-chromosome complement. It is not known whether this is confined to lymphocytes or also occurs in other types of cell. The relation of this phenomenon to aging is not known.

LYON'S HYPOTHESIS

The One Inactive X Hypothesis

One of the interesting cytogenetic developments is Lyon's hypothesis, i.e., that in normal females, one of the two X chromosomes in each cell becomes genetically inactivated early in embryonic life [10]. In addition, this X chromosome replicates its DNA late in the synthesis phase of the mitotic cycle, and is dark-staining (heteropyknotic) during the mitotic prophase and condensed during the interphase, when it forms the sex chromatin body. The relations between these properties and genetic inactivity are not known. This inactivation of an X chromosome does not make the individual uniformly isoallelic for X-borne traits, since it affects the paternal and maternal X at random, but once the inactivation has occurred for an X, whatever its origin, all the descendants of that cell will abide by the "decision." The hypothesis rests on the observed effects of mutant genes carried by one member of the X pair.

It has been demonstrated that females heterozygous for a pair of contrasting alleles are mosaics of two types of cells, one with the maternal X locus active and the other with the paternal X locus active. Studies of single cell clones of cultured fibroblasts from women heterozygous for the X-linked gene for glucose-6-phosphate dehydrogenase have shown that each clone produced only one of the two electrophoretic enzyme variants, either the paternal or the maternal one, while uncloned cultures yielded both variants [11]. Other examples of human X-linked genes in which cloning of cultured fibroblasts has shown populations with different gene activity in heterozygous females are those for hypoxanthine-guanine phosphoribosyl transferase (PRT) activity [12] and an X-linked mucopolysaccharidosis, Hunter's syndrome [13]. On the other hand, X inactivation of the Xg blood group locus has been in doubt, since ordinary agglutination techniques have failed to demonstrate two types of erythrocytes in Xg^a heterozygotes [14]. More recently the two populations of red blood cells of a woman heterozygous for an X-linked anemia, one normal, the other microcytic and hypochromic, were separated and tested for their X-linked blood group antigen. Normal erythrocytes were found to have the Xg phenotype, while the abnormal ones were Xg^a [15].

The hypothesis has recently been reexamined, particularly by Gruneberg [16–18] and by Back and Dormer [19]. Much of the original evidence mustered by Lyon depended on gene effects expressed in mammals by cells visible on the surface of the body, such as skin, eyes, and teeth. Gruneberg has questioned whether the phenotype of females heterozygous for X-linked genes studied from this point of view follows the patterns one would anticipate from X lyonization. As pointed out by Lyon [20], Gruneberg's argument is inconclusive, and at least some of his objections can be overcome. Thus, the differentiation of the two X's is fixed throughout the further development of any cell line, but between the time of embryonic X inactivation and the time of postnatal observation ample variation in the appearance of the phenotype may be expected as a result of differences in the rate of multiplication of the types of cells, their migration and mingling, and their interaction with other cells.

Recently a phenomenon termed *metabolic cooperation* has been described, whereby measurable enzyme activity appears in defective mutant cells which are in contact with normal cells [21]. Radioautographs taken after growth on labeled hypoxanthine of fibroblasts cultured from female carriers of the Lesch-Nyhan syndrome (an X-linked hereditary neurologic disorder with lack of hypoxanthine-guanine PRT) have demonstrated the two types of cells predicted by Lyon's hypothesis, one with and one without PRT activity, but, in addition, there was a third type of cell with intermediate degrees of PRT activity [22]. The persistence of this intermediate category after removal of the cells from contact with other cells in the cultures suggests mediation of the effect by macromolecules rather than by uptake of the end product, inosinic acid. Failure of heterozygotes to show clinical evidence of PRT deficiency may reflect attenuation of the metabolic defect by such metabolic cooperation. If valid, this might also explain the occurrence of large areas of uniformly intermediate fur-color phenotype in heterozygotes for an X-linked coat mutant, a fact put forward by Gruneberg [16] as invalidating Lyon's hypothesis. Gruneberg has proposed another hypothesis to explain the behavior of X-linked genes, i.e., that "partial inhibition of gene action happens in both X chromosomes of mouse females and presumably the females of other mammals" [17]. Though this concept would also explain the dosage compensation of X-borne gene products (females with pairs of X-borne alleles do not seem to manufacture more enzymes than the hemizygous males with one single locus), it would conflict with the evidence concerning the condensation, heteropyknosis, and late nucleic acid replication of one only of the X chromosomes.

The criticism of the one inactive X hypothesis made by Back and Dormer [19] is of a different kind. A lack of synthesis of messenger RNA should characterize inactive chromatin, but these authors found that all chromosomes in cultured lymphocytes, including both X chromosomes, incorporated ^{3}H uridine at prophase. As argued by Lyon, there is a possibility that this RNA may not be messenger RNA only, and may comprise other RNA molecules, possibly also produced by the inactive X. Reduced RNA labeling over the sex chromatin body of the condensed X at interphase was reported by Comings [23], who thought that the overall DNA labeling at metaphase was due to adherence of RNA to chromosomes at this stage [24]. At this moment it seems wise to consider X inactivation as a hypothesis, albeit an exciting one, which is in agreement with, but not necessarily established by, an aggregate of the facts presently in hand.

ABNORMAL HUMAN KARYOTYPES

As discussed in a recent review [25], chromosome aberrations may be manifested by changes in the structure or number of the chromosomes, or both. An alteration is said to be balanced if a complete set of genes is retained. Haploid gametes and polyploid liver cells are examples of normal changes in chromosome number in which chromosome balance, or euploidy, is maintained. Loss of chromosome balance may occur in several ways. The addition of a single chromosome to a diploid set results in trisomy. For example, E_{18} trisomy and G trisomy refer to the presence, respectively, of an extra eighteenth chromosome or an extra G-group member. If a single chromosome is removed, or if part of a chromosome is deleted from a diploid set, complete or partial monosomy is the result. A ring is a special class of deletion chromosome in which both ends of the chromosome have been lost and the broken ends have fused to form a ring structure. These alterations, which disturb gene balance, result in aneuploidy.

The term *translocation* refers to an exchange or transfer of genetic material between nonhomologous chromosome regions. Reciprocal translocation involves an exchange of chromosome arms, or parts thereof, between nonhomologous chromosome regions, whereas insertional translocation is the insertion of a piece of one chromosome into another chromosome arm. The broken end of a chromosome will not heal or fuse with the intact end of another chromosome (known as the *telomere*). Therefore, not less than two breaks are required for a reciprocal translocation, and not less than three for an insertional translocation. Complex translocations involve exchanges between more than two chromosomes.

Other types of chromosomal rearrangement include duplications and inversions. At a genic level, extensive evidence suggests that linear gene duplication has been an exceedingly important mechanism for the evolution of useful genes and gene systems in man [25]. Furthermore, the extensive alterations in chromosome number that have accompanied speciation may have been associated with the wholesale duplication of genes and chromosomes, which differentiated subsequently. Inversions are characterized by reversal of a segment along the length of a chromosome and may be pericentric or paracentric, depending upon whether or not the reversed segment includes the centromere. Evidence from lower organisms suggests that inversions may be quite common in wild populations.

Chromosomal rearrangements may not in themselves cause aneuploidy, but they can alter gene function, even in the absence of aneuploidy. In rearrangement, the intense pairing affinity of homologous chromosome regions results in unusual and complex synapsis during meiosis. In reciprocal translocations, pairing of homologous regions of the two chromosomes involved in the translocation and of their homologues occurs at the first meiotic division. This pairing results in the formation of a translocation cross, composed of the four doubled chromosomes, instead of the normal two-by-two pairing. If the translocation complex separates in such a way that the resulting gametes contain only the two translocation chromosomes or the two normal homologues, euploidy will be maintained. Other types of segregation are possible, and do occur, leading to the formation of aneuploid gametes. Pericentric inversions, duplications, and insertional translocations (depending upon the orientation of the inserted segment) also can give origin to aneuploid gametes as a consequence of crossing-over within the chromosomal regions involved (recombinational aneuploidy) [26]. Chromosomal rearrangements may be viewed collectively as events which in themselves may not be harmful, but which may lead to a genetic instability that predisposes the bearer to the formation of aneuploid cells. Depending largely on the extent and the particular genes involved in the resulting aneuploidy, this genetic instability might manifest itself as a high mutation rate at a single genetic locus, semisterility, repeated abortion, multiple defective children, or a predisposition to malignancy [25].

Balanced Structural Heterozygosity

In Mitotic Cells

The frequencies and distribution of the various types of balanced structural rearrangements in population studies are still poorly documented. The different forms reported may be arranged in two classes depending on whether the relevant chromosome breaks are confined to one autosome or whether more than one autosome is involved.

Intrachange

This category comprises aberrations following the interaction of broken ends confined to one autosome. It includes two classes of abnormality detectable in mitotic preparations, namely, deletions and pericentric inversions where the points of breakdown have not been equidistant from the centromere. Only pericentric inversions represent balanced rearrangements.

Interchanges

Simple Translocations Involving Two Autosomes

This category includes abnormalities which follow the reciprocal exchange of material between two autosomes without a subsequent reduction in chromosome number (Fig. 3-2). Most of these follow single breaks in nonhomologous autosomes, with interaction of the broken ends to produce a reciprocal exchange of material. More rarely, given three breaks in suitable circumstances, an interstitial segment of the arm of an autosome may be translocated into an arm of a nonhomologous autosome to produce a shift. An example of the latter type of translocation has not yet been described in human material. Since most instances of reciprocal translocations have been detected in studies of mitotic cells, the limitations to the identification of translocations by these methods should be kept in mind.

Centric Fusion of Two Acrocentric Chromosomes

Translocations in which both chromosomes are broken close to their centromere form a special category of rearrangement [27]. If two morphologically similar acrocentrics are involved, with a break just proximal to the centromere in one chromosome and just distal to it in the other, the products of a reciprocal translocation are a metacentric chromosome, composed of the long-arm material of the two participating chromosomes, and a much smaller chromosome consisting of the short-arm material. The smaller chromosome is almost inevitably lost, resulting in a reduction of the chromosome number by one (Fig. 3-3). This type of rearrangement may have occurred rather frequently in the phylogeny of many

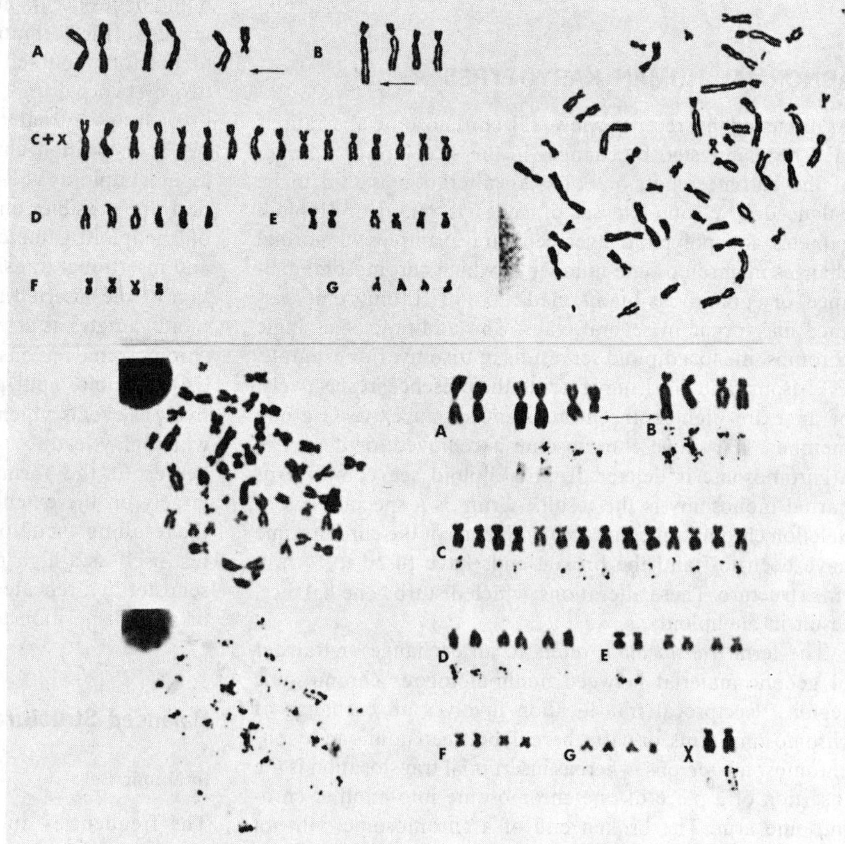

Figure 3-2. (*Top*) 46,XX,t (3?−; Bq+). Reciprocal exchange between one arm of an A_3 member (abbreviated) and the long arm of a B member (much lengthened). (*Bottom*) The ^{3}H-thymidine differential labeling pattern of DNA-replicating chromosomes, as shown by an autoradiograph. Radioactive thymidine, which is incorporated at the late stage of chromosome replication (S period), results in a label distribution, the terminal labeling pattern, which is characteristic for certain chromosomes and allows their identification from other morphologically similar chromosomes. For example chromosome Nos. 4 and 5 are differentially labeled, since the long arms of 4 have a greater concentration than those of 5, while the short arms of 5 are much more labeled than those of 4. This characteristic labeling pattern is recognizable on the above autoradiograph, indicating that one of the chromosomes involved in the interchange was a member of pair No. 4 of group B.

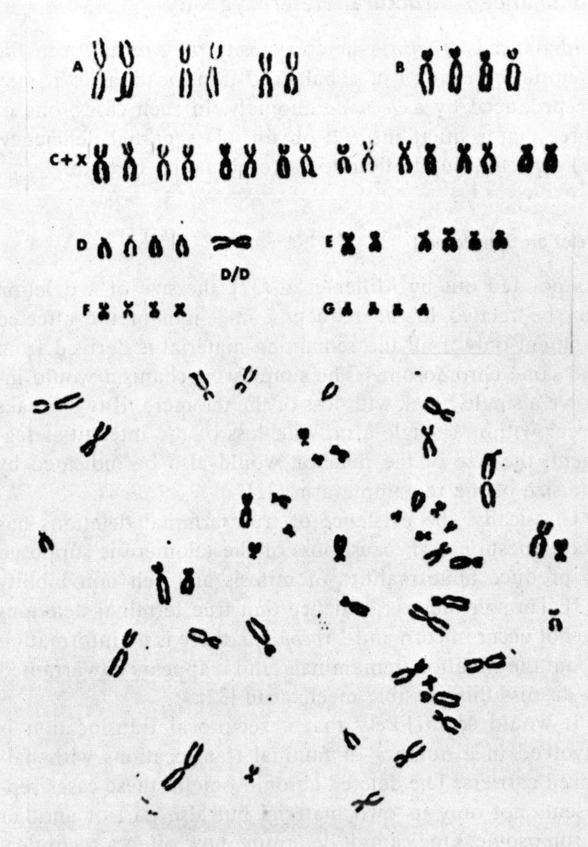

Figure 3-3. 45,XX,D–,D–,t(DqDq)+. Centric fusion (D/D) between two D chromosomes in a woman.

groups of animals. In man, centric-fusion translocations involving two large acrocentrics, or two small acrocentrics, or a large and a small acrocentric have now been described on many occasions. They are most conveniently described using the nomenclature of Patau [28], as D/D, D/G, or G/G translocations, and restricting this terminology to this special category of centric-fusion anomalies. D/D translocations involving nonhomologous autosomes are of considerable interest because they seem to represent the commonest type of translocation found in the study of mitotic cells of the general population [6]. However, the most frequent reports of translocations resulting from centric fusion are those of the D/G type. The reason for this is the association of this translocation with an increased frequency of conception of mongols (for review, see Penrose and Smith [29]).

In Meiotic Cells

Pericentric Inversions

In order to achieve complete synapsis at meiosis, one of the chromosomes of the involved pair of homologues has to form a reversed loop. In these circumstances the consequences of crossing-over depend on whether chiasma formation takes place within the loop. If we consider a chromosome pair represented as AB-CD, and AC-BD, with a pericentric inversion in one homologue, then with a single crossover within the loop, gametes of types AB-CD, AC-BD, AB-CA, and DB-CD will be produced, two of these types being unbalanced because of a duplication deficiency. In fact, individuals heterozygous for a pericentric inversion are likely to produce a high proportion of unbalanced gametes unless the chiasma frequency within the loop is very small or even zero, or unless reciprocal crossing-over occurs. If the inverted region involves almost the whole chromosome, then the noninverted terminal regions will be very small, and it might be possible that their absence or duplication would not be harmful. In general, it may be anticipated that duplication deficiencies will lead to the death of the affected gametes or will be lethal if involved in the formation of zygotes.

Reciprocal Translocations

If discordant meiotic orientation is ignored, then after concordant orientation three types of segregation are possible (alternate, adjacent nonhomologous, and adjacent homologous), which should result in six classes of gametes [30].

In balanced centric fusion of the t(DqGq) type (D/G in Patau's classification), two of these classes have not been detected [31]. These are the complementary G–,t(DqGq)+ and D– classes, and this type of adjacent segregation may not occur. A third class of gamete, G–, has never been detected, although it must be produced because, as pointed out by Hamerton, it is complementary to the D–,t(DqGq)+ class [31]. In male heterozygotes the absence of the G– class could be accounted for by the degeneration of nullisomic G secondary spermatocytes or spermatids; in female heterozygote cells of this class could be preferentially included in the first polar body.

For all practical purposes, therefore, three classes of gametes are formed by a balanced t(DqGq) heterozygote. These are (1) the normal 23,X or 23,Y; (2) the balanced 22,X or Y,D–,G–,t(DqGq)+ types, which are complementary and which result from alternate segregation; and (3) the 23,X or Y,D–,t(DqGq)+ class resulting from one form of adjacent segregation which leads to Down's syndrome (Fig. 3-4). If random segregation of the trivalent is assumed, then these three types of gamete should be produced with equal frequencies, so that among the progeny of balanced heterozygous parents we should observe equal numbers of normal subjects (46,XX or XY), balanced heterozygotes (45,XX or XY, D–,G–,t(DqGq)+), and unbalanced subjects affected with Down's syndrome (46,XX or XY, D–,t(DqGq)+). The same arguments apply to both t(DqGq) and t(21q22q) [31]. These assumptions, therefore, form the basis of the comparisons of observed with expected frequencies. In both t(DqGq) and t(DqDq) there is a sig-

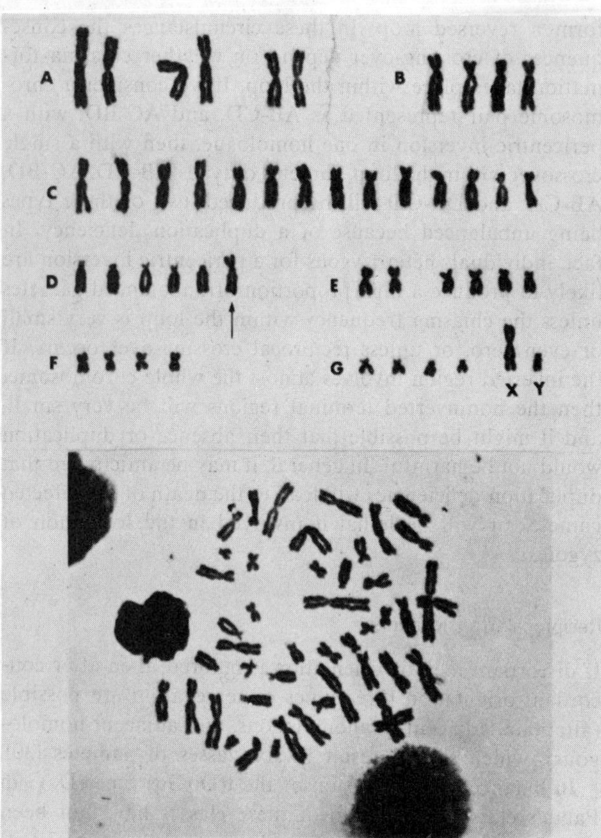

Figure 3-4. 46,XY,D−,t(DqGq)+ (or D/G translocation, Down's syndrome). The supernumerary G material is fused to the centromeric area of one of the six D members (arrow).

nificant excess of balanced heterozygotes over chromosomally normal progeny among the children of male heterozygotes, and this is considered to provide further evidence for some form of prezygotic selection or meiotic drive (defined as the preferential recovery of one or more of the classes of gametes resulting from meiosis in a structural heterozygote) in man, the most probable mechanism being the preferential recovery of certain classes of spermatozoa. There is also a deficiency of unbalanced progeny, which to some extent differs from translocation to translocation and may depend on the sex of the heterozygote. The risk of a female t(DqGq) heterozygote having affected abnormal offspring with Down's syndrome would seem to be nearly five times as high as that of a male heterozygote, but even so, it is probably nearer 10 percent than the theoretical 33 percent [31]. Balanced t(DqDq) heterozygotes have a low risk (probably less than 1 percent) of having affected progeny, and there is no evidence of any sex difference. Balanced t(21q22q) heterozygotes also have a low risk, perhaps less than 10 percent, but the numbers are so small that these figures are suspect. Again, there is little evidence of any sex difference.

Unbalanced Structural Heterozygosity

Unbalanced structural heterozygosity may result from the meiotic segregation of a balanced translocation, or it may be produced by a *de novo* anomaly. In such cases, one of three major situations will obtain: (1) a partial deficiency, (2) a partial duplication, (3) a combination of both.

Deletion Syndromes

As pointed out by Miller et al [32], the size of a deletion can be related to the reduction in length of the affected segment only if all the remaining material is derived from the same chromosome. The simplest mechanism would involve a single break with loss of the telomere. If two breaks occur within a single arm, with loss of the interstitial segment, the size of the deletion would also be indicated by the size of the remaining arm [32].

Classically, the existence of true terminal deletions has been questioned, because loss of the telomere is supposed to produce abnormalities of mitosis and cell nonviability [33]. Though there is evidence that true terminal deletions do not occur in corn and *Drosophila,* there is no information about the situation in mammals, and it appears unwarranted to dismiss this possible mechanism [32].

It would seem likely that a reciprocal translocation is involved in a number of familial translocations with balanced carriers. The deleted chromosome in these cases represents not only its own material but also part of another chromosome. One cannot determine how often a reciprocal translocation occurring at a premeiotic stage in gametogenesis has occurred in cases with karyotypically normal parents since the cytologic distinction between a deleted chromosome which has been self-repaired and one which has the terminal segment of another chromosome is not possible [31].

In cases where a deletion arises as a result of a reciprocal translocation in a premeiotic stage, every individual with clinical signs of the deletion should also be trisomic for part of another chromosome. Unless the same chromosome is repeatedly involved in translocation with the deleted arm, this might lead to variability in the phenotype. Variability could also arise from differences in the size and position of the deleted segment, as well as from differences in the gene loci present in the remaining hemizygous segment of the normal homologue. Despite these possible sources of variation, there is a surprising amount of consistency in the clinical findings of patients with deletions, as discussed below.

B_5 Short-arm Deletion—B_{5p-} (Cri-du-chat Syndrome)

This condition [34–36] owes its name to the peculiar cry of affected infants, which has been compared to the cry of a kitten in distress. The laryngeal abnormalities have been particularly studied by Ward et al. [37]. Children examined

Table 3-1. MAIN CLINICAL FINDINGS IN PATIENTS WITH B_5 SHORT-ARM DELETION

Abnormal cry	16/16*
Mental retardation	16/16
Growth failure	15/15
Hypertelorism	15/15
Microcephaly	14/15
Epicanthus	13/14
Abnormal dermatoglyphics	13/14
Low-set ears	12/13
Hypotonia	12/13
Oblique palpebral fissures	11/13
Rounded facies	10/14
Abnormal larynx	6/7
Strabismus	7/12
Micrognathia	8/15

* Numerator = number of cases in which feature is present; denominator = number of cases in which presence or absence was specifically reported.

Table 3-3. CLINICAL FEATURES IN PARTIAL DELETION OF THE SHORT-ARM OF CHROMOSOME 18—E_{18p-} (14 PATIENTS)

Sex (♂/total)	4/14*	Flat nose bridge	5/5
Maternal age (> 30)	6/13	Tooth decay	5/6
Paternal age (> 30)	9/11	Micrognathia	5/6
Mental retardation	11/12	Web neck	3/5
Small size	8/9	Short fingers	2/2
Eyes:		Abnormal hands	2/2
Hypertelorism	5/6	Abnormal feet	3/3
Epicanthus	4/5	Abnormal toes	3/3
Ptosis	4/4	Dermatoglyphics	High ridge count
Strabismus	2/2	Parental transmission	(3)
Ears			
Low-set	2/3		
Other abnormality	7/8		

* Numerator = number of cases in which feature is present; denominator = number of cases in which presence or absence was specifically reported.

had laryngomalacia, and the larynx had a distinctive appearance. The long, curved flappy epiglottis, the narrow diamond-shaped appearance of the vocal cords during inspiration, and the anterior approximation of the vocal cords with an abnormally large air space in the posterior commissure area during phonation were thought to be responsible for the stridor and the catlike cry. Table 3-1 lists the main clinical features encountered in patients described in the literature [34–36].

Table 3-2. CLINICAL FEATURES IN PARTIAL DELETION OF LONG-ARM CHROMOSOME 18—E_{18q-} (19 PATIENTS)

Sex (♂/total cases)	7/17*	Eyes:	
Birth weight (⩽ 3 kg)	10/13	Nystagmus	6/12
Maternal age (> 30)	7/14	Epicanthus	8/13
Paternal age (> 30)	6/14	Hypertelorism	9/12
Mental retardation	17/19	Fundus anomaly	13/15
Small size	14/17	Tapering fingers:	10/13
Hypotonia	13/15	Abnormal toes	6/10
Microcephaly	15/17	Skeletal:	
Mid-face retraction	14/16	Additional ribs	5/5
"Carp" mouth	9/10	Talipes	2/2
Prominent chin	7/8	Skin rash	2/5
Ears:		Low voice	6/10
Low-set	7/13	Cardiac anomaly	8/15
Curled helix	6/11	Genital anomaly	8/12
Prominent antihelix	6/9	Dermatoglyphics:	
Prominent antitragus	9/15	Whorls (3)	14/16
Atretic canals	8/15	Transverse line	3/9
Dimples:		Distal triradius	6/8
Acromial	7/12	Edema: foot	4/8
Metacarpal	8/9	Parent translocation: 3 families	

* Numerator = number of cases in which feature is present; denominator = number of cases in which presence or absence was specifically reported.

Another B short-arm deletion involving a member of pair No. 4 (B_{4p-}) which replicates later than pair No. 5 has also been recognized [35]. This deletion syndrome includes a number of signs rarely if ever seen in the B_{5p-} condition. These signs are cleft lip or palate, coloboma, internal hydrocephalus, seizures, hypospadias, heart defects, and central scalp defects.

E_{18} Long-arm Deletion—E_{18q-}

Table 3-2 includes the chief physical and clinical anomalies observed in the first 19 cases reported [38–41] since de Grouchy et al. [38] called attention to features accompanying this chromosome deficiency. As in the B short-arm deficiency, the amount of deletion may be variable and tends to involve only part of an arm length.

E_{18} Short-arm Deletion—E_{18p-}

Loss of the short arm of an E_{18} chromosome was the first autosomal deletion observed in man [42]. At least 14 instances of the condition have now been recorded. Careful comparison of these patients does not yield sufficient clues for establishing a clinical diagnosis [43, 44]. Nevertheless a number of malformations appear to be common to several patients and to involve similar organs (Table 3-3). In addition, other anomalies have been reported in isolated cases, such as microcephaly, hip luxation, hepatosplenomegaly, congenital alopecia, and hypothyroidism in two patients, one with familial transmission.

Ring for Chromosome 18—E_{18r} [45, 46]

The presence of a ring chromosome implies a deletion at both ends of a chromosome. Patients with an E_{18} ring chromosome show some of the signs which belong more particularly either to the E_{p-} or E_{q-} conditions. Table 3-4 lists the

Table 3-4. CLINICAL FEATURES IN RING CHROMOSOME 18—E_{18r} (11 PATIENTS)

Sex (♂/total cases)	5/11*	Widely set nipples	4/6
Maternal age (>30)	0/9	Acromial dimple	0/3
Paternal age (>30)	3/8	High-arched palate	3/4
Encephalopathy	9/10	Harelip	2/6
Epilepsy	2/7	Heart defect	3/5
Hypotrophy-hypotonia	6/6	Hands:	
Microcephaly	7/8	Short fingers	3/7
Eyes:		Spindle-shaped fingers	2/6
Hypertelorism	5/9	Tapered fingers	1/6
Epicanthus	5/8	Abnormal thumb implantation	4/7
Oblique palpebral fissures	2/6	Dermatoglyphics:	
Strabismus	1/7	Single palmar line	1/6
Low-set ears	5/7	Whorls	5/6
Abnormal ears	3/9	High triradius	3/6
Deafness, middle-ear atresia	3/6	Abnormal feet	4/8
Pterygium coli	2/4	Hip luxation	1/6
Low hairline	2/3	Renal anomalies	1/4
		Genital anomalies	1/8

* Numerator = number of cases in which feature is present; denominator = number of cases in which presence or absence was specifically reported.
Source: From Grouchy et al. [45, 46].

main features encountered in 11 patients presumed to have an E_{18r}.

G Monosomy: 46,G_r or 45,G−

Partial G monosomy, usually due to the formation of a ring chromosome, and apparent total monosomy of a G autosome have been observed in a few instances [47–51]. In patients with complete lack of a G autosome it is possible that undetected somatic mosaicism or an unrecognizable translocation of part at least of the missing small autosome exists. Such a translocation on an F member was identified in one of our patients, a 12-year-old girl with G monosomy and a 45 chromosome modal number [51]. From studies of the children of t(DqGq) balanced translocation carriers, it seems reasonable to postulate that gametes or zygotes resulting from adjacent meiotic segregants with G nullisomy are nonviable. Therefore, partial and apparent total G monosomies will be considered as a single group. Table 3-5 includes some of the common findings among those patients.

Other Chromosome Deficiencies

Sporadic instances of partial deficiencies of an autosome have been observed in all chromosome subgroups. They occurred either through fertilization of an aneuploid segregant formed by a balanced translocation carrier or through *de novo* deletion in one gamete or zygote. These instances have recently been reviewed by Polani [52]. They are extremely rare, but reporting will increase with time, and phenotype correlation between patients with deficiencies affecting similar regions of morphologically and autoradiographically identical chromosomes will undoubtedly disclose new rare deficiency syndromes. In other studies as well as in our own [51], cases have been found with 46,C_{p-} patterns and, on this still scant evidence, some striking similarities are occasionally seen. One of our patients with a sporadic D_{q-} deficiency had a general appearance similar to that reported in a previous case [53]. Hand roentgenograms of both patients showed an association of a Y-type synostosis between the fifth and the fourth metacarpals and extreme hypoplasia of the middle phalanx of the fifth finger. By contrast, the three cases of C_{p-} known to us [54] did not bear any resemblance, and one would assume that different C autosomes were affected in these subjects.

Partial Chromosomal Duplications

Partial duplications have resulted from the presence of supernumerary fragments of chromosomes sometimes identified as part of a D or an E or a G chromosome [55]. In other cases the origin of these fragments has remained undetermined [56]. There are still questions as to whether the presence of a minute extra metacentric found in some cases has a deleterious effect on the bearers of this anomalous chromosome [57].

Table 3-5. SIGNS COMMONLY OBSERVED IN G (PARTIAL) MONOSOMY

Antimongoloid slant
Prominent nose bridge
Small jaw
Large ears
Elongated skull
Hypertonicity
Hypertrophic pyloric stenosis

Partial chromosomal duplications carried as translocations are likely to form a group which will elude sound clinical classification for a long time. Enlargement of a chromosome arm cannot give any indication of the origin of the added material unless the aberration results from a balanced rearrangement between two identifiable chromosomes in one parent. Even in this case, and excluding the particular case of carriers with centric fusion of chromosomes, it remains improbable that the same type of balanced heterozygosis will often recur in different families and produce consistency among their unrelated affected offspring. It is therefore by no means surprising that patients affected with superficially similar intercalary or terminal arm enlargements of a particular chromosome have not displayed clinical similarities [51].

Autosomal Trisomies

Most instances of autosomal trisomies probably result from meiotic nonsegregation, although other mechanisms may lead to a similar imbalance. Thus, meiosis, which, through synapsis and diakinesis, is central to recombination, segregation, and assortment of Mendelizing genes, inevitably carries the risk of an abnormal gametal distribution of homologous chromosomes. In man three major viable autosomal trisomies have been identified [58–60].

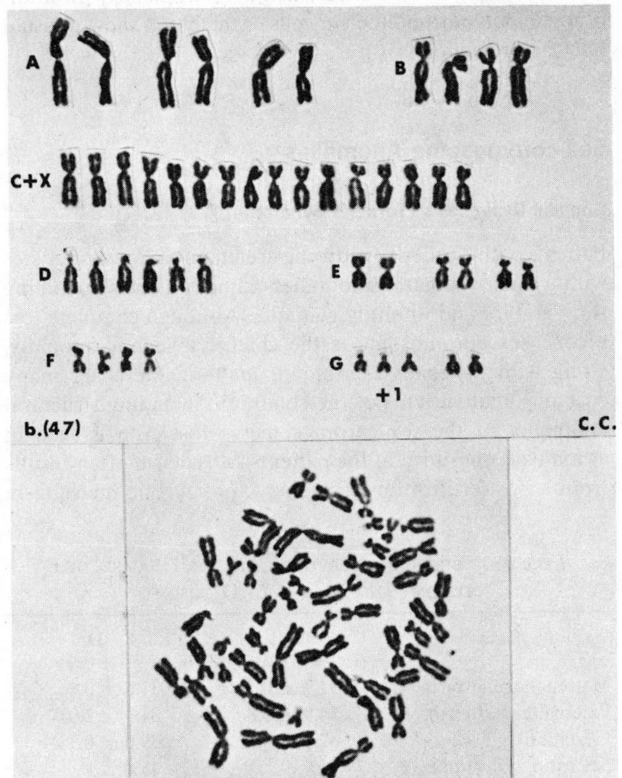

Figure 3-5. 47,XX,G+. The "regular" G-trisomy pattern of Down's syndrome in a female.

Table 3-6. MAJOR CLINICAL SIGNS IN DOWN'S SYNDROME (G TRISOMY)

Over 50 percent of cases	Under 50 percent of cases
Mental retardation	Malformed ears
Slanting eyes	Palmar line
Hyperextensible joints	Conical lateral incisors
Flat occiput	Flat nose
Small ear lobule	Furrowed tongue
Rough scaly cheeks	Gap between toes
High-arched palate	Crowded teeth
Short, broad hands	Blepharitis
Curved fifth finger	Broad lips
Hypotonic muscles	Dry lips
Red cheeks	Protruding tongue
Flat nose bridge	Speckling of iris
Mouth open constantly	Large tongue
Small teeth	Heart murmur
Fissured lips	Widely spaced teeth
Small nose	Strabismus and/or nystagmus
Narrow palate	One flexion furrow in finger no. 5
Epicanthus	
Prominent ears	

Down's Syndrome—47,XX or XY,G+ (Mongolism) (Fig. 3-5)

The condition is too well known to require extensive description. Table 3-6 shows some of the more common (over 50 percent) and rarer (below 50 percent) signs encountered in this trisomy [55, 61].

Incidence and Relation to Maternal Age

Various surveys in communities of European origin have indicated frequency figures for Down's syndrome between 1:636 and slightly less than 1:1,000 births [62]. The incidence does not seem to vary much among races [63]. As pointed out by Penrose [62], up to a maternal age of 29 the distribution curve of mongolian births does not rise appreciably more rapidly than the distribution curve for all births in the population, and the incidence is close to 1:2,000 births. After this point the distribution for all births falls, while that for mongols continues to rise. While the incidence is in the range of 1:1,000 for a maternal age of 30 to 34, it nears 1:300 for mothers between 35 and 39, is close to 1:100 between maternal ages of 40 and 44, and is 1:50 at age 45 and thereafter.

Irregular Patterns

A proportion of patients have Down's syndrome because of an unbalanced translocation with extra G material which is sometimes inherited from a balanced carrier parent [62, 64, 65]. Mikkelsen [66] has studied the frequency of these cases and contributed her own extensive series to a survey of cases previously reported. From the compiled data, about 8 percent of a group of almost 1,000 mongols born to young

Table 3-7. RELATIVE FREQUENCY OF MAJOR CLINICAL ABNORMALITIES IN E AND D TRISOMIES

Abnormality	E+, percent	D+, percent
Feeding difficulty	96.0	92.0
Failure to thrive	96.0	87.0
Developmental retardation	96.0	100.0
Arches on finger tip	*96.0**	33.0
Elongated skull	*93.0*	16.0
Micrognathia	92.0	84.0
Flexion deformity of fingers	89.0	68.0
Low-set, malformed ears	88.0	80.0
Congenital heart disease	85.0	73.0
Ocular hypertelorism	81.0	92.0
Prominent calcaneus	*77.0*	28.0
Short dorsiflexed big toe	*75.0*	24.0
Short sternum	68.0	12.5
Limited hip abduction	*68.0*	19.0
Hypoplastic nails	*63.0*	37.0
Short neck	62.0	79.0
Single palmar crease	61.0	69.0
Distal triradius	57.0	74.0
Extra skin of nape	56.0	59.0
Calcaneovalgus	*52.0*	8.7
Distally implanted thumbs	*52.0*	12.0
Retroflexible thumbs	*50.0*	25.0
Hypertonia	*50.0*	26.0
Jitteriness, apnea	*46.0*	58.0
Epicanthic folds	40.0	56.0
Hypotonia	36.0	48.0
Presumptive deafness	33.0	50.0
Catlike cry	*33.0*	4.4
Partial syndactyly	*32.0*	12.0
Webbed neck	*31.0*	0.0
Microphthalmos	29.0	*76.0*
Eye defect	29.0	*88.0*
Jaundice	23.0	42.0
Seizures	23.0	25.0
Hernias (inguinal, umbilical)	22.0	43.0
Capillary hemangiomas	19.0	*72.0*
Long, hyperconvex nails	16.0	*68.0*
Abnormal shoulder abduction	*12.5*	4.8
Cleft palate	11.0	*69.0*
Equinovarus	8.0	*17.0*
Polydactyly	7.7	*76.0*
Microcephaly	8.0	*64.0*
Fibulars	5.0	*39.0*
Strabismus	4.4	6.7
Harelip	3.7	*58.0*
Low-set normal ears	3.8	*12.0*
Iris colobomas	0.0	*33.0*
Undescended testes	100.0	93.0

Note: The percent figures for features prevailing in either E or D trisomy are in italic.
Source: After A. Taylor [67].

mothers (below 30) carry a G translocation, whereas barely more than 1 of the 668 cases born to older mothers (over 30) showed this pattern. In the group from younger mothers, t(DqGq) and t(GqGq) translocation were found in equal number. Whereas half the t(DqGq) unbalanced genotypes had derived from a carrier parent, most t(GqGq) cases were sporadic as a result of *de novo* accidents. It appears that 2 percent of all mongols born to young mothers have a t(DqGq) unbalanced translocation which can be traced to a balanced carrier parent. In this parental age group the proportion of mongol births is estimated at 1 per 2,000, so that one expects one t(DqGq) unbalanced proband whose anomaly was inherited familially in 100,000 live births.

E and D Trisomies—47,E+ and 47,D+

There is much overlap between the clinical and anatomic findings in D and E trisomies. Accordingly, both conditions will be considered together in an attempt to compare the frequency of the same features as documented in the large series of both disorders contributed by a single group of investigators [67]. Table 3-7, inspired by a recent publication by A. Taylor, lists the many characteristics encountered in both trisomies.

The principal birth and survival data appear in Table 3-8, and the chief autopsy findings are listed in Table 3-9 (from Taylor [67]).

Two further signs may help in delineating both trisomies. In the D trisomy some of the infants carry a small amount of embryonic hemoglobin and a still larger number show relatively high levels of fetal hemoglobin [68, 69]. In addition, the polymorphonuclear cells of the blood show unusual nuclear projections [70].

Sex-chromosome Anomalies

Gonadal Dysgenesis (Turner's Syndrome) [71, 72]

Patients with Turner's syndrome are unambiguously females with various somatic anomalies, almost always including short stature and infantile genitalia. Although complete loss of one sex chromosome is the chief cytogenetic anomaly, along with a negative chromatin pattern, there are many chromosomal variants of the condition, including structural anomalies of the sex chromosomes. Mosaicism is seen in as many as one-third of the patients. Mosaicism often results from a postfertilization accident. A postzygotic mechanism

Table 3-8. BIRTH AND SURVIVAL DATA FOR 153 CASES OF E TRISOMY AND 74 CASES OF D TRISOMY

Data	E	D
Maternal age at birth, yr	31.7 ± 0.7	31.6 ± 0.8
Paternal age at birth, yr	34.9 ± 0.8	31.9 ± 1.0
Gestation age, weeks	42.2 ± 0.8	39.0 ± 0.3
Sex ratio, ♂ to total	21%	45%
Birth weight, gm	2,243.0 ± 35.0	2,609.9 ± 86.7
Survival, days	70.85 ± 21.5	89.2 ± 29.9

Source: After Taylor [67].

Table 3-9. OCCURRENCE OF MAJOR AUTOPSY FINDINGS IN 18 CASES OF E TRISOMY AND 21 CASES OF D TRISOMY

Finding	E, percent	D, percent
Superficially normal brain	*92.0**	27.0
Renal anomaly	62.0	48.0
Persistent ductus arteriosus	53.0	63.0
Ventricular septal defect	47.0	48.0
Thin diaphragm, eventration	*40.0*	0.0
Normal renal tract	33.0	48.0
Major atrial septal defect	31.0	40.0
Normal heart	29.0	24.0
Pyloric stenosis	*25.0*	5.0
Horseshoe kidney	*23.0*	0.0
Hydronephrosis-hydroureter	*23.0*	9.5
Malrotation of intestine	17.0	14.0
Polycystic renal cortex	15.0	*33.0*
Dextroposed heart	13.0	18.0
Meningomyelocele	*12.0*	0.0
Coarctation of aorta	6.2	9.5
Absent olfactory bulbs	0.0	*70.0*
Biseptate uterus	0.0	*42.0*
Pyelon duplex	0.0	*14.0*

* The percent figures for features prevailing in either E or D trisomy are in italic.
Source: After Taylor [67].

Table 3-10. CONGENITAL ABNORMALITIES IN 24 PATIENTS WITH A CHROMATIN-NEGATIVE PATTERN AND 15 PATIENTS WITH CHROMATIN-POSITIVE PATTERN AND SEX CHROMOSOME ANOMALIES

Abnormality	Chromatin −	Chromatin +
Height (<60 in.)	23/24*	14/15
Webbed neck	10/21	1/15
Cubitus valgus	14/17	7/13
Pectus excavatum	6/12	0/9
Coarctation of aorta	3/20	0/14
Congenital lymphedema	10/12	0/2
Lymphedema, adult	. . .	6/12
Many nevi	12/18	9/10
Low hairline	16/21	10/11
Low-set ears	14/21	7/11
Malformed ears	10/17	3/8
Strabismus	11/16	4/7
Refractive error	8/13	2/7
Ptosis	10/15	3/10
Blue sclerae	4/10	2/7
Long, thin hands	4/17	2/11
Short metacarpals	3/18	2/10
Short second phalanx	12/19	3/7
Hypothenar pattern	8/18	7/11
Distal triradius	9/18	7/11
Single palmar line	4/18	2/10
Low intelligence	8/22	5/12

*Numerator = number of cases in which feature is present; denominator = number of cases in which presence or absence is specifically reported.
Source: From Engel and Forbes [72].

Table 3-11. GONADAL DYSGENESIS (TURNER'S SYNDROME). ACQUIRED DISORDERS IN 24 PATIENTS WITH CHROMATIN-NEGATIVE PATTERN AND 15 PATIENTS WITH CHROMATIN-POSITIVE PATTERN

Disorder	Chromatin −	Chromatin +
Seborrheic dermatitis	4/11*	1/10
Deafness	11/15	5/8
Otitis media	10/18	5/10
Cholesteatoma or polyp	4/15	1/10
Corneal or scleral disease	4/15	2/8
Cataract	3/15	5/10
Progeria	9/16	7/12
Osteoporosis	9/11	4/8
Hypertension (diastolic 10)	6/22	4/14
Obesity	14/16	8/12
Arcus senilis	4/12	5/8
Thin hair	7/17	8/10
Diabetes mellitus	2/19	4/9
Thyroid disease (thyroiditis, focal or generalized)	4/5	3/4
Thyroglobulin antibodies (titer >1/20)	9/15	5/12
Achlorhydria	3/7	5/7
Psychiatric disturbance	4/15	1/11

*Numerator = number of cases in which feature is present; denominator = number of cases in which presence or absence is specifically reported.
Source: From Engel & Forbes [72].

is further suggested in a number of patients by a high incidence of identical twinning among the sibs of the proband [73]. In some patients the gonadal failure is not absolute and, since some estrogenic function may exist, a degree of sexual maturation, and at least temporarily menses, can occur, but sterility remains the rule. Table 3-10 compares some of the main physical features in patients, all with a sex-chromosome anomaly. They are arbitrarily separated in two groups, depending on whether there is a negative chromatin pattern (mostly 45,X cases) or a chromatin-positive one, mainly with X structural anomalies or mosaicism [72]. Table 3-11 lists some of the acquired disorders prevailing in these patients.

Tubular Dysgenesis (Klinefelter's Syndrome)

Patients with Klinefelter's syndrome are on the whole chromatin-positive and have an XXY genotype. The use of X markers, particularly in the X-linked Xg blood system, has conclusively established that most cases arise by a prefertilization accident, most frequently a chromosome missegregation at the first meiotic division. Mosaicism is somewhat less frequent in this group than in Turner's syndrome, and when noted appears as a superimposed mitotic error occurring at the expense of an abnormal zygote. The physical features of these patients are far less impressive than those of patients with ovarian dysgenesis. The only consistent finding is the presence of abnormally small testes, which reflect destruction and replacement of tubular structures by

Table 3-12. PHYSICAL FINDINGS AND CONGENITAL ABNORMALITIES IN 24 PATIENTS WITH TUBULAR DYSGENESIS

Tallness (>72 in.)	8/24*
Marked eunuchoidism	6/24
Gynecomastia	21/24
Clinodactyly	11/24
Cubitus valgus	4/24

*Numerator = number of cases in which feature is present; denominator = number of cases in which presence or absence is specifically reported.
Source: From Zuppinger et al. [74].

hyaline material. Sterility is the almost unfailing rule. Other physical features and pathologic trends are assigned in Tables 3-12 and 3-13.

Triple X Females (47,XXX)

Consistent physical findings have not been associated with the chromosome abnormality of triple X females. Ovarian changes and menstrual irregularities as well as normal menses and fertility have been described [75]. Finger abnormalities, webbed neck, and neurologic signs have been occasionally observed. The number of XXX females found within populations of institutionalized mentally defective females is significantly higher than the expected number as calculated from the frequency of triple X at birth. It is not known whether the presence of three X chromosomes may

Table 3-13. HORMONAL AND METABOLIC PATTERNS AND ACQUIRED DISORDERS IN TUBULAR DYSGENESIS

Increased urinary gonadotropins (>15 IU/24 hr)	22/24*
Low PBI (<3.5 μg/100 ml)	4/24
Low thyroid ^{131}I uptake (<20% at 24 hr)	8/24
Thyroglobulin antibodies (titer >20)	1/24
Overt diabetes mellitus	2/24
Latent diabetes (diabetic glucose tolerance test)	4/24
Hypercholesterolemia (>300 mg/100 ml)	6/24
Hyperlipemia (fasting serum triglyceride >150 mg/100 ml)	8/23
Obesity	10/24
Venous disease	8/24
Peptic ulcer	5/24
Cholelithiasis	4/24
Nephrolithiasis	4/24
Heberden's nodes	3/24
Recurrent pulmonary infection	2/24
Behavioral disturbances (chronically unemployed)	12/24

*Numerator = number of cases in which feature is present; denominator = number of cases in which presence or absence is specifically reported.
Source: From Zuppinger et al. [74].

lower the mean IQ or whether an increased susceptibility to agents or factors primarily responsible for the retardation may exist in these patients [76].

Some triple X females are fertile, and lack of even a single XXX or XXY child in their progeny probably indicates preferential segregation, with the XX secondary oocyte becoming a polar body while the balanced oocyte develops into the ovum [76].

XYY Males

The genotype-phenotype correlation in males with an XYY sex complement remains a puzzle. Systematic screening of male populations in high-security institutions has revealed a relatively high incidence of this genotype among a confined population. The pattern has emerged that the XYY male tends to be an inordinately tall, antisocial person of low mentality whose base instincts and other behavioral problems become overt at an early age [77, 78]. After the appearance of the first report [77], a number of studies selecting men on the basis of the fact that they were tall and had a criminal record have confirmed the high prevalence of this genotype among delinquents. Twelve XYY males were found among 50 such subjects in one particular report [79]. Other studies have failed to uncover such a high frequency. These differences may well reflect both the mode of referral to certain institutions and the personal bias of the investigators [78]. There is, however, little doubt that there is an excess of XYY genotypes among delinquents. The extent of this excess is not known, since the incidence of this genotype in the general population has not been established. From the results of several systematic studies of approximately 8,000 male neonates [57, 80], a frequency of 1 in about 600 male births seems indicated, but, there are large differences among series (4:1,066 in Sergovich et al. [81] and 0:1,322 in Walzer et al. [57]). Jacobs et al. found 9 XYY patients among the 315 karyotyped inmates of the high-security institution at Carstairs, Scotland [77], when, according to figures now available, one case might have been expected from twice as many unselected males. It may not be an overestimate to foresee that the incidence of double-Y males among hard-core recidivist delinquents will be somewhat above that found in the general population. While there is no doubt that some XYY patients have proved to be dangerous criminals, others seem to confine their antisocial activities to petty larceny accomplished with little skill for a small profit [78].

Structural Anomalies of One X Chromosome

A number of patients with structural anomalies of one member in the X pair have been reported, such as short-arm deletion (XXp−), long-arm deletion (XXq−), or long-arm isochromosomes (XXqi) (Fig. 3-6). Loss of short-arm material is crucial to the appearance of the somatic stigmata of Turner's syndrome, including dwarfism and many other

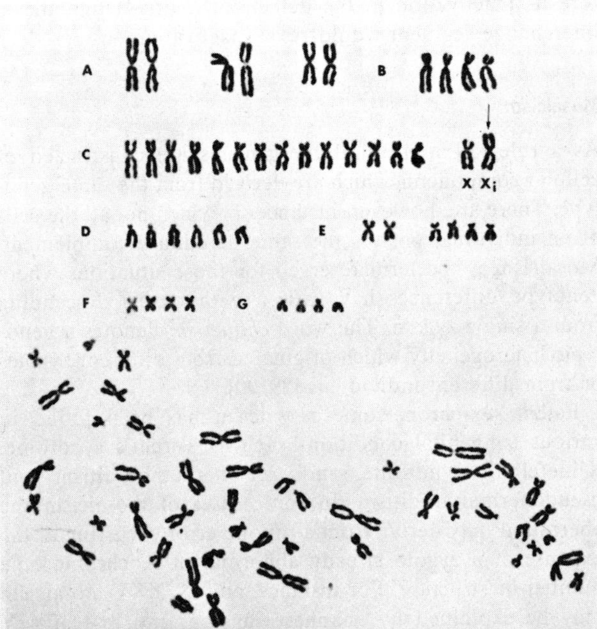

Figure 3-6. 46,XXqi. X long-arm isochromosome (arrow) in a patient with gonadal dysgenesis. The asymmetric X pair amounts to the presence of three X long arms and one X short arm.

features [82]. Deletions of either short- or long-arm material, on the other hand, leads to anomalies of gonadal development. Patients with an isochromosome of the long arm of the second X, which in fact is a duplication of long-arm and elimination of short-arm material, show most or all of the defects associated with Turner's syndrome. In addition, they appear more likely to develop some of the major metabolic disorders often associated with gonadal dysgenesis, such as diabetes mellitus [83] and autoimmune thyroiditis [84].

Structural Anomalies of the Y Chromosome

Structural anomalies of the human Y chromosome, such as short- and long-arm isochromosomes and dicentric formations, have been reported in a certain number of patients with aberrant sexual and gonadal differentiation [85]. While these anomalies should assist in establishing genotype-phenotype correlations and in mapping genes on the Y chromosome, their value, as "experiments of nature," has too often been obscured by the simultaneous occurrence of another cell line in which the defective Y chromosome is altogether deleted. From the scant evidence available several authors have suggested that genes responsible for testicular differentiation are located on the short arm of the Y chromosome [86]. Thus, when an isochromosome for the long arm of a Y is found, an anomaly which amounts to duplication of this arm and loss of the short-arm component, then no testicular tissue is found, whereas when the Y chromosome undergoes a pericentric inversion with conservation of at least some short-arm material, a degree, at least, of testicular development is achieved.

Xg Blood Groups and X Chromosome Nondisjunction [87]

The antigen Xg^a is an X-linked dominant character which in European communities is carried by the cells of almost exactly two-thirds of the hemizygous males. As a consequence of the gene frequency, approximately eight-ninths, or 88 percent, of females are either heterozygous or homozygous for the Xg^a allele, and, since the trait is dominant, they present a positive phenotype, as disclosed by agglutination of their red blood cells with the appropriate antiserum. Twelve percent of females totally lack the allele, and, being homozygous negative, they do not display the red blood cell agglutination with the antiserum [87].

The use of this blood-group system has proved invaluable as a marker for the origin of the X chromosome, particularly in patients with X chromosome aneuploidy [87]. For example, in the mating of an Xg^a male with an Xg female, all the female children must be phenotypically Xg^a because the Xg^a dominant locus is carried by the one X which females inherit from their father. All males born to this mating are Xg and negative for the antigen. If a child with the 45,X anomaly should result, the Xg blood system would indicate whether the paternal or maternal X is present, and by implication would disclose the parental origin of the missing sex chromosome. If a 45,X individual is Xg, then the X represented would be matroclinous (Xm), leaving the alternative that either an X or Y was lost from the father's gamete; should such a 45,X be Xg^a, this would indicate that one maternal X failed to be transmitted. In no instance would this tell whether the accident occurred at meiosis or after zygote formation. Similarly, if a 47,XXY should be Xg^a, then one of the 2 X's would have to be patroclinous, and this would indicate the presence of both an X and a Y from the father, instead of either X or Y alone. This type of nondisjunction could of course only arise at the first meiotic division or before that stage, during proliferation of the primitive germ cells. Xg negativity, on the other hand, would indicate an X duplication of maternal origin. Thus, used as a marker system, the Xg blood groups have taught us the following about the origin of X aneuploidy in major anomalies of the sex chromosome.

Klinefelter's Syndrome 47,XXY

Males with two X chromosomes do not quite show the Xg distribution of normal female populations and differ sharply from that expected of XY males [83]. A complete overlap with the female distribution of Xg alleles in XXY would result only if (1) one of the two X's came from the father and the other from the mother, as occurs in normal females, or (2) if both X's represented unchanged the X pair of the mothers of the proband. Thus the departure from the normal female ratio must derive from the fact that, in some cases, the X pair in the XXY complement is a duplicate copy of one of the two maternally derived X's. Incidentally, if the latter mechanism was the only one, Xg phenotype distribution in XXY patients would be the same as in normal males. Informative types of matings resulting in Klinefelter probands have indicated that the extra X is paternal in 40 percent of cases, and maternal in 60 percent. In the case of maternal nondisjunction, five of six instances suggest representation of both members of the maternal X pair, consistent with nondisjunction of these two chromosomes in the first meiotic division, while in one case in six, duplication of one only of the two maternal X's indicated second meiotic nondisjunction. Thus in the Klinefelter syndrome, when maternal, the nondisjunctional event, as analyzed from Xg systems, appears to take place chiefly at the first meiotic division and rarely at the second meiosis, whereas postzygotic mishap is almost ruled out.

Turner's Syndrome, 45,X

The distribution of 45,Xg group is the same as in normal males. Statistical analysis from informative matings after appropriate correction for biases in the efficiency of ascertainment shows that 74 percent of the patients have a maternal and 26 percent a paternal X chromosome.

Other Sex Chromosome Aneuploidies

In 48,XXXY and 49,XXXXY males the Xg group evidence points to nondisjunction at the first and second meiotic divisions of oogenesis. In XXYY individuals two informative studies indicated paternal contribution of a sperm with an X and two Y's, an error involving both meioses. In XXY/mosaics, most of whom are XXY/XY, the Xg group distribution disproves a mitotic accident involving a normal XY zygote and points to mitotic loss of an X by an XXY zygote in some cells. The testing of triple X females has not given evidence of the source of the extra X. 46,XX males form a rare, particular class. In three informative studies, both X's appeared to be of maternal origin, consistent with loss of the Y by XXY zygotes at some point after initiation of male development. The Xg testing of 20 XX propositi weighs against this interpretation, since they showed a predominantly male distribution, which might mean, if the trend is confirmed, that they only have one Xg locus for their X pair. One interpretation suggests that one X may have interchanged part of its length with a Y [88]. This would also explain testicular development in these exceptional XX males if one is willing to make a few of the following assumptions: (1) that this "Y-onized" X is not consistently "lyonized," in contrast to what seems to happen for structurally defective X chromosomes; or (2) that one segment of the second X is not inactivated and is the same as that into which the Y segment is incorporated; or (3) that the Y exchange would effect initial testicular development before its inactivation in the defective X; or (4) that the Y interchange segment would resist inactivation.

Mosaicism

As a rule, all multicellular organisms are constructed of cellular components which are derived from the same genotype. There are, however, instances in which not all the cells of an individual possess the same hereditary complement. Mosaicism is the term reserved for those situations where genotype differences have arisen within cells descending from a single zygote. The word *chimerism* denotes a genotypic heterogeneity which originated from different zygotes or from different individuals [89, 90].

Patent sex-chromosome mosaicism has been found in various congenital conditions such as Turner's syndrome, Klinefelter's syndrome, and true hermaphroditism and pseudohermaphroditism. In some cases of mosaicism the aberration may derive from a mitotic error occurring at the expense of a zygote already abnormal in its chromosome number or structure. For instance, an XX/XXY mosaicism may be explained by anaphase lagging, and loss of a Y chromosome by a daughter cell in an XXY zygote.

In other cases mosaicism seems to arise from an error occurring at the first cleavage of a normal diploid egg. Formulas such as XO/XXX and XO/XYY are likely to result from postzygotic nondisjunction, whereas anaphase lagging and ultimate loss of a Y chromosome by a daughter cell are almost certain in XO/XY patients.

In some cases of mosaicism different stem-lines lie adjacent, and some areas appear to contain almost exclusively one cell type, whereas others may be composed of another type. In others stem-lines seem intimately mixed. The im-

Table 3-14. ESTIMATES OF THE FREQUENCY OF THE MAIN VIABLE CHROMOSOME ANOMALIES

Autosomal anomalies	
45,D–,D–,t(DqDq)+	1–1.2 per 1,000 males and females [91]
Other centric fusions	0.05 per 1,000 males and females [92]
Interchanges	0.8 per 1,000 males and females [91]
46,B_{5p-}	0.02–0.01 per 1,000 males and females [52]
47,E+	0.15–0.30 per 1,000 males and females [52]
47,D+	0.10–0.15 per 1,000 males and females [52]
47,G+	1–1.50 per 1,000 males and females [62]
Sex-chromosome anomalies	
45,X	0.40 per 1,000 females [93]
47,XXX	1.40–1.80 per 1,000 females [75]
47,XXY	1.30 per 1,000 males [78]
47,XYY	1.5 per 1,000 males [80]

portance of the distribution of the stem-lines inside the body cannot yet be accurately assessed, but the pattern of distribution is perhaps significant in the phenotypical expression of mosaicism. This is suggested in the XO/XY group of patients. It seems probable that in patients with fair representation of the XY stem-line at the level of the gonad at least some testicular elements develop and undergo various degrees of male differentiation in utero to give signs of masculinization at puberty. The phenotype may be typically male. In other cases the phenotype is similar to that found in Turner's syndrome. There is merely a streak gonad, as if only the XO stem-line is present at this site.

Autosomal mosaicism of a generalized type is much more rarely seen than that involving the sex chromosomes. Localized chromosomal mosaicism affecting autosomes is almost unknown with the exception of malignant stem-lines and alterations due to irradiation.

Frequency of All Chromosome Anomalies (Human Population Cytogenetics)

At Birth

Table 3-14 shows the frequency of autosomal and sex-chromosome anomalies as obtained from aggregate data drawn from heterogeneous sources. These estimates rely on sex-chromatin screening or chromosome studies and, for some groups such as the mongols, on clinical criteria; they may be considered only as representing an order of magnitude, pending extensive prospective karyotypic studies of series of unselected neonates.

From the estimates of Table 3-14 it appears that 0.6 percent of all viable individuals are affected by one of the major structural or numerical chromosome disorders. The results of prospective chromosomal studies will have to be viewed in the light of ecologic and ethnic factors, since racial and geographic differences may be of importance [94]. In one survey involving 2,400 phenotypically normal healthy neonates (1,322 males and 1,068 females) 13 major abnormalities were observed [57]. These included four instances of the XXY karyotype, two instances of D/D centric fusion, one occurrence of a reciprocal translocation between a number 2 and a C chromosome, three examples of pericentric inversions (No. 2 once and the Y chromosome twice), and three instances of a small extra metacentric chromosome added to an otherwise normal karyotype. Thus 0.54 percent of these normal-appearing infants had a major anomaly.

In another relatively large survey in southwestern Ontario, 2,159 consecutive unselected newborn babies were studied and findings were obtained on 2,081 (1,066 males and 1,015 females), a 96.3 percent ascertainment [81]. Gross chromosome abnormalities were present in 0.48 percent. Among males there were four XYY, one XXY, and one with a D/D centric fusion. Among females there were two with trisomy 21, one with D/D centric fusion, and one with B short-arm deletion (cri-du-chat syndrome). Undoubtedly, the multiplication of such studies, possibly helped by automation, will unveil the spectrum of detectable chromosome anomalies in our species.

In Abortuses

The frequency and the nature of the major chromosome anomalies thought to be responsible for fetal wastage have also been studied to some extent. The data, reviewed by Inhorn [95], are impressive, although they still may underestimate the facts. Indeed, ascertainment through successful tissue cultivation of abortion products could introduce a bias in favor of those with less severely unbalanced cells, since more deleterious genotype defects might not be compatible with in vitro cell proliferation, not to mention initial embryonic survival. Of 466 spontaneously aborted specimens which were examined successfully, 120 revealed chromosome abnormalities. Of these, 55 were trisomies for an autosome; in 42, the trisomy was in the D, E, and G groups, with smaller numbers in the A, B, C, and F groups. In these studies no autoradiographic labelings were available to indicate whether the D trisomy affected a late DNA-synthesizing chromosome, as in Patau's syndrome, but a majority of the identifiable E errors were No. 16 trisomies, not No. 18 trisomies as in Edward's syndrome. The second largest group of abnormalities was monosomy for a sex chromosome, 45,X, found in 25 cases. Triploidy (3n cells) was observed in 22 cases, and tetraploidy (4n cells) accounted for 9 miscarriages. Only 4 possible structural aberrations and 3 autosomal monosomies were reported.

Estimates of spontaneous abortion rate in man have varied widely, but recent surveys would indicate a range of 10 to 20 percent. On the basis of these figures and assuming that one in five abortions is due to an embryonic chromosomal unbalance, then 2 to 4 percent of all conceptuses fail on account of a karyotypic abnormality, while another 0.5 percent are born with such an abnormality. Thus, the total load of chromosome abnormalities is in the range of a few percent (2.5 to 5 percent) of conceptuses, with 80 to 90 percent of them appearing as abortions. For 45,X, rejection may be even higher, and for trisomy 21 the rate could be 70 percent, assuming that all 47,G+ abortuses carry this specific chromosome [52].

Causes of Abnormal Chromosomes

Maternal Aging

Most trisomic individuals probably originate through the functioning of gametes carrying an extra chromosome as a result of faulty meiosis. Mitotic nondisjunction of sister chromatids during early cleavage(s) of the zygote will also produce trisomic and monosomic blastomeres, the latter perhaps unviable or selected against during embryonic development. Chromosome nondisjunction during the mitotic proliferation of gonial cells before meiotic divisions is another mechanism whereby abnormal gametes may be formed. Thus, in theory, premeiotic, meiotic, and postmeiotic errors may result in chromosome imbalance.

A prerequisite for an exact meiotic process is the regular pairing of homologous chromosomes (synapsis), the formation of chiasmata, the timely separation of homologous partners at diakinesis, and the proper orientation of the bivalents on the spindle. When considering both autosomal and sex-chromosome nondisjunction, four mechanisms at least must be mentioned, all bound to occur, although their relative importance is unknown. (1) Failure of homologues to pair in the first place. (2) Failure of the paired homologues to undergo firm association through chiasmata formation and crossing-over. (3) Failure of the chiasmata to persist long enough to preserve the bivalent arrangement of homologues throughout prophase and metaphase. All three mechanisms result in the falling apart of two chromosomes as univalents. Univalents can behave in different ways, but the overall consequence of their formation is their random migration to the poles, with the result that balanced as well as nullisomic or disomic gametes may be formed. (4) Failure of the partners of a bivalent to disjoin, so that instead of moving apart, both migrate together to a single pole.

The higher frequency of trisomic progenies of older women points to disturbances of anaphase separation during the meiotic divisions of the oocytes. As observed by Ohno et al. [96], in man the developmental sequence of oogenesis is very different from that of spermatogenesis. Oogonias cease to propagate while the female is in the fifth or sixth month of fetal life, and all oocytes complete the entire process of first meiotic prophase several weeks before the end of gestation. Thus, preparation for segregation of one haploid set from the other is completed in the female during prenatal life. Oocytes then enter the long interphase-like dictyotene stage during which the cytoplasm stores nutrients. When the estrus cycle begins, one or more oocytes at a time resume meiosis from diakinesis shortly before being ovulated into the fallopian tube. Second meiosis is usually completed only after an ovum has been fertilized. Thus, in females, at its shortest, the synapsis lasts about 12 years, until the first ovulation, and at its longest some 50 years, until the last. There should be almost 40 years of difference between the times that the first and the last oocytes enter the first meiotic metaphase from the dictyotene period. It seems possible that as time passes, chiasmata may be lost, either by rupture or by slipping off the chromosome ends. Thus, univalents would increase in frequency with increased maternal age and, as a result, so would also the risks of chromosome maldistribution. As pointed out by Patau [97], it seems that smaller chromosomes are more given to nondisjunction than larger ones, and this would be especially plausible if meiotic nondisjunction came about largely through failure or loss of chiasma formation. In this regard smaller chromosomes with perhaps only one chiasma should have a much narrower margin of safety than larger ones.

Interchromosomal Effects

Sturtevant made the unexpected discovery that heterozygous autosomal inversions may greatly increase the rate of nondisjunction of X chromosomes in *Drosophila* [98]. This observation is all the more surprising since suppression of crossing-over by means of inversions in either or both of the large autosomal pairs of female *Drosophila melanogaster* is accompanied by an increase in crossing-over in the X chromosomes. Cross-over X chromosomes rarely fail to segregate, whereas nondisjunctional X chromosomes are derived almost exclusively from non-cross-over pairs. To account for this paradox it has been suggested that interchromosomal effects on crossing-over are not actually increases per se, but are due rather to the elimination of low-cross-over chromosomes. The preferential retention of high-cross-over chromosomes would lead to an apparent increase, but selection rather than an increased rate of crossing-over would be the reason [99]. While there is no proof that such aberrations operate in a similar way in man, there is circumstantial evidence that this may be so [100].

Satellite Association

Nucleoli are organized at specific regions of specific chromosomes. In man nucleolus organizers are situated within the short arm of acrocentric chromosomes. At metaphase these regions stain poorly, and since they are located near the end of a chromosome, they appear as secondary constrictions or thin stalks terminated by small chromatic knobs, the satellites. The special property of adhesion of acrocentric chromosomes, exemplified by their close association at prophase and metaphase, may be related to the formation of nucleolar material. It was, therefore, tempting to postulate that satellite association could be one of the determining factors in the production of autosomal nondisjunction during meiotic and early division of the zygote [101, 102]. Along the same lines it was suggested that this type of association could increase the probability of reciprocal translocations between satellited chromosomes, if their breakage is facilitated by stretching of the satellite stalks which occurs normally at prophase. The role of satellite association in the cause of acrocentric chromosome nondisjuction remains conjectural.

Genetic Predisposition in Nondisjunction

A genetic predisposition to nondisjunction has been postulated as an explanation for the familial recurrence of cases of aneuploidy unaccounted for by translocation or secondary nondisjunction [103]. Genetic control of meiosis has been demonstrated in maize, corn, and *Drosophila;* it is obvious from the subtle and orderly sequence displayed by this complex phenomenon. A similar control must also account for the nonrandom organization of the genome of somatic cells, even during interphase [104], while its disruption would explain the recurrence of mosaicism, a prima facie post-zygotic mishap seen in certain kinships [105]. The claret gene in *Drosophila simulans* causes abnormal spindle formation and function during meiosis, and in addition to its effect on eye color, profoundly affects chromosome migration in the homozygous recessive female [106]. As pointed out by Hecht et al. [103], evidence for the participation of such mutant genes in human disorders is slight and rests primarily on the observation of increased consanguinity in the maternal grandparents of subjects with Down's syndrome.

Ionizing Radiation

In view of the relation between ionizing radiation and chromosomal aberrations, including nondisjunction in *Drosophila* and laboratory animals, and various types of alterations in human somatic chromosomes, a link between congenital aneuploidy and radiation has been considered a definite possibility [107]. The clinical data are conflicting, and while some retrospective studies point to a relationship between maternal radiation exposure and occurrence of G trisomy [107] and other trisomies [108], other studies have not found a connection. It may be relevant to stress that Schull and Neel [109] found no association in the data on children born to survivors of the atomic bomb explosions in Japan.

The average mutation rate in germ cells is of the order of one allele in 10^5 loci per generation [110]. Assuming that a zygote contains 20,000 loci, 10^4 per haploid set, one new mutation is expected to every five human zygotes. To put it another way, one in five individuals carries a new mutation. At the outset, these five individuals have together an average pool of perhaps 40 preexisting lethal equivalents, assuming eight such mutants in each genome [110]. Lethal equivalents are genes, each of which would be responsible in the homozygous state for death before reproduction. In short then, one new mutation occurs spontaneously in each generation for each 40 preexisting ones, or a *de novo* load of 2.5 percent. It is generally assumed that exposure to approximately 40 r will produce the same number of mutations as those occurring spontaneously. Therefore, it would take 400 r (an average of 80 r for each individual per generation) to increase our basic load in lethal equivalents by 25 percent and close to 1,600 (over 300 r per person per generation) to double it. Wolff has argued [111] that in mammals at least, the mutations observed under the effect of radiation are really chromosomal aberrations, rather than intragenic or true (point) mutations; by analogy one might argue that only staggering doses of radiation could possibly influence the background rate of viable nondisjunction in a population. Although, according to Wolff [111], the genetic changes seen in rodent experiments may be construed as chromosomal effects rather than as true mutations, it is obvious that not all damages induced by radiation are the consequence of chromosomal breakage and rejoining; this is well documented by studies of mutagenesis in microorganisms.

Infectious Agents

Stoller and Collman [112] suggested that Down's syndrome might be caused by an endemic or epidemic viral infection. They thought that peaks in the incidence of the syndrome could be correlated to the epidemiologic pattern of infectious hepatitis. This correlation was not confirmed in two subsequent studies [113, 114]. Robinson and Puck [115], however, observed a sharp increase of sex-chromosome aberrations in newborn infants during a rubella epidemic in Colorado.

Viruses are known to cause chromosomal damage in mitotically dividing cells, and it has been observed that cells infected in vitro by the SV_{40} agent may show preferential loss of acrocentric chromosomes in both the D and G subgroups [116]. Allison and Paton have shown that certain mycoplasmas recovered from the human female genital tract infected human fibroblasts in culture and produced certain structural anomalies, particularly loss of a G-group short arm and endoreduplication in a proportion of cells [117]. They concluded that the possibility that these agents may significantly contribute to congenital aneuploidy deserved further investigation. The meager evidence may be purely circumstantial; it needs to be greatly extended and highly refined before conclusions may be reached.

Autoimmunity

A tendency to form autoantibodies and to develop certain autoimmune disorders, particularly lymphocytic thyroiditis, has been reported in Down's syndrome [118] and in gonadal dysgenesis [84, 119–121]. These tendencies existed also among the parents and close relatives of the aneuploid probands. The clinical evidence points to a more than random association between disruption of immune homeostasis and the production of aneuploid children. Our initial suggestion that "chromosome nondisjunction occurs more frequently in families with genetic predisposition to autoimmunity" [122] has been further elaborated by Fialkow [123].

In addition, probands with Turner's syndrome and Klinefelter's syndrome and their close relatives were found to develop diabetes mellitus with relatively high frequency [83, 124]. An association between diabetes mellitus and autoimmune disorders has been found [125], and accordingly their concurrence in gonadal dysgenesis probands and their relatives is not surprising. Paradoxically, patients with the 47,XXY pattern do not show an excess of immune aberration [120], in spite of their liability to diabetes mellitus. The data pointing to an association between immune disturbances or diabetes mellitus or both and the occurrence of aneuploid offspring in certain families are impressive, particularly in gonadal dysgenesis, but they do not represent more than circumstantial evidence of a link between these conditions and faulty meiotic or mitotic division. A closer approach to the problem is clearly needed. Relevant is the observation of Vallotton and Forbes of the presence in a proportion of aneuploid probands and their kin of circulating antibodies which react in vitro with cytoplasmic components of mammalian ovarian germ cells [126].

An association between mother-child blood-group incompatibility for ABO and Rh alleles and chromosomal anomalies, particularly postzygotic ones, has also been suggested, but data supporting this view are scant [94].

Cytogenetic Anomalies and Gene Mapping

Increased levels of enzymes found in certain autosomal trisomy syndromes suggest that genes coding for these enzymes are located on the chromosomes involved. Thus, the alkaline phosphatase activity of polymorphonuclear cells from patients with Down's syndrome was significantly increased [127], while this enzyme activity was depressed in chronic myeloid leukemia [128], where there usually is partial monosomy for a G member, the Ph^1 anomaly. It was tempting to conclude that the locus for alkaline phosphatase was on the G chromosome, that three G loci resulted in an excess, and that only one G locus resulted in a deficit in enzyme production.

The findings that cultured fibroblasts from mongols show levels similar to those of normal controls [129], that blood cells in other trisomies also show increased alkaline phosphatase activity, and that the level of this enzyme is inversely related to the life-span of the cells have invalidated this correlation and generally discredited the conclusions based on such oversimplifications. Thus, increases in galactose-1-phosphate uridyl transferase [130] and phosphohexokinase [131] in the erythrocytes of G_{21}-trisomy patients must await another explanation, as must the increase of glucose-6-phosphate dehydrogenase in their leukocytes [132]. In the latter event the locus is clearly X-linked and the excess cannot be explained directly on the basis of gene-dosage effect.

Other interesting devices have been used to map certain genes on autosomes. Two independent studies have suggested linkage on autosome No. 1, between Un 1 and Duffy [133, 134]. The Un 1 is an uncoiler locus which induces an extended secondary constriction near the centromere of one arm of A1. The Duffy (Fy) locus appears to be linked to Cae, the locus for a congenital zonular pulverulent cataract. The study of chromosomal deletions has shed some light on the mapping of genes on autosomes, but no decisive conclusion can be reached for the moment. The haptoglobin locus, Hp, may be on chromosome 13, if anomalies of inheritance in patients with a 13 deletion may be taken as evidence in assigning a marker locus to a chromosome [135]. The same line of evidence has been used to assign a locus affecting Iga production to the long arm of E_{18} [136], as well as a locus for the production of factor XII (Hageman) to the short arm of a C autosome [137]. Pycnodysostosis is an extremely rare homozygous autosomal condition. The occurrence of this disorder in a patient with loss of part of one G chromosome may indicate that the pycnodysostosis locus is on the corresponding part of the homologous G chromosome made hemizygous by the G deletion [138]. A most elegant and promising method has recently indicated that the human locus for thymidine kinase production is on a chromosome E, either 17 or 18. A mouse heteroploid cell line in culture, lacking thymidine kinase, was hybridized with human fibroblasts lacking PRT and placed in a particular medium allowing survival and growth only of cells which would be complemented by the corresponding human locus. In time all the human chromosomes were lost by the mouse cells except the one supplying the locus for the missing enzyme product, identified as E_{17} or E_{18} [139].

Altogether, attempts at correlating known autosome anomalies and given biochemical defects have been extremely deceptive. In this respect chromosome anomalies might resemble the situation found in autosomal dominant mutations; in contrast to the situation in recessive mutations, it usually is difficult to pinpoint a specific enzyme defect as a central cause for the defective phenotype. As pointed out by Penrose [140], cytogenetic methods are so different from those of classical human genetics that advances in this field have not yet been closely integrated with defined quantitative and biochemical methodologies.

MENDELIAN INHERITANCE

At its simplest level, the phenotype of diploid organisms such as man is determined by the effect of a pair of genes. When the effect of one member of the pair is greater than that of the other, the effect is said to be dominant. A fully dominant gene achieves the effect regardless of the other member of the gene pair. A gene which promotes an effect which it cannot fully achieve is said to be incompletely dominant. Recessive genes are genes which do not express themselves at the level chosen for ascertainment. Since dominance is estimated on phenotype measurements, the notion ultimately depends on what is being measured and relates to gene products rather than to the gene per se. Thus, certain conditions may be viewed as dominant, codominant, or recessive, depending on the criteria used. A case in point is illustrated by sickle-cell anemia, a condition which is recessive when judged from the clinical picture, dominant when considered on the basis of a positive sickling test, and codominant when assessed by the detection of both normal and abnormal hemoglobin. *Penetrance* refers to the frequency with which any effect is shown in a population, and *expressivity* is the degree to which the effects are shown in an individual.

Autosomal Dominant Inheritance

A gene whose effect is recognized in the homozygous or heterozygous state is dominant. The risk that a child of an affected heterozygous and a normal parent will be affected is 50 percent, since, as a result of meiotic segregation, the affected parent may with equal probability give the normal gene or the mutant gene to any child regardless of its sex. The criteria for recognizing autosomal dominant inheritance are that every affected person has one affected parent, unless the abnormal gene is the result of a new mutation or shows great variability in penetrance and expressivity. Since the number of normal and affected children is on average equal, both sexes are equally likely to be affected unless there is sex limitation. Normal family members do not transmit the abnormality to their children.

Autosomal Recessive Inheritance

A gene with an effect recognizable only in the homozygous state is said to be recessive. In recessive conditions both parents are apparently normal, although each carries the gene for the trait in one of the relevant pair of chromosomes. The chance that a child will inherit a pair of chromosomes with the two mutant loci or the two normal loci from his heterozygous parents is respectively 1 in 4, whereas the probability of being heterozygous although unaffected is 1 in 2. Since homozygous children affected with recessive traits usually have phenotypically normal parents, the families recognized and studied are only those in which at least one affected child has occurred. This bias of ascertainment explains why the proportion of affected children among ascertained families is well above the theoretical one-fourth. Recessivity is often difficult or impossible to determine on the basis of a single pedigree because it is particularly difficult to distinguish a recessive from a dominant with low penetrance. The following features suggest recessive inheritance: consanguinity of the parents; most of the affected individuals having normal parents; a 3:1 ratio of normal to affected individuals in the sibship; appearance of the trait in all the children of two affected parents; and normal children usually resulting from marriage of a normal and an affected person.

X-linked Recessive Inheritance

A trait inherited as an X-linked recessive one is expressed by all males who carry the gene, since males have one X chromosome only and are hemizygous for all the X loci. Females are affected only if they are homozygous. Consequently, the incidence of the trait is much higher in males than in females. The trait is passed on from an affected man through all his daughters to half their sons; the trait is never directly transmitted from father to son, but from unaffected carrier mothers who may often be recognized by having affected brothers, fathers, or uncles.

X-linked Dominant Inheritance

Affected males transmit the trait to all their daughters and none of their sons. Affected females who, as a rule are heterozygous, transmit the condition to half their children of either sex, and transmission by females follows the pattern shown by an autosomal dominant characteristic. Thus, sex-linked dominant inheritance cannot be distinguished from autosomal dominant inheritance by the progeny of affected females, but only by the progeny of affected males. Catalogues of autosomal dominant and recessive and X-linked phenotypes have been prepared by McKusick [141].

Identification of Heterozygous Carriers

Heterozygous carriers of a number of recessive conditions have been detected by various means, including careful clinical scrutiny, measurements of gene products and gene-dosage effects, assessment by direct cytology, and phenotypic studies of cultured cells of suspected carriers. There are increasing hopes that an objective elucidation of the phenotype with respect to known allelic systems will progressively replace the statistical approach in the study of potential heterozygotes.

Gene-dosage or Gene-product Effects

A recessive mutation for one member of a gene pair may decrease, abolish, or alter the end product or end effect of this allele. In autosomal recessive conditions the heterozygote may manifest its genotype by producing a lesser amount of a normal enzyme or protein or by manufacturing both a normal and an abnormal product which can be distinguished qualitatively and thus identified. Similar criteria may be used for the detection of heterozygous females carrying an X-linked trait.

Direct Cytology

Direct microscopic studies of cellular material from definite or suspected heterozygotes may reveal cellular alterations which can assist in substantiating the nature of the genotype. Thus, erythrocyte sickling may be observed in otherwise clinically unaffected heterozygotes for the sickle-cell trait. In X-linked conditions, because of the mosaicism brought about by the inactivation of X chromosome material, two populations of cells can be found with respect to a particular trait in some heterozygous females.

Histo- and Biochemistry of Cultured Cells

Cultured cells may show phenotype variations which can be assessed by histochemical or biochemical means and used as a clue to the diagnosis of heterozygosity. This is illustrated by both autosomal and X-linked recessive conditions such as Hurler's and Hunter's syndromes in which the presence

Table 3-15. SOME GENETIC ABNORMALITIES AFFECTING SPECIFIC MOLECULES AND DEMONSTRABLE BY BIOCHEMICAL TECHNIQUES IN CULTURED HUMAN CELL STRAINS

Disease or Variant	Enzyme	Type of inheritance pattern
Acatalasia I (Japanese variant)	Catalase	Autosomal recessive
Acatalasia II (Swiss variant)	Catalase	Autosomal recessive
Familial nonspherocytic hemolytic anemia	Glucose-6-phosphate dehydrogenase	Sex-linked
Electrophoretic variants of G-6-PD (asymptomatic)	Glucose-6-phosphate dehydrogenase	Sex-linked codominant
G-6-PD deficiency (Mediterranean type)	Glucose-6-phosphate dehydrogenase	Sex-linked recessive
G-6-PD deficiency (Negro type)	Glucose-6-phosphate dehydrogenase	Sex-linked recessive
Galactosemia	UDP galactose transferase	Autosomal recessive
Hunter's syndrome	Uncertain*	Sex-linked recessive
Hunter's syndrome	Uncertain*	Autosomal recessive
Electrophoretic variants of lactic dehydrogenase	Lactic acid dehydrogenase	Autosomal codominant
Branched-chain ketonuria	Uncertain†	Autosomal recessive
Niemann-Pick disease	Uncertain‡	Autosomal recessive
Orotic aciduria	Orotidine-5′-monophosphate pyrophosphorylase and orotidine-5′-monophosphate decarboxylase	Autosomal recessive
Electrophoretic variant of phosphoglucomutase (asymptomatic)	Phosphoglucomutase	Autosomal codominant
Electrophoretic variants of 6-phosphoglucuronic acid dehydrogenase	6-Phosphoglucuronic acid dehydrogenase	Autosomal codominant
Citrullinemia	Argininosuccinate synthetase	Autosomal recessive
Glycogen storage disease (Cori's Type II)	Lysosomal α-1,4-glucosidase	Autosomal recessive
Lesch-Nyhan syndrome	Hypoxanthine-guanine phosphoribosyl transferase	Sex-linked recessive
Chediak-Higashi syndrome	Uncertain§	Autosomal recessive
Cystinosis	Uncertain¶	Autosomal recessive

*Cytoplasmic metachromasia.
†Loss of decarboxylase activity.
‡Excessive sphyngomyelin P content.
§Cytoplasmic inclusions.
¶Excessive free-cystine content.
Note: G-6-PD, glucose-6-phosphate dehydrogenase; UDP, uridine diphosphate.
Source: From Krooth et al. [143].

of metachromatic granules can be demonstrated [142]. Table 3-15, from Krooth et al., lists some biochemical products which can be studied in cultured human cell strains [143].

Detection of Balanced Carriers with Chromosome Heterozygosis

The detection of balanced carriers of chromosomal translocations is particularly important among couples in which a young mother has borne a child with Down's syndrome, since in 2 percent of these cases a familial translocation is the source of the unbalanced translocation affecting the offspring, and the risks of recurrence are high. The usefulness of chromosome studies of couples with repeated abortion cannot be overstressed, since unbalanced genomes may be the cause of repeated fetal death as a result of a balanced translocation in one parent (Fig. 3-2).

Antenatal Detection of Hereditary Disorders

Amniocentesis has been used as a diagnostic aid for several decades, but it is not until recently that the technique has given useful results [144, 145]. Amniotic fluid cells can be obtained in the third month of pregnancy or earlier, and their cultivation allows both a study of the fetal karyotype (Fig. 3-7) and a search for certain differences in the cell phenotype in women at high risk of producing abnormal

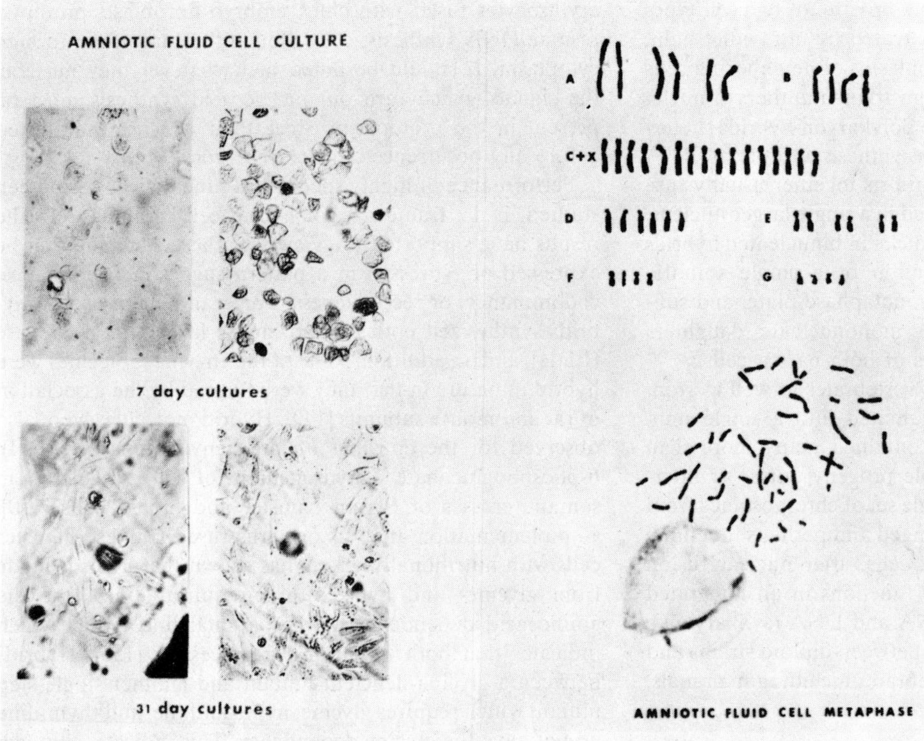

Figure 3-7. Live cultures of human amniotic fluid cells at 7 and 31 days (*left*). Metaphase spread and karyotype (normal 46,XX) from such a culture (*right*).

children. A list of the enzymes which have been studied in amniotic fluid cells has recently been compiled by Nadler [145]. See Table 3-16.

It is evident that detecting quantitative or qualitative variations of these enzymes can greatly assist in prenatal diagnosis [145]. For example, failure to demonstrate measurable levels of galactose-1-phosphate uridyl transferase has led to the correct anticipation of a diagnosis of galactosemia. Cells lacking hypoxanthine-guanine phosphoribosyl transferase (PRT), a defect responsible for X-linked uric aciduria, have also been identified in a fetus. The in utero diagnosis of a mucopolysaccharidosis was established using the technique of Danes and Bearn and demonstrating the presence of metachromatic granules in cultivated amniotic fluid cells. The familial metabolic disorders which have been identified in cultivated amniotic fluid cells are listed in Table 3-16.

SOMATIC CELL HYBRIDIZATION

It would be beyond our scope to review all the experimental procedures being developed and applied to the elucidation of the mechanisms of genetic expression and regulation of mammalian cells. Cell hybridization is one particular area in this quest which has been extremely productive and bears on many biologic problems.

Hybridization of somatic cells in vitro was first described in 1960 by Barski, Sorieul, and Cornefert [146]. In 1965, Harris and Watkins were able to produce heterokaryons and mononucleated hybrid cells following exposure of the cells to ultraviolet-inactivated Sendai virus [147]. These developments, by permitting the study of cellular interaction at the intimate level of cell fusion, have opened the way for a number of cytologic and physiologic studies on a variety of hybrid combinations.

Table 3-16. ENZYMES STUDIED IN HUMAN AMNIOTIC FLUID CELL CULTURES

Acid phosphatase	Glucocerebrosidase
Alkaline phosphatase	Glucose-6-phosphate dehydrogenase
α-Glucosidase	Hypoxanthine-guanine phosphoribosyl transferase (PRT)
α-Keto-isocaproate decarboxylase	Lactate dehydrogenase
β-Glucuronidase	Phytanic acid hydroxylase
Cystathionine synthetase	6-Phosphogluconic dehydrogenase
Galactose-1-phosphate uridyl transferase	Sphingomyelinase
	Valine-transaminase

Source: After Nadler [145].

When a suspension containing a mixture of two cell types is treated with Sendai virus inactivated by ultraviolet light, the cells clump together, the cytoplasms of neighboring cells coalescing so that cells containing varying numbers of nuclei are formed (polykaryons). These polykaryon hybrids (heterokaryons) are able to perform the synthesis of proteins, RNA and DNA. Nuclei which enter mitosis together usually fuse in the process and are reconstituted in a single larger nucleus. Synchronous mitosis of the two nuclei in binucleated hybrids commonly results in the formation of a single spindle; chromosomes line up in a single metaphase plate, and subsequent division produces two mononucleate daughters containing the chromosomal sets of both parent cells.

Cells from different species of vertebrates as well as from the same species can be amalgamated into a single unit. Though cells which originally contained many more than two nuclei do not produce viable progeny, intra- or interspecific hybrids comprising a single set of chromosomes from each parent are capable of prolonged and perhaps indefinite multiplication. These composite cells, after nuclear fusion has taken place, carry out their functions in an integrated way and synthesize proteins, RNA and DNA (synkaryons). Synkaryons have been produced between diploid strains and heteroploid lines of various vertebrates including mammals, birds, and amphibians.

Hybrid Cells and Genetic Regulation

Hybrids Made from Differentiated Cells

Interspecific hybrids can be made between a cell in which the synthesis of RNA or DNA or both is partially or wholly suppressed and a cell which is normally capable of RNA synthesis, DNA synthesis, and multiplication [148]. For example, rabbit macrophages synthesize RNA, but neither in the peritoneal cavity (where they can be obtained in large numbers by certain procedures) nor in vitro do they synthesize DNA or undergo mitosis. Only a fraction of the small lymphocytes of the rat obtained from the thoracic duct can synthesize RNA, and they do not normally synthesize DNA. Differentiated hen erythrocytes, unlike mammalian erythrocytes, remain nucleated throughout their life cycle but do not synthesize measurable amounts of RNA, nor do they synthesize DNA or undergo mitosis. It has been shown by Harris et al. [148] that these three types of cells—rabbit macrophages, rat lymphocytes, and hen erythrocytes—while restricted in their ability to synthesize one or both species of nucleic acid, resume these abilities when fused with cells which, like Hela cells, do not have such restrictions. Sometimes as early as 24 hr after fusion they begin to incorporate both RNA- and DNA-labeled precursors. This resumption of activity cannot be regarded as a nonspecific reaction to foreignness, since in macrophage-lymphocyte heterokaryons which are formed from nuclei which are incapable of DNA synthesis, there is no return of DNA synthesis. Also, chick erythrocytes fused with chick embryo fibroblasts promptly resume DNA synthesis, even though they are not in foreign cytoplasm. It should be noted that whatever they may be, the signals which turn on nucleic acid synthesis must be present in the protoplasm, since their effect is manifested before any occurrence of nuclear fusion.

Performance of highly specialized functions has also been studied in the framework of hybrid cell combination. The results have supported the view that these functions can be expressed or repressed in a pattern suggesting dominance, codominance, or recessiveness. For example, mouse-rat hybrids synthesized both rat and mouse lactic dehydrogenase (LDH), and, in addition, some of the enzyme molecules were hybrid in nature in that they were formed by the association of rat and mouse subunits [149]. Hybrid molecules were also observed for the enzymes malate dehydrogenase (MDH), 6-phosphogluconate dehydrogenase (6PGD), and LDH in somatic crosses of Syrian hamster and mouse cells [150]. Complementation analysis on virus-fused Chinese hamster cells with nutritional markers has shown that hybrids made from glycine- and hypoxanthine-requiring lines lose the amino acid dependency of the parental line, a fact which indicates that both mutations are recessive [150]. Hybrids between a glycine-deficient mutant and another single-step mutant which requires glycine, hypoxanthine, and thymidine do not have the glycine dependency. This indicates that two different loci are associated with the glycine dependence. In the same series of experiments, Kao et al. showed that the mutation to the triple-supplement requirement as well as another for proline were recessive as well [151]. Crosses between a hamster melanoma line which produced pigment and a mouse line which did not, remained unpigmented [152], and hybrids of two mouse lines no longer had the ability to cause tumors, a feature characterizing one of the two cell types prior to cell fusion [153]. On the other hand, hybrids of two mouse lines retained the ability to produce hyaluronic acid and collagen, a character possessed by only one of the two parental types initially mated [154]. It thus can readily be seen that cell hybridization provides a system which permits conclusions about dominance and recessiveness, gene-dosage effects, and linkage studies of genetic markers.

The use of cell-fusion systems also indicates that mechanisms other than the operator-regulator model intervene in gene expression and regulation of eukaryote cells. In higher organisms none of the essential components of bacterial genetic controls have been demonstrated [155, 156]. In order to study whether diffusible repressors modulate the synthesis of enzymes in mammalian cells, Littlefield hybridized wild-type hamster lines with mutant hamster sublines which produced up to 150 times the average amount of folate reductase [157]. This overproduction, if dependent on the loss of diffusible repressors, would have been corrected through complementation by the wild-type parent cells of the hybrid cross. Instead, the resulting hybrid clones contained intermediate levels of reductase activity; thus the excess of folate reductase was not due to lack of repression. In a series of elegant experiments Harris and his colleagues have shown that nucleoli play a decisive role in the transfer of information from nucleus to cytoplasm [158]. When hen erythrocyte nuclei are introduced into the cytoplasm of human or mouse cultured cells, they resume synthesis of large amounts of polydisperse RNA. This polydisperse RNA does not leave the erythrocyte nucleus until a nucleolus is formed. As the nuclei develop nucleoli, some of their RNA is transferred to the cell cytoplasm, and only then is the synthesis of hen-specific surface antigens resumed [158]. It appears, therefore, that some nucleolar component, perhaps a ribosomal RNA subunit or a specific protein(s), is essential for the transfer of mRNA to the cytoplasm. A mechanism of this sort might determine whether RNA synthesized on the genes is translated in the cytoplasm or merely degraded in the nucleus, and it could play a major role in the selection of gene expression in mammalian cells.

Karyotypic Evolution of Synkaryons

In a proportion of hybrid cells, cytoplasmic fusion is followed by nuclear fusion. These mononucleates are the only ones fitted for multiplication, and since they originate prin-

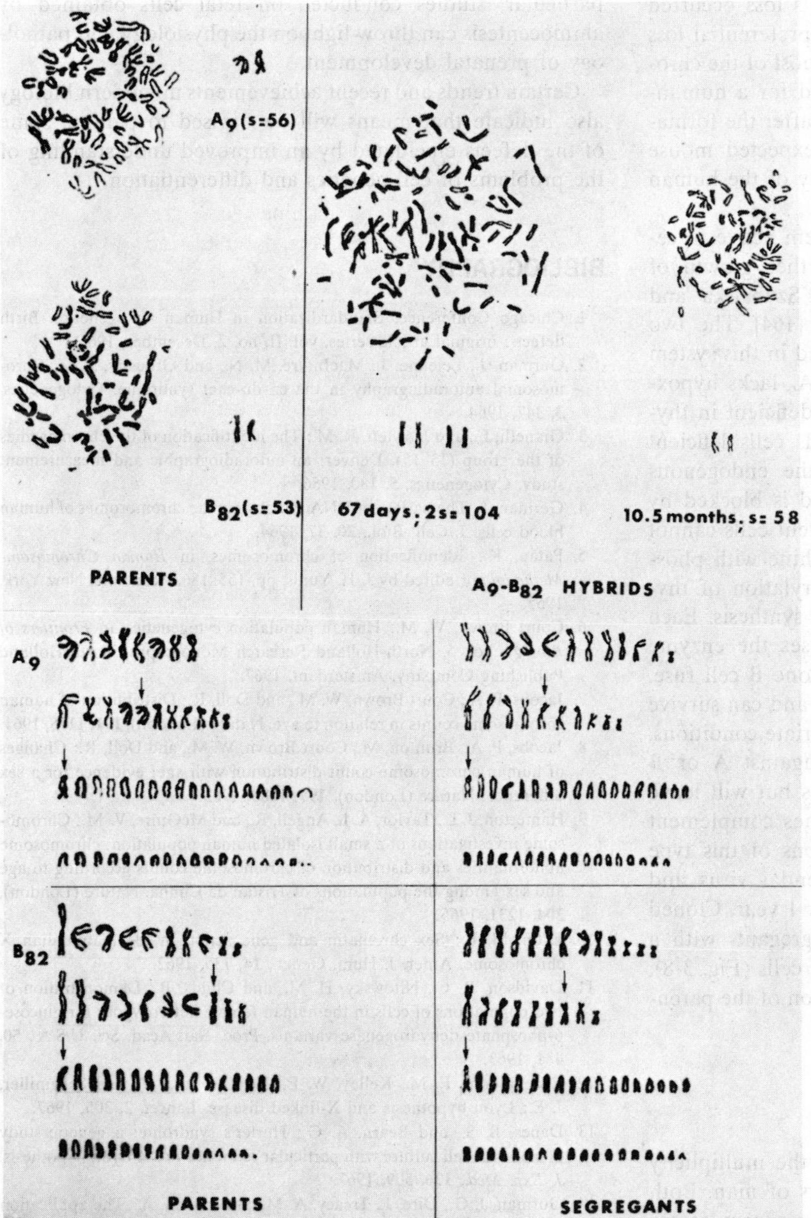

Figure 3-8. (*Top, left*) The chromosomes of A_9 and B_{82} cells. (*Top, middle*) A 2s hybrid containing most of the chromosomes of the two parent cells. (*Top, right*) An s segregant showing a loss of chromosomes equivalent to one parental set. Marker chromosomes of the two parent cells are present in pairs in the 2s hybrid, but singly in the segregant. (*Bottom, left*) The karyotypes of the A_9 and B_{82} parent cells. (*Bottom, right*) Karyotypes of two hybrid segregants, which are indistinguishable from those of the parent cells except that minute "dot"-like chromosomes are absent. Arrows show marker chromosomes.

cipally from fusion of two nuclei, initially they combine a set of the chromosomes of each parental line. These mononucleated hybrids are liable to chromosome changes. Their karyotypic evolution seems to depend on both the nature and origin of the cells involved. Littlefield [159], for instance, has reported that two spontaneous intraspecific mouse hybrid lines lost about 10 percent of their chromosomes over a 1-year period; a similar observation was made for another type of intraspecific (mouse) hybrid by Ephrussi et al. [160]. The karyotype of one series of interspecific hybrids resulting from a cross of normal diploid rat cells with heteroploid cells of a permanent mouse line showed loss of 5 to 10 percent of the chromosomes during an eight-month period of growth [161]. Most of this loss occurred during the first few months, and there was preferential loss of rat chromosomes. Rapid elimination of most of the chromosomes of one set has also been reported for a human-mouse line [162]. Twenty generations or so after the formation of hybrids, all or nearly all of the expected mouse chromosomes were present while a minority of the human chromosomes remained.

Aside from cloning, the only major system active in selecting for hybrids and in preventing further growth of individual parental cells was devised by Szybalska and Szybalski [163] and applied by Littlefield [164]. The two clonal sublines, A_9 and B_{82}, which were used in this system were derived from Earle's murine L line. A_9 lacks hypoxanthine phosphoribosyl transferase; B_{82} is deficient in thymidine kinase. In contrast to wild-type L cells, cells deficient in either enzyme do not survive when the endogenous biosynthesis of purines and thymidylic acid is blocked by aminopterin. Under these conditions, deficient cells cannot effect either the condensation of hypoxanthine with phosphoribosyl pyrophosphate or the phosphorylation of thymidine, steps in the pathway of nucleotide synthesis. Each of the two cell types, A_9 and B_{82}, possesses the enzyme lacking in the other, so that if one A and one B cell fuse, the resulting hybrid contains both enzymes and can survive exposure to aminopterin. Under the appropriate conditions, a medium with aminopterin will select against A or B mutants as well as AA or BB mating types but will leave unaffected AB heterokaryons whose enzymes complement each other. We have followed heterokaryons of this type produced by the action of inactivated Sendai virus and continuously maintained in culture for over 1 year. Cloned populations of these hybrids produced segregants with a karyotype very similar to that of the parent cells (Fig. 3-8), but these segregants showed complementation of the parental enzymatic defects [165].

SUMMARY

Studies in the last 10 years have revealed the multiplicity and diversity of the chromosomal disorders of man. Both numerical and structural alterations of the chromosomes affect a definite proportion of all the zygotes formed. Although most of these alterations lead to early embryonic death, it is clear that defects of chromosome integrity greatly contribute to human morbidity and mortality. The main anomalous patterns for both the autosomes and gonosomes of man have been presented.

Cytogenetic techniques and allied disciplines also provide the opportunity of studying genetic defects at the cell level, and some of their metabolic or enzymatic consequences can be demonstrated before as well as after birth. Thus an era has begun in which refined phenotypic studies on cells separated from the whole organism and grown in vitro provide a new and objective approach to genetic diagnosis and prognosis in an increasing number of genetic conditions. In particular, studies conducted on fetal cells obtained by amniocentesis can throw light on the physiology and pathology of prenatal development.

Certain trends and recent achievements in modern biology also indicate that means will be devised to palliate some of the defects elucidated by an improved understanding of the problems of cell genetics and differentiation.

BIBLIOGRAPHY*

1. Chicago Conference: Standardization in Human Cytogenetics. Birth defects: original article series, vol. II, no. 2, December, 1966.
2. German, J., Lejeune, J., MacIntyre, M. N., and Grouchy, J. de: Chromosomal autoradiography in the cri-du-chat syndrome. Cytogenetics, **3**, 347, 1964.
3. Gianelli, F., and Howlett, R. M.: The identification of the chromosomes of the group (13–15). Denver: an autoradiographic and measurement study. Cytogenetics, **5**, 180, 1966.
4. German, J.: The pattern of DNA syntehsis in the chromosomes of human blood cells. J. Cell. Biol., **20**, 37, 1964.
5. Patau, K.: Identification of chromosomes, in *Human Chromosome Methodology,* edited by J. H. Yunis, pp. 155–186. Academic, New York, 1965.
6. Court Brown, W. M.: Human population cytogenetics, in *Frontiers of Biology,* vol. 5, North-Holland Research Monographs. North-Holland Publishing Company, Amsterdam, 1967.
7. Jacobs, P. A., Court Brown, W. M., and Doll, R.: Distribution of human chromosome counts in relation to age. Nature (London), **191,** 1178, 1961.
8. Jacobs, P. A., Brunton, M., Court Brown, W. M., and Doll, R.: Changes of human chromosome count distribution with age: evidence for a sex difference. Nature (London), **197,** 1080, 1963.
9. Hamerton, J. L., Taylor, A. I., Angell, R., and McGuire, V. M.: Chromosome investigations of a small isolated human population: chromosome abnormalities and distribution of chromosome counts according to age and sex among the populations of Tristan da Cunha. Nature (London), **204,** 1231, 1965.
10. Lyon, M. F.: Sex chromatin and gene action in the mammalian X chromosome. Amer. J. Hum. Genet., **14,** 135, 1962.
11. Davidson, R. C., Nitowsky, H. M., and Childs, B.: Demonstration of two populations of cells in the human female heterozygous for glucose-6-phosphate dehydrogenase variants. Proc. Nat. Acad. Sci. U.S.A., **50,** 481, 1963.
12. Rosenbloom, F. M., Kelley, W. E., Henderson, J. F., and Seegmiller, J. E.: Lyon hypothesis and X-linked disease. Lancet, **2,** 305, 1967.
13. Danes, B. S., and Bearn, A. G.: Hurler's syndrome: a genetic study of clones in cell culture with particular reference to the Lyon hypothesis. *J. Exp. Med.,* **126,** 509, 1967.
14. Gorman, J. G., Dire, J., Treacy, A. M., and Cahan, A.: The application

*The survey of literature for this review was concluded in July, 1969.

of Xg^a antiserum to the question of red cell mosaicism in female heterozygotes. J. Lab. Clin. Med., **61**, 642, 1963.
15. Lee, G. R., MacDiarmid, W. D., Cartwright, G. E., and Wintrobe, M. M.: Hereditary, X-linked, sideroachrestic anemia. The isolation of two erythrocyte populations differing in Xg^a blood type and porphyrin content. Blood, **32**, 59, 1968.
16. Gruneberg, H.: More about the tabby mouse and about the Lyon hypothesis. J. Embryol. Exp. Morph., **16**, 569, 1966.
17. Gruneberg, H.: Gene action in the mammalian X-chromosome. Genet. Res., **9**, 343, 1967.
18. Gruneberg, H.: Sex-linked genes in man and the Lyon hypothesis. Ann. Hum. Genet., **30**, 239, 1967.
19. Back, F., and Dormer, P.: X-chromosome activity in lymphocytes. Lancet, **1**, 385, 1967.
20. Lyon, M. F.: Chromosomal and subchromosomal inactivation, in *Annual Review of Genetics,* edited by H. L. Roman, vol. 2, pp. 31–52. Annual Reviews, Inc., Palo Alto, Calif., 1968.
21. Subak-Sharpe, H., Bürk, R. R., and Pitts, J. D.: Metabolic cooperation between biochemically marked mammalian cells in tissue culture. J. Cell Sci., **4**, 353, 1969.
22. Fujimoto, W. Y., and Seegmiller, J. E.: Hypoxanthine-guanine phosphoribosyltransferase deficiency: activity in normal, mutant, and heterozygote cultured human skin fibroblasts. Program, American Society for Clinical Investigation, Abstr. 85, p. 27, 1969.
23. Comings, D. E.: Uridine 5-H^3 radioautography of the human sex chromatin body. J. Cell. Biol., **28**, 437, 1966.
24. Comings, D. E.: H^3 uridine autoradiography of human chromosomes. Cytogenetics, **5**, 247, 1966.
25. Nance, W. E., and Engel, E.: Human cytogenetics: a brief review and presentation of new findings. J. Bone Joint Surg., **49**, 1436, 1967.
26. Grouchy, J. de, Aussannaire, M., Brissaud, H. E., and Lamy, M.: Aneusomie de recombinaison: three further examples. Amer. J. Hum. Genet., **18**, 467, 1966.
27. White, M. J. D.: *Animal Cytology and Evolution,* 2d ed. Cambridge, London, 1954.
28. Patau, K.: Chromosome identification and the Denver Report. Lancet, **1**, 933, 1961.
29. Penrose, L. S., and Smith, G. F.: *Down's Anomaly.* Churchill, London, 1966.
30. Hamerton, J. L.: Chromosome segregation in three human interchanges in *Chromosomes Today,* edited by C. P. Darlington and K. R. Lewis, vol. 1, pp. 237–252. Oliver & Boyd, Edinburgh, 1966.
31. Hamerton, J. L.: Robertsonian translocation in man: evidence for prezygotic selection. Cytogenetics, **7**, 260, 1968.
32. Miller, D. A., Warburton, D., and Miller, O. J.: Clustering in deleted short-arm length among 25 cases with a Bp– chromosome. Cytogenetics, **8**, 109, 1969.
33. Sturtevant, A. H., and Beadle, G. W.: *An Introduction to Genetics.* Dover, New York, 1962.
34. Lejeune, J., Lafourcade, J., Berger, R., Vialatte, J., Boeswillwald, M., Seringe, P., and Turpin, R.: Trois cas de délétion partielle du bras court d'un chromosome 5. C. R. Acad. Sci. [D] (Paris) **257**, 3098, 1963.
35. Miller, O. J., Breg, W. R., Warburton, D., Miller, D. A., Firschein, I. L., and Hirschhorn, K.: Alternative DNA replication patterns associated with long arm length of chromosomes 4 and 5 in the cri-du-chat syndrome. Cytogenetics, **5**, 137, 1966.
36. Silber, D. L., Engel, E., and Merrill, R. E.: So-called "cri-du-chat syndrome." Amer. J. Ment. Defic., **71**, 486, 1966.
37. Ward, P. M., Engel, E., and Nance, W. E.: The larynx in the cri-du-chat (cat cry) syndrome. Trans. Amer. Acad. Ophthal. Otolaryng., **72**, 90, 1968.
38. Grouchy, J. de, Roger, P., Salmon, C., and Lamy, M.: Délétion partielle des bras longs du chromosome 18. Path. Biol. (Paris), **12**, 579, 1964.
39. Lejeune, J., Berger, E., Lafourcade, J., and Rethore, M. O. La délétion partielle du bras long du chromosome 18. Individualisation d'un nouvel état morbide. Ann. Genet. (Paris), **9**, 32, 1966.
40. Nance, W. E., Higdon, S. H., Chown, R., and Engel, E.: Partial E-18 long-arm deletion. Lancet, **1**, 303, 1968.
41. Wadia, R.: Deletion of part of long arm of chromosome 18, in *The First Conference on the Clinical Delineation of Birth Defects,* pp. 186–189. The Johns Hopkins Hospital, March of Dimes, National Foundation, 1968.
42. Grouchy, J. de, Lamy, M., Thieffry, S., Arthuis, M., and Salmon, C.: Dysmorphie complexe avec oligophrénie: délétion des bras courts d'un chromosome 17–18. Ann. Genet. (Paris), **9**, 19, 1966.
43. Grouchy, J. de, Bonnette, J., and Salmon, C.: Délétion du bras court du chromosome 18. Ann. Genet. (Paris), **9**, 19, 1966.
44. Grouchy, J. de, Rossier, A., and Joab, N.: Une nouvelle observation d'aberration chromosomique 18 p–. Ann. Genet. (Paris), **10**, 221, 1967.
45. Grouchy, J. de, Herrault, A., and Cohen-Solal, J.: Une observation de chromosome 18 en anneau (18r). Ann. Genet. (Paris), **11**, 33, 1968.
46. Wald, S., Engel, E., Nance, W. L., Davies, J., Puyau, F. A., and Sinclair-Smith, B. C.: "E-ring" chromosome with persistent left superior vena cava and hypertrophic subaortic stenosis. J. Med. Genet., **6**, 328, 1969.
47. Lejeune, J., Berger, R., Rethore, M. O., Archambault, L., Jerome, H., Thieffry, S., Aicardi, J., Broyer, M., Lafourcade, J., Cruveiller, J., and Turpin, R.: Monosomie partielle pour un petit-acrocentrique. C. R. Acad. Sci. [D] (Paris), **259**, 4187, 1964.
48. Reisman, L. E., Kasahara, S., Chung, C. Y., Darnell, A., and Hall, B.: Antimongolism: studies in an infant with a partial monosomy of the 21 chromosome. Lancet, **1**, 394, 1966.
49. Al-Aish, M. S., de la Cruz, F., Goldsmith, L. A., Volpe, J., Mella, G., and Robinson, J. C.: Autosomal monosomy in man. New Eng. J. Med., **277**, 777, 1967.
50. Engel, E., Hastings, C. P., Merrill, R. E., McFarland, R. S., and Nance, W. E.: Apparent cri-du-chat and "antimongolism" in one patient. Lancet, **1**, 1130, 1966.
51. Moore, M. K., and Engel, E.: Clinical, cytogenetic and autoradiographic studies in 10 cases with rare chromosome disorders. Ann. Genet. (Paris) (in press).
52. Polani, P. E.: Autosomal unbalance and its syndromes. Brit. Med. Bull., **25** (1), 81, 1969.
53. Laurent, C., Cotton, J. B., Nivelon, A., and Preycon, M.: La Délétion partielle du bras long d'un chromosome du groupe D (13–15): Dq-. Ann. Gent. (Paris), **10**, 25, 1967.
54. Laurent, C., Nivelon, A., Hartman, E., and Guerrier, G.: Monosomie partielle d'un chromosome du groupe C: (Cp-). Ann. Genet. (Paris), **11**, 231, 1968.
55. Moore, K. M., and Engel, E.: G chromosome trisomy: five cases with syndromes other than classical Down's. Southern Med. J., **61**, 146, 1968.
56. Engel, E., Haddow, J. E., Lewis, J. F., Tipton, R. E., Overall, J. C., McGee, B. J., Levrat, O. J., and Engel-de Montmollin, M.: Three unusual trisomic patterns in children. Amer. J. Dis. Child., **113**, 322, 1967.
57. Walzer, S., Breau, G., and Gerald, P. S.: A chromosome survey of 2,400 normal new born infants. J. Pediat., **74**, 438, 1969.
58. Lejeune, J., Gauthier, M., and Turpin, R.: Étude des chromosomes somatiques de neuf infants mongoliens. C. R. Acad. Sci. [D] (Paris), **248**, 1721, 1959.
59. Patau, K., Smith, D. W., Therman, E., Inhorn, S. L., and Wagner, H. P.: Multiple congenital anomaly caused by an extra autosome. Lancet, **1**, 790, 1960.
60. Edwards, J. W., Harnden, D. C., Cameron, A. H., Crosse, V. M., and Wolff, O. N.: A new trisomic syndrome. Lancet, **1**, 787, 1960.
61. Benda, C. E.: *The Child with Mongolism.* Grune & Stratton, New York, 1960.
62. Penrose, L. S.: Mongolism. Brit. Med. Bull., **17** (5), 184, 1961.
63. Kashgarians, M., and Rendtorff, R. C.: Incidence of Down's syndrome in American Negroes. J. Pediat., **74**, 468, 1969.
64. Hamerton, J. L., Briggs, S., Giannelli, F., and Carter, C. O.: Chromosome studies in detection of parents with high risk of second child with Down's syndrome. Lancet, **2**, 788, 1951.
65. Day, R. W., and Wright, S. W.: Down's syndrome at young maternal ages: chromosomal and family studies. J. Pediat., **66**, 764, 1965.
66. Mikkelsen, M.: Down's syndrome at young maternal age: cytogenetical and genealogical study of eighty-one families. Ann. Hum. Genet., **31**, 51, 1967.
67. Taylor, A.: I. Autosomal trisomy syndromes: a detailed study of 27 cases

of Edward's syndrome and 27 cases of Patau's syndrome. J. Med. Genet., **5**, 227, 1968.

68. Huehns, E. R., Hecht, F., Kerl, J. V., and Motulsky, A. G.: Developmental hemoglobin anomalies in a chromosomal triplication: D_1 trisomy syndrome. Proc. Nat. Acad. Sci. U.S.A., **51**, 89, 1964.
69. Powars, D., Rohde, R., and Graves, D.: Foetal haemoglobin and neutrophil anomaly in the D_1- trisomy syndrome. Lancet, **1**, 1363, 1964.
70. Huehns, E. R., Lutzner, M., and Hecht, F.: Nuclear abnormalities of the neutrophils in D_1 (13–15) trisomy syndrome. Lancet, **1**, 589, 1964.
71. Lindsten, J.: *The Nature and Origin of X Chromosome Aberrations in Turner's Syndrome: A Cytogenetical and Clinical Study of 57 Patients,* edited by Almquist and Wissel. Stockholm, 1963.
72. Engel, E., and Forbes, A. P.: Cytogenetic and Clinical findings in 48 patients with congenitally defective or absent ovaries. Medicine (Balt.), **44**, 135, 1965.
73. Nance, W. E., and Uchida, I.: Turner's syndrome, twinning and an unusual variant of glucose-6-phosphate dehydrogenase. Amer. J. Hum. Genet., **16**, 380, 1964.
74. Zuppinger, K., Engel, E., Forbes, A. P., Mantooth, L., and Claffey, J.: Klinefelter's syndrome, a clinical and cytogenetic study in twenty-four cases. Acta Endocr. (Kobenhavn), **54**, suppl. 113, 1–47, 1967.
75. Day, R. W., Larson, W., and Wright, S. W.: Clinical and cytogenetic studies on a group of females with XXX sex chromosome complements. J. Pediat., **64**, 24, 1964.
76. Miller, O. J.: The sex chromosome anomalies. Amer. J. Obstet. Gynec., **90**, 1078, 1964.
77. Jacobs, P. A., Brunton, M., Melville, M. M., Brittain, R. P., and McClermont, W. F.: Aggressive behavior, mental subnormality and the XYY male. Nature (London), **208**, 1351, 1966.
78. Court Brown, W. M.: Males with an XYY sex chromosome complement. J. Med. Genet., **5**, 341, 1968.
79. Casey, M. D., Blank, C. E., Street, D. R. K., Segall, L. J., McDougall, J. H., McGrath, P. J., and Skinner, J. L.: YY chromosomes and antisocial behavior. Lancet, **2**, 850, 1966.
80. Marinello, M. J., Berkson, R. A., Edwards, J. A., and Bannerman, R. M.: A study of the XYY syndrome in tall men and juvenile delinquents. J.A.M.A., **208**, 321, 1969.
81. Sergovich, F., Valentine, G. H., Chen, A. T. L., Kinch, R. A. H., and Smout, M. S.: Chromosome aberrations in 2159 consecutive newborn babies. New Eng. J. Med., **280**, 851, 1969.
82. Ferguson-Smith, M. A.: Karyotype-phenotype correlation in gonadal dysgenesis and their bearing on the pathogenesis of malformations. J. Med. Genet., **2**, 142, 1965.
83. Forbes, A. P., and Engel, E.: The high incidence of diabetes mellitus in 41 patients with gonadal dysgenesis and their close relatives. Metabolism, **12**, 428, 1963.
84. Williams, E. D., Engel, E., and Forbes, A. P.: Thyroiditis and gonadal dysgenesis. New Eng. J. Med., **270**, 805, 1964.
85. Ferrier, P. E., Ferrier, S. A., and Biel, A. W.: A male pseudohermaphrodite with a dicentric Y chromosome. Humangenetik, **6**, 131, 1968.
86. Jacobs, P. A., and Ross, A.: Structural abnormalities of the Y chromosome in man. Nature (London), **210**, 352, 1966.
87. Race, R. R., and Sanger, R.: Xg and sex-chromosome abnormalities. Brit. Med. Bull., **25** (1), 99, 1969.
88. Ferguson-Smith, M. A.: X-Y chromosomal interchange in the aetiology of true hermaphroditism and of XX Klinefelter's syndrome. Lancet, **2**, 475, 1966.
89. Ferrier, P. E.: Mosaiques et chimères. Schweiz Med. Wschr., **98**, 881, 1968.
90. Ford, C. E.: Mosaics and chimaeras. Brit. Med. Bull., **25** (1), 104, 1969.
91. Court Brown, W. M., and Smith, P. G.: Human population cytogenetics. Brit. Med. Bull., **25** (1), 74, 1969.
92. Polani, P. E., Hamerton, J. L., Giannelli, F., and Carter, C. O.: Cytogenetics of Down's syndrome (Mongolism). III. Frequency of interchange trisomies and mutation rate of chromosome interchanges. Cytogenetics, **4**, 193, 1965.
93. MacLean, N., Harnden, D. G., Court Brown, W. M., Bond, J., and Mantle, D. J.: Sex-chromosome abnormalities in newborn babies. Lancet, **1**, 286, 1964.
94. Chandra, H. S.: Mother-child incompatibilities for ABO and Rh alleles: possible association with certain types of chromosomal aberrations. New Eng. J. Med., **272**, 566, 1965.
95. Inhorn, S. L.: Chromosomal studies of spontaneous human abortions, in *Advances in Teratology,* edited by D. H. M. Woolam, vol. 2, pp. 37–99. Logos Press, Academic, New York, 1967.
96. Ohno, S., Klinger, H. P., and Atkin, N. B.: Human oogenesis, Cytogenetics, **1**, 42, 1962.
97. Patau, K.: The origin of chromosomal abnormalities. Path. Biol., **11**, 1163, 1963.
98. Morgan, T. H., and Sturtevant, A. H.: Maintenance of a *Drosophila* stock center, in connection with investigations on the constitution of the germinal material in relation to heredity. Carnegie Inst. Wash. Year Book, **43**, 164, 1944.
99. Cooper, K. W., Zimmering, S., and Krivshenko, J.: Interchromosomal effects and segregation. Proc. Nat. Acad. Sci. U.S.A., **41**, 911, 1955.
100. Grouchy, J. de, Thieffry, S., Arthuis, M., Gerbeaux, J., Poupinet, S., Salmon, C., and Lamy, M.: Chromosomes marqueurs familiaux et aneuploidie: rôle possible de l'interaction chromosomique. Ann. Genet., **7**, 76, 1964.
101. Ferguson-Smith, M., and Handmaker, S. D.: Observations on the satellited human chromosomes. Lancet, **1**, 638, 1961.
102. Ohno, S., Trujillo, J. M., Kaplan, W. D., and Kinosibar, R.: Nucleolus-organisers in the causation of chromosomal anomalies in man. Lancet, **2**, 123, 1961.
103. Hecht, F., Bryand, J. S., Gruber, D., and Townes, P. L.: The nonrandomness of chromosomal abnormalities. New Eng. J. Med., **271**, 1081, 1964.
104. Comings, D. E.: The rationale for an ordered arrangement of chromatin in the interphase nucleus. Amer. J. Hum. Genet., **20**, 440, 1968.
105. Green, J. R., Krovetz, L. J., and Taylor, W. J.: Two generations of 13–15 chromosomal mosaicism: possible evidence for a genetic defect in the control of chromosomal replication. Cytogenetics, **1**, 286, 1968.
106. Wald, H.: Cytologic studies on the abnormal development of the eggs of the claret mutant type of *Drosophila simulans.* Genetics, **21**, 264, 1936.
107. Sigler, A. T., Lilienfeld, A. M., Cohen, B. H., and Westlake, J. E.: Radiation exposure in parents of children with mongolism (Down's syndrome). Bull. Johns Hopkins Hosp., **117**, 374, 1965.
108. Townes, P. L., DeHart, K., and Ziegler, N. A.: Trisomy 17–18: an evaluation of preconceptional parental iradiation as a possible etiologic factor. J. Pediat., **65**, 870, 1964.
109. Schull, W. J., and Neel, J. V.: Maternal radiation and mongolism. Lancet, **1**, 537, 1962.
110. Porter, I. H.: *Heredity and Disease.* McGraw-Hill, New York, 1968.
111. Wolff, S.: Radiation genetics, in *Annual Review of Genetics,* edited by H. L. Roman, pp. 221–244. Annual Reviews, Inc., Palo Alto, 1967.
112. Stoller, A., and Collman, R. D.: Incidence of infective hepatitis followed by Down's syndrome. Lancet, **2**, 1221, 1965.
113. Stark, C. R., and Fraumeni, J. F.: Viral hepatitis and Down's syndrome. Lancet, **1**, 1036, 1966.
114. Leck, I.: Incidence and epidemicity of Down's syndrome. Lancet, **2**, 457, 1966.
115. Robinson, A., and Puck, T. T.: Sex chromatin in newborn: presumptive evidence for external factors in human nondisjunction. Science, **148**, 83, 1965.
116. Moorhead, P. S., and Saksela, E.: Non-random chromosomal aberrations in SV_{40}-transformed human cells. J. Cell. Comp. Physiol., **62**, 57, 1963.
117. Allison, A. C., and Paton, G. R.: Chromosomal abnormalities in human diploid cells infected with mycoplasma and their possible relevance to the aetiology of Down's syndrome (mongolism). Lancet, **2**, 1229, 1966.
118. Mellon, J. P., Day, B. Y., and Green, D. M.: Mongolism and thyroid autoantibodies. J. Ment. Defic. Res., **7**, 31, 1963.
119. Sparkes, R. S., and Motulsky, A. G.: Hashimoto's disease in Turner's syndrome with isochromosome X. Lancet, **1**, 947, 1963.
120. Vallotton, M. B., and Forbes, Anne P.: Autoimmunity in gonadal dysgenesis and Klinefelter's syndrome. Lancet, **1**, 648, 1967.

121. Engel, E., Northcutt, R. C., and Bunting, K. W.: Diabetes and hypothyroidism with thyroid auto antibodies in a patient with a long arm X-isochromosome. J. Clin. Endocr., **29,** 130, 1969.
122. Engel, E., and Forbes, A. P.: Further observations on the association of Hashimoto's thyroiditis and thyroid antibodies with Turner's syndrome. Harper Hosp. Bull., **21,** 83, 1963.
123. Fialkow, P. J.: Autoimmunity: a predisposing factor to chromosomal aberrations? Lancet, **1,** 474, 1964.
124. Nielsen, J.: Diabetes mellitus in parents of patients with Klinefelter's syndrome. Lancet, **1,** 1376, 1966.
125. Pettit, M. D., Landing, B. H., and Guest, G. M.: Antithyroid antibodies in juvenile diabetics. J. Clin. Endocr., **21,** 209, 1961.
126. Vallotton, M. B., and Forbes, A. P.: Antibodies to cytoplasm of ova. Lancet, **2,** 264, 1966.
127. Alter, A. A., Lee, S. L., Pourfar, M., and Dobkin, M.: Studies of leukocyte alkaline phosphatase in mongolism: a possible chromosome marker. Blood, **22,** 169, 1963.
128. Valentine, W. N., and Beck, W. S.: Biochemical studies on leukocytes: I. Phosphatase activity in health, leukocytosis and myelocytic leukemia. J. Lab. Clin. Med., **38,** 39, 1951.
129. Nadler, H. L., Inouye, T., and Hsia, D. Y. Y.: Enzymes in cultivated human fibroblasts derived from patients with autosomal trisomy syndrome. Amer. J. Hum. Genet., **19,** 94, 1967.
130. Brandt, N. J., Froland, A., Mikkelsen, M., Nielsen, A., and Tolstrup, N.: Galactosemia locus and the Down's syndrome chromosome. Lancet, **2,** 700, 1963.
131. Baikie, A. G., Brownwen, Loder P., de Gruchy, G. C., and Pitt, D. B.: Phosphohexokinase activity of erythrocytes in mongolism. Lancet, **1,** 412, 1965.
132. Mellman, W. J., Oshi, F. A., Tedesco, T. A., Maciera-Coelho, A., and Harris, H.: Leucocyte enzymes in Down's syndrome. Lancet, **2,** 674, 1964.
133. Donahue, R. P., Bias, W. B., Renwick, J. H., and McKusick, V. A.: Probable assignment of the Duffy blood group locus to chromosome 1 in man. Proc. Nat. Acad. Sci. U.S.A., **61,** 949, 1968.
134. Ying, I. A., and Ives, E.: Asymmetry of chromosome number 1 pair in three generations of a phenotypically normal family. Canad. J. Genet. Cytol., **10,** 575, 1968.
135. Gerald, P. S., Warner, S., Singer, J. D., Corcoran, P. A., and Umansky, I.: A ring D chromosome and anomalous inheritance of haptoglobin type. J. Pediat., **70,** 172, 1967.
136. Stewart, J., Go, S., Ellis, E., and Robinson, A.: IgA and partial deletions of chromosome 18. Lancet, **2,** 779, 1968.
137. Grouchy, J. de, Veslot, J., Bonnette, J., and Roidot, M.: A case of ?6p – chromosomal aberration. Amer. J. Dis. Child., **115,** 93, 1968.
138. Nance, W. E., and Engel, E.: Autosomal deletion mapping in man. Science, **155,** 692, 1967.
139. Miegon, B. R., and Miller, C. S.: Human mouse somatic cell hybrids with single human chromosome (group E): link with thymidine kinase activity. Science, **162,** 1005, 1968.
140. Penrose, L. S.: New aspects of human genetics: introduction. Brit. Med. Bull., **25**(1), 1, 1969.
141. McKusick, V. A.: *Mendelian Inheritance in Man. Catalogue of Autosomal Dominant, Autosomal Recessive and X-linked Phenotypes.* Johns Hopkins, Baltimore, 1966.
142. Danes, B. S., and Bearn, A. G.: Hurler's syndrome: a genetic study in cell culture. J. Exp. Med., **123,** 1, 1966.
143. Krooth, R. S., Darlington, G. A., and Velazquez, A. A.: The genetics of cultured mammalian cells, in *Annual Review of Genetics,* edited by H. L. Roman, vol. 2, pp. 141–164. Annual Reviews, Inc., Palo Alto, 1968.
144. Jacobson, C. B., and Barter, R. H.: Intrauterine diagnosis and management of genetic defects. Amer. J. Obstet. Gynec., **99,** 796, 1967.
145. Nadler, H. L.: Prenatal detection of genetic defects. J. Pediat., **74,** 132, 1969.
146. Barski, G., Sorieul, S., and Cornefert, F.: Production, dans des cultures in vitro de deux souches cellulaires en association, de cellules de caractère hybrid. C. R. Acad. Sci. [D] (Paris), **251,** 1825, 1960.
147. Harris, H., and Watkins, J. F.: Hybrid cells derived from mouse and man: artificial heterokaryons of mammalian cells from different species. Nature (London), **205,** 640, 1965.
148. Harris, H., Watkins, J. F., Ford, C. E., and Schoell, A. I.: Artificial heterokaryons of animal cells from different species. J. Cell Sci., **1,** 1, 1966.
149. Weiss, M. C., and Ephrussi, B.: Studies of interspecific (rat + mouse) somatic hybrids. II. Lactate dehydrogenase and β-glucuronidase. Genetics, **54,** 1111, 1966.
150. Migeon, B. R.: Hybridization of somatic cells derived from mouse and Syrian hamster: evolution of karyotype and enzyme studies. Biochem. Genet., **1,** 305, 1968.
151. Kao, F-T., Johnson, R. T., and Puck, T. T.: Complementation analysis on virus-fused Chinese hamster cells with nutritional markers. Science, **164,** 312, 1969.
152. Davidson, R. L., Ephrussi, B., and Yamamoto, K.: Regulation of pigment synthesis in mammalian cells, as studied by somatic hybridization. Proc. Nat. Acad. Sci. U.S.A., **56,** 1437, 1966.
153. Finch, B., and Ephrussi, B.: Retention of multiple developmental potentialities by cells of a mouse testicular teratocarcinoma during prolonged culture in vitro and their extinction upon hybridization with cells of permanent line. Proc. Nat. Acad. Sci. U.S.A., **57,** 615, 1967.
154. Green, H., Ephrussi, B., Yoshida, M., and Hamerman, D.: Synthesis of collagen and hyaluronic acid by fibroblast hybrids. Proc. Nat. Acad. Sci., U.S.A., **55,** 41, 1966.
155. Harris, H.: *Nucleus and Cytoplasm.* Clarendon Press, Oxford, 1968.
156. Clever, U.: Regulation of chromosome function, in *Annual Review of Genetics,* edited by H. L. Roman, vol. 2, pp. 11–30. Annual Reviews, Inc., Palo Alto, 1968.
157. Littlefield, J. W.: Hybridization of hamster cells with high and low folate reductase activity. Proc. Nat. Acad. Sci. U.S.A., **62,** 88, 1969.
158. Harris, W., Sidebottom, E., Grace, D. M., and Bramwell, M. E.: The expression of genetic information: a study with hybrid animal cells. J. Cell Sci., **4,** 499, 1969.
159. Littlefield, J. W.: The use of drug resistant markers to study the hybridization of mouse fibroblasts. Exp. Cell Res., **41,** 190, 1965.
160. Ephrussi, B., Stenchever, M. A., and Scaletta, L. J.: Hybridization as a tool for cell genetics, in *International Congress on Congenital malformations,* edited by M. Fishbein, pp. 85–93. International Medical Congress, Ltd., New York, 1964.
161. Weiss, M. C., and Ephrussi, B.: Studies of interspecific (rat + mouse) somatic hybrids. I. Isolation, growth and evolution of the karyotype. Genetics, **54,** 1095, 1966.
162. Weiss, M. C., and Green, H.: Human-mouse hybrid cell lines containing partial complements of human chromosomes and functioning human genes. Proc. Nat. Acad. Sci. U.S.A., **58,** 1104, 1967.
163. Szybalska, E. H., and Szybalski, W.: Genetics of human cell lines. IV. DNA-mediated heritable transformation of a biochemical trait. Proc. Nat. Acad. Sci. U.S.A., **48,** 2026, 1962.
164. Littlefield, J. W.: Selection of hybrids from matings of fibroblast in vitro and their presumed recombinants. Science, **145,** 709, 1964.
165. Engel, E., McGee, B. J., and Harris, H.: Recombination and segregation in somatic cell hybrids. Nature (London), **223,** 152, 1969.

PART TWO

DISEASES PRIMARILY MANIFEST AS DISORDERS OF CARBOHYDRATE METABOLISM

CHAPTER FOUR

DIABETES MELLITUS*

Albert E. Renold, Werner Stauffacher, and George F. Cahill, Jr.

Though future developments will surely justify the decision of the editors to consider diabetes mellitus an inborn error of metabolism (or possibly the result of several such errors), there is equally little reason to deny that the nature of this error (or these errors) remains unknown. Why, then, discuss this ancient disorder in a text whose title implies some degree of knowledge about the nature of the inherited metabolic aberrations to be discussed? Justification may perhaps be derived from at least two considerations:

1 Diabetes mellitus is indeed a familial disorder, and the susceptibility to diabetes mellitus is conditioned—at least in part—by inherited, genetic factors. It may thus quite properly be termed *inborn.*

2 Diabetes mellitus is a complex, widespread disorder of metabolism, intimately related in history to the development of understanding of the metabolism of carbohydrate, protein, and fat. It is clearly influenced by both environmental and genetic factors, which mutually influence each other, each being in itself multiple and complex. Its prevalence among all human races and societies is high. Though these are all complicating features for its study, they may well equally apply to other entities of the next major frontier of metabolic inherited disease, that of the metabolic and genetic aspects of degenerative diseases and of aging. The disorder may thus provide an example of the many approaches, difficulties, failures, and only very partial successes associated with a concentrated and long-lasting attempt to discover the primary metabolic defect or defects involved not only in diabetes mellitus but also in other equally complex yet practically important and widespread diseases.

Published evidence concerning every aspect of diabetes mellitus is so extensive as to preclude any attempt to provide complete coverage of possible topics, or of any single topic. Accordingly the authors have, *volens nolens,* exercised arbitrary selectiveness, with emphasis on concepts and on attempted synthesis and organization, rather than on erudition and documentation. Major omissions will be noted by all, and these we regret, although without apology.

Rather than provide an abbreviated historical introduction, we refer to the remarkable monographs of Allen [1, 2] for the preinsulin period, and to the monographs of Jensen [3] and of Wrenshall, Hetenyi, and Feasby [4] for the period which led to the discovery and application of insulin.

*The authors express their appreciation to the Fonds National Suisse de la Recherche Scientifique and the Howard Hughes Medical Institute.

DEFINITION AND CLASSIFICATION OF DIABETES MELLITUS

Although Dobson [5] concluded from his experiments, published in 1776, that the saccharine matter secreted by the kidney in diabetes was "not formed by the secretory organ, but previously existed in the serum of the blood," Ambrosiani is credited with having first recorded in 1835 that the blood of diabetic patients contains more sugar than that of nondiabetic individuals [3], and thus with having established what is still accepted as the only essential sign of the disorder, i.e., *hyperglycemia.* The severity and duration of hyperglycemia (with or without provocation) required to establish the diagnosis of the disease vary from medical center to medical center; widely accepted sets of criteria are those established by Joslin and his group [6], those proposed by the British Diabetic Association [7], and those recommended by an expert committee of the World Health Organization [8].

Whereas hyperglycemia inappropriate to the existing environmental and nutritional state remains, whether we like it or not, the only generally accepted definition of diabetes mellitus, it is equally accepted that this sign is but one of many endocrine and metabolic alterations present in clinically overt diabetes mellitus. Furthermore, it is possible that the future will bring the definition of abnormalities which are closer to the still legendary "primary" inherited defect(s) and thus better suited for diagnostic definition. Two such candidates have received more serious consideration already: thickening of capillary basement membranes, as studied in muscle [9, 10], and the delay in the initial secretion of insulin during glucose stimulation [11, 12]. Both these suggestions will be discussed more completely further on.

In the meantime, it would be unfair to consider that the definition of diabetes mellitus derives exclusively from inappropriate hyperglycemia, and it must be emphasized that this applies only to early and borderline cases, or to studies of its prevalence and, more generally, of its epidemiology. The large amount of clinical and experimental work which has gone into the scrutiny of diabetes mellitus has indeed resulted in the much more complex yet perfectly clear and unequivocal definition of at least two major syndromes associated with the general concept of diabetes, and these must be considered as part of the clinical definition of the disorder.

Acute Diabetic Syndrome

Within this syndrome are grouped all those manifestations more or less readily explained as derived from the cardinal manifestation—hyperglycemia. With increasing hyperglycemia, after the renal tubular capacity for glucose reabsorption is exceeded, glycosuria and, with it, polyuria result. Loss of water and glucose leads to increased thirst and hunger. Glucose loss, by draining the carbohydrate supplies of the organism, results in increased need for mobilization and catabolism of proteins and fats. This results in weight loss and, when the mobilization of fats becomes excessive, in the accumulation of ketone bodies in the blood and urine, i.e., ketonemia and ketonuria. Since the ketone bodies are primarily anionic, cations accompany their urinary excretion. When the blood levels of ketone bodies become excessive, ketoacidosis and (by still unclear mechanisms) coma and death result. The sequence is frequently rather rapid (several hours to several days), although *it may remain transiently or permanently arrested at any stage,* even at that of moderate hyperglycemia alone. The causal relationships assumed in the sequence of events just described are convenient and likely, but in many aspects still hypothetical. More will be said on this subject below during consideration of the metabolic consequences of insulin lack.

Chronic Diabetic Syndrome

This syndrome groups the many clinical manifestations which, in addition to some or all of the signs of the acute diabetic syndrome, are associated with diabetes of long duration. These manifestations may affect any system or organ, although the organs most frequently affected are the kidneys, eyes, heart muscle, and parts of the nervous system, including the peripheral nerves. Many of these signs appear to have a vascular basis, sometimes interpreted as accelerated vascular aging, although more specific alterations of capillaries, arterioles, and venules are frequently present, particularly in the eyes and kidneys. The frequent presence of abnormal deposits of glycogen, mucopolysaccharides, and glycoproteins in diabetic cells, in general, and in the basement membrane of capillaries, in particular, has led to the suggestion that a metabolic aberration of small-vessel walls might be at the origin of many pathologic and clinical manifestations of the chronic diabetic syndrome [13–16]. Indeed, as already mentioned, the "primary" nature of the capillary basement membrane defect is seriously considered by some investigators [9, 10]. Whether the acute and the chronic diabetic syndromes are directly related causally, or whether they both result from one or more separate primary anomalies, must be considered uncertain, at least at present.

Most of the following discussion will be limited to the acute diabetic syndrome. Whether or not the manifestations of the chronic syndrome are related to an inborn error of metabolism and, if so, whether or not the error is that responsible for the acute syndrome are considerations as yet so hypothetic as to preclude useful discussion in this text.

Classification of Early Stages of Diabetes

It is often necessary to define the basis of the diagnosis of diabetes mellitus, particularly in its early stages. The most generally applicable classification is, in our opinion, that proposed by the British Diabetic Association [17]. *Potential* diabetics exhibit glucose tolerance levels within normal limits but are considered at significantly greater risk of developing diabetes than the general population. Among potential diabetics are the identical twin of a diabetic, the offspring of two diabetic parents, other persons with diabetes in several close relatives, and women with a suggestive obstetric history [a live or stillborn child weighing 10 lb (4.5 kg) or more, or a stillborn child showing hyperplasia of the islets of Langerhans not due to rhesus incompatibility]. *Latent* diabetics have normal glucose tolerance but are known to have had a diabetic glucose tolerance in the past, usually during a pregnancy, an infection, some other type of stress, or when obese. Persons with an otherwise normal glucose tolerance which becomes abnormal during tests combining glucose with other provocative measures—e.g., the cortisone-augmented glucose tolerance test—are similarly considered to have latent diabetes. *Asymptomatic* (or *subclinical,* or *chemical*) diabetics are persons with inappropriate hyperglycemia but without significant glycosuria and without any other symptom, sign, or complication of the disease. In the presence of any of the latter, diabetes becomes *clinical,* or *overt.*

Prediabetes is a retrospective classification, defining the period in the life of a diabetic before a diagnosis can be made. In the United States, the term prediabetes is often used as synonymous with either potential or, in certain instances, latent diabetes [18].

GENETIC CONSIDERATIONS

Prevalence

Overall prevalence of diabetes mellitus is difficult to ascertain, because of lack of precision in its definition. Blood glucose levels, either postabsorptive or at varying intervals after glucose or a meal, continue as the only practical index for such estimations. Since it has been quite clearly demonstrated that the distribution of blood glucose levels in the population, with or without tolerance, is unimodal, albeit skewed, any dividing line between normality and disease must be arbitrary [19–22]. Furthermore, the disease may declare itself late in life and may go unrecognized for many years. Finally, the arbitrary blood glucose level above which diabetes is considered to be present should increase with age, particularly when tolerance conditions are being used for diagnosis [23, 24].

Despite these shortcomings, and using criteria similar to those already mentioned [6–8], a sufficient number of populations have by now been surveyed to permit reasonable confidence about the order of magnitude of present estimates. The first such prevalence survey was that of Wilkerson and Krall, who, in 1947, tested 3,516 of 4,983 inhabitants of a New England community (Oxford, Massachusetts) with an age distribution closely approximating that of the United States as a whole [25]. They found 40 known and 30 previously unknown diabetic patients, i.e., a prevalence of 2.0 percent of those tested, or a projected 1.7 percent of the entire population of the town. Follow-up studies indicated that the total incidence of the disease in the original population, if persons were followed to old age or death, will be at the very least double that of the prevalence initially found, i.e., 3.5 percent or, more likely, higher [26]. The reliability of prevalence estimates carried out with the techniques used by this group is attested to by the remarkably similar results obtained by the same unit in this relatively stable population over a total interval of 17 years [27]. In 1969, the United States Public Health Services estimated, on the basis of a number of individual population surveys and the overall United States National Health Interview survey, that the prevalence of diabetes in the United States in the year 1965–1966 was 2.3 percent, of which 0.8 percent was as yet unrecognized [28]. A general prevalence figure probably acceptable to most might be about 2 percent in the United States and Western Europe, recently somewhat higher in the former and often somewhat lower in the latter. Individual population surveys, using similar yet somewhat different criteria, have been adequately summarized elsewhere [29–32].

Since diabetes is usually recognized in adults, particularly between the ages of 50 and 75 years, it is evident that the prevalence of the disorder increases with age. For example, in the survey published in 1969 for the United States as a whole [28], the prevalence of diabetes in persons under the age of 25 was 0.16 percent, but it was 6.4 percent in the 65 to 75 age group. This increasing prevalence with age may well also be responsible, at least in part, for the reported increased prevalence of diabetes during the last several decades, although environmental factors which might also be at fault will be considered below. Of course, the fertility of juvenile diabetics, which was negligible or small prior to the discovery of insulin, has considerably increased with the advent of insulin treatment. However, the numbers involved are likely to be relatively small and probably did not significantly affect prevalence so far, as indicated also by the longitudinal Oxford survey [27].

A final but important reservation must be made: if the major physiologic variable controlling differences in blood glucose levels is variable tolerance for a glucose load, then the best prevalence figures should result from population analyses with complete glucose tolerance tests. Indeed, an important study carried out in the United Kingdom by a working party of the College of General Practitioners in 1963 suggests that routine screening with a glucose tolerance test would result in a prevalence figure on the order of 7.8 percent for the same group where standard surveying practices had resulted in a prevalence figure much closer to that previously mentioned, namely 1.3 percent. Although this is an observation of great interest, its interpretation remains difficult, particularly since even complete glucose tolerance tests do not ensure definitive classification: considerable variations may be observed from month to month or year to year even when the tests are carried out in the same persons by the same group and under identical conditions, but a few months or years apart [31, p. 49, and 33, 34].

For populations within the general area of the Western world, it is reasonable to assume today that the true prevalence of diabetes is somewhere within the range of 1 to 8 percent, discrepancies being due to age compositions of the groups surveyed, methods employed for the detection of inappropriate hyperglycemia, and to the value arbitrarily selected as dividing abnormal from normal.

Regional Variations in Diabetes Prevalence

An important and largely unexpected by-product of population surveys, has been the demonstration of much greater variability among racially or environmentally, as well as geographically, distinct populations than might have been expected from the general range of prevalence just described. To be sure, comparison is difficult between countries and groups which differ according to level of education (and therefore of understanding) and as to social taboos and medical outlook, in addition to differing as to environment and heredity. Reference is made here to some recent reviews [30, p. 188, and 35] and important original surveys [36–44], but our prejudice is that there is little which suggests a genetic basis for the striking geographic differences reported, while their relevance to environmental factors is much more likely and warrants discussion together with the more general consideration of environmental factors in diabetes.

Evidence for the Hereditary Nature of the Diabetic Potential

That the potentiality (or predisposition) to develop diabetes mellitus is inherited has been surmised for several centuries [45] and may be considered an established fact. This conclusion rests primarily upon (1) the greater frequency of diabetic persons among close relatives of known diabetic patients than among suitable control populations, and (2) the even more frequent occurrence of diabetes in the similar twins of diabetics. With regard to the first point, only one representative study among many will be mentioned [46]. The study concerns 1,307 diabetics and 859 nondiabetic controls. Of the diabetics, 21 percent were found to have a first-degree relative with diabetes, as compared with 7.5

percent for the nondiabetics. In other words, the frequency of diabetes in close relatives was approximately three times greater for diabetics than for nondiabetics. A particularly interesting feature of this study was the demonstration that this difference between diabetics and controls was more marked early in life than later, principally because young nondiabetics had very few first-degree relatives with diabetes, whereas older nondiabetics had almost half as many first-degree diabetic relatives as did the diabetics of the same age.

Although the degree of concordance in dissimilar twins should not be greater than that between other sibs, concordance in similar twins should approach 100 percent. In actual fact, concordance was present in 16 of 33 homozygous twin pairs observed in Boston [47], in 36 of 76 pairs reported from Denmark [48], and in 23 of 45 pairs reported from the United Kingdom [49]. The overall degree of concordance in these three studies thus was 75 of 154 twin pairs, or 48 percent, being quite similar in these three geographically separate and distant locations. For dissimilar twins, the concordance was 2 of 63 pairs in the Boston study, and 22 of 238 in Denmark, the combined concordance rate being 24 of 301, or 8 percent.

These studies leave no doubt about the presence of a major genetic component in the transmission of diabetes. They also indicate that what is transmitted is only the predisposition to diabetes and that identical twins of diabetics may remain normal for many years after the onset of diabetes in the affected member of the pair. The explanation usually given is that the *penetrance* (i.e., the likelihood that a gene will receive its morphologic or functional expression) of the diabetic trait is incomplete and, very likely, variable. Incomplete penetrance may result from the dependence for expression upon associated genetic factors, or from dependence upon associated environmental factors. In the similar twins, the importance of associated environmental factors for penetrance of the diabetic trait would seem more probable.

It is to be hoped that a sign or symptom more directly related to the genetic trait, or traits, responsible for predisposition to diabetes will in due time be found. Already, recent studies of the nondiabetic similar twins of diabetics have revealed anomalies other than those required for the diagnosis of clinical diabetes. Thus, Pyke and Taylor [50] have reported that while glucose tolerance in such nondiabetic similar twins of diabetics was within the normal range, it nonetheless differed significantly from the glucose tolerance of an appropriate control group, blood glucose levels being higher and serum immunoreactive insulin (IRI) levels being lower than in the controls. Cerasi and Luft [51], on the other hand, have clearly demonstrated that the pattern of variations of serum IRI in response to a glucose infusion in nonaffected similar twins of diabetics strikingly resembled the diabetic profile, in spite of glucose levels within the normal range.

Inheritance Pattern(s)

In the second edition of this text we reported that the then most prevalent opinion assigned to the predisposition for diabetes mellitus a *simple Mendelian recessive mode of inheritance,* although some serious reservations were also mentioned. Several geneticists expert in diabetes continue to favor autosomal recessive inheritance, involving one or several loci, as the most probable single explanation [53–55]. In our opinion, however, the intervening years have considerably eroded this relatively simple hypothesis in favor of a *multifactorial* one [19–22, 56–59]. In its most general form this hypothesis states that there are alleles at an unspecified number of different loci which by their combined action produce a diabetic predisposition, and that the precise combination of alleles responsible for the disposition may vary from one diabetic to the next. The nongeneticists can no longer decide from the available information what the most likely mode or modes of inheritance of diabetes mellitus might be, and the authors consider that the best presently available evaluation is that recently published by Neel [60].

As stated by Neel, an inherent difficulty even for expert geneticists is *the near-impossibility of deciding whether a relatively common trait is due to a recessive gene with incomplete penetrance or to multifactorial inheritance.* Nevertheless, at least two specific difficulties resulting from the attempt to explain what is known on the basis of simple autosomal recessive inheritance should be mentioned. (1) The unimodal distribution of blood sugar values in both the general population and among the offspring of selected types of matings suggests polygenic or multifactorial inheritance, even though underlying multimodality for any given set of data is always difficult to exclude. (2) The data on the children of conjugal diabetics is much more compatible with multifactorial than with simple recessive inheritance: if the mode of inheritance of diabetes were a simple recessive one, then all children of two diabetic parents should be homozygous for the predisposition to diabetes and the number developing clinical diabetes should be comparable to the rate of concordance of diabetes in similar twins. In fact, however, the overall prevalence of diabetes in three North American and one British series of offsprings of diabetic couples approximates 5 percent [61–64]. The interpretation of this rather small excess of diabetics, when compared with the prevalence of the disease in the general population, requires many age and sex adjustments in order to reach conclusions as to the percent occurrence of the diabetic predisposition in this group. Though some investigators have argued that the data are compatible with 100 percent predisposition in the children of conjugal diabetics [62], others have interpreted their findings as clearly indicating a mode of inheritance more complex than a simple autosomal recessive one [63, 64]. Thus Neel [60] concludes:

If the proportion of predisposed children in the marriage of conjugal diabetics is only some 50 percent, then this is evidence against an etiology based on a single recessive gene, or on many, equally frequent, different recessive genes. On the other hand, the data are consistent with expectation if there were a small number of relatively common recessive genes, with or without a few rare genes, or multifactorial inheritance.

Additional arguments in favor of complex or multifactorial inheritance result from the observation that the prevalence of diabetes is significantly greater in the offspring of diabetic couples whose diabetes started early in life than in the offspring of couples who become diabetic later [31, 63], and from the observation in twins that concordance of asymptomatic or chemical diabetes is very much greater in dissimilar twins than is true for overt or clinical diabetes [52].

Finally, there is published evidence favoring the *dominant* transmission of the diabetic trait [65] or of an antagonist to insulin action which has been implicated in diabetic pathogenesis [66].

The only conclusion that we would draw at this time is that the bulk of present evidence suggests either that the predisposition to diabetes mellitus is transmitted by a simple autosomal recessive gene(s), or that the mode of its genetic transmission is multifactorial. Indeed, it is still entirely possible that the genetic basis for diabetes in man may be heterogeneous, involving a mixture of simple and complex modes of inheritance. In other words, the same or similar phenotypes may well be controlled by any one of several distinct genotypes.

Etiologically Distinct Forms of Diabetes

The multifactorial mode of inheritance which is favored by the authors of this chapter allows for varying combinations of alleles responsible for the predisposition to diabetes in different diabetics. Indeed, one of the attractive features of the multifactorial hypothesis is that it may ultimately make it possible to account for the variable clinical manifestations of diabetes mellitus in man. It would be useful to find at least some degree of genetic segregation of the major clinically distinct syndromes, such as *juvenile-onset* and *adult-onset* diabetes. For the time being, however, it is quite generally accepted that such a genetic separation has not been demonstrated. Indeed both these major clinical types of diabetes frequently occur within the same family [6, 30–32, 53, 54], even though a few opinions to the contrary have been recorded [67, 68]. The widespread prevalence of the diabetic trait, or traits, in the general population clearly adds to the difficulty of establishing the presence or absence of genetic separation of different diabetic syndromes, particularly in highly mobile and mixed population groups.

We have already referred to *regional variations* in the prevalence of diabetes. Similarly, regional variations have been described with respect to distinct features of the regionally predominant syndromes and to the relative frequency of juvenile-onset or adult-onset types [35–44]. Although it is entirely possible that some of these differences are of genetic origin, environmental influences are just as likely and will be discussed below.

Lipoatrophic diabetes is a rare syndrome in which diabetes is usually preceded by either congenital or acquired complete atrophy of adipose tissue. The presently known cases probably comprise several types, one or more of which may be genetically distinct [69–74]. Another etiologically distinct but rare form of diabetes is *congenital temporary diabetes,* a disorder presenting with a severe acute diabetic syndrome, although frequently without ketosis, at or shortly after birth [75–77]. As a rule, there is no family history of diabetes, and hyperglycemia and glycosuria disappear permanently after a few months. The syndrome may be related to persistence of poor insulin-secretory capacity characteristic of fetal life.

Diabetes and Associated Conditions

The association of diabetes either with other diseases or with simple genetic characteristics might yield valuable pathogenetic leads or genetic markers useful for a better definition of the disorder, or of one of its parts. Diabetes is found in about half the cases of Werner's syndrome [78], which is probably inherited as an autosomal recessive trait and is characterized by features suggesting premature aging. An increased prevalence has also been reported in association with Friedreich's ataxia, Klinefelter's and Turner's syndromes, optic atrophy, Refsum's syndrome, Laurence-Biedl syndrome, the Prader-Labhart-Willi syndrome, and other rare hereditary syndromes. It remains unclear whether the association of diabetes and gout is or is not significant. A relationship has also been suggested of diabetes mellitus with pernicious anemia, as well as with hypothyroidism; these questions will be discussed further when dealing with the antigenicity of insulin and the hypothesis of an autoimmune component in the pathogenesis of diabetes mellitus. Although preferential association of diabetes mellitus with certain blood groups had been claimed, the position is confused, as is that of the possible association of diabetes with other well-defined proteins of serum or tissues. Further discussion of these associations would remain purely hypothetical and seems unwarranted within the scope of this chapter. They are amply discussed in specialized texts dealing exclusively with diabetes [30–32].

Hereditary Diabetes Mellitus in Animals

The preceding sections have clearly demonstrated that the predisposition to human diabetes mellitus is inherited, although it is not known whether all cases of human diabetes

Table 4-1. SYNDROMES ASSOCIATED WITH INAPPROPRIATE HYPERGLYCEMIA OR OBESITY IN MICE (*Mus musculus*)

Name	Gene symbol(s)	Transmission	Type of diabetes		Obesity	References
			MOD*	JOD†		
Yellow and variants	A^y, A^{vy}, A^{iy}	Autosomal dominant	++	...	++	[79, 86, 87]
Obese	*ob*	Autosomal recessive	++	...	++	[79, 88–90]
Adipose	*ad*	Autosomal recessive	++	...	++	[79]
Diabetes	*db*	Autosomal recessive	+	++	+	[79, 91–93]
New Zealand obese (NZO)	....	Inbred strain	+	...	++	[79, 94, 95]
KK	....	Inbred strain	+	...	+	[79, 84, 96, 97]
$C_3Hf \times IF$ hybrids (Wellesley)	....	Offspring of two inbred strains	+	...	++	[79, 98, 99]

*MOD, "maturity-onset diabetes type."
†JOD, "juvenile-onset diabetes type."
Note: + designates strains in which the corresponding feature occurs (++ in all animals).
− designates strains in which the corresponding feature does not occur.

have an inherited component, nor what the nature of the genetic lesion(s) or the mode of its transmission might be. Similarly, as we will see below, environmental factors are of considerable importance in either enhancing or obscuring the expression of the diabetic trait. Since it is impossible to control the genetic background of human populations, and difficult to control chronic environmental conditions, it would seem that the practical obstacles to a full definition of the factors involved in the pathogenesis of human diabetes are indeed formidable and might even prove insurmountable. Because of this, considerable attention is presently being devoted to a possible means of bypassing this deadlock through the investigation of spontaneous diabetes and related disorders in animals. Here, genetics and environment may be perfectly and separately controlled, the natural history of the syndromes may be studied in minute detail, and, among smaller rodents, many generations may be studied over relatively short periods. From a careful scrutiny of these spontaneous animal syndromes specific and testable leads and hypotheses might be derived and might then be applied to the investigation of diabetes in man [79–82].

The genetic aspects of the syndrome presently known to be associated with inappropriate hyperglycemia or obesity or both in laboratory rodents are shown in Tables 4-1 and 4-2. Inappropriate hyperglycemia clearly is a genetically controlled abnormality, and the precise mode of inheritance of the defect involved has been established in several syndromes of mice and in that of the Chinese hamster. Thus, the tendency to develop inappropriate hyperglycemia appears to be inherited as a dominant trait in yellow obese mice, and as a recessive trait in *dbdb* (diabetic), *obob* (obese), and *adad* (adipose) mice, while transmission is probably multifactorial in the inbred KK and NZO (New Zealand obese) strains of mice, and is certainly multifactorial in the $C_3Hf \times I$ hybrids and in Chinese hamsters. The multifactorial nature of the defect is most directly apparent in the $C_3Hf \times I$ hybrids, since colonies of neither inbred parent strain tend to have inappropriate hyperglycemia, while the anomaly suddenly appears in a large proportion of the progeny resulting from matings of the two strains.

Clearly the major observation here is that *inappropriate hyperglycemia in a single species may result not from one but from several distinct mutations,* some of which may be transmitted as dominant and others as recessive traits. In addition, inappropriate hyperglycemia may be selected from mixed genetic material through inbreeding, and considerable evidence suggests that the syndromes so selected are of multigenic or multifactorial origin.

Table 4-2. SYNDROMES ASSOCIATED WITH INAPPROPRIATE HYPERGLYCEMIA OR OBESITY IN RODENTS OTHER THAN MICE

Species	Transmission	Type of diabetes		Obesity	References
		MOD*	JOD†		
Acomys cahirinus (spiny mouse)	.....	++	+	+	[79, 100–102]
Ctenomys talarum (tuco-tuco)	.....	++	...	+	[79, 103]
Psammomys obesus (sand rat)	.....	++	+	+	[79, 104–107]
Cricetulus griseus (Chinese hamster)	Multifactorial	++	+	−	[79, 80, 81, 83–85]
"Fatty" rat	Autosomal recessive	−	−	++	[79, 108]

*MOD, "maturity-onset diabetes type."
†JOD, "juvenile-onset diabetes type."

The observations made in Chinese hamsters deserve particular attention with possible reference to diabetes in man. Butler, Gerritsen, and Dulin [83–85] have analyzed the records of several thousand Chinese hamsters maintained in a controlled environment over many generations, allowing for the analysis of a number of genetic sublines. All animals were tested at regular intervals throughout life for the presence of glycosuria. Although recognizing possible additional interpretations, Butler et al. came to the convincing conclusion that *in the Chinese hamster the inheritance of glycosuria is controlled by four recessive genes.* Any pair of the genes, when homozygous, will produce glycosuria, and whenever three of the genes are homozygous, ketotic diabetes results. In addition to the four recessive genes, a number of modifier genes may control the severity, duration, and constancy of the glycosuria. When these conclusions were applied to their breeding program, a remarkable degree of predictability of the incidence and type of diabetes in the offspring was achieved.

ENVIRONMENTAL CONSIDERATIONS

If a major genetic component contributing to the pathogenesis of diabetes is an accepted fact, it is equally unquestioned that environmental components are also significantly involved. Although such environmental actions may in rare instances exert a primary influence on the development of diabetes, as with certain *viral infections* which may selectively damage the pancreatic islets [109–111], a more frequent type of environmental effect is probably that modifying the duration of the period during which diabetes remains latent, thereby modifying the "penetrance" of the diabetic genotype(s). Again, this modifying effect may directly concern the insulin-producing β cells if, for example, it results in temporary damage with release of *autoantigens,* which might secondarily lead to an *autoimmune syndrome,* a possibility which will be discussed more at length below.

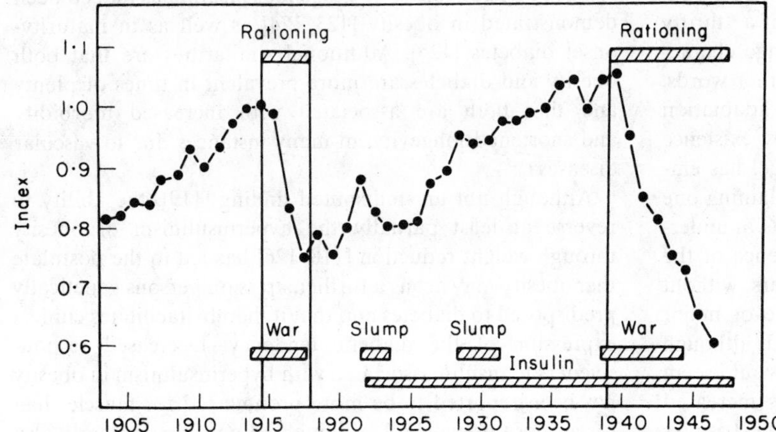

Figure 4-1. Comparative diabetes mortality indices (basis, 1938) for England and Wales. (*From Himsworth* [112], *as illustrated in Oakley et al.* [30].)

Effects of Dietary Regimen and Physical Exercise

These are probably the principal environmental factors involved in altering the "penetrance" of the diabetic genotype(s). Figure 4-1, taken from a review of this subject by Himsworth [112], will serve to illustrate the data upon which present thinking is based. The death rates from diabetes in England and Wales varied greatly during and after the First and Second World Wars, and the recorded changes correlated better with the duration of rationing than with the duration of the wars themselves. Similar observations were made during and after the Second World War in Japan [113] and in Germany [114], while Bouchardat was perhaps the first to comment extensively on the decrease in the prevalence of diabetes during the prolonged siege of Paris in the Franco-Prussian war of 1870 [115]. Though such observations clearly establish that, given a particular genotype, the prevalence of the overt disorder may be altered by changes in the environment, they do not by themselves suffice to define their dietary origin. During periods of war and rationing, environmental changes do not concern diet alone; other factors such as physical work and exercise, emotional tension, and many others may be just as strikingly involved. Indeed, we consider it impossible, for the time being, to differentiate between the influence of changes in diet and that of changes in the amount of physical exercise, because the data for such a differentiation are simply not available. Hence the frequent use of the collective "diet and exercise" in the present text.

We have already mentioned that much interest has centered on attempting to analyze the relative roles of environment and heredity through population surveys among different racial groups and in widely varying geographic locations. The majority of such studies have concerned large populations with reasonably long-term stability of environment and similar prevalence rates for diabetes, varying between 1 and 2 percent. This suggests that the genotype(s) favoring the development of diabetes is (are) not preferentially associated with race or with differing yet *stable* environmental conditions such as climate or individual foods.

An entirely different situation was encountered when the surveys concerned populations having been exposed relatively recently to major changes in their environmental conditions as to diet and need for physical exercise. Thus, an exceptionally high prevalence of diabetes, and also of obesity, has been observed in the Indian populations of South African cities such as Durban [116], in New Zealand Maoris [43], and in the North American Seneca, Cocopah, and Pima [35, 37] Indian tribes. In the Pima Indians, for example, the incidence of abnormal glucose tolerance in those over 50 years of age has been reported to be well in excess of 50 percent. All these populations had been transferred to relatively abundant Caucasian-type diets during the last generation or two, often with a recent increase in refined carbohydrates and fat. Furthermore all these population groups are characterized by a relatively recent decrease in the amount of physical activity required not only for survival but to maintain acceptable living standards. By contrast, an extremely low prevalence of diabetes has been reported in Alaskan Eskimos and in Athabaskan Indians. These groups are genetically unrelated, and both continue to lead a rugged type of existance, with considerable physical exercise, on a high-protein, low-carbohydrate, and moderate-fat diet.

The "Thrifty-genotype" Hypothesis of Neel

The environmental and hereditary components of both diabetes mellitus and obesity have been linked by Neel [117] in a hypothesis suggesting that in a population characterized by an excessive prevalence of inappropriate hyperglycemia, the major environmental event may have been a relatively sudden change *from* conditions preexisting over many generations and requiring hard physical work with overall restricted and irregular availability of food, *to* conditions of essentially unrestricted food availability throughout the year and greatly decreased need for physical activity. He suggested that, in such instances, diabetes mellitus, usually with obesity, might represent the detrimental aspect of a "thrifty genotype" unmasked by an environmental change characterized by unrestricted availability of food. In other words, diabetes and obesity might represent failures of adaptation to the relatively sudden transition to a sedentary existence combined with relatively high caloric intake. Neel has emphasized the usefulness of such a concept in explaining one of the major difficulties encountered by geneticists in understanding diabetes mellitus: the apparent persistence of the abnormal genotype over several thousands of years, without evidence suggesting a decrease in its prevalence or major variation from population to population. Indeed, although statistically valid information is not available, it would seem more likely that the prevalence of diabetes has increased rather than decreased through history. Neel [60, 117] argues that if diabetes mellitus were the result of a single disadvantageous mutation, it should be gradually eliminated under conditions allowing for the free expression of selective advantages or disadvantages. Accordingly, he suggests that one should consider the possibility that the particular genotype(s) associated with diabetes and obesity might have resulted in a selective advantage as long as availability of food was restricted and irregular, while under the presently prevailing condition in developed countries, only its disadvantages are perceived. Of course, the applicability of such a concept is exceedingly difficult to prove, but the evidence of spontaneous diabetes mellitus in animals tends to give it additional support, as detailed below.

Obesity and Diabetes

In considering how diet or exercise might influence the prevalence of diabetes or the "penetrance" of diabetic genotype(s), one is logically led to consider the effects of food intake on the secretion of insulin and also on its effectiveness. Though this will be discussed in some detail under Insulin, we should like to consider here the evidence linking diabetes and obesity, since obesity clearly is the result of food intake in excess of physiologic needs.

The existence of a link between diabetes and obesity is unquestioned, and the prevalence of obesity in adult diabetes has been reported as high as 60 percent [30, 32, 118], while the prevalence of impaired glucose tolerance in obesity has been estimated at around 60 percent as well [32, 119]. Obesity without diabetes is characterized by fasting hyperinsulinism and gross relative hyperinsulinism in response to glucose or other stimuli [120, 121]. When diabetes and obesity occur together, the immunoreactive insulin response to glucose or other stimuli is less than in nondiabetic obese, but may still be greater than in nonobese and nondiabetic controls [121, 122]. The coexistence of hyperinsulinism (as compared with the nonobese state) with either hyperglycemia or normoglycemia implies relative ineffectiveness of the circulating, endogenous immunoreactive insulin, and relative ineffectiveness of exogenous insulin has indeed been demonstrated in obesity [123, 124] as well as in maturity-onset diabetes [125]. Additional similarities are that both obesity and diabetes are more prevalent in times of plenty and that both are associated with increased morbidity and shortened longevity, in many instances due to vascular diseases.

Although not an undisputed finding [119], the ability to reverse at least partially the hyperinsulinism of obesity through weight reduction [118, 126] has led to the postulate that obesity may act as a further stress on persons genetically predisposed to diabetes and that it thereby facilitates clinical expression of the diabetic tendency. Decreased responsiveness to insulin associated with hyperinsulinism in obesity has been reported to be more pronounced for muscle than for adipose tissue [127], although adipose tissue clearly also responds less to insulin with increasing obesity [126]. The hyperinsulinism of obesity may therefore tend to favor insulin action on adipose tissue relative to its action on muscle and thus further the accumulation of fat.

Environmental Factors in Spontaneous Diabetes Mellitus and Obesity in Animals

As in human diabetes, we have already discussed the evident importance of genetic factors in *animal* diabetes. The influence of environment, more specifically of dietary factors, is equally well established, and dietary effects on the incidence and severity of the syndromes of inappropriate hyperglycemia have been demonstrated in almost all types of animal diabetes listed in Tables 4-1 and 4-2. These syndromes provide a spectrum extending from diabetes without obesity, in the Chinese hamster, through various degrees of severity in the association of hyperglycemia and obesity, to the "fatty" mutation in the rat, where obesity is associated with hyperlipemia and hypercholesterolemia but where carbohydrate intolerance is not seen. A summary of our present interpretation of the available information on the clinical courses of all syndromes associated, at least at some point, with inappropriate hyperglycemia is shown in Table 4-3. The syndromes may be subdivided quite generally into three groups [79]. The first of these comprises the severest form of the hyperglycemic syndrome, associated with pronounced resistance to insulin action, modest obesity, and degeneration of more or less hypertrophic and hyperplastic β cells of the islets of Langerhans (*dbdb* mice, spiny mice, and sand rats). In some instances, obesity may be pronounced but transient. Obesity always precedes the development of ketosis, which is then associated with weight loss and eventually leads to death.

Inappropriate hyperglycemia is much more benign in the second and largest group of syndromes, characterized by more or less pronounced resistance to insulin action, modest or marked obesity, and quite definite evidence for hypersecretion of insulin and elevated serum IRI. When both obesity and resistance to insulin are most severe, there is decided hyperplasia of the β cells of the islets of Langerhans. This group comprises *obob,* yellow, and most inbred strains of mice (NZO, KK, and the $C_3Hf \times I$ hybrids). Characteristic of the group is the previously best known of all hyperglycemic syndromes in rodents, that associated with the *ob* mutation and previously referred to under the name "obese hyperglycemic" syndrome. During the second half of the life expectancy of these animals, there may be not only lack of progression toward ketosis, but even significant regression.

The third category comprises only one syndrome, that in the Chinese hamster. This syndrome stands alone in that obesity never develops and courses of greatly varying severity and rate of progression are exhibited. Prolonged equilibrium may be reached, with intermittent, mild or severe glycosuria, and while progression to ketosis and death is more frequent in animals with severe, persistent glycosuria, it is not an inevitable sequela. Except at the earliest stages, there is little evidence for hyperinsulinism or even increased secretion rates of the hormone. Pancreatic insulin is almost uniformly lower in hyperglycemic animals of all types than in normoglycemic ones. Several features of this variable and polygenic syndrome clearly derive from genetic similarities or dissimilarities, as already discussed. Thus, the incidence of ketosis in the offspring of matings between two frankly ketotic parents approaches 100 percent.

At present, a possible sequence of events [79, 82, 128] might be postulated in most of the animal syndromes, per-

Table 4-3. FEATURES OF THE COURSE OF SYNDROMES ASSOCIATED WITH INAPPROPRIATE HYPERGLYCEMIA IN RODENTS*

Syndrome	Obesity	Elevated serum IRI†	Hypersecretion of insulin	"Resistance" to insulin	Progression to ketoacidosis
Yellow	+	+	+	+	−
Obese (*obob*)	++	++	++	++	−
Adipose (*adad*)	++				−
Diabetes (*dbdb*)	+	((+))	+++	((+))	++
NZO mice	+	+	+	+	−
KK mice	+	+	+	+	−
$C_3Hf \times I$ hybrids	+	+	++	(++)	−
Spiny mice	+	++	+	+	+
Sand rats	+	(++)	++	(++)	+
Tuco-tuco	+				
Chinese hamster	−	((+))		((+))	++

*This summary represents our interpretation of the information available to date. When no symbol is shown, no pertinent information is known to us. When the symbol is surrounded by a single pair of parentheses, the anomaly has been reported as transient over several months; a double pair of parentheses indicates transience over days or 2 to 3 weeks at most.

†IRI, immunoreactive insulin.

haps with the exception of that in Chinese hamsters. The syndromes would begin with decreased responsiveness to insulin as a primary event, a decreased responsiveness which may be spontaneous (as in *obob* or *dbdb*) or diet-induced (as in sand rats or $C_3Hf \times I$ hybrids). In some instances, this decreased responsiveness to insulin may be more pronounced in certain tissues: striated muscle appears to be particularly resistant to insulin action in *obob* and NZO mice [129], for example, while hepatic tissue has been suggested as a preferential site of decreased insulin effectiveness for *dbdb* mice [91]. Decreased effectiveness of insulin is almost invariably associated with hyperinsulinemia, which may be either very transient, as in Chinese hamsters, or long-lasting, as in *obob* mice. Insulin resistance is usually most pronounced in adult or middle-aged animals, and may decrease later. Both hypertrophy and hyperplasia of the β cells of the islets of Langerhans are frequently present at least at some point during the life history of most of the syndromes, with the notable exception of the syndrome in Chinese hamsters and that in *dbdb* mice. In the last instance, there is, however, excellent evidence for an early phase of attempted regeneration of islet cells from ductular epithelial cells, and mitoses in the β cells of these mice have been reported [130]. It would seem that whenever hypertrophy and hyperplasia are sufficient in degree and can be maintained for sufficient periods to allow for a new equilibrium to be reached, near-normalization or compensated diabetes together with hyperinsulinism is the result. Whenever the potential for hypertrophy and hyperplasia is limited, either in degree or in duration, however, diabetes progresses and decompensation occurs. *In all instances, this course may be markedly accelerated or delayed by manipulation of the diet.*

The emphasis given in this chapter to animal syndromes derives from our opinion that they illustrate more clearly than is so far possible for human diabetes the interdependence of genetic factors and of the environment in contributing to multifactorial diabetic syndromes exhibiting decided and understandable differences in their major clinical features as well as in their "penetrance."

The Thrifty-genotype Hypothesis in Animals

The applicability of Neel's hypothesis to human diabetes has already been presented. It is therefore of interest that some of the spontaneous syndromes in animals provide an excellent fit with the hypothesis as well. Indeed, zoologists have long known that many rodent species transferred from their wild environment to caged living conditions tend to become obese. This is particularly pronounced when the normal habitat is the desert or semidesert, arid regions. More specifically, the inappropriate hyperglycemia associated with obesity, which is so characteristic a feature of sand rats transferred from the Egyptian desert to a laboratory environment, exhibits several features predicted by Neel's concept [104–107]. Thus, diabetes is most severe in animals directly transferred and in the very first generations raised in the laboratory, and is often associated with life-threatening ketosis. The hyperglycemic syndrome then tends to become milder and disappear in subsequent laboratory-raised generations. Even in the directly transferred animals, diabetes may be entirely prevented by simple manipulation of the diet. Similar observations have been reported in the South American rodent tuco-tuco [103] and in the Eastern Mediterranean spiny mouse, *Acomys cahirinus* [100–102], although the case for a failure of adaptation as a principal cause of the high incidence of inappropriate hyperglycemia in the latter is less strong.

Pregnancy and Parity

Among environmental factors, particular importance may attach to the *environment of the fetus in utero.* Since diabetic mothers have been enabled to carry pregnancies to term only relatively recently, statistically fully adequate comparison of the incidence of diabetes in the offspring of diabetic mothers and in the offspring of diabetic fathers has not as yet been made; a greater incidence in the former has been suggested [131], but also questioned [132], while the incidence of large babies is more probable when the mother was the diabetic or prediabetic partner [133]. Even mild and unsuspected diabetes during pregnancy greatly increases fetal wastage, and the pathologic anatomic aberrations include hypertrophy of the fetal islet of Langerhans and interstitial, especially peri-insular eosinophilic infiltration [32, 134–138]. Accordingly, it would not be surprising if time were to substantiate the claim that the metabolic state of the mother during gestation influences the incidence of overt diabetes in the offspring, or at least the timing of its onset. Experimental models in animals have been suggested, although their validity remains to be established [139–141].

Whereas maternal metabolism must be of importance to the fetus, it is well established that the metabolic changes of *pregnancy* (for the mother) frequently uncover the existence of a previously latent diabetic trait [142, 143]. It has been strongly suggested that the acceleration of the metabolic decompensation process accompanying pregnancy may become permanent [142]. The reported increased incidence of diabetes in multiparous women over 40 years of age (when compared with men or with women not having borne children) supports this contention [30, 144, 145]. This relation between parity and development of diabetes after the age of 40 is not universally accepted [132].

EXPERIMENTAL DIABETES

The major endocrine defect in diabetes mellitus is considered to be absolute or relative insulin deficiency. It should be pointed out at the outset that this does not necessarily imply a *primarily* defective insulin-producing tissue.

Understanding of the nature of the major endocrine defect is, first of all, based on observations concerning the production of experimental diabetes and goes back to the demonstration by von Mering and Minkowski, in 1889, that removal of the pancreas in dogs produces a syndrome grossly similar to the acute diabetic syndrome in man. Experimental diabetes mellitus can be produced by one of the following procedures: (1) the surgical removal of all or at least a large portion of the pancreas; (2) the chemical destruction of all or at least a large portion of the β cells of the islets of Langerhans, a destruction which can be achieved by substances such as alloxan, dehydroascorbic acid, dithizone, or streptozotocin, all of which, in appropriate doses, produce a selective necrosis of the β cells [147–151]; (3) the inactivation of circulating insulin by the administration to animals of one species of antibody effective against its own insulin and obtained by immunizing other animals. This type of diabetic syndrome was first described by Moloney [152] in mice injected with antibodies to pig insulin obtained in guinea pigs; it has received its most extensive and convincing confirmation in the studies of Wright [153] in rabbits, rats, and sheep injected with antibodies to beef or pig insulin obtained in guinea pigs (Fig. 4-2). As might be anticipated, this type of diabetes is reversible with discontinuation of the administration of these species-specific insulin antibodies. (4) Finally, transient diabetes may also be produced by administering pharmacologic agents capable of inhibiting insulin release, such as mannoheptulose [145, 154, 155] or diazoxide [156].

It would seem almost impossible to produce a better biologic correlation between the experimental production of the diabetic syndrome, on the one hand, and interference with insulin production or effectiveness, on the other. If, in addition, one considers that the administration of insulin is capable of reversing completely all known features of the acute diabetic syndrome, the weight of evidence seems almost overwhelming. There are, however, additional experimental diabetic syndromes in animals in which the relationship to the insulin-producing cells of the pancreas is less evident. Among these are (5) the prolonged administration of anterior pituitary extract [157] or of purified pituitary growth hormone [158] preparations, as well as, in suitably prepared animals, of certain adrenocortical [159, 160] and thyroid hormones [161] or glucagon [162]. It has been postulated that the metabolic effects of these hormones create conditions leading to persistently increased insulin requirement and secretion [163] and thereby to eventual inadequacy of the insulin-secreting cells. A similar mechanism has been postulated for the production of a diabetic syndrome by (6) the prolonged administration of glucose in quantities sufficient to maintain a greatly elevated pancreatic arterial blood glucose level throughout the greater part of the 24-hr period [164]. This type of experimental diabetes has been reproducibly obtained in only one species, the cat.

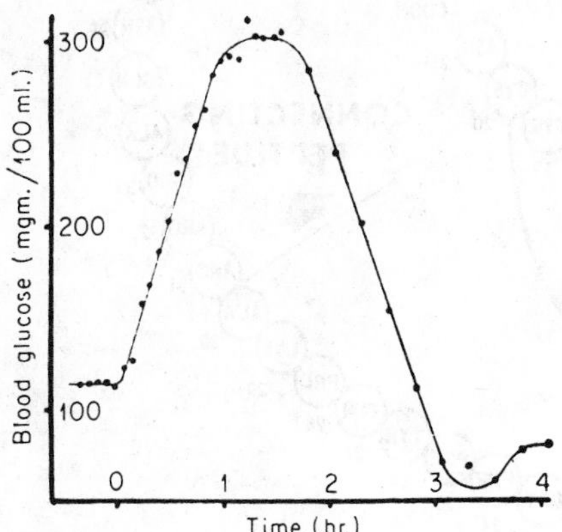

Figure 4-2. Concentration of glucose in the blood of a conscious female rabbit (2.65 kg) following the intravenous injection at zero time of serum (2.7 ml) from guinea pigs sensitized to bovine insulin. (*From Wright* [153].)

There is an evident, but as yet poorly understood relation between sex hormones and pancreatic diabetes in at least some species [165], including man [145, 166]. Temporary diabetes (as defined by more than just transient hyperglycemia) may be induced by a number of toxic substances and stressful stimuli which appear to act either by interference with cellular utilization of glucose or by eliciting sympathetic discharges at various levels of the central nervous system. Indeed it is quite likely that the central nervous system modulates both sensitivity to insulin and the reactivity of insulin-secreting cells by mechanisms of which the detailed nature remains to be described.

INSULIN

Although the nature of the primary, inherited defect, or defects, responsible for the subsequent development of diabetes is not yet known, much of the available evidence points to the important and probably early participation of insulin biosynthesis, storage, release, or effectiveness in the pathogenesis of diabetes mellitus. Accordingly, it is necessary to define in considerable detail the normal mechanisms by which insulin availability to its target tissues is controlled, to serve as base-line information for the exploration of possible anomalies in the human diabetic syndrome.

Chemistry

Insulin was the first naturally occurring protein to be completely analyzed with respect to its amino acid sequence [167, 168]. This remarkable achievement by Sanger was followed and fully confirmed by the no less remarkable accomplishment of the complete chemical synthesis of the hormone [169–171]. These advances reflected the astonishing methodologic evolution of both analytic and synthetic protein chemistry over the last two decades. Finally, the three-dimensional structure of insulin crystals has now been re-

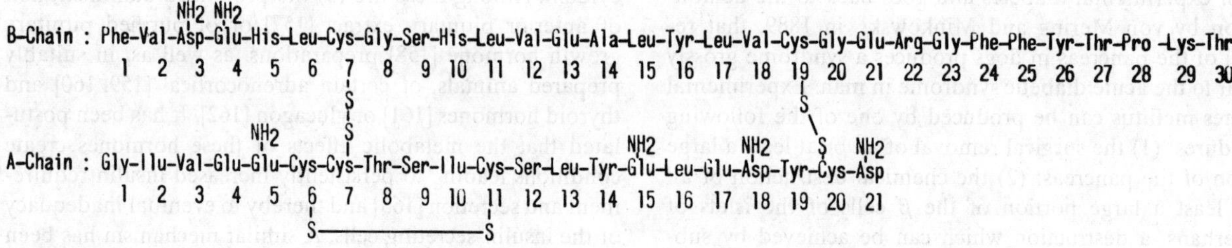

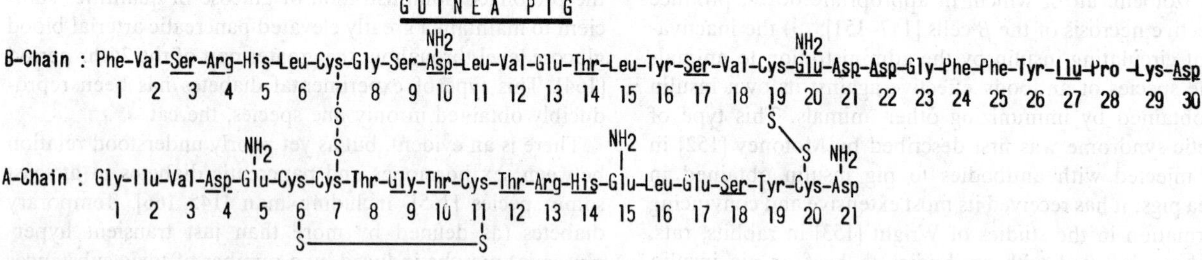

Figure 4-3. Amino acid sequences of two structurally distinct mammalian insulins, that of man and that of the guinea pig. In the latter, the 17 amino acid residues differing from those present in the same positions in human insulin are underlined.

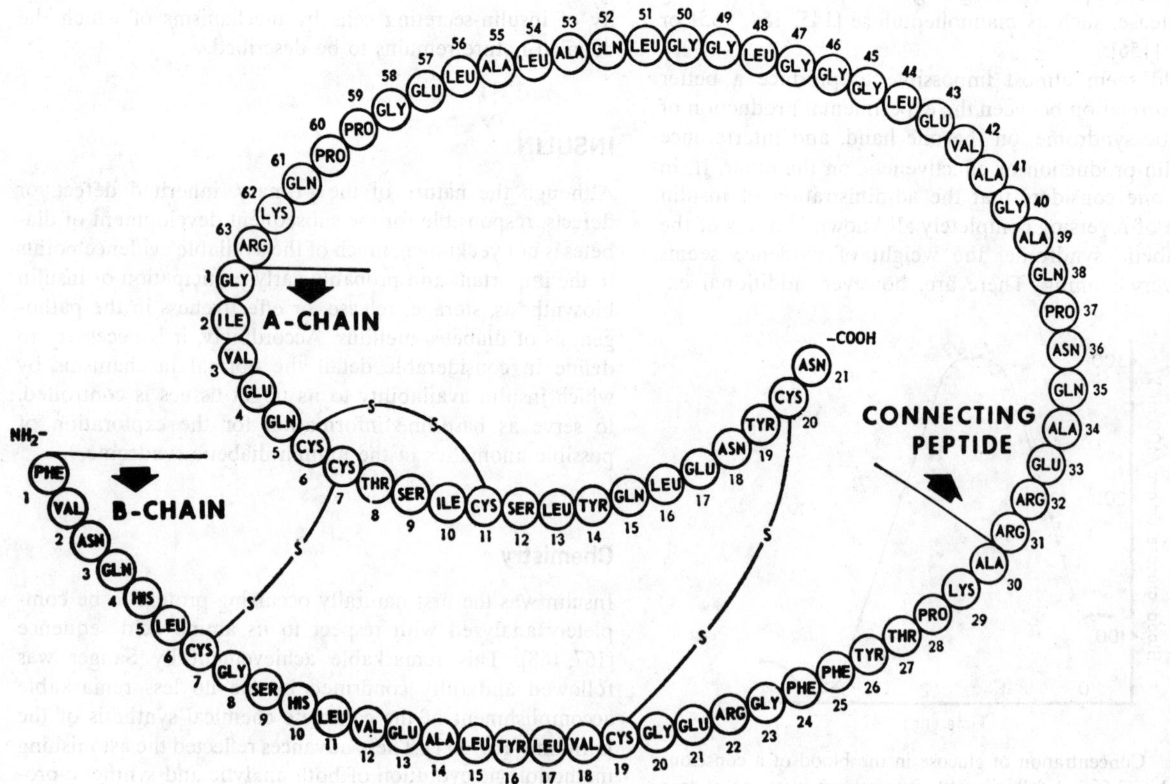

Figure 4-4. Amino acid sequence of porcine proinsulin. (*From Chance et al.* [183].)

ported by Hodgkin [172]. The amino acid sequences of two structurally distinct mammalian insulins (human and guinea pig) are shown in Fig. 4-3. Insulin is a relatively small protein molecule consisting of two peptide chains which comprise 21 (A-chain) and 30 (B-chain) amino acids, respectively. The two chains are linked by two disulfide bridges between positions 7 of both chains and between positions 20 of the A and 19 of the B chain. In addition, there is an intrachain disulfide bridge between the cysteine residues occupying positions 6 and 11 in the A chain. The structural analysis of insulins of various species has shown considerable species-specific variation in the amino acid sequence, in that the residues of no less than 29 of the 51 positions may be replaced, depending on the species examined [173]. It would appear that the amino acids comprised in the internal ring of the A chain (positions 8 to 10) and those immediately adjacent to it on its C-terminal side (positions 12 to 14), as well as the N- and C-terminal parts of the B chain, are most frequently involved in molecular differentiation between species. Although an attempt has been made to establish evolutionary patterns on the basis of these differences [173], the postulated evolutionary sequences remain purely hypothetical. Indeed, species as diverse as the pig, the dog, and two types of whale have structurally identical insulins, from which that of man differs only by one amino acid, while the differences between guinea pig insulin and that of all other mammals thus far studied are greater than the differences between mammalian and chicken insulins, and as great as those between insulins of mammals and fish! In addition to these compositional variations, small variations in chain length have been observed, in that in all fishes examined so far, residue B-30 is missing, and in some an extra residue is found at the N-terminal end of the B chain. For several types of fish and small rodents the existence within the same pancreas of two structurally distinct insulin molecules has been established [173, 174].

The structural feature most important for the biologic activity of insulin appears to be its molecular configuration governed by the spatial relationship of the three disulfide bridges [173, 175–177], while differences in the amino acid sequence are probably responsible for the variable biologic potency of certain insulins when they are assayed in homologous or heterologous test systems [178]. In addition, the compositional characteristics of the central part of the A chain and those of the N- and C-terminal portions of the B chain may be most important for the antigenic properties of a given insulin molecule [179]. Other portions of the two chains, as well as certain genetic determinants of the organism used to produce the antibodies, may be of equal importance in this respect [180, 181].

Biosynthesis

The discovery by Steiner of *proinsulin,* a precursor of insulin [182], and its subsequent structural analysis and identification as a single-chain molecule, with the A and B chains linked by a "connecting peptide" of variable length and amino acid composition (Fig. 4-4), is undoubtedly the most striking advance of diabetes research during the last few years [183, 184]. The importance of proinsulin for the biosynthesis of insulin is that its primary structure directs the folding of the polypeptide chain so as to allow for the formation of inter- and intrachain disulfide bridges at the correct sites. This facilitates the achieving of the tertiary structure necessary for biologic activity. Proinsulin is then cleaved to yield insulin by a process involving an enzyme probably related to but not identical with trypsin, since tryptic digestion of proinsulin yields insulin from which the C-terminal B-chain amino acid is missing. Proinsulin has lower biologic activity than insulin, and its affinity to antiinsulin serum is relatively weak. The amino acid sequence of the "connecting peptide" appears to be more species-specific than that of the corresponding insulin molecule. For a detailed summary of our current knowledge concerning proinsulin, its physiologic and potential pathogenetic importance, the reader is referred to a comprehensive review by Steiner [184].

Figure 4-5, a schematic representation of a β cell, may serve to formulate current concepts of the biosynthesis,

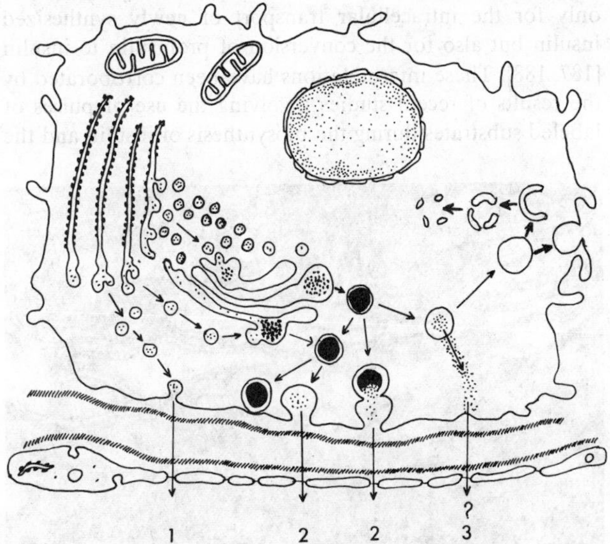

Figure 4-5. Schematic representation of a β cell showing insulin biosynthesis and secretion. *Top,* nucleus and two mitochondria. *Below,* from *left to right,* the lamellae of rough endoplasmic reticulum, with microvesicles budding off its smooth membranous portions; then the larger Golgi cisternae containing material, presumably proinsulin, undergoing packaging into β granules, which are represented at the *lower right,* where different possible release mechanisms are also outlined: 1, direct release of newly synthesized insulin transported in microvesicles; 2, emiocytosis of β granules, either as single granules or as rows of granules as suggested by Lacy [186]; 3, release of previously modified granular content, a mechanism that might include release into the cytoplasm. *Upper right,* disposal of empty granular sacs. (*Modified from Orci et al.* [187].)

storage, and release of insulin. These concepts derive from and extend those resulting from the pioneering work of Lacy and his collaborators [185, 186]; they have recently been reviewed in considerable detail [187, 188]. There is no reason to think that insulin synthesis differs fundamentally from that of other mammalian proteins. Amino acids entering the cell or synthesized within it are activated, transferred to soluble RNA, and assembled to form peptide chains on messenger RNA of ribosomes attached to the rough endoplasmic reticulum (RER). The synthesis of insulin involves both the RER and the Golgi complex. With the electron microscope, amorphous material can be detected in the cisternae of the RER and maturing secretory granules within the cisternae of the Golgi complex (Figs. 4-6 and 4-7). These observations are currently interpreted as indicating that proinsulin synthesized by the ribosomes attached to the RER is transferred to the cisternae of the latter and subsequently "packaged" in the Golgi complex to form typical β granules. Also, it would appear that the transfer of the material synthesized in the RER to the Golgi cisternae is a complex, discontinuous process involving the formation of microvesicular structures derived from the RER (Figs. 4-6 and 4-7). On the basis of morphologic evidence it has been suggested that these microvesicles may be of importance not only for the intracellular transport of newly synthesized insulin but also for the conversion of proinsulin to insulin [187, 188]. These interpretations have been corroborated by the results of recent studies involving the use of pulses of labeled substrates during the biosynthesis of insulin and the

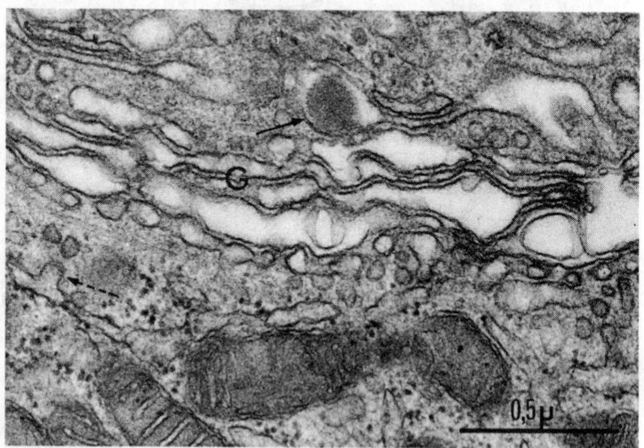

Figure 4-6. Electron microscopic appearance of part of a β cell of a rat having received glybenclamide intravenously 23 hr previously. The β cells of such animals show intensive evidence of new synthesis. Illustrated here is the Golgi region, with the Golgi cisternae in the median part of the micrograph, the solid arrow pointing to a maturing secretory granule within a cisternal space. The broken arrow points to the budding area of a granule-free portion of endoplasmic reticulum, probably representing the formation of a microvesicle. Two microvesicles are seen immediately adjacent and others throughout the region intermediate between cytoplasm with mitochondria and rough endoplasmic reticulum, on the one hand, and Golgi lamellae, on the other.

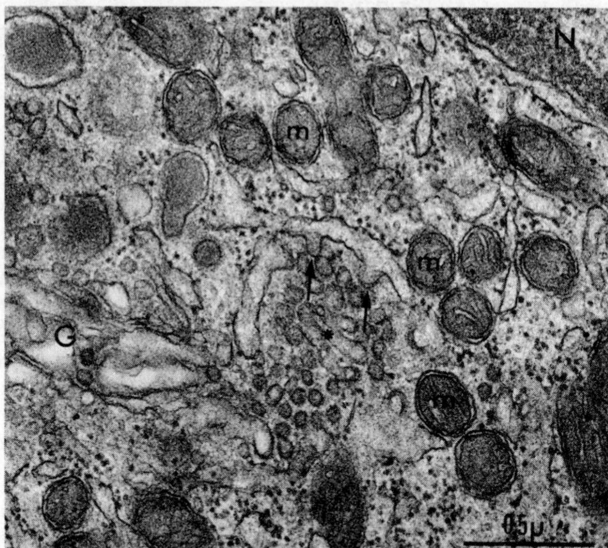

Figure 4-7. Electron micrograph of the perinuclear region of a β cell from the same animal as in Fig. 4-6. Note again the great richness in mitochondria of the transition zone from rough endoplasmic reticulum to the Golgi area. The arrows point to buds clearly originating from a smooth portion of endoplasmic reticulum with, beneath, numerous microvesicles (*) which are, in turn, closely associated with the Golgi cisternae (*G*); *m*, mitochondria; *N*, nucleus.

subsequent localization of the radioactive label, either by electron microscopic autoradiography [189] or by cell fractionation and the identification of labeled proinsulin or insulin associated with organelles separated by differential ultracentrifugation [184, 189, 190]. From all these studies it would now seem reasonable to accept that the biosynthesis of insulin first involves the synthesis of the single-chain precursor proinsulin by RER, then its transfer to the Golgi complex where packaging of the typical β granules takes place. Since the latter predominantly contain insulin rather than proinsulin [184], it is likely that the conversion of proinsulin to insulin occurs at some stage between synthesis in the RER and the formation of mature granules, i.e., near the Golgi complex or within it.

Our knowledge of the regulation of the rate of insulin synthesis is still limited. This is not surprising, since the normal pancreas contains considerable stores of insulin which greatly add to the difficulties of measuring small fluctuations of insulin content. However, the use in vitro of preparations of fetal rat pancreases harvested at a time when insulin content is relatively small yet insulin biosynthesis is going on at a rapid rate [191, 192] may well contribute to the elucidation of the regulatory mechanisms involved. At present, only glucose and, to a minor extent, growth hormone have been shown to accelerate the incorporation of amino acids into the insulin molecule [193–195], while agents known to promote insulin secretion such as tolbutamide, ACTH, or glucagon as well as pentoses were ineffective [195].

Storage

The pancreas of normal man contains amounts of insulin considerably in excess of immediate needs. The daily insulin output in man is estimated at about 30 to 50 units, which is the amount required to maintain normoglycemia in patients after total pancreatectomy [196, 197]. The insulin content of the normal human pancreas averages 4 units per gram, i.e., as much as about 200 units per pancreas. Since insulin is freely soluble at the pH encountered within cells and since β granules appear to contain insulin rather than proinsulin, the hormone must be stored in a form which prevents its sudden release and the resulting potential hypoglycemic disaster. All available information suggests that β granules are this storage form, but recent work performed on β granules isolated by differential ultracentrifugation [198–201] has failed to answer the question as to whether the granule membrane encloses free, biologically active insulin, an intermediate cleavage product of proinsulin [184], insulin associated with a specific protein [202], or insulin aggregates involving the presence of zinc [203].

The physicochemical properties of the storage form of insulin are not the only uncertainties regarding insulin storage and its physiologic meaning. While the usefulness of immediately available hormone stores is evident and unquestioned, it may well be that the hitherto generally accepted notion that all insulin is first stored in β granules and then released when needed is an oversimplification of reality. Indeed, it has long been suggested [204, 205] that some insulin, synthesized by free ribosomes, might leave the β cell directly without ever being incorporated into the granular pool of stored insulin. More recently, convincing evidence has been presented indicating that, under certain conditions, newly synthesized insulin [194, 206], possibly even uncleaved proinsulin [184, 207], may be secreted in preference to previously stored hormone. It may well be, therefore, that insulin storage may comprise more than one compartment and that these several compartments may be separately involved in glucose homeostasis [206, 208, 209]. Although the existence of such a pluricompartmental storage system may be considered probable, its individual components are neither morphologically nor functionally defined. At present, our conclusion must be that previous models of insulin storage will probably be revised in favor of more complex ones which, although still incompletely understood, will more closely approach reality.

Ultrastructural Changes Accompanying Insulin Release

As with insulin biosynthesis and storage, it now appears that the structures and mechanisms responsible for insulin release from β cells may be more complex than previously thought. Emiocytosis, i.e., the migration of β granules to the plasma membrane, and the fusion of their limiting membrane with the plasma membrane, followed by emptying of the granule content into the extracellular space, remains the best established mechanism for the release of stored insulin [185]. This mechanism is numbered 2 in Fig. 4-5. Just how granule migration toward the periphery is initiated and directed is still unknown. Lacy has suggested the possible participation of microtubular, contractile elements in this process [186]. In addition, observations made during strong stimulation of insulin release suggest that β granules may undergo modifications of the physicochemical nature of their contents, leading to disintegration and solubilization without evidence for disruption of the granular membrane [187, 210]. This process may initiate the sequence of events designated by 3 in Fig. 4-5, involving either the intracellular discharge and transcytoplasmic transport of solubilized insulin, or emiocytosis of such structurally altered β granules, or both. Finally, the emiocytosis of microvesicles, referred to as 1 in Fig. 4-5, may be the morphologic expression of the apparent preferential release of newly synthesized insulin or proinsulin under certain conditions, both in vitro and in vivo (184, 194, 206, 207, 209, 211).

Interpretation of the increasing morphologic complexity of insulin biosynthesis, storage, and release, well illustrated by Fig. 4-5, probably still represents gross oversimplification. It may well serve to help understand, however, the similarly increasing complexity of physiologic and biochemical entities required for the understanding of what is already known about the dynamics of insulin secretion: two or more storage pools [206, 208, 209], differential responsiveness to multiple stimuli, and the likely existence of parallel although not necessarily independent stimulatory mechanisms [188].

Insulin-releasing Effects of Metabolic Substrates and Intermediates

Quite generally, insulin release appears to be regulated by the coordinated interaction of the availability of *nutrients* and *substrates* with *hormonal* and *central nervous* settings. This is the framework which will be used in discussing present knowledge of the regulation of insulin release, in preference to the lengthy enumeration of the many agents now known to increase or diminish the production of insulin in vivo and in vitro.

Traditionally, insulin has been primarily considered a hormone regulating carbohydrate utilization and storage. More recently, principally as a result of studies in animals for which glucose is not a major food-derived metabolic substrate, it has become apparent that other and usually abundantly available nutrients may be just as potent stimuli for insulin release as glucose, or even more potent. Glucose remains the most probable principal stimulus in man [212–214], but amino acids are probably more potent in toadfish living on rotting mollusks and other semidegraded proteins [215, 216], and short-chain fatty acids and their derivatives in adult ruminants such as sheep [217, 218].

Though in any one of these species, the main exogenous substrate may be the most potent stimulator of insulin secretion, other substrates may also directly or indirectly enhance insulin release [218–222]. It is therefore likely that substrates derived from nutrients alter insulin release both by substrate-specific and less specific mechanisms. The latter may involve both indirect stimulation triggered by food intake, as outlined below, and local stimulation mediated through the production of a metabolite common to all three substrate groups (sugars, amino acids, and fats): pyruvate, citrate, or, possibly, as fundamental a metabolite as ATP (adenosine triphosphate) [188]. Substrate-specific stimulation, on the other hand, is more likely to result from specific metabolic intermediates such as those arising from the direct oxidation of glucose-6-phosphate [223], or from the structure of certain substrates themselves, as suggested for amino acids by experiments with nonmetabolized amino acid analogues [224].

These observations add further support to the concept that insulin is not to be considered as a hormone of carbohydrate storage, but rather as a hormone more generally related to the storage of metabolic fuels, whatever their nature. They also suggest that, since insulin would appear to be the principal fuel storage hormone in many species living under very different conditions of substrate availability, insulin itself, as well as the mechanisms involved in its secretion, must possess considerable evolutionary adaptability to differing environmental conditions. That this adaptability may not be restricted to phylogenetic evolution over thousands of years, but may also occur within days or weeks in the course of ontogenesis, is well illustrated by the evidence indicating that the role of the principal stimulator of insulin release may shift from glucose to fatty acids in lambs at the time of weaning [225], and from amino acids to glucose during the perinatal period in man [226]. Whether the excessive leucine-induced insulin release observed in certain instances of hypoglycemia in infants or in patients with insulin-secreting pancreatic tumors results from the persistence or the reappearance of an originally physiologic but transient pattern of β-cell responsiveness remains unknown.

Hormones, Gastrointestinal Signals, and Insulin Release

A variety of hormones have been shown to alter insulin secretion directly or indirectly, both in vivo and in vitro. Some of these stimulatory or inhibitory effects are, some may be, and others probably are not of physiologic importance. For more detailed discussions of this topic recent reviews may be consulted [30, 227–230]. We shall limit ourselves to a few specific instances where hormonal effects play a major physiologic role in the regulation of insulin release. The most important of these probably concern the hormones produced by endocrine cells located in or close to the gastrointestinal mucosa: others are related to the effects exerted by epinephrine and its derivatives. Although epinephrine-induced decrease of insulin release is seen in situations of acute stress and in patients with pheochromocytoma, it is obvious that the functional integrity of the autonomic α- and β-receptor systems is involved and that epinephrine effects are best considered together with the role of autonomic nervous stimulation which will be discussed separately below.

Although it was demonstrated as early as in 1896 that much smaller amounts of glucose are required to induce glycosuria by the intravenous than by the oral routes [231], and although hypoglycemic effects of duodenal extracts were tentatively related to the endocrine secretion of the pancreas as long as 40 years ago [232–234], it is only during the last decade that the importance of the gastrointestinal tract for the regulation of insulin release has become recognized. Thus it was shown that the disappearance of intravenously injected glucose was accelerated when its administration was preceded by that of an oral glucose load or accompanied by the intravenous injection of secretin [235], or that, for comparable blood glucose concentrations, serum IRI (immunoreactive insulin) rose to higher levels when glucose or amino acids were administered orally than after their intravenous injection. All this suggested gastrointestinal tract mediation in nutrient-stimulated insulin release [236–240]. So far no individual factor suffices to explain such a gastrointestinal function, and, indeed, it is more probable that several interdependent mechanisms are involved. *Vagal* stimulation is regularly associated with food intake and may enhance insulin release [241]. Several of the already known gastrointestinal hormones have been shown to stimulate insulin secretion either in vivo or in vitro or both [242, 243]. They include *secretin, pancreozymin,* and *gastrin,* the latter possibly exerting its action through a stimulatory effect on secretin release. While these hormones are themselves directly involved in the facilitation of the absorption of ingested food, an additional gastrointestinal hormone, *enteroglucagon,* structurally related to but not necessarily identical with glucagon and probably synthesized within the gastrointestinal mucosa, may also contribute to stimulation of insulin secretion in response to food [243–245].

Taken together, these findings suggest that at least the upper part of the gastrointestinal tract and the different types of endocrine and exocrine cells associated with it—including the pancreas—form a complex system responsible not only for the partial degradation and subsequent absorption of ingested food, but also for the initiation of the processes involved in its distribution, utilization, and storage.

The Autonomic Nervous System and Insulin Release

Since denervation of the pancreas or its transplantation to other anatomic sites within the organism does not appear to interfere with short-term glucose homeostasis, the nervous system has long been considered of only minor importance for the regulation of insulin release. However, the enhanced insulin secretion in response to direct vagal stimulation, the profound effects of pharmacologic α- or β-adrenergic stimulators in vivo, and the direct effect of these agents in vitro now clearly suggest that the autonomic nervous system may well be involved in the regulation of insulin release [241, 246–249]. This view is strongly supported by the excellent evidence for the presence of autonomic nerve endings in the endocrine pancreas of several species and their close relation to the surface of β cells [250]. In addition, the observation that ganglion cells and autonomic nerve endings exist and even develop in vitro in cultured explants of fetal rat pancreas [251] suggests that a considerable degree of nervous autonomy of the pancreas may allow for a relative independence of its peripheral receptor system from intact central connections, thereby explaining the persistence of some degree of regulation and coordination even after denervation or transplantation to other sites.

Although the detailed mechanisms by which autonomic nervous stimulation affects insulin release are still unknown, it appears quite generally that cholinergic or β-adrenergic stimulation enhances insulin release, while when α-adrenergic and β-adrenergic stimulation are applied simultaneously, the α-receptor–mediated suppressive effect predominates over the stimulatory β-adrenergic effect.

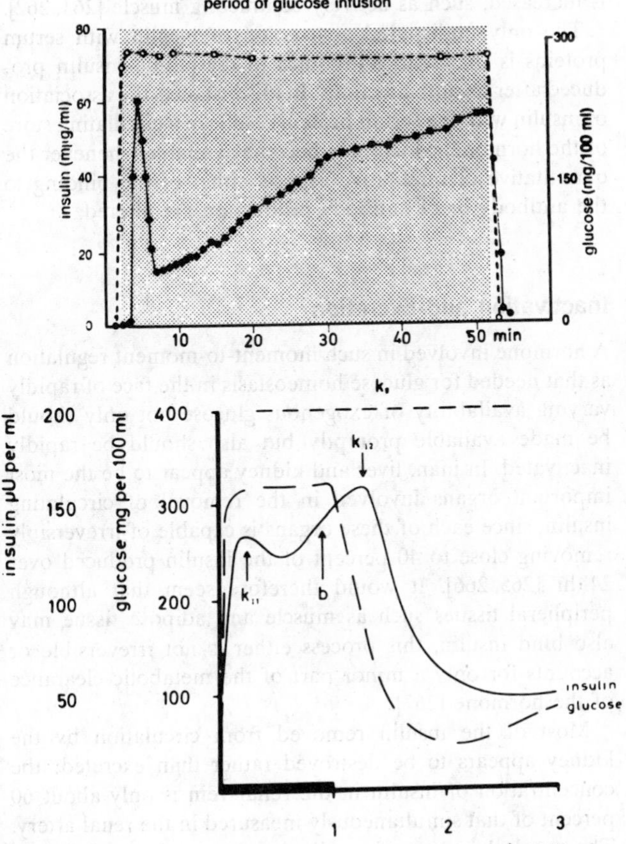

Kinetics of Insulin Release

When the β cell is subjected to prolonged (approximately 1 hr) and constant stimulation by a substrate such as glucose, insulin release does not increase linearily. As shown in Fig. 4-8, a remarkably similar profile is obtained both in vitro and in vivo [208, 252]: there is a first, rapid phase of insulin release, lasting but a few minutes (up to 15 or so), followed by slowing to about two to three times the nonstimulated rate, followed again by a gradual increase which may reach the initial stimulated-release rate by about 1 hour. This is the pattern which led to the concept of two insulin storage pools, already mentioned, and also that which serves as basis for the comparisons with potential, latent, and subclinical diabetes which will be discussed below. Although the two studies shown in the figure are the clearest ones and those most often referred to, other studies have yielded comparable results, and these profiles may be considered as securely established in normal organisms or pancreases [209, 253, 254]. Perhaps the autonomic nervous system, particularly the β receptors, are of special importance for the occurrence of the early peak of insulin secretion [255], whereas the secondary, or late, increase in insulin release may depend, at least in part, on active insulin synthesis [206], and it is during this phase that newly synthesized insulin or proinsulin

Figure 4-8. Insulin-release profile in vitro, above, and in vivo, below. The in vitro data are from Grodsky and collaborators, [252], and the in vivo derived profile is from Cerasi [208]. In both instances, the glucose concentration in the perfusion medium, in vitro, or in circulating blood, in vivo, was rapidly increased to 300 mg per 100 ml and again rapidly decreased after 50 min, in vitro, or 60 min, in vivo. Additional information is given in the text.

is released from the pancreas, at least in certain circumstances [184, 190, 207, 211].

Insulin-release Mechanisms

The intimate mechanisms responsible for the initiation of insulin mobilization and its final release are still unknown. Current knowledge allows us to consider the following features as the minimum number of the important components of the ultimate responsive system.

1 There seems to be no doubt that the adenyl cyclase-3′5′-cyclic-AMP system participates in insulin release, possibly irrespective of the nature of the initial stimulus, although the precise mechanism of this participation is still unknown [192, 227, 256].

2 The final common pathway of insulin release is characterized by an absolute requirement for Ca^{++} ions in order to respond to any stimulus [222, 257, 258]. In addition, other cations such as Na^+ and K^+ and their relative concentrations play an important, yet still ill-defined role which may be related either to the accumulation of cyclic-3′5′-AMP or to modifications in the functional state of membranous structures such as the plasma membrane of the β cells or the membrane surrounding the β granules [222, 259].

3 It appears that optimal conditions for insulin release are achieved by the combination of stimulation by a substrate with that more directly mediated through cyclic AMP. Stimulation by either one of these two types of agents alone is always less effective than that achieved in the presence of both. This suggests the probable importance of a synergism between endogenous (cyclic AMP—mediated stimulation by the nervous system or hormones) and exogenous (substrate-mediated stimulation) factors in the regulation of insulin release.

4 As outlined before, substrate-mediated stimulation of insulin release is most likely the result of (*a*) the presence of a metabolite common to all three major classes of fuels, and may well involve the substrate-dependent production of ATP, either as a precursor for cyclic AMP or by another mechanism. (*b*) In addition, in any given species or in specific metabolic states, certain substrates are considerably more effective than others, and it is likely that these specific substrate effects result either from the structural characteristics of the substrate involved or from the production of specific metabolites.

Insulin Transport

Although considerable evidence has been recorded indicating that a portion of endogenous insulin or of the radioactivity of labeled injected insulin may be associated with fractions of serum protein, predominantly related to α and β globulins, it is questionable whether any of these associations is truly significant, in that it might represent the transport form of the hormone [260]. Since much of the evidence is still conflicting and contradictory, we prefer to reserve judgment, while recognizing that significant pathogenetic anomalies may yet be proved to occur during insulin transport.

At least a fraction of serum "insulin" resembles crystalline pancreatic insulin sufficiently to react with antibodies produced against the latter. In addition, measurements of both immunoreactive insulin (IRI) and biologic insulin-like activity (ILA) in the lymph of the thoracic duct and of the liver and legs before, during, and after pancreatic stimulation with glucose strongly suggest that the bulk of secreted insulin circulates as a free molecule not bound to protein [261]. Apart from IRI, however, several serum fractions have been shown to exhibit insulin-like biologic activity not suppressible by antiinsulin serum [262–264]. These fractions, often referred to as "bound insulin," "atypical insulin," and "nonsuppressible insulin-like activity" (NSILA), have not yet been sufficiently characterized to allow for definitive judgment as to their function or as to their relationship to the hormone. Since NSILA appears to circulate in a form which prevents its transfer through normal peripheral capillary walls, it has been suggested that it might represent a circulating, rapidly available reserve of insulin-like activity which could reach tissue sites where capillary permeability is increased, such as actively contracting muscle [261, 262].

The only undisputed association of insulin with serum proteins is that with antibodies to crystalline insulin produced after insulin injections. In this instance, the association of insulin with the serum protein results in a circulating store of the hormone, which may become available whenever the quantitative or qualitative aspects either of the binding to the antibody or of antibody production are altered.

Inactivation and Excretion

A hormone involved in such moment-to-moment regulation as that needed for glucose homeostasis in the face of rapidly varying availability of exogenous glucose not only should be made available promptly but also should be rapidly inactivated. In man, liver and kidney appear to be the most important organs involved in the removal of circulating insulin, since each of these organs is capable of irreversibly removing close to 40 percent of the insulin produced over 24 hr [265, 266]. It would therefore seem that although peripheral tissues such as muscle and adipose tissue may also bind insulin, this process either is not irreversible or accounts for only a minor part of the metabolic clearance of the hormone [267].

Most of the insulin removed from circulation by the kidney appears to be destroyed rather than excreted: the concentration of insulin in the renal vein is only about 60 percent of that simultaneously measured in the renal artery. The renal clearance of insulin has been calculated to approximate 200 ml per min, whereas the urinary clearance is only 0.3 to 0.5 ml per min. Since the urinary clearance remains constant over a wide range of plasma insulin concentrations, measurements of urinary insulin reflect variations in plasma insulin concentrations [265]. Although the renal clearance of insulin is somewhat smaller than its hepatic clearance, under physiologic circumstances the insulin-destroying system of the kidney appears to be operating well below capacity, whereas that of the liver may be closer to saturation. This may explain why severe impairment of kidney function affects the rate of disappearance of circulating insulin more than does liver disease in man or hepatectomy in experimental animals [266, 268, 269]. Since neither total metabolic clearance nor that by liver and kidney changes appreciably over the range of physiologically occurring insulin concentrations, it would seem likely that excretion and inactivation of insulin are of minor importance in the regulation of availability of the hormone.

The destruction of insulin by liver and kidney is initiated by the reductive cleavage of its functionally essential disulfide bridges by glutathione-insulin transhydrogenase, with subsequent cleavage of the individual chains by peptidases [270, 271]. Binding to antibodies in patients treated with insulin leads to decreased metabolic clearance of the hormone, a complicating feature likely to interfere with the evaluation of insulin removal in such patients.

Metabolic Effects of Insulin

Although insulin has been shown to affect directly a large number of tissues, discussion of the metabolic consequences of its action will be limited to the three tissues principally concerned with glucose homeostasis and energy storage, i.e., adipose tissue, muscle, and liver. The principal metabolic characteristic of each of these tissues will be outlined briefly in order to facilitate understanding of the multiple direct and indirect effects of insulin on specific metabolic processes and of their repercussions on the metabolic state of the organism as a whole. For a detailed description of the metabolic pathways involved, the reader is referred to textbooks of biochemistry.

Adipose Tissue

Adipose-tissue metabolism is centered around the task of storing fuel in the form of fat at times of abundance and of releasing it when exogenous fuel is lacking. It is specialized for the synthesis of fatty acids, the storage of endogenous or exogenous fatty acids in the form of triglycerides, and the release of free fatty acids from its triglyceride stores into the bloodstream for further metabolism by other tissues. The outstanding energetic importance of the small, rapidly exchanging pool of circulating free fatty acids as substrates for practically all tissues, including brain, has recently been reemphasized on the basis of extensive studies in man [272] and will be discussed in another section of this chapter.

Glucose is the most important substrate required by adipocyte for its anabolic functions: glucose furnishes the α-glycerophosphate for the glycerol moiety of triglycerides; through catabolism to acetyl CoA it furnishes the two-carbon fragments from which fatty acids can be synthesized; through its partial oxidation in the pentose-phosphate pathway, as well as through the pyruvate-oxaloacetate-citrate-oxaloacetate-pyruvate shuttle, it may be the source of reduced pyridine nucleotides, principally NADPH, required for the reductive environment needed for fatty acid synthesis. Glucose enters the fat cell through "facilitated diffusion," a process implying the existence within the cell membrane of a mobile glucose carrier system [273]. After penetration into the cell, glucose is phosphorylated, and its oxidation then proceeds both through the pentose and the Embden-Meyerhof pathways.

In addition to locally synthesized fatty acids, the adipocyte can incorporate exogenous fatty acids which reach adipose tissue in the form of particulate triglycerides, i.e., chylomicrons of intestinal origin and lipoproteins of hepatic origin. Somewhere between the capillary endothelium and the surface of the adipocyte these triglycerides are cleaved by lipoprotein lipase to yield glycerol and free fatty acids (FFA), the latter then being taken up by the fat cell and incorporated into the triglyceride pool after esterification with the α-glycerophosphate resulting from glucose catabolism.

The triglyceride pool of adipose tissue is not an inert mass, but is constantly subjected to lipolytic and anabolic influences, resulting in a continuous turnover of at least part of the pool, with concomitant production of glycerol and FFA. The latter may be either liberated into the bloodstream or reesterified if α-glycerophosphate is available. The glycerol liberated during lipolysis is released into the bloodstream, since normal white adipose tissue is virtually incapable of metabolizing free glycerol.

Net lipolysis occurs in fat cells when glucose metabolism is sufficiently decreased to prevent the production of the α-glycerophosphate required to maintain the reesterification of FFA resulting from continuously occurring base-line lipolysis. Lipolysis may also be stimulated by several hormones such as epinephrine and, in some species, pituitary peptides and glucagon. Lipolytic agents are active through the activation of cell membrane–bound adenyl cyclase, the cyclic-3′5′-adenosine monophosphate (AMP), which then activates a "hormone-sensitive lipase" of adipocytes (for a detailed bibliography see [256]).

On the basis of current knowledge, the effects of insulin on adipose-tissue metabolism may be summarized as follows: (1) The hormone accelerates the transport of glucose across the cell membrane [273], although the exact mechanism of this action is as yet unknown. (2) The capacity of the cell to phosphorylate glucose is enhanced by insulin. It is currently not known with certainty whether this effect is mediated through substrate activation of hexokinase or whether it results from a direct modification by insulin of the specific activity or synthesis of the enzyme [274, 275]. Through its effects on glucose uptake and phosphorylation, insulin accelerates and facilitates glucose metabolism (and thereby fatty acid and triglyceride synthesis) and suppresses the net lipolysis resulting from intracellular glucose deprival. (3) Insulin directly alters lipolysis, probably through reduction of intracellular cyclic AMP concentrations and consequent inhibition of hormone-sensitive lipase [276]. Just how it decreases 3′5′-cyclic AMP is not yet understood, but decreased activity of adenyl cyclase is considered more likely than acceleration of the phosphodiesterase-mediated catabolism of cyclic AMP. The effect of insulin on cyclic AMP and on hormone-sensitive lipase is independent of that on glucose transport [256]. (4) The activity of lipoprotein lipase is increased in situations associated with accelerated glucose utilization and fat storage by adipose tissue; whether this increase in activity is a direct consequence of the action of insulin is still unknown [277].

Thus, the overall effect of insulin on adipose tissue is an increase in the availability of glucose and of endogenous substrate for triglyceride synthesis, as well as a reduction of net lipolysis resulting from both a direct antilipolytic effect and one secondary to the availability of α-glycerophosphate. It is evident that insulin is of prime importance for the maintenance of the anabolic, fat-storing function of the adipocyte and of adipose tissue as a whole.

Muscle

The metabolic pathways predominantly functional in muscle are determined by the need to provide energy for the complex process of contraction and to maintain both the contractile as well as the supporting protein structures of the muscle cell. Storage functions, which predominate in adipose tissue, are limited to the relatively small amount of glycogen synthesized from glucose taken up from the extracellular space. When large amounts of glucose are available, glucose may be the main metabolic fuel of muscle tissue; when its supply is limited, in situations such as starvation and in the normal postabsorptive state, or during exercise, muscle tissue predominantly oxidizes FFA taken up from the blood in proportion to its prevailing concentration or that cleaved from triglycerides through the action of muscle lipoprotein lipase.

Apart from its indirect effect on muscle metabolism through its regulation of the concentration of circulating FFA, insulin directly affects the metabolism of striated muscle by three possibly independent mechanisms. (1) It accelerates the carrier-mediated glucose transport across the cell membrane [278]. (2) It favors glycogen synthesis through a still insufficiently defined effect on UDPG (uridine-diphosphoglucose-glycogen) transferase, an effect apparently independent of that exerted on glucose transport [279]. (3) It increases protein synthesis by muscle ribosomes independently of its accelerating effects on the transport of either glucose or amino acids across the cell membrane [280]. Thus insulin provides muscle with the fuel required for its contractile activity at times when glucose is abundantly available. In addition it favors the storage of glycogen and may well be one of the main factors responsible for the maintenance of the functionally essential contractile and supportive protein structures of this tissue.

Liver

The importance of the liver for the regulation of carbohydrate metabolism was recognized and defined well over 100 years ago by Claude Bernard. It is capable of storing carbohydrate in the form of glycogen and of releasing it when needed in the form of glucose. It is also capable of converting noncarbohydrate substrates (amino acids, pyruvate, and lactic acid) to glucose and glycogen through gluconeogenesis. Thus, to some extent together with the kidney, the liver may supply glucose-dependent organs with their metabolic substrate at times when exogenous glucose is not available. The quantitative importance and the fine regulation of hepatic and renal gluconeogenesis in man have recently been studied in great detail; the reader is referred to these sources for more extensive discussions [281, 282].

At blood glucose concentrations of about 120 mg per 100 ml, the liver shows neither net uptake nor net release of glucose into the bloodstream; below this level glucose release, and above this level glucose uptake predominate. Therefore, regulatory mechanisms, capable of adapting the directional flow of glucose metabolism, must exist within the liver. In contrast to what occurs in muscle and adipose tissue, glucose transport into the liver, although also carrier-mediated, is apparently not influenced by insulin [283, 284]. Phosphorylation of glucose within the liver cell may be mediated both by hexokinase and glucokinase, but only the latter appears to be of importance for the regulatory adaptation of glucose phosphorylation to prevailing metabolic conditions.

Figure 4-9 shows the metabolic steps most revelant to the regulation of the bidirectional flow of hepatic glucose metabolism. Several of the reactions indicated in that figure are reversible and governed by a single enzyme. Three pairs of reactions are suitable for directional control since they are irreversible and each is governed by two separate enzymes. Specifically, these are: (1) glucose phosphorylation and dephosphorylation governed by glucokinase and glucose-6-phosphatase, respectively; (2) the phosphorylation of fructose-6-phosphate to fructose-1,6-diphosphate and the dephosphorylation of the latter to fructose-6-phosphate, these steps being catalyzed by phosphofructokinase and fructose-1,6-diphosphatase, respectively; (3) the dephosphorylation of phosphoenolpyruvate and the phosphorylation of pyruvate to phosphoenolpyruvate. As indicated in the figure, this last reaction is complex and occurs through the carboxylation of pyruvate to oxaloacetate, either directly or indirectly through malate. Oxaloacetate is subsequently

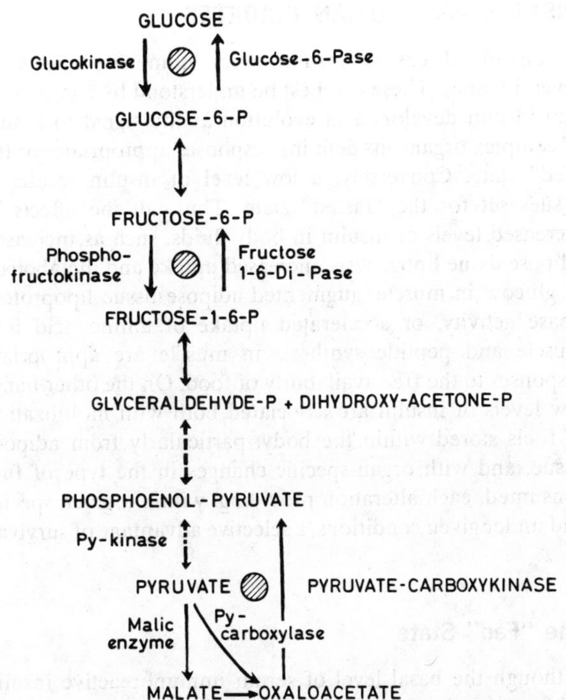

Figure 4-9. Schematic representation of hepatic glycolysis, indicating the steps most relevant for the regulation of bidirectional flow of glucose metabolism. Further comments are given in the text.

decarboxylated and phosphorylated in the presence of phosphoenolpyruvate-carboxykinase, a reaction which yields phosphoenolpyruvate.

The enzymes governing the three steps of glucose metabolism which are best suited to directional regulation are usually referred to as "glycolytic key enzymes" and "gluconeogenic key enzymes." The activity of the glycolytic key enzymes is increased when exogenous glucose is available, while that of the gluconeogenic key enzymes is increased in situations of glucose need, such as fasting. There is no doubt but that the flow of glucose metabolism in either direction is at least in part subject to hormonal regulation, since hormones such as glucagon and glucocorticoids stimulate gluconeogenesis, while insulin enhances glycolysis. Accordingly, and depending on the prevailing endocrine-metabolic state, the activities of the glycolytic or gluconeogenic enzymes are increased or suppressed, but the exact mechanisms by which these activities are regulated are still a matter of some controversy, in that directly hormone-induced or cyclic AMP–mediated enzyme activation, as well as *de novo* synthesis or substrate activation, may all be involved [256, 285, 286]. Under normal physiologic conditions, lactate produced by tissues such as muscle, as well as food-derived amino acids, provide the bulk of the carbon required for glucose synthesis; in situations of glucose need (e.g., starvation), amino acids mobilized from the protein pool of muscular tissue contribute to a major extent [272].

Glucose synthesis is a reductive process and requires the continued formation of reduced cofactors. In situations in which gluconeogenesis in the liver predominates, such as starvation and diabetes, the oxidation of fatty acids mobilized from adipose tissue represents the major source of these cofactors. Although high concentrations of FFA, their CoA derivatives, or keto acids within the liver cell may favor and accelerate gluconeogenesis [287], they are probably not directly involved in the short-term regulation of hepatic gluconeogenesis [288].

Whatever the exact mechanisms and the precise sites of action, there is no doubt that insulin profoundly affects hepatic glucose metabolism, although it has apparently no influence on the transport of glucose across the membrane of the liver cell. It reduces the rate of both glycogenolysis and gluconeogenesis and increases that of glycogen synthesis. In addition to effects of the hormone which are probably direct, it is evident that the metabolic pattern of the liver at any given time is largely governed by the available metabolic substrates, whether glucose or amino and fatty acids, and that insulin also exerts important indirect effects on liver metabolism through its influence on muscle and adipose tissue.

Mechanism of Insulin Action

As already stated, not all insulin effects can be explained on the basis of an acceleration of glucose transport across the cell membrane. In particular, the antilipolytic effect is seen in the absence of glucose; similarly, insulin-induced modifications of the activity or possibly the rate of *de novo* synthesis of hepatic glucokinase, of adipose tissue hexokinase, and of enzymes involved in glycogen synthesis, both in muscle and in liver, are independent of the glucose transport effect; finally, the stimulation of ribosomal protein synthesis in muscle is attributed to a "direct" action of insulin on the system involved in the transfer and translation of genetic information into the sequential assembly of amino acids into proteins [280]. Some of these effects may not be membrane-related, while the antilipolytic action probably is [289, 290]. More directly membrane-related insulin effects which are not secondary to the transport of glucose include the acceleration of the active transport of certain amino acids across the membranes of muscle cells and adipocytes [291, 292].

All concepts of the exact mode of action of the hormone are still hypothetical and concerned with the central question as to whether *all* effects will ultimately be related to its generally accepted action on the cell membrane. The experimental evidence accumulated most recently tends to re-emphasize the prime importance for many insulin effects of an interaction between the hormone and the plasma membrane of the responding cell. This might then result in overall modifications of the physical properties of the plasma membrane, leading in turn to easier access to a number of specific transport systems, to modifications in the transmembrane concentration gradients of critical cations such as Na^+, K^+, and Ca^{++}, and to alterations of the functional state of cell membrane–bound enzymes such as adenyl cyclase [256, 293]. This concept of a single, yet complex, "allosteric," primary action of insulin on the plasma membrane derives from experimental evidence indicating, for example, that effects on transmembrane inward transport, as well as the glucose-independent antilipolytic effect, and even accelerated protein synthesis may all be mimicked by exposure of at least the fat cell membrane to the controlled action of phospholipase or trypsin, enzymes which may alter the physicochemical state of the membrane [290, 293]. Furthermore, since the adenyl cyclase–mediated production of cyclic AMP or its suppression through hormonal action may profoundly affect intracellular processes such as *de novo* synthesis of enzyme proteins, as well as the specific activation of enzymes [256], and since the activation of genetic units, as well as the translocation and translation of their product, is profoundly affected by prevailing intracellular conditions, a predominantly cell membrane–located modification may perfectly well be thought of as initiating a multitude of directly as well as less and less directly membrane-related processes. A strong argument in favor of this view is the general dependence of practically all insulin-induced effects on an intact cell membrane at some time during the initiation of hormone action, even when the effect measured is clearly an intracellular, e.g., a ribosomal, one [280, 293]. Disrupted cell membrane particles retain the functional alterations induced by insulin only when they were induced *before* cell disruption [294], while certain cell "ghosts," which consist principally of empty but still structurally intact cell membrane saccules, remain hormone-sensitive with respect to both their transport systems and membrane-bound adenyl cyclase [293]. Many insulin effects also appear to require the presence of a locally synthesized membrane peptide with a rapid turnover: brief treatments of fat cells with trypsin have been reported to interfere with both the binding and the action of insulin, while both activities are restored by further incubation in vitro in the absence of trypsin, unless protein synthesis is inhibited by agents such as puromycin [295].

Analogous observations have been made with other hormones which similarly seem to affect membrane-bound adenyl cyclase (glucagon, epinephrine, thyroid hormone). The apparent contradiction between the individual specificity of these hormones and their common target in the membrane-bound adenyl cyclase system of the respective responsive tissues involved has led Rodbell to define receptor systems located within the cell membrane in terms of a hormone-specific discriminator (peptide), a nonspecific transducer (probably lipid) responsible for the transmission of the hormone-mediated signal to the third component of the system, the effector, which may be membrane-bound adenyl cyclase [295].

INSULIN AND HUMAN DIABETES

As already discussed, insulin exerts numerous effects on several tissues. These can best be understood by considering that insulin developed in evolution as the signal to tissues of complex organisms defining responses appropriate for the "fed" state. Conversely, a low level of insulin results in tissues set for the "fasted" state. Thus, all the effects of increased levels of insulin in body fluids, such as increased adipose tissue lipogenesis, increased uptake and metabolism of glucose in muscle, augmented adipose tissue lipoprotein lipase activity, or accelerated uptake of amino acid into muscle and peptide synthesis in muscle are appropriate responses to the free availability of food. On the other hand, low levels of insulin are associated both with mobilization of fuels stored within the body, particularly from adipose tissue, and with organ-specific changes in the type of fuel consumed, each alteration providing, within a given species and under given conditions, a selective advantage of survival.

The "Fed" State

Although the basal level of serum immunoreactive insulin (IRI) varies considerably from individual to individual in the postabsorptive state, and even more so after ingestion or administration of carbohydrate or protein (or amino acids), the bulk of available data suggests that a *rapid* insulin

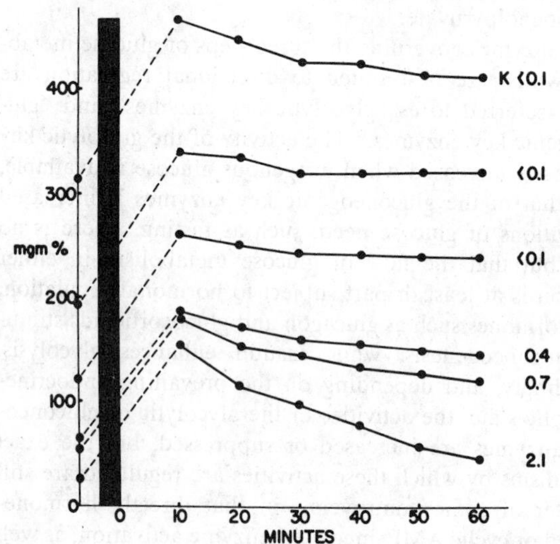

Figure 4-10. Utilization of intravenously administered blood glucose (0.5 gm/kg) in a juvenile diabetic whose initial, postprandial blood glucose level was adjusted through manipulation of the daily dose of long-acting insulin only. Note that normal glucose disposal rate was approached only when severe postabsorptive hypoglycemia occurred.

response is the best correlate to normal glucose tolerance [296]. In other words, the greater the proportion of insulin released from the β cells which appears in the circulation *early* after stimulation, the more efficient the disposition of glucose [297]. This observation concurs with the earlier studies of Conard [298], showing that a single intravenous injection of insulin resulted in a change in the exponential of glucose disappearance after about 10 min, as if the glucose removal system had been reset at a higher level by this "pulse" injection of insulin. Further support for the need for a *rapid* alteration in insulin level in man to achieve normal glucose tolerance derives from studies shown in Fig. 4-10. Administration of *long-acting* insulin to an individual lacking endogenous insulin, even in amounts sufficient to maintain subnormal fasting levels of glucose, was quite inadequate to provide even nearly normal tolerance for glucose. Only when the dose of long-acting insulin was grossly excessive, such that severe fasting hypoglycemia resulted, did glucose assimilation become normal. Similarly, the patient with mild diabetes may well exhibit decreased glucose tolerance as a result of relative or absolute β cell inertia. This inertia may become even more apparent when the diabetic is further penalized by the insulin resistance associated with obesity [254, 299]. Additional support for β cell inertia as the cause of carbohydrate intolerance in mild diabetes may be derived from the decreased responses observed after other stimuli such as oral sulfonylureas [300] or amino acids [301].

The "Fasted" State

The preceding paragraph summarizes in simple terms some current thinking on the physiology of the "fed" state as it relates to mild glucose intolerance in man. To understand metabolism in the more severe form of diabetes, the juvenile or ketosis-prone syndrome, the role of insulin in fasting man must also be defined. Before doing so, however, some general principles of fuel metabolism will be considered.

Man, similar to other terrestrial (or airborne) animals, all of whom depend on mobility, uses lipid storage for fasting survival, because of the high energy content and capacity for water-free deposition of triglyceride [302]. When proteins and carbohydrates (glycogen) are stored they require intracellular accumulation of water and electrolytes, resulting in only 1 to 2 cal per gm of additional stored fuel, by contrast with the 6 to 9 cal which may be stored in each gram of triglyceride-containing tissue [303]. Thus, in times of nutritional plenty, insulin first facilitates expansion of glycogen and protein reserves if they have been previously depleted, then favors the conversion of all excess calories into lipid stored as such. Normal man carries only a few hundred grams of glycogen, a very small caloric reserve when compared to the many kilograms of adipose tissue triglyceride. Also, there is an upper limit to the expansion of body protein, and normal, well-fed man usually has reached this limit.

During fasting, survival depends on the efficiency of the organism's drawing on its lipid stores so as to spare carbohydrate and protein, primarily muscle protein. In other words, whereas optimal conversion to lipid is of prime importance during "feasting," during fasting optimal (i.e., not too slow and not too fast) mobilization and utilization of lipid provide an overriding selective advantage.

Fuel Metabolism in Fasting Man

When data are pooled from many studies using radioactive-substrate turnover, selective catheterization of regional areas, total metabolic balance, and indirect calorimetry, an approximate scheme for substrate utilization in normal fasted man emerges [272]. This scheme is shown in Fig. 4-11. Of note is the predominant glucose utilization by brain (over 100 gm per 24 hr). Other tissues such as the red blood cells, white blood cells, platelets, peripheral nerve, and, to a much lesser extent, skeletal muscle also use glucose, the total amount approximating 36 gm per 24 hr, or one-fifth of the glucose turnover; in this second group of tissues glucose is mainly glycolyzed to lactate (and pyruvate) and returned to the circulation for removal by liver and kidney and reincorporation into glucose [304]. Figure 4-11 also illustrates that glucose utilization by the remainder of the body or carcass is very close to nil. In other words, in the fasting state the main bulk of the body is excluding glucose as fuel, using FFA and keto acids instead. This exclusion of glucose results from many factors, of which the low circulating insulin levels are of special importance, but elevated plasma fatty acids, keto acids, and probably other factors also play a role [305]. The liver uses amino acids, derived mainly from muscle protein, as substrate for gluconeogenesis but not for its own energy requirements. Approximately one-fourth of the flux of FFA derived from adipose tissue is metabolized by liver for its own energy needs, the remainder going directly to carcass. For the first few days of fasting, liver glycogen contributes slightly to the glucose being produced; thereafter, gluconeogenesis is its sole source.

With more prolonged starvation, brain diminishes its glucose consumption and substitutes keto acids as its major fuel supply [306]. Although long ignored, this fact is both evident and mandatory for survival, since withdrawal of 75 gm protein per day from muscle for gluconeogenesis and glucose consumption by brain would limit fasting survival to some 2 to 3 weeks of life, whereas total starvation has been maintained in obese individuals for many months. Thus, with prolonged starvation, even brain begins to use principally substrates that consist of fat or are fat-derived, as shown in Fig. 4-12; only a moderate amount of glucose is

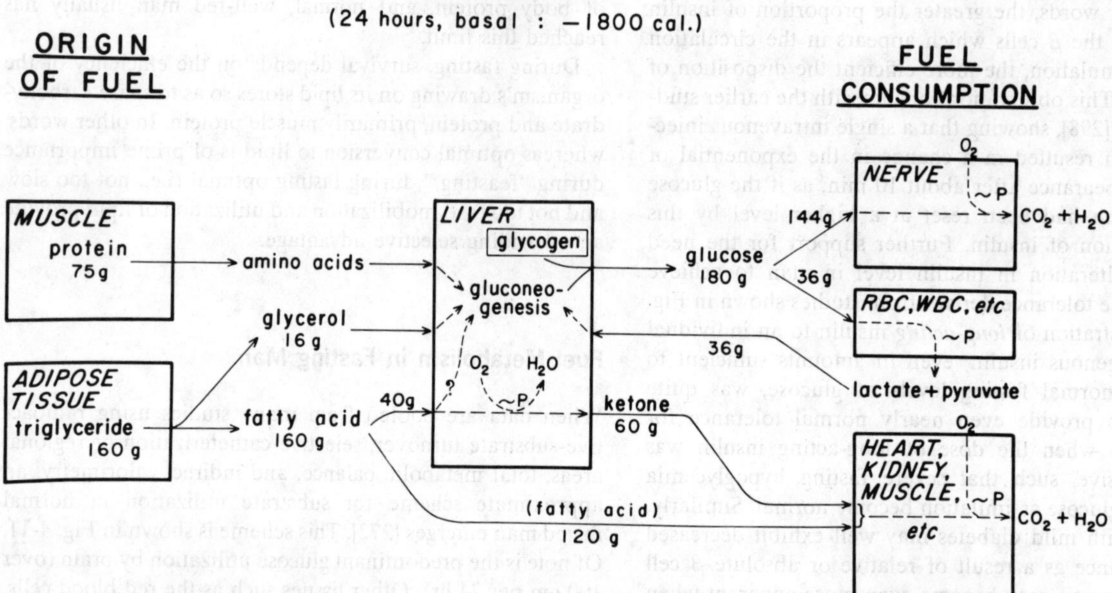

Figure 4-11. Schematic representation of substrate metabolism in man after a short period of fasting (36 hr). (*From Cahill et al.* [272].)

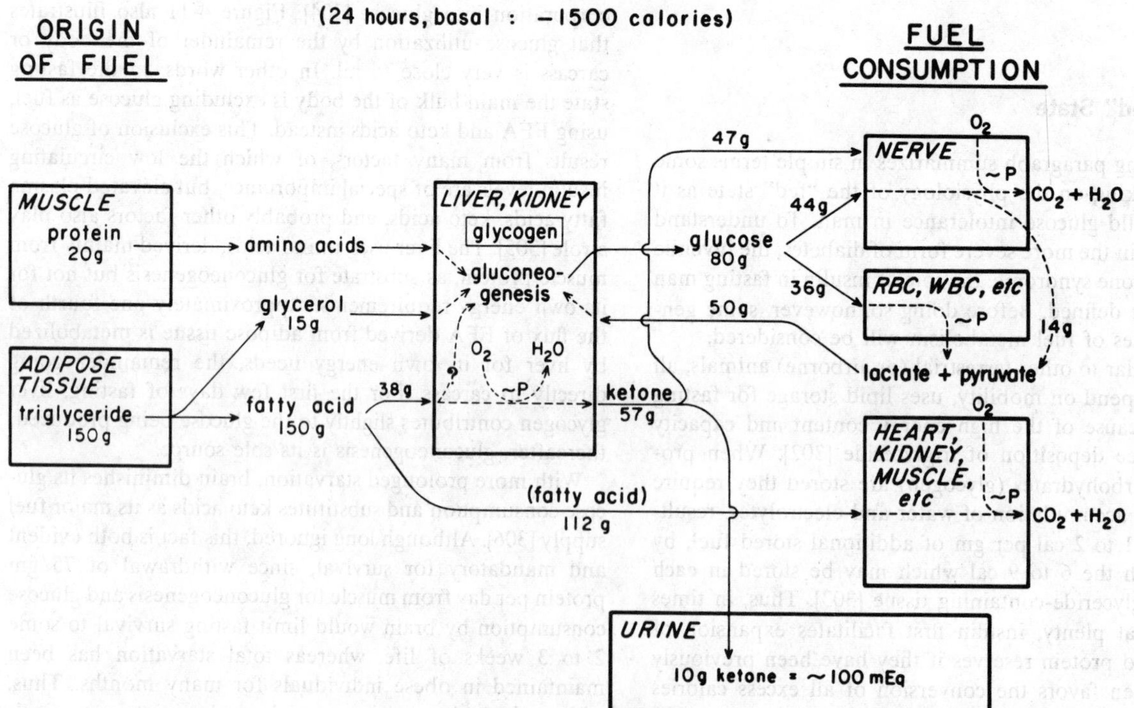

Figure 4-12. Schematic representation of substrate metabolism in man after a prolonged period of fasting (5 to 6 weeks). (*From Cahill et al.* [272].)

used, some of which is glycolyzed only to lactate and pyruvate and returned to the liver for glucose resynthesis [281]. It should be pointed out also that this cycle serves as an energy shuttle, using fat-derived calories in liver for the energy needed to convert lactate to glucose, calories which are then used by tissues which perform obligatory glycolysis whenever glucose is again metabolized to lactate.

Plasma insulin levels in fasting man fall to about one-half those seen in the postabsorptive state [304]. Levels of growth hormone, adrenal glucocorticoids, and catecholamines are variable. Glucagon, on the other hand, increases, and the level either remains elevated or subsequently decreases again toward normal with more prolonged starvation [307, 308]. In any case, glucagon relative to insulin is much higher than in the postabsorptive state, although its physiologic role remains to be defined. Returning to Fig. 4-12, it should be pointed out that the low plasma levels of insulin still suffice to regulate the rate of release of amino acids from muscle and that of free fatty acids from adipose tissue, since even very low levels of insulin may suppress free fatty acid release from adipose tissue and reduce the rate of release of amino acid from human muscle during fasting [309]. In other words, even after a prolonged fast it is still the low but significant amounts of insulin which control fuel metabolism. Also to be emphasized is the role of plasma keto acids as a normal physiologic intermediate. In fact, it has been suggested that their teleologic *raison d'être* may be to provide a water-soluble, fat-derived product capable of crossing the blood-brain barrier, thereby sparing gluconeogenesis and body protein [310]. As shown in Table 4-4, the blood levels of keto acids are sufficiently elevated to result in a mild metabolic acidosis and minimal ketonuria of about 10 gm per 24 hr.

Fuel Metabolism with Basal Insulin Deficiency

Whenever basal plasma insulin levels become inadequate for the maintenance of the well-integrated flux of substrates shown in Figs. 4-12 and 4-13, mobilization of free fatty acids from adipose tissue, and of amino acids from muscle, further and strikingly increases, resulting in enhanced gluconeogenesis. Since there is no compensatory increase of glucose utilization by brain or carcass, hyperglycemia and glycosuria result, together with weight loss, polydypsia, polyuria, and increased keto acid production.

Benedict and Joslin [311] and later Atchley et al. [312] in their classical metabolic studies on juvenile diabetes equated the development of ketoacidosis with the degree of net negative carbohydrate balance. Conversion of pyruvate to glucose in liver requires energy, which is derived from keto acid generation from long-chain fatty acid, and Wierzuchowski [313] demonstrated in phlorizinized dogs that ketoacidosis was directly related to the severity of glycosuria. Figure 4-13 illustrates the energy balance and flow of substrates in a diabetic. Gluconeogenesis is greatly increased, and the excess synthesized glucose is lost in the urine. Of more significance, there is an increase in keto acid production, and the balance between production and utilization is disturbed. Indeed, evidence from experimental animals suggests that in severe insulin lack, muscle utilization of acetoacetate may be diminished [314]. The plasma levels of keto acids rise, and the amount lost in urine increases precipitously, occasionally to as much as 50 to 75 gm (500 to 750 mEq) per day [311].

The rate of transition from the fed (hyperinsulinized) state to that with low levels of insulin is of considerable importance. Normal man develops progressive ketonuria as keto

Table 4-4. TYPICAL CONCENTRATIONS OF VARIOUS FUELS AND OF INSULIN IN BLOOD OR PLASMA OF MAN AFTER FEEDING, AFTER AN OVERNIGHT FAST (POSTABSORPTIVE STATE), AFTER SEVERAL WEEKS OF STARVATION, AND IN DIABETIC ACIDOSIS

Fuels and insulin	Fed state	Postabsorptive state	Starvation	Diabetic acidosis
Blood:				
Glucose, mg/100 ml	120	80	65	500
Glycerol, μM	50	100	100	200
Free fatty acid, μM	300	600	1,500	2,500
β-Hydroxybutyrate, mM	...	0.01	6	16
Acetoacetate, mM	...	0.01	1.5	4
Alanine, μM	400	400	100	300
Insulin, μU/ml	100	15	7	<5
Bicarbonate, mM	25	25	16	5
Urine:				
Glucose, gm/24 hr	<0.2	<0.2	<0.2	100*
β-Hydroxybutyrate, mM/24 hr	<0.1	<0.1	100	200
Acetoacetate, mM/24 hr	<0.1	<0.1	10	20

*This amount of glucose may be much greater if the subject has received exogenous glucose. Here, it represents net negative carbohydrate balance or that amount synthesized by gluconeogenesis.

Source: Data pooled from references [272, 281, 304, 306, 311, 312].

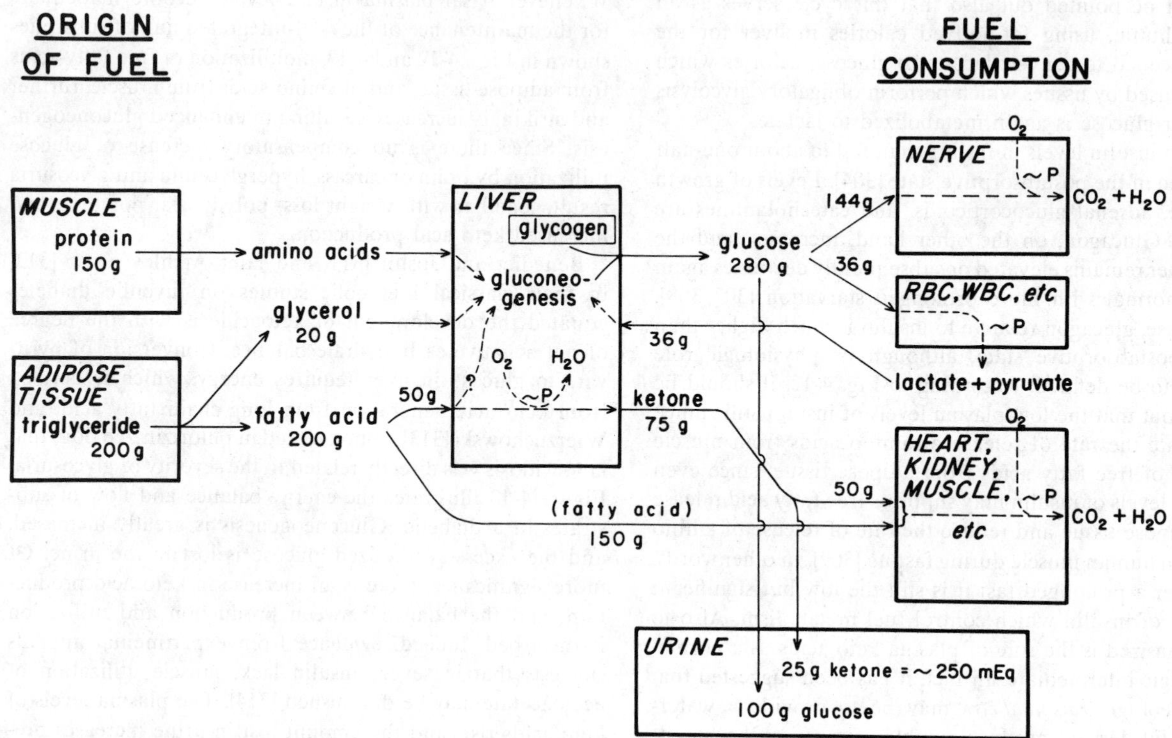

Figure 4-13. Schematic representation of substrate metabolism in man during severe insulin deficiency. (*From Cahill et al.* [272].)

acids increase in the blood during the first week of starvation, and approximately at the same rate as that at which the kidney adapts its ammoniagenic capacity [315]. Also, although not yet directly studied, adaptation of brain to keto acid utilization appears to require at least several days of starvation. In diabetic acidosis, Kety [316] found practically no brain uptake of keto acids, perhaps because the duration of preexisting ketosis was too brief, or perhaps because the brain does not adapt in the presence of hyperglycemia. In either case the severity of ketosis would be more extreme. Thus, the diabetic patient on insulin is uniquely liable to decompensated ketoacidosis if insulin is withdrawn or its metabolic effect inhibited. Similarly, a rat rendered diabetic with alloxan will usually not develop fatal ketoacidosis; but if it is treated with insulin and the insulin is then stopped, decompensated ketoacidosis and death occur rapidly. In the preinsulin era, the limited survival of juvenile diabetics was achieved primarily by maintaining the patient in a state of near-starvation with supplementation of electrolytes, particularly sodium bicarbonate [2].

In summary, normal man fluctuates easily between the fed and fasted states in large part as a result of his ability to alter the circulating levels of insulin. In the individual with mildly compromised insulin secretion, the rapid adaptation to the fed state is disturbed. With more severe degrees of insulin lack, particularly when the lack is acute, the homeostasis characteristic of the fasted state becomes grossly disturbed, with overproduction of fuels into the blood, excessive ketogenesis and gluconeogenesis, ketonuria, glycosuria, dehydration, acidosis, hypovolemia, and if the condition remains uncorrected, death.

Pancreatic β Cells in Human Diabetes

The discussion on diabetes mellitus presented in this chapter is built on the assumption that the central endocrine defect in diabetes is absolute or relative insulin deficiency, and the preceding detailed analysis of serum insulin and of fuel metabolism in fed, fasted, and diabetic man has in no way weakened this assumption. It is equally true that the cause underlying such an absolute or relative insulin deficiency is still unknown, and we have therefore emphasized exact knowledge of normal insulin biosynthesis, secretion, and effectiveness as the necessary basis for present and future progress and understanding. From the very complexity of the morphologic and functional system described (a complexity probably still greatly underestimated as a result of our still fragmentary, naive state of information [188]), it quite logically follows that many single defects, or possibly combined and multiple defects, might be involved in creating such absolute or relative insulin deficiency. Thus, it is evident that insulin deficiency need not be based on a subnormal total mass or number of pancreatic islets or even of insulin-producing β cells. Deficiency could equally well result from a normal number of cells normal in size but abnormal in their ability to synthesize normal insulin, or inadequately equipped with noninsulin constituents required for insulin storage, or insufficiently effective in releasing insulin from its storage form when required. Also, all or part of the insulin synthesized or released could be abnormal, a situation possibly involving an increased or a decreased secretion of proinsulin or of other insulin precursors as well [317, 318].

As far as *total β cell mass or pancreatic insulin content* is concerned, both may be said to be decreased in the great majority of instances in which autopsy took place after two or more years of preexisting diabetes [134, 319–322]. The decrease in both cell mass and insulin content is very much greater in youth-onset than in maturity-onset diabetes. Indeed, whereas the insulin content of pancreases of many persons with maturity-onset diabetes may be well within the normal range even after many years of preexisting diabetes, the pancreatic insulin content of patients with youth-onset diabetes is, as a rule, reduced to 5 percent or less of normal values. When death occurs in patients with youth-onset diabetes within a few weeks of the onset of symptoms (usually from nonrelated causes), however, a normal β-cell mass and significant amounts of extractable pancreatic insulin may be found [321, 323].

Levels of pancreatic insulin, extractable at autopsy, need not, of course, reflect the secretory ability of the pancreatic islets. Indeed, this measurement is more likely to relate to the adequacy of insulin storage. The more recent functional approach to insulin secretory capacity in human diabetics has tended to confirm the conclusions based on pancreatic β cell structure and insulin content. In juvenile diabetes of some duration, insulin response to stimulation with glucose or other stimuli is practically absent [228, 260, 324]. In maturity-onset diabetes, response is usually delayed, although high circulating levels of serum insulin may be reached during the secondary or late phase of insulin response to stimulation with, for example, glucose [325]. This is particularly true of persons with maturity-onset diabetes who are also obese. In general, plasma insulin response to glucose is almost invariably less in persons with maturity-onset diabetes than in controls of the same weight and age [238, 254].

Although the hypothesis of an abnormal insulin's being synthesized, stored, and secreted in at least some diabetics is most attractive, and although some supporting evidence has been presented [326], it is our interpretation that the evidence so far available is inconclusive.

Delayed Early Phase of Insulin Secretion in Potential Diabetes and Early Diabetes

An important aspect of insulin secretion, both in vivo and in vitro, is its biphasic nature, with a prompt primary peak and a more delayed and gradual secondary rise (Fig. 4-8). In many situations this early response may be of particular importance, as already illustrated by the impossibility of achieving normal glucose tolerance in patients with severe diabetes with the exclusive use of long-acting insulins (Fig. 4-10). In human diabetes, the earliest detectable anomaly of insulin secretion appears to be a decrease or indeed a disappearance of the primary, rapid secretory peak [327, 328]. This has been best defined by Cerasi and Luft [12], who further showed that this same early delay may be observed in as yet nondiabetic identical twins of diabetics [51]. It seems reasonable to say today that this anomaly of the early phase of insulin secretion and response to glucose is the most likely general and obligatory, genetically controlled component of human diabetes mellitus pertaining to insulin secretion, although it is quite evident that the anomaly by itself is insufficient to cause diabetes. Absence of the first peak is found not only in as yet *nondiabetic* identical twins of diabetics, but also in approximately 15 percent of the general population, both in adults and in children [12]. Cerasi and Luft have speculated that the organism may adapt to this delayed response by increased sensitivity to insulin, clinical diabetes resulting when this increased sensitivity can no longer be maintained. They have also shown that the abnormal early phase of insulin secretion in persons with potential diabetes may be influenced by drugs such as theophylline, which probably facilitates the intracellular accumulation of 3′,5′-AMP [329].

The abnormal profile of insulin release in diabetics might also be related to a physical phenomenon, such as greater difficulty encountered by insulin in passing through one of the several membranous structures separating the β granules from the bloodstream, as early emphasized by Lacy and Hartroft [330]. This hypothesis has received considerable support from the impressive evidence accumulated by Siperstein, evidence indicating that capillary basement membrane thickening in muscle may precede glucose intolerance in the life history of most diabetics [9, 10]. For the time being this remains a hypothesis only.

Immunologic β-cell Damage

Autoimmune mechanisms have been implicated in the pathogenesis of disorders of other endocrine cells, as in primary myxedema, thyrotoxicosis, and the idiopathic form of hypoadrenocorticism. It would be unreasonable to rule out *a priori* the possible participation of an autoimmune process in the pathogenesis of endocrine pancreatic disorders as well. At present, the evidence is inconclusive, but further consideration and testing of the concept are warranted.

What evidence there is about this possibility came initially from the observation that a specific immune-insulitis may be experimentally induced [331, 332]. In at least one species, the rabbit, experimental insulitis was associated with glucose intolerance [333]. Furthermore, eosinophilic infiltrations have been described in the pancreatic islets of approximately 30 percent of newborn infants of diabetic mothers [334], while striking lymphocytic infiltrations were seen in a large proportion of the small group of patients with severe youth-onset diabetes who came to autopsy within the first 2 weeks or months following the onset of symptoms [319, 335, 336]. Also, although circulating antibodies to insulin have usually not been found in previously untreated diabetics and potential diabetics, a few exceptions have been recorded [331], as well as binding of insulin to basement membrane material prominent in diabetic vascular lesions [337]. Finally, an increased prevalence of thyroid and gastric autoantibodies in diabetic populations [338, 339], as well as relatively frequent association of diabetes with hypofunction of the thyroid and the adrenal cortex [340] and of diabetes with idiopathic adrenocortical insufficiency [341], have been reported.

Inhibitors and Antagonists of Insulin Action

It is certainly true that variations in sensitivity to insulin action, resulting in variations of insulin effectiveness, contribute significantly to blood glucose and, more generally, fuel metabolism homeostasis in both normal and diabetic persons. Experimentally, this fact was established by Houssay when he showed the differences in effectiveness of insulin in normal and hypophysectomized toads, and most strikingly in animals either pancreatectomized or both pancreatectomized and hypophysectomized. By 1939 Himsworth had already clearly defined an insulin-sensitive and an insulin-insensitive type of diabetes in man [125]. Both concepts are still with us, as are thoughts about the possible pathogenetic importance in diabetes of increased or abnormal secretions of hormones leading to decreased insulin sensitivity, such as growth hormone, ACTH, glucocorticoids, glucagon, or epinephrine. It has become increasingly probable that at least some of these hormones exert their insulin-antagonistic action indirectly, either through mobilization of metabolites such as free fatty acids which then compete with glucose metabolites for oxidation [342], or through the production or maintenance of specific humoral agents such as the synalbumin antagonist of Vallance-Owen [343], or the food-induced inhibitor of insulin action described by Young [344], to cite but two examples.

Again, even recent studies continue to confirm the considerable differences among different types of diabetics as to their sensitivity to insulin [345, 346], and we have similarly commented above on a major variation in sensitivity to insulin which may be observed in animals, both normal and diabetic (Table 4-3). At present it is impossible to evaluate precisely the role of insulin inhibition or antagonism in the pathogenesis of human diabetes. A relationship between decreased sensitivity to insulin and atherosclerosis as well as microangiopathy has also been suggested [346–348].

SUMMARY

1 Diabetes mellitus is a metabolic disorder characterized by blood glucose levels greater than the range empirically considered appropriate for any given set of environmental and nutritional conditions. Although emphasis must remain on blood glucose levels, since the diagnosis of diabetes still cannot be made in the absence of inappropriate hyperglycemia, it is certain that the latter is but one of many derangements of metabolism occurring in clinically overt diabetes, derangements which affect protein and fat metabolism at least as much as they do carbohydrate metabolism. The diabetic manifestations which are readily explained as derived from altered intermediary metabolism in the tissues principally responsible for overall energy balance—adipose tissue, liver, and muscle—are referred to as the acute diabetic syndrome. The chronic diabetic syndrome further includes manifestations which develop only in the course of the disease, frequently appear to have a microvascular as well as a metabolic basis, and may or may not be pathogenetically related to the acute syndrome.

2 Although inappropriate hyperglycemia is not present from birth in the great majority of instances, excellent evidence indicates that the potentiality to develop diabetes mellitus is inherited. Thus, the prevalence of diabetes is certainly greater among close relatives of patients known to have diabetes than in suitable control populations, and diabetes occurs even more frequently in similar twins born of diabetic parents than when the twins are fraternal. More precise genetic analysis is greatly hampered by uncertainty as to even the operational definition of diabetes, by its age-related incidence, and by the very frequency of its occurrence in most economically developed populations today. Even in similar twins of diabetics, or in children of two diabetic parents, clinically overt diabetes may occur many years later than in the affected twin, or perhaps not at all. It has been customary to explain such difficulties by stating that the "penetrance" of the genetic tendency to develop diabetes is low, and furthermore that it may be variable.

3 Although a simple, autosomal, recessive mode of inheritance may yet prove true, present evidence suggests that it is becoming less and less likely. In our opinion, it is much more probable that the mode of inheritance of the disorder will in time be shown to be polygenic or multifactorial, opening the way to the definition of phenotypically similar yet genetically different diabetic syndromes.

4 Environmental influences certainly contribute to defining the period during which diabetes remains latent, thereby modifying the "penetrance" of the diabetic genotype(s). While such direct influences as viral infections or the eliciting of autoimmune mechanisms may be involved in some instances, perhaps especially in young diabetics, the principal environmental effects to be considered are dietary regimen, physical exercise, and intercurrent infections or other forms of "stress," including emotional ones. The best-documented instances concern changes in the prevalence of diabetes in populations undergoing major changes in their living conditions, such as food rationing during and after wars, or migration from food-restricted conditions with need for considerable physical exercise to an environment with abundant availability of food and demanding less physical exertion.

5 The environmental conditions leading to an increased prevalence of diabetes mellitus are likely also to lead to an increased prevalence of obesity. Though the two metabolic disorders may also be genetically linked, the environmental connection is surely evident and may well be secondary to the food-related decreased insulin effectiveness associated with the increased insulin secretion characteristic of obesity, and also seen in some diabetics. As long as life expectancy averaged 30 years or so, when man was frequently called upon to withstand prolonged periods of starvation often associated with cold exposure, ability to develop obesity rapidly whenever possible may well have been a selective survival advantage. This is no longer true in the economically developed countries of the world, and the adaptation imbalance so produced within relatively few decades has been described by Neel in his entirely novel hypothesis of a previously beneficial *thrifty genotype recently rendered detrimental by "progress,"* a genotype perhaps preferentially associated with many instances of diabetes mellitus or obesity or both.

6 Both the genetic diversity of phenotypically similar diabetic syndromes and the probable importance of environmental factors in controlling manifestations of a diabetic tendency have received considerable support from observations on spontaneous animal syndromes associated with inappropriate hyperglycemia, with or without concurrent obesity. Seven distinct genotypes associated with inappropriate hyperglycemia are now known in just the one species, the laboratory mouse! In Chinese hamsters, complete genetic analysis has yielded the near-certainty of a multifactorial basis for inheritance of glycosuria, with four pairs of alleles needed to explain the extensive observations made.

7 Evidence derived from the study of experimental diabetes in animals, from those instances where disease led to the necessary surgical removal of the pancreas in man, or to its inflammatory and fibrotic destruction, and from careful measurements of the mass of the β cells of the islets of Langerhans in patients suffering from diabetes, suggests that the acute diabetic syndrome is the result of absolute or relative deficiency of the hormone produced by the pancreatic β cells, i.e., insulin. Similarly, all the symptoms and signs of the acute diabetic syndrome may be reversed by the administration of insulin.

8 Whereas absolute or relative insulin deficiency must be considered a likely important pathogenetic link in the production of the acute diabetic syndrome, the mechanism producing this deficiency is as yet unknown. Possibilities which have to be considered include anomalies of the mechanisms of insulin synthesis, storage, release, and secretion, of insulin transport or destruction, and either directly or indirectly of altered insulin effectiveness at the tissue level. This is why so much effort has been devoted and continues to be devoted to the acquisition of detailed knowledge and information about all the complex components and processes which are or might be involved. Only their intimate understanding will some day make it possible to define the nature of the variant(s) which may be properly thought responsible for the anomaly ultimately resulting in diabetes mellitus.

9 At the time of writing this chapter, a genetically determined depression of the *early* phase of insulin release in response to glucose and other stimuli may well be considered an early and possibly an obligatory component of diabetic genotype(s). This anomaly is not in itself sufficient to cause diabetes to become clinically apparent, since it is also present in potential diabetics and, indeed, in about 15 percent of the limited random population samples tested so far. The primary pathogenetic importance of accelerated accumulation of capillary basement membrane material, at least in muscle, is also under scrutiny but is considered by us at this time to be a less likely possibility.

10 While the search for the precise and primary metabolic basis of diabetes mellitus continues to be fraught with numerous and complex difficulties, similar difficulties may well apply equally to other complex and chronic metabolic disorders with unquestioned yet complex hereditary components, such as atherosclerosis, connective tissue diseases, and, indeed, aging. Accordingly, much that might be learned from diabetes mellitus may prove applicable some day to the study of these anomalies which, with cancer, now represent perhaps the major frontier of biomedical research, at least in terms of practical importance.

BIBLIOGRAPHY

1. Allen, F. M.: *Studies Concerning Glycosuria and Diabetes.* Leonard, Boston, 1913.
2. Allen, F. M., Stillman, E., and Fitz, R.: *Total Dietary Regulation in the Treatment of Diabetes,* Monograph 11. Rockefeller Institute for Medical Research, New York, 1919.
3. Jensen, H. F.: *Insulin, Its Chemistry and Physiology.* Commonwealth Fund, New York, 1938.
4. Wrenshall, G. A., Hetenyi, G., Jr., and Feasby, W. R.: *The Story of Insulin.* Bodley Head, London, 1962.

5. Dobson, M.: Experiments and observations on the urine in diabetes. Med. Observations Inquiries, **5,** 298, 1776.
6. Joslin, E. P., Root, H. F., White, P., and Marble, A.: *Treatment of Diabetes Mellitus,* 10th ed. Lea & Febiger, Philadelphia, 1959.
7. Report of a working party appointed by the College of General Practitioners: A diabetes survey. Brit. Med. J., **1,** 1497, 1962; and report of a working party appointed by the College of General Practitioners: Glucose tolerance and glycosuria in the general populations. Brit. Med. J., **2,** 655, 1963.
8. World Health Organization Expert Committee: *Diabetes Mellitus.* W.H.O. Technical Report Series, No. 310, World Health Organization, Geneva, 1965.
9. Siperstein, M. D., Unger, R. H., and Madison, L. L.: Studies of muscle capillary basement membranes in normal subjects, diabetic, and prediabetic patients. J. Clin. Invest., **47,** 1973, 1968.
10. Siperstein, M. D.: The relationship of carbohydrate derangements to the microangiopathy of diabetes, in *Proc. Nobel Symposium XIII: On the Pathogenesis of Diabetes Mellitus,* p. 81. Wiley Interscience Div., New York, 1970.
11. Luft, R.: Studies on the pathogenesis of diabetes mellitus, in *Diabetes,* Suppl., Proc. 6th Congress of the International Diabetes Federation, p. 3, International Congress Series 172S. Excerpta Medica Foundation, Amsterdam, 1969.
12. Cerasi, E., and Luft, R.: The pathogenesis of diabetes mellitus, a proposed concept, in *Proc. Nobel Symposium XIII: On the Pathogenesis of Diabetes Mellitus,* p. 17. Wiley Interscience Div., New York, 1970.
13. LeCompte, P. M.: Vascular lesions in diabetes mellitus. J. Chron. Dis., **2,** 178, 1955.
14. Bloodworth, J. M. B., Jr.: Diabetic microangiopathy. Diabetes, **12,** 99, 1963.
15. Beaven, D. W.: Diabetic angiopathy. Aust. Ann. Med., **14,** 65, 1965.
16. Marble, A.: Angiopathy in diabetes, an unsolved problem. Diabetes, **16,** 825, 1967.
17. FitzGerald, M. G., and Keen, H.: Diagnostic classification of diabetes. Brit. Med. J., **1,** 1568, 1964.
18. Fajans, S. S., and Conn, J. W.: Prediabetes, subclinical diabetes and latent clinical diabetes: interpretation, diagnosis and treatment, in *On the Nature and Treatment of Diabetes,* edited by B. S. Leibel and G. A. Wrenshall, p. 641. Excerpta Medica Foundation, Amsterdam, 1965.
19. Mimura, G., Oshiro, S., Koganemaru, K., Haraguchi, Y., Jinnouchi, T., and Hashiguchi, J.: Studies on the heredity of diabetes mellitus in Japan. II. Inheritance of the fasting blood sugar value and the blood sugar value two hours after meal in Uto and Tomiai inhabitants. Kumamoto Med. J., **17,** 50, 1964.
20. Gordon, T.: Glucose tolerance of adults, United States, 1960–1962. National Center for Health Statistics, Public Health Service, U.S. Department of Health, Education and Welfare. Series 11, No. 2, p. 25, 1964.
21. Neel, J. V., Fajans, S. S., Conn, J. W., and Davidson, R. T.: Diabetes mellitus, in *Genetics and the Epidemiology of Chronic Diseases,* edited by J. V. Neel, M. W. Shaw, and W. J. Schull, pp. 105–132. Public Health Service Publication 1163, Washington, 1965.
22. Thompson, G. S.: Genetic factors in diabetes mellitus studied by the oral glucose tolerance test. J. Med. Genet., **2,** 221, 1965.
23. Butterfield, W. J. H.: The Bedford Diabetes Survey. Proc. Roy. Soc. Med., **57,** 196, 1964.
24. Streeten, D. H. P., Gerstein, M. M., Marmor, B. M., and Doisy, R. J.: Reduced glucose tolerance in elderly human subjects. Diabetes, **14,** 579, 1965.
25. Wilkerson, H. L. C., and Krall, L. P.: Diabetes in New England town: study of 3,516 persons in Oxford, Mass. J.A.M.A., **135,** 209, 1947.
26. Wilkerson, H. L. C., Krall, L. P., and Butler, F. K.: Diabetes in a New England town. III. A comprehensive baseline study in Oxford, Mass. J.A.M.A., **169,** 910, 1959.
27. O'Sullivan, J. B.: Population retested for diabetes after 17 years: new prevalence study in Oxford, Mass. Diabetologia, **5,** 211, 1969.
28. *Diabetes Source Book,* Public Health Service Publication 1168, revised 1968.
29. Walker, J. B.: in *Aetiology of Diabetes Mellitus and Its Complications,* p. 5, Ciba Colloquium. Churchill, London, 1964.
30. Oakley, W. G., Pyke, D. A., and Taylor, K. W.: *Clinical Diabetes and Its Biochemical Basis.* Blackwell Scientific Publications, Ltd., Oxford, 1968.
31. Malins, J.: *Clinical Diabetes Mellitus.* Eyre and Spottiswoode (Publishers), Ltd., London, 1968.
32. Marble, A., et al.: *Joslin's Textbook of Diabetes Mellitus,* 11th ed. Lea & Febiger, Philadelphia, 1970.
33. McDonald, G. W., Fisher, G. F., and Burnham, C.: Reproducibility of the oral glucose tolerance test. Diabetes, **14,** 473, 1965.
34. Unger, R. H.: The standard two-hour oral glucose tolerance test in the diagnosis of diabetes mellitus in subjects without fasting hyperglycemia. Ann. Intern. Med., **47,** 1138, 1957.
35. Pyke, D. A.: The geography of diabetes. Postgrad. Med. J., **45,** 796, suppl., December, 1969.
36. Cohen, A. M.: Prevalence of diabetes among different Jewish groups in Israel. Metabolism, **10,** 50, 1961.
37. Genuth, S. M., Bennett, P. H., Miller, M., and Burch, T. A.: Hyperinsulinism in obese diabetic Pima Indians. Metabolism, **16,** 1010, 1967.
38. Mouratoff, G. J., Carroll, N. V., and Scott, E. M.: Diabetes mellitus in Athabaskan Indians in Alaska. Diabetes, **18,** 29, 1969.
39. Tulloch, J. A.: *Diabetes Mellitus in the Tropics.* E. and S. Livingstone, Edinburgh and London, 1962.
40. West, K. M., and Kalbfleisch, J. M.: Glucose tolerance, nutrition and diabetes in Uruguay, Venezuela, Malaya and East Pakistan. Diabetes, **15,** 9, 1966.
41. Zammitt Maempel, J. V.: Diabetes in Malta. Lancet, **2,** 1197, 1965.
42. Murray, J. T., Hannah, E. E., Laing, J. K., Cotter, A. P., Ferrar, R. H., Jepson, L. F., and Beaven, D. W.: Diabetes mellitus in European New Zealanders. New Zeal. Med. J., **69,** 271, 1969.
43. Prior, I. A. M., and Davidson, F.: The epidemiology of diabetes in Polynesians and Europeans in New Zealand and the Pacific. New Zeal. Med. J., **65,** 375, 1966.
44. Rudnick, P. A., and Anderson, P. S.: Diabetes mellitus in Hiroshima, Japan. Diabetes, **11,** 533, 1962.
45. Ref. [6], p. 48.
46. College of General Practitioners: The family history of diabetes. Brit. Med. J., **1,** 960, 1965.
47. Ref. [6], p. 49.
48. Harvald, B., and Hange, M.: Hereditary factors elucidated by twin studies. U.S. Public Health Service Publication 1163, 1965.
49. Ref. [30], p. 214.
50. Pyke, D. A., and Taylor, K. W.: Glucose tolerance and serum insulin in unaffected identical twins of diabetics. Brit. Med. J., **2,** 21, 1967.
51. Cerasi, E., and Luft, R.: Insulin response to glucose infusion in diabetic and non-diabetic monozygotic twin pairs. Genetic control of insulin response? Acta Endocr. (Kobenhavn), **55,** 330, 1967.
52. Gottlieb, M. S., and Root, H. F.: Diabetes mellitus in twins. Diabetes, **17,** 693, 1968.
53. Steinberg, A. G.: Heredity in diabetes mellitus. Diabetes, **10,** 269, 1961.
54. Nilsson, S. E.: On the heredity of diabetes mellitus and its interrelationship with some other diseases. Acta Genet. (Basel), **14,** 97, 1964.
55. Steinberg, A. G., Rushforth, N. B., Bennett, P. H., Burch, T. A., and Miller, M.: On the genetics of diabetes mellitus, in *Proc. Nobel Symposium XIII: On the Pathogenesis of Diabetes Mellitus,* p. 237. Wiley Interscience Div., New York, 1970.
56. Mimura, G.: On the mode of inheritance of diabetes mellitus in Japan. Kumamoto Med. J., **15,** 154, 1962.
57. Lamy, M., Frézal, J., and Rey, J.: Hérédité du diabète sucré. Journées Ann. Diabét. Hôtel-Dieu, **2,** 5, 1961.
58. Simpson, N. E.: The genetics of diabetes: A study of 233 families of juvenile diabetics. Ann. Hum. Genet., **26,** 1, 1962.
59. Falconer, D. S.: The inheritance of liability to diseases with variable age of onset, with particular reference to diabetes mellitus. Ann. Hum. Genet., **31,** 1, 1967.
60. Neel, J. V.: Current concepts of the genetic basis of diabetes mellitus and the biological significance of the diabetic predisposition, in *Diabe-*

tes, p. 68. International Congress Series, vol. 72S. Excerpta Medica Foundation, Amsterdam, 1969.

61. West, K. M.: Response to cortisone in prediabetes: glucose- and steroid-glucose tolerance in subjects whose parents are both diabetic. Diabetes, **9,** 379, 1960.
62. Post, R. H.: An approach to the question, does all diabetes depend upon a single genetic locus? Diabetes, **11,** 56, 1962.
63. Simpson, N. E.: Multifactorial inheritance: a possible hypothesis for diabetes. Diabetes, **13,** 462, 1964.
64. Cooke, A. M., FitzGerald, M. G., Malins, J., and Pyke, D. A.: Diabetes in children of diabetic couples. Brit. Med. J., **2,** 674, 1966.
65. Pavel, I., and Pieptea, R.: Problèmes que pose l'hérédité diabétique. Journées Ann. Diabét. Hôtel-Dieu, **6,** 217, 1965.
66. Vallance-Owen, J.: The inheritance of essential diabetes mellitus from studies of the synalbumin insulin antagonist. Diabetologia, **2,** 248, 1966.
67. Harris, H.: Familial distribution of diabetes mellitus: study of relatives of 1241 diabetic propositi. Ann. Eugen., **15,** 95, 1950.
68. Cammidge, P. J.: Heredity as a factor in the aetiology of diabetes mellitus. Lancet, **1,** 393, 1934.
69. Lawrence, R. D.: Lipodystrophy and hepatomegaly with diabetes, lipemia and other metabolic disturbances. Lancet, **250,** 724, 1946.
70. Senior, B.: Lipodystrophic muscular hypertrophy. Arch. Dis. Child., **36,** 426, 1961.
71. Schwartz, R., Schafer, I. A., and Renold, A. E.: Generalized lipoatrophy, hepatic cirrhosis, disturbed carbohydrate metabolism and accelerated growth (lipoatrophic diabetes): longitudinal observation and metabolic studies. Amer. J. Med., **28,** 973, 1960.
72. Louis, L. H., Conn, J. W., and Minick, M. C.: Lipoatrophic diabetes: characterization and isolation of an insulin antagonist from urine. Metabolism, **12,** 867, 1963.
73. Craig, J. W., and Miller, M.: Lipoatrophic diabetes, in *Diabetes,* edited by R. H. Williams, p. 600. Hoeber-Harper, New York, 1960.
74. Seip, M., and Trygstad, O.: Generalized lipodystrophy. Arch. Dis. Child., **38,** 447, 1963.
75. Brunzell, J. D., Shankle, S. W., and Bethune, J. E.: Congenital generalized lipodystrophy accompanied by cystic angiomatosis. Ann. Intern. Med., **69,** 501, 1968.
76. Kitselle, J. F.: Ein Fall von Diabetes bei einem Kinde. J. Kinderkrankh., **18,** 313, 1852.
77. Hutchison, J. H., Keay, A. J., and Kerr, M. M.: Congenital temporary diabetes mellitus. Brit. Med. J., **2,** 436, 1962.
78. Epstein, C. J., Martin, G. M., Schultz, A. L., and Motulsky, A. G.: Werner's syndrome. Medicine (Balt.), **45,** 177, 1966.
79. Renold, A. E.: Spontaneous diabetes and/or obesity in laboratory rodents, edited by R. Levine and R. Luft. Advances Metab. Dis., **3,** 49, 1968.
80. Renold, A. E., and Dublin, W. E. (editors): Brook Lodge Workshop on spontaneous "diabetes" in animals. Diabetologia, **3,** 63, 1967.
81. Renold, A. E., Cahill, G. F., Jr., and Gerritsen, G. (editors): Second Brook Lodge Workshop on spontaneous "diabetes" in animals. Diabetologia, **6,** 1970.
82. Renold, A. E., Burr, I., and Stauffacher, W.: On the pathogenesis of diabetes mellitus: possible usefulness of spontaneous hyperglycemic syndromes in animals, in *Proc. Nobel Symposium XIII: On the Pathogenesis of Diabetes Mellitus,* p. 215. Wiley Interscience Div., New York, 1970.
83. Butler, L.: The Inheritance of Diabetes in the Chinese hamster. Diabetologia, **3,** 124, 1967.
84. Butler, L., and Gerritsen, G. C.: A comparison of the modes of inheritance of diabetes in the Chinese hamster and the KK mouse. Diabetologia, **6,** 163, 1970.
85. Gerritsen, G. C., Needham, L. B., Schmidt, F. L., and Dulin, W. E.: Studies on the prediction and development of diabetes in offspring of diabetic Chinese hamsters. Diabetologia, **6,** 158, 1970.
86. Weitze, M.: Hereditary adiposity in mice and the cause of this anomaly. Store Nord. Videnskabsboghandel, 1940.
87. Carpenter, K. J., and Mayer, J.: Physiologic observations on yellow obesity in the mouse. Amer. J. Physiol., **193,** 499, 1958.
88. Ingalls, A. M., Dickie, M. M., and Snell, G. D.: Obese, new mutation in the house mouse. J. Hered., **41,** 317, 1950.
89. Hellman, B.: Some metabolic aspects of the obese-hyperglycemic syndrome in mice. Diabetologia, **3,** 222, 1966.
90. Westman, S.: Pathogenetic aspects of the obese-hyperglycemic syndrome in mice (genotype *obob*): I. Function of the pancreatic β-cells. Diabetologia, **6,** 279, 1970.
91. Hummel, K. P., Dickie, M. M., and Coleman, D. L.: Diabetes, a new mutation in the mouse. Science, **153,** 490, 1964.
92. Coleman, D. L., and Hummel, K. P.: Studies with the mutation diabetes, in the mouse. Diabetologia, **3,** 238, 1967.
93. Chick, W. L., and Like, A. A.: Studies in the diabetic mutant mouse: III. Physiological factors associated with alterations in beta cell proliferation. Diabetologia, **6,** 243, 1970.
94. Bielschowsky, M., and Bielschowsky, F.: A new strain of mice with hereditary obesity. Proc. Univ. Otago Med. Sch., **31,** 29, 1953.
95. Sneyd, J. G. T.: Pancreatic and serum insulin in the New Zealand strain of obese mice. J. Endocr., **28,** 163, 1964.
96. Nakamura, M.: A diabetic strain of the mouse. Proc. Japan. Acad., **38,** 348, 1962.
97. Nakamura, M., and Yamada, K.: Studies on a diabetic (KK) strain of the mouse. Diabetologia, **3,** 212, 1967.
98. Cahill, G. F., Jr., Jones, E. E., Lauris, V., Steinke, J., and Soeldner, J. S.: Studies on experimental diabetes in the Wellesley hybrid mouse. II. Serum insulin levels and response of peripheral tissues. Diabetologia, **3,** 171, 1967.
99. Gleason, R. E., Lauris, V., and Soeldner, J. S.: Studies on experimental diabetes in the Wellesley hybrid mouse. III. Dietary effects and similar changes in a commercial Swiss-Hauschka strain. Diabetologia, **3,** 175, 1967.
100. Gonet, A. E., Stauffacher, W., Pictet, R., and Renold, A. E.: Obesity and diabetes mellitus with striking congenital hyperplasia of the islets of Langerhans in spiny mice (*Acomys cahirinus*). Diabetologia, **1,** 162, 1965.
101. Pictet, R., Orci, L., Gonet, A. E., Rouiller, C., and Renold, A. E.: Ultrastructural studies of the hyperplastic islets of Langerhans of spiny mice (*Acomys cahirinus*) before and during the development of hyperglycemia. Diabetologia, **3,** 188, 1967.
102. Stauffacher, W., Orci, L., Amherdt, M., Burr, I. M., Balant, L., Froesch, E. R., and Renold, A. E.: Metabolic state, pancreatic insulin content and β-cell morphology of normoglycemic spiny mice: indications for an impairment of insulin secretion. Diabetologia, **6,** 330, 1970.
103. Weir, B., Wise, P. H., and Hime, J. M.: Hyperglycaemia and cataract in the tucotuco. J. Endocr., **43,** 7 (abstract), 1969.
104. Schmidt-Nielsen, K., Haines, H. B., and Hackel, D. B.: Diabetes mellitus in the sand rat induced by standard laboratory diets. Science, **143,** 689, 1964.
105. Hackel, D. B., Mikat, E., Lebovitz, H. E., Schmidt-Nielsen, K., Horton, E. S., and Kinney, T. D.: The sand rat (*Psammomys obesus*) as an experimental animal in studies of diabetes mellitus. Diabetologia, **3,** 130, 1967.
106. Miki, E., Like, A. A., Steinke, J., and Soeldner, J. S.: Diabetic syndrome in sand rats. II. Variability and association with diet. Diabetologia, **3,** 135, 1967.
107. Like, A. A., and Miki, E.: Diabetic syndrome in sand rats. IV. Morphologic changes in islet tissue. Diabetologia, **3,** 143, 1967.
108. Zucker, L. M.: Hereditary obesity in the rat associated with hyperlipemia. Ann. N.Y. Acad. Sci., **131,** 447, 1965.
109. From, G. L. A., Craighead, J. E., McLane, M. F., and Steinke, J.: Virus-induced diabetes in mice. Metabolism, **17,** 1154, 1968.
110. Hinden, E.: Mumps followed by diabetes. Lancet, **1,** 1381, 1962.
111. Pedini, B., Avellini, G., Morettini, B., and Comodo, N.: Diabetes mellitus after foot and mouth disease in cattle. Atti Soc. Ital. Sci. Vet., **16,** part 2, 443, 1963.
112. Himsworth, H. P.: Diet in the etiology of human diabetes. Proc. Roy. Soc. Med., **43,** 323, 1949.
113. Goto, Y., Nakayama, Y., and Yagi, T.: Influence of world war II food shortage on the incidence of diabetes mellitus in Japan. Diabetes, **7,** 133, 1958.

114. Schliack, V.: Mangelernährung und Diabetes-Morbidität, Z. Klin. Med., **151,** 382, 1954.
115. Bouchardat, A.: *De la glycosurie ou diabète sucré.* Germer-Baillière, Paris, 1883.
116. Campbell, G. D.: Diabetes in Asians and Africans in and around Durban. S. Afr. Med. J., **37,** 1195, 1963.
117. Neel, J. V.: Diabetes mellitus: a "thrifty" genotype rendered detrimental by progress. Amer. J. Hum. Genet., **14,** 353, 1962.
118. Newburgh, L. H., and Conn, J. W.: A new interpretation of hyperglycemia in obese middle-aged persons. J.A.M.A., **112,** 7, 1939.
119. Boshell, B. R., Chandalia, H. B., Kreisberg, R. A., and Roddam, R. F.: Serum insulin in obesity and diabetes mellitus. Amer. J. Clin. Nutr., **21,** 1419, 1968.
120. Karam, J. H., Grodsky, G. M., and Forsham, P. H.: Excessive insulin response to glucose in obese subjects as measured by immunochemical assay. Diabetes, **12,** 197, 1963.
121. Perley, M., and Kipnis, D. M.: Plasma insulin responses to oral and intravenous glucose in normal and diabetic subjects. J. Clin. Invest., **46,** 1954, 1967.
122. Bagdade, J. D., Porte, D., and Bierman, E. L.: The interaction of diabetes and obesity on the regulation of fat mobilization in man. Diabetes, **18,** 759, 1969.
123. Rabinowitz, D., and Zierler, K. L.: Forearm metabolism in obesity and its response to intra-arterial insulin. Characterization of insulin resistance and evidence for adaptive hyperinsulinism. J. Clin. Invest., **41,** 2173, 1962.
124. Butterfield, W. J. H., Hanley, T., and Whichelow, M. J.: Peripheral metabolism of glucose and free fatty acids during oral glucose tolerance tests. Metabolism, **14,** 851, 1965.
125. Himsworth, H. P., and Ken, R. B.: Insulin sensitive and insulin insensitive types of diabetes. Clin. Sci., **4,** 119, 1939.
126. Salans, L. B., Knittle, J. L., and Hirsch, J.: The role of adipose cell size and adipose tissue insulin sensitivity in the carbohydrate intolerance of human obesity. J. Clin. Invest., **47,** 153, 1968.
127. Shreeve, W. W., Hoshi, M., Oji, N., Shigeta, Y., and Abe, H.: Insulin and the utilization of carbohydrates in obesity. Amer. J. Clin. Nutr., **21,** 1404, 1968.
128. Renold, A. E., Orci, L., Stauffacher, W., Junod, A., and Rouiller, Ch.: Remarks on pancreatic β-cells in spontaneous and experimental diabetes in small laboratory rodents, in *Structure and Function of Pancreatic Islets, II,* edited by B. Hellman, S. Falkmer, and I. Täljedal. Pergamon, London, p. 497, 1970.
129. Stauffacher, W., and Renold, A. E.: Effect of insulin in vivo on diaphragm and adipose tissue of obese mice. Amer. J. Physiol., **216,** 98, 1969.
130. Like, A. A., and Chick, W. L.: Mitotic divisions in pancreatic beta cells. Science, **163,** 941, 1969.
131. Ditzel, J., White, P., and Sargeant, L.: A follow-up study of children of young diabetic mothers. Acta Genet. (Basel), **7,** 101, 1957.
132. Steinberg, A. G.: Inheritance and anticipation in diabetes mellitus in relation to carbohydrate metabolism during pregnancy. Diabetes, **4,** 126, 1955.
133. Jackson, W. P. U.: The prediabetic syndrome: large babies and the (pre)diabetic father. J. Clin. Endocr., **14,** 177, 1954.
134. Warren, S., LeCompte, P. M., and Legg, M. A.: *The Pathology of Diabetes Mellitus,* 2d ed. Lea & Febiger, Philadelphia, 1966.
135. Van Beek, C. C.: Kan men aan een doodgeborene de diagnose diabetes mellitus der moeder stellen? Nederl. T. Geneesk., **83,** 5973, 1939.
136. D'Agostino, A. N., and Bahn, R. C.: A histopathologic study of the pancreas of infants of diabetic mothers. Diabetes, **12,** 327, 1963.
137. Lazarus, S. S., and Volk, B. W.: *The Pancreas in Human and Experimental Diabetes.* Grune & Stratton, New York, 1962.
138. Silverman, J. L.: Eosinophilic infiltration in the pancreas of infants of diabetic mothers, a clinico-pathological study. Diabetes, **12,** 528, 1963.
139. Okamato, K.: Experimental pathology of diabetes mellitus. II. Tohoku J. Exp. Med., **61,** suppl. III, 1, 1955.
140. Okamoto, K.: Induction of a diabetic disposition and of spontaneous diabetes in the descendants of diabetic animals. Tonyobyo, **3,** 33, 1960.
141. Spergel, G., Levy, L. J., and Goldner, M. G.: Impaired glucose tolerance in progeny of rats with induced latent diabetes. J. Clin. Invest., **48,** 799, 1969.
142. Hoet, J. P.: Carbohydrate metabolism during pregnancy. Diabetes, **3,** 1, 1954.
143. O'Sullivan, J. B.: Gestational diabetes: unsuspected, asymptomatic diabetes in pregnancy. New Eng. J. Med., **264,** 1082, 1961.
144. Pyke, D. A.: Parity and diabetes. Lancet, **2,** 818, 1956.
145. FitzGerald, M. G., Malins, J. M., O'Sullivan, D. J., and Wall, M.: The effect of sex and parity on the incidence of diabetes mellitus. Quart. J. Med., **30,** 57, 1961.
146. Mering, J. von, and Minkowski, O.: Diabetes mellitus nach Pankreasexstirpation. Arch. Exp. Path. Pharmakol., **26,** 371, 1890.
147. Dunn, J. S., Sheehan, H. L., and McLetchie, N. G. B.: Necrosis of the islets of Langerhans produced experimentally. Lancet, **1,** 484, 1943.
148. Lukens, F. D. W.: Alloxan diabetes. Physiol. Rev., **28,** 304, 1948.
149. Frerichs, H., and Creutzfeldt, W.: Diabetes durch Beta-Zytotoxine, in *Handbuch des Diabetes Mellitus,* edited by E. F. Pfeiffer, vol. 1, p. 811. Lehmanns, Munich, 1969.
150. Goldner, M. G.: Drug-induced diabetes, in *Diabetes,* p. 140, International Congress Series 172S. Excerpta Medica Foundation, Amsterdam, 1969.
151. Junod, A., Lambert, A. E., Stauffacher, W., and Renold, A. E.: Diabetogenic action of streptozotocin: relationship of dose to metabolic response. J. Clin. Invest., **48,** 2129, 1969.
152. Moloney, P. J., and Coval, M.: Antigenicity of insulin: diabetes induced by specific antibodies. Biochem. J., **59,** 179, 1955.
153. Wright, P. H.: The production of experimental diabetes by means of insulin antibodies. Amer. J. Med., **31,** 892, 1961.
154. Simon, E., and Kraicer, P. F.: The blockade of insulin secretion by mannoheptulose. Israel J. Med. Sci., **2,** 785, 1966.
155. Froesch, E. R., Jakob, A., Zahnd, G. R., and Simon, E.: Suppressible, immunoreactive and non-suppressible insulin-like activities in rats after administration of glucose and induction of hyperglycemia by mannoheptulose. Diabetologia, **2,** 265, 1966.
156. New York Acad. Sci.: Symposium on Diazoxide and the treatment of hypoglycemia. Ann. N.Y. Acad. Sci., **130,** 191, 1967.
157. Young, F. G.: Permanent experimental diabetes produced by pituitary (anterior lobe) injections. Lancet, **2,** 372, 1937.
158. Keterer, B., Randle, P. J., and Young, F. G.: The pituitary growth hormone and metabolic processes, in *Ergebnisse der Physiologie, biologischen Chemie und experimentellen Pharmakologie,* p. 127. Springer, Berlin, 1957.
159. Long, C. N. H.: The influence of the adrenal cortex on carbohydrate metabolism, in *Hormonal Factors in Carbohydrate Metabolism,* p. 136. Little, Brown, Boston, 1953.
160. Thorn, G. W., Renold, A. E., and Cahill, G. F., Jr.: The adrenal and diabetes. Diabetes, **8,** 337, 1959.
161. Houssay, B. A.: Thyroid and diabetes. Vitamins Hormones (N.Y.), **4,** 187, 1946.
162. Salter, J. M., Davidson, I. W. F., and Best, C. H.: The pathologic effects of large amounts of glucagon. Diabetes, **6,** 248, 1957.
163. Lukens, F. D. W., Dohan, F. C., and Wolcott, M. W.: Pituitary-diabetes in the cat: recovery following phlorizin treatment. Endocrinology, **32,** 475, 1943.
164. Dohan, F. C., and Lukens, F. D. W.: Lesions of pancreatic islets produced in cats by administration of glucose. Science, **105,** 183, 1947.
165. Houssay, B. A.: Other hormones, in *Diabetes,* edited by R. H. Williams, p. 233. Hoeber-Harper, New York, 1960.
166. Malins, J. M., FitzGerald, M. G., and Wall, M.: A change in the sex incidence of diabetes mellitus. Diabetologia, **1,** 121, 1965.
167. Sanger, F., Thompson, E. O. P., and Kitai, R.: The amide groups of insulin. Biochem. J., **59,** 509, 1955.
168. Sanger, F.: Chemistry of insulin. Science, **129,** 1340, 1959.
169. Meienhofer, J., Schnabel, E., Brinkoff, O., Zabel, R., Sroka, W., Klostermeyer, H., Brandenburg, D., Okuda, T., and Zahn, H.: Synthese der Insulinketten und ihre Kombination zu insulinaktiven Präparaten. Z. Naturforsch. [B], **18b,** 1120, 1963.

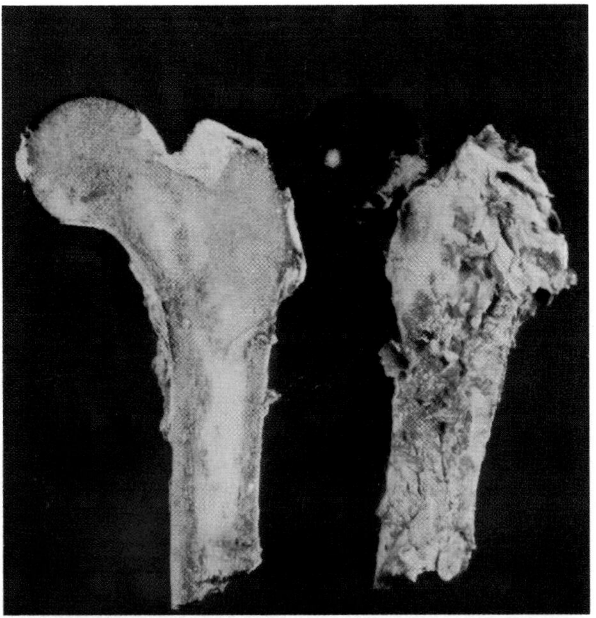

1 Ochronotic pigmentation of the femur of a 56-year-old alcaptonuric subject. (*See Fig. 13-4.*)

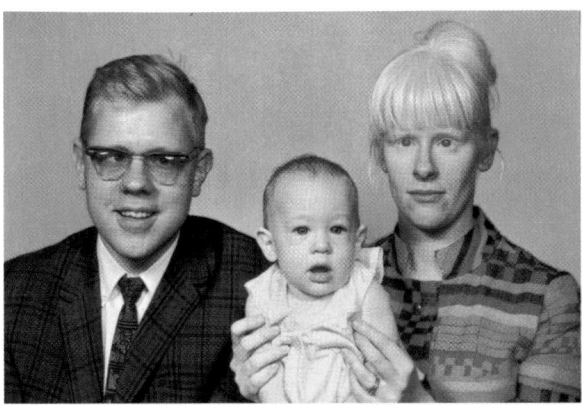

2 In this family, the mother has the tyrosinase-negative type of oculocutaneous albinism; her hair and skin are very light, and her irides are pale blue. The father has the tyrosinase-positive type of albinism; his hair is light brown, and his skin and irides are darker than those of his wife. Their child has normal pigmentation of the skin, hair, and eyes, and has no evidence of ocular albinism. (*See Chapter 14.*) (Photograph kindly provided by Victor A. McKusick, M.D.)

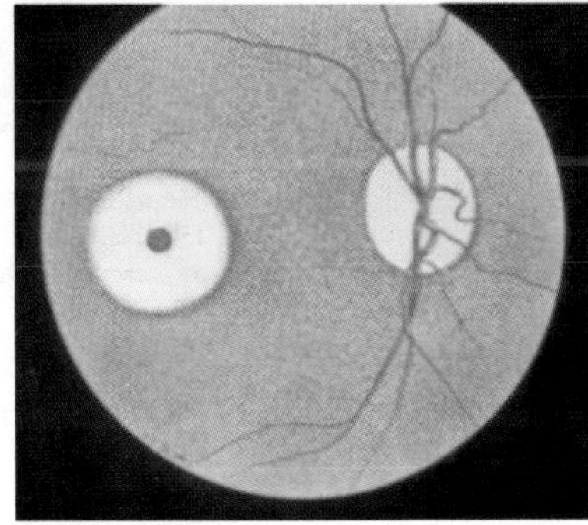

3 The cherry red spot in Tay-Sachs disease. (*See Fig. 29-3.*)

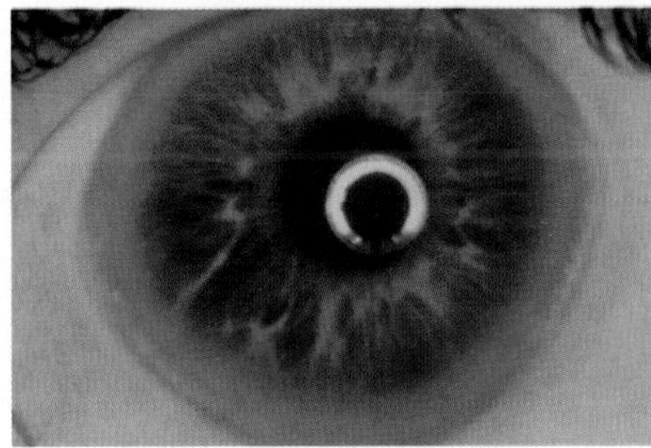

4 Infiltrates in the cornea of a patient with familial lecithin:cholesteryl acyl transferase deficiency. (*See Fig. 27-1.*)

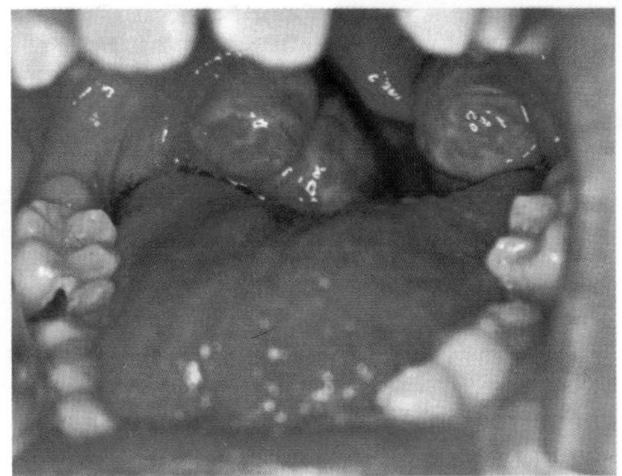

5 Tonsils in Tangier disease. (*See Chapter 26.*)

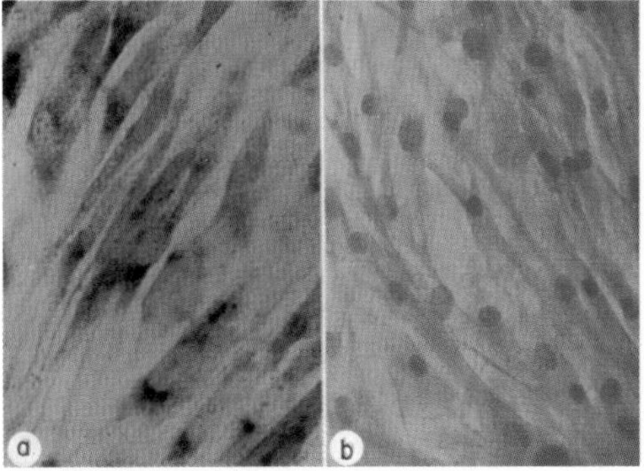

6 Histochemical assay for β-galactosidase activity in cultured skin fibroblasts. A. Normal cells contain blue granules. B. Cells from patient with G_{M1}-gangliosidosis Type 1 contain no granules (see p. 646). (*Courtesy Dr. H. R. Sloan.*)

PLATE II

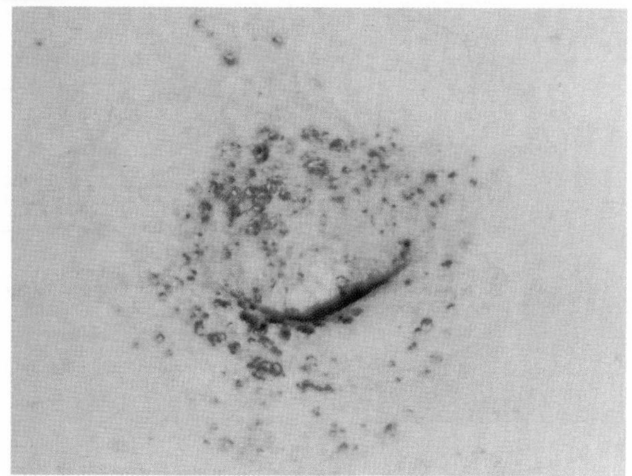

1 The dark red telangiectases of Fabry's disease. *(See Fig. 31-2.)*

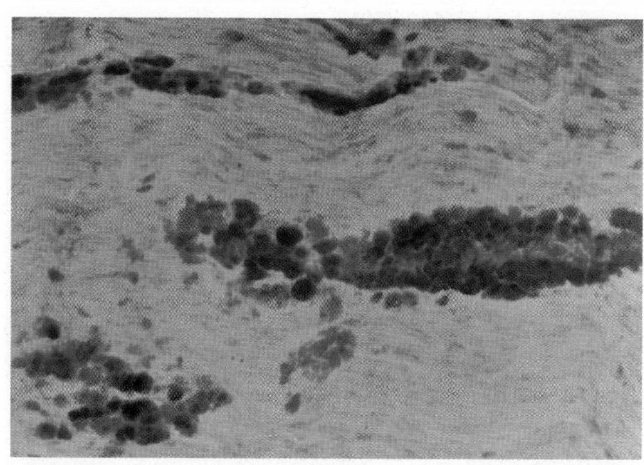

2 The metachromatic granules within Schwann cells and macrophages in a sural nerve biopsy from metachromatic leukodystrophy. *(See Fig. 32-23.)*

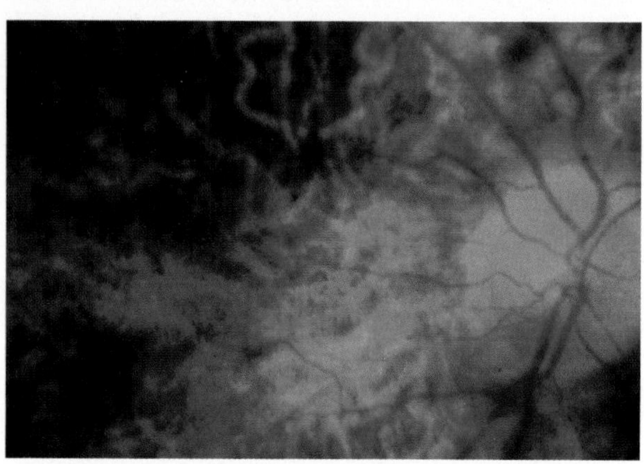

3 Retinitis pigmentosa in a patient with phytanic acid storage disease. *(See Chapter 37.)*

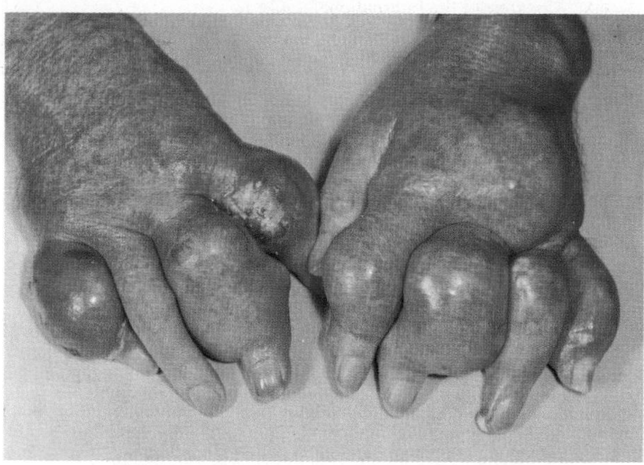

4 Chronic tophaceous gout of severe degree. *(See Chapter 39.) (Courtesy of Dr. R. Wayne Rundles.)*

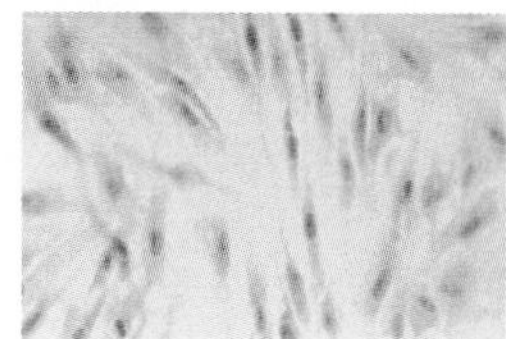

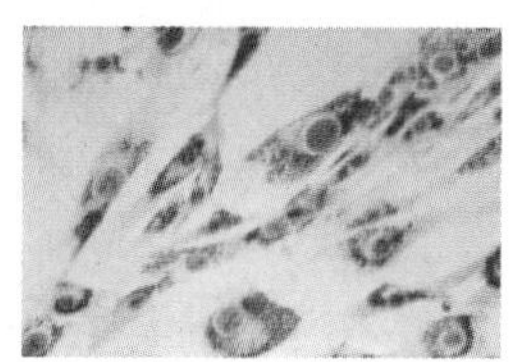

5 Normal and Hurler cultured fibroblasts stained with toluidine blue O (normal on left, Hurler on right). *(See page 1152.)*

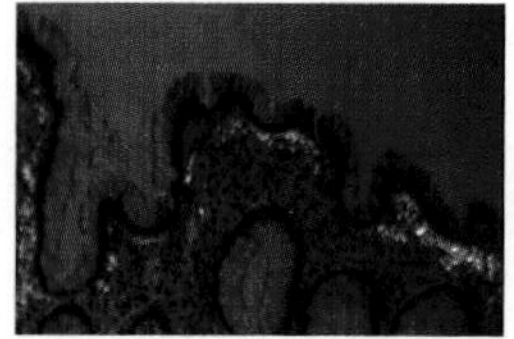

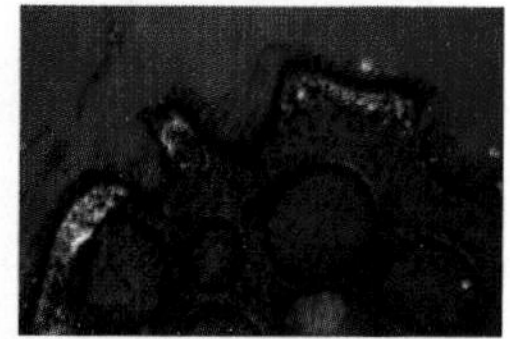

6 Light micrograph of a rectal biopsy demonstrating the green birefringence of amyloid in a patient with secondary amyloidosis. *(See Fig. 50-7.)*

170. Katsoyannis, P. G.: The synthesis of the insulin chains and their combination to biologically active material. Diabetes, **13,** 339, 1964.
171. Institute of Biochemistry, Academia Sinica; Department of Chemistry, Peking University; Institute of Organic Chemistry, Academia Sinica: The total synthesis of crystalline insulin. Kexue Tongbao, **17,** 241, 1966.
172. Adams, M. G., Blundell, T. L., Dodson, E. J., Dodson, G. G., Vijayan, M., Baker, E. N., Harding, D. C., Hodgkin, D. C., Rimmer, B., and Sheat, S.: Structure of rhombohedral 2 zinc insulin crystals. Nature (London), **224,** 491, 1969.
173. Smith, L.: Species variation in the amino acid sequence of insulin. Amer. J. Med., **40,** 662, 1966.
174. Humbel, R.: Personal communication.
175. Markus, G.: Electrolytic reduction of the disulfide bonds of insulin. J. Biol. Chem., **239,** 4163, 1964.
176. Carpenter, F. H.: Relationship of structure to biological activity of insulin as revealed by degradative studies. Amer. J. Med., **40,** 750, 1966.
177. Wilson, S.: Discussion of G. H. Dixon, Recombination of insulin α and β chains, hybrid insulins and synthetic insulin, in *On the Nature and Treatment of Diabetes Mellitus,* edited by B. S. Leibel and G. A. Wrenshall, p. 85. Excerpta Medica Foundation, Amsterdam, 1965.
178. Falkmer, S., and Wilson, S.: Comparative aspects of the immunology and biology of insulin. Diabetologia, **3,** 519, 1967.
179. Wilson, S.: The antigenic loci of insulin, in *Diabetes,* Proceedings of the Sixth Congress of the International Diabetes Federation, Stockholm, 1967, edited by J. Östman, p. 403. Excerpta Medica Foundation, Amsterdam, 1969.
180. Arquilla, E. R., Ooms, H., and Finn, J.: Genetic difference of combining sites of insulin antibodies and importance of C-terminal portion of the A-chain to biological and immunological activity of insulin. Diabetologia, **2,** 1, 1966.
181. Arquilla, E. R., and Bromer, W. W.: Conformation of antigenic determinants on insulin and biologic activity of insulin, in *Diabetes,* Supplement to Proceedings of the Sixth Congress of the International Diabetes Federation, Stockholm, 1967, edited by J. Östman, p. 28. Excerpta Medica Foundation, Amsterdam, 1969.
182. Steiner, D. F., Cunningham, D., Spigelman, L., and Aten, B.: Insulin biosynthesis: evidence for a precursor. Science, **157,** 697, 1967.
183. Chance, R. E., Ellis, R. M., and Bromer, W. W.: Porcine proinsulin: characterization and amino acid sequence. Science, **161,** 165, 1968.
184. Steiner, D. F., Clark, J. L., Nolan, C., Rubenstein, A. M., Margoliash, E., Aten, B., and Oyer, P. E.: Proinsulin and the biosynthesis of insulin. Recent Progr. Hormone Res., **25,** 207, 1969.
185. Lacy, P. E.: The pancreatic beta cell: structure and function. New Eng. J. Med., **276,** 187, 1967.
186. Lacy, P. E., Howell, S. L., Young, D. A., and Fink, C. J.: New hypothesis of insulin secretion. Nature (London), **219,** 1177, 1968.
187. Orci, L., Stauffacher, W., Beaven, D., Lambert, A. E., Renold, A. E., and Rouiller, Ch.: Ultrastructural events associated with the action of tolbutamide and glybenclamide on pancreatic β-cells in vivo and in vitro. Acta Diabet. Lat., **6,** suppl. 1, 271, 1969.
188. Renold, A. E.: Insulin biosynthesis and secretion, a still unsettled topic. New Eng. J. Med., **282,** 173, 1970.
189. Howell, S. L., Kostianovsky, M., and Lacy, P. E.: Beta granule formation in isolated islets of Langerhans. J. Cell Biol., **42,** 695, 1969.
190. Sorensen, R. L., Steffes, W., and Lindall, A. W.: Subcellular localization of proinsulin to insulin conversion in isolated rat islets. Endocrinology, **86,** 88, 1970.
191. Clark, W. R.: The synthesis and accumulation of insulin in the rat embryo during development. Thesis, University of Washington, Seattle, 1968.
192. Lambert, A. E., Junod, A., Stauffacher, W., Jeanrenaud, B., and Renold, A. E.: Organ culture of fetal rat pancreas. I. Insulin release induced by caffeine and by sugars and some derivatives. Biochim. Biophys. Acta, **84,** 529, 1969.
193. Taylor, K. W., Parry, D. G., and Smith, G. H.: Biosynthetic labelling of mammalian insulins in vitro. Nature (London), **203,** 1144, 1964.
194. Howell, S. L., and Taylor, K. W.: Secretion of newly synthetized insulin in vitro. Biochem. J., **102,** 1967.
195. Taylor, K. W.: The biosynthesis of insulin in vitro. Diabetologia, **4,** 279, 1968 (abstract).
196. Goldner, M. G., and Clark, D. E.: The insulin requirement of man after total pancreatectomy. J. Clin. Endocr., **4,** 194, 1944.
197. Whitfield, A. G. W., Crane, C. W., French, J. M., and Bayley, T. J.: Life without a pancreas. Lancet, **1,** 675, 1965.
198. Lazarow, A., Bauer, G. E., and Lindall, A.: Protein synthesis in islet tissue, in *The Structure and Metabolism of the Pancreatic Islets,* edited by S. E. Brolin, B. Hellman, and H. Knutson, p. 203, Pergamon, New York, 1964.
199. Howell, S. L., Young, D. A., and Lacy, P. E.: Isolation and properties of secretory granules from rat islets of Langerhans. III. Studies of the stability of the isolated beta granules. J. Cell Biol., **41,** 167, 1969.
200. Coore, H. G., Hellman, B., Pihl, E., and Taljedal, I. B.: Physicochemical characteristics of insulin secretion granules. Biochem. J., **111,** 107, 1969.
201. Sorensen, R. L., Lindall, A. W., and Lazarow, A.: Studies on the isolated goosefish insulin secretion granule. Diabetes, **18,** 129, 1969.
202. Lindner, F.: Ueber ein genuines Depot-Insulin Präparat (Nativ-Insulin). Med. Chem. (Basel), **4,** 248, 1940.
203. Maske, M.: Interaction between insulin and zinc in the islets of Langerhans. Diabetes, **6,** 335, 1957.
204. Haist, R. E.: Effects of changes in stimulation on the structure and function of islet cells, in *On the Nature and Treatment of Diabetes,* edited by B. S. Leibel and G. A. Wrenshall, p. 12. Excerpta Medica Foundation, Amsterdam, 1965.
205. Logothetopulos, J., Davidson, J. K., Haist, R. E., and Best, C. H.: Degranulation of beta cells and loss of pancreatic insulin after infusions of insulin antibodies or glucose. Diabetes, **14,** 493, 1965.
206. Grodsky, G. M., Curry, D., Landahl, M., and Bennet, L. L.: Further studies on the dynamic aspects of insulin release in vitro with evidence for a two-compartmental storage system. Acta Diabet. Lat., **6,** suppl. I, 554, 1969.
207. Burr, I. M., Stauffacher, W., Balant, L., Renold, A. E., and Grodsky, G. M.: Dynamic aspects of proinsulin release from perifused rat pancreas. Lancet, **2,** 882, 1969.
208. Cerasi, E.: An analogue computer model for the insulin response to glucose infusion. Acta Endocr. (Kobenhavn), **55,** 163, 1967.
209. Porte, D., Jr., and Pupo, A. A.: Insulin response to glucose: evidence for a two pool system in man. J. Clin. Invest., **48,** 2309, 1969.
210. Orci, L., Lambert, A. E., Kanazawa, Y., Renold, A. E., and Rouiller, Ch.: Organ culture of fetal rat pancreas: III. Ultrastructural changes occurring in β-cells during stimulation of insulin release. Chem. Biol. Interactions, **1,** 341, 1969/70.
211. Gorden, P., and Roth, J.: Plasma insulin: Fluctuations in the "big" insulin component in man after glucose and other stimuli. J. Clin. Invest., **48,** 2225, 1969.
212. Randle, P. J., and Taylor, K. W.: Insulin, in *Hormones in Blood,* edited by Ch. Gray and A. L. Bacharach, p. 11. Academic, New York, 1961.
213. Metz, R.: The effects of blood glucose concentration on insulin output. Diabetes, **9,** 89, 1960.
214. Grodsky, G. M., Batts, A., Bennet, L. L., Vcella, C., Mc. Williams, N. B., and Smith, D. F.: Effects of carbohydrate on secretion of insulin from isolated rat pancreas. Amer. J. Physiol., **205,** 638, 1963.
215. Tashima, L., and Cahill, G. F., Jr.: Role of glucagon and insulin in the carbohydrate metabolism of the toadfish. Excerpta Med. Int. Congr. Ser., **74,** 140, 1964.
216. Cahill, G. F., Jr.: Discussion in *On the Nature and Treatment of Diabetes,* edited by B. S. Leibel and G. A. Wrenshall, p. 116. Excerpta Medica Foundation, Amsterdam, 1965.
217. Manns, J. G., Boda, J. M., and Willes, R. F.: Probable role of propionate and butyrate in control of insulin secretion in sheep. Amer. J. Physiol., **212,** 756, 1967.
218. Horino, M., Machlin, L. J., Hertelendy, F., and Kipnis, D. M.: Effect of short chain fatty acids on plasma insulin in ruminant and non-ruminant species, Endocrinology, **83,** 118, 1968.
219. Greenough, W. B., III, Crespin, S. R., and Steinberg, D.: Hypoglycemia and hyperinsulinemia in response to raised free fatty acid levels. Lancet, **2,** 1334, 1967.

220. Crespin, S. R., Greenough, W. B., III, and Steinberg, D.: Stimulation of insulin secretion by infusion of free fatty acids. J. Clin. Invest., **48,** 1934, 1969.
221. Fajans, S. S.: Amino acids and insulin secretion, in *Diabetes,* Proceedings of the Sixth Congress of the International Diabetes Federation, edited by J. Östman, p. 151. Excerpta Medica Foundation, Amsterdam, 1969.
222. Milner, R. D. G., and Hales, C. N.: The role of calcium and magnesium in insulin secretion from rabbit pancreas studied in vitro. Diabetologia, **3,** 47, 1967.
223. Montague, W., and Taylor, K. W.: Pentitols and insulin release by isolated rat islets of Langerhans. Biochem. J., **109.** 333, 1968.
224. Christensen, H. N., and Cullen, A. N.: Behavior in the rat of a transport specific, bicyclic amino acid: hypoglycemic action. J. Biol. Chem., **244,** 1521, 1969.
225. Manns, J. G., and Boda, J. M.: Insulin release by acetate, propionate, butyrate and glucose in lambs and adult sheep. Amer. J. Physiol., **212,** 747, 1967.
226. Grasso, S., Saporito, N., Messina, A., and Reitano, G.: Serum insulin response to glucose and amino acids in the premature infant. Lancet, **2,** 755, 1968.
227. Malaisse, W.: Étude de la sécrétion insulinique in vitro. Ed. Arscia, Brussels, 1969.
228. Stauffacher, W., and Renold, A. E.: Pathophysiology of diabetes mellitus, in ref. [32].
229. Williams, R. H., and Ensinck, J. W.: Secretion, fates and actions of insulin and related products. Diabetes, **15,** 623, 1966.
230. Taljedal, I-B. (editor): *The Structure and Function of the Islets of Langerhans, II.* Pergamon, London, 1970.
231. Biedl, A., and Krans, R.: Über intravenöse Traubenzuckerinfusionen am Menschen. Wien. Klin. Wschr., **9,** 55, 1896.
232. Zunz, E., and La Barre, J.: Hyperinsulinémie consécutive à l'injection de solution de sécrétine non-hypotensive. C. R. Soc. Biol. (Paris), **98,** 1435, 1928.
233. La Barre, J., and Ledrut, J.: À propos de l'action hypoglycémiante des extraits duodénaux. C. R. Soc. Biol. (Paris), **115,** 750, 1934.
234. Laughton, N. B., and Macallum, A. B.: The relation of the duodenal mucosa to the internal secretion of the pancreas. Proc. Roy. Soc. [Biol.], **111,** 37, 1932.
235. Dupré, J.: An intestinal hormone affecting glucose disposal in man. Lancet, **2,** 672, 1964.
236. McIntyre, N., Holdsworth, C. D., and Turner, D. S.: Intestinal factor in the control of insulin secretion. J. Clin. Endocr., **25,** 1317, 1965.
237. Elrick, H., Stimmler, L., Hlad, C. J., Jr., and Arai, Y.: Plasma insulin response to oral and intravenous glucose administration. J. Clin. Endocr., **24,** 1076, 1964.
238. Perley, M. J., and Kipnis, D. M.: Plasma insulin responses to oral and intravenous glucose: studies in normal and diabetic subjects. J. Clin. Invest., **46,** 1954, 1967.
239. Dupré, J., Curtis, J. D., Waddell, R. W., and Beck, J. C.: Alimentary factors in the endocrine response to administration of arginine in man. Lancet, **2,** 28, 1969.
240. Pfeiffer, E. F.: Introduction: Intestinal function in relation to insulin secretion, sec. VIII in *Diabetes,* edited by J. Östman and R. D. G. Milner, International Congress Series, vol. 172, p. 419. Excerpta Medica Foundation, Amsterdam, 1969.
241. Frohman, L. A., Ezdinli, E. Z., and Javid, R.: Effect of vagotomy and vagal stimulation on insulin secretion. Diabetes, **16,** 443, 1967.
242. Chisholm, D. J., Young, J. D., and Lazarus, L.: The gastrointestinal stimulus to insulin release: I. Secretin. J. Clin. Invest., **48,** 1453, 1969.
243. Unger, R. H., Ketterer, H., Dupré, J., and Eisentraut, A. M.: Effects of secretin, pancreozymine and gastrin on insulin and glucagon secretion in anesthetized dogs. J. Clin. Invest., **46,** 630, 1967.
244. Unger, R. H., Ohneda, A., Valverde, I., Eisentraut, A. M., and Exton, J.: Characterization of the response of circulating glucagon-like immunoreactivity to intraduodenal and intravenous administration of glucose. J. Clin. Invest., **47,** 48, 1968.
245. Orci, L., Pictet, R., Forssmann, W. G., Renold, A. E., and Rouiller, Ch.: Structural evidence for glucagon producing cells in the intestinal mucosa of the rat. Diabetologia, **4,** 56, 1968.
246. Porte, D., Jr.: Stimulation of insulin release by beta-adrenergic receptor. Diabetes, **15,** 543, 1966.
247. Porte, D., Jr., Graber, A. L., Kuzuya, T., and Williams, R. H.: The effect of epinephrine on immunoreactive insulin levels in man. J. Clin. Invest., **45,** 228, 1966.
248. Malaisse, W., Malaisse-Lagae, F., Wright, P. H., and Ashmore, J.: Effects of adrenergic and cholinergic agents upon insulin secretion in vitro. Endocrinology, **80,** 975, 1967.
249. Kaneto, A., Kajinuma, H., Kosaka, K., and Nakao, K.: Stimulation of insulin secretion by parasympathicomimetic agents. Endocrinology, **80,** 530, 1967.
250. Luse, S. A., Caramia, F., Gerritsen, G., and Dulin, W. E.: Spontaneous diabetes mellitus in the Chinese hamster: an electron microscopic study of the islets of Langerhans. Diabetologia, **3,** 97, 1967.
251. Orci, L., Lambert, A. E., Kanazawa, Y., Renold, A. E., and Rouiller, C.: Development of fetal rat pancreas in organ culture: a morphological and biochemical study. J. Cell Biol., in press.
252. Curry, D. L., Bennett, L. L., and Grodsky, G. M.: Dynamics of insulin secretion by the perfused rat pancreas. Endocrinology, **83,** 572, 1968.
253. Soeldner, J. S., and Slone, D.: Critical variables in the radioimmunoassay of serum insulin using the double antibody technique. Diabetes, **14,** 771, 1965.
254. Bagdade, J. D., Bierman, E. L., and Porte, D., Jr.: The significance of basal insulin levels in the evaluation of the insulin response to glucose in diabetic and non-diabetic subjects. J. Clin. Invest., **46,** 1549, 1967.
255. Cerasi, E., Effendic, S., and Luft, R.: Role of adrenergic receptors in glucose-induced insulin secretion in man. Lancet, **2,** 301, 1969.
256. Turtle, J. R., and Kipnis, D. M.: An adrenergic receptor mechanism for the control of cyclic 3′5′-adenosine monophosphate synthesis in tissues. Biochem. Biophys. Res. Commun., **28,** 797, 1967.
257. Grodsky, G. M., and Bennet, L. L.: Cation requirement for insulin secretion in the isolated perfused pancreas. Diabetes, **15,** 910, 1966.
258. Sutherland, E. W., and Robinson, G. A.: The role of cyclic AMP in the control of carbohydrate metabolism. Diabetes, **18,** 797, 1969.
259. Lambert, A. E., Jeanrenaud, B., Junod, A., and Renold, A. E.: Organ culture of fetal rat pancreas. II. Insulin release induced by amino- and organic acids, by hormonal peptides, by cationic alterations of the medium and by other agents. Biochim. Biophys. Acta, **184,** 540, 1969.
260. Berson, S. A., and Yalow, R. S.: Insulin in blood and insulin antibodies. Amer. J. Med., **40,** 676, 1966.
261. Rasio, E., and Conard, V.: The distribution of insulin in body fluids, in *Diabetes,* Proceedings of the Sixth Congress of the International Diabetes Federation, Stockholm, edited by J. Östman and R. D. G. Milner, p. 193. Excerpta Medica Foundation, Amsterdam, 1969.
262. Froesch, E. R., Bürgi, H., Müller, W. A., Humbel, R. E., Jakob, A., and Labhart, A.: Nonsuppressible insulinlike activity of human serum: Purification, physicochemical and biological properties and its relation to total serum ILA. Rec. Progr. Hormone Res., **23,** 565, 1967.
263. Samaan, N., Fraser, R., and Dempster, W. J.: The "typical" and "atypical" forms of serum insulin. Diabetes, **12,** 339, 1963.
264. Antoniades, H. N., Bougas, J. A., Camerini-Davalos, R., and Pyle, H. M.: Insulin regulatory mechanisms and diabetes mellitus. Diabetes, **13,** 230, 1964.
265. Samols, E., and Ryder, J. A.: Studies on tissue uptake of insulin in man using a differential immunoassay for endogenous and exogenous insulin. J. Clin. Invest., **40,** 2092, 1961.
266. Rubenstein, A. H., and Spitz, I.: Role of the kidney in insulin metabolism. Diabetes, **17,** 161, 1968.
267. Sonksen, P. H., McCormick, J. R., Egdahl, R. H., and Soeldner, J. S.: Studies on the distribution and binding of insulin in the dog hind limb. Diabetologia, **6,** 65, 1970 (abstract).
268. Rabkin, R., Simon, N. M., Steiner, S., and Colwell, J. A.: Effect of renal disease on renal uptake and excretion of insulin in man. New Eng. J. Med., **282,** 182, 1970.
269. Silvers, A., Swenson, R. S., Farquhar, J. W., and Reaven, G. M.:

Derivation of a three compartment model describing disappearance of plasma insulin-^{131}I in man. J. Clin. Invest., **48,** 1461, 1969.
270. Tomizawa, H. H., and Varandani, P. T.: Glutathione-insulin transhydrogenase of human liver. J. Biol. Chem., **240,** 3191, 1965.
271. Varandani, P. T., and Nafz, M. A.: Glutathione-insulin transhydrogenase of human kidneys. Diabetes, **18,** 176, 1969.
272. Cahill, G. F., Jr., and Owen, O. E.: Some observations on carbohydrate metabolism in man, in *Carbohydrate Metabolism and Its Disorders,* edited by F. Dickens, P. J. Randle, and W. J. Whelan, p. 497. Academic, New York, 1968.
273. Crofford, O. B., and Renold, A. E.: Glucose uptake by incubated rat epididymal adipose tissue. Characteristics of the glucose transport system and action of insulin. J. Biol. Chem., **240,** 3237, 1965.
274. Katzen, H. M., and Schimke, R. T.: Multiple forms of hexokinase in the rat: tissue distribution, age dependency and properties. Proc. Nat. Acad. Sci. U.S.A., **54,** 1218, 1965.
275. Hansen, R. J., Pilkis, S. J., and Krahl, M. E.: Effect of insulin on the synthesis in vitro of hexokinase in rat epididymal adipose tissue. Endocrinology, **86,** 57, 1970.
276. Sneyd, J. G. T., Corbin, J. D., and Park, C. R.: The role of cyclic AMP in the action of insulin, in *Pharmacology of Hormonal Polypeptides and Proteins,* edited by N. Back, L. Martini, and R. Paoletti, p. 367. Plenum, New York, 1968.
277. Bagdade, J. D., Porte, D., Jr., and Bierman, E. L.: Acute insulin withdrawal and the regulation of plasma triglyceride removal in diabetic subjects. Diabetes, **17,** 127, 1968.
278. Park, C. R., Reinwein, D., Henderson, M. J., Regen, D. M., Cadenas, E., and Morgan, H. E.: The action of insulin on the transport of glucose through the cell membrane. Amer. J. Med., **26,** 674, 1959.
279. Villar-Palasi, C., and Larner, J.: The hormonal regulation of glycogen metabolism in muscle. Vitamins Hormones, **26,** 65, 1967.
280. Wool, I. G., Stirewalt, W. S., Kurihara, K., Low, R. B., Bailey, P., and Oyer, D.: Mode of action of insulin in the regulation of protein biosynthesis in muscle. Recent Progr. Hormone Res., **24,** 139, 1968.
281. Owen, O. E., Felig, Ph., Morgan, A. P., Wahren, J., and Cahill, G. F., Jr.: Liver and kidney metabolism during prolonged starvation. J. Clin. Invest., **48,** 574, 1969.
282. Goodman, A. D., Fuisz, R. E., and Cahill, G. F., Jr.: Renal gluconeogenesis in acidosis, alkalosis and potassium deficiency: its possible role in the regulation of renal ammonia production. J. Clin. Invest., **45,** 612, 1966.
283. Williams, T. F., Exton, J. H., Park, C. R., and Regen, D. M.: Stereospecific transport of glucose in the perfused rat liver. Amer. J. Physiol., **215,** 1200, 1968.
284. Cahill, G. F., Jr., Ashmore, J., Earle, A. S., and Zottu, S.: Glucose penetration into liver. Amer. J. Physiol., **192,** 491, 1968.
285. Ray, P. D., Foster, D. O., and Lardy, H. A.: Mode of action of glucocorticoids. I. Stimulation of gluconeogenesis independent of synthesis de novo of enzymes. J. Biol. Chem., **239,** 3396, 1964.
286. Weber, G., Singhal, R. L., and Srivastava, S. K.: Action of glucocorticoids as inducer and insulin as suppressor of biosynthesis of hepatic gluconeogenic enzymes. Advances Enzyme Regulat., **3,** 43, 1965.
287. Wieland, O.: Ketogenesis and its regulation, in *Advances in Metabolic Disorders,* vol. 3, p. 1. Academic, New York, London, 1968.
288. Exton, J. H., Corbin, J. G., and Park, C. R.: Control of gluconeogenesis in liver. IV. Differential effects of fatty acids and glucagon on ketogenesis and gluconeogenesis in the perfused rat liver. J. Biol. Chem., **244,** 4095, 1969.
289. Renold, A. E.: The mechanism of insulin action, an attempted synthesis, in *Handbuch des Diabetes mellitus,* edited by E. F. Pfeiffer, p. 553, 1969.
290. Rodbell, M.: in *Role of Adenyl Cyclase and Cyclic AMP in Biological Processes,* edited by M. Rodbell and P. Condliffe. Washington, in press.
291. Kipnis, D. M., and Noall, M. W.: Stimulation of aminoacid transport by insulin in the isolated rat diaphragm. Biochim. Biophys. Acta, **28,** 226, 1958.
292. Touabi, M., and Jeanrenaud, B.: α-Aminoisobutyric acid uptake in isolated mouse fat cells. Biochim. Biophys. Acta, **173,** 128, 1969.
293. Rodbell, M.: The fat cell in mid-term: its past and future, in *Hormone and Metabolic Research,* suppl. 2, edited by B. Jeanrenaud and D. Hepp, p. 1, 1970.
294. Martin, D. B., and Carter, J. R., Jr.: Insulin-stimulated uptake by subcellular particles from adipose tissue cells. Science, **167,** 873, 1970.
295. Kono, T.: Destruction and restoration of the insulin effector system of isolated fat cells. J. Biol. Chem., **244,** 5777, 1969.
296. Seltzer, H. S., Allen, E. W., and Henon, A. L.: Insulin secretion in response to glycemic stimulus: relation of delayed initial release to carbohydrate intolerance in mild diabetes mellitus. J. Clin. Invest., **46,** 323, 1967.
297. Soeldner, J. S., Tobin, J. D., and Gleason, R. E.: Interrelationships between glucose disappearance and serum insulin responses during intravenous glucose tolerance tests in normal and prediabetic man. Diabetes, **18,** 373, 1969.
298. Conard, V.: Mesure de l'assimilation du glucose. Acta Med. Belg., pp. 37–53, 1955.
299. Karam, J. H., Grodsky, G. M., and Forsham, P. H.: The relationship of obesity and growth hormone to serum insulin levels. Ann. N.Y. Acad. Sci., **131,** 374, 1965.
300. Unger, R. H., and Madison, L. L.: A new diagnostic procedure for mild diabetes mellitus: evaluation of an intravenous tolbutamide response test. Diabetes, **7,** 455, 1958.
301. Fajans, S. S., Floyd, J. C., Knopf, R. F., and Conn, J. W.: Effect of amino acids and proteins on insulin secretion in man. Recent Progr. Hormone Res., **23,** 617, 1967.
302. Renold, A. E., and Cahill, G. F., Jr.: Adipose tissue, in *Handbook of Physiology,* sec. 5. Williams & Wilkins, Baltimore, 1965.
303. Fenn, W. O., and Haege, L. F.: The deposition of glycogen with water in the livers of cats. J. Biol. Chem., **136,** 87, 1940.
304. Cahill, G. F., Jr., Herrera, M. G., Morgan, A. P., Soeldner, J. S., Steinke, J., Reichard, G. A., Jr., and Lipnis, D. M.: Hormone-fuel interrelationships during fasting. J. Clin. Invest., **45,** 1751, 1966.
305. Pogson, C. I.: Interactions of metabolism and the physiological role of insulin. Recent Progr. Hormone Res., **22,** 1, 1966.
306. Owen, O. E., Morgan, A. P., Kemp, H. G., Sullivan, J. M., Herrera, M. G., and Cahill, G. F., Jr.: Brain metabolism during prolonged starvation. J. Clin. Invest., **46,** 1589, 1967.
307. Aguilar-Parada, E., Eisentraut, A. M., and Unger, R.: Effects of starvation on plasma pancreatic glucagon in normal man. Diabetes, **18,** 717, 1969.
308. Marliss, E. B., Aoki, T. T., Ungar, R. H., Soeldner, J. S., and Cahill, G. F., Jr.: Glucagon: levels and metabolic effects in prolonged-fasted man. J. Clin. Invest., **49,** 2256, 1970.
309. Pozefsky, T., Felig, P., Tobin, J., Soeldner, J. S., and Cahill, G. F., Jr.: Amino acid balance across tissues of the forearm in post-absorptive man. Effects of insulin at two dose levels. J. Clin. Invest., **48,** 2273, 1969.
310. Cahill, G. F., Jr.: Starvation in man. New Eng. J. Med., in press, 1971.
311. Benedict, F. G., and Joslin, E. P.: A study of metabolism in severe diabetes. Carnegie Inst. Washington Year Book, **176,** 136, 1912.
312. Atchley, D. W., Loeb, R. F., Richards, D. W., Benedict, E. M., and Driscoll, M. E.: On diabetic acidosis: a detailed study of electrolyte balances following the withdrawal and reestablishment of insulin therapy. J. Clin. Invest., **12,** 297, 1933.
313. Wierzuchowski, M.: Intermediary carbohydrate metabolism. II. Ketosis in phlorizin diabetes. J. Biol. Chem., **73,** 417, 1927.
314. Beatty, C. H., Peterson, R. D., Bocek, R. M., and West, E. S.: Acetoacetate and glucose uptake by diaphragm and skeletal muscle from control and diabetic rats. J. Biol. Chem., **234,** 11, 1959.
315. Sartorius, O. W., Roemmelt, J. C., and Pitts, R. F.: The renal regulation of acid-base balance in man. IV. The nature of the renal compensations in ammonium chloride acidosis. J. Clin. Invest., **28,** 423, 1949.
316. Kety, S. S.: The general metabolism of the brain *in vivo,* in *The Metabolism of the Nervous System,* p. 221. Pergamon, New York, 1957.
317. Melani, F., Rubenstein, A. H., and Steiner, D. F.: Human serum proinsulin. J. Clin. Invest., **49,** 497, 1970.

318. Gorden, P., and Roth, J.: Circulating insulins: "big" and "little." Arch. Intern. Med., **123,** 237, 1969.
319. Gepts, W.: Pathologic anatomy of the pancreas in juvenile diabetes mellitus. Diabetes, **14,** 519, 1965.
320. Maclean, N., and Ogilvie, R. F.: Quantitative estimation of the pancreatic islet tissue in diabetic subjects. Diabetes, **4,** 1, 1955.
321. Ogilvie, R. F.: The endocrine pancreas in human and experimental diabetes, in *Aetiology of Diabetes Mellitus and Its Complications,* p. 49, Ciba Colloquium. Churchill, London, 1964.
322. Wrenshall, G. A., Bogoch, A., and Ritchie, R. C.: Extractable insulin of pancreas: correlation with pathological and clinical findings in diabetic and nondiabetic cases. Diabetes, **1,** 87, 1952.
323. Wrenshall, G. A.: Assays for insulin in the pancreas, in *Diabetes,* edited by R. H. Williams, p. 436. Hoeber-Harper, New York, 1960.
324. Soeldner, J. S.: in ref. [32].
325. Yalow, R. S., and Berson, S. A.: Plasma insulin concentrations in nondiabetic and early diabetic subjects. Diabetes, **9,** 254, 1960.
326. O'Brien, D.: Evidence for an abnormal insulin in diabetes mellitus, in *Early Diabetes,* edited by R. Camerini-Davalos and H. S. Cole, p. 135. Academic, New York, 1970.
327. Seltzer, H. S.: Evidence that the primary lesion in familial diabetes mellitus is an inherited defect of the β cell, in *Early Diabetes,* edited by R. Camerini-Davalos and H. S. Cole, p. 105. Academic, New York, 1970.
328. Camerini-Davalos, R., and Cole, H. S.: *Early Diabetes.* Academic, New York, 1970.
329. Cerasi, E., and Luft, R.: The effect of theophylline on the insulin response to glucose in prediabetic and diabetic patients. Hormone Metabolic Res., **1,** 162, 1969.
330. Lacy, P. E., and Hartroft, W. S.: Electron microscopy of the islets of Langerhans. Ann. N.Y. Acad. Sci., **82,** 287, 1959.
331. Renold, A. E., Gonet, A. E., and Vecchio, D.: Immunopathology of the endocrine pancreas, in *Textbook of Immunopathology,* edited by P. Miescher, vol. 2, p. 595. Grune & Stratton, New York, 1968.
332. Renold, A. E., Steinke, J., Soeldner, J. S., Smith, R. E., and Antoniades, H. N.: Immunologic responses of heifers to the administration of porcine and bovine (homologous) insulin. J. Clin. Invest., **45,** 702, 1966.
333. Grodsky, G. M., Feldman, R., Toreson, W. E., and Lee, J. C.: Diabetes mellitus in rabbits immunized with insulin. Diabetes, **15,** 579, 1966.
334. Steinke, J., and Driscoll, S. G.: The extractable insulin content of pancreas from fetuses and infants of diabetic and control mothers. Diabetes, **14,** 573, 1965.
335. Meyenburg, H., von: Ueber "Insulitis" bei Diabetes. Schweiz. Med. Wschr., **70,** 554, 1940.
336. LeCompte, P. M.: "Insulitis" in early juvenile diabetes. Arch. Path., **66,** 450, 1958.
337. Berns, A. W., Owens, C. T., Hirata, Y., and Blumenthal, H. T.: The pathogenesis of diabetic glomerulosclerosis. II. A demonstration of insulin-binding capacity of the various histopathological components of the disease by fluorescence microscopy. Diabetes, **11,** 308, 1962.
338. Moore, J. M., and Neison, J. M. E.: Antibodies to gastric mucosa and thyroid in diabetes mellitus. Lancet, **2,** 645, 1963.
339. Pettit, M. D., Landing, B. H., and Guest, G. M.: Antithyroid antibody in juvenile diabetics. J. Clin. Endocr., **21,** 209, 1961.
340. Carpenter, C. C. J., Solomon, N., Silverberg, S. G., Bledsoe, T., Northcutt, R. C., Klinenberg, J. R., Bennett, L. L., and Harvey, A.: Schmidt's syndrome: a review of the literature and a report of 15 new cases including ten instances of coexisting diabetes mellitus. Medicine, **43,** 153, 1964.
341. Irvine, W. J., Stewart, A. G., and Scarth, L.: A clinical and immunological study of adrenocortical insufficiency (Addison's disease). Clin. Exp. Immun., **2,** 31, 1967.
342. Randle, P. J.: The glucose fatty acid cycle, in *Aetiology of Diabetes Mellitus and Its Complications,* Ciba Colloquium, p. 192. Churchill, London, 1964.
343. Vallance-Owen, J.: Synalbumin insulin antagonism, in *Diabetes,* edited by J. Östman and R. D. G. Milner, International Congress Series 172, p. 243. Excerpta Medica Foundation, Amsterdam, 1969.
344. Young, D. A. B.: A serum inhibitor of insulin action on muscle: its detection and properties. Diabetologia, **3,** 287, 1967.
345. Martin, F. I. R., and Stocks, A. E.: Insulin sensitivity and ^{131}I-insulin metabolism in juvenile-type diabetics. Aust. Ann. Med., **16,** 289, 1967.
346. Martin, F. I. R., and Stocks, A. E.: Insulin sensitivity and vascular disease in insulin-dependent diabetics. Brit. Med. J., **2,** 81, 1968.
347. Waddell, W. R., and Field, R. A.: Carbohydrate metabolism in atherosclerosis. Metabolism, **9,** 900, 1967.
348. Kingsbury, K. J.: Glucose tolerance, age and atherosclerosis. Postgrad. Med. J., **44,** suppl., 944, 1968.

CHAPTER FIVE

PENTOSURIA *

Howard H. Hiatt

The first six decades which followed the original description by Salkowski and Jastrowitz in 1892 of an individual with essential pentosuria [1] produced much information concerning the clinical aspects of this condition but virtually none that cast light on the nature of the biochemical lesion. Clinical and laboratory studies in the ensuing 18 years, however, led to identification of the metabolic defect. As a result, and perhaps even more significantly, important information was uncovered concerning the operation in normal individuals of a previously unknown pathway of carbohydrate metabolism. Such an elucidation of a normal mechanism by studies of an accident of nature led Garrod [2] 43 years ago to stress "the lessons of rare maladies," and prompted Harvey [3] 300 years earlier to note that "nature is nowhere accustomed more openly to display her secret mysteries than in cases where she shows traces of her workings apart from the beaten path."

A consideration of essential pentosuria requires its separation from other conditions in which a five-carbon sugar is excreted in the urine. Essential pentosuria, or chronic essential pentosuria, is the only member of the group in which a genetic defect accounts for the melituria. It may be further defined as an innocuous condition, presumably present from birth, in which a relatively constant amount of the pentose L-xylulose appears in the urine. It has no apparent relation to diabetes mellitus and has been described almost exclusively in Jews. It is the result of an impairment in the metabolism of glucuronic acid and may easily be distinguished from several other situations in which much smaller quantities of certain pentoses other than L-xylulose are found in the urine (Table 5-1). The structure of some of the urinary pentoses follows:

L-Xylulose	D-Ribose	D-Ribulose	L-Xylose	L-Arabinose
H_2COH	HC=O	H_2COH	HC=O	HC=O
C=O	HCOH	C=O	HOCH	HCOH
HCOH	HCOH	HCOH	HCOH	HOCH
HOCH	HCOH	HCOH	HOCH	HOCH
H_2COH	H_2COH	H_2COH	H_2COH	H_2COH

Alimentary pentosuria is the term applied to the excretion of small amounts of arabinose or xylose[1] following the ingestion of unusually large quantities of such fruits as plums, cherries, and grapes, and fruit juices [4–6]. Small amounts of D-ribose are often present in urine from healthy persons, and slightly larger quantities may be found in the urine of some patients with muscular dystrophy [7], presumably as a result of the excessive breakdown of ribose-containing nucleotide in degenerating muscle. Finally, traces of L-xylulose [8, 9] and of D-ribulose [9] may be found in the urine of normal individuals. It is essential pentosuria with which this review will be primarily concerned.

HISTORICAL SURVEY

In 1887 Kiliani [10] demonstrated that arabinose, the sugar of gum arabic, was a member of a hitherto undescribed class of sugars containing, in contrast to the hexoses, only five carbon atoms. Shortly thereafter, the wood sugar xylose was identified as another member of this group. The biologic significance of this class of sugars was strengthened by the report by Salkowski and Jastrowitz of a human being in whose urine a pentose was consistently excreted [1]. This

*This work was supported in part by funds from the American Cancer Society, Inc., and the Public Health Service.

The author is most grateful to Dr. Margaret W. Lasker and Dr. J. H. Renwick for their very helpful suggestions.

[1] Although L-arabinose and L-xylose are said to be the alimentary pentoses [4, 5], the evidence for this chemical identification is not convincing.

Table 5-1. TYPES OF PENTOSURIA

Type	Urine pentose	Amount excreted, gm/24 hr	Cause	Origin of pentose
Essential	L-Xylulose	1.0–4.0	Metabolic error	D-Glucuronic acid
Alimentary	L-Arabinose L-Xylose	Less than 0.100	Excessive fruit intake	Dietary fruit
"Ribosuria"	D-Ribose	Up to 0.030	Muscular dystrophy	Muscle coenzymes (?)
Normal	L-Xylulose D-Ribose D-Ribulose	Up to 0.060 Up to 0.015 Traces		

sugar was not fermented by yeast, was optically inactive, and yielded an osazone with a melting point of 159°C. The latter observation led these authors to suggest that the sugar was a pentose. Several similar case reports appeared in the German literature during the next decade, and in 1906 Janeway [11], in a paper entitled "Essential Pentosuria in Two Brothers," recorded the first instances in an American publication. Although Janeway acknowledged that in many of the previous reports in the literature neurasthenic symptoms were prominent, he stressed that no harmful effects of the disorder were known. He emphasized that the most important responsibility of the physician was to explain carefully to the patient the difference between his ailment and diabetes mellitus and to effect "the removal of any dietetic restrictions he may have been subjected to." Although more than a half century has elapsed since Janeway's report, his advice still points out an essential function of any physician confronted by a person with pentosuria. Two years after Janeway's paper, in his classic Croonian lectures of 1908 Garrod [12] reviewed 30 recorded cases of essential pentosuria, and he assigned this abnormality along with cystinuria, alcaptonuria, and albinism to a category which he labeled as "inborn errors of metabolism." He stressed the differences between essential pentosuria and the alimentary variety. Garrod noted the incidence of essential pentosuria in Jews, and the tendency for the condition to occur in several members of the same family. A prevalent early impression that pentosuria frequently accompanies diabetes mellitus [13] has not been borne out.

Much of the present knowledge concerning the clinical aspects of pentosuria, its genetic transmission, and the nature of the urinary sugar is derived from the careful observations of Enklewitz and Lasker [14–20]. More than half their 70 subjects with pentosuria were followed for periods in excess of 16 years. Fifty years following the first description of pentosuria, Derivaux [21] was able to collect 163 case reports from the literature, and in a 1958 review of the subject this figure exceeded 200 [22].

For many years controversy existed concerning the nature of the sugar in pentosuric urine. The first chemical identification was that of Neuberg [23], who in 1900 reported that the sugar present in the urine of one case was racemic arabinose. Five additional individuals with arabinosuria were subsequently described by Cammidge and Howard [24], and single similar cases were noted by a number of authors, including Aron [25], Luzzatto [26], and Schüler [27]. Zerner and Waltuch [28] in 1913 presented convincing evidence that the urinary pentose was optically active and that it was not arabinose. The following year Levene and LaForge showed that the urinary sugar in a case of pentosuria was L-xylulose[2]

[2] The early reports of "D-xyloketose" excretion were published prior to the adoption of the current practice of classifying sugars according to their structural relation to D- and L-glyceraldehyde. Throughout this review the present convention will be followed, regardless of the terminology applied in the original reports.

[29]. Their identification was based on the following observations:

1 An osazone of the urinary sugar had a melting point of 160 to 163°C; when it was mixed with an osazone of D-xylose, the melting point was increased by 40°.
2 The initial optical rotation of the osazone was lower than the equilibrium rotation; this is characteristic of xylosazone but not of arabinosazone.
3 The foregoing observations indicated that the urinary pentosazone was a xylosazone. On the basis of the optical rotation of the urinary sugar ($\alpha_D^{20} = +33.1°$), the character of its *p*-bromphenylhydrazone, and its behavior in oxidation experiments, Levene and LaForge concluded that the urinary pentose could only have been L-xylulose.

In the same year Zerner and Waltuch [30] isolated the sugar from the urine of two patients with pentosuria and also concluded that it was L-xylulose. A similar conclusion concerning the pentose in their cases was reached by Hiller [31], Greenwald [32], and Enklewitz and Lasker [15]. Some of the early reports of arabinosuria were subsequently corrected. For example, a patient of Solis Cohen was first described in 1909 as having arabinosuria [33]. At that time the author assumed from previously reported cases that arabinose was the urinary sugar excreted in pentosuria. However, the patient was followed for almost three decades, and in a follow-up report which appeared in 1936 [34], the same author indicated that he had identified the urinary sugar as L-xylulose, and that his earlier impression had been in error. Similarly, a patient reported as having arabinosuria in 1913 [25] was reexamined 40 years later; paper chromatography of his urine revealed the major sugar component to be L-xylulose, and no evidence of arabinose was found [35].

The question of arabinosuria was considered at length in 1950 by Lasker [19], who indicated that she had identified L-xylulose in the urine of 72 individuals with pentosuria but had never seen a patient with arabinosuria. She further stated that no case of arabinosuria had been reported since 1928 and that since in early reports the arabinose was always identified by the same method, this impression may have been in error. Studies with paper chromatographic techniques have provided further corroboration that L-xylulose is the only sugar excreted in substantial amount in pentosuria. In addition to L-xylulose a small quantity of L-arabitol has been isolated from the urine of one pentosuric patient [36]; other reports that pentosuric patients excrete more than one pentose [35, 37] will be considered below.

The constancy of the amount of urine pentose excreted by individuals with pentosuria has long been recognized. Enklewitz and Lasker [16] found that the excretion in five adults varied from 1.1 to 3.7 gm per 24 hr, but that the daily variation in any given subject never exceeded 0.9 gm. The excretion is independent of dietary variations: early reports by Janeway [11] and Klercker [13] that the amount of urinary pentose can be altered by changes in dietary nucleic acid or protein have not been substantiated. Margolis noted a marked increase in pentose excretion in pentosuric subjects following aminopyrine ingestion [38]. When Enklewitz and Lasker observed a similar stimulation not only following the intake of certain other drugs, including borneol, antipyrine, and menthol, but also after the administration of glucuronic acid [16], they ascribed the effect of the drugs to their glucuronogenic action. The metabolic interrelations of glucuronic acid and L-xylulose, however, remained obscure, and there was no experimental evidence for Everett's postulate that an abnormal enzyme system existed in pentosuric patients which decarboxylated glucuronic acid to L-xylulose [39]. The identification of L-xylulose as an intermediate in the metabolism of glucuronic acid [40, 41], the elucidation of the reactions involved in the further metabolism of L-xylulose [42, 43], and the demonstration of xylitol metabolism by erythrocytes [44, 45] were followed by the localization of the biochemical defect [46]. Much of the present concept stems from the careful studies of Touster and his associates [40–43]. Further contributions have come from the laboratories of Ashwell [47–51], Burns [52], Lehninger [53], the author [75, 88, 89, 95], Wang and van Eys [46], and others. Not only have these studies permitted insight into the biochemical aberration in pentosuria, but they have also provided important information concerning the operation of the glucuronic acid oxidation pathway in normal individuals.

PENTOSE METABOLISM IN MAN

Several five-carbon sugars are known to be present in man. Some, such as ribose and deoxyribose, are present as part of more complex substances, including the nucleic acids and certain coenzymes. Others, including D-xylulose, D-ribulose, and L-xylulose, are intermediates in metabolic pathways and normally are not detectable in body fluids, or are present only in trace quantity. Finally, there are those which are not known to be synthesized by man but which occasionally may be ingested and thereafter are excreted in the urine. These include arabinose and xylose.

Many pathways of carbohydrate metabolism involve pentoses as key intermediates (for a summary see [54]). A consideration of these pathways is essential to understanding of the several varieties of pentosuria that have been described, including essential pentosuria.

The Pentose Phosphate Pathway [55]

Ribose, the sugar moiety found in all ribonucleic acids and several coenzymes, may be synthesized from glucose by either the oxidative or the nonoxidative reactions of the pentose phosphate pathway (Fig. 5-1). In the oxidative reactions glucose-6-phosphate is converted successively to 6-phosphogluconolactone, 6-phosphogluconic acid, and, following oxidative removal of its first carbon atom, ribulose-5-phosphate. The latter may be isomerized to ribose-5-phosphate. In this series of reactions, for every molecule of pentose phosphate synthesized from hexose phosphate, two molecules of nicotinamide adenine dinucleotide phosphate (NADP) are reduced to NADPH. Much information has accumulated indicating that the conversion of the coenzyme from its oxidized to its reduced form is as important a function of these reactions as pentose production [54]. This conclusion is based on the evidence for the NADPH requirement of a variety of reductive synthetic reactions, and on observations which suggest that the oxidative reactions of the pentose phosphate pathway are the principal means available to the cell for NADP reduction.

Ribose may also be produced nonoxidatively from hexose phosphate via the transketolase and transaldolase reactions. In these reactions the first two carbon atoms of one molecule of fructose-6-phosphate may be cleaved and condensed with a molecule of triose phosphate, under the influence of the enzyme transketolase. This results in the formation of one molecule of xylulose-5-phosphate and one of erythrose-4-phosphate. The latter, together with another molecule of fructose-6-phosphate, may then participate in the transaldolase reaction, resulting in the production of a molecule of sedoheptulose-7-phosphate and one of triose phosphate. In another reaction catalyzed by transketolase these products may undergo conversion to xylulose-5-phosphate and ribose-5-phosphate. The xylulose-5-phosphate may be epimerized to ribulose-5-phosphate, which, as already noted, can be isomerized to ribose-5-phosphate. Thus, in this series of reactions there is no net loss of carbon, and two molecules of hexose phosphate and one of triose phosphate may be converted to three molecules of pentose phosphate. Available data indicate that in animals [56, 57] and in man [58] ribose is normally synthesized from hexose by way of both the oxidative and the nonoxidative reactions of the pentose phosphate pathway. The fact that thiamine pyrophosphate is a cofactor for the enzyme transketolase [59] accounts for the block in ribose synthesis by way of the nonoxidative sequence of reactions in the thiamine-deficient animal [60].

In contrast to the oxidative reactions, which afford only a mechanism for pentose production from hexose, the transketolase-transaldolase sequence is reversible and provides a means for the interconversion of hexose and pentose [61]. Evidence has been presented demonstrating that the nonoxidative reactions mediate the conversion of ribose to hexose in man [62]. It has also been shown that ribose may participate directly in riboside [60] and nucleic acid [63] synthesis. Thus, mechanisms exist for the disposition of any ribose released in nucleic acid or coenzyme breakdown.

Small quantities (up to 2.8 μmoles per 24 hr per kg body weight) of ribose have been reported in normal human urine [7]. This presumably represents either newly synthesized ribose or pentose released from nucleic acids or coenzymes which escapes further metabolism. It has been asserted that ribose excretion is slightly but significantly increased in

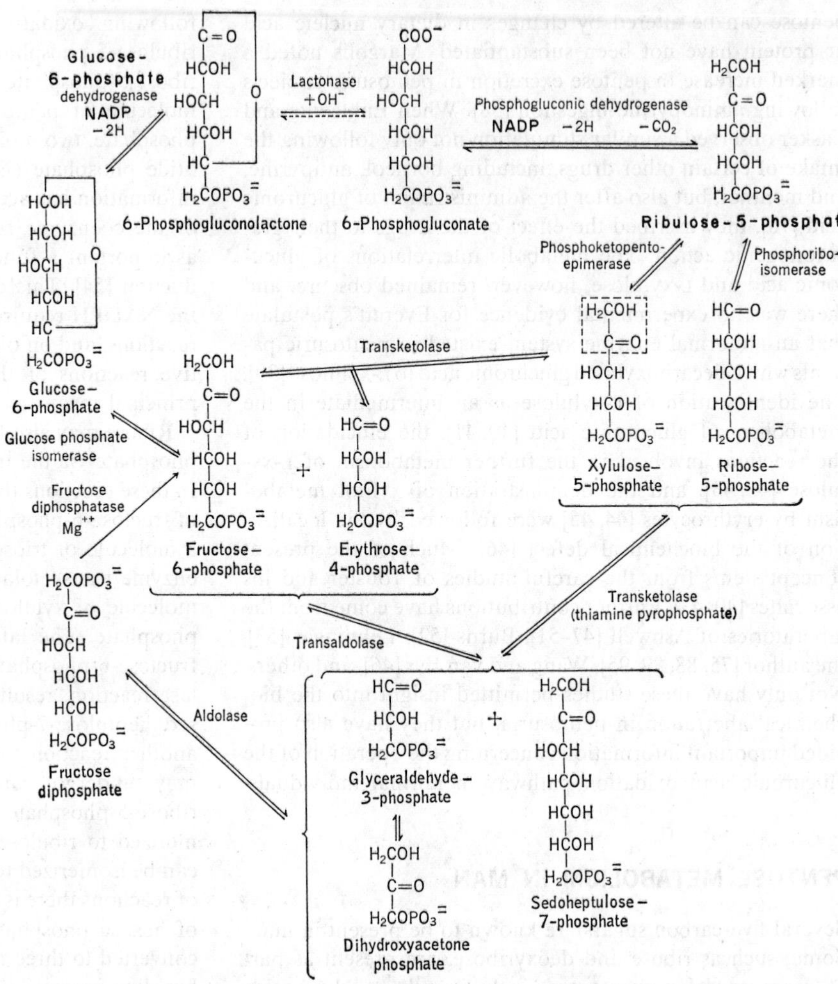

Figure 5-1. The phosphogluconate-oxidative pathway. (*By permission of B. L. Horecker and H. H. Hiatt* [54].)

patients with myopathies, presumably because of the increased breakdown of ribose-containing compounds in diseased muscle [7], but this observation has not met universal acceptance [64]. A metabolite of histamine, imidazoleacetic acid, is excreted by the rat [65, 66] and by man [58] in part as the riboside. Ribulose, a trace constituent of normal urine [9], is presumably excreted following hydrolysis of the phosphate ester, which is an intermediate in the pentose phosphate pathway.

Deoxyribose, the sugar component of deoxyribonucleic acid, is apparently synthesized by way of direct reduction of the ribose molecule at the nucleoside diphosphate level [67].

The Glucuronic Acid Oxidation Pathway

The pentoses L-xylulose and D-xylulose and the pentitol xylitol are intermediates in the glucuronic acid oxidation pathway (Fig. 5-2). The carbon skeleton of D-glucuronic acid is known to originate in glucose [68, 69], and uridine nucleotides are involved as intermediates [70, 71]. As has been noted, the studies of Touster [40–43], Ashwell [47–51], Burns [52], and Lehninger [53], and their associates have provided much information concerning the further metabolism of D-glucuronic acid. A reductive reaction involving NADPH as a cofactor results in the conversion of D-glucuronic acid to L-gulonic acid. L-Gulonolactone has been shown to be an intermediate in the synthesis of ascorbic acid in most animal species, but in primates and in the guinea pig this transformation cannot take place. L-Gulonic acid, however, may in all animal species examined be oxidized to β-keto-L-gulonic acid [50], which, in turn, is enzymatically decarboxylated to L-xylulose [49, 51]. In the latter reaction the atom corresponding to the sixth carbon atom of the parent glucose molecule is oxidized to CO_2. Carbon atom 1 of L-xylulose is derived from the fifth carbon atom of glucose. Touster has prepared two enzymes from guinea pig liver, one of which catalyzes the reduction of L-xylulose to the sugar alcohol xylitol and the other of which promotes the oxidation of xylitol to D-xylulose [42, 43]. These reactions require NADPH and nicotinamide adenine dinucleotide (NAD), respectively. It is noteworthy that in contrast to other schemes of intermediary carbohydrate metabolism in which only phosphate esters participate, these reactions involve the

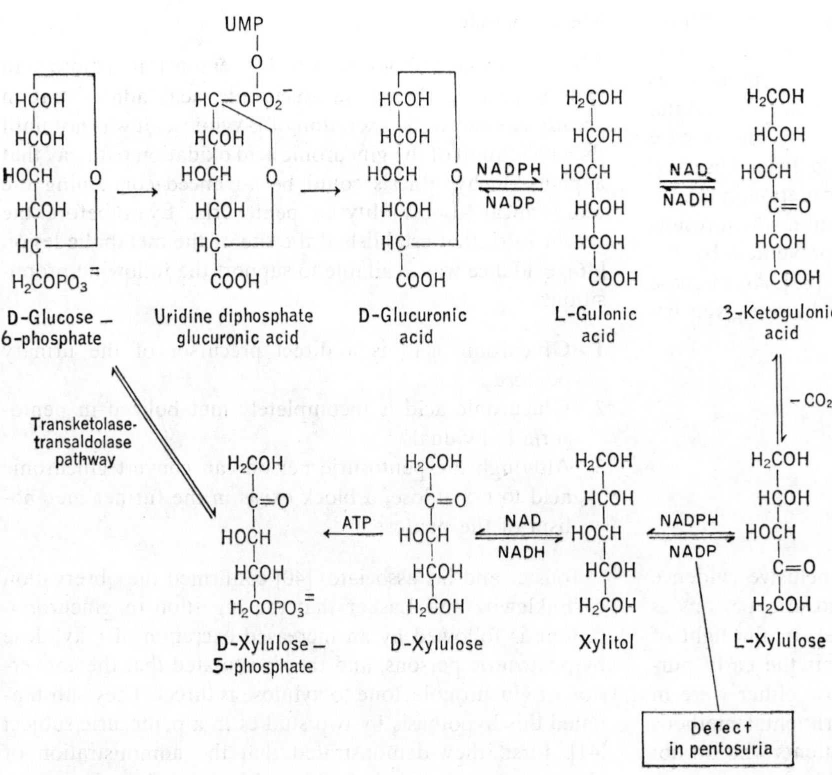

Figure 5-2. The glucuronic acid oxidation pathway.

free sugars. Hickman and Ashwell [48] have described a kinase for D-xylulose in mammalian liver. D-Xylulose-5-phosphate will be recognized as an intermediate in the pentose phosphate pathway and may, of course, be converted to ribose-5-phosphate and to hexose phosphate. A kinase for L-xylulose has been purified from bacteria [72], but there is no evidence for this enzyme in mammalian tissues. Evidence has been presented [72a] suggesting that the pathway is operative in rat adipose tissue, and that activity is increased in tissue from starved or diabetic animals and in human diabetics [73].

The elucidation of the reactions involved in glucuronic acid metabolism provides insight not only into the origin of the L-xylulose found in trace amount in normal urine, but also into the site of the defect in individuals with chronic essential pentosuria. Further, it explains the hitherto poorly understood increase in L-xylulose excretion by pentosuric subjects given glucuronic acid.

The glucuronic acid oxidation pathway does not play an indispensable role in human metabolism, for individuals with pentosuria, in whom the pathway is blocked, suffer no ill effects from the abnormality. It does appear to be responsible for *myo*-inositol catabolism [74]. Although the reactions of the glucuronic acid oxidation pathway together with those of the pentose phosphate pathway provide a potential mechanism for ribose biosynthesis from hexose (i.e., hexose phosphate → glucuronic acid → xylulose → xylulose phosphate → ribose phosphate), animal studies indicate that little ribose is normally produced by way of this sequence of reactions [75]. In most mammalian species the early reactions of the pathway are required for the production of L-gulonic acid, a precursor of ascorbic acid [76]. In primates and the guinea pig, however, ascorbic acid cannot be synthesized.[3] Thus, in man the pathway serves to return a portion of glucuronic acid carbon to the mainstream of carbohydrate metabolism.

Effects of Drugs

The basis for the effect of drugs and hormones on the glucuronic acid oxidation pathway remains a fascinating but poorly understood area. Margolis' early observation that aminopyrine stimulates the excretion of L-xylulose by individuals with pentosuria [38] was followed by reports indicating that this drug and others, such as Chloretone and barbital, stimulate free glucuronic acid [78] and ascorbic acid [79] excretion in animals. The drug effect is apparently not related to any known detoxification mechanism, since barbital is excreted unchanged. Studies of Burns and his associates indicate that the drugs enhance the production of glucuronic acid, as well as ascorbic acid (and presumably L-xylulose in pentosuria) from glucose [80] and from galactose [81]. Increased levels of uridine diphosphate glucose dehydrogenase have been found in livers of animals treated with

[3] A report of the urinary excretion of radioactive ascorbic acid following administration of radioactive glucuronolactone [77] requires confirmation and amplification.

some of [82, 83], but not all [83], the drugs known to stimulate ascorbic acid production. Hormonal involvement in this process is indicated by the observation of Burns and his associates that the administration of Chloretone or barbital to hypophysectomized rats is not followed by an increase in ascorbic acid excretion [78]. It has also been observed that thyroid hormone stimulates pentose excretion in the rat [84], and that the increase in pentose excretion which results from exposure to low temperatures is prevented by the administration of thyroid-blocking agents [85]. An increase in L-xylulose excretion by normal human beings given triiodothyronine has been reported [86].

THE BIOCHEMICAL ABNORMALITY IN ESSENTIAL PENTOSURIA

Nature of the Urinary Sugar

As has been pointed out, there is now conclusive evidence that the urinary sugar excreted by pentosuric persons is L-xylulose (L-xyloketose, L-threopentulose). In the light of present knowledge one must conclude that the early purported demonstrations of urinary arabinose either were in error because of deficiencies in the experimental methods employed or else were concerned with patients who do not fit into this category. L-Xylulose is excreted in fairly constant amount, ranging between 1.0 and 4.0 gm per 24 hr. The excretion is increased following the intake of glucuronic acid and of certain drugs, but it is unaffected by diet and is not altered by insulin administration.

Much smaller quantities of other sugars in addition to L-xylulose have been reported in pentosuric urine. Touster and his associates [36] found arabitol and suggested that this sugar alcohol may be derived from L-xylulose reduction. Wolfson, Cohn, and Devaney [37] observed a second unidentified component following chromatography of pentosuric urine, and Barnes and Bloomberg [35] found small amounts of several substances in addition to large quantities of L-xylulose following chromatography of deionized urine from several pentosuric subjects. Since one substance which appeared in all the urines examined by Barnes and Bloomberg had a chromatographic mobility similar to that of xylose, some of the author's unpublished observations seem pertinent. Following the procedure of Barnes and Bloomberg, the author, too, found a xylose-like component in the urine of two pentosuric subjects. This material was eluted from paper chromatograms and was found by Ashwell [87] to behave like L-xylose in several enzymatic reactions. However, this substance was not present in pentosuric urine subjected to paper chromatography *without* prior exposure to ion-exchange resins. In addition, normal urine to which only L-xylulose was added and which was then deionized and chromatographed on paper also exhibited the xylose spot. Accordingly, the author has concluded that the appearance of L-xylose in chromatograms of pentosuric urine is an artifact attributable to the preparative procedure.

Site of the Defect

Although Enklewitz and Lasker [16] demonstrated more than twenty years earlier that glucuronic acid administration greatly enhanced the excretion of L-xylulose, it was not until the elucidation of the glucuronic acid oxidation pathway that a plausible hypothesis could be advanced concerning the biochemical abnormality in pentosuria. Even before the recent work that established the site of the metabolic lesion [46], evidence was available to support the following propositions:

1 Glucuronic acid is a direct precursor of the urinary pentose.
2 Glucuronic acid is incompletely metabolized in pentosuric individuals.
3 Although the pentosuric person can convert glucuronic acid to L-xylulose, a block exists in the further metabolism of the pentose.

Touster and his associates [40] confirmed the observation of Enklewitz and Lasker that the ingestion of glucuronolactone is followed by an increased excretion of L-xylulose by pentosuric persons, and they postulated that the conversion of glucuronolactone to xylulose is direct. They substantiated this hypothesis by two studies in a pentosuric subject [41]. First, they demonstrated that the administration of glucuronolactone labeled with ^{13}C in its sixth carbon atom (the carboxyl carbon) was followed by the excretion of nonisotopic L-xylulose. Second, they showed that the ingestion of glucuronolactone 1-^{13}C was followed by the urinary excretion of heavily labeled pentose, the isotope of which was predominantly in the fifth carbon atom. These data indicate that the carboxyl carbon of glucuronic acid is lost in the conversion to L-xylulose but that the rest of the molecule is preserved intact. Touster also demonstrated that some normal human beings and guinea pigs excrete traces of L-xylulose and that this excretion is slightly augmented following glucuronolactone ingestion. These observations strengthened the concept that L-xylulose is a metabolic intermediate in normal subjects.

The following study from Hiatt's laboratory supported the hypothesis that a defect in glucuronic acid metabolism exists in pentosuria. Let us postulate that a pentosuric person can remove carbon atom 6 of glucuronolactone with unimpaired efficiency, but that he is incapable of metabolizing the remainder of the carbon chain. Then, following the administration of glucuronolactone uniformly labeled with ^{14}C, there should be six times as much $^{14}CO_2$ in the expired air of a normal person as is present in that of a pentosuric person. These expectations were fulfilled in an experiment that is shown in Fig. 5-3. In this study 5 microcuries of glucuronolactone uniformly labeled with ^{14}C (obtained through the generosity of Dr. N. Artz, Corn Products Refining Co., Argo, Ill.) was given intravenously to a 16-year-old male with essential pentosuria and to a 22-year-old female with no abnormality of carbohydrate metabolism. Samples of expired air were collected at intervals for 6 hr thereafter and

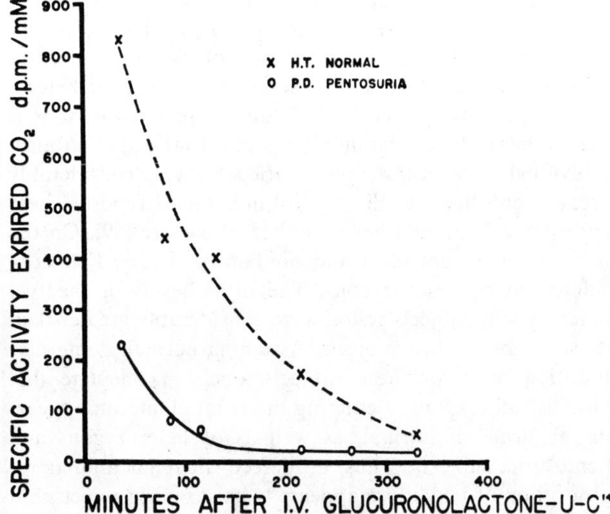

Figure 5-3 $^{14}CO_2$ excretion in the expired air following the intravenous administration of glucuronolactone uniformly labeled with ^{14}C to a normal subject and to a pentosuric individual.

were analyzed for CO_2 and for radioactivity. In this period of time 16 percent of the administered ^{14}C appeared in the expired air of the normal subject and 2.6 percent in that of the pentosuric subject, almost exactly the sixfold difference that was predicted. In the first 12 hr, 57 percent of the administered radioactivity appeared in the urine of the normal individual and 76 percent in that of the pentosuric person. Thus, the total ^{14}C excretion in urine and expired air of the normal and pentosuric subjects during the intervals measured was in excess of 73 and 79 percent, respectively.

Further Isotope Experiments

The foregoing study strongly supports the view that glucuronic acid metabolism is impaired in pentosuria. Some information concerning the site of the defect was deduced from the results of a published experiment [88], which will be briefly summarized. Using a "ribose-trapping" technique suggested by the observations of Tabor and Hayaishi [65] and of Karjala [66] that imidazoleacetic acid is excreted in the urine in part as a riboside, Hiatt demonstrated ribose synthesis from hexose in man by way of the oxidative and nonoxidative reactions of the pentose phosphate pathway [58]. If the glucuronic acid oxidation pathway were operative in normal individuals, it would afford a mechanism for the conversion of glucuronolactone carbon to ribose in this way: glucuronolactone → L-xylulose → D-xylulose → D-xylulose-5-phosphate → D-ribose-5-phosphate. (For an outline of the reactions involved, see Fig. 5-2.) Thus, the administration of imidazoleacetic acid and of glucuronolactone uniformly labeled with ^{14}C should be followed by the excretion of imidazoleacetic acid riboside containing ribose-^{14}C. On the other hand, if this pathway were blocked in pentosuria at a site beyond L-xylulose, then a pentosuric subject might be expected to excrete radioactive L-xylulose but nonisotopic riboside ribose. (Since there is no reason to postulate an impairment in the pentose phosphate pathway in pentosuria, the synthesis and excretion of the riboside ribose should proceed normally.) The results of such an experiment are described in Table 5-2. The significant ^{14}C incorporation in the urinary riboside ribose of the normal subject is consistent with the conversion of glucuronolactone to ribose by way of the reactions of the glucuronic acid oxidation and the pentose phosphate pathways (Fig. 5-2). The pentosuric subject excreted ribose in an amount comparable to that excreted by the normal individual, but the virtual absence of radioactivity indicated that it was derived from sources other than glucuronolactone. The large quantity of isotope in the urinary L-xylulose is in agreement with Touster's demonstration that glucuronic acid is a direct precursor of the pentose. This experiment not only provides information concerning the impairment in pentosuria, but also helps to establish the concept that the glucuronic acid oxidation pathway is operative in normal individuals.

Knox pointed out that impaired L-xylulose reabsorption by the renal tubule could be the defect present in pentosuria [22]. An experiment which was cited in support of this possibility is that of Enklewitz and Lasker [14], who gave 5 gm L-xylulose by mouth to a pentosuric subject and found only 0.5 gm "additional" L-xylulose in the urine. This suggested metabolism of the pentose. However, in the absence of information concerning the efficiency of L-xylulose absorption from the human gastrointestinal tract, the Enklewitz and Lasker experiment cannot be thus interpreted. Indeed, there are published studies which indicate that although parenteral administration of L-xylulose to animals is fol-

Table 5-2. URINARY L-XYLULOSE AND RIBOSE IN NORMAL AND PENTOSURIC SUBJECTS GIVEN IMIDAZOLEACETIC ACID (ImAA) AND D-GLUCURONOLACTONE UNIFORMLY LABELED WITH ^{14}C

	Normal person	Pentosuric subject
D-Glucuronolactone administered, counts/min	1.57×10^7	7.85×10^6
μmoles	370	185
ImAA hydrochloride administered, μmoles	2,000	1,000
Urinary L-xylulose (0–10 hr), μmoles	0.5	3,950
Relative molar activity, counts/min/μmole	....	85
Total ^{14}C content, counts/min	300*	3.36×10^5
Percent administered ^{14}C	0.002*	4.3
Ribose from urinary ImAA riboside (0–10 hr), μmoles	275	208
Percent administered ImAA	14	21
Relative molar activity, counts/min/μmole	33	
Total ^{14}C content, counts/min/μmole	9,100	190*
Percent administered ^{14}C	0.058	0.002*

* Significance doubtful because of small quantity of radioactivity.

lowed by extensive metabolism [40, 90, 91], the pentose orally administered is not glycogenic in rats [92]. Moreover, even if considerable absorption takes place, the possibility exists that the absorbed pentose might inhibit endogenous L-xylulose production by way of a feedback mechanism.

Following the publication of Knox's review, three studies appeared which convincingly excluded the renal abnormality hypothesis. Bozian and Touster [93] found in the plasma of a pentosuric subject, but not of two normal individuals, a sugar which was identified as xylulose by paper chromatographic techniques. (Flynn [94] had previously demonstrated xylulose in pentosuric plasma by chromatography.) After glucuronolactone administration, the serum xylulose level in a pentosuric subject of Bozian and Touster reached 11 mg per 100 ml. Simultaneous with the Bozian and Touster study, Freedberg, Feingold, and Hiatt [95] used the specific enzymatic assay of Hickman and Ashwell [96] to measure L-xylulose levels in the serum and urine of several non-Jewish controls, three pentosuric persons, and four close relatives of pentosuric persons (Table 5-3). This work was later extended [89], and one additional relative is included in Table 5-3. From the latter work, several points merit emphasis. Fasting serum L-xylulose levels in all three pentosuric persons were in excess of 1 mg per 100 ml, while in the serums of all but one of the other individuals no L-xylulose was detectable in the fasting state. In all but two subjects D-glucuronolactone led to a rise in serum L-xylulose levels, with a peak generally reached within 1 hr of feeding. The rise in serum pentose level was accompanied by a marked increase in urinary pentose in the pentosuric persons and by the appearance of urinary pentose in all other subjects tested. The serum levels of four heterozygotes (D and H in Table 5-3 are the parents of A; E is the mother of B; G's mother has pentosuria) and of a fourth individual, F, with three pentosuric sibs, were considerably greater than those of the control individuals reported here and of the large number described elsewhere [89]. On the basis of his serum level and his family history, F is considered to be heterozygous. The urine levels of the two heterozygous subjects tested were considerably greater than those of the control subjects. Assuming normal glomerular filtration rates for these subjects, one can calculate that virtually all L-xylulose entering the renal glomeruli appears in the urine of normal, as well as of heterozygous and pentosuric, subjects. Thus, a "defect" in renal tubular reabsorption of L-xylulose appears to exist in *all* subjects, but it is clearly not the metabolic error which distinguishes the pentosuric from the normal person.

Unequivocal proof that a block in the glucuronic acid oxidation pathway is the metabolic lesion in pentosuria has recently been provided by Wang and van Eys [46]. These workers found in the erythrocytes of three subjects homozygous for pentosuria a marked decrease in activity of the NADP-linked xylitol dehydrogenase, the enzyme involved in the conversion of L-xylulose to xylitol. Two activities, one "normal" and one "abnormal," were found in the erythro-

Table 5-3. SERUM AND URINE L-XYLULOSE LEVELS BEFORE AND AFTER ORAL ADMINISTRATION OF D-GLUCURONOLACTONE

Subject	Amount of glucuronolactone, gm	*Serum L-xylulose*			*Urine L-xylulose*		
		Fasting, mg/100 ml	Maximal, mg/100 ml	Time after glucuronolactone, min	Fasting, mg/hr	Maximal, mg/hr	Time after glucuronolactone, hr
Pentosuric subjects:							
A	5	1.2	7.2	60	....	320	1–2
B	10	1.3	9.9	60	106	549	1–2
C	10	1.7	14.7	30	88	450	1–2
Relatives of pentosuric subjects:							
D	25	*	1.26	60	*	....	....
E	25	*	3.9	30	*	....	....
F	25	0.18	0.71	30	*	81	0–1
G	25	*	1.41	30	0.1	63	0–1
H	25	*	0.77	30			
Control subjects:							
I	25	*	*	...	*	9	0–1
J	25	*	*	...	*	22	0–1
K	25	*	0.22	90	*	16	0–1
L	25	*	0.29	90	0.6	13	0–1
M	25	*	0.15	60	0.3	18	1–2

* Less than 0.1 mg per 100 ml.

cytes of a heterozygous subject. In contrast, activity of the NAD-linked xylitol dehydrogenase, which catalyzes the interconversion of xylitol and D-xylulose, was normal in both homozygous and heterozygous subjects.

CLINICAL CONSIDERATIONS

Manifestations

Pentosuria can be classified with those inborn errors of metabolism in which no disturbance of function has been demonstrated to result from the genetic abnormality. Indeed, the most frequent difficulty encountered by pentosuric subjects is consequent to a mistaken diagnosis of diabetes mellitus and the institution thereafter of dietary and insulin "therapy." A number of reports in the literature indicate that only after an episode of insulin-induced hypoglycemia has the correct diagnosis been made. No abnormality of glucose metabolism is demonstrable, except in those rare instances in which pentosuria and diabetes mellitus coincide. Several authors have commented on the frequency and severity of psychologic disturbances encountered in subjects with pentosuria, but a causal relationship between such disturbances and the error in carbohydrate metabolism has not been established, and the suggestion is often made that at least some neurotic complaints may be related to the conflicting medical opinions to which many patients have been subjected. Lasker has followed 40 pentosuric individuals for periods in excess of 16 years and has found no decrease in life expectancy as compared with normal individuals [20]. Some typical clinical considerations may best be presented by citing a report of a case of pentosuria first diagnosed in 1958.

P.D., a 16-year-old high school sophomore, was first seen in the Out-Patient Department of the Beth Israel Hospital in February, 1958. One year previously a physician had found a reducing substance in the patient's urine and had placed him on a low-carbohydrate diet. Despite his faithful adherence to this regimen, the urine continued consistently to show a 1+ reaction in the Benedict test. For this reason his physician suggested instituting insulin therapy, and the patient's father brought him to the Beth Israel Hospital to seek additional opinion. The patient had never noted polydipsia, polyuria, or polyphagia, and during the 6 months prior to admission he had gained 8 lb in weight. The father could not recall a single negative urine sugar test during this period, but at no time did he find more than a 1+ reduction. There was a family history of diabetes mellitus in a paternal great uncle, but not of other known disturbances of carbohydrate metabolism. The patient was an only child of Austrian-born Jewish parents, who were not consanguineous and whose forebears had come from Poland. His past medical history was not contributory except in two important respects. Ten years and six years previously the patient had been seen in the Pediatric Clinic of the Beth Israel Hospital for upper respiratory infections. Urinalyses carried out on both occasions were recorded as having shown a 1+ positive Benedict test. In addition, he had frequently been seen by psychiatrists during the previous decade because of problems of behavior. During the year prior to admission his emotional disturbances were apparently magnified by his concern over his condition and also by his resentment at the dietary restrictions to which he had been subjected.

Physical examination revealed a well-developed, well-nourished young male who appeared in good health. Vital signs were normal, and no significant abnormalities were found on examination. Laboratory studies revealed a normal hemogram, a 2-hr postprandial blood sugar of 95, and a urinalysis that was normal except for a 1+ positive test for a reducing substance. The urine, however, did not give a positive reaction with Testape (an enzyme-impregnated paper, which reacts specifically with glucose). The urine sugar was shown to be L-xylulose by preparation of the osazone and by paper chromatography in n-butanol-ethanol-water (50:10:40) with authentic L-xylulose as a standard, followed by staining with the orcinol-trichloroacetic acid reagent [97]. A glucose tolerance test (50 gm glucose by mouth) showed a fasting blood sugar level of 80 mg per 100 ml and blood glucose levels at 30, 60, 120, 180, and 240 min of 120, 110, 95, 80, and 60 mg per 100 ml, respectively. The patient's 24-hr urinary excretion of L-xylulose was found to be 2 gm, and this rose to 4 gm during the 24 hr following the ingestion of 5 gm of D-glucuronolactone. Studies of L-xylulose levels in the patient (A in Table 5-3), his mother (D), and his father (H) before and after glucuronolactone administration strengthen the assumption that the parents are heterozygous for the aberration apparent in the son. The patient and his parents were reassured concerning the benign nature of this disturbance in carbohydrate metabolism, and specifically concerning the absence of any relationship of his condition to diabetes mellitus. He was returned to an unrestricted diet and, according to his parents, within a month many of the behavioral disturbances which had been present during the previous year were greatly diminished.

Diagnostic Measures

A diagnosis of pentosuria should be suspected in any person, and particularly in a Jewish person, who has none of the symptoms of diabetes mellitus but in whose urine a small quantity of a reducing substance is consistently found. This possibility is strengthened in those instances in which the urine does not give a positive test with any of the enzymatic methods specific for glucose. The measures which have proved most useful in establishing the diagnosis of pentosuria may be summarized as follows:

1 *Reduction of Benedict's reagent at low temperature* [15]. L-Xylulose is a strong reducing substance and in contrast

to glucose and most other urinary sugars will reduce Benedict's reagent at 55°C in 10 min or at room temperature in 3 hr. (Fructose will also reduce Benedict's reagent at low temperature.)

2 *Paper chromatography.* On paper chromatography L-xylulose can be readily distinguished from other sugars. For example, with a mixture of *n*-butanol, ethanol, and water (50:10:40) as the solvent, L-xylulose has a characteristic mobility ($R_F = 0.26$) which exceeds those of other commonly observed urinary sugars [97] and gives a red color on staining with the orcinol-trichloroacetic acid reagent [98]. Chromatography is the most convenient means of establishing an unequivocal diagnosis.

3 *Cysteine-carbazole test* [99].

4 *Behavior of osazone* [29]. The phenylosazone of L-xylulose has a melting point of about 160°C. When it is mixed with the osazone of D-xylose, the crystalline appearance is radically altered, and the melting point rises approximately 40°.

5 *Demonstration of the enzymatic defect* in erythrocytes [46] can be carried out only in a laboratory in which special facilities are available.

GENETICS

Estimates of the incidence of pentosuria vary. The most widely accepted figure, 1 in 40,000 to 50,000, is derived from examinations of applicants for life insurance in the United States [92, 100]. All these cases were found in Jews; thus, the occurrence in American Jews is considered to be about 1:2,000 to 2,500. Mizrahi and Ser reported an incidence of pentosuria of 1:5,000 in Israeli Jews; their 18 cases, 8 males and 10 females, were all born in Eastern European countries [101]. The vast majority of pentosuric persons are Jews at present resident in widely dispersed areas, but the antecedents of a substantial number have been traced to Eastern Europe [102]. Two sisters of Lebanese descent with xylulosuria have been found in South Africa [35], and further study of four generations of the same family revealed an additional 8 cases in 127 members [103]. In this study individuals were reported to show pentosuria weeks to years after negative urine examinations. Twelve cases of pentosuria were found in 60 members of three other well-studied Lebanese families—these in Lebanon [104]. Among them was an infant with xylulosuria from at least the second week of life. The earlier reports that pentosuria occurs predominantly in males [12] are not substantiated by studies of the families of pentosuric persons, in which the incidence seems evenly divided between the sexes.

Garrod first proposed that a homozygous state was required for the expression of pentosuria [12], and this thesis has been amply supported by the very careful family studies of Lasker [18, 102]. The latter [102] has found 31 of 122 sibs (excluding propositi) to have pentosuria when both parents were negative. When one parent had the disturbance, however, 17 of 31 sibs were afflicted. The incidence of consanguinity in 79 marriages which produced pentosuric offspring was 12.6 percent.

The sensitivity of the enzymatic assay for L-xylulose, which permits measurement of serum levels far below those found in individuals with pentosuria, has made possible the demonstration of a partial lesion in parents and children of pentosuric individuals [95]. This provides unequivocal confirmation of the theories of Garrod and Lasker concerning a homozygous genotype in pentosuria. Relatives of pentosuric individuals with one normal and one abnormal gene apparently have sufficient competent enzyme to deal with the products of normal metabolism. However, when the glucuronic acid oxidation pathway is stressed, as occurs during the "loading test" with glucuronolactone, the pentosuria heterozygote is not able to metabolize the extra L-xylulose produced as efficiently as is the normal individual. The data in Table 5-3 demonstrate that following glucuronolactone administration, both parents of one pentosuric, the mother of a second, and the child of a third all had serum levels of L-xylulose significantly higher than those of control subjects, but far below those of pentosurics. Thus, it is apparent that while the presence of two abnormal genes is required to produce the clinical picture of essential pentosuria, the consequences of one abnormal gene are recognizable not only by enzyme studies [46], but also under the special conditions which prevail following glucuronolactone administration.

SUMMARY

1 Essential pentosuria is an inborn error of metabolism in which 1.0 to 4 gm of the pentose L-xylulose is excreted in the urine each day. It is a benign disturbance which occurs principally in Jews, and which behaves genetically as an autosomal recessive characteristic.

2 This disorder bears no relationship to diabetes mellitus and is easily distinguished from several other varieties of pentosuria in which milligram quantities of a number of pentoses other than L-xylulose appear in the urine.

3 Essential pentosuria is the result of a defect in the glucuronic acid oxidation pathway. In this route of carbohydrate metabolism the carboxyl carbon atom of D-glucuronic acid is removed in a series of reactions, giving rise to the pentose L-xylulose. The latter may then be converted to its stereoisomer, D-xylulose, which, in turn, may be phosphorylated. D-Xylulose-5-phosphate may participate in reactions of the pentose phosphate pathway which lead to its conversion to hexose phosphate. (Glucuronic acid → gulonic acid → L-xylulose → xylitol → D-xylulose → pentose phosphate pathway → hexose phosphate.) The glucuronic acid oxidation pathway serves no essential function in man.

4 The block results from reduced activity of the NADP-linked xylitol dehydrogenase, the enzyme that catalyzes the conversion of L-xylulose to xylitol.

5 The heterozygote can be recognized either by demonstrating an intermediate level of erythrocyte activity of the xylitol dehydrogenase, or increased urinary or serum L-xylulose, or both, in a glucuronolactone-loading test.

BIBLIOGRAPHY

1. Salkowski, E., and Jastrowitz, M.: Ueber eine bisher nicht beobachtete Zuckerart im Harn., Zbl. med. Wiss., **30**, 337, 1892.
2. Garrod, A. E.: The lessons of rare maladies. Lancet, **1**, 1055, 1928.
3. *The Works of William Harvey, M.D.,* translated by Robert Willis, p. 616. Syndenham, London, 1847. (Cited in ref. 2.)
4. Peters, J. P., and Van Slyke, D. D.: *Quantitative Clinical Chemistry. Interpretations,* vol. I. Williams & Wilkins, Baltimore, 1946.
5. Hawk, P. B., Oser, B. L., and Summerson, W. H.: *Practical Physiological Chemistry,* pp. 844–845. McGraw-Hill, New York, 1954.
6. Johnstone, R. W.: Pentosuria, chronic and alimentary. Edinburgh Med. J., **20**, 138, 1906.
7. Tower, D. B., Peters, E. L., and Pogorelskin, M. A.: Nature and significance of pentosuria in neuromuscular disease. Neurology, **6**, 37, 125, 1956.
8. Touster, O., Hutcheson, R. M., and Reynolds, V. H.: The formation of L-xylulose in mammals and its utilization by liver preparations. J. Amer. Chem. Soc., **76**, 5005, 1954.
9. Futterman, S., and Roe, J. H.: The identification of ribulose and L-xylulose in human and rat urine. J. Biol. Chem., **215**, 257, 1955.
10. Kiliani, H.: Ueber die Zusammensetzung und Constitution der Arabinose carbonsaüre bezw. der Arabinose. Ber. Deutsch. Chem. Ges., **20**, 339, 1887.
11. Janeway, T. C.: Essential pentosuria in two brothers. Amer. J. Med. Sci., **132**, 423, 1906.
12. Garrod, A. E.: Inborn errors of metabolism. Lancet, **2**, 217, 1908.
13. Klercker, K. O.: Studien über die Pentosurie. Nord. Med. Ark., **38**, 1, 1905.
14. Enklewitz, M., and Lasker, M.: Studies in pentosuria: a report of 12 cases. Amer. J. Med., Sci., **186**, 539, 1933.
15. Lasker, M., and Enklewitz, M.: A simple method for the detection and estimation of L-xyloketose in urine. J. Biol. Chem., **101**, 289, 1933.
16. Enklewitz, M., and Lasker, M.: The origin of L-xyloketose (urine pentose). J. Biol. Chem., **110**, 443, 1935.
17. Enklewitz, M., and Lasker, M.: Pentosuria in twins. J.A.M.A., **105**, 958, 1935.
18. Lasker, M., Enklewitz, M., and Lasker, G. W.: The inheritance of L-xyloketosuria (essential pentosuria). Hum. Biol., **8**, 243, 1936.
19. Lasker, M.: The question of arabinosuria. Am. J. Clin. Path., **20**, 485, 1950.
20. Lasker, M.: Mortality of persons with xyloketosuria. Hum. Biol., **27**, 294, 1955.
21. Derivaux, R. C.: Essential pentosuria (xyloketosuria). Southern Med. J., **36**, 587, 1943.
22. Knox, W. E.: Sir Archibald Garrod's inborn errors of metabolism. IV. Pentosuria. Amer. J. Hum. Genet., **10**, 385, 1958.
23. Neuberg, C.: Ueber die Harnpentose ein optisch inactives natürlich vorkomnendes Kohlehydrat. Ber. Deutsch. Chem. Ges., **33**, 2243, 1900.
24. Cammidge, P. J., and Howard, H. A. H.: Seven cases of essential pentosuria. Brit. Med. J., **2**, 777, 1920.
25. Aron, H.: Einfall von Pentosuria im frühen Kindesalter. Mschr. Kinderheilk., **1**, 177, 1913.
26. Luzzatto, R.: Recherches dans un cas de pentosurie chronique. Arch. Ital. Biol., **51**, 469, 1909.
27. Schüler, L.: Ueber inaktive und rechtsdrehende Arabinose ausscheidung im Harn. Berlin Klin. Wschr., **47**, 1322, 1910.
28. Zerner, E., and Waltuch, R.: Ein Beitrag zur Kenntnis der Pentosurie vom chemischen Standpunkt. Mschr. Chem., **34**, 1639, 1913.
29. Levene, P. A., and LaForge, F. B.: Note on a case of pentosuria. J. Biol. Chem., **18**, 319, 1914.
30. Zerner, E., and Waltuch, R.: Zur Frage des Pentosuriezuckers. Biochem. Z., **58**, 410, 1913.
31. Hiller, A.: The identification of the pentose in a case of pentosuria. J. Biol. Chem., **30**, 129, 1917.
32. Greenwald, I.: The nature of the sugar in four cases of pentosuria. J. Biol. Chem., **88**, 1, 1930.
33. Solis Cohen, S.: Essential pentosuria. Amer. J. Med. Sci., **139**, 349, 1910.
34. Solis Cohen, S., and Gershenfeld, L.: Supplemental report of a case of essential pentosuria of twenty-eight years' standing. Amer. J. Med. Sci., **192**, 610, 1936.
35. Barnes, H. D., and Bloomberg, B. M.: Paper chromatography of the urinary sugar in essential pentosuria. South African J. Med. Sci., **18**, 93, 1953.
36. Touster, O., and Harwell, S.: The isolation of L-arabitol from pentosuric urine. J. Biol. Chem., **230**, 1031, 1958.
37. Wolfson, W. G., Cohn, C., and Devaney, W. A.: An improved apparatus and procedure for ascending chromatography on large size filter paper sheets. Science, **109**, 541, 1949.
38. Margolis, J. I.: Chronic pentosuria and migraine. Amer. J. Med. Sci., **177**, 348, 1929.
39. Everett, M. R.: *Medical Biochemistry.* p. 312. Hoeber-Harper, New York, 1942.
40. Touster, O., Hutcheson, R. M., and Rice, L.: The influence of D-glucuronolactone on the excretion of L-xylulose by humans and guinea pigs. J. Biol. Chem., **215**, 677, 1955.
41. Touster, O., Mayberry, R. H., and McCormick, D. B.: The conversion of 1-^{13}C-D-glucuronolactone to 5-^{13}C-L-xylulose in a pentosurine human. Biochim. Biophys. Acta, **24**, 196, 1957.
42. Touster, O., Reynolds, V. H., and Hutcheson, R. M.: The reduction of L-xylulose to xylitol by guinea pig liver mitochondria. J. Biol. Chem., **221**, 697, 1956.
43. Hollman, S., and Touster, O.: The L-xylulose-xylitol enzyme and other polyol dehydrogenases of guinea pig liver mitochondria. J. Biol. Chem., **225**, 87, 1957.
44. Bässler, K. H., and Reimold, W. V.: Lactatbildung aus Zuckern und Zuckeralkoholen in Erythrocyten. Klin. Wschr., **43**, 169, 1965.
45. Asakura, T., Adachi, K., Minakami, S., and Yoshikawa, H.: Non-glycolytic sugar metabolism in human erythrocytes. I. Xylitol metabolism. J. Biochem., **62**, 184, 1967.
46. Wang, Y. M., and van Eys, J.: The enzymatic defect in essential pentosuria. New Eng. J. Med., **282**, 892, 1970.
47. Ashwell, G.: Enzymatic degradation of D-galacturonic and D-glucuronic acid. Fed. Proc., **16**, 146, 1957.
48. Hickman, J., and Ashwell, G.: Purification and properties of D-xylulokinase in liver. J. Biol. Chem., **232**, 737, 1958.
49. Ashwell, G., Kanfer, J., and Burns, J. J.: Studies of the mechanism of L-xylulose formation by kidney enzymes. J. Biol. Chem., **234**, 472, 1959.
50. Smiley, J. D., and Ashwell, G.: Purification and properties of β-L-hydroxy acid hydrogenase. II. Isolation of β-keto-L-gulonic acid, an intermediate in L-xylulose biosynthesis. J. Biol. Chem., **236**, 357, 1961.
51. Winkelman, J., and Ashwell, G.: Enzymic formation of L-xylulose from β-keto-L-gulonic acid. Biochim. Biophys. Acta, **52**, 170, 1961.
52. Burns, J. J., and Kanfer, J.: Formation of L-xylulose from L-gulonolactone in rat kidney. J. Amer. Chem. Soc., **79**, 3604, 1957.
53. ul Hassan, M., and Lehninger, A. L.: Enzymatic formation of ascorbic acid in rat liver extracts. J. Biol. Chem., **223**, 123, 1956.
54. Horecker, B. L., and Hiatt, H. H.: Pathways of carbohydrate metabolism in normal and neoplastic cells. New Eng. J. Med., **258**, 177, 225, 1958.
55. Horecker, B. L., and Mehler, A. H.: Carbohydrate metabolism. Ann. Rev. Biochem., **24**, 207, 1955.
56. Marks, P. A., and Feigelson, P.: Biosynthesis of nucleic acid ribose and of glycogen glucose in the rat. J. Biol. Chem., **226**, 1001, 1957.
57. Hiatt, H. H.: Studies of ribose metabolism. II. A method for the study of ribose synthesis *in vivo.* J. Biol. Chem., **229**, 725, 1957.
58. Hiatt, H. H.: Studies of ribose metabolism. VI. Pathways of ribose synthesis in man. J. Clin. Invest., **37**, 1461, 1958.

59. Horecker, B. L., and Smyrniotis, P. Z.: The coenzyme function of thiamine pyrophosphate in pentose phosphate metabolism. J. Amer. Chem. Soc., **75**, 1009, 1953.
60. Hiatt, H. H.: Studies of ribose metabolism. V. Factors influencing *in vivo* ribose synthesis in the rat. J. Clin. Invest., **37**, 1453, 1958.
61. Horecker, B. L., Gibbs, M., Klenow, H., and Smyrniotis, P. Z.: The mechanism of pentose phosphate conversion to hexose monophosphate. I. With a liver enzyme preparation. J. Biol. Chem., **207**, 393, 1954.
62. Hiatt, H. H.: Studies of ribose metabolism. III. The pathway of ribose carbon conversion to glucose in man. J. Clin. Invest., **37**, 651, 1958.
63. Hiatt, H. H.: Studies of ribose metabolism. I. The pathway of nucleic acid ribose synthesis in a human carcinoma cell in tissue culture. J. Clin. Invest., **36**, 1408, 1957.
64. Perkoff, G. T., and Tyler, F. H.: Studies in disorders of muscle. XI. The problem of pentosuria in progressive muscular dystrophy. Metabolism, **5**, 563, 1956.
65. Tabor, H., and Hayaishi, O.: The excretion of imidazoleacetic acid riboside following the administration of imidazoleactic acid or histamine to rats. J. Amer. Chem. Soc., **77**, 505, 1955.
66. Karjala, S. A.: The partial characterization of a histamine metabolite from rat and mouse urine. J. Amer. Chem. Soc., **77**, 504, 1955.
67. Reichard, P.: Enzymatic synthesis of deoxyribonucleotides. I. Formation of deoxycytidine diphosphate from cytidine diphosphate with enzymes from *Escherichia coli.* J. Biol. Chem., **237**, 3513, 1962.
68. Mosbach, E. H., and King, C. G.: Tracer studies of glucuronic acid biosynthesis. J. Biol. Chem., **185**, 491, 1950.
69. Eisenberg, F., Jr., and Gurin, S.: The biosynthesis of glucuronic acid from 1-C^{14}-glucose. J. Biol. Chem., **195**, 317, 1952.
70. Ginsburg, V., Weissbach, A., and Maxwell, E. S.: Formation of glucuronic acid from uridinediphosphate glucuronic acid. Biochim. Biophys. Acta, **28**, 649, 1958.
71. Pogell, B. M., and Leloir, L. F.: Nucleotide activation of liver microsomal glucuronidation. J. Biol. Chem., **236**, 293, 1961.
72. Anderson, R. L., and Wood, W. A.: Purification and properties of L-xylulokinase. J. Biol. Chem., **237**, 1029, 1962.
72*a.* Winegrad, A. I., and Shaw, W. N.: Glucuronic acid pathway activity in adipose tissue. Amer. J. Physiol., **206**, 165, 1964.
73. Winegrad, A. I., and Burden, C. L.: Hyperactivity of the glucuronic acid pathway in diabetes mellitus. Trans. Ass. Amer. Physicians, **78**, 158, 1965.
74. Hankes, L. V., Politzer, W. M., Touster, O., and Anderson, L.: Myoinositol catabolism in human pentosurics: the predominant role of the glucuronate-xylulose-pentose phosphate pathway. Ann. N. Y. Acad. Sci., **165**, 564, 1969.
75. Hiatt, H. H., and Lareau, J.: Studies of ribose metabolism. VII. An assessment of ribose biosynthesis from hexose by way of the C-6 oxidation pathway. J. Biol. Chem., **233**, 1023, 1958.
76. Isherwood, F. A., Chen, Y. T., and Mapson, L. W.: Synthesis of L-ascorbic acid in plants and animals. Biochem. J., **56**, 1, 1954.
77. Baker, E. M., Sauberlich, H. E., Wolfskill, S. J., Wallace, W. T., and Dean, E. E.: Tracer studies of vitamin C utilization in men: metabolism of D-glucuronolactone-6-C^{14}, D-glucuronic-6-C^{14} acid and L-ascorbic-1-C^{14} acid. Proc. Soc. Exp. Biol. Med., **109**, 737, 1962.
78. Burns, J. J., Evans, C., Trousof, N., and Kaplan, J.: Stimulatory effect of drugs on excretion of L-ascorbic acid and non-conjugated D-glucuronic acid. Fed. Proc., **16**, 286, 1957.
79. Longenecker, H. E., Fricke, H. H., and King, C. G.: The effect of organic compounds upon vitamin C synthesis in the rat. J. Biol. Chem., **135**, 497, 1940.
80. Burns, J. J., Evans, C., and Trousof, N.: Stimulatory effect of barbital on urinary excretion of L-ascorbic acid and non-conjugated D-glucuronic acid. J. Biol. Chem., **227**, 785, 1957.
81. Evans, C., Conney, A. H., Trousof, N., and Burns, J. J.: Metabolism of D-galactose to D-glucuronic acid, L-gulonic acid, and L-ascorbic acid in normal and barbital-treated rats. Biochim. Biophys. Acta, **41**, 9, 1960.
82. Conney, A. H., Bray, G. A., Evans, C., and Burns, J. J.: Metabolic interactions between L-ascorbic acid and drugs. Ann. N.Y. Acad. Sci., **92**, 115, 1961.
83. Hollmann, S., and Touster, O.: Alterations in tissue levels of uridine diphosphate glucose dehydrogenase, uridine diphosphate glucuronic acid pyrophosphatase, and glucuronyl transferase induced by substances influencing the production of ascorbic acid. Biochim. Biophys. Acta, **62**, 338, 1962.
84. Roe, J. H., and Coover, M. O.: Role of the thyroid gland in urinary pentose excretion in the rat. Proc. Soc. Exp. Biol. Med., **75:** 818, 1950.
85. Coover, M. O., Feinberg. L. J., and Roe, J. H.: Effect of cold, adrenocorticotropic and thyroid hormones on urinary excretion of pentose in the rat. Proc. Soc. Exp. Biol. Med., **74**, 146, 1950.
86. Baker, E. M., Plough, I. C., and Bierman, E. L.: Alternate pathways of glucose metabolism in man: factors influencing the excretion of ketopentose. Clin. Res. Proc., **6**, 406, 1958.
87. Ashwell, G.: Personal communication.
88. Hiatt, H. H.: Studies of ribose metabolism. IV. The metabolism of D-glucuronolactone in normal and pentosuric subjects. Biochim. Biophys. Acta, **28**, 645, 1958.
89. Kumahara, Y., Feingold, D. S., Freedberg, I. M., and Hiatt, H. H.: Studies of pentose metabolism in normal subjects and in patients with pentosuria and pentosuria trait. J. Clin. Endocr. **21**, 887, 1961.
90. Greenwald, I.: The possible significance of L-xyloketose (urine pentose) in normal metabolism. J. Biol. Chem., **91**, 731, 1931.
91. Larson, H. W., Chambers, W. H., Blatherwick, N. R., Ewing, M. E., and Sawyer, S. D.: The metabolism of D- and L-xylulose in the depancreatized dog. J. Biol. Chem., **129**, 701, 1939.
92. Larson, H. W., Blatherwick, N. R., Bradshaw, P. J., Ewing, M. E., and Sawyer, S. D.: The metabolism of L-xylulose. J. Biol. Chem., **138**, 353, 1941.
93. Bozian, R. C., and Touster, O.: Essential pentosuria: renal or enzymic disorder. Nature (London), **184**, 463, 1959.
94. Flynn, F. V.: Essential pentosuria. Brit. Med. J., **1**, 391, 1955.
95. Freedberg, I. M., Feingold, D. S., and Hiatt, H. H.: Serum and urine L-xylulose in pentosuric and normal subjects and in individuals with pentosuria trait. Biochem. Biophys. Res. Commun., **1**, 328, 1959.
96. Hickman, J., and Ashwell, G.: A sensitive and stereospecific enzymatic assay for xylulose. J. Biol. Chem., **234**, 758, 1957.
97. Lederer, E., and Lederer, M.: *Chromatography.* Elsevier, Amsterdam, 1955.
98. Hough, L., Jones, J. K. N., and Wadman, W. H.: Quantitative analysis of mixtures of sugars by the method of partition chromatography. Part V. Improved methods for the separation and detection of the sugars and their methylated derivatives on the paper chromatogram. J. Chem. Soc., 1702, 1950.
99. Dische, Z., and Borenfreund, E.: A new spectrophotometric method for the detection and determination of keto sugars and trioses. J. Biol. Chem., **192**, 583, 1951.
100. Wright, W. T.: Incidence of pentosuria. New Eng. J. Med., **265**, 1154, 1961.
101. Mizrahi, O., and Ser, I.: Essential pentosuria, in *Genetics of Migrant and Isolate Populations,* edited by E. Goldschmidt, p. 300. Williams & Wilkins, Baltimore, 1963.
102. Lasker, M.: Personal communication.
103. Politzer, W. M., and Fleischmann, H.: L-Xylulosuria in a Lebanese family. Amer. J. Hum. Genet., 14, **256**, 1962.
104. Khachadurian, A. K.: Essential pentosuria. Amer. J. Hum. Genet., **14**, 249, 1962.

CHAPTER SIX

ESSENTIAL FRUCTOSURIA AND HEREDITARY FRUCTOSE INTOLERANCE*

E. Rudolf Froesch

For many years one harmless inherited disturbance of fructose metabolism, i.e., essential fructosuria, was known. In 1957 a second disorder of fructose metabolism was described which differs from essential fructosuria in that fructose administration causes severe hypoglycemia and vomiting. This was termed *hereditary fructose intolerance,* and it was later shown that essential fructosuria and hereditary fructose intolerance are distinct from each other not only in symptoms but also with respect to the primary enzyme disorder. The subject was reviewed by Froesch in 1966 [1]. In 1960 and in 1970 two other disturbances of fructose metabolism were described.

In order to understand these four conditions, their symptoms, and their biochemical abnormalities, it is necessary first to discuss the normal metabolism of fructose.

METABOLISM OF FRUCTOSE

Occurrence of Fructose

The ketohexose fructose is widely distributed among plants and is an important source of dietary carbohydrate. It is present in fruits and vegetables as the free monosaccharide and as part of the disaccharide sucrose, which consists of one molecule of glucose and one of fructose. The relative content of these sugars in various comestibles has been studied by Hardinge et al. [2], among others. The average daily intake of fructose is of the order of 50 to 100 gm. Inulin, a polymer of fructose, is present in vegetables such as chicory and sweet potatoes. It may be hydrolyzed to fructose in acid at high temperature, but only insignificant quantities are split and absorbed as fructose in the intestine under physiologic circumstances. Fructose is also present in the trisaccharide raffinose and in the tetrasaccharide stachyose, but these play no role in human nutrition. Sorbitol, a sugar alcohol which is sometimes used as an ingredient of "diabetic" chocolate and as a substitute for sugar in infusion solutions because of its chemical stability, is quantitatively converted to fructose by the liver and metabolized as fructose.

Laboratory Methods for the Detection and Measurement of Fructose

The reducing capacity of fructose is approximately 98 percent of that of glucose. It is detected by all reactions based on the reducing properties of sugars. The older term *levulose* points to its optical levorotatory power. Fructose is fermented by yeast, but it is not attacked by glucose oxidase. The Seliwanoff reaction, based on the conversion of fructose to hydroxymethylfurfural and condensation with resorcinol in hot acid, was adapted by Roe et al. [3] and by Higashi and Peters [4] for the quantitative determination of fructose in blood and urine. It is not entirely specific for fructose. The best quantitative and entirely specific assay for fructose makes use of the enzymes hexokinase, phosphoglucose isomerase, and glucose-6-phosphate dehydrogenase. After the conversion of glucose to 6-phosphogluconate, phosphoglucose isomerase is added to the incubation mixture, allowing fructose-6-phosphate to be converted to 6-phosphogluconate and to be measured by the stoichiometric reduction of NADP to NADPH. Polysaccharides containing fructose, such as inulin, are quantitatively hydrolyzed and give the same color reaction. Pentoses, and to a lesser extent glucose, may also interfere. The removal of glucose by incubation with glucose oxidase has proved valuable for the accurate determination of fructose [5]. The osazones of fructose and of glucose are identical.

In order to prove that a reducing substance which gives a positive Seliwanoff reaction is fructose, one must resort to identification by paper chromatography [6].

Fructose Utilization

Fructose is utilized faster than glucose in the intact organism. In normal adult subjects the half-life of fructose averages 18 min [7, 8], whereas that of glucose averages 43 min [9]. At constant infusion rates of 0.5, 1.0, and 1.5 gm per kg per hr, only 2, 5, and 5.7 percent, respectively, of the administered doses was excreted in the urine [10]. Levels of blood lactate, pyruvate, α-ketoglutarate, and citrate rise more rapidly and higher after intravenous administration of fructose than after glucose [11]. Accumulation of lactic acid in blood, exacerbating acidosis in patients with ketoacidotic diabetes, has been described during rapid infusion of large amounts of fructose [12]. The fall of inorganic serum phosphorus level is more pronounced and is shorter-lived [13, 14]. These observations indicate a rapid phosphorylation of fructose. Fructose utilization is proportional to the fructose concentration in blood [7].

Patients with diabetes mellitus utilize fructose normally [7], but they convert more to glucose in the liver than normal subjects and may spill glucose into the urine [15–17]. Insulin does not enhance fructose removal from blood in the normal or diabetic subject [7, 16].

A large part of a given fructose load is utilized by the liver by way of the specific fructose-1-phosphate pathway

*The studies of the author related to hereditary fructose intolerance and to fructose metabolism in general were supported by grants from the Public Health Service (AM 05387) and the Schweizerische Nationalfonds.

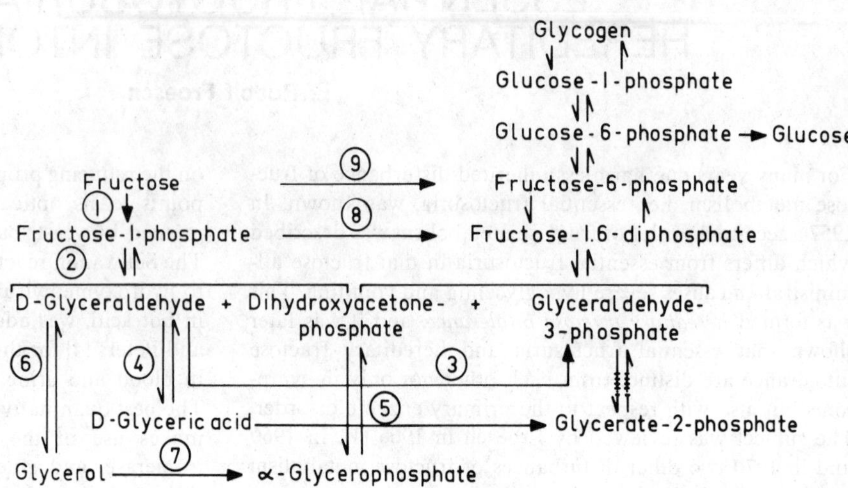

Figure 6-1. Enzymes and pathways of fructose metabolism.

shown in Fig. 6-1. Estimates vary between 23 [18] and 85 percent [19] of the administered dose. Bollman and Mann [20], Deuel [21], and Reinecke [22] have furnished conclusive evidence that the intestine and kidney also utilize fructose, converting some of it to glucose and releasing it as such into the blood. The quantitative relation of fructose disposal among these three organs is not known.

Enzymes and Pathways of Fructose Metabolism

The major pathway of fructose metabolism involves Reactions 1 to 7 of Fig. 6-1. The enzymes responsible for these reactions have been located in the liver, kidney, and small intestine.

Reaction 1

Fructose is first phosphorylated in the 1 position in the presence of ATP, potassium, and magnesium ions, by the relatively specific enzyme fructokinase (Reaction 1) [23, 24]. Fructokinase does not attack glucose or any other aldose, but two other ketohexoses, L-sorbose and D-tagatose, the pyranoid ketose L-galaheptulose, and the furanoid L-arabinulose are also phosphorylated [25]. A fructokinase which appears to catalyze phosphorylation of fructose in position 1 has also been detected in muscle [26], but this appears to be a minor side activity of phosphofructokinase [27].

Reaction 2

Fructose-1-phosphate is split to D-glyceraldehyde and phosphodihydroxyacetone by fructose-1-phosphate aldolase (Reaction 2) [28, 29]. It has been established that liver aldolase is responsible for three activities, the splitting of fructose-1-phosphate, fructose-1,6-diphosphate and the condensation of the trioses to fructose-1,6-diphosphate [29, 30, 31]. The K_m of liver aldolase for fructose-1-phosphate is 100 times that for fructose-1,6-diphosphate [29]. Muscle aldolase has only a feeble activity on fructose-1-phosphate [31, 32]. Liver and muscle aldolase are composed of four subunits which can be dissociated and subsequently may combine to form hybrids with intermediate activities for fructose-1- and fructose-1,6-diphosphate, respectively [33, 34].

Studies with specifically labeled fructose indicate that Reactions 1 and 2 lie on the major route of fructose metabolism in liver [35], kidney, and small intestine [36]. ^{14}C-fructose labeled in the first carbon atom is incorporated into liver glycogen in positions 1 (60 percent) and 6 (30 percent) of the glucose constituents [35]. This finding indicates that the fructose molecule is broken down into the trioses and that randomization between carbon atoms 1 and 6 takes place during isomerization by the enzyme triose isomerase before the trioses are recondensed to form fructose-1, 6-diphosphate.

Reactions 3 to 7

The fate of D-glyceraldehyde has not yet been completely elucidated. The most important reaction involves phosphorylation of D-glyceraldehyde to glyceraldehyde phosphate by the enzyme triose kinase (Reaction 3), which is located in the cytoplasm [29, 37]. In human liver, triose kinase is particularly active [38]. Oxidation of D-glyceraldehyde to glyceric acid by glyceraldehyde dehydrogenase [39] (Reaction 4) and subsequent phosphorylation of glyceric acid to 2-phosphoglyceric acid by the enzyme D-glycerate kinase (Reaction 5) [40, 41] has been demonstrated in liver mitochondria. Oxidation of D-glyceraldehyde to glycerol by glycerol dehydrogenase (Reaction 6) [42] (identical to alcohol dehydrogenase) and subsequent phosphorylation to α-glycerophosphate by glycerokinase (Reaction 7) no longer appears to be an important route of D-glyceraldehyde metabolism in liver.

Reaction 8

The phosphorylation of fructose-1-phosphate to fructose-1, 6-diphosphate by the enzyme 1-phosphofructokinase (Reaction 8) plays no role in the specific metabolic pathway of fructose [27]. Muscle extracts seem to phosphorylate fructose-1-phosphate to fructose-1, 6-diphosphate in the presence of ATP (adenosine triphosphate) and magnesium, but the reaction proceeds toward fructose-1-phosphate at a rate of only one-tenth that toward fructose-6-phosphate [26]. In view of the findings of Villar-Palasi and Sols [27], who showed that fructokinase activity of muscle is only a minor side activity of phosphofructokinase, it would appear rather unlikely that the major route of fructose metabolism in muscle proceeds by way of fructose-1-phosphate. In brain and adipose tissue neither fructokinase nor 1-phosphofructokinase activities could be demonstrated [26, 43].

Reaction 9

In brain [26], in red and white blood cells, and in adipose tissue [43, 44], fructose is phosphorylated by hexokinase to fructose-6-phosphate (Reaction 9). This reaction is competitively inhibited by glucose, since hexokinase has a 10 to 20 times greater affinity for glucose than for fructose [26, 43]. In spite of this unfavorable affinity of hexokinase for fructose, this enzyme reaction seems to play a major role in the metabolism of fructose in adipose tissue and possibly also in muscle and other tissues. Mention should be made of the metabolic pathway by which the accessory glands of the male reproductive tract and the placenta synthesize fructose from glucose by way of sorbitol. Hers has detected two enzymes catalyzing these reactions, i.e., sorbitol dehydrogenase and aldose reductase [45].

Fructose Transport

Fructose and glucose enter the hepatic cell freely and are present in the cell water in approximately the same concentration as in the surrounding fluid [46]. An active transport mechanism for fructose has been described in the erythrocytes, where free fructose accumulates intracellularly [47]. Erythrocytes and leukocytes metabolize fructose at approximately the same rate as glucose when the latter is absent from the medium [44, 48]. Fructose metabolism is almost completely suppressed by glucose because of competitive inhibition at the hexokinase level.

In adipose tissue fructose utilization depends on the fructose concentration in the medium. The relative rates of fructose utilization, expressed as the percentage of the simultaneous glucose utilization, are 47 percent at a concentration of 50 mg per 100 ml, 93 percent at 200 mg per 100 ml, and 165 percent at 800 mg per 100 ml [44]. At no hexose concentration in the medium is there any significant inhibition of fructose utilization by glucose. Fructose uptake is enhanced by insulin only in the absence of glucose. The enzymes of the specific fructose pathway (Reactions 1 and 2 of Fig. 6-1) have not been detected in adipose tissue.

The rapid rate of fructose utilization in adipose tissue is believed to be the result of a specific transport system for fructose which seems to operate independently of glucose and of insulin [44]. Once fructose has passed the barrier of the cell membrane, it appears to be phosphorylated to fructose-6-phosphate by hexokinase. No inhibition by glucose occurs at this stage, since hexose transport is the rate-limiting step of hexose metabolism, with the result that free glucose is not present in the adipose tissue cells under normal circumstances [44, 49].

It has been suggested by Froesch and Ginsberg [44] that adipose tissue might be an important site of fructose utilization in the intact organism. In severely decompensated diabetic persons the free fatty acid levels fall after fructose administration, whereas there is no longer such a response to glucose. This finding favors the hypothesis that fructose is utilized by adipose tissue in vivo in an insulin-independent way, leading to decreased fatty acid release from adipose tissue.

Muscle uses little fructose compared to glucose [50]. Fructose oxidation to CO_2 and incorporation into glycogen by the rat diaphragm in vitro proceeds at a rate of one-eighth to one-fourth that of glucose. Fructose metabolism by the diaphragm does not appear to be inhibited in the presence of small concentrations of glucose alone or together with insulin [44, 51, 52]. Fructose metabolism of muscle is inhibited only when glucose accumulates intracellularly because of an acceleration of glucose transport. This interpretation of results obtained with diaphragm is supported by the finding of Morgan et al. [53], who showed that there is no glucose in the cells of heart muscle at normal blood sugar concentrations.

Earlier experiments with the perfused hind-limb preparation indicated a greater fructose utilization by muscle than did those employing the isolated diaphragm. Fructose utilization was proportional to fructose concentration in perfusion fluid but was independent of the presence of glucose and insulin [54]. In view of the recent findings of a relatively active fructose metabolism in adipose tissue one wonders whether adipose tissue might not have contributed to fructose utilization in the hind-limb preparation.

Insulin lowers the blood glucose level appreciably and appears to affect markedly the conversion of glucose-^{14}C (from fructose-^{14}C) to diaphragm glycogen. This is also true to a lesser extent for adipose tissue, although less apparent since the basal fructose uptake of adipose tissue in animals treated with antiinsulin serum is considerable. If these results are extrapolated to the total muscle mass, it becomes evident that under the influence of insulin, most of the fructose may end up in muscle after conversion to glucose by the liver. These data also strengthen the in vitro observations that uptake of fructose by adipose tissue is insulin-independent (unpublished observation).

Pearson and Rimer [55] observed marked improvement of muscular work capacity in patients with McArdle's syndrome (see Chap. 7) during fructose infusions, and they suggested fructose utilization by skeletal muscle. These authors failed to consider blood lactate and pyruvate levels, which normally rise to very high levels during fructose infusions. These metabolites are readily available fuel for

Table 6-1. BLOOD GLUCOSE AND INCORPORATION OF FRUCTOSE-^{14}C INTO TOTAL LIPIDS OF FAT PAD AND INTO GLYCOGEN OF DIAPHRAGM AND LIVER 30 MIN AFTER INTRAVENOUS INJECTION OF FRUCTOSE-U-^{14}C TOGETHER WITH ANTI-INSULIN SERUM OR INSULIN

	Blood glucose, mg/100 ml	*Incorporation, in counts per min, of* ^{14}*C from fructose*-U-^{14}C *into*		
		Total lipids	Glycogen	
			Liver	Diaphragm
Antiinsulin serum, 0.05 ml/rat	162 ± 3	340 ± 32	740 ± 107	23 ± 5
Insulin, 18 mU/rat	79 ± 8	871 ± 105	789 ± 42	1,028 ± 219
p <	0.001	0.001	n.s.	0.001

muscle. It may be concluded that muscle can utilize fructose but that fructose utilization is small compared to glucose utilization. However, insulin greatly enhances the incorporation of glucose into glycogen of muscle and may thus, through conversion of fructose to glucose by the liver, influence fructose utilization to a considerable degree (Table 6-1).

Fructose is utilized to a considerable extent by brain slices as long as glucose is not in the incubation medium. Fructose does not alleviate hypoglycemic symptoms and therefore does not appear to be able to replace glucose in the metabolism of brain. Park et al. [56] have indicated that this discrepancy between utilization of fructose by brain in vivo and in vitro must be attributed to the fact that fructose does not pass the blood-brain barrier.

Absorption of Fructose by Intestine and Kidney

Fructose is absorbed from the intestine at a rate approximately 43 percent that of glucose [57]. Unlike glucose, absorption of fructose is not inhibited by phlorizin, dinitrophenol, fluoride, and cyanide, although some of these compounds diminish the conversion of fructose to glucose [58, 59]. It appears that fructose absorption requires no energy and that it conforms to the properties of a simple diffusion process, whereas the conversion of fructose to glucose requires energy. The conversion of fructose to glucose by the intestine occurs by phosphorylation to fructose-1-phosphate, splitting of this ester into trioses, and recondensation to fructose-1,6-diphosphate [60]. The rate of fructose conversion to glucose by the intestine depends on the amount of ingested fructose [59] and varies considerably from species to species. In man a relatively rapid rise of the fructose concentration in the portal blood after fructose ingestion was observed. Later the glucose concentration rose, possibly because of conversion of a portion of the ingested fructose to glucose (Fig. 6-2).

Fructose is actively reabsorbed by the renal tubule, and its reabsorption is decreased by phlorizin and inhibited by glucose [61]. The renal threshold for fructose is 10 to 20

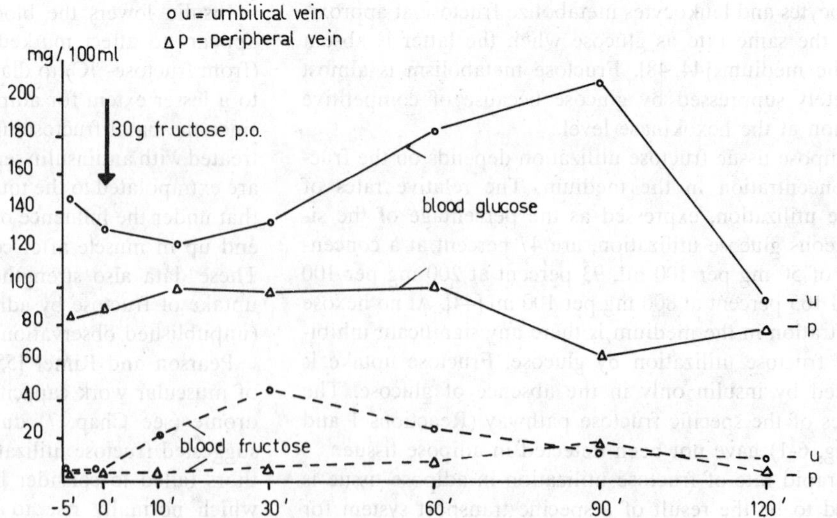

Figure 6-2. Oral fructose tolerance test with measurement of blood glucose and fructose in peripheral and portal (umbilical) veins.

mg per 100 ml [10]. The kidney converts fructose to glucose by way of fructose-1-phosphate.

ESSENTIAL FRUCTOSURIA

Historical Note and Definition

Essential fructosuria is a relatively rare disorder of metabolism. Sachs, Sternfeld, and Kraus [62] reviewed 57 cases of fructosuria reported until 1942. Twelve of these patients were Jewish. Marble [63] reported only 4 cases among 29,000 cases of mellituria seen at the Joslin Clinic, and Lasker [64] estimated the incidence in the general population at approximately 1 in 130,000. The actual incidence of essential fructosuria may well be considerably higher, since this disorder is harmless and asymptomatic and may not come to medical attention. The criteria for the diagnosis of fructosuria may be simply stated:

1 The reducing sugar in the urine must be identified as fructose; it is fermentable by yeast, yields a positive Seliwanoff reaction, does not react with glucose oxidase, and is levorotatory. Its identity should be confirmed by paper chromatography.
2 The condition is harmless and asymptomatic and is usually diagnosed on routine urine examinations.
3 Fructosuria is present only after ingestion of foods containing fructose. During oral fructose tolerance tests blood fructose rises to abnormally high levels, i.e., above 25 mg per 100 ml.
4 Glucose and galactose metabolism is normal, and fructosuria after fructose ingestion remains unchanged after insulin treatment.

Biochemical Findings

Fructose is found only in small quantities, if at all, in the blood of fasted normal subjects and of patients with essential fructosuria. The small blank value of fructose-equivalent material in the serum of fasted subjects, which amounts only to 1 to 6 mg per 100 ml when determined with Seliwanoff's reaction, is not attributable solely to the presence of free fructose [65]. After oral administration of fructose to normal subjects, the levels in serum do not exceed 15 to 25 mg per 100 ml, but in patients with essential fructosuria fructosemia may rise to 100 mg per 100 ml. The fall of the blood fructose concentration occurs more slowly than in normal subjects [63, 66, 68]. Between 10 and 20 percent of the administered dose of fructose is excreted in the urine, compared to 1 to 2 percent in normal subjects [62]. The rise of the RQ (respiratory quotient) in fasted patients with essential fructosuria after fructose ingestion is less than in normal subjects. This indicates a slower than normal utilization of fructose [69, 71]. The blood lactic and pyruvic acid concentrations remain unchanged [67, 70, 71], a finding which is in contrast to the sharp and rapid rise of these metabolites after oral or intravenous fructose administration to normal subjects.

Hypoglycemic symptoms have never been recorded in patients with essential fructosuria after fructose ingestion, although a slight decrease of blood glucose, formerly determined as the difference between total reducing substances and blood fructose, has been reported. This fall of the blood glucose level has not been substantiated by Steinitz et al. [70], who have used better and more specific methods for the measurement of blood glucose (Fig. 6-3). The serum phosphorus concentration remains unchanged, a further sign of deficient fructose utilization by the liver [70, 72]. D-Sorbitol is converted to fructose as in normal subjects, but a larger fraction is lost in the urine as fructose [66].

Primary Enzyme Disorder

The hypothesis that a primary lack of hepatic fructokinase underlies the metabolic abnormalities of essential fructosuria has been verified experimentally by Schapira et al. [73]. These authors found that uniformly labeled fructose-^{14}C is not taken up from the incubation medium by homogenates of liver tissue obtained at biopsy from patients with essential fructosuria. This is rather indirect and yet the best possible way to measure fructokinase in small tissue samples, and strongly indicates that fructokinase is deficient in hepatic tissue of patients with essential fructosuria. Thus the block appears to be as follows:

$$\textbf{Fructose} \underset{\textbf{Hepatic fructokinase}}{\not\rightleftharpoons} \textbf{Fructose-1-phosphate}$$

The activity of fructokinase measured by the same method was found to be within normal limits in patients with hereditary fructose intolerance (see below), where the second enzyme of the specific fructose pathway, the fructose-1-phosphate-aldolase, is deficient.

Genetics

The most careful study of the mode of inheritance of essential fructosuria is that of Lasker [64]. After reviewing the literature and her own cases, she concluded that the disorder is inherited as an autosomal recessive trait. Her arguments are as follows:

1 Of the 19 families on whom adequate data are available, 10 show the defect in more than one sib. In 15 families where there is information on the total size of the sibship, 40 brothers and sisters of the original patients were tested for fructosuria and 7 were found to be positive.
2 The defect is not found in any of the parents or offspring of the affected subjects.

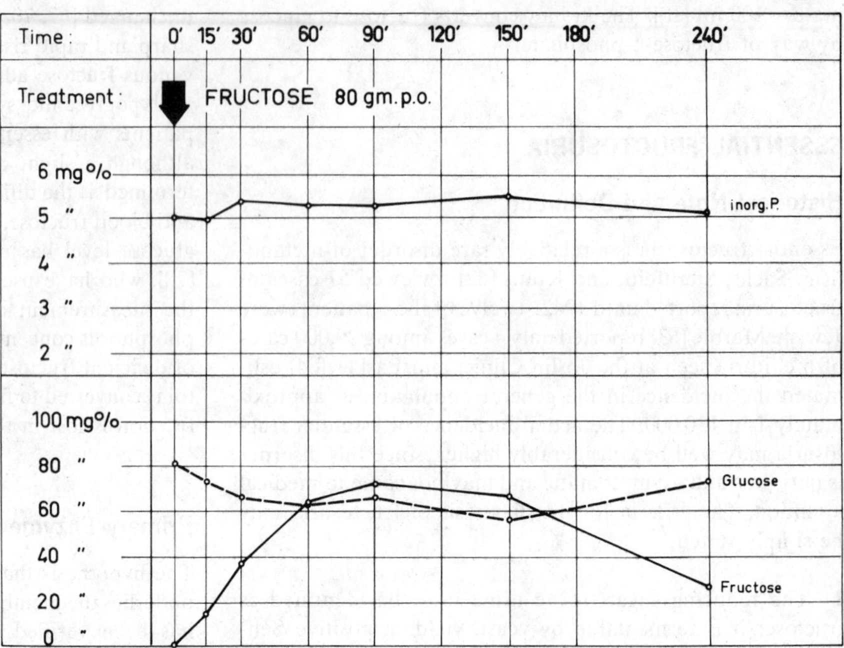

Figure 6-3. Oral fructose tolerance test in a patient with essential fructosuria. (*The author is indebted to Dr. H. Steinitz for permission to reproduce these results from* [70].)

3 In six of seven families where the facts are known, the parents of the patients are related in some manner.

HEREDITARY FRUCTOSE INTOLERANCE

Historical Note and Definition

In 1956 Chambers and Pratt described briefly a case of "idiosyncrasy to fructose" in a 24-year-old woman whose only complaints were feelings of anxiety and attacks of nausea and vomiting after eating food containing fruit or cane sugar [74]. Froesch, Prader, et al. [75] reported the typical syndrome of hereditary fructose intolerance in 1957 in two sibs and two relatives. They recognized that this disorder of fructose metabolism was inherited and distinct from essential fructosuria. Up to 1964, 25 families with hereditary fructose intolerance from 7 European countries and from the United States have come to our attention [74–86]. Since then, many more cases have been reported, so that the complete survey of the literature becomes more and more difficult [87–115]. The following features are characteristic:

1 The disorder is dominated by the syndrome of hypoglycemia and vomiting shortly after ingestion of fructose-containing food. The clinical picture of chronic fructose poisoning in small children consists of failure to thrive, hepatomegaly, vomiting, jaundice, hyperbilirubinemia, albuminuria, and aminoaciduria. A strong aversion for fruit and sweets is characteristic of older children and adults with hereditary fructose intolerance.

2 Fructosuria is present only after fructose ingestion. Abnormally high blood fructose levels are reached during oral fructose tolerance tests.

3 The rise in blood fructose level is accompanied by a marked and sustained fall of blood glucose to severely hypoglycemic levels, by a failure of the blood glucose level to rise adequately after glucagon administration, by a marked fall of serum inorganic phosphorus, and by a rise of serum magnesium [100]. Reactions to glucose and galactose tolerance tests are normal. Infusion of galactose together with fructose prevents hypoglycemia, whereas glycerol and dihydroxyacetone are ineffective in this respect [90].

4 The primary enzyme defect is a deficiency of fructose-1-phosphate aldolase. A protein (presumably fructose-1-phosphate aldolase) is detectable in the liver of patients with hereditary fructose intolerance by immunologic means (20 to 30 percent of normal), whereas its biologic activity is more drastically reduced (2 to 5 percent of normal) [106, 107].

5 The genetic findings are compatible with an autosomal recessive trait.

Clinical Findings (Table 6-2)

Infants and adult patients with hereditary fructose intolerance are perfectly healthy and without any symptoms as long as they do not ingest any food containing fructose [75–85]. The first symptoms begin when the infant is taken off the breast and when sucrose or fructose is added to the diet. As a rule, the firstborn child with the disease either dies or suffers more than the following children, who profit from the experience gathered by their parents and physicians with the first [75, 83, 85–100]. Figure 6-4 shows the typical lag of weight gain in a newborn with hereditary fructose intoler-

Table 6-2. SIGNS AND SYMPTOMS OF HEREDITARY FRUCTOSE INTOLERANCE

Beginning 20 min after oral administration of fructose	Chronic syndrome most often beginning during weaning upon addition of sucrose to regimen
Sweating	Failure to thrive
Trembling	Jaundice
Dizziness	Hepatomegaly
Nausea	Vomiting
Vomiting	Dehydration
Various degrees of disturbed consciousness to deep coma	Edema
	Ascites
Fructosuria	Seizures
Hypophosphatemia	Fructosuria
Fructosemia (not excessive)	Fructosemia
Aminoaciduria	Hypophosphatemia
Hyperbilirubinemia	Hyperbilirubinemia
Rise of serum levels of hepatic enzymes	Rise of serum levels of hepatic enzymes
	Fibrosis or cirrhosis of liver
	Aversion toward sweet food
	Lack of dental caries

ance receiving fructose from birth and the subsequent rapid recovery after introduction of a fructose-free diet [97]. Later the children develop a strong aversion to all sweets and fruit and thereby protect themselves against the noxious factor [75, 83, 85–100]. This distaste for sugar is probably due to the dramatic events which immediately succeed the ingestion of small amounts of fructose, and it explains why the chronic picture of the disease does not exist in adult patients as it does in infants.

In small children the leading symptoms are failure to thrive, protracted vomiting, frequent attacks of hypoglycemia with occasional unconsciousness and fits, hepatosplenomegaly, jaundice, albuminuria, and aminoaciduria. Cachexia may result in death. In a $1\frac{1}{2}$-month-old child edema and ascites disappeared after 2 weeks of a fructose-free diet [83]. Liver damage may be accompanied by increased serum enzyme levels during chronic fructose ingestion [83]. A marked rise of the fructose-1,6-diphosphate aldolase, glutamic-oxaloacetic transaminase, and glutamic-pyruvic transaminase in the serum was noted as early as $1\frac{1}{2}$ hr after a single large dose of fructose. At this time after fructose ingestion histologic alterations of hepatocytes were observed by electron microscopy. "Glycogen-associated membrane arrays" and "myelin-like figures" were interpreted as "cytolysomes" in various stages of development. They may represent lysosomes taking up fructose-1-phosphate and attempting to get rid of this toxic agent by acid hydrolysis [99]. On histologic examination the livers of two children with hereditary fructose intolerance were found to have lesions compatible with those seen in an early stage of cirrhosis. The pathogenesis of the acute and chronic liver cell damage due to fructose ingestion has not been studied in any detail. In galactosemia excessive intracellular galactose-1-phosphate accumulation has been incriminated as the cause of liver damage. In analogy to galactosemia, raised intracellular concentrations of fructose-1-phosphate, the metabolism of which is blocked, might be held responsible for liver toxicity. However, this is not likely to be the only cause of the acute liver cell damage. The energy metabolism of the liver cell would appear to be greatly disturbed, a hypothesis supported by the proved block of glucose release and by the acute hypophosphatemia which might well reflect intracellular ATP and inorganic phosphorus depletion.

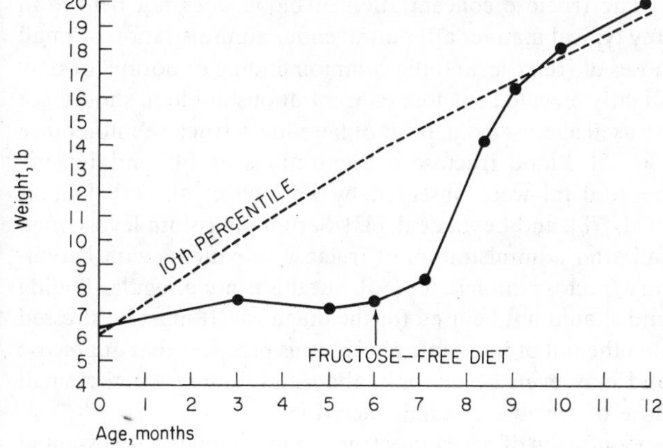

Figure 6-4. Weight chart showing the effect of the introduction of a fructose-free diet. (*From Black et al.* [97].)

Hypoglycemia develops at about the same rate whether fructose is taken by mouth or administered intravenously [85]. Nausea and vomiting seem to be more pronounced after oral ingestion of fructose. This suggests a disturbance of its metabolism in the intestine [85]. The absence of fructose-1-phosphate aldolase in the jejunum of patients with hereditary fructose intolerance has been proved (personal observation), and it is likely that fructose-1-phosphate accumulates after fructose ingestion. Hypoglycemia develops faster and after relatively smaller doses of fructose in children (in whom it reaches its maximum after 45 to 60 min) than in adults, who show the most profound hypoglycemia after 60 to 90 min [85].

The most striking and abrupt deterioration of renal function after fructose administration is the loss of the ability to acidify the urine. During ammonium chloride–induced acidosis the pH of the urine rises above 6 when fructose is administered to patients with hereditary fructose intolerance. Phosphate reabsorption is impaired. Fructose induced "renal tubular acidosis" is normalized as soon as the exposure to fructose ceases [104, 105]. In one patient hereditary fructose intolerance was associated with true renal tubular acidosis, hypokalemia and nephrocalcinosis [103]. Aminoaciduria and proteinuria develop rapidly when patients with hereditary fructose intolerance are treated with fructose [75, 78–80, 83–105]. These findings of pathologic renal function must be regarded as consequences of a severe derangement of metabolism of the proximal tubules, due to excessive accumulation of fructose-1-phosphate. The absence of fructose-1-phosphate aldolase from the renal tubules has been proved [112]. Blood amino acid nitrogen is increased as in other derangements of hepatic function. Thus, an overflow mechanism may be an additional cause of aminoaciduria.

The teeth of patients with hereditary fructose intolerance are, as a rule, in extraordinarily good condition [82, 85, 87, 100, 113, 114, 130]. It would seem that hereditary fructose intolerance protects the patients from caries. This observation may be taken as a proof that a diet low in mono- and disaccharides is unfavorable to the development of dental caries.

The intelligence of the older children and of all adult patients examined was normal [75, 82, 83, 85, 100]. The frequent hypoglycemic attacks do not seem to cause any serious brain damage. The derangements of liver and kidney function appear to be entirely reversible, since adult patients do not present any pathologic organic manifestations [74, 85, 100].

Diagnosis, Therapy, and Prognosis

The diagnosis of hereditary fructose intolerance should be made by means of an intravenous fructose tolerance test (Fig. 6-5) [85]. The intravenous dose is best administered by one rapid injection. The smallest dose which always produces the typical symptoms without causing nausea and vomiting is 0.25 gm per kg body weight in adults or 3 gm per m² surface area in children [85]. The metabolic indices which invariably are typical and therefore best suited to make the diagnosis are the blood glucose and the serum inorganic phosphorus levels. A marked and prolonged fall of these regularly occurs [76, 83, 85, 100]. In one child the diagnosis was almost missed because of a negative diagnostic fructose tolerance test with 3 gm per m² surface area. The

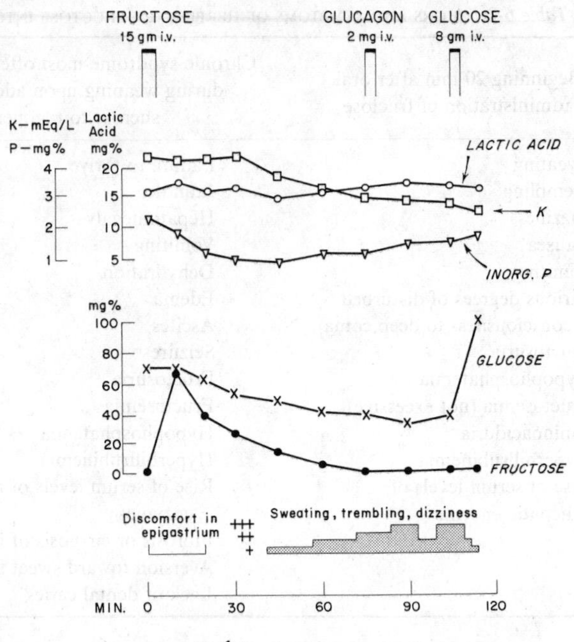

Figure 6-5. Intravenous fructose tolerance test with 0.25 gm per kg in a patient with hereditary fructose intolerance [85].

infant had a large liver and a severe disturbance of liver function. There was a reaction typical for the disease when the dose of fructose was doubled. Within 1 month after starting a fructose-free diet the child responded with severe hypoglycemia to the regular small test dose of 3 gm per m². Thus, the recommended diagnostic dose of 3 gm should be doubled or tripled in small infants with severe derangement of liver function resulting from prolonged exposure to fructose.

Transient fructose intolerance may be present in newborn infants, possibly because the liver aldolase is not yet matured [92].

The fructose concentration of blood does not behave in any typical manner after intravenous administration of small doses of fructose, and the common finding of normal or only slightly elevated fructose concentrations in blood should not be used against a diagnosis of hereditary fructose intolerance [76, 85]. Blood fructose concentrations of 145 and 160 mg per 100 ml were observed by Froesch et al. [75], Dubois et al. [78], and Levin et al. [83]. Serum potassium levels often fall after administration of fructose to patients with hereditary fructose intolerance [85], but this is not a regular finding and should not be used for the diagnosis. It must be stressed that the fall of inorganic phosphorus precedes that of glucose and may even be the only abnormal finding when a small dose of fructose is administered [85].

Confusion of hereditary fructose intolerance with essential fructosuria is hardly possible. Both disorders have only two signs in common: fructosemia and fructosuria after fructose ingestion. Hypoglycemic symptoms, nausea and vomiting, and a fall of inorganic serum phosphorus level have not been encountered in patients with essential fructosuria. The syndrome of combined galactose and fructose intolerance [116], which resembles hereditary fructose intolerance in several respects, will be discussed later.

A diet containing no fructose whatever is the only sensible therapeutic measure. It has been stressed that potatoes contain rather large quantities of fructose and that their intake must be reduced or forbidden in the event that omission of sucrose, fruits, and vegetables, does not suffice [108].

Biochemical Findings

Hypoglycemia

Fructose-induced hypoglycemia in hereditary fructose intolerance is not due to hyperinsulinism [76]. Insulin-like activity and immunologically determined serum insulin level were found to be unchanged or lowered during fructose-induced hypoglycemia when compared to the fasting value [85, 98, 117, 118]. Dubois et al. [78] determined that the coefficient of glucose assimilation, which increases after insulin administration, was decreased during the development of fructose-induced hypoglycemia. Furthermore, D-sorbitol provokes hypoglycemia before significant amounts of fructose are released into the blood. This proves that fructose as such is not the cause of hypoglycemia, particularly since similar and even higher blood fructose concentrations after intravenous administration of small amounts of fructose were insufficient to produce hypoglycemia [85].

Several lines of evidence point to a block of glucose release from the liver as the cause of fructose-induced hypoglycemia. The fall of blood glucose level is slower than that seen after insulin administration, and spontaneous recovery takes place in due time only when the dose of fructose is small. In one instance, in which 35 gm of fructose was given to a 7-year-old girl weighing 17.7 kg, a blood sugar level of 10 mg per 100 ml was maintained over a period of 6 hr [75]. Furthermore, glucagon, which normally counteracts insulin hypoglycemia by accelerating glycogenolysis in the liver, does not influence the hypoglycemia caused by fructose in these patients (Fig. 6-5) [83, 85, 117]. It may be of interest that the hypoglycemic symptoms were alleviated for a short period of time after glucagon administration in spite of a complete lack of a blood glucose response (Fig. 6-5) [85]. Dubois et al. [78] administered tracer amounts of glucose-1-^{14}C to their infant patient and followed the specific activity of blood glucose before and after fructose administration (Fig. 6-5). Before fructose was given, the specific activity of blood glucose fell off steadily, while the blood sugar level remained constant. Shortly after injection of fructose, the decline in specific activity ceased completely for a period of 60 min while hypoglycemia developed. The initial slope of the fall of the specific activity of blood glucose was resumed only when the blood glucose ceased to fall and began to rise again (Fig. 6-6). Thus, when fructose was given, dilution of the labeled blood glucose by unlabeled glucose

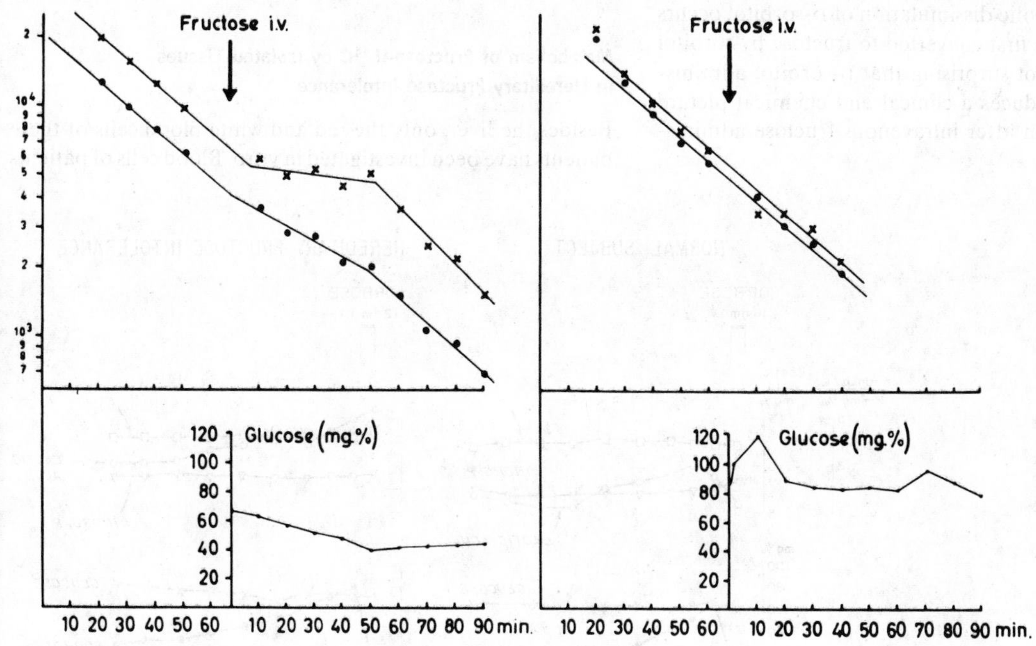

Figure 6-6. Total radioactivity of blood glucose-1-^{14}C (·) (in counts per minute per milliliter of blood) and specific activity of blood glucose (×) (in counts per milligram of blood glucose) before and after intravenous injection of fructose to a patient with hereditary fructose intolerance (*left*) and a normal subject (*right*). (*From Dubois et al.* [78].)

from the liver ceased. This does not appear to happen in insulin-induced hypoglycemia. The specific activity of the blood glucose reaches a plateau only during the first minutes after insulin administration or not at all [119, 120].

Hypophosphatemia

When large doses of fructose are administered intravenously to normal subjects, a short-lived fall in serum inorganic phosphorus level is observed [8, 13, 14]. The marked and long-lasting fall in inorganic phosphorus in patients with hereditary fructose intolerance may be explained by binding and sequestration of phosphorus in the form of fructose-1-phosphate in the liver [76, 91]. A simple calculation shows that if fructose-1-phosphate accumulates intracellularly, such a fall in serum inorganic phosphorus level might indeed be expected. When, for instance, 6.6 mmoles of fructose is administered to an infant patient weighing 8.8 kg, the fructose given exceeds the amount of inorganic phosphorus present in the entire extracellular fluid [85]. Although fructose is phosphorylated with ATP and not directly with inorganic phosphorus, the liver cell has to take up phosphorus from the serum if fructose-1-phosphate remains unavailable for tissue metabolism and accumulates intracellularly [85]. Excessive accumulation of fructose-1-phosphate in the liver of patients with hereditary fructose intolerance has been demonstrated [91].

Metabolism of D-Sorbitol and L-Sorbose

Since the major metabolic dissimulation of D-sorbitol occurs in the liver, where it is first converted to fructose by sorbitol dehydrogenase, it is not surprising that D-sorbitol administered intravenously induces a clinical and chemical picture identical with that seen after intravenous fructose administration [85].

The disappearance of L-sorbose from the blood of normal subjects is somewhat slower than that of fructose, as would be expected from the results of Kuyper [25], who showed that liver fructokinase phosphorylates fructose faster than sorbose and in preference to this ketose. The half-life of sorbose calculated from data of the author et al. [85] lies between 24 and 29 min. In two normal subjects about 30 percent of the administered dose of L-sorbose was excreted in the urine, compared to 1 to 2 percent in the case of fructose (Fig. 6-7) [85]. In patients with hereditary fructose intolerance, the sorbose level rose higher and fell more slowly, with a half-life of approximately 64 min, and accordingly these patients excreted over 80 percent of the administered sorbose in the urine within 24 hr. Although the ability to assimilate sorbose obviously was greatly impaired, the patients did not exhibit any symptoms whatever, and the blood glucose as well as the inorganic phosphorus level did not change. Furthermore, prior administration of sorbose did not alter or delay the response of patients with hereditary fructose intolerance to subsequent administration of fructose [85]. One might consider that, because of the relatively small affinity of fructokinase for sorbose, only a small amount of sorbose-1-phosphate might accumulate in the liver cells, and the intracellular concentration of this ester might be too small to inhibit fructose phosphorylation by fructokinase and insufficient to cause secondary inhibition of glycolytic enzymes responsible for development of hypoglycemia, as in fructose-1-phosphate accumulation [85]. Clearly, the interpretation of these results is purely speculative.

Metabolism of Fructose-U-^{14}C by Isolated Tissues in Hereditary Fructose Intolerance

Besides the liver, only the red and white blood cells of these patients have been investigated in vitro. Blood cells of patients

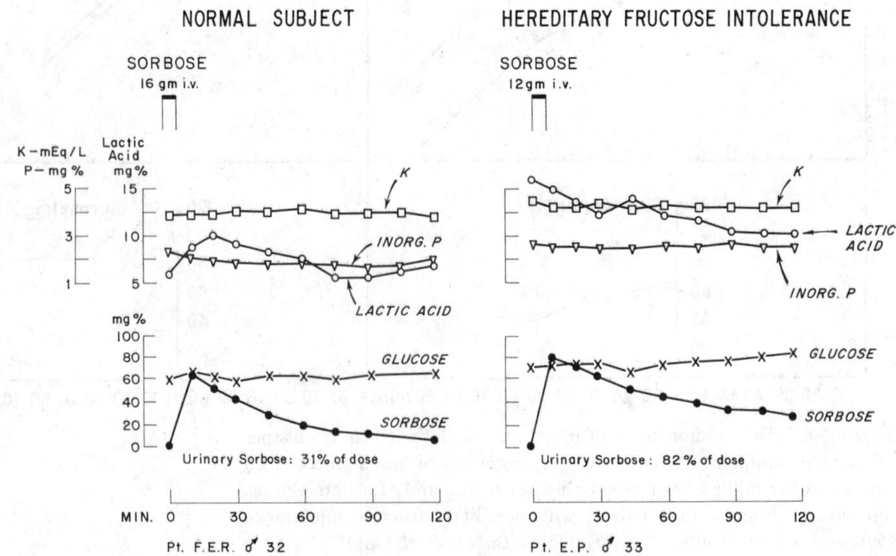

Figure 6-7. Intravenous L-sorbose tolerance test (0.20 gm per kg) in a normal subject (*left*) and in a patient with hereditary fructose intolerance (*right*) [85].

Table 6-3. METABOLISM OF FRUCTOSE-U-^{14}C BY LIVER BIOPSY TISSUE OF TWO PATIENTS WITH HEREDITARY FRUCTOSE INTOLERANCE AND OF FIVE NORMAL SUBJECTS*

Subject	Oxidation to $^{14}CO_2$	Incorporation into glycogen
Normal subjects	1.75 (0.60–2.56)	14.66 (8.6–23.1)
Case 1	0.109	0.151
Case 2	0.078	0.812

* Fructose-U-^{14}C and unlabeled glucose were present in the incubation medium in a concentration of 100 mg per 100ml. The figures represent micromoles of fructose carbon incorporated into glycogen or oxidized to $^{14}CO_2$ per gram of tissue per total incubation period. In the normal subjects, the mean and range are indicated. In each experiment with liver tissue of patients with hereditary fructose intolerance, tissue of normal subjects was also incubated.
Source: From Froesch et al. [85].

with hereditary fructose intolerance metabolize fructose normally, as would be expected on the basis of the finding that these cells do not contain fructokinase or fructose-1-phosphate aldolase activity [85]. Metabolism of fructose in blood cells occurs only by way of hexokinase.

Oxidation of fructose-U-^{14}C to $^{14}CO_2$ and incorporation into glycogen by liver tissue of patients with hereditary fructose intolerance incubated in vitro in the presence of unlabeled glucose is reduced to 1 to 6 percent of normal (Table 6-3) [85]. Thus, the utilization of fructose by liver tissue of patients with hereditary fructose intolerance appears to be almost completely defective. Whether the small amount of fructose which is metabolized to carbon dioxide and glycogen in spite of the enzyme defect enters the glycolytic scheme by way of fructokinase or by some other pathway cannot be decided from the available data. The amount of fructose utilized by the liver of these patients appears to be too small to explain why as much as 90 percent of an administered fructose load is assimilated. It has been suggested that adipose tissue is the main locus of fructose utilization in patients with hereditary fructose intolerance and also in patients with essential fructosuria [44, 85, 117].

Primary Enzyme Defect

The primary enzyme defect in hereditary fructose intolerance is a lack of fructose-1-phosphate aldolase (Table 6-4). Assays of fructose-1-phosphate aldolase activity in patients with hereditary fructose intolerance have varied in different laboratories from 0 to 12 percent of normal activity [81, 85, 115, 121]. A reduction of the activity of the fructose-1, 6-diphosphate aldolase to 25 percent of normal was reported by Hers and Joassin [121]. Froesch et al. [85] found activities of 55 and 87 percent of normal. Schapira et al. [73, 115] pointed out that the ratio of the activity of fructose-1, 6-diphosphate aldolase to the activity of fructose-1-phosphate aldolase, which is normally approximately 1, is greater than 6 in patients with hereditary fructose intolerance. The results of the aldolase activities found by various investigators are summarized in Table 6-4. The activity of liver fructokinase is normal in hereditary fructose intolerance [73, 121]. In one patient aldolase activities were determined in jejunal mucosa, and fructose-1-phosphate activity was deficient, whereas the activity toward fructose-1,6-diphosphate was normal. In renal biopsies of patients with hereditary fructose intolerance the ratio of fructose-diphosphate to fructose-1-phosphate aldolase activity was approximately 5 as compared with 1 to 1.5 in normal human kidney [112].

The interpretation of the significance of the deficiency of fructose-1-phosphate aldolase in hereditary fructose intolerance still is controversial [122]. The almost complete absence of fructose-1-phosphate aldolase in the presence of a mod-

Table 6-4. FRUCTOSE-1-PHOSPHATE AND FRUCTOSE-1,6-DIPHOSPHATE LIVER ALDOLASE ACTIVITIES* IN PATIENTS WITH HEREDITARY FRUCTOSE INTOLERANCE AND NORMAL SUBJECTS

Bibliographical reference no.	128, 129	85		1	127		86, 73†				83	127		126	
Normal subjects	x														
Hereditary fructose intolerance:															
Adults	. . . .	x	x												
Infants below 1 year	. . . .	. . .	. . .	x	x	x	x	x	x	x	x	x	x	x	x
Fructose-1,6-diphosphate-aldolase	229 ± 107 s.d.	125	200	50	170	137	55	63	102 (190)	55 (83)	187	1.5	2.1	6.5	2.7
Fructose-1-phosphate-aldolase	164 ± 76 s.d.	12	19	0	27	22	5	9	16 (28)	11 (16)	5	0.2	0	0	1.0
Ratio Fru-DP-/Fru-1-P-splitting activity	1.4	10.4	10.5	. . .	6.2	6.2	11.0	6.7	6.2 (6.7)	5.0 (5.2)	37.4	7.5	. . .	. . .	2.7

* Results of enzyme activities are expressed as Bücher units per gram of tissue, except those of [126 and 127], which are in micrograms triose ester formed per mg per 15 min, and μg of substrate used per mg per min, respectively.
† Cases of [86] were also studied by the authors of [73], whose results are given in parentheses.

erate reduction in activity of fructose-1,6-diphosphate aldolase is in good agreement with the theory of Leuthardt and Wolf [32] that fructose-1-phosphate and fructose-1,6-diphosphate are split by two different enzymes. In hereditary fructose intolerance, fructose-1-phosphate aldolase would be deficient, whereas the other aldolase would be present as in normal liver. The reduction of the activity of fructose-1,6-diphosphate aldolase could well be explained by the lack of fructose-1-phosphate aldolase, since this latter enzyme has an appreciable activity on fructose-1,6-diphosphate, as well [30]. Hers, who has not succeeded in separating different aldolase activities, has put forward two hypotheses according to which the residual aldolase in hereditary fructose intolerance might be the result of enzyme adaptation or of the survival of a fetal enzyme [121]. Muscle and liver aldolase appear, in fact, to have a number of properties in common, and Rutter et al. [123] and Drechsler et al. [124] have recently shown that even slight alterations of the aldolase molecule, such as splitting off an end-terminal amino acid group, may change the ratio of its affinity for both substrates quite markedly. Aldolases are composed of four subunits which may recombine in various ways to form hybrid aldolases with enzymatic properties between fructose-1-phosphate aldolase and fructose-1,6-diphosphate aldolase [33]. Gürtler and Leuthardt [34] have since crystallized liver aldolase and they have also shown that both enzymatic activities are attributable to a single liver aldolase.

Antibodies against fructose-1-phosphate aldolase react to an extent of 30 percent of normal with a protein of the liver of patients with hereditary fructose intolerance. It appears that these patients do in fact produce a certain percentage of an aldolase with the immunologic properties of hepatic fructose-1-phosphate aldolase but that this enzyme is biologically inactive [106]. On the basis of these results these authors suggested that a mutation of the structural gene is responsible for the abnormality of fructose-1-phosphate aldolase in hereditary fructose intolerance.

Biochemical Consequences of Fructose-1-phosphate Aldolase Deficiency

Figure 6-8 illustrates the present concepts about the mechanism by which hypoglycemia and hypophosphatemia may be induced. Fructosemia and fructosuria appear to be due to inhibition of fructokinase by its reaction product, fructose-1-phosphate. Thus, nearly complete inhibition of fructose phosphorylation by normal liver homogenate was obtained when fructose-1-phosphate was present in the incubation medium in a concentration of $1 \times 10^{-2} M$ [76].

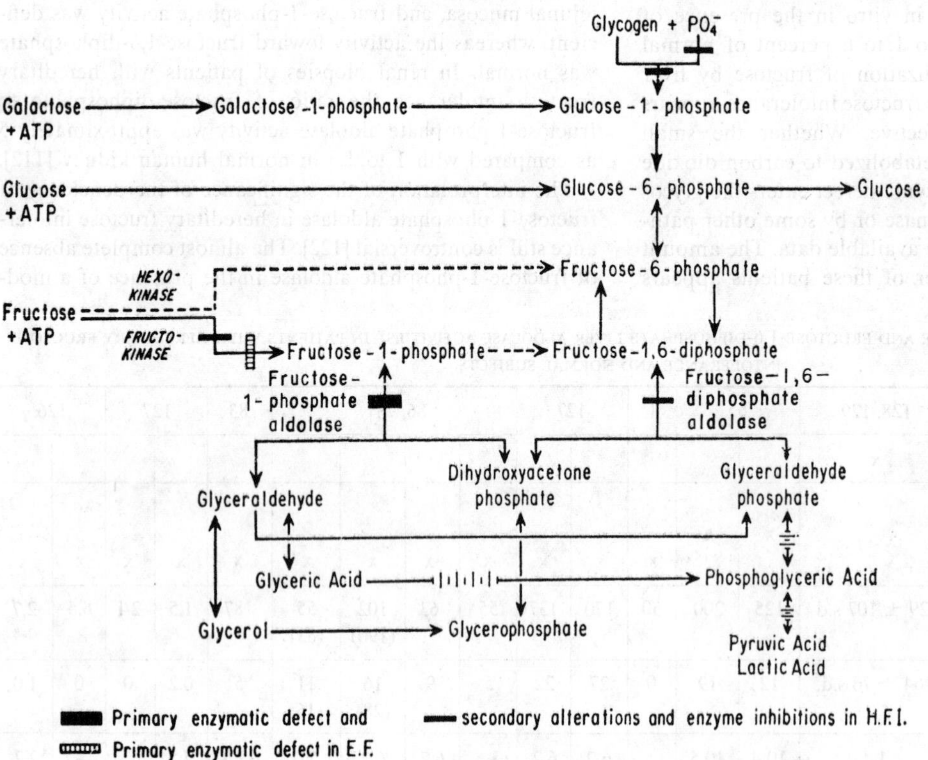

Figure 6-8. Primary enzyme defect in essential fructosuria and hereditary fructose intolerance and postulated secondary alterations and enzyme inhibitions in hereditary fructose intolerance. (*From Froesch et al.* [85], *reprinted with permission.*)

Whether the intracellular accumulation of this ester may ever reach values of that order of magnitude is uncertain, but there is evidence for it from two sources: (1) Kjerulf-Jensen [125] has measured concentrations of fructose-1-phosphate of this order of magnitude in the liver of rabbits after oral administration of fructose; (2) the K_m of normal liver aldolase for fructose-1-phosphate is of the order of magnitude of $10^{-2}M$ [32]. This indicates that its turnover may become appreciable only at high intracellular concentrations of fructose-1-phosphate. Since fructose is phosphorylated at a rapid rate, a steady state removal of fructose would be expected to occur at relatively high concentrations of fructose-1-phosphate.

It is tempting to search for a similar mechanism for the explanation of fructose-induced hypoglycemia. Fructose-1-phosphate has been shown to inhibit competetively fructose-1,6-diphosphate muscle aldolase, with an enzyme inhibitor dissociation constant of $0.91 \times 10^{-2}M$ [76]. This would impair new formation of glucose by the liver. In fact, fructose-induced hypoglycemia is not prevented by the simultaneous infusions of gluconeogenic precursors such as dihydroxyacetone or glycerol [90]. This was actually proved by incubating a liver biopsy specimen with glycerol-^{14}C with and without fructose. Whereas oxidation of glycerol to $^{14}CO_2$ was unaffected by fructose, the latter completely inhibited the conversion of glycerol-^{14}C to glucose-^{14}C (unpublished observations). Glycerol and dihydroxyacetone do not prevent fructose-induced hypoglycemia when infused simultaneously.

Using crystalline human liver aldolase, Bally and Leuthardt [131] have recently shown that fructose-1-phosphate does not interfere with the condensation of trioses to fructose-1,6-diphosphate. Under certain conditions, this condensation was actually activated by the simultaneous splitting of fructose-1-phosphate, indicating one single active site for all three reactions of normal human liver aldolase. In contrast, the condensation reaction was inhibited by fructose-1-phosphate in a liver homogenate from a patient with hereditary fructose intolerance. In this respect, the liver aldolase of patients with hereditary fructose intolerance again closely resembles normal muscle aldolase. However, when galactose is administered together with fructose to patients with hereditary fructose intolerance, hypoglycemia is less pronounced and lasts not as long as if fructose is given alone. This finding suggests that galactose is readily converted to glucose during fructose-induced hypoglycemia and, hence, that the activity of phosphoglucomutase under these circumstances in vivo is normal [82, 90]. Thus, a defect in the phosphorolysis of glycogen to glucose-1-phosphate must be incriminated in the failure of glucagon-induced glycogenolysis to repair hypoglycemia. According to Nivelon et al. [98] fructose-1-phosphate in a concentration of $8 \times 10^{-2}M$ almost completely inhibits phosphorolysis of glycogen by crystalline muscle phosporylase. Inhibition of glycogen breakdown by fructose-1-phosphate could not be demonstrated in liver homogenates.

Another important cause of diminished glycogenolysis might be a lack of inorganic phosphorus within the liver cell, reflecting the marked and prolonged fall of the serum inorganic phosphorus level. This hypothesis has been contested on the basis that phosphate infusions do not alter the hypoglycemic reaction in any way [98, 102]. In all fairness it must be said that a high level of inorganic phosphorus in the plasma can in no way indicate whether or not inorganic phosphorus is present at the site in the liver cell where phosphorylase splits off end-terminal glucose from glycogen. Furthermore, an intracellular ATP depletion might result from rapid fructose phosphorylation and deficient fructose oxidation due to the aldolase block. Data of Levin et al. [83, 100] on the magnesium levels in patients with hereditary fructose intolerance favor this hypothesis. Since ATP is needed for gluconeogenesis, a lack of ATP might be responsible for decreased or absent hepatic glucose formation. Since galactose does prevent fructose-induced hypoglycemia, this hypothesis appears rather unlikely. But again, ATP may be present in some cellular compartments and not in others. Obviously a discussion of the mechanism involved in the production of hepatic hypoglycemia must still be speculative.

Genetics

The pedigree of one large family with consanguineous ancestors (Fig. 6-9) shows that this form of fructose intolerance is a hereditary disorder. Most of the reported family histories are compatible with the hypothesis of an autosomal recessive inheritance on the basis of the following two criteria: (1) the patients belong to both sexes, and (2) sibs are affected, whereas the parents and offspring of the patients are always healthy. Consanguinity among the ancestors was present in two families.

There are three families in which parents with clear-cut hereditary fructose intolerance have had children with the same disorder. These families do not fit into the usual pattern of autosomal recessive inheritance, but rather suggest dominant inheritance [1, 77, 84]. One of the following two explanations for this finding must be considered:

1 These cases might be explained on the basis of recessive heredity if the affected homozygous child is an offspring of an affected homozygous father and a healthy but heterozygous mother.

2 The families may represent a different genotype with true dominant inheritance. Froesch et al. have found the typical fructose-1-phosphate aldolase defect in one patient whose father also had typical hereditary fructose intolerance [1].

Fructose tolerance test results in the parents of patients with hereditary fructose intolerance are normal, although this has been contested [109]. This problem has been settled by the findings of Raivio et al. [111], who found entirely

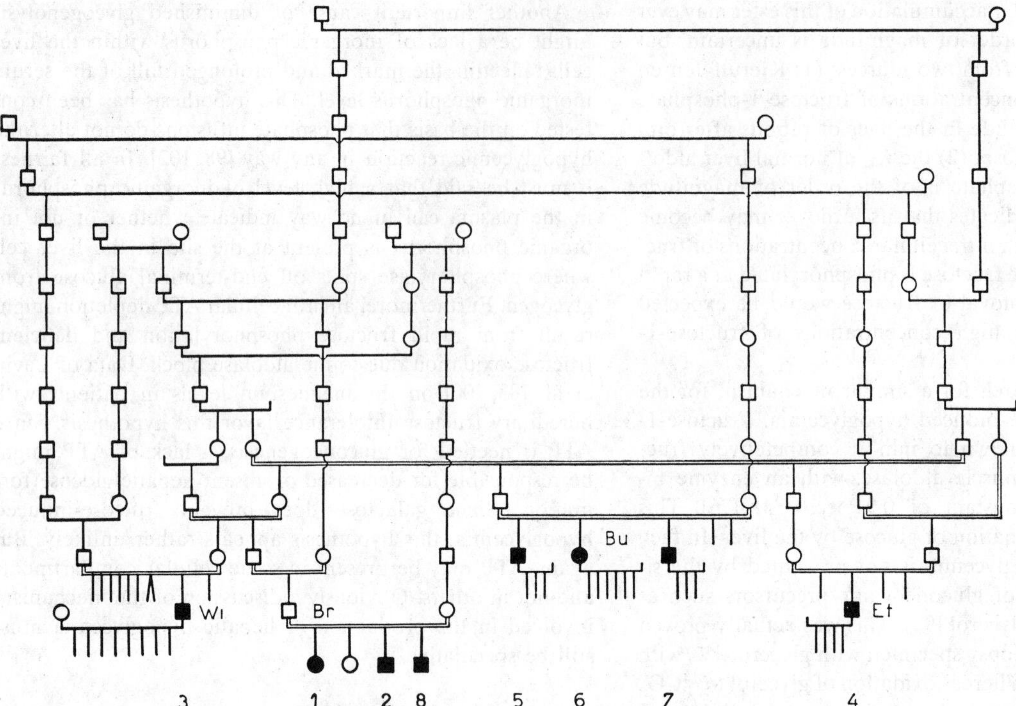

Figure 6-9. Pedigree of the largest documented family with hereditary fructose intolerance. Note the consanguineous marriages. The diagnosis was established by fructose tolerance tests in Cases 1, 2, 4, and 8, and is based on the case histories in the remaining patients [85]. The letters refer to family names. The vertical terminal lines indicate normal sibs.

normal fructose-1-phosphate aldolase activities in five parents of patients with hereditary fructose intolerance. This finding is compatible only with an autosomal recessive trait in which the fructose-1-phosphate aldolase of heterozygous carriers of hereditary fructose intolerance is functionally entirely intact [111].

FAMILIAL GALACTOSE AND FRUCTOSE INTOLERANCE

In 1961 Dormandy and Porter [116] reported the occurrence of a combination of fructose and galactose intolerance in two sisters. The symptoms in these patients are distinct from those of hereditary fructose intolerance, inasmuch as both patients were fond of sweets, sugar, and chocolate, and never showed nausea or vomiting after fructose ingestion. Both fructose and galactose induced severe hypoglycemia, with blood sugar levels below 20 mg per 100 ml. Clinical symptoms responded promptly to intravenous administration of glucose. The fall of blood glucose level was slower after intravenous galactose administration. As in hereditary fructose intolerance, there was a fall of the serum phosphorus concentration after fructose administration.

Galactose-1-phosphate uridyl transferase activity in the red blood cells of these patients was within the normal range. Studies of liver enzymes were not carried out in these patients. Samols and Dormandy [118] determined immunologically active insulin in both patients and found elevated fasting values that were in the same range as those of patients with islet cell adenomas. As in typical hereditary fructose intolerance, there was a fall of serum insulin level during the development of fructose-induced and of galactose-induced hypoglycemia. Serum insulin rose to extremely high levels after oral glucose administration, but the blood sugar curves were normal. It is impossible, at the present time, to find a link between the disturbance of fructose and galactose metabolism on the one hand and between these metabolic disturbances and the well-documented hyperinsulinism on the other hand.

HEREDITARY FRUCTOSE-1,6-DIPHOSPHATASE DEFICIENCY

This is a new genetic disorder described in one infant by Baker and Winegrad [132]. Another child of the healthy parents had died earlier of the same condition. Hereditary fructose-1,6-diphosphatase deficiency is characterized by hepatomegaly, spontaneous fasting hypoglycemia precipitated by stress such as acute infectious diseases and by fructose-induced hypoglycemia. In contrast to hereditary fructose intolerance, this child does not vomit after fructose ingestion and has developed normally both in growth and mentality despite regular intake of sucrose. Glucagon tests gave rise to a normal blood sugar increase only shortly after meals, whereas blood sugar failed to respond to glucagon after prolonged fasting. Normal blood sugar was maintained for 16 hours after the last meal, after which time it fell precipitously to low levels. It was concluded that the child could store glycogen normally after meals, but that gluconeogenesis was deficient. In fact, fructose-1,6-diphosphatase was demonstrated to be absent in liver biopsy specimens from this child. The mechanisms by which fructose and glycerol precipitate hypoglycemia is not entirely clear. It is likely that fructose-1-phosphate and fructose-1,6-diphosphate accumulate, leading to an intracellular depletion of inorganic phosphorus and to an inhibition of phosphorylase.

SUMMARY

1 Fructose accounts for one-sixth to one-third of the total carbohydrate intake. It is metabolized to more than 50 percent by way of a specific fructose pathway. Fructose may also be utilized through hexokinase if glucose is not present within the cell. This pathway is found in adipose tissue.
2 Essential fructosuria is a benign asymptomatic metabolic anomaly. The first enzyme of the specific fructose pathway, fructokinase, is deficient. Following ingestion of fructose, an abnormally high concentration of fructose appears in the blood, and blood lactate and the respiratory quotient fail to rise. In spite of this complete block of the specific fructose pathway, 80 to 90 percent of the fructose administered to patients with essential fructosuria is metabolized.
3 Hereditary fructose intolerance is characterized by severe hypoglycemia and vomiting shortly after ingestion of fructose. Prolonged periods of fructose ingestion in small children lead to failure to thrive, vomiting, jaundice, hepatomegaly, albuminuria, aminoaciduria, and finally to cachexia and death. The patients develop a strong distaste for sweets and fruit. The chronic picture of this syndrome is, therefore, encountered only in young children. Hepatic fructose-1-phosphate aldolase is deficient, and fructose-1-phosphate accumulates intracellularly. Hypoglycemia is due to a block of glucose release from the liver, not to hyperinsulinism. Both essential fructosuria and hereditary fructose intolerance appear to be inherited as autosomal recessive traits.
4 Another form of fructose intolerance has been described in association with galactose intolerance and hyperinsulinism. The pathogenesis of this syndrome, which is distinct from hereditary fructose intolerance, is not yet understood.
5 Hereditary hepatic fructose-1,6-diphosphatase deficiency is characterized by severe hypoglycemia during prolonged fasting. Hypoglycemia is also precipitated by ingestion of fructose, which, however, does not lead to vomiting. Mental development and growth remain normal despite fructose intake.

BIBLIOGRAPHY

1. Froesch, E. R.: Essential fructosuria and hereditary fructose intolerance, in *The Metabolic Basis of Inherited Disease,* 2d ed., edited by J. B. Stanbury, J. B. Wyngaarden, and D. S. Fredrickson, p. 124. Mc-Graw-Hill, New York, 1966.
2. Hardinge, M. G., Swarner, Julia, B., and Crooks, Hulda: Carbohydrates in foods. J. Amer. Diet. Ass., **46,** 197, 1965.
3. Roe, J. H., Epstein, J. H., and Goldstein, N. P.: A photometric method for the determination of inulin in plasma and urine. J. Biol. Chem., **178,** 839, 1949.
4. Higashi, A., and Peters, L.: A rapid colorimetric method for the determination of inulin in plasma and urine. J. Lab. Clin. Med., **35,** 475, 1950.
5. Froesch, E. R., Reardon, J. B., and Renold, A. E.: The determination of inulin in blood and urine using glucose oxidase for the removal of interfering glucose. J. Lab. Clin. Med., **50,** 918, 1957.
6. Lederle, E., and Lederle, M.: *Chromatography: A Review of Principles and Applications,* 2d ed., p. 245. Elsevier, Amsterdam, 1957.
7. Smith, L. H., Jr., Ettinger, R. H., and Seligson, D.: A comparison of the metabolism of fructose and glucose in hepatic disease and diabetes mellitus. J. Clin. Invest., **32,** 273, 1953.
8. Engelhardt-Goelkel, A., and Betz, B.: Ueber das Verhalten der Blutphosphate nach Glucose und Fructosebelastungen. Z. Ges. Exp. Med., **126,** 214, 1955.
9. Conard, V.: Mesure de l'assimilation du glucose: bases théoriques et applications cliniques. Acta Gastroent. Belg., **18,** 655, 1955.
10. Zöllner, N., Heuckenkamp, P. U., and Nechwatal, W.: Ueber die Verwertung und renale Ausscheidung von Fructose während ihrer langdauernden intravenösen Zufuhr. Klin. Wschr., **46,** 1300, 1968.
11. Craig, J. W., Miller, M., Mackenzie, M. S., and Woodward, H., Jr.: The influence of dietary carbohydrate deprivation on the metabolism of intravenously administered fructose and glucose in man. J. Clin. Invest., **37,** 118, 1957.
12. Bergström, J., Hultmann, E., and Roch-Norlund, A. E.: Lactic acid accumulation in connection with fructose administration. Acta Med. Scand., **184,** 359, 1968.
13. Pletscher, A., Fahrlaender. H., and Staub, H.: Zum Kohlenhydratstoffwechsel. III. Fructoseumsatz bei Gesunden, Diabetikern und Leberkranken. Helv. Physiol. Pharmacol. Acta, **9,** 46, 1951.
14. Miller, M., Drucker, W. R., Owens, J. E., Craig, J. W., and Woodward, H., Jr.: Metabolism of intravenous fructose and glucose in normal and diabetic subjects. J. Clin. Invest., **31,** 115, 1952.
15. Felber, J. P., Renold, A. E., and Zahnd, G. R.: The comparative metabolism of glucose, fructose, galactose and sorbitol in normal subjects and disease states. Mod. Probl. Pediat., **4,** 467, 1959.
16. Miller, M., Craig, J. W., Drucker, W. R., and Woodward, H., Jr.: The metabolism of fructose in man. Yale J. Biol., **29,** 355, 1956.
17. Metz, R., Mako, M., and Franklin, J.: The metabolism of fructose in diabetes mellitus. J. Lab. Clin. Med., **69,** 494, 1967.
18. Mendeloff, A. J., and Weichselbaum, T. E.: The role of the human liver in the assimilation of intravenously administered fructose. Metabolism, **2,** 450, 1953.
19. Levine, R., and Huddleston, B.: The comparative action of insulin on the disposal of intravenous fructose and glucose. Fed. Proc., **6,** 151, 1947.
20. Bollman, J. L., and Mann, C. F.: The physiology of the liver. XIX. The utilization of fructose following complete removal of the liver. Amer. J. Physiol., **96,** 683, 1931.
21. Deuel, H. J.: Intermediary metabolism of fructose and galactose. Physiol. Rev., **16,** 173, 1936.
22. Reinecke, R. M.: The kidney as a locus of fructose metabolism. Amer. J. Physiol., **141,** 669, 1944.

23. Leuthardt, F., and Testa, E.: Ueber die Phosphorylierung der Ketosen. Helv. Physiol. Pharmacol. Acta, **8,** 67, 1950.
24. Hers, H. G.: La fruktokinase du foie. Biochim. Biophys. Acta, **8,** 416, 1952.
25. Kuyper, Ch. M. A.: Studies on fructokinase. I. Substrate specificity. Koninkl. Nederl. Akad. Wetenschap. Proc. ser. B, **62,** 137, 1959.
26. Slein, M. W., Cori, G. T., and Cori, C. F.: Comparative study of hexokinase from yeast and animal tissue. J. Biol. Chem., **186,** 763, 1950.
27. Villar-Palasi, C., and Sols, A.: Phosphorylation du fructose par la phosphofructokinase du muscle. Bull. Soc. Chim. Biol., **39,** suppl. 2, 71, 1957.
28. Leuthardt, F., Testa, E., and Wolf, H. P.: Der enzymatische Abbau des Fructose-1-phosphats in der Leber. III. Mitteilung über den Stoffwechsel der Fructose in der Leber. Helv. Chim. Acta, **36,** 227, 1953.
29. Hers, H. G., and Kusaka, T.: Le métabolisme du fructose-1-phosphate dans le foie. Biochim. Biophys. Acta, **11,** 427, 1953.
30. Kaletta-Gmuender, U., Wolf, H. P., and Leuthardt, F.: Chromatographische Trennung von I-Phosphofructoaldolase und Diphosphofructoaldolase der Leber. Helv. Chim. Acta, **40,** 1027, 1957.
31. Peanasky, R. J., and Lardy, H. A.: Bovine liver aldolase. I. Isolation, crystallization and some general properties. II. Chemical and physical measurements on the crystalline enzymes. J. Biol. Chem., **233,** 365, 371, 1958.
32. Leuthardt, F., and Wolf, H. P.: Ueber die Spezifität der Aldolasen. Helv. Chim. Acta, **37,** 1734, 1954.
33. Penkoet, E., Rajkumar T., and Rutter, W. J.: Multiple forms of fructose diphosphate aldolase in mammalian tissues. Proc. Nat. Acad. Sci. U.S.A., **56,** 1275, 1966.
34. Gürtler, B. and Leuthardt, F.: Ueber die Heterogenität der Aldolase. Helv. Chim. Acta, **53,** 654, 1970.
35. Hers, H. G.: The conversion of fructose-1-C^{14} and sorbitol-1-C^{14} to liver and muscle glycogen in the rat. J. Biol. Chem., **214,** 373, 1955.
36. Salomon, L. L., and Johnson, J. E.: Transfer of fructose and glucose across surviving guinea pig intestine. Arch. Biochem. Biophys., **82,** 179, 1959.
37. Heinz, F., and Lamprecht, W.: Anreicherung und Charakterisierung einer Triosekinase aus Leber. Zur Biochemie des Fructosestoffwechsels. III. Z. Physiol. Chem., **324,** 88, 1961.
38. Heinz, F., Lamprecht, W., and Kirsch, J.: Enzymes of fructose metabolism in human liver. J. Clin. Invest., **47,** 1826, 1968.
39. Lamprecht, W., and Heinz, F.: Isolierung von Glycerin-aldehydehydrogenase aus Rattenleber. Zur Biochemie des Fructosestoffwechsels. Z. Naturforsch., **13b,** 464, 1958.
40. Holzer, H., and Holldorf, A.: Anreicherung, Charakterisierung und biologische Bedeutung einer D-glycerat-kinase aus Rattenleber. Biochem. Z., **329,** 283, 1957.
41. Ichihara, A., and Greenberg, D. M.: Studies on the purification and properties of D-glyceric acid kinase. J. Biol. Chem., **225,** 949, 1957.
42. Wolf, H. P., and Leuthardt, F.: Ueber die Glycerindehydrogenase der Leber. Helv. Chim. Acta, **36,** 1463, 1953.
43. Ginsberg, J. L.: Fruktosestoffwechsel des Fettgewebes. II. Abbauwege der Fruktose im epididymalen Fettgewebe der Ratte. Z. Ges. Exp. Med., **139,** 101, 1965.
44. Froesch, E. R., and Ginsberg, J. L.: Fructose metabolism of adipose tissue. I. Comparison of fructose and glucose metabolism in epididymal adipose tissue of normal rats. J. Biol. Chem., **237,** 3317, 1962.
45. Hers, H. G.: L'aldose-réductase: le mécansime de la formation du fructose séminal et du fructose foetal. Biochim. Biophys. Acta, **37,** 120, 127, 1960.
46. Cahill, G. F., Jr., Ashmore, J., Earle, A. S., and Zottu, S.: Glucose penetration into liver. Am. J. Physiol., **192,** 491, 1958.
47. LeFevre, P. G., and Davies, R. I.: Active transport into the human erythrocytes: evidence from comparative kinetics and competition among monosaccharides. J. Gen. Physiol., **34,** 515, 1951.
48. Froesch, E. R., Ginsberg, J. L., and Semenza, G.: Fructose metabolism of adipose tissue, in Fourth International Congress of the International Diabetes Federation, p. 607. Médecine et Hygiène, Geneva, 1962.
49. Crofford, O. B., and Renold, A. E.: Glucose uptake by incubated epididymal adipose tissue. Rate limiting steps and site of insulin action. J. Biol. Chem., **240,** 14, 1965.
50. Renold, A. E., and Thorn, G. W.: Clinical usefulness of fructose. Amer. J. Med., **19,** 163, 1955.
51. Mackler, B., and Guest, G. M.: Effects of insulin and glucose on utilization of fructose by isolated rat diaphragm. Proc. Soc. Exp. Biol. Med., **83,** 327, 1953.
52. Froesch, E. R.: Fructose metabolism of adipose tissue of normal and diabetic rats, in *Handbook of Physiology,* vol. on Adipose Tissue, edited by A. E. Renold and G. F. Cahill, Jr., p. 281. American Physiology Society, Washington, 1965.
53. Morgan, H. E., Henderson, M. J., Regen, D. M., and Park, C. R.: Regulation of glucose uptake in muscle. I. The effects of insulin and anoxia on glucose transport and phosphorylation in the isolated perfused heart of normal rats. J. Biol. Chem., **236,** 253, 1961.
54. Gammeltoft, A., Kruhohher, P., and Lundsgaard, E.: Insulin and the assimilation of fructose. Acta Physiol. Scand., **8,** 162, 1944.
55. Pearson, C. M., and Rimer, D. G.: Evidence of direct utilization of fructose in working muscle. Proc. Soc. Exp. Biol. Med., **100,** 671, 1959.
56. Park, C. R., Johnson, L. H., Wright, J. H., Jr., and Batsel, H.: Effect of insulin on transport of several hexoses and pentoses into cells of muscle and brain. Amer. J. Physiol., **191,** 13, 1957.
57. Cori, C. F.: The fate of sugar in the animal body. I. The rate of absorption of hexoses and pentoses from the intestinal tract. J. Biol. Chem., **66,** 691, 1925.
58. Crane, R. K.: Intestinal absorption of sugars. Physiol. Rev., **40,** 789, 1960.
59. Darlington, W., and Quastel, J. H.: Absorption of sugars from isolated surviving intestine. Arch. Biochem., **43,** 194, 1953.
60. Ginsburg, V., and Hers, H. G.: On the conversion of fructose to glucose by guinea pig intestine. Biochim. Biophys. Acta, **38,** 427, 1960.
61. Gammeltoft, A., and Kjerulf-Jensen, K.: Mechanism of renal excretion of fructose and galactose in rabbit, cat, dog, and man (with special reference to phosphorylation theory). Acta Physiol. Scand., **6,** 368, 1943.
62. Sachs, B., Sternfeld, L., and Kraus, G.: Essential fructosuria: its pathophysiology. Amer. J. Dis. Child., **63,** 252, 1942.
63. Marble, A.: Diagnosis of less common glycosurias, including pentosuria and fructosuria. Med. Clin. N. Amer., **31,** 313, 1947.
64. Lasker, M.: Essential fructosuria. Hum. Biol., **13,** 51, 1941.
65. Wallenfels, K.: Ueber das Vorkommen freier Fructose im menschlichen Blut. Naturwissenschaften, **38,** 238, 1951.
66. Silver, S., and Reiner, M.: Essential fructosuria: report of 3 cases with metabolic studies. A.M.A. Arch. Intern. Med., **54,** 412, 1934.
67. Edhem, Erden, F., and Steinitz, K.: Etudes sur un cas de lévulosurie essentielle. Acta Med. Scand., **97,** 455, 1938.
68. Steinitz, H.: Untersuchungen zur Pathologie des Fructose-Stoffwechsels: reine Fructosurie bei Geschwistern: Diabetes und Fructose-Stoffwechsel. Gastroenterologia, **64,** 334, 1939.
69. Heeres, P. A., and Vos, H.: Fructosuria. A.M.A. Arch. Intern. Med., **44,** 47, 1929.
70. Steinitz, H., Steinitz, K., and Mizrachi, O.: Essentielle Fructosurie: Untersuchungen des intermediären Stoffwechsels bei intravenöser Fructosebelastung. Schweiz. Med. Wschr., **93,** 756, 1963.
71. Baylon, H., Schapira, F., Wegmann, R., Dreyfus, J. C., Moulias, R., Poyart, C., and Coumel, Ph.: Note préliminaire sur l'étude clinique, biologique, histochimique et enzymatique de la fructosurie familiale essentielle. Rev. Franç. Étud. Clin. Biol., **7,** 531, 1962.
72. Laron, Z.: Essential benign fructosuria. Arch. Dis. Child., **36,** 273, 1961.
73. Schapira, F., Schapira, G., and Dreyfus, J. C.: La Lésion enzymatique de la fructosurie bénigne. Enzym. Biol. Clin. (Basel), **1,** 170, 1961/1962.
74. Chambers, R. A., and Pratt, R. T. C.: Idiosyncrasy to fructose. Lancet, **2,** 340, 1956.
75. Froesch, E. R., Prader, A., Labhart, A., Stuber, H. W., and Wolf, H. P.: Die hereditäre Fructoseintoleranz, eine bisher nicht bekannte kongenitale Stoffwechselstörung. Schweiz. Med. Wschr., **87,** 1168, 1957.
76. Froesch, E. R., Prader, A., Wolf, H. P., and Labhart, A.: Die hereditäre Fructoseintoleranz. Helv. Paediat. Acta, **14,** 99, 1959.

77. Wolf, H., Zschokke, B., Wedenmeyer, F. W., and Huebner, W.: Angeborene hereditäre Fructoseintoleranz. Klin. Wschr., **37**, 693, 1959.
78. Dubois, R., Loeb, H., Ooms, H. A., Gillet, P., Bartman, J., and Champenois, A.: Etude d'un cas d'hypoglycémie fonctionelle par intolérance au fructose. Helv. Paediat. Acta, **16**, 90, 1961.
79. Lelong, M., Alagille, D., Gentil, C., Colin, J., Tupin, J., and Bouguier, J.: Cirrhose hépatique et tubulopathie par absence congenitale de l'aldolase hépatique: intolérance héréditaire au fructose. Bull. Soc. Méd. Hop. Paris, **113**, 58, 1962.
80. Jeune, M., Planson, E., Cotte, J., Bonnefoy, S., Nivelon, J. L., and Skosowsky, J.: L'Intolérance héréditaire au fructose, à propos d'un cas. Pédiatrie, **16**, 605, 1961.
81. Perheentupa, J., Pitkänen, E., Nikkilä, E. A., Somersalo, O., and Hakosalo, J.: Hereditary fructose intolerance, a clinical study of 4 cases. Ann. Paediat. Fenn, **8**, 221, 1962.
82. Cornblath, M., Rosenthal, I. M., Reisner, S. H., Wybregt, S. H., and Crane, R. K.: Hereditary fructose intolerance. New Eng. J. Med., **269**, 1271, 1963.
83. Levin, B., Oberholzer, V. G., Snodgrass, G. J. A. I., Stimmler, L., and Wilmers, M. J.: Fructosemia: an inborn error of fructose metabolism. Arch. Dis. Child., **38**, 220, 1963.
84. Auricchio, S., and Prader, A.: Personal communication.
85. Froesch, E. R., Wolf, H. P., Baitsch, H., Prader, A., and Labhart, A.: Hereditary fructose intolerance: an inborn defect of hepatic fructose-1-phosphate splitting aldolase. Amer. J. Med., **34**, 151, 1963.
86. Hers, H. G.: Augmentation de l'activité de la glucose-6-phosphatase dans l'intolérance au fructose. Rev. Int. Hépat., **12**, 6, 1962.
87. Hübschmann, K., and Cobet, G.: Beitrag zur hereditären Fructose-intoleranz. Deutsch. Med. Wschr., **89**, 938, 1964.
88. Sacrez, R., Juif, J.-G., Metais, P., Sofatzis, J., and Dourof, N.: Un cas mortal d'intolérance héréditaire au fructose. Etude biochimique et enzymatique. Pédiatrie, **17**, 875, 1962.
89. Royer, P., Lestradet, H., Habib, R., Lardinois, R., and Desbuquois, B.: L'Intolérance héréditaire au fructose. Bull. Soc. Med. Hop. Paris, **115**, 805, 1964.
90. Gentil. C., Colin, J., Valetta, A. M., Alagille, D., and Lelong, M.: Etude du métabolisme glucidique au cours de l'intolérance héréditaire au fructose. Essai d'interprétation de l'hypoglucosemia. Rev. Franç. Etud. Clin. Biol., **9**, 596, 1964.
91. Milhaud, G.: Téchnique nouvelle de mise en évidence d'erreurs congénitales du métabolisme chez l'homme. Arq. Brasil Endocr., **13**, 49, 1964.
92. Schwartz, R., Gamsu, H., Mulligan, P. B., Reisner, S. H., Wybregt, S. H., and Cornblath, M.: Transient intolerance toward fructose in the newborn. J. Clin. Invest., **43**, 333, 1964.
93. Dahlqvist, A., and Crane, R. K.: The influence of the method of assay on the apparent specificity of rabbit-liver aldolase. Biochim. Biophys. Acta, **85**, 132, 1964.
94. Gmyrek, D., Hübschmann, K., and Klimmt, G.: Diagnostische und therapeutische Probleme bei der hereditären Fructoseintoleranz. Mschr. Kinderheilk., **116**, 16, 1968.
95. Swales, J. D., and Smith, A. D. M.: Adult fructose intolerance. Quart. J. Med., **35**, 455, 1966.
96. Hübschmann, K., Gobet, G., and Friedel, E.: Untersuchungen zur hereditären Fructoseintoleranz. Paediat. Grenzgeb., **4**, 107, 1965.
97. Black, J. A., and Simpson, K.: Fructose intolerance. Brit. Med. J., **4**, 138, 1967.
98. Nivelon, J. L., Mathieu, M., Kissin, C., Collombel, C., Cotte, J., and Béthenod, M.: Intolérance au fructose. Observation et mécanisme physiopathologique de l'hypoglucosémie. Ann. Pédiat., **43**, 817, 1967.
99. Philips, M. J., Path, M. C., Little, J. A., and Ptak, T. W.: Subcellular pathology of hereditary fructose intolerance. Amer. J. Med., **44**, 910, 1968.
100. Levin, B. Snodgrass, G. J. A. I., Oberholzer, V. G., Burgess, E. Ann, and Dobbs, R. H.: Fructosemia: observation on seven cases. Amer. J. Med., **45**, 826, 1968.
101. Cotte, J., Mathieu, M., Nivelon, J. L., Bethenod, M., Kissin, C., and Collombel, C.: Contribution à l'étude du mécanisme de l'hypoglycémie dans l'intolérance au fructose. Clin. Chim. Acta, **19**, 215, 1968.
102. Desbuquois, B., Lardinois, R., Gentil, C., and Odievre, M.: Effets d'une surcharge en phosphate de sodium sur l'hypoglucosémie dans onze observations d'intolérance héréditaire au fructose. Arch. Franç. Pédiat., **26**, 21, 1969.
103. Mass, R. E., Smith, W. R., and Walsh, J. R.: The association of hereditary fructose intolerance and renal tubular acidosis. Amer. J. Med. Sci., **251**, 516, 1966.
104. Morris, R. C., Jr.: An experimental renal acidification defect in patients with hereditary fructose intolerance. I. Its resemblance to renal tubular acidosis. J. Clin. Invest., **47**, 1389, 1968.
105. Morris, R. C., Jr.: An experimental renal acidification defect in patients with hereditary fructose intolerance. II. Its distinction from classical renal tubular acidosis; its resemblance to the renal acidification defect associated with the Fanconi syndrome of children with cystinosis. J. Clin. Invest., **47**, 1648, 1968.
106. Nordmann, Y., Shapira, F., and Dreyfus, J. C.: A structurally modified liver aldolase in fructose intolerance: immunological and kinetic evidence. Biochem. Biophys. Res. Commun., **31**, 884. 1968.
107. Shapira, F., Nordmann, Y., and Dreyfus, J. C.: La Lésion biochimique de l'intolérance héréditaire au fructose. Détection immunologique d'une aldolase modifiée. Rev. Franç. Etud. Clin. Biol., **13**, 267, 1968.
108. Klimmt, G., Hübschmann, K., and Gmyrek, D.: Untersuchungen zur Verminderung des Fructosegehalts der Kartoffel. Ein Beitrag zur diätetischen Behandlung der hereditären Fructoseintoleranz. Mschr. Kinderheilk., **116**, 21, 1968.
109. Beyreiss, K., Willgerodt, H., and Theile, H.: Untersuchungen bei heterozygoten Merkmalsträgern für Fructoseinterolanz. Klin. Wschr., **46**, 465, 1968.
110. Fiehring, C., and Braun, W.: Hereditäre Fructoseintoleranz. Paediat. Prax., **7**, 73, 1968.
111. Raivio, K., Perheentupa, J., and Nikkilä, E. A.: Aldolase activities in the liver in parents of patients with hereditary fructose intolerance. Clin. Chim. Acta, **17**, 275, 1967.
112. Morris, R. C., Jr., Ueki, I., Loh, D., Eanes, R. Z., and Melin, P.: Absence of renal fructose-1-phosphate aldolase activity in hereditary fructose intolerance. Nature (London), **214**, 920, 1967.
113. Marthaler, T. M., and Froesch, E. R.: Hereditary fructose intolerance. Dental status of eight patients. Brit. Dent. J., **123**, 597, 1967.
114. Marthaler, T. M., and Froesch, E. R.: Ist Weissbrot kariogen? Schweiz. Mschr. Zahnheilk., **77**, 630, 1967.
115. Shapira, F., and Dreyfus, J. C.: L'Aldolase hépatique dans l'intolérance au fructose. Rev. Franç. Etud. Clin. Biol., **12**, 486, 1967.
116. Dormandy, T. L., and Porter, R. J.: Familial fructose and galactose intolerance. Lancet, **1**, 1189, 1961.
117. Froesch, E. R.: Fructosurie und Fructoseintoleranz, in *Genetic Defects of Biologically Active Proteins,* edited by F. Linneweh, p. 242. Urban & Schwarzenberg, Munich, 1962.
118. Samols, E., and Dormandy, T. L.: Insulin response to fructose and galactose. Lancet, **1**, 478, 1963.
119. Schambye, P., and Tarding, F.: Changes induced by insulin and tolbutamide in the glucose output of the liver. Ann. N.Y. Acad. Sci., **74**, 557, 1959.
120. Shoemaker, W. C., Mahler, R., and Ashmore, J.: The effect of insulin on the hepatic glucose metabolism in the unanesthetized dog. Metabolism, **8**, 494, 1959.
121. Hers, H. G., and Joassin, G.: Anomalie de l'aldolase hépatique dans l'intolérance au fructose. Enzym. Biol. Clin., **1**, 4, 1961.
122. Wolf, H. P., and Froesch, E. R.: Ueber Aldolasen. IV. Mitteilung. Enzymaktivitäten in der Leber bei hereditärer Fructoseintoleranz. Biochem. Ztschr., **337**, 328, 1963.
123. Rutter, J. W., Richards, O. C., and Woodfin, B. M.: Comparative studies of liver and muscle aldolase. I. Effect of carboxypeptidase on catalytic activity. J. Biol. Chem., **236**, 3193, 1961.
124. Drechsler, E. R., Boyer, P. D., and Kowalesky, A. G.: The catalytic activity of carboxypeptidase-degraded aldolase. J. Biol. Chem., **234**, 2627, 1959.

125. Kjerulf-Jensen, K.: The phosphate esters formed in the liver tissue of rats and rabbits during assimilation of hexoses and glycerol. Acta Physiol. Scand., **4,** 249, 1942.

126. Nikkilä, E. A., Somersalo, O., Pitkänen, E., and Perheentupa, J.: Hereditary fructose intolerance, an inborn deficiency of liver aldolase complex. Metabolism, **11,** 727, 1962.

127. Pitkänen, E., and Perheentupa, J.: Eine biochemische Untersuchung über zwei Fälle von Fructoseintoleranz. Ann. Paediat. Fenn., **8,** 236, 1962.

128. Schmidt, E., Schmidt, F. W., and Wildhirt, E.: Vergleichende Aktivitäts-Bestimmungen von Enzymen des energieliefernden Stoffwechsels in der menschlichen und in der Rattenleber. Klin. Wschr., **36,** 172, 1958.

129. Schmidt, E., Schmidt, F. W., and Wildhirt, E.: Fermentaktivitäts-Bestimmungen in der menschlichen Leber. 6. Mitteilung. Klin. Wschr., **37,** 1221, 1959.

130. Auerswald, W., and Kupetz, G.-W.: Beitrag zur Klinik der hereditären Fruktoseintoleranz. Sonderdruck Deutsch. Gesundh., **19,** 875, 1969.

131. Bally, C., and Leuthardt, F.: Aldolase and hereditary fructose intolerance. In preparation.

132. Baker, L., and Winegrad, A. I.: Fasting hypoglycemia and metabolic acidosis associated with deficiency of hepatic fructose-1,6-diphosphatase activity. Lancet, **ii,** 13, 1970.

CHAPTER SEVEN

THE GLYCOGEN STORAGE DISEASES*

R. Rodney Howell

The dramatic physical findings which often accompany the glycogen storage diseases led to the clinical and pathologic recognition of these disorders as early as 1929 [1]. It was evident early that there were patients with prominent liver involvement ("hepatic" glycogen storage disease or von Gierke's disease) and other patients with a more generalized storage of glycogen, with striking cardiac involvement [2].

Until 1952 only these two general types of glycogen storage disease were differentiated. In that year the Coris [3] demonstrated a specific deficiency of glucose-6-phosphatase in a patient with the hepatic form of glycogen storage. As further enzyme studies have been performed on tissues from patients with the glycogen storage diseases, it has become clear that deficiencies of a variety of enzymes involved in glycogen synthesis and degradation can produce diseases which are not distinguishable clinically. On the other hand it is also remarkable that genetic abnormalities in glycogen metabolism can produce such a vast spectrum of clinical disorders. The glycogen storage diseases may present themselves primarily as disorders of the liver, heart, or musculoskeletal system. We now are aware of eight groups of inherited abnormalities in glycogen metabolism in man which can be defined clinically or biochemically; additional abnormalities will undoubtedly be defined in the future.

GLYCOGEN

Structure and Function

Glycogen is the principal storage form of carbohydrate in the animal and is found in varying concentrations in virtually all cells. Starches, the storage carbohydrates of plants, contain both amylose (which has exclusively 1,4 linkages between its constituent glucose molecules) and amylopectin (which has in addition 1,6 branch points). Glycogens have many more 1,6 linkages, which permit a highly branched polymeric structure. The highly branched molecule of mammalian glycogen imparts considerably greater solubility to glycogen than is possessed by the starches. Glycogens are simpler molecules than proteins or nucleic acids, since glucose is their only building block [4]. Glycogen differs from most other important macromolecules in man in that it is quite polydisperse and lacks a fixed molecular weight [5].

There is controversy about the exact macromolecular structure of glycogen. French has pointed out that it is particularly difficult to construct a physical model of glycogen based on a more or less regularly rebranched pattern when the molecular size becomes large [6]. If one begins at the reducing end and increases molecular size by elongating the straight chain and branching it, there is ample room to spare. But as the molecule increases in size, there comes a point at which the periphery is so densely packed that it is sterically impossible to continue regular branching. Since virtually all models with extensive branching would allow adequate space in the interior of the molecule, it is assumed that glycogen does indeed have many chains which terminate in the interior. These buried chains might well be resistant to enzymes because of steric protection. French has pointed out also that formation of the 1,6 (branch) points at the expense of 1,4 links is highly favored thermodynamically [6]. Since glycogen has less than 10 percent of glucose residues in 1,6 linkage (branch points), the branching enzyme must be severely hindered sterically (Fig. 7-1).

Glycogen extracted under gentle conditions in cold water has molecular weights ranging from a few million to well over several hundred million [7]. Physical evidence (such as viscosity measurements) suggests that glycogen is nearly spherical and is extensively hydrated. If the molecule has any regular branching structure and any hydration at all, a molecular weight of greater than 5 to 6 million would be about the largest possible. This consideration has led to the suggestion that the extraordinarily large-molecular-weight species are in reality aggregates of molecules of smaller size [6]. The exact nature of the forces holding the large molecules together is not known, but it appears that conven-

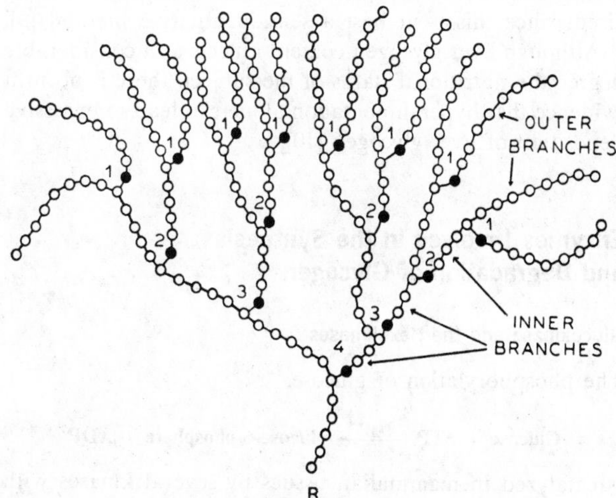

Figure 7-1. Schematic representation of a part of a glycogen molecule. Each circle represents a glucose molecule; the open circles represent the linear portions of glycogen with the glucoses in α-1,4 linkage. Branch points in the glycogen (α-1,6 linkage) are represented by closed circles. R = reducing end group. The terminal glucose in the outer branches is nonreducing. (*From G. T. Cori, with permission* [178].)

*Certain of the author's studies were supported by Grant No. AM09251 from the National Institutes of Health.

tional covalent or hydrogen bonds are not involved. When visualized under the electron microscope, these large particles appear to have single units that range in size from several million up to 5 million. It would appear, therefore, that glycogen as it exists in vivo is composed of small, nearly spherical, highly branched units which have molecular weights of several million. These in turn are aggregated by forces which are currently not clearly understood.

Glycogen Content of Human Tissues

There is limited information on the glycogen content of normal, fresh human liver and muscle. Preparation for biopsy often includes prolonged fasts and infusions of glucose. In addition, a wide variety of physiologic stimuli affect tissue glycogen concentration. Certain of the glycogen storage diseases may on occasion have normal or near-normal tissue glycogen content. The usual concentration of glycogen in liver is below 5 to 7 gm per 100 gm wet weight; muscle glycogen is usually under 2 gm per 100 gm wet weight.

Human fetal liver begins to accumulate glycogen during the final trimester of pregnancy [8]. The usual amount of branching is found at the earliest times investigated. Liver glycogen level falls rapidly in the newborn period, in association with increase in phosphorylase activity [8]. Adult levels are reached by 2 to 3 weeks of age.

In view of these findings measurement of tissue glycogen content may fail to extablish or rule out a diagnosis of a glycogen storage disease except when high concentrations or abnormal glycogen structure are encountered. As Öckerman has wisely emphasized, if tissue staining is used for glycogen quantitation, even greater caution must be exercised, since this is at best a semiquantitative method [9].

Although liver glycogen content reflects to a considerable degree the nutritional status of the subject, there is no firm evidence that hyperalimentation alone can lead to excessive deposition of liver glycogen [10].

Enzymes Involved in the Synthesis and Degradation of Glycogen

Glucokinase and the Hexokinases

The phosphorylation of glucose,

$$\textbf{Glucose} + \textbf{ATP} \xrightarrow{Mg^{++}} \textbf{glucose-6-phosphate} + \textbf{ADP}$$

is catalyzed in mammalian tissues by several kinases with different distributions and properties. In liver there is a highly specific glucokinase, in addition to other hexokinases. The glucokinase activity of liver falls dramatically during fasting and in alloxan diabetes. Treatment with insulin (in diabetes) or refeeding (after fasting) causes a prompt increase in glucokinase [11]. Adrenalectomy, cortisone, or thyroid hormone has no effect on glucokinase activity [12].

Muscle contains only the less specific hexokinase, and has no detectable specific glucokinase activity [13]. Certain of the properties of glucokinase and the hexokinases are summarized in Table 7-1 [14]. The rate of phosphorylation of glucose by liver is well correlated with glucokinase activity. As its activity is affected by a series of physiologic stimuli, its role in the regulation of glycogen synthesis is apparent. It is estimated that in the normal well-fed animal glucokinase accounts for 80 percent of hepatic phosphorylation of glucose [15].

Phosphoglucomutase

Phosphoglucomutase catalyzes the reversible transfer of a phosphate group between the 1 and 6 positions of glucose (see Fig. 7-2). There is no known complete deficiency of this enzyme in man. This is the only reversible step in glycogen synthesis and breakdown; its central position suggests that total deficiency of the enzyme might be lethal.

At 30°C, the equilibrium lies far towards glucose-6-phosphate (94 to 95 percent). The enzyme mechanism has been established as [16, 17]:

$$\alpha\textbf{-Glucose-1-P} + \textbf{phosphoenzyme}$$
$$\Updownarrow$$
$$\alpha\textbf{-Glucose-1,6 diphosphate} + \textbf{dephosphoenzyme}$$
$$\Updownarrow$$
$$\alpha\textbf{-Glucose-6-phosphate} + \textbf{phosphoenzyme}$$

The requirement for glucose-1,6-diphosphate is well established; it functions as a "primer," or as a true coenzyme and is required only in catalytic amounts [16]. This enzyme is not thought to be a site of physiologic regulation of glycogen synthesis or degradation [18].

Uridine Diphosphate (UDP) Glucose Pyrophosphorylase

Liver is extremely rich in this enzyme activity. As much as 0.3 percent of the extractable protein (from calf liver) has pyrophosphorylase activity [19]. The reaction catalyzed by the enzyme is (Fig. 7-2):

$$\textbf{Glucose-1-phosphate} + \textbf{UTP} \longrightarrow \textbf{UDP glucose} + \textbf{PP}_i$$

It provides UDP glucose for glycogen synthetase. The pyrophosphate can use other nucleoside sugars as substrates but at much lower rates.

This large enzyme (molecular weight 400,000) is competitively inhibited by uridine diphosphate. The large quantity of this enzyme in liver, in addition to its low Michaelis constant for UTP (uridine triphosphate) ($2.2 \times 10^{-4} M$), and glucose-1-phosphate ($5.5 \times 10^{-5} M$), and the high turnover number (83,000) indicate that this enzyme would rarely be limiting in glycogen formation [19]. Since UDP is inhibitory, it must be removed (by conversion to UTP or by further

Table 7-1. COMPARATIVE PROPERTIES OF GLUCOKINASE AND HEXOKINASES IN RAT LIVER

Property	Glucokinase	Hexokinases
Michaelis constant for glucose	10 mM	0.01–0.1 mM
Allosteric inhibition by glucose-6-P	No	Yes
Ability to phosphorylate fructose	Poor	Good
Ability to phosphorylate glucosamine	None	Good
Molecular weight	50,000	96,000
Typical activity in normal fed animals, μmoles/gm liver/min, at 30°C	3	1
Activity in starved animals	Decreased	Normal

Source: Data from Sols et al. [14].

degradation). There are no known deficiencies of this enzyme in man.

Glycogen Synthetase (UDP-glucose-glycogen Glucosyl Transferase)

It was once contended that phosphorylase is active in both the synthesis and degradation of glycogen. This enzyme is primarily responsible for the phosphorolysis of glycogen by breaking terminal 1,4 linkages to release glucose-1-P (see below). The difficulty in this concept was in understanding what might control the direction of this reaction so that it would go toward either synthesis or degradation. The reaction is in equilibrium when the ratio of inorganic phosphate to glucose-1-phosphate is 3.5 at pH 7. At higher ratios glycogen degradation occurs. In rat diaphragm the ratio is about 300. Also, agents which are known to activate phosphorylase (e.g., epinephrine and glucagon) always induce glycogenolysis.

In 1957, Leloir and Cardini [20] first demonstrated synthesis of glycogen in liver extracts incubated with uridine

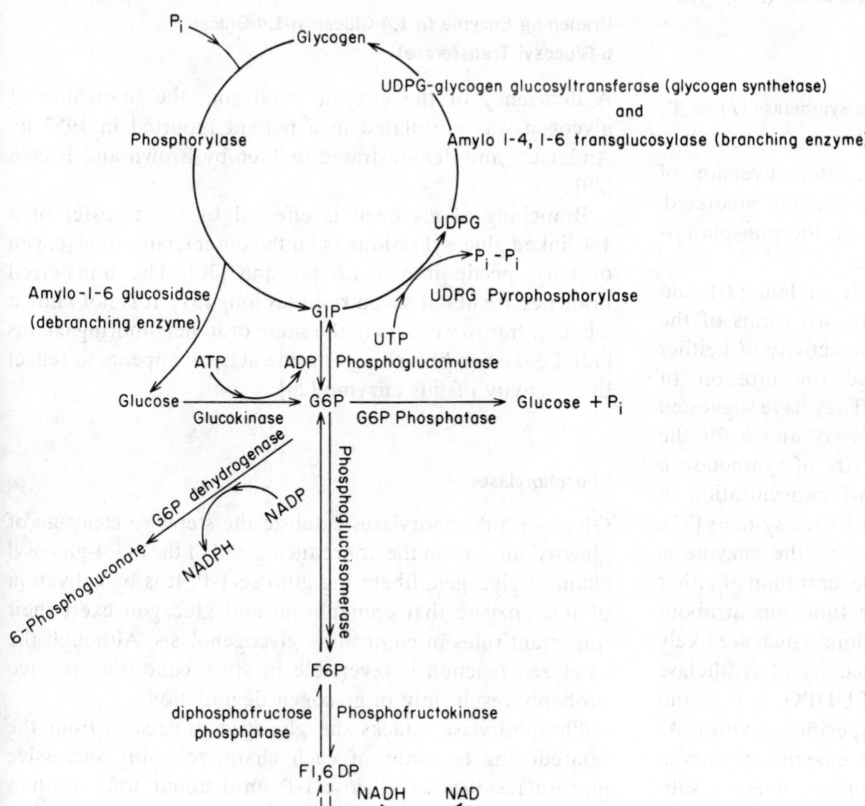

Figure 7-2. Major pathways in the synthesis and degradation of glycogen. The broken line indicates several steps which have been omitted between fructose-1,6-diphosphate and pyruvate. (*Modified from Bueding and Colacci* [179].)

diphosphate glucose (UDPG). Synthesis of glycogen in human muscle, not involving phosphorylase, was first clearly shown in studies of patients lacking muscle phosphorylase (McArdle's disease). The reaction catalyzed by glycogen synthetase is (Fig. 7-2):

$$\textbf{UDPG} + \textbf{G}_n \textbf{ (glycogen primer)} \longrightarrow \textbf{G}_{(n+1)} + \textbf{UDP}$$

The equilibrium of this reaction strongly favors glycogen synthesis.

Activity of the most highly purified glycogen synthetase is wholly dependent on the addition of glycogen as primer [21]. Although the enzyme does not require a metal ion, it is stimulated twofold by $MgCl_2$.

Pioneering studies from Larner's laboratories have clearly shown that glycogen synthetase exists in two distinct forms, termed *D* (dependent) and *I* (independent) [22]. This nomenclature refers to the fact that the *I* form is little stimulated in vitro by G-6-P whereas the *D* form is dependent on G-6-P for activity. The following interconversions occur between the *D* and *I* forms of glycogen synthetase:

$$\textbf{Glycogen synthetase } (I) + {}_n\textbf{ATP} \xrightarrow[\textbf{Mg}^{++}]{\textbf{kinase}} \textbf{glycogen synthetase } (D) + {}_n\textbf{ADP}$$

$$\textbf{Glycogen synthetase } (D) \xrightarrow{\textbf{phosphatase}} \textbf{glycogen synthetase } (I) + {}_n\textbf{P}_i$$

Larner and his group showed that the interconversion of the *I* to *D* form of the enzyme is enzymatically mediated. Unlike phosphorylase (as described later), the phosphorylated (*D*) form of the enzyme is inactive.

Mersmann and Segal suggest that dependent (*D*) and independent (*I*) are poor terms for the two forms of the enzyme [23]. Their studies show that the activity of neither form is significantly affected by changed concentrations of G-6-P, which are likely to occur in vivo. They have suggested that *a* be used for the form active in vivo, and *b* for the physiologically inactive form. The activity of synthetase *a* is highly responsive to changes in G-6-P concentration in the physiologic range (*ca.* 0.06 mM) in cell-free systems [23]. In the presence of G-6-P *and* P_i, however, the enzyme is relatively insensitive to changes in the concentration of either of these ligands. Therefore, the *a* form functions at about one-half to full capacity under all conditions which are likely to exist in vivo. If one compares the activity of synthetase *a* and *b* at physiologic concentrations of UDPG, G-6-P, and P_i, one finds a ratio of about 15:1 in specific activities. As extracted from normal, fed animals, the enzyme appears to be entirely in the *b* (inactive) form. Insulin converts a substantial portion to the *a* form; this effect is reversed by glucagon [24].

De Wulf and Hers [25, 26] have found that intravenous administration of glucose stimulates fifteen- to twentyfold the conversion of glucose to glycogen by liver. This is associated with a sharp increase in glycogen synthetase activity. The rate of glycogen synthesis is not correlated with liver glucose content but is highly correlated with the glycogen synthetase activity.

During glycogen breakdown adenosine-3′,5′-cyclophosphate (cyclic AMP) exerts control by activating phosphorylase *b* kinase (see below). This cyclic nucleotide also stimulates the kinase which converts the independent (active) form of glycogen synthetase to the dependent (inactive) form [27]. Huijing and Larner [27] suggest that Mg^{++} causes an allosteric activation of glycogen synthetase *I* kinase and that cyclic AMP increases the degree of affinity of the allosteric site of the enzyme for Mg^{++}. In this way cyclic AMP would impair glycogen synthesis.

Glycogen synthetase exists bound to particulate glycogen (as does phosphorylase) and is primarily associated with the smooth endoplasmic reticulum [28]. On fasting there is a progressive decrease in glycogen synthetase activity associated with the smooth endoplasmic reticulum. The enzyme responsible for converting the *a* form of glycogen synthetase to the *b* form, glycogen synthetase kinase, is also contained in the smooth endoplasmic reticulum fraction of liver.

Branching Enzyme (α-1,4-Glucan:α-1,4-Glucan 6-Glucosyl Transferase)

A deficiency of the enzyme catalyzing the branching of glycogen was postulated in a patient reported in 1952 by Andersen, and demonstrated in 1966 by Brown and Brown [29].

Branching of glycogen is effected by the transfer of a 1,4-linked glucosyl residue from the outer chains of glycogen or amylopectin into a 1,6 position [30]. The transferred branches are about seven residues long [31]. It is not known whether transfer occurs to the same or to neighboring chains [30]. Leukocyte branching enzyme activity appears to reflect liver activity of this enzyme [29].

Phosphorylases

Glycogen phosphorylases catalyze the stepwise cleavage of glucosyl units from the nonreducing end of the α-1,4-glucosyl chain of glycogen, liberating glucose-1-P. It is by activation of this enzyme that epinephrine and glucagon exert their important roles in controlling glycogenolysis. Although the catalyzed reaction is reversible in vitro, conditions in vivo probably result only in glycogen degradation.

Phosphorylase attacks the glycogen molecules from the nonreducing terminus of each chain, releasing successive glucose residues as glucose-1-P until about four residues remain on each branch. Phosphorylase can proceed no further until the α-1,4 trisaccharide is removed from the 1,6-linked glucose by an oligo-1,4 → 1,4-glucan transferase.

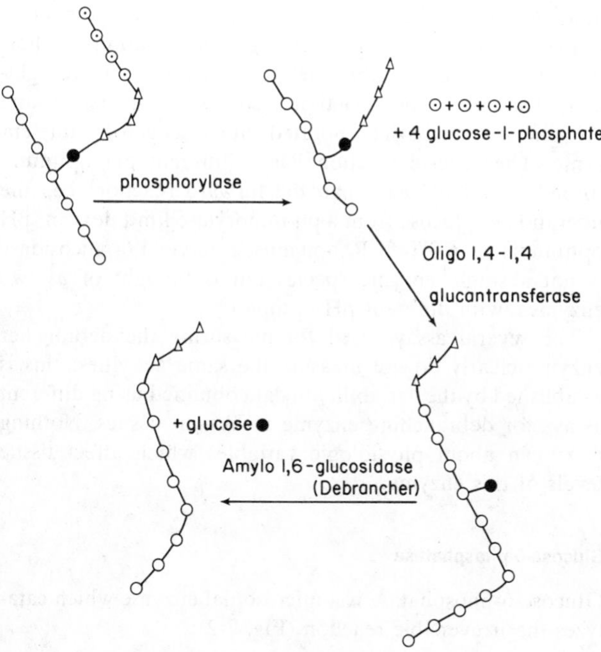

Figure 7-3. Schematic representation of the enzymatic debranching of glycogen. Only a small segment of a glycogen molecule is represented. In order for debrancher to work, the three glucose residues attached to the branched glucose (α-1,6-linked) after phosphorylase action must be transferred by an oligo-1,4 → 1,4-glucan transferase. Note that the debrancher yields free glucose while phosphorylase produces glucose-1-phosphate.

Removal of the glucose attached in a 1,6 linkage by an amylo-1,6-glucosidase permits phosphorylase to continue until the next branch point is reached [32] (Fig. 7-3). Since liver and muscle phosphorylases are distinct proteins [33], they will be considered separately.

Muscle Phosphorylase

Muscle phosphorylase, first crystallized from the rabbit, exists in an active (phosphorylase *a*) and inactive (phosphorylase *b*) form. Phosphorylase in resting muscle is predominately in the *b* (inactive) form [34]. The conversion of the *b* to *a* form of phosphorylase occurs as:

$$\textbf{Phosphorylase } b + 4\,\textbf{ATP} \xrightarrow[\textbf{Mg}^{2++}]{\textbf{active phosphorylase kinase}} \textbf{phosphorylase } a + 4\,\textbf{ADP}$$

This phosphorylation of the inactive enzyme in the presence of ATP is catalyzed by a specific kinase, phosphorylase *b* kinase. This kinase also exists in an active and inactive form and is activated by 3′,5′-cyclic adenylic acid. The activation of phosphorylase by epinephrine (and glucagon in liver) is mediated through changes in tissue levels of 3′,5′-cyclic adenylic acid.

The reverse reaction (phosphorylase dephosphorylation and inactivation) is catalyzed by a highly specific phosphatase [35] which is inhibited by AMP in concentrations as low as $10^{-5}M$.

Tryptic peptide analyses of phosphorylase have shown that seryl residues undergo phosphorylation during phosphorylase activation [36]. This seryl phosphate residue is in a different amino acid sequence depending on whether the phosphorylase is isolated from liver or from muscle.

AMP is required for any activity in vitro of phosphorylase *b*, and it stimulates phosphorylase *a* about 30 to 40 percent [36]). By light scattering there is no change in the molecular weight of phosphorylase *b* in the presence of AMP. Since the sedimentation constant of the inactive (nonphosphorylated) enzyme is changed in the presence of AMP, this nucleotide probably produces conformational changes in the protein.

At one time it was thought that the active muscle phosphorylase *a* exists solely as a tetramer with a molecular weight of 500,000, and that phosphorylase *b* is a dimer with a molecular weight of 250,000. Treatment of the enzymes with SH-binding reagents forms subunits with a molecular weight of 125,000. The tetrameric form of phosphorylase *a* contains four phosphate groups, four groups of pyridoxal-5′-phosphate, and binds four AMP units.

Recent studies have shown that phosphorylase *a* at high protein concentrations exists in equilibrium between a high-activity and a low-activity form and that the *active* form is a *dimer* with a molecular weight of about 250,000. The tetrameric form of phosphorylase *a* (molecular weight 500,000) cannot bind to glycogen, and therefore the only active form of phosphorylase *a* is the dimer [37].

Although aggregation of phosphorylase into a tetramer appears to follow phosphorylation closely, the exact relationship is unclear. Tryptic digests of phosphorylase *a* show that the peptide chain at the site of phosphorylation is highly charged positively. It is suggested that aggregation follows phosphorylation by neutralizing the charges at the positive site. This would allow interaction between interpeptide chains previously statically repulsed [38]. Aggregation would also be favored by high protein concentrations.

At high ionic strength and low protein concentrations the tetrameric form of phosphorylase *a* dissociates into a dimeric species of higher catalytic activity [39]. It has also been shown that the conversion of the dimeric species of phosphorylase *a* into the tetrameric form (inactive) is effectively blocked by glycogen [40, 41].

There is considerable difficulty in the determination of molecular weights of associating-dissociating systems such as phosphorylase. The molecular weights of phosphorylase *a* and *b* have been reinvestigated by Seery et al. [41*a*], using a variety of conditions favoring association and dissociation. They found a molecular weight of 185,000 to 188,000 for phosphorylase *b*, and 370,000 for phosphorylase *a*. Their data fit more closely than previous data with regard to stoichiometry of pyridoxal-5′-phosphate.

Liver Phosphorylase

Liver phosphorylase likewise exists in an active and inactive form. Similarly, the activation of phosphorylase is accomplished by phosphorylation (in a protein-phosphate covalent bond) of the enzyme by a highly specific phosphokinase which requires ATP and Mg^{++}.

Unlike muscle phosphorylase, liver phosphorylase does not appear to undergo molecular-weight change during activation. It has a molecular weight of about 237,000 in either the active or inactive condition [42].

Liver phosphorylase is inactivated by a highly specific phosphatase. The dephosphorylated liver phosphorylase is not activated by the addition of AMP [43]. Phosphorylated liver phosphorylase activity is increased up to 40 percent by AMP. Although cysteine and reduced glutathione do not stimulate phosphorylase activity, they do protect against inhibition by mercuric and other metal ions [43]. Liver phosphorylase is activated by both glucagon and epinephrine through their stimulatory effect on phosphorylase kinase, while the muscle phosphorylase is activated only by epinephrine.

The phosphorylase kinase activation by glucagon is effected by increasing the tissue concentrations of cyclic AMP. The plasma membrane of hepatic parenchymal cells contains an adenyl cyclase system which is stimulated by glucagon [44]. Epinephrine and ACTH do not stimulate this adenyl cyclase. This suggests that glucagon exerts its regulatory action in liver by stimulating adenyl cyclase activity in the plasma membrane [44]. This would in turn increase tissue levels of cyclic AMP, which would activate phosphorylase kinase and thereby produce the active form of the phosphorylase.

Amylo-1,6-glucosidase (Debrancher)

After extensive phosphorylase action on glycogen, the molecule contains four glucose residues in α-1,4-glucosidic bonds attached by a 1,6 link to the glycogen molecule (see Fig. 7-3). This molecule is called the phosphorylase limit dextrin, or LD [45]. In order for amylo-1,6-glucosidase (debrancher) to act on this molecule, three of these glucose residues must be removed to expose the 1,6-linked glucose at the branch point. This is accomplished by an *oligo-1,4 → 1,4-glucan transferase,* which transfers these three glucose residues (probably as a unit) to another glycogen chain, with resynthesis of the α-1,4 bond [46] (Fig. 7-3). The most highly purified preparations of amylo-1,6-glucosidase contain significant oligo-1,4 → 1,4-glucan transferase activity, and this enzyme has appropriately been called a glucosidase transferase. During purification and heat inactivation these enzyme activities remain in a constant ratio [47].

The action of debrancher on the limit dextrin yields free glucose. Since there are about 8 percent branch points (1-6 links) in glycogen, extensive glycogen degradation by phosphorylase and debrancher yields about 8 percent free glucose. The debrancher reaction is somewhat reversible, and ^{14}C-glucose can be incorporated into glycogen by this enzyme. The reverse reaction has a different pH optimum (broad, about pH 8.0) than the forward reaction, i.e., the liberation of glucose from a phosphorylase limit dextrin (pH optimum near 6.0) [45]. Rabbit muscle amylo-1,6-glucosidase is not a single enzyme species but is thought of as two enzymes, with different pH optima [48].

The several assays used for measuring the debrancher enzyme clearly do not measure the same activities; this is established by the variability in data obtained using different assays for debranching enzyme in human tissues. Nothing is known about physiologic variables which affect tissue levels of this enzyme.

Glucose-6-phosphatase

Glucose-6-phosphatase is a microsomal enzyme which catalyzes the irreversible reaction (Fig. 7-2):

$$\textbf{Glucose-6-P} + \textbf{H}_2\textbf{O} \longrightarrow \textbf{glucose} + \textbf{P}_i$$

As with most microsomal enzymes, it has not been highly purified and its molecular properties are not known. Although not absolutely specific for glucose-6-phosphate, none of the alternative hexose phosphates is hydrolyzed at a rate of more than one-fifth that of glucose-6-phosphate [49].

Incubation for several minutes at pH 5, 37°C, destroys the ability of this enzyme to hydrolyze glucose-6-phosphate without loss of the nonspecific hydrolase activity [49, 50]. This finding has been of practical value in correcting for nonspecific phosphatase activity when assaying liver tissues from patients.

This enzyme is normally present in human liver, kidney, and intestinal mucosa. By histochemical techniques it has also been demonstrated in the pancreatic β cells, localized specifically in the cisternae of the endoplasmic reticulum and the nuclear membrane [51].

Glucose-6-phosphatase possesses at least two other enzymatic properties [52]:

1. The ability to cleave inorganic pyrophosphate hydrolytically
2. The ability to transfer phosphate from inorganic pyrophosphate to glucose, thereby forming glucose-6-phosphate

In animals a 300 percent increase in glucose-6-phosphatase activity is seen after 48 hr of fasting [53]. With continued fasting, activity returns to near-basal levels by 124 hr. Alloxan-diabetic rats have increased liver glucose-6-phosphatase activity, which returns to normal during insulin treatment [54]. The increase in liver glucose-6-phosphatase which occurs on a diet rich in fructose and proteins can be blocked by including 1 percent ethionine in the diet [50].

Feeding of 1 percent ethionine in order to block protein synthesis for 4 days does not result in a fall in basal activity of glucose-6-phosphatase in liver; this suggests that this microsomal enzyme is synthesized and degraded slowly. This assumes that protein synthesis is effectively blocked under these conditions [50].

Hydrocortisone administration increases activity of this enzyme in rat liver [55]. There is also a large increase in liver glucose-6-phosphatase activity in hereditary fructose intolerance, in which there is a deficiency of aldolase activity [50].

Phosphofructokinase

This enzyme catalyzes the irreversible conversion of fructose-6-phosphate to fructose-1,6 diphosphate. At normal tissue substrate concentrations phosphorylation of F-6-P is a controlling step in glycolysis [56].

Citrate and ATP are inhibitors for liver and brain phosphofructokinase. Inhibition by ATP and citrate can be overcome by fructose diphosphate (FDP), P_i, F-6-P, AMP, 3′,5 AMP, or ADP. A fall in ATP, or a rise in P_i or AMP within the cell would activate phosphofructokinase and therefore enhance glycolysis [56]. At usual levels of ATP in the cell, phosphofructokinase is in an inactive state (as long as P_i, AMP, and FDP are at low levels) [56]. This enzyme, which has a molecular weight of about 360,000, exhibits kinetics typical for allosteric inhibition in the presence of high concentrations of ATP [57].

α-1,4-Glucosidase (Acid Maltase)

The potential importance of the activity of this enzyme was realized only after it was found by Hers [58] to be deficient in generalized glycogenosis. α-1,4-Glucosidase is compartmentalized within the lysosome and sediments during cell fractionation in the lysosome-rich, light mitochondrial fraction. In human liver the α-glucosidase activity at neutral pH is only one-tenth to one-third that at pH 4 [59]. The enzyme in human liver and muscle has optimal activity at pH 4 [59]. It hydrolyzes maltose and other linear oligosaccharides, as well as the outer branches of glycogen, to yield free glucose [50].

Many hydrolytic enzymes have the same distribution during ultracentrifugation and the same structure-linked latency pattern (e.g., acid ribonuclease, acid deoxyribonuclease, cathepsins, aryl-sulfatases, β-galactosidase, and β-*n*-acetylglucosaminidase). The lysosomal localization of acid maltase has been confirmed by equilibration centrifugation in a density gradient, by its structure-linked latency and by its release under controlled damage [60].

Widespread distribution of this activity in human tissues, including fibroblasts growing in vitro as well as leukocytes, has made it relatively easy to establish diagnoses of genetic deficiencies of this enzyme.

GENETIC ABNORMALITIES IN GLYCOGEN METABOLISM

In 1952, the Coris [3] demonstrated directly a deficiency of liver glucose-6-phosphatase in patients with von Gierke's disease. This, the first demonstrated inherited deficiency of a liver enzyme in man, marked the beginning of such studies on a variety of hereditary diseases. There is now a series of inherited defects involving glycogen metabolism in liver, muscle, and other tissues. The Coris began a system of numbering these diseases sequentially, and this will be followed here, but with each disease the enzyme deficiency associated with the disease will be listed, and the eponyms will also be given, for historic completeness.

Type I Glycogen Storage Disease: Glucose-6-phosphatase Deficiency (Hepatorenal Glycogen Storage Disease, von Gierke's Disease)

Clinical Features

Children with this disorder have short stature without disproportion of head, limbs, or trunk length. The abdomen is huge and rotund because of massive enlargement of the liver. Liver enlargement is found in the newborn and persists throughout life (Fig. 7-4). As the patients grow older, the abdomen becomes less prominent. There is a tendency to adiposity, with generous accumulations of fat in the cheeks, buttocks, and subcutaneous tissues. The musculature is flabby and poorly developed [61]. Although the kidneys are enlarged, they cannot be palpated because of the massive hepatic enlargement. Radiographically, the kidney enlargement is readily appreciated (Fig. 7-5). The spleen is not enlarged. Fine, Wilson, and Donnell [62] have reported multiple, bilateral, symmetric, yellowish, discrete paramacular lesions in the fundi of three of five patients with Type I glycogen storage disease. Osteoporosis is usually present and possibly is secondary to the negative calcium balance related to the chronic acidosis.

Xanthomas appear commonly over the extensor surfaces of the extremities. Since these patients always have hyperuricemia, gouty tophi must be distinguished from xanthomas, which may have similar distribution.

Bleeding may be a major clinical problem. Frequent, severe nosebleeds and persistent oozing of blood after surgery are troublesome. Although a variety of hemostatic problems have been reported [63], several of our patients who have had bleeding episodes have had extensive clotting studies which proved to be normal [61, 64]. Often an abundance of small superficial vessels is visible in the skin of these patients.

Although steatorrhea occurs in some patients [65], we found no abnormality in fat absorption in one of our patients suspected of malabsorption [61]. Liver function test results (transaminases, bromsulphalein conjugation) are normal.

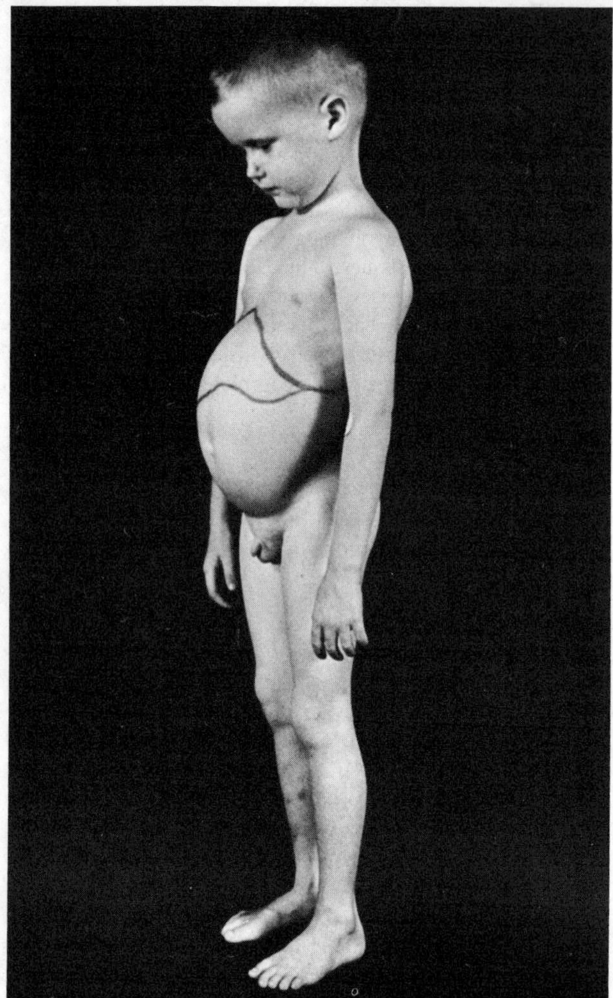

Figure 7-4. Seven-year-old boy (D.M.) with Type I (glucose-6-phosphatase deficiency) glycogen storage disease. The massive liver is outlined on the protuberant abdomen. In addition to short stature, there are generous fat deposits in the cheeks. We have previously published biochemical data on this boy [61].

In addition to fasting hypoglycemia and unresponsiveness to epinephrine and glucagon, there is a striking elevation in levels of blood lactate, pyruvate, triglycerides, phospholipids, cholesterol, ketones, and uric acid [61]. The degree of hypoglycemia is variable. The disease is compatible with a reasonably long life, and a number of adult patients are known [66, 67].

Convulsions accompanying severe hypoglycemia may occur during the first years of life; in others profound hypoglycemia is seen without clinical symptoms [66]. Patients may be asymptomatic with blood glucose concentrations of under 10 mg per 100 ml. It may be suggested that these patients, like starved obese patients [68], have replaced glucose with β-hydroxybutyrate and acetoacetate as the primary fuel of the brain.

Fanconi's syndrome (aminoaciduria, glucosuria, and phosphaturia) sometimes occurs in patients with Type I glycogen storage disease [69]. Three instances of both disorders are known. In normal mammals glucose-6-phosphatase is found in the proximal and distal convoluted tubules. In these patients glucose-6-phosphatase is deficient in the kidney, and glycogen accumulates there. If this enzyme were essential for energy-requiring renal processes, problems in renal transport would be expected.

The Mechanisms of the Lipid Abnormalities

Hyperlipemia may be a dominant feature in these patients [61, 70]. The operation of the glycolytic pathway and Krebs cycle results in production of NADH, while that of the oxidative pathway results in production of NADPH. Reduction of pyruvate to lactate requires either NADH or NADPH; fatty acid synthesis requires both these nucleotide

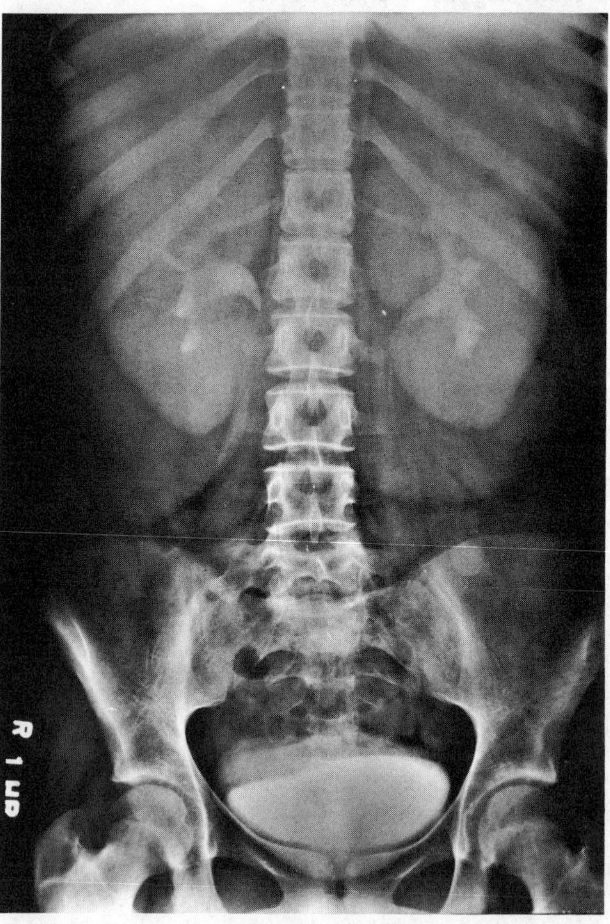

Figure 7-5. Abdominal roentgenogram, taken during an intravenous pyelogram, of young woman with Type I (glucose-6-phosphatase deficiency) glycogen storage disease. The nephrogram shows the large kidneys. The outline of the enormous liver can be seen bilaterally just above the pelvis; it is clear from this film why the enlarged kidneys are rarely palpable.

cofactors. Ketone body synthesis requires NADH, and NADPH is required in cholesterol synthesis, where it may indeed be the rate-limiting factor. Fatty acid, ketone, and cholesterol synthesis require acetyl CoA, which is produced in abundance from the pyruvate generated by glycolysis. Thus the substrates and the reduced coenzymes necessary for synthesis of lactate, ketones, fatty acids, and cholesterol are made available in quantity by high-level operation of the glycolytic and oxidative pathways, and these synthetic processes in turn regenerate the oxidized coenzymes necessary for sustaining active operation of these carbohydrate pathways. Thus, the elevated levels of serum triglycerides, phospholipids, ketone bodies, and cholesterol are possible consequences of glycogenolytic and gluconeogenetic responses to hypoglycemia in liver containing abundant glycogen, a block in glucose-6-phosphatase function, and active glycolytic and phosphogluconic oxidative pathways [61].

The elevation of free fatty acid levels in serum is probably a direct consequence of hypoglycemia. A reciprocal relationship between blood glucose and free fatty acid concentrations in serum has been noted on several occasions. Hypoglycemia is a potent stimulus to release of free fatty acids by adipose tissue, and the high free fatty acid levels observed probably reflect mobilization from the periphery [61]. Öckerman [71, 72] has also observed that serum concentrations of glycerol are elevated in these patients.

Glucose Tolerance and Insulin Output

Results of glucose tolerance tests in these patients are characteristically diabetic in type [61]. Earlier it was thought that this was due to the known inhibition of hexokinase by glucose-6-phosphate, which was thought to accumulate in the liver. Although liver glucose-6-phosphate concentration is moderately elevated [73], this would probably not inhibit hexokinase. More important, glucokinase, which is probably responsible for most hepatic glucose phosphorylation, is not inhibited by glucose-6-phosphate. In a recent study [74] basal plasma insulin levels were approximately 50 to 60 percent of normal in five older patients with Type I glycogen storage disease. Three well-known stimuli for secretion of insulin in normal man (glucose, glucose plus a protein meal, and arginine infusion) resulted in outputs of insulin significantly less than normal in these patients (Fig. 7-6).

The Mechanisms of the Hyperuricemia

Hyperuricemia in association with Type I glycogen storage disease has been reported in at least 38 patients since the association was first described by Kolb et al., in two patients in 1955 [75]. In these patients hyperuricemia appears in early infancy, but rarely becomes symptomatic before the end of the first decade of life. Although other symptoms from Type I glycogen storage disease diminish with age, acute gouty arthritis, gouty nephropathy, and chronic tophaceous gout often become major problems in adulthood.

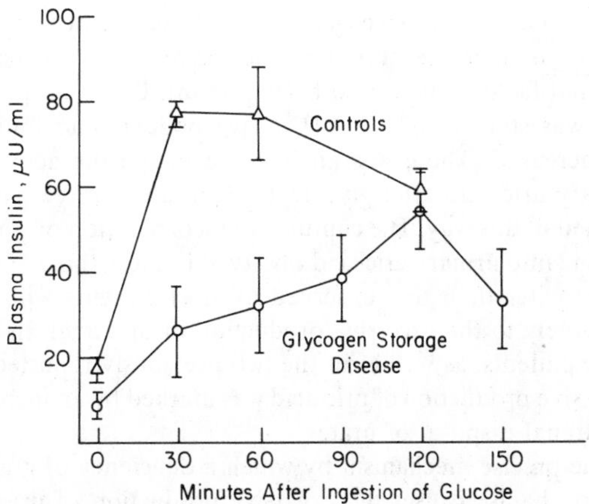

Figure 7-6. Plasma insulin levels after the ingestion of glucose in 15 normal subjects and 5 adolescent or adult patients with Type I glycogen storage disease. Values are the means ± standard errors of the means. The reduced insulin output in this group of patients with Type I glycogen storage disease is clear. (*From Lockwood et al.* [74].)

Hyperuricemia in this disease was originally attributed to a decreased excretion of uric acid because of competitive inhibition of renal tubular urate secretion by lactate [61, 76], which so frequently is elevated in the serum. This suggestion was supported by the demonstration of a reduced urate clearance in these patients [61], while renal function was normal as measured by other parameters. Fine et al. [77] and Alepa et al. [67] studied urate clearances in five patients with Type I glycogen storage disease and found that lowering serum lactic acid concentrations with glucose infusions increased the clearance of uric acid.

At least one additional factor probably contributes to the reduced renal clearance of uric acid in this disorder. These patients have serum ketone concentrations which may be elevated to several times normal. Studies by Goldfinger et al. [78] have shown that infusion of β-hydroxybutyrate or acetoacetate into control patients causes a significant renal retention of uric acid. Ketonemia has not been studied as an independent variable in the renal clearance of uric acid in glycogen storage disease.

In the course of renal clearance studies, both Fine et al. [77] and Alepa et al. [67] observed an increase in urate clearance when glucose was infused, but at a time when serum lactic acid had not changed detectably. Fine et al. suggested that since renal glucose-6-phosphatase was deficient in these patients, glucose was unavailable to the renal tubules as an energy source. Accordingly glucose infusion might increase urate clearance by making glucose available to the kidney tubule. An equally plausible explanation is that the glucose, by reducing the degree of ketonemia, might improve urate clearance. Since serum ketone concentrations were not monitored, this explanation can be neither confirmed nor excluded.

The finding by Jeune et al. [79] that several patients with

hyperuricemia and glycogen storage disease actually had a normal or increased uric acid clearance indicated that extrarenal factors might also be important. Uric acid production was studied [67, 80, 81] in five patients and found to be increased. There was an increase in specific activity of urinary uric acid after glycine-1-^{14}C in all of three patients studied in this way. The cumulative incorporation of isotopic glycine into urinary uric acid observed in these three patients was greater than that observed in most patients with gout due solely to the excessive production of uric acid. In these three patients, as well as in the two previously reported, the excessive production of uric acid was marked by an increased extrarenal disposal of urate.

The precise mechanism by which a deficiency of glucose-6-phosphatase causes the excessive production of uric acid remains unknown. It has been suggested that an increased synthesis of phosphoribosylpyrophosphate (PP-ribose-P) results from a deficiency of glucose-6-phosphatase [82, 83]. This might arise from a greater fraction of the glucose-6-phosphate being converted to ribose because one of its other major pathways is blocked. Increased production of PP-ribose-P, the substrate for the first specific irreversible, and rate-limiting step of purine synthesis, might lead to an increased rate of purine biosynthesis *de novo.*

Excessive uric acid production in certain other patients is associated with a complete or partial deficiency of an enzyme of purine metabolism, hypoxanthine-guanine phosphoribosyl transferase. This enzyme activity was normal in erythrocytes from three patients with Type I glycogen storage disease [81].

Functional Tests

Characteristically, these patients have a much diminished rise in blood glucose after administration of glucagon or epinephrine, as would be anticipated with a deficiency of glucose-6-phosphatase activity. The fact that the major product of glycogenolysis in these patients is lactic acid, rather than glucose, has been stressed by Lowe et al. [84]. Glucagon and epinephrine tolerance tests are rarely completely "flat"; this is probably related to the fact that in glycogenolysis, the 1,6-linked glucosyl residues are released as free glucose by debrancher activity.

Galactose Tolerance Test

Schwartz et al. [85] suggested that the inability of these patients to convert galactose (as well as other carbohydrates) to glucose would be useful as a diagnostic test. Figure 7-7 shows the results of a galactose infusion in a normal infant and in an infant with Type I glycogen storage disease. The inability to form glucose from galactose is obvious; in the patient with glycogen storage disease the galactose is rapidly converted to lactate. Fructose infusions produce similar results but are not as well tolerated clinically.

Biochemical Diagnosis

In all instances in which a glycogen storage disease is suspected, final diagnosis should be made by direct assay of appropriate tissue. In Type I glycogen storage disease, a liver

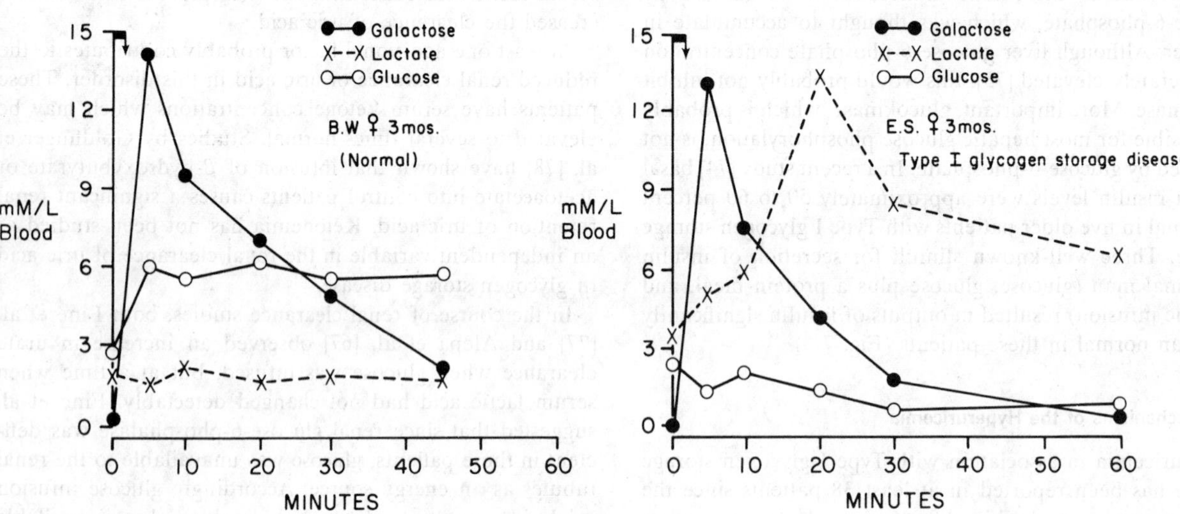

Figure 7-7. Intravenous galactose tolerance test in a normal infant and in an infant with absent glucose-6-phosphatase (Type I glycogen storage disease). One gram of galactose per kilogram of body weight was given. In the normal infant considerable galactose is converted to glucose, while in the patient with glycogen storage disease, blood glucose actually decreased while lactate increased briskly. (*Redrawn from Schwartz et al. with permission* [85].)

biopsy is desirable. Although a diagnosis can be made on needle biopsy material, an open biopsy is preferred except under unusual circumstances. The open biopsy affords adequate tissue for glycogen determination, glycogen structure analyses, and replicate assays of the various enzymes. More importantly, direct vision permits control of bleeding should any occur. Enzyme analysis should be done on freshly frozen, unfixed tissue in a laboratory in which these assays are well established. Glycogen content is usually elevated and has a normal structure. Glucose-6-phosphatase activity should be totally absent.

Genetics

There are many examples of this disorder among sibs, both male and female, whose parents are clinically normal. In addition, several patients affected with Type I glycogen storage disease (both male and female) have had phenotypically normal children [66, 67, 86]. Studies on intestinal glucose-6-phosphatase activity in patients with Type I glycogen storage disease and their families support an autosomal recessive inheritance scheme [87–89]. Field and Drash [89], who studied the parents of five children with Type I glycogen storage disease, found that all had reduced intestinal glucose-6-phosphatase activity. In one family the maternal grandfather and one of his brothers had reduced intestinal glucose-6-phosphatase, while another brother and the maternal grandmother had normal values.

Hsia and Kot [90] reported that erythrocyte sugar phosphate concentrations were increased in patients and families with this disease and concluded that they could ascertain the heterozygotes, but this has not been substantiated in erythrocytes or other tissues [50, 73].

Treatment

Glucagon and thyroxine have been suggested for treatment of this disease, but they appear to be of questionable benefit [61]. Frequent feedings are helpful if there is hypoglycemia. Since these patients have a limited capacity for converting amino acids to free glucose, a high-protein diet is not of special value.

Diazoxide (which increases blood sugar by increasing glycogenolysis, depressing insulin release, and inhibiting glucose uptake by the liver) has been used in two patients with Type I glycogen storage disease [92]. Since they were found to have higher fasting blood sugar levels, this drug may have some promise.

Portacaval transpositions or portacaval shunts have been performed in four patients with hepatic glycogen storage diseases. Three of these were Type I patients [93–97]. The rationale for this treatment was that Starzl and associates [94] had shown that portacaval shunts in animals reduce liver glycogen by over 50 percent. An additional benefit might be the delivery of glucose-rich blood to peripheral tissues before it reaches the liver. Two of the three patients with Type I disease apparently benefited from surgery, as shown by a growth spurt and reduction in liver size. The third patient (who had a portacaval transposition) died in the postoperative period with severe portal hypertension. Surgical procedures are probably worthy of future cautious evaluation. Probably the most promising surgical procedure would be the portacaval shunt [96].

Animal Models

Erickson et al. [98] have studied albino mice with four radiation-induced alleles, which were fatal in the newborn period if present in the homozygous state. These mice lack glucose-6-phosphatase activity in the liver and kidney. Liver glycogen was lower in the affected animals (1.9 gm per 100 ml) than in controls (5.9 gm per 100 ml). The short life of these mice makes interpretation of this finding difficult. Like patients with Type I glycogen storage disease, the mice also lacked inorganic pyrophosphatase activity, thought to be the same as glucose-6-phosphatase.

There is a report of glycogen storage disease (Types I, II, and III) in dogs, but the diagnosis has not been established at a tissue level [99].

Type II Glycogen Storage Disease: α-1,4-Glucosidase (Acid Maltase) Deficiency (Pompe's Disease, Generalized Glycogenosis)

The clinical manifestations of this disease contrast sharply with the other glycogen storage diseases. The usual presenting symptom of the child with this disorder is profound hypotonia during the first year of life (Fig. 7-8). The muscles

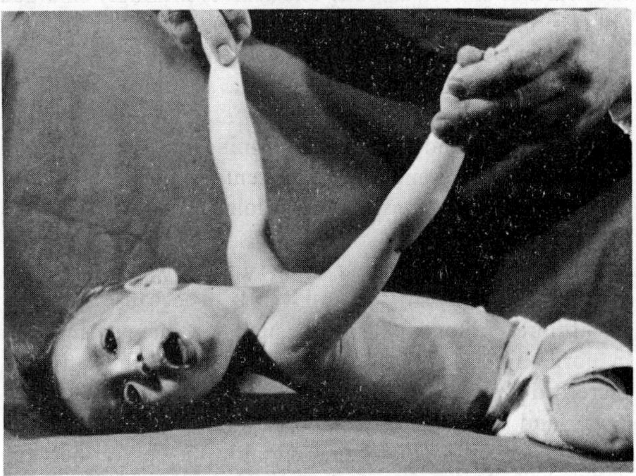

Figure 7-8. Seven-month-old female infant (D.B.) with generalized glycogenosis (Type II glycogen storage disease). The profound hypotonia is evident. Studies of a muscle biopsy in our laboratory showed increased glycogen (10 gm per 100 gm wet weight of tissue) of normal structure, normal phosphorylase and debrancher activity, and absent α-1,4-glucosidase activity. (*Photograph courtesy of Dr. M. Museles.*)

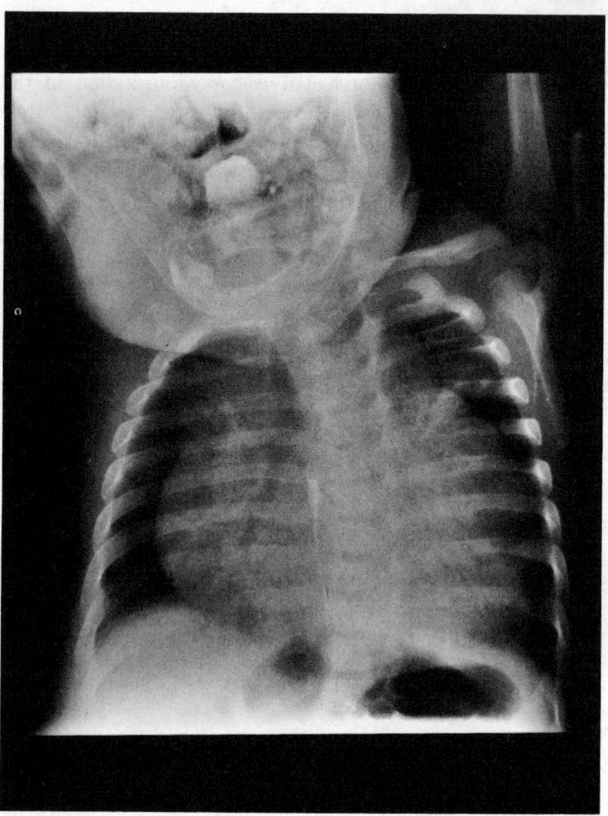

Figure 7-9. Chest roentgenogram of 4-month-old female infant (A.M.) with generalized glycogen storage disease (Type II). The massive heart dominates the film with a cardiothoracic index of 80 to 85.

are firm and of normal mass. The heart is strikingly enlarged (Fig. 7-9). The electrocardiogram shows the specific changes of gigantic QRS complexes in all leads and a shortened P-R interval [100, 101] (Fig. 7-10). Cardiac failure without cyanosis is common in the first year of life. Pulmonary vasculature is normal, and there are no significant murmurs [100]. Blood sugar, lipid and ketone concentrations are all within normal limits. Responses to glucagon and epinephrine are also normal.

Symptoms usually appear by age 2 months, and the average age at death is 5½ months [101]. The cause of death is cardiorespiratory failure. At autopsy a massive increase in normally structured glycogen is found in most tissues. Increased glycogen concentrations are found in muscle, liver, heart, and (histologically) in occasional glial cells of the brain. The most extensive deposition in the central nervous system is in the motor nuclei of the brain stem and anterior horn cells of the spinal cord [102]. About one-fifth of the patients have endocardial thickening compatible with a diagnosis of endocardial fibroelastosis [103, 104] (Fig. 7-11).

Rarely, the presenting clinical findings are severe muscular weakness and wasting, with minimal or no cardiac problems [102, 105, 106]. The prognosis in this group appears to be much better, and some have survived for at least 15 years [102, 107].

The usual enzymes of glycogen synthesis and degradation are normal in these patients, and it has been only recently that there has been any biochemical understanding of the disease. In 1961, Hers [58] demonstrated that tissues from normal persons contain an acid α-1,4-glucosidase (acid maltase) and that this enzyme activity is absent in patients with Type II glycogen storage disease. In normal tissues the enzyme has a pH optimum of 4, sediments with lysosomes during tissue fractionation, and is considered to be a lysosomal enzyme.

Baudhuin et al. [108], in an elegant electron-microscopic study of the liver of a child affected with Type II glycogenosis, demonstrated that there is a dual localization of glycogen in the parenchymal cells. As in normal liver, a part of the glycogen was freely dispersed within the cell, but in this liver specimen a large fraction was segregated in vacuoles surrounded by a single membrane (Fig. 7-12). The diameter of the vacuole was as long as 8 microns. The vacuoles had various shapes, and they are not seen in the parenchymatous cells of liver in other types of glycogenosis [108].

The simultaneous absence of a lysosomal α-glucosidase and the finding of an intravacuolar accumulation of glycogen indicate that there is a causal relationship between these two findings and strongly suggest that the vacuoles are lysosomes engorged with glycogen [109].

Presumably, during lysosomal development cell compo-

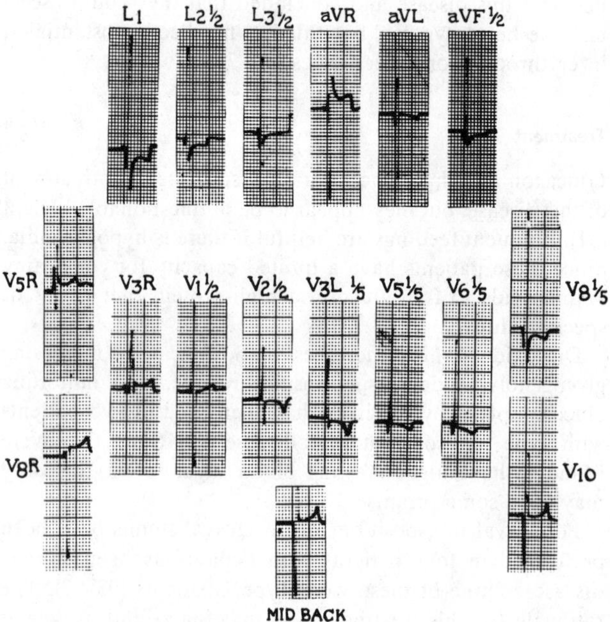

Figure 7-10. Electrocardiogram of the patient A.M. There are gigantic complexes, here reduced to one-fifth, in leads V_5, V_6, and V_8. This suggests massive biventricular hypertrophy. The P-R interval (0.04 sec) is short.

nents which accumulate within lysosomes are degraded by the enzymes which are localized therein. In Type II glycogen storage disease, glycogen may accumulate because of a deficiency of the lysosomal acid maltase, while other cell components (e.g., RNA, protein) are degraded. The lysosomal glycogen, enclosed by a membrane, would not be accessible to the other glycogenolytic enzymes, which are present at normal activities within the cytoplasm.

Garancis [110] found the lysosomal glycogen most abundant in liver and kidneys, and only a few engorged lysosomes in muscle and myocardium. This suggested another defect rather than that of the α-1,4-glucosidase, but no direct evidence supports this.

Diagnosis

In a patient with appropriate clinical symptoms, the diagnosis is established by the demonstration of an increased tissue glycogen concentration of normal structure in association with an α-1,4-glucosidase deficiency. Muscle biopsies are usually studied. Huijing et al. [111] found a virtual absence of leukocyte α-1,4-glucosidase in a patient with Type II glycogenosis. Steinitz et al. [112], while confirming this observation, found a second patient with only moderate reduction in leukocyte α-1,4-glucosidase. Therefore, the presence of the leukocyte enzyme does not preclude this diagnosis.

Normal urine is rich in acid α-1,4-glucosidase activity [113]. This probably arises from shed disrupted renal cells. It is possible that a deficiency of urinary acid α-1,4-glucosidase in these patients might be useful diagnostically. Steinitz et al. [112], however, found acid maltase in the kidney of patients with Type II glycogen disease. It is possible that the kidney enzyme differs from the α-1,4-glucosidase which is deficient in Type II glycogen storage disease.

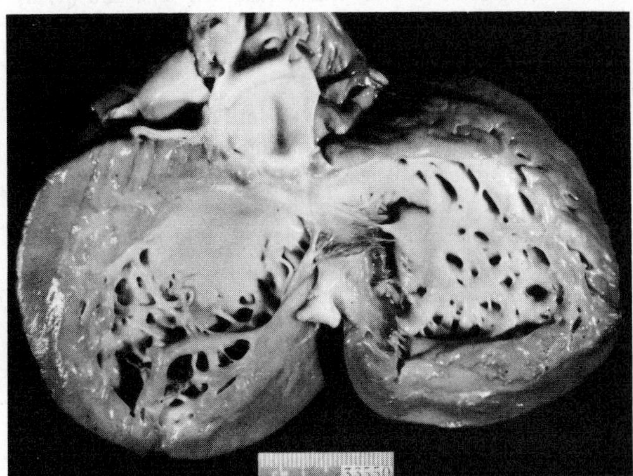

Figure 7-11. The heart of patient A.M. (see Figs. 7-9 and 7-10) at autopsy (age at death, 5 months). The heart is greatly enlarged, with thickened ventricles, due to extensive glycogen infiltration. There is some endocardial thickening.

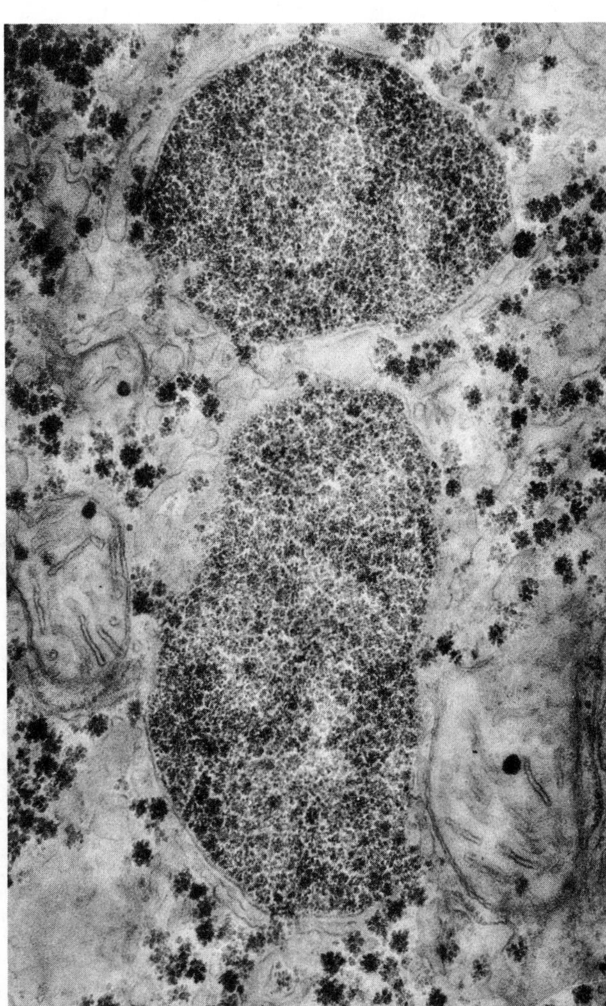

Figure 7-12. Electron micrograph of a portion of an hepatic parenchymatous cell from a liver biopsy of a patient with Type II glycogenosis. Two vacuoles filled with glycogen are seen at magnification ×69,000. A membrane can be followed around most of the periphery of the vacuoles. (*From P. Baudhuin, H. G. Hers, and H. Loeb, with permission* [108].)

Genetics

All the studies of families with affected children suggest autosomal recessive inheritance. Leukocyte α-1,4-glucosidase assays have been done in several groups of parents [112, 114, 115]. Some parents (both fathers and mothers) have had reductions in this enzyme activity, whereas others have been normal.

Enzyme activity in fibroblasts developed from skin biopsies of one patient and from two families with children affected with Type II glycogenosis were compatible with autosomal recessive inheritance. Presumed heterozygotes had reduced but detectable fibroblast α-1,4-glucosidase activity [115]. There is an interesting and unexplained preponderance of affected males [86]. Considerable variability in the tissue distribution of the enzyme deficiency has been seen. One father of an affected child had normal liver but reduced muscle enzyme activity [116]. Variability in the leukocytes already has been mentioned. Those few patients who have normal hearts might not lack the enzyme in the myocardium; direct assays have not been performed. Since this enzyme deficiency is demonstrable in the placenta and cord of affected infants [103], these tissues can be used diagnostically in infants known at birth to be at risk.

Treatment

As with other diseases in which materials accumulate within the lysosome, drugs which increase the lability of lysosomes (e.g., vitamin A) have been tried [106]. No benefit has come from this treatment. Purified acid maltase isolated from *Aspergillus niger* has been administered without clinical success [108, 117, 118]. The technical and theoretical problems arising from the infusion of purified enzymes are great. It seems possible that administered enzymes might get into lysosomes. The problems of administering purified enzymes for life are indeed formidable and currently not a promising answer to this problem.

Since α-1,4-glucosidase appears in fibroblasts developed from normal amniotic fluid cells obtained by amniocentesis in early gestation, prenatal diagnosis (with abortion if indicated) can be performed in this disorder [119]. With such a bleak outlook this is the optimum current management for women at risk of having affected infants.

Type III Glycogen Storage Disease: Amylo-1,6-glucosidase (Debrancher) Deficiency (Limit Dextrinosis, Cori's Disease)

In this form of glycogen storage disease, a polysaccharide accumulates which has a structure resembling the limit dextrin produced by degradation of glycogen by phosphorylase which is free of debrancher (amylo-1,6-glucosidase) activity [49]. By physical examination alone these patients usually cannot be distinguished from patients with Type I glycogen storage disease. Early in life hepatomegaly and growth retardation may be striking. In contrast to patients with Type I, moderate enlargement of the spleen is sometimes seen [120].

Glycogen of abnormal structure frequently accumulates in muscle as well as in the liver, and in older patients may cause a chronic progressive myopathy [121]. Glycogen may also accumulate in the heart, and moderate cardiomegaly [122] is sometimes seen, as are nonspecific ECG (electrocardiogram) changes [120]. Clinical cardiac difficulties are not reported.

Generally the clinical course of this disease is milder than that of Type I. Severe hypoglycemia and convulsions may appear [123]. Although remarkable and difficult to explain, it is well documented that the liver size returns to normal at puberty [49, 124] in at least some of these patients [Fig. 7-13]. There is no renal enlargement in this disease [120].

Lipid levels are variably elevated in serum; serum uric acid is usually but not always normal. Adult patients [124] have not had symptoms suggestive of gout. Serum transaminase levels are consistently elevated in young children, and normal in adults [124]. Cirrhosis, usually mild, has been seen in this disease [94, 120].

Function Studies

Galactose and fructose are readily converted to glucose; similarly, protein and amino acid mixtures given orally induce a small and prolonged rise in blood glucose level [123]. The rise in blood sugar level after epinephrine and glucagon is variable. Hug et al. [125] found a normal glucagon response 2 hr after feeding, and no response after a 14-hr fast. This was interpreted as indicating availability of glucose from the elongated outer branches (after feeding), which could be degraded by phosphorylase, in the absence of debranching activity. It is not a consistent finding in all patients.

Biochemical Investigations

Liver glycogen concentration is often much higher (up to 17.4 gm per 100 gm tissue) in this disorder [49]. By various techniques the glycogen is found to have short outer branches and resembles a phosphorylase limit dextrin.

A series of techniques is available for measuring debrancher activity. These assays do not measure the same enzyme activity. Methods currently used are (1) liberation of glucose from a phosphorylase limit dextrin, (2) incorporation of ^{14}C-glucose into glycogen, (3) 1,4 → 1,4 transfer of an oligoglucan (glucan transferase activity), and (4) hydrolysis of singly branched oligosaccharides, such as the glucosyl-Schardinger dextrin or the 6^3-α-glucosyl maltotetraose.

Using these various methods, Hers and associates [126, 127] have described a series of biochemical subtypes of Type III glycogen disease. These are summarized in Table 7-2.

Some of the patients studied by van Hoof and Hers (e.g., subtypes IIIB, IIIE, IIIF in Table 7-2) had normal muscle glycogen content, in contrast to the patients with IIIA, who have had elevated muscle glycogen concentration. When structural analyses were done on muscle biopsies, short outer branches were found [127]. Brown and Brown [49] found both glycogen content and structure normal in 7 of 29 muscle biopsies from their patients with Type III disease.

Sidbury et al. [128] demonstrated that a marked elevation in erythrocyte glycogen with abnormally short outer branches is specific for Type III glycogen disease. This has been repeatedly observed [129] but is not invariable [129, 130].

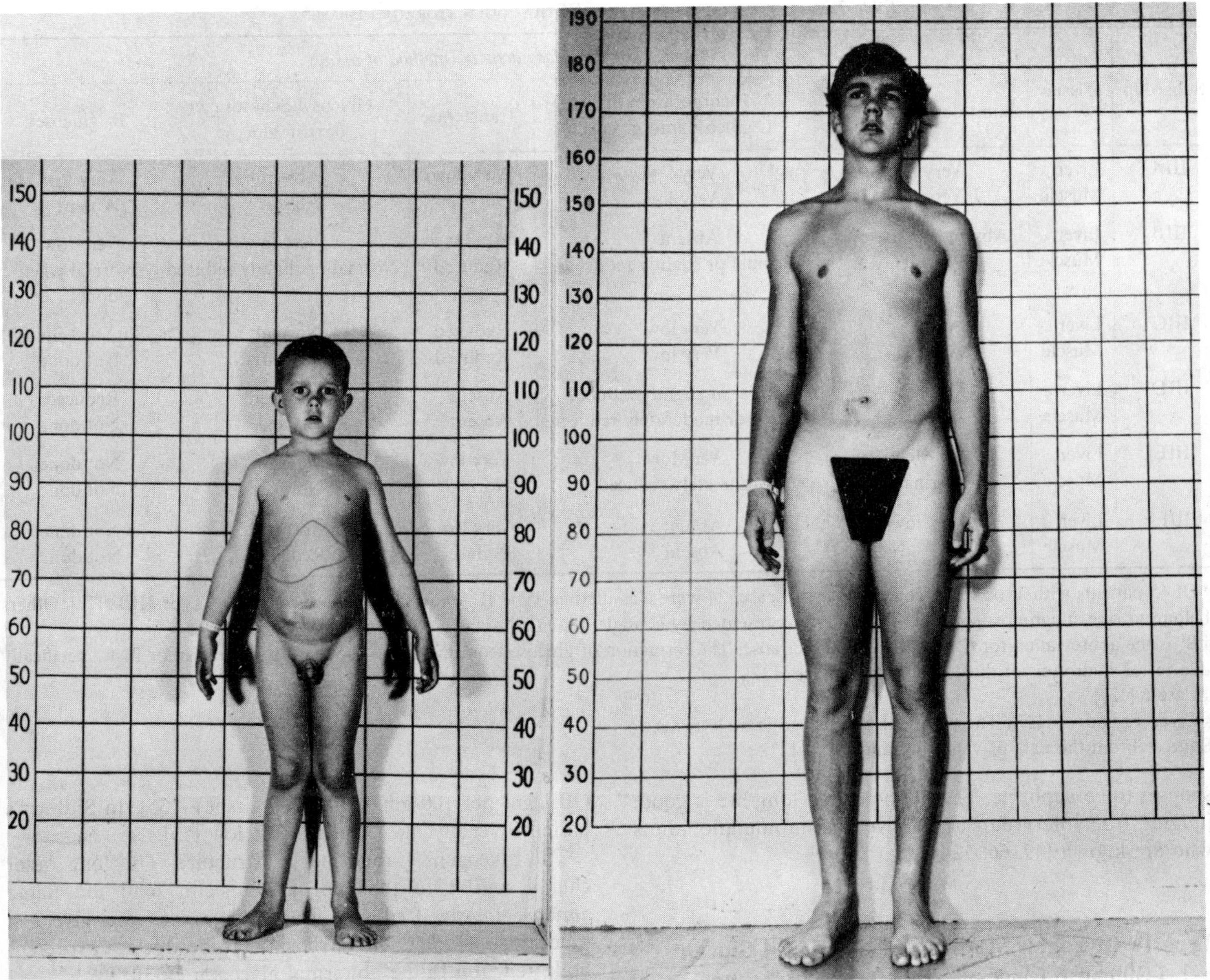

Figure 7-13. Growth and development in a young man (R.G.) with Type III glycogen storage disease. (Left) The patient at age 7 years with the enlarged liver outlined on the abdomen. The abdomen at age 7 was not as protuberant as when the patient was younger. (Right) The same patient at age 17 years. Growth has been completely normal, the liver is now not enlarged, and the patient is asymptomatic. (*Photographs courtesy of Dr. Harriet G. Guild.*)

Genetics

All the data available suggest an autosomal recessive inheritance of this disease. Some investigations have shown intermediate levels of leukocyte debrancher in presumed heterozygotes [130, 131], while others have not been able to identify heterozygotes [132]. There is widespread variability in tissue enzyme activity even within single affected families [89, 130]. Some discrepancies undoubtedly arise from the use of different assay techniques.

In Israel this disease accounts for 73 percent of the glycogen storage disorders. It is found to have a minimal incidence of 1:5,420 in a non-Ashkenazi Jewish community which originated in North Africa. No Type III glycogen storage disease has been seen in the Ashkenazi Jews [122].

Treatment

Frequent feedings and a high-protein diet are indicated for the child with symptoms [123]. The single patient who has had a portacaval transposition apparently benefited from this procedure [94]. The young man shown in Fig. 7-13 is now asymptomatic, has no hypoglycemia, and has normal re-

Table 7-2. THE SUBGROUPS OF TYPE III GLYCOGEN STORAGE DISEASE*

Subgroup	Tissue	*Amylo-1,6-glucosidase activity (method of assay)*				
		Limit dextrin glucose	Incorporation of ^{14}C glucose into glycogen	Transferase	Glucosyl-Schardinger dextrin glucose	B_5 glucose†
IIIA	Liver	Very low	Very low	Very low	Absent	Very low
	Muscle	Very low	Very low	Very low	Absent	Absent
IIIB	Liver	Absent or very low	Absent	Absent	Very low	Very low
	Muscle	Absent	Normal or slightly reduced	Reduced	Normal or slightly reduced	Normal when done
IIIC	Liver	Absent	Very low	Reduced	Normal	Slightly reduced
	Muscle	Absent	Very low	Reduced	Very low	Not done
IIID	Liver	Very low	Normal or slightly reduced	Absent	Reduced	Reduced
	Muscle	Absent	Normal or moderately reduced	Absent	Normal	Not done
IIIE‡	Liver	Very low	Very low	Very low	Very low	Not done
	Muscle	Normal	Moderately reduced	Normal	Normal	Not done
IIIF§	Liver	Very low	Absent	Very low	Absent	Not done
	Muscle	Very low	Absent	Reduced	Reduced	Not done

*Of 45 patients with Type III glycogen storage disease, 34 were classified as Type IIIA and 6 probably fit best into Type IIIB [127]. Others belong to rare subgroups; some subgroups are represented by a single patient.
† B_5 is the abbreviation for 6^3-α-glucosyl maltotetraose. The formation of glucose from the glucosyl-Schardinger dextrin or B_5 is specifically due to the hydrolysis of the 1,6-glucosyl linkage [127].
‡Case 6 [127].
§Cases 10 and 11 [127]. These patients are dizygotic male twins.
Source: From the data of van Hoof and Hers [127].

sponses to epinephrine. The outlook for a long life is good, judging from the group of relatively asymptomatic adults who are known [49, 66, 124].

Type IV Glycogen Storage Disease: α-1,4-Glucan: α-1,4-Glucan 6-Glucosyl Transferase (Brancher) Deficiency (Amylopectinosis; Andersen's Disease)

Seven infants have now been reported with this rare form of glycogen disease [55, 133–137]. The clinical histories of these children are similar; they appeared normal at birth, but soon failed to thrive. Hepatomegaly is seen in the first few months of life. There is poor weight gain, hypotonia, and increasing size of liver and spleen (Fig. 7-14). The clinical picture is that of progressive cirrhosis of the liver, with death in the second year of life. Only one child has survived until age 4 years. Nonspecific ECG abnormalities are found, but clinically significant heart disease does not appear during their short lives.

There are increases in serum transaminase activities, as would be expected in such active severe liver disease. Glucose tolerance test results are normal; epinephrine and glucagon tests have been variable. It might be expected that these functional tests would be abnormal in severe liver disease, even without a basic defect in glycogen metabolism.

The glycogen concentration is usually not increased in any tissues. In only one patient has liver glycogen been increased (10.7 gm per 100 gm wet-weight tissue) [135]. In Sidbury's patient liver glycogen content was low [55].

The glycogen is abnormal in structure. The long outer chains similar to those of amylopectin lend the name *amylopectinosis.* Reduced branching makes the glycogen much less soluble. The cirrhosis may be due to a foreign-body reaction to the abnormal glycogen [133].

Clinically this form of glycogen disease is distinctive because of the early cirrhosis with liver failure and the splenomegaly. A young boy with Type IV glycogenosis whom we have recently studied is shown in Fig. 7-14.

Biochemical Studies

Illingworth and Cori, after studying the glycogen in Andersen's original case [138], suggested that there was a deficiency of the branching enzyme. Brown and Brown [29] have recently shown brancher deficiency in liver and leukocytes of a 15-month-old Indian girl with Type IV disease. Similarly, Fernandes and Huijing [135] demonstrated leukocyte brancher deficiency in their patient. The patient, shown in Fig. 7-14, also lacks leukocyte brancher activity.

Glycogen from these patients has an abnormal iodine spectrum (with λ max around 525mμ, like amylopectin), as well as an increased degradation by amylase. These findings indicate long outer branches. Brown and Brown [29] found that muscle glycogen was normal in content and structure in their patient. If the branching enzyme is absent, how does

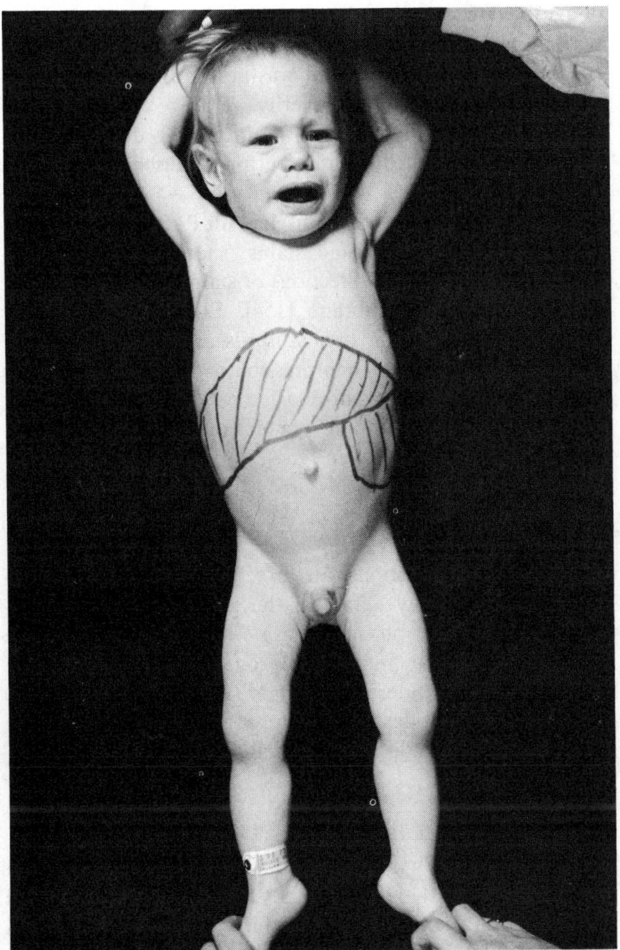

Figure 7-14. Fifteen-month-old boy with Type IV glycogen storage disease. The patient has marked hepatomegaly (with cirrhosis histologically) and considerable splenic enlargement. The liver and spleen are outlined. Venous distension was prominent over the abdomen but is not visible here. Brancher activity in the leukocytes of this patient was less than 10 percent of normal values.

the branching which is present arise? It has been suggested that there might be two branching activities with different substrate requirements [29, 137]. Also, branching enzyme activity could have been present during fetal development which is no longer active [31].

Genetics

Of the seven patients in the literature and two others known to the author, seven are male and two are female. This distribution probably reflects simply the small number of patients known. Two pairs of sibs are reported, and consanguinity is known to exist in at least two families. The parents of Levin's patient [136] and of our patient (Fig. 7-14) had normal leukocyte brancher activity. Howell et al. have recently found brancher activity in normal skin fibroblasts but found it deficient in skin fibroblasts derived from the patient of Fig. 7-14 [139]. Brancher activity in fibroblasts from the skin of both parents was below controls. This strongly suggests autosomal recessive inheritance [139].

Treatment

The treatment is that of liver failure and ascites. Parenteral administration of α-1,4-glucosidase from *Aspergillus niger* [135] was tried without benefit, although liver glycogen content decreased. One patient died 24 hr after portacaval transposition [136]. The identity of the defect in fibroblasts developed from skin suggests that prenatal diagnosis may prove possible [139].

Type V: Muscle Phosphorylase Deficiency (McArdle's Disease)

The 27 patients who have been reported with deficiency of muscle phosphorylase have given a striking history of limitation of ability to perform strenuous exercise because of painful muscle cramps [140–142]. Myoglobinuria has appeared in over half these patients following episodes of exercises and muscle cramps. This disorder was delineated clinically by McArdle in 1951 [143]. He studied a patient who during ischemic exercise had no increase in venous lactate from that extremity; McArdle suggested a defect in the degradation of glycogen to lactate. Momaerts et al. [143*a*] and Schmid et al. [144, 145] demonstrated in clinically similar patients a lack of muscle phosphorylase (<0.5 percent of normal), high muscle glycogen concentrations, and normal muscle phosphorylase kinase activities. Other studies in these patients showed normal activity of other glycogen enzymes in muscle [146]. Pearson et al. [147] found no rise in venous lactate (Fig. 7-15) and an absence of muscle phosphorylase. All these patients tolerated moderate exercise normally.

Clinically, these patients are normal and well developed and have no abnormalities at rest. Liver phosphorylase presumably is normal. Since, as discussed earlier, muscle and liver phosphorylase differ in many properties, it is not surprising that these two phosphorylases are under separate genetic control. These patients are not hypoglycemic and have a normal response to glucagon.

During muscular exercise the use of ATP increases perhaps several hundredfold [147]. Aerobic metabolism generates ATP as rapidly as possible but is limited by the diffusion rates of fuel and oxygen. The additional ATP required for sustained vigorous exercise must come from glycogenolysis (by way of phosphorylase); only during stressful exercise is muscle phosphorylase essential and its lack clinically evident. These patients have not had clinical cardiac problems, but electrocardiographic abnormalities have been recorded [147–149].

Rowland et al. [140] have pointed out that the profusion

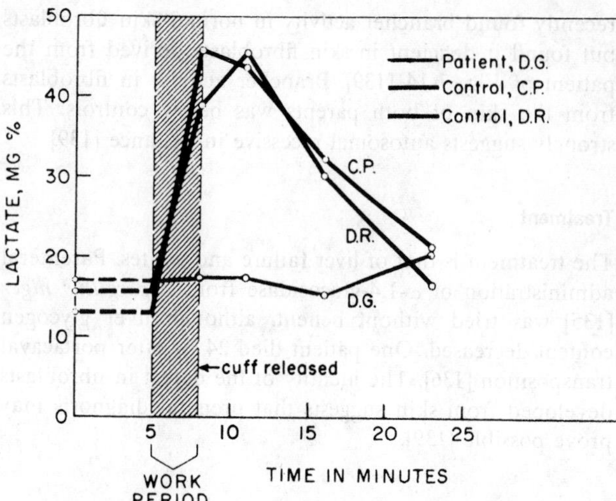

Figure 7-15. Blood lactate concentrations obtained from antecubital vein after ischemic forearm muscle work. Patient, D.G., has McArdle's disease (muscle phosphorylase deficiency) and has no rise in level of venous lactate. (*From Pearson et al, with permission* [147].)

of muscle-action potentials characteristic of muscle cramps in other situations is absent during the painful contractures experienced by these patients.

ATP is required for muscle relaxation in two different reactions. Rowland et al. studied tissue ATP concentrations in order to see whether a deficiency in tissue ATP levels might be responsible for the painful contractures characteristic of this disorder [150]; normal ATP concentrations were found.

If an exercising subject with McArdle's syndrome can sustain the exercise after symptoms appear, symptoms will lessen or disappear; this has been called the "second wind" phenomenon [144, 151]. Pernow et al. [151] found that this phenomenon is closely related to the prevailing levels of free fatty acids and increased blood flow to muscle, and postulated that these changes improve energy sources for the muscle.

Within hours after strenuous exercise, lactate dehydrogenase, aldolase, and creatine phosphokinase activities in serum increase dramatically [152]. This need not imply tissue death, but may be due only to reversible metabolic conditions within the muscle which compromise the ability of the cell to maintain membrane competence [153].

It is remarkable that this defect, although undoubtedly present from birth, produces either mild or no symptoms whatever during childhood. Indeed, it has been diagnosed in only one patient before 10 years of age (at 4 years), and that was due to his being a part of a family study [140]. Some affected children have tolerated extraordinary exercise (basketball, lacrosse) without symptoms [140].

The clinical history has been arbitrarily but usefully divided into three phases [144]. The first is childhood and adolescence, when one finds increased fatigability and few other symptoms. During the second period (20 to 40 years of age) severe cramps and myoglobinuria appear. In the third period (beginning at about age 40) cramps and myoglobinuria are less conspicuous and wasting and weakness begin to appear with increasing severity.

The single functional test of value is the demonstration that venous lactate from a limb performing ischemic exercise fails to increase.

Histologic studies of the muscle with PAS (periodic acid–Schiff) and Best's carmine stains, show numerous well-defined round or oval collections of staining material under the sarcolemmal membrane [154]. Electron micrographs display disorganization of myofibrils at the level of the *I* band. This is because of compression of myofibrils by excess glycogen in the intermyofibrillar space [154]. After exercise, some mitochondria contain vacuoles or collections of particles that resemble glycogen [154].

Biochemical Studies

It is important to demonstrate directly a deficiency of phosphorylase, since any defect in the glycolytic pathway, including a defect in phosphorylase *b* kinase, could generate superficially similar findings. Glycogen of normal structure accumulates in moderate amounts (up to 4.0 gm per 100 gm) in muscle. Modest depressions of other muscle enzyme activities occur [145], but are usually secondary defects.

Genetics

A large pedigree with well-studied patients was collected by Dawson et al. [142]. It strongly supported an autosomal recessive inheritance. Certain family members, who could have been heterozygotes, had cramps after exercise. The preponderance of males suggested heterogeneity. Many of the patients were not studied well enough to permit the ruling out of deficient phosphorylase *b* kinase. In mice this muscle enzyme is located on the X chromosome [155]; deficiency of the enzyme is not symptomatic but is accompanied by an increase in muscle glycogen concentration [156].

Treatment

Avoidance of extreme exercise is the best treatment. Administration of oral glucose and fructose (to increase muscle-energy supplies) has given variable results. Pernow [151] reported some success with isoproterenol. This drug increases the serum concentration of free fatty acids and blood flow to the muscle.

Type VI (Hers' Disease)

In a study of a large group of patients with hepatic forms of the glycogen storage diseases, Hers [157] segregated certain patients with increased hepatic glycogen and a reduction to about 25 percent of normal of hepatic phosphorylase activity. These patients clinically were like those with mild forms of Type I glycogen storage disease [158]. Although some were deficient in leukocyte phosphorylase [159], not all were [160]. Leukocyte phosphorylase activities in family members were variable and somewhat confusing with regard to genetic transmission. It may be noted that there is a major problem in assaying total liver phosphorylase activity in that the amount of active phosphorylase is variable and the activation of phosphorylase *b* by AMP is not complete.

Illingworth and Brown [161] do not equate Type VI with liver phosphorylase deficiency. They put all their patients with liver glycogen disease who fail to fit into another well-defined group in this one.

Hers [162], after studying many patients with the hepatic glycogenoses, is of the opinion that classification on the basis of low phosphorylase level is not adequate and that low phosphorylase is not a constant finding even among sibs [162]. Those investigators who have most studied tissues from patients with the glycogen diseases [161, 162] place patients with hepatomegaly, growth retardation (sometimes with ketosis), and increased concentrations of liver glycogen in Type VI. Some of these patients have reduced liver phosphorylase. This is not a very informative classification and is obviously heterogeneous from every standpoint. Hers has suggested that Type VI is a "waiting room" from which new diseases will be separated in the future [162]. This group is retained, but it is not to be inferred that all patients in this group are deficient in liver phosphorylase activity. Since this classification was established for patients with liver phosphorylase deficiency, it should be retained for patients who will be shown in the future to have this defect.

Type VII: Muscle Phosphofructokinase Deficiency

Tarui and his colleagues [163] recently reported a new muscular glycogen storage disease from Japan. They studied three sibs with clinical histories identical to McArdle's (muscle phosphorylase deficiency) disease. One had experienced myoglobinuria. Ischemic exercise caused no rise in venous lactate level. These patients showed marked increases in the concentrations of glucose-6-phosphate and fructose-6-phosphate in their muscles but had low muscle fructose-1,6-diphosphate. Muscle phosphofructokinase activity was 1 to 3 percent of normal. The increased activity both of glycogen synthetase and of UDPG pyrophosphorylase in the muscles contributed to glycogen storage in the muscle [164]. A fourth patient from the United States with similar clinical and biochemical findings has been studied by Layzer et al. [165]. In addition to demonstrating phosphofructokinase deficiency, Layzer et al. [165] found no component in the biopsy of their patient which reacted with an antibody which they had prepared against purified human muscle phosphofructokinase.

The four patients have had erythrocyte phosphofructokinase activity which was about 50 percent normal. Three parents who were studied had a similar reduction [163, 165]. Immunologic studies by Tauri et al. [165*a*] showed at least two components of erythrocyte phosphofructokinase. About 50 percent of the total activity is attributable to a form of the enzyme immunologically identical to muscle phosphofructokinase. They attribute the reduced erythrocyte lifespan (13 to 16 days by ^{51}Cr labeling) to erythroid hyperplasia, and the reticulocytosis (3.8 to 6.5 percent) seen in their patients to the deficiency of the muscle form of phosphofructokinase in the erythrocyte, which results in 50 percent reduction of total erythrocyte phosphofructokinase activity [165*a*]. The occurrence in sibs of both sexes, with consanguinity in one set of parents, suggests autosomal recessive inheritance. The reduction of erythrocyte phosphofructokinase activity in the parents also supports this view.

Type VIII: Hepatic Phosphorylase Kinase Deficiency

Phosphorylase requires specific enzymes for both activation and inactivation. The finding of a low phosphorylase activity in a biopsy might therefore arise from phosphorylase deficiency per se or from deficiency of the enzyme which activates phosphorylase.

Patients deficient in phosphorylase *b* kinase have recently been described. They have reduced liver and leukocyte phosphorylase and clearly can now be removed from the heterogeneous group of Type VI glycogen disease.

Hug et al. have reported [166] five children with no symptoms except hepatomegaly and increased liver glycogen concentration. Slow activation of phosphorylase was found in vitro, and it was inferred that there was about a 90 percent deficiency of phosphorylase *b* kinase. These findings are difficult to reconcile with the normal response to glucagon and the observation that there was shrinkage of the liver in response to glucagon.

By direct assay, Huijing [167] found low activity of phosphorylase *b* kinase in the leukocytes of a group of patients with "phosphorylase" deficiency. Huijing and Fernandes [168] have recently collected histories of 32 patients with phosphorylase *b* kinase deficiency. Enzyme data and the extensive pedigree of these patients support the theory of an X-linked inheritance (Fig. 7-16). These patients have had only mild symptoms. Three females with large livers and moderately reduced leukocyte enzyme concentrations were considered to be heterozygotes; they showed minimal manifestations of the disease [168]. Low leukocyte phosphorylase *b* kinase activity seems to reflect low activity of this enzyme in liver [168*a*].

Other Possible Inherited Defects in Glycogen Metabolism

Lewis, Spencer-Peet, and Stewart [169–171] described identical twins with profound hypoglycemia, low (but not absent) liver glycogen, and absence of liver glycogen synthetase.

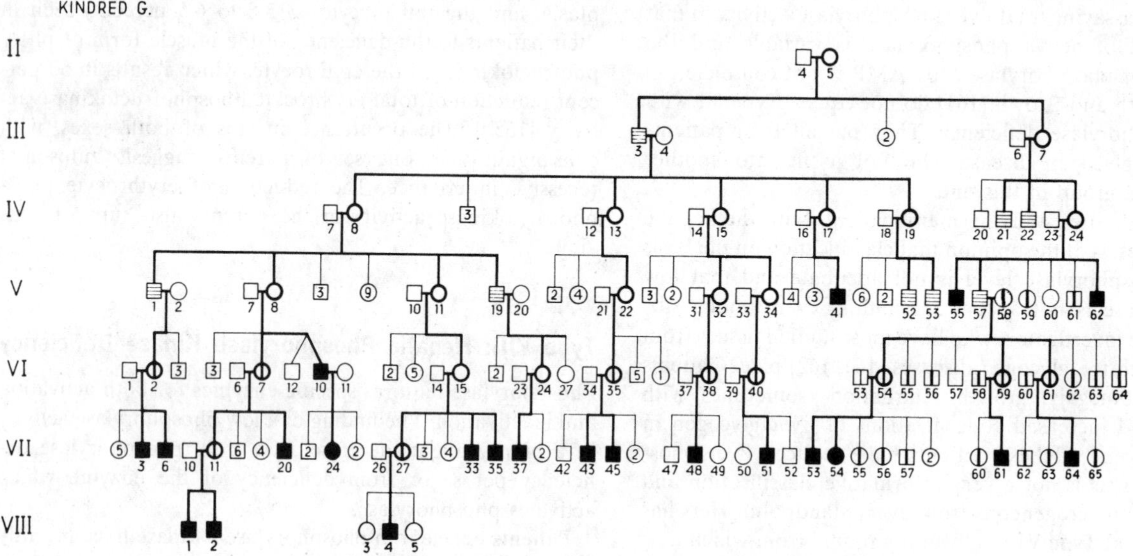

Figure 7-16. Pedigree with cases of liver glycogenosis due to hepatic phosphorylase *b* kinase deficiency (Type VIII glycogenosis). These data suggest an X-chromosomal inheritance; the two females with mild symptoms and moderate reduction in enzyme activity are thought to be heterozygotes. (*From F. Huijing and J. Fernandes with permission* [168].)

These children had diabetic-type glucose tolerance test results. The hypoglycemia appeared only after long fasting. When the children were in a fed state response to glucagon was normal. When the infants were hypoglycemic after fasting, glucagon produced no rise in blood sugar level. These patients clearly were able to synthesize glycogen, as proved by the presence of glycogen in the liver and a normal response to glucagon when fed.

Clinically the findings in these children fit well with the syndrome of ketotic hypoglycemia, a poorly understood but relatively common form of hypoglycemia in children. It appears that ketotic-hypoglycemic patients (and Lewis' patients) have a defect involving gluconeogenesis, rather than a primary disorder of glycogen metabolism. Some patients with ketotic hypoglycemia have extremely low concentrations of liver glycogen and low serum insulin values [172, 173]. Since glycogen synthetase is regulated by insulin, low liver glycogen synthetase activity would be expected to accompany low serum insulin concentrations. In addition, Hers has emphasized the lability of glycogen synthetase when isolated in the presence of low tissue concentrations of glycogen [174]. One would not expect that glycogen synthetase activity would be deficient in all children with ketotic hypoglycemia. It would probably occur with some frequency in that group with very low serum insulin concentrations. Although inherited deficiencies of glycogen synthetase may be documented in the future, existing data do not establish such an entity.

Individual patients with a partial deficiency of phosphoglucomutase in liver and muscle [161] and in muscle [149] have been reported. No direct assay was made in the patient with the muscular form of the disease. Some of these reports are brief but substantial [161]. The defect, either in muscle or in liver, may well require individual classification in the future.

Multiple Enzymatic Defects

Many examples of multiple enzymatic defects have been reported in glycogen storage disease. They have been summarized by Auerbach and DiGeorge [175]. Many may be artifactual because of improper handling of tissues and inadequate assays [50, 86]. In some instances, there is evidence that different enzyme deficiencies occurred in sibs [176, 177].

There are several examples of the simultaneous occurrence of debrancher deficiency along with marked reductions of glucose-6-phosphatase activity in the same family or same individual [49, 86]. Reductions of glucose-6-phosphatase and debrancher activities are seen together with some frequency. One of these is probably the primary genetic event, the other being secondary or adaptive. In order to prove a double genetic defect in an individual, one would require the demonstration that both parents are heterozygotes for *both* defects. This would occur with great rarity, even in highly inbred kindreds. It is perhaps surprising that multiple defects are not found more frequently, since the tissues are so frequently disorganized by glycogen and lipid deposition. The genetic implications of multiple enzyme deficiencies are so important that reports should be examined critically.

SUMMARY

Inherited defects may affect many enzymes involved in the synthesis and degradation of glycogen. A broad clinical spectrum is presented by the eight recognized clinical types of glycogen storage disease.

1 Type I glycogen storage disease, also called von Gierke's disease, is caused by a deficiency of glucose-6-phosphatase. The disorder is characterized by massive hepatomegaly, failure to thrive, and severe hypoglycemia, particularly during infancy. There are ketosis and increased plasma concentration of lactic acid and of all lipid fractions. Administration of epinephrine or glucagon causes a subnormal rise in blood glucose, but even further increases in blood lactate. Hyperuricemia occurs regularly, and all patients have developed clinical gout in young adulthood. Renal enlargement is seen roentgenographically. Inheritance is autosomal recessive. Treatment is symptomatic. The diagnosis is established by demonstrating an increased content of normal glycogen in a liver biopsy and absent glucose-6-phosphatase activity.

2 Infants with Type II glycogen disease have massive cardiomegaly, and hypotonia but no muscle wasting. The disease is inherited as an autosomal recessive trait. Diagnosis is made by finding an increased concentration of glycogen of normal structure in virtually all tissues and by demonstrating an absence of lysosomal α-1,4-glucosidase (acid maltase) activity. Cardiorespiratory failure causes death by age 2 years. In a much less common form of the disease there is no cardiac involvement and the patients survive much longer. This disease can be diagnosed in utero by amniocentesis and enzyme studies on the cultured amniotic fluid cells.

3 Type III glycogen storage disease is caused by deficiency of the debrancher enzyme. The clinical course is similar to that in Type I but is usually milder. Massive hepatomegaly present in the young children, diminishes with age, and some older patients lack hepatic enlargement. Hypoglycemia is variable, as are responses to epinephrine and glucagon. A variety of biochemical subtypes based on tissue variability of the enzyme defect is described in this condition. Muscle, liver, and erythrocyte glycogen is elevated, and the glycogen has abnormally short outer branches. Deficiency of the debrancher enzyme is inherited in an autosomal recessive fashion.

4 A deficiency of branching enzyme in Type IV glycogen storage disease produces an accumulation of abnormal glycogen with long outer branches. Clinically there is progressive cirrhosis with hepatosplenomegaly and ascites. Death from liver failure occurs usually before 2 years of age in this rare form of glycogen storage disease. It is inherited as an autosomal recessive.

5 Limitation of strenuous exercise by painful cramps is the presenting feature in patients with McArdle's disease—Type V glycogen storage disease. These symptoms do not usually appear until 20 years of age. Myoglobinuria occurs in half the patients after strenuous exercise. Findings on physical examination are normal. There is no hypoglycemia. Muscular exercise fails to cause an increase in venous lactate. Muscle biopsy shows absent phosphorylase activity and increased glycogen content. Inheritance is autosomal recessive.

6 Type VI glycogen storage disease was established for patients considered to have liver phosphorylase deficiency, but this category is now occupied by a heterogeneous group of patients who have increased liver glycogen and do not fit into any other well-defined group. Some, but not all, have reduced liver phosphorylase activity. This group is considered a "waiting room" from which patients will be removed when new defects are found. The classification is retained for patients who eventually will prove to have liver phosphorylase deficiency.

7 Patients with Type VII glycogen storage disease are clinically identical to those with Type V glycogen storage disease. After exercise these patients have painful cramps and sometimes myoglobinuria. Muscle biopsies are deficient in phosphofructokinase activity and have increased glycogen. Inheritance appears to be autosomal recessive.

8 A deficiency of liver phosphorylase *b* kinase characterizes Type VIII glycogen storage disease. Symptoms and findings include mild hepatomegaly, increased liver glycogen, and mild hypoglycemia. Diagnosis is made by the demonstration of deficient leukocyte phosphorylase *b* kinase. The disease is X-linked and is fully manifest only in males.

BIBLIOGRAPHY

1. von Gierke, E.: Hepato-nephromegalia glykogenia (Glykogenspeicherkrankhei den Leber und Nieren). Beitr. Path. Anat., **82,** 497, 1929.
2. Pompe, J. C.: Over idiopatische hypertrophie van het hart. Nederl. T. Geneesk., **76,** 304, 1932.
3. Cori, G. T., and Cori, C. F.: Glucose-6-phosphatase of the liver in glycogen storage disease. J. Biol. Chem., **199,** 661, 1952.
4. Cori, G. T.: Glycogen structure and enzyme deficiencies in glycogen storage disease. Harvey Lect., **48,** 145, 1954.
5. Stetten, DeW., Jr., and Stetten, M. R.: Glycogen metabolism. Physiol. Rev., **40,** 505, 1960.
6. French, D.: Structure of glycogen and its amylolytic degradation, in *Control of Glycogen Metabolism,* edited by W. J. Whelan, p. 7. Little, Brown, Boston, 1964.
7. Orrell, S. A., Jr., Bueding, E., and Reissig, M.: Physical characteristics of undegraded glycogen, in *Control of Glycogen Metabolism,* edited by W. J. Whelan, p. 29. Little, Brown, Boston, 1964.

8. Dawes, G. S., and Shelley, H. J.: Physiologic aspects of carbohydrate metabolism in the fetus and newborn, in *Carbohydrate Metabolism and Its Disorders,* edited by F. Dickens, P. J. Randle, and W. J. Whelan, p. 87. Academic, New York, 1968.
9. Öckerman, P. A.: The diagnosis of glycogen storage disease in clinical practice. Israel J. Med. Soc., **3,** 494, 1967.
10. Field, R. A.: Glycogen deposition diseases, in *The Metabolic Basis of Inherited Disease,* edited by J. B. Stanbury, J. B. Wyngaarden, and D. S. Frederickson. McGraw-Hill, New York, 1966.
11. Sols, A., Salas, M., and Vinuela, E.: Induced biosynthesis of liver glucokinase, in *Advances in Enzyme Regulation,* edited by George Weber, vol. 2, p. 177. Macmillan, New York, 1964.
12. Sharma, C., Manjeshwar, R., and Weinhouse, S.: Hormonal and dietary regulation of hepatic glucokinase, in *Advances in Enzyme Regulation,* edited by George Weber, vol. 2, p. 189. Macmillan, New York, 1964.
13. Sols, A.: Hexokinase and glucokinase, in *Control of Glycogen Metabolism,* edited by W. J. Whelan, p. 301. Little, Brown, Boston, 1964.
14. Sols, A.: Phosphorylation and glycolysis, in *Carbohydrate Metabolism and Its Disorders,* edited by F. Dickens, P. J. Randle, and W. J. Whelan, vol. 1, p. 53. Academic, New York, 1968.
15. London, W. P.: A theoretical study of hepatic glycogen metabolism. J. Biol. Chem., **241,** 3008, 1966.
16. Smith, E. E., Taylor, P. M., and Whelan, W. J.: Enzymic processes in glycogen metabolism, in *Carbohydrate Metabolism and Its Disorders,* edited by F. Dickens, P. J. Randle, and W. J. Whelan, vol. 1, p. 89. Academic, New York, 1968.
17. Ray, W. J., Jr., and Roscelli, G. A.: The phosphoglucomutase pathway. J. Biol. Chem., **239**(11), 3935, 1964.
18. White, A., Handler, P., and Smith, E. M.: *Principles of Biochemistry,* 4th ed., p. 424. McGraw-Hill, New York, 1968.
19. Albrecht, G. J., Bass, S. T., Seifert, L. L., and Hansen, R. G.: Crystallization and properties of uridine diphosphate glucose pyrophosphorylase from liver. J. Biol. Chem., **241**(12), 2968, 1966.
20. Leloir, L. F., and Cardini, C. E.: Biosynthesis of glycogen from uridine diphosphate glucose. J. Amer. Chem. Soc., **79,** 6340, 1957.
21. Hauk, R., and Brown, D. H.: Preparations and properties of uridine diphosphoglucose-glycogen transferase from rabbit muscle. Biochim. Biophys. Acta, **33,** 556, 1959.
22. Friedman, D. L., and Larner, J.: Studies on UDPG-α-glucan transglucosylase.III. Interconversion of two forms of muscle UDPG-α-glucan transglucosylase by a phosphorylation-dephosphorylation reaction sequence. Biochemistry, **2,** 669, 1963.
23. Mersmann, H. J., and Segal, H. L.: An on-off mechanism for liver glycogen synthetase activity. Proc. Nat. Acad. Sci. U.S.A., **58,** 1688, 1967.
24. Bishop, J. S., and Larner, J.: Rapid activation-inactivation of liver uridine diphosphate glucose-glycogen transferase and phosphorylase by insulin and glucagon *in vivo.* J. Biol. Chem., **242,** 1354, 1967.
25. De Wulf, H., and Hers, H. G.: The stimulation of glycogen synthesis and of glycogen synthetase in the liver by the administration of glucose. Europ. J. Biochem., **2,** 50, 1967.
26. Hers, H. G., and De Wulf, H.: The regulation of glycogen synthesis in the liver, in *Control of Glycogen Metabolism,* edited by W. J. Whelan, p. 65. Academic, New York, 1968.
27. Huijing, F., and Larner, J.: On the mechanism of action of adenosine 3′,5′ cyclophosphate. Proc. Nat. Acad. Sci. U.S.A., **56,** 647, 1966.
28. Meddaiah, V. T., and Madsen, N. B.: Studies on the biological control of glycogen metabolism in liver. III. Subcellular distribution of glycogen metabolizing enzymes. Canad. J. Biochem., **46,** 521, 1968.
29. Brown, B. I., and Brown, D. H.: Lack of an α-1,4-glucan: α-1,4-glucan-6-glucosyl transferase in a case of type IV glycogenosis. Proc. Nat. Acad. Sci. U.S.A., **56,** 725, 1966.
30. Verhue, W., and Hers, H. G.: A study of the reaction catalysed by the liver branching enzyme. Biochem. J., **99,** 222, 1966.
31. Manners, D. J.: Branching enzymes, in *Control of Glycogen Metabolism,* edited by W. J. Whelan, p. 83. Academic, New York, 1968.
32. White, A., Handler, P., and Smith, E. M.: *Principles of Biochemistry,* 4th ed., p. 436. McGraw-Hill, New York, 1968.
33. Henion, W. F., and Sutherland, E. W.: Immunological differences of phosphorylases. J. Biol. Chem., **224,** 477, 1957.
34. Fischer, E. H., and Krebs, E. G.: The isolation and crystallization of rabbit skeletal muscle phosphorylase *b.* J. Biol. Chem., **231,** 65, 1958.
35. Keller, P. J., and Cori, G. T.: Purification and properties of the phosphorylase-rupturing enzyme. J. Biol. Chem., **214,** 127, 1955.
36. Fisher, E. H., Appleman, M. M., and Krebs, E. G.: The structure of phosphorylases, in *Control of Glycogen Metabolism,* edited by W. J. Whelan, p. 94. Little, Brown, Boston, 1964.
37. Metzger, B., Helmreich, E., and Glaser, L.: The mechanism of activation of skeletal muscle phosphorylase *a* by glycogen. Proc. Nat. Acad. Sci. U.S.A., **57,** 994, 1967.
38. Fisher, E. H., Graves, D. J., Crittenden, E. R. S., and Krebs, E. G.: Structure of the site phosphorylated in the phosphorylase *b* to *a* reaction. J. Biol. Chem., **234,** 1698, 1959.
39. Wang, J. H., and Graves, D. J.: The relationship of the dissociation to the catalytic activity of glycogen phosphorylase *a.* Biochemistry, **3,** 1437, 1964.
40. Wang, J. H., Shonka, M. L., and Graves, D. J.: Influence of carbohydrates on phosphorylase structure and activity. I. Activation by preincubation with glycogen. Biochemistry, **4,** 2296, 1965.
41. Helmreich, E., Michaelides, M. C., and Cori, C. F.: Effects of substrates and a substrate analog on the binding of 5′-adenylic acid to muscle phosphorylase *a.* Biochemistry, **6,** 3695, 1967.
41*a*. Seery, V. L., Fischer, E. H., and Teller, D. C.: A reinvestigation of the molecular weight of glycogen phosphorylase. Biochemistry, **6**:3315, 1967.
42. Sutherland, E. W., and Wosilait, W. D.: The relationship of epinephrine and glucagon to liver phosphorylase. I. Liver phosphorylase: preparation and properties. J. Biol. Chem., **218,** 459, 1956.
43. Wosilait, W. D., and Sutherland, E. W.: The relationship of epinephrine and glucagon to liver phosphorylase. II. Enzymatic inactivation of liver phosphorylase. J. Biol. Chem., **218,** 469, 1956.
44. Pohl, S. L., Birnbaumer, L., and Rodbell, M.: Glucagon-sensitive adenyl cyclase in plasma membrane of hepatic parenchymal cells. Science, **164,** 566, 1969.
45. Hers, H. G., Verhue, W., and Mathieu, M.: The mechanism of action of amylo-1,6-glucosidase, in *Control of Glycogen Metabolism,* edited by W. J. Whelan, p. 151. Little, Brown, Boston, 1964.
46. Abdullah, M., Taylor, P. M., and Whelan, W. J.: The enzymic debranching of glycogen and the rôle of transferase, in *Control of Glycogen Metabolism,* edited by W. J. Whelan, p. 123. Little, Brown, Boston, 1964.
47. Brown, D. H., and Illingworth, B.: The rôle of oligo-1,4 → 1,4-glucantransferase and amylo-1,6-glucosidase in the debranching of glycogen, in *Control of Glycogen Metabolism,* edited by W. J. Whelan, p. 139. Little, Brown, Boston, 1964.
48. Taylor, P. M., and Whelan, W. J.: Rabbit muscle amylo-1,6-glucosidase: Properties and evidence of heterogeneity, in *Control of Glycogen Metabolism,* edited by W. J. Whelan, p. 101. Academic, New York, 1968.
49. Brown, B. I., and Brown, D. H.: The glycogen storage diseases, types I, III, IV, V, VII, and unclassified glycogenoses, in *Carbohydrate Metabolism and Its Disorders,* edited by W. J. Whelan, vol. II, p. 123. Academic, New York, 1968.
50. Hers, H. G.: Glycogen storage disease, in *Advances in Metabolic Diseases,* edited by R. Levine and R. Luft, vol. I, p. 1. Academic, New York, 1964.
51. Lazarus, S. S., and Barden, H.: Specificity and ultrastructural localization of pancreatic β cell glucose-6-phosphatase. Diabetes, **14**(3), 146, 1965.
52. Stetten, M. R., and Taft, H. L.: Metabolism of inorganic pyrophosphate. II. The probable identity of microsomal inorganic pyrophosphatase, pyrophosphate phosphotransferase and glucose 6-phosphatase. J. Biol. Chem., **239,** 4041, 1964.
53. Arion, W. J., and Nordlie, R. C.: Liver glucose-6-phosphatase and pyrophosphate-glucose phosphotransferase: effects of fasting. Biochem. Biophys. Res. Commun., **20,** 606, 1965.
54. Nordlie, R. C., and Arion, W. J.: Liver microsomal glucose-6-phosphatase, inorganic pyrophosphatase, and pyrophosphate-glucose phosphotransferase. J. Biol. Chem., **240,** 2155, 1965.
55. Sidbury, J. B., Jr., Mason, J., Burns, W. B., Jr., and Ruebner, B. H.: Type IV glycogenosis. Report of a case proven by characterization of

glycogen and studied at necropsy. Bull. Johns Hopkins Hosp., **111**, 157, 1962.

56. Passonneau, J. V., and Lowry, O. H.: The role of phosphofructokinase in metabolic regulation, in *Advances in Enzyme Regulation,* edited by George Weber, vol. 2, p. 265. Macmillan, New York, 1964.
57. White, A., Handler, P., and Smith, E. M.: *Principles of Biochemistry,* 4th ed., p. 395. McGraw-Hill, New York, 1968.
58. Hers, H. G.: α-Glucosidase deficiency in generalized glycogen storage disease (Pompe's disease). Biochem. J., **86,** 11, 1963.
59. Hers, H. G., and van Hoof, F.: Lysosomal α-1,4-glucosidase, in *Carbohydrate Metabolism and Its Disorders,* edited by F. Dickens, P. J. Randle, and W. J. Whelan, vol. II, p. 151. Academic, New York, 1968.
60. Lejeune, N., Thines-Sempoux, D., and Hers, H. G.: Tissue fractionation studies. 16. Intracellular distribution and properties of α-glucosidases in rat liver. Biochem. J., **86,** 16, 1963.
61. Howell, R. R., Ashton, D. M., and Wyngaarden, J. B.: Glucose-6-phosphatase deficiency glycogen storage disease. Studies on the interrelationships of carbohydrate, lipid and purine abnormalities. Pediatrics, **29,** 553, 1962.
62. Fine, R. N., Wilson, W. A., and Donnell, G. N.: Retinal changes in glycogen storage disease type I. Amer. J. Dis. Child., **115,** 328, 1968.
63. Lowe, C. U., Ambrus, J. L., Ambrus, C. M., Mosovich, L. L., Mink, I. B., and Sokal, J. E.: Bleeding diathesis in children with liver glycogen disease and in their parents. J. Clin. Invest., **39,** 1007, 1960.
64. Levin, J., and Howell, R. R.: Unpublished observations.
65. Sidbury, J. B., Jr., and Heick, H. M. C.: Glycogen storage disease: A review with emphasis on gastrointestinal manifestations. Southern Med. J., **61,** 915, 1968.
66. van Crevald, S.: Clinical course of glycogen storage disease. Chemi. Weekblad, **57,** 445, 1961.
67. Alepa, F. P., Howell, R. R., Klinenberg, J. R., and Seegmiller, J. E.: Relationships between glycogen storage disease and tophaceous gout. Amer. J. Med., **42,** 58, 1967.
68. Owen, O. E., Morgan, A. P., Kemp, H. G., Sullivan, J. M., Herrera, M. G., and Cahill, G. F., Jr.: Brain metabolism during fasting. J. Clin. Invest., **46**(10), 1589, 1967.
69. Lampert, F., Mayer, H., Tocci, P. M., and Nyhan, W. L.: Fanconi syndrome in glycogen storage disease, in *Amino Acid Metabolism and Genetic Variation,* edited by W. L. Nyhan. McGraw-Hill, New York, 1967.
70. Jakovcic, S., Khachadurian, A. K., and Hsia, D. Y. Y.: The hyperlipidemia in glycogen storage disease. J. Lab. Clin. Med., **68**(5), 769, 1966.
71. Öckerman, P. A.: Glucose, glycerol and free fatty acids in glycogen storage disease type I. Blood levels in the fasting and non-fasting state. Effect of glucose and adrenalin administration. Clin. Chim. Acta, **12,** 370, 1965.
72. Öckerman, P. A.: In vitro studies of adipose tissue metabolism of glucose, glycerol and free fatty acids in glycogen storage disease type I. Clin. Chim. Acta, **12,** 383, 1965.
73. Öckerman, P. A.: Assay by a spectrofluorimetric method of glucose-6-phosphate in the liver in glycogen storage disease type I. Clin. Chim. Acta, **12,** 445, 1965.
74. Lockwood, D. H., Merimee, T. J., Edgar, P. J., Greene, M. L., Fujimoto, W. Y., Seegmiller, J. E., and Howell, R. R.: Insulin secretion in type I glycogen storage disease. Diabetes, **18,** 755, 1969.
75. Kolb, F. O., De Lalla, O. F., and Gofman, J. W.: The hyperlipidemias in disorders of carbohydrate metabolism: Serial lipo protein studies in diabetic acidosis with xanthomatosis and in glycogen storage disease. Metabolism, **4,** 310, 1955.
76. Jeandet, J., and Lestradet, H.: L'hyperlactacidemie, cause probable de l'hyperuricemie dans la glycogenose hepatique. Rev. Franc. Etud. Clin. Biol., **6,** 71, 1961.
77. Fine, R. N., Strauss, J., and Donnell, G. N.: Hyperuricemia in glycogen storage disease type I. Amer. J. Dis. Child., **112,** 572, 1966.
78. Goldfinger, S., Klinenberg, J. R., and Seegmiller, J. E.: Renal retention of uric acid induced by infusion of beta-hydroxybutyrate and acetoacetate. New Eng. J. Med., **272,** 351, 1965.
79. Jeune, M., François, R., and Jarlot, B.: Contribution a l'étude des polycories glycogeniques du foie. Rev. Int. Hepat., **1,** 1, 1959.
80. Jakovcic, S., and Sorensen, L. B.: Studies of uric acid metabolism in glycogen storage disease associated with gouty arthritis. Arthritis Rheum., **10,** 129, 1967.
81. Kelley, W. N., Rosenbloom, F. M., Seegmiller, J. E., and Howell, R. R.: Excessive production of uric acid in type I glycogen storage disease. J. Pediat., **72,** 488, 1968.
82. Howell, R. R.: The interrelationship of glycogen storage disease and gout. Arthritis Rheum., **8,** 780, 1965.
83. Howell, R. R.: Hyperuricemia in childhood. Fed. Proc., **27,** 1078, 1968.
84. Lowe, C. U., Sokal, J. E., Mosovich, L. L., Sarcione, E. J., and Doray, B. H.: Studies in liver glycogen disease. Amer. J. Med., **33,** 4, 1962.
85. Schwartz, R., Ashmore, J., and Renold, A. E.: Galactose tolerance test in glycogen storage disease. Pediatrics, **19,** 585, 1957.
86. Sidbury, J. B.: The genetics of the glycogen storage diseases. Progr. Med. Genet., **4,** 32, 1965.
87. Williams, H. E., Johnson, P. L., Fenster, L. F., Laster, L., and Field, J. B.: Intestinal glucose-6-phosphatase in control subjects and relatives of a patient with glycogen storage disease. Metabolism, **12,** 235, 1963.
88. Field, J. B., Epstein, S., and Egan, T.: Studies in glycogen storage diseases. I. Intestinal glucose-6-phosphatase activity in patients with von Gierke's disease and their parents. J. Clin. Invest., **44,** 1240, 1965.
89. Field, J. B., and Drash, A. L.: Studies in glycogen storage disease. II. Heterogeneity in the inheritance of glycogen storage diseases. Trans. Ass. Amer. Physicians, **80,** 284, 1967.
90. Hsia, D. Y. Y., and Kot, E. G.: Detection of heterozygous carriers in glycogen storage disease of the liver. Nature (London), **183,** 1331, 1959.
91. Gitzelmann, R.: Glukogonprobleme bei den glykogenspeicherkrankheiten. Helv. Paediat. Acta, **12,** 425, 1957.
92. Rennert, O. M., and Mukhopadhyay, D.: Diazoxide in von Gierke's disease. Arch. Dis. Child., **43,** 358, 1968.
93. Riddell, A. G., Davies, R. P., and Clark, A. D.: Portacaval transposition in the treatment of glycogen storage disease. Lancet, **2,** 1146, 1966.
94. Starzl, T. E., Marchioro, T. L., Sexton, A. W., Illingworth, B., Waddell, W. R., Faris, T. D., and Hermann, T. J.: The effect of portacaval transposition on carbohydrate metabolism: experimental and clinical observations. Surgery, **57,** 687, 1965.
95. Hermann, R. E., and Mercer, R. D.: Portacaval shunt in the treatment of glycogen storage disease: report of a case. Surgery, **65,** 499, 1969.
96. Starzl, T. E., Brown, B. I., Blanchard, H., and Brettschneider, L.: Portal diversion in glycogen storage disease. Surgery, **65,** 504, 1969.
97. Riddell, A. G., and Davies, R. P.: Glycogen storage disease treated by portacaval transposition. Proc. Roy. Soc. Med., **59,** 484, 1966.
98. Erickson, R. P., Gluecksohn-Waelsch, S., and Cori, C. F.: Glucose-6-phosphatase deficiency caused by radiation-induced alleles at the albino locus in the mouse. Proc. Nat. Acad. Sci. U.S.A., **59,** 437, 1968.
99. Bardens, J. W.: Glycogen storage disease in puppies. Vet. Med., **61,** 1174, 1966.
100. Ruttenberg, H. D., Steidl, R. M., Carey, L. S., and Edwards, J. E.: Glycogen-storage disease of the heart. Amer. Heart J., **67**(4), 469, 1964.
101. Ehlers, K. H., and Engle, M. A.: Glycogen storage disease of myocardium. Amer. Heart J., **65**(2), 145, 1963.
102. Smith, J., Zellweger, H., and Afifi, A. K.: Muscular form of glycogenosis, type II (Pompe). Neurology, **17**(6), 1967.
103. Dincsoy, M. Y., Dincsoy, H. P., Kessler, A. D., Jackson, M. A., and Sidbury, J. B., Jr.: Generalized glycogenosis and associated endocardial fibroelastosis. J. Pediat., **67**(5), 728, 1965.
104. Hernandez, A., Jr., Marchesi, V., Goldring, D., Kissane, J., and Hartmann, A. F., Jr.: Cardiac glycogenosis. J. Pediat., **68**(3), 400, 1966.
105. Smith, H. L., Amick, L. D., and Sidbury, J. B., Jr.: Type II glycogenosis. Report of a case with four-year survival and absence of acid maltase associated with an abnormal glycogen. Amer. J. Dis. Child., **111,** 475, 1966.
106. Roth, J. C., and Williams, H. E.: The muscular variant of Pompe's disease. J. Pediat., **71**(4), 567, 1967.
107. Zellweger, H., Brown, B. I., McCormick, W. F., and Tu, J. B.: A mild

form of muscular glycogenosis in two brothers with alpha-1,4-glucosidase deficiency. Ann. Paediat., **205**(6), 413, 1965.
108. Baudhuin, P., Hers, H. G., and Loeb, H.: An electron microscopic and biochemical study of type II glycogenosis. Lab. Invest., **13**, 1139, 1964.
109. Hers, H. G.: Inborn lysosomal diseases. Gastroenterology, **48**, 625, 1965.
110. Garancis, J. C.: Type II glycogenosis. Amer. J. Med., **44**(2), 289, 1968.
111. Huijing, F., van Creveld, S., and Losekoot, G.: Diagnosis of generalized glycogen storage disease (Pompe's disease). J. Pediat., **63**(5), 984, 1963.
112. Steinitz, K., and Rutenberg, A.: Tissue α-glucosidase activity and glycogen content in patients with generalized glycogenosis. Israel J. Med. Sci., **3**,(3), 411, 1967.
113. Franzini, C., and Bonini, P. A.: Alpha-glucosidases in human urine. Clin. Chim. Acta, **17**, 505, 1967.
114. Williams, H. E.: α-Glucosidase activity in human leucocytes. Biochim. Biophys. Acta, **124**, 34, 1966.
115. Nitowsky, H. M., and Grunfeld, A.: Lysosomal α-glucosidase in type II glycogenosis; activity in leukocytes and cell cultures in relation to genotype. J. Lab. Clin. Med., **69**(3), 472, 1967.
116. Hug, G., Garancis, J. C., Schubert, W. K., and Kaplan, S.: Glycogen storage disease, types II, III, VIII, and IX. Amer. J. Dis. Child., **111**, 457, 1966.
117. Hug, G., and Schubert, W. K.: Lysosomes in type II glycogenosis. Changes during administration of extract from *Aspergillus niger.* J. Cell Biol., **35**, C1, 1967.
118. Lauer, R. M., Mascarinas, T., Racela, A. S., and Diehl, A. M.: Administration of a mixture of fungal glucosidases to a patient with type II glycogenosis (Pompe's disease). Pediatrics, **42**, 672, 1968.
119. Nadler, H. L.: Prenatal detection of genetic defects. J. Pediat., **74**, 132, 1969.
120. Brandt, I. K., and DeLuca, V. A., Jr.: Type III glycogenosis. A family with an unusual tissue distribution of the enzyme lesion. Amer. J. Med., **40**(5), 779, 1966.
121. Illingworth, B.: Glycogen storage disease. Amer. J. Clin. Nutr., **9**, 683, 1961.
122. Levin, S., Moses, S. W., Chayoth, R., Jagoda, N., and Steinitz, K.: Glycogen storage disease in Israel. Israel J. Med. Sci., **3**, 397, 1967.
123. Fernandes, J., and van de Kamer, J. H.: Hexose and protein tolerance tests in children with liver glycogenosis caused by a deficiency of the debranching enzyme system. Pediatrics, **41**(5), 935, 1968.
124. van Creveld, S., and Huijing, F.: Glycogen storage disease. Amer. J. Med., **38**, 554, 1965.
125. Hug, G., Krill, C. E., Jr., Perrin, E. V., and Guest, G. M.: Cori's disease (amylo-1,6-glucosidase deficiency). New Eng. J. Med., **268**, 113, 1963.
126. Hers, H. G.: Amylo-1,6-glucosidase activity in tissues of children with glycogen storage disease. Biochem. J., **76**, 69, 1960.
127. van Hoof, F., and Hers, H. G.: The subgroups of type III glycogenosis. Europ. J. Biochem., **2**, 265, 1967.
128. Sidbury, J. B., Jr., Cornblath, M., Fisher, J., and House, E.: Glycogen in erythrocytes of patients with glycogen storage disease. Pediatrics, **27**, 103, 1961.
129. van Hoof, F.: Amylo-1,6-glucosidase activity and glycogen content of the erythrocytes of normal subjects, patients with glycogen storage disease and heterozygotes. J. Biochem., **2**, 271, 1967.
130. Williams, C., and Field, J. B.: Studies in glycogen storage disease. III. Limit dextrinosis: a genetic study. J. Pediat., **72**(2), 214, 1968.
131. Williams, H. E., Kendig, E. M., and Field, J. B.: Leukocyte debranching enzyme in glycogen storage disease. J. Clin. Invest., **42**(5), 656, 1963.
132. Huijing, F., Klein Obbink, H. J., and van Creveld, S.: The activity of the debranching enzyme system in leucocytes. Acta Genet. (Basel), **18**, 128, 1968.
133. Andersen, D. H.: Familial cirrhosis of the liver with storage of abnormal glycogen. Lab. Invest., **5**, 11, 1956.
134. Holleman, L. W. J., van der Haar, J. A., and de Vaan, G. A. M.: Type IV glycogenosis. Lab. Invest., **15**(1), 357, 1966.
135. Fernandes, J., and Huijing, F.: Branching enzyme-deficiency glycogenosis: Studies in therapy. Arch. Dis. Child., **43**, 347, 1968.
136. Levin, B., Burgen, E. A., and Mortimer, P. E.: Glycogen storage disease type IV, amylopectinosis. Arch. Dis. Child., **43**(231), 548, 1968.
137. Reed, G. B., Jr., Dixon, J. F. P., Neustein, H. B., Donnell, G. N., and Landing, B. H.: Type IV glycogenosis patient with absence of a branching enzyme α-1,4-glucan α-1,4-glucan 6-glycosyl transferase. Lab. Invest., **19**, 546, 1968.
138. Illingworth, B., and Cori, G. T.: Structure of glycogens and amylopectins. III. Normal and abnormal human glycogen. J. Biol. Chem., **199**, 653, 1952.
139. Howell, R. R., Brown, B. I., and Kaback, M. M.: Brancher activity in normal skin fibroblasts and its deficiency in fibroblasts derived from patients with type IV glycogen storage disease. J. Pediat. (In Press.)
140. Rowland, L. P., Lovelace, R. E., Schotland, D. L., Araki, S., and Carmel, P.: The clinical diagnosis of McArdle's disease. Neurology, **16**, 93, 1966.
141. McArdle, B.: Metabolic myopathies. Amer. J. Med., **35**, 661, 1963.
142. Dawson, D. M., Spong, F. L., and Harrington, J. F.: McArdle's disease. Lack of muscle phosphorylase. Ann. Intern. Med., **69**, 229, 1968.
143. McArdle, B.: Myopathy due to a defect in muscle glycogen breakdown. Clin. Sci., **10**, 13, 1951.
143*a*. Mommaerts, W. F. H. M., Illingworth, B., Pearson, C. M., Guillory, P. J., and Seraydarian, K.: A functional disorder of muscle associated with the absence of phosphorylase. Proc. Nat. Acad. Sci. U.S.A., **45**, 791, 1959.
144. Schmid, R., and Mahler, R.: Chronic progressive myopathy with myoglobinuria: demonstration of a glycogenolytic defect in the muscle. J. Clin. Invest., **38**, 2044, 1959.
145. Schmid, R., Robbins, P. W., and Traut, R. R.: Glycogen synthesis in muscle lacking phosphorylase, Proc. Nat. Acad. Sci. U.S.A., **45**, 1236, 1959.
146. Larner, J., and Villar-Palasi, C.: Enzymes in a glycogen storage myopathy. Proc. Nat. Acad. Sci. U.S.A., **45**, 1234, 1959.
147. Pearson, C. M., Rimer, D. G., and Mommaerts, W. F. H. M.: A metabolic myopathy due to absence of muscle phosphorylase. Amer. J. Med., **30**, 502, 1961.
148. Salter, R. H.: The muscle glycogenoses. Lancet, **1**, 1301, 1968.
149. Thomson, W. H. S., MacLaurin, J. C., and Prineas, J. W.: Skeletal muscle glycogenosis: an investigation of two dissimilar cases. J. Neurol. Neurosurg. Psychiat., **26**, 60, 1963.
150. Rowland, L. P., Araki, S., and Carmel, P.: Contracture in McArdle's disease. Arch. Neurol., **13**, 541, 1965.
151. Pernow, B. B., Havel, R. J., and Jennings, D. B.: The second wind phenomenon in McArdle's syndrome. Acta Med. Scand., suppl., **472**, 294, 1967.
152. Hammett, J. F., Bale, P., Basser, L. S., and Neale, F. C.: McArdle's disease: three cases in an Australian family. Proc. Aust. Ass. Neurol., **4**, 21, 1966.
153. Howell, R. R.: The diagnostic value of serum enzyme measurements. J. Pediat., **68**, 121, 1966.
154. Schotland, D. L., Spiro, D., Rowland, L. P., and Carmel, P.: Ultrastructural studies of muscle in McArdle's disease. J. Neuropath. Exp. Neurol., **24**, 629, 1965.
155. Lyon, J. B., Jr., Porter, J., and Robertson, M.: Phosphorylase *b* kinase inheritance in mice. Science, **155**, 1550, 1967.
156. Lyon, J. B., Jr., and Porter, J.: The relation of phosphorylase to glycogenolysis in skeletal muscle and heart of mice. J. Biol. Chem., **238**, 1, 1963.
157. Hers, H. G.: Études enzymatiques sur fragments hépatiques. Rev. Int. Hepat., **9**(1), 35, 1959.
158. Lamy, M., Dubois, R., Rossier, A., Frezal, J., Loeb, H., and Blancher, G.: La Glycogenose par deficience en phosphorylase hépatique. Arch. Franc. Pediat., **17**, 14, 1960.
159. Williams, H. E., and Field, J. B.: Further studies on leukocyte phosphorylase in glycogen storage disease. Metabolism, **12**(5), 464, 1963.
160. Öckerman, P. A., Jelke, H., and Kaijser, K.: Glycogenosis type 6 (liver phosphorylase deficiency). Acta Paediat. Scand., **55**, 10, 1966.
161. Illingworth, B., and Brown, D. H.: Glycogen storage diseases, types III, IV, and VI, in *Control of Glycogen Metabolism,* edited by W. J. Whelan, p. 336. Little, Brown, Boston, 1964.

162. Hers, H. G., and van Hoof, F.: Glycogen storage diseases: type II and type VI glycogenosis, in *Carbohydrate Metabolism and Its Disorders,* edited by F. Dickens, P. J. Randle, and W. J. Whelan, p. 151. Academic, New York, 1968.

163. Tarui, S., Okuno, G., Ikura, Y., Tanaka, T., Suda, M., and Nishika, M.: Phosphofructokinase deficiency in skeletal muscle. A new type of glucogenosis. Biochem. Biophys. Res. Commun., **19**, 517, 1965.

164. Okuno, G., Hizukuri, S., and Nishikawa, M.: Activities of glycogen synthetase and UDPG-pyrophosphorylase in muscle of a patient with a new type of muscle glycogenosis caused by phosphofructokinase deficiency. Nature (London), **212**, 1490, 1966.

165. Layzer, R. B., Rowland, L. P., and Ranney, H. M.: Muscle phosphofructokinase deficiency. Arch. Neurol., **17**, 512, 1967.

165*a*. Tauri, S., Kono, N., Nasu, T., and Nishikawa, M.: Enzymatic basis for the coexistence of myopathy and hemolytic disease in inherited muscle phosphofructokinase deficiency. Biochem. Biophys. Res. Commun., **34**, 77, 1969.

166. Hug, G., Schubert, W. K., and Chuck, G.: Deficient activity of dephosphophorylase kinase and accumulation of glycogen in liver. J. Clin. Invest., **48**, 704, 1969.

167. Huijing, F.: Phosphorylase kinase in leukocytes of normal subjects and patients with glycogen storage disease. Biochim. Biophys. Acta, **148**, 601, 1967.

168. Huijing, F., and Fernandes, J.: X-chromosomal inheritance of liver glycogenosis with phosphorylase kinase deficiency. Amer. J. Hum. Genet., **21**, 275, 1969.

168*a*. Huijing, F., and Sandberg, D. H.: Phosphorylase kinase defect: a generalized disorder. Southern Med. J., **63**, 1482, 1970.

169. Lewis, G. M., Spencer-Peet, J., and Stewart, K. M.: Infantile hypoglycemia due to inherited deficiency of glycogen synthetase in liver. Arch. Dis. Child., **38**, 40, 1963.

170. Lewis, G. M., Stewart, K. M., and Spencer-Peet, J.: Absence of the liver enzyme, UDPG-glycogen 1,4 transglucosylase, as a cause of infantile hypoglycemia, Biochem. J., **84**, 115p, 1962.

171. Spencer-Peet, J., Lewis, G. M., and Stewart, K. M.: Glycogen synthetase deficiency, in *Control of Glycogen metabolism,* edited by W. J. Whelan, p. 377. Little, Brown, Boston, 1964.

172. Kogut, M. D., Blaskovics, M., and Donnell, G. N.: Idiopathic hypoglycemia: a study of twenty-six children. J. Pediat., **74**, 853, 1969.

173. Sauls, H. S.: Ketotic hypoglycemia: Quantitation of ketosis and liver glycogen during the ketogenic test diet. Program, Society for Pediatric Research, Atlantic City, N.J., 1966, p. 190.

174. Hers, H. G.: Comments, in *Control of Glycogen Metabolism,* edited by W. J. Whelan, p. 386. Little, Brown, Boston, 1964.

175. Auerbach, V. H., and DiGeorge, A. M.: Genetic mechanisms producing multiple enzyme defects. A review of unexplained cases and a new hypothesis. Amer. J. Med. Sci., **249**, 718, 1965.

176. Calderbank, A., Kent, P. W., Lorber, J., Manners, D. J., and Wright, A.: Biochemical investigation of a case of glycogen-storage disease (von Gierke's disease). Biochem. J., **74**, 223, 1960.

177. Eberlein, W. R., Illingworth, B. A., and Sidbury, J. B.: Heterogeneous glycogen storage disease in siblings and favorable response to synthetic androgen administration. Amer. J. Med., **33**, 20, 1962.

178. Cori, G. T.: Biochemical aspects of glycogen deposition diseases. Mod. Probl. Paediat., **3**, 344, 1957.

179. Bueding, E., and Colacci, A. V.: Enzymes of glycogen metabolism in mammalian fetal liver, in *Intrauterine Development,* edited by Allen C. Barnes, p. 233. Lea & Febiger, Philadelphia, 1968.

CHAPTER EIGHT

DISORDERS OF GALACTOSE METABOLISM*

Stanton Segal

The name *galactosemia* has been given to a toxicity syndrome associated with the administration of galactose to patients with an inherited disorder of galactose utilization [1–5]. The constellation of nutritional failure, liver disease, cataracts, and mental retardation results from a deficiency of galactose-1-phosphate uridyl transferase [6], one of several enzymes in the galactose metabolic pathway. Another inherited syndrome of elevated plasma galactose concentration associated with galactosuria and juvenile cataracts has now been described as resulting from galactokinase deficiency [7]. The possibility exists that disorders of other enzymes in the galactose metabolic sequence could also result in "galactosemia." The use of the term galactosemia, therefore, has become inadequate. Also the name *galactose diabetes* for galactokinase deficiency [8] seems inappropriate. It appears reasonable to qualify the descriptive term, galactosemia, with the appropriate enzyme fault. The two known syndromes of disordered galactose metabolism will be designated *transferase deficiency galactosemia* and *galactokinase deficiency galactosemia* and will be discussed as such in this chapter.

THE BIOCHEMISTRY AND PHYSIOLOGY OF GALACTOSE UTILIZATION

The Uridine Nucleotide Pathway

The main dietary source of galactose is the disaccharide, lactose, the principal carbohydrate of mammalian milk. Hydrolysis of lactose by the galactosidase, lactase, of the intestinal microvillae results in release of the monosaccharides, glucose and galactose. These two sugars differ only by the configuration of the hydroxyl group about the fourth carbon (Fig. 8-1). The main pathway of galactose metabolism in man is the conversion of galactose to glucose, without disruption of the carbon skeleton, by the epimerization of the hydroxyl group of carbon-4. This requires several enzymatic steps, as elucidated by Leloir and associates [9–11] and Kalckar and coworkers [12], and is shown in Fig. 8-2.

*Supported by Grant AM 10894 from the National Institutes of Health.

Galactokinase

This enzyme has been described in yeast [9, 13, 14], bacteria [15, 16], and mammalian tissues [10]. Galactose reacts with ATP to form galactose-1-phosphate and ADP; Mg^{++} is required. The equilibrium is far in the direction of sugar phosphorylation but the reaction is reversible [17]. The *Escherichia coli* enzyme has been purified, the amino acid composition found, and the molecular weight determined to be 40,000 [16]. The reaction of the bacterial enzyme is of the random bimolecular type [18]. Protection by thiols is a property common to the bacterial and liver enzyme. The mammalian enzyme has been partially purified and studied in some detail in rat [19, 20] and pig liver [21], as well as in human red cells [22, 23]. Liver enzyme reacts with galactosamine and 2-deoxygalactose, while the yeast enzyme is more specific for galactose. In the rat, activity of the liver enzyme increases after birth to a maximum at about 5 days of age, followed by a progressive decrease until adult levels are reached (Fig. 8-3) [19, 20].

The developmental changes in liver activity do not appear to be regulated by dietary galactose. Galactokinase activity is higher in red blood cells from newborn and human infants than in cells from adults [22]. Both substrate and product inhibition have been observed [19]. This type of regulation

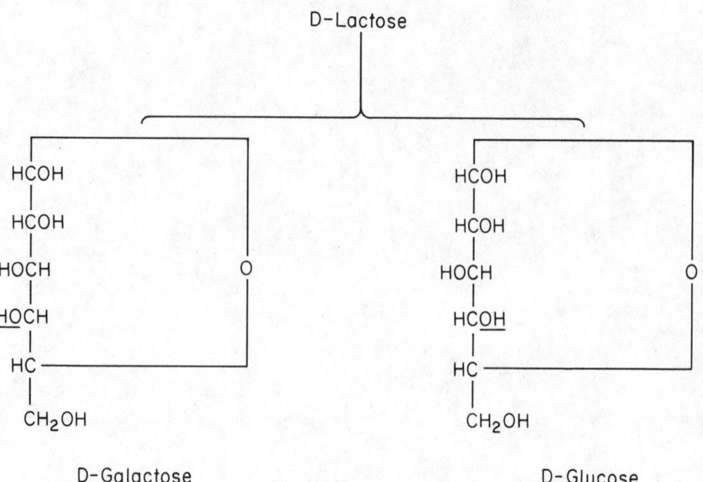

Figure 8-1. Structure of galactose and glucose, the monosaccharides in lactose. Note the difference in the spatial relation of the hydroxyl group on the fourth carbon.

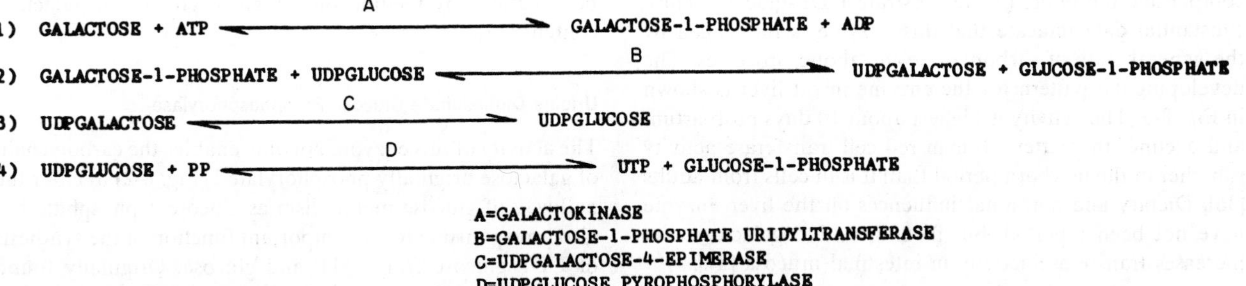

Figure 8-2. Reactions of the pathway of galactose metabolism responsible for the galactose-glucose interconversion.

would tend to decrease the formation of galactose-1-phosphate, a possible toxic metabolite. Although stimulation of *E. coli* galactokinase has been observed with 3′, 5′ cyclic adenosine monophosphate [24], no influence of this compound on the mammalian enzyme has been reported.

Galactose-1-Phosphate Uridyl Transferase

This enzyme catalyzes the second step in the galactose-glucose interconversion in which the product of the galactokinase reaction, galactose-1-phosphate, reacts with uridine diphosphate glucose (UDP-glucose) to give UDP-galactose and glucose-1-phosphate [12]. The enzyme is present in bacteria [25] and most mammalian tissues [26]. Bacterial transferase has been purified to homogeneity and consists of two structural subunits of 40,000 mol. wt [27]. Calf [28, 29] and human liver [30], and human red cell enzymes [31] have been partially purified. The biochemical properties of rat liver [26] and several human tissues including red cells [32], leucocytes [33], cultured fibroblasts [33], intestinal mucosa [34], and liver [30] have been examined. The mammalian enzyme is closely similar in most tissues, with a pH optimum of about 8.5 and a partial requirement for sulfhydryl compounds. Liver transferase has a K_m for UDP-glucose of 0.1 to 0.2 m*M*, a value within the physiological range of liver UDP-glucose concentration [35]. Thus the rate of the reaction may be regulated by substrate concentration, and limited by UDP-glucose substrate inhibition of the transferase observed at higher levels. Glucose-1-phosphate is a potent inhibitor of the enzyme [26] and evidence recently obtained in the author's laboratory indicates that uridine nucleotides such as uridine di- and triphosphate are extremely powerful

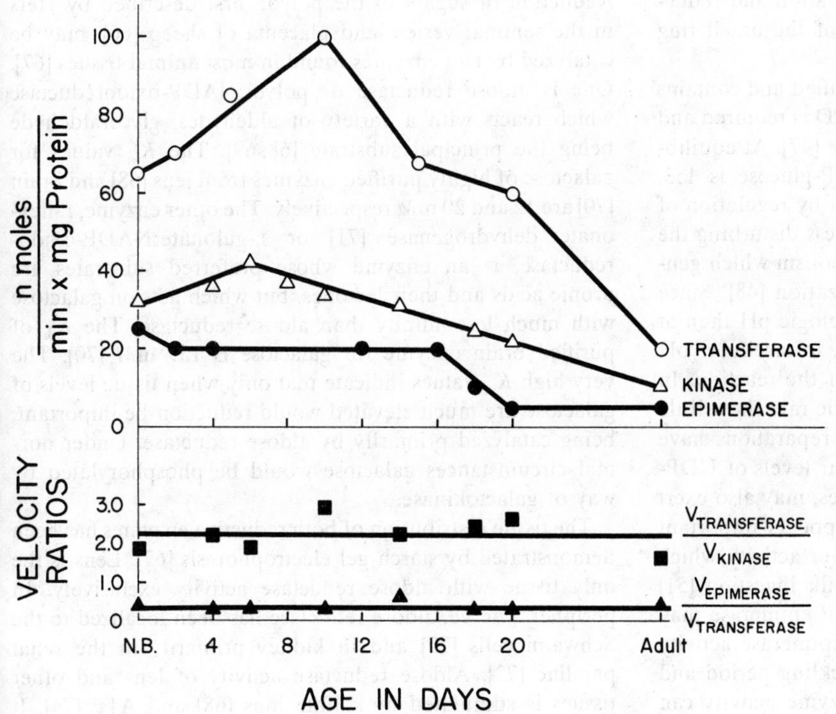

Figure 8-3. The activity of galactokinase, galactose-1-phosphate uridyl transferase and epimerase in rat liver as a function of age. (*From P. Cuatrecasas and S. Segal [19], D. Bertoli and S. Segal [26], and R. Cohn and S. Segal [51].*)

competitive inhibitors of the substrate UDP-glucose. Thus, substantial data indicate that this enzyme is influenced by the general state of carbohydrate metabolic processes. The developmental pattern for the enzyme in rat liver is shown in Fig. 8-3. The activity is highest about 10 days postpartum and declines thereafter. Human red cell transferase activity is higher in the newborn period than it is in cells from adults [36]. Dietary and hormonal influences on the liver enzyme have not been reported, but feeding a high galactose diet increases transferase activity in intestinal mucosa [37].

Uridine Diphosphate Galactose-4-epimerase

This enzyme is responsible for the inversion of the hydroxyl group at the fourth carbon of the hexose chain to form glucose from galactose and has a much broader biological significance than merely the catabolism of galactose. It is also important for the conversion of UDP-glucose to UDP-galactose in those situations where only glucose is available to the organism and where galactose is a constituent of complex polysaccharides. The enzyme is specific for UDP-glucose and UDP-galactose [38] and has been highly purified from bacteria [39, 40] and yeast [41, 42] in which a polymeric structure of the enzyme has been found. In these organisms 1 mole of NAD is bound to the enzyme, which in the presence of uridine nucleotides and galactose exhibits fluorescence and conformational changes [43, 44]. The mechanism of the inversion has generated considerable interest. Kalckar [45] has reviewed the data which indicate that neither hydrogen from water nor NAD is exchanged with hydroxyl hydrogen at carbon-4. ^{18}O from isotopic water is not involved. A novel mechanism for oxidation and reduction at carbon-4 involving the hydrogen of the uracil ring of UDP-glucose has been proposed [46].

The liver enzyme has been partially purified and contains no bound NAD coenzyme. Exogenous NAD is required and NADH is a potent inhibitor of the enzyme [47]. At equilibrium the ratio of UDP-galactose to UDP-glucose is 1:3. Metabolic control of galactose metabolism by regulation of liver epimerase activity is likely. Any process disturbing the NAD/NADH ratio, such as ethanol metabolism which generates NADH, will impair galactose utilization [48]. Since greater NADH inhibition occurs at physiologic pH than at the alkaline pH optimum of the enzyme, intracellular pH may be an important factor in the rate of the reaction. In this regard intact cells with a high glycolytic rate show little epimerase activity, whereas broken cell preparations have considerable enzyme function [49]. Cellular levels of UDP-glucose, as well as other uridine nucleotides, may also exert rate-regulating effects [50]. Animal age appears important since the liver of newborn rats has a higher activity which remains elevated during the period of milk ingestion [51] (Fig. 8-3). The data of Fig. 8-3 suggest that epimerase may be the rate-limiting enzyme in rat liver. Epimerase activity of intestinal mucosa is low during the suckling period and increases with age [51]. The intestinal enzyme activity can be enhanced by feeding diets high in glucose or galactose content [37].

Uridine Diphosphate Glucose Pyrophosphorylase

The activity of this enzyme not only enables the carbon chain of galactose originally phosphorylated (Fig. 8-2) to enter the pathway of glucose metabolism as glucose-1-phosphate but also is responsible for the important function of the synthesis of UDP-glucose from UTP and glucose. Originally found in yeast [52, 53], it is abundant in mammalian liver from which it has been crystallized [54]. A polymeric subunit structure has been determined [55]. The crystalline enzyme from human liver reacts to some extent with other sugar nucleotides besides UDP-glucose, including UDP-galactose. Bovine mammary gland enzyme is inhibited by galactose-1-phosphate [56]. Although no mutations of this enzyme have been observed in man, certain *E. coli* strains with defective galactose metabolism have been shown to have an absence of this enzyme [57, 58].

Alternate Pathways of Galactose Metabolism

Reduction to Galactitol

The presence of galactitol in the tissues of animals fed galactose [59–61] and in the tissues [62, 63] and urine of patients with both transferase [64] and galactokinase deficiency galactosemia [65] demonstrates the importance of the reduction of galactose in mammalian metabolism (Fig. 8-4). Reduction of sugars to the polyol, first described by Hers in the seminal vesicle and placenta of sheep [66], may be catalyzed by two enzymes found in most animal tissues [67]. One is aldose reductase or polyol:NADP-oxidoreductase which reacts with a variety of aldehydes, glyceraldehyde being the principal substrate [68, 69]. The K_m values for galactose of highly purified enzymes from lens [68] and brain [70] are 12 and 20 m*M* respectively. The other enzyme, L-hexonate dehydrogenase [71] or L-gulonate:NADP-oxidoreductase, is an enzyme whose preferred substrates are uronic acids and their lactones, but which acts on galactose with much less affinity than aldose reductase. The K_m of purified brain enzyme for galactose is 159 m*M* [70]. The very high K_m values indicate that only when tissue levels of galactose are much elevated would reduction be important, being catalyzed primarily by aldose reductase. Under normal circumstances galactose would be phosphorylated by way of galactokinase.

The tissue distribution of both reductive enzymes has been demonstrated by starch-gel electrophoresis [67]. Lens is the only tissue with aldose reductase activity exclusively. In peripheral nerve, aldose reductase has been localized to the Schwann cells [72] and in kidney primarily in the renal papillae [73]. Aldose reductase activity of lens and other tissues is stimulated by sulfate ions [68] and ATP [74]. It

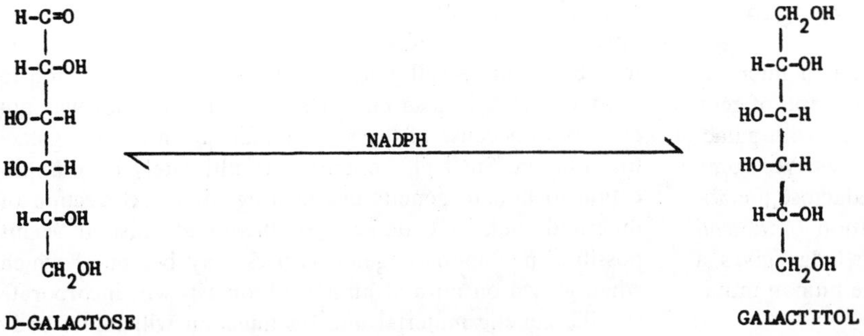

```
H-C=O                                              CH2OH
  |                                                  |
H-C-OH                                             H-C-OH
  |                                                  |
HO-C-H                                             HO-C-H
  |                NADPH                             |
HO-C-H     ----------------------->                HO-C-H
  |                                                  |
H-C-OH                                             H-C-OH
  |                                                  |
  CH2OH                                              CH2OH

D-GALACTOSE                                        GALACTITOL
```

Figure 8-4. The conversion of galactose to galactitol by aldose reductase.

is inhibited by various keto and fatty acids [67] and ADP [74]. Increased enzyme activity has been observed in rat brain after birth [75].

Oxidation of Galactose to Galactonate

A pathway of galactose metabolism in rat liver has been described in which galactose reacts with NAD to form galactonic acid [76]. The latter compound is then oxidized to form β-ketogalactonic acid which undergoes decarboxylation to D-xylulose, a sugar capable of further metabolism. The initial enzyme, galactose dehydrogenase, which exists in the soluble cell fraction has been partially purified [77] and its kinetic properties analyzed [78]. The K_m for galactose was 26 m*M*. Srivastava and Beutler [79] studied the formation of galactose-6-phosphate and showed its subsequent oxidation to 6-phosphogalactonic acid but, in their animals, failed to demonstrate the oxidation of galactose to galactonic acid. The evidence derived from the oxidation of galactose-1-^{14}C and galactose-2-^{14}C in normal man suggests that an oxidative pathway plays an insignificant role in galactose catabolism [80]. The data from similar studies in patients with transferase deficiency galactosemia indicate that this pathway may play a role in metabolism if the sugar nucleotide pathway is blocked [80].

Uridine Diphosphate Galactose Pyrophosphorylase

This enzyme, first detected in yeast [12] and subsequently identified in mammalian liver [81, 82], catalyzes the reaction of galactose-1-phosphate with uridine triphosphate to form UDP-galactose and pyrophosphate. Function of this enzyme could circumvent the block in galactose metabolism due to transferase deficiency and indeed, preliminary data indicated this could be the case [81]. Recent evidence, however, seems conclusive that the activity of this enzyme in human liver is low and does not increase with age [83]. There is now considerable doubt that catalysis is due to an enzyme with a unique affinity for galactose-1-phosphate. It is probable that the enzyme performing this function is UDP-glucose pyrophosphorylase [54].

Physiological Aspects of Galactose Metabolism

Man is capable of metabolizing large quantities of galactose given orally or intravenously, as demonstrated by the rapid elimination of galactose from blood [84] and the oxidation of radioactive galactose to $^{14}CO_2$ [85]. A rise in plasma glucose is found after galactose loading, due to the conversion of galactose to glucose through the sugar nucleotide pathway. When tracer amounts of radioactive galactose are given intravenously to normal subjects, 50 percent of the radioactivity may be found in the body glucose pools within 30 min. Curves of $^{14}CO_2$ excretion in expired air closely resemble those seen after the administration of radioactive glucose itself [85]. Plasma galactose is so rapidly removed by the liver that the measurement of galactose clearance is a measure of hepatic blood flow [86]. The mechanism appears to be saturated at plasma levels of 50 mg per 100 ml. Tygstrup estimates that the capacity of hepatic elimination corresponds to the limits of the ability of galactokinase to phosphorylate the sugar [87]. Urinary elimination is not a significant factor in the disposition of galactose loads [88]. Studies of the resorption of galactose by the human kidney reveal a low and incomplete threshold at plasma levels of 10 to 20 mg per 100 ml.

Galactose tolerance tests have been used to estimate impaired liver function [89] and have shown that clearance of intravenously administered galactose is slow in the presence of liver damage [90]. Ethanol administration slows galactose elimination from blood in both man [84, 85, 91] and rat [92], the effect presumably being due to tissue elevation of NADH and inhibition of UDP-galactose-4-epimerase [48].

Age may have some influence on galactose metabolism. Maximal utilization of galactose by rat liver in vitro occurs in tissue from the newborn and young [93]. This corresponds to the elevated enzyme levels shown in Fig. 8-3. Haworth and Ford [94] and Mulligan and Schwartz [95] have demonstrated that human neonates have a higher elevation of blood glucose after galactose administration than adults. The elimination of intravenous galactose in the neonate has been reported by some to be slower than in the adult [95, 96], while others report no difference [97]. Vink and Kroes reported the elimination rate to be faster in young children than in adults [98].

Galactose Enzymes and Mutations in Microorganisms

Studies of metabolism and genetic regulation in microorganisms have contributed greatly to modern concepts of gene function and enzyme synthesis. The work done with galactose mutants in bacteria, especially *E. coli,* deserves some mention in a consideration of disorders of galactose metabolism in man. Although the direct application of *E. coli* genetics cannot be made to man, the knowledge gives a greater conceptual framework for viewing the human mutations.

Normally the ability of *E. coli* to metabolize galactose is inducible, that is, incubation in solutions containing galactose is followed by the appearance of high levels of the enzymes of the sugar nucleotide pathway, galactokinase, galactose-1-phosphate uridyl transferase, and UDP-Gal-4-epimerase [99–101]. Numerous mutants have been described which are unable to metabolize galactose, the so-called Gal^- mutants [102]. Analysis of these mutants has shown an absence of one or more of the enzymes of the pathway. In addition, Gal^- mutants have been described with defective UDP-glucose pyrophosphorylase [57, 58]. Constitutive mutants have been described in which galactose no longer needs to be added to the media in order that the enzymes be present [103]. Genetic mapping of the galactose genes on the *E. coli* chromosome has been done. The sequence of the genes is kinase, transferase, epimerase, and operator (K-T-E-O) [104–106]. The UDP-glucose pyrophosphorylase maps in a different position on the *E. coli* chromosome. The K-T-E-O genes function as an operon, with a regulator gene which is not linked to the Gal region being present elsewhere on the chromosome [103]. Some constitutive mutations are located at the regulator gene site, but one has been described which is a mutation in the terminal region of the epimerase gene. This is a so-called operator constitutive mutation which no longer recognizes the ability of the product of the regulator gene to repress initiation of enzyme synthesis [103]. The works of Wilson and Hogness characterizing the protein structure of *E. coli* galactokinase [16] and UDP-galactose-4-epimerase [40] suggest that the genes are made up of 1,100 base pairs.

The effects of galactose on mutants with various enzyme deficiencies have been studied [107, 108]. The presence of galactose does not impair the growth of galactokinase deficient organisms but does impede the growth of transferase deficient organisms. Galactose-1-phosphate accumulates in the latter bacteria, and this inhibits glycerolkinase formation [109]. Epimerase [110, 111] and UDP-glucose pyrophosphorylase [57, 58] deficient organisms have marked alterations in the composition of polysaccharides in their cell walls.

Perhaps the most fascinating aspect of *E. coli* galactose operon genetics is that a lysogenic bacteriophage called λ may incorporate the whole or a part of the galactose region of the *E. coli* chromosome into its own gene complement [112]. These phage particles have been termed λ dg. The λ dg phage is able to tranduce the genes of the galactose operon into *E. coli* Gal^- mutants [113]. That is, the λ dg may bring into a cell genetic material that will function to produce the galactose enzymes which the mutant was not able to do because of the genetic makeup in its own galactose operon. Such phenomena may ultimately have application to human genetic engineering for the correction of inherited metabolic defects. In theory at least, it seems possible that nonpathogenic viruses may be found which when grown on normal human fibroblasts will incorporate specific genetic material and on injection will infect body cells with reparative genes.

TRANSFERASE DEFICIENCY GALACTOSEMIA

Clinical Aspects

The first detailed description of this first of the galactosemia syndromes by Mason and Turner in 1935 [1] was followed over the ensuing 25 years by numerous case descriptions which clearly established the clinical entity. The first reports of large groups of patients followed over a period of time appeared in 1961, when Hsia and Walker [114] discussed the variable clinical manifestations in 45 patients and Donnell et al. [115] described the growth of 24 affected children. The findings in 55 patients have been recently reported by Nadler and associates [116], and in 39 patients by Donnell et al. [117]. In 1970 Komrower and Lee reported a long-term follow-up of the 60 known cases of the disease in Great Britain [118].

The most common initial clinical symptom is failure to thrive. This occurs in almost all cases (Fig. 8-5). Vomiting or diarrhea was found in 52 out of 55 cases, usually starting within a few days of milk ingestion [116]. Signs of deranged liver function, either jaundice or hepatomegaly, are present almost as frequently after the first week of life. The jaundice of intrinsic liver disease may be accentuated by the severe hemolysis which may occur in some patients. Indeed, the peripheral blood picture may resemble that of erythroblastosis. Ascites may develop and is usually found in those infants who succumb. Cataracts have been observed within a few days of birth. These may be found only on slit-lamp examination by the ophthalmologist and are missed with an ophthalmoscope, since they consist of punctate lesions in the fetal lens nucleus. Retarded mental development may be apparent in those first observed after the first several months of life.

Occasionally, patients found to be homozygous for the disorder in the course of genetic studies have been asymptomatic while ingesting milk. These patients, in many instances, are Negro and may be capable of metabolizing galactose [119]. There may be other patients who do not present a failure-to-thrive syndrome and are seen months after birth with motor retardation, hepatomegaly, and cata-

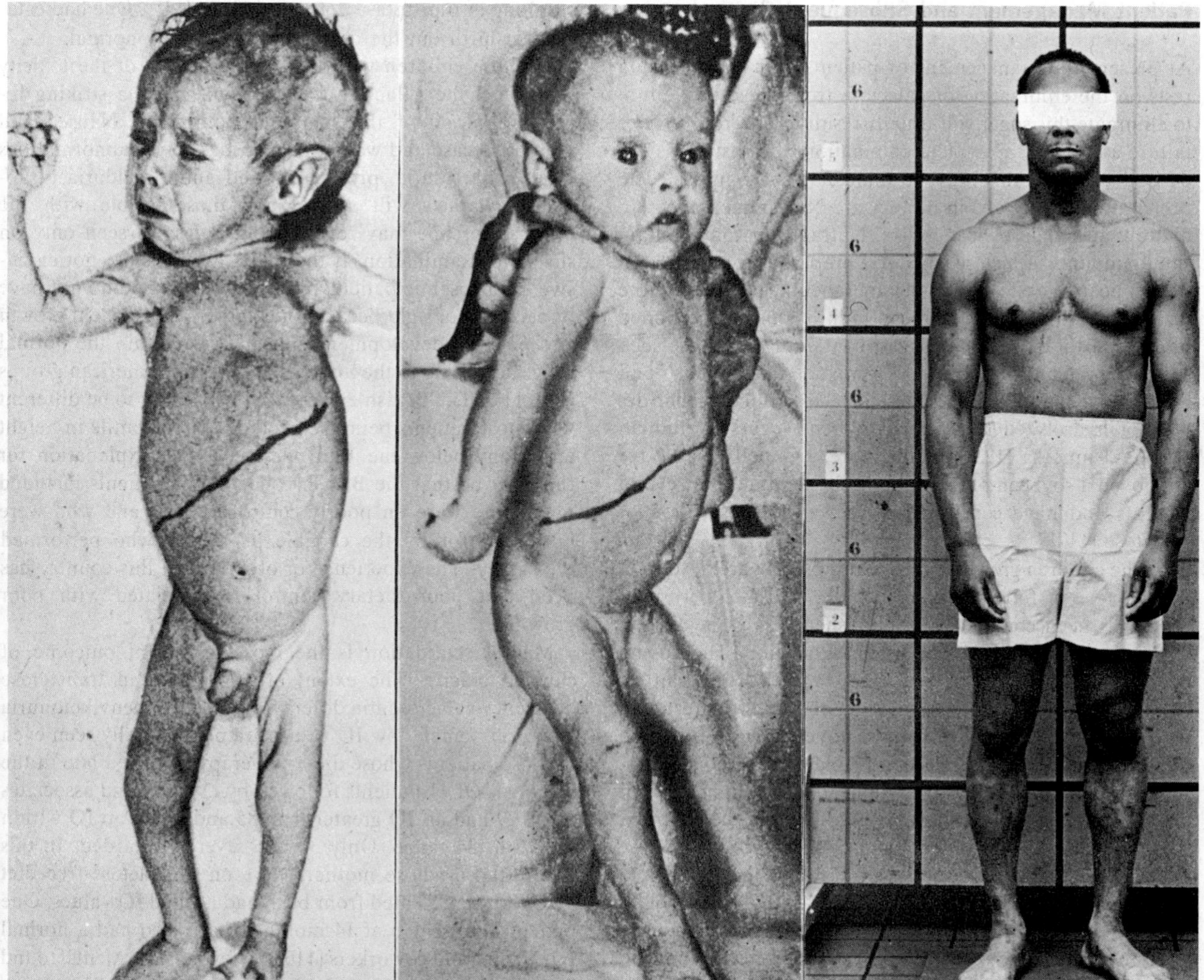

Figure 8-5. Patients with galactose-1-phosphate uridyl transferase deficiency. The left picture shows a 3½-month old child with inanition and hepatomegaly. In the middle is the same child after galactose restriction for 3 months. On the right is a 30-year old man diagnosed in infancy by Mason and Turner [1].

racts. The physician may be confronted with a child several years old with mental retardation and cataracts who proves to have this disorder. These children frequently have a history of partial treatment with milk substitutes and reduced milk intake instituted because of vomiting on milk formulas.

The chemical findings, besides those of deranged liver function tests, include elevated blood galactose, galactosuria, hyperchloremic acidosis, albuminuria, and amino aciduria [2, 3]. On rare occasions, there may be a depression of blood glucose concentration. Hyperchloremic acidosis may be secondary to the gastrointestinal disturbance and poor food intake but can be a result of renal tubular dysfunction and a defect in urine acidification mechanisms [2]. The albuminuria [3] and the generalized renal amino aciduria [120, 121] are manifestations of a renal toxicity syndrome. The galactosuria may be intermittent because of poor food intake or may disappear within 3 or 4 days with the use of intravenous glucose feeding. The finding of a urinary reducing substance which does not react in a glucose oxidase test is the alerting sign for considering a diagnosis of galactosemia. Yet these latter findings do not establish the diagnosis, since lactosuria also occurs in intestinal lactase deficiency, and severely impaired liver function due to viral or other causes may be accompanied by diminished galactose metabolism and galactosuria and be confused with galactosemia. The liver of affected patients has a characteristic acinar formation, so that liver biopsy on occasion has been helpful in establishing the diagnosis [122].

Patient Management and Subsequent Course

At present the management of patients with galactosemia rests on the elimination of galactose from the diet. Failure to eliminate this sugar will usually result in progressive liver failure and death. Complete elimination of the sugar is the desired goal but this may be difficult to accomplish. The preparations employed in infancy are Nutramigen, a casein hydrolysate, and soybean milks. Nutramigen may contain small amounts of lactose since it is prepared from milk, but this appears not to affect the therapeutic efficacy of the preparation. The use of soybean milk has been questioned because of the presence of sugars containing galactose such as raffinose and stachyose. However, Gitzelmann and Auricchio have shown that these galactose oligosaccharides are not hydrolyzed to their component sugars by human intestinal mucosa [123]. Furthermore, Donnell et al. have employed a soybean preparation in the treatment of several patients and have concluded there was no absorption of galactose [117].

As the children grow it is important to be aware of sources of galactose in foods other than milk. A list of permitted foods has been compiled and published [124]. The success of the procedure depends on parent education. There is no good evidence that at a prescribed age the diet can be relaxed. In childhood the ingestion of milk will result in gastrointestinal symptoms. It has frequently been observed that after puberty milk ingestion is tolerated without symptoms. Such findings have been interpreted as indication of the development of a metabolic capability. On the contrary, there are data to suggest that the patient with transferase deficient galactosemia does not develop the ability to metabolize galactose as he increases in age [119]. In older patients, there may be psychological problems associated with the adherence to stringent galactose restriction and permission to include cakes, bread, and similar food should be considered. Milk restriction should be maintained. Schwarz [125] and Donnell and associates [117, 126] have advocated assays of erythrocyte galactose-1-phosphate for monitoring adherence to the diet.

There is no evidence that dietary galactose restriction is harmful. Since the UDP-galactose-4-epimerase reaction is reversible and UDP-glucose can be converted to UDP-galactose, the body is able to provide adequately for the galactose component for brain cerebrosides and complex polysaccharides. Human intestinal lactase, the presence of which may be dependent on continued lactose ingestion, does not appear to be diminished in patients with galactosemia who have not ingested lactose for many years [127].

Recently attention has focused on the restriction of dietary galactose during the pregnancies of women who have had children with galactosemia. This has stemmed from observations that the galactosemic syndrome is present at birth [114], from experimental evidence that the pups of pregnant rats fed high galactose diets are born with cataracts, and from other findings of galactose toxicity [128, 129]. Donnell et al. have carried out this restriction in 11 pregnancies resulting in transferase deficient infants [117]. One had cataracts at birth but the other 10 were entirely normal.

In those children with the manifestations of the toxicity syndrome, the galactose-free diet will cause a striking regression of all of the symptoms and signs. Nausea and vomiting cease and weight gain ensues. Liver abnormalities clear; galactosuria, proteinuria and amino aciduria disappear. Cataracts will regress and those visible with the ophthalmoscope may revert to small lesions seen only on slit-lamp examination. If the initial cataracts are not extensive, galactosemic patients who are well treated do not have impairment of sight because of cataracts. Subsequent growth and physical development appear to be within the normal range according to the findings in the large American groups [116, 117]. The British experience [118] seems to be different with most patients being below the 50th percentile in height and many below the 10th percentile. The explanation for this may be that the British collection of patients included many who were on poorly controlled diets and who were not cared for by the capable physicians who performed the survey. The experience of observers in this country has been that poor dietary control is associated with poor growth.

Mental retardation is the most significant outcome of clinical toxicity. The extent of retardation in transferase deficiency galactosemia differs from that of phenylketonuria in that extremely low IQ values are not generally seen even in those patients whose dietary therapy is started late in the first year. Of 41 patients followed by Donnell and associates [117], 29 had an IQ greater than 85 and 7 had an IQ within the 70 to 84 range. Only 3 were severely retarded. In this group, those whose mothers were on a galactose-free diet and who were treated from birth had normal IQ values. One patient first treated at 14 months of age also had a normal IQ. Nadler and coworkers [116], reviewing 44 patients, found 8 with IQs below 70 and 10 with IQs between 71 and 89. Those in the normal range as a group had lower IQs than their sibs. The correlation with time of institution of therapy and IQ was not clear in this series (Fig. 8-6). In the British experience the average IQ of 32 patients on a good diet was 84 and of 22 patients on a moderately or poorly galactose-restricted diet was 77. Komrower and Lee [118] seem pessimistic about the outcome of dietary therapy. The eventual level of intelligence may be influenced by varying degrees of intrauterine damage due to fetal exposure to galactose. The best results are those of Donnell's group in whom intrauterine exposure to galactose was prevented by restricting lactose intake during pregnancy [117].

The actual measurement of IQ does not reveal the entire mental picture of these patients. Many with normal IQs are one or more grades behind in school and have specific learning disability involving spatial relationships and mathematics. Behavioral problems are frequent due to short attention span. Psychological problems seem to be prevalent, with inadequate drive, shyness, and withdrawal [116, 118]. These children may perform much better with close teacher supervision.

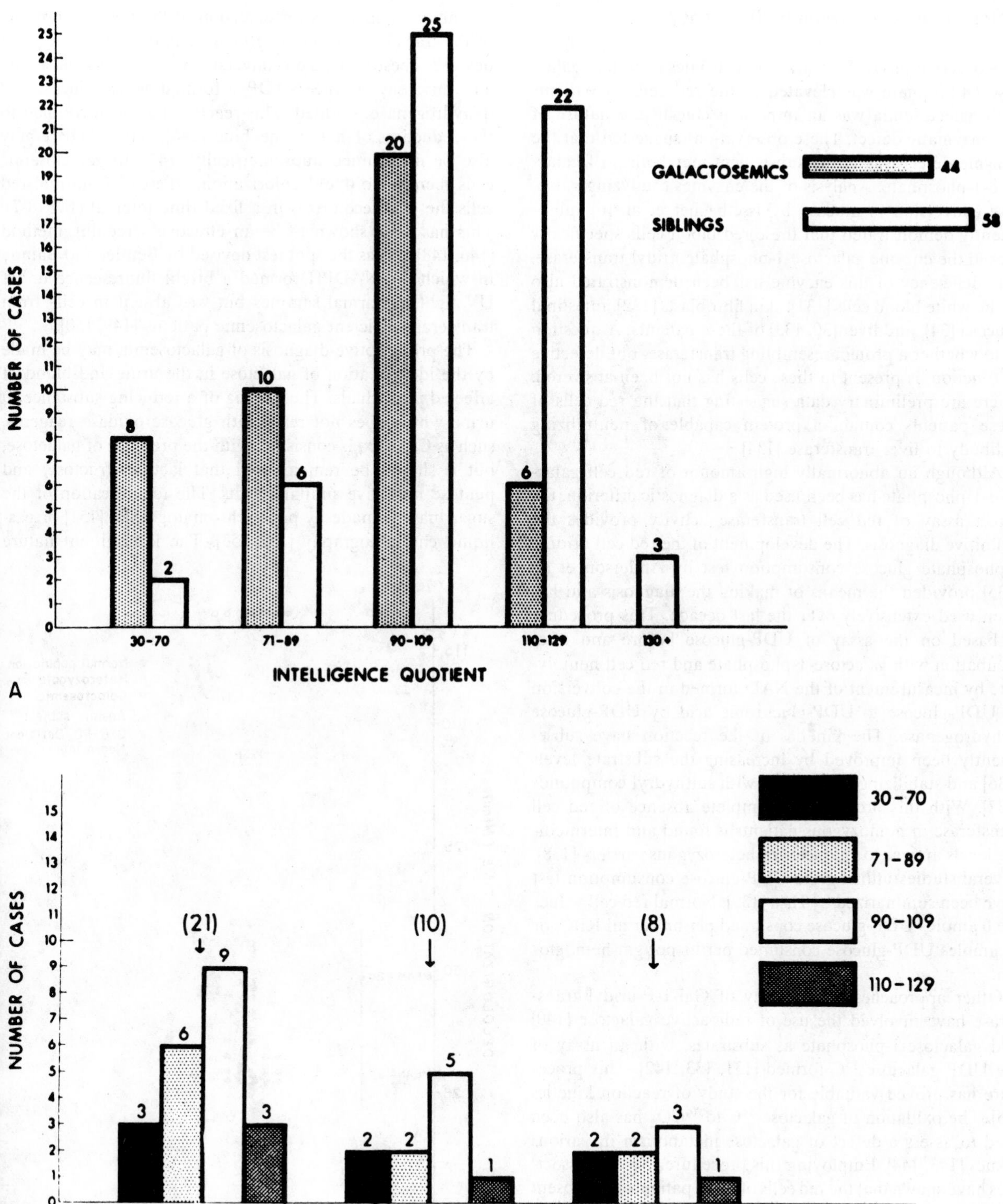

Figure 8-6. Intelligence of transferase deficient galactosemic patients. A. Galactosemic patients and their sibs grouped according to intelligence quotient. B. Age of starting galactose restriction, shown below the bars, compared with intelligence quotient, depicted by the shading of the bars. (*From H. L. Nadler, T. Inouye, and D. Y. Y. Hsia* [116].)

Detection of the Enzymatic Deficiency

The observations of Schwarz and associates [130] that galactose-1-phosphate was elevated in the red cells of patients with galactosemia was an important clue to the nature of the enzymatic defect. These observations suggested that the enzyme defect was in the subsequent metabolism of galactose-1-phosphate. Analysis of the enzymes catalyzing galactose conversion to glucose by Isselbacher et al. [6] subsequently demonstrated that these red blood cells specifically lacked the enzyme galactose-1-phosphate uridyl transferase. The deficiency of this enzyme has been demonstrated also in the white blood cells [131], skin fibroblasts [132], intestinal mucosa [34], and liver [30, 133] of these patients. A question as to whether a protein resembling transferase, but defective in function, is present in these cells has not been answered. There are preliminary data suggesting that the red cells of these patients contain a protein capable of neutralizing antibody to liver transferase [134].

Although an abnormally high amount of red cell galactose-1-phosphate has been used as a diagnostic criterion, the direct assay of red cell transferase activity provides the definitive diagnosis. The development of the red cell uridine diphosphate glucose consumption test by Anderson et al. [135] provided the means of making the diagnosis and has been used extensively over the last decade. This procedure is based on the assay of UDP-glucose before and after incubation with galactose-1-phosphate and red cell hemolysate by measurement of the NAD formed in the conversion of UDP-glucose to UDP-glucuronic acid by UDP-glucose dehydrogenase. The kinetics of the reaction have subsequently been improved by increasing the substrate levels [136] and stabilizing the enzyme with sulfhydryl compounds [137]. With this procedure a complete absence of red cell transferase in homozygous patients is found and intermediate levels appear to characterize heterozygous carriers [138]. Several studies utilizing the UDP-glucose consumption test have been summarized by Hsia [139]. Normal red cell values are 6 μmoles UDP-glucose consumed per hr per ml RBC, or 25 μmoles UDP-glucose consumed per hr per gm hemoglobin.

Other approaches to the assay of Gal-1-P-uridyl transferase have involved the use of radioactive galactose [140] and galactose-1-phosphate as substrates, with an assay of the UDP-galactose-^{14}C formed [131, 133, 142]. This procedure has proved valuable for the study of reaction kinetics [26]. The oxidation of galactose-^{14}C to $^{14}CO_2$ has also been used to assess a defect of galactose metabolism in various tissues [143, 144]. Employing this procedure, Ng and associates have shown that the red cells of three patients with absent transferase by the UDP-glucose consumption test had detectable $^{14}CO_2$ liberation and formation of small amounts of labeled UDP-galactose [145]. This type of test does not specifically determine a deficiency of transferase and may give abnormal results in galactokinase deficiency or any other deficient step in the series of reactions by which galactose is converted to CO_2.

Numerous methods for detection of the reaction product of the transferase reaction, glucose-1-phosphate, have been devised. These depend on conversion to glucose-6-phosphate and an assay of the NADPH formed when glucose-6-P dehydrogenase is added. This reaction has been coupled to the reduction of methylene blue [146], but NADPH may also be determined fluorometrically [147]. In galactosemic cells there is no dye decolorization, whereas in normal red cells the dye decolorizes in a fixed time interval (Fig. 8-7). This has been shown to be an effective screening method [146, 148], as has the spot test devised by Beutler and Baluda in which the NADPH formed a bright fluorescence under UV light in normal samples but was absent in cells from transferase deficient galactosemic patients [149, 150].

The presumptive diagnosis of galactosemia may be made by the identification of galactose in the urine and blood of affected individuals. The finding of a reducing substance in urine which does not react with glucose oxidase reagents, such as Clinistix, is consistent with the presence of galactose, but it should be remembered that lactose, fructose, and pentose may give similar results. The identification of the sugar may be made by paper chromatography [151] or gas-liquid chromatography [152, 153]. The intermittent nature

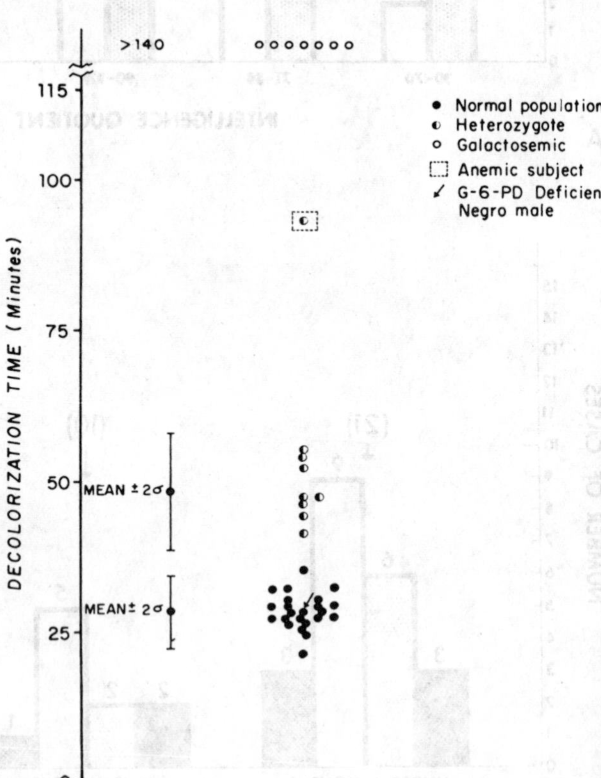

Figure 8-7. Reduction of methylene blue by venous blood samples as a detection method for transferase deficiency. Methylene blue is converted to its leuko form by the formation of NADPH resulting from the transferase assay procedure. The color change is detected visually. (*From E. Beutler, M. Baluda, and G. N. Donnell [146].*)

of the galactosuria may be a hazard in detecting galactosuria, and the sugar may not be detected in extremely dilute urine. Perhaps a greater hazard is the fact that many hospital laboratories routinely test urine only for glucose with commercial glucose oxidase preparations which will not detect galactose. The unwary physician may believe the urine to be sugar free. The same possibility holds for missing high blood galactose levels in hospital laboratories where a blood glucose test is performed by glucose oxidase methods. Recently, relatively specific methods for determining galactose in blood and urine with the use of galactose oxidase [90, 154–156] and galactose dehydrogenase [157] have been introduced. Dahlqvist has devised a paper impregnated with galactose oxidase which is very sensitive and when dipped in urine will detect abnormal amounts of galactose [157, 158]. This appears to be useful in routine screening for galactosuria. It should be pointed out that many normal infants [157, 159], and especially premature infants [157, 160], in the postnatal period have a physiologic mellituria. Normal newborns have up to 60 mg galactose per 100 ml urine in the first 5 days of life, while this level may be detected well into the second week of life in premature infants [157]. Some children with a high consumption of milk may have galactosuria [161]. The demonstration of galactosemia and galactosuria by the performance of a galactose tolerance test is not desirable as a diagnostic procedure.

Galactose Metabolism in Patients with Transferase Deficiency

Early attempts to measure the ability of galactosemic patients to metabolize galactose depended upon determination of the fraction of ingested galactose excreted in the urine. This ranged from 15 to 60 percent in 24 hr; the remainder presumably was stored in the body or metabolized [3, 162].

A more accurate quantitative assessment has been devised in which the conversion of intravenously administered galactose-^{14}C to $^{14}CO_2$ is measured for a period of 5 hr [80, 119, 163]. Of a group of 14 patients so studied, 9 converted the sugar slowly to $^{14}CO_2$, excreting 0 to 8 percent of the administered ^{14}C; and 5 oxidized the sugar in near-normal rates (Fig. 8-8). The ability to metabolize galactose to CO_2 was not related to sex, age, or puberty (Table 8-1). Those patients in the first group were reevaluated at intervals over a period of several years and did not develop greater ability to carry out the conversion. All of these patients were Caucasian. The 5 subjects who oxidized significant amounts of galactose in spite of an absence of red cell transferase were all Negro. One of these was the patient reported by Mason and Turner in 1935 [1] in the first careful delineation of the galactosemic syndrome associated with transferase deficiency (Fig. 8-5). One of these Negro subjects was asymptomatic while ingesting galactose and was detected only by family screening [163]. A similar Negro patient has been described by Hsia [139].

The group of Negro patients has been extensively studied. The ability of one subject to metabolize 10 gm given intravenously was limited, but he could ingest 40 gm of galactose per day for 5 days without developing elevated blood galactose levels [164]. This patient converted galactose to blood glucose [119], demonstrated ethanol inhibition of galactose metabolism [119], and oxidized galactose-1-^{14}C and galactose-2-^{14}C in a normal pattern [80]. These observations are consistent with the function of the sugar nucleotide pathway. Liver biopsy specimens from two Negro patients oxidized galactose-1-^{14}C to $^{14}CO_2$ [163, 165]. Assay for the transferase activity of intestinal mucosa [34] and liver tissue [30] from Negro subjects has disclosed levels of about 10 percent of normal (Table 8-2). Caucasian patients have no enzyme detectable in these tissues. The findings strongly indicate that the capacity of Negro patients with galactosemia to metabolize limited amounts of galactose is based on residual trans-

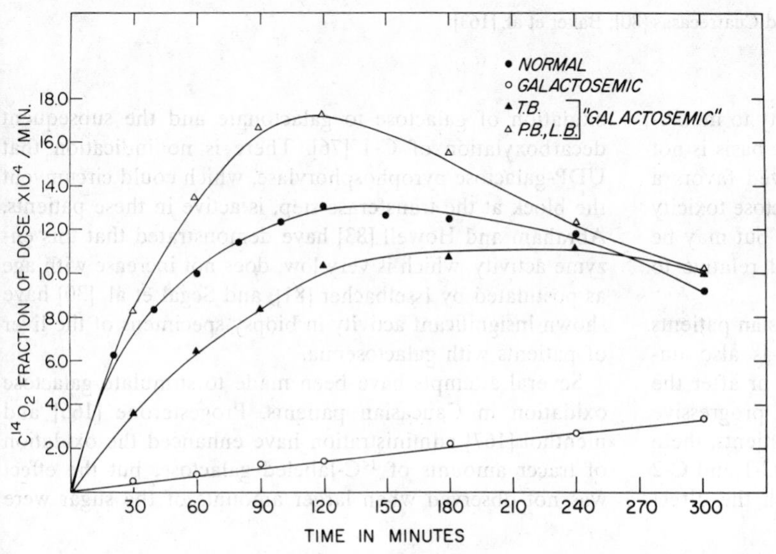

Figure 8-8. The excretion of $^{14}CO_2$ in expired air by normal subjects and patients with transferase deficiency after intravenous administration of 1-gm quantities of sugar containing galactose-1-^{14}C. (*From S. Segal, A. Blair, and H. Roth* [119].)

Table 8-1. THE OXIDATION OF INTRAVENOUS GALACTOSE-1-^{14}C BY NORMAL SUBJECTS AND PATIENTS WITH TRANSFERASE DEFICIENCY GALACTOSEMIA

Subject	Age, years	Sex	Race*	Amount* gm	Administered ^{14}C in expired $^{14}CO_2$ in 5 hr, percent injected†
Patients					
W.Wa	3	M	N	TR	21
	8			1.0	27
J.O	6	M	C	TR	1
M.Wa	7	M	N	1.0	28
B.A.	7	M	C	1.0	8
L.F.	7	F	C	TR	8
E.W.	9	M	C	TR	0
P.R.	9	F	C	TR	3
	11			1.0	7
	15			1.0	7
P.Br.	10	F	N	TR	45
				1.0	42
L.J.	11	M	C	TR	1
	15			TR	5
	19			1.0	11
L.Br.	11	M	N	TR	36
				1.0	35
H.T.	14	M	C	TR	5
	17			1.0	5
J.S.	16	M	C	1.0	2
J.D.	16	M	C	TR	3
				1.0	5
T.B.	30	M	N	TR	19
				1.0	26
				2.0	28
				10.0	19
Normals‡					
3	18–21	M	C	TR	30–35
2	25–35	M	C	1.0	31–33
1	18	M	C	10.0	29
3	18–21	M	C	20.0	25–27

* TR represents tracer, 1 to 5 mg. N is Negro. C is Caucasian.
† Patients received 1 to 3 microcuries of ^{14}C sugar; normals 5 microcuries.
‡ Total number of normal subjects studied.
Source: S. Segal, A. Blair, and H. Roth [119]; Segal and Cuatrecasas [80]; Baker et al. [163]; and some unpublished data of the author.

ferase activity in visceral tissue. While the ability to metabolize galactose is correlated with race, a genetic basis is not truly established. The fact that sibs are involved favors a genetic origin. Why the Negro may have a galactose toxicity syndrome in the neonatal period is not known but may be due to the large amount of galactose ingested relative to the limited enzyme capacity.

Why any galactose oxidation is seen in Caucasian patients when no transferase is detectable in tissues is also unanswered. Measurements of $^{14}CO_2$ for up to 9 hr after the administration of labeled sugar have shown a progressive increase in the amount oxidized [80]. In these patients, there is a different pattern and yield of $^{14}CO_2$ when C-1 and C-2 labeled sugar are given. This is consistent with the direct oxidation of galactose to galactonate and the subsequent decarboxylation of C-1 [76]. There is no indication that UDP-galactose pyrophosphorylase, which could circumvent the block at the transferase step, is active in these patients. Abraham and Howell [83] have demonstrated that this enzyme activity, which is very low, does not increase with age as postulated by Isselbacher [81], and Segal et al. [30] have shown insignificant activity in biopsy specimens of the liver of patients with galactosemia.

Several attempts have been made to stimulate galactose oxidation in Caucasian patients. Progesterone [166] and menthol [167] administration have enhanced the oxidation of tracer amounts of ^{14}C-labeled galactose, but the effect was not observed when larger amounts of the sugar were

Table 8-2. ACTIVITY OF HUMAN LIVER AND INTESTINAL GALACTOSE-1-PHOSPHATE URIDYL TRANSFERASE

Subject	Age, years	Race	Sex	Transferase activity, mμmoles/min/mg/protein	
				Liver	Intestine
Controls					
B	41	C	F	11.8	
S	37	C	F	17.2	
C	2	C	F	16.1	
K	9	C	M	14.7	
U	4 months	C	F	15.0	
S	23	C	M		15.2
D	21	C	M		12.2
H	22	C	F		8.9
M	22	C	F		12.3
L	22	C	M		15.8
Galactosemia*					
L.W.	7 months	N	F	...	1.0
W.Wa	9	N	M	1.3	0.5
M.Wa	8	N	M	1.8	1.6
C.Wi	5	C	F	Nondetectable	Nondetectable
F.R.	2	C	M	Nondetectable	Nondetectable

* Nondetectable red blood cell transferase.
Source: S. Segal, S. Rogers, and P. G. Holtzapple, [30]; S. Rogers, P. G. Holtzapple, W. J. Mellman, and S. Segal [34].

given [168]. Corticosteroids in high dosage cause no acceleration of impaired galactose metabolism [168]. Administration of orotic acid has been reported to be therapeutic when given to children showing galactose toxicity [169]; but under experimental conditions the oral administration of orotic acid seemed to have no influence on ^{14}C-galactose oxidation [170].

The alternate route which is clearly functioning is that in which galactose is reduced by the enzyme aldose reductase to form the sugar alcohol, galactitol [68, 69]. Galactitol has been isolated from the tissues and urine of patients [62–64], and radioactive galactose given to a patient was converted to galactitol [171]. The sugar alcohol is not further metabolized or converted to carbon dioxide. After the administration of ^{14}C-galactitol to normal subjects all of the label is excreted in the urine, with none appearing as $^{14}CO_2$ [172]. Galactitol excretion in the urine continues for several days after galactosuria disappears. This seems to be the main route of elimination. Tissue accumulation of galactitol may be important in galactose toxicity.

In 1962 Inouye et al. demonstrated the presence of galactose-6-phosphate in galactosemic erythrocytes [173]. Presumably this ester could be formed from galactose-1-phosphate by the action of phosphoglucomutase. The galactose-6-phosphate can be oxidized further to 6-phosphogalactonate by an enzyme, hexose-6-phosphate dehydrogenase, found in red cells [174] and liver [79, 175]. The significance of this pathway is unknown.

Genetics

Numerous investigations of red and white cell transferase of family members have indicated that the disorder is transmitted as an autosomal recessive gene [176–180]. Obligate heterozygotes have about 50 percent of normal activity [138, 140, 141, 146, 176–180]. The detection of the genotype in cultured fibroblasts and leukocytes is more accurate if the transferase to galactokinase ratio is determined [181]. In 1965 Beutler and associates [182], employing more sensitive methods, described another mutation at the transferase locus, termed the *Duarte* variant, which results in diminished red cell transferase activity but no clinical disorder. While screening a large number of blood samples for transferase activity, a number of specimens were found in which the enzyme level was 50 percent of normal. This was suggestive of heterozygosity for galactosemia, but pedigree studies revealed that the red cells of parents of these propositi had about 75 percent of normal enzyme levels. This was inconsistent with the genetics of the standard form of transferase deficiency galactosemia [183] (Fig. 8-9). Subsequent investigation of the enzyme of this variant showed it to be indistinguishable from normal with regard to the pH optimum, thermal stability, and Michaelis constant [32], but it migrates faster on starch-gel electrophoresis [184]. Ng et al. [185] have demonstrated two distinct enzyme bands for the Duarte red cell enzyme, which migrate faster on gel-electrophoresis than the single normal enzyme band. The

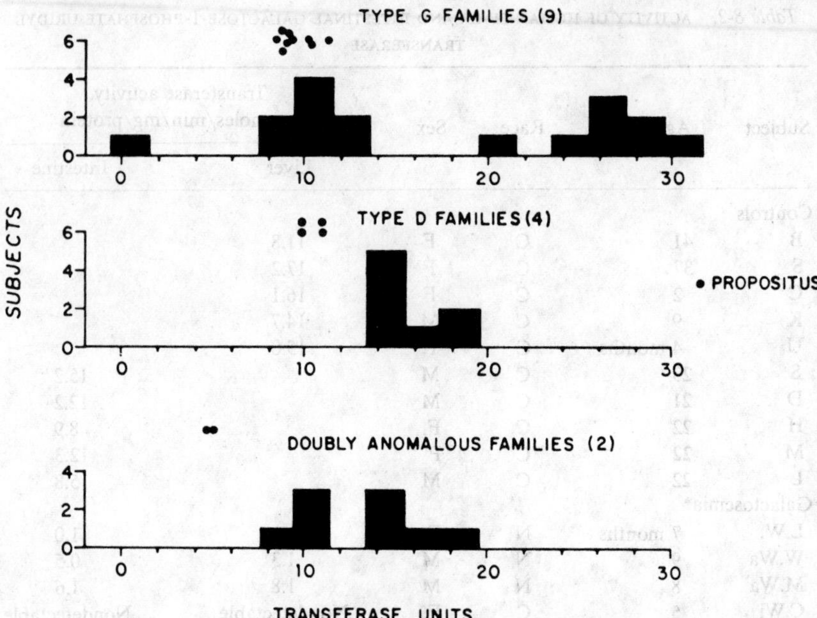

Figure 8-9. Distribution of transferase enzyme activity in parents and children of families with the galactosemia gene, who are designated type G, and the Duarte gene, who are called type D. In type G the propositi are heterozygous carriers for galactosemia (Gt^+/gt) and in type D the propositi are presumably homozygous for the Duarte variant (Gt^D/Gt^D). In the doubly anomalous families the propositi are thought to be heterozygous for both abnormal genes (Gt^D/gt). (*From E. Beutler [261].*)

enzyme activity of a sample from a parent of a subject homozygous for the Duarte variant reveals three bands, the normal and two bands for the variant enzyme.

All of the data are consistent with the Duarte gene being allelic with the normal and galactosemic gene. Indeed, Beutler et al. [183], Mellman and associates [186], and Gitzelmann and coworkers [187] have described individuals with lower levels of red cell transferase than the 50 percent of normal of either the galactosemic heterozygote or the Duarte homozygote. These subjects with 25 percent of normal enzyme activity are mixed heterozygotes, with one Duarte gene and one galactosemia gene (Fig. 8-9). The mixed heterozygote, although low in enzyme activity does not have galactose toxicity. One of these subjects was a medical student while another was a healthy 38-year-old female. A healthy infant shown to be of mixed genotype had detectable plasma galactose and elevated erythrocyte galactose-1-P but no galactosuria [187].

Estimates of the prevalence of transferase deficient galactosemia based on the detection of heterozygote in Wales [188], Denmark [189], and the United States [183, 187, 190] range from 1 in 18,000 to 1 in 50,000. The birth incidence has been 1 in 70,000 in the British Isles [177]. A large-scale screening program in New York State involving 141,000 infants has detected a birth incidence of 1 in 35,000 [191]. Population studies have indicated that from 0.9 to 1.25 percent are heterozygous for the galactosemic gene and 8 to 13 percent carry the Duarte gene [183, 186].

The location of the gene for transferase activity was postulated by Brandt et al. [192] to be on human chromosome 21, since patients with Down's syndrome and trisomy 21 had transferase activity in whole blood specimens which was about 40 percent higher than normals. Hsia et al. [193] found raised transferase activity in the white but not the red blood cells of patients with Down's syndrome. Rosner et al. [194], on the contrary, found elevation of the enzymes in red cells. A deletion of the long arm of chromosome 21, the so-called Philadelphia chromosome, is not associated with a decrease in transferase activity [195]. The finding that other leukocyte enzymes, such as galactokinase [196], acid phosphatase [197], and X-linked glucose-6-phosphate dehydrogenase [197] are elevated in Down's syndrome has prompted the interpretation that the enzyme changes are secondary to a generalized derangement of white cells in this disease. Dahlqvist et al. [198] have found transferase elevations not only in trisomy 21 but also in patients with other trisomy syndromes, as well as in patients with the Cornelia de Lange syndrome without chromosomal aberration. From the evidence, it seems premature to assign the transferase gene to a specific chromosome.

The screening of the newborn for transferase deficiency galactosemia has been effectively carried out at relatively little cost [191] and appears to be a worthwhile approach to a better salvage rate in these patients. Nadler et al. have reported the use of amniocentesis for the intrauterine diagnosis of the homozygote [116]. This procedure has less significance here than for the potentially lethal and untreatable metabolic diseases, since the placement of pregnant heterozygous women on galactose-free diets and the dietary treatment of the infant has resulted in normal children.

Pathogenesis of Galactose Toxicity

The patient with transferase deficiency who is never exposed to galactose should have no abnormalities. The manifestations of the disorder are entirely secondary to the deranged metabolism of galactose. The fact that galactose-1-phosphate is the metabolite which accumulates behind the metabolic block has suggested that high levels of this substance cause derangements of cellular metabolism [199]. With the discovery that galactitol, the product of an alternate route, also accumulates in tissues, the emphasis has shifted to the toxic effects of this polyol. The biochemical cause for the toxicity in any organ may differ and be dependent on its own peculiar metabolic patterns and structure. Investigation of the underlying disruption of cellular processes has depended mainly on changes induced in animals, especially young rats [128, 129, 200, 201] and chicks [202–205] which are fed diets abnormally high in galactose. In making use of these animal models, one must not lose sight of the fact that the enzymes of the sugar nucleotide pathway are present but in limiting quantity. Since the kinetics of the multienzyme galactose pathway and the rate-limiting step have not been clearly delineated, the situation is not entirely analogous to a complete metabolic block at the transferase step. For example, UDP-glucose appears to be depleted and UDP-galactose elevated in tissues of these galactose-fed animals, a situation which may not obtain in the human disease [206, 207].

The Lens

Investigations to elucidate the cause of the cataract provide an almost panoramic view of research in this field. The feeding of a 40 to 50 percent galactose diet to weanling rats uniformly induces cataracts within 2 to 3 weeks [166, 200, 208]. The amount of galactose in the diet and the age of the rat are critical, cataracts being induced most readily in the fetal rats whose mother is fed a high galactose diet [128] and with greater difficulty in older rats. Diets below 30 percent galactose may induce cataracts only in some weanling rats and only after prolonged feeding [166]. A high fat diet [209], progesterone administration [166], and hypophysectomy [210] decrease the incidence of cataract induced by galactose. Galactose-1-phosphate is elevated in the lens of the rat fed galactose [211], as well as in the lens of patients with galactosemia [212]. Early observations by Lerman [213] attempted to explain the cataract as a result of the inhibition by galactose-1-phosphate of glucose-6-phosphate dehydrogenase with a consequent decrease in glucose metabolism, but this has not been confirmed.

The demonstration by Van Heningen [59] that galactitol accumulates in the lens of rats fed galactose was followed by the work of Kinoshita and his associates who demonstrated the presence of aldose reductase in the lens [68] and also demonstrated that the cataracts were closely associated with the imbibition of water by the lens as galactitol accumulated [214, 215]. Galactitol is formed within the lens and becomes osmotically active because it diffuses from the lens with difficulty. Experiments with the lens in vitro have shown that balancing the osmolality of the incubation media to the osmotic properties of galactitol prevents cataract formation. In experiments with an inhibitor of aldose reductase, 3,3-tetramethyleneglutaric acid, Kinoshita et al. found that prevention of polyol accumulation blocked the water accumulation and resulted in a transparent lens after 3 days incubation in galactose [216] (Fig. 8-10). Many biochemical alterations occur concurrently in the lens undergoing galactose-induced cataract formation. These include alteration in protein synthesis [217], amino acid transport [218–220], ion fluxes [221, 222], inositol content [220, 223, 224], carbohydrate enzymes [225], and glutathione reductase [226]. The

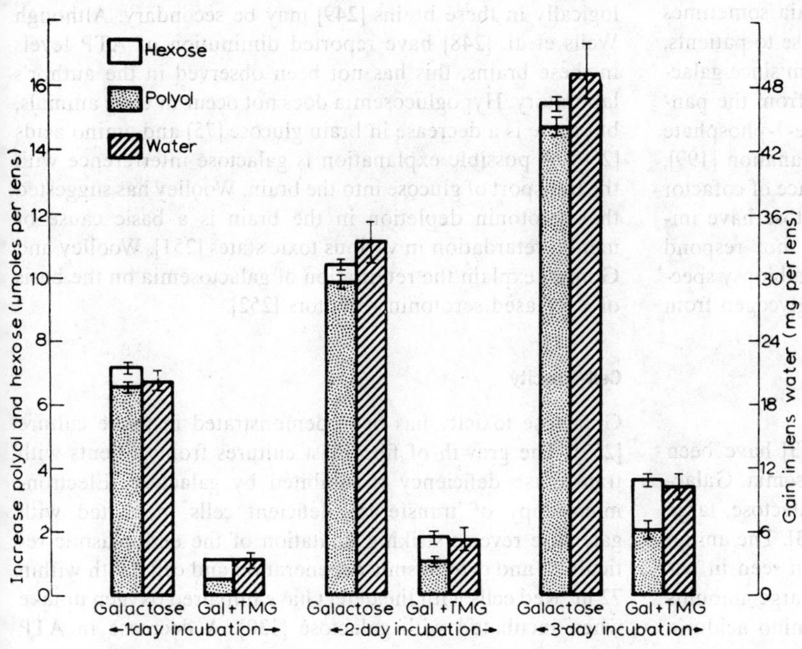

Figure 8-10. Prevention of galactitol formation and water accumulation by rabbit lens incubated with galactose. In 30 m*M* galactose solution the lens incubated for 3 days with 10 m*M* 3.3-tetramethylene glutaric acid (TMG), an aldose reductase inhibitor, remain clear. (*From J. H. Kinoshita, D. Dvornik, M. Kraml, and K. H. Gabbay [216].*)

change which appears first after the increased fluid uptake is a marked decrease in lens glutathione [215]. ATP changes occur late in the process and do not appear to be involved with the fundamental changes [227]. Glycolysis and respiration of the lens are reduced about 30 percent after 2 days of galactose feeding and remain at this level until cataracts occur [225]. It seems conclusive that the initiator of the cataractous process in rats is galactitol and not galactose-1-P, the latter accumulating only late in the process. Substantiating evidence is found in patients with galactokinase deficiency who have cataracts in the absence of galactose-1-phosphate formation [7].

Liver

If the cause of cataracts seems clear, the reason for toxicity in the liver remains obscure. The severe liver damage seen in transferase deficiency is not observed in rats fed a high galactose diet. Although the liver of children with galactosemia has elevated galactose-1-phosphate [125] and galactitol [63], the livers of rats fed galactose accumulate galactose-1-phosphate but not galactitol [60]. Chicks fed galactose accumulate large amounts of galactitol without severe liver damage [61]. Patients with galactokinase deficiency who ingest large quantities of galactose and who form galactitol have no liver damage [7]. It may be that an as yet unknown metabolite is responsible for the liver damage. In this regard, galactosamine is known to induce liver damage in animals [228, 229].

While microscopic liver damage is not seen in animals given galactose, biochemical abnormalities have been observed. In rats there is a decrease in liver glycogen [230] and diminished hexose phosphorylation [230], and in chicks an abnormal glycogen-containing galactose [231]. No decrease in ATP levels occurs. The hypoglycemia sometimes seen clinically and induced by feeding galactose to patients, may be related to deranged hepatic metabolism since galactose does not stimulate the release of insulin from the pancreas [232, 233]. Sidbury postulated galactose-1-phosphate inhibition of phosphoglucomutase as an explanation [199], but this can only be shown in vitro in the absence of cofactor glucose-1-6-diphosphate. Patients given galactose have impaired hepatic glucose output [234] and do not respond normally to glucagon administration [235]. In a biopsy specimen from a single patient, the formation of glycogen from glucose was impaired [236].

Kidney

Galactose-1-phosphate [125] and galactitol [63] have been detected in the kidney of patients with galactosemia. Galactitol accumulates in the kidney of rats fed galactose, large quantities being found in the renal papillae [73]. The amino aciduria of transferase deficiency has not been seen in patients with galactokinase deficiency, by whom large amounts of galactitol are excreted in the urine [7]. Amino aciduria has been induced in rats fed a high galactose diet [237] and in normal human subjects to whom galactose was given intravenously [238]. The incubation of slices of kidney cortex with galactose produces impairment of amino acid accumulation by tubule cells [239]. The inhibition, which is noncompetitive in nature, has been observed also in the intestinal mucosa of rats [240], a tissue which accumulates galactose-1-phosphate during galactose feeding [241].

Brain

The one manifestation of galactose toxicity which may not be reversible is mental retardation. In patients with transferase deficiency, galactitol is found in the brain [62], and in rats fed galactose, galactitol accumulates to a greater extent in the brain than in any other tissue except the lens [60]. Enzymes of galactitol formation are active in nerve tissue [70]. The weanling or adult rat develops no apparent brain abnormality when fed galactose, but the fetuses of pregnant rats fed galactose have decreased brain development [242] and decreased amounts of brain DNA, especially in the cerebrum [243]. Wells and Wells have shown an impaired conversion of glucose to inositol in brain slices from newborn rats exposed to galactose in utero [244]. Some of the effects on brain development may reflect the smaller body weight and placentas which occur in this model [128]. Decreased nerve conduction has been reported in toxic rats [245].

The chick given galactose in water develops ataxia, convulsions, and death [61, 202–205, 246–248]. The findings are more severe in females and in certain strains and are associated with both galactose-1-phosphate [247] and galactitol accumulation in brain [61]. They are reversible if the galactose is removed. This suggests that the changes seen pathologically in these brains [249] may be secondary. Although Wells et al. [248] have reported diminution of ATP levels in these brains, this has not been observed in the author's laboratory. Hypoglucosemia does not occur in toxic animals, but there is a decrease in brain glucose [75] and amino acids [250]. A possible explanation is galactose interference with the transport of glucose into the brain. Woolley has suggested that serotonin depletion in the brain is a basic cause of mental retardation in various toxic states [251]. Woolley and Gommi explain the retardation of galactosemia on the basis of decreased serotonin receptors [252].

Cell Toxicity

Galactose toxicity has been demonstrated in tissue culture [253]. The growth of fibroblast cultures from patients with transferase deficiency is inhibited by galactose. Electron-microscopy of transferase deficient cells incubated with galactose reveals striking dilatation of the endoplasmic reticulum, and cytoplasmic degeneration and cell death within 72 hr. Red cells with the defect have impaired oxygen uptake when incubated with galactose [130]. A decrease in ATP described under these conditions [254] has not been confirmed [255]. The fact that mutants of *E. coli* deficient in transferase have an impaired growth in galactose media, while galactokinase mutants do not, implies that galactose-1-phosphate is related to the toxicity in bacteria [107, 108].

GALACTOKINASE DEFICIENCY GALACTOSEMIA

Clinical Aspects

This disorder has been described only recently [7, 8]. The author is aware of seven cases: adult sibs aged 44, 62, and 64 [7], a 9-year-old [256], twins aged 4 months [257], and a newborn infant [258]. The wealth of knowledge garnered about the transferase deficiency disorder over the past two decades has not yet been duplicated in galactokinase deficiency.

The first patient recognized to have galactokinase deficiency was a male 44 years old at the time of biochemical diagnosis by Gitzelmann [78]. Galactosuria after milk ingestion was detected when he was treated for cataracts in 1932 at the age of 9. Investigations at that time led to a report of the patient by Fanconi as a case of "galactose diabetes" [259]. His sisters had been seen in 1909 at ages 5½ and 7½ by ophthalmologists because of cataracts, but mellituria had not been recognized. The impression by physicians was that both girls were mentally retarded. Dietary restrictions were never imposed and the patients developed recurrent cataracts, poor vision, and blindness. Both females married and had several children. When studied recently the 44-year-old male was ingesting 3 qt of milk a day without obvious effects. He was blind and complained of weakness and pain in his extremities which was attributed to neurofibromatosis. No IQ tests were performed on any of these patients, but the impression was that, while illiterate, intelligence as adults was normal. There was never any evidence of jaundice or liver disease, and no amino aciduria or proteinuria was detected [7].

The newborn with this disorder reported by Thalhammer et al. [258] was an apparently normal female who on a routine screen of capillary heel blood at 7 days of life was found to have 100 mg galactose per 100 ml blood. Routine examination at the time revealed no hepatosplenomegaly or gastrointestinal disturbance. At 17 days of age while still on milk feedings, the liver and spleen were felt just below the costal margin. Ophthalmologic examination revealed circumscript opacities along the posterior lens suture but they were not thought to be abnormal. Jaundice was not present. Total serum bilirubin was 2.0 mg per 100 ml (direct 1.2 mg per 100 ml). Serum enzyme tests of liver function were normal. The infant was placed on a galactose-free diet on day 20 and at age 4½ months was found to be thriving without other abnormalities.

The 9-year-old child reported by Monteleone et al. [256] had cataracts and red cells deficient in galactokinase, but no evidence of liver or renal disease or mental retardation. The two 4-month-old twins of McVie et al. [257] were admitted to hospital for hernia repair and were discovered incidentally to have high blood galactose levels, high urinary galactitol, but no liver disease or amino aciduria.

Diagnosis

The absence of inanition, gastrointestinal dysfunction, and jaundice in the newborn period and the appearance of cataracts in the older patients on unrestricted diets differentiate this disorder from transferase deficiency galactosemia. In the absence of severe manifestations it is apparent that the diagnosis in early infancy will depend upon the routine screening of blood and urine for galactose. Since cataracts may be the first and only abnormality, this disorder should be suspected in any child with cataracts.

The presence of a reducing substance in the urine may be identified as galactose by the methods described above for transferase deficiency. Thalhammer and coworkers [258] indicate that high blood galactose levels are best detected after milk feedings and may be low in morning fasting specimens. The diagnosis can be made by the finding of normal amounts of galactose-1-phosphate uridyl transferase and an absence of galactokinase in the red blood cells [7]. Like transferase deficient red cells, those with absence of galactokinase will be unable to oxidize galactose ^{14}C to $^{14}CO_2$ [7]. All young patients with cataracts should have the urine examined for sugar with methods other than those using glucose oxidase and should also have an assay of the red cells for the defect. Therapy should be aimed at galactose restriction as in transferase deficiency.

Galactose Metabolism in Galactokinase Deficiency

Gitzelmann studied the 44-year-old male with this disorder by milk loading and found that large quantities of ingested galactose were excreted as galactitol [7]. After ingesting 360 gm galactose over a period of 5 days without ill effects, he excreted 192 gm as galactose and 48 gm as galactitol. On most test procedures the urinary galactitol to galactose ratio was about 1:4.

The author, in collaboration with Dr. Gitzelmann and Dr. H. J. Wells, has studied the metabolism of galactose in the same male patient by injection of radioactive galactose and determination of $^{14}CO_2$ expired over a 5-hr period. After injection of galactose-1-^{14}C only 5 percent of the label appeared in expired air, an amount similar to that seen in Caucasian transferase deficient patients (Table 8-1). Essentially no label was excreted as CO_2 after the injection of ^{14}C-galactitol or galactonate. The low yield of $^{14}CO_2$ from galactose indicated that galactokinase deficiency exists in tissues other than the peripheral blood cells, the only type of cells directly assayed. This finding indicates that lack of severe galactose-induced toxicity is not due to a situation similar to that seen in Negro subjects with transferase deficiency, where the subjects lack the enzyme in the blood cells but have residual enzyme activity in the liver (Table 8-2) and can metabolize the sugar (Table 8-1 and Fig. 8-8). The lack of galactitol oxidation and almost total excretion of the labeled galactitol in urine are consistent with galactitol being an end product in galactose metabolism.

Genetics and Screening

Gitzelmann's erythrocyte assay for galactokinase among the kindred of the three adult patients revealed several members with values intermediate between the patients and a group of 100 normals [7]. Mays and Guthrie [260] have screened the red blood cells of 642 persons for galactokinase and have found the cells in 6 of them to have half the normal activity. Their data are consistent with an autosomal recessive inheritance. The estimate of heterozygotes is 1:107 and for homozygous births is about 1:40,000. The newborn described by Thalhammer and colleagues with complete deficiency was the first detected with galactosemia after the analysis of 35,770 blood samples for galactose. It is interesting that the first four patients described were members of unrelated gypsy families.

Screening programs in the United States have employed blood tests designed for easy transferase assay and would not detect this new entity. The assay for galactokinase [7, 260] is not yet applicable to mass screening. The screening of blood for galactose by the growth inhibition test of Guthrie [258] or of urine for galactose by galactose oxidase impregnated paper appear to be the procedures of choice [157, 158].

Toxicity Factors

The basis of the galactose toxicity syndromes has been discussed above under transferase deficiency. The topic is considered again here because of the contribution to the understanding of galactose-induced toxicity by the discovery of galactokinase deficiency. It seems clear that cataracts are the chief result of failure to phosphorylate galactose, with the reduction of galactose to galactitol through an alternative metabolic route. The absence of liver and kidney damage in galactokinase deficiency and the presence of damage to these organs in transferase deficiency make it likely that toxicity is in some way associated with galactose-1-phosphate formation. Not enough information is at hand to dissociate conclusively the mental retardation from galactokinase deficiency, although the evidence suggests that retardation is not a feature. If this is true, then brain damage in transferase deficiency would be the result of galactose phosphorylation and of the failure of galactose-1-phosphate to be further metabolized.

SUMMARY

1 Two inherited disorders of galactose metabolism have been delineated. They are transmitted by autosomal recessive inheritance.

2 The genetic disturbance is expressed as a cellular deficiency either of galactokinase or galactose-1-phosphate uridyl transferase, the enzymes catalyzing the first and second reactions in the unique pathway by which galactose is converted to glucose.

3 The clinical manifestations are toxicity syndromes resulting from exposure of the patients to galactose. Toxicity in galactokinase deficiency is milder and is mainly manifest by cataracts. In transferase deficiency, galactose ingestion is characterized by inanition, failure to thrive, vomiting, liver disease, cataracts, and mental retardation.

4 The diagnosis is suggested by detection of galactose in the blood or urine and is established by demonstration of the enzyme deficiency in the peripheral blood cells. Adequate procedures are available for screening large populations for transferase deficiency.

5 In these disorders, there is an alternative metabolic route of galactose metabolism through reduction to galactitol. Galactitol is not further metabolized but is excreted by the kidney. Transferase deficiency is associated with the accumulation of galactose-1-phosphate in the tissues in addition to galactitol accumulation.

6 Most patients with galactose-1-phosphate uridyl transferase deficiency can oxidize only a small fraction of galactose to carbon dioxide. This ability does not increase with age, and it seems unlikely that alternative metabolic pathways involving sugar nucleotides develop to circumvent the block in galactose conversion to glucose. There is, however, a group of galactosemic patients, all of whom are Negro, who in spite of the absence of transferase in the red cells can oxidize limited amounts of galactose. These patients have about 10 percent of normal transferase activity in the liver and intestine.

7 The cause of the entire toxicity syndrome in transferase deficiency is uncertain. On present evidence, it is reasonable to conclude that the cataract formation in both disorders of galactose metabolism is secondary to galactitol formation in the lens.

BIBLIOGRAPHY

1. Mason, H. H., and Turner, M. E.: Chronic galactosemia. Amer. J. Dis. Child., **50**, 359, 1935.
2. Komrower, G. M., Schwarz, V., Holzel, A., and Golberg, L.: A clinical and biochemical study of galactosemia. Arch. Dis. Child., **31**, 254, 1956.
3. Holzel, A., Komrower, G. M., and Schwarz, V.: Galactosemia. Amer. J. Med., **22**, 703, 1957.
4. Isselbacher, K. J.: Galactose metabolism and galactosemia. Amer. J. Med., **26**, 715, 1959.
5. Holzel, A.: Galactosemia. Brit. Med. Bull., **17**, 213, 1961.
6. Isselbacher, K. J., Anderson, E. P., Kurahashi, K., and Kalckar, H. M.: Congenital galactosemia, a single enzymatic block in galactose metabolism. Science, **123**, 635, 1956.

7. Gitzelmann, R.: Hereditary galactokinase deficiency, a newly recognized cause of juvenile cataracts. Pediat. Res., **1**, 14, 1967.
8. Gitzelmann, R.: Deficiency of erythrocyte galactokinase in a patient with galactose diabetes. Lancet, **2**, 670, 1965.
9. Caputto, R., Leloir, L. F. and Trucco, R. E.: Lactase and lactose fermentation in *S. fragilis.* Enzymologia, **12**, 350, 1948.
10. Cardini, C. E., and Leloir, L. F.: Enzymatic phosphorylation of galactosamine and galactose. Arch. Biochem. Biophys., **45**, 55, 1953.
11. Leloir, L. F.: Enzymatic transformation of uridine diphosphate glucose into galactose derivative. Arch. Biochem. Biophys., **33**, 186, 1951.
12. Kalckar, H. M., Braganca, B., and Munch-Petersen, A.: Uridyl transferases and the formation of uridine diphosphate galactose. Nature (London), **172**, 1038, 1953.
13. Wilkinson, J. F.: The pathway of the adaptive fermentation of galactose by yeast. Biochem. J., **44**, 460, 1949.
14. Heinrich, M. R.: The purification and properties of yeast galactokinase. J. Biol. Chem., **239**, 50, 1964.
15. Sherman, J. R., and Adler, J.: Galactokinase from *E. coli.* J. Biol. Chem., **238**, 874, 1963.
16. Wilson, D., and Hogness, D.: The enzymes of the galactose operon in *E. coli.* III. The size and composition of galactokinase. J. Biol. Chem., **244**, 2137, 1969.
17. Atkinson, M., Barton, R., and Morton, R.: Equilbrium constant of phosphoryl transfer from adenosine triphosphate to galactose in the presence of galactokinase. Biochem. J., **78**, 813, 1961.
18. Gulbinsky, J., and Cleland, W.: Kinetic studies of *Escherichia coli* galactokinase. Biochemistry, **7**, 566, 1968.
19. Cuatrecases, P., and Segal, S.: Mammalian galactokinase. J. Biol. Chem., **240**, 2382, 1965.
20. Walker, D. G., and Khan, H. H.: Some properties of galactokinase in developing rat liver. Biochem. J., **108**, 169, 1968.
21. Ballard, F. J.: Purification and properties of galactokinase from pig liver. Biochem. J., **98**, 347, 1966.
22. Ng, W. G., Donnell, G. N., and Bergren, W. R.: Galactokinase activity in human erythrocytes of individuals at different ages. J. Lab. Clin. Med., **66**, 115, 1965.
23. Mathai, C., and Beutler, E.: Biochemical characteristics of galactokinase from adult and fetal human red cells. Enzymologia, **33**, 14, 1967.
24. Tao, M., and Schweiger, M.: Stimulation of galactokinase synthesis in *Escherichia coli* by adenosine 3′, 5′ cyclic monophosphate. J. Bact., **102**, 138, 1970.
25. Kurahashi, K., and Sugimura, A.: Purification and properties of galactose-1-phosphate uridyl transferase from *E. coli.* J. Biol. Chem., **235**, 940, 1960.
26. Bertoli, D., and Segal, S.: Developmental aspects and some characteristics of mammalian galactose-1-phosphate uridyl transferase. J. Biol. Chem., **241**, 4023, 1966.
27. Saito, S., Ozutsumi, M., and Kurahashi, K.: Galactose 1-phosphate uridyl-transferase of *E. coli.* J. Biochem., **242**, 2362, 1967.
28. Kurahashi, K., and Anderson, E.: Galactose-1-phosphate uridyl transferase, its purification and application. Biochim. Biophys. Acta, **29**, 498, 1958.
29. Mayes, J. S., and Hanson, R. G.: Galactose-1-phosphate uridyl transferase, in *Methods of Enzymology,* edited by W. A. Wood, vol. 9, p. 708, Academic, New York, 1966.
30. Segal, S., Rogers, S., and Holtzapple, P. G.: Liver galactose-1-phosphate uridyl transferase: Activity in normal and galactosemic subjects. J. Clin. Invest., **50**, 500, 1971.
31. Riabov, S., Inouye, T., Parker, D., and Hsia, D.: Partial purification of hexose-1-phosphate uridyltransferase from human red cells. Biochim. Biophys. Acta, **99**, 173, 1963.
32. Beutler, E., and Baluda, M.: Biochemical properties of human red cell galactose-1-phosphate uridyl transferase (UDP glucose: α-D-galactose-1-phosphate uridyl transferase) from normal and mutant subjects. J. Lab. Clin. Med., **67**, 947, 1966.
33. Tedesco, T. A., and Mellman, W. J.: The UDPglucose consumption assay for gal-1-P uridyl transferase, in *Galactosemia,* edited by D. Y. Y. Hsia, p. 66. Charles C Thomas, Springfield, Ill., 1969.
34. Rogers, S., Holtzapple, P. G., Mellman, W. J. and Segal, S.: Characteristics of galactose-1-phosphate uridyl transferase in intestinal mucosa of normal and galactosemic humans. Metabolism, **19**, 701, 1970.
35. Keppler, D., Frohlich, J., Reuter, W., Wieland, O., and Decker, K.: Changes in uridine nucleotides during liver perfusion with D-galactosamine. Fed. Europ. Biol. Soc. Letters, **4**, 278, 1969.
36. Ng, W., Bergren, W., Donnell, G., and Hodgman, J.: Galactose-1-phosphate uridyl transferase activity in hemolysates of newborn infants. Pediatrics, **39**, 293, 1967.
37. Stifel, F. B., Herman, R. H., and Rosensweig, N. S.: Dietary regulation of galactose metabolizing enzymes: Adaptive changes in rat jejunum. Science, **162**, 692, 1968.
38. Salo, W., Nordin, J., Peterson, D., Bevill, R., and Kirkwood, S.: The specificity of UDP-glucose 4-epimerase from the yeast *Saccharomyces fragilis.* Biochim. Biophys. Acta, **151**, 484, 1968.
39. Wilson, D., and Hogness, D.: The enzymes of the galactose operon in *E. coli.* I. Purification and characterization of uridine diphosphogalactose-4-epimerase. J. Biol. Chem., **239**, 2469, 1964.
40. Wilson, D., and Hogness, D.: The enzymes of the galactose operon in *E. coli.* II. The subunits of uridine diphosphoglucose-4-epimerase. J. Biol. Chem., **244**, 2132, 1969.
41. Darrow, R., and Rodstrom, R.: Subunit association and catalytic activity of uridine diphosphate galactose-4-epimerase from yeast. Proc. Nat. Acad. Sci. USA, **55**, 205, 1966.
42. Darrow, R., and Rodstrom, R.: Uridine diphosphate galactose 4-epimerase from yeast. J. Biol. Chem., **245**, 2036, 1970.
43. Bertland, A., Bugge, B., and Kalckar, H.: Fluorescence enhancement of uridine diphosphogalactose 4-epimerase induced by specific sugars. Arch. Biochem. Biophys., **116**, 280, 1966.
44. Bertland, A., and Kalckar, H.: Reversible changes of ordered polypeptide structures in oxidized and reduced epimerase. Proc. Nat. Acad. Sci. USA, **61**, 629, 1968.
45. Kalckar, H. M.: Uridine diphosphogalactose metabolism, enzymology and biology. Advances Enzym. **20**, 111, 1958.
46. de Robichon-Szulmajster, H.: Sur un noveau mécanisme d'oxydo-réduction, appliqué á la réaction d'epimérisation: uridinediphosphogalactose uridine diphosphoglucose. J. Molec. Biol., **3**, 253, 1961.
47. Maxwell, E.: The enzymic interconversion of uridine diphosphogalactose and uridine diphosphoglucose. J. Biol. Chem., **229**, 139, 1957.
48. Isselbacher, K. J., and Krane, S. M.: Studies on the mechanism of the inhibition of galactose oxidation by ethanol. J. Biol. Chem., **236**, 2394, 1961.
49. Robinson, E., Kalckar, H., and Troedson, H.: Metabolic inhibition of mammalian uridine diphosphate galactose-4-epimerase in cell cultures and in tumor cells. J. Biol. Chem., **241**, 2737, 1966.
50. Cohn, R., and Segal, S.: Regulation of mammalian liver uridine diphosphogalactose-4-epimerase by pyrimidine nucleotides. Biochim. Biophys. Acta, **222**, 533, 1970.
51. Cohn, R., and Segal, S.: Some characteristics and developmental aspects of rat uridine diphosphogalactose-4-epimerase. Biochim. Biophys. Acta, **171**, 333, 1969.
52. Munch-Petersen, A., Kalckar, H., Cutolo, E., and Smith, E.: Uridyl transferases and the formation of uridine triphosphate. Nature (London), **172**, 1036, 1953.
53. Munch-Petersen, A.: Investigations of the properties and mechanism of the uridine diphosphate glucose pyrophosphorylose reaction. Acta Chem. Scand., **9**, 1523, 1955.
54. Knop, J., and Hansen, R.: Uridine diphosphate glucose pyrophosphorylase. IV. Crystallization and properties of the enzyme from human liver. J. Biol. Chem., **245**, 2499, 1970.
55. Levine, S., Gillett, T. A., Hogeman, E., and Hansen, R. G.: Uridine diphosphate glucose pyrophosphorylase. II. Polymeric and subunit structure. J. Biol. Chem., **244**, 5729, 1969.
56. Steelman, V. S., and Ebner, K. E.: The enzymes of lactose biosynthesis. I. Purification and properties of UDPG pyrophosphorylase from bovine mammary tissue. Biochim. Biophys. Acta, **128**, 92, 1966.
57. Sundararajan, T. A., Rapin, A. M., and Kalckar, H. M.: Biochemical observations on *E. coli* mutants defective in uridine diphosphoglucose. Proc. Nat. Acad. Sci USA, **48**, 2187, 1962.

58. Fukasawa, T., Jokura, K., and Kurahashi, H.: Mutations in *E. coli* that affect uridine diphosphate glucose pyrophosphorylase activity and galactose fermentation. Biochim. Biophys. Acta, **74,** 608, 1963.
59. Van Heyningen, R.: Formation of polyols by the lens of the rat with "sugar" cataracts. Nature (London), **184,** 194, 1959.
60. Quan-Ma, R., and Wells, W.: The distribution of galactitol in tissues of rats fed galactose. Biochem. Biophys. Res. Commun., 20, 486, 1965.
61. Wells, H., and Segal, S.: Galactose toxicity in the chick: Tissue accumulation of galactose and galactitol. Fed. Europ. Biol. Soc. Letters, **5,** 121, 1969.
62. Wells, W., Pittman, T., Wells, H., and Egan, T.: The isolation and identification of galactitol from the brains of galactosemia patients. J. Biol. Chem., **240,** 1002, 1965.
63. Quan-Ma, R., Wells, H., Wells, W., Sherman, F., and Egan, T.: Galactitol in the tissues of a galactosemic child. Amer. J. Dis. Child., **112,** 477, 1966.
64. Wells, W., Pittman, T., and Egan, T.: The isolation and identification of galactitol from the urine of patients with galactosemia. J. Biol. Chem., **239,** 3192, 1964.
65. Gitzelmann, R., Curtius, H. C., and Muller, M.: Galactitol excretion in the urine of a galactokinase deficient man. Biochem. Biophys. Res. Commun., **22,** 437, 1966.
66. Hers, H. G.: L'Aldose-reductase. Biochim. Biophys. Acta, **37,** 120, 1960.
67. Clements, R., Weaver, J., and Winegrad, A.: The distribution of polyol: NADP oxidoreductase in mammalian tissues. Biochem. Biophys. Res. Commun., 37, 347, 1969.
68. Hayman, S., and Kinoshita, J. H.: Isolation and properties of lens aldose reductase. J. Biol. Chem., **240,** 877, 1965.
69. Hayman, S., Lou, M., Merola, L., and Kinoshita, J. H.: Aldose reductase activity in the lens and other tissues. Biochim. Biophys. Acta, **128,** 474, 1966.
70. Moonsammy, G., and Stewart, M.: Purification and properties of brain aldose reductase and L-hexonate dehydrogenase. J. Neurochem., **14,** 1187, 1967.
71. Mano, Y., Suzuki, K., Yamata, K., and Schimazono, N.: Enzymic studies on TPN L-hexonate dehydrogenase from rat liver. J. Biochem. (Tokyo), **49,** 618, 1961.
72. Gabbay, K., and O'Sullivan, J.: The sorbitol pathway: Enzyme localization and content in normal and diabetic nerve and cord. Diabetes, **17,** 239, 1968.
73. Gabbay, K., and O'Sullivan, J.: The sorbitol pathway in diabetes and galactosemia: Enzyme and substrate localization and changes in kidney. Diabetes, **17,** 300, 1968.
74. Clements, R., and Winegrad, A.: Modulation of mammalian polyol: NADP oxidoreductase activity by ADP and ATP. Biochem. Biophys. Res. Commun., **36,** 1006, 1969.
75. Wells, W. W.: Galactitol metabolism, in *Galactosemia,* edited by D. Y. Y. Hsia, p. 227. Charles C Thomas, Springfield, Ill., 1969.
76. Cuatrecasas, P., and Segal, S.: Galactose conversion to D-xylulose: An alternate route of galactose metabolism. Science, **153,** 549, 1966.
77. Cuatrecasas, P., and Segal, S.: Mammalian galactose dehydrogenase. I. Identification and purification in rat liver. J. Biol. Chem., **241,** 5904, 1966.
78. Cuatrecasas, P., and Segal, S.: Mammalian galactose dehydrogenase. II. Properties, substrate specificity and developmental changes. J. Biol. Chem., **241,** 5910, 1966.
79. Srivastava, S. K., and Beutler, E.: Auxiliary pathways of galactose metabolism. J. Biol. Chem., **244,** 6377, 1969.
80. Segal, S., and Cuatrecasas, P.: The oxidation of C^{14} galactose by patients with congenital galactosemia. Amer. J. Med., **44,** 340, 1968.
81. Isselbacher, K. J.: Evidence for an accessory pathway of galactose metabolism in mammalian liver. Science, **126,** 652, 1957.
82. Isselbacher, K.: A mammalian uridinediphosphate galactose pyrophosphorylase. J. Biol. Chem., **232,** 429, 1958.
83. Abraham, H., and Howell, R.: Human hepatic uridine diphosphate galactose pyrophosphorylase. J. Biol. Chem., **244,** 545, 1969.
84. Stenstam, T.: Peroral and intravenous galactose tests; comparative study of their significance in different conditions. Acta Med. Scand., suppl. 177, 1946.
85. Segal, S., and Blair, A.: Some observations on the metabolism of D-galactose in normal man. J. Clin. Invest., **40,** 2016, 1961.
86. Tygstrup, N., and Winkler, K.: Galactose blood clearance as a measure of hepatic blood flow. Clin. Sci., **17,** 1, 1958.
87. Tygstrup, N.: Determination of the hepatic elimination capacity (Lm) of galactose by single injection. Scand. J. Clin. Lab. Invest., **18,** suppl. 92, 118, 1966.
88. Tygstrup, N.: The urinary excretion of galactose and its significance in clinical intravenous galactose tolerance tests. Acta Physiol. Scand., **51,** 263, 1961.
89. Colcher, H., Patek, A. J., and Kendall, F. E.: Galactose disappearance from the blood stream: Calculation of a galactose removal constant and its application as a test of liver function. J. Clin. Invest., **25,** 768, 1946.
90. Tengström, B.: An intravenous galactose tolerance test with an enzymatic determination of galactose: A comparison with other diagnostic aids in hepatobiliary diseases. Scand. J. Clin. Invest., **18,** 132, 1966.
91. Tygstrup, N., and Lundquist, F.: The effect of ethanol on galactose elimination in Man. J. Lab. Clin. Med., **59,** 102, 1962.
92. Salaspuro, M. P., and Salaspuro, A. E.: The effect of ethanol on galactose elimination in rats with normal and choline-deficient fatty livers. Scand. J. Clin. Lab. Invest., **22,** 49, 1968.
93. Segal, S., Roth, H., and Bertoli, D.: Galactose metabolism by rat liver tissue: Influence of age. Science, **142,** 1311, 1963.
94. Haworth, J. C., and Ford, J. D.: Variation of the oral galactose tolerance test with age. J. Pediat., **63,** 276, 1963.
95. Mulligan, P. B., and Schwartz, R.: Hepatic carbohydrate metabolism in the genesis of neonatal hypoglycemia. Pediatrics, **30,** 125, 1962.
96. Hjelm, M., and Sjölin, S.: Changes in the elimination rate from blood of intravenously injected galactose during the neonatal period. Scand. J. Clin. Invest., **18,** suppl. 92, 126, 1966.
97. Theodore, G. M., Ford, J. D., and Haworth, J. C.: The intravenous galactose tolerance test in infancy. Arch. Dis. Child., **39,** 505, 1964.
98. Vink, C. D. L., and Kroes, A. A.: Liver function and age. Clin. Chim. Acta, **4,** 674, 1959.
99. Jordan, E., Yarmolinsky, M. B., and Kalckar, H. M.: Control of inducibility of enzymes of the galactose sequence in *Escherichia coli.* Proc. Nat. Acad. Sci. USA, **48,** 32, 1962.
100. Buttin, G.: Mecanismes regulateurs dans la biosynthese des enzymes du metabolisme du galactose chez *E. coli* K-12: I. La biosynthese induite de la galactokinase et l'induction simultanée de la sequence enzymatique. J. Molec. Biol., **7,** 183, 1963.
101. Wu, H. C. P., and Kalckar, H. M.: Endogenous induction of the gal operon in *E. coli* K-12. Proc. Nat. Acad. Sci. USA, **55,** 622, 1966.
102. Kalckar, H. M., Kurahashi, K., and Jordan, E.: Hereditary defects in galactose metabolism in *E. coli* mutants. 1. Determination of enzyme activities. Proc. Nat. Acad. Sci. USA, **45,** 1776, 1959.
103. Buttin, G.: Mecanismes regulateurs dans la biosynthese des enzymes du metabolisme du galactose chez *E. coli* K-12. II. Le determinisme genetique de la regulation. J. Molec. Biol., **7,** 183, 1963.
104. Morse, M. L.: Preliminary genetic map of seventeen galactose mutations in *E. coli* K-12. Proc. Nat. Acad. Sci. USA, **48,** 1314, 1962.
105. Buttin, G.: Sur la structure de l'opéron galactose chez *E. coli* K-12. C. R. Acad. Sci. (Paris), **255,** 1233, 1962.
106. Adler, J., and Kaiser, A. D.: Mapping of the galactose genes of *Escherichia coli* by transduction with phage Pl. Virology, **19,** 117, 1963.
107. Kurahashi, K., and Wahba, A. J.: Interference with growth of certain *E. coli* mutants by galactose. Biochim. Biophys. Acta, **30,** 298, 1958.
108. Yarmolinsky, M. B., Wiesmeyer, H., Kalckar, H. M., and Jordan, E.: Hereditary defects in *E. coli* mutants. II. Galactose induced sensitivity. Proc. Nat. Acad. Sci. USA, **45,** 1786, 1959.
109. Sundararajan, T. A.: Interference with glycerokinase induction in mutants of *E. coli* accumulating Gal-1-P. Proc. Nat. Acad. Sci. USA, **50,** 463, 1963.
110. Fukasawa, T., and Nikaido, H.: Galactose sensitive mutants of Salmonella. I. Metabolism of galactose. Biochim. Biophys. Acta, **48,** 460, 1961.
111. Fukasawa, T., and Nikaido, H.: Galactose sensitive mutants of *Salmonella.* II. Bacteriolysis induced by galactose. Biochim. Biophys. Acta, **48,** 470, 1961.

112. Morse, M. L., Lederberg, E. M., and Lederberg, J.: Transduction in *E. coli* K-12. Genetics, **41**, 142, 1956.
113. Adler, J., and Templeton, B.: The amount of galactose genetic material in λ dg bacteriophage with different densities. J. Molec. Biol., **7**, 710, 1963.
114. Hsia, D. Y. Y., and Walker, F. A.: Variability in the clinical manifestations of galactosemia. J. Pediat., **59**, 872, 1961.
115. Donnell, G. N., Collado, M., and Koch, R.: Growth and development of children with galactosemia. J. Pediat., **58**, 836, 1961.
116. Nadler, H. L., Inouye, T., and Hsia, D. Y. Y.: Clinical galactosemia: A study of fifty-five cases, in *Galactosemia,* edited by D. Y. Y. Hsia, p. 127. Charles C Thomas, Springfield, Ill., 1969.
117. Donnell, G. N., Koch, R., and Bergren, W. R.: Observations on results of management of galactosemic patients, in *Galactosemia,* edited by D. Y. Y. Hsia, p. 247. Charles C Thomas, Springfield, Ill., 1969.
118. Komrower, G. M., and Lee, D. H.: Long term follow-up of galactosemia. Arch. Dis. Child., **45**, 367, 1970.
119. Segal, S., Blair, A., and Roth, H.: The metabolism of galactose by patients with congenital galactosemia. Amer. J. Med., **38**, 62, 1965.
120. Holzel, A., Komrower, G. M., and Wilson, V. K.: Aminoaciduria in galactosemia. Brit. Med. J., **1**, 194, 1952.
121. Cusworth, D. C., Dent, C. E., and Flynn, F. V.: The aminoaciduria in galactosemia. Arch. Dis. Child., **30**, 150, 1955.
122. Smetana, H. F., and Olen, F.: Hereditary galactose disease. Amer. J. Clin. Path., **38**, 3, 1962.
123. Gitzelmann, R., and Auricchio, S.: The handling of soya alpha galactosides by a normal and a galactosemic child. Pediatrics, **36**, 231, 1965.
124. Koch, R., Acosta, P., Donnell, G. N., and Lieberman, E.: Nutritional therapy of galactosemia. Clin. Pediat. (Phila.), **4**, 571, 1965.
125. Schwarz, V.: The value of galactose phosphate determinations in the treatment of galactosemia. Arch. Dis. Child., **35**, 428, 1960.
126. Donnell, G. N., Bergren, W. R., Perry, G., and Koch, R.: Galactose-1-phosphate in galactosemia. Pediatrics, **31**, 802, 1963.
127. Kogut, M. D., Donnell, G. N., and Sharo, K. N. F.: Studies of lactose absorption in patients with galactosemia. J. Pediat., **71**, 75, 1967.
128. Segal, S., and Bernstein, H.: Observations on cataract formation in the newborn offspring of rats fed a high-galactose diet. J. Pediat., **62**, 363, 1963.
129. Spatz, M., and Segal, S.: Transplacental galactose toxicity in rats. J. Pediat., **67**, 438, 1965.
130. Schwarz, V., Goldberg, L., Komrower, G. M., and Holzel, A.: Some disturbances of erythrocyte metabolism in galactosemia. Biochem. J., **62**, 34, 1956.
131. Inouye, T., Nadler, H. L., and Hsia, D. Y. Y.: Galactose-1-phosphate uridyl transferase in red and white blood cells. Clin. Chim. Acta., **19**, 169, 1968.
132. Krooth, R., and Weinberg, A. N.: Studies on cell lines developed from the tissues of patients with galactosemia. J. Exp. Med., **113**, 1155, 1861.
133. Anderson, E. P., Kalckar, H. M., and Isselbacher, K. J.: Defect in the uptake of galactose-1-phosphate into liver nucleotides in congenital galactosemia. Science, **125**, 113, 1957.
134. Mayes, J. S.: Thesis for the Ph.D. degree, Michigan State Univ., 1965. Quoted by Hansen, R. G.: Some chemical aspects of galactosemia, in *Galactosemia,* edited by D. Y. Y. Hsia, p. 55. Charles C Thomas, Springfield, Ill., 1969.
135. Anderson, E. P., Kalckar, H. M., Kurahashi, K., and Isselbacher, K. J.: A specific enzymatic assay for the diagnosis of congenital galactosemia. J. Lab. Clin. Med., **50**, 569, 1957.
136. Beutler, E., and Baluda, M. C.: Improved method for measuring galactose-1-phosphate uridyl transferase activity of erythrocytes. Clin. Chim. Acta., **13**, 369, 1966.
137. Mellman, W. J., and Tedesco, T. A.: An improved assay of erythroctye and leukocyte galactose-1-phosphate uridyl transferase: Stabilization of the enzyme by a thiol protective reagent. J. Lab. Clin. Med., **66**, 980, 1965.
138. Donnell, G. N., Bergren, W. R., Bretthauer, M. S., and Hansen, R. G.: The enzymatic expression of heterozygosity in families of children with galactosemia. Pediatrics, **25**, 572, 1960.
139. Hsia, D. Y. Y.: Clinical variants of galactosemia. Metabolism, **16**, 419, 1967.
140. Robinson, A.: The assay of galactokinase and galactose-1-phosphate uridyl transferase activity in human erythrocytes. J. Exp. Med., **118**, 359, 1963.
141. Ng, W. G., Bergren, W. R., and Donnell, G. N.: Galactose-1-phosphate uridyltransferase assay by use of radioactive galactose-1-phosphate. Clin. Chim. Acta, **10**, 337, 1964.
142. Ng, W. G., Bergren, W. R., and Donnell, G. N.: An improved procedure for the assay of hemolysate galactose-1-phosphate uridyl transferase activity by the use of ^{14}C labeled galactose-1-phosphate. Clin. Chim. Acta, **15**, 489, 1967.
143. Weinberg, A. N.: Detection of congenital galactosemia and the carrier state using galactose C^{14} and blood cells. Metabolism, **10**, 728, 1961.
144. Eggermont, E., and Hers, H. G.: Une nouvelle methode de détection de la galactosémie congénitale. Clin. Chim. Acta, **7**, 437, 1962.
145. Ng, W. G., Bergren, W. R., and Donnell, G. N.: Galactose-1-phosphate uridyl transferase activity in galactosaemia. Nature (London), **203**, 845, 1964.
146. Beutler, E., Baluda, M., and Donnell, G. N.: A new method for the detection of galactosemia and its carrier state. J. Lab. Clin. Med., **64**, 694, 1964.
147. Copenhaver, J. H., Bausch, L. C., and Fitzgibbons, J. F.: A fluorometric procedure for estimation of galactose-1-phosphate uridyltransferase activity in red blood cells. Anal. Biochem., **30**, 327, 1969.
148. Gatti, R., Manfield, P., and Hsia, D. Y. Y.: Screening for galactosemia in the newborn. J. Pediat., **69**, 1126, 1936.
149. Beutler, E., and Baluda, M. C.: A simple spot screening test for galactosemia. J. Lab. Clin. Med., **68**, 137, 1966.
150. Nelson, K., and Hsia, D. Y. Y.: Screening for galactosemia and glucose-6-phosphate dehydrogenase deficiency in newborn infants. J. Pediat., **71**, 582, 1967.
151. Haworth, J. C., and Barchuk, N. H.: A simple chromatographic screening test for the detection of galactosemia in newborn infants. Pediatrics, **39**, 608, 1967.
152. Wells, W. W., Chin, T., and Weber, B.: Quantitative analysis of serum and urine sugars by gas chromatography. Clin Chim. Acta, **10**, 352, 1964.
153. Copenhaver, J. H.: Quantitative analysis of plasma galactose and glucose by gas-liquid chromatography. Anal. Biochem., **17**, 76, 1966.
154. de Verdier, C. H., and Hjelm, M.: A galactose oxidase method for the determination of galactose in blood plasma. Clin. Chim. Acta, **7**, 742, 1962.
155. Roth, H., Segal, S., and Bertoli, D.: The quantitative determination of galactose—an enzymatic method using galactose oxidase with application to blood and other biological fluids. Anal. Biochem., **10**, 32, 1965.
156. Tengstrom, B.: Enzymatic determination of glucose and galactose in urine. Scand. J. Lab. Invest., **18**, suppl. 92, 104, 1966.
157. Dahlquist, A., and Svenningsen, N. W.: Galactose in the urine of newborn infants. J. Pediat., **75**, 454, 1969.
158. Dahlquist, A.: Test paper for galactose in urine. Scand. J. Clin. Lab. Invest., **22**, 87, 1968.
159. Bickel, H.: Mellituria, a paper chromatographic study. J. Pediat., **59**, 641, 1961.
160. Haworth, J. C., and MacDonald, M. S.: Reducing sugars in urine and blood of premature babies. Arch. Dis. Child., **32**, 417, 1952.
161. Hall, W. K., Cravey, C. E., Chen, P. T., Ostendorff, M. E., Hollowell, J. G., Jr., and Thevaos, T. G.: An evaluation of galactosuria. J. Pediat., **77**, 625, 1970.
162. Bruck, E., and Rapoport, S.: Galactosemia in an infant with cataracts: Clinical observations and carbohydrate studies. Amer. J. Dis. Child., **70**, 267, 1945.
163. Baker, L., Mellman, W. J., Tedesco, T. A., and Segal, S.: Galactosemia: symptomatic and asymptomatic homozygotes in one Negro sibship. J. Pediat., **68**, 551, 1966.
164. Segal, S.: The Negro variant of congenital galactosemia, in *Galactosemia,* edited by D. Y. Y. Hsia, p. 176. Charles C Thomas, Springfield, Ill., 1969.
165. Topper, Y. J., Laster, L., and Segal, S.: Galactose metabolism: Phenotype differences among tissues of a patient with congenital galactosemia. Nature (London), **196**, 1106, 1962.
166. Pesch, L. A., Segal, S., and Topper, Y. J.: Progesterone effects on

galactose metabolism in prepubertal patients with congenital galactosemia and in rats maintained on high galactose diets. J. Clin. Invest., **39**, 178, 1960.

167. Elder, T. D., Segal, S., Maxwell, E. S., and Topper, Y. J.: Some steroid hormone like effects of menthol. Science, **132**, 225, 1960.
168. Segal, S.: Isotopic studies of galactose oxidation in galactosemia, in *Galactosemia,* edited by D. Y. Y. Hsia, p. 42. Charles C Thomas, Springfield, Ill., 1969.
169. Tada, K., Kudo, Z., Ohno, T., Akabone, J., and Chica, R.: Congenital galactosemia and orotic acid therapy with promising results. Preliminary report. Tohoku J. Exp. Med., **77**, 340, 1962.
170. Segal, S., Roth, H., and Blair, A.: Observations of orotic acid on galactose metabolism in congenital galactosemia. J. Pediat., **68**, 135, 1966.
171. Egan, T. J., and Wells, W. W.: Alternate metabolic pathway in galactosemia. Amer. J. Dis. Child., **111**, 400, 1966.
172. Weinstein, A. N., and Segal, S.: The metabolic fate of 1-^{14}C galactitol in mammalian tissue. Biochim. Biophys. Acta, **156**, 9, 1968.
173. Inouye, T., Tannenbaum, M., and Hsia, D. Y. Y.: Identification of galactose-6-phosphate in galactosemic erythrocytes. Nature (London), **193**, 67, 1962.
174. Inouye, T., Schneider, J. A., and Hsia, D. Y. Y.: Enzymatic oxidation of galactose-6-phosphate. Nature (London), **204**, 1304, 1964.
175. Ohno, S., Payne, H. W., Morrison, M., and Beutler, E.: Hexose-6-phosphate dehydrogenase found in human liver. Science, **153**, 1015, 1966.
176. Kirkman, H. N., and Bynum, E.: Enzymatic evidence of a galactosemic trait in parents and galactosemic children. Ann. Hum. Genet., **23**, 117, 1959.
177. Schwarz, V., Wells, A. R., Holzel, A., and Komrower, G. M.: A study of the genetics of galactosemia. Ann. Hum. Genet., **25**, 179, 1961.
178. Hugh-Jones, K., Newcomb, A. L., and Hsia, D. Y. Y.: The genetic mechanism of galactosemia. Arch. Dis. Child., **35**, 521, 1960.
179. Walker, F. A., Hsia, D. Y. Y., Slatis, H. M., and Steinberg, A. G.: Galactosemia: A study of 27 kindreds in North America. Ann. Hum. Genet., **25**, 287, 1962.
180. Gitzelmann, R., and Hodorn, B.: Zur biochemischen genetik der galaktosämie. Helv. Paediat. Acta, **16**, 1, 1961.
181. Mellman, W. J., and Tedesco, T. A.: Galactose-1-phosphate uridyltransferase and galactokinase activity in cultured human diploid fibroblasts and peripherial blood leukocytes. J. Clin. Invest., **48**, 2391, 1969.
182. Beutler, E., Baluda, M. C., Sturgeon, P., and Day, R. W.: A new genetic abnormality resulting in galactose-1-phosphate uridyl transferase defeciency. Lancet, **1**, 353, 1965.
183. Beutler, E., Baluda, M. C., Sturgeon, P., and Day, R. W.: The genetics of galactose-1-phosphate uridyl transferase deficiency. J. Lab. Clin. Med., **68**, 646, 1966.
184. Mathai, C. K., and Beutler, E.: Electrophoretic variation of galactose-1-phosphate uridyl transferase. Science, **154**, 1179, 1966.
185. Ng, W. G., Bergren, W. R., Field, M., and Donnell, G. N.: An improved electrophoretic procedure for galactose-1-phosphate uridyl transferase: Demonstration of multiple activity bands with the Duarte variant. Biochem. Biophys. Res. Commun., **37**, 354, 1969.
186. Mellman, W. J., Tedesco, T. A., and Feigl, P.: Estimation of the gene frequency of the Duarte variant of galactose-1-phosphate uridyl transferase. Ann. Hum. Genet., **32**, 1, 1968.
187. Gitzelmann, R., Poley, J. R., and Prader, A.: Partial galactose-1-phosphate uridyltransferase deficiency due to a variant enzyme. Helv. Paediat. Acta, **22**, 252, 1967.
188. McGuiness, R., and Saunders, R. A.: Erythrocyte galactose-1-phosphate uridyl transferase and glucose-6-phosphate dehydrogenase activity in the population of Rhonda Foch. Clin. Chim. Acta, **16**, 221, 1967.
189. Brandt, N. J.: Frequency of heterozygotes for hereditary galactosemia in a normal population. Acta Genet. (Basel), **17**, 289, 1967.
190. Hansen, R. G., Bretthauer, R. K., Mayes, J., and Nordin, J. H.: Estimation of frequency of occurrence of galactosemia in the population. Proc. Soc. Exp. Biol. Med., **115**, 560, 1964.
191. Kelly, S., Katz, S., Burns, J., and Boylan, J.: Screening for galactosemia in New York State. Public Health Rep., **85**, 575, 1970.
192. Brandt, N. J., Forland, A., Mikkelsen, M., Nielsen, A., and Tolstrup, N.: Galactosaemia locus and the Down's syndrome chromosome. Lancet, **2**, 700, 1963.
193. Hsia, D. Y. Y., Inouye, T., Wong, P., and South, A.: Studies on galactose oxidation in Down's syndrome. New Eng. J. Med., **270**, 1085, 1964.
194. Rosner, F., Ong, B. H., Paine, R. S., and Mahanand, D.: Biochemical differentiation of trisomic Down's syndrome (mongolism) from that due to translocation. New Eng. J. Med., **273**, 1356, 1965.
195. Wang, M. Y. F. W., and Desforges, J. F.: The Philadelphia chromosome and galactose-1-phosphate uridyl transferase. Blood, **29**, 790, 1967.
196. Krone, W., Wolf, U., Goedde, H. W., and Baitsch, H.: Untersuchungen über die aktivität der galaktokinase im blut von normal personen und von patienten mit G_{DO}-trisomie. Hum. Genet., **1**, 279, 1965.
197. Mellman, W. J., Oski, F. A., Tedesco, T. A., and Harris, H.: Leucocyte enzymes in Down's syndrome. Lancet, **2**, 674, 1964.
198. Dahlquist, A., Hall, B., and Källén, B.: Blood galactose-1-phosphate uridyl transferase activity in dysplastic patients with and without chromosomal aberrations. Hum. Heredity, **19**, 628, 1969.
199. Sidbury, J. B., Jr.: The role of galactose-1-phosphate in the pathogenesis of galactosemia, in *Molecular Genetics and Human Disease,* edited by L. E. Gardner, p. 61. Charles C Thomas, Springfield, Ill., 1960.
200. Mitchell, H. S.: Cataract in rats fed on galactose. Proc. Soc. Exp. Biol. Med., **32**, 971, 1935.
201. Craig, J., and Maddock, C.: Observations on nature of galactose toxicity in rats. A.M.A. Arch. Path., **55**, 118, 1953.
202. Dam, H.: Galactose-poisoning in chicks. Proc. Soc. Exp. Biol. Med., **55**, 57, 1944.
203. Rutter, W. J., Krichevsky, P., Scott, H. M., and Hansen, R.G.: The metabolism of lactose and galactose in the chick. Poult. Sci., **32**, 706, 1953.
204. Perry, J., Moore, A., Thomas, D., and Hird, F.: Galactose intolerance: Observations on an experimental animal. Acta Paediat., **45**, 228, 1956.
205. Nordin, J. H., Wilken, D. R., Bretthauer, R. K., Hansen, R. G., and Scott, H. M.: A consideration of galactose toxicity in male and female chicks. Poult. Sci., **39**, 802, 1960.
206. Hansen, R. G., Freeland, R. A., and Scott, H. M.: Lactose metabolism. V. The uridine nucleotides in galactose toxocity. J. Biol. Chem., **219**, 391, 1956.
207. Klethi, J., and Mandel, P.: Uridine diphosphate hexoses of lens from rats on a galactose rich diet. Biochim. Biophys. Acta, **57**, 379, 1962.
208. Patterson, J. W.: Cataractogenic sugars. Arch. Biochem., **58**, 24, 1955.
209. Patterson, J. W., Patterson, M. E., Kensey, V. E., and Reddy, D. V. N.: Lens assay on diabetic and galactosemic rats receiving diets that modify cataract development. Invest. Ophthal., **4**, 98, 1965.
210. Cotlier, E.: Hypophysectomy effect on lens epithelium mitosis and galactose cataract development in rats. Arch. Ophthal., (Chicago), **67**, 476, 1962.
211. Schwarz, V., and Goldberg, L.: Galactose-1-phosphate in galactose cataract. Biochim. Biophys. Acta, **18**, 310, 1955.
212. Gitzelmann, R., Curtius, H. C., and Schneller, I.: Galactitol and galactose-1-phosphate in the lens of a galactosemic infant. Exp. Eye Res., **6**, 1, 1967.
213. Lerman, S.: Pathogenic factors in experimental cataract part I. Arch. Ophthal. (Chicago), **63**, 128, 1960.
214. Kinoshita, J. H., and Merola, L. O.: Hydration of the lens during the development of galactose cataract. Invest. Ophthal., **3**, 577, 1964.
215. Sippel, T. O.: Changes in the water, protein and glutathione contents of the lens in the course of galactose cataract development in rats. Invest. Ophthal., **5**, 568, 1966.
216. Kinoshita, J. H., Dvornik, D., Kraml, M., and Gabbay, K. H.: The effect of aldose reductase inhibition on the galactose exposed rabbit lens. Biochim. Biophys. Acta, **158**, 472, 1968.
217. Dische, Z., Zelmenis, G., and Youlous, J.: Studies on protein and protein synthesis—during the development of galactose cataract. Amer. J. Ophthal., **44**, 332, 1957.
218. Kinoshita, J. H., Merola, L. O., and Hayman, S.: Osmotic effects on the amino acid concentration mechanisms in the rabbit lens. J. Biol. Chem., **240**, 310, 1965.

219. Reddy, D.: Amino acid transport in the lens in relation to sugar cataracts. Invest. Ophthal., **4,** 700, 1965.
220. Kinoshita, J. H., Barber, G. W., Merola, L. O., and Tung, B.: Changes in levels of free amino acids and myo-inositol in the galactose-exposed lens. Invest. Ophthal., **8,** 625, 1969.
221. Cotlier, E., and Becker, B.: Rubidium 86 accumulation and dulcitol distributions in lens of galactose-fed rats. Exp. Eye Res., **4,** 340, 1965.
222. Kinoshita, J. H., Merola, L. O., and Tung, B.: Changes in cation permeability in the galactose-exposed rabbit lens. Exp. Eye Res., **7,** 80, 1968.
223. Brockhuyse, R.: Changes in myo-inositol permeability in the lens due to cataractous condition. Biochim. Biophys. Acta, **163,** 269, 1968.
224. Stewart, M., Kurien, M., Sherman, W., and Cotlier, E.: Inositol changes in nerve and lens of galactose fed rats. J. Neurochem., **15,** 941, 1968.
225. Sippel, T. O.: Enzyme of carbohydrate metabolism in developing galactose cataracts of rats. Invest. Ophthal., **6,** 59, 1967.
226. Korc, I.: Biochemical studies on cataracts in galactose fed rats. Arch. Biochem., **94,** 196, 1961.
227. Sippel, T. O.: Energy metabolism in the lens during development of galactose cataract in rats. Invest. Ophthal., **5,** 576, 1966.
228. Keppler, D., Rudiqier, J., Reutter, W., Lesch, R., and Decker, K.: Orotate prevents galactosamine hepatitis. Hoppe Seyler. Z. Physiol. Chem., **35,** 102, 1970.
229. Keppler, D., and Decker, K.: Studies on the mechanism of galactosamine hepatitis. Europ. J. Biochem., **10,** 219, 1969.
230. Landau, B., Hastings, A., and Zotta, S.: Studies on carbohydrate metabolism in rat liver slices. J. Biol. Chem., **233,** 1257, 1958.
231. Nordin, J., and Hansen, R. G.: Isolation and characterization of galactose from hydrolysates of glycogen. J. Biol. Chem., **238,** 489, 1963.
232. Grodsky, G. M., Batts, A. A., Bennett, L. L., Vcella C., McWilliams, N. B., and Smith, D. F.: Effects of carbohydrates on secretion of insulin from isolated rat pancreas. Amer. J. Physiol., **205,** 638, 1963.
233. Gitzelmann, R., and Illig, R.: Inability of galactose to metabolize insulin in galactokinase deficient individuals. Diabetologia, **5,** 143, 1969.
234. Dubois, R., Loeb, H., and Ooms, H. A.: Etude de métabolisme glucidique dans la galactosémie et la fructosémie. Rev. Franc. Etud. Clin. Biol., **7,** 509, 1962.
235. Gentil, C., Vallette, A. M., Lemonnier, A., Colin, J., Odievre, M., Leluc, R., Thuong, Trilu C., and Alagille, D.: Etude de métabolisme glucidique au cours de la galactosémie congenitale. Arch. Franc. Pediat., **23,** 509, 1966.
236. Tada, K: Glycogenesis and glycolysis in the liver from congenital galactosemia. Tohoku J. Exp. Med., **82,** 168, 1964.
237. Rosenberg, L., Weinberg, A., and Segal, S.: The effect of high galactose diets on urinary excretion of amino acids in the rat. Biochim. Biophys. Acta, **48,** 500, 1961.
238. Fox, M., Thier, S., Rosenberg, L., and Segal, S.: Impaired renal tubular function induced by sugar infusion in man. J. Clin. Endocr., **24,** 1318, 1964.
239. Thier, S., Fox, M., Rosenberg, L., and Segal, S.: Hexose inhibition of amino acid uptake in the rat-kidney-cortex slice. Biochim. Biophys. Acta, **93,** 106, 1964.
240. Saunders, S., and Isselbacher, K. J.: Inhibition of intestinal amino acid transport by hexoses. Biochim. Biophys. Acta, **102,** 397, 1965.
241. Diedrich, D., and Anderson, L.: Galactose 1-phosphate in the intestinal tissue of the rat during galactose absorption. Biochim. Biophys. Acta, **43,** 490, 1960.
242. Haworth, J. C., Ford, J. D., and Younoszai, M. K.: Effect of galactose toxicity on growth of the rat fetus and brain. Pediat. Res., **3,** 441, 1969.
243. Haworth, J. C., Ford, J. D., and Ho, H. K.: The effect of galactose toxicity on growth of the developing rat brain. Brain Res., **21,** 385, 1970.
244. Wells, H. J., and Wells, W. W.: Galactose toxicity and myoinositol metabolism in developing rat brain. Biochemistry (Wash.), **6,** 1168, 1967.
245. Gabbay, K. H., and Snider, J. J.: Galactosemic neuropathy: A model for diabetic neuropathy. Diabetes, **19,** 357, 1970.
246. Kozak, L. P., and Wells, W. W.: Effect of galactose on energy and phospholipid metabolism in the chick brain. Arch. Biochem. Biophys., **135,** 371, 1969.
247. Mayes, J. S., Miller, L. R., and Myers, F. K.: The relationship of galactose-1-phosphate accumulation and uridyltransferase activity to the differential galactose toxicity in male and female chicks. Biochem. Biophys. Res. Commun., **39,** 661, 1970.
248. Wells, H. J., Gordon, M., and Segal, S.: Galactose toxicity in the chick: Oxidation of radioactive galactose. Biochim. Biophys. Acta, **222,** 327, 1970.
249. Rigdon, R. H., Couch, J. R., Creges, C. R., and Ferguson, T. M.: Galactose intoxication pathologic study in the chick. Experientia, **19,** 349, 1963.
250. Carver, M. J.: Disturbances by galactose of the free amino acids of fetal rat brain. Biochim. Biophys. Acta, **130,** 514, 1966.
251. Woolley, D. W.: *Biochemical Basis of Psychosis or the Serotonin Hypothesis About Mental Diseases.* Wiley, New York, 1962.
252. Woolley, D. W., and Gommi, B. W.: Serotonin receptors. IV. Specific deficiency of receptors in galactose toxicity and its possible relationship to the idiocy of galactosemia. Proc. Nat. Acad. Sci. USA, **52,** 14, 1964.
253. Miller, L. R., Gordon, G. B., and Bench, K. G.: Cytologic alterations in hereditary metabolic disorders. I. The effects of galactose on galactosemic fibroblasts *in vitro.* Lab. Invest., **19,** 428, 1968.
254. Pennington, J. S., and Prankerd, T. A. J.: Studies of erythrocyte phosphate ester metabolism in galactosemia. Clin. Sci., **17,** 385, 1958.
255. Zipursky, A., Rowland, M., Ford, J. D., Haworth, J. C., and Israels, L. G.: Erythrocyte metabolism in galactosemia. Pediatrics, **35,** 126, 1965.
256. Monteleone, J. A., Beutler, E., Monteleone, P. H., Vtz, C. L., and Casey, E. C.: Cataracts galactosuria and hypergalactosemia due to galactokinase deficiency in a child: Studies of a kindred. *Abstr. Soc. Pediat. Res., 40th Annual meeting,* 1970, p. 123.
257. McVie, R., Deutsche, M. A., Olambiwonnu, N. O., Frasier, S. D., and Donnell, G. N.: Galactokinase deficiency: Clinical and biochemical studies in identical twins. Abstract submitted to the Western Soc. Pediat. Res., communicated personally.
258. Thalhammer, O., Gitzelmann, R., and Pantlitscho, M.: Hypergalactosemia and galactosuria due to galactokinase deficiency in a newborn. Pediatrics, **42,** 441, 1968.
259. Fanconi, G.: Hochgradige galaktose-Intoleranz (galaktose-Diabetes) bei einem Kinde mit Neurofibromatosis Recklinghausen. Jb. Kinderheilk., **138,** 1, 1933.
260. Mayes, J. S., and Guthrie, R.: Detection of heterozygotes for galactokinase deficiency in a human population. Biochem. Genet., **2,** 219, 1968.
261. Beutler, E.: The Duarte variant in galactosemia, in *Galactosemia,* edited by D. Y. Hsia, p. 163. Charles C Thomas, Springfield, Ill., 1969.

CHAPTER NINE

PRIMARY HYPEROXALURIA *

Hibbard E. Williams and Lloyd H. Smith, Jr.

Primary hyperoxaluria is a general term for two rare genetic disorders of glyoxylate metabolism which are characterized by recurrent calcium oxalate nephrolithiasis, chronic renal failure, and early death in uremia [1–4]. Nephrocalcinosis and extrarenal deposits of calcium oxalate, termed *oxalosis,* characterize the pathologic findings in this disorder. Patients with the major form of this disease (Type I, also called *glycolic aciduria*) excrete in the urine excessive amounts of oxalic, glycolic, and glyoxylic acids. The biochemical basis of the disease is a defect in glyoxylate metabolism, which leads to increased synthesis and excretion of oxalic acid. The pattern of inheritance of primary hyperoxaluria (Type I) suggests its transmission as an autosomal recessive trait.

Recently, a second type of primary hyperoxaluria has been described. Although the clinical findings do not distinguish this variant, there are differences in the pattern of urinary organic acids and in the basic metabolic defect [5]. In this new disorder, termed *L-glyceric aciduria* (or primary hyperoxaluria Type II), oxalic and glyceric acids are excreted in excess in the urine, but glycolic acid excretion is normal. A defect in hydroxypyruvate metabolism has been demonstrated. The disorder is presumably transmitted by an autosomal recessive mode of inheritance.

In this report emphasis will be placed on the biochemical pathogenesis and classification of these genetic disorders. Oxalate metabolism will be reviewed as it pertains to the biochemical basis for continued hyperoxaluria.

HISTORY

Oxalate was recognized in certain plants as early as the eighteenth century, but it was not until 1839 that calcium oxalate crystals were identified in urine [6]. Somewhat earlier certain renal stones were found to contain calcium oxalate [7]. Methods for the measurement of oxalate content of urine were introduced early in this century and led to an interest in the "oxalate diathesis," which was thought to be related to many cases of rheumatism, neurasthenia, and dyspepsia. Unfortunately, the plethora of such disorders described exceeded the reliability of the oxalate measurements.

Primary hyperoxaluria, first described by Lepoutre in 1925 [8], was rarely reported until the 1950s, when the clinical and pathologic entity was accurately characterized. Despite these early studies, there was disagreement about the relationship between oxalosis and hyperoxaluria as recently as 1960 [9]. It is now agreed that oxalosis is simply the tissue-storage complication of excessive oxalate synthesis (and presumed increased concentration), comparable to sodium urate deposits in tophaceous gout.

The first detailed report of a case of oxalosis appeared in 1950 [10]. This child had had renal stones and nephrocalcinosis beginning at the age of 2 years and died of renal failure at age 12. At post-mortem examination numerous calcium oxalate crystals were found in the bones and kidneys. Primary hyperoxaluria was first diagnosed during life in 1953, when a child with recurrent nephrolithiasis was found to have an increased urinary excretion of oxalate [11]. In 1954 the report of hyperoxaluria and oxalosis in identical twins dying of chronic renal failure emphasized the familial nature of the disease [12]. Since these early cases, primary hyperoxaluria has been reported with increasing frequency, and in 1964 an extensive review summarized data on 63 typical and 42 atypical cases [3]. Reports emphasizing the clinical and biochemical heterogeneity of this disorder have appeared mostly during the past few years [3, 4, 13, 14].

CLINICAL FEATURES

Patients with primary hyperoxaluria typically develop the initial symptoms of the disease at an early age. The onset of symptoms may occur before the age of 5 (approximately 65 percent of patients) or even before the age of 1 (12 percent). There appears to be no significant difference in the sex incidence of reported cases, the male to female ratio being 1.3 : 1.

Initial symptoms generally relate to the presence of calcium oxalate nephrolithiasis, with typical renal colic or asymptomatic gross hematuria being the most common. Less frequently patients may pass large numbers of small renal calculi with little discomfort. In a few male infants urethral meatotomy has been necessary for relief of blockage by small concretions.

In a minority of patients symptoms secondary to uremia may be the initial clinical manifestations of the disease. In such patients growth retardation is a frequent finding, and some patients with short stature have had features suggestive of secondary renal tubular acidosis. Symptoms are present for less than 10 years in over 90 percent of patients who die of the disease. Over 80 percent of patients die of renal failure before they reach the age of 20. This high mortality rate may reflect the method of ascertainment.

Other rarer clinical manifestations of primary hyperoxaluria include acute arthritis and symptoms referable to cardiac involvement. Attacks of joint pain have been diagnosed as gout [15, 16], supported in part by hyperuricemia, which is found frequently in this disease. Although this

* Many of the studies referred to in this chapter were supported by Research Grant AM-09406 from the Public Health Service. The authors express their appreciation to Drs. James B. Wyngaarden and T. David Elder for permission to incorporate in this revision some material from their chapter in the previous editions.

feature has been observed most commonly after the onset of the uremic phase of the disease, some patients have had both hyperuricemia and joint symptoms before renal insufficiency has appeared [12]. Sodium urate microcrystals in joint fluid from patients with primary hyperoxaluria have not yet been demonstrated. Since calcium oxalate crystals have been found in synovial membranes, it has been suggested that joint symptoms in these patients may be secondary to calcium oxalate crystallization in joint fluid. In two patients with primary hyperoxaluria [17, 18] the development of complete atrioventricular block was thought to be related to the deposition of calcium oxalate crystals near the myocardial conduction system, a pathologic feature which has been substantiated in one report [17].

A number of patients with hyperoxaluria do not show the typical pattern of onset or progression of the disease [3, 13]. In these patients the disease may become manifest initially in adult life, even after the age of 40, the renal damage progressing less rapidly. Urinary oxalate excretion has been measured reliably in some but not all of these patients, so that the diagnosis of primary hyperoxaluria has not always been established conclusively. A few of these cases may be examples of pyridoxine deficiency (see below). Another group of suspected hyperoxaluric subjects have died before the age of 1, with renal insufficiency, nephrocalcinosis, and, in some, extrarenal oxalate deposition. As in the former group, the diagnosis of primary hyperoxaluria has been presumptive but unproved in these infants because of the absence of data on urinary oxalate excretion. Such reports have raised the question of both clinical and biochemical heterogeneity in the definition of primary hyperoxaluria.

Recently, a second distinct type of primary hyperoxaluria, termed L-*glyceric aciduria,* has been reported. This disorder differs from the previously described form (termed *Type I primary hyperoxaluria*) [5, 19]. In three of the four known patients calcium oxalate nephrolithiasis developed before the age of 2. In the remaining patient the first symptoms of the disease did not develop until age 24. All four patients have had intermittent microscopic hematuria, but in none has renal insufficiency developed, in spite of symptoms for over 10 years in two. In the oldest patient insulin-requiring diabetes mellitus developed at age 34. Differences in the excretion of urinary organic acids and the site of the metabolic defect in L-glyceric aciduria will be described below.

There are no specific physical findings in patients with primary hyperoxaluria. Growth retardation reflects renal failure, and acute arthritis and atrioventricular block are extremely rare. In the early stages of the disease the development of hydronephrosis may lead to palpable renal enlargement. Calcium oxalate crystals in the eye have been reported in one patient, but they may have represented exudates of uremic retinopathy [20]. Many patients have been examined carefully for such crystals with negative results.

Roentgenographic features of primary hyperoxaluria are confined largely to the genitourinary tract and to the skeletal system. Urolithiasis and nephrocalcinosis are the abnormalities most frequently encountered. Radiopaque calcium oxalate densities may be observed both in the collecting system of the kidneys and within the renal parenchyma. In the uremic phase of the disease secondary hyperparathyroidism may develop and lead to the roentgenographic bone changes of that disorder and to other forms of renal osteodystrophy.

PATHOLOGIC FEATURES

Nephrectomy specimens [9] from patients with hyperoxaluria have revealed nephrolithiasis, hydronephrosis, acute and chronic pyelonephritis, and tubular deposits of calcium oxalate. Nephrocalcinosis may not be present, and decreased renal function may be secondary to chronic obstruction and infection.

At post-mortem examination [21] the kidneys are usually found to be small and to have thickened capsules which strip with difficulty. The surfaces are granular and contain focal depressed scars. They usually cut with noticeably increased resistance, and in most cases there is a gritty sensation, as though one were cutting through sand. On the cut surface the cortex is thin, and the pelves frequently contain calculi. Small crystals may sometimes be seen in the parenchyma with the naked eye.

On microscopic examination interstitial fibrosis and interstitial nephritis may be found. Refractile crystals of various sizes are seen, primarily in the proximal convoluted tubules (Fig. 9-1). The tubular epithelium may be compressed or destroyed (Fig. 9-2), and the crystals may extend into the interstitial spaces [18, 21]. At times large crystalline masses,

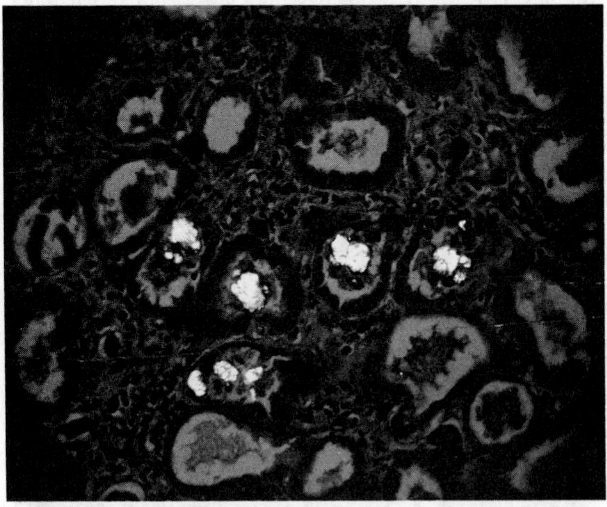

Figure 9-1. Calcium oxalate crystals in the proximal convoluted tubules of a 34-year-old male dying of oxalosis and renal insufficiency. (Polarization microscopy, ×175.) (*The authors are indebted to Dr. David Porter for permission to publish this photomicrograph.*)

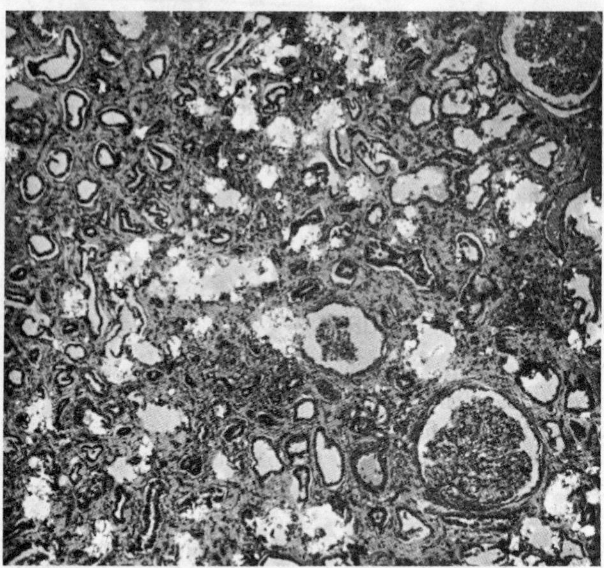

Figure 9-2. Oxalate nephrocalcinosis from a patient with primary hyperoxaluria and oxalosis. Most of the calcium oxalate crystals are related to the remains of renal tubules. (Half-crossed Nicol prisms, ×70.) (*From Scowen et al.* [21], *with permission of the authors and publisher.*)

accompanied by heavy scarring, are found in the tunica media and adventitia of small renal arteries and arterioles. The glomeruli are usually normal except for moderate pericapsular fibrosis and a rare hyalinized glomerulus.

Extrarenal deposits of calcium oxalate are variable in location and extent. The major sites of predilection are bone, heart, and the male urogenital system. In bone, crystal deposits occur in both the Haversian system and the marrow (Fig. 9-3) [10, 12, 21, 22]. They may also occur in cartilage (Fig. 9-4) [23]. The myocardium may contain scattered deposits of calcium oxalate crystals and rarely may be heavily involved [18, 23]. The testis is a common site of extrarenal deposits. Crystals are frequently found in the walls of veins, arteries, and arterioles in this location and elsewhere. There appears to be a predilection for sites of tissue injury, such as foci of fibrosis or of chronic granulomatous inflammation in lungs or lymph nodes, but calcium oxalate crystals may also occur in these sites in subjects without hyperoxaluria. In addition, deposits have been described in the thyroid, spleen, liver, thymus, pituitary, adrenal, pancreas, and parathyroids [1, 3, 9–12, 18, 22–26]. Often these deposits are limited to the arterial and arteriolar walls within these organs. In one fulminating case of primary hyperoxaluria, deposits were found within the central nervous system [21]. At death the concentration of oxalate in the spinal fluid may be elevated [27].

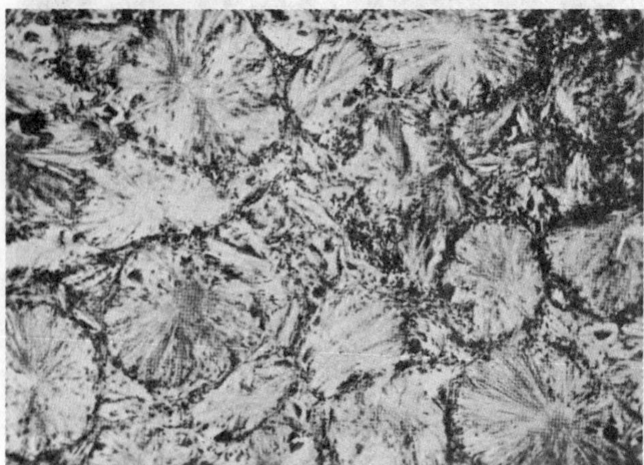

Figure 9-3. Calcium oxalate crystals in vertebral bone marrow from a patient with oxalosis (×150). (*From Dunn* [22], *with permission of the author and publisher.*)

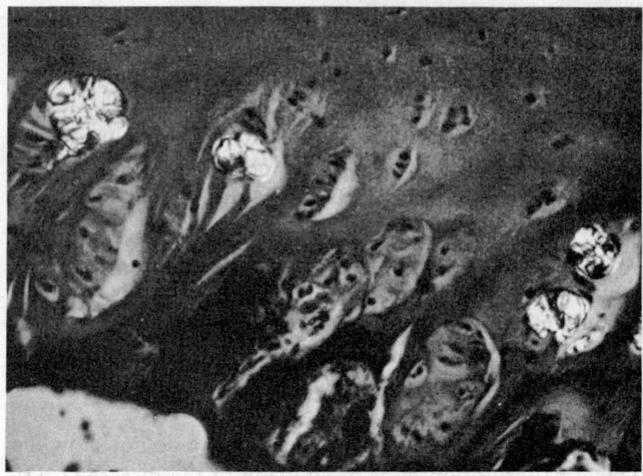

Figure 9-4. Calcium oxalate crystals in costochondral cartilage of a patient with primary hyperoxaluria and oxalosis, visualized under partial polarization (×175). (*From Godwin et al.* [23], *with permission of the authors and publisher.*)

On microscopic examination the crystals appear round and globular or rhomboidal in shape and have a radial rosette-like pattern. They have a slightly yellowish tinge and are doubly refractile under polarized light (Fig. 9-5). They do not stain with hematoxylin and eosin or, generally, with special techniques such as that of Von Kossa, unless calcium carbonate or phosphate has coprecipitated with oxalate [1, 22, 25, 26, 28].

The crystals may be identified in histologic sections by various chemical techniques. They are soluble when unstained deparaffinized sections are tested with concentrated hydrochloric or sulfuric acid, and are insoluble with lithium carbonate, glacial acetic acid, concentrated ammonium hydroxide, or concentrated potassium hydroxide. When the crystals are dissolved in concentrated sulfuric acid, small needle-like crystals of calcium sulfate may occasionally form [28]. If paraffin sections of tissue are first incinerated at 450°C for 30 min, calcium oxalate is oxidized to the carbonate, and small bubbles of carbon dioxide may be seen

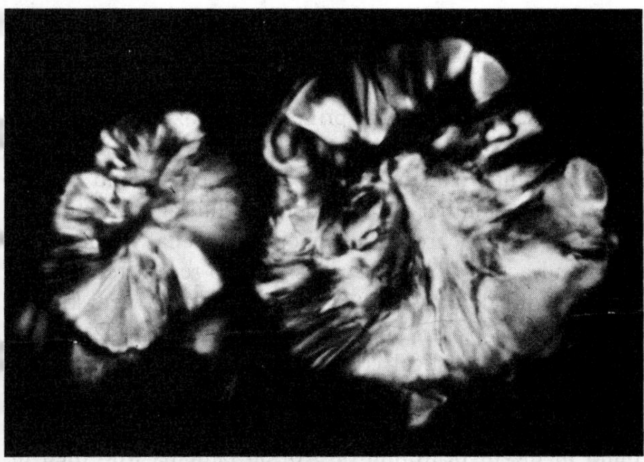

Figure 9-5. Calcium oxalate crystals from the lung of the patient of Fig. 9-1. (Polarization microscopy, × 1,500.) (*Courtesy of Dr. David Porter.*)

microscopically when concentrated sulfuric acid is allowed to run under the cover slip [29].

The crystals may be identified as calcium oxalate monohydrate by optical examination. The average width of single-needle crystals is 0.005 mm, and the average length is 0.05 mm. They have a birefringence of about 0.15 and an extinction angle of approximately 30° with respect to the length of the crystal. Calcium oxalate crystals have also been identified by x-ray diffraction in several cases of oxalosis [22–24, 28, 30].

DIAGNOSIS

The diagnosis of primary hyperoxaluria is based largely on the measurement of urinary oxalate excretion. Routine urinalysis is rarely of help in suggesting the diagnosis. Although calcium oxalate crystalluria is common in patients with hyperoxaluria, identical crystals occur in the urine of normal subjects, patients with calcium oxalate stones due to other causes, and patients with a variety of other renal abnormalities. Other nonspecific findings include microscopic hematuria, evidence of urinary tract infection, and (when renal failure supervenes) proteinuria and hyposthenuria.

The single most consistent laboratory finding in primary hyperoxaluria is an increased amount of urinary oxalate in the absence of pyridoxine deficiency or the excessive ingestion of oxalate or one of its immediate precursors (Fig. 9-6). Urinary oxalate excretion in normal man varies between 10 and 55 mg per 24 hr. When corrected for body surface area, the excretion of oxalate in children is comparable to that in adults [31, 32]. In patients with primary hyperoxaluria, urinary oxalate excretion has averaged 240 mg per 24 hr and has exceeded 400 mg per 24 hr in some patients [31]. In our experience it has been distinctly unusual to find urinary oxalate levels of less than 100 mg per 24 hr in patients with this disorder in the absence of renal failure. After renal failure develops, urinary oxalate excretion decreases, and in the late stages of the disease it may fall within the normal range. Consequently, the diagnosis of primary hyperoxaluria in the terminal uremic stage of the disease may be difficult to document by current methods.

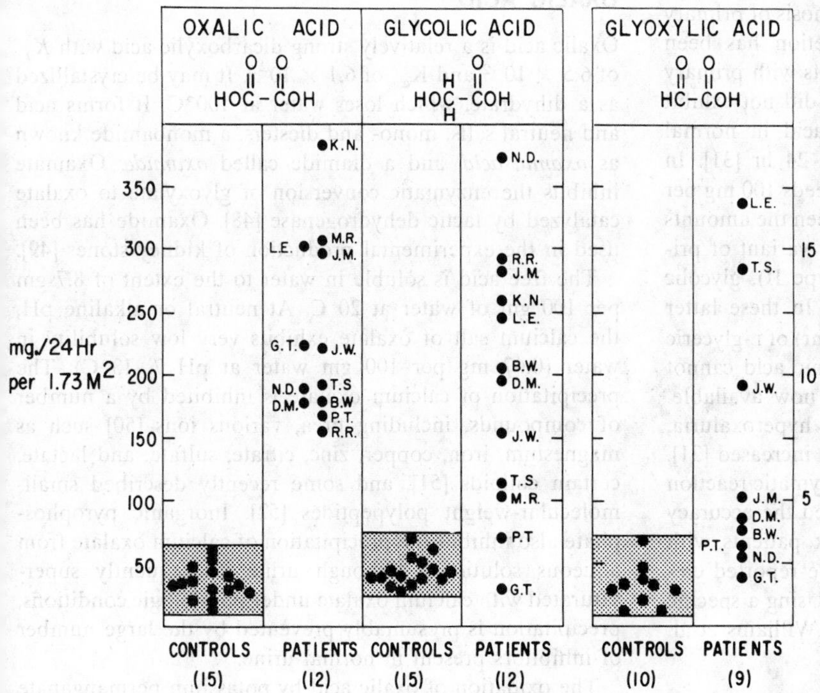

Figure 9-6. Urinary metabolites in primary hyperoxaluria. Patients P.T. and G.T. are siblings with L-glyceric aciduria (primary hyperoxaluria, Type II). (*From Hockaday et al.* [3] *with permission of the publishers.*)

Numerous reports of the oxalate content of human plasma have appeared in the past 35 years, with wide variations in the absolute values found. An early permanganate-titration method gave levels of 2 to 4 mg per 100 ml. [33]. Using more demanding extraction methods, Barber and Gallimore [34] found plasma oxalate levels of 0.4 to 0.6 mg per 100 ml. In 1961 Crawhall and Watts [35], utilizing a preparation of *Collybia velutipes* oxalic acid decarboxylase, found normal plasma oxalate concentrations to be less than 0.8 mg per 100 ml, the lower limit of sensitivity of the method. These investigators were able to measure elevated levels of plasma oxalate in patients with primary hyperoxaluria only during the terminal oliguric phase of the disease. Zarembski and Hodgkinson [36], using a fluoriometric method, found that serum oxalate levels in 17 normal adults ranged from 344 to 687 μg per 100 ml. In only one of six subjects with primary hyperoxaluria was serum oxalate increased above this normal range. A more recent report by these investigators records the concentration of serum oxalate in 15 normal adults as 135 to 280 μg per 100 ml [37]. Assuming no protein binding of oxalic acid, the plasma concentration of serum oxalate in normal subjects, studied with continuous intravenous infusion of isotopic oxalate, has been calculated as being approximately 15 μg per 100 ml [38].* These latter values approach more closely those calculated on the basis of the total miscible pool of oxalate (assuming homogeneous distribution of oxalate throughout body water) of 7 to 15 μg per 100 ml [39]. It is evident than an accurate method for the measurement of plasma oxalate would be very useful in the diagnosis of primary hyperoxaluria, especially after the development of renal failure.

The determination of the quantity of other urinary organic acids may be helpful in establishing the diagnosis of primary hyperoxaluria. Urinary glycolic acid excretion has been uniformly increased in all nonuremic patients with primary hyperoxaluria Type I, i.e., the patients who did not exhibit L-glyceric aciduria. Excretion of glycolic acid in normal subjects varies between 15 and 60 mg per 24 hr [31]. In primary hyperoxaluria Type I, it usually exceeds 100 mg per 24 hr. There is no constant relationship between the amounts of oxalic and glycolic acids excreted. In the variant of primary hyperoxaluria, L-glyceric aciduria (Type II), glycolic acid excretion is within the normal range. In these latter patients large amounts (200 to 600 mg per 24 hr) of L-glyceric acid are found in the urine [40]. This organic acid cannot be measured in normal urine by methods now available. In some but not all patients with primary hyperoxaluria, glyoxylic acid excretion in the urine may be increased [31]. The lability of this compound and its nonenzymatic reaction with other urinary constituents have impaired the accuracy and usefulness of its determination. In six patients with primary hyperoxaluria Zarembski et al. have reported elevations in urinary lactic acid excretion [14]. Using a specific isotope dilution method for urinary lactate, Williams et al. have not been able to confirm this finding in five patients with Type I primary hyperoxaluria [41].

*See also Williams, Johnson, and Smith [118].

Extrarenal deposition of calcium oxalate crystals is a frequent accompaniment of primary hyperoxaluria, but such crystals cannot be considered pathognomonic of these diseases. Calcium oxalate crystals have been found in the kidney in a number of disorders, including chronic glomerulonephritis, chronic pyelonephritis, renal tubular acidosis, and acute tubular necrosis. In two recent reports the incidence of calcium oxalate crystals in post-mortem kidney specimens was 6.4 and 6.2 percent, respectively [42, 43]. In one study no statistical correlation was observed between the presence of crystalline deposits of oxalate in the kidney and the existence of renal disease [42]. Crystals have been found in the myocardium of 5 of 50 patients who died in uremia [44]. Deposition of calcium oxalate may occur in other extrarenal sites, particularly in damaged tissues, in the absence of any disorder of oxalate metabolism [45–47]. Although oxalosis may be much more extensive in patients with primary hyperoxaluria, in the individual patient it is difficult to utilize this pathologic feature as a diagnostic criterion of the disease.

The recent elucidation of the specific enzyme defects in patients with the two genetic variants of primary hyperoxaluria may allow the diagnosis to be made with greater specificity and accuracy in the future [4]. At the present time these techniques for enzymatic assay are not readily available. The pattern of urinary excretion or organic acids remains the major basis for diagnosis.

OXALIC ACID

Oxalic acid is a relatively strong dicarboxylic acid with K_{a_1} of 6.5×10^{-2} and K_{a_2} of 6.1×10^{-5}. It may be crystallized as a dihydrate, which loses water at 100°C. It forms acid and neutral salts, mono- and diesters, a monoamide known as *oxamic acid,* and a diamide called *oxamide.* Oxamate inhibits the enzymatic conversion of glyoxylate to oxalate catalyzed by lactic dehydrogenase [48]. Oxamide has been used in the experimental production of kidney stones [49].

The free acid is soluble in water to the extent of 8.7 gm per 100 gm of water at 20°C. At neutral or alkaline pH, the calcium salt of oxalate exhibits very low solubility in water (0.67 mg per 100 gm water at pH 7, 13°C). The precipitation of calcium oxalate is inhibited by a number of compounds, including urea, various ions [50] such as magnesium, iron, copper, zinc, citrate, sulfate, and lactate, certain colloids [51], and some recently described small-molecular-weight polypeptides [52]. Inorganic pyrophosphate also inhibits the precipitation of calcium oxalate from aqueous solutions. Although urine is frequently supersaturated with calcium oxalate under physiologic conditions, precipitation is presumably prevented by the large number of inhibitors present in normal urine.

The oxidation of oxalic acid by potassium permanganate

has been used for its quantitative determination. In the presence of zinc and sulfuric acid, oxalic acid is successively and quantitatively reduced to glyoxylic and glycolic acids. A specific enzyme, oxalic acid decarboxylase, catalyzes the conversion of oxalate to carbon dioxide and formate [53]. Calcium oxalate is a common constituent of renal stones, being found in approximately 67 percent of all calculi [54]. In calculi it occurs as both the mono- and dihydrate, and rarely as the trihydrate. Calcium oxalate monohydrate, or Whewellite, is the most common form found in stones [54]. The typical ditetragonal pyramid crystals, or "envelope" crystals, found commonly in urine samples represent the dihydrate form (Weddellite) [54].

Absorption of Oxalate

Although oxalic acid is found in high concentration in certain plants (e.g., spinach and rhubarb), its biochemical function in plants has not been established. Oxalate is present in a normal diet, being found in highest concentration in spinach, rhubarb, parsley, cocoa, and tea. Smaller amounts are found in beans, carrots, and celery [55]. The content of oxalate in a typical diet has been reported as 930 mg and 97 mg [55–57]. This wide discrepancy calls for further study. Ingested oxalate is poorly absorbed from the gastrointestinal tract; only 2.3 to 4.5 percent of ingested sodium oxalate (800 to 3,200 mg) was absorbed by normal subjects as judged by the resulting increases in urinary oxalate [56], and similar percentages have been reported in two patients with hyperoxaluria [58]. Calcium oxalate is less well absorbed than sodium oxalate. No studies have been reported concerning the mechanism of absorption by intestinal mucosa.

Biosynthesis of Oxalate

In mammalian systems the synthesis of oxalic acid occurs through two separate pathways: (1) as an end product in the oxidative metabolism of ascorbic acid, and (2) by oxidation of glyoxylic acid. Although oxalate may be formed from a number of other precursors in microorganisms, particularly oxaloacetate, oxalosuccinate, and β-ketoadipate [59], in mammalian systems the major precursor of oxalate is glyoxylate. Evidence suggests that glyoxylate is formed primarily from glycine, glycolic acid, and α-keto-γ-hydroxyglutamic acid in man, although other precursors have not been excluded. In microorganisms isocitric acid is the major source of glyoxylic acid, its cleavage being catalyzed by isocitrate lyase [60]. This enzyme has not yet been identified in mammalian systems. Although tryptophan has been described as a source of oxalate in man [61], it is likely that such a conversion occurs through interconversion with serine and eventually glyoxylate. There is no evidence that tryptophan is of quantitative importance as an oxalate precursor. In the rat, phenylalanine and tyrosine give rise to oxalate, presumably by autooxidation of their respective α-keto analogues [62].

Ascorbic Acid Pathway

Ascorbic acid is a precursor of urinary oxalate in several laboratory animals and in man [63–66]. In vivo studies with isotopic ascorbate indicate that oxalate is derived from carbon atoms 1 and 2 of the parent compound. The pathways of ascorbic acid metabolism in man are not thoroughly understood. Although some controversy exists, it seems probable from recent studies that ascorbic acid is not metabolized significantly to respiratory carbon dioxide in man [67]. Ascorbate is probably first oxidized to dehydroascorbate and then hydrolyzed to 2,3-diketogulonic acid, with subsequent conversion of this compound to oxalate and L-threose [67]. There is some evidence, however, that 2,3-diketogulonic acid is not an intermediate in ascorbate metabolism and that cleavage of the C2—C3 bond may occur enzymatically while the ascorbate lactone ring is still intact [67]. The question of whether glyoxylate is an intermediate in ascorbate metabolism is unresolved, but the absence of $^{14}CO_2$ after administration of ascorbate-^{14}C to man makes this possibility unlikely.

Ascorbic acid has been established as an oxalate precursor by isotope techniques as noted, accounting for perhaps 35

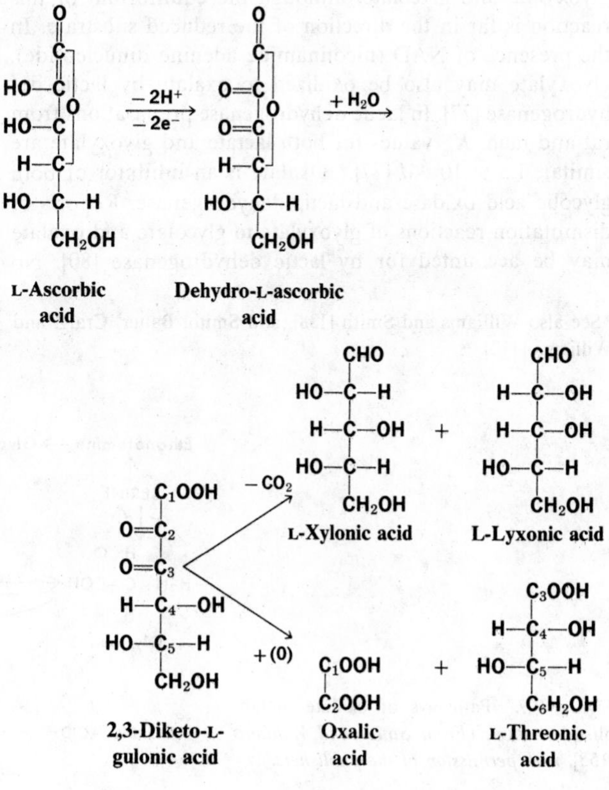

L-Ascorbic acid $\xrightarrow{-2H^+,\ -2e^-}$ Dehydro-L-ascorbic acid $\xrightarrow{+H_2O}$ 2,3-Diketo-L-gulonic acid

2,3-Diketo-L-gulonic acid $\xrightarrow{-CO_2}$ L-Xylonic acid + L-Lyxonic acid

2,3-Diketo-L-gulonic acid $\xrightarrow{+(0)}$ Oxalic acid + L-Threonic acid

to 50 percent of that normally excreted. Synthesis of oxalate from ascorbate must be maximally operative under normal conditions, since ingestion of large amounts of ascorbic acid (4 gm) does not increase urinary oxalate [68, 69]. The mechanisms of control of oxalate synthesis from ascorbic acid have not been studied.

Glyoxylic Acid Pathway

The conversion of glyoxylate to oxalate may be catalyzed by three enzymes—glycolic acid oxidase, xanthine oxidase, and lactic dehydrogenase. The first enzyme, a flavoprotein, catalyzes both the conversion of glycolate to glyoxylate [70, 71] and of glyoxylate to oxalate [72]. This latter step is functionally irreversible. Xanthine oxidase, also a flavoprotein which has been studied extensively in man [73], similarly catalyzes the oxidation of glyoxylate to oxalate in mammalian tissues [74]. Recent studies of this reaction in human liver tissue indicate that xanthine oxidase plays only a minor role, if any, in the overall production of oxalate from glyoxylate in the intact human subject [75]. Administration of the xanthine oxidase inhibitor allopurinol to gouty subjects did not alter the daily excretion of oxalate [75], and two patients with hereditary xanthinuria, with a genetic deficiency of xanthine oxidase, have had normal oxalate excretion [75].

Glyoxylate is a substrate for lactic dehydrogenase [76–79]. This enzyme can bring about the reversible conversion of glyoxylate and glycolate, although the equilibrium of this reaction is far in the direction of the reduced substrate. In the presence of NAD (nicotinamide adenine dinucleotide), glyoxylate may also be oxidized to oxalate by lactic dehydrogenase [77]. In lactic dehydrogenase preparations from rat and man, K_m values for both lactate and glyoxylate are similar, $1.5 \times 10^{-3}M$ [77].* Oxalate is an inhibitor of both glycolic acid oxidase and lactic dehydrogenase. Reports of dismutation reactions of glyoxylate to glycolate and oxalate may be accounted for by lactic dehydrogenase [80]. No specific mutase for glyoxylate has been demonstrated. Some dismutation of glyoxylic acid to oxalic and glycolic acids occurs nonenzymatically in vitro at neutral pH.

*See also Williams and Smith [138], and Smith, Bauer, Craig, and Williams [112].

Precursors of Glyoxylate

Three immediate precursors of glyoxylate in man are known: glycine, glycolic acid, and α-keto-γ-hydroxyglutarate (Fig. 9-7). Although other pathways may exist, they have not as yet been described. Glycine is a major precursor of oxalate and therefore presumably of glyoxylate in man. In an important study, Crawhall et al. administered glycine-1-^{13}C every 6 hr to a control subject over a period of 4 days and in this manner obtained constant isotopic enrichment of the free glycine pool, as judged by the isotopic content of urinary glycine [81]. At equilibrium urinary oxalate was approximately 40 percent as highly labeled as urinary free glycine (Fig. 9-8). If urinary free glycine is a valid sample of the first glycine pool, these data indicate that a similar percentage of oxalate normally derives from glycine. Glycine-^{14}C has also been demonstrated as an oxalate precursor in five normal subjects, approximately 0.051 percent of that administered appearing in urinary oxalate [39]. In a more recent study by Dean and coworkers [82], the conversion of both glycine-1-^{13}C and glycine-2-^{13}C into urinary oxalate was studied in a single patient with primary hyperoxaluria. Estimations based on the degree of isotope dilution between free urinary glycine and urinary oxalate indicated that about 10 percent of oxalate derived from glycine. The rate of disappearance of ^{13}C from urinary oxalate could be resolved into a single exponential component following glycine-1-^{13}C administration, and into two exponential components following glycine-2-^{13}C administration. These studies were thought to be consistent with the operation of two metabolic pathways in the conversion of glycine to oxalate, one by direct conversion of glycine to glyoxylate and oxalate, and a second involving the interconversion of glycine with serine, followed by the formation of ethanolamine, glycolaldehyde, glycolate, glyoxylate, and oxalate (Fig. 9-7).

Although glycine is an important source of urinary oxalate, it is unlikely that a large proportion of glycine is metabolized by way of the glyoxylate pathway. In a 72-kg normal subject,

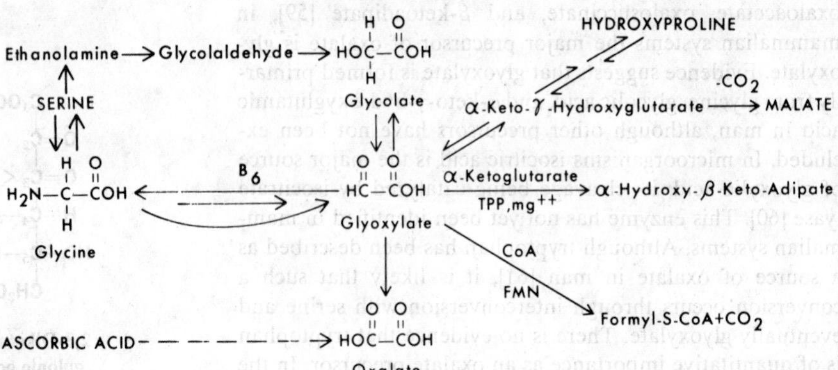

Figure 9-7. Pathways of oxalate metabolism in man. (*From Smith and Williams* [155], *with permission of the publishers.*)

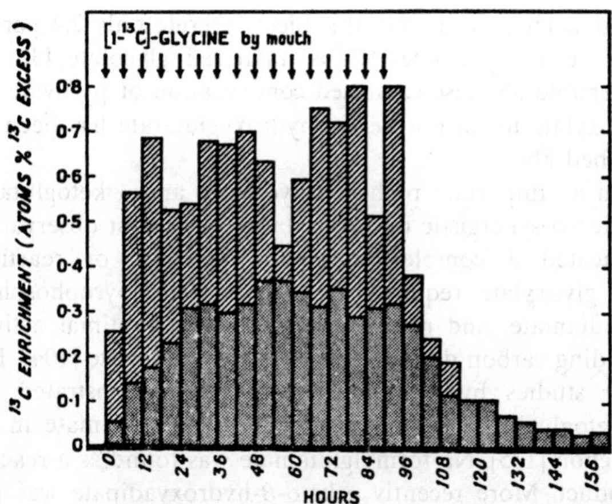

Figure 9-8. ^{13}C content of urinary oxalate (height of stippled columns) and of urinary glycine (combined heights of hatched and stippled columns) of a patient with primary hyperoxaluria. (*From Crawhall et al.* [81], *with permission of the authors and publishers.*)

a first glycine pool of 5.8 gm was found, with a turnover rate of 0.5 to 1.0 gm glycine per kg per day [83]. It can be calculated, with certain assumptions discussed elsewhere [3], that not more than 0.5 to 1.0 percent of the turnover of glycine is accountable by glyoxylate formation. This is consistent with the minimal changes in oxalate excretion which occur in normal subjects or in patients with primary hyperoxaluria when glycine is administered [58].

Glycine can be converted directly to glyoxylate by oxidative deamination catalyzed by glycine oxidase, or by transamination of glycine with a number of keto acids. It may be indirectly converted to glyoxylate by the serine-glycolate pathway (Fig. 9-7). Glycine oxidase, originally described in 1944 in mammalian liver and kidney preparations [84], oxidizes glycine to glyoxylate in the presence of flavin adenine dinucleotide. Evidence based on parallel activities during purification procedures suggests that this is the same enzyme as D-amino acid oxidase [85]. It belongs to the class of aerobic oxidases and yields H_2O_2 as a by-product.

$$\underset{\textbf{Glycine}}{\begin{array}{c}COOH\\|\\CH_2NH_2\end{array}} + O_2 + H_2O \longrightarrow \underset{\textbf{Glyoxylic acid}}{\begin{array}{c}COOH\\|\\CHO\end{array}} + NH_3 + H_2O_2$$

Although in theory glycine may also be converted to glyoxylate by reversible transamination reactions, all cases so far described have equilibria far in the direction of glycine synthesis. This is consistent with the finding that deficiency of pyridoxine, a cofactor in these reactions as pyridoxal phosphate, leads to increased rather than decreased oxalate synthesis [86, 87]. The transamination reactions of glyoxylate to form glycine will be described further below.

Glycolic acid is both a precursor and a product of glyoxylate. It is formed early in photosynthesis and so is present in plants, where it is the probable precursor of oxalate, glycine, and serine [88]. Administration of glycolic acid to the rat may lead to oxalosis and death in uremia [89]. The normal occurrence of glycolate in urine has been noted above (Fig. 9-6). Following the intravenous administration of a trace amount of glycolate-^{14}C, two normal control subjects excreted 1.03 percent as oxalate and 2.4 percent as unchanged glycolate over the subsequent 24 hr [3]. The only metabolic fate established for glycolate is its oxidation to glyoxylate and subsequent participation in the reactions summarized in Fig. 9-7. This oxidation is catalyzed by glycolic acid oxidase, a flavoprotein present in animals, plants, and microorganisms [70, 71]. In mammals the only known precursor of glycolate, other than glyoxylate, is glycolaldehyde. Glycolaldehyde may be formed from serine by way of ethanolamine [71] or from hydroxypyruvate catalyzed by pyruvate oxidase [90]. Glycolaldehyde also exists as a cofactor-bound intermediate in the transketolase reaction of the pentose-phosphate shunt pathway [91]. Oxidation of ethylene glycol, demonstrated as a component of a complex mammalian lipid [92], probably proceeds by way of glycolaldehyde. The oxidation of glycolaldehyde to glycolic acid is catalyzed by both aldehyde oxidases and dehydrogenases. The quantitative importance of the glycolaldehyde → glycolate → glyoxylate → oxalate pathway in man has not been determined.

In addition to glycine and glycolic acid, α-keto-γ-hydroxyglutarate is an immediate precursor of glyoxylate in mammalian systems (Fig. 9-7). This compound, formed during hydroxyproline catabolism, is reversibly converted to glyoxylate and pyruvate catalyzed by a specific aldolase [93]. It may also undergo oxidative decarboxylation to form malate [94]. Hydroxyketoglutarate aldolase activity is present but in low activity in human tissues [95]. In conditions associated with increased protein turnover and hydroxyprolinuria, no increase in urinary oxalate excretion has been observed, and administration of large doses of hydroxyproline to hyperoxaluric subjects failed to increase oxalate excretion [96]. In summary, current evidence does not suggest that hydroxyproline is an important precursor of glyoxylate and therefore of oxalate.

Pathways of Glyoxylate Metabolism

The alternate pathways of glyoxylate metabolism are important as they relate to possible mechanisms for in vivo accumulation of this oxalate precursor. Glyoxylate is an extremely versatile metabolic intermediate (Table 9-1), although not all its reactions can be demonstrated in mammalian systems. The oxidation of glyoxylate to oxalate has already been discussed. Glyoxylate may undergo transamination to glycine, with pyridoxal phosphate as a cofactor, a reaction or group of reactions extensively studied in preparations from animals, plants, and microorganisms [97, 98]. It has been reported that the most active amino donor in rat liver is glutamate, and partial purification of glutamate-

Table 9-1. ENZYMATIC REACTIONS IN GLYOXYLATE METABOLISM*

1. Glyoxylate + [0] ⟶ oxalate
2. Glyoxylate + L-glutamate $\xrightleftharpoons{B_6}$ glycine + α-ketoglutarate
3. Glyoxylate + L-ornithine $\xrightleftharpoons{B_6}$ glycine + glutamic-γ-semialdehyde
4. Glyoxylate + other amino acids $\xrightleftharpoons{B_6}$ glycine + keto acid
5. Glyoxylate $\xrightleftharpoons[-H]{+H}$ glycolate
6. Glyoxylate + α-ketoglutarate $\xrightarrow{TPP}$ α-hydroxy-β-ketoadipate
7. Glyoxylate + pyruvate ⇌ 2-keto-4-hydroxyglutarate
8. Glyoxylate + CoA $\xrightarrow{FMN}$ formyl-S-CoA + CO_2
9. Glyoxylate + acetyl CoA ⟶ malate + CoA
10. Glyoxylate + glyoxylate $\xrightarrow{TPP}$ tartronic semialdehyde + CO_2
11. Glyoxylate + urea ⟶ glyoxylurea
12. Glyoxylate + glycine ⟶ β-hydroxyaspartate
13. Glyoxylate + propionyl CoA ⟶ α-hydroxyglutarate + CoA
14. Glyoxylate + butyryl CoA ⟶ β-ethylmalate + CoA
15. Glyoxylate + valeryl CoA ⟶ β-η-propylmalate + CoA
16. Glyoxylate + succinate ⇌ isocitrate
17. Glyoxylate + pyruvate ⟶ lactaldehyde

* The first eight reactions have been found in mammalian systems. The remaining reactions have been described so far only in microorganisms or plants.

Source: From [4] with permission of the publishers.

glycine transaminase from human liver has been obtained [99]. In studies on transamination reactions of glyoxylate in human liver and kidney preparations from the laboratory of Williams and Smith, alanine was found to be the most active amino donor in both supernatant and particulate fractions [100]. Glyoxylate-ornithine transaminase was found only in the particulate fraction. Other amino acids, such as glutamine, arginine, and methionine, may be amino donors. In all these reactions the equilibrium lies far in the direction of glycine synthesis.

Glyoxylate may be reversibly reduced to glycolate (Fig. 9-7) in reactions catalyzed by three separate enzymes: lactic dehydrogenase [78], a NADH-linked glyoxylate reductase [101], and a separate NADPH-linked glyoxylate reductase [102]. The presence of specific glyoxylate reductases in man has not been established. Lactic dehydrogenase catalyzes a dismutation of glyoxylate, with partial reduction to glycolate and partial oxidation to oxalate [103]. It may account for the demonstrated conversion in vivo of glyoxylate-^{14}C to glycolate-^{14}C in human subjects. An average of 3.7 percent of administered glyoxylate-^{14}C was excreted as urinary glycolate-^{14}C within 24 hr in three control subjects [3]. This does not establish the percentage of glyoxylate normally reduced to glycolate, since control subjects excrete only 2.4 percent of injected glycolate-^{14}C as unaltered glycolate [3]. The reversible aldolase-catalyzed condensation of pyruvate and glyoxylate to form α-keto-γ-hydroxyglutarate has been described above.

In an important pathway glyoxylate and α-ketoglutarate undergo synergistic decarboxylation. The first observations indicated a complex enzymatic reaction, or reactions, for glyoxylate requiring NAD, thiamine pyrophosphate, L-glutamate, and manganese (Mn^{++}) for optimal activity, yielding carbon dioxide and N-formylglutamate [104]. Further studies by Crawhall and Watts demonstrated that α-ketoglutarate was more effective than glutamate in this reaction [105]. No formylglutamate was found as a reaction product. More recently α-keto-β-hydroxyadipate was proposed as the primary product of this carboligase reaction, with decarboxylation of α-ketoglutarate [106]. A partially purified enzyme from pig liver mitochondria catalyzed the synergistic decarboxylation of glyoxylate and α-ketoglutarate, but the products of the reaction were not identified [107]. Koch and coworkers have developed an assay for the activity of α-ketoglutarate:glyoxylate carboligase and have characterized the product as α-hydroxy-β-ketoadipate [108]. Activity was present in rat liver mitochondria and in cytoplasmic and mitochondrial fractions of human liver, kidney, and spleen. Both the cytoplasmic and mitochondrial enzymes had a similar pH optimum (6.5) and both required thiamine pyrophosphate and Mg^{++} for full activity. Lower levels of enzyme activity could also be detected in soluble and particulate fractions of skeletal muscle and in the particulate fraction of disrupted human leukocytes. The subsequent reactions and the purpose of the α-hydroxy-β-ketoadipate pathway have not been established.

Glyoxylate may react with CoA in the presence of flavin mononucleotide (FMN) to form formyl-S-CoA and carbon dioxide. This reaction, much less active in rat liver mitochondria than the carboligase reaction described in the previous paragraph [109], has not as yet been demonstrated in human tissue preparations.

Control of Oxalate Synthesis

Oxalate is a metabolic end product in man. All of the oxalate that is synthesized is excreted in the urine (see below). It has no known function even in leafy plants, where its concentration may reach levels of 14 gm per 100 gm of dry weight [57]. Its synthesis in mammalian systems appears to be the infortuitous result of the substrate versatility of glyoxylate for oxidation by enzymes with other primary catalytic functions: lactic dehydrogenase [76–79], glycolic acid oxidase [72], and xanthine oxidase [74]. As previously noted, the quantitative significance of these enzymes (or even the presence or absence of others) in glyoxylate oxidation has not been established. Recent studies of oxalate synthesis from glyoxylate in a dialyzed erythrocyte hemolysate preparation indicate that lactic dehydrogenase is the major enzyme responsible for this conversion in this in vitro preparation [110*a*]. Xanthine oxidase seems of least importance, since oxalate excretion is normal in hereditary xanthinuria [75] and allopurinol administration does not reduce oxalate excretion [75]. In three normal subjects only a small fraction, 11.7 percent, of intravenously administered glyoxylate-^{14}C was converted to oxalate, as judged by the urinary excretion of oxalate-^{14}C over the subsequent 24 hr. An increased percentage of glyoxylate is oxidized to oxalate when the glyoxylate pool is expanded in vitro, as demonstrated in the early studies of Nakada and Weinhouse [98], or in vivo as seen in primary hyperoxaluria (see below).

Oxalate exhibits product inhibition of its synthesis from glyoxylate catalyzed by partially purified glycolic acid oxidase [72] or by lactic dehydrogenase [48, 110*b*]. The recently described oxalate inhibition of oxalate synthesis in human erythrocytes may reflect oxalate inhibition of lactic dehydrogenase [111]. Oxalate inhibition of glyoxylate oxidation by glycolic acid oxidase is competitive in nature, with a K_i of 3.1×10^{-3} at pH 7.3 [72]. Inhibition of lactic dehydrogenase by oxalate demonstrates more complex kinetics, suggesting competition and also the formation of an inactive complex [48]. Pharmacologic agents which inhibit oxalate synthesis will be described below.

The oxidation of glyoxylate to oxalate by lactic dehydrogenase may be enhanced by pyruvate [103] or by hydroxypyruvate [112]. It is likely that this occurs through the reoxidation of the LDH (lactate dehydrogenase)-NADH complex. Enhancement of oxalate synthesis from glyoxylate by intact human erythrocytes, erythrocyte hemolysates, and rat liver supernatant can be demonstrated by the addition of hydroxypyruvate to the medium [112]. In partially purified lactic dehydrogenase preparations in the presence of NADH, both hydroxypyruvate and pyruvate increase the synthesis of oxalate from glyoxylate [112]. This may be the mechanism of the increased oxalate synthesis in L-glyceric aciduria (see below).

Catabolism of Oxalate

Oxalate may be further metabolized in microorganisms by direct decarboxylation [113] or by the intermediate formation of oxalyl-coenzyme A [114]. In man it is a nonessential end product of metabolism. Radioactive oxalate administered to rats is excreted unchanged in urine and feces, and respiratory CO_2 and urinary hippurate are not labeled [64, 115, 116]. Small amounts of oxalate may be stored in bone following large doses. Oxalate-^{14}C given intravenously to normal man does not label respiratory carbon dioxide, and 89 to 99 percent is recovered unchanged in the urine [39]. It is possible that a small amount of oxalate may be excreted in succus entericus and bile, with subsequent bacterial degradation in the intestinal lumen, a mechanism analogous to that of urate degradation. If so, the amounts destroyed must be small. The normal synthetic rate of oxalate can be calculated from its pool size (3.5 to 6.1 mg) and turnover rate (biologic half-time of 2.2 to 2.8 hr) as being 24 to 46 mg per day [39]. This figure agrees closely with the normal urinary excretory rate.

Excretion of Oxalate

In man, oxalate is excreted almost exclusively in the urine. Studies of the renal clearance of oxalate in man and laboratory animals have led to different conclusions. In the dog, using isotopic oxalate, Cattell and coworkers [117] have demonstrated three mechanisms in the renal excretion of oxalate: glomerular filtration, secretion in the proximal part of the nephron, and reabsorption by passive back diffusion. Net tubular secretion of oxalate was demonstrated with an oxalate/inulin clearance ratio averaging 1.28. Clearance of oxalate was reduced by caronamide, probenecid, and para-aminohippurate, but was unaffected by urine pH. In contrast to these findings, Zarembski and Hodgkinson [36] reported the renal clearance of oxalate in normal adults to be 3.4 to 5.0 ml per min and found an oxalate clearance of 12.4 to 51.3 ml per min in seven hyperoxaluric subjects, with oxalate/creatinine clearance ratios varying between 0.23 and 0.94. These studies have suggested a renal tubular defect in the reabsorption of oxalate in primary hyperoxaluria, but such a defect alone could not account for accumulation of calcium oxalate in the body in the face of excessive excretion. Recently, the renal clearance of oxalate in normal adults and patients with primary hyperoxaluria (Types I and II) has been restudied by Williams et al. [118], using an isotopic oxalate method similar to that used by Cattell and coworkers in the dog [117]. With this technique the calculated clearance of oxalate in man averaged 169 ml per min, with an oxalate/inulin clearance ratio of 1.6. In patients with both types of primary hyperoxaluria, the renal clearance of oxalate and the ratio of oxalate clearance to inulin clearance were not significantly different from those in normal subjects [118]. These differences in the reported oxalate clearance in man appear to be related to differences in methods of study. The results with isotopic oxalate in man, consistent with previous studies in the dog, raise questions concerning the accuracy of current methods for determining plasma oxalate.

THE PATHOGENESIS OF PRIMARY HYPEROXALURIA TYPE I (GLYCOLIC ACIDURIA)

Excessive accumulation of oxalate, or for that matter of any metabolite in the body, could result from one or a combination of the four variables listed in Table 9-2: increased absorption, decreased excretion, decreased catabolism, or increased biosynthesis.

Two patients with primary hyperoxaluria absorbed 1.2 to 5.4 percent of administered sodium oxalate, amounts com-

Table 9-2. METABOLIC DERANGEMENTS WHICH MIGHT RESULT IN OXALATE ACCUMULATION, CONTRASTED WITH CONDITION IN PRIMARY HYPEROXALURIA

Derangement	Primary Hyperoxaluria
1. Increased gastrointestinal absorption of oxalate	Normal gastrointestinal absorption
2. Decreased excretion of oxalate	Persistent hyperoxaluria
3. Decreased catabolism of oxalate	Not metabolized in man
4. Increased biosynthesis of oxalate	Increased biosynthesis

parable to those in a control series [58]. If recent figures of dietary content of oxalate are correct, even complete absorption could not account for the excessive amounts excreted in primary hyperoxaluria [3]. Reduction in excretion cannot primarily account for the accumulation of oxalate, since continued excessive excretion is the diagnostic hallmark of these genetic disorders. Reduced excretion may exacerbate oxalosis after renal failure occurs. Although increased clearance of oxalate has been reported in patients with primary hyperoxaluria [36], recent results obtained in the laboratory of Williams and Smith have demonstrated normal renal clearances in this disorder [118]. Furthermore, increased clearance of oxalate could not account for its pathologic accumulation as oxalosis. Oxalate is not normally catabolized in man, as reviewed above. Therefore, the continued excessive excretion of oxalate characteristic of primary hyperoxaluria must result from its increased rate of biosynthesis.

As reviewed above, the only known immediate precursors of oxalate in man are ascorbate and glyoxylate. In an important study using ascorbic acid-1-^{13}C, Atkins and coworkers demonstrated that the pool size, turnover rate, and metabolic conversion of ascorbate to urinary oxalate were similar in a control subject and in two patients with primary hyperoxaluria [119]. Less than 10 percent of the urinary oxalate in the patients derived from the oxidation of ascorbate, the absolute amount of ascorbate converted to oxalate being normal. Administration of large amounts of ascorbate to patients with primary hyperoxaluria failed to increase urinary oxalate [68, 69]. An abnormality of ascorbic acid metabolism cannot, therefore, be implicated as contributing to the excessive oxalate synthesis in these genetic disorders. By elimination, increased oxidation of glyoxylate offers the most likely explanation for enhanced oxalate synthesis in primary hyperoxaluria. Such increased synthesis might result from (1) an increased activity of the enzymes which oxidize glyoxylate to oxalate, or (2) an increased concentration of glyoxylate, most probably secondary to a block in an alternate pathway of metabolism.

Quantitative in vitro studies of the activities of enzymes which oxidize glyoxylate to oxalate in man are complicated by lack of information concerning their relative importance. [110*a*]. Within these limitations it has been demonstrated that glyoxylate conversion to oxalate is not enhanced in preparations of liver mitochondria [105], whole homogenates of liver and kidney [2], or in erythrocytes [111] from patients with primary hyperoxaluria Type I (glycolic aciduria). In addition no abnormality in oxalate inhibition of oxalate synthesis from glyoxylate was found in erythrocytes from hyperoxaluric patients. Secondary enhancement of enzyme activity may be the proximate cause of increased oxalate synthesis in L-glyceric aciduria, as noted below, but does not appear to contribute to that of glycolic aciduria. The evidence for accumulation of glyoxylate secondary to its impaired metabolism in vivo and in the in vitro studies of the site of the enzymatic defect will now be reviewed briefly.

In Vivo Studies of Glyoxylate Metabolism in Primary Hyperoxaluria

Early studies of the pathogenesis of primary hyperoxaluria were directed toward establishing the presence of glyoxylate accumulation in the disease and compiling evidence for its impaired metabolism. The measurement of glyoxylate in biologic fluids was found to be unreliable because of its nonenzymatic reactivity with a number of other normal metabolites [31]. Within these limitations the excretion of glyoxylate was found to be elevated above the normal range (0.5 to 4.4 mg per 1.73 m^2 per 24 hr) in 6 of 7 patients with primary hyperoxaluria Type I (Fig. 9-6). Reports to the contrary not withstanding [120], in the opinion of Williams and Smith no reliable method is now available for measuring glyoxylate in blood or plasma. It was reasoned that if the glyoxylate pool were expanded, increased reduction to glycolate might occur, in line with its increased oxidation to oxalate. As described above, hyperglycolic aciduria was found to be as characteristic of the disorder as hyperoxaluria (Fig. 9-6) [31]. In fact its demonstration is the most direct method for the diagnosis of the Type I variant of the disease.

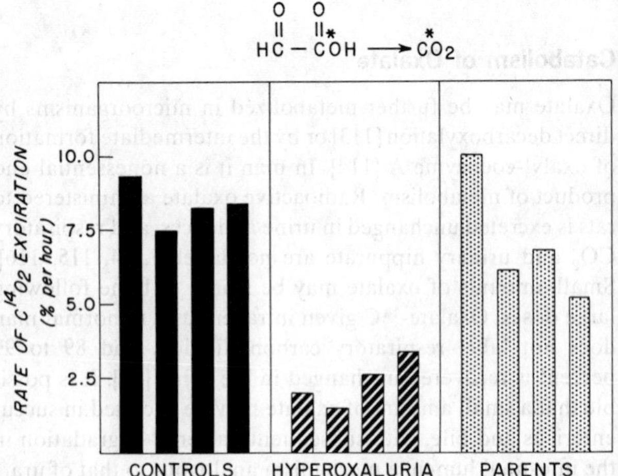

Figure 9-9. Metabolism of carboxyl-labeled glyoxylic acid-^{14}C. (*From Frederick et al.* [121], *with permission of the publishers.*)

Table 9-3. INCORPORATION OF GLYOXYLATE-1-^{14}C INTO URINARY OXALATE AND GLYCOLATE

Subjects	Percentage of isotope administered					
	Urinary oxalate			Urinary glycolate		
	0–2 hr	2–24 hr	0–24 hr	0–2 hr	2–24 hr	0–24 hr
Controls (3)	5.3	6.4	11.7	3.0	0.7	3.7
Parents (4)	14.1	6.1	20.2	2.7	0.5	3.2
Patients (4)	9.7	15.6	25.3	5.4	9.4	14.8

Source: From Frederick, Rabkin, Richie, and Smith [121].

The metabolism of glyoxylate-1-^{14}C (1 μmole per kg body weight intravenously) is altered in primary hyperoxaluria, with a diminished rate of conversion to respiratory carbon dioxide (Fig. 9-9) and increased excretion as urinary oxalate and glycolate (Table 9-3) [121]. In these same studies three of four parents of patients with primary hyperoxaluria demonstrated rates of carbon dioxide production from glyoxylate-^{14}C less than those of the control subjects. This suggested a partial defect in these presumed heterozygotes [121]. One of the parents metabolized glyoxylate at a normal rate. A similar impairment of glyoxylate-^{14}C metabolism to carbon dioxide, together with increased urinary excretion as glycolate and oxalate, was found during constant intravenous infusion of the isotope over a 6-hr period in order to obtain equilibrium rates [3].

Because of the close precursor-product relationship of glycolate with glyoxylate, similar in vivo studies of glycolate metabolism were performed in patients with primary hyperoxaluria [3]. In confirmation of the results with glyoxylate, the metabolism of intravenously administered glycolate-1-^{14}C to respiratory carbon dioxide was reduced, while its conversion to urinary oxalate and its excretion as unaltered glycolate-^{14}C were increased when compared with control subjects (Table 9-4).

The contribution of glycine to urinary oxalate has been studied by two different methods in patients with primary hyperoxaluria [39, 81]. Glycine-1-^{13}C was administered over 4 days in order to obtain constant isotope enrichment of the free glycine pool, as reflected in the isotopic content of urinary glycine [81]. At equilibrium the fractions of urinary oxalate derived from glycine were 50 and 32 percent, respectively, in two patients with primary hyperoxaluria, values comparable to that found in a control subject (40 percent). In another patient with primary hyperoxaluria the cumulative incorporation of glycine-^{14}C (given as a single oral tracer dose) into urinary oxalate was 0.22 percent, a value about four times higher than that found in five control subjects (0.051 percent) [39]. Because the degree of the increased incorporation of isotope approximated the degree of hyperoxaluria, the interpretation was made that the fractional contribution of glycine to oxalate synthesis was unchanged in the patient with primary hyperoxaluria. This observation, confirmatory of the glycine-^{13}C studies cited above, would be more consistent with a defect in the further metabolism of glyoxylate than with a selective overproduction of glyoxylate from one of its precursors.

In the studies with glyoxylate-^{14}C and glycolate-^{14}C the incorporation of isotope into urinary glycine was found to be diminished (Table 9-4) [3]. It has been established that pyridoxine deficiency results in hyperoxaluria in experimental animals [86] and in man [87]. This presumably represents a block in one or more of the transamination reactions which convert glyoxylate to glycine and in which pyridoxal phosphate serves as a cofactor. On the basis of these in vivo studies it seemed most likely that the enzymatic defect would be found in one of the transamination reactions, representing biochemically the apoenzyme equivalent of pyridoxine deficiency. As noted below, this has not been confirmed.

In Vitro Studies of the Enzymatic Defect in Glyoxylate Metabolism

In vitro studies of glyoxylate metabolism have been carried out using tissue preparations of liver, kidney, spleen, erythrocytes, and leukocytes from patients with primary hyperoxaluria Type I. Because of the in vivo studies outlined above, particular attention has been directed to the transamination reactions (with various amino donors) for the conversion of glyoxylate to glycine. Studies from two laboratories have failed to demonstrate any impairment of glycine synthesis from glyoxylate in whole homogenates, or soluble or particulate preparations from liver specimens

Table 9-4. DISPOSITION OF GLYCOLATE-1-^{14}C IN HYPEROXALURIC AND CONTROL SUBJECTS

Subjects	Percentage of isotope administered												
	Expired CO_2	Urinary oxalate			Urinary glyoxylate			Urinary hippurate			Urinary glycolate		
	0–2 hr	0–2 hr	2–24 hr	0–24 hr	0–2 hr	2–24 hr	0–24 hr	0–2 hr	2–24 hr	0–24 hr	0–2 hr	2–24 hr	0–24 hr
Controls (2)	18.2	0.9	0.13	1.03	0.09	0.03	0.12	2.50	0.48	2.98	2.3	0.1	2.4
Parent (1)	20.5	1.1	0.07	1.17	0.16	0	0.16	5.8	0.42	6.22	2.8	0.1	2.9
Patients (2)	2.6	4.1	13.4	17.5	0.27	0.12	0.39	0.29	0.22	0.51	12.2	26.0	38.2

Source: From Hockaday et al. [3] with permission of the publishers.

obtained from patients with primary hyperoxaluria [2, 105, 122]. These studies were carried out using glutamic acid and alanine as amino donors. More recently Dean et al. have reported reduced glycine synthesis from glyoxylate in kidney homogenates from two patients with primary hyperoxaluria [123, 124], one of whom had normal hepatic glyoxylate transaminase activity [124]. Low levels of renal transaminase activity were similarly found in kidney preparations from three patients by Williams et al., but control specimens from uremic patients demonstrated equally reduced activities [100]. It is clear that the enzymatic defect of primary hyperoxaluria cannot be confined to the kidneys, since excessive oxalate synthesis continues following bilateral nephrectomy in association with renal transplantation [125]. Williams and Smith conclude that no defect in glyoxylate transamination has been firmly established in vitro. It is possible that the wrong amino donors have been used or that a defect in the kinetics of the reaction(s) has been overlooked. The partial reversal of hyperoxaluria by excess pyridoxine (see below) may represent cofactor enzyme induction or stabilization, or possibly may indicate another pyridoxine dependency syndrome [126]. The requirement for added pyridoxal phosphate could not be demonstrated in vitro. In view of the demonstrated defect in the soluble carboligase reaction to be described, it seems most probable that the in vivo studies indicating reduced conversion of glyoxylate-^{14}C to urinary glycine-^{14}C reflect the expanded glyoxylate pool together with the small amount of the daily glycine pool which is excreted ($<$1 percent).

The reaction of glyoxylate with α-ketoglutarate to form α-hydroxy-β-ketoadipate has been described above (Fig. 9-7). This reaction sequence leads to the synergistic decarboxylation of glyoxylate and α-ketoglutarate. No abnormality in the activity of this pathway was found in liver mitochondria from three patients with primary hyperoxaluria by Crawhall and Watts [122]. Subsequently Koch et al. studied the activity of α-ketoglutarate: glyoxylate carboligase in cytoplasmic and mitochondrial preparations from liver, kidney, and spleen from five patients with primary

2-OXO-GLUTARATE: GLYOXYLATE CARBOLIGASE

$$\mathrm{OHC{-}COOH} \xrightarrow[\text{TPP, } Mg^{++}]{\alpha KG} \mathrm{HOC(=O){-}CH_2{-}CH_2{-}C(=O){-}CHOH{-}COOH} + CO_2$$

	LIVER C	LIVER PH	SPLEEN C	SPLEEN PH	KIDNEY C	KIDNEY PH

ENZYME ACTIVITY nmoles/mg·protein^{-1}xhr^{-1} (0, 25, 50, 75, 100)

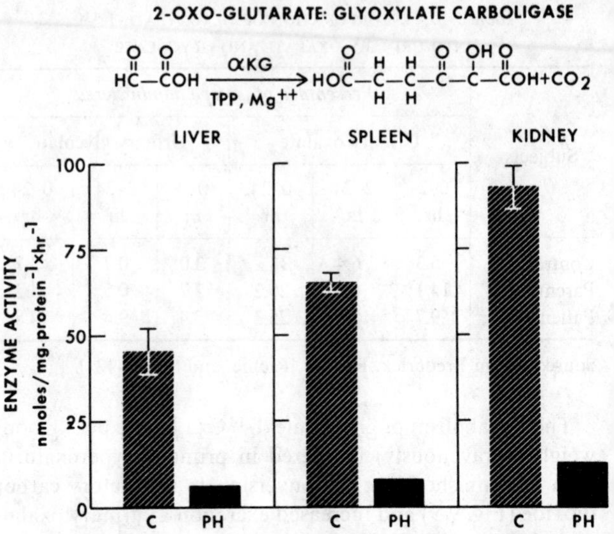

Figure 9-10. α-Ketoglutarate: glyoxylate carboligase activity in tissues from patients with primary hyperoxaluria, Type I (*PH*), and control subjects (*C*). (*From Williams and Smith* [4], *with permission of the publishers.*)

hyperoxaluria compared with control subjects undergoing renal homotransplantation because of uremia secondary to chronic glomerulonephritis [108]. In confirmation of the work of Crawhall and Watts, enzyme activity in mitochondria was found to be within the control range. In contrast, the activity of soluble α-ketoglutarate: glyoxylate carboligase was reduced markedly in all three organs (Fig. 9-10). No inhibition of activity was found on mixing hyperoxaluric and control enzyme preparations, nor was carboligase activity inhibited by oxalate or glycolate, which are overproduced in primary hyperoxaluria [3]. These data indicate a specific defect in the cytoplasmic carboligase, presumably an isoenzyme of the mitochondrial enzyme, as the cause of glyoxylate accumulation in primary hyperoxaluria. This concept of the disease is illustrated in Fig. 9-11. The consequences of this

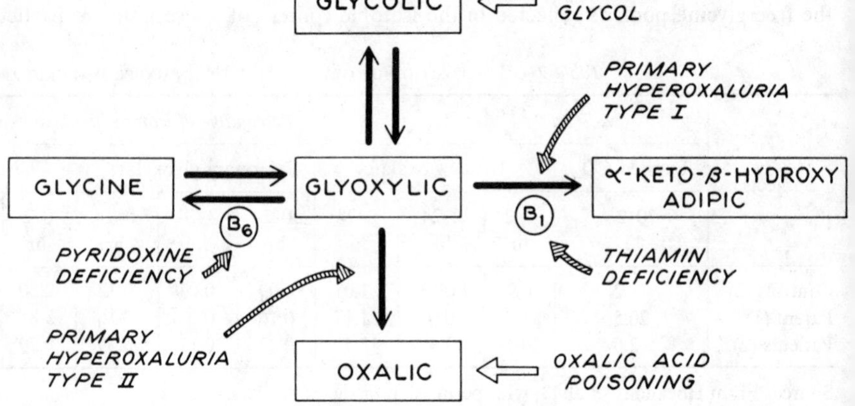

Figure 9-11. Disorders of oxalate metabolism in man. The open arrows indicate exogenous causes of hyperoxaluria. The cross-hatched arrows indicate the known acquired and hereditary enzyme defects or mechanisms leading to hyperoxaluria. (*From Williams and Smith* [4], *with permission of the publishers.*)

defect suggest that the cytoplasmic carboligase is of major importance in the further metabolism of glyoxylate. At the present time no studies have been carried out on the activity of soluble α-ketoglutarate: glyoxylate carboligase in preparations from presumed heterozygotes of primary hyperoxaluria.

Recently Bourke et al. [127] found normal activity of α-ketoglutarate: glyoxylate carboligase in both mitochondrial and soluble cytoplasmic fractions of skeletal muscle from a 10-year-old patient with Type I primary hyperoxaluria. Although other tissues were not examined in this patient, Bourke et al. suggested that this finding indicated further biochemical heterogeneity in primary hyperoxaluria.

THE PATHOGENESIS OF PRIMARY HYPEROXALURIA TYPE II (L-GLYCERIC ACIDURIA)

Recently, four patients (three of them sibs) were found to have excessive excretion of oxalate but normal excretion of glycolate. By chromatographic techniques a new organic acid was found in their urine, which was identified as L-glyceric acid by color reaction with chromotropic acid, quantitative conversion to glyoxylate by periodate oxidation, purification to constant specific activity after the addition of glycerate-^{14}C, substrate specificity with D-glyceric dehydrogenase and lactic dehydrogenase, and optical rotatory dispersion curves [5]. By an isotope-dilution method, L-glycerate excretion was found to be between 225 and 638 mg per 24 hr per 1.73 m^2 in the urine of patients with this disorder [40]. No L-glycerate was found in normal urine using this isotope-dilution technique. Urinary glyoxylate level was not elevated in the two patients studied [3]. A consideration of the pathogenesis of L-glyceric aciduria requires a brief review of glyceric acid and hydroxypyruvic acid metabolism.

Glyceric Acid and Hydroxypyruvic Acid Metabolism

Glyceric acid is a relatively weak acid, with many properties similar to those of lactic and glycolic acids. The L- form of glyceric acid forms calcium salts which are soluble in water to the extent of 1 gm in 10 ml water. The D- form also forms calcium salts, which are somewhat less soluble. The free acid is soluble in water, alcohol, and acetone. It can be prepared either by oxidation of glyceraldehyde or by the action of nitrous acid on serine.

The major source of glyceric acid in both plants and mammals is hydroxypyruvic acid (Fig. 9-12). D-Glyceric acid is produced from hydroxypyruvate by the enzyme D-glycerate dehydrogenase (hydroxypyruvate reductase). This enzyme has been studied extensively in plant, animal, and microbial systems [128–130]. The enzyme purified from calf liver utilizes NADH and NADPH equally well as hydrogen donors [130]. L-Glycerate, L-lactate, and glycolate will not serve as substrates for the enzyme. Glyoxylate is reduced to glycolate by this enzyme but more slowly than is hydroxypyruvate. The relative K_m values are: hydroxypyruvate—$4.5 \times 10^{-5}M$ (with NADH) and $2.0 \times 10^{-5}M$ (with NADPH), glyoxylate—$1.4 \times 10^{-4}M$ (with NADH) and $2.5 \times 10^{-4}M$ (with NADPH). The equilibrium of the reaction between hydroxypyruvate and glycerate strongly favors the reduced product, although the oxidative reaction is shifted to favor hydroxypyruvate synthesis at pH 9 in the presence of carbonyl-trapping reagents. D-Glycerate dehydrogenase purified from spinach leaves differs from the mammalian enzyme in its specificity for NADH [131]. Similar to the calf-liver enzyme, the spinach preparation utilizes both hydroxypyruvate and glyoxylate as substrates, but the maximal rate of reduction of hydroxypyruvate is four to five times that observed with glyoxylate. Crystalline D-glycerate dehydrogenase prepared from *Pseudomonas acidovorans* utilizes only hydroxypyruvate as substrate; no activity is observed with either pyruvate or glyoxylate [132]. A flavoprotein enzyme, D-α-hydroxy acid dehydrogenase, has been reported in yeast and mammalian liver and kidney mitochondria [133]. This enzyme has a wide specificity for many hydroxy acids, including D-glycerate, D-lactate, D-α-hydroxybutyrate, and D-malate.

Evidence in plants and bacteria has suggested the similarity of D-glycerate dehydrogenase and the NADH-linked glyoxylate reductase [131]. This latter enzyme has activity

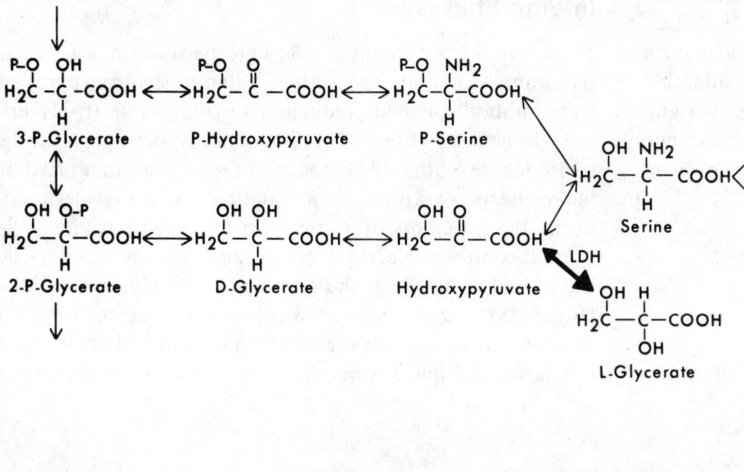

Figure 9-12. Pathways of serine and glycerate metabolism in mammalian systems. *LDH,* lactic dehyrogenase. (*From Williams and Smith* [40], *with permission of the publishers.*)

with both glyoxylate and hydroxypyruvate as substrates, but the maximal rate of activity with glyoxylate is three times that with hydroxypyruvate. In *Pseudomonas* preparations, D-glycerate dehydrogenase has many of the properties of glyoxylate reductase, including stimulation at high ionic strength, similar pH optimum, and inhibition with dihydroxyfumarate [132]. At the present time, the question of whether glyoxylate reductase and D-glycerate dehydrogenase represent different enzymes in mammalian systems has not been resolved.

In mammalian systems L-glyceric acid is the product of the reduction of hydroxypyruvate by lactic dehydrogenase in the presence of NADH [128]. L-Glycerate is as effective a substrate as L-lactate for the lactate dehydrogenases of skeletal and heart muscle [134]. The equilibrium of the oxidation-reduction of L-glycerate and hydroxypyruvate catalyzed by lactic dehydrogenase favors the reduced product.

As discussed above, hydroxypyruvate is a substrate for both D-glyceric acid and lactic dehydrogenase. It is the only known immediate precursor of L-glycerate. The major source of hydroxypyruvate is serine, an interconversion catalyzed by an alanine:hydroxypyruvate transaminase described in mammalian liver preparations, including adult and fetal human liver [135]. Glutamine has also been described as an effective amino donor for this enzyme.

Hydroxypyruvate is an important intermediate in both the synthesis and metabolism of serine (Fig. 9-12). In animals both phosphorylated and nonphosphorylated pathways exist for serine biosynthesis, the relative activity of the enzymes involved in these pathways varying widely in the species studied [136]. The regulation of these pathways, which has been studied extensively in animals, involves dietary factors, pyruvate, and product inhibition [129, 136]. In rats fed high-protein diets, depression of 3-phosphoglycerate dehydrogenase and phosphoserine dehydratase activities has been observed [129]. On low-protein diets an inverse relationship of these enzymes exists. With dietary manipulations no change in D-glycerate dehydrogenase was observed. In contrast, cortisone treatment of rats produced a 60 percent decrease in D-glycerate dehydrogenase activity and an 80 percent decrease in 3-phosphoglycerate dehydrogenase activity [137]. These studies have suggested that in the rat, the phosphorylated pathway is more important for serine biosynthesis and the nonphosphorylated pathway for gluconeogenesis and serine catabolism. Similar findings have been reported in beef and chicken liver, although considerable serine biosynthesis occurs by both pathways in pig liver and dog kidney [136]. The relative importance of these two pathways for the biosynthesis of serine in man has not been fully resolved (see below).

In Vivo Studies

The excretion of excessive amounts of L-glyceric acid in primary hyperoxaluria Type II suggested an abnormality in hydroxypyruvate metabolism with its secondary reduction catalyzed by lactic dehydrogenase. This would be analogous to the excessive reduction of glyoxylate to glycolate in primary hyperoxaluria Type I. In order to determine precursor-product relationships, hydroxypyruvate-1-^{14}C was given intravenously to a patient with L-glyceric aciduria [5]. Approximately 15 percent of the injected isotope was recovered in urinary L-glycerate, establishing hydroxypyruvate as a glycerate precursor in vivo. In this study none of the isotope was found in urinary oxalate. Accumulated hydroxypyruvate in the Type II disorder is not a direct precursor of oxalate, as is glyoxylate in the Type I variant.

In order to determine if any precursor-product relationship exists between glyoxylate and hydroxypyruvate, glyoxylate-1-^{14}C was given intravenously to a patient with L-glyceric aciduria [5]. Comparative studies were conducted in normal subjects and patients with hyperoxaluria Type I. The patient with L-glyceric aciduria incorporated excessive amounts of glyoxylate-1-^{14}C into urinary oxalate, a finding similar to that in patients with primary hyperoxaluria with glycolic aciduria (Table 9-3). In contrast, decreased amounts of isotope were recovered in urinary glycolate when compared with normal subjects and patients with primary hyperoxaluria and glycolic aciduria. This finding implies a partial defect in the conversion of glyoxylate to glycolate in L-glyceric aciduria. No isotope incorporation from glyoxylate-1-^{14}C into urinary L-glycerate was found in the patient with L-glyceric aciduria. This latter finding, together with the absence of any incorporation from hydroxypyruvate-1-^{14}C into urinary oxalate, suggested the lack of a close precursor-product relationship between glyoxylate and hydroxypyruvate in L-glyceric aciduria.

The studies carried out in vivo are consistent with a defect in hydroxypyruvate metabolism, although they fail to explain the mechanism of the accompanying increased oxalate synthesis. No method for measuring hydroxypyruvate in urine or blood has been developed. The lability of hydroxypyruvate interferes with such studies. Attention was therefore directed toward the demonstration in vitro of a defect in hydroxypyruvate metabolism.

In Vitro Studies

Hydroxypyruvate might accumulate because of a block in its transamination to serine (alanine:hydroxypyruvate transaminase) or in its reduction to D-glycerate (D-glyceric dehydrogenase) (Fig. 9-12). The activity of D-glyceric dehydrogenase with NADP as a cofactor was measured in leukocyte preparations from 4 patients with L-glyceric aciduria, the 2 parents of 3 sibs with this disorder, and in 14 normal control subjects [5]. No enzyme activity was detectable in leukocytes from the 4 patients with glyceric aciduria (Fig. 9-13). Enzyme activity was low in leukocytes from the mother, but was within the normal range in leukocytes from the father of the 3 sibs with L-glyceric aciduria. In one

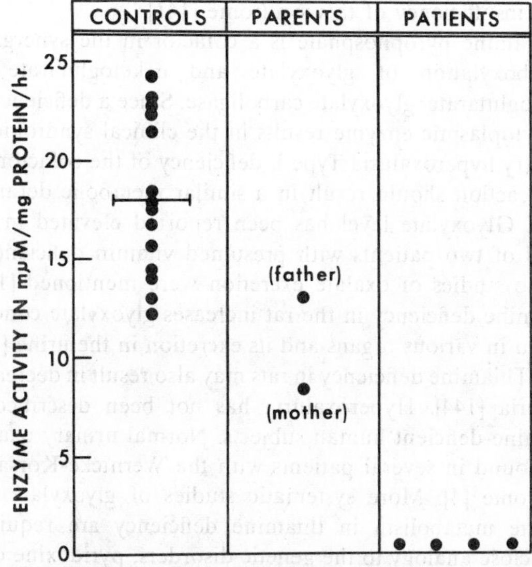

Figure 9-13. D-Glyceric dehydrogenase activity in leukocytes from four patients with L-glyceric aciduria (primary hyperoxaluria, Type II), parents of three sibs with this syndrome, and control subjects. (*From Williams and Smith* [5], *with permission of the publishers.*)

patient with primary hyperoxaluria and glycolic aciduria, leukocyte D-glyceric dehydrogenase activity was within the normal range. The presence of an enzyme inhibitor in patients with L-glyceric aciduria was ruled out by the failure of inhibition of normal enzyme activity in leukocyte preparations from patients mixed with preparations from normal subjects.

This enzyme defect in L-glyceric aciduria allows an explanation for the excessive synthesis and excretion of L-glyceric acid, presumably arising from hydroxypyruvate (Fig. 9-12). The cause of the hyperoxaluria in these patients is not directly clarified by this enzyme defect. As noted above there is some evidence in plants and bacteria to suggest the similarity of D-glyceric dehydrogenase and glyoxylate reductase [131]. It was postulated that the enzyme defect in L-glyceric aciduria may account for a block in the reduction of glyoxylate to glycolate as well as for a block in the reduction of hydroxypyruvate to D-glycerate. Such a parallel defect in these two metabolic pathways might explain the observed combination of L-glyceric aciduria and hyperoxaluria in the absence of hyperglycolic aciduria. A primary defect in glyoxylate metabolism leading to excessive hydroxypyruvate synthesis by some interconnecting pathway seems unlikely in view of the in vivo and in vitro studies. The possibility that hydroxypyruvate or L-glycerate accumulation might inhibit glyoxylate metabolism has not been fully investigated, but no inhibition of α-ketoglutarate : glyoxylate carboligase by hydroxypyruvate or glycerate was demonstrated [5].

The above speculations are based on the assumption that deficiency of D-glyceric dehydrogenase with hydroxypyruvate accumulation (reflected one step removed by L-glyceric aciduria) is somehow linked with a block in glyoxylate metabolism. A second mechanism to explain the relationship of hydroxypyruvate accumulation to increased oxalate synthesis should also be considered. As noted earlier in this chapter, an increased activity of the enzyme or enzymes which oxidize glyoxylate to oxalate might also result in increased synthesis of oxalate in the absence of glyoxylate accumulation. Urinary glyoxylate level was not elevated in either patient with L-glyceric aciduria in whom it was determined. Metabolism of glyoxylate-1-^{14}C to respiratory carbon dioxide was not as impaired in a patient with L-glyceric aciduria as in four patients with primary hyperoxaluria Type I, in spite of an even greater shunting of isotope into oxalate [5]. In recent studies in human erythrocytes and leukocytes and in partially purified LDH preparations it has been demonstrated that hydroxypyruvate enhances oxalate synthesis and diminishes glycolate synthesis from glyoxylate, presumably through reduction of lactic dehydrogenase–NADH (Fig. 9-14) [138]. It seems most likely, therefore, that the increased oxalate synthesis of D-glyceric dehydrogenase deficiency is the indirect consequence of coupled oxidation-reduction of glyoxylate and hydroxypyruvate through their common nonspecific reactivity with certain enzymes, especially lactic dehydrogenase.

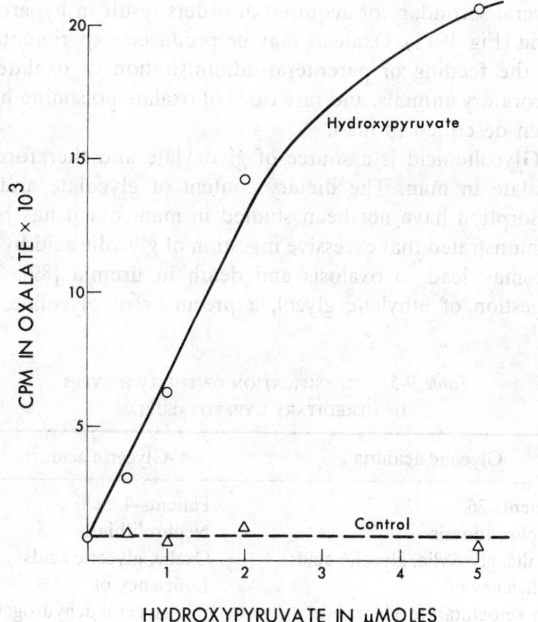

Figure 9-14. The effect of hydroxypyruvate on oxalate-^{14}C synthesis from glyoxylate-^{14}C catalyzed by lactic dehydrogenase.

The study of D-glyceric dehydrogenase deficiency in patients with L-glyceric aciduria has implications relating to the pathway of serine biosynthesis in man. Both phosphorylated and nonphosphorylated pathways for serine biosynthesis have been found in mammalian preparations [136]. In one patient with L-glyceric aciduria, serine was found in normal concentrations in plasma and urine [5]. The accumulation of hydroxypyruvate rather than D-glycerate in this disorder and the normal concentration of serine support the concept that the nonphosphorylated pathway of serine metabolism normally operates in the direction of gluconeogenesis in man (Fig. 9-12), serine biosynthesis occurring by way of the phosphorylated pathway.

CLASSIFICATION OF HYPEROXALURIC STATES

Hyperoxaluria in man may be divided into primary (or genetic) and secondary types, the latter related to an abnormal nutritional state. Strictly speaking, primary hyperoxaluria is also "secondary," since the increased production of oxalate in Type I results indirectly from a block in glyoxylate metabolism. It is analogous to the accumulation of phenylpyruvate, phenyllactate, and phenylacetate in phenylketonuria. In the Type II disease hyperoxaluria seems most likely to be "secondary" to enhanced shunting of glyoxylate to oxalate through coupled oxidation-reduction with hydroxypyruvate. Table 9-5 compares these two genetic disorders as studied by Williams and Smith. Other forms of genetic hyperoxaluria may exist.

In addition to these genetically determined conditions several secondary or acquired disorders result in hyperoxaluria (Fig. 9-11). Oxalosis may be produced experimentally by the feeding or parenteral administration of oxalate to laboratory animals, and rare cases of oxalate poisoning have been described in man.

Glycolic acid is a source of glyoxylate and therefore of oxalate in man. The dietary content of glycolate and its absorption have not been studied in man, but it has been demonstrated that excessive ingestion of glycolic acid by the rat may lead to oxalosis and death in uremia [89]. The ingestion of ethylene glycol, a precursor of glycolate, increases urinary oxalate in experimental animals and in man [139, 140]. Excessive ingestion of ethylene glycol leads to extensive crystallization of calcium oxalate in renal tubules and within the renal parenchyma [140]. Fatal cases of ethylene glycol poisoning in man exhibit similar pathologic lesions in the kidney, and this probably accounts for the acute renal insufficiency of this syndrome [141].

Table 9-5. CLASSIFICATION OF THE TWO TYPES OF HEREDITARY HYPEROXALURIA

Glycolic aciduria	L-Glyceric aciduria
Patients-26	Patients-4
Nephrolithiasis	Nephrolithiasis
Oxalic, glyoxylic, glycolic acids	Oxalic, glyceric acids
Deficiency of α-ketoglutarate: glyoxylate carboligase	Deficiency of D-glyceric dehydrogenase

Source: From [5] with permission of the publishers.

Thiamine pyrophosphate is a cofactor in the synergistic decarboxylation of glyoxylate and α-ketoglutarate by α-ketoglutarate: glyoxylate carboligase. Since a deficiency of the cytoplasmic enzyme results in the clinical syndrome of primary hyperoxaluria Type I, deficiency of the cofactor for this reaction should result in a similar metabolic derangement. Glyoxylate level has been reported elevated in the blood of two patients with presumed vitamin deficiencies, but no studies of oxalate excretion were mentioned [120]. Thiamine deficiency in the rat increases glyoxylate concentration in various organs and its excretion in the urine [142, 143]. Thiamine deficiency in rats may also result in decreased oxaluria [144]. Hyperoxaluria has not been described in thiamine-deficient human subjects. Normal urinary oxalate was found in several patients with the Wernicke-Korsakov syndrome [4]. More systematic studies of glyoxylate and oxalate metabolism in thiamine deficiency are required.

In close analogy to the genetic disorders, pyridoxine deficiency in experimental animals leads to hyperoxaluria and oxalosis, presumably because of the reduced transamination of glyoxylate to glycine [86]. The induction of pyridoxine deficiency in man also results in a progressive increase in urinary oxalate [87]. In in vivo studies, pyridoxine-deficient rats converted labeled ethanolamine and ethylene glycol to oxalate to a greater extent than normal controls [145]. Surprisingly, these studies did not show greater conversion of glyoxylate-^{14}C into labeled urinary oxalate in pyridoxine-deficient animals. In liver and kidney homogenates, oxalate synthesis from glycolate was similar in control and pyridoxine-deficient animals. Carbon dioxide production from glyoxylate-^{14}C was impaired in kidney but not in liver homogenates from pyridoxine-deficient animals [145]. The possibility that some previously described cases of hyperoxaluria represent pyridoxine deficiency has been emphasized. It is of interest that patients with pyridoxine-responsive seizures have no abnormality of oxalate metabolism.

Reduction in oxalate excretion during treatment of patients with primary oxaluria with excess pyridoxine has been noted (Fig. 9-15). The interrelationships of these abnormalities in oxalate metabolism are shown diagramatically in Fig. 9-11.

Recently, hyperoxaluria and recurrent calcium oxalate nephrolithiasis in the absence of hyperglycolic or L-glyceric aciduria has been seen in a group of patients with ileal resection [146*a*, *b*]. Isotope incorporation studies utilizing cholyl-glycine-^{14}C have suggested a role for bile salts in this disorder [146*b*]. The finding that taurine administration (4 gm per day) leads to a reduction of oxalate excretion into the normal range and a disappearance of new stone formation

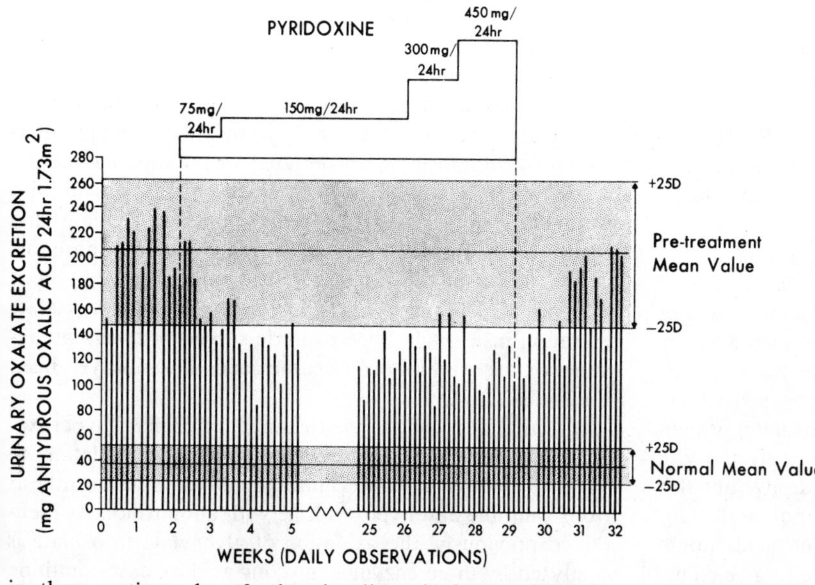

Figure 9-15. The effect of pyridoxine hydrochloride therapy on daily urinary oxalate excretion in a patient with primary hyperoxaluria, Type I. (*From Gibbs and Watts* [157], *with permission of the authors and publishers.*)

in these patients has further implicated abnormalities in bile salt metabolism in this syndrome [146*a*]. The relationship between the hyperoxaluria and bile salt malabsorption has not been completely defined. Studies to date suggest a role for both increased absorption of glyoxylate as a breakdown product of glycocholate metabolism by gut bacteria, and increased diversion of glyoxylate into oxalate synthesis and away from glycolate synthesis—a finding similar to that seen in primary hyperoxaluria, Type II.

INHERITANCE

On the basis of a number of family studies, Type I primary hyperoxaluria appears to be inherited as an autosomal recessive character. In at least 16 families hyperoxaluria has been documented in 2 or more sibs without evidence of the disease in their parents [3]. The incidence of consanguine marriages is ten- to twentyfold that found in the general population. In 13 families in which the disease was present, 30 sibs had hyperoxaluria and 29 had no evidence of the disease [3]. This deviation in the expected ratio of 1:3 in recessive transmission is probably related to bias in case selection.

The heterozygous state cannot be determined in Type I primary hyperoxaluria. In nearly all instances in which it has been studied urinary oxalate excretion has been normal in parents of patients with the disease [3]. Studies of α-ketoglutarate: glyoxylate carboligase activity have not been reported in presumed heterozygotes for Type I primary hyperoxaluria.

Although an autosomal recessive mode of inheritance seems most likely in this disorder, dominant inheritance has been suggested by some studies. This suggestion is based on the noted 1:1 ratio of sib involvement and by the occasional modestly increased oxalate excretion in parents of patients with the disorder [147–149]. In at least four instances hyperoxaluria has been detected in successive generations, and in one family, possibly in three generations [147–150]. These findings have suggested possible genetic heterogeneity in primary hyperoxaluria.

The inheritance pattern of Type II primary hyperoxaluria is difficult to determine because of the small number of cases reported. The disease has been found in three sibs (both sexes) whose parents did not show increased excretion of either oxalic or glyceric acids. Leukocyte D-glyceric dehydrogenase studies of two parents have demonstrated a definite reduction in enzyme activity in the mother's leukocytes; enzyme activity in the leukocytes of the father was at the lower range of normal [5]. Although it seems likely that Type II primary hyperoxaluria is transmitted as an autosomal recessive character, further study of a larger series of patients is necessary before definite conclusions can be reached.

Although oxalate is a component of nearly two-thirds of all renal calculi, the vast majority of patients with recurrent stones do not have hyperoxaluria [151]. A diurnal variation in oxalate excretion has been reported to be more evident in patients with renal calculi than in normal subjects [152]. Since normal urine is often supersaturated with calcium oxalate, it is not surprising that oxalate stone disease is so common. In an extensive study of familial calcium oxalate stone disease, Resnick et al. found higher frequencies of renal calculi among 625 parents and sibs of 106 subjects with recurrent calcium oxalate stones when compared with corresponding relatives of spouses of the propositi [153]. Analysis of the data ruled out monogenic inheritance, but the findings were compatible with inheritance by a polygenic system, with a lesser risk for females. One implication of these data suggested by Resnick et al. is that no single biochemical variable will be found that will account for calcium oxalate stone diathesis.

TREATMENT

Because of the progressive renal failure that eventually develops in most patients with primary hyperoxaluria, early diagnosis is essential if therapeutic measures are to prevent early demise. The major approaches to therapy have been directed either toward reduction in oxalate synthesis and excretion or toward prevention of calcium oxalate stone formation at a given level of urinary oxalate. Both methods have apparently met with some success, but long-term studies are necessary to evaluate fully the effects of any therapeutic program.

A number of attempts to reduce oxalate synthesis and excretion have been undertaken, with variable degrees of success. Reduction of the availability of glycine, a major precursor of oxalate, by dietary protein restriction or by trapping glycine as hippurate with benzoate has been attempted [9, 58]. Because of the extremely high turnover rate and low fractional conversion of glycine to oxalate, protein restriction has not met with success. Trapping of glycine with benzoate may reduce oxalate excretion modestly, but this effect has been temporary and, therefore, not useful for long-term treatment [154]. Although D-amino acids might competitively inhibit the oxidation of glycine to glyoxylate, large oral doses of D,L-glutamate and D,L-histidine have failed to reduce urinary oxalate levels in patients with primary hyperoxaluria [155].

Because hyperoxaluria has been observed to accompany pyridoxine deficiency, several attempts have been made to utilize this vitamin in the treatment of primary hyperoxaluria. In experimental animals pyridoxine administration may increase the transamination of glyoxylate to glycine, presumably by inducing synthesis of the transaminase apoenzyme or inhibiting its catabolism [156]. The administration of pyridoxine to normal subjects and mentally deficient patients without hyperoxaluria has been reported to reduce urinary oxalate excretion [144, 155].

Studies by Smith and Williams [155] and by Gibbs and Watts [157] have demonstrated a definite decrease in the excretion of urinary oxalate in patients with primary hyperoxaluria given large doses of pyridoxine (Fig. 9-14). A similar finding has been reported by Giertz in a single hyperoxaluric subject given 400 mg per day of pyridoxine [158]. This promising approach should receive more extensive evaluation with larger numbers of patients.

The use of aldehyde dehydrogenase inhibitors to reduce oxalate synthesis and excretion was introduced by Solomons and coworkers in 1967 [125]. These investigators reported a significant reduction in urinary oxalate with calcium carbimide in a 12-year-old patient with primary hyperoxaluria undergoing renal transplantation. These authors subsequently commented on the successful use of this drug in two other patients and postulated that the effect on oxalate synthesis was due to inhibition of glycolaldehyde conversion to glycolate [159]. Zarembski and coworkers [160] were unable to demonstrate a consistent reduction in urinary oxalate in three hyperoxaluric subjects treated with calcium carbimide. Other workers have also failed to confirm the effectiveness of aldehyde dehydrogenase inhibitors in reducing oxalate excretion in primary hyperoxaluria [161]. Gibbs and Watts [162] found no effect of disulfiram on oxalate excretion in a single patient when the drug was given alone or in combination with allopurinol. Similarly, in in vitro studies disulfiram did not inhibit the oxidation of glyoxylate to oxalate in human erythrocytes [111], the supernatant fraction of human liver [162], or the supernatant and particulate fractions of liver obtained from a patient with primary hyperoxaluria [162]. In the opinion of Williams and Smith the usefulness of aldehyde dehydrogenase inhibitors in the treatment of primary hyperoxaluria has not been established. The report of a 40 percent reduction in oxalate excretion in a single hyperoxaluric subject with the monamine oxidase inhibitor, isocarboxazid, has not yet been confirmed [127].

A similar approach to the treatment of primary hyperoxaluria has been the inhibition of glyoxylate oxidation to oxalate, analogous to the inhibition of uric acid synthesis from xanthine and hypoxanthine with allopurinol. As mentioned previously, the oxidation of glyoxylate to oxalate is catalyzed by three enzymes: glycolic acid oxidase, xanthine oxidase, and lactic dehydrogenase. Oxalate excretion is not affected by allopurinol, nor is oxalate excretion increased in patients with hereditary xanthinuria [75, 163].

Several compounds inhibit the oxidation in vitro of glyoxylate to oxalate by glycolic acid oxidase. The most active are hydroxymethanesulfonic acid and hydroxymethanesulfinic acid [164, 165]. Inhibition of oxalate synthesis from glyoxylate in human liver particulate and supernatant fractions with the former compound has been reported by Gibbs and Watts [162]. In erythrocyte hemolysates the synthesis of oxalate from glyoxylate can be inhibited by oxamate [112]. Since this compound is a potent inhibitor of lactic dehydrogenase, the inhibition of oxalate synthesis in this system is probably related to the effect of oxamate on lactic dehydrogenase, rather than glycolic acid oxidase. In addition, a number of other analogues of oxalate are potent inhibitors of lactic dehydrogenase-catalyzed oxalate synthesis [112]. Diminished oxidation of glyoxylate to oxalate by a partially purified glycolic acid oxidase preparation from rat liver and human erythrocytes has been observed with hydroxymethanesulfonic acid [112]. Attempts to demonstrate reduction of urinary oxalate in laboratory animals with the use of this compound in vivo has not been successful [165]. Oral administration of tris-hydroxymethylaminomethane (THAM) to two normal subjects and one patient with primary hyperoxaluria failed to alter significantly urinary oxalate excretion [166], in spite of the effectiveness of this compound as an inhibitor of glycolic acid oxidase in vitro [167]. The use of such agents would be a logical method for the treatment of patients with primary hyperoxaluria as well as of other patients with recurrent idiopathic calcium oxalate nephrolithiasis. Further studies of their effectiveness in vivo and their possible toxicity are necessary in order to establish the usefulness of this pharmacologic approach.

A second approach to the treatment of hyperoxaluria has been directed toward reducing the tendency to calcium oxalate stone formation at any given level of urinary oxalate concentration. As with other causes of recurrent nephrolithiasis, maintenance of large urine volumes is important. Restriction of dietary calcium may be of some help, but urinary calcium in nonhypercalciuric patients is affected relatively little by variations in dietary calcium [168, 169]. Several studies have emphasized the inhibitory effect of various metal ions, particularly magnesium, on kidney stone formation. Lyon and coworkers [170, 171] found inhibition of calcium oxalate stone formation in rats made hyperoxaluric by pyridoxine deficiency with the use of magnesium supplements, although occasional magnesium acid phosphate stones were found in the bladder of animals given the high magnesium intake. Recently, Gershoff and Prien [172] have reported the successful use of daily MgO and pyridoxine in patients with recurrent calcium oxalate nephrolithiasis. No recurrence of stones was found in 30 of 36 patients, for periods up to 5 years, and urine obtained from treated subjects had an increased capacity to maintain calcium oxalate in solution. No systematic trial of magnesium therapy in primary hyperoxaluria has been reported.

Several recent studies have emphasized the usefulness of a high phosphate intake in the treatment of recurrent calcium oxalate stone disease [173–175]. This therapeutic program has been supported by the demonstration that oral administration of orthophosphate to patients with recurrent kidney stone disease inhibits the ability of their urine to mineralize rachitic rat cartilage. Although the mechanism of this inhibition has not been clearly established, factors such as reduction of urinary calcium, increase in urinary pyrophosphate, and increase in certain protective polypeptides may play a role. As with oral magnesium therapy, no long-term control studies with this high-phosphate program in hyperoxaluric subjects have appeared. The supplementary phosphate program has seemed to reduce new stone formation in the series of patients with this serious disorder followed by Williams and Smith for the past several years.

Finally, renal transplantation has been used in the treatment of several uremic patients with primary hyperoxaluria. Two reports have recorded lack of success with this procedure, apparently related to the rapid reaccumulation of oxalate crystals in the transplanted kidney [176, 177]. Three other patients with primary hyperoxaluria known to Williams and Smith died shortly after renal transplantation. In one English patient a successful transplant has been maintained for more than 6 months without evidence of renal insufficiency [178]. Until successful methods for inhibition of oxalate synthesis become available, renal homotransplantation from a surviving donor does not seem indicated in primary hyperoxaluria. The advent of chronic dialysis programs for patients with chronic renal failure may obviate the need for transplantation in these patients. No studies of chronic dialysis in patients with primary hyperoxaluria have appeared.

SUMMARY

1 Primary hyperoxaluria is a general term for two rare genetic disorders characterized clinically by recurrent calcium oxalate nephrolithiasis and nephrocalcinosis, frequently leading to progressive renal insufficiency and death before the age of 20. Symptoms of renal stone disease begin usually before the age of 5, although there are variations in age of onset and in severity of clinical symptoms. Calcium oxalate deposits may be found in extrarenal tissues, a pathologic condition termed *oxalosis.*

2 The disease is characterized biochemically by the continuous excessive synthesis and excretion of oxalic acid. The demonstration of different patterns of urinary organic acid excretion has allowed classification of this disease into two specific types. In Type I (glycolic aciduria) excessive amounts of glyoxylic and glycolic acids are also found in the urine. In Type II (L-glyceric aciduria) large amounts of L-glyceric acid but normal amounts of glyoxylic and glycolic acids are excreted.

3 In Type I primary hyperoxaluria the excessive synthesis of oxalate and glycolate results from a block in the metabolism of their immediate precursor, glyoxylate. In five patients with this disorder a deficiency of a soluble α-ketoglutarate:glyoxylate carboligase has been demonstrated in preparations from liver, spleen, and kidney.

4 In Type II primary hyperoxaluria a defect in hydroxypyruvate metabolism results in its excessive reduction to L-glyceric acid, catalyzed by lactic dehydrogenase. A deficiency of leukocyte D-glyceric dehydrogenase has been demonstrated in four patients with this disorder.

5 The cause of excessive oxalate synthesis in primary hyperoxaluria Type II has not been completely clarified. Recent studies suggest that hydroxypyruvate accumulation, secondary to D-glyceric dehydrogenase deficiency, may indirectly increase oxalate synthesis from glyoxylate. The reduction of hydroxypyruvate to L-glycerate enhances the oxidation of glyoxylate to oxalate in a coupled reaction catalyzed by lactic dehydrogenase.

6 The inheritance of both types of primary hyperoxaluria is presumed to be autosomal recessive. This conclusion is based on genetic analyses in Type I and on limited leukocyte enzyme studies in Type II heterozygotes. No consistent test for heterozygosity is available for the Type I disease.

7 Treatment of primary hyperoxaluria is directed toward decreasing oxalate excretion by inhibition of oxalate synthesis and toward increasing calcium oxalate solubility at a given urinary concentration of oxalate. Pyridoxine in large doses has been successful in reducing oxalate synthesis in some patients with primary hyperoxaluria. Inhibitors of oxalate synthesis from glyoxylate have been effective in in vitro systems, but their efficacy has not been established in vivo. The use of phosphate or magnesium or both, agents which increase calcium oxalate solubility in vivo, may reduce the rate of new stone formation. Renal homotransplantation has not proved successful in the management of chronic renal insufficiency complicating primary hyperoxaluria.

BIBLIOGRAPHY

1. Archer, H. E., Dormer, A. E., Scowen, E. F., and Watts, R. W. E.: Primary hyperoxaluria. Lancet, **2**, 320, 1957.
2. Wyngaarden, J. B., and Elder, T. D.: Primary hyperoxaluria and oxalosis, in *The Metabolic Basis of Inherited Disease,* 2d ed., edited by J. B. Stanbury, J. B. Wyngaarden, and D. S. Fredrickson, p. 189. McGraw-Hill, New York, 1966.
3. Hockaday, T. D. R., Clayton, J. E., Frederick, E. W., and Smith, L. H., Jr.: Primary hyperoxaluria. Medicine, **43**, 315, 1964.
4. Williams, H. E., and Smith, L. H., Jr.: Disorders of oxalate metabolism. Amer. J. Med., **45**, 715, 1968.
5. Williams, H. E., and Smith, L. H., Jr.: L-Glyceric aciduria: a new genetic variant of primary oxaluria. New Eng. J. Med., **278**, 233, 1968.
6. Donné, M. A.: Tableau de différents dépôts de matières salines et de substance organisées qui se font dans les urines, presentant les caractères propre a les distinguer entre eux et a reconnaitre leure nature. C. R. Acad. Sci. [D] (Paris), **6**, 419, 1838.
7. Wollaston, W. H.: On cystic oxide, a new species of urinary calculus. Phil. Trans., London, **100**, 223, 1810.
8. Lepoutre, C.: Calculs multiples chez un enfant. Infiltration du parenchyme rénal par des cristaux. J. Urol., **20**, 424, 1925.
9. Daniels, R. A., Michels, R., Aisen, P., and Goldstein, G.: Familial hyperoxaluria. Amer. J. Med., **29**, 820, 1960.
10. Davis, J. S., Klingberg, W. G., and Stowell, R. E.: Nephrolithiasis and nephrocalcinosis with calcium oxalate crystals in kidneys and bones. J. Pediat., **36**, 323, 1950.
11. Newns, G. H., and Black, J. A.: A case of calcium oxalate nephrocalcinosis. Great Ormond St. J., **5**, 40, 1953.
12. Aponte, G. E., and Fetter, T. R.: Familial idiopathic oxalate nephrocalcinosis. Amer. J. Clin. Path., **24**, 1363, 1954.
13. Cochran, M., Hodgkinson, A., Zarembski, P. M., and Anderson, C. K.: Hyperoxaluria in adults. Brit. J. Surg., **55**, 121, 1968.
14. Zarembski, P. M., Hodgkinson, A., and Cochran, M.: Urinary excretion of lactic acid and other organic acids in patients with primary hyperoxaluria, in *Renal Stone Research Symposium,* edited by A. Hodgkinson and B. E. C. Nordin, p. 319. Churchill, London, 1969.
15. McLaurin, A. W., Beisel, W. R., McCormick, G. J., Scalettar, R., and Herman, R. H.: Primary hyperoxaluria. Ann. Intern. Med., **55**, 70, 1961.
16. Smith, L. H., Jr.: Unpublished cases.
17. Antoine, B., Slama, R., Josso, F., de Montera, H., Habib, R., and Richet, G.: La destruction du parenchyme rénal par envahissement de cristaux d'oxalates de calcium. Deux nouvelles observations d'oxalose rénale. Presse Méd., **68**, 803, 1960.
18. Stauffer, M.: Oxalosis. Report of a case, with a review of the literature and discussion of the pathogenesis. New Eng. J. Med., **263**, 386, 1960.
19. Williams, H. E., and Smith, L. H., Jr.: L-Glyceric aciduria, in *Renal Stone Research Symposium,* edited by A. Hodgkinson and B. E. C. Nordin, p. 309. Churchill, London, 1969.
20. Buri, J.-F.: l'Oxalose. Helvet. paediat. acta, **17**, suppl. 11, 1, 1962.
21. Scowen, E. F., Stansfield, A. G., and Watts, R. W. E.: Oxalosis and primary hyperoxaluria. J. Path. Bact., **77**, 195, 1959.
22. Dunn, H. G.: Oxalosis: report of a case with review of the literature. Amer. J. Dis. Child., **90**, 58, 1955.
23. Godwin, J. T., Fowler, M. F., Dempsey, E. F., and Henneman, P. H.: Primary hyperoxaluria and oxalosis: report of a case and review of the literature. New Eng. J. Med., **259**, 1099, 1958.
24. Chisholm, G. D., and Heard, B. E.: Oxalosis. Brit. J. Surg., **50**, 78, 1962.
25. Burke, E. C., Baggenstoss, A. H., Owen, C. A., Jr., Power, M. H., and Lohr, O. W.: Oxalosis. Pediatrics, **15**, 383, 1955.
26. Neustein, H. R., Stevenson, S. S., and Krainer, L.: Oxalosis with renal calcinosis due to calcium oxalate. J. Pediat., **47**, 624, 1955.
27. Hall, E. G., Scowen, E. F., and Watts, R. W. E.: Clinical manifestations of primary hyperoxaluria. Arch. Dis. Child., **35**, 108, 1960.
28. Edwards, D. L.: Idiopathic familial oxalosis. Arch. Path., **64**, 546, 1957.
29. Johnson, F.: A method for demonstrating calcium oxalate in tissue sections. J. Histochem. Cytochem., **4**, 404, 1956.
30. Marshall, V. F., and Horwith, M.: Oxalosis. J. Urol., **82**, 278, 1959.
31. Hockaday, T. D. R., Frederick, E. W., Clayton, J. E., and Smith, L. H., Jr.: Studies on primary hyperoxaluria. II. Urinary oxalate, glycolate and glyoxylate measurement by isotope dilution method. J. Lab. Clin. Med., **65**, 677, 1965.
32. Gibbs, D. A., and Watts, R. W. E.: The variation of urinary oxalate excretion with age. J. Lab. Clin. Med., **73**, 901, 1969.
33. Merz, W., and Maugeri, S.: Über das Vorkommen und die Bestimmung der Oxalsäure im Blut. Hoppe-Seyler Z. Physiol. Chem., **201**, 31, 1931.
34. Barber, H. H., and Gallimore, E. J.: The metabolism of oxalic acid in the animal body. Biochem. J., **34**, 144, 1940.
35. Crawhall, J. C., and Watts, R. W. E.: The oxalate content of human plasma. Clin. Sci., **20**, 357, 1961.
36. Zarembski, P. M., and Hodgkinson, A.: The renal clearance of oxalic acid in normal subjects and in patients with primary hyperoxaluria. Invest. Urol., **1**, 87, 1963.
37. Zarembski, P. M., and Hodgkinson, A.: Fluorimetric determination of oxalic acid in blood and other biological material. Biochem. J., **96**, 717, 1965.
38. Williams, H. E. and Smith, L. H., Jr.: Unpublished data.
39. Elder, T. D., and Wyngaarden, J. B.: The biosynthesis and turnover of oxalate in normal and hyperoxaluric subjects. J. Clin. Invest., **39**, 1337, 1960.
40. Williams, H. E., and Smith, L. H., Jr.: Identification and determination of glyceric acid in human urine. J. Lab. Clin. Med., **71**, 495, 1968.
41. Williams, H. E., Johnson, G., and Morris, R. C.: To be published.
42. Bennington, J. L., Haber, S. L., Smith, J. V., and Warner, N. E.: Crystals of calcium oxalate in the human kidney: studies by means of electron-microprobe and X-ray diffraction. Amer. J. Clin. Path., **41**, 8, 1964.
43. Fanger, H., and Esparza, A.: Crystals of calcium oxalate in the kidney in uremia. Amer. J. Clin. Path., **41**, 597, 1964.
44. Bennett, B., and Rosenblum, C.: Calcium oxalate crystals in the myocardium in uremic patients. Lab. Invest., **10**, 947, 1961.
45. Gross, S.: Granulomatous thyroiditis with anisotropic crystalline material. Arch. Path., **59**, 412, 1955.
46. Cogan, D. G., Kuwabara, T., Silbert, J., Kern, H., McMurray, V., and Hurlbert, C.: Calcium oxalate and calcium phosphate crystals in detached retinas. Arch. Ophthal., **60**, 366, 1958.
47. Glynn, L. E.: Crystalline bodies in tunica media of middle cerebral artery. J. Path. Bact., **51**, 445, 1940.
48. Novoa, W. B., Winer, A. D., Glaid, A. J., and Schwert, G. W.: Lactic dehydrogenase. V. Inhibition by oxamate and by oxalate. J. Biol. Chem., **234**, 1143, 1959.
49. Vermeulen, C. W., and Lyon, E. S.: Mechanisms of genesis and growth of calculi. Amer. J. Med., **45**, 684, 1968.
50. Elliot, J. S., and Eusebio, E.: Calcium oxalate solubility: the effect of trace metals. Invest. Urol., **4**, 428, 1967.
51. Maclagan, N. F., and Anderson, A. J.: Some observations on urinary colloids in relation to renal calculi. Brit. J. Urol., **30**, 269, 1958.
52. Howard, J. E., and Thomas, W. C., Jr.: Control of crystallization in urine. Amer. J. Med., **45**, 693, 1968.
53. Jakoby, W. B.: Oxalate decarboxylation: Oxalate $\rightarrow$ formate + CO_2, in *Methods in Enzymology,* vol. 5, *Preparation and Assay of Enzymes,* edited by S. P. Colowick and N. O. Kaplan, p. 637. Academic, New York, 1962.
54. Prien, E. L., and Prien, E. L., Jr.: Composition and structure of urinary stone. Amer. J. Med., **45**, 654, 1968.
55. Zarembski, P. M., and Hodgkinson, A.: The oxalic acid content of English diets. Brit. J. Nutr., **16**, 627, 1962.
56. Archer, H. E., Dormer, A. E., Scowen, E. F., and Watts, R. W. E.: Studies on the urinary excretion of oxalate by normal subjects. Clin. Sci., **16**, 405, 1957.
57. Zarembski, P. M., and Hodgkinson, A.: The determination of oxalic acid in food. Analyst, **87**, 698, 1962.
58. Archer, H. E., Dormer, A. E., Scowen, E. F., and Watts, R. W. E.: The aetiology of primary hyperoxaluria. Brit. Med. J., **1**, 175, 1958.
59. Kornberg, H. L., and Elsden, S. R.: The metabolism of 2-carbon compounds by microorganisms, in *Advances in Enzymology,* edited by F. F. Nord, p. 401. Interscience, New York, 1961.

60. Madsen, N. B.: Test for isocitritase and malate synthetase in animal tissues. Biochim. Biophys. Acta, **27**, 199, 1958.
61. Faragalla, F. F., and Gershoff, S. N.: Occurrence of C^{14}-oxalate in rat urine after administration of C^{14}-tryptophane. Proc. Soc. Exp. Biol. Med., **114**, 602, 1963.
62. Cook, D. A., and Henderson, L. M.: The formation of oxalic acid from the side chain of aromatic amino acids in the rat. Biochim. Biophys. Acta, **184**, 404, 1969.
63. Curtin, C. O., and King, C. G.: The metabolism of ascorbic acid-1-^{14}C and oxalic acid-^{14}C in the rat. J. Biol. Chem., **216**, 539, 1955.
64. Banay, M., and Dimant, E.: On the metabolism of L-ascorbic acid in the scorbutic guinea-pig. Biochim. Biophys. Acta, **59**, 313, 1962.
65. Abt, A. F., von Schuching, S., and Enns, T.: L-Ascorbic-1-C^{14} acid catabolism in the rhesus monkey. Nature (London), **193**, 1178, 1962.
66. Hellman, L., and Burns, J. J.: Metabolism of L-ascorbic acid 1-^{14}C in man. J. Biol. Chem., **230**, 923, 1958.
67. Baker, E. M., Saari, J. C., and Tolbert, B. M.: Ascorbic acid metabolism in man. Amer. J. Clin. Nutr., **19**, 371, 1966.
68. Lambden, M. P., and Chrystowski, G. A.: Urinary oxalate excretion by man following ascorbic acid ingestion. Proc. Soc. Exp. Biol. Med., **85**, 190, 1954.
69. Takenouchi, K., Aso, K., Kawase, K., Ichikawa, H., and Shiomi, T.: On the metabolites of ascorbic acid, especially oxalic acid, eliminated in urine, following the administration of large amounts of ascorbic acid. J. Vitamin. (Kyoto), **12**, 49, 1966.
70. Clagett, C. O., Tolbert, N. E., and Burris, R. H.: Oxidation of α-hydroxy acids by enzymes from plants. J. Biol. Chem., **178**, 977, 1949.
71. Kun, E., Dechary, J. M., and Pitot, H. C.: The oxidation of glycolic acid by a liver enzyme. J. Biol. Chem., **210**, 269, 1954.
72. Richardson, K. E., and Tolbert, N. E.: Oxidation of glyoxylic acid to oxalic acid by glycolic acid oxidase. J. Biol. Chem., **236**, 1280, 1961.
73. Engelman, K., Watts, R. W. E., Klinenberg, J. R., Sjoerdsma, A., and Seegmiller, J. E.: Clinical, physiological and biochemical studies of a patient with xanthinuria and pheochromocytoma. Amer. J. Med., **37**, 839, 1964.
74. Booth, V. H.: The specificity of xanthine oxidase. Biochem. J., **32**, 494, 1938.
75. Gibbs, D. A., and Watts, R. W. E.: An investigation of the possible role of xanthine oxidase in the oxidation of glyoxylate to oxalate. Clin. Sci., **31**, 285, 1966.
76. Krakow, G., and Vennesland, B.: The stereospecificity of glyoxylate reduction in leaves. Biochem. Z., **338**, 31, 1963.
77. Sawaki, S., Hattori, N., and Yamada, K.: Reduction of nicotinamide adenine dinucleotide by glyoxylate in animal organs. J. Vitamin. (Kyoto), **12**, 303, 1966.
78. Banner, M. R., and Rosalki, S. B.: Glyoxylate as a substrate for lactate dehydrogenase. Nature (London), **213**, 726, 1967.
79. Sawaki, S., Hattori, N., Morikawa, N., and Yamada, K.: Oxidation and reduction of glyoxylate by lactate dehydrogenase. J. Vitamin. (Kyoto), **13**, 93, 1967.
80. Kleinzeller, A.: Oxidation of acetic acid in animal tissues. Biochem. J., **37**, 674, 1943.
81. Crawhall, J. C., Scowen, E. F., and Watts, R. W. E.: Conversion of glycine to oxalate in primary hyperoxaluria. Lancet, **2**, 806, 1959.
82. Dean, B. M., Watts, R. W. E., and Westwick, W. J.: The conversion of [1-^{13}C] glycine and [2-^{13}C] glycine to [^{13}C] oxalate in primary hyperoxaluria: evidence for the existence of more than one metabolic pathway from glycine to oxalate in man. Clin. Sci., **35**, 325, 1968.
83. Watts, R. W. E., and Crawhall, J. C.: The first glycine metabolic pool in man. Biochem. J., **73**, 277, 1959.
84. Ratner, S., Nocito, V., and Green, D. E.: Glycine oxidase. J. Biol. Chem., **152**, 119, 1944.
85. Neims, A. H., and Hellerman, L.: Specificity of the D-amino acid oxidase in relation to glycine oxidase activity. J. Biol. Chem., **237**, 976, 1962.
86. Gershoff, S. N., Faragalla, F. F., Nelson, D. A., and Andrus, S. B.: Vitamin B_6 deficiency and oxalate nephrocalcinosis in the cat. Amer. J. Med., **27**, 72, 1959.
87. Faber, S. R., Feitler, W. W., Bleiler, R. E., Ohlson, M. A., and Hodges, R. E.: The effects of an induced pyridoxine and pantothenic acid deficiency on excretions of oxalic and xanthurenic acids in the urine. Amer. J. Clin. Nutr., **12**, 406, 1963.
88. Whittingham, C. P., and Pritchard, G. G.: The production of glycollate during photosynthesis in *Chlorella.* Proc. Roy. Soc. [Biol.], **157**, 366, 1963.
89. Silbergeld, S., and Carter, H. E.: The toxicity of glycolic acid in male and female rats. Arch. Biochem., **84**, 183, 1959.
90. Da Fonseca-Wollheim, F., Bock, K. W., and Holzer, H.: Preparation of "active glycolic aldehyde" [2-(1,2-dihydroxyethyl) thiamine pyrophosphate] from hydroxypyruvate and thiamine pyrophosphate with a preparation of pyruvic oxidase from pig-heart muscle. Biochem. Biophys. Res. Commun., **9**, 466, 1962.
91. Holzer, H., Katterman, R., and Busch, D.: A thiamine pyrophosphate-glycoladehyde compound ("active glycolaldehyde") as intermediate in the transketolase reaction. Biochem. Biophys. Res. Commun., **7**, 167, 1962.
92. Carter, H. E., Johnson, P., Teets, D. W., and Yu, R. K.: Isolation of ethylene glycol from the lipids of beef lung. Biochem. Biophys. Res. Commun., **13**, 156, 1963.
93. Dekker, E. E., and Maitra, U.: Conversion of γ-hydroxyglutamate to glyoxylate and alanine; purification and properties of the enzyme system. J. Biol. Chem., **237**, 2218, 1962.
94. Hockaday, T. D. R., Clayton, J. E., and Smith, L. H., Jr.: The metabolic error in primary hyperoxaluria. Arch. Dis. Childhood, **40**, 485, 1965.
95. Payes, B., and Laties, G. G.: The enzymatic conversion of γ-hydroxy-α-ketoglutarate to malate: a postulated step in the cyclic oxidation of glyoxylate. Biochem. Biophys. Res. Commun., **13**, 179, 1963.
96. Smith, L. H., Jr.: Unpublished observations.
97. Cammarata, P. S., and Cohen, P. P.: The scope of the transamination reaction in animal tissues. J. Biol. Chem., **187**, 439, 1950.
98. Nakada, H. I., and Weinhouse, S.: Non-enzymatic transamination with glyoxylic acid and various amino-acids. J. Biol. Chem., **204**, 831, 1953.
99. Thompson, J. S., and Richardson, K. E.: Isolation and characterization of a glutamate-glycine transaminase from human liver. Arch. Biochem., **117**, 599, 1966.
100. Williams, H. E., Wilson, K. M., and Smith, L. H., Jr.: Studies on primary hyperoxaluria. III. Transamination reactions of glyoxylate in human tissue preparations. J. Lab. Clin. Med., **70**, 494, 1967.
101. Zelitch, I.: Oxidation and reduction of glycolic and glyoxylic acids in plants. II. Glyoxylic acid reductase. J. Biol. Chem., **201**, 719, 1953.
102. Zelitch, I., and Gotto, A. M.: Properties of a new glyoxylate reductase from leaves. Biochem. J., **84**, 541, 1962.
103. Romano, M., and Cerra, M.: The action of crystalline lactate dehydrogenase from rabbit muscle on glyoxylate. Biochim. Biophys. Acta, **177**, 421, 1969.
104. Nakada, H. I., and Sund, L. P.: Glyoxylic acid oxidation by rat liver. J. Biol. Chem., **233**, 8, 1958.
105. Crawhall, J. C., and Watts, R. W. E.: The metabolism of glyoxylate by human and rat liver mitochondria. Biochem. J., **85**, 163, 1962.
106. Kawasaki, H., Okuyama, M., and Kikuchi, G.: α-Ketoglutarate-dependent oxidation of glyoxylic acid in rat mitochondria. J. Biochem., **59**, 419, 1966.
107. Stewart, P. R., and Quayle, J. R.: The synergistic decarboxylation of glyoxylate and 2-oxoglutarate by an enzyme from mammalian liver. Biochem. J., **98**, 43p, 1966.
108. Koch, J., Stokstad, E. L. R., Williams, H. E., and Smith, L. H., Jr.: Deficiency of 2-oxoglutarate: glyoxylate carboligase activity in primary hyperoxaluria. Proc. Nat. Acad. Sci. U.S.A., **57**, 1123, 1967.
109. Koch, J., and Stokstad, E. L. R.: Personal communication.
110*a*. Smith, L. H., Jr., Bauer, R. L., and Williams, H. E.: Oxalate and glycolate synthesis by hemic cell. J. Lab. Clin. Med., **78**, 245, 1971.
110*b*. Zewe, V., and Fromm, H. J.: Kinetic studies of rabbit muscle lactate dehydrogenase. II. Mechanism of the reaction. Biochemistry, **4**, 782, 1965.
111. Fisher, V., and Watts, R. W. E.: The metabolism of glyoxylate in blood from normal subjects and patients with primary hyperoxaluria. Clin. Sci., **34**, 97, 1968.

112. Smith, L. H., Jr., Bauer, R. L., Craig, J. C., and Williams, H. E.: Inhibition of oxalate synthesis: In vitro studies using analogues of oxalate and glycolate. Biochem. Med. (In Press.)
113. Shimazono, H., and Hayaishi, O.: Enzymatic decarboxylation of oxalic acid. J. Biol. Chem., **227,** 151, 1957.
114. Quayle, J. R., Keech, D. B., and Taylor, G. A.: Carbon assimilation by *Pseudomonas oxalaticus* (OXI). 4. Metabolism of oxalate in cell-free extracts of the organism grown on oxalate. Biochem. J., **78,** 225, 1961.
115. Weinhouse, S., and Friedmann, B.: Metabolism of labeled 2-carbon acids in the intact rat. J. Biol. Chem., **191,** 707, 1951.
116. Brubacher, G., Just, M., Bodur, H., and Bernhard, K.: Zur Biochemie der Oxalsaure. Z. Physiol. Chem., **304,** 173, 1956.
117. Cattell, W. R., Spencer, A. G., Taylor, G. W., and Watts, R. W. E.: The mechanism of the renal excretion of oxalate in the dog. Clin. Sci., **22,** 43, 1962.
118. Williams, H. E., Johnson, G. A., and Smith, L. H., Jr.: The renal clearance of oxalate in normal subjects and patients with primary hyperoxaluria. Clin. Sci. **41,** 213, 1971.
119. Atkins, G. L., and Dean, B. M., Griffin, W. J., Scowen, E. F., and Watts, R. W. E.: Quantitative aspects of ascorbic acid metabolism in patients with primary hyperoxaluria. Clin. Sci., **29,** 305, 1965.
120. Buckle, R. M.: The glyoxylic acid content of human blood and its relationship to thiamine deficiency. Clin. Sci., **25,** 207, 1963.
121. Frederick, E. W., Rabkin, M. T., Richie, R. H., Jr., and Smith, L. H., Jr.: Studies on primary hyperoxaluria. I. *In vivo* demonstration of a defect in glyoxylate metabolism. New Eng. J. Med., **269,** 821, 1963.
122. Crawhall, J. C., and Watts, R. W. E.: The metabolism of [1-^{14}C]-glyoxylate by the liver mitochondria of patients with primary hyperoxaluria and non-hyperoxaluric subjects. Clin. Sci., **23,** 163, 1962.
123. Dean, B. M., Griffin, W. J., and Watts, R. W. E.: Primary hyperoxaluria. Lancet, **1,** 406, 1966.
124. Dean, B. M., Watts, R. W. E., and Westwick, W. J.: Metabolism of [1-^{14}C] glyoxylate, [1-^{14}C] glycollate, [1-^{14}C] glycine and [2-^{14}C] glycine by homogenates of kidney and liver tissue from hyperoxaluric and control subjects. Biochem. J., **105,** 701, 1967.
125. Solomons, C. C., Goodman, S. I., and Riley, C. M.: Calcium carbimide in the treatment of primary hyperoxaluria. New Eng. J. Med., **276,** 207, 1967.
126. Scriver, C. R., and Hutchinson, J. H.: The vitamin B_6 deficiency syndrome in human infancy: biochemical and clinical observations. Pediatrics, **31,** 240, 1963.
127. Bourke, E., Frindt, G., Flynn, P., and Schreiner, G. E.: Primary hyperoxaluria with normal α-ketoglutarate: glyoxylate carboligase activity. Ann. Int. Med., **76,** 279, 1972.
128. Dawkins, P. D., and Dickens, F.: Oxidation of D- and L-glycerate by rat liver. Biochem. J., **94,** 353, 1965.
129. Fallon, H. J., Hackney, E. J., and Byrne, W. L.: Serine biosynthesis in rat liver: regulation of enzyme concentration by dietary factors. J. Biol. Chem., **241,** 4157, 1966.
130. Willis, J. E., and Sallach, H. J.: Evidence for mammalian D-glyceric dehydrogenase. J. Biol. Chem., **237,** 910, 1962.
131. Sallach, H. J.: D-Glycerate dehydrogenase of liver and spinach, in *Methods in Enzymology,* vol. 9, *Carbohydrate Metabolism,* edited by W. A. Wood, p. 221. Academic, New York, 1966.
132. Kohn, L. D., and Jakoby, W. B.: Hydroxypyruvate reductase (D-glycerate dehydrogenase; crystalline) *Pseudomonas,* in *Methods in Enzymology,* vol. 9, *Carbohydrate Metabolism,* edited by W. A. Wood, p. 229. Academic, New York, 1966.
133. Cremona, T., and Singer, T. P.: D-α-Hydroxy acid dehydrogenase, in *Methods in Enzymology,* vol. 9, *Carbohydrate Metabolism,* edited by W. A. Wood, p. 327. Academic, New York, 1966.
134. Anderson, S. R., Florini, J. R., and Vestling, C. S.: Rat liver lactate dehydrogenase. III. Kinetics and specificity. J. Biol. Chem., **239,** 2991, 1964.
135. Cheung, G. P., Cotropia, J. P., and Sallach, H. J.: Comparative studies of enzymes related to serine metabolism in fetal and adult liver. Biochim. Biophys. Acta, **170,** 334, 1968.
136. Walsh, D. A., and Sallach, H. J.: Comparative studies on pathways for serine biosynthesis in animal tissues. J. Biol. Chem., **241,** 4068, 1966.
137. Fallon, H. J., and Byrne, W. L.: Depression of enzyme activity by cortisone: an effect on serine metabolism. Endocrinology, **80,** 847, 1967.
138. Williams, H. E. and Smith, L. H., Jr.: Possible pathogenic mechanism for hyperoxaluria in L-glyceric aciduria. Science, **171,** 390, 1971.
139. Pohl, J.: Ueber den oxydativen Abbau der Fettkörper im thierischen Organismus. Arch. Exp. Path. Pharmkol., **37,** 413, 1896.
140. Lyon, E. S., Borden, T. A., and Vermeulen, C. W.: Experimental oxalate lithiasis produced with ethylene glycol. Invest. Urol., **4,** 143, 1966.
141. Friedman, E. A., Greenberg, J. B., Merrill, J. P., and Dammin, G. J.: Consequences of ethylene glycol poisoning. Amer. J. Med., **32,** 891, 1962.
142. Liang, C.: Studies on experimental thiamine deficiency. Trends of keto-acid formation and detection of glyoxylic acid. Biochem. J., **82,** 429, 1962.
143. Takasaki, E.: The urinary excretion of oxalic acid in vitamin B_1 deficient rats. Invest. Urol., **7,** 150, 1969.
144. Gershoff, S. N.: Vitamin B_6 and oxalate metabolism. Vitamins Hormones (N.Y.), **22,** 581, 1964.
145. Runyan, T. J., and Gershoff, S. N.: The effect of vitamin B_6 deficiency in rats on the metabolism of oxalic acid precursors. J. Biol. Chem., **240,** 1889, 1965.
146*a*. Admirand, W., Earnest, D., and Williams, H. E.: Hyperoxaluria and bowel disease. Trans. Ass. Am. Phys. **84,** 307, 1972.
146*b*. Smith, L. H., Jr., Hofmann, A. F., McCall, J. T., and Thomas, P. J.: Secondary hyperoxaluria in patients with ileal resection and oxalate nephrolithiasis. Clin. Res. **18,** 541, 1970.
147. de Toni, G., and Durand, P.: Observations on two opposite clinical situations: renal acidosis and alkalosis. Ann. Paediat., **193,** 257, 1959.
148. Lagrue, G., Laudat, M. H., Meyer, P., Sapir, M., and Milliez, P.: Oxalose familiale avec acidose hyperchlorémique secondaire. Sem. Hôp. Paris, **35,** 2023, 1959.
149. Öigaard, H., Sóderhjelm, L., Hóglund, N.-J., and Werner, I.: Familial oxalosis. II. Acta Soc. Med. Upsal., **68,** 55, 1963.
150. Shepard, T. H., II, Lee, L. W., and Krebs, E. G.: Primary hyperoxaluria. II. Genetic studies in a family. Pediatrics, **25,** 869, 1960.
151. Hodgkinson, A., and Zarembski, P. M.: Oxalic acid metabolism in man: a review. Calcif. Tissue Res., **2,** 115, 1968.
152. Zarembski, P. M., and Hodgkinson, A.: Some factors influencing the urinary excretion of oxalic acid in man. Clin. Chim. Acta, **25,** 1, 1969.
153. Resnick, M., Pridgen, D. B., and Goodman, H. O.: Genetic predisposition to formation of calcium oxalate renal calculi. New Eng. J. Med., **278,** 1313, 1968.
154. Swartz, D., and Israels, S.: Primary hyperoxaluria. J. Urol., **90,** 94, 1963.
155. Smith, L. H., Jr., and Williams, H. E.: Treatment of primary hyperoxaluria. Mod. Treatm., **4,** 522, 1967.
156. Greengard, O., and Gordon, M.: The cofactor-mediated regulation of apoenzyme levels in animal tissues. I. The pyridoxine-induced rise of rat liver tyrosine transaminase level *in vivo.* J. Biol. Chem., **238,** 3708, 1963.
157. Gibbs, D. and Watts, R. W. E.: The action of pyridoxine in primary hyperoxaluria. Clin. Sci. **38,** 277, 1970.
158. Giertz, G.: [Hyperoxaluria.] Urologists' Correspondence Club (Karolinska Sjukhuset, Stockholm 60, Sweden), Jan. 2, 1970.
159. Solomons, C. C., Goodman, S. I., and Riley, C. M.: Treatment of hyperoxaluria. New Eng. J. Med., **277,** 1425, 1967.
160. Zarembski, P. M., Hodgkinson, A., and Cochran, M.: Treatment of primary hyperoxaluria with calcium carbimide. New Eng. J. Med., **277,** 1000, 1967.
161. Smith, L. H., Jones, J. D., and Keating, F. R., Jr.: Primary hyperoxaluria, in *Renal Stone Research Symposium,* edited by A. Hodgkinson and B. E. C. Nordin, p. 297. Churchill, London, 1969.
162. Gibbs, D. A., and Watts, R. W. E.: Oxalate formation from glyoxylate in primary hyperoxaluria: studies on liver tissue. Clin. Sci., **32,** 351, 1967.
163. King, J. S., Jr., and Wainer, A.: Glyoxylate metabolism in normal and stone-forming humans and the effect of allopurinol therapy. Proc. Soc. Exp. Biol. Med., **128,** 1162, 1968.

164. Frederick, E. W., Rabkin, M. T., and Smith, L. H., Jr.: Primary hyperoxaluria: a defect in glyoxylate metabolism. J. Clin. Invest., **41**, 1358, 1962.
165. Bauer, R., Williams, H. E., and Smith, L. H., Jr.: Unpublished observations.
166. Williams, H. E., and Smith, L. H., Jr.: Unpublished observations.
167. Baker, A. L., and Tolbert, N. E.: Glycolate oxidase (ferredoxin-containing form), in *Methods in Enzymology,* vol. 9, *Carbohydrate Metabolism,* edited by W. A. Wood, p. 338. Academic, New York, 1966.
168. Hodgkinson, A., and Pyrah, L. N.: The urinary excretion of calcium and inorganic phosphate in 344 patients with calcium stone of renal origin. Brit. J. Surg., **46**, 10, 1958.
169. Peacock, M., Knowles, F., and Nordin, B. E. C.: Effect of calcium administration and deprivation on serum and urine calcium in stone-forming and control subjects. Brit. Med. J., **2**, 729, 1968.
170. Lyon, E. S., Borden, T. A., Ellis, J. E., and Vermeulen, C. W.: Calcium oxalate lithiasis produced by pyridoxine deficiency and inhibition with high magnesium diets. Invest. Urol., **4**, 133, 1966.
171. Borden, T. A., and Lyon, E. S.: The effects of magnesium and pH on experimental calcium oxalate stone disease. Invest. Urol., **6**, 412, 1969.
172. Gershoff, S. N., and Prien, E. L.: Effect of daily MgO and vitamin B_6 administration to patients with recurrent oxalate kidney stones. Amer. J. Clin. Nutr., **20**, 393, 1967.
173. Howard, J. E., Thomas, W. C., Jr., Mukai, T., Johnston, R. A., Jr., and Pascoe, B. J.: Calcification of cartilage by urine, and a suggestion for therapy in patients with certain kinds of calculi. Trans. Ass. Amer. Physicians, **75**, 301, 1962.
174. Howard, J. E., and Thomas, W. C., Jr.: Control of crystallization in urine. Amer. J. Med., **45**, 693, 1968.
175. Thomas, W. C., Jr., and Miller, G. H., Jr.: Inorganic phosphates in the treatment of renal calculi. Mod. Treatm., **4**, 494, 1967.
176. Deodhar, S. D., Tung, K. S. K., Zühlke, V., and Nakamoto, S.: Renal homotransplantation in a patient with primary familial oxalosis. Arch. Path., **87**, 118, 1969.
177. Klauwers, J., Wolf, P. L., and Cohn, R.: Failure of renal transplantation in primary oxalosis. J.A.M.A., **209**, 551, 1969.
178. Cameron, S.: Personal communication.

PART THREE

DISEASES RELATED PRIMARILY TO DISORDERS OF AMINO ACID METABOLISM

CHAPTER TEN

FAMILIAL GOITER*

John B. Stanbury

This chapter is concerned with the metabolic aspects of familial goiter. The patients to be discussed often but not always have retarded mental or skeletal development and, if untreated, show the outward appearance of thyroid hormone deficiency. Goiter may be present at birth but more commonly becomes noticeable during childhood. Sibs may be similarly afflicted. Several reviews have appeared [1–7] since the first cases were reported by Osler in 1897 [8].

Laboratory investigations of many subjects with familial goiter have made it possible to classify some of their conditions according to specific and identifiable biochemical lesions. Nodular goiter, Graves' disease, and Hashimoto's thyroiditis may also be familial, but will not be considered in this chapter. In each of the categories reviewed here, the lesion is specific and distinct, but the net effect is the same: synthesis and delivery of thyroid hormones are inadequate. Before considering these groups individually it is appropriate to survey the principal metabolic pathways of iodine, as they seem relevant to the subject of this chapter. These are illustrated in Fig. 10-1. Competent general reviews are available elsewhere [9–15].

METABOLISM OF IODINE

Absorption and Distribution

Iodide[1] is absorbed through the gastrointestinal tract as inorganic iodide and is rapidly distributed throughout the extracellular fluid of the body. Free iodine and the iodine of most organic compounds are reduced to iodide during digestion and absorption. The volume of distribution is approximately 28 percent of body weight at 1 hr. Iodide penetrates the red blood cell water to approximately the plasma concentration and also enters the bones to a detectable degree. Iodinated thyronines and tyrosines may be absorbed intact, but the latter are largely deiodinated prior to absorption. Soon after absorption, thyroxine (T_4) and 3,5,3′-triiodothyronine (T_3) are confined to the vascular compartment because of binding to carrier proteins in the plasma. Certain iodinated dyes, such as those used in the roentgenographic visualization of the biliary tree, are also absorbed unchanged.

Except in the postprandial state, the iodide concentration of the plasma is less than 0.5 μg per 100 ml. The inorganic iodide of the plasma is removed almost entirely by the kidney and the thyroid. The relative rates of clearance by these two organs determine the value of the routine radioactive iodine–uptake test for thyroid function. Renal clearance of iodide is normally about 35 ml per min and is independent of the iodine supply in man. Thyroidal clearance varies widely, depending on the functional state of the gland, but normally it lies between 10 and 35 ml per min. The small quantities of iodide removed from the plasma by the salivary and gastric glands are returned to the plasma after absorption in the small intestine. Small amounts of iodide are removed by the mammary glands during lactation. Losses of inorganic iodide in the feces, sweat, and expired air are small.

Iodide Transport

Iodide which enters the thyroid is retained momentarily as dialyzable inorganic iodide. Less than 1 percent of the iodine in the gland fails to precipitate with trichloroacetic acid. This small amount is in much higher concentration than is the iodide of the plasma, but it is in free exchange with the plasma iodide. This iodide pool in the gland may be conveniently referred to as the *readily exchangeable pool* [16].

The concentration of readily exchangeable iodine in the normal thyroid in terms of whole tissue or of tissue water may be 20 to 40 or more times that in the serum (T/S ratio); but if the gland is stimulated by thyrotropic hormone, by iodine deprivation, or by administration of a drug which impairs hormone synthesis, then the concentration in the exchangeable pool rises and may reach values several hundred times that in the plasma. Thus the potential quantity of iodine in the exchangeable pool varies with the overall physiologic activity of the gland. In addition, the T/S ratio may be regulated in part by the quantity of stored iodine within the gland itself [17, 18]. Interestingly, iodide accumulation is enhanced by actinomycin D, but because of a slowed rate of loss of iodide from the gland rather than because of increased transport [19, 20].

The readily exchangeable iodine pool can be isolated from further processes of hormone synthesis by administration of one of the thiocarbamide drugs. Under this circumstance, if ^{131}I is given, the labeled iodine in the thyroid can be quickly discharged by administration of stable I^-, or by any of several inorganic ions, of which thiocyanate (SCN^-) is the prototype. This iodide is presumed to be inorganic in nature [21]. Iodide accumulation is also isolated from further processes of hormonogenesis by relatively large doses of iodide [22, 23], at a stage in the development of the chick embryo [24], in a transplantable rat thyroid tumor studied by Wolff et al. [25], in certain patients with iodide goiter

*This work was supported in part by Grant AM 10992 from the Public Health Service.

[1] In this chapter *iodine* is used in a generic sense to encompass all forms and oxidation states unless otherwise indicated. Similarly, *labeled iodine* is used generically to indicate the iodine which is marked by a radioactive isotope of iodine. *Iodide* always indicates the reduced ionic form of the element.

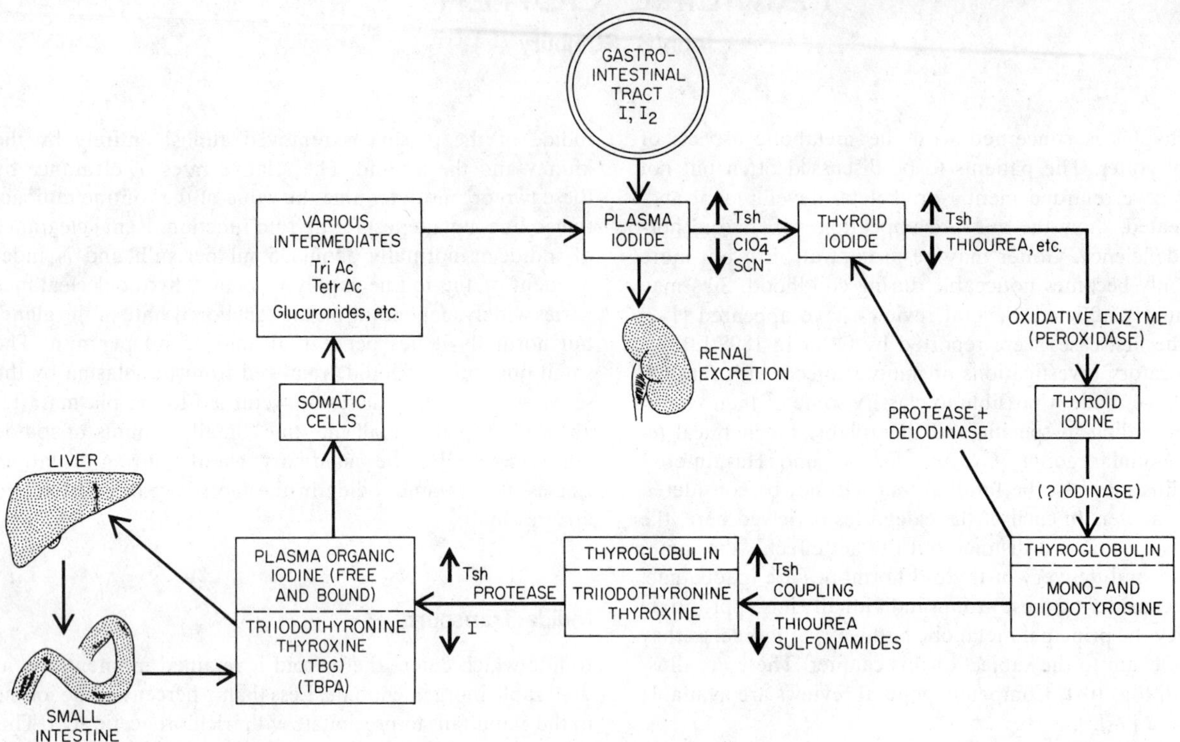

Figure 10-1. Schema of the metabolism of iodine in normal man. TriAc and TetrAc are the acetic acid analogues of tri- and tetraiodothyronine, respectively. *TBG,* thyroxine-binding globulin; *TBPA,* thyroxine-binding prealbumin.

[26], in a certain type of cretinism [27], and in a human thyroid tumor [28].

Transport in Other Tissues

Transport of iodine has been demonstrated in the salivary glands, the gastric mucosa, the mammary glands, the ciliary body, and the placenta [14, 29, 30]. The concentration ratios attained by the salivary gland and the stomach are of the same order as that attained by the thyroid. While the T/S ratio of the thiocarbamide-blocked thyroid can be stimulated to higher values by thyrotropic hormone (TSH) or by provoking intrinsic secretion of this hormone, the ratio between the concentration of iodine in other tissues to that in the plasma is not changed [16, 31]. SCN^-, which displaces inorganic iodide from the thyroid, impairs salivary and gastric transport also, but while SCN^- is much more concentrated in the gastric and salivary fluids than in the plasma [32, 33], it is not concentrated by the thyroid [16, 34]. The capacity of the iodide transport system of the gastric mucosa is higher than that of the salivary or thyroid gland [16, 35]. Thus, while there are iodide transport systems in the salivary glands and the gastric mucosa, as well as in the thyroid, there are certain interesting and as yet unexplained differences of behavior among them [16].

The salivary and gastric secretory cells make no stable organic compound of iodide. After a brief period of equilibration following a single dose of ^{131}I, the concentration in those secretions parallels that in the plasma, and the net rate at which its concentration falls is governed by the total clearance rate of iodide from the plasma.

Ion Competition

Several univalent anions in addition to SCN^- can displace iodide from the readily exchangeable pool, and some of these are selectively concentrated by the thyroid. Of the members of Group VII of the periodic table, F^- and Cl^- are not concentrated by the gland, and Br^- is concentrated only to a slight degree if at all [36]. Astatine (At^-) achieves a high T/S ratio [37], and much of it can be discharged with SCN^- [37]. Manganese, technetium, and rhenium are also concentrated by the thyroid, probably in the form of MnO_4^-, TeO_4^-, and ReO_4^- [38–41]. Selenocyanate ($SeCN^-$) is also transported into the thyroid cell and bound in a —S—S_e— linkage [42]. Nitrate impairs the accumulation of iodide. The most potent of the various anions in discharging iodide or interfering with its entry into the thyroid is ClO_4^-. This ion is approximately ten times as effective in preventing uptake of ^{131}I as is iodide or SCN^- [43, 44]. Labeled with both ^{18}O and ^{36}Cl, ClO_4^- is accumulated by the propylthiouracil-blocked thyroid to approximately the same degree as iodide. It is not metabolized, and it appears ultimately in the urine unchanged. Observations of Anbar et al. [45] led them to postulate that the competition between ClO_4^- and iodide ions might be due to their similar charge and ionic volume [46]. Accordingly, they tested several other ion species for their ability to impair the uptake of iodide. Several with similar charge and ionic volume were effective; among them were monofluorosulfonate, difluorophosphate, and fluoroborate [46, 47]. The last of these labeled with ^{18}F accumulated in the thyroid like iodide. It was suggested that the transport mechanism "involved a certain specially adapted protein in the thyroid cell or cell membrane, having a spatial arrangement that will specifically chelate all monovalent ions which might fulfill certain requirements of size and thus be adaptable into its spatial structure" [47]. These results have been confirmed and extended by Maurey and Wolff [48].

Intrathyroidal Iodide

If the thyroid of a rat that has been given propylthiouracil is excised within 15 min after intravenous administration of ^{131}I, the isotope is found to be not only already present in the parenchymal cells but suffused throughout the colloid. When a similar study was done on salivary gland, no iodide was found in the secretory cells [49, 50]. This transport of iodide into the readily exchangeable pool is active, i.e., against an electrochemical gradient. Woodbury and Woodbury [51] have demonstrated that the potential between the thyroid follicular lumen and the interstitial fluid is zero, and that the cellular potential is 50 mv negative to both lumen and interstitial fluid. Thus it appears that iodide must be transported into the cell against an electrochemical barrier and that it flows with an electrochemical gradient from the cell into the follicular lumen. The locus of the potential differences and several other lines of evidence place the site of active transport at the base of the thyroid follicular cell [14]. Inorganic iodide is also transported into the lumen of the stomach by the mucosa against a concentration and electrical gradient [52].

It may be assumed that much or all of the energy for iodide transport is derived from high-energy phosphate bonds. The transport system fails upon storage at 5°C [53], or on the addition of agents such as DNP, which uncouple oxidation from the generation of high-energy phosphate bonds [52]. Accumulation is also impaired by agents which impair intracellular aerobic metabolism, such as cyanide, azide, sulfide, and *p*-phenylenediamine [54, 55].

A second compartment of inorganic iodide within the thyroid is now recognized [14, 55–58]. This iodide is not discharged by ClO_4^-, and it appears to be functionally distinct from the iodide of the readily exchangeable pool. Presumably it is derived from deiodination of monoiodotyrosine (MIT) and diiodotyrosine (DIT) in the gland. The size of this pool becomes vanishingly small when the gland is depleted of iodine [58]. The precise role of this compartment in iodine economy in health and disease remains to be established.

Cations and ATPase

The cells of the body contain much more K^+ and much less Na^+ than the extracellular fluid, and these gradients are the result of active transport processes. The thyroid is unusual in that it is high both in Na^+ and in K^+ concentration. The entry of Na^+ into the gland is stimulated by TSH [59]. Digitoxin, digoxin, strophanthin, and several other glycosides and aglycones impair the transport of sodium and potassium across the red blood cell membrane [60]. Both Na^+ and K^+ are required to activate a Mg^{++}-dependent ATPase in erythrocyte membranes [61], and this activation is also blocked by the glycosides.

Wolff and colleagues have found that these glycosides also impair the transport of iodide into the thyroid [60, 62]. They have found a close correspondence between the biologic and biochemical behavior of iodide transport both in the thyroid and in other iodide-transporting tissues, and the Na^+-K^+–activated Mg^{++}-dependent ATPase activity of these same tissues. They reached the conclusion the ATPase activity is *indirectly* involved in iodide transport.

Turkington [63] has demonstrated a Mg^{++}-activated Na^+-K^+-dependent ATPase activity in thyroid cell membranes, and has found that this can be inhibited by ouabain. Just how the ATPase activity of the thyroid cell membrane is related to iodide transport is not clear, but it is of interest that Vilkki has demonstrated a chloroform-soluble iodide phospholipid complex in the thyroid, which conceivably could be an iodide receptor or carrier [64, 65], and a crude phospholipase has been shown to impair iodide transport, but not necessarily by phospholipase activity [66]. There is also an active kinase in the thyroid which can transfer the terminal phosphate from ATP to a phosphoprotein [67]. It seems probable that iodide transport is parasitic upon the energy supply of the Na^+-K^+ pump; certainly both require ATP. An increase in ouabain-sensitive ATPase is not required for TSH stimulation of iodide transport [68]. Amphotericin B inhibits iodide transport without impairing ATPase activity. This dissociation of effect is further evidence that operation of the cation-activated ATPase system is not in itself a sufficient condition for iodide transport [69].

Oxidation and Organification of Iodide

The next step in hormone synthesis is the oxidation of iodide and its displacement of hydrogen from the 3 position of tyrosyl residues in peptide linkage. This step may simply be an oxidation of iodide, with iodination of tyrosyl residues proceeding *pari passu,* or there may be an intermediate form of iodine which requires a transferring enzyme in order to facilitate the iodination of tyrosyl residues. Free or peptide-linked tyrosine is iodinated by iodine nonenzymatically in vitro, but it is entirely possible that the rate of this process is governed enzymatically in the gland.

Role of Peroxidase

Inorganic iodide must lose an electron before it can displace hydrogen from tyrosyl residues. Iodide is oxidized by slices in vitro, by cell-free homogenates, and by preparations of thyroid particulates [70–72], and this oxidation is abolished by heat. There seems to be good evidence that peroxidase is concerned in iodide oxidation. Not only has peroxidase activity been demonstrated many times in thyroid tissue [73–81], but also the oxidation of iodide, which proceeds rather specifically in thyroid tissue, is inhibited by catalase [70, 82]. Also, a variety of substances which inhibit organification of iodide in vivo or by thyroid slices, such as thiourea and resorcinol, either inhibit the peroxide-peroxidase system or act as competitive substrates for it [83, 84]. Furthermore, there is a small but nonetheless necessary oxygen requirement. Finally, there are ample sources for peroxide in tissues, but the precise source in thyroid in vivo is unsettled, as is the role of copper ion. Other electron carriers, such as cytochrome C, NADP, NAD, ferricyanide, and methylene blue [85], fail to stimulate MIT formation in thyroid particulate preparations but may do so in whole homogenates [86]. Thus it has been established that the conditions for iodide oxidation exist within the thyroid, but the specificity of the system for in vivo utilization of iodide in hormonogenesis has not been settled. The finding by Alexander [87] that a riboflavin-activated system in thyroid and salivary homogenates promotes the peroxidation of iodide and bromide whereas thyroid does not peroxidize bromide suggests that the peroxidase in the thyroid gland is iodide specific.

A complex which acts both as iodide-peroxidase and tyrosine iodinase has been solubilized and highly concentrated from sheep thyroid cell particles [88–90]. The complex has no cytochrome oxidase activity. It is thermolabile and requires a source of H_2O_2. It iodinates tyrosine and tyrosyl residues in peptide linkage to form MIT and a little DIT. The ratio of MIT to DIT formed is higher if the amount of iodide is small with respect to the available tyrosine. Small amounts of this complex can be recovered from rat spleen and salivary gland. It is inhibited by thiocarbamides, SCN^-, and CN^-, but not by ClO_4^- or by $10^{-3}M$ I^-. The iodide peroxidase also serves as a reduced pyridine nucleotide peroxidase, and this depends on the presence of iodide in the reaction mixture [88]. An interesting feature of this enzyme is that it is protected by iodide. DeGroot and Davis [89, 91] have suggested that this soluble enzyme complex is the peroxidase-iodinase portion of an iodinating system which normally exists in cell particles and which also generates peroxide by means of a reduced pyridine nucleotide–flavin nucleotide system. A similar and probably identical system which iodinates tyrosyl residues in the presence of thyroid particulates has been studied by others [87, 92–94]. The system described by Klebanoff et al. [93] formed thyroxine, and that of Suzuki et al. [94] iodinated thyroglobulin and was stimulated by thyrotropic hormone.

Actually, it is not established that an "iodinase" is required in order to promote the iodination of tyrosyl and MIT residues in vivo, but it seems probable. It is clear from the studies of Klebanoff et al. [93] that a single enzyme, a peroxidase, can catalyze the complete synthesis of iodotyrosines. If a thyroid iodinase exists, its lack should be marked by an expansion of the intrathyroidal iodide pool, which would be discharged by SCN^- or ClO_4^-, and by a slowed rate of hormonogenesis, but not a complete block. On the other hand, an absence of an iodide-peroxidase might be expected to block iodide oxidation and hormonogenesis quite completely.

Formation of iodoamino acids, especially MIT, can be readily demonstrated in tissue slices. Synthesis of organic iodine is abolished by azide, cyanide, and sulfide, substances which inhibit cytochrome oxidase, but this is by no means proof that cytochrome oxidase is involved, for this enzyme participates in many highly critical reactions which could be secondarily involved in iodide oxidation. Also, these chemical agents are all reducing substances and might simply donate electrons to I^0 nonenzymatically. The thiocarbamide drugs also inhibit formation of organic iodine, possibly by maintaining the iodide in the reduced state, but these are also inhibitors of thyroid tissue peroxidase [95] (see below).

Iodide is incorporated into organic form by thyroid cells in suspension [96, 97]. These produce MIT and possibly DIT. If albumin or thyroglobulin is present in the suspending medium, it is iodinated, but otherwise thyroglobulin is not synthesized [96].

Iodine Metabolism in Subcellular Preparations

Iodide is also used by whole tissue homogenates and by particulate preparations [95–101]. Formation of organoiodine is inhibited in thyroid particulate preparations by catalase, by the thiocarbamide drugs, and by azide, sulfide, cyanide, and SCN^- but not by ClO_4^-, as has already been mentioned. The process is stimulated by addition of FAD (flavin adenine dinucleotide), riboflavin, flavin mononucleotide (FMN) [102–104], and Cu^{++}, but addition of these substances is not required for organification of iodine. These preparations are thermolabile and require oxygen. The anomalous action of SCN^- may be due to its effect on peroxidase or the fact that it is a reducing agent rather than to its specific effect on iodide transport, which it shares with ClO_4^- [95]. A soluble system (unsedimented at $105,000 \times g$) requiring Cu^{++} which synthesized MIT from tyrosine and iodide has been prepared from homogenized salivary gland [105], and a soluble fraction has been obtained from thyroid homogenate which after dialysis iodinates tyrosine [93].

Homogenate preparations probably also produce small

amounts of DIT, as well [100–106]. In addition, two iodinated compounds of unknown structure and significance appear [106]. Formation of all these compounds is much enhanced by addition of flavin nucleotides to the system [106], but an effect of pyridine nucleotides is not established [100, 107]. NAD appears to stimulate the production of still another unidentified iodinated component [106]. The MIT formed in homogenate systems is in peptide linkage and is released as the free amino acid by proteolytic hydrolysis. The poor yield of DIT has suggested that a different iodinating system is required for the iodination of MIT than for the formation of MIT [108].

Iodination in homogenate preparations appears to be dependent upon, and regulated by, intermediary carbohydrate metabolism [86]. The rate is determined in part by NADP-linked dehydrogenation or by the presence of an endogenous inhibitor. The inhibitor has not been identified with certainty, but it is probably reduced glutathione (GSH) [93]. Ascorbic acid may contribute, as well [93, 106]. Inhibition of the sulfhydryl group of GSH by Cu^{++} could account for the stimulating effect of Cu^{++} on iodide organification in homogenates, as reported by others [100].

The Substrate of Iodination and Its Location

Iodination of protein in the thyroid occurs primarily in the numerous microvillae which extend into the colloid from the internal surfaces of the follicular cells [109]. Radioautographs of glands shortly after administration of radioiodine show the protein-bound iodine (PBI) at or near the cell-colloid interface, but later the bound iodine moves into the interior of the colloid. Addition of iodine to the molecule occurs after the thyroglobulin has been formed [110]. Iodination and thyroxine formation can proceed in the presence of puromycin. This indicates that iodination is not necessarily coupled to protein synthesis, and that preformed substrate can be iodinated [111]. Normally the principal substrate of iodination is thyroglobulin, and a conformational change occurs in the molecule as it becomes iodinated. Other proteins of the thyroid may also be iodinated, but only to a limited extent except in certain pathologic states [112].

Action of Thiocarbamide Drugs

Thiouracil and related antithyroid drugs of the thiocarbamide group block organification of iodine. These are reducing substances. They might act to maintain iodide in the reduced state or to reduce it, or as competing substrates. A mould chloroperoxidase studied by Morris and Hager [113] converts thiouracil to its disulfide through formation of an intermediate, sulfenyl iodide (^{-}SI), in the presence of iodide and peroxide. Hypothetically, in this way iodide might be diverted from its normal pathway by the antithyroid drug, and the inhibitor would compete for the thyroid peroxidase. Thiouracil labeled with ^{14}C binds to β-lactoglobulin and to thyroid microsomal protein in the presence of peroxide and iodide [114, 115]. The reaction evidently is with sulfenyl iodide groups found in the proteins. These findings suggest that sulfenyl iodide is a key intermediate in the iodination reaction [116], and that the thiocarbamide drugs react at these sites to prevent further transiodination from sulfenyl iodide to tyrosyl residues.

Iodothyronine Formation

The formation of T_4 in protein-free solutions was first observed by von Mutzenbecher [117, 118] and has been amply confirmed [119]. The reaction proceeds in alkaline solution under oxidizing conditions, is enhanced in the presence of hypoiodite or peroxide [120], and is inhibited by reducing substances such as sulfite. It is much enhanced if both the carboxyl and amino groups are covered, as, for example, in N-acetyldiiodotyrosylglutamic acid [121]. Diiodotyrosine reacts with diiodohydroxyphenylpyruvic acid (DIHPPA) to form T_4, and if the pyruvate derivative is produced from DIT by the deaminase of snake venom in the presence of catalase, then yields of 12 to 16 percent and more of T_4 can be obtained [122]. T_4 is also formed by iodination of casein, with milk used as the source of xanthine oxidase, xanthine as substrate, and iodide [123]. Roche and Michel [124] have proposed the scheme shown in Fig. 10-2, based largely on studies of Harington, for the in vitro synthesis of T_4 from diiodotyrosine [125], and subsequent studies have largely supported this general pattern. Coupling may involve oxidative formation of a quinoid which pairs with a phenoxide ion, both formed from iodotyrosyl residues, which splits out an alanine group to form iodothyronine. Alternative but similar schemes are reviewed elsewhere [14, 126, 127].

Triiodothyronine and thyroxine are doubtlessly formed in the thyroid by condensation of iodotyrosyl residues or their derivatives. Thyronine itself has never been isolated from the thyroid and, accordingly, could not serve as a substrate for iodination. Free labeled MIT, DIT, and iodothyronines can be extracted only in small amounts from gland homogenates which have been recently or remotely labeled by ^{131}I. The possibility that free MIT or DIT or a derivative serves as a precursor for iodothyronines, linking with a residue in peptide linkage, has not been excluded. Ljunggren [128, 129] has obtained ^{131}I-labeled 2,6-diiodohydroquinone from the thyroid gland and has suggested that this DIT derivative may be the intermediate coupling component. The specific activity of the free T_4 in the gland is lower than that of thyroglobulin, a fact indicating that it is a product of thyroglobulin rather than a precursor [130].

The nature of the coupling reaction may or may not be identical in cell preparations and in proteins or protein-free solutions in vitro, for iodination of tyrosyl residues does not always permit formation of T_4. Silk fibroin, for example,

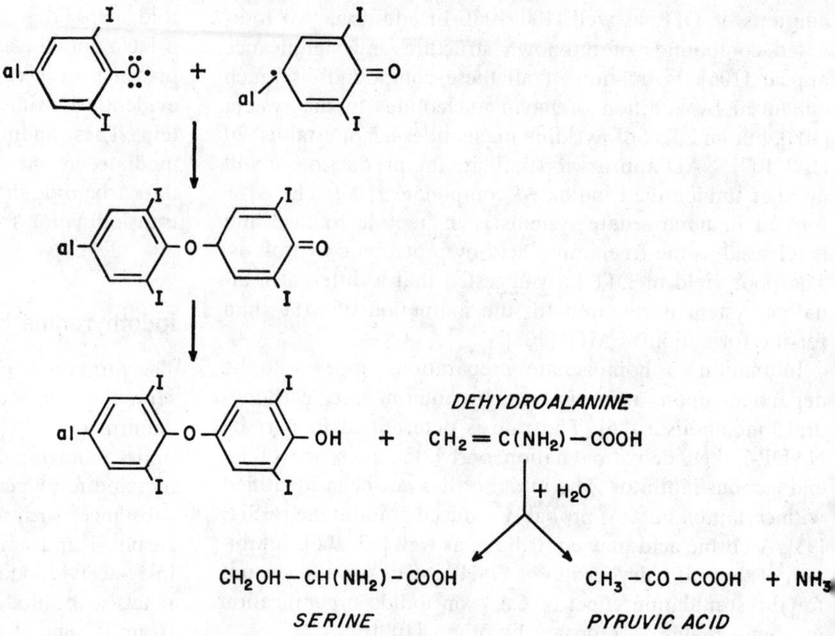

DEHYDROALANINE
$CH_2=C(NH_2)-COOH$
$+ H_2O$
$CH_2OH-CH(NH_2)-COOH$ SERINE
$CH_3-CO-COOH + NH_3$ PYRUVIC ACID

Figure 10-2. Scheme of iodothyronine synthesis as proposed by Roche and Michel [124], based largely on the studies of Harington [125].

is high in tyrosine, but iodination leads to formation of only traces of T_4, and the scleroproteins of certain invertebrates may contain huge amounts of iodotyrosine but no iodothyronine. Traces of I_2 catalyze the coupling reaction in vitro, as do other mild oxidizing conditions, and coupling is impaired by the thiocarbamides. The whole problem of iodination of proteins and T_4 synthesis has been exhaustively reviewed elsewhere [14, 126, 131, 132].

Failure of coupling to proceed in cell-free homogenate systems, whereas T_4 forms fairly readily in slices incubated with ^{131}I, strongly suggests that T_4 formation in vivo either is enzymatically controlled or requires a high degree of cellular organization. Addition of a wide variety of nucleotide and other cofactors to homogenates has failed to promote the formation of T_3 or T_4 [88, 100, 107].

It seems probable that not all tyrosyl residues in thyroglobulin are susceptible to iodination and coupling into iodothyronine residues. Only a small fraction of the tyrosyl residues ever become iodinated, and only some of these proceed to form iodothyronine. Of the approximately 140 tyrosyl residues in thyroglobulin, only an average of ten or so may be iodinated to MIT, five or ten to DIT, and one to four to T_4, even when the supply of iodine is ample. Steric factors in the thyroglobulin molecule, especially its tertiary structure, may govern the rate and degree of iodothyronine formation. In this regard the finding of Dunn that serine is the nearest neighbor of thyroxine in the thyroglobulin molecule doubtless has important implications with respect to the nonrandomness of iodothyronine formation [133].

The amount of iodothyronine which is formed is dependent in part on the available iodine. When the concentration of iodine in thyroglobulin is low, the ratio of triiodothyronine to thyroxine rises and the fraction of iodothyronine relative to iodotyrosine is low [134, 135]. Some molecules of thyroglobulin may contain no iodothyronine at all when the iodine content of the gland is unusually low. Thus there may be heterogeneity of the thyroglobulin [136]. Also the conformational state of the molecule determines the distribution of the iodoamino acids and the amount of coupling which takes place [137, 138].

Hormone synthesis may be summarized as follows. Iodotyrosines, probably in peptide linkage, are the precursors of iodothyronines in the thyroid gland. Though the precise mechanism of the coupling reaction either in vivo or in vitro remains to be disclosed, it seems established that oxidizing conditions are required. Peroxidase and systems for generating H_2O_2 are present in the thyroid, and there is some evidence for specificity of a tissue peroxidase for the iodide oxidation and iodination reactions. There is no proof that different sets of oxidizing conditions such as different sources of H_2O_2 or different peroxidases are needed for iodide oxidation and coupling. There is no direct evidence that DIHPPA is an intermediate in iodothyronine synthesis in vivo, but it has been identified in the thyroid [139]. Also, there is evidence that diiodohydroquinone is an intermediate. Among the possible mechanisms for coupling which have been suggested are the following:

1. Simple dismutation between iodotyrosyl residues
2. Free radical interaction, with formation of a diphenyl ether bridge and extrusion of dehydroalanine
3. Free radical displacement, with extrusion of alanine
4. Reaction between MIHPPA or DIHPPA and an iodo-

tyrosyl residue by dismutation or by free radical interaction
5. Reaction between an iodotyrosyl residue and a β-hydroxy derivative of an iodotyrosyl residue or of DIHPPA
6. Sequential degradation of the side chain through DIHPPA or MIHPPA, to benzaldehyde and quinone, followed by iodothyronine synthesis through coupling with an iodotyrosyl residue.

While there is no question but that model systems will form T_4 from iodotyrosyl precursors nonenzymatically, the possibility that the coupling reaction in vivo takes place enzymatically either directly or indirectly has been neither proved nor excluded. Several years ago Sir Charles Harington [140] wrote that all that is required for T_4 formation in the thyroid is thyroglobulin and conditions capable of oxidizing iodide. There can be no question about this, but whether these are sufficient conditions for the process in vivo will have to be settled in the future.

Hormone Storage and Release

T_4 and T_3 are retained in the thyroid gland in storage form within the colloid as peptide-linked residues within the specific thyroid protein, thyroglobulin. Thyroglobulin is a glycoprotein which has a molecular weight of approximately 650,000 and an isoelectric point of 4.5. Human thyroglobulin is salted out of phosphate buffer between 1.6 and 1.95*M* concentration. It is comprised of four polypeptide chains. Approximately 8 percent of the molecule is carbohydrate. The hexose subunits are added after synthesis of the peptide chain is completed [141, 142]. Ultrastructural studies have disclosed that the molecule has the shape of a flexible helix with two turns, a length of about 220 Å, and a maximal diameter of the coiled part of the molecule of about 110 Å [143].

When labeled leucine is used to follow the course of synthesis of thyroglobulin, it is incorporated successively into peptides with 3S to 8S, 12S, 17S to 18S, and 19S sedimentation constants [144]. Iodine is required for completion of the molecules to the 19S native thyroglobulin protein [145, 146]. The 19S units may be further aggregated into 27S and 32S units, and dissociated into 12S subunits for cross-species hybridization experiments [147]. The unit length of the RNA messenger of thyroglobulin subunit synthesis is not yet established [148–150]. The relative number of large polyribosomes in the thyroid is not appreciably greater than in other tissues, in spite of the predominant synthesis of a very large molecule. If the minimal thyroglobulin subunit is approximately 165,000 (four subunits per molecule), then by comparison with other well-characterized systems the polysomes should contain 40 to 50 ribosomes. Present evidence is that they contain less, perhaps 20 to 30; the ordinary thyroglobulin subunit may be smaller than 165,000 [149].

Thyroglobulins from many species have been studied [151, 152]. They have virtually the same molecular weight but may differ immunologically. The iodine content varies widely. There is a 12S subunit normally present in guinea pig thyroids which contains only about 10 percent of the iodine of thyroglobulin but which hybridizes with 12S subunits obtained from 19S thyroglobulin [147]. Synthesis of thyroglobulin is well established in the human fetus by the twenty-ninth day of development [153]. Small amounts can be detected in the plasma of adult man by radioimmunoassay [154, 155].

Thyroglobulin is the principal iodinated component of the thyroid, but at least two other iodinated components are present in much smaller concentration [156–159]. One of these is water-soluble and has a sedimentation constant of approximately 4. It has been termed the S-1 protein and has the electrophoretic, ultracentrifugal, and solubility characteristics of serum albumin. It may contain normally up to 4 percent of the total iodine in the gland. Another iodoprotein is closely attached to the cellular debris of thyroid homogenates and sediments with the nuclear fraction by conventional fractionation techniques. It may be distributed through at least three differently sedimenting fractions, and is clearly not attached to the cell nuclei [156]. The roles of these two components in normal thyroid physiology are entirely unknown at present, but there are interesting variations in disease states.

Proteolysis and Hormone Release

The strongly stimulated thyroid gland may secrete newly formed thyroid hormones rapidly into the blood [160], but under normal circumstances T_4 and T_3 are released as needed from the thyroglobulin pool. Degradation of thyroglobulin is brought about through a sequence of lytic enzymes [161–164], whose action may be stimulated by TSH [165, 166]. The proteases and peptidases which have been extracted from the thyroid lack specificity for thyroglobulin. One of the proteases has a pH optimum of 3.5 and is much more effective against hemoglobin than thyroglobulin. It has been purified to 500 times its original activity by cellulose column chromatography [167]. Another protease with a pH optimum of 5.7 has been identified [167]. Presumably these enzymes break thyroglobulin into large fragments, which are then hydrolyzed into the constituent amino acids by peptidases [168, 169]. Pastan and Almqvist [170] have described a potent thyroglobulin protease obtained from thyroid particulates; they point out that it probably does not function in vivo since it is located in the mast cells of the gland. This finding suggests caution in the interpretation of proteolytic activity found in preparations from thyroid homogenates.

Proteolysis releases T_4 and T_3 for diffusion into the blood. MIT and DIT, also present in the thyroglobulin, are also released but are deiodinated by a potent deiodinase which is present in the thyroid parenchymal cells [171, 172]. This deiodinase is a microsomal enzyme which requires NADPH [173–175]. Deiodination is stimulated by flavin nucleotide and nicotinamide [176, 177]. A soluble deiodinase, thought to be an isoenzyme, has also been described [178]. The removal of the first iodine from DIT occurs less rapidly than does the deiodination of MIT. The end products of the reaction are iodide and tyrosine. The freed iodide presumably is conserved for reutilization by the parenchymal cells, but some also leaks into the blood. Iodotyrosine deiodinase has also been demonstrated in liver, kidney, and other tissues. The presence of this enzyme in the thyroid cells prevents the appearance of MIT and DIT in the peripheral blood. Inhibitors of deiodinase, such as dinitrotyrosine, permit MIT and DIT to escape from the thyroid [179, 180]. Deiodination is inhibited by substances such as menadione which suppress NADPH oxidation [181]. What purpose, if any, is served by this enzyme in organs other than the thyroid is not apparent. In an assay for this enzyme in 39 glands from patients with familial goiter, Carr et al. found that the K_m was normal, except in the specimens from eight cancers of the thyroid, where the K_m was found to be low [182].

Kinetic analyses of thyroid function have shown repeatedly that in both the normal and in many abnormal states of thyroid activity there is a leak of iodide, or at least of a substance which is rapidly degraded to iodide from the gland into the blood [14, 15, 183–186]. The source of this iodide is presumably MIT and DIT which are deiodinated as they are released during proteolysis of thyroglobulin. Reuse of this iodide within the gland is blocked by the thiocarbamide drugs. It is the source of the so-called second iodide pool.

Hormone Transport and Fate

T_4 is carried in the plasma principally in association with a carrier protein (T_4-binding globulin, TBG) which has an electrophoretic mobility close to that of α_2-globulin [187]. In addition, a small amount of T_4 is carried with albumin, and with a component found in the prealbumin region. This carrier, called *prealbumin* (TBPA), may carry four times as much T_4 at pH 8.6 but carries much less at physiologic pH [188, 189]. T_3 is also carried by the thyroid-binding protein, but not by TBPA. It is less tightly bound and is found also in association with other plasma proteins [190]. TBG has been highly purified [191]. Its concentration in the blood falls from infancy to the fourth or fifth decade, and then rises again [192]. Reciprocal changes occur in the thyroxine bound by TBPA. Prednisone causes an increase in TBPA and a decrease in TBG [193]. It is interesting that genetic variation in the amount of binding protein in the plasma has little if any influence on thyroid function or metabolic state [194–196].

The equilibrium between free and bound iodothyronines determines the amount of hormone which actually impinges upon cells to give the characteristic metabolic stimulating effect. The amount of effective, or free, hormone is a function of the amount of hormone in the blood and the amount of carrier protein. The concentration of free T_4 iodine in normal serum is approximately 1.8 ng per 100 ml, or about one one-thousandth the concentration of the bound hormone.

The binding sites in the tissues which are effective in vivo are poorly defined. Some may be soluble [197] and some particulate [198]. Administration of phenobarbital to rats results in increased binding of thyroxine by intrahepatic microsomes and increased turnover of the thyroxine [199, 200]. The smooth endoplasmic reticulum contains important binding sites for thyroxine, and these proliferate under phenobarbital administration [201]. The binding by liver and kidney is to a degree reversible [202, 203].

The thyroid hormones are degraded in the peripheral tissues through several pathways. Small amounts appear as glucuronides in the bile [204, 205]. Isselbacher has found that these are formed by a liver microsomal enzyme which requires a uridine nucleotide [206]. The sulfate derivative may also be formed. Deamination and decarboxylation products have been demonstrated in brain tissue [207]. Conversion of T_4 to T_3 may take place in kidney slices in vitro [208] and also in isolated cell particulate preparations of liver, kidney, and other tissues [209]. T_3 is demonstrable in the serum in significant amounts after intravenous administration of T_4 [210]. Wynn et al. have described a liver microsomal system which degrades T_4 rapidly [211, 212]. Deiodination in their system requires initial oxygen-dependent fixation of the T_4 into a complex, and this can be inhibited by a large number of substances which can form phenoxyl free radicals, such as 2,6-diiodo-1,4-hydroquinone. Several other deiodinating systems for T_4 have been described, and this field remains in a confusing and uncertain state [213–217]. Some of the pitfalls in studies of deiodination reactions have been identified [218].

Thyroxine is deiodinated by peripheral tissues in vivo. Pittman and her colleagues [219, 220] have observed the fate of thyroxine labeled in various positions with radiocarbon, radioiodine, and tritium. Most of the thyroxine is deiodinated and excreted as various derivative components with the diphenyl ether bridge intact. In the rat most of the thyronyl derivatives are recovered in the feces. In man most of the iodine of injected thyroxine appears in the urine; the fate of the thyronyl nucleus is unknown. In the rat the deiodinating activity of the livers of riboflavin-deficient animals is much reduced, whereas it is increased in vitamin E–deficient animals [221].

The thyroid hormones cross the placenta to enter the fetal circulation. Transfer of thyroxine is slow and limited, presumably because of the tight binding to TBG. Triiodothyronine crosses more readily but fails to reach a concentration in cord blood as high as that in the maternal circulation even if an increase in maternal blood concentration has been present for as long as 3 weeks [222].

Peripheral Action of Thyroid Hormones

It is not possible within the scope of this chapter to examine critically the various theories which have been proposed to account for the stimulating effect of thyroid hormones on the oxygen consumption of cells. An attempt will be made only to mention the leading directions of investigation and to cite a few papers from the profuse literature on this subject.

Effects of Structure

The peripheral action of thyromimetic substances is intimately related to structure. An ether or thioether bridge between the two rings is necessary. The *p*-hydroxyl substituent can be replaced by a methoxy group, and the alanine side chain can be radically altered, with reduction but not deletion of action. Various substitutions of nitro, amino, alkyl, halogen, and hydroxyl groups can be made for the iodines, but almost always with diminution of activity [223–225]. Removal of one iodine from the 5 position enhances activity [226], and in general removal of the 5′ substituent from substances with thyromimetic activity enhances the activity. The relationships of structure to function are further complicated by the fact that a structural alteration may have differing metabolic effects, depending on which of several assays is employed. This is not surprising when one considers that a structural change may alter absorption, protein binding, cell penetrance, or degradation of the compound, and that different assays may measure different effects of the substances in question.

The iodothyronine which ultimately affects the machinery of the cell has not been identified. The in vivo latency of several hours in the effect of T_4 has suggested that it undergoes a structural alteration before it is active. The shorter latency of T_3 and the still shorter one of the acetic acid analogue of T_3 indicate a possible pathway of metabolism toward the effective substance. There is no proof at present that any such pathway is required. Still another interesting unsolved problem is that the thyroid hormones stimulate metabolic activity in some tissues, such as liver and muscle, and not in others, such as adult brain.

Effects on Peripheral Enzyme Activity

Cellular enzymes of various tissues are influenced by thyroid administration or in thyrotoxicosis [226–229]. The activity of succinic oxidase, amino acid oxidases, carbonic anhydrase, ascorbic oxidase, cytochrome oxidase, NADPH–cytochrome C reductase, arginase, muscle hexokinase, amylase, flavokinase, FAD pyrophosphorylase, and others varies with the thyroid dosage. Plasma pseudocholinesterase varies inversely. Some of these effects may be the result of binding of metals by iodothyronines. T_4 complexes with Cu^{++}, Co^{++}, Zn^{++}, Mg^{++}, Fe^{++}, and Mn^{++}. Adenylosuccinate synthetase, the enzyme of the first step in the conversion of inosine monophosphate to AMP, is stimulated twofold in rat liver at a concentration of $10^{-9}M$ triiodothyronine [230]. Cardiac phosphorylase activity is increased by thyroxine, and this effect is potentiated by corticosterone [231]. Thyroid hormone is necessary for cholinesterase activity in the developing rat brain [232].

T_4 and several analogues inhibit a number of NAD-dependent dehydrogenases in vitro. Among these are malic, glutamic, lactic, triosephosphate, inosine monophosphate, yeast alcohol, and yeast glucose-6-P dehydrogenases [233, 234]. All these enzymes contain zinc. With the possible exception of malic dehydrogenase, the concentration for T_4 effect ($\sim 10^{-5}M$) is above the physiologic range by two or three orders of magnitude. This inhibition of malic dehydrogenase accounts for the apparent stimulation of succinic oxidation by T_4, since succinic dehydrogenase is inhibited by oxaloacetate, which is formed by the malic dehydrogenase. The α-glycerophosphate and the liver malic enzyme are stimulated by administration of thyroxine in vivo [235]. Oxaloacetate is increased in the liver of hypothyroid rats and decreased in thyroid-fed rats [236]. This action of *l*-T_4 on dehydrogenases is shared by the *d*-isomer and by other substances which do not have T_4-like activity [237]. Inhibition of NAD-linked dehydrogenases has been attributed to a deleterious effect on mitochondria (which swell under the influence of T_4 [238]) that permits leakage of NAD from these structures [239]. This may be one way in which dehydrogenase activity is inhibited, but Wolff and Wolff found the inhibition in a system which was free of particulate material [234]. T_4 dissociates glutamic dehydrogenase into subunits and also reacts with the enzyme at the active site of the enzyme and at the position involved in its activation [240].

Steroid metabolism is intimately related to thyroid function. Patients with thyrotoxicosis dispose of administered steroids, such as cortisone, more rapidly than normal, and those with myxedema less rapidly [241]. This has been traced to control by T_4 of the capacity of the liver to reduce ring A of the steroid [242]. Not only does treatment of rats with T_4 increase the availability in liver homogenate of NADPH for ring reduction, but with prolonged treatment there is an increase in the microsomal reducing enzyme as well [243]. Similar results have been obtained for testosterone, hydrocortisone, progesterone, and others [244].

Administration of thyroxine to rats causes an increase of incorporation of phosphate into mitochondrial phospholipid and an increase in mitochondrial content of phospholipid [245]. Triiodothyronine enhances the effect of epinephrine in releasing glycerol and free fatty acids from the epididymal fat pad [246]. Thyroxine causes an increased utilization by heart of long-chain fatty acids and decreased use of glucose [247]. Large doses of thyroxine may have an antioxidant function in the fat stores, but this is probably a pharmacologic effect [248].

Effects on Oxidative Phosphorylation

Most of the chemical energy used by the body is channeled through high-energy phosphate bonds, especially ATP. The ratio of bonds formed (phosphate uptake) to oxygen used (P/O ratio) is a measure of the efficiency of oxygen utilization.

A significant advance in the understanding of thyroid hormones in relation to cellular physiology was the finding that there is a fall in the P/O ratio (uncoupling) of mitochondrial preparations in vitro when T_4 or any of a number of analogues is added, or in tissues removed from animals pretreated with T_4. Many other chemical substances, such as dinitrophenol, also uncouple [249–251].

The explanation of T_4 action as an uncoupler of oxidative phosphorylation has been an attractive one. The principal arguments advanced against it are that (1) many substances uncouple oxidative phosphorylation which are not effective in the treatment of hypothyroidism; (2) uncoupling fails to explain the "beneficial" effect of T_4; (3) the concentrations of thyromimetic substances necessary for uncoupling are somewhat higher than those existing in vivo; and (4) whereas T_4 may uncouple, this takes place largely at the expense of phosphate bond formation but with little, if any, increase in oxygen consumption. These objections have been largely answered by Lardy and Maley [252], who have proposed a mechanism for the central and most difficult problem, namely, that of the specific "beneficial" effect of T_4. They propose that T_4 and analogues in low concentration act at a specific biochemical locus to uncouple a rate-limiting step in a chain of energy-yielding reactions. In this way, subsequent steps proceed more rapidly and without significant overall loss in efficiency. Larger concentrations of T_4 cause the uncoupling effect to spread to other reactions and lower the overall efficiency. In support, oxidative phosphorylation may be stimulated in mitochondrial preparations prepared from animals given T_4 [251, 253, 254], and stimulation of oxidation of succinate by mitochondria has been observed without change in the P/O ratio in the presence of 5×10^{-7} M T_4 if these were prepared from thyroidectomized rats [255]. It may be said at present that the mechanism of action of T_4 as an uncoupler of oxidative phosphorylation is not entirely satisfactory but comes closer to explaining the facts than any other which has been proposed.

Other Hormone Effects

T_4 both in vivo and in vitro increases ATPase activity [256]. This not only increases the dissipation of high-energy phosphate bonds, either as work or as heat, but also provides ADP, which stimulates glycolysis. T_4 also inhibits transhydrogenation from NADPH to NADH and in this way inhibits production of ATP from processes dependent upon NADH [257]. All these observations may be related to the uncoupling effect of T_4 on oxidative phosphorylation.

Another interesting effect of T_4 is mitochondrial swelling [258–260]. This can be reversed by ATP. It has been suggested that swelling may be the primary effect and that uncoupling may be a secondary event. Similar phenomena can be shown with cyanogen iodide [259, 260], and it has been considered that the role of T_4 may be simply that of a carrier to move iodine into the mitochondria. Tata has suggested that the fundamental action of T_4 may be on protein synthesis, or on the genetic information transfer, for he finds no effect on respiration in the presence of inhibitors such as actinomycin D [261, 262]. Tata's findings would appear to shift the whole emphasis in T_4 action away from energy metabolism and the mitochondria and toward the control of protein synthesis in the cell. A stimulating effect of thyroxine on protein synthesis has been shown in several tissues, including the immature rat brain and cell-free preparations of muscle [263–265]. It has been suggested that stimulation of protein synthesis is the primary end-organ effect of thyroid hormone, but the concentrations required for an effect are well above those prevailing in vivo.

The thyroid hormones profoundly affect development. Induction of metamorphosis in the amphibian has been extensively studied. Hormone effects on brain lipid and motor activity can be detected prior to development of the homeothermic state in the perinatal rat [266]. Moss and Ingram have demonstrated a switch from synthesis of the component chains of fetal hemoglobin to those of adult hemoglobin in the amphibian undergoing thyroxine-induced metamorphosis [267]. Embryonic chicks deprived of thyroid hormone by an injection of propylthiouracil show specific lesions of the sensory hair cells of the acoustic papillae and of the cochlear spinal ganglia [268]. DNA-dependent RNA polymerase activity of rat liver is stimulated by thyroid hormones [269, 270].

Control of Thyroid Function

The activity of the thyroid gland is largely under the control of the anterior lobe of the adenohypophysis, which secretes thyrotropic hormone (TSH). Removal of the hypophysis reduces but does not entirely eliminate thyroid function. Development of a reliable sensitive and specific radioimmunoassay for TSH has confirmed and extended many observations on pituitary-thyroid control relationships painstakingly made in the past. Extensive critical reviews are available [271–273]. TSH in high concentration is found in human pituitary venous sinusoidal blood [274]. Secretion is rapidly suppressed upon administration of thyroxine and triiodothyronine, and resumes when they are withdrawn and blood levels fall below normal. Uptake of amino acids and glucosamine by the pituitary is stimulated by withdrawal of thyroid hormones and suppressed by their administration [275, 276]. Normal pituitary-thyroid feedback control may require a normal balance between triiodothyronine and thyroxine [277]. Release of TSH can be stimulated in vitro by cyclic 3′,5′-adenosine monophosphate (cyclic AMP), by theophylline (which inhibits cyclic AMP breakdown), and by epinephrine [278].

A major recent advance in thyroid physiology has been the discovery and characterization of the TSH-releasing factor (TRF). TRF arises in the hypothalamus and reaches the pituitary through the hypothalamic-portal system [278*a*]. It is effective when infused directly into the pituitary [279], and has been demonstrated to stimulate TSH release in man [280]. It is a remarkably potent tripeptide with the structure pyroglutaminylhistidylprolineamide [281, 282]. TRF probably arises from the ventromedial hypothalamus, and this center is probably under the influence of neural afferents arising elsewhere [283]. The thyroid hormones and TRF interact at the hypophyseal cell level to control TSH release; inhibitors of protein and RNA synthesis prevent T_3 inhibition but not the TRF-release response [284, 285]. The TSH-release response of the pituitary to cold is mediated through TRF [286].

A huge literature concerns the interaction between TSH and its target cell in the thyroid [286*a*, 286*b*]. All functions of the cell are stimulated, including cell division, but the time of appearance of various responses varies widely. Oxidation of glucose, for example, is stimulated within minutes, whereas other changes may not appear for many hours [275]. The effect on glucose oxidation may be demonstrated even if the TSH is washed from the tissue preparation immediately after exposure, but is blocked with antiserum to TSH [287]. This observation indicates that the initial interaction is a rapid, firm binding to a component of the plasma membrane. Other effects may arise because of deeper penetration of TSH into the cell, or because of products of the interaction of the plasma membrane and the TSH. Among the effects of TSH on the thyroid cell are stimulation of amino acid incorporation [288], creatine phosphokinase and lactic dehydrogenase activity [289], NAD kinase activity [290], and NADP synthesis [291], increased turnover of phosphorous in the acidic phosphoglycerides [292], stimulation of proteolysis [293], and depletion of gland serotonin [294]. TSH also stimulates iodide uptake, organification and coupling into hormones [295], and secretion of hormones. The TSH effect on secretion is inhibited by iodide [296].

Synthesis of cyclic AMP by the thyroid is stimulated by TSH within a 1-min incubation period presumably through an interaction with the thyroid cell plasma membrane [297, 298]. This does not involve an adrenergic receptor system, as does the TSH effect on adipose tissue which seems to be mediated through cyclic AMP. Cyclic AMP stimulates iodide uptake and organification by thyroid cells as well as protein and phospholipid synthesis [299]. Thus there is strong evidence that TSH may exert most of its effects on the thyroid by activation of adenyl cyclase [299*a*]. Oxidation of glucose is mediated in this way in the dog thyroid, but not in the bovine thyroid [300]. Thus there appear to be species differences. Some other effects of TSH such as that in phospholipogenesis may not be mediated by cyclic AMP [301].

Two other peptide substances stimulate the thyroid under special circumstances. The long-acting thyroid stimulator (LATS) is a 7S γ-globulin which appears in the blood of many patients with Graves' disease. It has many, if not all, of the effects of TSH on the thyroid cell [302–305]. It appears to be synthesized by lymphocytes [306]. It or a similar substance can be induced by immunization with thyroid microsomes [307], and it interacts with thyroid particulates [308, 309]. It is inactivated by antiserums against the kappa and lambda chains of immunoglobulin [310]. A thyrotropic substance has also been obtained from the placenta. It is distinct from TSH and LATS [311, 312].

The concentration of T_4 in the plasma may exert a measure of control directly on the thyroid [313]. Thyroid function and growth were influenced by the amount of T_4 given to hypophysectomized rats maintained on constant doses of TSH. The possibility that disposal of the TSH was influenced by the T_4 was not excluded in these experiments. The rate of hormone synthesis in the thyroid is controlled in part by the amount of stored iodine within the gland [16, 314]. There is no satisfactory explanation for this mechanism of control. It may be noted in passing that in the rat there may be a small amount of extrathyroidal synthesis of thyroxine [315].

Other Cellular Activities

Quite apart from its role in producing, storing, and secreting the thyroid hormones, the thyroid cell carries out many other less specific functions of other cells. For example, many of the enzymes of the Embden-Meyerhof and the Krebs cycle have been identified in the thyroid [316, 317]. Their activity in the normal gland is somewhat less per milligram of potassium than in some other structures, such as the liver. Both Dumont [318] and Field et al. [319, 320] have demonstrated an active hexose monophosphate shunt pathway in the thyroid. This pathway yields NADPH, and this nucleotide is important in protein and lipid synthesis. In this regard it is of particular interest that an early effect of TSH on the thyroid is a stimulation of the hexose monophosphate shunt [320, 321].

Protein is actively synthesized by the thyroid, and at least one product in subcellular particulate preparations has been identified as thyroglobulin [322]. Nadler et al. [323] have demonstrated incorporation of ^{3}H-labeled leucine into thyroid protein, and Seed and Goldberg [324] have demonstrated synthesis of thyroglobulin by thyroid slices. They found that synthesis proceeded even in the presence of actinomycin D and concluded that messenger RNA for thyroglobulin is quite stable.

Phosphate is incorporated into lipid by thyroid slices and in vivo [325, 326]. RNA is actively synthesized by the thyroid, and formate incorporation into RNA is stimulated by TSH in concentrations which are in the physiologic range.

The thyroid cell has an active electron transport system which seems to be in general much like that of other cells. Cytochrome B, A, and A_3 have been identified, and C is quite certainly present [327]. Many of the enzymes which mediate the transfer of electrons from substrate through pyridine nucleotides, flavoproteins, and down through the cytochromes to oxygen have been identified and measured in the thyroid [91, 328]. Well-coupled oxidative phosphorylation is a property of the normal gland [329].

TYPES OF FAMILIAL GOITER

The preceding pages have made it evident that there are many steps in the synthesis, storage, and secretion of the thyroid hormones. Many, if not all, of these steps depend on the functional integrity of specific enzymatic systems. Conceivably, thyroid disease could arise from defective function of any one of these steps; should a step be blocked or ineffective, production of thyroid hormones would be diminished or absent. Compensatory growth and increased activity of the gland might or might not restore an adequate supply of hormones.

Several types of familial goiter are now recognized which may be classified with more or less certainty according to specific failure of a normal physiologic process related to thyroid function. Clinical and laboratory criteria may be given for assignment of appropriate patients to each category. There are many reports of patients who doubtlessly belong in one or the other of these categories or variants of one of them but who cannot be classified because of the meager data available. Still other categories surely remain to be defined.

Familial Goiter from Failure to Transport Iodide (Iodide-transport Defect)

Case Studies

Only a single patient has been encountered by the author who had a defect in the transport of iodide into the thyroid [330]. He had only one sib, who was normal. The family was closely intermarried, and several members of both the paternal and maternal forebears had had goiter (Fig. 10-3).

The patient was a 15-year-old male at the time of study. Birth was at full term after a normal pregnancy. Birth weight was 4.3 kg. A small umbilical hernia noticed at birth was surgically repaired at 3 years of age. Early milestones of development were normal, but his progress in school was slow for the first 3 years. At age 8 the basal metabolic rate (BMR) was found to be minus 29 percent, and the serum cholesterol level was 560 mg per 100 ml. Roentgenograms of the bones disclosed a delay in maturation of 3 years. He responded well to 65 mg thyroid daily, and his growth and school performance became normal. Puberty was normal. Three months before admission, a small goiter was observed, and thyroid was discontinued. He quickly became lethargic, gained 9 kg, and became constipated.

Initial Findings

The skin was dry and moderately pigmented. Axillary and pubic hair and genitalia were normal. The thyroid was about three times normal size and contained numerous small

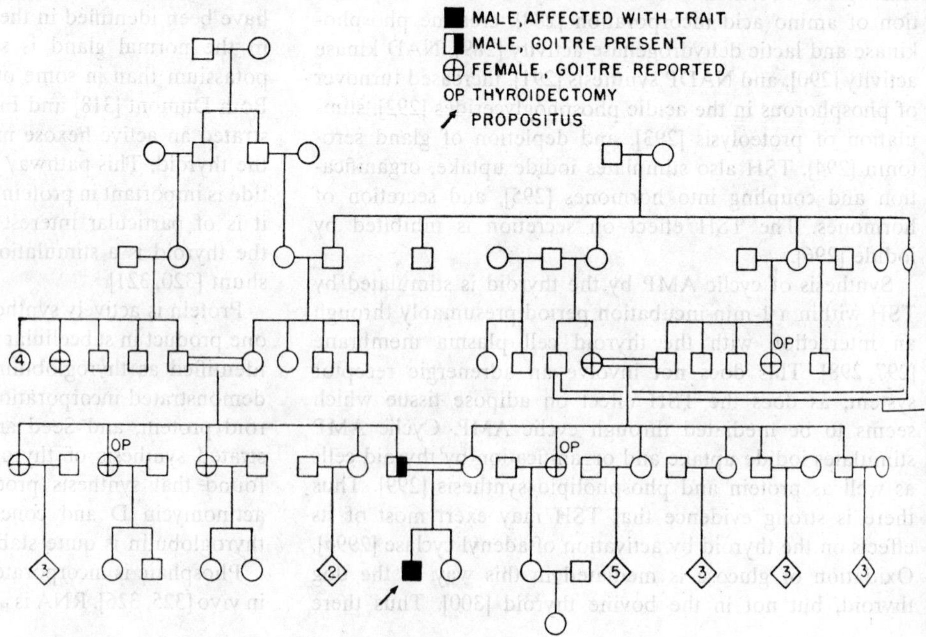

Figure 10-3. Family history of a 15-year-old male with failure of iodide transport. Note the several consanguine marriages.

nodules. The BMR was minus 39 percent. Total serum iodine concentration was 1.5 μg per 100 ml, and protein-bound iodine 0.5 μg per 100 ml. Serum-cholesterol concentration was 320 mg per 100 ml. Results of routine blood and urine tests were normal. The sella turcica was at the upper limits of normal or slightly larger than normal size, but there was no erosion of the clinoid processes. Bone age was consistent with the chronological age. Biopsy of the thyroid disclosed numerous small nodules. Some were cystic but most were cellular. There was intense hyperplasia of the parenchymal elements. Scarcely any colloid could be seen.

Investigations

Twenty-four hours after an oral dose of ^{131}I, 11.4 percent was in the gland, and at 48 hr, 7.8 percent was in the gland. A significant proportion of this may be assumed to have been in the vascular space of the hyperplastic thyroid and in the other vascular structures of the neck. Sixty-seven percent of the administered ^{131}I appeared in the urine within the first 24 hr, and 86.3 percent in the first 48 hr. Chromatography of samples of serum and urine obtained during the first 24 hr showed that inorganic iodide was the only ^{131}I-labeled substance.

The concentration of iodide in the saliva was not significantly different from that in the serum (S/P ratio). These results appear in Table 10-1, together with those obtained from several relatives of the patient and from a series of subjects with various other conditions. Both parents, a sister, and a maternal aunt of the patient had S/P ratios comparable to those of the control subjects.

Table 10-1. THE CONCENTRATION RATIOS BETWEEN SALIVA AND SERUM OF IODIDE, THIOCYANATE, AND CHLORIDE IN A PATIENT (A) WITH THE IODIDE TRANSPORT DEFECT, IN SEVERAL MEMBERS OF HIS FAMILY, AND IN CONTROL SUBJECTS

Patients	Sex	Age, yr	Diagnosis	Time after ^{131}I, hr	S/P†		
					^{131}I*	SCN⁻	Cl⁻
A	M	15	Goiter, hypothyroid	48	0.89	1.0	0.21
				1	1.46		
				2	1.64		
				3	1.31	1.6	0.40
				4	1.78		
				5	1.07		
B‡	M	50	Nodular goiter	2	64.3	10.2	0.15
C	F	21	Normal	2	29.7	13.0	0.15
D	F	54	Normal	2	53.4	26.0	0.46
E	F	49	Normal	1	21.4	10.0	0.10
				2	43.0	13.0	0.69
F	M	59	Thyrotoxicosis	2	10.9	8.9	0.14
G	F	42	Normal	2	27.7	4.1	0.11
H	F	43	Thyroid carcinoma	2	28.3	16.0	0.18
I	M	67	Normal	2	33.3	6.5	0.15
J	F	45	Previous thyrotoxicosis	2	30.8	17.2	0.10
K	F	60	Previous thyrotoxicosis	2	22.6	13.0	0.22
L	F	11	Hashimoto's thyroiditis	6	47.1		
				24	15.5		
				48	59.0	14.8	0.11
M	M	42	Hypothyroid	2	25.9	15.5	0.16
N	M	51	Myxedema	2	48.1	12.5	
O	F	52	Normal	2	70.2	9.0	0.33
P	F	28	Previous thyrotoxicosis	2	44.1	20.2	0.16
Q	M	30	Goitrous cretin§	2	35.7	8.1	0.17
R	F	39	Euthyroid	2	22.7	13.3	
S	F	41	Simple goiter	2	19.1	11.8	0.14
				4	32.4	16.0	0.12

* The ^{131}I ratio is based on trichloroacetic acid–soluble ^{131}I.

† S, concentration in saliva; P, concentration in serum.

‡ B is the father of A; C, sister of A; D, maternal aunt of A; E, mother of A. F through S are unrelated.

§ Previously reported.

The S/P ratio for Cl^- was consistently less than 1 and was comparable to values found in other subjects. On the other hand, the S/P ratios for SCN^- indicated little, if any, active concentration by the salivary glands. The level of SCN^- in the plasma of the patient was 0.4 mg per 100 ml, a normal value. The ratio of ^{131}I in gastric fluid collected 5 hr after administration of the ^{131}I and ½ hr after introduction of a gastric tube to that of the plasma was 0.8. The pH of the gastric fluid was 2.

Tissue slices cut at random from the biopsy fragments failed to accumulate ^{131}I from a medium in which they were incubated. On the other hand, a small amount of protein-bound ^{131}I initially present in the slices was formed from the two tracer doses of ^{131}I administered several days before biopsy. Approximately three-quarters of the protein-bound iodine (PBI) was MIT, and one-quarter DIT. Little, if any, iodothyronine was detected. Over 90 percent of the ^{131}I which was present in the supernatant after centrifuging the homogenate at 100,000 $\times$ *g* was precipitated between 1.6 and 1.95*M* phosphate. These are the conditions of thyroglobulin precipitation.

Concentrations of total and protein-bound iodine were 4.43 and 4.23 μg ^{127}I per gm wet weight, and 4.85 and 3.53 in two fragments. Assuming a total gland weight of 60 gm, one may estimate a total thyroid iodine of approximately 250 μg. The normal thyroid contains several milligrams of iodine.

Subsequent to biopsy the patient was discharged on a dose of 1 mg potassium iodide three times daily. Within 4 weeks the BMR had risen steadily to 8+, and his thyroid enlargement had virtually disappeared. He has remained well and euthyroid on this program for the intervening 9 years.

Interpretation

The physiologic abnormality in this patient may be interpreted as a missing essential component of the iodide transport system, a component common to the transport systems of the thyroid, the salivary gland, and the gastric mucosa. It is possible that some undetected inhibitor of the transport process is present. If so, it could not be SCN^-, because the amount of SCN^- in the saliva was less than normal.

The defect must be one which is fairly specific for transport of iodide and related anions and at the same time one which is not essential to more general transport processes in the cell and their energy sources, because apart from iodide transport those cells seem to be functioning quite normally. It may be assumed that the defect is not of the Na^+-K^+-activated cell membrane–ATPase membrane transport system, because significant defects in this system would doubtless be catastrophic for the cell. One interpretation is that the iodide gradient is dependent on a specific binding substance whose structure or orientation is maintained by an expenditure of cell energy, and that the defect in this patient was in this component which binds iodide and other anions of similar size and shape. No such substance has been described, except possibly the iodinated lipid of Vilkki [65].

Relatives of the patient who also had goiter failed to show any defect in salivary iodide transport even when heavily loaded with iodide. Possibly transport of iodide is more limited in the thyroid than in other structures.

Similar Cases Reported by Others

This form of familial goiter seems to be quite rare. Federman et al. [331] in 1958 reported a 19-month-old infant with cretinism and a goiter who failed to accumulate iodine in the gland. They surmised that the thyroid of their patient might be unable to take iodide from the blood. Later studies on this same patient confirmed this surmise and support the findings in the patient described above [332].

Two brothers whose parents were not consanguine have been reported by Gilboa et al. [333]. One was age 14. Myxedema had been diagnosed at age 1 month, and in the intervening years thyroid had been given and development had been normal. A goiter had appeared. Five weeks after withdrawal of medication the patient had the signs and symptoms of myxedema. An ^{131}I uptake was 11.5 percent at 24 hr. Tissue slices from a thyroid biopsy failed to concentrate iodide from the suspending medium. Administration of Lugol's solution was followed by a prompt disappearance of the findings of hyperthyroidism, but continued medication resulted in the appearance of thyrotoxicosis. When the dosage was reduced to 1 drop daily, the patient became quite normal. The 24-year-old brother had a large goiter. He had always taken thyroid and became critically hypothyroid when this was withdrawn. His ^{131}I uptake at 4 hr was only 3 percent 3 weeks after medication was discontinued. A mentally retarded 9-year old male with goiter has been described who appeared to have a partial defect in iodide transport [333*a*].

Genetics

The consanguinity of the parents of our patient and the appearance of the disorder in brothers in the family reported by Gilboa suggests autosomal recessive inheritance. Three of the reported patients are males and one is female. Nothing further can be said about inheritance from such limited data.

Diagnosis

Identification of this defect depends essentially on demonstration of low iodide clearance by the thyroid, hypothyroidism, and hyperplastic goiter. Diagnostic criteria appear in Table 10-2.

Table 10-2. DIAGNOSTIC CRITERIA FOR THE IODIDE-TRANSPORT DEFECT

Required	Helpful and confirmatory
1. Goiter; hypothyroid or compensated hypothyroid 2. Little if any uptake of radioiodine 3. No concentration of iodide by salivary glands	1. No concentration of iodide by gastric mucosa 2. No concentration of thiocyanate by salivary glands 3. Thyroid biopsy: *a.* Hyperplasia *b.* Low iodine content and concentration 4. Metabolic response to iodide medication

Familial Goiter from Failure to Form Organic Iodine (Organification Defect; Peroxidase Defect)

Case Studies

Five cretins with goiter who have a common defect in organification of iodine have been studied by Stanbury [27, 334, 335]. Four were sibs from a family of seven children. Three older sibs were normal and without thyroid disease, and now have a number of normal children. The parents were mixed Caucasian and American Indian and were first cousins on the Indian side of the family. Both pairs of grandparents were also first cousins. Growth and development of the affected children were considered normal during the first few months of life but thereafter became slowed. Thyroid medication was begun in all between the ages of a few months and 2 years, but was intermittent. A mass was observed in the neck of each between the ages of 7 and 13 years and slowly increased in size until they were seen in the hospital.

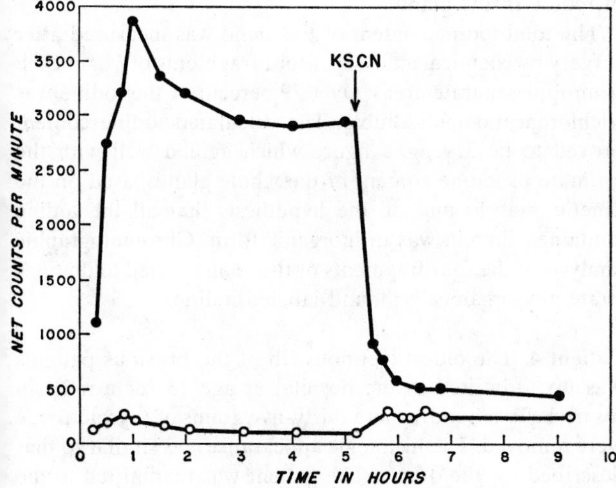

Figure 10-4. Discharge of iodide from the thyroid gland of a patient with cretinism and goiter, caused by administration of thiocyanate. ^{131}I was given at zero time. Thiocyanate was given orally as indicated by the vertical arrow.

Patient 1. This female patient was 16 years old in 1949 at the time of initial studies. She was dwarfed and grossly retarded mentally. The thyroid was enlarged five or six times normal size; it was nodular and firm. A bruit and thrill were present, and the skin over the thyroid felt warm to touch. The PBI concentration of the blood was 1.0 μg per 100 ml.

When the patient had been without thyroid medication for 3 weeks, ^{131}I was given orally. The labeled iodine in the gland reached a plateau in less than 2 hr. Twenty-seven hours later, 1.0 gm KSCN was given by mouth. This caused an immediate and striking fall in the concentration of labeled iodine in the gland (Fig. 10-4). At the end of 2 hr the counts had fallen to 25 percent of the previous level.

At thyroidectomy the gland weighed 97 gm. There was intense hyperplasia, coupled with cystic degeneration and fibrosis (Fig. 10-5). An analysis of the tissue disclosed a concentration of thyroid inorganic iodide of 29.3 μg per 100 gm and of protein-bound thyroid iodine of 1.4 μg per 100 gm. The normal thyroid gland weighing about 20 gm contains from 4 to 15 mg iodine, of which 1 to 2 percent at most is inorganic.

One of the normal sibs of this patient was similarly studied. A tracer dose of ^{131}I-labeled iodine slowly accumulated in the thyroid and reached a maximum value in approximately 24 hr. Oral administration of 2 gm KSCN caused no discharge of labeled iodine from the gland.

Patient 2. A 23-year-old cretinous male sib of Patient 1 was brought to the hospital because of a huge goiter and increasing difficulty in breathing (Fig. 10-6). A PBI determination of the serum was zero. The patient was given a tracer dose of 100 microcuries ^{131}I 5 months after he had last taken desiccated thyroid. Four and one-half hours later, when the counts over the thyroid had reached a plateau, he was given 2 gm KSCN by mouth. There was an immediate rapid fall in the recorded counts over the gland and a rise in the radioactivity recorded over the lower back. After 2 hr the counts in the neck had fallen by 70 percent.

The removed thyroid weighed 497 gm. Pathologic examination showed findings similar to those in Patient 1, above. In many areas there was a paucity of acinus formation characteristic of fetal adenoma, and in others disorganization of cellular pattern and fibrosis were found. The total in-

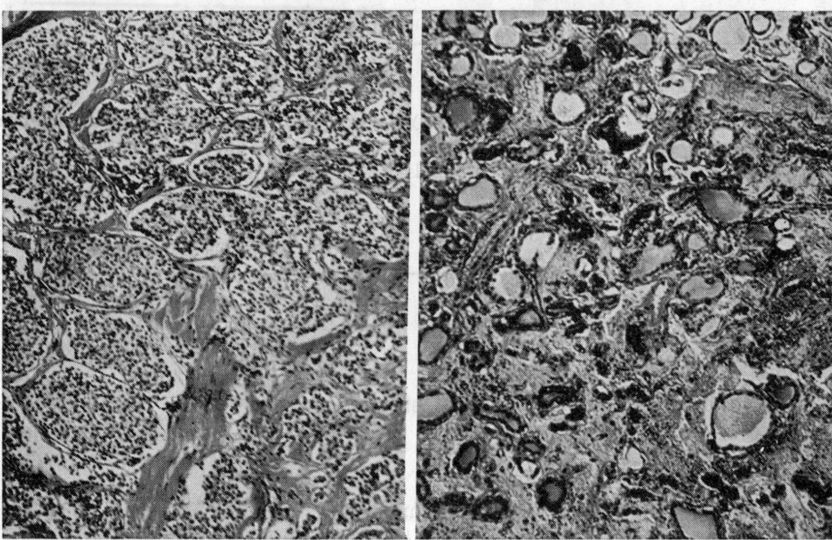

Figure 10-5. Histologic pattern from two areas of a thyroid gland removed from a patient with congenital goiter. Note the hyperplasia.

organic iodine was 173 μg per 100 gm, and the thyroid PBI was 15 μg per 100 gm.

Patient 3. This patient was a 13-year-old goitrous male sib of the previous two patients. His intellectual attainments were somewhat beyond those of his cretinous sibs. He had learned to feed himself and to walk but had never gone to school.

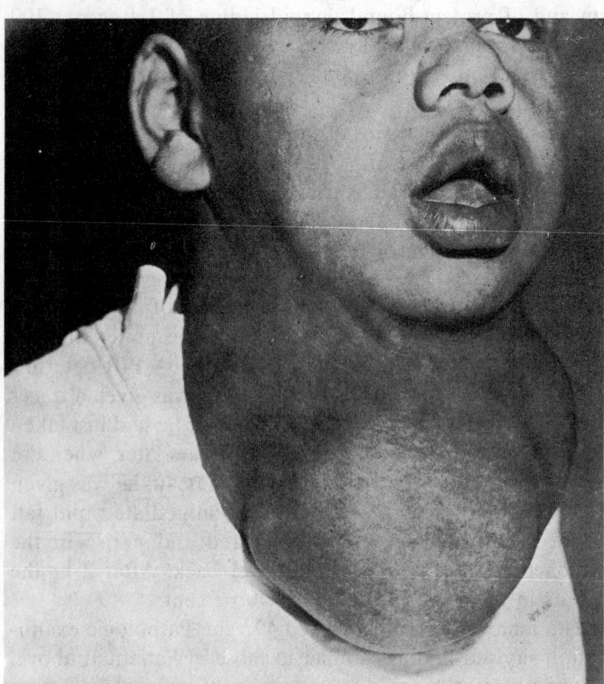

Figure 10-6. A 23-year-old cretinous male with goiter (Patient 2 of text). (*By permission of The Journal of Clinical Endocrinology and Metabolism.*)

Labeled iodine accumulated rapidly in the thyroid during the first hour after administration, and then slowly declined. Administration of 2 gm KSCN orally caused an immediate discharge of the labeled iodine from the thyroid. By 1 hr the counts were approximately 10 percent of the previous level. The concentration of PBI in the serum was 1.4 μg per 100 ml. The excretion of iodine in the urine varied from 86 to 232 μg for 24 hr (normal).

This patient was studied again 4 years later. The PBI concentration of the serum was 0.9 μg per 100 ml. The thyroid gland was fully five times normal size and was multinodular. Kinetic analysis of iodine metabolism was entirely consistent with the concept of a large intrathyroidal pool of readily exchangeable iodide and no organification of iodide in the gland.

The total iodine content of the gland was measured after surgery by chemical analysis of four fragments of ½ gm each from four separate areas. Over 99 percent of the iodine was trichloroacetic acid–soluble. The calculated iodine content proved to be 319 μg, a figure which agreed well with the estimate of iodine content of the whole gland based on the kinetic analysis and on the hypothesis that all the iodine contained therein was in inorganic form. Chromatographic analysis of the four fragments of tissue also failed to demonstrate any organically bound labeled iodine.

Patient 4. The oldest cretinous sib of the previous patients was first admitted to the hospital at age 13 for a mass in his neck. Two hundred and thirty-five grams of thyroid tissue were removed. The histologic appearance was similar to that described for the others. The patient was readmitted to the hospital at age 27 because of regrowth of the goiter and pressure symptoms causing respiratory difficulty. An emergency tracheotomy was required, and this was followed by a total thyroidectomy. Approximately 175 gm thyroid tissue was removed. In addition to the same histologic pattern which was evident at the time of the earlier thyroidectomy, there was an area of vascular and capsular invasion which was considered to be diagnostic of malignant change. No other laboratory investigations were made on this patient.

Patients 1 through 4 died in a fire which destroyed their home in 1962.

Patient 5. This 13-year-old female was unrelated to the previous patients. A diagnosis of cretinism was made at the age of 5 months, and thyroid medication was given until several weeks before admission. Enlargement of the thyroid was noticed 1 year prior to admission. Serum PBI concentration was 0.4 and 0.4 μg per 100 ml on successive analyses.

Radioactive iodine accumulated rapidly in the region of the thyroid and reached a maximal value at 1 hr. Two grams KSCN were given by mouth. Shortly, thereafter there was a rapid disappearance of the labeled iodine from the region of the thyroid gland. Subsequently the thyroid was removed. The gland was composed of adenomas of varying degrees of cellular differentiation. Some were solid masses of large thyroid cells in packed clusters and cords. Others showed evidence of acinus formation with colloid production. The degree of hyperplasia in many areas was intense and exaggerated. The excised gland contained 0.62 μg total iodine per gram of wet tissue and 0.07 μg precipitable iodine per gram of wet tissue.

Similar Cases Reported by Others

There have been sporadic reports of other patients with the same pattern of iodide metabolism as that described above.

Haddad and Sidbury [336] took advantage of an opportunity to study a homogenate prepared from the thyroid of a 15-year-old male with an identical defect. In contrast to findings with normal human thyroid tissue, no organification of iodide took place in this homogenate. There was no organoiodine formation when they added an H_2O_2-generating system which augmented the formation of organic iodine in homogenates from normal thyroid. The authors were unable to decide whether the defect in the abnormal gland was in the iodide-peroxidase (formation of active iodine), in iodinase activity, or was a defective receptor protein, but their results seemed to favor the absence of an iodinase. What their observations proved was that enzymatically generated peroxide failed to stimulate iodination, but this finding is also entirely consistent with absence of an iodide peroxidase, provided that the physiologically significant peroxidation of iodide is specific to the thyroid.

Schultz, Flink, Kennedy, and Zieve [337] reported a 34-year-old male cretin with a huge, lobular thyroid gland. Three cretinous sibs were not available for study. PBI concentration in the serum was 1.4 μg per 100 ml. ^{131}I uptake reached maximum values at 1½ hours. When 2 gm KSCN was given orally, there were a precipitous fall in the labeled iodine of the thyroid and a rise in the ^{131}I concentration of the serum.

Clayton, Smith, and Leiser [338] studied a family of six Negro children, four of whom were goitrous. The parents were not consanguine, nor did they have thyroid disease. A maternal great-aunt and uncle had goiter. The goitrous members of this family differed from those described above in that they were euthyroid. One had a PBI concentration above normal but a normal butanol-extractable iodine (BEI). Another had an abnormally wide difference between the BEI and the PBI. The four goitrous sibs demonstrated a release of labeled iodine when given KSCN. One of the normal sibs failed to show any effect of KSCN in releasing labeled iodine, but further uptake was inhibited. Two goitrous sibs with small goiters showed definite but slight discharge of labeled iodine following KSCN. T_4 and iodide were found in the peripheral serum, and T_3 as well. No MIT or DIT was found. A biopsy specimen from one of these patients disclosed a variegated appearance. Some areas showed intense hyperplasia, whereas others showed colloid involution.

Three members of a family of five euthyroid sibs from Brazil had goiter and elevated radioiodine uptake [339]. They were not deaf. Thiocyanate ordered a partial discharge of radioiodine from the thyroids of these three patients but not from their parents or sibs, and there was a corresponding rise in serum iodine. These observations of Clayton et al. and those on the Brazilian family suggest that there may be heterogeneity in the peroxidase defect.

Similar or identical patients have been reported [340–344, 414], and a thyroid tumor has been described which concentrated iodine without organification [345]. Neel et al. [346] surveyed 50 sibships containing at least one patient with congenital hypothyroidism and found only one family with an organification defect as demonstrated by a significantly positive SCN^- test. In another study from the same laboratory positive SCN^- tests were found in 7 of 56 Michigan cretins [347].

Interpretations

The common denominator of the patients in this group is the release of labeled iodine from the thyroid gland upon the administration of KSCN. The clinical findings have not been uniform. The majority have had a severely cretinous condition, with profound retardation of structural and intellectual development. Those reported by Clayton et al. [338] were clinically euthyroid, as confirmed by laboratory examination. Release of iodide from the thyroid by SCN^- or ClO_4^- has been abnormal in a few patients with lingual goiter [348, 349].

The release of labeled iodine from the thyroid by SCN^- indicates a store of inorganic iodide in the gland which can be readily displaced. Normally, virtually none of the accumulated iodine can be displaced in this way. Those patients who showed a SCN^- release of labeled iodine appear to have a metabolic defect which makes them unable to convert

Table 10-3. DIAGNOSTIC CRITERIA FOR THE PEROXIDASE DEFECT

Required	Helpful and confirmatory
1. Goiter; hypothyroid or compensated hypothyroid 2. Mental retardation usually 3. Accumulation and turnover of radioiodine 4. Rapid discharge of radioiodine from thyroid after administration of SCN^- or ClO_4^- 5. Low to absent PBI and $PB^{131}I$	1. Thyroid biopsy: *a.* Hyperplasia *b.* Low iodine content and concentration *c.* Little if any organic iodine *d.* Absent peroxidase activity 2. In vivo iodine kinetics consistent with only inorganic iodide pools

accumulated iodide to organically bound iodine. Since this limits or prevents hormone synthesis, compensatory hypertrophy and hyperplasia of the thyroid occur, as well as the consequences of an insufficient hormonal supply. Support of this interpretation has come from chromatographic and analytic studies.

The biochemical lesion in the thyroid of these patients seems established inferentially but not directly. Unquestionably, there is interference or failure in the step where iodide becomes oxidized to iodine and displaces a proton from a tyrosyl residue. The enzyme or enzymes which may be involved have been discussed earlier. The evidence is in accord with an absence of the specific oxidative enzymatic process, presumably a peroxidase, in the thyroid gland which is responsible for conversion of iodide ion to an iodinating species. If this process should fail to occur, no iodination of tyrosine residues could occur and no hormone could be formed.

Minimal diagnostic criteria for clinical and laboratory ascertainment of this disorder appear in Table 10-3.

Genetics

If one excludes the cases of Clayton et al. on the grounds that their patients were not cretinous, then 11 affected patients have been reported in 5 families of 30 children. The sex of 3 of the affected persons is not given, but 2 are female, and 6 are male. Although in the sibships reported to date there is a slight excess of affected persons, the data are not inconsistent with inheritance as a simple autosomal recessive character. This interpretation is also consistent with the consanguinity in the family of Patients 1 to 4.

The genetic interpretation of Clayton's patients who were not hypothyroid is difficult. It seems unlikely that they could be heterozygous for the same gene for which other members of this group are homozygous, because parents of other sibships have not shown evidence of thyroid disease and yet were obligate heterozygotes. As already mentioned, it is possible that oxidation of iodide to iodine and fixation to tyrosyl residues is a complex rather than a single-step process, and that the response to SCN^- might be similar in patients having different defects in hormone synthesis. It is also entirely possible that there is genetic heterogeneity in this defect.

Baschieri et al. [350] have tested a large number of patients with thyroid disease and their relatives with ClO_4^- after administration of ^{131}I. A significant number of normal relatives of patients who had positive-discharge test results also had positive test results, whereas no relatives of patients with negative results had positive results. The authors suggested that by this method of ascertainment the character has dominant transmission.

Familial Goiter and Deaf-mutism (Pendred's Syndrome)

Case Studies

A 67-year-old retired craftsman with familial goiter and deafness had always been well [351]. A goiter was found incidentally. A sister, also a deaf-mute, had a thyroidectomy for a large goiter many years previously, and within the past year had developed metastatic carcinoma in a cervical lymph node, which was not identifiable as of thyroid origin by histologic examination. No other source for this tumor has appeared.

Five of eight sibs have been deaf (compare Fig. 10-7). One died at 6 months of age, before any clinical abnormality in hearing or thyroid function was suspected. One died of rheumatic heart disease. One died recently, presumably from arteriosclerotic heart disease. One sister, already mentioned,

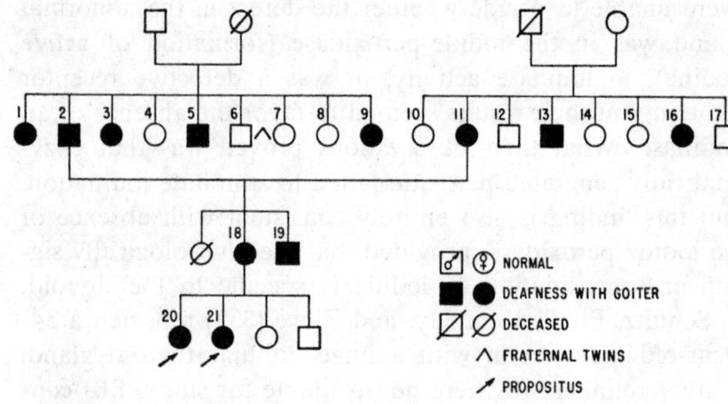

Figure 10-7. Inheritance of deafness and goiter in an intermarried family studied by Johnsen [353]. (*Redrawn and printed by permission from Acta Oto-laryngologica.*)

has had a biopsy diagnosis of carcinoma in a cervical lymph node. Only two sibs are normal. The parents were not consanguine. They emigrated from Ireland but not from the same community.

The patient was intelligent. The thyroid was diffusely enlarged to about three times normal size. No nodules were felt. The prostate was enlarged. There was no clinical suggestion of hypothyroidism.

Findings from routine clinical laboratory studies were within normal limits, except for mild glucose intolerance. Hearing loss was in the range of 95 to 100 decibels in both ears and was sensoneural in type.

A thyroid biopsy weighing 8.3 gm was obtained. Histologic examination disclosed a variable pattern of small nodules. Follicles varied in size and contained colloid. The epithelium was infolded slightly in focal areas, and the cell height indicated moderate hyperplasia.

A 62-year-old brother also had findings typical of Pendred's syndrome. His health had always been good. Physical examination disclosed normal findings except for deafness and a diffuse goiter enlarged two to three times. Routine clinical laboratory findings, chest roentgenogram, and electrocardiogram were within normal limits. Hearing loss was complete and was sensoneural in type.

Measurements of PBI, BEI, and total and free thyroxine were low-normal. ^{131}I uptake was 22.7 percent at 4 hr and 41.6 percent at 24 hr. Serum PB^{131}I at 48 hr (0.078 percent) was normal. The conversion ratio was 79.6 percent. The half-life of labeled thyroxine ^{125}I was normal (7.2 days). The plasma TSH level was normal. Antithyroid antibodies were absent. TBG and TBPA capacities proved to be slightly lower than normal (15.2 μg per 100 ml and 210 μg per 100 ml, respectively).

Sodium perchlorate given 2 hr after ^{131}I resulted in a 25 percent fall in the counting rate over the thyroid by 30 min, and in a 31 percent fall by 60 min.

Maximal thyroid uptake (46.8 percent) was reached in 4 days. The labeled trichloracetic acid–precipitable iodine in the plasma reached a peak of 0.138 percent of the dose on the fifth day. The disappearance rate of ^{131}I from the gland was accelerated during administration of perchlorate alone and of perchlorate with methimazole. The net release rate was not significantly changed by the addition of methimazole. Administration of perchlorate induced a threefold increase in urinary ^{131}I over the control rate, and was not further increased during methimazole.

Thyroid uptake of ^{131}I was inhibited for 4 days after a single 1-gm dose of perchlorate, and was significantly decreased for another 16 days after a second dose of perchlorate given simultaneously with 20 mg methimazole. Three months later perchlorate inhibition of uptake was again tested. Uptake was inhibited to the same degree as on the earlier occasions.

Studies on the patient's brother (who also had Pendred's syndrome) were normal except that the result of the perchlorate discharge test was positive.

Recovery from the blocking effect of a single 900-mg dose of perchlorate was studied in the brother, a normal sister, five control euthyroid subjects, and one hyperthyroid patient. Recovery was delayed in the brother and in the euthyroid sister as compared with the other subjects.

Analysis of the thyroid biopsy disclosed that more than 90 percent of ^{131}I and ^{125}I was in the soluble fraction. The MIT/DIT ratio for the soluble fraction was 5.36 for ^{131}I, given 19 days before surgery, and 4.95 for ^{125}I, given 2 days before the biopsy. Not more than 3 percent of the labeled iodine was present as iodothyronines. T_3 probably represented about a third of the thyroxine fraction.

Most of the protein (79.6 percent) and ^{127}I (81.2 percent) were found in the soluble fraction. Iodine concentration per gram of wet thyroid tissue was low (67.2 μg per gm). Starch-gel electrophoresis of the soluble fraction showed a principal protein zone corresponding to the radioactive peak and identical in mobility with normal 19S human thyroglobulin. Another band moved at the position of albumin, but there were no counts in excess of background in that region. The labeled iodoprotein began to salt out as the phosphate buffer reached 1.6*M*, reached 50 percent at 1.9*M*, and then was 80 percent precipitated at 2.3*M*. Thus, the salting-out curve of the $10^5 \times g$ supernatant was largely in the range of normal thyroglobulin.

The principal component, as determined in a 5 to 20 percent sucrose density gradient, was a 19S protein, and all the labeled iodine sedimented with this component. More than 80 percent of the total soluble iodoproteins could be identified as the 19S component. All the labeled iodine of this fraction was precipitable with a high-titer anti-human thyroglobulin pool of serum from patients with Hashimoto's thyroiditis.

Cases Reported by Other Investigators

Since Brain reported five families with congenital goiter and deafness in 1927 [352], many other families have been reported with this association of diseases. With few exceptions the clinical pattern has been uniform. Goiter has been apparent either at birth or within the first decade or two of life, and nerve deafness has been present from birth or has developed during childhood. Intelligence and growth have usually, but not always, been normal. Vestibular function has been normal or somewhat impaired, and the tympanic membranes have been intact.

These patients have usually not had huge goiters. Thyroid function, as assessed by the usual clinical and laboratory data, has been normal in most of them. The serum concentrations of PBI in most of the affected persons of Johnsen's three kindreds were distinctly low [353], and the mean PBI value of the 15 patients of Thould and Scowen [354] was 3.36 μg per 100 ml. Two of the four affected members of the sibship of Elman [355] had developed invasive adenocarcinoma, and Roberts' patient [356] had localized histologic change suggestive of malignant alteration. Two of the four patients in Thieme's sibship also had local malignant change without evidence of distant extension [357].

The literature on the Pendred syndrome was searched by Nilsson et al. in 1964 [358]. They found 224 case reports and added 11 of their own. In one of their kindreds some patients had goiter without deafness, while others had the reverse. Medeiros-Neto et al. have reported three patients with congenital goiter and deafness from Brazil [359]. Two of the thyroids became available for study. Both showed a large fraction of the iodine present as a dense particulate iodoprotein. Less than 15 percent of the iodine was present as 19S protein. A euthyroid female with deafness and a huge goiter, studied by Shane et al. [360], demonstrated the expected radioiodine discharge with thiocyanate. No T_3 or T_4 was found in the thyroid protein, and a defect both in organification of iodine and in iodotyrosine coupling was considered.

Thyroid Function Studies

A number of laboratory observations have sought to clarify the thyroid function of these patients [361–364]. Morgans and Trotter [361] first showed that ClO_4^- causes an appreciable discharge of iodide from the thyroids of these patients, and this abnormality has become a hallmark of this disease. The fraction of the radioiodine which accumulates in the thyroid within the first hour or two and which is discharged with ClO_4^- is usually 25 to 50 percent; discharge is not so complete as in the patients with the organification defect described in the preceeding paragraphs.

There have been only a few opportunities for study of thyroid specimens from these patients. The usual histologic pattern has been that of nodular goiter. Some of the findings are at variance with one another. The principal iodoprotein of our patient was a 19S soluble component, while that of Medeiros-Neto et al. was an insoluble complex. A patient of Ljungren and Vecchio [362] with typical findings of Pendred's syndrome had only a minute amount of 19S iodoprotein in the thyroid. Both our patient and that of Shane et al. had a high ratio of MIT to DIT. Our patient had T_4 in the gland, whereas Shane et al. found none. Our patient and his brother with Pendred's syndrome seemed unusually sensitive to perchlorate; this finding needs to be sought in other patients.

Suggested diagnostic criteria appear in Table 10-4.

Physiologic Interpretation

The patients of the Pendred group appear to differ from those with the full organification defect in several particulars. They are not myxedematous, and most of them are euthyroid, whereas the patients with the full organification defect (who are not deaf) are usually cretinous. The patients with Pendred's syndrome usually do not have large goiters. The discharge of labeled iodine from the gland is neither so precipitous nor so complete. It is tempting to suggest that the patients with the full organification defect lack an iodide peroxidase and accordingly have a complete block in hormone synthesis, whereas those of the Pendred-syndrome group lack an iodase, a condition which might permit a slow synthesis of hormone, as can be demonstrated in vitro when a source of elemental iodine is incubated with many proteins. The reason for the prolonged inhibition of iodine uptake after perchlorate, if indeed it should prove to be a feature of this disease, is unexplained at present.

Genetics

Fraser, Morgans, and Trotter [363] summarized their studies up to 1960. They found 113 affected patients among 72 families. Johnsen's two families included 24 members, of whom 21 were personally examined [353]. Of these, 12 exhibited goiter and deafness. Four of his patients were the result of intermarriage of two affected members of two families. Four of seven sibs of Elman's sibship were affected. Deraemaeker [365] in Belgium found 3 affected males in a sibship of 12 from a first-cousin marriage.

In Johnsen's kindred the disease appeared in successive generations, and Fraser et al. [363] reported the appearance of the disease among the children of a marriage between two persons with Pendred's syndrome. The disease has appeared only within a single generation in all other recorded instances.

The inheritance of this disease is not entirely clear from the family charts available. Approximately one-half the sibs in the reported families have been afflicted, but if a correction is applied for inadequate ascertainment, then the ratio of affected to nonaffected is very nearly 1:3 and accordingly fits the pattern of autosomal recessive inheritance [366]. The only discordant note is provided by Patient 18 of Johnsen's family, and we do not know whether or not her husband had Pendred's syndrome. It is well known that the social

Table 10-4. DIAGNOSTIC CRITERIA FOR PENDRED'S SYNDROME

Required	Helpful and confirmatory
1. Goiter and nerve deafness; no iodide deficiency 2. Mild hypothyroid or compensated hypothyroid condition, usually 3. Partial discharge of radioiodine from thyroid by SCN^- or ClO_4^- 4. Hypersensitivity to ClO_4^- (?) (see text)	1. Thyroid biopsy: *a.* Normal to slight hypoplasia *b.* Low concentration of iodine *c.* MIT/DIT ratio high; iodotyrosine/iodothyronine ratio high *d.* Thyroglobulin present and normal

intimacy among the deaf and blind often leads to marriage. It is by no means clear why the thyroid and VIIIth nerve are both involved. Close linkage of the relevant genes could obtain, or both goiter and deafness could be the result of pleiotropic action of a single gene. The effects of antithyroid drugs on the development of the cochlea of the developing chick have already been mentioned.

Cretinism with Failure of Coupling of Iodotyrosines

Case Study

Defective coupling of MIT and DIT into T_3 and T_4 appeared to be the cause of hypothyroidism and goiter in a 25-year-old retarded female [367]. A diagnosis of hypothyroidism was made at age 4; desiccated thyroid was prescribed but taken only intermittently. A goiter was first observed at age 17. At 22 the PBI was 3.5 μg per 100 ml. The daily excretion of ^{127}I was normal at a time when the patient had ingested no desiccated thyroid for the previous 8 weeks. Measurements of the BMR and PBI were normal at the time of study. A total thyroidectomy was performed at the completion of studies. Microscopically the specimen displayed extreme hyperplasia.

There were two first-cousin marriages (Fig. 10-8) in the immediate antecedents. A sister, 4 years older, suffered from an identical disorder. The PBI was 6.1 μg per 100 ml. She had undergone an uneventful subtotal thyroidectomy because of rapid growth of the gland. Pathologic examination disclosed multinodular goiter with extreme hyperplasia and almost no colloid formation within the follicles. Earlier studies on both sisters had shown an unusually rapid uptake of ^{131}I to values in excess of 95 percent. The labeled iodine

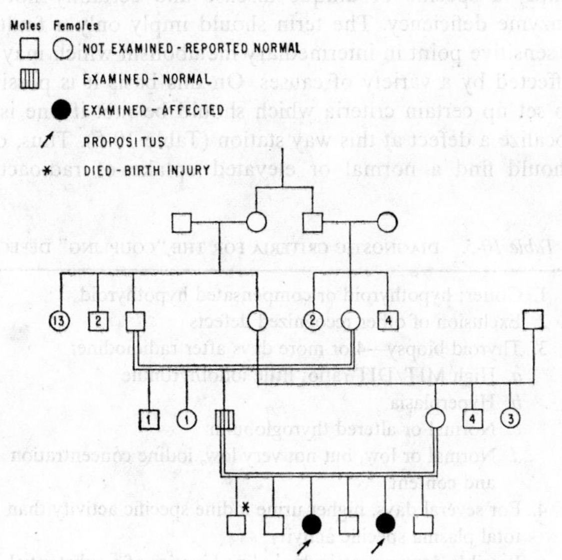

Figure 10-8. Inheritance pattern of a family with two siblings with congenital goiter (see text). Note the two consanguine marriages.

in the thyroid was not dislodged in either patient by administration of KSCN.

Studies included measurements of the uptake, retention, and release of labeled iodine and the excretion of stable iodine, and chemical examination of the histologic specimen at the time of surgery. Radioiodine uptake reached a maximum of 99.3 percent within the first 2 hr. Thereafter it was released at a rate approaching 3.0 percent per day. When methimazole was given, there was a sharp increase to 7.3 percent per day. Iodine clearance by the kidney was 30.5 ml per min. The renal excretion rate of labeled iodine rose sharply upon administration of methimazole; also the daily excretion of stable iodine rose from normal values to a mean daily ^{127}I excretion of 203 μg per day above mean control values. The labeled iodine in the plasma fell sharply soon after administration of ^{131}I, but began to rise after a few hours and reached a maximum on the fifth day of 0.52 percent per liter and then fell slowly.

Chromatographic analysis of serial serum samples taken between the seventh and seventy-ninth hours after administration of ^{131}I disclosed T_4 and T_3 in all samples. Yet in spite of heavy labeling of the gland and rapid turnover of iodine by the gland, it was impossible to demonstrate either T_4 or T_3 in four tissue specimens obtained at operation, although iodide and abundant MIT and DIT were demonstrated with ease. The specimens were obtained 79 hr after the administration of ^{131}I. One hundred and thirty grams of tissue were homogenized, hydrolyzed, and analyzed for T_4 by the method of Gross and Pitt-Rivers [368]. Pitt-Rivers was unable to demonstrate more than a trace of T_4.

Pathophysiologic Formulation

Two lines of investigation indicated that the primary fault in the thyroid gland of this patient was an impaired ability to couple MIT and DIT into T_3 and T_4. Serial chromatographic analyses of the serum for many hours after the administration of ^{131}I demonstrated the early appearance of T_4 and of T_3, whereas analysis of the glandular tissue failed to disclose labeled T_4 or T_3. Only when the whole gland was subjected to chemical analysis was it possible to identify a trace of T_4. Yet at the same time abundant quantities of MIT and DIT were found. In the normal thyroid gland at least 20 percent, if not more, of the labeled iodine is in the form of labeled T_4 by 79 hr. Thus it appeared that while this hyperplastic gland was making ample MIT and DIT and was storing them in large amounts in the gland, the T_4 and T_3 which were produced were immediately released into the blood. There was evidence, therefore, of an abundant formation of hormone precursors in the form of iodotyrosines, but of virtually no storage of iodothyronines.

Supporting information was obtained from kinetic studies of iodine metabolism. For the details of these observations and their interpretation the reader may consult the original publication [367]. It was possible to measure the rate at which iodine was leaving this gland in two ways: during administration of methimazole the specific activity of the labeled iodine which appeared in the urine was extremely high. This proved to be 17 percent per mg, at a time when the specific activity of the whole gland was only 2.9 percent per mg. This finding could only be interpreted as indicating that methimazole was blocking the reutilization of labeled iodine derived from a pool of high specific activity, whereas most of the labeled iodine in the thyroid was in a pool of low specific activity.

The amount of unlabeled iodine leaving the gland daily and entering the extrathyroidal iodine compartments was estimated. The calculated value was at least 1 mg. The normal amount of hormonal iodine secreted per day lies between 50 and 150 μg. Only a small fraction of the iodine leaving the gland could have been in the form of thyroid hormone, because otherwise the patient would have been thyrotoxic. Accordingly, the thyroid must have been releasing iodide or a readily metabolized iodinated substance which was quickly broken down, either by the gland itself or in the periphery, to yield iodide.

The simplest formulation to account for the facts was that the coupling of DIT to yield T_4 took place only to a limited degree. The T_4 which was formed was rapidly secreted. In this way it is possible to account for the almost complete absence of T_4 from the gland, in spite of a normal concentration in the peripheral blood. The highly stimulated gland maintained an exceedingly rapid flux of some of its iodine. Some went on to form hormone, some was retained for storage as MIT and DIT, and a large fraction—perhaps in the form of MIT—was formed and released for deiodinization either in the gland or in the periphery, or both.

Similar Cases Reported

A number of patients with strikingly similar clinical and biochemical findings have been reported. A 5-year-old male with hypothyroidism and goiter who has been studied in Stanbury's laboratory is like the patients described above in virtually all particulars [369].

Choufoer et al. [370] studied a 37-year-old female with MIT and DIT but only a trace of T_4 in the gland removed 7 days after administration of ^{131}I. Mosier et al. [371] studied two hypothyroid retarded females with large goiters. PBI was low and uptake of ^{131}I was rapid in both.

Chromatographic analysis of thyroid tissue disclosed that the labeled iodine was in the form of MIT and DIT; almost none was present as labeled T_4, although T_4 had been demonstrated in the peripheral blood. Mosier et al. concluded that the metabolic defect in these two patients was a block in the coupling of iodotyrosines into T_4 and T_3.

Similar patients have been described by Joseph and Job [372]. Two females from a sibship of 10 were hypothyroid and had goiter. Each patient had a high uptake of ^{131}I and prolonged retention in the gland. Chromatographic analysis of a biopsy specimen disclosed that 60 to 70 percent of the labeled iodine was in the form of DIT and 21 to 25 percent in the form of MIT. The rest was present as iodide; if T or other iodothyronines were present, they were in a concentration of less than 1 percent of the total.

There are numerous reports in the literature of patient who conform to the pattern of these patients clinically and who also have rapid and high uptake levels of radioactive iodine [372–379]. The cretinous brothers studied by Lerman et al. [375] were of particular interest, because they were the first to be studied physiologically and because of the intense hyperplasia which the glands displayed.

Interpretations and Diagnostic Criteria

Coupling defect is an abused term which has been applied to certain conditions with goiter and a reduced rate of thyroid hormone synthesis but no impairment in formation of mono- or diiodotyrosine. It has been inferred that these findings arise from defective coupling of hormone precursors into finished hormone. Coupling is a complex biochemical event which is poorly understood at best. Biochemical models have been constructed, and they work very well in producing thyroxine from iodotyrosyl precursors, but there is no certainty that they have an in vivo counterpart. No method has been devised for measuring the efficiency of the coupling reaction in vivo. While it seems highly likely that iodotyrosyl coupling is enzymatically controlled in vivo, no such enzyme or system has been identified. Thyroglobulin itself may be a coupling enzyme. The reaction is complex and surely vulnerable. Furthermore, coupling is impaired by anything which dilutes the iodine in the thyroglobulin molecule. A paradigm of this, as well pointed out by Ermans et al., is severe iodide deficiency [381].

From the foregoing it appears that one should speak of the coupling defect only in general terms and should not imply a specific or unique disease and certainly not an enzyme deficiency. The term should imply only a fault at a sensitive point in intermediary metabolism which may be affected by a variety of causes. On this basis it is possible to set up certain criteria which should be met if one is to localize a defect at this way station (Table 10-5). Thus, one should find a normal or elevated uptake of radioactive

Table 10-5. DIAGNOSTIC CRITERIA FOR THE "COUPLING" DEFECT

1. Goiter; hypothyroid or compensated hypothyroid
2. Exclusion of other recognized defects
3. Thyroid biopsy—4 or more days after radioiodine:
   a. High MIT/DIT ratio; little iodothyronine
   b. Hyperplasia
   c. Normal or altered thyroglobulin
   d. Normal or low, but not very low, iodine concentration and content
4. For several days, higher urine iodine specific activity than total plasma specific activity
5. Possible demonstration by iodine kinetics of a substantial iodide "leak" and a rapid intrathyroidal recycling of iodine

iodine. Turnover should be rapid, and hormone synthesis, as reflected in the PBI, should be barely sustained, if at all. Since the hyperplastic gland is making and degrading mono- and diiodotyrosine at a rapid rate and since the iodide from this cycling exchanges with iodide of the plasma, the specific activity of iodide in the urine should be higher than the specific activity of the plasma, at least for the first several days.

Because this disease could be easily confused with iodide deficiency, it should be shown that ample stores of iodine are available to the subject and that the quantity of iodine in the thyroid is within normal limits. The latter criterion might not be met if hyperplasia resulting from inadequate synthesis of thyroid hormone has resulted in a lowered concentration of iodine in the gland. This in its own right might accentuate a coupling defect by physically separating iodinated residues in the thyroglobulin molecule.

It has been shown that certain thyroids "leak" iodide in nonhormonal form and claimed that this constitutes a disease, *sui generis.* Whether indeed there is a condition uniquely characterized by a failure to conserve intrathyroidally generated iodide from the iodotyrosyl pools has not been proved, but if it were so this would only be another mechanism whereby a coupling defect could be generated. Indeed any pathophysiologic process which reduces the concentration of iodine in the thyroglobulin molecule impairs coupling and, *mutatis mutandis,* hormone synthesis.

The point of the argument is that the coupling reaction is critical, complex, and sensitive, and is almost surely the focal point of several inborn and acquired errors of the thyroid. The question, rather, is how frequent is this category of inborn error of the thyroid. It may prove to be the most common of all.

Genetics

Little can be said regarding the genetics of this group. Stanbury's two patients had no family history of thyroid disease except for their own sibship, but there were two first-cousin marriages among their antecedents. The family described by Joseph and Job [382], with 2 afflicted members out of 10 in the sibship, suggests simple autosomal recessive inheritance. All 6 of the patients who seem to conform most closely to the criteria for diagnosis are female.

Cretinism from Failure of Iodotyrosine Deiodinase Activity

Case Studies

In 1953 McGirr and Hutchison [383] reported 12 patients from Glasgow, Scotland, who were cretinous and hypothyroid. Four of these were sibs, and three, plus one subsequently described [384], were from the same kindred. These eight patients were of itinerant tinker stock, an isolated group of people living a nomadic existence in Argylshire and the Isle of Selay. Two others of the cretins were half-sibs and were also of tinker stock, but from Perthshire and Angus.

The tinker cretins were all goitrous. The uptake of ^{131}I of all but two was high, and the maximum value was quickly reached. Most of the glands lost a large fraction of the accumulated labeled iodine within a few hours after maximum uptake. Only two failed to show a high concentration of $PB^{131}I$ in the peripheral blood at 48 hr. Analyses of the serum of three of these patients disclosed an organic butanol-extractable substance. This component was not identified, but the possibility was entertained that it might be DIT. Chromatographic studies of the serum of one patient failed to identify the component as an iodothyronine.

Three similar patients were studied in Leiden in 1955 [385, 386]. The first of these was a 27-year-old male (Patient A) who had a goiter at birth. Thyroid medication was given for many years but was discontinued 4 years prior to entry to the hospital because of tuberculosis. From that time the goiter increased relentlessly in size. The serum concentration of PBI was 0.5 μg per 100 ml. His parents were not consanguineous and were normal, as was an older brother, but a younger brother (Patient B), who was also available for study, had a goiter at birth and was retarded, both physically and mentally. A third, unrelated patient (Patient C) was a 12-year-old female cretin with a huge multinodular goiter, short stature, and mental deficiency.

The initial study of Patient A concerned the fate of an administered dose of ^{131}I [385]. Labeled iodine accumulated unusually rapidly in the thyroid (Fig. 10-9). Within 70 min, 74 percent had appeared in the neck region, and during this time there was a rapid fall in the serum concentration of labeled iodine. After 70 min the labeled iodine began to leave the thyroid and to appear in the blood as a component which was partially precipitable with trichloracetic acid. By 48 hr, only 25 percent of the administered dose remained in the gland. The serum concentration of labeled iodine had

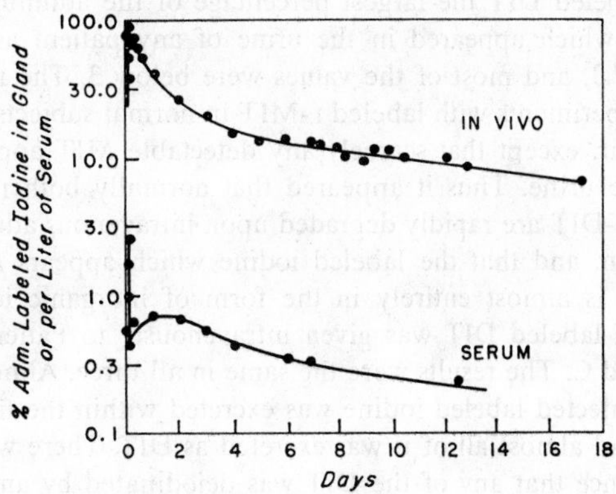

Figure 10-9. Metabolism of iodine in Patient A. ^{131}I was given orally at zero time, and serial counts were made over the thyroid and in the serum.

risen to 0.5 percent per liter, and from that point it slowly fell during succeeding days. Nearly identical in vivo retention and release curves were obtained from Patients B and C [386].

Specimens of serum obtained at 2, 4, 8, 16, and 22 hr were extracted with butanol and chromatographed in a butanol-dioxane-ammonia solvent system. In successive specimens there were increasing amounts of labeled iodine, which had the chromatographic mobility of MIT and DIT. Moderate amounts of T_4 and T_3 were also found.

The gland was removed because of pressure symptoms. The histologic pattern was that of intense hyperplasia, but some areas showed a tendency to form colloid, and there were also areas of cystic degeneration and fibrosis. The gland weighed 198 gm at operation; 3.4 percent of the labeled iodine was recovered as T_4, and the remainder in small amounts as iodine and in large amounts as MIT and DIT.

These findings were duplicated in Patient B. Large amounts of organic labeled iodine appeared in the serum. Several iodinated components were present on chromatograms of urine specimens. Labeled iodine was prominently present at the MIT and DIT zones. A component near the origin was readily hydrolyzed into MIT by treatment with dilute acid.

Observations on Patient C were more limited in scope initially but were later extended; they conformed to the findings in Patients A and B. The in vivo thyroidal uptake reached 70 percent in 1 hr and then fell rapidly. The same iodinated components in approximately the same proportion were found in successive urine specimens as were found in specimens from Patient B.

The fate of injected labeled MIT and DIT was observed in Patients A, B, and C, and in several relatives of Patient C, as well as in a group of 15 normal subjects [387]. The results confirmed the earlier studies of Albert and Keating [388], who found that after intravenous administration of ^{131}I-labeled DIT to normal subjects, only a small fraction of the labeled iodine is removed and excreted in the urine as free iodide. During the first few hours after administration of labeled DIT the largest percentage of the administered dose which appeared in the urine of any patient as DIT was 7.3, and most of the values were below 3. The results of experiments with labeled L-MIT in normal subjects were similar, except that scarcely any detectable MIT appeared in the urine. Thus it appeared that normally both L-MIT and L-DIT are rapidly degraded upon intravenous administration, and that the labeled iodine which appears in the urine is almost entirely in the form of inorganic iodide.

^{131}I-labeled DIT was given intravenously to Patients A, B, and C. The results were the same in all three. Almost all the injected labeled iodine was excreted within the first 24 hr, and almost all of it was excreted as DIT. There was no evidence that any of the DIT was deiodinated by any one of these three patients, and there was little evidence of conjugation or deamination. A small and questionably significant zone of labeled iodine was found near the solvent front. In the first 24 hr after administration, 78.6, 78.1, and 66.2 percent of the injected labeled DIT was recovered unchanged in the urine of Patients A, B, and C.

Limited but similar studies were permitted on the sister mother, two maternal aunts, and one maternal cousin of Patient C. The sister, age 20, was entirely normal, except for a moderately firm enlargement of her thyroid gland to about twice normal size. The mother of Patient C, age 43, had had a subtotal thyroidectomy at age 27 for progressive thyroid enlargement; there had been recurrent growth of the gland to about five times normal size at the time of study. The patient otherwise was normal, and her serum concentration of PBI was normal. One of the maternal aunts had had a thyroidectomy for an enlarged thyroid gland, which had been diagnosed as Graves' disease. The other maternal aunt was said to have had a goiter in the past, but this had disappeared. One of her daughters (cousin of Patient C) had had a surgical thyroidectomy at age 20 and had a recurrent goiter of about four times normal size at the time of study. A sib (cousin of Patient C) had died at age 9 on the day prior to a scheduled thyroidectomy for "Basedow's disease." In each of the five members of the kindred, a dose of labeled DIT was given and the excretion rate was measured during the subsequent 4 hr. The results were compared with those obtained from the 15 patients without thyroid disease discussed earlier. It was found that the mean excretion rate of unchanged labeled DIT was significantly higher than in the control group, although a large fraction of the DIT was deiodinated (Table 10-6).

The thyroid gland of Patient B was removed because of pressure symptoms. Calf thyroid tissue slices were incubated for 6 hr in the presence of ^{131}I-labeled L-DIT. Approximately 60 percent of the substrate was deiodinated. Similar findings were obtained with slices from normal human thyroids.

The thyroid gland of Patient B was studied similarly and with simultaneous human control tissue from a patient with nodular goiter. A normal amount of deiodination was demonstrated in the nodular goiter, but the thyroid tissue slices from Patient B failed to deiodinate the substrate DIT [389]. Later the thyroid of Patient C became available. Slices from it, too, failed to deiodinate DIT [370].

Detailed analytic studies of two of the tinker cretins of

Table 10-6 EXCRETION RATE OF UNCHANGED LABELED DIT IN PATIENTS WITH CONGENITAL GOITER, THEIR RELATIVES, AND CONTROL PATIENTS

Subjects	Percent injected dose DIT excreted as DIT		
	0–1 hr	0–2 hr	0–4 hr
15 control patients	1.8	2.4	2.8
3 patients with congenital goiter	29.2	46.2	62.3
5 relatives of one of above patients	4.6	6.2	7.1

Table 10-7. DIAGNOSTIC CRITERIA FOR THE DEHALOGENASE DEFECT

Required	Helpful and confirmatory
1. Goiter; hypothyroid or compensated hypothyroid 2. Mental retardation, usually 3. Rapid and high uptake of radioiodine; rapid turnover (unless compensated by therapy) 4. MIT, DIT and conjugates, and derivatives in plasma and urine 5. No deiodination of injected MIT or DIT	1. Thyroid biopsy: *a.* No deiodination of MIT or DIT *b.* Hyperplasia; normal thyroglobulin *c.* Abundant MIT and DIT; little or no iodothyronine 2. Temporary restoration of normal thyroid hormone production by thyroid or iodide medication

McGirr et al. [390, 391] have clearly shown that they have the same type of thyroid disorder as patients A, B, and C. Chromatograms of serum samples of one of their patients disclosed MIT and DIT, as well as iodothyronines.

Almost simultaneously with the publication of the studies on patients A, B, and C, Horst [392] published a brief account of his observations on two goitrous cretins. MIT and DIT were identified in serum samples. The same interpretation was offered as for those already described.

Other patients with the dehalogenase defect have been described [370, 393–403*a*]. Administration of desiccated thyroid [404] and of iodide [397] has induced remissions that have persisted long after withdrawal of medication.

The in vivo curves obtained on two unrelated retarded goitrous subjects by Bernheim and Berger [405] are similar to those on Patients A, B, and C. Burrell and Gairdner [406] suggested that their three cretinous sibs (one with goiter) might be secreting DIT. The thyroid glands of their patients had strong avidity for ^{131}I, and the serum concentration of PB^{131}I was much elevated at 48 hr. Kusakabe and Miyake [407] studied six patients with simple goiter in Japan who appeared to have partial defects in deiodination in the thyroid and in other organs. Four others had defective deiodination in other organs, but deiodination of three of these, as ascertained by thyroid biopsy, was normal. They have also reported three sisters from a first-cousin marriage who were goitrous but otherwise normal [408]. Diiodotyrosine was deiodinated by the thyroid glands but not in other organs. Dissociation of deiodinating capacity between the thyroid and other tissues has not been reported elsewhere.

Physiologic Interpretations

Patients in this category share a defect in their capacity to deiodinate MIT and DIT. The deiodinating enzyme occurs normally not only in the thyroid but in liver, kidney, and other organs. The metabolic defect is both intra- and extrathyroidal, for not only are the afflicted patients unable to deiodinate MIT and DIT in their thyroid glands, but when these substances are administered either before or after thyroidectomy or to the patient receiving full doses of desiccated thyroid, the labeled iodotyrosine appears almost qualitatively in an unchanged form in the urine, or (in the case of MIT) as conjugates.

The suggestion has been made on several occasions that a lack of deiodinase in the thyroid should not per se prevent T_4 synthesis, and that accordingly there must be some additional defect [409]. This additional hypothesis is unnecessary. Continued leakage of hormone precursors from the gland and from the body depletes the iodine stores and sets up a vicious cycle of thyroid hyperplasia, increasing synthesis and secretion of hormone precursors. Hypothetically it should be possible to restore hormone synthesis and put the gland at rest by supplying it with a large excess of T_4 or iodide. This has been done, and the expected results were achieved [370, 397, 403].

Diagnostic criteria appear in Table 10-7.

Genetics

An unusual opportunity to study the genetics of this kind of goitrous cretinism has been beautifully exploited by Hutchison and McGirr [390]. They have traced the complex family history of the Scottish patients through 160 years. The original male member came from Ireland and married his full cousin. There has been little marriage subsequently outside the tinker group, but close intermarriage within the group has been extremely frequent (Fig. 10-10). Ten goitrous cretins are known to have appeared among 31 persons in four sets of sibs.

A study of the family tree shows that this form of cretinism with goiter behaves as a simple autosomal recessive trait. There is no sex predilection. The marriages which resulted in afflicted persons were all consanguine, but in no case was a parent afflicted. The inheritance ratio was somewhat in excess of the expected 1:3, in that there were 10 afflicted sibs and 21 normal children in four sibships, but Hutchison and McGirr point out that undoubtedly a number of unafflicted sibs were lost to genetic study [390]. There have been no marriages of the afflicted members of this kindred, so that there has been no opportunity to test inheritance from phenotypes.

It seems a reasonable assumption that the cases of cretinism with goiter described from the Netherlands and from Scotland are homozygotes. The defect observed in these patients was quite complete. There is no evidence whatsoever of any deiodination of DIT. On the other hand, five relatives of one of the Netherlands patients and five nongoitrous and

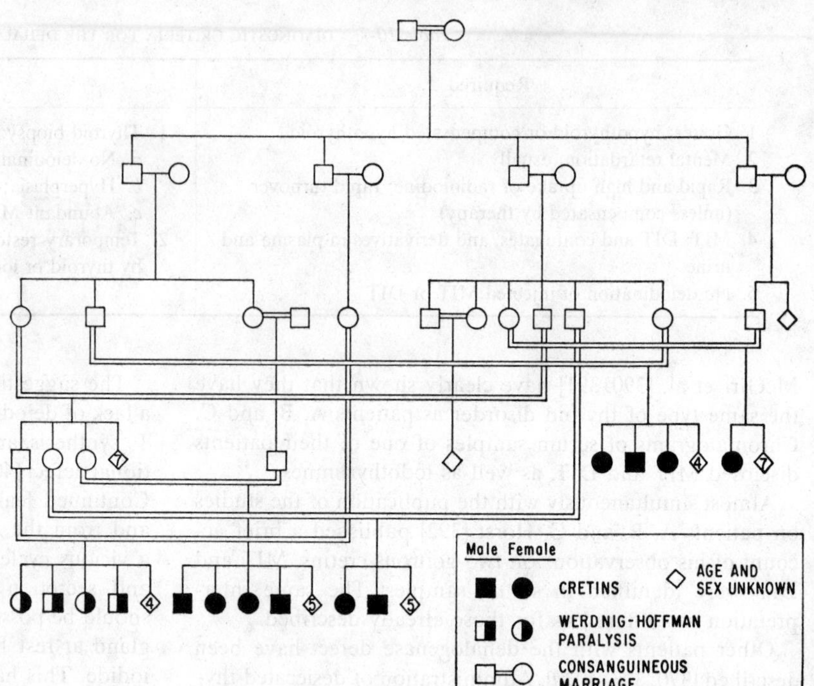

Figure 10-10. Pattern of heredity of cretinism with goiter as found by McGirr in a group of itinerant Scottish tinkers. Note particularly the remarkable number of consanguine marriages. (*From The American Journal of Medicine,* 22, 712, 1957, *with permission.*)

euthyroid relatives of a Scottish patient [402] demonstrated defective DIT deiodinase activity, and all had evidence of thyroid disease but without mental or skeletal retardation. It follows that these relatives represent the heterozygous condition.

Familial Goiter with Diminished or Altered Thyroglobulin Synthesis

Thyroglobulin is a large complex protein which is synthesized exclusively in the thyroid. It is entirely probable that there are errors in thyroglobulin structure, just as there are errors in hemoglobin structure, which are at the root of human disease, but no error of thyroglobulin structure has been identified at the molecular level. An extreme form of error would be one in which no identifiable protein would be produced. A presumed defect in thyroglobulin synthesis is illustrated in the following account [410].

Case Report

Three members of a sibship of four had goiter. The parents had no clinical sign of thyroid disorder, but by scanning it was found that the gland of the mother was twice normal size and that the father was one and one-half times normal. They are not consanguine. ^{131}I uptake by the thyroid glands of both parents was normal.

The oldest sib was a 20-year-old male. An enlarged thyroid was noted shortly after birth. Growth and development were normal, and he has attended college. The thyroid was estimated to weigh 100 gm. A 12-year-old female sib developed normally. There was no significant enlargement of the thyroid, and uptake of ^{131}I was normal. A 7-year-old male sib was hypothyroid. The thyroid was estimated to weigh 40 gm. Bone age at age 6 was 2½ years. PBI was normal, but free T_4 was low and ^{131}I uptake was high. The serum concentration of TSH was high by radioimmunoassay and by bioassay. Rapid improvement followed T_4 therapy.

The principal subject of investigation was a 16-year-old female who had an enlarged thyroid at birth. It had slowly increased in size over the years. Growth and development were probably within normal limits, but walking and talking seemed slightly delayed. There were no clinical signs of hyper- or hypothyroidism. Skin texture was normal. The pulse was 104. The thyroid was estimated to weigh 150 gm. A bruit was heard over the gland. When treated with L-thyroxine, the patient became tense and nervous and lost 5 lb. Serum protein-bound iodine and serum free thyroxine were normal; radioiodine uptake by the thyroid was elevated. Serum TSH concentration was normal, both by bioassay and by radioimmunoassay. Twenty-five percent of plasma labeled iodine was not extracted into acid butanol. On a second occasion during thyroxine therapy over 40 percent of the serum iodine was not butanol-extractable. Serum thyroxine-binding globulin level and triiodothyronine resin uptake were within normal limits.

A total thyroidectomy was performed. The specimen was a large multinodular goiter. Histologic examination disclosed large follicles, with cuboidal to columnar epithelium. The surgical specimen was homogenized and separated into conventional fractions. An aliquot of each fraction was hydrolyzed by trypsin under toluene for 48 hr at pH 8, and amounts of labeled thyroxine and triiodothyronine were estimated by chromatography.

Most of the iodine was in the soluble fraction. The MIT/DIT ratios were approximately 0.3 in the centrifugal fractions. Significant labeling above background was associated with thyroxine in the chromatograms of the trypsin digests of the soluble fraction.

Sucrose density gradient centrifugation of the soluble fraction showed only one absorbance peak in the 4S position. There were no peaks at the 12S or 19S positions, whereas these were clearly apparent in the curves obtained with normal thyroglobulin. Most of the labeled iodine coincided with the absorbance peak at 4S, but there was a small rise in amount of labeled iodine between the 12S and 19S positions. Thus, there appeared to be a virtual absence of stable thyroglobulin from the gland and little if any labeled thyroglobulin.

The salting-out curves with phosphate showed no sharp zone of precipitation as is seen with thyroglobulin between 1.6 and 1.9*M*. Starch-gel electrophoresis of the soluble supernatant showed no detectable staining in the band customarily occupied by thyroglobulin.

The soluble fraction gave a strong reaction against rabbit anti-human albumin antiserum on Ouchterlony plates, but none of the labeled iodine was precipitated by incubation with a sample of human serum containing a high titer of anti-human thyroglobulin.

Interpretation

Thyroglobulin might be undetectable in the thyroid because of failure of synthesis, rapid turnover, escape or degradation of subunits before aggregation into the tetrameric structures, or failure of subunits to undergo normal aggregation. Several findings suggested that fast turnover was not the cause of the absence of thyroglobulin from this gland. The follicular spaces at the time of surgery were amply large, and the gland did not resemble others in which metabolic blocks cause hyperplasia of the cells to such a degree as to fill the space normally occupied by the colloid. If turnover were unusually rapid, then one would not expect to find an ample follicular space. The low MIT/DIT ratio (0.3) also was not compatible with rapid synthesis and turnover of the iodoamino acids. Iodine deficiency and other causes of thyroid hyperplasia are generally associated with an MIT/DIT ratio higher than 1. Furthermore, serial in vivo measurements over the thyroid, extending over several days gave no evidence of unusually rapid turnover.

A number of reports have suggested absence of thyroglobulin from the thyroid glands of man and animals, or that thyroglobulin had altered characteristics; in others the predominant iodinated component was some other iodinated protein, such as iodoalbumin [411–414]. Iodide deficiency alters the distribution of the iodoamino acids in thyroglobulin [381] and is responsible for a conformational change in the molecule which changes its sedimentation constant. Iodoalbumin may comprise a substantial fraction of the total soluble iodoprotein of sporadic goiter. McGirr and his associates [415] demonstrated an abnormal iodinated protein in a patient with familial goiter which was resistant to trypsin and chymotrypsin. In three large thyroids from hypothyroid patients Michel et al. [416] found abnormal soluble iodoproteins. One of these was less soluble in ammonium sulfate than is thyroglobulin. Robbins et al. [417, 418] found an abnormal thyroglobulin in the thyroids of cattle with congenital goiter which reacted with antithyroglobulin antibody but had different physical characteristics. Its sedimentation constant and immunologic properties differed from the iodoprotein characterizing the thyroid of the patient described above. Other descriptions of abnormal thyroglobulins in diseased human thyroids have appeared [419, 420].

Inefficient or impaired biosynthesis of thyroglobulin has been reported. A 15-year-old euthyroid female with a congenital goiter had no detectable thyroglobulin in the thyroid, but a small amount of ^{131}I-labeled 4S protein [428]. The gland was intensely hyperplastic. A large amount of labeled iodine sedimented with the cell nuclei. Thyroglobulin was not detected by electrophoretic, ultracentrifugal, or immunologic methods. Pittman and Pittman reported two goitrous and cretinous sibs with low plasma thyroxine concentrations and evidence of thyroid hyperplasia [421]. Less than 8 percent of the labeled protein in the thyroid was thyroglobulin. The principal component was iodoalbumin. A deficiency in thyroglobulin synthesis was suggested as the definitive defect. Other reports have appeared since then with similar observations in man and in animals. Falconer, studying tissue slices from congenitally goitrous sheep, found impaired incorporation of labeled amino acids into the soluble fraction sedimenting between 35 and 42 percent ammonium sulfate (i.e., thyroglobulin fraction) [422, 423]. Similar findings in sheep have been reported by Rac et al. [424]. As in the case of the patient described here, administration of thyroxine to the sheep did not result in storage of thyroglobulin-like protein in the thyroid.

The findings on the patient described above are similar to those from a patient studied by Lissitzky et al. [400]. Their patient was an 8-year-old euthyroid girl. The thyroid contained no more than 10 percent of the iodoprotein as thyroglobulin. A large fraction of the iodoprotein was immunoprecipitable as albumin. The presence of free MIT and DIT in blood and urine suggested that the patient had the dehalogenase defect and that hyperplasia and rapid intrathyroidal turnover may have been responsible for the findings.

It is apparent that this category of thyroid disease is heterogeneous. Diagnosis rests principally on laboratory examination of a thyroid tissue specimen. Suggested diagnostic criteria appear in Table 10-8.

Table 10-8. DIAGNOSTIC CRITERIA FOR IMPAIRED THYROGLOBULIN SYNTHESIS

1. Goiter; hypothyroid or compensated hypothyroid
2. Radioiodine uptake normal or high
3. Rigorous exclusion of other defects
4. Thyroid biopsy:
   a. Colloid spaces present; cell hyperplasia
   b. No thyroglobulin
   c. Abnormal light iodoproteins present
   d. Thyroglobulin 3S to 8S subunits demonstrated immunologically (type of Robbins and Van Zyl)

Cretinism with Abnormal Iodinated Polypeptides in the Serum

This group of patients with goiter and hypothyroidism is less well defined, and the biochemical mechanisms are less well perceived, than some of those already discussed. The patients are characterized by the appearance in the blood of iodinated amino acids which are in peptide linkage and which are not extractable into acid butanol, as are the iodinated thyronines which normally appear in the peripheral blood.

Case Studies

The first of these patients to come to my attention were two sisters in the clinic of McGirr at the Royal Infirmary in Glasgow [425]. Both were in their early twenties, were retarded mentally, were hypothyroid, and had large nodular goiters. Each had been given a tracer of ^{131}I, and samples of serum had been obtained serially for many hours. The peculiarity of the samples was that the labeled iodine of the serum was incompletely extractable into butanol. When the samples were acidified to pH 2, it was possible to extract only 50 to 60 percent, whereas 85 to 95 percent is readily extractable from normal serums. These studies were not pursued further at that time.

In 1956, Whitelaw et al. reported in an abstract an 8½-year-old female cretin with a PBI concentration of 11.2 and 11.3 μg per 100 ml [373]. There was no goiter. The 24-hr ^{131}I uptake approached 100 percent. Chromatographic analyses of samples of serum—performed in the laboratory of Werner, Block, and Mandl [426]—disclosed a variety of iodinated compounds, but it was of particular interest that in three separate samples a large fraction of the labeled iodine was in the form of an unidentified iodoprotein.

In the following year DiGeorge and Paschkis described a 7½-year-old retarded girl who had a high uptake and retention of ^{131}I [427]. There was a small goiter. The serum concentration of PBI was 7.7 and 9.6 μg per 100 ml. Chromatographic analyses were performed by J. Gross. In two successive samples of serum, 85 and 63 percent of the labeled iodine failed to extract into butanol. That which did extract was identified as T_4. The authors suggested that a calorigenically inefficient product was being secreted by the gland and that it was an iodoprotein. In an addendum they briefly reported another similar case.

A short while later, Werner et al. [426] reported a 40-year-old-female with signs and symptoms suggestive of hypothyroidism, but without goiter. PBI was 4.2 μg per 100 ml, and the 24-hr ^{131}I uptake was 28 percent. Approximately one-third of the labeled iodine in the serum failed to extract into butanol. Upon hydrolysis in the presence of strong acid MIT and DIT were reported in chromatograms of serum samples.

Several patients with an abnormal iodinated component in their serums, which is poorly soluble in butanol, have been studied by DeGroot et al. [428]. The following case report is typical.

Case Report

This patient was a 28-year-old cretinous female. A large nodular goiter which was removed 10 years previously had shown hyperplasia on histologic examination. There was moderate regrowth of the thyroid when thyroid medication was discontinued several weeks prior to study in 1957.

The significant findings were a high uptake of ^{131}I and an iodinated fraction in the serum which was not extractable into butanol when the serum was acidified to pH 2. Only inorganic iodide was demonstrable in the urine.

Particular interest centered on the abnormal iodinated component in the serum. Extractability into butanol was increased by treatment of the serum with proteolytic enzymes, such as trypsin, chymotrypsin, or pepsin. Chromatograms of these serum hydrolysates revealed MIT and DIT in addition to iodide, T_4, and T_3.

The abnormal iodinated component of the serum was transported differently from T_4. It was found as a single zone associated with the peak and the advancing limb of the albumin fraction on electrophoresis. When ^{131}I-labeled T_4 was added to the serum of this patient it was more than 90 percent extractable under conditions which gave only a 60 or 65 percent extractability of the iodinated components of the patient's serum labeled in vivo. Thus there was no abnormality of the thyroid-binding protein of the serum.

A retarded patient, the product of a first-cousin marriage, has been reported by Derome et al. [429]. Observations quite similar to those on the patient described above were obtained. The labeled iodine in the serum was poorly extractable into butanol, and on electrophoresis it moved with albumin. Six similar patients with large amounts of butanol-insoluble plasma iodine have been reported by McGirr et al. [415] and by others as well [430–433].

Lissitzky et al. [434] have studied a 39-year-old female with goiter since age 4; there was a large fraction of an iodinated component in the thyroid, which had an electrophoretic mobility just greater than albumin (prealbumin). This component also appeared in the plasma and differed from the iodoalbumin found in thyrotoxicosis and other conditions in its electrophoretic behavior and in containing more DIT than MIT. The goiter was probably familial in origin.

Furth et al. [434*a*] have described a 35-year-old cretinous patient with iodinated albumin and prealbumin in the serum and thyroglobulin and iodoalbumin in the thyroid. They suggested that the primary defect in their patient was an inability to hydrolyze and release biologically active thyronines from thyroglobulin and that the iodination of albumin and prealbumin was an aberrant pathway of iodination because of the block in the normal route.

Interpretations

The differences observed among the patients in this category may possibly be attributable to variations existing among patients who have in common certain fundamental abnormal characteristics. Most of them show evidence of hypothyroidism, and all have goiter which appears at an early age. All, in addition, have an iodinated component in the blood which is identified by labeling with ^{131}I and which is not extractable from the acidified serum into *n*-butanol. One patient from whom thyroid tissue was available had no thyroglobulin in the gland, and another had an increased amount of a component with an S°_{20},w equal to 4. Upon hydrolysis with trypsin or chymotrypsin, the circulating iodinated component in the plasma yields iodinated MIT, DIT, T_3, and T_4.

The available data do not permit an exact interpretation of the abnormality. The thyroid is secreting an abnormal iodinated component into the blood which is calorigenically ineffective. This component is hydrolyzable with crude trypsin, chymotrypsin, and pepsin to release iodotyrosines and iodothyronines.

The significant question regards the reason for the production and secretion of an abnormal polypeptide. A similar and perhaps identical albumin-like protein has been identified in the plasma of certain patients with endemic goiter [435], Hashimoto's disease [436], cancer of the thyroid [437], Graves' disease [438], and nodular goiter [439]. Strong evidence identifying it as iodoalbumin has been obtained in Graves' disease, and evidence contrary to its identity with albumin has been obtained in cancer of the thyroid [440].

It seems probable that the synthesis of this protein, or family of proteins, or that of a precursor is a normal event in the thyroid, and that under special circumstances, perhaps as a result of hyperplasia, it spills into the blood perfusing the gland. This might occur *pari passu* with increased metabolic activity of the gland from any cause, or as a result of any block in normal synthesis through the thyroglobulin pathway. It has been suggested that these abnormal plasma iodoproteins may be precursors of thyroglobulin in the gland or a fragment of thyroglobulin which escapes into the blood. The remarkable resemblance to serum albumin would be surprising if either of these possibilities were true. The possibility is by no means excluded that the plasma component is plasma albumin iodinated as it passes through the thyroid, or perhaps albumin that diffuses into the thyroid cell, becomes iodinated, and then diffuses out again. The latter seems more probable [400]. Thus it is by no means clear whether the plasma albumin-like iodoprotein appears in the blood because of a block in synthesis, or in degradation, of thyroglobulin, or simply because the gland is hyperplastic and vascular, or for other undisclosed reasons. Clearly a case should never be put into this diagnostic category until all other types of familial goiter have been excluded.

Genetics

Too few patients have been studied to permit the genetics of this disease or group of diseases to be characterized. The two sibships of McGirr [415] and the two brothers in the clinic of Courvoisier [431] strongly suggest that the disease is heredofamilial. Insofar as is known, no affected parents have been found in the kindred of any one of these patients, except that the mother of one had an asymptomatic goiter.

Cretinism with Impaired Thyroid Response to Thyrotropin

Case Study

An 8-year-old boy appeared normal at birth [441]. When he was about 6 months of age his mother realized that intellectual development was slow. A diagnosis of hypothyroidism was first made at 2 years of age. Desiccated thyroid (between 15 and 60 mg per day) was given until the age of 8. The IQ at age 7 was said to have been 50.

Investigation at age 6 disclosed a PBI of 2.5 μg and a serum thyroxine concentration of 0.7 μg per 100 ml. ^{131}I uptake was 25 percent at 48 hr. A thiocyanate test showed a discharge of radioactivity from 19 percent at 2 hr to 14 percent 1 hr later.

The parents are free of thyroid disease. They are first cousins once removed. They have three normal children and one other who is said to be retarded but who has a "normal PBI."

The patient was 110 cm in height at both admissions (below the 3rd percentile). He weighed 19.3 kg. He was able to feed and dress himself and to say a few intelligible words. The bone age was 3½ years. The face was typically cretinoid (Fig. 10-11). Hearing was normal. The isthmus and right lobe of the thyroid gland were easily palpable but not enlarged. Reflex relaxation was strikingly slow. Excretion of ^{127}I in the urine was normal.

The PBI concentration was 1.0 μg per 100 ml at one study and 2.4 μg at another. Uptake of ^{131}I at 24 hr was 37 percent during a first study and 27 percent during a second. Administration of 1 gm of sodium perchlorate 5 hr after administration of ^{131}I induced a 22 percent discharge from the thyroid gland in 30 min. Five units of thyrotropin (Armour's Thytropar) administered intramuscularly for 4 days failed to increase the PB^{131}I uptake. There was no evidence of any

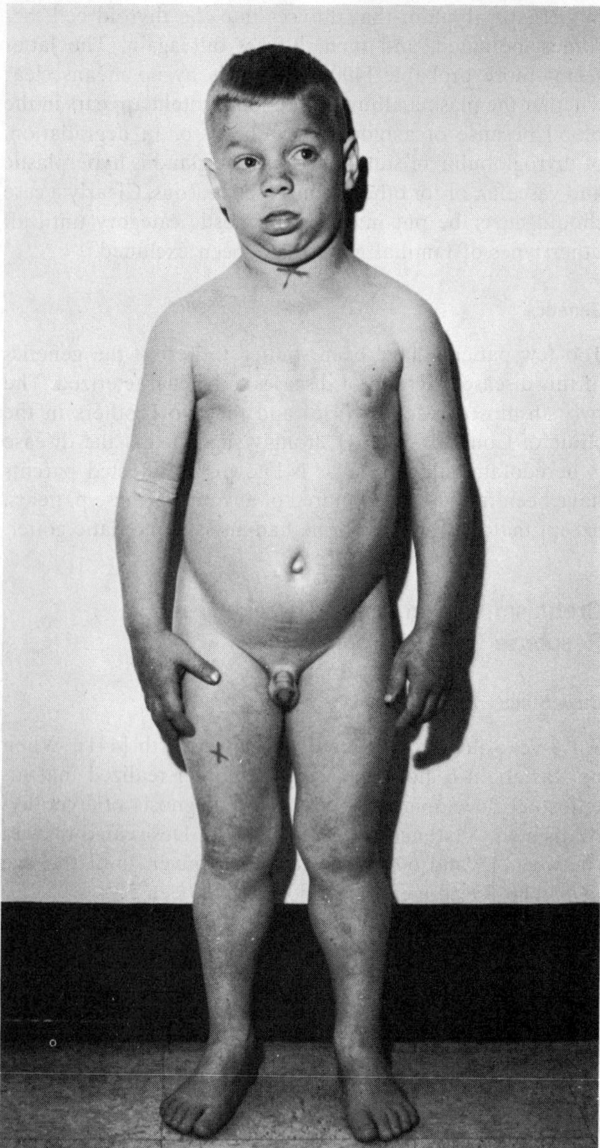

Figure 10-11. Eight-year-old male with cretinism and hypothyroidism. The thyroid failed to respond to thyrotropin.

response to TSH in terms of either ^{131}I uptake or net rate of loss of iodine from the gland. There was normal degradation of DIT. No labeled iodine corresponding to any component other than iodide was found in the urine after administration of radioiodine.

The thyroxine (T_4)-binding globulin capacity was slightly low. Thyroxine-binding prealbumin capacity and resin triiodothyronine uptake were normal. Assay for TSH by the McKenzie method showed 393 $\pm$ 56 percent of control at 2 hr and 340 $\pm$ 34 percent at 8 hr. The concentration of TSH by radioimmunoassay was 145 microunits per ml (normal, 1.5 to 20).

The thyroid weighed about 5 gm. It was normally vascularized. Slices from a biopsy were incubated in buffer containing L-^{14}C-glucose and Armour's TSH (1 unit). Evolution of labeled carbon dioxide was approximately the same in control flasks containing slices of thyroid from a calf and from the patient. The calf slices were stimulated by TSH but there was no stimulation of the slices from the patient's thyroid gland. The total amount of iodine in the gland was somewhat low. DIT/MIT ratios were high.

Salting-out of the soluble fraction from a homogenate of the biopsy specimen showed no pattern consistent with thyroglobulin. Sucrose gradient centrifugation disclosed two protein peaks. One of these, by far the larger, had a sedimentation constant of 3.5 to 4. The other was at the barrier between the applied sample and the sucrose. There was no peak corresponding to thyroglobulin. No zone of precipitation developed in Ouchterlony diffusion plates between the soluble fraction and a high-titer human antithyroglobulin serum. Starch-gel electrophoresis of the soluble fraction failed to disclose a zone corresponding to thyroglobulin.

The microscopic picture was unusual. There was a diffuse increase in the stroma. Between the thickened fibrous septums the follicles were generally small to medium in size but displayed a wide variation in the lining cells. Some follicles filled with colloid had cells that were very flat and involuted or even atrophic. Other follicles, often adjacent to the inactive ones, were lined with hypertrophied large cuboidal cells typical of reactive hyperplasia. There was a heterogeneous mixture of these two follicular patterns. Another feature of interest was the frequency of atypical nuclear forms, often bizarre in shape and hyperchromatic.

Interpretation

The patient displayed certain unusual features. In spite of severe clinical hypothyroidism and a low serum PBI concentration, the avidity of the thyroid for iodine was normal. Although the TSH level in the blood was high and there was much cellular hypertrophy in the biopsy specimen, there was no goiter. No evidence for a protein resembling thyroglobulin could be found. The labeled iodine of the soluble fraction was distributed between MIT and DIT and a small amount of iodothyronine in a protein that had a sedimentation constant of approximately 4.

Many of the abnormalities encountered in this patient indicated a failure of the thyroid gland to respond adequately to TSH. There was a high concentration of TSH in the blood without hypertrophy of the gland or increase above normal of ^{131}I uptake, and administration of TSH caused no change in glandular function. Thus, the epithelial cells appeared to be unable to respond to TSH in two ways that are specific to the hormone-gland interaction: cell division and synthesis of the organ-specific protein, thyroglobulin.

There are at least two other situations in mammalian cells in which cytoplasmic growth occurs together with impaired cell division. The megakaryocyte in pernicious anemia does not divide, probably because vitamin B_{12} is required for synthesis of new DNA. Also, after radiation, although thyroid cells may become hypertrophic, cell division may be impaired. The only known prior radiation of this patient was a tracer dose of ^{131}I one year earlier, but his thyroid disease dated from infancy. Also, fibrosis as seen in the biopsy specimen is not a feature of the thyroid gland damaged by radiation, although focal cellular hypertrophy is.

There are doubtless other hypotheses to explain the thyroid disorder exhibited by this patient. At present the theory is offered that the basic defect is a disorder that has impaired the responses of the thyroid cells to the tropic hormone that stimulates them uniquely, and that this resulted in impairment concordant with their specialized nature: cell division and the synthesis of the organ-specific protein, thyroglobulin.

A suggested set of diagnostic criteria appears in Table 10-9.

Table 10-9. DIAGNOSTIC CRITERIA FOR THYROTROPIN INSENSITIVITY

1. Hypothyroid; no goiter; thyroid in normal position
2. Normal or low-normal ^{131}I uptake
3. No in vivo response to TSH
4. Plasma TSH high by bioassay
5. Thyroid biopsy:
   a. Little colloid; no thyroglobulin
   b. Epithelial cells abnormal; no cell division
   c. No response of slices to TSH

Hypothyroidism with Possible Target-organ Refractoriness to Thyroid Hormone

Case Study

A family with thyroid disease seemingly resulting from reduced responsiveness of the tissues to thyroid hormones has been described by Refetoff et al. [442].

Attention was first directed to the family when a 6-year-old girl deaf from birth was referred. A skeletal roentgenographic survey disclosed stippling of the major secondary ossification centers. The epiphyses appeared to have developed from multiple centers. The thyroid gland was normal to palpation. The child had no symptoms or signs of hyper- or hypothyroidism. The PBI was 19.8 μg per 100 ml, and the BEI was 12.8 μg per 100 ml.

An older brother was also deaf from birth. Radiologic survey showed similar stippling of the major secondary ossification centers. The PBI and BEI were 14.6 and 9.2 μg per 100 ml, respectively.

There is no history of goiter, deafness, or other congenital abnormality in the family. The father and mother were first cousins once removed. Three half-sibs from a previous marriage of the mother are normal. Both parents are third-generation Americans of Mexican extraction. Only two of the sibship present the complete syndrome of deaf-mutism, stippled epiphyses, goiter, and abnormally high PBI. Two others are normal.

The oldest child is a 12½-year-old male. Early development was somewhat delayed, and deafness was noted during early infancy. At school he was above average in general performance. He had normal body proportions and normally erupted teeth. The thyroid gland was diffusely enlarged and was estimated to be about four times normal size. Findings on otoscopic examination were normal. There were no stigmata suggestive of thyroid dysfunction.

An 8½-year-old sister, deaf from early infancy, was delayed in early development and was small. School performance was average. Body proportions and teeth were normal. The resemblance of her facial features to those of her brother was striking. The thyroid was diffusely enlarged to approximately three times normal size. Findings on otoscopic examination were normal. A brisk Achilles reflex, elevated pulse rate, and slight hyperactivity were the sole physical findings compatible with hyperthyroidism. An 8-week-old male was the youngest of the sibs. He apparently was deaf, and had stippled epiphyses.

The striking finding was the discrepancy between the euthyroid clinical state and the clinical laboratory evidence consistent with hyperthyroidism. The initial mean PBI levels were 14.0, 20.8, and 19.3 μg per 100 ml for the three patients. These results were confirmed on repeated determinations, and similar values were obtained from different laboratories. The PBI of the mother during the last trimester of gestation was 8.1 μg per 100 ml. Measurements of BEI and T_4 by column chromatography confirmed the PBI values. The 24-hr uptake of ^{131}I fell within the hyperthyroid range in one of the patients (70 percent) and was borderline for the other two (49 and 51 percent, respectively). This finding was a reflection of a rapid iodine turnover within the gland. Scans of the neck in the three subjects showed somewhat irregular distribution of radioiodine throughout symmetric thyroid glands.

Cholesterol levels were normal. Electrocardiograms and chest and skull roentgenograms were all within normal limits except for the epiphyseal dysgenesis. Serum protein electrophoretic pattern was normal. The antithyroglobulin titers were negative at 1:16 dilution. Results of thyroxine-binding globulin assays were normal. Result of a perchlorate test on one patient was normal.

In order to obtain data on iodine metabolism and the secretion of thyroid hormone, an iodide kinetic study was performed on one of the patients. The distribution space of iodide was increased, thyroid iodide clearance from plasma was elevated, and renal clearance was normal. The disappearance rate of labeled iodine from the serum was increased, as was the thyroid uptake fraction. Serum inorganic iodine was unusually high. The rate of release of iodine from the thyroid was well above the average of control subjects. Absolute iodine uptake was high. Serum $PB^{131}I$ at 48 hr was normal, but the conversion ratio was high.

Interpretation

The data obtained in the course of studies on these three subjects indicated that the diet contained adequate iodine, that the thyroid accumulation of iodine was several times the normal level, that the thyroid concentrated and bound iodine adequately and, in fact, appeared to have established a remarkably high organic iodine store, that the gland secreted iodine at an excessive rate, and finally that the main secretory product was thyroxine. Even so, at no time did the patients show signs of hyperthyroidism. In fact, hypothyroidism was suggested on the basis of the roentgenographic findings of the bones.

It seems highly improbable that these patients were hyperthyroid. They had none of the cutaneous, neural, or cardiac manifestations. Peripheral resistance to thyroid hormone seems a more reasonable explanation. There was no abnormality of hormone binding or in concentration of free thyroxine to explain the remarkable elevation in plasma hormone level, and all available chemical evidence was consistent with the principal iodinated species contributing to the high PBI being authentic thyroxine. Perhaps the best explanation for the disorder is a disturbance in transport of hormone into the cell or of binding within the cell.

On the basis of the account of Refetoff et al. [442], a set of diagnostic points appears in Table 10-10.

Other Types of Familial Thyroid Disease with Hypothyroidism

A number of case reports have appeared from time to time concerning individuals or families of patients with thyroid disease and hypothyroidism which do not fall conveniently into any of the groups delineated earlier in this chapter. In each instance the disease is presumably the result of an inborn error in one of the metabolic pathways of the thyroid, and in each case the error has defied precise definition.

An unusual family has been described by Murray et al. [443], in which nontoxic goiter occurred in five generations and in four of five members of the sibship of the propositus. The thyroid glands were characterized by nodularity and by calcification which was strikingly evident on roentgenographic examination. None of the recognized abnormalities of thyroid function was present. There was evidence of increased uptake and turnover of iodine, and distribution of iodoamino acids in these thyroid glands was normal.

Two cretinous patients among 12 children of a consanguine marriage had no demonstrable uptake in the neck region when radioactive iodine was used, but when technetium scanning was employed, a thyroid in normal position was detected in each [444]. Thus the thyroid was present in each patient, but with minimal function. Because the salivary/plasma ratio of radioactive iodine was normal, it was concluded that there was no defect in iodide transport. Other causes of hypothyroidism with goiter were ruled out. The patients improved with thyroxine medication.

Greig et al. [445] have reported two pairs of monozygotic twins, of which one pair was athyreotic and the other had ectopic thyroid tissue. They also reported a mother-daughter pair who were athyreotic. There are a number of reports of genetic alterations in the thyroxine-binding globulin and thyroxine-binding prealbumin, but these abnormalities are not associated with clinical disease [194–196, 446, 447]. Diminished thyroid protease activity has been suggested as a cause of familial goiter [448]. Uncertainty regarding the exact nature of the proteases of the thyroid which are concerned with hormone mobilization has limited exploration of this promising possibility for definition of additional metabolic errors of the thyroid.

Table 10-10. DIAGNOSTIC CRITERIA FOR SYNDROME OF THYROID HORMONE UNRESPONSIVENESS

1. Hypothyroid or compensated hypothyroid; small goiter
2. Nerve deafness
3. Stippled femoral epiphyses
4. High plasma thyroxine level; normal plasma thyroxine-binding proteins
5. Subnormal response to large doses of thyroxine or triiodothyronine; lack of response to normal thyroid suppression test
6. Rigorous exclusion of endemic goiter and of iodine deficiency

Diagnosis

There are few distinguishing clinical features among the various types of familial goiter with hypothyroidism, except for that group which has an associated nerve deafness. Differential diagnosis of the various types must depend on laboratory tests. Diagnostic criteria have been presented in the foregoing pages in tabular form.

The most useful preliminary observation is the uptake and retention of labeled iodine by the thyroid. Characteristically these patients, except those with the transport defect and TSH unresponsiveness, have an unusually rapid uptake curve, which reaches high levels within the first hour or two following administration. Measurements of turnover and of the effects of ClO_4^- and methimazole may give further clues to diagnosis. Analysis of the pattern of metabolism of the iodoamino acids in the peripheral blood also may be helpful. Most important is histologic and biochemical analysis of the thyroid itself.

The discussion thus far has centered largely on the diagnosis in patients who have a complete defect, i.e., homozygous expression. An important problem, and a more difficult one from many points of view, is the diagnosis of a specific genetic defect in patients who may be heterozygous for that defect. From studies done to date it is clear that in the deiodinase-defect group the heterozygous state may cause disease. In one study it was possible to show that various goitrous members of the family of a patient with fully expressed cretinism and deiodinase defect were less able to deiodinate injected DIT than normal persons. There is also evidence that heterozygotes for the transport and organification defects may also have goiter. Clearly, much further research is needed in order that heterozygotes may be detected and in order that the contribution of the heterozygous state of these defects to mild thyroid disease can be determined.

Treatment

Satisfactory treatment of familial goiter depends on the stage of development of the local disease and the degree to which irreversible changes have occurred in the skeleton and central nervous system. Remarkable shrinkage of the goiter may be expected from treatment with L-thyroxine or desiccated thyroid in usual maintenance doses, provided irreversible changes of degeneration, cyst formation, and fibrous replacement have not taken place. The goiter will inevitably recur if medication is discontinued.

Care should be exercised in treating medically a familial goiter in view of the tendency of some of them to undergo malignant change. In general it would be wise to remove any nodule which fails to shrink after several weeks of replacement therapy. Unfortunately, this will often be the case with well-established goiters, so that more often than not these patients eventually require surgery. Desiccated thyroid is required after thyroidectomy, unless it is desirable to maintain the patient in a hypothyroid state.

Unless treatment is begun early within the first few weeks of life, there is considerable risk of permanent retardation of intellectual development of skeletal growth. There is reason to suspect that damage may occur in utero, so that no amount of replacement therapy may prevent developmental arrest and permanent retardation. Carr et al. [449] have demonstrated the desirability of treating a mother, who has already given birth to a cretin, with large doses of desiccated thyroid during a subsequent pregnancy.

Medication should be sufficient. Perhaps a safe rule is to give increasing doses of desiccated thyroid until the first signs of overdosage appear (tachycardia, hyperactivity) and then to reduce the dosage slightly. Particular attention should be paid to newborn sibs of patients who have familial goiter.

Management of the patient with fully developed goiter, hypothyroidism, and permanent retardation is unsatisfactory. Little is accomplished in the adult by replacement therapy, and as often as not unacceptable aggressiveness or other undesirable behavior may be the result of full thyroid medication. In these patients the dosage is best adjusted to that which keeps the patient active and comfortable without arousing unwanted side effects.

A few patients with familial goiter, such as some of those who have associated VIIIth nerve deafness, appear to manufacture adequate amounts of hormone and to develop normally. They require thyroid substance only to prevent growth of the small goiters to which they are predisposed.

SUMMARY

1 The synthesis, storage, secretion, delivery, and utilization of the thyroid hormones involve a complex sequence of metabolic events, each of which is probably dependent upon specific enzymatic activity. Thyroid disease may result from blockage at many steps in this metabolic process.

2 Familial goiter and hypothyroidism may occur when there is failure of the thyroid cell to transport iodide and maintain a favorable concentration gradient inside the follicle iodide transport defect). The salivary and gastric glands of these patients are also unable to concentrate iodide.

3 Familial goiter may also result from failure to convert inorganic iodide into iodine in the thyroid gland (organification defect). Accumulated iodide is precipitously discharged from the gland upon the administration of SCN^-. A group of closely related patients have goiter and congenital nerve deafness (Pendred's syndrome). Labeled iodine in the gland is partially discharged upon the administration of SCN^-.

4 Several families of patients have now been studied who have a defect in the coupling of iodotyrosines into iodothyronines (coupling defect). The disease can be demonstrated with certainty only when it is shown that iodothyronines fail to appear in biopsy specimens of thyroid tissue which has a normal or nearly normal concentration of iodine.

5 Several family groups are known to be unable to deiodinate iodotyrosines (iodotyrosine deiodinase defect). Loss of hormone precursors from the gland and into the urine accounts for hypothyroidism and compensatory goiter. Goitrous but otherwise normal relatives of one such patient have been shown to deiodinate DIT less well than normal individuals. The condition is most convincingly diagnosed by the demonstration that intravenously administered labeled DIT is excreted intact in the urine.

6 Familial goiter may occur in man and sheep because of impaired synthesis of thyroglobulin. Some of these patients may iodinate other proteins within the thyroid cell. Other thyroids may synthesize abnormal forms of thyroglobulin.

7 A syndrome of familial goiter, nerve deafness, and stippled epiphyses has been described. The results of investigations are consistent with an impaired ability of the cells of the body to respond adequately to thyroid hormone.

8 Studies of one cretinous patient from a consanguine marriage have indicated a limited response to thyrotropin, both in synthesis of the specific thyroid protein thyroglobulin and in cell growth and division.

9 Certain patients with congenital goiter have been found with a circulating butanol-insoluble iodinated component in the serum (plasma iodoprotein disorder). Certain differences among patients suggest that this group may be heterogeneous.

BIBLIOGRAPHY

1. Wilkins, L., Clayton, G. W., and Berthong, M.: Development of goiters in cretins without iodine deficiency: hypothyroidism due to apparent inability of the thyroid gland to synthesize hormone. Pediatrics, **13**, 235, 1954.
2. Joseph, R., Tubiana, M., and Job, J.-C.: L'Hypothyroïdie par anomalie congénitale de la thyroxinogenèse. Rev. Franç. Étud. Clin. Biol., **3**, 167, 1958.
3. Stanbury, J. B.: The metabolic errors in certain types of familial goiter. Recent Progr. Hormone Res., **19**, 547, 1963.
4. Stanbury, J. B.: Classification and diagnostic criteria of the inborn errors of the thyroid. Presented at the North African Thyroid Association Meeting, Algiers, Algeria, Apr. 27–30, 1969. In press.
5. Collaço, F. M.: Bocio por dishormonogenesis. Rev. Clin. Esp., **108**, 490, 1968.
6. Hutchison, J. H.: Familial goitrous hypothyroidism, in *Endocrine and Genetic Diseases of Childhood,* edited by L. I. Gardner, p. 253. Saunders, Philadelphia, 1969.
7. Stanbury, J. B., and DeGroot, L. J.: The clinical chemistry and pathologic physiology of thyroid tissue. Clin. Chem., **13**, 542, 1967.
8. Osler, W.: Sporadic cretinism in America. Trans. Congr. Amer. Physicians Surg., **4**, 169, 1897.
9. Berson, S. A.: Pathways of iodine metabolism. Amer. J. Med., **20**, 653, 1956.
10. Riggs, D. S.: Quantitative aspects of iodine metabolism in man. Pharmacol. Rev., **4**, 284, 1952.
11. Ingbar, S. H., and Woeber, K. A.: The thyroid gland, in *Textbook of Endocrinology,* edited by R. H. Williams, p. 105. Saunders, Philadelphia, 1968.
12. Roche, J., and Michel, R.: Nature, biosynthesis, and metabolism of thyroid hormones. Physiol. Rev., **35**, 583, 1955.
13. Wayne, E. J., Koutras, D. A., and Alexander, W. D.: *Clinical Aspects of Iodine Metabolism,* Davis, Philadelphia, 1964.
14. DeGroot, L. J.: Current views on formation of thyroid hormones. New Eng. J. Med., **272**, 243, 1965.
15. DeGroot, L. J.: Kinetic analysis of iodine metabolism. J. Clin. Endocr., **26**, 149, 1966.
16. Halmi, N. S.: Thyroidal iodide transport. Vitamins Hormones, **19**, 133, 1961.
17. VanderLaan, W. P., and Caplan, R.: Observations on a relationship between total thyroid iodine content and the iodide-concentrating mechanism of the thyroid gland of the rat. Endocrinology, **54**, 437, 1954.
18. Socolow, E. L., Dunlap, D., Sobel, R. A., and Ingbar, S. H.: A correlative study of the effect of iodide administration in the rat on thyroidal iodide transport and organic iodine content. Endocrinology, **83**, 737, 1968.
19. Halmi, N. S., Nissen, W. M., and Scranton, J. R.: The kinetics of the enhancement of thyroidal iodide accumulation after actinomycin D administration. Endocrinology, **84**, 943, 1969.
20. Halmi, N. S., Gifford, T. H., and Glesne, R. E.: Further observations concerning the effect of actinomycin D on thyroidal iodide transport in rats. Endocrinology, **81**, 893, 1967.
21. VanderLaan, J. E., and VanderLaan, W. P.: The iodide concentrating mechanism of the rat thyroid and its inhibition by thiocyanate. Endocrinology, **40**, 403, 1947.
22. Raben, M. S.: The paradoxical effects of thiocyanate and of thyrotropin on the organic binding of iodine by the thyroid in the presence of large amounts of iodide. Endocrinology, **45**, 296, 1949.
23. Wolff, J., Chaikoff, I. L., Goldberg, R. C., and Meier, J. R.: The temporary nature of the inhibitory action of excess iodide on organic iodine synthesis in the normal thyroid. Endocrinology, **45**, 504, 1949.
24. Wollman, S. H., and Zwilling, E.: Radioiodine metabolism in the chick embryo. Endocrinology, **52**, 526, 1953.
25. Wolff, J., Robbins, J., and Rall, J. E.: Iodide trapping without organification in a transplantable rat thyroid tumor. Endocrinology, **64**, 1, 1959.
26. Paris, J., McConahey, W. M., Owen, C. A., Woolner, L. B., and Bahn, R. C.: Iodide goiter. J. Clin. Endocr., **20**, 57, 1960.
27. Stanbury, J. B., and Hedge, A. N.: A study of a family of goitrous cretins. J. Clin. Endocr., **10**, 1471, 1950.
28. Valenta, L.: Metastatic thyroid carcinoma in man concentrating iodine without organification. J. Clin. Endocr., **26**, 1317, 1966.
29. Harden, R. McG., Mason, D. K., and Buchanan, W. W.: Quantitative studies of iodide excretion in saliva in euthyroid, hypothyroid and thyrotoxin patients. J. Clin. Endocr., **25**, 957, 1965.
30. Fellinger, K., Höfer, R., and Vetter, H.: Salivary and thyroidal radioiodide clearances of plasma in various states of thyroid function. J. Clin Endocr., **16**, 449, 1956.
31. Taurog, A., Potter, G. D., and Chaikoff, I. L.: The effect of hypophysectomy and of TSH on the mouse submaxillary iodide pump. Endocrinology, **64**, 1038, 1959.
32. Logothetopoulos, J. H., and Myant, N. B.: Concentration of radio-iodide and ^{35}S-labelled thiocyanate by the stomach of the hamster. J. Physiol., **133**, 213, 1956.
33. Logothetopoulos, J. H., and Myant, N. B.: Concentration of radio-iodide and ^{35}S-thiocyanate by the salivary glands. J. Physiol., **134**, 189, 1956.
34. Wollman, S. H., Reid, J. C., and Reed, F. E.: Nonconcentration of thiocyanate-C^{14} by the thyroid gland of the mouse, Amer. J. Physiol., **193**, 83, 1958.
35. Halmi, N. S., and Stuelke, R. G.: Comparison of thyroidal and gastric iodide pumps in rats. Endocrinology, **64**, 103, 1959.
36. Yagi, Y., Michel, R., and Roche, J.: Sur le métabolisme des bromures radioactifs (^{82}Br). Bull. Soc. Chim. Biol. (Paris), **35**, 289, 1953.
37. Shellabarger, C. J., Durbin, P. W., Parrott, M. W., and Hamilton, J. G.: Effects of thyroxine and KSCN on capacity of rat thyroid gland to accumulate astatine^{211}. Proc. Soc. Exp. Biol. Med., **87**, 626, 1954.
38. Baumann, E. J., Searle, N. Z., Yalow, A. A., Siegel, E., and Seidlin, S. M.: Behavior of the thyroid toward elements of the seventh periodic group. Amer. J. Physiol., **185**, 71, 1956.
39. Bruner, H. D., Perkinson, J. D., and Hayes, R. L.: Deposition of Mn in the thyroid using Mn^{52-54}. Fed. Proc., **12**, 305, 1953.
40. Schindler, W. J., McHorse, T. S., and Krause, D. M.: Use of technetium-99m in studying thyroid physiology in the mouse: double label experiment with technetium-99m and iodine-125. Endocrinology, **79**, 281, 1966.
41. Shimmins, J., Hilditch, T., Hardin, R. McG., and Alexander, W. D.: Thyroidal uptake and turnover of the pertechnetate ion in normal and hyperthyroid subjects. J. Clin. Endocr., **28**, 575, 1968.
42. Wolff, J., and Maurey, J. R.: Thyroidal iodide transport. IX. The accumulation and metabolism of selenocyanate. Endocrinology, **79**, 795, 1966.
43. Wyngaarden, J. B., Stanbury, J. B., and Rapp, B.: The effects of iodide, perchlorate, thiocyanate, and nitrate administration upon the iodide concentrating mechanism of the rat thyroid. Endocrinology, **52**, 568, 1953.
44. Wyngaarden, J. B., Wright, B. M., and Ways, P.: The effect of certain anions upon the accumulation and retention of iodide by the thyroid gland. Endocrinology, **50**, 537, 1952.
45. Anbar, M., Guttmann, S., and Lewitus, Z.: The mode of action of perchlorate ions on the iodine uptake of the thyroid gland. Int. J. Appl. Radiat., **7**, 87, 1960.
46. Anbar, M., Guttmann, S., and Lewitus, Z.: The accumulation of fluoroborate ions in thyroid glands of rats. Endocrinology, **66**, 888, 1960.
47. Lewitus, A., Anbar, M., and Guttmann, S.: *Advances in Thyroid Research,* edited by R. Pitt-Rivers, p. 235. Pergamon, New York, 1961.
48. Maurey, J. R., and Wolff, J.: The partial molal volumes of OCN^-, $SeCN^-$, ReO_4^-, BF_4^-, SO_3F^-, SO_3NH_2. J. Inorg. Nuclear Chem., **25**, 312, 1963.
49. Doniach, I., and Logothetopoulos, J. H.: Radioautography of inorganic iodide in the thyroid. J. Endocr., **13**, 65, 1956.
50. Pitt-Rivers, R., and Trotter, W. R.: The site of accumulation of iodide in the thyroid of rats treated with thiouracil. Lancet, **2**, 918, 1953.
51. Woodbury, D. M., and Woodbury, J. W.: Correlation of micro-electrode potential recordings with histology of rat and guinea-pig thyroid glands. J. Physiol., **169**, 553, 1963.
52. Schackter, D., and Britten, J. S.: Active transport on non-electrolytes and the potential gradients across intestinal segments in vitro. Fed. Proc., **20**, 137, 1961.

53. Slingerland, D. W.: The influence of various factors on the uptake of iodine by the thyroid. J. Clin. Endocr., **15,** 131, 1955.
54. Freinkel, N., and Ingbar, S. H.: Effect of metabolic inhibitors upon iodide transport in sheep thyroid slices. J. Clin. Endocr., **15,** 598, 1955.
55. Halmi, N. S., and Pitt-Rivers, R.: The iodide pools of the rat thyroid. Endocrinology, **70,** 660, 1962.
56. Halmi, N. S.: The accumulation and recirculation of iodide by the thyroid, in *The Thyroid Gland,* vol. 1, edited by R. Pitt-Rivers and W. R. Trotter, p. 71. Butterworth, London, 1964.
57. DeCostre, P. L., Phair, R. D., Dingwell, I. W., and DeGroot, L. J.: A thyroid model and its analysis by computer, in *Endemic Goiter,* edited by J. B. Stanbury, p. 49. World Health Organization, Washington, D.C., 1969.
58. Ohtaki, S., Moriya, S., Suzuki, H., and Horiuchi, Y.: Nonhormonal iodine escape from the normal and abnormal thyroid gland. J. Clin. Endocr., **27,** 728, 1967.
59. Solomon, D. H.: Effects of thyrotropin on thyroidal water and electrolytes in the chick. Endocrinology, **69,** 939, 1961.
60. Wolff, J.: Thyroidal iodide transport. I. Cardiac glycosides and the role of potassium. Biochim. Biophys. Acta, **38,** 316, 1960.
61. Stanbury, J. B., Wicken, J. V., and Lafferty, M. A.: Preparation and properties of thyroid cell membranes. J. Membrane Biol. **1,** 459, 1969.
62. Wolff, J., and Halmi, N. S.: Thyroidal iodide transport. V. The role of Na^+-K^+-activated, ouabain-sensitive adenosinetriphosphatase activity. J. Biol. Chem., **238,** 847, 1963.
63. Turkington, R. W.: The effect of ouabain on thyrotropin stimulated respiration of thyroid slices. J. Biol. Chem., **238,** 3463, 1963.
64. Vilkki, P.: In vitro studies on phospholipid metabolism of the thyroid, in *Advances in Thyroid Research,* edited by R. Pitt-Rivers, p. 231. Pergamon, New York, 1961.
65. Vilkki, P.: An iodide-complexing phospholipid. Arch. Biochem., **97,** 425, 1962.
66. Larsen, P. R., and Wolff, J.: Iodide transport: inhibition by agents reacting at the membrane. Science, **155,** 335, 1967.
67. Stanbury, J. B., and Hughes, V.: The initial step in thyroid hormone biosynthesis. Medicine, **43,** 407, 1964.
68. Brunberg, J. A., and Halmi, N. S.: The role of ouabain-sensitive adenosine triphosphatase in the stimulating effect of thyrotropin on the iodide pump of the rat thyroid. Endocrinology, **79,** 801, 1966.
69. Shishiba, Y., and Solomon, D. H.: Effect of amphotericin B on thyroidal iodide concentration. Endocrinology, **81,** 467, 1967.
70. Wyngaarden, J. B., and Stanbury, J. B.: The formation of monoiodotyrosine and an intermediate iodine complex by thyroid homogenates. J. Biol. Chem., **212,** 151, 1955.
71. Taurog, A., Potter, G. C., Tong, W., and Chaikoff, I. L.: Formation of I-131-monoiodotyrosine from I-131-iodide by isolated particulate fractions of non-thyroid tissues. Endocrinology, **58,** 132, 1956.
72. Tong, W., and Chaikoff, I. L.: Stimulating effects of cytochrome C and quinones on I^{131} utilization by cell-free sheep thyroid gland preparations. Biochim. Biophys. Acta, **46,** 259, 1961.
73. DeRobertis, E., and Garro, R.: Peroxidase activity of the thyroid gland under normal and experimental conditions. Endocrinology, **38,** 137, 1946.
74. Hosoya, T., Kondo, Y., and Ui, N.: Peroxidase activity in the thyroid gland and partial purification of the enzyme. J. Biochem. (Tokyo), **52,** 180, 1962.
75. Alexander, N. M.: Mechanism of iodination reactions in thyroid glands. Endocrinology, **68,** 671, 1961.
76. Alexander, N. M.: Iodide peroxidase in rat thyroid and salivary glands and its inhibition by antithyroid compounds. J. Biol. Chem., **234,** 1530, 1959.
77. Alexander, N. M., and Corcoran, B. J.: Reversible dissociation of thyroid iodide peroxidase into apoenzyme and prosthetic group. J. Biol. Chem., **237,** 243, 1962.
78. DeGroot, L. J., and Davis, A. M.: Studies on the biosynthesis of iodotyrosines: a soluble thyroidal iodide-peroxidase tyrosine-iodinase system. Endocrinology, **70,** 492, 1962.
79. Ljunggren, J.-G., and Åkeson, Å.: Solubilization, isolation and identification of a peroxidase from the microsomal fraction of beef thyroid. Arch. Biochem. Biophys., **127,** 346, 1968.
80. Niepomniszcze, H., Altschuler, N., Korob, M. H., and Degrossi, O. J.: Iodide-peroxidase activity in human thyroid. 1. Studies on non-toxic nodular goiter. Republica Argentina Comisión Naçional de Energía Atómica, Buenos Aires, 1969.
81. Hosoya, T., and Morrison, M.: The isolation and purification of thyroid peroxidase. J. Biol. Chem., **242,** 2828, 1967.
82. Serif, G. S., and Kirkwood, S.: Enzyme systems concerned with the synthesis of monoiodotyrosine. J. Biol. Chem., **233,** 109, 1958.
83. Rosenberg, I. N.: The antithyroid activity of some compounds that inhibit peroxidase. Science, **116,** 503, 1952.
84. Randell, L. O.: Reaction of thiol compounds with peroxidase and hydrogen peroxide. J. Biol. Chem., **164,** 521, 1946.
85. Tong, W., and Chaikoff, I. L.: Stimulating effects of cytochrome C and quinones on ^{131}I utilization by cell-free sheep thyroid gland preparations. Biochim. Biophys. Acta, **46,** 259, 1961.
86. Schussler, G. C., and Ingbar, S. H.: The role of intermediary carbohydrate metabolism in regulating organic iodinations in the thyroid gland. J. Clin. Invest., **40,** 1394, 1961.
87. Alexander, N. M.: The mechanism of iodination reactions in thyroid glands, in *Advances in Hormone Research,* edited by R. Pitt-Rivers, p. 215. Pergamon, New York, 1961.
88. DeGroot, L. J., and Davis, A. M.: Studies on the biosynthesis of iodotyrosines: reduced pyridine nucleotide peroxidation by a thyroidal-iodinating enzyme. Biochim. Biophys. Acta, **59,** 581, 1962.
89. DeGroot, L. J., and Davis, A. M.: Studies on the biosynthesis of iodotyrosines: a soluble thyroidal iodide-peroxidase tyrosine-iodinase system. Endocrinology, **70,** 492, 1962.
90. DeGroot, L. J., and Davis, A. M.: Studies on the biosynthesis of iodotyrosines: the relationship of peroxidase, catalase and cytochrome oxidase. Endocrinology, **70,** 505, 1962.
91. DeGroot, L. J., and Davis, A. M.: Studies on the biosynthesis of iodotyrosines. J. Biol. Chem., **236,** 2009, 1961.
92. Alexander, N. M., and Corcoran, B. J.: Catalase inhibition of the peroxidatic reaction in thyroid tissue. Biochem. Biophys. Res. Commun., **4,** 248, 1961.
93. Klebanoff, S. J., Yip, C., and Kessler, D.: The iodination of tyrosine by beef thyroid preparations. Biochim. Biophys. Acta, **58,** 563, 1962.
94. Suzuki, M., Nagashima, M., and Yamamoto, K.: Studies on the mechanism of iodination by the thyroid gland: iodide-activating enzyme and an intracellular inhibitor of iodination. Gen. Comp. Endocr., **1,** 103, 1961.
95. Alexander, N. M.: Iodide peroxidase in rat thyroid and salivary glands and its inhibition by antithyroid compounds. J. Biol. Chem., **234,** 1530, 1959.
96. Pastan, I.: Certain functions of isolated thyroid cells. Endocrinology, **68,** 924, 1961.
97. Tong, W., Kerkof, P., and Chaikoff, I. L.: Iodine metabolism of dispersed thyroid cells obtained by trypsinization of sheep thyroid glands. Biochim. Biophys. Acta, **60,** 1, 1962.
98. Alexander, N. M.: The mechanism of iodination reactions in thyroid glands. Endocrinology, **68,** 671, 1961.
99. Igo, R. P., and Mackler, B.: Isolation of a particulate iodide metabolizing system from thyroid mitochondria. Arch. Biochem., **95,** 12, 1961.
100. Lamberg, B.-A., Matovinovic, J., and Stanbury, J. B.: The in vitro formation of iodinated compounds by thyroid slices and homogenate preparations. Acta Endocr., **29,** 33, 1958.
101. Taurog, A., Potter, G. D., and Chaikoff, I. L.: Conversion of inorganic I^{131} to organic I^{131} by cell-free preparations of thyroid tissue. J. Biol. Chem., **213,** 119, 1955.
102. Robbins, J., Wolff, J., and Rall, J. E.: Iodoproteins in normal and abnormal human thyroid tissue and normal sheep thyroid. Endocrinology, **64,** 37, 1959.
103. Freinkel, N.: The intermediary metabolism of thyroid tissue, in *The Thyroid Gland,* edited by R. Pitt-Rivers and W. R. Trotter, vol. 1, p. 131. Butterworth, London, 1964.

104. Tong, W., Taurog, A., and Chaikoff, I. L.: Activation of the iodinating system in sheep thyroid particulate fractions by flavin cofactors. J. Biol. Chem., **227,** 773, 1957.
105. Cunningham, B. A., and Kirkwood, S.: Enzyme systems concerned with the synthesis of monoiodotyrosine. III. Ion requirements of the soluble system. J. Biol. Chem., **236,** 485, 1961.
106. Fawcett, D. M., and Kirkwood, S.: The synthesis of organically bound iodine by cell-free preparations of thyroid tissue. J. Biol. Chem., **205,** 795, 1953.
107. Weiss, B.: Utilization of radioactive iodine by cell-free preparations of beef thyroid tissue. J. Biol. Chem., **201,** 31, 1953.
108. Pitt-Rivers, R., Galton, V. A., and Halmi, N. S.: Nature of radioiodine not dischargeable with perchlorate in the thyroid glands of thiouracil-treated rats. Endocrinology, **63,** 699, 1958.
109. Benabdeljlil, C., Michel-Béchet, M., and Lissitzky, S.: Isolation and iodinating ability of apical poles of sheep thyroid epithelial cells. Biochem. Biophys. Res. Commun., **27,** 74, 1967.
110. Nunez, J., Mauchamp, J., Macchia, V., and Roche, J.: Biosynthèse in vitro d'hormones doublement marquées dans des coupes de corps thyroïde. II. Biosynthèse d'une préthyroglobuline non iodée. Biochim. Biophys. Acta, **107,** 247, 1965.
111. Tishler, P. V., and Ingbar, S. H.: Correlative effects of puromycin on ^{131}I metabolism and amino acid incorporation by calf thyroid slices. Endocrinology, **76,** 295, 1965.
112. de Crombrugghe, B., Edelhoch, H., Beckers, C., and De Visscher, M.: Thyroglobulin from human goiters. Effects of iodination on sedimentation and iodoamino acid synthesis. J. Biol. Chem., **242,** 5681, 1967.
113. Morris, D. R., and Hager, L. P.: Mechanism of inhibition of enzymatic halogenation by antithyroid agents. J. Biol. Chem., **241,** 3582, 1966.
114. Jirousek, L.: The reaction of thiouracil with β-lactoglobulin sulfenyl iodide. Biochim. Biophys. Acta, **170,** 152, 1968.
115. Jirousek, L., and Cunningham, L. W.: Stimulation of thiouracil binding and the iodination system in beef thyroid microsomes. Biochim. Biophys. Acta, **170,** 160, 1968.
116. Cunningham, L. W.: The reaction of β-lactoglobulin sulfenyl iodide with several antithyroid agents. Biochemistry, **3,** 1629, 1964.
117. Ludwig, W., and von Mutzenbecher, P.: Die Darstellung von Thyroxin, Monojodtyrosin und Dijodtyrosin aus jodiertem Eiweib. Z. Physiol. Chem., **258,** 195, 1939.
118. von Mutzenbecher, P.: Über die Bildung von Thyroxin aus Dijodtyrosin. Z. Physiol. Chem., **261,** 253, 1939.
119. Johnson, T. B., and Tewksbury, L. B.: The oxidation of 3,5-diiodotyrosine. Proc. Nat. Acad. Sci. U.S.A., **28,** 73, 1942.
120. Harington, C., and Pitt-Rivers, R.: The chemical conversion of di-iodotyrosine into thyroxine. Biochem. J., **39,** 157, 1945.
121. Pitt-Rivers, R.: The oxidation of diiodotyrosine derivatives. Biochem. J., **43,** 223, 1948.
122. Shiba, T., and Cahnmann, H. J.: Conversion of 3,5-diiodotyrosine to thyroxine by rattlesnake venom. Biochim. Biophys. Acta, **58,** 609, 1962.
123. Keston, A. S.: The Schardinger enzyme in biological iodinations. J. Biol. Chem., **153,** 335, 1944.
124. Roche, J., and Michel, R.: Natural and artificial iodoproteins. Advances Protein Chem., **6,** 253, 1951.
125. Harington, C. R.: Newer knowledge of the biochemistry of the thyroid gland. J. Chem. Soc., 193, 1944.
126. Stanbury, J. B.: Iodothyronine synthesis and the so-called "coupling defect" in familial goitre. Memoirs of the Society for Endocrinology, No. 15, p. 107. Cambridge, London, 1967.
127. Pitt-Rivers, R., and Cavalieri, R. R.: Thyroid hormone biosynthesis, in *The Thyroid Gland,* edited by R. Pitt-Rivers and W. R. Trotter, vol. 1, p. 87. Butterworth, London, 1964.
128. Ljunggren, J.-G.: The isolation and identification of 2,6-diiodohydroquinone from the thyroid gland. Acta Chem. Scand., **15,** 1772, 1961.
129. Ljunggren, J.-G.: The oxidation of 3,5-diiodotyrosine by peroxidase and hydrogen peroxide. Acta Chem. Scand., **17,** 567, 1963.
130. Gross, J., and Leblond, C. P.: The presence of free iodinated compounds in the thyroid and their passage into the circulation. Endocrinology, **48,** 714, 1951.
131. Pitt-Rivers, R.: The biosynthesis of thyroid hormones. J. Clin. Path. **20,** 318, 1967.
132. Taurog, A.: The biosynthesis of thyroxine. Mayo Clin. Proc., **39,** 569 1964.
133. Dunn, J. T.: The amino acid neighbors of thyroxine in thyroglobulin. J. Biol. Chem., **245,** 5954, 1970.
134. Inoue, K., and Taurog, A.: Acute and chronic effects of iodide on thyroid radioiodine metabolism in iodine-deficient rats. Endocrinology, **83,** 279, 1968.
135. Heninger, R. W., and Albright, E. C.: Effect of iodine deficiency on iodine-containing compounds of rat tissues. Endocrinology, **79,** 309, 1966.
136. Mates, G. P., and Shulman, S.: Studies on thyroid proteins. V. Immunochemical heterogeneity of human thyroglobulin. Immunochemistry, **4,** 475, 1967.
137. van Zyl, A., and Edelhoch, H.: The properties of thyroglobulin. XV. The function of the protein in the control of diiodotyrosine synthesis. J. Biol. Chem., **242,** 2423, 1967.
138. Inoue, K., and Taurog, A.: Freezing-induced alterations in thyroglobulin from iodine deficient and iodine sufficient rats. Endocrinology, **83,** 833, 1968.
139. Surks, M. I., Weinbach, S., and Volpert, E. M.: On the identification of 4-hydroxy-3,5-diiodophenylpyruvic acid in rat thyroid glands. Endocrinology, **82,** 1156, 1968.
140. Harington, C. R.: Twenty-five years of research on the biochemistry of the thyroid gland. Endocrinology, **49,** 401, 1951.
141. Spiro, R. G., and Spiro, M. J.: Glycoprotein biosynthesis: studies on thyroglobulin. Characterization of a particulate precursor and radioisotope incorporation by thyroid slices and particle systems. J. Biol. Chem., **241,** 1271, 1966.
142. Cheftel, C., and Bouchilloux, S.: Glycoprotein biosynthesis in sheep thyroid slices incubated with radioactive glucosamine and leucine. I. Polysomes, microsomes and postmicrosomal fraction. Biochim. Biophys. Acta, **170,** 15, 1968.
143. Bloth, B., and Bergquist, R.: The ultrastructure of human thyroglobulin. J. Exp. Med., **128,** 1129, 1968.
144. Thomson, J. A., and Goldberg, I. H.: Biosynthesis of thyroglobulin and its subunits *in vivo* in the rat thyroid gland. Endocrinology, **82,** 805, 1968.
145. Simon, C., Roques, M., Torresani, J., and Lissitzky, S.: Effect of propylthiouracil on the iodination and maturation of rat thyroglobulin. Acta Endocr., **53,** 271, 1966.
146. Morais, R., and Goldberg, I. H.: Cell-free synthesis of thyroglobulin. Biochemistry, **6,** 2538, 1967.
147. Salvatore, G., Aloj, S., Salvatore, M., and Edelhoch, H.: Hybridization of half molecules of guinea pig thyroglobulin. J. Biol. Chem., **242,** 5002, 1967.
148. Kondo, Y., De Nayer, P., Salabe, G., Robbins, J., and Rall, J. E.: Function of isolated bovine thyroid polyribosomes. Endocrinology, **83,** 1123, 1968.
149. Kondo, Y., De Nayer, P., Labaw, L. W., Robbins, J., and Rall, J. E.: Properties of bovine thyroid ribosomes and polyribosomes. Endocrinology, **83,** 1117, 1968.
150. Lecocq, R. E., and Dumont, J. E.: Polysomes from thyroids incubated in vitro. Biochim. Biophys. Acta, **129,** 421, 1966.
151. Derrien, Y., Michel, R., Pederson, K. O., and Roche, J.: Recherches sur la préparation et sur les propriétés de la thyroglobuline pure. II. Biochim. Biophys. Acta, **3,** 436, 1949.
152. Roche, J., Salvatore, G., Sena, L., Aloj, S., and Covelli, I.: Thyroid iodoproteins in vertebrates: ultracentrifugal pattern and iodination rate. Comp. Biochem. Physiol., **27,** 67, 1968.
153. Gitlin, D., and Biasucci, A.: Ontogenesis of immunoreactive thyroglobulin in the human conceptus. J. Clin. Endocr., **29,** 849, 1969.
154. Roitt, I. M., and Torrigiani, G.: Identification and estimation of undegraded thyroglobin in human serum. Endocrinology, **81,** 421, 1967.
155. Torrigiani, G., Doniach, D., and Roitt, I. M.: Serum thyroglobulin levels in healthy subjects and in patients with thyroid disease. J. Clin. Endocr., **29,** 305, 1969.
156. Smith, D. W. E., Robbins, J., and Rall, J. E.: Iodine containing subcellular particles in thyroid tissue. Endocrinology, **69,** 510, 1961.

157. Robbins, J., Wolff, J., and Rall, J. E.: Iodoproteins in normal and abnormal human thyroid tissue and in normal sheep thyroid. Endocrinology, **64**, 37, 1959.
158. Medeiros-Neto, G. A., Manzano, E., and Cintra, A. B. U.: Intrathoracic goiter in a euthyroid patient: localization with ^{125}I and study of thyroidal iodoproteins. J. Clin. Endocr., **29**, 183, 1969.
159. Boat, T. F., and Halmi, N. S.: Studies of particulate iodoproteins in the rat thyroid. Endocrinology, **77**, 537, 1965.
160. Stanbury, J. B., Brownell, G. L., Riggs, D. S., Perinetti, H., Itoiz, J., and del Castillo, E. B.: *Endemic Goiter: The Adaptation of Man to Iodine Deficiency.* Harvard, Cambridge, Mass., 1954.
161. Laver, W. G., and Trikojus, V. M.: Complex nature of the proteolytic system of the thyroid gland. Biochim. Biophys. Acta, **20**, 444, 1956.
162. Weiss, B.: Peptidase and proteinase activity of beef thyroid tissue. J. Biol. Chem., **205**, 193, 1953.
163. Alpers, J. B., Robbins, J., and Rall, J. E.: The hydrolysis of rat thyroglobulin by thyroidal enzymes. Endocrinology, **56**, 110, 1955.
164. Dopheide, T. A. A., Menzies, C. A., McQuillan, M. T., and Trikojus, V. M.: Studies with purified pig thyroglobulin and thyroid enzymes. Biochim. Biophys. Acta, **181**, 105, 1969.
165. Konno, N., Murthy, P. V. N. and McKenzie, J. M.: Stimulation of proteolysis in the mouse thyroid gland by thyrotropin and the long-acting thyroid stimulator: Comparison of intact lobe and homogenate. Endocrinology, **87**, 1062, 1970.
166. Taurog, A., and Thio, D. T.: TSH-induced thyroxine release from puromycin-blocked thyroid glands of intact rabbits. Endocrinology, **78**, 103, 1966.
167. Haddad, H. M., and Rall, J. E.: Purification of thyroid proteases by cellulose column chromatography. Endocrinology, **67**, 413, 1960.
168. McQuillan, M. T., Mathews, J. D., and Trikojus, V. M.: Proteolysis of thyroglobulin by thyroid enzymes. Nature (London), **192**, 333, 1961.
169. Litonjua, A. D.: Thyroglobulin. Nature (London), **191**, 356, 1961.
170. Pastan, I., and Almqvist, S.: Hydrolysis of thyroglobulin by a mast cell enzyme present in rat thyroid homogenates. Endocrinology, **78**, 350, 1966.
171. Hartmann, N.: Über den Abbau von Dijodtyrosin im gewebe. Z. Physiol. Chem., **285**, 1, 1950.
172. Roche, J., Michel, R., Michel, O., and Lissitzky, S.: Sur la déshalogenation enzymatique des iodotyrosines par le corps thyroïde et sur son rôle physiologique. Biochim. Biophys. Acta, **9**, 161, 1952.
173. Stanbury, J. B.: The requirement of monoiodotyrosine deiodinase for triphosphopyridine nucleotide. J. Biol. Chem., **228**, 801, 1957.
174. Stanbury, J. B., and Morris, M. L.: Deiodination of diiodotyrosine by cell-free systems. J. Biol. Chem., **233**, 106, 1958.
175. Matsuzaki, S., and Suzuki, M.: Deiodination of iodinated amino acids by pig thyroid microsomes. J. Biochem., **62**, 746, 1967.
176. Rosenberg, I. N., and Ahn, C. S.: Enzymatic deiodination of diiodotyrosine; possible mediation by reduced flavin nucleotide. Endocrinology, **84**, 727, 1969.
177. Maayan, M. L.: Effect of injection of nicotinamide, nicotinic acid and L-tryptophan upon deiodination of diiodotyrosine by thyroid and liver homogenates of normal and hypophysectomized rats. Endocrinology, **77**, 32, 1965.
178. Kusakabe, T., and Miyake, T.: Iodotyrosine deiodinase isozymes in the normal and in thyroid diseases. J. Clin. Endocr., **26**, 615, 1966.
179. Greer, M. A., and Grimm, Y.: Changes in thyroid secretion produced by inhibition of iodotyrosine deiodinase. Endocrinology, **83**, 405, 1968.
180. Green, W. L.: Inhibition of thyroidal iodotyrosine deiodination by tyrosine analogues. Endocrinology, **83**, 336, 1968.
181. Bastomsky, C. H., and Rosenberg, I. N.: Inhibition of thyroidal deiodination of diiodotyrosine by compounds which enhance NADPH oxidation. Endocrinology, **79**, 505, 1966.
182. Carr, E. A., Beierwaltes, W. H., Spafford, N. R., Duncan, L. L., and Stambaugh, R. A.: Activity of iodotyrosine deshalogenase in normal and diseased human thyroids. J. Clin. Endocr., **19**, 1282, 1959.
183. Ermans, A. M., Dumont, J. E., and Bastenie, P. A.: Thyroid function in a goitrous endemic. II. Nonhormonal iodine escape from the goitrous gland. J. Clin. Endocr., **23**, 550, 1963.
184. Rosenberg, I. N., Athans, J. C., Behar, A., and Ahn, C. S.: Thyrotropin-induced release of iodide from the thyroid, in *Advances in Thyroid Research,* edited by R. Pitt-Rivers, p. 194. Pergamon, New York, 1961.
185. Berman, M., Hoff, E., Barandes, M., Becker, D. V., Sonenberg, M., Benua, R., and Koutras, D. A.: Iodine kinetics in man—a model. J. Clin. Endocr., **28**, 1, 1968.
186. Ohtaki, S., Moriya, S., Suzuki, H., and Horiuchi, Y.: Nonhormonal iodine escape from the normal and abnormal thyroid gland. J. Clin. Endocr., **27**, 728, 1967.
187. Oppenheimer, J. H.: Role of plasma proteins in the binding, distribution and metabolism of the thyroid hormones. New Eng. J. Med., **278**, 1153, 1968.
188. Hollander, C. S., Odak, V. V., Prout, T. E., and Asper, S. P., Jr.: An evaluation of the role of pre-albumin in the binding of thyroxine. J. Clin. Endocr., **22**, 617, 1962.
189. Woeber, K. A., and Ingbar, S. H.: The contribution of thyroxine-binding prealbumin to the binding of thyroxine in human serum, as assessed by immunoadsorption. J. Clin. Invest., **47**, 1710, 1968.
190. Zaninovich, A. A., Farach, H., Ezrin, C., and Volpé, R.: Lack of significant binding of L-triiodothyronine by thyroxine-binding globulin *in vivo* as demonstrated by acute disappearance of ^{131}I-labeled triiodothyronine. J. Clin. Invest., **45**, 1290, 1966.
191. Marshall, J. S., and Pensky, J.: Studies on human thyroxine-binding globulin (TBG). I. Purification of TBG and immunologic studies on the relationship between TBG from normal persons and those with TBG "deficiency." J. Clin. Invest., **48**, 508, 1969.
192. Braverman, L. E., Dawber, N. A., and Ingbar, S. H.: Observations concerning the binding of thyroid hormones in sera of normal subjects of varying ages. J. Clin. Invest., **45**, 1273, 1966.
193. Oppenheimer, J. H., and Werner, S. C.: Effect of prednisone on thyroxine-binding proteins. J. Clin. Endocr., **26**, 715, 1966.
194. Beierwaltes, W. H., and Robbins, J.: Familial increase in the thyroxine-binding sites in serum alpha globulin. J. Clin. Invest., **38**, 1683, 1959.
195. Nikolai, T. F., and Seal, U. S.: X-chromosome linked inheritance of thyroxine-binding globulin deficiency. J. Clin. Endocr., **27**, 1515, 1967.
196. Refetoff, S., Robin, N. I., and Asper, C. A.: Genetic polymorphism of thyroxine-binding prealbumin (TBPA) in the rhesus (Macaca mulatta). Presented at the 51st Meeting of the Endocrine Society, New York, June 27–29, 1969.
197. Hamada, S., Torizuka, K., Miyake, T. and Fukase, M.: Specific binding proteins of thyroxine and triiodothyronine in liver soluble proteins. Biochim. Biophys. Acta, **201**, 479, 1970.
198. Tata, J. R., Ernster, L., and Suranyi, E. M.: Interaction between thyroid hormones and cellular constituents. I. Binding to isolated sub-cellular particles and sub-particulate fractions. Biochim. Biophys. Acta, **60**, 461, 1962.
199. Schwartz, H. L., Bernstein, G., and Oppenheimer, J. H.: Effect of phenobarbital administration on the subcellular distribution of ^{125}I-thyroxine in rat liver: importance of microsomal binding. Endocrinology, **84**, 270, 1969.
200. Oppenheimer, J. H., Bernstein, G., and Surks, M. I.: Increased thyroxine turnover and thyroidal function after stimulation of hepatocellular binding of thyroxine by phenobarbital. J. Clin. Invest., **47**, 1399, 1968.
201. Lissitzky, S.: Métabolisme cellulaire des hormones thyroïdiennes et désiodation. Bull. Soc. Chim. Biol., **42**, 1187, 1960.
202. Gorman, C. A., Flock, E. V., Owen, C. A., Jr., and Paris, J.: Factors affecting exchange of thyroid hormones between liver and blood. Endocrinology, **79**, 391, 1966.
203. Hasen, J., Bernstein, G., Volpert, E., and Oppenheimer, J. H.: Analysis of the rapid interchange of thyroxine between plasma and liver and plasma and kidney in the intact rat. Endocrinology, **82**, 37, 1968.
204. Roche, J., Michel, R., and Tata, J.: Sur l'excrétion biliaire et la glycuroconjugaison de la 3:5:3′-triiodothyronine. Biochim. Biophys. Acta, **11**, 543, 1953.
205. West, C. D., Simons, E. L., Gortatowski, M. J., and Kumagai, L. F.: The metabolism of ring-labeled L-thyroxine-C^{14} in vivo. J. Clin. Invest., **42**, 1134, 1963.

206. Isselbacher, K. J.: Enzymatic mechanisms of hormone metabolism. II. Mechanism of hormonal glucuronide formation. Recent Progr. Hormone Res., **12,** 134, 1956.
207. Tata, J. R., Rall, J. E., and Rawson, R. W.: Metabolism of L-thyroxine and L-3:5:3′-triiodothyronine by brain tissue preparations. Endocrinology, **60,** 83, 1957.
208. Larson, F. C., Tomita, K., and Albright, E. C.: The deiodination of thyroxine to triiodothyronine by kidney slices of rats with varying thyroid function. Endocrinology, **57,** 338, 1955.
209. Albright, E. C., Tomita, K., and Larson, F. C.: *In vitro* metabolism of triiodothyronine. Endocrinology, **64,** 208, 1959.
210. Braverman, L. E., Ingbar, S. H., and Sterling, K.: In vivo conversion of thyroxine (T_4) to triiodothyronine (T_3) in man. Presented at the 51st Meeting of the Endocrine Society, New York, June 27–29, 1969.
211. Wynn, J., Gibbs, R., and Royster, B.: Thyroxine degradation. I. Study of optimal reaction conditions of a rat liver thyroxine-degrading system. J. Biol. Chem., **237,** 1892, 1962.
212. Wynn, J., and Gibbs, R.: Thyroxine degradation. III. Competitive inhibition of thyroxine degradation: relationship of structure to inhibition. J. Biol. Chem., **238,** 3490, 1963.
213. Stanbury, J. B., Morris, M. L., Corrigan, H. J., and Lassiter, W. E.: Thyroxine deiodination by a microsomal preparation requiring Fe^{++}, oxygen, and cysteine or glutathione. Endocrinology, **67,** 353, 1960.
214. Stanbury, J. B.: Deiodination of the deiodinated amino acids. Ann. N.Y. Acad. Sci., **86,** 417, 1960.
215. Galton, V. A., and Ingbar, S. H.: A photoactivated flavin-induced degradation of thyroxine and related phenols. Endocrinology, **70,** 210, 1962.
216. Reinwein, D., Rall, J. E., and Durrer, H. A.: Deiodination of thyroxine by a hydrogen peroxide generating system. Endocrinology, **83,** 1023, 1968.
217. Galton, V. A., and Ingbar, S. H.: Observations on the nature of the heat-resistant thyroxine deiodinating system of rat liver. Endocrinology, **78,** 855, 1966.
218. Jolin, T., de Escobar, G. M., and del Ray, F. E.: Pitfalls in studies of *in vitro* deiodination of thyroxine. Endocrinology, **78,** 7, 1966.
219. Pittman, C. S., Maruyama, T., and Chambers, J. B., Jr.: Metabolism of the diiodotyrosyl moiety of specifically labeled thyroxines. Endocrinology, **83,** 489, 1968.
220. Pittman, C. S., and Chambers, J. B., Jr.: Carbon structure of thyroxine metabolites in urine. Endocrinology, **84,** 705, 1969.
221. Galton, V. A., and Ingbar, S. H.: Effects of vitamin deficiency on the *in vitro* and *in vivo* deiodination of thyroxine in the rat. Endocrinology, **77,** 169, 1965.
222. Dussault, J., Row, V. V., Lickrish, G., and Volpé, R.: Studies of serum triiodothyronine concentration in maternal and cord blood: transfer of triiodothyronine across the human placenta. J. Clin. Endocr., **29,** 595, 1969.
223. Selenkow, H. A., and Asper, S. P.: Biological activity of compounds structurally related to thyroxine. Physiol. Rev., **35,** 426, 1955.
224. Money, W. L., Meltzer, R. I., Young, J., and Rawson, R. W.: The effect of change in chemical structure of some thyroxine analogues on the metamorphosis of *Rana pipiens* tadpoles. Endocrinology, **63,** 20, 1958.
225. Money, W. L., Kumaoka, S., and Rawson, R. W.: Comparative effects of thyroxine analogues in experimental animals. Ann. N. Y. Acad. Sci., **86,** 512, 1960.
226. Barker, S. B.: Mechanism of action of thyroid hormone. Physiol. Rev., **31,** 205, 1951.
227. Nikkilä, E. A., and Pitkänen, E.: Liver enzyme pattern in thyrotoxicosis. Acta Endocr., **31,** 573, 1959.
228. Lindsay, S., and Jenks, P. R.: Enzymatic histochemistry of the rat thyroid gland, in *Advances in Thyroid Research,* edited by R. Pitt-Rivers, p. 215. Pergamon, New York, 1961.
229. Rivlin, R. S., and Langdon, R. G.: Effects of thyroxine upon biosynthesis of flavin mononucleotide and flavin adenine dinucleotide. Endocrinology, **84,** 584, 1969.
230. Ackerman, C. J., and Al-Mudhaffar, S.: Stimulation of adenylosuccinate synthetase by thyroid hormones *in vitro.* Endocrinology, **82,** 905, 1968.
231. Hess, M. E., Aronson, C. E., Hottenstein, D. W., and Karp, J. S.: Effects of adrenal cortical hormones and thyroxine on phosphorylase activity in muscle. Endocrinology, **84,** 1107, 1969.
232. Geel, S. E., and Timiras, P. S.: Influence of neonatal hypothyroidism and of thyroxine on the acetylcholinesterase and cholinesterase activities in the developing central nervous system of the rat. Endocrinology, **80,** 1069, 1967.
233. Al-Mudhaffar, S., and Ackerman, C. J.: Inhibition of inosine monophosphate-dehydrogenase by thyroid hormones *in vitro,* Endocrinology, **82,** 912, 1968.
234. Wolff, J., and Wolff, E. C.: The effect of thyroxine on isolated dehydrogenases. Biochim. Biophys. Acta, **26,** 387, 1957.
235. Ruegamer, W. R., Newman, G. H., Richert, D. A., and Westerfeld, W. W.: Specificity of the α-glycerophosphate dehydrogenase and malic enzyme response to thyroxine. Endocrinology, **77,** 707, 1965.
236. Schapiro, S., and Percin, C. J.: Thyroid hormone induction of α-glycerophosphate dehydrogenase in rats of different ages. Endocrinology, **79,** 1075, 1966.
237. Wolff, E. C., and Ball, E. G.: The action of thyroxine on oxidation of succinate and malate. J. Biol. Chem., **224,** 1083, 1957.
238. Tapley, D. F., Cooper, C., and Lehninger, A. L.: The action of thyroxine on mitochondria and oxidative phosphorylation. Biochim. Biophys. Acta, **18,** 597, 1955.
239. Emmelot, P., and Bos, C. J.: Thyroxine-mediated release of diphosphopyridine nucleotide from mitochondrial dehydrogenases. Exp. Cell Res., **14,** 132, 1958.
240. Wolff, J.: The effect of thyroxine on isolated dehydrogenases. III. J. Biol. Chem., **237,** 236, 1962.
241. Peterson, R. E.: The influence of the thyroid on adrenal cortical function. J. Clin. Invest., **37,** 736, 1958.
242. Yates, F. E., Urquhart, J., and Herbst, A. L.: Effect of thyroid hormones on ring A reduction of cortisone by liver. Amer. J. Physiol., **195,** 373, 1958.
243. McGuire, J., and Tomkins, G.: Effect of thyroxin administration on the rate and steric course of enzymatic reduction of steroids. Nature (London), **182,** 261, 1958.
244. Bradlow, H. L., Fukushima, D. K., Zumoff, B., Hellman, L., and Gallagher, T. F.: Influence of thyroid hormone on progesterone transformation in man. J. Clin. Endocr., **26,** 831, 1966.
245. Nelson, D. R., and Cornatzer, W. E.: Role of the thyroid in the synthesis of heart, liver and kidney mitochondrial phospholipids. Endocrinology, **77,** 37, 1965.
246. Vaughan, M.: An in vitro effect of triiodothyronine on rat adipose tissue. J. Clin. Invest., **46,** 1482, 1967.
247. Bressler, R., and Wittels, B.: The effect of thyroxine on lipid and carbohydrate metabolism in the heart. J. Clin. Invest., **45,** 1326, 1966.
248. Wynn, J.: Antioxidant function of thyroxine *in vivo.* Endocrinology, **83,** 376, 1968.
249. Maley, G. F., and Lardy, H. A.: Efficiency of phosphorylation in selected oxidations by mitochondria from normal and thyrotoxic rat livers. J. Biol. Chem., **215,** 377, 1955.
250. Martius, G., and Hess, B.: The mode of action of thyroxin. Arch. Biochem., **33,** 486, 1951.
251. Hoch, F. L., and Lipmann, F.: The uncoupling of respiration and phosphorylation by thyroid hormones. Proc. Nat. Acad. Sci. U.S.A., **40,** 909, 1954.
252. Lardy, H. A., and Maley, G. F.: Metabolic effects of thyroid hormones in vitro. Recent Progr. Hormone Res., **10,** 129, 1954.
253. Bronk, J.: Some actions of thyroxine on oxidative phosphorylation. Biochim. Biophys. Acta, **37,** 327, 1960.
254. Dallam, R. D., and Howard, R. B.: Thyroxine-enhanced oxidative phosphorylation of rat-liver mitochondria. Biochim. Biophys. Acta, **37,** 188, 1960.
255. Bronk, J. A., and Bronk, M. S.: The influence of thyroxine on oxidative phosphorylation in mitochondria from thyroidectomized rats. J. Biol. Chem., **237,** 897, 1962.
256. Lardy, H. A., and Maley, G. F.: Metabolic effects of thyroid hormones in vitro. Recent Progr. Hormone Res., **10,** 129, 1954.

257. Ball, E. G., and Cooper, O.: The oxidation of reduced triphosphopyridine nucleotide as mediated by the transhydrogenase reaction and its inhibition by thyroxine. Proc. Nat. Acad. Sci. U.S.A., **43,** 357, 1957.
258. Lehninger, A. L.: Reversal of thyroxine-induced swelling of rat liver mitochondria by adenosine triphosphate. J. Biol. Chem., **234,** 2187, 1959.
259. Roche, J., Michel, R., Rall, J. E., Michel, O., Girard, M., and Varrone, S.: Action de la L-thyroxine et de l'iodure de cyanogène sur la morphologie mitochondriale et les phosphorylations oxydatives. Biochim. Biophys. Acta, **71,** 494, 1963.
260. Rall, J. E., Michel, R., Roche, J., Michel, O., and Varrone, S.: Action and metabolism of thyroid hormones and iodine-donating substances. J. Biol. Chem., **238,** 1848, 1963.
261. Tata, J. R.: Inhibition of the biological action of thyroid hormones by actinomycin D and puromycin. Nature (London), **197,** 1167, 1963.
262. Tata, J. R., Ernster, L., Lindberg, O., Arrhenius, E., Pedersen, S., and Hedman, R.: The action of thyroid hormones at the cell level. Biochem. J., **86,** 408, 1963.
263. Adamson, L. F., and Ingbar, S. H.: Some properties of the stimulatory effect of thyroid hormones on amino acid transport by embryonic chick bone. Endocrinology, **81,** 1372, 1967.
264. Buchanan, J., and Tapley, D. F.: Stimulation by thyroxine of amino acid incorporation into mitochondria. Endocrinology, **79,** 81, 1966.
265. Kandemir, N., Eich, E., Alfano, J., and Greif, R. L.: Some effects of thyroxine on mitochondria from livers of newborn and partially hepatectomized rats. Endocrinology, **78,** 505, 1966.
266. Schapiro, S.: Metabolic and maturational effects of thyroxine on the infant rat. Endocrinology, **78,** 527, 1966.
267. Moss, B., and Ingram, V. M.: Hemoglobin synthesis during amphibian metamorphosis. II. Synthesis of adult hemoglobin following thyroxine administration. J. Molec. Biol., **32,** 493, 1968.
268. Bargman, G. J., and Gardner, L. I.: Otic lesions and congenital hypothyroidism in the developing chick. J. Clin. Invest., **46,** 1828, 1967.
269. Tata, J. R., and Widnell, C. C.: Ribonucleic acid synthesis during the early action of thyroid hormones. Biochem. J., **98,** 604, 1966.
270. Widnell, C. C., and Tata, J. R.: Additive effects of thyroid hormone, growth hormone and testosterone on deoxyribonucleic acid-dependent ribonucleic acid polymerase in rat-liver nuclei. Biochem. J., **98,** 621, 1966.
271. Utiger, R. D.: Radioimmunoassay of human plasma thyrotropin. J. Clin. Invest., **44,** 1277, 1965.
272. Odell, W. D., Wilber, J. F., and Utiger, R. D.: Studies of thyrotropin physiology by means of radioimmunoassay. Recent Progr. Hormone Res., **23,** 47, 1967.
273. Dumont, J. E.: LeMécanisme d'action de l'hormone thyréotrope. Bull. Soc. Clin. Biol., **50,** 2401, 1968.
274. Conway, L. W., Schalch, D. S., Utiger, R. D., and Reichlin, S.: Hormones in human pituitary sinusoid blood: concentration of LH, GH and TSH. J. Clin. Endocr., **29,** 446, 1969.
275. Tonoue, T., and Yamamoto, K.: Stimulation by thyroidectomy and suppression by thyroxine administration of amino acid uptake by the rat pituitary gland. Endocrinology, **81,** 101, 1967.
276. Wilber, J. F., and Utiger, R. D.: Thyrotropin incorporation of ^{14}C-glucosamine by the isolated rat adenohypophysis. Endocrinology, **84,** 1316, 1969.
277. Yamada, T., and Lewis, A. E.: An essential role of thyroxine and triiodothyronine balance in establishing normal pituitary-thyroid feedback control in goitrogen-treated rats. Endocrinology, **82,** 91, 1968.
278. Wilber J. F., Peake, G. T., and Utiger, R. D.: Thyrotropin release *in vitro*: stimulation by cyclic 3′,5′-adenosine monophosphate. Endocrinology, **84,** 758, 1969.
278*a*. Wilber, J. F. and Porter, J. C.: Thyrotropin and growth hormone releasing activity in hypophysial portal blood. Endocrinology, **87,** 807, 1970.
279. Averill, R. L. W.: Responses to thyrotropin-releasing factor (TRF) by intrapituitary infusion of hypothalamic extracts. Endocrinology, **84,** 514, 1969.
280. Bowers, C. Y., Schally, A. V., Hawley, W. D., Gual, C., and Parlow, A.: Effect of thyrotropin-releasing factor in man. J. Clin. Endoc., **28,** 978, 1968.
281. Folker, K., Chang, J.-K., Currie, B. L., Bowers, C. Y., Weil, A. and Schally, A. V.: Synthesis and relationship of L-glutaminyl-L-histidyl-L-prolinamide to the thyrotropin releasing hormone. Biochem. Biophys. Res. Commun., **39,** 110, 1970.
282. Schally, A. V., Nair, R. M. G., Barrett, J. F., Bowers, C. Y. and Folkers, K.: The structure of hypothalamic thyrotropin-releasing hormone. Abstract. Fed. Proc., **29,** 470, 1970.
283. Halász, B., Florsheim, W. H., Corcorran, N. L., and Gorski, R. A.: Thyrotrophic hormone secretion in rats after partial or total interruption of neural afferents to the medial basal hypothalamus. Endocrinology, **80,** 1075, 1967.
284. Bowers, C. Y., Lee, K. L., and Schally, A. V.: A study on the interaction of the thyrotropin-releasing factor and L-triiodothyronine: effects of puromycin and cycloheximide. Endocrinology, **82,** 75, 1968.
285. Bowers, C. Y., Lee, K.-L., and Schally, A. V.: Effect of actinomycin D on hormones that control the release of thyrotropin from the anterior pituitary glands of mice. Endocrinology, **82,** 303, 1968.
286. Yamada, T., Kajihara, A., Onaya, T., Kobayashi, I., Takemura, Y., and Shichijo, K.: Studies on acute stimulatory effect of cold on thyroid activity and its mechanism in the guinea pig. Endocrinology, **77,** 968, 1965.
286*a*. Liberti, P. and Stanbury, J. B.: The pharmacology of substances affecting the thyroid gland. Ann. Rev. Pharm. (in press).
286*b*. Dumont, J. E., Neve, P. and Otten, J.: Recent advances in the knowledge of the control of thyroid growth and function. In *Endemic Goiter,* edited by J. B. Stanbury, (chap. 2), p. 14, World Health Organization, Washington, D.C., 1969.
287. Pastan, I., Roth, J., and Macchia, V.: Binding of hormone to tissue: the first step in polypeptide hormone action. Proc. Nat. Acad. Sci. U.S.A., **56,** 1802, 1966.
288. Tong, W.: TSH stimulation of ^{14}C-amino acid incorporation into protein by isolated bovine thyroid cells. Endocrinology, **80,** 1101, 1967.
289. Graig, F. A.: Thyrotropin and propylthiouracil-induced stimulation of thyroidal creatine phosphokinase and lactic dehydrogenase in the rat. Endocrinology, **81,** 708, 1967.
290. Zakarija, M., Bastomsky, C. H., and McKenzie, J. M.: Effect of thyrotropin on thyroid pyridine nucleotides *in vivo.* Endocrinology, **84,** 1310, 1969.
291. Oka, H., and Field, J. B.: Pyridine nucleotides in the thyroid gland. VIII. Effect of thyroid-stimulating hormone on nicotinic acid-^{14}C incorporation into NAD, NADP and NADPH. Endocrinology, **81,** 1291, 1967.
292. Scott, T. W., Jay, S. M., and Freinkel, N.: Further studies on the action of pituitary thyrotropin on the individual phosphatides of thyroid tissue. Endocrinology, **79,** 591, 1966.
293. Deiss, W. P., Jr., Balasubramaniam, K., Peake, R. L., Starrett, J. A., and Powell, R. C.: Stimulation of proteolysis in thyroid particles by thyrotropin. Endocrinology, **79,** 19, 1966.
294. Clayton, J. A., and Szego, C. M.: Depletion of rat thyroid serotonin accompanied by increased blood flow as an acute response to thyroid-stimulating hormone. Endocrinology, **80,** 689, 1967.
295. Shimoda, S.-I., Kendall, J. W., and Greer, M. A.: Acute effects of thyrotropin on thyroid hormone biosynthesis in the rat. Endocrinology, **79,** 921, 1966.
296. Ochi, Y., and DeGroot, L. J.: TSH- or LATS-stimulated thyroid hormone release is inhibited by iodide. Endocrinology, **84,** 1305, 1969.
297. Kaneko, T., Zor, U., and Field, J. B.: Thyroid-stimulating hormone and prostaglandin E_1 stimulation of cyclic 3′,5′-adenosine monophosphate in thyroid slices. Science, **163,** 1062, 1969.
298. Zor, U., Bloom, G., Lowe, I. P., and Field, J. B.: Effects of theophylline, prostaglandin E_1 and adrenergic blocking agents on TSH stimulation of thyroid intermediary metabolism. Endocrinology, **84,** 1082, 1969.
299. Wilson, B., Raghupathy, E., Tonoue, T., and Tong, W.: TSH-like actions of dibutyryl-cAMP on isolated bovine thyroid cells. Endocrinology, **83,** 877, 1968.

299*a*. Schell-Frederick, E. and Dumont, J. E.: Mechanism of action of thyrotropin. In *Biochemical Actions of Hormones,* vol. 1, chap. 10, p. 415, Academic Press, New York, 1970.
300. Levey, G. S., Roth, J., and Pastan, I.: Effect of propranolol and phentolamine on canine and bovine responses to TSH. Endocrinology, **84,** 1009, 1969.
301. Burke, G.: Failure of theophylline to potentiate stimulated thyroidal glucose oxidation and phospholipogenesis. Endocrinology, **84,** 1055, 1969.
302. Scott, T. W., Good, B. F., and Ferguson, K. A.: Comparative effects of long-acting thyroid stimulator and pituitary thyrotropin on the intermediate metabolism of thyroid tissue *in vitro.* Endocrinology, **79,** 949, 1966.
303. Burke, G.: Comparison of early effects of thyrotropin and long-acting thyroid stimulator on thyroidal phospholipogenesis. Endocrinology, **83,** 1210, 1968.
304. Pinchera, A., Liberti, P., DeSantis, R., Grasso, L., Martino, E., and Baschieri, L.: Relationship between the long-acting thyroid stimulator and circulating thyroid antibodies in Graves' disease. J. Clin. Endocr., **27,** 1758, 1967.
305. Field J. B., Remer, A., Bloom, G., and Kriss, J. P.: In vitro stimulation by long-acting thyroid stimulator of thyroid glucose oxidation and ^{32}P incorporation into phospholipids. J. Clin. Invest., **47,** 1553, 1968.
306. Miyai, K., Fukuchi, M., Kumahara, Y., and Abe, H.: LATS production by lymphocyte culture in patients with Graves' disease. J. Clin. Endocr., **27,** 855, 1967.
307. Beall, G. N., and Solomon, D. H.: Thyroid-stimulating activity in the serum of rabbits immunized with thyroid microsomes. J. Clin. Endocr., **28,** 503, 1968.
308. Beall, G. N., and Solomon, D. H.: Inhibition of long-acting thyroid stimulator by thyroid particulate fractions. J. Clin. Invest., **45,** 552, 1966.
309. Wong, E. T., and Litman, G. W.: Interaction of purified long-acting thyroid stimulator (LATS) and thyroid microsomes *in vitro.* J. Clin. Endocr., **29,** 72, 1969.
310. Kriss, J. P.: Inactivation of long-acting thyroid stimulator (LATS) by anti-kappa and anti-lambda antisera. J. Clin. Endocr., **28,** 1440, 1968.
311. Hennen, G., Pierce, J. G., and Freychet, P.: Human chorionic thyrotropin: further characterization and study of its secretion during pregnancy. J. Clin. Endocr., **29,** 581, 1969.
312. Hershman, J. M., and Starnes, W. R.: Extraction and characterization of a thyrotropic material from the human placenta. J. Clin. Invest., **48,** 923, 1969.
313. Cortell, R., and Rawson, R. W.: The effect of thyroxin on the response of the thyroid gland to thyrotropic hormone. Endocrinology, **35,** 488, 1944.
314. Braverman, L. E., and Ingbar, S. H.: Changes in thyroidal function during adaptation to large doses of iodide. J. Clin. Invest., **42,** 1216, 1963.
315. Taurog, A., and Evans, E. S.: Extrathyroidal thyroxine formation in completely thyroidectomized rats. Endocrinology, **80,** 915, 1967.
316. Weiss, B.: Carbohydrate utilization by beef thyroid tissue. J. Biol. Chem., **193,** 509, 1951.
317. Dumont, J. E.: Carbohydrate metabolism in the thyroid gland. J. Clin. Endocr., **20,** 1246, 1960.
318. Dumont, J. E.: Hexose monophosphate pathway in thyroid tissue. Biochim. Biophys. Acta, **40,** 354, 1960.
319. Field, J. B., Pastan, I., Johnson, P., and Herring, B.: In vitro stimulation of the hexose monophosphate pathway in thyroid by thyroid-stimulating hormone. Biochem. Biophys. Res. Commun., **1,** 284, 1959.
320. Field, J. B., Pastan, I., Johnson, P., and Herring, B.: Stimulation in vitro of pathways of glucose oxidation in thyroid by thyroid-stimulating hormone. J. Biol. Chem., **235,** 1863, 1960.
321. Dumont, J. E.: Effect in vitro of thyroid-stimulating hormone on the hexose monophosphate pathway in thyroid. Biochim. Biophys. Acta, **46,** 195, 1961.
322. Nunez, J., Mauchamp, J., Jérusalmi, A., and Roche, J.: Synthèse acellulaire de la thyroglobuline et site d'iodation. Biochim. Biophys. Acta, **145,** 127, 1967.
323. Nadler, N. J., Young, B. A., Leblond, C. P., and Mitmaker, B.: Elaboration of thyroglobulin in the thyroid follicle. Endocrinology, **74,** 333, 1964.
324. Seed, R. W., and Goldberg, I. H.: Biosynthesis of thyroglobulin: relationship to RNA-template and precursor protein. Proc. Nat. Acad. Sci. U.S.A., **50,** 275, 1963.
325. Barzolatto, J., Murray, I. P. C., and Stanbury, J. B.: Effects of gamma radiation on oxygen utilization, iodine metabolism and leucine incorporation by surviving sheep thyroid tissue slices. Endocrinology, **70,** 328, 1962.
326. Freinkel, N.: Pathways of thyroid phosphorus metabolism: the phospholipids of sheep thyroid. Biochem. J., **68,** 327, 1958.
327. DeGroot, L. J., Thompson, J. E., and Dunn, A. D.: Studies on an iodinating enzyme from calf thyroid. Endocrinology, **76,** 632, 1965.
328. Suzuki, M., and Nagashima, M.: Studies on the mechanism of iodination by the thyroid gland. 3. Concentration of catalase, flavine and cytochrome *C* oxidase in the pig thyroid gland and other tissues. Gunma J. Med. Sci., **10,** 168, 1961.
329. Turkington, R. W., and Nordwind, B.: Oxidative phosphorylation and respiratory control in mitochondria from normal, adenomatous, and hyperplastic thyroid glands. J. Clin. Invest., **41,** 1725, 1962.
330. Stanbury, J. B., and Chapman, E. M.: Congenital hypothyroidism with goitre: absence of an iodide-concentrating mechanism. Lancet, **1,** 1162, 1960.
331. Federman, D., Robbins, J., and Rall, J. E.: Some observations on cretinism and its treatment. New Eng. J. Med., **259,** 610, 1958.
332. Wolff, J., Thompson, R. H., and Robbins, J.: Congenital goitrous cretinism due to absence of iodide-concentrating ability. J. Clin. Endocr., **24,** 699, 1964.
333. Gilboa, V., Ber, A., Lewitis, Z., and Hasenfratz, J.: Goitrous myxedema due to iodide trapping defect. Arch. Int. Med., **112,** 212, 1963.
333*a*. Papadopoulos, S. N., Vagenakis, A. G., Moschos, A., Koutras, D. A., Matsaniotis, N. and Malamos, B.: A case of a partial defect of the iodide trapping mechanism. J. Clin. Endocr., **30,** 302, 1970.
334. Stanbury, J. B.: Cretinism with goiter: a case report. J. Clin. Endocr., **11,** 740, 1951.
335. Stanbury, J. B., Ohela, K., and Pitt-Rivers, R.: The metabolism of iodine in 2 goitrous cretins compared with that in 2 patients receiving methimazole. J. Clin. Endocr., **15,** 54, 1955.
336. Haddad, H. M., and Sidbury, J. B., Jr.: Defect of the iodinating system in congenital goitrous cretinism: report of a case with biochemical studies. J. Clin. Endocr., **19,** 1446, 1959.
337. Schultz, A., Flink, E. B., Kennedy, B. J., and Zieve, L.: Exchangeable character of accumulated I^{131} in the thyroid gland of a goitrous cretin. J. Clin. Endocr., **17,** 441, 1957.
338. Clayton, G. W., Smith, J. D., and Leiser, A.: Familial goiter with defect in intrinsic metabolism of thyroxine without hypothyroidism. J. Pediat., **52,** 129, 1958.
339. Furth, E. D., Carvalho, M., and Vianna, B.: Familial goiter due to an organification defect in euthyroid siblings. J. Clin. Endocr., **27,** 1137, 1967.
340. Lelong, M., Joseph, R., Canlorbe, P., Job, J.-C., and Plainfosse, B.: L'hypothyroïdie par anomalie congénitale de l'hormonogénèse (cinq observations). Arch. Franç. Pédiat., **13,** 1, 1956.
341. Gardner, J. V., Hayles, A. B., Woolner, L. B., and Owen, C. A.: Iodine metabolism in goitrous cretins. J. Clin. Endocr., **19,** 638, 1959.
342. König, M. P., Baumann, Th., Schärer, K., and Herren, Ch.: Familiäre, kongenitale Störung der Schilddrüsenhormonsynthese: fehlerhafte Oxydation von anorganischem zu organischem Jod. Schweiz. Med. Wschr., **94,** 319, 1964.
343. Jackson, A. D. M.: Non-endemic goitrous cretinism. Arch. Dis. Child., **29,** 571, 1954.
344. Penã, J., Belmonte, A. V., and Tojo, R.: Hipotiroidismo bocioso por defecto en el proceso de organificación del iodo. Una observación en gemelos. Rev. Esp. Pediat., **21,** 103, 1965.
345. Valenta, L.: Metastatic thyroid carcinoma in man concentrating iodine without organification. J. Clin. Endocr., **26,** 1317, 1966.
346. Neel, J. V., Carr, E. A., Beierwaltes, W. H., and Davidson, R. T.: Genetic studies on the congenitally hypothyroid. Pediatrics, **27,** 269, 1961.

47. Carr, E. A., Beierwaltes, W. H., Neel, J. V., Davidson, R., Lowry, G. G. Dodson, V. N., and Tanton, J. H.: The various types of thyroid malfunction in cretinism and their relative frequency. Pediatrics, **28,** 1, 1961.

48. Ferrini, O., and Biassoni, P.: Criptotiroidismo enzimopenico. Folia Endocr. (Roma), **19,** 313, 1966.

49. Smith, J. D., Cagas, C. R., Seely, J. R., and Neeman, J.: Defective iodide organification in "'cryptothyroidism." Southern Med. J., **59,** 1478, 1966.

50. Baschieri, L., Benedetti, G., de Luca, F., and Negri, M.: Evaluation and limitations of the perchlorate test in the study of thyroid function. J. Clin. Endocr., **23,** 786, 1963.

51. Milutinovic, P. S., Stanbury, J. B., Wicken, J. V., and Jones, E. W.: Thyroid function in a family with the Pendred syndrome. J. Clin. Endocr., **29,** 962, 1969.

352. Brain, W. R.: Heredity in simple goitre. Quart. J. Med., **20,** 303, 1927.

353. Johnsen, S.: Familial deafness and goitre in persons with a low level of protein-bound iodine. Acta Otolaryng (Stockholm), suppl. **140,** 168, 1958.

354. Thould, A. K., and Scowen, E. F.: The syndrome of congenital deafness and simple goitre, in *Advances in Thyroid Research,* edited by R. Pitt-Rivers, p. 22. Pergamon, New York, 1961.

355. Elman, D. S.: Familial association of nerve deafness with nodular goiter and thyroid carcinoma. New Eng. J. Med., **259,** 219, 1958.

356. Roberts, K. D.: Thyroid carcinoma in childhood in Great Britain. Arch. Dis. Child., **32,** 58, 1957.

357. Thieme, E. T.: A report of the occurrence of deaf-mutism and goiter in four of six siblings of a North American family. Ann. Surg., **146,** 941, 1957.

358. Nilsson, L. R., Borgfors, N., Gamstorp, I., Holst, H.-E., and Lidén, G.: Nonendemic goitre and deafness. Acta Paediat., **53,** 117, 1964.

359. Medeiros-Neto, G. A., Nicolau, W., Kieffer, J., and Cintra, A. B. U.: Thyroidal iodoproteins in Pendred's syndrome. J. Clin. Endocr., **28,** 1205, 1968.

360. Shane, S. R., Jones, J. E., and Flink, E. B.: Familial goiter and congenital nerve deafness. J. Clin. Endocr., **25,** 1085, 1965.

361. Morgans, M. E., and Trotter, W. R.: Association of congenital deafness with goitre. Lancet, **1,** 607, 1958.

362. Ljungren, J.-G., and Vecchio, G.: Studies on a patient with congenital deafness, nodular goitre, positive perchlorate test, abnormal biosynthesis of thyroglobulin and a high total concentration of thyroid peroxidase. Presented at 7th Acta Endocrinologia Congress, Stockholm, 1969.

363. Fraser, G. R., Morgans, M. E., and Trotter, W. R.: The syndrome of sporadic goitre and congenital deafness. Quart. J. Med., **29,** 279, 1960.

364. McGirr, E. M., Hutchison, J. H., and Clement, W. E.: Sporadic goitre due to dyshormonogenesis: impaired utilization of trapped iodide. Scottish Med. J., **4,** 107, 1959.

365. Deraemaeker, R.: Congenital deafness and goiter. Amer. J. Hum. Genet., **8,** 253, 1956.

366. Trotter, W. R.: The association of deafness with thyroid dysfunction. Brit. Med. Bull., **16,** 92, 1960.

367. Batsakis, J. G., and Nishiyama, R. H.: Deafness with sporadic goiter. Pendred's syndrome. Arch. Otolaryng. (Chicago), **76,** 401, 1962.

368. Gross, J., and Pitt-Rivers, R.: 3:5:3'-triiodothyronine. I. Isolation from thyroid gland and synthesis. Biochem. J., **53,** 645, 1953.

369. Stanbury, J. B., Riccabona, G., and Janssen, M.-A.: Iodotyrosyl coupling defect in congenital hypothyroidism with goitre. Lancet, **1,** 917, 1963.

370. Choufoer, J. C., Kassenaar, A. A. H., and Querido, A.: The syndrome of congenital hypothyroidism with defective dehalogenation of iodotyrosines: further observations and discussion of the pathophysiology. J. Clin. Endocr., **20,** 983, 1960.

371. Mosier, H. D., Blizzard, R. M., and Wilkins, L.: Congenital defects in the biosynthesis of thyroid hormone: report of two cases. Pediatrics, **21,** 248, 1958.

372. Joseph, R., and Job, J.-C.: Les Hypothyroidies par troubles congénitaux de l'hormonogénèse. Vie Méd., **42,** 1259, 1961.

373. Whitelaw, M. J., Thomas, S., and Reilly, W. A.: A nongoitrous cretin with a high level of serum PBI and thyroidal I^{131} uptake. J. Clin. Endocr., **16,** 983, 1956 (abstract).

374. Leszynsky, H. E.: Metabolic defects of thyroid hormone synthesis in a case of infantilism without clinical evidence of thyroid pathology (thyrogenic infantilism). Acta endocr., **36,** 221, 1961.

375. Lerman, J., Jones, H. W., and Calkins, E.: Studies on two sporadic cretinous brothers with goiter, together with some remarks on the relation of hyperplasia to neoplasia. Ann. Intern. Med., **25,** 677, 1946.

376. Hamilton, J. G., Soley, M. H., Reilly, W. A., and Eichorn, K. B.: Radioactive iodine studies in childhood hypothyroidism. A.M.A. J. Dis. Child., **66,** 495, 1943.

377. Pickering, D. E., Sheline, G. E., and Crane, J. T.: Sporadic familial goitrous hypothyroidism. A.M.A. J. Dis. Child., **93,** 510, 1957.

378. Zondek, H., Leszynsky, H. E., and Zondek, G. W.: Triiodothyronine in myxedema and familial sporadic cretinism with goiter. Acta Endocr., **18,** 117, 1955.

379. Hubble, D.: Familial cretinism. Lancet, **1,** 1112, 1953.

380. Werner, S. C., Block, R. J., Mandl, R. H., and Kassenaar, A. A. H.: Pathogenesis of a case of congenital goiter with abnormally high levels of SPI and with mono- and diiodotyrosine in the serum. J. Clin. Endocr., **17,** 817, 1957.

381. Ermans, A. M., Kinthaert, J., and Camus, M.: Defective intrathyroidal iodine metabolism in nontoxic goiter: inadequate iodination of thyroglobulin. J. Clin. Endocr., **28,** 1307, 1968.

382. Joseph, R., and Job, J.-C.: L'Hypothyroïdie congénitale avec anomalie de la condensation des iodotyrosines. Arch. Franç. Pédiat., **15,** 1, 1958.

383. McGirr, E. M., and Hutchison, J. H.: Radioactive iodine studies in non-endemic goitrous cretins. Lancet, **1,** 1117, 1953.

384. Hutchison, J. H., and McGirr, E. M.: Hypothyroidism as an inborn error of metabolism. J. Clin. Endocr., **14,** 869, 1954.

385. Stanbury, J. B., Kassenaar, A. A. H., Meijer, J. W. A., and Terpstra, J.: The occurrence of mono- and diiodotyrosine in the blood of a patient with congenital goiter. J. Clin. Endocr., **15,** 1216, 1955.

386. Stanbury, J. B., Meijer, J. W. A., and Kassenaar, A. A. H.: The metabolism of iodotyrosines. II. The metabolism of mono- and di-iodotyrosine in certain patients with familial goiter. J. Clin. Endocr., **16,** 848, 1956.

387. Stanbury, J. B., Kassenaar, A. A. H., and Meijer, J. W. A.: The metabolism of iodotyrosines. I. The fate of mono- and di-iodotyrosine in normal subjects and in patients with various diseases. J. Clin. Endocr., **16,** 735, 1956.

388. Albert, A., and Keating, F. R., Jr.: Metabolic studies with I^{131}-labeled thyroid compounds: distribution and excretion of radiodiiodotyrosine in human beings. J. Clin. Endocr., **11,** 996, 1951.

389. Querido, A., Stanbury, J. B., Kassenaar, A. A. H., and Meijer, J. W. A.: The metabolism of iodotyrosines. III. Di-iodotyrosine deshalogenating activity of human thyroid tissue. J. Clin. Endocr., **16,** 1096, 1956.

390. Hutchison, J. H., and McGirr, E. M.: Sporadic nonendemic goitrous cretinism. Lancet, **1,** 1035, 1956.

391. McGirr, E. M., Clement, W. E., Currie, A. R., and Kennedy, J. S.: Impaired dehalogenase activity as a cause of goitre with malignant changes. Scottish Med. J., **4,** 232, 1959.

392. Horst, W.: Radiojoddiagnostik van Struma und Schilddrüsenkrebs und Untersuchungen zur Frage einer Jodfehlverwertung in deren Pathogenese. Verh. d. 4 Jahrestagung des Deutschen Zentralaus-Schusses für Krebsbekämfung und Krebsforschung, edited by A. Dietrich. Sonderbd. zur Strahlentherapie, **34,** 150, 1956.

393. McGirr, E. M., Hutchison, J. H., and Clement, W. E.: Sporadic goitrous cretinism. Dehalogenase deficiency in the thyroid gland of a goitrous cretin and in heterozygous carriers. Lancet, **2,** 823, 1959.

394. Lobo, L. C., Rodrigues, J., and Fridman, J.: Hipotireoidismo congenito por defeito na sintese hormonal. J. Brasil. Med., **3,** 17, 1960.

395. Béraud, Th., Dorta, T., and Vannotti, A.: Étude du métabolisme de la diiodotyrosine en pathologie humaine. J. Suisse Méd., **89,** 980, 1959.

396. Vague, J., Lissitzky, S., Simonin, R., Codaccioni, J. L., Miller, G., Boyer, J., and Audibert, G.: Hypothyroïdie infantile avec goitre. Identification de mono-et de diiodotyrosines dans le sang et les urines resultant favorable du traitment par l'iode. Ann. Endocr., **23,** 213, 1962.

397. Vague, J., Lissitzky, S., Codaccioni, J.-L., Simonin, R., Miller, G., Boyer, J., Audibert, G., and Nicolino, J.: Hypothyroïdie infantile avec goitre par defaut de la desiodation des iodotyrosines, traitée avec succes par l'iode. Presse Méd., **70,** 2497, 1962.

398. Vague, J., Lissitzky, S., Codaccioni, J.-L., Simonin, R., Miller, G., Boyer, J., and Audibert, G.: Infantile Hypothyroidism with goitre and defect of deiodination of iodotyrosines: treatment with Lugol's solution. Lancet, **1,** 1070, 1962.

399. Lissitzky, S., Comar, D., Rivière, R., and Codaccioni, J.-L.: Étude quantitative du métabolisme de l'iode dans un cas d'hypothyroïdie avec goitre due à un défaut d'iodotyrosine-déshalogénase. Rev. Franç. Études Clin. Biol., **10,** 631, 1965.

400. Lissitzky, S., Bismuth, J., Codaccioni, J.-L., and Cartouzou, G.: Congenital goiter with iodoalbumin replacing thyroglobulin and defect of deiodination of iodotyrosines. Serum origin of the thyroid iodoalbumin. J. Clin. Endocr., **28,** 1797, 1968.

401. Niall, H. D., Wellby, M. L., Hetzel, B. S., Hudson, B., and Chenoweth, R. A.: Biochemical and clinical studies in familial goitre caused by an iodotyrosine deiodinase defect. Aust. Ann. Med., **17,** 89, 1968.

402. Murray, P., Thomson, J. A., McGirr, E. M., and Wallace, T. J.: Absent and defective iodotyrosine deiodination in a family some of whose members are goitrous cretins. Lancet, **2,** 183, 1965.

403. Harden, R. McG., Alexander, W. D., Papadopoulos, S., Harrison, M. T., and Macfarlane, S.: The influence of the plasma inorganic iodine concentration on thyroid function in dehalogenase deficiency. Acta Endocr., **55,** 361, 1967.

403*a*. Jaffiol, C., Khalil, R., Pastorello, R., Baldet et Mirouze, J.: Goitre sporadique tardif de l'adulte, avec déficit enzymatique en deshalogénase. Étude clinique, biochimique, isotopique. Rev. Franc. Endoc. Clin., **10,** 67, 1969.

404. Choufoer, J. C.: Further observations on congenital hypothyroidism with defective dehalogenation of iodotyrosines, in *Advances in Thyroid Research,* edited by R. Pitt-Rivers, p. 36. Pergamon, New York, 1961.

405. Bernheim, M., and Berger, M.: Le Diagnostic et le mécanisme de l'insuffisance thyroïdienne de l'enfant études à la faveur des épreuves au radioiode. Semaine hôp. Paris, **30,** 3575, 1954.

406. Burrell, C. D., and Gairdner, D. M. T.: Cretinism in three siblings. Proc. Roy. Soc. Med., **48,** 1026, 1955.

407. Kusakabe, T., and Miyake, T.: Defective deiodination of I^{131}-labeled L-diiodotyrosine in patients with simple goiter. J. Clin. Endocr., **23,** 132, 1963.

408. Kusakabe, T., and Miyake, T.: Thyroidal deiodination defect in three sisters with simple goiter. J. Clin. Endocr., **24,** 456, 1964.

409. Gardner, J. U., Hayles, A. B., Woolner, L. B., and Owen, C. A., Jr.: Iodine metabolism in goitrous cretins. J. Clin. Endocr., **19,** 638, 1959.

410. Riddick, F. A., Jr., Desai, K. B., Stanbury, J. B., and Murison, P. J.: Familial goiter with diminished synthesis of thyroglobulin. Z. Exp. Med., **150,** 203, 1969.

411. Stanbury, J. B.: The iodoproteins of the normal and abnormal thyroid gland. 6th International Congress of Clinical Chemistry, Munich, 1966. Advances Clin.-Biochem. Res., **4,** 5, 1968.

412. Lizarralde, G., Jones, B., Seal, U. S., and Jones, J. E.: Goitrous cretinism with chromosomal aberration and defect in thyroglobulin synthesis. J. Clin. Endocr., **26,** 1227, 1966.

413. Alexander, N. M. and Burrow, G. N.: Thyroxine biosynthesis in human goitrous cretinism. J. Clin. Endocr., **30,** 308, 1970.

414. Mouriz, J., Riesco, G., and Usobiaga, P.: Thyroid proteins in a goitrous cretin with iodide organification defect. J. Clin. Endocr., **29,** 942, 1969.

415. McGirr, E. M., Hutchison, J. H., Clement, W. E., Kennedy, J. S., and Currie, A. R.: Goitre and cretinism due to the production of an abnormal iodinated thyroid compound. Scottish Med. J., **5,** 189, 1960.

416. Michel, R., Rall, J. E., Roche, J., and Tubiana, M.: Thyroidal iodoproteins in patients with goitrous hypothyroidism. J. Clin. Endocr., **24,** 352, 1964.

417. Robbins, J., Van Zyl, A., and Van Der Walt, K.: Abnormal thyroglobulin in congenital goiter of cattle. Endocrinology, **78,** 1213, 1966.

418. Van Zyl, A., Schulz, K., Wilson, B., and Pansegrouw, D.: Thyroidal iodine and enzymatic defects in cattle with congenital goiter. Endocrinology, **76,** 353, 1965.

419. Ramagopal, E., Spiro, M. J., and Stanbury, J. B.: Some properties of the soluble iodoproteins from normal and certain abnormal thyroid glands. J. Clin. Endocr., **25,** 742, 1965.

420. Wiener, J. D., and Linderboom, G. A.: The possible occurence of two inborn errors of iodine metabolism in one patient. Acta Endocr., **47,** 385, 1964.

421. Pittman, C. S., and Pittman, J. A., Jr.: A study of the thyroglobulin thyroidal protease and iodoproteins in two congenital goitrous cretins. Amer. J. Med., **40,** 49, 1966.

422. Falconer, I. R.: Biochemical defect causing congenital goitre in sheep. Nature (London), **205,** 978, 1965.

423. Falconer, I. R., Roitt, I. M., Seamark, R. F. and Torrigiani, G.: Studies of the congenitally goitrous sheep. Iodoproteins of the goitre. Biochem. J., **117,** 417, 1970.

424. Rac, R., Hill, G. N., Pain, R. W., and Mulhearn, C. J.: Congenital goitre in merino sheep due to an inherited defect in the biosynthesis of thyroid hormone. Vet. Sci., **9,** 209, 1968.

425. Stanbury, J. B., and McGirr, E. M.: Sporadic or nonendemic familial cretinism with goiter. Amer. J. Med., **22,** 712, 1957.

426. Werner, S. C., Block, R. J., and Mandl, R. H.: Circulating iodoprotein in a nongoitrous adult with primary amenorrhea, bony deformities, and normal levels of serum precipitable iodine and thyroidal I^{131} uptake. J. Clin. Endocr., **17,** 1141, 1957.

427. DiGeorge, A. M., and Paschkis, K. E.: Sporadic hypothyroidism associated with goiter. J. Clin. Endocr., **17,** 645, 1957.

428. DeGroot, L. J., and Stanbury, J. B.: The syndrome of congenital goiter with butanol-insoluble serum iodide. Amer. J. Med., **27,** 586, 1959.

429. Derome, G., Mahaux, J., and Henry, A.: Iodoprotéinémie anormale chez un enfant porteur d'un goitre congénital. Ann. Endocr., **19,** 873, 1958.

430. Kahn, A., Cogan, S. R., and Berger, S.: Circulating iodoprotein in two patients with autonomous thyroid nodules. J. Clin. Endocr., **22,** 1, 1962.

431. Courvoisier, B., DeGroot, L. J., Stanbury, J. B., Béraud, Th., and Koralnik, L.: Insuffisances thyroïdiennes par anomalies congénitales de la synthèse hormonale. J. Suisse Méd., **89,** 973, 1959.

432. Chavarria, C., Monos-Ferreira, G., Guevara, G., Rupp, J. J., and Paschkis, K. E.: Butanol-insoluble iodinated compound in the plasma of a goitrous cretin. J. Clin. Endocr., **20,** 894, 1960.

433. Katznelson, D., and Sack, J.: Congenital hypothyroidism probably due to an abnormal iodoprotein. Proc. Tel-Hashomer Hosp., Tel Aviv, **5,** 36, 1966.

434. Lissitzky, S., Codaccioni, J.-L., Cartouzou, G., and Mante, S.: Eumetabolic goitrous adult with iodoprealbumin in thyroid tissue and blood. J. Clin. Endocr., **24,** 305, 1964.

434*a*. Furth, E. D., Agrawal, R. B. and Propp, R. P.: Secretion of iodoalbumin and iodoprealbumin by a congenital goiter containing thyroglobulin and the iodoalbumins. J. Clin. Endocr., **31,** 60, 1970.

435. Lamberg, B.-A., Hintze, G., and Karlsson, R.: Non-butanol extractable iodine in the serum of eumetabolic adult goitre patients. Acta Endocr., **44,** 291, 1963.

436. Owen, C. A., Jr., and McConahey, W. M.: An unusual iodinated protein of the serum in Hashimoto's thyroiditis. J. Clin. Endocr., **16,** 1570, 1956.

437. Robbins, J., Rall, J. E., and Rawson, R. W.: A new serum iodine component in patients with functional carcinoma of the thyroid. J. Clin. Endocr., **15,** 1315, 1955.

438. Stanbury, J. B., and Janssen, M.-A.: Labeled iodoalbumin in the plasma in thyrotoxicosis after I^{125} and I^{131}. J. Clin. Endocr., **23,** 1056, 1963.

439. Greenspan, F. S., Lowenstein, J. M., Spilker, P., and Craig, S.: Abnormal iodoprotein in nontoxic goiter. New Eng. J. Med., **269,** 830, 1963.

440. Tata, J. R., Rall, J. E., and Rawson, R. W.: Studies on an iodinated protein in the serum of subjects with cancer of the thyroid. J. Clin. Endocr., **16,** 1554, 1956.

441. Stanbury, J. B., Rocmans, P., Buhler, U. K., and Ochi, Y.: Congenital hypothyroidism with impaired thyroid response to thyrotropin. New Eng. J. Med., **279,** 1132, 1968.

442. Refetoff, S., DeWind, L. T., and DeGroot, L. J.: Familial syndrome combining deaf-mutism, stippled epiphyses, goiter and abnormally high PBI: possible target organ refractoriness to thyroid hormone. J. Clin. Endocr., **27,** 279, 1967.

443. Murray, I. P. C., Thomson, J. A., McGirr, E. M., Macdonald, E. M., Kennedy, J. S., and McLennan, I.: Unusual familial goiter associated with intrathyroidal calcification. J. Clin. Endocr., **26,** 1039, 1966.

444. Cross, H. E., Hollander, C. S., Rimoin, D. L., and McKusick, V. A.: Familial agoitrous cretinism accompanied by muscular hypertrophy. Pediatrics, **41,** 413, 1968.

445. Greig, W. R., Henderson, A. S., Boyle, J. A., McGirr, E. M., and Hutchison, J. H.: Thyroid dysgenesis in two pairs of monozygotic twins and in a mother and child. J. Clin. Endocr., **26,** 1309, 1966.

446. Jones, J. E., and Seal, U. S.: X-chromosome linked inheritance of elevated thyroxine-binding globulin. J. Clin. Endocr., **27,** 1521, 1967.

447. Nicoloff, J. T., Dowling, J. T., and Patton, D. D.: Inheritance of decreased thyroxine-binding by the thyroxine-binding globulin. J. Clin. Endocr., **24,** 294, 1964.

448. Reinwein, D.: Hormonsynthese und Enzymspektrum bei Erkrankungen der menschlichen Schildrüsse. Acta Endocr., **47,** suppl. 94, 1964.

449. Carr, E. A., Beierwaltes, W. H., Raman, G., Dodson, V. N., Tanton, J., Betts, J. S., and Stambaugh, R. A.: The effect of maternal thyroid function on fetal thyroid function and development. J. Clin. Endocr., **19,** 1, 1959.

CHAPTER ELEVEN

PHENYLKETONURIA *

W. Eugene Knox

"The study of phenylpyruvic amentia may throw light on the whole problem of mental deficiency. . . ." This statement by Jervis [1] emphasizes the major problem left to be solved in connection with phenylketonuria. This chapter aims to collect and codify the considerable knowledge of this disease in the hope that it will serve as a basis primarily for the future study of the mental defect in phenylketonuria, an endeavor which has the potential of furnishing insight into the nature and mechanism of development of the intellectual functions.

HISTORY AND DEFINITION

Garrod's recognition of the relationship between gene, enzyme, and clinical abnormality [2], 25 years before the first case of phenylketonuria was described by Følling [3], provided the conceptual basis for the disorder. Indeed phenylketonuria was the first of these inherited metabolic disorders for which the postulates of Garrod were unequivocally demonstrated.

In 1934 Følling described 10 patients, several of them sibs, who excreted phenylpyruvic acid and were mentally deficient. Jervis [1] then proved that the condition was inherited through a single autosomal recessive gene, a double dose of which produces the disease, and showed that large amounts of phenylalanine accumulated in these patients [4]. He located the metabolic error as the inability to oxidize phenylalanine to tyrosine [5]. In 1953 Jervis demonstrated that the phenylalanine hydroxylase of the liver was inactive in these patients [6]. A rational therapy, best described as an effective preventive regimen, consisting of a low-phenylalanine diet, was then developed [7, 8]. Tests for distinguishing the heterozygotes of phenylketonuria followed [9], and then an effective neonatal screening test that was broadly utilized [10]. These salient facts provide the means for understanding and controlling phenylketonuria. Many cogent reviews of this disease have appeared [11–20], as well as a classified bibliography [21]. The condition has been variously termed *imbecillitas phenylpyruvica, Følling's disease,* and *phenylpyruvic oligophrenia.* The term *phenylketonuria,* first introduced by Penrose and Quastel [22], has now been generally adopted, even though treatment may temporarily eliminate the excretion of phenylketones.

The uniform manifestations and the precision with which phenylketonuria can be identified allow it to be defined exactly. It is required that both parents of a patient have the defective form of one of the two genes controlling phenylalanine hydroxylase. An apparent reduction in phenylalanine hydroxylase activity can be detected in the parents, but there is no serious known consequence of this inadequacy. On the average, one out of four offspring from two heterozygous parents has both genes defective; in these offspring there is no active phenylalanine hydroxylase, and phenylketonuria results. Both sexes are affected equally often.

The disability is first manifested in the weeks after birth, initially by elevation of plasma phenylalanine level to 30 times normal and by the excretion of phenylpyruvic acid. After 6 months, retardation of mental development is evident. Seizures and other neurologic abnormalities, diluted pigmentation of hair and skin, and eczema may occur. In older children and adults the process remains stationary, but life expectancy is reduced. The majority of patients are idiots, a few are imbeciles, and rare patients have borderline intellectual development.

The incidence of the disease is approximately 1 in 20,000 among mixed populations stemming from Northern European countries. Most of the patients are found in institutions, where they make up about 1 percent of the mentally defective population. The disease is readily diagnosed by the olive-green color produced in the urine upon addition of $FeCl_3$. This color is due to phenylpyruvic acid.

CHARACTERISTICS

Incidence

The primary data for calculating the incidence of phenylketonuria consist of its frequency among institutionalized mentally defective individuals. Surveys of a total of 48,536 defective patients examined in 12 different countries were compiled by Jervis [12]. A total of 312 phenylketonuric patients was found, or an average incidence of 0.64 percent of the worldwide institutionalized defective population. The problems raised by these data are whether the disease is evenly distributed among peoples, and the numerical relation between the defective populations and the populations from which they are drawn. The incidence in single institutions varied from 0 percent in French Canada to 2.7 percent in England. From the figure of 0.64 percent as the incidence of phenylketonuria in the defective population, and an estimate of somewhat less than 1 percent as the incidence of defectives in the general population (estimated for the United States), Jervis calculated that the incidence of phenylketonuria in the general population was below 6 per

*This work was done under U.S. Atomic Energy Commission Contract AT(30-1)-3779 with the New England Deaconess Hospital, by Public Health Service Grant AM 00567, by Research Career Award AM-K6-2018 from the National Institute of Arthritis and Metabolic Diseases of the National Institutes of Health, and by Children's Bureau Grant CB-250 from the Department of Health, Education, and Welfare.

100,000. He accepted 4 per 100,000 as the order of the real figure. It is clear that better estimates of the incidence could be obtained only for specific populations.

Other local and independent estimates of the incidence of phenylketonuria are therefore of interest. Munro [23] calculated the incidence in England to be between 2 and 6 per 100,000. For a south Swedish region comprising nearly half the Swedish population, Larson [24] similarly calculated an incidence of 3.5 per 100,000. There were first-cousin marriages among 12.5 percent of the parents of the Swedish phenylketonuria probands. From Larson's [25] later estimate of 1.7 percent frequency of first-cousin marriages in this population, a similar incidence of phenylketonuria can be calculated.

Methods which approach complete ascertainment in localized populations have given similar figures. Armstrong and Low [26] calculated an incidence of 1 in 20,400 in Utah. They noted that all except 3 of the 18 phenylketonuric persons born in Utah and known to them were under 16 years of age. They suspected that this unusual age distribution might be due to a high death rate among phenylketonuric patients. It should be noted that Larson's [24] estimate of the incidence of phenylketonuria in Sweden included a correction for the higher mortality rate among low-grade defectives. The mass screening of all babies born in a locality as a means of case finding for early treatment will give more precise figures. The first surveys found 21 cases among a total of 215,000 infants [10, 27–29], but in some cases the diagnosis was not later confirmed. During 1967, 89 percent of the registered live births in the United States were screened, showing 222 confirmed cases of elevated phenylalanine among 3,138,000 live births, or 1 in 14,100 [30]. Surveys of half as many births during the two previous years (1966 and 1965) gave similar results that were subsequently investigated in detail [31]. About one-quarter of the cases had only smaller elevations of plasma phenylalanine ($<$1.2 mM = $<$20 mg per 100 ml), not associated with mental deficiency, and without familial association with phenylketonuria. When these cases were subtracted, 55 cases of authentic phenylketonuria were found in 1,014,024 births, an incidence of 1 in 18,500. These incidences, based on tests of millions of individuals, are so close to that estimated from mentally defective populations that there is no longer the possibility that any large number of untreated phenylketonurics with normal intelligence can exist in the population.

The survey by Jervis [12] indicated that phenylketonuria was most common in Northern European or Scandinavian countries and in populations derived from this stock. The conclusion was heavily weighted by the high proportion of surveys from such countries. Jervis noted that of all the groups represented in his United States sample of mentally defective patients, phenylketonuria was uncommon only among Jews and Negroes [32]. Surveys in Israel confirmed this rarity among the Ashkenazi ethnic group of Jews, though it occurred in the oriental (Sephardic) Jews [33]. The reported cases in American Negroes were reviewed in 1964 [34], and 3 cases were added later [35, 36], for a total of 11. This incidence is about the number expected solely from white admixture [37]. African and other populations are still unsurveyed. The disease has been found in Japan [38–40], and the expected incidence is found in Czechoslovakia [41], Hungary [42], and in Arabs and Armenians in the Middle East [43]. Two anomalous incidences are the very low one in Finland [44] and the very high one in Eire (1 in 4,000) [45]. The latter was anticipated from surveys showing a higher incidence in Celtic populations [46].

It is of interest that many more cases of phenylketonuria are known than of other comparably rare hereditary diseases. The fact that they were concentrated into institutions, and later that there was a possibility of treatment, stimulated case finding. In populations where mental defectives are not in institutions or particularly where phenylketonuric persons of normal intelligence are sought, only enormous surveys could find these rare individuals.

Age Distribution and Cause of Death

The age distributions of all sizable series of patients show deficiencies in the numbers of those under 5 years and of those over 35 years of age. The former reflects tardy diagnosis plus a period when patients may be kept at home, since the majority of reports come from institutions. The scarcity of older patients may be only the result of the higher death rate common to institutionalized persons and particularly to those who are mentally defective. The graphed age-incidence curves of phenylketonuric patients, constructed by Lang [14] from the ages of 500 reported patients, indicate that half died by 20 years of age, and three-quarters by 30 years of age. This tendency was confirmed by a survey in Czechoslovakia which found phenylketonuric persons seven times as frequently among juvenile as among adult populations of mental defectives [41]. Partington's comparisons showed no significant difference in the age distribution of phenylketonuric and other types of patients with mental defects in the same institutions, although both were deficient in older members compared with the population at large (Fig. 11-1) [47]. The ages and causes of death for 41 patients recorded before there was active experimental interest in these patients [48, 47] confirm that most deaths were of young people, who died usually with the infectious diseases common to institutionalized populations (Table 11-1). No unusual causes for these early deaths were evident, beyond those expected among severely defective individuals.

Sex

There was no difference in incidence between the sexes in the massive compilation by Jervis [12]: 237 females (51 percent) and 228 males (49 percent). The characteristics of the disease in the two sexes are not different, but there is

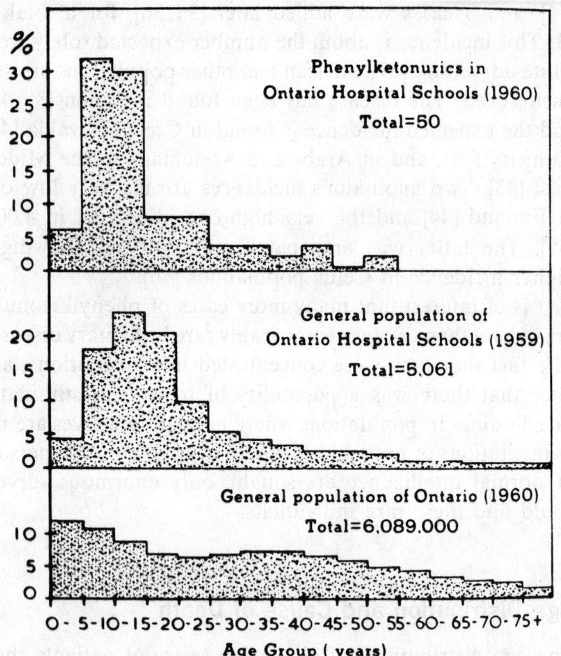

Figure 11-1. Age distribution of institutionalized phenylketonuric persons and mental defectives and of the general population in Ontario, Canada. (*By permission of M. W. Partington* [47].)

apparently a higher death rate among affected males [14, 47]. More males than females have been found with elevated phenylalanine levels by neonatal screening, but as noted above, these include some who are ultimately recognized not to have phenylketonuria [251].

Intelligence

Figure 11-2 reveals starkly the severe effect of untreated phenylketonuria on mental performance. This distribution of IQ in a total of 434 patients from two independent studies [12, 49, 51] was confirmed in another 75 patients over the age of 2 years [52]. These IQ scores for phenylketonurics, the majority of them institutionalized, fall considerably below those of the whole population in institutions for the mentally retarded [50]. This supports the general concept that cases in the population of severe retardation result mainly from pathologic processes, while the majority of cases of mild retardation represent the lower end of the normal distribution of scores for the population [53]. In human terms phenylketonuria produces mainly idiots (IQ < 50). About one-third cannot walk or control excretory sphincters and about two-thirds cannot talk.

Before complete ascertainments were available of the prevalence of phenylketonuria in populations, it was uncertain whether institutionalized patients such as those described by Fig. 11-2 were representative of phenylketonuria. Such a severe degree of retardation could result from selection. It was possible that only persons with the most severe cases of phenylketonuria were institutionalized or that significant deterioration occurred in institutions, and that a large number of phenylketonuric patients without mental defect might exist in the normal population. This would weaken the postulated association between defective phenylalanine metabolism and mental function, and weaken, as well, the evidence for the effectiveness of treatment.

However, institutionalized patients appeared to be generally representative of the disease for several reasons. Admission policies of institutions were such that they mostly admitted even less defective patients than the phenylketonuric ones (Fig. 11-2). Repeated determinations in institutionalized patients over periods as long as 29 years showed a remarkable stability of mental age [12, 20, 54, 55]. Progressive deterioration of mental age (not simply a "fall in IQ" with increased age) is so unusual in phenylketonuria as to suggest another concurrent disease process. The general shape of the IQ distribution curve, with progressively fewer

Table 11-1. CAUSES AND DECADE OF DEATH IN PHENYLKETONURIA

Decade	No. of deaths	Cause	No. of deaths
1	15	Pneumonia	14
2	9	Tuberculosis	8
3	13	Nephritis	4
4	1	Liver disease	3
5	0	Perforated ulcer	3
6	2	Septicemia	2
7	1	Carcinoma	1
		Miscellaneous, 1 each	6
Total	41	Total	41

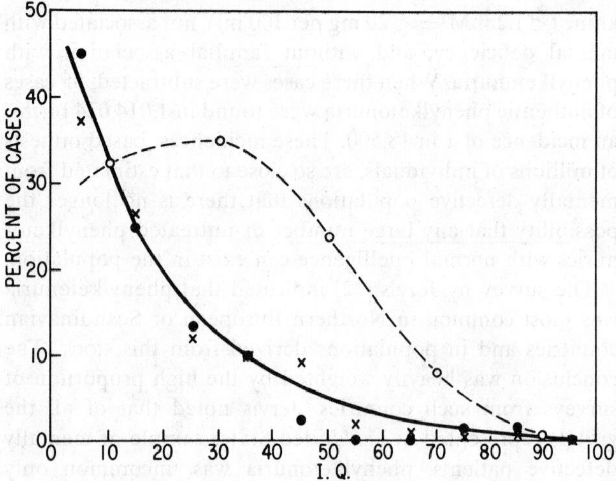

Figure 11-2. Frequency distribution of IQ scores among 330 [12] and 104 [49] patients with phenylketonuria (•, ×). The distribution for all patients in California state hospitals for the mentally retarded (approximately 12,000 in 1960 [50]) is shown for comparison (--o--).

patients at the higher levels, both relatively and in absolute numbers, has been confirmed by investigations of the frequencies in special populations. An incidence close to 1 percent among populations including the seriously retarded has been firmly established by the screening of most United States institutions. Yet only 0.57 percent were found among 5,872 "trainable" (IQ 25 to 49), and 0.13 percent among 15,240 "educable" (IQ 50 to 70) school children in California [56]. The relatively low latter incidence among the mildly retarded was established earlier when only 0.07 percent of phenylketonurics was found among a total of 5,493 morons tested in Sweden, Germany, and England [24, 57, 58]. Enormous surveys of intellectually normal populations [12, 59], most of them as yet unpublished, have failed to reveal any cases of phenylketonuria. They do exist, but they are rare. In the earlier editions of this book figures on these patients were tabulated from published reports up to 1963. They numbered 30 with IQs above 60. This total necessarily included those with lower phenylalanine levels than are now accepted as typical for the disease. The number decreased progressively at the higher IQ levels, clearly so if those with the milder chemical abnormality were omitted, as predicted by the curve in Fig. 11-2. Assuming that the reportage of these unusual patients with mild phenylketonuria was at least as complete as that of the usual kind of phenylketonuric patient, it appeared that they comprised only a tiny fraction of the total. Subsequently, additional cases have continued to be reported at about the expected rate for this rare variety. They constitute merely the statistical extreme of the distribution curve of IQ in this disease. They would nevertheless be of great interest if they could reveal which factors ameliorate the usual disease effects. Further study of such cases is complicated because recent surveys have included patients without typical phenylketonuria who cannot be clearly distinguished by the data provided.

Clinical Features

Development

There is almost universal agreement that the infant with phenylketonuria is not clinically abnormal at birth. Even later, the signs and symptoms are not sufficiently characteristic to make an unaided specific clinical diagnosis. The first patients were recognized because the mother complained of their musty odor [60], now known to be referable to the phenylacetic acid in the excretions of these patients and associated with the "hyperhidrosis" often described. In addition, the mother of five phenylketonuric children is reported to have diagnosed the condition in the fourth when it was still at an early age [61]. Partington found a history of vomiting in early life in nearly half of his 36 patients, 4 of whom were operated on for pyloric stenosis [62]. Kang et al. [63] were impressed with the number of obstetric complications among mothers of their patients. Saugstad made similar observations in Oslo [64]. But in the main there are no consistent neonatal abnormalities for the first month or two, after which the usual developmental milestones are often delayed. These delays are progressively prolonged, so that at the latest ages that the performance could normally be expected, 35 percent could not walk and 63 percent could not talk. Independent locomotion may cease, as well as efforts to talk. In the latter half of the first year convulsions may supervene, along with the other features described later for the full-blown disease picture.

The transformation of an apparently normal baby into a severely defective one during the first year or so of life is the most striking clinical characteristic of the disease. It is borne out repeatedly by longitudinal reports on the same individual in numerous case studies. Quantitative information about the rate and extent of this change is needed. Bickel and Bremer presented an idealized diagram of this change: a precipitous loss of IQ during the first year and more gradual losses thereafter [65]. Enough actual data have now accumulated to permit construction of such an average curve. There is resistance, usually for irrelevant reasons, to such use of developmental (DQ) or intelligence (IQ) quotients to score the performance of these infants. The early tests depend largely on motor behavior, instead of relying on cognition, as later tests do. They are not precise or reproducible enough to predict the same subtle differences among normal or superior children that can be found in such a group by later tests [66]. Infant tests do, however, correlate well with later tests when significant differences from normal are involved. The more abnormal the infant, the higher the correlation with later tests [67, 68]. Early test performances are also familiar, objective, and readily scaled measures, in part of neurologic integrity, that are clinically useful even to pediatricians, who can make their own remarkably accurate appraisals [69]. Early test results, therefore, offer a way to quantify the transformation that occurs in phenylketonuria during early life.

The earliest test results in a significant number of patients in relation to age were collected and graphed in Fig. 11-3. The data show an even more dramatic transformation than expected. Though based on cross-sectional studies (i.e., studies of different patients at each age) by different investigators and with different means of ascertainment, there is notable agreement. The variance is constant throughout the range of age. Average quotients decline precipitously and almost linearly for the first 10 months, then very slowly until the third year, and show no significant loss thereafter. The whole curve, as well as that of the mental age on which it is based, does not fit a simple formula. If there is an initial flat period before the precipitous fall, it lasts no more than a month. The test results used were referred to the sometimes earlier age when treatment was begun. Only if scores continued to fall while the patient was receiving treatment, which is not generally observed, would the actual curve be somewhat less steep than that shown. A curve for 70 patients with the same shape was presented by Koch et al. [79]. These results, then, provide an objective basis for more precise analysis of the disease process, and for evaluation of treatment effects.

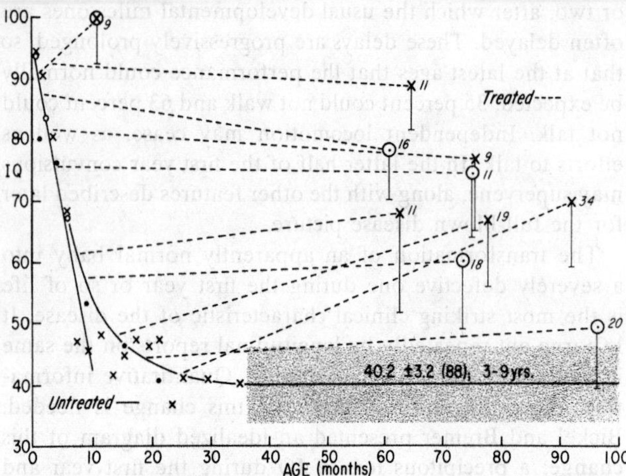

Figure 11-3. Loss of IQ with age in 392 untreated phenylketonuric patients (—) and preservation of IQ in 158 patients treated with a low-phenylalanine diet (---). Points represent mean IQ and age of more than six patients of similar ages who were grouped together. The ages of untreated patients are the earlier ones, either at the first IQ test or at start of treatment. Some groups were assessed by a single psychologist (● [70]), and some were ascertained from affected sibs (o [71]) or by neonatal screening and medical complaints (× [1, 54, 72–83]). There was no further change in average IQ with age in the 88 patients 36 to 108 months of age. These are represented by the mean line with shading 2 s.e. above and below it. The straight line from 0 to 10 months was drawn by least squares through values for 144 individuals. Its equation is IQ (est.) = 94.7 − 5.24 months, with a standard error of estimate of ±18.67, and $r = -0.680$.

Treated patients were taken from sizable series including only individuals treated for 3 years or more except in one group (⊗). They were grouped according to the age at start of treatment (mean starting age in at left origin of dashed line), and the final mean IQ and age are plotted at the right (⊗, ⊙, ×). The number of patients and a bracket extending 2 s.e. below its mean are shown for each group. The short-treatment group was thoroughly evaluated at one institution (⊗ [35]); others were evaluated by a collaborative study (× [84]). The remaining groups were compiled from several series (⊙ [52, 74, 77, 85–89]).

Apart from the central nervous system, developmental abnormalities have been reported only of the skin (eczema), teeth, and bones. The latter includes microcephaly, found in over half the cases [49]. Head circumference averages nearly 2 cm smaller than normal [90]; microcephaly is more marked in low-grade patients. Prominent maxillae, with consequent widening of the interdental spaces, have also been described [20, 91, 92]. In about half the patients of some series, beginning in infancy calcified spicules extended from the long bones into the cartilage, persisting later as dense, vertical striations into the diaphysis [93]. In other series these changes were not seen [94]. It is attractive to associate the abnormalities of skin, teeth, and brain, since all are of ectodermal origin. At least the latter two also undergo postnatal development simultaneously. It was confirmed that enamel hypoplasia [72] is significantly more common in phenylketonuric persons (60 percent) than i those with other types of mental deficiency [95]. There wa however, no difference in the incidence of malocclusion. I other respects, physical development is entirely normal ex cept for a tendency toward smallness [49], which may b secondary to the effect of retardation on food intake.

Appearance

Useful and independent clinical descriptions are provide by the reports of 50 cases by Jervis [32], 41 by Følling, Moh and Ruud [11], 15 by Cowie [96], 21 by Wright and Tarja [20], 106 by Paine [49], and 12 by Kratter [55]. I have use these as well as those in my own experience as the bas for evaluating smaller series or single cases. A tabulatio of findings is given in Table 11-2.

SKIN LESIONS. "Eczema," usually beginning in infancy occurred in 19 percent of Paine's cases [49]. In the majorit it persisted to adolescence or adulthood. The incidence wa 34 percent in Knox's survey of 104 published cases. I one-third the eczema was said to be severe, and one patier died with generalized eczema. It is sometimes the presentin medical complaint [77].

A dry or rough skin was often noted. Some of these ski manifestations can be attributed to unhygienic condition and to a light and sensitive skin. Følling et al. [11] empha sized the frequency of the same affections in normal ind viduals. The first published dermatologic study [97] demon strated that phenylketonuric skin was normally tanned b

Table 11-2. MAJOR CLINICAL FINDINGS IN PHENYLKETONURIA*

Finding	Incidence, percent	Occurrence in low-grade patients
Agitated behavior	90–32	+
EEG abnormalities	80	−†
Muscular hypertonicity	75	+
Microcephaly	68	+
Hyperactive reflexes	66	+
Blond hair, blue eyes	62	−
Inability to talk	63	+
Hyperkinesis	50	+
Inability to walk (and usually incontinence)	35	+
Tremors	30	+
Eczema	19–34	−
Seizures	26	+

*Percentages of incidences are approximately those reported i the major series, adjusted for redefinition of signs as given in tex Those findings occurring more frequently or severely in the low grade patients are marked +.

†The incidence of EEG abnormalities is not different in high- an low-grade patients, but the latter may have more obviously ab normal tracings.

the sun and was not abnormally sensitive to sunlight. Later studies suggest that eczema has been overemphasized as a sign of phenylketonuria [98, 62].

A large number of rare associated conditions have been described, each in one or a few cases. Among these are scleroderma in several cases [99].

PIGMENTATION. Deficient pigmentation with blond hair and blue eyes is characteristic of phenylketonuria, but the coloration is not abnormal in type and was not noted in Følling's original description from Oslo, where most individuals have a similar coloration. In Paine's cases from the Northeastern United States, 64 percent had blue eyes and 17 percent brown eyes. Sixty percent had blond hair, and the remainder had light brown or brown [49]. Berg and Stern [100] demonstrated a significantly lighter iris color in 26 phenylketonuric mentally defective patients than in controls, and lighter irides in 12 phenylketonuric patients than in 23 of their unaffected sibs. There was no relation to IQ. The dilution of hair color in phenylketonuric patients compared with their unaffected relatives has been demonstrated by reflecting spectrophotometry [96]. Striking instances of blond phenylketonuric patients in darkly pigmented families of Sicilian [1] or Spanish [101] origin have been reported. Other striking cases are mulattos, less pigmented than their parents and with sandy-blond hair and blue eyes but negroid fundi [36, 102]. Phenylketonuric Japanese patients have brown hair [38, 40]. The correct generalization is that each patient has a relatively lighter complexion than other members of his family. The normally pigmented areas of the brain, such as the substantia nigra and locus ceruleus, may lack pigmentation [103, 104].

Nervous System

The vast majority of patients show a series of typical neurologic changes which run parallel to the degree of mental defect and in general are worse in severely defective individuals. Traces of the same abnormalities are evident in the high-grade patients.

EPILEPSY. A history of convulsive seizures appears in 26 percent of Paine's series plus the 418 cases reported by Jervis [12, 49]. Seizures usually began between 6 and 18 months of age [77], and stopped spontaneously before adulthood. The incidence of seizures was higher and the attacks were more severe in the severely defective patients. Recurrent episodes of staring or inattentiveness after 6 months of age are very frequently recorded. The incidence of these petit mal attacks plus overt convulsions gives an overall incidence of abnormal cerebral activity which is probably over 50 percent. The epilepsy may be resistant to the usual therapy as well as to treatment with a low-phenylalanine diet [20, 64]. This incidence is not necessarily higher than in other types of mental retardation [15].

ELECTROENCEPHALOGRAM. The majority of phenylketonuric patients have abnormal EEG patterns regardless of whether they have had seizures. The incidence is approximately the same with low- or high-grade defective patients. Paine [49] found 78 percent abnormal recordings in 33 cases (75 percent were abnormal in 24 of these patients who had never had seizures). Fois, Rosenberg, and Gibbs [105] reported 95 percent abnormal tracings in 19 patients. Their investigation included the technique of sleep recording, by means of which disorders of this type are best seen. The abnormalities consist of spike and wave complexes, dysarrhythmia, and the "petit mal variant" type (even in some individuals without epilepsy). The most common finding is a mixture of high-voltage fast and slow waves occurring more irregularly than in petit mal. Fois et al. likened the disorganized sleep patterns to those seen in hydrocephalus with injury to the thalamus or hypothalamus. These abnormalities are not pathognomonic, but they do suggest deep midline brain damage. High-grade phenylketonuric patients also have abnormal EEGs [106] which can be intensified by phenylalanine [107].

BEHAVIOR. The statement of Wright and Tarjan [20] is most apt: "None could be described as friendly, placid or happy." Apart from the completely helpless, bedridden idiots, they are restless, jerky, and fearful individuals. Their behavior ranges from that of the shy, anxious, and restless high-grade patient to the destructive and noisy psychotic episodes observed in 10 percent of the patients. Night terrors beset the higher-grade patients. Uncontrollable temper tantrums are common (32 percent in Paine's series). The hyperactivity, irritability, and uncontrollable temper are the usual reasons given for admitting these patients to institutions. These characteristics in high-grade patients may provide the indication for therapy [108].

Profile ratings by teachers of school behavior disclosed that phenylketonuric children (mildly retarded after treatment) were significantly more clumsy and awkward, more talkative, and more hypersensitive than matched controls [88]. Explicit tests of manual dexterity showed that only those on a normal diet performed significantly more poorly than controls [85]. A "pithicoid" stance is sometimes seen, and in severely defective patients a "tailorwise" sitting position, or *Schneidersitz* [91], is typical (Fig. 11-4).

MUSCULAR HYPERTONICITY. Jervis found increased muscle tone in 70 percent of patients, and Wright and Tarjan in 76 percent. The patients seem always ready to jump. This unrelaxed attitude may be responsible for the awkward or even rigid, short-stepped gait with few associative movements that is seen in 20 percent of the low-grade group. Approximately 20 percent are described as having hypotonic muscle tone. Jervis also described cog-wheel rigidity. This finding is particularly difficult to evaluate in these patients.

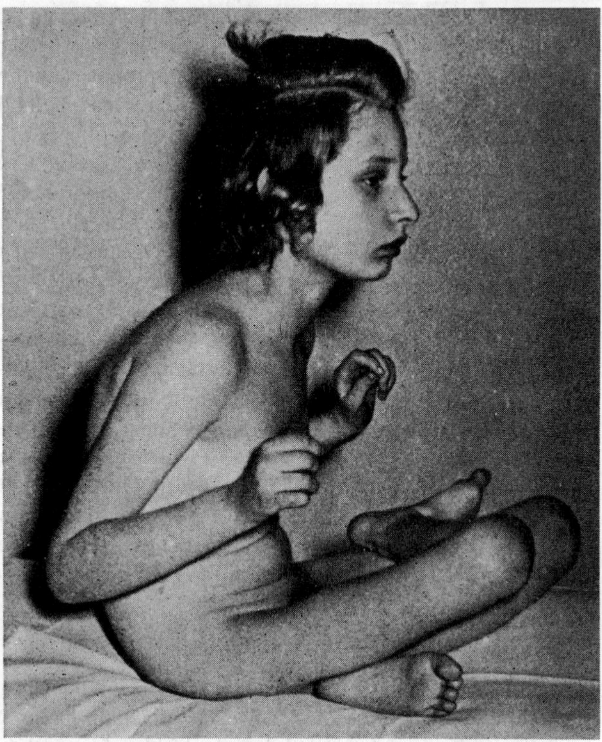

Figure 11-4. The characteristic "Schneidersitz" of severely defective phenylketonuria patients. (*By permission of K. Lang* [14]). Incessant rhythmic motions complete the usual picture [91].

HYPERACTIVE TENDON REFLEXES. Two-thirds of all patients show abnormally brisk tendon reflexes, and in a sizable fraction ankle and patellar clonus can be elicited. Clonus persists continuously in some patients. Half of a group of patients had lowered stimulus thresholds with persistence of infantile reflex patterns like those seen in congenital lesions of the descending tracts [109].

ADVENTITIOUS HYPERKINESIS. A great variety of abnormal body movements has been described. Each patient has his own favored motions out of the infinite variety possible. The important point is his restless movement. There are voluntary, purposeless, and repetitive motions of the whole or a part of the body. There may be inconspicuous fiddling movements of the fingers or violent body swinging which continues for hours. The persistent ankle clonus may be of this type. Each patient has a limited repertoire of these movements, but if one motion is suppressed, others occur. They contribute a great deal to the picture of behavioral unrest and agitation. Because of their combination with muscular rigidity, they are often described as choreiform or athetoid.

TREMORS. A fine, rapid, and irregular tremor of the outstretched hands was seen in 30 percent of Paine's series. It may become stronger on volition, and may spread to other parts of the body. Together with increased tendon reflexes and jerky rigidity, it is one of the reasons for suspecting extrapyramidal disease in these patients, even though true spasticity may not be present.

OTHER NEUROLOGIC FINDINGS. A small percentage of phenylketonuric patients has signs of severe brain disease in association with severe mental defect. These are the patients described by Jervis [32] as the 4 percent with "stationary severe cerebral-palsy with diplegia, contractures and pyramidal signs" and by Paine [49] as 5 percent with spastic para- or tetraplegia. There are rare reports of positive Babinski or Hoffman signs [38, 96]. The relationship of these findings to phenylketonuria is not clear. The patients may have other concurrent diseases, or the signs may represent the ultimate degree of cerebral defect caused by phenylketonuria. The latter possibility is supported by the occurrence of leukodystrophy in several patients [103].

PNEUMOENCEPHALOGRAPHS. Pneumoencephalographs of patients have shown evidence of diffuse cortical atrophy [32, 110].

Pathologic Findings

No relevant pathologic changes occur outside the central nervous system in phenylketonuria. Until recently, the changes in the central nervous system which had been observed did not account for the mental deficiency. About 25 cases have been examined, and the findings collected [48, 111]. One frequent finding was that the weight of the brains was about two-thirds of normal.

In some of the patients, especially the youngest, a deficient myelination was observed [112, 113], but not in others. Nevertheless, on review, defective myelination could be suggested as the underlying process [48], and this has now been established. Poser and Van Bogaert [114] described the widespread deficient myelination with secondary fibrillary gliosis in the brain of their 18-year-old patient and mobilized the evidence in favor of a pathogenetic mechanism involving "dysmyelination" in the early years of life, with secondary gliosis, and ultimate formation of a small, atrophic, but superficially normal-appearing brain. Substantially the same findings were made by Crome and Pare [111]. They found microencephaly, fibrous gliosis of the white matter, and, in two of their four young patients, pallor of myelin staining. Chemical analysis for the galactocerebroside components by Crome, Tymms, and Woolf [115] revealed the deficient myelination more clearly than did the density of staining under a light microscope (Fig. 11-5). The picture emerging is one of nonspecific alterations in white matter progressing in severity with age to active diffuse or focal demyelination accompanied by intense gliosis and myelin breakdown products (sudanophilic lipids) [116, 117].

It is a major but limited advance to establish that there are pathologic changes in the brains of patients with phenylketonuria. Brain changes must be closely related to the

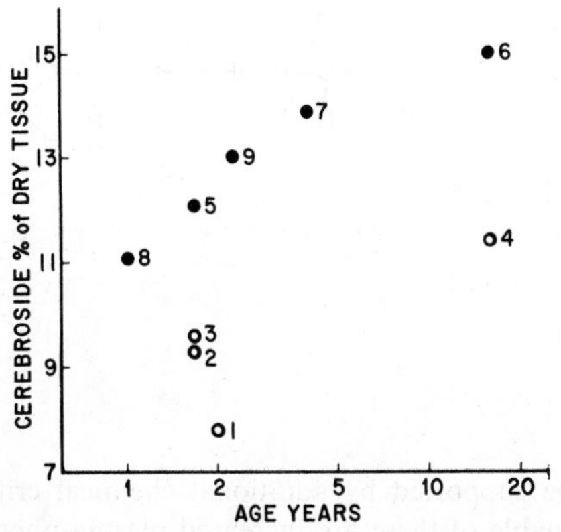

Figure 11-5. Cerebroside content of white matter plotted against age (log scale) of normal controls (•) and phenylketonuric subjects (o). (*By permission of L. Crome et al.* [115].)

functional defects of the brain. These mental defects develop appropriately in the first years of life when myelination is also occurring. But myelination is a complex process of the glial cell–myelin sheath system, involving stepwise elaboration of several complex lipids and their lamination in lipoprotein layers about the nerves [118]. It is premature to suggest how phenylalanine excess can derange this process. While the primary abnormality of the brain is defective myelin *formation* and not the more familiar demyelination, the latter has also been recognized (Schilder's disease) in 4 young adults among the first 26 patients autopsied [103]. Not only may the myelin formation in phenylketonuria be deficient, but also the myelin itself may be defective, so that it ultimately breaks down. The significant structural abnormalities, nevertheless, must occur contemporaneously with the onset of functional defect in the first 10 months of life (Fig. 11-3). They are sufficiently subtle to require chemical rather than histologic recognition. Indications point to anomalies of cerebral lipids, particularly of the proteolipids [117, 119, 120].

BIOCHEMICAL ABNORMALITIES

The normal oxidation of L-phenylalanine to tyrosine in the liver is almost completely stopped in phenylketonuria. The evidence is quite complete that hereditary inactivity of the enzyme for this reaction, phenylalanine hydroxylase, is the primary phenotypic lesion in this disease. The failure to convert the essential amino acid phenylalanine to tyrosine causes directly and indirectly a host of biochemical, physiologic, and pathologic repercussions.

Not only is there accumulation of the phenylalanine, which is constantly fed into the organism by the diet and which must seek the other avenues of removal (and a relative deficiency of tyrosine, which becomes an essential dietary amino acid), but a variety of intracellular systems are called upon to adjust their function to this new metabolic state. The renal tubular transport system, which normally reabsorbs relatively small amounts of phenylalanine, is faced with the reabsorption of amounts approaching its maximum transfer capacity. Amino acids that are normally concentrated in cells for purposes of growth and metabolism must continue to be taken up in appropriate amounts despite the high concentration of phenylalanine seeking entry. Each amino acid residue must continue to be incorporated accurately into the myriad proteins synthesized by the cells regardless of the distorted pattern of free amino acids in the intracellular pool. It is remarkable indeed that so few of the functions of the body are seriously impaired in phenylketonuria. The relative lack of damage indicates that all processes but one are intact, and that biologic processes have great adaptability for meeting new conditions.

Preliminary Considerations

The metabolic flow of phenylalanine and tyrosine appears in Fig. 11-6. The amino acids are continuously supplied from the diet and are incorporated into the body protein of the different cells. Phenylalanine is also oxidized in the liver to tyrosine. The reverse reaction does not occur.

Tyrosine undergoes further reactions in various specialized tissues. The largest dissimulative reaction of tyrosine occurs in the liver; there is a small reaction in the kidney. This is oxidative ring fission to components of the citric acid cycle. In this way tyrosine is eliminated as an aromatic compound. The amount of tyrosine handled in other ways is very much smaller, though no exact quantitative comparisons can be made. These smaller amounts of tyrosine are metabolized

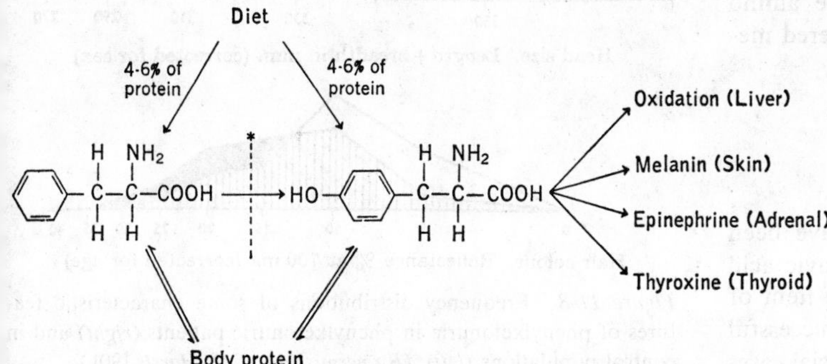

Figure 11-6. Normal metabolic flow of phenylalanine and tyrosine and the location of the reaction blocked in phenylketonuria (∗).

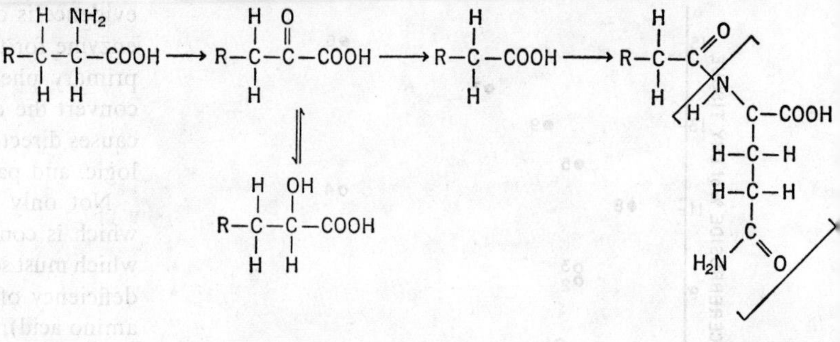

Figure 11-7. A common nonspecific pathway of amino acid degradation through keto and lactic acids, acetic acids, and conjugates of the latter. Such secondary pathways account for many of the metabolites in phenylketonuria.

in specialized organs such as the skin, adrenal glands, and thyroid.

D-Phenylalanine Metabolism

The unnatural form of phenylalanine, like most other D-amino acids, is oxidatively deaminated by D-amino acid oxidase. This reaction forms phenylpyruvic acid, which is identical with the typical metabolite of phenylketonuria. This has been known since the early work of Kotake, Masai, and Mori [121]. However, Følling found only L-phenylalanine in blood and urine in phenylketonuria, and this was confirmed by the microbiologic assays of Prescott et al. [122]. This route of phenylpyruvic acid formation may confuse experiments when DL-phenylalanine is used, but it is otherwise unrelated to the reactions primarily involved here.

The Common Pathway of Amino Acid Metabolism

Nearly every amino acid has a highly individual pathway by which it is metabolized. Since most amino acids also participate in oxidative deaminations by the L- or D-amino acid oxidases, and in transaminations to the α-keto acids, there is also potentially a common pathway of degradation through the keto acids to the next lower carboxylic acids, as shown in Fig. 11-7. The major metabolites found in phenylketonuria find representation in such sequences of reactions [13]. Thus the parent amino acid, phenylalanine, gives rise to phenylpyruvate, phenyllactate, phenylacetate, and the glutamine conjugate of phenylacetate. Because the excess phenylalanine in some way disturbs the metabolism of tryptophan and tryosine, small amounts of some of the analogous derivatives of these amino acids are also excreted in phenylketonuria. Inhibited absorption of these amino acids in the intestine accounts mainly for their altered metabolism [123, 124].

Biochemical Diagnostic Criteria and Methods

The vast majority of phenylketonuric patients have been recognized solely by their excretion of phenylpyruvic acid as identified by the simple $FeCl_3$ test. This single item of qualitative information has been extraordinarily successful in distinguishing phenylketonuria. Diagnosis of crucial cases should be supported by additional chemical criteria. The most valuable of these are increased plasma phenylalanine concentration and the excretion of *o*-hydroxyphenylacetic acid.

The need for complete reliance upon chemical criteria for the diagnosis of phenylketonuria can be seen from the frequency distribution of certain characteristics of phenylketonuria measured in normal and phenylketonuric populations (Fig. 11-8). Only the biochemical criterion furnishes absolute discrimination between normal and phenylketonuric persons, even though the two populations differ significantly with respect to certain of the overlapping characteristics.

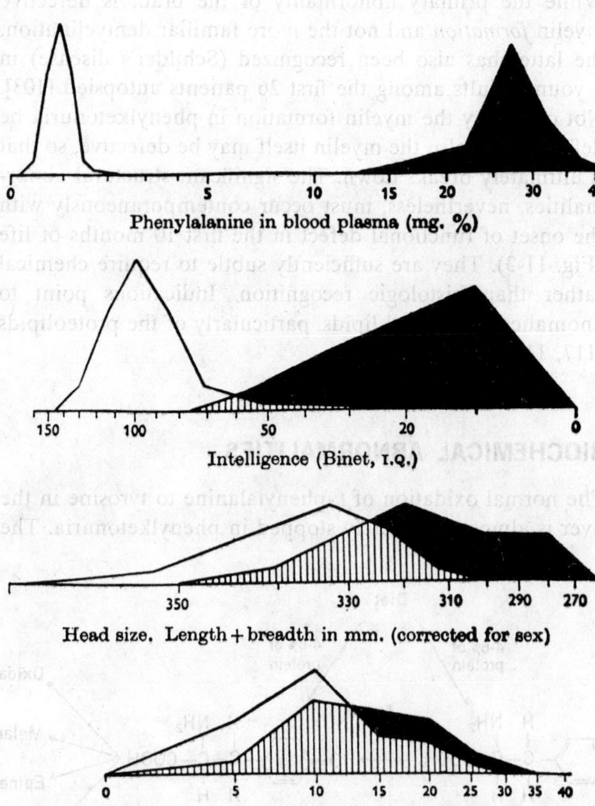

Figure 11-8. Frequency distributions of some characteristic features of phenylketonuria in phenylketonuric patients (*right*) and in control populations (*left*). (*By permission of H. Harris* [90].)

The $FeCl_3$ test: The addition of several drops of 5 percent $FeCl_3$ to 5 ml fresh urine first produces some precipitation of phosphates; then as more is added to positive specimens, there appears, after 2 or 3 min, an olive-green color which fades slowly over the next hour or two. Acidification is not necessary.

The test is sometimes negative in phenylketonuria when the urinary concentration of phenylpyruvic acid is less than 0.2 mg per ml. This occurs in very dilute urines, in rare individuals with low phenylpyruvic acid output, with low protein intake, or in day-old urine after the relatively labile phenylpyruvic acid has decomposed. Gibbs and Woolf [29] give 0.05 mg per ml as the limit of detection with ferric chloride. The color results from the chelation of Fe^{3+} with the enol group of the phenylpyruvic acid. The analogous reaction of Fe^{3+} with acetoacetic acid is used as a standard clinical test. Acetoacetic acid and salicylic acid give distinctive colors in this test that are not confused with the typical green reaction of phenylpyruvic acid. A green color similar to that given by phenylpyruvic acid occurs with a metabolite of chlorpromazine [125], and at times in urines containing bile, or in urine of patients with histidinemia. Ephemeral green colors caused by *p*-hydroxyphenylpyruvate were found in urines of 7 out of 1,141 infants screened by Gibbs and Woolf [29]. The presence of phenylpyruvic acid is confirmed by extracting it from acid solution with ether and repeating the $FeCl_3$ test [126] or by forming the insoluble 2,4-dinitrophenylhydrazone [22]. Both tests can be used for quantitative determinations. Conditions for increasing the sensitivity of the ferric chloride test were described by Saifer and Harris [127]. Stabilized ferric test papers (Phenistix, Ames Co.) are available which are sensitive and convenient for qualitative tests [128].

Characteristic Metabolites

There are no abnormal metabolites in phenylketonuria, only normal metabolites in abnormal amounts. Følling [3] isolated and identified phenylpyruvic acid as part of the original description of the disease. Later [129] he found elevated amounts of L-phenylalanine and probably phenyllactic acid in urine, and L-phenylalanine in serum. The true significance of the elevated plasma phenylalanine, indicating a block in the metabolism of the phenylalanine itself, became clear with the confirmation of the high phenylalanine levels by Jervis, Block, Bolling, and Kanze [4]. Jervis [5] then demonstrated the block by showing that no rise in blood tyrosine level occurs in the plasma of phenylketonuric patients after a dose of phenylalanine. It then became clear that phenylalanine is the primary metabolite which accumulates and that the other metabolites are derivatives of it. Later other compounds (derivatives of tyrosine and tryptophan) were recognized as arising secondarily from separate metabolic reactions. The compounds now known to be present in abnormal amounts are described below and listed in Tables 11-3 and 11-4.

PHENYLALANINE. Probably the most accurate plasma phenylalanine concentrations are those determined by column chromatography, which gives the lowest values of the several methods. Slightly higher values are obtained with the specific enzyme decarboxylase method, and still higher ones with the microbiologic and paper-chromatographic methods. The method of choice for sensitivity and simplicity is the fluorimetric procedure of McCaman and Robins [138]. Accepted normal values are under 0.1 μmole per ml (1.65 mg per 100 ml). Blood concentrations are expressed preferably as millimolarity (1 mM = 1 μmole per ml) instead of milligrams per 100 ml. Much higher concentrations in normal persons are given by the Kapeller-Adler chemical method (0.18 to 0.30 μmoles per ml or 3 to 5 mg per 100 ml), which has frequently been used to measure the high levels found in phenylketonuric patients [153]. It is not recommended for the lower normal values [154, 155].

Plasma phenylalanine concentrations in heterozygotes of phenylketonuria are definitely higher than those in normal persons as determined by the same method, but the difference is small and demonstrable only with the most precise methods of analysis.

Higher phenylalanine values were found in phenylketonuric children under 2 years of age, as is shown in Table 11-3.

The phenylalanine level in cerebrospinal fluid is approximately one-fourth that in the plasma, and the level in sweat is still lower.

PHENYLPYRUVIC ACID. Jervis [143] was able to measure phenylpyruvic acid in the plasma of phenylketonuric patients, but he was unable to detect it in normal plasma. The low concentration in plasma is referable to renal excretion, which may occur in part by active tubular secretion. The evidence for this is that probenecid, an inhibitor of renal transport, decreased the renal excretion of phenylpyruvic acid by one-half and simultaneously increased the blood level of this compound [143]. The compound may also be actively secreted by the skin, since the concentration of phenylpyruvic acid in sweat is substantially higher than in plasma.

OTHER COMPOUNDS IN BLOOD: PHARMACODYNAMIC AMINES. Most of the other metabolites formed in abnormal amounts by phenylketonuric patients have been detected only in urine. Mention should be made of the pharmacologically active substances which occur in concentrations an order of magnitude lower than those described. These include 5-hydroxytryptamine, which is lower than normal in the plasma in phenylketonuria [144], epinephrine, which is lower than normal in the plasma of all mental defectives [156], and the still hypothetic intermediate, *o*-tyramine. The last, a probable precursor of *o*-hydroxyphenylacetic acid [157], can be formed from *o*-tyrosine and concentrated in brain

Table 11-3. BLOOD CONCENTRATIONS OF METABOLITES

Metabolite	No. of patients	Mean ± s.d., μmoles/ml	Range, μmoles/ml	Method	Reference
Phenylalanine:					
Normal:					
Plasma	14	0.051	0.040–0.064	Column chromatography	[130] [131] [132]
Plasma	10	0.054 ± 0.003	0.042–0.074	Column chromatography	[133]
Plasma	106	0.078 ± 0.015	0.040–0.115	Enzyme	[134]
Plasma	17	0.058 ± 0.003 (s.e.)	0.036–0.079	Microbiology	[122]
		0.084 ± 0.019		Microbiology	[135]
Plasma	17	0.120 ± 0.024	0.067–0.240	Microbiology	[136]
Plasma	10	0.097 ± 0.036	0.061–0.151	Paper chromatography	[137]
Plasma	19 (infants)	0.090 ± 0.008 (s.e.)	. . . .	Fluorimetry	[138]
Heterozygote:					
Plasma	22	0.103 ± 0.016	0.075–0.205	Enzyme	[134]
Plasma	10	0.151 ± 0.054	0.085–0.254	Paper chromatography	[137]
Phenylketonuric:					
Plasma (serum)	1	1.42	. . . .	Column chromatography	[132]
Plasma	14	1.52 ± 0.23	1.18–1.96	Column chromatography	[133]
	18	1.68	1.15–2.12	Microbiology	[139]
Plasma	34	1.78	1.03–2.81	Enzyme	[51]
Plasma	12 (<11 mos)	3.26 ± 0.85	. . . .	Enzyme	[140]
Plasma	62 (>1 yr)	1.83 ± 0.36	. . . .	Enzyme	[140]
Plasma (serum)	12 (<2 yr)	4.05	2.18–6.00	Kapeller-Adler	[26]
Plasma (serum)	24 (>2 yr)	2.48	1.33–3.21	Adler	[26]
Plasma (serum)	18 (all ages)	2.54	1.33–3.82	Adler	[141]
Plasma	6	2.01 ± 0.16		Fluorimetry	[138]
Spinal fluid	9	0.44	0.37–0.50	Microbiology	[139]
Sweat	10	0.20	0.085–0.108	Microbiology	[142]
Phenylpyruvic acid:					
Phenylketonuric:					
Plasma	39	0.043 ± 0.015	0.019–0.108	$FeCl_3$ extract	[143]
Sweat	10	1.55	0.36–3.40	Phenylhydrazone	[142]
5-Hydroxytryptamine (serum)					
Other mental deficiency	32	283 mμg/ml	77–608	Uterus assay	[144]
Phenylketonuric	49	71.2 mμg/ml	8–120	Uterus assay	[144]

and to a lesser extent in liver. Though no amines could be detected in the cerebrospinal fluid of phenylketonuric patients given an inhibitor of monamine oxidase [158], significant amounts of phenylethylamine were formed and excreted under these conditions by phenylketonuric subjects but not by normal individuals [159].

Quantities of Urinary Metabolites

Many of the values recorded in the literature for the metabolites excreted in abnormal amounts in phenylketonuria are not useful. There is great difficulty in collecting all urine for a given period from these patients. There is also uncertainty about body size and protein intake of the patients in many reports. In Table 11-4, only the urinary excretion values which give a basis for comparison, such as the urinary nitrogen or creatinine have been included.

PHENYLPYRUVIC ACID. The phenylpyruvic acid excretions recorded by Jervis [142] have been expressed per 15 gm urinary nitrogen to approximate the daily output of an adult. The remarkable constancy within this group, which included children as well as adults, shows that phenylpyruvic acid excretion in these patients is largely a function of protein intake. The larger variation seen in the series of Armstrong and Low [26], which is expressed as per gram creatinine,

Table 11-4. AMOUNTS OF URINARY METABOLITES IN PHENYLKETONURIA

Compound*	No.	Mean	Range	Reference
Phenylpyruvic acid	20	2.13	1.68–2.72 gm/15 gm N	[142]
	27	2.27	0.8–5.6 gm/gm creatinine	[26]
Phenyllactic acid	20	0.95	0.60–1.35 gm/15 gm N	[142]
Phenylalanine	20	0.45	0.30–0.75 gm/15 gm N	[142]
Phenylalanine	25	0.45	Gm/gm creatinine	[145]
N-Acetylphenylalanine	18	0.054	0.016–0.140 gm/gm creatinine	[146]
o-Hydroxyphenylacetic acid	12	0.22	0.10–0.40 gm/gm creatinine	[147]
Indolepyruvic acid	3	.....	0.11–0.17 gm/day (normals, average = 0.042 gm/day)	[148]
Indolelactic acid	15	.....	0.02–0.15 gm/gm creatinine	[149]
Indoleacetic acid	..	.....	Amount uncertain	
Indican	10	0.244	0.090 gm/gm creatinine	[150]
5-Hydroxyindoleacetic acid:				
Other mental deficiency	32	7.2	1.6–8.0 mg/gm creatinine	[144]
Phenylketonuria	49	2.2	1.6–3.6 mg/gm creatinine	[144]
Phenylacetylglutamine	6	.....	0.30–2.4 gm/day	See text
Phenylacetic acid	..	.....	Amount uncertain	[151]
p-Hydroxyphenyllactic acid	..	.....	Traces reported	[152]

*Other compounds, for which data are not available: *p*-hydroxyphenylpyruvic acid and *p*-hydroxyphenylacetic acid.

may be the result of varying protein intakes. Creatinine excretion reflects body size but not intake, although the two are roughly parallel under usual circumstances. One patient, who excreted only 0.3 gm phenylpyruvic acid per gm creatinine and who was a high-grade defective (Case C. W. [160]), has been omitted from the second series in Table 11-4.

PHENYLLACTIC ACID. Zeller [161] isolated and identified phenyllactic acid from phenylketonuric urine. Few measurements have been reported, but it is excreted in quantities intermediate between those of phenylpyruvic acid and phenylalanine.

PHENYLALANINE. Normally phenylalanine is excreted in amounts of 10 to 15 mg per gm creatinine, as determined by column chromatography [162], although children under 1 year excrete several times as much of this. It can be a sensitive indicator of the blood level if careful measurements are made, since the excretion is greatly elevated in phenylketonuria [145]. A significant fraction is excreted in acetylated form [146], and about 5 percent after fission of benzoic acid is excreted as hippuric acid [163].

o-HYDROXYPHENYLACETIC ACID. Armstrong, Shaw, and Robinson [147] discovered this unexpected metabolite of phenylalanine in phenylketonuric urine. Amounts less than 1 mg per day are normally excreted. The excretion of a high-grade patient (Case C. W. [160]) was the lowest in the series of measurements used for Table 11-4 (0.08 gm per gm) and has been omitted.

INDOLEPYRUVIC, INDOLELACTIC, AND INDOLEACETIC ACIDS. Indolelactic and indoleacetic acids were discovered in abnormal amounts in phenylketonuric urine by Armstrong and Robinson [149] and confirmed by Jepson [164]. Schreier and Flaig [148] completed this group with the discovery of the very labile pyruvic acid derivative. These arise from tryptophan metabolism. Indoleacetic acid is said to be excreted in larger amounts than indolelactic acid, but no figures are available [149]. The diversion of tryptophan from its usual metabolism is also indicated by the three times normal excretion of indican [150].

5-HYDROXYINDOLEACETIC ACID. 5-Hydroxyindoleacetic acid excretion was first found to be slightly low in phenylketonuria by Armstrong and Robinson [149]. This was confirmed by Ferrari, Campagnari, and Guida [165]. The measurements by Pare et al. [166] shown in Table 11-4 accompanied the demonstration of low serum 5-hydroxytryptamine (serotonin) cited in Table 11-3.

PHENYLACETYLGLUTAMINE AND PHENYLACETIC ACID. Woolf [151] detected phenylacetic acid, for which no satisfactory methods of measurement are available, and also its principal conjugation product with glutamine. Small amounts are said to be conjugated with glucuronic acid [12]. The normal excretion of phenylacetylglutamine is significant (250 to 500 mg per day [167]). The amount excreted in phenylketonuria is about double this and is not quantitatively related to the intelligence of the patients [168].

Quantitative Interrelationships of Metabolites

There are clear correlations between the quantities of various metabolites in phenylketonuria but there is none between these amounts and the severity of the intellectual defect. The plasma level of phenylalanine reflects the amount in the diet. It is elevated, for example, with the relatively high intake of infants in their first year [140] and lowered by the therapeutic low phenylalanine levels. All other metabolites are in turn proportional to the phenylalanine plasma level [26, 147, 169, 170]. Normal amounts of these are restored when the plasma phenylalanine is lowered by treatment. This includes the secondary abnormalities, such as the elevation to normal of 5-hydroxytryptamine [144] and the reduction of the extra indican excretion [150].

The urinary concentrations of three compounds, phenylpyruvic acid, *o*-hydroxyphenylacetic acid, and phenylalanine, have been tested as indicators of the plasma phenylalanine concentration during treatment of patients. Phenylpyruvic acid excretion ceases at phenylalanine plasma levels below 0.6 μmoles per ml (10 mg per 100 ml) [171] or 0.90 μmoles per ml (15 mg per 100 ml) [7]. The latter value is probably high. *o*-Hydroxyphenylacetic acid excretion was detected at plasma phenylalanine levels above 0.48 or 0.67 μmoles per ml (8 or 11 mg per 100 ml) [171, 172]. At the critical lower levels the excretion of phenylalanine itself may be superior to either acid [145, 171]. Since these substances occur in urine in proportion to the plasma phenylalanine, their determination supports only indirectly a diagnosis based on the qualitative $FeCl_3$ test. Quantitative determination of the plasma phenylalanine itself is preferable to all urine tests.

Quantitative Relations of Metabolites to Intelligence

Except for rare atypical cases (see Differential Diagnosis, further on) there exists no causal correlation between intelligence and amounts of any of the metabolites measured. But it must be remembered that chemical measurements have generally been made on phenylketonuric patients of all ages, and not at the time when the mental damage was done. The rare high-grade patient with a relatively low phenylalanine level may be an exception to this generalization.

Tabulated plasma phenylalanine levels and IQs for 18 patients [139], for another 18 patients [141], and for 34 patients [5] showed that there is no relationship. There was also no relation between IQs of 8 patients and their cerebrospinal fluid levels of phenylalanine [139]. Jervis [142] found that the higher urine phenylpyruvic acid levels were associated with higher IQs and with better nutritional status in 34 patients. He attributed the low levels of the severely defective patients to their chronic malnutrition. 5-Hydroxytryptamine levels were independent of the IQs of 49 patients [144].

Since no relation between intelligence as measured by the IQ test and plasma phenylalanine concentrations exists, none would be expected with the urinary metabolites that are formed in proportion to the plasma phenylalanine. This has been borne out in a number of studies [57, 92, 142, 144, 147].

There is no evidence that any of the metabolites of phenylalanine are toxic to the brain in the amounts occurring in phenylketonuria. Great emphasis has therefore been given to deficiencies or excesses of certain pharmacodynamic amines which might offer some connection between the known metabolic defect in liver and the unknown functional defect in brain (see Other Biochemical Abnormalities, below).

Partington and Lewis [140] called attention to the fact that phenylalanine levels in phenylketonuria were more than twice as high during infancy as later (Table 11-3). Any effect of phenylalanine or its metabolites could therefore be greater at this period than later, even independently of an increased sensitivity of the brain at that age. Detailed comparisons should then show parallelism between the loss of IQ (Fig. 11-3) and phenylalanine levels at those ages.

Origin of Metabolites

Figure 11-9 indicates by double arrows the major metabolic pathways of phenylalanine, tyrosine, and tryptophan under normal conditions. As a consequence of the block in the normal conversion of phenylalanine to tyrosine, phenylalanine must detour through the other little used but not abnormal pathways, as indicated.

It has been suggested that there is inhibition of some of the steps in the normal metabolism of tryptophan and of tyrosine in phenylketonuria. The evidence is indirect, but there is indeed an accumulation of derivatives of the α-keto acids of phenylalanine, *o*-tyrosine, tyrosine, and tryptophan. The keto acids are the parent substances which can give rise to the standard series of metabolites already listed: the related pyruvic, lactic, acetic, and conjugated acetyl forms. The individual enzyme reactions on which this metabolic map (Fig. 11-9) is based are described below, and elsewhere for tyrosine (Chap. 13, Alcaptonuria) and tryptophan (Chap. 61, Hartnup Disease). Each step in the map has been numbered for convenience in discussion.

Phenylalanine Hydroxylase (A1)

The original isotopic demonstration of the phenylalanine hydroxylase reaction was in rats. Deuterium-labeled phenylalanine was metabolized to labeled tyrosine isolated from the tissue proteins [173]. The observation was then repeated in phenylketonuric patients with ^{14}C-phenylalanine [174]. Less than 10 percent, or none [175], of the usual amount of tyrosine was formed from phenylalanine. Any small amount formed could be attributed to other unknown reactions, or to residual activity of the genetically distorted enzyme protein. Residual activity has not been detected in studies of the enzyme in phenylketonuric liver. Direct studies of the enzyme from patients were first reported by Jervis [5] and later by others [176–178]. Phenylalanine hydroxylase assays in liver from normal controls and seven phenylketonuric patients proved that the enzyme was present in specimens from normal man but that there was no detectable activity in phenylketonuric liver.

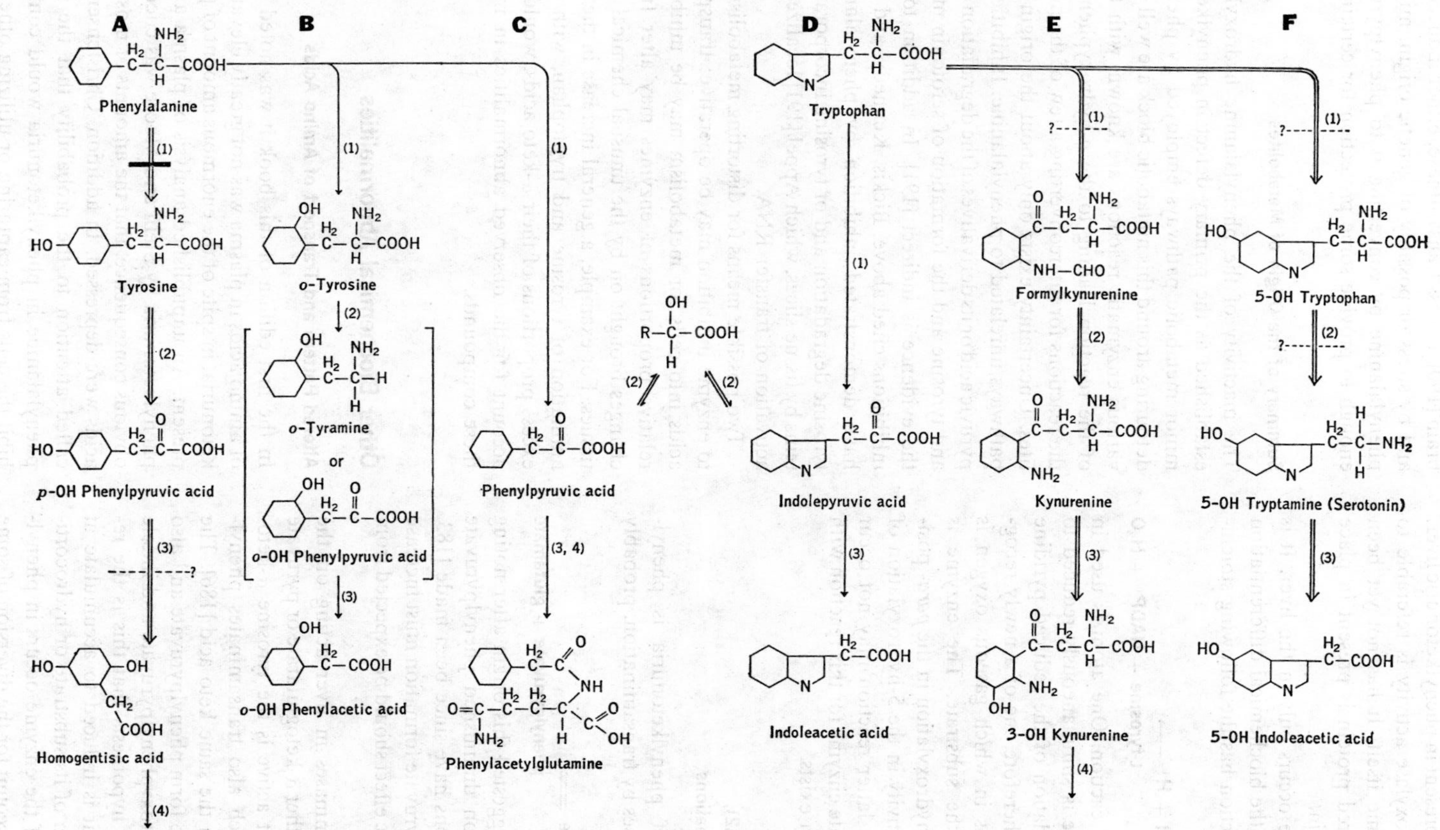

Figure 11-9. Map of the main normal metabolic routes of phenylalanine, tyrosine, and tryptophan (double arrows), the location of the real and apparent blocks in phenylketonuria, and the alternate routes (single arrows) giving rise to the metabolites characteristic of the disease. The individual reactions are described in the text.

The enzyme requires for activity a second protein fraction which is widely distributed in the body, either reduced NAD or NADP, and a new coenzyme related to folic acid [179]. All these cofactors are present in phenylketonuric liver. Lack of phenylalanine hydroxylase activity is referable to a fault of the specific enzyme itself. It has not yet been determined whether an altered protein is present in place of the normal enzyme protein.

Phenylalanine hydroxylase occurs only in the liver. It is found in the liver only after the biochemical differentiation following birth [180]. Its reaction has the following stoichiometry:

$$\text{L-Phenylalanine} + O_2 + \text{NADPH} + H^+ \longrightarrow \text{L-tyrosine} + \text{NADP}^+ + H_2O$$

Oxygen is required for the reaction. One atom is used in the *p*-hydroxylation, and one is simultaneously reduced to water by the associated oxidation of the reduced pyridine nucleotide. The reaction is therefore one of a newly recognized group of oxygenations in which gaseous oxygen is incorporated directly into the substrate. The enzyme is specific for L-phenylalanine hydroxylation in the *para-* position, but it also has weak activity in the 5-hydroxylation of L-tryptophan [181, 182]. The latter reaction may not occur physiologically since a separate enzyme for this reaction with a different tissue distribution exists.

Phenylalanine (C1), Tyrosine (A2), and Tryptophan (D1) Transaminations

The cardinal metabolite of phenylketonuria is phenylpyruvate. It undoubtedly arises by transamination, probably with α-ketoglutarate:

$$\text{Phenylalanine} + \alpha\text{-ketoglutarate} \rightleftharpoons \text{phenylpyruvate} + \text{glutamate}$$

Utena and Saito [40] first suggested this origin after noting that glutamate administration diminished phenylpyruvate excretion. Similar observations have since been made [183, 184]. Since lessened phenylpyruvate formation must increase phenylalanine, no therapeutic effect should be expected from this treatment.

There are several transaminases in liver acting on the aromatic amino acids with either α-ketoglutarate or pyruvate as acceptors [185]. The most active is the tyrosine α-ketoglutarate transaminase, which also transaminates phenylalanine and tryptophan with the same keto acid [186]. The same enzyme could therefore form phenylpyruvate and also the minor metabolites *p*-hydroxyphenylpyruvate and indole pyruvate. It is an attractive hypothesis that this is the responsible enzyme, because it is induced to accumulate at high levels by administration of its substrate or hydrocortisone [187]. If a high level of the enzyme occurs in phenylketonuria, this alone could account for the diversion of some tyrosine and tryptophan to their keto acids and subsequent metabolites. In addition, the enzyme appears only after birth in the livers of rats [188], and a similar delayed appearance in man could account for the delay, sometimes until the age of 1 month, of the excretion of phenylpyruvate in phenylketonuric infants [189]. A very similar enzyme is present in brain [190]. Excess transaminase, either induced hormonally and by stress or possibly of genetic origin, might eliminate phenylalanine by converting it to phenylpyruvate rapidly enough to provide some protection for certain patients.

Summary of the Origin of Metabolites

The inactivity of the phenylalanine hydroxylase is firmly established as the primary defect in phenylketonuria. The minor metabolic pathways employed by phenylalanine in detouring around this metabolic block are well outlined. The various enzymatic reactions are known, with the exception of the reaction leading to the *o*-hydroxyphenyl series and the reactions for interconverting a few of the minor metabolites. Uncertainty exists only about the origin of defects in pathways unrelated to phenylalanine. Inhibition by phenylpyruvic acid or its derivatives of the degradation of tryptophan and tyrosine and the formation of serotonin may occur, but the evidence is indirect [191]. In addition to the enzyme inhibitions cited above, Bickis, Kennedy, and Quastel [192] have demonstrated inhibition by phenylalanine both of tyrosine degradation and of tyrosine incorporation into proteins by tissue slices, which Appel [191] localized to inhibited activation of transfer RNA.

Two possible means for distorting metabolism in addition to enzyme inhibition may be operative: transport of amino acids into cells for metabolism may be inhibited, and the relative proportions of enzymes may alter from adaptive changes brought on by the unusual chemical milieu of the tissues. For example, a general increase in the rate of transamination of tyrosine and tryptophan, with formation of excess proportions of their α-keto acids, would equally well account for the observed abnormalities in metabolism of these compounds.

Other Biochemical Abnormalities

Altered Pattern and Transport of Amino Acids

In the first edition of this book it was noted that the total of amino acids in plasma was not greatly elevated in phenylketonuria, in spite of the enormous amount of phenylalanine present. An unpublished analysis of plasma amino acids in phenylketonuria by Stein and Moore was cited to show the obvious consequence, that the amounts of most other amino acids were depressed. In addition, Christensen in 1953 had called attention to the probability that the high level of phenylalanine in phenylketonuria would competitively inhibit the cells from capturing or utilizing other amino acids [193]. These facts are now established, and they offer a reasonable pathogenetic mechanism by which the liver defect can produce a defective maturation of the brain.

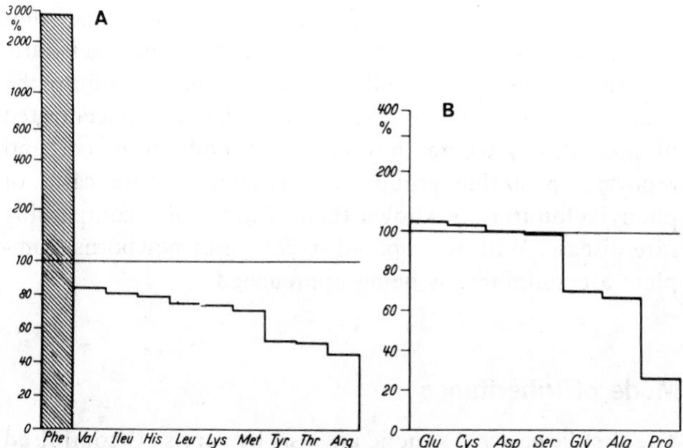

Figure 11-10. Average quantities of plasma essential (A) and non-essential (B) amino acids in phenylketonuria as percentage of normal controls. (*By permission of F. Linneweh and M. Ehrlich* [133].)

Linneweh and Ehrlich [194] first confirmed that the total of amino acids other than phenylalanine is low in phenylketonuria and then analyzed the individual amino acids in patients and controls to show the statistically significant depressions of the essential amino acids and most others (Fig. 11-10). The nutritional problem of cells in such a deficient medium is intensified by the high phenylalanine present. Chirigos, Greengard, and Udenfriend [195] had already shown that phenylalanine inhibits transport of tyrosine and other amino acids into brain. This was confirmed for the transport of a number of amino acids in brain slices [196, 197], including 5-hydroxytryptophan, the precursor of serotonin [198]. There is no substantial intracellular concentration of phenylalanine above that of plasma for the whole body in phenylketonuria [199], but intracellular amino acid patterns in some tissues must be distorted. Linneweh et al. [200] demonstrated that the inhibitory effect of phenylalanine on amino acid transport extended also to absorption from the intestine. The defect occurred in phenylketonuria and was eliminated by the low phenylalanine treatment (Fig. 11-11). The same inhibition of tryptophan absorption occurs [123, 124]. Thus it can be hypothesized that damage to the brain occurs in phenylketonuria and in diseases with similar amino acid imbalances, like maple syrup urine disease, when the immature brain is presented with an abnormal and deficient pattern of amino acids from which it cannot correctly construct its essential and permanent components [201, 202]. There is now direct evidence of the complex distortions of the amino acid patterns in cerebrospinal fluid and in brain [252, 253].

Pharmacodynamic Amines

Emphasis has been placed on certain real or postulated abnormalities of aromatic amine metabolism in phenylketonuria in the hope of establishing some functional connection between the defect of liver chemistry and the defect of brain function in this disease. The possibilities both of excesses of pharmacodynamic amines derived from phenylalanine and of deficiencies of others such as serotonin have been canvassed. Some illogicality has been unavoidable in the present state of our ignorance about the roles of these amines in brain function. This is especially so, given the fact that after early childhood the phenylketonuric brain has been irreversibly damaged during its development. Possible roles for aromatic amines in brain maturation are vague indeed.

There is a rapidly reversible pharmacologic component in the disease, seen even in the high-grade patients, especially when comparing behavior at high and low phenylalanine levels. Attention span increases, irritability and destructiveness decrease, and behavioral improvements are such as to promote learning when phenylalanine is reduced [52, 203, 204]. To these promptly reversible abnormalities a disturbed aromatic amine metabolism might contribute.

The Conversion of Tyrosine to Melanin Pigment

The decreased pigmentation in phenylketonuria is accounted for by competitive inhibition of phenylalanine on the tyrosinase system. Dancis and Balis [205] first demonstrated competition between phenylalanine and tyrosine with a mushroom tyrosinase system. Miyamoto and Fitzpatrick [206] confirmed this with mammalian tyrosinase. An unusually clear demonstration of the phenomenon of competitive inhibition under physiologic conditions is provided by the darkening of new-grown hair of phenylketonuric patients when either tyrosine intake is increased [207] or phenylalanine intake is lowered [7]. Boylen and Quastel [208] provided evidence that the phenylalanine concentration in phenylketonuria is adequate to inhibit melanin formation.

Hemoglobin Synthesis

The possibility of an error in the synthesis of one protein, hemoglobin, in the presence of the high concentration of

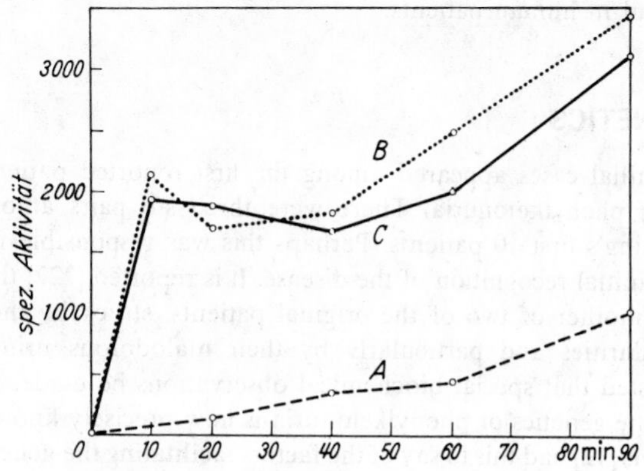

Figure 11-11. Rates of absorption into serum of tritiated L-leucine after oral dosage in a 3-year-old normal control (C) and in a 7-year old phenylketonuric patient before treatment (A) and after low-phenylalanine diet (B). (*By permission of F. Linneweh et al.* [200])

phenylalanine was excluded by the precise analysis by Allen and Schroeder [209]. The incorporation of phenylalanine into hemoglobin by a phenylketonuric subject was correct to within less than one residue per molecule. Thus protein synthesis may be remarkably accurate even in abnormal conditions.

Cerebral Oxygen Consumption

Oxygen arteriovenous differences in the cerebral circulation were lower in nine phenylketonuric patients than in other comparable mentally defective patients [210, 211]. Since blood flow measurements were not made, it is not known whether cerebral oxygen uptake was actually decreased. The oxygen uptake per gram may still be normal because of the reduced brain weight of these patients.

Experimental Phenylketonuria

An experimental approach to this disease was opened by Auerbach, Waisman, and Wycoff [212], whose phenylalanine-fed rats showed some retardation of learning ability. In subsequent work, Waisman et al. have produced mental deficiency by long-continued overfeeding of infant monkeys with L-phenylalanine [213]. Decreased performance and lowered brain serotonin were also produced in rats fed excess L-phenylalanine [214]. These models depend upon flooding the organism with phenylalanine in excess of the amount that can be degraded. Coleman's discovery that the diluted lethal gene in mice was associated with diminished phenylalanine hydroxylase activity [215] offered a second type of model of the human disease. A third type utilizes hamsters with normally low phenylalanine hydroxylase activity, or inhibition of the enzyme in rats by analogues of its coenzyme or its substrate [216, 217]. Recent studies emphasize the biochemical differences between these models and the human disease [218–221]. Nevertheless, these models will facilitate studies on the developing brain defect in the experimental disease, which cannot be examined in similar detail in human patients.

GENETICS

Familial cases appeared among the first reported patients with phenylketonuria. There were three sib pairs among Følling's first 10 patients. Perhaps this was responsible for the initial recognition of the disease. It is reported [222] that the mother of two of the original patients, struck by their similarities and particularly by their malodorous urines, insisted that special biochemical observations be made.

The genetics of phenylketonuria is now precisely known. Jervis [12] had this to say of the factors facilitating the genetic study: "(1) The identification of this condition is simple and exact, being made by a chemical test; (2) the character segregates sharply, affected individuals being entirely different biochemically from nonaffected ones; (3) the disease fulfills the requirement of being a unit in a biological (biochemical) sense." It should be added that the disease is rare, for this permits some simplified assumptions in handling the distribution data. These rare cases are largely concentrated in institutions, where they can be found, observed, and reported in sizable groups. Consequently, more cases of phenylketonuria are known than of any other comparably rare disease. With widespread screening of newborns, complete ascertainment is being approached.

Mode of Inheritance

The first large-scale genetic analysis by Jervis [1] comprised 213 patients and indicated that the disease is transmitted by a single autosomal gene, a double dose of which produces the disease. His definitive review [12] included data from 146 personally observed families, 46 families of Munro [23], 22 families of Følling, Mohr, and Ruud [11], and 52 other families reported in the world literature up to 1954. In the 266 families were 1,094 siblings, 433 (39.6 percent) with phenylketonuria. On the hypothesis of a single autosomal recessive gene, 25 percent would be affected. Corrections for the method of ascertainment by the methods of Weinberg and Lenz, which allowed for the uncounted families with only normal children, gave corrected percentages with standard errors of affected children as 27.37 ± 2.57 (sib method), 22.38 ± 2.66 (proband method), and within one-third of the standard error of the hypothetic 25 percent by the Lenz a priori method. There was no significant difference in the sex incidence. The evidence for autosomal recessive transmission was further substantiated by the occurrence of parental consanguinity in 8.33 percent of 206 of these families from the United States, England, and Norway. This is the incidence expected for a recessive disease occurring once in 25,000 times in a population that has approximately 1 percent cousin marriages. The precision with which the inheritance of phenylketonuria conforms to expectations lends considerable weight to the simple mathematic calculation of the risk of this disease in different types of matings, as shown in Table 11-5.

In the vast majority of families the parents are normal, are often related, and rarely have affected relatives. A typical pedigree is shown in Fig. 11-12. It is probable that in the few twin pairs reported the monozygotic pairs are concordant while the dizygotic pairs are either concordant or discordant, as expected (Table 11-6). Sixty-five half-sibs of affected individuals were all normal as expected, except for two whose father had married two sisters and produced a phenylketonuric offspring in each union [12].

Records exist of matings of affected individuals, usually females [168, 228, 229]. The few phenylketonuric offspring of some of these matings may be explained adequately by presumed heterozygosity of spouses. Births of normal children from phenylketonuric mothers establish the fact that intrauterine damage need not be done to the fetus by the

Table 11-5. FREQUENCY OF PHENYLKETONURIC OFFSPRING IN VARIOUS MATINGS*

Marital partners A: Carrier status	A: Chances of carrying gene	Marital partners B: Carrier status	B: Chances of carrying gene	Theoretic frequency of affected children if both partners were carriers	Chances of affected children from such a mating
Unknown	1:80	Unknown	1:80	1:4	1:25,600
Unknown	1:80	Normal sibling of phenylketonuric	2:3	1:4	1:480
Unknown	1:80	Parent of phenylketonuric	1	1:4	1:320
Unknown	1:80	Phenylketonuric	1	1:2	1:160
Normal sibling of phenylketonuric	2:3	Normal sibling of phenylketonuric	2:3	1:4	1:9
Normal sibling of phenylketonuric	2:3	Parent of phenylketonuric	1	1:4	1:6
Normal sibling of phenylketonuric	2:3	Phenylketonuric	1	1:2	1:3
Parent of phenylketonuric	1	Parent of phenylketonuric	1	1:4	1:4
Parent of phenylketonuric	1	Phenylketonuric	1	1:2	1:2
Phenylketonuric	1	Phenylketonuric	1	1	1

* Calculated on prevalence rate of disease as approximately 4:100,000, as suggested by Jervis [1].
Source: Wright et al. [20].

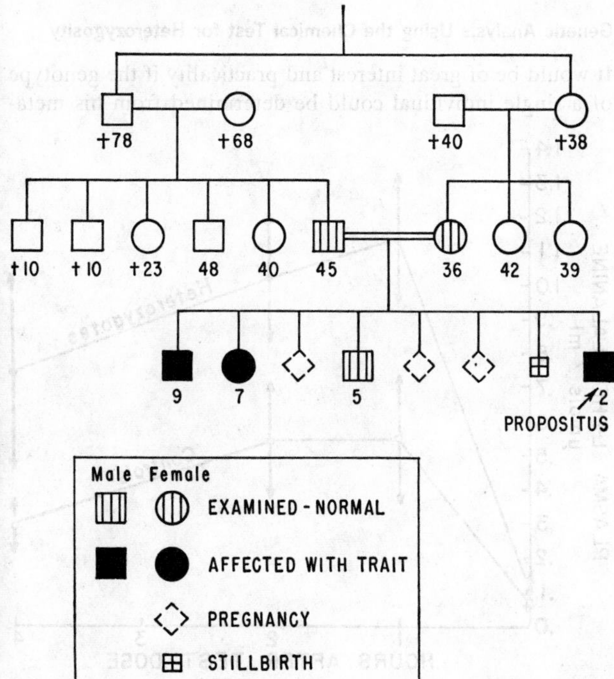

Figure 11-12. Pedigree of a Japanese family with phenylketonuria illustrating parental consanguinity, parental normality, and multiple siblings affected [38]. Age in years and deaths (+) are indicated. Other symbols are standard.

mother's metabolites. However, the frequency of mental retardation and congenital anomalies in these children is so high, especially in women with phenylalanine levels above 1.2 mM (> 20 mg per 100 ml), as to make it clear that phenylalanine or its derivatives can affect intrauterine development. Control of phenylalanine levels during pregnancy will be necessary to avoid such effects on offspring of phenylketonuric mothers.

Heterozygote Characteristics

A recessively inherited disease, of which phenylketonuria is typical, does not develop in individuals possessing only one of the defective genes (heterozygous individuals). Yet some signs of the defect might be expected. Evidences for less than the normal amount of phenylalanine hydroxylase can be found in many such individuals. There are no known clinical effects of this deficiency in these substantially normal individuals. Suppositions that the incidence of mental disease might be increased were guardedly denied from a survey in Sweden [15], and disproved in a well-designed study by Blumenthal [230].

Chemical Identification of Heterozygotes of Phenylketonuria

With Jervis' direct proof that phenylalanine hydroxylase activity is missing from the livers of patients with phenyl-

Table 11-6. PHENYLKETONURIA IN TWINS*

Authors and cases	Diagnosis		Sexes	Zygosity	Ref.
	Phenylketonuria	Normal			
Jervis, 1939, Nos. 185, 186	2	...	?	Mono- (probably)	[1]
Jervis, 1939, Nos. 21, 22	2	...	?	Mono- (?)	[1]
Wright and Tarjan, 1957	2	...	F,F	Mono- (probably)	[20]
Herrlin, 1962	2	...	M,M	Mono-	[224]
Szabó et al., 1965	2	...	M,M	Mono-	[225]
Mardens et al., 1967, Nos. 1, 2	2	...	M,M	Mono-	[223]
Mardens et al., 1967, Nos. 4, 5	2	...	M,M	Mono-	[223]
Jervis, 1939, Nos. 158, 159	2	...	?	Di- (probably)	[1]
Jervis, 1939, No. 1	1	1	?	Di- (probably)	[1]
Følling et al., 1944	1	1(?)	F,F	?	[11]
Thompson, 1957	1	1	M,M	?	[226]
Woolf et al., 1958	1	1	F,F	Di-	[82]
Renwick et al., 1960	1	1	M,F	Di-	[227]
Partington, 1961	1	1	M,F	Di-	[47]

* The compilation and evaluations are those of Mardens et al. [223].

ketonuria [6], and his final proof that this is a recessive disease [14], it was considered possible that the heterozygous carriers with one defective gene would have less than the normal complement of phenylalanine hydroxylase, as suggested by King [231] during the discussion following the presentation of Jervis' classic review. Følling and Closs [232] hinted that there might be increased phenylalanine in the urine of heterozygotes. Waelsch could find no abnormality in phenylalanine level in the blood in 10 pairs of parents [233], and it is clear in retrospect that the small difference that does exist could not then be detected.

This question was reinvestigated by Hsia, Driscoll, Troll, and Knox [9], who gave standard doses of L-phenylalanine and followed the plasma concentration of phenylalanine by a specific enzymatic method. Parents of known phenylketonuric patients were the heterozygotes. Their phenylalanine concentrations were higher and more sustained after the given dose than those of control individuals. The results are shown graphically in Fig. 11-13. The same distinction between 10 heterozygotes and 10 controls was confirmed by Berry, Sutherland, and Guest [137].

Further investigation disclosed that more detailed measurements could detect a subtle abnormality even under basal conditions. Knox and Messinger [134] were able to show that a group of heterozygotes had a significantly higher mean fasting level than a control group (Fig. 11-14). The phenylalanine concentration of the heterozygote group was about 1.5 to 2.5 times the normal, both in the fasting state and after the loading dose.

Only a reduced capacity of heterozygotes to metabolize phenylalanine was demonstrated, but the phenylalanine hydroxylase reaction is the one deficient in heterozygotes because less tyrosine is formed. Jervis [235] proved this by the smaller rise in tyrosine in plasma after a large dose of phenylalanine.

Other chemical abnormalities were investigated which might possibly permit discrimination between normal individuals and heterozygotes. Since all other metabolites, except tyrosine, occur in proportion to the plasma phenylalanine, their determination offers no improvement over the usual tolerance test.

Genetic Analysis Using the Chemical Test for Heterozygosity

It would be of great interest and practicality if the genotype of a single individual could be determined from his meta-

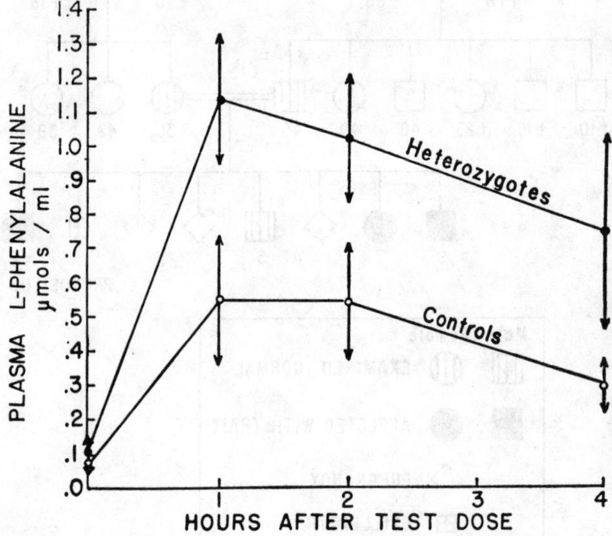

Figure 11-13. Plasma L-phenylalanine levels in normal and heterozygous persons following oral doses of 0.1 gm L-phenylalanine per kg body weight. Each line represents the mean value from 19 persons. The length of the arrows represents 1 s.d. above and below the mean [234].

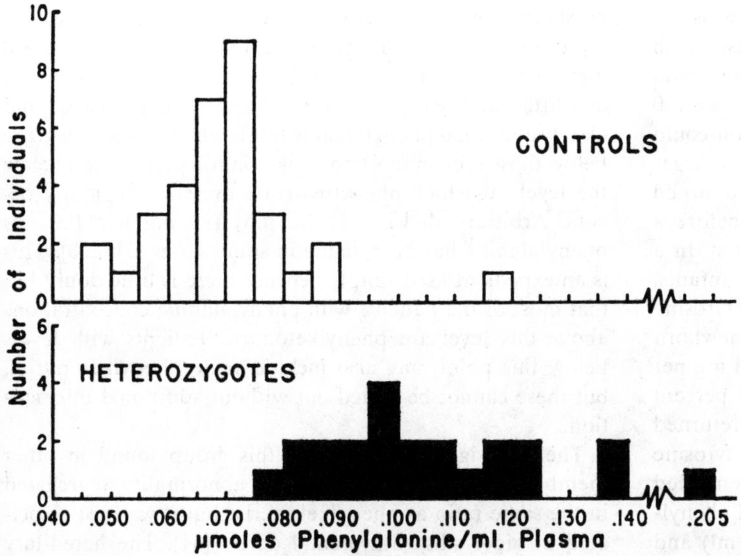

Figure 11-14. Distributions of plasma phenylalanine levels in 33 controls and 23 heterozygous individuals [134].

bolic phenotype. The discrimination described was only between sizable groups of heterozygotes and normal homozygotes, and about 15 percent of the groups overlapped. In connection with searches for linkage between the phenylketonuric gene and blood group genes, large numbers of phenylalanine tolerance tests were reported [236, 227], and the probabilities were evaluated statistically of correctly assigning an individual condition by the various values in this test. Highest discrimination utilizes intravenously administered phenylalanine and measurement of kinetics of its disappearance [237, 238]. It is clear that even in known phenylketonuric families decisions must be made with great caution, for any results might affect individual lives.

DIFFERENTIAL DIAGNOSIS

Phenylketonuria as described here represents the vast majority of cases seen and validated after infancy. It is common experience that any abnormality becomes subdivided upon intensive study. Phenylketonuria remains more homogeneous than most diseases studied in comparable detail. But when radically new means of ascertaining significant numbers of patients were employed, a few cases were found that conformed only in some respects to the picture of phenylketonuria. Differential diagnosis then became an important problem and has not yet been clearly solved. The nature and extent of the problem must be understood to keep it in perspective. The accepted homogeneity of phenylketonuria with the characteristics described here is based on study of patients primarily identified by mental retardation (or of sibs of such patients) and in whom the condition was confirmed by the $FeCl_3$ test for excretion of phenylpyruvate. The latter is sufficiently unambiguous so that cases have often been diagnosed with it alone, including a few without significant mental impairment but with the usual other chemical defects. As mentioned above, phenylpyruvate excretion merely reflects the plasma phenylalanine level. Phenylpyruvate excretion is recognized only at plasma phenylalanine levels above the approximate values of 0.6 to 0.9 mM (10 to 15 mg per 100 ml).

In order to find patients so they could be treated as early as possible, various forms of screening of newborn infants were undertaken. With present family sizes, about half the patients are younger sibs of an older phenylketonuric child. The simplest form of screening is the intensive examination of subsequent children born to a family in which phenylketonuria has already been recognized. Such examination would permit detection of about half the patients early enough so that they could be treated; possibly more patients could be detected early if detailed family histories were utilized. To find, as well, the other half of the patients at an early age, another dimension of effort is required. In place of one family known to be at risk, 10,000 must be screened to find the other half of these patients who will be born. Geographic areas were screened in this way with one of the forms of the familiar $FeCl_3$ test on urines. Though tedious and administratively awkward, these surveys produced for about every 20,000 negative tests the expected positive one. Coverage was considerably less than complete [239], and some technicians did not see a positive test in years, if ever [75]. Since the criterion was an established one, no diagnostic difficulties arose. When a new criterion, the elevation of plasma phenylalanine, was chosen, enabling more efficient screening procedures [10, 240], diagnostic difficulties began to arise in direct proportion to the use of the new methods [31].

In place of the "simple and exact" [12] qualitative distinction between positive and negative urine test results for diagnosis of phenylketonuria, the rare cases of newborn infants with persistently elevated phenylalanine concentration in plasma were distributed without a break in frequency above and below the level expected to give rise to phenylpyruvate excretion (Fig. 11-15) [31]. Of cases with more than 0.36 mM (6 mg per 100 ml) phenylalanine, about 12 percent fell in the range below 0.9 mM (15 mg per 100 ml) where negative tests of phenylpyruvate excretion could be expected at least some of the time. In addition, a larger number of patients had transient elevations that returned to normal in the first few weeks of life, usually before a second measurement could be made for confirmation. In a small fraction of these patients, mostly premature infants, phenylalanine was accompanied by elevation of tyrosine level [241, 242]. In Cahalane's series, 1 in 1,000 newborn infants had phenylalanine levels above 0.25 mM (4 mg per 100 ml) in the first week of life. When retested, 71 percent of these children had a phenylalanine level that had returned to normal, and 6.5 percent, who had had an elevated tyrosine level as well, later also returned to normal. There remained 14 children (22.5 percent) with persistently elevated phenylalanine levels, all above 0.6 mM (10 mg per 100 ml) and all but 3 with levels of 1.2 mM (20 mg per 100 ml) or higher [45]. This distribution is similar to that of Fig. 11-15. As expected, about half the new patients had older sibs with phenylketonuria.

Screening for phenylketonuria at an early age by use of blood analysis has introduced new classifications of patients for differential diagnosis, and even more new names to increase the confusion. The screening itself need not be more discriminative; its purpose is merely to permit a preliminary selection of patients for diagnosis, as admission to institutions for the mentally retarded formally did. It is not itself a diagnostic test, although this has not always been understood. The majority of the patients indicated by screening have only transiently elevated levels of phenylalanine, and they soon reveal themselves to be normal. Safe criteria for

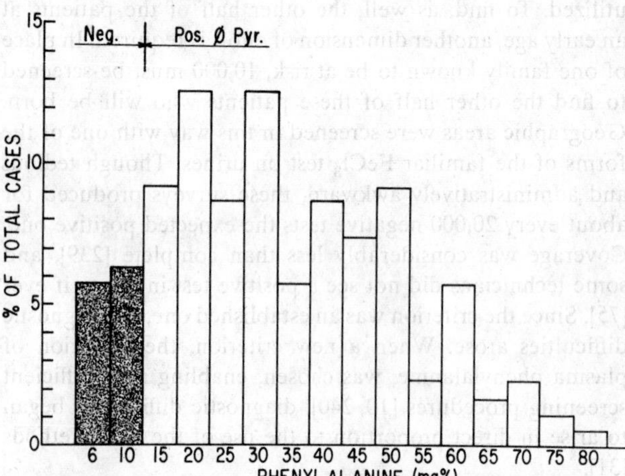

Figure 11-15. Distribution of phenylalanine plasma levels in 174 cases, 122 of which were ascertained by newborn screening. (*Calculated from Table 1 of Berman et al.* [31].) Shaded bars indicate the concentrations not regularly associated with phenylpyruvate excretion [7, 171].

persistence will be elevations lasting longer than a few months; periodic challenges of treated patients with normal diets are necessary. The problematic patients are about one-fifth (or less) of the total—those with persistent and clearly abnormal phenylalanine levels which nevertheless are below those seen in most phenylketonuric persons and below the levels at which phenylpyruvate excretion regularly occurs. Arbitrary division at 1.2 mM (20 mg per 100 ml) phenylalanine has been made in some series [31, 228]. This is an expedient used simply because there is little doubt but that most of the patients with phenylalanine concentrations above this level are phenylketonuric. Patients with levels below this point may also include some phenylketonurics, but these cannot be sorted out without additional information.

The first significant study of this group found in other members of a family the same mild abnormality, segregated in the same ratio as phenylketonuria, but it was not associated in older sibs with mental defect [31]. The hereditary pattern, lack of mental defect, and mild chemical disorder are similar to the "third-allele" disease characterized by Woolf et al. [238]. This is a variant form of phenylketonuria in which the gene from one parent codes for an enzyme that appears to be abnormally sensitive to inhibition by excess phenylalanine.

Clinicians have the immediate problem of deciding whether or not to treat a patient, irrespective of the final decision about the nature of the disease. Treatment will not substantially lower the phenylalanine levels in a patient with less than 0.6 mM (10 mg per 100 ml); this patient runs little risk of preventable mental retardation in any event. Levels above 1.2 mM (20 mg per 100 ml) carry a substantial risk and should be lowered. For the moderate, intermediate levels, a balance must be sought between the disturbance to child and family caused by treatment and the risk of mental retardation. The principles are that substantially elevated phenylalanine level is particularly harmful during the first year of life, and that the treatment is relatively safe, but only preventive. To provide treatment only when development slows is to provide it too late.

TREATMENT

The therapy of phenylketonuria is considered here only for the confirmation it provides that phenylalanine accumulation is the primary cause of disability in this disease. The earlier and useless treatments, employing various types of diets and vitamin, mineral, and hormone supplements, will not be considered. Attention need be given only to the low-phenylalanine regimen. The principle of this treatment is to provide only the amount of phenylalanine needed for growth and repair, and to avoid its accumulation.

Phenylalanine limitation was first attempted by Dent (unpublished) and by Armstrong and Tyler [7] with diets in which protein was replaced by a costly mixture of pure amino acids. L. I. Woolf (unpublished) suggested a practical method of preparation of casein hydrolyzate with phenylalanine removed by charcoal treatment. Bickel et al. [8], in 1951, maintained a 3-year-old girl for 6 weeks on a diet based on this preparation. Reversal of the major biochemical abnormalities was demonstrated at that time, but a larger number of cases and longer periods of treatment have been necessary to evaluate the effect of this diet on the clinical symptoms. These experiments have been possible only because essentially normal growth and development of infants and children can be maintained on this regimen, while at the same time the level of phenylalanine in the body is held at nearly normal concentration. Limitation of phenylalanine intake with more normal diets low in protein has not been successful in either lowering the phenylalanine concentrations or maintaining adequate nutrition [216, 243].

The most common difficulty encountered in limiting phenylalanine intake is dietary insufficiency, with loss of body protein, cessation of growth, and flooding of the tissues with phenylalanine released from the body protein. Frank phenylalanine deficiency and starvation occurred in a few early patients, sometimes with disastrous results, before the principles of control were worked out. Adequate control depends on meeting but not exceeding the phenylalanine requirement, and on meeting the caloric and other nutritional requirements. The requirement for phenylalanine during the rapid growth of phenylketonuric infants decreases from 50 to 70 mg per kg daily to less than 20 mg at 3 years of age [65, 244]. A provisional but authoritative guide for treatment and dietary requirements was the subject of a report to the Medical Research Council [17]. It includes the reminder that diagnosis must be confirmed by elevated plasma phenylalanine level before starting treatment and subsequently, and that the degree of control, also measured by phenylalanine levels, must be known in order to evaluate the results of treatment.

The observed relations between phenylalanine intake and plasma levels in 10 young treated children whose condition was under good control are shown in Fig. 11-16 [245].

"Overtreatment," a euphemism for at least mild phenylalanine deficiency, is most likely to occur in young, rapidly growing infants with higher phenylalanine requirements and in infants with only transiently elevated phenylalanine levels as they begin to metabolize it normally. Phenylalanine values are depressed well into the normal range, and in the latter type of patient remain so in the face of successively increased intakes until the diet can obviously be abandoned. Growth is frequently somewhat retarded with the stringent control [35, 77, 93, 246], but is normal with levels above 0.2 mM (3.3 mg per 100 ml) [74, 244]. There is no reason to suppose that such a small increase in phenylalanine is harmful, while malnutrition might be [77], so exactly normal levels are not insisted upon.

Reversal of Biochemical Abnormalities

All the major biochemical abnormalities of phenylketonuria are reversed by the low-phenylalanine diet. Figure 11-16 [169] shows the dramatic effects observed in the first treated patient. Also illustrated were preliminary periods of treatment showing the effects of several other dietary regimens. Besides the decrease of phenylalanine and phenylpyruvic acid, *o*-hydroxyphenylacetic acid [153], phenylacetylglutamine, phenyllactic acid, indolelactic acid, and indoleacetic acid [82] decreased to normal values. The peculiar odor of the urine vanished. There are no reports of the effect of treatment on the supposed excretion of *p*-hydroxyphenyl derivatives or on the sensitivity of these patients to epinephrine. The amount of 5-hydroxyindoleacetic acid in urine was unchanged, but the serotonin in blood rose during treatment [144]. The abnormal components, which occurred in the β-globulin fraction of plasma in about half the cases, disappeared with treatment and reappeared when phenylalanine was restored to the diet [141].

Skin and Pigment Changes

The eczema of patients with this disturbance usually cleared up promptly during treatment [110, 153, 247], only to recur if treatment was stopped. Hair (and possibly skin) pigmentation has increased with treatment in many individuals. This is best seen in the zone of new growth at the hair roots. The darkening can also be produced without lowering the phenylalanine level, simply by increasing the tyrosine intake

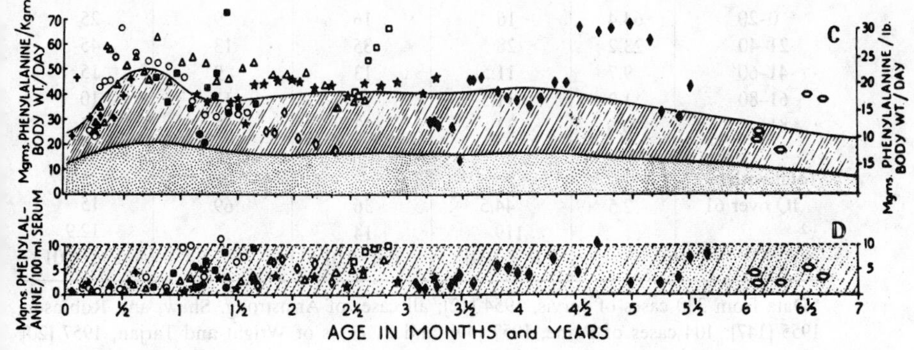

Figure 11-16. Daily dietary intakes of phenylalanine during treatment in 10 young phenylketonuric patients (upper curve) and serum phenylalanine levels. Note increased requirement during the first year of life, and the degree of control. (*By permission of W. R. Centerwall et al.* [245].)

to overcome the competitive inhibition of tyrosinase by phenylalanine.

Neurologic Signs

Treatment ameliorates most of the neurologic signs of phenylketonuria with the exception of structural defects and those produced by severe brain damage [153]. A prompt effect on the behavior is usually observed. The patient becomes less restless and irritable, and attention span increases [51]. An unmanageable child, for example, may develop appropriate fear of approaching automobiles. Motor performance improves, and hyperactive reflexes, hyperkinesis, and tremors lessen. The muscular hypertonicity also decreases. When phenylalanine is administered the abnormalities promptly return, and large doses intensify this effect. These prompt effects were described above as pharmacologic ones, independent of irreversible (structural) damage.

Seizures and Electroencephalograms

Treatment almost always improves or normalizes the EEG and lessens or eliminates the seizures when continued for a sufficient period. EEGs became normal in 9 of the 10 treated cases in Fig. 11-16 [73]. The exceptions to this rule are those patients with the most severe neurologic impairment. Even in these patients, conventional drug therapy may become more effective. Except for those with seizures as a complication developing early in treatment, no seizures have developed for the first time during therapy. Treatment may affect favorably other neurologic signs within weeks, but the full effect on the EEG and on seizure frequency is achieved only after months.

Intelligence

The most important evidence that phenylalanine accumulation is the basic physiologic abnormality in phenylketonuria is the effect of phenylalanine deprivation on the intelligence of these patients. Reversal of intellectual impairment of older patients has not been realized, but the low-phenylalanine diet can prevent intellectual impairment expected during the first few years of life and may reverse recently established impairment [51, 72, 78, 82, 153]. This conclusion is based on the evaluation of the first published results in adults [51] and in the first 43 patients treated at less than 3 years of age [248]. The results are shown in Table 11-7 [248]. Although the degree of control was often poor in these first cases, the same study showed a statistically significant effect of the age when treatment was started [248]. Delay of treatment beyond the first few weeks of life resulted in irreversible intellectual impairment which worsened with time.

Subsequent studies of significant numbers of patients confirmed that adequate treatment before impairment occurs will prevent or ameliorate the development of the expected defect. A long time was needed for separate institutions to accumulate and evaluate properly significant numbers of these rare cases. The weight of recently published studies [17, 35, 63, 73, 74, 77, 79, 80, 84, 86, 87, 89, 244, 246, 249] should quiet ill-founded allegations that treatment was useless or harmful. The small proportion of cases in which diagnosis might be in doubt (even after years of study) could

Table 11-7. IQ DISTRIBUTION IN UNTREATED AND TREATED PATIENTS WITH PHENYLKETONURIA

*Untreated (all ages)**		*Treated under 3 years of age*			
IQ	% of 466	Total, % of 43	Tested after 2 years of age, % of 31	Treated before age 16 months, % of 23	Treated after age 16 months, % of 20
0–20	64.4	16	16	9	25
21–40	23.2	28	35	13	45
41–60	9.7	11.5	13	9	15
61–80	1.9	11.5	13	13	10
81–	0.6	33	23	56	5
Total with IQ over 61	2.5	44.5	36	69	15
x^2	....	119 $P \ll 0.01$	14 $P < 0.01$	..	12.9 $P < 0.01$

*Data from 330 cases of Jervis, 1954 [12]; all cases of Armstrong, Shaw, and Robinson, 1955 [147]; 104 cases of Paine, 1957 [49], and 21 cases of Wright and Tarjan, 1957 [20].

be subtracted without significantly lowering the appraisal of results. Baumeister [250] demonstrated the same substantial correlation first reported [248] between age at which diet was initiated and final IQ for 167 of these patients, as had most of the individual authors. There was significant correlation between the degree of chemical control and the final IQ, though this is not yet clear in most smaller studies. There was no correlation between duration of treatment and final IQ, which is consistent with the damage occurring precipitously in the first 10 months (Fig. 11-3) [63], and with the relative well-being of older patients taken off the diet [61, 89]. The optimum degree of chemical control and duration of treatment are still to be achieved.

The effects of treatment are in complete accord with the view that the phenylketonuric infant is normal at birth and that in the first months of life retardation begins and becomes progressively more severe. The results also indicate that this retardation is largely irreversible, but is prevented or arrested by lowering phenylalanine. A graphic demonstration of this effect is shown in Fig. 11-3, which gives the results in treated groups of the same age, all at least 3 years after the start of treatment. It is apparent that the most significant effect of treatment is not to be evaluated by the extent of the return to a normal IQ range or by the gain in IQ, but by the contrast with what happens to an untreated group of the same age in the same time period. A particularly well-studied and homogeneous group evaluated at about 1 year of age [35] is included to show how this type of analysis makes possible a rapid evaluation of treatment results.

SUMMARY

1 The major biochemical changes in phenylketonuria can be traced through known chemical reactions to the accumulation in the tissues of that part of the dietary L-phenylalanine which would normally be converted to tyrosine. These changes are reversed when phenylalanine accumulation is avoided. The accumulation occurs because the specific liver enzyme, phenylalanine hydroxylase, is missing or inactive.

2 The disease is inherited as an autosomal recessive character. The phenylalanine concentration of the serum of heterozygotes may be elevated, but there are no definite deleterious phenotypic consequences of the heterozygous state.

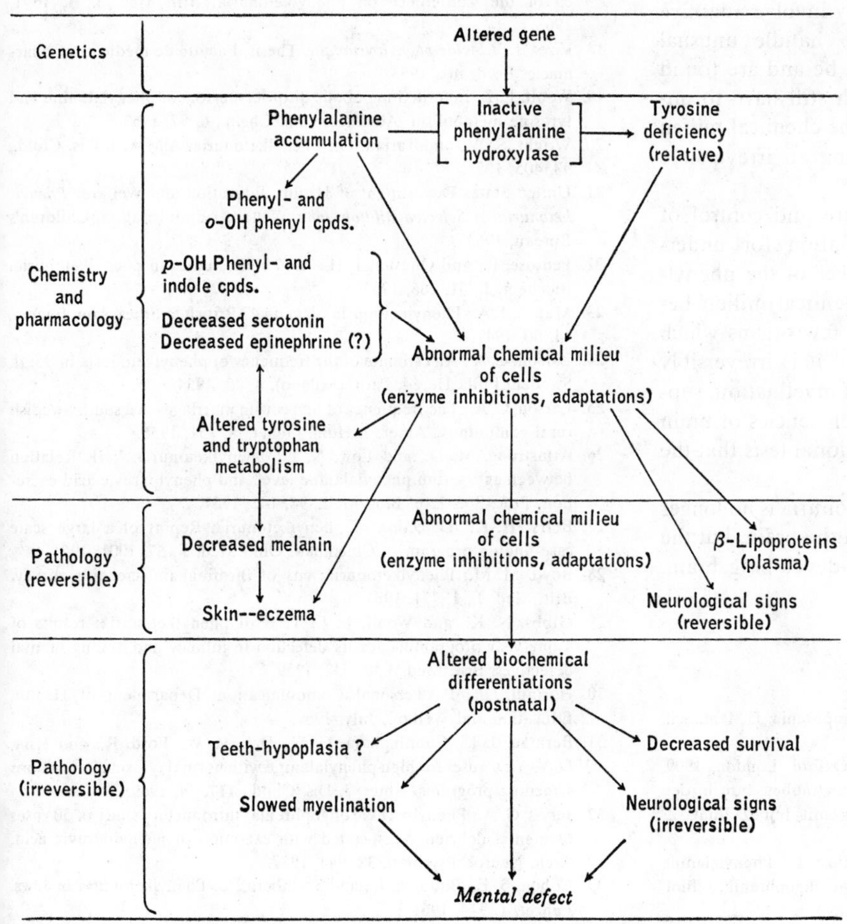

Figure 11-17. Scheme of pathogenesis in phenylketonuria. Irreversible changes such as the mental defect are considered to result from altered biochemical differentiation of the immature brain.

3 The pathologic changes of skin and mind in phenylketonuria are also referable to the accumulation of phenylalanine, since they are either reversed or prevented when the accumulation is avoided by a low-phenylalanine diet. In this sense the disease phenylketonuria, but not the primary defect of the enzyme, is acquired. It is evident that treatment must be started early and continued at least until biochemical differentiation is complete. The stepwise pathogenesis of the serious and permanent mental deficiency and other defects is less well understood than the biochemical disturbances. One of the abnormalities, melanin deficiency, is clearly referable to competitive enzyme inhibition. Pharmacologic effects of the abnormal metabolites, especially derivatives of *o*-tyrosine and serotonin, may contribute to the symptoms. The pathogenesis, involving the chemical derangements and the reversible and irreversible pathologic changes, is summarized in Fig. 11-17. The most obvious abnormality of the chemical milieu of the cells results from the disturbance of amino acid transport into cells by the high phenylalanine levels.

4 The consequences of the defect are best considered as the results of accumulation of (internal) environmental abnormalities which affect the tissues of the developing child. Some of these may be enzyme-inhibitory and pharmacologic effects on preformed systems. Others may involve adaptive changes in the capacity of systems to handle unusual amounts of metabolites. All these should be and are found to be reversible, but those systems which still have to undergo biochemical differentiation when the chemical milieu becomes abnormal may be directed along an irreversible series of abnormal changes.

5 Too little is now known of the nature and control of embryologic and biochemical differentiation for understanding the intimate cellular consequences of the phenylketonuric abnormality, but when the chemical milieu becomes abnormal, the brain is one of the few organs which must still differentiate biochemically, and it is irreversibly altered by this disease. The retardation of myelination, supported by chemical measurements and deficiencies of brain weight, is the only evidence besides functional tests that the brain is affected.

6 The outstanding problem in phenylketonuria is no longer the effect of the abnormal metabolism on the brain, but the nature of the alterations induced in the developing brain.

BIBLIOGRAPHY

1. Jervis, G. A.: The genetics of phenylpyruvic oligophrenia. J. Ment. Sci., **85**, 719, 1939.
2. Garrod, A. E.: *Inborn Errors of Metabolism.* Oxford, London, 1909.
3. Følling, A.: Über Ausscheidung von Phenylbrenztraubensäure in den Harn als Stoffwechselanomalie in Verbindung mit Imbezzillität. Z. Physiol. Chem., **227**, 169, 1934.
4. Jervis, G. A., Block, R. J., Bolling, D., and Kanze, L.: Phenylalanine content of blood and spinal fluid in phenylpyruvic oligophrenia. J. Biol. Chem., **134**, 105, 1940.
5. Jervis, G. A.: Studies of phenylpyruvic oligophrenia: the position of the metabolic error. J. Biol. Chem., **169**, 651, 1947.
6. Jervis, G. A.: Phenylpyruvic oligophrenia: deficiency of phenylalanine oxidizing system. Proc. Soc. Exp. Biol. Med., **82**, 514, 1953.
7. Armstrong, M. D., and Tyler, F. H.: Studies on phenylketonuria. I. Restricted phenylalanine intake in phenylketonuria. J. Clin. Invest., **34**, 565, 1955.
8. Bickel, H., Gerrard, J., and Hickmans, E. M.: Influence of phenylalanine intake on the chemistry and behavior of a phenylketonuric child. Acta Pediat., **43**, 64, 1954.
9. Hsia, D. Y.-Y., Driscoll, K., Troll, W., and Knox, W. E.: Detection by phenylalanine tolerance tests of heterozygous carriers of phenylketonuria. Nature (London), **178**, 1239, 1956.
10. Guthrie, R., and Susi, A.: A simple phenylketonuria screening method for newborn infants. Pediatrics, **32**, 338, 1963.
11. Følling, A., Mohr, O. L., and Ruud, L.: *Oligophrenia Phenylpyruvica, a Recessive Syndrome in Man.* I. Mat.-Naturv. Klasse, 1944, vol. 2, no. 13. Skrifter Norske Videnskaps-Akad., Oslo, 1945.
12. Jervis, G. A.: Phenylpyruvic oligophrenia (phenylketonuria). Res. Publ. Ass. Res. Nerv. Ment. Dis., **33**, 259, 1954.
13. Knox, W. E., and Hsia, D. Y.-Y.: Pathogenetic problems in phenylketonuria. Amer. J. Med., **22**, 687, 1957.
14. Lang, K.: Die phenylpyruvische Oligophrenie. Ergebn. inn. Med. Kinderheilk., **6**, 78, 1955.
15. Larson, C. A.: Phenylketonuria, in *De Genetica medica,* part IV, edited by L. Gedda, p. 122. Istituto Gregorio Mendel, Rome, 1962.
16. Lyman, F. L. (ed.): *Phenylketonuria.* Charles C Thomas, Springfield, Ill., 1963.
17. Treatment of phenylketonuria. Report to the Medical Research Council of the Conference on Phenylketonuria. Brit. Med. J., **1**, 1691, 1963.
18. Vizet, J.: *L'Acide phenylpyruvique.* Thesis, Faculté de médicine et pharmacie, Bordeaux, 1953.
19. Woolf, L. I.: Inherited metabolic disorders: errors of phenylalanine and tyrosine metabolism. Advances Clin. Chem., **6**, 97, 1963.
20. Wright, S. W., and Tarjan, G.: Phenylketonuria. A.M.A. J. Dis. Child., **93**, 405, 1957.
21. United States Department of Health, Education and Welfare: *Phenylketonuria: A Selected Bibliography.* Welfare Administration, Children's Bureau, 1963.
22. Penrose, L., and Quastel, J. H.: Metabolic studies in phenylketonuria. Biochem. J., **31**, 266, 1937.
23. Munro, T. A.: Phenylketonuria: data on 47 British families. Ann. Eugen., **14**, 60, 1947.
24. Larson, C. A.: An estimate of the frequency of phenylketonuria in South Sweden. Folia Héréd. Path. (Milano), **4**, 40, 1954.
25. Larson, C. A.: The frequency of first cousin marriages in a south Swedish rural community. Amer. J. Hum. Genet., **8**, 151, 1956.
26. Armstrong, M. D., and Low, N. L.: Phenylketonuria. VIII. Relation between age, serum phenylalanine level, and phenylpyruvic acid excretion. Proc. Soc. Exp. Biol. Med., **94**, 142, 1957.
27. Berry, H. K.: Detection of phenylketonuria. Report of a large scale case-finding program in Cincinnati. Ohio Med. J., **57**, 1001, 1961.
28. Boyd, M. M.: Phenylketonuria: city of Birmingham screening survey. Brit. Med. J., **1**, 771, 1961.
29. Gibbs, N. K., and Woolf, L. I.: Tests of phenylketonuria: results of a one-year programme for its detection in infancy and among mental defectives. Brit. Med. J., **2**, 532, 1959.
30. Hormuth, R. P.: Personal Communication. Department of Health, Education and Welfare, July, 1969.
31. Berman, J. L., Cunningham, G. C., Day, R. W., Ford, R., and Hsia, D. Y.-Y.: Causes for high phenylalanine with normal tyrosine in newborn screening programs. Amer. J. Dis. Child., **117**, 54, 1969.
32. Jervis, G. A.: Phenylpyruvic oligophrenia: introductory study of 50 cases of mental deficiency associated with excretion of phenylpyruvic acid. Arch. Neurol. Psychiat., **38**, 944, 1937.
33. Cohen, B. E., Bodonyi, E., and Szeinberg, A.: Phenylketonuria in Jews. Lancet, **1**, 344, 1961.

34. Katz, H. P., and Menkes, J. H.: Phenylketonuria occurring in an American Negro. J. Pediat., **65,** 71, 1964.
35. Castells, S., and Brandt, I. K.: Phenylketonuria: evaluation of therapy and verification of diagnosis. J. Pediat., **72,** 34, 1968.
36. Graw, R. G., Jr., and Koch, R.: Phenylketonuria in two American Negroes. Amer. J. Dis. Child., **114,** 412, 1967.
37. Glass, B., and Li, C. C.: The dynamics of racial intermixture: an analysis based on the American Negro. Amer. J. Hum. Genet., **5,** 1, 1953.
38. Kobayashi, T., Saito, S., Kawamura, K., and Koga, B.: Oligophrenia pyruvica: three cases in one family. Shônika Rinshô, **5,** 6, 1952.
39. Tanaka, K., Matsunaga, E., Handa, Y., Murata, T., and Takehara, K.: Phenylketonuria in Japan. Jap. J. Hum. Genet., **6,** 65, 1961.
40. Utena, H., and Saito, T.: On the Phenylpyruvic oligophrenia. Psychiat. Neurol. Jap., **53,** 365, 1951.
41. Blehová, B.: Phenylketonuria in Czechoslovakia. J. Ment. Defic. Res., **4,** 116, 1960.
42. Szabó, L., Tóth, G., and Molnár, L.: A phenylketonuriáról (adatok hazai gyakoriságához és terápiájához). Orv. Hetil., **102,** 1361, 1961.
43. Salam, M.: Phenylketonuria in a child from the Middle East. Amer. J. Dis. Child., **105,** 102, 1963.
44. Visakorpi, J. K.: Personal communication, July, 1969.
45. Cahalane, S. F.: Phenylketonuria: mass screening of newborns in Ireland. Arch. Dis. Child., **43,** 141, 1968.
46. Carter, C. O., and Woolf, L. I.: The birthplaces of parents and grandparents of a series of patients with phenylketonuria in south-east England. Ann. Hum. Genet., **25,** 57, 1961.
47. Partington, M. W.: Observations on phenylketonuria in Ontario. Canad. Med. Ass. J., **84,** 985, 1961.
48. Knox, W. E.: Phenylketonuria, in *The Metabolic Basis of Inherited Disease,* 1st ed., edited by J. B. Stanbury, J. B. Wyngaarden, and D. S. Fredrickson, p. 321. McGraw-Hill, New York, 1960.
49. Paine, R. S.: The variability in manifestations of untreated patients with phenylketonuria (phenylpyruvic aciduria). Pediatrics, **20,** 290, 1957.
50. Kleinman, D. S.: Phenylketonuria, a review of some deficits in our information. Pediatrics, **33,** 123, 1964.
51. Hsia, D. Y.-Y., Knox, W. E., Quinn, K. V., and Paine, R. S.: A one-year, controlled study of the effect of low-phenylalanine diet on phenylketonuria. Pediatrics, **21,** 178, 1958.
52. Partington, M. W.: Variations in intelligence in phenylketonuria. Canad. Med. Ass. J., **86,** 736, 1962.
53. Anderson, V. E.: Genetics in mental retardation, in *Mental Retardation,* edited by H. A. Stevens and R. F. Haber, p. 348. The University of Chicago Press, Chicago, 1964.
54. Bruhl, H. H., Arnesen, J. F., and Bruhl, M. G.: Effect of a low-phenylalanine diet on older phenylketonuria patients (long range controlled study). Amer. J. Ment. Defic., **69,** 225, 1964.
55. Kratter, F. E.: The physiognomie, psychometric, behavioral and neurological aspects of phenylketonuria. J. Ment. Sci., **105,** 421, 1959.
56. Williamson, M., Koch, R., and Henderson, R.: Phenylketonuria in school age retarded children. Amer. J. Ment. Defic., **72,** 740 (1968).
57. Schöenenberg, H., Schmidt, D., and Wönckhaus, I.: Der phenylbrenz Traubensäureschwachsinn, Z. Kinderheilk., **77,** 363, 1955.
58. Coates, S., Norman, A. P., and Woolf, L. I.: Phenylketonuria with normal intelligence and Gowen's muscular dystrophy. Arch. Dis. Child. **32,** 313, 1957.
59. Larson, C. A.: The absence of phenylketonuria in 8,220 individuals not known to be mental defectives, in *Novant' anni delle Leggi Mendeliane,* p. 311. Istituto Gregorio Mendel, Rome, 1956.
60. Centerwall, W. R., and Centerwall, S. A.: Phenylketonuria (Følling's disease): the story of its discovery. J. Hist. Med., **16,** 292, 1961.
61. Murphy, D.: Termination of dietary treatment of phenylketonuria. Irish J. Med. Sci., **452,** 355, 1963.
62. Partington, M. W.: The Early symptoms of phenylketonuria. Pediatrics, **27,** 465, 1961.
63. Kang, E. S., Kennedy, J. L., Gates, L., Burwash, I., and McKinnon, A.: Clinical observations in phenylketonuria. Pediatrics, **35,** 932, 1965.
64. Saugstad, L. F.: Develop. Med. Child, Neurol., in press, 1970.
65. Bickel, H., and Bremer, H. J.: Über die Phenylketonurie. Deutsch. Med. Wschr., **92,** 700, 1967.
66. Bailey, N.: Consistency and variability in the growth of intelligence from birth to eighteen years. J. Genet. Psychol., **75,** 165, 1949.
67. Knobloch, H., and Pasamanick, B.: Factors affecting human development, before and after birth. Pediatrics, **26,** 210, 1960.
68. Knobloch, H., and Pasamanick, B.: The developmental behavioral approach to the neurologic examination in infancy. Child Develop., **33,** 181, 1962.
69. Korsch, B., Cobb, K., and Ashe, B.: Pediatricians' appraisals of patients' intelligence. Pediatrics, **27,** 990, 1961.
70. Fuller, R.: Treated phenylketonuria: analysis of psychological results, in *International Association for the Scientific Study of Mental Deficiency,* edited by B. W. Richards. Jackson, Reigate, England, 1968.
71. Berman, P. W., Waisman, H. A., and Graham, F. K.: Effectiveness of dietary treatment in phenylketonuria—What is proof? Develop. Med. Child Neurol., **9,** 411, 1967.
72. Blainey, J. D., and Guilliford, R.: Phenylalanine-restricted diets in the treatment of phenylketonuria. Arch. Dis. Child., **31,** 452, 1956.
73. Centerwall, W. R., Centerwall, S. A., Armon, V., and Mann, L. B.: Phenylketonuria. II. Results of treatment of infants and young children: a report of 10 cases. J. Pediat., **59,** 102, 1961.
74. Clayton, B., Moncrieff, A., and Roberts, G. E.: Dietary treatment of phenylketonuria: a follow-up study. Brit. Med. J., **3,** 133, 1967.
75. Farquhar, J. W., Richmond, J., and Tait, H. P.: Phenylketonuria in pediatric practice. Clin. Pediat., **2,** 504, 1963.
76. Gruttner, R., Muller, F., and Wallis, H.: Evaluation of the success of dietetic treatment with casein hydrolysate low in phenylalanine in phenylpyruvic oligophrenia. Mschr. Kinderheilk., **106,** 41, 1958.
77. Hackney, I. M., Hanley, W. B., Davidson, W., and Linsao, L.: Phenylketonuria: mental development, behavior, and termination of low phenylalanine diet. J. Pediat., **72,** 646, 1968.
78. Horner, F. A., Streamer, C. W., Clader, D. E., Hassell, L. L., Binkley, E. L., and Dumars, K. W., Jr.: Effect of phenylalanine-restricted diets in phenylketonuria. II. A.M.A. J. Dis. Child., **93,** 615, 1957.
79. Koch, R., Acosta, P., Fishler, K., Schaeffler, G., and Wohlers, A.: Clinical observations on phenylketonuria. Amer. J. Dis. Child., **113,** 6, 1967.
80. O'Flynn, M. E., and Hsia, D. Y.-Y.: Some observations on the dietary treatment of phenylketonuria. J. Pediat., **72,** 260, 1968.
81. Pergamit, L. D.: Phenylketonuria. Northwest Med., **64,** 353, 1965.
82. Woolf, L. I., Griffiths, R., Moncrieff, A., Coates, S., and Dillistone, F.: Dietary treatment of phenylketonuria. Arch. Dis. Child., **33,** 167, 1958.
83. Zellweger, H. U.: Enzyme deficiency diseases. J. Amer. Diet. Ass., **34,** 1045, 1958.
84. Dobson, J., Koch, R., Williamson, M., Spector, R., Frankenburg, W., O'Flynn, M., Warner, R., and Hudson, F.: Cognitive development and dietary therapy in phenylketonuric children. New Eng. J. Med., **278,** 1142, 1968.
85. Anderson, V. E., Siegel, F. S., Tellegen, A., and Fisch, R. O.: Manual dexterity in phenylketonuric children. Percept. Motor Skills, **26,** 827, 1968.
86. Berman, P. W., Waisman, H. A., and Graham, F. K.: Intelligence in treated phenylketonuric children—a developmental study. Child Develop., **37,** 731, 1966.
87. Cohen, B. E., Szeinberg, A., Aviad, Y., and Costeff, H.: Evaluation of dietary treatment in phenylketonuria: a proposed methodology. Develop. Med. Child. Neurol., **11,** 96, 1969.
88. Siegel, F. S., Balow, B., Fisch, R. O., and Anderson, V. E.: School behavior profile ratings of phenylketonuric children. Amer. J. Ment. Defic., **72,** 937, 1968.
89. Solomons, G., Kelescke, L., and Opitz, E.: Evaluation of the effects of terminating the diet in phenylketonuria. J. Pediat., **69,** 596, 1966.
90. Harris, H.: *An Introduction to Human Biochemical Genetics,* Eugenics Laboratory Memoirs, 37. Cambridge, New York, 1955.
91. Lang, K.: Über phenylpyruvische Oligophrenie. Z. Kinderheilk., **75,** 132, 1954.
92. Woolf, L. I., and Vulliamy, D. G.: Phenylketonuria with a study of the effect upon it of glutamic acid. Arch. Dis. Child., **26,** 487, 1951.

93. Fisch, R. O., Graven, H. J., and Feiberg, S. B.: Growth and bone characteristics of phenylketonurics. Amer. J. Dis. Child., **112,** 3, 1966.
94. Sutherland, B. S., Umbarger, B., and Berry, H. K.: The clinical management of phenylketonuria. Family Physician, **12,** 61, 1967.
95. Myers, H. M., Duman, M., and Ballhorn, H. B.: Dental manifestations of phenylketonuria. J. Amer. Dent. Ass., **77,** 586, 1968.
96. Cowie, V.: Phenylpyruvic oligophrenia. J. Ment. Sci., **97,** 505, 1951.
97. Hassel, C. W., and Brunsting, L. A.: Phenylpyruvic oligophrenia. A.M.A. Arch. Derm., **79,** 458, 1959.
98. Fleisher, T. L., and Zeligman, I.: Cutaneous findings in phenylketonuria. A.M.A. Arch. Derm., **81,** 898, 1960.
99. Jablonska, S., Stachow, A., and Suffczynska, M.: Skin and muscle indurations in phenylketonuria. Arch. Derm. (Chicago), **95,** 443, 1967.
100. Berg, J. M., and Stern, J.: Iris color in phenylketonuria. Ann. Hum. Genet., **22,** 370, 1958.
101. Turpin, R., Dagand, H., Duchene, H., and Delbarre, F.: Présentation clinique d'un malade atteint d'oligophrénie phénylpyruvique. Ann. Medicopsychol. (Paris), **105,** 65, 1947.
102. Stadler, H. E., Meyer, H., and Leland, H.: Phenylpyruvic oligophrenia in a mulatto: probable manifestation of the pleiotropic effect. J. Nerv. Ment. Dis., **124,** 205, 1956.
103. Crome, L.: The association of phenylketonuria with leucodystrophy. J. Neurol. Neurosurg. Psychiat., **25,** 149, 1962.
104. Fellman, J. H.: Epinephrine metabolites and pigmentation in the central nervous system in a case of phenylpyruvic oligophrenia. J. Neurol. Neurosurg. Psychiat., **21,** 58, 1958.
105. Fois, A., Rosenberg, C., and Gibbs, F. A.: The electroencephalogram in phenylpyruvic oligophrenia. Electroenceph. Clin. Neurophysiol., **7,** 569, 1955.
106. Allen, R. J., and Gibson, R. M.: Phenylketonuria with normal intelligence. Amer. J. Dis. Child., **102,** 115, 1961.
107. Woolf, L. I., Ounsted, C., Lee, D., Humphrey, M., Cheshire, N. M., and Steed, G. R.: Atypical phenylketonuria in sisters with normal offspring. Lancet, **2,** 464, 1961.
108. Sutherland, B. S., Berry, H. K., and Shirkey, H. C.: A syndrome of phenylketonuria with normal intelligence and behavior disturbances. J. Pediat., **57,** 521, 1960.
109. French, J. H., Clark, D. B., Butler, H. G., and Teasdall, R. D.: Phenylketonuria: some observations on reflex activity. J. Pediat., **58,** 16, 1961.
110. Braude, H.: Phenylketonuria—a case report in a European child treated with low phenylalanine diet. South African Med. J., **30,** 83, 1956.
111. Crome, L., and Pare, C. M. B.: Phenylketonuria: a review and a report of the pathological findings in four cases. J. Ment. Sci., **106,** 862, 1960.
112. Alvord, E. C., Stevenson, L. D., Vogel, F. S., and Engle, R. L., Jr.: Neuropathological findings in phenylpyruvic oligophrenia. J. Neuropath. Exp. Neurol., **9,** 298, 1950.
113. Scholz, W.: Contribution à l'anatomie pathologique du systeme nerveux central dans l'oligophrénie phenylpyruvique. Encéphale, **46,** 668, 1957.
114. Poser, C. M., and Van Bogaert, L.: Neuropathologic observations in phenylketonuria. Brain, **82,** 1, 1959.
115. Crome, L., Tymms, V., and Woolf, L. I.: A chemical investigation of the defects of myelination in phenylketonuria. J. Neurol. Neurosurg. Psychiat., **25,** 143, 1962.
116. Malamud, N.: Neuropathology of phenylketonuria. J. Neuropath. Exp. Neurol., **25,** 254, 1966.
117. Menkes, J. H.: Cerebral proteolipids in phenylketonuria. Neurology (Minneap.), **18,** 1003, 1968.
118. Folch-Pi, J.: Composition of the brain in relation to maturation, in *Biochemistry of the Developing Nervous System,* edited by H. Waelsch, p. 121. Academic, New York, 1955.
119. Gerstl, B., Malamud, N., Eng. L. F., and Hayman. R. B.: Lipid alterations in human brains in phenylketonuria. Neurology (Minneap.), **17,** 51, 1967.
120. Menkes, J. H.: The pathogenesis of mental retardation in phenylketonuria and other inborn errors of amino acid metabolism. Pediatrics, **39,** 297, 1967.
121. Kotake, Y., Masai, Y., and Mori, Y.: Über das Verhalten des Phenylalanine im tierschen Organismus. Z. Physiol. Chem., **122,** 195, 1922.
122. Prescott, A. B., Borek, E., Brecher, A., and Waelsch, H.: Studies on oligophrenia phenylpyruvica. I. Microbiological determination of L- and D-phenylalanine and phenyllactic acid. J. Biol. Chem., **181,** 273, 1949.
123. Anderson, J. A., Bruhl, H., Michaels, A. J., and Doeden, D.: Tryptophan oxidation in phenylketonuria. Pediat. Res., **1,** 372, 1967.
124. Vassella, F., Colombo, J. P., Humbel, R., and Rossi, E.: L-Tryptophan metabolism in phenylketonuria. Helv. Paediat. Acta, **23,** 22, 1968.
125. Fellman, J. H.: Detection of phenylpyruvic oligophrenia. J. Nerv. Ment. Dis., **123,** 575, 1956.
126. Berry, J. P., and Woolf, L. I.: Estimation of phenylpyruvic acid. Nature (London), **169,** 202, 1952.
127. Saifer, A., and Harris, A.: Studies on the photometric determination of phenylpyruvic acid in urine. Clin. Chem., **5,** 203, 1959.
128. Woolf, L. I.: Tests for phenylketonuria. Cereb. Palsy J., **3,** 249, 1961.
129. Følling, A., Closs, K., and Gamnes, T.: Vorläufige Schlussfolgerungen aus Belastungversuchen mit Phenylalanin an Menschen und Tieren. Z. Physiol. Chem., **256,** 1, 1938.
130. Stein, W. H., Bearn, A. G., and Moore, S.: The amino acid content of the blood and urine in Wilson's disease. J. Clin. Invest., **33,** 410, 1954.
131. Evered, D. F.: The excretion of amino acids by the human. Biochem. J., **62,** 416, 1956.
132. Stein, W. H., and Moore, S.: The free amino acids of human blood plasma. J. Biol. Chem., **211,** 915, 1954.
133. Linneweh, F., and Ehrlich, M.: Zur Pathogenese des Schwachsinns bein Phenylketonurie. Klin. Wschr., **40,** 225, 1962.
134. Knox, W. E., and Messinger, E.: The detection of the metabolic effect of the recessive gene for phenylketonuria. Amer. J. Hum. Genet., **10,** 53, 1958.
135. Hier, S. W., and Bergeim, O.: The microbiological determination of certain free amino acids in human and dog plasma. J. Biol., Chem., **163,** 129, 1946.
136. Harper, H. A., Hutchin, M. E., and Kimmel, J. R.: Concentrations of 19 amino acids in plasma and urine of fasting normal males. Proc. Soc. Exp. Biol. Med., **80,** 768, 1952.
137. Berry, H., Sutherland, B. S., and Guest, G. M.: Phenylalanine tolerance tests on relatives of phenylketonuric children. Amer. J. Hum. Genet., **9,** 310, 1957.
138. McCaman, M. W., and Robins, E.: Fluorimetric method for the determination of phenylalanine in serum. J. Lab. Clin. Med., **59,** 885, 1962.
139. Borek, E., Brecher, A., Jervis, G. A., and Waelsch, H.: Oligophrenia phenylpyruvica: constancy of the metabolic error. Proc. Soc. Exp. Biol. Med., **75,** 86, 1950.
140. Partington, M. W., and Lewis, E. J. M.: Variations with age in plasma phenylalanine and tyrosine levels in phenylketonuria. J. Pediat., **62,** 348, 1963.
141. Brown, D. M., Armstrong, M. D., and Smith, E. D.: Studies on phenylketonuria. IV. Serum proteins in phenylketonuria. Proc. Soc. Exp. Biol. Med., **89,** 367, 1955.
142. Jervis, G. A.: Excretion of phenylalanine and derivatives in phenylpyruvic oligophrenia. Proc. Soc. Exp. Biol. Med., **75,** 83, 1950.
143. Jervis, G. A.: Studies on phenylpyruvic oligophrenia: phenylpyruvic acid content of blood. Proc. Soc. Exp. Biol. Med., **81,** 715, 1952.
144. Pare, C. M. B., Sandler, M., and Stacey, R. S.: Decreased 5-hydroxytryptophan decarboxylase activity in phenylketonuria. Lancet, **2,** 1099, 1958.
145. Berry, H. K., Umbarger, B., and Livingston, B.: Excretion of phenylalanine by normal children and by patients with phenylketonuria. J. Pediat., **63,** 954, 1963.
146. Goldstein, F. B.: Studies on phenylketonuria. II. The excretion of N-acetyl-L-phenylalanine in phenylketonuria. Biochim. Biophys. Acta, **71,** 204, 1963.
147. Armstrong, M. C., Shaw, K. N. F., and Robinson, K. S.: Studies on phenylketonuria. II. The excretion of *o*-hydroxyphenylacetic acid in phenylketonuria. J. Biol. Chem., **213,** 797, 1955.
148. Schreier, K., and Flaig, H.: Urinary excretion of indole-pyruvic acid in normal conditions and in Følling's disease. Klin. Wschr., **34,** 1213, 1956.

149. Armstrong, M. D., and Robinson, K. S.: On the excretion of indole derivatives in phenylketonuria. Arch. Biochem., **52**, 287, 1954.
150. Bessman, S. P., and Tada, K.: Indicanuria in phenylketonuria. Metabolism, **9**, 377, 1960.
151. Woolf, L. I.: Excretion of conjugated phenylacetic acid in phenylketonuria. Biochem. J., **49**, ix, 1951.
152. Bickel, H. Boscott, R. J., and Gerrard, J.: Observations on the biochemical error in phenylketonuria and its dietary control, in *Biochemistry of the Developing Nervous System,* edited by H. Waelsch, p. 417. Academic, New York, 1955.
153. Armstrong, M. D., Low, N. L., and Bosma, J. F.: Studies on phenylketonuria. IX. Further observations on the effect of phenylalanine-restricted diet on patients with phenylketonuria. Amer. J. Clin. Nutri., **5**, 543, 1957.
154. Henry, R. J., Sobel, C., and Chiamori, N.: Method for determination of serum phenylalanine with use of the Kapeller-Adler reaction. A.M.A. J. Dis. Child., **94**, 604, 1957.
155. Zahn, H., and Marstaller, H.: Phenylalanine in serum. Z. Physiol. Chem., **310**, 44, 1958.
156. Weil-Malherbe, H.: The concentration of adrenaline in human plasma and its relation to mental activity. J. Ment. Sci., **101**, 733, 1955.
157. Mitoma, C., Posner, H. S., Bogdanski, D. F., and Udenfriend, S.: Biochemical and pharmacological studies on *o*-tyrosine and its meta- and para-analogues; a suggestion concerning phenylketonuria. J. Pharmacol. Exp. Ther., **120**, 188, 1957.
158. Perry, T. L., Shaw, K. N. F., and Walker, D.: Apparent absence of amines in cerebrospinal fluid of phenylketonurics. Nature (London), **189**, 926, 1961.
159. Oates, J. A., Nirenberg, P. Z., Jepson, J. B., Sjoerdsma, A., and Udenfriend, S.: Conversion of phenylalanine to phenylethylamine in patients with phenylketonuria. Proc. Soc. Exp. Biol. Med., **112**, 1078, 1963.
160. Low, N. L., Armstrong, M. D., and Carlisle, J. W.: Phenylketonuria: two unusual cases. Lancet, **2**, 917, 1956.
161. Zeller, E. A.: Isolierung von Phenylmilchsäure und Phenyltraubensäure aus Harn bei Imbecillitas phenylpyruvica. Helv. Chim. Acta, **26**, 1614, 1943.
162. Fowler, D. I., Norton, P. M., Cheung, M. W., and Pratt, E. L.: Observations on urinary amino acid excretion in man: the influence of age and diet. Arch. Biochem., **68**, 452, 1957.
163. Grümer, H.-D.: Formation of hippuric acid from phenylalanine labelled with carbon-14 in phenylketonuric subjects. Nature (London), **189**, 63, 1961.
164. Jepson, J. B.: Paper chromatography of urinary indoles. Lancet, **2**, 1009, 1955.
165. Ferrari, V., Campagnari, F., and Guida, A: Oligofrenia fenilpiruvica: nuovi reperti chimicopathologici. Minerva Med., **46**, 119, 1955.
166. Pare, C. M. B., Sandler, M., and Stacey, R. S.: The relationship between decreased 5-hydroxyindole metabolism and mental defect in phenylketonuria. Arch. Dis. Child., **34**, 422, 1959.
167. Stein, W. H., Paladini, A. C., Hirs, C. H., and Moore, S.: Phenylacetylglutamine as a constituent of normal human urine. J. Amer. Chem. Soc., **76**, 2848, 1954.
168. Knox, W. E.: Phenylketonuria, in *The Metabolic Basis of Inherited Disease,* 2d ed., edited by J. B. Stanbury, J. B. Wyngaarden, and D. S. Fredrickson, p. 258. McGraw-Hill, New York, 1966.
169. Doolan, P. D., Harper, H. A., Hutchin, M. E., and Shruve, W. W.: Renal clearance of 18 individual amino acids in human subjects. J. Clin. Invest., **34**, 1247, 1955.
170. Russo, H. F., Wright, L. D., Skeggs, H. R., Tillson, E. K., and Beyer, K. H.: Renal clearances of essential amino acids: threonine and phenylalanine. Proc. Soc. Exp. Biol. Med., **65**, 215, 1947.
171. Berry, H. K., Sutherland, B. S., Guest, G. M., and Umbarger, B.: Chemical and clinical observation during treatment of children with phenylketonuria. Pediatrics, **21**, 929, 1958.
172. Cullen, A. M., and Knox, W. E.: *o*-Hydroxyphenylacetic acid excretion in the phenylalanine tolerance test for carriers of phenylketonuria. Proc. Soc. Exp. Biol. Med., **99**, 219, 1958.
173. Moss, A. R., and Schoenheimer, R.: The conversion of phenylalanine to tyrosine in normal rats. J. Biol. Chem., **135**, 415, 1940.
174. Udenfriend, S.: The hydroxylation of phenylalanine and antipyrine in phenylpyruvic oligophrenia. J. Biol. Chem., **203**, 961, 1953.
175. Grümer, H.-D., Koblet, H., and Woodard, C.: Phenylalanine metabolism in the phenylpyruvic condition. II. An attempt to calculate the daily incorporation of phenylalanine into proteins. J. Clin. Invest., **41**, 61, 1962.
176. Kaufman, S.: Phenylalanine hydroxylation cofactor in phenylketonuria. Science, **128**, 1506, 1958.
177. Mitoma, C., Auld, R. M., and Udenfriend, S.: On the nature of enzymic defect in phenylpyruvic oligophrenia. Proc. Soc. Exp. Biol. Med., **94**, 634, 1957.
178. Wallace, H. W., Moldave, K., and Meister, A.: Studies on conversion of phenylalanine to tyrosine in phenylpyruvic oligophrenia. Proc. Soc. Exp. Biol. Med., **94**, 632, 1957.
179. Kaufman, S.: On the structure of the phenylalanine hydroxylation cofactor. J. Biol. Chem., **237**, 2712, 1962.
180. Kenney, F. T., Reem, G. H., and Kretchmer, N.: Development of phenylalanine hydroxylase in mammalian liver. Science, **127**, 86, 1958.
181. Freedland, R. A.: Factors affecting the activity *in vitro* of the tryptophan- and phenylalanine-hydroxylating systems. Biochim. Biophys. Acta, **73**, 71, 1963.
182. Renson, J., Weissbach, H., and Udenfriend, S.: Hydroxylation of tryptophan by phenylalanine hydroxylase. J. Biol. Chem., **237**, 2261, 1962.
183. Bowman, G. H., and King, F. J.: Effects of glutamine and asparagine supplements in the dietary regimen of three phenylketonuric patients. Nature (London), **190**, 417, 1961.
184. Meister, A., Udenfriend, S., and Bessman, S. P.: Diminished phenylketonuria in phenylpyruvic oligophrenia after administration of L-glutamine, L-glutamate, or L-asparagine. J. Clin. Invest., **35**, 619, 1956.
185. Lin, E. C. C., Pitt, B. M., Civen, M., and Knox, W. E.: The assay of aromatic amino acid transaminations and keto acid oxidation by the enol borate-tautomerase method. J. Biol. Chem., **233**, 668, 1958.
186. Jacoby, G. A., and LaDu, B. N.: Nonspecificity of tyrosine transaminase: an explanation for the simultaneous induction of tyrosine, phenylalanine, and tryptophan transaminase activities in rat liver. Biochem. Biophys. Res. Commun., **8**, 352, 1962.
187. Lin, E. C. C., and Knox, W. E.: Specificity of the adaptive response of tyrosine-α-ketoglutarate transaminase in the rat. J. Biol. Chem., **233**, 1186, 1958.
188. Auerbach, V. H., and Waisman, H. A.: Tryptophan peroxidase-oxidase, histidase and transaminase activity in the liver of the developing rat. J. Biol. Chem., **234**, 304, 1959.
189. Armstrong, M. D., Centerwall, W. R., Horner, F. A., Low, N. L., and Weil, W. B.: The development of biochemical abnormalities in phenylketonuric infants, in *Chemical Pathology of the Nervous System,* edited by J. Folch-Pi, p. 38. Pergamon, New York, 1961.
190. Haavaldsen, R.: Transamination of aromatic amino-acids in nervous tissue. Nature (London), **196**, 577, 1962.
191. Appel, S. H.: Inhibition of brain protein synthesis: an approach to the biochemical basis of neurological dysfunction in the amino acidurias. Trans. N.Y. Acad. Sci., **29**, 63, 1966.
192. Bickis, I. J., Kennedy, J. P., and Quastel, J. H.: Phenylalanine inhibition of tyrosine metabolism in the liver. Nature (London), **179**, 1124, 1957.
193. Christensen, H. N.: Amino acid metabolism. Ann. Rev. Biochem., **22**, 235, 1953.
194. Linneweh, F., and Ehrlich, M.: Die renalen und prärenalen Störungen des Aminosäuren-stoffwechsels bei phenylalaninearmer Ernährung. Klin. Wschr., **38**, 904, 1960.
195. Chirigos, M. A., Greengard, P., and Udenfriend, S.: The uptake of tyrosine by rat brain *in vivo.* J. Biol. Chem., **235**, 2075, 1960.
196. Guroff, G., King, W., and Udenfriend, S: The uptake of tyrosine by rat brain *in vitro.* J. Biol. Chem., **236**, 1773, 1961.
197. Neame, K. D.: Phenylalanine as inhibitor of transport of amino-acids in brain. Nature (London), **192**, 173, 1961.

198. McKean, C. M., Schanberg, S. M., and Giarman, N. J.: A mechanism of the indole defect in experimental phenylketonuria. Science, **137**, 604, 1962.
199. Grümer, H.-D., Koblet, H., and Woodard, C.: Phenylalanine metabolism in the phenylpyruvic condition. I. Distribution, pool size, and turnover rate in human phenylketonuria. J. Clin. Invest., **40**, 1758, 1961.
200. Linneweh, F., Ehrlich, M., Graul, E. H., and Hundeshagen, H.: Über den Aminosäuren-transport bein phenylketonurischer Oligophrenie. Klin. Wschr., **41**, 253, 1963.
201. Knox, W. E.: Pathogenetic effects of elevated plasma phenylalanine in phenylketonuria, in *Chemical Pathology of the Nervous System,* edited by J. Folch-Pi, p. 32. Pergamon, New York, 1961.
202. Menkes, J. H.: The effect of branched-chain alpha-keto acids on the utilization of other branched-chain compounds by *Lactobacillus casei:* a suggestion for the mechanism of central nervous system damage in maple syrup disease and phenylketonuria. Neurology, **12**, 860, 1962.
203. Langdell, J. I.: Phenylketonuria (eight year evaluation of treatment). Arch. Gen. Psychiat., **12**, 363, 1965.
204. Poser, C. M.: Ten-year follow-up of treatment of two phenylketonuric brothers. Arch. Neurol., **16**, 658, 1967.
205. Dancis, J., and Balis, M. E.: A possible mechanism for disturbance in tyrosine metabolism in phenylpyruvic oligophrenia. Pediatrics, **15**, 63, 1955.
206. Miyamoto, M., and Fitzpatrick, T. B.: Competitive inhibition of mammalian tyrosinase by phenylalanine and its relationship to hair pigmentation in phenylketonuria. Nature (London), **179**, 199, 1957.
207. Snyderman, S. E., Norton, P., and Holt, L. E., Jr.: Effect of tyrosine administration in phenylketonuria. Fed. Proc., **14**, 450, 1955.
208. Boylen, J. B., and Quastel, J. H.: Effects of phenylalanine and sodium phenylpyruvate on the formation of melanin from L-tyrosine in melanoma. Nature (London), **193**, 376, 1962.
209. Allen, D. W., and Schroeder, W. A.: A comparison of the phenylalanine content of hemoglobin of normal and phenylketonuric individuals determined by ion exchange chromatography. J. Clin. Invest., **36**, 1343, 1957.
210. Himwich, H. E., and Fazekas, J. F.: Cerebral metabolism in mongolian idiocy and phenylpyruvic oligophrenia. A.M.A. Arch. Neurol. Psychiat., **44**, 1213, 1940.
211. Himwich, H. E., and Fazekas, J. F.: Cerebral arterio-venous oxygen difference. II. Mental deficiency. A.M.A. Arch. Neurol. Psychiat., **51**, 73, 1944.
212. Auerbach, V. H., Waisman, H. A., and Wycoff, L. B.: Phenylketonuria in the rat associated with decreased temporal discrimination learning. Nature (London), **182**, 871, 1958.
213. Waisman, H. A., Wang, H. L., Palmer, G., and Harlow, H. F.: Phenylketonuria in infant monkeys. Nature (London), **188**, 1124, 1960.
214. Yuwiler, A., and Louttit, R. T.: Effects of phenylalanine diet on brain serotonin in the rat. Science, **134**, 831, 1961.
215. Coleman, D. L.: Phenylalanine hydroxylase activity in dilute and nondilute strains of mice. Arch. Biochem., **91**, 300, 1960.
216. Karrer, R., and Cahilly, G.: Experimental attempts to produce phenylketonuria in animals: a critical review. Psychol. Bull., **64**, 52, 1965.
217. Lipton, M. A., Gordon, R., Guroff, G., and Udenfriend, S.: *p*-Chlorophenylalanine-induced chemical manifestations of phenylketonuria in rats. Science, **156**, 248, 1967.
218. Dolan, G., and Godin, C.: Phenylketonuria in rats: a model for biochemical studies. Nature (London), **213**, 916, 1967.
219. McKean, C. M., Schanberg, S. M., and Giarman, N. J.: Aminoacidemias: effects on maze performance and cerebral serotonin. Science, **157**, 213, 1967.
220. Polidora, V. J., Cunningham, R. F., and Waisman, H. A.: Dosage parameters of a behavioral deficit associated with phenylketonuria in rats. J. Comp. Physiol. Psychol., **61**, 436, 1966.
221. Zannoni, V. G., Weber, W. E., Van Valen, P., Rubin, A., Berstein, R., and LaDu, B. N.: Phenylalanine metabolism and "phenylketonuria" in dilute-lethal mice. Genetics, **54**, 1391, 1966.
222. Centerwall, S. A., and Centerwall, W. R.: The discovery of phenylketonuria, in *Phenylketonuria,* edited by F. L. Lyman, p. 3. Charles C Thomas, Springfield, Ill., 1963.
223. Mardens, Y., Dumon, J., Hayez, F., Vrydagh, S., Cools, A., and Myle, G.: Observation de deux paires de jumeaux monozygotiques atteints de phenylcetonurie. J. Genet. Hum., **16**, 42, 1967.
224. Herrlin, K. M.: A clinician and electroencephalographic study of a pair of monozygotic twins with phenylketonuria. Acta Paediat., **51**, 88, 1962.
225. Szabó, L., Durkó, I., Nagy, M. E., and Obál, F.: Biochemische und EEG-Untersuchungen bei einem an Phenylketonurie leideuden eineiigen Zwillingspaar. Acta Paediat. Acad. Sci. Hung., **6**, 227, 1965.
226. Thompson, T. H.: Relatives of phenylketonuric patients. J. Ment. Defic. Res., **1**, 67, 1957.
227. Renwick, J. H., Lawler, S. D., and Cowie, V. A.: Phenylketonuria: a linkage study using phenylalanine tolerance tests. Amer. J. Hum. Genet., **12**, 287, 1960.
228. Frankenburg, W. K., Duncan, B. R., Dofflet, R. W., Koch, R., Coldwell, J. G., and Son, C. D.: Maternal phenylketonuria: implications for growth and development. J. Pediat., **73**, 560, 1968.
229. Mabry, C. C., Denniston, J. C., and Coldwell, J. G.: Mental retardation in children of phenylketonuric mothers. New Eng. J. Med., **275**, 1331, 1966.
230. Blumenthal, M. D.: Mental illness in parents of phenylketonuric children. J. Psychiat. Res., **5**, 59, 1967.
231. King, C. G.: Discussion of paper by G. A. Jervis (ref. 12).
232. Følling, A., and Closs, K.: Über das Vorkommen von L-Phenylalanin in Harn und Blut bei Imbecillitas phenylpyruvica. Z. Physiol. Chem., **254**, 115, 1938.
233. Waelsch, H.: Discussion of L. S. Penrose, Biochemical genetics as an approach to mental disease and defect, in *Biochemistry of the Developing Nervous System,* edited by H. Waelsch, p. 414. Academic, New York, 1955.
234. Hsia, D. Y.-Y., Knox, W. E., and Paine, R. S.: A case of phenylketonuria with borderline intelligence. A.M.A. J. Dis. Child., **94**, 33, 1957.
235. Jervis, G. A.: Detection of heterozygotes for phenylketonuria. Clin. Chem. Acta, **5**, 471, 1960.
236. Hsia, D. Y.-Y., and Steinberg, A. G.: Studies on linkage between phenylketonuria and the blood groups. Amer. J. Hum. Genet., **12**, 277, 1960.
237. Woolf, L. I., Cranston, W. I., and Goodwin, B. L.: Genetics of phenylketonuria. Nature (London), **213**, 882, 1967.
238. Woolf, L. I., Goodwin, B. L., Cranston, W. I., Wade, D. N., Woolf, F., Hudson, F. P., and McBean, M. S.: The third allele at the phenylalanine-hydroxylase locus in mild phenylketonuria (hyperphenylalaninaemia). Lancet, **1**, 114, 1968.
239. Woolf, L. I.: Mass screening of the newborn for metabolic disease. Arch. Dis. Child., **43**, 137, 1968.
240. Hill, J. B., Summer, G. K., Pender, M. W., and Roszel, N. O.: An automated procedure for blood phenylalanine. Clin. Chem., **11**, 541, 1965.
241. Bremer, H. J., Tosberg, P., and Hönscher, U.: Untersuchungen über die Tyrosin-Stoffwechselstörung Frühgeborener. Ann Paediat., **206**, 12, 1966.
242. Hsia, D. Y.-Y.: Phenylketonuria, 1967. Develop. Med. Child. Neurol., **9**, 531, 1967.
243. Meyer, H., Mertz, E. T., Stadler, H. E., Leland, H., and Calandro, J.: Psychometabolic changes in phenylketonuria treated with low-phenylalanine diet. A.M.A. Arch. Intern. Med., **101**, 1094, 1958.
244. Kennedy, J. L., Wortelecki, W., Gates, L., Sperry, B. P., and Cass, V. M.: The early treatment of phenylketonuria. Amer. J. Dis. Child., **113**, 16, 1967.
245. Centerwall, W. R., Centerwall, S. A., Acosta, P. B., and Chinnock, R. F.: Phenylketonuria. I. Dietary management of infants and young children. J. Pediat., **59**, 93, 1961.
246. Berry, H. K., Sutherland, B. S., Umbarger, B., and O'Grady, D.: Treatment of phenylketonuria. Amer. J. Dis. Child., **113**, 2, 1967.
247. Murphy, D.: The dietetic treatment of phenylketonuria. Irish J. Med. Sci., **391**, 335, 1958.

248. Knox, W. E.: An evaluation of the treatment of phenylketonuria with diets low in phenylalanine. Pediatrics, **26,** 1, 1960.
249. Brimblecombe, F. S. W., Blainey, J. D., Stoneman, M. E. R., and Wood, B. S. B.: Dietary biochemical control of phenylketonuria. Brit. Med. J., **2,** 793, 1961.
250. Baumeister, A. A.: Effects of dietary control on intelligence in phenylketonuria. Amer. J. Ment. Defic., **71,** 840, 1967.
251. Knox, W. E., and Kang, E. S.: Excess of males among false positives screened for phenylketonuria. New Eng. J. Med. **283,** 102, 1970.
252. McKean, C. M., and Peterson, N. A.: Glutamine in the phenylketonuric central nervous system. New Eng. J. Med. **283,** 1364, 1970.
253. Knox, W. E.: What's new in PKU. New Eng. J. Med. **283,** 1404, 1970.

CHAPTER TWELVE

TYROSINOSIS AND TYROSINEMIA*

Bert N. La Du and Leiv R. Gjessing

During the past 45 years a number of hereditary metabolic disorders have been observed that have been characterized by abnormalities in the metabolism of tyrosine and the excretion of tyrosyl compounds in the urine.

In 1927, Medes et al. [1, 71] found an unusual reducing substance in the urine of a patient with myasthenia gravis. The reducing compound was later isolated and identified as *p*-hydroxyphenylpyruvic acid, the α-keto acid of tyrosine, and this condition was named *tyrosinosis* by Medes [2]. Other patients with myasthenia gravis were not found to excrete *p*-hydroxyphenylpyruvic acid, and no particular clinical symptoms were observed in the tyrosinosis patient which could be attributed to the excretion of the α-keto acid. Without doubt, tyrosinosis must be a very rare disease. A search for additional cases made by Blatherwick among more than twenty thousand persons with a weakly positive reduction test result for glucose in the urine failed to uncover any additional cases [3].

Other familial disorders of tyrosine metabolism associated with cirrhosis of the liver and defective renal tubular reabsorption have been reported and given the name *hereditary tyrosinemia, atypical tyrosinosis, genuine tyrosyluria,* or simply, *tyrosinemia.* While there are enough cases with common features to describe acute and chronic forms of a reasonably well-defined "disease," it would be preferable to continue to use less precise terms, such as *symptom-complex* and *syndrome.* We still are not sure that these patients share a common biochemical deficiency, nor that the primary genetic defect affects one of the enzymes of tyrosine catabolism. The obvious disturbance in tyrosine metabolism may be secondary to some other, undiscovered hereditary disorder. We will first consider the interesting studies on the patient with tyrosinosis and then review the more complicated status of hereditary tyrosinemia.

METABOLIC STUDIES IN A TYROSINOSIS PATIENT

It is indeed fortunate that the unique case of tyrosinosis was in the hands of the capable investigator Grace Medes; her classic paper in 1932 [2] still remains the key source of information on this disease. The patient with tyrosinosis was a male Russian Jew, 49 years old at the time. Initial metabolic balance studies clearly showed that the excretion of *p*-hydroxyphenylpyruvic acid and the other tyrosine metabolites increased proportionately to increases in dietary phenylalanine and tyrosine. The pattern of urinary metabolites found after placing the patient on various dietary and experimental feeding regimens is given in Table 12-1.

*The authors are grateful to Dr. Sverre Halvorsen for his help in preparing this chapter.

It should be noted that *p*-hydroxyphenylpyruvic acid was excreted continually, even during fasting or on a diet of very low tyrosine content. Under both these conditions, about 1.6 gm of the α-keto acid was excreted per day. Medes pointed out that this is a reasonable figure for the amount expected from tyrosine derived from the catabolism of endogenous protein, and she concluded that the metabolic defect was essentially complete. When the patient was placed on a regular diet, the amount of urinary *p*-hydroxyphenylpyruvic acid doubled, and tyrosine could then also be isolated from the urine. At still higher levels of tyrosine intake, *p*-hydroxyphenyllactic acid was also excreted.

One of the most remarkable findings in the studies with this patient was the observation that feeding large amounts of tyrosine also led to the excretion of 3,4-dihydroxyphenylalanine (dopa). In fact, the identification of dopa in the urine of this patient has been cited as one of the most convincing pieces of evidence that dopa is a normal metabolic product of phenylalanine and tyrosine in the higher animals [5]. It is assumed that in tyrosinosis the main pathway for tyrosine metabolism is blocked, and therefore much more of this amino acid must be metabolized by alternative pathways than under normal conditions.

On the basis of the metabolites excreted in the urine of this patient, and in order to emphasize the excretion of *p*-hydroxyphenylpyruvic acid, perhaps a more appropriate name for this condition would be "tyrosyluria" [6]. One might refer to the case described by Medes as one of *essential* or *idiopathic tyrosyluria,* to distinguish it from a number of other conditions in which tyrosyluria has been observed, such as scurvy [7–9], pernicious anemia [10], and a variety of other diseases [11].

Spontaneous excretion of *p*-hydroxyphenylpyruvic acid was reported by Felix et al. [12] in two patients with liver diseases and a splenectomy. In these patients, however, the amount of the α-keto acid excreted was regularly less than 50 mg per day, and the amount exceeded this value only slightly when extra tyrosine was fed. Although the excretion of the α-keto acid in these patients is of considerable theoretical interest, the amount excreted is much less than that found in the patient studied by Medes. It is a different type of metabolic abnormality and should not be classed as an additional case of tyrosinosis [6].

On the basis of the pattern of the urinary metabolites found in the urine of this patient, Medes proposed that the metabolic defect in tyrosinosis was a failure of the enzymatic step in which *p*-hydroxyphenylpyruvic acid is oxidized to homogentisic acid [2, 71]. It was believed that the excretion of *p*-hydroxyphenylpyruvic acid represented an inability to metabolize this α-keto acid and that as a consequence of this defect the earlier steps were also partially impaired, thus leading to the excretion of the closely related compounds

Table 12-1. METABOLIC STUDIES WITH TYROSINOSIS PATIENT

Diet and supplement	Compounds excreted in the urine			
	p-Hydroxyphenylpyruvic acid, gm/day	Tyrosine, gm/day	*p*-Hydroxyphenyllactic acid, gm/day	3,4-Dihydroxyphenylalanine
Fasting	1.54	0	0	0
Tyrosine-free diet	1.64, 1.43	0	0	0
Mixed hospital diet	2.8	0.38	0	0
High-protein diet	3.2	0.80	Trace	0
High-protein diet + 15 gm L-tyrosine	4.64	2.17	0.32	+ Urine turned black with alkali
High-protein diet + 15 gm L-tyrosine	5.17	2.52	0.73	+ 30 mg dopa isolated
Tyrosine-free diet + 2 gm *p*-hydroxyphenyllactic acid	No increase	0	1.78 (4 days)	0
Tyrosine-free diet + 4 gm *p*-hydroxyphenylpyruvic acid on 2 consecutive days	Immediate increase, continued for several days	0	Increase after 2 days for several days	0
Tyrosine-free diet + 2 gm L-3,4-dihydroxyphenylalanine	Delayed increase, maximum on 4th day*	0.100†	0	Nearly 0.800 gm recovered (incomplete)

*The unusual 2-day delay before an increase in *p*-hydroxyphenylpyruvic acid was found and the rapid rate at which dopa is known to be metabolized [4] suggest that this increase may have been due to variation in the dietary intake of tyrosine rather than the test substance.

†It was suggested that the oxidation of tyrosine to dopa is reversible since some tyrosine was excreted after feeding dopa, but this is not supported by more recent studies [8]. Dehydroxylation of dopa to meta-tyrosine has been reported in rabbits [13] but not in man [5].

Source: G. Medes [2].

when extra tyrosine was fed. The demonstration that administered homogentisic acid was metabolized completely, even when given in relatively large amounts, indicated that the defect must be located earlier in the pathway of tyrosine metabolism than it is in alcaptonuria (see Chap. 13).

The general scheme of tyrosine metabolism has undergone relatively little modification in recent years, but the component enzymatic steps have been isolated and intensively investigated [14]. Therefore, it is of interest to look again at the evidence upon which these interpretations were made over 40 years ago and see whether, in view of present understanding of the metabolic pathway, the same conclusions would be reached today.

BIOCHEMICAL ASPECTS

Recent progress in understanding the metabolism of phenylalanine and tyrosine has been largely due to the successful isolation and purification of the enzymes catalyzing each of the reactions. The enzymatic steps pertinent to this discussion are summarized in Fig. 12-1. Since several excellent reviews summarize these reactions [6–8, 14–16], only a few points will be mentioned here. It is clear that most of the phenylalanine ingested is catabolized via its oxidation to tyrosine and that this hydroxylation step is essentially irreversible. For this reason, experiments carried out with administered phenylalanine should be equivalent to those in which tyrosine is given if the defect under study involves one of the steps in tyrosine metabolism.

The main pathway for tyrosine metabolism in mammals is indicated in Fig. 12-1. The first step, a transamination reaction with α-ketoglutarate to yield *p*-hydroxyphenylpyruvic acid, appears to be the rate-limiting step of the tyrosine oxidation pathway [17, 18]. At present, it is believed that most of the *p*-hydroxyphenylpyruvic acid derived from tyrosine is formed via transamination. This transamination reaction is catalyzed by a specific transaminase which has been purified from dog liver [19, 20], and from rat liver [21, 22]. Pyridoxal phosphate is the coenzyme, and neither pyruvate nor oxaloacetate can replace the requirement for α-ketoglutarate. The enzyme is not specific for L-tyrosine. Activity is found with phenylalanine, 3,4-dihydroxyphenylalanine, tryptophan, and several tyrosine analogues [23]. The transaminase is inhibited by sulfhydryl reagents such as iodoacetate and *p*-chloromercuriphenylsulfonate, but it is not inhibited by metal-binding agents such as α,α'-dipyridyl, diethyldithiocarbamate, and 8-hydroxyquinoline.

The next enzyme, *p*-hydroxyphenylpyruvic acid oxidase, is the one proposed by Medes as defective in tyrosinosis. It catalyzes the oxidation of *p*-hydroxyphenylpyruvic acid to homogentisic acid and is present in the liver of various

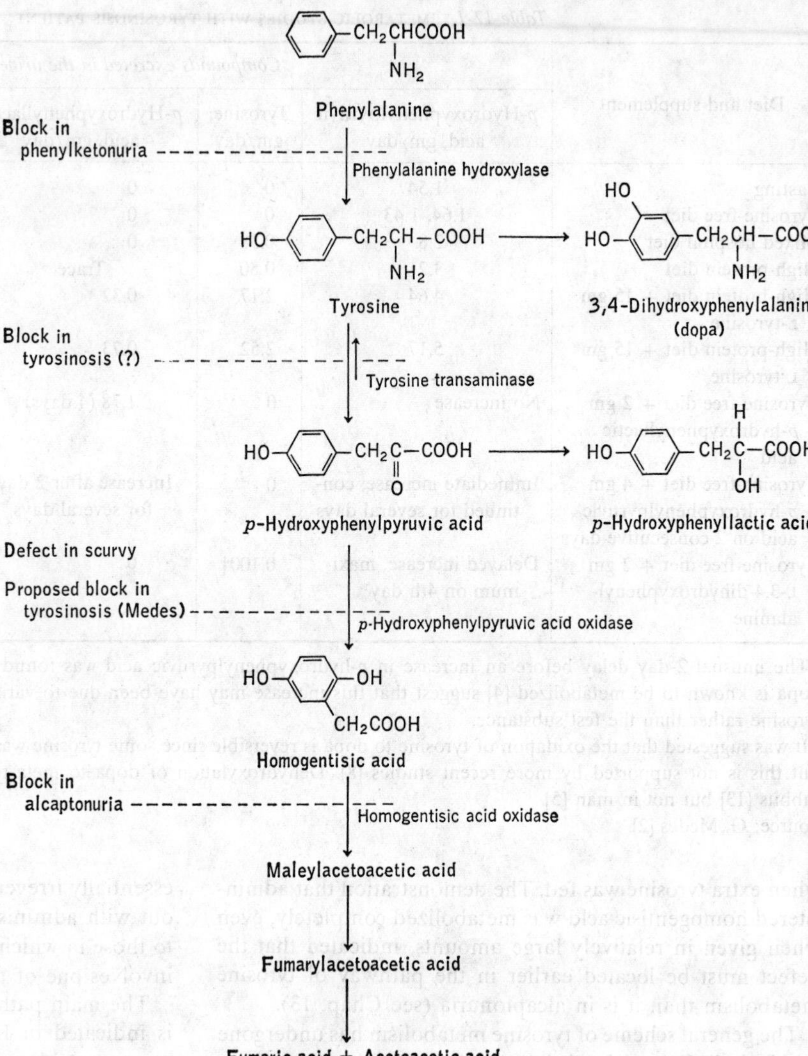

Figure 12-1. Metabolic blocks in the oxidation of phenylalanine and tyrosine.

mammalian species, including hog, rabbit, rat, dog, and man. It has also been detected, though with lower activity, in the kidney of some of, if not all, these species. Purified *p*-hydroxyphenylpyruvic acid oxidase has been prepared from beef [24], pig [24, 25], and dog liver [26–28], and properties of the purified enzyme have been described. The conversion of phenylpyruvate to *o*-hydroxyphenylacetic acid may be catalyzed by this enzyme [29], and the ratio of phenylpyruvate oxidase and *p*-hydroxyphenylpyruvate oxidase activities remains constant during purification [30].

The conversion of *p*-hydroxyphenylpyruvic acid to homogentisic acid requires two atoms of oxygen and the liberation of one molecule of CO_2. The reaction is complex; it involves hydroxylation of the aromatic ring, migration of the side chain, and oxidation and decarboxylation of the pyruvate to an acetate side chain. No intermediary compound has been identified in this reaction; 2,5-dihydroxyphenylpyruvic acid was considered a possible intermediate in the past [31] but this acid is not a substrate for *p*-hydroxyphenylpyruvic acid oxidase [24, 26], nor is it converted to homogentisic acid when incubated with homogenates of normal human liver [18].

p-Hydroxyphenylpyruvic acid oxidase requires either ascorbic acid or one of the group of compounds which can replace the vitamin, such as the reduced form of 2,6-dichlorophenolindophenol in vitro [15]. These agents are required in considerably less than stoichiometric amounts and appear to function by preventing a gradual inhibition of the enzyme by its substrate, which would occur in the absence of the protective agent [26–28, 32], and ascorbic acid seems to act in this protective capacity in vivo [33]. Although it was proposed several years ago that ascorbic acid acted as a coenzyme for *p*-hydroxyphenylpyruvic acid oxidase [34, 35], its function in this reaction now seems to be much less specific [15, 36, 37] and unlike the coenzyme functions associated with the members of the B vitamins.

The enzyme can be inhibited by relatively low concentrations of diethyldithiocarbamate [26] and by sulfhydryl-binding agents such as p-chloromercuribenzoic acid [24]. In view of the known affinity of diethyldithiocarbamate for copper, a search has been made for this metal in the purified enzyme, but there is no evidence that it is a copper-containing protein [24, 26].

The occurrence of homogentisic acid as a normal metabolite was subject to some dispute in the past, but there is now general agreement that most of the tyrosine is degraded via p-hydroxyphenylpyruvic acid and homogentisic acid.

METABOLIC DEFECT IN TYROSINOSIS

Medes proposed [2], on the basis of the tyrosine metabolites found in the urine, that the defect in tyrosinosis must be the lack of p-hydroxyphenylpyruvic acid oxidase activity. The constant excretion of the α-keto acid, accompanied by closely related compounds, when tyrosine was fed suggested that the primary difficulty was in metabolizing this acid and that, as a consequence, the preceding steps were secondarily impaired.

It is of interest to reexamine the balance study data from the tyrosinosis patient in view of current understanding of tyrosine metabolism. There is no reason to doubt that the metabolic defect occurs early in tyrosine metabolism. There are, however, several observations not in accord with the localization of the defect at the p-hydroxyphenylpyruvic acid oxidase step. These are the finding that the predominant metabolite was p-hydroxyphenylpyruvic acid with very little p-hydroxyphenyllactic acid; the apparent completeness of the block at low levels of tyrosine intake, yet its incompleteness at moderate or high levels of tyrosine intake; and the excretion of dopa when tyrosine was fed.

There is a striking difference in the tyrosyluria found in the patient with tyrosinosis from that present in other conditions in which the excretion of p-hydroxyphenylpyruvic acid has been observed. In tyrosinosis, *only* p-hydroxyphenylpyruvic acid was excreted (except on a diet high in tyrosine), whereas in the other conditions, p-hydroxyphenyllactic acid was a major tyrosyl product in the urine. For example, premature infants fed extra tyrosine [9] were found to excrete several times as much p-hydroxyphenyllactic acid as p-hydroxyphenylpyruvic acid. Scorbutic guinea pigs [38] and children [39] also excrete appreciable quantities of the lactic derivative. This difference in the tyrosyluria was not due to an inability of the tyrosinosis patient to reduce the α-keto acid, since he excreted a small amount of p-hydroxyphenyllactic acid when the diet contained large amounts of tyrosine (Table 12-1). Furthermore, when the patient was given p-hydroxyphenylpyruvic acid, a considerable portion of it was excreted as p-hydroxyphenyllactic acid. The latter acid was isolated from the urine and found to be optically active, and it was presumed to arise by the enzymatic reduction of p-hydroxyphenylpyruvic acid. Meister [40] has reported that p-hydroxyphenylpyruvic acid is reduced by the lactic acid dehydrogenase of muscle. However, an aromatic α-keto acid reductase has been described which also catalyzes the reduction of phenylpyruvate and p-hydroxyphenylpyruvate [41, 42].

On the basis of these results, one would expect that if p-hydroxyphenylpyruvic acid were circulating in the tissues of the tyrosinosis patient, much more reduction and excretion of the lactic acid analogue would take place. It is difficult to understand why only the α-keto acid was excreted if the defect were the lack of liver p-hydroxyphenylpyruvic acid oxidase activity.

On the other hand, the urinary metabolites found in the urine in premature infants and in scorbutic guinea pigs and man are those one would expect to find with an impaired activity of liver p-hydroxyphenylpyruvic acid oxidase. Evidence that this enzyme is relatively deficient in premature infants has been obtained by Kretchmer et al. [43, 44]. It has also been recently shown that about one-half of liver p-hydroxyphenylpyruvic acid oxidase activity is inhibited by the administration of p-hydroxyphenylpyruvic acid to scorbutic guinea pigs. Under these conditions, the activities of tyrosine transaminase and homogentisic acid oxidase are not affected [33].

Attempts have been made to induce experimental tyrosinosis in guinea pigs by inhibiting p-hydroxyphenylpyruvic acid oxidase with diethyldithiocarbamate [45]. The administration of this compound results in almost complete inhibition of the oxidase in vivo. Animals so treated were injected with p-hydroxyphenylpyruvic acid intraperitoneally, and even under these conditions very little of the α-keto acid was excreted unchanged. The main tyrosyl product in the urine was p-hydroxyphenyllactic acid [46].

It appears, therefore, that in the various conditions in which liver p-hydroxyphenylpyruvic acid oxidase is known to be impaired, one finds a relatively large amount of p-hydroxyphenyllactic acid in addition to p-hydroxyphenylpyruvic acid in the urine.

In view of these observations, the different pattern of tyrosyluria found in the patient with tyrosinosis raises the possibility that this metabolic disorder may not be due to a defect in p-hydroxyphenylpyruvic acid oxidase. It also seems unlikely that p-hydroxyphenylpyruvic acid was circulating in the tissues, except when the intake of tyrosine was very high, since the ability to reduce the α-keto acid to p-hydroxyphenyllactic acid was demonstrated to be present in this patient (Table 12-1).

One possibility is that the metabolic error in tyrosinosis is much like that found in phenylketonuria, with the primary defect a failure to metabolize the amino acid in liver, even though the corresponding α-keto acid is the main abnormal urinary metabolite. If tyrosinosis were analogous to phenylketonuria, one should find a high level of circulating tyrosine but not of p-hydroxyphenylpyruvic acid. The α-keto acid, rather than tyrosine or p-hydroxyphenyllactic acid, would be the expected main metabolite in the urine, just as was found. In addition, an elevated tissue level of tyrosine would be more likely to lead to extra dopa being synthesized than would a block in the oxidation of *p*-hydroxyphenylpyruvic acid. If the keto acid which was excreted arose by the metabolism of tyrosine within the kidney (analogous to the keto acid from phenylalanine in phenylketonuria), it would not be surprising to find this mechanism saturated at moderate levels of tyrosine intake. This is in accord with the apparent incompleteness of the block when high dosages of tyrosine were given to the patient.

If another patient with tyrosinosis should ever be found, it would be particularly important to determine the plasma levels of tyrosine and *p*-hydroxyphenylpyruvic acid. Fortunately, a number of microenzymatic methods are now available for these determinations [47, 48]. The ultimate proof that a particular enzyme is missing in tyrosinosis will, of course depend upon the availability of suitable tissues from a patient with this disease.

TYROSINEMIA

The first description of tyrosinemia is that of Baber [49] in 1956. She established the clinical syndrome in a case with congenital cirrhosis of the liver, renal tubular defects with amino aciduria of a distinctive type, and vitamin D–resistant (hypophosphatemic) rickets. In 1957–59 Sakai et al. [50–52] reported on another patient with similar clinical symptoms, under the heading "an atypical case of tyrosinosis," with pronounced *p*-hydroxyphenyllactic aciduria. These investigators focused attention on the metabolism of tyrosine and found it to be abnormal. There were hypertyrosinemia, tyrosyluria, and very low activity of liver *p*-hydroxyphenylpyruvic acid oxidase.

Since then, nearly 100 cases of tyrosinemia have been reported [53–103] and the disorder has been discussed at meetings in Oslo [71–76] in 1965, and in Toronto [84–95] and Chicago [79–83] in 1966. Although presenting the same general features, the illness of these patients has been given various names, among which are *tyrosyluria* and *hypermethioninemia* in an infant with hepatic cirrhosis and nodular hyperplasia [61], *hypermethioninemia* [62, 67], *tyrosinosis* [63, 82], *tyrosinose congenitale* [77], *tyrosinemia* [72], *hereditary tyrosinemia* [81], and *inborn hepatorenal dysfunction* [74].

Clinical Features

The leading symptoms in hereditary tyrosinemia are failure to thrive, vomiting, diarrhea, enlargement of the abdomen, and dyspnea combined with hemorrhages, edema, ascites, rickets, and hepatosplenomegaly. Slight or moderate mental retardation has been noted in some of the patients, but mental deficiency is not a constant or typical feature of the disorder.

In some cases the course is more *acute* [68], and the symptoms appear during the first month of life. These patients frequently die within the first 3 to 8 months with sign of liver failure.

In other cases the course is more *chronic* [78], with a later onset and longer life-span, with or without acute exacerbations.

Laboratory Findings

The dominating symptom is rickets combined with hyperphosphaturia and hypophosphatemia due to reduced tubular reabsorption of phosphorus. Other signs of renal dysfunction are glucosuria, proteinuria, and hyperamino aciduria.

The coagulation factors produced in the liver are reduced and there is a moderate anemia. In the acute stage, shortly before death, hypoproteinemia, hyperbilirubinemia, and collapse of liver functions prevail. In the chronic phase, leukopenia and thrombocytopenia are usually present [101].

Gentz et al. [98] noted that two patients with hereditary tyrosinemia had attacks of severe pain in the abdomen and legs and a polyneuropathy which resembled crises in patients with acute intermittent porphyria. They measured the excretion of δ-aminolevulinic acid, porphobilinogen, and porphyrins in these and four other patients with tyrosinemia. The urinary δ-aminolevulinic acid was one hundred times normal, but porphobilinogen and porphyrins were within the normal range or slightly elevated. Recently, Gaull et al [104] have found elevated δ-aminolevulinic acid excretion in two of three of their tyrosinemic patients.

Histologically, the major finding is liver cirrhosis with advanced fibrosis and marked regeneration of liver cells, sometimes developing into hepatoma. The renal tubular cells are swollen and show sign of degeneration. The islands of Langerhans are hyperplastic. In the basal ganglia of the brain the astroglial cells show pathologic changes [78].

Biochemically, in the chronic phase of this disease, the serum concentration of tyrosine is elevated, and sometimes methionine is also increased. There is a generalized amino aciduria, and the pattern of the urinary amino acids is of a distinct type. The amino acids excreted in excessive amounts, in decreasing order, are tyrosine (64 to 150 times normal), proline (10 to 125), threonine (10 to 37), alanine (9 to 30), glycine (8 to 20), phenylalanine (8 to 16), α-aminobutyric acid (7 to 30), isoleucine (5 to 24), serine (5 to 8), leucine and aspartic acid (3 to 10), methionine (2 to 14), and ethanolamine (1 to 5). This pattern is very different from the Fanconi syndrome in cystinosis and in maple syrup disease [103].

The excretion of *p*-hydroxyphenolic acids is markedly increased, particularly *p*-hydroxyphenyllactic acid. The latter metabolite, as a reduced product from *p*-hydroxyphenylpyruvic acid, indicates a deficiency in *p*-hydroxyphenylpyruvate oxidase activity in these patients. This conclusion is supported by enzymatic studies of liver tissue obtained at biopsy or autopsy which show reduced activity of the above mentioned oxidase [52, 64, 66, 83] (Table 12-2). In addition, Gaull et al. [96, 104] found a reduced activity of

Table 12-2. ACTIVITY OF TYROSINE TRANSAMINASE AND *p*-HYDROXYPHENYLPYRUVATE OXIDASE IN LIVER BIOPSY SAMPLES FROM PATIENTS WITH HEREDITARY TYROSINEMIA AND CIRRHOSIS (POST-HEPATITIS)

Patient	Diagnosis	Dietary treatment‡	Source	*Tyrosine transaminase*				*p-Hydroxyphenylpyruvate oxidase*			
				Activity based on liver wet weight*	Percent of normal	Activity based on liver soluble protein†	Percent of normal	Activity based on liver wet weight*	Percent of normal	Activity based on liver soluble protein†	Percent of normal
5 yr ♂	Tyrosinemia	2 yr	Aronsson [75]	4.7	23	75.2	376	2.0	3	32	53
9 mo ♀	Tyrosinemia	3 mo	R. C. Harris	2.6	13	3.0	15	3.0	5	3.8	6
2 mo ♂	Tyrosinemia	1 mo	V. Shih	1.5	7.5	3.0	15	3.3	5.5	6.6	11
9 yr ♀	Tyrosinemia	2 yr	E. Kang	7.1	35.5	5.9	29	12.0	20	10.0	17
8 mo ♂	Tyrosinemia	3 mo	Silverberg	<0.1	No significant activity	....	....	<0.5	No significant activity	....	....
5 yr ♂	Cirrhosis (post-hepatitis)	....	R. C. Harris	4.1	20	7.2	36	4.5	7.5	8.0	13
4 yr ♂	Cirrhosis (post-hepatitis)	....	R. C. Harris	6.7	33.5	9.4	47	10.5	17.5	14.6	24
	Normal			20	100	20	100	60	100	60	100

* Activity = μmoles oxidized per hour per gm wet weight liver at 27°C.

† Activity = μmoles oxidized per hour adjusted to 12 mg soluble protein in supernatant fraction ($10{,}000 \times g$) from 10 percent liver homogenate. The 10 percent supernatant fraction from normal liver contains approximately 12 mg protein per milliliter; cirrhotic liver contains less soluble protein.

‡ Patients on diets low in phenylalanine and tyrosine before biopsy for time indicated in the table.

Source: B. N. La Du and V. G. Zannoni, previously unpublished data.

both the methionine-activating enzyme and the cystathionine synthetase, and this is consistent with the raised serum level of methionine.

In the acute stage, not only are tyrosine and methionine increased in the serum but also hydroxyproline, threonine, serine, proline, alanine, cystathionine, phenylalanine, ethanolamine and histidine [84, 103].

The amino aciduria of the acute stage is similar to that of the chronic stage, except that it is much more pronounced, and in addition to the 12 amino acids mentioned above, lysine, histidine, methylhistidines, ornithine, and hydroxyproline are excreted in increased amounts [103].

The pattern of amino acids in the serum and urine in acute hereditary tyrosinemia is very different from prolinemia, methylmalonic aciduria, homocystinuria, and maple syrup disease [103]. On the other hand, the amino acid pattern in hereditary tyrosinemia is very similar to Perry's case of hypermethioninemia [67] (which might have been a case of acute tyrosinemia).

The pattern of urinary tyrosine and phenolic acids in tyrosinemic patients is similar to that in infants with transitory hypertyrosinemia. The latter is a relatively common, benign condition in infants with low birth weight. It may be due to several causes, such as delayed development of *p*-hydroxyphenylpyruvate oxidase, increased protein load, or a deficiency of ascorbic acid. These infants, however, have no cirrhosis or renal tubular defects and their response to a phenylalanine load is also different from that of patients with hereditary tyrosinemia [99].

Although the above clinical description applies reasonably well to the majority of tyrosinemic patients, a few unusual patients should be specifically mentioned with entirely different clinical manifestations. These exceptional cases must be thought of when considering the probable relationships between the biochemical disturbances and the clinical and pathologic features of this metabolic disease.

Wadman et al. [105] investigated an 18-year-old girl who was mentally retarded and probably had tyrosinemia and tyrosyluria from birth. Plasma tyrosine was about 10 times normal and the urinary metabolites were mainly *p*-hydroxyphenyllactic acid, *p*-hydroxyphenylpyruvic acid, *p*-hydroxyphenylacetic acid, and *p*-hydroxymandelic acid. The patient developed bilateral cataracts at age 17 years but showed no indications of either liver disease or renal tubular defects. The authors concluded that *p*-hydroxyphenylpyruvic acid and its metabolites do not have toxic effects on the liver and kidney.

Another patient, a 10½-year-old boy with IQ less than 25 was studied recently in Boston [106]. His plasma tyrosine concentration varied from 16 to 25.6 mg per 100 ml, and the tyrosyluria was similar to that of the above patient. Again, there was no evidence of renal or liver disease.

A third patient, a 33-year-old man in Australia, is reported to be retarded and have an elevated serum tyrosine concentration, about 24 mg per 100 ml [107]. Studies on his urinary metabolites have not yet been completed but the Phenistix test was positive and phenylketonuria was excluded. He has no clinical features of tyrosinemia.

One patient is of particular interest. This is a 5-year-old boy with multiple congenital anomalies and mental retardation with an elevated concentration of tyrosine in the plasma (20 to 50 mg per 100 ml) who excreted large amounts of the usual tyrosyl acids and *N*-acetyltyrosine in the urine [108]. Studies on a liver biopsy sample revealed normal *p*-hydroxyphenylpyruvic acid oxidase activity and normal mitochondrial tyrosine transaminase activity. However, soluble tyrosine transaminase activity was negligible [109]. Tyrosinemia and tyrosyluria in the presence of normal liver *p*-hydroxyphenylpyruvic acid oxidase and a deficiency of soluble tyrosine transaminase may appear paradoxical, but defective tyrosine transamination in the liver would be expected to produce hypertyrosinemia, and this might favor conversion of tyrosine to *p*-hydroxyphenylpyruvic acid and additional metabolites in other tissues. Medes's case of tyrosinosis seems most likely to have been a variation of this type of enzymatic deficiency, rather than a lack of *p*-hydroxyphenylpyruvic acid oxidase, as discussed earlier.

Diagnosis

Tyrosinemia in the *chronic* stage is clearly characterized by liver cirrhosis, tyrosinemia, methioninemia, tyrosyluria with *p*-hydroxyphenyllactic acid as the major metabolite, generalized amino aciduria of a distinct type, glucosuria, proteinuria, and hyperphosphaturia with rickets.

In the *acute* stage the diagnosis is more difficult; biochemically and clinically, fructosemia closely resembles transitory hypertyrosinemia combined with liver disease [100–103]. Therefore it is necessary to differentiate one from the other by fructose, galactose, ascorbic acid, and phenylalanine loading tests [99, 102].

Treatment

In a few cases of chronic [63, 75, 76, 78–80, 101, 103] and acute [81, 82, 84, 93, 96, 97, 99] hereditary tyrosinemia, a synthetic diet, restricted in phenylalanine and tyrosine, has been given. The dietary treatment has generally been found to successfully counteract the renal tubular lesion: hyperphosphaturia, hyperamino aciduria, glucosuria, proteinuria, and the pathologic urinary sediments disappeared. Often the rickets was cured, a growth spurt occurred, and the general condition improved remarkably, with disappearance of acidosis and ascites.

Addition of tyrosine to the diet had a deleterious effect on the renal tubules, and phosphorus excretion increased [63].

The effect of the special diet on the liver is uncertain in chronic cases [63, 101], but in one acute case [97] repeated biopsies showed regression of fibrosis and infiltrations. Other acute cases [81, 82, 99] did not respond so well.

Etiology and Pathogenesis

The association of hypertyrosinemia and tyrosyluria with liver and kidney disturbances in patients with hereditary tyrosinemia has encouraged the conclusion that a hereditary deficiency of *p*-hydroxyphenylpyruvic acid oxidase accounts for both the biochemical and clinical findings. Numerous liver biopsy and autopsy reports confirm the expectation that a deficiency of the oxidase occurs in these patients. The clinical improvement in patients on a diet low in phenylalanine and tyrosine, at least as far as the renal tubular defects, supports the assumption that aromatic amino acid derivatives may exert a toxic effect on the liver and kidney, and the failure of the diet to correct all of the liver pathology has been attributed to extensive, only partly reversible pathology.

Nevertheless, there has been an increasing doubt over the past few years that the above hypothesis is correct, and suggestions have been made that the primary metabolic defect in hereditary tyrosinemia is something other than a lack of *p*-hydroxyphenylpyruvic acid oxidase. Woolf questioned the hypothesis at the symposium on tyrosinosis in Norway in 1965 [74], and the etiology was debated during the conference on hereditary tyrosinemia in Toronto in 1966 [110]. Gaull et al. [96, 104] stated that a specific deficiency of *p*-hydroxyphenylpyruvic acid oxidase is not the primary defect, and that hypermethioninemia, which occurs in some of these patients, is not due to a loss of functioning liver tissue but to the decrease in both the methionine-activating enzyme and cystathionine synthetase. They believe that all of these enzymatic deficiences are secondary manifestations of an unknown hereditary metabolic disease.

The lack of hepatic and renal pathology in infants with transitory hypertyrosinemia and tyrosyluria has been one reason to question the *p*-hydroxyphenylpyruvic acid oxidase hypothesis [74]. The finding that a few patients have had persistant hypertyrosinemia and tyrosyluria for years without signs of renal and liver disease is further evidence that the disturbance in tyrosine metabolism need not produce pathologic changes in these organs. Whether these metabolites have an adverse effect on the central nervous system is less certain, but transitory tyrosinemia seems to lead to no permanent mental impairment [120, 121]. The beneficial effects of the low phenylalanine and tyrosine diet on renal reabsorption, and the improved synthesis of proteins in the liver might both result from the removal of aromatic metabolites which further compound and aggravate the unknown metabolic disorder.

Experimental work in animals has not yet produced a model disease like hereditary tyrosinemia. Boctor and Harper [111] found that rats fed large amounts of tyrosine or *p*-hydroxyphenylpyruvic acid had hypertyrosinemia, but these treatments did not decrease liver tyrosine transaminase or *p*-hydroxyphenylpyruvic acid oxidase. Rats, of course, can synthesize ascorbic acid, and quite different results are found if excess tyrosine is fed to vitamin C–deficient guinea pigs [83]. *p*-Hydroxyphenylpyruvic acid oxidase is inhibited and hypertyrosinemia and tyrosyluria follow as a result of the reduced oxidase activity. Perry et al. [112] fed tyrosine to newborn guinea pigs on a vitamin C–deficient diet and found the expected disturbance in tyrosine metabolism without renal or hepatic pathology. However, feeding methionine produced a syndrome in some animals resembling hereditary tyrosinemia in some respects; these animals showed hypertyrosinemia, tyrosyluria, hypermethioninemia, generalized amino aciduria, hypoglycemia, and pancreatic islet cell degeneration. These experiments suggest that abnormal methionine metabolism may be an important factor and contribute to the pathologic features of hereditary tyrosinemia. On the other hand, Daniel and Waisman [113] recently studied the effect of excess methionine on the free amino acids of serum, liver, brain, and urine of weanling rats. They found only an increase of methionine, taurine, and alanine but not of tyrosine in the serum. There was an amino aciduria, but the quantitative profile of the amino acids excreted was very different from that in chronic and acute tyrosinemia [103].

It should be mentioned that patients with fructosemia show many of the same clinical and biochemical features as those with hereditary tyrosinemia, but the enzymatic defect in fructosemia is neither in tyrosine nor methionine metabolism [100–103]. Figure 12-2 is a hypothetical model of hereditary tyrosinemia, fructosemia, and galactosemia to illustrate common features in these metabolic disorders. In fructosemia [114] and in galactosemia [115] the inherited lack of specific enzymes leads to specific metabolites; in tyrosinemia the critical metabolites are still unknown. Presumably liver cirrhosis, the disturbances in tyrosine and methionine metabolism, and the renal reabsorption defects all result from the primary enzymatic disturbance and the metabolic changes it produces. Aromatic amino acid metabolites seem to intensify the renal dysfunction and bring about multiple proximal tubular reabsorption defects. These, in turn, may exaggerate liver dysfunction, and a vicious cycle is established which can be disrupted by a diet low in phenylalanine and tyrosine. Defective renal reabsorption of amino acids and other constituents might be explained by an abnormal metabolite which acts like maleic acid [116, 117], or by inhibition of enzyme systems of the kidney that provide energy for reabsorption. Liver glycogen is very low in patients with tyrosinemia, but the series of enzymes required to convert glucose to liver glycogen seem to be present [118]. In the chronic stage of tyrosinemia it is not surprising to find a reduced ability to metabolize tyrosine since cirrhosis from other causes impairs tyrosine metabolism [119].

The weight of evidence, at present, is against the *p*-hydroxyphenylpyruvic acid oxidase hypothesis, and we believe that further investigations on tyrosinemia should include a search for other possible biochemical defects which might be responsible for the clinical and pathologic features of this hereditary metabolic disease.

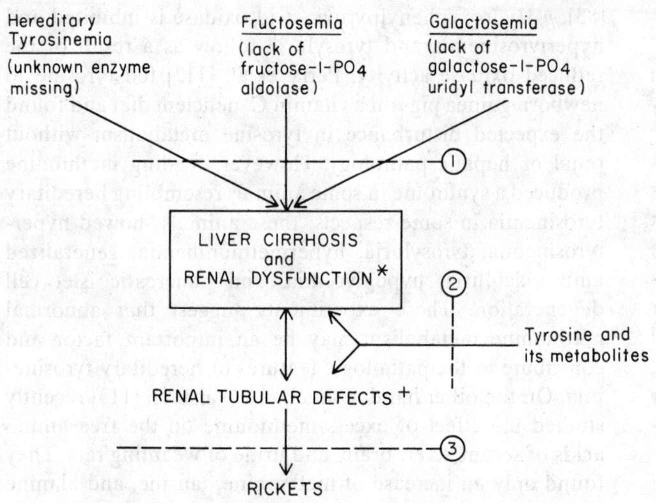

Figure 12-2. Model for the etiology and pathogenesis of hereditary tyrosinemia.

Genetic Considerations

Several investigators have shown that both acute and chronic types of tyrosinemia are inherited as an autosomal recessive trait [64, 94]. It is of interest that the estimated frequency of heterozygous carriers of tyrosinemia in the Chicoutimi region of northeastern Quebec is 5.05 percent to 3.24 percent, that is, one carrier for every 20 to 31 persons [95].

No biochemical test has been developed to detect heterozygous carriers of the disorder.

SUMMARY

1 Tyrosinosis, a rare metabolic disease of tyrosine metabolism is characterized by the excretion of *p*-hydroxyphenylpyruvic acid. Other tyrosyl metabolites are also excreted when large amounts of this amino acid are given. Only one case of the disease has ever been found and the inheritance of the condition has not been demonstrated.

2 It is generally assumed that the enzyme system defective in tyrosinosis is *p*-hydroxyphenylpyruvic acid oxidase. However, the defect may well be in the preceding step, tyrosine transaminase. Evidence supporting the localization of the defect in each of these steps is discussed.

3 The term hereditary tyrosinemia, is being applied to a disorder characterized by a complex set of clinical and laboratory findings: hepatosplenomegaly, nodular cirrhosis of the liver, abnormal tyrosine and methionine metabolism with pronounced *p*-hydroxyphenyllactic aciduria, multiple renal tubular defects with hyperphosphaturia, rickets, mellituria, proteinuria, and an amino aciduria of a distinct type. Treatment with a diet restricted in phenylalanine and tyrosine has a beneficial effect on the renal tubular defects and seems to improve the general condition of the patient.

4 The inherited enzymatic deficiency in hereditary tyrosinemia is unknown, but it is probably not in *p*-hydroxyphenylpyruvic acid oxidase and may not be in an enzyme of either tyrosine or methionine metabolism. Tyrosinemia is probably inherited as an autosomal recessive trait.

BIBLIOGRAPHY

1. Medes, G., Berglund, H., and Lohmann, A.: An unknown reducing urinary substance in myasthenia gravis. Proc. Soc. Exp. Biol. Med., **25**, 210, 1927.
2. Medes, G.: A new error of tyrosine metabolism: tyrosinosis. The intermediary metabolism of tyrosine and phenylalanine. Biochem. J., **26**, 917, 1932.
3. Blatherwick, N. R.: Tyrosinosis: a search for additional cases. J.A.M.A., **103**, 1933, 1934.
4. Axelrod, J. E.: The metabolism of adrenalin and other sympathomimetic amines. Physiol. Rev., **39**, 751, 1959.
5. Shaw, K. N. F., McMillan, A., and Armstrong, M. D.: The metabolism of 3,4-dihydroxyphenylalanine. J. Biol. Chem., **226**, 255, 1957.
6. Kretchmer, N., and Etzwiler, D. D.: Disorders associated with the metabolism of phenylalanine and tyrosine. Pediatrics, **21**, 445, 1958.
7. Dalgliesh, C. E.: Metabolism of the aromatic amino acids. Advances Protein Chem., **10**, 31, 1955.
8. Lerner, A. B.: Metabolism of phenylalanine and tyrosine. Advances Enzym., **14**, 73, 1953.
9. Levine, S. Z.: Tyrosine and phenylalanine metabolism in infants and the role of vitamin C. Harvey Lect., ser. **42**, 303, 1947.
10. Swendseid, M. E., Wandruff, B., and Bethell, F. H.: Urinary phenols in pernicious anemia. J. Lab. Clin. Med., **32**, 1242, 1947.
11. Gros, H., and Kirnberger, E. J.: Spontanausscheidung von *p*-Oxyphenylbrenztraubensäure im Harn. Klin. Wschr., **32**, 115, 1954.

12. Felix, K., Leonhardi, G., and Glasenapp, I.: Über Tyrosinosis. Ztschr. physiol. Chem., **287,** 141, 1951.
13. DeEds, F., Booth, A. N., and Jones, F. T.: Methylation and dehydroxylation of phenolic compounds by rats and rabbits. J. Biol. Chem., **225,** 615, 1957.
14. Meister, A.: *Biochemistry of the Amino Acids.* Academic, New York, 1965.
15. Knox, W. E.: The metabolism of phenylalanine and tyrosine, in *A Symposium on Amino Acid Metabolism,* edited by W. D. McElroy and H. B. Glass. Johns Hopkins, Baltimore, 1955.
16. Mason, H. S.: Mechanisms of oxygen metabolism. Advances Enzym., **19,** 79, 1957.
17. Lin, E. C. C., and Knox, W. E.: Specificity of the adaptive response of tyrosine-α-ketoglutarate transaminase in the rat. J. Biol. Chem., **233,** 1186, 1958.
18. La Du, B. N., Zannoni, V. G., Laster, L., and Seegmiller, J. E.: The nature of the defect in tyrosine metabolism in alcaptonuria. J. Biol. Chem., **230,** 251, 1958.
19. Canellakis, Z. N., and Cohen, P. P.: Purification studies of tyrosine-α-ketoglutaric acid transaminase. J. Biol. Chem., **222,** 53, 1956.
20. Canellakis, Z. N., and Cohen, P. P.: Kinetic and substrate specificity study of tyrosine-α-ketoglutaric acid transaminase. J. Biol. Chem., **222,** 63, 1956.
21. Kenney, F. T.: Induction of tyrosine-α-ketoglutaurate transaminase in rat liver. II. Enzyme purification and preparation of antitransaminase. J. Biol. Chem., **237,** 1605, 1962.
22. Valeriote, F. A., Auricchio, F., Tomkins, G. M., and Riley, D.: Purification and properties of rat liver tyrosine aminotransferase. J. Biol. Chem., **244,** 3618, 1969.
23. Jacoby, G. A., and La Du, B. N.: Studies on the specificity of tyrosine-α-ketoglutarate transaminase. J. Biol. Chem., **239,** 419, 1964.
24. Hager, S. E., Gregerman, R. I., and Knox, W. E.: *p*-Hydroxyphenylpyruvate oxidase of liver. J. Biol. Chem., **225,** 935, 1957.
25. Roka, L., König, G., and Rübner, H.: Die fermentative Oxydation von *p*-Hydroxyphenylbrenztraubensäure zu Homogentisinsäure. Ztschr. physiol. Chem., **313,** 87, 1958.
26. La Du, B. N., and Zannoni, V. G.: The tyrosine oxidation system of liver. II. Oxidation of *p*-hydroxyphenylpyruvic acid to homogentisic acid. J. Biol. Chem., **217,** 777, 1955.
27. La Du, B. N., and Zannoni, V. G.: The tyrosine oxidation system of liver. III. Further studies on the oxidation of *p*-hydroxyphenylpyruvic acid. J. Biol. Chem., **219,** 273, 1956.
28. Zannoni, V. G., and La Du, B. N.: The tyrosine oxidation system of liver. IV. Studies on the inhibition of *p*-hydroxyphenylpyruvic acid oxidase by excess substrate. J. Biol. Chem., **234,** 2925, 1959.
29. Taniguchi, K., and Armstrong, M. D.: The enzymatic formation of *o*-hydroxyphenylacetic acid. J. Biol. Chem., **238,** 4091, 1963.
30. Taniguchi, K., Kappe, T., and Armstrong, M. D.: Further studies on phenylpyruvate oxidase. J. Biol. Chem., **239,** 3389, 1964.
31. Neubauer, O.: Über den Abbau der Aminosäuren im gesunden und kranken Organismus. Deutsches Arch. klin. Med., **95,** 211, 1909.
32. La Du, B. N., and Zannoni, V. G.: The role of ascorbic acid in tyrosine metabolism. Ann. N.Y. Acad. Sci., **92,** 175, 1961.
33. Zannoni, V. G., and La Du, B. N.: Studies on the defect in tyrosine metabolism in scorbutic guinea pigs. J. Biol. Chem., **235,** 165, 1960.
34. Sealock, R. R., and Goodland, R. L.: Ascorbic acid, a coenzyme in tyrosine oxidation. Science, **114,** 645, 1951.
35. Sealock, R. R., Goodland, R. L., Sumerwell, W. N., and Brierly, J. M.: The role of ascorbic acid in the oxidation of L-tyrosine by guinea pig liver extracts. J. Biol. Chem., **196,** 761, 1952.
36. La Du, B. N., and Greenberg, D. M.: Ascorbic acid and the oxidation of tyrosine. Science, **117,** 111, 1953.
37. Knox, W. E.: Coenzyme functions of ascorbic acid. Symposium on Vitamin Metabolism, in *Proc. IVth International Congress of Biochemistry,* Vienna, 1958, vol. XI. Pergamon Press, Ltd., London.
38. Sealock, R. R., and Silberstein, H. E.: The excretion of homogentisic acid and other tyrosine metabolites by the vitamin C-deficient guinea pig. J. Biol. Chem., **135,** 251, 1940.
39. Huisman, T. H. J., and Jonxis, J. H. P.: Some investigations on the metabolism of phenylalanine and tyrosine in children with vitamin C deficiency. Arch. Dis. Child., **32,** 77, 1957.
40. Meister, A.: Reduction of α,γ-diketo and α-keto acids catalyzed by muscle preparations and by crystalline lactic dehydrogenase. J. Biol. Chem., **184,** 117, 1950.
41. Zannoni, V. G. and Weber, W. W.: Isolation and properties of aromatic α-keto acid reductase. J. Biol. Chem., **241,** 1340, 1966.
42. Weber, W. W., and Zannoni, V. G.: Reduction of phenylpyruvic acids to phenyllactic acids in mammalian tissues. J. Biol. Chem., **241,** 1345, 1966.
43. Kretchmer, N., Levine, S. Z., McNamara, H., and Barnett, H. L.: Certain aspects of tyrosine metabolism in the young. I. The development of the tyrosine oxidizing system in human liver. J. Clin. Invest., **35,** 236, 1956.
44. Kretchmer, N., Levine, S. Z., and McNamara, H.: The *in vitro* metabolism of tyrosine and its intermediates in the liver of the premature infant. Am. J. Diseases Children, **93,** 19, 1957.
45. La Du, B. N., and Zannoni, V. G.: Tyrosinosis in guinea pigs induced by diethyldithiocarbamate. Fed. Proc., **17,** 260, 1958.
46. La Du, B. N., and Zannoni, V. G.: Unpublished observations.
47. Knox, W. E., and Pitt, B. M.: Enzymic catalysis of the keto-enol tautomerization of phenylpyruvic acids. J. Biol. Chem., **225,** 675, 1957.
48. La Du, B. N., Howell, R. R., Michael, B. S., and Sober, E. K.: A quantitative micromethod for the determination of phenylalanine and tyrosine in blood and its application in the diagnosis of phenylketonuria in infants. Pediatrics, **31,** 39, 1963.
49. Baber, M. D.: A case of congenital cirrhosis of the liver with renal tubular defects akin to those in the Fanconi syndrome. Arch. Dis. Child., **31,** 335, 1956.
50. Sakai, K., and Kitawaga, T.: An atypical case of tyrosinosis. Part I. Clinical and laboratory findings. Jikeikai M. J., **4,** 1, 1957.
51. Sakai, K., and Kitagawa, T.: An atypical case of tyrosinosis. II. A research on the metabolic block. Jikeikai M. J., **4,** 11, 1957.
52. Sakai, K., Kitagawa, T., and Yoshioka, K.: An atypical case of tyrosinosis. III. The outcome of the patient: pathological and biochemical observations on the organ tissues. Jikeikai M. J., **6,** 15, 1959.
53. Fritzell, S., Jagenburg, R., and Schnürer, L.-B.: Studium av aminosyreomsättningen i fall av Fanconio-syndrom med levercirrhos. Nord. Med. **61,** 410, 1959.
54. Jagenburg, O. R.: The urinary excretion of free amino acids and other amino compounds by the human. Scand. J. Clin. Lab. Invest. **11,** Suppl. 43, 1959.
55. Lelong, M., Alagille, D., Tan Vinh, L., Colin, J., Roux, M., Gentil, C., and Gabilan, J.-C.: Cirrhose congénitale et familiale rachitisme vitamino-résistant avec diabète glucophosphoaminé, hépatome terminal. Pediatrie, **16,** 221, 1961.
56. Royer, P., Bernard, R., Boissiere, H., Maestraggi, P., and Roussel, A.: Cirrhose hépatique avec rachitisme secondaire et tyrosinurie. Pediatrie **16,** 510, 1961.
57. Bernheim, M., Monnet, P., Francois, R., Larbre, F., and Fleurette, M.: Cirrhose congenitale familiale avec tubulopathic. Pediatrie **17,** 561, 1962.
58. Lelong, M., Alagille, D., Gentil, C., Colin, J., Le Tan Vinh, and Gabilan, J.-C.: Cirrhose congenitale et familiale avec diabète phospho-glucoaminé rachitisme vitamino-résistant et tyrosinurie massive. Etude métabolique et anatomique. Rev. Franc. Etudes Clin. Biol. **8,** 37, 1963.
59. Woolf, L. I.: Phenylalanine and tyrosine metabolism. Advances Clin. Chem. **6,** 175, 1963.
60. Fritzell, S., Jagenburg, O. R., and Schnürer, L. B.: Familial cirrhosis of the liver, renal tubular defects with rickets and impaired tyrosine metabolism. Acta Pediat. **53,** 18, 1964.
61. Sass-Kortsak, A., Jackson, S. H., and Scriver, C.: Tyrosyluria and hypermethioninemia in an infant with hepatic cirrhosis and nodular hyperplasia. Abstr. Amer. Ped. Soc., 74th Ann. Meet., p. 74, 1964.
62. Greenberg, R. E., Chase, H. P., Lovrien, E., Hurwitz, R., and Efron, M. L.: Hypermethioninemia. Abstr. Amer. Ped. Soc., 74th Ann. Meet., p. 142, 1964.

63. Halvorsen, S., and Gjessing, L. R.: Studies on tyrosinosis: I. Effect of low-tyrosine and low-phenylalanine diet. Brit. Med. J., **2,** 1171, 1964.
64. Gentz, J., Jagenburg, R., and Zetterström, R.: Tyrosinemia. An inborn error of tyrosine metabolism with cirrhosis of the liver and multiple renal tubular defects (de Toni-Debre-Fanconi syndrome). J. Pediat., **66,** 670, 1965.
65. Poinso, R., Lissitzki, S., Bernard, P.-M., Fenasse, F., Laurent, M., and Mme. Duveau: A propos d'un de tyrosinémie avec cirrhose congénitale et tubulopathie. Bull. Mém. Soc. Méd. Hôp. Paris, **116,** 1357, 1965.
66. Taniguchi, K., and Gjessing, L. R.: Studies on tyrosinosis: 2, Activity of the transaminase, parahydroxyphenyl-pyruvate oxidase, and homogentisic-acid oxidase. Brit. Med. J. **1,** 968, 1965.
67. Perry, T. L., Hardwick, D. F., Dixon, G. H., Dolman, C. L., and Hansen, S.: Hypermethioninemia: a metabolic disorder associated with cirrhosis, islet cell hyperplasia, and renal tubular degeneration. Pediatrics **36,** 236, 1965.
68. Gjessing, L. R., and Halvorsen, S.: Hypermethioninaemia in acute tyrosinosis. Lancet **2,** 1132, 1965.
69. Scriver, C. R., Clow, C. L., and Siverberg, M.: Hypermethioninaemia in acute tyrosinosis. Lancet **1,** 153, 1966.
70. Odievre, M.: Glycogénose hépatorénale avec tubulopathie complexe. Deux observations d'une entité nouvelle. Rev. Intern. Hepatol. **16,** 1, 1966.
71. Medes, G.: Tyrosinosis. In *Symposium on Tyrosinosis.* In Honour of Dr. Grace Medes 2–3 June 1965. Edited by L. R. Gjessing. Universitetsforlaget, Oslo, 1966, pp. 13–23.
72. Jagenburg, R.: The effect of low tyrosine and low phenylalanine diet on the amino acid metabolism in a case of tyrosinemia. In *Symposium on Tyrosinosis.* In Honour of Dr. Grace Medes, 2–3 June 1965. Edited by L. R. Gjessing. Universitetsforlaget, Oslo, 1966, pp. 37–49.
73. Gjessing, L. R.: Studies on the aromatic pyruvic acid metabolism in Fölling's disease, tyrosinosis, and neuroblastoma. In *Symposium on Tyrosinosis.* In Honour of Dr. Grace Medes, 2–3 June 1965. Edited by L. R. Gjessing, Universitetsforlaget, Oslo, 1966, pp. 55–71.
74. Woolf, L. I.: Inborn hepato-renal dysfunction. In *Symposium on Tyrosinosis.* In Honour of Dr. Grace Medes, 2–3 June 1965. Edited by L. R. Gjessing. Universitetsforlaget, Oslo, 1966, pp. 82–91.
75. Aronsson, S., Englesson, G., Jagenburg, R., and Palmgren, B.: Clinical effects of low-tyrosine–low-phenylalanine diet in a case of tyrosinemia. In *Symposium on Tyrosinosis.* In Honour of Dr. Grace Medes, 2–3 June 1965. Edited by L. R. Gjessing. Universitetsforlaget, Oslo, 1966, pp. 101–104.
76. Halvorsen, S., and Gjessing, L. R.: Clinical studies of dietary treatment of tyrosinosis. In *Symposium on Tyrosinosis.* In Honour of Dr. Grace Medes, 2–3 June 1965. Edited by L. R. Gjessing. Universitetsforlaget, Oslo, 1966, pp. 105–110.
77. Tron, P.: Tyrosinose congenitale. Arch. Franc. Pediat. **23,** 935, 1966.
78. Halvorsen, S., Pande, H., Christie Loken, A., and Gjessing, L. R.: Tyrosinosis. Arch. Dis. Child. **41,** 238, 1966.
79. Gentz, J., Lindbald, B., Lindstedt, S., Levy, L., Shasteen, W., and Zetterstrom, R.: Dietary treatment in tyrosinemia (tyrosinosis). Amer. J. Dis. Child. **113,** 31, 1967.
80. Halvorsen, S.: Dietary treatment of tyrosinosis. Amer. J. Dis. Child. **113,** 38, 1967.
81. Scriver, C. R., Larochelle, J., and Silverberg, M.: Hereditary tyrosinemia and tyrosyluria in a French Canadian geographic isolate. Amer. J. Dis. Child. **113,** 41, 1967.
82. Kogut, M. D., Shaw, K. N., and Donnell, G. N.: Tyrosinosis. Amer. J. Dis. Child. **113,** 47, 1967.
83. La Du, B. N.: The enzymatic deficiency in tyrosinemia. Amer. J. Dis. Child. **113,** 54, 1967.
84. Scriver, C. R., Silverberg, M., and Clow, C. L.: Hereditary tyrosinemia and tyrosyluria: clinical report on four patients. Canad. Med. Ass. J. **97,** 1047, 1967.
85. Larochelle, J., Mortezai, A., Belanger, M., Tremblay, M., Claveau, J. C., and Aubin, G.: Experience with 37 infants with tyrosinemia. Canad. Med. Ass. J. **97,** 1051, 1967.
86. Prive, L.: Pathological findings in patient with tyrosinemia. Canad. Med Ass. J. **97,** 1054, 1967.
87. Sass-Kortsak, A., Ficici, S., Paunier, L., Kooh, S. W., Fraser, D., and Jackson, S. H.: Clinical and biochemical study of three patients with tyrosyluria. Canad. Med. Ass. J. **97,** 1056, 1967.
88. Partington, M. W., and Haust, M. D.: A patient with tyrosinemia and hypermethioninemia. Canad. Med. Ass. J. **97,** 1059, 1967.
89. Perry, T. L.: Tyrosinemia associated with hypermethioninemia and islet cell hyperplasia. Canad. Med. Ass. J. **97,** 1067, 1967.
90. Scriver, C. R.: The phenotypic manifestations of hereditary tyrosinemia and tyrosyluria: a hypothesis. Canad. Med. Ass. J. **97,** 1073, 1967.
91. Scriver, C. R., and Davies, E.: Investigation *in vivo* of the biochemical defect in hereditary tyrosinemia and tyrosyluria. Canad. Med. Ass. J. **97,** 1076, 1967.
92. Sass-Kortsak, A., Ficici, S., Paunier, L., Kooh, S. W., Fraser, D., and Jackson, S. H.: Secondary metabolic derangements in patients with tyrosyluria. Canad. Med. Ass. J. **97,** 1079, 1967.
93. Sass-Kortsak, A., Ficici, S., Paunier, L., Kooh, S. W., Fraser, D., Jackson, S. H.: Observations on treatment in patients with tyrosyluria. Canad. Med. Ass. J. **97,** 1089, 1967.
94. Dallaire, L.: Genetic aspects of tyrosinemia. Canad. Med. Ass. J. **97,** 1098, 1967.
95. Laberge, C., and Dallaire, L.: Genetic aspects of tyrosinemia in the Chicoutimi region. Canad. Med. Ass. J. **97,** 1099, 1967.
96. Gaull, G. E., Rassin, D. K., and Sturman, J. A.: Significance of hypermethioninaemia in acute tyrosinosis. Lancet **1,** 1318, 1968.
97. Tada, K., Wada, Y., Yazaki, N., Yokoyama, Y., Nakagawa, H., Yoshida, T., Sato, T., and Arakawa, T.: Dietary treatment of infantile tyrosinemia. Tohoku J. Exp. Med. **95,** 337, 1968.
98. Gentz, J., Johansson, S., Lindblad, B., Lindstedt, S., and Zetterström, R.: Excretion of δ-aminolevulinic acid in hereditary tyrosinemia. Clin. Chim. Acta **23,** 257, 1969.
99. Bodegård, G., Gentz, J., Lindblad, B., Lindstedt, S., Zetterström, R.: Hereditary tyrosinemia. III. On the differential diagnosis and the lack of effect of early dietary treatment. Acta Paediat. Scand. **58,** 37, 1969.
100. Lindemann, R., Gjessing, L. R., Merton, B., and Halvorsen, S.: Fructosaemia, "acute-tyrosinosis." Lancet **1,** 891, 1969.
101. Halvorsen, S., and Gjessing, L. R.: Tyrosinosis. In *Symposium on Phenylketonuria. Present status and future developments.* Editor, H. Bickel. In press.
102. Lindemann, R., Gjessing, L. R., Merton, B., Christie Löken, A., and Halvorsen, S.: Amino acid metabolism in fructosemia. Acta Paediat. Scand. **59,** 141, 1970.
103. Gjessing, L. R., Vellan, E. J., Borud, O., and Halvorsen, S.: Unpublished observations.
104. Gaull, G. E., Rassin, D. K., Solomon, G. E., Harris, R. C., and Sturman, J. A.: Biochemical observations on so-called hereditary tyrosinemia. Pediat. Res. **4,** 337, 1970.
105. Wadman, S. K., Van Sprang, F. J., Maas, J. W., and Ketting, D.: An exceptional case of tyrosinosis. J. Ment. Defic. Res. **12,** 269, 1968.
106. Holston, J. L., Jr., Levy, H. L., Tomlin, G. A., Atkins, R. J., Patton, T. H., and Hosty, T. S.: Tyrosinosis: a patient without liver or renal disease. Pediatrics. In press.
107. Levy, H. L., and Pitt. D.: Personal communication.
108. Kennaway, N. G., and Buist, N. R. M.: Metabolic studies in a patient with hepatic soluble tyrosine aminotransferase deficiency. Pediat. Res. In press.
109. Fellman, J. H., Vanbellinghen, P. J., Jones, R. T., and Koler, R. D.: Soluble and mitochondrial forms of tyrosine aminotransferase. Relationship to human tyrosinemia. Biochemistry **8,** 615, 1969.
110. Partington, M., Scriver, C. R., and Sass-Kortsak, A. (eds.): *Conference on Hereditary Tyrosinemia.* Canad. Med. Ass. J. **97,** 1045, 1967.
111. Boctor, A. M. and Harper, A. E.: Tyrosine toxicity in the rat: effect of high intake of *p*-hydroxyphenylpyruvic acid and of force-feeding high tyrosine diet. J. Nutrition **95,** 535, 1968.
112. Perry, T. L., Hardwick, D. F., Hansen, S., Pohlmann, L., and Warrington, P. D.: Methionine induction of experimental tyrosinaemia. J. Ment. Defic. Res. **11,** 246, 1967.

113. Daniel, R. G., and Waisman, H. A.: The influence of excess methionine on the free amino acids of brain and liver and of the weanling rat. J. Neurochem. **16,** 787, 1969.

114. Froesch, E. R.: Essential fructosuria and hereditary fructose intolerance. In *The Metabolic Basis of Inherited Disease.* J. B. Stanbury, J. B. Wyngaarden, D. S. Fredrickson (eds.), 2d ed., p. 124. McGraw-Hill, New York, 1966.

115. Isselbacher, K. J.: Galactosemia. In *The Metabolic Basis of Inherited Disease.* J. B Stanbury, J. B. Wyngaarden, D. S. Fredrickson (eds.), 2d ed., p. 178. McGraw-Hill, New York, 1966.

116. Rosenberg, L. E., and Segal, S.: Maleic acid-induced inhibition of amino acid transport in rat kidney. Biochem. J. **92,** 345, 1964.

117. Kramer, H. J., and Gonick, H. C.: Experimental Fanconi syndrome I. Effect of maleic acid on renal cortical Na-K-ATPase activity and ATP levels. J. Lab. Clin. Med. **76,** 799, 1970.

118. Silverberg, M. *In* General discussion on hereditary tyrosinemia. Canad. Med. Ass. J. **97,** 1086, 1967.

119. Levine, R. J. and Conn, H. O.: Tyrosine metabolism in patients with liver disease. J. Clin. Invest. **46,** 2012, 1967.

120. Menkes, J. H., Chernick, V., and Ringel, B.: Effect of elevated blood tyrosine on subsequent intellectual development of premature infants. J. Pediat. **69,** 583, 1966.

121. Partington, M. W., Delahaye, D. J., Masotti, R. E., Read, J. H., and Roberts, B.: Neonatal tyrosinaemia: a follow-up study. Arch. Dis. Child. **43,** 195, 1968.

CHAPTER THIRTEEN

ALCAPTONURIA

Bert N. La Du

Alcaptonuria is a rare hereditary metabolic disease in which the enzyme homogentisic acid oxidase is missing. Because of this defect, homogentisic acid produced during the metabolism of phenylalanine and tyrosine cannot be further metabolized; it therefore accumulates and is excreted in the urine.

If urine containing homogentisic acid is allowed to stand for some time, it gradually turns dark as the acid is oxidized to a melanin-like product. The polymerization is speeded by alkali; this explains why washing diapers of alcaptonuric infants with soap tends to make the stains more intense instead of removing them.

It is not surprising that such an obvious sign as dark urine led to the early recognition of this disease. Several persons reported in the medical literature of the sixteenth and seventeenth centuries who continually passed dark urine are presumed to have had alcaptonuria (see Garrod [1]). The first patient in whom the diagnosis was made with certainty was one described by Boedeker in 1859 [2]. He recognized that the reducing properties of this patient's urine were different from those of one containing glucose (e.g., it did not reduce bismuth hydroxide), and he observed the darkening of the urine when alkali was added. He used the property of avid oxygen uptake in alkaline solution to give the substance a name. ". . . *in alkalischer Lösung bei gewöhnlicher Temperature den Sauerstoff begierig zu verschlucken und nannte ihn danach Alcapton* (*freilich recht barbarisch zusammengesetzt aus dem arabischen* alkali *und dem griechischen καπτεῖν, begierig verschlucken.*)" [2, p. 139]. Two years later [4], Boedeker spelled it "Alkapton," and since then this condition has been known as *Alkaptonurie* in the German literature and as *alcaptonurie* in the French. Both "c" and "k" have been used by writers in English.[1]

Boedeker precipitated homogentisic acid from alcaptonuric urine as the lead salt [2, 4], but he was unable to obtain enough material to purify it and determine its exact chemical structure. He did point out the similarity of its behavior in alkali with that of known hydroxyphenols.

During the following 30 years there was considerable confusion as to the chemical structure of "alkapton." It was variously reported by different groups to be catechol [5, 6], protocatechuic acid [7], "glycosuric acid" [8], and uroleucic acid [9]. The various claims and disputes about its composition during this period are well summarized in a review by Knox [10]. The controversy ended and the chemical structure of "alcapton" was firmly established in 1891 by the excellent work of Wolkow and Baumann [11]. They identified it as 2,5-dihydroxyphenylacetic acid and named it *homogentisic acid,* because of its close structural relationship to gentisic acid (2,5-dihydroxybenzoic acid). The earlier reports of other substances, such as uroleucic acid in alcaptonuric urine were shown to be the result of analytic errors from contamination with various normal urinary constituents [12].

Once the aromatic structure of homogentisic acid was known, it was not long before various suggestions were made as to the source of this unusual urinary product. The known aromatic substances in proteins, tyrosine and phenylalanine were, of course, the primary suspects (Fig. 13-1). Wolkow and Baumann demonstrated in 1891 [11] that feeding either extra tyrosine or a diet high in protein greatly increased the amount of homogentisic acid excreted by an alcaptonuric patient. Even though they were incorrect in believing that the formation of homogentisic acid was due to the activity of bacteria in the intestine, their important observation initiated a number of studies by clinical investigators of that time, who used the metabolic defect in alcaptonuric individuals to determine the pathway by which phenylalanine and tyrosine are metabolized to homogentisic acid. Numerous compounds which were possible intermediary substances in the formation of homogentisic acid were fed to alcaptonuric patients. It was expected that compounds in the metabolic sequence would increase the excretion of homogentisic acid but that those which were not intermediates would fail to do so. On the basis of such studies Neubauer suggested a preliminary scheme of tyrosine metabolism in 1909 [13], the first such scheme for any of the amino acids. In 1928 [14] he revised it to incorporate the results obtained during the intervening years (Fig. 13-2). Although a few changes have been made since then, the basic scheme which he postulated has remained essentially unchanged during the last 40 years.

Studies on alcaptonuria have been of general importance in the development of ideas about diseases of metabolism. As a result of his studies on alcaptonuria, Sir Archibald Garrod developed his whole concept of inheritable metabolic diseases. In 1908 he discussed alcaptonuria in one of the Croonian Lectures [1], and in the following year he expanded his ideas more completely in his classic book *Inborn Errors of Metabolism* [12]. He thought of alcaptonuria as a metabolic "freak," or "sport," comparable to a structural abnormality, rather than as a disease in the usual sense. He felt that patterns of metabolism varied in each individual according to his hereditary background and that alcaptonuria and the other inborn errors of metabolism represented extreme examples of such variant possibilities [15]. He sus-

[1]Several medical dictionaries erroneously assume alkapton to be derived from "alkali" and the Greek root ἅπτω meaning to seize, to possess, the combination, therefore, meaning, "to have an affinity for alkali." *The Oxford English Dictionary* [3] gives the correct origin and indicates that the "k" of alkaptonuria comes from the Greek root καπτω rather than from alkali. Transliteration of the "k" to "c" therefore follows the same pattern used in many words derived from similar Greek roots.

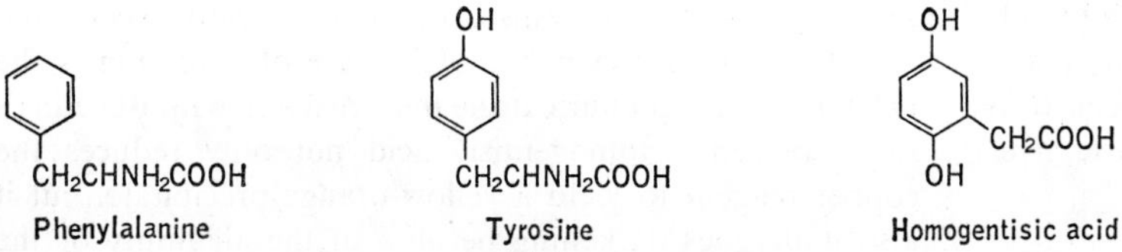

OH
OH
CH_2CHNH_2COOH Phenylalanine
CH_2CHNH_2COOH Tyrosine
CH_2COOH
OH
Homogentisic acid

Figure 13-1. Formulas of phenylalanine, tyrosine, and homogentisic acid.

pected that these variations ultimately might depend upon differences in the activity of specific enzymes, thus anticipating by many years the conclusion of Beadle and Tatum [16] that a single defective gene is correlated with a metabolic block in one enzymatic reaction.

In 1909 Garrod [12] wrote of the probable defect in alcaptonuria:

We may further conceive that the splitting of the benzene ring in normal metabolism is the work of a special enzyme, that in congenital alcaptonuria this enzyme is wanting, whilst in disease its working may be partially or even completely inhibited. The experiments of G. Embden and others upon perfusion of the liver suggest that organ as the most probable seat of the change.

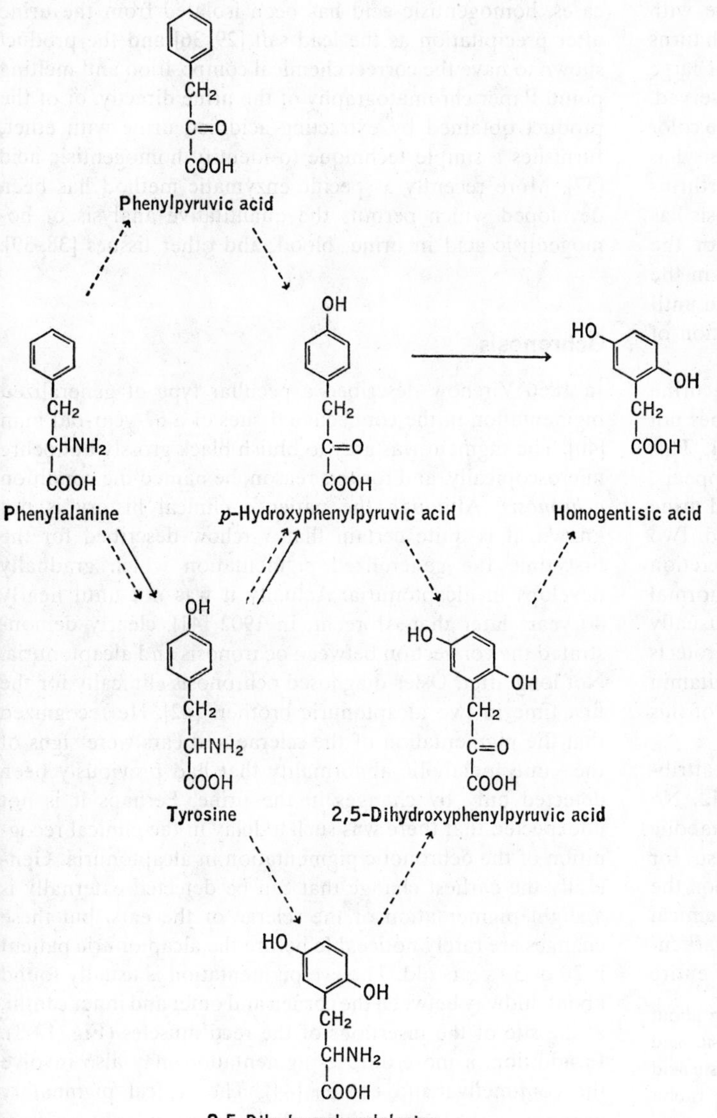

Figure 13-2. Scheme of phenylalanine and tyrosine metabolism to homogentisic acid based upon feeding experiments with alcaptonuric patients [14]. The dotted arrows show various pathways considered possible by Neubauer; the solid arrows indicate the pathway as it is viewed today.

Garrod's supposition that a specific enzyme is missing in alcaptonuria has been supported through the years by many types of circumstantial evidence and recently has been confirmed by direct biochemical assay of alcaptonuric liver preparations [17].

CLINICAL FEATURES

The cardinal features of alcaptonuria are signs due to the presence of homogentisic acid in the urine, pigmentation of cartilage and other connective tissues, and nearly always, in later years, arthritis [18].

Urinary Changes

According to the usual textbook description, people with alcaptonuria give a history of dark urine or urine which turns dark on standing. It should be emphasized that in a large number of alcaptonuric patients this finding is not observed. Many patients have never noted any abnormality in the color of the urine during childhood [19–21], and diagnosis has been made only after they sought treatment for arthritis during their later years [20–25]. In some cases diagnosis has followed a false positive test for diabetes [20, 24] or the finding of the unusual and distinctive x-ray changes in the spine [26]. In others the disease has not been suspected until a surgical procedure has revealed marked pigmentation of the cartilage [27].

Alcaptonuric individuals on a normal diet void a urine which at first is not an abnormal color, and which does not darken for many hours if it remains at an acid pH. This is true even for patients with extensive ochronosis. It appears, therefore, that in those instances where freshly voided urine turns dark quickly, additional factors must be involved. Two factors that would favor rapid darkening are the excretion of an alkaline urine and a lower concentration than normal of vitamin C and possibly other reducing agents usually present in the urine. It is well known that vitamin C protects homogentisic acid against oxidation, and in the past vitamin C has been suggested as a therapeutic agent because of this property [28].

The unusual findings in alcaptonuric urine can all be attributed to one abnormal constituent, homogentisic acid. No abnormal amino acid pattern [19] or other tyrosine metabolic products are found [29].[2] The various diagnostic tests for alcaptonuria by urinalysis, therefore, are all based upon the detection of homogentisic acid through its unusual chemical properties. Its ease of oxidation results in a gradual darkening of the urine downward from the surface until the entire sample is dark brown; this darkening is greatly accelerated by alkali. Further evidence of its ease of oxidation is the behavior of alcaptonuric urine in its reaction with Benedict's sugar reagent. Homogentisic acid not only reduces the copper reagent to yield a yellow-orange precipitate, but it also undergoes darkening because of the alkalinity of the reagent. The net effect is an orange precipitate in a muddy-brown solution. The reduction of molybdate is the basis of the Brigg's test, commonly used to follow the urinary excretion of homogentisic acid [33]. Reduction of silver in photographic paper emulsion has been used as a qualitative test [34] and as the basis of a quantitative method to measure this acid [35]. Homogentisic acid is not fermented by yeast, and it does not fluoresce under ultraviolet light.

A presumptive diagnosis of alcaptonuria can be made on the basis of the results of these nonspecific tests, but a more specific means for its identification is desirable. In many cases, homogentisic acid has been isolated from the urine after precipitation as the lead salt [29, 36] and the product shown to have the correct chemical composition and melting point. Paper chromatography of the urine directly, or of the product obtained by extracting acidified urine with ether, furnishes a simple technique to identify homogentisic acid [37]. More recently a specific enzymatic method has been developed which permits the quantitative analysis of homogentisic acid in urine, blood, and other tissues [38, 39].

Ochronosis

In 1866 Virchow described a peculiar type of generalized pigmentation in the connective tissues of a 67-year-old man [40]. The pigment was gray to bluish black grossly but ochre microscopically, and for this reason, he named the condition *ochronosis.* Although the patient's clinical history is not known, it is quite certain that Virchow described for the first time the generalized pigmentation which gradually develops in alcaptonuria. Actually it was not until nearly 40 years later that Albrecht, in 1902 [41], clearly demonstrated the connection between ochronosis and alcaptonuria. Not long after, Osler diagnosed ochronosis clinically for the first time in two alcaptonuric brothers [42]. He recognized that the pigmentation of the sclerae and ears were signs of the same metabolic abnormality that had previously been detected only by changes in the urine. Perhaps it is not unexpected that there was such a delay in the clinical recognition of the ochronotic pigmentation in alcaptonuria. Generally the earliest change that can be detected externally is a slight pigmentation of the sclerae or the ears, but these changes are rarely noticeable before the alcaptonuric patient is 20 or 30 years old. The eye pigmentation is usually found about midway between the cornea and outer and inner canthi, at the site of the insertions of the recti muscles (Fig. 13-3). In addition, a more diffuse pigmentation may also involve the conjunctiva and cornea [44]. The typical pigmentary changes in the ear cartilages similarly occur only in long-

[2] It has been reported that an alcaptonuric patient excreting about 7 gm homogentisic acid also excreted about 0.5 mg gentisic acid per day [30]. The conversion of small amounts of homogentisic acid to gentisic acid has been demonstrated in homogenates of rabbit liver [31, 32].

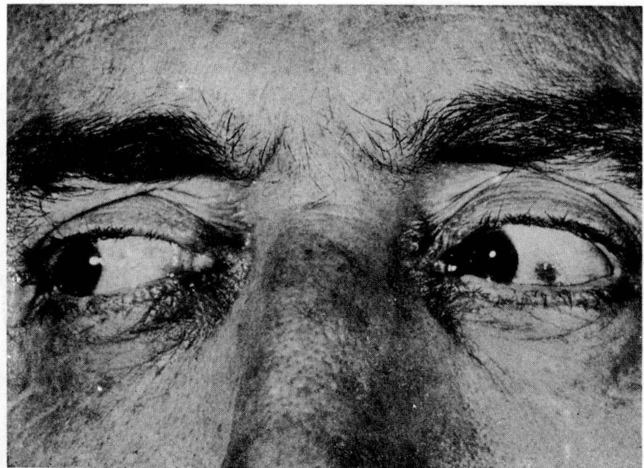

Figure 13-3. The bilateral deposition of ochronotic pigment in the sclerae, best seen in the left eye [43].

standing alcaptonuria. The cartilage is slate blue or gray and feels irregular and thickened. It is first seen in the concha and the antihelix, and later in the tragus. It is sometimes reported that a dusky discoloration, corresponding to the underlying tendons, can be seen through the skin over the hands. The prominence of this pigmentation is variable, and in many instances it is scarcely evident at all. The pigment appears in perspiration; clothing near the axillary regions may be stained, and the skin may have a brownish discoloration in the axillary and genital regions [26].

In contrast to these rather minimal findings, the pigmentation observed in the tissues of an elderly alcaptonuric patient at operation or at post mortem is indeed striking [40, 45–48]. Cartilage in many areas, particularly the costal, laryngeal, and tracheal cartilage, is densely pigmented and is described as being coal black in some areas. Pigmentation is also present throughout the body in fibrous tissues, fibrocartilage, tendons, and ligaments (Fig. 13-4). To a lesser degree it is also found in the endocardium, the intima of the larger vessels, in various organs such as kidney and lung, and in the epidermis. Microscopic examination shows the pigment to be deposited both intercellularly and intracellularly, and it may be either granular or homogeneous. Like melanin, the ochronotic pigment is bleached when treated for 24 hr with hydrogen peroxide, and it is soluble in alkali, but only slightly soluble in hydrochloric acid. Thus, in many of its chemical characteristics the ochronotic pigment resembles melanin arising from 3,4-dihydroxyphenylalanine (dopa). Unfortunately there is no specific stain to distinguish the ochronotic pigment of alcaptonuria from melanin derived from other sources. Although Fitzpatrick and Lerner [49] state that Becker's silver stain for melanin is not darkened by ochronotic pigment and that the latter is stained intensely black with polychrome methylene blue, Cooper and Moran [47] compared the staining properties of ochronotic pigment and melanin, employing a number of special stains. They concluded that no specific differentiation can be made with any of the stains used. Both pigments were best detected by the Nile blue stains of Lillie [50]. Variations with trichrome, cresyl violet, and the periodic acid–Schiff (PAS) stains seemed to depend mainly upon the differences in the amount of pigment present rather than the type of pigment represented.

The pigment deposited in ochronosis is presumably a polymer derived from homogentisic acid, but its exact chemical structure has not yet been determined. It is possible that some other constituents, in addition to homogentisic acid, are included in the product, just as melanin obviously contains more than a polymerized dopa unit, i.e., a considerable quantity of sulfur [51].

The formation of the pigment in the tissues may be entirely nonenzymatic, like the darkening of alcaptonuric urine. Solutions of pure homogentisic acid, made alkaline and aerated with air or oxygen, form a dark-brown product which has an ultraviolet absorption peak at 250 mμ (Milch et al. [52]). Unfortunately, the pigment deposited in the tissues of an alcaptonuric patient with ochronosis has not been analyzed in the same way, and so the relevance of the model polymerization to the in vivo process has not been established. Milch and Titus [53] have suggested that since polymerization of pure homogentisic acid solutions does not proceed at neutral pH and low partial pressure of oxygen (as occurs in cartilage), it is likely that if molecular oxygen is involved in vivo, it involves the participation of an enzyme system present locally. This conclusion assumes not only that the composition and steps of formation of the ochronotic

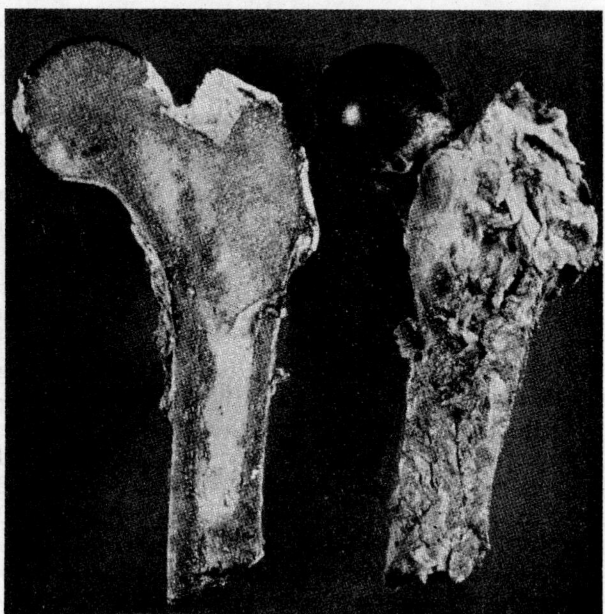

Figure 13-4. Ochronotic pigmentation of the femur of a 56-year-old alcaptonuric subject. See also Plate I-1 for a version of this picture in color. (*Courtesy of Dr. H. W. Edmonds of the Washington Hospital Center, Washington, D.C.*)

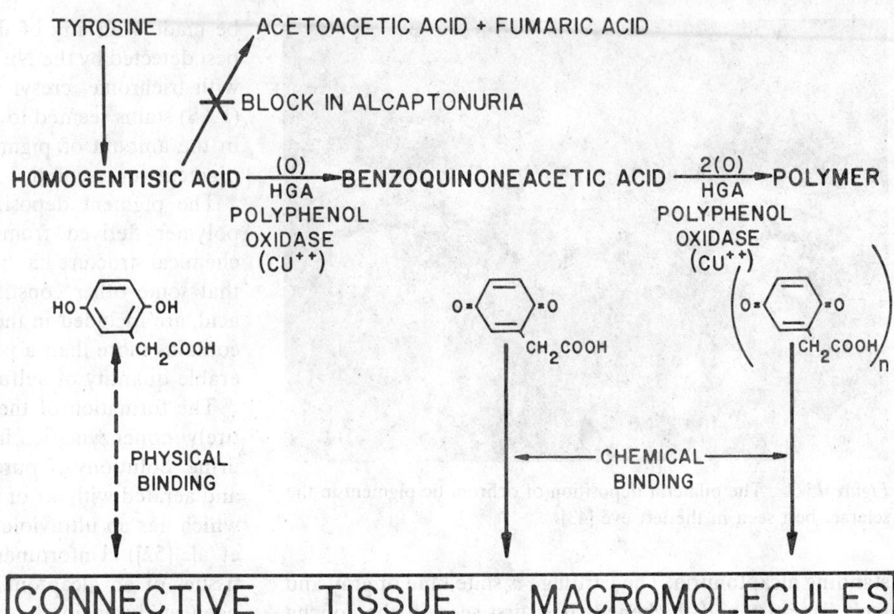

Figure 13-5. Postulated scheme for the formation of ochronotic pigment in alcaptonuria [54].

pigment would be the same in vivo as in solutions of pure homogentisic acid but that the pigment is both formed and deposited within the cartilage. It is not possible today to say to what degree enzymes play a role in the synthesis of the ochronotic pigmentation in alcaptonuria, although on the basis of their specificity it seems reasonable to exclude the enzymes involved in the synthesis of melanin by way of dopa.

Mammalian (human, rabbit, and guinea pig) skin and cartilage contain an enzyme called *homogentisic acid polyphenol oxidase* which catalyzes the oxidation of homogentisic acid to an ochronotic-like pigment [54]. Benzoquinoneacetic acid has been identified as an intermediary metabolite in the oxidation. The enzyme is a copper-protein, but it is clearly distinguished from tyrosinase by the finding that tyrosine, dopa, and other catechols are not substrates for the polyphenol oxidase. Earlier studies by La Du and Zannoni [55] demonstrated that *p*-quinones, such as benzoquinoneacetic acid, can form 1,4 addition products with sulfhydryl groups, and Stoner and Blivaiss [56] observed similar derivatives with the amino groups of glycine. Binding and chemical reactions of benzoquinone (or polymers derived from the acid) with the connective tissues may produce important chemical changes that alter tissue constituents and lead to ochronosis and ochronotic arthritis [57]. A possible scheme for the enzymatic oxidation of homogentisic acid and the formation of ochronotic pigment in the connective tissues of alcaptonuric patients is given in Figure 13-5.

Ochronosis Not Due to Homogentisic Acid

Clinically, ochronosis due to alcaptonuria might possibly be confused with the pigmentation of the skin, nail beds, conjunctivas, and cartilage seen in persons who have taken Atabrine for many months [58, 59]. Of course the history and the failure to find homogentisic acid in the urine should establish the diagnosis.

Another type of acquired ochronosis is that which is secondary to the prolonged use of carbolic acid dressings for chronic cutaneous ulcers [60–65]. This pigmentation is reversible and recedes after the medication is discontinued. Since this agent is rarely used today, nearly all the cases of ochronosis seen now are secondary to alcaptonuria. There are, however, a few puzzling cases of ochronosis in the literature in which exogenous agents, such as phenol, can probably safely be excluded as causative agents and in which the urine is reported to contain no homogentisic acid [66, 67]. In the case described by Oppenheimer and Kline [66], a determined effort to isolate homogentisic acid from the urine was made by Janney [68]. He concluded that this was an example of ochronosis secondary to a melanuria, but no aromatic metabolite related to dopa was identified in the urine. He was able to isolate a melanin-like pigment from the urine and from a prostatic calculus which had, by elementary analysis, much the same values as those reported by Mörner [51] for melanin obtained from the urine and tumor tissue of a patient with a melanosarcoma. It is possible that melanotic tumors might cause a generalized ochronosis also, but it is unlikely that a patient with such a condition would survive long enough for this complication to become evident [61]. In one case of alcaptonuria the ochronotic pigment in the eye was misdiagnosed as a melanosarcoma, and the eye was removed (69).

On the other hand, instances in which alcaptonuria, unaccompanied by ochronosis, has been diagnosed with certainty are extremely rare. From the nature and completeness of the metabolic defect one would expect that all alcaptonuric patients would develop ochronosis to some degree if they live to middle age. The two patients with alcaptonuria who did not have ochronosis at autopsy [70, 71] had extensive tuberculosis. No mention was made of ochronotic changes in their connective tissues, but it is unlikely that if they were present to the degree found in most alcaptonuric patients, they would have gone unnoticed.

Arthritis

"Ochronotic arthritis" is a manifestation of longstanding alcaptonuria. From the case reports in the literature, it appears that alcaptonuric arthritis occurs at an earlier age and is more severe in males than in females [72], even though the sex incidence of alcaptonuria is roughly equal. This sex difference in ochronotic arthritis is reminiscent of the similar preponderance of gouty arthritis in males. Hench [73] has stated that ochronotic arthritis resembles rheumatoid arthritis clinically but resembles osteoarthritis roentgenographically. The earliest symptoms observed are usually some degree of limitation of motion of the hip, knee joints, or occasionally the shoulders. There are nearly always periods of acute inflammation which may resemble rheumatoid arthritis, and later there is usually rather marked limitation of motion and ankylosis in the lumbosacral region.

X-rays may reveal changes considered almost pathognomonic of alcaptonuria [26]. The vertebral bodies of the lumbar spine show degeneration of the intervertebral disks with a narrowing of the space and dense calcification of the remaining disk material (Fig. 13-6). This is accompanied to a variable degree by fusion of the vertebral bodies. From the x-ray changes in the lumbar spine alone, it is often possible to be reasonably certain of the diagnosis of alcaptonuria. In contrast to rheumatoid spondylitis, little osteophyte formation and minimal calcification of the intervertebral ligaments are present. The large peripheral joints involved also differ from osteoarthritis in that the degenerative joint changes in ochronotic arthritis are most commonly in the shoulder and hip, whereas such joints as the sacroiliac may be completely spared.

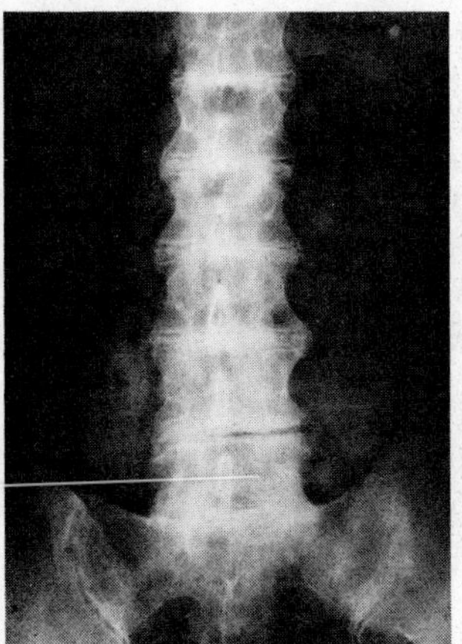

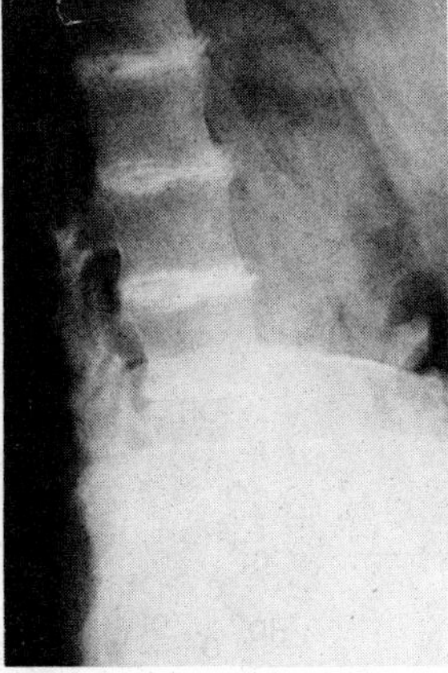

Figure 13-6. Roentgenograms of the spine showing the typical narrowing and calcification of the intervertebral disks [43].

Calcification of the ear cartilage is another sign of the disease that may be observed by x-ray. The large joints affected generally show degenerative osteoarthritic changes with calcified deposits most commonly in the muscle tendons around the large joints. Occasionally free intra-articular bodies are found [74]. By contrast, the smaller joints usually show little or no abnormality.

The common occurrence of arthritis in the general population and the long period before its onset in patients with alcaptonuria no doubt account for the failure of the earlier investigators to appreciate the association of arthritis with alcaptonuria. The first case described by Boedeker was reported to have neuralgia of the lower lumbar spine. The early investigators considered alcaptonuria a completely benign disease without symptoms and of clinical importance only in that it might be misdiagnosed as diabetes. A review of the earlier case reports shows that in most instances osteoarthritis was mentioned and, indeed, nearly all alcaptonuric patients develop arthritis during their later years. The arthritic complications are often severe and painful and may lead to a completely bedridden existence in later life.

The relationship between the deposition of pigment in the connective tissue and the degenerative changes which occur in some areas of the connective tissues, particularly the cartilage and the intervertebral disks, remains unknown. It has been proposed that the pigment acts as a chemical irritant to accelerate a degenerative process in the cartilage, leading to changes similar to those in osteoarthritis [23, 74]. The intra-articular injection of homogentisic acid into the knee joints of rabbits produced local lesions in cartilage and the soft tissues resembling those seen in alcaptonuria [75]. It is also possible that either the ochronotic pigment or homogentisic acid itself might inhibit some of the enzyme systems involved in cartilage metabolism. Greiling [76] has shown that low concentrations of the pigment prepared by treating homogentisic acid with alkali inhibit the action of hyaluronidase on chondroitin sulfuric acid and on hyaluronic acid, but homogentisic acid does not act as an inhibitor at the same concentrations. More recently, Dihlmann et al., [77] have extended these studies and noted the inhibition of several additional enzymes, particularly glutamic dehydrogenase, hexokinase, and malate dehydrogenase by the oxidized, polymerized product of homogentisic acid.

Other Findings in Alcaptonuria

In addition to the features mentioned above, other complications seem to occur in alcaptonuric patients with a greater frequency than might be anticipated in the general population. The relationship between ochronosis and cardiovascular disease is not clearly established, but a review of the case histories of alcaptonuric patients indicates that there is a high incidence of heart disease [24]. In 1910 Beddard

[63] tabulated the autopsy findings in 11 cases of ochronosis (none due to treatment with phenol) and found that 8 had chronic mitral and aortic valvulitis, 1 had an aortic aneurysm, and 1 an aneurysm of the left ventricle. Other investigators [45, 78] have noted generalized arteriosclerosis, and calcification in the heart valves and of the annulus of the aortic and mitral valves [46]. Myocardial infarction is a common cause of death in this group.

Other complications reported in alcaptonuric patients are ruptured intervertebral disks [79], and prostatitis [19, 24, 66, 80] or renal stones (see Young [80]). Clinical case reports on new cases of alcaptonuria should be encouraged in order that additional phenomena related to this metabolic disease may be revealed. One case of alcaptonuria with polycythemia [81] and one with severe renal disease, called "ochronotic nephrosis" [47], remain isolated examples, presumably because of chance association with other diseases. It should be kept in mind that conditions which favor the expression of alcaptonuria, such as consanguineous marriages, would also favor the manifestation of other recessive but unrelated traits.

SYNTHESIS AND DEGRADATION OF HOMOGENTISIC ACID

Biosynthesis

In mammals most of the dietary phenylalanine and tyrosine is oxidized to acetoacetic acid by enzyme systems localized primarily in the liver and kidney. The scheme of this metabolic pathway is shown in Fig. 13-7. Several excellent reviews

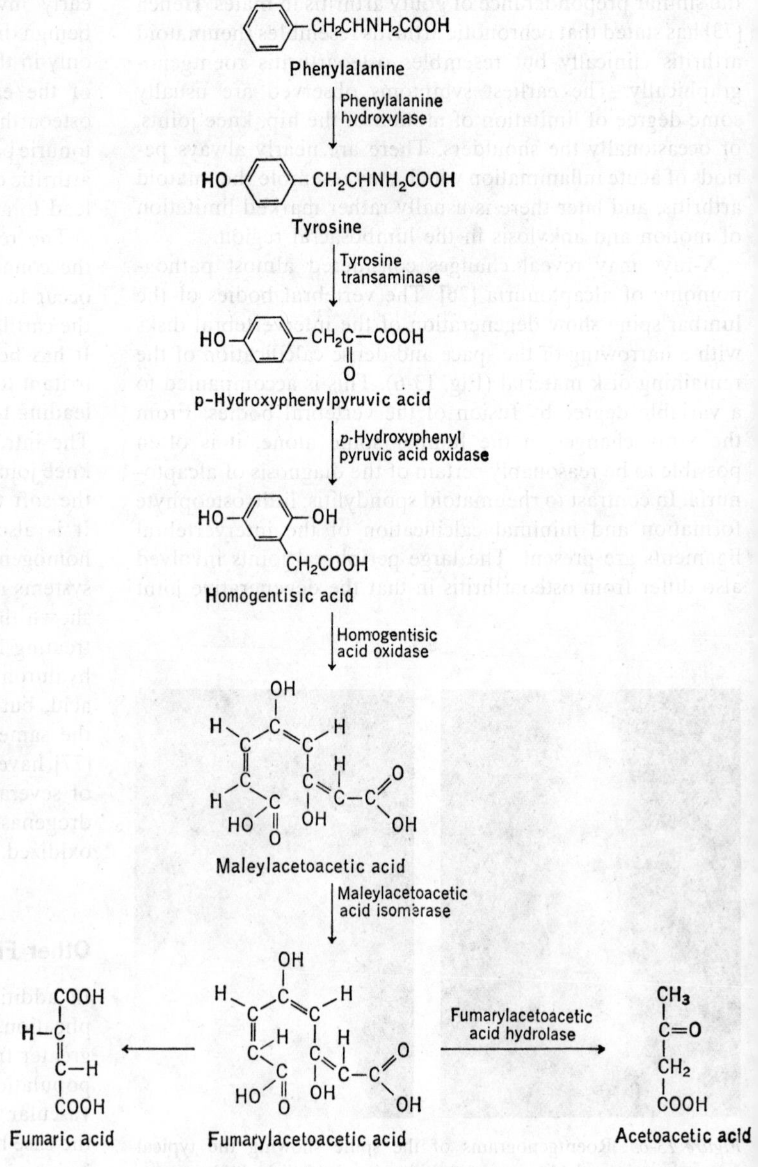

Figure 13-7. Enzymatic steps in the oxidation of phenylalanine and tyrosine to acetoacetic acid.

Phenylalanine (C_6H_5–CH_2CHNH_2COOH)
↓ Phenylalanine hydroxylase
Tyrosine (HO–C_6H_4–CH_2CHNH_2COOH)
↓ Tyrosine transaminase
p-Hydroxyphenylpyruvic acid (HO–C_6H_4–$CH_2C(=O)COOH$)
↓ *p*-Hydroxyphenyl pyruvic acid oxidase
Homogentisic acid
↓ Homogentisic acid oxidase
Maleylacetoacetic acid
↓ Maleylacetoacetic acid isomerase
Fumarylacetoacetic acid
→ Fumarylacetoacetic acid hydrolase →
Fumaric acid + Acetoacetic acid (CH_3COCH_2COOH)

of phenylalanine and tyrosine metabolism have appeared [82–85]. These may be consulted for the detailed experimental evidence supporting each of the steps in this scheme. As mentioned above, the scheme is based upon the earlier studies with alcaptonuric patients and many animal experiments in vivo. It has been revised and extended particularly during the past 20 years, by a large number of experiments on tyrosine metabolism in vitro.

In some of these in vitro studies, isotopically labeled phenylalanine and tyrosine were used to determine the fate of each of the carbon atoms in the aromatic ring and of the side chain [86–90]. The labeled amino acids were incubated with liver slices, and the distribution of the isotope was determined in the products CO_2, acetoacetic acid, and fumaric acid. These experiments showed that two of the four carbon atoms of acetoacetic acid were derived from carbon atoms 2 and 3 of the side chain and that the other two came from the ring. Furthermore, the position of the isotope from the ring carbon atoms indicated that the side chain must have migrated during the oxidation (Fig. 13-8). The isotopic evidence was entirely in agreement with the scheme postulated earlier by Neubauer [14] (Fig. 13-2), to account for the 2,5-dihydroxyphenyl intermediary product, homogentisic acid, from the 4-hydroxyphenyl substrates. This rearrangement was believed to involve a quinol intermediate with a migration of the side chain much like the migration of the methyl group in the oxidation of *p*-cresol [91] (Fig. 13-9). This unusual migration in the oxidation of *p*-hydroxyphenylpyruvic acid to homogentisic acid is, even today, the least understood step of any in the scheme shown in Fig. 13-7. So far, it has not been possible to identify a free intermediate in this step. It appears as though the hydroxylation of the ring and the migration and oxidative decarboxylation of the side chain all take place as a complicated single step. This reaction is discussed in more detail in the chapter on tyrosinosis (Chap. 12).

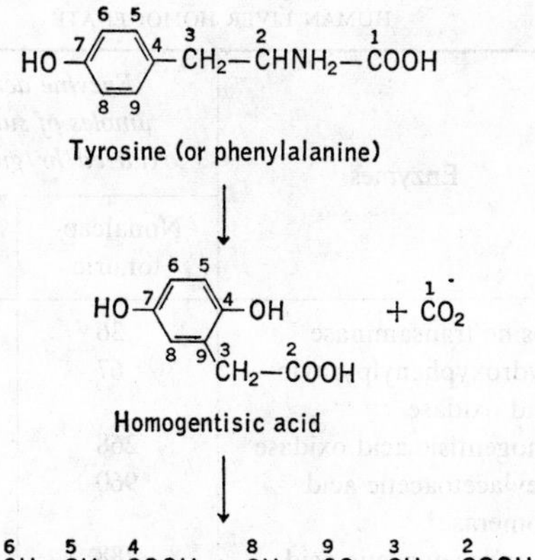

Figure 13-8. Fate of each of the carbon atoms of phenylalanine or tyrosine based upon experiments with the amino acids labeled with isotopic carbon.

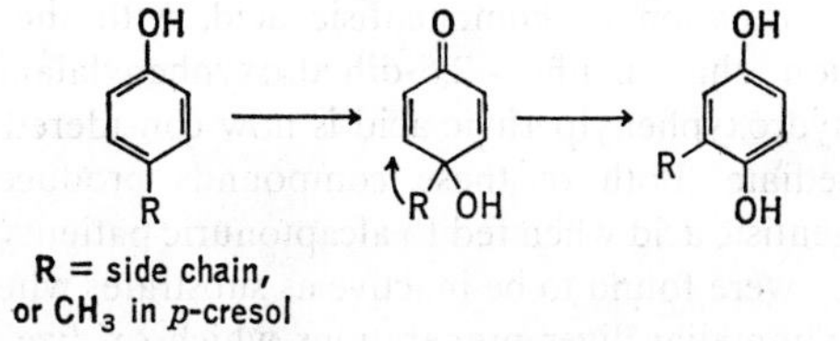

Figure 13-9. Formation of quinol intermediate and migration of the substituent (CH_3 in *p*-cresol or side chain) in *p*-hydroxyphenylpyruvic acid oxidation.

Homogentisic Acid a Normal Intermediate

The presence of homogentisic acid as a normal intermediate in the scheme deserves further comment. It should be recalled that in 1911 Dakin [92] suggested that not only was homogentisic acid an abnormal urinary product but its formation resulted from the metabolism of tyrosine by an abnormal pathway in alcaptonuria. The main support for this proposal was that when he fed animals and an alcaptonuric patient [93, 94] derivatives of phenylalanine and tyrosine (*p*-methylphenylalanine and *p*-methoxyphenylalanine) which, because of their *para*- substituent, could not form quinol intermediates, he found them to be well metabolized (in his view, by the normal pathway of tyrosine metabolism). He also found that these compounds caused an increase in acetoacetic acid when perfused through dog liver, as did phenylalanine and tyrosine. Although Dakin's results remained unexplained, through the years more and more evidence has accumulated that homogentisic acid is indeed a normal intermediate. For example, it was shown that some homogentisic acid accumulated from tyrosine in rat liver homogenates under certain experimental conditions [37, 83]; more recently, it was shown that homogentisic acid accumulated quantitatively from tyrosine or *p*-hydroxyphenylpyruvic acid in dog liver [95] and human liver [17] preparations in the presence of α,α'-dipyridyl, an inhibitor of homogentisic acid oxidase. Homogentisic acid oxidase is widely distributed in nature, and where it occurs it is associated with the other enzymes involved in the oxidation of tyrosine to acetoacetic acid.

There still remained the problem of explaining Dakin's results. In 1957 Pirrung et al. [96] reinvestigated the ketogenic effect of the tyrosine analogues. They found that *p*-methoxy-DL-phenylalanine is not ketogenic and that neither the L- form nor *p*-methoxyphenylalanine was metabolized, although the D- isomer was deaminated in dog liver. They attributed the earlier results of Wakeman and Dakin [94] to the ketogenic effect of the ammonium ion released by the deamination of the D- component. (The ketogenic effect of ammonium ion [97] was not known in 1911.) It must also be inferred from these results that Dakin did not have sufficiently sensitive methods to detect the excretion of the unchanged compounds in the urine. The present scheme of tyrosine oxidation (Fig. 13-7) is therefore very much like that of Neubauer (Fig. 13-2) in the steps leading to the formation of homogentisic acid, with the notable exception that neither 2,5-dihydroxyphenylalanine nor 2,5-dihydroxyphenylpyruvic acid is now considered a likely intermediate. Both of these compounds produced extra homogentisic acid when fed to alcaptonuric patients [13, 29], but they were found to be inactive as substrates when tested with mammalian liver preparations which oxidize tyrosine or *p*-hydroxyphenylpyruvic acid to homogenistic acid [17, 37, 95, 98]. These results also exclude the alternative pathway suggested by Neuberger in 1947 in which tyrosine would be oxidized first to 2,5-dihydroxyphenylalanine and then either through 2,5-dihydroxyphenylpyruvic acid or 2,5-dihydroxyphenylethylamine to homogentisic acid [99].

Metabolic Defect in Alcaptonuria

Even though Garrod suggested in 1908 [12] that the metabolic defect in alcaptonuria was the absence of the liver enzyme catalyzing the oxidation of homogentisic acid, other possible explanations have been offered from time to time by other workers. At the time Garrod presented his theory, it was quite generally believed that alcaptonuria was due to the formation of homogentisic acid by intestinal organisms. This opinion was based upon an assumption of Wolkow and Baumann [11] that the synthesis of homogentisic acid from tyrosine or phenylalanine was too complicated to be accomplished by human tissues and therefore must have resulted from the action of bacteria in the intestine.

In 1914 Gross [100] presented evidence for an enzymatic defect in alcaptonuria. He reported that homogentisic acid did not disappear when it was incubated with the serum from an alcaptonuric patient, whereas it did disappear when incubated with the serum from normal individuals, presumably because of the presence in normal serum of a homogentisic acid-oxidizing enzyme. A few years later Katsch and Stern [101] suggested that the results of Gross were due not to an enzyme that was missing in alcaptonuric serum but to the presence of an inhibitor in alcaptonuric blood. Both these findings were disputed by Lanyar and Lieb [102], who pointed out that the previous workers had not controlled the experimental conditions satisfactorily, particularly the pH, and that autooxidation of homogentisic acid probably accounted for their results. Unfortunately, the report that Gross found an enzyme missing in alcaptonuric blood is still widely quoted in medical texts. It is now certain that his results were in error, since plasma contains no detectable homogentisic acid oxidase [38].

Another proposal as to the nature of the defect was that of Dakin [92], as discussed above, in which he considered that the whole pathway to homogentisic acid in alcaptonuric patients is abnormal. Neuberger et al. [29] suggested that perhaps the alcaptonuric kidney differs from the normal kidney in having the capacity to secrete homogentisic acid actively while the normal kidney might not, and that this unusual renal defect might account for the abnormal urinary product (see Dent [103]). However, throughout the last 55 years, Garrod's suggestion that a liver enzyme is missing has been generally considered the most reasonable hypothesis. It was obvious that the net effect would be the same whether the enzyme itself or a vital cofactor is missing or whether there is an inhibitor of the enzyme in alcaptonuric liver.

A careful analysis of the enzymes involved in tyrosine metabolism in normal and alcaptonuric liver showed that only homogentisic acid oxidase is missing in alcaptonuric liver and that all the other enzymes involved in tyrosine metabolism to acetoacetic acid are present and have about the same activity as in normal liver [17, 43] (Table 13-1). Evidence was also obtained that the lack of activity is not due to the presence of inhibitor or to the lack of any known cofactor [17]. It now seems reasonable to define the defect in alcaptonuria as the failure to synthesize active homogentisic acid oxidase, and to attribute all the findings in alcaptonuria to this specific enzymatic defect. Whether these individuals form a catalytically inactive protein, differing perhaps only slightly in structure from active homogentisic acid oxidase, or whether they produce no protein at all resembling the enzyme is still unknown.

Later, the opportunity to obtain at autopsy samples of kidney tissue from two alcaptonuric patients made it possible to show that homogentisic acid oxidase is also absent in alcaptonuric kidney, but that the other enzymes involved in the oxidation of tyrosine to acetoacetic acid can be easily detected [104]. Homogentisic acid oxidase could be demonstrated in nonalcaptonuric human kidney autopsy samples. Thus, the genetic defect in alcaptonuria is not limited to the synthesis of homogentisic acid oxidase in liver; it appears to affect the synthesis of the enzyme wherever it is normally present. This is of theoretical interest, from the viewpoint

Table 13-1. ACTIVITY OF TYROSINE OXIDATION ENZYMES IN ALCAPTONURIC AND NONALCAPTONURIC HUMAN LIVER HOMOGENATE

Enzymes	*Enzyme activity, µmoles of substrate oxidized/hr/gm of liver*	
	Nonalcaptonuric	Alcaptonuric
Tyrosine transaminase	36	32
p-Hydroxyphenylpyruvic acid oxidase	67	46
Homogentisic acid oxidase	268	<0.048
Maleylacetoacetic acid isomerase*	960	780
Fumarylacetoacetic acid hydrolase	288	222

* Units calculated as Δ log optical density per hr per 0.1 gm wet weight of liver [105].
Source: From La Du et al. [17].

of the genetic control and tissue specificity of enzymes [106, 107], and it may be of some practical value in the detection of the carrier trait in relatives of alcaptonuric patients. It might be possible to show a decreased amount of enzyme in carriers of the trait by a direct assay of the enzyme in a tissue more accessible than liver or kidney. This would perhaps be a more accurate means to measure the enzyme than to determine it indirectly by the rate of metabolism of homogentisic acid in a tolerance test.

Carboxyl-^{14}C-labeled homogentisic acid injected intravenously in two alcaptonuric patients was over 90 percent excreted in the urine without change. In contrast, only 3.2 percent was excreted by a control patient, and over 95 percent was oxidized to $^{14}CO_2$ within 12 hr [108]. The results support the conclusions from earlier enzymatic studies in vitro and metabolic balance studies in vivo that the enzymatic block is essentially complete in alcaptonuria.

The metabolic abnormality in alcaptonuria is present essentially from birth. Garrod noted in 1901 [109] that staining of the diapers was scarcely evident 38 hr after birth, although after 52 hr they were deeply stained and continued to be thereafter. The reason for the delay in the excretion of homogentisic acid in newborn alcaptonuric patients is probably that the enzyme systems involved in tyrosine oxidation are not completely developed at birth and that they increase in activity during the next few days [110]. Once established, the defect continues relentlessly throughout life. No therapeutic agent has been found which substantially alters the degree of the defect. The amount of homogentisic acid excreted per day is usually from 4 to 8 gm; it can be altered by changing the content of phenylalanine and tyrosine in the diet. In starvation there is a marked decrease in homogentisic acid excretion [111], as would be expected, although Mittlebach [112] showed that on a diet very low in protein, the alcaptonuric patient continued to excrete some homogentisic acid, presumably from the breakdown of tissue proteins.

Homogentisic Acid Oxidase

The enzymatic step which is missing in alcaptonuria is the further metabolism of homogentisic acid by an oxidative cleavage of the ring to yield maleylacetoacetic acid [113], which in turn is isomerized enzymatically to fumarylacetoacetic acid [105, 114, 115] (Fig. 13-7). The next step is hydrolysis to fumaric and acetoacetic acids by an enzyme which appears to be the same as that shown to hydrolyze a number of α,γ-diketo acids by Meister and Greenstein [116] and to hydrolyze triacetic acid [117, 118].

In 1951, Suda and Takeda [119] solubilized an enzyme from a strain of *Pseudomonas* adapted to tyrosine which catalyzed the oxidation of homogentisic acid; they named it *homogentisicase.* They then studied the properties of a similar enzyme from rabbit liver [120]. Homogentisicase, or, as it is more generally called, homogentisic acid oxidase, has been purified to some degree in several laboratories, and many of its properties have been described [113, 121–123]. It belongs to the class of oxygenases. In the cleavage of the benzene ring, both oxygen atoms come from atmospheric oxygen, as indicated in experiments with ^{18}O [124]. The enzyme contains essential sulfhydryl groups and requires ferrous iron [120, 125], as do several of the other oxygenases involved in ring cleavage reactions, such as pyrocatechase [126, 127], hydroxyanthranilate oxidase [128], and protocatechuic acid oxidase [129, 130] (see Mason [131], p. 126). No other cofactors have been clearly implicated in this reaction. Although evidence that one did exist was presented by Suda and Takeda [120] in 1950, it now appears that a protective effect of glutathione may account for the earlier results [132]. There is also general agreement that the previously suggested requirement for ascorbic acid in this enzyme system [133] is an indirect one due to the requirement for ferrous iron. The only function that has been demonstrated for ascorbic acid in this reaction is to maintain iron in the reduced form [120, 134]. Homogentisic acid oxidase is inhibited by various quinones [122], by sulfhydryl-binding agents [125], and by metal-chelating agents such as α,α'-dipyridyl and *o*-phenanthroline [135], which reacts with ferrous iron.

Homogentisic acid oxidase activity can be measured manometrically, since the oxidation requires the uptake of two atoms of oxygen [113, 136], or it can be measured spectrophotometrically [113] by following the absorption of the product maleylacetoacetic acid at 330 mμ, provided the product is stable under the assay conditions. The enzyme is found in the soluble fraction of liver and kidney [137], as are all the mammalian enzymes involved in the conversion of tyrosine to acetoacetic acid [138]. Homogentisic acid oxidase activity is highest in liver; there is less activity in kidney, and no significant activity has been found in any of the other tissues so far examined [123, 139], such as blood, salivary glands, germinal epithelium, and muscle. This general distribution pattern has been found in rat, rabbit, guinea pig, and pigeon [123]. In man, too, it is highest in liver [17], and appreciable activity is also present in kidney [104]. The liver of the toad, *Buffo marinus,* has as high homogentisic acid oxidase activity as that found in mammalian liver [140]. The presence of the enzyme in some microorganisms adapted to tyrosine has been previously mentioned [119, 141].

The optimal pH for this enzyme is about 7 [120, 121], and it is specific for homogentisic acid. Closely related compounds, such as *o*-hydroxyphenylacetic acid, *p*-hydroxyphenylacetic acid, and gentisic acid are not oxidized [121], nor are homogentisic acid ethyl ester and homogentisic acid lactone. The quinone formed by oxidizing homogentisic acid [142] does not appear to be an intermediate in the oxidation [121], and, in fact, this quinone is an inhibitor of the enzyme [121, 143]. The requirement for ferrous iron is apparently specific, since other bivalent metals, such as Co^{++}, Zn^{++}, Mg^{++}, and Mn^{++}, cannot replace it [120, 143].

A report in the German literature [144] that gentisic acid was less well metabolized in an alcaptonuric patient than in the normal person led Garrod to conclude that the enzyme system defective in alcaptonuria must catalyze the oxidation of some other 2,5-dihydroxyphenyl compounds, as well as homogentisic acid [1]. The specificity of the enzyme rules out this possibility, and the reason for the results in the original study is not known. It is possible that a larger percentage of gentisic acid is excreted as the free acid and less as conjugated derivatives in the alcaptonuric patient because of some inhibitory effect of homogentisic acid on the conjugation of gentisic acid and that for this reason less gentisic acid appeared to be metabolized. However, in one attempt to confirm this finding, the excretion of free gentisic acid was found to be about the same in an alcaptonuric patient as in nonalcaptonuric persons [145].

Intermittent Alcaptonuria

There are a few reports in the literature of intermittent alcaptonuria, or instances in which it is reported that alcaptonuria has spontaneously disappeared (see Galston et al. [45]). In view of the finding that alcaptonuria is associated with the lack of a specific enzyme, it is difficult to imagine how this hereditary condition would undergo intermittent exacerbations and remissions or a spontaneous cure. Perhaps some of these cases of "alcaptonuria" are misdiagnosed and have some other reducing substance present in the urine. Other cases may be examples in which some agent such as those described below, which can induce experimental alcaptonuria in animals, has altered the activity of the enzymes in this pathway, with resultant homogentisic acid excretion. Any further cases of alcaptonuria of this type should be carefully investigated with the specific methods now available, to establish beyond any doubt that homogentisic acid is the reducing substance excreted in the urine. In 1948 Fishberg reported [146] that a patient with autotoxic enterogenous cyanosis excreted up to ½ gm per day of benzoquinone acetic acid, the quinone corresponding to homogentisic acid. The amount excreted varied in inverse ratio to the ascorbic acid excretion. She also found, on the basis of nonspecific tests, that patients with rheumatic fever and with scurvy excrete a similar quinone capable of producing methemoglobinemia. These results have been questioned by Consden et al. [147], who found no benzoquinone acetic acid excreted in scorbutic guinea pigs or in patients with rheumatic fever. They suggest that bacterial activity in the urine leading to nitrite formation may have been responsible for the results of the qualitative tests employed by Fishberg. The excretion of benzoquinone acetic acid in the case of enterogenous cyanosis cannot be explained in this way. They suggest that the product might have been homogentisic acid which was oxidized to the quinone by nitrite arising from bacterial activity. Others have found nitrite in the urine and blood of patients with enterogenous cyanosis [148].

Metabolism of Homogentisic Acid

Under normal conditions no homogentisic acid is present in the urine, and none can be detected in plasma by the methods now available [83]. Leaf and Neuberger [149] found that feeding as much as 5 gm homogentisic acid to normal adults produced no homogentisic aciduria. However, they found a transitory alcaptonuria following the intravenous injection of 0.3 or 1.0 gm homogentisic acid. In these experiments the plasma concentration never rose above 15 mg per 100 ml plasma, and it returned to normal values within 30 min.

One might expect to find elevated plasma levels of homogentisic acid in alcaptonuric patients in view of the large quantity of this acid excreted per day. Neuberger et al. [29] found, however, that in a 7-year-old alcaptonuric girl, the fasting plasma level was not more than about 3 mg per 100 ml plasma and that this level did not increase significantly following the oral administration of 3 gm L-phenylalanine. Nevertheless, within 6 hr approximately 85 percent of the given amino acid could be accounted for as homogentisic acid in the urine. Neuberger et al. made a very significant observation regarding the excretion of homogentisic acid during this investigation. The plasma clearance data indicated that unless a large fraction of the urinary homogentisic acid were both synthesized and excreted within the kidney, glomerular filtration alone could not begin to account for the rate of homogentisic acid excretion. In fact, the clearance approached 400 to 500 ml per min, about equal to the renal blood flow. Even though it is most unusual for a normally occurring intermediate to be actively secreted by the kidney, this seems to be true of homogentisic acid. This conclusion is in agreement with the earlier observation of Katsch and Metz [150] that intravenous homogentisic acid given to an alcaptonuric subject did not increase the plasma concentration significantly.

Experiments in La Du's laboratory [38] using an enzymatic assay to estimate plasma homogentisic acid have confirmed these conclusions. Alcaptonuric and nonalcaptonuric individuals were found to excrete homogentisic acid rapidly after oral administration, and the renal clearance data indicated active secretion by the kidney. The possibility [29, 103] that there might be an important difference in the renal handling of homogentisic acid between normal individuals and alcaptonuric patients can be dismissed.

It appears that two factors serve to keep the plasma, and presumably the tissue, concentrations of homogentisic acid at a low level: the great capacity to metabolize this acid in the liver and kidney, and the rapid renal tubular secretion of homogentisic acid. Even in the alcaptonuric patient, the renal mechanism is capable of effectively lowering the plasma level when homogentisic acid is given. This defense mechanism may be highly significant in view of the many years required for ochronosis to appear. It is quite possible that in the alcaptonuric person the tissues are only occasionally flooded with homogentisic acid and that this event has to be repeated many times over a period of years before tissue pigmentation occurs to a significant extent. Benzoquinone acetic acid may be an intermediate in this process [151].

Experimental Alcaptonuria and Ochronosis

Spontaneous alcaptonuria has not been found in any species except man. Although there is a report by Lewis [152] of a rabbit with urine that darkened upon exposure to air and gave some of the qualitative tests for homogentisic acid, the latter was never isolated or positively identified, and the rabbit died without offspring. There are also reports of generalized ochronosis in the bones and connective tissues of cattle, dogs, and horses in which the tissues are described as being black as coal, but again homogentisic acid has never been identified in the urine with certainty [22, 152, 153].

Experimental alcaptonuria has been produced in rats and mice by feeding large quantities of phenylalanine or tyrosine (see Table 13-2). It is also reported that vitamin C–deficient guinea pigs fed extra phenylalanine [134, 158] or tyrosine [134] excreted homogentisic acid, as well as *p*-hydroxyphenylpyruvic acid and *p*-hydroxyphenyllactic acid. Other workers, however, have found only the latter two compounds and no homogentisic acid in similar experiments with vitamin C–deficient guinea pigs [165]. It should be noted that in some experiments of this type the claim has been made that homogentisic acid was excreted, even though the analytic methods employed would not distinguish between *p*-hydroxyphenylpyruvic acid and homogentisic acid [166].

Experimental alcaptonuria has been produced in rats and mice by feeding large quantities of phenylalanine and tyrosine (see Table 13-2). There is also a report of transitory homogentisic acid excretion after feeding a human volunteer large amounts of L-tyrosine [160].

Another type of experimental alcaptonuria has been induced in rats by a diet deficient in the sulfur-containing amino acids [161]. This was not corrected by giving ascorbic acid but was reversed by giving cysteine [162]. In this type of experimental alcaptonuria, proportionately less *p*-hydroxyphenylpyruvic acid is excreted than in the type that responds to ascorbic acid [134].

In addition to the above methods, the finding that homogentisic acid oxidase requires ferrous iron and can be inhibited by α,α'-dipyridyl was used by Suda and Takeda [120] to induce experimental alcaptonuria in guinea pigs. They injected α,α'-dipyridyl and fed extra tyrosine. The excretion of homogentisic acid in these animals was not corrected by administration of vitamin C.

In another investigation, it was found that human volunteers on a vitamin C–deficient diet for several months with frank scorbutic symptoms did not excrete increased amounts of urinary phenols when given 20 gm tyrosine orally [167]. This is further evidence that there is no direct requirement for ascorbic acid in homogentisic acid oxidation. It can be concluded that the majority of instances of experimental alcaptonuria are either the result of direct inhibition of homogentisic acid oxidases or are due to an imbalance in the various enzyme reactions sufficient to cause an accumulation of homogentisic acid and its urinary excretion.

Lin and Knox [159] have reported that in experimental alcaptonuria in rats induced by a diet supplemented with extra tyrosine, no homogentisic acid was excreted for the first 3 or 4 days. Following this initial lag period, the degree of homogentisic acid excretion increased during the next

Table 13-2. METHODS OF PRODUCING EXPERIMENTAL ALCAPTONURIA

Agent	Species	Comment	Reference
Feeding L-phenylalanine	Rats	....	[154–156]
	Mice	....	[157]
	Guinea pigs	Excreted HGA and PHPP on vitamin C–deficient diet; defect corrected by vitamin C [134]	[158, 134]
Feeding L-tyrosine	Rats	Believed by authors to be due to adaptive increase in tyrosine transaminase activity, but decrease in homogentisic acid oxidase activity also found	[159]
	Guinea pigs	On vitamin C–deficient diet; other workers find only PHPP, PHPL, no HGA [165]	[133, 134]
		Defect corrected by ascorbic acid [134] or folic acid [171, 172]	
	Human beings	Large doses over 1 day; 50 gm; 150 gm. Little or no HGA excreted	[160]
Diet deficient in sulfur amino acids	Rats	Effects reversed by cysteine—not by ascorbic acid	[161, 162]
Diet deficient in tryptophan	Rats	Effects reversed by tryptophan	[163]
α,α'-Dipyridyl	Guinea pigs	Defect not altered by ascorbic acid	[120, 164]

Note: HGA = homogentisic acid, PHPP = *p*-hydroxyphenylpyruvic acid, PHPL = *p*-hydroxyphenyllactic acid.

several weeks. They attribute these findings of the gradual increase in intensity of the alcaptonuria to an adaptive increase in tyrosine transaminase activity. They believe that this type of alcaptonuria occurs because the relative rate of homogentisic acid formation overbalances the rate of homogentisic acid degradation. Their data also show a significant decrease in liver homogentisic acid oxidase in the experimental group; the decrease may be an important contribution to the resulting alcaptonuria.

It is of interest to recall that the activity of the enzymes in the pathway following homogentisic acid oxidase was approximately normal in alcaptonuric liver (Table 13-1). Since the only known endogenous source of maleylacetoacetic acid is the oxidation of homogentisic acid, it appears that normal levels of the isomerase are produced in the absence of its substrate. Thus it is a constitutive rather than an adaptive enzyme.

Further studies should be mentioned in connection with the "adaptive" changes in the activity of liver tyrosine transaminase. Lin and Knox [168] found that the level of this transaminase could be increased several-fold by injecting rats intraperitoneally with L-tyrosine. Under these conditions the activity of the enzymes later in the pathway was not changed significantly. This adaptation is unusual, since it can also be produced by injecting hydrocortisone, by certain other amino acids, and by propylene glycol [139]. They also found that injections of L-tyrosine were not effective in adrenalectomized animals unless hydrocortisone was also given.

Most attempts to produce experimental alcaptonuria and ochronosis in animals by feeding special diets have met with very limited success. In most instances the inhibition of homogentisic acid oxidase has been inadequate, and only a small fraction of the normal activity is sufficient to prevent the accumulation of the acid and deposition of ochronotic pigment. More recently, prolonged feeding of L-tyrosine has produced some degree of ochronotic pigmentation of the connective tissues in animals. Bondurant and Henry [169] maintained rats on a diet supplemented with 12 percent tyrosine for 40 days. Gross examination of the dissected knee and hip joints revealed no structural abnormalities, but these tissues showed the deposition of pigment in the articular cartilage of the head of the femur and in opposing tibial and patellar surfaces of the knee joint. Microscopic examination showed focal accumulations of dark brown pigment in the cytoplasm of chondrocytes in the epiphyseal cartilage in some animals.

Blivaiss et al., [170] induced experimental ochronosis in 4-week-old rats by supplementing their diet with 8 percent tyrosine for as long as 28 months. After this time there were ochronotic-like pigment deposits in cartilage, such as the joint capsules, condyles, sternum, and trachea. Pathologic changes were found in the articular cartilage which included abnormal alignment of chrondrocytes with pigment inclusion, fibrillation, and fragmentation, as well as bone denudation. By histochemical techniques, they found an increase in nonsulfated acid mucopolysaccharides in the connective tissues. The histochemical changes were similar to those observed in the patella from a patient with alcaptonuria.

HEREDITARY ASPECTS

The first paper describing the inheritance of alcaptonuria was that of Garrod in 1902 [15], in which he presented evidence that this condition is congenital and familial and that it occurs more often in families in which there are consanguineous marriages. He suggested that alcaptonuria might be transmitted as a single recessive Mendelian trait. He believed that homogentisic acid arose in the normal course of tyrosine metabolism and that consanguineous marriages brought to light a recessive defect in this metabolic process. In 1902 Bateson and Saunders [173] also suggested that the inheritance of a rare recessive factor might explain the incidence of alcaptonuria. These studies on the mode of transmission of alcaptonuria were among the first on hereditary metabolic diseases.

Although in the years immediately following, examples were recorded in which direct transmission (i.e., parent and offspring affected) of alcaptonuria occurred, Garrod believed that these were examples of a heterozygous individual mating with a homozygote. As more family histories were described, the general opinion of the recessive nature of the disease remained unchallenged. In 1932 Hogben et al. [174] carefully summarized all the known cases of alcaptonuria reported up to that time. Again the recessive character of the disease was confirmed in nearly all the families, and it was observed that at least half the affected individuals were the offspring of consanguineous matings. Although there was an unequal sex distribution in their cases—100 males and 46 females—they did not consider this an indication that the condition was semilethal in females. They noted that males were more often the probands in affected families and suggested that the higher incidence in males might be because of the more frequent examination of males. They also noted that among infants there were slightly more females than males, which was in agreement with this explanation. Nevertheless, it is frequently stated in medical texts that the incidence of alcaptonuria is twice as high in males as in females. The paper by Hogben et al. is obviously the source of this information.

Among the families reviewed by Hogben et al., there were some in which a dominant form of alcaptonuria had to be considered. In a family studied by Pieter [175], the author felt compelled to conclude that a dominant type of alcaptonuria existed. In the end, this conclusion depended upon the predicted opportunity for marriage between homozygous and heterozygous individuals, and the frequency of the heterozygote in the general population, or perhaps more exactly, the incidence of the heterozygote within a selected population. The incidence of alcaptonuria in the general population can be only roughly estimated. At least 600 cases have been described, but this is a conservative number, since new cases are generally not reported unless there are some other special features present. It is reasonably certain, however, that alcaptonuria is less rare than was believed 30 years ago. It is reported [10] that in a study in Northern Ireland by A. C. Stephenson, the incidence of alcaptonuria was from 3 to 5 per million individuals. This would give a considerably higher incidence of heterozygous individuals in the general population than assumed by Hogben et al. [174].

It is important to recall that in the families in which direct transmission of alcaptonuria has been found, the number of consanguineous marriages is very high. One of the best examples of this is the kindred described by Khachadurian and Abu Feisal [176]. In this Lebanese family, there was a total of eight alcaptonuric patients in five successive generations (Fig. 13-10). Careful investigation, however, showed that the grandmothers of the propositus were first cousins and that at least three consanguineous marriages existed in this family. This pedigree is particularly instructive because it illustrates how a recessive trait could appear to be a dominant one unless the entire family pedigree is known.

At present most, if not all, cases appear to represent the inheritance of a single autosomal recessive gene. This is supported by the biochemical finding that a single enzyme system is inactive in this condition and that only one clinical form of alcaptonuria is known. The few cases in which it has been considered as possibly a dominant form have not shown any clinical differences from the majority of cases.

The suggestion by Milch [177, 178] that alcaptonuria is inherited as a dominant gene with incomplete penetrance seems unnecessarily complicated to explain the data at hand (see Knox [10]). In fact, while the possibility of a dominant type of alcaptonuria cannot be excluded, it should be pointed out that no convincing evidence for it has yet been presented.

The fact that a rare disease with recessive inheritance may be encountered more frequently in selected inbred populations complicates the estimation of the incidence of heterozygotes in the general population. It would be most helpful if a diagnostic test were available to detect the carrier state. In view of the nature of the enzymatic defect in alcaptonuric individuals, one might hope to find approximately one-half of the normal amount of enzyme in the tissues of heterozygous individuals, as is apparently the situation in phenylketonuria [179–181] and galactosemia [182, 183]. However, heterozygous carriers of alcaptonuria do not excrete homogentisic acid after an oral loading dose of L-tyrosine [184], and measurements of the ability to metabolize homogentisic acid by an oral homogentisic acid tolerance test have so far shown no difference between relatives of alcaptonuric patients and normal controls [185]. These results may be due to the tremendous capacity of the liver (see Table 13-1) to metabolize this acid. Perhaps even if this reserve were reduced to one-half, it might not be detected by an oral tolerance test. In fact, assuming a liver weight of 1,500 gm and assuming that the liver homogentisic acid oxidase is as efficient in vivo as under assay conditions in vitro, it can be calculated that the normal adult liver can metabolize over 1,600 gm homogentisic acid per day.

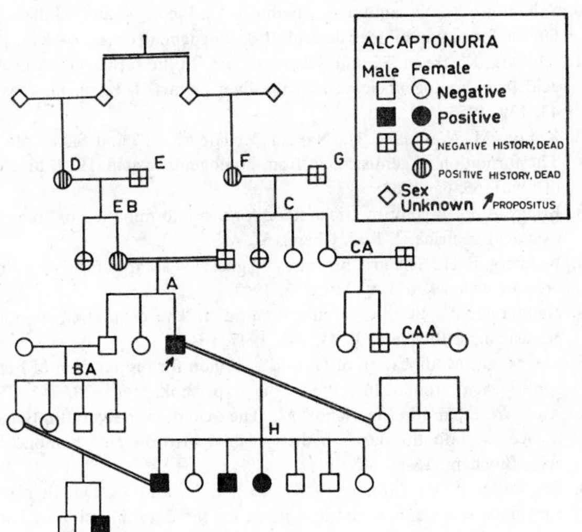

Figure 13-10. Alcaptonuria in a Lebanese family reported by Khachadurian and Abu Feisal. (*By permission of A. Khachadurian and K. Abu Feisal* [176].)

TREATMENT

Attempts to treat alcaptonuria have been directed either toward correcting the underlying metabolic defect or preventing or reversing the pigmentation and arthritic changes. Galdston et al. [45] administered several vitamins, brewers' yeast, tyrosinase, insulin, and adrenocortical extract without altering the amount of homogentisic acid excreted by an alcaptonuric patient. Several groups have studied the effectiveness of vitamin C [28, 29, 45, 186, 187]. Although it corrects the alcaptonuria induced in guinea pigs by feeding large amounts of tyrosine [133], it does not change the hereditary type of alcaptonuria.

Other agents, such as vitamin B_{12} [188], cortisone [21, 189, 190], and phenylbutazone [191], are without influence on the metabolic defect. A confusing report by Cope and Kassander [67] that cortisone corrected the metabolic error is difficult to interpret, since the authors claim this was a case of ochronosis without homogentisic acid in the urine.

Now that it is certain that the basic defect is the lack of a specific enzyme, replacement of the missing enzyme is theoretically a therapeutic measure to consider, but this is not practical at present. Even if pure homogentisic acid oxidase were available in large quantities, its administration might very well cause an antibody response capable of inactivating the enzyme. It is possible that a synthetic chemical compound might be found which could replace the missing enzyme, but no such catalyst is now available.

In the past it has been suggested that dietary phenylalanine and tyrosine be reduced to decrease the output of homogentisic acid. A severe restriction of the intake of these amino acids is not practical except for brief periods and might be dangerous to the patient if continued over a long time.

Since from a practical standpoint the importance of the metabolic defect is mainly that it leads to pigmentation and arthritic changes, therapeutic measures could be aimed primarily at preventing or correcting these complications of the disease. It is possible, as Sealock et al. have pointed out, that large amounts of ascorbic acid might prevent the deposition of ochronotic pigment [28] even though this does not alter the metabolic defect.

SUMMARY

1 Alcaptonuria is a rare, hereditary, metabolic disease in which homogentisic acid, an intermediary product in the metabolism of phenylalanine and tyrosine, cannot be further metabolized. The metabolic defect causes a characteristic triad of homogentisic aciduria, ochronosis, and arthritis.

2 The cause of the disease is a constitutional lack of the enzyme homogentisic acid oxidase. This enzyme normally exists primarily in the liver and kidney. It requires oxygen, ferrous ion, and sulfhydryl groups for opening the ring of homogentisic acid.

3 The condition is inherited as an autosomal recessive disease. No method for the detection of heterozygotes has been devised.

4 The relationships between the metabolic defect and the complications, ochronosis and arthritis, remain a challenging research problem of the future. Even though the lack of homogentisic acid oxidase is no doubt the ultimate cause of these complications, the mechanisms which bring them about are unknown.

BIBLIOGRAPHY

1. Garrod, A. E.: The Croonian lectures on inborn errors of metabolism. Lecture II. Alkaptonuria. Lancet, **2,** 73, 1908.
2. Boedeker, C.: Ueber das Alcapton; ein neuer Beitrag zur Frage: welche Stoffe des Harns können Kupferreduction bewirken? Z. Rat. Med., **7,** 130, 1859.
3. *The Oxford English Dictionary, Supplement,* p. 15. Oxford, New York, 1933.
4. Boedeker, C.: Das Alkapton; ein Beitrag zur Frage: welche Stoffe des Harns Können aus einer alkalischen Kupferoxydlösung Kupferoxydul reduciren? Ann. Chem. Pharm., **117,** 98, 1861.
5. Ebstein, W., and Müller, J.: Brenzkatechin in dem Urin eines Kindes. Arch. Path. Anat., **62,** 554, 1875.
6. Fürbringer, P.: V. Nachtrag über Alkaptonurie. Berlin klin. Wschr., **12,** 390, 1875.
7. Smith, W. G.: On the occurrence of protocatechuic acid in urine. Dublin J. Med. Sci., **73,** 465, 1882.
8. Marshall, J.: A preliminary notice of a crystalline acid in urine possessing more powerful reducing properties than glucose. Med. News (Philadelphia), **50,** 35, 1887.
9. Kirk, R.: On a new acid found in human urine which darkens with alkalies. J. Anat. Physiol., London, **23,** 69, 1889.
10. Knox, W. E.: Sir Archibald Garrod's "inborn errors of metabolism." II. Alkaptonuria. Amer. J. Hum. Genet., **10,** 95, 1958.
11. Wolkow, M., and Baumann, E.: Über das Wesen der Alkaptonurie. Z. Physiol. Chem., **15,** 228, 1891.
12. Garrod, A. E.: *Inborn Errors of Metabolism.* Frowde, Hodder and Stoughton, London, 1909.
13. Neubauer, O.: Über den Abbau der Aminosäuren im gesunden und kranken Organismus. Deutsch. Arch. Klin. Med., **95,** 211, 1909.
14. Neubauer, O.: Intermediärer Eiweisstoffwechsel. Handb. Norm. Path. Physiol., **5,** 671, 1928.
15. Garrod, A. E.: The incidence of alkaptonuria: a study in chemical individuality. Lancet, **2,** 1616, 1902.
16. Beadle, G. W., and Tatum, E. L.: Genetic control of biochemical reactions in neurospora. Proc. Nat. Acad. Sci., U.S.A., **27,** 499, 1941.
17. La Du, B. N., Zannoni, V. G., Laster, L., and Seegmiller, J. E.: The nature of the defect in tyrosine metabolism in alcaptonuria. J. Biol. Chem., **230,** 251, 1958.
18. O'Brien, W. M., La Du, B. N., and Bunim, J. J.: Biochemical, pathological and clinical aspects of alcaptonuria, ochronosis and ochronotic arthropathy. Amer. J. Med., **34,** 813, 1963.
19. Cooper, P. A.: Alkaptonuria with ochronosis. Proc. Roy. Soc. Med., **44,** 917, 1951.
20. Minno, A. M., and Rogers, J. A.: Ochronosis: report of a case. Ann. Intern. Med., **46,** 179, 1957.
21. Yules, J. H.: Ochronotic arthritis: report of a case. Bull. New Eng. Med. Center, **16,** 168, 1954.
22. Martin, W. J., Underdahl, L. O., and Mathieson, D. R.: Alkaptonuria: report of 3 cases. Proc. Staff Meet. Mayo Clin., **27,** 193, 1952.
23. Crissey, R. E., and Day, A. J.: Ochronosis: a case report. J. Bone Joint Surg., **32A,** 688, 1950.
24. Smith, H. P., and Smith, H. P., Jr.: Ochronosis: report of two cases. Ann. Intern. Med., **42,** 171, 1955.
25. Hammond, G., and Powers, H. W.: Alkaptonuric arthritis: report of a case. Lahey Clin. Bull., **11,** 18, 1958.
26. Pomeranz, M. M., Friedman, L. J., and Tunick, I. S.: Roentgen findings in alcaptonuric ochronosis. Radiology, **37,** 295, 1941.
27. Rose, G. K.: Ochronosis. Brit. J. Surg., **44,** 481, 1957.
28. Sealock, R. R., Gladston, M., and Steele, J. M.: Administration of ascorbic acid to an alkaptonuric patient. Proc. Soc. Exp. Biol. Med., **44,** 580, 1940.
29. Neuberger, A., Rimington, C., and Wilson, J. M. G.: Studies on alcaptonuria. II. Investigations on a case of human alcaptonuria. Biochem. J., **41,** 438, 1947.
30. Sakamoto, Y., Nakamura, K., Inamori, K., Ikeda, S. and Ichihara, K.: On the formation of gentisic acid. II. J. Biochem. (Tokyo), **44,** 849, 1957.
31. Ichihara, K., Ikeda, S., and Sakamoto, Y.: On the formation of gentisic acid from homogentisic acid by the liver extract. J. Biochem. (Tokyo), **43,** 129, 1956.
32. Kanda, M., Watanabe, H., Nakata, Y., Higashi, T., and Sakamoto, Y.: The formation of gentisic acid from homogentisic acid. IV. J. Biochem. (Tokyo), **55,** 65, 1964.
33. Briggs, A. P.: A colorimetric method for the determination of homogentisic acid in urine. J. Biol. Chem., **51,** 453, 1922.
34. Fishberg, E. H.: The instantaneous diagnosis of alkaptonuria on a single drop of urine. J.A.M.A., **119,** 882, 1942.
35. Neuberger, A.: Studies on alcaptonuria. I. The estimation of homogentisic acid. Biochem. J., **41,** 431, 1947.
36. Medes, G.: Modification of Garrod's method for preparation of homogentisic acid from urine. Proc. Soc. Exp. Biol. Med., **30,** 751, 1933.
37. Knox, W. E., and LeMay-Knox, M.: The oxidation in liver of L-tyrosine to acetoacetate through *p*-hydroxyphenylpyruvate and homogentisic acid. Biochem. J., **49,** 686, 1951.
38. Seegmiller, J. E., Zannoni, V. G., Laster, L., and La Du, B. N.: An enzymatic spectrophotometric method for the determination of homogentisic acid in plasma and urine. J. Biol. Chem., **236,** 774, 1961.
39. La Du, B. N., O'Brien, W. M., and Zannoni, V. G.: Studies on ochronosis. I. The distribution of homogentisic acid in guinea pigs. Arthritis Rheum., **5,** 81, 1962.

40. Virchow, R.: Ein Fall von allgemeiner Ochronose der Knorpel und knorpelähnlichen Theile. Arch. Path. Anat., **37,** 212, 1866.
41. Albrecht, H.: Ueber Ochronose. Z. Heilk., **23,** 366, 1902.
42. Osler, W.: Ochronosis: the pigmentation of cartilages, sclerotics and skin in alkaptonuria. Lancet, **1,** 10, 1904.
43. Bunim, J. J., McGuire, J. S., Jr., Hilbish, T. F., Laster, L., La Du, B. N., Jr., and Seegmiller, J. E.: Alcaptonuria: clinical staff conference at the National Institutes of Health. Ann. Intern. Med., **47,** 1210, 1957.
44. Smith, J. W.: Ochronosis of the sclera and cornea complicating alkaptonuria: review of the literature and report of four cases. J.A.M.A., **120,** 1282, 1942.
45. Galdston, M., Steele, J. M., and Dobriner, K.: Alcaptonuria and ochronosis with a report of three patients and metabolic studies in two. Amer. J. Med., **13,** 432, 1952.
46. Lichtenstein, L., and Kaplan, L.: Hereditary ochronosis: pathological changes observed in two necropsied cases. Amer. J. Path., **30,** 99, 1954.
47. Cooper, J. A., and Moran, T. J.: Studies on ochronosis. A.M.A. Arch. Path., **64,** 46, 1957.
48. O'Brien, W. M., Banfield, W. G., and Sokoloff, L.: Studies on the pathogenesis of ochronotic arthropathy. Arthritis Rheum., **4,** 137, 1961.
49. Fitzpatrick, T. B., and Lerner, A. B.: Biochemical basis of human melanin pigmentation. A.M.A. Arch. Derm., **69,** 133, 1954.
50. Lillie, R. D.: A Nile blue staining technic for the differentiation of melanin and lipofuscins. Stain Techn., **31,** 151, 1956.
51. Mörner, K. A. H.: Zur Kenntnis von den Farbstoffen der melanotischen Geschwülste. Z. Physiol. Chem., **11,** 66, 1887.
52. Milch, R. A., Titus, E. D., and Loo, T. L.: Atmospheric oxidation of homogentisic acid: spectrophotometric studies. Science, **126,** 209, 1957.
53. Milch, R. A., and Titus, E. D.: Studies of alcaptonuria: absorption spectra of homogentisic acid–chondroitin sulfate solutions. Arthritis Rheum., **1,** 566, 1958.
54. Zannoni, V. G., Lomtevas, N., and Goldfinger, S.: Oxidation of homogentisic acid to ochronotic pigment in connective tissue. Biochim. Biophys. Acta, **177,** 94, 1969.
55. La Du, B. N., and Zannoni, V. G.: Oxidation of homogentisic acid catalyzed by horse-radish peroxidase. Biochim. Biophys. Acta, **67,** 281, 1963.
56. Stoner, R., and Blivaiss, B. B.: Homogentisic acid metabolism: A 1,4-addition reaction of benzoquinone-2-acetic acid with amino acids and other biological amines. Fed. Proc., **24,** 656, 1965.
57. La Du, B. N., and Zannoni, V. G.: in *Pigments in Pathology,* edited by M. Wolman, p. 465. Academic, New York, 1969.
58. Sugar, H. S., and Waddell, W. W.: Ochronosis-like pigmentation associated with the use of atabrine. Illinois Med. J., **89,** 234, 1946.
59. Ludwig, G. D., Toole, J. F., and Wood, J. C.: Ochronosis from quinacrine (atabrine). Ann. Intern. Med., **59,** 378, 1963.
60. Pick, L.: Ueber die Ochronose. Berlin. Klin. Wschr., **43,** 591, 1906.
61. Reid, E., Osler, W., and Garrod, A. E.: On ochronosis. Quart. J. Med., **1,** 199, 1908.
62. Pope, F. M.: A case of ochronosis: with a note on the relationship of alkaptonuria to ochronosis by A. E. Garrod. Lancet, **1,** 24, 1906.
63. Beddard, A. P.: Ochronosis associated with carboluria. Quart. J. Med., **3,** 329, 1910.
64. Beddard, A. P., and Plumtre, C. M.: A further note on ochronosis associated with carboluria. Quart J. Med., **5,** 505, 1912.
65. Brogren, N.: Case of exogenetic ochronosis from carbolic acid compresses. Acta Dermatovener., **32,** 258, 1952.
66. Oppenheimer, B. S., and Kline, B. S.: Ochronosis, with a study of an additional case. Arch. Intern. Med., **29,** 732, 1922.
67. Cope, C. B., and Kassander, P.: Cortisone in ochronotic arthritis. J.A.M.A., **150,** 997, 1952.
68. Janney, N. W.: A study of ochronosis. Amer. J. Med. Sci., **156,** 59, 1918.
69. Skinsnes, O. K.: Generalized ochronosis: report of an instance in which it was misdiagnosed as melanosarcoma, with resultant enucleation of an eye. Arch. Path., **45,** 552, 1948.
70. Fürbringer, P.: Beobachtungen über einen Fall von Alkaptonurie. Berlin. Klin. Wschr., **12,** 330, 1875.
71. Moraczewski, W. von: Ein Fall von Alkaptonurie. Centr. Inn. Med., **XVII,** 177, 1896.
72. Harrold, A. J.: Alkaptonuric arthritis. J. Bone Joint Surg., **38B,** 532, 1956.
73. Hench, P. S.: Rheumatism and arthritis: review of American and English literature of recent years. 9th Rheumatism Review. Ann. Intern. Med., **28,** 310, 1948.
74. Sutro, C. J., and Anderson, M. E.: Alkaptonuric arthritis: cause for free intraarticular bodies. Surgery, **22,** 120, 1947.
75. Moran, T. J., and Yunis, E. J.: Studies on ochronosis. 2. Effects of injection of homogentisic acid and ochronotic pigment in experimental animals. Am. J. Path., **40,** 359, 1962.
76. Greiling, H.: Beitrag zur Entstehung der Ochronose bei Alkaptonurie. Klin. Wschr., **35,** 889, 1957.
77. Dihlmann, W., Greiling, H., Kisters, R., and Stuhlsatz, H. W.: Biochemische und radiologische Untersuchungen zur Pathogenese der Alkaptonurie. Deutsche Med. Wschr., **95,** 839, 1970.
78. Coodley, E. L., and Greco, A. J.: Clinical aspects of ochronosis, with report of a case. Amer. J. Med., **8,** 816, 1950.
79. Eisenberg, H.: Alkaptonuria, ochronosis, arthritis and ruptured intervertebral disk. A.M.A. Arch. Intern. Med., **86,** 79, 1950.
80. Young, H. H.: Calculi of the prostate associated with ochronosis and alkaptonuria. J. Urol., **51,** 48, 1944.
81. Rosenbaum, H., and Reveno, W. S.: Polycythemia and alkaptonuria. Harper Hosp. Bull., **10,** 36, 1952.
82. Dalgliesh, C. E.: Metabolism of the aromatic amino acids. Advances Protein Chem., **10,** 31, 1955.
83. Knox, W. E.: The metabolism of phenylalanine and tyrosine, in *A Symposium on Amino Acid Metabolism,* edited by W. D. McElroy, and H. B. Glass. Johns Hopkins, Baltimore, 1955.
84. Lerner, A. B.: Metabolism of phenylalanine and tyrosine. Advances Enzym., **14,** 73, 1953.
85. Meister, A.: *Biochemistry of the Amino Acids.* Academic, New York, 1957.
86. Schepartz, B., and Gurin, S.: The intermediary metabolism of phenylalanine labeled with radioactive carbon. J. Biol. Chem., **180,** 663, 1949.
87. Weinhouse, S., and Millington, R. H.: Ketone body formation from tyrosine. J. Biol. Chem., **175,** 995, 1948.
88. Weinhouse, S., and Millington, R. H.: Ketone body formation from tyrosine. J. Biol. Chem., **181,** 645, 1949.
89. Dische, R., and Rittenberg, D.: The metabolism of phenylalanine-4-C^{14}. J. Biol. Chem., **211,** 199, 1954.
90. Lerner, A. B.: On the metabolism of phenylalanine and tyrosine. J. Biol. Chem., **181,** 281, 1949.
91. Bamberger, E.: Über das Verhalten paraalkylierter Phenole gegen das Carosches Reagens. Ber. Deutsch. Chem. Ges., **36,** 2028, 1903.
92. Dakin, H. D.: The chemical nature of alkaptonuria. J. Biol. Chem., **9,** 151, 1911.
93. Dakin, H. D.: Experiments relating to the mode of decomposition of tyrosine and of related substances in the animal body. J. Biol. Chem., **8,** 11, 1910.
94. Wakeman, A. J., and Dakin, H. D.: The catabolism of phenylalanine, tyrosine and of their derivatives. J. Biol. Chem., **9,** 139, 1911.
95. La Du, B. N., and Zannoni, V. G.: The tyrosine oxidation system of liver. II. Oxidation of *p*-hydroxyphenylpyruvic acid to homogentisic acid. J. Biol. Chem., **217,** 777, 1955.
96. Pirrung, J., Gottesman, L., and Crandall, D. I.: The metabolism of *p*-methoxyphenylalanine and *p*-methoxyphenylpyruvate. J. Biol. Chem., **229,** 199, 1957.
97. Recknagel, R. O., and Potter, V. R.: Mechanism of the ketogenic effect of ammonium chloride. J. Biol. Chem., **191,** 263, 1951.
98. Edwards, S. W., Hsia, D. Y.-Y., and Knox, W. E.: The first oxidative enzyme of tyrosine metabolism, *p*-hydroxyphenylpyruvate oxidase. Fed. Proc., **14,** 206, 1955.
99. Neuberger, A.: Synthesis and resolution of 2:5-dihydroxyphenylalanine. Biochem. J., **43,** 599, 1948.
100. Gross, O.: Über den Einfluss des Blutserums des Normalen und des Alkaptonurikers auf Homogentisinsäure. Biochem. Z., **61,** 165, 1914.
101. Katsch, G., and Stern, G.: Zur Theorie der alkaptonurischen Stoffwechselstörung. Deutsch. Arch. Klin. Med., **151,** 329, 1926.

102. Lanyar, F., and Lieb, H.: Die quantitative Bestimmung der Homogentisinsäure im Blutserum und in der Milch des Alkaptonurikers. Z. Physiol. Chem., **203,** 135, 1931.
103. Dent, C. E. (editor): Symposium on inborn errors of metabolism. Amer. J. Med., **22,** 671, 1957.
104. Zannoni, V. G., Seegmiller, J. E., and La Du, B. N.: Nature of the defect in alcaptonuria. Nature (London), **193,** 952, 1962.
105. Knox, W. E., and Edwards, S. W.: The properties of maleylacetoacetate, the initial product of homogentisate oxidation in liver. J. Biol. Chem., **216,** 489, 1955.
106. Henion, W. F., and Sutherland, E. W.: Immunological differences of phosphorylases. J. Biol. Chem., **224,** 477, 1957.
107. Schlamowitz, M.: Immunochemical studies on alkaline phosphatase, in Symposium on Enzymes in Blood. Ann. N.Y. Acad. Sci., **75,** 373, 1958.
108. Lustberg, T. J., Schulman, J. D., and Seegmiller, J. E.: Metabolic fate of homogentisic acid-1-^{14}C (HGA) in alcaptonuria and effectiveness of ascorbic acid in preventing experimental ochronosis. Arthritis & Rheumat., **12,** 678, 1969.
109. Garrod, A. E.: About alkaptonuria. Lancet, **2,** 1484, 1901.
110. Kretchmer, N., Levine, S. Z., McNamar, H., and Barnett, H. L.: Certain aspects of tyrosine metabolism in the young. I. The development of the tyrosine oxidizing system in human liver. J. Clin. Invest., **35,** 236, 1956.
111. Braid, F., and Hickmans, E. M.: Metabolic study of an alkaptonuric infant. Arch. Dis. Child., **4,** 389, 1929.
112. Mittelbach, F.: Ein Beitrag zur Kenntnis der Alkaptonurie. Deutsch. Arch. Klin. Med., **71,** 50, 1901.
113. Knox, W. E., and Edwards, S. W.: Homogentisate oxidase of liver. J. Biol. Chem., **216,** 479, 1955.
114. Edwards, S. W., and Knox, W. E.: Homogentisate metabolism: the isomerization of maleylacetoacetate by an enzyme which requires glutathione. J. Biol. Chem., **220,** 79, 1956.
115. Ravdin, R. G., and Crandall, D. I.: The enzymatic conversion of homogentisic acid to 4-fumarylacetoacetic acid. J. Biol. Chem., **189,** 137, 1951.
116. Meister, A., and Greenstein, J. P.: Enzymatic hydrolysis of 2,4-diketo acids. J. Biol. Chem., **175,** 573, 1948.
117. Witter, R. F., and Stotz, E.: The metabolism *in vitro* of triacetic acid and related diketones. J. Biol. Chem., **176,** 501, 1948.
118. Connors, W. M., and Stotz, E.: The purification and properties of a triacetic acid-hydrolyzing enzyme. J. Biol. Chem., **178,** 881, 1949.
119. Suda, M., and Takeda, Y.: Metabolism of tyrosine. I. Application of successive adaptation of bacteria for the analysis of the enzymatic breakdown of tyrosine. J. Biochem. (Tokyo), **37,** 375, 1950.
120. Suda, M., and Takeda, Y.: Metabolism of tyrosine. II. Homogentisicase. J. Biochem. (Tokyo), **37,** 381, 1950.
121. Crandall, D. I.: Homogentisic acid oxidase. II. Properties of the crude enzyme in rat liver. J. Biol. Chem., **212,** 565, 1955.
122. Schepartz, B.: Inhibition and activation of the oxidation of homogentisic acid. J. Biol. Chem., **205,** 185, 1953.
123. Crandall, D. I., and Halikis, D. N.: Homogentisic acid oxidase. I. Distribution in animal tissues and relation to tyrosine metabolism in rat kidney. J. Biol. Chem., **208,** 629, 1954.
124. Crandall, D. I., Yasunobu, K., Krueger, R. C., and Mason, H. S.: Oxygen transfer by homogentisate oxidase. Fed. Proc., **17,** 207, 1958.
125. Crandall, D. I.: in *Symposium on Amino Acid Metabolism,* edited by W. D. McElroy and H. B. Glass, p. 867. Johns Hopkins, Baltimore, 1955.
126. Suda, M., Hashimoto, K., Matsuoka, H., and Kamahora, T.: Further studies on pyrocatecase. J. Biochem. (Tokyo), **38,** 289, 1951.
127. Stanier, R. Y., and Ingraham, J. L.: Protocatechuic acid oxidase. J. Biol. Chem., **210,** 799, 1954.
128. Long, C. L., Hill, H. N., Weinstock, I. M., and Henderson, L. M.: Studies of the enzymatic transformation of 3-hydroxyanthranilate to quinolinate. J. Biol. Chem., **211,** 405, 1954.
129. Mac Donald, D. L., Stanier, R. Y., and Ingraham, J. L.: The enzymatic formation of β-carboxymuconic acid. J. Biol. Chem., **210,** 809, 1954.
130. Dagley, S., and Patel, M. D.: Microbial oxidation of *p*-cresol and protocatechuic acid. Biochem. J., **60,** XXXV, 1955.
131. Mason, H. S.: Mechanisms of oxygen metabolism. Advances Enzym., **19,** 79, 1957.
132. Suda, M.: Homogentisic acid oxidizing enzyme. Med. J. Osaka Univ., **8,** suppl.: 57, 1958.
133. Sealock, R. R., and Silberstein, H. E.: The control of experimental alcaptonuria by means of vitamin C. Science, **90,** 571, 1939.
134. Sealock, R. R., and Silberstein, H. E.: The excretion of homogentisic acid and other tyrosine metabolites by the vitamin C-deficient guinea pig. J. Biol. Chem., **135,** 251, 1940.
135. Schepartz, B.: Intermediate steps in tyrosine metabolism. Fed. Proc., **12,** 265, 1953.
136. Edwards, S. W., and Knox, W. E.: in *Methods in Enzymology,* edited by S. P. Colowick and N. O. Kaplan, vol. 2, p. 292. Academic, New York, 1955.
137. Crandall, D. I.: L-Tyrosine oxidation in rat kidney. Fed. Proc., **13,** 195, 1954.
138. Knox, W. E.: in *Methods in Enzymology,* edited by S. P. Colowick and N. O. Kaplan, vol. 2, p. 287. Academic, New York, 1955.
139. Lin, E. C. C., and Knox, W. E.: Specificity of the adaptive response of tyrosine-α-ketoglutarate transaminase in the rat. J. Biol. Chem., **233,** 1186, 1958.
140. La Du, B. N., and Zannoni, V. G.: Unpublished observations.
141. Jones, J. D., Smith, B. S., and Evans, W. C.: Homogentisic acid, an intermediate in the metabolism of tyrosine by the aromatic ring-splitting microorganisms. Biochem. J., **51,** XI, 1952.
142. Mörner, C. T.: Weitere Beiträge zur Chemie der Homogentisinsäure. Z. Physiol. Chem., **78,** 306, 1912.
143. Crandall, D. I.: Properties and distribution of homogentisic acid oxidase. Fed. Proc., **12,** 192, 1953.
144. Neubauer, O., and Falta, W.: Über das Schicksal einiger aromatischer Säuren bei der Alkaptonurie. Z. Physiol. Chem., **42,** 81, 1904.
145. La Du, B., et al.: Unpublished observations.
146. Fishberg, E. H.: Excretion of benzoquinoneacetic acid in hypovitaminosis C. J. Biol. Chem., **172,** 155, 1948.
147. Consden, R., Forbes, H. A. W., Glynn, L. E., and Stanier, W. M.: Observations on the oxidation of homogentisic acid in urine. Biochem. J., **50,** 274, 1951.
148. Evans, A. S., Enzer, N., Eder, H. A., and Finch, C. A.: Hemolytic anemia with paroxysmal methemoglobinemia and sulfhemoglobinemia. A.M.A. Arch. Intern. Med., **86,** 22, 1950.
149. Leaf, G., and Neuberger, A.: The preparation of homogentisic acid and of 2:5-dihydroxyphenylethylamine. Biochem. J., **43,** 606, 1948.
150. Katsch, G., and Metz, E.: Der Nachweis der Homogentisinsäure im Serum des Alkaptonurikers. Deutsch. Arch. Klin. Med., **157,** 143, 1927.
151. Zannoni, V. G., Malawista, S. E., and La Du, B. N.: Studies on ochronosis. II. Studies on benzoquinoneacetic acid, a probable intermediate in the connective tissue pigmentation of alcaptonuria. Arthritis Rheum., **5,** 547, 1962.
152. Lewis, J. H.: Alcaptonuria in a rabbit. J. Biol. Chem., **70,** 659, 1926.
153. Poulsen, V.: Über Ochronose bei Menschen und Tieren. Beitr. Path. Anat., **48,** 346, 1910.
154. Papageorge, E., and Lewis, H. B.: Experimental alcaptonuria in the white rat. J. Biol. Chem., **123,** 211, 1938.
155. Butts, J., Dunn, M. S., and Hallman, L. F.: Studies in amino acid metabolism. IV. Metabolism of dl-phenylalanine and dl-tyrosine in the normal rat. J. Biol. Chem., **123,** 711, 1938.
156. Lanyar, F.: Über experimentelle Alkaptonurie bei der weissen Ratte. Z. Physiol. Chem., **278,** 155, 1943.
157. Lanyar, F.: Über experimentelle Alkaptonurie bei der weissen Maus. Z. Physiol. Chem., **275,** 225, 1942.
158. Sealock, R. R., Perkinson, J. D., Jr., and Basinski, D. H.: Further analysis of the role of ascorbic acid in phenylalanine and tyrosine metabolism. J. Biol. Chem., **140,** 153, 1941.
159. Lin, E. C. C., and Knox, W. E.: Role of enzymatic adaptation in production of experimental alkaptonuria. Proc. Soc. Exp. Biol. Med., **96,** 501, 1957.
160. Abderhalden, E.: Bildung von Homogentisinsäure nach Aufnahme grosser Mengen von 1-Tyrosin per os. Z. Physiol. Chem., **77,** 454, 1912.

161. Glynn, L. E., Himsworth, H. P., and Neuberger, A.: Pathological states due to deficiency of the sulfur-containing amino-acids. Brit. J. Exp. Path., **26**, 326, 1945.
162. Neuberger, A., and Webster, T. A.: Studies on alcaptonuria. 3. Experimental alcaptonuria in rats. Biochem. J., **41**, 449, 1947.
163. Woodford, V. R., Quan, L., and Cutts, F.: Experimental alkaptonuria in the rat induced by tryptophan deficiency. C. J. Biol. Chem., **45**, 791, 1967.
164. Suda, M., Takeda, Y., Sujishi, K., and Tanaka, T.: Metabolism of tyrosine. III. Relation between homogentisicase, ferrous ion and L-ascorbic acid in experimental alcaptonuria of guinea pig. J. Biochem. (Tokyo), **38**, 297, 1951.
165. Painter, H. A., and Zilva, S. S.: The influence of L-ascorbic acid on the disappearance of the phenolic group of L-tyrosine in the presence of guinea pig-liver suspensions. Biochem. J., **46**, 542, 1950.
166. Malakar, M. C., and Banerjee, S. N.: Effect of glycine or choline chloride on the excretion of homogentisic acid by the tyrosine-fed and scorbutic guinea pigs. Ann. Biochem. Exp. Med., **15**, 69, 1955.
167. Bartley, W., Krebs, H. A., and O'Brien, J. R. P.: Vitamin C requirement of human adults. Medical Research Council, Special Report Series, No. 280, p. 27. H. M. Stationery Office, London, 1953.
168. Lin, E. C. C., and Knox, W. E.: Adaptation of the rat liver tyrosine-α-ketoglutarate transaminase. Biochim. Biophys. Acta, **26**, 85, 1957.
169. Bondurant, R. E., and Henry, J. B.: Pathogenesis of ochronosis in experimental alkaptonuria of the white rat. Lab. Invest., **14**, 62, 1965.
170. Blivaiss, B. B., Rosenberg, E. F., Kutuzov, H., and Stoner, R.: Experimental ochronosis. Induction in rats by long-term feeding with L-tyrosine. A.M.A. Arch. Path., **82**, 45, 1966.
171. Woodruff, C. W., Cherrington, M. E., Stockell, A. K., and Darby, W. J.: The effect of pteroylglutamic acid and related compounds upon tyrosine metabolism in the scorbutic guinea pig. J. Biol. Chem., **178**, 861, 1949.
172. Woodruff, C. W., and Darby, W. J.: An *in vivo* effect of pteroylglutamic acid upon tyrosine metabolism in the scorbutic guinea pig. J. Biol. Chem., **172**, 851, 1948.
173. Bateson, W., and Saunders, E. R.: *Report of the Evolution Committee of the Royal Society* (*London*), No. 1, p. 133, 1902. Cited by Garrod (ref. 14).
174. Hogben, L., Worrall, R. L., and Zieve, I.: The genetic basis of alkaptonuria. Proc. Roy. Soc. Edinburgh, **52**, 264, 1932.
175. Pieter, H.: Une famille d'alcaptonuriques. Presse méd., **33**, 1310, 1925.
176. Khachadurian, A., and Abu Feisal, K.: Alkaptonuria: report of a family with seven cases appearing in four successive generations with metabolic studies in one patient. J. Chron. Dis., **7**, 455, 1958.
177. Milch, R. A.: Direct inheritance of alcaptonuria. Metabolism, **4**, 513, 1955.
178. Milch, R. A.: Inheritance of alcaptonuria. Bull. Hosp. Joint Dis., **18**, 103, 1957.
179. Hsia, D. Y-Y., Driscoll, K. W., Troll, W., and Knox, W. E.: Detection by phenylalanine tolerance tests of heterozygous carriers of phenylketonuria. Nature (London), **178**, 1239, 1956.
180. Hsia, D. Y-Y., and Paine, R. S.: Phenylketonuria: detection of the heterozygous carrier. J. Ment. Defic. Res., **1**, 53, 1957.
181. Knox, W. E., and Messinger, E. C.: The detection in the heterozygote of the metabolic effect of the recessive gene for phenylketonuria. Amer. J. Hum. Genet., **10**, 53, 1958.
182. Holzel, A., and Komrower, G. M.: A study of the genetics of galactosaemia. Arch. Dis. Child. **30**, 155, 1955.
183. Kirkman, H. N., and Bynum, E.: Enzymic evidence of a galactosemic trait in patients of galactosemic children. Ann. Hum. Genet., **23**, 117, 1959.
184. Roth, M., and Felgenhauer, W.-R.: Recherche de l'excrétion d'acide homogentisique urinaire chez des hétérozygotes pour l'alcaptonurie. Enzymol. Biol. Clin., **9**, 53, 1968.
185. La Du, B., et al.: Unpublished observations.
186. Mosonyi, L.: A propos de l'alcaptonurie et de son traitement. Presse Méd., **47**, 708, 1939.
187. Díaz, C. J., Mendoza, H. C., and Rodríguez, J. S.: Alkapton, Aceton und Kohlehydratmangel. Klin. Wschr., **18**, 965, 1939.
188. Flaschenträger, B., Halawani, A., and Nabeh, I.: Alkaptonurie und Vitamin B_{12}. Klin. Wschr., **32**, 131, 1954.
189. Black, R. L.: Use of cortisone in alkaptonuria. J.A.M.A., **155**, 968, 1954.
190. Suzman, M. M.: The clinical application of corticotropin and cortisone therapy: a report of 247 cases. South African Med. J., **27**, 195, 1953.
191. Biggs, T. G., Jr., and Cannon, E., Jr.: Ochronosis: report of a case. J. Louisiana State Med. Soc., **105**, 395, 1953.

CHAPTER FOURTEEN

ALBINISM*

Thomas B. Fitzpatrick and
Walter C. Quevedo, Jr.

HISTORICAL INTRODUCTION

Albinism is a heritable disorder of the melanin pigmentary system, found throughout the animal kingdom. It is characterized by decrease or absence of melanin in the skin, hair, and eyes. Historical reviews of albinism can be found in the comprehensive monographs by Pearson, Nettleship, and Usher [1] and in more recent summaries by Froggatt [2, 3] and Witkop [4]. It is believed that the term *albino* is derived from the Latin adjective *albus,* "white," and was first applied by Balthazar Tellez to certain "white" Negroes whom he observed on the west coast of Africa [1]. The essential clinical features of albinism are well summarized in the following description published in 1699 by Lionel Wafer [5]:

> *There is one complexion so singular . . . that I never saw nor heard of any like them in any part of the world. . . . They are white . . . 'tis rather a milk-white, lighter than the colour of any* Europeans, *and much like that of a white horse. . . . From their seeing so clear as they do in a moon-shiny night, we us'd to call them moon-ey'd. For they see not very well in the sun, poring in the clearest Day; their eyes being but weak, and running with water if the sun shine towards them; so that in the day-time they care not to go abroad. . . . When moon-shiny night's come, they are all life and activity, running abroad, and into the woods, skipping about like wild-bucks; and running as fast by moon-light, even in the gloom and shade of the woods, as the other* indians *by Day, being as nimble as they, tho' not so strong and lusty. . . . Neither is the child of a man and woman of these white* indians, *white like the parents, but copper-colour'd as their parents were. . . . They were but short-liv'd.*

Outstanding characteristics are the "milk-white" color and photophobia, with "eyes being but weak, and running with water if the sun shine towards them." The recessive inheritance is suggested by "neither is the child of a man and woman of these white *indians,* white like the parents, but copper-colour'd." The striking contrast of albino skin with the normal darkly pigmented skin of Indians and Negroes sets them apart, and many myths were conjured up about these strange "moon-ey'd" people. Several albino heroes are prominent in the mythology of the Cuna tribe of Indians residing on the San Blas Islands off the coast of Panama.

Sir Archibald Garrod [6] included albinism among the inborn errors of metabolism. His speculations about the nature of the metabolic defect in albinism and the mechanism of melanin formation are truly remarkable. In 1908, when enzyme chemistry was in its infancy and there was no knowledge of a melanin-synthesizing enzyme in the skin, Garrod wrote:

> *Three possible explanations of the phenomenon of albinism suggest themselves. We might suppose that the cells which usually contain pigment fail to take up melanins formed elsewhere; or that the albino has an unusual power of destroying these pigments; or again that he fails to form them. . . . It is very unlikely that the melanin is conveyed to the pigmented cells and there deposited, for all the evidence available indicates that the pigment is formed* in situ, *probably by the action of intracellular enzymes. . . . Only certain specialised cells appear to have the power of forming melanin. . . . Taking all the known facts into consideration, the theory that what the albino lacks is the power of forming melanin which is normally possessed by certain specialised cells is that which has most in its favour and is probably the true one. If so, an intracellular enzyme is probably wanting in the subjects of this anomaly, an explanation which . . . brings albinism into line with some other inborn metabolic errors, of which a similar explanation is at least a possible one.*

This chapter, devoted to albinism in man, reexamines Garrod's [6] brilliant proposal in the light of recent research in pigment-cell biology.

Albinism is found in fishes, amphibians, reptiles, and birds, as well as in man and other mammals [7–10]. It is the gross manifestation of a heritable defect in the pigment-cell (melanocyte) system; because of this defect, the melanocytes fail to produce normal amounts of melanin. Melanin may never be completely absent in human albinism, although it may be undetectable in certain animals, e.g., the albino mouse.

DEFINITION

Melanocytes are distinctive, specialized, dendritic cells in which the biosynthesis of melanin takes place. During the embryonic development of mice, precursor melanocytes (melanoblasts), except in the retinal pigment epithelium,

*Dr. Fitzpatrick's work was supported by Grant CA05010 from the National Cancer Institute, Public Health Service. Dr. Quevedo's work was supported in part by PHS Research Grant CA-06097 from the National Cancer Institute, Training Grant GM-00582 from the Division of General Medical Sciences, Public Health Service, and American Cancer Society Grant PS-42.

arise in the neural crest and actively migrate to peripheral sites.[1] In man, mature melanocytes are normally present in certain characteristic regions: *skin* (hair bulbs, dermis, and dermoepidermal junction), *mucous membranes, nervous system* (piarachnoid), and *eye* (uveal tract and retinal pigment epithelium). Melanin pigment is synthesized on specialized cytoplasmic organelles called *melanosomes*. The enzymic conversion of the amino acid tyrosine to melanin is catalyzed by the aerobic oxidase, *tyrosinase*. The major features of melanogenesis will be summarized later in this chapter. All melanocytes, with the curious exception of those in the hair bulbs and retinal pigment epithelium, appear to have the ability to form malignant melanomas.

The metabolic defect that is manifested as albinism may involve the entire melanocyte system (oculocutaneous albinism) or the melanocytes at a specific site (ocular albinism). The terminology used in the classification of the different types of albinism should clearly reflect the extent and, when possible, the nature of pigmentary involvement. Recently, and unfortunately, the term albinism has been applied to an increasing number of heritable conditions of hypopigmentation in spite of the demonstration that many differ significantly in their genetic control and developmental expression. One goal of human genetics is to relate specific variations in expressed characteristics (phenotype) to the hereditary information coded within the genome. Genetic terminology should reflect the precision of this knowledge. Use of the term albinism should be restricted to congenital heritable hypomelanosis that is limited to the eye (ocular albinism) or that involves the eye and integument (oculocutaneous albinism) and in which the basic defect is a partial or total reduction of melanin deposition on melanosomes. This definition would, for example, exclude circumscribed (spotty) hypomelanosis of the skin, which has been called *cutaneous albinism* but should more correctly be called *piebaldism*. The justification for this restriction of terminology is to be found in a number of recent studies with the electron microscope and with enzyme histochemistry.

CLASSIFICATION

Although not perfect, the proposed classification (Table 14-1) provides some advantages over any used previously.

[1] The melanocytes of the retinal pigment epithelium are derived from the outer layer of the optic cup and differ morphologically from the melanocytes present in other sites. Electron micrographs show that the fine structure of the melanosomes of retinal pigment epithelium is similar to that of melanosomes of the hair bulb. The melanocytes of the retinal pigment epithelium contain high levels of tyrosinase only during the early stages of embryonic development; no tyrosinase activity is demonstrable in the postnatal retinal pigment epithelium [11].

Table 14-1. CLASSIFICATION AND CLINICAL FEATURES OF HUMAN ALBINISM

Recommended terminology	Present terminology	Inheritance
Tyrosinase-positive oculocutaneous albinism	Oculocutaneous albinism	Autosomal recessive
Tyrosinase-negative oculocutaneous albinism	Oculocutaneous albinism	Autosomal recessive
Ocular albinism	Ocular albinism	X-linked recessive

Oculocutaneous Albinism

In all races of man, oculocutaneous albinism is characterized by a marked hypomelanosis of the hair, skin, and eyes [1–3, 12]. Witkop and his associates [4] have helped to clarify the genetic basis for variations in the phenotypic expression of oculocutaneous albinism. Two forms have been clearly identified, on the basis of the ability of follicular melanocytes to synthesize melanin when plucked hair bulbs are incubated in solutions containing tyrosine [4, 13]. In one type of oculocutaneous albinism, the presence of tyrosinase is indicated by a darkening of the hair bulbs when they are incubated in tyrosine solutions; this type is therefore called "tyrosinase-positive" oculocutaneous albinism. In the other type the hair bulbs fail to darken in tyrosine solutions; this type is therefore called "tyrosinase-negative" oculocutaneous albinism. There are characteristic differences in the extent of hypomelanosis in the two types [4]. The tyrosinase-positive and tyrosinase-negative types (see Plate I-2) are each inherited as simple recessive traits, and each is the result of the action of two nonallelic autosomal genes [4]. The basis for this statement will be discussed later.

Paralleling the marked reduction in melanin pigmentation throughout the body, there is a susceptibility to solar radiation which is shared by individuals with either type of oculocutaneous albinism. The sensitivity to solar exposure is greatest in the tyrosinase-negative type [4]. When albinotic skin is repeatedly exposed to sunlight, it acquires folds and wrinkles caused by changes in the dermal connective tissue [14], and there is also a high frequency of solar keratosis and basal cell and squamous cell carcinomas of the skin of the exposed areas [15–17]. Malignant melanomas have been found in persons with oculocutaneous albinism [18–23].

The skin of persons with tyrosinase-positive oculocutaneous albinism contains benign pigmented nevi and, in addition, large deeply pigmented "freckles" in the light-exposed areas [4]. Whether pigmented lesions may also occur in the skin of persons with tyrosinase-negative oculocutaneous albinism remains to be established [4].

Visual acuity in both types of oculocutaneous albinism is impaired, and there is evidence of astigmatism, hypermetropia, and myopia [24, 25]. Congenital ocular abnormalities associated with albinism include absence of the sphincter muscle, partial aniridia, absence of the pupillary membrane, atrophy of the optic disk, and colobomas of the mesodermal tissue of the iris [25].

It is generally believed, but not statistically confirmed, that the intelligence of persons with oculocutaneous albinism is normal [26]. Indeed, the disorder is compatible with high intelligence; the Rev. W. A. Spooner (1844–1930), a distinguished scholar (also famous for "spoonerisms") and warden of New College, Oxford University, is reputed to have had oculocutaneous albinism.

Tyrosinase-negative Oculocutaneous Albinism

The skin and hair of Negroids and Caucasoids with tyrosinase-negative oculocutaneous albinism (as determined by the negative reaction of the hair bulb) are strikingly white [4]. The eye color may range from gray to blue. Examination of the retina reveals no pigment, and the color of the hair, skin, and eyes does not increase with age [4]. There is a pronounced red reflectance of the fundus of the eye (incorrectly called "red reflex") in both children and adults; nystagmus, translucence of the iris, and photophobia are pronounced [4]. There is also an abnormal degree of translucence of the iris in all Caucasoid and some Negroid carriers (heterozygotes) of tyrosinase-negative oculocutaneous albinism [4].

Tyrosinase-positive Oculocutaneous Albinism

Pigmentation of the skin and hair in tyrosinase-positive oculocutaneous albinism varies with age and race [4, 14]. Negroids with tyrosinase-positive albinism may be darker than are blond Caucasoids. In contrast with tyrosinase-negative oculocutaneous albinism, there is a tendency for pigmentation of the hair, skin, and eye to increase with advancing age. "Freckles" on the exposed areas and pigmented nevi are frequent [4]. Although a red reflectance is readily demonstrated in all infants with this disorder, it is not often observed in the albinotic older children and adults of heavily pigmented races [4]. It may occur in adult tyrosinase-positive albino Caucasoids [4]. Funduscopic observations reveal an absence of pigment in infants and young children, whereas adults, particularly in dark-skinned races, show increased pigmentation [4]. In both Negroids and Caucasoids, pigmentation of the iris increases with age [27]. Nystagmus, photophobia, and iris translucence are present but are probably less pronounced than in persons with tyrosinase-negative oculocutaneous albinism. In some cases the severity of the eye abnormalities decreases with age. Some persons with oculocutaneous albinism do not have nystagmus [3]; these persons probably have the tyrosinase-positive type.

Ocular Albinism

Pigmentation is normal in the hair and skin in ocular albinism, but there is hypomelanosis of the eye. It is inherited as an X-linked recessive trait. In hemizygous males and homozygous females there is slight pigmentation of the iris and, because of hypomelanosis of the fundus, the choroidal vessels are visible. Defects in vision, nystagmus, and head nodding may occur in combination or singly. Translucent irides and a mosaic pattern of pigmentation may be found in the fundi of females who are carriers (heterozygotes) [28–32]. This mosaicism appears to be the result of X inactivation [33]. In some retinal melanocytes the X chromosome bearing the allele for ocular albinism is active and, as a consequence, melanin synthesis is subnormal, whereas in others the X chromosome bearing the normal allele is active, and normal melanin synthesis takes place. Forsius and Eriksson [34] have described an X-linked type of ocular albinism in which the female carrier has an absence of mosaic pigmentation of the fundus and a slight disturbance in ocular discrimination; the male carrier is partially colorblind (protanomalous, i.e., there is reduced sensitivity to red).

PEDIGREE STUDIES

Two pedigrees supplemented by physiologic testing clearly demonstrate the separate gene loci for the tyrosinase-positive and tyrosinase-negative varieties of oculocutaneous albinism.

The North Carolina family studied by Witkop et al. [35] unequivocally demonstrates that a mating of two individuals manifesting the two different types of oculocutaneous albinism produces normal children. The family consisted of Negroid parents with oculocutaneous albinism and their normally pigmented daughter. The father exhibited striking hypopigmentation of the hair, skin, and eyes, with marked red reflectance, photophobia, and nystagmus. General pigmentation had not increased with advancing age. A hair test indicated tyrosinase-negative oculocutaneous albinism. The mother, although clearly an albino, showed more evidence of pigmentation. The hair was light golden brown and the skin cream-colored. The skin showed less solar degeneration (solar keratosis, wrinkling) of the exposed areas than did that of her husband. The fundus was lightly pigmented. There were moderate photophobia and nystagmus but no red reflectance. The irides of the mother were light blue in color, contrasting with the gray of the father. The mother had a positive hair test for tyrosinase. The child had a normal Negroid appearance, with black hair and light-brown skin. There was no evidence of a mosaic pattern of pigmentation in the fundus, and the irides were dark brown. Visual acuity was normal, and there was no nystagmus, photophobia, or red reflectance.

Similar observations were made by Witkop et al. [35] when they reexamined an English Caucasoid family reported by Trevor-Roper [36, 37]. The husband and wife with oculocutaneous albinism each had normally pigmented parents. The general pigmentary features and the hair test of the wife indicated tyrosinase-negative oculocutaneous albinism, while the husband had tyrosinase-positive oculocutaneous albinism. The couple had four normally pigmented children.

Both these pedigrees are consistent with autosomal recessive inheritance and indicate nonallelism between the genes conditioning the tyrosinase-positive and tyrosinase-negative forms of oculocutaneous albinism.

INCIDENCE

Tyrosinase-negative oculocutaneous albinism occurs among Negroids and Caucasoids with a frequency of about 1:34,000 to 36,000 persons [4]. Froggatt [3] estimated that the total incidence of oculocutaneous albinism is about 1:10,000 in Northern Ireland. Basing his conclusions on Froggatt's estimates of the frequency of iris translucence among heterozygotes, Witkop proposed that the frequency of tyrosinase-negative albinism is approximately 1:15,000 in Ireland. The estimated mutation rate for albinism is 3.3×10^{-5} to 7.0×10^{-5} per gene per generation in the population of Ireland.

Tyrosinase-positive oculocutaneous albinism occurs more frequently among Negroids than among Caucasoids [4]. Among Negroids, it occurs at a frequency of about 1:14,000; among Caucasoids, the frequency is approximately 1:60,000 [4]. Oculocutaneous albinism also occurs with high frequency among Amerindians (Tule Cuna Indians, 1:143; Hopi, 1:227; Jemez, 1:140; Zuni, 1:247; Navajo, 1:3,750) [4]. Ocular albinism has a frequency of 1:54,000 persons in Denmark [38].

METABOLIC BASIS OF THE PIGMENTARY DEFECT

A review of the biology of the melanin pigmentary system is necessary for an understanding of the pathogenesis of human and animal albinism.

Normal Melanin Biosynthesis

The major structural basis for color in the mammalian epidermis is the *melanosome.* These granular cytoplasmic organelles containing chromoprotein impart various hues to the epidermis. The isolated epidermis without melanin is a transparent, grayish-white membrane. The wide range of tan-to-black hues in the skins of the various races of man is attributable to variations in the number, packaging, and distribution of melanosomes throughout the epidermis [39]. Melanosomes are synthesized by melanocytes in the basal layer of the epidermis and transported by keratinocytes. Melanin pigmentation expresses the integration of structural and functional elements at a number of discrete levels of biologic organization that range in complexity from the specific molecules relevant to melanin synthesis to the skin as a fully unified, pigmented organ (Fig. 14-1). Several

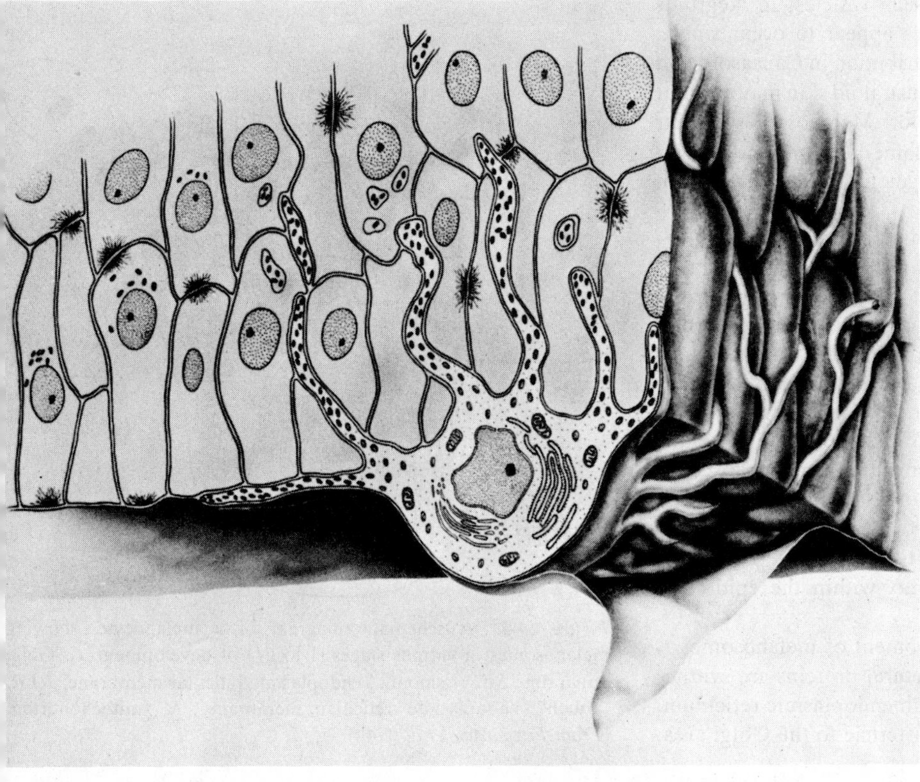

Figure 14-1. The epidermal melanin unit, showing the relationship of a basal melanocyte, a "high-level" Langerhans cell, and the keratinocytes in mammalian epidermis. (*From Quevedo* [73].)

general reviews of melanin pigmentation have been published recently [39–42].

The levels of organization at which the process of melanin pigmentation may be examined include:

Organ:	Epidermis and melanocytes with their melanin content, as seen clinically
Multicellular unit:	Partnership of melanocytes and keratinocytes, *the epidermal melanin unit* (Fig. 14-2), as seen by light microscopy
Cell:	The *melanocyte,* the secretory unicellular gland
Organelle:	The *melanosome,* the metabolic unit of melanin synthesis
Macromolecules:	(1) *Tyrosinase,* the enzyme, and (2) *melanoprotein,* the end product
Molecule:	*Tyrosine,* the precursor

The degree of melanin pigmentation in the skin directly reflects the color and the size of melanosomes and their number and distribution within melanocytes and keratinocytes. After synthesis of melanosomes by the melanocyte, melanosomes are delivered to keratinocytes. Keratinocytes acquire melanosomes either by direct transfer or by phagocytosis of portions of the dendrites of melanocytes. Melanosomes have been observed as aggregates in lysosome-like vesicles within the keratinocytes. These aggregates have been called *melanosome complexes.* In the skin of man, melanosomes of Caucasoids and Mongoloids usually occur in groups of three or more within such vesicles; in Negroids and Australoids, the melanosomes appear to occur singly. This difference in melanosome distribution in Caucasoid and Mongoloid *vis à vis* Negroid and Australoid skin may account in part for differences in skin color. Melanosomes appear to be degraded within the lysosome-like structures, with subsequent release of melanin fragments into the cytoplasm of keratinocytes.

Clear evidence of close interrelationship between melanocytes and keratinocytes has led to the concept of a functional and structural pigment unit known as the epidermal melanin unit [39, 42, 43]. It is composed of an epidermal melanocyte and a group of keratinocytes with which it maintains functional contact and to which it supplies melanosomes. The concept of the epidermal melanin unit proposes that there is an integration of melanocytes and keratinocytes at a level of biologic organization which transcends that of the individual cells. It is not known at this time just exactly how the genes, hormones, or ultraviolet exposure that influence melanocyte activity affect the process of melanosomal synthesis and delivery within the epidermal melanin units [39, 42].

The present view of the development of melanosomes is that tyrosinase and, possibly, structural proteins are synthesized on the ribosomes of the rough endoplasmic reticulum, and then transferred through its cisternae to the Golgi area, where the proteins are segregated within membrane-limited vesicles (Fig. 14-2) [44]. An alternative or additional possibility for melanosome formation was advanced by Novikoff et al. [45], Maul [46], and Toda and Fitzpatrick [47]. These authors proposed that melanosomes may develop in the cisternae of the endoplasmic reticulum closely adjacent to the Golgi apparatus.

The earliest stage in melanosome formation was designated by Toda and Fitzpatrick [44] as Stage I (Fig. 14-3). Within the Stage I melanosome the basic fibrous protein units consist of tyrosinase and, probably, the structural elements of the protein matrix. An ordered pattern is gradually developed within the melanosome to form the fully developed inner membranous structure of the Stage II melanosome, which shows no evidence of melanin deposition. Melanin deposition signals the onset of Stage III: melanin gradually accumulated on the inner membranes, obscuring the characteristic periodicity of their fibrillar components. Finally, the deposited melanin transforms the melanosome into a uniformly dense particle without visible internal structure: this is the Stage IV melanosome (Fig. 14-3). To recapitulate, the definitions of the stages (Fig. 14-3) in the ontogeny of melanosomes are as follows:

STAGE I: A spherical, membrane-delineated vesicle (or perhaps dilated cisternae of the Golgi-associated smooth endoplasmic reticulum) that either (1) can be shown to contain tyrosinase by electron-microscope histochemistry, or

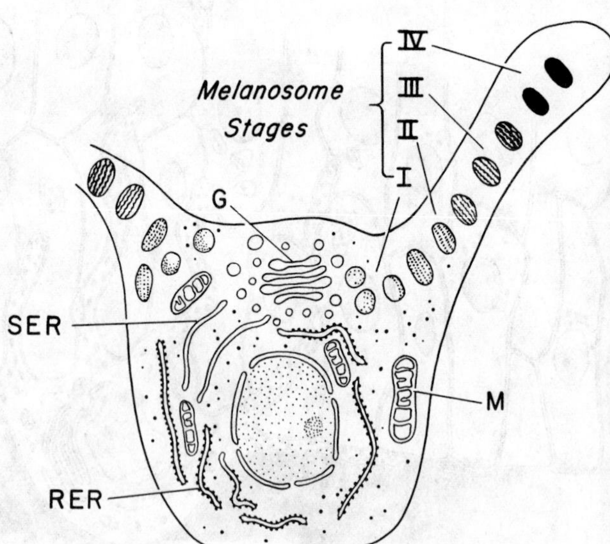

Figure 14-2. A schematic diagram of a melanocyte, showing melanosomes in various stages (I to IV) of development. *G,* Golgi apparatus; *SER,* "smooth" endoplasmic reticular membrane; *RER,* "rough" endoplasmic reticular membrane; *M,* mitochondrion. (*From Fitzpatrick et al.* [74].)

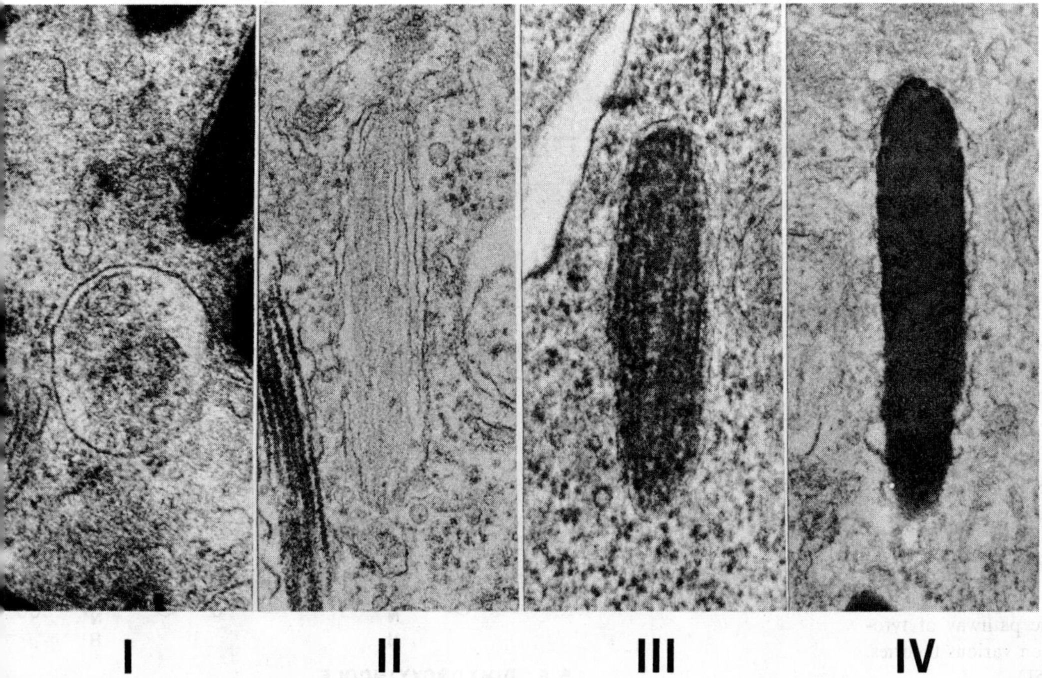

Figure 14-3. Stages in the development of the melanosome. (From *Fitzpatrick et al.* [74].)

(2) contains filaments that have the distinctive periodicity of the melanosomal inner membrane

STAGE II: An oval organelle that shows numerous membranous filaments with or without cross-linking, and with distinctive periodicity

STAGE III: An oval organelle, of which the internal structure, characteristic of melanosomes of Stage II, is partly obscured by electron-dense material

STAGE IV: An oval organelle which, because of deposition of melanin, has become electron-opaque without discernible internal structure in routine preparations

The application of the term melanosome to all stages of the development of the organelle follows Moyer's suggestion [48]. He divided melanosome development into four stages, similar to those described above. This terminology differs somewhat from the definitions offered at the Sixth International Pigment Cell Conference [49], where it was proposed that the term melanosome be applied only to the completely melanized organelle. The term melanosome as used by most investigators usually refers to all stages in the ontogeny of the melanosome. The use of "stages" to indicate the structural events in the ontogeny of the melanosome provides a precise designation of each step.

Melanin in human tissues always occurs in the form of a melaninoprotein complex resulting from a combination of the large melanin polymer with proteins of the matrix. The melanin polymer is derived from tyrosine by the action of tyrosinase according to the metabolic pathway outlined in Fig. 14-4. Until recently, indole-5,6-quinone was considered to be the sole monomer polymerized in the formation of melanin. New evidence clearly indicates that other compounds formed as intermediates in the synthesis of indole-5,6-quinone may copolymerize with it during melanogenesis. Melanin in man, then, may be defined as an insoluble copolymerizate of tyrosine-derived pigmentary intermediates (Fig. 14-5), particularly 5,6-dihydroxyindole, which are formed by the copper-containing aerobic oxidase, tyrosinase. This enzyme is confined to melanocytes and is usually active only within the melanosome. This definition of melanin excludes the pigmented particles found in the pigmented nuclei of the midbrain. These are also derived from tyrosine, by way of the pathway that produces catecholamines. The enzyme catalyzing the hydroxylation of tyrosine to dopa in the nervous system is not tyrosinase but tyrosine hydroxylase [50]. It is therefore not surprising that the pigmented granules present in the substantia nigra and the locus caeruleus are not changed in oculocutaneous albinism [51].

The nature of genetic control of pigmentation in mammals has been clarified in some details by study of the laboratory mouse. Numerous sites of gene action in the origin, distribution, and differentiation of melanoblasts during embryonic

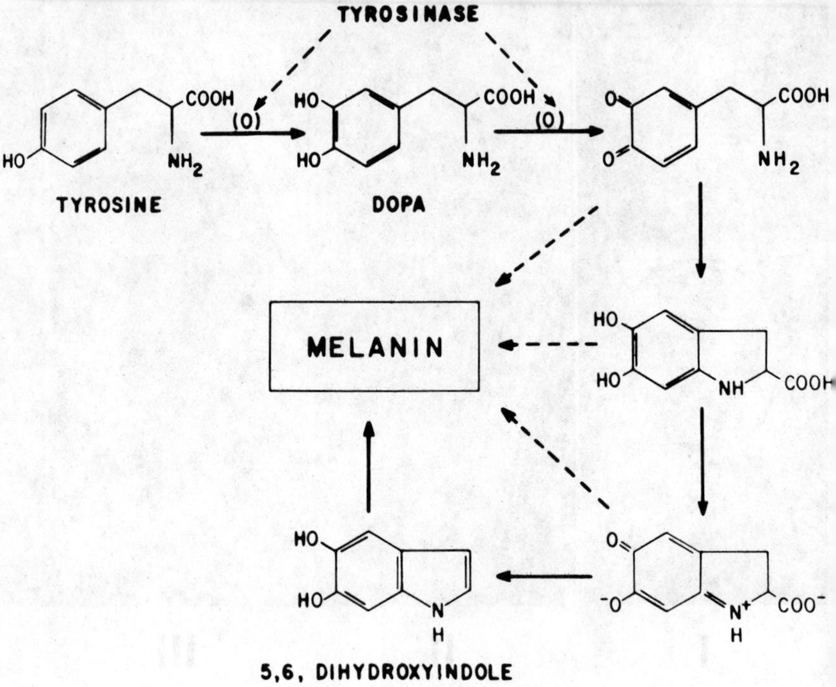

TYROSINASE

TYROSINE

DOPA

MELANIN

5,6, DIHYDROXYINDOLE

Figure 14-4. Metabolic pathway of tyrosine to melanin, based on various theories. (*From Duchon et al.* [75].)

development have been identified in this species. In addition, it is now possible to outline in a preliminary fashion the biochemical pathways that translate hereditary information coded within the genome into the specialized pigmented organelles (melanosomes) elaborated by melanocytes [52–54]. In view of the structural similarity of the melanocytes and melanosomes of mouse and man, it is highly probable that the basic features of the genetic mechanisms that regulate melanocyte performance in the two species are also comparable.

Many of the numerous gene mutations associated with altered hair and skin color in mice have been preserved by selective breeding and thereby provide a valuable source of material for experimental analysis. Approximately 70 genes at 40 loci are now known to influence coloration in mice [54]. Four factors have been demonstrated to be of paramount importance in determining melanocyte form and function: (1) the genotype of the melanoblast; (2) the genotype of the environmental cells; (3) the environmental history of the melanocyte; and (4) the characteristics of the differentiated environmental cells [55, 56]. These factors, acting singly or in combination, influence such diverse events as the origin and differentiation of melanoblasts; melanocyte structure and number; size, shape, and color of melanosomes; specific stages in the biosynthesis of tyrosinase and melanosome assembly; and the patterns of transport of melanosomes within receptor cells. Detailed morphologic and biochemical analyses of numerous coat-color mutants of the house mouse have provided a clear insight into the step-by-step action of genes in morphogenesis of pigment patterns.

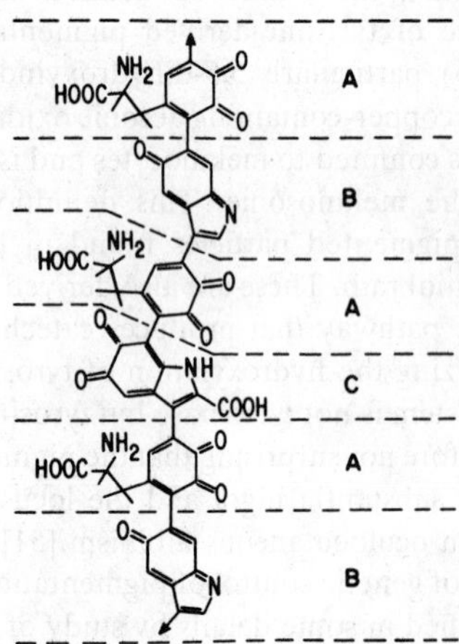

Figure 14-5. The structure of melanin, as proposed by Hempel [76]. *A*, dopa-quinone; *B*, indole-5,6-quinone; *C*, indole-5,6-quinone-2-carboxylic acid. (*From Duchon et al.* [75].)

Attention will be focused here on selected alleles at two gene loci that not only affect the pigmentation of mice but have relevance to the problem of albinism in man. Table 14-2 summarizes the nature and action of various genes on pigment in the mouse.

The *c* locus in the mouse is of particular importance because the manifestations of its activities have parallels in human tyrosinase-negative oculocutaneous albinism. Alleles at this locus appear to regulate the structure of tyrosinase, and, consequently, the overall intensity of pigmentation. The dominant allele at the *c* locus permits formation of the full color appropriate to the remaining genotype. The lowest

Table 14-2. SELECTED GENES INFLUENCING MELANOGENESIS IN MICE

Locus	Gene symbols	Name of genes	Site of action	Influence on melanocyte form and function
a	A^y	Yellow	Hair follicle	Morphology of melanosomes; chemical composition of melanin (eumelanin and phaeomelanin)
	A^{vy}	Viable yellow	Melanocyte environment	
	A^w	White-bellied agouti		
	A	Agouti		
	a^t	Black-and-tan		
	a	Nonagouti		
	a^e	Extreme nonagouti		
b	*B*	Black	Within the melanoblast	Polymerization of melanin; melanosome structure
	B^{lt}	Light		
	b^c	Cordovan		
	b	Brown		
c	*C*	Colored	Within the melanoblast	Tyrosinase structure; melanosome number
	c^{ch}	Chinchilla		
	c^h	Himalayan		
	c^e	Extreme dilution		
	c	Albino		
d	*D*	Nondilute	Within the melanoblast (but expressed only in suitable tissue environments)	Melanocyte morphology ("stubby dendrites")
	d	Dilute		
	d^l	Dilute-lethal		
ln	*Ln*	Nonleaden	Within the melanoblast (but expressed only in suitable tissue environments)	Melanocyte morphology ("stubby dendrites")
	ln	Leaden		
p	*P*	Colored eye	Within the melanoblast	Melanosome structure; melanin synthesis in melanosome
	p	Pink-eyed dilution		
Mo	*Mo*	Mottled	Within the melanoblast (based on X-chromosome-inactivation hypothesis)	(Action unknown)
	Mo^{br}	Brindled		
	Mo^{dp}	Dappled		

Source: Reproduced from Fitzpatrick et al. [39].

allelic member, when present in the homozygous state (*c/c*), produces albinism with absence of melanin pigment in the hair, skin, and eyes. The intermediate alleles bring about gradations of coat pigmentation between albinism and full color. Albino mice produce melanosomes within which no melanin is deposited. These pseudo-Stage II melanosomes appear normal with respect to their structural proteins, but active tyrosinase is lacking. Albino melanocytes transfer these melanosomes to the keratinocytes of the hair follicle [57]. It appears that alleles at the *c* locus, through their influence on the structure of tyrosinase, ultimately regulate the number and size of melanosomes and the amount of melanin deposited on each [54]. Recent studies with radioactive tyrosine in vivo and in vitro have demonstrated that tyrosinase activity increases within the melanosome when allelic substitutions are made progressively from *c/c* to *C/C* [58].

A recessive allele at the *p* locus brings about a reduction in the amount of melanin within the eyes and hair coat, the absolute amount of pigment being determined by other gene loci. In overall features, the pink-eyed dilution mutation shows considerable resemblance to tyrosinase-positive oculocutaneous albinism in man. The *p/p* melanosomes in retinal melanocytes are abnormal in structure as a result of a defective alignment and cross-linkage of many compound fibers. Sidman and Pearlstein [59], on the basis of in vitro studies, concluded that the restricted melanin deposition within *p/p* melanosomes is caused primarily by limitations in the amount of tyrosine available for melanin synthesis, not by an impaired tyrosinase (enzyme) system. Presumably, in mice expressing pink-eyed dilution, tyrosine is "drained off" by competing metabolic reactions, with the result that the rate of melanogenesis is limited by the low availability of melanogenic substrate. In contrast with *p/p* retinal melanocytes [48], the *p/p* follicular melanocytes appear to contain melanosomes with essentially normal matrices [60].

Abnormal Melanin Biosynthesis

The general or local absence of melanin pigmentation in human skin theoretically may result from the absence of melanocytes because of a failure of melanoblasts to invade or survive within specific areas of skin (mechanism A); the failure of melanoblasts to differentiate into melanocytes by initiating the production of melanosomes (mechanism B); the failure of melanocytes to deposit melanin within melanosomes as the result of a tyrosinase defect (mechanism C); the failure of melanocytes to deposit melanin within melanosomes owing to a substrate defect (mechanism D); the dilution of pigmentation by abnormal "packaging" of melanosomes within melanocytes or keratinocytes or both (mechanism E); the destruction of newly synthesized melanosomes (mechanism F); or various combinations of the foregoing mechanisms (mechanism G).

There is clearly a normal distribution of melanocytes in oculocutaneous albinism. In 1952, Becker et al. [61] reported the identification of amelanotic melanocytes in human albino skin by the gold-impregnation technique. Hu et al. [62] confirmed the presence of melanocytes in sheets of epidermis from a person with oculocutaneous albinism. Similar findings were reported by Kugelman and Van Scott [63] and by Mishima and Loud [64].

Witkop and his associates concluded that one form of oculocutaneous albinism results from mechanism C (tyrosinase deficiency) and a second from mechanism D (tyrosine deficiency) [4]. As already stated, melanocytes in depilated hair bulbs in tyrosinase-negative oculocutaneous albinism fail to deposit melanin on incubation in a buffered solution of tyrosine. This finding indicates little or no activity of tyrosinase. Electron microscope examination of skin and hair bulbs from persons with tyrosinase-negative oculocutaneous albinism reveals that the melanocytes contain Stage I and Stage II melanosomes without evidence of melanin deposition. The molecular basis for the defect in tyrosinase function is not known. The defect seems to persist throughout life, inasmuch as skin and hair of "tyrosinase-negative" individuals are reported not to darken significantly with advancing age. In view of the variation in eye color from translucent gray to blue in tyrosinase-negative oculocutaneous albinism, it is probable that melanin is present in the eye, but this assumption needs to be confirmed histologically.

The plucked hair bulbs in tyrosinase-positive oculocutaneous albinism darken on incubation in buffered tyrosine solution [4], and accordingly have active tyrosinase. In tyrosinase-positive albinism, the amount of pigment in skin, hair, and eyes varies significantly with race and age. Pigment in the skin and eye may increase with advancing age. Negroids with tyrosinase-positive albinism in some cases may be darker than are blond Caucasoids (see Plate I-2). Electron microscope observations of hair bulbs in tyrosinase-positive oculocutaneous albinism indicate the presence of numerous Stage II and Stage III melanosomes [4]. Rarely do melanocytes contain the fully mature (Stage IV) melanosomes. Available data indicate that the failure of melanogenesis results from a restriction in the amount of tyrosine within melanosomes (mechanism D). Elevation of blood levels of tyrosine by dietary supplementation fails to modify the pigmentation in oculocutaneous albinism [4]. In vivo pigmentation has been induced in tyrosinase-positive oculocutaneous albinos, however, by application of wet tyrosine packs to epidermis stripped of the cornified layer. As one possibility it has been proposed that a "permease" necessary for the penetration of tyrosine into melanosomes is lacking or reduced in oculocutaneous albinos, with the consequence that less tyrosine is available for incorporation into melanin [4]. Stripping of the epidermis and presentation of tyrosine by an unusual route may disturb this relationship. Some support for the "permease" hypothesis comes from the observations that the tyrosine in saliva secreted by the parotid gland is lower in concentration in individuals with tyrosinase-positive oculocutaneous albinism that it is in normal individuals [65]. This lower concentration of tyrosine suggests a defect in permease activity of the cell membrane and an associated reduced transport of tyrosine from the blood. It is not known how this relates to the melanogenic activity of melanocytes in tyrosinase-positive oculocutaneous albinism. Moreover, the presence of inhibitors and reduced amounts of tyrosinase cannot be ruled out as the primary cause of the pigmentary defect in tyrosinase-positive albinism. Breathnach and Robins [66] have reported the occurrence of abnormal matrices in some melanosomes in oculocutaneous albinism, but they did not specify the type of oculocutaneous albinism involved.

In ocular albinism there is characteristic depigmentation of the iris and fundus. Although the amount of pigment is reduced, the ultrastructural appearance of melanosomes and the biochemical basis for the lesions are not known. It is possible that a mechanism comparable with that in tyrosinase-positive oculocutaneous albinism (mechanism D) is operative, but no evidence is available to date. It is noteworthy that females heterozygous for the gene often have a mosaic pattern of pigmentation in the fundus. This presumably is the result of X inactivation during early embryonic development, and thus some retinal pigment cells possess an active X chromosome with the recessive ocular-albinism allele, whereas the others possess an active X chromosome containing the normal allele.

OTHER HERITABLE HYPOMELANOSES UNRELATED TO ALBINISM

In the past, other hypopigmentary disorders have been included under the general heading of albinism, although there now appears to be no justification for this practice. *Piebaldism* is inherited as a dominant autosomal trait. In almost all patients, a triangular white forelock is present on the scalp, and the hair of this region is depigmented, as is the skin below it [67]. In addition, there are variable patterns of symmetrical circumscribed hypomelanosis on the extremities and anterior surface of the trunk [67]. Pigmented islands may occur within the hypomelanotic areas. Electron microscope studies indicate that melanocytes are absent from the epidermis [67, 68] and hair follicles [69] of the white-forelock region. Melanocytes abnormal in structure have been observed in the depigmented skin of the trunk and extremities of some patients, whereas in others, melanocytes are absent from the depigmented regions [67]. The general histologic features of piebaldism suggest a neural crest defect (mechanism A) leading to abnormal melanocyte performance quite distinct from that in ocular or oculocutaneous albinism.

Chédiak-Higashi syndrome, a fatal childhood disease, involves hypopigmentation resulting from the operation of mechanisms E and F [70]. Melanin is deposited within abnormal giant melanosomes, unusual groups of melanosomes are transferred to keratinocytes, and certain of the giant melanosomes undergo degeneration within melanocytes. This disease is inherited as a recessive autosomal trait and is characterized by a dilution of eye, skin, and hair pigmentation, with a positive hair test for tyrosinase [4]. Skin color varies from a light cream to a slate gray; the slate-gray color is most often in the exposed areas. Hair color varies from blond to brunette and frequently possesses a gray sheen. Afflicted individuals often burn readily on exposure to sunlight. Most patients have photophobia, nystagmus, and pale-blue translucent irides [70]. Some have dark eyes and do not have photophobia, nystagmus, or translucent irides [70]. The blood is characterized by the presence of giant peroxidase-positive granules, which are presumably derived from lysosomes, in leukocytes [70]. Death in young children with the Chédiak-Higashi syndrome usually is the result of infection. Children and adolescents (5 to 18 years) frequently die with lymphoma-like infiltrations. Although some patients have lived until their twentieth year, most die before adulthood [71]. The pattern of cellular infiltration may involve almost every organ of the body. Although many histiocytes are in evidence, the dominant cell type in the infiltrate is an immature lymphoid cell [71]. The abnormal giant granules in the blood leukocytes and the dilution of pigment in the hair, eye, and skin permit an early diagnosis. Inasmuch as the skin, hair, and eye changes of tyrosinase-positive oculocutaneous albinism and Chédiak-Higashi syndrome may be almost identical, persons with clinical features suggesting oculocutaneous albinism should be screened for the presence of giant peroxidase-positive granules in the leukocytes.

ALBINISM IN THE PERSPECTIVE OF EVOLUTIONARY BIOLOGY

The diverse groups of mammals are presumed to have arisen from related ancestral stocks in the distant past, and thus may share genes in common. Though it is impossible to identify homologous genes in members of different species by standard breeding tests, it is possible to demonstrate gene homology at the molecular (DNA) level [72]. The evidence indicates the existence of considerable genic homology among the various classes of vertebrates [72].

Oculocutaneous albinism is broadly distributed among mammals [9]. It is possible that the similarities of expression of tyrosinase-negative oculocutaneous albinism in man and in the mouse may reflect the existence of gene loci maintained in common by both species throughout broad periods of evolutionary diversification. Studies of the nature of tyrosinases in a variety of mammals lend some support to this possibility. As with other functions of the body, evolution may have acted conservatively in the preservation of many genes central to the control of pigmentation and somewhat radically in the case of a more-limited number of other genes. This interpretation explains the similarities of the features of melanogenesis in many mammalian species. The variations may reflect gene selection in adaptation to specialized modes of life.

SUMMARY

1 Albinism is the clinical manifestation of a heritable metabolic defect in the pigment-cell (melanocyte) system of the eye and skin or of the eye alone. The metabolic defect may involve melanocytes in the system as a whole (as in oculocutaneous albinism) or only those melanocytes in one part of the system (as in ocular albinism).

2 Ocular albinism is inherited as an X-linked recessive trait. The metabolic defect in ocular albinism is unknown. Oculocutaneous albinism exists in two forms, tyrosinase-positive oculocutaneous albinism, and tyrosinase-negative oculocutaneous albinism. Each is controlled by a separate gene locus and is inherited as an autosomal recessive trait. In tyrosinase-negative oculocutaneous albinism, there appears to be a tyrosinase defect. In tyrosinase-positive oculocutaneous albinism, there may be a limitation in the availability of tyrosine, the melanogenic substrate of tyrosinase.

3 The phenotypic frequency of tyrosinase-positive oculo-

cutaneous albinism is about 1:14,000 among Negroids and about 1:60,000 among Caucasoids [4]. Tyrosinase-negative oculocutaneous albinism has an incidence of about 1:34,000 to 36,000 among both groups of peoples [4].

4 It is recommended that the term albinism be restricted to the tyrosinase-positive and tyrosinase-negative forms of oculocutaneous albinism and to ocular albinism. Piebaldism, a hypomelanotic condition often included as a form of albinism (and called "partial albinism"), is specifically excluded from this category. In piebaldism, the secretory melanocytes in the skin are absent, with resultant hypomelanosis; in oculocutaneous albinism, the secretory melanocytes and melanosomes are present, but there is a marked reduction in the melanization of the melanosomes, with resultant hypomelanosis.

BIBLIOGRAPHY

1. Pearson, K., Nettleship, E., and Usher, C. H.: *A Monograph on Albinism in Man.* Drapers' Company Research Memoirs, Biometric Series VI, VIII, and IX; parts I, II, and IV. Dulau, London, 1911–1913.
2. Froggatt, P.: "Albinism: a statistical, genetical and clinical appraisal based upon a complete ascertainment of the condition in Northern Ireland." Thesis presented at Trinity College, Dublin, December, 1957.
3. Froggatt, P.: Albinism in northern Ireland. Ann. Hum. Genet., **24,** 213, 1960.
4. Witkop, C. J., Jr.: Albinism, in *Advances in Human Genetics,* edited by H. Harris and K. Hirschhorn, vol. 2. Plenum Press, New York, in press.
5. Wafer, L.: *New Voyage and Description of the Isthmus of America, Giving an Account of the Author's Abode There,* p. 134. London, 1699 (cited by Pearson et al., text part I, pp. 17–18).
6. Garrod, A. E.: Inborn errors of metabolism, Croonian Lectures, Lecture I. Lancet, **2,** 1–7, 1908.
7. Shufeldt, R. W.: Albinism in American animals. Proc. Zool. Soc. London, 540, 1916.
8. Little, C. C.: Coat color genes in rodents and carnivores. Quart. Rev. Biol., **33,** 103, 1958.
9. Searle, A. G.: *Comparative Genetics of Coat Colour in Mammals.* Logos, London (Academic, New York), 1968.
10. Noble, G. K.: *The Biology of the Amphibia,* p. 577. Dover, New York, (1931) 1954.
11. Miyamoto, M., and Fitzpatrick, T. B.: On the nature of the pigment in retinal pigmented epithelium. Science, **126,** 449, 1957.
12. Waardenburg, P. J.: Uveal membrane, in *Genetics and Ophthalmology,* vol. 1, pp. 645–846 ("Albinism," pp. 714–741), by P. J. Waardenburg, A. Franceschetti, and D. Klein. Royal Van Gorcum, Assen, Netherlands, 1961.
13. Witkop, C. J., Jr., Van Scott, E. J., and Jacoby, G. A.: Evidence for two forms of autosomal recessive albinism in man, in *Proceedings of the IInd International Congress of Human Genetics, Rome, 1961,* pp. 1064–1065. Istituto Gregorio Mendel, Rome, 1963.
14. Barnicot, N. A.: Albinism in southwestern Nigeria. Ann. Eugen., **17,** 38, 1952.
15. Hadida, E., Sayag, J., and Tasso, F.: Albinos de 25 ans. Peau rhomboidale, lésions kératosiques, dégénérescence epithéliomateuse. Bull. Soc. Franc. Derm. Syph., **73,** 294, 1966.
16. Curban, G. V.: Multiple cutaneous carcinomatosis in 2 albino brothers. Rev. Paul. Med., **39,** 440, 1951.
17. Shapiro, M. P., Keen, P., Cohen, L. and Murray, J. F.: Skin cancer in the South African Bantu. Brit. J. Cancer, **7,** 45, 1953.
18. Bhende, Y. M.: Malignant amelanotic melanoma of the skin in an albino. Indian J. Med. Sci., **6,** 755, 1952.
19. Young, T. E.: Malignant melanoma in an albino. A.M.A. Arch. Path., **64,** 186, 1958.
20. Leonardi, R., and Grasso, S.: Melanoblastoma in albino: histological findings, Minerva Derm., **33,** 24, 1958.
21. Oettle, A. G.: Skin cancer in Africa, in First International Conference on the Biology of Cutaneous Cancer, U.S. National Cancer Institute, Monograph No. 10, edited by F. Urbach, p. 197. U.S. National Cancer Institute, Washington, 1963.
22. Duron, R. A.: Malignant melanoma in albinos. Rev. Med. Honduras **33,** 149, 1965.
23. Garrington, G. E., Scofield, H. H., Cornyn, J., and Lacy, G. R.: Intraoral malignant melanoma in a human albino. Oral Surg., **24,** 224, 1967.
24. Edmunds, R. T.: Vision of albinos. Arch. Ophthal. (Chicago), **42,** 755, 1949.
25. Wallner, A., and Rudens, M. C.: Report on an unusual family. Amer J. Ophthal., **33,** 785, 1950.
26. Beckham, A. S.: Albinism in Negro children. J. Genet. Psychol., **66,** 199, 1946.
27. Clark, C. P.: Albinism with coexisting anomalies of the central nervous system. Trans. Amer. Ophthal., Soc., **42,** 250, 1944.
28. Vogt, A.: The iris in albinismus solum bulbi, in *Handbook and Atlas of the Slit Lamp Microscopy of the Living Eye,* vol. 3, p. 844-847. Schweizer Druck-und Verlagshaus, Zurich, 1941.
29. Falls, H. F.: Sex-linked ocular albinism displaying typical fundus changes in the female heterozygote. Amer. J. Ophthal., **34,** 41, 1951.
30. Francois, J., and Deweer, J. P.: Albinisme oculaire lié au sexe et altérations caractéristiques du fond d'oeil chez les femmes heterozygotes Ophthalmologica, **126,** 209, 1953.
31. Waardenburg, P. J., and van den Bosch, J.: X-chromosomal ocular albinism in Dutch family. Ann. Hum. Genet., **21,** 101, 1956.
32. Gillespie, F. D.: Ocular albinism with report of a family with female carriers. Arch. Ophthal., (Chicago) **66,** 774, 1961.
33. Lyon, M. F.: Sex chromatin and gene action in the mammalian X-chromosome. Amer. J. Hum. Genet., **14,** 135, 1962.
34. Forsius, H., and Eriksson, A. W.: Ein neues Augensyndrom mit X-chromosomaler Transmission: eine Sippe mit Fundusalbinismus Foveahypoplasie, Nystagmus, Myopie, Astigmatismus und Dyschromatopsie. Klin. Mbl. Augenheilk., **144,** 447, 1964.
35. Witkop, C. J., Jr., Nance, W. E., Rawls, R. F., and White, J. G.: Autosomal recessive oculocutaneous albinism in man: evidence for genetic heterogeneity. Amer. J. Hum. Genet., **22,** 55, 1970.
36. Trevor-Roper, P. D.: Marriage of two complete albinos with normally pigmented offspring. Brit. J. Ophthal., **36,** 107, 1952.
37. Trevor-Roper, P. D.: Albinism. Proc. Roy. Soc. Med. Sec. Ophthal., **56,** 21, 1963.
38. Norn, M. S.: Ocular albinism. Acta Ophthal., **44,** 20, 1966.
39. Fitzpatrick, T. B., Quevedo, W. C., Jr., Seiji, M., and Szabó, G.: Biology of the melanin pigmentary system, in *Dermatology in General Medicine* edited by T. B. Fitzpatrick, K. A. Arndt, W. H. Clark, Jr., A. Z. Eisen E. J. Van Scott, and J. H. Vaughan, McGraw-Hill, New York, 1971.
40. Duchon, J., Fitzpatrick, T. B., and Seiji, M.: Melanin, 1968: Some definitions and problems, in the *Year Book of Dermatology 1967–68,* edited by A. W. Kopf and R. Andrade, pp. 6–33. Year Book Medical Publishers, Inc., Chicago, 1968.
41. Quevedo, W. C., Jr.: The control of color in mammals. Amer. Zool., **9,** 531, 1969.
42. Breathnach, A. S.: Normal and abnormal melanin pigmentation of the skin, in *Pigments in Pathology,* edited by M. Wolman, p. 353. Academic Press, New York, 1969.
43. Fitzpatrick, T. B., and Breathnach, A. S.: Das epidermale Melanin-Einheit-System. Derm. Wschr., **147,** 481, 1963.
44. Toda, K., and Fitzpatrick, T. B.: Isolation of the intermediate "vesicles" during ontogeny of melanosomes in embryonic chick retinal pigmented epithelium. Fed. Proc., **27,** 722, 1968.
45. Novikoff, A. B., Albala, A., and Biempica, L.: Ultrastructural and cytochemical observations on B-16 and Harding-Passey mouse melanoma J. Histochem. Cytochem., **16,** 299, 1968.

46. Maul, G.: Golgi-melanosome relationship in human melanoma *in vitro*. J. Ultrastruct. Res., **26**, 163, 1969.
47. Toda, K., and Fitzpatrick, T. B.: Ultrastructural and biochemical studies of the formation of melanosomes in the embryonic chick retinal pigment epithelium (ECRPE). J. Invest. Derm., **54**, 99, 1970 (abstract).
48. Moyer, F. H.: Electron microscope observations on the origin, development and genetic control of melanin granules of the mouse eye, in *The Structure of the Eye. Proc. Symposium April 11–13, 1960, during the 7th International Congress of Anatomists, New York,* edited by G. K. Smelser, pp. 469–486. Academic, New York, 1961.
49. Fitzpatrick, T. B., Quevedo, W. C., Jr., Levene, A. L., McGovern, V. J., Mishima, Y., and Oettle, A. G.: Terminology of vertebrate melanin-containing cells: 1965. Science, **152**, 88, 1966.
50. Nagatsu, T., Levitt, M., and Udenfriend, S.: Tyrosine hydroxylase: the initial step in norepinephrine biosynthesis. J. Biol. Chem., **239**, 2910, 1964.
51. Marsden, C. D.: Brain melanin, in *Pigments in Pathology,* edited by M. Wolman, p. 395. Academic, New York, 1969.
52. Billingham, R. E., and Silvers, W. K.: The melanocytes of mammals. Quart. Rev. Biol., **35**, 1, 1960.
53. Foster, M.: Mammalian pigment genetics. Advances Genet., **13**, 311, 1965.
54. Wolfe, H. G., and Coleman, D. L.: Pigmentation, in *Biology of the Laboratory Mouse,* 2d ed., edited by E. L. Green, p. 405. McGraw-Hill, New York, 1966.
55. Markert, C. L., and Silvers, W. K.: The effects of genotype and cell environment on melanoblast differentiation in the house mouse. Genetics, **41**, 429, 1956.
56. Silvers, W. K.: Genes and the pigment cells of mammals. Science, **134**, 368, 1961.
57. Parakkal, P. E.: Transfer of premelanosomes into the keratinizing cells of albino hair follicle. J. Cell Biol., **35**, 473, 1967.
58. Coleman, D. L.: Effect of gene substitution on the incorporation of tyrosine into the melanin of mouse skin. Arch. Biochem. Biophys., **96**, 562, 1962.
59. Sidman, R. L., and Pearlstein, R.: Pink-eyed dilution (*p*) gene in rodents: increased pigmentation in tissue culture. Develop. Biol., **12**, 93, 1965.
60. Rittenhouse, E.: Genetic effects on fine structure and development of pigment granules in mouse hair bulb melanocytes. II. The *c* and *p* loci, and *ddpp* interaction. Develop. Biol., **17**, 366, 1968.
61. Becker, S. W., Jr., Fitzpatrick, T. B., and Montgomery, H.: Human melanogenesis: cytology of human pigment cells (melanodendrocytes). A.M.A. Arch. Derm. Syph., **65**, 511, 1952.
62. Hu, F., Fosnaugh, R. P., and Lesney, P. F.: Studies on albinism. The demonstration of dopa-positive melanocytes in albino skin. Arch. Derm. (Chicago), **83**, 723, 1961.
63. Kugelman, T. P., and Van Scott, E. J.: Tyrosinase activity in melanocytes of human albinos. J. Invest. Derm., **37**, 73, 1961.
64. Mishima, Y., and Loud, A. V.: The ultrastructure of unmelanized pigment in cells in induced melanogenesis. Ann. N.Y. Acad. Sci., **100**, 497, 1963.
65. Zipkin, I., Hawkins, G. R., and Mazzarella, M.: The tyrosine, tryptophan and protein content of human parotid saliva in oral and systemic disease. Use of ultraviolet absorption technics, in *Salivary Glands and Their Secretions,* edited by L. M. Sreebny and J. Meyer. Macmillan, New York, 1964.
66. Breathnach, A. S., and Robins, J.: Ultrastructure of melanocytes and melanosomes in human oculocutaneous albinism. J. Anat., **103**, 387, 1968.
67. Breathnach, A. S., Fitzpatrick, T. B., and Wyllie, L. M.: Electron microscopy of melanocytes in human piebaldism. J. Invest. Derm., **45**, 28, 1965.
68. Comings, D. E., and Odland, G. F.: Partial albinism. J.A.M.A., **195**, 510, 1966.
69. Kinebuchi, S., Hori, Y., Toda, K., Fitzpatrick, T. B., and Kobori, T.: unpublished data.
70. Windhorst, D. B., Zelickson, A. S., and Good, R. A.: A human pigmentary dilution based on a heritable subcellular structural defect—the Chédiak-Higashi syndrome. J. Invest. Derm., **50**, 9, 1968.
71. Dent, P. B., Fish, L. A., White, J. G., and Good, R. A.: Chédiak-Higashi syndrome: Observations on the nature of the associated malignancy. Lab. Invest., **15**, 1634, 1966.
72. Hoyer, B. H., Bolton, E. T., McCarthy, B. J., and Roberts, R. B.: The evolution of polynucleotides, in *Evolving Genes and Proteins,* edited by V. Bryson and H. J. Vogel. Academic, New York, 1965.
73. Quevedo, W. C., Jr.: The control of color in mammals. Amer. Zool., **9**, 531, 1969.
74. Fitzpatrick, T. B., Quevedo, W. C., Jr., Seiji, M., and Szabó, G.: Biology of the melanin pigmentary system, in *Dermatology in General Medicine,* edited by T. B. Fitzpatrick, K. A. Arndt, W. H. Clark, Jr., A. Z. Eisen, E. J. Van Scott, and J. H. Vaughan. McGraw-Hill, New York, 1971.
75. Duchon, J., Fitzpatrick, T. B., and Seiji, M.: Melanin, 1968: Some definitions and problems, in *1967–68 Year Book of Dermatology.,* pp. 1–33. Year Book Medical Publishers, Inc., Chicago, 1968.
76. Hempel, K.: Investigation of the structure of melanin in malignant melanoma with H^3- and C^{14}-DOPA labelled at different positions, in *Structure and Control of the Melanocyte,* edited by G. Della Porta and O. Mühlbock, pp. 162–175. Springer-Verlag, Berlin, 1966.

CHAPTER FIFTEEN

HISTIDINEMIA

Bert N. La Du

Histidinemia is a rare hereditary metabolic disorder first recognized in 1961. Ghadimi et al. [1] found elevated levels of histidine in the blood and urine of two sisters, one of whom had a speech defect, and it was concluded that these cases represented a new inborn error of histidine metabolism. In 1962, a report of a similar disorder of histidine metabolism was presented by Auerbach et al. [2]. Their patient was a 5-year-old girl with retardation of speech and an elevation of histidine in the blood and urine. The urine from their patient, as from the two patients of Ghadimi et al. [1], reacted with ferric chloride to give a green color similar to that observed in patients with phenylketonuria. The abnormal urinary metabolite responsible for the reaction in histidinemia was identified as imidazolepyruvic acid [3, 4], the α-keto acid corresponding to histidine, rather than phenylpyruvic acid, the metabolite excreted in phenylketonuria.

Auerbach et al. [2] obtained evidence that the metabolic disorder in their patient was an inability to metabolize histidine to urocanic acid, and they proposed that histidinemia resulted from the lack of histidase* activity. They suggested that the metabolic disorder be called *histidinemia,* rather than *histidinuria,* to distinguish it clearly from conditions in which increased urinary excretion of histidine is not associated with an elevated concentration of blood histidine.

In 1962, the author and his associates [5] studied two additional cases of histidinemia, and by direct enzymatic assays they demonstrated that histidase activity was missing from the skin of these patients. In 1967, Auerbach et al. [59] found a complete absence of histidase in liver biopsy specimens from two patients with histidinemia, one of these was Case 3 (see Table 15-1). The inherited defect in histidinemia thus appears to be a deficiency of histidase, and the pathologic biochemical findings associated with the metabolic disorder can be reasonably well explained by the absence of this enzyme.

Since 1962 the number of additional cases of histidinemia reported has gradually increased to at least 54 in 1970. Some of the earlier reports (with subsequent observations noted) are summarized in Table 15-1.

* *Histidase* was the name originally given to the "enzyme" discovered by Edlbacher [55] and by György and Röthler [56] in 1926 which was thought to catalyze the hydrolysis of histidine to α-formaminoglutamic acid and ammonia. These workers were probably studying a mixture of histidine α-deaminase, urocanase, and other enzymes as well. There is no evidence for a "histidase" such as Edlbacher described. Today, both *histidase* and *histidine α-deaminase* refer to the enzyme which catalyzes the nonoxidative deamination of histidine to urocanic acid (see Fig. 15-1).

CLINICAL ASPECTS

The incidence of histidinemia is not known, but it must be a relatively rare metabolic disorder. In the newborn urine screening program in Massachusetts, ten new cases of histidinemia were found among 141,903 infants tested. An incidence of one in 14,190 is similar to the frequency of phenylketonuria in that population [77]. A few adults with histidinemia have been found in recent years. They include a 38-year old male of Japanese lineage with mental retardation and spastic diplegia [62], and a histidinemic mother and two aunts of the propositus in the kindred studied by Bruckman et al. [74]. Most of the patients so far described are less than 8 years old. Some of the main clinical features of the reported cases of histidinemia are summarized in Table 15-1.

The birth weight and very early development of histidinemic individuals has generally been found to be entirely normal. About one-third of the cases (Table 15-1) were described as slow or retarded in general physical development. In four (Cases 1, 6, 8, and 20) there were recurrent infections, and another child, presumed to have histidinemia, died in infancy of a staphylococcal infection [8, 66]. Nevertheless, it has not been definitely established that individuals with histidinemia are more susceptible to infectious diseases. Although hemoglobin is rich in histidine and metabolites of histidine contribute to the synthesis of purines and pyrimidines, patients with histidinemia show no metabolic disturbance in these synthetic functions. The bone age generally approximates the chronological age, although slight retardation was noted in the children described by Auerbach et al. [2] (Case 3) and by Berlow [9] (Case 8). In several of the earlier reports it was noted that affected children had blond hair and a fair complexion. While this suggested that this metabolic condition might occur more frequently in this group, additional cases have been described in dark-complexioned individuals. So far there are no specific clinical features which are characteristic of histidinemia. Some of the affected children are completely normal except for the disturbance in histidine metabolism. They were detected only because they were tested as siblings of other histidinemic individuals [1, 59].

Of the first six cases of histidinemia, only one was reported to be mentally retarded, and this child (Case 3) was probably not a typical histidinemic subject, since several other congenital anomalies were present. At that time it appeared probable that, unlike phenylketonuria, histidinemia would not be generally associated with mental retardation [5]. As additional cases of histidinemia were described during mid 1960's the proportion with mental retardation has been high. In fact, among the next 14 cases (Table 15-1) nearly all were retarded to a mild or severe degree. Among the most recent case reports (Table 15-1, footnote 4), there are many more, over half, with normal intelligence. It is accordingly difficult to predict the expectancy or the degree of mental retardation which can be anticipated in new cases of histidinemia on the basis of the present limited number of case reports.

The electroencephalographic pattern has been variable in the few patients examined. No abnormalities were observed in Cases 4 and 5 [10], but abnormal wave patterns were found in at least 5 of the other cases summarized in Table 15-1 and in additional patients [74].

Of the 40 patients old enough to be evaluated for speech development, 23 have shown some degree of retardation or abnormality. The type of speech defect varies even in histidinemic sibs [10], but careful evaluation of these children (Cases 4 and 5) indicated that both had a short auditory memory span but no hearing defect [60]. The functional defect in histidinemia might be a short auditory memory leading to delayed speech development, and short auditory memory has been noted in other patients [74, 77]. Quantitative assessment of the speech defect and memory span in other histidinemic patients would be helpful in further studies to determine whether these findings are coincidental or directly related to the metabolic disorder. Most histidinemic patients with mental retardation also have shown abnormal speech patterns or retardation in speech development. On the other hand, several children have had speech defects without mental retardation (Cases 1, 4, and 5, and others [71, 74]).

Lott et al. [77] believe that speech and language difficulties in histidinemic patients may result from cultural deprivation, mental subnormality, or hearing loss, rather than from a central nervous system disturbance secondary to the metabolic disorder. Garvey and Gordon [78] also feel that there is no direct evidence that the disorders of speech are directly related to the metabolic disease. Reports that 10 children with hereditary stammering had positive ferric chloride tests on their urine and excreted increased amounts of histidine, imidazolepyruvic acid, and imidazoleacetic acid [79] might suggest a further connection between speech difficulties and histidine metabolism. However, Auerbach [59] found histidinuria but normal plasma histidine values in samples sent from one of the Polish patients. Witkop [80] has raised the possibility that one reason why children who recover from kwashiorkor have short auditory memory and decreased visual tracking ability may be the depression of certain enzymes, particularly histidase and phenylalanine hydroxylase, during the period of protein malnutrition.

The wide variation in the clinical features in patients with histidinemia makes any claim about the consequences of the metabolic disease open to question, and the need for more careful observations and study of additional patients is obvious.

Other physical findings reported singly in patients with histidinemia could be mentioned, but it is unlikely that they are associated with the metabolic disorder. For example, Case 8 had precocious development of puberty, dislocation of the patellas, and hemivertebrae [9]; Case 4 had elevated serum uric acid [10]; one child had congenital hypoplastic anemia [73] and another had idiopathic thrombocytopenic purpura [75].

Patients do not show unusual sensitivity to light, chemicals, or topical agents. Eczema, rashes, or other indications of unusual skin sensitivity have not been noted, although one histidinemic patient had atopic dermatitis [71] which responded to the usual treatment, and the patient's minimal erythema was normal. Ghadimi et al. [13] found a normal reaction to intradermal histamine in Case 2.

LABORATORY FINDINGS

Blood

The consistent and most characteristic biochemical finding in histidinemia is a marked elevation in the level of blood histidine. The average concentration of histidine in the blood of 12 normal children from 3 to 11 years old was found by Ghadimi et al. [13] to be 1 mg per 100 ml (range 0.41 to 1.90). Average normal values in milligrams per 100 milliliters for adults reported from several laboratories have been 1.15 [14], 0.91 to 1.38 [1], 1.15 [2], and 1.3, with a range 0.3 to 2.6 [15]. From the available data, it appears that blood histidine concentrations above 3 mg per 100 ml must be considered above normal, and fasting values in adults above 2.5 mg per 100 ml are probably elevated.

Several methods have been employed to determine histidine in the blood in investigations on histidinemic patients and their families. The method of Hunter [16], based upon the Knoop reaction with bromine, was used by Ghadimi et al. [13]. Auerbach et al. [2] and the present author and his associates [10] used snake venom L-amino acid oxidase at pH 7.8 to convert histidine to imidazolepyruvic acid and determined the latter as the enolborate complex spectrophotometrically at 292 mμ. Baldridge and Greenberg [15] have recently published a method for the determination of histidine in blood based upon this principle.

Fasting blood histidine levels in patients with histidinemia (Table 15-1) have varied from 4 to 10 times the normal level, and the degree of elevation depends to a considerable extent upon the dietary protein intake. The highest plasma concentrations of histidine reported in histidinemic subjects have been reached following an oral loading dose of L-histidine, and the values have approached 40 mg per 100 ml under these conditions [2]. It should be pointed out that the histidinemic patient described by Davies and Robinson [12] maintained a relatively low level of histidine, about 9 mg per 100 ml. This 5-year-old boy excreted imidazolepyruvic acid (indicated by a positive ferric chloride test result) after he was fed extra histidine but not at other times.

Ghadimi et al. [13] analyzed the amino acid pattern in the plasma of their first patient (Case 1) by column chroma-

Table 15-1. SUMMARY OF 20 CASES OF HISTIDINEMIA

Case no.	Age, years	Sex	Intel-ligence	Speech	Weight and height	Blood histidine, mg/100 ml	Urine histidine, mg/24 hr	Skin histidase	Comments	References
1	3	♀	IQ 85	Slurred	Normal	9.01	616	Absent	EEG normal, hearing normal	[1, 13, 57, 58]
2	4	♀	Normal	Normal	Normal	7.13	819	Absent	Sib of Case 1	[1, 13, 57, 58]
3	4 4/12	♀	IQ 83	Delayed, slurred	Below normal	15.8	500	NR; assumed to be absent*	Reexamined at 9½ yr; short stature, IQ 85–90, minor speech abnormalities	[2, 3, 59]
4	6 9/12	♀	Normal	Retarded, articulation defects	Normal	17.3	378	Absent	Blond, blue eyes; mirror writing	[5, 10, 60, 61]
5	5	♂	Normal	Retarded, articulation defects	Normal	13.4	850	Absent	Sib of Case 4	[5, 10, 60, 61]
6	5	♂	Slightly retarded	Normal	Below normal	9.0	312,578	NR	Normal bone age, $FeCl_3$ test on urine positive only after oral histidine. Frequent infections	[12]
7	13	♀	IQ 50	Retarded	Approx. normal	4.5–5.3	340–680†	Very low or absent	Mild cerebellar ataxia	[7, 62]
8	8 8/12	♀	IQ 60	Retarded	Normal	15.0	709	Very low or absent	Hemivertebrae, dislocation of patellas, precocious puberty, convulsions	[9, 20, 62]
9	6 mo	♂	Retarded	Retarded	Retarded develop-ment	14.0	218	Absent	On low histidine diet from 7th mo until 4th yr when patient died from broncho-pneumonia; there was little progress in development after first year	[6, 43, 63, 64]
10	3	♂	Retarded no speech at 3 yr	Retarded no speech	Retarded	8	600	NR	Obese, showed clinical signs of degenerative brain disease; died at 3 yr 8 mo	[8, 65, 66]
11	10 6/12	♀	IQ 85	Speech defect	NR	10.4	NR	NR	Had mild hydrocephalus, arrested at early age. At 13 yr showed severe emo-tional disturbances	[8, 65, 66]
12	2	♀	NR	NR	NR	12.6	112	NR	$FeCl_3$ test of urine not con-sistently positive	[52, 53]
13	13	♀	Retarded IQ 54	Retarded	Below normal	11.2	599	Absent	Height and weight at approxi-mately third percentile; speech was immature	[67]
14	10	♂	Retarded IQ 52	Retarded articulation defect	Normal	3.9‡ 6.5§	900†	Present	Slow development; bone de-velopment normal, ab-normal EEG; sweat urocanic acid normal	[11]

Table 15-1. SUMMARY OF 20 CASES OF HISTIDINEMIA

Case no.	Age, years	Sex	Intelligence	Speech	Weight and height	Blood histidine, mg/100 ml	Urine histidine, mg/24 hr	Skin histidase	Comments	References
15	8	♂	Retarded IQ 47	Articulation defect	Normal	5.2‡ 5.0§	868†	Present	At 2¾ yr developed generalized convulsive disorder; sweat urocanic acid normal	[11]
16	6	♀	Retarded IQ 53	Retarded articulation defect	Normal	3.1‡ 5.6§	413†	Present	At 3½ yr developed convulsive disorder; sweat urocanic acid not determined	[11]
17	10	♀	Retarded	Retarded articulation defect	Below normal	8.1–10.3	495–† 590	NR	Slow early physical and mental development	[68]
18	13	♀	Retarded	NR	Normal	7.4	771†	NR	Slow early development, convulsions	[68]
19	3	♀	Retarded	Retarded	Normal	12.6–18.0	1409–† 2629	NR	Diagnosed at 4 mo of age; treated with low histidine diet at 1 yr	[68, 69]
20	18 mo	♂	Normal	Normal	Below normal	4.9	79– 112	Absent	Recurrent infections, convulsive disorder, delayed bone age, $FeCl_3$ test positive only with histidine load; no sweat urocanic acid	[70]

NR = no report.

* Patient (R.M.) had no detectable urocanic acid in sweat; liver biopsy showed complete absence of histidase activity [59].

† Values, mg histidine per gram creatinine.

‡ Values by enol-borate method.

§ Values by paper chromatography.

Note: Additional cases of suspected histidinemia are described as follows:

1. A 5½-year-old girl with speech retardation and possible mental retardation probably had histidinemia. She, her sister (7 years old, asymptomatic), and mother all had a positive urinary ferric chloride test. Oral histidine load caused a prolonged elevation of plasma histidine levels in the patient, and an elevation to a lesser degree in sister and mother [54].
2. Two younger sisters of Case 10 had elevated plasma histidine values; one, with values between 9.2 and 11.5 mg per 100 ml, died at 1 year of pneumonitis; the other had levels about 5 mg per 100 ml at 5 days, which fell to normal levels by 1 year. The latter had a normal response to histidine load, but was unable to speak and was retarded in motor development [66].
3. A 1-month-old baby (sex not stated) reported to have elevated blood histidine [53].
4. Thirty additional cases of histidinemia have been reported: 6 cases, [59]; 3 cases, [62]; 1 case, [71]; 4 cases, [72]; 1 case, [73]; 9 cases, [74]; 1 case, [75]; 1 case [76], and 4 cases, [77].

tography and found histidine to be the only amino acid elevated in histidinemia. Elevated alanine concentrations were reported by Auerbach et al. [59] and by Carton et al. [75].

Imidazolepyruvic acid is excreted in substantial quantities in the urine of histidinemic subjects, but no significant concentration of this acid is present in the blood [17]. Other imidazole metabolites of histidine, such as imidazolelactic acid and imidazoleacetic acid, have not been measured quantitatively in the blood of histidinemic patients.

It is of interest that in the three cases of histidinemia in which serotonin levels have been determined, the values were found to be below normal. The values found by Auerbach et al. were approximately half the normal, and 0.012 μg per ml versus 0.10 μg per ml for the normal were found by Holton [6]. Both these histidinemic patients were mentally retarded. Corner et al. [63] found that depressed platelet serotonin levels were restored to normal after their patient (case 9) was treated with a low histidine diet. Serotonin analyses in other histidinemic patients would be of value. Ghadimi and Zischka [57] noted reduced platelet but normal serum serotonin levels in their two patients.

Urine

Increased urinary excretion of histidine is also a characteristic finding in histidinemia, but it is not as specific an indicator of this disorder as an elevation of blood histidine. The amount excreted per day in cases of histidinemia is given in Table 15-1. In those instances in which the intake of protein was controlled or was known, it has been observed that the daily histidine excretion is directly related to the protein intake. Although some of the data are reported as milligrams of histidine excreted per gram of creatinine, it can be calculated that the daily excretion varies from 300 to 900 mg per day, depending upon the diet and the age of the patient. The increase in excretion represents a six- to tenfold increase over the normal values [13].

Imidazolepyruvic acid is present in normal urine in only very small amounts. Auerbach et al. [2] found the normal values to be 0 to 11 mg per day, with a mean of 3.2 mg per day. In two histidinemic patients the excretion of imidazolepyruvic acid was found to be 26 to 150 mg per day [2] (Case 3), and 65 to 264 mg per day, an average of 155 mg, over a 7-day period [10] (Case 4). Imidazolepyruvic acid in the urine has been determined quantitatively as the enol-borate complex by Auerbach et al. [2] and by the author and his associates [10], and the acid was identified qualitatively by paper chromatography with the Pauly reagent by Ghadimi et al. [13]. The latter investigators reported that imidazolepyruvic acid is relatively unstable when subjected to paper chromatography and that only a weak Pauly test is given unless at least 100 to 200 μg are applied. It was observed [18] that if borate is added to the mixture being chromatographed, the keto acid is protected, and only 5 to 10 μg is needed to obtain a discrete spot with the Pauly reagent. In addition, borate facilitates a separation of the keto acid from histidine in the propanol-ammonia solvent system of Ames and Mitchell [19].

Imidazolepyruvic acid has been regularly identified in the urine of histidinemic subjects. Other imidazole metabolites of histidine which are usually found in the urine by chromatographic methods are imidazolelactic acid and imidazoleacetic acid.

Several groups have reported the absence of urocanic acid from the urine in histidinemia [2, 6, 11, 13, 75] but the values in normal urine are often low, and methods of detection lack specificity. Imidazolepropionic acid [2] and hydantoin propionic acid [20], metabolites of urocanic acid (see Fig. 15-1), also are not found in the urine of histidinemic subjects [2], and the absence of formiminoglutamic acid (FIGlu) has been noted by several investigators [2, 6, 10, 20], but not all [74].

Analysis of the urinary amino acids by two-dimensional chromatography by Ghadimi et al. [1] has shown that the only amino acid excreted in great excess is histidine. They, and others have noted a moderate increase in alanine and a slight increase in several other amino acids [59, 75].

Cerebrospinal Fluid

Analyses of cerebrospinal fluid in patients with histidinemia have been made in 5 cases. In Case 1, Ghadimi et al. [1] first reported that the histidine concentration was elevated, but in a later publication [13] the level was considered to be at the upper limits of the normal range. They found a low concentration of glutamic acid—glutamine. The α-amino nitrogen value in the cerebrospinal fluid was 0.83 mg per 100 ml, which is at the lowest limit of normal found in their control group of 50 children. Shaw et al. [7] found a spinal fluid histidine level of 0.75 mg per 100 ml, which they considered to be about three times the normal concentration, and Wadman et al. [68] found a tenfold elevation in one patient (case 19) on two occasions. Berlow [9] found that the histidine concentration was not definitely increased in his patient, but by paper chromatographic analysis he found a decrease in the glutamic acid—glutamine concentration. In contrast, Holton [6] found no abnormality in the concentration of glutamic acid or glutamine by chromatographic analysis in his 6-month-old patient with severe mental retardation.

METABOLISM OF HISTIDINE

Histidine is an essential amino acid for growth in the rat, dog, mouse, and chick [21]. Adult male rats appear to require dietary histidine to maintain both weight and nitrogen balance [22–24], although an earlier study with female rats suggested that histidine was not essential for the older ani-

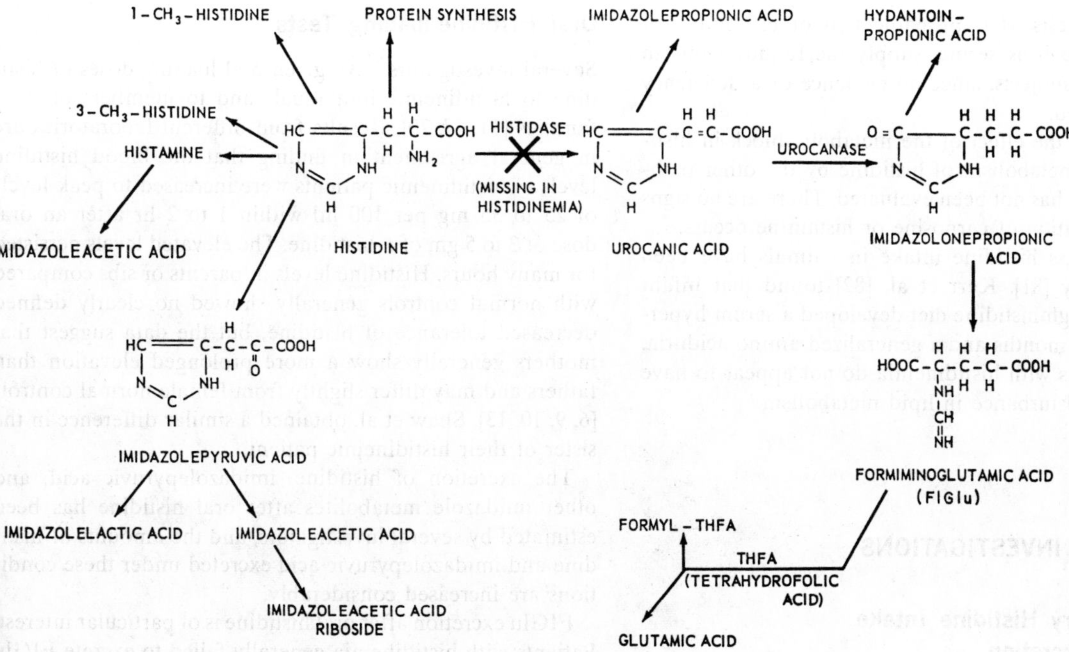

Figure 15-1. Pathways of histidine metabolism and the enzymatic defect in histidinemia.

mals [25]. Histidine has not been considered essential for man since three male adults remained in nitrogen balance on a synthetic diet free of histidine for 8 days [26]. On the other hand a careful study of the histidine requirements of young male infants by Snyderman et al. [27] indicated that this amino acid is required for growth. Infants on a diet lacking histidine had a reduced rate of gain in weight and less retention of nitrogen than normal controls. In addition, a rash appeared during periods of histidine withdrawal [27a]. Based upon their experience, the dietary requirement of histidine was estimated to be somewhat less than 35 mg per kg per day.

The effect of low dietary histidine on older infants and adults over longer periods remains uncertain. The capacity to synthesize histidine has not been established, and it is possible that human subjects vary in their ability to synthesize this amino acid. The sequential steps involved in the synthesis of histidine in microorganisms has been investigated by Ames and coworkers [28–30] and by others [31–33]. A scheme, based upon known mutant strains deficient in particular enzymatic steps of histidine biosynthesis, is given below:

P-ribose-P → 5′-phosphoribosyl-ATP → "III" → imidazoleglycerol phosphate → imidazoleacetol phosphate → L-Histidinol phosphate → L-histidinol → L-histidinal → L-histidine

Whether a similar synthetic pathway is utilized in man is not known. Particular intermediary compounds in the synthetic pathway (above) have not been administered to histidinemic subjects to determine whether an increased concentration of histidine in blood or urine would result.

The metabolism of histidine in mammalian tissue is much better understood than its synthesis (see Meister [34]) [35–37]. Among the various pathways available to histidine are:

1 Utilization in protein synthesis
2 Formation of carnosine (β-alanylhistidine)
3 Methylation to 1- or 3-methylhistidine
4 Decarboxylation to histamine
5 Deamination or transamination to imidazolepyruvic acid
6 Deamination to urocanic acid and further metabolism to FIGlu and glutamic acid.

The pathway by way of urocanic acid to glutamic acid (Fig. 15-1) has received relatively more attention since it has been generally assumed to be the major route of histidine degradation in mammalian tissue. However, the pathway through imidazolepyruvic acid is shown to be of considerable importance by the extent to which it is utilized by histidinemic subjects. Imidazolepyruvic acid, formed by deamination or transamination [38, 39] of histidine, is excreted in the urine of histidinemia patients in amounts approaching half the amount of histidine excreted. This represents a low estimate of the amount of imidazolepyruvic acid formed, since part is further metabolized to imidazolelactic acid and imidazoleacetic acid and the latter partly conjugated and excreted as the riboside.

It might be suspected that a block in histidine metabolism by way of the urocanic acid pathway would lead to clinical symptoms because of a lack of FIGlu, an important donor of formyl groups to tetrahydrofolic acid for purine and pyrimidine synthesis. It is probable that other sources of formyl groups, such as serine, supply the requirements in the histidinemic subjects, since no evidence of a deficiency has been observed.

Unfortunately, the effect of the metabolic block in histidinemia on the metabolism of histidine by the other pathways listed above has not been evaluated. There are no signs that excess formation of carnosine or histamine occurs.

Effects of excess histidine intake in animals have been reviewed recently [81]. Kerr et al. [82] found that infant monkeys fed a high histidine diet developed a serum hyperlipemia in 3 to 4 months and a generalized amino aciduria. However, patients with histidinemia do not appear to have any significant disturbance in lipid metabolism.

BIOCHEMICAL INVESTIGATIONS

Effect of Dietary Histidine Intake on Histidine Excretion

In several investigations attempts have been made to study the effect of dietary histidine intake on the blood concentration of histidine and the urinary excretion of histidine and its metabolites. Ghadimi et al. [13] found that either a high-protein diet or the addition of histidine as an oral load produced a marked increase in histidine excretion. On one occasion, the histidine excretion was 3.67 gm per 24 hr (Case 1). Plasma histidine levels varied with dietary histidine intake and decreased from a range of 6.4 to 9.0 mg per 100 ml on a regular diet to 2.0 mg per 100 ml when no protein was ingested for 24 hr. They also observed that the daily output of histidine slightly exceeded the calculated dietary intake during a short period while the intake was low. They proposed that the excess histidine excreted was contributed by body tissues other than plasma acting as a reservoir.

In similar studies by the author and his associates [10] a histidinemic patient (Case 5) was placed on a diet low in histidine for 4 days (calculated to contain approximately 90 mg histidine per day). The average daily histidine excretion was 405 mg per day. Fasting histidine values in the blood remained high, at approximately 15 mg per 100 ml, and were not reduced significantly below the values found when the daily histidine intake had been approximately 2 gm per day. These data suggest that this patient synthesized histidine, at least to a limited degree. Cain and Holton [70] found no significant decrease in the blood histidine concentration in their patient (Case 20) on a diet containing 40 mg per kg per day of histidine. Most dietary studies, however, have obtained a prompt reduction in plasma histidine [59, 63, 66, 69, 72]. It appears that histidinemic patients differ in their response to a reduction of dietary histidine.

Oral Histidine-loading Tests

Several investigators have given oral loading doses of histidine to histidinemic individuals and to members of their families [11, 67, 70]. Results from different laboratories are in general agreement in finding that the blood histidine levels in histidinemic patients were increased to peak levels of 25 to 35 mg per 100 ml within 1 to 2 hr after an oral dose of 3 to 5 gm of L-histidine. The elevated levels persisted for many hours. Histidine levels in parents or sibs compared with normal controls generally showed no clearly defined decreased tolerance of histidine, but the data suggest that mothers generally show a more prolonged elevation than fathers and may differ slightly from female normal controls [6, 9, 10, 13]. Shaw et al. obtained a similar difference in the sister of their histidinemic patient.

The excretion of histidine, imidazolepyruvic acid, and other imidazole metabolites after oral histidine has been estimated by several investigators, and the amounts of histidine and imidazolepyruvic acid excreted under these conditions are increased considerably.

FIGlu excretion after oral histidine is of particular interest. Patients with histidinemia generally failed to excrete FIGlu after oral histidine [2, 6, 10, 70], and parents of histidinemic subjects were found to excrete less FIGlu than normal controls (Table 15-2).

Administration of Urocanic Acid

The metabolism of urocanic acid following its administration to histidinemic patients has been studied by three groups of investigators [2, 6, 10]. In the first study, Auerbach et al [2] showed that both FIGlu and urocanic acid were excreted in the urine after 1 gm urocanic acid (sodium salt) had been given slowly by intravenous infusion, whereas neither acid was excreted during the preceding control period. Another metabolite, imidazolepropionic acid, also appeared in the

Table 15-2. EXCRETION OF FORMIMINOGLUTAMIC ACID FOLLOWING ORAL L-HISTIDINE LOAD*

Subject	*FIGlu excretion, μmoles*				
	0–1 hr	1–2 hr	2–3 hr	3–4 hr	0–4 hr
Histidinemic (W. B.)	0	0	0	0	0
Father (E. B.)	1.11	1.94	2.33	3.48	8.86
Mother (R. B.)	0.31	1.20	1.57	1.83	4.91
Normal controls (4)	2.14	6.66	7.60	5.89	22.3 (16.3–28.7)

* 0.1 gm per kg body weight of L-histidine monochloride given orally.

Source: B. N. La Du et al. [10].

urine of the histidinemic patient only following the urocanic acid loading. Excretions of imidazolepyruvic acid, imidazolelactic acid, and imidazoleacetic acid were not increased by urocanic acid administration. Similar results have been observed in other histidinemic patients by the author and his associates [10] and by Holton et al. [6].

Enzymatic Defect in Histidinemia

In 1961 Ghadimi et al. [1] suggested that the metabolic disorder in histidinemia was a defect in an early enzymatic step in histidine metabolism, either histidase or urocanase. In 1962, Auerbach et al. [2] demonstrated that urocanic acid was metabolized to FIGlu by their histidinemic patient and concluded that the defect was a deficiency of histidase. They did not verify their hypothesis by direct enzymatic assay.

In 1962, La Du et al. [5] determined the distribution of histidase in mammalian tissues, including man, and found high histidase activity in the epidermal layer of the skin as well as liver. These results were in agreement with those obtained by Schwarz [40], who found labeled histidine to be degraded to urocanic acid by guinea pig skin homogenates. Enzymatic assay methods have been developed [41, 62, 83] for the determination of histidase activity in homogenates of stratum corneum of human skin by modifying the method of Tabor and Mehler for liver histidase [42], which was based upon the rate of urocanic acid formation at 277 mμ. A lack of histidase activity in skin samples (stratum corneum) from two histidinemic siblings and decreased activity in members of their family compared to normal controls is illustrated in Table 15-3. Direct demonstration of the lack of histidase furnished the additional evidence needed to establish that histidinemia is characterized by a deficiency of a specific enzyme.

Skin histidase is absent or very low in patients with histidinemia (Table 15-1, [62, 72, 74, 75, 76]), but normal values have been found in the three cases of Woody [11]. Woody's cases differ from the usual patients with histidinemia in having lower concentrations of histidine in the blood, and the response to an oral load of histidine was less pronounced. The genetic defect in these patients may represent a variant form of histidinemia.

Skin and Sweat Urocanic Acid

It has been proposed by Zenisek et al. [44], by Hais and Zenisek [45], and by Everett et al. [46] that urocanic acid, a normal constituent of sweat, protects the skin from ultraviolet irradiation by acting as a physiologic sun screen. The urocanic acid in sweat probably is not a product of the sweat glands but is present because of diffusion from the epithelial skin cells [84]. Exposure of skin to solar radiation increases the concentration of urocanic acid [86]; ultraviolet light

Table 15-3. HISTIDASE ACTIVITY IN THE STRATUM CORNEUM OF A FAMILY WITH HISTIDINEMIA AND OF NORMAL INDIVIDUALS

Subjects	*Epidermal histidase activity,* μg of urocanic acid formed/hr/gm fresh weight*
Histidinemic family:	
W. B., 6 years, ♀, histidinemia	0 (<1.5)
E. B., Jr., 5 years, ♂, histidinemia	0 (<1.5)
Sister (L. B.), 4 years	276 (264–295)
Father (E. B.), 31 years	193 (166–219)
Mother (R. B.), 25 years	318 (305–335)
Controls:†	
Children (8)	740 (579–910)
Adult male (12)	413 (249–731)
Adult female (12)	502 (263–732)

* The results are given as means with the ranges in parentheses. Values were determined at least three times with each member of the histidinemic family.
† Numbers in parentheses represent the number of individuals.
Source: B. N. La Du et al. [10]; obtained by enzymatic assay [41].

converts the trans isomer to the cis form of the acid [88]. Baden and Pathak [89] suggest that isomerization of urocanic acid is an effective mechanism for the absorption and dissipation of solar radiation energy. It is, therefore, of interest that the skin and sweat of histidinemic individuals have no urocanic acid, yet they show no unusual sensitivity to sunlight, nor do they have any cutaneous sensitivities. Urocanic acid may provide some special protective effect in the skin, but it apparently is not vital for healthy skin.

Histidine is concentrated in keratohyalin granules of the skin, and this amino acid has been implicated in the keratinization process [71, 85, 86]. Histidase is present in benign epidermal tumors but low or absent in basal and squamous cell carcinomas; the concentration of urocanic acid in these tumors reflects their level of histidase activity [90].

DIAGNOSIS

Diagnosis of histidinemia is based upon finding an elevation of histidine in the blood and an increased excretion of histidine in the urine. In addition, the abnormal urinary metabolite, imidazolepyruvic acid, can usually be detected by the ferric chloride test or by the Phenistix test. The green color obtained is very similar to that observed with urine from a phenylketonuric subject. In histidinemia the color usually develops more slowly and remains longer than in phenylketonuria, but this difference is not sufficiently specific to use as a differential diagnostic test. Occasionally tests for imidazolepyruvic acid in histidinemic urine may be only weakly positive or, at times, negative. Cases 6 and 12 (Table

15-1) had a positive ferric chloride test result following an oral load of histidine but were negative at other times. Variation in the test seems to be greater in histidinemia than in phenylketonuria, perhaps because the excretion of the keto acid is more closely related to the intake of protein in the former condition.

Increased excretion of histidine occurs in conditions other than histidinemia, and a diagnosis cannot be made based upon this finding alone. The increased excretion of histidine in pregnancy is well known [47–50]. It also occurs in a hereditary imidazole amino aciduria associated with cerebromacular degeneration described by Bessman and Baldwin [51]. Histidinuria in the latter condition appears to be inherited as a dominant trait and is apparently a failure to reabsorb histidine by the kidney tubules since the blood histidine concentration is not elevated.

Histidinemia can be diagnosed during the neonatal period [77], and screening programs for the detection of hereditary disorders of amino acid metabolism now generally include tests for histidinemia.

Other findings which aid in establishing the diagnosis are the lack of urocanic acid in the sweat, the lack of histidase activity in skin biopsies, and the absence of FIGlu in the urine even after an oral load of histidine. It should be mentioned that an absence of histidase in the skin may not be characteristic of all cases of histidinemia [11], since in some patients the enzymatic defect might possibly be restricted to liver histidase. It would seem unwise to require that the absence of skin histidase activity be established to confirm a diagnosis of histidinemia. Absence of FIGlu from the urine can not be an absolute requirement for diagnosis, either. The histidinemic members of the family studied by Bruckman et al. [74] had little or no detectable skin histidase, but they excreted low concentrations of FIGlu.

Differential diagnostic problems are mainly to distinguish this metabolic disorder from phenylketonuria and to rule out other causes of histidinuria. It is of interest that several of the cases of histidinemia were first presumed to be phenylketonuria, and the first case, reported by Ghadimi et al. [13] had been placed on a low-phenylalanine diet before the correct diagnosis was established. Quantitative blood levels of phenylalanine and histidine should clearly differentiate the two conditions.

TREATMENT

It is not known whether a restriction of the dietary intake of histidine would be beneficial in those cases of histidinemia with mental retardation or speech difficulties. There are many similarities in the metabolic disorder in histidinemia and phenylketonuria, and it is not surprising that a diet low in histidine would be employed in selected cases of histidinemia.

Waisman [66] tested the effects of a low-histidine diet for a month when his patient (Case 10) was about 2 years old, and again, at 3½ years of age. There was no clinical improvement either time, although the plasma histidine concentration decreased to approximately one-half of its previous value.

Another patient (Case 3) [59] was given a histidine-free diet for a month. The plasma histidine concentration fell but the alanine remained elevated and there were no signs of clinical improvement.

Longer experience with low-histidine diets was obtained in the treatment of Cases 9 [63] and 19 [69]. The special diet was started when Case 9 was 7 months old. At first, there was better growth and development, but at 20 months this stopped and it was difficult to balance nutritional needs with the low intake of histidine necessary to maintain a low plasma level of the amino acid. There was no improvement in the patient's mental capacity and the child died of pneumonia in the fourth year. Treatment of Case 19 started at 1 year and the blood histidine level decreased from 17 to 2.2 mg per 100 ml within 2 weeks. Growth was inadequate, however, and the diet had no beneficial effects on the speech, mental retardation, or motor function.

Case 20 [70] was treated for 11 months with a diet containing 40 mg of histidine per kg per day. Blood histidine remained high but there was less gain in weight and no acceleration of general development.

Two additional histidinemic children were given a low-histidine diet for approximately 3 months [72]. The blood histidine concentrations fell but growth was retarded by the diet and no changes were noted in the clinical features.

From these few reports it can be concluded that diets low in histidine can usually reduce the concentration of histidine in the blood, but this requires a diet which is inadequate for proper growth and development. No favorable effects of dietary treatment have been observed, though biochemical control was achieved and serotonin levels were restored [43, 63].

GENETIC CONSIDERATIONS

Cases of histidinemia have been found in the United States, Canada, Great Britain, and Australia, but the limited number precludes any generalization on the geographic areas or racial groups in which this metabolic disorder may occur most frequently. More than one sib is affected in several families, and in only one of the pedigrees has the disorder been detected in more than one generation [74].

In only one histidinemic family has a consanguineous marriage been noted, and in this family the relationship is several generations removed [11]. The incidence of histidinemia is approximately equal in both sexes, and it is probable that the disorder is transmitted as a single autosomal recessive trait.

Bruckman et al. [74] suggest an autosomal dominant pattern of inheritance in their family. The father of three affected sibs was very carefully studied and classified as normal rather than a heterozygous carrier of histidinemia.

Ghadimi et al. [1, 13] studied the family of their first two histidinemic patients to determine whether an increased excretion of histidine might be found in some of the relatives. Although none showed histidinuria to the extent of the affected children, the mother and five more distant relatives excreted histidine in amounts considered to be at the upper limits of normal. The concentration of histidine in the blood of both parents was within normal limits, the mother's value being at the upper limit of the normal range.

Attempts have been made to detect the heterozygous carrier of histidinemia (assuming that the disorder is inherited as an autosomal recessive trait) by the response to an oral loading dose of L-histidine. Results of the tolerance tests on the levels of histidine in the blood have not permitted a clear differentiation between parents of affected children and normal controls. Holton [6] observed that the mother of his patient had a persistent elevation of blood histidine and excreted a greater fraction of the oral dose than the father. Shaw et al. [7] reported that a sister of their histidinemic patient also maintained a higher blood histidine level than was expected following an oral loading dose. Ghadimi et al. [13] found that the parents excreted more of the administered oral histidine (7.9 and 13.2 percent) than adult controls (1.2, 2.1, and 5.7 percent).

The author and his associates [10] measured the excretion of FIGlu following an oral load of L-histidine and found that less was excreted by both parents than by normal controls (Table 15-2). These results are not inconsistent with the findings that blood histidine levels during tolerance tests do not differ significantly in parents and controls. Alternative pathways, particularly through imidazolepyruvic acid, would

Table 15-4. HISTIDASE ACTIVITY IN THE STRATUM CORNEUM OF HISTIDINEMIC PATIENTS, THEIR PARENTS, AND CONTROLS*

Patient		Father	Mother	Controls			References
				Children	Adult male	Adult female	
Case 1 (Case 4, Table 15-1)	<0.01	1.4	2.3	**(8)** 5.4 (1.7–8.8)	**(17)** 3.7 (1.9–6.4)	**(14)** 3.1 (1.8–5.3)	[41, 83]
Case 2 (Case 5, Table 15-1)	<0.01						
Case 1 (Case 1, Table 15-1)	0	0.81	0.65	For controls, same data as above			[57]
Case 2 (Case 2, Table 15-1)	0						
Case 1, 12 yr ♀	<0.1	0.74	0.54				[73]
Case 1 (Case 9, Table 15-1)	0	0.50	0.40	....	**(12)** 1.9 (1.0–2.7)	**(12)** 2.0 (1.4–2.7)	[64]
Case 1 (Case 20, Table 15-1)	0	0.24	1.99	....	(1.4–2.7)	(1.0–2.7)	[70]
Case 1, 5 yr ♀	<0.1	....	0.27	(7) 2.8 (0.73–4.8)	(7) 1.1 (0.41–1.8)		[72]
Case 2, 1 7/12 yr ♀	<0.1						
Case 3, 6 yr ♂	<0.1						
Case 4, 11 yr ♀	<0.1						
Case 1, 6 9/12 yr ♂	0	1.4	0†	....	(7) (1.5–3.2)		[74]
Case 2, 8 9/12 yr ♀	0						
Case 3, 12 9/12 yr ♀	0.3						
Case 6, 44 yr ♂	0†						
Case 1 (Case 7, Table 15-1)	0.12	3.22	1.61	....	**(46)** 3.39		[62]‡
Case 2 (Case 8, Table 15-1)	0.45	....	2.03	....	**(46)** 3.39		[62]
Case 3, L_1, 4 yr ♀	0.11	1.26	0.12§	....	**(46)** 3.39		[62]
Case 4, T_1, 38 yr ♂	0.12	1.56	1.44	....	**(46)** 3.39		[62]
Case 1 (Case 14, Table 15-1)	2.2	1.9	1.6	....	(7) (0.8–2.8)		[11]
Case 2 (Case 15, Table 15-1)	4.3						
Case 3 (Case 16, Table 15-1)	3.7						

*Activity is measured in μmoles of urocanic acid formed per hour per gram wet weight; activity less than 0.10 μmoles per hour per gram wet weight is considered undetectable. In the control columns figures in bold type refer to numbers of individuals; figures in lightface type in parentheses are ranges of activity; figures without parentheses are mean values.

†Mother and Case 6 (aunt of Cases 1, 2 and 3) are sisters; both have histidinemia.

‡Recalculated from activity per gram of protein.

§Mother had normal blood histidine and normal response to histidine loading test.

still be available to heterozygous carriers. The amount of histidine metabolized by way of urocanic acid and FIGlu might be reduced if there were a partial deficiency of histidase activity in heterozygotes, and the decreased amount of FIGlu excreted may indicate a decrease of liver histidase activity. Further investigation of FIGlu excretion as a means of detecting the carrier should be made in other histidinemic families.

Of course, direct determination of histidase would theoretically be the most promising means of obtaining a clear distinction between carriers of histidinemia and normal controls, and the level of histidase in skin (stratum corneum) might be of value with further refinement of the assay method. At the present time there is a high risk of error in assigning a specific genotype (except for affected homozygotes) even though parents, as a group, show a mean histidase value significantly below that of normal controls [61, 62, 64] (Table 15-4). The activity of histidase in the skin may not always reflect the level of histidase activity in liver, since its activity may be modified by hormones and other environmental factors. Thus, although the skin assay is a simple and convenient enzyme assay, there is no assurance that it will give an unequivocal answer. Experience in the detection of heterozygous carriers of histidinemia by several groups of investigators has been summarized by Bruckman et al. [74].

Histidase activity has been demonstrated in human foreskin epithelial cells and in epithelial cells growing from explants of this tissue; fibroblast-like cells in serial culture do not have measurable histidase activity [91]. It is suggested that the presence or absence of histidase could be used as an index of the state of differentiation of these epithelial cells in culture.

SUMMARY

1 Histidinemia, a rare metabolic disorder of histidine metabolism first described in 1961, is characterized by an elevation of the histidine concentration of the blood and excretion of histidine, imidazolepyruvic acid, and other imidazole metabolites in the urine.

2 About 54 cases of histidinemia are known, most of the affected individuals being less than 8 years old. Over half of the histidinemic subjects are mentally retarded, and more than half of the cases have a defect, or retarded development, of speech.

3 The biochemical disturbance in histidinemia is believed to be the lack of the enzyme histidase. Direct demonstration of this enzymatic deficiency has been made in skin and liver biopsies from affected children.

4 Histidinemia is probably inherited as an autosomal recessive trait. One kindred may be an example of histidinemia inherited as an autosomal dominant condition.

BIBLIOGRAPHY

1. Ghadimi, H., Partington, M. W., and Hunter, A.: A familial disturbance of histidine metabolism. New Eng. J. Med., **265**, 221, 1961.
2. Auerbach, V. H., DiGeorge, A. M., Baldridge, R. C., Tourtellotte, C. D., and Brigham, M. P.: Histidinemia: a deficiency in histidase resulting in the urinary excretion of histidine and of imidazolepyruvic acid. J. Pediat., **60**, 487, 1962.
3. Auerbach, V. H., DiGeorge, A. M., Baldridge, R. C., Tourtellotte, C. D., and Brigham, M. P.: Histidinemia: a deficiency in liver histidase resulting in the urinary excretion of histidine and of imidazolepyruvic acid. Clin. Res., **9**, 334, 1961.
4. Baldridge, R. C., and Auerbach, V. H.: The metabolism of histidine. VI. Histidinemia and imidazolepyruvic aciduria. J. Biol. Chem., **239**, 1557, 1964.
5. La Du, B. N., Howell, R. R., Jacoby, G. A., Seegmiller, J. E., and Zannoni, V. G.: The enzymatic defect in histidinemia. Biochem. Biophys. Res. Commun., **7**, 398, 1962.
6. Holton, J. B., Lewis, F. J. W., and Moore, G. R.: Biochemical investigation of histidinaemia. J. Clin. Path., **17**, 671, 1964.
7. Shaw, N. F. K., Boder, E., Gutenstein, M., and Jacobs, E. E.: Histidinemia. J. Pediat., **63**, 720, 1963.
8. Waisman, H. A.: Personal communication.
9. Berlow, S., Arends, R., and Harries, C.: Studies in histidinemia. J. Lancet **85**, 241, 1965.
10. La Du, B. N., Howell, R. R., Jacoby, G. A., Seegmiller, J. E., Sober, E. K., Zannoni, V. G., Canby, J. P., and Ziegler, L. K.: Clinical and biochemical studies on two cases of histidinemia. Pediatrics, **32**, 216, 1963.
11. Woody, N. C., Snyder, C. H., and Harris, J. A.: Histidinemia. Amer. J. Dis. Child. **110**, 606, 1965.
12. Davies, H. E., and Robinson, M. J.: A case of histidinaemia. Arch. Dis. Child., **38**, 80, 1963.
13. Ghadimi, H., Partington, M. W., Hunter, A.: Inborn error of histidine metabolism. Pediatrics, **29**, 714, 1962.
14. Stein, W. H., and Moore, S.: The free amino acids of human plasma. J. Biol. Chem., **211**, 915, 1954.
15. Baldridge, R. C., and Greenberg, N.: A method for the determination of histidine in blood. J. Lab. Clin. Med., **61**, 700, 1963.
16. Hunter, A.: Determination of urinary histidine. Fed. Proc., **18**, 251, 1959.
17. Zannoni, V. G., and La Du, B. N.: Unpublished observations.
18. Zannoni, V. G.: Unpublished observations.
19. Ames, B. N., and Mitchell, H. K.: The paper chromatography of imidazoles. J. Am. Chem. Soc., **74**, 252, 1952.
20. Snyder, S. H., Myron, P., Kies, M. W., and Berlow, S.: Metabolism of 2-C^{14}-labeled L-histidine in histidinemia. J. Clin. Endocrinol., **23**, 595, 1963.
21. Meister, A.: *Biochemistry of the Amino Acids*, p. 99. Academic, New York, 1957.
22. Frazier, L. E., Wissler, R. W., Steffee, C. H., Woolridge, R. L., and Cannon, P. R.: Studies in amino acid utilization. I. The dietary utilization of mixtures of purified amino acids in protein-depleted adult albino rats. J. Nutrition, **33**, 65, 1947.
23. Wissler, R. W., Steffee, C. H., Frazier, L. E., Woolridge, R. L., and Benditt, E. P.: Studies in amino acid utilization. III. The role of the indispensable amino acids in maintenance of the adult albino rat. J. Nutrition, **36**, 245, 1948.
24. Benditt, E. P., Woolridge, R. L., Steffee, C. H., and Frazier, L. E.: Studies in amino acid utilization. IV. The minimum requirements of the indispensable amino acids for maintenance of the adult well-nourished male albino rat. J. Nutrition, **40**, 335, 1950.
25. Burroughs, E. W., Burroughs, H. S., and Mitchell, H. H.: The amino acids required for the complete replacement of endogenous losses in the adult rat. J. Nutrition, **19**, 363, 1940.
26. Rose, W. C., Haines, W. J., Warner, D. T., and Johnson, J. E.: The amino acid requirements of man. II. The role of threonine and histidine. J. Biol. Chem., **188**, 49, 1951.
27. Snyderman, S. E., Boyer, A., Roitman, E., Holt, L. E., Jr., and Prose, P. H.: The histidine requirement of the infant. Pediatrics, **31**, 786, 1963.

27a. Snyderman, S.: An eczematoid dermatitis in histidine deficiency. J. Pediat. **66,** 212, 1965.
28. Ames, B. N., and Mitchell, H. K.: The biosynthesis of histidine. Imidazoleglycerol phosphate, imidazoleacetol phosphate and histidinol phosphate. J. Biol. Chem., **212,** 687, 1955.
29. Ames, B. N., Garry, B., and Herzenberg, L. A.: The genetic control of the enzymes of histidine biosynthesis in *Salmonella typhimurium.* J. Gen. Microbiol., **22,** 369, 1960.
30. Ames, B. N., Martin, B. G., and Garry, B. J.: The first step of histidine biosynthesis. J. Biol. Chem., **236,** 2019, 1961.
31. Moyed, H. S., and Magasanik, B.: The biosynthesis of the imidazole ring of histidine. J. Biol. Chem., **235,** 149, 1960.
32. Adams, E.: Synthesis and properties of an α-amino aldehyde, histidinal. J. Biol. Chem., **217,** 317, 1955.
33. Klopotowski, T., Luzzati, M., and Slonimski, P. P.: Evidence for a new step between ATP and 5-amino 4-imidazolcarboxamide ribotide in the cyclic process of histidine biosynthesis. Biochem. Biophys. Res. Commun., **3,** 150, 1960.
34. Meister, A.: *Biochemistry of the Amino Acids,* p. 328. Academic, New York, 1957.
35. Baldridge, R. C., and Tourtellotte, C. D.: The metabolism of histidine. III. Urinary metabolites. J. Biol. Chem., **233,** 125, 1958.
36. Brown, D. D., Silva, O. L., McDonald, P. B., Snyder, S. H., and Kies, M. W.: The mammalian metabolism of L-histidine. III. The urinary metabolites of L-histidine-C^{14} in the monkey, human and rat. J. Biol. Chem., **235,** 154, 1960.
37. Peterkofsky, A.: The mechanism of action of histidase: amino-enzyme formation and partial reactions. J. Biol. Chem., **237,** 787, 1962.
38. Lin, E. C. C., Pitt, B. M., Civen, M., and Knox, W. E.: The assay of aromatic amino acid transaminations and keto acid oxidation by the enol boratetautomerase method. J. Biol. Chem., **233,** 668, 1958.
39. Spolter, P. D., and Baldridge, R. C.: The metabolism of histidine. V. On the assay of enzymes in rat liver. J. Biol. Chem., **238,** 2071, 1963.
40. Schwarz, E.: Abbau von Histidin zu Urocaninsäure in der Epidermis. Biochem. Ztschr., **344,** 415, 1961.
41. Zannoni, V. G., and La Du, B. N.: Determination of histidine α-deaminase in human stratum corneum and its absence in histidinaemia. Biochem. J., **88,** 160, 1963.
42. Tabor, H., and Mehler, A. H.: Histidase and urocanase, in *Methods in Enzymology,* edited by S. P. Colowick and N. O. Kaplan, vol. II, p. 228. Academic, New York, 1955.
43. Holton, J. B.: Histidinaemia. *First Meeting Abstracts, Federation of European Biochemical Societies,* p. 117, London, 1964.
44. Zenisek, A., Kral, J. A., and Hais, I. M.: Sunscreening effect of urocanic acid. Biochem. Biophys. Acta, **18,** 589, 1955.
45. Hais, I. M., and Zenisek, A.: Urocanic acid, a physiological sunscreen. Am. Perfumer Aromatics, **73,** 26, 1959.
46. Everett, M. A., Anglin, J. H., Jr., and Bever, A. T.: Ultraviolet induced biochemical alterations in skin. Arch. Dermat., **84,** 59, 1961.
47. Voge, C. I. B.: A simple chemical test for pregnancy. Brit. Med. J., **2,** 829, 1929.
48. Page, E. W.: The mechanism of the histidinuria of pregnancy. Am. J. Obst. Gynec., **51,** 553, 1946.
49. Page, E. W., Glendening, M. B., Dignam, W., and Harper, H. A.: The causes of histidinuria in normal pregnancy. Am. J. Obst. Gynec., **68,** 110, 1954.
50. Page, E. W., Glendening, M. B., Dignam, W., and Harper, H. A.: The reasons for decreased histidine excretion in pre-eclampsia. Am. J. Obst. Gynec., **70,** 766, 1955.
51. Bessman, S. P., and Baldwin, R.: Imidazole amino-aciduria in cerebromacular degeneration. Science, **135,** 789, 1962.
52. Roberts, E. E. G., and Ireland, J. T.: Personal communication.
53. Hudson, F. P., Dickinson, R. A., and Ireland, J. T.: Experiences in the detection and treatment of phenylketonuria. Pediatrics, **31,** 47, 1963.
54. Andrews, B. F., Crosby, P. F., and Angel, C. R.: Histidinemia: a new metabolic disorder. South. Med. J., **55,** 1326, 1962.
55. Edlbacher, S.: Zur Kenntnis des intermediären Stoffwechsels des Histidins. Hoppe-Seyler's Ztschr. physiol. Chem., **157,** 106, 1926.
56. György, P., and Röthler, H.: Über Bedingungen der autolytischen Ammoniakbildung in Geweben. Biochem. Ztschr., **173,** 334, 1926.
57. Ghadimi, H., and Zischka, R.: Histidinemia, in *Amino Acid Metabolism and Genetic Variation,* edited by W. L. Nyhan, p. 133. McGraw-Hill, 1967.
58. Ghadimi, H. and Partington, M. W.: Salient features of histidinemia. Amer. J. Dis. Child., **113,** 83, 1967.
59. Auerbach, V. H., DiGeorge, A. M., and Carpenter, G. G.: Histidinemia, in *Amino Acid Metabolism and Genetic Variation,* edited by W. L. Nyhan, p. 145. McGraw-Hill, 1967.
60. Witkop, C. J., and Henry, F. V.: Sjögren-Larssen syndrome and histidinemia. Hereditary biochemical diseases with defects of speech and oral functions. J. Speech Hearing Dis., **28,** 109, 1963.
61. La Du, B. N.: Histidinemia. Amer. J. Dis. Child., **113,** 88, 1967.
62. Kihara, H., Boggs, D. E., Lassila, E. L., and Wright, S. W.: Histidinemia: Studies on histidase activity in stratum corneum. Biochem. Med., **2,** 243, 1968.
63. Corner, B. D., Holton, J. B., Norman, R. M., and Williams, P. M.: A case of histidinemia controlled with a low histidine diet. Pediatrics, **41,** 1074, 1968.
64. Holton, J. B.: Skin L-histidine ammonia-lyase activity in the family of a child with histidinaemia. Clin. Chim. Acta, **11,** 193, 1965.
65. Gerritsen, T.: Histidinemia and mental retardation, in *International Copenhagen Conference on the Scientific Study of Mental Retardation,* edited by J. Oster, vol. I, p. 94. Statens Andssvageforsorg, Copenhagen, 1964.
66. Waisman, H. A.: Variations in clinical and laboratory findings in histidinemia. Amer. J. Dis. Child., **113,** 93, 1967.
67. Clarance, G. A., and Bowman, J. K.: Further case of histidinaemia. Brit. Med. J., **1,** 1019, 1966.
68. Wadman, S. K., van Sprang, F. J., van Stekelenburg, G. J., and de Bree, P. K.: Three new cases of histidinemia. Clinical and biochemical data. Acta Paediat. Scand., **56,** 485, 1967.
69. van Sprang, F. J., and Wadman, S. K.: Treatment of a patient with histidinemia. Acta Paediat. Scand., **56,** 493, 1967.
70. Cain, A. R. R. and Holton, J. B.: Histidinaemia: a child and his family. Arch. Dis. Child., **43,** 62, 1968.
71. Society Transactions: Histidinemia and atopic dermatitis. Arch. Derm., **98,** 317, 1968.
72. Gatfield, P. D., Knights, R. M., Devereux, M., and Pozsonyi, J. P.: Histidinemia: Report of four new cases in one family and the effects of low-histidine diets. Canad. Med. Ass. J., **101,** 71, 1969.
73. Gilman, P. A., and Howell, R. R.: The simultaneous occurrence of histidinemia and congenital hypoplastic anemia. J. Pediat., **75,** 878, 1969.
74. Bruckman, C., Berry, H. K., Dasenbrock, R. J.: Histidinemia in two successive generations. Amer. J. Dis. Child., **119,** 221, 1970.
75. Carton, D., Dhondt, F., de Schrijver, F., Samyn, W., Kint, J., Delbeke, M. J., and Hooft, C.: Histidinemia. Helv. Paediat. Acta, **25,** 127, 1970.
76. Kibel, M. A., and Levy, H. L.: A further case of histidinaemia: clinical and biochemical aspects. S. Afr. Med. J., **44,** 242, 1970.
77. Lott, I. T., Wheelden, J. A., and Levy, H. L.: Speech and histidinemia: Methodology and evaluation of four cases. Develop. Med. Child Neurol., **12,** 596, 1970.
78. Garvey, A. M., and Gordon, N.: Histidinaemia and speech disorders. Brit. J. Disorders Commun., **4,** 146, 1969.
79. Galamon, T., Szulc-Kuberska, J., and Tronczynska, J.: The disturbances in histidine metabolism in hereditary stammering. Folia phoniat. (Basel), **21,** 449, 1969.
80. Witkop, C. J., Jr.: Histidinemic-like symptoms in children recovering from kwashiorkor. In *Genetic, Metabolic and Developmental Aspects of Mental Retardation,* edited by R. F. Murray, Jr., and P. L. Rosser. Thomas, Springfield. In press.
81. Harper, A. E., Benevenga, N. J., and Wohlhueter, R. M.: Effects of ingestion of disproportionate amounts of amino acids. Physiol. Rev., **50,** 428, 1970.
82. Kerr, G. R., Wolf, R. C., and Waisman, H. A.: A disorder of lipid metabolism associated with experimental hyperhistidinemia in *macaca mulatta,* in *Some Recent Developments in Comparative Medicine* (*Symp. Zool. Soc. London*), p. 371. Academic, New York, 1966.

83. La Du, B. N.: L-Histidine ammonia-lyase (Human stratum corneum), in *Methods in Enzymology,* edited by H. Tabor, vol. 17b. Academic, New York, in press.
84. Brusilow, S. W., and Ikai, K.: Urocanic acid in sweat: an artifact of elution from the epidermis. Science, **160,** 1257, 1968.
85. Reaven, E. P. and Cox, A. J.: Histidine and keratinization. J. Invest. Derm., **45,** 422, 1965.
86. Nagy-Vezekényi, C.: On the histidine content of human epidermis. Brit. J. Derm., **81,** 685, 1969.
87. Hais, I. M., and Strych, A.: Increase in urocanate concentration in human epidermis following insolation. Experientia, **24,** 231, 1968.
88. Anglin, J. H., Bever, A. T., Everett, M. A., and Lamb, J. H.: Ultraviolet-light-induced alterations in urocanic acid *in vivo.* Biochim. Biophys. Acta, **53,** 408, 1961.
89. Baden, H. P., and Pathak, M. A.: The metabolism and function of urocanic acid in the skin. J. Invest. Derm., **48,** 11, 1967.
90. Baden, H. P., Mittler, B., Sviokla, S., and Pathak, M. A.: Urocanic acid in benign and malignant human epidermal tumors. J. Nat. Cancer Inst., **38,** 205, 1967.
91. Barnhisel, M. L., Priest, R. E., and Priest, J. H.: Histidase function in human epithelial cells. J. Cell. Physiol., **76,** 7, 1970.

CHAPTER SIXTEEN

DISORDERS OF PROLINE AND HYDROXYPROLINE METABOLISM*

Charles R. Scriver and
Mary L. Efron†

HYDROXYPROLINEMIA

Hydroxyprolinemia is a metabolic disorder characterized by a considerable elevation of the concentration of free hydroxyproline in plasma and urine and normal excretion of hydroxyproline-containing peptides. The disease has been reported in only one patient thus far [1], and it is suspected that the parents of that patient are sibs. This, combined with evidence that there is a deficiency of an enzyme which catalyzes one step in hydroxyproline degradation, suggests that the disorder is inherited. The affected child is severely retarded mentally.

Clinical Features

History and Physical Findings

At the time of examination the patient was 12 years old and was hyperactive, aggressive, and severely retarded in mental development. The IQ had ranged from 17 to 32 using the Cattell Infant Scale and later the Stanford Binet LM form, 1960 revision. The patient appeared physically normal except for small size (below the tenth percentile for height and weight) and mild strabismus.

She was a premature infant weighing 4 lb 7 oz at birth. The delivery and neonatal course were uneventful. There was no feeding difficulty. There was no history of serious illness and no history of fracture, poor wound healing, or other evidence of collagen disease, in spite of the excretion of large amounts of hydroxyproline, a major constituent of collagen. Mental retardation was noted in the first few months of life, and she was late in reaching all milestones.

Laboratory and X-ray Findings

Results of routine blood counts, serum calcium, phosphorus and alkaline phosphatase, protein-bound iodine, serum proteins, transaminases, blood sugar, and liver function studies were normal. The only abnormality detected by routine laboratory tests was persistent hematuria, without proteinuria, pyuria, or casts, even in catheterized urine specimens. Renal function as estimated by blood urea nitrogen (BUN), nonprotein nitrogen (NPN), intravenous pyelogram (IVP), renal concentrating power, and creatinine clearance was normal. Because of the hematuria, the child was investigated for deafness and photogenic epilepsy, both of which have been present in patients with the related disorder hyperprolinemia. An audiogram was normal, and the EEG showed no abnormality, other than poorly developed alpha rhythm. Photic stimulation had no effect. The cerebrospinal fluid (CSF) was normal. Bone roentgenograms were normal, and bone age was estimated at 9½ years when the child was 11½; this was consistent with her size. Mucopolysaccharide excretion was normal [2]. This and the normal bone roentgenograms are further evidence that the child has no collagen disease. Steroid excretion was studied because it is known that cortisone causes accumulation of free hydroxyproline in chick embryos [3], but urinary 17-ketosteroid and 11-oxysteroid excretion was normal.

Repeated amino acid analyses of urine have shown a persistent excretion of large amounts of free hydroxyproline (average 2,037 μmoles, or 267 mg per day; the normal excretion is below the limit of detection by the methods used). The plasma concentrations of free hydroxyproline have varied from 0.20 to 0.41 μmole per ml (normal less than 0.06 μmole per ml) [4–7]. Hydroxyproline accumulation was accounted for by the natural form, L-hydroxyproline; D-, allo-, and 3-hydroxyproline were not present [2].

The plasma hydroxyproline concentration was not altered by a hydroxyproline-free diet, by supplementation of the diet with proline, or by withdrawal of all drugs [2]. The cerebrospinal fluid hydroxyproline concentration was below the limit of detection. The concentration of other amino acids in the CSF was normal. Except for hydroxyproline, all other amino acids in blood and urine were within normal limits.

Family History and Genetics

The patient was the illegitimate offspring of a mother who was institutionalized for much of her life because of mental retardation. The father is unknown, but there is reason to suspect that he is a sib of the mother.

The mother, like her daughter, was aggressive and hyperactive while in the institution; her IQ has averaged about 50. The mother had no hematuria, and her plasma and urine amino acids, including hydroxyproline, were normal. Three sibs of the mother are living and are of normal intelligence; they have not been available for study. The parents of the mother were not related. One was from Greece and the other from Albania.

*The authors' studies were supported by grants from the Public Health Service, the John A. Hartford Foundation, and the Medical Research Council of Canada.

†Deceased.

The information available is too limited for any analysis of the genetics of the disorder. It is not known whether the mental retardation is related to the biochemical defect. Since the mother is also retarded but has no obvious abnormality in hydroxyproline metabolism, it is by no means certain that the mental retardation in the mother and in the child is in any way related to the defect in hydroxyproline metabolism.

The disease is probably very rare. No case was observed in a survey of 37,000 newborn infants [8] in whom persistent hydroxyprolinemia was sought by specific tests, nor has the condition been described again in any of the surveys for aminoacidopathies among many thousands of mentally retarded subjects in institutions around the world. It may be that the apparent rarity of the condition in disabled subjects reflects a very low frequency of a trait which may, in fact, be harmless, and which may appear with equal frequency in disabled and normal populations. No large surveys have actually been performed on normal children and adults to investigate this point.

HYDROXYPROLINE METABOLISM

Hydroxyproline and Collagen

Hydroxyproline constitutes about 14 percent of collagen [5], and this is at present the only known role of hydroxyproline in mammals. The hydroxyproline in collagen is not derived from plasma hydroxyproline [9]. Collagen synthesis proceeds by two mechanisms [10–16]. The first involves synthesis of a polypeptide of high molecular weight called *protocollagen* [10]; the second involves hydroxylation of selected peptide-bound proline residues in the protocollagen. The two events are independent of each other but occur consecutively. Incorporation of ^{14}C-proline into intracellular protocollagen in embryonic cartilage may proceed when hydroxylation of proline is inhibited [10]. Protocollagen need not be attached to sRNA in order for it to be hydroxylated [11]. The hydroxyproline-deficient, collagenase-degradable protocollagen is hydroxylated by a collagen-proline hydroxylase. This enzyme has been isolated and is active in cell-free systems prepared from sources such as fetal rat skin, adult rat liver, guinea pig granuloma, and chick embryo [12]. Hydroxylation can occur on proline and lysine residues [13]. The hydroxylase requires several cofactors and substrates [13, 14]. There is an absolute requirement for ferrous iron, α-ketoglutarate, and atmospheric oxygen [15], and a preferential requirement for ascorbic acid, which can be partially replaced by reduced pteridines [14]. The apparent K_m values at low concentrations of proline-^{14}C-labeled protocollagen were: ferrous iron, $1.5 \times 10^{-6} M$; α-ketoglutarate, $5 \times 10^{-6} M$; ascorbic acid, $10^{-4} M$; and protocollagen (molecular weight about 100,000), $8 \times 10^{-9} M$ [13]. Hydroxylation occurs on the second proline after glycine in the sequence gly-pro-pro [16], to give a tripeptide sequence, gly-pro-hypro. The term *protocollagen, ascorbate:oxygen oxidoreductase* (*proline and lysine hydroxylating*) (EC 1.14.2 class) has been suggested for this enzyme [13]. The equivalent trivial name is *protocollagen hydroxylase.*

The product of these reactions is soluble collagen. The rate of its synthesis is enhanced by growth hormone, which acts at the stage of protein synthesis, not on the hydroxylation step [17]. Synthesis of soluble collagen is inhibited at the hydroxylation step by ascorbic acid deficiency. Soluble collagen may either be converted to insoluble collagen, or degraded to smaller subunits by collagenase-mediated depolymerization. These hydroxyproline-containing subunits may have two fates. They may be reaggregated to form new soluble collagen [18], or they may be degraded to free amino acids (including hydroxyproline) and low-molecular-weight peptides [19, 20]. The turnover of insoluble collagen and its subsequent degradation to free amino acids and small peptides is enhanced by growth hormone [17].

Hydroxyproline appears in body fluids after release from a bound pool. About 75 percent of the hydroxyproline released from this pool is in the free form and is normally oxidized to CO_2 [20]. The remaining 25 percent is retained in peptide linkage and is excreted in the urine [20].

A number of peptides containing hydroxyproline are found in human urine [21–23]. The principal species which escape from proteolysis are prolyl-hydroxyproline and glycyl-prolyl-hydroxyproline. The integrity of these oligopeptides may be attributed to poor uptake into cells [24] and a slow rate of hydrolysis by prolidase [20, 25]. Under some conditions in which the amount of released peptide-bound hydroxyproline is abnormally increased, the excretion of the dipeptide, glycyl-proline, is also increased [26, 27]. This peptide is poorly transported [27] and presumably escapes dipeptidase activity; the attendant free hydroxyproline which has been released from the initial tripeptide, glycyl-prolyl-hydroxyproline, is efficiently oxidized to CO_2 in subjects who have normal hydroxyproline oxidase.

The excretion of bound hydroxyproline [20] has been the object of intense study in the past decade. Excretion levels have been defined for the full age range of normal human subjects [28–30] (Fig. 16-1). Excretion is elevated under those conditions which enhance the rate of synthesis and turnover of soluble collagen or the turnover and degradation of insoluble collagen [31]. Thus, periods of rapid growth and tissue involution (e.g., the post-partum state) and disorders of connective tissue (e.g., bone disease, various endocrinopathies, and Marfan's syndrome) are all accompanied by increased excretion in urine of bound hydroxyproline and degradation of free hydroxyproline.

Degradative Pathway

There are no published data on the degradation of hydroxyproline in human subjects. In animals the degradative pathway has been well defined [32–37]. It is believed to proceed according to the scheme shown in Fig. 16-2, which is taken from Goldstone and Adams [35].

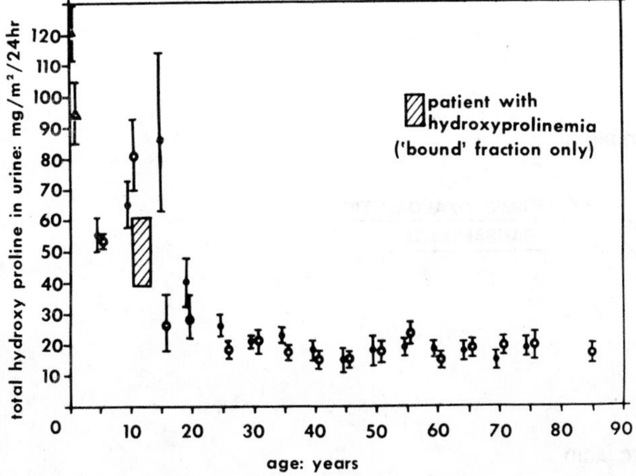

Figure 16-1. Excretion (mean $\pm$ s.e.) of total (free + peptide-bound) hydroxyproline by 166 subjects [30] (male, ●; female, o), divided into 5-year age groups, and by 14 male infants aged 120 to 200 days (▲) and 5 male infants aged 250 to 580 days (Δ) [28]. Free hydroxyproline comprises only a small or negligible percentage of total excretion in all age groups. The excretion of bound hydroxyproline by the patient with hydroxyprolinemia [1, 2] is normal for her age and accounts for only one-sixth of the total excretion of this imino acid.

The production of Δ^1-pyrroline-3-hydroxy-5-carboxylate (HPC), γ-hydroxyglutamic acid (HGA), and α-keto-γ-hydroxyglutaric acid (HKG) has been observed in homogenates of human liver and kidney incubated with hydroxyproline [2]. It is clear, therefore, that the metabolic pathway outlined in Fig. 16-2 is present in man as well as in animals.

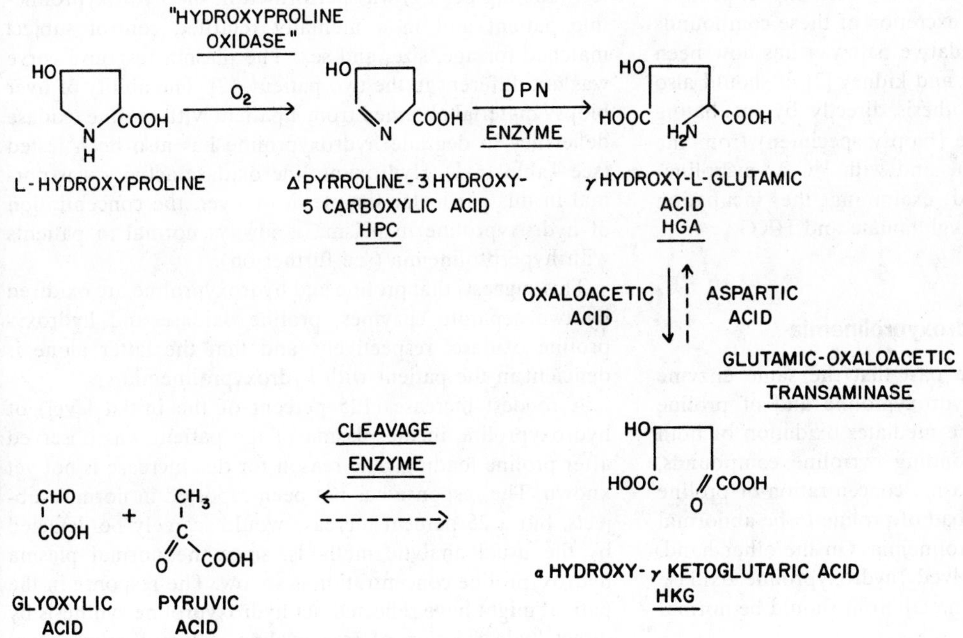

Figure 16-2. Degradative pathway of L-hydroxyproline.

Biosynthetic Pathway

Goldstone and Adams produced evidence for a biosynthetic pathway for free hydroxyproline in mammals [38]. Hydroxyproline is synthesized from glyoxylate and pyruvate, which is the reverse of the degradative pathway shown in Fig. 16-2 but with different enzymes (Fig. 16-3). The reason for the survival of this apparently "useless" biosynthetic pathway is not clear, since free hydroxyproline itself has no known role in human metabolism.

Site of the Metabolic Block in Hydroxyprolinemia

Normal fasting human subjects do not excrete detectable quantities of the products of degradation of hydroxyproline [2]. Following ingestion of 100 mg per kg L-hydroxyproline, however, HPC, HGA, and HKG are detectable in the urine of the normal person. The maximum excretion of these compounds is observed in urine collected between 1 and 2 hr after ingestion of the oral load of hydroxyproline.

In contrast, the child with hydroxyprolinemia, following ingestion of a similar load of L-hydroxyproline and even after the ingestion of 200 mg per kg, excreted no detectable HPC, HGA, or HKG. Figure 16-4 shows the excretion of HPC in the urine of 10 normal subjects and the hydroxyprolinemic patient after ingestion of 200 mg per kg L-hydroxyproline. HPC was measured by the *o*-amino benzaldehyde reaction [39]. It is postulated, therefore, that this child has a block in the degradation of hydroxyproline and that the block is probably in the first step, i.e., that there is a deficiency of the enzyme mediating the oxidation of hydroxyproline to HPC.

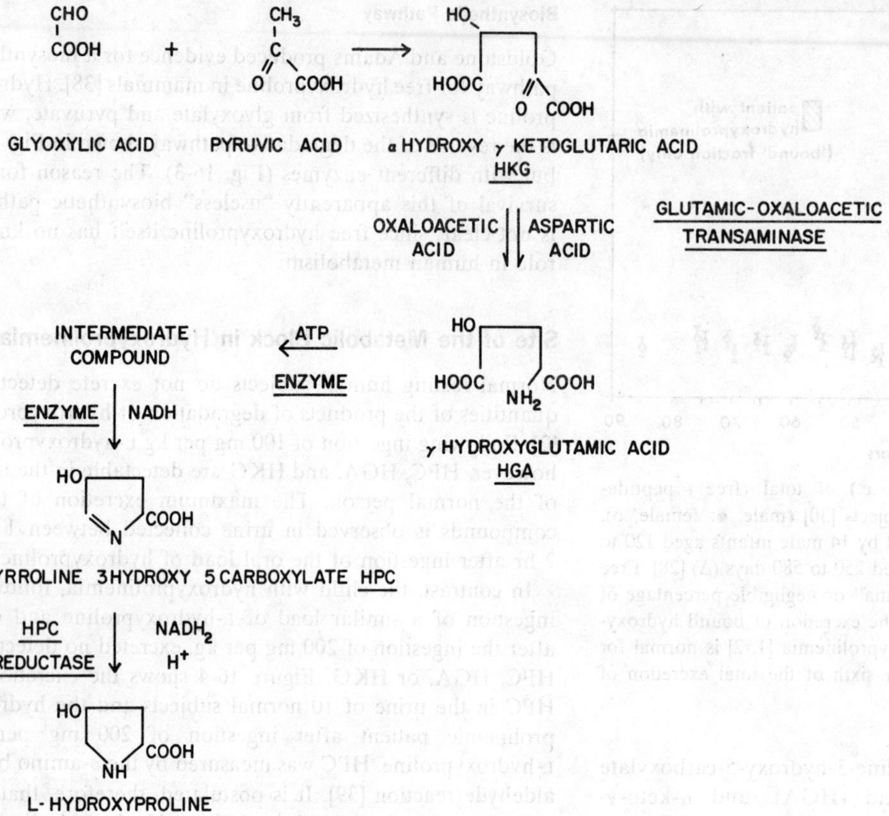

Figure 16-3. Biosynthetic pathway of L-hydroxyproline.

This could be tested by administration of HPC to the child. If the hypothesis is correct, one would then expect production of HGA and HKG and excretion of these compounds in the urine. Since the degradative pathway has now been demonstrated in human liver and kidney [2], it should also be possible to test this hypothesis directly by incubating aliquots of liver homogenate (biopsy specimen) from the child with ^{14}C-hydroxyproline and with ^{14}C-Δ^1-pyrroline-3-hydroxy-5-carboxylate, and examining the incubation mixture for labeled γ-hydroxyglutamate and HKG.

Proline Metabolism in Hydroxyprolinemia

It has been suspected in the past that the same enzyme catalyzes the oxidation of hydroxyproline and of proline [32–35, 39, 40]. If one enzyme mediates oxidation of both imino acids to their corresponding pyrroline compounds, then one might expect the plasma concentration of proline and the tolerance to an oral load of proline to be abnormal in the patient with hydroxyprolinemia. On the other hand, if separate enzymes are involved (hydroxyproline oxidase and proline oxidase), proline metabolism should be normal in the patient.

The concentration of proline in plasma was normal on all occasions in the patient [1, 2]. An oral proline tolerance test (100 mg per kg) was performed in the hydroxyprolinemic patient and in a mentally retarded control subject matched for age, size, and sex. The plasma response curve was not different in the two patients [2]. The ability of liver biopsy material obtained from a patient with proline oxidase deficiency to degrade hydroxyproline has also been tested (see Table 16-1). Hydroxyproline oxidase activity was normal in this particular sample. Moreover, the concentration of hydroxyproline in plasma is always normal in patients with hyperprolinemia (see further on).

This suggests that proline and hydroxyproline are oxidized by two separate enzymes, proline oxidase and hydroxyproline oxidase, respectively, and that the latter alone is deficient in the patient with hydroxyprolinemia.

A modest increase (125 percent of the initial level) of hydroxyproline in the plasma of the patient was observed after proline loading. The reason for this increase is not yet known. The response has not been reported in normal subjects, but a 25 percent increase would scarcely be detected by the usual analytic methods, since the normal plasma hydroxyproline concentration is so low. The response in the patient might have reflected net hydroxyproline synthesis by direct hydroxylation of free proline, a hypothetical event which in this instance accounted for at least 5 percent of proline conversion. A reaction of this apparent importance has not yet been documented in mammalian tissues. It is more probable that the plasma response of hydroxyproline to proline loading reflected a change in the distribution of hydroxyproline across cell membranes through interaction and exchange with proline during transport; this type of interaction has been well shown in mammalian tissues [41, 42].

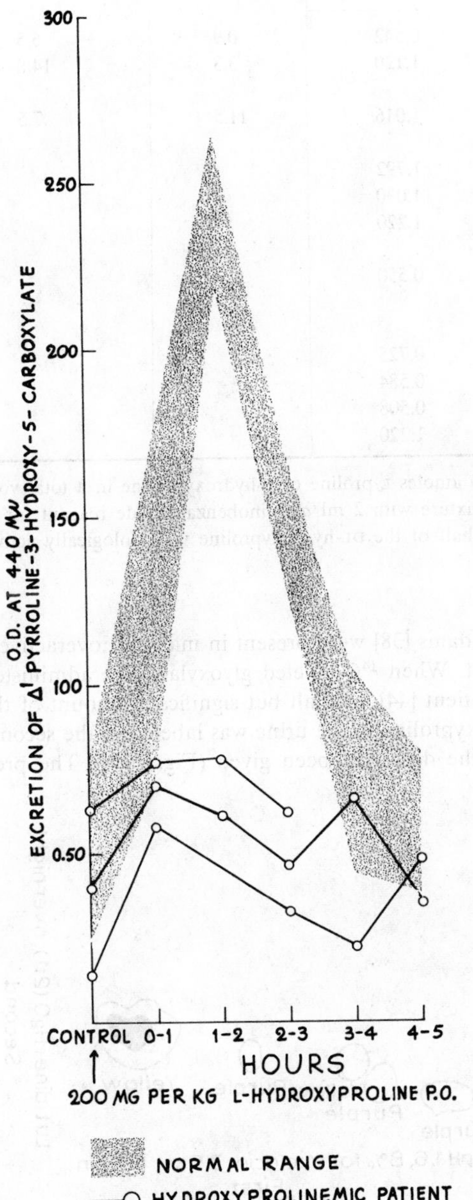

Figure 16-4. Excretion of Δ^1-pyrroline-3-hydroxy-5-carboxylate (HPC) in the hydroxyprolinemic patient and in normal subjects. HPC was measured by treatment of urine (1-min vol in 2 ml) with 2 ml 0.5 percent *o*-aminobenzaldehyde and 5 percent trichloracetic acid in ethanol.

Origin of Excess Hydroxyproline in Hydroxyprolinemia

Hydroxyproline is present in all foods containing collagen or gelatin [43]. Dietary hydroxyproline is apparently not a significant source of the elevated hydroxyproline in this child. After 3 weeks on a low-hydroxyproline diet [43] (the hydroxyproline concentration of the diet was below the limit of detection using an automatic amino acid analyzer), the plasma concentration was almost identical with that on a normal mixed diet (control plasma hydroxyproline concentration, 0.28 μmole per ml; after 3 weeks on a low-hydroxyproline diet, 0.27 μmole per ml).

The patient usually received a variety of drugs. In order to be certain that a drug did not alter her hydroxyproline metabolism, the child was maintained on a drug-free regimen for 3 weeks. There was no change in blood hydroxyproline concentration.

Since another possible source of free plasma hydroxyproline is collagen breakdown, the contribution from the pool of bound hydroxyproline to the expanded free pool was investigated in the patient with hydroxyproline oxidase

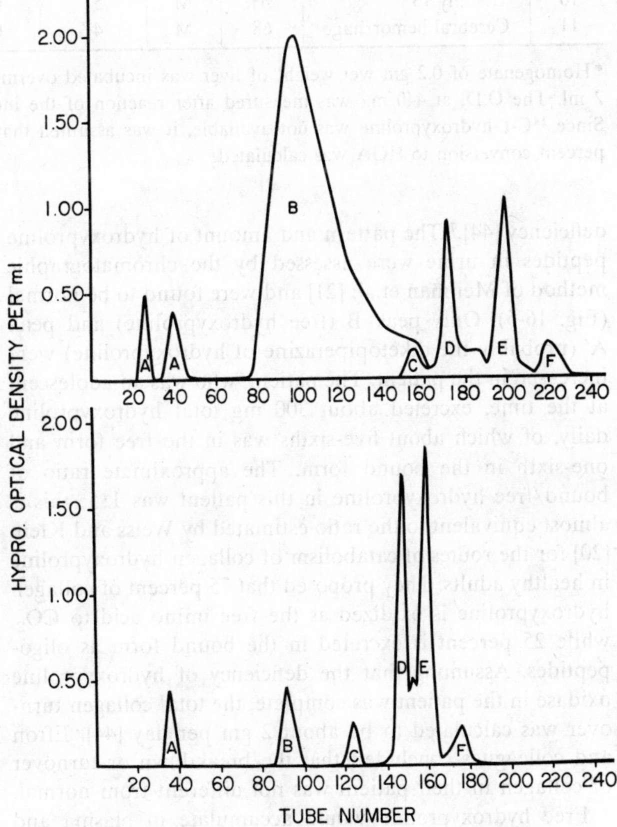

Figure 16-5. Urinary hydroxyproline-containing peptides in hydroxyprolinemia (*top*) compared to the normal excretion (*bottom*). (*The normal pattern is taken from* Fig. 2 *of Meilman et al.* [21], *reproduced by permission of the Journal of Clinical Investigation.*)

Table 16-1. L-PROLINE AND L-HYDROXYPROLINE DEGRADATION IN HYPERPROLINEMIC AND CONTROL LIVER HOMOGENATES*

No.	Patient, cause of death	Age	Sex	Hours dead	Production of PC from proline	Production of HPC from hydroxyproline	Percent conversion ^{14}C-proline to ^{14}C-glutamic acid	Percent conversion ^{14}C-hydroxyproline to ^{14}C-hydroxyglutamic acid
					O.D. 440 mμ			
1	Propositus, Family B	33	M	1	0.016	0.542	0.9	6.5
2	Father, Family B (jaundice)	69	M	Biopsy	0.520	1.120	3.3	14.8
3	Neuroblastoma (jaundice)	5	M	5	1.024	1.016	11.5	7.5
4	Cholecystitis	71	M	Biopsy	1.525	1.792		
5	Cholecystitis	65	F	Biopsy	0.400	1.030		
6	Uremia, glomerulonephritis	64	M	4½	0.403	1.220		
7	Uremia, hereditary nephropathy, deafness	19	M	1	0.265	0.550		
8	Trauma	73	M	10	1.000	0.725		
9	Trauma	43	M	3	0.578	0.584		
10	Trisomy 13	3/12	M	5	0.572	0.508		
11	Cerebral hemorrhage	68	M	4½	0.389	1.220		

*Homogenate of 0.2 gm wet weight of liver was incubated overnight with 60 μmoles L-proline or L-hydroxyproline in a total volume of 2 ml. The O.D. at 440 mμ was measured after reaction of the incubation mixture with 2 ml *o*-aminobenzaldehyde reagent for 30 min. Since ^{14}C-L-hydroxyproline was not available, it was assumed that only one-half of the DL-hydroxyproline was biologically active when percent conversion to HGA was calculated.

deficiency [44].[1] The pattern and amount of hydroxyproline peptides in urine were assessed by the chromatographic method of Meilman et al. [21] and were found to be normal (Fig. 16-5). Only peak B (free hydroxyproline) and peak A′ (probably the diketopiperazine of hydroxyproline) were increased in the patient. The patient, who was an adolescent at the time, excreted about 300 mg total hydroxyproline daily, of which about five-sixths was in the free form and one-sixth in the bound form. The approximate ratio of bound/free hydroxyproline in this patient was 1:5; this is almost equivalent to the ratio estimated by Weiss and Klein [20] for the routes of catabolism of collagen hydroxyproline in healthy adults. They proposed that 75 percent of collagen hydroxyproline is oxidized as the free imino acid to CO_2, while 25 percent is excreted in the bound form as oligopeptides. Assuming that the deficiency of hydroxyproline oxidase in the patient was complete, the total collagen turnover was calculated to be about 2 gm per day [44]. Efron and colleagues concluded that the breakdown or turnover of collagen in their patient was not different from normal.

Free hydroxyproline would accumulate in plasma and urine if the biosynthetic pathway proposed by Goldstone and Adams [38] were present in man and overactive in the patient. When ^{14}C-labeled glyoxylate was administered to the patient [44], a small but significant amount of the free hydroxyproline in the urine was labeled in the second hour after the dose had been given (Fig. 16-6). The precursor

[1] This paper was published posthumously through the devoted efforts of Dr. Efron's colleagues.

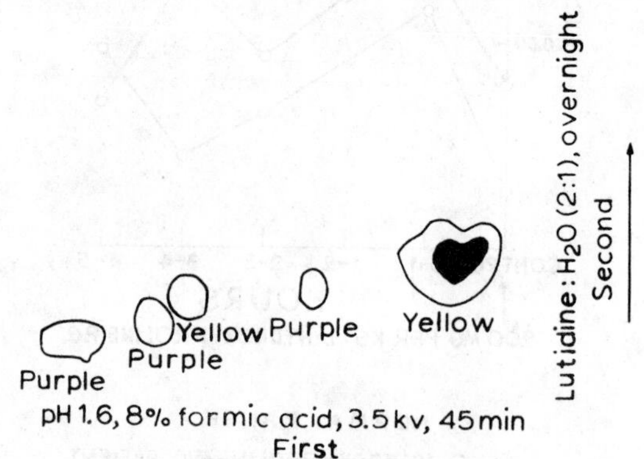

Figure 16-6. Radioautogram showing radioactivity (black) in position of hydroxyproline in urine collected 62 to 88 min after intravenous injection of ^{14}C-glyoxalate into a patient with "hydroxyproline oxidase" deficiency. (*Reproduced from Efron et al.* [44] *by permission of the Biochimica et Biophysica Acta.*)

substances, γ-hydroxyglutamic and α-hydroxy-γ-ketoglutaric acid, were also labeled at the same time. These findings indicate that the postulated biosynthetic pathway [38] exists in man. However, its activity was so small in the patient (with only one-thousandth of the injected glyoxalate appearing as hydroxyproline) that it seems unlikely that overproduction through biosynthesis could account for the amount of hydroxyproline retained by the patient. The most reasonable explanation for the excess of hydroxyproline in the patient is a deficiency of hydroxyproline oxidase activity in the presence of normal collagen turnover and breakdown.

Mechanism of Iminoaciduria in Hydroxyprolinemia

Free hydroxyprolinuria occurred in the patient. This is a normal finding in man only in the newborn (see Chap. 63, Familial Iminoglycinuria). No other amino acids were excreted in excess in the urine. The renal clearance of hydroxyproline was 0.35 ml per min [1]. The venous plasma threshold for hydroxyprolinuria in normal subjects under infusion conditions is about 0.4 μmole per ml [42], or about 40 times the normal concentration in plasma of mature subjects. The concentration in the plasma of the patient was 0.20 to 0.47 [2], an amount sufficient to produce the specific iminoaciduria.

Hydroxyproline interacts with proline and glycine at a shared membrane site serving their tubular absorption [41, 42]. When this happens, proline and glycine absorption is inhibited competitively and all three compounds are excreted in the urine. The absence of prolinuria and hyperglycinuria in the patient with hydroxyprolinuria can be attributed to an insufficient amount of the imino acid for initiating competitive inhibition at the shared site. The concentration of hydroxyproline in plasma must exceed 0.4 mM before the more complex pattern of iminoglycinuria appears in man [42]. This level was significantly exceeded by the patient only once in 14 occasions [2].

Hydroxyprolinemia and Mental Retardation

In this laboratory no hydroxyproline oxidase activity could be demonstrated either in rat or in human brain [2]. It has been shown that γ-hydroxyglutamate is decarboxylated in rat brain to α-hydroxy-γ-aminobutyrate [45]. This reaction may be mediated by glutamic acid decarboxylase, which is present in brain but not in liver. The hydroxyprolinemic patient had no detectable hydroxyproline in the CSF.

The absence of hydroxyproline oxidase in brain, and the presence of mental retardation in the mother, who had normal plasma hydroxyproline concentration, suggest that the biochemical defect and the mental retardation might not be directly related.

Diagnosis

Hydroxyprolinemia is easily detected by paper chromatography of urine. There is a ninhydrin-yellow spot in the position of hydroxyproline, and no other abnormalities in the urinary amino acid pattern.

If hydroxyprolinuria is suspected on the basis of this chromatogram, a second chromatogram should be prepared and stained with isatin (0.2 percent in acetone containing 5 percent glacial acetic acid). This gives a robin's egg blue color with hydroxyproline. The same chromatogram is then dipped in Ehrlich's aldehyde reagent (*p*-dimethylaminobenzaldehyde 10 percent w/v in concentrated HCl, diluted 1:4 with acetone just before use). After about 1 min a red-purple spot of increasing intensity appears if hydroxyproline is present, and this slowly changes to a permanent dull purple. This reaction apparently is specific for hydroxyproline and allohydroxyproline [46]. It is negative for a different compound, 3-hydroxyproline, recently discovered to be a constituent of collagen [47]. The stain is sensitive to 0.1 μg per cm^2 of hydroxyproline and may be positive even when the isatin stain is negative [46].

To confirm that the hydroxyprolinuria is associated with hydroxyprolinemia, 10 μl of serum (not deproteinized) [48] is placed on filter paper and a one-dimensional chromatogram made in butanol–acetic acid–water (12:3:5). The chromatogram is stained with isatin followed by Ehrlich's aldehyde reagent [46]. Normal serum gives no purple color. If the serum hydroxyproline concentration is greater than about 0.08 μmole per ml, the test result will be positive. Figure 16-7 shows diagrammatically the position of hydroxyproline on such a chromatogram.

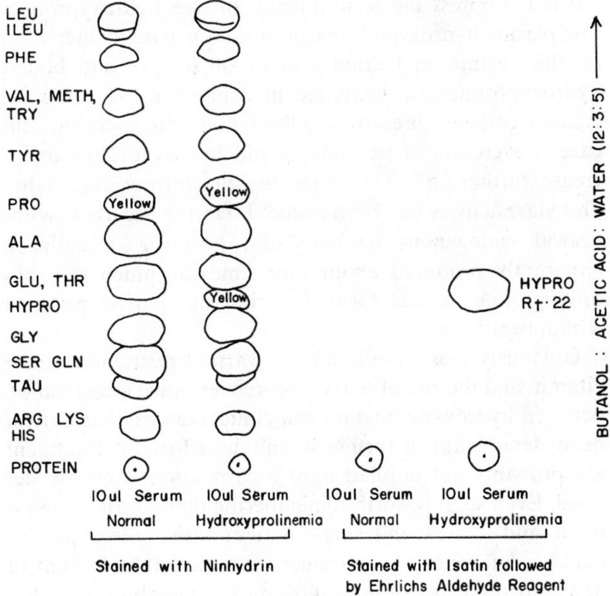

Figure 16-7. Simple chromatographic method for detection of hydroxyprolinemia using undeproteinized serum.

Hydroxyproline can also be detected in blood and urine by specific chemical methods [5-7], but these are more tedious than paper chromatography.

The concentration of hydroxyproline in the plasma of normal adults is about 0.01 μmole per ml. Newborn infants (premature and full-term) have considerably higher levels (0.03 to 0.1 μmole per ml) during the first few weeks of life [49]. These levels might suggest a diagnosis of hydroxyprolinemia without further investigation [8]. Neonatal hydroxyprolinemia in man probably reflects a transient impairment of hydroxyproline catabolism [8, 49], as well as increased collagen turnover during growth [17, 49]. Support for the proposal is found in measurements of hydroxyproline oxidase activity in liver homogenates from fetal newborn rats [49]. The activity is about one-third of that found in mature animals.

Therapy

The prospects of therapy in this disease are not encouraging [44, 50]. A diet free of hydroxyproline does not lower the concentration of hydroxyproline in body fluids [2]. Since collagen breakdown is the principal endogenous source of free hydroxyproline [20, 44], plasma hydroxyproline is not lowered by dietary limitations. A prolonged scorbutogenic regime has been attempted in the patient with hydroxyproline oxidase deficiency [44, 50] on the premise that ascorbic acid–deficient guinea pigs excrete less hydroxyproline than normal animals [51] and because ascorbic acid is a cofactor for hydroxylation of protocollagen [13, 14]. Nonetheless, withdrawal of dietary ascorbic acid for 5 months did not suppress the accumulation of free hydroxyproline. The plasma hydroxyproline concentration actually increased on this regime, and urinary excretion of free and bound hydroxyproline also increased in a manner indicating increased collagen breakdown. Repletion with ascorbic acid caused excretion of free and bound hydroxyproline to increase further still. This suggested that protocollagen hydroxylase activity had been restored. During ascorbate withdrawal endogenous synthesis and turnover of collagen apparently produced about four times as much free hydroxyproline as was formed during the period prior to withdrawal.

Obviously these results do not warrant restriction of the vitamin and the risk of scurvy. Moreover, since a correlation between hydroxyprolinemia and clinical disease has not yet been demonstrated, further strenuous efforts at treatment are probably not justified until a correlation is clearly defined. Even so, it is worth remembering that efforts to investigate and to treat this single patient with hydroxyproline oxidase deficiency have produced a remarkable amount of new and important information on the metabolism of hydroxyproline in man.

HYPERPROLINEMIA

Hyperprolinemia is an inborn error of metabolism which is characterized by elevation of the plasma proline concentration and a specific aminoaciduria marked by increased excretion, not only of proline, but also of hydroxyproline and glycine. In some cases, when the plasma proline level is below 0.8 to 1.0 μmole per ml, there is no aminoaciduria, and the disorder can be detected only by measurement of plasma proline.

There is evidence for two different types of hyperprolinemia. In Type I, deficiency of the enzyme proline oxidase has been demonstrated in liver. In Type II, the metabolic block is in the same pathway of proline catabolism but the second enzyme, Δ^1-pyrroline-5-carboxylate-dehydrogenase, appears to be abnormal. Δ^1-Pyrroline-5-carboxylic acid (PC) and proline both accumulate in body fluids in this latter trait. The enzyme defect has not yet been demonstrated in vitro in Type II hyperprolinemia.

A direct relationship between the biochemical abnormality and any particular clinical phenotype has not yet been proved. Several different types of renal disease have been associated with Type I hyperprolinemia, but many subjects with hyperprolinemia are quite healthy. Type II hyperprolinemia has been associated with seizures in four of the five known patients.

Clinical Features

Hyperprolinemia was first discovered during investigation of the disease of a 5-year-old boy with deafness and renal failure [52]. Partition chromatography disclosed a specific hyperaminoaciduria comprising proline, hydroxyproline, and an excess of glycine. There was a fourfold increase of the proline concentration of the plasma (Fig. 16-8). From these initial observations there evolved a more extensive analysis of the pedigree [53], in which it was observed that the renal disease, which resembled Alport's syndrome, was inherited as a dominant trait, while the disorder of proline metabolism appeared as an autosomal recessive trait. In spite of the discordance shown by analysis of the pedigree and the emphasis in the report [53] on the independent inheritance of the renal disease and the aminoacidopathy, this pedigree launched a popular misconception that hyperprolinemia and the nephropathy are closely related as cause and effect.

The association of renal disease with hyperprolinemia in members of several pedigrees subsequently reported (Table 16-2) has persuaded physicians that hyperprolinemia may offer an explanation for the puzzling nephropathy. Renal disease has a high frequency in medical practice. Physicians have asked us more often to search for this particular disorder of amino acid metabolism in their patients with renal disease than for any other trait. This bias in ascertainment

Table 16-2. PHENOTYPIC ASPECTS OF PROPOSITI WITH HYPERPROLINEMIA AND OF THEIR RELATIVES

Pedigree	Reference	*Propositus and relevant clinical features*								*Relatives*			
		Age, yr	Sex	Plasma proline, mg/100 ml/*	Enzyme defect (type)†	Renal disease	Deafness	Mental retardation	Seizures	Consanguinity in parents	Proline defect (alone)	Clinical disease (alone)	Both traits
A	Schafer et al. [52, 53]	5	M	7.8, 7.9	I	+	+	+	+	0	0	19	3
B	Kopelman et al. [54]	13	M	5.9	I(?)	+	?	0	0	?	2	(1)?	1
C	Efron [55]	33	M	13.4–20.1	I	+	0	+	0	0	0	5	3
D‡	Berlow and Efron [55–57]	1 7/12	M	42.4	II	0	0	+	+	0	0	0	0
E	Perry et al. [58]	3	M	9.1–14.5	I	+	0	+	0	+	5	3	5
F	Similä and Visakorpi [59, 103]	½	M	45.6	II	0	0	+	+	+	0	?	1
G	Emery et al. [60]	18	F	20–30	II	0	0	+	+	+	0	0	(1)?
H	Goyer et al. [61]	14	F	8.8, 9.3	I(?)	+	+	0	0	+	0	10	2
I	Piesowicz [62, 63]	½	M	25–30	I	0	0	+	+	0	2	0	0
J	Fontaine [64, 104]	¾	F	8.2–11.7	I	0	0	0	0	0	6	0	0
K	Woody et al. [65]	¼	M	15.0–21.3	I	+	?	0	+	+	4	Many	3
L	Jeune et al. [105]	4/12	M	5.4–13.8§	II	0	?	+	+	0	0	0	1 (only sib)
M	Goodman [106]	9	F	19	II	0	0	0	0	0	0	0	0
N	Mollica, Pavone, Artener [107]	1 8/12	F	10.8–11.7	I	0	0	0	0	0	6	0	0
O	Applegarth [108]	13	M	359	II	0	0	0	0¶	0	?	0	?

*Normal values (range) for all ages, infant to adult—1.15–5.0 mg per 100 ml [66]. Results obtained by quantitative analysis by elution chromatography on ion-exchange resin columns, except in pedigrees B and K, where direct chemical methods were used for proline analysis.

†Type I = block at proline oxidase; Type II = block at Δ^1-pyrroline-5-carboxylic acid (PC dehydrogenase); ? = PC excretion not mentioned, defect presumed to be Type I.

‡An additional patient with Type II hyperprolinemia and convulsions is mentioned by Efron elsewhere [50]. No details on this patient have been obtained except that the proline concentration was about 40 mg per 100 ml in plasma.

§Coexistent leucine transaminase defect proposed since the proband also had hyperleucine-isoleucinemia. He thus had a double aminoacidopathy.

¶One seizure with fever at 2 years of age. EEG was mildly abnormal at 13 years, suggesting epileptic disorder without localizing features.

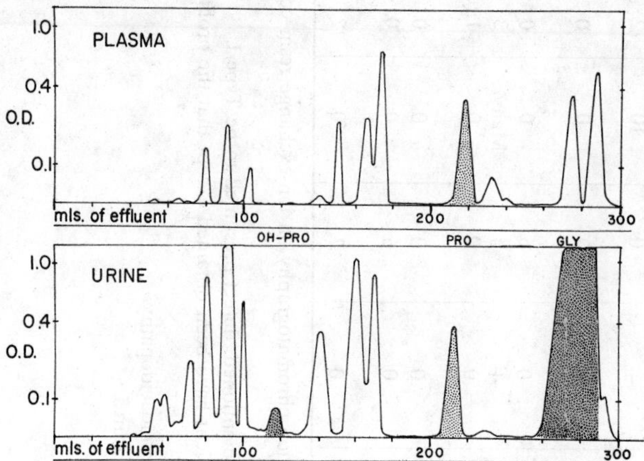

Figure 16-8. Amino acids in plasma and urine of the propositus [52, 53] with hyperprolinemia. The urine contains an excess of hydroxyproline, proline, and glycine (iminoglycinuria). The plasma shows an excess of proline alone. Analysis was performed by elution chromatography on ion-exchange resin columns as described in the text [53].

may explain why the condition has been found so frequently in families carrying a nephropathic trait. Many pedigrees with nephropathies of various types, including Alport's syndrome, have been screened and found free of the hyperprolinemia trait (cited in [53]). This fact has been underplayed in discussions of this topic.

There are now at least 11 families with hyperprolinemia in which one or more members have been studied (Table 16-2). A number of features become evident from inspection of the table and the reports upon which it is based.

1 There are two biochemical phenotypes of hyperprolinemia. Type I is accompanied by an accumulation of proline alone among the metabolites in the degradative pathway of L-proline. Type II is characterized by accumulation of proline and proline Δ^1-pyrroline-5-carboxylic acid (PC). The latter is formed by proline oxidase, the first step in proline degradation, and is degraded by PC dehydrogenase, the second enzyme in the catabolic pathway.

2 Type I hyperprolinemia is often associated with renal disease in the propositus. This was so in the original patient (pedigree A of [53]) and also in proband C (Fig. 16-9 [55]). Renal disease occurred also in the patients of pedigrees B, E, H, and K, all of whom came to the attention of investigating physicians because of renal disease in the propositus.

In this context pedigrees I [62, 63] and J [64] in particular are important. Fontaine [64] discovered hyperprolinemia in the proband of a pedigree (Fig. 16-10) during systematic screening of infants in his community. Subsequent studies uncovered hyperprolinemia in several sibs and in the parents of the proband. All members of this family with hyperprolinemia are healthy. The proband of pedigree I had hypocalcemia, developmental retardation, and steatorrhea.

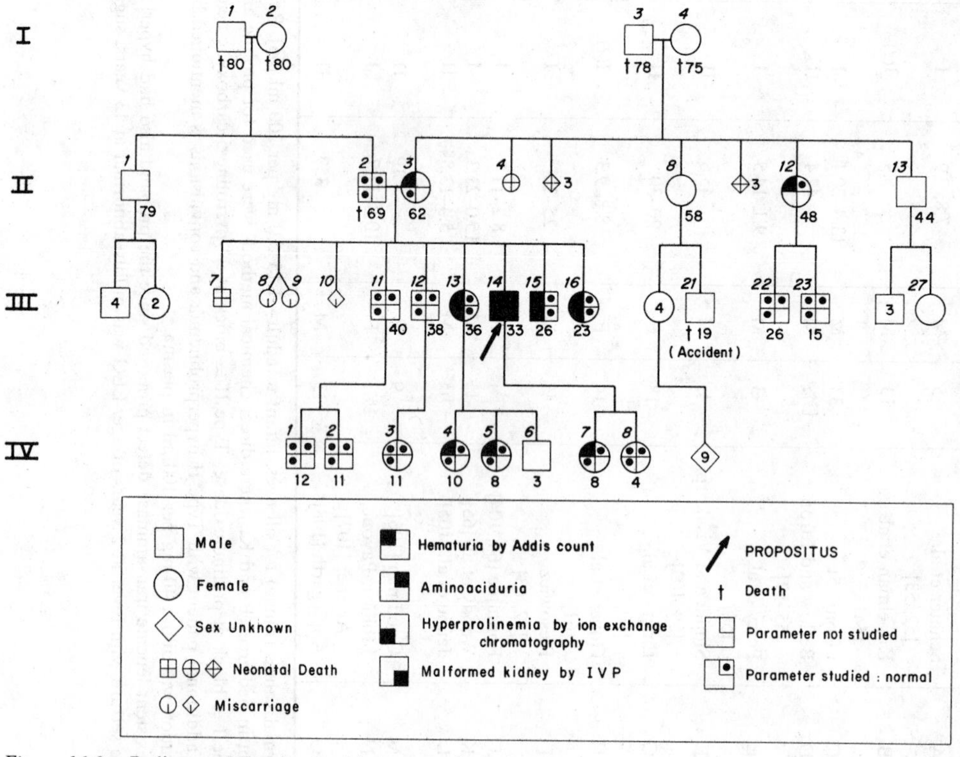

Figure 16-9. Pedigree of Family C with hyperprolinemia.

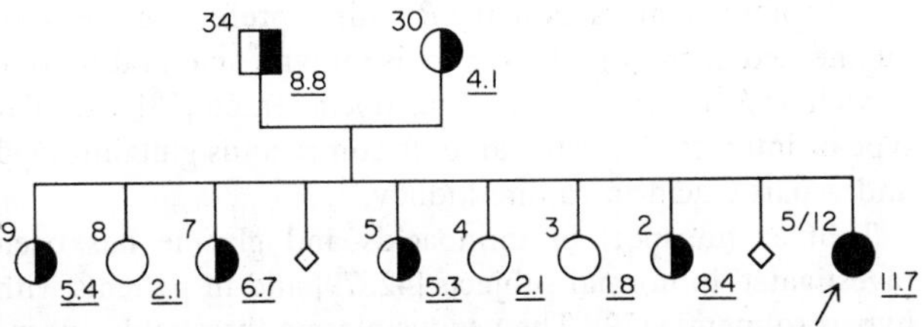

Figure 16-10. An Algerian family with Type I hyperprolinemia [64]. The proband was discovered in a community screening program for aminoacidopathies. All members of the pedigree are otherwise healthy. The underlined numbers indicate the proline concentration in plasma; the age in years of the subject is given in numbers above the symbols. A completely filled symbol indicates presumed homozygote; semifilled symbols indicate presumed heterozygote; open symbols are presumed normal homozygotes. The designation of a genotype on the basis of the plasma proline concentration is obviously arbitrary.

An obstructive uropathy of the lower part of the urinary tract without renal decompensation was an incidental finding.

Two of the eight propositi with Type I hyperprolinemia listed in Table 16-2 do not have a nephropathy. In the six who do, the type of nephropathy varies. In pedigree A [53] the nephropathy included congenital hypoplasia as well as a disorder resembling Alport's syndrome [67, 68]. A nephrotic syndrome brought the propositus of pedigree B [54] to the physician's attention. Uremia secondary to bilateral congenital obstruction occurred in the propositus of pedigree C [55]. A Wilms' tumor was found 8 months after the incidental discovery of hyperprolinemia during investigation of the retarded development of the propositus of pedigree E [58], and a nephropathy compatible with Alport's syndrome brought the H pedigree [61] to the investigator's attention. Pyelonephritis in the 3-month-old proband of pedigree K [65] was apparently incidental and terminal.

Two other reports not included in Table 16-2 have been cited in support of a relationship between renal disease and hyperprolinemia. Fuhrmann [69] found Alport's syndrome in a pedigree; the propositus, a sib, and the mother had "iminoglycinuria," but plasma proline concentrations were not reported. Rokkones and Løken [70] described a single infant, the product of a consanguine mating, in whom congenital nephropathy, retarded development, retinal dysplasia, and iminoaciduria were found. Hyperprolinemia was not proved. They used their findings to support a correlation between the occurrence of hyperprolinemia and renal disease, an interpretation not justified in the absence of any proof of hyperprolinemia. Iminoglycinuria may occur for other reasons (see Chap. 63), and even occurs in renal failure per se in some patients (see addendum to [55]).

Another line of evidence also impugns the supposed relationship between hyperprolinemia and renal disease. In pedigrees B, E, I, J, and K the propositi have sibs and other relatives with hyperprolinemia but without any associated clinical abnormality. Conversely, there are other relatives in these and other pedigrees with the index nephropathy who do not have hyperprolinemia. Finally, patients with Type II hyperprolinemia do not have renal disease in spite of a remarkable degree of hyperprolinemia.

Thus within pedigrees and between pedigrees there is no constant relationship between hyperprolinemia and nephropathy.

3 Type II hyperprolinemia is characterized by two distinctive biochemical features. There is excretion in the urine of PC (a compound which reacts with *o*-aminobenzaldehyde [39]), and the concentration of proline in plasma is usually much higher in the propositi (pedigrees D [56–57], F [59], and G [60] in Table 16-2) than in subjects with the Type I trait.

4 Propositi in four different families with Type II hyperprolinemia were mentally retarded and had a convulsive disorder [50, 55–57, 59, 60]. This does not prove a cause-and-effect relationship. The sib of one patient [59] does not have seizures even though he has hyperprolinemia. Disorders of the central nervous system also occurred in three (A, I, and K of Table 16-2) of eight probands with Type I hyperprolinemia. This suggests that hyperprolinemia may adversely affect the function of the central nervous system. Further studies are needed to confirm or deny this apparent relationship. Proline participates in brain metabolism [71], but an interdependence between normal metabolism of proline and normal function of brain has not yet been documented. The concentration of proline may be elevated in the cerebrospinal fluid of patients with Type II hyperprolinemia [60]. This is a function of the degree to which proline accumulates in body fluids, and it is not an exclusive feature of the Type II trait, since proline also accumulates in the cerebrospinal fluid of patients with Type I hyperprolinemia [55].

One fact cited in Table 16-2 may explain, in part, the frequency with which hyperprolinemia and clinical abnormalities appear together in a given pedigree. In 5 of 10 pedigrees where the information is recorded, there is consanguinity in parents of the propositus.[2]

Mechanism of the Aminoaciduria

Propositi with hyperprolinemia are usually discovered because they have a specific hyperaminoaciduria comprising prolinuria, hydroxyprolinuria, and hyperglycinuria (iminoglycinuria) (Fig. 16-8). The point of interest is that three compounds appear in excess in the urine while only one of them is present in excess in plasma. This finding provoked the proposal that the iminoacids and glycine share a common membrane transport system in the renal tubule [52]. Subse-

[2] Rokkones and Løken [70] also reported consanguinity in the parents of their patient with congenital anomalies and iminoglycinuria.

quent work has borne out this suggestion (see Chap. 63).

Tubular absorption of amino acids in man is a physiologic process which has been extensively studied [72]. Binding by the membrane of an organic solute such as an amino acid occurs during the transfer of the solute across the membrane. Membrane transport is a mediated process; it is finite, it obeys Michaelis kinetics, and it has specificity with regard to the binding of the substrate. The mediation of this transport process is accomplished by transport proteins [73] which are present in the lipid matrix of the membrane [74] and which accomplish transfer of the solute across the membrane by some as yet undisclosed energy and ion-dependent process [73, 74].

Hyperaminoaciduria reflects perturbation of the normal process of solute transport. If the solute is present in excess in the glomerular filtrate, a larger number of molecules will escape binding to the transport site (protein) and will appear in the urine ("overflow" or saturation mechanism). If the tubular membrane site is so modified that it does not bind its substrate(s) efficiently, more molecules will escape absorption and appear in the urine (specific "renal" aminoaciduria). If transfer across the membrane is inhibited, fewer molecules will be absorbed and more will appear in the urine (renal aminoaciduria which is usually generalized in character). It follows that if several substrates usually share a site, and one species fills that site, the other species will be displaced. Both "saturation" and "renal" mechanisms coexist, and a *combined* mechanism is said to account for the hyperaminoaciduria. The iminoglycinuria of hyperprolinemia (Fig. 16-8) is an example of a combined hyperaminoaciduria. When proline is present at sufficient concentration, it can compete with and displace more molecules of hydroxyproline and glycine from the site normally shared by these three substrates.

The transport sites at which amino acids are transported in kidney have been mapped, and a series of common sites has been identified [41, 75]. Several types of combined aminoaciduria are known. Patients with hyperlysinemia [76] or with raised arginine levels in plasma [77] excrete lysine, arginine, and ornithine in excess [76]. This reflects interaction at a shared site for the transport of cationic amino acids. Hyper-β-alaninemia in man (see Chap. 25) is accompanied by competitive interaction at a β-amino–preferring site, with augmented excretion of β-aminoisobutyric acid and taurine as well as β-alanine. Webber has documented [78] a similar type of interaction for the anionic compounds glutamic acid and aspartic acid in canine kidney.

Tubular transport of iminoacids and glycine has been investigated in normal subjects [42, 79] and in patients with hyperprolinemia [79]. The venous plasma threshold concentration at which prolinuria occurs in normal subjects is about 0.8 mM and is similar in hyperprolinemic subjects. Prolinuria (and the accompanying hydroxyprolinuria and hyperglycinuria) does not usually appear in subjects with plasma proline concentrations below this value.[3]

The maximum rate of tubular absorption of proline (T_m proline) is 160 to 300 μmoles per min per 1.73 m^2 in normal subjects. On the basis of the available evidence the T_m proline appears to be normal in hyperprolinemic patients. Proline at high concentrations displaces hydroxyproline and glycine competitively from renal transport sites in vivo and in vitro [41], and in normal man this produces iminoglycinuria [79]. Iminoglycinuria occurs in normal and in hyperprolinemic subjects when the plasma proline concentration exceeds 0.8 mM (9.2 mg per 100 ml).

Thus, tubular transport of the iminoacids and glycine in subjects with hyperprolinemia caused by impaired proline catabolism (either Type I or Type II) is not different from transport in normal subjects in whom the proline concentration in plasma is raised artificially.

Normal Metabolism of L-Proline

The Interconversion of Proline and Glutamic Acid

Proline is not an essential amino acid. Nutritional, bacteriologic and isotopic carbon studies have shown that proline is readily synthesized from glutamic acid and that it is degraded to glutamic acid [40, 80–89]. Not all the steps have been precisely defined, but the available data suggest that this interconversion occurs through a series of irreversible steps, according to the scheme taken from Strecker [39] (Fig. 16-11).

The Biosynthetic Pathway

Studies on *Escherichia coli* mutants lend support to the metabolic scheme shown in Fig. 16-11. Two variants of *E. coli* mutants which require proline for growth have been well studied [88, 89]. One of them (called strain 55-25) lacks the enzyme which catalyzes the first step of the reaction.

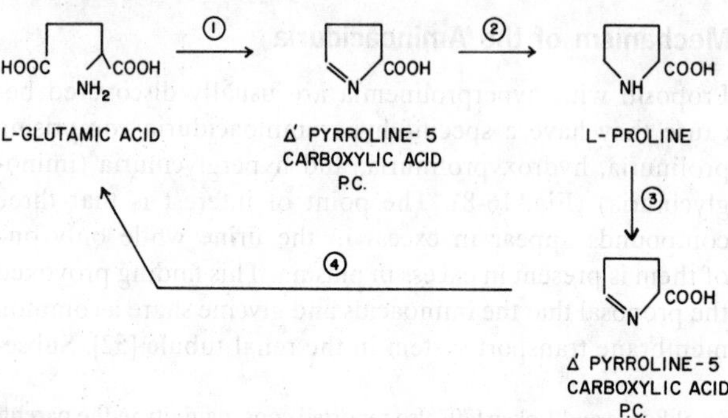

Figure 16-11. Interconversion of glutamic acid and proline. (*From Strecker* [39].)

[3] Kopelman et al. [54] described iminoglycinuria in patients whose proline in plasma did not exceed 0.5 mM. They measured proline in plasma by a direct chemical method, whereas the iminoglycinuria was detected by chromatographic procedures. The estimates of proline by these investigations are not equivalent to those obtained by elution chromatography on ion-exchange resin columns.

This organism will grow only in a medium containing Δ^1-pyrroline-5-carboxylate (PC) or proline. The other mutant lacks Δ^1-pyrroline-5-carboxylic acid reductase, which catalyzes step 2. This organism accumulates large quantities of PC and will grow only if proline is added to the medium. The accumulation of PC is enhanced if glutamic acid is added. This indicates that glutamic acid is a precursor of PC. A third mutant (strain 22-64) will grow on glutamic acid, on PC, or on amounts of proline which are much larger than those required for growth of strains 55-1 and 55-25. It appears that this mutant can make glutamic acid from proline (by way of steps 3 and 4 in Fig. 16-11) but in no other way. The proline requirement of this organism is about equal to the glutamic acid requirement.

Step 1 (Fig. 16-11) has been demonstrated in vitro in mammalian tissue [85], and the corresponding step in hydroxyproline biosynthesis has recently been demonstrated in rat liver [38]. Step 2 has been observed in rat and beef liver. The enzyme is dependent on NADH (nicotinamide adenine dinucleotide) [86, 89].

The Degradative Pathway

As far as is known, the only pathway for degradation of proline is through steps 3 and 4 (Fig. 16-11). It is known from animal studies that isotopic proline is converted to isotopic aspartic acid, alanine, ornithine, arginine, γ-aminobutyric acid, and glutamic acid [71, 85]. Figure 16-12 shows the pathways from proline to glutamic acid and on to the other compounds in the urea and Krebs cycles. Recent evidence indicates that proline oxidase is located in the inner membrane of the mitochondria in rat liver and that PC dehydrogenase is present in the mitochondrial matrix and in the supernatant fraction [109].

Sporn, Dingman, and DeFalco injected ^{14}C-proline intracisternally into rats and recovered ^{14}C in the amino acids enumerated above after isolation of the amino acids from brain protein [71]. The finding of ^{14}C-ornithine and arginine after proline administration was the first clue that the brain, like the liver, can synthesize urea. Obviously steps 3 and 4 must exist in the brain, and this has been demonstrated directly in vitro in rat and human brain [55].

The conversion of proline to glutamic acid by way of PC has now been demonstrated in human liver and kidney [55]. Proline also is incorporated into protein, both as proline itself and as the hydroxyproline of collagen [90]. When labeled proline is administered to an animal, the collagen hydroxyproline becomes labeled, but collagen hydroxyproline does not become labeled after administration of labeled hydroxyproline.

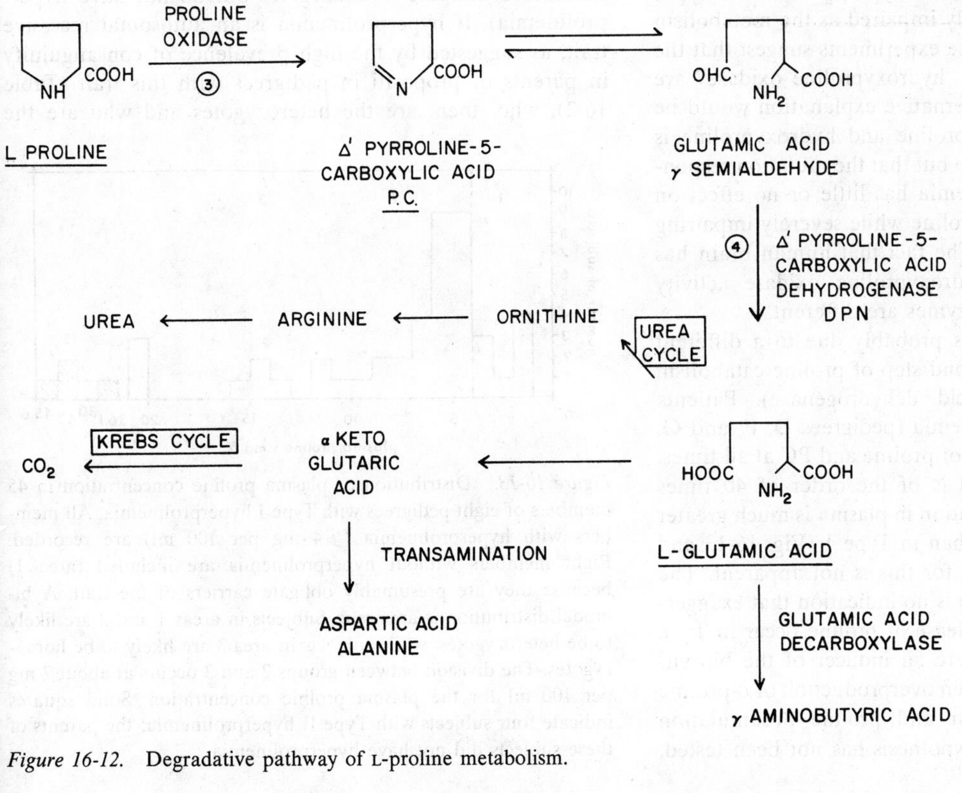

The Metabolic Block

It was postulated that Type I hyperprolinemia is secondary to a block in the degradation of proline to glutamic acid [53, 55]. Since no Δ'-pyrroline-5-carboxylate is accumulated in blood or urine in these patients, it seems probable that

PROLINE OXIDASE
③
COOH
NH
L PROLINE
COOH
N
Δ' PYRROLINE-5-CARBOXYLIC ACID
P.C.
OHC
COOH
NH_2
GLUTAMIC ACID
γ SEMIALDEHYDE
④
Δ' PYRROLINE-5-CARBOXYLIC ACID DEHYDROGENASE
DPN
UREA ← ARGININE ← ORNITHINE
UREA CYCLE
KREBS CYCLE
CO_2 ←
α KETO GLUTARIC ACID
HOOC
COOH
NH_2
L-GLUTAMIC ACID
TRANSAMINATION
ASPARTIC ACID
ALANINE
GLUTAMIC ACID DECARBOXYLASE
γ AMINOBUTYRIC ACID

Figure 16-12. Degradative pathway of L-proline metabolism.

the hyperprolinemia is due to a deficiency of the enzyme proline oxidase, which oxidizes proline to PC.

Liver from propositus C (Table 16-2) was obtained at autopsy approximately 1 hr postmortem [55]. It was homogenized according to the method of Adams and Goldstone [32]. Aliquots of the homogenate were incubated with L-proline and L-hydroxyproline and assayed for production of PC and HPC by the *o*-aminobenzaldehyde reaction [39]. Other aliquots were incubated with ^{14}C-L-proline and ^{14}C-DL-hydroxyproline, and the recovery of ^{14}C in isolated glutamic acid and γ-hydroxyglutamic acid, respectively, was measured by means of a scintillation counter. The results are presented in Table 16-1 together with those obtained from control subjects and from the father of the propositus of Family C (II 2). As a control for the father, who had obstructive jaundice, autopsy liver from a patient who had died of tumor and obstructive jaundice (patient 3, Table 16-1) was incubated with proline and hydroxyproline at the same time as the biopsy specimen from the father.

It is apparent that the degradation of proline to glutamic acid was much less efficient in liver from the hyperprolinemic subject than in the controls. The block apparently is in the first step of proline degradation, i.e., in the production of PC from proline.

Since there was considerable variation in proline oxidase activity in control patients, both in biopsy and in autopsy specimens (see Table 16-1), it was not possible to determine whether the father, as might be anticipated, carried a reduced complement of enzyme.

The metabolism of hydroxyproline, on the other hand, was normal or near normal in the hyperprolinemic subject; certainly it was not so severely impaired as the metabolism of proline. The results of these experiments suggest that the enzyme proline oxidase and "hydroxyproline oxidase" are not the same in man. An alternative explanation would be that the oxidation of both proline and hydroxyproline is mediated by the same enzyme but that the mutation responsible for Type I hyperprolinemia has little or no effect on the metabolism of hydroxyproline while severely impairing the metabolism of proline. The fact that human brain has proline oxidase but no hydroxyproline oxidase activity strongly suggests that the enzymes are different.

Type II hyperprolinemia is probably due to a different type of block, one at the second step of proline catabolism (Δ^1-pyrroline-5-carboxylic acid dehydrogenase). Patients with this type of hyperprolinemia (pedigrees D, F, and G, Table 16-1) excrete an excess of proline and PC at all times. The amount of PC excreted is of the order of 40 times normal [60]. Proline accumulation in plasma is much greater in Type II hyperprolinemia than in Type 1 (Fig. 16-13 and Table 16-1). The explanation for this is not apparent. The cause is not dietary, and there is no indication that exaggerated tissue catabolism and release of proline occur in Type II hyperprolinemia. If PC were an inducer of the biosynthetic pathway (Fig. 16-11), then overproduction of L-proline from glutamate would occur and proline accumulation would be augmented. This hypothesis has not been tested, since tissue has not yet become available for study of proline (and hydroxyproline) metabolism in vitro.

Genetics

Previous discussion of the genetics of Type I hyperprolinemia [57] relied on two published pedigrees [53, 55]. Hyperprolinemia appeared as an autosomal recessive trait without expression in presumed heterozygotes, while clinical manifestations (e.g., renal disease) behaved as dominant traits (see Fig. 16-9). Six new pedigrees (Table 16-2) have both simplified and confused the picture. As discussed above, the clinical disorders in hyperprolinemic pedigrees seem to bear no direct relationship to the iminoacidopathy, and the latter may appear without any associated clinical abnormality (Fig. 16-10). "Factor interaction" was proposed earlier [57] to explain the appearance of hyperprolinemia in one sibship out of a large pedigree, in which another trait occurred in several generations as well as in one of the parents of hyperprolinemic sibs. Nevertheless, it is no longer possible to invoke factor interaction if one believes that hyperprolinemia will occur when one or more mutant alleles are expressed at a gene locus controlling a step in proline degradation. The associated clinical disease(s) merely reflect the independent expression of mutant allele(s) at other loci.

A review of Type I hyperprolinemic pedigrees clearly reveals variability in the expression of the hyperprolinemic allele. This is summarized in Fig. 16-13, which shows the plasma proline concentration in all hyperprolinemic subjects found in these pedigrees (including individuals who are considered obligate heterozygotes but do not have hyperprolinemia). If hyperprolinemia is an autosomal recessive trait, as suggested by the high prevalence of consanguinity in parents of propositi in pedigrees with this trait (Table 16-2), who, then, are the heterozygotes and who are the

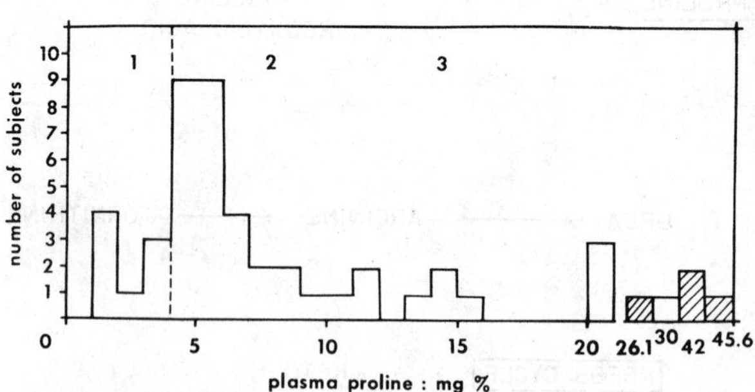

Figure 16-13. Distribution of plasma proline concentration in 45 members of eight pedigrees with Type I hyperprolinemia. All members with hyperprolinemia (>4 mg per 100 ml) are recorded. Eight members without hyperprolinemia are included (area 1) because they are presumably obligate carriers of the trait. A bimodal distribution is apparent. Subjects in areas 1 and 2 are likely to be heterozygotes, while subjects in area 3 are likely to be homozygotes. The division between groups 2 and 3 occurs at about 7 mg per 100 ml for the plasma proline concentration. Solid squares indicate four subjects with Type II hyperprolinemia; the parents of these subjects did not have hyperprolinemia.

mutant homozygotes if both genotypes exhibit hyperprolinemia? The assignment of symbols designating genotype (see Fig. 16-10) can only be arbitrary under these circumstances. Moreover, assay of proline oxidase in liver apparently cannot, by itself, segregate heterozygotes from normal homozygotes (see Table 16-1). Only if data on the in vitro enzyme assay and on the plasma proline concentration are available together is it possible to assign the genotype and phenotype with any certainty. Mutant homozygotes have hyperprolinemia and negligible enzyme activity at low substrate concentrations. Normal homozygotes must have a normal plasma proline concentration and easily demonstrable proline oxidase activity in liver. Heterozygotes might have normal or slightly reduced enzyme activity in vitro. If they had modest hyperprolinemia, their status would be obvious, but if they were not hyperprolinemic and hepatic proline oxidase activity was not clearly deficient, then there would be no way to distinguish them from normal subjects. Thus, resolution of heterozygote from mutant homozygote is feasible, but segregation of the former from the normal population is difficult.

Identification of hyperprolinemic subjects in successive generations of several pedigrees (B, E, H, J, and K of Table 16-2) suggests that a single hyperprolinemic gene may be expressed as hyperprolinemia, while the data from pedigrees A and C also indicate that a single dose is not always expressed. Plasma proline values in all hyperprolinemic subjects in the eight Type I pedigrees are plotted in Fig. 16-13 as a frequency distribution. Eight subjects who could be considered as "obligate heterozygotes" but who have normal plasma proline levels in pedigrees A, C, and E are also plotted (area 1). There are 22 subjects (group 2) with a plasma proline concentration above 4 mg per 100 ml (taken as the limit of normal in mature subjects [53]) but less than 7 mg per 100 ml. There are another 15 subjects whose proline concentration exceeds 7 mg per 100 ml (group 3). The distribution of these subjects is thus bimodal. The ratio of persons with modest hyperprolinemia ($<$7 mg per 100 ml) to those with severe hyperprolinemia ($>$7 mg per 100 ml) is thus about 2:1. This suggests that the lower range of values represents heterozygotes and the higher range is compatible with the homozygous phenotype. Segregation of homozygotes from heterozygotes is not as simple as this in practice, because there are presumed homozygotes in these pedigrees with proline levels in plasma lower than 7 mg per 100 ml and presumed heterozygotes with values which are higher. Nonetheless, the conclusion that heterozygotes may have modest hyperprolinemia is supported by similar interpretations of specific pedigrees by Perry et al. [58] and by Woody and coauthors [65].

Variation in the degree of hyperprolinemia in the Type I trait may also reflect genetic heterogeneity (heteroallelism) at the gene locus for proline oxidase. This possibility cannot be investigated until more precise evaluation of enzyme activity in the mutant phenotype can be undertaken. Tissue culture techniques may provide this opportunity.

The existing evidence indicates that phenotypic differences in Type II hyperprolinemia (Table 16-2 and Fig. 16-13), which also behaves as an autosomal recessive trait, are accountable to alleles at the gene locus controlling PC dehydrogenase activity in proline catabolism, rather than to different alleles at the Type I (proline oxidase) locus. The presumed homozygotes with the Type II trait have high proline accumulation compared with patients who have Type I hyperprolinemia. The corresponding obligate heterozygotes do not have hyperprolinemia [57, 59, 60]. The Finnish investigators [91] have studied both parents, the maternal grandparents, and two female sibs of their Type II hyperprolinemic proband, by means of intravenous L-proline loading tests (230 mg per kg per 10-min infusion). The mother, her parents, and both sibs had normal fasting proline levels; however, each had a reduced ability to clear the plasma of the injected proline, and the highest concentration of proline reached in their plasma was greater than in the five control subjects. These relatives of the propositus also excreted some Δ^1-pyrroline-5-carboxylic acid in urine after loading, whereas the five control subjects did not. The paternal phenotype was not abnormal under the same conditions of investigation. It thus seems that the heterozygous phenotype is variably expressed. It is also possible that paternal and maternal Type II hyperprolinemic mutations in this pedigree were not allelic.

Diagnosis

In all three families the accumulation of proline was first detected in the urine by paper chromatography. Proline can be easily detected if the chromatogram is stained with isatin (0.2 percent in butanol containing 5 percent acetic acid; heat 10 min at 110°C). Most other amino acids also stain with isatin, but proline is obvious by its bright blue color. The paper is then dipped into 1*N* HCl and, while still damp, washed with water. Only the bright blue proline spot persists [92]. This is a very sensitive test and appears to be specific for proline. Since the isatin complexes formed with other amino acids wash out of the paper, a simple screening test can be performed with a drop of urine on paper, even without separation of the proline by chromatography.

To determine whether the plasma proline concentration is elevated, unidimensional chromatographic analysis of serum may be made with 10 μl, exactly as described earlier in this chapter under "Hydroxyprolinemia." Proline is clearly separated from other serum amino acids in this system and can be readily recognized by its blue color with isatin. The proline concentration can be roughly measured by application of standard quantities of proline to the same paper and by visual comparison of the intensity of the spots.

A microbiologic method is also available for quantitation of proline [88]. Since this method uses mutants which grow only when L-proline is added to the medium, confirmation also is obtained that the substance accumulated is L-proline.

There are several chemical methods for measurement of proline [93–96]. These are reasonably satisfactory for plasma, but the presence of proline-containing peptides which yield free proline by hydrolysis during the determination may give falsely high results, particularly in urine. This disadvantage can be partially overcome by treatment of the urine with charcoal to remove some of the peptides or by partial purification of the proline by ion-exchange chromatography before proceeding with the chemical method.

Since some patients with hyperprolinemia have only a moderately elevated plasma proline concentration and no iminoglycinuria, it is important that the analysis be as accurate as possible. For this reason column chromatographic procedures or more precise chemical methods [96] are preferable for family studies in hyperprolinemia, even though they are more tedious and expensive.

Type II hyperprolinemia is distinguished by the excretion of PC in the urine. This compound may be specifically identified by the yellow color produced by reaction with a 2-ml volume of a mixture containing *o*-aminobenzaldehyde (0.5 percent w/v) and trichloracetic acid (5 percent v/v) in alcohol and a 1-min volume of urine diluted to 2 ml. The optical density of this reaction mixture is read at 440 mμ and corrected for the urine blank [39, 40, 55]. PC may also be identified by partition chromatography and staining with acid ninhydrin or isatin [39].

When the concentration of proline in plasma is greater than 4 mg per 100 ml, it is usually considered to be abnormal [53]. This assumption is based on published values for the mean, s.d., and range of proline concentration in human plasma [66]. The newborn infant may have a slightly higher normal value (up to 5 mg per 100 ml) for a few weeks after birth. Proline oxidation is depressed in tissues of the newborn rat [97] when compared with the adult animal, and the same circumstance may be true of man.

Therapy

Proline is not an essential amino acid and is freely synthesized from glutamic acid. Nearly all protein contains proline (lactalbumin is an exception) [98]. Accordingly, one anticipates that dietary management by protein restriction would be difficult and probably not effective. Piesowicz and colleagues have attempted dietary restriction of proline accumulation in a 9-month-old patient with Type I hyperprolinemia [62, 63]. The proline intake was reduced to 1.5 mg per kg per day (normal intake is about 500 mg per kg per day); within 24 hr the plasma proline level fell from 62 to 7 mg per 100 ml and later to 2 mg per 100 ml. After several days the plasma concentration stabilized at 6 to 8 mg per 100 ml. When dietary proline was introduced again in large amounts, the plasma proline returned to the former level and remained high. Reduction of proline intake a second time was followed immediately by a fall in proline accumulation. At present the child's diet contains 130 mg per kg per day of proline. Plasma proline level is moderately elevated, and reasonable growth is proceeding. Clinical symptoms (convulsions, hypocalcemia, steatorrhea, and osteoporosis) had all begun to improve prior to initiation of the diet. The diet did not retard this improvement.

Goyer and his associates have also studied the effect of dietary restriction of proline [99] in the proband of a pedigree with hyperprolinemia and multiple inherited clinical abnormalities [61]. The proband had advanced renal failure in addition to hyperprolinemia. The diet employed to restrict proline intake was also of such composition as to ameliorate the uremia. Proline accumulation fell, as did accumulations of ornithine, lysine, and histidine. Thus they demonstrated that a diet restricted in nitrogen and proline reduces proline accumulation in renal failure.

Berlow and colleagues [100] prescribed a diet free of meat, eggs, cheese, and milk for their patient with Type II hyperprolinemia, beginning in the sixth year of life. The plasma proline concentration was held between 1.5 and 2.0 μmoles per ml (10 times normal) for 12 months on this dietary regime, which provided about 100 to 200 mg proline per kg per day. No control plasma values were obtained just prior to treatment to indicate the effect of diet; hence, the only indications that this diet helped to reduce proline accumulation are the data showing much higher plasma proline levels long before the diet was begun and immediately after it was relaxed and the intake of proline increased. The abnormal prolinuria also disappeared on the dietary regime. The concentration of other amino acids remained in the normal range while the special diet was used. Whether use of this dietary regime early in life will control seizure activity or prevent mental retardation is unknown, and will not be known until the relation of these problems to Type II hyperprolinemia is further clarified.

Is a low-proline diet worth the effort? If Type I hyperprolinemia is harmless, then treatment is unnecessary. If Type II hyperprolinemia is eventually proved to have some effect on brain development, then there appears to be some hope that dietary treatment would be useful. The forthcoming published details on the composition and use of the diet of Piesowicz and colleagues [62, 63] will be important in this respect.

ADDENDUM

The following new information has appeared since preparation of this chapter.

Hydroxyprolinemia

Dr. Noel Raine of The Children's Hospital, Birmingham, England, has written [101] to describe a new patient with hydroxyprolinemia. She is the second of three sibs born to parents who were not consanguine. Only the proband has hydroxyprolinemia; all other members of the family are healthy. The proband's early infancy was uneventful, but the parents suspected retarded development when she was 6 months of age. Careful examinations at 4 and 5 years confirmed obvious retardation. Hyperactivity, temper tantrums, rhythmic behavior, and vacant spells characterized a behavior pattern with almost psychotic features. There were no abnormal physical signs, and growth was normal. An electroencephalogram showed an atypical spike and slow-wave pattern with focal signs in the right temporal region. Hydroxyprolinemia was discovered when the patient was $5\frac{9}{12}$ years old. Two values of 0.5 μmole per ml were reported. The plasma concentration fell to 0.22 μmole per ml during a 5-day period when glycine (10 gm, three times daily at meals) was added to the diet. This caused an increase in plasma glycine from 0.3 to 2.8 μmoles per ml (normal <0.5 μmole per ml) [66]. The plasma hydroxyproline level rose slightly, to 0.25 μmole per ml, over the next 2 weeks, while the glycine concentration fell steadily to 1.0 μmole per ml.

This history suggests, as did the first report on hydroxyprolinemia [1, 2], that this condition may be associated with mental retardation. The treatment regime and the clinical response must be documented in detail before the significance of the plasma changes can be assessed.

A third case of hydroxyprolinemia was reported from Finland in 1970 [102]. The propositus was a 31-year-old woman whose brother also had hydroxyprolinemia. One of the five children born to these individuals also had a slight elevation of the urinary free hydroxyproline concentration. All three subjects were healthy with the exception of a nodular goiter in the propositus, for which a urinary hydroxyproline assay had been done, leading to the diagnosis of the iminoacidopathy. A deficiency of hydroxyproline oxidase was proposed; Δ^1-pyrroline-3-hydroxy-5-carboxylic acid was absent in the urine of the three patients. The significance of "mild" hydroxyprolinuria in only the one child, who was 4 years old, among the five born to parents with hydroxyprolinemia is unknown since the plasma hydroxyproline concentration was not measured in these children. Each of these children is an obligate heterozygote presumably. It would be interesting to know whether a single dose of the mutant allele is expressed as it may be in the hyperprolinemia trait. The expression of the single mutant allele in the young subject in the Finnish pedigree may be related to the normal ontogeny of hydroxyproline oxidase in men. The authors suggested that the apparent rarity of recognized hydroxyprolinemia reflects the truly benign nature of the condition, it being another example of autosomal recessive "nondisease." They used the trait to confirm the existing belief that about 90 percent of peptide bound hydroxyproline released from collagen is degraded via the free hydroxyproline route.

Hyperprolinemia

New reports of this condition have appeared. Similä [103] has published the details of Pedigree F (Table 16-1), an example of the Type II trait. Fontaine and colleagues [104] have published their observations in Type I hyperprolinemia in Pedigree J (Table 16-2). Four new cases of hyperprolinemia [104–108] have been reported in correspondence to Scriver (see Pedigrees L to O in Table 16-2). These new cases support the belief that the hyperprolinemias are not necessarily associated with clinical disease. When the data on plasma proline concentration in members of these pedigrees are examined with respect to Figure 16-13, it is seen that the distribution pattern in this figure is not altered by the new material.

SUMMARY

1 One disorder of hydroxyproline and two of proline catabolism have now been described.

2 Hydroxyprolinemia, characterized by accumulation of free hydroxyproline in blood and urine, may be associated with mental retardation. Studies in vivo indicate a deficiency of the enzyme which oxidizes hydroxyproline to Δ^1-pyrroline-3-hydroxy-5-carboxylic acid.

3 Hyperprolinemia is caused by at least two different enzyme defects. These disorders are characterized by elevated plasma proline concentration and by hyperaminoaciduria comprising proline, hydroxyproline, and glycine.

4 One type of hyperprolinemia (Type I) is apparently caused by a deficiency of the enzyme proline oxidase. Type II is accompanied by accumulation of Δ^1-pyrroline-5-carboxylic acid. This suggests impairment of the second step of proline degradation, which is performed by the enzyme Δ^1-pyrroline-5-carboxylic acid dehydrogenase. The enzyme defect in Type I hyperprolinemia has been demonstrated in vitro; this has not yet been done for Type II.

5 That a relationship other than coincidental exists between Type I hyperprolinemia and nephropathy is unproved. Nine pedigrees have now been examined. Renal disease, if present at all and if hereditary, is inherited independently of the mutant allele causing hyperprolinemia. Type II hyperprolinemia is not consistently associated with disturbed function of the central nervous system (seizures, mental retardation, abnormal electroencephalogram).

6 Both types of hyperprolinemia are inherited as autosomal recessive traits. Modest hyperprolinemia is usually found in Type I heterozygotes, but the trait is not expressed in Type II heterozygotes. Proline accumulation in the Type II homozygotes is usually much greater than in Type I homozygotes. The two traits are presumably the result of mutant alleles at different gene loci. The presence of more than one mutant allele at the individual loci has not been ruled out.

7 A successful form of treatment for hydroxyproline accumulation has not yet been found. Dietary restriction of proline has been tried in two patients with a reasonable degree of success in preventing Type I hyperprolinemia. Results of dietary treatment have not been reported for Type II patients. This approach might be of value in those patients who have neurologic disturbances.

BIBLIOGRAPHY

1. Efron, M. L., Bixby, E. M., Palattao, L., and Pryles, C. V.: Hydroxyprolinemia associated with mental deficiency. New Eng. J. Med., **267**, 1193, 1962.
2. Efron, M. L., Bixby, E. M., and Pryles, C. V.: Hydroxyprolinemia: II.

A rare metabolic disease due to a deficiency of the enzyme "hydroxyproline oxidase." New Eng. J. Med., **272,** 1299, 1965.

3. Roberts, E., Kernofsky, D. A., and Frankel, S.: Influence of cortisone on free hydroxyproline in the developing chick embryo. Proc. Soc. Exp. Biol. Med., **76,** 289, 1961.
4. Øye, I.: Amount of free hydroxyproline in human blood serum. Scand. J. Clin. Lab. Invest., **14,** 259, 1962.
5. Neumann, R. E., and Logan, M. A.: The determination of hydroxyproline. J. Biol. Chem., **184,** 299, 1950.
6. Martin, C. J., and Axelrod, A. E.: Modified method for determination of hydroxyproline. Proc. Soc. Exp. Biol. Med., **83,** 461, 1953.
7. Morrow, G., III., Kivirikko, K. I., and Prockop, D. J.: Hydroxyprolinemia and increased excretion of free hydroxyproline in early infancy. J. Clin. Endocr., **26,** 1012, 1966.
8. Clow, C. L., Scriver, C. R., and Davies, E.: Results of mass screening for hyperaminoacidemias in the newborn infant. Amer. J. Dis. Child., **117,** 48, 1969.
9. Stetten, M. R.: Some aspects of the metabolism of hydroxyproline studied with the aid of isotopic nitrogen. J. Biol. Chem., **181,** 31, 1949.
10. Juva, K., Prockop, D. J., Cooper, G. W., and Lash, J. W.: Hydroxylation of proline and the intracellular accumulation of a polypeptide precursor of collagen. Science, **152,** 92, 1966.
11. Lukens, L. N.: The size of the polypeptide precursor of collagen hydroxyproline. Proc. Nat. Acad. Sci., **55,** 1235, 1966.
12. Hutton, J. J., Jr., and Udenfriend, S.: Soluble collagen proline hydroxylase and its substrates in several animal tissues. Proc. Nat. Acad. Sci., **56,** 198, 1966.
13. Kivirikko, K. I., and Prockop, D. J.: Enzymatic hydroxylation of proline and lysine in protocollagen. Proc. Nat. Acad. Sci., **57,** 782, 1967.
14. Hutton, J. J., Jr., Tappel, A. L., and Udenfriend, S.: Cofactor and substrate requirements of collagen proline hydroxylase. Arch. Biochem. Biophys., **118,** 231, 1967.
15. Prockop, D., Kaplan, A., and Udenfriend, S.: Oxygen-18 studies on the conversion of proline to collagen hydroxyproline. Arch. Biochem. Biophys., **101,** 499, 1963.
16. Kivirikko, K. I., and Prockop, D. J.: Hydroxylation of proline in synthetic polypeptides with purified protocollagen hydroxylase. J. Biol. Chem., **242,** 4007, 1967.
17. Aer, J., Halme, J., Kivirikko, K. I., and Laitinen, O.: Action of growth hormone on the metabolism of collagen in the rat. Biochem. Pharmacol., **17,** 1173, 1968.
18. Klein, L., and Weiss, P. H.: Induced connective tissue metabolism in vivo: reutilization of pre-existing collagen. Proc. Nat. Acad. Sci., **56,** 277, 1966.
19. Hurych, J., and Chvapil, M.: The role of free hydroxyproline in the biosynthesis of collagen. Biochim. Biophys. Acta, **107,** 91, 1965.
20. Weiss, P. H., and Klein, L.: The quantitative relationship of urinary peptide hydroxyproline excretion to collagen degradation. J. Clin. Invest., **48,** 1, 1969.
21. Meilman, E., Urivetzky, M. M., and Rapaport, C.: Urinary hydroxyproline peptides. J. Clin. Invest., **42,** 40, 1963.
22. Mechanic, G., Skupp, S. J., Saifer, L. B., and Kibrick, A. C.: Isolation of two peptides containing hydroxyproline from urine of a patient with rheumatoid arthritis. Arch. Biochem., **86,** 71, 1960.
23. Kibrick, A. C., Hashiro, C. Q., and Saifer, L. B.: Hydroxyproline peptides in urine in arthritic patients and controls on a collagen-free diet. Proc. Soc. Exp. Biol. Med., **109,** 473, 1962.
24. Christensen, H. N., and Rafn, M. L.: Uptake of peptides by a free-cell neoplasm. Cancer Res., **12,** 495, 1952.
25. Smith, E. L., David, N. C., Adams, E., and Spackman, D. H.: The specificity and mode of action of two metal-peptidases, in *The Mechanism of Enzyme Action,* edited by W. D. McElroy and B. Glass, p. 291. Johns Hopkins, Baltimore, 1954.
26. Seakins, J. W. T.: Peptiduria in an unusual bone disorder. Arch. Dis. Child., **38,** 215, 1963.
27. Scriver, C. R.: Glycyl-proline in urine of humans with bone disease. Canad. J. Physiol. Pharmacol., **42,** 357, 1964.
28. Younoszai, M. K., Andersen, D. W., Filer, L. J., Jr., and Fomon, S. J.: Urinary excretion of endogenous hydroxyproline by normal male infants. Pediat. Res., **1,** 266, 1967.
29. Jones, C. R., Bergman, M. W., Kittner, P. J., and Pigman, W. W.: Urinary hydroxyproline excretion in normal children and adolescents. Proc. Soc. Exp. Biol. Med., **115,** 85, 1964.
30. Anderson, J., Bannister, D. W., and Tomlinson, R. W. S.: Total urinary hydroxyproline excretion in normal human subjects. Clin. Sci., **29,** 583, 1965.
31. Smiley, J. D., and Ziff, M.: Urinary hydroxyproline excretion and growth. Physiol. Rev., **44,** 30, 1964.
32. Adams, E., and Goldstone, A.: Hydroxyproline metabolism: enzymatic preparation and properties of Δ^1-pyrroline-3-hydroxy-5-carboxylate. J. Biol. Chem., **235,** 3492, 1960.
33. Adams, E., and Goldstone, A.: Hydroxyproline metabolism: enzymatic synthesis of hydroxyproline from Δ^1-pyrroline-3-hydroxy-5-carboxylate. J. Biol. Chem., **235,** 3499, 1960.
34. Adams, E., and Goldstone, A.: Hydroxyproline metabolism: enzymatic synthesis of gamma hydroxyglutamate from Δ^1-pyrroline-3-hydroxy-5-carboxylate. J. Biol. Chem., **235,** 3504, 1960.
35. Goldstone, A., and Adams, E.: Metabolism of gamma hydroxyglutamic acid. J. Biol. Chem., **237,** 3476, 1962.
36. Bouthillier, L. P., Binette, Y., and Pouliot, G.: Transformation de l'acide gamma hydroxyglutamique en alanine et en acide glyoxylique. Canad. J. Biochem. Physiol., **39,** 1596, 1961.
37. Benoiton, L., and Bouthillier, L. P.: The metabolism of gamma hydroxyglutamic αC^{14} acid in the intact rat. Canad. J. Biochem. Physiol., **34,** 661, 1956.
38. Goldstone, A., and Adams, E.: Further metabolic reactions of hydroxyglutamate: amidation to hydroxyglutamine; possible reduction to hydroxyproline. Biochem. Biophys. Res. Commun., **16,** 71, 1964.
39. Strecker, H. J.: The interconversion of glutamic acid and proline. I. The formation of Δ^1-pyrroline-5-carboxylic acid from glutamic acid in *Escherichia coli.* J. Biol. Chem., **225,** 825, 1957.
40. Strecker, H. J.: The interconversion of glutamic acid and proline. II. The preparation and properties of Δ^1-pyrroline-5-carboxylic acid. J. Biol. Chem., **235,** 2045, 1960.
41. Wilson, O. H., and Scriver, C. R.: Specificity of transport of neutral and basic amino acids in rat kidney. Amer. J. Physiol., **213,** 185, 1967.
42. Scriver, C. R., and Goldman, H.: Renal tubular transport of proline, hydroxyproline and glycine. II. Hydroxy-L-proline as substrate and as inhibitor in-vivo. J. Clin. Invest., **45,** 1357, 1966.
43. Ziff, M., Kibrick, A., Dresner, E., and Gribetz, H. J.: Excretion of hydroxyproline in patients with rheumatic and non-rheumatic diseases. J. Clin. Invest., **35,** 579, 1956.
44. Efron, M. L., Bixby, E. M., Hockaday, T. D. R., Smith, L. M., Jr., and Meshover, E.: Hydroxyprolinemia. III. The origin of free hydroxyproline in hydroxyprolinemia. Collagen turnover. Evidence for a biosynthetic pathway in man. Biochim. Biophys. Acta, **165,** 238, 1968.
45. Bouthillier, L., and Binette, Y.: Decarboxylation of gamma hydroxyglutamate to α hydroxy gamma aminobutyrate in rat brain. Canad. J. Biochem. Physiol., **39,** 1595, 1961.
46. Jepson, J. B., and Smith, I.: Multiple dipping procedures in paper chromatography: specific test for hydroxyproline. Nature (London), **172,** 1100, 1953.
47. Ogle, J. D.: 3-Hydroxyproline, a new amino acid of collagen, J. Biol. Chem., **237,** 3667, 1962.
48. Culley, W. J., Luce, M. W., Calandio, J. M., and Jolly, D. H.: Paper chromatographic estimation of phenylalanine and tyrosine using finger tip blood. Clin. Chem., **8,** 266, 1962.
49. Morrow, G., III, Kivirikko, K. I., and Prockop, D. J.: Catabolism and excretion of free hydroxyproline in infancy. J. Clin. Endocr., **27,** 1365, 1967.
50. Efron, M. L.: Treatment of hydroxyprolinemia and hyperprolinemia. Amer. J. Dis. Child., **113,** 166, 1967.
51. Martin, G. R., Mergenhagen, S. E., and Prockop, D. J.: Influences of scurvy and lathyrism (odoratism) on hydroxyproline excretion. Nature (London), **191,** 1008, 1961.
52. Scriver, C. R., Schafer, I. A., and Efron, M. L.: A new renal tubular

amino acid transport system and a new hereditary disorder of amino acid metabolism. Nature (London), **192,** 672, 1961.

53. Schafer, L. A., Scriver, C. R., and Efron, M. L.: Familial hyperprolinemia, cerebral dysfunction and renal anomalies occurring in a family with hereditary nephropathy and deafness. New Eng. J. Med., **267,** 51, 1962.
54. Kopelman, H., Asatoor, A. M., and Milne, M. D.: Hyperprolinaemia and hereditary nephritis. The Lancet, **2,** 1075, 1964.
55. Efron, M. L.: Familial hyperprolinemia. Report of a second case, associated with congenital renal malformations, hereditary hematuria and mild mental retardation, with demonstration of an enzyme defect. New Eng. J. Med., **272,** 1243, 1965.
56. Berlow, S., and Efron, M. L.: A new cause of hyperprolinemia associated with the excretion of Δ^1-pyrroline-5-carboxylic acid (Abstract) Proceedings of the Society for Pediatric Research, p. 43, 34th Annual Meeting, Seattle, Washington, 1964.
57. Efron, M. L.: Disorders of proline and hydroxyproline metabolism, in *The Metabolic Basis of Inherited Disease,* 2d edition, edited by J. B. Stanbury, J. B. Wyngaarden, and D. S. Fredrickson, p. 376. McGraw-Hill, New York, 1966.
58. Perry, T. L., Hardwick, D. F., Lowry, R. B., and Hansen, S.: Hyperprolinemia in two successive generations of a North American Indian family. Ann. Hum. Genet., **31,** 401, 1968.
59. Simila, S., and Visakorpi, J. K.: Hyperprolinemia without renal disease (abstract). Acta Paediat. Scand. suppl., **177,** 122, 1967.
60. Emery, F. A., Goldie, L., and Stern, J.: Hyperprolinaemia Type 2. J. Ment. Defic. Res., **12:**187, 1968.
61. Goyer, R. A., Reynolds, J., Burke, J., and Burkholder, P.: Hereditary renal disease with neurosensory hearing loss, prolinuria and ichthyosis. Amer. J. Med. Sci., **256,** 166, 1968.
62. Piesowicz, A. T.: Hyperprolinaemia. British Paediatric Association, Proceedings of the Thirty-ninth Annual Meeting (Abstract). Arch. Dis. Child., **43,** 748, 1968.
63. Piesowicz, A. T., and Seakins, J. T.: Personal communication, May, 1969.
64. Fontaine, G.: Personal communication, May, 1969.
65. Woody, N. C., Snyder, C. H., and Harris, J. A.: Hyperprolinemia: clinical and biochemical family study. *Pediatrics,* **44,** 554, 1969.
66. Rosenberg, L. E., and Scriver, C. R.: Amino acid metabolism, in *Duncan's Textbook of Diseases of Metabolism.* 6th ed., edited by P. Bondy, 1969, pp. 366–515.
67. Alport, A. C.: Hereditary familial congenital hemorrhagic nephritis. Brit. Med. J., **1,** 504, 1927.
68. Cohen, M. M., Cassady, G., and Hanne, B. L.: A genetic study of hereditary renal dysfunction with associated nerve deafness. Amer. J. Hum. Genet., **13,** 379, 1961.
69. Fuhrmann, W.: Das Syndrom der erblichen Nephropathie mit Innenohrschwerhorigkeit (Alport-syndrom). Deutch. Med. Wschr., **88,** 525, 1963.
70. Rokkones, T., and Løken, A. C.: Congenital renal dysplasia, retinal dysplasia and mental retardation associated with hyperprolinuria and hyper-OH-prolinuria. Acta Paediat. Scand., **57,** 225, 1968.
71. Sporn, M. B., Dingman, W., and DeFalco, A.: A method for studying metabolic pathways in the brain of the intact animal: the conversion of proline to other amino acids. J. Neurochem., **4,** 141, 1959.
72. Scriver, C. R.: Use of human genetic variation to study membrane transport of amino acids in kidney. Amer. J. Dis. Child., **117,** 4, 1969.
73. Pardee, A. B.: Membrane transport proteins. Science, **162,** 632, 1968.
74. Korn, E. D.: Current concepts of membrane structure and function. Fed. Proc., **28,** 6, 1969.
75. Scriver, C. R., and Hechtman, P.: Human genetics of membrane transport with emphasis on amino acids. Advances Hum. Genet., **1,** 211, 1970.
76. Woody, N. C.: Lysinemia. Amer. J. Dis. Child., **108,** 543, 1964.
77. Dent, C. E.: Argininosuccinicaciduria and maple syrup urine disease. Bull. Schweiz. Akad. Med. Wiss., **17,** 329, 1961.
78. Webber, W. A.: Characteristics of acidic amino acid transport in mammalian kidney. Canad. J. Biochem. Physiol., **41,** 131, 1963.
79. Scriver, C. R., Efron, M. L., and Schafer, I. A.: Renal tubular transport of proline, hydroxyproline and glycine in health and in familial hyperprolinemia. J. Clin. Invest., **43,** 374, 1964.
80. Rose, W. C., Osterling, M. J., and Womack, M.: Comparative growth on diets containing ten and nineteen amino acids, with further observations upon the role of glutamic and aspartic acids. J. Biol. Chem., **176,** 753, 1948.
81. Weil-Malherbe, H., and Krebs, H. A.: Metabolism of amino acids. V. The conversion of proline into glutamic acid in kidney. Biochem. J., **29,** 2077, 1935.
82. Roloff, M., Ratner, S., and Schoenheimer, R.: The biological conversion of ornithine into proline and glutamic acid. J. Biol. Chem., **136,** 561, 1940.
83. Stetten, M. R.: Mechanism of the conversion of ornithine into proline and glutamic acid in vivo. J. Biol. Chem., **189,** 499, 1951.
84. Lang, K., and Schmidt, G.: Über Prolinoxydase. Biochem. Z., **322,** 1, 1951.
85. Stetten, M. R., and Schoenheimer, R.: The metabolism of L-proline studied with the aid of deuterium and isotopic nitrogen. J. Biol. Chem., **153,** 113, 1944.
86. Smith, M. E., and Greenberg, D. M.: Characterization of an enzyme reducing Δ^1-pyrroline-5-carboxylate to proline. Nature (London), **177,** 1130, 1952.
87. Strecker, H. J.: The interconversion of glutamic acid and proline. III. Δ^1-Pyrroline-5-carboxylic acid dehydrogenase. J. Biol. Chem., **235,** 3218, 1960.
88. Vogel, H. J., and Davis, B. D.: Glutamic acid γ-semialdehyde and Δ^1-pyrroline-5-carboxylic acid, intermediates in the biosynthesis of proline. J. Amer. Chem. Soc., **74,** 109, 1952.
89. Yura, T., and Vogel, H. J.: On the biosynthesis of proline in *Neurospora crassa:* enzymatic reduction of Δ^1-pyrroline-5-carboxylate. Biochim. Biophys. Acta, **17,** 582, 1955.
90. Green, N. M., and Lowther, D. A.: Formation of collagen hydroxyproline in vivo. Biochem. J., **71,** 55, 1959.
91. Visakorpi, J. P., and Simila, S.: Unpublished manuscript sent as personal communication, September, 1969.
92. Pasieka, A. E., and Morgan, J. F.: Specific determination of proline in biological materials. Proc. Soc. Exp. Biol. Med., **93,** 54, 1956.
93. Chinard, F. P.: Photometric estimation of proline and ornithine. J. Biol. Chem., **199,** 91, 1952.
94. Troll, W., and Lindsley, J. A.: Photometric method for the determination of proline. J. Biol. Chem., **215,** 655, 1955.
95. Messer, M.: Interference by amino acids and peptides with the photometric estimation of proline. Anal. Biochem., **2,** 353, 1961.
96. Summers, G. K., and Hawes, J. A.: Determination of free proline in serum. Proc. Soc. Exp. Biol. Med., **112,** 402, 1963.
97. Baerlocher, K., Scriver, C. R., and Mohyuddu, F.: Ontogeny of iminoglycine transport in mammalian kidney. Proc. Nat. Acad. Sci., **65,** 1009, 1970.
98. Block, R. J., and Bolling, D.: *The Amino Acid Composition of Proteins and Foods.* Charles C. Thomas, Springfield, Ill., 1951.
99. Goyer, R. A., Mitchell, B. J., and Leonard, D. L.: Dietary reduction of hyperprolinemia. J. Lab. Clin. Med., **73,** 819, 1969.
100. Berlow, S., Lepp, P., Sellcoe, D., and Efron, M.: Hyperprolinemia, Type II: Δ^1-pyrroline-5-carboxylic acid dehydrogenase deficiency. Unpublished manuscript sent as personal communication, September, 1969.
101. Raine, D. N.: Personal communication, July, 1969.
102. Pelhonen, R., and Kivirikko, K. I.: Hydroxyprolinemia. An apparently harmless familial metabolic disorder. New Eng. J. Med., **283,** 451, 1970.
103. Similä, S.: Hyperprolinemia Type II. Ann. Clin. Res., **2,** 143, 1970.
104. Fontaine, G., Farniaux, J. P. et Dautrevaux, M.: L'hyperprolinemie de Type I. Etude d'une observation familiale. Helv. Paediat. Acta, **25,** 165, 1970.
105. Jeune, M., Collambel, C., Michel, M., David, H., Guibaud, P., Guerrer, G., et Albert, J.: Hyperleucin-isoleucinemie par defaut partiel de transamination associée à une hyperprolinemic de Type 2. Observation familiale d'une double aminoacidopathie. Ann. Pediat., **46,** 349, 1970.
106. Goodman, S. I.: Personal communication, November, 1970.
107. Mollica, F.: Personal communication, December, 1970.
108. Applegarth, D., and Hingston, J.: Personal communication, 1970.
109. Brunner, G., and Newport, W.: Localization of proline oxidase and Δ^1-pyrroline-5-carboxylic acid dehydrogenase in rat liver. FEBS Letters, **3,** 283, 1969.

CHAPTER SEVENTEEN

UREA CYCLE DISORDERS*

Vivian E. Shih
Mary L. Efron†

The urea cycle is the only known metabolic pathway of urea synthesis and is the major pathway of ammonia detoxication in man. Deficiencies of the enzyme activities in this cycle have usually been associated with hyperammonemia, intolerance to protein ingestion, and mental deficiency. Hyperammonemia has also been found in several other familial diseases or apparent inborn errors of metabolism in which the basic defects have not yet been defined. All the presently defined disorders manifested by hyperammonemia will be discussed in this chapter.

THE UREA CYCLE

There are five steps in the biosynthesis of urea [1–14], as shown in Fig. 17-1. The relative activities of each enzyme of the urea cycle in human liver (Table 17-1) indicate that the rate-limiting steps are at carbamylphosphate (CP) synthetase and the argininosuccinic acid–synthesizing and –cleavage enzymes, while the ornithine carbamyl transferase (OCT) and arginase activities are much greater. Similar results have been obtained in rat liver [15].

There appear to be two CP synthetases. The CP synthetase in mitochondria requires acetylglutamate as a cofactor and is involved in urea synthesis [6]. CP synthetase in the soluble fraction of liver is distinguishable from that in mitochondria by its location. It utilizes glutamine instead of ammonia as the nitrogen donor [16]. This latter enzyme is presumably involved in pyrimidine synthesis (see Chap. 42).

*We wish to thank Dr. Sarah Ratner for her critical review of the manuscript.
†Deceased.

Ammonia* + bicarbonate + 2ATP $\xrightarrow[\text{carbamyl phosphate synthetase}]{Mg^{++};\ \text{acetylglutamate}}$ **carbamyl phosphate + 2ADP + Pi (1)**

Carbamyl phosphate + ornithine $\xrightarrow[\text{ornithine transcarbamylase}]{}$ **citrulline + Pi (2)**

Citrulline* + aspartate + ATP $\xrightarrow[\text{argininosuccinic acid synthetase (condensing enzyme)}]{}$ **argininosuccinic acid + AMP + PP (3)**

Argininosuccinic acid* $\xrightleftharpoons[\text{argininosuccinase (cleavage enzyme)}]{}$ **arginine + fumaric acid (4)**

Arginine + water $\xrightarrow[\text{arginase}]{Mn^{++}}$ **urea + ornithine (5)**

Figure 17-1. The urea cycle.

Liver is the major site of CP synthetase and OCT activity [17]. Very low activity was demonstrated in all other human tissues investigated by Reichard [18] except for the small intestine, which contained about one-tenth the OCT activity of liver per unit weight.

Liver is believed to be the only organ containing the complete urea cycle. Brain can synthesize arginine and urea from citrulline but cannot convert ornithine to citrulline [19–23]. The argininosuccinic acid (ASA) synthetase, ASase, and arginase activities of the brain are much lower than those of liver [19, 20]; thus it appears unlikely that the brain contributes significantly to total urea production. The kidney can synthesize arginine from citrulline but contains relatively little arginase; the arginine formed is normally used for guanidinoacetic acid synthesis [24]. Human skin fibroblasts cultured in vitro as well as heteroploid human cell cultures are also able to utilize citrulline but not ornithine in place of arginine for growth [25, 26]. This indicates the presence of ASA synthetase and ASase.

Metabolic errors have been discovered which involve each of the five steps of the urea cycle. These disorders have been named after the compound which is accumulated in blood and urine as a result of a block of the enzyme activity which mediates each of these steps.

The discovery of these metabolic errors has stimulated investigation into urea synthesis in these metabolic abnormalities in man. Activities of the five urea cycle enzymes have been studied in tissue obtained at both biopsy and autopsy by investigators who have collected data mainly to serve as controls for patients with suspected urea cycle disorders. The difficulties in obtaining human tissue have limited the number of measurements in each series. It should be noted that indications of enzyme activities based on examination of post-mortem liver are in general lower than those for liver obtained at biopsy. The effect of post-mortem changes on enzyme activity is difficult to estimate. The two synthetases appear to be particularly labile. For example, when one biopsy specimen in Levin's series [27] was frozen for 1 day before assay, the CP synthetase activity was only half that of two specimens assayed immediately [28].

Nuzum and Snodgrass [29] obtained eight liver biopsies from healthy adults on an average dietary protein intake. These individuals had no evidence of liver disease, and the histologic characteristics of the liver specimens were normal. Their data are probably the most representative of normal urea cycle activity in human adults (Table 17-1).

Findings concerning enzyme activity may vary depending on the method employed. Overall arginine synthesis has often been used to measure the ASA synthetase activity [1]. Liver homogenate is incubated with citrulline, aspartic acid,

Table 17-1. ACTIVITIES OF UREA CYCLE ENZYMES IN LIVER OBTAINED SURGICALLY FROM EIGHT NORMAL ADULTS, AGE 30 TO 70, WITH AN AVERAGE PROTEIN INTAKE (1 TO 1.5 GM/KG/DAY)

Enzymes	µmoles/hr/gm wet weight, mean ± s.d.	µmoles/hr/mg protein, mean ± s.d.	Ratio
CPS	279 ± 66	1.91 ± 0.27	3
OCT	6,600 ± 1,580	44.2 ± 7.8	70
ASA synthetase	90.0 ± 12.3	0.62 ± 0.14	1
ASase	220 ± 26.3	1.49 ± 0.27	2
Arginase	85,600 ± 9,280	579 ± 106	(1000)

Note: CPS, carbamylphosphate synthetase; OCT, ornithine carbamyl transferase; ASA, argininosuccinic acid.

Source: From Nuzum and Snodgrass [29]; assayed by method modified from Schimke [15].

and arginase, and the urea produced is measured colorimetrically. No ASase is added to the reaction mixture, on the assumption that there is ample ASase activity in a given sample of liver to measure the rate-limiting step. It is found, however, that in the absence of added ASase the rate of urea synthesis is 50 to 60 percent below that in the presence of added ASase [15]. The estimation of overall arginine synthesis as carried out with the liver homogenate unsupplemented with ASase would usually give less than maximal value for ASA synthetase.

The urea cycle enzymes are adaptive, to a degree, to various levels of dietary protein. Schimke [15] found that the total quantities of all the urea cycle enzymes of the liver were directly proportional to the daily consumption of protein in rats. Similar changes of lesser extent were observed recently in primates [29]. It may be inferred that the urea cycle in man is also adaptive; this may explain in part the wide range of enzyme activities reported in the literature. In fact, ASase activity was found to be lower in liver biopsies taken from children with protein malnutrition as compared with values obtained after their recovery [30].

Schimke [31] has also studied various other factors that affect the levels of urea cycle enzymes in rat liver and found that physiologic states, e.g., starvation or corticosteroid administration, which lead to protein breakdown and resultant increased urea excretion, increase all five urea cycle enzymes in proportion to the increase in urea synthesis. Adrenalectomy, on the other hand, results in a 70 to 80 percent decrease in arginase activity, whereas decreases in the other four enzymes are at most 30 percent. When rats are fed an arginine-free diet, the specific activities of the four enzymes involved in arginine biosynthesis (steps 1 through 4) are increased up to twofold over levels predicted on the basis of urea excretion, whereas arginase activity is unchanged.

Activities of urea cycle enzymes in human fetal liver are detectable as early as the fiftieth day of pregnancy and are increased toward the end of pregnancy [32, 33].

The three urea cycle amino acids—citrulline, ornithine, and arginine—are normally present in the blood and cerebrospinal fluid, but only very small amounts are excreted in the urine. Table 17-2 gives the normal ranges of these three amino acid concentrations [34, 35] and that of the ammonia concentration [36]. The ammonia concentration in cerebrospinal fluid is related to that in venous blood [37]; their relationship could be approximated by the equation: CSF ammonia = (0.69) (blood ammonia) − 20.

Table 17-2. UREA CYCLE AMINO ACIDS AND AMMONIA IN PLASMA AND CEREBROSPINAL FLUID (CSF)

Amino acids and ammonia	*Plasma*		*CSF*	
	µmole/ml (N = 10)	mg/100 ml (N = 10)	µmoles/100 ml (N = 18)	mg/100 ml (N = 18)
Ornithine	0.089 ± 0.018	1.18 ± 0.24	0.20 ± 0.08	0.035 ± 0.014
Citrulline	0.029 ± 0.012	0.51 ± 0.21	0.57 ± 0.18	0.075 ± 0.024
Arginine	0.076 ± 0.033	1.32 ± 0.58	2.01 ± 0.58	0.350 ± 0.101
		µg/100 ml (N = 20)		µg/100 ml (N = 7)
Ammonia		55.6 (44–71)		6.4 (0–14.7)

Source: Values taken from references [34–36].

Blood Urea and Urea Excretion in Urea Cycle Disorders

Studies of patients with disorders of the urea cycle have provided opportunities to investigate ammonia metabolism and the control of urea synthesis. It is of interest that patients with urea cycle enzyme deficiency states have had normal plasma concentrations of urea and excreted substantial amounts of urea in the urine even though there was an enzymatic block in the only known biosynthetic pathway of urea. The origin of urea in these patients is of considerable interest. Three possibilities for this anomaly have been suggested: (1) that there is an alternative pathway; (2) that the urea cycle enzymes in different organs are under different genetic controls and that the biochemical defect involves one or more, but not all, organs; and (3) that the enzyme defect is only partial. Evidence regarding these hypotheses will be discussed next.

The Hypothesis of an Alternative Pathway for Urea Synthesis

Although alternative pathways for urea synthesis have been suggested from time to time, none has yet been proved. A recent study [38] showed that rats injected with α-methylaspartic acid, an inhibitor of ASA synthetase, continued to excrete urea, and ASA synthetase activity could not be detected in the liver homogenate. The authors proposed another urea synthetic pathway, but their observations were not confirmed by two independent groups of investigators [39–41].

The Hypothesis of Different Genetic Controls for Urea Cycle Enzyme Activities in Different Organs

In patients with argininosuccinic aciduria, the concentration of ASA in the cerebrospinal fluid is higher than it is in the blood. The presence of ASA in the cerebrospinal fluid is difficult to explain, unless the synthesis of this highly polar substance takes place in the brain [19]. Dent speculated that the enzymatic block was present only in the brain and that the liver system was functioning normally [42]. Ratner, on the other hand, found that the total activity of ASA synthetase in the brain is relatively small and far too low to account for the massive amounts of ASA excreted by these patients [19]. ASA synthetase activity in the kidney, at least for some of the animal species investigated, is comparable to that in the liver [24]. Ratner therefore proposed the possibility that ASase in the brain and kidney were inactive in the patient, whereas that in the liver functioned normally. In argininosuccinic aciduria a deficiency of ASase activity has been found in several organs, including brain, liver, kidney, red blood cells, and skin fibroblasts. Unfortunately, in none of these patients was the ASase activity studied in all of these organs. It has been shown, however, that the ASase activity in one patient was deficient in the brain and normal in the kidney. This finding supports the hypothesis that the defect may be present in one or more but not i all organs of the body. Nevertheless, the resolution of th problem will require thorough studies of different tissu from the same patient.

The Hypothesis of a Partial Enzyme Defect

A complete block in one of the steps of the urea cycle woul probably be incompatible with life. It has been suggeste that only one-fifth to one-fourth of the potential ability c the liver for urea synthesis is used under normal circum stances [14, 43]. On the basis of this estimate a 20 perce residual enzyme activity in a patient with a defect in on of the enzymes of the urea cycle would be accompanie by no significant reduction in urea excretion. After the a ministration of ^{14}C-citrulline in a patient with ASA sy thetase deficiency, McMurray and coworkers [44] studied th fate of ^{14}C-citrulline in their citrullinemic patient who ha a residual liver ASA synthetase activity between 4 and percent of the control, and found that only 11 percent c the injected dose was excreted unchanged in the urine, an 31 percent was metabolized to urea in the first 24 hr. Ure formation from administered ^{15}N-labeled ammonium lacta has also been studied in a patient with ASA deficiency [45 The labeled isotope excreted as urea in 3 days was 34 percer of the given dose, less than half the amount obtained fro the control. These data indicate that a substantial urea e cretion would still be possible in patients with a significa reduction of enzyme activity.

Since liver is the major source of CP synthetase and OC activity, the hypothesis of a partial enzyme defect in patien with congenital hyperammonemia Types 1 and 2 is plausib in the absence of an alternative pathway of urea synthesi

PATHOGENESIS OF NEUROLOGIC ABNORMALITIES

The pathogenesis of mental retardation in amino acid meta bolic disease in general is still unknown. The accumulatio of the involved amino acid and its metabolites, either actin as an inhibitor of other important enzymatic actions c interfering with the transport of other amino acids into th cells, has been considered directly or indirectly responsib for the cerebral defect. This may be true in urea cyc disorders. For instance, in deficiencies of the ASA-synthe sizing and -cleavage enzymes, citrulline and ASA, which ar produced in huge amounts, may be toxic. Moreover, markedly increased blood ammonia level is the prominer feature in both CP synthetase and OCT deficiency. In fac blood ammonia elevation, although in different degrees, i a finding common to all urea cycle disorders. In additio to mental retardation in this group of patients, a charac teristic symptom complex is seen, and these symptoms im prove with lowering of blood ammonia levels. These ob servations suggest that high blood ammonia levels either pla

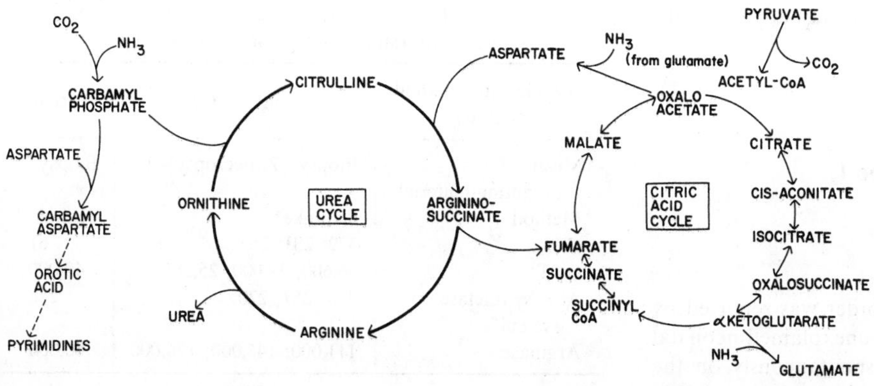

Figure 17-2. The relationship of the urea cycle to the citric acid cycle and pyrimidine biosynthesis.

an important role in the pathogenesis of the clinical symptoms or are at least partially responsible for them. Ammonia intoxication has also been considered as a contributing factor to such neurologic abnormalities as encephalopathies in acquired liver diseases [46] or following portacaval shunt [47] and in Reye's syndrome [48]. The episodic stupor and coma seen in the first two conditions are similar to the attacks in urea cycle disorders. These adult patients may have a specific neuropsychiatric syndrome [49]. The neuropathologic changes in these patients are similar to those that have been found in the congenital forms of ammonia intoxication.

When the high blood ammonia level occurs early in life, it is likely to be more injurious than when it occurs later. Cerebral atrophy has been found not infrequently in patients with urea cycle disorders [50–52]. Slow mental development may be a nonspecific reaction of the developing brain to any toxic agent or injury, since it is seen in many inborn errors of metabolism.

In the brain the major mechanism for the removal of ammonia is glutamine formation. Berl et al. [53] administered ^{15}N-ammonia to cats by carotid infusion and found that most of the injected ammonia was present as free ammonia. The next largest pool in the cerebral cortex was in the amide group of glutamine, followed by the α-amino group. Glutamine is the only amino acid in the brain that is considerably increased in amount as a result of ammonia infusion; this increase occurs without a corresponding decrease in the glutamic acid concentration. It is therefore concluded that the glutamic acid of the newly formed glutamine is synthesized in the brain and is from a small and metabolically active compartment.

Little is known about the cerebral ammonia metabolism in urea cycle disorders. With the information available on metabolic studies in hepatic encephalopathy and the data from animal experiments, a number of hypotheses concerning the mechanism of ammonia intoxication have been put forward [54]. Most of them explain the effect of high ammonia levels on brain function on the basis of interference with cerebral energy metabolism at some step in the citric acid cycle or a related reaction. The citric acid cycle is connected to ammonia nitrogen metabolism by a number of reactions. The former supplies oxaloacetate in the production of aspartate, which then condenses with citrulline to form ASA. Alpha-ketoglutarate forms glutamate by transamination with other amino acids. A popular hypothesis is that an increased demand for glutamate formation would result in depletion of α-ketoglutarate and in impairment of the citric acid cycle, and a consequent decrease in ATP [55] (Figs. 17-2 and 17-3).

Although many observations have been made in animal experiments, both in vivo and in vitro, it should be emphasized that detailed knowledge about ammonia metabolism, the control of the urea cycle, and its relation with other metabolic pathways in human beings is still lacking. The mechanism of ammonia intoxication may be manyfold.

CONGENITAL HYPERAMMONEMIA TYPES I AND II
(CP synthetase deficiency and OCT deficiency)

A metabolic block at either the first or second step in the urea cycle usually results in a severe degree of hyperammonemia and in clinical syndromes characterized by episodic vomiting and stupor and by psychomotor retardation. In addition, a patient with hyperammonemia Type I had ketoacidosis and neutropenia. Intermittent hepatomegaly and SGOT (serum glutamic oxaloacetic transaminase) elevation are frequently noted in Type II. Symptoms and signs respond to a restricted protein intake. The glutamine content of the blood and urine is often increased.

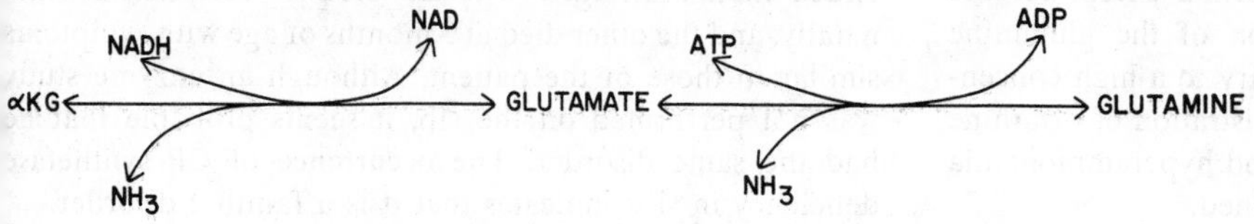

Figure 17-3. Glutamine synthesis from α-ketoglutarate (αKG).

Metabolites of the pyrimidine pathway may appear in the urine of patients with Type II.

Congenital Hyperammonemia Type I (CP Synthetase Deficiency)

Clinical Features

The one known patient with this disorder was reported by Freeman in 1964 [56]. The infant had unexplained neonatal hyperbilirubinemia, which subsided spontaneously on the fifth day of life. Vomiting, lethargy, dehydration, and flaccidity appeared on the tenth day. The symptoms recurred each time the child was fed a proprietary milk formula and promptly subsided following the administration of protein-free fluids. During periods of lethargy, a marked increase in blood ammonia (480 μg per 100 ml) and cerebrospinal fluid ammonia (550 μg per 100 ml) was noted. With the restriction of protein intake, both the ammonia level and the neurologic status of the patient returned to normal. On a diet containing 0.8 to 1.0 gm protein per kg per day, the patient failed to gain weight, and hypoalbuminemia (2.6 gm per 100 ml) and marked osteoporosis developed. On one occasion while receiving this diet, the patient, for no apparent reason, began to vomit and became markedly acidotic. The blood ammonia level at this time was in the upper range of normal. While the patient was receiving a regular diet, liver function test results were normal and the blood urea nitrogen (BUN) concentration was 12 mg per 100 ml. When the patient was on a low-protein diet, the BUN was 2 to 4 mg per 100 ml. A mild metabolic acidosis was present at all times. Cyclic neutropenia, with at times as few as four neutrophils per 100 leukocytes, was observed but it appeared to have no causal relationship to the clinical condition.

After an open liver biopsy the patient developed severe ketoacidosis and hyperlipemia and died at 5 months of age. Pathologic examination of the liver specimen showed fatty infiltration. No significant abnormalities were found in the brain.

Biochemical Findings and the Enzyme Defect

A mild hyperglycinemia (3.4 to 5.1 mg per 100 ml) and an increased glutamine concentration were the only abnormalities of the plasma amino acids. The urinary excretion of glycine was also increased. The reason for glycine elevation in the blood and urine is not clear. Amino acids in the cerebrospinal fluid were essentially normal except for the increased glutamine content. Elevation of the glutamine level in body fluid is a finding secondary to a high concentration of blood ammonia. Oral administration of ornithine and citrulline, 1 gm each per day, caused hyperammonemia [57]; this response could not be explained.

Table 17-3. LIVER UREA CYCLE ENZYME ACTIVITY IN HYPERAMMONEMIA TYPE I, μMOLES/GM PROTEIN/HR

Enzymes and method of study	Controls (3)	Patient
Means of obtaining material	Biopsy—2; necropsy—1	Biopsy
Method	Schimke*	Schimke*
CPS	372; 281; 253	61
OCT	36,600; 29,000; 25,200	40,000
ASA synthetase system	433; 257; 220	288
Arginase	111,000; 145,000; 126,000	80,000

* From Schimke [15].

Note: CPS, carbamylphosphate synthetase; OCT, ornithine carbamyl transferase; ASA, argininosuccinic acid.

Source: From Freeman et al. [57].

CP synthetase activity in the liver obtained at biopsy was low, as shown in Table 17-3; activities of other enzymes of the urea cycle were normal [57].

The findings of acidosis, neutropenia, and mild hyperglycinemia are similar to those seen in ketotic hyperglycinemia [58] and in a patient with mild hyperglycinemia and hyperammonemia who was reported by Soriano [59]. In neither study were the urea cycle enzymes recorded.

Diagnosis

The only amino acid abnormality in this disorder is the nonspecific finding of increased glycine and glutamine concentration in blood and urine. The normal range of urinary glycine excretion is very wide. With routine amino acid screening, a small increase of glycine in the urine or blood may not be obvious on the paper chromatogram. Glutamine is an unstable compound and may deteriorate if the urine specimen is allowed to stand at room temperature. Diagnosis of this disorder by the usual amino acid screening method is not possible. Measurement of blood ammonia 2 hr after a protein meal is the preferred diagnostic test and should be performed on any patient who has a history of protein intolerance.

Genetics

The family history of this patient is quite remarkable [54]. A maternal great-aunt and maternal aunt died of convulsions in the neonatal period. Three pregnancies of the mother ended in miscarriages. One sib died of convulsions neonatally, and the other died at 5 months of age with symptoms similar to those of the patient. Although an enzyme study was not performed on the sib, it seems probable that he had the same disorder. The occurrence of CP synthetase deficiency in sibs indicates that it is a familial disorder.

A Case of Multiple Enzyme Deficiency Including CP Synthetase Deficiency

An infant has recently been described by Hommes et al. [60] as having CP synthetase deficiency. The problems in this patient were complicated: she had a deficiency in both the glycolytic enzymes and the urea cycle enzymes, and hyperammonemia was not documented.

She was first admitted to the hospital at 20 days of age because of poor feeding, lethargy, irregular eye movements, and slight convulsions. On admission she was extremely lethargic and had no Moro's reflex. Bilateral papilledema was present. Liver and spleen were not enlarged. Her EEG showed convulsive activity when she was 2 months old and generalized paroxysmal high-voltage complexes at 7 months. A mild metabolic alkalosis was present. She responded at first to a low-protein diet with an improvement in her general condition but later began to deteriorate until she died at 7½ months of age. BUN values were low on several occasions: 1 mg per 100 ml when she had a protein intake of 2 gm per kg per day, and 2 mg per 100 ml on a protein intake of 1 gm per kg per day. Her blood ammonia concentrations of 25 to 75 μg per 100 ml on a low-protein diet were well within the normal range. Levels were not recorded while she was on the higher protein intake. SGOT and SGPT (serum glutamic pyruvic transaminase) were normal. The plasma amino acid pattern was normal except for a low-arginine content.

Fasting blood glucose levels varied between 100 and 150 mg per 100 ml. A blood pyruvate concentration of 1.3 mg per 100 ml, a lactate concentration of 3 mg per 100 ml, and an overall oxygen consumption of 5 ml per kg per min were low, suggesting a low capacity for glycolysis. Moreover, the patient failed to respond to leucine and arginine stimulation for insulin production. Activities of the glycolic enzymes were measured in liver tissue which was obtained with a needle biopsy. When the patient was 31 days of age, low activities of hexokinase and glucokinase were found. A subsequent liver biopsy when she was 56 days of age following insulin administration showed an increase of both enzyme activities.

The urea cycle enzymes were also studied in the liver and brain of this patient [60]. The activities of their control liver CP synthetase of 0.67 and OCT of 9.23 μmoles per min per gm wet weight were very low when compared with other reported values (Table 17-1). The patient had a liver CP synthetase activity of 0.28 and an OCT activity of 12 μmoles per min per gm wet weight, the former being about 40 percent of the one control value and the latter being higher than the control. The significance of this reduction of CP synthetase activity is uncertain.

The findings by Hommes et al. [60] of a significant amount of CP synthetase and OCT activity in the brain are at variance with those of several other groups of investigators. There has been no evidence for the presence of the first two steps of the urea cycle in the brain [19–23].

The primary cause of the metabolic derangement in this patient is far from clear.

Congenital Hyperammonemia Type II (OCT Deficiency)

Clinical Features

Russell et al. [61] described the first two patients in one family.

Patient 1. A girl, age 20 months, had been ill since the fifth week of life, when episodic vomiting began. Subsequently, she had more severe vomiting attacks, characterized also by screaming and agitation, and followed by lethargy and stupor. The child did not thrive. The head circumference increased only 1.5 cm in 15 months. There appeared to be some limited mental development up to age 6 months, and there had been a regression of mental function and a decline in vision at 20 months. She showed persistently neutral or alkaline urine, with normal or slightly low plasma CO_2-combining capacity.

Patient 2. A first cousin of Patient 1 was one of apparently monozygotic twins. She also was retarded in early development. At age 2 she developed attacks of vomiting accompanied by screaming, headache, slurring of speech, and confusion, followed by lethargy and stupor. During the recovery phase she had ataxia and ptosis. An IQ at age 6 measured 60 (Merrill-Palmer Scale). The head circumference at age 6 was only 51 cm. Pneumoencephalography in both patients showed cortical atrophy and radiotranslucencies suggestive of cerebromalacia [50]. The excretion of ammonium ion in the urine of both Patients 1 and 2 was greater than normal. In both children the levels of ammonia in the blood (980 and 480 μg per 100 ml) and in the cerebrospinal fluid (360 and 320 μg per 100 ml) were exceedingly high. These levels fell to normal limits when the protein intake was drastically reduced.

Patient 3. Apparently the *identical* twin of Patient 2 was well until 9 years of age, when she began to complain of headache, malaise, and lethargy [27]. Growth and development were normal. Clinical symptoms were mild as compared with those of her twin sister, Patient 2, and of her cousin, Patient 1. Fasting blood ammonia levels were only mildly elevated, ranging from 60 to 109 μg per 100 ml, and the glutamine content in her cerebrospinal fluid was within normal limits. Her tolerance to protein ingestion or ammonia loading was diminished, as shown by a prolonged rise of blood ammonia level after loading.

The mothers of Patients 1, 2, and 3 were sisters. Both disliked protein-rich food and had high fasting blood ammonia concentrations and abnormal ammonia tolerance tests [62].

Patient 4. This patient was the daughter of unrelated parents [51]. Growth and development were normal until 7 months of age, when she was weaned and given a variety of milk feedings, whereupon she became increasingly irritable, hypotonic, and less alert, vomited frequently, and failed to gain weight. Initial examination at 10 months of age showed pronounced hypotonia. The head circumference was in the third percentile (44 cm). The liver was enlarged to 4 cm below the right costal margin. At 13 months of age she was readmitted to the hospital with similar symptoms. She was listless and vomited intermittently. Her condition rapidly deteriorated, and she became comatous when given a high-protein diet. Hypertonia, multifocal clonic twitching of the extremities, and swelling of the optic disks developed. She failed to recognize her parents or to focus or follow visually. She improved on intravenous fluid therapy, but the symptoms recurred when oral feeding was started again.

The blood ammonia concentration increased to 430 and 730 μg per 100 ml on two occasions (normal <60). The SGOT level was only mildly elevated, to 100 Sigma-Frankel units, and BSP (Bromsulphalein) retention was 1 percent in 45 min. Repeated blood urea estimations were between 18 and 21 mg per 100 ml. Amino acid analyses showed that glutamine was increased in blood and urine, and lysine was slightly increased in blood. Pneumoencephalography showed mild to moderate generalized ventricular dilatation.

The patient was then started on a low-protein diet (1.5 gm per kg per day) and was given neomycin orally. Clinical improvement paralleled the falling ammonia levels. Vision and recognition of parents returned after 1 month of treatment, but swelling of the optic disks persisted for 6 weeks. Since there was no elevation of the intracranial pressure, the optic swelling was attributed to optic neuritis rather than to papilledema. While the patient was receiving this dietary therapy, the liver returned to normal size and liver function tests were normal. The electroencephalogram (EEG) showed a relatively normal pattern within 1 month of starting treatment.

Shortly after an elective open biopsy of the liver at 18 months of age, the patient deteriorated rapidly, with vomiting, coma, respiratory depression, convulsions, and increase in blood ammonia (1,000 μg per 100 ml). Only temporary improvement was gained by peritoneal dialysis [63].

Patient 5. This girl was asymptomatic, with normal growth and development, until 3½ years of age [64]. She then showed progressive intermittent behavioral changes, such as crying, screaming, nightmares, and aggressiveness. There were periods of lethargy, vomiting, abdominal pain, and inappropriate speech. Intellectual function was in the low-normal range, and there was evidence of a visual-perceptual disturbance. By age 4 she had hepatomegaly and bilateral slowing on the EEG; gait disturbance and ataxia later developed. During the next 1½ years she was hospitalized four times; each time she had behavioral changes, vomiting, ataxia, lethargy (often progressing to coma), and hepatomegaly. Intermittent elevations of blood ammonia concentrations to 1,200 μg per 100 ml, of SGOT to 2,200 units, of SGPT to 2,600 units, and of lactic dehydrogenase (LDH) to 2,500 units, and depression of prothrombin time to 52 percent were observed and were correlated with her protein intake. During one comatous episode the ammonia concentration was 550 μg per 100 ml in blood, and 166 μg per 100 ml in CSF. Limitation of protein intake during each of her episodic attacks resulted in a significant decrease in blood ammonia concentration and clinical improvement. At age 5½ her weight, height, and bone age were those of a 3½-year-old child. She had right hemiparesis and bilateral Babinski signs. The EEG continued to show bilateral slowing. Intellectual function was in the low-normal range, with evidence of a visual-perceptual disturbance.

A laparotomy was performed while she was on a diet containing 0.5 gm protein per kg per day. The microscopic examination of the liver showed it to be normal except for a slight increase in glycogen content. The patient recovered from the operation.

Patient 6. Recently Levin et al. [65] reported the sixth family with hyperammonemia in which both mother and child were investigated. The child (Patient 6) was breast-fed for 3 weeks and then given cow's milk. She then began to vomit after each feeding. By 3½ months of age she was vomiting persistently, and renal tubular acidosis was suspected because the plasma bicarbonate was 18 mEq per liter when the corresponding urine was pH 9. A diagnostic oral ammonium chloride loading test was performed. After 2 days of receiving ammonium chloride medication the patient refused feedings and became drowsy, hypotonic, and mildly dehydrated. The liver became enlarged to 4 cm below the costal margin. Twelve hours later the patient collapsed and became comatose, had myoclonic convulsions with episodes of apnea, and was found to have multifocal EEG abnormalities. Symptoms improved in 3 days, but recurred when milk feeding was reintroduced. Ammonia levels were high in both fasting (865 μg per 100 ml) and postprandial blood (1,240 μg per 100 ml). The level in the CSF was 435 μg per 100 ml. The liver became enlarged during these episodic bouts of unconsciousness and convulsions and decreased in size during recovery. At 5 months of age the histologic findings from a biopsy of the liver were normal.

At 8 months of age the infant had residual spasticity of the lower limbs and lay in an opisthotonic position with clenched hands. There was evidence of gross brain damage. Growth was retarded; there had been no increase in height or head circumference since 5 months of age. A brain biopsy was performed. The brain was greatly reduced in size and showed "virtual disintegration of the cerebral cortex with proliferation of astrocytes and lipophages."

The mother of this child was found to have reduced OCT activity in the liver (Table 17-4). She was 23 years of age and mentally and physically normal. The only complaint was aversion to protein foods; ingestion of these foods

Table 17-4. LIVER UREA CYCLE ENZYMES IN HYPERAMMONEMIA TYPE II

Enzymes	Levin [27, 65, 67]						Hopkins et al. [51]		Sunshine et al. [64]		Corbeel et al. [66]	
	Controls	Patient 1	Patient 2	Patient 6	Mother of Patient 6	Patient 8	Control	Patient 4	Controls	Patient 5	Controls	Patient 7
Method of obtaining material	Biopsy and necropsy	Biopsy	Necropsy	Biopsy	Biopsy	Biopsy	Necropsy	Biopsy	Biopsy	Biopsy	Not stated	Biopsy
No. of studies		1	1	1	1	1	1	1	3	1	12	1
CPS	320 (182–615)	112	199	152	153	250	448	159	540–1,250	535	7.8–28.8	4.14
OCT at pH 8	5,787 (3,900–9,090)	250	370	1,051	2,288	4,332	6,550	249	29,000–50,000	2,320	105–131	38.7
OCT at pH 7	5,183 (3,950–6,650)			432	415	1,228						
ASA synthetase	37	21	44	37	41	37	33	18	58–62	62		
ASase	177	100	178	122	190	177	144	87	115–202	178	21–50	34.3
Arginase	38,400 (24,600–56,380)	9,000	16,480	45,100	56,300	38,420	12,000	15,350	48,000–82,000	54,000	2,610–6,134	9,060

Note: All investigators measured enzyme activity in micromoles per gram wet weight per hour, except that Sunshine et al. used micromoles per gram of protein per hour. The method used by all was modified from that of Brown and Cohen [1].
CPS, carbamylphosphate synthetase; OCT, ornithine carbamyl transferase; ASA, argininosuccinic acid.

caused lethargy and sometimes induced vomiting. Her usual protein intake was less than 0.5 gm per kg per day. The fasting plasma ammonia level was 116 μg per 100 ml, and there was a rise to 209 μg per 100 ml 2 hr after a protein feeding [65].

Patient 7. Reported by Corbeel et al. [66], Patient 7 began to have episodes of vomiting at the age of 14 days and was hospitalized at 1 month of age because she could not be awakened. The only abnormal findings were a diffuse slow-wave pattern on the EEG and a slight increase in urinary amino acids shown on paper chromatography. The patient remained in a coma for 48 hr and recovered with intravenous fluid therapy. Following discharge from the hospital her development was slow. Vomiting recurred repeatedly and was associated with lethargy and refusal of food: these episodes increased in frequency after the age of 1 year. She was again admitted to the hospital at 18 months of age because of failure to thrive and mild mental retardation. Her height and weight were in the 25th percentile. She was hypotonic and slightly microcephalic; the head circumference was 43 cm. On the eighth day of hospitalization vomiting increased suddenly, and the patient went into a coma. The liver became slightly enlarged. Blood ammonia concentration was 300 μg per 100 ml (normal range, up to 120 μg per 100 ml), and the SGOT was increased to 176 units. She was treated with intravenous fluids and after 24 hr she returned to consciousness; at that time the blood ammonia level decreased to normal. She was put on a low-protein diet and did well on this over the next 9 months. Mental retardation, however, was not improved.

Patient 8. This boy was recently described as having a variant type of OCT deficiency [67]. The clinical features, while relatively mild, were clearly those of protein intolerance and ammonia intoxication. The boy began to have occasional vomiting at 6 months of age and ceased to gain weight. When admitted to the hospital at 6½ months of age he had slowly developed drowsiness and had become feverish. The liver was found to be enlarged. Immediately after a lumbar puncture the patient collapsed, became comatose, and had convulsions. He remained in this condition for more than 36 hr. The fontanel was tense and bulging, and the EEG was grossly abnormal. An air ventriculogram showed no abnormality. His condition began to improve shortly after intravenous glucose infusion, and consciousness returned within 24 hr. More than 48 hr after the infusion the plasma ammonia concentration was 182 μg per 100 ml. A diagnosis of an enzyme defect in the urea cycle was then made by liver biopsy. A low-protein diet was begun and the infant became normal within a few days except for persisting enlargement of the liver, which gradually returned to normal during the next 4 weeks. All subsequent electroencephalograms have been normal. The patient has done well on a diet containing about 2 gm protein per kg per day. At 2 years of age his growth and development were normal.

Summary of Clinical Findings

A summary of the findings is presented in Table 17-5. Patients usually have a history of intolerance to formula feeding or protein food. In the severe cases recurrent vomiting and irritability begin in the early weeks of life and may progress to lethargy, coma, and seizures. During these episodes patients develop muscular rigidity, opisthotonos, and hepatomegaly and have marked hyperammonemia and abnormal liver function. The EEG is often abnormal, showing diffuse slow-wave patterns or multifocal abnormalities indi-

Table 17-5. SOME CLINICAL FEATURES OF CONGENITAL HYPERAMMONEMIA TYPE II*

Patient's No.	Ref.	Sex	Age at onset of symptoms	Slow development	Seizures	Abnormal EEG	Hepatomegaly	SGOT	Other findings
1	[62]	F	5 wk†	+	0	+	−	−	Cerebral atrophy
2	[62]	F	3 yr†	+	0	+	−	−	Cerebral atrophy
3	[27]	F	9 yr	0	0	−	−	−	−
4	[51]	F	7 mo†	+	+	+	+	↑	Hypotonia Dilated ventricles Optic disk swelling
5	[64]	F	3½ yr	Low normal	0	+	+	↑	Hemiparesis
6	[65]	F	3 wk	+	+	+	+	↑	Spasticity and opisthotonos
7	[66]	F	14 days	+	0	+	+	↑	Microcephaly
8	[67]	M	6 mo	0	+	+	+	↑	−

* Features in addition to episodic vomiting, irritability, and lethargy, which are present in all patients.
† Died.
Note: + = present; 0 = absent; − = not mentioned; ↑ = elevated.

cating diffuse metabolic disturbances of the brain. This metabolic imbalance can be precipitated by infection or by subjecting the patient to anesthesia and surgery. With intravenous fluid infusion these symptoms and signs return to normal. Mental retardation is common and may be associated with dilatation of the ventricles and microcephaly.

The onset of symptoms may be as late as 9 years of age. Patients with the milder form have only intolerance to protein food and after eating may complain of headache or lethargy. They stay on a self-regulated low-protein diet and are mentally normal.

Biochemical Findings and Enzyme Defects

There is no consistent abnormality of the amino acids in the blood, urine, or CSF except for a very high glutamine content. The increased glutamine content is attributable to increased synthesis secondary to hyperammonemia, which is usually of severe degree. The blood ammonia level may be over 1,000 μg per 100 ml during the episodic attacks. The level in the CSF is correspondingly increased. Blood ornithine levels are notably within normal limits. The blood urea nitrogen concentrations were normal in all cases. Ketoacidosis has not been observed in this type of hyperammonemia.

One might expect to find a high ornithine level in body fluid in this disorder, and it is surprising that the plasma ornithine concentration is not elevated. There is a type of defect, however, in which blood ornithine level is greatly increased (see below).

Of the six instances (Patients 1, 2, 3, 6, 7, 8) in which excretion of metabolites of the pyrimidine pathway was looked for, urinary orotic acid and uracil were found to be greatly increased in five. Uridine excretion was increased in four instances (Patients 1, 2, 6, 8). Patient 7 had only orotic aciduria. In Patient 8, the presence of uracil in the urine was the clue leading to the investigation of the urea cycle enzymes.

Orotic acid may form crystals in the urine. The amount of these metabolites decreased when the protein intake was lowered. The reason for the presence of the intermediate metabolites in the pyrimidine biosynthesis pathway is not known. CP, the product of the first enzymatic step in the urea cycle, is also involved in pyrimidine synthesis (Fig. 17-2). One might speculate that the block in the urea cycle may have shunted this compound to the latter pathway.

The blood ammonia levels of normal individuals are not affected by protein ingestion, and they rise slightly with ammonia loading. Significant and prolonged elevations of blood ammonia level have been observed in patients with hyperammonemia II after a protein meal or a loading test with ammonium chloride. Oral alanine loading in one patient resulted in a similar rise in blood ammonia. The simultaneous administration of arginine did not abolish this hyperammonemic response as it does in patients with familial protein intolerance [67]. Moreover, arginine infusion in one patient with hyperammonemia Type II [66] led to prolonged elevations of blood ammonia levels; this is contrary to the previous finding of arginine protection in ammonia intoxication [68, 69].

The OCT activity of the liver was virtually absent (less than 5 percent of normal) in four patients (Patients 1, 2, 4, and 5). In Patient 6 the enzyme deficiency was milder (25 percent residual activity), and her mother, who also had hyperammonemia, had 50 percent of normal activity in a liver biopsy. The activity of CP synthetase tends to be lower in these patients than in controls.

Levin et al. [67] have measured OCT activity in the liver homogenate of Patient 8 at pH 8 and pH 7 and found a significant reduction of OCT at pH 7 in comparison with the controls. They thus postulated that this patient represents a variant type of OCT deficiency. The significance of this observation awaits further studies in other patients and further investigation into the properties of the enzyme.

Intestinal mucosa has OCT activity [18]. The jejunal mucosa can be more easily biopsied for diagnostic enzyme studies than can liver. Reduced OCT activity in intestinal mucosa has been shown in a patient (Patient 1) with liver OCT deficiency and in the mother of Patient 2 [62].

OCT activity in the normal serum is either absent or very low, and its measurement is not useful in the diagnosis of OCT deficiency. The finding of an elevated OCT activity in serum usually accompanies hepatocellular injury and suggests that OCT is present in the liver.

Diagnosis

As in hyperammonemia Type I, paper chromatography for routine amino acid screening is not useful in diagnosing this disorder. The finding of high glutamine content in blood or urine should arouse the suspicion of hyperammonemia. Measurement of blood ammonia is recommended for any patient with a history suggestive of protein intolerance. Orotic acid and other pyrimidine metabolites in the urine would be another indication to measure blood ammonia.

The prognosis of these patients is poor. Three of the eight patients have died. Early diagnosis and early treatment are therefore of great importance.

Genetics

The occurrence of OCT deficiency in eight patients in six families indicates that this disease is inherited. In one family both twins and their first cousin were affected.

Studies concerning ammonia metabolism were carried out in five mothers and three fathers. Three mothers who had a history of aversion to protein food and high fasting blood ammonia levels had abnormal ammonia tolerance tests. In one family the child (Patient 6) had 25 percent and her mother approximately 50 percent of mean normal activity of OCT by liver biopsy. The mother of Patients 2 and 3 had an intestinal biopsy which showed marked OCT deficiency. Results of investigations in the fathers, including fasting blood ammonia levels [62, 66], ammonia tolerance test [62], and liver urea cycle enzyme study [65], were all normal.

The results of these studies indicate that the mother but not the father showed both clinical and biochemical abnormalities. It is also worth noting that all reported patients with OCT deficiency, except the one with the possible variant type (Patient 8), are female. Thus OCT deficiency may be sex-limited, at least in its expression.

The mode of inheritance of this disorder will become apparent when more cases and families are studied.

CITRULLINEMIA

Citrullinemia is a metabolic disorder characterized by mental retardation, marked accumulation of citrulline in the blood, CSF, and urine, and by elevation of the blood ammonia concentration in the postabsorptive state. To date there are only two known patients with this disorder. A metabolic block at the conversion of citrulline to ASA mediated by ASA synthetase has been demonstrated.

Clinical Features

The first reported patient [52, 70], a boy, was the product of a normal pregnancy and delivery. The parents were first cousins. Early growth and development seemed normal. The boy sat alone at 6 months, and at 9 months crawled and began to imitate sounds. At 9 months he began to have attacks of vomiting but continued to gain weight normally. At 13 months he was hospitalized in an alkalotic, semicomatose condition following a severe bout of vomiting. Generalized convulsions developed while he was in the hospital. The electroencephalogram was diffusely abnormal. The CSF was normal. Radiologic examination of the skull revealed separation of the suture lines. The child improved slowly and was discharged from the hospital.

During the next 5 months, hospitalization was required on two occasions because of vomiting and developmental regression. The child became irritable, limp, and unable to raise his head without difficulty or to sit up. He no longer paid attention to his environment and was obviously severely retarded. He was hospitalized again at age 18 months and appeared quite ill, irritable, and dehydrated. There was evidence of a recent marked weight loss. The liver was enlarged. There was a coarse Parkinsonian tremor of head and hands, hyperactive deep-tendon reflexes, equivocal plantar responses, and hypotonia. Abnormal tests included a cephalin flocculation of 3+, a serum protein-bound iodine level of 3.8 μg per 100 ml, and a ^{131}I uptake of 14 percent rising to 28 percent after ACTH stimulation. The SGOT was normal. The electroencephalogram was grossly abnormal, with low-voltage slow waves. A skull roentgenogram was normal. A pneumoencephalogram showed generalized cortical atrophy.

The patient was treated with desiccated thyroid and improved considerably. He became more alert, and vomiting decreased. Later, at 27 months of age, his protein intake was moderately restricted to 1 gm per lb per day. There was no further improvement in his condition except that vomiting ceased. The bone age was 9 months at a chronological age of 20 months. When he was 2⅓ years of age his IQ measured less than 20. His fasting blood ammonia concentration was twice normal and rose significantly after a protein meal, reaching 1,020 μg per 100 ml. No further attacks of vomiting or convulsions have been observed, and he has been more responsive and less irritable.

Patient 2 [71] was a girl born out of wedlock with a history similar to that of the first patient. Recurrent vomiting began at 4½ months of age. She became less interested in her surroundings, and her growth became retarded. Changing her formula at 6 months of age from a high-protein mixture to a different high-protein soy preparation resulted in some temporary relief of symptoms. Vomiting then resumed and persisted until hospitalization. Hospital admission at 8 months was occasioned by hematemesis, hematuria, purpura, and melena. She was an irritable child, with weight and height in the 10th percentile. The head circumference was below the 10th percentile. A grand mal seizure in the hospital resulted in temporary right hemiparesis and a permanent tremor of the right arm. A diagnosis of citrullinemia was established. Since then the child has been maintained on a low-protein diet of 1.1 to 1.5 gm per kg per day. She is greatly improved but is still moderately retarded at 21 months of age. At this age she walks unsteadily and her vocabulary consists of four words. Her performance on the Cattell Intelligence Scale was at approximately the 8½-month level. The Vineland Social Maturity Scale placed her at the 12-month level.

Initial abnormal laboratory tests indicated an elevated SGOT level of 1,280 Sigma-Frankel units, a plasma BUN concentration of 6 mg per 100 ml, and a PTC (plasma thromboplastin component) deficiency. These findings, indicative of hepatic dysfunction, improved on the low-protein diet. This suggests that the abnormal liver function might be related to ammonia intoxication. Radiologic examination of the bones showed severe osteoporosis.

The fasting blood ammonia nitrogen concentration obtained on admission of the child to the hospital was 87 μg per 100 ml, i.e., in the upper-normal range. The postprandial rise in blood ammonia level to 260 μg per 100 ml when the patient's diet contained 2.9 gm protein per kg per day was much less severe than in McMurray's patient [52]. The hyperammonemic response was even less when the protein intake was restricted. The CSF ammonia concentrations were less than 40 μg per 100 ml during protein restriction.

Trials of triiodothyronine, arginine, pyridoxine, and neomycin administration had no effect on the clinical condition or the biochemical findings.

Biochemical Investigations

Identification and Quantitation of Citrulline in Urine, Plasma, and Cerebrospinal Fluid

Citrulline was first detected in the urine of Patient 1 at age 18 months by means of paper chromatography, and the identity of the urinary amino acid was confirmed by chemical analysis after isolation of this compound. The 24-hr excretion of citrulline is between 1 and 2 gm in both patients. Normal persons excrete less than 1 mg per day. The excretion of some of the neutral and acidic amino acids by Patient 1 was slightly elevated, but this elevation was insignificant when compared with the massive increase in citrulline in the urine. Citrulline is believed to share the same renal transport system as the neutral amino acids [72], and the small increase in excretion of other amino acids can be adequately explained by competition for the pathway which mediates transport in the proximal tubule of the kidney.

In both patients the plasma level of citrulline was greatly increased, to 20 to 30 mg per 100 ml, a figure at least 40 times normal. The plasma concentrations of all amino acids other than citrulline were normal or near normal.

The citrulline concentration in cerebrospinal fluid is also markedly increased, ranging between 2 to 6 mg per 100 ml (normal = less than 0.05 mg per 100 ml). The citrulline levels in the CSF have been lower than that in the blood. This is in contrast to argininosuccinic aciduria, in which the ASA in the cerebrospinal fluid is greater than that in the blood. It is not yet clear whether the increase in CSF is merely a reflection of the increased plasma concentration or whether citrulline is accumulated in the brain as a result of a deficiency of ASA synthetase activity in the brain as well as in the liver.

The citrulline and urea levels in the blood and urine are correlated with the protein intake. As expected, a low-protein diet lowered the excretion of citrulline and urea and a high protein diet increased it.

Studies of Urea Synthesis

Morrow et al. [71] investigated urea synthesis in their patient (Patient 2) by means of a nitrogen balance study. The urea excretion was approximately 20 percent of the total nitrogen excretion when the patient was on a diet containing 1.5 gm protein per kg per day, and it increased to 44 percent when the protein intake was increased to 2.9 gm per kg per day. They commented that most of the increase in urea excretion was of dietary origin and suggested that the block in the urea cycle was quite severe. On the other hand McMurray et al. [44] investigated the fate of citrulline-ureido ^{14}C that had been injected intravenously into Patient 1. Roughly one-half the total was recovered in the urine; only 11 percent of the citrulline that had been injected was excreted unchanged in the urine, while 31 percent had been metabolized to urea during the first 24 hr. These findings indicate that the block in the urea cycle of this patient was incomplete.

It was found that in the postprandial state, the blood ammonia concentration in Patient 1 rose dramatically to values of the order of 1,000 μg per 100 ml, a value comparable to those in the cases of hyperammonemia Types I and II and exceeding the values found in hepatic coma [37]. This dramatic finding suggests a lack of a reserve capacity for removal of ammonia from the blood both in citrullinemia and in hyperammonemia. Although the blood urea is "normal" and substantial amounts of urea are produced, it appears that the removal of ammonia is not adequate. This is reflected in the elevated blood ammonia concentration after protein loading.

The Enzyme Defect

The primary biochemical defect in citrullinemia is in the synthesis of ASA (step 3). Deficiency of hepatic ASA synthetase activity in the first patient (Table 17-6) was demonstrated by McMurray et al. [44]. Tedesco and Mellman [25] found an altered enzyme in the extract of fibroblasts cultured from the skin of Patient 2; the K_m for ASA synthetase of the patient (between 10 and 100 $\times 10^{-3}M$) was at least 25 times normal ($4 \times 10^{-4}M$). In the presence of excess citrulline concentration of 10 mmoles, ASA synthesis in the cell extract of the patient was similar to that of the controls, ranging from 0.01 to 0.03 μmole urea formed per hour per 10^6 cells.

Diagnosis

Citrullinemia can be diagnosed by the detection of a ninhydrin-positive spot in the position of citrulline by paper chromatography or by high-voltage paper electrophoresis, in the absence of any other amino aciduria. The identity of the spot as citrulline is confirmed by dipping the paper in Ehrlich's aldehyde reagent (*p*-dimethylaminobenzaldehyde 10 percent w/v in concentrated HCl, diluted 1:4 with acetone just before use). This reagent gives a bright yellow or pink color with citrulline and will stain over ninhydrin.

One must be careful not to confuse citrulline with homocitrulline. Homocitrulline is commonly found in the urine of infants and small children who are fed sterilized cow's milk or evaporated milk [73]. Gerritsen et al. showed that homocitrulline is produced from lysine during sterilization or preparation of canned formulas [74].

Homocitrulline occupies a different position on the chromatogram from citrulline. Since it has an additional CH_2 group, the R_f in butanol-acetic acid-water, butanol-pyridine-water, lutidine-water, and in most other chromatographic solvents is higher than that of citrulline. Homocitrulline also stains with Ehrlich's aldehyde reagent. The diagnosis of citrullinemia must not be made in an infant or small child unless the spot on the chromatogram is in the same position as that of authentic citrulline. The diagnosis can be confirmed on an amino acid analyzer; the citrulline peak is far removed from that of homocitrulline when examined by column chromatography [75].

A Case of Citrullinuria Associated with Other Amino Acidurias

A possible third case of citrullinemia has been reported by Visakorpi [76, 77]. The patient developed normally until age 3 years, after which time mental development ceased. At age 10 he was placed in an institution for the mentally retarded. At age 16 he began to have periods of unconsciousness. His IQ at that time measured 32. At age 18 he died in status epilepticus. Necropsy revealed cerebral edema and fatty infiltration of the liver. A urinary amino acid chromatogram at age 15 revealed a large spot in the position of citrulline which stained with ninhydrin and Ehrlich's reagent. The excretion of citrulline measured approximately 500 mg per 24 hr as estimated by elution of the spot and ninhydrin color determinations. This is only about one-quarter of the amount of citrulline excreted by McMurray's patient. Plasma citrulline was not measured.

The interpretation of this finding is confusing because the patient had, in addition to citrulline, large amounts of cystine, lysine, arginine, and ornithine in the urine; this is the pattern typical of cystinuria. Milne et al. have shown that in cystinuria there is incomplete and slow absorption of the

Table 17-6. LIVER UREA CYCLE ENZYME ACTIVITY IN CITRULLINEMIA AND ARGININOSUCCINIC ACIDURIA, μMOLES/GM WET WEIGHT/HR

Enzymes	*Citrullinemia (McMurray [44])*		*Argininosuccinic aciduria*					
			Miller and McLean [91]		*Solitare et al. [95]*		*Levin [125]*	
	Controls	Patient	Controls	Patient	Controls	Patient	Controls	Patient
Means of obtaining material	Necropsy	Biopsy	Necropsy	Necropsy	Necropsy	Necropsy	Biopsy	Biopsy
No. of studies	2	1	5	1	3	1	3	1
Method	Schimke*	Schimke*	Modified Brown and Cohen†	Modified Brown and Cohen†	Modified Schimke*	Modified Schimke*	Modified Brown and Cohen†	Modified Brown and Cohen†
CPS	65; 151	82	156 ± 29	195	299; 301; 81	52	209–615	222
OCT	4,200; 5,000	5,500	4,388 ± 537	3,295	6,825; 3,560; 3,280	3,600	4,050–6,650	9,720
ASA synthetase	17; 35	1.4	75 ± 9	87	117; 93; 46	42	41–44	122
ASase	256; 422	290	276 ± 39	<13	216; 252; 98	32	177	0
Arginase	24,000; 21,000	59,000	33,600 ± 7,535	20,600	51,700; 38,000; 15,000	12,000	28,500–30,000	24,600

* Reference [15].
† Reference [1].
Note: CPS, carbamylphosphate synthetase; OCT, ornithine carbamyl transferase; ASA, argininosuccinic acid.

dibasic amino acids from the intestine [78, 79]. *Streptococcus faecalis* is a potent source of arginine desiminase [80], and this enzyme is capable of producing considerable amounts of citrulline from arginine, particularly in the presence of constipation, which is common in institutionalized mentally retarded patients [79]. Citrulline can then be absorbed from the colon and excreted in the urine. The amount of citrulline excreted by Visakorpi's patient was considerably higher than that usually found in cystinuria, but the question of whether the citrullinuria was the result of bacterial action in the intestine or of a metabolic block could have been answered only by enzyme studies or by sterilization of the intestine and subsequent determination of urinary citrulline. McMurray's patient did not have cystinuria, and, as predicted by Milne [79], sterilization of the intestine produced no change in plasma citrulline [52, 81]. The case is instructive in that it points out that caution must be exercised in the interpretation of citrulline excretion in the urine in the presence of cystinuria or any other amino aciduria of which arginine is a component, particularly if urinary tract infection is present. If there is any doubt about the diagnosis, it should be determined that the citrullinemia and citrullinuria persist after sterilization of the intestine.

Genetics

Citrullinemia is probably a recessively inherited disorder. Two patients with citrullinemia from two families are known. The parents of Patient 1 were first cousins, and those of Patient 2 were supposedly unrelated. Both the father and the mother of Patient 2 have normal plasma citrulline levels of 0.61 and 0.73 mg per 100 ml, respectively, and low-normal plasma arginine levels of 0.46 and 0.27 mg per 100 ml, respectively [71].

ARGININOSUCCINIC ACIDURIA

Argininosuccinic aciduria, a rare, hereditary disease, is characterized clinically by mental retardation, seizures, intermittent ataxia, hepatomegaly, and accumulation of large amounts of argininosuccinic acid in the blood, urine, and CSF. This amino acid is usually present in higher concentrations in the CSF than in the blood. This disorder is frequently associated with friable, tufted hair, known as *trichorrhexis nodosa* (Figs. 17-4, 17-5). A total of 22 patients are now known; their clinical and biochemical findings are summarized in Table 17-7.

Analysis of the symptoms and the mode of onset of this disease in 22 patients show that it may be divided into two types:* (1) Late-onset type. Slow development, seizure, and intermittent ataxia usually become noticeable in the second year of life. (2) Early-onset type. Failure to thrive, recurrent vomiting and coma, and hepatomegaly in the early months of life are characteristic. The course is malignant and usually results in early death. Absence or reduced activity of the argininosuccinic acid cleavage enzyme (step 4 in Fig. 1) has been demonstrated in the brain, liver, kidney, red blood cells, and cultured fibroblasts.

Clinical Features

The Late-onset Type

Neurologic abnormalities are the main features of the patients in this group. There may be a history of irritability in infancy and feeding difficulties. Delayed psychomotor development is usually evident until the second year of life. Seizures (in 6 of 15 patients), abnormal EEG (in 9 of 15), and intermittent ataxia (in 6 of 15) are not infrequent. The histories of the first two reported patients [82] are representative of this type: A $3\frac{5}{12}$-year-old girl, who was normal in the neonatal period, had a moderate amount of vomiting in the first few months of life. There was no delay in reaching the early developmental milestones, but speech was retarded. She had several convulsions over a 1-week period around $2\frac{8}{12}$ years of age, without a known precipitating cause. This was followed by unsteadiness in hand movement for about 2 weeks. At age $3\frac{5}{12}$ more seizures were followed by ataxia and incoordination resembling chorea, so severe that the child could not stand up or feed herself. These symptoms lasted for a few days. An older brother had a similar history of delayed speech development, but he had no seizures or ataxia. Physical findings in both children were normal except for obvious mental retardation, "rough skin," and abnormal hair. The hair was light brown, dry, and friable. Its growth seemed to be irregular, giving a tufted, almost matted appearance. The ends were frayed and seemed to break off easily. Both sibs had a heart murmur, presumably caused by ventricular septal defects. Abnormal laboratory test results included an elevated serum alkaline phosphatase level and an abnormal EEG.

Patients in this late-onset group have been identified primarily by amino acid screening among children with convulsive disorders or mental retardation. It is therefore not surprising to find that all but one have been mentally retarded (IQ: 20 to 75). Since data on the amino acid-excretion patterns in apparently normal persons are lacking, the true incidence of mental retardation in patients with argininosuccinic aciduria cannot be assessed. Of particular interest is the family history reported briefly by Carson and Neill [84]. There was no history of mental retardation or neurologic disease in this family except for the index patient and her sibs. The index patient (Patient 4), one of seven sibs, was mentally retarded and unsteady but had normal hair. Examination of the urine of the parents and the sibs disclosed normal amino acid excretory patterns except for one sister. This sister had borderline normal intelligence (IQ: 92), normal hair, and excreted argininosuccinic acid. Cerebellar signs or cranial nerve palsies or both were found in

*See Ref. 136 for late-arriving data modifying these categories.

Table 17-7. SUMMARY OF CLINICAL FEATURES IN ARGININOSUCCINIC ACIDURIA

Patient's No.	Ref.	Sex	Age at diagnosis, yr.	IQ	Seizures	Abnormal EEG	Ataxia	Hepatomegaly	Abnormal liver function	Abnormal hair	Other findings	Postprandial blood ammonia
1	[82]	F	$3\frac{6}{12}$	32	+	+	+	0	Alkaline phosphatase	+	Heart murmur, ventricular septal defect	–
2	[82]	M	$6\frac{3}{12}$	50	0	+	0	0	Alkaline phosphatase	+	Heart murmur	–
3	[82]	M	23 (days)	Retarded	+	0	0	+	Alkaline phosphatase	+	Edema of feet and ankles; dry, rough skin	–
4	[84]	F	2	51	0	0	+	0	–	0	0	–
5	[84]	F	4	92	0	0	0	0	–	+	0	–
6	[85]	F	$6\frac{3}{12}$	20	+	0	–	0	N	0	Pyramidal tract signs	–
7	[85]	M	$1\frac{9}{12}$	75	0	0	0	0	–	0	Hypotonicity; strabismus	–
8	[86]	F	2	40	+	+	0(?)	+	–	+	47 chromosomes; poor coordination; hyperactivity	–
9	[87]	F	18	45	0	–	0	0	–	0	Poor coordination; hyperactivity	–
10	[87]	F	15	67	0	–	0	0	–	0	0	–
11	[88]	F	$\frac{9}{12}$	Approx. 60	+	0	0	+	SGOT	+	0	↑
12	[89]	F	8	30–50	0	+	+	0	Alkaline phosphatase	+	Small stature	↑
13	[90]	M	15	30–40	+	+	+	0	SGOT	0	0	↑
14	[90]	M	$3\frac{6}{12}$	40–50	–	0	0	0	N	0	0	↑
15	[91]	M	16	Retarded	+	+	+	0	Alkaline phosphatase	+	Partial deafness	–
16	[92]	F	$7\frac{6}{12}$	40–50	+	+	+	0	–	0	Wide-base gait; skeletal anomalies; trivial aortic stenosis	–
17	[93]	M	5 (days)	?	+	–	–	+	SGOT	–	0	–
18	[94]	F	20	57	+	+	0	0	N	+	Hypoparathyroidism; prematurity	↑
19	[94]	F	8	Retarded	+	+	0	0	N	+	Hyperactivity	↑
20	[95]	F	$\frac{8}{12}$	Retarded	+	–	–	+	Alkaline phosphatase SGOT	+	Patent foramen; annular pancreas	↑
21	[96]	F	4 (days)	?	+	–	–	0	–	–	Respiratory distress; hypotonia	–
22	[97]	F	6 (wk)*	N	–			–	N	–	Tachypnea	↑

* = detected by routine newborn screening [105].
Note: + = present; 0 = absent; – = not mentioned; N = normal; ↑ = elevated.

four other sibs, two of whom were mentally retarded, but none excreted argininosuccinic acid. In this particular family the neurologic abnormalities did not correlate with the excretion of ASA.

The Early-onset, or Malignant, Type

Of the 22 patients with argininosuccinic aciduria, 6 were of the early-onset type. Vomiting, failure to thrive, hepatomegaly, and seizures are common during early infancy. Two had seizures and respiratory distress and died in the neonatal period. Rapid respiratory rates without good explanation were observed in 2 infants [83, 96]. All were retarded in intellectual development. An illustrative case history follows:

Patient 20. A girl, the product of a normal pregnancy and delivery, was well for the first 5 weeks of life, when a gradually enlarging liver was first observed [95]. The patient was thought to be blind, deaf, and severely retarded in both growth and development. The hair was rather brittle and rubbed off easily. A loud systolic murmur was detected at this time, and an ECG showed right ventricular hypertrophy. A liver biopsy disclosed no significant microscopic abnormalities. The patient sustained a linear skull fracture while in the hospital, but no neurologic abnormality resulted from it. At 7½ months of age she was put on high-protein feedings but ate poorly and exhibited increasing lethargy and fussiness. A generalized tonicoclonic seizure associated with high fever occurred 10 days later. When admitted to the hospital at 8 months of age, the infant was small and poorly nourished, with decerebrate posturing and occasional twitching of all extremities. Head circumference was 38 cm, less than the 3d percentile. A loud blowing systolic murmur was again heard. The liver was enlarged to near the iliac crest; the tip of the spleen could also be palpated. Abnormal laboratory test results included elevated blood ammonia concentration (350 μg per 100 ml) and high alkaline phosphatase (350 units) and SGOT levels (248 units). The child died shortly thereafter. The diagnosis of argininosuccinic aciduria was made by paper chromatographic screening of a urine specimen collected the day before death.

Patients 17 and 21. The two newborn infants (Patients 17 and 21) who died of this disease had a rapid downhill course. The infant reported by Baumgartner et al. [93] became lethargic and apathetic, nursed poorly, and had feeble reflexes soon after birth, when feeding began. When she was 4 days old, generalized seizures, increasing respiratory distress, and progressive somnolence appeared. The infant died on the eighth day of life. Carton et al. [96] described two sisters who died after a similar course of respiratory distress and seizures in the neonatal period. An amino acid study was performed on one of them, and argininosuccinic aciduria was detected.

Experience with these patients indicates that argininosuccinic aciduria should be considered in the differential diagnosis of neonatal convulsive disorders or in any infant with failure to thrive and hepatomegaly.

Biochemical Investigations and Enzyme Defect

Argininosuccinic acid, which is normally absent from the urine, is excreted by these patients in large quantity. Most of them have excreted several grams a day, and the amount varies with protein intake.

Argininosuccinic acid is present in the blood of patients, ranging from 3.5 to 4.4 mg per 100 ml, except in the two newborns (Patients 17 and 21), who had much higher levels of 10 and 11.4 mg per 100 ml, respectively. In almost all patients the ASA was higher in the cerebrospinal fluid than in the blood except in the two patients who excreted very little ASA in the urine and who had none detectable in the CSF. ASA is a highly polar substance, and its penetration from blood to CSF would be expected to be extremely poor. The presence of ASA in CSF and brain matter [95] indicates that the enzymatic block is present in the brain.

The level of citrulline, the precursor of ASA, was shown to be moderately elevated in the blood, urine, and cerebrospinal fluid.

Postprandial hyperammonemia has been observed. The elevation is not so high as in congenital hyperammonemia or citrullinemia. This may be explained by the fact that the enzymatic block in argininosuccinic aciduria is at least two metabolic steps removed from those involving ammonia directly. A mild elevation of blood glutamine level may be found and is probably related to the high blood ammonia concentration. The blood alanine concentration was greatly increased in a newborn patient [93] and mildly increased on occasion in an older patient [90]. This is unexplained. Hyperalaninemia has been observed in pyruvate decarboxylase deficiency [98]. The blood pyruvate level was not measured in these argininosuccinic aciduric patients with hyperalaninemia.

Decreased ammonia tolerance was shown in one patient by an oral ammonia loading test [90]. The peripheral venous ammonia level rose rapidly and returned to near normal in 3 hr, a pattern similar to that seen in patients with liver cirrhosis. The ammonia level in CSF was higher than that in blood at 2 hr. A protein loading test in the same patient [90] resulted in a slower but more persistent rise in ammonia in both blood and CSF.

Alkaline phosphatase and SGOT activities have been elevated in several patients; the activities have fluctuated and have had a positive correlation with blood ammonia levels.

Patients with argininosuccinic aciduria have normal blood urea and excrete substantial amounts of urea in the urine. Urea synthesis from orally administered ^{15}N-labeled ammonium lactate has been studied in a 17-year-old patient with argininosuccinic aciduria [45]. Maximum labeling of the blood urea occurred later and was less than in a control. At the end of the 3-day period the control subject excreted 80 percent of the dose as urea, while the patient excreted only 35 percent. This result correlates with the current thinking that enzyme deficiency is partial and that in the presence of the residual enzyme, urea synthesis proceeds at a significant rate.

Tomlinson and Westall [99] demonstrated the presence of ASase in red blood cells from 54 normal subjects and its absence from the blood cells of 3 patients with argininosuccinic aciduria. This enzyme was not detectable in blood cells in 7 other patients studied (Table 17-8). The ASase activity in red blood cells is in the range of 3.5 ± 1 μmole per gm hemoglobin [99]. Assuming 12 gm hemoglobulin per 100 ml blood, the ASase activity in 1 pint blood is approximately equal to that in 1 gm liver. The contribution of red blood cells to total urea production is therefore negligible.

A marked deficiency of ASase activity in liver (Table 17-6) and in brain (less than 2.7 percent of the mean of the controls, 17.1 ± 7.4 nmoles per mg protein per hour [96, 100]) has been demonstrated. This enzyme in the kidney was studied in two patients and was found to be deficient in one. Interestingly, the rapid fatal courses of these two patients are indistinguishable [96, 101].

Table 17-8. ARGININOSUCCINASE ACTIVITY IN BLOOD CELLS, μMOLES UREA/GM HEMOGLOBIN/HR

Ref.	Case no.	Patient	Father	Mother	Sibs	Normal subjects (N = number)
[82]	1, 2	0; 0	1.6	1.8	1.6; 1.1; 3.0	3.4 ± 1.2 (1.9–6.5) (N = 54)
[83]	3	0	?	?	?	?
[89]	12	0	?	1.3	?	2.2–5.6 (N = 7)
[90]	13, 14	0; 0	2.1	2.1	2.6	3.8 ± 1.1 (2.6–6.9) (N = 17)
[94]	18, 19	0; 0	"Decreased"	"Decreased"	?	?
[96]	21	0	1.4	1.3	1.6	4.2 (N = 1)
[97]	22	0	2.2	1.9	?	3.8 ± 1.1 (2.6–6.9) (N = 17)

Pathology

Pathologic findings in argininosuccinic aciduria are reported in only four cases. In an 8-day-old infant who died with argininosuccinic aciduria the most severe pathologic changes were observed in liver, kidney, myocardium, and brain [93]. Focal necrosis in several organs was similar to that in many toxic conditions. Multiple necrotic foci were especially prominent in the liver parenchyma. Degenerative alterations, including multiple tubular casts, were seen in the kidney. The myocardium also displayed extensive necrosis. Spongy alteration of the white and gray matter of the brain was found, as well as a deficiency in myelinization and degeneration of the myelin sheaths. The histologic findings suggest a process that began in fetal life.

Pathologic examination of the patient who died on the sixth day of life [96] revealed a diffuse bilateral pneumonia, anoxemic subepicardial, subpleural, and subarachnoidal bleeding, and depletion of thymocytes from the thymus. Microscopic examination of the brain showed only a discrete congestion.

Another patient, who died at 8 months of age [95], had a patent foramen ovale and acute focal bronchopneumonia. The enlarged liver was not accompanied by any significant microscopic abnormality other than vascular congestion and foci of acute pericentral necrosis. The spleen was acutely congested. The brain weighed approximately 840 gm. The principal neuropathologic changes consisted of extensive regions in which myelin had not been formed and a prominent degree of astrocytic nuclear swelling with numerous astrocytes of Alzheimer's type II, particularly among the neurons of the basal ganglia, pontine nuclei, and Purkinje's cell layer of the cerebellar cortex.

There is no anatomic basis for liver enlargement in the severe form of argininosuccinic aciduria. A liver biopsy in the two patients who had an enlarged liver showed no significant microscopic abnormalities [86, 95].

In a fourth patient, who died at age 16 [102], the general pathologic condition was not remarkable except that the liver was enlarged, with increased fat deposition. The brain was swollen, with flattening of gyri and narrowing of sulci. Atypical astrocytic nuclei, resembling Alzheimer's type II cells, were found in the cerebral cortex, basal ganglia, and dentate nucleus.

In summary, the general pathologic status of various organs was nonspecific, and the anatomic basis for the enlarged liver was not evident. Neuropathologic changes are, however, most important. Many Alzheimer type II cells were found in the cerebral cortex, basal ganglia, and cerebellar nuclei of the two older patients (8 months and 16 years of age) but were not found in the two neonates. Alzheimer's type II cell has been seen consistently in both the familial and acquired forms of hepatocerebral degeneration [49]. The common denominator of argininosuccinic aciduria and hepatocerebral degeneration is the increased ammonia content in the blood. The appearance of this type of abnormal astrocytes has also recently been shown to correlate with the plasma ammonia level in experimental rats [103]. One might, therefore, expect to find similar neuropathologic changes in all urea cycle disorders and other types of hyperammonemia.

Spongy degeneration of the brain white matter, as seen in one infant [93], has been described in infants with other amino acid disorders [104] and is apparently a nonspecific change.

Diagnosis

ASA is excreted in massive amounts in the urine even in the absence of clinical symptoms [105]. Accordingly, the disgnosis is readily made by a two-dimensional chromato-electrophoresis commonly used for screening urine for amino aciduria [106]. Paper chromatograms of these specimens often show not one but two or three abnormal spots when the urine is not fresh. This is because of a tendency for ASA to form cyclic anhydrides, particularly in acid solution. The properties of the two anhydrides have been studied by Westall [107], and by Ratner and Kunkemueller [108].

Very little ASA is reabsorbed by the renal tubule. The renal clearance as measured in Patient 2 was 105 ml per min per 1.75 m^2, a value quite comparable to the glomerular filtration rate [109]. The amount of ASA present in the blood may not be obvious on the one-dimensional paper chromatogram prepared from blood-spots [110], commonly used as a screening procedure.

Quantitative measurement of ASA, using an amino acid analyzer, is complicated by the instability of free ASA. It is best to convert the ASA to its anhydrides before analysis. This is done by allowing the solution that contains ASA to stand at room temperature for 48 hr at pH 2 [111] or, better, by boiling the acidified (pH 2) urine for 2½ hours [87]. An anion exchange column chromatographic method described by Ratner and Kunkemueller [108] separates ASA from other amino acids and is a useful method for the identification of ASA and its anhydrides. Alternatively, ASA can be isolated from the urine by precipitation as barium salt for chemical analysis [12, 83, 107].

Quantitative measurement of ASase activity in the red blood cells, as described by Tomlinson and Westall [99], is easy to set up for confirmation of the diagnosis. A simple bacterial auxiotroph assay using filter paper blood spots had been devised by Murphy and Guthrie [112]. This latter test can be used in large-scale screening, particularly of the newborn population. Since this test measures ASase activity, not the accumulation of ASA, it can be performed on cord blood for early detection and early treatment.

Cultured fibroblasts from the skin of normal persons contain ASase, while those derived from the skin of patients (Patients 13, 14, 18, 19, and 22) with argininosuccinic aciduria are deficient in this enzyme [113]. The fact that this enzyme is also present in cultivated amniotic fluid cells may make possible the prenatal diagnosis of this disorder by means of amniocentesis [114].

Genetics

The available information about the patients and their family members is compatible with the conclusion that ASase deficiency is inherited as an autosomal recessive trait.

Results of studies on the red blood cell ASase activity in seven families are shown in Table 17-8. Homozygous patients had no detectable activity. Parents who are obligate heterozygotes had in general only half as much activity as the control subjects. Three sibs were also in the heterozygote range.

The excretion of a small amount of ASA was found in both parents and relatives in four families. In the family reported by Coryell et al. [86], 10 apparently heterozygous relatives of the propositus were found to excrete from 4 to 29 mg ASA per gm creatinine. The mother of this patient excreted more ASA after being given a citrulline load than did two controls. This family lived in an isolated area where a large proportion of the population is at least indirectly related. Both the propositus and the mother, who was also mentally retarded, had 47 chromosomes with an extra metacentric chromosome in group C. This abnormal karyotype appears to be an incidental finding, since six other patients with argininosuccinic aciduria whose chromosomes were studied had normal karyotypes [90, 94, 115].

It may be of significance that there is a sex difference in the incidence of argininosuccinic aciduria. Including the three presumptive patients who were sisters of patients with proved cases (Table 17-7), there have been 18 female and 7 male patients.

ASA in Relation to Diseases of the Hair

The abnormality of the hair called *trichorrhexis nodosa* (Figs. 17-4 and 17-5) has been observed in approximately half the patients with argininosuccinic aciduria, but not in those with other disorders of the urea cycle enzymes. The pathogenesis is not clear. This defect can be produced even in normal hair by frequent trauma [116, 117]. It may be a manifestation of arginine deficiency, since human hair normally contains 7.5 to 10 percent arginine [118]. Patients who are unable

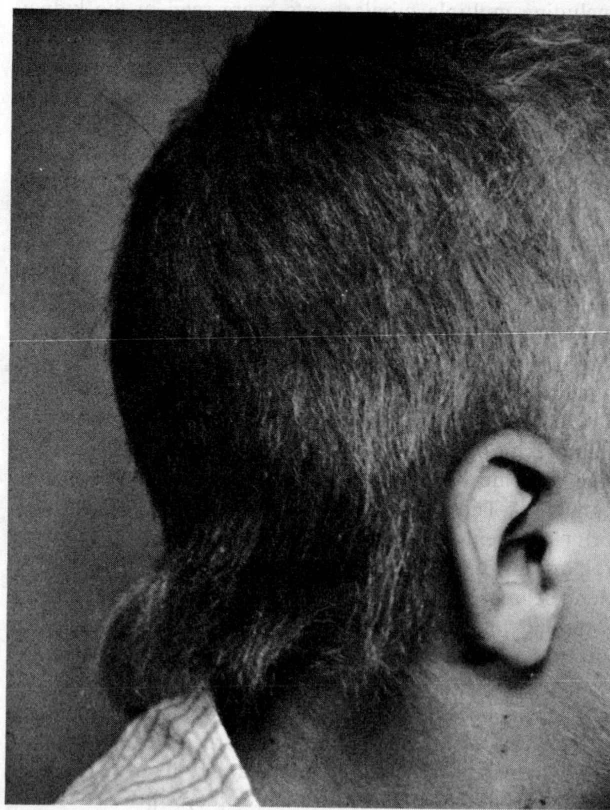

Figure 17-4. Patient with argininosuccinic aciduria, showing dry, breakable, and short hair (*From Farrell et al.* [94], *with permission of the author and publisher.*)

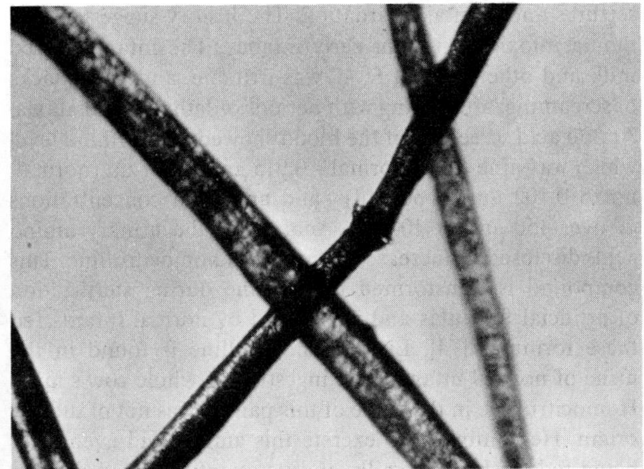

Figure 17-5. Microscopic appearance of hair from a patient with argininosuccinic aciduria. This illustrates classical trichorrhexis nodosa, a condition in which minute nodes are formed in the shafts of the hairs, the latter splitting and breaking incompletely at these points (*From Farrell et al.* [94], *with permission of the author and publisher.*)

to make arginine from ASA depend on dietary intake for the supply of arginine. Coryell et al. [86] reported that the hair of their patient became normal after institution of a good high-protein diet. However, the follow-up of the two original patients disclosed that the general appearance of the hair was also much improved without any therapy [119].

Because of the high frequency of abnormal hair in patients with argininosuccinic aciduria, ASA has been sought in the urine of patients with different types of hereditary hair disease. Small amounts of ASA were found in some patients. Grosfeld [120] reported the presence of ASA in the urine of patients with monilethrix and suggested that this disease might be due to ASase deficiency in the hair follicles or skin. The same urine was studied again by Efron and Hoefnagel [121], using three different methods, including electrophoresis and paper and column chromatography. It was proved that the ninhydrin-positive compounds in the urine were not ASA. Urine specimens from three brothers in another family with the characteristic findings of monilethrix were also analyzed for ASA but none was found. Shelley and Rawnsley [122] screened a series of 56 patients with various types of hair disorders and found two patients, both with hair loss resulting from breakage, who excreted from 10 to 20 mg ASA per day. One patient had much reduced ASase activity in the blood cells; the other had slightly lower than normal activity. Trace amounts of ASA were detected in occasional first-morning urine specimens of six patients with unclassified hair loss. In a recent study of 22 patients with hereditary hair diseases and their relatives, Winther and Bundgaard [123] found trace amounts of ASA in some patients and relatives. The relationship of ASA to the hair abnormality is not clear.

HYPERARGININEMIA

Arginase deficiency resulting in hyperargininemia is the most recently discovered urea cycle disorder. A preliminary report by Terheggen et al. [124] described two sisters, 18 months and 5 years of age, with spastic diplegia, epileptic seizures, and mental retardation. Both showed hyperammonemia and increases in blood and CSF arginine concentrations. Arginase activity in the red blood cells was low: 120 μmoles per hr per gm hemoglobin in one patient and none detectable in the other (normal range, 793 to 1,330). The father and mother both had lower-than-normal activities (573 and 743 μmoles per hr per gm hemoglobin, respectively). Liver enzyme activity was not measured. The urinary amino acid pattern of these patients resembled that of lysine-cystinuria. This pattern could be explained on the basis of reduced renal absorption of these compounds in the presence of high arginine concentrations (cf. Chap. 62).

A low-protein diet resulted in a lowering of blood ammonia levels and the disappearance of the lysine-cystinuria pattern.

TREATMENT

The clinical features of the urea cycle disorders and other types of congenital hyperammonemia are remarkably similar. There is evidence that the high blood NH_3 level in these patients is a result of protein intolerance and is responsible for the clinical symptoms. Patients improve on a restricted protein diet. The current concept of management of these patients is therefore oriented toward limitation of protein intake and lowering of blood ammonia level.

The ordinary American infant is fed a diet containing at least 3 to 5 gm protein per kg per day. A low-protein diet may be achieved by reducing the intake to 1.0 to 1.5 gm per kg per day. The possibility of protein malnutrition and growth failure must be considered if the intake is less than 1 gm per kg per day. One is faced with the problem of keeping a balance between biochemical control of the disease and allowance of sufficient protein for growth. The protein requirement is the highest in the first few months of life and gradually decreases as the child grows older. Diet therapy may be guided by frequent measurement of blood ammonia and the growth curve. A blood ammonia level of less than 100 μg per 100 ml, or no more than twice the normal level, is compatible with clinical well-being. The amount of protein intake should be adjusted to meet the individual requirement. It is also important that the intake of essential amino acids, calories, vitamins, and minerals be adequate.

One might expect that a block in any of the five steps in the urea cycle would result in a decrease in the biosynthesis of arginine. On this hypothesis, Dent gave supplementary arginine [126] to his patient with argininosuccinic aciduria, but there was no improvement. Since the child was

8 years old, brain damage was probably irreversible. Argininosuccinic aciduria was detected in one infant [105] in a routine newborn screening program. The child was asymptomatic; she was started on a low-protein diet in combination with an arginine supplement at 6 weeks of age and is doing well, with normal growth and development at age 10 months [97]. Although it is still too early to draw any conclusion about the effect of this treatment, this regimen appears to be reasonable and promising.

Since it is known that a protein load may cause a rise in blood ammonia level, the diet should be divided into frequent small feedings to minimize such responses.

Glutamine synthesis is an important mechanism for the detoxication of ammonia. In hyperammonemia the glutamine content of the blood is much increased. Alpha-ketoglutarate combines with ammonia to form, first, glutamic acid and then glutamine. Shunting of this compound from Krebs' tricarboxylic cycle has been suggested as the cause of clinical symptoms [55]. Therapy with citric acid, the stable precursor of α-ketoglutaric acid, at 2 to 4 gm per day, has been attempted in congenital hyperammonemia Type II [27, 65], with varying degrees of success. Large intake of juices of citrus fruit appears to be advisable, since the juices contain abundant citric acid.

Viral or bacterial infections may precipitate a symptomatic hyperammonemic episode. Anorexia and lowered food intake during illness suggest that the breakdown of tissue protein may be a contributing factor. Adequate caloric intake during this illness would be advisable. Surgery or other stresses may also have an adverse effect on the metabolic homeostasis of these patients. Two infants with congenital hyperammonemia died shortly after a laparotomy [51, 56].

During digestion of protein some of the amino acids are subjected to bacterial deamination. Ammonia thus formed is absorbed from the intestine and carried to the liver by way of the portal vein. Sterilization of the gut in an attempt to decrease the ammonia production caused by bacteria has not been effective in lowering blood NH_3 levels in patients with urea cycle enzyme deficiencies [71, 90].

DISORDERS OF UNKNOWN METABOLIC DEFECT ASSOCIATED WITH HYPERAMMONEMIA

A number of disorders, apparently familial in nature, with elevated concentrations of ammonia in the blood have been described in the literature. In some there is no apparent rationale for the metabolic anomaly; in others the abnormality can be explained. Among the latter is congenital lysine intolerance, described in Chap. 18. Others are mentioned below.

Hyperornithinemia

In a single case report, Shih et al. [34] described a 3-year-old boy who was first seen at 16½ months of age with myoclonic seizures and mental retardation. The history suggested ammonia intoxication from early infancy. The infant refused milk and other protein food, was irritable, and had attacks of screaming, alternating with periods of lethargy and ataxia. Amino acid screening of the blood showed an ornithine level which was nine times normal—0.915 μmole per ml (normal, up to 0.102 μmole per ml)—and ammonia concentrations of over 150 μg per 100 ml. Analysis of the urinary amino acids disclosed an increased excretion of homocitrulline. This compound is transformed from lysine during sterilization of artificial formulas and is excreted by normal infants fed these formulas [74]. Little homocitrulline is found in the urine of normal infants after ingestion of whole cow's milk. Homocitrulline in the urine of this patient was not of dietary origin. He continued to excrete this amino acid even after being fed fresh cow's milk, and its quantity varied directly with the level of dietary protein intake.

There was a dramatic clinical response to a low-protein diet. The seizures and irritability disappeared, and the blood ammonia level fell to near normal on an intake of 1.5 gm protein per kg per day. Disposal of ornithine was slow following oral loading, suggesting a block in the ornithine metabolic pathway. The basic defect in this syndrome is not yet defined.

Bickel et al. [127] reported a different type of hyperornithinemia, which was shown to be hepatic ornithine-ketoacid transaminase deficiency, i.e., a block in the pathway from ornithine to proline and glutamic acid. Both his patients had evidences of liver disease and renal tubular dysfunction. One was moderately retarded, the other only slightly so. The blood ornithine level was only three times normal; the postprandial blood ammonia concentration was not elevated. This type of hyperornithinemia is distinguishable from the type reported by Shih et al. [34] by clinical findings. The ornithine-ketoacid transaminase activity in cultured skin fibroblasts of the latter patient is within the normal range.

Hyperglycinemia, Ketoacidosis, and Hyperammonemia

The clinical syndrome of hyperglycinemia and ketoacidosis in early infancy, first described in ketotic hyperglycinemia [58], has now been found in several other metabolic disorders. These include CP synthetase deficiency [56], vitamin B_{12}-responsive and vitamin B_{12} unresponsive methylmalonic acidemia [128], and propionyl CoA carboxylase deficiency [129]. In CP synthetase deficiency and vitamin B_{12}-unresponsive methylmalonic acidemia, elevation of blood ammonia level is also present.

Hyperglycinemia appears to be a nonspecific finding and is not causally related to clinical symptoms. Observations in these patients suggest that there is a close relationship between the metabolisms of glycine, ammonia, and short-chain fatty acids.

The case of a patient recently described by Kirkman et al. [130] illustrates this point. The infant was hospitalized at

1 month of age with severe growth failure, tremulousness, and a history suggesting pyloric stenosis. Hyperammonemia (356 μg per 100 ml), acidosis, and neutropenia were found. When the patient was put on a restricted protein diet of 1.5 gm per kg per day, the blood ammonia concentration decreased to 80 to 260 μg per 100 ml. Further studies disclosed mild hyperglycinemia, high blood and urinary lysine levels on a high-protein diet, and increased excretion of methylmalonic acid (MMA) which was unresponsive to vitamin B_{12} therapy. Liver CP synthetase activity proved to be deficient. Kirkman commented that deficiency of CP synthetase activity is probably secondary to MMA inhibition, and animal experiments are now in progress to test this hypothesis [131].

It cannot be overemphasized that investigations in these various aspects of metabolism should be included in the work-up of a patient with an elevation of blood glycine level.

Familial Protein Intolerance with Deficient Transport of Basic Amino Acids

Perheentupa et al. [132] in 1965 reported three patients with a new syndrome characterized by a combination of protein intolerance and deficient transport of basic amino acids. This observation has now been extended to include 10 patients in 7 families [68], and the condition is considered a clinical syndrome of unknown cause. All patients tolerated breast milk but began to have vomiting and diarrhea after weaning. There was a strong aversion to protein food in the older children. Vomiting and diarrhea and elevated blood ammonia concentrations were associated with a protein-rich diet. Growth failure was severe, and the patients were dwarfed. Except in two patients, intelligence was normal. All had enlarged livers in at least some stage of the disease; some had a palpable spleen. Histologic changes in the liver were mainly in the portal tract, varying from cellular infiltrates to incipient diffuse cirrhosis. Neutropenia was present in half the patients; this has been found in patients with other types of hyperammonemia. The histologic picture of the small-intestinal mucosa was that of a normal villous structure and epithelial pattern but with round-cell infiltration of the lamina propria. Plasma on study showed reduced concentrations of lysine, arginine, leucine, and tyrosine; amounts of alanine, citrulline, and serine were slightly increased. Urinary excretion of amino acids was normal except for an increased lysine excretion. Arginine excretion increased with protein ingestion. Renal reabsorption of lysine, and to a lesser extent of arginine, was reduced. Activities of the urea cycle enzyme were normal in the liver [133], but that of ornithine-ketoacid transaminase was low in one patient [134]. After oral alanine loading, blood ammonia concentration rose markedly in all patients except one; arginine abolished the hyperammonemic responses, while lysine augmented them. Five patients were treated with arginine supplements on the assumption that the plasma arginine concentration was low and because the amount of arginine might be a limiting factor in urea synthesis. The clinical condition of three of the five patients improved. Though arginine deficiency may have contributed to the hyperammonemia, the cause of the arginine deficiency remains to be explained. If the slight increase in the renal clearance of arginine is the cause of arginine deficiency, why does one not see this syndrome in homozygous cystinuria patients, who lose much more arginine in the urine? The basic defect of this syndrome is still far from clear.

Cerebroatrophic Syndrome and Hyperammonemia

In a survey of 6,000 mentally retarded children, Rett [135] found 30 girls with a neurologic and psychiatric syndrome and hyperammonemia. The pneumoencephalogram showed cerebral atrophy. No good explanation was offered.

SUMMARY

1 The urea cycle is the only known metabolic pathway of urea synthesis and is the major pathway of ammonia detoxication in man. It is known to involve five sequential enzymatic reactions. The relative activity of each enzyme of the urea cycle in mammalian liver indicates that step 1 (carbamylphosphate synthetase) and steps 3 and 4 (the argininosuccinic acid–synthesizing and –cleavaging enzymes) are the rate-limiting steps, while the ornithine transcarbamylase (step 2) and arginase (step 5) activities are much greater.

2 A disorder associated with deficiency of each of the five enzymes in this cycle has been described. All these disease states are associated with ammonia intoxication. As would be expected, blood ammonia levels are greatly increased when the blocks are at steps 1 and 2, and are only moderately elevated when the block is further removed from the step that involves ammonia.

3 The clinical symptoms that are seen in all the urea cycle disorders include dislike of protein foods, vomiting in infancy, episodes of intermittent ataxia, irritability, lethargy, and coma; and mental retardation. In addition, ketoacidosis, cyclic neutropenia, and mild hyperglycinemia have been observed in the patient with hyperammonemia Type I, carbamyl phosphate synthetase deficiency.

4 Hyperammonemia Type II is due to ornithine carbamyl transferase deficiency. The glutamine content in the blood, cerebrospinal fluid, and urine is elevated. All reported patients except one are female. Mothers of the patients may have hyperammonemia and a history of aversion to protein food.

5 Citrullinemia is characterized by an elevated level of citrulline in the blood, cerebrospinal fluid, and urine. A deficiency of the liver argininosuccinic acid synthetase activity was found in one patient, and an abnormal enzyme which required unusually high concentrations of its substrate was demonstrated in the cultured skin fibroblasts of another.

6 Argininosuccinic aciduria may be divided into early-onset and late-onset types (but see Ref. 136). In the first there may be neonatal seizures, apathy, respiratory distress, and a rapid fatal course; some vomit, fail to thrive, and develop hepatomegaly in the first months of life; death may occur during a severe attack of hyperammonemia. In the late-onset type, symptoms of ammonia intoxication and slow development become noticeable in the second year of life. Hepatomegaly is absent, and survival into adulthood is common. A hair abnormality, trichorrhexis nodosa, has been observed in both types of patients. Argininosuccinic acid is present in greater quantities in the cerebrospinal fluid than in the blood. A deficiency of argininosuccinase activity has been demonstrated in the brain, liver, kidney, red blood cells, and cultured skin fibroblasts. In one patient the enzyme deficiency was found in the brain but not in the kidney. Proof of heterogeneity of this disease may be expected.

7 The blood urea concentration is usually within normal limits in these disorders in spite of the marked deficiency of the enzymes which mediate synthesis of urea. The explanation for this is not clear, but there is evidence that the enzyme defect is only partial and that some urea synthesis continues.

8 Neuropathologic and biochemical findings suggest that ammonia intoxication plays an important role in the pathogenesis of the neurologic abnormalities. A low-protein diet usually results in simultaneous clinical improvement and lowering of blood ammonia levels. This indicates that restriction of protein intake is beneficial in preventing the severe brain damage that is seen in these patients.

BIBLIOGRAPHY

1. Brown, G. W., Jr., and Cohen, P. P.: Comparative biochemistry of urea synthesis. I. Methods for the quantitative assay of urea cycle enzymes in liver. J. Biol. Chem., **234**, 1769, 1959.
2. Cohen, P. P., and Sallach, H. J.: Nitrogen metabolism of amino acids, in *Metabolic Pathways*, edited by D. Greenberg, vol. 2, p. 1. Academic, New York, 1961.
3. Krebs, H. A.: Urea synthesis, in *The Enzymes*, edited by J. B. Sumner and K. Myrbach, vol. 2, part 2, p. 866. Academic, New York, 1951.
4. Ratner, S.: Urea synthesis and metabolism of arginine and citrulline. Advances Enzym., **15**, 319, 1954.
5. Metzenberg, R. L., Hall, L. M., Marshall, M., and Cohen, P. P.: Studies on the biosynthesis of carbamyl phosphate. J. Biol. Chem., **229**, 1019, 1957.
6. Metzenberg, R. L., Marshall, M., and Cohen, P. P.: Carbamyl phosphate synthesis: studies on the mechanism of action. J. Biol. Chem., **233**, 1560, 1958.
7. Grisolia, S., and Cohen, P. P.: The catalytic role of glutamate derivatives in citrulline biosynthesis. J. Biol. Chem., **204**, 753, 1953.
8. Jones, M. E., Spector, L., and Lipmann, F. J. J.: Carbamyl phosphate, the carbamyl donor in enzymatic citrulline synthesis. J. Amer. Chem. Soc., **77**, 819, 1955.
9. Reichard, P.: Ornithine carbamyl transferase from rat liver. Acta Chem. Scand., **11**, 523, 1957.
10. Burnett, G. H., and Cohen, P. P.: Studies of carbamyl phosphate-ornithine transcarbamylase. J. Biol. Chem., **229**, 337, 1957.
11. Ratner, S., and Petrack, B.: Biosynthesis of urea. IV. Further studies in arginine synthesis from citrulline. J. Biol. Chem., **200**, 161, 1953.
12. Ratner, S., Petrack, B., and Rochovansky, O.: Biosynthesis of urea. V. Isolation and properties of argininosuccinic acid. J. Biol. Chem., **204**, 95, 1953.
13. Ratner, S., Anslow, W. P., Jr., and Petrack, B.: Biosynthesis of urea. VI. Enzymatic cleavage of argininosuccinic acid to arginine and fumaric acid. J. Biol. Chem., **204**, 115, 1953.
14. Kennan, A. L., and Cohen, P. P.: Ammonia detoxication in liver from humans. Proc. Soc. Exp. Biol. Med., **106**, 170, 1961.
15. Schimke, R. T.: Adoptive characteristics of urea cycle enzymes in the rat. J. Biol. Chem., **237**, 459, 1962.
16. Hager, S. E., and Jones, M. E.: A glutamine-dependent enzyme for the synthesis of carbamyl phosphate for pyrimidine biosynthesis in fetal rat liver. J. Biol. Chem., **242**, 5674, 1967.
17. Jones, M. E., Anderson, A. D., Anderson, C., and Hodes, S.: Citrulline synthesis in rat tissues. Arch. Biochem., **95**, 499, 1961.
18. Reichard, H.: Ornithine carbamyl transferase activity in human tissue homogenates. J. Lab. Clin. Med., **56**, 218, 1960.
19. Ratner, S., Morell, H., and Carvalho, E.: Enzymes of arginine metabolism in brain. Arch. Biochem., **91**, 280, 1960.
20. Tomlinson, S., and Westall, R. G.: Argininosuccinase activity in brain tissue. Nature (London), **188**, 235, 1960.
21. Sporn, M. B., Dingman, W., Defalco, A., and Davies, R. K.: The synthesis of urea in the living rat brain. J. Neurochem., **5**, 62, 1959.
22. Kemp, J. W., and Woodbury, D. M.: Synthesis of urea-cycle intermediates from citrulline in brain. Biochim. Biophys. Acta, **3**, 23, 1965.
23. Buniatian, H. Ch., and Davtian, M. A.: Urea synthesis in brain. J. Neurochem., **13**, 743, 1966.
24. Ratner, S., and Petrack, B.: The mechanism of arginine synthesis from citrulline in kidney. J. Biol. Chem., **200**, 175, 1953.
25. Tedesco, T. A., and Mellman, W. J.: Argininosuccinate synthetase activity and citrulline metabolism in cells cultured from a citrullinemic subject. Proc. Nat. Acad. Sci., **57**, 169, 1967.
26. Eagle, H.: Amino acid metabolism in mammalian cell cultures. Science, **130**, 432, 1959.
27. Levin, B., and Russell, A.: Treatment of hyperammonemia. Amer. J. Dis. Child., **113**, 142, 1967.
28. Levin, B.: Personal communication.
29. Nuzum, C. T., and Snodgrass, P. J.: Urea cycle enzyme adaptation to dietary protein in primates. Fed. Proc., **29**, 293, 1970.
30. Waterlow, J. C.: Observations on the mechanism of adaptation to low protein intake. Lancet, **2**, 1091, 1968.
31. Schimke, R. T.: Studies on factors affecting the levels of urea cycle enzymes in rat liver. J. Biol. Chem., **238**, 1012, 1963.
32. Colombo, J. P., and Richterich, R.: Urea cycle enzymes in the developing human fetus. Enzym. Biol. Clin. (Basel), **9**, 68, 1968.
33. Raiha, N. C. R., and Suihkonen, J.: Development of urea-synthesizing enzymes in human liver. Acta Paediat. Scand., **57**, 121, 1968.
34. Shih, V. E., Efron, M. L., and Moser, H. W.: Hyperornithinemia, hyperammonemia, and homocitrullinuria. A new disorder of amino acid metabolism associated with myoclonic seizures and mental retardation. Amer. J. Dis. Child., **117**, 83, 1969.
35. Dickinson, J. C., and Hamilton, P. B.: The free amino acids of human spinal fluid determined by ion exchange chromatography. J. Neurochem., **13**, 1179, 1966.
36. McDermott, W. V., Jr., Adams, R. D., and Riddell, A. G.: Ammonia levels in blood and cerebrospinal fluid. Proc. Soc. Exp. Biol. Med., **88**, 380, 1955.
37. Moore, E. W., Strohmeyer, G. W., and Chalmers, T. C.: Distribution of ammonia across the blood-cerebrospinal fluid barrier in patients with hepatic failure. Amer. J. Med., **35**, 350, 1963.
38. Cedrangolo, F., Pietra, G. D., Cittadini, D., Pappa, S., and DeLorenzo, F.: Urea synthesis in rats treated with alpha-D,L-methylaspartic acid. Nature (London), **195**, 708, 1962.

39. Rochovansky, O., and Ratner, S.: Effects of analogues of aspartic acid on enzymes of urea synthesis. Arch. Biochem., **127,** 688, 1968.
40. Crokaert, R., Baroen, J. P., and Wiesenfeld, M.: Biosynthase de l'urée chez le rat. II. Inhibition *in vitro* par les acides alpha-ET-beta-methylaspartique. Bull. Soc. Chim. Biol., **47,** 701, 1965.
41. Crokaert, R., and Wiesenfeld, M.: Biosynthase de l'urée chez le rat. III. Essais d'inhibition *in vivo* par les acides alpha-ET-beta-methylaspartique. Bull. Soc. Chim. Biol., **47,** 1235, 1965.
42. Dent, C. E.: Argininosuccinic aciduria. A new form of mental deficiency due to metabolic causes. Proc. Roy. Soc. Med., **52,** 885, 1959.
43. Roberge, A., Dorval, G., and Charbonneau, R.: Le Métabolism de l'ammoniaque. IV. Effet in vivo d'injections prolongées de sulfate d'ammonium et d'arginine sur l'activité specifique des enzymes du cycle de l'urée. Rev. Canad. Biol., **28,** 119, 1969.
44. McMurray, W. C., Mohyuddin, F., Bayer, S. M., and Rathbun, J. D.: Citrullinuria: a disorder of amino acid metabolism associated with mental retardation. International Copenhagen Congress on the Scientific Study of Mental Retardation. Denmark, 7–14 August, 1964.
45. Crane, C. W., Gay, W. M., and Jenner, F. A.: Urea production from labelled ammonia in argininosuccinic aciduria. Clin. Chim. Acta, **24,** 445, 1969.
46. Stahl, J.: Studies of the blood ammonia in liver disease: its diagnostic, prognostic, and therapeutic significance. Ann. Intern. Med., **58,** 1, 1963.
47. McDermott, W. V., and Adams, R. D.: Episodic stupor associated with an Eck fistula in the human with particular reference to the metabolism of ammonia. J. Clin. Invest., **33,** 1, 1954.
48. Huttenlocher, P. R., Schwartz, A. D., and Klatskin, G.: Reye's syndrome: ammonia intoxication as a possible factor in the encephalopathy. Pediatrics, **43,** 443, 1969.
49. Victor, M., Adams, R. D., and Cole, M.: The acquired (non-Wilsonian) type of chronic hepatocerebral degeneration. Medicine, **44,** 345, 1965.
50. Starer, F., and Couch, R.: Cerebral atrophy in hyperammonaemia. Clin. Radiol., **14,** 353, 1963.
51. Hopkins, I. J., Connelly, J. F., Dawson, A. G., Hird, F. J. R., and Maddison, T. G.: Hyperammonaemia due to ornithine transcarbamylase deficiency. Arch. Dis. Child., **44,** 143, 1969.
52. McMurray, W. C., Rathbun, J. C., Mohyuddin, F., and Koegler, S. J.: Citrullinuria. Pediatrics, **32,** 347, 1963.
53. Berl, S., Takagaki, G., Clarke, D. D., and Waelsch, H.: Metabolic compartments *in vivo*. Ammonia and glutamic acid metabolism in brain and liver. J. Biol. Chem., **237,** 2562, 1962.
54. Gabuzda, G. J.: Ammonium metabolism and hepatic coma. Gastroenterology, **53,** 806, 1967.
55. Bessman, S. P., and Bessman, A. N.: The cerebral and peripheral uptake of ammonia in liver disease with a hypothesis for the mechanism of hepatic coma. J. Clin. Invest., **34,** 622, 1955.
56. Freeman, J. M., Nicholson, J. F., Masland, W. S., Rowland, L. P., and Carter, S.: Ammonia intoxication due to a congenital defect in urea synthesis. J. Pediat., **65,** 1039, 1964.
57. Freeman, J. M., Nicholson, J. F., Schimke, R. T., Rowland, L. P., and Carter, S.: Congenital hyperammonemia. Arch. Neuro (Chicago), **23,** 430, 1970.
58. Childs, B., Nyhan, W. L., Borden, M., Bard, L., and Cooke, R. E.: Idiopathic hyperglycinemia and hyperglycinuria: a new disorder of amino acid metabolism. I. Pediatrics, **27,** 522, 1961.
59. Soriano, J. R., Taitz, L. S., Finberg, L., and Edelmann, C. M., Jr.: Hyperglycinemia with ketoacidosis and leukopenia: metabolic studies on the nature of the defect. Pediatrics, **39,** 818, 1967.
60. Hommes, F. A., DeGrott, C. J., Wilmink, C. W., and Jonxis, J. H. P.: Carbamylphosphate synthetase deficiency in an infant with severe cerebral damage. Arch. Dis. Child., **44,** 688, 1969.
61. Russell, A., Levin, B., Oberholzer, V. G., and Sinclair, L.: Hyperammonemia, a new instance of an inborn enzymatic defect of the biosynthesis of urea. Lancet, **2,** 699, 1962.
62. Levin, B., Oberholzer, V. G., and Sinclair, L.: Biochemical investigations of hyperammonaemia. Lancet, **2,** 170, 1969.
63. Herrin, J. T., and McCredie, D. A.: Peritoneal dialysis in the reduction of blood ammonia levels in a case of hyperammonaemia. Arch. Dis. Child., **44,** 149, 1969.
64. Sunshine, P., Lindenbaum, J. E., Levy, H. L., and Freeman, J. M.: Hyperammonemia due to a defect in hepatic ornithine transcarbamylase. Submitted for publication.
65. Levin, B., Abraham, J. M., Oberholzer, V. G., and Burgess, E. A.: Hyperammonaemia: a deficiency of liver ornithine transcarbamylase. Occurrence in mother and child. Arch. Dis. Child., **44,** 152, 1969.
66. Corbeel, L. M., Colombo, J. P., VanSande, M., and Weber, A.: Periodic attacks of lethargy in a baby with ammonia intoxication due to a congenital defect in ureogenesis. Arch. Dis. Child., **44,** 681, 1969.
67. Levin, B., Dobbs, R. H., Burgess, E. A., and Palmer, T.: Hyperammonaemia. A variant type of deficiency of liver ornithine transcarbamylase. Arch. Dis. Child., **44,** 162, 1969.
68. Kekomäki, M., Visakorpi, J. K., Perheentupa, J., and Saxen, L.: Familial protein intolerance with deficient transport of basic amino acids. An analysis of 10 patients. Acta Pediat. Scand., **56,** 617, 1967.
69. Salvatore, F., Cimino, F., d'Ayello-Caracciolom, and Cittadini, D.: Mechanism of the protection by L-ornithine-L-aspartate mixture and by L-arginine in ammonia intoxication. Arch. Biochem., **107,** 499, 1964.
70. McMurray, W. C., Mohyuddin, F., Rossiter, R. J., Rathburn, J. C., Valentine, G. H., Koegler, S. J., and Zarfas, D. E.: Citrullinuria: a new aminoaciduria associated with mental retardation. Lancet, **1,** 138, 1962.
71. Morrow, G., Barness, L. A., and Efron, M. L.: Citrullinemia with defective urea production. Pediatrics, **40,** 565, 1967.
72. Webber, W. A.: Interaction of neutral and acidic amino acids in renal tubular transport. Amer. J. Physiol., **202,** 577, 1962.
73. Gerritsen, T., Lipton, S. H., Strong, F. M., and Waisman, H. A.: On the isolation and identification of homocitrulline from urine. Biochem. Biophys. Res. Commun., **4,** 379, 1961.
74. Gerritsen, T., Vaughn, J. G., and Waisman, H. A.: The origin of homocitrulline in the urine of infants. Arch. Biochem., **100,** 298, 1963.
75. Hamilton, P. B.: Ion-exchange chromatography of amino acids. A single column, high resolving, fully automatic procedure. Anal. Chem., **35,** 2055, 1963.
76. Visakorpi, J. K.: Citrullinuria. Lancet, **1,** 1357, 1962.
77. Visakorpi, J. K., and Hyrske, J.: Urinary amino acids in mentally retarded patients. Ann. Paediat. Fenn., **6,** 112, 1960.
78. Milne, M. D., Asatoor, A. M., Edwards, K. D. G., and Loughridge, L. W.: The intestinal absorption defect in cystinuria. Gut, **2,** 323, 1961.
79. Milne, M. D., London, D. A., and Asatoor, A. M.: Citrullinuria in cases of cystinuria. Lancet, **2,** 49, 1962.
80. Roche, J., and Lacombe, G.: Sur l'argininedesiminase et sur la formation enzymatique de citrulline par les levures. Biochem. Biophys. Acta, **9,** 687, 1952.
81. McMurray, W. C., and Mohyriddin, F.: Citrullinuria. Lancet, **2,** 352, 1962.
82. Allan, J. D., Cusworth, D. C., Dent, C. E., and Wilson, V. K.: A disease, probably hereditary, characterized by severe mental deficiency and a constant gross abnormality of amino acid metabolism. Lancet, **1,** 182, 1958.
83. Levin, B., Mackay, H. M. M., and Oberholzer, V. G.: Argininosuccinic aciduria. An inborn error of amino acid metabolism. Arch. Dis. Child., **36,** 622, 1961.
84. Carson, N. A. J., and Neill, D. W.: Metabolic abnormalities detected in a survey of mentally backward individuals in Northern Ireland. Arch. Dis. Child., **37,** 505, 1962.
85. Wallis, K., Beer, S., and Fischl, J.: A family affected by argininosuccinic aciduria. Helv. Paediat. Acta, **4,** 339, 1963.
86. Coryell, M. E., Hall, W. K., Thevaos, T. G., Welter, D. A., Gatz, A. J., Horton, B. F., Sisson, B. D., Looper, J. W., Jr., and Farrow, R. T.: A familial study of a human enzyme defect, argininosuccinic aciduria. Biochem. Biophys. Res. Commun., **14,** 307, 1964.
87. Armstrong, M. D., and Stemmermann, M. G.: An occurrence of argininosuccinic aciduria. Pediatrics, **33,** 280, 1964.
88. Schreier, K., and Leuchte, G.: Argininbernsteinsäure-Krankheit. Deutsch. Med. Wschr., **90,** 864, 1965.

89. Edkins, E., and Hockey, A.: A case of argininosuccinic-aciduria. 4th Annual Interstate Conference on Mental Deficiency, p. 54. Melbourne, October, 1965.
90. Moser, H. W., Efron, M. L., Brown, H., Diamond, R., and Neumann, C. G.: Argininosuccinic aciduria. Report of two cases and demonstration of intermittent elevation of blood ammonia. Amer. J. Med., **42**, 9, 1967.
91. Miller, A. L., and McLean, P.: Urea cycle enzymes in the liver of a patient with argininosuccinic aciduria. Clin. Sci., **32**, 385, 1967.
92. Moore, P. T., Martin, M. C., Coffey, V. P., and Stokes, B. M.: Argininosuccinicaciduria—a case report on a rare condition. J. Irish Med. Ass., **61**, 172, 1968.
93. Baumgartner, R., Scheidegger, S., Stalder, G., and Hottinger, A.: Neonatal death due to argininosuccinic aciduria. Helv. Paediat. Acta, **23**, 77, 1968.
94. Farrell, G., Rauschkolb, E. W., Moure, J., Headlee, R. E., and Moser, H.: Argininosuccinic aciduria. Texas Med., **65**, 90, 1969.
95. Solitare, G. B., Shih, V. E., Nelligan, D. J., and Dolan, T. F., Jr.: Argininosuccinic aciduria: clinical, biochemical, anatomical and neuropathological observations. J. Ment. Defic. Res., **13**, 153, 1969.
96. Carton, D., DeSchrijver, F., Kint, J., Van Durme, J., and Hooft, C.: Case report. Argininosuccinic aciduria. Neonatal variant with rapid fatal course. Acta Paediat. Scand., **58**, 528, 1969.
97. Shih, V. E.: Early dietary management in an infant with argininosuccinase deficiency. Preliminary report, J. Ped., **80**: 645, 1972.
98. Landsdale, D., Faulkner, W. K., Price, J. W., and Smeby, R. R.: Intermittent cerebellar ataxia associated with hyperpyruvic acidemia, hyperalaninemia, and hyperalaninuria. Pediatrics, **43**, 1025, 1969.
99. Tomlinson, S., and Westall, R. G.: Argininosuccinic aciduria: argininosuccinase and arginase in human blood cells. Clin. Sci., **26**, 261, 1964.
100. Kint, J., and Carton, D.: Deficient argininosuccinase activity in brain in argininosuccinicaciduria. Lancet, **2**, 635, 1968.
101. Colombo, J. P., and Baumgartner, R.: Argininosuccinate cleavage enzyme of the kidney in ASAciduria, in *Proceedings of 6th Symposium of the Society for the Study of Inborn Errors of Metabolism, Zurich, June 24–25, 1968,* p. 119. E. & S. Livingstone, Ltd., Edinburgh, 1969.
102. Lewis, P. D., and Miller, A. L.: ASAciduria. Case report with neuropathological findings, Brain, **93**, 413, 1970.
103. Cavanagh, J. B., and Kyu, M. H.: Colchicine-like effect on astrocytes after portocaval shunt in rats. Lancet, **2**, 620, 1969.
104. Donohue, W. L.: Lesions in the central nervous system associated with inborn errors of amino acid metabolism. Acta Paediat., **56**, 116, 1967.
105. Levy, H. L., Shih, V. E., Madigan, P. M., and Karolkewicz, V.: Screening for metabolic disorders in Massachusetts by urine chromatography of newborns. Abstract in the Program of the Society for Pediatric Research Fortieth Annual Meeting, Atlantic City, N.J., April 29–30, 1970.
106. Efron, M. L.: High voltage paper electrophoresis, in *Chromatographic and Electrophoretic Techniques,* edited by Ivor Smith, vol. 2, *Zone Electrophoresis,* chap. 5, p. 166. Interscience, New York, 1968.
107. Westall, R. G.: Argininosuccinic aciduria: identification and reactions of the abnormal metabolite in a newly described form of mental disease, with some preliminary metabolic studies. Biochem. J., **77**, 135, 1960.
108. Ratner, S., and Kunkemueller, M.: Separation and properties of argininosuccinate and its two anhydrides and their detection in biological materials. Biochemistry, **5**, 1821, 1966.
109. Cusworth, D. C., and Dent, C. E.: Renal clearance of amino acids in normal adults and in patients with aminoaciduria. Biochem. J., **74**, 550, 1960.
110. Efron, M. L., Young, D., Moser, H. W., and MacCready, R. A.: A simple chromatographic screening test for the detection of disorders of amino acid metabolism. New Eng. J. Med., **270**, 1378, 1964.
111. Cusworth, D. C., and Westall, R. G.: Determination of argininosuccinic acid by ion-exchange chromatography. Nature (London), **192**, 555, 1961.
112. Murphy, W. H., and Guthrie, R.: Personal communication.
113. Shih, V. E., Littlefield, J. W., and Moser, H. W.: Argininosuccinase deficiency in fibroblasts cultured from patients with argininosuccinic aciduria. Biochem. Genet., **3**, 81, 1969.
114. Shih, V. E., and Littlefield, J. W.: Lancet, **2**, 45, 1970.
115. Wallis, K., and Beer, S.: Karyotype in two cases of argininosuccinuria. Ann. Paediat., **206**, 9, 1966.
116. Chernosky, M. E., and Owens, D. W.: Trichorrhexis nodosa: clinical and investigative studies. Arch. Derm. (Chicago), **94**, 577, 1966.
117. Owens, D. W., and Chernosky, M. E.: Trichorrhexis nodosa: *in vitro* reproduction. Arch. Derm. (Chicago), **94**, 586, 1966.
118. Rothman, S.: *Physiology and Biochemistry of the Skin,* p. 352. University of Chicago Press, Chicago, 1954.
119. Westall, R. G.: Treatment of argininosuccinic aciduria. Amer. J. Dis. Child., **113**, 160, 1967.
120. Grosfeld, J. C. M., Mighorst, J. A., and Moolhuysen, T. M. G. F.: Argininosuccinic aciduria in monilethrix. Lancet, **2**, 789, 1964.
121. Efron, M. L., and Hoefnagel, D.: Argininosuccinic acid in monilethrix. Lancet, **1**, 321, 1966.
122. Shelley, V. B., and Rawnsley, H. M.: Aminogenic alopecia. Trans. Ass. Amer. Physician, **47**, 146, 1966.
123. Winther, A., and Bundgaard, L.: Argininosuccinic aciduria in hereditary hair diseases. Acta Dermatovener. (Stockholm), **48**, 567, 1968.
124. Terheggen, H. G., Schwenk, A., Lowenthal, A., Van Sande, M., and Colombo, J. P.: Argininaemia with arginase deficiency. Lancet, **2**, 748, 1969.
125. Levin, R.: Argininosuccinic aciduria. Amer. J. Dis. Child., **113**, 162, 1967.
126. Dent, C. E.: Argininosuccinic aciduria and maple syrup urine disease. Bull. Schweiz. Akad. Med. Wiss., **17**, 329, 1961.
127. Bickel, H., Feist, D., Müller, H., and Quadbeck, G.: Ornithinämie, eine weiter Aminosäurenstoff-wechselstörung mit Hirnschädigung. Deutsch. Med. Wschr., **47**, 2247, 1968.
128. Morrow, G., III, Barress, L. A., Auerbach, V. H., DiGeorge, A. M., Ando, T., and Nyhan, W. L.: Observations on the coexistence of methylmalonic acidemia and glycinemia. J. Pediat., **74**, 688, 1969.
129. Hsia, Y. E., Scully, K. J., and Rosenberg, L. E.: Defective propionate carboxylation in ketotic hyperglycinemia. Lancet, **1**, 757, 1969.
130. Kirkman, H. N., and Kiesel, J. L.: Congenital hyperammonemia. Presented at the Society for Pediatric Research. Thirty-ninth Annual Meeting, Atlantic City, N.J., May 2–3, 1969.
131. Kirkman, H. N.: Personal communication.
132. Perheentupa, J., and Visakorpi, J. K.: Protein intolerance with deficient transport of basic amino acids. Lancet, **2**, 813, 1965.
133. Kekomäki, M., Räihä, N. C. R., and Perheentupa, J.: Enzymes of urea synthesis in familial protein intolerance with deficient transport of basic amino acids. Acta Paediat. Scand., **56**, 631, 1967.
134. Kekomäki, M. P., Räihä, N. C. R., and Bickel, H.: Ornithine-ketoacid aminotransferase in human liver with reference to patients with hyperornithinaemia and familial protein intolerance. Clin. Chim. Acta, **23**, 203, 1969.
135. Rett, A.: Über ein cerebral-atrophisches Syndrom bei Hyperammonämie. Mschr. Kinderheilk., **116**, 310, 1968.
136. Two new case reports have come to our attention. In the first family (Levin and Dobbs, Proc. Roy. Soc. Med., **61**, 773, 1968) all three siblings died on the fourth day of life with massive pulmonary hemorrhage. Large amounts of ASA and glutamine were found in blood and urine of the third sibling. Blood ammonia was elevated to 850 μg per 100 ml. Argininosuccinase activity was not detectable in either red blood cells or the liver. In the second family (W. H. Murphey, personal communication) one child was normal and four others died within days of birth. The disorder in the last child was diagnosed as ASase deficiency by the bacterial auxiotroph assay [112], and ASA was found in blood and urine. Enzyme assays of liver and kidney tissue obtained at necropsy were markedly deficient in ASase activity.

CHAPTER EIGHTEEN
THE HYPERLYSINEMIAS*

H. Ghadimi

Reports concerning disturbances in lysine metabolism reflect wide variation both in clinical and in biochemical findings. Obviously, more than one disease is involved. To put this chapter in perspective, a brief review of lysine metabolism is in order. Lysine (a diaminomonocarboxylic acid) is an essential amino acid; our knowledge of its metabolism is still in many respects fragmentary and controversial.

THE METABOLISM OF LYSINE

The principal degradative product of lysine metabolism is acetyl CoA (Fig. 18-1). Higashino et al. [1] found that in the presence of an excess of α-ketoglutaric acid, lysine proceeds through saccharopine [ε-N-(L-glutaryl-2)-L-lysine] to α-aminoadipic acid. Ghadimi and Zischka [2], using fresh specimens of healthy human liver, also found that the major catabolic pathway of lysine is by way of saccharopine formation. Hutzler and Dancis [3] confirmed this finding. They partially purified the enzyme "lysine-ketoglutarate reductase" from human liver, and found it in kidney, heart, adrenal gland, thyroid gland, brain, and skin, in order of decreasing activity.

Lysine also enters pathways to homocitrulline and homoarginine, but these are quantitatively minor [4]. It also may be metabolized to pipecolic acid. Rothstein and Miller [5], studying this route, trapped pipecolic acid in the urine of rats by the metabolic overloading technique. They identified the pipecolic acid and concluded that lysine metabolism proceeds with cyclization of α-keto-ϵ-aminocaproic acid to Δ^1-piperideine-2-carboxylic acid, which in turn is reduced to pipecolic acid. Paik et al. [6, 7] suggested that acetylation of the ϵ-amino group would enhance deamination for the cyclization step. This pathway progresses through many steps, including α-aminoadipic acid, to acetyl CoA and CO_2. Burgi et al. [8] showed that human liver homogenate degrades lysine by oxidative deamination, provided that NAD (nicotinamide-adenine dinucleotide) is present as coenzyme. The finding of pipecolic acid in human urine [9–11] implies the presence of this catabolic pathway in man; but our own experience with lysine metabolites in man has not supported the cyclization path to pipecolic acid as a major route [2]. Further degradation of pipecolic acid through the saccharopine pathway, i.e., conversion to Δ^1-piperideine-6-carboxylic acid, remains to be proved.

Pertinent to hyperlysinemias is the observation of Hunter and Downs [12] that the activity of arginase in the Krebs urea cycle can be inhibited by naturally occurring L-amino acids. Lysine and ornithine are the most potent competitive inhibitors of arginase, and the affinity of arginase for lysine is 1.6 times greater than that for arginine. Competitive inhibition in man could interfere with ammonia elimination through the Krebs urea cycle, if the lysine concentration in the body greatly exceeds physiologic levels. In vivo inhibition of urea formation by intravenously administered L-lysine supports this hypothesis [13, 14]. In studies of competitive inhibition of arginase, red blood cells can be used as a source of the enzyme [15–17] in order to avoid liver biopsy.

If it is assumed that the original observation of lysine inhibition of arginase holds true for man in vivo, then the hyperlysinemias may be conveniently divided into two groups:

1. Periodic hyperlysinemia associated with hyperammonemia
2. Persistent hyperlysinemia

PERIODIC HYPERLYSINEMIA ASSOCIATED WITH HYPERAMMONEMIA

Hyperlysinemia with crises of ammonia intoxication associated with normal or high-protein intake was originally described by Colombo et al. in 1964 [18, 19]. The crises were ameliorated by fluid therapy and could be prevented by restricting the daily protein intake to 1.5 gm per kg body weight. Their patient, a 3-month-old female, had no evidence of advanced parenchymal liver disease, and the liver function test results did not notably depart from normal values. The activities of the urea cycle enzymes and enzymes of ammonia detoxication were normal as compared with those of controls. The increased plasma concentrations of lysine and arginine indicated that the hyperammonemia was a result of inhibition of arginase, which, in turn, interfered with ammonia elimination via the urea cycle. Following lysine loading, the blood ammonia level rose to 680 μg per 100 ml, and the patient became comatose. It was concluded that an inborn error in the catabolism of lysine was the primary cause of the clinical entity.

Clinical Features

The original case described by Colombo and coworkers still remains the only well-documented report of periodic hyperlysinemia associated with hyperammonemia. The first clinical manifestation was vomiting. This began early in the neonatal period and progressively worsened. The patient was hospitalized at 2½ months of age in a state of severe dehydration and coma. She was spastic. The temperature was

*This work was supported by Grant No. 1 RO1 HD-03992-01 from the National Institute of Child Health and Human Development.

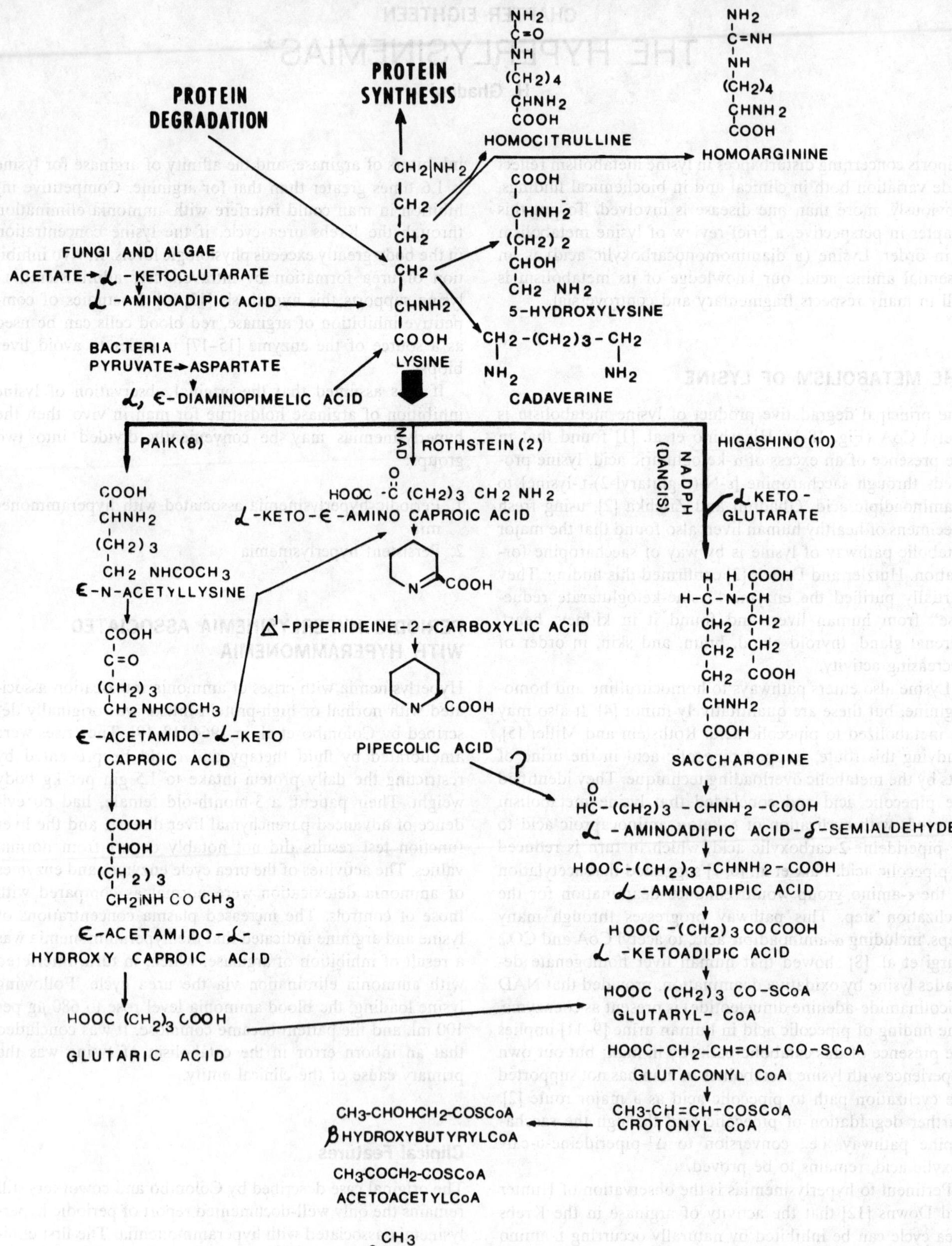

Figure 18-1. Schematic representation of lysine metabolism.

normal. The EEG was diffusely abnormal. Tests of the spinal fluid and blood disclosed no abnormalities.

With fluid therapy the patient recovered within a week and was discharged from the hospital with a normal EEG. Two weeks later, she was readmitted because of another episode of vomiting, spasticity, convulsions, and coma. Her weight was 4,560 gm (normal, 4,850 to 6,360 gm) and her length was 56 cm (normal, 57 to 62 cm). Speedy recovery again followed fluid therapy, but vomiting and coma recurred on a diet containing 3 gm protein per kg. When 3 gm of protein per kg per day was administered, a similar episode of coma developed after 3 weeks. On 1.5 gm per kg there was a dramatic improvement in general condition and no further episodes of coma occurred.

During coma the blood ammonia concentration varied between 500 and 600 μg per 100 ml. The highest value for spinal fluid ammonia was 165 μg per 100 ml. Other significant findings during the crises were increased plasma concentrations of lysine and arginine.

An EEG taken during an episode showed low voltage with high waves over the right hemisphere. These disappeared as the plasma ammonia level fell. The liver was normal in size, color, and consistency, as judged at laparotomy performed for a wedge biopsy. Microscopic examination of the liver tissue showed no necrosis or inflammation but a "slight, fatty infiltration." In the same operation, the possibility of a portacaval shunt as an explanation for the hyperammonemia was excluded. Except for slightly elevated glutamic-pyruvic transaminase and alkaline phosphatase, liver function test results were normal. The serum protein concentration remained around 5.3 gm per 100 ml, and the blood urea nitrogen value was 8.3 mg per 100 ml. Results of renal function tests and excretion of free amino acids were normal.

The patient was discharged from the hospital at 10 months of age with definite evidence of retardation. Weight was 6.8 kg (normal, 7.5 to 10 kg), and length was 63 cm (normal, 67 to 73 cm). She could not sit or hold her head up, and her extremities were spastic.

Biochemical Findings

At this juncture Colombo et al. had established a relationship of the protein in the diet to the hyperammonemia and the clinical manifestations, and had excluded parenchymal liver disease or a portacaval shunt as a cause for the hyperammonemia.

The possibility of an enzymic defect in the urea cycle, resulting in impaired ammonia disposal, was considered. In vitro studies on liver biopsy material showed normal activities for carbamylphosphate synthetase, ornithine carbamyl transferase, argininosuccinase, and arginase. The activities of enzymes for the other biochemical routes of ammonia detoxication, glutamate dehydrogenase, glutamate oxaloacetate transaminase, glutamic-pyruvic transaminase, and glutaminase were also comparable to control values.

When the daily protein intake was 3 gm per kg or more, the plasma concentrations of lysine and arginine were significantly increased. On one occasion, for example, values of 470 μmoles lysine per liter and 360 μmoles arginine per liter contrasted to corresponding control values of 103 and 180 μmoles per liter, respectively. Since the competitive inhibition of arginase by lysine [12] was well known, the investigators concluded that the increased concentration of lysine disturbed the last step of urea formation. This, in turn, resulted in impaired elimination of ammonia and increased the concentration of arginine.

The effects of separate loading doses (300 mg per kg) of L-lysine, L-arginine, and L-leucine were studied in the patient, her parents, and a healthy child of the same age. The loading dose of L-leucine was expected to reveal whether L-amino acids other than lysine inhibit arginase activity and to provide a means for the patient to act as her own control. The biochemical indicators studied at various time intervals after administration were blood ammonia, red blood cell arginase activity, blood urea nitrogen, and plasma α-amino nitrogen. In addition, plasma lysine was determined at 0 and 3 hr after the lysine load and proved to be 5.6 mg per 100 ml at 0 hr and 16 mg per 100 ml at 3 hr. The response of the patient to the lysine load was in sharp contrast to both her own responses to arginine or leucine and to the responses of the controls to any of the three amino acids.

Clinically the response was also in accord with the biochemical data. The patient became comatose 1 hr after ingestion of the lysine, while the control child remained well throughout the test. The L-arginine and L-leucine doses resulted in slight elevation of the patient's blood ammonia level but did not affect the clinical condition.

With development of coma the blood ammonia level rose from a fasting value of 240 to 700 μg per 100 ml at 3 hr, and then fell to 480 μg per 100 ml at 4 hr. There was a parallel decrease in the arginase activity of the red blood cells. This fell from 227 to 54 μmoles per hr per gm hemoglobin at 3 hr, and then to no activity at 4 hr. The blood urea nitrogen and α-amino nitrogen were not significantly changed.

The biochemical responses of the parents to the lysine loading test gave no indication as to the mode of inheritance.

The high concentration of lysine in the plasma was attributed to a partial block in the catabolic pathway of lysine. The activity of the deaminating enzyme, L-lysine NAD oxidoreductase, was measured in the liver biopsy specimen. In nine control specimens, the range of activity of the enzyme was 2.24 to 2.44 μmoles per min per gm protein, while the activity in the patient's sample was 0.524 μmole per min per gm protein.

The explanation for the sequence of events in periodic hyperlysinemia offered by Colombo et al. is attractive, but it has been challenged, and certain objections remain unanswered. As the investigators have pointed out, the competitive inhibition of arginase by lysine fails to explain the decreasing activity of the enzyme in the red blood cells during the loading test. A large excess of arginine substrate (250 μmoles) added to assay tubes should have overcome lysine inhibition, since the affinity of arginase for lysine is only 1.6 times its affinity for arginine. Moreover, high relative specific activity of arginase compared to that of other enzymes of the Krebs urea cycle has been reported [20, 21]. In light of these considerations, the implication that arginase activity is the limiting factor seems questionable.

As with certain inborn errors related to the Krebs urea cycle, i.e., ornithine transcarbamylase deficiency, citrullinemia, and argininosuccinic aciduria, in periodic hyperlysinemia associated with hyperammonemia the blood urea concentration is within the normal range. Development of ammonia intoxication in the face of a normal blood urea concentration remains difficult to explain.

The possibility of a qualitative difference in the arginase of the patient from that of controls was ruled out by the investigator by determination of the K_m of the red blood cell arginase [19].

Since in vivo conditions cannot be fully reproduced in vitro, measurement of enzymic activity in vitro cannot be taken as a full representation of the intracellular situation. The conventional pH of 9.5 and the excessive amount of Mn^{++} ions used for in vitro experiments are not conditions which prevail in the cell. It should be borne in mind that the intracellular concentration of most amino acids is 2 to 21 times larger than the concentration in plasma [22]. The ability of red blood cells of the patient to concentrate amino acids may be abnormal.

It is not known why patients with persistent hyperlysinemia [9, 23–25] show no clinical sign or biochemical evidence of hyperammonemia. It is possible that excessive intracellular concentrations of some metabolites of lysine may inhibit arginase with greater efficiency than lysine itself. Obviously, depending on the site of the block, different lysine metabolites would accumulate in the cell. Moreover, the concentrations of metabolites of subsidiary pathways, e.g., homocitrulline and homoarginine, are governed by the efficiency of the functioning pathways. Studies of the possible inhibitory effect of different lysine metabolites on arginase and determination of the intracellular concentrations of these metabolites may explain the difference in the two hyperlysinemias regarding the development of hyperammonemia.

Diagnosis

Although only one authentic case of periodic hyperlysinemia associated with hyperammonemia has been described, similar symptoms are encountered rather frequently, and the disease may have been often overlooked. Conventional fluid therapy generally includes restriction of protein intake. If reinstitution of a diet containing 3 gm or more protein per kilogram should trigger ammonia intoxication, with vomiting and failure to thrive, then the diagnosis is suggested. The amount of plasma lysine should be measured under such circumstances. The effect of a loading test with L-lysine should confirm the diagnosis in instances where hyperammonemia is associated with hyperlysinemia. Studies of the arginase of the red blood cells obtained during lysine loading tests would confirm the diagnosis.

Failure to thrive, feeding difficulties, and vomiting in early life, proceeding to convulsion and coma, are not uncommon clinical manifestations of inborn errors of metabolism. These signs and symptoms when associated with hyperammonemia suggest one of the following:

1. Ornithine transcarbamylase deficiency—"hyperammonemia"
2. Citrullinemia
3. Argininosuccinic aciduria
4. Hyperornithinemia [26]
5. Periodic hyperlysinemia

Enzymes of the Krebs urea cycle are relatively inactive in the first three conditions. Hyperornithinemia [26] associated with ammonia intoxication has been found in a 3-year-old boy with psychomotor retardation, infantile spasms, irritability, and ataxia. Restriction of daily dietary protein intake to 1.5 gm per kg lowered the blood ammonia and ornithine levels and led to clinical improvement. Ornithine transcarbamylase of the liver was not studied, but repeated measurement of the activity of the enzyme in plasma gave consistently high values. By inference, the authors concluded that the enzyme in the liver was normal.

Periodic hyperlysinemia associated with hyperammonemia has little in common with "cerebral atrophy and chronic hyperammonemia," as described by Rett [27], or with "familial protein intolerance with deficient transport of basic amino acids," reported by Perheentupa and Visakorpi [28]. The hyperammonemia in the three children with the latter condition was not associated with hyperlysinemia. Although these patients refused milk and other animal protein, they nevertheless continued to have attacks of vomiting and diarrhea. Severe growth failure, hepatomegaly with normal liver function tests, and a tendency to low blood granulocyte count were also observed in these patients. The authors suggested that the hyperammonemia was due to arginine deficiency, since arginine was low in the diet, was absorbed poorly from the gut, and was excreted excessively in the urine. Seven additional cases were reported later [29].

"Hereditary hyperlysinemia and lysine-induced crises" were reported by Ghadimi et al. [30] in a 14-year-old male. The patient had repeated attacks of abdominal pain, vomiting, ptyalism, profound muscle weakness, and lethargy. There appeared to be no relation between protein intake and these attacks. The blood ammonia concentration during the crises was only slightly elevated (260 μg per 100 ml). At the time of this writing, the patient is healthy and has experienced only one episode in the past 18 months.

PERSISTENT HYPERLYSINEMIA

Persistent hyperlysinemia is a rare metabolic anomaly with varied clinical manifestations, judging from four reports [9, 23–25] of seven patients. The common biochemical denominator is persistence of hyperlysinemia and hyperlysinuria, without hyperammonemia. The original reports were presented simultaneously and independently by Woody [31] and Ghadimi et al. [32].

Clinical Features

Table 18-1 summarizes the salient clinical features of persistent hyperlysinemia, as described in the four reports. The patients reported by Armstrong et al. [23] and Ghadimi et al. [25] were profoundly retarded. The initial patient of Woody was "severely retarded," but her sister and a cousin with normal physical and mental development had persistent hyperlysinemia [33]. The IQ of the patient reported by Carson et al. [24] was estimated at 67. Physical retardation occurred in three patients. Synophrys was seen in five. The oldest patient, 27 years of age, was grossly retarded (Fig. 18-2), with an IQ estimated at 13. He learned to walk at the age of 2 years, but was thought to be normal during early infancy. His mother was described by a local physician as mentally defective. The single blood specimen obtained from her also showed hyperlysinemia in the range of 7.5 mg per 100 ml. One of the patient's sibs had a speech defect, and the father and three other sibs had borderline intelligence. There was no history of consanguinity.

At present the patient cannot talk or walk, is not toilet-trained, and cannot dress himself. Weight is 31.8 kg, and physical development is at the level of a 9- or 10-year-old. The jaw is protruding, and maxillae are wide and high. The outer and middle thirds of the eyebrows are raised and have scanty hair, and there is a pad of soft tissue between the eyebrows. Other notable features are protruding tongue, open mouth, and high palate. Secondary sexual characteristics are absent. Skeletal maturation is much delayed. The EEG is compatible with petit mal epilepsy. There have been no noteworthy clinical changes during 9 years of follow-up. The patient described by Armstrong et al. [23] had similar facial features.

There has been a high incidence of consanguinity among the parents of these patients, and the familial occurrence of the biochemical anomaly is noteworthy. Routine clinical laboratory studies of all patients have disclosed no significant abnormalities other than a mild anemia observed in Woody's index patient and in Ghadimi's two patients.

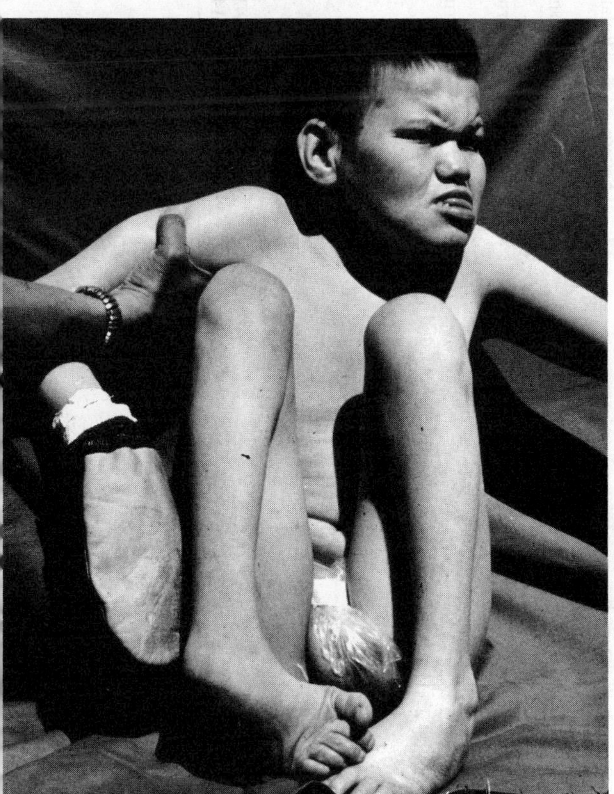

Figure 18-2. Patient 1 with persistent hyperlysinemia.

Biochemical Findings

Blood

The concentration of plasma lysine in persistent hyperlysinemia is not so high as that of plasma phenylalanine in phenylketonuria (Table 18-2). The levels are generally above the upper limit of normal, and sometimes as high as four to five times the upper values for controls. The combined range is 2.4 to 22.5 mg per 100 ml. The three patients of Woody contribute the highest figures. There is no correlation between the plasma lysine level and the degree of retardation or other clinical manifestations.

Carson [24] reported small quantities of saccharopine and homocitrulline in the serum of her patient. Saccharopine completely overlaps cystine in certain column chromatographic techniques. It is possible that small quantities of saccharopine were present in the biologic fluids of other patients but were masked by the cystine normally present.

Cerebrospinal Fluid

The lysine concentration in the CSF was measured in only three patients. In two, when quantitative techniques were used, the range was found to be 0.8 to 2.2 mg per 100 ml, compared with 0.3 to 0.7 mg per 100 ml in 10 controls.

Carson found saccharopine in the CSF of her patient [24].

Table 18-1. CLINICAL FEATURES OF PERSISTENT HYPERLYSINEMIA

Author and ref. no.	Case no.	Age, yr	Sex	Consanguinity of parents	Clinical manifestations: Familial occurrence	Mental development	Physical development	Lax ligaments	Synophrys	Convulsions: History	Convulsions: EEG	Other characteristics
Ghadimi et al. [2]	1	27	M	?	3 sibs and father mildly retarded; 1 sib with speech retardation; mother mentally subnormal	IQ 13	Height, 132 cm Weight, 31.5 kg Head circumference, 53 cm (all 3d percentile)	Yes	Yes	No	Petit mal type	Absence of secondary sexual characteristics; prognathous jaw; high maxilla; sunken root of nose; slightly webbed fingers; mild anemia
	2	2	M	Incest	NS	Severe retardation	Height, 30 cm Weight, 9.6 kg (both 3d percentile)	Yes	No	Yes	Petit mal type	Undescended testicle; strabismus; mild hepatosplenomegaly; mild anemia
Woody et al. [9, 32]	3	4½	F	Yes	Yes	Severe retardation	Retardation	Yes	Yes	Yes	Normal	Mild anemia
	4	2	F	Yes	Sister of Case 3	Normal	Normal	No	Yes	No	Normal	Slightly webbed toes
	5	11	F	Yes	Cousin of Cases 3 and 4	Normal	Normal	No	Yes	No	NR	Obese
Armstrong et al. [23]	6	3¾	M	No	2 half-sibs retarded; mother and 5 sibs (3M, 2F) all retarded; maternal grandmother retarded	IQ 32	Normal	No	Yes	No	Normal	Facial features similar to those of Case 1; simian line in one hand
Carson et al. [24]	7	22	F	No	No	IQ 67	Short stature (145 cm)	No	No	No	Abnormal	

Note: NS, not studied; NR, not reported.

Table 18-2. FINDINGS IN BIOLOGIC FLUIDS IN PERSISTENT HYPERLYSINEMIA

Case no.*	Plasma lysine, mg/100 ml	CSF lysine, mg/100 ml	*Urine*														Other findings
			Lysine, mg/24 hr	Lysine, μmole/mg creatinine	Saccharopine	Pipecolic acid	α-Aminoadipic acid	ε-N-Acetyllysine, mg/24 hr	ε-N-Acetyllysine, μmole/mg creatinine	Homocitrulline, mg/24 hr	Homocitrulline, μmole/mg creatinine	Homoarginine, mg/24 hr	Homoarginine, μmole/mg creatinine	Ornithine, mg/24 hr	Citrulline, mg/24 hr	γ-Aminobutyric acid	
1	3.5–8.4	0.8, 2.2	177.2	NS	NR	NR	NR	NR	NS	59	NS	8	NS	Occasionally high	Normal	None	
2	4.5–8.6	1.2	24.4–65.1	NS	NR	NR	NR	NR	NS	5.4–38.9	NS	NS	NS	Normal	Normal	None	
3†	13.0–22.5	High‡	NS	42.5	NR	"Excess"	"Excess"	NR	0.6	NR	0.6	NR	0.6	High	NR	High	α-Ketoglutarate-high arginine "periodically"
4†	10.0–15.0	NR	NS	23.8	NR	NR	NR	NR	0.6	NR	0.7	NR	1.4	NR	NR	NR	
5†	13.6–16	NR	"Elevated"	"Elevated"	NR	NR	NR	NR	NR	NR	NR	NR	NR	NR	NR	NR	
6 Uncontrolled diet	1.8–5.1	NR	193	7.68, 7.05	NR	NR	NR	3.4	0.09; 0.1	4.2	0.14; 0.10	2.4	0.06; 0.09	NR	NR	None	α-N-Acetyllysine 0.07, 0.06 μmole/mg creatinine
Loading conditions		NR	335	11.60	NR	NR	NR	4.9	0.131	9.0	0.241	3.4	0.093				
7	4–5 times normal	NR	"Excessive"	"Excessive"	Present	NR	Present	NR	NR	Present	Present	Present	Present	NR	Excessive	NR	
Controls	1.3–4.4 [34–38] 1.2–4.7 [25]	0.29–0.71 [25]	7–57 [39–42] 2.1–15.0 [25]	11 [23]	NR	NR	Trace [23]	NR	0.025 [23]	None [23]		ca. 0.0025 [23]		10 [36]	10 [36]	NR	α-N-Acetyllysine 0.018 μmole/mg creatinine

* Cases listed in same order as in Table 18-1.
† Not all values determined by column chromatography.
‡ 80 mg/100 ml by paper chromatography.
Note: NR, not reported; NS, not studied.

Urine

As shown in Table 18-2, all patients have hyperlysinuria. The hyperlysinemia is not associated with increased urinary output of the three other basic amino acids, cystine, arginine, and ornithine.

The metabolites in the major catabolic pathway of lysine, saccharopine, pipecolic acid, α-aminoadipic acid, and ε-N-acetyllysine were studied in some of the patients. Woody [9] reported "elevated levels" of pipecolic acid and α-aminoadipic acid in his original paper. Later, he confirmed the presence of ε-N-acetyllysine in the urine of his index case and her sister [43]. Armstrong et al. [23] and Ghadimi et al. [25] failed to find pipecolic acid or α-aminoadipic acid in the urine of their patients. Ghadimi examined urine samples from premature infants in an attempt to verify the presence of pipecolic acid, as reported by Jagenburg [10] for that age group. Even application of exceedingly large volumes (2 ml) to paper chromatograms and staining with both ninhydrin and isatin failed to disclose a trace of pipecolic acid in the urine of premature infants, patients with generalized amino aciduria, or two patients with hyperlysinemia (Cases 1 and 2). On the other hand, Woody [9] reported pipecolic acid in "elevated concentrations" in the urine of Case 3, as confirmed by different paper chromatographic and staining techniques.

Armstrong et al. [23] reported finding ε-N-acetyllysine in concentrations of 3.4 mg per 24 hr on an uncontrolled diet, and 4.9 mg per 24 hr under loading conditions. On the other hand, Carson et al. [24] observed saccharopine in the urine (as well as in the CSF) of their patient. They also reported the presence of α-aminoadipic acid, but no pipecolic acid.

Metabolites of subsidiary pathways, such as homocitrulline and homoarginine, were detected in the urine of all patients where they were sought.

High concentrations of ornithine, citrulline, γ-aminobutyric acid (GABA), α-ketoglutarate, and arginine have been occasionally reported.

Loading Tests

Lysine loading tests were performed by oral administration of 150 mg L-lysine per kg body weight in Ghadimi's two patients [32] and two comparable controls, and in Armstrong's [23] patient. The load was administered after an overnight fast. The results are presented graphically in Fig. 18-3. The responses of phenylketonuric patients to an analogous loading test with phenylalanine [44] and of histidinemic patients to loads of L-histidine [34] are also shown for purposes of comparison.

In Ghadimi's patients [32] the fasting values, even after 48 hr on a low protein diet, were still above the corresponding values for controls. The peaks for the three patients in Fig. 18-3 were three to five times higher than those for controls. The results from the patients show lysine tolerance curves significantly different from those of control subjects and similar to those of patients with phenylketonuria and histidinemia.

The percentage of the dose recovered in a 24-hr urinary collection following administration of the test dose was calculated for Patients 2 and 6. In the two control subjects recovery did not exceed 1 percent of the administered dose. Patient 2 failed to utilize 43 percent of the administered dose and excreted it in urine in the next 24 hr; the corresponding value for Patient 6 was 6 percent.

The occasional high concentration of ornithine in the blood of Patient 1 and the structural similarity of ornithine to lysine suggested the desirability of an ornithine loading test. Accordingly, the patient and two control subjects were given an oral dose of 150 mg per kg body weight. The patient's response was similar to those of the controls.

Patient 1, as well as an appropriate control subject and two monkeys, were given 150 mg DL-pipecolic acid per kilogram [25]. The slow clearances of the substance from the blood of the patient, of the control, and of the monkeys were similar.

Studies with ^{14}C Lysine

Several findings have suggested that these hyperlysinemic patients have an inborn error of lysine metabolism. Among these findings are the prevalence of consanguinity of the parents, the familial incidence of the disease, the persistence of the hyperlysinemia regardless of the amount of protein in the diet, the resulting hyperlysinuria, the much-increased lysine concentration in the cerebrospinal fluid, the abnormal responses to loading tests with lysine, the excessive urinary output of the administered dose, and the presence of metabolites of subsidiary catabolic pathways of lysine.

In order to locate the site of the metabolic block further studies were carried out with uniformly labeled ^{14}C L-lysine. Patient 1 and two control subjects were given intravenous injections of 0.5 to 1 microcuries of ^{14}C L-lysine [2]. Blood samples were obtained at various times and analyzed for both radioactivity and free amino acids by the use of an amino acid analyzer connected to a liquid-flow scintillation counter. The samples from the two control subjects showed peaks at the positions of α-ketoglutarate and acetate. These two early peaks were also observed in most of the blood samples taken from dogs in similar studies [2]. The sample from the patient failed to show any radioactive peak at the positions of α-ketoglutarate or acetate. In contrast, the patient's radiochromatogram revealed three peaks; one ^{14}C-containing metabolite masked by ammonia, another in the area of arginine, and a third eluted at 180 min which did not correspond to any ninhydrin-positive substance. These results confirmed previous findings and suggested that the patient metabolized lysine in an entirely different way from the control subjects. These studies failed to reveal the site of the block.

Expired CO_2 was also collected for 3 hr in the patient

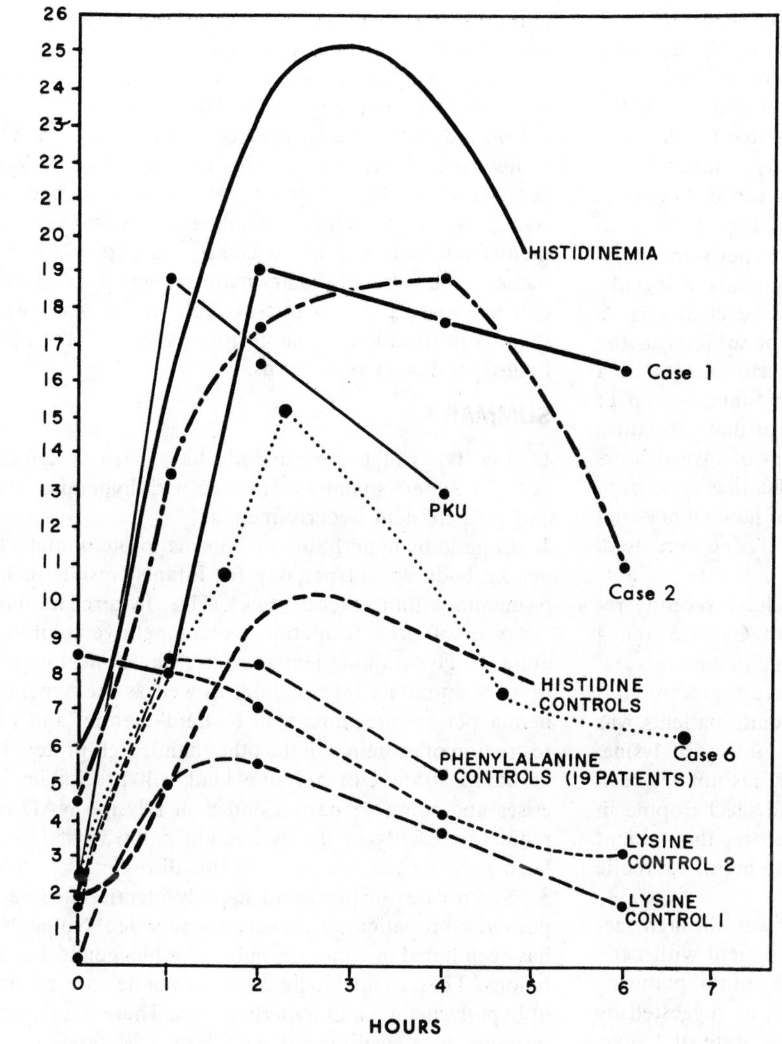

Figure 18-3. Loading tests with lysine, histidine, and phenylalanine in patients and controls.

and in one of the control subjects by the use of a face mask connected to a CO_2 trap. Constant struggling of the patient under the mask resulted in unusually heavy breathing. The determination of $^{14}CO_2$ showed that the patient exhaled 1.5 percent of the administered dose within the first 3 hr, and the control subject exhaled 2.5 percent. The difference was not significant. Without knowledge of the exact size of the lysine and bicarbonate pools, and the rate of the turnover of the latter, it was not possible to interpret accurately the result of this study.

Nevertheless, the indication is that the block in lysine metabolism is in the catabolic pathway, since $^{14}CO_2$, the end product of lysine breakdown, was produced much less by the patients than by controls. This contention is supported more convincingly by similar studies by Woody, Hutzler, and Dancis [33]. They measured the percentage of radioactivity exhaled as $^{14}CO_2$ during 6 hr following the administration of uniformly labeled ^{14}C L-lysine. They studied two hydrocephalic control subjects on two occasions and Patients 3 and 4 on one occasion each. The two control patients on the second occasion were primed by the oral administration of a load of lysine-free base in order to bring their lysine pools to a level comparable to those of the patients. The load consisted of 150 mg per kg body weight of L-lysine which was administered 45 min before subcutaneous injection of the labeled lysine. The percentage of radioactivity exhaled by the two control subjects on the first occasion amounted to 7 and 9 percent; after priming, the corresponding figures rose to 18 and 23 percent. In sharp contrast, their two hyperlysinemic patients (Cases 3 and 4), with lysine pools comparable to those of the primed controls, exhaled 0.4 and 0.6 percent of the total dose within the same period. The priming of the control subjects with a load of lysine created a temporary pool of this substance, which, in turn, resulted in greater dilution of the labeled injected amino acid. Considering this dilution factor, the control subjects when primed should have eliminated a much lower percentage of the administered radioactivity than in the nonprimed state. On the other hand, the major catabolic pathway is not fully utilized under normal conditions of life, and, therefore, can greatly expand on demands created by loading conditions. This capacity for expansion on demand of the major catabolic pathway not only compensated for the dilution factor, but indeed resulted in an output in excess of that in the nonprimed state. This makes the contrast between control subjects and patients far more striking.

These results suggest that the block in hyperlysinemia is in the major catabolic pathway. If the major catabolic pathway were intact, exhaled $^{14}CO_2$ would have reached a figure comparable to that exhaled by the control subjects in the primed state. In any event, significant accumulation of a substrate does not occur without a block in a metabolic path which plays a major role in the economy of that substance. In comparing the results of the two groups of investigators in respect to $^{14}CO_2$ studies, additional difficulties arise from the fact that the routes of administration of labeled material were different, and two different batches of lysine were used, probably with different impurities.

Dancis, Hutzler, Cox, and Woody [45] have recently reported that cultures of skin fibroblasts of Cases 3 and 4 converted radioactive lysine to saccharopine in amounts less than 10 percent that of controls. They have therefore concluded that the block in their hyperlysinemic patients was in the first step of the major catabolic pathway of lysine. The site of the block in the other patients has not yet been verified. Carson's patient, Case 7 [24], had saccharopine in her urine and cerebrospinal fluid. Therefore, this patient cannot have a block in the first step of the major catabolic pathway, as in Woody's patients.

Assuming that the major catabolic pathway through saccharopine [10, 11] is intact in Colombo's patient with periodic hyperlysinemia, a *partial* block in a minor pathway, i.e., L-lysine NAD oxidoreductase activity, as suggested by Colombo et al. [19], can hardly explain a state of hyperlysinemia occurring with normal protein intake. It is possible that the label "persistent hyperlysinemia" is being given to a heterogeneous group of diseases. Studies of these patients may help in defining the various metabolic pathways open to lysine, as well as their relative importance.

Diagnosis

The diverse clinical signs of hyperlysinemia are not suggestive of the metabolic anomaly. At one end of the scale there have been two normal-appearing children (Cases 4 and 5); at the other end is a severely retarded patient with an IQ of 13. There was no correlation between the degree of retardation and the lysine concentration in biologic fluids. Persistent hyperlysinemia, unlike periodic hyperlysinemia associated with hyperammonemia, is not reported to have elevated blood ammonia concentrations or to have produced clinical manifestations of hyperammonemia even during loading tests with L-lysine. The indications for screening for hyperlysinemia, therefore, are similar to those for many inborn errors of amino acid metabolism, i.e., mental retardation of unknown origin, especially occurring in the children of consanguineous marriages.

The present limited information suggests an autosomal recessive pattern of inheritance. The incidence of the disease is low, judged by the number of reported cases. The value of low-lysine treatment remains in doubt. Two of Woody's patients who were related to his index case had hyperlysinemia without clinical manifestations, suggesting that mental retardation is not necessarily a part of the clinical picture. The value of dietary management is therefore difficult to prove, and it is questionable at this stage whether there is justification for subjecting patients to the rigors of long-term dietary restrictions.

SUMMARY

1 Two types of hyperlysinemia have been described: (*a*) periodic hyperlysinemia associated with hyperammonemia, and (*b*) persistent hyperlysinemia.

2 In periodic hyperlysinemia, normal protein intake (3 gm per kg body weight per day for infants) results in hyperlysinemia within several weeks. This, in turn, inhibits the last step of urea formation by competitive inhibition of arginase. Hyperammonemia ensues. The clinical manifestations of ammonia intoxication, as well as the hyperammonemia per se, are amenable to fluid therapy and dietary restriction of protein. On the other hand, high-protein intake or administration of a lysine load will precipitate severe crises and coma. A partial defect in L-lysine NAD oxidoreductase activity in the cyclization pathway of lysine has been suggested as the cause of this disorder.

3 Seven cases of persistent hyperlysinemia have been reported. Four patients were severely retarded. No periodicity has been noted in either the clinical or biochemical manifestations. The salient biochemical anomalies are persistence of hyperlysinemia and hyperlysinuria. There is an abnormal response to a loading test with lysine. Metabolites of the subsidiary pathway of lysine metabolism may appear in biologic fluids, and hyperammonemia does not appear even under the stress of lysine-loading conditions.

BIBLIOGRAPHY

1. Higashino, K., Tsukada, K., and Lieberman, I.: Saccharopine, a product of lysine breakdown by mammalian liver. Biochem. Biophys. Res. Commun., **20**, 285, 1965.
2. Ghadimi, H., and Zischka, R.: Hyperlysinemia and lysine metabolism, in *Amino Acid Metabolism and Genetic Variation,* edited by W. K. Nyhan, p. 227. McGraw-Hill, New York, 1967.
3. Hutzler, J., and Dancis, J.: Conversion of lysine to saccharopine by human tissues. Biochim. Biophys. Acta, **158**, 62, 1968.
4. Ryan, W. I., and Wells, I. C.: Homocitrulline and homoarginine synthesis from lysine. Science, **144**, 1122, 1964.
5. Rothstein, M., and Miller, L. L.: The conversion of lysine to pipecolic acid in the rat. J. Biol. Chem., **211**, 851, 1954.
6. Paik, W. K., and Benoiton L.: Purification and properties of hog kidney L-lysine acylase. Canad. J. Biochem., **41**, 1643, 1963.
7. Kim, S., Benoiton, L., and Paik, W. K.: L-Alkyllysinase: purification and properties of the enzyme. J. Biol. Chem., **239**, 3790, 1964.
8. Burgi, W., Richterich, R., and Colombo, J. P.: L-Lysine dehydrogenase deficiency in a patient with congenital lysine intolerance. Nature (London), **211**, 854, 1966.

9. Woody, N. C.: Hyperlysinemia. Amer. J. Dis. Child., **108,** 543, 1964.
10. Jagenburg, O. R.: Urinary excretion of free amino acids and other amino compounds by humans. Scand. J. Clin. Lab. Invest., **11,** suppl. 43, 1, 1959.
11. Gatfield, P. D., Taller, E., Hinton, G. G., Wallace, A. C., Abdelnour, G. M., and Houst, M. D.: Hyperpipecolatemia: a new metabolic disorder associated with neuropathy and hepatomegaly. Canad. Med. Ass. J., **99,** 1215, 1968.
12. Hunter, A., and Downs, C. E.: The inhibition of arginase by amino acids. J. Biol. Chem., **157,** 427, 1945.
13. Sen, K. D.: Uremia and its treatment by arginase inhibitor. Nature (London), **184,** 459, 1959.
14. Wilson, L., and Klystra, J. A.: Effect of L-lysine monohydrochloride upon urea formation in two patients with chronic renal failure. Med. J. Aust., **51,** 232, 1963.
15. Cabello, J., Basilio, C., and Prajoux, V.: Kinetic properties of erythrocyte and liver arginase. Biochim. Biophys. Acta, **48,** 148, 1961.
16. Edlbacher, S., Krause, S., and Merz, D. W.: Beitrage zur Kenntnis der Arginase. V. Mitteilung. Das Vorkommen der Arginase in Blut und die Beeinflussung ihrer Wirkung durch Serum. Hoppe Seyler Z. Physiol. Chem., **170,** 68, 1927.
17. Moore, T. W., Rodarte, J., and Smith, L. H.: Urea synthesis by hemic cells. Clin. Chem., **10,** 1059, 1964.
18. Colombo, J. P., Richterich, R., Donath, A., Spahr, A., and Rossi, E.: Congenital lysine intolerance with periodic ammonia intoxication. Lancet, **1,** 1014, 1964.
19. Colombo, J. P., Burgi, W., Richterich, R., and Rossi, E.: Congenital lysine intolerance with periodic ammonia intoxication: a defect in L-lysine degradation. Metabolism, **16,** 910, 1967.
20. McLean, P., Reid, E., and Gurney, M. W.: Effect of azo-dye carcinogenesis on enzymes concerned with urea synthesis in rat liver. Biochem. J., **91,** 464, 1964.
21. Kennan, A., and Cohen, P. P.: Ammonia detoxication in liver from humans. Proc. Soc. Exp. Biol. Med., **106,** 170, 1961.
22. Christensen, H. V.: Free amino acids and peptides in tissues, in *Mammalian Protein Metabolism,* edited by N. N. Munro and J. B. Allison, vol. 1, p. 105. Academic, New York, 1964.
23. Armstrong, M. D., and Robinow, A. M.: A case of hyperlysinemia: biochemical and clinical observations. Pediatrics, **39,** 546, 1967.
24. Carson, N. A., Scally, B. G., Neill, D. W., and Carre, J. J.: Saccharopinuria: a new inborn error of lysine metabolism. Nature (London), **218,** 679, 1968.
25. Ghadimi, H., Binnington, V. I., and Pecora, P.: Hyperlysinemia associated with retardation. New Eng. J. Med., **273,** 723, 1965.
26. Shih, V. E., Efron, M. L., and Moser, H. W.: Hyperornithinemia, hyperammonemia, and homocitrullinuria. Amer. J. Dis. Child., **117,** 83, 1969.
27. Rett, A.: *Ueberein cerebral-atrophistiches Syndrom bei Hyperammonamie.* Verlag Hollinek, Vienna, 1966.
28. Perheentupa, J., and Visakorpi, J. K.: Protein intolerance with deficient transport of basic amino acids. Lancet, **1,** 813, 1965.
29. Kekomaki, M., Visakorpi, J. K., Perheentupa, J., and Saxen, L.: Familial protein intolerance with deficient transport of basic amino acids. Acta Paediat. Scand., **56,** 617, 1967.
30. Ghadimi, H., Kottmeier, P., Achs, R., Prabhu, R., and Jaffe, B.: Hereditary hyperlysinemia and lysine-induced crisis (Abstract 68), 35th Annual Meeting, Society for Pediatric Research, Philadelphia, May, 1965.
31. Woody, N. C.: Hyperlysinemia (abs.), in *Proceedings of the American Pediatric Society,* p. 33, 74th Annual Meeting, Seattle, 1964.
32. Ghadimi, H., Binnington, V. I., and Pecora, P.: Hyperlysinemia associated with mental retardation (abs.), in *Proceedings of the Society for Pediatric Research,* p. 41, 34th Annual Meeting, Seattle, 1964.
33. Woody, N. C., Hutzler, J., and Dancis, J.: Further studies of hyperlysinemia. Amer. J. Dis. Child., **112,** 577, 1966.
34. Ghadimi, H., Partington, M. W., and Hunter, A.: Inborn error of histidine metabolism. Pediatrics, **29,** 714, 1962.
35. Stein, W. H., and Moore, S.: Free amino acids of human blood plasma. J. Biol. Chem., **211,** 915, 1954.
36. Grundig, E.: (Separation process for quantitative determination of keto and amino acids in small amounts of cerebrospinal fluids). Clin. Chem. Acta, **1,** 498, 1962.
37. Stein, W. H., Bearn, A. G., and Moore, S.: Amino acid content of blood and urine in Wilson's disease. J. Clin. Invest., **33,** 410, 1954.
38. Krampitz, G., and Doempfmer, R.: Determination of free amino acids in human ejaculate by ion exchange chromatography. Nature (London), **194,** 684, 1962.
39. Iob, V., McMath, M., and Coon, W. W.: Intra-individual and inter-individual variations in plasma free amino acids in normal adults. J. Surg. Res., **3,** 185, 1963.
40. Soupart, P.: Urinary excretion of free amino acids in normal adult men and women. Clin. Chem. Acta, **4,** 265, 1959.
41. Gross, B., Comfort, M. W., and Ulrich, J. A.: Abnormalities of serum and urinary amino acids in hereditary and non-hereditary pancreatitis. Trans. Ass. Amer. Physicians, **70,** 127, 1957.
42. Evered, D. F.: Excretion of amino acids by human quantitative study with ion exchange chromatography. Biochem. J., **62,** 416, 1956.
43. Woody, N. C., Ong, E. B., and Pupene, M. B.: Paths of lysine degradation in patients with hyperlysinemia. Pediatrics, **40,** 986, 1967.
44. Hsia, D.-Y. Y., Paine, R. S., and Driscoll, K. W.: Phenylketonuria: detection of the heterozygous carrier. J. Ment. Defic. Res., **1** (part 1), 53, 1957.
45. Dancis, J., Hutzler, J., Cox, R., and Woody, N. C.: The metabolic defect in familial hyperlysinemia (abstract), 79th Annual Meeting, American Pediatric Society, May, 1969.

CHAPTER NINETEEN

HOMOCYSTINURIA

Cystathionine Synthase Deficiency

Theo Gerritsen and Harry A. Waisman*

Homocystinuria, an inborn error of sulfur amino acid metabolism, was discovered at about the same time in the United States and in Northern Ireland. Two sibs with homocystinuria, ages 4 and 6 years, were discovered in 1962 by Carson and Neill [1] in a survey of mentally backward persons in Northern Ireland. At the same time a mentally retarded infant with congenital anomalies and failure to thrive was described and homocystine identified in the urine by Gerritsen, Vaughn, and Waisman [2]. More complete descriptions of clinical and laboratory findings in these three patients appeared subsequently [3, 4], and now more than 100 such patients have been reported from all over the world. The disorder may produce only minimal mental or physical abnormality and may be detected first in early adult life.

Homocystinuria may now be considered the second most common inborn error of amino acid metabolism, the first being phenylketonuria. Among adults entering a general medical service it is the most common. The disease is caused by the absence of or a defect in the activity of the liver enzyme cystathionine synthase (E.C. 4.2.1.13) [5]. The multiplicity of clinical signs and symptoms, of which ectopia lentis, mental retardation, thromboembolic phenomena, and the excretion of homocystine are the most outstanding, can be treated with a diet which must at least be low in methionine and supplemented with cystine. Two types of homocystinuria are known, a vitamin B_6–sensitive and a non-vitamin B_6–sensitive form; both types of the disease are inherited as autosomal recessive traits.

*Deceased

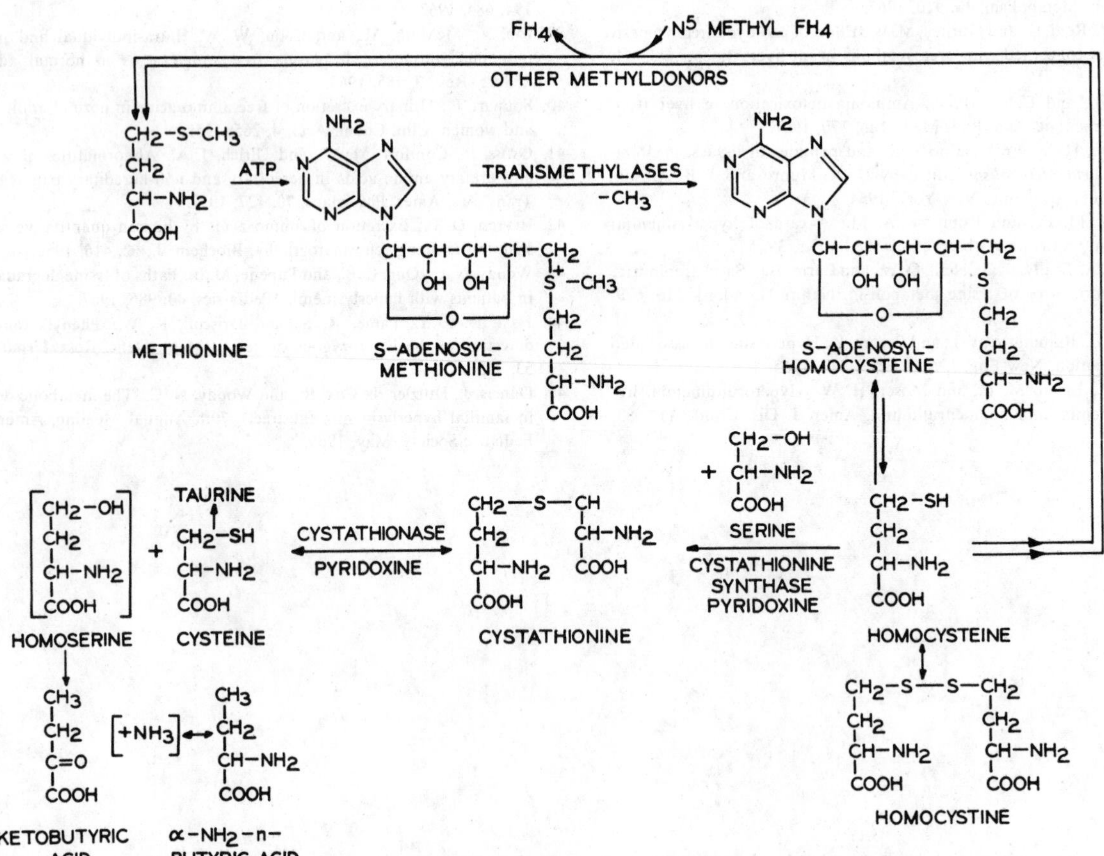

Figure 19-1. Metabolism of methionine in mammals. The formulas in parentheses refer to co-products of the essential reactions which do not take further part in the metabolic pathway under discussion.

METABOLISM OF METHIONINE

The pathways of methionine metabolism are discussed in some detail in Chap. 20. Apart from its structural role in protein synthesis, the amino acid has two major functions in metabolism: as S-adenosylmethionine it is the methyl group donor in the synthesis of compounds such as choline, creatine, N-methylnicotinamide, and epinephrine, and it is also the precursor of cysteine (Fig. 19-1). The intermediate by-product of the various transmethylation reactions is S-adenosylhomocysteine [6]. This compound is hydrolyzed by a specific enzyme to homocysteine and adenosine. The equilibrium of this reaction greatly favors the synthesis of S-adenosylhomocysteine [7]. Two enzymic reactions are known which resynthesize methionine from homocysteine [7*a*] in mammals. Betaine-homocysteine methyltransferase [E.C. 2.1.1.5] requires betaine, a derivative from choline in the 1-carbon cycle, as methyl donor. The methyl groups of choline are derived from methionine, and this vitamin B_{12}-requiring reaction is inhibited by its reaction products, dimethylglycine and methionine. The second reaction which remethylates homocysteine to methionine uses N^5-methyltetrahydrofolate as methyl donor, and seems to be of greater importance than the methylating reaction requiring betaine. This reaction also requires vitamin B_{12}. The main intermediate in the pathway between homocysteine and cysteine is cystathionine, formed from homocysteine and serine with the aid of cystathionine synthase [8]. The equilibrium of this reaction greatly favors cystathionine synthesis. In view of the equilibria of the reactions which form or metabolize homocysteine, it is understandable that under normal conditions little or no free homocysteine accumulates. Cystathionine is cleaved by the vitamin B_6-dependent cystathionase [9] into cysteine and homoserine, and the latter is then deaminated to α-ketobutyrate and ammonia.

Cystine formation from cysteine can be accomplished by cytochrome oxidase, but it is not known whether this enzyme also participates in the formation of homocystine from homocysteine. Homocystine can be formed in vitro by aerobic oxidation of a solution of homocysteine thiolactone. The latter is in equilibrium in acid solution with free homocysteine, the equilibrium being greatly in favor of the lactone. At a neutral or slightly alkaline pH, three products are formed: cystine, homocystine, and the mixed disulfide. The last was identified by Frimpter [10] in the urine of cystinuric patients and is also present in the urine of homocystinuric persons. Since no homocystine is found in the urine of cystinuric persons [10], it is unlikely that the mixed disulfide is formed by oxidation of a cysteine-homocysteine mixture in the body, and it is also improbable that the mixed disulfide is formed by interchange between cystine and homocystine.

Table 19-1. CLINICAL ASPECTS OF HOMOCYSTINURIA

I. Ocular abnormalities
  A. Primary: Ectopia lentis
  B. Secondary
    1. Glaucoma
    2. Myopia
    3. Retinal detachment
    4. Cataracts
II. Skeletal manifestations
  A. Consistently observed
    1. Osteoporosis
    2. Genu valgum
  B. Frequently observed
    1. Dolichostenomelia
    2. Pes cavus
    3. Flatfoot
    4. Scoliosis
    5. Pectus excavatum
III. Central nervous system signs
  A. Frequently observed: Mental retardation
  B. Occasionally observed:
    1. Seizures
    2. Abnormal EEG
    3. Spasticity
IV. Cardiovascular system abnormalities (frequently observed)
  A. Arterial and venous thrombosis
  B. Malar flush
  C. Livedo reticularis
V. Abnormal hair (light, sparse, brittle)
VI. Usual cause of death: Thromboembolic phenomena

CLINICAL ASPECTS

In spite of the variable clinical manifestations of homocystinuria in patients of all ages, certain key signs and symptoms must be considered characteristic of this disease; these are listed in Table 19-1. They fall into three main classes: the connective tissue features (osseous and ocular), the central nervous system manifestations including mental retardation, and the thrombotic features.

Ocular Abnormalities

Ectopia lentis is typically found in homocystinuric patients, usually with downward displacement. Interestingly, dislocated lenses are also found in patients with Marfan's syndrome, but the latter patients may be clearly differentiated from those with homocystinuria. Schimke et al. [11] pointed out that a "small but significant proportion of cases of presumed Marfan's Syndrome have homocystinuria." The ocular changes of homocystinuria probably cannot be distinguished from those of true Marfan's syndrome, since myopia and glaucoma secondary to displaced lenses and retinal detachment may occur in both diseases. Some adults with homocystinuria have no disease manifestations other than ectopia lentis prior to the occurrence of thrombosis. McKusick [11*a*] points out two differences in the lens dislocation between homocystinuria and Marfan's syndrome. In homocystinuria the lens tends to be dislocated downward, and it is an acquired and progressive abnormality. In Marfan's syndrome lens dislocation is usually upward, and the feature is probably congenital.

Johnston [12] has discussed pupil-block glaucoma in homocystinuria and has recommended extraction of the lens for patients with this condition. Not all those with homocystinuria develop glaucoma or need lens extraction. Interestingly, Gaull and Gaitonde [13] were able to demonstrate cystathionine synthase activity in the lens of a patient with homocystinuria, although the enzyme was absent from the liver and brain of the patient. Curtius et al. [14] determined the presence of free amino acids in the aqueous humor of normal subjects and patients with homocystinuria and found that free amino acid concentrations in the aqueous humor were similar to those found in plasma. In patients with homocystinuria considerable amounts of homocystine and markedly elevated levels of methionine were present. Only small traces of cystathionine could be detected in homocystinuric patients, but none was found in controls.

The pathogenesis of the subluxation of the lens in homocystinuria is unexplained. Arnott and Greaves [15] suggested that the zonule of Zinn fails to develop normally because of deficiency of cystine, since the zonular fibers are probably comprised of collagen. It is also possible that the large amount of methionine in the aqueous humor interferes directly with protein metabolism or synthesis in the lens.

Cardiovascular System

Arterial or venous thromboses may be a lethal complication of homocystinuria. Although fibrotic changes have been observed in both the intimal and medial vessels, there is no known explanation for intravascular thrombosis. McDonald et al. [16] found abnormal platelet "stickiness" in patients with homocystinuria, and demonstrated that homocystine enhances platelet stickiness. Other workers failed to find any abnormality in either platelet adhesiveness or platelet survival in homocystinuria. It is of interest that L-homocystine activates Hageman factor, as demonstrated by its capacity to initiate clotting and to form plasmakinins. Intravascular thrombosis may occur in most arteries or veins. Reports include coronary and carotid occlusion, renal artery stenosis with hypertension, inferior vena caval and portal vein thrombosis, and generalized multiple arterial or venous thrombosis [11, 17]. Malar flush is present in most patients, and livedo reticularis of the trunk and extremities is frequent [11].

Central Nervous System

Mental retardation was originally thought to be characteristic of homocystinuria, but later reports indicate that nearly half of affected individuals have normal intelligence [17]. A slight correlation exists between normal intelligence and absence of high blood methionine levels, but this may be accidental. Abnormal EEG patterns and seizures are frequently found but may result from cerebral thrombosis. Histories of psychosis or severe behavioral disorders and schizophrenia appear to be more frequent among relatives of patients with homocystinuria [18]

Skeletal Manifestations

Generalized osteoporosis is present in all patients with homocystinuria. This is unusual in Marfan's syndrome and is a point for differentiating between the two diseases. Long, thin extremities with a decreased upper segment/lower segment ratio, scoliosis, pectus excavatum, genu valgum, vertebral changes, and susceptibility to bone fractures are present in many patients. A peculiar gait because of flatfoot and a wide-based stance is almost specific. Tooth problems are frequent. The palate is highly arched, and the teeth are crowded.

Other Abnormalities

Lighter coloration of hair, eyes, and skin is apparent when the patient is compared with parents or healthy sibs. The hair is sparse and fine and breaks easily. Price [19] described a homocystinuric patient with telangiectasia around scars, abnormal skin crease over terminal interphalangeal joints of the fingers, and abnormal nail-fold capillaries. In general the skin in older patients is coarse, with wide pores. Minor congenital anomalies have been reported in approximately half the patients. The amounts of homocystine excreted in the urine are not high enough to cause urinary stone formation as in cystinuria or cystinosis.

A Clinically Mild Form of Homocystinuria

McKusick et al. [11*a*] have recently reported on four families with a total of eight patients with a mild form of homocystinuria. With one exception these individuals were not mentally retarded (one has a doctorate in psychology), some developed eye problems (ectopia lentis, glaucoma) at a later age, and all had some mild clinical manifestations which became obvious only at ages varing from 3 to about 20 years. Clinically and biochemically all these patients reacted favorably to pyridoxine in amounts up to 400 mg per day. It is improbable, however, that pyridoxine acts by increasing the residual activity of cystathionine synthase [57]. The difference in metabolic defects between this form and the classic form of cystathionine synthase deficiency has not yet been elucidated.

DIAGNOSTIC STUDIES

Qualitative Urine Tests

Urine specimens from patients with homocystinuria give a positive reaction to the cyanide nitroprusside test. (*Test:* 2 ml urine is mixed with 1 ml 5 percent NaCN solution and left to react at room temperature for 10 min. On addition of a few drops of a 5 percent sodium nitroprusside solution, a positive reaction is indicated by development of a beet-red color.) A positive test result indicates that further investigation of the patient is necessary; a negative test excludes the diagnosis of homocystinuria. A modification of the standard cyanide nitroprusside test which is specific for homocystine in the presence of cystine was reported by Spaeth and Barber [20]. This so-called silver nitroprusside test is based on the difference in reactivity of homocystine and cystine to the dismutative action of the silver diamine ion. Urine specimens or aqueous extracts of filter paper strips, which are soaked in urine, dried, and stored for later testing, can be used for this sensitive test.

The presence of homocystine, before or after oxidation to homocysteic acid, can be further confirmed by the usual techniques of two-dimensional paper chromatography, high-voltage electrophoresis, or thin-layer chromatography.

Quantitative Urine and Plasma Tests

The most reliable, simple method for the quantitative estimation of homocystine in urine, and of methionine and homocystine in plasma, is column chromatography using an automatic amino acid analyzer. These analyses will provide quantitative values for homocystine, homocysteine, methionine, cystathionine, cystine, and HCD (homocysteine-cysteine disulfide), and often homolanthionine will be detected. HCD is eluted from the column between leucine and isoleucine. Those who use the new accelerated systems of amino acid analysis or the recently developed beaded resins should ascertain whether proper separation of β-aminoisobutyric acid, homocystine, and β-alanine takes place. In order to estimate the total homocysteine excretion, the homocystine, homocysteine, and half of the HCD amounts should be added together.

A fast, reliable method for determining total homocysteine and total cysteine takes advantage of their oxidation products, homocysteic acid and cysteic acid. This method employs a 20- by 0.9-cm column of an anion-exchange resin (Biorad AG 2-X10) and 0.1*M* chloroacetic acid as eluant [4]. The elution can be performed in only 3 hr and will separate quantitatively the homocysteine of the urine from the cysteine. An accelerated method for determining the homocystine in urine on an automatic amino acid analyzer but without accurate estimation of the other amino acids has been reported by Benson et al. [21].

The urine of normal persons usually does not contain detectable amounts of homocystine. In infants under 1 year of age about 1 mg methionine, 2 mg cystine, 1 mg cystathionine, and 20 mg taurine are excreted daily.

Estimation of Enzyme Activity in Liver Biopsies

Cystathionine synthase activity can be determined in extracts of liver obtained by needle biopsy, according to Mudd et al. [5, 22]. The assay should be performed immediately after the biopsy is obtained. An amount of enzyme extract containing 0.1 to 0.5 mg protein is incubated in Tris buffer at pH 8.3 in a medium containing pyridoxal phosphate, L-homocysteine, L-serine-3-^{14}C, and L-cystathionine. After incubation for 135 min at 37°, the serine and cystathionine are separated by column chromatography, and the radioactivity of the cystathionine is determined. In extracts of homocystinuric livers, no activity was obtained. It is interesting that parents of patients, presumably heterozygous for the metabolic defect, showed about 40 percent of the cystathionine synthase activity found in controls when the enzyme activity was determined in this way [23].

In a later report, Mudd [7*a*] stressed that extracts of homocystinuric liver biopsies have a small residual activity of cystathionine synthase, of the order of 1 to 2 percent of the mean control value. Mudd calculated that this residual activity is sufficient to metabolize a major portion of the homocysteine arising from the normal dietary intake of methionine, and should not be neglected in attempts to decide by which pathways methionine is being metabolized by patients with homocystinuria.

Tissue Culture Studies

Cystathionine synthase activity could not be demonstrated in leukocytes, erythrocytes, platelets, or skin biopsies, but Uhlendorf and Mudd [24] showed that the enzyme is easily detectable in fibroblasts cultivated from the skin and from cells in amniotic fluid. Skin from homocystinuric patients produced fibroblast lines with low or undetectable cystathionine synthase activity. This finding indicates that tissue culture of amniotic cells can be used to predict whether the child in utero is homocystinuric.

BIOCHEMICAL ABNORMALITIES AND THE METABOLIC DEFECT

Amino Acid Abnormalities

Investigations of many patients with homocystinuria have demonstrated that the characteristic biochemical findings are the excretion of homocystine in the urine and the occurrence of homocystine and of elevated concentrations of methionine in the plasma. Since homocystine has a high renal clearance, plasma levels are usually low. The presence of homocysteine can be demonstrated only in fresh plasma, and this is easier after oxidation of the compound to S-carboxymethylhomocysteine with iodoacetic acid [25]. Methionine blood levels in homocystinuria can go as high as 30 mg per 100 ml, while homocystine blood levels of 5 mg per 100 ml are considered high and are seen only in severe, untreated cases [25, 26]. In order to calculate the total urinary excretion of homocyst(e)ine one must add together the homocysteine (if present), homocystine, and the homocysteine part of the cysteine–homocysteine mixed disulfide (HCD). When the total excretion of homocyst(e)ine is estimated in this way, it may come to 300 mg homocystine per day in a homocystinuric patient.

The Enzyme Defect

In 1964 Mudd et al. [5] demonstrated that the metabolic defect in homocystinuria is the absence or deficiency of the enzyme cystathionine synthase in the liver. This enzyme, which is not identical with the L-serine hydrolyase in mammals [27], was not found in skin, leukocytes, erythrocytes, or platelets of rats or normal man, but activity could be demonstrated, together with activity of the so-called methionine-activating enzyme [adenosine triphosphate (ATP): L-methionine, S-adenosyl transferase; E.C. 2.4.2.13], in homogenates of liver obtained by needle biopsy or at autopsy. In a liver biopsy from a patient with homocystinuria, the methionine-activating enzyme was found to be of normal or even increased activity, but no cystathionine synthase activity could be demonstrated. This finding has now been confirmed by many workers. Finkelstein et al. [23] reported that in several presumed heterozygotes the cystathionine synthase activity was about 40 percent of the level of control subjects.

The result of the enzyme deficiency is a lack of cystathionine synthesis at the cellular level. The importance of cellular synthesis of cystathionine is unknown: insufficient knowledge is available about the physiologic role which cystathionine plays in the metabolism of cells, especially those of the central nervous system. The cystathionine content of normal human brain is surprisingly high [28], but Gerritsen and Waisman [29] failed to find cystathionine in the brain of a homocystinuric child examined at autopsy. This has been confirmed by others [30]. It is therefore of great interest that Wong et al. [31] discovered that it is possible for a homocystinuric patient to synthesize cystathionine from homoserine and cysteine, probably by the enzyme cystathionase. Some of the metabolic consequences of cystathionine synthase deficiency were explored by Laster et al. [32]. As expected, they found an impaired capacity to convert methionine sulfur into urinary inorganic sulfate, but formation of inorganic sulfate from cystine was normal. Strangely, upon administration of methionine to a homocystinuric patient, there was no marked increase of homocystine excretion. Large amounts of methionine and methionine sulfoxide accumulated in the plasma and were excreted in the urine for several days after discontinuation of the methionine supplement. The amounts of other sulfur-containing compounds in the urine, some of which were unidentified, exceeded by far the quantity of homocystine found.

Only a small fraction of the daily dietary intake of methionine in a patient with homocystinuria can be accounted for in the excretion of known sulfur-containing compounds and the amount which is used for protein synthesis. It was therefore of great importance when Perry et al. [33, 34] discovered several sulfur-containing compounds in the urine of homocystinuric patients and isolated and analyzed at least four of them. These were S-adenosylhomocysteine, homolanthionine, and 5-amino-4-imidazolecarboxamide-5′-S-homocysteinylribonucleoside (AICHR), the formulas of which are shown in Fig. 19-2, and α-hydroxy-γ-mercaptobutyrate-homocysteine disulfide,

$$HOOC{-}CH(OH){-}CH_2{-}CH_2{-}S{-}S{-}CH_2{-}CH_2{-}CH(NH_2){-}COOH$$

which has recently been identified [34*a*]. The presence of S-adenosylhomocysteine is not unexpected, but this was the first time that it was detected in physiologic fluids in man. The enzyme which hydrolyzes S-adenosylhomocysteine to adenosine and homocysteine can also condense these two substances to S-adenosylhomocysteine [7], a reaction which greatly favors the formation of the latter compound. Homolanthionine, a higher homologue of cystathionine, could be formed by the condensation of homocysteine and homoserine. It would be interesting if it could be demonstrated that in homocystinuric patients the enzyme cystathionine synthase is not absent but only slightly altered in order to permit the condensation of homocysteine with homoserine instead of serine [33]. The metabolic origin of AICHR has not yet been clarified. One further compound isolated by Perry from the urine of homocystinuric patients remains unidentified, and there may be others which have not yet been detected. Identification of these compounds may provide more knowledge about the normal and abnormal metabolism of methionine and perhaps yield clues to the causation of the signs and symptoms of the disease. Several homocystinuric patients are thriving on a diet low in methionine without supplements of cystathionine or homoserine. From this observation one may conclude that the lack of cystathionine in the brain is not directly related to the clinical manifestations of homocystinuria.

Reference to this disease by the name, *cystathionine syn*

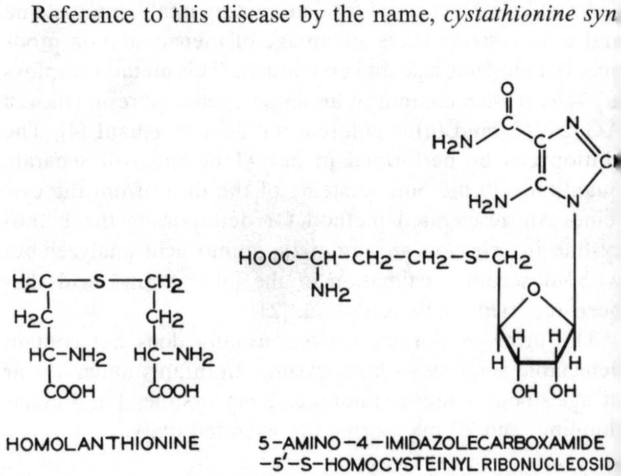

HOMOLANTHIONINE

$$\begin{array}{ccc} H_2C & -S- & CH_2 \\ | & & | \\ H_2C & & CH_2 \\ | & & | \\ HC{-}NH_2 & & HC{-}NH_2 \\ | & & | \\ COOH & & COOH \end{array}$$

5-AMINO-4-IMIDAZOLECARBOXAMIDE-5′-S-HOMOCYSTEINYL RIBONUCLEOSIDE

$$HOOC{-}CH(NH_2){-}CH_2{-}CH_2{-}S{-}CH_2{-}\text{ribose (H, H, H, H; OH OH)}{-}\text{imidazole}(C(=O)NH_2,\ H_2N)$$

Figure 19-2. Structural formulas of unusual S-containing amino acids isolated from the urine of homocystinuric patients by Perry [33, 34]. The formula of S-adenosylhomocysteine can be seen in Fig. 19-1.

thase deficiency, will prevent confusion with other defects in which homocystine is also excreted. An example of such a disease is N^5-methyltetrahydrofolate-methyltransferase deficiency. In this metabolic error, homocystinuria is accompanied by excessive concentrations of cystathionine in plasma and urine and low methionine plasma levels [7*a*].

PATHOLOGY

Autopsy findings in eight patients with homocystinuria have been reported [35–39]. Characteristically, recurrent arterial and venous thromboses were found in almost any part of the body and accounted for the varied clinical features, such as "encephalitis," "meningitis," pyelonephritis, diffuse myocardial fibrosis, and so on. Surgery should always be considered hazardous in homocystinuric patients.

Komrower and Wilson reported a pulmonary embolus and an ante-mortem thrombus in the right femoral vein of their patient [35]. Chou and Waisman [36] demonstrated spongy degeneration of the central nervous system as a prominent finding in the first known American case of homocystinuria [4]. Widespread vacuolization in the subcortical white matter of the cerebrum and a defective myelin pattern throughout were seen in this study, as were micropolygyric areas in the cortex.

In a well-documented review of 10 cases by Carson et al. [37], the autopsy findings on a 9½-year-old girl revealed these major findings: patchy fibrosis of the intima of blood vessels, degeneration of the elastic fibers of arteries, degenerative changes of the zonular fibers of the eye lens, many old and recent thromboemboli, and fatty changes in the liver. The most obvious alteration in the brain was in the gray matter, with the most striking focal necrosis and gliosis in the midbrain.

Gibson et al. [38] reported autopsy findings on a 7-year-old boy who died of infarction of the left kidney secondary to left renal artery thrombosis. Findings in all other organs were similar to those reported by Carson et al. [37]. Henkind and Ashton [38*a*] showed histologically that the zonular fibers in homocystinuric eyes had recoiled to the surface of the ciliary body where they lay matted and retracted into a feltwork which fused with a greatly thickened ciliary epithelium. Under electron microscopy the fibers appeared disorganized and granular.

In an extensive clinical and pathologic study of nine patients in six families Carey et al. [39] reported on the autopsy findings in an 11-year-old girl who died of coronary occlusion after surgery for thrombosis of an aortic bifurcation. The patient had encephalomalacia from recurrent cortical venous thromboses. The kidneys showed fresh infarcts. There were recent thromboses in the large arteries, but no macroscopic cross-ridging of the aorta and major vessels, as has been reported by others. In the other eight living patients, the authors mention several conditions not found before in homocystinuria: chronic pyelonephritis, gluten enteropathy, chronic cor pulmonale, and "tissue-paper" scarring of the skin. A variable degree of mild hepatocellular dysfunction was commonly found. In four of the nine cases serum fibrinogen levels were elevated.

In a study of 20 families with 38 homocystinuric patients by Schimke et al. [11] autopsy was performed on 3 of the 10 who died. In these three, severe medial changes, with dilatation and thrombosis, were present in various large arteries. The media were thin, and the muscle fibers of the media were wildly separated by expansion of the intracellular ground substance. In at least two cases extensive left atrial endocardial fibroelastosis was found. All autopsied cases showed fatty degeneration of the liver.

GENETICS

Homocystinuria has been found in persons of Northern and Western European, Italian, Russian, Negro, Jewish, Japanese, and Spanish-American parentage [17]. From the clinical reports of a large number of patients since the disease was discovered in 1962, one may conclude that the homocystinuria gene is present in rather high frequency. A rough estimate of the incidence is one in 20,000 to 40,000 live births, as compared with one in 15,000 for phenylketonuria.

Because the enzyme cystathionine synthase is deficient in the liver and the brain of patients with homocystinuria, it was of interest that Gaull and Gaitonde [13] found enzyme activity in the lens of the eye of their patient. This may be an example of multiplicity of gene control of the synthesis of cystathionine synthase.

In 1967 Schimke et al. [17] reported an extended study on 68 patients with homocystinuria in a total of 36 families. There were several affected sibs, and the sex distribution was approximately equal. There were several cases of suspected consanguinity and occasional instances in which it was proved. No evidence of two-generation transmission was found. Segregation analysis of the available pedigrees according to standard genetic techniques, combined with the other evidence, is compatible with autosomal recessive inheritance. There is also biochemical support for this mode of inheritance from the finding of intermediate enzyme activity values in a number of parents of homocystinuric patients, indicative of single-gene dosage effect in presumed heterozygotes.

Under normal conditions it is impossible to distinguish heterozygotes from controls using the methionine or homocystine blood levels, or the excretion of homocystine in the urine. More data are needed to permit decision as to whether methionine loading tests are of value. Carson found occasional excretion of homocystine in the urine, or abnormally elevated plasma methionine levels with delayed clearance, after administration of methionine loads to parents of homocystinurics. This test had not been consistent enough for the determination of heterozygosity among sibs of affected persons. Up to now the best way to do this is by estimation of cystathionine synthase activity from a liver biopsy [23]. In a heterozygote this enzyme should have an activity of about 40 percent of the levels found in controls [40]. An alternative to the use of a liver biopsy is the estimation of enzyme activity in fibroblasts obtained by culturing of skin tissue [7*a*].

DIETARY TREATMENT

The problem of dietary treatment of homocystinuria is much more complex than that of phenylketonuria, histidinemia, or even branched-chain ketoaciduria. Although it is not yet known which biochemical products cause the brain damage and other anatomic abnormalities in homocystinuria, the dietary treatment has to deal with the following facts. When patients with homocystinuria are fed a normal diet, methionine and homocystine accumulate in their body fluids and tissues. Also, the enzyme block prevents the normal formation of cystathionine [29, 30] and cystine, and patients with homocystinuria require cystine as an essential amino acid [41]. Furthermore it may be possible that in certain cases the enzyme block is due to a decreased affinity of the apoenzyme for the coenzyme pyridoxine phosphate. With these factors in mind, one might prescribe one of the following possible diets for a homocystinuric patient:

1 A diet low in methionine
2 A diet high in cystine
3 A low-methionine diet to which cystine is added
4 A low-methionine diet to which cystine and cystathionine or homoserine are added
5 A diet, very low in methionine, to which cystine and massive doses of the methyl-group donor choline are added
6 A normal diet with massive doses of pyridoxine

It seems inappropriate to decrease the methionine intake without providing the "essential" amino acid cystine or to add cystine to a normal diet without preventing the formation of large amounts of homocystine from methionine. Therefore, the first two diets would seem unwise on purely biochemical grounds. The third diet, one low in methionine (20 to 40 mg per kg per day) but supplemented with L-cystine or the more soluble Ca-cystinate (100 to 200 mg per kg per day), was successfully used by Perry et al. [42] and by Komrower et al. [43], starting shortly after the patient's birth. The patient of Komrower et al. had normal intelligence and was healthy after 2 years of this treatment, and the patient of Perry et al. at age 5 was also normal. Both groups were of the opinion that the patients should be kept on the diet indefinitely since at any later age cessation of the diet might cause difficulty. Evaluation of diet therapy is made difficult, however, by the fact that many untreated patients show normal intelligence, and that some may reach early adult life with only ectopia lentis or asymptomatic osteoporosis.

The fourth program, a low-methionine diet with supplemental cystathionine, has been considered by us [44] but should be discarded for several reasons: (1) Cystathionine, apart from its function as an intermediate in the methionine pathway, has no known role in human metabolism. It is present in brain tissue, but it is not known whether it plays a role in the functioning of this organ. (2) It is known to have a high kidney clearance. (3) Its cost would undoubtedly prevent long-term high-dosage administration to a patient. Wong et al. [31] discovered that homocystinuric patients have a normally active cystathionase system and can synthesize cystathionine from homoserine and cystine. They suggest adding homoserine to the low-methionine, cystine-supplemented diet, since this might permit synthesis of cystathionine at the cellular level and in this way possibly prevent tissue damage.

The fifth dietary variation for the treatment of homocystinuria, the addition of a methyl donor to a diet low in methionine and supplemented with cystine, is based on the assumption that most of the clinical manifestations of the disease are caused by the high homocystine levels in the plasma or by its metabolites, and that the high methionine levels are of secondary importance. Carey et al. [45] attempted to promote remethylation of homocysteine to methionine by the use of folic acid, after they had demonstrated low serum folate levels in eight homocystinuric children. Serum homocystine levels were apparently lowered by this treatment Perry et al. [46] report on the use of a diet providing only 10 mg methionine per kg per day supplemented by *l*-cystine (1.5 gm per day) and large doses of choline (up to 10 gm per day). Choline, the precursor of betaine and dimethylglycine, provides active methyl groups for the enzymic remethylation of homocysteine to methionine (Fig. 19-1). The administration of choline to the patients who were on a low-methionine diet caused a rise in plasma methionine concentration (from about 3 mg per 100 ml to pretreatment levels of 6 to 18 mg per 100 ml) and further reduction in plasma homocystine to less than one-third of the original levels. It is not known whether this method of reducing homocystine and increasing methionine concentrations in the blood of an already damaged patient with homocystinuria will still improve health and prolong life.

Addition of massive doses of vitamin B_6 or pyridoxine to a normal diet has been reported from several centers. Barber and Spaeth [47] completely reversed the biochemical abnormalities in three patients with confirmed homocystinuria with dosages of 250 and 500 mg pyridoxine daily. Hooft et al. [48] obtained good biochemical results with 500 mg pyridoxine daily in a 10-year-old patient, but in another patient these investigators failed to lower homocystine blood levels, although the methionine levels decreased to almost normal. Turner [49] was unable to confirm any effect by pyridoxine on the biochemistry of two unrelated patients, aged 4 and 9, who had previously been on a restricted protein diet. The variability was explained by the possibility that there are different genetic expressions of the disease. Gaull [50] had an opportunity to investigate the two pyridoxine-responsive sibs described by Barber and Spaeth [47]; he confirmed that biochemical control could be obtained with 200 mg pyridoxine on a diet containing 105 mg methionine per kg per day. Methionine loading tests before and after pyridoxine treatment suggested that the metabolism of methionine was improved but was still abnormal and that pyridoxine exerted its effect more on the metabolism of homocystine than on methionine. They also proved by in vitro experiments on liver biopsies from these patients that pyridoxine did not improve or restore the absent cystathionine synthase activity. Gaull et al. [50] concluded that the added pyridoxine did not have a direct effect on the cystathionine synthase activity, but that in some patients it has an unexplained effect on the homocystine and methionine blood levels. Hollowell et al. [51] reported that administration of vitamin B_{12} and folic acid also resulted in a decrease in excretion of homocystine, although not to such a degree as with pyridoxine. Carson and Carré [52] treated 11 patients with high doses of oral pyridoxine; 6 patients responded biochemically as shown by the return of the plasma amino acid pattern to near-normal. Five patients showed no response. The type of biochemical response was uniform in all affected members of one family. Carson suggested that in those patients who respond biochemically to pyridoxine treatment, the disorder may be another example of "a pyridoxine-dependency syndrome." The clinical effectiveness of pyridoxine treatment in newborn infants with homocystinuria has not been investigated.

Sufficient experience has already shown that newborn patients with homocystinuria can be kept on a diet low in methionine and supplemented by cystine for extended periods with good results. Also, sufficient data have been obtained with treatment of homocystinuria with pyridoxine to warrant a closely supervised trial period on a normal protein diet supplemented with pyridoxine. In this way it may be possible to ascertain whether the patient belongs to the "pyridoxine-sensitive" group. The value of the addition of choline to the diet can be judged only after comparison with the use of choline-free diets. The value of adding homoserine to the diet is uncertain, but increasing the cellular cystathionine level can certainly not be harmful.

SUMMARY

1 The disease homocystinuria is the result of an inborn error in the metabolism of methionine. Patients with this disease excrete homocystine in the urine and have increased levels of methionine in the plasma. The most important clinical manifestations are ectopia lentis, osteoporosis, thromboembolic phenomena, and in a majority of patients mental retardation.

2 The basic defect is an inactivity of hepatic cystathionine synthase, which prevents formation of cystathionine from homocysteine and serine. The deficiency of cystathionine synthase activity can be demonstrated in liver.

3 Diagnosis is based on the urinary excretion of up to 300 mg homocysteine + homocystine per 24 hr, and in most cases on an increased level of methionine in the blood.

4 In all patients who came to autopsy recurrent arterial and venous thromboses were found.

5 The mode of inheritance of homocystinuria is autosomal recessive.

6 The clinical and pathologic consequences of homocystinuria can be prevented by a diet, which should be started as early in life as possible. This diet should be low in methionine and high in cystine.

7 At least two types of homocystinuria have been recognized. One is pyridoxine-sensitive: the other fails to respond to addition of pyridoxine to the diet.

BIBLIOGRAPHY

1. Carson, N. A. J., and Neill, D. W.: Metabolic abnormalities detected in a survey of mentally backward individuals in Northern Ireland. Arch. Dis. Child., **37**, 505, 1962.
2. Gerritsen, T., Vaughn, J. G., and Waisman, H. A.: The identification of homocystine in the urine. Biochem. Biophys. Res. Commun., **9**, 493, 1962.
3. Carson, N. A. J., Cusworth, D. C., Dent, C. E., Field, C. M. B., Neill, D. W., and Westall, R. G.: Homocystinuria: a new inborn error of metabolism associated with mental deficiency. Arch. Dis. Child., **38**, 425, 1963.
4. Gerritsen, T., and Waisman, H. A.: Homocystinuria: an error in the metabolism of methionine. Pediatrics, **33**, 413, 1964.
5. Mudd, S. H., Finkelstein, J. D., Irreverre, F., and Laster, L.: Homocystinuria: an enzymatic defect. Science, **143**, 1443, 1964.
6. Cantoni, G. L., and Scarano, E.: The formation of S-adenosylhomocysteine in enzymatic transmethylation reactions. J. Amer. Chem. Soc., **76**, 4744, 1954.
7. De la Haba, G., and Cantoni, G. L.: The enzymatic synthesis of S-adenosyl-L-homocysteine from adenosine and homocysteine. J. Biol. Chem., **234**, 603, 1959.

7*a*. Mudd, S. H.: Homocystinuria: the known causes, in *Inherited Disorders of Sulphur Metabolism,* Proc. 8th Symposium of the Society for the Study of Inborn Errors of Metabolism, Belfast, 1970, edited by N. A. J. Carson and D. N. Raine, Livingstone, London, 1971.

8. Binkley, F.: Synthesis of cystathionine by preparation from rat liver. J. Biol. Chem., **191**, 531, 1951.
9. Matsuo, Y., and Greenberg, D. M.: A crystalline enzyme that cleaves homoserine and cystathionine. J. Biol. Chem., **230**, 545, 561, 1958.
10. Frimpter, G. W.: The disulfide of L-cysteine and L-homocysteine in urine of patients with cystinuria. J. Biol. Chem., **236**, PC51, 1961.
11. Schimke, R. M., McKusick, V. A., Huang, T., and Pollack, A. D.: Homocystinuria. Studies of 20 families with 38 affected members. J. Amer. Med. Ass., **193**, 711, 1965.

11*a*. McKusick, V. A., Hall, J. G., and Char, F.: The clinical and genetic characteristics of homocystinuria, in *Inherited Disorders of Sulphur Metabolism,* Proc. 8th Symposium of the Society for the Study of Inborn Errors of Metabolism, Belfast, 1970, edited by N. A. J. Carson and D. N. Raine. Livingstone, London, 1971.

12. Johnston, S. S.: Pupil-block glaucoma in homocystinuria. Brit. J. Ophthal., **52**, 251, 1968.
13. Gaull, G., and Gaitonde, M. K.: Homocystinuria: an observation on the inheritance of cystathionine synthetase deficiency. J. Med. Genet., **3**, 194, 1966.

14. Curtius, H-CH, Martenet, A. C., and Anders, P. W.: Bestimmung von freien Aminosaüren im Augenkammerwasser des Menschen bei Homocystinurie—Patienten und Kontrollfallen. Clin. Chim. Acta, **19,** 469, 1968.
15. Arnott, E. J., and Greaves, D. P.: Ocular involvement in homocystinuria. Brit. J. Ophthal., **48,** 688, 1964.
16. McDonald, L., Bray, C., Field, C., Love, F., and Davies, B.: Homocystinuria, thrombosis and the blood-platelets. Lancet, **1,** 745, 1964.
17. Schimke, R. M., McKusick, V. A., and Weilbaecher, R. G.: Homocystinuria, in *Amino Acid Metabolism and Genetic Variation,* edited by W. L. Nyhan. McGraw-Hill, New York, 1967.
18. Dunn, H. G., Perry, T. L., and Dolman, C. L.: Homocystinuria: a recently discovered cause of mental defect and cerebrovascular thrombosis. Neurol., **16,** 407, 1966.
19. Price, J., Vickers, C. F. H., and Brooker, B. K.: A case of homocystinuria with noteworthy dermatological features. J. Ment. Defic. Res., **12,** 111, 1968.
20. Spaeth, G. L., and Barber, G. W.: Prevalence of homocystinuria among the mentally retarded: evaluation of a specific screening test. Pediatrics, **40,** 586, 1967.
21. Benson, J. V., Carmick, J., and Patterson, J. A.: Accelerated chromatography of amino acids associated with phenylketonuria, leucinosis (maple syrup urine disease) and other inborn errors of metabolism. Analyt. Biochem., **18,** 481, 1967.
22. Mudd, S. H., Finkelstein, J. D., Irreverre, F., and Laster, L.: Transsulfuration in mammals. Microassays and tissue distribution of three enzymes in the pathway. J. Biol. Chem., **240,** 4382, 1965.
23. Finkelstein, J. D., Mudd, S. H., Irreverre, F., and Laster, L.: Homocystinuria due to cystathionine synthetase deficiency: the mode of inheritance. Science, **146,** 785, 1964.
24. Uhlendorf, B. W., and Mudd, S. H.: Cystathionine synthetase in tissue culture, derived from human skin: enzyme defect in homocystinuria. Science, **160,** 1007, 1968.
25. Perry, T. L., Hansen, S., MacDougall, L., and Warrington, P. D.: Sulfur-containing amino acids in the plasma and urine of homocystinurics. Clin. Chim. Acta, **15,** 409, 1967.
26. Werder, E. A., Curtius, H. C., Tancredi, F., Anders, P. W., and Prader, A.: Homocystinurie. Helv. Paediat. Acta, **21,** 1, 1966.
27. Finkelstein, J. D.: Methionine metabolism in mammals: effects of age, diet and hormones on three enzymes of the pathway in rat tissues. Arch. Biochem. Biophys., **122,** 583, 1967.
28. Tallan, H. H., Moore, S., and Stein, W. H.: L-Cystathionine in human brain. J. Biol. Chem., **230,** 707, 1958.
29. Gerritsen, T., and Waisman, H. A.: Homocystinuria: absence of cystathionine in the brain. Science, **145,** 588, 1964.
30. Brenton, D. P., Cusworth, D. C., and Gaull, G. E.: Homocystinuria: biochemical studies of tissues including a comparison with cystathioninuria. Pediatrics, **35,** 50, 1965.
31. Wong, P. W. K., Schwarz, V., and Komrower, G. M.: The biosynthesis of cystathionine in patients with homocystinuria. Pediat. Res., **2,** 149, 1968.
32. Laster, L., Mudd, S. H., Finkelstein, J. D., and Irreverre, F.: Homocystinuria due to cystathionine-synthetase deficiency: the metabolism of L-methionine. J. Clin. Invest., **44,** 1708, 1965.
33. Perry, T. L., Hansen, S., and MacDougall, L.: Homolanthionine excretion in homocystinuria. Science, **152,** 1750, 1966.
34. Perry, T. L.: Unsolved problems in homocystinuria, in *Amino Acid Metabolism and Genetic Variation,* edited by W. L. Nyhan. McGraw-Hill, New York, 1967.
34*a*. Perry, T. L.: Unusual sulphur containing amino acids in homocystinuria, in *Inherited Disorders of Sulphur Metabolism,* Proc. 8th Symposium of the Society for the Study of Inborn Errors of Metabolism, Belfast, 1970, edited by N. A. J. Carson and D. N. Raine. Livingstone, London, 1971.
35. Komrower, G. M., and Wilson, V. K.: Homocystinuria. Proc. Roy. Soc. Med., **56,** 996, 1963.
36. Chou, S. M., and Waisman H. A.: Spongy degeneration of the central nervous system: case of homocystinuria. Arch. Path., **79,** 357, 1965.
37. Carson, N. A. J., Dent, C. E., Field, C. M. B., and Gaull, G. E.: Homocystinuria: clinical and pathological review of ten cases. J. Pediat., **66,** 565, 1965.
38. Gibson, J. B., Carson, N. A. J., and Neill, D. W.: Pathological findings in homocystinuria. J. Clin. Path., **17,** 427, 1964.
38*a*. Henkind, P. and Ashton, N.: Ocular pathology in homocystinuria. Trans. Ophthal. Soc. UK, **85,** 21, 1965.
39. Carey, M. C., Donovan, D. E., Fitzgerald, O., and McAuley, F. D.: Homocystinuria. I. A clinical and pathological study of nine subjects in six families. Amer. J. Med., **45,** 7, 1968.
40. Laster, L., Spaeth, G. L., Mudd, S. H., and Finkelstein, J. D.: Homocystinuria due to cystathionine synthetase deficiency. Ann. Intern. Med., **63,** 1117, 1965.
41. Brenton, D. P., Cusworth, D. C., Dent, C. E., and Jones, E. E.: Homocystinuria: clinical and dietary studies. Quart. J. Med., **35,** 325, 1966.
42. Perry, T. L., Dunn, H. G., Hansen, S., MacDougall, L., and Warrington, P. D.: Early diagnosis and treatment of homocystinuria, Pediatrics, **37,** 502, 1966.
43. Komrower, G. M., Lambert, A. M., Cusworth, D. C., and Westall, R. G.: Dietary treatment of homocystinuria. Arch. Dis. Child., **41,** 66, 1966.
44. Waisman, H. A.: Some theoretical considerations in the treatment of homocystinuria. Amer. J. Dis. Child., **113,** 101, 1967.
45. Carey, M., Fennelly, J. J., and Fitzgerald, O.: Homocystinuria. II. Subnormal serum folate levels, increased folate clearance and effects of folic acid therapy. Amer. J. Med., **45,** 26, 1968.
46. Perry, T. L., Hansen, S., Love, D. L., Crawford, L. E., and Tischler, B.: Treatment of homocystinuria with a low methionine diet, supplemental cystine, and a methyl donor. Lancet, **2,** 474, 1968.
47. Barber, G. W., and Spaeth, G. L.: Pyridoxine therapy in homocystinuria. Lancet, **1,** 337, 1967.
48. Hooft, C., Carton, D., and Samyn, W.: Pyridoxine treatment in homocystinuria. Lancet, **1,** 1385, 1967.
49. Turner, B.: Pyridoxine treatment in homocystinuria. Lancet, **2,** 1151, 1967.
50. Gaull, G. E., Rassin, D. K., and Sturman, J. A.: Pyridoxine-dependency in homocystinuria. Lancet, **2,** 1302, 1968.
51. Hollowell, J. G., Coryell, M. E., Hall, W. K., Findley, J. K., and Thevaos, T. G.: Homocystinuria as affected by pyridoxine, folic acid and vitamin B_{12}. Proc. Soc. Exp. Biol. Med., **129,** 327, 1968.
52. Carson, N. A. J., and Carré, I. J.: Treatment of homocystinuria with pyridoxine. Arch. Dis. Child., **44,** 387, 1969.

CHAPTER TWENTY

CYSTATHIONINURIA, SULFITE OXIDASE DEFICIENCY, AND "β-MERCAPTOLACTATE-CYSTEINE DISULFIDURIA"*

George W. Frimpter

This chapter is concerned with three rare disorders of the metabolism of the sulfur-containing amino acids: cystathioninuria, sulfite oxidase deficiency, and a disorder with β-mercaptolactate-cysteine disulfide in the urine. Only a single occurrence of each of the latter two disorders has been recorded. These diseases have little in common, either clinically or biochemically, with other disturbances of the metabolic pathways of the sulfur-containing amino acids such as homocystinuria and cystinuria.

CYSTATHIONINURIA

Incidence

Familial cystathioninuria has now been described in several patients [1–10]. The major clinical features are summarized in Table 20-1. In addition to these patients, subjects who are probably heterozygotes for cystathioninuria have been detected in kindreds with cystinuria by Frimpter [11], and with iminoaciduria by Scriver [12]. Schneiderman described a family with varying degrees of cystathioninuria as determined by paper chromatography after methionine loading [13]. Some of the family members were mentally retarded. It is possible that these patients are heterozygotes; the lack of quantitative measurements of cystathionine limits interpretations. Schneiderman screened 50 mentally retarded patients and 50 healthy volunteers with a methionine tolerance test. From the former he identified the two brothers in his study, and also found two brothers among the healthy subjects who excreted some cystathionine after the load. This limited sample indicates an overall incidence of the trait of about 4 percent. If one assumes that the affected individuals are heterozygotes, then the incidence of homozygous persons would be much higher (i.e., about 4 per 10,000) than has been generally believed.

Table 20-1 reveals that the patients homozygous for cystathioninuria thus far discovered have had very little in common. There are a few with mental retardation, developmental defects, endocrinopathy, and thrombocytopenia, but no consistent clinical picture has emerged. Two patients (9 and 10) are normal physically and mentally. These children, although biochemically abnormal, indicate the wide variation which is present within the phenotype.

Other Occurrences of Cystathioninuria

Cystathionine may appear in the urine as a manifestation of other disease; this not only is a potential problem in differential diagnosis, but bears on the biochemical mechanism of the familial type. Cystathioninuria has been described in cretinism by Fourman, Summerscales, and Morgan [14], and during a thyroxine load by Gjessing [15], as well as in certain functional neoplasms of neural tissue, especially neuroblastomas [16]. Gjessing observed that the degree of cystathioninuria seems to be related to the amount of malignant tissue which is present [17]. The production of cystathionine by these tumors is probably related to the high concentration which normally occurs in human nervous tissue (see further on).

Identification in Reported Cases

Elaborate techniques were used by investigators of the first few patients to identify cystathionine in the urine. Harris, Penrose, and Thomas [1] used paper chromatography, and after preparative chromatography on heavy paper, they treated the eluted material with Raney nickel. Two-dimensional paper chromatography yielded equimolar amounts of α-alanine and α-aminobutyric acid.

Frimpter, Haymovitz, and Horwith [2] used various ion-exchange resins as well as paper chromatography. The compound was purified from the urine by ion-exchange resins according to the method of Hope [18]. The isolated material was recrystallized three times from 50 percent ethanol, treated with cyanide to remove traces of disulfide [19], further recrystallized, and finally passed through Dowex 2 (acetate) to remove traces of chloride and resins picked up during the preparatory work [20]. In this way several hundred milligrams of pure material was obtained. Elemental analysis was compatible with cystathionine, as follows [21]:

Calculated for										
($C_7H_{14}N_2O_4S$):	C	37.82	H	6.35	H	12.61	O	28.79	S	14.43
Found:		37.52		6.37		12.50		28.78		14.15

The specific rotation in 1*N* HCl was +23.4°. Since cystathionine has two α-amino groups, it has four possible stereoisomeric configurations, as follows:

*The writer's studies were supported in part by Grants H-04148, FR-47, AM-08404, and AM-13923, from the National Institutes of Health, Public Health Service; by a grant from The National Foundation; and by an Established Investigatorship of The American Heart Association and a Senior Research Fellowship of The New York Heart Association, both at Cornell University Medical College.

Table 20-1. SUMMARY OF PATIENTS WITH CYSTATHIONINURIA

Patient's no.	Author	Age, yr	Sex	Clinical features	Mental status	Family involvement	Response to vitamin B_6	Liver enzyme
1	Harris et al., 1959 [1]	64	Female	Talipes calcaneo valgus, hypo-pituitarism	Imbecilic	Yes		
2	Frimpter et al., 1963 [2]	44	Male	Defects about ears, heart murmur, thrombocytopenia, acromegaly	"Aberrations"	Yes; brother of Patient 4	Yes	Low (64) Increased with PLP*
3	Berlow, 1966 [3]	14	Male	Regression, grand mal epilepsy, hypothyroid	IQ, 35–50		Yes	Low (65, 66)
4	Frimpter, 1966 [4]	49	Female	Heart disease, died of "stroke"	Paranoid(?)	Yes; sister of Patient 2		
5	Mongeau et al., 1966 [5]	1½	Male	Thrombocytopenia, renal calculi	Normal	Yes	Yes	Low (64) Increased with PLP*
6	Shaw et al., 1967 [6]	10	Female	Phenylketonuria	Retarded		Yes	
7	Perry et al., 1967 [7]	1	Male	Nephrogenic diabetes insipidus, Anemia, vitamin B_6 responsive	Retarded	Nephrogenic diabetes insipidus	Yes	
8	Haraguchi et al., 1968 [8]	13	Female	Abnormal EEG	Normal		Yes	
9	Perry et al., 1968 [9]	8	Female	Normal	Normal	Yes; sister of Patient 10	Yes	
10	Perry et al., 1968 [9]	2	Male	Normal	Normal	Yes; brother of Patient 9	Yes	
11	Tada et al., 1968 [10]	¾	Male	Normal	Retarded	Yes	No	Low (10) No increase with PLP*

* Pyridoxal phosphate.

```
      COOH              COOH
       |                 |
  H2N—C—H           H—C—NH2
       |                 |
      CH2               CH2
       |                 |
      CH2               CH2
       |                 |
       S                 S
       |                 |
      CH2               CH2
       |                 |
      HC—NH2        H2N—CH
       |                 |
      COOH              COOH
  L-Cystathionine   D-Cystathionine

      COOH              COOH
       |                 |
      HC—NH2        H2N—CH
       |                 |
      CH2               CH2
       |                 |
      CH2               CH2
       |                 |
       S                 S
       |                 |
      CH2               CH2
       |                 |
      HC—NH2        H2N—CH
       |                 |
      COOH              COOH
L-Allocystathionine  D-Allocystathionine
```

Anslow, Simmonds, and du Vigneaud reported the specific rotations for the four stereoisomers as follows: L-allocystathionine, −25.0°; D-allocystathionine, +24.5°; D-cystathionine, −23.5°; and L-cystathionine, +23.7°—all 1 percent in 1*N* HCl [22]. Thus, the specific rotation of the component obtained from the urine was nearly identical to that found by Anslow et al. for L-cystathionine. The possibility of D-allocystathionine, which has a similar rotation, was eliminated by ion-exchange chromatography at 50° with pH 3.25 buffer throughout. This separates the L- and D-allocystathionines from L-cystathionine [23, 24].

Since the early reports of cystathioninuria these elaborate measures for identifying the amino acid have not been necessary. There is no reason to doubt the diagnosis in any of the published reports. In most systems of ion-exchange chromatography cystathionine is eluted in a nonspecific area. Accordingly it is desirable to employ multiple systems and to compare an eluted aliquot with an authentic sample by paper chromatography for identification of non-disulfide sulfur [25]. These methods are within the capability of any laboratory.

Cystathionine

Chemical Properties

The thio ether S-(β-amino-β-carboxyethyl)-homocysteine

```
 O   H   H       H   H   H   O
  \\ |   |       |   |   |  //
   C—C———C—S—C———C———C———C
  /  |   |       |   |   |   \
HO  NH2  H       H   H  NH2   OH
```

was first called *cystathionine* for convenience by Binkley and du Vigneaud [26]. It is a "neutral" amino acid, relatively stable, and sparingly soluble in water. About 80 mg of the white powder, composed of very fine crystals, will dissolve in 100 ml water with some difficulty, but it is soluble in urine to at least 200 mg per 100 ml.

The four possible stereoisomeric forms of cystathionine were first synthesized by Anslow, Simmonds, and du Vigneaud [22]. Later Armstrong described a simpler method of preparing L-cystathionine and L-allocystathionine, using a series of recrystallizations for resolving a mixture of stereoisomers [19]. The former method has been used for synthesis of radioactive cystathionine [27, 28].

Intermediary Metabolism

As far as is known, cystathionine is involved in but a single biochemical process, the transfer of sulfur from methionine to cysteine. The historical aspects of the elaboration of the cystathionine pathway are of considerable interest and have been reviewed in detail by du Vigneaud [29]. Briefly, there was evidence from several sources that methionine sulfur is transferred to cysteine. In effect this shortens the distance from the α-amino group to the sulfur atom by one methylene ($-CH_2-$) group. This evidence came largely from feeding experiments in rats, in which it was shown that methionine is necessary for growth and can substitute entirely for cysteine [30]. It was later found that homocysteine substituted for methionine (provided there was an adequate source of methyl groups) [31]. An interesting series of observations, illustrating the use of patients with a metabolic disorder to demonstrate a basic biochemical principle, was made by Brand and coworkers. They found that feeding methionine and homocysteine [32, 33] to patients with cystinuria (Chap. 62) resulted in increased excretion of cystine. Direct evidence that the methionine sulfur becomes cystine sulfur in the rat was provided by Tarver and Schmidt using methionine labeled with ^{35}S [34].

Several theories were proposed for the mechanism of transfer of methionine sulfur to cystine. Brand and coworkers postulated a transfer of sulfur by way of the compound which later was called *cystathionine* [33]. du Vigneaud, Kilmer, Rachele, and Cohn found evidence for this mechanism in rats on a cystine-free diet, when they fed methionine labeled with ^{34}S and with ^{13}C in the β and γ positions [35]. When cystine isolated from hair was found to contain isotopic sulfur but no isotopic carbon, the pathway seemed clear. Cystathionine was then synthesized and was found to substitute in the diet for methionine [22]. Later it was observed that cystathionine labeled with ^{35}S is metabolized to cystine ^{35}S in animals [27]. du Vigneaud and colleagues demonstrated that this system also applies to man when they gave methionine ^{35}S [36] and later cystathionine ^{35}S [37] to a patient with cystinuria.

These experiments were a few of the stepping-stones in the elaboration of the scheme of transsulfuration and the cystathionine pathway (Fig. 20-1).

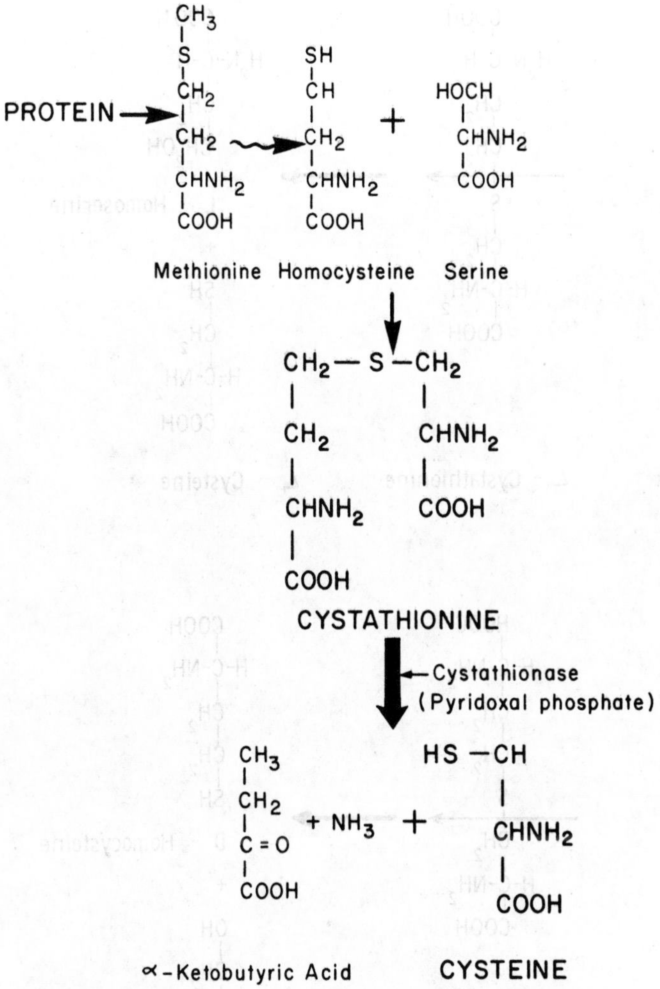

Figure 20-1. Abbreviated transsulfuration pathway. The complete pathways for sulfur amino acid metabolism are considerably more complex. (*Reproduced from Frimpter et al.* [78], *with permission of The American Journal of Diseases of Children.*)

The Cystathionine-cleaving Enzyme

Binkley, Anslow, and du Vigneaud reported in 1942 that rat liver slices and saline extracts of liver formed cysteine when incubated with cystathionine [26]. Binkley later published a comprehensive study on the specificity of the enzyme. It was found to split other thio ethers, including L-allocystathionine, lanthionine, and djenkolic acid [38]. It was further demonstrated that while L-cystathionine is split to yield L-cysteine and L-homoserine, L-allocystathionine is split on the other side of the sulfur to yield L-serine and D-homocysteine (Fig. 20-2).

Matsuo and Greenberg succeeded in purifying and crystallizing cystathionase [39]. Yellowish when in combination with pyridoxal phosphate [40], the enzyme was white when the coenzyme was split off. The molar ratio of the enzyme to pyridoxal phosphate in the active combination is 1:4.

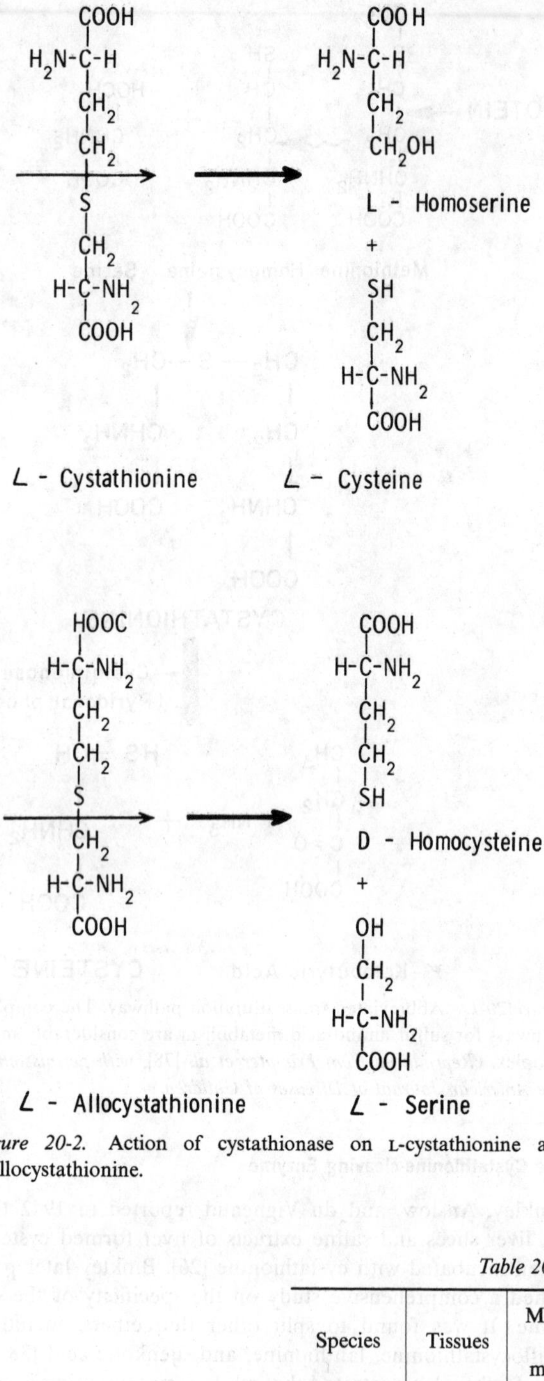

L - Cystathionine → L - Homoserine + L - Cysteine

L - Allocystathionine → D - Homocysteine + L - Serine

Figure 20-2. Action of cystathionase on L-cystathionine and L-allocystathionine.

Loiselet and Chatagner purified rat liver cystathionase by precipitation and chromatography [41]. Molecular weight determined by ultracentrifugation was 194,000 for the complete enzyme and 142,000 for a dialyzed sample with coenzyme removed. These authors confirmed the relative nonspecificity of the enzyme by showing that it attacks various thioethers, as previously suggested by Binkley [38]. It was found that the chromatographically pure protein possessed the activities of L-cystathionase, L-cysteine desulfurase, and L-homoserine dehydrase [41]. In a later paper Loiselet and Chatagner reported the amino acid composition of rat liver cystathionase, and that it increased in activity after the rats had been fed ethionine [42]. From amino acid analysis a minimum molecular weight, calculated from the relative occurrence of the "rare" amino acids, was about 85,200. When considered with the other data, this suggested that the protein may be a "dimer" with a molecular weight approximating 170,500.

Distribution

One of the most arresting facts of cystathionine metabolism is the high concentration in the human brain. Tallan, Moore, and Stein [23] found that human liver, kidney, and muscle contained 0.8, 0.7, and 0.8 mg per 100 gm, but five human brain specimens contained from 22.5 to 56.6 mg per 100 gm tissue. Duck and chicken brains contained 0.2 and 0.6 mg, while those of the guinea pig, rat, cat, and cow contained 1.2 to 3.9 mg per 100 ml. A monkey brain was intermediate between these animals and man, with 12.8 mg per 100 gm.

Mudd, Finkelstein, Irreverre, and Laster performed a comprehensive comparative study of the occurrence of cystathionase and related enzymes in several animals and in man [43]. The methionine-activating enzyme, cystathionine synthetase, and cystathionase all showed a considerable variation in activity (Table 20-2). The authors stated that the relative activities of cystathionine synthetase to cystathionase ". . . may explain, in part, the accumulation by human and monkey cerebral cortex, but it fails to explain the lesser cystathionine concentration of rat brain."

Table 20-2. CONCENTRATION OF ENZYMES IN LIVER AND BRAIN

Species	Tissues	Methionine-activating enzymes, mμmoles/mg/60 min	Cystathionine synthetase, mμmoles/mg/135 min	Cystathionase, mμmoles/mg/30 min
Rat	Liver	34.0	415	54.00
	Brain	3.3	84	0.11
Monkey	Liver	37.0	323	28.00
	Brain	4.0	68	0.32
Human	Liver	9.7	252	16.00
	Brain	1.6	22	0.15

Source: From Mudd et al. [43]. (Reproduced from *The Journal of Biological Chemistry,* with permission of the author and publisher.)

Normal human urine and blood plasma contain traces of cystathionine too small for accurate measurement by ion-exchange column chromatography [2]. Normal daily excretion is less than 10 mg.

Animal Studies

An unexpected ninhydrin-positive spot on paper chromatograms of urine from pyridoxine-deficient rats was first noted by Blashko, Datta, and Harris [44]. These experiments were repeated by Hope, and the substance was identified as L-cystathionine [18]. It is noteworthy that cystathioninuria developed in rats of the hooded Lister strain but not in Wistar albino rats. Hope demonstrated elevation of cystathionine concentration in the brain and liver of pyridoxine-deficient rats and concluded that transsulfuration must normally proceed at a rapid rate [45]. A metabolic block leading to an accumulation of cystathionine has been observed in *Neurospora crassa* [46] and *Aerobacter aerogenes* [47] mutants.

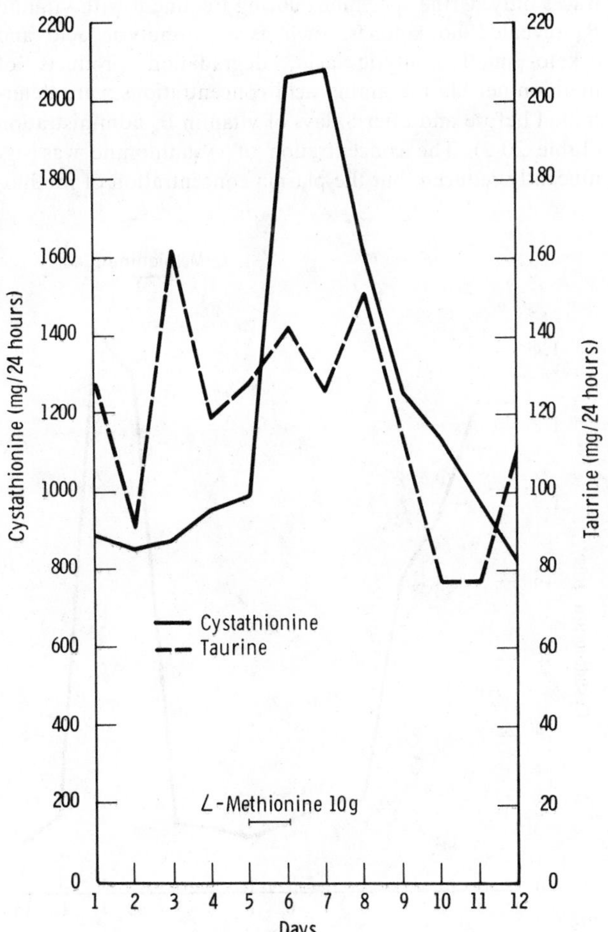

Figure 20-3. Cystathionine and taurine excretion following an oral load of L-methionine.

Frimpter, George, and Andelman [48] attempted to interfere with the production of hepatic cystathionase or its affinity for pyridoxal phosphate by treating young vitamin B_6-deficient rats with puromycin. While no significant difference was found between puromycin-treated and control animals, the results suggested that cystathionase is not turned over rapidly.

Ressler, Nelson, and Pfeffer [49] found that β-cyanoalanine, one of the toxic compounds of *Lathyrus* seeds, produces cystathioninuria when administered to rats.

Administration of Methionine

Feeding of a methionine load to several patients produced, as expected, an increase in plasma concentration and in urinary excretion of cystathionine [1, 3]. A typical result is shown in Fig. 20-3. Frimpter compared the effect of administration of a load of D-methionine to that of L-methionine. About half as much cystathionine and some methionine were excreted after feeding the D-stereoisomer. No allocystathionine was detected in the urine. This indicated that racemization of methionine was necessary prior to either cystathionine synthesis or methionine activation, or both. Methionine racemization (D- to L-) capacity was considerable, but not unlimited [50].

Effect of Pyridoxine (Vitamin B_6)

The effect of administration of vitamin B_6 to one of Frimpter's patients is shown in Fig. 20-4. Cystathionine excretion fell dramatically. Excretion of methionine, cystine, and taurine was not altered. The possibility that the patient was deficient in vitamin B_6 was unlikely, since the diet contained adequate amounts of this vitamin and there was no clinical evidence of deficiency. Furthermore, urinary kynurenine, kynurenic acid, and xanthurenic acid were normal after a test dose of 4 gm L-tryptophan. The values did not change when the test was repeated during administration of vitamin B_6 [2, 51].

The effect of vitamin B_6 was not achieved by other components of the vitamin B complex, including thiamine, nicotinamide, folic acid, and riboflavin. A course of tetracycline was given to inhibit any possible abnormal gastrointestinal flora that might have contributed to the disorder by the production of cystathionine, but this had no effect.

Wilson and du Vigneaud [52] and Kuchinskas, Horvath, and du Vigneaud [53] found that administration of L-penicillamine arrested the growth of rats and that this effect was prevented by either vitamin B_6 or ethanolamine. Because of these observations, 30 gm ethanolamine hydrochloride was given orally to Frimpter's patient daily for 3 days, but there was no effect on cystathionine excretion.

In one experiment the patient was given vitamin B_6 intramuscularly for several days. The cystathionine excretion fell and within 4 days stabilized at a lower level, which was still abnormal but was less than one-tenth the original level.

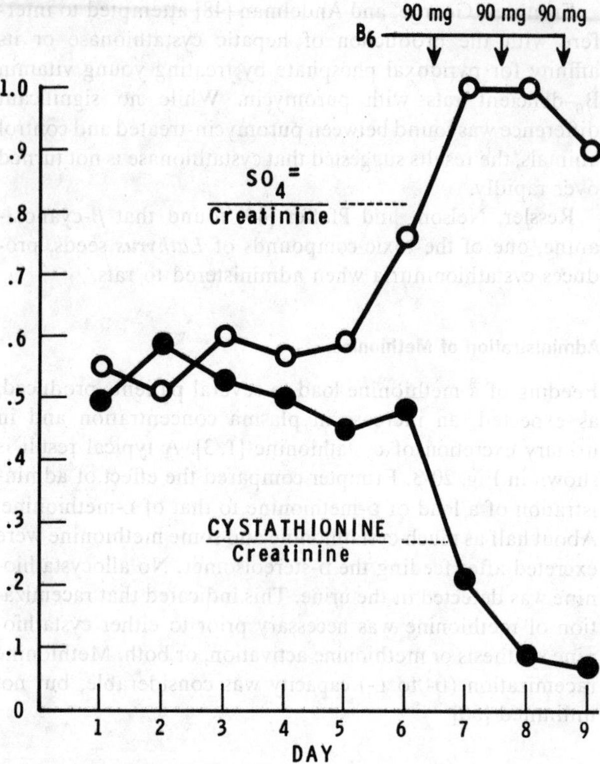

Figure 20-4. Effect of high doses of vitamin B_6 on cystathionine excretion in patient with cystathioninuria. (*Reproduced from Frimpter et al.* [2], *with permission of The New England Journal of Medicine.*)

Administration of 120 mg pyridoxine hydrochloride daily was continued for 8 days. An oral load of 10 gm L-methionine over a 24-hr period resulted in a large increase in cystathionine excretion in spite of continued high dosage of vitamin B_6 (Fig. 20-5). This experiment seemed to rule out vitamin B_6 deficiency as the primary defect, since if the coenzyme pyridoxal phosphate were missing, then a deficiency would have been restored by the massive doses of vitamin B_6. The prompt return of the cystathionine excretion to low levels several days after the methionine loading might be used as an argument that the apoenzyme itself was present in effective amounts.

What explanation is there for the observed effect of vitamin B_6 administration? There are few situations in biology where administration of a coenzyme will result in increased activity of the enzyme. LaDu and Zannoni have postulated that ascorbic acid protects *p*-hydroxyphenylpyruvic acid oxidase from inhibition by its substrate [54]. They observed that protection occurred only when large amounts of tyrosine were metabolized. It is possible that there is a parallel here, since the patient's diet, which consisted largely of dairy products, contained considerable methionine. Efforts to explore this possibility were frustrated. The patient was placed on a diet calculated to contain 418 mg methionine per day. He lost 3.34 kg during 8 hospital days on this diet, but the cystathionine excretion did not change. Thus the hypothesis that enzyme activity was inhibited by large amounts of substrate was not confirmed, for if this had been the cause of the cystathioninuria, then an abrupt decrease in the excretion of the amino acid would have been expected. Nevertheless, it is possible that the continued high cystathionine excretion could be from large extravascular stores of cystathionine such as were found at autopsy in the patient of Harris, Penrose, and Thomas [1].

The question arises as to whether vitamin B_6 causes the reduction in cystathioninuria through increased activity of the cleaving enzyme or whether there is a deviation of sulfur away from the normal transsulfuration pathway. Pyridoxine is involved in many biochemical reactions [55], and cystathionine is known to be involved only in transsulfuration. It is possible, for example, that cystathionine was destroyed by deamination or decarboxylation. On the other hand, methionine is involved in several reactions, and it is possible that it was channeled into some other pathway. The excretion of taurine in the urine was unchanged by vitamin B_6, and cystine has been present in the urine of this patient in traces only. Urine specimens during treatment with vitamin B_6 revealed no ketones, such as α-ketobutyric acid and α-keto-γ-methiolbutyric acid, degradation products of methionine. Plasma amino acid concentrations were determined before and after 8 days of vitamin B_6 administration (Table 20-3). The concentration of cystathionine was significantly reduced, but the plasma concentration of methio-

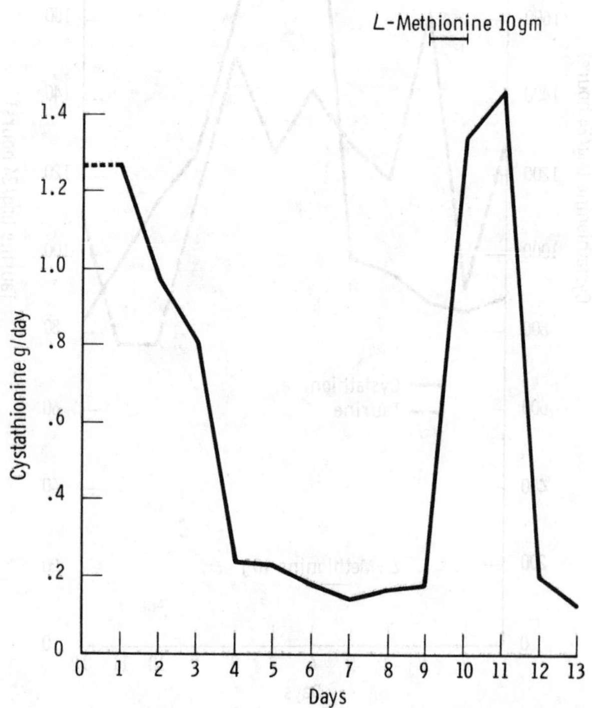

Figure 20-5. Effect of pyridoxine and methionine. A methionine load was superimposed upon the effect of vitamin B_6. See text.

Table 20-3. PLASMA AMINO ACID CONCENTRATIONS BEFORE AND AFTER ADMINISTRATION OF PYRIDOXINE,* MG/100 ML

Amino acid	Before	After
Taurine	0.96	0.88
Cystine†	1.59	1.57
Cystathionine	0.69	0.11
Methionine	0.45	0.53
α-Amino-*n*-butyric acid	0.12	0.33

* Pyridoxine HCl, 30 mg intramuscularly every 6 hr for 8 days.
† Includes cysteine.

nine actually increased slightly. There was no significant change in either cystine or taurine concentration (intermediates between cystathionine and inorganic sulfate). A significant rise in α-amino-*n*-butyric acid concentration was compatible with cleavage of cystathionine [56], but this rise might also have been derived from methionine, as has been demonstrated in bacterial systems.

Degradation of methionine to α-ketobutyric acid by certain bacteria requires pyridoxal phosphate [57]. Homocysteine (demethylated methionine) may also undergo alternate metabolism. A homocysteine desulfurase yielding hydrogen sulfide and unidentified products has been described in liver, kidney, and pancreas [58]. Kallio has shown that a homocysteine desulfhydrase system of *Proteus morganii* requires pyridoxal phosphate in a reaction which yields α-ketobutyric acid [59].

There may be some similarity in the effect of vitamin B_6 in cystathioninuria and its effect in the excretors of excessive kynurenine, oxykynurenic acid, and xanthurenic acid described by Knapp [60]. In this inherited disorder vitamin B_6 also temporarily corrected the defect. Greengard and Gordon showed that vitamin B_6 may stimulate the production of rat liver tyrosine α-ketoglutarate transaminase in vivo [61]. These authors suggested that the coenzyme may function to regulate the production of apoenzyme. The principle would seem *not* to apply to cystathioninuria, because the defect is manifest in the presence of normal amounts of vitamin B_6.

One possible explanation is that the binding of coenzymes by the apoenzyme might be defective. Thus, greater activity might occur when the amount of the active combination is increased by high concentrations of coenzyme. Bonner and coworkers have discussed the possible occurrence of mutation giving rise to change in the requirement for coenzyme [62].

Evidence was provided for this possibility by the incubation of liver homogenates from two patients with L-cystathionine-^{3}H [63]. When compared with what occurred in normal controls, the substrate cystathionine was split minimally. When an excess of pyridoxal phosphate was added, the production of radioactive cysteine, separated as cystine by ion-exchange chromatography, approached that of the normal controls (Table 20-4). These data were interpreted as compatible with a genetically determined defective binding of the apoenzyme to the cofactor pyridoxal phosphate to form the active complex.

Previous studies [64], described later in detail by Finkelstein et al. [65], using a somewhat different assay system, had shown a low cystathionase activity in a liver biopsy specimen obtained from Berlow's patient. They were unable to demonstrate any noteworthy increase in enzymatic activity upon addition of pyridoxal phosphate. Finkelstein and coworkers [66] later discussed the discrepancy between their result and Frimpter's. One possibility is that their study was performed while the patient was receiving vitamin B_6, while Frimpter's patients were not.

Finkelstein et al. suggested a nonenzymatic degradation of cystathionine by pyridoxal phosphate [65]. Evidence for such an effect in the presence of a protein and certain metallic ions had been provided by Binkley and Boyd [67]. Gaull and coworkers have described the formation of a "chemical adduct" between homocysteine and pyridoxal phosphate in order to explain the apparent vitamin B_6 dependency in some patients with homocystinuria [68]. The same or a similar mechanism could be present in cystathioninuria. Rosenberg et al. attributed vitamin B_{12}-dependent

Table 20-4. CYSTATHIONASE ACTIVITY IN LIVER FROM TWO PATIENTS WITH CYSTATHIONINURIA AND FIVE CONTROL SUBJECTS

Pyridoxal phosphate, mg	Cystine (dpm × 10^3)	Cystine (dpm × 10^3), mg protein
Patient B:		
0	2.3	0.6
0.1	8.8	2.4
Patient D:		
0	0.8	0.2
0.1	34.7	9.9
Normal 1:		
0	28.6	13.0
0.1	35.6	16.8
Normal 2:		
0	36.1	10.3
0.2	87.8	25.1
Normal 3:		
0	28.2	8.0
0.2	51.6	14.7
Normal 4:		
0	35.2	5.2
0.008	45.3	6.7
0.02	38.0	5.6
0.2	36.8	5.0
0.4	59.0	7.5
Normal 5:		
0	97.3	14.5
0.2	120.0	18.0

Source: From Frimpter [63]. (Reproduced with permission of *Science*. Copyright, 1965, by the American Association for the Advancement of Science.)

methylmalonic aciduria [69] to failure of transformation of vitamin B_{12} to an active coenzyme form. Similarly, failure to metabolize pyridoxine to pyridoxal may be the cause of cystathioninuria. The fact that patients with cystathioninuria do not have evidence of faulty function in other biochemical systems and also have normal responses to tryptophan loads is evidence against such an explanation for cystathioninuria. Mudd, Levy, and Abeles recently described a patient with methylmalonic aciduria, homocystinuria, and cystathioninuria which appeared to be due to a deficiency in methylfolate-H_4 methyltransferase deficiency [70]. Normal activities of cystathionine synthase and cystathionase were found. This observation may not be immediately relevant to the question of the molecular explanation for the cystathioninuria seen in most patients, i.e., those with the "vitamin B_6-dependent" type.

Tada et al. described an infant whose liver showed no response to vitamin B_6 either in vivo or in vitro with a specimen obtained by biopsy [10]. They concluded that their patient had a different type of cystathioninuria, one that was due to a different mutation from that of the other reported patients. The broader significance of this observation is that it would seem to eliminate the theory that vitamin B_6 in one form or another can by itself and without an enzyme effect a reduction in the cystathionine concentration of plasma and urine.

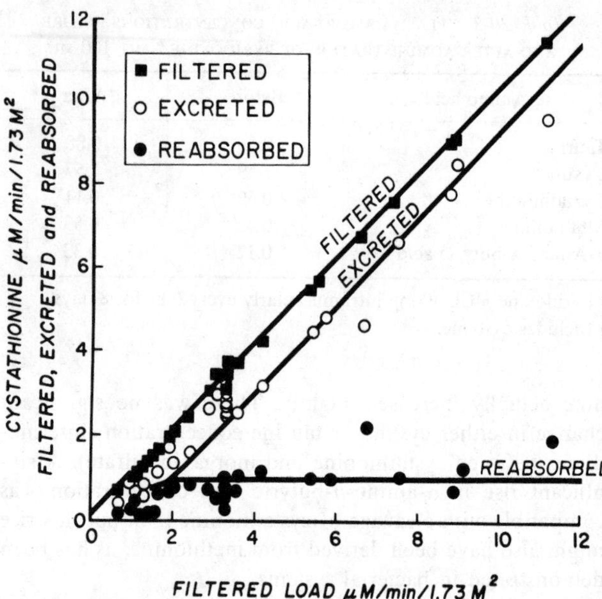

Figure 20-6. Excretion of cystathionine by normal subjects, two patients with homozygous cystathioninuria, one with heterozygous cystathioninuria, and one with homozygous cystinuria. There are no apparent differences among these individuals. See text. (*Reproduced from Frimpter and Greenberg* [72], *with permission of The Journal of Clinical Investigation.*)

Other Sulfur Compounds

Kodama et al. found S-(carboxymethyl) homocysteine, S-(2-hydroxy-2-carboxyethyl) homocysteine, S-(3-hydroxy-3-carboxyethyl) homocysteine, S-(3-hydroxy-3-carboxy-*n*-propyl) cysteine, and S-(β-carboxyethyl) cysteine in the urine of a patient with cystathioninuria [71]. These compounds could be degradation products of cystathionine. The effect of high doses of vitamin B_6 upon the excretion of these compounds would be of considerable interest.

Cystathionine and the Kidney

Frimpter and Greenberg studied the excretion of cystathionine in two patients with homozygous cystathioninuria, one heterozygous parent, one patient with homozygous cystinuria, and four normal subjects [72]. The two patients with homozygous cystathioninuria were studied at endogenous plasma concentrations. The plasma and urinary cystathionine concentrations in the heterozygous parent were elevated to measurable levels by feeding 1 gm L-methionine every 4 hr for 4 days, and in the patient with cystinuria and the normal subjects by infusing L-cystathionine. No essential differences were observed among these groups, as seen in Fig. 20-6. It is apparent that cystathionine is rapidly cleared from the plasma. It has a low tubular maximum (T_m), on the order of 1 μmole per 1.73 m^2 body surface area per minute. The importance of this is that screening of plasma samples for cystathioninuria may fail to detect a slightly elevated concentration. Examination of urine should be more fruitful.

In a detailed study of cystathionine excretion in dogs, Strickler and Frimpter offered evidence that renal tubular secretion of cystathionine may occur under special circumstances, and probably occurs in the distal tubule [73].

Therapy

The beneficial effect of vitamin B_6 in most of the patients has led to the inclusion of cystathioninuria among the "vitamin B_6-dependent" syndromes [74]. Thus, like familial xanthurenic aciduria [75], vitamin B_6-responsive anemia [76], and vitamin B_6-dependent convulsions [77], cystathioninuria may respond to treatment with massive doses of vitamin B_6. The relationship of the varied clinical findings in the reported patients to the enzymatic defect is not clear. Perhaps the two "normal" patients of Perry and coworkers [9] indicate that the biochemical disorder and the various clinical findings are coincidental, or perhaps the normal individuals are only variations within the phenotype [48]. Prolonged administration of high doses of vitamin B_6 to a child with homocystinuria and thrombocytopenia had no beneficial effect [5]. Further, L-cystathionine had no in vitro effect on platelet functions [5]. Though it is possible that vitamin B_6 therapy might benefit a patient or prevent progression of associated clinical findings, even in utero [78],

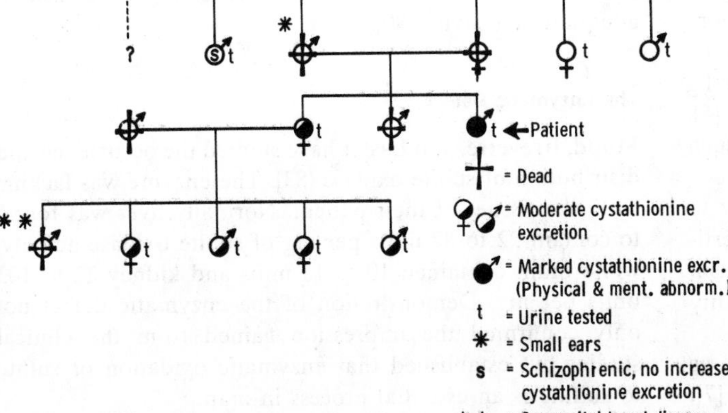

Figure 20-7. Pedigree of the second reported family manifesting cystathioninuria. (*Reproduced from Frimpter et al.* [2], *with permission of The New England Journal of Medicine; modified by addition of new information.*)

there is scant evidence at present that this therapy is worthwhile.

Genetics

All the patients for whom adequate family information is available conform to a pattern of an autosomal recessive inheritance. Two representative pedigrees are shown in Figs. 20-7 and 20-8. Presumptive heterozygotes may have a slightly elevated cystathionine excretion as demonstrated by ion-exchange chromatography. Excretion of the amino acid in these patients probably reflects a balance between multiple factors, including enzyme activity, metabolic requirements for methionine and cystine (or cysteine), and dietary intake of these amino acids and vitamins, particularly vitamin B_6.

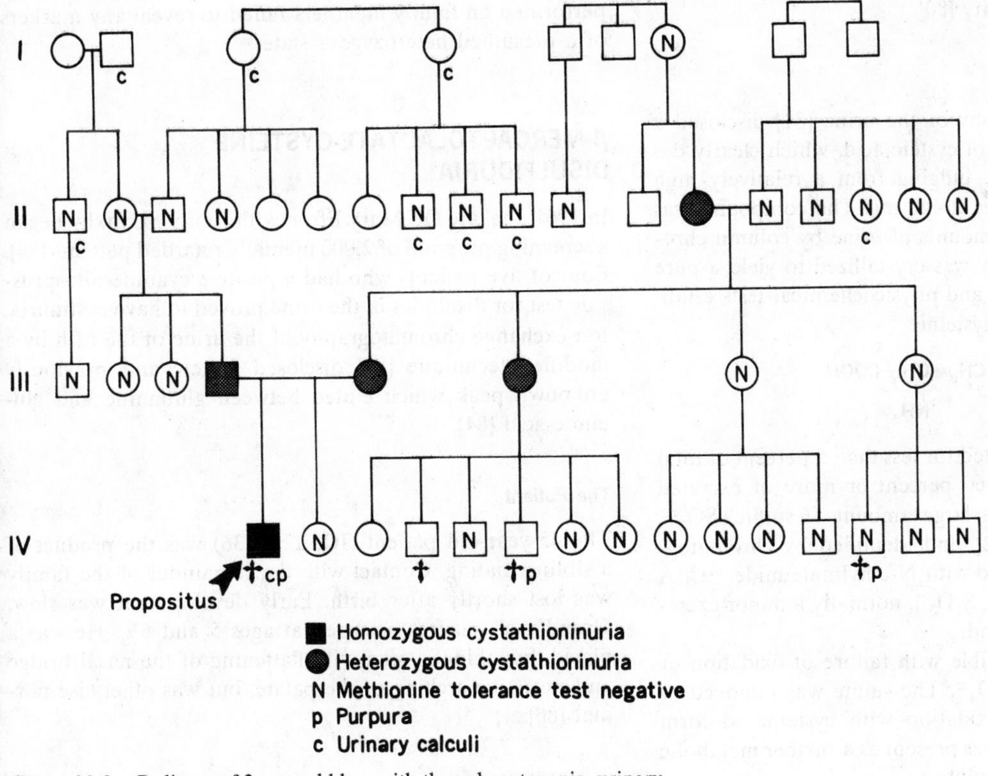

Figure 20-8. Pedigree of 2-year-old boy with thrombocytopenia, urinary calculi, and cystathioninuria. The tests in generations I and II were performed outside the United States, specimens having been submitted by mail. (*Reproduced from Mongeau* [5], *with permission of Pediatrics; modified by new data.*)

Since the amount of cystathionine excreted by heterozygous persons may be low, heterozygosity may be determined more convincingly by a methionine tolerance test. This can be conveniently done by giving 100 mg L-methionine per kg orally and determining the excretion of cystathionine [5]. The methionine can be easily suspended in a vehicle such as fruit juice. The test seems to be harmless.

Further genetic data are urgently required, not only to clarify the problem of possible phenotype, but also to estimate the incidence of the disorder. The absence of cousin marriages in reported pedigrees suggests that the abnormality may not be rare.

The association of other inherited conditions, such as phenylketonuria [6] and nephrogenic diabetes insipidus [7], may reflect only the population examined for the disease.

SULFITE OXIDASE DEFICIENCY

In 1967 Laster, Irreverre, Mudd, and Heizer reported their studies on a 2½-year-old boy with severe brain damage, mental retardation, and dislocated ocular lenses [79]. The patient died on the forty-sixth hospital day. Studies conducted during his brief hospitalization contain the maximum amount of information available about the only known example of this abnormality [80].

Chemistry

Amino acid chromatography of the urine [81] disclosed a large peak at the position of cysteic acid, which clearly did not represent cysteic acid, judging from a relatively high spectrophotometric reading at 440 mμ. The compound was concentrated from large amounts of urine by column chromatography and eventually was crystallized to yield a pure product. Various chemical and physicochemical tests established its identity as sulfocysteine:

$$HO_3S{-}S{-}CH_2{-}\underset{\displaystyle NH_2}{\underset{|}{CH}}{-}COOH$$

Inorganic sulfate accounted for less than 5 percent of total sulfur excreted; normally 60 percent or more of excreted sulfur is sulfate. Instead, a large amount of sulfite, $SO_3^{=}$, was found by spot test [82], and identified by chromatography of the adduct formed with N-ethylmaleimide ^{14}C. A large amount of thiosulfate, $S_2O_3^{=}$, normally a minor excretion product, was also found.

These data were compatible with failure of oxidation of sulfite, $SO_3^{=}$, to sulfate, $SO_4^{=}$. The sulfite was removed or "detoxified" in part by oxidation with cysteine to form sulfocysteine. Thiosulfate was present as a further metabolic product of the remaining sulfite.

Plasma and Tissue Concentrations

Studies with the small amounts of plasma available suggested an elevated plasma concentration of sulfocysteine, but extracts of tissues did not, probably owing to a lack of adequate sensitivity [80].

The Enzymatic Defect

Mudd, Irreverre, and Laster have studied the occurrence and distribution of sulfite oxidase [83]. The enzyme was lacking from the tissues of their patient. Normally liver was found to contain 22 to 87 units per mg of sulfite oxidase activity, while brain contained 10 to 13 units and kidney 22 to 103 units per mg. Demonstration of the enzymatic defect not only confirmed the impression gained from the clinical studies but established that enzymatic oxidation of sulfite to sulfate is an essential process in man.

Genetics

The mother of the patient was Scotch and Irish, and the father was of Italian descent. There was no consanguinity. The parents had at least average intelligence. The patient had four normal living sibs, aged 11, 9, 7, and 1. Three sibs had died in the first few days of life with neurologic signs. A maternal aunt who died at age 8 was severely retarded. Post-mortem examination of these patients disclosed no important pathologic similarities. Various chemical tests performed on family members failed to reveal any markers of a presumed heterozygous state.

β-MERCAPTOLACTATE-CYSTEINE DISULFIDURIA

In 1961, the late Dr. Mary Efron with Emily M. Bixby began a screening program of 2,000 mentally retarded patients [84]. Four of five patients who had a positive cyanide-nitroprusside test for disulfides in the urine proved to have cystinuria. Ion-exchange chromatography of the urine of the fifth by a modified technique [85] disclosed a new and previously unknown peak which eluted between glutamine and glutamic acid [84].

The Patient

The 45-year-old patient (IQ, 22 to 36) was the product of a sibling mating. Contact with the remainder of the family was lost shortly after birth. Early development was slow. Grand mal seizures occurred at ages 5 and 6½. He was a placid, hypokinetic man with flattening of the nasal bridge and excessive arching of the palate, but was otherwise normal [86].

Chemistry

The unknown compound was isolated by ion-exchange chromatography and high-voltage electrophoresis [87]. Reduction of the disulfide yielded only one ninhydrin-positive substance; it proved to be cysteine [87]. Working largely with infrared spectrophotometry, Crawhall and coworkers [88] determined that the compound was the disulfide of β-mercaptolactate and cysteine [87, 88].

```
                NH2
                |
S—CH2—CH—COOH
|
S—CH2—CH—COOH
                |
                OH
```

Significance

The β-mercaptolactate-cysteine disulfide could arise from β-mercaptopyruvate [87]. Crawhall and coworkers [88] speculated on alternative possibilities and offered the intriguing suggestion that β-mercaptopyruvate may play a role in formation of thionucleotides in man as it does in *Escherichia coli* [89].

β-Mercaptolactate might be present in excessive amounts because of a defect in a mechanism for its normal disposal. Subsequent reaction with cysteine would give the new mixed disulfide. Alternately, the mixed disulfide itself might be a normal intermediate, disposal of which is defective.

Further studies are necessary to determine the role of the compound in metabolism, the exact nature of the defect, and the role of the defect, if any, in production of mental retardation.

Genetics

A formal inheritance pattern cannot be derived from this one instance. The sibling mating is exceeded only by a parent-child cross in closeness of inbreeding. The risk is 0.04 that the child of a sibling mating will be homozygous for an autosomal recessive trait present in a grandparent, whereas it is 0.125 for the child of a parent-child cross if the parent has the recessive trait.

SUMMARY

1 Cystathioninuria is an uncommon disorder of metabolism with uncertain clinical manifestations. Some patients have had developmental defects or mental retardation, but others have been clinically normal. Cystathioninuria may be a benign disorder of metabolism.

2 The biochemical defect is low activity of the cystathionine-cleaving enzyme. This causes an increase in blood and tissue concentrations of cystathionine and a high urinary excretion of the amino acid because of its high rate of renal clearance.

3 Except for one patient who may have a genetically different type of cystathioninuria, a consistent feature has been a remarkable reduction in plasma and urine concentrations of cystathionine after high doses of vitamin B_6. There is in vitro evidence that this reflects a genetic abnormality in the binding of pyridoxal phosphate by a cystathionine apoenzyme to form the active combination necessary for cystathionine cleavage.

4 Cystathioninuria is inherited as an autosomal recessive trait. A methionine tolerance test may aid in the identification of heterozygous persons.

5 A single example of a severely retarded patient with failure to oxidize sulfite to sulfate has been studied in detail. This occurrence represents another block in the metabolism of sulfur, this one at the final stage in disposal of sulfur. The enzyme defect, lack of sulfite oxidase, is probably inherited as a recessive trait.

6 A mentally defective patient, a product of a sibling mating, has been described with β-mercaptolactate-cysteine disulfide in the urine. The metabolic implications, nature of the defect, and true incidence of the abnormality remain obscure.

BIBLIOGRAPHY

1. Harris, H. L., Penrose, L. S., and Thomas, D. H. H.: Cystathioninuria. Ann. Hum. Genet., **23**, 442, 1959.
2. Frimpter, G. W., Haymovitz, A., and Horwith, M.: Cystathioninuria. New Eng. J. Med., **268**, 333, 1963.
3. Berlow, S.: Studies in cystathioninemia. Amer. J. Dis. Child., **112**, 135, 1966.
4. Frimpter, G. W.: Cystathioninuria, in *The Metabolic Basis of Inherited Disease,* 2d ed., edited by J. B. Stanbury, J. B. Wyngaarden, and D. S. Fredrickson. McGraw-Hill Book Company, New York, 1966.
5. Mongeau, J.-G., Hilgartner, M., Wortehn, H. G., and Frimpter, G. W.: Cystathioninuria: study of an infant with normal mentality, thrombocytopenia, and renal calculi. J. Pediat., **69**, 1113, 1966.
6. Shaw, K. N. F., Lieberman, E., Kock, R., and Donnell, G. N.: Cystathioninuria. Amer. J. Dis. Child., **113**, 119, 1967.
7. Perry, T. L., Robinson, G. C., Teasdale, J. M., and Hansen, S.: Concurrence of cystathioninuria, nephrogenic diabetes insipidus, and severe anemia. New Eng. J. Med., **276**, 721, 1967.
8. Haraguchi, H., Iwatani, E., Yamashita, F., and Nagayama, T.: Studies on cystathioninuria. Igakunoayumi, **61**, 72, 1967.
9. Perry, T. L., Hardwick, D. F., Hansen, S., Love, D. L., and Israles, S.: Cystathioninuria in two healthy siblings. New Eng. J. Med., **278**, 590, 1968.
10. Tada, K., Yoshida, T., Yokoyama, Y., Sato, T., Nakagawa, H., and Arakawa, T.: Cystathioninuria not associated with vitamin B_6 dependency: a probably new type of cystathioninuria. Tohoku J. Exp. Med., **95**, 235, 1968.
11. Frimpter, G. W.: Cystathioninuria in cystinuria. Amer. J. Med., **46**, 823, 1969.
12. Whelan, D. T., and Scriver, C. R.: Cystathioninuria and renal iminoglycinuria in a pedigree. New Eng. J. Med., **278**, 924, 1968.
13. Schneiderman, L. J.: Latent cystathioninuria. J. Med. Genet., **4**, 260, 1967.
14. Fourman, P., Summerscales, J. W., and Morgan, D. M.: Cystathioninuria from pyridoxine deficiency complicating treatment of hypercalcaemia in a cretin. Arch. Dis. Child., **41**, 273, 1966.
15. Gjessing, L. R.: Cystathioninuria during a load of thyroxine. Scand. J. Clin. Lab. Invest., **16**, 680, 1964.
16. Gjessing, L. R.: Studies of functional neural tumors. II. Cystathioninuria. Scand. J. Clin. Lab. Invest., **15**, 474, 1963.
17. Gjessing, L. R.: Studies of functional neural tumors. III. Cystathionine in the tumor tissues. Scand. J. Clin. Lab. Invest., **15**, 479, 1963.
18. Hope, D. B.: L-Cystathionine in the urine of pyridoxine deficient rats. Biochem. J., **66**, 486, 1957.
19. Armstrong, M. D.: A preparation of L-cystathionine and L-allocystathionine. J. Org. Chem., **16**, 433, 1951.

20. Hirs, C. W. H., Moore, S., and Stein, W. H.: The chromatography of amino acids on ion exchange resins: use of volatile acids for elution. J. Amer. Chem. Soc., **76,** 6063, 1954.
21. Frimpter, G. W.: Unpublished observations.
22. Anslow, W. P., Jr., Simmonds, S., and du Vigneaud, V.: The synthesis of the isomers of cystathionine and a study of their availability in sulfur metabolism. J. Biol. Chem., **166,** 34, 1946.
23. Tallan, H. H., Moore, S., and Stein, W. H.: L-Cystathionine in human brain. J. Biol. Chem., **230,** 707, 1958.
24. Frimpter, G. W., Ohmori, S., and Mizuhara, S.: Ion-exchange chromatography of sulfur amino acids and the separation of diastereoisomers. J. Chromatogr., **10,** 439, 1963.
25. Toennies, G., and Kolb, J. J.: Techniques and reagents for paper chromatography. Anal. Chem., **23,** 823, 1951.
26. Binkley, F., Anslow, W. P., Jr., and du Vigneaud, V.: The formation of cysteine from L-L-S-(β-amino-β-carboxyethyl) homocysteine by liver tissue. J. Biol. Chem., **143,** 559, 1942.
27. Rachele, J. R., Reed, L. J., Kidwai, A. R., Ferger, M. F., and du Vigneaud, V.: Conversion of cystathionine, labeled with S^{35} to cystine in vivo. J. Biol. Chem., **185,** 817, 1950.
28. Murray, A., III, and Williams, D. L.: *Organic Synthesis with Isotopes,* part II, pp. 1962–1964. Interscience, New York, 1958.
29. du Vigneaud, V.: *A Trail of Research in Sulfur Chemistry and Metabolism and Related Fields.* Cornell, Ithaca, N.Y., 1952.
30. Womack, M., Kemmerer, K. S., and Rose, W. C.: The relation of cystine and methionine to growth. J. Biol. Chem., **121,** 403, 1937.
31. du Vigneaud, V., Chandler, J. P., Moyer, A. W., and Keppel, D. M.: The effect of choline on the ability of homocysteine to replace methionine in the diet. J. Biol. Chem., **131,** 57, 1939.
32. Brand, E., Cahill, G. F., and Harris, M. M.: Cystinuria. II. The metabolism of cystine, cysteine, methionine, and glutathione. J. Biol. Chem., **109,** 69, 1935.
33. Brand, E., Cahill, G. F., and Block, R. J.: Cystinuria. IV. The metabolism of homocysteine and homocystine. J. Biol. Chem., **110,** 399, 1935.
34. Tarver, H., and Schmidt, C. L. A.: The conversion of methionine to cystine: experiments with radioactive sulfur. J. Biol. Chem., **130,** 67, 1939.
35. du Vigneaud, V., Kilmer, G. W., Rachele, J. R., and Cohn, M.: On the mechanism of the conversion in vivo of methionine to cystine. J. Biol. Chem., **155,** 645, 1944.
36. Reed, L. J., Cavallini, D., Plum, F., Rachele, J. R., and du Vigneaud, V.: The conversion of methionine to cystine in a human cystinuric. J. Biol. Chem., **180,** 783, 1949.
37. Wilson, J. E., Plum, F., Reed, L. J., Rachele, J. R., and du Vigneaud, V.: Unpublished observations, cited in V. du Vigneaud, *A Trail of Research in Sulfur Chemistry and Metabolism and Related Fields,* p. 53. Cornell, Ithaca, N.Y., 1952.
38. Binkley, F.: Enzymatic cleavage of thioethers. J. Biol. Chem., **186,** 559, 1942.
39. Matsuo, Y., and Greenberg, D. M.: A crystalline enzyme that cleaves homoserine and cystathionine. I. Isolation procedures and some physiochemical properties. J. Biol. Chem., **230,** 545, 1958.
40. Matsuo, Y., and Greenberg, D. M.: A crystalline enzyme that cleaves homoserine and cystathionine. II. Prosthetic group. J. Biol. Chem., **230,** 561, 1958.
41. Loiselet, J., and Chatagner, F.: Purification et étude de quelques propriétés de la cystéine désulfurase "soluble" (cystathionase) du foie de rat. Bull. Soc. Chim. Biol., **47,** 33, 1965.
42. Loiselet, J., and Chatagner, F.: Amino acid composition of "ethionine-induced" cystathionase of rat liver. Biochim. Biophys. Acta, **130,** 180, 1966.
43. Mudd, S. H., Finkelstein, J. D., Irreverre, F., and Laster, L.: Transsulfuration in mammals. J. Biol. Chem., **240,** 4382, 1965.
44. Blashko, H., Datta, S. P., and Harris, H.: Pyridoxine deficiency in the rat: liver L-cysteic acid decarboxylase activity and urinary amino acids. Brit. J. Nutr., **7,** 364, 1953.
45. Hope, D. B.: Cystathionine in brain and liver from pyridoxine deficient rats. J. Physiol., **141,** 31P, 1958.
46. Horowitz, N. M.: Methionine synthesis in *Neurospora:* the isolation of cystathionine. J. Biol. Chem., **171,** 255, 1947.
47. Harold, F. M.: Accumulation of cystathionine in a homocysteine-requiring mutant of *Aerobacter aerogenes.* J. Bacteriol., **84,** 382, 1962.
48. Frimpter, G. W., George, W. F., and Andelman, R. J.: Cystathioninuria and B_6 dependency. Ann. N.Y. Acad. Sci., **166,** 109, 1969.
49. Ressler, C., Nelson, J., and Pfeffer, M.: A pyridoxal-β-cyanoalanine relation in the rat. Nature (London), **203,** 1286, 1964.
50. Frimpter, G. W.: Unpublished observations.
51. Kowlessar, O. D., Haeftner, L. J., Benson, G., and Sleisenger, M. H.: Evidence for deficiency of vitamin B_6 in nontropical sprue. J. Clin. Invest., **40,** 1055, 1961.
52. Wilson, J. E., and du Vigneaud, V.: Inhibition of growth of the rat by L-penicillamine and its prevention by aminoethanol and related compounds. J. Biol. Chem., **184,** 63, 1950.
53. Kuchinskas, E. J., Horvath, A., and du Vigneaud, V.: Anti-vitamin B_6 action of L-penicillamine. Arch. Biochem., **68,** 175, 1961.
54. LaDu, B. N., and Zannoni, V. G.: Role of ascorbic acid in tyrosine metabolism. Ann. N.Y. Acad. Sci., **92,** 175, 1961.
55. Meister, A.: *Biochemistry of the Amino Acids,* 2d ed., p. 376. Academic, New York, 1965.
56. Carroll, W. R., Stacy, G. W., and du Vigneaud, V.: α-Ketobutyric acid as a product in the enzymatic cleavage of cystathionine. J. Biol. Chem., **180,** 375, 1949.
57. Kallio, R. E., and Larson, A. D.: Methionine degradation by a species of *Pseudomonas,* in *A Symposium on Amino Acid Metabolism,* edited by W. D. McElroy and H. B. Glass. Johns Hopkins, Baltimore, 1955.
58. Fromageot, C., and Desneuelle, P.: La Décomposition anérobic de l'homocystéine-désulfurase par différents systèmes biologiques: existence d'une homocystéine désulfurase. C. R. Acad. Sci. [D] (Paris), **214,** 647, 1942.
59. Kallio, R. E.: Function of pyridoxal phosphate in desulfhydrase systems of *Proteus morganii.* J. Biol. Chem., **192,** 371, 1951.
60. Knapp, A.: Über eine neue, hereditäre, von-Vitamin-B_6 abhängige Storung Tryptophan-stoffwechsel. Clin. Chim. Acta, **5,** 6, 1960.
61. Greengard, O., and Gordon, M.: The cofactor-mediated regulation of apoenzyme levels in animal tissues. I. The pyridoxine-induced rise of rat liver tyrosine transaminase level in vivo. J. Biol. Chem., **238,** 3708, 1963.
62. Bonner, D. M., Suyama, Y., and Demoss, J. A.: Genetic fine structure and enzyme formation. Fed. Proc., **19,** 926, 1960.
63. Frimpter, G. W.: Cystathioninuria: nature of the defect. Science, **149,** 1095, 1965.
64. Laster, L., Spaeth, G. L., Mudd, S. H., and Finkelstein, J. D.: Homocystinuria due to cystathionine synthase deficiency. Ann. Intern. Med., **63,** 1117, 1965.
65. Finkelstein, J. D., Mudd, S. H., Irreverre, F., and Laster, L.: Deficiencies of cystathionase and homoserine dehydratase activities in cystathioninuria. Proc. Nat. Acad. Sci. U.S.A., **55,** 865, 1966.
66. Finkelstein, J. D., Mudd, S. H., Irreverre, F., and Laster, L.: Cystathioninuria. Amer. J. Dis. Child., **115,** 388, 1968.
67. Binkley, F., and Boyd, M.: Catalytic cleavage of thioamino acids. J. Biol. Chem., **217,** 67, 1955.
68. Gaull, G. K., Rassin, D. K., and Sturman, J. A.: Pyridoxine-dependency in homocystinuria. Lancet, **2,** 1302, 1968.
69. Rosenberg, L. E., Lilljeqvist, A.-C., Hsia, Y. E., and Rosenbloom, F. M.: Vitamin B_{12}–dependent methyl malonic aciduria: defective cobamide coenzyme metabolism in cultured fibroblasts. J. Clin. Invest., **48,** 70a, 1969.
70. Mudd, S. H., Levy, H. L., and Abeles, R. H.: A derangement in B_{12} metabolism leading to homocystinuria, cystathioninemia, and methylmalonic aciduria. Biochem. Biophys. Res. Commun., **35,** 121, 1969.
71. Kodama, H., Yao, K., Kobayashi, K., Hirayama, K., Fujii, Y., Mizuhara, S., Haraguchi, H., and Hirosawa, M.: New sulfur-containing amino acids in the urine of cystathioninuria patients. Physiol. Chem. Physics, **1,** 72, 1969.
72. Frimpter, G. W., and Greenberg, A. J.: Renal clearance of cystathionine in homozygous and heterozygous cystathioninuria, cystinuria, and the normal state. J. Clin. Invest., **46,** 975, 1967.
73. Strickler, J. C., and Frimpter, G. W.: Renal excretion of cystathionine in dogs. Amer. J. Physiol., **217,** 1199, 1969.

74. Scriver, C. R.: Vitamin B_6 deficiency and dependency in man. Amer. J. Dis. Child., **113**, 109, 1967.
75. Tada, K., Yokayama, Y., Nakagawa, H., Yashida, T., and Arakawa, T.: Vitamin B_6 dependent xanthurenic aciduria. Tohoku J. Exp. Med., **93,** 115, 1967.
76. Horrigan, D. L., and Harris, J. W.: Pyridoxine responsive anemia: analysis of 62 cases. Advances Intern. Med., **12,** 103, 1964.
77. Hunt, A. D., Jr., Stokes, J., Jr., McCrory, W. W., and Stroud, H. D.: Pyridoxine dependency: report of a case of intractable convulsions in an infant controlled by pyridoxine. Pediatrics, **13,** 140, 1954.
78. Frimpter, G. W., Greenberg, A. J., Hilgartner, M., and Fuchs, F.: Cystathioninuria: management. Amer. J. Dis. Child., **113,** 115, 1967.
79. Laster, L., Irreverre, F., Mudd, S. H., and Heizer, W. D.: A previously unrecognized disorder of metabolism of sulfur-containing compounds—abnormal urinary excretion of S-sulfo-L-cysteine, sulfite and thiosulfate in a severely retarded child with ectopia lentis. J. Clin. Invest., **46,** 1082, 1967 (abstract).
80. Irreverre, F., Mudd, S. H., Heizer, W. D., and Laster, L.: Sulfite oxidase deficiency: studies of a patient with mental retardation, dislocated ocular lenses, and abnormal urinary excretion of S-sulfo-L-cysteine, sulfite, and thiosulfate. Biochem. Med., **1,** 187, 1967.
81. Spackman, D. H., Stein, W. H., and Moore, S.: Automatic recording apparatus for use in the chromatography of amino acids. Anal. Chem., **30,** 1190, 1958.
82. Feigl, F.: *Spot Tests in Inorganic Analysis,* 5th ed., p. 307. Elsevier, New York, 1958.
83. Mudd, S. H., Irreverre, F., and Laster, L.: Sulfite oxidase deficiency in man: demonstration of the enzymatic defect. Science, **156,** 1599, 1967.
84. Moser, H. W.: Editorial comment. Amer. J. Dis. Child., **117,** 66, 1969.
85. Efron, M. L.: The quantitative estimation of amino acids in physiological fluids using technicon amino acid analyzer: a modified technique with improved separation of amino acids and a simplified method for preparation of blood samples, in *Proceedings of the Technicon Symposium on Automation in Analytical Chemistry,* pp. 637–642, New York, Sept. 8, 1965. Mediad, Inc., New York, 1966. Cited by Ampola et al. [86].
86. Ampola, M. G., Efron, M. L., Bixby, E. M., and Meshorer, E.: Mental deficiency and a new aminoaciduria. Amer. J. Dis. Child., **117,** 66, 1969.
87. Kun, E.: The reaction of β-mercaptopyruvate with lactic dehydrogenase of heart muscle. Biochem. Biophys. Acta, **25,** 135, 1957.
88. Crawhall, J. C., Parker, R., Sneddon, W., and Young, E. P.: β-Mercaptolactate-cysteine disulfide in the urine of a mentally retarded patient. Amer. J. Dis. Child., **117,** 71, 1969.
89. Lipsett, M. N., Norton, J. S., and Peterkofsky, A.: A requirement for β-mercaptopyruvate in the in vitro thiolation of transfer ribonucleic acid. Biochemistry, **6,** 855, 1967.
90. Tallan, H. H., Pascal, T. A., Gillam, B. M., and Gaull, G. E.: Homolanthionine synthesis by human liver cystathionase. Biochem. Biophys. Res. Communications, **43,** 303, 1971.

ADDENDUM

Tallan, Pascal, Schneidman, Gillam, and Gaull described purification of cystathionase from human liver and noted several differences between rat and human liver cystathionases. These included pH optima, isoelectric points, and chromatographic behavior. Rabbit antibody to rat liver enzyme did not inhibit cystathionase or homoserine dehydratase activity of the human enzyme preparation [90].

CHAPTER TWENTY-ONE

ABNORMALITIES OF BRANCHED-CHAIN AMINO ACID METABOLISM

Hypervalinemia, Branched-chain Ketonuria (Maple Syrup Urine Disease), Isovaleric Acidemia

Joseph Dancis and Mortimer Levitz

In 1954 Menkes, Hurst, and Craig described a family in which four of six infants died during the first weeks of life [1]. The prominent signs were vomiting, muscular hypertonicity, and a maple syrup odor to the urine. In 1957 Westall, Dancis, and Miller reported an infant with brain damage, a similar odor to the urine, and increased levels of the branched-chain amino acids in the blood and urine [2]. Since these initial observations, our knowledge concerning maple syrup urine disease has rapidly increased, and at least three additional abnormalities of branched-chain amino acid metabolism have been recognized. In this chapter we shall consider hypervalinemia, maple syrup urine disease and its variants, and isovaleric acidemia.

METABOLISM OF THE BRANCHED-CHAIN AMINO ACIDS

The essential amino acids valine, leucine, and isoleucine are referred to as the branched-chain amino acids because each contains a methyl group which is not part of the longest carbon-to-carbon chain. The degradation of these amino acids involves sequentially (1) transamination, (2) oxidative decarboxylation of the resulting keto acid to the homologous branched-chain fatty acid, and (3) metabolism of the fatty acid. Since recent investigations have uncovered metabolic errors centering on each of these steps in the degradation of at least one of these branched-chain amino acids, a detailed discussion of the relevant enzymology is indicated.

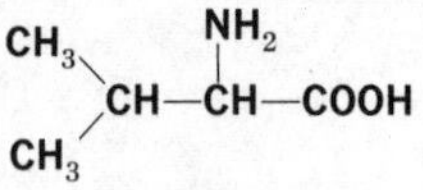

$$(CH_3)_2CH{-}CH(NH_2){-}COOH$$

Valine

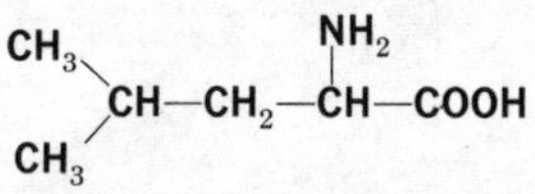

$$(CH_3)_2CH{-}CH_2{-}CH(NH_2){-}COOH$$

Leucine

$$CH_3{-}CH_2{-}CH(CH_3){-}CH(NH_2){-}COOH$$

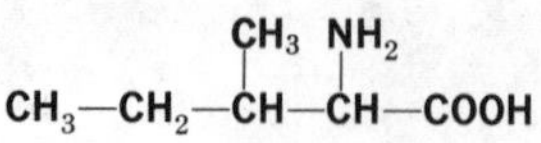

Isoleucine

Transamination

The catabolism of valine, leucine, and isoleucine is initiated by the loss of the amino group, either by oxidative deamination (Reaction 1) or by transamination (Reaction 2). In oxidative deamination, L-amino oxidase catalyzes the liberation of ammonia to form the corresponding α-keto acid. The branched-chain amino acids are relatively good substrates for L-amino acid oxidase, but the low enzymatic activity and the limited distribution of the enzyme make this pathway insignificant in mammals [3].

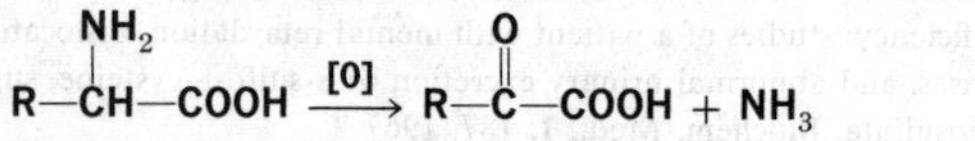

$$R{-}CH(NH_2){-}COOH \xrightarrow{[O]} R{-}C({=}O){-}COOH + NH_3 \qquad (1)$$

$$R{-}CH(NH_2){-}COOH + R'{-}C({=}O){-}COOH \rightleftharpoons R{-}C({=}O){-}COOH + R'{-}CH(NH_2){-}COOH \qquad (2)$$

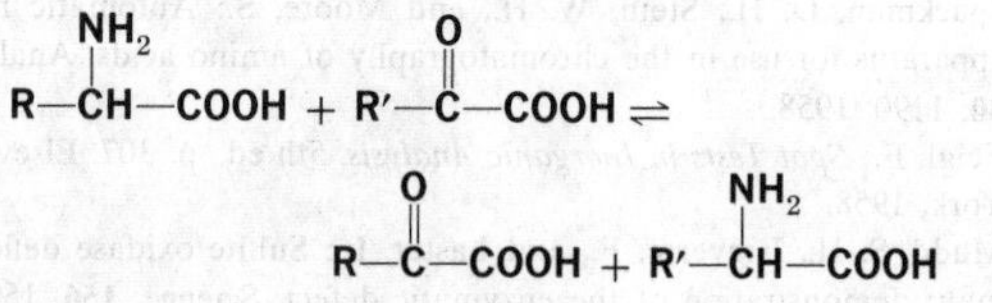

Transamination occurs in most animal tissues, and virtually all the natural amino acids participate [4]. Transamination differs from oxidative deamination in that ammonia is not liberated [5]. The cofactor which mediates transamination is vitamin B_6 in either the pyridoxal or the pyridoxamine form [6]. A plausible mechanism for coenzymatic participation of the vitamin is shown in Reaction 3 [6, 7]. A reversible enzymatic reaction between pyridoxal phosphate and the amino acid on the enzyme surface produces the Schiff base [1]. Hydrogen and double-bond shifts result in the isomeric Schiff base [11], which then splits into the keto acid and pyridoxamine phosphate. The reversibility of the reaction permits the regeneration of pyridoxal phosphate.

Alpha-ketoglutarate is the most common of several α-keto acids which may function as an NH_2 acceptor in enzymatic transamination. It couples effectively with valine, leucine, and isoleucine, converting them to the corresponding α-keto acids—α-ketoisovaleric acid, α-ketoisocaproic acid, and α-keto-β-methylvaleric acid [8]. The literature on the specificity of the transaminases is too extensive and, at times, too contradictory to be reviewed here. It would appear that some transaminases are effective against several amino acids, while others are more specific [9]. Even the more specific transaminases may retain activity when the receptor or donor is replaced by a substrate of similar structure [8].

Careful studies by two groups of investigators [10, 11] have led to the conclusion that a single transaminase from pig heart accepts the three branched-chain amino acids as substrates. Homogeneity was demonstrated by ultracentrifugation. In addition, in one of the studies [10] the relative activities toward valine, leucine, and isoleucine remained constant during seven purification stages. It is difficult to

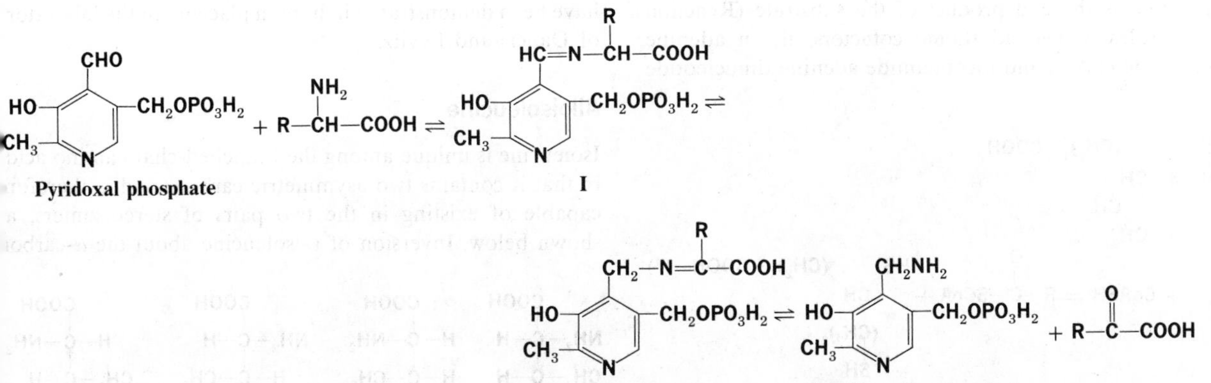

Pyridoxal phosphate + $R-CH(NH_2)-COOH \rightleftharpoons$ I $\rightleftharpoons$ (3)

II $\rightleftharpoons$ Pyridoxamine phosphate + $R-CO-COOH$

reconcile these data with the results obtained with a patient with hypervalinemia [12] (see below). The leukocytes of the patient were incapable of transaminating valine, whereas normal transamination of leucine and isoleucine was effected. A number of speculative alternatives can be offered to explain the anomalous behavior of the mutant leukocyte and the possibility of the existence of separate transaminases for the three branched-chain amino acids merits further consideration.

Oxidative Decarboxylation of the Branched-chain Keto Acids

Following transamination the α-keto acids are degraded further by oxidative decarboxylation (Reaction 4). This reaction is involved in the metabolic block in maple syrup urine disease and therefore requires detailed attention. Although the mechanism of the reaction has been deduced from studies with bacteria using pyruvate and α-ketoglutarate as substrates [13], there is ample evidence that the same mechanism prevails for enzymes derived from mammalian sources [14]. It seems reasonable that the branched-chain keto acids are decarboxylated in a similar manner.

$$R-\overset{O}{\overset{\|}{C}}-COOH \xrightleftharpoons{[O]} R-COOH + CO_2 \quad (4)$$

Decarboxylation is effected by a high-molecular-weight multienzyme complex, the components of which may be dissociated and reconstituted. Each component is responsible for one step of the pathway [14]. The initial step in the oxidative decarboxylation of the α-keto acids is commonly written as shown in Reaction 5. Thiamine pyrophosphate (TPP) mediates the elimination of carbon dioxide and becomes covalently bound to the decarboxylated fragment. The reaction appears to be reversible. If pig heart homogenate is fortified with TPP, increased incorporation of ^{14}C from $^{14}CO_2$ into the α-keto acid is observed [15], but the forward reaction is highly favored. The branched-chain keto acids are also substrates for the exchange reaction when incubated with guinea pig liver homogenate [16]. This suggests that these acids, too, may undergo initial decarboxylation. Breslow [17] has presented convincing arguments for the structure of the TPP complex as hydroxyethyl thiamine pyrophosphate (when pyruvate is the substrate). Carlson and Brown [18] isolated this compound from microorganisms and demonstrated its formation from TPP and pyruvate in the presence of wheat germ decarboxylase.

$$R-\overset{O}{\overset{\|}{C}}-COOH + TPP \rightleftharpoons \left[R-\overset{O}{\overset{\|}{C}}\cdot TPP\right]_{H} + CO_2 \quad (5)$$

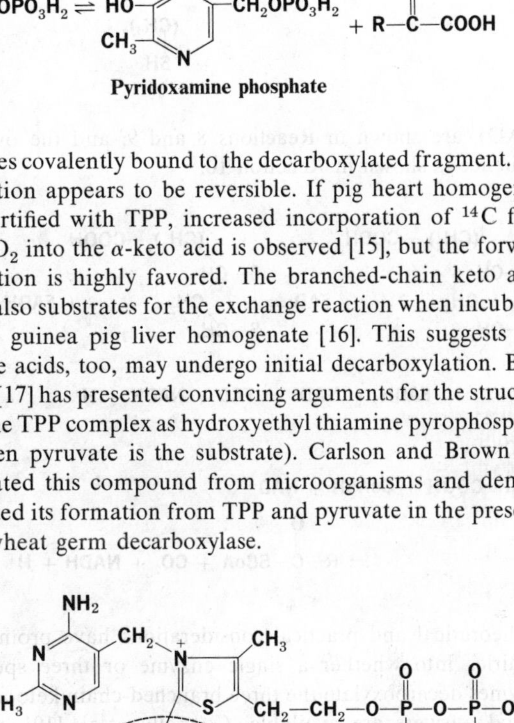

Hydroxyethyl thiamine pyrophosphate

The next step in the decarboxylation of the α-keto acids is the oxidation of the TPP complex by lipoic acid catalyzed by a second enzyme of the multienzyme system. Reduced lipoic acid is covalently bound to the decarboxylated acid, and TPP is liberated (Reaction 6).

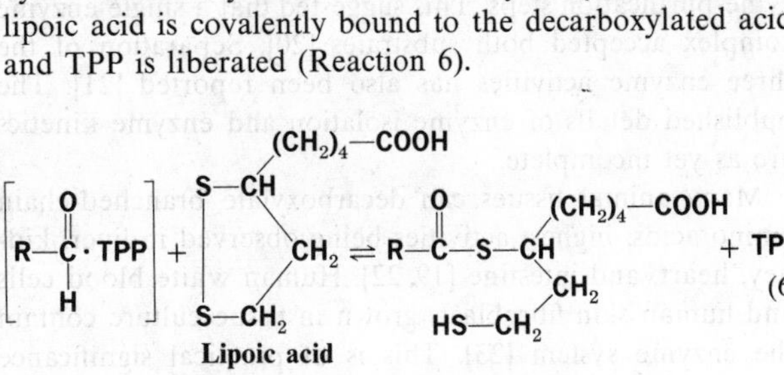

$$\left[R-\overset{O}{\overset{\|}{C}}\cdot TPP\right]_{H} + \text{Lipoic acid} \rightleftharpoons R-\overset{O}{\overset{\|}{C}}-S-CH((CH_2)_4-COOH)-CH_2-CH_2-SH + TPP \quad (6)$$

A third cofactor, coenzyme A (CoASH), displaces reduced lipoic acid to form the CoA derivative of the decarboxylated acid, which is the end product of the substrate (Reaction 7). The roles of two additional cofactors, flavin adenine dinucleotide (FAD) and nicotinamide adenine dinucleotide

$$\mathrm{R{-}\overset{O}{\overset{\|}{C}}{-}S{-}CH(CH_2)_4{-}COOH;\ {-}CH{-}CH_2{-}CH_2{-}SH} + \mathrm{CoASH} \rightleftharpoons \mathrm{R{-}\overset{O}{\overset{\|}{C}}{-}SCoA} + \mathrm{HS{-}CH((CH_2)_4{-}COOH){-}(CH_2)_2{-}SH} \quad (7)$$

(NAD), are shown in Reactions 8 and 9, and the overall sequence is shown in Reaction 10.

$$\mathrm{HS{-}CH((CH_2)_4{-}COOH){-}CH_2{-}CH_2{-}SH} + \mathrm{FAD} \rightleftharpoons \mathrm{\underset{S{-}CH_2{-}CH_2}{S{-}CH((CH_2)_4{-}COOH)}} + \mathrm{FADH_2} \quad (8)$$

$$\mathrm{FADH_2 + NAD^+ \rightleftharpoons FAD + NADH + H^+} \quad (9)$$

$$\mathrm{R{-}\overset{O}{\overset{\|}{C}}{-}COOH + CoASH + NAD^+ \rightleftharpoons R{-}\overset{O}{\overset{\|}{C}}{-}SCoA + CO_2 + NADH + H^+} \quad (10)$$

Theoretical and practical considerations have prompted inquiries into whether a single enzyme or three specific enzymes decarboxylate the three branched-chain keto acids. Partial answers are available. Connelly et al. [19], using ultracentrifugation, separated a complex with α-ketoisocaproic: α-keto-β-methylvaleric acid decarboxylase activity from a fraction with α-ketoisovaleric decarboxylase activity, the source of the enzymes being bovine liver. In a subsequent investigation, it was shown that the relative decarboxylase activities toward α-ketoisocaproic and α-keto-β-methylvaleric acids remained constant through a number of enzyme-purification steps. This suggested that a single enzyme complex accepted both substrates [20]. Separation of the three enzyme activities has also been reported [21]. The published details of enzyme isolation and enzyme kinetics are as yet incomplete.

Many animal tissues can decarboxylate branched-chain amino acids, highest activities being observed in liver, kidney, heart, and intestine [19, 22]. Human white blood cells and human skin fibroblasts grown in tissue culture contain the enzyme system [23]. This is of practical significance because these are cells which are easily obtained. Human placenta and muscle are reported to be devoid of detectable activity [22], but recently traces of decarboxylase activity have been demonstrated in human placenta in the laboratory of Dancis and Levitz.

Alloisoleucine

Isoleucine is unique among the branched-chain amino acids in that it contains two asymmetric carbons and is therefore capable of existing in the two pairs of stereoisomers, as shown below. Inversion of L-isoleucine about the α-carbon

L-Isoleucine	D-Isoleucine	L-Alloisoleucine	D-Alloisoleucine
$COOH$	$COOH$	$COOH$	$COOH$
$NH_2{-}C{-}H$	$H{-}C{-}NH_2$	$NH_2{-}C{-}H$	$H{-}C{-}NH_2$
$CH_3{-}C{-}H$	$H{-}C{-}CH_3$	$H{-}C{-}CH_3$	$CH_3{-}C{-}H$
CH_2	CH_2	CH_2	CH_2
CH_3	CH_3	CH_3	CH_3

produces D-alloisoleucine, while inversion at the β carbon results in L-alloisoleucine.

Interest in alloisoleucine was intensified when Norton et al. [24], using the modified ion-exchange column of Piez and Morris [25], found that alloisoleucine rather than methionine, with which it travels in the standard amino acid column chromatogram, was elevated in the plasma in a patient with maple syrup urine disease. Alloisoleucine is not normally found in animal tissue but may be formed in vivo when the level of isoleucine is increased.

Drastic conditions are required for the in vitro conversion of isoleucine to alloisoleucine. For example, an equal mixture of L-isoleucine and D-alloisoleucine is produced after heating L-isoleucine in barium hydroxide at 180°C for 20 hr [26]. L-Isoleucine is unaffected by refluxing with 20 percent hydrochloric acid [27]. L-Isoleucine is converted partially to D-alloisoleucine by treatment with pyridoxal and ferric ammonium sulfate at 100°C. The milder conditions for this conversion suggest a role of vitamin B_6 in the in vivo conversion [28].

Norton et al. [29] have indirect evidence that it is the L-form of alloisoleucine that is found in the plasma of the patient with maple syrup urine disease. The administration of a single dose of L-isoleucine resulted in the appearance of alloisoleucine in the plasma, and it persisted for several days. This is characteristic of L-alloisoleucine and is in contrast to D-alloisoleucine, which is rapidly cleared from the blood.

A mechanism for the conversion of L-isoleucine to L-alloisoleucine is shown in Reaction 11. The fact that D-α-keto-β-methylvaleric acid promotes growth (although at a lower rate than with the L- isomer) in the rat lends support to the hypothesis that the D- and L- isomers are interconverted in vivo [30]. The interconversion of isomers is somehow facilitated in vivo, because in vitro no noticeable racemization occurs below pH 8.4 [31]. The specific L-transaminase would then convert the mixture of keto acids to either L-isoleucine or L-alloisoleucine.

$$\underset{\text{L-Isoleucine}}{\begin{array}{c}COOH\\ |\\ NH_2-C-H\\ |\\ CH_3-C-H\\ |\\ CH_2\\ |\\ CH_3\end{array}} \rightleftharpoons \underset{\text{L-}\alpha\text{-Keto-}\beta\text{-methylvaleric acid}}{\begin{array}{c}COOH\\ |\\ O=C\\ |\\ CH_3-C-H\\ |\\ CH_2\\ |\\ CH_3\end{array}} \rightleftharpoons \begin{array}{c}COOH\\ |\\ HOC\\ \|\\ CH_3-C\\ |\\ CH_2\\ |\\ CH_3\end{array} \rightleftharpoons \underset{\text{D-}\alpha\text{-Keto-}\beta\text{-methylvaleric acid}}{\begin{array}{c}COOH\\ |\\ O=C\\ |\\ H-C-CH_3\\ |\\ CH_2\\ |\\ CH_3\end{array}} \rightleftharpoons \underset{\text{L-Alloisoleucine}}{\begin{array}{c}COOH\\ |\\ NH_2-C-H\\ |\\ H-C-CH_3\\ |\\ CH_2\\ |\\ CH_3\end{array}} \quad (11)$$

Isovaleric Acid

A metabolic disease characterized by the accumulation of isovaleric acid was first reported by Tanaka et al. [32]. Since Reaction 10 indicates that the coenzyme A derivative of isovaleric acid is the product of oxidative decarboxylation of α-ketoisocaproic acid, the metabolism of isovaleric acid is crucial to the understanding of this disease.

Rat liver, chicken liver, and pig heart are the main enzyme sources which revealed the catabolic route of isovaleric acid. The first step is dehydrogenation to yield β-methylcrotonyl-CoA (Reaction 12) [33]. This in turn is carboxylated to form β-methylglutaconyl-CoA [34]. The carboxylase is biotin-dependent [35]. A hydrating enzyme converts β-methylglutaconyl-CoA to β-hydroxy-β-methylglutaryl-CoA [36]. The latter is then split to acetoacetic acid and acetyl CoA [37, 38]. This reaction provides an explanation for the ketogenic effect of leucine.

$$\underset{\text{Isovaleryl-CoA}}{(CH_3)_2CH-CH_2-C(=O)-SCoA} \rightleftharpoons \underset{\beta\text{-Methylcrotonyl-CoA}}{(CH_3)_2C=CH-C(=O)-SCoA}$$

$$\underset{\beta\text{-Hydroxy-}\beta\text{-methylglutaryl-CoA}}{(HOOC-CH_2)(CH_3)COH-CH_2-C(=O)-SCoA} \rightleftharpoons \underset{\beta\text{-Methylglutaconyl-CoA}}{(HOOC-CH_2)(CH_3)C=CH-C(=O)-SCoA} \quad (12)$$

$$\underset{\text{Acetoacetic acid}}{CH_3-C(=O)-CH_2-COOH} + \underset{\text{Acetyl-CoA}}{CH_3-C(=O)-SCoA}$$

The catabolism of the other two branched-chain fatty acids, isobutyric acid and α-methylbutyric acid, does not appear to be involved in metabolic diseases within the scope of this chapter and will not be discussed here. Excellent reviews of these pathways are available [39, 40].

HYPERVALINEMIA

Incidence

To date, only one child with hypervalinemia has been recognized [41]. The parents were not related, and results of their valine loading tests were normal [42].

The Metabolic Error

Elevation of the blood level of valine in the absence of ketoaciduria strongly suggested a defect in the transamination of valine (see Fig. 21-1). This was confirmed by an investigation of the metabolism of the peripheral leukocytes (Table 21-1).

The defect in transamination appears to be specific for valine. The leukocytes of the patient converted the remaining two branched-chain amino acids and methionine and phenylalanine to their respective keto acids. This strongly suggests that the transamination of valine is effected primarily by a specific transaminase in this patient.

As already noted, two groups of investigators have concluded that there is a single transaminase in pig heart that will accept the three branched-chain amino acids [10, 11]. It is possible that the mammal synthesizes a specific transaminase, as well as one that is less specific, a feature that is commonly noted in transport systems. If so, the observations in the hypervalinemic patient strongly suggest that the major degradative pathway involves the specific pathway. It is also possible that one protein, functioning as the transaminase for the three branched-chain amino acids, has an active site that is specific for valine, and that only this site is defective in hypervalinemia. It is perhaps risky to generalize too broadly from a single case.

Clinical Findings

The one reported case occurred in a Japanese infant who, shortly after birth, was noted to suck poorly and to vomit

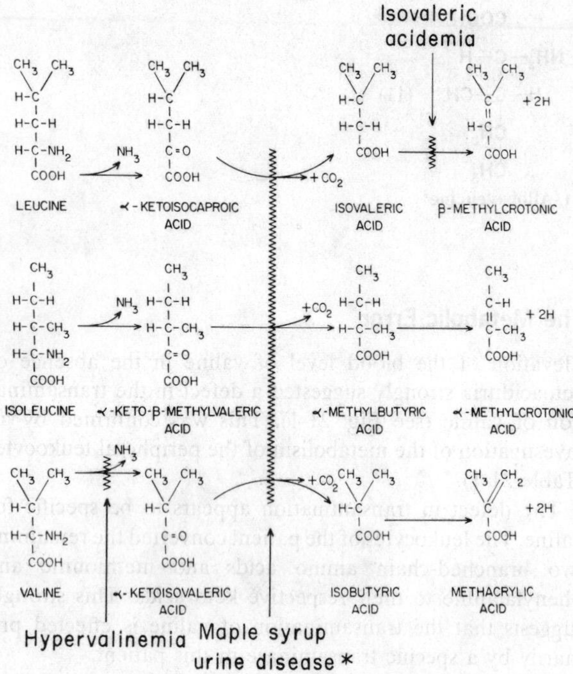

Figure 21-1. Degradative pathway of the branched-chain amino acids, indicating the metabolic defects that have been so far described. Asterisk denotes block found at the same metabolic step in both classic and variant forms. (*From Dancis et al.* [98]; *reprinted by permission.*)

frequently. Severe mental and physical retardation rapidly became evident. When last reported, the child was 3 years old and living at home.

With experience limited to one case, it is not possible to be certain as to which of the manifestations are directly related to the hypervalinemia. The cessation of vomiting, improved weight gain, and reduced hyperkinesia when a low-valine diet was started suggest that these symptoms may be so related. Mental retardation commonly leads to a search for abnormalities in amino acid metabolism, and the mental retardation in this patient may be only coincidental.

Table 21-1. TRANSAMINATION OF SELECT AMINO ACIDS BY LEUKOCYTES OF A PATIENT AND CONTROL SUBJECTS

Amino acid	Hypervalinemia	Control A	Control B
Valine	0	134	71
Isoleucine	346	268	222
Leucine	387	183	143
Methionine	198	98	55
Phenylalanine	48	32	42

Leukocytes were incubated with one of the following substrates: 4 μmoles (0.4 microcurie) of DL-valine-1-^{14}C, DL-leucine-1-^{14}C, DL-phenylalanine-1-^{14}C, or 2 μmoles (0.2 microcurie) of L-isoleucine-U-^{14}C or L-methionine-methyl-^{14}C. The radioactive keto acids are reported in disintegrations per minute.
Source: From Dancis et al. [12].

Diagnosis

Hypervalinemia in the absence of ketoaciduria is probably sufficient to establish the diagnosis. Demonstration of the enzyme defect in peripheral leukocytes will provide confirmation. Diagnostic methods are basically the same as those used in maple syrup urine disease (see Metabolism of Leucocytes, under Methods, later in this chapter).

Conversion of valine to α-ketoisovaleric acid may be assessed in the peripheral leukocytes as follows [12]. Radioactive valine is incubated with leukocytes as described for the diagnosis of maple syrup urine disease. The incubation medium contains L-valine-^{14}C 0.25 μmole (1 microcurie), and sodium α-ketoisovalerate, 0.5 μmole, in Krebs-Ringer phosphate buffer, pH 7.4, with a total volume of 1 ml. Incubation is for 75 min at 37°C, with agitation. The incubation is terminated with one drop of 1*N* hydrochloric acid, and the leukocytes are removed by centrifuging. To the supernatant is added 0.5 ml of 0.2 percent 2,4-dinitrophenylhydrazine in 2*N* HCl, and the hydrazones are then extracted sequentially into 5 ml *m*-xylene, 3 ml of 10 percent Na_2CO_3, and, following acidification with HCl, into 5 ml toluene. The toluene is transferred to the scintillant solution for assay of the labeled 2,4-dinitrophenylhydrazone of α-ketoisovaleric acid.

The radioactivity in the reagent blank is greatly reduced if the stock valine-^{14}C solution is first reacted with 0.1 ml of the dinitrophenylhydrazine solution. The solution is then extracted six or more times with peroxide-free ether. The remaining traces of ether are removed with nitrogen, and the solution is neutralized with sodium hydroxide.

MAPLE SYRUP URINE DISEASE (Branched-chain Ketonuria; Leucinosis)

Incidence

Approximately 50 patients have been reported in the literature [1, 43–62]. This provides only a rough indication of the frequency of the disease. Undoubtedly the diagnosis is often missed if death occurs early. In recent years these patients are frequently not reported unless there is some unusual aspect to be described. A better indication of the incidence may eventually be derived from screening programs. In the Massachusetts program, 508,000 newborn infants have been tested for elevated blood leucine levels by means of a bacterial-inhibition assay devised by Guthrie; two cases of maple syrup urine disease have been detected [63]. In New York City blood samples of newborn infants have been analyzed by paper chromatography, and two cases have been found in 190,000 tested [64].

The mutation has been found in many ethnic groups, including the Negro [50] and Japanese [49]. Because of the difficulties in diagnosis, case reports have been limited to the medically advanced countries.

Genetics

The lack of large lineages has impeded determination of the inheritance pattern. The clinical histories are consistent with an autosomal recessive pattern. Multiple cases have appeared in families, and both males and females are affected. The parents appear normal but in at least three instances have been related.

Biochemical investigations of parents have been undertaken to determine whether they are heterozygotes. Leucine or α-ketoisocaproic acid has been administered orally, and the blood levels have been followed, but the results have been inconclusive. Studies using the metabolism of the blood cells in vitro have been more successful. In evaluating reports of measurements on parents and sibs which purport to document the accuracy of the assay method, one must eliminate from consideration the results with the sibs unless their genetic status can be independently ascertained.

Three laboratories have reported that the parents of propositi have appeared, on the basis of assay tests, to be heterozygotes. Linneweh and his colleagues incubated whole blood of four parents and nine normal subjects with leucine-1-^{14}C and found lower decarboxylase activities in the parents of the patients [65]. A more extensive study sufficient for statistical evaluation was done with the peripheral leukocytes of 18 parents and 19 normal adults [66]. The metabolism of sodium α-ketoisocaproate-2-^{14}C was compared to that of sodium isovalerate-1-^{14}C, the latter providing a control for the number of cells and their metabolic status. A significantly reduced ratio was found in the fathers; the mean in the mothers was also reduced but did not reach a level of statistical significance. Goedde and Keller [67] have reported a high degree of accuracy in identifying the individual heterozygote. They have also measured the decarboxylase activity of peripheral leukocytes, using a standardized number of cells. More recently, Goedde [68] has suggested that accuracy may be further increased by studying only the lymphocytes.

Table 21-2. PLASMA LEVELS OF AMINO ACIDS IN UNTREATED CASES OF MAPLE SYRUP URINE DISEASE

	Normal	L. O'C.*	G. B.†	C. O'C.‡
Alanine	3.0–4.8	0.5	0.6	1.47
Arginine	......	....	0.8	
Asparagine plus glutamine	6.0–8.0	3.5	2.0	1.96
Aspartic acid	0.1–0.2	0.1	0.04	0.14
Cystine	1.0–1.5	0.2	0	0
Glutamic acid	1.0–1.5	0.1	0.9	0.5
Glycine	1.0–2.0	1.4	1.5	0.9
Histidine	......	......	0.7	0.8
Isoleucine	0.8–1.5	17.9	2.2	8.5
Leucine	1.5–3.0	52.4	14.5	21.1
Lysine	......	....	1.1	0.7
Methionine plus alloisoleucine	......	4.0	2.7	3.9
Ornithine	......	....	0.5	
Phenylalanine	1.0–1.7	1.5	0.8	0.9
Proline	1.5–3.0	0.1	0.9	
Serine	1.3–2.2	1.2	0.9	1.2
Taurine	0.9–1.8	0.4	0.4	
Threonine	1.2–1.6	1.0	0.3	0.9
Tryptophan	......	......	0	
Tyrosine	1.5–2.3	2.0	0.7	0.8
Valine	2.0–3.0	23.9	13.1	14.5

* Six days old [86].
† Eighteen months old [43].
‡ Eight months old [93].

The Metabolic Error

The metabolic defect has been localized in two ways: (1) identification of the metabolites accumulated in the disease has indicated indirectly the step at which normal metabolism is interrupted; (2) study of the peripheral leukocytes by enzymatic methods has demonstrated the enzymatic defect directly.

The demonstration that plasma levels of leucine, isoleucine, and valine are extremely elevated in maple syrup urine disease suggested that there is an interruption in the catabolic pathway of these amino acids (Table 21-2) [2]. Because the keto acids were also present in excess, it was evident that the amino acids were being effectively transaminated [69, 70]. Lack of elevation of the branched-chain fatty acids [43] suggested that the metabolic pathway was interrupted at the point of oxidative decarboxylation of the branched-chain keto acids (see Fig. 21-2).

Investigation of the enzymatic activity of the peripheral leukocytes has confirmed the locus of the block. Leukocytes from patients with maple syrup urine disease can transaminate the branched-chain amino acids but cannot decarboxylate the resulting keto acids [71]. Localization of the defect has been completed by the demonstration that isovaleric acid, which is distal to the block, is metabolized normally [66].

Studies with the peripheral leukocytes were performed when dietary therapy had restored the blood levels of the amino acids to normal. This virtually excluded the possibility that the metabolism of only one amino acid was defective and that excess of this amino acid or its metabolites was secondarily depressing the degradation of the others.

Recent evidence that the branched-chain amino acids may have specific decarboxylases has revived the suggestion that only one of the decarboxylases may be involved primarily [19, 20]. In order to reinvestigate this possibility under carefully controlled conditions, the metabolism of fibroblasts grown in tissue culture from the skin of a patient with maple syrup urine disease and from a patient with intermittent branched-chain ketonuria has been studied [72]. In both instances, the decarboxylation of the three branched-chain amino acids was greatly reduced or absent. It appears that in maple syrup urine disease the activity of three decarboxylases is depressed. This must be reconciled with the evidence

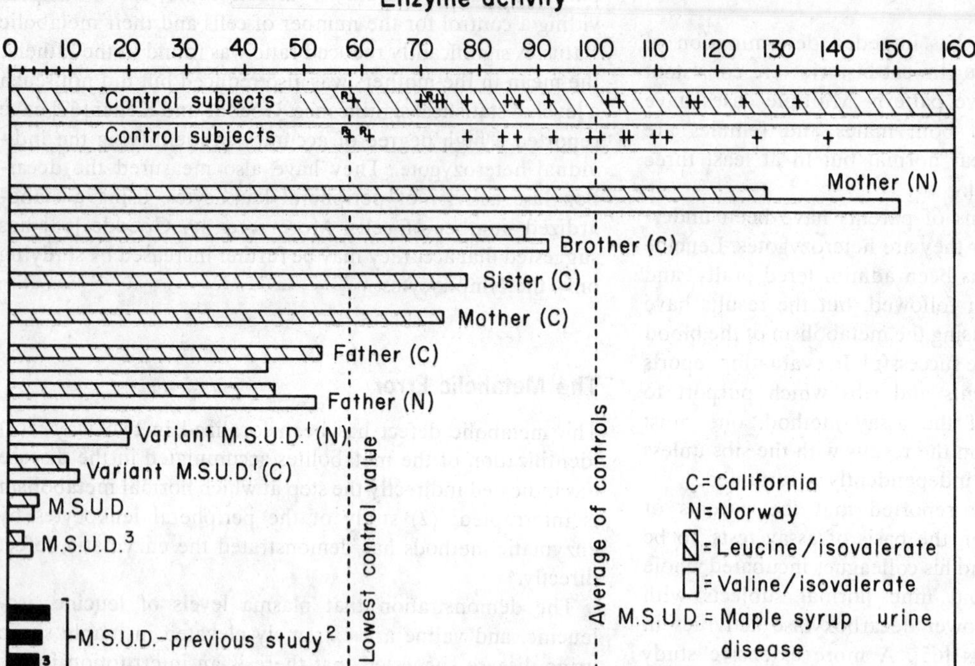

Figure 21-2. Branched-chain keto acid decarboxylase activity of leukocytes. The leucine/isovaleric acid and valine/isovaleric acid ratios are adjusted so that the average of the normal values (1.84 and 1.92, respectively) equals 100. The determination on one normal subject was repeated and these results are identified by R. 1, average of two determinations; 2, α-ketoisocaproic acid/isovaleric acid ratios; 3, determinations on the same subject. (*From Dancis et al.* [98]; *reprinted by permission.*)

that there may be more than one branched-chain keto acid decarboxylase. According to current genetic concepts, a plausible explanation is that a polypeptide under the control of one gene is common to the enzymes, to some portion of the enzyme complex, or to some factor involved in their regulatory control.

Earlier a peak on the amino acid chromatogram was thought to represent methionine, and this could not be reconciled with a primary block in the metabolism of the branched-chain amino acids. This peak has since been identified as alloisoleucine [24]. The alloisoleucine is probably derived from the abnormal excess of isoleucine (see Metabolism of the Branched-chain Amino Acids, earlier in this chapter).

Other Metabolites

The hydroxyacids of the branched-chain amino acids have been identified in the urine [44, 45]. They probably arise by reduction of the keto acids. An excess of indoleacetic acid, as in phenylketonuria, has also been reported.

Pathology

Several reports of autopsy examinations have now appeared [1, 47, 48, 53, 56, 73]. The findings probably reflect in part the terminal illnesses, malnutrition, and infection. The pathologic change in the brain has been qualitatively consistent and probably is more directly related to the metabolic defect.

If the patient dies during the first weeks of life, no morbid changes may be evident, except possibly a sponginess of the white matter, which is generally attributed to edema. If the patient lives for some months, a deficiency in myelin and an astrocytosis are seen. The absence of degradative products of myelin suggests that the lack of myelin results from an interruption in postnatal synthesis. If the patient has been successfully treated by diet, there may be no deficiency in myelinization [53].

Similar changes have been reported in phenylketonuria and in patients dying with no recognized metabolic anomaly. It is a matter of speculation as to what may be the common mechanism in these varied entities.

Chemical analyses of the brain have been reported by

several investigators [53, 74–77]. In general, there have been edema and a reduction in the total lipids, including both cerebrosides and proteolipids. This is the chemical parallel to the reduction in myelin noted histologically. Prensky and Moser [77] have suggested that the primary feature may be a reduced synthesis of proteolipids resulting from the elevations of the branched-chain amino acids in the brain. This, in turn, may interfere with the normal myelin synthesis. They have also reported a reduction in glutamic acid, glutamine, and γ-aminobutyric acid in the brain. The brains of patients in whom dietary therapy has been initiated early in their disease have normal lipid composition [76, 78].

The relation of the pathologic findings to symptoms is not clear. The deficiency in myelin could contribute to the chronic mental and neurologic signs but cannot explain the acute episodes in patients who lapse transiently from dietary control (see Treatment, later in this chapter). Even the chronic symptoms cannot be completely explained by the deficiency in myelin. One patient died at 3 years of age with normal brain lipids [76]. Dietary treatment had not been instituted until the patient was 35 days old, and the child had remained mentally retarded.

The "Toxic Agent"

The favorable response to diets low in the branched-chain amino acids suggests that the deleterious effects result from the abnormal accumulation of metabolites proximal to the metabolic block, rather than an insufficiency of metabolites distal to the block. The acute onset and relief of symptoms such as ataxia, convulsions, and coma in patients under dietary treatment and in patients with intermittent branched-chain ketonuria (see below) indicate a "toxic agent" that directly interferes with brain function.

Clinical observations indicate that these acute symptoms are more directly related to excess of leucine than to excess of the remaining two branched-chain amino acids [79]. It is not clear whether it is the excess of the amino acids, their keto acids, or some other metabolite that is most significant.

Elevated levels of the branched-chain amino acids may disturb transport of other amino acids and distort the free amino acid pools [80]. This could interfere with function, inhibit protein synthesis [81], and reduce proteolipid and myelin formation [77]. Rats fed diets containing 5 percent leucine developed smaller brains with lower concentrations of serotonin [82]. The branched-chain keto acids competitively inhibit glutamic acid decarboxylation [83], a reaction considered important in brain function. Oxygen consumption of brain slices is reduced in the presence of α-ketoisocaproic acid or valine [84]. These varied observations suggest the possibility that multiple factors contribute to the signs and symptoms.

The metabolite responsible for the maple syrup odor is unknown. Keto acids often contain trace contaminants that smell like maple syrup. The oral administration of isoleucine to a patient under dietary control reproduced the odor, whereas leucine and valine did not [79].

If the keto acids are toxic, the transaminases of the branched-chain amino acids in brain tissue [43] would facilitate their formation directly at the site of greatest sensitivity. The keto acids in spinal fluid [45] may originate directly in the brain rather than from the blood.

Clinical Findings

The infant appears normal at birth but by the end of the first week usually feeds poorly and may vomit and become lethargic. Muscular hypertonicity and convulsions may appear. The maple syrup odor has been detected in the urine as early as the fifth day, but it is often missed until much later. Death is usually caused by an intercurrent infection.

The disease varies widely in the rapidity of its course. Death may occur during the first week of life and has usually occurred during the first year. It is rare for a patient to survive past the second year. The disease is much more lethal than phenylketonuria. If the patient lives long enough, severe brain damage is always evident.

Hypoglycemic episodes occur [45, 47, 48]. They are probably caused by the excessively high levels of leucine, which depress blood glucose levels even in the normal subject [85].

Diagnosis

A familial history of neurologic disease with mental retardation and convulsions, or of unexplained death in infancy, should alert the physician to the possibility of a genetic defect. The only clinically distinctive feature of maple syrup urine disease is the odor. For physicians unfamiliar with maple syrup (maple syrup is not generally available in Europe), the odor may be compared to that of burned sugar.

Though the odor is virtually pathognomonic of the disease, the diagnosis must be verified in the laboratory. Two patients have come to our attention in whom reliable observers had noted an odor similar to maple syrup, but in whom laboratory studies excluded the diagnosis. In both instances the odor was transient.

The untreated patient has a large excess of branched-chain amino acids (Table 21-2) and keto acids in the blood and urine. The diagnosis is relatively simple if any of the methods described below is used. If the patient is under dietary treatment, these signs of biochemical abnormality disappear, but the enzyme defect is still demonstrable in the peripheral leukocytes.

Our experience with maple syrup urine disease at birth is limited to three patients. The following generalizations appear reasonable: At birth, analysis of blood and urine is not likely to reveal significant abnormalities. The maternal plasma, which serves as the source of the fetal amino acids, has normal concentrations of the branched-chain amino acids. Thus, an excess is not likely to accumulate in the fetus prior to birth. At birth the diagnosis can probably be made only by demonstration of the enzyme defect. By the end of the first week there should be sufficient accumulation of the amino acids and keto acids to permit diagnosis by the usual methods. Paper chromatographic examination of plasma on the fourth day [86] and of blood on the fifth day [87] has been adequate to demonstrate elevation of the branched-chain amino acids.

The keto acids in maple syrup urine disease accumulate early, whereas in phenylketonuria the keto acid (phenylpyruvic acid) may not be demonstrable until the third week of life. The reason for this is that in maple syrup urine disease the keto acids lie in the major metabolic pathway of the branched-chain amino acids, while phenylpyruvic acid is normally a minor metabolite and the pathway appears to be poorly developed at birth.

METHODS

Analysis for Amino Acids

1 Paper chromatography. The characteristic pattern of elevations in valine, leucine, and isoleucine has been demonstrated using 10 μl of either blood or plasma as early as the fourth or fifth day of life. A one-dimensional chromatogram with the solvent system *n*-butanol–acetic acid–water (12:3:5) is adequate [87].

2 Column chromatography. This form of separation is most convenient for the quantitative determination of the branched-chain amino acids. The modified technique of Piez and Morris [25] is superior in that alloisoleucine is separated from methionine. The method permits confirmation of the diagnosis and evaluation of the effects of the dietary regimen.

3 Microbiologic assay. A microbiologic assay for the branched-chain amino acids, intended as a screening procedure, has been described [88].

Analysis for Keto Acids

1 Qualitative demonstration of excess keto acids.

a. To 1 ml urine add 4 ml 0.2 percent 2,4-dinitrophenylhydrazine in 2*N* hydrochloric acid. In a positive test a yellow precipitate forms.

b. After 10 min extract with peroxide-free ether.

c. Remove the ether layer and extract it with 5 ml of 10 percent sodium carbonate. The yellow 2,4-dinitrophenylhydrazones of the keto acids enter the water phase and develop a deep red color after addition of an equal volume of 1*N* sodium hydroxide.

2 Identification of keto acids and quantitative analysis. The 2,4-dinitrophenylhydrazones of the branched-chain keto acids can be identified by chromatography, and may then be eluted and assayed spectrophotometrically if a quantitative analysis is desired. Paper chromatography has been widely used. Details may be found in a review by Neish [89]. Thin-layer chromatography offers advantages over paper chromatography in providing a more rapid and discrete separation [90] (see Table 21-3).

The keto acids may also be identified and quantitated by gas-phase chromatography [91]. Another approach is to hydrogenate the hydrazones [92]. This converts the keto acid to its respective amino acid, which can then be identified by standard methods.

Normal values: In blood in milligrams per 100 ml: α-ketoglutaric acid, 0.13; pyruvic acid, 0.65; α-ketoisovaleric acid, 0.13; α-ketoisocaproic plus α-keto-β-methylvaleric acids, 0.38 [102].

In urine, the branched-chain keto acids are ordinarily not present in significant amounts.

The values for the branched-chain keto acids in an untreated infant with maple syrup urine disease at age 8 months were 12.3 mg per 100 ml in plasma and 64 mg per 100 ml in urine [93].

Metabolism of Leukocytes

The demonstration that the enzyme defect in maple syrup urine disease is present in the white blood cells of the peripheral blood forms the basis of a diagnostic test [71]. The leukocytes are incubated with leucine-1-^{14}C, and the liberated $^{14}CO_2$ provides an assay of decarboxylase activity.

1 Mix freshly drawn heparinized blood with 2 volumes of 3 percent dextran (molecular weight 200,000 to 300,000) in 0.15*M* sodium chloride.

2 After about 45 min of sedimentation, remove the supernatant containing the leukocytes.

Table 21-3. THIN-LAYER CHROMATOGRAPHY* OF 2,4-DINITROPHENYLHYDRAZONES OF KETO ACIDS†

Keto acid	R_F
α-Ketoglutaric	0
Acetoacetic	9
Pyruvic (isomer II)‡	11
Phenylpyruvic (isomer II)	22
α-Ketoisocaproic (isomer II)	22
Pyruvic acid (isomer I)	28
α-Keto-γ-methiolbutyric	34
α-Ketoisovaleric	42
Phenylpyruvic (isomer I)	46
α-Keto-β-methylvaleric	48
α-Ketoisocaproic (isomer I)	48

* Plates (100 × 200 mm, 0.3 mm thickness of Silica Gel G) were developed with isoamyl alcohol—0.25*M* NH_4OH (20:1).

† Several α-keto acids give rise to isomeric 2,4-dinitrophenylhydrazones.

‡ By convention the isomer with the greater mobility is denoted isomer I.

Source: From Dancis [90].

3 Mix to distribute the leukocytes evenly. Place aliquots in incubation flasks and centrifuge at 1,200 × *g* for 20 min. Small Erlenmeyer flasks equipped with center-wells are satisfactory. We have also used small glass vials (Kimble No. 60957) and inserted glass cups for center wells (Kontes, K-882320-9001).

4 Carefully remove the supernatant by aspiration and immediately add the incubation media: L- branched-chain amino acid-1-^{14}C, 1 μmole, 0.1 microcurie;[1] thiamine · HCl, 0.5 mg; and Krebs-Ringer phosphate buffer, pH 7.4, 0.8 ml.

5 Charge the center well with 0.1 ml of 1 percent potassium hydroxide solution. Flush with oxygen, stopper securely, and incubate 90 min at 37°C with agitation.

6 Transfer the center-well contents quantitatively to a scintillation-counting vial containing toluene-methanol-phenylethylamine (2:1:1) and scintillants. Determine the radioactivity.

Alternatively, the $^{14}CO_2$ may be precipitated as $BaCO_3$ and counted in a gas-flow counter.

In a positive test result the center-well is virtually devoid of radioactivity. Control leukocytes form easily measurable amounts of $^{14}CO_2$.

In order to identify either the heterozygote of patients with partial defects, such as those with intermittent branched-chain ketonuria, it may be necessary to have a more quantitative assay of decarboxylase activity. Incubation of a separate aliquot of leukocytes with isovaleric acid-1-^{14}C provides a suitable base line which reflects the number of leukocytes and their metabolic status [66]. Relating the decarboxylase activity to the total leukocyte or lymphocyte counts may be just as satisfactory [68].

The radioactive keto acid is, theoretically, the better substrate to use, but it is not commercially available, and when prepared, it yields a relatively high background of volatile radioactive products. In practice we have preferred to use the radioactive amino acid. Transamination does not appear to be a limiting step in the degradation of the branched-chain amino acids by the leukocyte.

Treatment

The success of low-phenylalanine diets in phenylketonuria suggested a similar approach in maple syrup urine disease. For the success of a dietary approach, it is necessary that the infant be born undamaged and that the subsequent damage be due to the accumulation of metabolites proximal to the metabolic block, rather than to a deficiency of the products distal to the block. Although experience with maple syrup urine disease is still limited, there has been sufficient success to indicate that both requirements are probably met.

[1] The stock amino acid should be freed of volatile radioactive contaminants prior to use. The solution is adjusted to pH 3 to 4, flushed with nitrogen, and stored below 0°C.

The principles of treatment are simple. When the diagnosis is established, the patient is placed on an amino acid diet from which the branched-chain amino acids are omitted, together with supplements of carbohydrate, fat, vitamins, and minerals. When the plasma levels of the branched-chain amino acids have fallen to normal, these amino acids are restored to the diet in amounts to maintain the levels at, or a little above, normal. When the patient's condition has been stabilized, milk and then other foods are added in amounts adequate to supply but not exceed the requirements for the branched-chain amino acids. The remaining requirements for amino acids are supplied as the purified substances. The purpose of adding natural foods is to avoid omission of unrecognized essential dietary components.

In practice, the dietary treatment in maple syrup urine disease is far more difficult than in phenylketonuria. The reasons are multiple:

1 Three amino acids are involved in the disease, and the requirements for each must be determined individually. This requires close laboratory supervision.

2 There are no simple methods for the analysis of the branched-chain amino acids. At present major reliance must be placed on column chromatography. Early in the disease dietary adjustments must be frequent. It is necessary to avoid both excess and insufficiency of the branched-chain amino acids. Insufficiency of these amino acids will interfere with growth and, if extreme, may even lead to a degradation of tissue protein and a secondary elevation of the branched-chain amino acids.

3 Relapses from control occur during minor infections, particularly in the early months of infancy. These may be serious and require vigorous and intelligent treatment. They are usually heralded by anorexia and a return of the maple syrup odor, followed shortly by ataxia, lethargy, and convulsions. The provocative factor in these attacks is probably catabolism of body proteins with a high content of branched-chain amino acids, and an acute accumulation of the keto acids.

4 Most foods have a high content of the branched-chain amino acids, and there is no simple way for removing them, as there is for phenylalanine. Thus diets must make liberal use of purified amino acids.

Snyderman, Holt, and their colleagues have reported their experience with dietary treatment in seven patients [79]. They have stressed the importance of early initiation of treatment, careful biochemical monitoring, and the early introduction of natural foods. Westall has had excellent success with a child in whom treatment was started at 5 days of age [93].

There is no indication as to when, if ever, dietary restrictions may be eased. The experience with children with intermittent branched-chain ketonuria dictates extreme caution (see below). A fatal outcome has been associated with acute elevation of the branched-chain amino acids as late as 8 years of age.

The Acute Episode

Frequently, at the time the diagnosis is initially made, the levels of the branched-chain amino acids and keto acids are extremely elevated in blood and urine. The patient may be comatose and having convulsions, and life may be threatened. A similar picture occurs episodically in patients on the prescribed diet or with intermittent branched-chain ketonuria (see below). Usually, parenterally administered fluids containing glucose and electrolytes followed by an amino acid diet in which the branched-chain amino acids are omitted will reverse the findings. On occasion, the response to the standard regimen may be unsatisfactory. Under this circumstance, exchange transfusion or peritoneal dialysis may be lifesaving [94]. Both the branched-chain keto acids and amino acids equilibrate rapidly throughout the body compartments and with the dialysis fluid. Large amounts of the excess metabolites may be rapidly removed.

INTERMITTENT BRANCHED-CHAIN KETONURIA (A Variant of Maple Syrup Urine Disease)

Clinical Findings

Two unrelated families have been reported, each with two children who have presented an interesting variation in the classical picture of maple syrup urine disease [95–97]. The common features were initial manifestations months or years after birth, intermittent attacks of neurologic symptoms associated with a maple syrup odor and elevations of the branched-chain amino acids and keto acids in blood and urine, and normal mental and physical development. One patient in each family has died during an acute attack. These patients will be described in some detail to illustrate the significant features.

W.T. seemed normal until $10\frac{1}{2}$ months old, when, during a mild respiratory infection, he became irritable and ataxic and excreted large amounts of branched-chain amino acids and keto acids, associated with the characteristic odor. Subsequently, occasional mild ataxia was noted until the child was 19 months old, when his milk intake was increased because of thirst during a lengthy cross-country trip. Probably because of the large protein intake, he relapsed, became semicomatose, and required hospitalization and parenteral therapy. He remained irritable and ataxic during the next 6 months and irreversible damage was suspected, but when protein intake was reduced and foods were selected that were low in leucine, the symptoms disappeared.

At $4\frac{1}{2}$ years of age, he was admitted to the hospital for tonsillectomy. Peripheral collapse because of hemorrhage required transfusion. He became comatose, had high blood levels of the branched-chain amino and keto acids, and failed progressively until he died on the seventh day. Autopsy revealed cerebral edema.

B.F., an 8-year-old boy, was admitted to the hospital with a presumptive diagnosis of meningitis following a 3-day history of fever, headache, vomiting, and lethargy. There was a "curry-like" odor to the urine. An elevation in level of serum valine and leucine-isoleucine was demonstrated by paper chromatography, and the respective keto acids were found in the urine. In spite of intravenous infusions of fluid and electrolytes, he lapsed into coma and died 5 days after admission to the hospital. Autopsy disclosed spongy degeneration of the cortex and necrosis of the granule cell layer of the cerebellum. Before this hospital admission he had been considered physically normal and mentally bright.

Besides the four cases mentioned above, two other cases described in the literature may fit in this category [48, 99].

Metabolic Defect

Two surviving children with intermittent branched-chain ketonuria have been studied. Examination of the peripheral leukocytes has revealed a considerably reduced decarboxylase activity for leucine and valine, the only amino acids that were tested [98]. Assay of the fibroblasts grown in tissue culture from E.T. has demonstrated a reduction in the activity for all three branched-chain amino acids [72]. In this respect the metabolic anomaly parallels that of maple syrup urine disease.

The enzyme activity as measured in the leukocytes is distinctly greater than in maple syrup urine disease. A relatively modest increase in activity (about 3 percent of normal in maple syrup urine disease and 12 to 18 percent in the variant), if representative of the levels in the liver and other tissues, is sufficient to meet the usual requirements for metabolism of the branched-chain amino acids, and thereby to alter radically the clinical picture.

There is suggestive evidence that the genetic defects in the two families may not be identical. The defect seems somewhat more severe in family T. In that family the first findings appeared during infancy and the protein intake had to be reduced to keep the children symptom-free. Enzyme activity in the surviving child was lower than in family F.

Genetics

The variant form of the disease appears to be genetically distinct from classical maple syrup urine disease. In clinical terms, one would not expect a child with classical maple syrup urine disease to be born to a family with a child with intermittent branched-chain ketonuria. The heterozygous condition for maple syrup urine disease is also distinct from the variant form. Parents of children with maple syrup urine disease, who may be assumed to be heterozygous, are asymptomatic and have enzyme levels that are higher than those in the two children with the variant disease.

The data are insufficient to permit certainty about the genetic pattern. The fact that the parents are symptom-free suggests an autosomal recessive type of inheritance. The enzyme levels in both fathers were below normal, but the mothers had normal levels (Fig. 21-2). A similar anomalous and unexplained disparity between mothers and fathers was reported in a study of children with maple syrup urine disease, a clearly recessive disease [65].

ISOVALERIC ACIDEMIA

Clinical Findings

In 1966, two sibs, aged 2½ and 4 years, were reported who had a persistent odor to their breath and body fluids described as "cheesy" or "like sweaty feet" [32]. Recurrent episodes of vomiting, acidosis, and coma were precipitated by excessive protein ingestion or intercurrent infections. The peculiar odor intensified during attacks. Both children have mild mental retardation [100].

In 1967 [101], a third infant was described with what appears to have been the same metabolic anomaly. This baby died at 2 days of age following an operation for intestinal obstruction. Metabolic acidosis associated with twitching led to coma. The urine and serum had the characteristic odor of short-chain fatty acids. Gas-phase chromatography disclosed an isovaleric acidemia of 100 mg per 100 ml.

Metabolic Error

Serum levels of isovaleric acid during an attack in the two children described by Tanaka et al. [32] were 30 mg and 6 mg per 100 ml, compared to normal levels of approximately 0.06 mg per 100 ml. Between attacks the levels remained two to three times normal. Lack of any increase in the blood level of β-methylcrotonic acid localized the defect to the isovaleric acid dehydrogenase (Reaction 12 and Fig. 21-1). Identification of the organic acids was by gas-phase chromatography.

Further evidence for an interruption in the normal pathway for the degradation of leucine was obtained by load tests which caused a sharp elevation in level of isovaleric acid. There was no accumulation of leucine or its keto acid, probably because decarboxylation of the keto acid is virtually irreversible. Diminished production of radioactive CO_2 has been demonstrated following incubation of leukocytes with isovaleric acid-1-^{14}C.

Diagnosis

The diagnosis is suggested by the distinctive odor. The demonstration of an isovaleric acidemia with normal or reduced plasma concentration of β-methylcrotonic acid establishes the diagnosis. The organic acids are most accurately identified by gas-phase chromatography. Amino acid analysis is of no value, since the significant compounds do not react with ninhydrin.

A simple method for demonstrating a defect in the degradation of isovaleric acid is the incubation of the radioactive compound with peripheral leukocytes from the patient and measurement of the radioactive CO_2 released. The method is basically the same as that described earlier for maple syrup urine disease. In this instance, however, the demonstration of a degradative defect does not localize the metabolic block because several enzymatic steps precede the evolution of CO_2.

Treatment

The dramatic increases in isovaleric acid induced by oral loads of leucine suggest that dietary control may be helpful to these patients. As yet there has been no report of the results of such an approach.

SUMMARY

Metabolic anomalies have been identified for three degradative steps of the branched-chain amino acids, leucine, valine, and isoleucine.

1 Hypervalinemia associated with a deficiency in valine transamination has been reported in a Japanese child. Transamination of leucine and isoleucine was normal. The child is mentally and physically retarded.

2 Maple syrup urine disease (branched-chain ketonuria) has been reported in approximately 50 children. There is a deficiency in the oxidative decarboxylation of the three branched-chain keto acids. Diets that are low in leucine, isoleucine, and valine offer promise of prolonging life and preventing neurologic damage.

A variant form of maple syrup urine disease, intermittent branched-chain ketonuria, has been described. Signs and symptoms may not appear for months or years after birth and are intermittent in character. The children develop normally but may die during an attack.

3 Isovaleric acidemia, probably a result of a defect in the conversion of isovaleryl coenzyme A to β-methylcrotonyl coenzyme A, has been recognized in three children in two families. The presenting symptoms are the distinctive odor and relatively mild mental retardation.

BIBLIOGRAPHY

1. Menkes, J. H., Hurst, P. L., and Craig, J. M.: New syndrome: progressive familial infantile cerebral dysfunction associated with an unusual urinary substance. Pediatrics, **14**, 462, 1954.
2. Westall, R. G., Dancis, J., and Miller, S.: Maple sugar urine disease. A.M.A. J. Dis. Child., **94**, 571, 1957.

3. Blanchard, M., Green, D. E., Nocito, V., and Ratner, S.: L-Amino acid oxidase of animal tissue. J. Biol. Chem., **155,** 421, 1944.
4. Cammarata, P. S., and Cohen, P. P.: The scope of the transamination reaction in animal tissues. J. Biol. Chem., **187,** 439, 1950.
5. Needham, D. M.: A quantitative study of succinic acid in muscle—glutamic and aspartic acids as precursors. Biochem. J., **24,** 208, 1930.
6. Meister, A., Sober, H. A., and Peterson, E. A.: Studies on the coenzyme activation of glutamic-aspartic apotransaminase. J. Biol. Chem., **206,** 89, 1954.
7. Braunstein, A. E.: Transamination and the integrative functions of the dicarboxylic acids in nitrogen metabolism. Advances Protein Chem., **111,** 1, 1947.
8. Meister, A.: Transamination. Advances Enzymol., **16,** 185, 1955.
9. Green, D. E., Leloir, L. F., and Nocito, V.: Transaminases. J. Biol. Chem., **161,** 559, 1945.
10. Taylor, R. T., and Jenkins, W. T.: Leucine aminotransferase. II. Purification and characterization. J. Biol. Chem., **241,** 4396, 1966.
11. Aki, K., Ogawa, K., Shirai, A., and Ichihara, A.: Transaminase of branched chain amino acids. III. Purification and properties of the mitochondrial enzyme from hog heart and comparison with the supernatant enzyme. J. Biochem. (Tokyo), **62,** 610, 1967.
12. Dancis, J., Hutzler, J., Tada, K., Wada, Y., Morikawa, T., and Arakawa, T.: Hypervalinemia: a defect in valine transamination. Pediatrics, **39,** 813, 1967.
13. Gunsalus, I. C.: Oxidative and transfer reaction of lipoic acid. Fed. Proc., **13,** 715, 1954.
14. Ishikawa, E., Oliver, R. M., and Reed, L. J.: α-Keto acid dehydrogenase complexes. V. Macromolecular organization of pyruvate and α-ketoglutarate dehydrogenase complexes isolated from beef kidney mitochondria. Proc. Nat. Acad. Sci. U.S.A., **56,** 534, 1966.
15. Goldberg, M., and Sanadi, D. R.: Incorporation of labeled carbon dioxide into pyruvate and α-keto-glutarate. J. Am. Chem. Soc., **74,** 4972, 1952.
16. Dancis, J., Hutzler, J., and Levitz, M.: The exchange of $^{14}CO_2$ with branched-chain keto acids by guinea pig liver. Biochim. Biophys. Acta, **78,** 90, 1963.
17. Breslow, R.: On the mechanism of thiamine action. IV. Evidence from studies on model systems. J. Am. Chem. Soc., **80,** 3719, 1958.
18. Carlson, G. L., and Brown, G. M.: The natural occurrence, enzymatic formation, and biochemical significance of a hydroxyethyl derivative of thiamine pyrophosphate. J. Biol. Chem., **236,** 2099, 1961.
19. Connelly, J. L., Danner, D. J., and Bowden, J. A.: I. Isolation, purification, and partial characterization of bovine liver α-ketoisocaproic: α-keto-β-methylvaleric acid dehydrogenase. J. Biol. Chem., **243,** 1198, 1968.
20. Bowden, J. A., and Connelly, J. L.: Branched chain α-keto acid metabolism. II. Evidence for the common identity of α-ketoisocaproic acid and α-keto-β-methylvaleric acid dehydrogenases. J. Biol. Chem., **243,** 3526, 1968.
21. Goedde, H. W., and Keller, W.: Metabolic pathways in maple syrup urine disease, in *Amino Acid Metabolism and Genetic Variation,* edited by W. L. Nyhan, p. 191. McGraw-Hill Book Company, New York, 1967.
22. Dancis, J., Hutzler, J., and Levitz, M.: Tissue distribution of branched chain keto acid decarboxylase. Biochim. Biophys. Acta, **52,** 60, 1961.
23. Dancis, J., Jansen, V., Hutzler, J., and Levitz, M.: The metabolism of leucine in tissue culture of skin fibroblasts of maple syrup urine disease. Biochim. Biophys. Acta, **77,** 523, 1963.
24. Norton, P. M., Roitman, E., Snyderman, S. E., and Holt, L. E., Jr.: A new finding in maple syrup urine disease. Lancet, **1,** 26, 1962.
25. Piez, K. A., and Morris, L.: A modified procedure for the automatic analysis of amino acids. Anal. Biochem., **1,** 187, 1960.
26. Ehrlich, F.: Ueber das naturliche Isomere des Leucins. Chem. Ber., **37,** 1809, 1904.
27. Levene, P. A., and Van Slyke, D. D.: The leucine fraction of proteins. J. Biol. Chem., **6,** 391, 1909.
28. Olivard, J., Metzler, D. E., and Snell, E. E.: Catalytic racemization of amino acids by pyridoxal and metal salts. J. Biol. Chem., **199,** 669, 1952.
29. Norton, P. M., Roitman, E., Snyderman, S. E., and Holt, L. E., Jr.: Further studies on alloisoleucine in maple syrup urine disease. Fed. Proc., **22,** 549, 1962.
30. Meister, A., and White, J.: Growth response of the rat to the keto analogues of leucine and isoleucine. J. Biol. Chem., **191,** 211, 1951.
31. Meister, A.: Studies on D- and L-α-keto-β-methylvaleric acids. J. Biol. Chem., **190,** 269, 1951.
32. Tanaka, K., Budd, M. A., Efron, M. L., and Isselbacher, K. J.: Isovaleric acidemia: a new genetic defect of leucine metabolism. Proc. Nat. Acad. Sci. U.S.A., **56,** 236, 1966.
33. Bachhawat, B. K., Robinson, W. G., and Coon, M. J.: Enzymatic carboxylation of β-hydroxyisovaleryl coenzyme A. J. Biol. Chem., **219,** 539, 1956.
34. del Campillo-Campbell, A., Dekker, E. E., and Coon, M. J.: Carboxylation of β-methylcrotonyl coenzyme A by a purified enzyme from chicken liver. Biochim. Biophys. Acta, **31,** 290, 1959.
35. Lynen, F., Knappe, I., Lourch, E., Jiiting, G., and Ringelmann, E.: Die biochemische Funktion des Biotins. Angew. Chem. (Eng.), **71,** 481, 1959.
36. Hilz, H., Knappe, J., Ringelmann, E., and Lynen, F.: Methylglutaconase, eine neue Hydratase, die am Stoffwechsel verzweigter Carbonsäuren beteiligt ist. Biochem. Z., **329,** 477, 1958.
37. Bachhawat, B. K., Robinson, W. G., and Coon, M. J.: The enzymatic cleavage of β-hydroxy-β-methylglutaryl coenzyme A to acetoacetate and acetyl coenzyme A. J. Biol. Chem., **216,** 727, 1955.
38. Lynen, F., Henning, U., Bublitz, C., Sörbo, B., and Kröplin-Rueff, L.: Der chemische Mechanismus der Acetessigsäurebildung in der Leber. Biochem. Z., **330,** 269, 1958.
39. Greenberg, D. M.: Carbon catabolism in amino acids, in *Metabolic Pathways,* edited by D. M. Greenberg, vol. II, p. 79. Academic, New York, 1961.
40. Meister, A.: *Biochemistry of the Amino Acids,* vol. II, p. 729, Academic, New York, 1965.
41. Wada Y., Taka, K., Minagawa, A., Yoshida, T., Morikawa, T., and Okamura, T.: Idiopathic hypervalinemia: probably a new entity of inborn error of valine metabolism. Tohoku J. Exp. Med., **81,** 46, 1963.
42. Wada, Y.: Idiopathic hypervalinemia: valine and alpha keto acids in blood following an oral dose. Tohoku J. Exp. Med., **87,** 322, 1965.
43. Dancis, J., Levitz, M., and Westall, R. G.: Maple syrup urine disease: branched chain keto-aciduria. Pediatrics, **25,** 72, 1960.
44. Patrick, A. D.: Maple syrup urine disease. Arch. Dis. Child., **38,** 269, 1961.
45. Mackenzie, D. Y., and Woolf, L. I.: Maple syrup urine disease: an inborn error of the metabolism of valine, leucine and isoleucine associated with gross mental deficiency. Brit. Med. J., **1,** 90, 1959.
46. Lane, M. R.: Maple syrup urine disease. J. Pediat., **58,** 80, 1961.
47. Silberman, J., Dancis, J., and Feigin, I. H.: Neuropathological observations in maple syrup urine disease: branched chain ketoaciduria. Arch. Neurol., **5,** 351, 1961.
48. Lonsdale, D., Mercer, R. D., and Faulkner, W. R.: Maple syrup urine disease: report of two cases. Amer. J. Dis. Child., **106,** 258, 1963.
49. Tada, K., Wada, Y., and Okamura, T.: A case of maple sugar urine disease. Tohoku J. Exp. Med., **79,** 142, 1963.
50. Woody, N. C., Woody, H. B., and Tilden, T. D.: Maple syrup urine disease in a Negro infant. Amer. J. Dis. Child., **105,** 381, 1963.
51. Abrams, R. M.: Maple syrup urine disease: a case report. Clin. Proc. Child. Hosp., **21,** 189, 1965.
52. Mueller, W., and Schreier, K.: Die Ahorn-sirup Krankheit. Deutsch. Med. Wschr., **87,** 2479, 1962.
53. Linneweh, F., and Socher, H.: Über den Einflut diätetischer Prophylaxie auf die Myelogenese bei der Leucinose. Klin. Wschr., **43,** 926, 1965.
54. Jimenez, A. I., Sifontes, J. E., and Sanchez-Longo, L. P.: Maple syrup urine disease. Report of the first case in Puerto Rico, Bol. Asoc. Med. P. Rico, **55,** 463, 1963.
55. Voyce, M. A., Montgomery, J. N., Lynch, G. A. C., and Bowman, J. K.: Maple syrup urine disease. Brit. Med. J., **1,** 1293, 1964.
56. Schmidt, G. W., Benecke, G. and Peiffer, J.: Über einen diätetisch langfristeg behandelten Sängling mit Valin-Leucin-Urie und Delibität (Ahorn Sirup Urinkrankheit). Helv. Paediat. Acta, **20,** 147, 1965.

57. Frezal, J., Gabilan, J. C., Rey, J., Vis, H., Roy, C., Olivennes, M., and Lamy, M.: Deux observations de leucinose. Arch. Franc. Pediat., **22,** 1226, 1965.
58. Cerrutti, M.: Un cas di malattia dello sciroppo d'acero ("maple syrup urine disease"). Minerva Pediat., **18,** 1969, 1966.
59. Hooft, C., Timmermans, J., van Werveke, S., deHawere, R., Roels, H., and van der Recken, H.: La Maladie du sirop d'érable. Étude biochimique et morphologique. Ann. Pediat. (Paris), **13,** 83, 1966.
60. Spahr, A., and Kaeser, H.: Un cas de maple syrup urine disease (maladie de l'urine: sirop d'érable). Ann. Paediat. Fenn., **206,** 224, 1966.
61. Kamraj-Mazurkiewicz, K., and Szelozynska, K.: Przypadek choroby syropu klonowego. Pediat. Pol., **40,** 337, 1966.
62. Masingue, Michel: La Leucinose à propos d'une observation. Thèse pour le Doctorat en Médicin, Lille, 1967.
63. Levy, H. L., Shih, V. E., Karolkewicz, V., and MacCready, R. A.: Personal communication.
64. Snyderman, S.: Personal communication.
65. Linneweh, F., Ehrlich, M., Graul, E. H., and Hundeshagen, H.: Ein weiterer heterozygoten—Test für die Ahornsirupkrankheiten (maple syrup urine disease). Klin. Wschr., **41,** 941, 1963.
66. Dancis, J., Hutzler, J., and Levitz, M.: Detection of the heterozygote in maple syrup urine disease. J. Pediat., **66,** 595, 1965.
67. Goedde, H. W., and Keller, W.: Metabolic pathways in maple syrup urine disease, in *Amino Acid Metabolism and Genetic Variation,* edited by W. L. Nyhan. McGraw-Hill Book Company, New York, 1967.
68. Goedde, H. W., Langenbeck, U., and Brackertz, D.: Detection of heterozygotes in maple syrup urine disease: role of lymphocyte count. Humangenetik, **6,** 189, 1968.
69. Dancis, J., Levitz, M., Miller, S., and Westall, R. G.: "Maple syrup urine disease." Brit. Med. J., **1,** 91, 1959.
70. Menkes, J. H.: Maple syrup urine disease: isolation and identification of organic acids in the urine. Pediatrics, **23,** 348, 1959.
71. Dancis, J., Hutzler, J., and Levitz, M.: The diagnosis of maple syrup urine disease (branched chain ketoaciduria) by the *in vitro* study of the peripheral leucocyte. Pediatrics, **32,** 234, 1963.
72. Dancis, J., Hutzler, J., and Cox, R. P.: Enzyme defect in skin fibroblasts in intermittent branched-chain ketonuria and in maple syrup urine disease. Biochem. Med., **2,** 407, 1969.
73. Diezel, P. B., and Martin, K.: Die Ahornsirup Krankheit mit familiären Befall. Virchows Arch. Path. Anat., **337,** 425, 1964.
74. Woolf, L. I.: Recent work on phenylketonuria and maple syrup urine disease (leucinosis). Proc. Roy. Soc. Med., **55,** 824, 1962.
75. Menkes, J. H., Philippart, M., and Fiol, R. E.: Cerebral lipids in maple syrup disease. J. Pediat., **66,** 584, 1965.
76. Prensky, A. L., Carr, S., Moser, H. W.: Development of myelin in inherited disorders of amino acid metabolism. Arch. Neurol., **19,** 552, 1968.
77. Prensky, A. L., and Moser, H. W.: Brain lipids, proteolipids and free amino acids in maple syrup urine disease. J. Neurochem., **13,** 863, 1966.
78. Menkes, J. H., and Solcher, H.: Maple syrup urine disease: effects of diet therapy on cerebral lipids. Arch. Neurol., **16,** 486, 1967.
79. Snyderman, S. E., Norton, P. M., Roitman, E., and Holt, L. E., Jr.: Maple syrup urine disease, with particular reference to dietotherapy. Pediatrics, **34,** 454, 1964.
80. Carver, M. J.: Free amino acids of fetal brain. Influence of the branched chain amino acids. J. Neurochem., **16,** 113, 1969.
81. Appel, S. H.: Inhibition of brain protein synthesis: an approach to the biochemical basis of neurological dysfunction in the aminoacidurias. Ann., N.Y., Acad. Sci., **291,** 63, 1966.
82. Yuwiler, A., and Geller, E.: Serotonin depletion by dietary leucine. Nature (London), **208,** 83, 1965.
83. Tashian, R. E.: Inhibition of brain glutamic decarboxylase by phenylalanine, leucine and valine derivatives: a suggestion concerning the neurological defect in phenylketonuria and branched chain keto aciduria. Metabolism, **10,** 393, 1961.
84. Howell, R. K., and Lee, M.: Influence of α-keto acids on the respiration of brain *in vitro.* Proc. Soc. Exp. Biol. Med., **113,** 660, 1963.
85. DiGeorge, A. M., Auerbach, V. H., and Mabry, C. C.: Leucine-induced hypoglycemia. II. The blood glucose depressant action of leucine in normal individuals. J. Pediat., **63,** 295, 1963.
86. Westall, R. G.: Dietary treatment of a child with maple syrup urine disease (branched chain keto-aciduria). Arch. Dis. Child., **38,** 485, 1963.
87. Efron, M., Young, D., and Moser, H.: Personal communication.
88. Berry, H. K., Scheel, C., and Marks, J.: Microbiological test for leucine, valine and isoleucine using urine sample dried on filter paper. Clin. Chem., **8,** 242, 1962.
89. Neish, W. J. P.: in *Methods of Biochemical Analysis,* edited by D. Glick, vol. 5, p. 154. Interscience, New York, 1957.
90. Dancis, J., Hutzler, J., and Levitz, M.: Thin-layer chromatography and spectrophotometry of α-keto acid hydrazones. Biochim. Biophys. Acta, **78,** 85, 1963.
91. Greer, M., and Williams, C. M.: Diagnosis of branched-chain ketonuria (maple syrup urine disease) by gas chromatography. Biochem. Med., **1,** 87, 1967.
92. Meister, A., and Abendschein, P. A.: Chromatography of α-keto acid, 2,4-dinitrophenylhydrazones and their hydrogenation products. Anal. Chem., **28,** 171, 1956.
93. Dent, C. E., and Westall, R. G.: Studies in maple syrup urine disease. Arch. Dis. Child., **38,** 259, 1961.
94. Gaul, G. E.: Maple syrup urine disease: observations using peritoneal dialysis in treatment of coma. Annual meeting of Society for Pediatric Research, Atlantic City, May 3–4, 1969.
95. Morris, M. D., Lewis, B. D., Doolan, P. D., and Harper, H. A.: Clinical and biochemical observations on an apparently non-fatal variant of branched chain ketoaciduria (maple syrup urine disease). Pediatrics, **28,** 918, 1961.
96. Kiil, R., and Rokkones, T.: Late manifesting variant of branched-chain ketoaciduria (maple syrup urine disease). Acta Paediat. Scand., **53,** 356, 1964.
97. Morris, M. D., Fisher, D. A., and Fiser, R.: Late-onset branched-chain ketoaciduria (maple syrup urine disease). Journal-Lancet (Minneapolis), **86,** 149, 1966.
98. Dancis, J., Hutzler, J., and Rokkones, T.: Intermittent branched chain ketonuria. Variant of maple-syrup-urine disease. New Eng. J. Med., **276,** 84, 1967.
99. Durand, P., Lamedica, E. M., and Martino, A. M.: La Leucinose: une variante de la céto-acidurie à chaîne ramifiée. Pediatrie, **20,** 147, 1965.
100. Efron, M. L.: Isovaleric acidemia. Amer. J. Dis. Child., **113,** 74, 1967.
101. Newman, C. G. H., Wilson, B. D. R., Callaghan, P., and Young, L.: Neonatal death associated with isovaleric acidaemia. Lancet, **2,** 439, 1967.
102. Käser, H., Käser, R., and Lestradet, H.: Separation and quantitative estimation of new alpha keto-acids in human blood by paper chromatography. Metabolism, **9,** 926, 1960.

CHAPTER TWENTY-TWO

DISORDERS OF PROPIONATE, METHYLMALONATE, AND VITAMIN B_{12} METABOLISM

Leon E. Rosenberg

Methylmalonic acid and its immediate precursor, propionic acid, are detectable in normal human blood, urine, and cerebrospinal fluid only in trace amounts. The miniscule quantities of these compounds in extracellular fluids have obscured, until recently, the key role that these acids play in human metabolism. Biochemists interested in animal nutrition have explored propionate catabolism for nearly 10 years since it was found that ruminants derive most of their energy requirements from the oxidation of propionate and acetate produced by bacterial fermentation in their rumens [1]. Although propionate and methylmalonate are of little quantitative importance in man as direct sources of energy, these acids, found intracellularly largely as their coenzyme A (CoA) esters, are vital intermediates in the catabolism of fat and protein.

Several independent, and seemingly unrelated, lines of evidence drew the attention of the physician and the clinical investigator to the study of propionate and methylmalonate metabolism. In 1959 and 1960, several groups reported that 5′-deoxyadenosylcobalamin, one of the coenzyme forms of vitamin B_{12}, is an essential cofactor in the enzymatic conversion of methylmalonyl CoA to succinyl CoA [2–4]. Shortly thereafter, patients with acquired vitamin B_{12} deficiency were shown to excrete large amounts of methylmalonic acid in the urine [5, 6]. The methylmalonic aciduria was rapidly reversed by administration of physiologic doses of vitamin B_{12}, and was attributed to an acquired block in methylmalonate catabolism caused by inadequate amounts of the needed vitamin B_{12} coenzyme.

In 1961, Childs, Nyhan, and their associates [7] described a young boy with recurrent attacks of severe ketoacidosis who had elevated concentrations of glycine and several other amino acids in his blood and urine. A series of detailed metabolic studies demonstrated that the attacks were precipitated by protein feeding and more specifically by ingestion of the branched-chain amino acids methionine and threonine. Since elevation in plasma glycine level was the most striking biochemical abnormality, the disorder was called "ketotic hyperglycinemia." Recent evidence indicates that this disorder is caused by an inherited defect in the catabolism of propionate, *not* by a primary abnormality in glycine utilization or biosynthesis [8, 9].

Since 1967, a number of critically ill children have been described who draw these seemingly disparate observations together and focus attention on the enzymes and coenzymes which regulate the pathway responsible for the conversion of propionate to succinate. Oberholzer [10], Stokke [11], and their colleagues described infants with profound metabolic acidosis and hyperglycinemia (or hyperglycinuria) who excreted huge amounts of methylmalonic acid in the urine but who were not vitamin B_{12}–deficient. Subsequently, Rosenberg and his colleagues [8] reported that urine from the index patient with "ketotic hyperglycinemia" and from his affected sister contained *no* methylmalonic acid. This observation indicated that primary methylmalonic aciduria and "ketotic hyperglycinemia" were different disorders with identical clinical manifestations [8].

The latter group and Lindblad et al. [12, 13] also described children with ketoacidosis and methylmalonic aciduria who were not vitamin B_{12}–deficient but who responded to administration of pharmacologic doses of vitamin B_{12} or its coenzyme with a marked fall in concentration of urinary methylmalonic acid. This unique vitamin B_{12} dependency appears to be caused by abnormalities in vitamin B_{12} coenzyme biosynthesis [14, 15], not by a mutation of the apoenzyme which converts methylmalonate to succinate.

These observations, and others which will be discussed in detail subsequently, emphasize that inherited abnormalities in the metabolic pathway for propionate and methylmalonate occur, and that these defects lead to profound illness and, in many cases, death due to disturbed acid-base balance. The study of these disorders has led to important insights in our understanding of the role of this pathway in man, and has illustrated, once again, that a group of clinically identical disorders can be produced by several different mutations affecting the synthesis of related apoenzymes and coenzymes.

BIOCHEMICAL PATHWAYS

Propionate Metabolism

Formation of Propionate and Methylmalonate

Most of the propionic acid utilized by ruminant animals is formed by bacterial fermentation in the rumen [1]. By contrast, nonruminant mammals derive nearly all their propionate from the catabolism of lipid and protein. As noted in Fig. 22-1, catabolism of the branched-chain amino acid isoleucine leads to the formation of propionyl CoA, as does the degradation of methionine and threonine [16]. Catabolism of these amino acids accounts for much of the propionate formed in man, but other sources are known. Beta oxidation of fatty acids with an odd number of carbon atoms ultimately leads to the formation of 1 mole of propionyl CoA per mole of fatty acid [17]. Degradation of the side

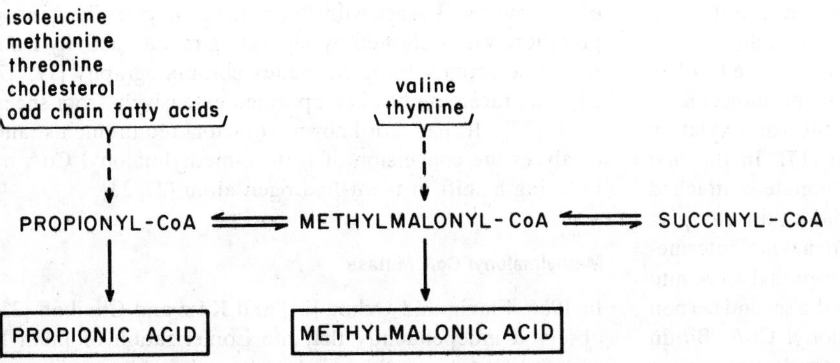

Figure 22-1. Major pathway of formation and catabolism of propionate and methylmalonate. Broken arrows indicate the presence of several reactions.

chain of cholesterol also leads to the synthesis of propionyl CoA, but this pathway appears to be of little quantitative significance [18].

Methylmalonyl CoA is synthesized from three sources (Fig. 22-1). Catabolism of thymine accounts for only a small amount of the intracellular methylmalonyl CoA compared to either the degradation of valine [16] or the carboxylation of propionyl CoA. Thus, protein catabolism ultimately yields propionate and methylmalonate directly, whereas lipid oxidation leads only to the formation of propionate.

Catabolism of Propionyl CoA

Propionate has long been known to be glycogenic in animals [19, 20], but the pathway by which propionate is converted to carbohydrate became clear only when Lardy and his colleagues demonstrated that liver mitochondria contain enzymes which synthesize succinate from propionate [19, 20]. The discovery in 1955 that methylmalonate is an intermediate in the formation of succinate from propionate (Fig. 22-1) provided an important further step in the characterization of this pathway [21, 22].

Ochoa and his coworkers have defined the individual steps of propionate catabolism in animal tissues and characterized the enzymes involved [17]. Propionyl CoA, formed either by the degradative reactions discussed above or by the enzymatic esterification of propionate itself [23], may be considered the precursor of this reaction sequence (Fig. 22-2).

Three enzymatic reactions are responsible for the conversion of propionyl CoA to succinyl CoA. (1) The first involves the carboxylation of propionyl CoA to methylmalonyl CoA [23, 24]. Although two diastereoisomers of methylmalonyl CoA are known, only the D- form is produced in the carboxylation reaction [25, 26]. (2) This isomer is not a substrate for the subsequent mutase reaction, and must be racemized to the L- configuration by another enzyme, methylmalonyl CoA racemase [27]. (3) The third reaction, catalyzed by methylmalonyl CoA mutase, isomerizes L-methylmalonyl CoA to succinyl CoA [28]. The latter compound enters the tricarboxylic acid cycle and is ultimately glycogenic because of its conversion to pyruvate by way of oxaloacetate. The net sum of all of these reactions may be written as follows:

$$\text{Propionate} + \text{ATP} \longrightarrow \text{pyruvate} + 4\text{H}^+ + \text{ADP} + \text{P}_i$$

In bacteria, propionate is formed from pyruvate by reversal of the reaction sequence just described [17], but in mammalian systems the equilibrium of the system is far in the direction of propionate catabolism rather than biosynthesis.

Propionyl CoA Carboxylase and Biotin

This enzyme has been crystallized from pig heart and characterized extensively [29]. It is found almost exclusively in mitochondria and has a molecular weight of approximately 700,000. Biotin has been shown to be a prosthetic group for the apoenzyme, four molecules of this cofactor being bound

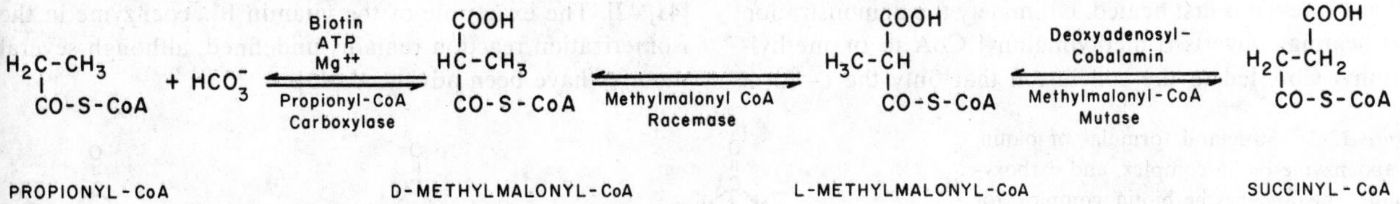

$H_2C{-}CH_3$ / $CO{-}S{-}CoA$ + HCO_3^- ⇌ (Biotin, ATP, Mg^{++}; Propionyl-CoA Carboxylase) $COOH$ / $HC{-}CH_3$ / $CO{-}S{-}CoA$ ⇌ (Methylmalonyl CoA Racemase) $COOH$ / $H_3C{-}CH$ / $CO{-}S{-}CoA$ ⇌ (Deoxyadenosyl-Cobalamin; Methylmalonyl-CoA Mutase) $COOH$ / $H_2C{-}CH_2$ / $CO{-}S{-}CoA$

PROPIONYL-CoA — D-METHYLMALONYL-CoA — L-METHYLMALONYL-CoA — SUCCINYL-CoA

Figure 22-2. Enzymatic details of major catabolic pathway for propionyl CoA and methylmalonyl CoA. Succinyl CoA has several metabolic fates, including oxidation through the tricarboxylic acid cycle and condensation with glycine to form δ-aminolevulinic acid. Two coenzymes act in this reaction sequence: biotin in the carboxylation of propionyl CoA, and 5′-deoxyadenosylcobalamin (dA B_{12}) in the isomerization of L-methylmalonyl CoA.

to one molecule of the apoprotein. This ratio and additional physicochemical studies with urea suggested that the enzyme is probably composed of four subunits of equal size (molecular weight 175,000), each of which binds one molecule of biotin [29]. Several groups showed that the carboxylation of propionyl CoA is a two-step reaction [17]. In the first step, which requires ATP and Mg^{++}, bicarbonate is attached to the ureido nitrogen of the apoenzyme-biotin complex (Fig. 22-3), forming a carboxybiotin-apoenzyme intermediate. This complex in turn reacts with propionyl CoA and transfers the carboxyl group from biotin to the second carbon of propionyl CoA, forming D-methylmalonyl CoA. Biotin is bound to the apoenzyme through an amide linkage involving its terminal carboxyl group and an epsilon amino group of a lysine residue on the protein. As is with several other biotin-catalyzed, carbon dioxide–fixation reactions, the biotin molecule is directly responsible for the transfer of the carboxyl group [30].

Biotin (Fig. 22-3) is widely distributed in plant and animal tissues and is readily synthesized by a variety of microorganisms. Spontaneous deficiency of biotin has not been reported in man, probably because intestinal microorganisms synthesize ample quantities of the cofactor for most needs, even in the absence of nutritional sources. Experimental biotin deficiency has been produced in animals and man by ingestion of large amounts of egg white, which contains avidin, a protein known to bind and inactivate biotin [31]. Under these conditions the experimental subjects developed cutaneous pallor, dermatitis, depression, lassitude, muscle pains, hyperesthesia, and finally anemia and electrocardiographic changes [32]. All these symptoms and signs were rapidly reversed by administration of 150 to 300 μg biotin daily for a few days. From studies in animals it has been estimated that the daily human requirement for biotin is approximately 10 μg.

Methylmalonyl CoA Racemase

This enzyme owes its discovery to the observation that methylmalonyl CoA, which has been synthesized chemically, is a substrate for the mutase reaction (Fig. 22-2), whereas the methylmalonyl CoA formed enzymatically from the carboxylation of propionyl CoA will not react with the mutase unless it is first heated. Ultimately the demonstration that heating converts D-methylmalonyl CoA to DL-methylmalonyl CoA led to the conclusion that only the L- form of the ester will react with the mutase enzyme. This interpretation was confirmed by separating mutase activity from racemase activity using Sephadex chromatography [17, 27, 33]. The racemase has been purified extensively from sheep liver [27]. It has no known cofactor requirements and catalyzes the conversion of D- to L-methylmalonyl CoA by inducing a shift in the α-hydrogen atom [27, 33].

Methylmalonyl CoA Mutase

In 1955, Flavin and Ochoa [21] and Katz and Chaikoff [22] observed independently that the isomerization of methylmalonyl CoA to succinyl CoA was catalyzed by an enzyme found in sheep kidney and rat liver. The chemical analogy between this isomerization reaction and the isomerization of glutamate to β-methylaspartate in bacteria [34], along with the demonstration by Barker and his colleagues [35, 36] that a coenzyme form of vitamin B_{12} was needed for the latter reaction, led to the finding in several laboratories that a vitamin B_{12} coenzyme is also required for the isomerization of methylmalonyl CoA [2–4]. This enzyme, originally called methylmalonyl CoA isomerase, but now designated methylmalonyl CoA mutase, has been crystallized from sheep kidney [37] and from bacteria [38, 39]. The mammalian holoenzyme has a molecular weight of 165,000 and appears to be composed of two equal-sized subunits. The enzyme, which has a pH optimum of 7, has a K_m of $2 \times 10^{-4}M$ for L-methylmalonyl CoA and a K_m of $6 \times 10^{-5}M$ for succinyl CoA. Although the isomerization reaction is reversible, equilibrium lies far in favor of succinyl CoA formation [37]. The apoenzyme binds its vitamin B_{12} coenzyme avidly, the K_m for coenzyme being $2 \times 10^{-8}M$. One molecule of coenzyme is bound per apoenzyme subunit, probably through a two-point attachment involving an apoenzyme sulfhydryl group [37]. The specific vitamin B_{12} coenzyme required for this reaction is 5′-deoxyadenosylcobalamin, a cofactor which will be discussed in detail subsequently.

It can be seen from Fig. 22-2 that the isomerization reaction could occur either by transfer of the free carboxyl group or by transfer of the coenzyme A–carboxyl radical. Studies using isotopically labeled methylmalonyl CoA demonstrated convincingly that it is the CoA carboxyl group which is transferred [40] through an intramolecular isomerization [41, 42]. The exact role of the vitamin B_{12} coenzyme in the isomerization reaction remains undefined, although several theories have been advanced [43].

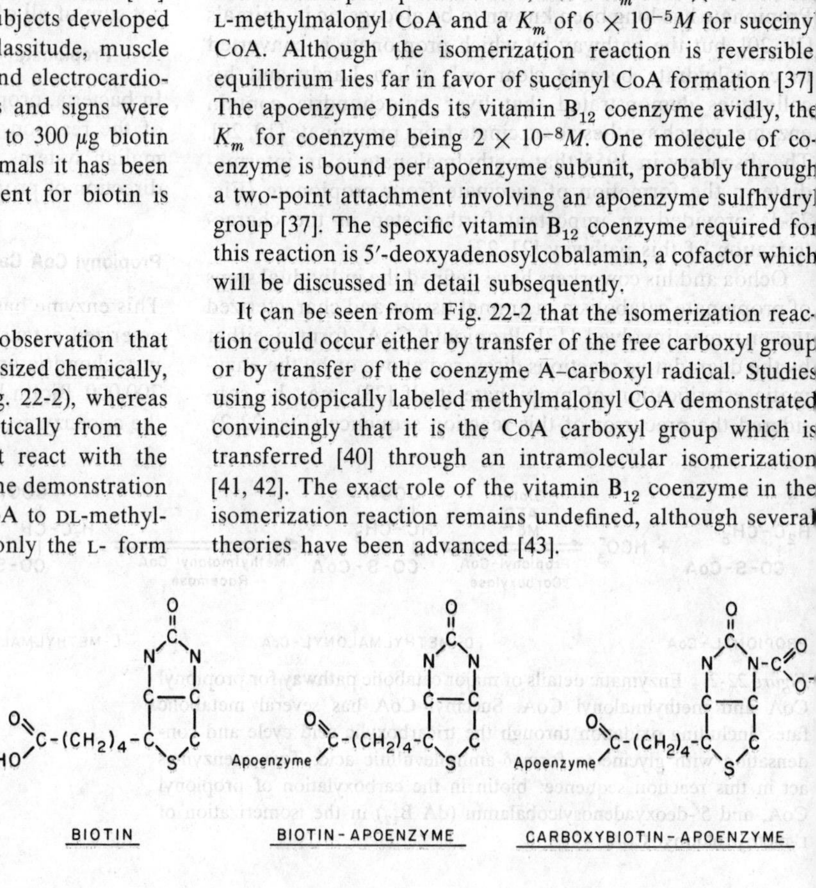

Figure 22-3. Structural formulas of biotin, an apoenzyme-biotin complex, and carboxybiotin. The apoenzyme-biotin complex for propionyl CoA carboxylase is formed through an amide linkage between the terminal carboxyl group of biotin and an epsilon amino group of a lysine residue of the apoenzyme. Bicarbonate has been demonstrated to be the active moiety in the formation of carboxybiotin.

BIOTIN BIOTIN-APOENZYME CARBOXYBIOTIN-APOENZYME

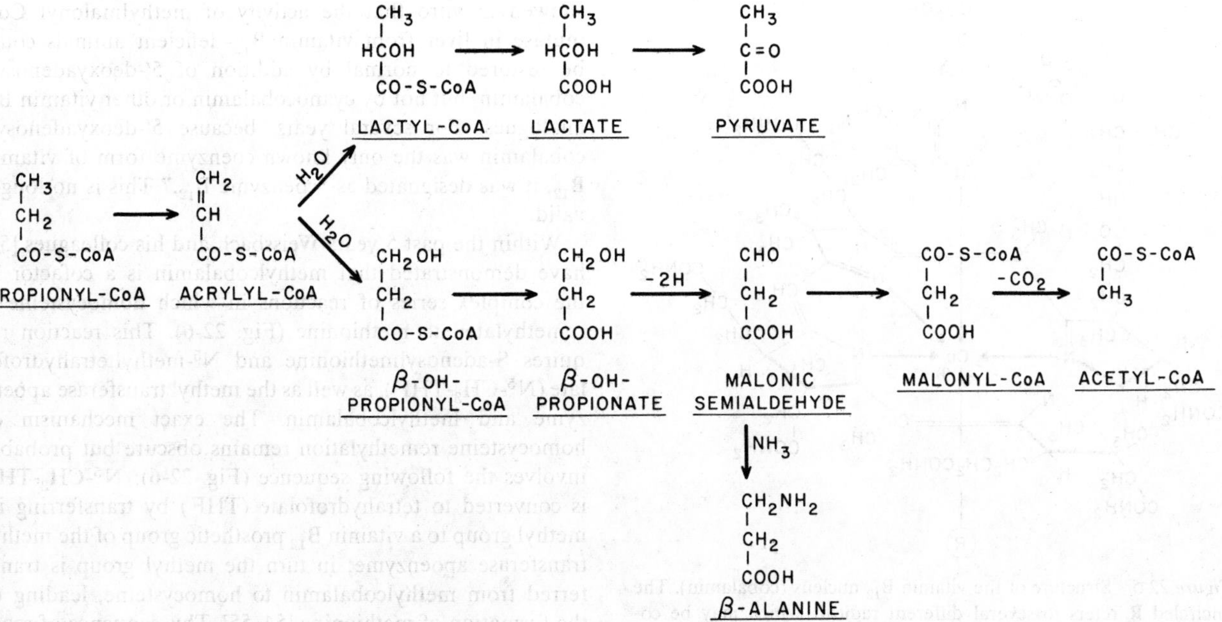

Figure 22-4. Minor pathways of propionate catabolism. Note that both pathways can ultimately generate acetyl CoA. The significance of these minor pathways is discussed in the text.

Alternate Pathways of Propionate Metabolism

Although the catabolism of propionate to succinate through methylmalonate is the major pathway for propionate utilization in mammalian systems, recent evidence suggests that alternate pathways exist. Propionyl CoA can replace acetyl CoA as a "primer" for long-chain fatty acid synthesis [41, 44], and lead to the formation of odd-chain fatty acids, notably heptanoate, nannonoate, and undecanoate [45]. There is also an alternate catabolic mechanism, which is described in Fig. 22-4 [17]. The first step in this reaction involves the formation of the α,β-unsaturated fatty acid, acrylyl CoA, which may be subsequently hydrated, leading to the formation of either lactyl CoA or β-OH-propionyl CoA. The former compound is hydrolyzed to lactate, thus providing a second means by which propionate may be converted to pyruvate. Catabolism of β-OH-propionyl CoA leads ultimately to the synthesis of acetyl CoA or β-alanine, compounds discussed elsewhere in this volume. These alternate pathways have been demonstrated in human leukocytes [46] and in man in vivo [47], but their quantitative significance remains undefined.

Vitamin B_{12}

The structure and function of vitamin B_{12} have intrigued students of human biology since 1926, when Minot and Murphy demonstrated that oral administration of crude liver extract was effective in the treatment of pernicious anemia [48]. In 1948, this "anti-pernicious anemia factor" was isolated from liver and kidney [49, 50] and was named vitamin B_{12}. Administration of as little as 1 μg of the vitamin daily was shown to prevent relapse of pernicious anemia. Although vitamin B_{12} is widely distributed in animal tissues, there is strong evidence that it is synthesized only in microorganisms found in soil, water, or in the rumen and intestine of animals.

Structural Features

The isolation of vitamin B_{12} culminated in the elucidation of its three-dimensional structure by Hodgkin and coworkers using x-ray crystallographic techniques [51]. Vitamin B_{12}, or as it has been officially designated, cobalamin, is composed of a central cobalt atom (Co) surrounded by a corrin ring (Fig. 22-5). The molecule also includes a complex side chain consisting of a 5,6-dimethylbenzimidazole group, a ribose molecule and a phosphate moiety. The benzimidazole is linked to the cobalt atom through one of its nitrogens, while the phosphate is bonded to the "D" member of the corrin ring. The molecule is completed by coordinate linkage of one of several different radicals to the cobalt nucleus. Thus, cyanocobalamin, or more strictly α-(5,6-benzimidazolyl)-cobamide cyanide, is formed by the attachment of a cyanide radical to the cobalt atom. Although this compound is the most common commercial form of the vitamin, it is almost surely an artifact of the chemical procedures used to isolate vitamin B_{12} and does not occur naturally in microorganisms, plants, or animal tissues. Many other cobalamins have been formed by replacement of the cyanide radical, but only three

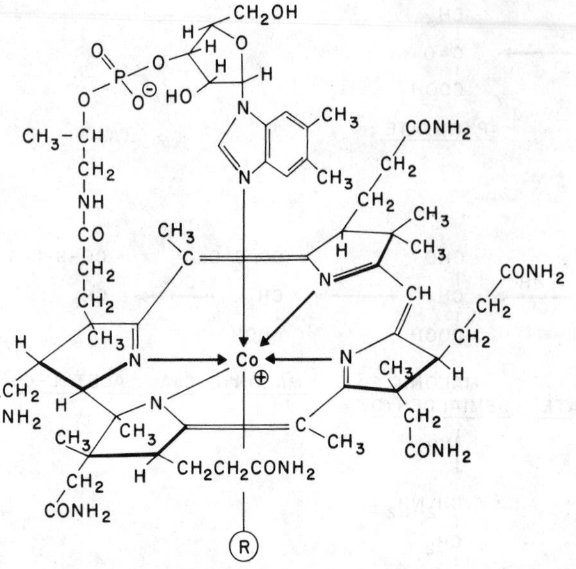

Figure 22-5 Structure of the vitamin B_{12} nucleus (cobalamin). The encircled R refers to several different radicals which may be coordinately linked to the cobalt atom, such as CN^-, CH_3, OH^-, and 5′-deoxyadenosyl.

have been isolated from mammalian tissues: hydroxocobalamin, methylcobalamin, and 5′-deoxyadenosylcobalamin. The latter two compounds are unique for two reasons: (1) they are the only two compounds in nature known to have a direct carbon-cobalt bond; (2) they are the only two forms of vitamin B_{12} which are known to act as specific coenzymes in mammalian systems.

The structure and nomenclature of vitamin B_{12} are further complicated by oxidation and reduction of the cobalt atom [43]. In hydroxocobalamin the cobalt atom is trivalent (Co^{3+}), and this compound has been called vitamin B_{12a}. When the cobalt is reduced to a divalent state (Co^{++}) the molecule is called vitamin B_{12r}, and in the monovalent state, vitamin B_{12s}. These oxidation-reduction states are important, since there appear to be specific reductase enzymes which sequentially convert vitamin B_{12a} to B_{12s}, with B_{12r} acting as an intermediate [52]. The cobalt atom is monovalent in methylcobalamin and 5′-deoxyadenosylcobalamin.

Vitamin B_{12} Coenzymes

In 1958, Barker and his colleagues demonstrated that the glutamate mutase reaction in *Clostridium tetanomorphum* required vitamin B_{12} [34] and, more specifically, that the active coenzyme form of the vitamin was 5′-deoxyadenosylcobalamin [35, 36]. One year later, Smith and Monty reported that the analogous isomerization of methylmalonyl CoA to succinyl CoA was defective in the liver of vitamin B_{12}–deficient rats [2]. They suggested that vitamin B_{12} was a cofactor for the latter isomerization system, a thesis born out by Gurnani et al. [3] and Stern and Friedmann [4], who showed in vitro that the activity of methylmalonyl CoA mutase in liver from vitamin B_{12}–deficient animals could be restored to normal by addition of 5′-deoxyadenosylcobalamin, but not by cyanocobalamin or other vitamin B_{12} analogues. For several years, because 5′-deoxyadenosylcobalamin was the only known coenzyme form of vitamin B_{12}, it was designated as "coenzyme B_{12}." This is no longer valid.

Within the past 5 years Weissbach and his colleagues [53] have demonstrated that methylcobalamin is a cofactor in the complex series of reactions in which homocysteine is remethylated to methionine (Fig. 22-6). This reaction requires S-adenosylmethionine and N^5-methyltetrahydrofolate (N^5-CH_3-THF), as well as the methyl transferase apoenzyme and methylcobalamin. The exact mechanism of homocysteine remethylation remains obscure but probably involves the following sequence (Fig. 22-6): N^5-CH_3-THF is converted to tetrahydrofolate (THF) by transferring its methyl group to a vitamin B_{12} prosthetic group of the methyl transferase apoenzyme; in turn the methyl group is transferred from methylcobalamin to homocysteine, leading to the formation of methionine [54, 55]. This sequence of reactions, which is relevant to the manifestations of vitamin B_{12} deficiency and to the interrelationships between folate and vitamin B_{12}, will be discussed in more detail subsequently.

It should be emphasized that the conversion of methylmalonyl CoA to succinyl CoA and the methylation of homocysteine to methionine are the only vitamin B_{12}–dependent reactions which have been demonstrated in mammalian systems. In microorganisms several other apoenzymes require vitamin B_{12} coenzymes: glutamate mutase [34]; diol dehydrase [56]; glycerol dehydrase [57]; and oligo-

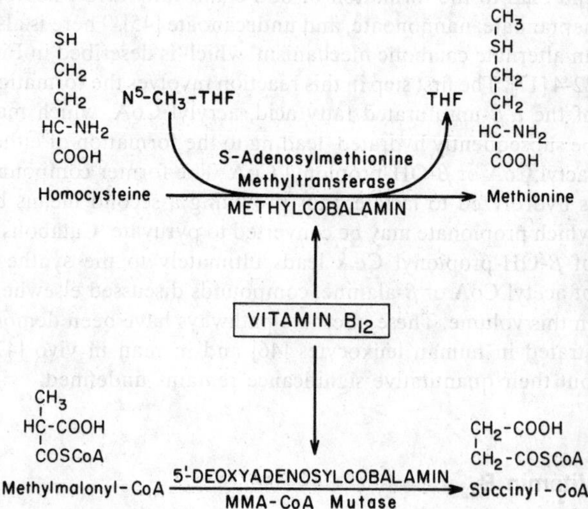

Figure 22-6. Reactions catalyzed by vitamin B_{12} coenzymes in mammalian systems. Note the specificity of 5′-deoxyadenosylcobalamin for the isomerization of methylmalonyl CoA and of methylcobalamin for the methylation of homocysteine. N^5-CH_3-THF denotes N^5-methyltetrahydrofolate.

nucleotide reductase [58]. In addition vitamin B_{12} catalyzes the formation of methane [59] and acetic acid [60] and the fermentation of lysine [61], but the specific enzymes which catalyze these reactions are not known.

Coenzyme Biosynthesis

Huennekens and his colleagues have demonstrated conclusively that vitamin B_{12} coenzymes are synthesized enzymatically in *Clostridium tetanomorphum* [52, 62]. Although no similar studies have been carried out in mammalian systems to date, it seems likely that a similar sequence also exists in higher organisms. The reaction sequence defined in clostridia is shown in Fig. 22-7. Hydroxocobalamin (vitamin B_{12a}) is the precursor compound and, as stated above, exists with its cobalt atom oxidized to a trivalent state (Co^{3+}). Vitamin B_{12a} is reduced to B_{12r} (Co^{++}) by an enzyme called vitamin B_{12a} reductase, a flavoprotein which uses NADH as the reductant [52]. A second flavoprotein, B_{12r} reductase, converts B_{12r} to B_{12s} (Co^{+}), NADH again acting as the reductant [52]. These two enzymes appear to be distinct, as shown by their thermal lability and their reductant specificity. Vitamin B_{12s}, but not B_{12a} or B_{12r}, is the substrate for the final enzymatic reaction leading to the synthesis of 5′-deoxyadenosylcobalamin [62]. ATP provides the adenosine moiety for this reaction, which is catalyzed by an adenosylating enzyme designated ATP: vitamin B_{12s} 5′-deoxyadenosyl transferase. This enzyme has been purified approximately 300-fold and has a pH optimum of 8, requires Mn^{++}, and has a K_m of $1 \times 10^{-5} M$ for vitamin B_{12s} and a K_m of $1.6 \times 10^{-5} M$ for ATP. No evidence has been obtained for reversal of the reaction.

The biosynthetic mechanisms for methylcobalamin synthesis have not been defined, but it does not appear to be an intermediate in the biosynthesis of 5′-deoxyadenosylcobalamin. Furthermore, the chemical form of vitamin B_{12} which attaches to the homocysteine methyl transferase is not known; it could be vitamin B_{12s}, 5′-deoxyadenosylcobalamin, or, as has been suggested by Ertel et al., sulfito-B_{12} [63].

Absorption and Distribution of Vitamin B_{12} and Its Coenzymes

Vitamin B_{12} has a unique and highly specialized mechanism of intestinal absorption. The ability to transport physiologic quantities of the vitamin depends on the combined action of gastric and ileal components. The gastric substance, called "intrinsic factor" (IF) by Castle, who first demonstrated its existence [64, 65], is a glycoprotein which binds vitamin B_{12} in the intestinal lumen. IF, which has been purified but not isolated, forms a complex with vitamin B_{12} which subsequently interacts with specific ileal receptor sites in the presence of calcium ions [66]. In this process the IF–vitamin B_{12} complex is dissociated by a "releasing enzyme" [67] and the vitamin B_{12} is actively transported across the ileal membrane into the portal blood. Once in the bloodstream, the free vitamin is bound by at least two different globulins, designated transcobalamin I and transcobalamin II. Transcobalamin I is an α-globulin which carries the majority of vitamin B_{12} found in plasma and appears to be concerned with storage of the vitamin in the circulation [67–69]. Transcobalamin II, a β-globulin, is probably the transport protein for newly absorbed vitamin B_{12}, as indicated by studies using Co^{57}–vitamin B_{12} which showed that vitamin B_{12} entering the body by either the oral or parenteral route was bound by transcobalamin II and subsequently transferred to transcobalamin I [69, 70]. This complex absorption and transport process appears to be specific for cyanocobalamin or hydroxocobalamin. The chloro-, nitro-, and thiocyanatocobalamin analogues are much less well absorbed [71].

The mechanisms by which vitamin B_{12} is released from serum proteins and taken up by tissues are under active investigation and appear to be analogous to its intestinal absorptive process. In vitro uptake of vitamin B_{12} by liver slices is enhanced by IF [72] and may depend on "transferase" enzymes. Once inside tissue cells, vitamin B_{12} is protein-bound, presumably to specific apoenzymes.

Lindstrand and Stahlberg have characterized the vitamin B_{12} components of human plasma and liver in a series of important studies [73–75]. They showed initially that the major vitamin B_{12} component of normal plasma is distinct from cyano-, hydroxo-, or 5′-deoxyadenosylcobalamin; they called this material "fourth factor" [73]. Lindstrand subsequently demonstrated that "fourth factor" was methylcobalamin [74]. This provided the first evidence for a role of this analogue in man. The amount of methylcobalamin in plasma far exceeded that of hydroxocobalamin [73]. Using purified plasma extracts and bioautography, these workers were unable to identify 5′-deoxyadenosylcobalamin in

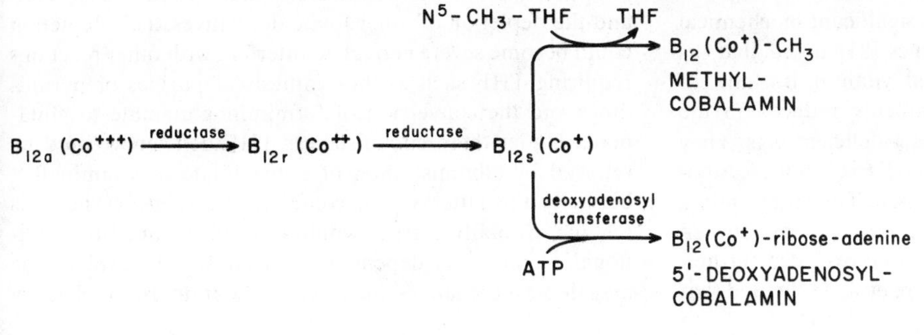

B_{12a} (Co^{+++}) —reductase→ B_{12r} (Co^{++}) —reductase→ B_{12s} (Co^{+})

B_{12s} + N^5-CH_3-THF → THF + $B_{12}(Co^{+})$-CH_3 METHYL-COBALAMIN

B_{12s} + ATP —deoxyadenosyl transferase→ $B_{12}(Co^{+})$-ribose-adenine 5′-DEOXYADENOSYL-COBALAMIN

Figure 22-7. Pathway of formation of vitamin B_{12} coenzymes in microbial systems. Vitamin B_{12a} is synonymous with hydroxocobalamin. Note the valence changes for the cobalt atom and the three enzymes required in the synthesis of 5′-deoxyadenosylcobalamin. This reaction sequence has not, thus far, been defined in mammalian systems.

plasma. Thus this coenzyme form of vitamin B_{12} may be confined to tissue spaces [73, 75].

Data obtained from needle biopsy specimens of human liver in controls and patients with vitamin B_{12} deficiency also provided valuable information [76]. Normal liver contained about 1 μg total vitamin B_{12} per gram wet weight and was fractionated as follows: 5′-deoxyadenosylcobalamin, 70 percent; hydroxocobalamin, 27 percent; and methylcobalamin, 3 percent. In patients with vitamin B_{12} deficiency the total vitamin B_{12} content was much reduced, to 0.02 to 0.126 μg per gm, and, interestingly, the ratio of 5′-deoxyadenosylcobalamin to methylcobalamin approached unity. The latter finding is unexplained but may reflect undefined and important relationships between vitamin B_{12} and folate which will be discussed subsequently.

The distribution and utilization of vitamin B_{12} have also been studied in man using parenteral administration of labeled vitamin B_{12} compounds [77–79]. These studies indicate that hydroxo- and 5′-deoxyadenosylcobalamin are taken up by the tissues in preference to cyanocobalamin.

Metabolic Abnormalities in Vitamin B_{12} Deficiency

As mentioned earlier, the biochemical aberrations in patients with vitamin B_{12} deficiency have been concentrated along the pathway from propionate to succinate. The first relevant observation in this context was the demonstration by Cox and White [5] and by Barness and his colleagues [6] that methylmalonic acid excretion in the urine was distinctly increased in vitamin B_{12}–deficient patients. The methylmalonic aciduria in these patients was reversed rapidly by administration of vitamin B_{12}. Thus repletion of vitamin B_{12} stores restored the methylmalonyl CoA mutase reaction to normal. Recently, Cox et al. reported that patients with vitamin B_{12} deficiency also have distinctly increased amounts of propionic acid in the urine, this abnormality again being reversed by vitamin B_{12} treatment [80]. Interestingly, they also found excessive amounts of acetic acid in the urine of vitamin B_{12}–deficient subjects. The mechanism of this abnormality is not clear, since acetate does not participate in the major pathway of propionate catabolism. The finding could, of course, reflect increased utilization of the alternate pathways of propionate metabolism in the face of a block in the major pathway, since each of the alternate routes leads eventually to the formation of acetyl CoA (Fig. 22-3).

Biochemical studies in an animal model, the vitamin B_{12}–deficient pig, have yielded other significant biochemical findings. Cardinale and his colleagues [81] noted that, as expected, the concentration of total vitamin B_{12} and of 5′-deoxyadenosylcobalamin was markedly reduced in the liver, kidney, and brain of vitamin B_{12}–deficient pigs. They also observed that the methylmalonyl CoA mutase apoenzyme content appeared to be increased. The latter finding suggests the possibility of a feedback control system between apoenzyme and coenzyme which must be explored further. Using the same model system, Seashore et al. [82] noted that propionate-3-^{14}C oxidation by leukocytes from vitamin B_{12}–deficient pigs was much impaired at a time when no abnormality in erythrocyte morphology or hemoglobin concentration was present. Such oxidation studies might provide a sensitive and early diagnostic test for vitamin B_{12} deficiency in man.

It should be pointed out that although vitamin B_{12} coenzymes are needed in mammalian systems for the formation of methionine from homocysteine, no data demonstrate any abnormality in sulfur amino acid metabolism in patients or animals with vitamin B_{12} deficiency. This negative result may reflect either insufficient study of sulfur amino acid metabolism in this clinical setting or the presence of alternate pathways for methionine biosynthesis which decrease the metabolic significance of the vitamin B_{12}–dependent pathway. Additional study in this area will be of considerable interest.

Vitamin B_{12} and Folic Acid

An interesting, important, and still puzzling aspect of vitamin B_{12} function concerns its relationship to folic acid. Several lines of evidence bear out this relationship: the appearance of megaloblastic anemia in either vitamin B_{12} or folate deficiency; the reversal of megaloblastic anemia in vitamin B_{12} deficiency by large doses of folate; the amelioration of megaloblastic changes in folic acid deficiency by pharmacologic doses of cyanocobalamin [83]; the increased plasma concentrations of N^5-CH_3-THF in patients with vitamin B_{12} deficiency [84]; the excretion of excessive amounts of formiminoglutamic acid (FIGLU) after histidine loading in patients with either vitamin B_{12} or folate deficiency [85, 86]; and the reduced amounts of total vitamin B_{12} in the liver of patients with folate deficiency [87]. A plausible explanation for most of these overlapping effects was proposed independently by Herbert [84], Noranha [88], Larrabee [89], and their colleagues, and is summarized in Fig. 22-8. The central cycle depicts the conversion of tetrahydrofolate (THF) via $N^{5,10}$-methylene-THF to N^5-CH_3-THF and the regeneration of THF as a result of the transfer of the methyl group to homocysteine to form methionine, a reaction catalyzed by a vitamin B_{12}–dependent methyl transferase. If methionine biosynthesis is the only quantitatively significant reaction using N^5-CH_3-THF, vitamin B_{12} deficiency will interfere with the folate cycle and, barring other control mechanisms, will lead to the accumulation of N^5-CH_3-THF and the depletion of other folate derivatives. This depletion could become severe enough to interfere with other reactions requiring THF such as the synthesis of purines or pyrimidines and the conversion of formiminoglutamate to glutamate. Under these circumstances THF deficiency could be relieved by administration of either folate or vitamin B_{12}, but only the latter would complete the folate cycle. This scheme, if totally correct, would obviate the need for additional vitamin B_{12}–dependent mechanisms to explain the megaloblastic changes observed in vitamin B_{12} deficiency

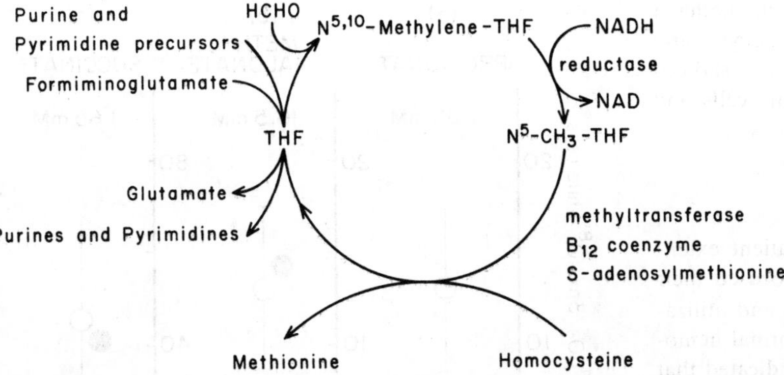

Figure 22-8. Schematic representation of the "folate cycle." THF denotes tetrahydrofolate; N^5-CH_3-THF, N^5-methyltetrahydrofolate. Of particular interest to this discussion is the methylation of homocysteine to methionine, in which N^5-CH_3-THF is converted to THF by transferring its methyl group to a vitamin B_{12} coenzyme. The function of S-adenosylmethionine in this reaction is not known.

and would account for the specific disorders of folate metabolism observed in vitamin B_{12}-deficient man. It does not explain the low vitamin B_{12} content of livers from folate-deficient subjects [87], nor the hematologic response of folate-deficient patients to vitamin B_{12} [83]. The latter observations suggest an alternate feedback regulatory system between folic acid and vitamin B_{12} which could be of great significance.

DISEASE STATES

A number of different inborn errors of metabolism may lead to metabolic ketoacidosis and protein intolerance or both during the neonatal period or infancy. Designations such as "idiopathic acidosis of infancy" and "idiopathic lactic acidosis" are giving way to specific etiologic diagnoses. The following inborn errors of carbohydrate, amino acid, or fatty acid metabolism must now be considered in the differential diagnosis of infantile metabolic ketoacidosis: glycogen storage disease (Type I) (see Chap. 7); isovaleric acidemia (see Chap. 21); branched-chain ketonuria (see Chap. 21); the "sweaty-feet" syndrome, characterized by accumulation of butyric acid and hexanoic acid in blood or urine; "ketotic hyperglycinemia"; propionic acidemia; and methylmalonic aciduria (or acidemia).

The present discussion will concern only the last three conditions. The term "ketotic hyperglycinemia" will be discarded because (1) elevated plasma glycine concentrations reported in patients with disorders of the urea cycle, with defective carboxylation of propionate, and with methylmalonic aciduria demonstrate that the hyperglycinemia is not a specific finding; (2) the term suggests a primary abnormality in glycine metabolism, which is clearly not the case; and (3) it may be confused with the disorder called "nonketotic hyperglycinemia," which is caused by a defect in glycine catabolism (see Chap. 24).

The disorders to be discussed herein will be grouped according to their most prominent and specific biochemical abnormalities, with full recognition that this classification may require modification in the light of future clinical or biochemical investigation.

Propionyl CoA Carboxylase Deficiency

In 1961, Childs et al. [7] described a male infant with episodic metabolic ketoacidosis, protein intolerance, and remarkably elevated plasma glycine concentration. More than a dozen children with closely similar clinical and biochemical findings have since been described [90]. Many of these children were found subsequently to have methylmalonic aciduria [91]. The observation that in at least four patients no methylmalonic acid was detected in the urine [8, 91] indicated that methylmalonic aciduria and "ketotic hyperglycinemia" were *not* identical diseases. Recently, Hommes [92], Hsia [9], and their colleagues have presented data which demonstrate that these children have a primary defect in propionyl CoA carboxylase, the enzyme which catalyzes the conversion of propionyl CoA to D-methylmalonyl CoA (Fig. 22-2). These children will be discussed next.

Clinical Manifestations

E. G., the patient described by Childs et al. [7, 93, 94] presented with dehydration, lethargy, and coma on the first day of life. He was found to be severely ketoacidotic, and responded slowly to massive alkali replacement. The clinical course was characterized by recurrent attacks of ketoacidosis, precipitated by infections or protein ingestion, and by developmental retardation, electroencephalographic abnormalities, and osteoporosis. The patient had episodic neutropenia and thrombocytopenia prior to death at age 7. A sister (A.G.) also became ketotic and acidotic during the first 4 days of life, but the course of her condition has been modified dramatically because of the extensive experience gained in studying her brother. Although she has had mild attacks of ketoacidosis during intercurrent infections, maintenance on a low-protein diet has resulted in normal somatic and mental development up to age 7 and little need for hospital care.

In 1968, Hommes and his colleagues [92] described a male infant with hyperventilation, areflexia, and grunting at age 60 hrs. There was a profound metabolic acidosis (arterial pH 6.98), but in spite of administration of massive amounts of sodium bicarbonate and Trishydroxyaminomethane (THAM), he died on the fifth day of life. Leukocytes and platelets were normal. Post-mortem examination showed only a fatty liver and degeneration of Purkinje cells and the granular layer of the cerebellum.

Biochemical Abnormalities

Childs and Nyhan [7, 93–95] studied their patient extensively. Because of the hyperglycinemia, they focused their attention on the pathways of glycine formation and utilization but found no consistent abnormalities. Normal hemoglobin concentration in the peripheral blood indicated that the pathway from glycine to δ-aminolevulinic acid was not blocked. Slices of the patient's liver incorporated glycine-^{14}C into protein and carbon dioxide as well as rat liver slices did. Salicylate and benzoate were normally conjugated with glycine, and the glutathione concentration of whole blood was normal. Although the rate of conversion of tritiated glycine to serine in vivo was slower than in controls, this difference may have reflected the enlarged glycine pool rather than a specific block in the conversion of glycine to serine [95].

Several observations suggested an abnormality in the catabolism of the branched-chain amino acids, methionine and threonine: Plasma concentrations of valine, isoleucine, and leucine were elevated intermittently (as were those of alanine, serine, and threonine). Administration of leucine, valine, isoleucine, threonine, and methionine each precipitated attacks of ketoacidosis, but no other amino acids were toxic. Menkes [96] reported that the urine contained large amounts of butanone (a four-carbon ketone which may be an intermediate in isoleucine catabolism) and the longer-chain ketones, pentanone and hexanone. These long-chain ketones were not detected in the urine of patients with ketosis due to diabetes, starvation, or ketogenic diets.

Since isoleucine, valine, threonine, and methionine are all precursors of either propionate or methylmalonate, a defect in propionate metabolism seemed likely. The urine contained no methylmalonic acid. The patient died before any other studies of propionate catabolism could be performed. Recently, Hsia et al. [9] demonstrated a striking defect in propionate catabolism in A.G., the affected sister of E.G. When leukocytes isolated from the peripheral blood were incubated with propionate-3-^{14}C, negligible quantities of $^{14}CO_2$ were evolved compared with the amount in controls (Fig. 22-9). These cells oxidized methylmalonate and succinate normally. Identical findings have also been obtained using fibroblasts grown in tissue culture [97]. These data indicate that the primary metabolic defect in E.G. and A.G. is in the conversion of propionyl CoA to D-methylmalonyl CoA, a reaction catalyzed by propionyl CoA carboxylase.

Hommes et al. [92] made two interesting observations on their child with lethal neonatal acidosis. They found that the serum propionic acid concentration was 40 mg per 100 ml (5.4 mM), a value more than 1,000 times that reported

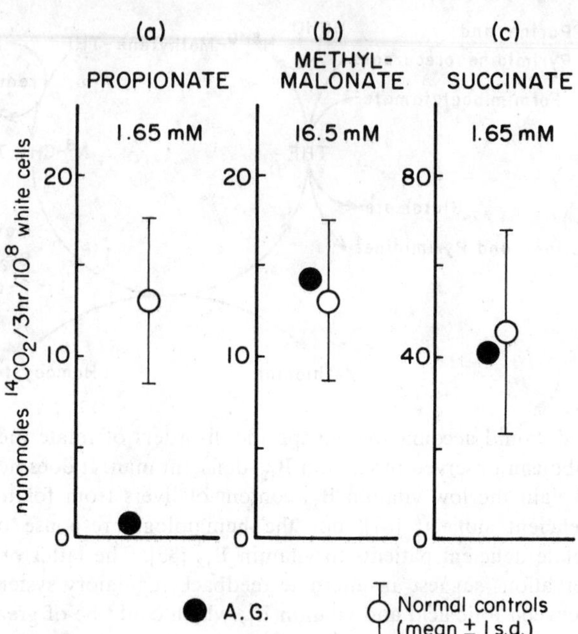

Figure 22-9. Oxidation of radioisotopically labeled propionate, methylmalonate, and succinate by leukocytes from A.G. and from healthy controls. Cells were incubated for 3 hr at 37°C in Krebs bicarbonate buffer. See discussion of defective propionate carboxylation for details. (*From Hsia et al.* [9].)

in normal infants (Fig. 22-10). They also noted that the liver of their patient contained fatty acids with 15 and 17 carbon atoms in addition to the even-chain fatty acids found in control livers (Fig. 22-11). From these data, Hommes postulated a defect in propionyl CoA carboxylation in their patient.

Pathologic Physiology

A defect in the carboxylation of propionate provides a satisfactory explanation for many of the findings reported by Childs [7], Hsia [9], Hommes [92], and their coworkers. This defect would be expected to lead to an elevated concentration of propionate in the blood and an inability of leukocytes to catabolize propionate to carbon dioxide. Since isoleucine, threonine, and methionine are precursors of propionate, such a block should also lead to the observed protein and specific amino acid intolerance which was observed. The appearance of long, odd-chain fatty acids in the liver suggests that when propionyl CoA carboxylation is blocked, odd-chain fatty acid biosynthesis may be augmented, because propionyl CoA is the "primer" for such compounds. Three salient features of the disease are not adequately explained by the proposed block in propionate catabolism. (1) The severe acidosis is not explained by the accumulation of propionate alone. It is possible that other fatty acids and, perhaps, lactic acid accumulate in front of the block in the major pathway of propionate catabolism,

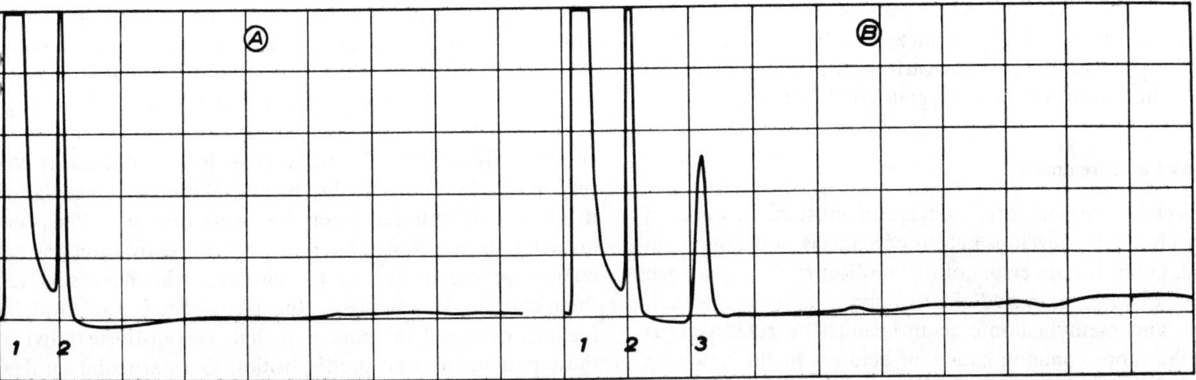

Fig. 22-10. Gas chromatograms of serum short-chain fatty acids from control (*A*) and from patient with propionic acidemia (*B*). 1 = solvent; 2 = formic acid; 3 = propionic acid. (*Reproduced from Hommes et al.* [92], *with permission of authors and publisher.*)

but there are no data at present to support such a thesis. (2) The ketosis produced by leucine and valine is not understood, since these amino acids are not catabolized to propionate. These two amino acids are ketogenic, however, and the mechanism of the intolerance might not be related to the block in propionate metabolism but could still lead to the same physiologic derangement. (3) There is no satisfactory explanation for the elevated plasma glycine concentrations which were so prominent in E.G. and A.G. In this regard it is noteworthy that the infant studied by Hommes et al. [92] did not have hyperglycinemia, a finding demonstrating that acidosis or elevated propionate concentration in body fluids (or both) does not always produce a rise in plasma glycine level. Since plasma glycine concentration may rise in sick children with negative nitrogen balance of many causes [98], the hyperglycinemia may be quite nonspecific.

Genetics

The onset of symptoms within the first few hours or days of life and the presence of two or more affected siblings of both sexes in several families suggested that propionyl-CoA carboxylase deficiency is inherited as an autosomal recessive trait. This suggestion has been confirmed by Hsia et al. [111] in the index family with this disorder. Propionyl-CoA carboxylase activity in cultured skin fibroblast extracts from both parents of E.G. and A.G. was about half the normal

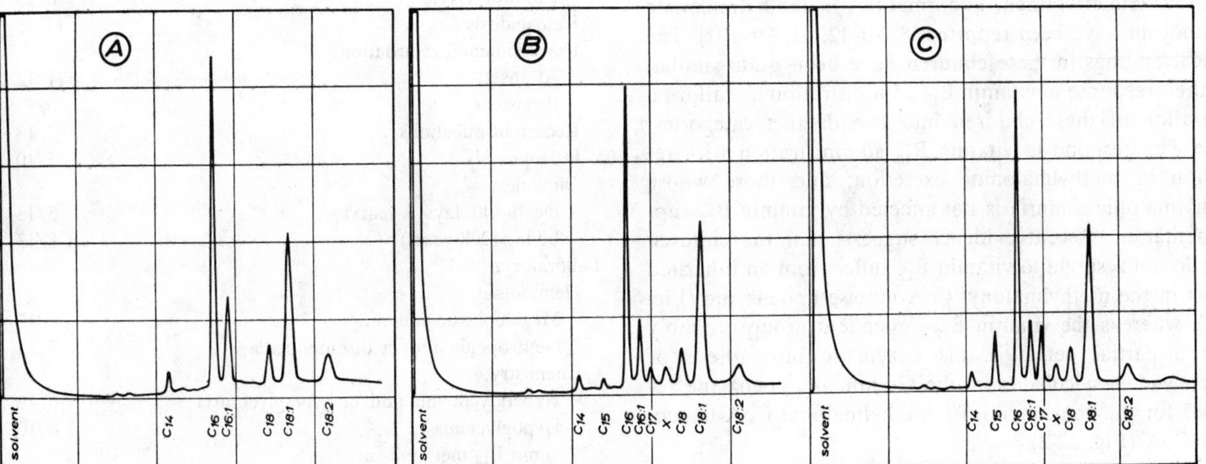

Figure 22-11. Gas chromatograms of methyl esters of fatty acids extracted from liver of control (*A*); patient with propionic acidemia (*B*); and patient with propionic acidemia plus added methyl esters of C_{15} and C_{17} fatty acids (*C*). C_{14}, C_{15}, etc., denotes chain length of fatty acids. (*Reproduced from Hommes et al.* [92], *with permission of authors and publisher.*)

value, while extracts from A.G.'s cells had no activity. These results indicate that A.G. is homozygous for a mutant allele which impairs propionyl-CoA carboxylase activity and that each of her parents is heterozygous for this trait.

Diagnosis and Treatment

A defect in propionate carboxylation must be considered in any child who develops ketosis or acidosis in the neonatal period. Other inborn errors of metabolism such as glycogen storage disease, branched-chain ketonuria, isovaleric acidemia, and methylmalonic aciduria must be ruled out, as must the more common causes of acidosis in the newborn period. Determinations of propionic acid in blood or urine and studies of propionate oxidation by leukocytes are necessary to make a specific diagnosis of defective propionate carboxylation.

A low-protein diet (0.5 to 1.5 gm per kg per day) appears to be the best treatment for the disorder at this time. This diet will minimize the number of attacks of ketoacidosis, although it may not prevent them entirely. Attacks of ketoacidosis should be treated vigorously by withdrawing all dietary protein and administering sodium bicarbonate parenterally. Since propionyl CoA carboxylase requires biotin as a coenzyme, it would be particularly interesting to give patients with this disorder large doses of biotin to determine if any of the affected children demonstrate an unusual requirement for this cofactor, as has been observed in the next disorder to be discussed, methylmalonic aciduria.

Methylmalonic Aciduria

Since 1967, 13 non-vitamin B_{12}-deficient infants or young children with prominent abnormalities in methylmalonate metabolism have been reported [8, 10–12, 91, 99–101]. The clinical findings in these children have been quite similar, but their response to vitamin B_{12} administration has allowed separation of these children into two distinct categories: those who respond to vitamin B_{12} administration with reduction in methylmalonate excretion; and those whose methylmalonic aciduria is not affected by vitamin B_{12} supplementation. Recent evidence suggests that the children who do not respond to vitamin B_{12} suffer from an inherited defect in the methylmalonyl CoA mutase apoenzyme (Fig. 22-2), whereas the vitamin B_{12}-dependent group probably have a partial defect in the enzymatic biosynthesis of 5′-deoxyadenosylcobalamin, the vitamin B_{12} coenzyme required for the conversion of L-methylmalonyl CoA to succinyl CoA (Fig. 22-2).

Clinical Findings

Signs and Symptoms

The clinical and laboratory abnormalities in these patients are summarized in Table 22-1. Six of the thirteen children were male. Seven children had the onset of their disease within the first month of life; the remainder developed signs or symptoms before the end of the first year. Life-threatening metabolic ketoacidosis has been the clinical hallmark in all these children. Arterial pH values of 6.9 to 7.1 have been documented in several, associated with serum bicarbonate concentrations of 5 mEq per liter or less. The acidosis was responsible for failure to thrive or developmental retardation in 11 of these children when they were first seen. Persistent growth failure or central nervous system retardation has not been observed in any of the children who have survived their episodic ketoacidosis. Recurrent bacterial or viral infections occurred in more than half (seven-thirteenths) of these patients, but no predisposition to a particular viral or bacterial agent has been noted. Osteoporosis was observed in 5 of 10 children who had appropriate x-ray studies. Five patients have died from their disease at ages 40 days to 3 years, death being secondary to uncontrolled acidosis or overwhelming infection. Eight patients are still alive; they range in age from 2 to 8 years. All five of the children who responded to vitamin B_{12} are still alive, whereas 4 of the 5 children who died did not respond biochemically to vitamin B_{12} supplementation.

Table 22-1. CLINICAL AND LABORATORY FEATURES OF PATIENTS WITH METHYLMALONIC ACIDURIA

Parameter	No. affected
Clinical:	
Sex:	
Male	6/13
Female	7/13
Age of onset:	
Birth–1 month	7/13
1 month–1 year	6/13
Ketoacidosis	13/13
Developmental retardation:	
At onset	11/12
Persistent	0/8
Recurrent infections	7/13
Osteoporosis	5/10
Outcome:	
Death (40 days–3 years)	5/13
Living (2–8 years)	8/13
Laboratory:	
Hematology:	
Megaloblastic anemia	0/10
Neutropenia and/or thrombopenia	7/13
Chemistry:	
Hyperglycinemia and/or hyperglycinuria	10/12
Hypoglycemia	4/10
Vitamin B_{12} metabolism:	
Decreased serum vitamin B_{12} concentration	0/5
Vitamin B_{12} dependent*	5/9

Source: Data derived from following references: [8, 10–13, 91, 100, 101].

* Vitamin B_{12} dependency defined as marked reduction in urinary methylmalonate following administration of cyanocobalamin or 5'-deoxyadenosylcobalamin.

Routine Laboratory Findings

Transient neutropenia or thrombocytopenia or both have appeared in 7 patients, but these abnormalities have disappeared with correction of the acidosis. Significantly, none of the children had megaloblastic anemia, nor was the serum vitamin B_{12} concentration reduced in any of 5 patients in whom it was measured. In spite of convincing absence of vitamin B_{12} deficiency, 5 of 9 children have responded to massive doses of vitamin B_{12} with marked decrease in urinary methylmalonate [100–102]. Hyperglycinemia or hyperglycinuria was noted in 10 of twelve patients, but no other reproducible abnormalities in blood or urine amino acids were found. The other noteworthy laboratory feature of this disease has been hypoglycemia, with blood sugar values of less than 30 mg per 100 ml in 4 of 10 patients in whom it was measured. The hypoglycemia has occurred coincident with the attacks of ketoacidosis and has not appeared in intercritical periods.

Biochemical Studies

Large amounts of methylmalonic acid have appeared in the urine of all reported patients. Normal children and adults excrete less than 5 mg of this dicarboxylic acid per day, but these children have excreted from 240 to 5,760 mg methylmalonate in a 24-hr period. Methylmalonate, normally undetectable in plasma, was found in concentrations ranging from 2.6 to 34 mg per 100 ml. In a few patients the cerebrospinal fluid concentration of methylmalonate was also determined and was found to be equal to that in plasma.

Vitamin B_{12}-unresponsive Patients

Oberholzer et al. [10] carried out extensive studies in a female patient who was alive and well at age 6 years, in spite of recurrent attacks of ketoacidosis. They noted that urinary methylmalonate ranged from 5,300 to 5,700 mg per day and that the plasma and cerebrospinal fluid concentrations were 18.6 and 18.3 mg per 100 ml, respectively. When this child was given oral loading tests with protein, valine, or sodium propionate, hypoglycemia and ketosis ensued. None of these stresses led to distinct changes in plasma methylmalonic acid concentration, but the propionate load was followed by a distinct rise in urinary methylmalonate.

Stokke and his colleagues [11] observed independently that protein and valine accentuated the biochemical disturbance in a female infant with methylmalonic aciduria. Their demonstration that parenteral administration of valine-^{14}C was followed by appearance of the radioisotope in urinary methylmalonate confirmed the thesis that valine is a precursor of methylmalonate in man. Small but detectable amounts of $^{14}CO_2$ were recovered in the expired air of this patient after valine-^{14}C administration. Thus either the block in methylmalonate catabolism was not complete, or, alternatively, there are routes of valine catabolism to carbon dioxide which do not go through the methylmalonate-succinate pathway.

These findings were interpreted by Oberholzer, Stokke, and their colleagues to indicate a block in the conversion of methylmalonate to succinate, a reaction catalyzed by methylmalonyl CoA mutase and 5′-deoxyadenosylcobalamin. In vitro confirmation of this thesis was provided by Oberholzer et al. in preliminary studies with leukocytes [10] and by Morrow, Barness, and their colleagues using leukocytes, cultured fibroblasts, and liver. The latter investigators observed that leukocytes and fibroblasts from patients with methylmalonic aciduria failed to convert propionate-^{14}C to $^{14}CO_2$ in vitro [99, 103]. They also measured mutase activity directly in liver biopsies and found almost none in three patients with the non-vitamin B_{12}-responsive form of methylmalonic aciduria [104]. It is particularly significant that addition of 5′-deoxyadenosylcobalamin in vitro failed to enhance methylmalonyl CoA mutase activity in the liver of these patients, in contrast to the results to be reported below in the vitamin B_{12}-dependent form of the disease.

Vitamin B_{12}-responsive Methylmalonic Aciduria

In 1968, Rosenberg and coworkers [8, 102] reported that a 1-year-old boy (R.P.) with episodic ketoacidosis and methylmalonic aciduria responded to parenteral administration of vitamin B_{12} (1,000 mg per day for 5 days) with a prompt fall in urinary methylmalonate level from 900 to 1,200 mg per 24 hr to 200 to 250 mg per day (Fig. 22-12). After the vitamin supplement was discontinued, urinary methylmalonate rose to pretreatment values within 30 days, but it fell again when vitamin B_{12} or 5′-deoxyadenosylcobalamin was administered [105]. Lindblad et al. [13] found independently that two Swedish infants with methylmalonic aciduria responded in a completely analogous way to parenteral administration of 5′-deoxyadenosylcobalamin. Recent studies by Walker [100], Sotos [101], and their colleagues have confirmed these observations.

The nature of the metabolic lesion in vitamin B_{12}-dependent methylmalonic aciduria has been studied in detail by Rosenberg and his colleagues [8, 14]. The following observations were made during a series of dietary perturbations. (1) Methylmalonic acid excretion increased markedly during protein loading and after administration of valine, isoleucine, methionine, and threonine but *not* with leucine. (2) Urinary methylmalonate dropped from 1,000 to 200 mg per 24 hr when the child was fasted for 1 day. These results confirm that amino acids which are catabolized to methylmalonate directly (valine) or through propionate (isoleucine, methionine, threonine) are the precursors for most of the methylmalonic acid in the urine. (3) Since more than 90 percent of an oral valine load could be accounted for as urinary methylmalonate, the block in methylmalonate catabolism was virtually complete. (4) When the child was given daily injections of vitamin B_{12}, valine failed to induce ketosis and only about 25 percent of the administered load could be accounted for as urinary methylmalonate. (5) The

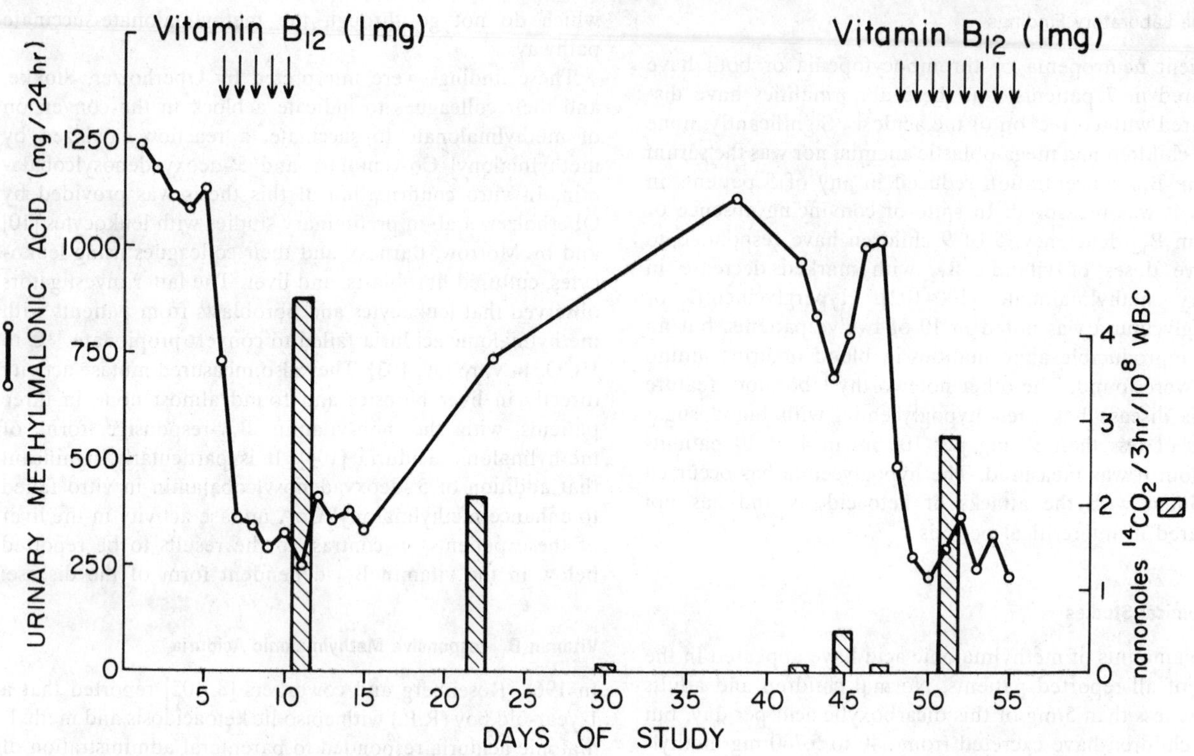

Figure 22-12. Effect of parenteral vitamin B_{12} administration on methylmalonic acid excretion (left ordinate) and on propionate-3-^{14}C oxidation by isolated leukocytes (right ordinate) in R.P., a patient with methylmalonic aciduria. Each arrow represents single daily injection of cyanocobalamin. Increasing the vitamin B_{12} dose to 4 mg per day failed to depress the urinary methylmalonate concentration further. (*From Rosenberg et al.* [102], *with permission.*)

excretion of butanone and hexanone, long-chain ketones which were detectable in the urine of this child during periods of ketosis or ketoacidosis, was accentuated by valine or isoleucine loading. Thus these unusual ketone products appeared to accumulate behind the block in methylmalonate catabolism.

These in vivo observations were supported and extended by studies in vitro [14, 102]. Leukocytes isolated from the peripheral blood of this boy converted negligible quantities of propionate-^{14}C or methylmalonate to $^{14}CO_2$, but oxidized succinate normally. In addition, incubation of leukocytes with propionate-^{14}C led to accumulation of methylmalonate and a much-reduced formation of succinate (Fig. 22-13). When the patient was receiving vitamin B_{12} supplements his leukocytes oxidized measurable amounts of propionate-^{14}C to $^{14}CO_2$, but still in amounts far lower than normal (Fig. 22-12) [102].

As seen in Fig. 22-14, the biochemical block in R. P. was also demonstrated in cultured fibroblasts. This ready source of tissue was then used by Rosenberg and colleagues [14] to define the mechanism of the vitamin B_{12} responsiveness. When fibroblasts were grown in medium containing 25 pg per ml of vitamin B_{12}, the cells of R. P. oxidized propionate-^{14}C poorly and contained only about 10 percent as much 5′-deoxyadenosylcobalamin as control cells (Fig. 22-15). When the cells were grown in 250,000 pg per ml of vitamin B_{12}, propionate oxidation approached normal, as did the concentration of coenzyme B_{12} in fibroblasts (Fig. 22-15). The marked reduction in 5′-deoxyadenosylcobalamin content of cells grown under standard conditions could reflect either abnormal biosynthesis of the coenzyme or defective binding of coenzyme by a mutant mutase apoenzyme. Accordingly, mutase activity was assayed directly in fibroblast homogenates. As can be seen in Table 22-2, no significant reduction in mutase activity was found in cells from R. P., either in the absence of added vitamin B_{12} coenzyme in vitro or in its presence. Furthermore, the K_m for vitamin B_{12} coenzyme was the same in the cells of R. P. as in those from two controls [106]. These findings lend strong support to the thesis that the basic defect in the vitamin B_{12}–dependent form of methylmalonic aciduria is in the enzymatic biosynthesis of 5′-deoxyadenosylcobalamin, *not* in the mutase apoenzyme per se. Studies of coenzyme biosynthesis in vitro have confirmed this thesis [15].

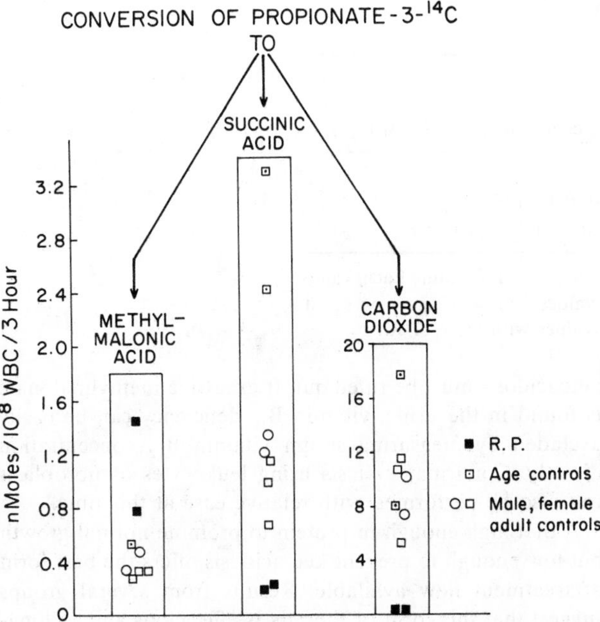

Figure 22-13. Conversion of propionate-3-^{14}C to methylmalonate, succinate, and $^{14}CO_2$ by leukocytes from R.P., a patient with vitamin B_{12}-dependent methylmalonic aciduria (solid squares), and healthy controls (open circles and squares). Note accumulation of methylmalonic acid and reduced formation of succinate and carbon dioxide. (*From unpublished observations of L. E. Rosenberg, A.-Ch. Lilljeqvist, and Y. E. Hsia.*)

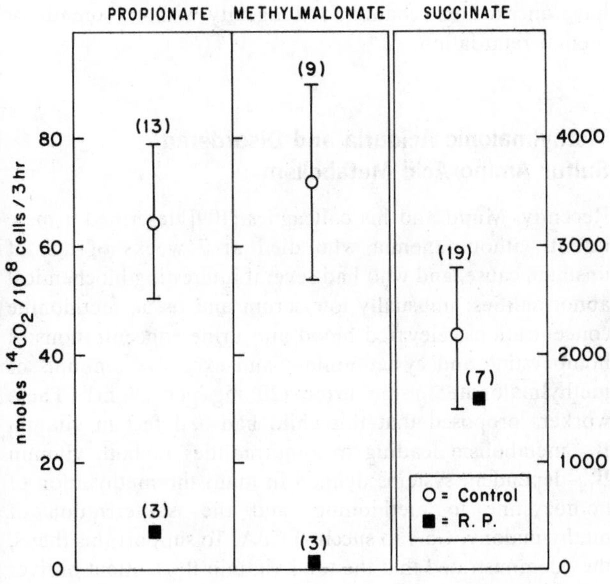

Figure 22-14. Oxidation of labeled propionate, methylmalonate, and succinate by cultured fibroblasts from controls (open circles) and from R.P. (closed squares), a child with vitamin B_{12}-dependent methylmalonic aciduria.

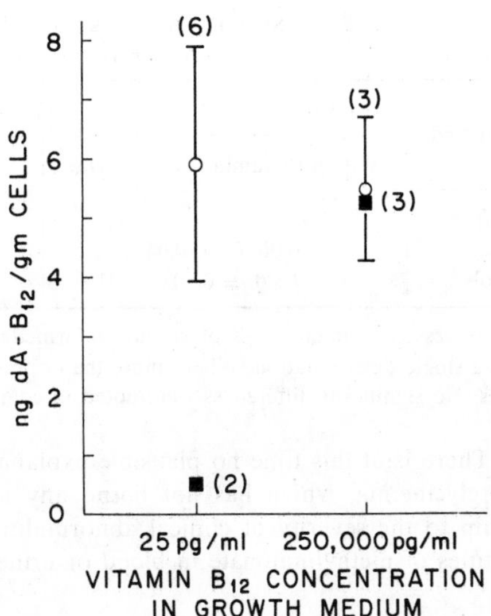

Figure 22-15. Concentration of 5′-deoxyadenosylcobalamin in fibroblasts from R.P., a patient with vitamin B_{12}-dependent methylmalonic aciduria (closed squares), and from controls (open circles). Note that increasing the vitamin B_{12} concentration of the growth medium failed to change the content of vitamin B_{12} coenzyme in control cells but produced a distinct increase in the mutant cell line. (*From Rosenberg et al.* [14].)

Pathophysiology

All the in vivo and in vitro studies in patients with methylmalonic aciduria indicate that the primary derangement is a block in the conversion of methylmalonyl CoA to succinyl CoA. This block explains admirably the accumulation of methylmalonate in blood and urine, the augmentation of methylmalonate excretion and the precipitation of ketosis by protein, amino acids, or propionate, and the excretion of long-chain ketones formed in the catabolism of branched-chain amino acids.

The primary block does not explain several important physiologic disturbances: the mechanism of the acidosis; the basis for the hypoglycemia; and the cause of the hyperglycinemia. Oberholzer et al. [10] pointed out that the concentration of methylmalonate in the blood (no more than 2 mM) could not alone explain the acidosis, and they suggested other possibilities. They proposed that an accumulation of coenzyme A "trapped" intracellularly as methylmalonyl CoA could lead to insufficient amounts of this widely utilized coenzyme and secondarily to impaired carbohydrate metabolism and subsequent acidosis. Alternatively they suggested that methylmalonyl CoA, which is a known inhibitor of pyruvate carboxylase [107], could interfere with gluconeogenesis and lead directly to hypoglycemia and indirectly to excessive catabolism of lipid, with ketosis and acidosis. It seems equally plausible that longer odd-chain fatty acids might accumulate behind the block in methylmalonate isomerization and lead directly to keto-

Table 22-2. CONVERSION OF DL-METHYL-^{3}H-MALONYL CoA TO SUCCINYL CoA BY FIBROBLAST HOMOGENATES

Subjects studied	Enzymatic activity*	
	Without vitamin B_{12} coenzyme	With vitamin B_{12} coenzyme ($2 \times 10^{-5} M$)
Patient:		
R.P.	0.06; 0.09; 0.04	1.40; 0.97; 1.07
Controls	$\bar{x} \pm 1$ s.d. = 0.10 ± 0.03	$\bar{x} \pm 1$ s.d. = 1.89 ± 1.1

*Activity expressed as micromoles of succinate formed per gram wet weight per 30 min. Each value represents a single determination. Where more than one value is given, values represent assays on serial subcultures. No significant differences were noted in comparing control values with these of R.P.

acidosis. There is at this time no plausible explanation for the hyperglycinemia, which has not borne any temporal relationship to the severity of clinical abnormalities or to the quantities of methylmalonate in blood or urine.

Genetics

The 13 children reported with methylmalonic aciduria were found in 13 different sibships, but in at least four of these families other children had died with similar findings and presumably suffered from the same illness. There is no suggestion of parent-to-child transmission, but none of the affected patients is old enough to test this hypothesis directly. Since both males and females have been found in about equal numbers in both the vitamin B_{12}–responsive and –unresponsive groups, there is little reason to consider X-chromosome linkage. The pedigree data are most consistent with autosomal recessive inheritance, but attempts to identify asymptomatic heterozygotes by measuring urinary methylmalonate, the response to propionate loading, or oxidation of propionate or methylmalonate by leukocytes have been singularly unrewarding. It seems likely that specific assays of mutase activity in leukocytes or fibroblasts from parents of children with the vitamin B_{12}–unresponsive form of the disease will provide a means of heterozygote detection in this group. In the vitamin B_{12}–dependent form, assays of vitamin B_{12}–coenzyme biosynthesis will probably be necessary.

It is significant that a relatively large number of patients from many different ethnic backgrounds (English, Swedish, Norwegian, Polish, American Indian) have been reported in less than 3 years, and that no instance of parental consanguinity has been documented. These findings suggest that the mutations in question are relatively frequent, but no incidence figures have been compiled.

Diagnosis and Treatment

Since simple colorimetric assays for urinary methylmalonate are now available [108], it should no longer be difficult to make a diagnosis of methylmalonic aciduria once this condition is considered. As was discussed with propionate carboxylase deficiency, other sources of neonatal or infantile ketoacidosis must be ruled out. If excessive methylmalonate is found in the urine, vitamin B_{12} deficiency can be easily excluded by measuring serum vitamin B_{12} concentration directly. Confirmatory tests using leukocytes or fibroblasts can also be performed with relative ease at this time.

A diet high enough in protein to promote normal growth but low enough to prevent ketoacidosis offers the best form of treatment now available. Results from several groups suggest that this form of therapy is efficacious and of long-term benefit, providing intercurrent infections do not supervene and progress to septicemia or cause uncontrollable acidosis. Vitamin B_{12} supplements should be tried in every patient with methylmalonic aciduria. Oral or parenteral administration of the vitamin should probably be continued for those who respond favorably, since data suggest that vitamin B_{12} may protect against protein or amino acid–induced ketoacidosis [105]. More long-term observations are needed, but present results suggest that patients with methylmalonic aciduria who survive the first 2 to 3 years of life have an excellent chance for longevity without somatic or mental retardation.

Methylmalonic Aciduria and Disordered Sulfur Amino Acid Metabolism

Recently, Mudd and his colleagues [109] described a male infant without anemia who died at 7 weeks of age of unstated cause, and who had several interesting biochemical abnormalities: unusually low serum and tissue methionine concentrations; elevated blood and urine concentrations of homocystine and cystathionine; and excessive amounts of methylmalonate in the urine (20 mg per 24 hr). These workers proposed that this child had a defect in vitamin B_{12} metabolism leading to abnormalities in both vitamin B_{12}–dependent systems defined in man: the methylation of homocystine to methionine, and the isomerization of methylmalonyl CoA to succinyl CoA. To support this thesis, they demonstrated that the total vitamin B_{12} content of liver and kidney was normal but that the concentration of 5′-deoxyadenosylcobalamin was very much reduced. Furthermore, they noted a defect in homocysteine methyl transferase activity in the tissues of their patient.

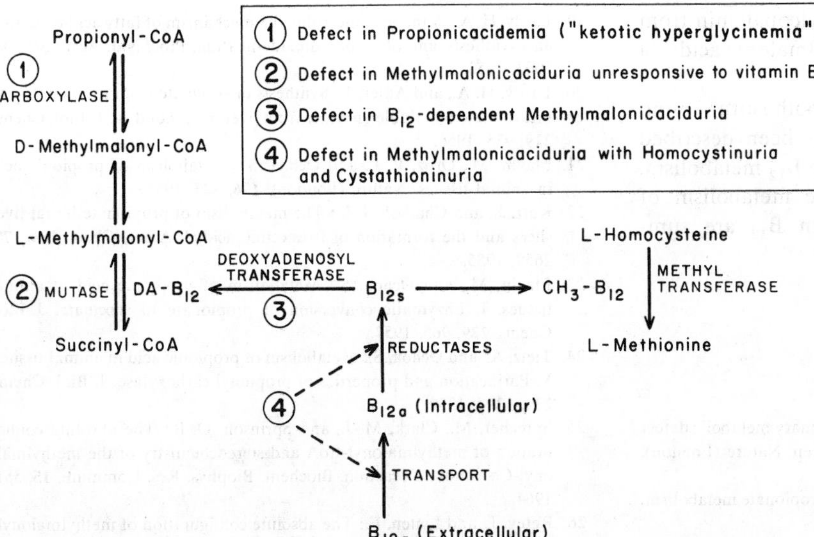

Figure 22-16. Hypothetical scheme of inherited defects of propionate, methylmalonate, and vitamin B_{12} metabolism. The data supporting defects at sites 1 and 2 are convincing. The exact nature of the defects in vitamin B_{12} metabolism remains unclear, but the available data are consistent with the proposed sites (3 and 4).

Unfortunately the child died before definitive therapy with vitamin B_{12} or B_{12} coenzyme could be tried, but the results obtained are important and raise some interesting questions. If this child has the same disorder as that described by Rosenberg et al. [8, 102], why did he excrete so little methylmalonate in the urine? Conversely, why did the child studied by Rosenberg demonstrate no abnormalities of sulfur amino acid metabolism in spite of repeated analyses of blood and urine? No satisfactory answers to these questions are currently available, but it seems likely that the two diseases are *not* identical and represent defects at different sites in the biochemical pathway of vitamin B_{12}–coenzyme biosynthesis (Fig. 22-16). Thus, it is possible that patients with vitamin B_{12}–dependent methylmalonic aciduria without disordered sulfur amino acid metabolism have a defect in the enzymatic conversion of vitamin B_{12s} to 5′-deoxyadenosylcobalamin, whereas patients with abnormalities of both methylmalonate and sulfur amino acids may have a defect earlier in the scheme which results in defective formation of a precursor common to both methylcobalamin and 5′-deoxyadenosylcobalamin.

Finally, it should be pointed out that there is an alternative explanation for the findings in the child described by Mudd et al. [109] which involves folate metabolism. Arakawa et al. [110] described a child who had megaloblastic anemia, elevated plasma folate levels, and defective N^5-methyltetrahydrofolate (N^5-CH_3-THF) methyl transferase activity in the liver. They proposed that this child had a primary defect in the transferase system which caused elevated N^5-CH_3-THF concentrations in blood and subsequently folate-deficient megaloblastosis. Since folate deficiency, per se, can affect vitamin B_{12} metabolism, as documented previously, it is conceivable that a primary block in folate metabolism or in the transferase apoenzyme could result in impairment of both methionine biosynthesis and methylmalonate catabolism. This hypothesis seems improbable and should be ruled out by appropriate study of methylmalonate excretion in patients or animals with pure folate deficiency.

SUMMARY

1 Propionic acid, formed in the catabolism of several amino acids, odd-chain fatty acids, and cholesterol, is metabolized primarily by enzymatic conversion to methylmalonic acid, which is subsequently isomerized to succinate. Propionyl CoA carboxylase, the enzyme which catalyzes the formation of methylmalonate, requires a biotin coenzyme, while 5′-deoxyadenosylcobalamin (a vitamin B_{12} coenzyme) is needed for the isomerization of methylmalonate to succinate.

2 Coenzymes formed from vitamin B_{12} are cofactors for only two known reactions in mammalian systems. Methylcobalamin acts as the methyl donor in the enzymatic remethylation of homocysteine to methionine. Another coenzyme form of vitamin B_{12}, 5′-deoxyadenosylcobalamin, co-catalyzes the formation of succinate from methylmalonate. These coenzymes are formed from precursor vitamin B_{12} species by specific enzymatic processes.

3 Propionyl CoA carboxylase deficiency is characterized chemically by accumulation of propionate in blood and by defective utilization of propionate by leukocytes. Clinically the disorder leads to neonatal ketoacidosis, which may prove lethal unless treated with vigorous alkali replacement and a low-protein diet.

4 Two forms of primary methylmalonic aciduria are described. The clinical hallmark in each is metabolic ketoacidosis, but the two conditions can be distinguished by their response to pharmacologic doses of vitamin B_{12}. The vitamin B_{12}–unresponsive patients have an abnormality in the apoenzyme portion of methylmalonyl CoA mutase. The patients with vitamin B_{12}-responsive methylmalonic aciduria appear

to be unable to synthesize 5′-deoxyadenosylcobalamin from its precursor vitamin. Both forms of methylmalonic aciduria respond to a protein-restricted diet.

5 A single patient with abnormalities of both sulfur amino acid and methylmalonate metabolism has been described who may have a different defect in vitamin B_{12} metabolism.

6 The postulated human defects in the metabolism of propionate, methylmalonate, and vitamin B_{12} are summarized in Fig. 22-16.

BIBLIOGRAPHY

1. Marston, H. R., Allen, S. H., and Smith, R. M.: Primary metabolic defect supervening on vitamin B_{12} deficiency in the sheep. Nature (London), **190,** 1085, 1961.
2. Smith, R. M., and Monty, K. J.: Vitamin B_{12} and propionate metabolism. Biochem. Biophys. Res. Commun., **1,** 105, 1959.
3. Gurnani, S., Mistry, S. P., and Johnson, B. C.: Function of vitamin B_{12} in methylmalonate metabolism. I. Effect of a cofactor form of B_{12} on the activity of methylmalonyl-CoA isomerase. Biochim. Biophys. Acta, **38,** 187, 1960.
4. Stern, J. R., and Friedmann, D. C.: Vitamin B_{12} and methylmalonyl-CoA isomerase. I. Vitamin B_{12} and propionate metabolism. Biochem. Biophys. Res. Commun., **2,** 82, 1960.
5. Cox, E. V., and White, A. M.: Methylmalonic acid excretion: Index of vitamin-B_{12} deficiency. Lancet, **2,** 853, 1962.
6. Barness, L. A., Young, D., Mellman, W. J., Kahn, S. B., and Williams, W. J.: Methylmalonate excretion in patient with pernicious anemia. New Eng. J. Med., **268,** 144, 1963.
7. Childs, B., Nyhan, W. L., Borden, M., Bard, L., and Cooke, R. E.: Idiopathic hyperglycinemia and hyperglycinuria: new disorder of amino acid metabolism. I. Pediatrics, **27,** 522, 1961.
8. Rosenberg, L. E., Lilljeqvist, A.-C., and Hsia, Y. E.: Methylmalonic aciduria: an inborn error leading to metabolic acidosis, long-chain ketonuria and intermittent hyperglycinemia. New Eng. J. Med., **278,** 1319, 1968.
9. Hsia, Y. E., Scully, K. J., and Rosenberg, L. E.: Defective propionate carboxylation in ketotic hyperglycinaemia. Lancet, **1,** 757, 1969.
10. Oberholzer, V. G., Levin, B., Burgess, E. A., and Young, W. F.: Methylmalonic aciduria: an inborn error of metabolism leading to chronic metabolic acidosis. Arch. Dis. Child., **42,** 492, 1967.
11. Stokke, O., Eldjarn, L., Norum, K. R., Steen-Johnsen, J., and Halvorsen, S.: Methylmalonic aciduria: a new inborn error of metabolism which may cause fatal acidosis in the neonatal period. Scand. J. Clin. Lab. Invest., **20,** 313, 1967.
12. Lindblad, B., Olin, P., Svanberg, B., and Zetterström, R.: Methylmalonic acidemia. Acta Paediat. Scand., **57,** 417, 1968.
13. Lindblad, B., Lindstrand, K., Svanberg, B., and Zetterström, R.: The effect of cobamide coenzyme in methylmalonic acidemia. Acta Paediat. Scand., **58,** 178, 1969.
14. Rosenberg, L. E., Lilljeqvist, A.-Ch., Hsia, Y. E., and Rosenbloom, F. M.: Vitamin B_{12} dependent methylmalonicaciduria: Defective B_{12} metabolism in cultured fibroblasts. Biochem. Biophys. Res. Commun., **37,** 607, 1969.
15. Mahoney, M. J., and Rosenberg, L. E.: Inherited defects of B_{12} metabolism. Amer. J. Med., **48,** 584, 1970.
16. Meister, A.: *Biochemistry of the Amino Acids,* pp. 674, 729, 753. Academic, New York, 1965.
17. Kaziro, Y., and Ochoa, S.: The metabolism of propionic acid. Advances Enzymol., **26,** 283, 1964.
18. Danielsson, H.: Present status of research on catabolism and excretion of cholesterol. Advances Lipid Res., **1,** 335, 1963.
19. Lardy, H. A.: A theory concerning the mechanism of fatty acid oxidation and synthesis, and of carbon dioxide fixation. Proc. Nat. Acad. Sci., **38,** 1003, 1952.
20. Lardy, H. A., and Adler, J.: Synthesis of succinate from propionate and bicarbonate by soluble enzymes from liver mitochondria. J. Biol. Chem., **219,** 935, 1956.
21. Flavin, M., Ortiz, P. J., and Ochoa, S.: Metabolism of propionic acid in animal tissues. Nature (London), **176,** 823, 1955.
22. Katz, J., and Chaikoff, I. L.: The metabolism of propionate by rat liver slices and the formation of isosuccinic acid. J. Amer. Chem. Soc., **77,** 2659, 1955.
23. Flavin, M., and Ochoa, S.: Metabolism of propionic acid in animal tissues. I. Enzymatic conversion of propionate to succinate. J. Biol. Chem., **229,** 965, 1957.
24. Tietz, A., and Ochoa, S.: Metabolism of propionic acid in animal tissues V. Purification and properties of propionyl carboxylase. J. Biol. Chem., **234,** 1394, 1959.
25. Sprecher, M., Clark, M. J., and Sprinson, D. B.: The absolute configuration of methylmalonyl-CoA and stereochemistry of the methylmalonyl-CoA mutase reaction. Biochem. Biophys. Res. Commun., **15,** 581, 1964.
26. Retey, J., and Lynen, F.: The absolute configuration of methylmalonyl-CoA. Biochem. Biophys. Res. Commun., **16,** 358, 1964.
27. Mazumder, R., Sasakawa, T., Kaziro, Y., and Ochoa, S.: Metabolism of propionic acid in animal tissues. IX. Methylmalonyl coenzyme A racemase. J. Biol. Chem., **237,** 3065, 1962.
28. Beck, W. S., Flavin, M., and Ochoa, S.: Metabolism of propionic acid in animal tissues. III. Formation of succinate. J. Biol. Chem., **229,** 997, 1957.
29. Kaziro, Y., Ochoa, S., Warner, R. C., and Chen, J.: Metabolism of propionic acid in animal tissues. VIII. Crystalline propionyl carboxylase. J. Biol. Chem., **236,** 1917, 1961.
30. Mistry, S. P., and Dakshinamurti, K.: Biochemistry of biotin. Vitamins Hormones N.Y., **22,** 1, 1964.
31. Fraenkel-Conrat, H., Snell, N. S., and Ducay, E. D.: Avidin. I. Isolation and characterization of the protein and nucleic acid. Arch. Biochem. Biophys., **39,** 80, 1952.
32. Sydenstricker, V. P., Singal, S. A., Briggs, A. P., and DeVaughn, N. M.: Preliminary observations on "egg white injury" in man and its cure with a biotin concentrate. Science, **95,** 176, 1942.
33. Overath, P., Kellerman, G. M., Lynen, F., Fritz, H. P., and Keller, H. J.: Zum Mechanismus der Umlagerung von Methylmalonyl-CoA in Succinyl-CoA. II. Versuche zur Wirkungsweise von Methylmalonyl-CoA-Isomerase und Methylmalonyl-CoA-Racemase. Biochem. Z., **335,** 500, 1962.
34. Barker, H. A., Smyth, R. D., Wawszkiewicz, E. J., Lee, M. N., and Wilson, R. M.: Enzymatic preparation and characterization of an α-L-β-methylaspartic acid. Arch. Biochem. Biophys., **78,** 468, 1958.
35. Barker, H. A., Weissbach, H., and Smyth, R. D.: A coenzyme containing pseudovitamin B_{12}. Proc. Nat. Acad. Sci. U.S.A., **44,** 1093, 1958.
36. Weissbach, H., Toohey, J., and Barker, H. A.: Isolation and properties of B_{12} coenzymes containing benzimidazole or dimethylbenzimadizole. Proc. Nat. Acad. Sci. U.S.A., **45,** 521, 1959.
37. Cannata, J. J. B., Focesi, A., Jr., Mazumder, R., Warner, R. C., and Ochoa, S.: Metabolism of propionic acid in animal tissues. XII. Properties of mammalian methylmalonyl coenzyme A mutase. J. Biol. Chem., **240,** 3249, 1965.
38. Overath, P., Stadtman, E. R., Kellerman, G. M., and Lynen, F.: Zum Mechanismus der Umlagerung von Methylmalonyl-CoA in Succinyl-CoA. III. Reinigung und Eigenschaften der Methylmalonyl-CoA-Isomerase. Biochem. Z., **336,** 77, 1962.
39. Kellermeyer, R. W., Allen, S. H. G., Stjernholm, R., and Wood, H. G.: Methylmalonyl isomerase. IV. Purification and properties of the enzyme from propionibacteria. J. Biol. Chem., **239,** 2562, 1964.
40. Eggerer, H., Stadtman, E. R., Overath, P., and Lynen, F.: Zum Mechanismus der durch Cobalamin-Coenzym katalysierten Umlagerung von Methylmalonyl-CoA in Succinyl-CoA. Biochem. Z., **333,** 1, 1960.

41. Kellermeyer, R. W., and Wood, H. G.: Methylmalonyl isomerase: a study of the mechanism of isomerization. Biochemistry (Wash.), **1,** 1124, 1962.
42. Phares, E. F., Long, M. V., and Carson, S. F.: An intramolecular rearrangement in the methylmalonyl isomerase reaction as demonstrated by positive and negative mass analysis of succinic acid. Biochem. Biophys. Res. Commun., **8,** 142, 1962.
43. Wagner, F.: Vitamin B_{12} and related compounds. Ann. Rev. Biochem., **35,** 405, 1966.
44. Lynen, F.: Biosynthesis of saturated fatty acids. Fed. Proc., **20,** 941, 1961.
45. Katz, J., and Kornblatt, J.: Propionate metabolism by slices of mammary gland and liver of lactating rat. J. Biol. Chem., **237,** 2466, 1962.
46. Dimitrov, N., and Stjernholm, R. L.: Metabolic deviations in lymphoproliferative disorders. Blood, **28,** 998, 1966.
47. Fish, M. B., Pollycove, M., and Wallerstein, R. O.: In vivo oxidative metabolism of propionic acid in human vitamin B_{12} deficiency. J. Lab. Clin. Med., **72,** 767, 1968.
48. Minot, G. R., and Murphy, L. P.: Treatment of pernicious anemia by a special diet. J.A.M.A., **87,** 470, 1926.
49. Smith, E. L.: Purification of anti-pernicious anemia factors from liver. Nature (London), **161,** 638, 1948.
50. Rickes, E. L., Brink, N. G., Koniuszy, F. R., Wood, T. R., and Folkers, K.: Crystalline vitamin B_{12}. Science, **107,** 396, 1948.
51. Hodgkin, D. C., Kamper, J., MacKay, M., Pickworth, J., Trueblood, K. N., and White, J. G.: Structure of vitamin B_{12}. Nature (London), **178,** 64, 1956.
52. Walker, G. A., Murphy, S., and Heunnekens, F. H.: Enzymatic conversion of vitamin B_{12} to adenosyl-B_{12}: Evidence for the existence of two separate reducing systems. Arch. Biochem. Biophys., **134,** 95, 1969.
53. Weissbach, H., and Taylor, R.: Role of vitamin B_{12} in methionine biosynthesis. Fed. Proc., **25,** 1649, 1966.
54. Taylor, R. T., and Weissbach, H.: Enzymatic synthesis of methionine: formation of a radioactive cobamide enzyme with N^5-methyl-^{14}C-tetrahydrofolate. Arch. Biochem. Biophys., **119,** 572, 1967.
55. Taylor, R. T., and Weissbach, H.: *Escherichia coli B* N^5-methyltetrahydrofolate-homocysteine vitamin-B_{12} transmethylase: Formation and photolability of a methylcobalamin enzyme. Arch. Biochem. Biophys., **123,** 109, 1968.
56. Abeles, R. H., and Frey, P. A.: Role of B_{12} coenzymes in the dioldehydrase reaction. Fed. Proc., **25,** 1639, 1966.
57. Abeles, R. H., Brownstein, A. M., and Randles, C. H.: β-Hydroxypropionaldehyde, an intermediate in the formation of 1,3-propanediol by *Aerobacter aerogenes.* Biochim. Biophys. Acta, **41,** 530, 1960.
58. Blakley, R. L.: B_{12}-dependent synthesis of deoxyribonucleotides. Fed. Proc., **25,** 1633, 1966.
59. Stadtman, T. C., and Blaylock, B. A.: Role of B_{12} compounds in methane formation. Fed. Proc., **25,** 1657, 1966.
60. Poston, J. M., Kuratomi, K., and Stadtman, E. R.: Methyl-vitamin B_{12} as a source of methyl groups for the synthesis of acetate by cell free extracts of *Clostridium thermoaceticum.* Ann. N.Y. Acad. Sci., **112,** 804, 1964.
61. Stadtman, T. C.: Cobamide coenzyme requirement for anaerobic degradation of lysine. Ann. N.Y. Acad. Sci., **112,** 728, 1964.
62. Vitols, E., Walker, G. A., and Huennekens, F. M.: Enzymatic conversion of vitamin B_{12} to a cobamide coenzyme, α(5,6-dimethylbenzimidazolyl) deoxyadenosylcobamide (adenosyl-B_{12}). J. Biol. Chem., **241,** 1455, 1966.
63. Ertel, R., Brot, N., Taylor, R., and Weissbach, H.: Studies on the nature of the bound cobamide in *E. coli* N^5-methyltetrahydrofolate-homocysteine transmethylase. Arch. Biochem. Biophys., **126,** 353, 1968.
64. Castle, W. B., Townsend, W. C., and Heath, C. W.: Observations on the etiologic relationship of achylia gastrica to pernicious anemia. III. The nature of the reaction between normal human gastric juice and beef muscle leading to clinical improvement and increased blood formation similar to the effect of liver feeding. Amer. J. Med. Sci., **180,** 305, 1930.
65. Castle, W. B., Heath, C. W., and Strauss, M. B.: Observations on the etiologic relationship of achylia gastrica to pernicious anemia. IV. A biologic assay of the gastric secretion of patients with pernicious anemia having free hydrochloric acid and that of patients without anemia or with hypochromic anemia having no free hydrochloric acid, and of the role of intestinal impermeability to hematopoietic substances in pernicious anemia. Amer. J. Med. Sci., **182,** 741, 1932.
66. Cooper, G. A., and Castle, W. B.: Sequential mechanisms in the enhanced absorption of vitamin B_{12} by intrinsic factor in the rat. J. Clin. Invest., **39,** 199, 1960.
67. Reisner, E. H.: Deficiency effects and physiology in man, in *The Vitamins,* edited by W. H. Sebrell, Jr., and R. S. Harris, 2d ed., vol. 2, p. 220. Academic, New York, 1968.
68. Mendelson, R. S., Watkin, D. M., Horbett, A. P., and Fahey, J. L.: Identification of the vitamin B_{12}-binding protein in the serum of normals and of patients with chronic myelocytic leukemia. Blood, **13,** 740, 1958.
69. Hall, C. A., and Finkler, A. E.: The dynamics of transcobalamin. II. A vitamin B_{12} binding substance in plasma. J. Lab. Clin. Med., **65,** 459, 1965.
70. Hom, B. L.: Plasma turnover of ^{57}cobalt-vitamin B_{12} bound to transcobalamin I and II. Scand. J. Haemat., **4,** 321, 1967.
71. Rosenblum, C., Davis, R. L., and Chow, B. F.: Comparative absorption of vitamin B_{12} analogues by normal humans. III. 5,6-Dichlorobenzimidazole, 5,6-desdimethylbenzimidazole and 5-hydroxybenzimidazole analogues. Proc. Soc. Exp. Biol. Med., **95,** 30, 1957.
72. Rachmilewitz, M., Moshkowitz, B., Lefton, F., and Gross, J.: The uptake of $Co^{57}B_{12}$ by rat liver slices. 1. Effect of calcium and intrinsic factor. 2. Demonstration of an intrinsic factor-like effect in human serum. Israel J. Med. Sci., **4,** 843, 1968.
73. Lindstrand, K., and Stahlberg, K. G.: On vitamin B_{12} forms in human plasma. Acta Med. Scand., **174,** 665, 1963.
74. Lindstrand, K.: Isolation of methylcobalamin from natural source material. Nature (London), **204,** 188, 1964.
75. Stahlberg, K. G.: Studies on methyl-B_{12} in man. Scand. J. Haemat., suppl. 1, p. 7, 1967.
76. Stahlberg, K. G., Radmer, S., and Norden, A.: Liver B_{12} in subjects with and without vitamin B_{12} deficiency: a quantitative and qualitative study. Scand. J. Haemat., **4,** 312, 1967.
77. Glass, G. B. J., Skeggs, H. R., Lee, D. H., Jones, E. L., and Hardy, W. W.: Hydroxocobalamin. I. Blood levels and urinary excretion of vitamin B_{12} in man after a single parenteral dose of aqueous hydroxocobalamin, aqueous cyanocobalamin and cyanocobalamin zinc–tannate complex. Blood, **18,** 511, 1961.
78. Yagir, Y.: On the metabolism of coenzyme B_{12}. II. Disappearance from blood and distribution in tissues of coenzyme B_{12} and hydroxocobalamin and the effect of intrinsic factor on the distribution of both cobamides in tissues following intravenous administration. J. Vitamin. (Kyoto), **13,** 210, 1967.
79. Boddy, K., and Adams, J. F.: Excretion of cobalamins and coenzyme B_{12} following massive parenteral doses. Amer. J. Clin. Nutr., **21,** 657, 1968.
80. Cox, E. V., Robertson-Smith, D., Small, M., and White, A. M.: The excretion of propionate and acetate in vitamin B_{12} deficiency. Clin. Sci., **35,** 123, 1968.
81. Cardinale, G. J., Dreyfus, P. M., Auld, P., and Abeles, R. H.: Experimental vitamin B_{12} deficiency. Its effect on tissue vitamin B_{12}-coenzyme levels and on the metabolism of methylmalonyl-CoA. Arch. Biochem. Biophys., **131,** 92, 1969.
82. Seashore, M., Durant, J. L., Hsia, Y. E., and Rosenberg, L. E.: Defective propionate metabolism in leukocytes of vitamin B_{12} deficient pigs (in preparation).
83. Zalusky, R., Herbert, V., and Castle, W. B.: Cyanocobalamin therapy effect in folic acid deficiency. Arch. Intern. Med., **109,** 545, 1962.
84. Herbert, V., and Zalusky, R.: Interrelations of vitamin B_{12} and folic acid metabolism: folic acid clearance studies. J. Clin. Invest., **41,** 1263, 1962.

85. Chanarin, I., Bennett, M. C., and Berry, V.: Urinary excretion of histidine derivatives in megaloblastic anemia and other conditions and a comparison with the folic acid clearance test. J. Clin. Path., **15**, 269, 1962.
86. Zalusky, R., and Herbert, V.: Urinary formiminoglutamic acid in test of folic-acid deficiency. Lancet, **1**, 108, 1962.
87. Joske, R. A.: The vitamin B_{12} content of human liver tissue obtained by aspiration biopsy. Gut, **4**, 231, 1963.
88. Noronha, J. M., and Silverman, M.: On folic acid, vitamin B_{12}, methionine and formiminoglutamic acid metabolism, in *Vitamin B_{12} and Intrinsic Factor,* edited by H. C. Heinrich. Verlag, Stuttgart, 1962.
89. Larrabee, A. R., Rosenthal, S., Cathow, R. E., and Buchanan, J. M.: Enzymatic synthesis of the methyl group of methionine. IV. Isolation, characterization, and role of 5-methyl tetrahydrofolate. J. Biol. Chem., **238**, 1025, 1963.
90. Nyhan, W. L., Ando, T., and Gerritsen, T.: Hyperglycinemia, in *Amino Acid Metabolism and Genetic Variation,* edited by W. L. Nyhan, p. 255. McGraw-Hill, New York, 1968.
91. Morrow, G., Barness, L. A., Auerbach, V. H., DiGeorge, A. M., Ando, T., and Nyhan, W. L.: Observations on the coexistence of methylmalonic acidemia and glycinemia. J. Pediat., **74**, 680, 1969.
92. Hommes, F. A., Kuipers, J. R. G., Elema, J. D., Jansen, J. F., and Jonxis, J. J. P.: Propionicacidemia, a new inborn error of metabolism. Pediat. Res., **2**, 519, 1968.
93. Nyhan, W. L., Borden, M., and Childs, B.: Idiopathic hyperglycinemia: a new disorder of amino acid metabolism. II. The concentrations of other amino acids in the plasma and their modification by the administration of leucine. Pediatrics, **27**, 539, 1961.
94. Childs, B., and Nyhan, W. L.: Further observations of a patient with hyperglycinemia. Pediatrics, **33**, 403, 1964.
95. Nyhan, W. L., and Childs, B.: Hyperglycinemia. V. The miscible pool and turnover rate of glycine and the formation of serine. J. Clin. Invest., **43**, 2404, 1964.
96. Menkes, J. H.: Idiopathic hyperglycinemia: isolation and identification of three previously undescribed urinary ketones. J. Pediat., **69**, 413, 1966.
97. Hsia, Y. E., and Rosenberg, L. E.: Unpublished observations.
98. Snyderman, S. E., Holt, C. E., Norton, P. M., Roitman, E., and Phansalkar, S. V.: The plasma aminogram. I. Influence of the level of protein intake and a comparison of whole protein and amino acid diets. Pediat. Res., **2**, 131, 1968.
99. Morrow, G., and Barness, L. A.: Studies in a patient with methylmalonic acidemia. Pediatrics, **74**, 691, 1969.
100. Walker, F. A., Agarwal, A. B., and Singh, R.: The importance of the falsely positive reaction. J. Pediat., **75**, 344, 1969.
101. Sotos, J. F., Romshe, C. A., Boggs, D. E., and Menking, M. F.: Methylmalonicaciduria B_{12} dependent, in *Abstracts of the Society for Pediatric Research,* p. 13, 1969 (abstract).
102. Rosenberg, L. E., Lilljeqvist, A.-C., and Hsia, Y. E.: Methylmalonic aciduria: metabolic block localization and vitamin B_{12} dependency. Science, **162**, 805, 1968.
103. Morrow, G., Mellman, W. J., Barness, L. A., and Dimitrov, N. V.: Propionate metabolism in cells cultured from a patient with methylanic acidemia. Pediat. Res., **3**, 217, 1969.
104. Morrow, G., Barness, L. A., Cardinale, G. J., Abeles, R. H., and Flaks, J. G.: Congenital methylmalonic acidemia: enzymatic evidence for two forms of the disease. Proc. Nat. Acad. Sci. U.S.A., **63**, 191, 1969.
105. Hsia, Y. E., Scully, K., Lilljeqvist, A.-Ch., and Rosenberg, L. E.: Vitamin B_{12} dependent methylmalonicaciduria. Pediatrics, **46**, 497, 1970.
106. Rosenberg, L. E., and Lilljeqvist, A.-Ch.: Unpublished observations.
107. Utter, M. F., Keech, D. B., and Scrutten, M. L.: A possible role for acetyl-CoA in the control of gluconeogenesis, in *Advances in Enzyme Regulation,* edited by G. Weber, vol. 2, p. 49. Pergamon, New York, 1964.
108. Giorgio, A. J., and Plaut, G. W. E.: Method for colorimetric determination of urinary methylmalonic acid in pernicious anemia. J. Lab. Clin. Med., **66**, 667, 1965.
109. Mudd, S. H., Levy, H. L., and Abeles, R. H.: A derangement in B_{12} metabolism leading to homocystinemia, cystathioninemia and methylmalonicaciduria. Biochem. Biophys. Res. Commun., **35**, 121, 1969.
110. Arakawa, T., Narisawa, K., Tanno, K., Ohava, K., Higashi, O., Honda, Y., Tamura, T., Wada, Y., Mizuno, T., and Hayashi, T.: Megaloblastic anemia and mental retardation associated with hyperfolic-acidemia: Probably due to N^5-methyltetrahydrofolate transferase deficiency. Tohoku J. Exp. Med., **93**, 1, 1967.
111. Hsia, Y. E., Scully, K. J., and Rosenberg, L. E.: Inherited proprionyl-CoA carboxylase deficiency in "ketotic hyperglycinemia." J. Clin. Invest. **50**, 127, 1971.

CHAPTER TWENTY-THREE

HYPERSARCOSINEMIA

Theo Gerritsen and Harry A. Waisman*

Hypersarcosinemia with sarcosinuria, an inborn error of amino acid metabolism, was first reported by Gerritsen and Waisman in 1965 [1, 2], and their two patients were extensively discussed by the same authors in 1966 [3]. A third case was reported by Hagge et al. in 1967 [4]. Since then, at least four more cases of this metabolic abnormality have been described. The disease has no specific clinical features, and although the original two patients were mentally backward, no proof existed that this was due to the hypersarcosinemia. Although the enzymic defect is presumed to be in sarcosine dehydrogenase, this has not been proved.

METABOLISM OF SARCOSINE

Sarcosine is the intermediate between dimethylglycine (DMG) and glycine in the one-carbon cycle [5] (Fig. 23-1). Hoskins and Mackenzie [6] demonstrated two different demethylating enzymes in liver mitochondria, one for the oxidative demethylation of DMG to form sarcosine, and one for the formation of glycine from sarcosine. The enzyme of the latter step, sarcosine dehydrogenase, contains tightly bound FAD (flavin adenine dinucleotide) [6] and requires an electron transfer flavoprotein for its dehydrogenating activity [5]. The total reaction from DMG to glycine accounts for the formation of two-thirds of the active methyl groups in man.

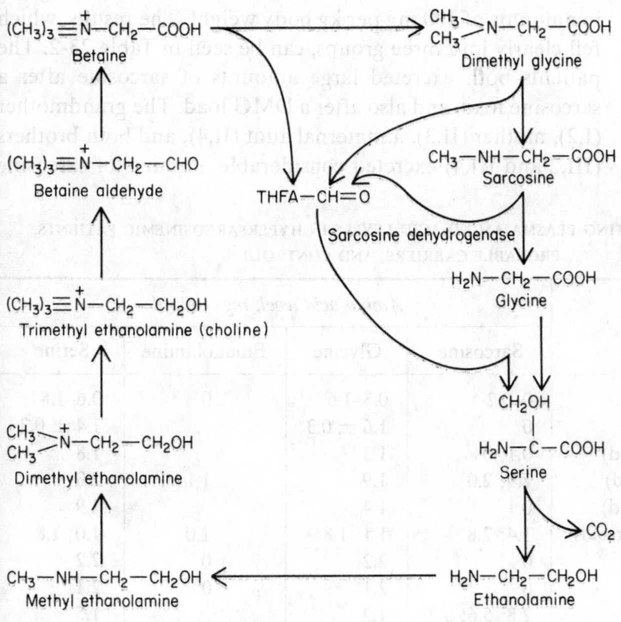

Figure 23-1. The one-carbon cycle and the position of sarcosine dehydrogenase.

Normal control subjects have fasting sarcosine plasma levels of 0 to 0.2 mg per 100 ml, and less than 2 mg sarcosine is excreted in the urine per 24 hr.

CLINICAL ASPECTS

The first patient (III,5[1]) with hypersarcosinemia was discovered during a screening program for abnormal urinary amino acids in all the patients within an institution for retarded children in Wisconsin.[2] There were few noteworthy clinical signs and symptoms in the proband; he was hypertonic and had tremors and difficulty in swallowing. There were no obvious congenital abnormalities. He did not thrive and was slow in all developmental milestones. On two different occasions the patient excreted 102 and 168 mg sarcosine per day. Fasting sarcosine blood levels were 1.4 and 2.8 mg per 100 ml on two separate occasions. Apart from a measurable amount of ethanolamine in the urine, all other amino acids in urine and plasma were normal. The patient had frequent episodes of pneumonitis, and died at age 1²⁄₁₂ years during a visit to his home. Autopsy was unfortunately performed only after embalming, and tissues that reached the laboratory were not completely satisfactory for pathologic study. From acceptable sections the diagnoses were pneumonitis, probably due to chronic aspiration; fat metamorphosis in the liver, with moderate hepatomegaly; and spongy degeneration in the brain.

The second patient (III,3) was the sister of the first and at the time of investigation was 6 to 7 years old. She had an IQ of 81 and was found on physical examination to be essentially normal. The third case of sarcosinemia was discovered in West Germany and reported by Hagge et al. [4]. This patient was the third child of parents who were first cousins; two other sibs died early in infancy. This child vomited frequently and had to be fed by gavage throughout the neonatal period. He developed a marked hepatosplenomegaly, but otherwise, findings on physical examination were normal. At age 3 months he excreted on one occasion 77 mg sarcosine in 24 hr. Sarcosine blood levels were 2.8, 5.6, and 3.2 mg per 100 ml. All other plasma amino acids were within normal limits. At age 8 months there were no signs of developmental retardation, but there has been no further opportunity to observe or examine this patient [7].

Two sibs, a boy born in 1962 and a girl born in 1968,

*Deceased.

[1]These numbers refer to the pedigree in Fig. 23-3.

[2]The cooperation and help of Drs. E. Kaveggia, J. Toussaint, and T. Shimaneck of the Central Wisconsin Colony and Training School are gratefully acknowledged.

were found to have hypersarcosinemia and sarcosinuria by a group of investigators in Belgium in 1968 [10]. Fasting serum sarcosine levels were 4.8 and 7.6 mg per 100 ml, respectively. Loading experiments on the parents and four other sibs demonstrated abnormal elevations of serum sarcosine values in both parents and two sibs, consistent with heterozygosity. The nonidentical twin brother of the younger patient was normal. The female patient showed sarcosinuria (3.32 μmoles/gm creatinine) and increased levels of sarcosine in feces, but no sarcosine was detected in the cerebrospinal fluid. The two patients and one of the heterozygote sibs had dwarfism, multiple anomalies, and mental retardation. The parents and the other sibs, including the other heterozygote and the twin, were physically and neurologically normal.

Glorieux et al. [11] reported on a 10-year-old, intelligent boy of small stature with hypersarcosinemia. Scott et al. [12], described details of clinical and cellular studies in an infant with sarcosinemia. This patient had mental and motor retardation but no specific physical abnormalities. His plasma sarcosine level was 0.31 to 0.54 mM (2.7 to 4.7 mg per 100 ml) and he excreted 3.35 to 5.57 mmoles (298 to 496 mg) sarcosine per 24 hr. Sarcosine tolerance tests on the patient, his parents, and controls gave results that were similar to those reported by Gerritsen and Waisman [3].

DIAGNOSTIC STUDIES

The two-dimensional paper chromatogram of the urine from the two sibs showed an unusual spot, caused by a substance that gave a reddish-purple color with ninhydrin, had an R_f value of 29 in BuAc (*n*-butanol/acetic acid/water = 150:10:50) and of 78 in Ph (phenol/water = 4:1). It could in no way be separated from synthetic sarcosine when the latter was added to the urine.

Quantitative determination of sarcosine was performed by column chromatography on an automatic amino acid analyzer. Amino acid analyses were performed on the fasting plasma of the patients, their sibs, and their parents. The blood levels of sarcosine in all these patients were increased, as were the levels of ethanolamine in the Wisconsin patients. The plasma levels of sarcosine, glycine, serine, and ethanolamine are compared with those of controls in Table 23-1. All amino acid levels not reported in this table were within the normal range.

Quantitative analyses of the urine for free amino acids were performed on 24-hr collections of both Wisconsin patients, the two brothers, the parents, aunts, uncles, the maternal grandmother and her sister, on the German patient and his parents, and on controls. The results of these analyses are listed in Table 23-2, under "Basal." Only the propositus (III,5), his sister (III,3), and patient W.P. excreted large amounts of sarcosine in the urine. The cerebrospinal fluid of patient B.K. showed no amino acid abnormalities. No samples were obtained from the other members of the family.

Apart from the sarcosine content of the brain and the liver, analysis for free amino acids in the organs from the propositus obtained at autopsy showed no abnormalities. The brain contained 5.8 mg sarcosine per 100 mg wet weight, and the liver 8.1 mg, as compared with only traces found in control specimens of these organs from subjects of various ages.

METABOLIC STUDIES

In order to evaluate the metabolism of sarcosine and its precursor DMG in the two Wisconsin patients and in other members of this family, sarcosine excretion was determined after loading with sarcosine and with DMG. Both were given in amounts of 100 mg per kg body weight. The results, which fell clearly into three groups, can be seen in Table 23-2. The patients both excreted large amounts of sarcosine after a sarcosine load, and also after a DMG load. The grandmother (I,2), mother (II,3), a maternal aunt (II,4), and both brothers (III,2 and III,4) excreted considerable amounts of sarcosine

Table 23-1. FASTING PLASMA AMINO ACID LEVELS IN HYPERSARCOSINEMIC PATIENTS, PROBABLE CARRIERS, AND CONTROLS

Subject	*Amino acid level, mg/100 ml*			
	Sarcosine	Glycine	Ethanolamine	Serine
Controls (9)	0–0.2	0.8–1.6	0	0.6–1.8
Controls (12)*	0	1.6 ± 0.3	...	1.4 ± 0.3
III,2 (brother, 7 yr old)	0.1; 0	1.3	...	1.8
III,3 (patient, 6 yr old)	2.9; 2.0	1.9	1.1	2.0
III,4 (brother, 5 yr old)	0.1	1.4	...	1.9
III,5 (propositus, 1 yr old)	1.4; 2.8	1.1; 1.8	1.0	1.0; 1.8
II,11 (father)	0	2.2	0	2.2
II,3 (mother)	0	2.1	0	2.1
Patient W.P.*	2.8; 5.6; 3.2	1.2	...	1.5

* From Hagge [4, 7].

Table 23-2. URINARY SARCOSINE EXCRETION BY HYPERSARCOSINEMIC PATIENTS, PROBABLE CARRIERS, OTHER MEMBERS OF THE AFFECTED FAMILY, AND CONTROLS

Subject	Sarcosine excretion		
	Basal, mg/24 hr	After sarcosine load,* mg/24 hr	After DMG load,* mg/24 hr
Controls, adult (14)	0–2.0	4–55	0–2†
Controls, 4–6 yr old (4)	0–2.0	2–15	0–2
I,2 (grandmother)	6.3	441	
I,3	1.3	45	
II,1 (aunt)	0	26	
II,2 (aunt)	0	38	
II,3 (mother)	0; 0	265; 247	17
II,4 (aunt)	1.0	298	
II,5 (uncle)	0	55	
II,6 (uncle)	0	6	
II,7 (uncle)	0	52	
II,8 (uncle)	0	46	
II,9 (aunt)	. .	47	
II,10 (husband of II,1)	0	10	
II,11 (father)	0; 8.0	19; 23	10
III,1 (cousin, 1 mo old)	0	5	0
III,2 (brother, 7 yr old)	0; 0	196; 93	58
III,3 (sister, 6 yr old)	703; 474	1,589; 1,660	1,858; 952
III,4 (brother, 5 yr old)	2.0; 0	73; 48	15
III,5 (propositus, 1 yr old)	102; 168	347	247
	mg/24 hr	mg/8 hr§	mg/8 hr§
Controls, adult (3)‡	0	11–29	6.0–8.4
Patient, 8 mo old‡	77	137	55
Father‡	0	171	15
Mother‡	0	102	17

* 100 mg/kg body weight.
† Three control subjects.
‡ From Hagge [4, 7].
§ Sarcosine estimations in 8-hr collections are comparable with estimations in 24-hr collections, as after a loading test in controls, practically all sarcosine is excreted within 8 hr. Therefore in the patient, the basal 24-hr excretion is not comparable with the sarcosine estimated in the 8-hr collections after the loading tests.

after a sarcosine load, when compared with control subjects of the same age group, but after a DMG load sarcosine excretion was only questionably increased in some of these individuals. Sarcosine loading tests on the rest of the family, including the father, gave results within the normal range. Hagge [4, 7] performed similar loading tests on the third patient and his parents, and as can be seen in the lower part of Table 23-2, his results were in good agreement with those from the Wisconsin kindred.

The patients were fed 100 mg sarcosine per kilogram body weight, and blood samples were obtained at various time intervals for sarcosine determination. These sarcosine blood tolerance curves appear in Fig. 23-2A and B. Although no statistical calculations were performed, the curves appear to fall into three different groups. In Fig. 23-2A the curves of the control subjects and of the father (No's. 4, 5, and 6) began at a level of 0 mg, reached a maximum of 1.5 to 3 mg after $1\frac{1}{2}$ to 2 hr, and returned to near-normal after 8 hr. The curves of the mother (II,3) and the brothers (III,2 and III,4) reached a maximum of 3.5 to 4.5 mg per 100 ml between $1\frac{1}{2}$ and 3 hr, whereas the patient with hypersarcosinemia (III,3) had a tolerance curve markedly above the two former groups. In Fig. 23-2B (Hagge [7]), the same three different groups can be distinguished, while here the tolerance curve of the mother does not reach the expected peak after $1\frac{1}{2}$ hr. The absolute values of the curves in Fig. 23-2A are generally lower than those in Fig. 23-2B, possibly because of differences in the methods used for the estimation of sarcosine. Similar loading experiments performed by Van Sande et al. [10] and Scott et al. [12] confirmed the former results.

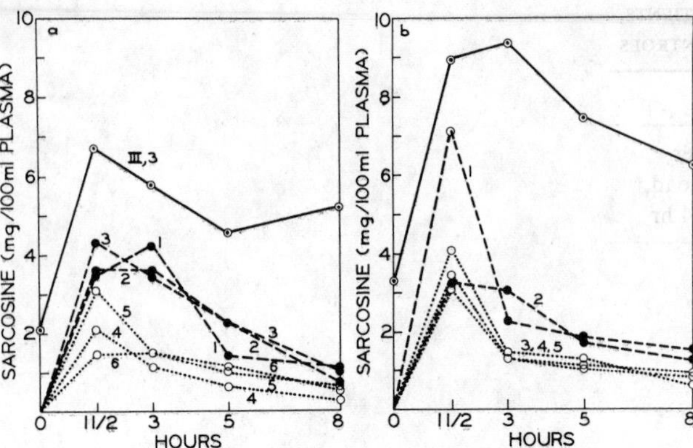

Figure 23-2. Sarcosine blood tolerance curves: A. Patient III,3: 1, mother; 2 and 3, brothers; 4, father; 5 and 6, controls. (*From Gerritsen and Waisman* [3].) B. Patient W.P.: 1, father; 2, mother; 3, 4, and 5, controls. (*From Hagge* [4, 7].)

THE METABOLIC DEFECT

Although no proof is available, it is assumed that in a patient with hypersarcosinemia, the activity of the sarcosine dehydrogenase in the liver mitochondria is greatly reduced. It is in fact the only way to account for the biochemical findings of accumulation of sarcosine in the organisms, increased blood levels, and excretion in the urine. Since all compounds of the one-carbon cycle before sarcosine would be expected to be present in increased amounts, this defect would also explain the increased levels of ethanolamine in the blood. Other one-carbon cycle compounds may have been present in increased amounts also but were not determined.

After developing a rapid and simple method to determine sarcosine dehydrogenase activity in tissue homogenates based on the isotope-dilution technique of Hoskins and Bjur [8], Rehberg and Gerritsen [9] attempted to create a model for hypersarcosinemia by feeding rats with diets high in sarcosine. Diets containing 5 and 7½ percent sarcosine caused elevated blood levels of sarcosine, glycine, and serine. This was not in agreement with the findings in the patients, who had high sarcosine levels only and no increased levels of glycine and serine. This difference could easily be explained by assuming a block at the sarcosine dehydrogenase level in the metabolism of the patients. Psychologic testing of the rats was not performed but probably was of little importance since the psychologic symptoms of the patients were ill-defined and of uncertain relevance.

No sarcosine dehydrogenase activity was detected in leukocytes and fibroblasts obtained from skin tissue cultures from normal controls [9, 11, 12]. Consequently lack of activity in a patient's fibroblasts is of no significance. Final confirmation of the enzyme defect will have to await direct assay of liver tissue from an affected patient.

GENETICS

The pedigree of the Wisconsin family appears in Fig. 23-3. As far as is known, the parents were not related. Both patients excreted large amounts of sarcosine while on a normal diet. When they were fed sarcosine or its precursor DMG, the excretion of this compound increased sharply. The fasting blood concentration of patient III,3 was 2.0 mg per 100 ml and was highly abnormal.

A modified biochemical response, which was different from that in the control subjects and the father, was demonstrated in the mother, a sister of the mother, the maternal grandmother, and the two sibs (III,2 and III,4). These family members excreted little or no sarcosine normally, but when sarcosine was fed, the excretion was far above control values. In addition, the blood tolerance curves of these patients were clearly distinguishable from the tolerance curve of the patient and from those of the controls. This phenomenon is probably best explained by a partial enzyme defect in heterozygotes. The pedigree of the German family supports the supposition that hypersarcosinemia is the homozygous expression of a recessive trait. Though the sarcosine tolerance curve of the mother does not show much less tolerance for this compound than that of the controls, it is not completely normal. Hagge [4] suggested that hypersarcosinemia is a recessive trait and that the parents react as heterozygotes. Nevertheless the genetics of this error of metabolism are not clear, since the father of the Wisconsin patients had a normal sarcosine tolerance curve, and his sarcosine excretions after loading with sarcosine or DMG were not different from normal. A likely interpretation is that the disease is transmitted as an autosomal recessive trait, but that the carrier state is highly variable in expression. Thus, the defect in the father was so slight that it could not be demonstrated with the loading tests as performed.

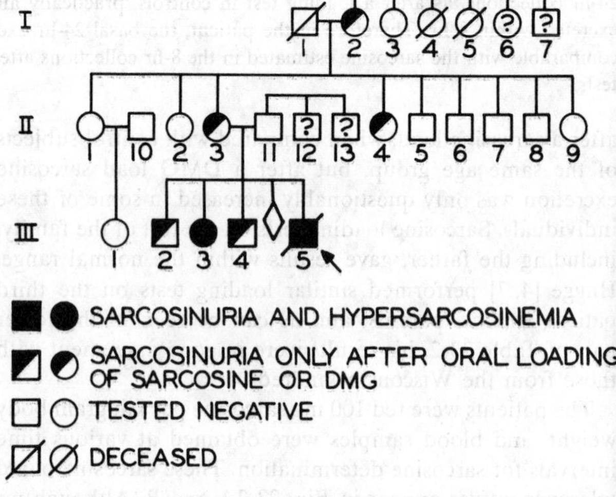

Figure 23-3. Pedigree of family with hypersarcosinemia [3]. The arrow indicates the propositus.

SUMMARY

1 Hypersarcosinemia has been described in two sibs and in a third unrelated child of a consanguine marriage. There is no certainty that the slight mental retardation and ill-defined symptoms of the patients were related to the hypersarcosinemia.

2 The metabolic defect in hypersarcosinemia is assumed to be reduced activity of sarcosine dehydrogenase, an enzyme which transforms sarcosine into glycine. This metabolic step does not appear to be essential in man.

3 Loading tests with sarcosine and with dimethylglycine, a sarcosine precursor, in family members of patients with hypersarcosinemia have suggested that some may be heterozygotes. The presumed inheritance pattern is autosomal recessive.

BIBLIOGRAPHY

1. Gerritsen, T., and Waisman, H. A.: Hypersarcosinemia, a new error of metabolism. Fed. Proc., **24,** 470, 1965.
2. Gerritsen, T., and Waisman, H. A.: Sarcosinemia and sarcosinuria: a new familial error of metabolism. Abstr. Amer. Pediat. Soc., p. 28, 1965.
3. Gerritsen, T., and Waisman, H. A.: Hypersarcosinemia: an inborn error of metabolism. New Eng. J. Med., **275,** 66, 1966.
4. Hagge, W., Brodehl, J., and Gellissen, K.: Hypersarcosinemia. Pediat. Res., **1,** 409, 1967.
5. Mackenzie, C. G., and Frisell, W. R.: Metabolism of dimethylglycine by liver mitochondria. J. Biol. Chem., **232,** 417, 1958.
6. Hoskins, D. D., and Mackenzie, C. G.: Solubilization and electron transfer flavoprotein requirement of mitochondrial sarcosine dehydrogenase and dimethylglycine dehydrogenase. J. Biol. Chem., **236,** 177, 1961.
7. Hagge, W.: Personal communication.
8. Hoskins, D. D., and Bjur, R. A.: The oxidation of N-methylglycines by primate liver mitochondria. J. Biol. Chem., **239,** 1856, 1964.
9. Rehberg, M. L., and Gerritsen, T.: Sarcosine metabolism in the rat. Arch. Biochem. Biophys., **127,** 661, 1968.
10. Van Sande, M., Hainaut, H., Hariga, J., Chapelle, P., Willems, C., and Heusden, A.: Personal communication from Dr. Van Sande to one of the authors (T. G.), 1969.
11. Glorieux, F. H., Mohyuddin, F., Whelan, D. T., and Scriver, C. R.: Hypersarcosinemia: new observations. Abstracts 80th Annual meeting, American Pediatric Society, p. 47, 1970.
12. Scott, C. R., Clark, S. H., Teng, C. C., and Svedberg, K. R.: Clinical and cellular studies of sarcosinemia. J. Pediat., **77,** 805, 1970.

CHAPTER TWENTY-FOUR

NONKETOTIC HYPERGLYCINEMIA

William L. Nyhan

Elevated concentrations of glycine are found in the blood in an increasing number of disorders. In most of these, large amounts of glycine are also present in other body fluids such as urine and cerebrospinal fluid. These conditions include some in which hyperglycinemia is clearly secondary. For example, hyperglycinemia may be present in methylmalonic acidemia [1], isovaleric acidemia [2], and in a disorder of the urea cycle in which the activity of carbamylphosphate synthetase is diminished [3].

The conditions we have called ketotic hyperglycinemia and nonketotic hyperglycinemia [4] are so named because the elevations of glycine are their most prominent chemical characteristic. It seems likely that both these categories are heterogeneous. A molecular product of a mutant gene has not yet been established within either category. In ketotic hyperglycinemia there is a defect in the oxidation of propionate [5]. There is also a defect in glycine oxidation in vivo [6]. These observations suggest the possibility of a primary defect in the synthesis of a common cofactor. Propionic acidemia, a different condition, recently described by Hommes and colleagues [7], is not characterized by high concentrations of glycine in the blood. Ketotic hyperglycinemia is considered in Chap. 22 under Disorders of Propionate Metabolism. Nonketotic hyperglycinemia probably represents a primary defect in glycine metabolism, and is, accordingly, considered separately in this chapter.

Recognition of the possibility of inborn errors of glycine metabolism began with the description of ketotic hyperglycinemia by Childs and colleagues [8] in 1961. The most prominent clinical characteristics of that disorder are recurrent episodes of ketoacidosis, precipitated by the intake of protein or by infection, eventuating in coma and death. The features which distinguish it clinically from nonketotic hyperglycinemia appear in Table 24-1.

Nonketotic hyperglycinemia was first described in detail by Gerritsen, Kaveggia, and Waisman [9]. Two sibs described in an abstract by Mabry and Karam [10] may have had the same disorder. Biochemical investigations of patients with nonketotic hyperglycinemia using ^{14}C-labeled glycine have indicated a defect in the oxidation of carbon-1 of glycine to CO_2 and in the conversion of carbon-2 of glycine to carbon-3 of serine [11]. It is now possible to characterize the hyperglycinemias according to whether they have this defect or not.

Table 24-1. CLINICAL MANIFESTATIONS OF HYPERGLYCINEMIA

Ketotic type	Nonketotic type
Mental retardation	Mental retardation
Neutropenia	Failure to thrive
Thrombocytopenia	Spastic paraplegia
Osteoporosis	Opisthotonos
Abnormal electroencephalogram; seizures	Seizures
Periodic ketosis with vomiting, dehydration, and coma	Hypooxaluria

GLYCINE METABOLISM

Glycine is the simplest of the amino acids. Its metabolism is complex. It is a nonessential amino acid that can be synthesized in a number of ways in man. It is present in high concentrations in collagen and gelatin and is abundant in most animal proteins. The daily intake for the average adult in the United States is 3 to 5 gm.

Glycine received a name reminiscent of sugar because of its sweet taste. It is a glycogenic amino acid. If one feeds a starved animal relatively large quantities of glycine, glycogen is laid down in the liver.

Synthetic Reactions Involving Glycine

Some synthetic roles are illustrated in Fig. 24-1. Probably the most important is the synthesis of proteins. In studies in which ^{15}N-labeled glycine was added to the diet of rats in nitrogen equilibrium, Schoenheimer [12] found that about 50 percent of the label remained in the body, most of it in protein. Approximately 10 percent was found in the body in nonprotein nitrogen, 40 percent was excreted directly in the urine, and 2 to 3 percent was found in the feces. Thus, about half the ingested glycine is involved in the synthesis of protein. In these experiments the label was widely dis-

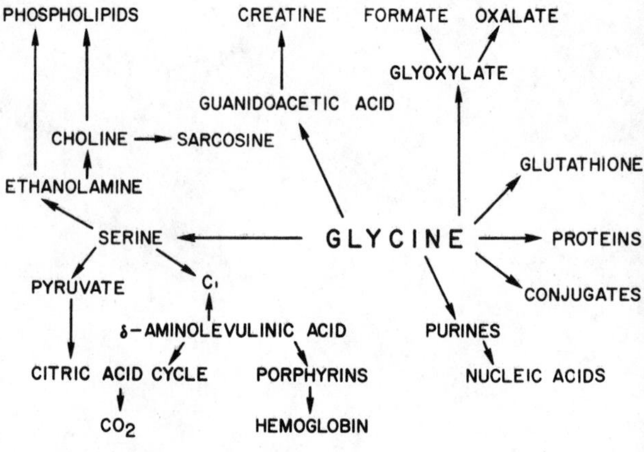

Figure 24-1. Metabolic pathways of glycine, concerned particularly with the synthesis of other molecules.

tributed among the proteins of the tissues of the body. Hydrolysis of liver proteins indicated that some of the label had been transferred to other amino acids such as glutamate and aspartate. Most of the label found in proteins following the administration of ^{14}C- or ^{15}N-labeled glycine is in glycine and serine. The extent of conversion to protein serine is about four times that of direct incorporation into protein glycine [13, 14]. These observations indicate the importance of the glycine-serine interconversion.

When labeled glycine is fed, there is a lag of 6 to 8 hr before glycogen is formed: the peak is at about 12 hr. This suggests that glycine must first be converted to other molecules, which are subsequently converted to glucose. Furthermore, there appears in glycogen twice as much of the α-carbon of glycine as of the carboxyl carbon. This suggests that there is first a conversion to serine. The nitrogen of glycine also appears in urinary urea. There is a lag of 6 to 8 hr before glycine appears in the urine as urea. This suggests further that glycine is to a considerable extent first involved in synthetic reactions which tie up the molecule.

Glycine plays an important role in the synthesis of purines. It is incorporated *in toto* into what become the 4, 5, and 7 positions of the purine ring, and it provides a source of 1-carbon units for *de novo* purine synthesis. Most of the purines of the body are made in this way. This pathway accounts for about a tenth of a percent of the glycine metabolized.

Glycine undergoes a series of reactions in which acyl derivatives are formed. The most prominent of these is hippuric acid. An amide bond is formed between benzoic acid and glycine which is like the peptide bonds in proteins. The acylation of glycine proceeds after formation of coenzyme A, a derivative of the carboxyl group of benzoic acid. A similar reaction serves in the detoxification of salicylates by formation of salicyluric acid, and bile acids are excreted into the intestine in the form of glycine conjugates. A large amount of isovalerylglycine has recently been found in the urine of a patient with isovaleric acidemia [2]. It appears that examination of the urine for isovalerylglycine is a much simpler and more reliable method for detection of that condition than is examination of the blood for isovaleric acid.

Glycine is also involved in the synthesis of heme, creatine, glutathione, ethanolamine, choline, and sarcosine.

Catabolism of Glycine

Many of the catabolic reactions may be in fact primarily synthetic in character. For example, the glycine-succinate reaction is primarily concerned with the synthesis of porphyrins, and probably plays no significant part in the degradation of glycine. Similarly, some reversible reactions may be more concerned with the synthesis of glycine itself than with its catabolism.

The Glycine-Serine Interconversion

The central features of this interconversion and certain related reactions are illustrated in Fig. 24-2. Definitive evidence for conversion of serine to glycine was first provided by Shemin [15], who fed rats serine labeled with ^{15}N and ^{13}C. He found that the ratio of ^{15}N to ^{13}C was the same in hippurate isolated from the urine as in the precursor. This was a strong indication that the conversion was direct. Similarly, in the studies of Winnick and colleagues [13], in which ^{14}C-labeled glycine was fed to rats, the protein of the liver was found to contain labeled serine, and the amount was about six times that of labeled glycine. Sakami [16] demonstrated the formation of serine from ^{13}C-labeled glycine and ^{14}C-labeled formate in the rat. Moreover, in man labeled serine appears in the blood promptly after the injection of ^{14}C-labeled glycine [11, 17]. All these observations indicate that glycine can be converted to serine, and that serine can be converted to glycine.

In studies in which glycine was labeled in the 2 position with carbon-14, the label was found in the 2 and 3 positions of serine [18]. The enzyme involved in this transformation is variously known as serine hydroxymethyl transferase, serine methylase, or serine aldolase [19, 20]. The proportions of carbon-2 of glycine converted to carbon-2 and carbon-3 of serine have generally been found to be about equal, but Arnstein and Neuberger [21] found this labeling pattern only when relatively large amounts of glycine were administered. In experiments in which labeled amino acids were fed for 20 to 40 days until a steady state pattern was developed, this labeling pattern was found when glycine constituted 2 percent of the diet, but with 0.5 percent glycine the specific activity of carbon-3 of serine was only 20 percent of that of carbon-2. Thus, experiments in which large loads of substrate are employed may demonstrate pathways which are operative only under those conditions. Arnstein and Neuberger found the turnover of serine to be 35 mmoles per kg in rats; that of glycine was 25 mmoles per kg. They interpreted these data as indicating that serine is generally the precursor of glycine and that glycine is converted to serine under conditions in which there is need for removal of large quantities of glycine. Actually this may be more than the data would imply, for under all conditions studied there was conversion of glycine to serine. One might interpret the glycine-to-serine conversion as an important physiologic pathway which is subject to stimulation by large amounts of glycine. It may be relevant to this argument that Newman and Magasanik [22] found that the enzyme system which converts glycine to single-carbon units is adaptive in *Escherichia coli;* it is induced by glycine and repressed by single-carbon units derived from other sources.

The system involved in the conversion of glycine to serine has been studied in avian liver by Richert and colleagues [23]. A close relationship was observed between the production of CO_2 and NH_3 and the synthesis of serine. Pyridoxal phosphate, NAD, and tetrahydrofolic acid were stimulatory.

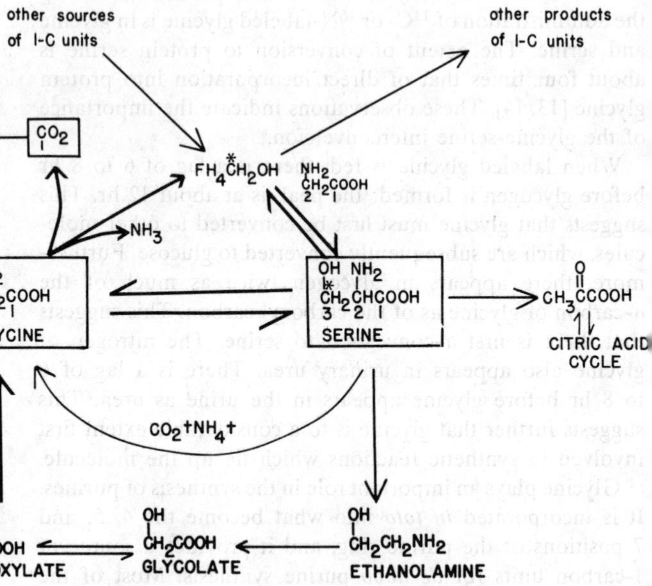

other sources of I-C units
other products of I-C units
Expired air
CO_2 1
$FH_4\overset{*}{C}H_2OH$
NH_2 CH_2COOH
NH_3
NH_2 $\overset{*}{C}H_2COOH$ 2 1 GLYCINE
OH NH_2 $\overset{*}{C}H_2CHCOOH$ 3 2 1 SERINE
$CH_3\overset{O}{C}COOH$
CITRIC ACID CYCLE
$CO_2 + NH_4^+$
$\overset{O}{C}HCOOH$ GLYOXYLATE
OH CH_2COOH GLYCOLATE
OH $CH_2CH_2NH_2$ ETHANOLAMINE

Figure 24-2. The interconversion of glycine and serine and related aspects of metabolism. The two arrows in the center connecting the glycine and serine boxes indicate that the two molecules are interconvertible and by a number of pathways, without specification as to type. The two carbons of glycine are numbered 1 and 2; in this way it is possible to see that carbon-1 and carbon-2 are incorporated directly into the corresponding 1 and 2 carbons of serine. Carbon-2 is also convertible to a tetrahydrofolate derivative, which then becomes carbon-3 of serine. The asterisk has been employed in order to follow this carbon through this reaction sequence. This reaction sequence is probably reversible. The CO_2-fixation reaction drawn with the curved arrow below, which produces two molecules of glycine from a molecule of serine, may take the same pathway, but it is drawn separately because the mechanism of that reaction has not yet been clarified. Abbreviations include: FH_4, tetrahydrofolic acid; 1-C unit, single-carbon unit. (*Reprinted with permission from Karger, Basel, New York,* 1968 [11].)

These observations are consistent with the pathway described by Sagers and Gunsalus [24] in *Peptococcus glycinophilus.* The following series of reactions has been proposed (FH_4 indicates tetrahydrofolic acid, and FH_4CH_2OH its hydroxymethyl derivative):

$$NH_2CH_2COOH + FH_4 + H_2O \longrightarrow FH_4CH_2OH + CO_2 + NH_3 \quad (1)$$

$$FH_4CH_2OH + NH_2CH_2COOH \longrightarrow HOCH_2CHNH_2COOH + FH_4 \quad (2)$$

The overall reaction for the synthesis of serine from glycine by this pathway is as follows:

$$2NH_2CH_2COOH + H_2O \longrightarrow HOCH_2CHNH_2COOH + CO_2 + NH_3 \quad (3)$$

As suggested in Fig. 24-2, there are many sources of the CH_2OH group of FH_4CH_2OH other than glycine. It derives from the so-called one-carbon pool. Reaction 1, therefore, is not required for the conversion of glycine to serine by way of Reaction 2. It is Reaction 2 that is catalyzed by serine hydroxymethyl transferase [20]. Reaction 1 requires NAD and pyridoxal phosphate as cofactors.

The mechanisms of this reaction and the enzymes involved have been extensively studied in *P. glycinophilus.* Four protein fractions, called P_1, P_2, P_3, and P_4 by Klein and Sagers, have been separated [25, 26]. The enzyme catalyzing the decarboxylation of glycine has been purified [26], and the reaction is reversible. We have designated the fractions E_1, E_2, E_3, and E_4 in Fig. 24-3. All four proteins are required to catalyze the overall conversion of glycine to CO_2, NH_3, and an FH_4 derivative. E_1 contains a bound pyridoxal phosphate. E_2 is a heat-stable protein. E_1 and E_2 are required for the formation of CO_2 from glycine. NAD and FH_4 are not required for this decarboxylation. E_3 is a flavoprotein which is reduced in the presence of E_2 and glycine and which transfers electrons to NAD [27]. E_4 functions in the presence of the rest of the system to transfer carbon-2 of glycine to FH_4. It is not known whether the system studied in avian liver [23] is the same as this bacterial system.

Recent investigations from Sendai, Japan, have clarified the glycine-serine interconversion in mammalian systems. It was first found [28] that rat liver mitochondria can synthesize glycine by a CO_2-fixation reaction in which serine and ammonia yield two molecules of glycine. The β-carbon of serine and bicarbonate carbon were incorporated in a 1:1 ratio into the α- and carboxyl carbons of glycine. The enzymes catalyzing this reaction were solubilized from an acetone powder

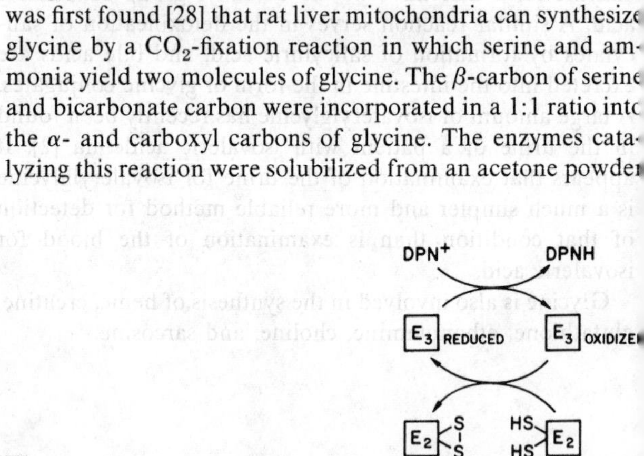

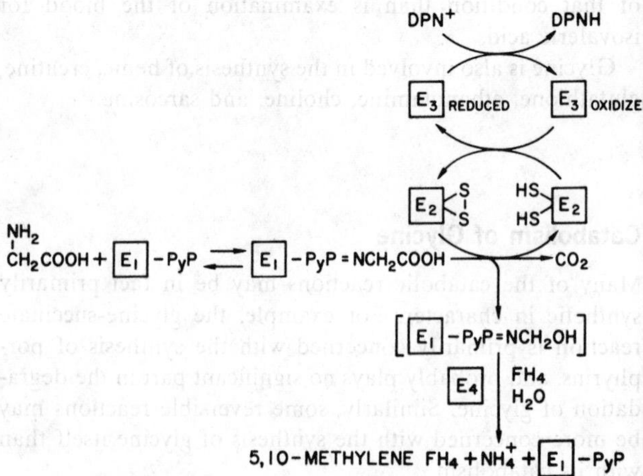

Figure 24-3. The glycine decarboxylase system.

of rat liver mitochondria [29]. Methylene-FH_4 was effective in replacing serine in the synthesis of glycine [30]. The enzyme preparation also catalyzed the decarboxylation of glycine; the glycine cleavage required FH_4. The extracts also catalyzed an exchange between the carboxyl carbon of glycine and CO_2. Pyridoxal phosphate is a component of the enzyme complex. More recently, the system has been fractionated and a hydrogen carrier protein isolated [33]. Two protein fractions were isolated from rat liver mitochondria which together catalyzed the cleavage of glycine and the exchange of carbon-1 of glycine and bicarbonate. The hydrogen carrier protein appeared to be analogous to E_2. It also catalyzed the reduction of dithionitrobenzoic acid (DTNB). These observations appeared to indicate the presence in rat liver of a system similar to that in *P. glycinophilus.*

Glycine Oxidase

The conversion of glycine to glyoxylate and NH_3 is catalyzed by an enzyme purified by Ratner et al. [34]. This enzyme, which is present in liver and kidney, is the same enzyme as D-amino acid oxidase [35]. It has a high K_m and is therefore thought not to play a major role in glycine degradation.

Transaminases

Glyoxylate may also be formed from glycine by transamination [36]. Pyruvate or α-ketoglutarate may be the amino group receptors. It is unlikely that these pathways serve significantly in the degradation of glycine. Thermodynamic considerations strongly favor the synthesis of glycine rather than its catabolism [37].

Amino Ketone Formation

Δ-Aminolevulinic acid is formed by the condensation of glycine and succinyl CoA. This is an essential step in the biosynthesis of porphyrins and heme [38].

$$\mathrm{HOOCCH_2CH_2CO{-}S{-}CoA + CH_2NH_2COOH} \rightarrow \mathrm{[HOOCCH_2CH_2COCHNH_2COOH]} \xrightarrow{-CO_2} \mathrm{HOOCCH_2CH_2COCH_2NH_2} \quad (4)$$

The α-carbon of glycine becomes the δ-carbon of δ-amino levulinic acid, and is a precursor of a C-1 unit which finds its way into methionine, purines, the β-carbon of serine, or, ultimately, CO_2. The rest of the compound yields α-ketoglutaraldehyde, which can be converted to α-ketoglutaric acid and succinate. Thus, this pathway could operate as a cycle providing the complete oxidation of glycine while regenerating succinate. Although this cycle has been proposed as a major route for the degradation of glycine, studies using ^{14}C-labeled glycine and δ-aminolevulinic acid disclosed that the rate of conversion of glycine to CO_2 was 25 times that of δ-aminolevulinic acid [39]. This finding is not consistent with the cycle as a major pathway.

A similar condensation of glycine and acetyl CoA would yield aminoacetone:

$$\mathrm{CH_3CO{-}S{-}CoA + CH_2NH_2COOH} \rightarrow \mathrm{[CH_3COCH_2NH_2COOH]} \xrightarrow{CO_2} \mathrm{CH_3COCH_2NH_2} \quad (5)$$

The intermediate, α-amino-β-ketobutyric acid, readily undergoes decarboxylation nonenzymatically. The aminoacetone synthesized can be converted by transamination or by action of monamine oxidase to methylglyoxal, which could then be converted through a glyoxalase reaction to lactate and then to pyruvate. Thus, the synthesis of this amino ketone could also lead to the complete metabolism of glycine, and this pathway could operate as a cycle.

Urata and Granick [40] found that aminoacetone was readily formed from acetyl CoA and glycine in guinea pig liver mitochondria. They calculated that conversion to aminoacetone could account for as much as one-fourth of the glycine metabolized each day [41]. If these calculations are valid, this would be a major pathway for the catabolism of glycine.

Aminoacetone may also be formed from threonine. It was identified by Elliott [42] as a metabolite of *Staphylococcus aureus* growing in the presence of threonine. An enzyme has been studied by Neuberger and Tait [43] in *Rhodopseudomonas spheroides* which converts threonine to aminoacetone [43]. Our own studies indicate that it is not a major route for the catabolism of glycine in man [44]. Following the administration of ^{14}C-labeled glycine there was no evidence of incorporation of label into aminoacetone. By contrast, there was significant conversion of the label of administered threonine to aminoacetone. Thus in man the source of urinary aminoacetone is threonine, not glycine.

The Synthesis of Glycine

Glycine is a nonessential amino acid which can be synthesized in a number of ways. These include transamination of glyoxylate and conversion from serine, as previously discussed. The CO_2-fixation reaction described by Kikuchi and colleagues [28–31] may be the major route for the formation of glycine. Glycine could also be synthesized from serine by way of ethanolamine:

$$\begin{array}{l}
\mathrm{HOCH_2CH(NH_2)COOH} \rightarrow \mathrm{HOCH_2CH_2NH_2} \rightarrow \mathrm{HOCH_2CH_2N^+(CH_3)_3} \quad (\rightarrow \text{lipids} \rightarrow \text{brain}) \\
\mathrm{HOCH_2CH_2NH_2} \rightarrow \mathrm{HOCH_2COOH} \rightarrow \mathrm{OHCCOOH} \rightarrow \mathrm{HOOCCH_2NH_2} \\
\mathrm{HOCH_2CH_2N^+(CH_3)_3} \rightarrow \mathrm{HOOCCH_2NH(CH_3)} \rightarrow \mathrm{HOOCCH_2NH_2}
\end{array} \quad (6)$$

Glycine may also derive from threonine. In this process threonine is degraded to glycine and acetaldehyde [45]. In the rat one-third to one-fifth of ingested threonine is converted to glycine [46].

The Turnover of Glycine

The rate of turnover of glycine has been measured in man and animals. Arnstein and Neuberger [21] calculated that in the rat about 2 gm glycine is synthesized per kilogram per day. In man, Watts and Crawhall [47] found a glycine turnover of 1 gm per kg per day. Similarly, in children, rates average about 1 gm per kg per day [17].

The plasma concentration of glycine as measured by column chromatography is approximately 1 mg per 100 ml [48]. In children 5 to 14 years of age a similar value has been found using a colorimetric method [8], while in children under 5 years of age the mean value was 0.65 mg per 100 ml. The average adult excretes approximately 100 mg glycine per 24 hr, with a range of 50 to 200 mg per 24 hr [49]. These values amount to 0.1 to 0.2 mg glycine per mg creatinine. Similar values have been found in children [8, 48]. The concentration of glycine in cerebrospinal fluid is approximately 0.1 gm per 100 ml [50].

CLINICAL FEATURES

All the patients described in the literature have had severe mental retardation. The patient reported by Gerritsen et al. [9] was listless, lacked spontaneous movements even in the neonatal period, failed to thrive physically, and failed to develop mentally. He did not sit up, roll over, or respond to his mother at 5 months of age. He was admitted at 9 months to the Central Wisconsin Colony and Training School, where he is still institutionalized. At 5 years of age he could only lie in a hyperextended position. He could hear, and he resisted manipulation. His cry was high-pitched and had a low volume. There was no adaptive or social behavior. Similarly, the patient described by Ziter and colleagues [51] was lethargic from the third day of life. By 33 months he was diffusely hypotonic, had severe developmental retardation, was unaware of his environment, had wandering, dysconjugate eye movements, and incessantly turned his head from side to side. At 36 months of age he was still unable to roll over or sit unassisted and was unresponsive to social stimulation.

A family has recently been reported by Stern [52] with three involved girls who appear to have the same metabolic defect but much less severe developmental retardation.

Convulsive seizures have been prominent in virtually all the reported patients with nonketotic hyperglycinemia [53]. Myoclonic seizures as well as grand mal convulsions have been observed. Most of the patients have had clinical evidence of spastic cerebral palsy. Opisthotonos is common and persistent. The patient described by Rampini and colleagues [53] was found to have a communicating internal hydrocephalus, as well as seizures and severe developmental retardation.

A patient with nonketotic hyperglycinemia has recently been reported [54] in whom the diagnosis was made in the first week of life. Treatment with a respirator was required. Except for myoclonic jerks, generalized seizures, and persistent hiccupping, there was no movement, nor was there spontaneous respiration. Exchange transfusion reversed most of these findings, but the patient promptly relapsed and his condition continued to degenerate (Fig. 24-4). At 7 months of age he was unaware of his surroundings, had only a few spontaneous movements, and showed no head control. Muscle tone was normal at rest but became hypertonic when he was disturbed. Tendon reflexes were exaggerated. The patient died shortly thereafter.

Patients with ketotic hyperglycinemia are often severely ill in the neonatal period, as are other patients with inborn metabolic disease, such as those with methylmalonic acidemia, isovaleric acidemia, propionic acidemia, and maple syrup urine disease. To this differential diagnosis of devastating illness in the first days or weeks of life one must now add nonketotic hyperglycinemia. Earlier we were of the

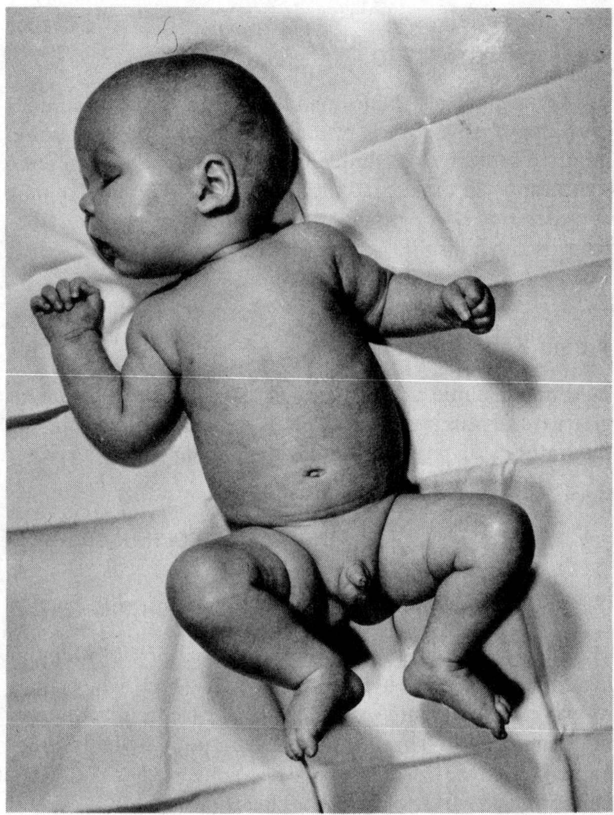

Figure 24-4. Patient R.H. at 5 months of age. The baby was essentially decerebrate and assumed a tonic neck-reflex posture. The patient has been reported by Baumgartner et al. [54]. The picture was kindly provided by Dr. Baumgartner.

Table 24-2. PROGNOSIS IN HYPERGLYCINEMIA

Case no.	Sex	Age at first symptoms	Age at death	Ref.
		Ketotic Hyperglycinemia		
1	M	18 hr	7 yr	[8]
2	M	4 mo	16 mo	[55]
3	F	3 days	4 days	[56]
4	?	12 days	2 mo	[57]
5	M	36 hr	4 days	[58]
6	F	5 days	4 mo	[53]
7	M	9 days	9 mo	[59]
8	F	1–4 wk	6 wk	[60]
9	F	6 days	3 wk	[60]
10	F	3 days	5+ yr	[60]
11	F	?	5+ yr	[61]
		Nonketotic Hyperglycinemia		
1	M	Early postnatal	9+ yr	[9]
2	?	4 mo	3+ yr	[10]
3	?	2 mo	8+ yr	[10]
4	F	2½ days	9+ days	[62]
5	?	24 hr	11 days	[63]
6	F	5 days	2+ yr	[64]
7	M	8 days	13+ mo	[53]
8	M	3 days	3+ yr	[51]
9	M	3 days	1 yr	[54]

NOTE: The + designation indicates that the patient was living at the time of the most recent report.

opinion that patients with hyperglycinemia who die early in life probably have ketotic hyperglycinemia [4]. This view is no longer tenable. A classification of reported patients with hyperglycinemia and an assessment of the prognoses appears in Table 24-2.

Neutropenia has been a characteristic finding in ketotic hyperglycinemia and is possibly related to the concentration of glycine itself [8, 48]. It has not generally occurred in nonketotic hyperglycinemia, but was observed in the patient reported by Baumgartner et al. [54]. In that patient the percentage of neutrophils in smears of peripheral blood seldom exceeded 20; the total neutrophil count was often under 2,000 per mm^3, and sometimes well under 1,000. The absence of neutropenia in other patients with nonketotic hyperglycinemia may reflect the fact that glycine in body fluids tends to be less in this condition than in ketotic hyperglycinemia.

BIOCHEMICAL CHARACTERISTICS

Plasma Concentrations

The concentration of glycine in the blood is elevated. In Gerritsen's patient the plasma concentration averaged 8.1 mg per 100 ml, with a range of 6.9 to 9.3 mg per 100 ml

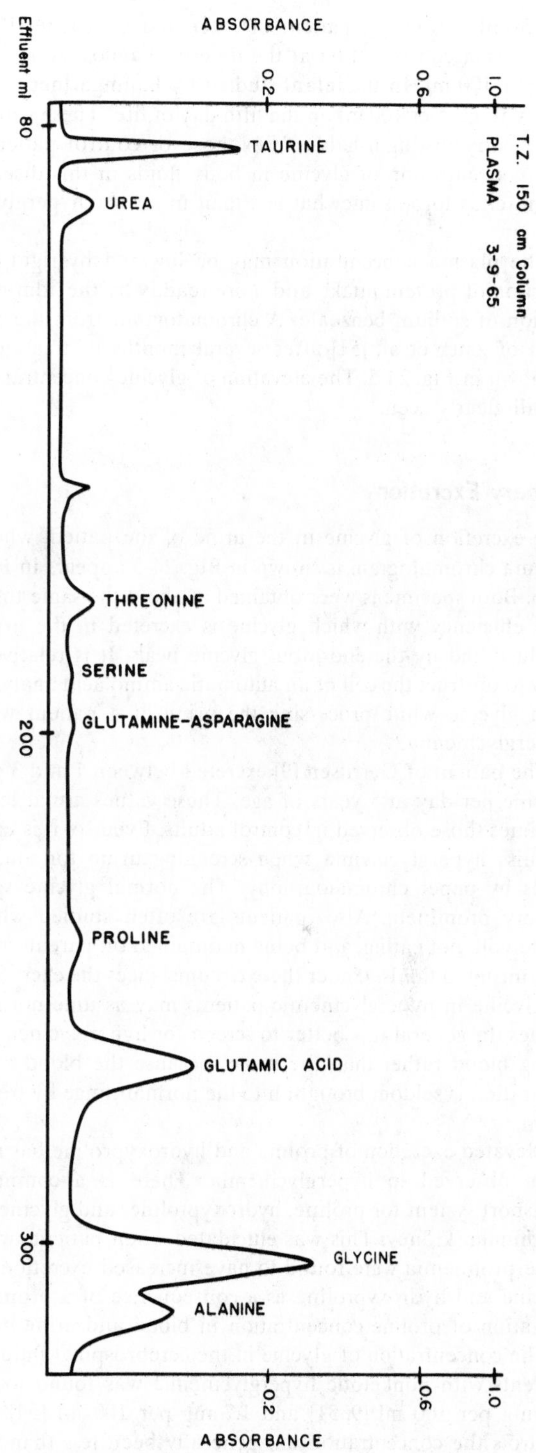

Figure 24-5. Chromatogram of the plasma of patient T.Z. Even though the plasma concentrations had been reduced by treatment with sodium benzoate for months, the elevation of glycine content is readily seen. The concentration was 5.3 mg per 100 ml plasma. At a sample volume which permitted a glycine peak of reasonable size and reasonable separation from alanine, amino acids such as threonine or serine, which are usually as large as the glycine peak or larger, are barely detectable.

[9]. Similarly, in the patient of Ziter and colleagues [51], the plasma concentration at the time of diagnosis was 11.3 mg per 100 ml. In the infant studied by Baumgartner et al. it was 12 mg per 100 ml on the fifth day of life. These values are clearly distinguishable from those of control patients. The concentration of glycine in body fluids in this disease often tends to be somewhat less than in ketotic hyperglycinemia.

The plasma concentration may be lowered by rigid restriction of protein intake and more readily by the administration of sodium benzoate. A chromatogram from the patient of Ziter et al. [51] after several months of treatment is shown in Fig. 24-5. The elevation of glycine concentration is still clearly seen.

Urinary Excretion

The excretion of glycine in the urine of the patient whose plasma chromatogram is shown in Fig. 24-5 appears in Fig. 24-6. Both specimens were obtained at about the same time. The efficiency with which glycine is excreted in the urine is illustrated by the enormous glycine peak. It is relatively easy to obstruct the coil of an automatic amino acid analyzer with glycine while processing the urine of a patient with hyperglycinemia.

The patient of Gerritsen [9] excreted between 1 and 3 gm glycine per day at 5 years of age. These values are at least 10 times those observed in control adults. Even so, it is easy to miss hyperglycinemia when screening urine for amino acids by paper chromatography. The normal glycine spot is very prominent. Also, patients are often studied when acutely ill, not eating, and being maintained on parenterally administered fluids. Under these circumstances the excretion of glycine in hyperglycinemic patients may assume normal values. In general it is better to screen for hyperglycinemias using blood rather than the urine, because the blood concentration is seldom brought into the normal range by treatment.

Elevated excretion of proline and hydroxyproline has not been observed in hyperglycinemia. There is a common transport system for proline, hydroxyproline, and glycine in the human kidney. This was elucidated when patients with hyperprolinemia were found to have increased excretion of glycine and hydroxyproline as a consequence of a primary elevation of proline concentration in blood and urine [65].

The concentration of glycine in the cerebrospinal fluid of patients with nonketotic hyperglycinemia was found to be 1.0 mg per 100 ml [9, 51] and 1.7 mg per 100 ml [54]. In controls the concentration has generally been less than 0.1 mg per 100 ml.

Oxalate Excretion

Hypooxaluria was initially described as a feature of this syndrome [9]. It is now clear that a diminished excretion

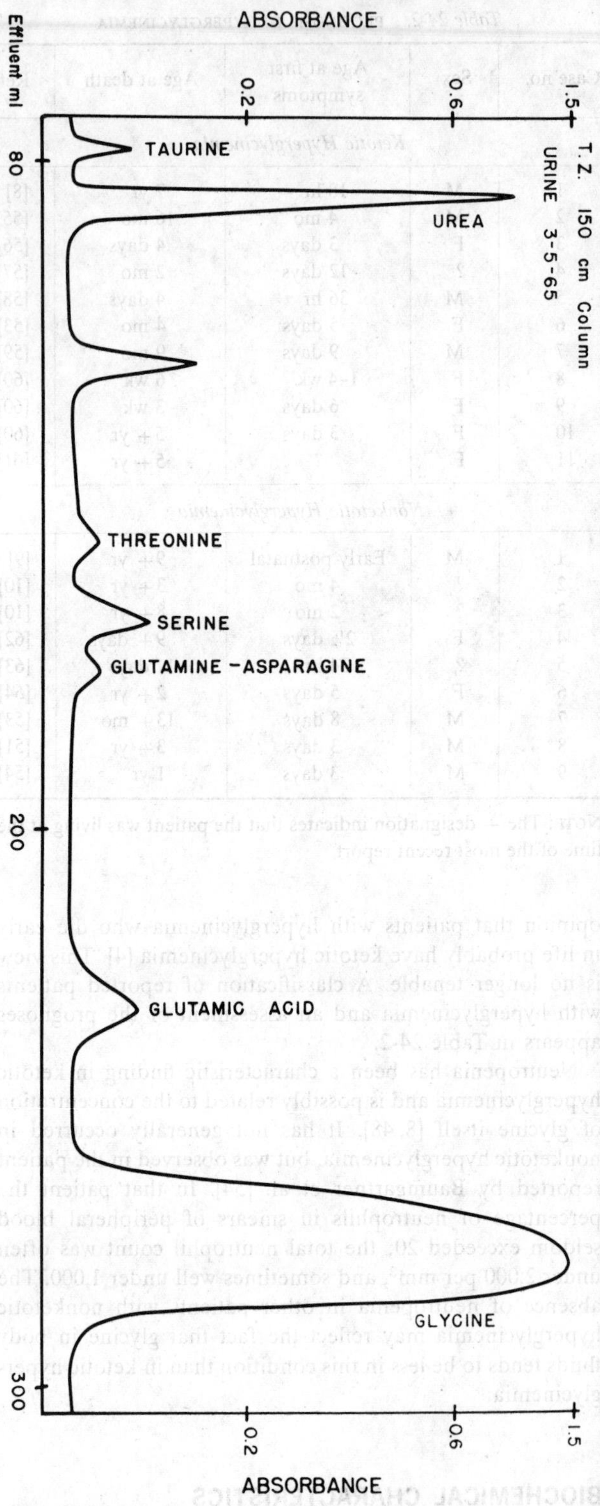

Figure 24-6. Chromatogram of the urine of a patient, T.Z., obtained on the Beckman Spinco Automatic Amino Acid Analyzer. He excreted 172 mg glycine on that day, as contrasted, for instance, with 3 mg threonine. The glycine excretion amounted to 2.39 mg per mg creatinine.

of oxalate is not characteristic of the disorder. Oxalate excretion was not decreased in the patients described by Rampini et al. [53] and by Baumgartner et al. [54]. Furthermore, the original patient has now been restudied, and the excretion of oxalate is well within the normal range [66]. Glyoxylate excretion was normal in this study [66]. These observations constitute evidence against the hypothesis of a defect in glycine oxidase, which at one time was postulated as the defect in this disorder.

Glycine Utilization

Delayed disappearance of glycine from plasma has been observed in the course of loading tests [19, 54]. During loading there was no appreciable increase in the plasma concentration of serine. On the other hand, there is abundant evidence of ready conversion of serine to glycine [9, 54]. A serine tolerance test is shown in Fig. 24-7. The prompt rise and fall in the concentration of serine indicated normal metabolism of serine. In contrast, the glycine concentration rose steadily over a 4-hr period of study. These data confirm a defect in the utilization of glycine.

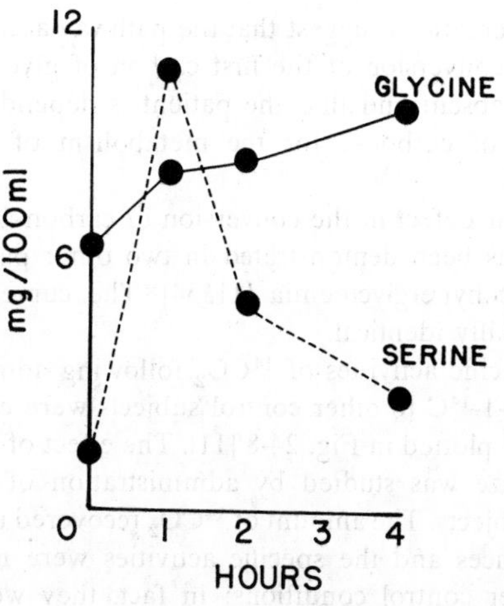

Figure 24-7. Serine loading test. The patient was 4 months old and was given a dose of 200 mg per kg. (*Reprinted with permission from the Journal of Pediatrics* [54].)

Studies of Glycine Metabolism

The metabolism of glycine has been assessed in three patients with nonketotic hyperglycinemia [11, 54]. The experiment was designed for evaluating separately the fates of carbon-1 and carbon-2 of glycine by separate experiments in which glycine-1-^{14}C or glycine-2-^{14}C was injected intravenously. Collection of expired air permitted measurement of the kinetics of conversion of glycine to CO_2. Blood was also drawn at intervals, and the glycine was isolated. In this way the specific activity of the glycine pool was known. The serine of the plasma was also isolated, and after the specific activity was measured the molecule was degraded and the β-carbon trapped. Control subjects were studied in the control state and during constant infusion of glycine at a rate which increased the pool to a level comparable to that of patients.

The formation of $^{14}CO_2$ from glycine is shown in Fig. 24-8. In the control subject (J.E.), the formation of CO_2 from glycine-1-^{14}C was rapid. There was a linear decline of specific activity from a maximum at the earliest time point, 5 min. By contrast, the conversion of CO_2 from glycine-2-^{14}C was much slower, showing a flat curve, as one might expect if conversion to serine and pyruvate and oxidation through the citric acid cycle is required for the release of this carbon as CO_2. In the patient the formation of $^{14}CO_2$ from glycine-1-^{14}C and glycine-2-^{14}C had a similar time course.

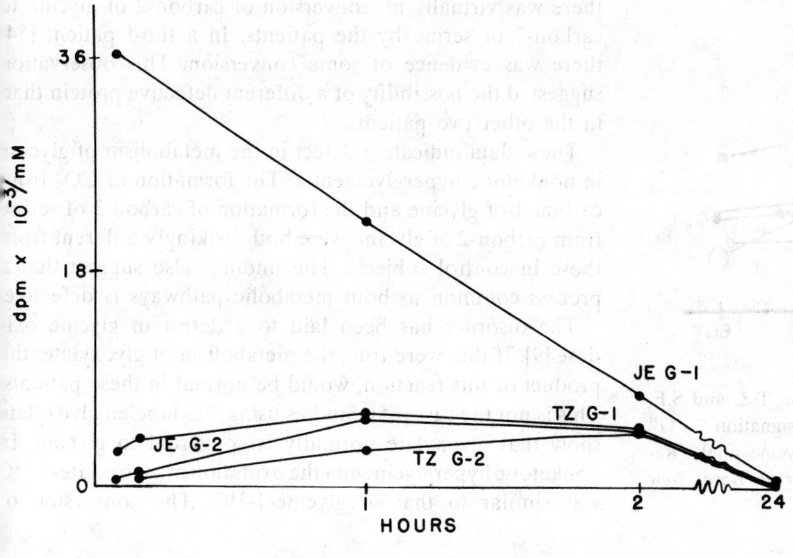

Figure 24-8. The conversion of glycine to CO_2. The data plotted are the specific activities of respiratory CO_2 collected following the intravenous injection of glycine. The curves are labeled with the initials of the subject T.Z. and of a control J.E., with G-1 for glycine-1-^{14}C and G-2 for glycine-2-^{14}C. (*Reprinted with permission from Nyhan et al.* [4].)

These observations suggest that the pathway accounting for the rapid conversion of the first carbon of glycine to CO_2 might be absent and that the patient is dependent on the oxidation of carbon-2 for the metabolism of the whole molecule.

A similar defect in the conversion of carbon-1 of glycine to CO_2 has been demonstrated in two other patients with nonketotic hyperglycinemia [11, 54]. The curves obtained were virtually identical.

The specific activities of $^{14}CO_2$ following administration of glycine-1-^{14}C to other control subjects were even higher than those plotted in Fig. 24-8 [11]. The effect of differences in pool size was studied by administration of glycine to control subjects. The amount of $^{14}CO_2$ recovered under these circumstances and the specific activities were not smaller than under control conditions; in fact, they were higher. Obviously, there was greater dilution of the label in a larger pool, but this was more than balanced by an increase in metabolism of glycine in the presence of large amounts of glycine. These findings are similar to those of Arnstein and Neuberger [21], who found increased conversion of glycine to serine in the rat when larger amounts of glycine were fed. Appreciable quantities of respiratory $^{14}CO_2$ were no longer detected 24 hr after the administration of labeled glycine.

The kinetics of the overall labeling of serine following administration of glycine was similar whether the glycine administered was glycine-1-^{14}C or glycine-2-^{14}C, as shown in Fig. 24-9. The specific activities of serine in the patients were considerably lower than those of control subjects for at least 30 min, and the curves of the patients were so flat that it appeared again that a different process was under study in patient and control.

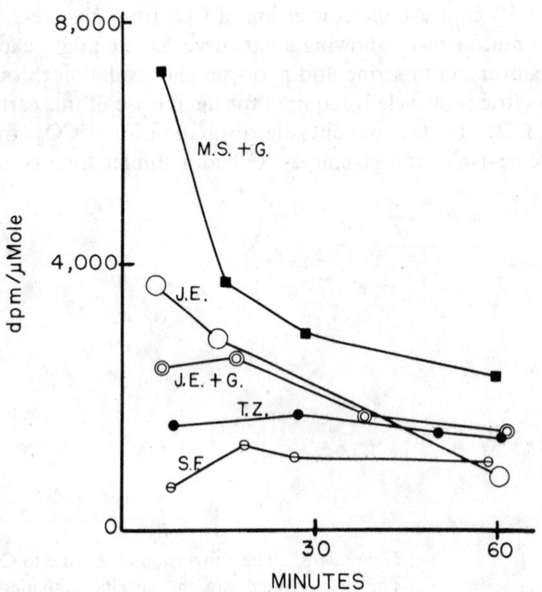

Figure 24-9. Conversion of glycine-2-^{14}C to serine. T.Z. and S.F. were patients; J.E. and M.S. were controls. The designation "+G" indicates the creation of an artificially elevated glycine pool. (*Reprinted with permission from Pediatric Research, Karger, Basel, New York,* 1968 [11].)

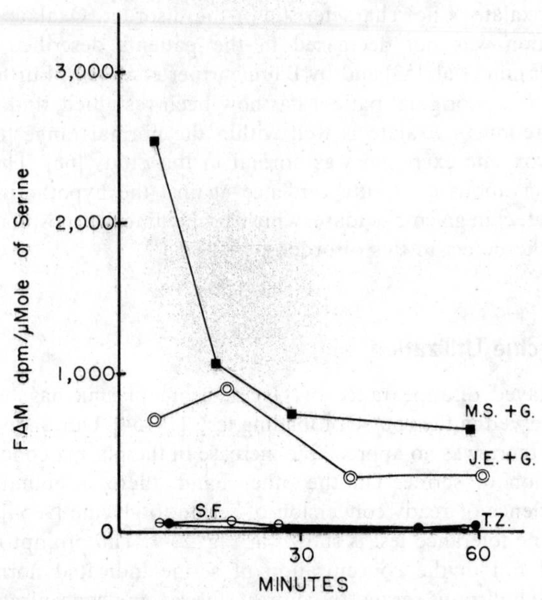

Figure 24-10. Conversion of glycine-2-^{14}C to carbon-3 of serine. Subjects as identified in Fig. 24-9. (*Reprinted with permission from Pediatric Research, Karger, Basel, New York,* 1968 [11].)

The process was elucidated through degradation of the serine isolated with periodate. This permitted the selective trapping of carbon-3 as the dimedon derivative. The specific activities of this β-carbon are shown in Fig. 24-10. In this experiment patients and control subjects had similar concentrations of glycine in the plasma. The conversion by the control subjects much exceeded that of the patients. In fact there was virtually no conversion of carbon-2 of glycine to carbon-3 of serine by the patients. In a third patient [54] there was evidence of some conversion. This observation suggested the possibility of a different defective protein than in the other two patients.

These data indicate a defect in the metabolism of glycine in nonketotic hyperglycinemia. The formation of CO_2 from carbon-1 of glycine and the formation of carbon-3 of serine from carbon-2 of glycine were both strikingly different from those in control subjects. The findings also suggest that a process common to both metabolic pathways is defective.

The disorder has been laid to a defect in glycine oxidase [9]. If that were true, the metabolism of glyoxylate, the product of this reaction, would be normal in these patients. This is not the case [65]. Studies using ^{14}C-labeled glyoxylate show that glyoxylate normally is converted to glycine. In nonketotic hyperglycinemia the oxidation of glyoxylate-1-^{14}C was similar to that of glycine-1-^{14}C. The conversion o glyoxylate-2-^{14}C to carbon-3 of serine was similar to that of glycine-2-^{14}C. These observations indicate no impairment in the interconversion of glycine and glyoxalate in this disease and accordingly rule out a defect in glycine oxidase and a defect in glycine-α-ketoglutarate transaminase as well.

We have postulated that the glycine decarboxylating system studied by Richert [23] in avian liver and by Sagers, Klein, and Gunsalus [24–26] in bacteria is present in man and that it is defective in nonketotic hyperglycinemia. The recent demonstration of the existence of this system in rat liver mitochondria by Sato, Kikuchi, and colleagues [29–33] has provided support for this hypothesis. This is that there is a block in the decarboxylation of glycine to give CO_2 and a methylene or hydroxymethyltetrahydrofolate derivative:

$$NH_2CH_2COOH + FH_4 + H_2O \longrightarrow FH_4CH_2OH + CO_2 + NH_3 \quad (7)$$

Glycine could still be converted to serine in the presence of FH_4CH_2OH, which can be provided from many sources other than glycine:

$$FH_4CH_2OH + H_2NCH_2COOH \longrightarrow HOCH_2CHNH_2COOH + FH_4 \quad (8)$$

There would not be a way to convert carbon-2 of glycine to carbon-3 of serine. Thus a defect in one enzyme accounts for the decrease in formation of CO_2 from carbon-1 as well as for the block in conversion of C-2 to C-3 of serine.

These conclusions have been supported recently by DeGroot and colleagues in the Netherlands [67]. These investigators studied the metabolism of glycine in vitro in liver homogenates obtained from three patients with nonketotic hyperglycinemia. The rates of conversion of glycine-2-^{14}C to serine were about equal to those of glycine-1-^{14}C. In contrast, in rat liver homogenate the rate of incorporation of glycine-2-^{14}C to serine was 1.6 times that of glycine-1-^{14}C. These data indicate that in the normal rat carbon-2 of glycine is converted to carbon-2 and -3 of serine, while in the patients carbon-2 of glycine is converted only to carbon-2 of serine.

Tada and colleagues [68] have recently studied a girl with nonketotic hyperglycinemia. They found that the conversion of glycine-1-^{14}C in vivo and in liver in vitro was extremely low as compared to that in controls. The rates of conversion of glycine-1-^{14}C and glycine-2-^{14}C to serine were also low. Furthermore, in control subjects the conversion of glycine-2-^{14}C to serine was almost twice that of glycine-1-^{14}C, whereas in the patient this ratio was close to unity. The activity of serine hydroxymethylase was normal. These findings are consistent with a defect in the conversion of glycine to CO_2, NH_3, and a one-carbon tetrahydrofolate compound.

GENETICS

The genetic transmission of this condition is not yet clear. Most of the case reports have been isolated. The experience is consistent with a rare autosomal recessive character. The family reported by DeGroot [67], in which two sisters had the disease, was consanguineous.

TREATMENT

Effective treatment has not been found. Exchange transfusion may be lifesaving in the neonatal period [54], but the improvement is only temporary. The plasma concentrations of glycine may be lowered by dietary restriction or by the administration of sodium benzoate [51, 54], but these measures have not appreciably altered the course of the disease. A temporary decrease in glycine concentration in serum was observed following the infusion of N^5-formyltetrahydrofolate (leucovorin) [67]. Treatment with methionine in order to provide one-carbon groups was reported by DeGroot et al. [67]. The glycine concentration of plasma was reduced to normal levels. It is not yet known whether the course of the disease can be altered in this way.

SUMMARY

1 Nonketotic hyperglycinemia is an inborn error of amino acid metabolism in which large amounts of glycine accumulate in the blood, urine, and cerebrospinal fluid.

2 The patients are mentally retarded and have seizure disorders. The disease may be life-threatening early in the postnatal period.

3 Glycine utilization is impaired, but serine is readily converted to glycine.

4 The most probable site of the metabolic block is in a glycine decarboxylase reaction, which converts glycine to CO_2, NH_3, and a single-carbon tetrahydrofolate derivative.

BIBLIOGRAPHY

1. Morrow, G., III, Barness, L. A., Auerbach, V. H., DiGeorge, A. M., Ando, T., and Nyhan, W. L.: Observations on the coexistence of methylmalonic acidemia and glycinemia. J. Pediat., **74**, 680, 1969.
2. Ando, T., Klingberg, W. G., and Nyhan, W. L.: Unpublished observations.
3. Freeman, J. M., Nicholson, J. F., Masland, W. S., Rowland, L. P., and Carter, S.: Ammonia intoxication due to a congenital defect in urea synthesis. Proc. Amer. Pediat. Soc., **74**, 36, 1964.
4. Nyhan, W. L., Ando, T., and Gerritsen, T.: Hyperglycinemia, in *Amino Acid Metabolism and Genetic Variation,* edited by W. L. Nyhan, p. 225. McGraw-Hill, New York, 1967.
5. Hsia, Y. E., Scully, K. J., and Rosenberg, L. E.: Defective propionate carboxylation in ketotic hyperglycinemia. Lancet, **1**, 787, 1969.

6. Ando, T., and Nyhan, W. L.: Unpublished observations.
7. Hommes, F. A., Kuipers, J. R. G., Elera, J. D., Jansen, J. F., and Jonxis, J. J. P.: Propionic acidemia, a new inborn error of metabolism. Pediat. Res., **2**, 519, 1968.
8. Childs, B., Nyhan, W. L., Borden, M., Bard, L., and Cooke, R. E.: Idiopathic hyperglycinemia and hyperglycinuria, a new disorder of amino acid metabolism. Pediatrics, **27**, 522, 1961.
9. Gerritsen, T., Kaveggia, E., and Waisman, H. A.: A new type of idiopathic hyperglycinemia with hypoxaluria. Pediatrics, **36**, 882, 1965.
10. Mabry, C. C., and Karam, A.: Idiopathic hyperglycinemia and hyperglycinuria, Southern Med. J., **56**, 1444, 1963.
11. Ando, T., Nyhan, W. L., Gerritsen, T., Gong, L., Heiner, D. C., and Bray, P. F.: Metabolism of glycine in the nonketotic form of hyperglycinemia. Pediat. Res., **2**, 254, 1968.
12. Ratner, S., Rittenberg, D., Keston, A. S., and Schoenheimer, R.: Studies in protein metabolism. XIV. The chemical interaction of dietary glycine and body proteins in rats. J. Biol. Chem., **134**, 665, 1940.
13. Winnick, T., Moring-Claesson, I., and Greenberg, D. M.: Distribution of radioactive carbon among certain amino acids of liver homogenate protein, following uptake experiments with labeled glycine. J. Biol. Chem., **175**, 127, 1948.
14. Bakay, B., and Nyhan, W. L.: Effects of thalidomide and chlorcyclizine on the biosynthesis of nucleic acids and proteins in fetal and maternal tissues of rats. J. Pharmacol. Exp. Ther. (in press).
15. Shemin, D.: The biological conversion of l-serine to glycine. J. Biol. Chem., **162**, 297, 1946.
16. Sakami, W.: The conversion of formate and glycine to serine and glycogen in the intact rat. J. Biol. Chem., **176**, 995, 1948.
17. Nyhan, W. L., and Childs, B.: Hyperglycinemia. V. The miscible pool and turnover rate of glycine and the formation of serine. J. Clin. Invest., **43**, 2404, 1964.
18. Sakami, W.: The conversion of glycine into serine in the intact rat. J. Biol. Chem., **178**, 519, 1949.
19. Kisliuk, R. L., and Sakami, W.: A study of the mechanism of serine biosynthesis. J. Biol. Chem., **214**, 47, 1955.
20. Schirch, L., and Ropp, M.: Serine transhydroxymethylase: affinity of tetrahydrofolate compounds for the enzyme and enzyme-glycine complex. Biochemistry, **6**, 253, 1967.
21. Arnstein, H. R. V., and Neuberger, A.: The synthesis of glycine and serine by the rat. Biochem. J., **55**, 271, 1953.
22. Newman, E. B., and Magasanik, B.: The relation of serine-glycine metabolism to the formation of single-carbon units. Biochim. Biophys. Acta, **78**, 437, 1963.
23. Richert, D. A., Amberg, R., and Wilson, M.: Metabolism of glycine by avian liver. J. Biol. Chem., **237**, 99, 1962.
24. Sagers, R. D., and Gunsalus, I. C.: Intermediary metabolism of *Diplococcus glycinophilus.* I. Glycine cleavage and one-carbon interconversions. J. Bact., **81**, 541, 1961.
25. Klein, S. M., and Sagers, R. D.: Flavin-linked glycine dehydrogenase from *Peptococcus glycinophilus,* Bact. Proc.: 103, 1966.
26. Klein, S. M., and Sagers, R. D.: Glycine metabolism. I. Properties of the system catalyzing the exchange of bicarbonate with the carboxyl group of glycine in *Peptococcus glycinophilus.* J. Biol. Chem., **241**, 197, 1966.
27. Baginski, M. L., and Huennekens, F. M.: Electron transport function of the heat-stable protein and a flavoprotein in the oxidative decarboxylation of glycine by *Peptococcus glycinophilus.* Biochem. Biophys. Res. Commun., **23**, 600, 1966.
28. Kawasaki, H., Sato, T., and Kikuchi, G.: A new reaction for glycine biosynthesis. Biochem. Biophys. Res. Commun., **23**, 227, 1966.
29. Sato, T., Kochi, H., Motokawa, Y., Kawasaki, H., and Kikuchi, G.: Glycine metabolism by rat liver mitochondria. I. Synthesis of two molecules of glycine from one molecule each of serine bicarbonate, and ammonia. J. Biochem., **65**, 63, 1969.
30. Sato, T., Motokawa, Y., Kochi, H., and Kikuchi, G.: Glycine synthesis by extracts of acetone powder of rat-liver mitochondria, Biochem. Biophys. Res. Commun., **28**, 495, 1967.
31. Motokawa, Y., and Kikuchi, G.: Glycine metabolism by rat liver mitochondria. II. Methylene tetrahydrofolate as the direct one carbon donor in the reaction of glycine synthesis. J. Biochem., **65**, 71, 1969.
32. Sato, T., Kochi, H., Sato, N., and Kikuchi, G.: Glycine metabolism by rat liver mitochondria. III. The glycine cleavage and the exchange of carboxyl carbon of glycine with bicarbonate. J. Biochem., **65**, 77, 1969.
33. Motokawa, Y., and Kikuchi, G.: Glycine metabolism by rat liver mitochondria. IV. Isolation and characterization of hydrogen carrier protein, an essential factor for glycine metabolism. Arch. Biochem. Biophys., **135**, 402, 1969.
34. Ratner, S., Nocita, V., and Green, D. E.: Glycine oxidase. J. Biol. Chem., **152**, 119, 1944.
35. Neims, A. H., and Hellerman, L.: Specificity of the D-amino acid oxidase in relation to glycine oxidase activity. J. Biol. Chem., **237**, PC976, 1962.
36. Nakada, H. I.: Glutamic-glycine transaminase from rat liver. J. Biol. Chem., **239**, 468, 1964.
37. Metzler, D. E., Olivard, J., and Snell, E. E.: Transamination of pyridoxamine and amino acids with glyoxylic acid. J. Amer. Chem. Soc., **76**, 644, 1954.
38. Shemin, D., and Russell, C. S.: Aminolevulinic acid. Its role in the biosynthesis of porphyrins and purines, J. Amer. Chem. Soc., **75**, 4873, 1953.
39. Nemeth, A. M., Russell, C. S., and Shemin, D.: The succinate-glycine cycle. II. Metabolism of δ-aminolevulinic acid. J. Biol. Chem., **229**, 415, 1957.
40. Urata, G., and Granick, S.: Biosynthesis of α-aminoketones and the metabolism of aminoacetone. J. Biol. Chem., **238**, 811, 1963.
41. Neuberger, A.: Aspects of the metabolism of glycine and of porphyrines, Biochem. J., **78**, 1, 1961.
42. Elliott, W. H.: Amino-acetone: its isolation and role in metabolism. Nature (London), **183**, 1051, 1959.
43. Neuberger, A., and Tait, G. H.: The enzymic conversion of threonine to aminoacetone. Biochim. Biophys. Acta, **41**, 164, 1960.
44. Ando, T., and Nyhan, W. L.: The excretion and formation of aminoacetone and δ-aminolevulinic acid in man. Tohoku J. Exp. Med., **99**, 189, 1969.
45. Karasek, M. A., and Greenberg, D. M.: Studies of the properties of threonine aldolases. J. Biol. Chem., **227**, 191, 1957.
46. Meltzer, H. L., and Sprinson, D. B.: The synthesis of 4-C^{14}, N^{15}-L-threonine and a study of its metabolism. J. Biol. Chem., **197**, 461, 1952.
47. Watts, R. W. E., and Crawhall, J. C.: The first glycine metabolic pool in man. Biochem. J., **73**, 277, 1959.
48. Nyhan, W. L., Borden, M., and Childs, B.: Idiopathic hyperglycinemia, a new disorder of amino acid metabolism. II. The concentrations of other amino acids in the plasma and their modification by the administration of leucine. Pediatrics, **27**, 539, 1961.
49. Stein, W. H.: A chromatographic investigation of the amino acid constituents of normal urine. J. Biol. Chem., **201**, 45, 1953.
50. Christensen, H. N., Cooper, P. F., Johnson, R. D., and Lynch, E. L.: Glycine and alanine concentrations of body fluids: experimental modification. J. Biol. Chem., **168**, 191, 1947.
51. Ziter, F. A., Bray, P. F., Madsen, J. A., and Nyhan, W. L.: The clinical findings in a patient with nonketotic hyperglycinemia. Pediat. Res., **2**, 250, 1968.
52. Stern, J., Nyhan, W. L., and Ando, T.: Unpublished observations.
53. Rampini, S., Vischer, D., Curtius, H. C., Anders, P. W., Tancredi, F., Frischknecht, W., and Prader, A.: Hereditäre Hyperglycinämie. Klinisches Bild und Bestimmung von Glyoxylsäure und Oxalsäure im Urin bei je einem Patienten mit der acidotischen und der nichtacidotischen Form. Helv. Paediat. Acta, **22**, 135, 1967.
54. Baumgartner, R., Ando, T., and Nyhan, W. L.: Nonketotic hyperglycinemia. J. Pediat., **75**, 1022, 1969.
55. Nyhan, W. L., Chisolm, J. J., Jr., and Edwards, R. L., Jr.: Idiopathic hyperglycinuria. III. Report of a second case, J. Pediat., **62**, 540, 1963.
56. Tada, K., Yoshida, T., Morikawa, T., Minakawa, A., and Wada, Y.: Idiopathic hyperglycinemia (the first case in Japan). Tohoku J. Exp. Med., **80**, 218, 1963.
57. Cochrane, W., Scriver, C. R., and Krause, V.: Hyperglycinemia-hyperglycinuria in a newborn infant. Proc. Soc. Pediat. Res., **33**, 102, 1963.

58. Visser, H. K. A., Veenstra, H. W., and Pik, C.: Hyperglycinemia and hyperglycinuria in a newborn infant. Arch. Dis. Child., **39**, 397, 1964.
59. Baerlocher, K., Baumgartner, R., and Hottinger, A.: Unpublished observations.
60. Nyhan, W. L.: Unpublished observations.
61. Donnell, G. N.: Unpublished observations.
62. Schreier, K., and Mueller, W.: Idiopathic hyperglycinämie (Glycinose), Deutsch. Med. Wschr., **89**, 1739, 1964.
63. Balfe, J. W., Levison, H., Hanley, W. B., Jackson, S. H., and Sass-Kortsak, A.: Hyperglycinemia and glycinuria in a newborn. Canad. Med. Ass. J., **92**, 347, 1965.
64. Corbeel, L.: Congenital hyperglycinemia and hyperglycinuria. Annual Meeting of the European Club for Pediatric Research, Athens, June, 1966.
65. Scriver, C. R.: Amino acid transport in the mammalian kidney, in *Amino Acid Metabolism and Genetic Variation,* edited by W. L. Nyhan, p. 327. McGraw-Hill, New York, 1967.
66. Gerritsen, T., Nyhan, W. L., Rehberg, M. L., and Ando, T.: Metabolism of glyoxylate in nonketotic hyperglycinemia, Pediat. Res., **3**, 269, 1969.
67. DeGroot, C. J., Troelstra, J. A., and Hommes, F. A.: The enzymatic defect of the nonketotic form of hyperglycinemia. Pediat. Res. (in press).
68. Tada, K., Narisawa, K., Yoshida, T., Konno, T., Yokoyama, Y., Nakagawa, H., Tanno, K., Mochizuki, K., and Arakawa, T.: Hyperglycinemia: a defect in glycine cleavage reaction. Tohoku J. Exp. Med., **98**, 289, 1969.

CHAPTER TWENTY-FIVE

DISORDERS OF β-ALANINE AND CARNOSINE METABOLISM*

Charles R. Scriver and Thomas L. Perry

Hyper-β-alaninemia has been reported in only one patient [1]. In that patient it appeared to be a metabolic disorder characterized by an elevation of the concentration of free β-alanine in plasma, cerebrospinal fluid, and urine, and a normal concentration in these fluids of peptide-bound β-alanine in the form of carnosine and anserine. The free β-amino compounds taurine and β-aminoisobutyric acid were also excreted excessively into urine, in amounts directly proportional to the amount of β-alanine. Interaction among β-amino compounds with a membrane transport system in the kidney presumably accounted for the β-amino aciduria. The tissue concentrations of carnosine and γ-aminobutyric acid (GABA) were also elevated, and GABA was present in elevated amounts in urine, plasma, and cerebrospinal fluid. The metabolic disorder was accompanied by somnolence and seizures. It is believed that the primary abnormality was a deficiency of β-alanine: α-ketoglutaric acid amino transferase. Certain features of the pedigree suggest that it was an inherited disease.

Carnosinemia (β-alanyl-L-histidinemia) is a disease of bound β-alanine. It is characterized by carnosine in blood and urine even when all sources of this dipeptide are excluded from the diet. The concentration of free β-alanine in body fluids is not abnormal in this disease. Carnosinemia is apparently associated with impaired function of the central nervous system. It has been described in only two unrelated patients at the time of this writing [2]. The finding of a specific deficiency of carnosinase suggests that the disease is inherited.

METABOLISM OF β-ALANINE, CARNOSINE, AND OTHER DIPEPTIDES

β-Alanine Metabolism

Free β-alanine forms an insignificant fraction of the free amino acid pool in human body fluids [3–5]. Liver and kidney, unlike other mammalian tissues which have been examined, contain a small amount of free β-alanine [1, 5*a*].

Synthesis

The principle endogenous sources of β-alanine in mammalian tissues are found in the metabolism of the pyrimidine, uracil, and the dipeptides, carnosine (β-alanyl-L-histidine) and anserine (β-alanyl-l-methyl-L-histidine) (Fig. 25-1).

Microorganisms can form β-alanine by alpha decarboxylation of aspartic acid, but this reaction does not occur in mammalian tissue. It is possible that the contents of the large intestine might serve as an exogenous source of β-alanine under appropriate conditions. Hydrolysis of dietary dipeptides which contain β-alanine will release β-alanine into the free pool.

Catabolism

β-Alanine can be removed from the free pool by two reactions in mammalian tissues. It may be degraded first to

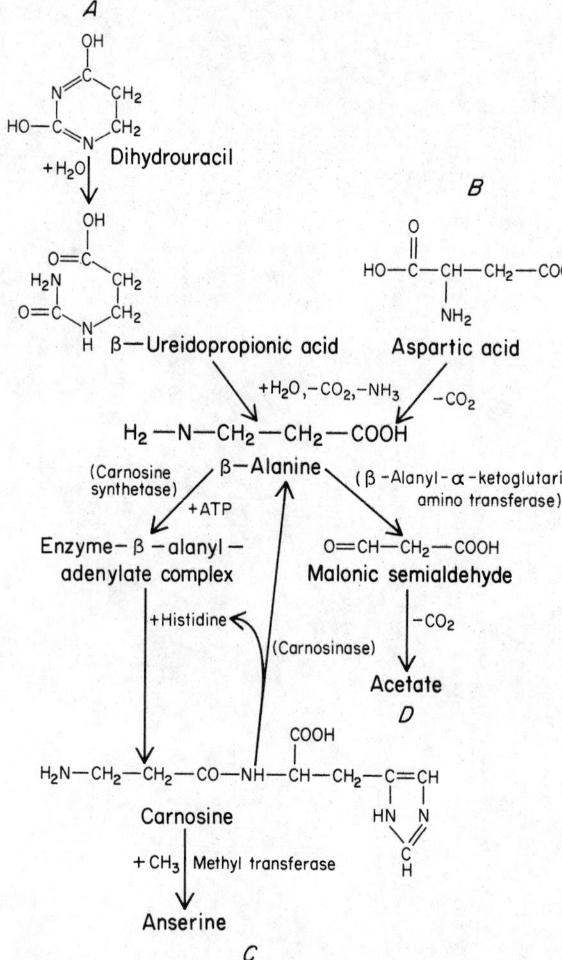

Figure 25-1. Simplified metabolic scheme for β-alanine and carnosine.

*This work was supported in part by grants from the Medical Research Council of Canada to the authors, and by an Associateship of the Medical Research Council to C.R.S.

malonic semialdehyde by the action of β-alanine-α-ketoglutarate amino transferase, an enzyme which has been well characterized in microorganisms [6]. Impairment of this enzyme as the result of mutation completely blocks oxidative catabolism of β-alanine in *Pseudomonas* [7]. Little is known about the characteristics of this initial step of β-alanine oxidation in human or other mammalian tissues. It has been suggested [8] that β-alanine, γ-aminobutyric, and β-amino-isobutyric acid may utilize the same transaminase. Decarboxylation of malonic semialdehyde to form acetate presumably occurs in human tissues, as it does in microorganisms [6], but the reaction has not been characterized in the former.

Incorporation

β-Alanyl-imidazole Dipeptides

The majority of β-alanine in the human body is bound in the dipeptide carnosine. The bound concentration in skeletal muscle may be 500 times greater than the free form. Incorporation of β-alanine into carnosine (Figs. 25-1 and 25-2) is an important reaction which has been studied intensively in the skeletal muscles of mammals and birds. Carnosine is not present in cardiac muscle [9, 10]. It is synthesized by carnosine synthetase, an enzyme which requires ATP during the formation of an enzyme-β-alanyl-adenylate complex [11–13]. L-Histidine is then united with β-alanine, and the dipeptide (β-alanyl-L-histidine) is released from the enzyme.

Skeletal muscle of birds and certain species of mammals, notably the rabbit, rat, and whale [14, 15], can also form anserine (β-alanyl-1-methyl-L-histidine) (Figs. 25-2 and 25-3). Anserine is absent from human skeletal muscle [2, 16]. The methyl group of anserine is added to the peptide after formation of carnosine by the enzyme S-adenosyl methionine: carnosine N-methyl transferase [13, 17]. Vitamin E deficiency causes impaired synthesis of anserine [18], and the dipeptides are lost from muscle.

The physiologic function of β-alanyl-imidazole dipeptides is not completely understood. Davey [15] has suggested that they may serve as buffers in stabilizing the pH of muscle contracting anaerobically. Avena and Bowen [19] have shown that carnosine and anserine serve in vitro as potent activators of myosin ATPase in concentrations comparable to those found in skeletal muscle.Anserine is most prominent in muscles and species where rapid contractile activity is a function of successful adaptation and survival (e.g., limb muscle of the rabbit and pectoral muscle of the bird, Fig. 25-3). Apparently anserine has some particular function apart from carnosine, which is worthy of the burden of the additional genetic and enzymatic apparatus in the cell.

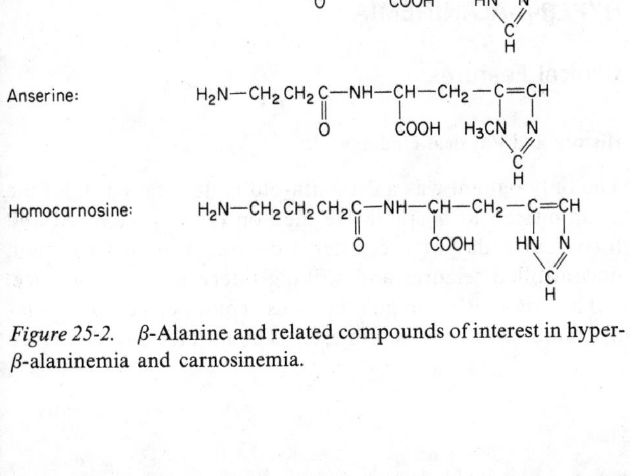

β-Alanine:
H2N—CH2CH2COOH
γ-Aminobutyric acid:
H2N—CH2CH2CH2COOH
Pantothenic acid:
HO—CH2—C(CH3)2—CHOH—C(O)—NH—CH2—CH2—COOH
Carnosine:
H2N—CH2CH2C(O)—NH—CH(COOH)—CH2—C=CH (HN N C H)
Anserine:
H2N—CH2CH2C(O)—NH—CH(COOH)—CH2—C=CH (H3CN N C H)
Homocarnosine:
H2N—CH2CH2CH2C(O)—NH—CH(COOH)—CH2—C=CH (HN N C H)

Figure 25-2. β-Alanine and related compounds of interest in hyper-β-alaninemia and carnosinemia.

Coenzyme A

β-Alanine is a constituent of coenzyme A in its pantothenate moiety (Fig. 25-2). Incorporation into pantothenic acid does not occur in mammalian tissues. Pantothenate is thus an essential human nutrient [20].

β-Alanyl-dipeptide Catabolism

Carnosine is hydrolyzed to β-alanine and histidine by the enzyme carnosinase, which has been found in the liver, spleen, and kidney of the rat [21], and has been isolated and purified from the kidney of swine [21, 22]. It is a metalloprotein, and although it is activated in vitro by both manganese and zinc ions, it is probable that zinc is the metal which occurs naturally in the enzyme in tissues [22]. Tissue carnosinase also hydrolyzes anserine to β-alanine and 1-methylhistidine [21]. The same enzyme, or at least one which is similar to that which hydrolyzes carnosine and anserine but not other imidazole dipeptides, is present in human serum [23].

Related Imidazole Dipeptides

Cetasine, or β-alanyl-3-methyl-L-histidine, as well as anserine, occurs in the muscle of fin and sei whales [24]. Homocarnosine, or γ-aminobutyryl-L-histidine (Fig. 25-2), was first isolated from bovine brain [25]; later it was also found in the brains of a number of other species of mammals, including man [26]. Kanazawa and Sano [27] have investigated the regional distribution of homocarnosine in human brain. The concentration varies in different areas from 15 to 60 μmoles per 100 gm. Like its precursor, γ-aminobutyric acid, homocarnosine is found in the central nervous system; to date it has not been found in other tissues. Homocarnosine may possibly be synthesized in brain by the same enzyme which forms carnosine in skeletal muscle, although carnosine synthetase has not yet been demonstrated in brain [26]. Homocarnosine is not hydrolyzed by the carnosinase present in human serum [23] but is hydrolyzed by carnosinase from swine kidney [25]. The physiologic role of homocarnosine in human brain remains unknown.

Carnosine also has been found in normal brain, but in much smaller amounts than homocarnosine [1, 26, 28, 29]. Additional related dipeptides that have been found in mammalian tissues are homoanserine (γ-aminobutyryl-L-1-methylhistidine) in bovine brain [30], α-(γ-aminobutyryl)-lysine in the brain of a number of mammalian species [31], and α-(β-alanyl)-lysine in rabbit muscle [32]. The physiologic roles of these peptides are unknown.

Imidazole Dipeptides in Physiologic Fluids and Relation to Diet

Carnosine and anserine are not detectable in the fasting plasma of normal persons, nor are they usually found in significant amounts in the urine of normal subjects who are consuming diets low in meat. Normal urine contains scores of unidentified ninhydrin-reacting compounds, some of which include β-alanine and imidazole in peptide linkage [33]. For this reason, qualitative identification of carnosine or anserine in the urine should first be made with paper chromatography or electrophoresis. If a large amount of either dipeptide is present, then the amino acid analyzer can properly be employed for quantitation.

Normal persons consuming considerable carnosine or anserine in their diet, as they do if they eat chicken or turkey [2, 16, 34–36], excrete part of these dipeptides unhydrolyzed in the urine. They have carnosine in the plasma 2 hr after a heavy meal of meat [2]. Since renal clearance of dipeptides is high, the urine reflects the endogenous appearance of these compounds better than plasma. All forms of meat and poultry, including soup stocks made from meat, contain carnosine. The most common dietary sources of anserine are chicken, turkey, duck, and rabbit. White meat of chicken or turkey seems to be one of the richest dietary sources of anserine [16, 34] (Fig. 25-3).

Subjects fed large amounts of carnosine or anserine may also excrete small amounts of free β-alanine in the urine [2, 16, 33]. The consumption of even modest amounts of anserine in the diet regularly leads to the appearance of 1-methylhistidine in the urine [16, 35, 36], except in patients with carnosinemia [2]. 1-Methylhistidine is irregularly detectable when fasting human plasma is chromatographed on the amino acid analyzer, and since it has no known endogenous source in man, its appearance probably indicates recent consumption of anserine-containing foods. Since renal clearance of 1-methylhistidine is rapid [37, 38], the urine is more likely to reflect its presence than plasma. Large amounts of 1-methylhistidinuria may give a green ferric chloride reaction when the reagent is added dropwise to the urine [16]. Dietary carnosinuria is found more frequently in young children than in adults, and presumably reflects a relatively lower level of serum carnosinase activity in children than in adults [23].

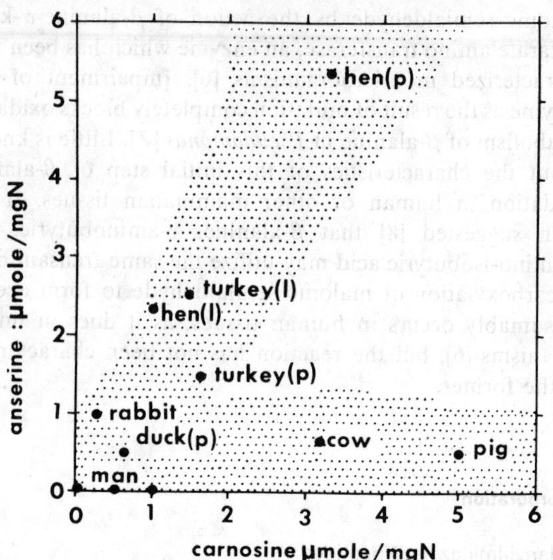

Figure 25-3. Carnosine and anserine content of muscle in various species. In all cases, skeletal muscle was analyzed [16]. *p*, pectoral muscle; *l*, leg muscle. Limb muscles examined where type not specified.

Homocarnosine is not detectable in the plasma or urine of normal subjects, but this dipeptide is routinely found in the gray matter of the brain [39] and in the cerebrospinal fluid of normal children [40]. It can sometimes be detected in the CSF of normal adults, and is found in greater amounts in the CSF of neurologically diseased adults. In 27 neurologically normal infants and children under the age of 3½ years, the mean homocarnosine concentration in the CSF was 0.8 μmole per 100 ml. The mean concentration in 11 adults who had a variety of neurologic disorders was 0.1 μmole per 100 ml [40].

HYPER-β-ALANINEMIA

Clinical Features

History and Physical Findings

The only patient was a 2-month-old male infant at the time of admission to hospital. He died on the one hundred and forty-fourth day of life, after a course of almost constant, uncontrolled seizures and striking intervening somnolence.

The mother's pregnancy was complicated by polyhydramnios in the last trimester. The mother also described very little intrauterine fetal activity. Delivery occurred, with normal vertex presentation, at 38 weeks. Persistent lethargy, accompanied by hyporeflexia which could not be attributed to prenatal medication or anesthesia, was observed in the infant beginning 30 min after delivery. This continued as a state of somnolence through the first 7 weeks of life, when the infant was admitted to hospital because of difficulties with feeding and fever. Grand mal seizures first occurred at this time. He was than transferred to a medical center where a diagnosis of hyper-β-alaninemia was reached and subsequent investigations were performed.

Already by the beginning of the second month of life the infant had grown poorly. Height, weight, and head circumference were all below the third percentile for his age. The most important physical findings were related to the nervous system. They included frequent grand mal seizures, impaired Moro and sucking reflexes, a poor response to painful stimuli, and muscular hypotonia between seizures. The other clinical feature which attracted attention was the angelic repose, interrupted only by seizures or the necessity for insertion of a gavage tube for nourishment.

A host of anticonvulsant medications (including phenobarbital, diphenylhydantoin, primidone, corticosteroids, acetazoleamide, and pyridoxine) and a ketogenic diet were without effect on the seizures or the somnolence. Bronchopneumonia, otitis media, and mastoiditis caused by *Pseudomonas* infection appeared, probably as a complication of the continual gavage feedings.

Pathology

Autopsy was performed within 2 hr of death. There were numerous areas of pneumonic consolidation. The brain weighed 470 gm (normal for age and habitus, 620 ± 71 gm). The ventricles were slightly dilated, and there was diffuse edema of the white matter and focal areas of vacuole formation. The demarcation between white and gray matter was blurred. Microscopic examination disclosed beading of the myelin sheaths, but a careful search revealed no significant neuronal abnormalities.

Laboratory Findings

Routine blood examinations and all routine analyses of urine and cerebrospinal fluids gave normal findings. Concentrations of blood glucose and urea nitrogen, serum sodium, chloride, potassium, total calcium, inorganic phosphorus, creatinine, and plasma CO_2 were normal. Examination of the urine for cytomegalic inclusion bodies and a search for evidence of toxoplasmosis were negative. An extensive search for pathogenic microorganisms in urine, blood, cerebrospinal fluid, and feces was unrewarding.

Roentgen ray examinations of chest and skull were normal prior to the terminal pneumonia. A pneumoencephalogram was normal, but repeated electroencephalographic studies in the third and fourth months of life revealed a diffuse disturbance of cerebral activity involving cortical and subcortical structures.

The most important laboratory finding was made initially on a urine specimen. Although a number of simple chemical screening tests [41, 42] were normal, a partition filter paper chromatogram of the urine revealed a striking abnormality in amino acid excretion (Fig. 25-4). A large amount of β-alanine was present; this substance is normally detected in human urine only in very small amounts [5, 33] during urinary putrefaction. In addition, the excretion of β-aminoisobutyric acid and of taurine was particularly prominent. Another unusual ninhydrin-reactive component was found (Fig. 25-4) and identified as GABA [1].

The concentrations of β-alanine and GABA were also increased in the plasma and in cerebrospinal fluid (Table 25-1). Neither substance is detected normally in cerebrospinal fluid [39, 43], and only β-alanine is present, in very small amounts, in normal plasma [3, 4, 38]. With the exception of the β-amino acids and GABA, the concentrations of all other free amino acids in plasma and urine were normal. The concentrations in body fluids of the dipeptides carnosine and anserine, and of pantothenic acid, were also normal at all times.

Family History and Inheritance

The patient was the fourth child of the second marriage of an Anglo-Canadian mother to a French Canadian (Fig. 25-5). A half-brother (II-1) and half-sister (II-2) of the patient are healthy. Four children were conceived by the second father; only the eldest (II-3) is alive and well. The second child (II-4) died with "breathing trouble" 4 hr after birth. The third pregnancy (II-5) terminated in a miscarriage at the third month. The mother had one further pregnancy in 1966 after the proband died; this child (II-7) was stillborn at term. There is no consanguinity between the parents, and they have no relatives with convulsive disorders, mental retardation, or chronic diseases. The available living members of the immediate family were investigated for β-alaninuria before and after a meat-containing meal, but the amino acid content of the urine was normal. The information is not sufficient for any definite statement concerning the presumed inheritance of hyper-β-alaninemia, but the circumstances of the pedigree suggest that the trait, if it is inherited, is autosomal recessive. The unusual incidence of stillbirth or early death in infancy (four of five offspring) arising from the second marriage of the mother may indicate the existence of such a trait, but this cannot be proved.

Hyper-β-alaninemia in liveborn infants is apparently a rare disease. It has been described only once, although many thousands of patients with manifestations of disordered function of the nervous system have been examined with reliable chromatographic methods throughout the world.

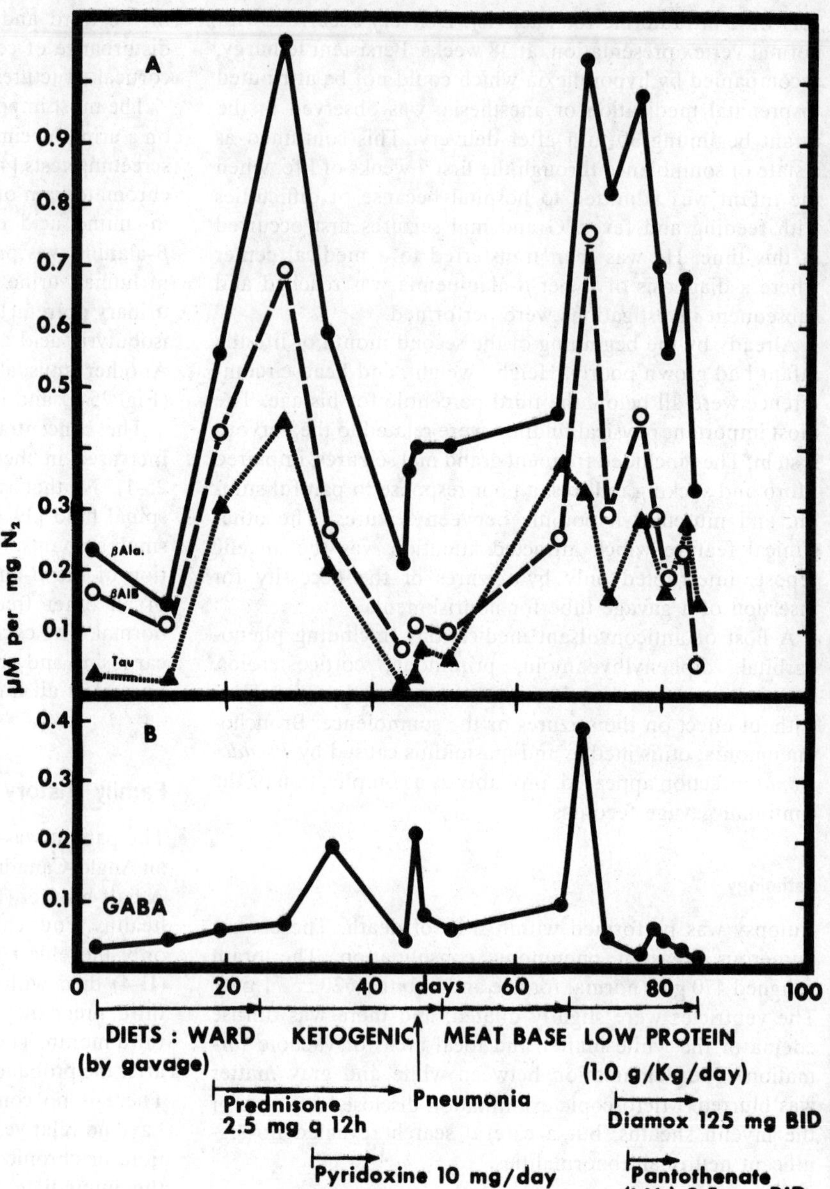

Figure 25-4. Excretion of β-amino compounds, β-alanine, taurine, and β-aminoisobutyric acid in urine of a patient with hyper-β-alaninemia under various conditions of diet and medication. Excretion of GABA, which is independent of the excretion of β-amino acids, is also shown. Excretion of two α-amino acids, threonine and α-alanine, is shown to indicate specificity of hyper-β-amino aciduria.

Table 25-1. CONCENTRATION OF β-ALANINE AND γ-AMINOBUTYRIC ACID IN BODY FLUIDS

Amino acid	Source*	*Plasma, μmoles/liter*		*Urine, μmoles/gm total nitrogen*		Cerebrospinal fluid, μmoles/liter
		Mean	Range	Mean	Range	
β-Alanine	Normal	...	<14	...	<10	0
	Patient	33	20–51	564	140–1,060	45
GABA	Normal	0	...	0	...	0
	Patient	4.4	1–7	81	25–400	1–2

*Normal values taken from Dickinson et al. [4], and from data cited and compiled elsewhere [3].

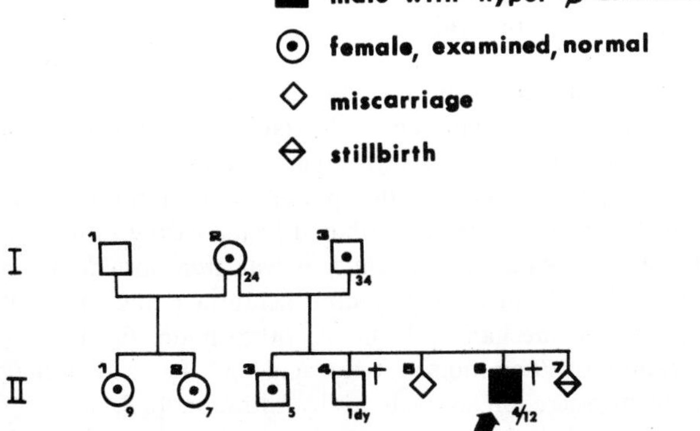

Figure 25-5. Pedigree of proband with hyper-β-alaninuria.

Proposed Site of Metabolic Defect in Hyper-β-alaninemia

The abnormal distribution of certain free amino acids in hyper-β-alaninemia (Table 25-1) is only part of the story. Tissues obtained within 2 hr of death [1] revealed another aspect of this disease. The concentration of carnosine in the tissues was six times greater than in the post-mortem tissues of age-matched controls (Table 25-2). The increase of carnosine was directly proportional to the excess of free β-alanine. The accumulation of carnosine cannot be attributed to deficient carnosinase activity, for when this occurs, as in carnosinemia [2, 23], carnosine is present in plasma and is also excreted in urine, yet the concentration of free β-alanine is normal. The accumulation of carnosine in tissues in hyper-β-alaninemia can therefore be attributed to overproduction of the dipeptide in the presence of an expanded free β-alanine pool.

Accumulation of homocarnosine was not recognized if it was present, but it is possible that it occurred as a result of the increased amount of GABA available for synthesis by a mechanism analagous to that proposed for the augmentation of brain carnosine in hyper-β-alaninemia.

There is no evidence that intestinal overproduction of β-alanine accounted for the disorder. Fecal amino acid content was normal, particularly with respect to β-alanine and aspartic acid [1]. Overproduction from uracil was not specifically investigated, but it seems an unlikely cause of hyper-β-alaninemia in man.

Impaired oxidation of β-alanine is the most probable cause of the abnormality. Malonic semialdehyde was not found in urine extracted with 2,4-dinitrophenylhydrazine [6, 44] and examined chromatographically. Furthermore, hydrogenation of the phenylhydrazine derivatives [45] did not produce detectable amounts of β-alanine. Thus, though these studies involved an unstable compound and were performed on acidified urine which had been frozen at −20°C for 4 months, there appeared to be no accumulation of malonic semialdehyde. A block in decarboxylation is accordingly unlikely.

If β-alanine oxidation was indeed impaired in the disorder, the defect was more likely at the stage of transamination. Two features point to this possibility:

1 The transaminase requires pyridoxal-5-phosphate as coenzyme. One trial of pyridoxine (10 mg per day) during the lifetime of the patient was accompanied by an abrupt fall in β-alanine excretion (Fig. 25-4). When administration of pyridoxine was stopped, β-alanine excretion rose sharply.

Table 25-2. CONCENTRATION OF β-ALANINE, CARNOSINE, AND GABA IN POST-MORTEM TISSUES OF A PATIENT WITH HYPER-β-ALANINEMIA

Tissue	Source*	β-Alanine, μmoles/gm wet wt	Carnosine, μmoles/gm wet wt	GABA, μmoles/gm wet wt
Brain	Patient	0.20	0.39	3.83†
	Control	0	<0.02	0.8†
Muscle‡	Patient	0.07–0.11	36.1–45.0	<0.02
	Control	<0.01	6.62–6.84	0
Liver	Patient	0.36	0	<0.02
	Control	0.16	0	0
Kidney	Patient	1.12	0	0.24
	Control	. . .	. . .	0.03–0.45§

*Post-mortem control is an age-matched, male patient with Werdnig-Hoffmann disease. Tissues from patient and control were obtained 2 and 3 hr respectively after death.
†Values indicate total (bound and free) GABA in occipital cortex, deproteinized with picric acid [1]. The patient's value is high for his age when compared with control and published data on infants and children [56]. The wide range of published control values [29, 39, 56] reflects techniques of tissue preparation and an age effect, since GABA content of brain increases during human infancy [56].
‡Deltoid and rectus abdominis.
§Values obtained from Whelan et al. [51] and Zachmann et al. [53].

The specificity of the response may be questioned, since fluctuation in β-alanine excretion occurred at times when pyridoxine intake did not vary. Unfortunately, because no clinical improvement accompanied it, this interesting biochemical response to the vitamin was not recognized until after the infant had died. Further investigation along this line was not undertaken.

2 The concentration of GABA, which is considered to be a neuroinhibitor substance [46, 47], was elevated in postmortem samples of brain and kidney (Table 25-1), and GABA was also detected in plasma, CSF, and urine (Table 25-1). Therefore, the metabolism of GABA also seems to have been impaired. Glutamic acid decarboxylase (GAD) and its product, GABA, which were once thought to be present only in brain [48–50], have now been identified in kidney as well [51–53]. This may explain the accumulation of GABA in the kidney. Free GABA is either bound to neuronal sites [50] or degraded by transamination, and GABA and β-alanine probably share the same transaminase [8, 54]. Loss of this transaminase might thus cause accumulation of β-alanine and GABA. On the other hand there is evidence [55] that β-alanine is not the natural substrate for GABA transaminase in brain, and that β-alanine is an inhibitor of its activity [53, 55]. Thus GABA accumulation might have reflected only a secondary effect of a deficiency in a specific β-alanine transaminase, which caused β-alanine accumulation and competitive inhibition of GABA transaminase.

Mechanism for β-Amino Aciduria in Hyper-β-alaninemia

A combined mechanism underlay the excretion of β-amino acids in hyper-β-alaninemia. β-Alanine concentration in plasma was elevated. Its own high excretion rate, which is directly proportional to the plasma concentration (Fig. 25-6A), can therefore be attributed to increasing saturation of the membrane site at which it was transported in the tubule. This form of hyperamino aciduria is the result of a saturation mechanism.[1] On the other hand, the urinary excretion of β-aminoisobutyric acid (βAIB), which may occur by secretion as well as by filtration [60], was not proportional to plasma concentration in the patient. Instead, βAIB excretion varied in direct proportion to the concentration of β-alanine in the plasma (Fig. 25-6B). Similarly, taurine excretion in urine varied more in relation to β-alanine in plasma than to its own plasma concentration (Fig. 25-6C). Therefore, βAIB and taurine were excreted in excess because of impaired tubular conservation of these two compounds. The determinant of this relationship presumably was the degree of hyper-β-alaninemia.

If one postulates that β-amino compounds are transported

[1] The terms *overflow* [57] and *prerenal* [58] are often used to describe hyperamino aciduria occurring by a saturation mechanism; they suggest the enzymatic nature of membrane transport of amino acids [59].

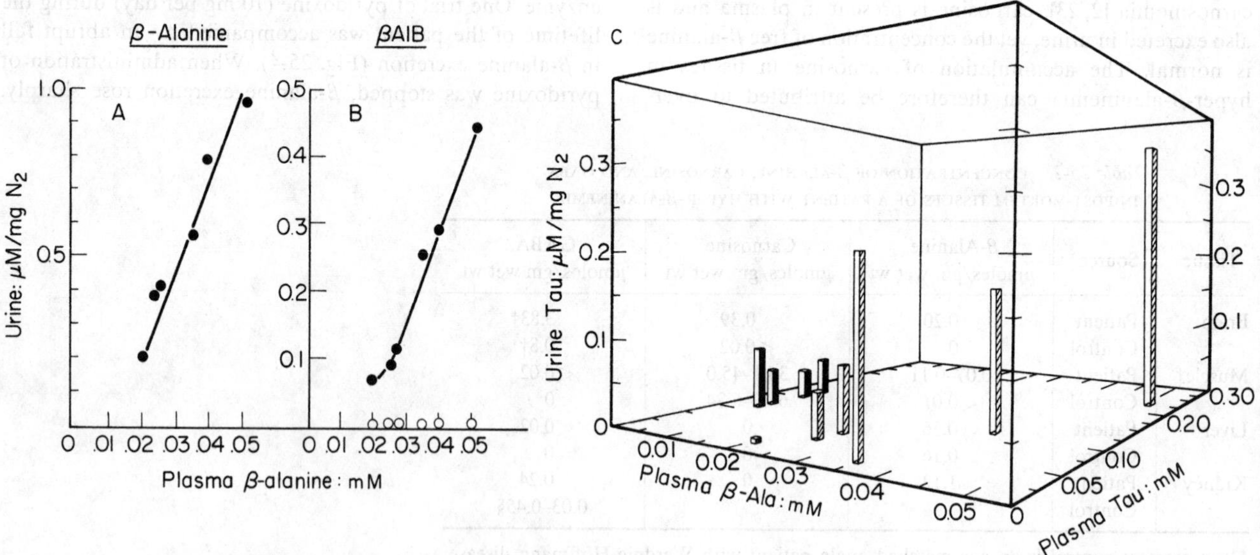

Figure 25-6. Excretion of β-amino compounds (A, β-alanine; B, β-aminoisobutyric acid; C, taurine) in relation to plasma concentration of β-alanine in the patient with hyper-β-alaninuria. The direct relationship indicates that hyper-β-amino aciduria reflects interaction at a tubular transport site selective for these compounds. This specific amino aciduria is of the "combined" type, representing overflow (β-alanine) and renal (βAIB and taurine) mechanisms, the latter by virtue of competitive inhibition by β-alanine.

at a common site with preference for these solutes over α-amino acids, then the mechanism of the hyper-β-amino aciduria becomes apparent. At the high concentrations of β-alanine which occurred in the patient the amino acid behaved as a competitive inhibitor at the membrane site shared by the other two substrates. The latter were displaced, appearing in the urine as if by a "renal" mechanism [57–59]. The selective hyperamino aciduria involving β-amino acids was therefore the result of combined overflow and renal mechanisms [60]. A similar mechanism accounts for the selective hyperamino aciduria (iminoglycinuria) of hyperprolinemia [61] (see Chap. 16).

Evidence for a membrane site with preference for β-amino acid transport has been found under other circumstances. Gilbert et al. [62] studied interactions between β-amino compounds in mouse kidney in vivo and found evidence for a tubular absorptive system. Wilson and Scriver [63] and Goldman and Scriver [64] studied interactions between β-amino compounds in the rat in vivo and found that β-amino acids interacted with one another but not with α-amino acids during tubular absorption. Christensen [65] has also found support for a β-amino–preferring transport system in another mammalian tissue, viz., the Ehrlich ascites tumor cell.

GABAuria

GABA and other ω-amino acids are poorly transported across cell membranes [66]. In the patient the GABAuria varied independently of the plasma β-alanine concentration (Fig. 25-4) but in direct proportion to the plasma level of GABA [1]. GABAuria was accordingly related to the initial impairment of GABA metabolism, not to any modulation in tubular transport.

Interpretation of Clinical Symptoms

Presumably, the seizures and somnolence were primarily related in some way to hyper-β-alaninemia and the consequent interference with GABA metabolism. This assumption is by no means proved, and until more cases of hyper-β-alaninemia are found and studied the possibility must be entertained that the biochemical disorder was discovered merely because the patient had seizures caused by some other abnormality. Nonetheless, β-alanine is a neuroinhibitory substance in cortex, brain stem, and spinal cord [67]. Clearly the depressed activity of the central nervous system could have been one manifestation of hyper-β-alaninemia.

GABA, too, is a neuroinhibitory substance [48, 68], and depletion of GABA in brain produces seizures [49]. GABA acts as a neuroinhibitor following binding at synaptic junctions, and β-alanine inhibits binding of GABA by brain [69]. Thus, although the total GABA was elevated in the brain of the patient with hyper-β-alaninemia, it is possible that the amount actually bound to the sites which mediate its neurochemical effect actually decreased. The seizures may have reflected this postulated imbalance.

GABA also participates in an "oxidative shunt" which has quantitative significance in brain metabolism [69*a*]. Any inhibition of GABA oxidation would depress the activity of this shunt and contribute to the pathogenesis of seizures in hyper-β-alaninemia by a metabolic, rather than a neurochemical, mechanism.

The significance of an elevated level of carnosine (and possibly of homocarnosine) in brain must also be considered [70, 70*a*]. Carnosinemia [2] and hyper-β-alaninemia are both accompanied by retarded development of the nervous system and a severe convulsive disorder. Only the latter has impaired metabolism of β-alanine and GABA; in both carnosinemia and hyper-β-alaninemia there is some abnormality of imidazole dipeptide metabolism. Thus, one might ask: Is too much carnosine (and homocarnosine) harmful to the central nervous system? Allen et al. [70*a*] have found that homocarnosine is present in excess in phenylketonuric brain and CSF. Further study of this facet of dipeptide metabolism is required before the question can be answered.

It is important to emphasize again that hyper-β-alaninemia and carnosinemia were discovered only because the patients were ill. This does not necessarily mean that the biochemical disorders caused the illness.

Diagnosis

The color of β-alanine on a partition chromatogram developed in Dent's system [71] and stained with ninhydrin is so unmistakable that diagnosis should not be missed in a simple preliminary chromatographic investigation. Urine is the preferred source of material for diagnosis, since it also contains the other β-amino compounds and GABA. The latter substance is not found in normal human urine [5, 33]. Since the plasma concentrations of β-alanine and GABA are low even if abnormally elevated, one cannot expect detection of the trait in the newborn by the simple screening methods which have been used to discover amino acidopathies in blood and plasma [72, 73]. These screening methods permit detection of β-alanine only when the concentration in plasma exceeds 0.1 mM; the concentration in the patient did not exceed 0.05 mM.

Acquired causes of β-alaninuria should be excluded and confirmatory investigations should be performed when the patient is not on a diet rich in foods containing carnosine or anserine. Certain drugs may also cause hyper-β-alaninuria. We have studied one patient who was being treated with isoniazid for a granulomatous disease. Prominent hyper-β-alaninuria was observed, and the plasma β-alanine concentration was 0.025 mM. The abnormality of β-alanine metabolism disappeared when pyridoxine was added. This form of β-alaninuria is probably caused by the inhibition of β-alanine transaminase that is induced by the depletion of pyridoxine brought about by isoniazid.

Treatment

No effective therapy was discovered during the lifetime of the patient. Many anticonvulsant drugs were tried; none controlled the seizures. Ketogenic, low-protein, and high-protein diets produced modulations in the degree of biochemical imbalance (Fig. 24-4), but none had any effect on the clinical course. Only one agent showed any particular therapeutic promise. Pyridoxine appeared to restore some degree of biochemical order in the patient, and this vitamin is a coenzyme for β-alanine transaminase. Although no clinical improvement accompanied the temporary reduction of β-alanine accumulation, it is possible that the biochemical disorder would respond to vitamin B_6 therapy, as have other inborn errors of amino acid metabolism [74]. If β-alanine accumulation is the cause of the clinical manifestations of the disease, future patients should be given a trial with a low-protein, low-pyrimidine diet and a high-pyridoxine intake in order to determine whether early and consistent reduction of β-alanine accumulation is of any benefit.

CARNOSINEMIA

Clinical Features

The Patients

Patient A is a 5-year-old boy of North European origin who is institutionalized for mental retardation. He appeared normal in early infancy but developed episodes of twitching at the age of 2 months, and myoclonic seizures at the age of 8 months. Electroencephalograms revealed a widespread dysrhythmia from this time on. Behavioral development was normal during the first year of life, but thereafter the child lost the ability to sit, crawl, and stand. He is now profoundly retarded mentally, is unable to sit alone or hold his head up, and does not follow objects with his eyes. The skeletal muscles are flaccid but not wasted. Myoclonic jerks are frequent, and there have been occasional grand mal seizures. No retinal abnormalities are apparent on ophthalmoscopic examination.

Patient B developed normally until the age of 2 months, when myoclonic seizures first appeared. Electroencephalograms were normal at 2 and 3 months of age, but by 4 months there was a widespread paroxysmal abnormality. The infant lost his ability to hold his head erect and to follow objects with the eyes after age 4 months. Grand mal seizures and generalized spasticity appeared, and by 8 months the patient was deaf and blind. The eye grounds were normal. The patient died at age 10 months.

Biochemical Investigations

Two-dimensional paper chromatography of urinary amino acids, performed as part of a routine investigation because of the neurologic disorder, disclosed the presence of large amounts of carnosine in the urine of Patient B. This dipeptide is occasionally found in the urine of mentally retarded children (and presumably in the urine of normal children as well) if a chromatographic solvent system is used which separates carnosine from histidine and other basic amino acids. An unusual feature in these two patients was the persistence of the carnosinuria after all sources of carnosine were withdrawn from the diet.

The amounts of carnosine and other imidazole dipeptides found in the physiologic fluids of Patient A on various occasions appear in Table 25-3. The dipeptides were identified qualitatively by means of paper chromatography, high-voltage paper electrophoresis, and by acid hydrolysis of the

Table 25-3. IMIDAZOLE DIPEPTIDES IN PHYSIOLOGIC FLUIDS OF CARNOSINEMIA, PATIENT A

Age, mo	Diet	Carnosine in plasma, μmoles/100 ml	Carnosine in urine, μmoles/mg creatinine	Anserine in plasma, μmoles/100 ml	Anserine in urine, μmoles/mg creatinine	Homocarnosine in CSF, μmoles/100 ml
11	Regular	...	0.83	...	0	
28	Regular	...	3.21	...	0	
29	Regular	0.5	1.28	0	0	
30	Regular	0.8	...	0	...	1.1
30	Meat-free, 72 hr	Trace	0.58	0	0	
30	Regular	...	1.30	...	0	
31	Meat-free, 72 hr	0.4	0.97	0	0	1.1
31	Chicken breast, 24 hr	5.3*	4.53	10.2*	8.59	
32	Regular	...	1.69	...	0	
33	Meat-free, 72 hr	0.1	0.54	...	0	1.1
57	Regular	0	...	0		
57	Regular	1.9*	...	0*		

* All plasma carnosine and anserine values were determined in the fasting state, except on these two occasions when blood was obtained 2 hr after a meal containing chicken or meat.

peptides followed by identification of their component amino acids [2]. Quantitation of the dipeptides was carried out on the automatic amino acid analyzer.

Carnosine has been readily demonstrable in the urine of Patient A on every occasion that it has been examined, even when the child had eaten no carnosine-containing foods for at least 72 hr. Carnosine has been detectable in low concentration in the fasting plasma on all occasions except one, and has been measurable in fasting plasma when the patient has been on a meat-free diet. Carnosine is normally not detectable in fasting plasma. Presumably the persistence of carnosine in the plasma and urine of patient A after exclusion of carnosine from the diet indicates that the dipeptide is discharged slowly from skeletal muscles into the circulation. In plasma obtained 2 hr after a meal of meat or chicken, much higher concentrations of carnosine (as well as anserine, after chicken) have been found. On three occasions the cerebrospinal fluid of Patient A has contained easily measurable amounts of homocarnosine, but not of carnosine. Although the concentration of homocarnosine in the CSF was originally thought to be elevated, since it was approximately ten times higher than had previously been reported [26], a subsequent investigation [40] has shown that infants and young children normally have concentrations of homocarnosine in the CSF similar to those found in Patient A.

Patient A excretes from 1 to 3 μmoles of carnosine per milligram of creatinine when he is on a regular diet, and about half this much when on a meat-free diet. Whenever he is given chicken breast, which is a good source of anserine as well as of carnosine, the former is readily identified on paper chromatograms of the urine. In spite of ingestion of large quantities of anserine, as demonstrated by its presence in the urine, Patient A does not excrete detectable amounts of 1-methylhistidine, one of the amino acids produced by the hydrolysis of anserine. By contrast, other children with the more common dietary form of carnosinuria, when fed enough chicken breast to cause excretion of anserine in the urine, also excrete large amounts of 1-methylhistidine [16, 35, 36].

Patient B also excreted large amounts of carnosine in the urine when on a regular diet, and both carnosine and anserine when fed chicken. No 1-methylhistidine was detectable in the urine on occasions when it contained large amounts of anserine. When on a meat-free diet, the patient excreted 0.2 to 0.3 μmole of carnosine per milligram of creatinine, about a quarter to a third the amount excreted by Patient A on a similar diet. In addition, carnosine could not be detected in fasting plasma, although it did appear in the plasma 2 hr after a meal containing carnosine.

The Enzyme Defect

The carnosinuria and anserinuria in both these patients, as well as the carnosinemia found during the postabsorptive state in Patient A, can be explained by a deficiency in carnosinase activity in the blood of these patients. A simple assay for carnosinase in serum was developed,[2] and the activity of this enzyme was determined in serums from normal adults, normal children, mentally retarded children, and from the two patients [23].

In the assay, 0.1 ml serum is preincubated at 37°C for 1 hr in tris buffer at pH 8 with manganese chloride. Twenty micromoles of L-carnosine is then added as substrate, and the incubation is continued for 16 hr at 37°C. The reaction is stopped and the solution deproteinized at the end of the incubation with sulfosalicylic acid. A blank containing tetrasodium ethylenediaminetetraacetate (EDTA) is run with each serum specimen. EDTA chelates the Mn^{++}ion which activates carnosinase. This blank can be used for eventual measurement of histidine which might be present in the serum, as a contaminant in the carnosine substrate, or possibly formed by nonenzymatic hydrolysis of carnosine. The amounts of histidine and β-alanine produced by the enzymatic hydrolysis of carnosine in each incubation tube are then estimated semiquantitatively on high-voltage paper electrophoretograms, and finally are quantitated on the amino acid analyzer. The peptidase in normal human serum readily hydrolyzes L-carnosine and L-anserine but shows no activity toward three other imidazole dipeptides—L-homocarnosine, β-L-aspartyl-L-histidine, and L-histidyl-L-proline [23].

The carnosinase activities of the two patients and their family members, as well as of various control subjects, are shown in Table 25-4. Patient A has consistently had little or no carnosinase activity in the serum. The carnosinase activity of his father's serum is within the normal range for adults, while his mother and his healthy sibling show serum carnosinase activity appreciably lower than that of healthy control subjects. It has not been possible to arrange a liver biopsy on Patient A, and no conclusions can be drawn regarding a possible deficiency in carnosinase in the tissues.

A low serum carnosinase activity was found on one occasion in Patient B a month before his death (Table 25-4). Activity was normal in his parents and three sibs. Heart blood was obtained by cardiac puncture 16 hr after death, but tissues could not be obtained until autopsy 34 hr after death. Serum carnosinase activity in the post-mortem heart blood was found to be as high as that in the serum of living adults. Carnosinase activity in liver and kidney was substantial, although lower than that found in the same organs of a control subject of comparable age who died of congenital heart disease. The paradoxical rise in serum carnosinase activity, from a very low value during life to a high value 16 hr after death, might have been due either to an agonal leakage of carnosinase from hepatic and renal cells into the circulation, or to post-mortem autolysis of cardiac muscle, causing contamination of heart blood with tissue carnosinase. (Cardiac muscle from a control infant at post-mortem examination was found to have appreciable carnosinase activity.)

[2] The assay for serum carnosinase was kindly suggested by Prof. Harry Harris.

Table 25-4. SERUM CARNOSINASE ACTIVITY OF CONTROL SUBJECTS AND OF TWO CARNOSINEMIA PATIENTS AND THEIR RELATIVES

Subjects and age	Condition	Carnosine hydrolyzed, μmoles/ml serum/16 hr
15 adults	Good health	19.3 ± 7.7; range, 7.7–31.2
9 children (1–8 yr)	Good health	11.4 ± 5.0; range, 6.0–22.3
14 children (6 mo–3½ yr)	Mental defectives, in hospital	5.5 ± 2.6; range, 1.7–11.8
Family A:		
Patient A:	Carnosinemia	0, 0, 0.5, 0.8
3½ yr	Carnosinemia	0.3
4½ yr	Carnosinemia	0.6
5 yr	Good health	12.0
Father	Good health	5.6
Mother	Good health	2.0
Brother (6 yr)	Carnosinemia	0.7
Family B:		
Patient B (9 mo)	Heart blood, 16 hr post mortem	21.4
Father	Good health	21.1
Mother	Good health	16.2
Brother (6 yr)	Good health	12.7
Sister (5 yr)	Good health	16.2
Sister (3 yr)	Good health	8.0

The carnosine concentration of skeletal muscle of Patient B at autopsy was approximately the same as that found in the skeletal muscle of a control infant at autopsy. Carnosine could not be detected in the cerebral cortex of Patient B, while the concentration of homocarnosine in the cortex of this child was comparable to that found in the brain of an adult who died without neurologic disease.

Diagnosis

The diagnosis of carnosinemia should be suspected when two-dimensional paper chromatography of urine discloses carnosine or anserine. When pyridine/acetone/ammonium hydroxide/water (45:30:5:20) is used as the first solvent, followed by isopropanol/formic acid/water (75:12.5:12.5) as the second solvent, and the sheets are sprayed with ninhydrin-lutidine [75], carnosine and anserine appear as yellow or tan-yellow spots close to and partially overlapping histidine. The two dipeptides can be conveniently identified if the chromatogram is then countersprayed with diazotized sulfanilic acid. When this is done, histidine turns from purple to orange-brown, carnosine turns red, anserine turns grayish blue, and all other ninhydrin-positive spots on the chromatogram are decolorized [2]. Carnosine and anserine can also be identified by their characteristic positions and colors with the same staining reagents, when the chromatogram is developed in a phenol-lutidine system [71].

To distinguish between true carnosinemia and the relatively common carnosinuria that follows consumption of large amounts of meat or poultry, the patient can be fed white meat of chicken or turkey, which serves as an inexpensive source of anserine. If urine collected after such a meal contains easily detectable 1-methylhistidine, the possibility of true carnosinemia is excluded. 1-Methylhistidine is conveniently identified by two-dimensional paper chromatography of urine.[3] If 1-methylhistidine is absent from the urine at a time when the urine contains anserine, determination of serum carnosinase is indicated; the finding of little or no carnosinase activity in blood confirms the diagnosis of carnosinemia. The absence of 1-methylhistidine from the urine if it contains anserine and carnosine also differentiates carnosinemia from the imidazoluria reported by Bessman and Baldwin [76], Levenson et al. [77], and Tocci and Bessman [78] in children with juvenile amaurotic idiocy (Spielmeyer-Vogt syndrome).

Therapy

In view of the present incomplete information about this metabolic disorder, no form of treatment is known for carnosinemia. It must be emphasized that there is no certainty that the degenerative neurologic disease found in the two patients so far reported was causally related to their deficiency in serum carnosinase activity. Tissue carnosinase activity was demonstrable in the liver and kidney of Patient B after death, and there was no excessive accumulation of carnosine in skeletal muscles, or of either carnosine or homocarnosine in brain. It does not seem likely that the periodic presence of carnosine in the blood could have caused the severe neurologic disorder. Patient A, who is still

[3]Described by Dent [71] as compounds 51 and 53 on his map. 1-Methylhistidine gives a characteristic green color after the paper chromatogram is stained with ninhydrin and heated to 105°C for a few minutes.

living, may or may not have exactly the same disorder as Patient B, since it is not known whether his lack of serum carnosinase is accompanied by a deficiency of carnosinase in the tissues.

More patients with carnosinemia will have to be discovered and studied before meaningful conclusions can be drawn as to the possible harmful effects of serum carnosinase deficiency, or as to the possibility that a mutant gene or genes produce *both* neurologic disease and an otherwise harmless serum carnosinase deficiency. It is well to stress again that if a biochemical error is searched for *only* in patients with neurologic disease, then all subjects having the biochemical trait will have neurologic disease! This logical trap has been demonstrated in a number of the inborn errors of metabolism [e.g., see Chap. 20 (cystathioninuria) and Chap. 63 (iminoglycinuria)].

Genetics

The parents of Patient A are first cousins. One child, a 6-year-old boy, is in good health. The other sib, a girl, became ill soon after birth, with excessive crying, vomiting, and rigidity, showed progressive neurologic deterioration, and died at the age of 3 months. Neither laboratory studies nor an autopsy was performed on this child.

Patient B was the son of Chinese parents. They were not consanguine. Three sibs are in good health.

It is reasonable to suspect that serum carnosinase deficiency is a genetically determined disorder. The biochemical findings in the two patients and in their close relatives, as well as the fact that the parents of one are first cousins, are consistent with an autosomal recessive form of inheritance. A more definitive answer must await discovery of further patients with the disorder.

SUMMARY

1 Two disorders of β-alanine metabolism have been identified. One involves free β-alanine catabolism (hyper-β-alaninemia), and the other the degradation of a peptide-bound form of β-alanine (β-alanyl-L-histidinemia, or carnosinemia).

2 Hyper-β-alaninemia has been reported in only one patient. The trait is probably autosomal recessive. The proband was affected from birth with severe depression of the central nervous system punctuated by uncontrollable seizures. He died in his fifth month. Three sibs died in utero or at birth, and it is possible that they also had the disease.

3 This disorder is accompanied by abnormal accumulation of β-alanine and γ-aminobutyric acid in plasma, cerebrospinal fluid, and urine. A deficiency in β-alanine-α-ketoglutarate amino transferase is the presumed enzymatic abnormality.

4 Excretion of the two natural β-amino metabolites, β-aminoisobutyric acid and taurine, is increased. The degree of β-amino aciduria is directly proportional to the plasma concentration of β-alanine. This amino aciduria reflects a combined saturation and competitive inhibition of a tubular transport system, with selective preference for β-amino compounds.

5 Tissue concentrations of β-alanine, γ-aminobutyric acid, and carnosine are elevated. Dipeptide accumulation presumably reflects increased endogenous synthesis in the presence of an expanded free β-alanine pool. The absence of carnosine from the urine distinguishes hyper-β-alaninemia from carnosinemia.

6 Carnosinemia is a rare metabolic error that has been described in two unrelated children. It was associated with a progressive neurologic disorder, myoclonic seizures, and profound mental retardation in both patients.

7 The enzymatic defect in carnosinemia is a deficiency in carnosinase activity in serum. In one of the two patients, carnosinase activity was found in liver and kidney obtained at autopsy.

8 The deficiency in serum carnosinase results in carnosinuria, and it may cause carnosine to rise in fasting plasma as well. Large amounts of carnosine and anserine appear in the urine when foods containing these dipeptides are consumed, but 1-methylhistidine, which is formed by the hydrolysis of anserine, is absent from the urine.

9 No effective therapy is known for either disorder. It is still unproved that either biochemical abnormality causes central nervous system dysfunction. The possibility that hyper-β-alaninemia can be controlled with pyridoxine needs further investigation.

ADDENDUM

Metabolism

β-Alanine transport is not achieved by β-amino-preferring systems in microorganisms. Hechtman and Scriver [79–81] have shown that β-alanine enters *Pseudomonas fluorescens* on an α-alanine permease.

The transport of β-alanine and carnosine by human intestine has been examined in normal subjects [82] and patients with Hartnup disease [83]. Dipeptide absorption is normally slower than for the constituent free amino acids, β-alanine and L-histidine [82]. The rate-limiting step was thought to be intracellular hydrolysis of the accumulated dipeptide in mucosal cells. Dipeptide transport was normal in Hartnup disease [83], which is an inborn error of transport known to affect transport of L-histidine but not of β-alanine.

The metabolism of GABA, which appears to be involved in hyper-β-alaninemia, has taken on new perspectives. Whereas GABA was thought to be limited to the nervous system, it has now been identified in many other tissues [51, 52, 85, 88]. Nonneural GABA appears to be synthesized by a decarboxylase with properties different from that in the CNS. GABA is oxidized to succinate in kidney [86], and this pathway may play a role for glutamate disposal and support of gluconeogenesis in ammoniagenesis [86].

If pyridoxine is truly an effective agent in preventing hyper-β-alaninemia [1], it may act to increase the residual amounts of mutant enzyme protein, which presumably is the apoaminotransferase for β-alanine in this case. Mudd and colleagues [87] have described this mechanism for pyridoxine responsiveness in cystathionine synthase deficiency.

The topic of carnosine and related substances in animal tissues was extensively reviewed in 1970 [89]. The concentration of carnosine in tissue is presented for a wide range of vertebrate species; the relative tissue distribution is also discussed. The possible role of the dipeptide and its derivatives has not yet been clearly defined in any particular circumstance.

New Patients

A Dutch patient with serum carnosinase deficiency has been documented [84]. The new proband was male. Obvious mental and motor retardation at $2\frac{8}{12}$ years and seizures had brought him to attention as early as the first year of life. Carnosinuria was discovered, in association with consistently low serum carnosinase activity. Carnosinase deficiency was proven in a brother at 4 weeks of age. The parents were consanguineous. The authors suggest that the term "carnosinemia" [2] be replaced by "deficiency of serum carnosinase activity coupled with carnosinuria," since their patient did not have carnosinemia. The parents of the proband both had dipeptiduria and modestly decreased serum carnosinase activity. The probability is great that the trait in this family was autosomal recessive. Whether it is the same as that described by Perry et al. [2], and whether it is a condition invariably associated with disease, has yet to be determined.

BIBLIOGRAPHY

1. Scriver, C. R., Pueschel, S., and Davies, E.: Hyper-β-alaninemia associated with β-aminoaciduria and γ-aminobutyricaciduria, somnolence and seizures. New Eng. J. Med., **274,** 636, 1966.
2. Perry, T. L., Hansen, S., Tischler, B., Bunting, R., and Berry, K.: Carnosinemia: a new metabolic disorder associated with neurologic disease and mental defect. New Eng. J. Med., **277,** 1219, 1967.
3. Rosenberg, L. E., and Scriver, C. R.: Amino acid metabolism, in *Duncan's Textbook on Diseases of Metabolism,* 6th ed., edited by P. Bondy, p. 366–515. Saunders, Phila., 1969.
4. Dickinson, J. C., Rosenblum, H., and Hamilton, P. B.: Ion exchange chromatography of the free amino acids in the plasma of the newborn infant. Pediatrics, **36,** 2, 1965.
5. Soupart, P.: Free amino acids of blood and urine in the human, in *Amino Acid Pools: Distribution, Formation and Function of Free Amino Acids,* edited by J. T. Holden, p. 220. Elsevier, Amsterdam, 1962.

5*a*. Roberts, E., and Simonsen, D. G.: Free amino acids in animal tissues, in *Amino Acid Pools: Distribution, Formation and Function of Free Amino Acids,* edited by J. T. Holden, p. 285. Elsevier, Amsterdam, 1962.

6. Hayaishi, O., Nishizuka, Y., Tatibana, M., Takeshita, M., and Kuno, S.: Enzymatic studies on the metabolism of β-alanine. J. Biol. Chem., **236,** 781, 1961.
7. Hechtman, P., and Scriver, C. R.: β-Alanine transport in a catabolically defective mutant of *Pseudomonas fluorescens.* Proc. Canad. Fed. Biol. Soc., **11,** 94, 1968.
8. Roberts, E., and Bregoff, H. M.: Transamination of γ-aminobutyric acid and β-alanine in brain and liver. J. Biol. Chem., **201,** 393, 1953.
9. Schmidt, G., and Cubiles, R.: Comparative studies on occurrence of carnosine-anserine fraction in skeletal muscle and heart. Arch. Biochem. Biophys., **58,** 227, 1955.
10. Reddy, W. J., and Hegsted, D. M.: Measurement and distribution of carnosine in rat. J. Biol. Chem., **237,** 705, 1962.
11. Kalyankar, G. D., and Meister, A.: Enzymatic synthesis of carnosine and related β-alanyl and γ-aminobutyryl peptides. J. Biol. Chem., **234,** 3210, 1959.
12. Stenesh, J. J., and Winnick, T.: Carnosine-anserine synthetase of muscle. 4. Partial purification of the enzyme and further studies of β-alanyl peptide synthesis. Biochem. J., **77,** 575, 1960.
13. McManus, I. R., and Benson, M. S.: Studies on the formation of carnosine and anserine in pectoral muscle of the developing chick. Arch. Biochem. Biophys., **119,** 444, 1967.
14. DuVigneaud, V., and Behrens, O.: Carnosine and anserine. Ergebn. Physiol., **41,** 917, 1939.
15. Davey, C. L.: Significance of carnosine and anserine in striated skeletal muscle. Arch. Biochem. Biophys. **89,** 303, 1960.
16. Davies, E., and Scriver, C. R.: 1-Methylhistidinuria in man: a festive index. Proceedings of the Society for Pediatric Research, N.J., Atlantic City, 1967, p. 134.
17. McManus, I. R.: Enzymatic synthesis of anserine in skeletal muscle by *N*-methylation of carnosine. J. Biol. Chem., **237,** 1207, 1962.
18. McManus, I. R.: Metabolism of anserine and carnosine in normal and vitamin E–deficient rabbits. J. Biol. Chem., **235,** 1398, 1960.
19. Avena, R. M., and Bowen, W. J.: Effects of carnosine and anserine on muscle adenosine triphosphatases. J. Biol. Chem., **244,** 1600, 1969.
20. Report of the Food and Nutrition Board, of the National Academy of Science & National Research Council on Recommended Daily Allowances. 7th rev. ed., Publication 1694, Washington, D.C., 1968.
21. Hanson, H. T., and Smith, E. L.: Carnosinase: enzyme of swine kidney. J. Biol. Chem., **179,** 789, 1949.
22. Rosenberg, A.: Purification and some properties of carnosinase of swine kidney. Arch. Biochem. Biophys., **88,** 83, 1960.
23. Perry, T. L., Hansen, S., and Love, D. L.: Serum-carnosinase deficiency in carnosinaemia. Lancet, **1,** 1229, 1968.
24. Nakai, T., and Tsujigado, N.: β-Alanyl dipeptide preparations from whale muscles made by several workers. J. Biochem., **57,** 812, 1965.
25. Pisano, J. J., Wilson, J. D., Cohen, L., Abraham, D., and Udenfriend, S.: Isolation of γ-aminobutyrylhistidine (homocarnosine) from brain. J. Biol. Chem., **236,** 499, 1961.
26. Abraham, D., Pisano, J. J., and Udenfriend, S.: The distribution of homocarnosine in mammals. Arch. Biochem. Biophys., **99,** 210, 1962.
27. Kanazawa, A., and Sano, I.: Method of determination and its distribution in mammalian tissues. J. Neurochem., **14,** 211, 1967.
28. Hosein, E. A., and Smart, M.: The presence of anserine and carnosine in brain tissue. Canad. J. Biochem. Physiol., **38,** 569, 1960.
29. Tallan, H. H.: A survey of the amino acids and related compounds in nervous tissue, in *Amino Acid Pools: Distribution, Formation and Function of Free Amino Acids,* edited by J. T. Holden, p. 471. Elsevier, Amsterdam, 1962.
30. Nakajima, T., Wolfgram, F., and Clark, W. G.: The isolation of homoanserine from bovine brain. J. Neurochem., **14,** 1107, 1967.
31. Nakajima, T., Kakimoto, Y., Kumon, A., Matsuoka, M., and Sano, I.: α-(γ-Aminobutyryl)-lysine in mammalian brain: its identification and distribution. J. Neurochem., **16,** 417, 1969.
32. Matsuoka, M., Nakajima, T., and Sano, I.: Identification of α-(β-alanyl)-lysine in rabbit muscle, Biochim. Biophys. Acta, **177,** 169, 1969.
33. Westall, R. G.: The amino acids and other ampholytes of urine. 3. Unidentified substances excreted in normal human urine. Biochem. J., **60,** 247, 1955.
34. Block, W. D., Hubbard, R. W., and Steele, B. F.: Excretion of histidine and histidine derivatives by human subjects ingesting protein from different sources. J. Nutr., **85,** 419, 1965.

35. Hubbard, R. W., and Block, W. D.: Urinary excretion of 1-methylhistidine and histidine in human subjects on low and high protein intake. Fed. Proc., **22,** 320, 1963.
36. Butts, J. H., and Fleshler, B.: Anserine, a source of 1-methylhistidine in urine of man. Proc. Soc. Exp. Biol. Med., **118,** 722, 1965.
37. Cusworth, D. C., and Dent, C. E.: Renal clearances of amino acids in normal adults and in patients with aminoaciduria. Biochem. J., **74,** 550, 1960.
38. Scriver, C. R., and Davies, E.: Endogenous renal clearance rates of free amino acids in pre-pubertal children. Pediatrics, **32,** 592, 1965.
39. Palo, J., Saifer, A., and Mazelis, F.: Free amino acids in Tay-Sachs and normal human brain gray matter. Clin. Chim. Acta, **22,** 327, 1968.
40. Perry, T. L., Hansen, S., Stedman, D., and Love, D.: Homocarnosine in human cerebrospinal fluid: an age-dependent phenomenon. J. Neurochem., **15,** 1203, 1968.
41. Perry, T. L., Hansen, S., and MacDougall, L.: Urinary screening tests in the prevention of mental deficiency. Canad. Med. Ass. J., **95,** 89, 1966.
42. Tocci, P. M.: The biochemical diagnosis of metabolic disorders by urinalysis and paper chromatography, in Nyhan, W. L. (ed), *Amino Acid Metabolism and Genetic Variation,* edited by W. L. Nyhan, p. 461. McGraw-Hill, New York, 1967.
43. Perry, T. L., and Jones, R. T.: The amino acid content of human cerebrospinal fluid in normal individuals and in mental defectives. J. Clin. Invest., **40,** 1363, 1961.
44. McArdle, B.: Quantitative estimation of pyruvic and α-oxoglutasic acids by paper chromatography in blood, urine and cerebrospinal fluid. Biochem. J., **66,** 144, 1957.
45. Smith, I., and Smith, M. J.: Keto acids, in *Chromatographic and Electrophoretic Techniques,* edited by I. Smith, vol. I, p. 261. Interscience, New York, 1960.
46. Roberts, E., and Frankel, S.: Glutamic acid decarboxylase in brain. J. Biol. Chem., **188,** 789, 1951.
47. Wingo, W. J., and Awapara, J.: Decarboxylation of L-glutamic acid by brain. J. Biol. Chem., **187,** 267, 1950.
48. Roberts, E. (ed.): *Inhibition of the Nervous System and γ-Aminobutyric Acid.* Pergamon Press, New York, 1960, 591 pp.
49. Roberts, E., Wein, J., and Simonsen, D. G.: γ-Aminobutyric acid (γABA), vitamin B_6 and neuronal function—a speculative synthesis. Vitamins Hormones, **22,** 503, 1964.
50. Elliott, K. A. C.: γ-Aminobutyric acid and other inhibitory substances. Brit. Med. Bull., **21,** 70, 1965.
51. Whelan, D. T., Scriver, C. R., and Mohyuddin, F.: Glutamic acid decarboxylase and gamma-aminobutyric acid in mammalian kidney. Nature **224,** 916, 1969.
52. Scriver, C. R., and Whelan, D. T.: Glutamic acid decarboxylase in mammalian tissue outside the central nervous system, and its possible relevance to hereditary vitamin B_6 dependency with seizures. Proc. N.Y. Acad. Sci., **166,** 83, 1969.
53. Zachmann, M., Tocci, P., and Nyhan, W. L.: The occurrence of γ-aminobutyric acid in human tissues other than brain. J. Biol. Chem., **241,** 1355, 1966.
54. Baxter, C. F., and Roberts, E.: Elevation of γ-aminobutyric acid in brain: selective inhibition of γ-aminobutyric-α-ketoglutaric acid transaminase. J. Biol. Chem., **236,** 3287, 1961.
55. Van Gelder, N. M.: The histochemical demonstration of γ-aminobutyric acid metabolism by reduction of a tetrazolium salt. J. Neurochem., **12,** 231, 1965.
56. Okamura, N., Otsuki, S., and Kameyama, A.: Studies on free amino acids in human brain. J. Biochem. (Tokyo), **47,** 315, 1960.
57. Dent, C. E., and Walshe, J. M.: Amino acid metabolism. Brit. Med. Bull., **10,** 249, 1954.
58. Efron, M. L.: Aminoaciduria. New Eng. J. Med., **272,** 1058 and 1107, 1965.
59. Scriver, C. R.: The use of human genetic variation to study membrane transport of amino acids in kidney. Amer. J. Dis. Child., **117,** 4, 1969.
60. Armstrong, M. D., Yates, K., Kakimoto, Y., Taniguchi, K., and Kappe, T.: Excretion of β-aminoisobutyric acid by man. J. Biol. Chem., **238,** 1447. 1963.
61. Scriver, C. R., Efron, M. L., and Schafer, I. A.: Renal tubular transport of proline, hydroxyproline and glycine in health and in familial hyperprolinemia. J. Clin. Invest., **43,** 374, 1964.
62. Gilbert, J. B., Ku, Y., Rogers, L. L., and Williams, R. L.: The increase in urinary taurine after intraperitoneal administration of amino acids to the mouse. J. Biol. Chem., **235,** 1055, 1960.
63. Wilson, O. H., and Scriver, C. R.: Specificity of transport of neutral and basic amino acids in rat kidney. Amer. J. Physiol., **213,** 185, 1967.
64. Goldman, H., and Scriver, C. R.: A transport system in mammalian kidney with preference for β-amino compounds. Pediat. Res., **1,** 212, 1967.
65. Christensen, H. N.: Relations in the transport of β-alanine and α-amino acids in the Ehrlich cell. J. Biol. Chem., **239,** 3584, 1964.
66. Christensen, H. N.: Reactive sites and biological transport. Advances Protein Chem., **15,** 239, 1960.
67. Krnjević, K.: Action of drugs on single neurones in the cerebral cortex. Brit. Med. Bull., **21,** 10, 1965.
68. Steiner, F. A.: L-Glutamic acid, GABA and pyridoxal-5'-phosphate at single unit level in brain. Proc. N.Y. Acad. Sci., **166,** 199, 1969.
69. Tsukada, Y., Nagata, Y., Hirano, S., and Matsutani, T.: Active transport of amino acids into cerebral cortex slices. J. Neurochem., **10,** 241, 1963.
69*a*. McKhann, G. M., Labers, R. W., Sokoloff, L., Mickelsen, O., and Tower, D. B.: The quantitative significance of the gamma-aminobutyric acid pathway in cerebral oxidative metabolism, in *Inhibitions of the Nervous System and γ-Aminobutyric Acid,* edited by E. Roberts et al., p. 169. Pergamon, London, 1960.
70. Scriver, C. R.: Carnosinaemia. (letter to the editor) Lancet, **1,** 1249, 1968.
70*a*. Allen, R. J., Tourtellotte, W. W., Adriaenssens, K., Lowenthal, A., and Mardens, Y.: (Letter to the Editor). Lancet, **1,** 1249, 1968.
71. Dent, C. E.: A study of the behaviour of some sixty amino acids and other ninhydrin reacting substances on phenol-"collidine" filter paper chromatograms with notes as to the occurrence of some of them in biological fluids. Biochem. J., **43,** 169, 1948.
72. Efron, M. L., Young, D., Moser, H. W., and MacCready, R. A.: A simple chromatographic screening test for the detection of disorders of amino acid metabolism: a technique using blood or urine collected on filter paper. New Eng. J. Med., **270,** 1378, 1964.
73. Scriver, C. R., Davies, E., and Cullen, A. M.: Application of a simple method to the screening of plasma for a variety of aminoacidopathies. Lancet, **2,** 230, 1964.
74. Scriver, C. R.: Vitamin B_6 deficiency and dependency in man. Amer. J. Dis. Child., **113,** 109, 1967.
75. Perry, T. L., Shaw, K. N. F., Walker, D., and Redlich, D.: Urinary excretion of amines in normal children. Pediatrics, **30,** 576, 1962.
76. Bessman, S. P., and Baldwin, R.: Imidazole aminoaciduria in cerebromacular degeneration. Science, **135,** 789, 1962.
77. Levenson, J., Lindahl-Kiessling, K., and Rayner, S.: Carnosine excretion in juvenile amaurotic idiocy. Lancet, **2,** 756, 1964.
78. Tocci, P. M., and Bessman, S. P.: Histidine peptiduria, in *Amino Acid Metabolism and Genetic Variation,* edited by W. L. Nyhan, p. 161. McGraw-Hill, New York, 1967.
79. Hechtman, P., Scriver, C. R., and Middleton, R. B.: Isolation and properties of a β-alanine transaminaseless mutant of *Pseudomonas fluorescens.* J. Bact., **104,** 851, 1970.
80. Hechtman, P., and Scriver, C. R.: Neutral amino acid transport in *Pseudomonas fluorescens.* J. Bact., **104,** 857, 1970.
81. Hechtman, P., and Scriver, C. R.: The isolation and properties of a β-alanine permeaseless mutant of *Pseudomonas fluorescens.* Biochim. Biophys. Acta, **219,** 428, 1970.
82. Asatoor, A. M., Bandoh, J. K., Lant, A. F., Milne, M. D., and Navab, F.: Intestinal absorption of carnosine and its constituent amino acids in man. Gut, **11,** 250, 1970.
83. Navab, F., and Asatoor, A. M.: Studies on intestinal absorption of amino acids and a dipeptide in a case of Hartnup disease. Gut, **11,** 373, 1970.
84. van Heeswijk, P. J., Trijbels, J. M. F., Schretlen, E. D. A. M., van Munster, P. J. J., and Monnens, L. A. H.: A patient with a deficiency of serum-carnosinase activity. Acta Paediat. Scand., **58,** 584, 1969.
85. Haber, B., Kuriyama, K., and Roberts, E.: An anion stimulated L-glutamic acid decarboxylase in non-neural tissues. Occurrence and subcellular localization in mouse kidney and developing chick brain. Biochem. Pharmacol., **19,** 1119, 1970.

86. Whelan, D. T., Scriver, C. R., and Mohyuddin, F.: A gamma aminobutyric acid "shunt" in kidney. Role in acidosis. J. Clin. Invest., **49,** 101A (June), 1970.

87. Mudd, S. H., Edwards, W. A., Loeb, P. M., Brown, M. S., and Laster, L.: Homocystinuria due to cystathionine synthase deficiency: the effect of pyridoxine. J. Clin. Invest., **49,** 1762, 1970.

88. Seiler, von N., und Wiechmann, M.: Zum workommen der γ-amino-buttersäure und der γ-amino-β-hydroxy-buttersäure in tierischen geweb[e]. Hoppe Seyler Z. Physiol. Chem., **350,** 1493, 1969.

89. Crush, K. G.: Carnosine and related substances in animal tissues. Comp. Biochem. Physiol., **34,** 3, 1970.

PART FOUR

DISORDERS CHARACTERIZED BY EVIDENCE OF ABNORMAL LIPID METABOLISM

CHAPTER TWENTY-SIX

FAMILIAL LIPOPROTEIN DEFICIENCY

(Abetalipoproteinemia, Hypobetalipoproteinemia, and Tangier Disease)

Donald S. Fredrickson, Antonio M. Gotto, Robert I. Levy

The plasma lipoproteins conventionally are divided into four families: chylomicrons: very low density or prebetalipoproteins; low density or β-lipoproteins; and high density or α-lipoproteins. In this and succeeding chapters these last three will usually be abbreviated VLDL, LDL, and HDL. All the families are interrelated; they consist of the same lipids in differing proportions complexed with proteins, some of which are also shared by different lipoproteins. The lipoproteins serve different metabolic functions, not all of which are known, and the plasma concentrations of each are subject to some independent controlling mechanisms. These in turn may be affected by one or more mutations.

There are three genetically determined disorders in which one or more of the lipoprotein families are absent from plasma or their concentrations are extremely low. The major manifestations are compared in Table 26-1. The first of these to be discovered was *abetalipoproteinemia,* in which chylomicrons, VLDL, and LDL are missing. This is accompanied by malabsorption of fat and later by severe degenerative changes in the nervous system. Many of the circulating erythrocytes have a thorny appearance (acanthocytosis). The probable inherited defect is one involving synthesis of the major protein moiety of LDL. Another disease is *hypobetalipoproteinemia* (*familial LDL deficiency*), in which no lipoproteins are missing but LDL concentrations are far below normal. Nervous system dysfunction and, possibly, acanthocytes may be present, but usually the patients appear to be well. There may be more than one form of hypobetalipoproteinemia. In one kindred, decreased LDL synthesis appears to be involved. The trait is dominant and is probably unrelated to abetalipoproteinemia. In the third disorder, *familial HDL deficiency* or *Tangier disease,* only a small amount of HDL circulates and this contains an abnormal proportion of the two major HDL apolipoproteins. A defect in the synthesis of one, called here apoHDL-threonine (or apoHDL-thr), is the probable locus affected by this rare mutation. Patients with Tangier disease store cholesteryl esters in most parts of the body and often have neuropathic changes, for reasons that are not understood. Their large orange tonsils form an unforgettable part of the syndrome.

All these diseases are usually detected initially because of a common manifestation, *hypocholesterolemia.* They can be readily differentiated, however, and most easily if one has a basic understanding of the plasma lipoprotein system. This system will be described before the disorders are separately discussed.

THE PLASMA LIPOPROTEINS

The plasma lipoproteins are macromolecular complexes of specific lipids and proteins in relatively fixed proportions. They represent the vehicles whereby water-insoluble lipids are maintained in a stable colloidal form and are transported in the blood. Their high content of lipid makes the lipoproteins lighter than the other plasma proteins, a property which is the basis for the commonly used method of isolation by flotation in salt solutions in the ultracentrifuge. The densities of the plasma lipoproteins, as defined in this discussion, are less than 1.21 gm per ml; the average densities of the other plasma proteins are 1.33 to 1.35 gm per ml. Classification of the plasma lipoproteins has been based mainly on differences in the size and charge of the complexes as defined by their rates of flotation[1] in the ultracentrifuge

[1] The most generally adopted system of ultracentrifugal classification of lipoproteins is based on their rates of flotation at 26°C and at densities of 1.063 and 1.21 gm per ml [1]. Flotation rates are measured in Svedberg units, designated S_f, which may be thought of as negative sedimentation coefficients.

Table 26-1. MANIFESTATIONS OF LIPOPROTEIN DEFICIENCY

Disease	Plasma chol	Plasma TG	Acanthocytes	Retinitis	Neurologic signs	Malabsorption	Abnormal tonsils	Key lipoprotein abnormality
Abetalipoproteinemia	Low	Low	+	+	+	+	0	LDL, VLDL, chylomicrons absent
Hypobetalipoproteinemia	Low	Low or normal	0	0	Rarely	0	0	LDL low
Tangier disease	Low	High, rarely normal	0	0	+ (sometimes absent)	0	+	HDL low and abnormal

Note: LDL, low density lipoproteins; VLDL, very low density lipoproteins; chol, cholesterol; TG, triglycerides; + = present, 0 = absent.

Table 26-2. MAJOR LIPOPROTEIN FAMILIES

Family name	Synonyms	Range of particle size, Å[1]	Electrophoretic definition[2]	Ultracentrifugal definition[3]
Chylomicrons	....	750–10,000	Remain at origin[4]	$D < 0.94$, $S_f > 400$
Very low density lipoproteins (VLDL)	Prebetalipoproteins	300–500	Pre-beta mobility	$0.94 < D < 1.006$, S_f 20–400
Low density lipoproteins (LDL)	β-lipoproteins	200–220	Beta mobility	$1.006 < D < 1.063$[5], S_f 0–20
High density lipoproteins (HDL)	α-lipoproteins	75–100	Alpha$_1$ mobility	$1.063 < D < 1.21$[6]

[1] As determined by electron microscopy.
[2] On paper and agarose-gel electrophoresis.
[3] Expressed as densities in gm/ml and in Svedberg flotation units, S_f, which may be thought of as negative sedimentation units. The S_f values are for a NaCl solution of D 1.063 at 26°C.
[4] On starch-block electrophoresis chylomicrons have alpha$_2$ mobility.
[5] LDL includes the subclasses of D 1.006–1.019 (S_f 12–20) and of D 1.019–1.063 (S_f 0–12).
[6] HDL includes the subclasses HDL_2 (1.063–1.12) and HDL_3 (D 1.12–1.21). It does not float at D 1.063.

[1] or by their electrophoretic mobilities [2]. Four major families of lipoproteins, which are separated by these methods (Tables 26-2 and 26-3), are discussed in the following sections. Many reviews may be consulted for details not provided here [3–6].

Chylomicrons

The largest of the lipoproteins, the chylomicrons, were originally described by Gage as "the free granules of the blood as shown by the dark-field microscope" [7, 8]. His definition was restricted to fat particles of dietary origin; the chylomicrons have subsequently been defined by their particle size (varying from 750 to 12,000 Å in diameter), by their S_f range (400 to 10^5), and by their density (less than 0.95 gm per ml). Chylomicrons do not migrate on paper or agarose-gel electrophoresis, but they move similarly to the very low density lipoproteins (see below) on cellulose acetate and starch block.

Chylomicrons are the most difficult of the lipoprotein families to isolate in an uncontaminated state and cannot be obtained free of other lipoproteins by a single centrifugation in an angle head rotor. Repeated washings introduce the possibility of altering structure and of causing artifacts. It is possible, with the use of a stabilizing density gradient and a swinging bucket rotor, to obtain uncontaminated chylomicrons in a single centrifugation [9].

The chemical composition of a chylomicron particle varies with the size of the particle and the conditions under which it is collected [10]. Chylomicrons from the thoracic duct change rapidly after entering the blood, especially in their fatty acid composition, their electrophoretic mobility, and their susceptibility to flocculation with solutions of poly-

Table 26-3. COMPOSITION OF THE LIPOPROTEIN FAMILIES, INCLUDING APOLIPOPROTEINS, PERCENT OF DRY WEIGHT

	Chylomicrons	VLDL	LDL	HDL
Lipoprotein constituents:				
Protein	1–2	10	25	45–55
Triglyceride	80–95	55–65	10	3–8
Unesterified cholesterol	1–3	10	8	3
Esterified cholesterol	2–4	5	37	15
Phospholipids	3–6	15–20	22	30
Carbohydrate	?	<1	~ 1	<1
Apoprotein constituents:*				
ApoLP-ala	Unknown	Major	Minor	Minor
ApoLP-val	Unknown	Major	Minor, if present	Minor
ApoLP-glu	Unknown	Major	Minor, if present	Minor
ApoLP-ser	Unknown	Major	Major	Absent
ApoLP-thr	Unknown	Minor, if present	Trace, if present	Major
ApoLP-gln	Unknown	Minor, if present	Trace, if present	Major

*The nomenclature used is described in the text. "Major" refers to proteins making up 10 percent or more of the total protein. See the addendum (p. 530) for qualifications about this nomenclature.

vinylpyrrolidine [11, 12]. Average values for the composition of chylomicrons are given in Table 26-3. They contain 80 to 95 percent (by weight) of triglyceride and only 1 to 2 percent of protein [9, 13]. The nature and functions of the protein components have not been elucidated. It has generally been found that if the particles are washed to the extent of reducing their protein content below 1 percent, they become unstable and can no longer be suspended [14, 15]. Evidence for the presence of HDL-protein in chylomicrons has been obtained by the fingerprinting technique [16] and by amino acid analysis [17], while immunologic studies have suggested that chylomicrons contain a protein similar to that in LDL [18].

Very Low Density Lipoproteins

The very low density family of lipoproteins (VLDL) are heterogeneous with respect to size (280 to 750 Å in diameter), density (0.95 to 1.006 gm per ml), and S_f rate (20 to 400). At the lower end of their density range, they overlap with chylomicrons; at the higher end they merge with the low density lipoproteins (LDL). The less-dense particles have relatively more triglyceride and less protein; the particles of higher density have more protein and less triglyceride [19]. VLDL have pre-beta mobility on paper or starch-block electrophoresis. Average values for the composition of VLDL, percent by weight, are triglyceride, 55; phospholipid, 20; cholesterol (about one-third is esterified), 15; and protein, 10 [20].

Apoproteins

The proteins of VLDL have recently been fractionated into four major constituents [21–24] (Table 26-3), although several other components, some possibly minor ones, have been found by Shore and Shore [22]. Oncley has suggested the designation of apolipoprotein, usually shortened to apoprotein, for the lipid-free protein components of the plasma lipoproteins [4]. The recent discovery of multiple proteins, the incomplete state of their characterization, and the possibility that others may yet be found have discouraged the establishment of a system of nomenclature for the apolipoproteins. In this chapter a temporary improvisation will be employed that corresponds to the shorthand designations used in most laboratories today.[2]

[2]The term apoLP for apolipoprotein is followed by the carboxyl-terminal amino acid residue and preceded by the amino-terminal residue, where that is known. If more than one apoprotein has the same carboxyl-terminal group, it is followed by a subscript, e.g., apoLP-ala$_1$, apoLP-ala$_2$. It is sometimes useful to indicate the lipoprotein family from which the apoprotein has been isolated and the species of origin, e.g., H for human, R for rat, etc. By these inventions the first apoprotein isolated from human VLDL which has N-terminal serine and C-terminal alanine is represented as ser-apoVLDL$_H$-ala$_1$ or ser-apoLP$_H$-ala$_1$. The subscripts and the N-terminal acid will frequently be dropped in this chapter.

The four major apoproteins of VLDL that have been isolated and partially characterized are glu-apoLP-ser, thr-apoLP-val, thr-apoLP-glu, and ser-apoLP-ala [21–24]. The first of these proteins, glu-apoLP-ser, appears to be identical with the major protein component of LDL and accounts for about 40 percent of the total protein of VLDL. The other three proteins make up approximately 50 percent of the VLDL protein [23]. Thr-apoLP-val is missing the amino acids tyrosine, histidine, cysteine, and cystine, and has a molecular weight of 7,000 daltons [24]. Thr-apoLP-glu does not contain histidine or cysteine and has a molecular weight of about 10,000 daltons [24]. Ser-apoLP-ala is devoid of isoleucine, cysteine, or cystine, and has a molecular weight of 9,800 daltons [24]. In addition to these four apoproteins, VLDL also may contain minor quantities of the major HDL apoproteins, apoHDL-thr and apoHDL-gln, as judged by immunochemical reactions [21].

Low Density Lipoproteins

By electron microscopy the low density lipoproteins (LDL) appear as homogeneous, spherical particles, 215 to 220 Å in diameter [25–27]. This family is usually defined by its density of 1.006 to 1.063 gm per ml (S_f 0 to 20) and by its beta mobility on electrophoresis. It contains immunochemical determinants distinct from those of the other lipoprotein families. The molecule contains about 75 percent lipid and 25 percent protein by dry weight [28]. Average percentage values for the lipid composition are phospholipid, 28; triglyceride, 13; unesterified cholesterol, 11; and cholesteryl ester, 47 [28]. The apoprotein residue contains about 4 to 5 percent carbohydrate [29, 30]. Ultracentrifugal measurements of the molecular weight are in the range of 2.1 to 2.6×10^6 [31–34].

Electron micrographs, prepared by the technique of negative staining, have recently been interpreted as showing subunit structure in LDL [35]. From an examination of these micrographs, Pollard and colleagues deduced an icosahedral symmetry compatible with a dodecahedral structure [35]. Twenty apoprotein subunits would occupy the apices of the dodecahedron. Phospholipids might occupy the 12 faces, and neutral lipids the central core. Such subunit structure was not noted by previous investigators using negative staining [25–27], and confirmation of this interesting suggestion is awaited.

ApoLDL

The protein moiety of LDL (apoLDL) has a subunit molecular weight that is variously estimated at 26,000 [36]; 27,500 [35]; 36,000 to 38,000 [32]; 42,000 or 64,000 [37]; and 80,000 [38]. The dodecahedral structure of Pollard et al. requires a molecular weight of 27,500 [35]. Since protein constitutes a weight of about 500,000 per gm mole of LDL, it is apparent that there must be a large number of subunits. Evidence has been obtained for nonidentical subunits [22, 36]. The

N-terminal amino acid of LDL is glutamic acid [16, 39–41]. For a number of years, it has been thought that serine is the C-terminal amino acid [41], but in a recent report [22] none could be identified. Although the nomenclature may prove to be inaccurate, the apoprotein of LDL will be called here glu-apoLP-ser, apoLP-ser, or simply apoLDL.

Structure

One of the major hindrances to the characterization of apoLDL is the insolubility of the protein once its complement of lipid is removed. A number of procedures have now been described for the solubilization of apoLDL, including the use of detergents [42, 43], urea or guanidine [36–38], incubation at pH 11.5 [44], and chemical derivatives [26, 32, 37, 45, 46]. When the apoprotein is solubilized with sodium decyl sulfate, the concentration of this detergent may conveniently be reduced to 0.2 to 0.5 mM by dialysis without loss of solubility [43]. ApoLDL prepared in this way has many of the optical and immunologic properties of native LDL, although some changes are detected in the absence of lipids [43, 46–48].

LDL and apoLDL have been found to contain a mixture of different conformations with a relatively high amount of pleated sheet or beta structure [47], in contrast to earlier reports that little or no beta structure was present [49]. The amounts of the various conformations are temperature-dependent, there being relatively more beta structure at higher than at lower temperatures [44, 50].

The High Density Lipoproteins

The high density lipoproteins (HDL) contain relatively more protein (45 to 55 percent by weight) and less lipid (Table 26-3) than any of the other families of the plasma lipoproteins [51]. HDL has α-electrophoretic mobility and floats between densities 1.063 and 1.21 gm per ml in the ultracentrifuge. It is usually subdivided into fractions of density 1.063 to 1.12 (HDL_2) and 1.12 to 1.21 (HDL_3) gm per ml [1]. HDL_3 contains relatively more protein, less total cholesterol, and higher ratios of cholesteryl ester to unesterified cholesterol and phosphatidyl choline to sphingomyelin than does HDL_2 [52]. ApoHDL contains about 3 percent carbohydrate by weight [53–55]. HDL contains antigenic determinants distinct from those of LDL.

Ultrastructural subunits may be seen in HDL_2 and HDL_3 with the electron microscope. In negatively stained preparations the overall particle diameters are 95 Å for HDL_2 and 65 Å for HDL_3 [27]. Subunit structure has been seen in particles of both HDL_2 and HDL_3 [27]. A molecular weight of 386,000 has been reported for HDL_2 [56], and one of 186,000 to 215,000 for HDL_3 [53, 56–58].

ApoHDL

It has been known for a number of years that apoHDL contains N-terminal aspartic acid [16, 39–41] and C-terminal threonine [41]. Recently, with the use of carboxypeptidase, both C-terminal threonine and glutamine have been identified [56, 59, 60]. It appears that the previous failure to demonstrate C-terminal glutamine was due to the formation of the γ-hydrazide of glutamic acid in the hydrazinolysis procedure [41]. ApoLP-thr and apoLP-gln have now been separated and isolated in relatively pure form by chromatography on DEAE-cellulose in 8*M* urea [59, 60]. The former contains N-terminal aspartic acid (asp-apoLP-thr); the latter appears to have a blocked N-terminus unidentifiable by the dansylation procedure [61]. Asp-apoLP-thr contains no cysteine, cystine, or isoleucine; apoLP-gln contains no cysteine, histidine, arginine, or tryptophan but does have cystine [60]. The ratio of asp-apoLP-thr to apoLP-gln in HDL_2 is about 3:1 [62, 63]. The subunit molecular weight of each protein is thought to be 14,000 to 15,000 [59, 60].

Scanu et al. have attempted to fractionate apoHDL by gel filtration in urea [62]. From the amino acid compositions of the fractions obtained it appears that this procedure does not achieve complete separation of the apoproteins. The fractions III and IV of Scanu et al. [62] probably contain primarily apoLP-thr and apoLP-gln, respectively; fraction V is a mixture of the apoproteins of VLDL, except for apoLP-ser.

Though asp-apoLP-thr and apoLP-gln are the principal apoproteins of HDL, they are not the only proteins found in this family of lipoproteins [59, 60, 62–64]. The major apoproteins found in VLDL, except for apoLDL, also occur as minor constituents in HDL [59, 64]. The quantity of the VLDL proteins found in HDL is greatly increased by the intravenous administration of heparin [64]. The normal presence of the VLDL apoproteins in HDL is a feature of significance in certain studies of abetalipoproteinemia, as will be seen presently.

Conformation

On the basis of the parameters observed with polypeptides and proteins of known conformation, the optical rotatory dispersion [65] and circular dichroic [66] spectrums of HDL are consistent with a high content of helical structure. After they have been isolated, and in the absence of urea, the two major apoproteins of HDL—apoLP-gln and asp-apoLP-thr—refold to conformations which differ significantly in their helical content, the latter containing 50 to 60 percent more helical structure than the former [67]. The significance of this difference and whether or not it exists in the native lipoprotein have not been established. These conformational differences in the isolated apoproteins have been confirmed by Scanu, who reports that the reduction and alkylation of apoLP-gln, which contains a disulfide linkage, leads to a further reduction in helicity [68].

Transfer of Apoproteins

When heparin is given in vivo, the so-called postheparin lipolytic activity (PHLA) appears in plasma. PHLA is a heterogeneous collection of enzymatic activities which catalyze the hydrolysis of glycerides in lipoproteins or micellar suspensions. It is specifically stimulated by the addition of apoLP-glu as a cofactor in the presence of phospholipid [69]. Recent evidence suggests at least three different activities, two toward triglycerides and another toward mono- or diglycerides [70–72]. It is now well established that the in vivo action of PHLA results in a decrease in the plasma concentration of VLDL and an increase in HDL [20, 30, 73, 74] and LDL [75]. Plasma concentrations of LDL and HDL are especially low in patients with Type I hyperlipoproteinemia, who have low levels of PHLA activity (see Chap. 28).

LCAT and HDL

Another plasma enzymatic activity which affects the composition of HDL is lecithin:cholesterol acyltransferase (LCAT) [76] (see Chap. 27). This enzyme is functionally related to HDL in that it catalyzes the transfer of an acyl fatty acid residue from phosphatidyl choline to the 3-OH position of unesterified cholesterol bound to HDL. In the inherited deficiency of LCAT, the plasma is practically devoid of esterified cholesterol and concentrations of HDL are extremely low [77, 78]. The interrelationships between LCAT and HDL also may be related to the pleomorphic abnormalities in Tangier disease that will be taken up later.

LCAT may be involved [79] in certain in vitro interconversions in which prolonged incubation of HDL leads to an increase in HDL_2, a decrease in HDL_3, and the production of a lipid-poor protein moiety but with a negligible net loss in lipid [80]. Similar results, not necessarily related to LCAT, have been found after either extraction or dehydration-rehydration [81, 82]. These observations may be relevant to two immunochemical forms of HDL, α-lipoprotein$_A$ and α-lipoprotein$_B$, described some years ago [83]. Each of these occurs in HDL_3, but only α-lipoprotein$_A$ is found in HDL_2. The common denominator of all these phenomena may be a dissociation-association process in which lipid is transferred from asp-apoLP-thr to apoLP-gln and to the apoproteins commonly found in VLDL.

Lipoprotein Reconstitution

Some light has been shed on the forces associating lipid and protein by recombination experiments, especially those involving the reassembly of HDL from its lipid and protein constituents. ApoHDL readily recombines with phospholipid in micellar suspensions or in petroleum ether [84, 85]. In the presence of phospholipid, unesterified cholesterol combines with apoHDL to the extent of 2 to 4 percent by weight, which is about one-half the ratio of cholesterol to protein in HDL [84]. In contrast to phospholipids and cholesterol, the neutral lipids—cholesteryl ester and triglycerides—combine with apoHDL to only a limited extent [84]. The recombination of phospholipid with apoHDL has been found to restore partially the circular dichroic spectrum to that of native HDL and to restore the ability to activate lipoprotein lipase [85]. However, the nuclear magnetic resonance spectrum of the recombined complex of apoHDL and phospholipid suggests a looser structure than in HDL [86], and the temperature dependence of the circular dichroism of the complex more closely resembles that of apoHDL than HDL [87]. Furthermore, the electron paramagnetic resonance spectrum of spin-labeled apoHDL differs in no way from the spectrum after recombination with phospholipid [88].

With the use of sonic energy it has been possible to effect the recombination of apoHDL with cholesteryl ester and triglyceride as well as phospholipids [87, 89]. Minor components produced by the procedure either floated at a density of 1.063 (apoLP-gln and the major apoproteins of VLDL) or sedimented at 1.21 gm per ml (asp-apoLP-thr). The circular dichroism of the major reconstituted lipoprotein had the same temperature stability as in native HDL [87]. The electron paramagnetic resonance spectrum of HDL, spin-labeled in its protein moiety, may be restored by sonication of the spin-labeled apoprotein in the presence of either HDL-lipids or both phospholipid and cholesteryl ester [90]. Triglyceride but not free cholesterol can replace the requirement for cholesteryl ester. Thus, with the use of sonication it is possible to solubilize neutral lipids with apoHDL and phospholipids, restoring a chemical composition and stability approximating that of the native lipoprotein. Similar experiments have not been done with LDL or other lipoproteins.

Sites of Origin of Plasma Lipoproteins

The chylomicrons originate in the intestinal mucosa to transport the glycerides which have been reassembled there after the digestion and absorption of fat. Most of the fatty acids come from the diet, but some are contributed by phospholipids in the bile [91, 92]. At least in certain pathologic states (see Type III hyperlipoproteinemia, Chap. 28), not all large particles having the behavior of chylomicrons necessarily arise in the intestine, and some of the dietary glycerides appear soon after absorption in particles of the density and electrophoretic behavior of VLDL [93].

The VLDL family transports triglyceride that has been synthesized endogenously. The major site of VLDL synthesis is the liver [94–97], but it has recently been shown in the rat that the intestine also produces VLDL [98–100]. From the Golgi apparatus of rat liver, particles of 300 to 1,000 Å in diameter have been isolated that have electron microscopic appearance and immunologic and chemical properties similar to those of circulating VLDL [101]. Lipoproteins isolated from the Golgi apparatus of the rat appear to contain apoproteins identical to VLDL apoproteins from rat plasma or liver perfusate [102]. Thus the very low density lipoproteins from these three sources contain the same major apoproteins, and it is concluded that this lipoprotein family is stored in the Golgi apparatus prior to its release into plasma. It is not known whether the lipoprotein is assembled at these sites or whether it is modified there by the addition of carbohydrate.

The origin of LDL remains an important and unanswered question. It is likely that LDL comes primarily from the liver. It is currently considered that much of the LDL may come from the metabolism of VLDL, i.e., after the removal of much of the glyceride and all the apoproteins except for apoLP-ser.

HDL synthesis is primarily independent of LDL, although it may occur in the same organs, the liver most probably being the principal site. The turnover of cholesteryl esters is much more rapid in HDL than in LDL [103]. This may be related to activity of the LCAT enzyme, and it has been suggested that lipid-poor HDL may emerge from the liver to be lipidated shortly thereafter in plasma (Chap. 27). The previously mentioned transfer of VLDL apoproteins to HDL while VLDL is being cleared indicates that a quantitatively small but significant portion of total circulating HDL comes from this source. The same is probably true of chylomicron metabolism. There are marked differences in the degree to which lipolysis and many other factors influence the respective concentrations of the HDL_2 and HDL_3 subclasses [75, 104]. The mechanisms underlying these changes will become clearer when more is known of the structure of HDL and its subfractions.

Recognition and Quantification of Lipoproteins

The methods of measuring plasma lipids and lipoproteins, as well as the usual concentrations, are described in detail in Chap. 28. The genetic deficiency states are frequently detected because of a low plasma cholesterol concentration (usually below 120 mg per 100 ml); triglyceride concentrations help to distinguish among various forms of hypocholesterolemia. A presumptive diagnosis can be made by the combination of the low lipid determinations and lipoprotein electrophoresis. It is also desirable to determine HDL by a simple precipitation technique [105] and to estimate LDL concentrations (see Chap. 28) in the instance of hypobetalipoproteinemia. Neither preparative nor analytic ultracentrifugal separation of the lipoproteins is essential for diagnosis, and, as will be seen, such separation can even be misleading.

Immunochemistry

The final diagnoses of abetalipoproteinemia and Tangier disease rest on immunochemical tests. The lipoproteins, especially LDL, are fairly powerful antigens. The major antigenic determinants reside in the apolipoproteins, and both the lipids and carbohydrate moieties are considered to be haptenes. Antiserums made to native LDL, for example, permit detection of some minor antigenic determinant not revealed by antiserums made to apoLDL [48]. Specific antiserums have been made in this and other laboratories to five of the six apolipoproteins shown in Fig. 26-3. One must be careful with commercial antiserums, for often they are not specific for a single lipoprotein species and contain antibodies to albumin and other plasma proteins; they should always be checked by examination for multiple precipitin reactions on immunoelectrophoresis against whole serum and, when possible, against different lipoprotein fractions. It is particularly important to remember that antiLDL serums react with VLDL and chylomicrons as well as with LDL, and that VLDL and HDL also share certain apoproteins and hence some antigenic determinants. The application of immunochemical methods for qualitative and quantitative measurement of lipoproteins has been described elsewhere [106, 107].

Genetic Polymorphism of LDL (see Chap. 69)

Among the lipoprotein families genetic polymorphism has thus far been described only for LDL. The first polymorphic form of LDL described was called the Ag antigen [108]. Antibodies to Ag were found in patients who had received multiple blood transfusions, especially in thalassemic patients. Antibodies specific for Ag have not been produced in animals, and there is no available information about the structural basis of this variant. A second polymorphic form has been called the Lp system [109]. The Lp antigen readily produces antibodies when injected into rabbits. Average densities of 1.064 to <1.12 have been reported for the lipoproteins carrying this determinant [110]. Other investigators [111] have found that the lipoprotein carrier may have a density as low as 1.040. In straddling the density boundary between LDL and HDL, the lipoprotein carrier resembles HDL_1, which forms a tail on the ultracentrifugal Schlieren pattern of some serums in the upper density range of LDL [1]. Recent structural studies have shown both similarities and differences between the apoprotein of the Lp determinant and apoLDL [112]. When antiserums to Lp antigen are absorbed with LDL or with apoLDL, they no longer form precipitin lines with these antigens but do continue to show activity with the Lp lipoprotein [111]. A frequency of 0.33 has been found for the Lp antigen in Caucasian populations [113]. However, it has now been found that the Lp antigen—Lp(a^+)—can be detected in the serums (11 out of 11) of individuals classified as Lp(a^-) [114]. This demonstration required a 120-fold concentration of the Lp(a^-) serums. The Lp lipoprotein was also shown to be present in these concentrated serums by immunoelectrophoresis and analytic ultracentrifugation.

The Lp antigen has recently been found [111] to be the same as "sinking pre-beta" [111, 115], a fraction of pre-beta-migrating lipoproteins that sediment rather than float at density 1.006 [115]. All the 10 percent of subjects with sinking pre-beta are also Lp(a+) [111]. Antiserums made to sinking pre-beta, which do not react with LDL, and antiserums to Lp antigen, form precipitin lines of identity when tested against Lp(a+) plasma [111]. The Lp(a+) determinants with the presence of sinking pre-beta are inherited as an autosomal dominant trait.

ABETALIPOPROTEINEMIA

Synonyms. Bassen-Kornzweig syndrome, acanthocytosis, congenital absence of β-lipoprotein or LDL, or familial low density or β-lipoprotein deficiency.

This rare disorder has five basic features: abetalipoproteinemia, malabsorption of fat, acanthocytosis, retinitis pigmentosa, and ataxic neuropathic disease. Abetalipoproteinemia [116] (ABL) is the preferred name. Several of the above synonyms under which it has been reported are inexact. Acanthocytosis [117] may occur in other diseases, in which lipoproteins are not deficient. In abetalipoproteinemia, LDL is absent, not merely deficient; the misconception concerning this point arose from the finding in the ultracentrifuge of lipoproteins which had the density but not the composition of LDL.

History

In 1950 Bassen and Kornzweig reported an 18-year-old girl who had a new syndrome featuring retinitis pigmentosa, ataxic neuropathic disease, and circulating erythrocytes that seemed to be crenated [118]. The younger brother who was similarly affected, was described later in detail by the same authors [123]. The second patient in the literature was described by Singer, Fisher, and Perlstein, under the name *acanthrocytosis* [119]. The important observation of hypocholesterolemia in this boy was first reported in 1958 by Jampel and Falls [120]. Druez then reported a case from Belgium [117] and suggested that the correct term for the deformed erythrocytes in the disease was *acanthocytosis.* In 1960 Salt et al. [116] demonstrated the absence of LDL from serum in an English child with apparently the identical syndrome. This important observation was made independently in the same year by Lamy et al. [121] and by Mabry, Di George, and Auerbach [122]. At the same time the unique changes in the small intestine and absence of plasma chylomicrons were reported [116, 122]. There are no less than 28 known examples of abetalipoproteinemia (Table 26-4). Nineteen of them were collected in the comprehensive surveys of Farquhar and Ways [128] and Kahlke [142]. One patient [143] listed in the latter review has been shown to have a different disorder [144, 145]. Four of the patients in

Table 26-4. SUMMARY OF PATIENTS WITH ABETALIPOPROTEINEMIA

Case no.	Patient	Sex	Ethnic origin	Year of birth	Reference
1 } Sibs	R.Kl.	F	Jewish	1932	[118]
2 } Sibs	L.Za.	M	Jewish	1938	[123]
3	....	M	Jewish	1938	[119]
4	R.C.	F	French	1927	[117]
5	C.S.	F	English	1958	[116]
6	N.S.	M	Jewish	1923	[124]
7	G.F.	M	French	1953	[121]
8 } Sibs	C.R.	F	Negro	1947	[122]
9 } Sibs	M.R.	M	Negro	1950	[125]
10	A.Co.	M	Jewish	1956	[126]
11	R.B.	M	Jewish	1956	[127]
12 } Sibs	J.V.	M	Italian	1953	[128, 128*a*]
13 } Sibs	A.V.	F	Italian	1957	[128]
14	M.S.	M	Jewish	1954	[129]
15	R.Is.	M	Italian	1953	[130]
16	A.L.	M	Scottish	1956	[131]
17	J.G.	M	American	1957	[128, 152]
18	A.E.	F	White, non-Jewish	1926	[132]
19	J.M.	M	Maori	1962	[133]
20 } Sibs	S.Sm.	F	Negro	1953	[134]
21 } Sibs	M.Sm.	M	Negro	1956	[134]
22	P.B.	M		1965	[135]
23	B.C.	F	American	1937	[136]
24	P.B.	M	......	1963	[137]
25	....	M	Dutch	1951	[138, 139]
26	....	M	British	ca. 1965	[140]
27	....	M	British	ca. 1967	[140]
28	R.H.	M	Caucasian, American, non-Jewish	1952	[141]

Table 26-4 have died (Nos. 2, 12, 18, 19). The excellent review of Farquhar and Ways appearing in the previous edition of this book [128] is incorporated into this chapter. Several other extensive reviews of abetalipoproteinemia are available [130, 142, 146, 147].

Clinical and Laboratory Findings

The first abnormalities to be noticed are likely to be steatorrhea and abdominal distension developing during infancy in a child who appeared normal at birth. Weight gain and growth are thereafter retarded. Presumably the plasma lipid and lipoprotein abnormalities are present at birth, and this may also be true of the acanthocytosis. Between the ages of 5 and 10, atypical retinitis pigmentosa and a neurologic picture resembling Friedreich's ataxia develop. Disability becomes progressively severe; death has occurred both in early childhood and as late as the age of 37 [132], but little is known of the course after the third decade.

Malabsorption of Fat

Moderate or severe steatorrhea occurs in early infancy, even before gluten has become part of the diet. The frequent, loose, pale, and bulky stools may be accompanied by vomiting and abdominal distension. By the fourth or fifth year of life, the steatorrhea becomes less marked. This is partly because of conditioned avoidance of fat intake; it is also possible that a pathway for transport of fatty acids from the gut to the liver through the portal vein, usually used only for short-chain fatty acids, becomes adapted to the handling of longer-chain fatty acids [128].

A barium meal gives the same roentgenogram of dilated intestine as seen in celiac disease [147] and cystic fibrosis of the pancreas; however the contents of the intestinal lumen, unlike the contents in celiac disease, also include normal amounts of bile acids and enzymes [116, 124, 128, 130]. Fat-balance studies indicate that 70 to 80 percent of ingested fat has been absorbed [116, 128].

Jejunal biopsy reveals a pathognomonic mucosal abnormality (Fig. 26-1). The mucosa is of normal thickness, and the villi are of normal shape and length and are readily distinguished, for example, from the atrophic villi of celiac disease. If the diet has contained long-chain glycerides within the previous 10 to 14 days, many droplets are visible throughout the cytoplasm of the mucosal cells, especially at the villous tips. Conventional stains indicate that these droplets contain lipid [150, 151], and chemical determinations affirm that most of it is triglyceride [128, 152]. Except in the intestinal lumen, there are no lipid *droplets* outside the mucosal cells, i.e., there are none in the intracellular spaces, in the villous cores, or in the lacteals [128, 153]. If all fat is removed from the diet, excess lipid may remain in the villous tips for more than a month [152]. Electron micrographs reveal none of the abnormalities of the cellular organelles seen in celiac disease [149, 154].

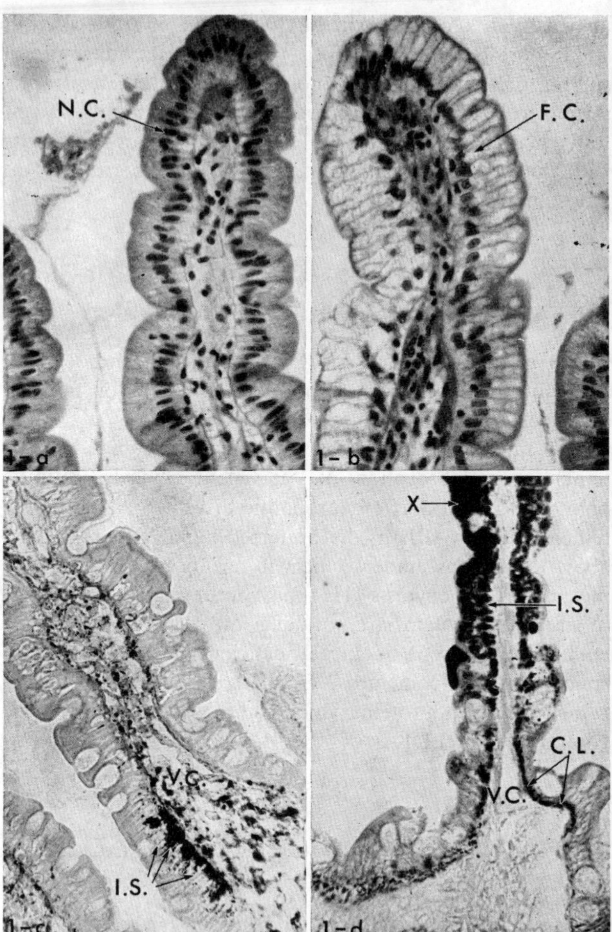

Figure 26-1. Photomicrographs of small-intestinal epithelial villi obtained by peroral biopsy. The upper figures are stained with hematoxylin-eosin. (*From Ways et al.* [148].) The lower figures are stained with oil-red-O. (*From Ahrens et al.* [149].) A. Upper villous tip from a normal subject. The cytoplasm of all the villous lining cells (*N.C.*) are of a homogeneous gray density. (×300.) B. Upper villous tip from a subject with abetalipoproteinemia. Note that the cytoplasm of every intestinal epithelial cell appears foamy and vacuolated (*F.C.*). This abnormal appearance is caused by the presence of abundant amounts of unstained lipid (see below). C. Middle and lower portions of villi from a normal subject. Lipid is generously distributed throughout the villous core (*V.C.*) and may be seen not only within some of the epithelial cells but indistinctly in some of the intercellular spaces (*I.S.*). Evidence for the precise location of lipid in these intercellular spaces comes from electron micrographs. (*From Ahrens et al.* [149].) D. Middle and lower portions of villi from a subject with abetalipoproteinemia. Note increasing amounts of lipid as the tip of a villus is approached (the tip, not shown, contained cells more heavily stained than those marked ×). In the region toward the base of the villus, where the epithelial cells are only partly filled with lipid, no lipid is seen in the intercellular spaces. Also, lipid in cells closest to the base of the villus (*C.L.*) appears abnormally concentrated toward the villous core. Finally, also in contrast to the normal (Fig. 26-1c), no lipid is present in the villous core (*Photographs from Farquhar and Ways* [128].)

The distinctive changes in abetalipoproteinemia are consistent with normal digestion and assimilation of fats into the intestinal mucosa and a defect in their removal from this site. Chylomicrons never appear in the plasma of the patient with abetalipoproteinemia [116, 135, 155]. There are conflicting published reports concerning the absorption of long-chain fatty acids in abetalipoproteinemia. It is well established that there is no increase in plasma triglyceride following a fatty meal [146, 152, 156, 157]. A transfusion with LDL-rich plasma does not lead to an increase in fat absorption [156, 158] in abetalipoproteinemia. In separate studies, neither fed isotopically labeled long-chain fatty acids [128], nor trimargarin (containing margaric acid, C 17:0) [146] could be detected in the plasma of patients. Though there is no net increase in plasma triglycerides following fat feeding in abetalipoproteinemia, there is considerable evidence that linoleic acid is absorbed [121, 152, 157] and that it is incorporated initially into plasma nonesterified fatty acids and subsequently into cholesteryl esters [157]. Some of the apparent discrepancies regarding fat absorption may be related to the composition of the fat that is fed. This is consonant with observations that polyunsaturated fats, specifically linoleic acid, are more efficiently absorbed than saturated fatty acids in both abetalipoproteinemic [121, 159] and normal persons [160].

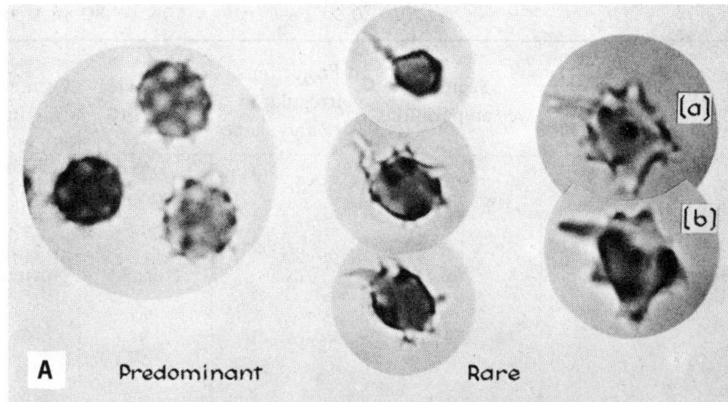

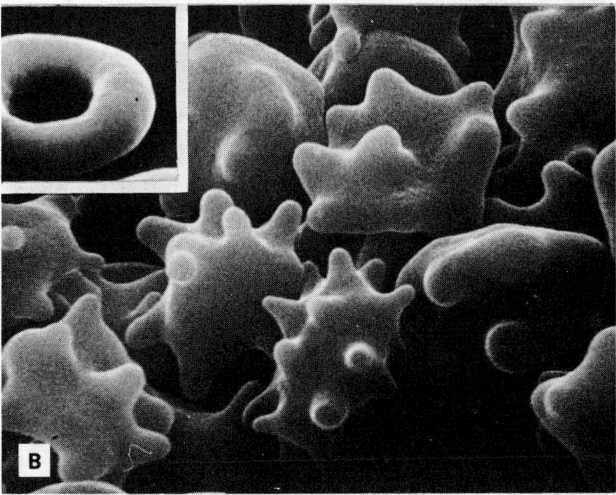

Figure 26-2. A. Light micrograph of examples of the *predominant* and the *rare* types of red blood cells found in fresh "wet" blood smears from patients with abetalipoproteinemia. On the far right, *a* and *b* are photographs of the same cell in different planes of focus. While all the cells may be termed *acanthocytes,* the "rare" cells (*center* and *right*) possess the long extending tentacles which distinguish acanthocytes from crenated erythrocytes present in other conditions or as artifacts (see text). (×200.) (*From Farquhar and Ways* [128].) B. Acanthocytes in abetalipoproteinemia as seen by the scanning electron microscope. A normal erythrocyte is seen in the insert (*upper left*). (×5,000.) (*Photographs supplied by Dr. Herbert Kayden and reprinted from Kayden and Bessis* [160a] *with permission of the authors and publishers.*)

Erythrocytes

Acanthocytes have been reported in patients as young as 17 months of age [116]. Most frequently they appear as crenated spheres with spiny excrescences (Fig. 26-2). Acanthocytes are compared with other abnormal erythrocytes in Table 26-5. Farquhar and Ways [128] have emphasized that rare cells with long tentacles found in the blood of patients with abetalipoproteinemia are most helpful in differentiating true acanthocytes from crenated cells which may occur in azotemia, in gastric cancer [161], or in blood from normal subjects after the cells have been washed with isotonic saline solution [162, 163] or exposed to traces of fatty acids [163].

A wet preparation of fresh blood suspended in Dacie's solution [164] is recommended for best visualization of the red blood cell defect [128]. The acanthocytes do not form rouleaux, and the sedimentation rate is low [116, 164]. Osmotic fragility is normal or slightly decreased; mechanical fragility is increased [147].

The average red blood cell is normal in size and is usually normochromic. The hemoglobin concentration is also usually normal, although anemia has been described [116–119]. A review of possible causes for anemia in the reported cases [128] does not indicate a common mechanism. Folic acid deficiency secondary to malabsorption of fat is one possible cause [116, 119]. There are reports of decreased red blood cell survival [126, 165], reticulocytosis [117, 126, 128, 130, 166], and hemolytic crises [128]. The Coombs' test is not positive; and other hemolytic antibodies [118, 119, 126, 166], abnormal hemoglobins [117, 126, 159, 166], or erythrocyte enzyme deficiencies [126, 166] have not been found. The bone marrow may be normal or may show some erythroid hyperplasia [117–119, 126, 128, 166]. Acanthocytes are not seen in the marrow. The leukocytes and platelets are normal.

Retinitis

Vision and retinal appearance are normal in early childhood; abnormalities usually are not seen until after adolescence. The deterioration of a normal-appearing retina has been observed between the ages of 13 and 19 years in one patient [119, 120] and in another between 18 months and 6 years of age [116, 167]. In the latter patient the first abnormalities were fine bluish pigment granules in the macular region.

Table 26-5. A COMPARISON OF SOME MORPHOLOGIC ABNORMALITIES IN ERYTHROCYTES

Type of cell	Seen in wet preparations	Projections irregular in size and shape	Mechanical fragility	Osmotic fragility	Sensitivity to lysolecithin	Autohemolysis	Condition associated with	Present in high proportion of cells
Acanthocytes	Yes	No	↑	Normal or ↓	↑	↑	Abetalipoproteinemia, neurologic disease with normal LDL	Yes, 50–100% in abetalipoproteinemia
Burr cells	Yes	Yes	Normal	Normal	Normal	Normal	Azotemia (BUN > 175), gastric carcinoma, bleeding peptic ulcer, microangiopathic anemia	No, accompanied by crescent- and helmet-shaped cells
Crenated red blood cells	No	No	....	....	....	Rapid	Rapid drying or preparation of smears in hyperosmotic solutions	
Spur cells	Yes	..	....	....			Hemolytic anemia, alcoholic cirrhosis	

Similar granules then appeared at the extreme periphery, along with minute, bright colloid bodies similar to those seen in retinitis punctata albescens [167]. At this time visual acuity and electroretinogram were normal, but rod function during dark adaptation was diminished.

By adolescence or early adulthood it is probable that all patients have some decrease in visual acuity, visual field defects, night blindness, and pigmentary degeneration of the retina, including the macular region. Lenticular opacities, "choroiditis" [124], ophthalmoplegia, and ptosis may also be present [124, 130]. The virtual absence of plasma carotenoids [118, 126, 128–130] and the usually low concentrations of vitamin A [167] may be related to the visual defect, although this assumption has not been proved. In one 6-year-old patient it was possible to maintain normal plasma levels of vitamin A by giving high oral doses of the vitamin [167]. However, maintenance of this therapy for 3 years did not prevent the onset of retinal deterioration. It was shown in this patient that β-carotene was converted to vitamin A, [168].

Neuromuscular Abnormalities

Diminished tendon reflexes are probably the earliest neurologic sign of abetalipoproteinemia, and these have been detected in the second year of life [133]. An accompanying decrease in position and vibratory sense is common and more pronounced in the lower extremities. The earliest symptom is unsteadiness in walking [130]. The manifestations developing between ages 2 and 17 years compiled from reports of 10 patients by Schwartz et al. [130], in order of their frequency, were areflexia, proprioceptive deficit, cerebellar signs (ataxia of gait, trunk, and extremities, with titubation and dysarthria), muscle weakness, kyphoscoliosis, ophthalmoparesis, Babinski's sign, and cutaneous sensory loss. Diminished pain and temperature sense has been reported in a few patients [128]. Thus there appears to be degeneration of the posterior and lateral columns of the spinal cord, the spinocerebellar pathways, and also of some peripheral nerves.

Muscular weakness may be severe in one affected sib, and the muscles may be quite normal in another [130]. There may or may not be muscle wasting; true fasciculations have not been reported. The pes cavus deformities of the feet, kyphoscoliosis, and other changes in posture and gait conceivably are all of neural origin; there is as yet no clear evidence for either primary skeletal or myopathic origin. Electromyographic findings have been normal in two patients [128, 130], and the result of a muscle biopsy was normal in one [130]. The neuromuscular changes are slowly progressive but in the adult the neuromuscular condition may remain apparently static for many years [124]. The ability to walk unassisted declines, and most patients are unable to stand by their thirtieth year [128]. Scoliosis may become so severe that spinal fixation is necessary.

Cerebral abnormalities are not definitely a part of abetalipoproteinemia. The intellectual status of the patients may be perfectly normal. Sluggish responses may be secondary to dysarthria rather than to intellectual impairment. Mental retardation has been reported in at least five patients [142]. Forsyth et al. [131] observed that this association occurred only when parental consanguinity was also noted.

Other Clinical Abnormalities

Dyspnea may be present. It is possibly related to decreased respiratory exchange due to thoracic and spinal abnormalities, but may have a cardiovascular origin. Cardiac enlargement with premature ventricular contractions and evidence of congestive heart failure preceded the death of one adult [132]. The second patient in the literature (No. 2 in Table 26-4) [123] had some cardiac enlargement [169]. He died suddenly at age 27; cardiac arrhythmia was suspected of being the cause of death [170]. Patient 4 (Table 26-4) had a cardiac arrhythmia [117], and Patient 12, a 10-year-old boy, may well have died from an arrhythmia [171]. In the latter child, the onset of palpitations was noted approximately 1 month before death. An electrocardiogram showed multifocal ventricular premature beats. It is perhaps noteworthy that the association of cardiac disturbances and spinocerebellar ataxia is common to both abetalipoproteinemia and Friedreich's ataxia. Extensive fibrosis of the ventricles and cardiomegaly may occur in Friedreich's ataxia [172], and major cardiac disease has been reported in 55 percent of patients with this disorder [173].

Lipids and Lipoproteins

Lipids

Plasma lipids in six examples are shown in Table 26-6. The plasma cholesterol concentration does not exceed 80 mg per 100 ml and is likely to be not higher than 50. This is accompanied by lower concentrations of triglycerides than are seen in any other disease. These are less than 20 mg per 100 ml, or below the limits of accurate detection. The total phospholipid concentration is also low, i.e., 100 mg per 100 ml or less. Both the phospholipid partition and the fatty acid composition of the plasma lipids are abnormal and are frequently reflected in similar abnormalities in erythrocytes and adipose tissue. Most prominent among these alterations are a decrease in the concentration of linoleic acid and a decrease in the ratio of phosphatidyl choline to sphingomyelin. The decrease in linoleic acid affects all plasma lipid fractions, including cholesteryl esters, phosphatidyl choline [151, 174], triglycerides [157], and nonesterified fatty acids [157]. There may be an increased proportion of palmitic, palmitoleic, and oleic acids [151, 174]. It is likely that these changes reflect a decrease in fat absorption and an increase in lipogenesis. The proportion of arachidonic acid is normal [157, 174]. One group has reported the presence of eicosatrienoic acid (C_{20}:3) [174], but others have failed to find this substance [157]. The percentage of the total phospholipid in sphingomyelin is 30 to 50, compared to 15 to 25 in the phospholipids of normal subjects [128]. The percentage of phosphatidyl choline is correspondingly decreased.

Table 26-6. PLASMA LIPIDS IN ABETALIPOPROTEINEMIA

Patients' no.	Age	Sex	C	Plasma PL	TG
1	37	F	52	83	2
2	26	M	72	96	10
10	23	M	46	76	10
15	12	M	35		2
20	9	F	54		2
21	7	M	50		1
Normal	1–19	M	120–230	155–265	10–140

Note: *C*, cholesterol; *PL*, phospholipids; *TG*, triglycerides. Patients are numbered as in Table 26-4. Values from patients are derived from Levy, Fredrickson, and Laster [155]; the control data are derived from sources identified in Chap. 28.

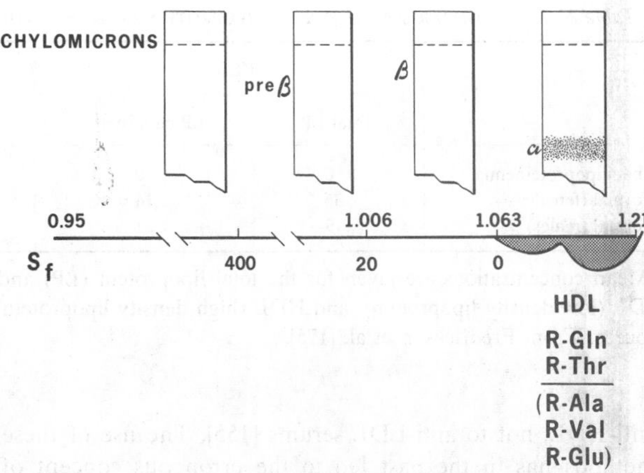

Figure 26-3. Schematic representation of plasma lipoproteins in abetalipoproteinemia as seen by the analytic ultracentrifuge and paper electrophoresis (*top*). Note that only HDL or α-lipoproteins are present. The apolipoproteins known to be present are shown at the bottom right. Ultracentrifuge data from Fredrickson et al. [175] may be compared with normal values in Fig. 28-1.

Lipoproteins

The extreme hypolipidemia is also qualitatively unique when translated into lipoprotein patterns as obtained by various methods. The abnormalities seen upon analytic ultracentrifugation and electrophoresis are shown in Fig. 26-3. With electrophoresis on paper, starch, agarose, cellulose acetate, or other media, no β-lipoproteins, prebetalipoproteins (or α_2-lipoproteins), or chylomicrons are present. Only α-lipoprotein is visible. In the analytic ultracentrifuge no lipoproteins of $S_f > 0$ are detectable. The HDL profile is also remarkable for its pronounced two-component concentration curve with a shift in the mean flotation rate of HDL to somewhat higher values than normal. Total HDL is low, and its lipid content reflects the same abnormalities seen in the total plasma lipids [174]. In addition to these changes, a decrease in the percentage of esterified cholesterol in HDL has been noted [174]. Since the normal pathway for synthesis of plasma cholesteryl ester involves the LCAT reaction [76] (see Chap. 27), a reduced concentration of the substrate phosphatidyl choline could possibly lead to a reduction in the extent of cholesterol esterification.

In the preparative ultracentrifuge (Table 26-7), there are sometimes small amounts of lipoproteins floating at a density of less than 1.063, the cutoff point usually employed for separating HDL from LDL. This "LDL" [155, 174] is immunochemically indistinguishable from normal HDL [155]. The total amount of HDL is usually below normal [155, 174, 175]. There are no lipoproteins of a density less than 1.006 [155].

When dextran, heparin-Mn^{++}, or other precipitation methods are used, a small amount of lipid is usually precipitated and sometimes interpreted as LDL. The material precipitated by heparin, however, contains reactivity only to

Table 26-7. A COMPARISON OF PLASMA LIPOPROTEIN CONCENTRATIONS,* MG PER 100 ML, IN ABETALIPOPROTEINEMIA AND NORMAL SUBJECTS

	VLDL		*LDL*		*HDL*	
	Total LP	LP cholesterol	Total LP	LP cholesterol	Total LP	LP cholesterol
Abetalipoproteinemia	0	0	0	1	145	37
Normal (females)	36	14	323	130	437	62
Normal (males)	119	21	409	128	275	49

*Mean concentrations are given for the total lipoprotein (LP) and for the total cholesterol of the VLDL (very low density lipoprotein), LDL (low density lipoprotein), and HDL (high density lipoprotein) families.
Source: From Fredrickson et al. [175].

anti-HDL, not to anti-LDL serums [155]. The use of these methods has in the past led to the erroneous concept of deficiency rather than absence of normal LDL in abetalipoproteinemia.

Immunochemical Methods

Even when serums from patients with abetalipoproteinemia are concentrated five- to tenfold, no material is found reacting to antiserums made to LDL, when tested by Ouchterlony plates (Fig. 26-4) or immunoelectrophoresis [155] (see also "Search for apoLDL," below).

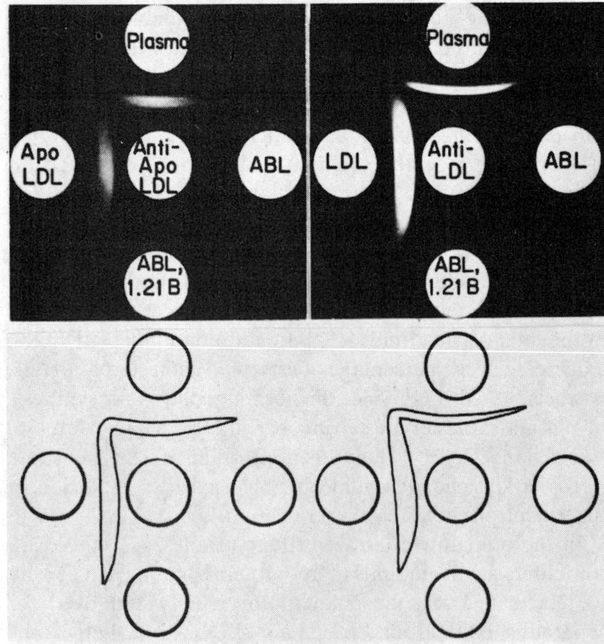

Figure 26-4. Immunochemical evidence that neither LDL (*right panel*) nor apoLDL (*left panel*) is detected in plasma in abetalipoproteinemia. Wells contain normal plasma (*top*), abetalipoproteinemia (ABL) plasma, and the infranatant layer after ultracentrifugation at density 1.21 ("1.21 B"), and the normal lipoprotein (LDL) or delipidated apoprotein (apoLDL). The antiserums in the center wells are to LDL or apoLDL.

Other Findings

Postheparin lipolytic activity (PHLA) is reduced in abetalipoproteinemia to ranges seen in Type I hyperlipoproteinemia or examples of severe malabsorption [157, 176, 177]. This deficiency could be a secondary consequence of fat malabsorption [178]. Although one patient had generalized aminoaciduria with normal amino acid concentrations in plasma [133], urinary amino acids have been normal in others [128, 130]. Patient 19 (Table 26-4) also had moderate azotemia, again not reported in others. A variety of other laboratory tests have been performed. None has demonstrated other consistent or specific abnormalities.

The Probable Defect

The Apolipoproteins

The primary defect in abetalipoproteinemia is most likely to be found among the lipoprotein apoproteins. In this regard, several of the points discussed in connection with lipoprotein structure deserve reemphasis. (1) One family of lipoproteins may utilize more than one carrier protein. (2) Different lipoprotein families may share in common certain protein carriers. (3) ApoLDL probably occurs in all the three lipoprotein families that are absent in abetalipoproteinemia and certainly is a major constituent of VLDL and LDL. Some obvious questions arise from these considerations. Is apoLDL (apoLP-ser) synthesized, and, if so, is it possibly abnormal? Are the three other major apolipoproteins associated with apoLP-ser in the transport of triglyceride in VLDL also missing? These apolipoproteins normally are also present as minor constituents in HDL (Table 26-3). For this reason and because the high density lipoproteins in this disease seem to be abnormal, the HDL apoproteins have been scrutinized. Finally, it has been suggested that the apoprotein of LDL circulates in a lipid-free state both in abetalipoproteinemia and in the normal state [135]; this possibility has been the subject of recent investigations.

Search for ApoLDL (ApoLP-ser)

The intriguing idea that an apolipoprotein may be present in blood devoid of its usual complement of lipid originated from the observation by Roheim and coworkers that the release of lipoprotein, mostly VLDL, could be effected by the perfusion of rat liver with the plasma fraction of density > 1.21 gm per ml [179]. Later, Lees suggested that the apoLDL of the 1.21 infranatant fraction (density > 1.21) may have an altered conformation or structure that in some way makes it similar to azo and acetyl derivatives of LDL prepared in the laboratory [135]. This suggestion is made partly because of the production of antibodies to these derivatives when the human density > 1.21 fraction is injected into rabbits. However, the density > 1.21 fraction from normal subjects or patients with abetalipoproteinemia does not elicit antibodies which form precipitin lines with soluble apoLDL [48]. Also antibodies to LDL and apoLDL do not form precipitin lines with the density > 1.21 fraction from normal subjects or patients with abetalipoproteinemia [48] (Fig. 26-4). Wilson and Lees have recently reported the purification from normal subjects of an apoLP from the density > 1.21 fraction [180]. The purified fraction reacts with antiserums to delipidated VLDL but not with antiserums to LDL and HDL. Therefore, while some apoproteins normally may occur in a form that is heavier than the density of conventional lipoproteins (density > 1.21), there is as yet no convincing evidence for the occurrence of lipid-free apoLDL.

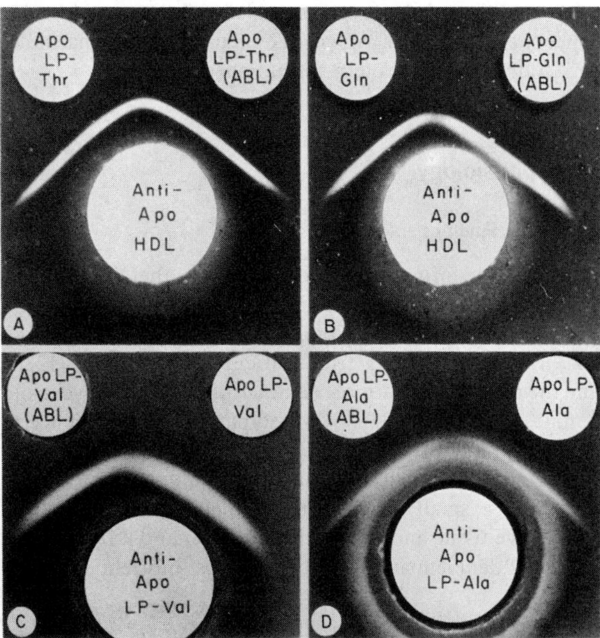

Figure 26-5. Evidence that apoLP-thr, -gln, -val, and -ala are isolable from abetalipoproteinemia plasma (ABL) and are apparently immunochemically identical with their normal counterparts. No antiserum was available for the fifth apoprotein, apoLP-glu, but it also has been tentatively identified as present. (Reprinted from [181] with permission of the authors and publishers.)

Presence of Other Apoproteins

Gotto et al. have examined the lipoprotein fraction (density < 1.21) from four patients with abetalipoproteinemia [181]. The lipoproteins were delipidated and examined with polyacrylamide-gel electrophoresis. The major protein components of VLDL (except for glu-apoLP-ser) and of HDL were identified [181]. From one patient, the three VLDL proteins—thr-apoLP-val, thr-apoLP-glu, and ser-apoLP-ala—were then isolated by a combination of gel-filtration and ion-exchange chromatography and were shown to be identical with their counterparts from normal VLDL (Fig. 26-5). The two major proteins of HDL (asp-apoLP-thr and apoLP-gln) were likewise isolated from abetalipoproteinemia plasma. They appear to be indistinguishable from their counterparts in normal plasma. Therefore, of the six plasma apolipoproteins that are consistently present in normal plasma, only apoLP-ser is apparently absent in abetalipoproteinemia.

The Selective Absence of ApoLDL

It is conceivable that LDL enters plasma in the form of VLDL and, possibly, chylomicrons. The evidence for this is presently confined to the rat liver, where the preformed very low density lipoproteins in the Golgi apparatus [182–184] appear to contain apoLDL [102]. Presumably this protein forms the protein moiety of LDL that is eventually derived from the processes of degradation and clearance of VLDL from plasma.

The weight of present evidence is toward the complete absence of apoLDL (apoLP-ser) from abetalipoproteinemia plasma. The other major VLDL apoproteins are present, although it is not known how they appear in plasma in the apparent absence of secretion of VLDL. Final proof of the selective absence of apoLDL in abetalipoproteinemia will need to include examination of both hepatic and intestinal cells for apoLP-ser and a demonstration that this protein can be detected in normal human tissues. Neither of these facts has been established.

For the present, the most likely genetic defect in abetalipoproteinemia is one deleting all synthesis of apoLDL. It is probable that a single amino acid substitution in this protein would neither affect its lipid-carrying capacity nor prevent its immunologic recognition as a cross-reacting material (CRM). Other possibilities remain. A glycopeptide has been isolated from apoLDL [185], and the essentiality of the glycoside chain for both the function and antigenicity of the apoprotein remains to be established. It is also conceivable that some process of assembly of apoLDL into lipoproteins is the locus of the defect. Finally, it has not been excluded that the primary defect lies in some other aspect of intracellular triglyceride metabolism and has nothing to do with lipoprotein formation per se.

Pathophysiology

Pathologic Findings

The available information about tissues in abetalipoproteinemia is limited to that obtained from three patients and consists of a sural nerve biopsy in Patient 2 (Table 26-4) [123, 130], autopsy data from Patient 12 (Fig. 26-6) [128*a*], and the published post-mortem description of the 37-year-old female, Patient 18 [132]. All three patients had evidence of neurologic impairment in life, and all had pathologic findings in nervous tissues. The sural nerve biopsy from Patient 2 showed a small increase in the quantity of endoneural connective tissue and of sheath cell nuclei and a remarkable degree of demyelination [130]. In the post-mortem examination of Patient 18, the brain and spinal cord were found to be grossly normal, but there was extensive demyelination of the anterior columns, spinocerebellar tract, and cerebellum, as well as focal demyelination of peripheral neurons [132]. There was an accompanying loss of nuclei of the cerebellar and anterior horn cells. Extensive macular atrophy of the retina was also present. Examination of the nervous tissues of Patient 12 was significant in the finding of large quantities of lipochrome pigment in the poles of neurons in the cerebral cortex (Fig. 26-6).

Both Patients 12 and 18 had electrocardiographic evidence of cardiac dysfunction, with ventricular premature beats. Patient 12 was thought to have died from an arrhythmia; Patient 18 developed florid congestive heart failure, with orthopnea, paroxysmal nocturnal dyspnea, and ankle edema. The latter patient died after treatment with diuretics and digitalis, and a digitalis-induced arrhythmia was suspected as the terminal event. On microscopic examination no evidence of myocarditis was found in Patient 18, and the coronary vessels appeared normal. The only positive finding in

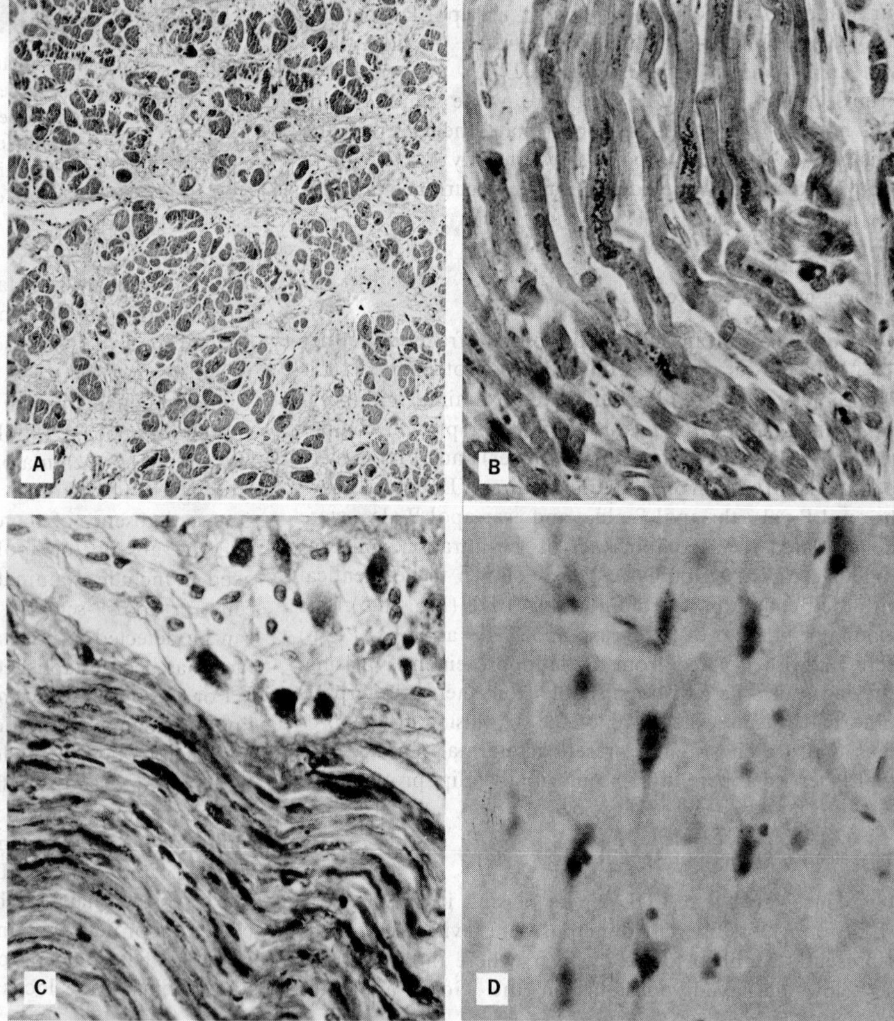

Figure 26-6. Pathologic changes in abetalipoproteinemia. A. Interstitial replacement fibrosis of left ventricular myocardium. (Hematoxylin and eosin stain ×100.) B. Coarse lipofuscin granules in core regions of ventricular myocardial fibers. (Acid-fast stain, ×400.) C. Clumps of ceroid pigment in smooth muscle of jejunum. Note involvement of ganglion cells in Meissner's submucosal plexus. (Periodic acid–Schiff stain, ×400.) D. Fine granules of ceroid pigment in neurons of cerebral cortex. (Oil-red-O stain, ×400.)

The establishment of inclusions as being either lipofuscin or ceroid is based on reactions obtained with PAS and other histochemical stains as well as the presence of autofluorescence under ultraviolet light. (*Photographs supplied by Dr. Philip Grimley, National Institutes of Health. The patient material was supplied by Dr. M. Erlandson, The New York Hospital.*) This patient (No. 12 in Table 26-4) is the subject of an autopsy report by Dische and Porro [128a].

the heart was an organizing mural thrombus in the left ventricle. In Patient 12, however, extensive replacement of myocardial tissue by fibrosis was seen in the myocardium (Fig. 26-6). In addition, a large quantity of lipochrome (ceroid) pigment was deposited in the myocardium, particularly in the atria. No mention was made of involvement of the conduction system in these two patients.

Functional Disturbances in Fat Transport

Whatever the altered mechanism in abetalipoproteinemia, there is a complete blockade of the normal means of removing long-chain glycerides from cells. Chylomicrons never enter the plasma, and net transport of endogenous glycerides in VLDL appears to be either absent or sustained at some unchanging minimum level. Heavy feeding of carbohydrate for days, which promotes a brisk rise in level of plasma glycerides and VLDL in patients with Tangier disease and in nearly all other subjects, fails to do so in patients with abetalipoproteinemia [155]. Detection of excess triglyceride in the liver in one patient [146] supports the concept that this lipid is available in the liver but cannot be secreted. In animals, inhibitors of protein synthesis block chylomicron formation and cause changes in the intestinal mucosa similar to those seen in abetalipoproteinemia [186]. These findings support the possibility that the defect in triglyceride formation may be due to apoprotein deficiency. On the other hand, intravenous infusion of plasma LDL, combined with oral fat ingestion, has not led to chylomicronemia or to increased plasma triglycerides in two patients [156, 159]. There is no evidence, however, that the infused LDL ever reaches the respective intracellular sites of chylomicron and VLDL synthesis, viz., the intestinal mucosal and hepatic cells. Recent animal studies with fluorescent antibodies suggest that the protein moiety of LDL remains extracellular in atherosclerotic plaques [187].

Changes in Erythrocyte and Neuronal Membranes

A cogent explanation is lacking for the acanthocytes and functional changes in neurons that occur in abetalipoproteinemia. There has been considerable speculation about the possibilities of (1) a defect in a protein common to intestine, liver, erythrocytes, and LDL; (2) a defect in phospholipid synthesis underlying changes in the structure of erythrocyte membranes, neuronal membranes, and lipoproteins; or (3) essential fatty acid deficiency arising from malabsorption of fat. Biochemical evidence permitting discussion of these possibilities is limited to the red blood cells. The erythrocyte abnormality is confined to circulating cells.

Possible Changes in the Erythrocyte

The cells contain relatively less phosphatidyl choline and more sphingomyelin but about the same total amounts of phospholipid as normal cells [129, 188]. The sterol content of the acanthocytes in abetalipoproteinemia has been reported to be normal [128] or elevated [189]. Red blood cells from patients with acanthocytosis and normal LDL also may have increased cholesterol [145, 190]. McBride and Jacob [189] have also described acanthocytosis and hemolytic anemia in a fat-deprived infant who had 20 percent of the normal level of LDL and in rats made abetalipoproteinemic by treatment with 1 percent orotic acid. In the orotic acid–treated rats, the erythrocytes progressed from normal concave cells to target cells to acanthocytes over a period of a month. Osmotic fragility and ^{51}Cr survival both decreased. The only detected abnormality of erythrocyte lipid was a 20 to 50 percent increase in the concentration of cholesterol. Identical changes were described after excessive cholesterol had been fed to rabbits [189]. In both orotic acid-fed rats and in human beings with abetalipoproteinemia, a 30 percent decrease in the efflux of ^{14}C-cholesterol from erythrocytes was observed. The incubation of rat erythrocytes in normal plasma restored the normal osmotic fragility and cholesterol content [189]. McBride and Jacob speculated that excessive cholesterol in the red blood cell membrane led to an increase in surface area and the appearance of thorny excrescences, and that the increased cholesterol was itself secondary to a deficiency of LDL.

This interesting explanation of acanthocytosis must still contend with some discordant evidence. One is the finding in LCAT deficiency (Chap. 27) of a marked increase in the concentration of unesterified cholesterol in both plasma and erythrocytes associated with target cells and hemolytic anemia, but not with acanthocytosis. The value of the acanthocyte for illuminating a possible function of LDL is also lessened by the occurrence of acanthocytes in some patients with normal concentrations of LDL; e.g., in alcoholic cirrhosis with hemolytic anemia [190], and in a pyruvate kinase deficiency with anemia [146]. Moreover, severe hypobetalipoproteinemia occurs without acanthocytosis (see below). Conversely, acanthocytes and varying degrees of neurologic impairment may occur with normal plasma LDL concentrations [144, 145].

Possible Effects of the Plasma Milieu

It has been inferred that the rigid, thorny excrescences on the red blood cells may be related to the nature of the plasma milieu rather than to an intrinsic cellular abnormality. The erythrocytes in abetalipoproteinemia can be returned to a normal shape by in vitro incubation in plasma or some other milieu containing surface-active agents [191], or in vivo by the intravenous injection of an emulsion of cottonseed oil [192]. More recently, partial or complete conversion of acanthocytes to a normal shape has been described after incubation in a 5 percent solution of albumin, or at pH 5.8 in buffer, or after treatment with cationic or nonionic detergents [128]. The nonionic detergents were required in higher concentrations and were effective only if they contained unsaturated long-chain fatty acids.

The findings of both a normal phospholipid content and ratio of phosphatidyl choline to sphingomyelin in the plasma of some patients with abetalipoproteinemia [130, 188] make it difficult to attach pivotal importance to the phospholipid changes that do occur. Nor can acanthocytosis be explained by a relative deficiency of known essential fatty acids, particularly linoleic acid, since this substance may be decreased in malabsorption syndromes or hemolytic anemias [193, 194] without the concomitant occurrence of acanthocytosis. Severe deficiency of essential fatty acids in the rat is also not accompanied by acanthocytosis or by a decrease in the phosphatidyl choline to sphingomyelin ratio of red blood cells [195]. The $C_{20}:3$ acid (eicosatrienoic) that characteristically accompanies deficiency of essential fatty acids in animals has been detected in some patients with abetalipoproteinemia whose fat intake was severely restricted [174]; it has not been observed in all patients [146, 157].

In summary, the mechanism of acanthocyte formation in abetalipoproteinemia remains unclear. Such formation cannot be clearly attributed to the altered lipid content of plasma or the cells themselves. One feels that it is more likely that LDL itself or some essential ingredient transported by LDL (or by chylomicrons and VLDL, since all are missing in this disorder) is the common link between structural changes in red blood cells and both structural and functional abnormalities in neural tissues. It may also be that changes in different tissues are brought about by inadequate transport of several different factors resulting from one defect. Two such factors that must be considered are vitamins A and E.

Vitamin A

Vitamin A is derived both from preformed vitamin in the diet and from the conversion of β-carotene in the intestine. Plasma levels of this vitamin may be quite low in abetalipoproteinemia. Vitamin A is transported in plasma complexed to a specific retinol binding protein [196, 197]. Plasma levels of this protein in abetalipoproteinemia are reduced to the same extent as the levels of vitamin A [198]. The carotenoid precursor of vitamin A circulates bound to lipoproteins, mainly LDL [199]. It is not likely that deficient carotenoid transport in abetalipoproteinemia is responsible for the low plasma concentrations of vitamin A; these are more probably related to malabsorption. It is not possible at this time to relate the altered levels of vitamin A to the retinopathy that occurs in abetalipoproteinemia. Many patients with retinitis pigmentosa have normal plasma vitamin A levels.

Vitamin E

Vitamin E (or α-tocopherol, its major active form) contains a substituted phenol that reacts with free radicals, making the substance a potent antioxidant. It also contains a long-chain fatty acid that imparts lipid solubility, and it has been established that vitamin E is normally transported in plasma in association with LDL [200]. The lowest plasma concentrations of the vitamin have been reported in abetalipoproteinemia [201]. When the erythrocytes from vitamin E–deficient rats or from vitamin E–deficient patients with abetalipoproteinemia are exposed to hydrogen peroxide, there is an increase in the quantity of substances that react with 2-thiobarbituric acid, presumably peroxides [202]. There is also a decrease in the content of polyunsaturated fatty acids, including linoleic acid, and of the phospholipids, phosphatidyl ethanolamine and phosphatidyl serine. Polyunsaturated fatty acids are much more susceptible than saturated acids to autoxidation [203]. Of the red blood cell phospholipids, phosphatidyl ethanolamine is the least stable to peroxidation, owing to its high content of polyunsaturated acids [204]. The susceptibility of the abetalipoproteinemic red blood cells to peroxidative hemolysis was reversed by treatment with vitamin E [202].

A deficiency of vitamin E is thus germane to the pathophysiology of abetalipoproteinemia. The primary changes in plasma and red blood cells in this disorder are decreased concentrations of linoleic acid, absolute decreases in the concentration of phosphatidyl choline, and a decrease in the ratio of phosphatidyl choline to sphingomyelin. These changes may all be produced by vitamin E deficiency and a consequent peroxidation of polyunsaturated fatty acids. In abetalipoproteinemia, however, the phosphatidyl ethanolamine content is usually less severely depressed than that of phosphatidyl choline. It has been observed that administration of vitamin E to patients with abetalipoproteinemia restored resistance to peroxidative hemolysis, but it did not correct the abnormalities of lipid distribution [202].

Of more pertinence is the possible relationship between vitamin E deficiency and the disease of the central nervous system and heart. The central nervous system appears particularly susceptible to peroxidation, owing to the low levels of glutathione peroxidase and catalase in this tissue [205]. Neurologic lesions may be experimentally produced in animals by vitamin E deficiency [206–208]. The large deposits of lipochrome or ceroid pigment demonstrated in the cerebral cortex and myocardium of Patient 12 are consistent with peroxidative changes. A deficiency of vitamin E is thought to play a key role in the accumulation of ceroid [209, 210], which is a highly insoluble pigment formed by the polymerization of oxidized unsaturated fats and containing both lipid and protein. Its exact pathologic role is uncertain. It has been thought to be related to the aging process and appears to be associated with free radical formation [211]. Defective vitamin E transport therefore is a possible common denominator of pleomorphic changes attendant upon abetalipoproteinemia.

Genetics

In the 24 families listed in Table 26-4, more than one sib was affected in 4. Seventy-one percent of the patients were males. Consanguinity was present in at least 7 of 18 of the affected families. About half of the known cases have occurred in Jews, but various ethnic groups, including blacks and the Maoris, have been affected.

Many of the parents and other first-degree relatives of patients with abetalipoproteinemia have been examined. Only Salt et al. [116] concluded that the parents of one patient had somewhat decreased β-lipoprotein. All the other relatives have normal concentrations of lipoprotein. Other manifestations of the disorder, including acanthocytosis, have been absent in relatives except for affected sibs. Lipids and fatty acid components of red blood cells and plasma have been normal.

If we assume that all 28 known patients have an identical mutation, the most likely mode of transmission is that of an autosomal defect nearly always requiring double dosage of the allele for detectable expression. The presumed heterozygotes for abetalipoproteinemia are not now detectable by any marker except parenthood of a child with abetalipoproteinemia. A gene frequency of 0.005 percent, or 1 in 20,000, has been calculated from the frequency of first-cousin parents of affected children [128]. A reduced but detectable level of the involved protein cannot be demonstrated in abetalipoproteinemia as it can in most protein or enzymatic defects on a genetic basis. This finding in all patients studied, taken in conjunction with the characteristic recurrent clinical features, permits the assumption that all examples of "abetalipoproteinemia" probably represent the same mutation.

Diagnosis

Abetalipoproteinemia should be considered in any patient with one of the following abnormalities: severe malabsorption of fat, retinitis pigmentosa or other macular degeneration, unexplained neurologic abnormalities resembling Friedreich's ataxia and including ataxic neuropathy, or acanthocytosis. The possibility of dysglobulinemia, producing antibodies to LDL, should also be kept in mind. The single most important laboratory test for screening is the plasma cholesterol determination. The finding of a subnormal value, as defined in Chap. 28, particularly any concentration below 100 mg per 100 ml, should be followed by a triglyceride determination and lipoprotein electrophoresis. The definitive diagnosis depends on immunochemical demonstration of the absence of LDL.

Treatment

During the first few years of life the major problem in management is to maintain adequate nutrition in a child who has a poor tolerance of fats. As the patient gets older, fat tolerance improves, but the acceptance of more than 10 percent of calories as fat is unusual until the patient passes adolescence. Some patients prefer many small feedings, and those who have tried medium-chain-length triglycerides (MCT) have generally found them palatable. No harmful effects of MCT, which is absorbed by way of the portal vein and is metabolized by the liver, have been discovered.

One of the more exciting findings of the past several years with regard to abetalipoproteinemia is the apparent reversal of some of the changes in macular degeneration or retinitis pigmentosa by vitamin A administration. This has been observed by National Eye Institute ophthalmologists working with a patient of Dr. Leonard Laster [170], and subsequently in Patient 15 when he was under the care of Fredrickson, Gotto, and Levy. A single parenteral dose of vitamin A (50,000 units) or larger amounts given orally appear subjectively to improve dark adaptation. Wolff et al. [167] obtained evidence in a long-term study with one patient that the administration of vitamin A did not prevent the development of retinitis. Maintenance therapy with vitamin A has not yet been established as an essential part of treatment for abetalipoproteinemia. Consideration should be given to supplementary administration of both vitamins A and E.

Two attempts to improve fat absorption by short-term infusion of plasma or LDL did not succeed in clearly altering fat absorption [156, 158].

As the patients become older, muscular and skeletal deformities become the major problem for most of them, and much care and understanding are necessary to assist them in adapting to progressive, severe disability.

HYPOBETALIPOPROTEINEMIA (Familial Low Density Lipoprotein Deficiency)

Apparently unrelated to abetalipoproteinemia is another genetic disorder, or group of similar ones, in which plasma LDL concentrations are roughly one-tenth of normal. Four affected families, a Dutch, a French, and two American, have been described. In one of these a single patient had central nervous system abnormalities and malabsorption, possibly akin to the changes accompanying the absence of LDL seen in abetalipoproteinemia. Hypobetalipoproteinemia is inherited as an autosomal dominant trait. As determined in one kindred, the defect is likely to be one of abnormal limitation on the rate of synthesis of LDL.

History

In 1966 van Buchem et al. described an asymptomatic 46-year-old Dutch male with hypobetalipoproteinemia discovered during a community screening of cholesterol levels [212]. The patient was repeatedly found to have low cholesterol concentrations (70 to 80 mg per 100 ml) associated with marked reduction in concentrations of LDL (β-lipoproteins), to about 10 percent of normal. Two of the patient's three healthy brothers also had hypocholesterolemia (plasma concentrations of 126 and 109 mg per 100 ml, respectively). Apparently because the two children of the propositus had normal cholesterol and lipoprotein concentrations the authors concluded that the deficiency of LDL was inherited as a Mendelian recessive trait. In 1969 Mars and coworkers in Cleveland reported a second family with genetic β-lipoprotein deficiency [213]. The propositus, a 37-year-old female, had a progressive demyelinating central nervous system disorder of adult onset. As in van Buchem's patients and in contrast to those with abetalipoproteinemia, the patient had detectable LDL (10 percent of normal). Eleven of 30 immediate blood relatives, including two brothers and all four of her children, had hypobetalipoproteinemia, and were asymptomatic. Mars et al. concluded that hypobetalipoproteinemia was a dominant trait.

The third family in the literature is that reported by Richet and colleagues in Paris [214]. The propositus, a 15-year-old boy, was initially examined because of proteinuria. His cholesterol concentration was 70 mg per 100 ml, and the triglyceride level was 45 mg per 100 ml. Three of his sibs, the mother, and a maternal aunt also had hypocholesterolemia; LDL was demonstrated in the plasma of each by immunoelectrophoresis and was shown to be deficient in several by ultracentrifugal analyses. The proteinuria in the propositus remained unexplained; all the other relatives had no other abnormalities.

Levy, Langer, Gotto, and Fredrickson have recently studied a fourth kindred with apparently the same disorder [215]. The propositus, a 30-year-old asymptomatic male, was referred to them because of persistently low plasma cholesterol concentrations. Intensive examinations revealed no associated hematologic, gastrointestinal, or neurologic abnormalities. His mother, his maternal aunt, and her son were similarly affected. Turnover studies in several members indicated a decreased synthesis of plasma LDL.

Clinical and Laboratory Findings

Disease-related Findings

No clinical abnormalities have been consistently found in all the patients with hypobetalipoproteinemia. In fact, most of the patients seem otherwise healthy. If we assume that any specific disability observed should resemble the abnormalities seen when LDL is completely absent (abetalipoproteinemia), then only the propositus of the second reported kindred has been so affected [213]. At the age of 36 years she developed progressive weakness, clumsiness, and dysesthesia in the lower extremities. Her gait was ataxic, there was objective weakness in the left leg, and she had an extensor plantar response and positive Hoffmann's and Chaddock's signs. No sensory deficiencies were present. Her retinas appeared normal, and there was no organomegaly. Biopsy material from the sural nerve was normal when examined by light microscopy. With the electron microscope some suggestion of localized delipidation of the myelin sheath was observed [213]. It may be pertinent that the neurologic symptoms in this patient began several years after her fourth child was born, and that her mother died of congestive heart failure at age 38 during her fifth pregnancy, having had an earlier history of difficulty in walking. She and several relatives also appeared to be relatively unresponsive to local anesthetics.

Malabsorption

An aversion to dietary fat has been noted in one kindred with hypobetalipoproteinemia [213]. The propositi of Kindreds 1, 2, and 4 were specifically shown to absorb test loads of fat, following which chylomicrons appeared transiently in plasma. A jejunal biopsy in the propositus of Kindred 2 after a 12-hr fast contained many droplets of fat beneath the lamina propria and within capillary endothelial cells; no pinocytotic vesicles were seen in a specimen taken after a 40-hr fast [213]. The jejunal biopsy in the propositus of Kindred 1 was unremarkable [212]. If there is any malabsorption of fat in hypobetalipoproteinemia it is minimal and difficult to ascertain.

Probably Unrelated Abnormalities

Three of the four propositi have had other disease or abnormalities that do not form any obvious pattern. The 46-year-old propositus of Kindred 1 had an earlier history of lymphadenopathy. He had slight splenomegaly, extensive pulmonary fibrosis, and probable hilar adenopathy as seen on a roentgenogram, a compensated hemolytic anemia with a positive Coombs' test, and scattered, fine, shiny dots on both optic fundi. The second propositus, the 36-year-old woman with evidence of a demyelinating process, had earlier had cholelithiasis. She also had a systolic murmur and for about 9 years prior to her neurologic symptoms had had paroxysmal atrial fibrillation. The propositus of Kindred 3, age 15, was first seen because of proteinuria [214]. Extensive examination failed to disclose a pathologic cause for this condition. The propositus of the fourth kindred was completely healthy and was discovered after a routine cholesterol determination.

Laboratory Findings

Plasma Lipids and Lipoproteins

The ranges of plasma lipids in the affected members of the four kindreds are given in Table 26-8. It is important to note that the plasma cholesterol concentrations (ranging from 55 to 146 mg per 100 ml) are occasionally as low as those seen in abetalipoproteinemia. The percentage of cholesterol esterified is normal. The triglyceride levels may be well within normal range, but sometimes are at the lower limits of accurate measurement. The phospholipid concentrations have varied from 110 to 170 mg per 100 ml and are usually

Table 26-8. RESULTS OF LABORATORY TESTS IN PATIENTS WITH HYPOBETALIPOPROTEINEMIA*

Kindred and ref.	Plasma concentrations				Acanthocytes	Vitamins A and E
	Cholesterol, mg/100 ml	Triglycerides, mg/100 ml	HDL	LDL		
1 [212]	70–126	25–44	Normal	Low	No	Low normal
2 [213]	55–146	25–106	Normal	Low	No	Borderline low
3 [214]	70–140	20–125	....	Low	No	Normal
4 [215]	75–140	20–140	Normal	Low	No	Low normal

*Includes propositi and affected relatives.
Note: LDL, low density lipoproteins; HDL, high density lipoproteins.

on the low-normal borderline in most patients. The ratio of sphingomyelin to phosphatidyl choline in plasma was considered to be slightly increased in one kindred [212] but was normal in another [213]. Vitamin A and E concentrations are normal or low but if low are not decreased to the level seen in abetalipoproteinemia.

Fatty Acid Composition

In the propositus and several affected relatives in Kindred 1, the fatty acids in the cholesteryl esters of plasma were deficient in relative content of linoleic acid [212]. The relative content of linoleic acid was also decreased in the phospholipids of the erythrocytes of the propositus but not in the total phospholipids of plasma. Linoleic acid was modestly decreased in plasma lipids in the propositus of Kindred 2 [213]. It is possible that these changes are related to the diet selected by the patients, particularly since members of Kindred 2 had an expressed aversion for fats. It should also be emphasized that the changes are relatively small and, in fact, are on the borderline of low-normal values reported by others [157]. The changes are only a small fraction of those seen in abetalipoproteinemia.

Lipoproteins

A faint β-lipoprotein band is visible on electrophoresis. HDL concentrations, as measured by precipitation, or in the preparative ultracentrifuge, or the analytic ultracentrifuge (Chap. 28), are normal. VLDL or prebetalipoproteins are usually modestly reduced in quantity but are present. Some persistence of a chylomicron band was observed in several members of Kindred 4 in samples obtained overnight after intake of high-fat meals on the preceding day. On a regular diet, chylomicrons are not present in the usual postabsorptive specimen.

LDL is present in immunoprecipitin tests based on immunodiffusion or immunoelectrophoresis. Titers have suggested concentrations of LDL that are one-eighth to one-sixteenth of normal, levels that are consistent with chemical or optical measurements of LDL concentrations. A variety of antiserums have failed to indicate any cross-reacting material suggestive of two populations of LDL, one altered in terms of antigenic determinants. In Kindred 4, lines of identity between the patients' LDL and normal LDL were obtained with 12 different specific antiserums.

Chemical Studies of LDL

LDL and its apoprotein moiety were isolated and studied from the propositus and an affected relative of Kindred 4. The lipid and protein composition of LDL were entirely normal, as reported by others [213], including the ratio of esterified cholesterol. The isolated apoprotein moiety was soluble at low concentration of detergent (0.5 mM sodium decyl sulfate; see earlier) and was indistinguishable from normal apoLDL in its circular dichroic spectrum, its amino acid composition, and its immunologic properties. When tested with antiserums to LDL or to apoLDL, the soluble apoprotein formed precipitin lines of complete identity with normal apoLDL.

Acanthocytes

The propositus of Kindred 2 had some poikilocytosis, and her cells became acanthocytes when added to tissue culture medium [213]. The abnormal appearance was corrected by the addition of hypercholesterolemic serum or triglyceride emulsions. Irregularities in the red blood cell ghosts of this patient were seen with the electron microscope. In neither this patient nor in any other patient with hypobetalipoproteinemia have acanthocytes been observed on repeated blood smears.

Other Hematologic Tests

The propositus of the Dutch kindred had splenomegaly and evidence of intravascular hemolysis, but the Coombs' test was only weakly positive and no warm or cold hemolysins were detectable [212]. This finding has not been present in other patients, in whom hemograms have been almost uniformly normal.

Findings from many other laboratory tests, including liver function tests, have been unremarkable.

Pathophysiology

Nature of the Defect

Either a decrease in synthesis or an increase in catabolism, with one or the other possibly being related to elaboration of an abnormal LDL, could lead to LDL deficiency. Evidence obtained in two kindreds that the LDL is chemically normal was summarized above. It is not possible to exclude all possible abnormalities, including alteration in the covalent structure of the apolipoprotein.

Measurement of the plasma turnover of ^{125}I-labeled isologous LDL has revealed the probable defect in Kindred 4 [215]. The technique consists of observing the die-away of a tracer amount of intravenous LDL tagged in the protein moiety. During experiments conducted in the steady state, the distribution and removal rate of LDL protein from the readily exchangeable pool are directly obtained; the synthetic rate is calculated. In the three patients, the distribution of the injected LDL was not remarkable and the fractional rate of disappearance of the rapidly exchangeable LDL (a mean of 0.47) was not abnormal. The synthetic rate, however, averaged only 17.0 mg of LDL per kg per day, compared to a mean value in 10 normal subjects of 58.4 mg per kg per day. The rate of entry of new LDL into the plasma pool thus seems to be limited severely, allowing maintenance of an LDL concentration at only about 10 percent of normal. Some corroboration of this conclusion by another approach is desirable. For the present, at least one kindred with this disorder may be considered to have a primary reduction in LDL synthetic rate. Molecular abnormalities in LDL too subtle to be detected by present techniques may lie behind this limitation in synthetic rate. It is puzzling also that in this apparently autosomal dominant disorder, the presumably normal allele is incapable of maintaining a rate of synthesis somewhat closer to one-half the normal. It has not been excluded that several different mutants may produce an apparently similar disorder.

Consequences of LDL Deficiency

The pleomorphic derangements that are associated with absence or deficiency of LDL were summarized in Table 26-1. If one attributes these derangements to the deficiency of lipoprotein, it must be concluded that patients with hypobetalipoproteinemia are close to the margin of adequate LDL but rarely will manifest pathologic changes. The only patient to have neurologic abnormalities, in the form of a demyelinating disorder, had first undergone four pregnancies, periods when demand for lipid transport is increased [213]. Her neurologic symptoms were also subject to frequent partial remissions. The levels of circulating vitamin A and E in this patient were low, but it is not known whether the concentrations of these and other substances transported by LDL were critically limiting. Several other affected patients in this and other kindreds (Fig. 26-7) also had children, without consequent difficulty; pregnancy is thus not a hazard for all women with hypobetalipoproteinemia.

The propositus of Kindred 1 developed fine, shiny, scattered dots on both optic fundi between the ages of 42 and 46, with an accompanying visual defect, including dark adaptation. He also had a mildly fatty liver, a condition present in abetalipoproteinemia [146], and attributed in that disease to inability to transport VLDL from the liver. In Kindred 4, however, it was shown that carbohydrate induction (a rise in VLDL following high-carbohydrate feeding; see Chap. 28) was normal in the patients with hypobetalipoproteinemia [215].

The propositus in Kindred 1 had changes in the fatty acid content of plasma cholesteryl ester and erythrocyte phospholipid similar to those in abetalipoproteinemia [212]. No acanthocytes were present. As in abetalipoproteinemia, the significance of this chemical change is not understood; it may be due only to marginal transport of essential fatty acids.

Undoubtedly there is considerable range of adaptation to LDL deficiency, but most of the patients with hypobetalipoproteinemia demonstrate that man seems to need less than 20 percent of the LDL normally seen in plasma. In this regard one cannot resist comparing hypobetalipoproteinemia with its converse, hyperbetalipoproteinemia (Type II in Chap. 28). In the latter disease, LDL concentrations are two to six times normal and are accompanied by premature atherosclerosis. No patient with the deficiency disease has come to autopsy; none has been described as having unequivocal coronary artery disease. Given the large number of factors contributing to atherogenesis, it may some day be possible to learn from hypobetalipoproteinemia the effect of maximum tolerable reduction in a single factor, that of circulating LDL.

Genetics

The significant portions of the four known kindreds with hypobetalipoproteinemia are reproduced in Fig. 26-7. If all the data are pooled, on the unproved assumption that each kindred has the same genetic error, the following facts emerge: (1) When both parents could be tested, each affected child had one affected parent; (2) 16 of the 27 patients found affected were females, and male-to-male transmission was observed in at least two different matings; (3) no consanguinity was noted in the four kindreds; and (4) of a total of 27 offspring examined who had an affected parent (excluding propositi), 16 (59 percent) were affected.

The pooled data and the evidence for each kindred considered individually are most consistent with the autosomal dominant mode of inheritance previously proposed [213–215]. The original suggestion of van Buchem et al. [212] that the mode was probably autosomal recessive or the conclusion [213] that hypobetalipoproteinemia is a *forme fruste* of abetalipoproteinemia—if the latter implies a genetic rela-

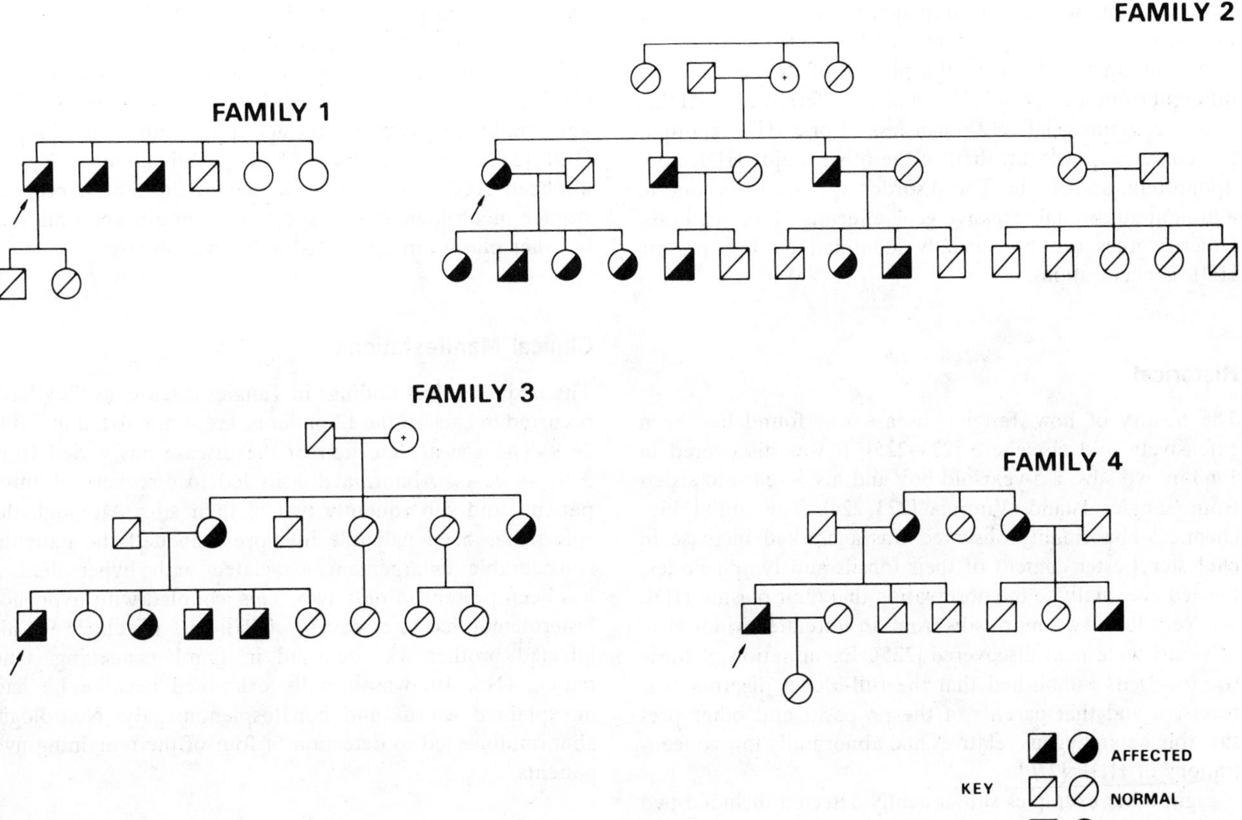

Figure 26-7. The four known kindreds with hypobetalipoproteinemia. They are numbered as in Table 26-8.

tionship—is not compatible with the apparent mode. Abetalipoproteinemia is clearly a recessive trait, leaving most presumed heterozygotes with no detectable abnormality. It is concluded that the gene loci affected in the two disorders are not the same.

Diagnosis and Treatment

The presence of hypobetalipoproteinemia will first be suspected because of a low cholesterol concentration in the absence of hypoglyceridemia. The criteria for definition of the genetic form should include the following: (1) LDL abnormally low but present and identifiable immunochemically, while concentrations of VLDL and HDL are normal, (2) absence of diseases to which hypobetalipoproteinemia may be secondary, and, to be certain, (3) detection of a similar pattern in a first-degree relative.

Hypobetalipoproteinemia may be secondary to acute and severe trauma [216], myocardial infarction [217, 218], hyperthyroidism [219], hepatic necrosis, anemia [220], infections [221], or malabsorption of fat, the latter sometimes being associated with abnormalities in the intestinal lacteals [222]. Usually HDL is also decreased in the secondary form, although during recovery from some of the disorders that lower concentrations of all lipoproteins the rates at which HDL and LDL concentrations return to normal may be different.

There is no treatment for hypobetalipoproteinemia. Plasma vitamin A and E levels should be monitored and supplements considered if concentrations are very low.

FAMILIAL HDL DEFICIENCY (Tangier Disease)

Tangier disease is a rare disorder named after the Chesapeake Bay island home of the first two patients. It is characterized by severe deficiency or absence of normal HDL in plasma and by storage of cholesteryl esters in many tissues throughout the body. The latter include liver, spleen, lymph nodes, thymus, the cornea, intestinal mucosa, skin, and, possibly, blood vessels. A combination of two features is pathognomonic; a low plasma cholesterol concentration in association with normal or elevated triglyceride levels and enlargement and distinctive orange-yellow coloration of the tonsils. Eight of the twelve patients known to have the disease have also had peripheral neuropathic changes. The small amounts of HDL in the plasma of the patients are different from the normal HDL and are referred to as HDL_T. HDL_T contains relatively much less of one HDL apolipoprotein, asp-apoLP-thr, than of the other major HDL apolipoprotein, apoLP-gln. The disorder appears to be due to a mutant autosomal recessive gene affecting HDL synthesis. Heterozygotes can be partially identified by low plasma HDL concentrations.

Historical

The history of how Tangier disease was found has been extensively told elsewhere [223–225]. It was discovered in 1960 in two sibs, a 5-year-old boy and his 6-year-old sister, from Tangier Island, Virginia [223, 224]. The initial biochemical abnormality observed was a marked increase in cholesteryl ester content of their tonsils and lymph nodes; this led eventually to the observation that their plasma HDL was very low. Two more sibs from an unrelated kindred in Missouri were next discovered [225]. Examination of these two kindreds established that the full-blown disorder was recessive and that parents of the propositi and other presumably heterozygous relatives had abnormally low concentrations of HDL [226].

Eight other examples subsequently detected included two adult sibs from Kentucky [227], a male in London [228], two sisters from Louisiana [229], another male in Bern [230], and a 3-year-old girl in Germany [230*a*, and *b*). The twelfth case was discovered in New Zealand [231] in a 47-year-old man. None of the affected families appear to be related. Neurologic symptoms were first observed independently by Kocen [228], Engel [229], and coworkers. All but one patient, an affected sib in the Kentucky kindred, are still alive.

Fredrickson, Gotto, and Levy have been fortunate in having the opportunity to study directly 8 of the 12 patients with Tangier disease, some for more than a decade, and to have examined plasma samples from all 12. The immunochemical difference between their HDL and the normal HDL was first reported by Levy and Fredrickson in 1966 [232]. In 1970, Lux and coworkers described the chemical abnormality observable in the apolipoproteins of the Tangier HDL [233]. The exact locus of the genetic abnormality has not been fixed, and still unexplained are the cholesteryl ester storage, neurologic disturbances, and certain abnormalities in other plasma lipoproteins in Tangier disease.

Clinical Manifestations

The major clinical findings in Tangier disease, as they have occurred in each of the 12 patients, are summarized in Table 26-9. The age at detection of the disease has varied from 3 to 48 years. Abnormal tonsils led to discovery of three patients and subsequently two of their sibs. Although the spleen has been palpable in more than half the patients, considerable enlargement associated with hypersplenism has been present in only two. This, coupled with hypocholesterolemia, led to discovery of Patient 5 (Table 26-9); his affected brother was detected in family screening. One patient (No. 10) was initially examined because he had unexplained icterus and hepatosplenomegaly. Neurologic abnormalities led to detection of four of the remaining five patients.

Tonsils

The unique appearance of the tonsils makes it possible to diagnose the disorder through examination of the oropharynx. The tonsils are large and lobulated and have a distinctive orange or yellowish-gray overlay of coloration on the normal red mucosa (Fig. 26-8). When the tonsils have been removed, small plaques or tags of mucosa having the same appearance will usually betray the diagnosis if one examines very carefully. Some patients have a history of recurrent "tonsillitis" and obstruction which has led to ton-

Table 26-9. CLINICAL FEATURES OF TANGIER DISEASE

Patient	Ref.	Sex	Age at detection, yr	Abnormal tonsils	Splenomegaly	Foam cells in marrow	Abnormal rectal mucosa	Skin deposition	Corneal deposits	Lymphadenopathy	Hepatomegaly	Neurologic abnormalities
1. T.La.	[223, 225]	M	5	+	+	+	−	+	0	+	+	+
2. E.La.	[223, 225]	F	6	+	0	+	−	0	0	0	0	+
3. Pe.Lo.	[223, 225]	F	8	+	+	0	−	+	0	0	0	0
4. Pa.Lo.	[223, 225]	F	12	+	+	0	−	+	0	0	0	0
5. C.No.	[227]	M	45	+	+	0	+	+	+	+	0	+
6. L.No.	[227]	M	48	+	+	+	+	−	+	0	0	−
7. P.Li.	[228]	M	37	+	+	+	+	−	0	0	0	+
8. J.Mi.	[229]	F	16	+	+	+	−	0	0	0	0	+
9. C.Mi.	[229]	F	24	0	0	0	+	0	+	0	0	+
10. E.Ri.	[230]	M	40	+	+	+	+	+	+	0	+	+
11. A.J.	[230*a*, *b*]	F	3	+	0	−	−	−	−	±	0	0
12. V.Ca.	[231]	M	47	−	+	−	+	−	0	0	+	+

Note: + = present; 0 = absent; − = not completely examined.

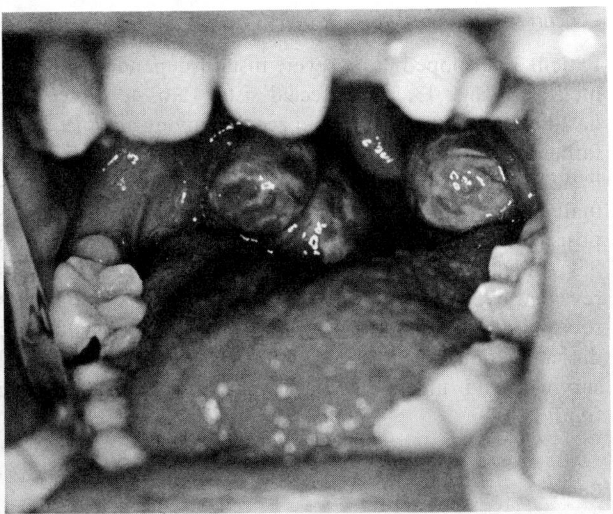

Figure 26-8. Tonsils in Tangier disease. Patient E.L., age 6. The lighter bands on the tonsils appear orange *in situ,* yellow-white after removal. (*From Fredrickson* [225].) (See also Plate I-5.)

sillectomy. The peculiar color of the tonsils is attributable to deposition of cholesteryl esters.

Cholesterol Deposition in Other Tissues

Reticulum cells in other sites also become enlarged and loaded with cholesteryl esters. In addition to moderate enlargement of the spleen, hepatomegaly may also occur. In one patient, the latter was shown to be accompanied by foamy reticulum cells scattered among the hepatocytes [230]. Most of the patients also have large, irregular foam cells in the marrow. Under phase microscopy these cannot be differentiated from storage cells seen in many other storage disorders. All patients who have been examined by sigmoidoscopy also have had foam cells in the rectal mucosa, which lend it a peculiar red-yellow cast, sometimes with prominent orange stippling. Deposits in the cornea present in four of the six adult patients appear as a hazily flocculent infiltration throughout the corneal stroma which can be resolved into many fine equidistant "dots" [227]. This is visible only by slit lamp and has not affected vision.

Lipid deposition has also been detected in the skin of five of eight patients examined by punch biopsy. Birefringent fat droplets are seen in the dermis, both in large histiocytes and fibroblasts and outside cells [234]. The overlying skin is usually normal, and the epidermis and sebaceous glands do not appear to be altered morphologically. A few lymph nodes have been moderately enlarged in two patients; biopsy of one revealed the typical cholesterol storage.

Neurologic Abnormalities

In five of the patients most recently discovered, peripheral neuropathy was added to the list of manifestations of Tangier disease, and similar abnormalities have now appeared in several of the patients who were discovered earlier. The degree of severity in the 8 of 12 patients so affected varies greatly. The disturbances are asymmetric and tend to fluctuate greatly. They include muscular weakness in either upper or lower extremities, sensory loss, paresthesias, diminished reflexes, and transient diplopia or ptosis.

The English patient of Kocen and colleagues [228] and the New Zealand patient of Hass and coworkers [231] have been the most seriously affected. The former (No. 7, Table 26-9) had a 10-year history of painless injuries on the arms and in his mouth. Later he could not close his eyes fully and noted weakness and wasting of his hands. He was considered to have syringomyelia and was treated with radiotherapy (1,000 r) to the cervical spinal cord. Two years later when the diagnosis of Tangier disease was established, he had normal motor function but impaired temperature and pain sensation over the distribution of the trigeminal nerve. There was weakness of the periorbital muscles, hands, and one forearm. Triceps and knee jerks were diminished. Ankle jerks were absent. Pain and temperature sensation was impaired over most of the body (Fig. 26-9), with the exception of the distal extremities. Other tactile and proprioceptive modalities were intact [228].

Patient 12 fractured a cervical vertebra at age 20 and a few weeks later noticed weakness and wasting of his arm muscles [231]. By age 35, he was unable to close his eyes. Moreover, all sense of pain was lost except in the lower

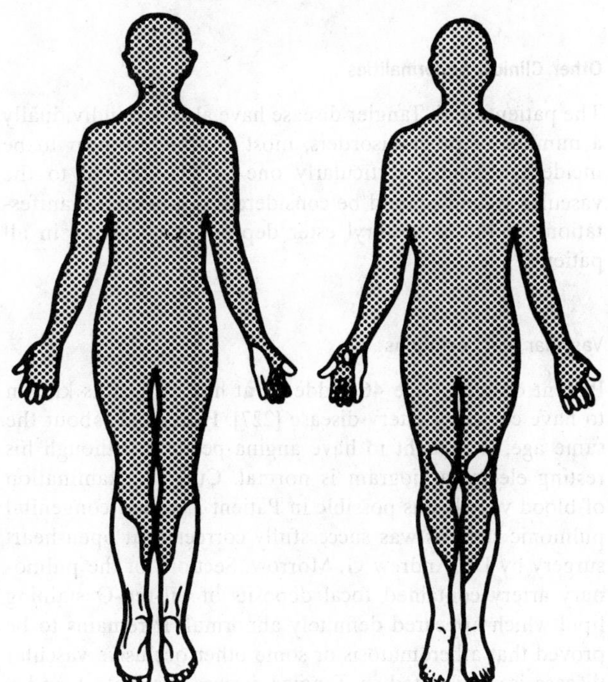

Figure 26-9. Shaded areas show the distribution of impaired pain and temperature sensation in Patient 7. (*Reprinted from Kocen et al.* [228] *with permission of the authors and publishers.*)

legs; tactile sensation remained intact. Later, touch also began to decrease, and by age 46 he had total body anesthesia except for the soles of his feet. Only pressure and vibration were perceptible. Deep reflexes were absent, and fasciculations were apparent in the upper and lower extremities.

Patients 8 and 9 had neurologic difficulties beginning at ages 8 and 12 years, respectively [229]. One started with asymmetric sensory symptoms and weakness in the lower extremities that led to laminectomy at age 14, and the use of braces for support. Then similar changes occurred in the upper limbs, and she developed diplopia. By age 15 all abnormalities had markedly improved. Her sister had varying numbness, tingling, and weakness in the lower extremities, and then in the upper ones. When examined at ages 16 and 24, respectively, both girls were much improved. Each had mild asymmetric muscle weakness, including the lateral rectus muscle of the eye. Sensory loss was minimal or absent at this time.

Patient 2, the girl in the original Tangier sibship, developed footdrop at age 16. This persisted for several months, was severe enough to require a brace, and then suddenly disappeared. Her brother also had some evidence of peripheral neuropathy at this time. Two years earlier both had had normal electromyograms [229].

Of the other patients, Nos. 5 and 7 to 10 also had abnormal myograms [228–230], and four had muscle biopsies interpreted as compatible with denervation. Patient 5 had scattered muscle weakness and decreased ankle jerks [229]; Patient 10 had slight muscle weakness in the toes [230].

Other Clinical Abnormalities

The patients with Tangier disease have also had individually a number of other disorders, most of which appear to be incidental. Some, particularly one or two related to the vascular system, should be considered as potential manifestations of the cholesteryl ester deposition occurring in all patients.

Vascular Manifestations

Patient 6 died at age 46 suddenly at home; he was known to have coronary artery disease [227]. Patient 12, about the same age, is thought to have angina pectoris, although his resting electrocardiogram is normal. Cursory examination of blood vessels was possible in Patient 3, whose congenital pulmonic stenosis was successfully corrected at open-heart surgery by Dr. Andrew G. Morrow. Sections of the pulmonary artery contained focal deposits of oil-red-O staining lipid which appeared definitely abnormal. It remains to be proved that atheromatosis or some other occlusive vascular disease is accelerated in Tangier disease. Patients 1 and 8 have had frequent atrial extrasystoles, and one has had transient bundle-branch block on repeated electrocardiograms.

Concurrent Disorders

Patient 3 developed fairly severe insulin-dependent diabetes mellitus at age 13. Her affected sister (No. 4, Table 26-9) has thalassemia trait with mild accompanying anemia. Their father has both thalassemia trait and adult-onset diabetes. Patient 9, having had ulcerative colitis for many years, eventually underwent total colectomy because of extensive polyposis. Patient 7 has goiter and proteinuria [228]. He also has some well-corticated cystic lesions in the fingers, as revealed by x-ray. Patient 10 has had nonprogressive icterus for two decades (total bilirubin, 2.6 to 4 mg per 100 ml; direct fraction, 0.25 to 1.85) with decreased red blood cell survival, and unexplained microaneurysms in the optic fundi [230].

Course

The prognosis in Tangier disease is not yet predictable. With the exception of the puzzling and episodic neurologic deficits, the general course in childhood is relatively benign. From the admittedly slender evidence that corneal infiltration has been visible only in adults, it seems probable that deposition of lipid progressively increases as the patients grow older. All the adults have had some rather serious disability, although not clearly attributable to the disease itself.

It is noteworthy that, in contrast to what occurs in LDL deficiency states, changes in visual acuity, retinitis, acanthocytes, and malabsorption of fat are not features of Tangier disease. Moreover, the neurologic abnormalities that are present involve primarily sensory pathways more peripheral than the cerebellar and long-tract changes found in all patients with abetalipoproteinemia.

Table 26-10. PLASMA LIPID CONCENTRATIONS IN TANGIER DISEASE, MG PER 100 ML

Patient	Age, yr	Cholesterol	Triglycerides	Phospholipids
1	5	101	225	144
2	6	77	205	101
3	8	112	224	137
4	12	72	151	104
8	16	84	138	
11	3	61	196	70
Normal subjects	1–19	120–230	10–140	155–265
9	24	94	164	
7	37	47	332	110
10	40	69	116	23
5	45	38	142	86
6	48	69	213	114
12	47	60	230	
Normal subjects	30–39	140–270	10–150	205–340

Note: Lipid concentrations for the patients are derived from case reports (see Table 26-9 for identification of patient and source reference). The normal ranges for cholesterol, triglyceride, and phospholipids are derived from Chap. 28.

Table 26-11. DISTRIBUTION OF PLASMA PHOSPHOLIPIDS IN TANGIER DISEASE

Patient*	Total plasma phospholipids, mg/100 ml	*Distribution of phospholipids, % of total phospholipids*†		
		Phosphatidyl choline	Sphingomyelin	Lysophosphatidyl choline
5	94	63	5	18
6	165	71	9	13
1	199	58	22	9
8	160	62	18	9
7	110	72	13	9
Normal No. 1	289	58	17	13
Normal No. 2	218	67	18	11

* As identified in Table 26-9.

† Values are less than 100 percent since phosphatidyl ethanolamine and minor constituents are not included.

It is justifiable to rank severe HDL deficiency as a lesser threat to life than abetalipoproteinemia. The life expectancy in Tangier disease, however, cannot now be considered entirely normal.

Laboratory Findings

Plasma Lipids

Among the lipoprotein deficiency states, and indeed among all known diseases, the combination of very low cholesterol and elevated triglyceride levels gives Tangier disease a unique signature. Some patients may have normal triglyceride levels, however, and may superficially resemble those with LDL deficiency. The total plasma cholesterol level ranges from about 30 to 125 mg per 100 ml (Table 26-10), within the range also observed in abetalipoproteinemia and LDL deficiency. The percentage of the cholesterol that is esterified appears to be within normal limits; in six patients the average was 70 percent (range, 64 to 72). The triglycerides are variable; the range of 150 to 330 mg per 100 ml shown in Table 26-10 is representative of the collection of patients. Variation in multiple samples from an individual patient is similar to that for single samples from the group.

The plasma phospholipid concentration is abnormally low [225, 228] (Tables 26-10 and 26-11). The distribution of lipid phosphorus among the several phospholipids varies in different patients (Table 26-11). The ratio of total phospholipids to cholesterol (PL/chol) in plasma and in the lipoproteins of density < 1.063 appears to be higher than in controls (Table 26-12), an anomaly discussed below in its relationship to lipoprotein structure.

Occasionally plasma carotene and vitamin A levels may be low [227, 231], but this is neither consistent nor characteristic.

Plasma Lipoproteins

A characteristic lipoprotein pattern attends the changes in lipid composition in Tangier disease; some of its salient features are shown in Fig. 26-10. As defined by several

Table 26-12. THE RELATIVE AMOUNTS OF PHOSPHOLIPID AND CHOLESTEROL—PHOSPHOLIPID/CHOLESTEROL (WET WEIGHT)—IN PLASMA AND THE LIPOPROTEIN FAMILIES IN TANGIER DISEASE

Subject	Age, yr	Whole plasma	D < 1.019	D 1.019–1.063	D 1.063–1.21
1	6	1.36	1.36	1.00	
2	7	1.34	1.04	1.31	>5
3	8	1.28	2.63	0.99	
4	12	1.43	3.08	0.81	3.0
7	37	2.34	1.76	2.25	3.12*
5	45	2.27	2.31	1.36	
6	48	2.08	2.12	1.77	3.0
Male controls	21–28	1.26	1.19	0.71	
Female controls	23–29	1.26	1.26	0.72	

* This value, obtained by Kocen et al. [228], represents all lipids of D (density) > 1.063; the control value for this fraction obtained by these same authors was 1.98.

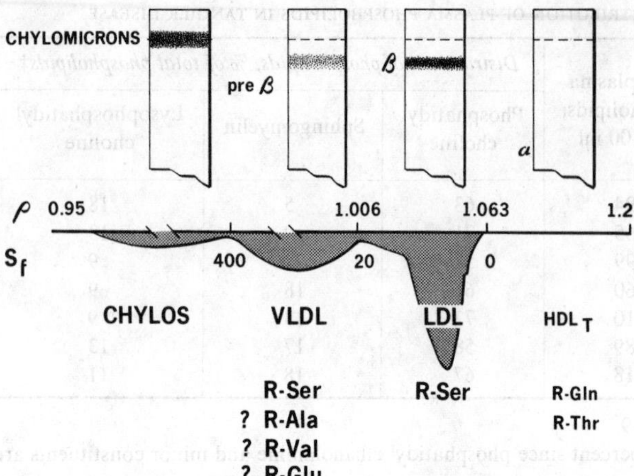

Figure 26-10. Plasma lipoprotein pattern in Tangier disease. By either paper electrophoresis (*top*) or analytic ultracentrifugation [175], the HDL, or α-lipoprotein, appears to be absent. The small amount of HDL_T is detected by preparative ultracentrifugation or immunochemical methods. Current knowledge of which apoproteins are present is shown at the bottom.

methods of analysis, these are: (1) Electrophoresis: The α-lipoproteins are absent, and the β-lipoprotein band appears broader than usual. No distinct pre-beta-band is formed in Tangier disease, and there are abnormal β-migrating lipoproteins in the VLDL fraction of plasma, an anomaly otherwise restricted so far to the disorder known as Type III hyperlipoproteinemia (Chap. 28). If the patient has eaten fat in the preceding 12 hr, a small chylomicron band is usually present. (2) Analytic ultracentrifugation (Fig. 26-10): High density lipoproteins (HDL_2 and HDL_3) are not detectable; the concentration of S_f 0 to 12 lipoproteins is decreased, and usually that of S_f 12 to 100 lipoproteins is increased [175]. (3) Preparative ultracentrifugation [225]: The lipoprotein fraction of density < 1.019 (VLDL + the LDL of S_f 12 to 20) is increased; that of density 1.019 to 1.063 (LDL of S_f 0 to 12) is decreased. Lipoproteins of density 1.063 to 1.21 (HDL) are markedly decreased, there being 1 to 4 mg per 100 ml of cholesterol instead of the usual 35 to 50 mg per 100 ml or more. The fraction of density > 1.21 contains about half the usual phospholipid, which, as in the normal subject, is mainly lysolecithin. (4) Precipitation of plasma by dextran or heparin-Mn^{++}: The lipid remaining in the supernatant is less than one-tenth of that in normal subjects. (5) Immunochemistry (Fig. 26-11): One or two very faint precipitation lines are formed with anti-HDL serums when either double diffusion or immunoelectrophoresis is employed. Precipitation with anti-LDL or anti-apoLDL serums is normal.

Other Laboratory Tests

Other routine laboratory test results are not typically abnormal in Tangier disease. The hemogram is normal unless hypersplenism has led to thrombocytopenia. No acanthocytes are present. Minor and nonspecific electroencephalographic changes have been observed [229]; electromyographic changes have already been described. Spinal fluid protein was slightly increased in two [229] of four patients with neuropathy.

Tissue Abnormalities

Morphology

Foam Cells

The bone marrow (Fig. 26-12), the reticuloendothelial system elsewhere, and the skin contain scattered foam cells. Massive sheets of such cells replace much of the tonsillar or thymic tissue. In supravital preparations or frozen sections, these cells appear to contain doubly refractile droplets (Fig. 26-12) that stain brightly with oil-red-O (neutral lipids) and Schultz's stain for cholesterol. There is no characteristic reaction with the periodic acid–Schiff stain or the Smith-Dietrich and Nile blue stains, typical of phospholipids. All reaction is removed by paraffin fixation. Many of the droplets seem to spill out of the foam cells, and very large, anisotropic crystals have been observed in thymus, skin, and other tissues. These take the same stain as the lipid in the cytoplasm of foam cells. There is no associated inflammatory or granulomatous change; the marked histiocytic proliferation seen in xanthoma disseminatum is likewise absent. Under the electron microscope the foam cells are seen to

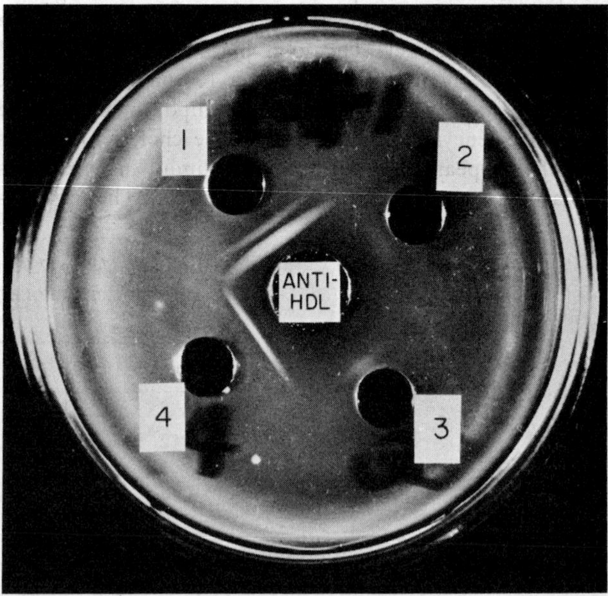

Figure 26-11. Immunoprecipitation lines formed by plasma from a normal subject (1), patients with Tangier disease (2) and (3), and a patient with abetalipoproteinemia (4) against anti-HDL serum. Only very faint lines are obtained with (2) and (3).

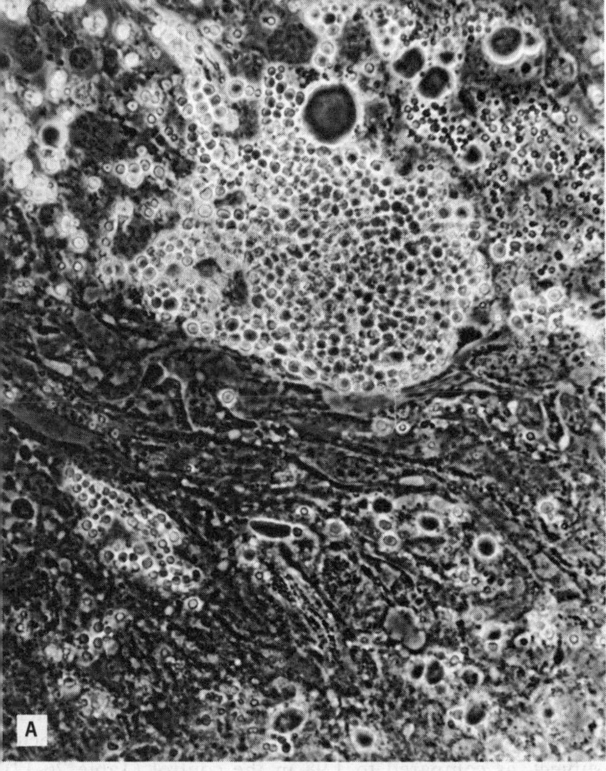

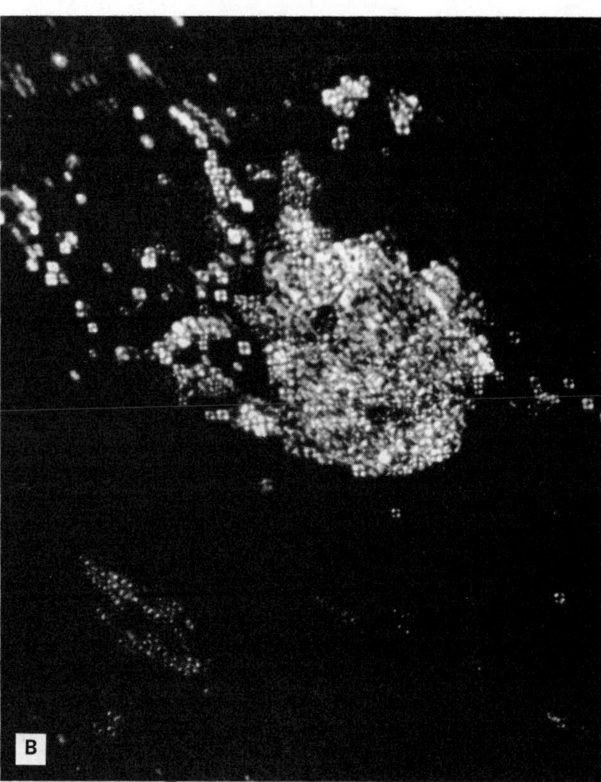

Figure 26-12. Foam cells in the bone marrow in Tangier disease. Supravital preparations are seen in phase contrast (A) and polarized light (B). Magnification can be judged from adjacent erythrocytes. (*Photomicrographs by courtesy of Dr. George Brecher.*)

contain large dense bodies full of a rather amorphous substance, but features distinct from those seen in other "foam cell disorders" have not been described [235].

Nervous Tissue

Biopsy of a superficial cutaneous branch of the left radial nerve in Patient 7 showed a great increase in amount of endoneural collagen, as well as extensive loss of myelin sheaths and axons. Cells containing Scharlach R–positive material were present close to nerve fibers [228]. Results of several nerve biopsies in two other patients were negative [229]. No amyloid was seen in any of the three biopsies.

Lipid Content

The content of tissue lipids first described in the Tangier kindred [223], now repeatedly confirmed in patients from other kindreds, has been described extensively elsewhere [225, 228, 230]. In tonsils, spleen, and lymph node, the sole characteristic abnormality has been an increase of 25- to 150-fold in the content of cholesteryl esters. The sterol has been identified as cholesterol [224]. Free cholesterol has been only slightly increased, if at all. There have been no clear-cut changes in total phospholipids, distribution among the major phospholipid classes, or triglycerides. The total neutral glycolipid content has also appeared to be normal, but analyses of specific glycolipids or tissue gangliosides [236] have not been made.

The fatty acids present in the cholesteryl esters in tonsils, lymph node, and spleen are predominantly 18 : 1 (oleic), the next most common acids being 16 : 0, 16 : 1, 18 : 2, and 20 : 4 [225]. The methods used would have detected phytanic acid [225, 228] had any been present. Chromatographic analyses for possible hydroxyacids have not been made. In general, the fatty acids appear quite similar to those of cholesteryl esters found in chylomicrons or deposited in tissues in eosinophilic granuloma [225] or atheromatous plaques [237].

Erythrocytes

Erythrocytes from four patients were interpreted as being probably not significantly different from normal erythrocytes in content of cholesterol, total phospholipids, phosphatidyl choline, sphingomyelin, or phosphatidyl ethanolamine [225]. Shacklady et al. [140] more recently published analyses of red blood cells from one additional adult which they interpret as indicating the lecithin to be increased and the sphingomyelin decreased. Comparison of the two sets of data [140, 225] suggests that minor changes in red blood cell lipids, opposite to those seen in abetalipoproteinemia, may be present in adults.

The Lipoprotein Abnormalities

Tangier HDL (HDL_T)

Immunochemical Recognition

A small quantity of lipoprotein may be isolated from Tangier plasma between the HDL density range of 1.063 to 1.21. The protein content of this fraction, referred to as Tangier HDL or HDL_T, is perhaps 1 to 2 percent of the normal amount. This lipoprotein fraction, like normal HDL, is not precipitated with heparin and manganese. It reacts with antiserums prepared to normal human HDL, but 14 of 16 such antiserums detected antigenic differences and formed lines of only partial identity between HDL and HDL_T on double diffusion experiments [232]. Differences in migration on immunoelectrophoresis are depicted in Fig. 26-13. If HDL_T is injected into rabbits, it elicits antibodies which react with normal HDL [232]. Thus, HDL and HDL_T are immunologically related but different.

A dramatic demonstration of HDL_T was possible in Patient 3, nearly all of whose blood was exchanged with normal blood in the course of open-heart surgery. Postoperatively, sequential immunoelectrophoretic analysis made possible the clear demonstration of HDL_T as it "reemerged," with the gradual disappearance of normal HDL [238]. The occurrence of HDL_T as a genetic variant has also been established in two obligate heterozygotes, in whom detection was facilitated by use of a high-carbohydrate diet to depress the concentration of normal HDL [238]. These findings provide strong evidence that HDL_T is a bona fide mutant lipoprotein, not an artifact secondary to altered concentrations of the plasma lipoproteins.

Composition of HDL_T

The amounts of HDL_T in Tangier homozygotes is estimated to be between one-twentieth and one-one hundredth of the amount of HDL normally present. Quantitation is uncertain because the amounts present are so small. It has been necessary to process large quantities of plasma obtained by plasmaphoresis to establish what is presently known about the chemical composition of the mutant lipoprotein.

As previously mentioned, the phospholipid/cholesterol ratio in plasma is not normal in Tangier disease. This is not necessarily ascribable simply to absence of normal HDL, for the ratio appears abnormal in several of the lipoprotein families (Table 26-12). In a previous study of two affected kindreds, the phospholipid/cholesterol ratios of the HDL present were believed to be within the range of that in controls [225]. In the study of Kocen et al. [228], in which a correction was not applied, the phospholipid/cholesterol ratio in the density $>$ 1.063 fraction was 3.12 in the affected subject, as compared to 1.98 in the control (Table 26-12). Further careful studies are needed to establish whether the lipoprotein present in the normal HDL density range in Tangier disease contains an unbalanced phospholipid/cholesterol ratio.

In Table 26-13 are shown preliminary studies by Dr. S. E. Lux of the neutral lipid content in HDL_T. The proportion

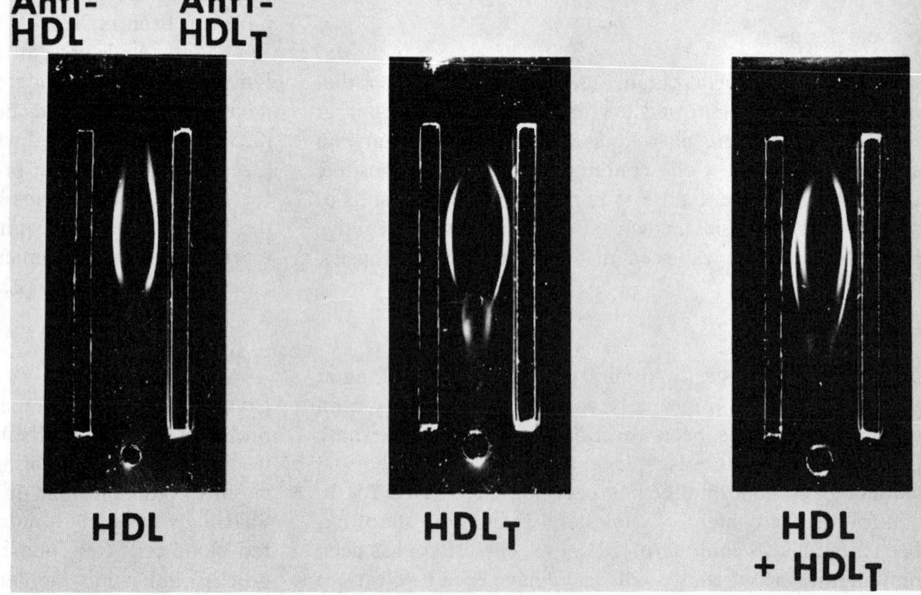

Figure 26-13. The immunoelectrophoresis of normal HDL, HDL_T, and the two combined. In the righthand panel, the line nearest the trough containing antiserum is HDL_T.

Table 26-13. DISTRIBUTION OF NEUTRAL LIPIDS WITHIN THE HDL (D 1.063–D 1.21 FRACTION) IN TANGIER DISEASE, MG LIPID PER 100 MG PROTEIN

Lipid	Patients 3 and 4 with Tangier disease	Normal control	Data from Scanu et al. [5]
Cholesterol:	20.8–21.5	31.1	36.0
Unesterified	6.7–7.3	7.2	6.0
Esterified	13.5–14.8	23.9	30.0
Triglyceride	29.3–44.8	5.4	12.0

Source: From Dr. S. E. Lux.

of cholesterol to protein is decreased, because of a marked decrease in the relative content of esterified cholesterol. Conversely, the ratio of triglycerides to protein is increased. The latter finding was first reported by Kocen et al. [228].

Apolipoproteins of HDL_T

As reviewed at the beginning of the chapter, HDL is believed to contain two major apoprotein subunits, designated apoLP-thr and apoLP-gln [59–60]. In normal HDL, the ratio of the LP-thr: LP-gln subunits is approximately 3:1 [62, 63]. For purposes of comparing HDL_T with normal HDL, the apolipoproteins in the density 1.063 to 1.21 fraction from Tangier homozygotes have been isolated, fractionated, and studied in parallel with the corresponding fraction from a normal control by Lux et al. [233]. ApoLP-thr and apoLP-gln are immunochemically different, and antiserums to native HDL detect both subunits in apoHDL, as shown by the formation of nonidentical precipitin lines on Ouchterlony plates. When an equal quantity of apoHDL_T was substituted for apoHDL in such immunochemical measurements, it was observed that anti-HDL serums formed a precipitin line with apoLP-gln, but apoLP-thr was not detected. The possibility that HDL_T contained at least trace amounts of apoLP-thr, however, was suggested by experiments in which an antiserum to HDL_T showed some reactivity toward pure apoLP-thr, although in very low titer. The same antiserum exhibited a high titer of reactivity with apoLP-gln. An antiserum to native HDL was then absorbed with HDL_T; reactivity with apoLP-gln was completely removed, while that with apoLP-thr was only slightly reduced. Absorption of the antiserum with the same quantity of native HDL totally abolished the activity toward both apolipoprotein subunits. In a more definitive experiment employing many times the usual amount of antigen and an absorbed antiserum specific for apoLP-thr, it was possible to prove that a small amount of antigen identical to apoLP-thr was present in apoHDL_T.

The results of the immunochemical experiments were confirmed in a qualitative way by electrophoresis on polyacrylamide gel at a pH of 8.9, where apoLP-thr and apoLP-gln differ in their relative mobilities. In normal apoHDL apoLP-thr produces a more intense band than apoLP-gln, consistent with the approximate ratio of 3:1 for these subunits in HDL. When the same quantity of apoHDL_T was examined under identical experimental conditions [233], there was an intensely staining band with the mobility of apoLP-gln and an extremely faint band in the region of apoLP-thr. With a very large load of apoHDL_T, it was possible to show that the band of mobility similar to apoLP-thr reacted with an absorbed antiserum specific for this subunit.

Identical amounts of apoHDL and apoHDL_T were further compared by chromatography on Sephadex G-200 in 8*M* urea-tris buffer, pH 8.2 [233] (Fig. 26-14). Peaks corresponding to apoLP-thr, apoLP-gln, and the major apoproteins specific for VLDL were obtained, with recoveries of >95 percent. The distribution of the proteins obtained is shown in Table 26-14. They confirm the impression that the ratio of apoLP-thr to apoLP-gln is inverted in the tiny amounts of HDL present in Tangier plasma. They also show that the "trace" apolipoproteins (of VLDL) are present in Tangier as well as normal HDL, for proteins with the electrophoretic mobilities of apoLP-val, apoLP-glu, and apoLP-ala

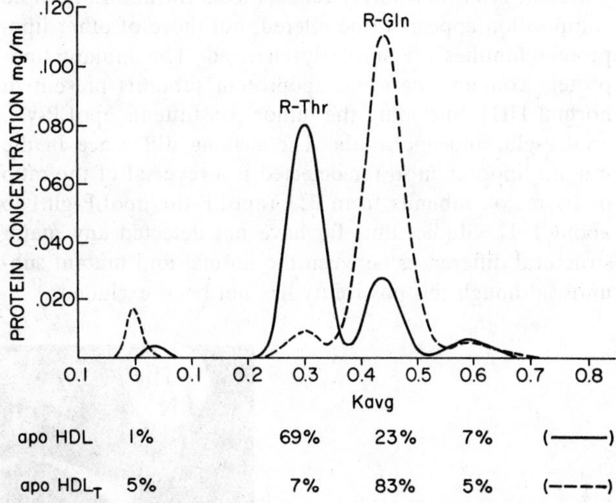

Figure 26-14. Separation of the two major protein components, apoHDL-thr (R-thr) and apoHDL-gln (R-gln), of normal apoHDL and of apoHDL_T. Chromatography is on Sephadex G-200 in 8*M* urea-tris buffer, pH 8.2 [238]. Identical amounts of normal apoHDL (solid line) and apoHDL_T (dashed line) were applied sequentially to the same column. The percentage of total protein in each peak is shown at the bottom.

Table 26-14. DISTRIBUTION OF APOPROTEINS IN CHROMATOGRAPHIC SEPARATIONS* OF ApoHDL AND ApoHDL$_T$, PERCENT OF TOTAL PROTEIN ELUTED

Sample	ApoLP-thr	ApoLP-gln	ApoLP-val, -glu, and -ala	Void volume
ApoHDL	69	23	7	1
ApoHDL$_T$	7	83	5	5

* Chromatography on Sephadex G-200 as described by Lux et al. [233] and shown in Fig. 26-14. The protein in the initial void volumes probably represented aggregates and was not further studied.

were present in the fourth peak of each chromatogram.

The apoLP-thr and apoLP-gln isolated from the Tangier HDL migrated on polyacrylamide-gel electrophoresis (at pH 8 to 9) to positions identical to those of their normal counterparts. They were also immunochemically identical, respectively, to apoLP-thr and apoLP-gln with five of five antiserums (Fig. 26-15). These apolipoprotein subunits were isolated from two Tangier homozygotes and were demonstrated by polyacrylamide-gel electrophoresis in a total of four subjects.

The decreased relative amount of apoLP-thr in the density 1.063 to 1.21 fraction of Tangier plasma could not be accounted for by a shift of the protein either to other portions of the lipoprotein density spectrum (the density 1.063 supernatant fraction) or elsewhere in the plasma (the density 1.21 infranatant). In one heterozygous subject, the ratio of apoLP-thr to apoLP-gln in his total apoHDL was decreased to approximately one-half the usual ratio.

Thus, Tangier disease is attended by the occurrence of a mutant HDL in severely reduced concentrations. Its lipid composition appears to be altered, but those of other lipoprotein families are similarly changed. The mutant lipoprotein contains the same apoprotein subunits present in normal HDL, including the minor constituents apoLP-val, apoLP-glu, and apoLP-ala. The striking difference in the mutant lipoprotein so far detected is a reversal of the ratio of its major subunits from 3:1 (apoLP-thr/apoLP-gln) to about 1:11. Studies thus far have not detected any major structural differences between the normal and mutant subunits, although this possibility has not been excluded.

Other Lipoprotein Families

Abnormalities in plasma lipoproteins other than HDL in Tangier disease have been already alluded to and were noted in the first several patients [225]. These are (1) decreased amounts of LDL of S_f 0 to 12 (density 1.019 to 1.063); (2) abnormal increases in VLDL and S_f 12 to 20 LDL; and (3) an increased phospholipid/cholesterol ratio in these lipoproteins (Table 26-12). In addition, the amount of glyceride relative to phospholipid seems to be increased [228]. In the patient of Kocen et al. [228], the proportion of triglyceride (calculated as triglyceride/triglyceride + cholesterol + phospholipid) was increased nearly twofold in the density < 1.019 fraction, and nearly sixfold in the density 1.019 to 1.063 fraction, presumably as a consequence of the mutant gene.

Chylomicrons

Patients with Tangier disease absorb fat well and form stable chylomicrons [225]. Earlier studies suggesting a delay in clearance of chylomicrons in several of the patients [225] have been confirmed only to the extent that "chylomicrons" seem unusually prominent in samples collected during the day and electrophoresed on paper. Still unexplained, but possibly gaining more importance in light of knowledge about odd lipid composition in other lipoproteins, is the observation of relative impoverishment of the free and esterified cholesterol content of Tangier chylomicrons [225].

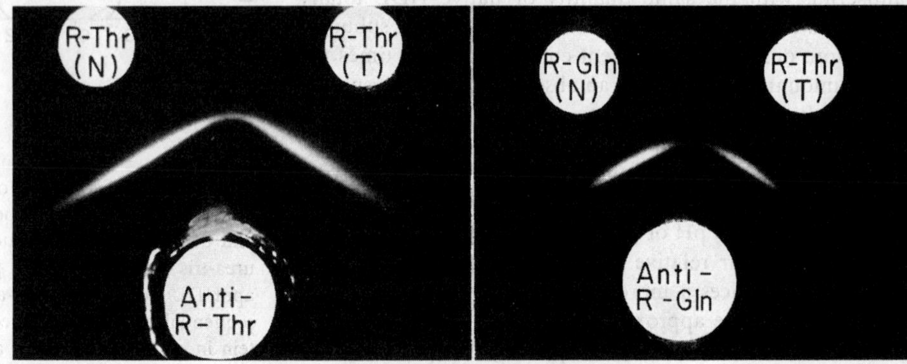

Figure 26-15. The immunochemical identity of isolated R-thr and R-gln from normal (*N*) and Tangier (*T*) HDL [233].

Pathophysiology

Many pieces of the puzzle of Tangier disease are still missing, even though more of the pattern has recently emerged with the establishment of a mutant HDL. Small amounts of this lipoprotein appear to represent the only semblance of HDL in the homozygote; the plasma of the obligate heterozygote contains roughly the same amounts of this HDL_T and about half the usual amounts of one of two major subunits of HDL protein, apoLP-thr. For the moment, the ranking supposition is that the mutation occurs in an allele regulating synthesis of apoLP-thr. A logical extension of this hypothesis is that the synthesis of the other subunit, apoLP-gln, is normal or potentially so. Presumably, without apoLP-thr, apoLP-gln is unable to sustain a stable HDL complex, and any mutant lipoprotein form is probably removed from plasma at a high rate. The possibility of abnormal structural features in either of the subunits cannot be completely ruled out until larger amounts of protein are available for study.

Even assuming that a deficiency of one of the apoproteins is the primary defect, we are left with many abnormalities to explain on the basis of inadequate circulating HDL. These include most prominently the inexorable and profound deposition of cholesteryl esters in reticuloendothelial tissues and the cornea, the neurologic abnormalities, and changes in the lipid composition and behavior of other lipoproteins. The task would be simpler if one knew the normal functions of HDL. Perhaps, as is often the case with genetic errors, these functions may become clear only when the mystery of the disease is unraveled. An example of how much related information is still needed is the explanation of why Tangier VLDL does not migrate normally on electrophoresis (Fig. 26-10). This was previously attributed to lack of apoHDL, whose positive charge was believed to increase the mobility of normal VLDL [20]. Recent attempts to demonstrate significant amounts of apoHDL in normal VLDL have not been successful, even though immunochemically it appears to be present.

The Cause of Cholesterol Storage

There are several possible theories to explain the selective storage of cholesteryl esters in Tangier disease. From evidence of peculiar composition of chylomicrons and VLDL in Tangier plasma it was suggested that these lipoproteins might be relatively unstable and might deposit much of their contents in reticuloendothelial macrophages [224]. Many studies of the lipids found in xanthomas and atheromas make it appear likely that cholesteryl esters are the last residue accumulating when a mixture of lipids is deposited in tissue sites. The discovery of mutant HDL offers the companion possibility that it is an unstable HDL, poor in apoLP-thr, that is rapidly removed from plasma and is the major contributor to the tissue excesses of cholesterol.

The third set of possibilities is somewhat more complicated. It involves the relationship between HDL and the enzyme lecithin:cholesterol acyl transferase (LCAT, Chap. 27). LCAT activity is present in Tangier plasma, as measured in vitro [239]. Nevertheless it is possible that, in vivo, the absence of an effective concentration of HDL could prove crippling to two actions of LCAT that have been postulated. One is the suggestion that LCAT activity maintains the concentrations of cholesterol in tissues by promoting its transfer to plasma HDL and thereby its transport to the liver for catabolism. The other action suggested for LCAT, in concert with HDL, relates to chylomicron and VLDL metabolism. It has been speculated that LCAT and HDL assist in the maintenance of a stable surface/volume ratio of these particles in the course of their degradation [37], by promoting exchange of cholesteryl esters from HDL and triglycerides from chylomicrons and VLDL [6]. Interference with this cycle could, indeed, result in the decreased ratio of cholesterol to phospholipid that is present in Tangier VLDL. It could also lead to instability of these particles and cause their removal from the plasma by macrophages. It is noteworthy that patients who have inheritable LCAT deficiency have foam cells in the marrow and kidneys and lipid deposition in the cornea. They do not have orange tonsils, however, or other evidence of cholesteryl ester storage as extensive as that seen in Tangier disease. It is likely that study of the turnover and fate of HDL_T will be the most direct route to further information bearing on the storage component of Tangier disease.

There is inadequate evidence that cholesteryl esters accumulate in the ganglion cells or myelin in Tangier disease. This makes it presently impossible to determine the basis for neuropathic changes in Tangier disease. Since cholesterol deposition seems to underlie all the other known abnormalities secondary to HDL deficiency in Tangier disease, it is possible that the neurologic changes will prove to be related to this phenomenon. It has not been excluded that HDL may be responsible for maintaining the nutrition or integrity of neurons in some other manner. The available evidence does not allow extension to Tangier disease of the possible deprivation of vitamins A and E discussed under abetalipoproteinemia. The diseases in which LDL is deficient have previously suggested that LDL is much more critical for maintenance of the normal neural structure and functions than is HDL.

Genetics

Studies undertaken in the first three kindreds to determine the mode of inheritance of Tangier disease [226, 227] were extensively summarized in the previous edition of this book [225]. They indicated that full expression of Tangier disease occurs in subjects homozygous for an autosomal mutant allele. They also demonstrated that obligate heterozygotes and other first-degree relatives of probands often have plasma HDL concentrations below the 5 percent limit for controls. All five available parents of the propositi had abnormally low values, although a general tendency for female obligate heterozygotes to have quite variable HDL concentrations on repeated testing was noted; and the mother of Patients 3 and 4 occasionally had HDL in the normal range. The parents and other heterozygotes, like the patients, tend to have hyperglyceridemia [175, 225].

Family data obtained in the next four affected kindreds are consistent with this mode of inheritance, although normal limits used by the English and Swiss workers [228, 230] do not correspond to those used in the American studies [225, 226]. Six of the eight parents were sampled; all had "low" HDL concentrations, as did some of their sibs. Thus all parents of Tangier patients examined to date have had low HDL levels. One of the propositi had two children by a woman with normal HDL levels [228]. The plasma HDL in one child was low; the other had normal HDL concentrations. Another example was reported earlier [227] of a child with normal HDL from a mating in which only heterozygotes were to be expected. It is quite possible that these apparent exceptions demonstrate the inaccuracies of measurement of HDL or the inadequacies of defining normal limits, rather than refute an otherwise consistent genetic mode.

Consanguinity has been demonstrated in two kindreds. In the first (Table 26-9), the parents were fourth cousins [226]. The parents of the German patient (No. 11) were first cousins [230*a*, 230*b*].

Detection of Heterozygotes

As discussed in detail elsewhere [225], the cutoff limits of HDL concentrations of 32 and 35 mg per 100 ml (as HDL cholesterol) in males and females, respectively, used in the early genetic studies do not provide reliable limits for detection of Tangier heterozygotes in the general population. This is particularly true because many patients with familial or acquired forms of hyperlipemia also have low HDL concentrations secondary to increases in VLDL or chylomicrons (Chap. 28). It is remotely possible that use of the analytic ultracentrifuge separately to quantify HDL_2 and HDL_3 might be more helpful in segregating Tangier heterozygotes from other patients with low HDL [175].

Of potentially greater significance is the finding that HDL_T is present in patients heterozygous for the trait [232]. This determination requires rather tedious immunochemical comparisons and is also not yet widely available on a practical basis. As polyacrylamide-gel electrophoresis and other methods are employed more extensively in analyses of lipoproteins, it is possible that better tests will be devised.

One parent of the first propositus also had foam cells in the bone marrow; this was not true in the other parent or in either of one other set of parents [225]. The tonsils of one heterozygote relative were also examined histochemically and by chemical analyses; there was no evidence of cholesterol storage [225].

Diagnosis

In any patient with unexplained hepatic or splenic enlargement, corneal deposits, or neuropathy, a close examination of the oropharynx and a plasma cholesterol determination are indicated. The finding of cholesterol level below about 125 mg per 100 ml must lead directly to triglyceride determination and lipoprotein electrophoresis. Triglyceride levels will usually be high in Tangier disease and normal or low in the several LDL deficiency states. Paper electrophoresis is helpful in enhancing suspicion of Tangier disease, but HDL levels below those producing a visible α-lipoprotein band can also occur in other conditions. HDL should be quantitatively determined by precipitation tests or ultracentrifugation (Chap. 28). The definitive diagnostic tests are immunochemical ones showing near-absence of HDL. At the same time minor antigenic differences between any trace of remaining HDL and the same lipoproteins from normal plasma should be sought (test for HDL_T).

In addition to LDL absence or deficiency, the following diseases must be excluded: (1) familial deficiency of lecithin:cholesteryl acyl transferase (LCAT) (Chap. 27). Here HDL is also very low, but plasma cholesterol is normal or high and most of the plasma cholesterol is unesterified. (2) Obstructive liver disease, in which the HDL pattern is sometimes highly distorted. In this disorder the cholesterol level is not low, but high, and cholesteryl esters are also deficient; appropriate liver function studies will usually permit the diagnosis; more specific tests for lipoprotein abnormalities in this condition are available [240]. (3) Severe malnutrition or liver parenchymal disease in which HDL is decreased; the decrease in cholesterol will also be associated with low triglyceride and LDL levels. (4) Acquired HDL deficiency due to dysglobulinemia, including possible development of antibodies to HDL. (5) Other storage diseases associated with foam cells and hepatosplenomegaly. HDL may be low in these conditions but not at the levels seen in Tangier disease [225]. In none of these diseases are the tonsils abnormal, nor is HDL_T present.

Treatment

There is no specific treatment. Theoretically, chronic infusions of HDL or apoLP-thr are possible; they have not been tried in any patient. The relative freedom of most of the patients from severe and sustained disability has not commended this potentially lifelong measure. It might be considered for short-term trial in possible future patients who have extreme neurologic disability. Splenectomy for hypersplenism in one patient was followed by a return of platelets to normal, and no worsening of his disease was noted up to 4 years subsequent to operation.

SUMMARY

1 The plasma lipoproteins may be separated into four major families according to their densities and electrophoretic mobilities. These are chylomicrons, very low density lipoproteins (VLDL), low density lipoproteins (LDL), and high density lipoproteins (HDL). Some of the specificity of lipoproteins is contributed by their protein portion, or apoproteins, here identified by their C-terminal amino acid. The specific apoprotein composition of chylomicrons has not been established. VLDL contain at least four. Three of these, apoLP-val, apoLP-glu, and apoLP-ala (50 percent of the VLDL protein), are also found in HDL as minor constituents. The rest of VLDL protein is apoLP-ser, which is also the major apoprotein of LDL. The major apoproteins of HDL are apoLP-thr and apoLP-gln.

2 In abetalipoproteinemia, chylomicrons, VLDL, and LDL are absent. The clinical manifestations are fat malabsorption, ataxic neuropathy, retinitis pigmentosa, and acanthocytosis. The usual mechanisms for transporting triglycerides from the intestine and liver to the circulation are abolished. ApoLP-ser is missing from plasma. All the other apoproteins are present in the remaining lipoprotein family, HDL. Deficient synthesis or utilization of apoLP-ser is the most probable metabolic defect. The relationship between the absence of apoLP-ser or of the several missing lipoproteins to the clinical manifestations has not been established. The inheritance is as an autosomal recessive.

3 In familial hypobetalipoproteinemia, LDL concentrations are decreased to as low as 10 to 20 percent of the normal level. In the four known affected kindreds, only one subject had malabsorption and central nervous system dysfunction. Otherwise the low concentrations of LDL are not associated with the clinical abnormalities seen in abetalipoproteinemia. The trait appears to be autosomal dominant. It has been related to a decrease in LDL synthesis in one kindred.

4 In familial deficiency of HDL, Tangier disease, normal HDL is absent and a small quantity of an aberrant HDL—"HDL_T"—circulates. HDL_T contains relatively less apoLP-thr and more apoLP-gln than does HDL, the ratio of apoLP-thr to apoLP-gln being 1:11 instead of the usual 3:1. An imbalanced synthesis of these two proteins may underlie this rare, autosomal recessive disease. The accumulation of cholesteryl esters in the reticuloendothelial system suggests failure to mobilize this lipid and accounts for the clinical signs of orange tonsils and hepatosplenomegaly. The pathophysiology of the accompanying neuropathy has not been explained. Heterozygotes have HDL_T in plasma and abnormally low HDL concentrations.

BIBLIOGRAPHY

1. deLalla, O. F., and Gofman, J. W.: Ultracentrifugal analysis of serum lipoproteins, in *Methods of Biochemical Analysis,* edited by D. Glick, p. 459. Interscience, New York, 1954.
2. Hatch, F. T., and Lees, R. S.: Practical methods for plasma lipoprotein analysis. Advances Lipid Res., **6,** 1, 1968.
3. Dole, V. P., and Hamlin, J. T.: Particulate fat in lymph and blood. Physiol. Rev., **42,** 674, 1962.
4. Oncley, J. L.: Lipid protein interactions, in Brain Lipids and Lipoproteins, and the Leukodystrophies, edited by J. Folch-Pi and H. Bauer, p. 1. Elsevier, Amsterdam, 1963.
5. Scanu, A. M.: Factors affecting lipoprotein metabolism. Advances Lipid Res., **3,** 63, 1965.
6. Schumaker, V. N., and Adams, G. H.: Circulating lipoproteins. Ann. Rev. Biochem., **38,** 113, 1969.
7. Gage, S. H.: The free granules (chylomicrons) of the blood as shown by the dark-field microscope. Cornell Vet., **10,** 154, 1920.
8. Gage, S. H., and Fish, P. A.: Fat digestion and assimilation in man and animals as determined by dark-field microscope, and fat-soluble dye. Amer. J. Anat., **34,** 1, 1924.
9. Lossow, W. J., Lindgren, F. T., Murchio, J. C., Stevens, G. R., and Jensen, L. C.: Particle size and protein content of six fractions of the S_f 20 plasma lipoproteins isolated by density gradient centrifugation. J. Lipid Res., **10,** 68, 1969.
10. Yokoyama, A., and Zilversmit, D. B.: Particle size and composition of dog lymph chylomicrons. J. Lipid Res., **6,** 241, 1965.
11. Bierman, E. L., Porte, D., O'Hara, D. D., Schwartz, M., and Wood, F. C.: Characterization of fat particles in plasma of hyperlipemic subjects maintained on fat-free high-carbohydrate diets. J. Clin. Invest., **44,** 261, 1965.
12. O'Hara, D. D., Porte, D., and Williams, R. H.: Use of constant composition polyvinylpyrrolidone columns to study the interaction of fat particles with plasma. J. Lipid Res., **7,** 264, 1966.
13. Zilversmit, D. B.: The composition and structure of lymph chylomicrons in dog, rat, and man. J. Clin. Invest., **44,** 1610, 1965.
14. Avigan, J.: Modification of human serum lipoprotein fractions by lipide extraction. J. Biol. Chem., **226,** 957, 1957.
15. Alaupovic, P., Sanbar, S. S., Furman, R. H., Sullivan, M. L., and Walraven, S. L.: Studies of the composition and structure of serum lipoproteins. Isolation and characterization of very high density lipoproteins of human serum. Biochemistry, **5,** 4044, 1966.
16. Rodbell, M., and Fredrickson, D. S.: The nature of the proteins associated with dog and human chylomicrons. J. Biol. Chem., **234,** 562, 1959.
17. Levy, R. S., Lynch, A. C., McGee, E. D., and Mehl, J. W.: Amino acid composition of the proteins from chylomicrons and human serum lipoproteins. J. Lipid Res., **8,** 463, 1967.
18. Middleton, E., Jr.: Immunochemical relationship of human plasma beta-lipoprotein and chylomicrons. Amer. J. Physiol., **185,** 309, 1956.
19. Gustafson, A., Alaupovic, P., and Furman, R. H.: Studies of the composition and structure of serum lipoproteins: isolation, purification, and characterization of very low density lipoproteins of human serum. Biochemistry, **4,** 596, 1965.
20. Levy, R. I., Lees, R. S., and Fredrickson, D. S.: The nature of pre-beta (very low density) lipoproteins. J. Clin. Invest., **45,** 63, 1966.
21. Brown, W. V., Levy, R. I., and Fredrickson, D. S.: Studies of the proteins in human plasma very low density lipoproteins. J. Biol. Chem., **244,** 5687, 1969.
22. Shore, B., and Shore, V.: Isolation and characterization of human serum lipoproteins. Biochemistry, **11,** 4510, 1970.
23. Brown, W. V., Levy, R. I., and Fredrickson, D. S.: Further separation of the apoproteins of the human plasma very low density lipoproteins. Biochim. Biophys. Acta, **200,** 576, 1970.
24. Brown, W. V., Levy, R. I., and Fredrickson, D. S.: Further characterization of apoproteins from the human plasma very low density lipoproteins. J. Biol. Chem., **245,** 6588, 1970.
25. Forte, G. M., Nichols, A. V., and Glaeser, R. M.: Structure of high density serum lipoproteins after partial or complete delipidation. Biophys. J., **9,** Society Abstracts A111, 1968.
26. Gotto, A. M., Levy, R. I., and Fredrickson, D. S.: Preparation and properties of an apoprotein derivative of human serum β-lipoprotein. Lipids, **3,** 463, 1968.

27. Forte, G. M., Nichols, A. V., and Glaeser, R. M.: Electron microscopy of human serum lipoproteins using negative staining. Chem. Phys. Lipids, **2**, 396, 1968.
28. Bragdon, J. H., Havel, R. J., and Boyle, E.: Human serum lipoproteins. I. Chemical composition of four fractions. J. Lab. Clin. Med., **48**, 36, 1956.
29. Ayrault-Jarrier, M., Chefter, R. I., and Polonovski, J.: Les Glucides de la β-lipoprotéine S_f 1.063 0–12 du serum sanguin humain. Bull. Soc. Chim. Biol., **43**, 811, 1961.
30. Marshall, N. B.: Gonadal hormones and lipid metabolism, in *Lipid Pharmacology,* edited by R. Paoletti, p. 325, Academic, New York, 1964.
31. Toro-Goyco, E.: Physical-chemical studies of the β_1-lipoproteins of human plasma. Ph.D. Thesis, Harvard University, 1958, 86 pp.
32. Scanu, A., Pollard, H., and Reader, J. W.: Properties of human serum low density lipoproteins after modification by succinic anhydride. J. Lipid Res., **9**, 342, 1968.
33. Adams, G. H., and Schumaker, V. N.: Rapid molecular weight estimates for low-density lipoproteins. Anal. Biochem., **29**, 117, 1968.
34. Lindgren, F. T., Jensen, L. C., Wills, R. D., and Freeman, N. K.: Flotation rates, molecular weights and hydrated densities of the low-density lipoproteins. Lipids, **4**, 337, 1969.
35. Pollard, H., Scanu, A. M., and Taylor, E. W.: On the geometrical arrangement of the protein subunits of human serum low-density lipoprotein: evidence for a dodecahedral model. Proc. Nat. Acad. Sci. U.S.A., **64**, 304, 1969.
36. Kane, J. P., Richards, E. G., and Havel, R. J.: Subunit heterogeneity in human serum beta lipoprotein. Proc. Nat. Acad. Sci. U.S.A., **66**, 1075, 1970.
37. Shore, B., and Shore, V.: The protein moiety of human serum β-lipoproteins. Biochem. Biophys. Res. Commun., **28**, 1003, 1967.
38. Day, C. E., and Levy, R. S.: Determination of the molecular weight of apoprotein subunits from low density lipoprotein by gel filtration. J. Lipid Res., **9**, 789, 1968.
39. Avigan, J., Redfield, R., and Steinberg, D.: N-Terminal residues of serum lipoproteins. Biochim. Biophys. Acta, **20**, 557, 1956.
40. Brown, R. K., Davis, R. E., Clark, B., and van Vunakis, H.: Clinical studies of the protein portion of human lipoproteins, in *The Blood Lipids and the Clearing Factor,* edited by R. Ruyssen, Proceedings of the 3rd International Conference on Biochemical Problems of Lipids (Brussels), July 26–28, 1956, pp. 104–112.
41. Shore, B.: C- and N-terminal amino acids of human serum lipoproteins. Arch. Biochem. Biophys., **21**, 1, 1957.
42. Granda, J. L., and Scanu, A.: Solubilization and properties of the apoproteins of the very low- and low-density lipoproteins of human serum. Biochemistry, **5**, 3301, 1966.
43. Gotto, A. M., Levy, R. I., Rosenthal, A. S., Birnbaumer, M. E., and Fredrickson, D. S.: The structure and properties of human beta-lipoprotein and beta-apoprotein. Biochem. Biophys. Res. Commun., **31**, 699, 1968.
44. Scanu, A., Pollard, H., Hirz, R., and Kothary, K.: On the conformational instability of human serum low-density lipoprotein: effect of temperature. Proc. Nat. Acad. Sci. U.S.A., **62**, 171, 1969.
45. Gotto, A. M., Levy, R. I., and Fredrickson, D. S.: Human serum beta-lipoprotein: preparation and properties of a delipidated, soluble derivative. Biochem. Biophys. Res. Commun., **31**, 151, 1968.
46. Gotto, A. M., Levy, R. I., Rosenthal, A. S., and Fredrickson, D. S.: Human serum beta-lipoprotein. Nature (London), **219**, 1157, 1968.
47. Gotto, A. M., Levy, R. I., and Fredrickson, D. S.: Observations on the conformation of human beta lipoprotein: evidence for the occurrence of beta structure. Proc. Nat. Acad. Sci. U.S.A., **60**, 1436, 1968.
48. Gotto, A. M., Levy, R. I., Birnbaumer, M. E., and Fredrickson, D. S.: Human serum beta lipoprotein and beta apoprotein. Nature (London), **223**, 835, 1969.
49. Scanu, A., and Granda, J. L.: Comparative optical properties of human serum low- and high-density lipoproteins before and after delipidation. Progr. Biochem. Pharmacol., **4**, 153, 1968.
50. Dearborn, G. D., and Wetlaufer, D. B.: Reversible thermal conformation changes in human serum low-density lipoprotein. Proc. Nat. Acad. Sci. U.S.A., **62**, 179, 1969.
51. Lindgren, F. T., and Nichols, A. V.: Structure and function of human serum lipoproteins in *The Plasma Proteins,* edited by F. W. Putnam, density lipoproteins. J. Lipid Res., **7**, 638, 1966.
52. Glomset, J. A., Janssen, E. T., Kennedy, R., and Dobbins, J.: Role of plasma lecithin: cholesterol acyltransferase in the metabolism of high density lipoproteins. J. Lipid Res., **7**, 638, 1966.
53. Scanu, A., Lewis, A., and Bumpus, M.: Separation and characterization of the protein moiety of human α_1-lipoprotein. Arch. Biochem. Biophys., **74**, 390, 1958.
54. von Schultze, H. E.: Über Glykoproteine. Deutsch. Med. Wschr., **83**, 1742, 1958.
55. Epstein, F. H., and Block, W. D.: Glycoprotein content of serum lipoproteins. Proc. Soc. Exp. Biol. Med., **101**, 740, 1959.
56. Scanu, A., Reader, W., and Edelstein, E.: Molecular weight and subunit structure of human serum high density lipoprotein after chemical modification by succinic anhydride. Biochim. Biophys. Acta, **160**, 32, 1968.
57. Oncley, J. L., and Allerton, S. E.: Characterization of the α_1-lipoproteins of human plasma. Vox Sang., **6**, 201, 1961.
58. Cox, A. C., and Tanford, C.: The molecular weights of porcine plasma high density lipoprotein and its subunits. J. Biol. Chem., **243**, 3083, 1968.
59. Shore, B., and Shore, V.: Heterogeneity in protein subunits of human serum high-density lipoproteins. Biochemistry, **7**, 2773, 1968.
60. Shore, V., and Shore, B.: Some physical and chemical studies on two polypeptide components of high-density lipoproteins of human serum. Biochemistry, **7**, 3396, 1968.
61. Lux, S. E.: Unpublished results.
62. Scanu, A., Toth, J., Edelstein, C., Koga, S., and Stiller, S.: Fractionation of human serum high density lipoprotein in urea solutions. Evidence for polypeptide heterogeneity. Biochemistry, **8**, 3309, 1969.
63. Scanu, A., Cump, E., Toth, J., Koga, S., Stiller, E., and Albers, L.: Degradation and reassembly of a human serum high-density lipoprotein: evidence for differences in lipid affinity among three classes of polypeptide chains. Biochemistry, **9**, 1327, 1970.
64. LaRosa, J. L., Brown, W. V., Levy, R. I., and Fredrickson, D. S.: Alterations in HDL protein composition after heparin-induced lipolysis. Amer. J. Physiol. **220**, 785, 1971.
65. Scanu, A.: Studies on the conformation of human serum high-density lipoproteins HDL_2 and HDL_3. Proc. Nat. Acad. Sci. U.S.A., **54**, 1699, 1965.
66. Scanu, A., and Hirz, R.: On the structure of human serum high-density lipoprotein: studies by the technique of circular dichroism. Proc. Nat. Acad. Sci. U.S.A., **59**, 890, 1968.
67. Gotto, A. M., and Shore, B.: Conformation of human serum high density lipoprotein and its peptide components. Nature (London), **224**, 69, 1969.
68. Scanu, A. M.: The effect of reduction and carboxymethylation on the circular dichroic spectra of two polypeptide classes of serum high density lipoprotein. Biochem. Biophys. Acta, **200**, 570, 1970.
69. LaRosa, J. C., Levy, R. I., Herbert, P., Lux, S. E., and Fredrickson, D. S.: A specific apoprotein cofactor for lipoprotein lipase. Biochem. Biophys. Res. Commun., **41**, 57, 1970.
70. Shore, B., and Shore, V.: Heparin-released lipolytic and esterolytic activities of human and rabbit plasmas. Amer. J. Physiol., **201**, 915, 1961.
71. Greten, H., Levy, R. I., and Fredrickson, D. S.: Evidence for separate monoglyceride hydrolase and triglyceride lipase in post-heparin human plasma. J. Lipid Res., **10**, 326, 1969.
72. LaRosa, J. C., Levy, R. I., Windmueller, H. G., and Fredrickson, D. S.: Evidence for two triglyceride lipases in post-heparin plasma J. Clin. Invest., **49**, 55*a*. 1970.
73. Gofman, J. W., deLallá, O., Glazier, F., Freeman, N. K., Lindgren, F. T., Nichols, A. V., Strishower, E. H., and Tamplin, A. R.: The serum lipoprotein transport system in health, metabolic disorders, atherosclerosis and coronary artery disease. Plasma, **2**, 413, 1954.
74. Gustafson, A., Alaupovic, P., and Furman, R. H.: Studies on composition and structure of serum lipoproteins: separation and characteriza-

tion of phospholipid protein residues obtained by partial delipidization of very low density lipoproteins of human serum. Biochemistry, **3**, 632, 1966.

75. Nichols, A. V., Strishower, E. H., Lindgren, F. T., Adamson, G. L., and Coggiola, E. L.: Analysis of change in ultracentrifugal lipoprotein profiles following heparin and ethyl-*p*-chlorophenoxyisobutyrate administration. Clin. Chim. Acta., **20**, 277, 1968.
76. Glomset, J. A.: The plasma lecithin: cholesterol acyltransferase reaction. J. Lipid Res., **9**, 155, 1968.
77. Norum, K. R., and Gjone, E.: Familial plasma lecithin: cholesterol acyltransferase deficiency. Biochemical study of a new inborn error of metabolism. Scand. J. Clin. Invest., **20**, 231, 1967.
78. Gjone, E., and Norum, K. R.: Familial serum cholesterol ester deficiency. Acta Med. Scand., **183**, 107, 1968.
79. Nichols, A. V.: Personal communication.
80. Hayashi, S., Lindgren, F., and Nichols, A. B.: Degradation of S_f 20–400 and high density lipoproteins of human sera by ethyl ether. J. Amer. Chem. Soc., **81**, 3793, 1959.
81. Nichols, A. V., Coggiola, E. L., Jensen, L. C., and Yokoyama, E. H.: Physical-chemical changes in serum lipoproteins during incubation of human serum. Biochim. Biophys. Acta, **168**, 87, 1968.
82. Lux, S., Nichols, A., Gong, E., Forte, G., and Levy, R. I.: Molecular transformations of high density lipoproteins. Circulation, **42**, suppl. III-7, A-21, 1970.
83. Levy, R. I., Fredrickson, D. S.: Heterogeneity of plasma high density lipoproteins. J. Clin. Invest., **44**, 426, 1965.
84. Sodhi, H. S., and Gould, R. G.: Combination of delipidized high-density lipoprotein with lipids. J. Biol. Chem., **242**, 1205, 1967.
85. Scanu, A.: Binding of human serum high density lipoprotein apoprotein with aqueous dispersions of phospholipids. J. Biol. Chem., **242**, 711, 1967.
86. Chapman, D., Leslie, R. B., Hirz, R., and Scanu, A. M.: High resolution NMR spectra of high-density serum lipoproteins. Biochim. Biophys. Acta, **176**, 524, 1969.
87. Scanu, A. M.: On the temperature dependence of the conformation of human serum high density lipoproteins. Biochim. Biophys. Acta, **181**, 268, 1969.
88. Gotto, A. M., Kon, H., and Birnbaumer, M. E.: Electron spin resonance studies of lipid-protein interaction in human serum lipoproteins. Proc. Nat. Acad. Sci. U.S.A., **65**, 145, 1968.
89. Hirz, R., and Scanu, A. M.: Reassembly *in vitro* of a serum high-density lipoprotein. Biochim. Biophys. Acta, **207**, 364, 1970.
90. Hirz, R., Lux, S., and Gotto, A. M.: Lipid-protein interactions in native and reconstituted high density lipoprotein studied with a spin label. Circulation, **42**, suppl. III-8, A-27, 1970.
91. Baxter, J. L.: Origin and characteristics of endogenous lipid in thoracic duct lymph in rat. J. Lipid Res., **7**, 158, 1966.
92. Shrivastava, B. K., Redgrave, T. G., and Simmonds, W. J.: The source of endogenous lipid in the thoracic duct. Quart. J. Exp. Physiol., **52**, 305, 1967.
93. Lees, R. S., and Fredrickson, D. S.: The differentiation of exogenous and endogenous hyperlipemia by paper electrophoresis. J. Clin. Invest., **44**, 1968, 1965.
94. Kay, R. E., and Entenman, C.: The synthesis of "chylomicron-like" bodies and maintenance of normal blood sugar levels by the isolated, perfused rat liver. J. Biol. Chem., **236**, 1006, 1961.
95. Robinson, P. S.: The uptake and release of lipids by the liver, in *Proceedings of an International Symposium on Lipid Transport,* edited by H. C. Meng, p. 194. Charles C Thomas, Springfield, Ill., 1964.
96. Heimberg, M., Weinstein, I., Dishmon, G., and Fried, M.: Lipoprotein lipid transport by livers from normal and CCl_4-poisoned animals. Amer. J. Physiol., **209**, 1053, 1965.
97. Windmueller, H. G., and Levy, R. I.: Total inhibition of hepatic β-lipoprotein production in the rat by orotic acid. J. Biol. Chem., **242**, 2246, 1967.
98. Windmueller, H. G., and Levy, R. I.: Production of β-lipoprotein by intestine in the rat. J. Biol. Chem., **243**, 4878, 1968.
99. Ockner, R. K., Hughes, F. B., and Isselbacher, K. J.: Very low density lipoproteins in intestinal lymph: origin, composition and role in lipid transport in the fasting state. J. Clin. Invest., **48**, 2079, 1969.
100. Ockner, R. K., and Jones, A. L.: An electron microscope and functional study of very low density lipoproteins in intestinal lymph. J. Lipid Res., **11**, 284, 1970.
101. Mahley, R. W., Hamilton, R. L., and LeQuire, V. S.: Characterization of lipoprotein particles isolated from the Golgi apparatus of rat liver. J. Lipid Res., **10**, 433, 1969.
102. Mahley, R. W., Bersot, T. P., LeQuire, V. S., Levy, R. I., Windmueller, H. G., and Brown, W. V.: Identity of very low density lipoprotein apoproteins of plasma and liver Golgi apparatus. Science, **168**, 380, 1970.
103. Goodman, D. S.: Cholesterol ester metabolism. Physiol. Rev., **45**, 747, 1965.
104. Gofman, J. W., and Tandy, R. K.: Lipid transport in hyperlipidemia, in *Atherosclerotic Vascular Disease* (Transactions of the 16th Hahnemann Symposium on Atherosclerotic Vascular Disease, Philadelphia, Apr. 27–30, 1966), edited by A. N. Brest and J. H. Moyer, p. 162. Appleton-Century-Crofts, New York, 1967.
105. Burstein, M., and Samaille, J.: Sur un dosage rapide du cholesterol lié aux α- et aux β-lipoprotéines du sérum. Clin. Chem. Acta, **5**, 609, 1960.
106. Eaton, R. P., and Kipnis, D. M.: Radioimmunoassay of beta lipoprotein-protein of rat serum. J. Clin. Invest., **48**, 1387, 1969.
107. Lees, R. S.: Immunoassay of plasma low-density lipoproteins. Science, **169**, 493, 1970.
108. Blumberg, B. S., Bernanke, D., and Allison, A. C.: Human lipoprotein polymorphism. J. Clin. Invest., **41**, 1936, 1962.
109. Berg, K.: New serum type system: Lp system. Acta Path. Microbiol. Scand., **59**, 369, 1963.
110. Schultz, J. S., Shreffler, D. C., and Harvie, N. R.: Genetics and antigenic studies and partial purification of a human serum lipoprotein carrying the Lp antigenic determinant. Proc. Nat. Acad. Sci. U.S.A., **61**, 963, 1968.
111. Rider, A. K., Levy, R. I., and Fredrickson, D. S.: "Sinking" pre-beta lipoprotein and the Lp antigen. Circulation **42**, suppl. III-10, A-34, 1970.
112. Wiegandt, H., von Lipp, K., and Wendt, G. G.: Identifizierung eines Lipoproteins mit Antigenwirksamkeit im Lp-system. Hoppe Seyler Z. Physiol. Chem., **394**, 489, 1968.
113. Berg, K.: "International Lp—Arbeitstangung am 3 und 4, Oktober 1966," pp. 1–45, in Institut für human Genetik der Philipps-Universität, Marburg/Lahn, 1966.
114. Harvie, N. R., and Schultz, J. S.: Studies of Lp-lipoprotein as a quantitative genetic trait. Proc. Nat. Acad. Sci. U.S.A., **66**, 99, 1970.
115. Sodhi, H. S.: New lipoprotein differing in charge and density from known plasma lipoproteins. Metabolism, **18**, 852, 1969.
116. Salt, H. B., Wolff, O. H., Lloyd, J. K., Fosbrooke, A. S., Cameron, A. H., and Hubble, D. V.: On having no beta-lipoprotein: a syndrome comprising a-beta-lipoproteinaemia, acanthocytosis, and steatorrhoea. Lancet, **2**, 325, 1960.
117. Druez, G.: Un nouveau cas d'acanthocytose: dysmorphie erythrocytaire congénitale avec retinité, troubles nerveux et stigmates dégénératifs. Rev. Hemat., **14**, 3, 1959.
118. Bassen, F. A., and Kornzweig, A. L.: Malformation of the erythrocytes in a case of atypical retinitis pigmentosa. Blood, **5**, 381, 1950.
119. Singer, K., Fisher, B., and Perlstein, M. A.: Acanthrocytosis: a genetic erythrocyte malformation. Blood, **7**, 577, 1952.
120. Jampel, R. S., and Falls, H. F.: Atypical retinitis pigmentosa, acanthrocytosis, and heredodegenerative neuromuscular disease. Arch. Ophthal., **59**, 818, 1958.
121. Lamy, M., Frezal, J., Polonovski, J., and Rey, J.: L'Absence congénitale de β-lipoprotéines. C. R. Soc. Biol. (Paris), **154**, 1974, 1960.
122. Mabry, C. C., Di George, A. M., and Auerbach, V. H.: Studies concerning the defect in a patient with acanthocytosis. Clin. Res., **8**, 371, 1960.
123. Kornzweig, A. L., and Bassen, F. A.: Retinitis pigmentosa, acanthrocytosis and heredodegenerative neuromuscular disease. Arch. Ophthal. (Chicago), **58**, 183, 1957.

124. Friedman, I. S., Cohn, J., Zymariss, M., and Goldner, M. G.: Hypocholesteremia in idiopathic steatorrhea. Arch. Intern. Med., **105,** 112, 1960.
125. Di George, A. M., Mabry, C. C., and Auerbach, V. H.: Cited by Farquhar and Ways, in [128].
126. Mier, M., Schwartz, S. O., and Boshes, B.: Acanthrocytosis, pigmentary degeneration of the retina and ataxia neuropathy: a genetically determined syndrome with associated metabolic disorder. Blood, **5,** 1586, 1960.
127. Wolff, J. A., and Bauman, W. A.: Studies concerning acanthocytosis: a new genetic syndrome with absent beta-lipoprotein (abstract). Amer. J. Dis. Child., **102,** 478, 1961.
128. Farquhar, J. W., and Ways, P.: Abetalipoproteinemia, in *The Metabolic Basis of Inherited Disease,* 2d ed., edited by J. B. Stanbury, J. B. Wyngaarden, and D. S. Fredrickson, p. 509. McGraw-Hill, New York, 1966.
128*a*. Dische, M. R., and Porro, R. S.: The cardiac lesions in Bassen-Kornzweig syndrome. Amer. J. Med., **49,** 568, 1970.
129. Ways, P., Reed, C. F., and Hanahan, D. J.: Red-cell and plasma lipids in acanthocytosis. J. Clin. Invest., **42,** 1248, 1963.
130. Schwartz, J. F., Rowland, L. P., Eder, H., Marks, P. A., Osserman, E. F., Hirschberg, E., and Anderson, H.: Bassen-Kornzweig syndrome: deficiency of serum β-lipoprotein. Arch. Neurol., **8,** 438, 1963.
131. Forsyth, C. C., Lloyd, J. K., and Fosbrooke, A. S.: A-β-lipoproteinaemia. Arch. Dis. Child., **40,** 47, 1965.
132. Sobrevilla, L. A., Goodman, M. L., and Kane, C. A.: Demyelinating central nervous system disease, macular atrophy and acanthocytosis (Bassen-Kornzweig syndrome). Amer. J. Med., **37,** 821, 1964.
133. Becroft, D. M. O., Costello, J. M., and Scott, P. J.: A-β-lipoproteinaemia (Bassen-Kornzweig syndrome). Arch. Dis. Child., **40,** 40, 1965.
134. Rosen, F.: Cited by Levy, Fredrickson, and Laster [155].
135. Lees, R. S.: Immunological evidence for the presence of B protein (apoprotein of β-lipoprotein) in normal and abetalipoproteinemic plasma. J. Lipid Res., **8,** 396, 1967.
136. Law, D., and Nance, W.: Personal communication.
137. Bach, C., Polonovski, J., and Polonovski, C.: Congenital absence of beta-lipoproteins: a further case. Arch. Franc. Pediat., **24,** 1093, 1967.
138. Hooghwinkel, G. J.: Disorders in the lipid pattern in a patient with acanthocytosis and in some of his family members. Nederl. T. Geneesk., **108,** 1831, 1964.
139. Hooghwinkel, G. J. M., and Bruyn, G. W.: Congenital lack of serum β-lipoproteins: a study of blood phospholipids in a patient and his family. J. Neurol. Sci., **3,** 374, 1966.
140. Shacklady, M. M., Djardjouras, E. M., and Lloyd, J. K.: Red-cell lipids in familial alphalipoprotein deficiency (Tangier disease). Lancet, **2,** 151, 1968.
141. Lourien, E. W.: Personal communication.
142. Kahlke, W.: A-β-lipoproteinemia, in *Lipids and Lipidoses,* edited by G. Schettler, p. 382. Springer-Verlag, New York, 1967.
143. Kuo, P. T., and Bassett, D. R.: Blood and tissue lipids in a family with hypo-beta-lipoproteinaemia. Circulation, **26,** 660, 1962.
144. Critchley, E. M. R., Clark, D. B., and Wikler, A.: An adult form of acanthocytosis. Trans. Amer. Neurol. Ass., **92,** 132, 1967.
145. Estes, J. W., Morley, T. J., Levine, I. M., and Emerson, C. P.: A new hereditary acanthocytosis syndrome. Amer. J. Med., **42,** 868, 1967.
146. Isselbacher, K. J., Scheig, R., Plotkin, G. R., and Caulfield, J. B.: Congenital β-lipoprotein deficiency: an hereditary disorder involving a defect in the absorption and transport of lipids. Medicine, **43,** 347, 1964.
147. Wolff, O. H.: A-beta-lipoproteinaemia. Ergebn. Inn. Med. Kinderheilk., **23,** 190, 1965.
148. Ways, P., Parmentier, C., Saunders, D., Dobbins, W., and Rubin, C. E.: Unpublished data.
149. Ahrens, E. H., Jr., Novikoff, A., and Spritz, N.: As cited by Farquhar and Ways [128].
150. Wolff, O. H.: A-beta-lipoproteinaemia, in *Erbliche Stoffwechselkrankheiten,* edited by F. Linneweh, p. 603. Urban & Schwarzenberg, Munich, 1962.
151. Lamy, M., Frezal, J., Polonovski, J., Druez, G., and Rey, J.: Congenital absence of beta-lipoproteins. Pediatrics, **31,** 277, 1963.
152. Ways, P. O., Parmentier, C. M., Kayden, H. J., Jones, J. W., Saunders, D. R., and Rubin, C. E.: Studies on the absorptive defect for triglyceride in abetalipoproteinemia. J. Clin. Invest., **46,** 35, 1967.
153. Dobbins, W. O., III: An ultrastructural study of the intestinal mucosa in congenital β-lipoprotein deficiency with particular emphasis upon the intestinal absorptive cell. Gastroenterology, **50,** 195, 1966.
154. Rubin, C. E., Brandborg, L. L., Phelps, P. C., and Taylor, H. C., Jr.: Studies of celiac disease. I. Apparent identical and specific nature of duodenal and proximal jejunal lesion in celiac disease and idiopathic sprue. Gastroenterology, **32,** 28, 1960.
155. Levy, R. I., Fredrickson, D. S., and Laster, L.: The lipoproteins and lipid transport in abetalipoproteinemia. J. Clin. Invest., **45,** 531, 1966.
156. Lees, R. S., and Ahrens, E. H., Jr.: Fat transport in abetalipoproteinemia: the effects of repeated infusions of beta-lipoprotein-rich plasma. New Eng. J. Med., **280,** 1261, 1969.
157. Barnard, G., Fosbrooke, A. S., and Lloyd, J. K.: Neutral lipids of plasma and adipose tissue in a-betalipoproteinemia. Clin. Chim. Acta, **28,** 417, 1970.
158. Frezal, J., Rey, J., Polonovski, J., Levy, G., and Lamy, M.: L'Absence congénitale de β-lipoprotéines: étude de l'absorption intestinale prés exsanguinotransfusion: mesure de la demi-vie lipoprotéines injectées. Rev. Franc. Clin. Biol., **6,** 677, 1961.
159. Rey, J.: *L'Absence congénitale de beta-lipoprotéines.* Foulon et Cie., Paris, 1961.
160. Fernandes, J., van De Kramer, J. H., and Weigers, H. A.: Differences in absorption of the various fatty acids studied in children with steatorrhea. J. Clin. Invest., **41,** 488, 1962.
160*a*. Kayden, H. J., and Bessis, M.: Morphology of normal erythrocyte and acanthocyte using Nomarski optics and the scanning electron microscope. Blood, **35,** 427, 1970.
161. Schwartz, S. O., and Motto, S. A.: The diagnostic significance of "burr" red blood cells. Amer. J. Med. Sci., **218,** 513, 1949.
162. Ponder, E.: *Hemolysis and Related Phenomena,* p. 40. Grune & Stratton, New York, 1948.
163. Trotter, W. D.: The slide-coverslip disc-sphere transformation in mammalian erythrocytes. Brit. J. Haemat., **2,** 65, 1956.
164. Dacie, J. V.: *Practical Haematology,* 2d ed., p. 15. New York Publishing Co., New York, 1956.
165. Druez, G., Lamy, M., Frezal, J. Polonovski, J., and Rey, J.: L'Acanthocytose: ses rapports avec l'absence congénitale de β-lipoprotéines. Presse Med., **69,** 1546, 1961.
166. Simon, E. R., and Ways, P.: Incubation hemolysis and red cell metabolism in acanthocytosis. J. Clin. Invest., **43,** 1311, 1964.
167. Wolff, O. H., Lloyd, J. K., and Tonks, E. L.: A-beta-lipoproteinaemia with special reference to the visual defect. Exp. Eye Res., **3,** 439, 1964.
168. Shearrer, A. C. I.: Absorption of β-carotene in human retinitis pigmentosa. Exp. Eye Res., **3,** 427, 1964.
169. Eder, H.: The medical grand rounds. Massachusetts General Hospital Case 525, acanthocytosis. Amer. Practitioner, **13,** 225, 1962.
170. Laster, L.: Personal communication.
171. Smith, C. H., and Erlandsen, M.: Personal communication.
172. Russell, D. S.: Myocarditis in Friedreich's ataxia. J. Path. Bact., **58,** 739, 1946.
173. Boyer, S. H., Chisholm, A. W., and McKusick, V. A.: Cardiac aspects of Friedreich's ataxia. Circulation, **25,** 493, 1962.
174. Jones, J. W., and Ways, P.: Abnormalities of high density lipoproteins in abetalipoproteinemia. J. Clin. Invest., **46,** 1151, 1967.
175. Fredrickson, D. S., Levy, R. I., and Lindgren, F. T.: A comparison of heritable abnormal lipoprotein patterns as defined by two different techniques. J. Clin. Invest., **47,** 2446, 1968.
176. Fredrickson, D. S., Ono, K., and Davis, L. L.: Lipolytic activity of post-heparin plasma in hyperglyceridemia. J. Lipid Res., **4,** 1963.
177. Kuo, P., Bassett, D., Di George, A., and Carpenter, C.: Lipolytic activity of post-heparin plasma in hyperlipemia and hypolipemia. Circulation Res., **16,** 221, 1965.

178. Slack, J., Nair, S., Traisman, H., Becker, G., Mohler, S., and Hsia, D. Y.: Lipoprotein lipase in cystic fibrosis. J. Lab. Clin. Med., **59,** 302, 1962.
179. Roheim, P. S., Miller, and Eder, H. A.: The formation of plasma lipoproteins from apoprotein in plasma. J. Biol. Chem., **240,** 2994, 1965.
180. Wilson, D. E., and Lees, R. S.: A free apolipoprotein in human plasma. Clin. Res., **18,** 467, 1970.
181. Gotto, A. M., Levy, R. I., John, K., and Fredrickson, D. S.: On the nature of the protein defect in abetalipoproteinemia. New. Eng. J. Med., **284,** 813, 1971.
182. Hill, R. B.: Participation of the Golgi complex in hepatic lipoprotein metabolism. J. Cell Biol., **27,** 43A, 1965.
183. Stein, O., and Stein, Y.: Fine structure of the ethanol induced fatty liver in the rat. Israel J. Med. Sci., **1,** 378, 1965.
184. Hamilton, R. L., Regen, D. M., Gray, M. E., and LeQuire, V. S.: Lipid transport in liver. I. Electron microscopic identification of very low density lipoproteins in perfused rat liver. Lab. Invest., **16,** 305, 1967.
185. Sloan, H. S. Kwiterovich, P. O., Levy, R. I., and Fredrickson, D. S.: Carbohydrate components of human plasma lipoproteins. Circulation **42,** III-8, A-28, 1970.
186. Sabesin, S. M., and Isselbacher, K. J.: Protein synthesis inhibition: mechanism for the production of impaired fat absorption. Science, **147,** 1149, 1965.
187. Walton, K. W., and Williamson, N.: Histological and immunofluorescent studies on the evolution of the human atheromatous plaque. J. Atheroscler. Res., **8,** 599, 1968.
188. Phillips, G. B.: Quantitative chromatographic analysis of plasma and red cell lipids in patients with acanthocytosis. J. Lab. Clin. Med., **59,** 357, 1962.
189. McBride, J. A., and Jacob, H. S.: Cholesterol loading of acanthocytic red cell membranes causing hemolytic anemia in experimental and genetic abetalipoproteinemia. J. Clin. Invest., **47,** 67*a*, 1968.
190. Smith, J. A., Lonergan, E. T., and Sterling, K.: Spur-cell anemia. New Eng. J. Med., **271,** 396, 1964.
191. Switzer, S., and Eder, H. A.: Interconversion of acanthocytes and normal erythrocytes with detergents (abstract), J. Clin. Invest., **41,** 1404, 1962.
192. Di George, A. M., Mabry, C. C., and Auerbach, V. H.: A specific disorder of lipid transport (acanthrocytosis): treatment with intravenous lipids. Amer. J. Dis. Child., **102,** 580, 1961.
193. de Gier, J., van Deenen, L. L. M., Verloop, M. C., and van Gastel, C.: Phospholipid and fatty acid characteristics of erythrocytes in some cases of anaemia. Brit. J. Haemat., **10,** 246, 1964.
194. van Deenen, L. L. M., and de Gier, J.: In *The Red Blood Cell,* edited by C. W. Bishop and D. M. Surgenor, p. 298. Academic, New York, 1964.
195. Watson, W. C.: The morphology and lipid composition of the erythrocytes in normal and essential-fatty-acid-deficient rats. Brit. J. Haemat., **9,** 32, 1963.
196. Kanai, M., Raz, A., and Goodman, D. S.: Retinol-binding protein: the transport protein for vitamin A in human plasma. J. Clin. Invest., **47,** 2025, 1968.
197. Smith, F. R., Raz, A., and Goodman, D. S.: Radioimmunoassay of human plasma retinol-binding protein. J. Clin. Invest., **49,** 1754, 1970.
198. Goodman, D. S.: Personal communication.
199. Krinsky, N. I., Cornwell, D. G., and Oncley, J. L.: Transport of vitamin A and carotenoids in human plasma. Arch. Biochem., **73,** 233, 1958.
200. McCormick, E. C., Cornwell, D. G., and Brown, J. B.: Studies on the distribution of tocopherol in human serum lipoproteins. J. Lipid Res., **1,** 211, 1960.
201. Kayden, H. J., and Silber, R.: The role of vitamin E deficiency in the abnormal autohemolysis of acanthocytosis. Trans. Ass. Amer. Physicians, **78,** 334, 1965.
202. Dodge, J. T., Cohen, G., Kayden, J. H., and Phillips, G. B.: Peroxidative hemolysis of red blood cells from patients with abetalipoproteinemia (acanthocytosis). J. Clin. Invest., **46,** 357, 1967.
203. Swern, D.: *Primary Products of Olefinic Autoxidations in Autoxidation and Antioxidants,* edited by W. O. Lundberg, vol. 1, p. 1. Interscience, New York, 1961.
204. Ways, P., and Hanahan, D.: Characterization and quantification of red cell lipids in normal man. J. Lipid Res., **5,** 318, 1964.
205. Cohen, G., and Hochstein, P.: Enzymatic mechanisms of drug sensitivity in the brain. Dis. Nerv. Syst. (suppl.), **24,** 44, 1963.
206. Pentschew, A., and Schwarz, K.: Systemic axonal dystrophy in vitamin E-deficient adult rats with implications in human neuropathology. Acta Neuropath. (Berlin), **1,** 313, 1962.
207. Lampert, P., Blumberg, J. M., and Pentschew, A.: An electron microscopic study of dystrophic axons in the gracile and cuneate nuclei of vitamin E-deficient rats. J. Neuropath. Exp. Neurol., **23,** 60, 1964.
208. Parnell-King, J.: Neuronal changes in spinal cord of mice on vitamin E and fat-deficient diet. Anat. Rec., **148,** 320, 1964.
209. Hartroft, W. F., and Porta, E. A.: Ceroid. Amer. J. Med. Sci., **250,** 326, 1965.
210. Binder, H. J., Herting, D. C., Hurst, V., Finch, S., and Spiro, H. M.: Tocopherol deficiency in man. New Eng. J. Med., **273,** 1289, 1965.
211. Chio, K. S., Reiss, U., Fletcher, B., and Tappel, A. L.: Peroxidation of subcellular organelles: formation of lipofuscin-like fluorescent pigments. Science, **166,** 1535, 1969.
212. van Buchem, F. S. P., Pol, G., de Gier, J., Bottcher, C. J. F., and Pries, C.: Congenital β-lipoprotein deficiency. Amer. J. Med., **40,** 794, 1966.
213. Mars, H., Lewis, L. A., Robertson, A. L., Jr., Butkus, A., and Williams, G. H., Jr.: Familial hypo-β-lipoproteinemia. Amer. J. Med., **46,** 886, 1969.
214. Richet, G., Durepaire, H., Hartmann, L., Ollier, M. -P., Polonovaki, J., and Maitrot, B.: Hypolipoprotéinemie familiale asymptomatique prédominant sur les beta-lipoprotéines: révélée lors de l'étude d'une protéinurie isolée. Presse Med., **77,** 2045, 1969.
215. Levy, R. I., Langer, T., Gotto, A. M., and Fredrickson, D. S.: Familial hypobetalipoproteinemia, a defect in lipoprotein synthesis. Clin. Res., **18,** 539, 1970.
216. Birke, G., Duner, H., Liljedahl, S. O., Pernow, B., Plantin, L. O., and Troell, L.: Histamine, catechol amines and adrenocortical steroids in burns. Acta Chim. Scand., **114,** 87, 1959.
217. Dodds, C., and Mills, G. L.: Influence of myocardial infarction on plasma-lipoprotein concentration. Lancet, **1,** 1160, 1959.
218. Fredrickson, D. S.: The role of lipids in acute myocardial infarction. Circulation, Suppl: IV, **39** and **40,** IV-99, 1969.
219. Walton, K. W., Scott, P. J., Dykes, P. W., and Davies, J. W. L.: Alterations of metabolism and turnover of I^{131} low density lipoproteins in myxoedema and thyrotoxicosis. Clin. Sci., **29,** 217, 1965.
220. Bazzano, G.: Effects of folic acid metabolism on serum cholesterol levels. Arch. Intern. Med., **124,** 710, 1969.
221. Gallin, J. I., Kaye, D., and O'Leary, W. M.: Serum lipids in infection. New Eng. J. Med., **281,** 1981, 1969.
222. Dobbins, W. O.: Hypo-β-lipoproteinemia and intestinal lymphangiectasia. Arch. Intern. Med., **122,** 31, 1968.
223. Fredrickson, D. S., and Altrocchi, P. H.: Tangier disease (familial cholesterolosis with high-density lipoprotein deficiency), in *Cerebral Sphingolipidoses,* edited by S. M. Aronson and B. W. Volk, p. 343. Academic, New York, 1962.
224. Fredrickson, D. S., Altrocchi, P. H., Avioli, L. V., Goodman, D. S., and Goodman, H. C.: Tangier disease. Ann. Intern. Med., **55,** 1016, 1961.
225. Fredrickson, D. S.: Familial high-density lipoprotein deficiency: Tangier disease, in *The Metabolic Basis of Inherited Disease,* edited by J. B. Stanbury, J. B. Wyngaarden, and D. S. Fredrickson, 2d ed., p. 486. McGraw-Hill, New York, 1966.
226. Fredrickson, D. S.: The inheritance of high density lipoprotein deficiency (Tangier disease). J. Clin. Invest., **43,** 228, 1964.
227. Hoffman, H. N., and Fredrickson, D. S.: Tangier disease (familial high density lipoprotein deficiency): clinical and genetic features in two adults. Amer. J. Med., **39,** 582, 1965.
228. Kocen, R. S., Lloyd, J. K., Lascelles, P. T., Fosbrooke, A. S., and Williams, D.: Familial α-lipoprotein deficiency (Tangier disease) with neurological abnormalities. Lancet, **1,** 1341, 1967.
229. Engel, W. K., Dorman, J. D., Levy, R. I., and Fredrickson, D. S.: Neuropathy in Tangier disease: α-lipoprotein deficiency manifesting as familial recurrent neuropathy and intestinal lipid storage. Arch. Neurol., **17,** 1, 1967.

230. Kummer, H., Laissur, J., Spiess, H., Pflugshaupt, R. and Bucher, U.: Familiäre analphalipoproteinämie (Tangier-Krankheit). Schweiz. Med. Wschr., **98,** 406, 1968.

230*a*. Kracht, J., Huth, K., Schoenborn, W., and Fuhrmann, W.: Hypo-α-lipoproteinämie (Tangier disease). Verh. Deutsch. Ges. Path., **54**, 355, 1970.

230*b*. Kracht, J., Huth, K., Schoenborn, W., and Fuhrmann, W.: Hypo-α-lipoproteinemia (Tangier disease). Verh. Deutsch. Ges. Path., **54,** 355, 1970.

231. Haas, L. F., Austad, W. I., and Bergin, J. D.: "Familial alpha-lipoprotein deficiency": report of a further case with neurologic abnormalities. Lancet (in press).

232. Levy, R. I., and Fredrickson, D. S.: Nature of the alpha lipoproteins in Tangier disease. Circulation, **34,** III-156, 1966.

233. Lux, S. E., Levy, R. I., Gotto, A. M., and Fredrickson, D. S.: Studies of the protein defect in Tangier disease, p. 26. Abstracts of the Society for Pediatric Research, 40th Annual Meeting, Atlantic City, Apr. 29–May 2, 1970.

234. Waldorf, D. S., Levy, R. I., and Fredrickson, D. S.: Cutaneous cholesterol ester deposition in Tangier disease. *Arch. Derm.* (Chicago), **95,** 161, 1967.

235. Tanaka, Y., Brecher, G., and Fredrickson, D. S.: Cellules de la maladie de Niemann-Pick et de quelques autres lipidoses (The storage cells of Niemann-Pick disease and some other lipidoses). Nouv. Rev. Franc. Hemat., **3,** 5, 1963.

236. Kwiterovitch, P. O., Sloan, H. R., and Fredrickson, D. S.: Glycolipids and other lipid constituents of normal human liver. J. Lipid Res., **11,** 322, 1970.

237. Böttcher, C. J. F., Woodford, F. P., Ter Haar Romeny-Wachter, C. Ch., Boelsma-Van Houten, E., and Van Gent, C. M.: Fatty acid distribution in lipids of the aortic wall. Lancet, **1,** 1378, 1960.

238. Levy, R. I., and Fredrickson, D. S.: In preparation.

239. Glomset, J. A.: Cited by Norum and Gjone [77].

240. Seidel, D., Alaupovic, P., and Furman, R. H.: A lipoprotein characterizing obstructive jaundice. I. Method for quantitative separation and identification of lipoproteins in jaundiced subjects. J. Clin. Invest., **48,** 1211, 1969.

241. Herbert, P. N.: Personal communication.

242. Kostner, G., and Alaupovic, P.: Studies of the composition and structure of plasmalipoproteins. C- and N-terminal amino acids of the two nonidentical polypeptides of human plasma apolipoprotein A. F.E.B.S. Letters, **15,** 320, 1971.

243. Brewer, H. B., Jr., Shulman, R., Herbert, P., Ronan, R., and Wehrly, K.: The complete amino acid sequence of an apolipoprotein obtained from human very low density lipoprotein (VLDL). Presented at the Fourth International Symposium on Drugs Affecting Lipid Metabolism Sept. 8-11, 1971, Philadelphia.

Addendum: Recent work has indicated that the carboxyl-terminal amino acids in two of apolipoproteins listed in Table 26-3 may be incorrect. ApoVLDL-val probably contains instead carboxyl-terminal serine [241]. It has been reported that "apoHDL-thr," contrary to earlier reports (see page 496), contains glutamine as the carboxyl-terminal amino acid [242]. Both major HDL apoproteins therefore may have the same C-terminal residues, and Kostner and Alaupovic suggest that "apoHDL-thr" and "apoHDL-gln" be designated apoA-I and apoA-II, respectively [242]. A more stable and completely acceptable convention is obviously needed for apolipoprotein nomenclature, and perhaps trivial, but more characteristic names will evolve as the complete structure and the functions of these proteins are uncovered. In this regard, it is encouraging that the complete amino acid sequence of one human apolipoprotein, apoLP-ala, has recently been determined [243].

CHAPTER TWENTY-SEVEN

FAMILIAL LECITHIN:CHOLESTEROL ACYL TRANSFERASE DEFICIENCY

Kaare R. Norum, John A. Glomset, and Egil Gjone

Familial lecithin:cholesterol acyl transferase deficiency (familial plasma cholesteryl ester deficiency) is characterized by corneal opacities, anemia, and proteinuria, by markedly reduced levels of plasma cholesteryl esters and lysolecithin, and by absent or very low levels of plasma lecithin:cholesterol acyl transferase (LCAT) activity. Seven afflicted individuals discovered in three Scandinavian families (Table 27-1) appear to be homozygotes, although no abnormalities have been detected in presumptive heterozygotes.

HISTORY

In June, 1966, a 33-year-old woman (A.R.) from western Norway was admitted to the University Hospital in Oslo. She had diffuse grayish corneal opacities, anemia, proteinuria, and hyperlipemia, and was presumed to have chronic nephritis. However, there was no history of acute nephritis, renal tubular function was normal, and the serum albumin level was only slightly reduced. Furthermore, both plasma triglycerides and cholesterol were increased, and most of the cholesterol was unesterified. Plasma lecithin was increased, plasma lysolecithin was decreased, and no pre-β- or α_1-lipoproteins could be detected on electrophoresis. In addition, a kidney biopsy, examined by Dr. Brynjulf Øystese, University Hospital, Oslo, was most unusual in that it showed foam cells in the glomerular tufts. Subsequently, the same clinical features and the same relative abnormalities in plasma cholesterol and phospholipid were found in two sisters (I.S. and M.R.), and further studies of all three sibs disclosed the absence of plasma LCAT activity. Because all three were afflicted and because none had a history of liver or kidney disease which could account for the abnormalities, it appeared that they suffered from a previously undiscovered inborn error of metabolism [1, 2, 3].

This interpretation was strengthened in 1968 when Dr. Bengt Hamnström of Karlstad, Sweden, brought to our attention a patient whom he had been studying for several years. This patient, a 45-year-old woman (M.L.), had corneal opacities, anemia, proteinuria, and hyperlipemia. Furthermore, a brother (B.B.) had developed the same symptoms and had died in uremia. When Dr. Hamnström's patient was admitted to the University Hospital in Oslo, she was found to have the same plasma lipid and lipoprotein abnormalities and the same LCAT abnormality previously observed in the three Norwegian sisters [4]. Finally, in 1968 a brother (L.G.) and sister (A.A.) from a third family were referred to us by Dr. Sigurd Börsting of Kristiansund, Norway. These last two patients live in the same general area of Norway as the three original patients and have the same symptoms, plasma lipid abnormalities, and LCAT deficiency [39].

CLINICAL MANIFESTATIONS

Corneal Opacity

The clinical sign most easily detectable is an infiltrate of numerous minute grayish particles distributed in all layers of the stroma (Fig. 27-1). It is most pronounced near the limbus, where it is annular and resembles a corneal arcus [5].

Table 27-1. CLINICAL FEATURES

Patient	Sex	Age detected, yr	Corneal opacity	Anemia	Foam cells in bone marrow	Proteinuria	Foam cells in kidney	Hyperlipemia	LCAT	Cholesteryl esters
Norway:										
M.R.	F	19	+	+	+	+	+	–	–	Low
I.S.	F	31	+	+	+	+	0	+	–	Low
A.R.	F	33	+	+	+	+	+	+	–	Low
Sweden:										
M.L.	F	47	+	+	–	+	0	+	–(+)	Low
B.B.	M	Post mortem	+	+	0	+	+	+	0	0
Norway:										
L.G.	M	35	+	+	–	+	0	+	–	Low
A.A.	F	42	+	+	–	+	0	+	–	Low

Note: – = not detected; 0 = not examined.

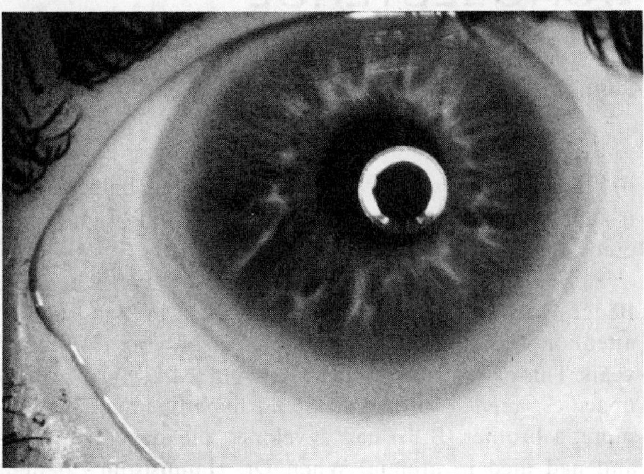

Figure 27-1. Corneal infiltrate in A.R. It is localized to the parenchyma, is composed of numerous minute dots, and is most prominent in the periphery, where it resembles a corneal arcus. (See also Plate I-4.)

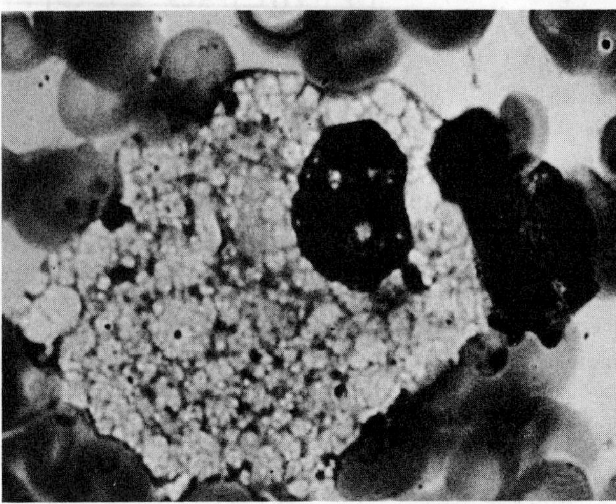

Figure 27-2. Foam cells in a bone marrow aspirate from A.R.

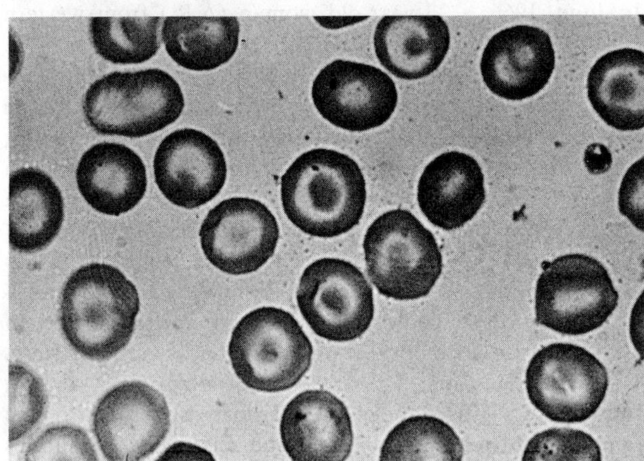

Figure 27-3. "Target cells" in peripheral blood from A.R. (*From E. Gjone, H. Torsvik, and K. Norum. Scand. J. Clin. Lab. Invest.*, **21**, 327, 1968.)

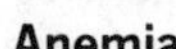

Anemia

The patients all have a moderate normochromic anemia with a hemoglobin concentration of about 10 gm per 100 ml. The hematologic data (Table 27-2) suggest that the anemia is due to a combination of decreased erythropoiesis and moderately increased erythrocyte destruction. Two findings are of special interest: (1) bone marrow aspirates from A.R., M.R., and I.S. (but not from M.L.) were unusual in that they contained "foam cells" (Fig. 27-2); (2) dry smears of the blood of all the patients showed "target cells" (Fig. 27-3). Both findings may be causally related to the anemia (see later discussion). Nevertheless, osmotic fragility of the erythrocytes is normal, and surface scanning after erythrocyte labeling has given no indication that the patients' spleens are particularly active in erythrocyte destruction.

Table 27-2. HEMATOLOGIC DATA

	Patients					
	A.R.	I.S.	M.R.	A.A.	L.G.	M.L.
Hemoglobin, gm/100 ml	8.7–10.5	9.5	10.5–11.5	8.9–10.9	11.2–12.2	10.5
Erythrocytes, $10^6/\mu l$	2.9–3.7	3.88	3.58–3.47	3.13	3.89–4.51	3.8
Mean cell hemoglobin, $\mu\mu g$	30–28	25	29–33	28–35	29–27	28
Reticulocytes (per 1,000 erythrocytes)	0.1–16	18	14	0	0	12–74
Serum iron, μg/100 ml	30–90	85	170	138	115	159
Transferrin (iron-binding capacity, μg/100 ml)	140	240	270	....	....	252
White blood cells, per μl	4,500–7,000	4,100–5,300	3,700–4,500	4,600	4,700	4,400
Platelets, $10^3/\mu l$	113–148	132–179	143	220	320	140
Osmotic fragility	Normal	Normal	Normal	0	0	Normal
Erythrocyte life-span (chromium) (days $t_{1/2}$)	16	....	....	....	....	17

Note: 0 = not examined.

Table 27-3. SOME PERTINENT LABORATORY FINDINGS

	Patients					
	A.R.	I.S.	M.R.	A.A.	L.G.	M.L.
Serum proteins, gm/100 ml	5.2–6.6	5.3	5.5	6.1	6.4	6.1
Serum albumin, gm/100 ml	2.3–2.9	3.1	3.1	3.5	3.7	3.8
Urea, mg/100 ml	45–65	44	30	41	50	32
Creatinine, mg/100 ml	1.0–1.3	1.1	0.9	0.9	0.9–1.5	0.9
Uric acid, mg/100 ml	8.6–10.3	4.6	3.9	8.8	10.6	4.9
Antistreptolysin (specific)	80–120	120	400	200	250	120
Antistreptolysin (nonspecific)*	72,000	30,000	25,000	2,100	15,000	8,500–72,000

Note: The data represent nonspecific antistreptolysin values obtained by the method of J. Hällen, Acta Path. Microbiol. Scand., **57,** 301, 1963, before precipitating the β-lipoproteins with dextran sulfate and calcium chloride.
*Data presented through the courtesy of Dr. Bengt Hamnström, Karlstad, Sweden.

Proteinuria

The urine of the patients contains protein, erythrocytes, and hyaline casts. Most of the urinary protein migrates in the position of albumin on electrophoresis; α_1- and α_2-migrating proteins are also present. The protein is moderately concentrated (about 0.5 to 1.5 mg protein per ml urine) in five of the six living patients. The proteinuria of the sixth patient (A.R.) was moderate when she was first studied, but recently has increased considerably. A seventh patient (B.B.), now deceased, also had moderate proteinuria, which increased a few months before he died in uremia.

All but one of the living patients have only slightly reduced serum albumin levels (Table 27-3). Recently, A.R. has developed a much-reduced level (1.5 gm per 100 ml), in association with increased proteinuria. All the living patients have normal serum creatinine and urea concentrations. Foam cells have been found in the glomerular tufts of the three patients (A.R., M.R., and B.B.) whose renal histology has been studied (Fig. 27-4).

Plasma Lipid and Lipoprotein Abnormalities

All the patients have abnormally low concentrations of plasma cholesteryl esters and abnormally high levels of plasma unesterified cholesterol. In all, the relative amounts of lecithin are increased and those of lysolecithin are decreased; in all but one patient the absolute amounts of lecithin are increased and those of lysolecithin are decreased. All but the youngest have hyperglyceridemia and pro-

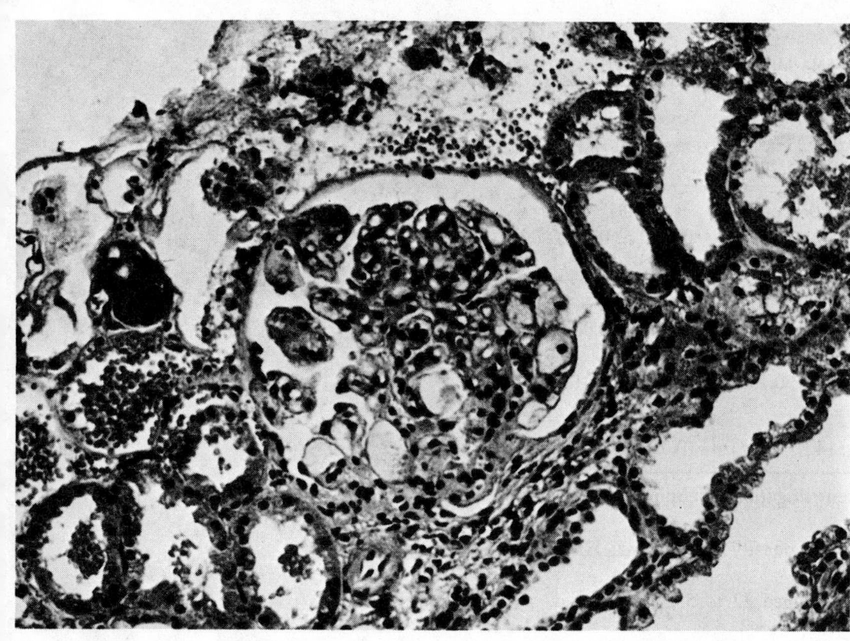

Figure 27-4. Foam cells in a glomerular tuft in a renal biopsy from A.R. (*Courtesy of Dr. Brynjulf Øystese, University Hospital, Oslo, Norway.*)

Table 27-4. PLASMA LIPIDS

Lipids	Patients					
	A.R.	I.S.	M.R.	A.A.	L.G.	M.L.
Total cholesterol, mg/100 ml	300–400	400–600	140–200	300–400	350	370
Cholesteryl ester mg/100 ml	15–40	30–80	10–25	20–30	30	100
Unesterified cholesterol, mg/100 ml	285–380	370–550	130–180	280–370	320	270
Triglycerides, mg/100 ml	300–500	570–700	120–180	400–1,800	1,500	533
Phospholipids, total, mg/100 ml	400–600	600–800	160–200	200–400	220	380
Phosphatidylcholine*	85	83	83	85	82	86
Phosphatidylethanolamine and phosphatidylserine*	3.9	3.6	3.6	3.9	7.4	3.3
Sphingomyelin*	9.7	11.3	11.6	8.8	7.8	8.8
Lysolecithin*	1.3	1.8	2.0	2.0	2.8	2.0

* Figures represent percentages of total phospholipid phosphorus.

nounced hyperlipemia (Table 27-4). The lipid content in the major plasma lipoprotein classes isolated by preparative ultracentrifugation shows corresponding changes (Tables 27-5 and 27-6). The ratio of cholesteryl ester to unesterified cholesterol is low in all the lipoprotein classes, and it *decreases* rather than increases with increasing lipoprotein density. Also, both the absolute concentrations of lecithin and unesterified cholesterol and the relative concentration of lecithin compared to sphingomyelin are increased in the LDL (low density lipoproteins). Only in the HDL (high density lipoproteins) is the concentration of lecithin below normal. Even the nonlipemic patient (M.R.) has less than 40 percent of the normal concentration of HDL lecithin.

Further lipoprotein abnormalities are disclosed by electrophoresis. No pre-β-lipoprotein band is seen in spite of the hyperlipemia, and there is no α_1-lipoprotein band (Fig. 27-5) even when the plasma is not hyperlipemic. The very low density lipoproteins (VLDL) isolated by preparative ultracentrifugation migrate in the β position, instead of the usual pre-β position. Most of the HDL migrate in the α_2 position instead of the usual α_1 position, but some migrate in the prealbumin position. Both the HDL and the unfractionated plasma react with anti-HDL serum, however, but form precipitin arcs in abnormal positions on immunoelectrophoresis (Fig. 27-6) [6].

Other Findings

Postheparin lipolytic activity [7] has been determined in three patients. The peak levels occurred about 30 min after the injection of 1 mg per kg body weight of heparin, and were 0.09, 0.32, and 0.35 mmole FFA per liter of plasma per minute in M.L., A.R., and A.A., respectively. The peak

Table 27-5. DISTRIBUTION OF LIPIDS IN PLASMA LIPOPROTEINS OF M.R.*

Lipoproteins†	Lecithin, μmoles/ml	Unesterified cholesterol, μmoles/ml	Triglyceride, μmoles/ml
VLDL	0.08 (0.077 ± 0.008)‡	0.11 (0.084 ± 0.074)	0.31 (0.220 ± 0.223)
LDL:			
D, 1.006–1.019	0.09 (0.009 ± 0.005)	0.15 (0.020 ± 0.008)	0.14 (0.009 ± 0.003)
D, 1.019–1.063	0.65 (0.336 ± 0.088)	0.93 (0.627 ± 0.134)	— (0.071 ± 0.012)
HDL	0.39 (1.07 ± 0.151)	0.40 (0.514 ± 0.085)	0.04 (0.052 ± 0.009)

* Plasma lipoproteins separated by serial ultracentrifugation in a Spinco preparative ultracentrifuge.

†VLDL, very low density lipoproteins; LDL, low density lipoproteins; HDL, high density lipoproteins; D, density, gm per ml.

‡Values in parentheses from six normal females aged 22 to 55. Mean ± s.d.

Source: J. A. Glomset, et al., [11].

Table 27-6. LIPID RATIOS IN PLASMA LIPOPROTEINS OF M.R.*

Lipoproteins	Lecithin/ sphingomyelin	Lecithin/ unesterified cholesterol	Cholesteryl ester/ unesterified cholesterol
VLDL	12.1 (8.00 ± 1.71)	0.72 (0.826 ± 0.151)	0.52 (0.755 ± 0.094)
LDL:			
D, 1.006–1.019	7.24 (5.89 ± 1.34)	0.60 (0.455 ± 0.087)	0.23 (1.30 ± 0.131)
D, 1.019–1.063	7.72 (2.21 ± 0.156)	0.70 (0.519 ± 0.039)	0.13 (2.16 ± 0.153)
HDL	7.83 (6.20 ± 0.998)	0.98 (2.11 ± 0.253)	0.08 (2.84 ± 0.202)

* Same experiment as shown in Table 27-5. Data from normal controls and abbreviations as in Table 27-5.
Source: J. A. Glomset, et al., [11].

level obtained in M.L. is far below normal, whereas peak levels obtained in A.R. and A.A. are in the normal range. Elevated serum uric acid concentrations have been found in three of the hyperlipemic patients (A.R., A.A., and L.G.). Finally, very high nonspecific antistreptolysin titers (up to 72,000 units) were found in all the patients when sheep erythrocytes were used as substrates, whereas normal titers were found when rabbit erythrocytes were used (Table 27-3).

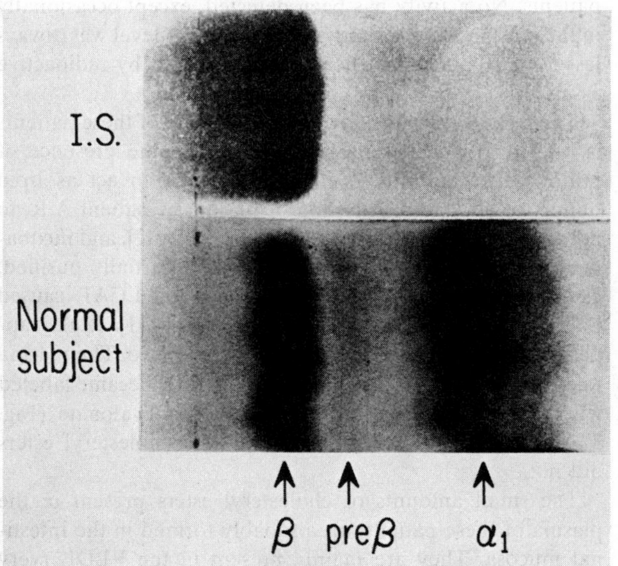

Figure 27-5. Paper electrophoresis of 50 μl plasma from I.S. and from a normal subject. No α_1- or pre-β-lipoproteins are seen in the plasma of I.S. upon staining with Sudan black. A faintly stained band in the α_2 region is probably caused by small amounts of abnormally migrating HDL. See text, and compare with Fig. 27-6. (*From K. Norum and E. Gjone. Scand. J. Lab. Clin. Invest.*, **20,** 231, 1967.)

CLINICAL COURSE

The earliest sign of the disease noted in any of the patients was proteinuria (discovered in M.L. at age 3 or 4 years). Corneal infiltrates were noticed at puberty, and in most cases anemia was discovered toward the end of the second decade. The earliest symptom directly attributable to the disease occurred in A.R. at the age of 33. At that time she was weak and tired, and had a hemoglobin concentration of 8.7 gm per 100 ml. At age 36 kidney function began to deteriorate and proteinuria with hyaline casts, severe hypoproteinemia, and edema developed. Hemoglobin concentration fell to

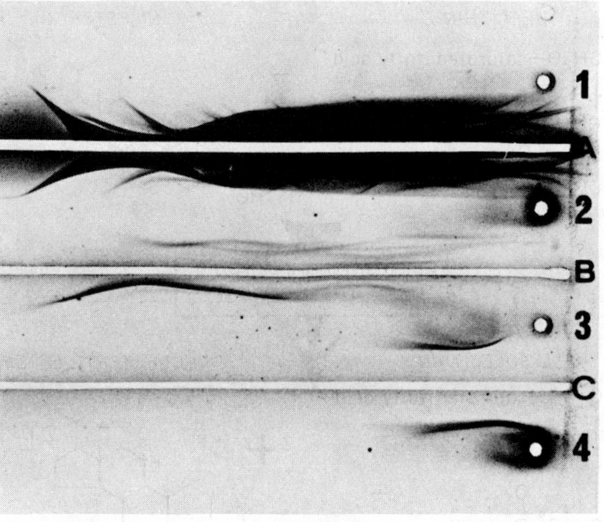

Figure 27-6. Immunoelectrophoresis in agar of serum from A.R. (wells 2 and 4) and from a normal subject (wells 1 and 3). The troughs contained: A, anti-human serum; B, anti-α_1-lipoprotein serum; C, anti-β-lipoprotein serum. The slide was stained for protein. (*From H. Torsvik. Scand. J. Clin. Lab. Invest.*, **24,** 187, 1969.)

about 7.5 gm per 100 ml. At age 37 urine production essentially ceased; since then she has been treated by dialysis. The oldest living patient, M.L., is 48 years old and still has only mild proteinuria. Her brother, who died in uremia at the age of 41, probably had the same disease. He had corneal opacities, anemia, proteinuria, and hyperlipemia at age 37, when endogenous creatinine clearance, serum nonprotein nitrogen, and an intravenous pyelogram were all normal. At autopsy extensive hyaline degeneration of the glomeruli was found, and foam cells similar to those shown in Fig. 27-4 were seen in the less-damaged glomerular tufts. Advanced atherosclerosis of the abdominal aorta was also found, with marked obstruction of both renal arteries.

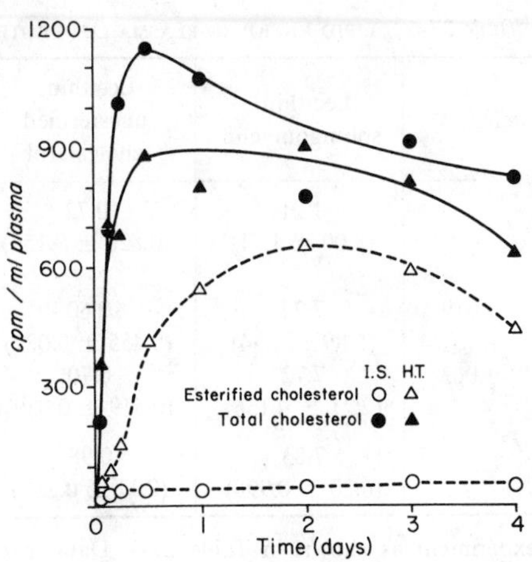

Figure 27-8. Labeled total and esterified cholesterol in the plasma of I.S. and a normal subject, H.T., after the intravenous injection of mevalonate-3-^{14}C.

LECITHIN:CHOLESTEROL ACYL TRANSFERASE

The Enzyme

The relatively low levels of cholesteryl ester and lysolecithin and the relatively high levels of unesterified cholesterol and lecithin in the plasma of these patients appear to be due to a deficiency of plasma lecithin:cholesterol acyl transferase (LCAT). This enzyme, discovered by Sperry in 1935 [8], is normally present in human plasma. For many years it was erroneously believed to be a cholesterol esterase, of no importance in plasma lipoprotein metabolism. Recent experiments by several investigators [9] have shown that the enzyme catalyzes the formation of cholesteryl esters by promoting the transfer of fatty acids from the lecithin to the cholesterol of plasma lipoproteins (Fig. 27-7). Also, evidence has been adduced that the acyl transferase reaction normally forms most of the cholesteryl esters of human plasma.

The presence of the enzyme can be demonstrated by incubating plasma at 37°C for several hours and then measuring the changes in plasma lecithin or cholesterol. Alternatively, plasma can be incubated with radioactive cholesterol, and the formation of radioactive cholesteryl esters measured [10]. Both procedures have been used in attempts to demonstrate LCAT activity in the plasma of the patients. No activity has been detected, except occasionally in the plasma of M.L., and then the enzyme level was always less than 10 percent of normal as measured by radioactive assay [4].

The lack of enzyme activity in the plasma of these patients is due to absence of the enzyme, not to the presence of inhibitors or inability of the lipoproteins to act as lipid donors or acceptors. Addition of plasma of patient A.R. to normal plasma did not inhibit LCAT activity [2], and incubation of the plasma of this patient with a partially purified, essentially lipoprotein-free preparation of LCAT caused esterification of the lipoprotein cholesterol [11]. It also appears that the enzyme is not functioning in vivo. The plasma unesterified cholesterol of patient I.S. rapidly became labeled when she was injected with radioactive mevalonate (Fig. 27-8). In contrast to normal, the plasma cholesteryl esters did not.

The small amounts of cholesteryl esters present in the plasma of these patients are probably formed in the intestinal mucosa. They are mainly present in the VLDL (very low density lipoproteins) (Table 27-5) and, like the chylomicrons in human thoracic duct lymph [12], contain large amounts of oleate and palmitate (Table 27-7). Also, they become labeled following the ingestion of radioactive cholesterol (Fig. 27-9) but not following the intravenous administration of labeled mevalonate, a precursor of cholesterol (Fig. 27-8).

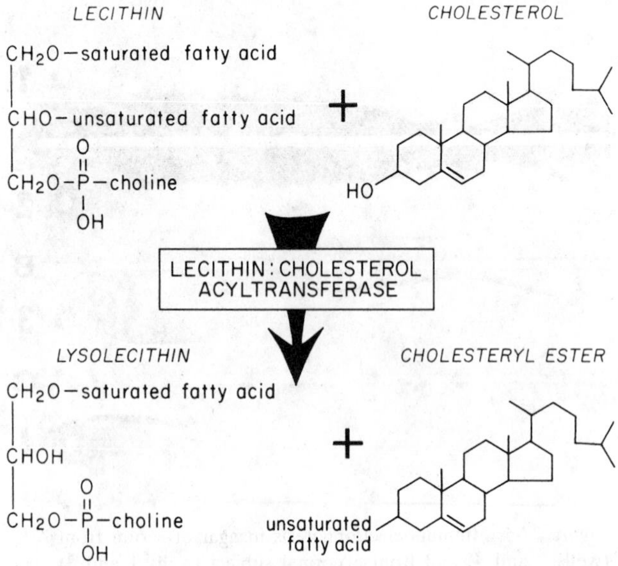

Figure 27-7. Principal lipid reactants in the plasma lecithin:cholesterol acyl transferase reaction. (*From J. Glomset, in Blood Lipids and Lipoproteins, edited by G. Nelson. Wiley, New York, in press.*)

Table 27-7. CHOLESTERYL ESTER FATTY ACIDS*

Patient	12:0	14:0	16:0	16:1	17:0	18:0	18:1	18:2	20:0	20:4
A.R.	2.0	2.4	20.5	4.7	1.7	12.8	41.4	14.1	...	0.3
I.S.	1.9	2.6	32.5	5.9	0.6	10.4	39.0	6.5	...	0.6
M.R.	...	2.4	23.3	5.3	1.0	8.7	40.2	15.5	2.4	1.0
A.A.	1.4	2.9	27.4	6.7	...	7.2	35.1	16.9		
L.G.	...	1.6	24.4	6.3	...	8.8	42.8	12.5	...	3.7
M.L.	3.5	1.6	13.0	6.2	...	4.3	35.6	33.6	1.4	0.8
Normal plasma†	0.3	1.2	12.4	6.1	...	2.4	18.4	47.8	...	5.3

* Values expressed as percent of total fatty acid methyl esters.
† From W. Schrade, R. Biegler, E. Boehle, and E. Harmuth. Lancet, **1,** 285, 1963.

High Density Lipoproteins and LCAT

The high density lipoproteins normally play an important role in the LCAT reaction. They form specific complexes with the enzyme [13], and are preferred substrates of the enzyme in vitro [14] and apparently in vivo [15]. Through them LCAT exerts important indirect effects on the composition of VLDL and LDL [16, 11]. Because of this special relationship, LCAT probably has a considerable influence on the properties of circulating HDL, and it is assumed that newly formed HDL differs considerably from HDL that has been exposed to the enzyme for several hours [17]. One might expect that the HDL of patients who lack LCAT would differ from most of the circulating HDL of normal individuals and would resemble recently formed normal HDL. Insufficient information is available concerning either such newly formed HDL or the lipoproteins of these patients for ascertaining whether such a resemblance actually exists. However, some suggestive evidence has been obtained by experimentation [11].

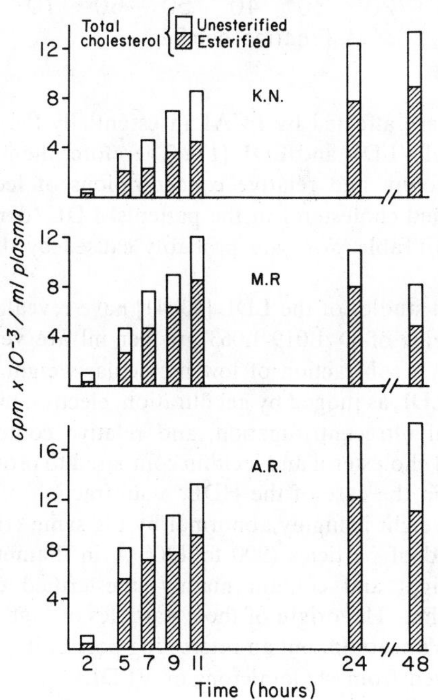

Figure 27-9. Labeled cholesterol in the plasma of A.R., M.R., and a normal subject, K.N., after the oral administration of cholesterol-3-^{14}C. Bars, total plasma labeled cholesterol; hatched segments, esterified cholesterol; open segments, unesterified cholesterol.

Plasma proteins of a density greater than 1.063 from patient M.R. were separated by gel filtration on Sephadex G 200 (Fig. 27-10), and compared with corresponding proteins from normal plasma (Fig. 27-11). The upper part of each figure shows the relative position of the HDL compared with the other plasma proteins. The lower part shows the relative lipid composition of the lipoprotein subfractions. The plasma of M.R. contained two distinct HDL subfractions, one apparently of larger and one of smaller molecular size than most of the HDL from normal plasma. Studies of the plasma of A.R. and A.A. have yielded similar results, except that in both of them the minor peak was smaller. Other experiments support the possibility that the minor peak has a counterpart in normal plasma. Thus, the position of the minor peak corresponds to that postulated [17] for recently secreted normal HDL. Furthermore, like the normal HDL that appear in this position, the lipoproteins in the minor peak from the plasma of M.R. reacted rapidly with LCAT (Fig. 27-12). The total cholesterol of these lipoproteins also increases dramatically when they are incubated with LCAT in the presence of erythrocyte membranes (Table 27-8). Whether the major peak also has a counterpart in normal plasma remains to be determined. One possibility is that it corresponds to HDL formed during the metabolism of VLDL. If so, its composition may be somewhat different from that of HDL normally formed in this way, because the lipid composition of the VLDL of the patients is abnormal. The reader may refer to Chap. 26 for a further discussion of the relationships between HDL and VLDL.

Recent studies [40, 41] of the HDL have substantiated the differences between the two subfractions. The subfraction of low molecular weight more nearly resembles normal HDL as judged by electron microscopy, analytical ultracentrifugation, and the relative content of unesterified cholesterol and lecithin compared to protein. The subfraction of high molecular weight is markedly abnormal by all these criteria.

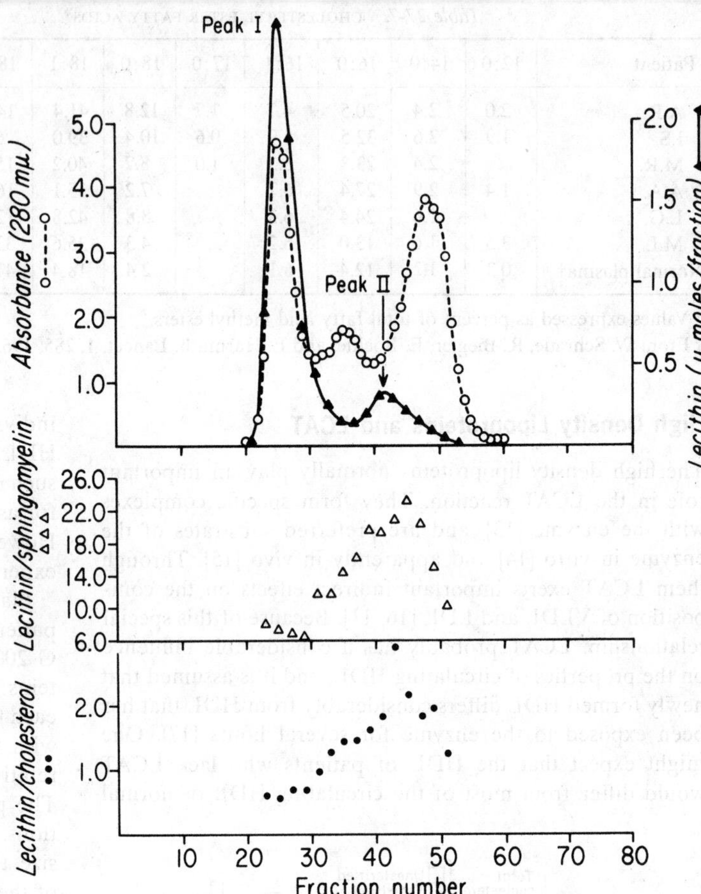

Figure 27-10. Separation of M.R.'s plasma proteins with density greater than 1.063 gm per ml, by gel filtration on Sephadex G 200. *Upper part,* position of the HDL; *lower part,* ratios of lecithin/sphingomyelin and lecithin/cholesterol in the HDL subfractions. (*From J. A. Glomset, K. R. Norum, and W. King,* J. Clin. Invest., **49,** 1827, 1970.)

Very Low Density Lipoproteins, Low Density Lipoproteins, and LCAT

Although LCAT preferentially esterifies the cholesterol of the HDL, it affects VLDL and LDL also. It does not directly esterify the cholesterol of the VLDL, but in the presence of HDL it indirectly increases the cholesteryl ester [16] and decreases the unesterified cholesterol, lecithin, and triglyceride [11, 16] of the VLDL. Apparently, it does this by directly catalyzing changes in HDL cholesterol and lecithin, which in turn promote nonenzymatic transfers of lipid between the HDL and VLDL. The enzyme has a similar indirect effect on the unesterified cholesterol and lecithin of LDL. Also, it directly catalyzes the esterification of LDL cholesterol by the mechanism shown in Fig. 27-7. Presumably, as lipoprotein lipase progressively removes the triglyceride of circulating VLDL in vivo, causing the formation of lipoproteins of greater density, the LCAT reaction both directly and indirectly changes the phospholipid and cholesterol of these lipoproteins [18]. This sequence of events would explain why in normal man the ratio of cholesteryl ester to unesterified cholesterol increases with increasing lipoprotein density in the VLDL-LDL classes while the ratio of lecithin to sphingomyelin decreases (Table 27-6) [11]. Experiments performed in vitro have indicated that VLDL and LDL of the patients are affected by LCAT in essentially the same way as normal VLDL and LDL [11]. Therefore, the abnormally high absolute and relative concentrations of lecithin and unesterified cholesterol in the patients' LDL (density 1.019 to 1.063) (Table 27-6) are probably caused by the enzyme lack.

Recent studies of the LDL [40, 41] have revealed that the lipoproteins of D 1.019-1.063 gm per ml are very heterogeneous. A subfraction of low molecular weight resembles normal LDL as judged by gel filtration, electron microscopy, analytical ultracentrifugation, and relative content of unesterified cholesterol and lecithin compared to protein. However, as in the case of the HDL, a subfraction of high molecular weight is highly abnormal by the same criteria. It is composed of particles (900 to 1200 Å in diameter) which scatter light and contain mainly unesterified cholesterol and lecithin. The origin of these particles of high molecular weight is uncertain, but an interesting possibility is that they are derived from chylomicrons or VLDL.

Erythrocytes and LCAT

Both the lecithin [19] and the unesterified cholesterol [20] of erythrocyte membranes can exchange with the lecithin

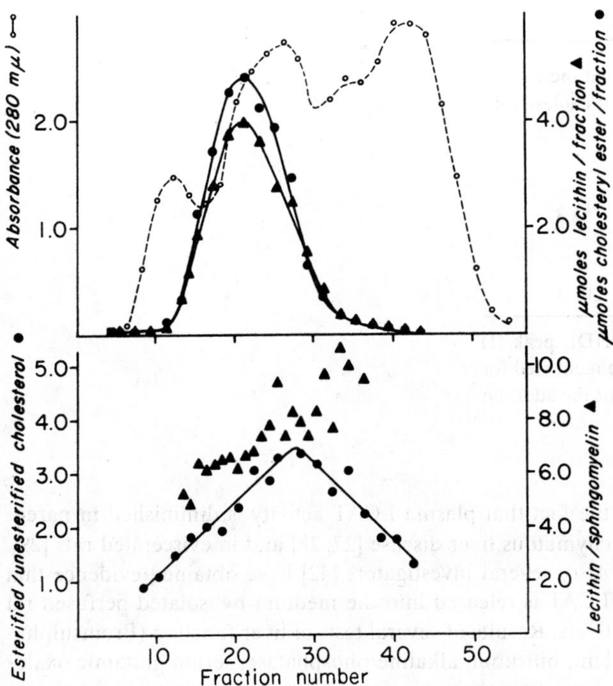

Figure 27-11. Separation of the plasma proteins with density greater than 1.063 gm per ml, of a normal subject, by gel filtration on Sephadex G 200. *Upper part,* position of the HDL; *lower part,* ratios of lecithin/sphingomyelin and cholesteryl ester/unesterified cholesterol in the HDL subfractions. (*From J. Glomset, F. Janssen, R. Kennedy, and J. Dobbins. J. Lipid Res.,* **7**, 639, 1966; *Rockefeller University Press, New York.*)

and unesterified cholesterol of plasma lipoproteins. Also, the unesterified cholesterol of erythrocyte membranes is decreased when erythrocytes are incubated with plasma in the presence of LCAT [21]. These findings suggest that the LCAT reaction may indirectly regulate the cholesterol and possibly the lecithin content of plasma membranes, a possibility which is supported by studies of erythrocytes of the patients. Dry smears of blood of the patients show the presence of target cells (Fig. 27-3) [22]. Also, the erythrocytes have an abnormal lipid composition (Table 27-9). Both the cholesterol content and the lecithin content per erythrocyte are nearly twice normal, although the total phospholipid is normal because the phosphatidylethanolamine and sphingomyelin are reduced. These erythrocyte abnormalities appear to be secondary to the abnormal plasma lipid composition. This is indicated by the fact that both the proportion of "target cells" and the cholesterol content per cell are diminished following incubation of the erythrocytes in normal plasma (Table 27-10). Furthermore, the cholesterol content of normal erythrocytes increases when the latter are incubated in plasma from the patients (Table 27-11) [23].

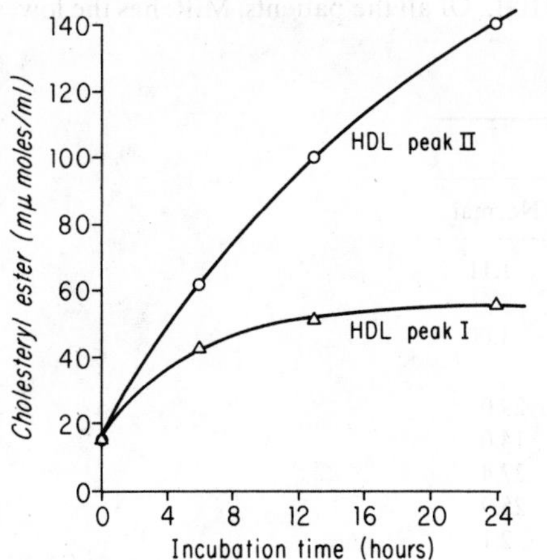

Figure 27-12. Reactivity of HDL peak I and HDL peak II, prepared as in Fig. 27-10, with LCAT. (*From J. A. Glomset, K. R. Norum, and W. King,* J. Clin. Invest., **49,** 1827, 1970.)

NATURE OF THE BIOCHEMICAL DEFECT

Plasma Lipids

At the present stage of knowledge concerning the biochemistry of the several processes affected, only a few features of the disease can be convincingly traced to the enzyme deficiency. One of these is the abnormal cholesterol and phospholipid composition of the plasma. The relatively high levels of unesterified cholesterol and lecithin and the relatively low levels of cholesteryl ester and lysolecithin can be ascribed to the absence of the enzyme, in view of the considerable evidence concerning the role of LCAT in forming plasma cholesteryl esters in man. The formation of the cholesteryl esters of human plasma in vivo is impressively similar to the formation of plasma cholesteryl esters by the LCAT reaction in vitro. The rates of plasma cholesteryl ester formation in vivo and in vitro appear to be identical: about 40 mg cholesterol per liter of plasma per hour is esterified in both cases [24, 25]. The composition of the cholesteryl esters of fresh plasma coincides with that of the esters formed by the LCAT reaction: nearly 90 pércent of the esters are comprised of mono-, di-, and tetraunsaturated fatty acids in both cases [14]. Finally, the relative incorporation of radioactive cholesterol into the cholesteryl esters of VLDL, LDL, and HDL is similar in vivo and in vitro. Both when radioactive mevalonate is injected intravenously [15] and when radioactive cholesterol is incubated with plasma [14], the order of lipoprotein cholesteryl ester specific activity is HDL $\gg$ VLDL $>$ LDL. In view of this evidence one would expect an increase in unesterified cholesterol and lecithin and a decrease in cholesteryl ester and lysolecithin in the plasma of subjects with absent or very low enzyme activity.

Similarly, one might expect changes in the physical properties of the lipoproteins carrying these lipids. In particular the HDL and LDL might be atypical. Speculation has already been mentioned that a minor HDL subfraction obtained from the plasma of M.R. by gel filtration (Fig. 27-10) may resemble normal HDL that have entered the plasma

Table 27-8. INCUBATION OF HDL SUBFRACTION FROM M.R.*

Subfraction	*Cholesterol, mμmoles per ml*			Percent increase in total cholesterol
	Unesterified	Esterified	Total	
HDL peak I	72.6	2.9	75.5	
HDL peak I + LCAT	57.4	58.3	115.7	
Δ			40.2	52.8
HDL peak II	61.2	4.3	65.5	
HDL peak II + LCAT	57.4	142.4	199.8	
Δ			134.3	205.3

* Lipoproteins corresponding to the major (HDL peak I) and minor (HDL peak II) subfractions prepared from plasma of patient M.R. by gel filtration were incubated for 24 hr in the presence of normal erythrocyte membranes, with and without the addition of partially purified LCAT from normal plasma.
Source: J. A. Glomset, et al., [11].

too recently to have reacted extensively with the enzyme. Nevertheless, it is far from clear that HDL abnormalities can be explained on this basis. It would appear that the apolipoproteins responsible for the α_1 mobility of normal HDL are altered or deficient. We presently do not know of a metabolic relationship between LCAT and apoHDL. HDL and LCAT are related functionally, and both proteins are probably synthesized in the liver [9, 26]. Therefore, it is conceivable that the biosynthesis of the enzyme and one or more of the HDL apoproteins (see Chap. 26) is at least partially regulated by a common control mechanism. If so, then a primary defect in LCAT formation might be associated with reduced synthesis of one or more of the HDL apoproteins, or vice versa. As knowledge of the interrelationships between apoproteins of HDL and VLDL accumulates it will also be easier to understand the concomitant VLDL abnormalities in LCAT deficiency. The fact that plasma of patients with Tangier disease (Chap. 26) contains LCAT activity (J. Glomset, unpublished results) indicates that the synthesis of LCAT is not absolutely dependent on the synthesis or elaboration of normal HDL.

Evidence for the hepatic origin of LCAT rests largely on the fact that plasma LCAT activity is diminished in parenchymatous liver disease [27, 28] and in eviscerated rats [29]. Also, several investigators [42] have obtained evidence that LCAT is released into the medium by isolated perfused rat livers. Results of several tests of liver function (Bromsulphalein, bilirubin, alkaline phosphatase, serum glutamic oxaloacetic transaminase, serum glutamic pyruvic transaminase, Thrombotest, and galactose tolerance) have been normal in the patients with familial LCAT deficiency, and sections of liver tissue from three patients (A.R., M.L., and B.B.) have a normal histologic appearance.

The hyperlipemia in LCAT deficiency also remains to be explained. Although all the older patients are hyperlipemic, the youngest (M.R.) was not hyperlipemic at age 19, but did have high plasma triglyceride levels, which have increased further since then. The hyperlipemia may be age-dependent. It does not seem to be related to obesity, since only one of the patients (A.A.) is overweight, nor has evidence of diabetes been found in the patients tested (glucagon and oral glucose tolerance tests were normal in M.R., A.R., and M.L.). It may be related to the low concentration of plasma HDL. Of all the patients, M.R. has the lowest plasma

Table 27-9. ERYTHROCYTE LIPIDS

Lipids	*Patients*						
	A.R.	I.S.	M.R.	A.A.	L.G.	M.L.	Normal
Cholesterol (10^{-10} mg/erythrocyte)	1.7–1.8	1.8	2.0	1.9	1.8	2.06	1.11
Total phospholipid phosphorus (10^{-11} mg/erythrocyte)	1.02	1.06	0.96	1.23	1.00	1.10	1.00
Phosphatidylethanolamine*	19.9	19.8	21.2	17.6	19.5	18.0	29.0
Phosphatidylserine*	14.8	12.5	11.9	12.6	10.0	11.6	14.0
Phosphatidylcholine*	46.2	49.6	51.4	53.2	53.7	52.1	27.4
Sphingomyelin*	15.9	16.7	14.3	14.6	11.0	14.9	25.9
Lysolecithin*	1.3	0.7	0.9	1.1	1.9	1.7	2.1
Phosphatidylinositol*	1.9	0.7	0.9	0.9	3.9	1.7	1.6

* Figures represent percentages of total phospholipid phosphorus.

Table 27-10. CHOLESTEROL, 10^{-10} MG PER CELL, IN ERYTHROCYTES FROM A.R. BEFORE AND AFTER INCUBATION IN NORMAL PLASMA

Plasma	Days of incubation			
	0	1	2	3
Normal plasma	1.84	1.56	1.48	1.32
Heat-inactivated normal plasma	1.84	1.73	1.62	1.56
Plasma from A.R.	1.84	....	....	1.93

Source: From K. Norum and E. Gjone. Scand. J. Clin. Lab. Invest., **22**, 94, 1968.

triglyceride level and the largest amount of the minor HDL subfraction. If her hyperlipemia progresses, it will be of particular interest to follow the changes in this component. It is entirely possible that the hyperlipemia is related to abnormal VLDL, and in turn related to the HDL abnormalities. In Tangier disease, hyperglyceridemia and VLDL abnormalities are associated with severe deficiency of HDL (Chap. 26).

Erythrocytes

The abnormal composition and shape of the erythrocytes are almost certainly caused by the changes in plasma milieu due to LCAT deficiency. The unesterified cholesterol and, to a somewhat lesser extent, the lecithin of plasma lipoproteins and erythrocytes may be considered parts of common pools of these lipids. The distribution of unesterified cholesterol within its pool probably depends on competitive binding of the lipid by the various participating plasma lipoproteins and plasma membranes. LCAT appears to participate in regulating the total quantity of unesterified cholesterol in this pool by converting unesterified cholesterol of the HDL and LDL to cholesteryl ester. When the unesterified cholesterol content of these lipoproteins drops, the unesterified cholesterol of plasma membranes is presumably redistributed by a net transfer from the membranes to the lipoproteins. This type of net transfer has been demonstrated for erythrocytes in vitro [21]. Also, transfusion experiments with A.R. (see "Treatment," further on) have shown that transfer can occur in vivo. Net changes in erythrocyte lecithin appear to occur less readily than net changes in erythrocyte cholesterol. No definite shift of erythrocyte lecithin was detected in either the in vitro or in vivo studies on patient A.R. Nevertheless, the LCAT reaction may have a slow indirect effect on erythrocyte lecithin levels. Presumably, neither the lipoprotein nor the plasma membrane binding sites for lecithin are absolutely specific. The lecithin of lipoproteins probably exchanges to a limited extent with the sphingomyelin and phosphatidylethanolamine of plasma membranes. If the proportion of lecithin in the plasma phospholipids is unusually high, an increase in the proportion of lecithin in plasma membrane phospholipids would be expected.

The fact that smears of the erythrocytes show "target cells" is probably due to the excessive amount of cholesterol present. When the cholesterol of these erythrocytes was reduced by incubation with normal plasma, the number of target cells decreased, and similar changes occurred in vivo when patient A.R. was given a transfusion of normal plasma. The target cell erythrocytes of patients with obstructive jaundice provide an interesting parallel to those of patients with familial LCAT deficiency. They, also, contain excessive amounts of unesterified cholesterol [30] and lecithin [31] in conjunction with high plasma levels of these lipids [32] and low levels of LCAT activity [28].

Anemia and Renal Changes

The causes of the defective erythrogenesis and proteinuria are not clear. It is tempting to speculate that both features of the disease are related to the accumulation of cholesterol in cell membranes, i.e., those of the bone marrow and glomeruli. It seems unlikely that the equilibrium existing between cholesterol in the plasma and the erythrocyte plasma membranes is unique. The cholesterol of other tissues can also exchange with the plasma unesterified cholesterol [33–36], and this unesterified cholesterol is probably similarly affected by changes in total pool size. Furthermore, when the plasma cholesterols of patients I.S., A.R., and M.R. were labeled in vivo and half-times calculated from the disap-

Table 27-11. CHANGES IN ERYTHROCYTE CHOLESTEROL IN VITRO*

Incubation medium	Cholesterol in incubation medium before incubation, mg/100 ml		Cholesterol, 10^{-10} mg/erythrocyte	
	Free	Ester	Before incubation	After incubation
Plasma from A.R.	299	32	1.30	1.72
Plasma from I.S.	323	21	1.30	1.60

*Concentration of cholesterol in normal erythrocytes before and after 24 hr of incubation in plasma from two patients (A.R. and I.S.) with familial LCAT deficiency.
Source: From K. Norum and E. Gjone. Scand. J. Clin. Lab. Invest., **22**, 94, 1968.

pearance curves, they were found to be 124, 130, and 155 days, respectively, whereas the corresponding half-time for a control subject was 59 days. These data are compatible with the possibility that the pools with which the plasma cholesterol exchanges are enlarged in LCAT deficiency. Therefore, plasma membrane cholesterol is probably increased in the bone marrow and glomeruli of the patients, and it is conceivable that this interferes with erythrogenesis and glomerular filtration. With progressively impaired kidney function, decreased erythropoietin secretion and a further diminution in erythrogenesis might be expected. On partial autopsy performed on B.B., advanced atherosclerosis of the abdominal aorta with marked obstruction of both the renal arteries was found (Dr. B. Hamnström, personal communication). These findings may explain the rapid onset of uremia in this patient.

Tissue Lipids

If the amount of tissue cholesterol of these patients is increased, it is interesting that more impairment of tissue function is not evident. The patients have foam cells in the bone marrow and glomeruli, but no xanthomatous deposits or signs of clinical heart disease, and they have no lymph gland enlargement or hepatosplenomegaly, as is seen in some patients with Tangier disease. The patient B.B. died before the nature of his disease was discovered. The lipids of the atherosclerotic abdominal aorta were not analyzed.

We cannot end this discussion of the biochemical defects in familial LCAT deficiency without pointing out that our fundamental assumption is that the principal function of the LCAT reaction is to regulate the level of unesterified cholesterol and lecithin in plasma lipoproteins and plasma membranes. Associated with this assumption is the concept that unesterified cholesterol in plasma lipoproteins and plasma membranes is readily exchangeable, while cholesteryl ester is not, and that an increase in membrane unesterified cholesterol can be harmful. According to this view, esterification within the plasma is a means of preventing cholesterol from accumulating in membranes. These concepts have yet to be proved, and alternative possibilities exist. One of these is that plasma cholesteryl esters have some specific, unknown function, and that the lack of this function is responsible for the clinical manifestations of familial LCAT deficiency.

GENETICS

Familial LCAT deficiency has been found in three Scandinavian families—two from the same area of Norway, and one from Sweden. Although no consanguinity has been demonstrated, all three families are from isolated communities where intermarriage has occurred frequently. In the first Norwegian family the three affected sisters are from a sibship of five females. In the second the affected brother and sister are from a sibship of two females and one male. In the Swedish family the affected brother and sister are from a sibship of two females and three males. No abnormalities have been found in the parents or children of the propositi. All appear to have normal plasma LCAT activity, normal cholesterol/cholesteryl ester ratios, and normal α_1-lipoprotein levels [4, 37]. Nevertheless, partially diminished biosynthesis of LCAT or HDL would not necessarily affect plasma levels of these proteins. The plasma levels probably depend at least as much on the rate at which the molecules are removed from the plasma as on the rate at which they are synthesized and secreted. Furthermore, the amount of LCAT in plasma probably depends on the amount bound to HDL. Thus the evidence favors the view that the disease is an expression of a homozygous autosomal recessive trait. The Swedish patient M.L. has some LCAT activity in the plasma; the Norwegian patients have none. It is presently not possible to determine whether different mutations might be involved in production of what appears to be the same phenotype.

TREATMENT

If failure to synthesize LCAT is the primary cause of the disease, it might be possible to treat the disease by injecting LCAT intravenously. The present method of purifying the enzyme is laborious and yields only small quantities of an unstable preparation. Therefore, a number of attempts have been made to treat the patients by transfusing whole plasma or blood. In one instance patient A.R. was given 450 ml blood and 500 ml plasma in a single transfusion [38]. This caused an immediate rise in her plasma cholesteryl esters, followed by a slower increase to a peak level at 6 days. The peak level considerably exceeded that caused by the cholesteryl esters of the transfused plasma, the plasma cholesteryl ester composition shifted toward one which more closely resembled that of normal plasma, and the plasma lysolecithin increased. Therefore the change in cholesteryl esters was probably caused by the transfused LCAT. Two weeks later the plasma cholesteryl esters had again diminished to the pretreatment level, probably reflecting the rate of decline of LCAT activity.

Both patients A.R. and M.L. have been treated with several successive plasma transfusions. Figure 27-13 shows the changes induced in A.R. during one such treatment period. The plasma cholesteryl ester increased from 35 to 310 mg per 100 ml, while the unesterified cholesterol decreased, but not so markedly. The latter may have been due to an influx of unesterified cholesterol from plasma membranes, because the erythrocyte cholesterol decreased from 1.8 to 1.3 mg per 10^{10} cells. The relative concentration of plasma lysolecithin increased from 1.8 to 3.4 percent, but no other changes in plasma phospholipid pattern were observed, nor did α_1-lipoproteins appear. Furthermore, the plasma triglycerides did not change significantly, although some lipoproteins of

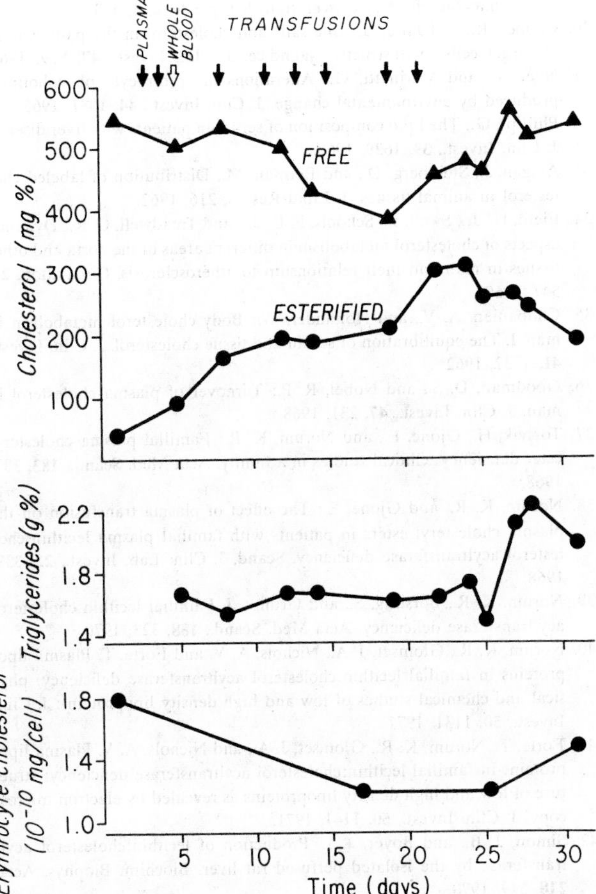

Figure 27-13. Effect of repeated transfusions of normal plasma on some plasma and erythrocyte lipids of A.R. (*Unpublished results from K. R. Norum and E. Gjone.*)

pre-β mobility appeared. Clinically, the edema cleared, but there was no apparent change in the anemia or proteinuria. In general the effects of transfusion in patients M.L. and M.R. have been similar. This suggests that treatment must be continued for much longer periods of time if plasma lipoprotein and plasma membrane defects, not to speak of the anemia and proteinuria, are to be corrected.

SUMMARY

1 Familial lecithin:cholesterol acyl transferase deficiency has been described in seven adult patients from three Scandinavian families. The disease is characterized by corneal infiltration, anemia, proteinuria, reduced plasma cholesteryl esters and lysolecithin, increased plasma unesterified cholesterol and lecithin, and absent or near-absent levels of the enzyme in plasma.

2 Blood smears show target cells. The erythrocytes contain increased amounts of cholesterol and lecithin. There are both decreased erythropoiesis and increased erythrocyte destruction. Foam cells appear in the glomerular tufts.

3 The plasma contains no pre-β-lipoprotein and no α_1-lipoprotein. The very low density lipoproteins of the plasma migrate in the β position, and the high density lipoproteins in the α_2 position.

4 The lack of enzyme activity in the plasma is attributable to lack of enzyme. The high concentrations of unesterified cholesterol and lecithin in the plasma are attributable to the lack of the transferase. The hyperlipemia in this disease is presently unexplained. The erythrocyte abnormality is presumably attributable to changes in the plasma environment resulting from the enzyme deficiency. Indeed many of the clinical features can presumably be traced to abnormalities in plasma membranes resulting from the plasma deficiency of transferase activity.

5 Though the genetic data are sparse, the disease appears to be an expression of the homozygous state of an autosomal recessive trait.

6 It is possible that treatment with multiple transfusions may be of value in reversing some of the changes attendant upon this disease.

BIBLIOGRAPHY

1. Norum, K. R., and Gjone, E.: Familial serum-cholesterol esterification failure: a new inborn error of metabolism. Biochim. Biophys. Acta, **144,** 698, 1967.
2. Norum, K. R., and Gjone, E.: Familial plasma lecithin:cholesterol acyltransferase deficiency. Biochemical study of a new inborn error of metabolism. Scand. J. Clin. Lab. Invest., **20,** 231, 1967.
3. Gjone, E., and Norum, K. R.: Familial serum-cholesterol ester deficiency: clinical study of a patient with a new syndrome. Acta Med. Scand., **183,** 107, 1968.
4. Hamnström, B., Gjone, E., and Norum, K. R.: Familial plasma lecithin: cholesterol acyltransferase deficiency: report of a Swedish family. Brit. Med. J., **2,** 283, 1969.
5. Gjone, E., and Bergaust, B.: Corneal opacity in familial plasma cholesterol ester deficiency. Acta Ophthal., **47,** 222, 1969.
6. Torsvik, H.: Presence of α_1-lipoprotein in patients with familial plasma lecithin:cholesterol acyltransferase deficiency. Scand. J. Clin. Lab. Invest., **24,** 187, 1969.
7. Boberg, J., and Carlson, L. A.: Determination of heparin-induced lipoprotein lipase activity in human plasma. Clin. Chim. Acta, **10,** 420, 1964.
8. Sperry, W. M.: Cholesterol esterase in blood. J. Biol. Chem., **111,** 467, 1935.
9. Glomset, J. A.: The plasma lecithin:cholesterol acyltransferase reaction. J. Lipid Res., **9,** 155, 1968.
10. Glomset, J. A., and Wright, J. L.: Some properties of a cholesterol esterifying enzyme in human plasma. Biochim. Biophys. Acta, **89,** 266, 1964.
11. Glomset, J. A., Norum, K. R., and King, W.: Plasma lipoproteins in familial lecithin:cholesterol acyltransferase deficiency: lipid composition and reactivity in vitro. J. Clin. Invest., **49,** 1827, 1970.
12. Blomstrand, R., Gürtler, J., and Werner, B.: Fatty acid esterification in man during fat absorption. Acta Med. Scand., **18,** 1019, 1964.
13. Akanuma, Y., and Glomset, J.: A method for studying the interaction between lecithin:cholesterol acyltransferase and high density lipoproteins. Biochem. Biophys. Res. Commun., **32,** 639, 1968.
14. Akanuma, Y., and Glomset, J.: *In vitro* incorporation of cholesterol-^{14}C into very low density lipoprotein cholesteryl esters. J. Lipid Res., **9,** 620, 1968.

15. Goodman, D.: The *in vitro* turnover of individual cholesteryl esters in human plasma lipoproteins. J. Clin. Invest., **43,** 2026, 1964.
16. Nichols, A., and Smith, L.: Effect of very low density lipoproteins on lipid transfer in incubated serum. J. Lipid Res., **6,** 206, 1965.
17. Glomset, J. A., Janssen, E. T., Kennedy, R., and Dobbins, J.: Role of plasma lecithin:cholesterol acyltransferase in the metabolism of high density lipoproteins. J. Lipid Res., **7,** 639, 1966.
18. Schumacher, U. N., and Adams, G. H.: Circulating lipoproteins. Ann. Rev. Biochem., **38,** 113, 1969.
19. Reed, C.: Phospholipid exchange between plasma and erythrocytes in man and dog. J. Clin. Invest., **47,** 749, 1968.
20. Gould, R., LeRoy, G., Okita, G., Kabora, J., Keegan, P., and Bergenstal, D.: The use of C^{14}-labeled acetate to study cholesterol metabolism in man. J. Lab. Clin. Med., **46,** 372, 1955.
21. Murphy, J.: Erythrocyte metabolism. III. Relationship of energy metabolism and serum factors to the osmotic fragility following incubation. J. Lab. Clin. Med., **60,** 86, 1962.
22. Gjone, E., Torsvik, H., and Norum, K. R.: Familial plasma cholesterol ester deficiency: a study of the erythrocytes. Scand. J. Clin. Lab. Invest., **21,** 327, 1968.
23. Norum, K. R., and Gjone, E.: The influence of plasma from patients with familial plasma lecithin:cholesterol acyltransferase deficiency on the lipid pattern of erythrocytes. Scand. J. Clin. Lab. Invest., **22,** 94, 1968.
24. Glomset, J.: The mechanism of the plasma cholesterol esterification reaction: plasma fatty acid transferase. Biochim. Biophys. Acta, **65,** 128, 1962.
25. Nestel, P., and Monger, E.: Turnover of plasma esterified cholesterol in normocholesterolemic and hypercholesterolemic subjects and its relation to body build. J. Clin. Invest., **46,** 967, 1967.
26. Scanu, A.: Factors affecting lipoprotein metabolism, in *Advances in Lipid Research,* edited by R. Paoletti and D. Kritchevsky, vol. III, p. 64. Academic, New York, 1965.
27. Turner, K., McCormack, G., Jr., and Richards, A.: The cholesterol-esterifying enzyme of human serum. I. In liver disease. J. Clin. Invest., **32,** 801, 1953.
28. Gjone, E., and Norum, K. R.: Plasma lecithin-cholesterol acyltransferase and erythrocyte lipids in liver disease. Acta Med. Scand., **187,** 153, 1970.
29. Brot, N., Lossow, W., and Chaikoff, I.: *In vitro* esterification of cholesterol by plasma: the effect of evisceration. J. Lipid Res., **3,** 413, 1962.
30. Cooper, R., and Jandl, J.: Bile salts and cholesterol in the pathogenesis of target cells in obstructive jaundice. J. Clin. Invest., **47,** 809, 1968.
31. Nye, W., and Marinetti, G.: Alterations in erythrocyte phospholipids produced by environmental change. J. Clin. Invest., **44,** 1081, 1965.
32. Phillips, G.: The lipid composition of serum in patients with liver disease. J. Clin. Invest., **39,** 1639, 1960.
33. Avigan, J., Steinberg, D., and Berman, M.: Distribution of labeled cholesterol in animal tissues. J. Lipid Res., **3,** 216, 1962.
34. Field, H., Jr., Swell, L., Schools, P. E., Jr., and Treadwell, C. R.: Dynamic aspects of cholesterol metabolism in different areas of the aorta and other tissues in man and their relationship to atherosclerosis. Circulation, **22,** 547, 1960.
35. Chobanian, A. V., and Hollander, W.: Body cholesterol metabolism in man. I. The equilibration of serum and tissue cholesterol. J. Clin. Invest., **41,** 1732, 1962.
36. Goodman, D. S., and Nobel, R. P.: Turnover of plasma cholesterol in man. J. Clin. Invest., **47,** 231, 1968.
37. Torsvik, H., Gjone, E., and Norum, K. R.: Familial plasma cholesteryl ester deficiency: clinical studies in a family. Acta Med. Scand., **183,** 387, 1968.
38. Norum, K. R., and Gjone, E.: The effect of plasma transfusion on the plasma cholesteryl esters in patients with familial plasma lecithin:cholesterol acyltransferase deficiency. Scand. J. Clin. Lab. Invest., **22,** 339, 1968.
39. Norum, K. R., Børsting, S., and Grundt, I. Familial lecithin:cholesterol acyltransferase deficiency. Acta Med. Scand., **188,** 323, 1970.
40. Norum, K. R., Glomset, J. A., Nichols, A. V. and Forte, T. Plasma lipoproteins in familial lecithin:cholesterol acyltransferase deficiency: physical and chemical studies of low and high density lipoproteins. J. Clin. Invest., **50,** 1131, 1971.
41. Forte, T., Norum, K. R., Glomset, J. A., and Nichols, A. V. Plasma lipoproteins in familial lecithin:cholesterol acyltransferase deficiency: structure of low and high density lipoproteins as revealed by electron microscopy. J. Clin. Invest., **50,** 1141, 1971.
42. Simon, J. B., and Boyer, J. L. Production of lecithin:cholesterol acyltransferase by the isolated perfused rat liver. Biochim. Biophys. Acta, **218,** 549, 1970.

CHAPTER TWENTY-EIGHT

FAMILIAL HYPERLIPOPROTEINEMIA

Donald S. Fredrickson and Robert I. Levy

This chapter is concerned with *primary familial hyperlipidemia,* which comprises heritable diseases whose characteristic expression is an increase in the plasma concentrations of cholesterol or triglycerides. It is most convenient to classify all the abnormalities meeting this generic definition into five major groups according to the plasma lipoprotein pattern as defined under certain conditions. This translation of hyperlipidemia into hyperlipoproteinemia does not imply that the diseases necessarily arise from mutations at loci regulating the structure or metabolism of lipoproteins per se. The latter are macromolecules or complexes whose concentrations and other behavior in the extracellular fluid are potentially under the control of many genomes that regulate diverse aspects of lipid, protein, or carbohydrate metabolism. The value of lipoprotein patterns for classification of hyperlipidemia devolves mainly from a limited but definite increase in specificity over that possible from measurements of plasma lipid concentrations alone. The further identification of phenotypes depends on the combination of lipoprotein pattern and other clinical information.

HISTORICAL ASPECTS

Familial hyperlipoproteinemia was initially discovered through one of its secondary and inconstant manifestations, the deposition of lipids in skin and tendons, called *xanthomatosis.* The first appearance of xanthomas in medical literature is in the atlas prepared by Rayer in 1835 [1], from the last page of which peers a pair of eyes with typical xanthelasmas. There is no explanatory comment on the patient. The second example is the report of Addison and Gull in 1851 [2], which initiated a lively interest in xanthomas and the coinage of terms to describe them. Between 1850 and 1875 this activity was popular particularly among British dermatologists, most notably at Guy's Hospital [3]. Practically all the patients who had florid and extensive xanthomas at that time appear to have had *secondary* hyperlipoproteinemia due to biliary obstruction. It was about the turn of the century that xanthomas occurring in the absence of jaundice were recognized. These fell into two major types: (1) *xanthoma tuberosum multiplex,* which consisted of tendon, tuberous, and plane xanthomas like those seen with jaundice, but which sometimes appeared in sibs and often was associated with vascular disease [4–8] (most of these patients probably were homozygous for what is here called familial Type II hyperlipoproteinemia); (2) *xanthoma diabeticorum* [2, 3, 9–12], which consisted of superficial, more evanescent lesions (eruptive and tuberoeruptive xanthomas) that first were noted in diabetics.

As early as 1873 it was suggested that xanthomas might arise from hyperlipidemia [13, 14], a supposition reinforced by histologic and chemical analyses of xanthomatous lesions in man and experiments in animals [15–21]. This was actually proved to be the case in "primary xanthoma tuberosum multiplex" in 1920 [22, 23]. About the same time, it was realized that "xanthoma diabeticorum" was always accompanied by *hyperlipemia* (lactescence due to hyperglyceridemia) and that it could also occur without diabetes [3, 12].

Attention gradually turned to measurement of the amount of plasma lipids in patients with xanthomas, and sometimes in their normal-appearing relatives [20, 24–40]. By 1950 xanthoma tuberosum multiplex had become *essential familial hypercholesterolemia* [41, 42]. *Idiopathic familial hyperlipemia* [43], now called *familial hyperchylomicronemia* (Type I) [44, 45], had also been recognized. Greater heterogeneity in familial hyperlipidemia was suspected, but new tools for separation were needed. Over the next 5 years, these emerged in the form of lipoprotein analyses [46–53] and the identification of the enzyme lipoprotein lipase [54]. By 1955, Gofman and his colleagues [49, 55, 56] and others [48, 53, 57–59] had laid the foundation for study of hyperlipidemia based on lipoprotein analyses. The application of these techniques to the investigation of more and more cases [60–63] made possible contemporary classification of genetically determined hyperlipoproteinemia.

The classification used in this chapter is derived from a study begun about 8 years ago in the Clinical Center at Bethesda. The aim was to use lipoprotein patterns, derived from techniques simpler and more available than the ultracentrifuge, to define various phenotypes among patients with familial hyperlipidemia. Paper electrophoresis provided the basis for classification [45, 64]. When quantitative steps were added and as experience grew, the definitions became sharper and one, that of Type III, was changed [65]. By March 1971, the number of probands with familial hyperlipoproteinemia whose kindreds had been partially screened exceeded 400 (Table 28-1). The present classification of hyperlipidemia and hyperlipoproteinemia has been recommended as an international standard by the World Health Organization [66]. It is apparent, however, that this system will be replaced by one based on etiology as new knowledge permits.

DEFINITIONS AND BASE LINES

The Index Sample

Though clinicians often prefer to know the plasma lipid and lipoprotein concentrations under the conditions in which a given patient chooses to live, the establishment of phenotypes requires that all patients be classified with plasma or

Table 28-1. PATIENTS WITH FAMILIAL HYPERLIPOPROTEINEMIA CLASSIFIED IN THE NATIONAL INSTITUTES OF HEALTH STUDY UP TO MARCH, 1971

Type	Patients	Kindreds
I	18	12
II	620	225
III	86	68
IV	171	82
V	71	34
Total	966	421

*This table does not include many patients with Type IV patterns detected during screening of families affected with other types of hyperlipoproteinemia (see text); nor does it reflect accurately the frequency of the various types in the American population, since patients were not selected at random.

serum samples taken under minimum standard conditions. These are (1) the subject should have not eaten for 12 to 14 hr before the blood is drawn, usually in the morning; (2) for 2 weeks prior to the sample he should not have gained or lost weight or have been on a diet unusual for his population group; and (3) he must not be taking medications known to affect plasma lipid or lipoprotein concentrations.

Normal Concentrations

Hyperlipidemia

Hyperlipidemia is defined in quantitative terms and, today, only in regard to the plasma concentrations of cholesterol and triglycerides. A vast amount of epidemiologic data gathered from highly industrialized and more agrarian cultures indicate that lipid concentrations that are "normal" in a statistical sense are not necessarily "healthy." Moreover, lipid and lipoprotein concentrations are subject to strong influences from diet and other environmental or cultural factors. Standards must be established for each different population.

It is usually necessary to set arbitrary statistical limits of normal concentrations, on the basis of examination of a sufficient number of healthy-appearing subjects of different ages. In them, the distribution of values is rarely gaussian; some investigators prefer to use log transformations to obtain a clearer mode [67]. The limits of normal also have to be set high to minimize the effect of variation due to environmental factors in presumed "genetically normal" subjects. This means that only the most obvious genetic variants will be recognized; and in the study of these obvious variants there may be a tendency to oversimplify apparent modes of genetic determination that are actually complex or polygenic.

The limit that we have used is the approximate upper 5 percent found in apparently healthy Caucasian Americans (Table 28-2). The limitations of this arbitrary definition have been further discussed elsewhere [65].

Cholesterol and triglyceride concentrations can be used to detect hyperlipoproteinemia. Over 95 percent of patients with hyperlipoproteinemia, as defined below, have "hyperlipidemia" [70]. The major exception is provided by patients with excessive amounts of low density lipoprotein (LDL) whose plasma cholesterol is kept within normal limits by a concomitant decrease in high density lipoprotein (HDL).

As described in Chap. 26, cholesterol is found in all the types of lipoproteins. From 50 to 75 percent is normally found in low density lipoproteins. The normal fraction of the total plasma cholesterol in high density lipoproteins is 20 to 35 percent in males and 25 to 45 percent in females. Only 5 to 10 percent is found in very low density lipoprotein (VLDL), where 1 mg cholesterol is usually accompanied by about 5 mg triglyceride; the amount in chylomicrons is usually negligible.

Triglycerides are mostly transported in VLDL and chylomicrons. VLDL contains glycerides that are mainly of endogenous origin. Most of the glycerides in chylomicrons come directly from the diet. It is because cholesterol and triglycerides are unevenly distributed in four major lipoprotein categories that hyperlipidemia is more usefully considered in terms of hyperlipoproteinemia.

Hyperlipoproteinemia

With one exception (Type III), hyperlipoproteinemia, too, is defined in quantitative terms. Arbitrary limits of lipoprotein concentrations have been established in a manner similar to that used for the lipid concentrations (Table 28-3).

The classification of hyperlipoproteinemia begins with the determination of the type of abnormal lipoprotein pattern, but it does not end with this step. Two other sequential ones are always required: (1) separation of hyperlipoproteinemia

Table 28-2. PLASMA LIPID CONCENTRATIONS, MG PER 100 ML, IN NORMAL* SUBJECTS

Age, yr	Cholesterol, mean and 90 percent limits	Triglyceride, mean and 90 percent limits
0–19	175 (120–230)	65 (10–140)
20–29	180 (120–240)	70 (10–140)
30–39	205 (140–270)	75 (10–150)
40–49	225 (150–310)	85 (10–160)
50–59	245 (160–330)	95 (10–190)

* The population sample is derived from a total of 511 normal subjects (279 males, 232 females) and includes the smaller sample previously described [65]; the criteria for acceptance of patients were no evidence of metabolic disease or family history of hyperlipoproteinemia, and plasma triglyceride levels less than 200 mg per 100 ml; all samples were obtained 12 to 16 hr after the last (evening) meal. Some significant differences between the sexes were ignored [49, 68, 69].

Table 28-3. PLASMA LIPOPROTEIN CONCENTRATIONS, MG PER 100 ML (MEAN ± 1 S.D.) IN NORMAL SUBJECTS*

Age, yr	Sex	VLDL cholesterol	LDL cholesterol	HDL cholesterol	No. of subjects
0–19	M	12 ± 8	103 ± 29	51 ± 13	72
	F	12 ± 8	103 ± 25	54 ± 18	71
	Combined	12 ± 8	103 ± 27	52 ± 13	143
20–29	M	16 ± 9	115 ± 24	49 ± 11	47
	F	16 ± 12	108 ± 33	56 ± 13	41
	Combined	16 ± 10	112 ± 29	52 ± 12	88
30–39	M	19 ± 8	130 ± 32	46 ± 11	38
	F	15 ± 11	119 ± 34	57 ± 17	29
	Combined	17 ± 9	126 ± 33	51 ± 15	67
40–49	M	22 ± 13	142 ± 27	48 ± 13	25
	F	17 ± 8	129 ± 32	65 ± 14	34
	Combined	19 ± 11	134 ± 30	58 ± 16	59
50–59	M	25 ± 7	156 ± 28	42 ± 8	14
	F	26 ± 16	167 ± 32	49 ± 13	10
	Combined	25 ± 11	161 ± 30	45 ± 11	24
		Suggested "Normal Limits"†			
				F	M
0–19	....	5–25	50–170	30–70	30–65
20–29	....	5–25	60–170	35–75	35–70
30–39	....	5–35	70–190	35–80	30–65
40–49	....	5–35	80–190	40–85	30–65
50–59	....	10–40	80–210	35–85	30–65

*The population is a subgroup of that described in the legend of Table 28-2.
†Based on 90 percent fiducial limits calculated for small samples; all values are rounded to the nearest 5 mg, and for practical purposes, differences between the sexes have been ignored except for HDL concentrations.
Note: Abbreviations: VLDL, very low density lipoproteins; LDL, low density lipoproteins; HDL, high density lipoproteins.

into primary and secondary forms. The secondary form is that caused by other known diseases, e.g., insulinopenic diabetes mellitus, which can result in secondary hyperlipoproteinemia manifesting itself in any of the five types of lipoprotein patterns; (2) differentiation of primary hyperlipoproteinemia into heritable and nonheritable forms. The manner of distinguishing these forms is taken up under each of the phenotypes.

Nearly all the patients with heritable hyperlipidemia have one of five abnormal lipoprotein patterns. These patterns are summarized in Table 28-4, where it will be observed that only three of the four lipoprotein families serve as determinants. These three families are chylomicrons (density < 1.006, $S_f > 400$), very low density lipoproteins (density < 1.006, S_f 20 to 400 and equivalent to prebetalipoprotein), and low density lipoproteins (density 1.006 to 1.063, S_f 0 to 20, and equivalent to β-lipoprotein). These lipoproteins are usually referred to here as chylomicrons, VLDL, and LDL. All the lipoprotein families are described in greater detail in Chap. 26.

The presence of chylomicrons 12 to 16 hr after a meal is considered abnormal and is a feature of two of the patterns (Types I and V). (Small amounts of chylomicrons are normally "present" in the fasting state but are not detectable by most methods.) Increased LDL of normal composition defines a third pattern (Type II), and the presence of LDL with abnormal flotation properties defines another (Type III). Increased concentration of normal VLDL is a feature of two more (Types IV and V). The fourth lipoprotein family is the high density lipoproteins (α-lipoprotein of density > 1.063, usually referred to as HDL). Increased concentration of HDL has not been proved to be familial; it is pathologic only in the presence of biliary obstruction [71]. Abnormal forms of HDL have been observed only in hypolipoproteinemia (see Chap. 26) and, possibly, LCAT deficiency (see Chap. 27). HDL concentrations, and often those of LDL, tend to be low in certain forms of hyperlipoproteinemia, especially in the presence of markedly increased quantities of chylomicrons or of very low density lipoproteins.

Table 28-4. ABNORMAL LIPOPROTEIN PATTERNS IN FAMILIAL HYPERLIPOPROTEINEMIA

Type	Defintive lipoprotein abnormalities	Appearance of plasma*	Usual changes in lipid concentrations†
I	1. Chylomicrons present and markedly increased 2. VLDL, LDL, HDL normal or decreased	Cream layer on top, clear below	C↑, TG↑ (C/TG < 0.2)
II	1. LDL increased‡ 2. VLDL normal (Type II*a*); or VLDL increased (Type II*b*)	Usually clear, may be slightly turbid	C↑, TG normal or ↑ (C/TG usually >1.5)
III	1. Presence of β-VLDL ("floating beta," LDL of abnormal lipid composition)	Usually turbid, often with faint cream layer	C↑, TG↑ (C/TG variable, often = 1)
IV	1. VLDL increased 2. Chylomicrons "absent" 3. LDL not increased	Usually turbid; no cream layer	C↑ or normal, TG↑ (C/TG variable)
V	1. Chylomicrons present 2. VLDL increased	Cream layer on top, turbid below	C↑, TG↑ (C/TG usually >0.15 and <0.6)

* After standing at 4°C for 18 hr or more.
† C, cholesterol; TG, triglycerides.
‡ "Increased" implies in excess of whatever cut-off limit is used.

METHODS OF LIPOPROTEIN ANALYSES

In order to define all the lipoprotein patterns seen in familial hyperlipoproteinemia one must have answers to the following questions: (1) Are chylomicrons present? (2) Is the concentration of VLDL excessive? (3) Is LDL with abnormal flotation properties present? and (4) Is the LDL concentration abnormally high? A measurement of HDL concentration is often made to assist in the estimation of LDL (see below). Most of the methods for differentiating the lipoprotein families are based on either electrophoresis or ultracentrifugation.

Ultracentrifugation

Analytic ultracentrifugation comes closest to the ideal of defining hyperlipoproteinemia by a single operation or, more accurately, a series of such operations [72–74]. As now adapted, the analytic ultracentrifuge has the ability to draw a continuous plot of the concentrations of lipoproteins in flotation (S_f) classes differing by very small density increments [75]. Examples of the Schlieren profiles obtained are shown in Fig. 28-1. The instrument is not generally available, and its use for the study of many patients is not practicable. It is also not necessary for defining the phenotypes that have been recognized thus far [76].

The preparative ultracentrifuge can also be used to obtain quantitative lipoprotein patterns [59, 62, 63]. To do so in a single plasma sample requires three or four serial runs and subsequent lipid determinations. When combined with electrophoresis, precipitation, and chemical analyses, one ultracentrifugal separation of plasma without adjustment of its salt density (1.006) is very helpful in defining lipoprotein patterns [65, 77]. The use of density gradients [78, 79] or continuous zonal ultracentrifugation [80, 81] is mainly restricted to provision of lipoprotein subfractions for experimental work.

Electrophoresis

There are now several useful methods for separating the four plasma lipoprotein families on the basis of their electrophoretic migration (Fig. 28-2). Electrophoresis is relatively rapid, simple, and inexpensive but does not have the resolution of the ultracentrifuge. It is also usually a semiquantitative technique, although quantification is possible by staining of the lipoprotein bands and measurement of intensity of staining by densitometry before or after elution [52, 82]. Electrophoresis on paper using albuminated buffer [83] or agar-agarose gel [84–88] provides easily interpretable and comparable patterns [89]. Paper electrophoresis takes longer but requires less preparation and, some investigators believe, less effort. Agar-agarose gel provides sharper bands than paper, and it more often resolves the pre-β-lipoprotein (VLDL) and α-lipoprotein (HDL) into several bands; no pathologic significance has yet been assigned to these subbands [84, 87, 88]. Cellulose acetate, a conventional medium for electrophoresis of most plasma proteins, is also used for lipoproteins [90–95], but in some preparations chylomicrons do not remain at the origin and migrate with pre-β-

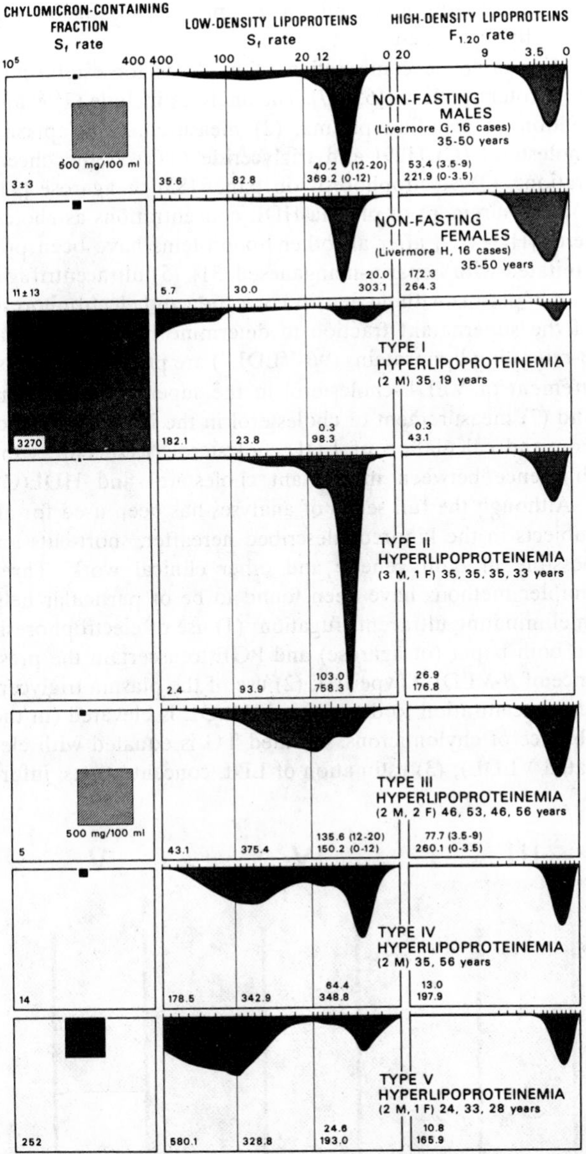

Figure 28-1. Plasma lipoprotein patterns as obtained in the analytic ultracentrifuge. The normal males and females were nonfasting. The pooled plasma samples from each of the five types of hyperlipoproteinemia were obtained under conditions described for "index samples" as explained in the test. Lipoprotein concentrations are given as milligrams per 100 ml of plasma. (*The data are replotted from Fredrickson et al.,* [76].)

lipoproteins as they do on free electrophoresis. Similar merger of chylomicrons and pre-β-lipoproteins, as well as the greater time and effort required, also makes starch-gel electrophoresis impractical for lipoprotein screening [96].

These electrophoretic systems mainly separate the lipoproteins by differences in charge and do not offer an assessment of other useful physical properties. They do not by themselves permit ready identification of several unusual kinds of lipoproteins. One is the β-migrating VLDL ("β-VLDL" or "floating beta") that defines the Type III lipoprotein pattern. Another is the apparently normal variant pre-β-lipoprotein that has a higher density than conventional VLDL. This "sinking pre-beta" has a density of 1.050 to 1.080 [97]. Conventional electrophoresis also does not usually permit recognition of "LpX," the lipoproteins rich in unesterified cholesterol and phospholipids that occur only in chronic biliary obstruction [98].

Polyacrylamide Gel

Polyacrylamide-gel electrophoresis (PGE) separates lipoproteins on the basis of both their size and charge [99] and has practical application in lipoprotein phenotyping [100]. This method is rapid, easily standardized, and sensitive. The migration of two of the lipoprotein families differs from that on other electrophoretic media (Fig. 28-2). On PGE, VLDL runs behind β-lipoproteins (LDL) and sometimes stays in the loading gel. The latter phenomenon, plus the prestaining technique used with PGE, often suggests the presence of chylomicrons not seen by other methods. On PGE, the β-VLDL characteristic of Type III migrates with the VLDL. So do all the normal β-lipoproteins (LDL) in the plasma of patients with Type III. It is not certain why this is so, but the anomaly is useful in diagnosis when PGE and paper or agarose are used concomitantly. In Type III, β-migrating lipoproteins appear on conventional electrophoresis but not in PGE. This "crossover" test permits identification of about 95 percent of patients with Type III [100].

Other Methods

Cohn fractionation [46], nephalometric measurements of light-scattering chylomicrons, VLDL, and LDL [101, 102], and precipitation methods employing dextran sulfate, amylopectin sulfate, heparin, or polyvinylpyrrolidone [103,

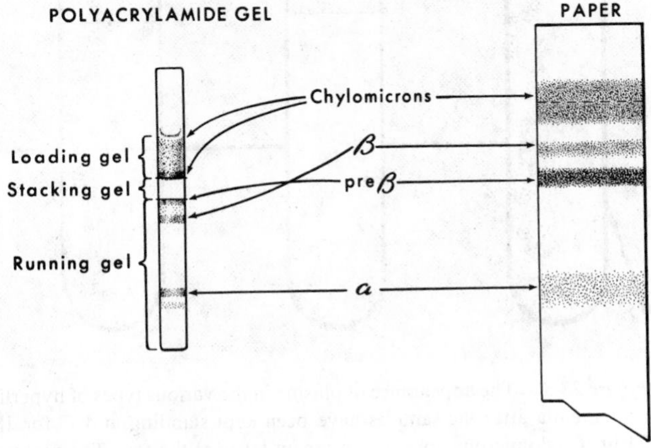

Figure 28-2. Migration of plasma lipoprotein families on polyacrylamide gel and paper electrophoresis.

104] are useful for determining portions of the lipoprotein pattern. Immunochemical methods provide sensitive measurement of LDL in plasma [105, 106] but are not yet used as routine procedures. Because VLDL and LDL share antigenic determinants, VLDL must be removed by ultracentrifugation before LDL can be quantified immunochemically.

Observation of Plasma

The simplest of all techniques is observation of plasma that has stood in the refrigerator, *unfrozen,* for 18 to 24 hr (Fig. 28-3 and Table 28-4). It is also the most sensitive for the detection of chylomicrons.

Combination of Methods

The definition of abnormal lipoprotein patterns does not depend on any single method for determining lipoproteins; in fact no one method is adequate. The combination of electrophoresis and cholesterol and triglyceride determinations has mainly been used to classify hyperlipidemia in many clinics around the world [107–120]. It has sometimes been modified by the addition of preparative ultracentrifugation [121–128]. In not permitting either estimation of LDL or ascertainment of the Type III anomaly, or both, the techniques employed have often fallen short of that necessary for definition of all known phenotypes of familial hyperlipoproteinemia.

We employ a combination of methods for establishing lipoprotein patterns [65, 77]. The analyses include (1) examination of standing plasma, (2) measurement of plasma cholesterol (C) [129] and triglyceride (TG) [130] concentrations, (3) electrophoresis on paper [83] or agarose [84], (4) measurement of plasma HDL concentrations as cholesterol [HDL(C)] after all other lipoproteins have been precipitated with heparin-manganese [131], (5) ultracentrifugation of plasma without density correction and electrophoresis of the supernatant fraction to determine if any abnormal β-migrating lipoproteins ("β-VLDL") are present, (6) measurement of VLDL-cholesterol in the supernatant fraction, and (7) measurement of cholesterol in the infranatant fraction and calculation of LDL cholesterol [LDL(C)] as the difference between infranatant cholesterol and HDL(C).

Although the full series of analyses has been used for all subjects in the kindreds described hereafter, short-cuts are possible in both genetic and other clinical work. Three simpler methods have been found to be of particular help in eliminating ultracentrifugation: (1) use of electrophoresis on both paper (or agarose) and PGE to ascertain the presence of β-VLDL (Type III); (2) use of the plasma triglyceride concentration to determine if VLDL is elevated (in the absence of chylomicrons, elevated TG is equated with elevated VLDL); (3) estimation of LDL concentrations, infor-

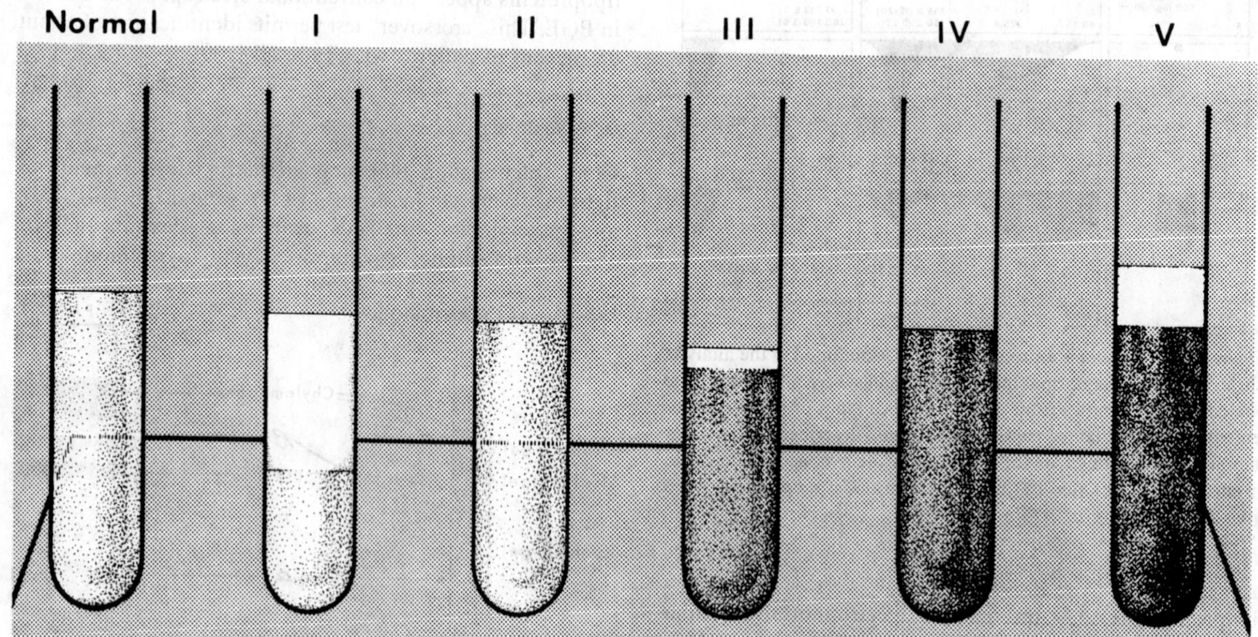

Figure 28-3. The appearance of plasma in the various types of hyperlipoproteinemia after the samples have been kept standing at 4°C for 18 to 24 hr. Chylomicrons appear as a cream layer at the top. The plasma or infranatant layers in Types III, IV, and V are turbid; those in Types I and II are clear.

mation that is essential for ascertainment of Type II. This can be obtained from the following formula:

$$\text{LDL(C)} = \text{plasma (C)} - [\text{HDL(C)} + \text{plasma TG}/5]$$

This formula gives LDL(C) values that correlate extremely well with ultracentrifugal analyses, provided that the plasma TG is not over 400 mg per 100 ml and that β-VLDL (Type III) is not present [132]. Harlan has proposed a nomogram for determination of lipoprotein patterns from cholesterol and triglycerides alone [133]. It does not correlate well with the types defined by estimations of lipoprotein concentrations.

Definition of Abnormal Patterns

The definitive criteria for establishment of the five abnormal lipoprotein patterns are shown in Table 28-4, along with other features that are helpful. The definitions are flexible in terms of the methods that may be used; the absolute concentrations of lipids and lipoproteins considered "abnormal" also need to be set for the particular population under study. The selection of limits for defining abnormality among Americans is further discussed under each phenotype.

Identification of Phenotypes

Under each type of familial hyperlipoproteinemia a definition of phenotype(s) is given. The *major criteria* are essential for the diagnosis. It is understood that the lipoprotein pattern specified has been obtained under the "index" conditions previously described and that all known diseases to which the pattern might be secondary have been excluded. Some *minor criteria* are also provided; they are not essential but may be helpful in ascertaining the phenotype.

TYPE I HYPERLIPOPROTEINEMIA: FAMILIAL LIPOPROTEIN LIPASE-DEFICIENT HYPERCHYLOMICRONEMIA

SYNONYMS: Familial hyperchylomicronemia, familial fat-induced hyperlipemia, hepatosplenomegale lipoidose—type Bürger-Grütz, and sometimes called idiopathic familial hyperlipemia, retention hyperlipemia, or essential hyperlipemia; the condition is referred to in this chapter as familial Type I hyperlipoproteinemia.

Definition

Familial Type I hyperlipoproteinemia is defined by the presence of massive amounts of chylomicrons while the patient is on a normal diet and by their complete disappearance within a few days after fat-free feeding is instituted. On a normal diet low density lipoproteins and high density lipoproteins are low; very low density lipoproteins are low or may appear to be slightly increased (Fig. 28-4). During fat-free feeding very low density lipoproteins increase modestly. The disease is due to a defect in removal of chylomicrons. The patients have decreased plasma postheparin lipoprotein lipase activity, and deficiency in tissue activity of this enzyme is believed to be the inheritable anomaly. The rare severe form of the disease is probably the expression of a double dose of a mutant autosomal allele. Parents and sibs sometimes have slight hyperglyceridemia and low plasma postheparin lipolytic activity (PHLA).

History

A young boy described by Bürger and Grütz in 1932 probably had the first reported example of this disease [134]. The earliest report of a definitely familial example was that of Holt, Aylward, and Timbres in 1939 [43] (Patient 1, Table 28-5). Eleven years old at that time, their patient (C.B.M.) was subsequently followed by Knittle and Ahrens [135] and was shown to have the typical PHLA deficiency [141]; she died at age 42 following repeated attacks of severe pancreatitis [136]. In the last 25 years many cases have been described as further examples, but in retrospect it is clear that most of them represented other forms of hyperlipoproteinemia. In the previous edition of this book [45], by employing strict criteria, 34 examples were selected from among all reported patients with hyperlipemia. It was inferred that this syndrome is rare and that its clinical manifestations are uniform and predictable.

In 1957 Havel [151] and Havel and Gordon [140] unequivocally demonstrated retardation of chylomicron clearance and decrease in PHLA in patients with familial Type I hyperlipoproteinemia. A study of many hyperlipemic patients with a standardized assay for PHLA confirmed this finding and suggested that it was unique for Type I among all familial forms of hyperlipoproteinemia [141]. It also was

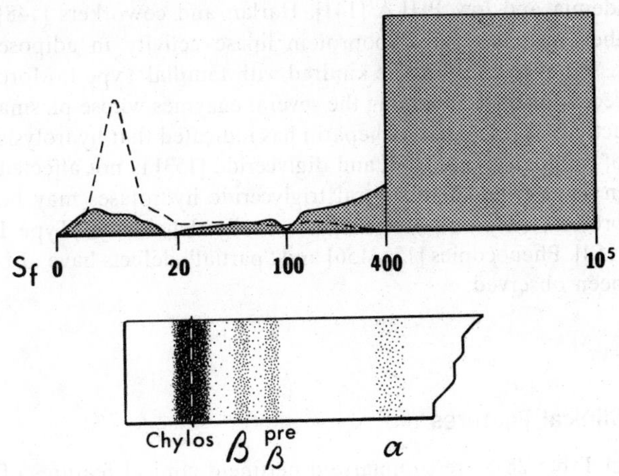

Figure 28-4. Type I hyperlipoproteinemia.

Table 28-5. CLINICAL FEATURES OF PATIENTS WITH TYPE I HYPERLIPOPROTEINEMIA*

Patient's No.	Kindred No.	Reference	Sex	Age at Detection, yr	Familial	Xanthoma	Hepatomegaly	Episodic abdominal pain	Pancreatitis	Abnormal glucose tolerance	PHLA
1	1	[43, 135, 136]	F	4	+	+	+	+	+	0	Low
2	1	[43, 135, 136]	M	8	+	0	+	+	+	0	–
3	2	[44, 137, 138]	M	8	+	0	+	+	0	–	Low
4	2	[137, 138]	F	4	+	–	+	+	0	0	Low
5	2	[137, 138]	F	<1	+	–	+	+	0	0	Low
6	3	[139–141]	M	<10	+	0	+	+	0	0	Low
7	3	[139–141]	M	8	+	0	+	+	0	0	Low
8	3	[139–141]	M	2	+	0	+	+	+	0	Low
9	4	[45, 141]	M	<1	+	+	+	+	+	0	Normal
10	4	[45, 141]	F	17	+	0	+	+	+	0	Low
11	5	[142]	F	1	+	+	+	+	0	0	Low
12	6	[135]	M	<1	0	+	+	0	0	0	Low
13	7	[135]	F	8	0	0	0	+	+	0	Low
14	8	[143]	F	2	+	+	+	0	0	0	–
15	8	[143]	M	11	+	+	+	+	0	0	Low
16	9	[142]	F	10	0	0	+	+	+	0	Low
17	10	[142]	F	<1	0	+	+	+	0	0	Low
18	11	[144]	F	4	–	0	0	+	+	0	Low
19	12	[145, 146]	F	16	–	+	+	+	0	–	Low
20	13	[147, 148]	F	24	+	+	+	+	+	–	–
21	13	[148]	F	16	+	+	+	+	0	0	Low
22	13	[148]	M	19	+	0	+	0	0	0	Low
23	14	[146]	M	4	0	+	+	+	0	0	Low
24	15	[149]	M	3	0	+	+	+	0	0	Low
25	16	[150]	F	<1	–	0	+	–	0	–	Low
26	17	[144*a*]	M	9	–	0	0	+	+	0	Low
27	18	[144]	M	33	+	0	0	0	0	0	Low
28	18	[144]	F	28	+	0	0	0	0	0	Low
29	19	[144]	M	<1	+	+	0	0	0	–	Low
30	19	[144]	F	4	+	+	0	0	0	–	Low
31	20	[144]	F	34	–	0	0	+	+	0	Low
32	21	[144]	M	22	–	0	+	+	+	+	Low

*The published data on many of these patients have been kindly supplied by their physicians. Symbols used: +, present; 0, absent; –, insufficient information.

shown that relatives of such patients may have hyperglyceridemia and low PHLA [141]. Harlan and coworkers [148] then described low lipoprotein lipase activity in adipose tissue of patients in one kindred with familial Type I. More recent distinction among the several enzymes whose plasma activity is increased by heparin has indicated that hydrolysis of monoglyceride [152] and diglyceride [153] is not affected in Type I, and that several triglyceride hydrolases may be present, only one of which is actually deficient in Type I [154]. Phenocopies [155, 156] and "partial" defects have also been observed.

Clinical Features

In Table 28-5 are summarized pertinent clinical features of 32 patients with familial Type I hyperlipoproteinemia from 21 kindreds. Only those patients are included who have been shown to meet the major criteria of the phenotype as described below. Some other examples in the literature have doubtless been excluded for lack of PHLA measurements or other information. These include the patient of Bürger and Grütz [134] and at least 20 others [157–176]. Another source of bias in case selection cannot be eliminated. This is the possibility that patients originally typical of Type I may have "converted" to an atypical lipoprotein pattern, especially Type V, through the superimposition of other disease or a complication of their hyperlipemia such as pancreatitis. This could account for the apparent uniformity in the clinical manifestations of the Type I syndrome, but long-term observation of a few patients suggests that this is not likely.

Two patients, a brother and sister described earlier [45, 141], are illustrative of the clinical course of the Type I syndrome.

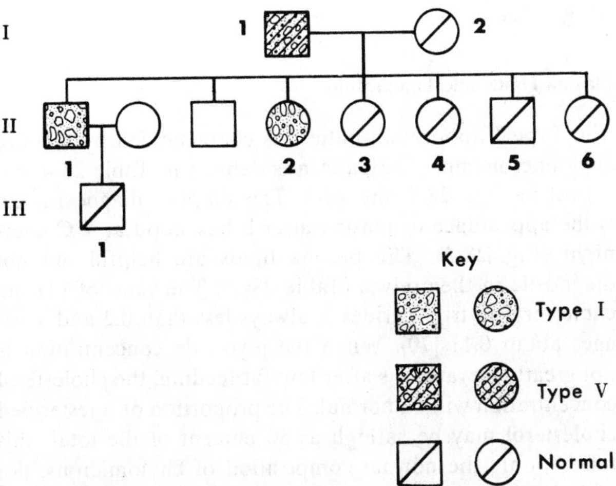

Figure 28-5. A family with Type I hyperlipoproteinemia; details about each member are given in Table 28-6.

L. Wy. (Patient 9 in Table 28-5, and II-1 in Fig. 28-5 and Table 28-6), a male, was born after an uneventful pregnancy and was breast-fed with formula supplements to the age of 4 months. At age 3 weeks he developed "numerous pale creamy plaques" over the skin of the trunk and lower extremities, surrounded by reddened areas. When he was 6½ months old his mother noted an abdominal mass, for which he was admitted at age 8 months to Vanderbilt University Hospital. The patient was noted there to be a well-developed infant with "yellowish-white patches on the hard palate and tonsillar fossa resembling those on the skin," lipemia retinalis, and moderate hepatosplenomegaly. His blood "looked like cream-of-tomato soup." The clinical impression was that of "idiopathic hyperlipemia" with eruptive xanthomas (proved by biopsy). His total plasma lipids were 4,300 mg per 100 ml, and the cholesterol level was over 1,000. Blood sugar level and oral glucose tolerance were normal. The remaining data were not remarkable except for roentgenographic changes consonant with "healing rachitic changes in the long bones." After a few days of low-fat diet, plasma total lipids fell, the skin eruptions and lipemia retinalis cleared up, and the hepatosplenomegaly decreased. On a return visit 3 months later the patient was well but was noted to have persistent lipemia.

About age 7 he had the first of many attacks of diffuse anterior abdominal pain. The pain was steady and excruciating and was often relieved only by narcotics or the passage of 1 to 3 days' time. The attacks were usually related to recent dietary intake of fat and occasionally were preceded by the appearance of eruptive xanthomas. There was no nausea, vomiting, or diarrhea. At age 19, he was first seen at the Clinical Center. Findings on physical examination were normal except for lipemia retinalis and palpable liver and spleen. At age 27 the patient's abdominal pain recurred more frequently and began to localize to the upper quadrant of the abdomen. He became dependent on narcotics for relief. A celiac angiogram was performed that revealed "multiple splenic infarcts." At exploratory laparotomy in 1969, the spleen was removed. It weighed 500 gm and contained small numbers of foam cells, but no infarcts were seen in multiple sections [177]. A 3- by 3-in. matted inflammatory mass was also observed in the tail of the pancreas and was considered evidence of chronic pancreatitis. In the year since splenectomy the patient has continued to experience severe intermittent anterior and left upper quadrant abdominal pain. His plasma PHLA has been in the normal range in at least 30 analyses by the Ediol method [141] over a 9-year period. This is in contrast to subnormal activity in his sister and all other Type I patients studied thus far. In 1969 more specific analyses indicated that the plasma postheparin monoglyceride hydrolase activity was normal but that triglyceride lipase activity was very low [152].

Table 28-6. PLASMA LIPIDS AND LIPOPROTEINS IN A TYPE I HYPERLIPOPROTEINEMIA KINDRED

Position in pedigree†	Age, yr	*Cholesterol, mg/100 ml*				Triglyceride plasma, mg/100 ml	Type
		Plasma	"VLDL"*	LDL	HDL		
I-1	50	245	144	83	18	854	V
2	51	249	. . .	. . .	. . .	109	N
II-1	25	436	386	34	16	2,850	I
2	27	302	266	22	14	3,374	I
3	16	130	. . .	. . .	. . .	40	N
4	14	129	. . .	. . .	. . .	54	N
5	12	157	. . .	. . .	. . .	62	N
6	10	149	. . .	. . .	. . .	62	N
III-1	0	138	. . .	. . .	. . .	48	N

* Includes both VLDL and chylomicrons.
† As shown in Fig. 28-5.
Note: N, normal lipoprotein pattern; other abbreviations as in Table 28-3.

All the triglyceride lipase activity was further shown to have the characteristics of a lipase other than lipoprotein lipase [154], as described below.

G.W.J. (Patient 10 in Table 28-5, and II-2 in Fig. 28-5 and Table 28-6), a younger sister of L.Wy., was discovered to have hyperglyceridemia at age 17 during family screening (Fig. 28-5). She had been in good health all her life except for several episodes of severe abdominal pain, and had never had xanthomas. When she was examined at the Clinical Center at ages 18 and 20, the only remarkable findings were lipemia retinalis, palpable liver and spleen, and a Type I lipoprotein pattern. All other routine laboratory tests, including an intravenous glucose tolerance test, gave normal results. Her plasma lipids are shown in Table 28-6, and their responses to various diets appear in Fig. 28-6. At age 25 after a holiday feast she required hospitalization because of severe "peritonitis" and was fed intravenously for 18 days. Now 27 years of age and carefully adhering to a diet moderately restricted in fat, she has been symptom-free for 2 years. She has borne two children without obvious difficulties; blood lipid analyses have not been obtained on either child. Her PHLA as ascertained by the Ediol method has always been abnormally low [141]. Like her brother, she has very low postheparin plasma triglyceride lipase activity and normal monoglyceride hydrolase activity.

Their father (I-1 in Fig. 28-5), now 50 years old, has mild Type V hyperlipoproteinemia (Table 28-6). He has normal PHLA and has never had abdominal pain.

Diagnosis

Plasma Lipids and Lipoproteins

The Type I lipoprotein pattern is characterized by massive chylomicronemia. The pattern is defined in Table 28-4 and shown in Figs. 28-1 and 28-4. The simplest diagnostic test is the appearance of plasma after it has stood at 4°C overnight (Fig. 28-3). The plasma lipids are helpful but not diagnostic in themselves (Table 28-7). The ratio of plasma cholesterol to triglycerides is always less than 0.2 and averages about 0.11 [70]. When the glyceride concentration is not greatly elevated, as after low-fat feeding, the cholesterol concentration will be normal. The proportion of unesterified cholesterol may be as high as 50 percent of the total; this reflects only the normal composition of chylomicrons, not hepatic disease.

The HDL and LDL concentrations are always markedly decreased in severe Type I (Table 28-7). Probably these lipoproteins aggregate with the chylomicrons and lose the flotation or electrophoretic properties by which they are usually defined. In familial Type I, however, the high density lipoproteins are always decreased, even when fat intake has been restricted for weeks. This is a yet-unexplained part of this disease.

It is sometimes difficult on any electrophoretic system to determine whether the very low density lipoproteins are increased or not in Type I. If they are modestly increased

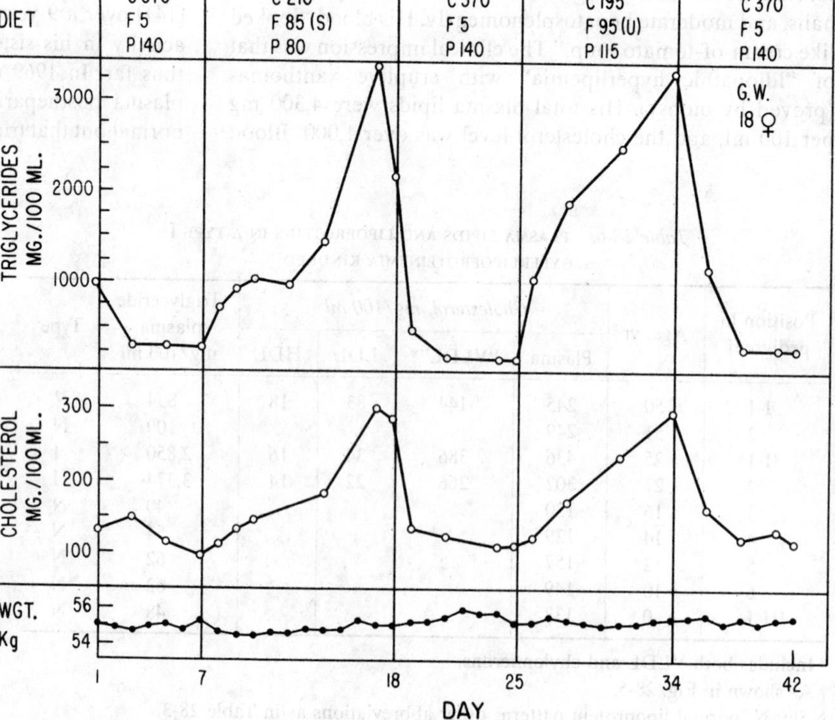

Figure 28-6. The response of plasma lipids to changes in diet in a subject with Type I familial hyperlipoproteinemia (G.W.J., Patient 10, Table 28-5). Small adjustments in caloric intake were made to maintain constant weight. *C, F,* and *P* refer respectively to the approximate grams of carbohydrate, fat, and protein in the daily diet. *F(S)* refers to provision of 95 percent of fat as butterfat, and *F(U)* to 95 percent of fat as corn oil. (*From Fredrickson et al.* [141]; *reprinted with permission of the Journal of Lipid Research.*)

Table 28-7. PLASMA LIPIDS AND LIPOPROTEINS IN TYPE I HYPERLIPOPROTEINEMIA

Patient's no.*	Age, yr	*Cholesterol, mg/100 ml*				Triglyceride plasma, mg/100 ml
		Plasma	"VLDL"†	LDL	HDL	
		Regular Diet				
6	32	238	202	24	12	2,964
7	36	434	392	28	14	4,400
8	24	336	306	21	9	7,100
16	10	224	185	21	18	2,880
9	27	302	266	22	14	3,374
10	24	388	360	14	14	3,510
Mean		320	285	22	12	4,035
		Fat-free Diet‡				
6	32	138	78	47	13	390
7	36	120	71	35	14	395
8	24	172	46	74	12	212
16	10	156	70	71	15	360
9	27	92	33	41	18	168
10	24	117	48	51	18	250
Mean		133	58	53	15	296

* Numbers as in Table 28-5.
† Includes both VLDL and chylomicrons.
‡ For 5 or more days.
Note: Normal values for comparison shown in Tables 28-2 and 28-3. Abbreviations as in Table 28-3.

(Fig. 28-1), the increase is proportionately far less than that of the chylomicrons. This helps distinguish the Type I from the Type V lipoprotein pattern (see below). Moreover, in familial Type I, the very low density lipoproteins do not increase beyond the level represented by a plasma triglyceride concentration of 400 mg per 100 ml after carbohydrate has been substituted for all fat in the diet (Table 28-7). This degree of "carbohydrate induction" is less than that which occurs in Type V.

Diet Response

After ascertainment of the Type I pattern, the next step is to remove all fat from the diet and watch for the rapid and extreme reduction of plasma lipids that is characteristic of familial Type I (Fig. 28-6). It is also useful to measure plasma free fatty acid (FFA) concentrations; these remain unusually low in familial Type I [45], and the normal rise after fat ingestion does not occur.

Lipoprotein Lipase Activity

In each patient suspected of having Type I, postheparin lipolytic activity (PHLA) should be measured. Normally there is little or no lipolytic activity against long-chain glycerides in plasma [178–180], as opposed to esterases which split short-chain substrates such as tributyrin (the "lipase" activity referred to in routine clinical tests). A small dose of intravenous heparin is followed immediately by a brief appearance of lipolytic activity in plasma. The peak is reached in about 10 min, and the die-away is rapid, unless delayed by hepatic disease [181]. A simple test for PHLA is described in Fig. 28-7. The postheparin enzymes are heterogeneous; recent studies indicating the need for more specific analyses for the lipoprotein lipase component are discussed later. Because PHLA, as measured in some methods, is decreased in subjects on diets severely restricted in fat [141], the patient should be fed as much of the normal fat intake as he can tolerate for 1 week prior to measurement of PHLA.

Identification of Phenotype

Homozygote

MAJOR (DIAGNOSTIC) CRITERIA. (1) Type I lipoprotein pattern; and (2) plasma postheparin triglyceride lipase (lipoprotein lipase) deficiency. There is no single absolute marker for phenotype. The definition presumes that all familial Type I is due to lipoprotein lipase deficiency and does not discriminate among possible different causes for this deficiency. Only the presumed homozygous abnormal subject appears to have clinically recognizable disease, and because sibs and other first-degree relatives will usually

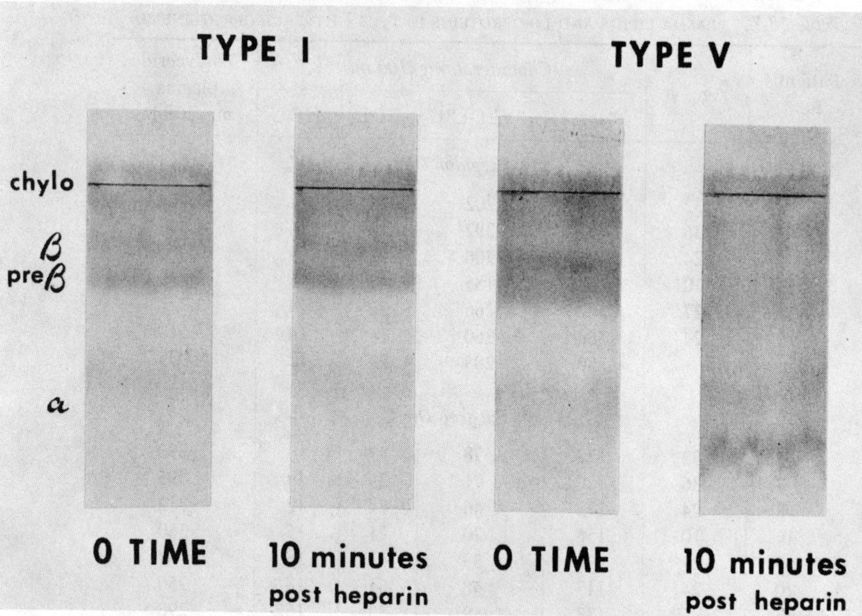

Figure 28-7. A simple qualitative test for postheparin lipolytic activity (PHLA) in plasma. Plasma obtained before and after heparin is electrophoresed on paper in albuminated buffer. In the Type V patient shown, the presence of PHLA is indicated by the increased mobility of α-, pre-β-, and β-lipoproteins. No change in migration is seen in the lipoprotein lipase-deficient Type I patient. (*Studies done in collaboration with Dr. John LaRosa.*)

appear normal, a presumption of genetic determination is made in all patients with a primary Type I pattern and PHLA deficiency.

MINOR (HELPFUL, BUT NOT DIAGNOSTIC) CRITERIA. (1) The Type I pattern in a close relative; (2) appearance of abdominal pain, eruptive xanthomas, or pancreatitis before age 20; (3) the following response to a fat-free diet: chylomicrons disappear by 5 days, very low density lipoproteins rise slightly, but plasma triglyceride does not exceed 400 mg per 100 ml; and, though high density lipoproteins may rise slightly, the level remains abnormally low; (4) exclusion of phenocopies.

Heterozygote

There are no absolute criteria to determine this phenotype; although parents are presumed to be heterozygotes, many have normal lipoprotein patterns and normal PHLA. The distribution of PHLA in relatives of homozygotes, as measured by a nonspecific method, is shown in Fig. 28-8.

Phenocopies

In the last few years imitations of familial Type I have been observed in several diseases. Prominent among these is dysglobulinemia, in which both the typical lipoprotein pattern and a deficient enzyme response to heparin may be present [155, 156]. Both electrophoresis of plasma proteins and lupus erythematosus tests are therefore *de rigueur* in diagnosis of familial Type I. Sometimes phenocopies may also be due to pancreatitis [182], uncontrolled diabetes [183], use of oral contraceptives [184], and hypothyroidism [185]. In all these instances, PHLA may be low although hyperglyceridemia is usually expressed in a lipoprotein pattern other than Type I. Gram-negative infections can also produce severe hyperglyceridemia [186].

Age at Detection

The defect in familial Type I hyperlipoproteinemia is believed to be expressed as soon as the infant takes fat. As indicated by Table 28-5, many patients come to the attention

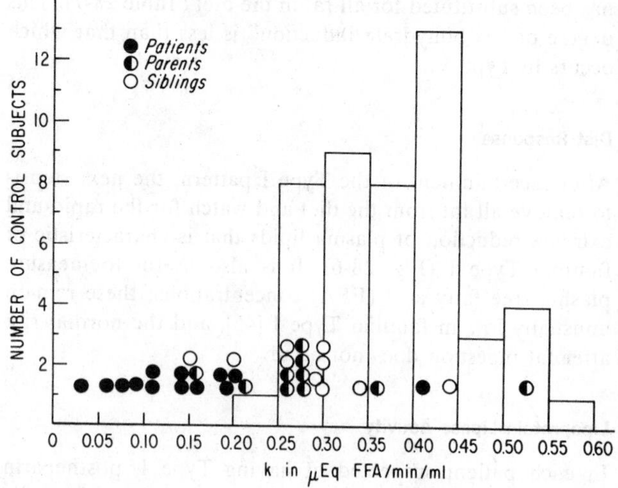

Figure 28-8. Postheparin lipolytic activity (PHLA) as measured in vitro [141] in normoglyceridemic subjects (frequency distribution shown in bars) and in patients with Type I hyperlipoproteinemia and their relatives. The symbols for the relatives represent a single determination; those for the patients represent the mean of 2 to 10 determinations. (*Data reprinted from Fredrickson and Lees* [45].)

of physicians before the age of 10 years. Rarely, a case may not be detected before the fourth decade. Hyperlipemia is usually discovered accidentally or because of eruptive xanthomas, bouts of abdominal pain, or hepatic and splenic enlargement. Occasionally the disease may be noted for the first time during examination of a patient presenting symptoms that suggest an acute "surgical" emergency with severe abdominal pain and signs of peritoneal irritation.

Characteristic Signs and Symptoms

Xanthomas

When present, xanthomas are of the eruptive type (Fig. 28-9). These lesions characteristically appear when the hyperlipemia is severe, and they disappear when it is reduced by a low fat intake. They suddenly arise when plasma triglyceride levels have been in the neighborhood of only 2,000 mg per 100 ml for a brief period. Some patients whose glyceride concentrations have chronically been in excess of 2,000 to 4,000 mg per 100 ml for many years never have xanthomas. In several patients small vesicles, which have broken down and exuded milky fluid, have also been described [43, 134]. Eruptive xanthomas may appear at any site, including the mucous membranes. They have a faint erythematous base, surmounted by a yellowish nodule. A few may coalesce to form larger lesions. After they begin to fade, the xanthomas usually disappear completely within a few weeks.

Abdominal Pain

Episodic abdominal pain may occur in all types of hyperglyceridemia [187] and is very common in the Type I syndrome. Pain may be generalized or localized to one quadrant and associated with tenderness of the spleen or liver. It is frequently in the epigastrium or midabdominal region, and sometimes radiates to the back. General malaise and anorexia are common, but nausea, vomiting, or collapse is not. Spasm, rigidity, rebound tenderness, leukocytosis, and fever may be present. Febrile "crises," associated with abdominal pain and prostration, sometimes occur; they resolve rapidly when the hyperlipemia suddenly decreases. The liver and spleen may enlarge as hyperlipemia dramatically clears up [43], but usually the liver and spleen become smaller after a few weeks of a fat-free diet.

Although attacks are usually preceded by excessive fat intake and are always associated with hyperlipemia, they are not precisely correlated with diet or triglyceride concentration. Patients have frequently undergone laparotomy, but the only abnormality usually observed is milky exudate in the peritoneal cavity.

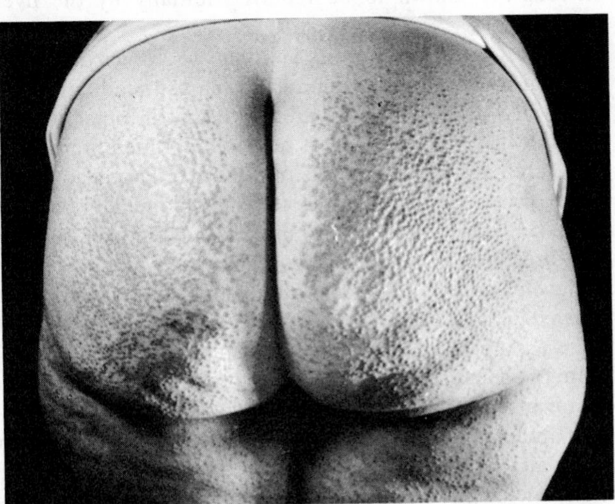

Figure 28-9. Eruptive xanthomas. (*Photograph kindly supplied by Prof. K. Polano, University of Leiden.*)

Pancreatitis

Serum lipase and amylase values often are elevated during the attacks of abdominal pain. There is no question that hyperlipemia can precede, and apparently cause, pancreatitis [165]. Unfortunately, the plasma lipid levels are usually not examined until after pancreatitis has occurred, and there is little solid evidence that pancreatitis initiates a chronic state of hyperglyceridemia. Either a Type I or Type V pattern is seen in patients with acute or chronic pancreatitis.

Lipemia Retinalis

Hyperglyceridemia may impart a pale cast to the retina, associated with a marked increase in light reflex of the vessels. Lactescence in plasma (hyperlipemia) is due to light scattering and is a function of both triglyceride concentration and of particle size. No absolute glyceride concentration is necessary, therefore, for lipemia retinalis to appear, and it is not specific for any one type of hyperlipoproteinemia.

Foam Cells

In severe hyperglyceridemia, foam cells may be found in biopsies of tissues rich in reticuloendothelial cells such as bone marrow, spleen, and liver [177, 188]. These large histiocytes are 10 to 90 microns in diameter and contain droplets of lipid, which give the cytoplasm a finely reticulated or "mulberry" appearance. Their morphologic appearance, by either phase or electron microscopy, is indistinguishable from that of foam cells seen in many other lipid storage diseases [188]. These foam cells are also identical to those early reported in the spleens of diabetic patients [189, 190]. Vacuolization of parenchymal as well as Kupffer and sinusoidal cells has been observed in biopsy specimens from the liver [164].

Other Clinical Features

Two clinical manifestations common in other forms of hyperglyceridemia do not appear to be unusually prevalent in Type I: (1) abnormal glucose tolerance (Table 28-5) [this may follow pancreatitis in Type I (patient No. 32 in Table 28-5) but is not a feature of the uncomplicated disease; nor is diabetes prominent in the available family histories]; (2) premature vascular disease. There is a noteworthy lack of evidence of premature ischemic heart disease or other forms of arteriosclerosis in Type I, although the patients are admittedly few and, as a group, rather young.

Autopsies have been performed on two adult women with familial Type I, both of whom died of pancreatitis [136, 147]. The first patient (C.B.M., Patient 1 in Table 28-5) died at 42 years of age [136]. Her coronary arteries were found to be fully patent, without any narrowing or significant atherosclerosis. There were some yellow plaques in the aorta, particularly in its branches, but the degree of atherosclerosis was not remarkable. There was no evidence of myocardial infarction in any of many sections made of the heart [136]. In the other patient, who died at age 24 [147], abnormalities in the pancreas were again more remarkable than changes in the blood vessels.

Laboratory Abnormalities

No routine laboratory test gives characteristically abnormal results in Type I hyperlipoproteinemia, although some assays having colorimetric end points are difficult to perform in the presence of hyperchylomicronemia. Thymol turbidity cannot be measured; other liver function tests have repeatedly given normal results. Anemia is not typical of familial Type I, and the hemolytic phenomena described with hyperglyceridemia by Zieve [191, 192] do not occur. Several young sibs with severe "malignant" hyperlipemia and coagulation abnormalities [193–195] have not been included in the compilation of Type I patients in Table 28-5.

Chylomicron Metabolism

Synthesis

As dietary fatty acids enter the intestinal mucosal cells, those of chain length C_{12} or greater are reassembled into glycerides that coalesce into particles called *chylomicrons.* These have a diameter of 100 to 1,000 mμ (Fig. 28-10). They acquire a stabilizing surface-active layer of phospholipid, cholesterol, and protein, which apparently is not part of a cellular membrane [197, 198]. The chylomicrons then move out into lymph channels, filter through lymph nodes [199], and eventually reach the plasma by way of the thoracic duct.

As indicated in Chap. 26, little of the new knowledge concerning the apolipoproteins found in other lipoprotein families has yet been extended to the chylomicrons. The particles react to antiserums made to LDL and HDL; it is not established whether the other apolipoproteins of VLDL (apoVLDL-ala, -glu, and -val, see Chap. 26) are also present. Evidence has been summarized in Chap. 26 supporting an absolute requirement for the apolipoprotein characteristic of LDL (apoLDL-ser) for the formation or release of chylomicrons from the intestines.

Removal of Chylomicrons

The mechanisms of removal of triglycerides from the blood are only partially understood; they have been the subject of a number of reviews [178, 199–201]. Chylomicrons are normally removed after only a brief stay in plasma [202–206]. Some of the fatty acids of the chylomicron glycerides are rapidly oxidized [204, 207]; most of them find their way into glycerides and phospholipids in cells located throughout the body, with the probable exception of the brain. Most of the fatty acids go to adipose tissue and skeletal muscle; a significant fraction appear in liver, and much lesser amounts in lung, spleen, kidney, heart, and other tissues [207–211]. During lactation, mammary gland uptake is proportionately very high [212, 213]. Precise localization of chylomicron clearance is subject to some uncertainty, introduced by the rapid transport of FFA released from glyceride in one organ which quickly reappear in another.

With the possible exception of the liver, it appears that most of the chylomicron glyceride is hydrolyzed during the removal process. Recent experiments suggest that some chylomicrons are degraded during removal in such a way that most of the fatty acid components of glycerides enter adjacent muscle or adipose tissue, while "remnants," relatively enriched in cholesterol, travel to the liver for clearance [214]. Most of the cholesterol and cholesteryl esters in chylomicrons are known to be removed initially by the liver [215, 216].

Part of the difference in mechanisms for chylomicron removal probably lies in the difference in structure of capillary walls in the liver compared with that in other tissues. In the liver capillaries there is no basement membrane, and there are gaps in the endothelium that are large enough to admit intact chylomicrons to the subendothelial space of Disse [217]. Kupffer cells also may protrude into the lumen and directly exercise their phagocytic capacity upon particles in the bloodstream [217]. In muscle, adipose tissue, and other organs, the spaces between endothelial cells are closed and there are no pores or gaps in the capillary walls [217].

In nonhepatic tissues, then, the process of chylomicron removal requires several steps. Some of these can be visualized and others imagined, as in Fig. 28-10. The chylomicron must attach itself or pass into the endothelial cell. Some chylomicrons, or parts of them, move beyond into pericytes and other macrophages below the basement membrane.

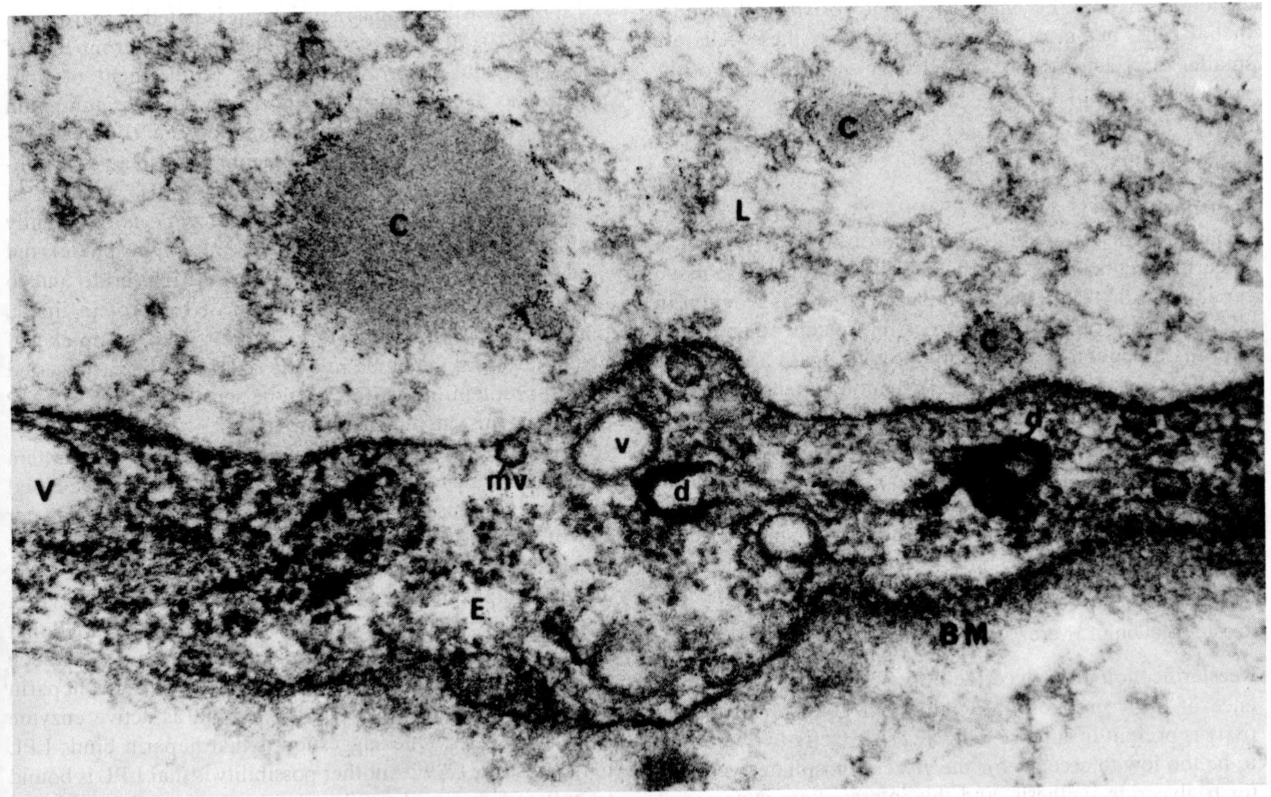

Figure 28-10. Electron photomicrograph of a capillary of the parametrial fat pad of a fed rat. The fat pad was perfused for 10 min with blood containing chylomicrons. After perfusion, the tissue was immediately fixed in glutaraldehyde and then incubated in a medium containing $CaCl_2$ (pH 8.3) for 1 hr and postincubated for 10 min in $Pb(NO_3)_2$. Hydrolysis of chylomicron triglyceride by lipoprotein lipase occurred during the incubation. The fatty acids released when trapped at the site of hydrolysis within the endothelial cell (*E*) form an insoluble calcium-lead-soap, which can be visualized as the electron-dense laminated deposits (*d*) in microvesicles (*mv*) and vacuoles (*V*). Unhydrolyzed chylomicrons (*C*) are present in the capillary lumen (*L*). The basement membrane is labeled *BM*. (×85,000.) (*Courtesy of Drs. E. J. Blanchette-Mackie and R. O. Scow, National Institutes of Health.*)

Within these several cells the glycerides are hydrolyzed [196, 201] (Fig. 28-10). The fatty acid products are mainly reincorporated into other glycerides or other esters. It is not known whether this reesterification occurs in the endothelial cell directly or whether the FFA first pass into other adjacent, extravascular sites. Some FFA from chylomicron glycerides return directly to the bloodstream for retransport on albumin to other sites of disposal [200, 204]. Perhaps these FFA come from hydrolysis occurring particularly close to the endothelial surface; it is generally believed that no significant hydrolysis occurs normally in the bloodstream in man, and now there is clear-cut evidence that it occurs within the endothelial cells themselves, at least in adipose tissue [201].

Cellular Uptake of Chylomicrons

A separateness of endothelial cell uptake of the chylomicron and hydrolysis of its glycerides is illustrated in the electron photomicrograph in Fig. 28-10. There is little intimate knowledge of the process of uptake and of how independent it may be of hydrolysis. It is apparent that cells having the potential for microphage formation, such as Kupffer cells, accumulate large fat droplets when bathed in blood rich in chylomicrons [218]. This is probably a secondary mechanism for chylomicron removal, dependent on phagocytosis of these lipoproteins in the same manner as any other particles and probably associated with degradation of the lipids by acid hydrolases in the lysosomes of the phagocyte. Whole chylomicrons may be engulfed (pinocytosis) by the endothelial cells, but most of the "vesicles" in these cells are smaller than chylomicrons, which suggests dispersion of the particles upon uptake.

Hydrolysis of Chylomicron Glyceride

Blanchette-Mackie and Scow (Fig. 28-10) have recently obtained clear-cut evidence that hydrolysis of chylomicron glyceride occurs in the endothelial cells of the adipose tissue capillary wall [196]. The enzyme catalyzing this reaction in adipose tissue capillaries, and possibly in all other tissues with the exception of liver, is lipoprotein lipase (see further on). This enzyme has not been demonstrated in hepatic tissue; the evidence that hepatic parenchymal cells do not take up glycerides without concomitant hydrolysis [219] indicates that other "hepatic lipases" serve this function in the liver. Some experiments have been interpreted as indicating that liver directly removes only a very small fraction of chylomicron glyceride fatty acids [220].

Reesterification of Hydrolysis Products

Reesterification of triglyceride fatty acids requires the presence of α-glycerophosphate. Although glycerol kinase activity is present in adipose tissue [221], its activity is believed to be too low to account for the glycerophosphate necessary for triglyceride synthesis, and this intermediate is provided mainly from glucose catabolism [200, 222].

Therefore, at least in adipose tissue, insulin activity may regulate the critical reesterification step in the process of chylomicron removal [222, 223]. Insulinopenia also decreases the activity of lipoprotein lipase [183, 224, 225]. Functionally, this linkage of insulin to control of both hydrolysis and esterification is valuable, for release of FFA in high concentrations could be seriously damaging to tissues unable to esterify them.

Lipoprotein Lipase

Lipoprotein lipase (LPL) is the name given by Korn [54] to one of several triglyceride lipases found in the body. The enzyme was discovered in research aimed at explaining the "clearing factor" which reduced lactescence in hyperlipemic plasma after heparin was injected [226]. LPL hydrolyzes the ester bonds in glycerides in chylomicrons, in other lipoproteins, and in artificial fat emulsions, provided the latter are first activated by the presence of serum. This ability to activate LPL was identified by Korn as residing primarily in the HDL fraction of human plasma [227]. Recent studies suggest that one or more of the apolipoproteins found in VLDL, and also present as minor constituents of apoHDL, are potent activators of LPL [228–230]. On a weight basis, the most active is apoVLDL-glu (Chap. 26), and the next most active is apoVLDL-ala; both are more effective in the presence of added phospholipid [230].

Lipoprotein lipase has never been isolated in pure form [231, 232]. Its activity is usually distinguished from that of pancreatic and other lipases by its requirement of lipoproteins as a "cofactor" and its rather selective inhibition by high NaCL concentrations, protamine, and sodium pyrophosphate [231, 232]. It is not epinephrine-activated, in contrast to the "hormone-sensitive" lipase also present in adipose tissue [233–235]. The latter enzyme is apparently regulated by cyclic AMP (adenosine monophosphate) and appears to catalyze hydrolysis of tissue triglyceride and to effect FFA release [236]. The action of lipoprotein lipase, on the other hand, appears to be restricted to uptake of glycerides from the blood into the cell. It has been suggested that lipoprotein lipase, too, may be sensitive to cyclic AMP [237], but this has not been proved.

A characteristic, but not unique, feature of lipoprotein lipase is its immediate and transient appearance in the blood after the administration of small quantities ($<$ 10 units per kg) of heparin or similar polyfunctional anions. There is no detectable LPL activity in preheparin plasma in man, and none appears when heparin is added to blood in vitro. Bacterial heparinase inactivates LPL, and it is presumed that heparin or one of its congeners is present as a prosthetic group in the enzyme [238]. It is not known how heparin causes LPL activity to appear in plasma as active enzyme from tissue sites. One suggestion is that heparin binds LPL to its substrate [239]. Another possibility is that LPL is bound to sulfated mucopolysaccharides in the vascular wall and is displaced by heparin. Heparin also causes activity of some other lipolytic enzymes [152, 240, 241] and histaminase [242] to appear briefly in plasma.

Tissue Localization of LPL

LPL activity is present in many organs and tissues; prominent among these are adipose tissue, the mammary gland, muscle, heart, and aorta [201, 231, 232]. It is also present in milk [243, 244]. Although arteriovenous measurements across the liver have been interpreted as indicating hepatic release of LPL [245, 246], little activity is extractable from this organ [54, 247]. Adipose tissue is especially rich in LPL [248]; some of the activity here may be present in the adipocytes themselves [248], but probably most of it is located in the capillary-rich stroma, where lipolysis within the endothelial cells is demonstrable histochemically [196] (Fig. 28-10). LPL activity also appears to be present in the endothelial cells of the mammary gland; during lactation chylomicrons readily attach themselves to the capillary walls or are engulfed by the endothelium and are hydrolyzed [249].

Control of LPL Activity

The turnover time of LPL in endothelial or other cells is probably very rapid. Activity is quickly induced or deinduced by many factors [231, 232]. These include caloric intake or intake of fat, insulin activity, and probably certain hormonal influences [185, 201, 250]. It is suggested, for example, that prolactin may control the increase in LPL activity in mammary gland during lactation and concomitantly may decrease activity of the enzyme in adipose tissue [201]. Possibly this interrelationship helps divert substrate to the mammary gland when it is secreting actively.

Inactivation of LPL

It was first suggested by Jeffries [251] that the liver inactivated LPL. Felts and coworkers have conducted a number of studies to determine the nature of hepatic inactivation [252, 253]. They believe the first step may be the removal of a heparin prosthetic group.

Estimation of LPL Activity

The activity of LPL in human adipose tissue is relatively low, and this tissue has been little used for assay in man [133, 254]. The measurement of tissue LPL activity as a clinical test remains the indirect one of determining lipolysis in plasma after heparin administration. Gross estimates of activity are obtained by allowing lipemic postheparin plasma to stand and either measuring the FFA released [140] or noting whether sufficient free fatty acids have been released to increase the electrophoretic migration of the plasma lipoproteins (Fig. 28-7). The inadequacies of these techniques for the measurement of reaction kinetics notwithstanding, they sometimes provide a better view of effective capacity for hydrolysis of chylomicron glyceride than does incubation of plasma with artificial glyceride substrates under more controlled conditions [141, 255, 256]. This is particularly true of emulsions like Ediol, which may give falsely high estimates of lipolytic activity in familial Type I [141].

The explanation for this fact lies in the heterogeneity of plasma PHLA and in the special "cofactor" requirements of lipoprotein lipase for optimal activity. After heparin injection, monoglyceride hydrolase (MGH) activity that is apparently distinct from LPL appears in plasma [152, 240, 257]. An experiment by Greten and coworkers with pure labeled substrates is shown in Fig. 28-11. It is apparent that MGH and triglyceride lipase activities rise and fall together after heparin, and that in familial Type I, MGH activity is normal while triglyceride lipase activity is reduced [152]. This remains the strongest evidence of the separateness of MGH and triglyceride lipase activities in PHLA. When fat emulsions, such as Ediol, that contain appreciable amounts of monoglycerides are used to measure PHLA, it is probable that the normal MGH activity provides a misleading estimate of LPL activity in Type I. Diglyceride-splitting activity in postheparin plasma is also normal in Type I [153]; it has not been established that the activity against di- and monoglycerides represents more than one enzyme. The failure of salt to inhibit much of the plasma PHLA in both Type I and normal subjects has also aroused suspicion of other heterogeneity in triglyceride lipase activity in postheparin plasma [141].

Heterogeneity of Triglyceride Lipases

Experiments by LaRosa et al. [154] provide strong evidence for the presence of at least two triglyceride lipases in postheparin plasma. The activity of one is identical to that of adipose tissue lipoprotein lipase in its sensitivity to salt and other inhibitors and in its requirement for lipoprotein (or apolipoproteins plus phospholipids) for maximal activity against artificial substrates. This lipase is effective in hydrolysis of chylomicrons under conditions approximating those in plasma. All triglyceride lipase activity in postheparin plasma is not inhibited by salt, however, and there seems to be another lipase present that is relatively inactive in catalyzing hydrolysis of glycerides in chylomicrons and other lipoproteins. Lipase having these properties has been obtained from heparin-containing perfusates of isolated rat livers [154]. Thus distinction between lipoprotein lipase and "hepatic" triglyceride lipase in PHLA can be made by measurements in the presence and absence of salt and in media containing a concentration of HDL comparable to that in plasma. Under these conditions, the lipoprotein lipase activity, and hence the effective capacity for hydrolysis of chylomicron triglycerides, appears to be markedly reduced in familial Type I [154].

Clearance of Glycerides in Other Lipoproteins

It is likely that glycerides in VLDL and other lipoproteins are handled in a manner similar to those in chylomicrons [200]. The sites and mechanisms for removal have not yet been established. The glycerides in VLDL are substrates for lipoprotein lipase. The rate of clearance of VLDL particles from plasma is slower than that of chylomicrons. This may be attributable to differences in size between chylomicrons and very low density lipoproteins, for larger chylomicrons are removed more rapidly than smaller ones [258].

The Defect in Familial Type I Hyperlipoproteinemia

Chylomicron Formation and Structure

There is no evidence that digestion and absorption of fat from the intestinal lumen into the mucosal villae or lacteals are abnormal in Type I hyperlipoproteinemia. Type I chylomicrons are good substrates for normal plasma PHLA [141] and for rat adipose tissue lipoprotein lipase. They are also cleared rapidly from the circulation of normal subjects [140].

Lipoprotein Lipase Deficiency

The sum of available evidence indicates that a deficiency of lipoprotein lipase activity is the metabolic defect in Type I. Deficiency of activity has been described in the adipose tissue of affected members of one family [148], but the

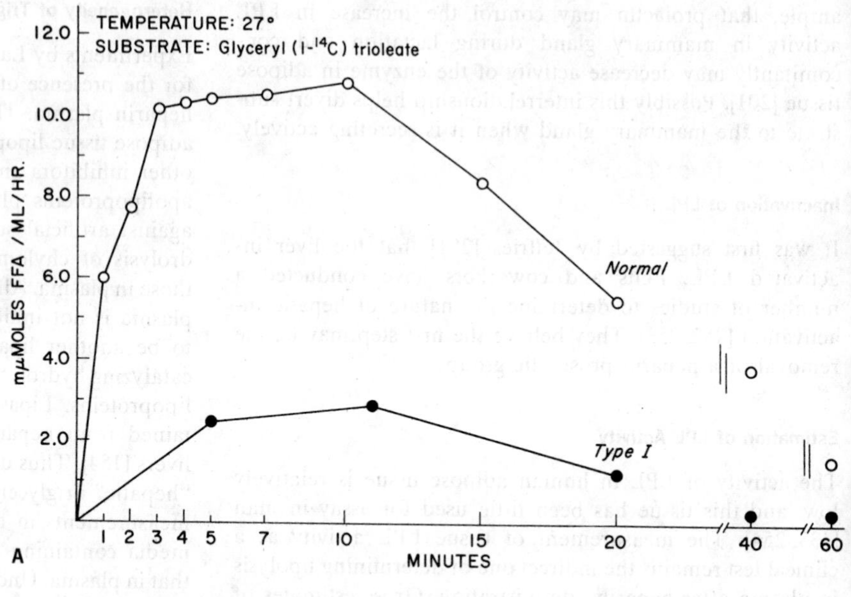

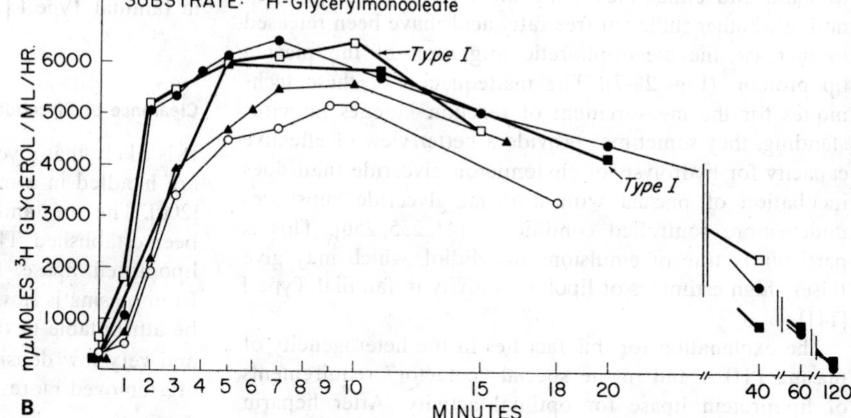

Figure 28-11. The time course of plasma triglyceride lipase activity (*A*) and monoglyceride hydrolase activity (*B*) after intravenous injection of heparin (100 units per kg body weight). Note that only the triglyceride lipase activity is low in the patient with Type I hyperlipoproteinemia (*Data from Greten et al.* [152]. *Reprinted with permission of the Journal of Lipid Research.*)

activity in human adipose tissue is normally quite low, and no attempts to confirm these experiments have been reported. All the patients listed in Table 28-5 have been deficient in plasma PHLA, as measured with Ediol, except for L.Wy., whose history was summarized above. In a few patients, the deficiency in PHLA has now been shown specifically to be in the activity of triglyceride lipase, not of monoglyceride or diglyceride hydrolase [152, 153]. Using several labeled substrates, Greten et al. [153] have concluded that the defect in Type I specifically involves the hydrolysis of the initial ester bond in triglycerides. In only two or three patients have the lipoprotein lipase and "hepatic" triglyceride lipase activities in postheparin plasma been differentiated [154]. In these patients, who include patient L.Wy., it appears that practically all the plasma PHLA in familial Type I represents activity of a lipase that is different from lipoprotein lipase and is directed toward artificial glyceride emulsions, as opposed to chylomicrons. An interesting distinction between familial Type I and its phenocopy produced by abnormal immunoglobulins that bind heparin has also been made [155, 156]. In these patients both monoglyceride and triglyceride lipase activity is depressed in postheparin plasma. Steiner has reported a patient with fat-induced hyperlipemia whose postheparin plasma could not hydrolyze chylomicrons but was active against fat emulsions [259].

A practical assay specific for plasma postheparin lipoprotein lipase activity has not yet been developed. The ideal conditions must include a triglyceride substrate activated by amounts of HDL and possibly other lipoproteins in a manner comparable to that obtaining for chylomicrons in normal plasma. Any dilution due to endogenous substrate in normal plasma must be compensated. Advantages of in vitro tests using the artificial emulsion Intralipid have been claimed [255, 256], but it has not been shown that these test systems meet all the above criteria. When a suitable test is developed, it will be of the utmost interest to apply it not only to Type I patients and their families but also to Type V and several of the secondary PHLA deficiency states such as those seen with pancreatitis [185] and insulinopenic diabetes [183]. No inhibitor of lipoprotein lipase has been demonstrated in the plasma of patients with familial Type I [138, 140, 141].

Alternative Hypotheses

A defect distal to the process of hydrolysis, as in the re-esterification of fatty acids, has not been unequivocally eliminated in familial Type I. It is conceivable that hydrolysis might be normal but rendered ineffective by some failure in disposal of FFA or chylomicron "remnants." The best, although indirect, argument against this is based on the low FFA concentrations in Type I, the opposite of that expected if FFA utilization were compromised.

The structure and metabolism of HDL need further examination in Type I. HDL concentrations are usually inversely proportional to the plasma triglyceride concentration, but in familial Type I they remain steadfastly low after all chylomicrons have disappeared as a result of a low-fat diet.

Another paradox requiring explanation is the unexpectedly small effect of fat-free, high-carbohydrate feeding on VLDL concentrations in familial Type I ("carbohydrate induction"). After a fat-free diet, the triglyceride concentrations in such patients (Table 28-7) are much less exaggerated than they are in patients with familial Type V hyperlipoproteinemia. It is likely that the defective hydrolysis of chylomicrons in Type I also applies to VLDL, and it is possible that secondary (phagocytic) mechanisms for removing glyceride-rich particles are so activated in Type I that they accelerate VLDL removal during carbohydrate induction.

One possible explanation of decreased lipoprotein lipase activity in familial Type I has recently been excluded, at least in two representative patients. This is a possible deficiency of the apoprotein activators of lipoprotein lipase [229, 230]. ApoVLDL from Patients 8 and 9 in Table 28-5 has been examined [260]. ApoVLDL-val, -glu, and -ala were present in amounts similar to those in VLDL from normal subjects. The apoVLDL-glu, in presence of phospholipid, was also found to activate adipose tissue lipoprotein lipase in vitro.

Partial Defects

A puzzling example of apparent relapsing or "intermittent" Type I was briefly described elsewhere [65]. Since that time we have observed two other patients with a partial or less-severe defect. One was a 26-year-old black woman, the other a 19-year-old Chinese woman. Both had a history of episodic abdominal pain and recurrent pancreatitis beginning in the second decade. When examined at the Clinical Center each had a florid Type I pattern and no evidence of a disease to which this might be secondary. They were placed on a fat-free diet for a week and then challenged with 50 to 80 gm fat per day. Both developed only modest chylomicronemia over a period of 1 week. PHLA was estimated by the crude test of electrophoretic mobility of lipoproteins after heparin injection. Activity was detected on some occasions and not on others. Each patient appeared to have a capacity for chylomicron clearance which was below normal and which was episodically exceeded during periods of high fat intake. None of the close relatives of either patient was available for examination.

Pathophysiology

The typical patient with familial Type I hyperlipoproteinemia has an extreme limitation in the rate of removal of chylomicrons from plasma. This is probably present and potentially recognizable from the time when fat first enters the diet in infancy. Because several different mutants may give rise to the same phenotype or because other factors may moderate gene expression, it is possible that some patients have more capacity than others to keep plasma glycerides from reaching the level of 10,000 mg per 100 ml or higher that may be present in this disorder. Most patients learn that fatty foods are related to their discomfort, but true rejection or intolerance of fat, similar to that seen in abetalipoproteinemia, is not typical of patients with familial Type I.

It is not known whether the chylomicrons in familial Type I attach themselves to, or are engulfed by, endothelial cells or other phagocytic cells near the capillary wall. Probably they are, for this has been known to occur in patients with Type V hyperlipoproteinemia, many of whom were deficient in plasma PHLA [261]. This has been demonstrated in the dermis, where fat particles appear in endothelial cells, perithelial cells, and reticulum cells and the glyceride content of these cells markedly increases. In the dermal cells, cholesterol and phospholipids also accumulate; some of this accumulation lies in cells and some in the extracellular space. In the skin there is an increase in vascularity or an inflammatory-like reaction, and papules with a yellow center and a reddish base (eruptive xanthomas) appear on the surface. As these lesions resolve, the glyceride content decreases and the trapped cholesterol is progressively esterified. Transesterification of the existing cholesteryl esters also occurs: the amount of saturated and monounsaturated fatty acids increases at the expense of the more polyunsaturated ones [261].

Reticuloendothelial cells in the spleen, liver, bone marrow, and elsewhere also take up fat and become foam cells. Although the cytoplasm is filled with residual bodies or secondary lysosomes and the cells resemble foam cells in other lipid storage diseases [177, 188], familial Type I is not a "lysosomal disorder," after the definition of Hers [262]. There is no evidence that the activity of a lysosomal enzyme is deficient. The pH optimum of lipoprotein lipase is far higher than that of the typical acid hydrolases in lysosomes. (See "Wolman's Disease," Chap. 36, for a disorder in which a lysosomal triglyceride lipase may be deficient.)

The liver and spleen often enlarge, but liver function is not impaired and hypersplenism has never been observed. Bone marrow function is also not affected by the foam cells. As in other hyperglyceridemic states, the fat content of erythrocytes may be abnormal [174, 263], but hemolysis or anemia is not characteristic of familial Type I.

The causes of the most serious complications, abdominal pain and pancreatitis, are unknown. Enlargement of the liver and spleen, with acute distension of their capsules [43], or temporary blockage of the thoracic duct by clumps of chylomicrons, with resultant distension due to serous effusions [264], has been suggested as a possible cause of pain. So has fat embolism, particularly within the pancreas [147]. Effusions of triglyceride-laden fluid in the vicinity of the pancreas, particularly, with its high content of lipase, could also lead to lipolysis, with irritating local increases in quantities of free fatty acids. At the autopsy of patient C.B.M., the prosector commented on several interesting findings [136], among which were the obliteration of the pericardial and lesser omental sacs by adhesions, and the presence of many parchment-like adhesions on the surface of the pancreas. This organ also contained many areas, from pinhead-to penny-sized, having a soapy or cheesy appearance, indicating fat necrosis.

Because of recurrent pancreatitis, the prognosis in familial Type I is not normal. A young child who apparently had the same disorder also died and was autopsied [265]. He may have succumbed to an intercurrent illness, and the autopsy was not revealing. The lack of evidence of any premature vascular disease has already been commented upon; most of those with known examples of the disease who are being followed, however, are under 40 years of age.

Genetics

Adequate family data are available from eight kindreds in which the diagnosis of Type I hyperlipoproteinemia in one or more members was based on both lipoprotein patterns and PHLA measurements. The information about four of these kindreds (Families 3, 4, 6, and 7 in Table 28-5) was summarized in the previous edition of this book [45]. Two other kindreds (Families 1 and 13 in Table 28-5) were separately reported by Holt [43] and Harlan [148] and their coworkers. The brother of C.B.M. reported by Holt, Aylward, and Timbres was later seen by Ahrens; the diagnosis of Type I appears established, although PHLA was not measured [136]. Findings on two others (Families 5 and 9) are previously unpublished.

There was a total of 31 sibs, including propositi, in these eight kindreds. Of these 12 had the full-blown Type I syndrome, 17 were normolipoproteinemic, 1 may have had mild hyperglyceridemia, and 1 was not tested. Of the 32 affected patients listed in Table 28-5, 17 were females. There is no documented instance of vertical transmission. The mother of C.B.M. had total lipid levels over 1,400 mg per 100 ml and a normal cholesterol level [43]; the father of the Wy. children (Fig. 28-5) has Type V hyperlipoproteinemia and a definite limitation of fat tolerance, but clearly not to the same extent as his affected children. The father of the Pr. children (Family 3 in Table 28-5), previously reported to have a plasma glyceride level of 180 mg per 100 ml [45], now has severe Type IV hyperlipoproteinemia; in addition he has insulin-dependent diabetes. There is no definite evidence of increased consanguinity in the Type I families.

The distribution of plasma PHLA measurements in Fig. 28-8 indicates that some sibs and parents, most of whom had normal plasma lipid concentrations, may have low or marginal PHLA values. Of five pairs of parents in whom PHLA has been measured (Families 3, 4, 6, 9, and 13 in Table 28-5), six parents have abnormally low values and only two have clearly normal ones.

All the available data are most consonant with the view that familial Type I is the expression of a double dose of an autosomal allele. It is possible that more than one similar mutant leads to the same phenotype. The presumed heterozygote usually has low PHLA, but no specific test for ascertainment of this phenotype is yet available.

The disorder has been observed in Caucasoids, Chinese, and black people. There is no estimate of the gene frequency, nor are there reliable data as to consanguinity. Type I is the rarest form of familial hyperlipoproteinemia.

Treatment

Familial Type I hyperlipoproteinemia is presently treated with dietary restriction. The aim is to reduce chylomicronemia to a minimum that is based on the patient's acceptance of a diet extremely low in the usual dietary fats. Whether the fat is saturated, monounsaturated, or polyunsaturated is not important. Most adult patients will restrict fat intake to between 40 and 60 gm per day. Medium-chain triglycerides (MCT) are absorbed by way of the portal circulation and do not appear as chylomicrons [266, 267]. They are recommended as supplements to the diet [44, 268]. The responses of the plasma triglycerides to experimental diets is shown in Fig. 28-6. Such dramatic success is not achieved in the outpatient clinic, where the patients' glycerides are frequently between 1,000 and 2,000 mg per 100 ml. Caloric restriction has not been carefully examined in Type I. The patients are usually not obese, and weight reduction probably has no effect.

TYPE II: FAMILIAL HYPERBETALIPOPROTEINEMIA

SYNONYMS: (Essential) familial hypercholesterolemia, essential (familial) hypercholesterolemic xanthomatosis; at one time also called xanthoma tuberosum, xanthoma tendinosum, familial xanthoma, and xanthoma tuberosum multiplex; referred to in this chapter as familial Type II hyperlipoproteinemia.

Definitions of Phenotypes

Familial Type II is the commonest single disorder characterized by an abnormality in plasma lipoprotein concentrations; it is also the oldest known and the most extensively studied. It is defined here as an inheritable increase in the plasma concentrations of low density lipoproteins, or β-lipoproteins (Fig. 28-12). Two phenotypes are recognized, although neither can yet be ascertained by single tests that unequivocally describe a homogeneous disease. The phenotypes are herein defined as follows:

Heterozygous Type II

MAJOR CRITERIA: (1) Type II hyperlipoproteinemia, and either (2) Type II in a first-degree relative, or (3) tendon xanthomas.

MINOR CRITERIA: (1) Plasma cholesterol concentration between 300 and 600 mg per 100 ml in adults, and between 230 and 500 in patients below 20 years of age; (2) plasma triglyceride level between 50 and 500 mg per 100 ml; (3) LDL concentration (as LDL cholesterol) greater than 210 mg per 100 ml in adults, and greater than 170 in children; (4) failure of LDL and cholesterol to become unequivocally normal on diet therapy alone; and (5) exclusion of phenocopies.

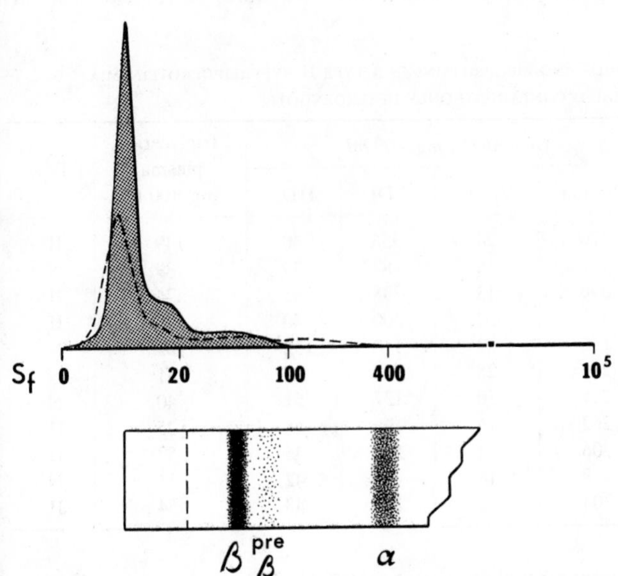

Figure 28-12. Type II hyperlipoproteinemia.

Homozygous Type II

MAJOR CRITERIA: (1) Type II pattern with an LDL concentration about twice that of heterozygotes in the same kindred, and (2) Type II pattern in both parents. The presence of Type II in the family line of an unavailable parent permits presumptive fulfillment of this criterion.

MINOR CRITERIA: (1) Plasma cholesterol concentration greater than 500 mg per 100 ml; (2) triglyceride level between 50 and 500 mg per 100 ml; (3) xanthomas appearing before the age of 10 years, including subcutaneous lesions of the palms, buttocks, knees, or other areas, as well as tendon xanthomas; (4) vascular disease before the age of 20; and (5) exclusion of phenocopies.

These definitions describe a disorder that always includes hyperlipoproteinemia and is sometimes associated with xanthomas and premature vascular disease. There is still confusion about separation of familial Type II from other forms of hyperlipoproteinemia; some of this confusion is due to limitations in defining the disease by lipid rather than lipoprotein analyses, and some of it is due to semantic issues that are more understandable as one considers the history of the disease.

History

The kinds of xanthomas that occur in familial Type II also can be features of secondary hyperlipoproteinemia. This was especially noteworthy in the literature of the latter half of the nineteenth century, in which many patients with biliary obstruction and "xanthoma tuberosum multiplex" were described [3]. Possibly as early as 1879 [5], similar lesions were seen in a rare patient without jaundice, and after 1900 a number of such instances had been recorded, some in close relatives [12, 20, 32, 37]. As noted earlier, the proof that a primary form of xanthoma tuberosum multiplex was always associated with hypercholesterolemia had to wait upon the availability of reliable measurements of plasma cholesterol, i.e., until about 1920 [22, 23]. From time to time during this period, patients with xanthoma disseminata, the cutaneous form of eosinophilic granuloma (in which plasma lipids are normal), were presented as a refutation of the obligatory presence of hypercholesterolemia in severe xanthomatosis [12]. Such confusion was gradually dispelled by the improved classification of the xanthomatous disorders that was developed between 1920 and 1950 [39, 269–273]. By 1940, sufficient data had been collected to indicate that the primary expression of xanthoma tuberosum multiplex was not skin lesions but hyperlipidemia [26, 28–30, 33–36]. There then ensued considerable debate concerning the genetic mode of transmission [33–36, 426, 274–287], much of this centering about the belief of some investigators [42, 286] that xanthomatosis was found only in homozygous abnormal subjects. This question has been generally resolved [45], with agreement that the disease is detectable in nearly every bearer of a mutant gene in single dosage and that he is likely to develop xanthomatosis in time. The homozygote has a greater degree of hyperlipidemia and more severe xanthomatosis, which also appears much earlier than in the heterozygote.

The name *familial* (or *essential* or *idiopathic*) *hypercholesterolemic xanthomatosis,* suggested by Thannhauser [40], emerged for a time as the most popular designation for the disease. Thannhauser considered hypercholesterolemia as a *forme fruste* of the disease. Gradually this term was supplemented by *essential familial hypercholesterolemia,* as suggested by Wilkinson and coworkers [41].

The transformation of the concept of the disease to *familial hyper-β-lipoproteinemia* began between 1950 and 1955. The specific lipoprotein class involved in Type II was suggested from analyses made by Cohn fractionation [48, 58] and by electrophoresis [58], and specific involvement of low density lipoproteins of a narrow density range was first established by Gofman, McGinley, and colleagues [49, 55, 56]. They showed that patients with xanthoma tendinosum, a fairly good but nonspecific marker for the disease, had discrete elevations in S_f 0 to 12 and 12 to 20 lipoproteins.

By the time the studies in the Clinical Center in Bethesda were under way, a number of patients with hyperglyceridemia in addition to hypercholesterolemia and tendon and tuberous xanthomas had also been observed in many other clinics. Some of these patients were then conclusively shown to have Type II hyperlipoproteinemia and some to represent a completely independent disorder (Type III) [65]. Plasma samples from over 600 patients with Type II in 225 kindreds have been analyzed at the Clinical Center (Table 28-1). This group is by far the largest to be segregated by lipoprotein analyses. Concepts of the disease derived from it are not always identical, but they conform in general to those derived from other genetic studies in which plasma lipids and xanthomas have usually provided the basis of segregation [60, 115, 123, 176, 281, 284, 287, 288–300]. Understanding of the homozygous phenotype of Type II has been greatly assisted by Khachadurian's extensive studies of an almost unique population in Lebanon [287]. The most recent developments in Type II relate to the discovery of its responsiveness to cholestyramine therapy [301–306].

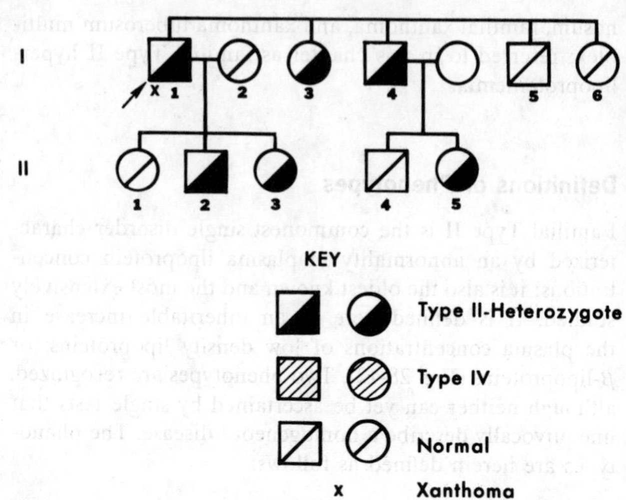

Figure 28-13. A family with Type II hyperlipoproteinemia (the Ja. family, Table 28-8).

Clinical Features

The following are summaries of the histories of typical patients who are heterozygous and homozygous, respectively, for familial Type II.

H.Ja. (I-1 in Fig. 28-13 and Table 28-8), a 34-year-old white male, became aware of nodules on the extensor sur-

Table 28-8. PLASMA LIPIDS AND LIPOPROTEINS IN A TYPE II HYPERLIPOPROTEINEMIA KINDRED CONTAINING ONLY HETEROZYGOTES

Position of subject in pedigree*	Age, yr	Cholesterol, mg/100 ml Plasma	VLDL	LDL	HDL	Triglyceride plasma, mg/100 ml	Type
I-1	34	420	24	356	40	149	II
2	27	142	16	87	39	39	N
3	45	396	13	338	45	74	II
4	41	362	22	300	40	103	II
5	36	192	22	118	52	102	N
6	31	220	28	125	67	61	N
II-1	8	218	30	137	51	40	N
2	6	262	16	198	48	25	II
3	3	306	4	257	45	57	II
4	16	128	16	70	42	31	N
5	19	304	22	234	48	54	II

* As shown in Fig. 28-13.

Note: N, normal lipoprotein pattern; other abbreviations as in Table 28-3.

faces of the hands and the Achilles, plantar, and subpatellar tendons at age 24. One of the plantar nodules was removed when he was 28 and was diagnosed as a "uric acid granuloma." When he was 30 angina pectoris appeared, a systolic murmur was heard, and his electrocardiogram was found compatible with a recent myocardial infarction. Plasma lipid levels were determined for the first time. In milligrams per 100 ml, the cholesterol was 516; phospholipids were 328; and triglycerides were 234. His glucose tolerance was normal. A tentative diagnosis of hypertrophic subaortic stenosis led to his admission to the Clinical Center for cardiac evaluation. The physical examination revealed only the heart murmur, corneal arcus, and the tendon xanthomas previously noted. The lipid and lipoprotein analyses are shown in Table 28-8. The uric acid was normal. The abnormalities found at cardiac catheterization were confined to the coronary angiogram, in which the right coronary artery appeared to be occluded proximally. It was filled below through anastomoses with the left anterior descending and circumflex arteries, which also were diffusely narrowed and irregular. No history of hyperlipoproteinemia existed in the Ja. family prior to the screening that was prompted by the patient's admission. Several other affected relatives (Fig. 28-13) and a disastrous family history of premature vascular disease were uncovered. The father had three myocardial infarctions between age 42 and his death at age 50. The mother had a cerebrovascular accident at age 30 and died at 48. One brother died of myocardial infarction at age 32.

H.Ja. was placed on a diet containing less than 300 mg cholesterol per day and 40 percent of calories as fat, the latter having an overall ratio of polyunsaturates to saturates (P/S) of 2. The results of the diet and subsequent trial of drugs are depicted in Fig. 28-21. The net effect of both diet and cholestyramine was a reduction in plasma cholesterol from 420 to 250 mg per 100 ml and of LDL cholesterol from 360 to 200 mg per 100 ml. Cholestyramine did not increase plasma triglycerides in H.Ja. as it sometimes does. Clofibrate was without significant effect on his lipid levels. His course has been followed for 2 years on an outpatient basis, and his cholesterol level has been maintained below 280 mg per 100 ml, by means of diet and cholestyramine, 24 gm per day. He continues to have occasional anterior chest pain, relieved by nitroglycerine.

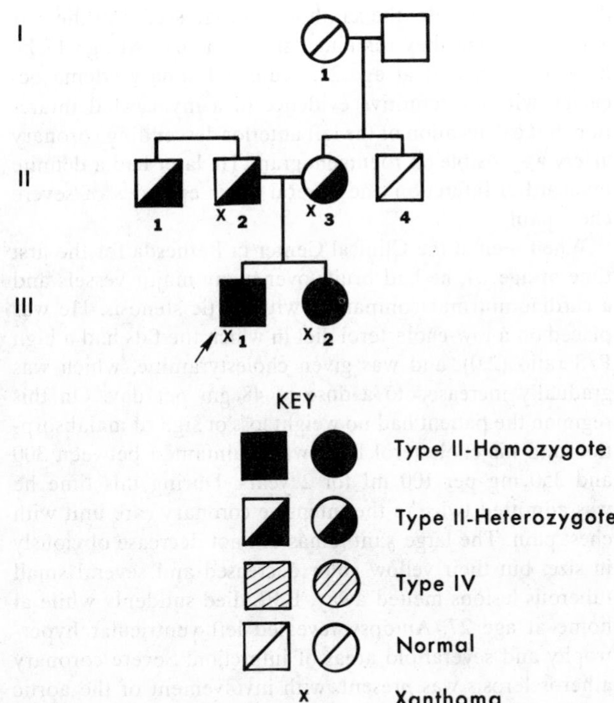

Figure 28-14. A family with Type II hyperlipoproteinemia, including both homozygotes and heterozygotes (the Fl. family, Table 28-9).

L.Fl. (III-1 in Fig. 28-14 and Table 28-9), a 27-year-old male, had multiple, large tendon and tuberous xanthomas over the elbows, dorsal aspects of the hands, buttocks, soles of the feet, and Achilles tendons for as long as he could remember; small xanthomas had been noticed as early as age 1 year. When he was 2 years old his left eye was enucleated for a suspected melanoma; the lesion proved to be a xanthoma. Although he had been on a low-cholesterol

Table 28-9. PLASMA LIPIDS AND LIPOPROTEINS IN A TYPE II HYPERLIPOPROTEINEMIA KINDRED CONTAINING HOMOZYGOTES

Position of subject in pedigree*	Age, yr	Cholesterol, mg/100 ml				Triglyceride plasma, mg/100 ml	Type
		Plasma	VLDL	LDL	HDL		
I-1	75	190	20	134	36	76	N
II-1	62	378	24	276	78	132	II
2	51	378	32	297	49	168	II
3	51	366	28	287	51	158	II
4	55	224	12	154	58	100	N
III-1	26	600	22	553	25	119	II^2
2	19	582	18	513	51	85	II^2

* As shown in Fig. 28-14.

Note: N, normal lipoprotein patterns; II^2, homozygote; other abbreviations as in Table 28-3.

diet most of his life, the xanthomas progressed until he was about 20, when they remained stable in size. At age 17 he developed angina; at age 22, acute pulmonary edema occurred without definitive evidence of a myocardial infarction, but calcification of the left anterior descending coronary artery was visible on roentgenogram. He later had a definite myocardial infarction and several other episodes of severe chest pain.

When seen at the Clinical Center in Bethesda for the first time at age 24, he had bruits over many major vessels and a cardiac murmur compatible with aortic stenosis. He was placed on a low-cholesterol diet in which the fats had a high P/S ratio (2.0), and was given cholestyramine, which was gradually increased to a dose of 48 gm per day. On this regimen the patient had no weight loss or sign of malabsorption and his cholesterol level was maintained between 300 and 350 mg per 100 ml for 2 years. During this time he was admitted twice to the intensive coronary care unit with chest pain. The large xanthomas did not decrease obviously in size, but their yellow color decreased and several small tuberous lesions melted away. L.Fl. died suddenly while at home at age 27. Autopsy revealed left ventricular hypertrophy and several old areas of infarction. Severe coronary atherosclerosis was present, with involvement of the aortic valve and extensive atherosclerosis of both the upper and lower aortas and the cerebral vessels (Fig. 28-20). The other findings, save for the xanthomas, were unremarkable.

His younger sister, age 19 (III-2 in Fig. 28-14), has had xanthomas since age 2, when she was found to have a cholesterol level above 600 mg. Although her lesions are not as large as her brother's, they also cover the extensor surfaces of the hands, the elbows, knees, and ankles. She has been on a low-cholesterol diet for many years. The mother and father both were found to have hypercholesterolemia 20 years ago. A paternal uncle of the proband died at age 20 of a heart attack. The paternal grandmother had diabetes, and both paternal grandparents died of heart disease. The occurrence of hyperlipoproteinemia and xanthomas in the Fl. family is shown in Fig. 28-14 and Table 28-9.

Plasma Lipids and Lipoproteins

LDL

Type II hyperlipoproteinemia is defined as an increase in LDL (Table 28-4). Typical patterns obtained in the analytic ultracentrifuge and by electrophoresis combined with preparative ultracentrifugation are shown in Figs. 28-1 and 28-12. The mean lipoprotein concentrations in the two phenotypes, defined according to the major criteria listed above, are shown in Table 28-10. The arbitrary cut-off limits selected to establish abnormal LDL, and hence the Type II pattern, are shown in Table 28-3.

As will be seen below, these limits appear to have been felicitous choices, for the ratio between normal subjects and heterozygotes is almost exactly 1 : 1. The separation of normal persons from heterozygotes by LDL concentrations is as apparent in the first decade as it is later [307]. It is clear, however, from the distribution of LDL values obtained in heterozygotes and normal relatives (Fig. 28-15) that a zone of uncertainty exists between LDL cholesterol concentrations of about 150 to 210 mg per 100 ml. Some "false positives" undoubtedly lie above this arbitrary limit of 170, and some "false negatives" below it. From the data in Fig. 28-15 we infer that an LDL cholesterol level of 150 mg per 100 ml would provide a better screen for more complete detection of *possible* abnormal levels in subjects under 30 years old. For older subjects, correction of LDL values is necessary because a sharp rise in LDL concentrations occurs around age 30 in normal subjects (Table 28-3).

The mean LDL concentration in homozygotes is roughly

Table 28-10. PLASMA LIPIDS AND LIPOPROTEINS IN TYPE II HYPERLIPOPROTEINEMIA

Age, yr	No. of patients	Cholesterol, mg/100 ml (mean ±1 s.d.)				Triglyceride plasma, mg/100 ml
		Plasma	VLDL	LDL	HDL	
Heterozygotes:						
1–19	117	310 ± 66	16 ± 8	249 ± 61	44 ± 12	83 ± 54
20–29	32	351 ± 87	15 ± 8	299 ± 91	40 ± 7	109 ± 41
30–39	38	371 ± 73	26 ± 13	298 ± 73	44 ± 14	126 ± 60
40–49	43	384 ± 85	28 ± 17	313 ± 84	43 ± 11	146 ± 98
50–59	19	434 ± 81	29 ± 15	354 ± 83	55 ± 17	141 ± 60
60+	13	433 ± 95	38 ± 29	341 ± 92	43 ± 17	173 ± 117
Homozygotes:						
1–19	10	678 ± 170	19 ± 8	625 ± 160	34 ± 10	101 ± 51

Note: Normal values for comparison are shown in Tables 28-2 and 28-3. Concentrations are expressed as means ±1 s.d. All values were obtained under the conditions described in the text for index samples. Except for the age group 1–19 years, the patients represent only a fraction of the total number of patients with Type II referred to in Table 28-1. Approximately equal numbers of males and females comprise the sample in each age group. Abbreviations as in Table 28-3.

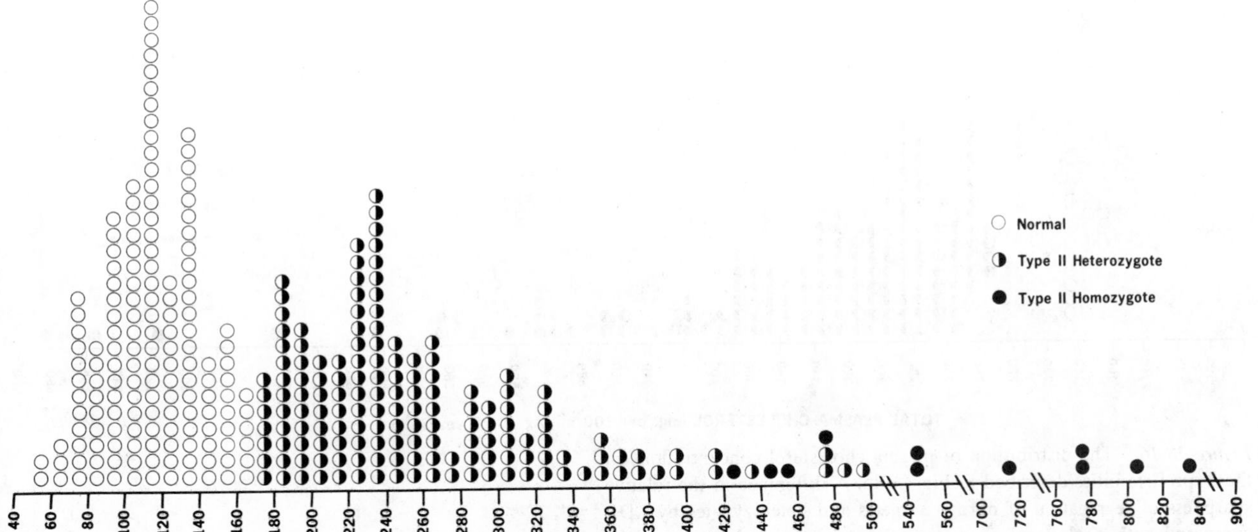

Figure 28-15. The distribution of plasma LDL concentrations in first-degree relatives of many kindreds affected with Type II hyperlipoproteinemia. The phenotypic designations are those described in the text. The cut-off limits for LDL given in Table 28-3 are the same up to age 29, and no age correction was made. The sample includes 151 subjects classified as normal, 154 heterozygotes, and 11 subjects considered homozygotes. Of the total, 117 patients were under 20 years of age and are reported separately by Kwiterovich et al. [307].

twice the mean of heterozygotes (Table 28-10 and Fig. 28-15), but variation is great between homozygotes in different kindreds.

Cholesterol

Most analyses of Type II kindreds have used cholesterol as the discriminant. It is somewhat less precise than LDL, even in younger patients (Figs. 28-15 and 28-16). We have found that 13 percent of heterozygotes of all ages who were defined by LDL have cholesterol concentrations within the upper 5 percent limits of normal (Table 28-2). Cholesterol is most reliable in subjects who have no accompanying increase in glycerides or very low density lipoproteins. The distribution of cholesterol levels in subjects under age 30 from many Type II kindreds is shown in Fig. 28-16. Discordance between plasma cholesterol and LDL levels is more common in subjects over age 30. From comparison of cholesterol and LDL concentrations, we have found that in order to "capture" all North American subjects with LDL concentrations above the upper 5 percent limit, one must be suspicious of a cholesterol concentration greater than 220 mg per 100 ml in subjects under age 30, 240 in subjects age 30 to 40, and 250 in subjects ages 40 to 50. Other workers have used the upper 1 percent of normal levels [290], or cholesterol concentrations between 280 and 325 mg per 100 ml in American or Western European adults [176, 278, 284, 295, 308, 309].

It is apparent that limits set for some cultures do not apply to others. Cut-off points used in North America, for example, are probably too high to detect heterozygotes among Japanese [299, 114] and are possibly too low for Finns [293, 310]. Khachadurian's studies of Lebanese families, including many homozygotes, have emphasized the differences in absolute cholesterol concentrations induced by cultural (mainly dietary) differences within the same country [287, 304]. Cholesterol and LDL are under polygenic influences, and an undetermined number of factors introduce intrakindred and interkindred variation in cholesterol or LDL concentrations in the abnormal phenotypes and their relatives. The criteria suggested for definition of Type II homozygotes take this into account.

Very Low Density Lipoproteins and Triglycerides

The virtue of defining Type II as hyperbetalipoproteinemia becomes especially apparent when plasma glycerides are also considered. Increased amounts of both triglycerides and VLDL occur in patients with Type II. This was recorded in ultracentrifugal studies some years ago [49, 60] and was emphasized in a revision of the Bethesda Clinical Center typing system in 1967 [65]. The possibility has not been excluded that increases in VLDL in addition to LDL may

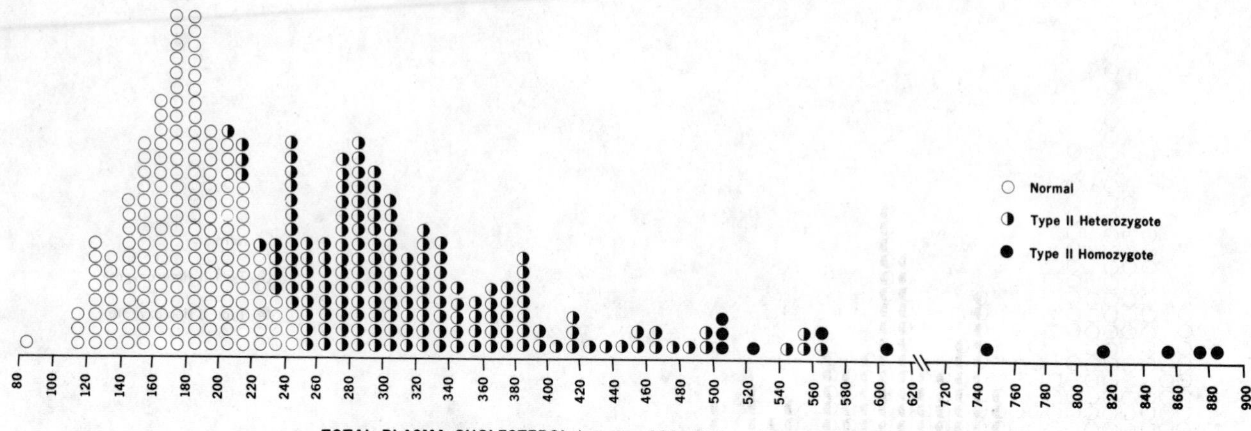

Figure 28-16. The distribution of plasma cholesterol concentrations in the Type II families described in Fig. 28-15. A difference in the relative sharpness of segregation of normal subjects and heterozygotes by LDL compared with cholesterol measurements can be seen by comparison with Fig. 28-15.

someday be discovered to indicate the presence of mutant alleles other than the gene(s) for familial Type II. At present, however, the patterns II*a* and II*b,* defined in Table 28-4, do not indicate different diseases.

The mean VLDL and triglyceride concentrations in a large sample of Type II heterozygotes are almost twice those in normal subjects (Table 28-10). The range extends from the low-normal to triglyceride values as high as the 600 to 900 mg per 100 ml that have been repeatedly observed in two heterozygotes among over 600 examined. Normal and abnormal VLDL concentrations have been observed by us in different relatives heterozygous for Type II in no less than in 79 kindreds. Discordance occurs in the same or in different generations. An increased amount of VLDL has been present in 12 percent of Type II heterozygotes under the age of 19. Some of the affected parents had normal VLDL levels. VLDL and triglyceride levels do not tend to be higher in homozygotes and often are normal.

Similar discordance between triglycerides in members of Danish families with Type II were observed by Jensen, Blankenhorn, and Kornerup [295], who also found no correlation between glycerides and the vascular manifestations of Type II. Nevin and Slack [176], who separated hypercholesterolemic kindreds into a group having normal glycerides (Type II) and a mixed group having glyceride elevations (possibly including Types II, III, and IV), also observed that the glyceride concentrations do not appear to provide good discrimination among different kindreds with possible Type II.

Other Lipids and Lipoproteins

The total concentration of phospholipids is usually increased in Type II [45], but to a lesser extent than that of cholesterol, in keeping with the distribution of the two lipids in LDL. No abnormalities within the phospholipid classes in the plasma [290] or their fatty acid components [311] have been detected. No remarkable changes in fatty acid composition of other plasma lipids have been observed [311].

It was reported by Gofman et al. [49] that HDL concentrations are decreased in Type II. This observation is borne out in the series of Fredrickson and Levy (Table 28-10), although the decrease in HDL is not as great. Chylomicrons are not present in the fasting state in Type II.

Age at Onset

Kwiterovich, Levy, and Fredrickson [307] have found that 7 of 15 offspring having one parent heterozygous for Type II had cord blood LDL concentrations more than 2 s.d. higher than the mean of controls (Table 28-11). One apparent false negative and possibly one false positive were observed in later follow-up [307]. This confirms and extends earlier indications that Type II heterozygotes can be detected at birth [312, 313] but that one may have to wait until the first year to be certain of the diagnosis [312, 314]. Possibly, expression might very rarely be delayed longer [315, 316]. As it does later in life, cord blood concentration of LDL provides a better discriminant of Type II than does the cholesterol concentration [307].

Xanthomatosis

The occurrence of xanthomas in familial Type II is a function of age and phenotype. The major determinants are severity and duration of the elevation in LDL, but local

Table 28-11. PLASMA LIPID AND LIPOPROTEIN CONCENTRATIONS IN CORD BLOODS FROM CHILDREN OF HETEROZYGOTES AND CONTROLS

	Cholesterol, mg/100 ml (mean ±1 s.d.)				Triglyceride plasma, mg/100 ml
	Plasma	VLDL	LDL	HDL	
Controls	74 ± 11 (36)	6 ± 4 (36)	31 ± 6 (36)	37 ± 8 (36)	37 ± 15 (36)
"Positives"*	104 ± 14 (7)	6 ± 3 (6)	65 ± 14 (6)	32 ± 4 (7)	37 ± 14 (7)
P	<0.001	NS	<0.001	NS	NS
"Negatives"*	72 ± 15 (8)	8 ± 3 (6)	28 ± 14 (6)	30 ± 11 (8)	40 ± 22 (8)
P	NS	NS	NS	NS	NS

* Cord bloods from children having one parent heterozygous for type II. "Positives" were defined by an LDL concentration greater than 2 s.d. above the mean in the controls [307].
Note: Numerals in parentheses indicate number of subjects studied. NS, not significantly different from controls.

factors, including motion [317] and other unknown influences, also dictate differences in the rate and location of tissue lipid deposition. The panoply of lesions seen in Type II is illustrated in Figs. 28-17 and 28-18. There are some differences in the kinds of xanthomas that occur in the homozygote (Fig. 28-18) and the heterozygote (Fig. 28-17). Both phenotypes may have palpebral xanthomas (xanthelasma), tendon xanthomas (especially in the Achilles tendons and the extensor tendons of the hand), and tuberous xanthomas, especially over the elbows. Both phenotypes also may have subperiosteal xanthomas, commonly below the knee and over the olecranon process. Soft, elevated orange-yellow planar lesions lying superficially in the skin over the extremities, buttocks, and hands are common in homozygotes and rare in the heterozygote.

A summation of the frequency of all xanthomas in heterozygotes of two age groups is shown in Table 28-12. The presence of tendon xanthomas in more than half of adults is consonant with other reports [41, 60, 281, 290]. As many as 80 percent of patients may have xanthomas before death [281]. There is a long lag period in heterozygotes before xanthomas usually appear. Only 3 of 117 heterozygotes between birth and 20 years of age who were examined by us had xanthomas [307].

The xanthomas in homozygotes are often very severe and are sometimes present at birth [287]. Occasionally, planar lesions on the palms may be confused with those considered otherwise typical for Type III. Many striking examples of xanthomatosis in those who are definitely or probably homozygotes are present in the recent literature [287, 291, 293, 296, 298–300, 304, 318–324], in addition to others cited in the earlier edition of this book [45].

The authors are aware of only one patient with tendon xanthomas and apparently *primary* Type II hyperlipoproteinemia in which familial involvement was clearly excluded, i.e., both parents were shown to be free of Type II. It is for this reason that the presence of typical xanthomas (not including xanthelasma) with primary Type II has been offered as a criterion for familial involvement if relatives are unavailable for testing. Tendon and tuberous xanthomas also accompany Type II hyperlipoproteinemia that is *secondary* to obstructive liver disease. They rarely may occur in the hyperlipoproteinemia associated with dysglobulinemia [325] and possibly with long-standing myxedema.

Xanthomas without Hyperlipidemia

There are also patients with familial tendon xanthomas without hyperlipoproteinemia [326–330]. Some of these also have intracerebral xanthomatosis and "cerebrotendinous xanthomatosis" [326, 327, 329, 330], a disorder unrelated to familial Type II. It now appears that the storage of cholestanol is a biochemical feature of this disease [327, 330] (see Chap. 36).

Table 28-12. CLINICAL FEATURES IN A SAMPLE OF PATIENTS WITH FAMILIAL TYPE II HYPERLIPOPROTEINEMIA

Age, yr	Ischemic heart disease	Claudication	Hypertension	Xanthelasma	*Xanthomas*			Arcus corneae	Hepato-splenomegaly	Hyper-uricemia
					Tendon	Tuberous	Planar			
Heterozygotes:										
1–29	4/135	0/133	0/118	1/129	8/130	4/129	0/130	5/40	0/127	1/45
>30	15/45	3/30	5/24	8/33	23/37	14/33	1/34	12/26	0/28	2/31
Homozygote:										
1–19	8/10	0/8	0/10	0/6	6/10	4/10	9/10	3/10	0/10	0/7

Note: Clinical data for adults among Type II patients shown in Fig. 28-1 are incomplete; the above represents only a small, nonrandom sample.

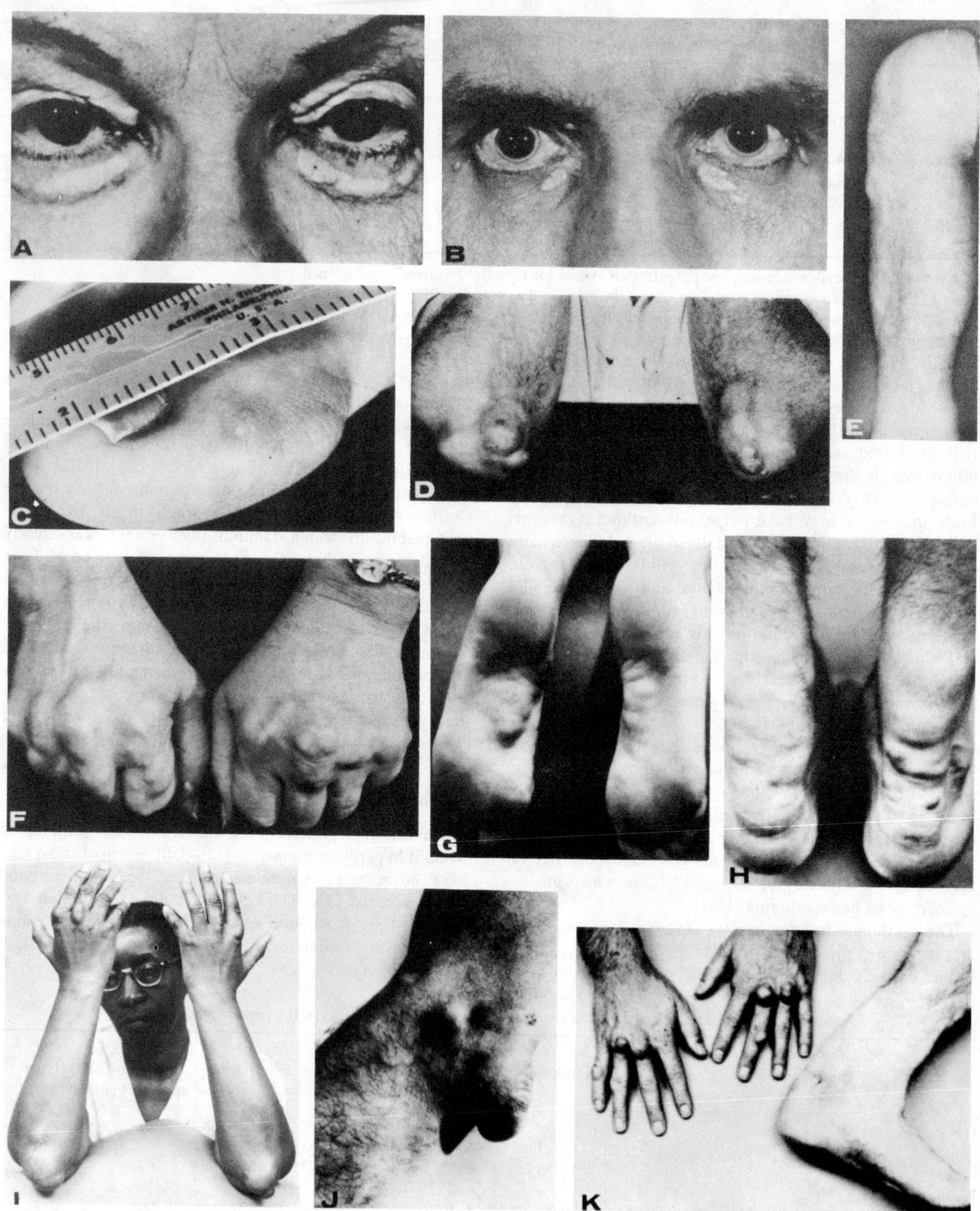

Figure 28-17. Forms of xanthomas and other lipid deposition frequently seen in patients heterozygous for Type II hyperlipoproteinemia. A, xanthelasma; B, arcus corneae and xanthelasma; E, subperiosteal xanthoma over the tibial tuberosity; I and J, fairly pure tuberous xanthomas; others are tendon or a combination of tendon and tuberous xanthomas.

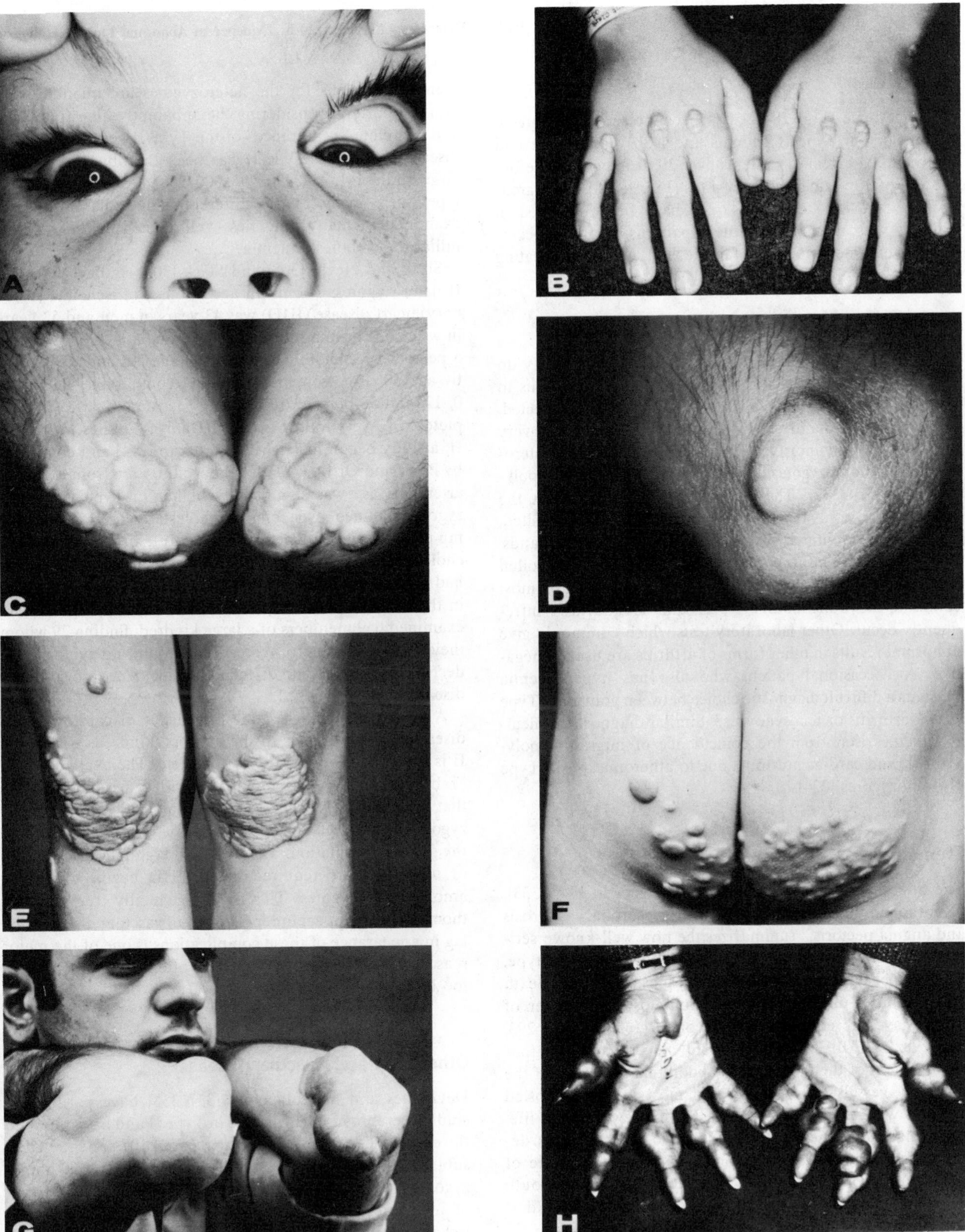

Figure 28-18. Xanthomas frequently seen in patients homozygous for Type II hyperlipoproteinemia. A, arcus corneae (appears earlier, but is otherwise similar to that seen in heterozygotes); B, C, E, and F, cutaneous "planar" xanthomas, usually having a bright-orange hue; D and G, tuberous xanthomas on the elbows; H, tendon and tuberous lesions on the hands. (*H reproduced through the courtesy of Dr. A. Khachadurian, American University, Beirut.*)

Arcus Corneae

Arcus corneae (Fig. 28-17) has been present in about 10 percent of our Type II patients under 30 years of age and in about 50 percent of patients over 30. It may occur before the age of 10 years in homozygotes (Fig. 28-18). Both arcus corneae and xanthelasma [49, 56] have been observed in patients with normal lipoprotein patterns. Such an occurrence sometimes appears in families in a manner indicating genetic determination.

Polyarthritis

There are few complications of xanthomas. Very rarely do osteolytic lesions appear beneath those lying contiguous to bone [331], and mobility of joints is almost never affected. One associated manifestation, however, is sometimes very troublesome. A minority of Type II patients, either heterozygotes or homozygotes, have recurrent attacks of "polyarthritis" [324, 332]. These most commonly occur in the ankles, usually only those in which xanthomas are deposited. They also frequently involve the knees, and rarely the hands. The joints are painful, hot, and tender, and may be swollen and inflamed. The attacks last a few days and are most common in young adults. Fever and leukocytosis infrequently occur. Other laboratory tests which commonly give abnormal results in other forms of arthritis are usually negative. An occasional patient who also has hyperuricemia presents a difficult diagnostic choice between gout and "Type II polyarthritis or tenosynovitis." Similar diagnostic difficulties have arisen from the coincidence of migratory polyarthritis and cardiac murmurs due to atheromatosis in Type II homozygotes [324].

Premature Vascular Disease

The title of a review by Cook and colleagues in 1947 [333], "Xanthoma tuberosum, aortic stenosis, coronary sclerosis and angina pectoris," summarizes the now well-known serious complications of the Type II homozygous phenotype. Their paper described 14 earlier examples of vascular death and disability in youth from atheromatosis; a number of others have subsequently been reported [163, 284, 287, 293, 296, 298, 299, 310, 321, 323, 334–336]. Severe atheromatous involvement of the thoracic and abdominal aorta and of the coronary vessels has been seen in most of the autopsied patients who have died, some in the first few years of life. Deformation of the aortic valve due to atheromatous deposits frequently leads to aortic stenosis. We are aware of one death from myocardial infarction in a white South African homozygous child 18 months of age. The oldest homozygote in our series was L.Fl., whose death at age 27 following his third myocardial infarction was described above. Probably very few homozygotes reach the fourth decade of life.

As serious as are these complications in the homozygote, their implications for the heterozygtoes are quantitatively more important, considering the apparently high frequency and complete "penetrance" of the Type II gene(s). Vascular disease in familial Type II has been the object of several large studies [41, 284, 290, 295, 300, 309], in which the phenotypes were fairly clearly differentiated. It has also been examined in many other less-well-defined studies of "familial hypercholesterolemia."

Slack and Nevin [308] and Slack [309] studied 104 Type II heterozygotes. The mean age at onset of ischemic (coronary) heart disease (IHD) was 43 years in men and 53 years in women. For men the chance of a first attack of IHD was 5 percent by age 30; 51 percent by age 50; and 85 percent by age 60. For women the risks at comparable ages were 0, 12, and 58 percent, respectively. Jensen et al. [295] completed a 20-year follow-up of 11 Danish families with Type II, a study begun in 1944 by Kornerup [274] and continued by Piper and Orrild [281]. The morbidity rate from coronary artery disease was significantly higher in Type II heterozygotes (defined by a plasma cholesterol level above 350 mg per 100 ml in subjects over age 15) than in their normocholesterolemic relatives. Over 32 percent of 181 patients had IHD, compared with a prevalence of only 1.3 percent in their normal relatives. Harlan, Graham, and Estes [290] examined 659 members of a large kindred, finding 79 whom they considered heterozygotes. They found no evidence for decreased longevity or of increased incidence of coronary disease in their kindred.

A large-scale survey of the prevalence of cardiovascular disease and xanthomas in the authors' kindreds with Type II is under way but is not yet complete. The available data (Table 28-12) are in accord with the widely accepted opinion that premature IHD occurs in both male and female heterozygotes at a much higher rate than would be expected in the general population. The data also highlight the 20 years or more that are required before IHD begins to appear among heterozygotes. This is also generally true for xanthomas, which appear independently of vascular disease. The lag in appearance of these complications is one of the major reasons why treatment of Type II is often begun many years too late.

Other Forms of Vascular Disease

DeGennes and his colleagues [337, 338] have particularly studied cerebrovascular disease in Type II and have reported the occurrence of strokes in 29 percent of 107 patients. Their subjects appear to include both heterozygotes and homozygotes. These investigators believe that nearly 70 percent of all subjects may have had small strokes or transient ischemic episodes. Although cerebrovascular disease has been observed in other series of Type II patients, the recorded incidence has not been as high; and in our patients IHD has been more common than overt cerebrovascular disease.

Peripheral vascular disease is, in our experience, also less prevalent than ischemic heart disease and is more typical of Type III hyperlipoproteinemia than of Type II. Obstructive lesions in vessels of the lower extremities and intermittent claudication, however, are not rare in Type II.

Other Abnormalities

CARBOHYDRATE INTOLERANCE. Most studies of Type II have agreed that the incidence of diabetes is not abnormal [41, 42, 290, 339]. Glueck, Levy, and Fredrickson [339] found that 33 percent of familial Type II heterozygotes had abnormal response to oral glucose tolerance tests using several standard criteria. This frequency was not significantly higher than that found in controls without hyperlipoproteinemia (28 percent), but was lower than the prevalence of glucose intolerance in patients with Types III, IV, or V hyperlipoproteinemia. Sixty-six percent of the Type II heterozygotes had normal insulin responses to glucose loading; 26 percent were judged to have low responses, and 8 percent to have hyperactive ones. Normal glucose tolerance and responses of FFA to glucose loads were also found in their Type II kindred by Harlan et al. [290].

HYPERURICEMIA. Jensen, Blankenhorn, and Kornerup have reviewed the evidence suggesting some association between gout and hypercholesterolemia [340]. They found no evidence of unusual hyperuricemia in 98 members of the Danish Type II kindreds mentioned earlier. This is in accord with our experience (Table 28-12) and that of Harlan et al. [290]. There is thus no evidence of a linkage between gout and familial Type II.

OTHER TESTS. The only other common laboratory test that usually gives abnormal results in severe familial Type II is the sedimentation rate; it is elevated, apparently because of the augmentation of LDL [341].

Phenocopies of Familial Type II

Familial Type II has many imitators, requiring stringent application of the major criteria for diagnosis stated above. There is at least one other familial disease in which the Type II pattern can occur in close relatives. This is porphyria [342]. Another potential cause is myxedematous familial goiter (Chap. 10). Other diseases causing secondary Type II and xanthomas are hepatic obstruction, dysglobulinemia (including possibly the autoimmune hyperlipoproteinemia described by Beaumont [325]), and (nonfamilial) myxedema. "Primary," but presumably nongenetic, Type II can occur in individuals or in families where the diet is unusually high in cholesterol and saturated fats. In our experience the LDL in the latter patients always falls to well within normal limits on a restricted diet. The response of patients with familial Type II is qualitatively similar, but far less dramatic. Except for a few very young heterozygotes, diet changes alone do not return LDL levels to unequivocally normal levels.

The Possible Defect in Familial Type II

The biochemical defect in familial Type II has not been discovered. It is quite possible that there is more than one defect and that different mutants cause the same apparent abnormalities. Basically, one must consider two major possibilities, overproduction or defective catabolism of LDL, and either of these may be derived from abnormal metabolism of the lipoprotein complex or of one of its components.

Chemical Components of LDL

The composition of LDL is described in Chap. 26. The three major components are cholesterol and cholesteryl esters, phospholipids, and the apolipoprotein(s). The subclass of LDL that is primarily elevated in familial Type II is the discrete one having an S_f of 0 to 12 and lying in the narrow density range of 1.019 to 1.063. These lipoproteins apparently have a single apolipoprotein, apoLDL-ser, although it may be an aggregate of more than one polypeptide. There are also almost always traces of other HDL and VLDL apolipoproteins present in any preparation of LDL, the degree of contamination being greater in the LDL subclass of S_f 12 to 20 [343].

The apoLDL-ser of a number of patients with familial Type II has been partially examined. No obvious abnormalities in total amino acid composition, conformation as judged by optical studies, or immunochemical behavior have been found [344]. ApoLDL-ser is a glycoprotein containing appreciable amounts of mannose, galactosamine, glucosamine, and neuraminic acid [345]. The glycoside moieties in normal and Type II LDL have not been compared. There remain possibilities of undiscovered abnormalities in the covalent structure of the LDL apoprotein in this disorder.

The lipids in LDL include small amounts of glycerides, glycolipids, carotenoids, and other trace components. At least 80 percent of the total consists of cholesterol and phospholipids. Although these lipid classes are also present in other lipoproteins, it is possible that a metabolic error affecting either could be reflected almost exclusively in LDL. This is especially true for cholesterol because much of the "physiologic" variation in plasma cholesterol concentration in man is rather selectively confined to variations in LDL concentrations. The plasma sterol that is increased in amount in "essential hypercholesterolemia" was shown by Schönheimer to be cholesterol [346]; this has been established by chemical analyses in a few other patients. Furthermore, no abnormality in composition of cholesteryl esters or of phospholipids in Type II has been discovered. We have also observed in our Type II patients a persistently normal proportion of cholesterol to protein in LDL, over a wide range of LDL concentrations as altered by diet [77].

Cholesterol Metabolism

Readers are referred to recent reviews [347–349] of this subject; no specific biochemical defect in cholesterol metabolism per se has yet been established in Type II. Overproduction of cholesterol, reflected in a lack of feedback control by fed sterol, has been suggested by Khachadurian [350]. His interesting in vivo experiments did not include sufficient control data to permit a firm conclusion about this possibility. The incorporation of labeled precursors into plasma cholesterol in patients has been found normal by some investigators [351, 352] and possibly abnormal by others [353].

The plasma turnover of labeled cholesterol has been measured in Type II patients by many investigators [294, 348, 354–359]. Such experiments now are usually analyzed on the basis of a two-compartment model [356]. The total exchangeable pool is increased in Type II patients with xanthomatosis; the rapidly exchangeable pool, of which the plasma cholesterol is a relatively small part, is not remarkably different from normal. The calculated rates of exchange between the two pools and the overall rates of input and removal from the total exchangeable mass do not appear to be abnormal in Type II. As Nestel, Whyte, and Goodman [357] were the first to point out, however, there is evidence that there is some impediment to the clearance or excretion of cholesterol from the plasma compartment.

It has been suggested that there may be defective conversion of cholesterol to bile acids [360]. A marked difference in the pattern of bile acid excretion between Type II patients and other hyperlipidemic patients was described by Kottke [361], but the Type II pattern was not necessarily abnormal. Grundy and Ahrens [348] did not find a definite abnormality in overall sterol balance in Type II patients studied in the steady state. In Type II there is a marked increase in bile acid turnover after cholestyramine treatment, even when the plasma cholesterol concentration does not change [358].

LDL Metabolism

Turnover studies of LDL labeled in the protein moiety have been made in normal subjects and in Type II patients [362–369] (Fig. 28-19). The experiments of Langer, Strober, and Levy [367] have included more than 30 subjects, most of them studied at two different plasma concentrations, before and upon treatment. They conclude that the intravascular-extravascular partition of labeled LDL is not different in Type II, nor is the calculated synthetic rate (60 mg LDL per kg body weight per day). The mean fractional catabolic rate (FCR) of the intravenous LDL pool in untreated Type II was 0.24, significantly lower than the mean of 0.46 in normal persons (Fig. 28-19). The mean biologic half-life of LDL was 4.7 days in Type II and 3.1 days in the normal subjects. The same abnormalities existed in Type II whether tracer amounts of labeled LDL from patients or from normal subjects were infused. In these studies it

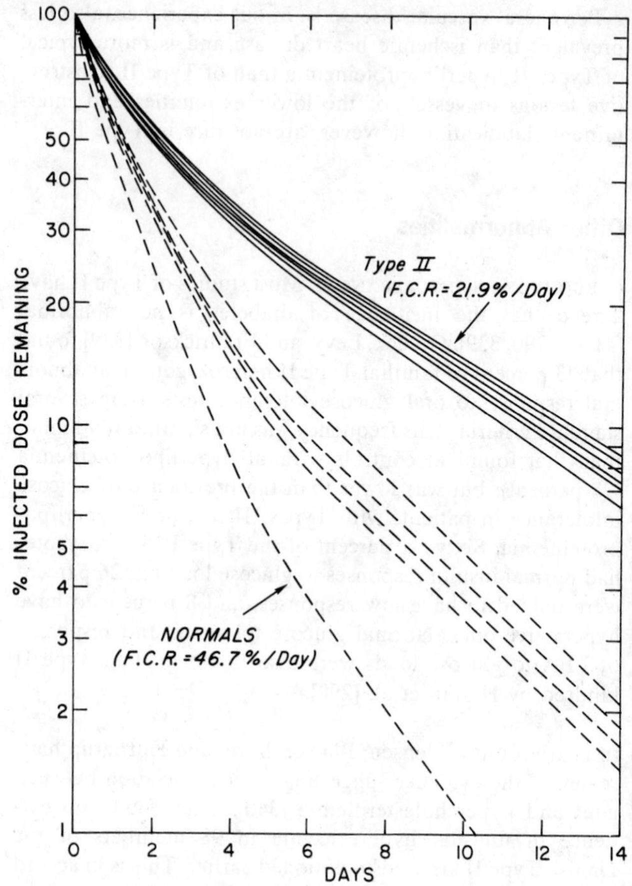

Fig. 28-19. Disappearance of ^{125}I-labeled LDL (protein) after intravenous injection in normal subjects and patients with familial Type II hyperlipoproteinemia. F.C.R., fractional catabolic rate of plasma LDL pool. (*Data from Langer et al.* [367].)

was found that the FCR of plasma LDL in normal subjects is an inverse function of pool size. When the expanded pool in Type II patients was decreased by lowering the LDL synthetic rate with nicotinic acid, however, the FCR remained abnormally low in Type II patients [370].

Scott and Hurley [366], using similar studies with protein-labeled LDL, have concluded that some hypercholesterolemic subjects may have increased synthesis rather than a decreased rate of catabolism of LDL. Their patients react differently from ours to treatment [305] and may have an unusual variant of Type II.

A Defect in LDL Catabolism

The data of Langer et al. [367] are among the most convincing evidence that the defect in some or all patients with familial Type II is a rate limitation in LDL catabolism. They are necessarily based on kinetic measurements in the steady state, require independent corroboration, and do not pinpoint the site or mechanism of such a defect. Although LDL cholesterol is degraded mainly in the liver, nothing is known about the normal removal or destruction of the LDL complex. No clear-cut evidence has been obtained showing that the protein moiety enters hepatic cells.

A most intriguing question concerning Type II is the manner in which apparently a double dose of the abnormal allele leads to almost precisely twice the limitation in catabolic rate induced by one abnormal allele. Enzyme-regulated catabolism rarely operates normally at maximum capacity, and heterozygotes for mutant enzymes often have decreased activity without evidence of net catabolic deficiency. It is possible that a nonenzymatic protein governing a site of catabolism of LDL is affected by the mutant. More information is awaited.

Pathophysiology

Whatever may be the cause or causes, hyperbetalipoproteinemia exists throughout the life of an untreated patient with familial Type II. In utero and at each of the usual changes in LDL concentrations—the abrupt rise after birth and the steeper rise at maturity—the Type II patient responds in a mode simulating the normal. But levels in the heterozygote are about twice that in his normal counterpart, and the homozygote has levels that are two or three times higher than his heterozygous sib. The xanthomatosis and premature atherogenesis associated with these differences in LDL concentrations are almost certainly caused by the hyperlipoproteinemia.

It is not appropriate to dwell here at length on the pathology of atherosclerosis per se and the valid objections to acceptance of this disease as being due solely to hypercholesterolemia. But that acceleration of this process is related to the plasma LDL level may be more dramatically demonstrated in familial Type II than in any other "natural experiment" in which man is the subject. Final proof of this rests on collection of adequate control data from normolipidemic relatives of Type II patients. It is still only an inadequately controlled impression that these relatives have no more proclivity toward premature vascular disease than normolipidemic nonrelatives in the same cultural group.

Xanthoma Formation

Histologically, the xanthomas in Type II are fairly simple lesions [371]. Lipids accumulate in the dermis in large macrophages and also lie free in the interstitial spaces where cholesterol clefts are frequently seen in cut sections. Sometimes a few giant cells are present, but inflammatory reaction is usually minor. Deposition of Sudan-positive lipid has also been reported in foam cells or extracellularly in lymph nodes or spleen [293, 299] or in the kidney, thymus, lungs, and Virchow-Robin's space in the brain [299] of homozygous children with plasma cholesterol levels exceeding 1,000 mg per 100 ml. Such tissue involvement is very rarely seen, if at all, in heterozygotes.

The evolution of cutaneous xanthomas, like the eruptive ones associated with hyperglyceridemia, has been subjected to better serial studies [261] than has the evolution of the deeper xanthomas more common to Type II. The accumulated lipids in tendinous and tuberous lesions include phospholipids, cholesterol, cholesteryl esters, and variable amounts of triglycerides [261, 317, 372–375]. There is evidence that cholesterol becomes esterified in xanthomas and that transesterification of fatty acids occurs in several of the lipid classes [261]. The net result is an increased content of 18:1 acids and a decline in more polyunsaturated ones. Tagged LDL protein appears in xanthomas [317]. Lipid accumulation occurs primarily because of increased circulating LDL concentrations, but there are local factors, such as friction and movement, that determine the sites of xanthoma formation.

Arcus Corneae

The net sum of studies on arcus corneae [376] indicates that the cornea so involved contains increased amounts of phospholipids, cholesterol, and triglycerides, and an unremarkable fatty acid composition. The increased amounts of lipids are presumably due to heightened infiltration, some of the lipids being deposited as critical concentrations are exceeded.

Atheromatosis

In heterozygotes the pathologic anatomy of the coronary [177] and cerebral [337–338] vessels does not appear different from the atherosclerosis seen in the general population and in other types of hyperlipoprotenemia. The extraordinary degree of atheroma formation in homozygotes (Fig. 28-20) has sometimes led observers to believe that a completely different disease entity is present [299]. The aorta is usually heavily studded with small or confluent yellow intimal plaques, which may contain cholesterol crystals and foam cells [293, 296, 299, 321, 324, 336]. These may fill the sinuses of Valsalva and partially occlude the orifices of the coronary arteries (Fig. 28-20). The plaques usually produce some deformation of the aortic valve cusps and lead often to aortic stenosis and sometimes to regurgitation. Similar involvement of the mitral valve occurs less commonly. The pulmonary arteries may also contain atheromas [296]. No evidence is available to support a presumption that the changes in the vessels of the homozygote represent anything other than an extreme exaggeration of the same atherosclerotic processes common to heterozygotes and other patients with ischemic heart disease. Probably the incidence of IHD in middle-aged patients with Type II is not far from that predicted from the observation that, in general, the incidence is a function (roughly the cube) of the plasma cholesterol concentration [377]. It is apparent, however, that the provocative influence of LDL concentrations on this process is not yet adequately

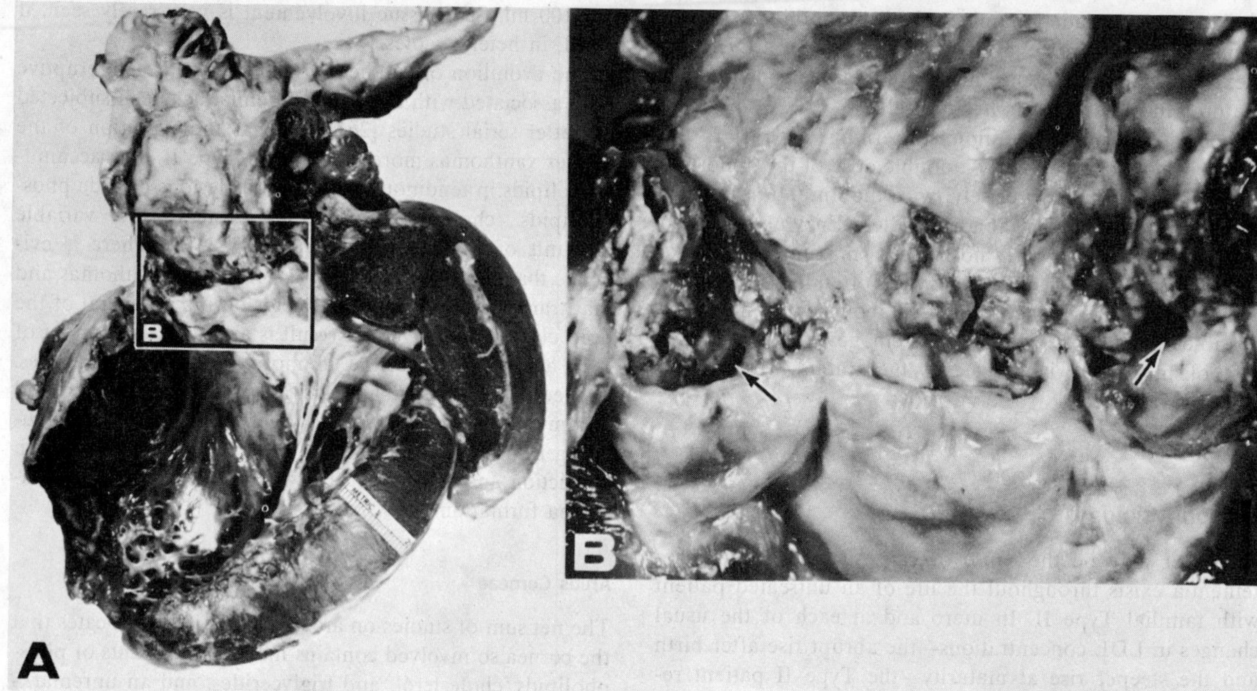

Figure 28-20. Heart of a 27-year-old patient homozygous for Type II hyperlipoproteinemia (Patient III-1 in Table 28-9). Severe atheromatous involvement of the aortic valve and ascending aorta is visible, as is narrowing of the ostiums of coronary vessels, indicated by arrows in B. (*Courtesy of Dr. W. C. Roberts, National Heart and Lung Institute.*)

explained. There may be initiatory factors that produce vascular damage by means other than the increase in concentration gradient for LDL or some of its components. Also, females with Type II retain some, but not all, of the unexplained protection that non-type II females seem to have from IHD prior to the menopause.

Familial Type II hyperlipoproteinemia is a model of great potential importance in the general public health problem of premature atherosclerosis. It is now possible to detect most heterozygotes in childhood and feasible to collect a large number of cases. In these patients, questions relative to the number and frequency of possible mutants may be determined, perhaps by using other markers showing linkages to some phenotypes and not to others. Most importantly, it may be possible to establish once and for all the effect of long-term treatment on the incidence or regression of premature IHD.

Genetics

Serious study of the genetics of Type II hyperlipoproteinemia began over 30 years ago [34, 35] and since has been the subject of many analyses [41, 60, 176, 274–278, 280–284, 286, 287, 290, 293, 300, 378]. The evolution of opinion concerning the genetic mode was reviewed earlier [45]. There is no longer much controversy over the concept that a single autosomal allele mutant for Type II confers on the bearer an almost 100 percent certainty that he will have hyperbetalipoproteinemia. It is also generally accepted that the homozygous abnormal subject will have elevations of LDL two to three times that of heterozygotes in the same family.

Nevin and Slack [176] examined 67 relatives of 16 male and 16 female index patients with "familial hypercholesterolemic xanthomatosis" (representing Type II patients selected by high cholesterol and normal glyceride levels). Thirty-seven were affected and 30 were considered normal. The Clinical Center series differs from the series of Nevin and Slack in that lipoprotein analyses have been used for definition, and hyperglyceridemic subjects with Type II have been included. The resultant cohort numbers over 800 first-degree relatives of probands in whom lipoprotein patterns have been determined (Table 28-13). The ratio of Type II to normal subjects among the first-degree relatives of propositi [379] is so close as to suggest that all the kindreds are representative of the same mutation or, at least, very similar ones as judged by the completeness of their "penetrance." The data in Table 28-13, however, are based on a phenotypic definition that *requires* demonstration of

Table 28-13. LIPOPROTEIN PATTERNS IN RELATIVES OF 175 PROPOSITI WITH TYPE II HYPERLIPOPROTEINEMIA

	N*	II	III	IV	Total
Parents	64	65	0	4	133
Siblings	126	143	0	8	277
Children	210	200	0	5	415
Total	400	408	0	17	825

* N, normal lipoprotein pattern.

familial involvement. It is more desirable that Mendelian ratios or penetrance be established in family members exclusive of not only the propositus but also the relative whose abnormal pattern established the familial nature of Type II in each kindred. Such an analysis has not been completed.

No example of Type III were found in these kindreds [77, 379], proving unequivocally the separateness of this mutant for "familial hypercholesterolemia" from the Type II mutant(s). The incidence of Type IV (VLDL increase without a rise in LDL) was 2 percent, in line with the 5 percent limits for plasma triglyceride used to define Type IV.

We have also studied eight families involving matings between two heterozygotes; these were all detected through homozygous propositi. Among the 25 progeny, 8 were normal, 5 were heterozygotes, and 12, including the propositi, were homozygotes. The number of such matings, in which parental phenotype was unequivocal, is still relatively small and does not offer a sufficient sample for confirmation of the predicted Mendelian ratios. Consanguinity has been referred to in some reports of Type II families, particularly of homozygotes. There did not appear to be any increase in consanguinity in the Clinical Center series or in the study of Nevin and Slack [176].

It has been suggested [278] that familial Type II is a trait determined by several genes. To the extent that the severity of its expression varies in different kindreds or in different members of the same kindred, this is very likely true. Distinctions between polygenic and monogenic determination also may depend on the trait in question, i.e., hyperlipoproteinemia or its associated manifestations. For all patients with familial Type II taken together, the range of abnormality in the LDL concentration is extremely great. There is also such wide variation in LDL among different "normal" subjects that the issue of multiple genic determinants will not be settled without much intensive, and longitudinal, analysis of various kindreds. Presently, the question of how many different single-mutant alleles might be responsible for apparently the same disorder is of equal interest.

If we assume that a single mutant is the cause of Type II, the gene frequency remains unknown. When the upper 1 percent of cholesterol levels is used as a discriminant [290], the gene frequency for familial Type II could be made to appear as high as 1:20 to 1:100. A preliminary report of a study by Glueck and coworkers has appeared [380] in which cholesterol level was determined in 1,660 children at birth. The parents of the 20 children with cord blood cholesterol > 100 mg per 100 ml were examined. Of the 10 complete parent pairs, at least one parent was a Type II heterozygote. These findings suggest a frequency of Type II of between 1 : 100 or 1 : 200.

It will be interesting to have such information not only in America but also in other countries, for Type II seems to be no respecter of ethnic groups or countries. It is frequent among both black and white peoples in North America. Among countries other than Britain and France, where it appears to be as common as in America, families have been reported from Sweden [381], Norway [291], Denmark [35, 113, 274, 281], Finland [293, 310], Poland [112], Czechoslovakia [292, 382], Spain [107], Germany [108, 109, 118, 383], Australia [297], New Zealand [317], Japan [299], Lebanon [287], Italy [384], and India [319, 385]. Although Type II was earlier thought to be more prevalent among Jews [279], we have observed no obvious increase in frequency among them.

No heterozygote advantage has yet been demonstrated for Type II. There is also no known linkage to other genetic traits or diseases. An interesting kindred in which all sibs affected with Type II have also had a form of amyotrophic lateral sclerosis has been reported [386]. Recent studies of the occurrence of the Lp antigen [387], or of "sinking pre-beta" anomaly, related forms of genetic polymorphism of LDL, have shown the same distribution in Type II as in normal families [97].

Treatment

The most significant advance in knowledge of familial Type II in the last 5 years is the unequivocal demonstration that treatment can effectively lower plasma cholesterol and LDL concentrations for long periods of time. If the relationship between LDL and premature vascular disease mentioned above is correct, the decrements in LDL achievable by therapy in patients with Type II theoretically should reduce their hazard no less than five-to tenfold.

The first principle of therapy is diet. Based on the work of many clinics, the presently most-used diet contains as high an amount of polyunsaturates (8 to 15 percent of total calories as linoleic acid) and as low an amount of saturates (<5 percent of calories) and cholesterol (<250 mg per day) as is practicable. Some investigators advocate lowering the cholesterol level and the intake of saturated fats without increasing intake of polyunsaturates. Polyunsaturates have been considered to have little effect in children [388], but an extensive comparison of both diets in familial Type II has not yet been made. Prepared diet instructions for patients with Type II are available from several sources [268, 389]. In our experience, the average response to the in-patient "Type II diet," after a base line obtained on the normal American diet, is a fall of 15 to 30 percent in plasma cholesterol level, all of this decrease representing cholesterol in LDL. The maximum effect of the diet takes 2 to 5 weeks. Type II heterozygotes rarely ever return to within the normal range on diet alone, and homozygotes never do.

Certain drugs produce an additive effect when combined with diet in treating familial Type II. Among those reported to have at least a short-term effect are clofibrate [115, 390], D-thyroxine [391–393], nicotinic acid [394–396], nicotinyl alcohol [397], dextran [115], and cholestyramine [301–306]. Of the two drugs with the lowest toxicity, clofibrate and cholestyramine, we have found the latter to be unquestionably superior [306, 398]. A typical therapeutic response in a Type II heterozygote is shown in Fig. 28-21. In 60 adult patients already on the "Type II diet" and followed up to 26 months, a dose of 16 to 24 gm per day of cholestyramine has produced an additional 25 to 35 percent lowering of LDL. Only a 6 percent fall was obtained with clofibrate [305]. The weight of evidence suggests that clofibrate is not very useful in familial Type II [305]; possibly it may be effective in some nonfamilial forms of Type II. Except for constipation, no significant toxicity has been obtained with one form of cholestyramine (Questran, Mead Johnson).

The results with cholestyramine in homozygotes are less predictable [304, 307, 358, 399]. Doses of up to 48 gm have been used. Usually there is some fall in level of LDL, but often there is a rebound, occasionally to pretreatment levels. Despite this, xanthomas may soften [304] and the total body cholesterol pool [358] appears to decrease. More recently, a combination of cholestyramine and nicotinic acid has been found to be more effective than one drug alone in homozygous patients. We have found homozygotes in several kindreds to be extremely sensitive to therapy that was only partially successful or not successful at all in other kindreds.

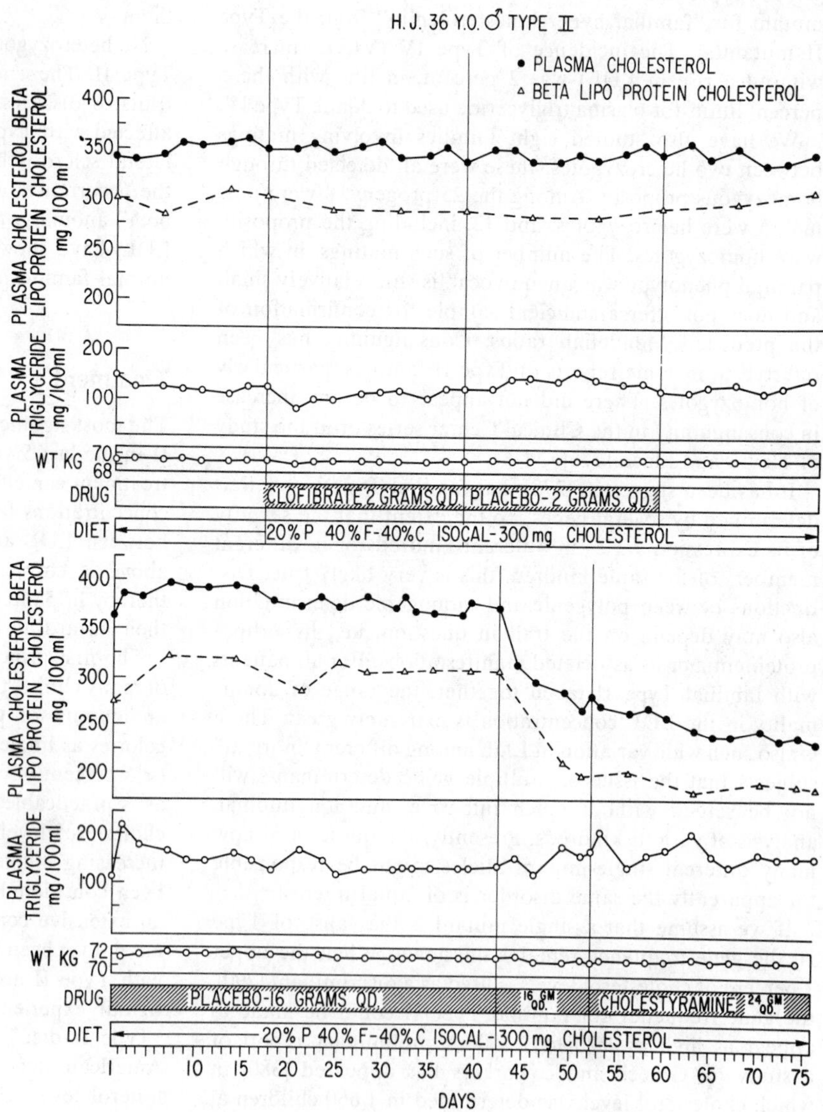

Figure 28-21. Response of a patient heterozygous for Type II hyperlipoproteinemia to clofibrate and cholestyramine while on a therapeutic diet. The clofibrate trial was performed double-blind, the cholestyramine trial was single-blind. Note the definite effect with cholestyramine, the lack of any effect with clofibrate. (*Reprinted from* [306] *through the courtesy of Post-graduate Medicine.*)

This may mean genetic heterogeneity of the responsible mutants.

The maximum effect of diet or any drug is achieved within 6 to 8 weeks. In the heterozygote there is no evidence that xanthomas will resolve unless cholesterol or LDL levels also decline; an ineffective regimen (producing less than a 15 percent reduction in cholesterol) is discontinued.

The success of bile acid sequestrants in Type II has led to trial of ileal bypass as a permanent, nonmedical means of achieving the same effect or of doing so more completely, particularly in homozygotes [298, 322, 400–403]. The largest series is that of Buchwald [401], who reported an average 39 percent reduction of cholesterol in 15 patients, some of whom appear to have had Type II. Other investigators have also observed sustained reduction [402], but with persistent steatorrhea. It presently seems unnecessary to consider ileal bypass in heterozygotes, and we believe that this form of therapy in homozygotes should be approached with considerable caution. Failure of this treatment in homozygotes has been recorded [298, 322].

Plasmapheresis [296], attempted as therapy in Type II, seems a heroic approach that is unlikely to win many advocates.

TYPE III: FAMILIAL "BROAD BETA" DISEASE

SYNONYMS. Familial Type III hyperlipoproteinemia or "floating beta" disorder; referred to in this chapter as familial Type III hyperlipoproteinemia. (Patients have also been described as having xanthoma tuberosum, idiopathic hypercholesterolemic xanthomatosis with hyperlipemia, familial hypercholesterolemic xanthomatosis with hypertriglyceridemia, or mixed hyperlipemia.)

Definition

Familial Type III hyperlipoproteinemia is an uncommon disorder characterized by the persistent presence of easily detectable amounts of plasma VLDL having abnormal composition. This VLDL should more accurately be called abnormal LDL, for it consists of LDL that contains a peculiarly high content of glycerides. The resulting lipoproteins have a density <1.006 (like normal VLDL) but also migrate in the beta region on most types of zonal electrophoresis; hence the term "floating beta." A "broad beta" band is sometimes visible on electrophoresis in paper, agarose, and cellulose acetate (Fig. 28-22). On starch-block electrophoresis the VLDL in Type III consists of two components, one of which migrates to a β position, abnormal for VLDL. The term "β-VLDL" refers to the anomalous lipoproteins found in Type III hyperlipoproteinemia. Although the Type III lipoprotein pattern may be secondary to severe insulinopenic diabetes and possibly to hypothyroidism and other diseases, it most commonly is "primary." In the kindreds of patients with the primary pattern, there may be others in one or more generations who are similarly affected. Familial Type III is rarely, if ever, seen in the first 20 years of life and is usually expressed earlier in men than in women. It is accompanied by an increased incidence of premature vascular disease. The accompanying hyperlipidemia can be eliminated by appropriate therapy, but some β-VLDL persistently remains.

History

The cholesterol and glyceride concentrations in familial Type III hyperlipoproteinemia are extremely variable and, like its accompanying cutaneous and vascular abnormalities, may overlap those seen in several other types of hyperlipoproteinemia. The present definition of the lipoprotein abnormality (β-VLDL) and the separateness of the disorder from other genetic diseases were not firmly established until 1967 [65]. For these reasons it is not possible to determine when the first example of Type III may have entered medical literature. In 1954, Gofman and coworkers [49, 55, 56] provided the first clear-cut separation by lipoprotein analyses of what they called "xanthoma tuberosum" (Type III) from "xanthoma tendinosum" (Type II). They studied 23 patients, as representatives of the former, who had xanthomas on the buttocks, extensor surfaces of the elbows and knees, the hands (especially the palmar surfaces), and the ankles. All had first noted their skin lesions in adulthood. Two of the patients were sibs, establishing a familial character to the syndrome. The lipoprotein pattern in these patients, featuring an excess of lipoproteins of S_f 12 to 20 (LDL) and of $S_f > 20$ (VLDL), and a depression of the S_f 0 to 12 class (LDL) [49], was confirmed 15 years later [76] in patients identified by the presence of β-VLDL. Borrie has recently noted [404] that several of his patients, earlier reported as having "idiopathic hypercholesterolemic xanthomatosis associated with hypertriglyceridemia" [405], are now recognized as having Type III; other probable examples are to be found in case reports in the period from 1950 to 1965 [58, 121, 123, 364, 406–410].

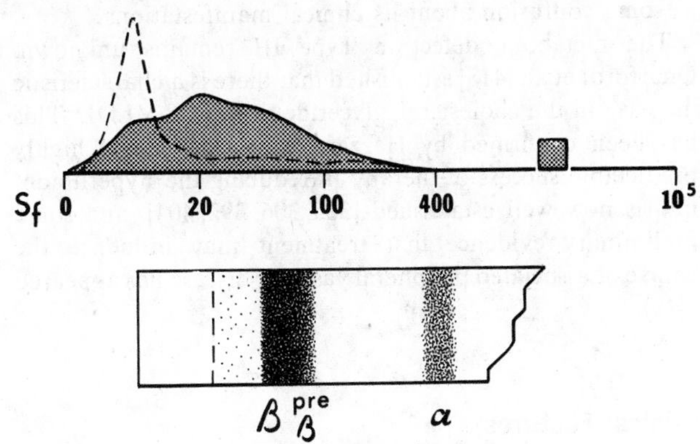

Figure 28-22. Type III hyperlipoproteinemia.

Table 28-14. PLASMA LIPIDS AND LIPOPROTEINS IN A TYPE III HYPERLIPOPROTEINEMIA KINDRED

Position in pedigree*	Age, yr	Cholesterol, mg/100 ml				Triglyceride plasma, mg/100 ml	Type
		Plasma	VLDL	LDL	HDL		
I-1	33	352	236	82	34	362	III
2	42	230	26	168	36	104	N
3	34	268	62	164	42	279	IV
4	28	199	8	142	49	39	N
5	31	660	545	81	34	828	III
II-1	5	147	1	77	69	17	N
2	7	142	14	87	41	25	N

* As shown in Fig. 28-23.
Note: N, normal lipoprotein pattern; other abbreviations as in Table 28-3.

Type III was rediscovered and clarified in the Clinical Center studies through a process of trial and error. The Type III pattern was first considered to be an increase in both β-lipoproteins (LDL) and prebetalipoproteins by electrophoresis [64]. The deficiencies in this definition, later consigned to Type II ("II*b*"), were only becoming apparent as the last edition of this book was written [45]. Consequently, several families, notably the St. kindred, were erroneously considered to have Type III and other now-apparent errors in definition were included [45]. The new definition of Type III was established in 1967 [65] according to the presence of "floating beta" (β-VLDL). At that time the description rested on 24 patients, a number which has increased to 86 patients in 68 kindreds at this writing. Much of the biochemical and genetic data on this, the largest collection of patients with Type III, has only recently been assembled [77, 379].

Many other patients in different countries have now been described as having "Type III" [94, 107–110, 112–119, 125–128, 176, 177, 297, 303, 308, 309, 366, 373, 375, 390, 392, 411–417]. Judging from the reported clinical and laboratory data, some represent Type III but the majority probably do not. Very few laboratories have checked their phenotypic assignments by determining the presence of the pathognomonic abnormal β-VLDL. As a result, there is currently considerable uncertainty about the prevalence of Type III, as well as some confusion about its clinical manifestations.

The metabolic defect in Type III remains unknown. Quarfordt et al. [418] established that there is a characteristic increase in the cholesterol/glyceride ratio in β-VLDL. This has been confirmed by Hazzard et al. [417]. The highly predictable success of therapy in reducing the hyperlipidemia is now well established [305, 306, 392, 404], and some preliminary evidence that treatment may influence the course of associated peripheral vascular disease has appeared [419].

Clinical Features

The following case summary illustrates some of the clinical features of familial Type III:

J.Tu. (I-1 in Fig. 28-23 and Table 28-14), a 44-year-old male accountant, noted the development of orange-yellow deposits in the creases of his palms and tuberous lesions on his elbows and buttocks, beginning at about age 22. These were diagnosed as xanthomas, and a fat-restricted diet was prescribed. At age 28 he had a probable myocardial infarction. At 33, intermittent claudication began in the left leg and he was evaluated at the Clinical Center in Bethesda. In milligrams per 100 ml, his cholesterol level was 370; phospholipids, 334; and triglycerides, 393. A femoral arteriogram revealed irregularity in the proximal popliteal artery on the right and complete occlusion of the comparable vessel on the left. The occluded portion of the left popliteal artery was replaced with a venous graft, and claudication disappeared.

The patient was not seen again until age 39, when he still had his xanthomas and in addition moderate claudication in both legs. The arterial pulses in both feet were absent. At this time his cholesterol level was 420 mg per 100 ml, that of triglycerides 450, and the diagnosis of Type III was established. His hyperlipidemia responded to reduction in

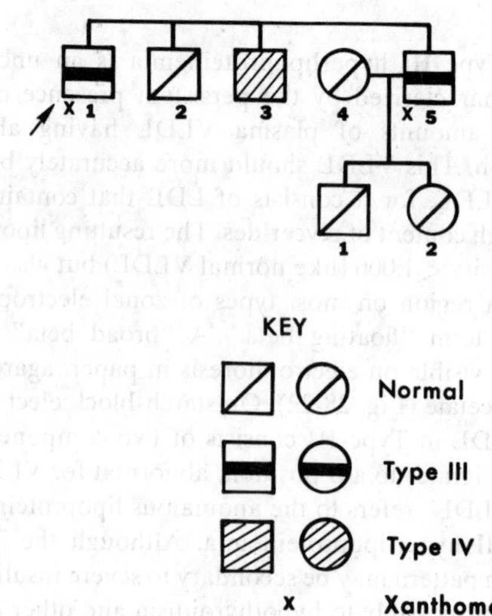

Figure 28-23. A family with Type III hyperlipoproteinemia (see Table 28-14).

body weight, maintenance of a diet moderately restricted in cholesterol, and added clofibrate, 2 gm per day (Fig. 28-29). In the ensuing 4 years, this combination therapy has lost none of its effectiveness. Even though the patient has not always followed the diet, all his xanthomas have completely disappeared. Pulses are now definitely present in the dorsalis pedis and posterior tibial arteries on the right and are weakly palpable on the left. The results of lipoprotein screening in the patient's family are shown in Fig. 28-23 and Table 28-14. His brother (I-5) had not noticed the planar xanthomas on his palms and had ignored the tuberoeruptive lesions on his elbows and knees before Type III was diagnosed. These lesions then disappeared with weight reduction and combined drug and dietary therapy. Another brother (I-3) who was found to have Type IV hyperlipoproteinemia later sustained a myocardial infarction at age 39.

Diagnosis

The diagnosis of familial Type III rests on unequivocal establishment of the characteristic lipoprotein pattern. The lipids and lipoproteins in 67 patients are summarized in Table 28-15. Suspicion of Type III should be entertained in any adult who manifests one or more of the following abnormalities: (1) hypercholesterolemia and hypertriglyceridemia that vary in severity from week to week, being particularly responsive to gain or loss of body weight; (2) a ratio of plasma cholesterol to triglyceride that is about 1 (this ratio may vary, however, from 0.3 to 1.5 in Type III); (3) planar xanthomas; or (4) the combination of peripheral vascular disease, hyperglyceridemia, and diabetes.

If only lipid analyses are available, the likelihood that Type III is present can be determined from an estimate of the ratio of cholesterol to glyceride in the patient's VLDL. In Type III, this ratio is much greater than the 1:5 proportion (weight by weight) that obtains in normal VLDL. The rule-of-thumb for this is to divide the plasma triglyceride concentration by 5 and subtract the dividend from the plasma cholesterol concentration. The balance in untreated Type III usually exceeds 250; in Type IV it should be less than 200, but the test is far from infallible.

Whenever possible, the diagnosis must be confirmed by lipoprotein analyses. The simplest is the combination of electrophoresis on polyacrylamide gel (PGE) and one other medium. Lack of β-migrating lipoproteins on PGE (Fig. 28-2) and their presence on paper, agarose, or cellulose acetate usually indicates Type III [100]. On these latter three media a "broad beta band" (Fig. 28-24) is present in about two-thirds of untreated patients with Type III. This is not an infallible test, and electrophoresis alone does not provide an absolute diagnosis of this type.

The one certain test is provided by preparative ultracentrifugation of plasma, without changing its density, for 16 hr at 100,000 g. The supernatant fraction is then electrophoresed on paper or other media. In Type III, β-migrating lipoproteins are present in the supernatant fraction [77]. The differentiation of such "floating beta" is depicted in Fig. 28-24. This anomaly is peculiar to Type III among all types of familial hyperlipoproteinemia. Determination of the relative content of cholesterol and triglyceride in the lipoproteins of density <1.006 isolated by the preparative ultracentrifuge can probably be used in place of electrophoresis of this fraction to make the diagnosis.

Analytic Ultracentrifuge

The pattern in the analytic ultracentrifuge is shown in Fig. 28-1. There is considerable variation among patients, but the main features are an inversion of the usual relationship between the concentrations of the S_f 0 to 12 and 12 to 20 subclasses of LDL and an increase in VLDL, especially of the subclass 20 to 100. Because it is possible to have a very similar pattern in some patients with Type IV hyperlipoproteinemia—in which "floating beta" is not present—the pattern obtained in the analytic ultracentrifuge does not provide an absolute test of Type III.

A peculiarity in Type III, but not a diagnostic feature, is the presence of small amounts of "chylomicrons" (Fig. 28-3); these are apparent whether the patient's diet contains fat or not. Probably these "chylomicrons" represent abnormally large particles of the β-VLDL characteristic of this disorder. Plasma PHLA is normal in Type III, and HDL concentrations are not remarkable.

Table 28-15. PLASMA LIPIDS AND LIPOPROTEINS IN 67 PATIENTS WITH TYPE III HYPERLIPOPROTEINEMIA

Age, yr	No.		*Cholesterol, mg/100 ml (mean ±1 s.d.)*				Triglyceride plasma, mg/100 ml
	M	F	Plasma	VLDL	LDL	HDL	
20–29	7	1	282 ± 71	153 ± 81	98 ± 20	98 ± 6	512 ± 267
30–39	18	1	477 ± 150	339 ± 168	102 ± 27	36 ± 10	752 ± 489
40–49	7	9	378 ± 138	222 ± 142	115 ± 36	45 ± 27	455 ± 235
50–59	7	9	435 ± 104	275 ± 119	119 ± 30	42 ± 10	602 ± 348
60+	3	5	434 ± 153	280 ± 149	113 ± 50	37 ± 11	568 ± 224

Note: Abbreviations and normal values for comparison are shown in Tables 28-2 and 28-3.

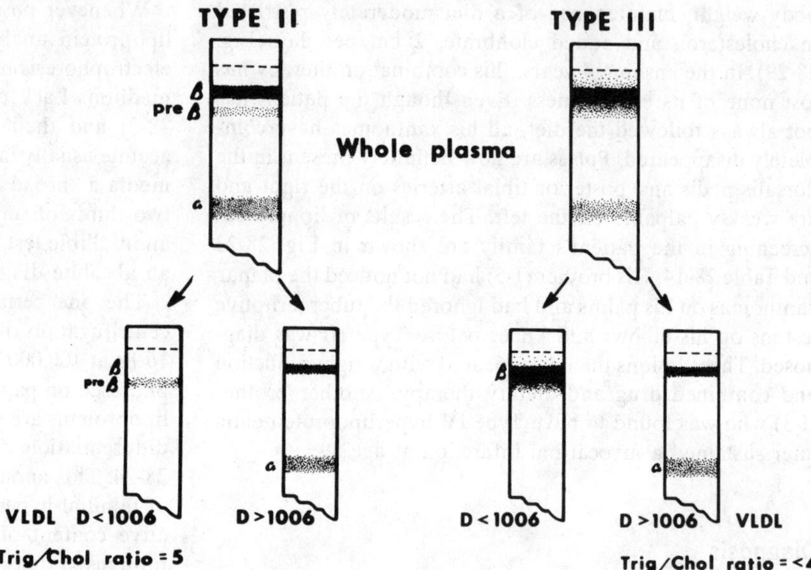

Figure 28-24. Schematic presentation of the distinction between Type III and all other forms of hyperlipoproteinemia (represented here by Type II). In Type III β-migrating lipoproteins also appear in the ultracentrifuge fraction of density <1.006. VLDL Trig/Chol = ratio of triglyceride to cholesterol in the very low density lipoprotein fraction of density < 1.006.

Identification of Phenotype

Major Criteria

The following criteria are considered diagnostic: (1) the Type III lipoprotein pattern, and (2) presence of Type III in a first-degree relative. Patients with an apparently identical phenotype may or may not have a similarly affected relative. A presumption of familial Type III is usually made in all who clearly satisfy the first criterion.

Minor Criteria

Helpful but not diagnostic criteria are (1) planar or "tubero-eruptive xanthomas;" (2) unusual lability in plasma cholesterol and triglyceride concentrations, these tending to rise precipitously with high carbohydrate or calorie intake and to fall rapidly with caloric restriction; (3) a Type IV pattern in adult first-degree relatives; and (4) exclusion of phenocopies.

Phenocopies

The Type III pattern may occur transiently in diabetic acidosis. It probably also occurs in occasional patients with dysglobulinemia, but this has not been adequately documented. Hypothyroidism markedly aggravates Type III hyperlipoproteinemia and may conceivably produce it. Conversely, hyperthyroidism may mask Type III by suppressing the cholesterol and triglyceride concentrations, which then rise rapidly upon return to a euthyroid state. The authors' experience with one such patient indicates that β-VLDL persists despite the normolipidemia maintained by hyperthyroidism.

Age at Detection

The mean age at detection of this disorder in our series of 67 patients was 40 years (Table 28-15). For the men, the mean age was 34, for women, it was much later, or 49 years. Although the youngest patient at the time of detection was a boy, age 20, he was asymptomatic and the case was detected because his mother had Type III. All the women whose disease was discovered before age 50 either were grossly obese or had undergone premature induction of the menopause. The patient discovered latest in life was a woman, 83 years old.

Borrie [404] describes 18 Type III patients defined by planar xanthomas, paper electrophoresis, and plasma lipid analyses. All were referred to him because of xanthomas; their ages at onset ranged from 24 to 53 years. Four were women, only one of whom was under 45 years of age at the onset of skin lesions. The mean age at which the males noted xanthomas was 31 years. Although many children and younger sibs of propositi have now been screened, the Type III pattern has not been observed in any subject under 20 years of age. The phenotypic expression is thus tied to determinants related to maturity and probably to the balance between estrogens and androgens.

Xanthomas

The cutaneous and subcutaneous lesions that often accompany Type III hyperlipoproteinemia are illustrated in Fig. 28-25. The most typical are yellowish elevations on the palmar surface of the hands and fingers, so-called planar xanthomas. These xanthomas may also accompany the severe hyperbetalipoproteinemia in Type II homozygotes and

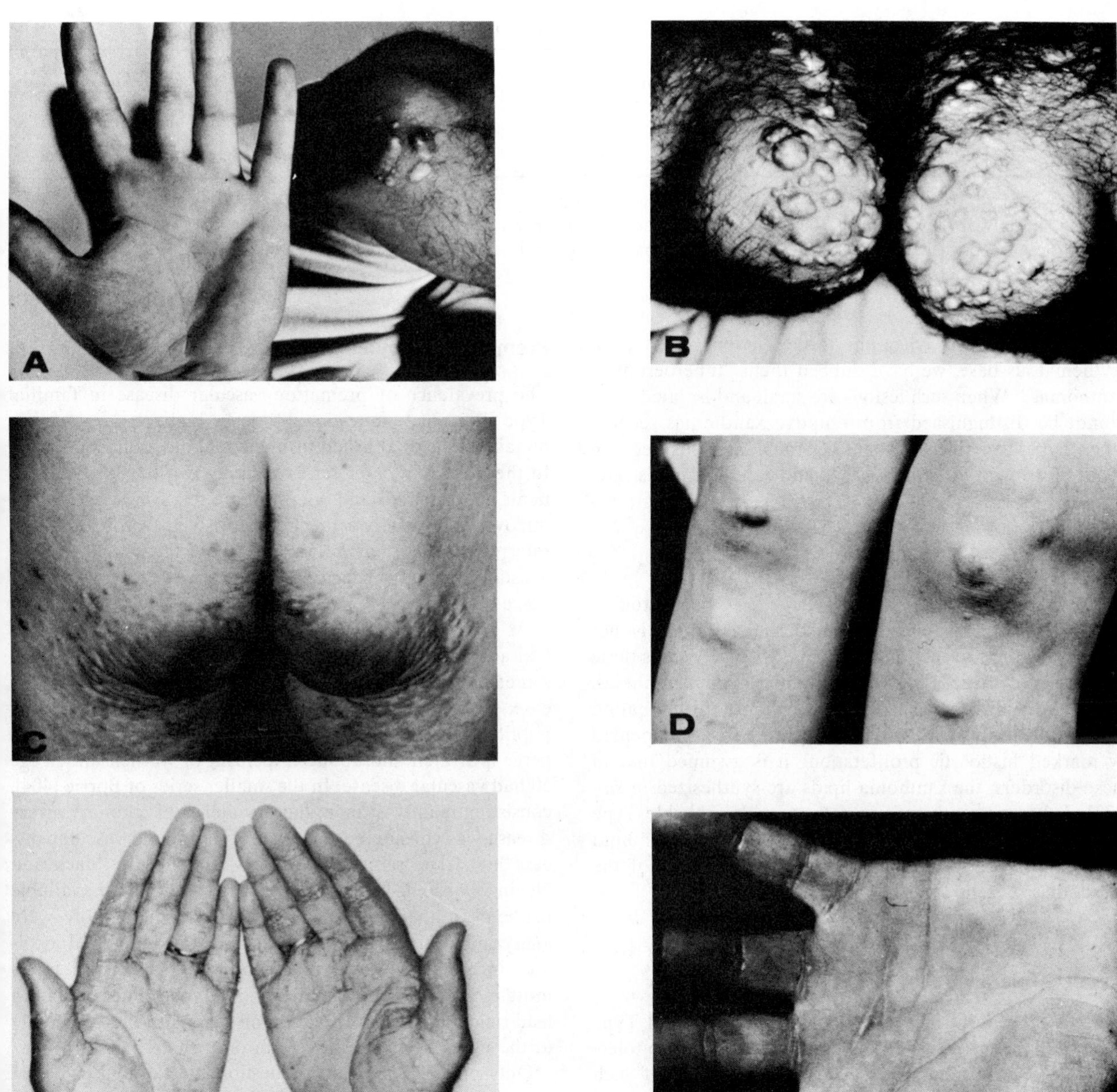

Figure 28-25. Xanthomas commonly seen in Type III hyperlipoproteinemia. A, B, C, and D include tuberoeruptive xanthomas on elbows, buttocks, or knees; D also displays subperiosteal xanthomas over the tibial tuberosities; A, E, and F demonstrate planar xanthomas in the creases and on other surfaces of the palms and fingers.

the variety of lipoprotein patterns seen in obstructive liver disease or dysglobulinemia. In the paraproteinemias, xanthomas may occur in the absence of hyperlipidemia [420, 421]. Planar xanthomas have been present in 65 percent of our patients (Table 28-16) and in 13 of Borrie's 18 patients [404]. According to Polano and coworkers [126–128] and Jepson and colleagues [390], such planar xanthomas also occur in primary Type IV hyperlipoproteinemia. Possible discrepancies in their definitions of Type III, however, leave this association unproved. Tendon xanthomas have been present in about 20 percent of our patients with Type III (Table 28-16). Tuberous and subperiosteal xanthomas (Fig.

Table 28-16. FREQUENCY OF CLINICAL FEATURES IN PATIENTS WITH TYPE III HYPERLIPOPROTEINEMIA*

Ischemic heart disease	Peripheral vascular disease	Fasting hyper-glycemia†	Abnormal glucose tolerance	Hyper-uricemia‡	Hepatospleno-megaly	Hyper-tension	Arcus corneae	Abdominal pain	Xanthelasma	*Xanthomas*			
										Planar	Tendon	Tuboeruptive	Eruptive
55	49	6.4	46	16	11	33	22	5.9	4	65	19	60	10

* Percentages of all 51 parents with Type III identification in Fig. 28-27.
† Fasting hyperglycemia was defined as a fasting blood sugar > 120 mg per 100 ml.
‡ Hyperuricemia was defined as a plasma uric acid of 7.2 and 7.6 mg per 100 ml in females and males, respectively.

28-25) are common; when the former lesions develop an erythematous base, we have dubbed them "tuberoeruptive xanthomas." When such lesions are small and isolated, they cannot be distinguished from eruptive xanthomas seen in other hyperglyceridemic states. Corneal arcus is seen in about 20 percent of patients [379], and xanthelasma is rare.

Pathology

The planar lesions in Type III have not been studied morphologically or reproduced experimentally. It is not known how the presence of circulating β-VLDL causes these rather characteristic lesions. When similar plane xanthomas, often widely distributed, occur in xanthoma disseminatum or reticuloendothelial neoplasias [422], they are accompanied by marked histiocytic proliferation; it is assumed that in these disorders, the xanthoma lipids are synthesized *in situ* [423]. Tuberous xanthomas in patients with probable Type III have been examined chemically [373–375]. Their lipid composition was not obviously different from that of the xanthomas seen in Type II hyperlipoproteinemia.

Glucose Tolerance

Roughly 40 percent of all our patients with familial Type III have diabetic responses to a standard oral glucose tolerance test. Borrie reports a much lower incidence of such a response [404]. None of our patients has been ketotic or has required insulin. In 31 Type III patients (22 men and 9 women), 39 percent of whom had abnormal glucose tolerance, Glueck, Levy, and Fredrickson [339] found that immunoreactive insulin responses were normal in 55 percent; the abnormal responses were equally divided between hypo- and hypersecretion. Compared with normolipidemic controls and patients with familial Type II in this same study, Type III patients appeared to have a somewhat greater prevalence of abnormal glucose tolerance, but the incidence of this abnormality was distinctly less than in patients with familial Type IV or Type V hyperlipoproteinemia. There is therefore no characteristic insulin response to an oral glucose load in Type III.

Premature Vascular Disease

The prevalence of premature vascular disease in familial Type III seems unquestionably to be high; the exact figure remains to be established firmly in a large unbiased sample. In the Clinical Center series, roughly two-thirds of the patients are probands and one-third are relatives subsequently discovered in family screening. Most of the probands were referred because of hyperlipidemia, but a few sought medical assistance initially because of xanthomas or symptoms of vascular disease.

As seen in Table 28-16, 27 of 51 patients with Type III had a history or signs of ischemic heart disease. Nearly the same percentage (49 percent) had peripheral vascular disease, as indicated by decreased pulses in the femoral, popliteal, or smaller leg arteries. In the aggregate, over 80 percent of men and about 25 percent of women under age 50 had vascular disease. In the smaller series of Borrie [404], consisting mainly of men, the prevalence of coronary artery disease was considered low, that of peripheral vascular disease high. The same conclusion was drawn by Slack and Nevin [308, 309]. The latter, however, did not have available to them an adequate test for Type III and therefore were analyzing a mixed group of Types III, IV, and V. All available information leaves no doubt that a history of intermittent claudication in a patient with hyperlipidemia should lead quickly to an examination of his palms and ultimately to the necessary test to ascertain or exclude Type III.

Only one patient with unquestionable familial Type III has come to autopsy. Death followed a myocardial infarction at age 56. The pathologist, Dr. William Roberts [177], found the deposition of highly sudanophilic foam cells immediately beneath the patient's endocardium to be unique in his experience. This was accompanied by grossly visible orange streaks on the endocardial surface and by extensive involvement of the coronary arteries and abdominal aorta by apparently "ordinary" atherosclerosis. There also were similar fat-laden foam cells in the spleen and other tissues [177]. The superficial deposits of lipid on the endocardium were reminiscent of the cutaneous xanthomas seen in Type III, leading to speculation as to whether such changes in the vascular system might respond as quickly and completely to therapy as do the skin lesions.

It is of considerable interest to determine whether changes in the capillary basement membrane described in diabetes [424] occur in Type III. This has not been reported in a clearly defined case of the disease.

Other Clinical Abnormalities

Between 15 and 20 percent of patients have hyperuricemia (Table 28-16) [379]. An elevated uric acid level is apparently less typical of this disorder than it is of Types IV and V (see below). None of the other routine chemical or hematologic laboratory tests give characteristically abnormal results. A single patient has been reported to have low thyroid-binding globulin [415].

The Lipoprotein Abnormality in Type III

Plasma very low density lipoproteins, isolated in the ultracentrifuge at density <1.006, normally migrate in advance of low density lipoproteins on all zonal electrophoretic systems except polyacrylamide gel. The composition of these pre-β or α_2 very low density lipoproteins is usually quite reproducible, consisting of about 10, 12, and 65 percent by weight of protein, cholesterol, and triglycerides, respectively (Chap. 26).

In Type III hyperlipoproteinemia, the very low density lipoproteins have unusual electrophoretic mobility, extending from the β to the α_2 zone on paper electrophoresis (the "broad beta band"). On starch-block electrophoresis they distribute in two distinct modes, so-called β-VLDL and α_2-VLDL (Fig. 28-26) [418]. The β-migrating VLDL ("β-VLDL") are seen in only one other form of dyslipoproteinemia, the homozygous phenotype for Tangier disease (Chap. 26), in which all the very low density lipoproteins have abnormal mobility. The various means of determining the presence of β-VLDL for purposes of diagnosis of Type III have been described earlier.

Lipid Composition of VLDL

The unique abnormalities in lipid composition of the VLDL in Type III are shown in Table 28-17. Separate analyses of β-VLDL and α_2-VLDL in Type III patients isolated by means of starch-block electrophoresis are compared with the total VLDL from patients with Type IV hyperlipoproteinemia in Table 28-18. The small relative increase in cholesterol content of the Type III α_2-VLDL may be due to contamination with β-VLDL [418]. The β-VLDL and α_2-VLDL in Type III do not differ significantly in the fraction of their cholesterol component that is esterified (about 60 percent), in the relative contributions of phosphatidyl choline and sphingomyelin to the total phospholipid component, or in the fatty acid composition of their isolated glycerides, cholesteryl esters, and phospholipids [418].

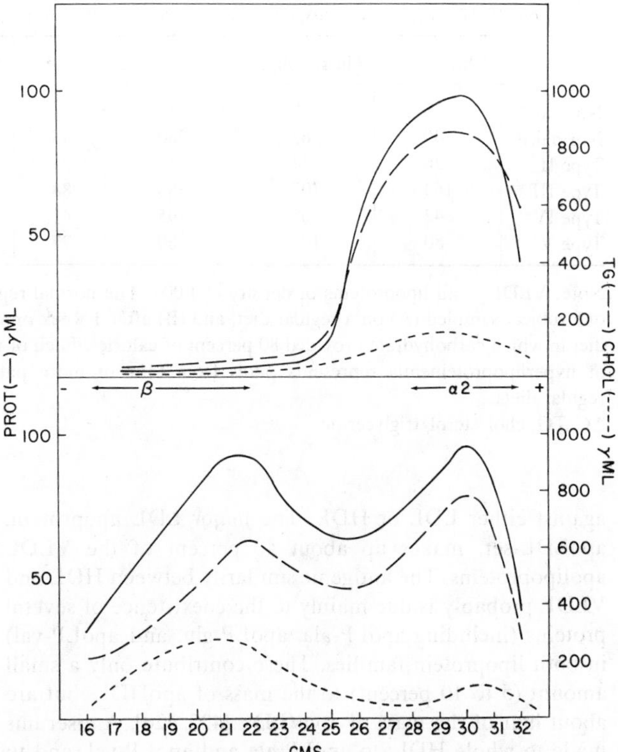

Figure 28-26. The distribution of the usual very low density lipoproteins (density <1.006) (*top*) compared with that of VLDL from Type III (*bottom*) as obtained on starch-block electrophoresis. The distributions of protein (*prot*), triglycerides (*TG*), and cholesterol (*chol*) are shown; *cms* = centimeters of distance along the block. Note the presence of a second component (β-VLDL) in Type III. (*Data from Quarfordt et al.* [418]; *reprinted by permission of the Journal of Clinical Investigation.*)

Flotation Characteristics of β-VLDL

In a single patient the isolated β-VLDL had a mean S_f of 25, and the α_2-VLDL had a mean S_f of 55 [418]. Though the bulk of β-VLDL thus may have a slightly higher density, analyses of isolated VLDL subfractions indicate that the abnormal lipid content is present in all VLDL from S_f 20 to 400 [417, 418]. Hazzard et al. report that β-VLDL is confined to the subfraction of S_f 20 to 60 [417], but Quarfordt et al. also found it in subfractions of S_f 60 to 100 and 100 to 400 [418].

Protein Content of β-VLDL

The apolipoprotein content of VLDL is normally heterogeneous, as described in detail in Chap. 26. When VLDL is delipidated, the proteins react with antiserums prepared

Table 28-17. CHEMICAL COMPOSITION OF VLDL, MG/100 ML PLASMA

	Cholesterol	Phospholipid	Triglyceride	Protein	C/TG*
Normal A	5	8	35	5	0.14
Normal B	49	62	260	48	0.19
Type II	26	37	120	25	0.22
Type III	163	107	380	88	0.43
Type IV	42	65	195	41	0.22
Type V	80	104	560	77	0.14

Note: VLDL = all lipoproteins of density < 1.006. The normal represented one subject sampled (A) on a regular diet, and (B) after 1 week on a fat-free diet in which carbohydrate provided 80 percent of calories. Each of the types of hyperlipoproteinemia represents pools from four or more patients on regular diets.
* C/TG, cholesterol/triglyceride.

against either LDL or HDL. The major LDL apoprotein, apoLDL-ser, makes up about 40 percent of the VLDL apolipoproteins. The antigenic similarity between HDL and VLDL probably is due mainly to the coexistence of several proteins (including apoLP-ala, apoLP-glu, and apoLP-val) in both lipoprotein families. These contribute only a small amount (5 to 10 percent) to the mass of apoHDL, but are about half of the mass of apoVLDL [425, 426]. Antiserums made to whole HDL, to apoLP-ala and apoLP-val, and to apoLDL all react with the delipidated α_2-VLDL from patients with familial Type III. The isolated β-VLDL, however, reacts only with anti-LDL serums [427]. The apoLDL in β-VLDL appears to be immunochemically identical with apoLDL from normal subjects [427]. The apoprotein (apoLDL) in β-VLDL from several Type III patients has also had a behavior on several gel filtration systems, optical properties, and an amino acid composition that are not significantly different from those of normal apoLDL [427].

It is still possible that subtle differences in structure of the apoprotein exist and will be discovered by more extensive analyses, but at present it appears that the β-VLDL in Type III is composed of normal apoLDL complexed with a complement of glyceride that is far greater than that in LDL. This peculiar lipid composition decreases the density of this "LDL" to such an extent that it has the flotation of VLDL.

Variations in β-VLDL in Type III

The distribution of the mass of VLDL between the β- and α_2-VLDL fractions in a given Type III patient can be radically changed by several means [418]. The total VLDL can be sharply increased by changing from a normal diet or one high in fat to a diet in which carbohydrate contributes 70 percent or more of calories. Type III is the most "carbohydrate-inducible" [428] of all types of familial hyperlipoproteinemia [339]; and under these conditions, the proportion of α_2-VLDL is greatly increased and the ratio of triglyceride to cholesterol in the total VLDL increases to the figure of 4 or 5 found in normal VLDL.

If the total VLDL concentration is then abruptly lowered, by either fasting or induction of lipolysis in blood by heparin injection, the ratio of β-VLDL to α_2-VLDL quickly rises. The ratio of triglyceride to cholesterol in the total plasma VLDL approaches unity, the ratio characteristic of β-VLDL. Fasting or postheparin lipolysis produces an effect on VLDL in Type III that differs from that in Type IV patients. In Type III the glyceride content declines much more rapidly that that of cholesterol or protein; in Type IV the glyceride and cholesterol content of VLDL decline together. No β-VLDL is observed in Type IV plasma during the clearance of VLDL. Even when plasma glycerides and total VLDL concentrations are well within normal limits, the Type III

Table 28-18. COMPOSITION OF VLDL IN TYPE III AND TYPE IV HYPERLIPOPROTEINEMIA, GM/100 GM

Type		Cholesterol	Triglyceride	Phospholipid	Protein
Type III:	β-VLDL*	33	39	19	9
	α_2-VLDL*	15	62	15	8
Type IV	Total VLDL†	11	68	13	8

* Means of nine analyses of samples from five patients, ages 33 to 61 years.
† Means of four analyses from four patients, ages 46 to 62 years.
Source: From Quarfordt et al. [418].

patient always has detectable amounts of β-VLDL, observed as β-migrating lipoproteins on paper electrophoresis of the ultracentrifugally isolated plasma lipoprotein fraction of density <1.006.

The Metabolic Defect in Type III

The earliest supposition [65] about the metabolic defect in Type III was that an abnormal species of apoLDL was present which had an unusual affinity for glycerides. The resulting complex (β-VLDL) was presumed to linger in plasma and to be difficult to remove. The failure of all attempts to date to uncover an abnormality in the apoLDL present in either the VLDL or LDL of patients with Type III does not yet exclude this possibility. It has, however, directed speculation to other possible mechanisms.

These speculations unfortunately suffer from lack of adequate knowledge of the normal metabolism of VLDL and LDL. One key question that is still unanswered is how much of the LDL in plasma originates from the catabolism of VLDL and, possibly, chylomicrons. It has been convincingly demonstrated that plasma very low density lipoproteins normally contain apoLDL (Chap. 26). Moreover, studies of particles in rat liver Golgi bodies indicate that the apoLDL is already present before discharge of VLDL into the blood [429, 430]. When very low density lipoproteins, labeled in the protein moiety, are injected intravenously in man, the label appears in the LDL [363, 431]. From estimates of LDL and VLDL turnover in plasma it can be calculated that normally all LDL might be derived from VLDL catabolism. The process of conversion of VLDL to LDL would require removal of most of the glyceride, and the removal or transfer of the VLDL apolipoproteins other than the carboxy-terminal-serine protein of apoLDL to HDL or other VLDL molecules. Rises in both HDL and LDL concentrations occur [49, 432], and apoVLDL-ala has been observed to increase in HDL when VLDL is subjected to postheparin lipolysis [433].

Missing from this construction of the possible origin of β-VLDL is demonstration of a discrete step in VLDL removal that normally produces particles containing triglyceride-rich LDL having an $S_f > 20$. The identification of such particles would imply a possible site for a specific metabolic error in Type III. It has been suggested [434], and is entirely possible, that β-VLDL does appear in normal plasma and has too rapid a turnover to permit its detection. Careful studies have yet to be made of the removal of VLDL tagged in the protein moiety, and no experiments have yet been made to compare the removal of β-VLDL as compared to α_2-VLDL.

The defect in familial Type III thus remains unknown. The likely defect is an extraordinary rate limitation in a late stage of VLDL catabolism, but at a step that has not yet been convincingly demonstrated to be a physiologic one. Whether a mutant form of VLDL or LDL lies at the root of the defect or whether some other metabolic process is affected must yet be determined.

Genetics

The mode of genetic transmission of the Type III defect also remains to be clarified. Most of the available data from which deductions may be made are displayed in Table 28-19 and Fig. 28-27. On the basis of their study of a heterogeneous population of patients containing an undefined number of Type III patients, Nevin and Slack [176] have suggested that the disorder may be inherited as an incomplete dominant trait. Matthews, studying hyperlipoproteinemic members of one large kindred [413], came to the conclusion that Type III and Type IV are different phenotypic expressions of the same mutant gene(s). Unfortunately, his criterion for Type III was the electrophoretic one [45], antedating the present definition [65], and his data do not provide a clear indication of which, if any, members of the family would today be considered to have the disorder.

All the probands and their relatives that have been sampled in the Clinical Center cohort (Fig. 28-27) have been classified by the test for β-VLDL that utilizes paper electrophoresis after ultracentrifugal separation of VLDL. A few of the 36 families shown in Fig. 28-27 are incomplete, but most of the close relatives of the probands have been classified by lipoprotein analyses.

The Coincidence of Type III and Type IV Patterns

Two abnormal lipoprotein patterns appear in the families of Type III probands. One is Type III, the other is Type IV. No Type II pattern has appeared in these families. It will be recalled that there also were no Type III patterns in the more than 200 Type II families described in the previous section.

The prevalence of Type IV hyperlipoproteinemia in all the relatives of Type III probands is about 14 percent (Table 28-19). This is significantly increased above the 5 percent prevalence that might be expected from the limits of normal used to define hyperglyceridemia. It is also far above the

Table 28-19. SUMMARY OF LIPOPROTEIN PATTERNS IN RELATIVES OF PROBANDS WITH TYPE III HYPERLIPOPROTEINEMIA SHOWN IN FIG. 28-27.

Relatives	N*	II	III	IV	Total
Parents	20	0	3	6	29
Siblings	35	0	10	14	59
Children	80	0	2	4	86
Total	135	0	15	24	174

* N, normal.

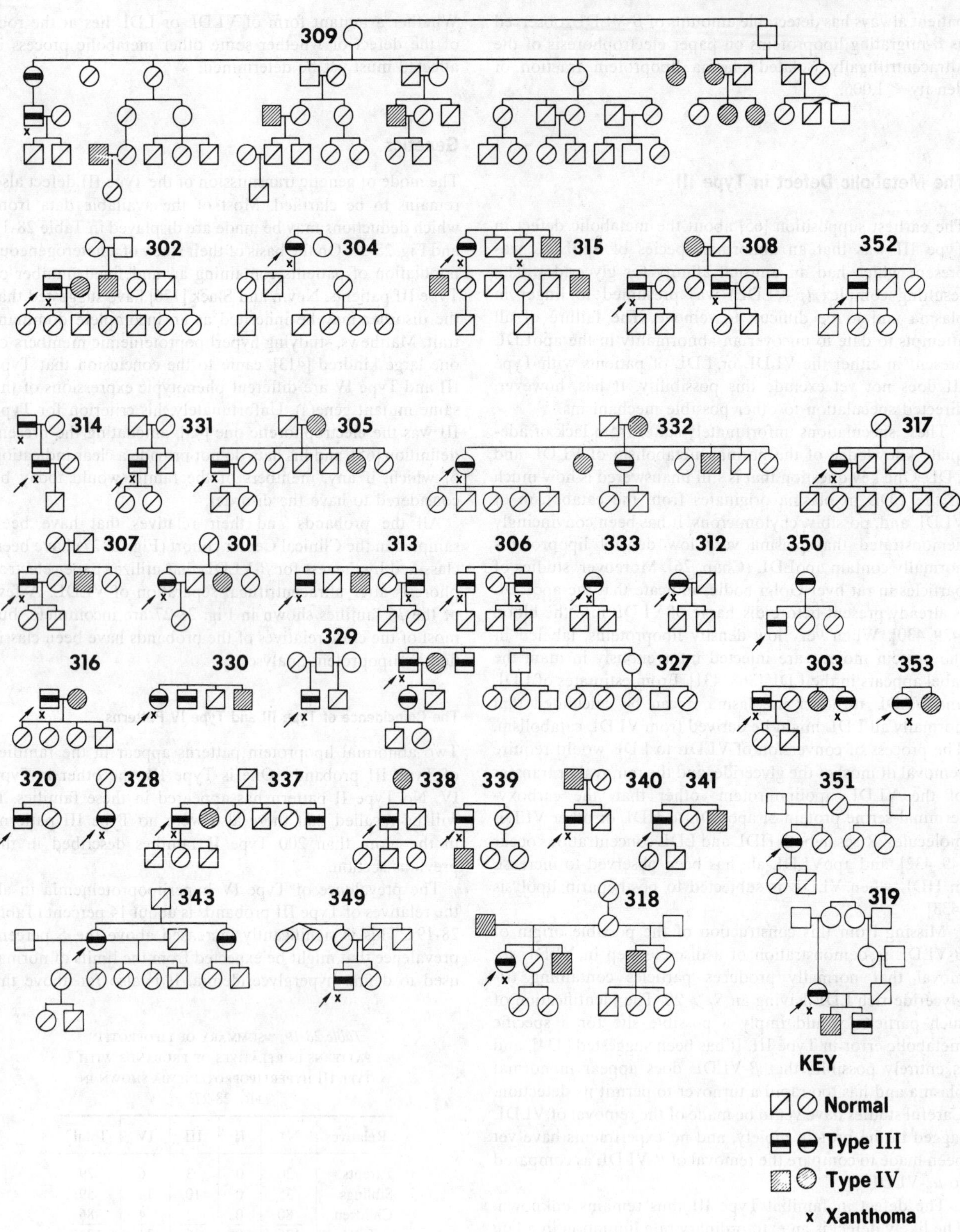

Figure 28-27. Thirty-six kindreds affected with Type III hyperlipoproteinemia.

2 percent prevalence in the Type II kindreds previously described. Because Type IV hyperlipoproteinemia is much more common in adults, children of probands can be excluded from the analyses. The prevalence of Type IV in parents or (adult) sibs of Type III probands is then 23 percent. In the adult relatives the prevalence of Type III patterns is about 15 percent. Slightly more than a third of the adult relatives, then, have either a Type III or Type IV pattern.

The association of these two patterns in these kindreds, and in the proportions observed, is undoubtedly significant. Type III is a rare pattern. We have seen it in less than 100 of some 3,000 individuals, the majority of whom were sampled because they or a relative had hyperlipoproteinemia. Type IV is a much more common pattern, and we have examined about 150 adult sibs or parents of Type IV probands without finding Type III in a single instance.

It is a reasonable conclusion that at least some of the bearers of the Type IV pattern in "Type III families" represent a special abnormality. Its nature is obscured by the lack of specificity implied by a pattern that is defined simply as an increase in VLDL. We have used a gross test, the comparison of estimated VLDL cholesterol with the total plasma glyceride [70], to see if an abnormal lipid composition might be detected in the Type IV relatives in these kindreds. None was seen, but a more sensitive test is needed. We have also never observed the peculiar planar xanthomas associated with Type III in any patient with Type IV, including the relatives under consideration here.

Possible Modes of Inheritance

If we assume that all forms of familial Type III are manifestations of the same disorder, the postulated mode of inheritance must be in accord with the following observations. The disease is subject to a long latent period before it is expressed. This is evident in failure thus far to find the disease in a patient less than 20 years old, even after intensive screening of relatives of probands. The earlier detection of the disease in men than in women could be due to an earlier manifestation of skin or vascular complications, rather than to an expression of the defect by lipoprotein pattern alone. This can be established only by the screening of a very large and unbiased selection of subjects. It will also be necessary in longitudinal studies to learn whether the Type IV relative in the Type III families ever "converts" to a Type III pattern.

Both parents of affected offspring may be normal, but vertical transmission has been observed in 5 of 36 families. One of these five represents the only family in which consanguinity has been established, the parents being first cousins. Male-to-male transmission occurs, and there is no evidence to support an X-linked mutant.

The possible modes of inheritance of the Type III pattern, in descending order of probability, would appear to be (1) autosomal dominance with markedly incomplete expression in many heterozygotes, (2) mixed heterozygosity for two or more different mutant alleles, or (3) double dosage of an autosomal recessive gene. All these modes could include the "Type IV pattern" as representing either a form of incomplete expression of the single dominant allele, or the phenotype of the heterozygote for the recessive gene, or of only one of two different mutants in a mode depending on mixed heterozygosity. In the latter instance one or more of the mutants might be relatively common gene(s), such as one related to diabetes. If the disorder is transmitted as an autosomal recessive allele, the frequency of vertical transmission observed would require the mutant to be more common than the present number of patients suggests. Perhaps it is, and the weaknesses of the data are derived from an inadequate and difficult test for ascertainment.

We have seen one black patient. All the rest have been Caucasians, about 5 percent of them being Jews and the majority being of European-Protestant origin. Adequate survey with appropriate tests for phenotype have not yet been made in any population. The examples of "Type III" cited under "History" (above) include patients from Britain, Western Europe, Scandinavia, Australia, New Zealand, and Japan.

Treatment

The therapy of Type III leads to the most gratifying response of plasma lipids seen in any form of familial hyperlipoproteinemia. It always involves diet control and usually the addition of one of several medications. The success of therapy is currently measured by the ability to maintain plasma cholesterol and triglyceride concentrations within normal limits.

Diet

If necessary, caloric intake is restricted until ideal body weight is achieved. We routinely then use a maintenance diet containing about 40 percent of calories from carbohydrate and 40 percent from fats. In selecting the latter, the amount of saturated fat is decreased and fats high in polyunsaturated acids are increased in a manner similar to, but not as severe as, that in the diet for Type II. Cholesterol is kept to about 300 mg per day, and alcohol intake is restricted [268]. Apart from a healthy respect for the sensitivity of Type III patients to induction of hyperglyceridemia on a very high carbohydrate intake, the prescription of low cholesterol and high polyunsaturated fat intake has been an arbitrary one; it remains for this to be established as necessary.

Drugs

Additional lowering of lipid levels is always achieved by adding clofibrate, 2.0 gm per day, to the regimen [305, 306].

Both nicotinic acid, 3.0 gm per day, and D-thyroxine, 4 to 8 mg per day, appear to have a similar effect. Cholestyramine does not lower blood lipid levels in Type III and may indeed increase triglyceride concentrations [412].

The effects of therapy on plasma lipids and lipoproteins are illustrated in Fig. 28-29. The cutaneous xanthomas disappear within a few weeks or months concomitant with the decline in lipid concentrations (Fig. 28-28). As mentioned earlier, detectable β-VLDL always remains. Zelis and colleagues [419] have described improvement in plethysmographic measurements of peripheral blood flow in Type III patients after several months of therapy. A number of patients have commented upon some decrease in angina or claudication after therapy has been instituted. Objective evidence of improvement or retardation in progression of vascular disease due to treatment of the lipoprotein pattern in still insufficient.

TYPE IV: FAMILIAL HYPERPRE-β-LIPOPROTEINEMIA, AND TYPE V: FAMILIAL HYPERPRE-β-LIPOPROTEINEMIA AND HYPERCHYLOMICRONEMIA

SYNONYMS FOR TYPE IV. Familial endogenous hyperglyceridemia (or hyperlipemia), carbohydrate-induced hyperlipemia, and essential or idiopathic hyperlipemia (archaic); in this chapter referred to as familial Type IV hyperlipoproteinemia.

SYNONYMS FOR TYPE V. Familial endogenous and exogenous hyperglyceridemia (or hyperlipemia), familial mixed hyperlipemia, and essential or idiopathic hyperlipemia (archaic); in this chapter referred to as familial Type V hyperlipoproteinemia.

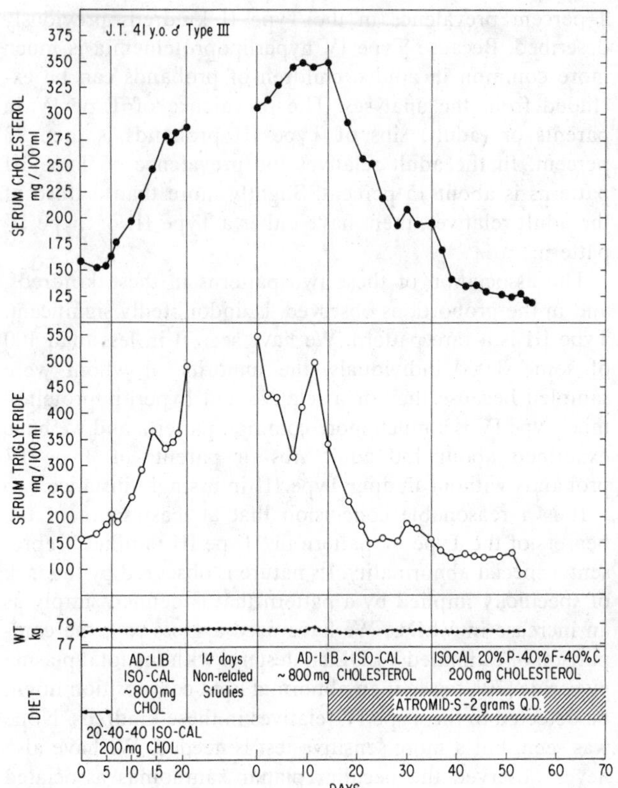

Figure 28-29. Response of plasma cholesterol and triglyceride to diet and clofibrate (Atromid-S) in a patient with Type III hyperlipoproteinemia. From left to right, it will be noted that (1) on an isocaloric diet low in cholesterol, cholesterol and triglyceride were well within normal range; (2) increasing the cholesterol and the amounts of saturated fat compared to polyunsaturated fat in the diet was followed by a prompt rise in cholesterol and triglyceride; (3) clofibrate then lowered cholesterol and triglyceride; (4) a small further decrement in these lipids was obtained when the initial diet was given with clofibrate. Weight changes during the study were negligible. (*Reprinted with permission of Plenum Press.*)

Figure 28-28. The complete resolution of tuberoeruptive xanthomas on the elbow of a patient with Type III hyperlipoproteinemia after 5 months of treatment with diet and clofibrate. (*Reprinted with permission of Plenum Press.*)

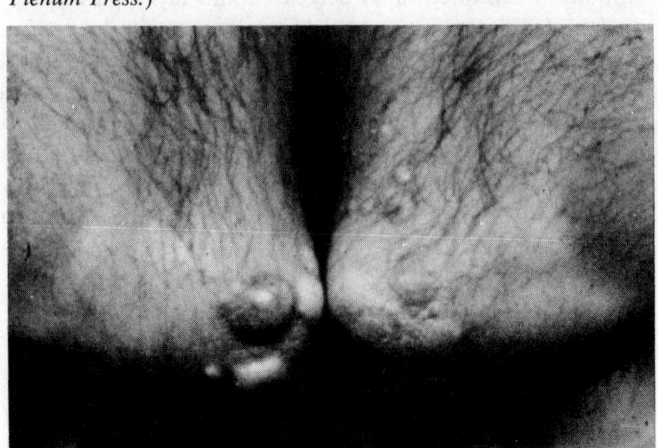

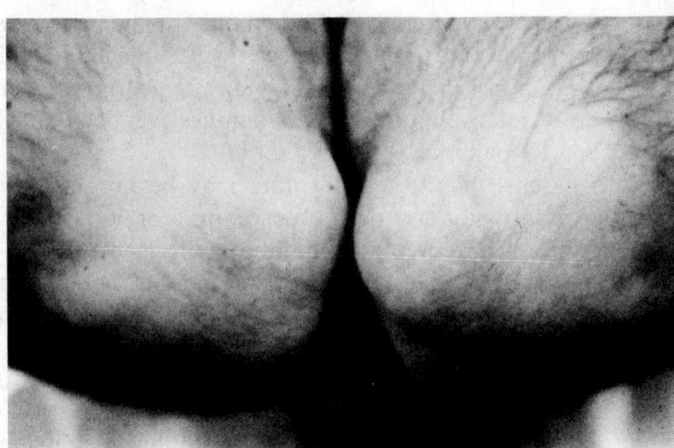

Definitions

Type IV hyperlipoproteinemia is the presence of increased very low density lipoproteins or pre-β-lipoproteins without chylomicronemia (Fig. 28-30). This is considered as endogenous hyperglyceridemia because the increased amounts of glycerides are synthesized in the liver and intestine from fatty acids that have not come directly from the diet. The VLDL concentrations are usually higher when the patient's intake of calories comes mainly from carbohydrate. Such "carbohydrate induction" [428] is a normal phenomenon that also occurs to a degree in all types of hyperlipoproteinemia [339]. Type IV may be called "carbohydrate-induced hyperlipemia" when it has been shown that the pattern is due to an exaggerated response to the usual carbohydrate content of the diet. If this is not certain, the broader or more generic term of "endogenous hyperlipemia" is more appropriate.

The Type V pattern (Fig. 28-31) is the combination of exogenous hyperglyceridemia (chylomicrons being present in the postabsorptive state) and endogenous hyperglyceridemia (increased VLDL). The distinction between "no" chylomicrons and a "few," and thus, the difference between Types IV and V, is a fine one. Moreover, if the VLDL concentration in a Type IV patient is greatly increased by high-carbohydrate feeding and he then eats several high-fat meals, his Type IV pattern can be converted to Type V. In the families of Type V probands there are usually one or more relatives with Type IV patterns. Finally, both lipoprotein patterns, perhaps particularly Type IV, are undoubtedly nonspecific, and both appear secondary to a variety of diseases.

There are arguments, nevertheless, for maintaining the separation between these two patterns. Some are clinical ones, consisting mainly of quantitative differences between Types IV and V in the degree of fat intolerance, the frequency of abdominal pain, pancreatitis, and glucose intolerance, all of which are much more exaggerated with Type V. The major argument is a genetic one; the distribution of IV and V patterns in affected families is not random, and though the genotype underlying Type V may be related to the genotype for Type IV, they are apparently not identical.

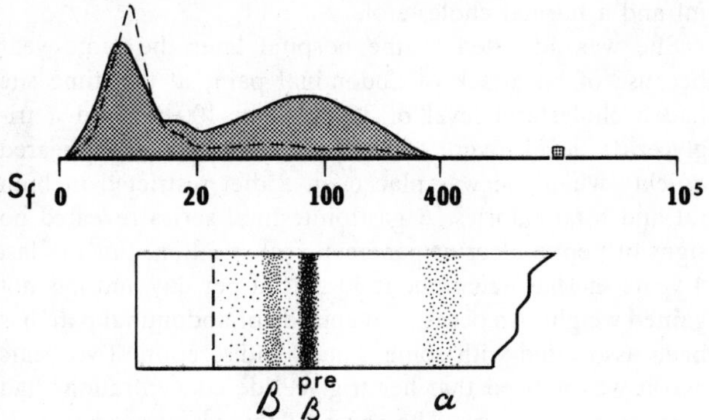

Figure 28-30. Type IV hyperlipoproteinemia.

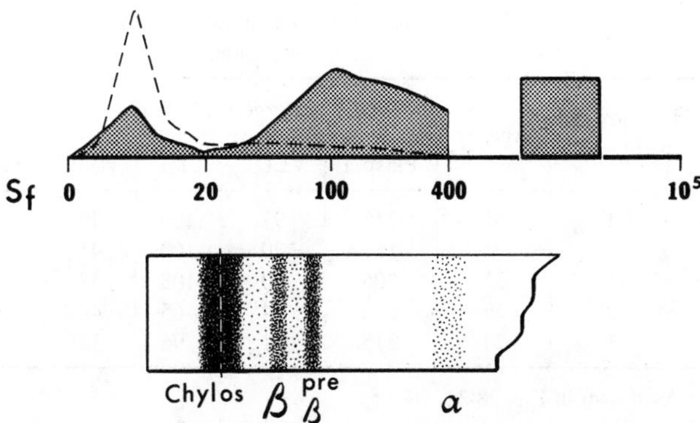

Figure 28-31. Type V hyperlipoproteinemia.

Primary hyperlipoproteinemia of either type should be considered to represent groups of disorders, rather than single diseases. The number of mutants responsible for the familial forms is potentially large. The expression of these mutants has some relationship with maturity, caloric balance, and diabetes. None of the specific biochemical defects due to such mutants has been identified.

History

As mentioned in the introduction to this chapter, the evolution of "xanthoma diabeticorum" to "essential hyperlipemia" began about the turn of this century and progressed little for about 50 years. This was especially true of the lesser degrees of hyperglyceridemia that had none of the more dramatic signs of Types I, II, and III to hold the attention of investigators. Around 1955, endogenous hyperglyceridemia became a popular subject. Smith and Besterman, in England, called attention to the frequency of pre-β-lipoprotein increases after myocardial infarction [435, 436]. Even earlier, in America, Gofman and coworkers had added certain subclasses of VLDL to their calculations of atherogenic index [437]. With very few exceptions [45, 406, 410, 438, 439], familial studies of endogenous hyperglyceridemia did not begin until about 1965, when methods for analyses of glycerides became widely available and efforts had been made to distinguish different types of hyperlipoproteinemia from the grouping of "essential hyperlipemia."

A number of kindreds with familial Type IV and V have now been studied [65, 411, 440–443]. In 1967, Fredrickson, Levy, and Lees drew some conclusions about inheritance from families of 22 probands with Type IV and 9 with Type V [65]. Type IV behaved as a "dominant" trait, with expression usually beginning in adulthood; Type V was thought to be possibly a mixed genotype, related to Type IV. The number of Type IV kindreds at least partially examined in the Clinical Center at Bethesda has risen to about 80, and the Type V kindreds to more than 30. The number of new insights into these genetic abnormalities has not grown proportionately, and Types IV and V remain at the frontier of studies of familial hyperlipoproteinemia.

Table 28-20. PLASMA LIPIDS AND LIPOPROTEINS IN A TYPE IV HYPERLIPOPROTEINEMIA KINDRED

Position in pedigree*	Age, yr	Cholesterol, mg/100 ml				Triglyceride plasma, mg/100 ml	Type
		Plasma	VLDL	LDL	HDL		
I-1	55	245	97	109	39	467	IV
2	54	165	20	100	45	109	N
II-1	23	206	50	108	48	242	IV
2	29	208	94	65	49	550	IV
3	24	215	81	96	38	393	IV

* As shown in Fig. 28-32.
Note: N, normal; other abbreviations as in Table 28-3.

Clinical Features

Case Histories

The following are case summaries of representatives of familial Type IV and familial Type V.

TYPE IV. J.Br., a 23-year-old medical student, the propositus in Fig. 28-32 and Table 28-20, was found to have an elevated triglyceride level of 300 mg per 100 ml, with a cholesterol level of 220 mg per 100 ml at a routine screening. Findings on physical examination were negative, as was the glucose tolerance test result and other laboratory determinations, including electrocardiogram, uric acid, and liver and renal function tests. With a reduction of 15 lb in weight and a limitation of alcohol in the diet, the patient's triglyceride level has been maintained just at the upper limits of normal for the past 3 years. When J.Br. was found to be hyperglyceridemic, his parents and two sibs were examined. The father, age 52, had a Type IV pattern (Table 28-20) and a history of mild labile hypertension and gout treated with salt restriction, colchicine, and probenemid. An oral glucose tolerance test result was abnormal, with a ½-hr value of 190 mg per 100 ml and a 2-hr value of 150. At age 56, J.Br., Sr., sustained an acute anterior myocardial infarction, from which he recovered uneventfully. Since that time he has been on a diet which first reduced and then maintained his body weight and is restricted in carbohydrates and alcohol. His cholesterol remains normal, and his triglyceride stays between 150 and 250 mg per 100 ml. The two sibs of the propositus, ages 27 and 24, also have Type IV and hyperuricemia. The oldest brother has an abnormally high 2-hr postprandial blood glucose concentration.

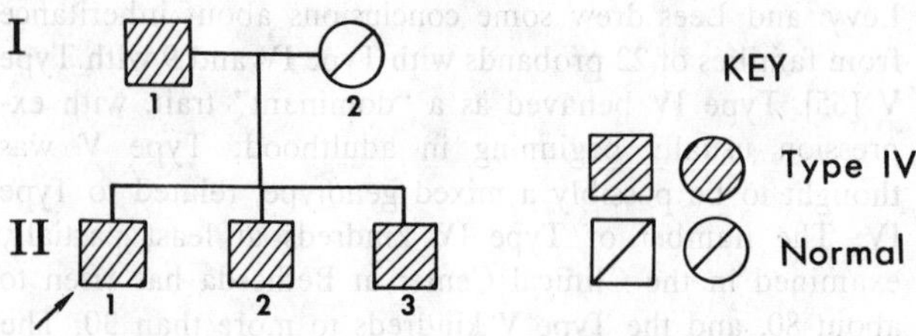

Figure 28-32. A family affected with Type IV hyperlipoproteinemia; details are presented in Table 28-20.

TYPE V. A.Pr., a 32-year-old woman (II-1 in Fig. 28-33 and Table 28-21), began to experience bouts of abdominal pain at age 22. They were associated with lethargy, nausea, and vomiting, occurred several times a year, lasted hours to days, and were associated with dietary excesses, especially of fatty foods. The pain was usually located in the left upper quadrant. Antacids prescribed for a peptic ulcer did not eliminate the attacks, and during hospitalization for one of these attacks when she was 26, her plasma cholesterol concentration was found to be greater than 400 mg per 100 ml. On another occasion, cholesterol was 1,320 mg per 100 ml and the total esterified fatty acids were 6,000 mg per 100 ml. She was referred to the National Institutes of Health at age 27. Her cholesterol level was 262 mg per 100 ml, that of the triglycerides was 1,410, and a Type V lipoprotein pattern was present. Except for obesity (89 kg; 163 cm), the findings on physical examination were negative. A 2-hr postprandial blood glucose level was 136 mg per 100 ml; the uric acid and other laboratory tests were normal. The patient was treated only by weight reduction and when discharged had a plasma triglyceride under 300 mg per 100 ml and a normal cholesterol.

She was admitted to the hospital later the same year because of an attack of abdominal pain; at this time she had a cholesterol level of 366 mg per 100 ml and a triglyceride level over 2,000. The symptoms disappeared quickly when she was placed on a diet restricted in both fat and total calories. A gastrointestinal series revealed no signs of peptic ulcer or pancreatic calcification. For the last 4 years she has eaten about 50 gm fat per day and has not gained weight. An occasional episode of abdominal pain has been associated with some dietary indiscretion. Two years ago it was noticed that her triglyceride concentrations had become much lower. The cause of this was traced to nor-

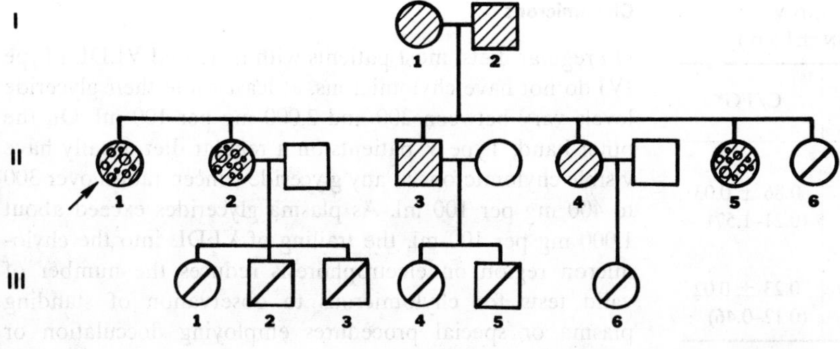

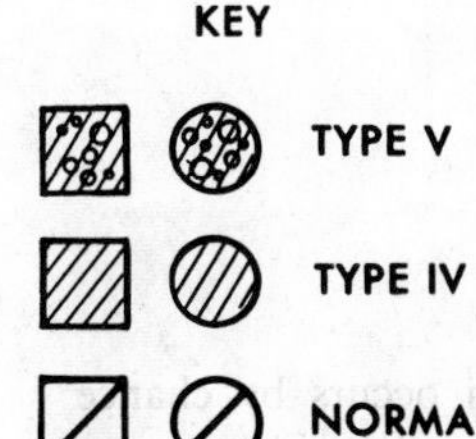

Figure 28-33. A family affected with Type V hyperlipoproteinemia; details are given in Table 28-21.

ethindrone acetate (Norlutate) prescribed for menorrhaghia and later shown to be effective in other women with Type V hyperlipoproteinemia [444]. Norlutate was stopped because of amenorrhea, and on the diet above, the patient's cholesterol level remains between 200 and 250 mg per 100 ml, and her triglyceride between 400 and 800. None of the affected relatives shown in Fig. 28-33 and Table 28-21 was aware of hyperlipoproteinemia prior to screening of the family prompted by the study of the proband. Both parents have abnormal glucose tolerance, and the mother has hyperuricemia. Both parents and the patient have low-normal plasma PHLA. A sister of the patient, who also has Type V, has subsequently been hospitalized on two occasions for treatment of severe abdominal pain.

Diagnosis

Lipids and Lipoproteins

The lipid concentrations seen in Types IV and V are shown in Table 28-22. The lipoprotein patterns are displayed in Figs. 28-1, 28-30, and 28-31.

Table 28-21. PLASMA LIPIDS AND LIPOPROTEINS IN A TYPE V HYPERLIPOPROTEINEMIA KINDRED

Position in pedigree*	Age, yr	*Cholesterol, mg/100 ml*				Triglyceride plasma, mg/100 ml	Type
		Plasma	VLDL	LDL	HDL		
I-1	60	286	114	124	48	591	IV
2	61	260	142	91	27	704	IV
II-1	27	764	708	31	25	4,188	V
2	34	472	424	23	25	3,320	V
3	30	232	49	136	47	249	IV
4	26	236	40	141	55	235	IV
5	24	568	386	129	53	2,184	V
6	21	166	24	64	78	76	N
III-1	12	126	10	71	45	70	N
2	10	162	2	103	57	35	N
3	9	150	6	86	58	54	N
4	5	168	...	...	...	61	N
5	4	150				54	N
6	4	168	4	117	47	61	N

* As shown in Fig. 28-33.
Note: N, normal lipoprotein pattern; other abbreviations as in Table 28-3.

Table 28-22. PLASMA LIPIDS IN TYPES IV AND V HYPERLIPOPROTEINEMIA, MG PER 100 ML (MEAN ±1 S.D.)

No. of subjects	Age, yr	Cholesterol	Triglyceride	C/TG*
		Type IV		
189	42.3 ± 7 (1–75)	257 ± 36 (158–708)	445 ± 37 (150–3,280)	0.86 ± 0.03 (0.21–1.57)
		Type V		
36	40.4 ± 2 (22–62)	452 ± 47 (147–1,320)	2425 ± 319 (428–6,450)	0.23 ± 0.02 (0.12–0.46)

* C/TG, cholesterol/triglyceride.
Source: From Fredrickson et al. [70].

Triglycerides

The initial detection of most propositi occurs by chance through observation of hyperlipemia. As glycerides are incorporated into routine screening tests, more patients are being detected by a postabsorptive triglyceride concentration out of the normal range. Concentrations of triglycerides are more variable than those of cholesterol, and it is reemphasized that plasma samples for phenotyping must be taken 12 to 14 hr after the last meal and while the subject has been maintaining weight on a diet that is usual for his population. It has been suggested that at least three glyceride analyses on separate days are needed to define differences among normal twins [445], and when concentrations are less than 200 mg per 100 ml, repeated samples are highly desirable in familial studies.

The selection of the upper limit of "normal" for glyceride concentrations is no less arbitrary than for other lipids or lipoproteins. In all adults, the limits used in the Clinical Center studies, and shown in Table 28-2, are above the 150 mg per 100 ml (5.2 mEq per liter) that is generally regarded as normal among North Americans and most Europeans [446–449].

VLDL

Unless the analytic ultracentrifuge is available, the quantity of very low density lipoproteins or pre-β-lipoproteins is assessed from the plasma triglyceride concentration. The underlying assumption is that any glyceride excess is carried in VLDL, provided chylomicrons are not increased. As mentioned earlier, "sinking pre-beta," which is glyceride-poor, will sometimes cause an apparent discrepancy between the intensity of the pre-β band and the plasma glyceride concentration [97]. Use of the glyceride level as an indicator, however, avoids labeling as Type IV the 10 percent of subjects who have detectable amounts of "sinking pre-beta," an apparently normal variant of lipoproteins having pre-β mobility.

Chylomicrons

On regular diets, most patients with increased VLDL (Type IV) do not have chylomicrons, at least while their glyceride levels vary between 200 and 2,000 mg per 100 ml. On the other hand, Type V patients on a regular diet usually have visible chylomicrons at any glyceride concentration over 300 to 400 mg per 100 ml. As plasma glycerides exceed about 1,000 mg per 100 ml, the trailing of VLDL into the chylomicron region on electrophoresis reduces the number of valid tests for chylomicrons to observation of standing plasma or special procedures employing flocculation or starch electrophoresis [450, 451].

Carbohydrate Induction

High-carbohydrate diets cause hyperglyceridemia in both normal subjects and patients with hyperlipoproteinemia [223, 339, 428, 452–470]. When all fat in the diet is replaced with carbohydrate and weight is held constant, the plasma triglyceride in patients with Type IV is roughly doubled in 1 week [339, 468], all of it in VLDL. The mean percentage increase is about the same as in normal subjects, but the base line begins at a higher level. The increase (ΔTG) in 20 familial Type IV patients so tested (mean base-line triglyceride of 280 ± 149 mg per 100 ml) ranged from 35 to 213 percent [339].

When the same test is applied to Type V patients, the chylomicrons disappear within 2 to 5 days, and the level of very low density lipoproteins rises. The net ΔTG in Type V may be positive or negative and may vary by 2,000 mg per 100 ml or more [339]. The increase in VLDL usually appears to exceed that seen in Type IV patients on fat-free diets. Most normal subjects reach their peak ΔTG in 1 week; many Type IV or Type V patients have sustained increases in VLDL as long as the high-carbohydrate diets have been maintained, but not enough patients have been carefully observed for more than 2 to 3 weeks on such a diet to establish the long-range peak or stability of carbohydrate induction. The degree of carbohydrate induction does not provide a very reliable separation of different kinds of hyperglyceridemia. Ideally, comparisons are valid only between patients starting at the same glyceride concentrations and when the excess glycerides are in the same lipoproteins, i.e., very low density lipoproteins or chylomicrons. These conditions are very hard to obtain.

Effect of Feeding Fat

Some patients with familial Type IV, whose base-line glycerides are 500 mg per 100 ml or more, have been found to tolerate as much as 200 gm fat per day without developing postabsorptive chylomicronemia. Under such a challenge, others develop chylomicronemia for a day or two and then appear to adapt. Conversely, patients with familial Type V will usually have a marked increase in chylomicrons the morning after high-fat feeding and show no signs of adaptation. It is unusually difficult to test for such adaptation in Type V because sustained high-fat diets are frequently interrupted by the occurrence of abdominal pain.

Thus, there appears to be a qualitative difference in the abilities of Type IV and Type V patients to handle dietary fat at comparable levels of circulating VLDL. As is the case with carbohydrate induction, the quantification of a difference in fat tolerance has been primitive and difficult to control. The vagaries of gastric emptying and absorption have nullified all attempts to define an oral test of fat tolerance. Human chylomicrons are not available for intravenous tolerance tests; several laboratories are experimenting with fat emulsions for this purpose. There is also the possibility that better diurnal observations of glyceride concentrations, as early suggested by Kuo and coworkers [457], may improve the diagnostic distinction between Types IV and V.

Other Lipoproteins

By definition (Table 28-4), LDL is not increased in either Types IV or V. An increase in both VLDL and LDL is considered to indicate a form of Type II (see above). Both LDL and HDL are usually decreased when very low density lipoproteins or chylomicrons are increased, and both LDL and HDL increase when the glyceride level is reduced by therapy. Strisower and colleagues [392] maintain that LDL may climb to pathologic levels on treatment of Type IV hyperlipoproteinemia. In about 40 percent of our familial Type IV's we have always observed a rise in LDL after VLDL is suppressed, but have never seen a sustained elevation above our upper limits of normal for LDL. Wilson and Lees [471] have reported that LDL composition, specifically its content of cholesterol relative to protein, may change in Types IV and V during carbohydrate induction or clofibrate administration. Apparently, LDL of the density range 1.006 to 1.063 was included in their measurements. If so, the admixture of LDL and VLDL present in the density range of 1.006 to 1.019 is undoubtedly changing during these manipulations and it is not possible to assess the significance of this finding.

FFA

Although fasting plasma free fatty acid concentrations [441, 472] and FFA turnover [45] have been reported to be elevated in Type IV and Type V, FFA may also be within the normal range and have the usual response to high-carbohydrate diets [45]. No comprehensive comparisons of average diurnal concentrations or flux of FFA or responses to diet and agents regulating FFA concentrations have been made between normal persons and patients with hyperglyceridemia.

Phenotypes

The diagnosis of familial Type IV or Type V hyperlipoproteinemia only begins with the establishment of the appropriate pattern in the absence of diseases to which it may be secondary. Because the patterns are believed to be nonspecific, it is necessary in every instance to explore familial involvement and to do so in adults, because expression of hyperglyceridemia is usually delayed beyond childhood. An additional complication in classifying affected kindreds is encountered by intermingling of Type IV and Type V patterns in certain families. Type IV patterns also occur, as previously described, in families affected with Types I, II, or III. The coincidence of Type IV patients in familial Type V kindreds is more frequent and undoubtedly of special significance. From data given further on (see "Genetics") one gains the expectation that among parents and adult sibs of a Type V patient there will be about equal proportions of Type IV, Type V, and normal patterns. In the general population, however, Type V is much less common than Type IV. About half of all first-degree adult relatives of a patient with primary Type IV hyperlipoproteinemia will also have Type IV. In 175 such relatives of 53 different propositi with Type IV not one relative with Type V was seen (Table 28-25). A Type IV patient can be expected, however, occasionally to lead the investigator to a "Type V family," i.e., a kindred in which at least one relative has Type V. Until tests more specific than the measurement of lipoproteins are developed for phenotyping, it is suggested that when this occurs, the Type V patient be considered the proband and the kindred be labeled "Type V." On this basis the following phenotypic definitions are offered.

Familial Type IV

MAJOR CRITERIA. (1) Type IV pattern; and (2) one or more first-degree relatives with Type IV patterns; and (3) no close relative with primary Type I, III, or V hyperlipoproteinemia. If a relative is found with one of the latter patterns, he becomes the propositus, and the proper designation of the original patient is "Type IV variant of familial Type I (or III or V)."

MINOR CRITERIA. (1) At least one parent and half the adult sibs will usually have Type IV; (2) the cholesterol level will be normal if triglyceride levels are less than 400 mg per 100 ml; (3) triglyceride level is usually less than 1,500 mg per 100 ml; (4) a family history of diabetes is common; and (5) phenocopies are excluded.

Familial Type V

MAJOR CRITERIA. (1) Type V pattern, and (2) Type IV or V patterns in one or more parents or adult sibs.

MINOR CRITERIA. (1) Usually each parent and about two-thirds of adult sibs have either Type IV or Type V; (2) cholesterol level is usually elevated, and triglyceride levels are usually greater than 400 mg per 100 ml, (3) there are bouts of abdominal pain, pancreatitis, or family history of diabetes, and (4) phenocopies are excluded.

Phenocopies

Either the Type IV or Type V pattern may be secondary to severe insulinopenic diabetes, the nephrotic syndrome or renal failure [473], paraproteinemias, hypothyroidism, alcoholic excess, and rarer conditions such as glycogen storage disease [474], idiopathic hypercalcemia, and Werner's syndrome. Pancreatitis occurs in hyperglyceridemic subjects [475, 476]; how often the pancreatitis antedates chronic hyperlipemia is not known, but Type V hyperlipoproteinemia is commonly seen in patients admitted to hospitals on repeated occasions because of pancreatitis suspected to be due to chronic alcoholism. As a rule, hyperglyceridemia is considered to be secondary to insulin-dependent (ketotic) diabetes. Well-controlled juvenile diabetes is not usually accompanied by hyperglyceridemia [468, 470]. Hyperglyceridemia frequently, but by no means invariably [263], accompanies nonketotic, maturity-onset diabetes. When it does, the hyperglyceridemia is presently considered "primary" for purposes of classifying hyperlipoproteinemia. Estrogens, either alone or in oral contraceptives, frequently seem to cause hyperglyceridemia [184, 477] and may particularly exacerbate familial Type IV or Type V. Secondary hyperglyceridemia can be associated with all the clinical features of the genetic forms of hyperlipemia.

Clinical Features

No large population representing all ages has been randomly surveyed for familial Type IV or V. The Clinical Center population has been derived from referrals, and the proportion of Type V families shown in Table 28-1 is exaggerated by preferential selection.

There are ample clinical impressions of the signs and symptoms that may coexist with hyperlipoproteinemia in patients with familial Type IV or V, but few data are available that show their prevalence in patients selected without bias. Such information from the kindreds of Fredrickson and Levy with these disorders is quite incomplete. That which is available from a total of 139 Type IV patients is displayed in Table 28-23, and a similar summary of findings in 22 probands with Type V is shown in Table 28-24.

Age at Detection

Primary Type IV has been described in a 12-year-old child, who may have had familial disease [472], but it is present in relatively few patients below age 21 years in either Type IV or V families. Children with primary Type IV tend to be obese and to have parents who both have hyperglyceridemia. The authors have seen one clear-cut example of familial Type V in a child of 13 years.

Glucose Intolerance

In a comparative study by Glueck et al. [339] abnormal oral glucose tolerance tests were present in 19 of 36 patients with familial Type IV (52 percent). A history of "diabetes" in Type IV patients was obtained less frequently (Table 28-23). More than 75 percent of patients with familial Type V have abnormal glucose tolerance [339] (Table 28-24). Because the prevalence of diabetes is greater in Type V it would be interesting to know whether the Type IV relatives in "Type V kindreds" have a higher tendency toward diabetes than the "usual" Type IV patient. This has not yet been determined.

Insulin

Hyperinsulinemia has been reported to be frequent in patients with primary Type IV and is sometimes considered to be the mechanism underlying endogenous hyperglyceridemia [223, 464, 466, 467, 478, 480]. In the same series of patients whose glucose tolerance was measured [339], a major-

Table 28-23. FREQUENCY OF CLINICAL FEATURES IN PATIENTS WITH TYPE IV HYPERLIPOPROTEINEMIA OVER 25 YEARS OF AGE AS OBTAINED FROM THE MEDICAL HISTORY*

Type IV patients	Total	Abnormal glucose tolerance	Ischemic heart disease	Claudication	Eruptive xanthomas	Hepatomegaly	Splenomegaly	Abdominal pain
In Type IV Families:								
Probands (A)	26	8/23	17/22	5/22	4/22	4/23	0/22	2/22
Relatives (B)	32	1/20	2/23	0/7	1/5	0/3	0/3	1/5
In Type V Families (C)	26	2/15	0/12	0/7	0/8	0/4	0/4	0/4
Type IV (not proved familial) (D)	55	5/20	11/21	4/18	3/19	8/18	1/18	5/19
Totals	139	16/78	30/78	9/54	8/54	12/48	1/47	8/50
Percent Positive		20	38	17	15	25	2	16

*Analyses of data from patients and relatives. Many were seen as outpatients, and information is incomplete. The percentage of patients in A, B, C, and D who were over 50 years of age was 31, 41, 31, and 36, respectively.

Table 28-24. CLINICAL ABNORMALITIES IN PATIENTS WITH TYPE V HYPERLIPOPROTEINEMIA, PERCENT

Fasting hyperglycemia	Abnormal glucose tolerance	Ischemic heart disease	Peripheral vascular disease	Eruptive xanthomas	Hepatosplenomegaly	Abdominal pain	Pancreatitis	Hyperuricemia
13.6	82	4.5	0	45	32	73	41	41

Note: Data were available under each rubric for all the 22 probands of the kindreds shown in Fig. 28-34. The upper limit of normal for fasting blood glucose was considered to be 120 mg/100 ml; for plasma uric acid, 7.2 and 7.6 mg/100 ml for females and males, respectively. The one subject with coronary artery disease was 59 years old. The ages of the probands were from 22 to 59 years; 8 of the 22 were females.

ity of those with Type V did have hyperinsulinemia. In Type IV, however, only 25 percent of patients had high insulin responses (compared with 22 percent in Type III and 8 percent in Type II), and a larger fraction (36 percent) had abnormally low insulin responses. Similar variability in insulin responses in hyperglyceridemia has been obtained by Nikkilä [223]. There is, therefore, no characteristic insulin response in either familial Type IV or V, as determined in patients whose disorders were of various degrees of severity and who were of both sexes and various ages. Moreover, carbohydrate induction is not well correlated with either glucose tolerance or the insulin responses [339].

PHLA

In Type V, some plasma postheparin lipolytic activity is present, as detected by the "quick" test illustrated in Fig. 28-7. In a number of patients normal levels have been obtained by the in vitro assay system employing Ediol [141]. With this or similar methods, PHLA in a few Type V patients may be as low as some of the levels obtained in Type I homozygotes [259, 444]. PHLA may also be low in secondary Type V [156, 182, 183, 261]. An inhibitor of PHLA has been suggested in secondary Type V [481]. Progestational steroids increase PHLA in Type V [444]. More specific measurements distinguishing between activity of lipoprotein lipase (LPL) and that of other triglyceride lipase or monoglyceride hydrolase in postheparin plasma [152, 154] have not yet been applied to enough Type V patients to determine whether there is a "true" deficiency of LPL activity in the familial syndrome.

In our series of familial Type IV patients [141] and in others with endogenous hyperglyceridemia described elsewhere [441, 442], PHLA has always been normal when tested. It has not been determined whether PHLA might be low in some of the "Type IV variants" who appear in Type V families. The entire issue of lipoprotein lipase activity in both Types IV and V awaits restudy with more specific assay methods.

Xanthomas

Eruptive xanthomas (Fig. 28-9) may occur in patients with Type IV or V. They usually appear only when glyceride concentrations are over 1,500 mg per 100 ml, and quickly disappear when the level is decreased. About 15 percent of Type IV patients have them at some time; they are about three times more common in Type V (Tables 28-23, 28-24). The mechanism of their formation is presumably the same as that mentioned under Type I. "Tuberoeruptive xanthomas" may occasionally occur; we have never seen planar xanthomas on the palms associated with primary Type IV or V. They have been reported by other investigators in Type IV patients [126–128, 390], but it was not definitely shown that their patients did not have Type III hyperlipoproteinemia.

Hyperuricemia

Hyperuricemia is common in patients who have hyperglyceridemia [482–484] and occurs in both familial Types IV and V [65, 441]. In our series, the uric acid was elevated in 9 of 22 Type IV probands and in 40 percent of Type V probands (Table 28-24). Either males or females may have hyperuricemia. Podagra occasionally occurs, although gouty arthritis is quite uncommon.

Abdominal Pain and Pancreatitis

About 75 percent of patients with Type V commonly have a history of episodic abdominal pain (Table 28-24). As a rule it usually begins about the third decade. The attacks begin later in life than in Type I, but are otherwise the same. A history of one or more surgical explorations of the abdomen is often obtained. The patient often recalls a period of dietary excess or weight gain a few days preceeding the attacks. Occasionally, they follow the onset of estrogen administration in postmenopausal women. About half the time the pancreatic lipase or amylase levels in blood or urine are normal despite severe abdominal discomfort, but frank and severe pancreatitis occurs often and can be life-threatening. Calcification of the pancreas has been sought by x-ray in many patients with Type V; it is usually not found.

Although we have observed a few patients with Type IV who develop abdominal pain on a high-fat diet, and as high as 16 percent of Type IV patients admit to a history of same (Table 28-23), by far the majority of patients with severe hyperlipemia who have abdominal distress at the time a lipoprotein pattern is obtained prove to have Type V.

Obesity

Many patients with either syndrome are lean and have normal ponderal indices. There is no doubt that obesity aggravates VLDL excess, but no certainty that it has any direct effect on exogenous fat tolerance beyond that possibly induced by very high VLDL levels. Abnormal glucose tolerance is almost always improved when the patient is placed on a reduction diet.

Premature Vascular Disease

A history of angina pectoris or myocardial infarction was recorded in an overall 38 percent of 78 patients with Type IV (Table 28-23). The prevalence was especially high in probands (Table 28-23), in whom the presence of ischemic heart disease (IHD) was corroborated by in-patient examination. Twelve of the 15 patients who were between ages 30 and 49 had IHD. It must be noted, however, that 9 of the 15 also had hypertension and some had abnormal glucose tolerance. A history of IHD was far less common in their Type IV relatives (2 of 23), even though their mean age was higher than that of the probands. Most of the relatives in Table 28-23 have not been examined extensively for IHD. The discrepancy in prevalence of vascular disease in probands and relatives is probably due mainly to the more frequent referral of patients with IHD for hospitalization.

Brown has summarized many studies that have shown that Type IV hyperlipoproteinemia is commonly found in patients with myocardial infarction [448, 485]. We have also recently found that two-thirds of a small sample of young adults with primary Type IV and angiographically proved IHD had familial hyperlipoproteinemia. It is very probable that familial Type IV carries a higher than normal hazard for premature IHD; the risk cannot yet be estimated accurately. Seventeen percent of 54 patients with Type IV in Table 28-23 had a history of claudication in the lower extremities.

The prevalence of premature IHD or peripheral vascular disease in patients with familial Type V patterns is not known accurately. The relatively low frequency of vascular disease in the small sample of probands in Table 28-24, however, is very interesting. One would expect any bias introduced by selection to be in the direction of overestimating vascular disease, as was apparently the case in Type IV (Table 28-23). The impression one gains in studying both Types I (see above) and V is that an excess of circulating chylomicrons does not have an adverse effect—and might even have some retarding influence—on the rate of atherogenesis.

Other Clinical Abnormalities

Lipemia retinalis and hepatosplenomegaly may be present in Type IV and are more common in Type V. Patients with the latter pattern sometimes complain of paresthesias of the arms or legs that resemble those seen in diabetic neuropathy. These are frequently disabling and only occasionally improve when the hyperglyceridemia is lowered by therapy.

Other Laboratory Abnormalities

Other laboratory test results are not characteristically abnormal. Kuo and colleagues [416, 486] report that examination of the gingival and nail-fold capillaries in Type IV reveals pericapillary hemorrhages and a "nondiabetic" type of microangiopathy. Siperstein and coworkers have examined the thickness of the muscle capillary basement membranes in at least one patient with primary Type V and found no changes similar to those seen in diabetics [424]. A larger survey of such families for this defect has not been reported.

Possible Biochemical Defects in Types IV and V

A recent excellent review by Nikkilä [223] summarizes the background related to the possible errors in endogenous hyperglyceridemia. The area in which these errors seem to lie includes the relationships between insulin activity, glucose utilization, the release and utilization of FFA, and the synthesis and catabolism of glycerides, as well as the structure and metabolism of the chylomicrons and very low density lipoproteins in which glycerides predominantly appear in plasma. There are many other reviews of these subjects, some of which [179, 199, 201, 222, 487–489] seem particularly pertinent, and their topics also have already been referred to under the sections on Type I and Type III and in Chap. 26.

In a functional sense, the rate of removal of glycerides from plasma is always inadequate when a Type IV or Type V lipoprotein pattern is present. Actually, of course, the removal mechanisms may be functioning normally, but are possibly frustrated by lipoproteins of abnormal structure or simply overwhelmed by endogenous overproduction of glycerides. Many experiments, most of them using isotopic techniques, have been performed to measure the rates of synthesis, release, and catabolism of plasma glycerides [223, 290–499]. The interpretations of the results vary; latter-day studies have tended to suggest a decreased rate of removal as the more common defect in patients having Type IV or Type V hyperlipoproteinemia. The patients examined have been heterogeneous, and no clear-cut genetic abnormality has been demonstrated. Such kinetic analyses are also difficult to extrapolate beyond a single patient examined at a particular state of compensation or adjustment to his underlying derangement. We are therefore restricted to a few generalizations about possible metabolic errors.

Structure of the Lipoproteins

In a few patients, very low density lipoproteins or chylomicrons have been reported to be resistant to lipolysis or otherwise to behave abnormally [259]. No structural defects in these lipoproteins in Type IV or V have been exposed.

For that matter, much of the work on the identification of the apoVLDL proteins has been done on plasma from Type IV patients [426, 427]. No obvious differences in the polypeptides obtained from a number of such donors and a few "normals" have yet been observed, but comparisons have been neither extensive nor sophisticated enough to exclude significant abnormalities. The large number of proteins in very low density lipoproteins and, presumably, in chylomicrons, offers many possibilities for mutations; and their potential exposure is one of the tantalizing barriers yet to be scaled in the study of hyperlipoproteinemia.

Control of Glyceride Synthesis

Very low density lipoproteins are assembled and discharged into the plasma or lymph from both the liver [200, 500] and the intestine [501–503]. The major precursors for hepatic glyceride synthesis are glucose and plasma FFA [200, 223]. The glycerophosphate required to form the glyceryl esters is derived both from glucose and from glycerol released by lipolysis in the periphery and transported to the liver in the blood. During the postabsorptive period, free fatty acids are the principal source of glyceride fatty acids [200], and the production of VLDL during this period involves a number of steps. Some of these that can be rate-limiting include the release of free fatty acids by lipolysis in adipose tissue, their reesterification in the liver, the assembly of glycerides into VLDL, and the secretion of the latter into plasma. Insulin probably controls directly only the first of these steps, by opposing many hormonal and other factors promoting lipolysis.

Carbohydrate in the diet has both acute and chronic effects on plasma glycerides [223]. Carbohydrate loads may acutely depress glyceride levels, possibly by first increasing insulin activity and then decreasing FFA flux. "Carbohydrate induction" may be a result of both a stimulation of glyceride synthesis or secretion of VLDL and a depression of clearance and oxidation of glycerides. Simple and complex carbohydrates seem to differ in respect to their effect on glyceride concentrations. Fructose, for example, is sometimes more potent than glucose. The difference has been postulated to be due to both a relatively greater promotion of glyceride synthesis and a weaker provocation of insulin response and, hence, to less induction of lipoprotein lipase activity required to clear glyceride from the plasma [223].

Control of Glyceride Catabolism

As discussed under Type I (earlier in this chapter), the mechanisms for removal of glycerides in very low density lipoproteins and chylomicrons are presumed, but not proved, to be identical. The removal sites are limited in capacity and become saturated at higher plasma triglyceride levels [206, 504]. The fractional removal rate thus decreases with increase in the total plasma glyceride pool. Here again, insulin has important influences on glyceride removal. Its regulation of glucose uptake and utilization promotes the reesterification necessary to complement the hydrolytic step critical for glyceride uptake in peripheral tissues. Insulin also promotes activation of LPL or depresses its synthesis. The latter may be accomplished by the lowering of FFA concentrations and may be separate from insulin effects on glucose uptake or metabolism.

Notable among determinants of hyperglyceridemia seem to be positive caloric balance and alcohol. Obesity is known to be accompanied by decreased sensitivity of the adipose tissue cell to insulin [505]. The improvement in glyceride levels in Type IV seems to occur immediately upon decrease in caloric intake, however, and before much loss in adipocyte cell size is likely to occur. Like obesity, alcohol may be a more important factor in secondary than familial hyperlipoproteinemia. A history of alcoholic excess is notoriously common among patients with Type V patterns and pancreatitis. Many of the effects of alcohol on FFA flux, synthesis, and release of glycerides are known [506], but their relationships in producing hyperglyceridemia are not clear.

Multiple Mechanisms

Unquestionably, two of the inconstant features of familial Types IV and V, abnormal glucose tolerance and hyperinsulinism, are important clues to the defects in these disorders. To be sure, hyperglyceridemia may itself decrease glucose tolerance [507], and the cause and the effect have not been separated in the disorders compounded of both diabetes and hyperglyceridemia. It seems particularly noteworthy, however, that Type V patients, as a group, have much higher prevalence of both glucose intolerance and hyperinsulinism than do Type IV patients, a discrepancy almost certainly not related alone to absolute triglyceride concentrations in the two groups.

The likelihood that abnormal response of plasma glycerides to dietary carbohydrate is the metabolic error in many cases of endogenous hyperglyceridemia is discounted by Nikkilä [223]. The failure of such patients to return to normal glyceride levels on subnormal caloric intake and the frequent failure to show an absolute abnormality in carbohydrate induction indicates that other explanations must be found.

The search for metabolic errors in Types IV and V requires refocusing. The probability of multiple defects is high, and better means to discriminate among different disorders has a high priority. It will also be necessary to obtain much more information about single patients; the plasma activity of insulin and specific assessment of LPL are among tests that need to accompany all clinical assessments and kinetic analyses. There is, too, the problem of overinterpreting variables determined in the steady state when glyceride levels are high and clearance mechanisms have all but decompensated. It may be that insights will be less obscured if attention is turned to those at genetic hazard for hyperglyceridemia, and before the time that their normal homeostasis is lost.

Genetics

Type IV

Familial Type IV, despite its probable heterogeneity, distributes itself in families as though it were the expression of a single autosomal allele with fairly complete penetrance in the adult. The data in Table 28-25 for relatives of 53 propositi are still consistent with the 1:1 proportion of normal subjects to those affected found in the smaller series previously described [65]. These data are also subject to the same bias discussed under the genetics of Type II, i.e., the requirement of familial involvement in the definition of the propositus. The ratio of affected to nonaffected relatives shown in Table 28-25 does not provide a valid basis for assuming that Type IV patterns are distributed as a trait behaving as a Mendelian dominant with a high degree of penetrance. Note that no Type V patterns were observed among these 175 relatives, a good indication of the relative infrequency of Type V compared to Type IV and an observation that takes on special significance when one notes the frequency of Type IV relatives in Type V families (see below). As was true in the earlier report [65], the distribution between the sexes of abnormal patterns is about equal. Braunsteiner et al. found about 40 percent abnormality in relatives of several small kindreds with Type IV [442]. Schreibman et al. [441] found 8 Type IV subjects among 22 relatives in three generations of the family of a 17-year-old Type IV propositus.

Usually one parent has Type IV; sometimes both do, and occasionally, neither one does. While the gene(s) usually may be expressed in presumed adult carriers, they are usually undetectable in childhood. Very few of the children under 12 years of age of either probands, or their abnormal sibs, are abnormal, and only an occasional child under 20 has Type IV. Sufficient children of parents who both have Type IV have not been sampled to determine whether the likelihood is greater that they will have Type IV, or whether this pattern might be expressed earlier.

Type V

In Fig. 28-34 are illustrated 22 kindreds with familial Type V; pertinent information from them is summarized in Table 28-26. Whenever both parents of the Type V probands could be examined, at least one was abnormal. Of the eight complete parental pairs, two were V-IV; two, IV-IV; two, V-normal; and two IV-normal. Thus, there were more IV than V patterns in the parents. The preponderance of males among probands may have been due to chance (Fig. 28-34). Sixty-five percent of the brothers were abnormal, 54 percent of the sisters. Approximately one-third each of these close adult relatives had normal, Type IV, and Type V patterns.

Table 28-25. DISTRIBUTION OF LIPOPROTEIN PATTERNS AMONG PARENTS AND ADULT SIBLINGS OF 53 PROPOSITI WITH TYPE IV HYPERLIPOPROTEINEMIA

Normal	II	III	IV	V
90	0	0	85	0

Table 28-26. DISTRIBUTION OF LIPOPROTEIN PATTERNS AMONG PARENTS AND ADULT SIBS OF 22 PROPOSITI WITH FAMILIAL TYPE V HYPERLIPOPROTEINEMIA*

Relative	N	IV	V	Other	Total
Fathers	2	6	2	0	10
Mothers	5	4	3	0	12
Brothers	13	12	13	0	38
Sisters	13	10	5	0	28
Totals	33	32	23	0	88

* As shown in Fig. 28-34.
Note: N, normal lipoprotein pattern.

The influence of parental phenotype is hard to assess. In no kindred were both parents Type V. Offspring with Type V were produced by marriages in which one partner was normal and by marriages in which neither partner had Type V. Conversely, normal (adult) offspring occurred among the progeny of IV-V marriages. Only 2 of the 20 children under 21 years of the Type V probands were abnormal; one had Type V, the other, Type IV. The patterns in relatives have not yet been correlated with body weight, age, or diabetes, factors already mentioned as possible determinants of phenotypic expression.

Consanguinity was known to be present in only one of the Type V families (No. 515, Fig. 28-34), in which the parents were first cousins. No obvious concentration among any particular ethnic groups was noted. All these families, however, were white; they included Protestants, Catholics, and Jews.

It is concluded that Type V patients are genotypically different from Type IV patients. They could represent mixed heterozygotes having an allele in common, but in combination with another mutant in Type V. The probable nonspecificity of the phenotype(s) currently recognized makes further speculation on the genetic mode unprofitable.

Treatment

Type IV

The initial step is reduction to ideal weight. The maintenance diet is concerned primarily with the content of carbohydrate and alcohol. We prescribe a diet containing between 35 and 40 percent of calories from carbohydrate, and avoidance of alcohol excess [268]. Other workers stress a somewhat lower carbohydrate content, using fat as a substitute, and also recommend substitution of complex for simple sugars, especially avoiding fructose [479]. Weight maintenance and avoidance of low fat—and therefore, a very high-carbohydrate intake—are paramount. If triglycerides are still over

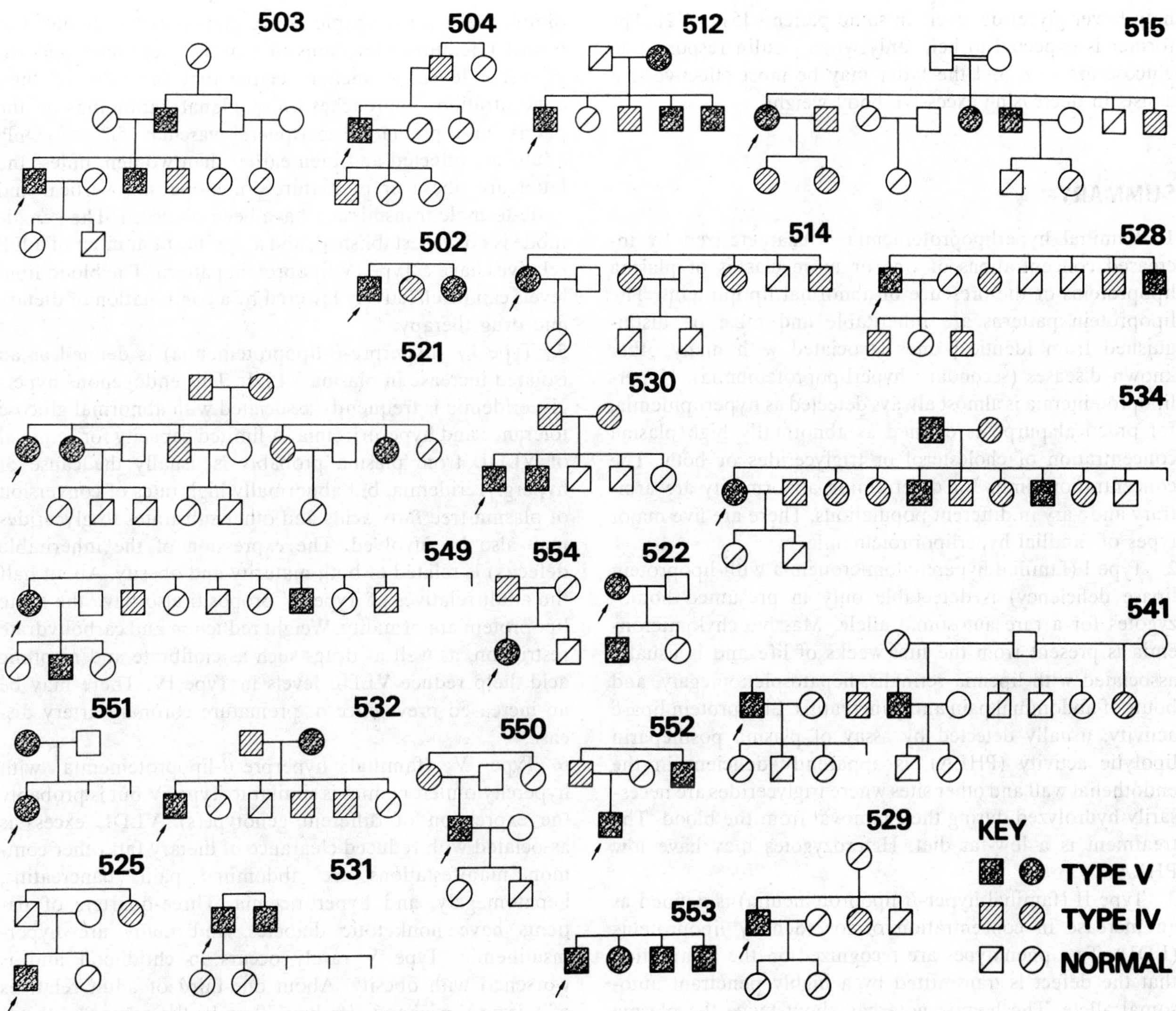

Figure 28-34. Twenty-two kindreds affected with Type V hyperlipoproteinemia. Propositi are denoted by arrows.

300 mg per 100 ml after 6 weeks of appropriate dietary regulation, clofibrate [305, 306, 391, 392, 508, 509] may be tried. In about half of familial Type IV patients clofibrate is not effective. Nicotinic acid, less pleasant to take, will usually lower glycerides. This drug is a potent inhibitor of FFA release [510], although its effect on hyperglyceridemia may be related to other mechanisms as well. If calorie restriction and weight maintenance do not return the triglycerides to completely normal values, drugs rarely will, and control, not "cure," becomes the highest expectation.

Type V

Maintenance of ideal weight is also important in treatment of this syndrome. If the patient is obese, the effect is usually a lowering of glyceride levels, but not to the same extent obtained in Type IV. The maintenance diet is developed empirically and often has to be as high in protein as possible, avoiding excess of either fat or carbohydrate [268]. Return from a high-carbohydrate diet to one normal in fat content must be made cautiously to avoid an abdominal crisis. Nicotinic acid, 3 to 6 gm daily, is the most effective drug and is often added to the diet for maintenance therapy [306]. Norethindrone acetate, 2.5 mg per day [444], may also be very helpful in improving fat tolerance in women. The effect is less in men.

During abdominal crises, oral intake of food is stopped, and fluids along with suction and other general measures for treatment of pancreatitis are employed until the symptoms have abated.

Insulin is not recommended unless the patient is insulinopenic. Tolbutamide and phenformin have been reported to help lower glyceride levels in some patients [511, 512]. The former is expected to help only when insulin responses to glucose are low, and the latter may be most effective if it assists in decreasing excessive body weight.

SUMMARY

1 Familial hyperlipoproteinemia is characterized by increased concentrations of one or more classes of plasma lipoproteins or the presence of abnormal lipoproteins. The lipoprotein patterns are inheritable and must be distinguished from identical ones associated with many other known diseases (secondary hyperlipoproteinemia). Hyperlipoproteinemia is almost always detected as hyperlipidemia, for practical purposes defined as abnormally high plasma concentration of cholesterol or triglycerides or both. The concentration limits for determining abnormality are arbitrary and vary in different populations. There are five major types of familial hyperlipoproteinemia.

2 Type I (familial hyperchylomicronemia with lipoprotein lipase deficiency) is detectable only in presumed homozygotes for a rare autosomal allele. Massive chylomicronemia is present from the first weeks of life and is usually associated with lipemia retinalis, hepatosplenomegaly, and bouts of abdominal pain and pancreatitis. Lipoprotein lipase activity, usually detected by assay of plasma postheparin lipolytic activity (PHLA), is apparently deficient in the endothelial wall and other sites where triglycerides are necessarily hydrolyzed during their removal from the blood. The treatment is a low-fat diet. Heterozygotes may have low PHLA.

3 Type II (familial hyper-β-lipoproteinemia) is defined as an increase in concentration of low density lipoproteins (LDL). Two phenotypes are recognized on the assumption that the defect is transmitted by a highly penetrant autosomal allele. The homozygote has about twice the plasma LDL and cholesterol concentrations of the heterozygote. Either may also have a modest increase in plasma triglyceride levels. Both develop tendon and tuberous xanthomas and premature coronary, cerebral, and peripheral vascular disease. These manifestations appear earlier and are more severe in the homozygote. The rate of removal of cholesterol and LDL from plasma is limited, the precise defect or defects being still unknown. The heterozygote frequently dies prematurely of vascular disease; the homozygote rarely survives to adulthood. Either phenotype can be detected in cord blood. LDL can be decreased by treatment consisting of diet and oral intake of cholestyramine, a bile acid–sequestering resin.

4 Type III ("broad beta disease") is characterized by the presence of complexes of LDL and glycerides that have the flotation properties of very low density lipoproteins (VLDL) and the electrophoretic mobility of LDL. The abnormal lipoproteins ("β-VLDL") are best detected by a combination of preparative ultracentrifugation and electrophoresis. Simpler tests for probable ascertainment are available. The disorder features elevations in plasma cholesterol and triglyceride levels to such a degree that the ratio of their concentrations approaches unity, planar xanthomas on the palms, and premature peripheral vascular disease. Only adults are affected and men earlier than women, unless the latter are obese or prematurely menopausal. Vertical and male-to-male transmission have been observed. The genetic mode is not yet established, and a significant number of adult relatives have a Type IV lipoprotein pattern. The blood lipid levels can be effectively lowered by a combination of dietary and drug therapy.

5 Type IV (hyperpre-β-lipoproteinemia) is defined as an isolated increase in plasma VLDL. This endogenous hyperglyceridemia is frequently associated with abnormal glucose tolerance and hyperuricemia. A limited capacity for removal of VLDL from plasma probably is usually the cause of hyperglyceridemia, but abnormally high rates of conversion of plasma free fatty acids and other substrates to glycerides may also be involved. The expression of the inheritable defect(s) is related to both maturity and obesity. About half the adult relatives of Type IV propositi also have the same lipoprotein abnormality. Weight reduction and carbohydrate restriction, as well as drugs such as clofibrate and nicotinic acid, help reduce VLDL levels in Type IV. There may be an increased prevalence of premature coronary artery disease.

6 Type V (familial hyperpre-β-lipoproteinemia with hyperchylomicronemia) is similar to Type IV but is probably the expression of different genotype(s). VLDL excess is associated with reduced clearance of dietary fat; other common manifestations are abdominal pain, pancreatitis, hepatomegaly, and hyperuricemia. Three-quarters of patients have nonketotic diabetes, and many are hyperinsulinemic. Type V rarely occurs in childhood and is worsened with obesity. About one-third of adult relatives of a Type V proband also have Type V; the other two-thirds have normal or Type IV patterns. There is no evidence of accelerated vascular disease. Treatment consists of a diet avoiding excesses of either carbohydrates or fat, and nicotinic acid.

BIBLIOGRAPHY

1. Rayer, P. F. O.: Traité théorique et pratiques des maladies de la peau. Paris, 1827.
2. Addison, T., and Gull, W.: On a certain affection of the skin, vitiligoidea (*a*) plana, (*b*) tuberosa, with remarks. Guy. Hosp. Rep., **7**, 265, 1851.
3. Jensen, J.: The story of xanthomatosis in England prior to the first world war. Clio. Med., **2**, 289, 1967.
4. Fagge, C. H.: General xanthelasma or vitiligoidea. Trans. Path. Soc., London, **24**, 242, 1872.
5. Fox, T. C.: A case of xanthelasma multiplex. Lancet, **2**, 688, 1879.
6. Poensgen, A.: Mittheilung eines seltenen Falles von Xanthelasma multiplex. Arch. Path. Anat. Physiol., **91**, 350, 1883.
7. Lehzen, G., and Knauss, K.: Über Xanthoma multiplex planum, tuberosum, mollusciforme. Arch. Path. Anat. Physiol., **116**, 85, 1889.

8. Arning, E.: Ein Fall von familiäre Xanthomatose. Arch. Derm. Syph., **105**, 290, 1910.
9. Bristow, J. S.: Case of keloid. Trans. Path. Soc., London, **17**, 414, 1866.
10. Proctor, W. J.: Xanthoma diabeticorum. Lancet, **2**, 1392, 1905.
11. Adamson, H. G.: A case of xanthoma diabeticorum. Westminster Hosp. Rep., **14**, 84, 1905.
12. Siemans, H. W.: Zur Kenntnis der Xanthoma. Arch. Derm. Syph., **136**, 159, 1921.
13. Quinquaud, M.: Recherches hematochimiques et dermatochimiques. Bull. Soc. Chim. Paris, France, p. 259, 1878.
14. Chauffard, A., and La Roche, G.: Pathogénie du xanthélasma. Sem. Méd., **30**, 241, 1910.
15. Bazin, cited by M. Hillairet: Vitiligoidea-xanthelasma-xanthoma. Bull. Acad. Med., ser. 2, **7**, 1166, 1878; cited by A. C. Curtis, U. J. Wile, and H. C. Eckstein. The involution of cutaneous xanthomata caused by diets low in calories. J. Clin. Invest., **7**, 249, 1929.
16. Mallassez, cited by E. Laraiddy: Étude sur le xanthelasma. Thèse de Paris, 1877, cited by U. J. Wile, H. C. Eckstein, and A. C. Curtis. Lipid studies in xanthoma. Arch. Derm. Syph., **19**, 35, 1929.
17. Carry, C. A.: Contribution à l'étude du xanthoma. Anal. Derm. Syph., ser. 2, **1**, 64, 1880.
18. Pincus, F., and Pick, L.: Zur Struktur und Genese der symptomatischen Xanthome. Deutsch. Med. Wschr., **34**, 1426, 1908.
19. Pick, L., and Pinkus, F.: Weitere Untersuchungen zur Xanthomfrage: die echten xanthomatosen Neubeldungen. Derm. Z., **36**, 1827, 1909.
20. Pollitzer, S., and Wile, U. J.: Xanthoma tuberosum multiplex. J. Cutan. Dis., **30**, 1912.
21. Anitschkow, N.: Über die Veränderungen der Kaninchenaorta bei experimenteller Cholesterinasteatose. Beitr. Path. Anat., **56**, 379, 1913.
22. Burns, F. S.: A contribution to the study of the etiology of xanthoma multiplex. Arch. Derm. Syph., **2**, 415, 1920.
23. Arning, E., and Lippmann, A.: Essentielle Cholesterinämie mit Xanthombildung. Z. Klin. Med., **89**, 107, 1920.
24. Morichau-Beauchant, R., and Bessonnet, R.: Le Xanthome héréditaire et familial: ses relations avec la diathèse biliaire. Arch. Gén. Med., **192**, 2313, 1903.
25. Gossage, A. M.: The inheritance of certain human abnormalities. Quart. J. Med., **1**, 331, 1907–08.
26. Schmidt, E.: Beiträge zur Xanthomfrage. Arch. Derm. Syph., **140**, 408, 1922.
27. Fasold, A.: Studien über Vererbung von Hautkrankheiten. VI. Xanthom (Cholesterosis cutis). Arch. Rass. Ges. Biol., **16**, 54, 1924.
28. Hufschmitt, M.: Un cas de xanthome familial. Presse Med., **32**, 99, 1924.
29. Llambias, J., and Celesia, A.: Xanthome familial. C. R. Soc. Biol. (Paris), **93**, 1011, 1925.
30. Harbitz, F.: Tumors of tendon sheaths, joint capsules and multiple xanthoma. Arch. Path. (Chicago), **4**, 507, 1927.
31. Wile, U. J., Eckstein, H. C., and Curtis, A. C.: Lipid studies in xanthoma. Arch. Derm. Syph., **20**, 489, 1929.
32. Wile, U. J., and Duemling, W. W.: Familial xanthoma. Arch. Derm. Syph., **21**, 642, 1930.
33. Müller, D.: Xanthomata, hypercholesterolemia, angina pectoris. Acta Med. Scand., suppl., **89**, 75, 1938.
34. Müller, C.: Angina pectoris in hereditary xanthomatosis. Arch. Intern. Med., **64**, 675, 1939.
35. Svendsen, M.: Are supernormal cholesterol-values in serum caused by a dominantly inherited factor? Report of a family investigation of 34 individuals. Acta Med. Scand., **104**, 235, 1940.
36. Bloom, D., Kaufman, S. R., and Stevens, R. A.: Hereditary xanthomatosis: familial incidence of xanthoma tuberosum associated with hypercholesteremia and cardiovascular involvement, with report of several cases of sudden death. Arch. Derm. Syph., **45**, 1, 1942.
37. Grenaud, M.: Les xanthomes familiaux (thèsis). Paris, 1927: cited by Bloom et al. [36].
38. Török, L.: De la nature des xanthomes (avec quelques remarques critiques sur la nature des tumeurs). Ann. Derm. Syph. (Paris), **4**, 1109, 1893: cited by Bloom et al. [36].
39. Thannhauser, S. J., and Magendantz, H.: The different clinical groups of xanthomatous diseases: a clinical physiological study of 22 cases. Ann. Intern. Med., **11**, 1662, 1938.
40. Thannhauser, S. J.: *Lipoidoses.* Oxford, New York, 1950.
41. Wilkinson, C. F., Hand, E. A., and Fliegelman, M. T.: Essential familial hypercholesterolemia. Ann. Intern. Med., **29**, 671, 1948.
42. Wilkinson, C. F.: Essential familial hypercholesterolemia: cutaneous metabolic and hereditary aspects. Bull. N.Y. Acad. Med., **26**, 670, 1950.
43. Holt, L. E., Jr., Aylward, F. X., and Timbres, H. G.: Idiopathic familial lipemia. Bull. Johns Hopkins Hosp., **64**, 279, 1939.
44. Furman, R. H., Howard, R. P., Brusco, O. J., and Alaupovic, P.: Effects of medium chain length triglyceride (MCT) on serum lipids and lipoproteins in familial hyperchylomicronemia (dietary fat-induced lipemia) and dietary carbohydrate–accentuated lipemia. J. Lab. Clin. Med., **66**, 912, 1965.
45. Fredrickson, D. S., and Lees, R. S.: Familial hyperlipoproteinemia, in *The Metabolic Basis of Inherited Disease,* 2d ed., edited by J. B. Stanbury, J. B. Wyngaarden, and D. S. Fredrickson, p. 429. McGraw-Hill, New York, 1966.
46. Cohn, E. J., Gurd, F. R. N., Surgenor, D. M., Barnes, B. A., Brown, R. K., Derouaux, G., Gillespie, J. M., Kahnt, F. W., Lever, W. F., Lin, C. H., Mittelman, D., Mouton, R. F., Schmid, K., and Uroma, E.: A system for the separation of the components of human blood: quantitative procedures for the separation of the protein components of human plasma. J. Amer. Chem. Soc., **72**, 465, 1950.
47. Lindgren, F. T., Elliott, H. A., and Gofman, J. W.: The ultracentrifugal characterization and isolation of human blood lipids and lipoproteins, with applications to the study of atherosclerosis. J. Phys. Colloid Chem., **55**, 80, 1951.
48. Barr, D. P., Russ, E. M., and Eder, H. A.: Protein-lipid relationships in human plasma. II. In atherosclerosis and related conditions. Amer. J. Med., **11**, 480, 1951.
49. Gofman, J. W., deLalla, O., Glazier, F., Freeman, N. K., Lindgren, F. T., Nichols, A. V., Strishower, E. H., and Tamplin, A. R.: The serum lipoprotein transport system in health, metabolic disorders, atherosclerosis and coronary artery disease. Plasma, **2**, 413, 1954.
50. Dangerfield, W. G., and Smith, E. B.: Investigation of serum lipids and lipoproteins by paper electrophoresis. J. Clin. Path., **8**, 132, 1955.
51. Bragdon, J. H., Havel, R. J., and Boyle, E.: Human serum lipoproteins. I. Chemical composition of four fractions. II. Some effects of their intravenous injection in rats. J. Lab. Clin. Med., **48**, 36, 1956.
52. Jencks, W. P., Hyatt, M. R., Jetton, M. R., Mattingly, T. W., and Durrum, E. L.: A study of serum lipoproteins in normal and atherosclerotic patients by paper electrophoretic techniques. J. Clin. Invest., **35**, 980, 1956.
53. Kunkel, H. G., and Trautman, R.: The α_2 lipoproteins of human serum: correlation of ultracentrifugal and electrophoretic properties. J. Clin. Invest., **35**, 641, 1956.
54. Korn, E. D.: Clearing factor, a heparin-activated lipoprotein lipase. I. Isolation and characterization of the enzyme from normal rat heart. J. Biol. Chem., **215**, 1, 1955.
55. McGinley, J., Jones, H., and Gofman, J.: Lipoproteins and xanthomatous diseases. J. Invest. Derm., **19**, 71, 1952.
56. Gofman, J. W., Rubin, L., McGinley, J. P., and Jones, H. B.: Hyperlipoproteinemia. Amer. J. Med., **17**, 514, 1954.
57. Nikkilä, E.: Studies on lipid-protein relationships in normal and pathological sera and effect of heparin on serum lipoproteins. Scand. J. Clin. Lab. Invest., **5** (suppl. 8), 1, 1953.
58. Lever, W. F., Smith, P. A. J., and Hurley, N. A.: Idiopathic hyperlipemia and primary hypercholesteremic xanthomatosis. I. Clinical data and analysis of the plasma lipids. J. Invest. Derm., **22**, 33, 1954.
59. Havel, R. J., Eder, H. A., and Bragdon, J. H.: The distribution and chemical composition of ultracentrifugally separated lipoproteins in human serum. J. Clin. Invest., **34**, 1345, 1955.
60. Guravich, J. L.: Familial hypercholesteremic xanthomatosis: a preliminary report. I. Clinical, electrocardiographic and laboratory considerations. Amer. J. Med., **26**, 8, 1959.
61. Fredrickson, D. S.: Essential familial hyperlipidemia, in *The Metabolic Basis of Inherited Disease,* 1st ed., edited by J. B. Stanbury, J. B. Wyngaarden, and D. S. Fredrickson, p. 489. McGraw-Hill, New York, 1960.

62. Furman, R. H., Howard, R. P., Lakshmi, K., and Norcia, L. N.: The serum lipids and lipoproteins in normal and hyperlipidemic subjects as determined by preparative ultracentrifugation. Amer. J. Clin. Nutr., **9,** 73, 1961.
63. Cornwell, D. G., Kruger, F. A., Hamwi, G. J., and Brown, J. B.: Studies on the characterization of human serum lipoproteins separated by ultracentrifugation in a density gradient. I. Serum lipoproteins in normal, hyperthyroid and hypercholesterolemic subjects. Amer. J. Clin. Nutr., **9,** 24, 1961.
64. Fredrickson, D. S., and Lees, R. S.: System for phenotyping hyperlipoproteinemia. Circulation, **31,** 321, 1965.
65. Fredrickson, D. S., Levy, R. I., and Lees, R. S.: Fat transport in lipoproteins—an integrated approach to mechanisms and disorders. New Eng. J. Med., **276,** 32, 94, 148, 215, and 273, 1967.
66. Beaumont, J. L., Carlson, L. A., Cooper, A. R., and Fredrickson, D. S.: Classification of hyperlipidaemias and hyperlipoproteinaemias. Bull. W. H. O. (in press).
67. Thomas, C. B., Murphy, E. A., and Bolling, D. R.: The precursors of hypertension and coronary disease: statistical consideration of distributions in a population of medical students. I. Total serum cholesterol. Bull. Johns Hopkins Hosp., **114,** 290, 1964.
68. Lewis, L. A., Olmstead, F., Page, I. H., Lawry, E. Y., Mann, G. V., Stare, F. J., Hanig, M., Lauffer, M. A., Gordon, T., and Moore, F. E.: Serum lipid levels in normal persons. Circulation, **16,** 227, 1957.
69. Schaefer, L. E.: Serum cholesterol-triglyceride distribution in a "normal" New York City population. Amer. J. Med., **36,** 262, 1964.
70. Fredrickson, D. S., Levy, R. I., Kwiterovich, P. O., and Jover, A.: The typing of hyperlipoproteinemia: a progress report (1968), in *Drugs Affecting Lipid Metabolism,* edited by W. L. Holmes, L. A. Carlson, and R. Paoletti, p. 307. Plenum, New York, 1969. (Proceedings of the Third International Symposium on Drugs Affecting Lipid Metabolism, Milan, Italy, Sept. 8–11, 1968.)
71. Smith, S. C., Scheig, R. L., Klatskin, G., and Levy, R. I.: Lipoprotein abnormalities in liver disease. Clin. Res., **15,** 330, 1967.
72. deLalla, O. F., and Gofman, J. W.: Ultracentrifugal analysis of serum lipoproteins, in *Methods of Biochemical Analysis,* edited by D. Glick, vol. 1, p. 459. Interscience, New York, 1954.
73. Ewing, A. M., Freeman, N. K., and Lindgren, F. T.: Analysis of human serum lipoprotein distributions. Advances Lipid Res., **3,** 25, 1965.
74. Lindgren, F. T., Jensen, L. C., Wills, R. D., and Freeman, N. K.: Flotation rates, molecular weights and hydrated densities of the low-density lipoproteins. Lipids, **4,** 337, 1969.
75. Jensen, L. C., Rich, T. H., and Lindgren, F. T.: Graphic presentation of computer-derived schlieren lipoprotein data. Lipids, **5,** 491, 1970.
76. Fredrickson, D. S., Levy, R. I., and Lindgren, F. T.: A comparison of heritable abnormal lipoprotein patterns as defined by two different techniques. J. Clin. Invest., **47,** 2446, 1968.
77. Levy, R. I., and Fredrickson, D. S.: Type II and Type III hyperlipoproteinemia. I. Chemical differentiation (in preparation).
78. Hatch, F. T., Freeman, N. K., Jensen, L. C., Stevens, G. R., and Lindgren, F. T.: Ultracentrifugal isolation of serum chylomicron-containing fractions with quantitation by infrared spectrometry and NCH elemental analysis. Lipids, **2,** 183, 1967.
79. Lossow, W. J., Lindgren, F. T., Murchio, J. C., Stevens, G. R., and Jensen, L. C.: Particle size and protein content of six fractions of the S_f 20 plasma lipoproteins isolated by density gradient centrifugation. J. Lipid Res., **10,** 68, 1969.
80. Viikari, J., Haahti, E., Helela, T.-T., Juva, K., and Nikkari, T.: Fractionation of plasma lipoproteins with preparative zonal ultracentrifugation. Scand. J. Clin. Lab. Invest., **23,** 85, 1969.
81. Wilcox, H. G., and Heimberg, M.: Isolation of plasma lipoproteins by zonal ultracentrifugation in the B14 and B15 titanium rotors. J. Lipid Res., **11,** 7, 1970.
82. Hatch, F. T., and Lees, R. S.: Practical methods for plasma lipoprotein analysis. Advances Lipid Res., **6,** 4, 1968.
83. Lees, R. S., and Hatch, F. T.: Sharper separation of lipoprotein species by paper electrophoresis in albumin-containing buffer. J. Lab. Clin. Med., **61,** 518, 1963.
84. Noble, R. P.: Electrophoretic separation of plasma lipoproteins in agarose gel. J. Lipid Res., **9,** 693, 1968.
85. McGlashan, D. A. K., and Pilkington, T. R. E.: A method of lipoprotein electrophoresis using agarose gel. Clin. Chim. Acta, **22,** 646, 1968.
86. Rapp, W., and Kahlke, W.: Lipoprotein-elektrophorese in agarosegel. Clin. Chim. Acta, **19,** 493, 1968.
87. Papadopoulos, N. M., and Kintzios, J. A.: Determination of human serum lipoprotein patterns by agarose gel electrophoresis. Anal. Biochem., **30,** 421, 1969.
88. Houtsmuller, A, J.: *Agarose-gel-electrophoresis of Lipoproteins, a Clinical Screening Test.* Van Gorcum, Assen, 1969.
89. Noble, R. P., Hatch, F. T., Mazrimas, J. A., Lindgren, F. T., Jensen, L. C., and Adamson, G. L.: Comparison of lipoprotein analysis by agarose gel and paper electrophoresis with analytical ultracentrifugation. Lipids, **4,** 55, 1969.
90. Colfs, B., and Verheyden, J.: Electrophoresis and sudan black staining of lipoproteins on gelatinized cellulose acetate. Clin. Chim. Acta, **18,** 325, 1967.
91. Chin, H. P., and Blankenhorn, D. H.: Separation and quantitative analysis of serum lipoproteins by means of electrophoresis on cellulose acetate. Clin. Chim. Acta, **20,** 305, 1968.
92. Chin, H. P., and Blankenhorn, D. H.: On the precision of lipoprotein electrophoresis on cellulose acetate and its use in the diagnosis of hyperlipoproteinemia. Clin. Chim. Acta, **23,** 239, 1969.
93. Farber, E., Batsakis, J., Giesen, P., and Thressen, M.: Lipoprotein electrophoresis: a comparison of cellulose acetate and paper techniques. Amer. J. Clin. Path., **51,** 523, 1969.
94. Winkelman, J., Ibbott, F. A., Sobel, C., and Wybenga, D. R.: Studies on the phenotyping of hyperlipoproteinemias: evaluation of cellulose acetate technique and comparison with paper electrophoresis. Clin. Chim. Acta, **26,** 33, 1969.
95. Fletcher, M. J., and Styliou, M. H.: A simple method for separating serum lipoproteins by electrophoresis on cellulose acetate. Clin. Chem., **16,** 362, 1970.
96. Lewis, L. A.: Screening for serum lipoprotein abnormalities: comparison of ultracentrifugal, paper and thin-layer starch-gel electrophoresis techniques. Lipids, **4,** 60, 1969.
97. Rider, A. K., Levy, R. I., and Fredrickson, D. S.: "Sinking" pre-beta lipoprotein and the Lp antigen. Circulation, **42:**III-10, 1970.
98. Seidel, D., Alaupovic, P., and Furman, R. H.: A lipoprotein characterizing obstructive jaundice. I. Method for quantitative separation and identification of lipoproteins in jaundiced subjects. J. Clin. Invest., **48,** 1211, 1969.
99. Pratt, J. J., and Dangerfield, W. G.: Polyacrylamide gels of increasing concentration gradient for the electrophoresis of lipoproteins. Clin. Chim. Acta, **23,** 189, 1969.
100. Masket, B. H., Levy, R. I., and Fredrickson, D. S.: The use of paper and polyacrylamide gel electrophoresis for phenotyping familial hyperlipoproteinemia. (in preparation).
101. Stone, M. C., and Thorp, J. M.: A new technique for the investigation of the low-density lipoproteins in health and disease. Clin. Chim. Acta, **14,** 812, 1966.
102. Meulendijk, P. N.: De directe Bepaling van "very low density"-lipoproteinen met de Nefelometer volgens Thorp. Nederl. T. Geneesk., **113,** 1348, 1969.
103. Cornwell, D. G., and Kruger, F. A.: Molecular complexes in isolation and characterization of plasma lipoproteins. J. Lipid Res., **2,** 110, 1961.
104. Burstein, M., and Moffin, R.: Precipitation of serum lipoproteins by anionic detergents in the presence of bivalent cations. Europ. J. Clin. Biol. Res., **15,** 109, 1970.
105. Eaton, R. P., and Kipnis, D. M.: Radioimmunoassay of beta lipoprotein-protein of rat serum. J. Clin. Invest., **48,** 1387, 1969.
106. Lees, R. S.: Immunoassay of plasma low-density lipoproteins. Science, **169,** 493, 1970.
107. Iglesias, A. M., Perez, P. R., Alonso, J. A. A., and Pascuau, F. J.: Consideraciones sobre los estados hiperlipémicos con aportación de dos casos. Rev. Clin. Esp., **103,** 32, 1966.

108. Knuchel, F.: Hyperlipidämien: Vorkommen, Bedeutung, Therapie. Med. Welt (Berlin), **32,** 1848, 1967.
109. Kahlke, W., Schettler, G., and Schlierf, G.: Die essentiellen Hyperlipämien. Deutsch. Med. J., **19,** 258, 1968.
110. Goto, Y., Katayama, T., and Nakamura, H.: Classification and etiology of hyperlipemia. Naika, **22,** 812, 1968.
111. Lloyd, J. K.: Disorders of the serum lipoproteins. II. Hyperlipoproteinemic states. Arch. Dis. Child., **43,** 505, 1968.
112. Ciswicka-Sznajderman, M.: Investigations on primary hyperlipoproteinemias. I. Clinical symptoms and serum lipid level. Pol. Med. J., **7,** 524, 1968.
113. Dyerberg, J.: Lipoproteinmønstret ved hyperlipidaemi. Ugeskr. Laeg., **130,** 359, 1968.
114. Goto, Y., and Nakamura, H.: Studies on hyperlipidemia among Japanese. Israel J. Med. Sci., **5,** 661, 1969.
115. Sanbar, S. S.: *Hyperlipidemia and Hyperlipoproteinemia.* Little, Brown and Company, Boston, 1969, 153 pp.
116. Loeper, J., Tricot, R., Loeper, J., and Rouffy, J.: Valeur du lipidogramme (technique de Lees et Hatch) pour le depistage et la classification des hyperlipoproteinémies. Presse Med., **77,** 171, 1969.
117. Galazka, A., Kayzer, Z., Plamieniak, Z., and Smolik, R.: Hiperlipoproteinemia pierwotna: two cases. Przegl. Lek., **25,** 430, 1969.
118. Forster, G.: Zur Klinik und Einteilung der Hyperlipidämien. Med. Welt. (Berlin), **28,** 1553, 1969.
119. Schatz, I. J.: Classification of primary hyperlipidemia: observations on 214 patients. J.A.M.A., **210,** 701, 1969.
120. Havel, R. J.: Typing of hyperlipoproteinemias. Atherosclerosis, **11,** 3, 1970.
121. de Gennes, J.-L., Polonovski, J., Ayrault-Jarrier, M., Bard, D., and Levy, G.: Étude analytique des lipoproteines par ultracentrifugation preparatrice dans 21 cas d'hyperlipidémies majeures. Rev. Franc. Étud. Clin. Biol., **9,** 273, 1964.
122. de Gennes, J.-L., and Bouchon, J.-P.: Les Hyperlipémies ou hyperglyceridémies idiopathiques. Rev. Pratn., **15,** 4095, 1965.
123. de Gennes, J.-L., and Maunand, B.: Les hypercholesterolémies familiales. Rev. Pratn., **15,** 4068, 1965.
124. de Gennes, J.-L., Bouchon, J.-P., Godeau, P., Betourne, C., Camus, J. P., Levy, R., and Siquier, F.: Confrontation aux conceptions classiques de 14 cas personnels d'hyperlipémie. Sem. Hop. Paris, **41,** 263, 1965.
125. Pries, C., Van Gent, C. M., Baes, H., Polano, M. K., Hulsman, H. A. M., and Querido, A.: Primary hyperlipoproteinemia: the clinico-chemical classification of the most common types. Clin. Chim. Acta, **19,** 181, 1968.
126. Baes, H., Polano, M. K., Pries, C., and Van Gent, C. M.: Distribution of various forms of xanthomata in three types of primary hyperlipoproteinemia. Dermatologica (Basel), **136,** 300, 1968.
127. Polano, M. K.: Cutaneous xanthomatosis in relation to the blood lipoprotein pattern. Brit. J. Derm., **81,** suppl. 2, 39, 1969.
128. Polano, M. K., Baes, H., Hulsmans, H. A. M., Querido, A., Pries, C., and van Gent, C. M.: Xanthomata in primary hyperlipoproteinemia: a classification based on the lipoprotein pattern of the blood. Arch. Derm., **100,** 387, 1969.
129. Total cholesterol procedure N-24b, in *Auto Analyzer Manual.* Technicon Instruments Corp., Chauncey, N.Y., 1964.
130. Kessler, G., and Lederer, H.: Fluorometric measurement of triglycerides: automation in analytical chemistry, in *Technicon Symposia, 1965,* edited by L. T. Skeggs, Jr., p. 341. Medial, Inc., New York, 1966.
131. Burstein, M., and Samaille, J.: Sur un dosage rapide du cholesterol lié aux α- et aux β-lipoprotéines du sérum. Clin. Chim. Acta, **5,** 609, 1960.
132. Friedewald, W. T., Levy, R. T., and Fredrickson, D. S.: In preparation.
133. Harlan, W. R., Jr.: A nomogram for determining types of hyperlipidemia. Arch. Intern. Med., **124,** 64, 1969.
134. Bürger, M., and Grütz, O.: Über Hepatosplenomegale lipoidose mit xanthomatösen Veränderungen in Haut und Schleimhaut. Arch. Derm. Syph., **166,** 542, 1932.
135. Knittle, J. L., and Ahrens, E. H., Jr.: Carbohydrate metabolism in two forms of hyperglyceridemia. J. Clin. Invest., **43,** 485, 1964.
136. Ahrens, E. H., Jr.: Personal communication.
137. Levy, B. M.: Idiopathic lipemia. J. Pediat., **29,** 367, 1946.
138. Bradford, R. H., and Furman, R. H.: Plasma post-heparin lipolytic activity in hyperchylomicronemia (fat-induced lipemia). Biochim. Biophys. Acta, **164,** 172, 1968.
139. Gaskins, A. L., Scott, R. B., and Kessler, A. D.: Report of three cases of idiopathic familial hyperlipemia: use of ACTH and cortisone. Pediatrics, **2,** 480, 1953.
140. Havel, R. J., and Gordon, R. S., Jr.: Idiopathic hyperlipemia: metabolic studies in an affected family. J. Clin. Invest., **39,** 1777, 1960.
141. Fredrickson, D. S., Ono, K., and Davis, L. L.: Lipolytic activity of postheparin plasma in hyperglyceridemia. J. Lipid Res., **4,** 24, 1963.
142. Levy, R. I. and Fredrickson, D. S.: Unpublished data.
143. Lloyd, J. K.: Personal communication.
144. Havel, R. J.: Personal communication.
144*a*. Havel, R. J.: Diagnosis of hyperlipoproteinemias. Calif. Med., **110,** 519, 1969.
145. Kuo, P. T., and Bassett, D. R.: Primary hyperlipidemias and their management. Ann. Intern. Med., **59,** 495, 1963.
146. Kuo, P., Bassett, D., DiGorge, A., and Carpenter, G.: Lipolytic activity of post-heparin plasma in hyperlipemia and hypolipemia. Circulation Res., **16,** 221, 1965.
147. Hudson, P., and Moon, J. H.: Discussants: H. P. Royster, A. J. Wasserman, and F. Davis, Clinicopathological conference, case historys. Va. Med. Mon., **92,** 321, 1965.
148. Harlan, W. R., Jr., Winesett, P. S., and Wasserman, A. J.: Tissue lipoprotein lipase in normal individuals and in individuals with exogenous hypertriglyceridemia and the relationship of this enzyme to assimilation of fat. J. Clin. Invest., **46,** 239, 1967.
149. Kuo, P. T.: Personal communication.
150. Farquhar, J. W.: Personal communication.
151. Havel, R. J.: Evidence for the participation of lipoprotein lipase in the transport of chylomicrons, in *Blood Lipids and the Clearing Factor,* Third International Conference on Biochemical Problems of Lipids, p. 265. K. Vlaamse Acad., Brussels, 1956.
152. Greten, H., Levy, R. I., and Fredrickson, D. S.: Evidence for separate monoglyceride hydrolase and triglyceride lipase in post-heparin human plasma. J. Lipid Res., **10,** 326, 1969.
153. Greten, H., Levy, R. I., Fales, H., and Fredrickson, D. S.: Hydrolysis of diglyceride and glyceryl monoester diethers with lipoprotein lipase. Biochim. Biophys. Acta, **210,** 39, 1970.
154. LaRosa, J. C., Levy, R. I., Windmueller, H. G., and Fredrickson, D. S.: Evidence for two triglyceride lipases in post-heparin plasma. J. Clin. Invest., **49,** 55a, 1970.
155. Glueck, C. J., Levy, R. I., Glueck, H. I., Gralnick, H. R., Greten, H., and Fredrickson, D. S.: Acquired type I hyperlipoproteinemia with systemic lupus erythematosus, dysglobulinemia and heparin resistance. Amer. J. Med., **47,** 318, 1969.
156. Glueck, C. J., Kaplan, A. P., Levy, R. I., Greten, H., Gralnick, H., and Fredrickson, D. S.: A new mechanism of exogenous hyperglyceridemia. Ann. Intern. Med., **71,** 1051, 1969.
157. Abegg, W.: Ein Fall von hochgradiger alimentärer "hepatogener" Fettretention im Blut bei einem ll-jährigen Kinde. Jahrb. Kinderheilk., **149,** 94, 1937.
158. Bernstein, S. S., Williams, H. H., Hummel, F. C., Shepherd, M. L., and Erickson, B. N.: Metabolic observations on a child with essential hyperlipemia. J. Pediat., **14,** 570, 1939.
159. Goodman, M., Shuman, J., and Goodman, S.: Idiopathic lipemia with secondary xanthomatosis, hepatosplenomegaly, and lipemic retinalis. J. Pediat., **16,** 596, 1940.
160. Hopgood, W. C.: Idiopathic hyperlipemia. New Eng. J. Med., **238,** 429, 1948.
161. Kennedy, R. L. J., and Collett, R. W.: Chronic relapsing pancreatitis and hyperlipemia. Amer. J. Dis. Child., **78,** 80, 1949.
162. Poulsen, H. M.: Familial lipaemia: a new form of lipoidosis showing increase in neutral fats combined with attacks of acute pancreatitis. Acta Med. Scand., **138,** 413, 1950.
163. Crocker, A. C.: Skin xanthomas in childhood. Pediatrics, **8,** 573, 1951.

164. Bruton, O. C., and Kanter, A. J.: Idiopathic familial hyperlipemia. Amer. J. Dis. Child., **82**, 153, 1951.
165. Klatskin, G., and Gordon, M.: Relationship between relapsing pancreatitis and essential hyperlipemia. Amer. J. Med., **12**, 3, 1952.
166. Hetzel, P. S.: Idiopathic hyperlipaemia: with a report of two cases occurring in one family, and a review of the literature. Med. J. Aust., **2**, 396, 1951.
167. Rausen, A. R., and Adlersberg, D.: Idiopathic (hereditary) hyperlipemia and hypercholesteremia in children. Pediatrics, **28**, 276, 1961.
168. Binkowska-Fellmann, K.: Hiperlipemia samoistna U 4-tygodniowego neimowlecia. Pediat. Pol., **33**, 325, 1958.
169. Bialkin, G., Zucker, S., Sklarin, B. S., Hirschhorn, K., and Davidson, M.: A genetic and metabolic study of a family with hyperlipemia. Pediatrics, **29**, 566, 1962.
170. Baba, N., and Volk, T. L.: Idiopathic hyperlipemia. Amer. J. Dis. Child., **108**, 633, 1964.
171. Rozynkowa, D., Paluszak, J., Borowczyk, T., and Rakowski, W.: Hiperlipidemia samoistna, poszukiwanie detektu metabolicznego jego rodzinnego pochodzenia. Pol. Arch. Med. Wewnet., **37**, 61, 1966.
172. Rozynkowa, D., Paluszak, J., Borowczyk, T., and Rakowski, W.: Idiopathic hyperlipidemia: search for a metabolic defect and its familial origin. Pol. Med. J., **6**, 429, 1967.
173. Braunsteiner, H., Berger, H., Sailer, S., and Sandhofer, F.: Utersuchungen bei einem Fall von fettinduzierter (exogener) Hypertriglyceridämie. Schweiz. Med. Wschr., **98**, 458, 1968.
174. Neerhout, R. C.: Erythrocyte stromal lipids in hyperlipemic states. J. Lab. Clin. Med., **71**, 448, 1968.
175. Vancsik, O., Vancsik, I., and Bolcas, D.: Consideratii pe marginea unui caz de hiperlipemie esentiala familiala la un sugar de 2 luni. Pediatria, **17**, 437, 1968.
176. Nevin, N. C., and Slack, J.: Hyperlipidaemic xanthomatosis. II. Mode of inheritance in 55 families with essential hyperlipidaemia and xanthomatosis. J. Med. Genet., **5**, 9, 1968.
177. Roberts, W. C., Levy, R. I., and Fredrickson, D. S.: Hyperlipoproteinemia, a review of the five types with first report of necropsy findings in type 3. Arch. Path., **90**, 46, 1970.
178. Robinson, D. S., Jeffries, G. H., and French, J. E.: Studies on the interaction of chyle and plasma in the rat. Quart. J. Exp. Physiol., **39**, 165, 1954.
179. Fredrickson, D. S., and Gordon, R. S., Jr.: Transport of fatty acids. Physiol. Rev., **38**, 585, 1958.
180. Robinson, D. S., and French, J. E.: Heparin, the clearing factor lipase, and fat transport. Pharmacol. Rev., **12**, 241, 1960.
181. Yoshitoshi, Y., Naito, C., Okaniwa, H., Usui, M., Mogami, T., and Tomono, T.: Kinetic studies on the metabolism of lipoprotein lipase. J. Clin. Invest., **42**, 707, 1963.
182. Kessler, J. I., Kniffen, J. C., and Janowitz, H. D.: Lipoprotein lipase inhibition in the hyperlipemia of acute alcoholic pancreatitis. New. Eng. J. Med., **269**, 943, 1963.
183. Bierman, E. L., Bagdade, J. D., and Porte, D., Jr.: Concept of pathogenesis of diabetic lipemia. Trans. Ass. Amer. Physicians, **79**, 348, 1966.
184. Hazzard, W. R., Spiger, M. J., Bagdade, J. D., and Bierman, E. L.: Studies on the mechanism of increased plasma triglyceride levels induced by oral contraceptives. New Eng. J. Med., **280**, 471, 1969.
185. Porte, D., Jr., O'Hara, D. D., and Williams, R. H.: Relation between postheparin lipolytic activity and plasma triglyceride in myxedema. Metabolism, **15**, 107, 1966.
186. Gallin, J. I., Kaye, D., and O'Leary, W. M.: Serum lipids in infection. New Eng. J. Med., **281**, 1981, 1969.
187. Bloomfield, A. L., and Shenson, B.: The syndrome of idiopathic hyperlipemia with crises of violent abdominal pain. Stanford Med. Bull., **5**, 185, 1947.
188. Tanaka, Y., Brecher, G., and Fredrickson, D. S.: Cellules de la maladie de Niemann-Pick et de quelques autres lipoïdoses. Nouv. Rev. Franc. Hemat., **3**, 5, 1963.
189. Schultze, W. H.: Über grosszellige Hyperplasie der Milz bei Lipoidaemie. Verh. Deutsch. Ges. Path., **15**, 47, 1912.
190. Warren, S., and Root, H. F.: Lipoid containing cells in the spleen in diabetes with lipemia. Amer. J. Path., **2**, 69, 1926.
191. Zieve, L.: Jaundice, hyperlipemia and hemolytic anemia: heretofore unrecognized syndrome associated with alcoholic fatty liver and cirrhosis. Ann. Intern. Med., **48**, 471, 1958.
192. Zieve, L.: Relationship between acute pancreatitis and hyperlipemia. Med. Clin. N. Amer., **52**, 1493, 1968.
193. Hagberg, B., Hultquist, G., Svennerholm, L., and Voss, H.: Malignant hyperlipemia in infancy. Amer. J. Dis. Child., **107**, 267, 1964.
194. Lusher, J., and Farber, S. D.: Another case of malignant hyperlipemia in infancy? Amer. J. Dis. Child., **108**, 211, 1964.
195. Campbell, S., and Carre, I. J.: Fatal haemolytic uraemic syndrome and idiopathic hyperlipaemia in monozygotic twins. Arch. Dis. Child., **40**, 654, 1965.
196. Blanchette-Mackie, E. J., and Scow, R. O.: Sites of lipoprotein lipase activity in perfused adipose tissue: electron microscopic, cytochemical study. J. Cell. Biol. (in press).
197. Zilversmit, D. B.: The composition and structure of lymph chylomicrons in dog, rat, and man. J. Clin. Invest., **44**, 1610, 1965.
198. Zilversmit, D. B.: The surface coat of chylomicrons: lipid chemistry. J. Lipid Res., **9**, 180, 1968.
199. Dole, V. P., and Hamlin, J. T., III: Particulate fat in lymph and blood. Physiol. Rev., **42**, 674, 1962.
200. Havel, R. J.: Metabolism of lipids in chylomicrons and very low density lipoproteins, in *Handbook of Physiology,* sect. 5, Adipose Tissue, edited by A. E. Renold and G. F. Cahill, Jr., p. 499. American Physiological Society, Washington, 1965, 824 pp.
201. Scow, R. O.: Transport of triglyceride: its removal from blood circulation and uptake by tissues, in *Parenteral Nutrition,* edited by H. C. Meng and D. H. Law, chap. 24, Charles C Thomas, Springfield, Ill., 1970.
202. Havel, R. J., and Fredrickson, D. S.: The metabolism of chylomicra. I. The removal of palmitic acid-l-C^{14} labeled chylomicra from dog plasma. J. Clin. Invest., **35**, 1025, 1956.
203. French, J. E., and Morris, B.: The removal of ^{14}C-labeled chylomicron fat from the circulation in rats. J. Physiol., **138**, 326, 1957.
204. Fredrickson, D. S., McCollester, D. L., and Ono, K.: The role of unesterified fatty acid transport in chylomicron metabolism. J. Clin. Invest., **37**, 1333, 1958.
205. Havel, R. J., and Goldfien, A.: The role of the liver and of extrahepatic tissues in the transport and metabolism of fatty acids and triglycerides in the dog. J. Lipid Res., **2**, 389, 1961.
206. Nestel, P. J.: Relationship between plasma triglycerides and removal of chylomicrons. J. Clin. Invest., **43**, 943, 1964.
207. Bragdon, J. H., and Gordon, R. S., Jr.: Tissue distribution of C^{14} after the intravenous injection of labeled chylomicrons and unesterified fatty acids in the rat. J. Clin. Invest., **37**, 574, 1958.
208. Borgström, B., and Jordan, P.: Metabolism of chylomicron glyceride as studied by C^{14}-glycerol-C^{14}-palmitic acid labeled chylomicrons. Acta Soc. Med. Upsal., **64**, 185, 1959.
209. Olivecrona, T.: Metabolism of chylomicrons labeled with ^{14}C-glycerol-^{3}H-palmitic acid in the rat. J. Lipid Res., **3**, 1, 1962.
210. Robinson, D. S.: The uptake and release of lipids by the liver, in *Proceedings of an International Symposium on Lipid Transport,* edited by H. C. Meng, J. G. Coniglio, V. S. LeQuire, G. V. Mann, and J. M. Merrill, p. 194. Charles C. Thomas, Springfield, Ill., 1964.
211. Olivecrona, T., and Belfrage, P.: Mechanisms for removal of chyle triglyceride from the circulating blood as studied with ^{14}C-glycerol and ^{3}H-palmitic acid labeled chyle. Biochim. Biophys. Acta, **98**, 81, 1965.
212. Barry, J. M., Bartley, W., Linzell, J. L., and Robinson, D. S.: The uptake from blood of triglyceride fatty acids of chylomicra and low-density lipoproteins by the mammary gland of the goat. Biochem. J., **89**, 6, 1963.
213. McBride, O. W., and Korn, E. D.: The uptake of doubly labeled chylomicrons by guinea pig mammary gland and liver. J. Lipid Res., **5**, 459, 1964.
214. Redgrave, T. G.: Formation of cholesteryl ester-rich particulate lipid during metabolism of chylomicrons. J. Clin. Invest., **49**, 465, 1970.
215. Goodman, DeW. S.: The metabolism of chylomicron cholesterol ester in the rat. J. Clin. Invest., **41**, 1886, 1962.
216. Quarfordt, S. H., and Goodman, DeW. S.: Metabolism of doubly-labeled chylomicron cholesteryl esters in the rat. J. Lipid Res., **8**, 264, 1967.

217. Majno, G.: Ultrastructure of the vascular membrane, in *Handbook of Physiology,* sec. 2, Circulation, edited by W. F. Hamilton and P. Dow, vol. 3, chap. 64, pp. 2293–2375. American Physiological Society, Washington, 1965.
218. DiLuzio, N. R., and Riggi, S. J.: The relative participation of hepatic parenchymal and Kupffer cells in the metabolism of chylomicrons. J. Reticuloendothelial Soc. (RES), **1,** 248, 1964.
219. Stein, O., and Stein, Y.: The role of the liver in the metabolism of chylomicrons, studied by electron microscopic autoradiography. Lab. Invest., **17,** 436, 1967.
220. Felts, J. M.: The metabolism of chylomicron triglyceride fatty acids by perfused rat livers and by intact rats. Ann. N.Y. Acad. Sci., **131,** 24, 1965.
221. Robinson, J., and Newsholme, E. A.: Glycerol kinase activities in rat heart and adipose tissue. Biochem. J., **104,** 20, 1967.
222. Levine, R., and Haft, D. E.: Carbohydrate homeostasis. New Eng. J. Med., **283,** 237, 1970.
223. Nikkilä, E. A.: Control of plasma and liver triglyceride kinetics by carbohydrate metabolism and insulin. Advances Lipid Res., **7,** 63, 1969.
224. Kessler, J. I.: Effect of diabetes and insulin on activity of myocardial and adipose tissue lipoprotein lipase of rats. J. Clin. Invest., **42,** 362, 1963.
225. Schnatz, J. D., and Williams, R. H.: Effect of acute insulin deficiency in the rat on adipose tissue lipolytic activity and plasma lipids. Diabetes, **12,** 174, 1963.
226. Hahn, P. F.: Abolishment of alimentary lipemia following injection of heparin. Science, **98,** 19, 1943.
227. Korn, E. D.: Clearing factor, a heparin-activated lipoprotein lipase. II. Substrate specificity and activation of cocoanut oil. J. Biol. Chem., **214,** 15, 1955.
228. Fielding, C. J., Lim, C. T., and Scanu, A. M.: A protein component of serum high density lipoprotein with co-factor activity against purified lipoprotein lipase. Biochem. Biophys. Res. Commun., **39,** 889, 1970.
229. Havel, R. J., Shore, V. G., Shore, B., and Bier, D. M.: Role of specific glycopeptides in the activation of lipoprotein lipase. Circ. Res., **27,** 595, 1970.
230. LaRosa, J. C., Levy, R. I., Herbert, P., Lux, S. E., and Fredrickson, D. S.: A specific apoprotein cofactor for lipoprotein lipase. Biochem. Biophys. Res. Commun. **41,** 57, 1970.
231. Korn, E. D.: The assay of lipoprotein lipase *in vivo* and *in vitro,* in *Methods of Biochemical Analysis,* vol. VII, p. 145. Interscience, New York, 1959.
232. Robinson, D. S.: The clearing factor lipase and its action in the transport of fatty acids between the blood and the tissues. Advances Lipid Res. **1,** 133, 1963.
233. Vaughan, M.: The metabolism of adipose tissue *in vitro.* J. Lipid Res., **2,** 293, 1961.
234. Vaughan, M., and Steinberg, D.: Glyceride biosynthesis, glyceride breakdown and glycogen breakdown in adipose tissue: mechanisms and regulation, in *Handbook of Physiology,* sec. 5, Adipose Tissue, edited by A. E. Renold and G. F. Cahill, Jr., chap. 24, pp. 239–251. American Physiological Society, Washington, 1965.
235. Ho, S. J., Ho, R. J., and Meng, H. C.: Comparison of heparin-released and epinephrine-sensitive lipases in rat adipose tissue. Amer. J. Physiol., **212,** 284, 1967.
236. Rizack, M. A.: Activation of an epinephrine-sensitive lipolytic activity from adipose tissue by adenosine 3′,5′-phosphate. J. Biol. Chem., **239,** 392, 1964.
237. Wing, D. R., and Robinson, D. S.: Clearing-factor lipase in adipose tissue: a possible role of adenosine 3′-5′-(cyclic)-monophosphate in the regulation of its activity. Biochem. J., **109,** 841, 1968.
238. Korn, E. D.: Inactivation of lipoprotein lipase by heparinase. J. Biol. Chem., **226,** 827, 1957.
239. Patten, R. L., and Hollenberg, C. H.: The mechanism of heparin stimulation of rat adipocyte lipoprotein lipase. J. Lipid Res., **10,** 374, 1969.
240. Shore, B., and Shore, V.: Heparin-released lipolytic and esterolytic activities of human and rabbit plasmas. Amer. J. Physiol., **201,** 915, 1961.
241. Vogel, W. C., and Zieve, L.: Post-heparin phospholipase. J. Lipid Res., **5,** 177, 1964.
242. Dahlback, O., Hansson, R., and Tibbling, G.: The effect of heparin on diamine oxidase and lipoprotein lipase in human lymph and blood plasma. Scand. J. Clin. Lab. Invest., **21,** 17, 1968.
243. McBride, O. W., and Korn, E. D.: The lipoprotein lipase of mammary gland and the correlation of its activity to lactation. J. Lipid Res., **4,** 17, 1963.
244. Robinson, D. S.: Changes in the lipolytic activity of the guinea pig mammary gland at parturition. J. Lipid Res., **4,** 21, 1963.
245. LeQuire, V. S., Hamilton, R. L., Adams, R., and Merrill, J. M.: Lipase activity in blood from the hepatic and peripheral vascular beds following heparin. Proc. Soc. Exp. Biol. Med., **114,** 104, 1963.
246. Boberg, J., Carlson, L. A., and Normell, L.: Production of lipolytic activity by the isolated perfused dog liver in response to heparin. Biochem. J., **92,** 43P, 1964.
247. Carter, J. R., Jr.: Hepatic lipase in the rat. Biochim. Biophys. Acta, **137,** 147, 1967.
248. Rodbell, M., and Scow, R. O.: Chylomicron metabolism: uptake and metabolism by perfused adipose tissue, in *Handbook of Physiology,* sec. 5, Adipose Tissue, edited by A. E. Renold and G. F. Cahill, Jr., chap. 49, p. 491. American Physiological Society, Washington, 1965.
249. Schoefl, G. I., and French, J. E.: Vascular permeability to particulate fat: morphological observations on vessels of lactating mammary gland and of lung. Proc. Roy. Soc. [Biol], **169,** 153, 1968.
250. Alousi, A. A., and Mallov, S.: Effects of hyperthyroidism, epinephrine, and diet on heart lipoprotein lipase activity. Amer. J. Physiol., **206,** 603, 1964.
251. Jeffries, G. H.: The site at which plasma clearing activity is produced and destroyed in the rat. Quart. J. Exp. Physiol., **39,** 261, 1954.
252. Whayne, T. F., Jr., Felts, J. M., and Harris, P. A.: Effect of heparin on the inactivation of serum lipoprotein lipase by the liver in unanesthetized dogs. J. Clin. Invest., **48,** 1246, 1969.
253. Naito, C., and Felts, J. M.: Influence of heparin on the removal of serum lipoprotein lipase by the perfused liver of the rat. J. Lipid Res., **11,** 48, 1970.
254. Diengott, D., and Kerpel, S.: Lipoprotein lipase in human adipose tissue. Israel J. Med. Sci., **1,** 1015, 1965.
255. Boberg, J., and Carlson, L. A.: Determination of heparin induced lipoprotein lipase activity in human plasma. Clin. Chim. Acta, **10,** 420, 1964.
256. Boberg, J.: Quantitative determination of heparin released lipoprotein lipase activity in human plasma. Lipids, **5,** 452, 1970.
257. Biale, Y., and Shafrir, E.: Lipolytic activity toward tri- and monoglycerides in postheparin plasma. Clin. Chim. Acta, **23,** 413, 1969.
258. Quarfordt, S. H., and Goodman, D. S.: Heterogeneity in rate of plasma clearance of chylomicrons of different size. Biochim. Biophys. Acta, **116,** 382, 1966.
259. Steiner, G.: Lipoprotein lipase in fat-induced hyperlipemia. New Eng. J. Med., **279,** 70, 1968.
260. Herbert, P., LaRosa, J., Krauss, R., Lux, S., Levy, R. I., and Fredrickson, D. S.: On the lipolytic defect in familial type I hyperlipoproteinemia. J. Clin. Invest. (abstract) (in press).
261. Parker, F., Bagdade, J. D., Odland, G. F., and Bierman, E. L.: Evidence for the chylomicron origin of lipids accumulating in diabetic eruptive xanthomas: a correlative lipid biochemical, histochemical and electron microscopic study. J. Clin. Invest. **49,** 2172, 1970.
262. Hers, H. G.: Inborn lysosomal diseases. Gastroenterology, **48,** 625, 1965.
263. Bagdade, J. D., and Ways, P. O.: Erythrocyte membrane lipid composition in exogenous and endogenous hypertriglyceridemia. J. Lab. Clin. Med., **75,** 53, 1970.
264. Ahrens, E. H., Jr.: Essential hyperlipemia (discussion 4a), in *Fat Metabolism,* edited by V. A. Najjar, p. 61. Johns Hopkins, Baltimore, 1954.
265. Chapman, F. D., and Kinney, T. D.: Idiopathic lipemia. Amer. J. Dis. Child., **62,** 1014, 1941.
266. Schizas, A. A., Creman, J. A., Latson, E., and O'Brien, R.: Medium-chain triglycerides—use in food preparation. J. Amer. Diet. Ass., **51,** 228, 1967.
267. Greenberger, N. J., and Skillman, T. G.: Medical progress, medium-chain triglycerides, physiologic considerations and clinical implications. New Eng. J. Med., **280,** 1045, 1969.
268. Fredrickson, D. S., Levy, R. I., Jones, E., Bonell, M., and Ernst, N.:

The Dietary Management of Hyperlipoproteinemia: A Handbook for Physicians. U.S. Dept. of Health, Education, and Welfare, Public Health Service, Washington, 1970, 83 pp.

269. Rowland, R. S.: Xanthomatosis and the reticuloendothelial system. Arch. Intern. Med., **42,** 611, 1928.
270. Urbach, E.: Lipoid Stoffwechsellerkrankungen der haut, in *Handbuch der Haut- und Geschlechtskrankheiten,* edited by J. Jadassohn, vol. 12, p. 238. Springer, Berlin, 1932.
271. Polano, K.: Über die Pathogenese der Cholesteren der Haut. Arch. Derm. Syph., **213,** 1936.
272. Montgomery, H., and Osterberg, A. I.: Xanthomatosis: correlation of clinical, histopathologic and chemical studies of cutaneous xanthoma. Arch. Derm. Syph., **37,** 373, 1938.
273. Thannhauser, S. J.: *Lipidoses: Diseases of the Cellular Lipid Metabolism,* 3d ed. Grune & Stratton, New York, 1958.
274. Kornerup, V.: *Familiaer Hypercholesteroaemia og Xanthomatose.* Kolding, Denmark, 1948, 211 pp.
275. Boas, E. P., Parets, A. D., and Adlersberg, D.: Hereditary disturbance of cholesterol metabolism: a factor in the genesis of atherosclerosis. Amer. Heart J., **35,** 611, 1948.
276. Stecher, R. M., and Hersh, A. H.: Note on the genetics of hypercholesterolemia. Science, **109,** 61, 1949.
277. Alvord, R. M.: Coronary heart disease and xanthoma tuberosum associated with hereditary hyperlipemia: study of 30 affected persons in family. Arch. Intern. Med., **84,** 1002, 1949.
278. Adlersberg, D.: Hypercholesteremia with predisposition to atherosclerosis: an inborn error of lipid metabolism. Amer. J. Med., **11,** 600, 1951.
279. Schaefer, L. E., Drachman, S. R., Steinberg, A. G., and Adlersberg, D.: Genetic studies on hypercholesteremia: frequency in a hospital population and in families of hypercholesteremic index patients. Amer. Heart J., **46,** 99, 1953.
280. Leonard, J. C.: Hereditary hypercholesterolaemic xanthomatosis. Lancet, **2,** 1239, 1956.
281. Piper, J., and Orrild, L.: Essential familial hypercholesterolemia and xanthomatosis: follow-up study of twelve Danish families. Amer. J. Med., **21,** 34, 1956.
282. Wheeler, E. O.: The genetic aspects of atherosclerosis. Amer. J. Med., **23,** 653, 1957.
283. Harris-Jones, J. N.: Hyperuricemia and essential hypercholesterolemia. Lancet, **1,** 857, 1957.
284. Epstein, F. H., Block, W. D., Hand, E. A., and Francis, T. F., Jr.: Familial hypercholesterolemia, xanthomatosis and coronary heart disease. Amer. J. Med., **26,** 39, 1959.
285. Osborne, R. H., Adlersberg, D., DeGeorge, F. W., and Wang, C.: Serum lipids, heredity and environment: a study of adult twins. Amer. J. Med., **26,** 54, 1959.
286. Hirschhorn, K., and Wilkinson, C. F.: The mode of inheritance in essential familial hypercholesterolemia. Amer. J. Med., **26,** 60, 1959.
287. Khachadurian, A. K.: The inheritance of essential familial hypercholesterolemia. Amer. J. Med., **37,** 402, 1964.
288. Meilman, E., Holtzman, C. M., and Samuel, P.: Familial hypercholesterolemia and xanthomatosis. Amer. J. Med., **36,** 277, 1964.
289. Vaillaud, J. C., Sabatini, R., Revol, A., Biot, N., Trouyez, R., and Sarrouy, Ch.: Xanthomatose hypercholestérolémique familiale. Lyon Med., **215,** 385, 1966.
290. Harlan, W. R., Jr., Graham, J. B., and Estes, E. H.: Familial hypercholesterolemia: a genetic and metabolic study. Medicine, **45,** 77, 1966.
291. Nitter-Hauge S.: "Juvenile" xanthomatosis—a recessive inherited disease? Acta Med. Scand., **179,** 71, 1966.
292. Sobra, J.: Inborn errors of lipid metabolism. XIII. Familial hypercholesterolemic xanthomatosis, a review of the genealogical tree of 142 patients. Acta Univ. Carol. [Med.] (Praha), **13,** 295, 1967.
293. Miettinen, M.: Familial hypercholesterolaemic xanthomatosis and coronary heart disease in a ten-year-old girl. Ann. Paediat. Fenn., **13,** 35, 1967.
294. Lewis, B., and Myant, N. B.: Studies in the metabolism of cholesterol in subjects with normal plasma cholesterol levels and in patients with essential hypercholesterolaemia. Clin. Sci., **32,** 201, 1967.
295. Jensen, J., Blankenhorn, D. H., and Kornerup, V.: Coronary disease in familial hypercholesterolemia. Circulation, **36,** 77, 1967.
296. de Gennes, J.-L., Touraine, R., Maunand, B., Truffert, J., and Laudat, M. P.: Formes homozygotes cutanéo-tendineuses de xanthomatose hypercholestérolémique dans une observation familiale exemplaire. Essai de plasmaphérèse à titre de traitement héroïque. Bull. Soc. Med. Hop. Paris, **118,** 1377, 1967.
297. Mishkel, M. A.: The diagnosis and management of the patient with xanthomatosis. An experience with thirty-five cases. Quart. J. Med., **36,** 107, 1967.
298. Buchwald, H., Lee, G. B., and Amplatz, K.: Severe atherosclerotic cardiovascular disease in a 14-year-old homozygous familial hypercholesterolemic. Minn. Med., **51,** 477, 1968.
299. Watanabe, T., Tanaka, K, Yanai, N.: Essential familial hypercholesteremic xanthomatosis—an autopsy case with special reference to the pathogenesis of cardiovascular lipidosis. Acta Path. Jap., **18,** 319, 1968.
300. Hould, F., Leclerc, R., and Marcoux, J.: Essential familial hypercholesterolemia with xanthomatosis. Pediatrics, **43,** 455, 1969.
301. Horan, J. M., DiLuzio, N. R., and Etteldorf, J. N.: Use of an anion exchange resin in treatment of two siblings with familial hypercholesterolemia. J. Pediat., **64,** 201, 1964.
302. Howard, R. P., Osvaldo, J. B., and Furman, R. H.: Effect of cholestyramine administration on serum lipids and on nitrogen balance in familial hypercholesterolemia. J. Lab. Clin. Med., **68,** 12, 1966.
303. Fallon, H. J., and Woods, J. W.: Response of hyperlipoproteinemia and cholestyramine. J.A.M.A., **204,** 1161, 1968.
304. Khachadurian, A. K.: Cholestyramine therapy in patients homozygous for familial hypercholesterolemia (familial hypercholesterolemic xanthomatosis). J. Atheroscler. Res., **8,** 177, 1968.
305. Levy, R. I., Quarfordt, S. H., Brown, W. V., Sloan, H. R., and Fredrickson, D. S.: The efficacy of clofibrate (CPIB) in familial hyperlipoproteinemias, in *Drugs Affecting Lipid Metabolism,* edited by W. L. Holmes, L. A. Carlson, and R. Paoletti, p. 377. Plenum, New York, 1969. (Proceedings of the Third International Symposium on Drugs Affecting Lipid Metabolism, Milan, Italy, Sept. 8–11, 1968.)
306. Levy, R. I., and Fredrickson, D. S.: The current status of hypolipidemic drugs. Postgrad. Med., **47,** 130, 1970.
307. Kwiterovich, P. O., Levy, R. I., and Fredrickson, D. S.: Early detection and treatment of familial type II hyperlipoproteinemia. Circulation, **42,** III-11, 1970.
308. Slack, J., and Nevin, N. C.: Hyperlipidaemic xanthomatosis. I. Increased risk of death from ischaemic heart disease in first degree relatives of 53 patients with essential hyperlipidaemia and xanthomatosis. J. Med. Genet., **5,** 4, 1968.
309. Slack, J.: Risks of ischaemic heart-disease in familial hyperlipoproteinaemic states. Lancet, **2,** 1380, 1969.
310. Burstein, J., and Malm, C. W.: Familial hypercholesterolemic xanthomatosis and coronary disease. Acta Med. Scand., **175,** 569, 1964.
311. Laudat, P., Lefevre, M., Saltiel, H., and DeGennes, J.: Preliminary note on plasma fatty acids composition of the various lipid fractions in essential familial hypercholesterolaemia. J. Atheroscler. Res., **6,** 192, 1966.
312. Sohar, E., Bossak, E. T., Wang, C. I., and Adlersberg, D.: Serum components in the newborn. Science, **123,** 461, 1956.
313. Lee, G. B., Culley, G. A., Lawson, M. J., Adcock, L. L., and Krivit, W.: Type II hyperlipoproteinemia in mother and twins. Circulation, **39,** 183, 1969.
314. Lewis, L. A., Brown, H. B., and Green, J. G.: Serum cholesterol and lipoprotein levels of familial hypercholesteremic infants (P). Circulation, suppl. II, **35** and **36,** II-24, 1967.
315. Sperry, W. M., and Schick, B.: Essential xanthomatosis: treatment with cholesterol-free diet in two cases. Amer. J. Dis. Child., **51,** 1372, 1936.
316. Schick, B., and Sperry, W. M.: Essential xanthomatosis: fifteen years' observation on a case occurring in a family with hypercholesteremia. Amer. J. Dis. Child., **77,** 164, 1949.
317. Scott, P. J., and Winterbourn, C. C.: Low-density lipoprotein accumulation in actively growing xanthomas. J. Atheroscler. Res., **7,** 207, 1967.
318. Davis, J. A., Johnston, I. D. A., Moutafis, C. D., and Myant, N. B.: Ileal bypass in hypercholesterolaemia. Lancet, **2,** 971, 1966.

319. Kumbhani, A. P., Daftary, V. G., Yawalkar, S. J., and Mehta, S. P.: Xanthomatous aortic stenosis in familial hypercholesterolemia. Indian Heart J., **19**, 171, 1966.
320. Orsini, A., Perrimond, H., and Vo Van, L.: (Essential hypercholesteremia with cutaneous and tendinous xanthomatosis in a 14-year-old child), Marseille Med., **103**, 317, 1966.
321. Mishkel, M. A., and Freeman, Z.: Hypercholesterolaemic xanthomatosis: a case studied for three years. Med. J. Aust., **3**, 794, 1966.
322. Johnston, I. D., Davis, J. A., and Moutafis, C. D.: Ileal by-pass in the management of familial hypercholesterolaemia. Proc. Roy. Soc. Med., **60**, 746, 1967.
323. Aerichide, N., Gilbert, G., and David, P.: Insuffisance coronarienne chez un enfant de ll ans atteint d'une xanthomatose hypercholesterolémique. Laval Med., **39**, 955, 1968.
324. Khachadurian, A. K.: Migratory polyarthritis in familial hypercholesterolemia (type II hyperlipoproteinemia). Arthritis Rheum., **11**, 385, 1968.
325. Beaumont, J.-L., Jacotot, B., and Beaumont, V.: L'hyperlipdémie par auto-anticorps une cause d'atherosclerose. Presse Med., **75**, 2315, 1967.
326. van Bogaert, L., Froelich, A., and Epstein, E.: Une deuxième observation de cholestérinose tendineuse symétrique avec symptoms cérébraux. Ann. Med., **42**, 79, 1937.
327. Menkes, J. H., Schimschock, J. R., and Swanson, P. D.: Cerebrotendinous xanthomatosis. Arch. Neurol., **19**, 47, 1968.
328. Harlan, W. R., Jr., and Still, W. J. S.: Hereditary tendinous and tuberous xanthomatosis without hyperlipidemia: a new lipid storage disorder. New Eng. J. Med., **278**, 416, 1968.
329. Schimschock, J. R., Alvord, E. J., Jr., and Swanson, P. D.: Cerebrotendinous xanthomatosis. Arch. Neurol., **18**, 688, 1968.
330. Philippart, M., and van Bogaert, L.: Cholestanolosis (cerebrotendinous xanthomatosis). Arch. Neurol., **21**, 603, 1969.
331. Brusco, O. J., Howard, R. P., Jarman, J. B., and Furman, R. H.: Osseous xanthomatosis and pathologic fractures in familial hyperlipemia (hyperglyceridemia). Amer. J. Med., **40**, 477, 1966.
332. Glueck, C. J., Levy, R. I., and Fredrickson, D. S.: Acute tendinitis and arthritis—a presenting symptom of familial type II hyperlipoproteinemia. J.A.M.A., **206**, 2895, 1968.
333. Cook, G. D., Smith, H. L., Giesen, C. W., and Berdez, G. L.: Xanthoma tuberosum, aortic stenosis, coronary sclerosis and angina pectoris. Amer. J. Dis. Child., **73**, 326, 1947.
334. Rigdon, R. H., and Willeford, G.: Sudden death during childhood with xanthoma tuberosum. J.A.M.A., **142**, 1268, 1950.
335. Maher, J. A., Epstein, F. H., and Hand, E. A.: Xanthomatosis and coronary heart disease: necropsy studies of two affected siblings. Arch. Intern. Med., **102**, 437, 1958.
336. Stanley, P., Chartrand, C., and Davignon, A.: Acquired aortic stenosis in a twelve-year old girl with xanthomatosis. New Eng. J. Med., **273**, 1378, 1965.
337. deGennes, J.-L., and Thervet, F.: Détection d'un terrain d'hyperlipidémie familiale chez deux femmes victimes, avant l'âge de 30 ans, d'un accident vasculaire cérébral sous traitements par contraceptifs hormonaux. Bull. Acad. Nat. Med. (Paris), **151**, 450, 1967.
338. deGennes, J.-L., Rouffy, J., and Chain, F.: Complications vasculaires cérébrales des xanthomatoses tendineuses hypercholesterolémiques familiales. Soc. Med. Hop. Paris, **119**, 569, 1968.
339. Glueck, C. J., Levy, R. I., and Fredrickson, D. S.: Immunoreactive insulin, glucose tolerance and carbohydrate inducibility in types II, III, IV and V hyperlipoproteinemia. Diabetes, **18**, 739, 1969.
340. Jensen, J., Blankenhorn, D. H., and Kornerup, V.: Blood-uric-acid levels in familial hypercholesterolaemia. Lancet, **1**, 298, 1966.
341. Khachadurian, A. K.: Persistent elevation of the erythrocyte sedimentation rate (ESR) in familial hypercholesterolemia. J. Med. Liban., **20**, 31, 1967.
342. Lees, R. S., Song, C. S., Levere, R. D., and Kappas, A.: Hyperbetalipoproteinemia in acute intermittent porphyria. New Eng. J. Med., **282**, 432, 1970.
343. Lee, D., and Alaupovic, P.: Studies of the composition and structure of plasma lipoproteins. Isolation, composition and immunochemical characterization of low density lipoprotein subfractions of human plasma. Biochemistry, **9**, 2244, 1970.
344. Gotto, A. M., Levy, R. I., and Fredrickson, D. S.: Unpublished data.
345. Sloan, H. S., Kwiterovich, P. O., Levy, R. I., and Fredrickson, D. S.: Carbohydrate components of human plasma lipoproteins. Circulation, **42**, III-8, 1970.
346. Schönheimer, R.: Über eine Störung der Cholesterin-Ausscheidung. Klin. Med., **132**, 749, 1933.
347. Goodman, D. S.: Cholesterol ester metabolism. Physiol. Rev., **45**, 747, 1965.
348. Grundy, S. M., and Ahrens, E. H., Jr.: Measurements of cholesterol turnover, synthesis, and absorption in man, carried out by isotope kinetic and sterol balance methods. J. Lipid Res., **10**, 91, 1969.
349. Dietschy, J. M., and Wilson, J. D.: Regulation of cholesterol metabolism. New Eng. J. Med., **282**, 1128, 1179, and 1241, 1970.
350. Khachadurian, A. K.: Lack of inhibition of hepatic cholesterol synthesis by dietary cholesterol in cases of familial hypercholesterolaemia. Lancet, **2**, 778, 1969.
351. Hellman, L., Rosenfeld, R. S., and Gallagher, T. F.: Cholesterol synthesis from C^{14}-acetate in man. J. Clin. Invest., **33**, 142, 1954.
352. Hellman, L., Rosenfeld, R. S., Eidinoff, M. L., Fukushima, D. K., Gallagher, T. F., Wang, C.-I., and Adlersberg, D.: Isotopic studies of plasma cholesterol of endogenous and exogenous origins. J. Clin. Invest., **34**, 48, 1955.
353. Gee, D. J., Goldstein, J., Gray, C. H., and Fowler, J. F.: Biosynthesis of cholesterol in familial hypercholesterolaemic xanthomatosis. Brit. Med. J., **2**, 341, 1959.
354. Nestel, P. J., Couzens, E., and Hirsch, E. Z.: Comparison of turnover of individual cholesterol esters in subjects with low and high plasma cholesterol concentrations. J. Lab. Clin. Med., **66**, 582, 1965.
355. Nestel, P. J., and Monger, E. A.: Turnover of plasma esterified cholesterol in normocholesterolemic and hypercholesterolemic subjects and its relation to body build. J. Clin. Invest., **46**, 967, 1967.
356. Goodman, D. S., and Noble, R. P.: Turnover of plasma cholesterol in man. J. Clin. Invest., **47**, 231, 1968.
357. Nestel, P. J., Whyte, H. M., and Goodman, D. S.: Distribution and turnover of cholesterol in humans. J. Clin. Invest., **48**, 982, 1969.
358. Moutafis, C. D., and Myant, N. B.: The metabolism of cholesterol in two hypercholesteremic patients treated with cholestyramine. Clin. Sci., **37**, 443, 1969.
359. Samuel, P., and Perl, W.: Long-term decay of serum cholesterol radioactivity: body cholesterol metabolism in normals and in patients with hyperlipoproteinemia and atherosclerosis. J. Clin. Invest., **49**, 346, 1970.
360. Miettinen, T. A., Pelkonen, R., Nikkila, E. A., and Heinonen, O.: Low excretion of fecal bile acids in a family with hypercholesterolemia. Acta Med. Scand., **182**, 645, 1967.
361. Kottke, B. A.: Difference in bile acid excretion. Primary hypercholesterolemia compared to combined hypercholesterolemia and hypertriglyceridemia. Circulation, **40**, 13, 1969.
362. Volwiler, W., Goldsworthy, P. D., MacMartin, M. P., Wood, P. A., Mackay, I. R., and Fremont-Smith, K.: Biosynthetic determination with radioactive sulfur of turn-over rates of various plasma proteins in normal and cirrhotic man. J. Clin. Invest., **34**, 1126, 1955.
363. Gitlin, D., Cornwell, D. G., Nakasato, D., Oncley, J. L., Hughes, W. L., Jr., and Janeway, C. A.: Studies on metabolism of plasma proteins in nephrotic syndrome. II. Lipoproteins. J. Clin. Invest., **37**, 172, 1958.
364. Walton, K. W., Scott, P. J., Verrier-Jones, J., Fletcher, R. F., and Whitehead, T.: Studies on low density lipoprotein turnover in relation to atromid therapy. J. Atheroscler. Res., **3**, 396, 1963.
365. Walton, K. W., Scott, P. J., Dykes, P. W., and Davies, J. W. L.: Alterations of metabolism and turnover of I^{131} low density lipoprotein in myxoedema and thyrotoxicosis. Clin. Sci., **29**, 217, 1965.
366. Scott, P. J., and Hurley, P. J.: Effect of clofibrate on low-density lipoprotein turnover in essential hypercholesterolaemia. J. Atheroscler. Res., **9**, 25, 1969.
367. Langer, T., Strober, W., and Levy, R. I.: Familial type II hyperlipoproteinemia: a defect of beta apoprotein catabolism. J. Clin. Invest., **48**, 49a, 1969.

368. Scott, P. J., White, B. M., Winterbourn, C. C., and Hurley, P. J.: Low density lipoprotein peptide metabolism in nephrotic syndrome: a comparison with patterns observed in other syndromes characterized by hyperlipoproteinemia. Aust. Ann. Med., **1**, 1, 1970.

369. Hurley, P. J., and Scott, P. J.: Plasma turnover of S_f 0-9 low-density lipoprotein in normal men and women. J. Atheroscler. Res., **11**, 51, 1970.

370. Langer, T., and Levy, R. I.: Effect of nicotinic acid on beta lipoprotein metabolism. Clin. Res., **18**, 458, 1970.

371. Fredrickson, D. S.: Plasma lipid abnormalities and skin lesions (xanthoma) in *Dermatology in General Medicine,* edited by T. B. Fitzpatrick, et al., McGraw-Hill, New York, 1971.

372. Wilson, J. D.: Studies on the origin of the lipid components of xanthomata. Circulation Res., **12**, 472, 1963.

373. Fletcher, R. F., and Gloster, J.: The lipids in xanthomata. J. Clin. Invest., **43**, 2104, 1964.

374. Jepson, E. M., Billimoria, J. D., and MacLagan, N. F.: Serum and tissue lipids in patients with familial xanthomatosis. Clin. Sci., **29**, 383, 1965.

375. Baes, H., Gent, C. M. Van, Pries, C.: Lipid composition of various types of xanthoma. J. Invest. Derm., **51**, 286, 1968.

376. Tschetter, R. T.: Lipid analysis of the human cornea with and without arcus senilis. Arch. Ophthal., **76**, 403, 1966.

377. Cornfield, J.: Joint dependence of risk of coronary heart disease on serum cholesterol and systolic blood pressure: a discriminant function analysis. Fed. Proc., **21**, part II, suppl. 11, 58, 1962.

378. Guravich, J. L., and Venegas, J.: Familial hypercholesterolemia. Fed. Proc., **21**, 44, 1962.

379. Fredrickson, D. S., and Levy, R. I.: Type II and Type III hyperlipoproteinemia II. Clinical and genetic features (in preparation).

380. Glueck, C. J., Heckman, F., Schonfeld, M., Steiner, P., and Pearce, W.: Neonatal familial type II hyperlipoproteinemia: cord blood cholesterol in 1660 births. Circulation, **42**, III-11, 1970.

381. Carlson, L. A., and Sterner, G.: Essential hypercholesterolaemia in two siblings. Acta Paediat., **49**, 168, 1960.

382. Vrana, J., Vykydal, M., and Pegrimova, E.: (Hypercholesterolemic xanthomatosis) (Cze). Cas. Lek. Cesk., **105**, 1383, 1966.

383. Kleinbaum, H., Zöllner, H., and Hessel, D.: Untersuchungen zur essentiellen Hypercholesterinämie im Kindesalter. Arch. Kinderheilk., **175**, 113, 1967.

384. Giampalmo, A.: Heredo-familial hypercholesterinemic xanthomatosis Minerva Med. Roma, **59**, 2125, 1968.

385. Gulati, P. D., and Vyas, P. B.: Hypercholesteraemic xanthomatosis. J. Indian Med. Ass., **48**, 500, 1967.

386. Quarfordt, S. H., De Vivo, D. C., Engel, W. K., Levy, R. I., and Fredrickson, D. S.: Familial adult-onset proximal spinal muscular atrophy. Arch. Neurol., **22**, 541, 1970.

387. Berg, K.: New serum type system: Lp system. Acta Path. Microbiol. Scand., **59**, 369, 1963.

388. Segall, M. M., Fosbrooke, A. S., Lloyd, J. K., and Wolfe, O. H.: Treatment of familial hypercholesterolaemia in children. Lancet, **1**, 641, 1970.

389. Stone, D. B., Connor, W. E., Lichty, J. A.: *A Low Cholesterol Diet Manual.* Dept. of Internal Medicine, College of Medicine, The University of Iowa, Iowa City, Iowa. Copyright, 1968, The University of Iowa.

390. Jepson, M., Fahmy, M. F. I., Torrens, P. E., Billimoria, J. D., and Maclagan, N. F.: Treatment of essential hyperlipidaemia. Lancet, **2**, 1315, 1969.

391. Best, M. M., and Duncan, C. H.: Effects of clofibrate and dextrothyroxine singly and in combination on serum lipids. Arch. Intern. Med., **118**, 97, 1966.

392. Strisower, E. H., Adamson, G., and Strisower, B.: Treatment of hyperlipidemias. Amer. J. Med., **45**, 488, 1968.

393. Bechtol, L. D., and Warner, W. L.: Dextrothyroxine for lowering serum cholesterol. Analysis of data on 6066 patients. Angiology, **20**, 565, 1969.

394. Parsons, W. B., and Flinn, J. H.: Reduction of serum cholesterol levels and beta-lipoprotein cholesterol levels by nicotinic acid. Arch. Intern. Med., **103**, 783, 1959.

395. Berge, K. G., Achor, R. W. P., Christensen, N. A., Mason, H. L., and Barker, N. W.: Hypercholesteremia and nicotinic acid—a long term study. Amer. J. Med., **31**, 24, 1961.

396. Carlson, L. A.: Effect of nicotinic acid treatment on the chemical composition of plasma lipoprotein classes in man, in *Drugs Affecting Lipid Metabolism,* edited by W. L. Holmes, L. A. Carlson, and R. Paoletti, p. 327. Plenum Press, New York, 1969. (Proceedings of the Third International Symposium on Drugs Affecting Lipid Metabolism, Milan, Italy, Sept. 8–11, 1968.)

397. Zöllner, N., and Gudenzi, M.: Behandlung der hypercholesterinämie mit Beta-pyridylkarbinol. Medsche. Klin., **61**, 1996, and 2036, 1966.

398. Fredrickson, D. S., and Levy, R. I.: Treatment of essential hyperlipidaemia. Lancet, **1**, 199, 1970.

399. Hashim, S. A., and Van Itallie, T. B.: Cholestyramine resin therapy for hypercholesterolemia. J.A.M.A., **192**, 289, 1965.

400. Buchwald, H., and Varco, R. L.: Ileal bypass in patients with hypercholesterolemia and atherosclerosis. J.A.M.A., **196**, 627, 1966.

401. Buchwald, H., and Varco, R.: Partial ileal bypass for hypercholesterolemia and atherosclerosis. Surg., Gynec., Obstet., **124**, 1231, 1967.

402. Strisower, E. H., Krodjian, R. M., Nichols, A. V., Coggiola, E., and Tsai, J.: Effect of ileal bypass on serum lipoproteins in essential hypercholesterolemia. J. Atheroscler. Res., **8**, 525, 1968.

403. Moore, R. B., Frantz, I. D., Jr., and Buchwald, H.: Changes in cholesterol pool size, turnover rate, and fecal bile acid and sterol excretion after partial ileal bypass in hypercholesteremic patients. Surgery, **65**, 98, 1969.

404. Borrie, P.: Type III hyperlipoproteinaemia. Brit. Med. J., **2**, 665, 1969.

405. Borrie, P.: Essential hyperlipaemia and idiopathic hypercholesterolaemic xanthomatosis. Brit. Med. J., **2**, 911, 1957.

406. Malmros, H., Swahn, B., and Truedsson, E.: Essential hyperlipaemia. Acta Med. Scand., **149**, 91, 1954.

407. Adlersberg, D.: Inborn errors of lipid metabolism: clinical, genetic, and chemical aspects. Arch. Path., **60**, 481, 1955.

408. Schettler, G., Eggstein, M., and Jobst, H.: Essential hyperlipaemia. German Med. Monthly, **3**, 310, 1958.

409. Carlson, L. A., and Olhagen, B.: Studies on a case of essential hyperlipemia: blood lipids, with special reference to the composition and metabolism of the serum glycerides before, during and after the course of a viral hepatitis. J. Clin. Invest., **38**, 854, 1959.

410. Jobst, H., Huber, H., and Schettler, G.: Essentielle familiäre hyperlipämie bei einem eineigen Zwillingspaar. Med. Klin., **58**, 710, 1963.

411. Braunsteiner, H., Herbst, M., Sailer, S., and Sandhofer, F.: Family studies in essential "carbohydrate-induced" hyperlipaemia. German Med. Monthly, **12**, 426, 1967.

412. Roe, D. A.: Essential hyperlipemia with xanthomatosis. Arch. Derm., **97**, 436, 1968.

413. Matthews, R. J.: Type III and IV familial hyperlipoproteinemia: evidence that these two syndromes are different phenotypic expressions of the same mutant gene(s). Amer. J. Med., **44**, 188, 1968.

414. Fleischmajer, R.: Familial hyperlipoproteinemia type III. Arch. Derm., **100**, 401, 1969.

415. Dyerberg, J.: Type III hyperlipoproteinemia with low plasma thyroxine binding globulin. Metabolism, **18**, 50, 1969.

416. Kuo, P. T., Feng, L. Y., and Pamintaun, J.: Study of nailfold capillaries in hypertriglyceridemia (types III and IV hyperlipoproteinemia). Circulation, **41**, 309, 1970.

417. Hazzard, W. R., Lindgren, F. T., and Bierman, E. L.: Very low density lipoprotein subfractions in a subject with broad-β disease (type III hyperlipoproteinemia) and a subject with endogenous lipemia (type IV) chemical composition and electrophoretic mobility. Biochim. Biophys. Acta, **202**, 517, 1970.

418. Quarfordt, S. H., Levy, R. I., and Fredrickson, D. S.: On the lipoprotein abnormality in type III hyperlipoproteinemia. J. Clin. Invest. **50**, 754, 1971.

419. Zelis, R., Mason, D. T., Braunwald, E., and Levy, R. I.: Effects of hyperlipoproteinemias and their treatment on the peripheral circulation. J. Clin. Invest., **49**, 1007, 1970.

420. Feiwel, M.: Xanthomatosis in cryoglobulinaemia and other paraproteinaemias with report of a case. Brit. J. Derm., **80**, 719, 1968.

421. Walker, A. E., and Sneddon, I, B.: Skin xanthoma following erythroderma. Brit. J. Derm., **80**, 580, 1968.

422. Altman, J., and Winkelmann, R. K.: Diffuse normolipemic plane xanthoma. Arch. Derm., **85**, 633, 1962.

423. Zemel, H., Deeken, J., Asel, N., and Packer, J.: The ultrastructural features of normolipemic plane xanthoma. Arch. Path., **89,** 111, 1970.
424. Siperstein, M. D., Norton, W., Unger, R. H., and Madison, L. L.: Muscle capillary basement membrane width in normal, diabetic and prediabetic patients. Trans. Ass. Amer. Physicians, **79,** 330, 1966.
425. Shore, B., and Shore, V.: Isolation and characterization of polypeptides of human serum lipoproteins. Biochemistry, **8,** 4510, 1969.
426. Brown, W. V., Levy, R. I., and Fredrickson, D. S.: Further separation of the apoproteins of the human plasma very low density lipoproteins. Biochim. Biophys. Acta, **200,** 573, 1970.
427. Brown, W. V., Levy, R. I., and Fredrickson, D. S.: A comparative study of the very low density lipoproteins in normal subjects and patients with types III, IV and V hyperlipoproteinemia. Circulation, **40,** 4, 1969.
428. Ahrens, E. H., Jr., Hirsch, J., Oette, K., Farquhar, J. W., and Stein, Y.: Carbohydrate-induced and fat-induced lipemia. Trans. Ass. Amer. Physicians, **74,** 134, 1961.
429. Mahley, R. W., Hamilton, R. L., and Lequire, V. S.: Characterization of lipoprotein particles isolated from the Golgi apparatus of rat liver. J. Lipid Res., **10,** 433, 1969.
430. Mahley, R. W., Bersot, T. P., Lequire, V. S., Levy, R. I., Windmueller, H. G., and Brown, W. V.: Identity of very low density lipoprotein apoproteins of plasma and liver Golgi apparatus. Science, **168,** 380, 1970.
431. Langer, T., Bilheimer, D., and Levy, R. I.: Plasma low density lipoprotein (LDL): a remnant of very low density lipoprotein (VLDL) catabolism? Circulation, **42,** III-7, 1970.
432. Nichols, A. V., Strisower, E. H., Lindgren, F. T., Adamson, G. L., and Coggiola, E. L.: Analysis of change in ultracentrifugal lipoprotein profiles following heparin and ethyl-*p*-chlorophenoxyisobutyrate administration. Clin. Chim. Acta, **20,** 277, 1968.
433. LaRosa, J. C., Levy, R. I., Brown, W. V., and Fredrickson, D. S.: Changes in high density lipoprotein protein composition after heparin-induced lipolysis. Amer. J. Physiol., **220,** 785, 1971.
434. Hazzard, W. R., Porte, J. D., and Bierman, E. L.: Heterogeneity of very low density lipoproteins in man: evidence for a functional role of a beta migrating fraction in triglyceride transport and its relation to broad-beta disease (type III hyperlipoproteinemia). J. Clin. Invest., **49,** 40a, 1970.
435. Smith, E. B.: Lipoprotein patterns in myocardial infarction. Lancet, **2,** 910, 1957.
436. Besterman, E. M. M.: Lipoproteins in coronary artery disease. Brit. Heart J., **10,** 503, 1957.
437. Gofman, J. W., Glazier, F., Tamplin, A., Strisower, B., and de Lalla, O.: Lipoproteins, coronary heart disease, and atherosclerosis. Physiol. Rev., **34,** 589, 1954.
438. Lees, R. S., Canellos, G. P., Rosenberg, I. H., and Hatch, F. T.: Myocardial infarction in one of a pair of twenty-seven-year-old identical male twins. Amer. J. Med., **34,** 741, 1963.
439. Spritz, N.: Carbohydrate-induced lipemia: report of a familial occurrence. New Eng. J. Med., **271,** 291, 1964.
440. Kuo, P. T.: Hyperglyceridemia in coronary artery disease and its management. J.A.M.A., **201,** 87, 1967.
441. Schreibman, P. H., Wilson, D. E., and Arky, R. A.: Familial type IV hyperlipoproteinemia. New Eng. J. Med., **281,** 981, 1969.
442. Braunsteiner, H., Herbst, M., Rhomberg, H., Sailer, S., and Sandhofer, F.: Familienuntersuchungen bei primärer Kohlenhydratinduzierter Hypertriglyzeridämie. Schweiz. Med. Wschr., **99,** 286, 1969.
443. Nixon, J. C., Martin, W. G., Kalab, M., and Monahan, G. J.: Type V hyperlipoproteinemia: a study of a patient and family. Clin. Biochem., **2,** 389, 1969.
444. Glueck, C. J., Brown, W. V., Levy, R. I., Greten, H., and Fredrickson, D. S.: Amelioration of hypertriglyceridaemia by progestational drugs in familial type V hyperlipoproteinaemia. Lancet, **1,** 1290, 1969.
445. Blankenhorn, D. H., Jensen, J., and Chin, H. P.: Familial likeness of normal serum triglyceride. Circulation, suppl. II, **35** and **36,** II-5, 1967.
446. Albrink, M. J.: Triglycerides, lipoproteins, and coronary artery disease. Arch. Intern. Med., **109,** 345, 1962.
447. Brown, D. F., Kinch, S. H., and Doyle, J. T.: Serum triglycerides in health and in ischemic heart disease. New Eng. J. Med., **273,** 947, 1965.
448. Brown, D. F.: Blood lipids and lipoproteins in atherogenesis. Amer. J. Med., **46,** 691, 1969.
449. Carlson, L. A., and Lindstedt, S.: The Stockholm prospective study 1: The initial values for plasma lipids. Acta Med. Scand., suppl., **493,** 1, 1968.
450. Gordis, E.: Demonstration of two kinds of fat particles in alimentary lipemia with polyvinylpyrrolidone gradient columns. Proc. Soc. Exp. Biol. Med., **110,** 657, 1962.
451. Bierman, E. L., Gordis, E., and Hamlin, J. T., III: Heterogeneity of fat particles in plasma during alimentary lipemia. J. Clin. Invest., **41,** 2254, 1962.
452. Watkins, D. M., Froeb, H. F., and Gutman, A. B.: Effects of diet in essential hypertension. II. Results with unmodified Kempner rice diet in fifty hospitalized patients. Amer. J. Med., **9,** 441, 1950.
453. Walker, W. J., Lawry, E. Y., Love, D. E., Mann, G. V., Levine, S. A., and Stare, F. J.: Effect of weight reduction and calorie balance on serum lipoprotein and cholesterol levels. Amer. J. Med., **14,** 654, 1953.
454. Hatch, F. T., Abell, L. L., and Kendall, F. E.: Effects of restriction of dietary fat and cholesterol upon serum lipids and lipoproteins in patients with hypertension. Amer. J. Med., **19,** 48, 1955.
455. Ahrens, E. H., Jr., Insull, W., Jr., Blomstrand, R., Hirsch, J., Tsaltas, T. T., and Peterson, M. L.: The influence of dietary fats on serum-lipid levels in man. Lancet, **1,** 943, 1957.
456. Nichols, A. V., Dobbin, V., and Gofman, J. W.: Influence of dietary factors upon human serum lipoprotein concentrations. Geriatrics, **12,** 7, 1957.
457. Kuo, P. T., and Carson, J. C.: Dietary fats and the diurnal serum triglyceride levels in man. J. Clin. Invest., **38,** 1384, 1959.
458. Antonis, A., and Bersohn, I.: The influence of diet on serum-triglycerides in South African white and Bantu prisoners. Lancet, **1,** 3, 1961.
459. Farquhar, J. W., Reaven, G. M., Gross, R., and Wagner, R.: Rate of plasma triglyceride synthesis in carbohydrate-induced lipemia. J. Clin. Invest., **42,** 930, 1963.
460. Kuo, P. T., and Bassett, D. R.: Dietary sugar in the production of hyperglyceridemia, Ann. Intern. Med., **62,** 1199, 1965.
461. Kuo, P. T.: Dietary sugar in the production of hyperglyceridemia in patients with hyperlipemia and atherosclerosis. Trans. Ass. Amer. Physicians, **78,** 97, 1965.
462. Kane, J. P., Longcope, C., Pavlatos, F. Ch., and Grodsky, G. M.: Studies of carbohydrate metabolism in idiopathic hypertriglyceridemia. Metabolism, **14,** 471, 1965.
463. Macdonald, I.: The lipid response of young women to dietary carbohydrates. Amer. J. Clin. Nutr., **16,** 458, 1965.
464. Farquhar, J. W., Frank, A., Gross, R. C., and Reaven, G. M.: Glucose, insulin, and triglyceride responses to high and low carbohydrate diets in man. J. Clin. Invest., **45,** 1648, 1966.
465. Kaufmann, N. A., Poznanski, R., Blondheim, S. H., and Stein, Y.: Comparison of effects of fructose, sucrose, glucose, and starch on serum lipids in patients with hypertriglyceridemia and normal subjects. Amer. J. Clin. Nutr., **20,** 131, 1967.
466. Ford, S., Jr., Bozian, R. C., and Knowles, H. C., Jr.: Interactions of obesity, and glucose and insulin levels in hypertriglyceridemia. Amer. J. Clin. Nutr., **21,** 904, 1968.
467. Sailer, S., Bolzano, K., Sandhofer, F., Spath, P., and Braunsteiner, H.: Plasma triglyceride and insulin concentration following oral glucose load in patients with primary carbohydrate-induced hypertriglyceridemia. Schweiz. Med. Wschr., **98,** 1512, 1968.
468. Bierman, E. L., and Porte, D., Jr.: Carbohydrate intolerance and lipemia. Ann. Intern. Med., **68,** 926, 1968.
469. Romhanyi, M., and Bajzik, E.: Hypertriglyceridemia caused by carbohydrate. Orv. Hetil., **110,** 1561, 1969.
470. Levy, R. I., and Glueck, C. J.: Hyperglyceridemia, diabetes mellitus and coronary vessel disease. Arch. Intern. Med., **123,** 220, 1969.
471. Wilson, D. E., and Lees, R. S.: Metabolic interrelationships between lipoproteins: effect of clofibrate treatment and carbohydrate induction. Circulation. **42,** III-25, 1970.
472. Segall, M. M., Fosbrooke, A. S., Lloyd, J. K., and Wolff, O. H.: Carbohydrate-induced hypertriglyceridaemia in a child. Arch. Dis. Child., **45,** 73, 1970.

473. Bagdade, J. D., Porte, D., Jr., and Bierman, E. L.: Hypertriglyceridemia: a metabolic consequence of chronic renal failure. New Eng. J. Med., **279,** 181, 1968.

474. Jakovcic, S., Khachadurian, A. K., and Hsia, D. Yi-Y.: The hyperlipidemia in glycogen storage disease. J. Lab. Clin. Med., **68,** 769, 1966.

475. Greenberger, N. J., Hatch, F. T., Drummey, G. D., and Isselbacher, K. K.: Pancreatitis and hyperlipemia: study of serum lipid alterations in 25 patients with acute pancreatitis. Medicine, **45,** 161, 1966.

476. Braunsteiner, H., Sandhofer, F., and Sailer, S.: Hyperlipämie und akute Pankreatitis. T. Gastroent, **1,** 32, 1969.

477. Wynn, V., Doar, J. W. H., Mills, G. L., and Stokes, T.: Fasting serum triglyceride, cholesterol and lipoprotein levels during oral contraceptive therapy. Lancet, **2,** 756, 1969.

478. Reaven, G. M., Lerner, R. L., Stern, M. P., and Farquhar, J. W. (with technical asst. of R. Nakanishi): Role of insulin in endogenous hypertriglyceridemia. J. Clin. Invest., **46,** 1756, 1967.

479. Kuo, P. T.: Current metabolic-genetic interrelationship in human atherosclerosis. With therapeutic considerations. Ann. Intern. Med., **68,** 449, 1968.

480. Tzagournis, M., Chiles, R., and Ryan, M. M.: Interrelationships of hyperinsulinism and hypertriglyceridemia in young patients with coronary heart disease. Circulation, **38,** 1156, 1968.

481. Kessler, J. I., Miller, M., and Barza, D.: Hyperlipemia in acute pancreatitis. Metabolic studies in a patient and demonstration of abnormal lipoprotein-triglyceride complexes resistant to the action of lipoprotein lipase. Amer. J. Med., **42,** 968, 1967.

482. Feldman, E. B., and Wallace, S. L.: Hypertriglyceridemia in gout. Circulation, **29,** 508, 1964.

483. Berkowitz, D.: Gout, hyperlipidemia, and diabetes interrelationships. J.A.M.A., **197,** 77, 1966.

484. Barlow, K. A.: Hyperlipidemia in primary gout. Metabolism, **17,** 289, 1968.

485. Brown, D. F., and Doyle, J. T.: Pre-beta lipoproteinemia: its bearing on the dietary management of serum lipid disorders as related to ischemic heart disease. Amer. J. Clin. Nutr., **20,** 324, 1967.

486. Cornog, J. L., Jr., Fitts, W. T., Jr., and Kuo, P. T.: Intramural and pericapillary distribution of lipids in gingival tissue of patients with carbohydrate-induced hyperglyceridemia. Circulation, **28,** 201, 1968.

487. Fritz, I. B.: Factors influencing the rates of long-chain fatty acid oxidation and synthesis in mammalian systems. Physiol. Rev., **41,** 52, 1961.

488. Steinberg, D.: Fatty acid mobilization: mechanisms of regulation and metabolic consequences. Biochem. Soc. Sympos., **24,** 111, 1963.

489. Adipose Tissue, in *Handbook of Physiology,* sect. 5, edited by A. E. Renold and G. F. Cahill, Jr. American Physiological Society, Washington, 1965.

490. Baker, N., and Schotz, M. C.: Use of multicompartmental models to measure rates of triglyceride metabolism in rats. J. Lipid Res., **5,** 188, 1964.

491. Ryan, W. G., and Schwartz, T. B.: Dynamics of plasma triglyceride turnover in man. Metabolism, **14,** 1243, 1965.

492. Farquhar, J. W., Gross, R. C., Wagner, R. M., and Reaven, G. M.: Validation of incompletely coupled two-compartment nonrecycling catenary model for turnover of liver and plasma triglyceride in man. J. Lipid Res., **6,** 119, 1965.

493. Reaven, G. M., Hill, D. B., Gross, R. C., and Farquhar, J. W.: Kinetics of triglyceride turnover of very low density lipoproteins of human plasma. J. Clin. Invest., **44,** 1826, 1965.

494. Sailer, S., Sandhofer, F., and Braunsteiner, H.: Umsatzraten für freie fettsäuren und triglyceride im Plasma bei essentieller Hyperlipämie. Klin. Wschr., **44,** 1032, 1966.

495. Baker, N., and Schotz, M. C.: Quantitative aspects of free fatty acid metabolism in the fasted rat. J. Lipid Res., **8,** 646, 1967.

496. Sandhofer, F., Bolizano, K., Sailer, S., and Braunsteiner, H.: Über den Einbau von Plasmaglucose-Kohlenstoff in Plasmatriglyceride bei Normalpersonen und Hyperlipamikern. Klin. Wschr., **46,** 158, 1968.

497. Porte, D., Jr., and Bierman, E. L.: The effect of heparin infusion on plasma triglyceride *in vivo* and *in vitro* with a method for calculating triglyceride turnover. J. Lab. Clin. Med., **73,** 631, 1969.

497*a.* Eaton, R. P., Berman, M., and Steinberg, D.: Kinetic studies of plasma free fatty acid and triglyceride metabolism in man J. Clin. Invest., **48,** 1560, 1969.

498. Havel, R. J., Kane, J. P., Balasse, E. O., Segel, N., and Basso, L. V.: Splanchnic metabolism of free fatty acids and production of triglycerides of very low density lipoproteins in normotriglyceridemic and hypertriglyceridemic humans. J. Clin. Invest., **49,** 2017, 1970.

499. Quarfordt, S. H., Frank, A., Shames, D. M., Berman, M., and Steinberg, D.: Very low density lipoprotein triglyceride transport in type IV hyperlipoproteinemia and the effects of carbohydrate-rich diets. J. Clin. Invest., **49,** 2281, 1970.

500. Havel, R. J., Felts, J. M., and Van Duyne, M.: Formation and fate of endogenous triglycerides in blood plasma of rabbits. J. Lipid Res., **3,** 297, 1962.

501. Ockner, R. K., Hughes, F. B., and Isselbacher, K. J.: Very low density lipoproteins in intestinal lymph: origin, composition, and role in lipid transport in the fasting state. J. Clin. Invest., **48,** 2079, 1969.

502. Windmueller, H. G., and Levy, R. I.: Production of β-lipoprotein by intestine in the rat. J. Biol. Chem., **243,** 4878, 1968.

503. Ockner, R. K., and Jones, A. L.: An electron microscopic and functional study of very low density lipoproteins in intestinal lymph. J. Lipid Res., **11,** 284, 1970.

504. Carlson, L. A., and Hallberg, D.: Studies on the elimination of exogenous lipids from the blood stream. The kinetics of the elimination of a fat emulsion and of chylomicrons in the dog after single injection. Acta Physiol. Scand., **59,** 52, 1963.

505. Salans, L. B., Knittle, J. L., and Hirsch, J.: The role of adipose cell size and adipose tissue insulin sensitivity in the carbohydrate intolerance of human obesity. J. Clin. Invest., **47,** 153, 1968.

506. Isselbacher, K. J., and Greenberger, N. J.: Metabolic effects of alcohol on the liver. New Eng. J. Med., **270,** 351, 1964.

507. Felber, J.-P., and Vannotti, A.: Effects of fat infusion on glucose tolerance and insulin plasma levels. Med. Exp., **10,** 153, 1964.

508. Symposium on Atromid: Proceedings of conference held in Buxton, England, June 5-6, 1963. J. Atheroscler. Res., **3,** 341, 1963.

509. Hunninghake, D. B., Tucker, D. R., and Azarnoff, D. L.: Long-term effects of clofibrate (Atromid-S) on serum lipids in man. Circulation, **39,** 675, 1969.

510. Carlson, L. A., and Oro, L.: Persistence of inhibitory effect of nicotinic acid on catecholamine-stimulated lipid mobilization during prolonged treatment with nicotinic acid. J. Atheroscler. Res., **5,** 436, 1965.

511. Morris, J. H., West, D. A., and Bolinger, R. E.: Effect of oral sulfonylurea on plasma triglycerides in diabetics. Diabetics, **13,** 87, 1964.

512. Schwartz, M. J., Mirsky, S., and Schaefer, L. E.: Phenformin, serum lipids, and diabetes mellitus. Lancet, **1,** 959, 1965.

CHAPTER TWENTY-NINE

G_{M2} GANGLIOSIDOSES: TAY-SACHS DISEASE

Howard R. Sloan and Donald S. Fredrickson

Tay-Sachs disease (G_{M2} gangliosidosis) is a biochemical abnormality of the nervous system that becomes clinically evident by 5 to 6 months of age and is characterized by progressive retardation in development, paralysis, dementia, and blindness associated with a cherry-red spot in the retina. It is invariably fatal, usually by the age of 3 to 4 years. The ganglion cells and, later, proliferating glial cells contain abnormally large amounts of gangliosides. Ganglioside is the trivial name for the most complex member of a family of lipids called *sphingolipids.* Most of the sphingolipids in animal tissues contain *ceramide* (N-acylsphingosine) as a structural unit; the nature of the group covalently bonded to ceramide determines the sphingolipid class. In this and later chapters on abnormal lipid metabolism, the accompanying schematic diagram will be employed to designate ceramide (Fig. 29-1). The ganglioside that accumulates in

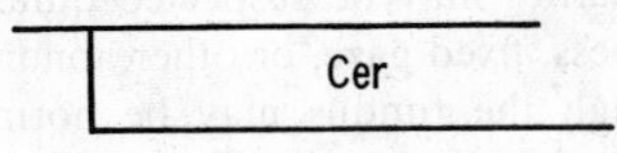

Figure 29-1. Ceramide.

Tay-Sachs disease is ganglioside G_{M2}, N-acetylgalactosaminyl-(N-acetylneuraminyl)-galactosylglucosyl-N-acylsphingosine (Fig. 29-2).

This compound normally constitutes only a very small fraction of brain gangliosides, and its excessive accumulation is accompanied by extensive myelin degeneration. The disease is due to a double dose of a mutant autosomal allele which is unusually frequent among Jews, particularly those of Northeastern European origin. The basic inheritable metabolic defect is deficient activity of a specific hexosaminidase, hexosaminidase A. There is no specific therapy for Tay-Sachs disease.

In the past, Tay-Sachs disease (TSD) was considered a variant of the amaurotic familial idiocies (AFI), a term which was originally introduced by Sachs [1] to designate specifically what is now known as Tay-Sachs disease. Age

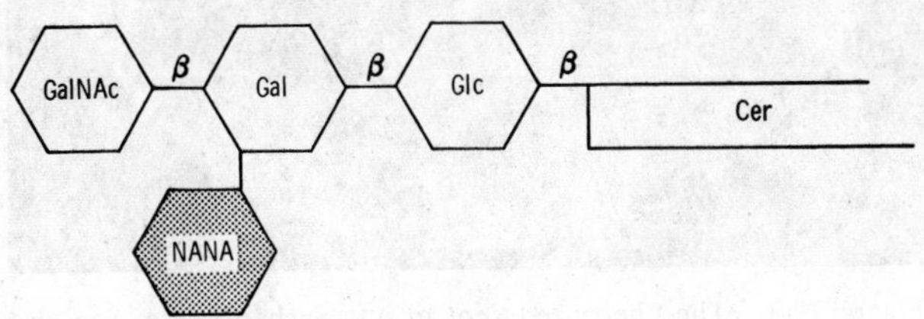

Figure 29-2. Ganglioside G_{M2}.

of onset, ethnic extraction of the patient, and other clinical symptoms were the basis for the subdivision of the AFI's into six variants. The six forms of amaurotic familial idiocy are congenital amaurotic idiocy (Norman-Wood disease) [2–4], infantile amaurotic idiocy (Tay-Sachs disease) [5–7], the late infantile group (Jansky-Bielschowsky disease) [8–10], the systemic late infantile type [11] (Chap. 30), the juvenile form (Vogt-Spielmeyer or Batten's disease) [12–15], and adult amaurotic idiocy (Kufs' or Hallervorden-Spatz disease) [6, 7, 16]. This array of eponyms is partially responsible for the confusion about the interrelationships among the amaurotic familial idiocies. It is clear that several of these variants are themselves heterogeneous [17, 18]. It has often been erroneously concluded that all the amaurotic idiocies are disorders of ganglioside metabolism, and indeed the two terms, *gangliosidosis* (ganglioside storage disease) and *amaurotic idiocy,* are frequently used interchangeably. Abnormal accumulation of gangliosides has been conclusively demonstrated, however, in only two of the variants of AFI: G_{M1} and G_{M2} gangliosidoses. For clinicians accustomed to the present subdivision of the amaurotic familial idiocies, the term retains some usefulness. As these diseases progressively yield to new definitions in biochemical terms, the confusing and erroneous concept of AFI as a group of closely related diseases is certain to be abandoned. In this book the term *gangliosidosis* will be used to refer to a disease in which abnormal ganglioside metabolism has been demonstrated.

A diagnosis of Tay-Sachs disease should not be made from morphologic or histochemical impressions alone. No stains are absolutely specific for gangliosides or glycolipids. Chemical and enzymatic analyses are necessary for the certain establishment of the diagnosis.

HISTORICAL ASPECTS

In 1881, Tay, a British ophthalmologist, described a cherry-red macular degeneration (cherry-red spot) in the fundus of an infant with marked weakness of the trunk and limbs [19]. Subsequently, he reported two additional patients in the same family [20] and a fourth in another family [21]. In 1887, Sachs, an American neurologist, reported clinical and pathologic observations of an infant with blindness and dementia [1, 22]. Within a few years he observed a total of eight patients with the typical retinal change and described the syndrome, using the name "amaurotic family idiocy" [1, 23]. It became more popularly known as Tay-Sachs disease as further reports appeared.

Well over 500 cases have been reported subsequently [24];

the typical and the extremes of clinical behavior have been recorded, and the genetic mode has been well established. Though children whose parents are both Jewish are much more likely to have the disease, non-Jewish patients began to appear by the turn of the century [25], and a considerable number have since been reported [26].

Between 1939 and 1942, Klenk and his colleagues [27–33] made the important discovery that the brain in Tay-Sachs disease contains greatly increased concentrations of gangliosides. In nearly 30 years of work by many investigators a more complete understanding of the lesion in G_{M2} gangliosidosis has been acquired. Several investigators noted that the ganglioside that accumulates in TSD ("Tay-Sachs ganglioside" or ganglioside G_{M2}) has different chromatographic behavior [34] and solubility properties [35–37] from the predominant normal brain gangliosides. In 1961, Svennerholm and Raal [38] reported the important finding that these brains contain abnormal amounts of monosialogangliosides (gangliosides with only one sialic acid residue). These were then shown by Svennerholm [39] and Klenk and coworkers [40] to be a ganglioside with the same structural formula as the major normal monosialoganglioside but lacking the terminal galactose. The correct structure of ganglioside G_{M2} was first reported by Makita and Yamakawa in 1963 [41]. Large amounts of another glycolipid, asialo-G_{M2} (G_{M2} minus the N-acetylneuraminic acid moiety), have also been observed in Tay-Sachs brains [38, 42–44].

In 1969, first Okada and O'Brien [45] and then Hultberg, Kolodny, Sandhoff, and their coworkers demonstrated that a specific hexosaminidase activity, hexosaminidase A, was deficient in Tay-Sachs disease [46–48]. Enzyme measurements have now been extended to tissue culture, and the intrauterine diagnosis of Tay-Sachs disease has recently been achieved [49].

CLINICAL MANIFESTATIONS

The largest personal experience with Tay-Sachs disease is that of Aronson and Volk and their coworkers at the Jewish Chronic Disease Hospital in Brooklyn, New York. Their reviews of the clinical and genetic features extend to both Jewish [24, 50, 51] and non-Jewish [26] infants. There are no remarkable differences between the manifestations in these two groups. There have been many other extensive reviews of TSD [5, 6, 52–56].

Onset

Tay-Sachs disease usually has its clinical beginning between birth and age 10 months, most commonly by 6 months of age. In most instances, the abnormality first noticed by the parents is an inability to sit by 8 months of age. Superficially the children previously appear healthy and normal, but in retrospect many parents recall that the child had always been quiet, apathetic, and somewhat listless. No significant correlation has been discovered between occurrence of the disease and order of birth or prenatal or early postnatal environmental influences.

Symptoms and Signs

The disease often begins insidiously, with listlessness or weakness, retardation in development, or difficulty in feeding. Hypotonia, particularly of the pectoral musculature, may be present before the fourth month. Spasticity is another early and consistent sign. The most common initial sign is an exaggerated extension response to sound that has frequently, but erroneously, been termed hyperacusis [26]. The initiating sound is more likely to be sharp rather than loud, and it elicits rapid extension of both arms and a startled expression ("startle reaction"). The motor response resembles decerebrate posturing and myoclonus. This reaction could be induced in 12 of 15 children with TSD [57, 58]. Four other common diagnostic features have been inability to sit up, listlessness or lack of awareness, inability to hold up the head, and abnormal limb movements [50].

Visual difficulties may be suspected quite early because of inattentiveness, fixed gaze, or other abnormal eye movements. Although the fundus may be normal in the first months of life, the changes in the macular region leading to the typical cherry-red spot soon become evident (Fig. 29-3). This lesion has been present in virtually every patient in whom the diagnosis has been confirmed by biochemical

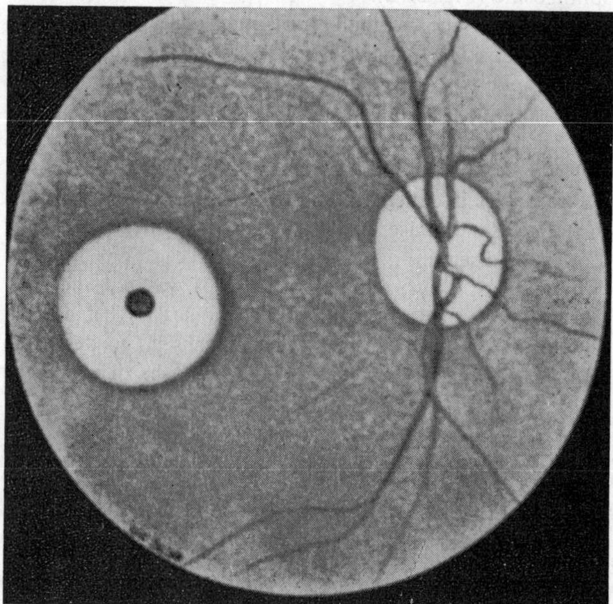

Figure 29-3. The cherry-red spot in Tay-Sachs disease. See also Plate I-3.

analysis. Blindness usually occurs between the twelfth and eighteenth months of life and appears to be of central rather than peripheral origin. The pupils of children who do not respond to visual stimuli will frequently react to light [58]. Optic atrophy, which may precede or follow blindness, is usually evident by 2 years of age; the pupillary response to light may be intact even in the terminal vegetative stage. Jampel [59] has provided a detailed description of the ophthalmologic observations at various stages of the disease.

In a few unusual cases, a child with TSD may sit without support, or even crawl. By 1 year of age, however, the retardation in motor activity is obvious. The infant no longer sits and is unable to hold or transfer objects; by 2 years of age there is usually little or no spontaneous motor activity.

Seizures before 1 year of age are rare [7]. As the neurologic symptoms increase in severity, epileptiform seizures occur. In the early stage convulsions are frequently associated with periods of abnormal laughter and episodes of autonomic dysfunction.

Course

The average duration of the disease is about 24 to 30 months, the survival of the child in part being related to the quality of nursing care and the treatment of intercurrent infections [52]. Survival up to 60 months has been reported [50]. The clinical course has been divided into several arbitrary time phases [50, 51] correlated with certain interesting morphologic changes which are observed as these children survive 15 months or longer. Up to that time the cranial measurements are normal and the brain is slightly subnormal in weight. Thereafter, the brain actually may increase in size because of reactive proliferation of glial cells, and by age 24 months the cranial measurements progressively become larger than normal. Children dying between the ages of 2 and 3 years may have brain weights nearly 50 percent greater than normal. Possibly because of hypothalamic involvement, precocious puberty may develop after the age of two. In the terminal stages of the illness the child is quiet and hypotonic and the startle reaction is much less prominent.

The only physical abnormality is megalocephaly; there is no hepatosplenomegaly. No specific roentgenologic abnormalities have been noted, although electrocardiographic abnormalities have been observed in the older children [60].

CLINICOPATHOLOGIC CORRELATIONS

Gross Pathology and Light Microscopy

Nervous System

The most striking pathologic changes in TSD occur in the nervous system.

Brain

The brain may vary greatly in size [52, 61, 62]. In patients dying at a very early age, the brain is diffusely atrophic, and moderate ventricular dilatation is often found. When the onset is later or the rate of progression slower, the cerebral expansion is associated with marked atrophy of the cerebellum and brain stem. If the ventricles were enlarged earlier, they now become smaller. Regardless of size, the brain is frequently firm or leathery in consistency.

CEREBRAL CORTEX. The ganglion cells of the cerebral cortex are enormously swollen, or "ballooned," and distorted. The cytoplasm appears pale and spongy, and in some patients it is vacuolated and filled with a material reacting with some, but not all, lipid stains (Fig. 29-4). The Nissl bodies gradually decrease in number until only a small zone, localized around the nucleus, remains [7, 63, 64]. This zone eventually disappears as well. Most of the ganglion cell nuclei are displaced to the periphery and may appear to be in various stages of disintegration. In the late stages of the disease there may

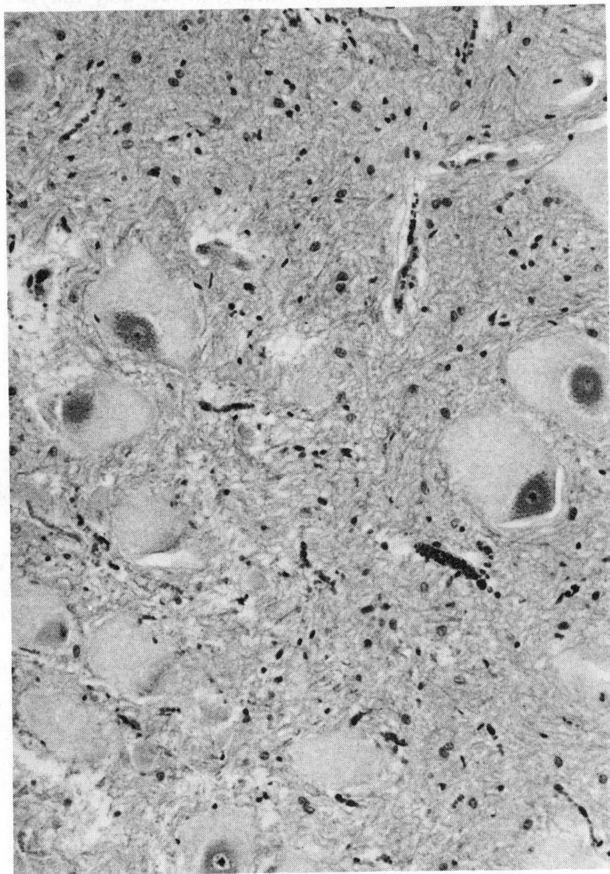

Figure 29-4. Ganglion cells from spinal cord of a patient with Tay-Sachs disease showing typical swelling and vacuolation; ×160. (*Courtesy of Dr. Allen Crocker.*)

be a significant loss of ganglion cells and the remaining cells have no nuclei and appear "washed-out."

Associated with the loss of ganglion cells is a concomitant decrease in the number of cortical axons. In the later stages of the disease the axons frequently demonstrate fusiform swellings which have been termed "torpedoes" and are associated with marked disturbance of the fibrillary structure [7]. The astrocytes and microglia proliferate and become hypertrophied during the later stages of the disease. The glial cells are distended and filled with large granules which have the same staining characteristics as the neurons. Demyelination is consistently found and may be quite extensive. In some patients there may be demyelination of almost the entire white matter [62, 65, 66]. Far-advanced disease is associated with extreme glial hyperplasia, patchy encephalomalacia, and meningeal fibrosis. In this late stage the leptomeninges may be swollen, gelatinous, and loaded with foam cells.

CEREBELLUM. Cerebellar neuronal lipid storage is similar to that observed in the cerebrum. The volume and weight of the cerebellum are normal. The most striking alteration is the marked loss of Purkinje cells; indeed they may be almost completely absent. Those that remain are distended with lipid and irregularly distributed, and they show significant variations in size and shape. The thickness of the external granular layer may be markedly decreased, and the folia are usually shrunken. The axons are only moderately decreased in number, and there is usually only minimal astrocytic and microglial reaction [67]. The myelin sheath may be almost completely destroyed.

Basal Ganglia, Brain Stem, and Spinal Cord

The nerve cells of the basal ganglia, brain stem, and spinal cord (Fig. 29-4) demonstrate abnormalities that are quite similar to those found in the cerebral cortex. The brain stem shows only a small loss of axons [68].

Peripheral Nerves and the Autonomic Nervous System

In one patient with TSD, the sciatic nerve and the extracerebral part of the oculomotor nerve showed loss of the myelin sheaths and "torpedo" formation in the axons [68].

Neurons throughout the autonomic nervous system show the same changes found in the central nervous system. Affected neurons may be found in the myenteric plexus of the intestine, the sympathetic ganglia, ganglion cells of the pancreas, the adrenal gland, and the wall of the urinary bladder [63, 69–72].

Retina

The cherry-red spot is produced by lesions in the cells in the retinal layers identical to those encountered in the ganglion cells in the brain [73–75]. The characteristic sign consists of a grayish or grayish-yellow zone in the macular region, in which the fovea is seen as a red spot. The grayish macula is thought to be due to edema and swelling of the internuclear layers on either side of the fovea [76], or to swelling and necrosis of the ganglion cells, which are most numerous in the region of the macula [77]. Demyelination and degeneration of the optic nerve also occur. The cherry-red spot is also seen frequently in G_{M1} gangliosidosis and in Niemann-Pick disease, and the histologic features of the retina in the latter disease are virtually identical to those in TSD [76]. Cherry-red spots have also been reported in Vogt-Spielmeyer disease [78] and in the myoclonic syndrome [79].

Other Tissues

Pick and Bielschowsky [80] precipitated a long debate with their opinion that TSD and Niemann-Pick disease are different manifestations of the same disease. There is no longer any question that these two diseases are genetically and biochemically different. Before the delineation of G_{M1} gangliosidosis as a distinct entity, several patients were described as having Tay-Sachs disease with visceral involvement [11, 81]. The morphology of nonneural tissue from patients with TSD under the light microscope is generally described as being unremarkable. In a few cases, however, careful examination has revealed the presence of lipid, staining positively with periodic acid–Schiff, in the parenchymal cells of the liver [63], and of lipid-laden foam cells in the spleen and lung [64].

Electron Microscopy

Careful study of the ultrastructure of biopsy specimens from Tay-Sachs brains has been made by Terry and Weiss in collaboration with Korey and coworkers [66, 82–84]. The ganglion cell nuclei are unchanged, although often displaced to the side of the cell. Mitochondria, ribosomes, and endoplasmic reticulum appear normal. In the cytoplasm of the ganglion cells, axis cylinders, glial cells, and perivascular tissue cells, there are numerous round or oval membranous cytoplasmic bodies (MCB) (Fig. 29-5), which measure 0.5 to 2.0 μ in diameter. The MCB consist of concentric layers of dense membranes, many of which surround a homogeneous or finely granular central zone. Membranous cytoplasmic bodies have been harvested [83]; they contain primarily gangliosides, cholesterol, phosphatides, and possibly other glycolipids. It has been shown that mixtures of lipids with a similar composition will form MCB in vitro [85]. Harcourt and Dobbs [86] showed that the ganglion cells of the retina and the cerebral cortex have quite similar morphologic changes. MCB have also been observed in postsynaptic terminals [87] and in neurons of the rectal mucosa [71].

Although light microscopy reveals only minimal abnor-

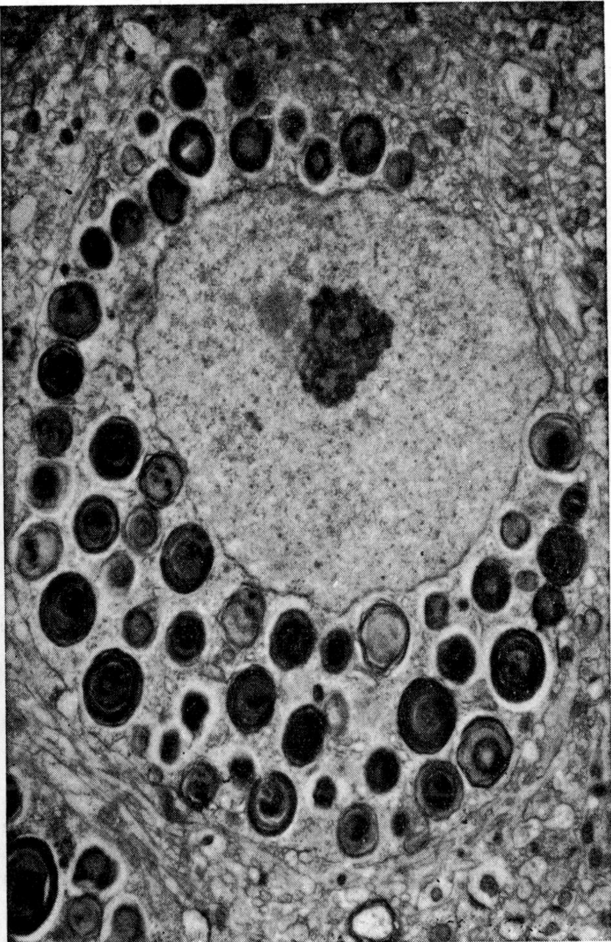

Figure 29-5. Electron micrograph of a neuron in Tay-Sachs disease. Note in the cytoplasm many membranous cytoplasmic bodies (MCB), 0.5 to 2.0 microns in diameter and consisting of closely packed, concentrically arranged electron-dense membranes. Methacrylate embedding: ×9,800. (*Courtesy Dr. Robert D. Terry, Albert Einstein College of Medicine; reprinted from* [66], *with permission of the publishers.*)

malities in the liver in TSD, abnormal and distinctly laminated bodies have been repeatedly observed with the electron microscope [66, 71, 88]. The laminated bodies in the liver parenchyma are readily differentiated from those found in ganglion cells; a few, however, have been observed that are quite similar to those present in neural tissue [88].

Histochemistry

Light Microscopy

The abnormal ganglion cells in the brain and spinal cord or outside the central nervous system cannot be distinguished by ordinary hematoxylin-eosin staining from those in Niemann-Pick, infantile Gaucher's, or Pfaundler-Hurler diseases. Even with the use of all available differential stains, it may be most difficult to distinguish gangliosides sufficiently well to provide a specific diagnosis [69, 70]. Schneck et al. have reported the staining characteristics of the intraneuronal material in TSD [7]. A modified Bial's test for neuraminic acid has been used in attempts to characterize gangliosides histochemically [89, 90]. The assumption that neuraminic acid in tissues is representative of gangliosides is unwarranted. Moreover, Svennerholm [91] has indicated the difficulty involved in correlating histochemical staining reactions and chemical structures.

Enzymatic histochemical assays have revealed the presence of large amounts of acid phosphatase in the neurons and glial cells of patients with TSD [92]. Friede and Allen [93] and Lazarus and his colleagues [92] have shown that in the neurons in TSD adenosinetriphosphatase, acetylcholinesterase, and several oxidative enzymes are confined to the perinuclear zone and to the periphery of the cell. They believe that this displacement is caused by the massive accumulation of lipid within the ganglion cells. Acid phosphatase activity has been observed in the perikaryon of affected neurons, where its distribution was almost identical to that of material staining strongly for lipid [92]. Lazarus and coworkers [92] suggested that this finding implies that the lipid-laden granules found in the ganglion cells of patients with TSD are lysosomes loaded with Tay-Sachs ganglioside.

Electron Microscopy

Wallace and her colleagues [94, 95] have identified the fine structural localization of acid phosphatase and thiolactate esterase activities in the cerebellum of children with TSD. MCB in the Purkinje, stellate, and astrocytic cells contained both enzymatic activities. Acid phosphatase activity was also observed in the laminated bodies found in the hepatocytes of patients with TSD [96]. Halaris and Jatzkewitz [97], employing Hale's stain, concluded that the gangliosides stored in the neurons in TSD are localized in the membranes of the MCB and probably also in the membranes of the nerve endings.

THE SPHINGOLIPIDS

We now turn to an examination of the sphingolipids in general and of the gangliosides in particular. Abnormalities of sphingolipid metabolism are involved not only in TSD but also in Niemann-Pick disease (Chap. 35), Gaucher's disease (Chap. 33), G_{M1} gangliosidosis (Chap. 30), metachromatic leukodystrophy (Chap. 32), Fabry's disease (Chap. 31), and Krabbe's disease (Chap. 34).

The sphingolipids derive their name from sphingosine, a long-chain base originally discovered and described by Thudichum in his classic studies of the chemical composition of the brain [98, 99]. It is not clear whether Thudichum derived the word *sphingosine* from the Greek *sphingein,* meaning to bind tight, i.e., tightly bound to brain tissue, or from the Sphinx of Thebes, whose riddle was so difficult to solve. The story of the controversy that surrounded Thudichum's research is fascinating reading [99].

The actual structure of sphingosine, 2-amino-4-octadecene-1,3-diol, was unknown to Thudichum and has only recently been elucidated by a number of studies which have been summarized by Carter and his colleagues [100, 101]. Proof of structure has been confirmed by total synthesis [102, 103].

The principal naturally occurring member of this family is D(+) erythro-1,3-dihydroxy-2-amino-4-transoctadecene:

$$\begin{array}{l} \phantom{CH_3(CH_2)_{12}CH=}{}^{4}\quad {}^{3}\quad {}^{2}\quad {}^{1} \\ CH_3(CH_2)_{12}CH{=}CH{-}\underset{OH}{CH}{-}\underset{NH_2}{CH}{-}CH_2OH \end{array}$$

Erythro refers to the configuration of the substitutions on carbon-2 and carbon-3; *trans* to the configuration of the 4,5 double bond; and D to the configuration of carbon-2. Over the last 30 years it has become clear that the sphingolipids do not always contain sphingosine as their basic component, but rather contain one of a group of closely related long-chain bases, all of which are aliphatic 2-amino-1,3-diols.

Many other members of this family of bases occur in nature. The term sphingosine is sometimes used generically to refer to all of them. In addition to the C_{18}-sphingosine shown above, sphingosines of longer chain length (C_{19} and C_{20}) [104–111], or shorter (C_{14}, C_{16}, or C_{17}) [109, 111, 112], have been found. Sphingosines in which the aliphatic portion of the molecule is branched (branched-chain sphingosines) have also been isolated. Another congener of sphingosine is dihydrosphingosine (saturated sphingosine) [106, 110, 113, 114].

$$CH_3(CH_2)_{12}CH_2CH_2{-}\underset{OH}{CH}{-}\underset{NH_2}{CH}{-}CH_2OH$$

Another common variation is phytosphingosine (C_3,C_4-dihydroxysphingosine) [115, 116].

$$CH_3(CH_2)_{12}CH_2{-}\underset{OH}{CH}{-}\underset{OH}{CH}{-}\underset{NH_2}{CH}{-}CH_2OH$$

The most complex congener of sphingosine is sphingadienine, in which there is an additional carbon-carbon double bond in the aliphatic portion of the molecule [112, 117].

Because the old nomenclature for sphingosine bases is confusing, a new scheme has been tentatively adopted internationally [112]. C_{18}-saturated- (or dihydro-) sphingosine, the reference compound in this system, is termed *sphinganine.* Higher and lower homologues are indicated by the appropriate prefix; e.g., C_{20}-dihydrosphingosine would be called *eicosasphinganine.* A double bond is indicated by the suffix -enine, and its position by a numerical prefix; sphingosine therefore becomes 4-sphingenine. The position of additional hydroxy- groups is also designated by a numerical prefix; phytosphingosine would, therefore, be called 4-hydroxysphinganine. The new nomenclature is not being used extensively, and throughout this book the older nomenclature will be used.

Ceramide

The basic unit of most sphingolipids is the N-acyl derivative of sphingosine or its congeners, in which a long-chain fatty acid is attached to the amino group on carbon-2 through an amide linkage. The generic term for this class of compounds is *ceramide.* Free ceramide has been isolated from several tissues [111, 118, 119].

Utilization of gas-liquid and thin-layer chromatography has demonstrated that a considerable variety of long-chain fatty acids, either saturated or unsaturated, having even- or odd-numbered carbon chains, and either normal or hydroxy, occur within almost every class of sphingolipids. In general, C_{20} to C_{24} fatty acids predominate in the neutral glycosphingolipids and the sphingomyelins, and stearic acid (C_{18}) is the major fatty acid of the neural gangliosides [111].

Sphingolipid Classes

All the major mammalian sphingolipids contain ceramide as a structural unit; the distinguishing feature of each is the moiety esterified to the C_1 of ceramide. In the sphingomyelins this group is phosphorylcholine, while in the neutral glycosphingolipids it is a mono- or oligosaccharide. The substituent is galactose-3-sulfate in the sulfatides and is an oligosaccharide containing sialic acid in the gangliosides (Table 29-1). The structure of the neutral glycosphingolipids, sulfatides, and sphingomyelins is discussed in detail in Chaps. 31, 32, and 35, respectively. Table 29-1 provides a schematic illustration of the structure of the major gangliosides.

Gangliosides

Structure

Gangliosides are glycosphingolipids that contain at least one molecule of sialic acid. The highest concentration of ganglioside is found in the gray matter of the brain, and only very small amounts are found in nonneural tissues [111, 131–134]. At the present time at least 15 different gangliosides have been isolated; more undoubtedly will be identified [111, 120, 126, 130, 135–144]. There is a distressingly large number of names for each ganglioside (Table 29-1), and in this chapter we will adhere to the most widely employed terminology, which was suggested by Svennerholm [120].

As mentioned earlier, the gangliosides were originally

Table 29-1. SYSTEMS OF NOMENCLATURE OF GANGLIOSIDES

Structure	Svennerholm [120]	Korey, Gonatas, et al. [82]	Kuhn, Wiegandt, et al. [121–123]	Klenk, et al. [124–126]	Burton [127]	Penick and McCluer [128–130]	*Normal distribution of gangliosides**			
							Gray matter		White matter	
							Newborn	Adult	Newborn	Adult
Cer ← 1 Glc 4 $\xleftarrow{\beta}$ 1 Gal 3 ← 2NANA	G_{M3}	G_6	G_{LACT}	B_2	B_1	HG-C	1.0	. . .	1.0	
Cer ← 1 Glc 4 $\xleftarrow{\beta}$ 1 Gal 4 $\xleftarrow{\beta}$ 1 GalNac 3 ↑ 2NANA	G_{M2}	G_5	G_{GNTr}II	A_1	B_2	HG-D	3.6	1.7	6.9	1.9
Cer ← 1 Glc 4 $\xleftarrow{\beta}$ 1 Gal 4 $\xleftarrow{\beta}$ 1 GalNac 3 3 ↑β ↑ 1 Gal 2NANA	G_{M1}	G_4	G_{GNT}I	A_2	B_3	HG-1	14.6	12.8	19.1	12.6
Cer ← 1 Glc 4 $\xleftarrow{\beta}$ 1 Gal 4 $\xleftarrow{\beta}$ 1 GalNac 3 3 ↑β ↑ 1 Gal 2NANA 3 ↑ NANA2	G_{D1a}	G_3	G_{GNT}II	B_1	B_4	HG-2	71.6	22.8	57.8	18.4
Cer ← 1 Glc 4 $\xleftarrow{\beta}$ 1 Gal 4 $\xleftarrow{\beta}$ 1 GalNac 3 3 ↑β ↑ 1 Gal 2NANA 8 ← 2NANA	G_{D1b}	G_2	G_{GNT}III	C_1	C_3	HG-4	1.8	23.5	2.1	30.4
Cer ← 1 Glc 4 $\xleftarrow{\beta}$ 1 Gal 4 $\xleftarrow{\beta}$ 1 GalNac 3 3 ↑β ↑ 1 Gal │ 3 │ ↑ │ NANA2 2NANA 8 ← 2NANA	G_{T1}	G_1	G_{GNT}IV	C_3	C_4		7.3	31.2	3.4	27.9

* Data from Martensson [111] and Suzuki et al. [157].

discovered by Klenk in the brain from a patient with Tay-Sachs disease [30, 32, 33]. He named them gangliosides because they appeared to be characteristic of ganglion cells. Similar, or possibly identical, products were isolated from brain by Folch-Pi and his colleagues [145] and by Rosenberg and Chargaff, who applied to them the names strandin [135, 146] and mucolipid [147, 148], respectively. The term *ganglioside* has become more generally accepted for this class of glycolipids.

Ceramide Moiety

Each ganglioside molecule contains one residue of sphingosine and fatty acid and one or more residues of both sialic acid and hexose; many gangliosides also contain one hexosamine moiety. The number and relative positions of the hexose and sialic acid residues are the distinguishing characteristics of each ganglioside.

The asialogangliosides are a family of molecules derived from the gangliosides by the removal of a sialic acid moiety, e.g., asialoganglioside G_{M2} is:

$$\text{GalNac 1} \xrightarrow{\beta} \text{4 Gal 1} \xrightarrow{\beta} \text{4 Glc 1} \xrightarrow{\beta} \text{Cer}$$

The structure of gangliosides has not yet been proved by chemical synthesis, but Shapiro and his colleagues have synthesized a significant portion of the ganglioside molecule [149].

In the gangliosides found in mammalian neural tissues, both C_{18} and C_{20} sphingosine bases are present. The relative amounts of the two vary with age. In fetal tissue, C_{18} sphingosine predominates [106–108, 110]; with increasing age, the relative concentration of C_{20} sphingosine increases until C_{20} sphingosine constitutes about 60 to 70 percent of the total bases in senile brain [106–108, 110]. Brain gangliosides also contain both C_{18} and C_{20} dihydrosphingosine; the C_{20}-saturated form also becomes relatively more abundant with increasing age [106, 110]. C_{18} sphingosine is the major long-chain base in extraneural tissue [150, 151]; many sphingosine congeners have been isolated from bovine kidney gangliosides.

The fatty acid composition of the gangliosides from neural tissue is quite different from that of other sphingolipids.

Most (80 to 90 percent) brain gangliosides contain stearic acid (C_{18}); the remainder are C_{16}, C_{20}, and C_{22} fatty acids [106, 111, 150, 152]. In fetal human brain, gangliosides contain more than 90 percent stearic acid; the adult composition is attained by 3 years of age [153]. Furthermore, most gangliosides contain very little if any hydroxy fatty acids [106, 111]; the only exception is the novel ganglioside isolated by Siddiqui and McCluer that contains approximately equal amounts of hydroxy and normal fatty acids [141]. The fatty acid composition of gangliosides from nonneural tissue has not been studied extensively; the composition seems to be similar to that of other nonneural sphingolipids, with a predominance of C_{22} and C_{24} fatty acids [150, 151].

Carbohydrate Components

Sialic acid is the common name for a group of complex carbohydrates, and N-acetylneuraminic acid and N-glycolylneuraminic acid are the two most common sialic acids. The sialic acid of brain gangliosides is N-acetylneuraminic acid [111]. It is also the predominant sialic acid in human spleen, liver, and erythrocytes [111, 131, 132, 134].

In addition to sialic acid there are four other carbohydrate constituents of the gangliosides. Glucose and galactose are found in all human gangliosides except for a sialosylgalactosylceramide recently isolated from brain [141]. Although N-acetylgalactosamine is present in most of the more complex gangliosides, N-acetylglucosamine has been found in only one human ganglioside [132].

Tissue Distribution

The highest concentration of gangliosides is present in nervous tissue, and there are significant variations in the concentration and relative composition of gangliosides in specific areas of the nervous system [111, 154–156]. In the gray matter of the brain they comprise about 6 percent of the lipids, or 2 percent of the dry weight; in white matter they constitute about 0.6 percent of the total lipids, or 0.4 percent of the dry weight. Much smaller concentrations of gangliosides have been found in liver [133, 134, 150, 157, 158], spleen [131, 132, 157–159], kidney [111, 113, 151, 159, 160], retina [161], erythrocytes [111, 162, 163], plasma [164], cardiac muscle [133, 165], alimentary tract [133], mammary gland [133], lung [133], placenta [166], human skin fibroblasts [167], and rat hepatoma cells [168].

Developmental Changes

Although the gangliosides are the largest glycolipid fraction in fetal brain, the concentration of other glycolipids increases much more rapidly in the neonatal period [111]. Between birth and the end of myelination there is a twofold increase in the concentration of brain gangliosides [111, 155]; developmental changes in the ganglioside concentration of nonneural tissues have not been investigated. There are also significant changes in the ganglioside pattern of brain between the fetus and the adult [111, 155, 169].

Cellular and Subcellular Localization

Significant concentrations of gangliosides have been observed in neuronal cell bodies [170], peripheral nerves [171], synaptosomes [172–174], axons [174], and nerve endings [170, 175–177]. Much smaller concentrations are found in glial cells [170]. The gangliosides in neural tissue appear to be structural lipids and are primarily localized in the microsomes, particularly in the light microsomes [172, 175]. Although Cumings et al. were unable to find gangliosides in myelin [178], Suzuki and his colleagues have presented convincing evidence for their presence in this substance [179–181].

Physical State of Gangliosides

It was originally proposed that gangliosides occur as high-molecular-weight polymers, but recent evidence leaves very little doubt that the isolated gangliosides form micelles in aqueous solutions with axial ratios of about 1.2 and with aggregate weights between 200,000 and 250,000 [182–184]. It is likely that the gangliosides *in situ* are bound to, or are associated with, other molecular species, probably lipids or lipoproteins. The gangliosides have been isolated from brain by various methods, and recent advances in chromatographic procedures have led to methods that provide good separation of the various members of this class of sphingolipids [120, 130, 159].

Physiologic Functions

The physiologic function of the sphingolipids is not understood. In general, they are primarily localized to membranes where it is assumed they have an important structural role. Gangliosides are present in the membranes of nerve endings, and it has been suggested that they are important in the transmission of nerve impulses at the synapse. Lowden and Wolfe have reported that the regional distribution of γ-aminobutyric acid, the presumed transmitter substance of inhibitory synapses, and that of gangliosides are quite similar [185]. This observation, combined with the finding that tetanus toxin both binds specifically to gangliosides and blocks inhibitory synapses [186, 187], suggests a role for gangliosides at such junctions. It has also been suggested that gangliosides serve as receptors for serotonin at synapses [188]. Lapetina et al. [172] and Dekirmenjian and his colleagues believe that gangliosides may interact with acetylcholine, serotonin, norepinephrine, dopamine, and histamine in synaptic membranes [174].

Immunochemical Properties

Antibodies have been produced against mixed brain gangliosides; the antigenicity of individual gangliosides has not been adequately evaluated. The nature and relative position of the carbohydrate residues appear to be important immunologic determinants. The immunochemical reactions of the gangliosides and the other sphingolipids have been extensively reviewed by Rapport and Graf [189].

Metabolism of the Gangliosides

The metabolism of gangliosides has been the object of active research in recent years. Studies of the turnover of gangliosides in rat brain have indicated that their half-life is between 20 and 24 days [127, 190, 191]. There appears to be a rapid turnover before and during myelination. It is not yet clear whether or not there is a precursor-product relationship between the various gangliosides [111, 192].

Many investigators have shown that radioactively labeled acetate, fatty acids, serine, and carbohydrates are incorporated into glycosphingolipids [111, 127, 191, 193, 194]. A combination of in vivo and in vitro techniques has clarified some of the pathways leading to the biosynthesis of the gangliosides.

Biosynthesis of Gangliosides

Sphingosine

The mechanisms involved in the biosynthesis of sphingosine and its congeners have been elucidated by Brady [195–197], Braun [198, 199], Snell [198], Stoffel [200], Fujino [201, 202], and their coworkers. The first step in the biosynthesis of sphingosine is the condensation of a 16-carbon unit, palmitoyl coenzyme A, with a 2-carbon fragment derived from serine:

$$CH_3(CH_2)_{14}\overset{O}{\overset{\|}{C}}{-}SCoA + H{-}\underset{NH_2}{\underset{|}{\overset{COOH}{\overset{|}{C}}}}{-}CH_2OH \xrightarrow[\text{Pyridoxal phosphate}]{Mn^{++}} CH_3(CH_2)_{14}\overset{O}{\overset{\|}{C}}{-}\underset{NH_2}{\underset{|}{CH}}{-}CH_2OH \quad (1)$$

Reaction 1 requires pyridoxal phosphate as a cofactor, and it is believed that a Schiff's base is an intermediate. It has been established [198, 199, 200] that the 3-ketodihydrosphingosine intermediate is reduced by NADPH (nicotinamide adenine dinucleotide phosphate reduced to dihydrosphingosine,

$$\underset{\text{3-Ketodihydrosphingosine}}{CH_3(CH_2)_{14}\overset{O}{\overset{\|}{C}}{-}\underset{NH_2}{\underset{|}{C}}HCH_2OH} + NADPH + H^+ \longrightarrow \text{dihydrosphingosine} + NADP^+ \quad (2)$$

The further pathway for sphingosine synthesis has not been established; it may be that 3-ketodihydrosphingosine is converted to sphingosine with 3-ketosphingosine as an intermediate [198]. Dihydrosphingosine is converted to phytosphingosine, 3-ketodihydrosphingosine again being an intermediate. The substitution of stearoyl CoA for palmitoyl CoA results in the formation of C_{20} sphingosines [199].

Ceramide

Radin and his colleagues have studied the formation of ceramide from acyl coenzyme A and long-chain base in mouse brain microsomal preparations [199, 203]. The facility with which individual fatty acyl CoA's were incorporated into ceramide approximately paralleled their distribution in brain sphingolipids [203].

Gangliosides

The pathways of ganglioside formation have not been firmly established. Roseman's group [204–209] has employed homogenates of embryonic chicken brain and has elucidated a system of glycosyl transferases that catalyzes the synthesis of gangliosides by the stepwise addition to ceramide of one monosaccharide unit at a time. Sialic acid is added through the intermediate, cytidine monophosphate-N-acetylneuraminic acid (CMP-NANA).

$$\text{UDP (uridine diphosphate)-glucose} + \text{ceramide} \longrightarrow \text{glucosyl ceramide} + \text{UDP-galactose} \longrightarrow \text{galactosylglucosyl ceramide} \quad (1)$$

$$\text{Galactosylglucosyl ceramide} + \text{CMP-NANA} \longrightarrow \text{ganglioside } G_{M3} \quad (2)$$

$$\text{Ganglioside } G_{M3} + \text{UDP-N-acetylgalactosamine} \longrightarrow \text{ganglioside } G_{M2} + \text{UDP} \quad (3)$$

$$\text{Ganglioside } G_{M2} + \text{UDP-galactose} \longrightarrow \text{ganglioside } G_{M1} + \text{UDP} \quad (4)$$

$$\text{Ganglioside } G_{M1} + \text{nCMP-NANA} \longrightarrow \text{higher gangliosides} \quad (5)$$

Several of the glycosyltransferases have also been described by other groups of investigators [173, 210, 211].

The sialyltransferase catalyzing Reaction 2 has also been detected in a microsomal fraction of mouse brain by Arce et al. [212]. The sialyltransferases of Reactions 2 and 5 appear to be distinct enzymes [209]. Employing cell-free preparations from rat kidney, Kanfer et al. [213] have obtained results that suggest that N-acetylgalactosaminylgalactosylglucosyl ceramide may serve as the receptor for N-acetylneuraminic acid in the formation of ganglioside G_{M2}. The later steps in this scheme were Reactions 4 and 5. The scheme proposed by Roseman and coworkers has thus not yet been established as the only route of ganglioside synthesis. It has been noted [111, 197] that the structure of several products has yet to be established. Some of the glycosyl transferases also lack absolute specificity. Kanfer and Richards [214] observed that the administration of puromycin to neonatal rats blocks both protein and ganglioside synthesis. This finding is difficult to reconcile with the notion that gangliosides are synthesized by an independent system of preformed glycosyl transferases and suggests that ganglioside synthesis may be dependent on the simultaneous synthesis of protein. Complete understanding of the biosynthesis of gangliosides will probably require further purification of the enzymes involved in the synthetic process.

Catabolism of Gangliosides

Oligosaccharide Unit

The catabolism of sphingolipids has been investigated extensively. The initial reactions in the catabolism of gangliosides are the removal of terminal monosaccharides by highly specific glycosyl hydrolases. The internal sugar residues are then sequentially cleaved by other specific glycosyl hydrolases until the ganglioside has been degraded to ceramide. Many of these enzymes have been partially purified and described in detail [111, 197, 215–218]. Neuraminidases, specific for the cleavage of sialic acid from gangliosides, have also been described [47, 216, 218–220]. Leibovitz and Gatt [220] observed a neuraminidase in calf brain that cleaved sialic acid from di- and trisialogangliosides but not from the monosialogangliosides, G_{M1} and G_{M2}.

There seems to be general agreement that the polysialogangliosides are first converted to ganglioside G_{M1} by neuraminidases. The next catabolic step is either the removal of the final sialic acid (Reaction 2, Fig. 29-6) or the terminal galactose (Reaction 1, Fig. 29-6), reactions yielding asialo-G_{M1} or ganglioside G_{M2}, respectively. Both reactions occur in human tissue [221]. Asialo-G_{M1} is then further degraded to ceramide, with asialo-G_{M2}, lactosyl ceramide, and glucosyl ceramide as sequential intermediates. Ganglioside G_{M2} is converted either to asialo-G_{M2} (Reaction 4, Fig. 29-6) or to ganglioside G_{M3} (Reaction 5). Both asialo-G_{M2} and ganglioside G_{M3} can be catabolized further to ceramide.

Ceramide

Gatt and his colleagues have partially purified from rat brain an enzyme that cleaves ceramide into sphingosine and fatty acid [222, 223]. Ceramidase activity has also been found in mouse brain [203] and in the intestine [224]. It has been claimed that the rat brain enzyme catalyzes both the synthesis and breakdown of ceramide. Morell and Radin [203] note that ceramide synthesis occurs primarily in microsomes,

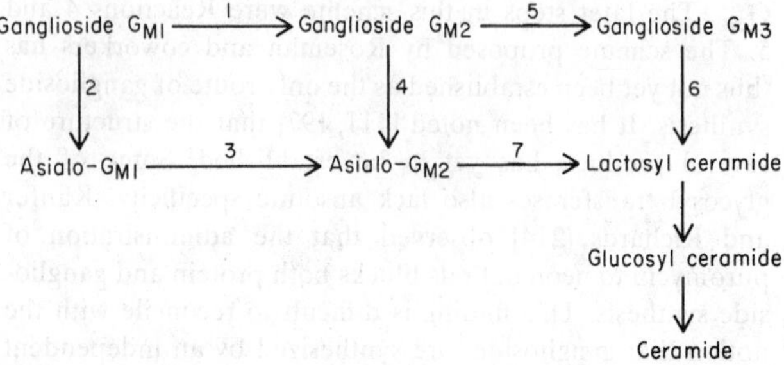

Figure 29-6. Steps in the catabolism of gangliosides. (*After Kolodny* [221].)

whereas ceramide hydrolysis is localized to lysosomes. They suggest that ceramidase has no significant synthetic activity.

Fatty Acids and Sphingosines

The fatty acids cleaved from ceramide are oxidized in the usual pathways for fatty acid catabolism. The complete catabolism of sphingosine is initiated by a series of reactions in which ethanolamine, a 2-carbon unit, is cleaved from sphingosine and its congeners. Sphingosine and dihydrosphingosine are converted to palmitic acid and ethanolamine [200, 225–230]; phytosphingosine is degraded to α-hydroxypalmitic acid and ethanolamine [200, 227, 228]; C_{20} sphingosine is converted in an analogous fashion to stearic acid and phosphorylethanolamine.

The enzymatic reactions involved in these conversions have been investigated. The first step appears to be a kinase reaction in which sphingosine and dihydrosphingosine are converted to the 1-phosphate derivatives [231, 232]. These are then cleaved in an aldolase type of reaction to a C_{16} aldehyde and phosphorylethanolamine [231, 233, 234]. It has also been suggested that sphingosine may first be oxidized to the 3-keto derivative and then cleaved to the aldehyde [235]; the studies with the sphingosine kinase system would suggest that this pathway, if it exists, is not of major importance in sphingosine metabolism. The palmitic acid derived from the catabolism of sphingosine is shunted into the fatty acid oxidation system or undergoes other reactions [226]. The α-hydroxypalmitic acid formed in the degradation of phytosphingosine is converted to a C_{15} fatty acid and then oxidized further [227, 228].

In brain the fatty acid and sphingosine composition of the gangliosides as a group differ entirely from that of the cerebrosides, sulfatides, and dihexosyl ceramides. This would indicate that these two groups are synthesized from different pools of fatty acids and sphingosines; perhaps even different cell types synthesize the two groups [111]. Dihexosyl ceramides appear to be both biosynthetic and catabolic intermediates in ganglioside metabolism [111]. Because of the marked differences in the fatty acid composition of gangliosides and dihexosyl ceramides, it is assumed that only a small part of brain dihexosyl ceramide is involved in ganglioside metabolism [111]. A similar interpretation may be applicable to the precursors of the other sphingolipids.

CHEMICAL ABNORMALITIES IN TAY-SACHS DISEASE

Brain

Tay-Sachs Ganglioside

The historic finding by Klenk that the NANA (ganglioside) content of the cortex of the Tay-Sachs brain is greatly increased [27, 28] has since been amply confirmed. The ganglioside that accumulates in patients with Tay-Sachs disease is ganglioside G_{M2}; it has frequently been termed Tay-Sachs ganglioside. The structure of ganglioside G_{M2} is shown schematically in Fig. 29-2. The presence of ganglioside G_{M2} in brain is not peculiar to Tay-Sachs disease; small amounts of ganglioside G_{M2} are also found in normal brain (Table 29-2). By contrast, G_{M2} represents approximately 90 percent of the total gangliosides in the Tay-Sachs brain, and indeed an increase in the G_{M2} content of brain is the primary basis for the diagnosis of the disease [34, 40, 41, 63, 150, 236–245]. The concentration of G_{M2} may be more than 70 times normal [63]. This abnormality is readily demonstrated by thin-layer chromatography (Fig. 29-7). The lipid composition, including ganglioside pattern, of cerebellar white matter and the basal ganglia is very similar to that of cerebral white matter. The accumulation of gangliosides is somewhat lower [63, 150].

The fatty acids of the gangliosides in Tay-Sachs brains are primarily C_{16} and C_{18} [150, 157] and are therefore similar to those found in normal brain gangliosides. The sphingosines of the G_{M2} in Tay-Sachs brains consist of the C_{18} and C_{20} forms and in the 4:1 ratio that is found normally in fetal and young infant brain gangliosides [150].

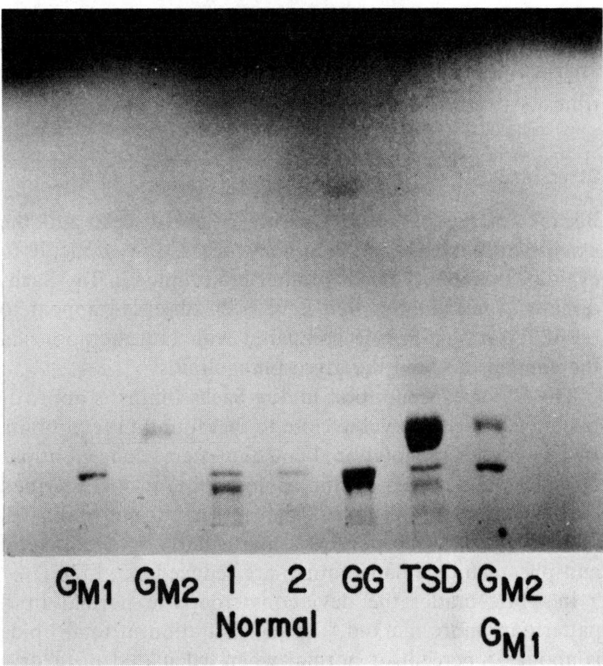

Figure 29-7. Thin-layer chromatogram of brain gangliosides prepared according to conventional methods [155, 157, 159]. The lanes are marked according to the following abbreviations: G_{M1}, ganglioside G_{M1}; G_{M2}, ganglioside G_{M2}; 1 and 2, ganglioside fraction extracted from normal brain; GG, gangliosides from brain of patient with G_{M1} gangliosidosis; TSD, gangliosides from brain of patient with G_{M2} gangliosidosis.

Glycosphingolipids

In addition to the Tay-Sachs ganglioside, there are elevated levels of neutral glycosphingolipids in Tay-Sachs brains. Gatt and Berman [43] and Svennerholm [42] first observed the abnormal accumulation of asialoganglioside G_{M2}, and the observation has been confirmed repeatedly [41, 63, 150, 157, 246]. Asialo-G_{M2} may constitute as much as 3 percent of the lipids of the brain [157, 246].

Elevated concentrations of tetrahexosyl ceramide [157, 246, 247], dihexosyl ceramide [43, 157, 246], and glucosyl ceramide [63, 157, 245, 246] have been observed in Tay-Sachs brains, but the concentration of galactosyl ceramide is less than normal [63, 157, 246]. Normal levels of di- and tetrahexosyl ceramides have been reported in whole brain of one patient with Tay-Sachs disease [63]. Because it has been noted that the abnormalities of glycolipid concentration are most striking in gray matter [157, 246], this discrepant finding may have been due to assay of heterogeneous brain substance.

The fatty acids of the mono-, di-, tri-, and tetrahexosyl ceramides in Tay-Sachs brains are primarily C_{16} and C_{18} rather than the usual C_{22} and longer chain lengths [111, 150, 157, 245]; the sphingosines of the glucosyl and trihexosyl ceramides are the C_{18} and C_{20} forms in a 4:1 ratio. These

Table 29-2. CONCENTRATION OF GANGLIOSIDE G_{M2} IN THE CEREBRUM IN TAY-SACHS DISEASE

Ref.	Age, mo	Gray matter, % of total NANA	White matter, % of total NANA	Whole cerebrum, mg/gm wet weight
[236]	39	73.3		
[63]	48	....	....	6.24
[155]	..	83.4		
[155]	..	88.4		
[155]	..	87.9		
[155]	..	84.1		
[157]	30	88.4	82.2	
[167]	38	....	....	5.72
Normal	4–48	2.3 [157]	1.5 [157]	0.11 [63]

similarities with the components of ganglioside G_{M2} suggest that a precursor-product relationship exists between ganglioside G_{M2} and the increased amounts of mono-, di-, and trihexosyl ceramide.

Other Lipids

Because of the progressive nature of the disease and the extensive demyelination that may occur, it is difficult to evaluate possible changes in other brain lipids in Tay-Sachs disease. Abnormalities that have been observed appear to be of lesser significance compared with the alterations in the gangliosides and the glycosphingolipids.

The water concentration in Tay-Sachs brains is approximately 90 percent, a value close to that found in fetal brain. In gray matter the total lipid and cholesterol concentrations are normal; 8 percent of the cholesterol is in the esterified form, compared with 1 to 2 percent in normal brain [63, 150, 157]. Total phospholipids, particularly sphingomyelin and phosphatidylethanolamine, are reduced [63, 157].

In white matter the deviations from the normal lipid pattern are more marked. The concentration of total lipids is about 55 percent of normal when calculated on a dry-weight basis [63, 157]; on a wet-weight basis the value is 25 to 35 percent of normal. Total phospholipids are reduced to about 50 percent of the normal value [63, 157]. Total cholesterol may be decreased to 50 percent of normal, and an unusually high percentage may be in the esterified form [63, 157]. These lipid values suggest the existence of a demyelinating process. The low values of galactosyl ceramide support the assumption.

Edgar observed an accumulation of nonlipid hexosamine in addition to ganglioside G_{M2} in the white matter from 10 patients with TSD. He suggested that G_{M2} and this hexosamine-containing material are derived from the same substance [248]. Bogoch and Belval reported that Tay-Sachs brains contained large amounts of a specific protein associated with sialic acid and hexose [249]. The importance of these two observations has not been established.

Spinal Cord, Spinal Roots, and Peripheral Nerves

Extensive chemical studies of neural tissue outside the cerebrum and cerebellum have not been reported in patients with Tay-Sachs disease. The available data are, however, in general agreement with those reported for cerebrum. The levels of ganglioside G_{M2} and asialo-G_{M2} are markedly elevated [63, 150].

Organs Outside the Central Nervous System

Liver, Spleen, and Heart

Eeg-Olofsson, Kristensson, Sourander, and Svennerholm were the first to demonstrate that in Tay-Sachs disease ganglioside G_{M2} accumulates in significant amounts not only in neural tissue but also in the viscera [63, 150]. They demonstrated the presence of elevated levels of ganglioside G_{M2} in the liver and spleen of a child who died with Tay-Sachs disease at 4 years of age. The G_{M2} isolated from the liver contained approximately equal amounts of C_{18} and C_{22} + C_{24} fatty acids. The fatty acid composition, therefore, resembled a mixture of normal brain and liver gangliosides. Sixteen percent of the sphingosine was C_{20}. Svennerholm and his colleagues interpreted the fatty acid and sphingosine composition as indicating that a portion of the ganglioside G_{M2} in the Tay-Sachs liver is synthesized in neural tissue and then transported to the liver; the remainder may be synthesized in the liver [63, 150]. Gregoire and his colleagues have confirmed the observation that ganglioside G_{M2} is stored in the Tay-Sachs liver [250]. Schneck et al. found an accumulation of ganglioside G_{M2} in the heart of one patient [165].

In an elegant study Suzuki and his colleagues confirmed and extended Svennerholm's quantitative data [157]. In the liver and spleen of three children with Tay-Sachs disease, Suzuki found abnormal concentrations of ganglioside G_{M2}. The patients were 33, 41, and 54 months old at the time of their death. The G_{M2} level in Tay-Sachs liver and spleen is elevated between four- and elevenfold [157]. The major ganglioside of human spleen and liver is normally ganglioside G_{M3} [134, 157]. In the liver and spleen of Suzuki's three patients, the concentration of ganglioside G_{M2} was as great as that of G_{M3} or greater [157]. Gregoire and his colleagues observed the presence of asialoganglioside G_{M2} in Tay-Sachs liver [250], but quantitative values were not provided.

In contrast to the above studies, Taketomi and Kawamura were not able to demonstrate an abnormal G_{M2} concentration in the liver and spleen of a child who died of Tay-Sachs disease at the age of 11 months [251]. This patient was much younger than those of Suzuki [157], Svennerholm [63, 150], and Gregoire [250], and the difference in ages may account for the discrepancy between the observations.

Cerebrospinal Fluid and Tissue Culture Cells

Bernheimer has reported abnormally high concentrations of ganglioside G_{M2} in the cerebrospinal fluid of a patient with Tay-Sachs disease [252].

Batzdorf and his colleagues have demonstrated that a tissue culture of the frontal lobe from a patient with Tay-Sachs disease contained increased amounts of ganglioside G_{M2} [236]. The authors believe that the cells that grew in culture were probably derived from pericytes of the brain parenchyma or from the leptomeninges.

Membranous Cytoplasmic Bodies

Employing the Hale stain, Halaris and Jatzkewitz concluded that gangliosides are localized in the membranes of the membranous cytoplasmic bodies [97]. Suzuki and his colleagues have isolated MCB from Tay-Sachs brains and determined their lipid composition [157, 253]. The gangliosides of the MCB were almost exclusively G_{M2}. A series of oligohexosyl ceramides were also present. Glucosyl ceramides made up 95 percent of the monohexosyl ceramides, and trihexosyl ceramides comprised 67 percent of the total neutral glycosphingolipids [157].

Blood

Edgar et al. reported that erythrocytes from patients with Tay-Sachs disease contained abnormally high levels of lipid-bound N-acetylneuraminic acid [254], but Booth was unable to confirm this observation [163]. Employing thin-layer chromatography, Sastry and Stancer found G_{M2} in whole blood from two patients with TSD; none was present in the blood of five controls [164]. This observation confirms the report of Rouser et al., who detected an increased concentration of ganglioside in erythrocytes from patients with Tay-Sachs disease [255].

Ancillary Clinical Findings

Electroencephalogram and Electroretinogram

The EEG is usually normal during the first year of life [7, 190, 256, 257]. During the second year the EEG is characterized by paroxysmal discharges of high-voltage, slow activity with single and occasionally multiple spike and sharp-wave complexes [7, 256]. These abnormalities are associated with frequent focal and generalized convulsions and myoclonic seizures. After 2 years of age there is a decrease in both the frequency of seizures and the frequency and voltage amplitude of the spike potentials [256]. Photic stimulation affected the EEG in only 1 of the 14 patients and never initiated a clinical seizure. Schneck describes abnormal laughter (which he terms "gelastic seizures") in 13 of 14 patients with TSD. These seizures began at about 10 months of age and usually preceded the onset of tonic-clonic seizures [256]. The electroretinogram usually becomes abnormal late in the disease [58].

Blood

Erythrocytes

A decrease in the sphingomyelin content of red blood cell stroma has been described by Balint et al. [258, 259]. Such abnormalities were found in all of the 6 patients with TSD and in 9 of the 12 apparently healthy parents. They were also noted in one patient with Niemann-Pick disease and in one with Gaucher's disease. Balint and Kyriakides observed increased amounts of protein, hexosamine, threonine, serine, and probably sialic acid in red blood cell stromal proteins from 9 patients with TSD [260]. This seemed to indicate increased amounts of a glycoprotein in the red blood cells, and that the defect in TSD affects glycoprotein metabolism. There is no obvious relationship of these abnormalities to the basic biochemical defect in TSD.

Leukocytes

Strouth and coworkers observed basophilic granulation in the leukocytes from two patients with TSD [261]. Rosner et al. were not able to confirm this finding [262]. Vacuolated lymphocytes have been seen occasionally in Tay-Sachs disease [263, 264]. No large lipid-containing cytoplasmic inclusions have been demonstrated by electron microscopy [264].

Plasma

Volk, Schneck, Aronson, and their colleagues have reported that the activity of serum lactic dehydrogenase (LDH) and that of glutamic oxaloacetic transaminase are frequently and markedly elevated in the early stages of Tay-Sachs disease. At the same time serum fructose-1-phosphate aldolase activity is frequently reduced [7, 265–267]. Children with TSD have a normal fructose tolerance test result and have readily measurable, although less than normal, fructose-1-phosphate aldolase activity in the liver [7]. A decrease in the serum activity of this enzyme was observed in 51 of 52 obligate heterozygotes [266]. Saifer et al. noted that the ratio of the LDH-3 and LDH-5 isoenzymes was abnormal in TSD [268]. They have also reported a shift of serum sialic acid from the albumin-bound to the globulin-bound form without an increase in the total sialic acid [269]. Spiegel-Adolf and her colleagues observed an increased level of serum lysolecithin in Tay-Sachs patients [270]. These changes have not been observed in all patients with TSD, and their precise meaning is not understood.

Cerebrospinal Fluid

The activity of a number of glycolytic enzymes, dehydrogenases and transaminases has been found abnormal in the spinal fluid of Tay-Sachs patients [265, 271, 272]. Tourtellotte and coworkers [273, 274] have reported that foam cells may be present in the spinal fluid. The significance of these results is uncertain.

Immunochemistry

Pascal and his colleagues reported that antibodies produced against Tay-Sachs brain gangliosides reacted specifically with ganglioside G_{M2}. Anti–normal brain ganglioside serum produced two to three bands with normal brain and only one with Tay-Sachs brain [275, 276]. This technique for establishing an excess of G_{M2} may be useful when only very small amounts of brain are available and may also permit the localization of gangliosides by the fluorescent antibody method.

THE METABOLIC DEFECT IN TAY-SACHS DISEASE

The significant biochemical feature of Tay-Sachs disease is the accumulation of a specific monosialoganglioside and its NANA-free product, a ceramide trisaccharide. These lipids seem to collect in progressively increasing quantities in the cytoplasm of ganglion cells, causing them to enlarge grotesquely and eventually to die. The lipid also appears to be extruded both from the cell bodies in the gray matter and from the axons in the white matter. It is phagocytosed by surrounding glia. The myelin undergoes concomitant or subsequent degeneration.

The key question is whether there is an increased synthesis of monosialoganglioside or whether this compound accumulates because of a block in a normal catabolic pathway for gangliosides.

Possible Increased Synthesis of Ganglioside G_{M2}

No studies have been made of the synthesis of ganglioside G_{M2} in patients with Tay-Sachs disease. The disease could be due to overproduction of ganglioside G_{M2}, but there is no evidence to support this hypothesis. It is counter to the finding of catabolic defects in many other similar diseases and is now rendered extremely unlikely with the finding of deficient activity of a specific hydrolase, as described below.

Possible Elaboration of an Abnormal Ganglioside

As mentioned earlier, the ganglioside G_{M2} that accumulates in TSD brains contains the same high ratio of C_{18} to C_{20} sphingosine that is found in normal fetal brain [150]. This feature probably reflects the failure of the Tay-Sachs brain to mature normally. The remainder of the molecule is indistinguishable from normal G_{M2} [242, 243].

Decreased Catabolism of Ganglioside G_{M2}

It is possible that further elaboration of gangliosides from precursor G_{M2} could be blocked by deficient activity of an enzyme such as UDP-(uridine diphosphate-) galactose transferase [206, 277]. Deficient activity of this enzyme, which catalyzes the reaction:

$$\text{Ganglioside } G_{M2} + \text{UDP-galactose} \longrightarrow \text{Ganglioside } G_{M1}$$

could account for the accumulation of G_{M2} in TSD. If this were the metabolic defect in TSD, one might expect a marked reduction in ganglioside G_{M1} content of Tay-Sachs brain. Suzuki has found, however, a normal or slightly increased level of G_{M1} in TSD [157].

The metabolic defect in all the disorders of sphingolipid metabolism that have thus far been defined is one of deficient activity of a catabolic enzyme; and such a defect in TSD has long been suggested by many investigators. Two possible sites for such a metabolic lesion exist: the point of attachment of the N-acetylneuraminyl residue or that of the N-acetylgalactosaminyl moiety. The former possibility was eliminated by the studies of Kolodny and coworkers, who showed that ganglioside G_{M2} neuraminidase activity was normal in muscle from patients with TSD [47].

Deficiency of N-acetylgalactosaminidase (hexosaminidase) activity, an alternative frequently considered, for some time appeared to be eliminated. When assayed with the artificial substrate, *p*-nitrophenyl-β-N-acetylgalactosaminide, Tay-Sachs brain and kidney contained greater than normal total hexosaminidase activity [45, 247]. Robinson and Sterling had found, however, that human tissue contains two hexosaminidase components, hexosaminidase A and B [278]. Taking advantage of this observation, Okada and O'Brien used starch-gel electrophoresis and artificial substrates to show that the A component of hexosaminidase is missing in Tay-Sachs tissues (Fig. 29-8). Hexosaminidase A activity was absent in brain, liver, kidney, skin, cultured fibroblasts, plasma, serum, and leukocytes from nine patients with Tay-Sachs disease [45, 279].

Sandhoff [48] and Hultberg [46] also separated two hexosaminidase components in normal human brain and liver by isoelectric focusing electrophoresis. The isoelectric points were pH 5 for the A form and pH 7 for the B form. Hexosaminidase A activity was absent in the liver and brain of Hultberg's patient with TSD and in the brain of three of Sandhoff's four patients with apparently proved TSD. The presence of hexosaminidase A activity in one of Sandhoff's patients cannot be explained; O'Brien has suggested that this patient may not have had TSD [280]. Noting that incubation with neuraminidase converted hexosaminidase A into a form that had the mobility of hexosaminidase B, Hultberg has suggested that the A variant may be the form in which the enzyme is transported in plasma [46]. Suzuki et al. have also

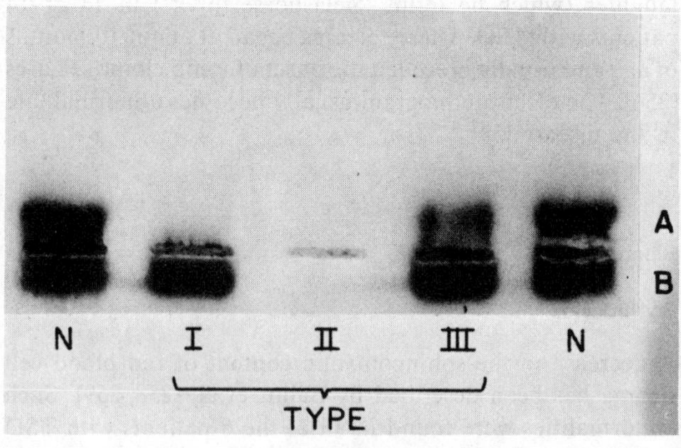

Figure 29-8. Starch-gel electrophoretogram of hexosaminidases from normal liver (N) and liver from patients with G_{M2} gangliosidases, types 1, 2, and 3. Homogenates of liver were prepared and electrophoresed as described elsewhere [45]. (*Courtesy of Dr. John O'Brien.*)

found deficient hexosaminidase A activity in the brain, liver, spleen, leukocytes, and cultured skin fibroblasts of five patients with TSD [281].

Kolodny et al. demonstrated that normal human skeletal muscle can hydrolyze the N-acetylgalactosaminyl residue from authentic Tay-Sachs ganglioside [47]. Ganglioside G_{M2}-hexosaminidase activity was absent in skeletal muscle from three patients with TSD [47]. These results, employing authentic substrate, demonstrate conclusively that the primary enzymatic defect in TSD is the failure to cleave the N-acetylgalactosamine residue from ganglioside G_{M2}.

The abnormalities in Tay-Sachs disease are not confined to the nervous system. It has now been observed that ganglioside G_{M2} accumulates in several organs (brain, liver, spleen, and heart) and that hexosaminidase activity is deficient in many tissues (brain, liver, kidney, skin, cultured fibroblasts, spleen, skeletal muscle, and extracellular fluids). The disorder is therefore a generalized gangliosidosis in the same sense as G_{M1} gangliosidosis (Chap. 30), but the extraneural manifestations of the latter disease are more prominent.

Ganglioside G_{M2} Precursors

Ganglioside G_{M2} is believed to be derived normally from the sequential removal of sialic acid and galactose from G_{M1} and more complex gangliosides. The ganglioside G_{M2} that accumulates in the brain in Tay-Sachs disease almost certainly arises from catabolism of brain gangliosides. That which accumulates in visceral organs may also, at least partially, be of neural origin [63, 150].

PATHOPHYSIOLOGY

There now seems to be no doubt that Tay-Sachs disease arises because the normal turnover of gangliosides is blocked at the step in which ganglioside G_{M2} normally loses hexosamine through action of a specific hexosaminidase. Not all the consequences of this block are understood; they are presently perceived as morphologic changes due to accumulation of G_{M2} and particularly as changes in the structures of the brain attending this storage. Ganglioside G_{M2} is stored throughout the nervous system and, to a much lesser extent, in visceral tissues. In the nervous system, storage occurs within the ganglion cells and axis cylinders of nerves. At the same time G_{M2} piles up in glial cells and in macrophages, some of them adjacent to the capillaries. All these cells become filled with secondary lysosomes or membranous cytoplasmic bodies (MCB). The lysosomal nature of the MCB is supported by their high content of acid phosphatase activity both on the membranes themselves and in the heterogeneous granular core within the membranes [92, 94]. The lipid composition of MCB as determined by Samuels [83] has been confirmed and extended by Suzuki and coworkers [157]. One-third of the dry weight of MCB in Tay-Sachs disease is ganglioside, and all of the ganglioside is G_{M2}.

The function of affected visceral cells is not obviously altered. The brain, however, is confined to a rigid space, and neurons are generally unable to regenerate damaged components. Critical spatial relationships between cells and even their organelles are undoubtedly distorted early in the storage process, and important changes in neural function may be occurring long before membranous cytoplasmic bodies appear. The progression of clinical symptoms has not yet been correlated with specific morphologic changes, nor has it been explained why some children survive longer than others. It does appear that the enlargement of the brain characteristic of the late stage is associated with massive gliosis.

Why Other Lipids Accumulate

It is characteristic of storage diseases that more than one chemical constituent accumulates in the affected tissues. Several sphingoglycolipids in addition to ganglioside G_{M2} are stored in Tay-Sachs disease. The concentration of asialoganglioside G_{M2} may be increased to 15 times the normal value [157]. Kolodny and coworkers have performed an interesting group of experiments that indicate two possible sources for asialo-G_{M2} in Tay-Sachs tissues [47, 221]. The first, shown in human tissues, is by action of a sialidase on ganglioside G_{M2} (Reaction 4, Fig. 29-6). The second, demonstrated in rat intestine, is the combined action upon ganglioside G_{M1} of a β-galactosidase (Reaction 1) and a sialidase (Reaction 2). Reaction 4 proceeds normally in Tay-Sachs brain [47], and presumably the activities of the enzymes regulating Reactions 2 and 3 also are not affected. Although asialo-G_{M2} can be further catabolized in both normal and Tay-Sachs brain [221, 247] (Reaction 7, Fig. 29-6), ganglioside G_{M2} inhibits this reaction in vitro [221]. It has not yet been demonstrated that the accumulated Tay-Sachs ganglioside is available to inhibit this reaction in the abnormal tissues.

The work of Kolodny et al. just referred to raises other questions concerning Tay-Sachs disease. Why, if G_{M2}-sialidase activity is normal, does ganglioside G_{M2} accumulate? Theoretically, the combination of sialidase and hexosaminidase activities shown for Reactions 4 and 7 in Fig. 29-6 should serve as a bypass route avoiding the normal pathways (Reactions 5 and 6). Two possible explanations are offered [221]. (1) The G_{M2}-sialidase reaction is one of the slowest reactions, and may be the rate-limiting step, in normal ganglioside metabolism. (2) Higher gangliosides, particularly ganglioside G_{D1a}, inhibit the sialidase reaction in vitro. Excess ganglioside G_{M2} may therefore overwhelm the slow and partially inhibited G_{M2} sialidase system. Ganglioside G_{D1a} is not elevated in TSD [157] and there is no evidence that the higher gangliosides inhibit the G_{M2} sialidase in vivo.

DIAGNOSIS

It is difficult to establish the diagnosis of Tay-Sachs disease in the first 6 months of life by clinical examination. The disorder should be considered in any infant with progressive psychomotor retardation, exaggerated extension response to sound, and visual difficulties. The presence of a cherry-red spot, hypotonia, and general apathy—in the absence of hepatosplenomegaly—strongly suggests the diagnosis. In patients in whom the diagnosis is suspected, a thorough examination of the nervous system, x-ray survey of the lungs, skull, and long bones, complete hemogram, and determination of plasma acid phosphatase and possibly fructose-1-phosphate aldolase activities are indicated. A bone marrow aspirate should also be examined under the phase microscope to exclude other similar storage diseases in which foam cells may appear. Such cells rarely, if ever, appear in Tay-Sachs disease. Sometimes early neural involvement may be detected upon examination of the autonomic ganglia obtained through transrectal biopsy [63, 69–72]. MCB have been observed in such ganglia [71]. Rectal biopsy does not provide a specific diagnosis.

Until recently a definitive diagnosis of TSD could not be obtained without brain biopsy. Should this heroic procedure be performed, the tissue obtained should be subdivided immediately [282]. A small aliquot is allotted to histologic examination, to include frozen, paraffin-fixed preparations and electron microscopy. A minimum microscopic examination requires staining with oil-red-O or other dyes for neutral lipids, Baker hematoxylin (or Smith-Dietrich stain), periodic acid–Schiff, Nile blue, Schultze, Bial, and Okamato reactions [7]. Formalin fixation rapidly alters both the concentration and composition of gangliosides [283, 284] and irreversibly inactivates enzymes. Most of the biopsy tissue should be aliquoted to separate plastic containers, immediately frozen to $-20°C$, and kept frozen at this temperature. The presence of massive amounts of G_{M2} in the tissue provides a definitive diagnosis of the disease (Fig. 29-7).

Tay-Sachs disease can now be diagnosed without brain biopsy through the observation of marked decrease in activity of hexosaminidase A in blood plasma, serum leukocytes, or cultured fibroblasts taken from skin (Fig. 29-8). Similar decrease in activity of the enzyme in brain, skeletal muscle, or other tissues such as liver, kidney, or spleen also provides a diagnosis.

TREATMENT

There is no specific therapy for Tay-Sachs disease. Treatment is entirely supportive. An intensive care unit skilled in handling such children can provide considerable help to parents and temporarily improve the immediate prognosis of the affected child [285]. No attempt to replace the deficient hexosaminidase has yet been made.

GENETICS

In few inheritable diseases is the genetic mode of transmission better substantiated than in Tay-Sachs disease. A high degree of penetrance, a consistent and unequivocal form of expression, and a relatively high frequency of the disease in an unusually available population have helped to make this possible. The thoroughness with which the data have been gathered and analyzed is also exceptional. Large numbers of cases have been collected and reviewed by Slome [286], Ktenidès [287], Kozinn et al. [288], Goldschmidt et al. [289, 290], and, in the largest series, Aronson and Volk [24, 26, 51]. Included in all these are about 550 different children with the disease [24]. Myrianthopoulos searched all deaths occurring in the United States in the 4-year period from 1954 to 1957 and found that 89 were due to Tay-Sachs disease [291]. His analyses of these data were in agreement with others that indicate the disease to be about 100 times more frequent in the Jewish population than among non-Jews in the United States. The exhaustive analyses of Aronson and Volk [24] have provided a particularly valuable review which needs only to be summarized here to give an adequate description of the genetics and demography of Tay-Sachs disease.

Tay-Sachs disease has been reported from every continent and in most ethnic groups. About 90 percent of affected children are of Jewish heritage. The remainder have come mainly from other Caucasian groups, but Singhalese, Chinese, Japanese, Hindu, Negro, Egyptian, and Lebanese-Syrian children have also been affected. The clinical and pathologic findings appear to be the same in Jewish and non-Jewish children, and the mode of inheritance is indistinguishable [24, 26].

The disease is unquestionably the expression of a double dose of an autosomal allele. Penetrance or certainty of clinical expression seems to be nearly complete, and comparisons of the frequency in many sibships approach the predicted figure of 0.25 for a Mendelian recessive trait. The sexes are equally affected.

The frequency of the Tay-Sachs gene in the Jewish population of New York City is estimated to be approximately 0.016, or a carrier rate of nearly 1:30 [24], compared with an estimated carrier rate of about 1:300 in non-Jewish Americans [24, 29]. Goldschmidt et al. have estimated the frequency of the Tay-Sachs gene as 1:60 in Ashkenazi Jews [290]. Aronson and Volk [24] have further shown that the highest carrier rate appears to lie in Jews whose antecedents lived in the Lithuanian and Polish provinces of Korno and Grodno in the late nineteenth century. Although the consanguinity rate (second-cousin marriages or closer) was not found to be significantly elevated among parents of Jewish children, it is predictably higher among affected non-Jewish marriages. One affected offspring of an incestuous father-daughter union has been reported [74]. As noted earlier, no relationship of incidence or clinical expression to birth order, length of gestation, pregnancy, labor, or other maternal factors has been uncovered [51].

Myrianthopoulos [291–293] and Knudson and Kaplan [294, 295] have discussed the interesting question of why the gene frequency for Tay-Sachs disease, and for others of the sphingolipidoses as well, appears to be so elevated in the Jewish population. They suggest that heterozygote advantage is the most plausible explanation and that the heterozygote may be more fertile [292, 293]. Shaw and Smith have suggested that the incidence of TSD may actually be increasing [296]. It seems likely that the high incidence of TSD in Eastern European Jews reflects both a high gene frequency and a high rate of intramarriage in this cultural group, and does not depend on a specific heterozygote advantage.

Heterozygote Detection

A technique for the certain detection of heterozygotes in the general population has not yet been established. Earlier attempts to do so utilized measurement of serum fructose-1-phosphate aldolase activity [7, 266] or of red blood cell lipids [258]. O'Brien and coworkers have developed an assay of serum hexosaminidase A activity for the purpose of heterozygote detection [279]. Obligate heterozygotes (parents of children with the disease) had enzyme activity that was somewhat lower than that in control subjects and much higher than that in affected children [279]. Although the activity in healthy controls was greater than that in any heterozygote, activity in many patients hospitalized with other diseases fell within the heterozygote range. Friedland et al. have recently reported that it may be possible to distinguish heterozygotes by assay of hexosaminidase A in white blood cells [279*a*].

Prenatal Diagnosis

The first attempt to diagnose TSD prenatally was that of Abood and Lipman, who noted that the usual rise in ceruloplasmin in maternal blood occurred earlier if the mother was carrying a fetus with Tay-Sachs disease [297]. The far more specific measurement of hexosaminidase A activity in fetal cell cultures offers much greater promise for accurate intrauterine diagnosis. Schneck et al. have reported one instance in which the level of hexosaminidase activity in amniotic fluid and uncultured fetal cells was barely detectable. Diagnosis of the disease was confirmed in the aborted fetus [49]. Hexosaminidase A activity was absent in the brain and liver, and the brain contained elevated quantities of ganglioside G_{M2}. The fetal brain also contained inclusions suggestive of membranous cytoplasmic bodies [49]. Because many of the cells in amniotic fluid may be dead or dying, it is desirable to measure enzyme activities in cultured cells from amniotic fluid for the purposes of prenatal diagnosis.

OTHER PHENOTYPES OF G_{M2} GANGLIOSIDOSIS

Type 2

An interesting variant of TSD has been reported by Sandhoff, Jatzkewitz, Pilz, and coworkers [218, 247, 298], in which hexosaminidase activity appeared to be totally absent. The disorder closely resembles Tay-Sachs disease, but visceral involvement, particularly in the kidney, is more prominent. In addition to accumulation of G_{M2}, there is much more pronounced storage of asialo-G_{M2} than in TSD. There is also storage of another glycolipid, N-acetylgalactosaminylgalactosylgalactosylglucosyl ceramide. This "kidney globoside" accumulates in kidney, spleen, and liver [218]. O'Brien has suggested that this disorder be called G_{M2} gangliosidosis, Type 2, to distinguish it from Type 1 (Tay-Sachs disease) [299]. Several other apparent examples of Type 2 have now been reported [299–301], and it is quite likely that many other reported cases of "Tay-Sachs disease" may have represented this variant. O'Brien has shown that both hexosaminidase A and B activity is absent in Type 2 [299].

Type 3

A third type of G_{M2} gangliosidosis has been reported by Bernheimer and Seitelberger [302, 303], Volk and coworkers [304–306], and Suzuki et al. [307]. These patients develop ataxia and progressive psychomotor retardation in the second [304] to fifth [307] year of life and die between about 5 and 15 years of age. Megalocephaly and the cherry-red spot have not occurred, although optic atrophy [303] or retinitis pigmentosa [305] may be present. Ganglioside G_{M2} and asialo-G_{M2} accumulate in brain [302, 306, 307], as does ganglioside G_{M2} in the liver and spleen [307]. Less lipid is stored in these organs than in classical Tay-Sachs disease. Electron microscopy reveals the presence of both MCB and less-well-defined lamellar structures that are reminiscent of those observed in TSD. O'Brien [299] has suggested that this disorder be called gangliosidosis G_{M2}, Type 3. He has demonstrated a partial deficiency of hexosaminidase A in the tissues of the patient described by Volk et al. [305]. This has been confirmed by Schneck and coworkers [305a].

OTHER POSSIBLE GANGLIOSIDOSES

G_{M3} Gangliosidosis

This disorder is possibly represented by one report in the literature. The patient was studied by Pilz [308] and Jörgensen [309] and their coworkers. The patient, who had nonspecific symptoms suggestive of degeneration of the central nervous system, died in the third year of life. The brain contained abnormally high concentrations of ganglioside G_{M3} and asialo-G_{M3} (galactosylglucosyl ceramide). The brain had long been stored in formalin, so that no enzymatic studies were possible; nor can it be excluded that the lipid changes in the brain may have been artifactual.

Higher Gangliosidoses

Schneck et al. [310] describe a 2½-year-old child with psychomotor deterioration, optic atrophy, and exaggerated extension response to sound. Chemical assays on a small piece of brain obtained at biopsy suggested the possible accumulation of a disialoganglioside. Further studies will be required to demonstrate that this is a type of gangliosidosis.

SUMMARY

1 Tay-Sachs disease is a fatal familial disease characterized by the presence of an increased concentration of ganglioside G_{M2} in nervous tissue. This compound contains sphingosine, fatty acid, hexose, hexosamine, and sialic acid. It accumulates in ganglion cells, where a large proportion of the ganglioside is stored within secondary lysosomes that are termed *membranous cytoplasmic bodies.* The eventual death of the ganglion cells is accompanied by proliferation and lipid loading of glial cells in the brain and by severe myelin degeneration.

2 The disease usually becomes evident between ages 4 to 6 months. Psychomotor retardation, exaggerated extension response to sound, visual difficulties, hypotonia, and general apathy are the most common initial signs. Dementia, motor loss, and blindness associated with a cherry-red spot in the retina develop progressively through several well-defined stages until death occurs by the age of 3 to 4 years. All the clinical symptoms are attributable to ganglion cell destruction, demyelination, and reactive gliosis.

3 In the classical form of the disease (Type 1), tissues are deficient in the activity of a specific enzyme, ganglioside G_{M2}-hexosaminidase, that catalyzes the cleavage of the terminal N-acetylgalactosamine moiety from ganglioside G_{M2}. This activity may be more conveniently evaluated with an artificial substrate and is then termed hexosaminidase A. Definitive diagnosis requires the demonstration of ganglioside G_{M2} accumulation in nervous tissue or, preferably, of deficient tissue hexosaminidase A activity.

4 The disease is completely expressed in children homozygous for a mutant autosomal allele. The frequency of heterozygotes is highest in Jewish subjects whose antecedents came from Northeastern Europe. About 10 percent of patients are non-Jewish, and the disease has been reported in most ethnic groups and throughout the world.

5 A reliable test for detection of heterozygotes is not yet available. Intrauterine diagnosis has been achieved by detecting deficient hexosaminidase A activity in fetal tissues.

6 There appear to be two other rare forms of G_{M2} gangliosidosis. Type 2 is similar to Tay-Sachs disease but there is a deficiency of hexosaminidases A and B. The clinical course in Type 3 is more protracted.

7 There is no specific therapy.

BIBLIOGRAPHY

1. Sachs, B.: A family form of idiocy, generally fatal, associated with early blindness. J. Nerv. Ment. Dis., **21**, 475, 1896.
2. Epstein, J.: Amaurotic family idiocy. N.Y. J. Med., **106**, 887, 1917.
3. Norman, R. M., and Wood, N.: A congenital form of amaurotic family idiocy. J. Neurol. Neurosurg. Psychiat., **4**, 175, 1941.
4. Hagberg, B., Hultquist, G., Ohman, R., and Svennerholm, L.: Congenital amaurotic idiocy. Acta Paediat. Scand., **54**, 116, 1965.
5. Fredrickson, D. S., and Trams, E. G.: Ganglioside lipidosis: Tay-Sachs' disease, in *The Metabolic Basis of Inherited Disease,* 2d ed., edited by J. B. Stanbury, J. B. Wyngaarden, and D. S. Fredrickson, p. 523. McGraw-Hill Book Company, New York, 1966.
6. Schettler, G., and Kahlke, W.: Gangliosidoses, in *Lipids and Lipidoses,* edited by G. Schettler, p. 213. Springer-Verlag, New York, 1967.
7. Schneck, L., Volk, B. W., and Saifer, A.: The gangliosidoses. Amer. J. Med., **46**, 245, 1969.
8. Jansky, J.: Über einen noch nicht beschriebenen Fall der familiären amaurotischen Idiotie mit Hypoplasie des Kleinhirns. Z. Erforsch. Behandl. Jugendl. Schwachsinns., **3**, 86, 1909–1910.
9. Bielschowsky, M.: Über spätinfantile familiäre amaurotische Idiotie mit Kleinhirnsymptomen. Deutsch. Z. Nervenheilk., **50**, 7, 1914.
10. Rouser, G., and Wade, R. R.: Amaurotic idiocy. Lipids, **4**, 176, 1969.
11. Norman, R. M., Urich, H., Tingey, A. H., and Goodbody, R. A.: Tay-Sachs disease with visceral involvement and its relationship to Niemann-Pick disease. J. Path. Bact., **78**, 409, 1959.
12. Jervis, G. A.: Familial idiocy due to neuronal lipidosis (the so-called late amaurotic idiocy). Amer. J. Psychiat., **107**, 409, 1950.
13. Jervis, G. A.: Juvenile amaurotic idiocy. A.M.A. J. Dis. Child., **97**, 663, 1959.
14. Zeman, W., and Donahue, S.: Studies on the substantia nigra in Batten's disease. Path. Europ., **3**, 332, 1968.
15. Zeman, W., and Dyken, P.: Neuronal ceroid-lipofuscinosis (Batten's disease): relationship to amaurotic family idiocy. Pediatrics, **44**, 570, 1969.
16. Rozdilsky, B., Cumings, J. H., and Huston, A. F.: Hallervorden-Spatz disease: late infantile and adult types, report of two cases. Acta Neuropath., **10**, 1, 1968.
17. Zeman, W.: What is amaurotic idiocy? Short communication. Lipids, **4**, 76, 1968.
18. Elfenbein, I. B., and Cantor, H. E.: Late infantile amaurotic idiocy with multilamellar cytosomes: an electron microscopic study. J. Pediat., **75**, 253, 1969.
19. Tay, W.: Symmetrical changes in the region of the yellow spot in each eye of an infant. Trans. Ophthal. Soc. U.K., **1**, 155, 1881.
20. Tay, W.: A third instance in the same family of symmetrical changes in the region of the yellow spot in each eye of an infant closely resembling those of embolism. Trans. Ophthal. Soc. U.K., **4**, 158, 1884.
21. Tay, W. A.: A fourth instance of symmetrical changes in the yellow spot region of an infant closely resembling those of embolism. Trans. Ophthal. Soc. U.K., **7**, 125, 1892.
22. Sachs, B.: On arrested cerebral development, with special reference to its cortical pathology. J. Nerv. Ment. Dis., **14**, 541, 1887.
23. Sachs, B., and Hausman, L.: *Nervous and Mental Disorders from Birth through Adolescence.* Hoeber, New York, 1926.
24. Aronson, S. M., and Volk, B. W.: Genetic and demographic considerations concerning Tay-Sachs disease, in *Cerebral Sphingolipidoses,* edited by S. M. Aronson and B. W. Volk, p. 375. Academic, New York, 1962.

25. Falkenheim, K.: Über familiäre amaurotische Idiotie. Jahrb. Kinderheilk., **54**, 123, 1901.
26. Aronson, S. M. Valsamis, M. P., and Volk, B. W.: Infantile amaurotic family idiocy: occurrence, genetic considerations and pathophysiology in the non-Jewish infant. Pediatrics, **26**, 229, 1960.
27. Klenk, E.: Beiträge zur Chemie der Lipoidosen. Niemann-Pick'sche Krankheit und amaurotische Idiotie. Hoppe Seyler. Z. Physiol. Chem., **262**, 128, 1939–1940.
28. Klenk, E.: Beiträge zur Chemie der Lipoidosen. Z. Physiol. Chem., **267**, 128, 1940.
29. Klenk, E., and Langerbeins, H.: Über die Verteilung der Neuraminsäure im Gehirn. Hoppe Seyler. Z. Physiol. Chem., **270**, 185, 1941.
30. Klenk, E.: Neuraminsäure, das Spaltprodukt eines neuen Gehirnlipoids. Hoppe Seyler. Z. Physiol. Chem., **268**, 50, 1941.
31. Klenk, E., and Rennkamp, F.: Über die Ganglioside und Cerebroside der Rindermilz. Hoppe Seyler. Z. Physiol. Chem., **273**, 253, 1942.
32. Klenk, E.: Über die Ganglioside des Gehirns bei der infantilen amaurotischen Idiotie von Typus Tay-Sachs. Ber. Deutsch. Chem. Ges., **75**, 1632, 1942.
33. Klenk, E.: Über die Ganglioside, eine neue Gruppe von zuckerhaltingen Gehirnlipoiden. Hoppe Seyler. Z. Physiol. Chem., **273**, 76, 1942.
34. Svennerholm, L.: The nature of the gangliosides in Tay-Sachs disease, in *Cerebral Lipidoses,* edited by L. van Bogaert, J. N. Cumings, and A. Lowenthal, p. 139. Blackwell, Oxford, 1957.
35. Rosenberg, A., and Chargaff, E.: Some observations on the mucolipids of normal and Tay-Sachs disease brain tissue. A.M.A. J. Dis. Child., **97**, 739, 1959.
36. Terry, R. D., and Korey, S. R.: Membranous cytoplasmic granules in infantile amaurotic idiocy. Nature (London), **188**, 1000, 1960.
37. Gatt, S., and Berman, E. R.: Studies on brain lipids in Tay-Sachs disease. II. Solubility properties of gangliosides. J. Neurochem., **10**, 65, 1963.
38. Svennerholm, L., and Raal, A.: Composition of brain gangliosides. Biochim. Biophys. Acta, **53**, 422, 1961.
39. Svennerholm, L.: The chemical structure of normal human brain and Tay-Sachs gangliosides. Biochem. Biophys. Res. Commun., **9**, 436, 1962.
40. Klenk, E., Liedtke, U., and Gielen, W.: Das Gangliosid des Gehirns bei der infantilen amaurotischen Idiotie vom Typ Tay-Sachs. Hoppe Seyler. Z. Physiol. Chem., **334**, 186, 1963.
41. Makita, A., and Yamakawa, T.: The glycolipids of the brain of Tay-Sachs disease. The chemical structures of a globoside and main ganglioside. Jap. J. Exp. Med., **33**, 361, 1963.
42. Svennerholm, L.: Some aspects of the biochemical changes in leucodystrophy, in *Brain Lipids and Lipoproteins and the Leucodystrophies,* edited by J. Folch-Pi, p. 104. Elsevier, Amsterdam, 1963.
43. Gatt, S., and Berman, E. R.: Studies on brain lipids in Tay-Sachs disease. I. Isolation of two sialic acid-free glycolipids. J. Neurochem., **10**, 43, 1963.
44. Gatt, S., and Berman, E. R.: Studies on brain lipids in Tay-Sachs disease. III. Incorporation of tritiated water into brain lipids. J. Neurochem., **10**, 73, 1963.
45. Okada, S., and O'Brien, J.: Tay-Sachs disease: generalized absence of a beta-D-N-acetylhexosaminidase component. Science, **165**, 698, 1969.
46. Hultberg, B.: N-Acetylhexosaminidase activities in Tay-Sachs disease. Lancet, **2**, 1195, 1969.
47. Kolodny, E. H., Brady, R. O., and Volk, B. W.: Demonstration of an alteration of ganglioside metabolism in Tay-Sachs disease. Biochem. Biophys. Res. Commun., **37**, 526, 1969.
48. Sandhoff, K.: Variation of β-N-acetylhexosaminidase-pattern in Tay-Sachs disease. FEBS Letters, **4**, 351, 1969.
49. Schneck, L., Valenti, C., Amsterdam, D., Friedland, J., Adachi, M., and Volk, B. W.: Prenatal diagnosis of Tay-Sachs disease. Lancet, **1**, 582, 1970.
50. Kanof, A., Aronson, S. M., and Volk, B. W.: Clinical progression of amaurotic family idiocy. A.M.A. J. Dis. Child., **97**, 656, 1959.
51. Aronson, S. M., Aronson, B. E., and Volk, B. W.: A genetic profile of infantile amaurotic family idiocy. A.M.A. J. Dis. Child., **98**, 50, 1959.
52. Aronson, S. M., Volk, B. W., and Epstein, N.: Morphologic evolution of amaurotic family idiocy. Amer. J. Path., **31**, 609, 1955.
53. Schneck, L., and Volk, B. W.: Clinical manifestations of Tay-Sachs disease and Niemann-Pick disease, in *Inborn Disorders of Sphingolipid Metabolism* (proceedings of the 3rd international symposium on the cerebral sphingolipidoses, 1965), edited by S. M. Aronson and B. W. Volk, p. 403. Pergamon, New York, 1967.
54. Landolt, R.: Biochemische-pathologische Aspekte der Sphingolipidosen. Bull. Schweiz. Akad. Med., **24**, 73, 1968.
55. Brady, R. O.: Genetics and the sphingolipidoses. Med. Clin. N. Amer., **53**, 827, 1969.
56. Allan, J. D., and Raine, D. N.: *Some Inherited Disorders of Brain and Muscle,* Proceedings of the Fifth Symposium of The Society for the Study of Inborn Errors of Metabolism, p. 82. Livingstone, Edinburgh and London, 1969.
57. Schneck, L., Maisel, J., and Volk, B. W.: The startle response and serum enzyme profile in early detection of Tay-Sachs' disease. J. Pediat., **65**, 749, 1964.
58. Schneck, L.: The clinical aspects of Tay-Sachs disease, in *Tay-Sachs' Disease,* edited by B. W. Volk, p. 16. Grune & Stratton, New York, 1964.
59. Jampel, R. S.: Eye movements in Tay-Sachs disease. Neurology, **14**, 1013, 1964.
60. Schneck, L., and Volk, B. W.: Clinical manifestations of Tay-Sachs disease and Niemann-Pick disease, in *Inborn Disorders of Sphingolipid Metabolism* (proceedings of the 3rd international symposium on the cerebral sphingolipidoses, 1965), edited by S. M. Aronson and B. W. Volk, p. 403. Pergamon, New York, 1967.
61. Aronson, S. M., Lewitan, A., Rabiner, A. M., Epstein, N., and Volk, B. W.: The megalencephalic phase of infantile amaurotic family idiocy: cephalometric and pneumoencephalic studies. Arch. Neurol. Psychiat., **79**, 151, 1958.
62. Aronson, S. M., and Volk, B. W.: Pathogenesis of white matter changes in Tay-Sachs disease, in *Cerebral Sphingolipidoses,* edited by S. M. Aronson and B. W. Volk, p. 15. Academic, New York, 1962.
63. Eeg-Olofsson, L., Kristensson, K., Sourander, P., and Svennerholm, L.: Tay-Sachs disease: a generalized metabolic disorder. Acta Paediat. Scand., **55**, 546, 1966.
64. Norman, R. M.: Observations on the neuropathology of the cerebral lipidoses. Path. Europ., **3**, 143, 1968.
65. Wenderowic, E., Sokolansky, G., and Klossowsky, B.: Beiträge zur Histopathologie der Tay-Sachsen Krankheit mit besonderer Berücksichtigung der dabei stattfindenden Faserveränderungen und ihrer Charakteristik. Mschr. Psychiat. Neurol., **78**, 305, 1931.
66. Terry, R. D., and Weiss, M.: Studies in Tay-Sachs disease. II. Ultrastructure of the cerebrum. J. Neuropath. Exp. Neurol., **22**, 18, 1963.
67. Volk, B. W.: Pathologic anatomy, in *Tay-Sachs Disease,* edited by B. W. Volk, p. 36. Grune & Stratton, New York, 1964.
68. Kristensson, K., Olsson, Y., and Sourander, P.: Peripheral nerve changes in Tay-Sachs and Batten-Spielmeyer-Vogt disease. Acta Path. Microbiol. Scand., **70**, 630, 1967.
69. Nakai, H., and Landing, B. H.: Suggested use of rectal biopsy in the diagnosis of neural lipidoses. Pediatrics, **26**, 225, 1960.
70. Bodian, M., and Lake, B. D.: The rectal approach to neuropathology. Brit. J. Surg., **50**, 702, 1963.
71. Volk, B. W., Wallace, B. J., and Aronson, S. M.: Some ultrastructural and histochemical aspects of lipidoses. Path Europ., **3**, 200, 1968.
72. Kamoshita, S., and Landing, B. H.: Distribution of lesions in myenteric plexus and gastrointestinal mucosa in lipidoses and other neurologic disorders of children. Amer. J. Clin. Path., **49**, 312, 1968.
73. Greenfield, J. G.: The retina in cerebrospinal lipidosis. Proc. Roy. Soc. Med., **44**, 686, 1951.
74. Duke, J. R., and Clark, D. B.: Infantile amaurotic familial idiocy (Tay-Sachs disease) in the Negro race. Amer. J. Ophthal., **53**, 800, 1962.
75. Manschot, W. A.: Retinal histology in amaurotic idiocies and tapetoretinal degenerations. Ophthalmologica, **156**, 28, 1968.
76. Goldstein, I., and Wexler, D.: Niemann-Pick's disease with cherry-red spots in the macula: ocular pathology. Arch. Ophthal. (Chicago), **5**, 704, 1931.

77. Frenkel, H., and Dide, M.: Rétinite pigmentaire avec atrophie papillaire et ataxie cérébelleuse familiales. Rev. Neurol. (Paris), **25,** 729, 1913.
78. Tamura, O., Matsubara, M., and Nagayama, A.: Tay-Sachs: a case of Vogt-Spielmeyer disease with ophthalmoscopic findings of Tay-Sachs disease. Folia Ophthal. Jap., **19,** 185, 1968.
79. Tittarelli, R., Giagheddu, M., and Spadetta, V.: Typical ophthalmoscopic picture of "cherry-red spot" in an adult with the myoclonic syndrome. Brit. J. Ophthal., **50,** 414, 1966.
80. Pick, L., and Bielschowsky, M.: Über lipoidzellige Splenomegalie (Typus Niemann-Pick) und amaurotische Idiotie. Klin. Wschr., **6,** 1631, 1927.
81. Attal, C., Farkas-Bargeton, E., Edgar, G. W. F., Huu-Trong, P., Girard, F., and Mozziconacci, P.: Idiotic amaurotique infantile familiale avec surcharge viscerale. Ann. Pediat. (Paris), **14,** 457, 1967.
82. Korey, S. R., Gomez, C. J., Stein, A., Gonatas, J., Suzuki, K., Terry, R. D., and Weiss, M.: Studies in Tay-Sachs disease. I. A. Methods, 1. Biochemical, 2. Electron microscopic. B. Clinical and pathologic descriptions. J. Neuropath. Exp. Neurol., **22,** 2 and 10, 1963.
83. Samuels, S., Korey, S. R., Gonatas, J., Terry, R. D., and Weiss, M.: Studies in Tay-Sachs disease. IV. Membranous cytoplasmic bodies. 1. Biochemistry. 2. Ultrastructure. J. Neuropath. Exp. Neurol., **22,** 81, 1963.
84. Terry, R. D., and Korey, S. R.: Studies in Tay-Sachs disease. V. The membrane of the membranous cytoplasmic body. J. Neuropath. Exp. Neurol., **22,** 98, 1963.
85. Samuels, S., and Gonatas, N.K.: Formation of the membranous cytoplasmic bodies of Tay-Sachs disease. Trans. Amer. Neurol. Ass., **88,** 267, 1963.
86. Harcourt, R. B., and Dobbs, R. H.: Ultrastructure of the retina in Tay-Sachs's disease. Brit. J. Ophthal., **52,** 898, 1968.
87. Gonatas, N. K., Baird, H. W., and Evangelista, I.: The fine structure of neocortical synapses in infantile amaurotic idiocy. J. Neuropath. Exp. Neurol., **27,** 39, 1968.
88. Volk, B. W., and Wallace, B. J.: The liver in lipidosis. An electron microscopic and histochemical study. Amer. J. Path., **49,** 203, 1966.
89. Diezel, P. B.: Histochemische Untersuchungen am primären Lipoidosen: amaurotische Idiotie, Gargoylismus, Niemann-Picksche Krankheit, Gauchersche Krankheit, mit besonderer Berücksichtigung des Zentralnervensystems. Arch. Path. Anat., **326,** 89, 1954.
90. Diezel, P. B.: Histochemical study of primary lipidoses, in *Cerebral Lipidoses,* edited by L. van Bogaert, J. N. Cumings, and A. Lowenthal, p. 11. Blackwell, Oxford, 1957.
91. Svennerholm, L.: Determination of gangliosides in nervous tissue, in *Cerebral Lipidosis,* edited by L. van Bogaert, J. N. Cummings, and A. Lowenthal, p. 122. Blackwell Scientific Publications, Ltd., Oxford, 1957.
92. Lazarus, S. S., Wallace, B. J., and Volk, B. W.: Neuronal enzyme alterations in Tay-Sachs disease. Amer. J. Path., **41,** 579, 1962.
93. Friede, R. L., and Allen, R. J.: Enzyme histochemical studies of Tay-Sachs disease. J. Neuropath. Exp. Neurol., **23,** 619, 1964.
94. Wallace, B. J., Volk, B. W., and Lazarus, S. S.: Fine structural localization of acid phosphatase activity in neurons of Tay-Sachs disease. J. Neuropath. Exp. Neurol., **53,** 676, 1964.
95. Wallace, B. J., Volk, B. W., Schneck, L., and Kaplan, H.: Fine structural localization of two hydrolytic enzymes in the cerebellum of children with lipidoses. J. Neuropath. Exp. Neurol., **25,** 76, 1966.
96. Wallace, B. J., Lazarus, S. S., and Volk, B. W.: Electron microscopic and histochemical studies of viscera in lipidoses, in *Inborn Disorders of Sphingolipid Metabolism* (proceedings of the 3rd international symposium on the cerebral sphingolipidoses, 1965), edited by S. M. Aronson and B. W. Volk, p. 107. Pergamon, New York, 1967.
97. Halaris, A., and Jatzkewitz, H.: Electron histochemical demonstration of gangliosides in normal and Tay-Sachs brain tissue. Acta Neuropath. (Berlin), **13,** 157, 1969.
98. Thudichum, J. L. W.: *Die chemische Konstitution des Gehirns des Menschen und der Tiere.* Verlag von Franz Pietzcker. Tübingen, 1901.
99. Drabkin, D. L.: *Thudichum, Chemist of the Brain.* University of Pennsylvania Press, Philadelphia, 1958.
100. Carter, H. E., Glick, F. J., Norris, W. P., and Phillips, G. E.: Biochemistry of the sphingolipids. III. Structure of sphingosine. J. Biol. Chem., **170,** 285, 1947.
101. Carter, H. E.: Sphingolipides, in *Chemistry of Lipids as Related to Atherosclerosis,* edited by I. H. Page, p. 82. Charles C Thomas, Springfield, Ill., 1958.
102. Grob, C. A., and Gadient, F.: Die Synthese des Sphingosins und seiner Stereoisomeren. Helv. Chim. Acta, **40,** 1145, 1957.
103. Shapiro, D., Segel, H., and Flowers, H. M.: The total synthesis of sphingosine. J. Amer. Chem. Soc., **80,** 1194, 1958.
104. Klenk, E., and Gielen, W.: Über ein chromatographisch einheitliches hexosaminhaltiges Gangliosides aus Menschengehirn. Hoppe Seyler. Z. Physiol. Chem., **326,** 158, 1961.
105. Sambasivarao, K., and McCluer, R. H.: Characterization of the long chain bases in gangliosides. Fed. Proc., **22,** 300, 1963.
106. Sambasivarao, K., and McCleur, R. H.: Lipid components of gangliosides. J. Lipid Res., **5,** 103, 1964.
107. Rosenberg, A., and Stern, N.: Changes in sphingosine and fatty acid components of the gangliosides in developing rat and human brain. J. Lipid Res., **7,** 122, 1966.
108. Svennerholm, L.: The patterns of gangliosides in mental and neurological disorders. Biochem. J., **98,** 20P, 1966.
109. Karlsson, K. A., Samuelsson, B. E., and Steen, G. O.: Structure and function of sphingolipids. 1. Difference in sphingolipid long-chain base pattern between kidney cortex, medulla and papillae. Acta Chem. Scand., **22,** 1361, 1968.
110. Smid, F., and Michalec, C.: Biochemistry of sphingolipids. XXIV. Long-chain base variations in gangliosides of developing human brain. Brain Res., **10,** 441, 1968.
111. Martensson, E.: Glycosphingolipids of animal tissue. Progress in the Chemistry of Fats and other Lipids, **10,** 367, 1969.
112. Panganamala, R. V., Geer, J. C., and Cornwell, D. G.: Long-chain bases in the sphingolipids of atherosclerotic human aorta. J. Lipid Res., **10,** 445, 1969.
113. Sweeley, C. C., and Moscatelli, E. A.: Qualitative microanalysis and estimation of sphingolipid bases. J. Lipid Res., **1,** 40, 1959.
114. Isaacson, E., and Moscatelli, E. A.: Sphingolipids of developing human central nervous tissue: changes in composition of sphingosine bases. J. Neurochem., **17,** 365, 1970.
115. Carter, H. E., and Hirschberg, C. B.: Phytosphingosines and branched sphingosines in kidney. Biochemistry, **7,** 2296, 1968.
116. Okabe, K., Keenan, R. W., and Schmidt, G.: Phytosphingosine groups as quantitively significant components of the sphingolipids of the mucosa of the small intestines of some mammalian species. Biochem. Biophys. Res. Commun., **31,** 137, 1968.
117. Renkonen, O., and Hirvisalo, E. L.: Structure of plasma sphingadienine. J. Lipid Res., **10,** 687, 1969.
118. Gatt, S.: Enzymatic hydrolysis and synthesis of ceramides. J. Biol. Chem., **238,** 3131, 1963.
119. Samuelsson, K.: On the occurrence and nature of free ceramides in human plasma. Biochim. Biophys. Acta. **176,** 211, 1969.
120. Svennerholm, L.: The gangliosides. J. Lipid Res., **5,** 145, 1964.
121. Kuhn, R., Egge, H., Brossmer, R., Gaube, A., Klesse, P., Lochinger, W., Röhm, R., Trischmann, H., and Tschampel, D.: Über die Ganglioside des Gehirns. Angew. Chem., **72,** 805, 1960.
122. Kuhn, R., and Wiegandt, H.: Die Konstitution der Ganglioside G_{II}, G_{III} and G_{IV}. Z. Naturforsch., **18b,** 541, 1963.
123. Wiegandt, H.: Ganglioside, in *Untersuchung und Bestimmung der Lipoide im Blut,* edited by N. Zöllner and D. Eberhagen, p. 19. Springer-Verlag, Berlin, Heidelberg, New York, 1965.
124. Klenk, E, and Gielen, W.: Zur Kenntnis der Ganglioside des Gehirns. Hoppe Seyler. Z. Physiol. Chem., **319,** 283, 1960.
125. Klenk, E., Gielen, W., and Padberg, G.: The structure of the gangliosides, in *Cerebral Sphingolipidoses,* edited by S. M. Aronson and B. W. Volk, p. 301. Academic, New York, 1962.
126. Klenk, E.: On cerebrosides and gangliosides. Progress in the Chemistry of Fats and other Lipids, **10,** 409, 1969.
127. Burton, R. M.: Biochemistry of sphingosine containing lipids, in *Lipids and Lipidoses,* edited by G. Schettler, p. 122. Springer-Verlag, Berlin, Heidelberg, New York, 1967.
128. Pennick, R. J., Meisler, M. H., and McCluer, R. H.: Thin-layer chro-

matographic studies of human brain gangliosides. Biochim. Biophys. Acta, **116,** 279, 1966.

129. Penick, R. J., and McCluer, R. H.: Quantitative determination of glucose and galactose in gangliosides by gas liquid chromatography. Biochim. Biophys. Acta, **116,** 288, 1966.

130. McCluer, R. H., and Penick, R. J.: Isolation and structural analysis of brain gangliosides, in *Inborn Disorders of Sphingolipid Metabolism* (proceedings of the 3rd international symposium on the cerebral sphingolipidoses, 1965), edited by S. M. Aronson and B. W. Volk, p. 241. Pergamon, New York, 1967.

131. Svennerholm, L.: Isolation of the major ganglioside of human spleen. Acta Chem. Scand., **17,** 860, 1963.

132. Wagner, A., and Weicker, H.: Untersuchungen an gangliosidartigen Substanzen aus menschlicher Milz. Z. Klin. Chem., **4,** 73, 1966.

133. Puro, K., Maury, P., and Huttunen, J. K.: Qualitative and quantitative patterns of gangliosides in extraneural tissues. Biochim. Biophys. Acta, **187,** 230, 1969.

134. Kwiterovich, P. O., Sloan, H. R., and Fredrickson, D. S.: Glycolipids and other lipid constituents of normal human liver. J. Lipid Res., **11,** 322, 1970.

135. Folch-Pi, J., Arsove, S., and Meath, J. S.: Isolation of brain strandin, a new type of large molecule tissue component. J. Biol. Chem., **191,** 819, 1951.

136. Klenk, E., and Gielen, W.: Untersuchungen über die Konstitution der Ganglioside aus Menschengehirn und die Trennung des Gemischs in die Komponenten. Hoppe Seyler Z. Physiol. Chem., **326,** 144, 1961.

137. Kuhn, R., and Weigandt, H.: Die Konstitution der Ganglio-N-Tetraose und des Ganglioside G_I. Chem. Ber., **96,** 866, 1963.

138. Handa, S., and Yamakawa, T.: Chemistry of lipids of posthemolytic residue or stroma of erythrocytes. XII. Chemical structure and chromatographic behaviour of hematosides obtained from equine and dog erythrocytes. Jap. J. Exp. Med., **34,** 293, 1964.

139. Leden, R.: The chemistry of gangliosides: A review. J. Amer. Oil Chem. Soc., **43,** 57, 1966.

140. Wiegandt, H.: Ganglioside. Ergebn. Physiol., **57,** 190, 1966.

141. Siddiqui, B., and McCluer, R. H.: Lipid components of sialosylgalactosylceramide of human brain. J. Lipid Res., **9,** 366, 1968.

142. Wiegandt, H., and Schulze, B.: Spleen gangliosides: "The structure of ganglioside $G_{LNnT}1$ (NGNA)." Z. Naturforsch., **24,** 945, 1969.

143. Leikola, E., Nieminen, E., and Teppo, Anna-Maija: New sialic acid-containing sulfolipid: "ungulic acid." J. Lipid Res., **10,** 440, 1969.

144. Hakomori, S.-I., and Saito, T.: Isolation and characterization of a glycosphingolipid having a new sialic acid. Biochemistry, **8,** 5082, 1969.

145. Folch-Pi, J., Meath, A., and Arsove, S.: Isolation of brain strandin, a new type of large molecule tissue component. J. Biol. Chem., **191,** 819, 1951.

146. Folch-Pi, J., and Lees, M.: Studies on the brain ganglioside strandin in normal brain and in Tay-Sachs disease. A.M.A. J. Dis. Child., **97,** 730, 1959.

147. Rosenberg, A., and Chargaff, E.: Nitrogenous constituents of an ox brain mucolipid. Biochim. Biophys. Acta. **21,** 588, 1956.

148. Rosenberg, A., and Chargaff, E.: A study of a mucolipid of ox brain. J. Biol. Chem., **230,** 1031, 1958.

149. Shapiro, D., and Archer, A. J.: Studies in the ganglioside series. III. Synthesis of 4-0-(2-Acetamide-2-deoxy-β-D-galactopyranosyl)-D-galactopyranose. J. Org. Chem., **35,** 229, 1970.

150. Svennerholm, L.: The metabolism of gangliosides in cerebral lipidoses, in *Inborn Disorders of Sphingolipid Metabolism* (proceedings of the 3rd international symposium on the cerebral sphingolipidoses, 1965), edited by S. M. Aronson and B. W. Volk, p. 169. Pergamon, New York, 1967.

151. Puro, K., and Keranen, A.: Fatty acids and sphingosines of bovine-kidney gangliosides. Biochim. Biophys. Acta, **187,** 393, 1969.

152. Kishimoto, Y., and Radin, N. S.: Determination of brain gangliosides by determination of ganglioside stearic acid. J. Lipid Res., **7,** 141, 1966.

153. Rosenberg, A.: The nature of the lipophilic portions of the brain gangliosides, in *Inborn Disorders of Sphingolipid Metabolism* (proceedings of the 3rd international symposium on the cerebral sphingolipidoses, 1965), edited by S. M. Aronson and B. W. Volk, p. 267. Pergamon, New York, 1967.

154. Suzuki, K.: The pattern of mammalian brain gangliosides. III. Regional and developmental differences. J. Neurochem., **12,** 969, 1965.

155. Suzuki, K.: Ganglioside patterns of normal and pathological brains, in *Inborn Disorders of Sphingolipid Metabolism* (proceedings of the 3rd international symposium on the cerebral sphingolipidoses, 1965), edited by S. M. Aronson and B. W. Volk, p. 215. Pergamon, New York, 1967.

156. Dominick, V. E., and Gielen, W.: Über unterschiedliche Gehalte einzelner Gehirnregionen an Gangliosiden. Hoppe Seyler. Z. Physiol. Chem., **349,** 731, 1968.

157. Suzuki, K., Suzuki, K., and Kamoshita, S.: Chemical pathology of G_{M2}-Gangliosidosis (generalized gangliosidosis). J. Neuropath. Exp. Neurol., **28,** 25, 1969.

158. Kamoshita, S., Aron, A., Suzuki, K., and Suzuki, K.: Original articles: Infantile Niemann-Pick Disease: a chemical study with isolation and characterization of membranous cytoplasmic bodies and myelin. Amer. J. Dis. Child., **117,** 379, 1969.

159. Wherrett, J. R., and Cumings, J. H.: Detection and resolution of gangliosides in lipid extracts by thin-layer chromatography. Biochem. J., **86,** 378, 1963.

160. Kawanami, J.: Glycolipids from rat kidney. J. Biochem., **64,** 625, 1968.

161. Handa, S., and Burton, R.: Lipids of Retina: 1. Analysis of gangliosides in beef retina by thin layer chromatography. Lipids, **4,** 205, 1969.

162. Wintzer, G., and Uhlenbruck, G.: Topochemische Anordnung von Gangliosiden in der Erythrozytenmembran. Z. Immunitätsforsch., **33,** 60, 1967.

163. Booth, D. A.: Erythrocyte lipids in Tay-Sachs disease. Lancet, **1,** 626, 1967.

164. Sastry, P. S., and Stancer, H. C.: Blood gangliosides in infantile amaurotic idiocy. Clin. Chim. Acta, **20,** 487, 1968.

165. Schneck, L., Kleinberg, W., and Volk, B. W.: Cardiac gangliosides in sphingolipidoses. Proc. Soc. Exp. Biol. Med., **130,** 404, 1969.

166. Svennerholm, L.: Gangliosides and other glycolipids of human placenta. Acta Chem. Scand., **19,** 1506, 1965.

167. Sloan, H. R.: Unpublished observations.

168. Brady, R. O., Borek, C., and Bradley, R. M.: Composition and synthesis of gangliosides in rat hepatocyte and hepatoma cell lines. J. Biol. Chem., **244,** 6552, 1969.

169. Svennerholm, L.: The distribution of lipids in the human nervous system: I. Analytical procedure. Lipids of foetal and newborn brain. J. Neurochem., **11,** 839, 1964.

170. Derry, D. M., and Wolfe, L. S.: Gangliosides in isolated neurons and glial cells. Science, **158,** 1450, 1967.

171. MacMillan, V. H., and Wherrett, J. R.: A modified procedure for the analysis of mixtures of tissue gangliosides. J. Neurochem., **16,** 1621, 1969.

172. Lapetina, E. G., Soto, E. F., and Robertis, E. de.: Gangliosides and acetylcholinesterase in isolated membranes of the rat-brain cortex. Biochim. Biophys. Acta, **135,** 33, 1967.

173. Den, H., and Kaufman, B.: Ganglioside and glycoprotein glycosyltransferases in synaptosomes. Fed. Proc., **27,** 346, 1968.

174. Dekirmenjian, H., Brunngraber, E. G., Johnston, N. L., and Larramendi, L. M. H.: Distribution of gangliosides, glycoprotein-NANA and acetylcholinesterase in axonal and synaptosomal fractions of cat cerebellum. Exp. Brain Res., **8,** 97, 1969.

175. Wiegandt, H.: The subcellular localization of gangliosides in the brain. J. Neurochem., **14,** 671, 1967.

176. Derry, D. M., and Wolfe, L. S.: Ganglioside analyses of serial cryostat sections through Ammon's horn and cerebellar folia. Exp. Brain Res., **5,** 32, 1968.

177. Wiegandt, H.: The structure and the function of gangliosides. Angew. Chem. (Eng.), **7,** 87, 1968.

178. Cumings, J. N., Thompson, E. J., and Goodwin, H.: Sphingolipids and phospholipids in microsomes and myelin from normal and pathological brains. J. Neurochem., **15,** 243, 1968.

179. Suzuki, K., Poduslo, S. E., and Norton, W. T.: Gangliosides in the myelin fraction of developing rats. Biochim. Biophys. Acta, **144,** 375, 1967.

180. Suzuki, K., Poduslo, J. F., and Poduslo, S. E.: Further evidence for a specific ganglioside fraction closely associated with myelin. Biochim. Biophys. Acta, **152**, 576, 1968.
181. Suzuki, K.: Formation and turnover of myelin gangliosides. J. Neurochem., **17**, 209, 1970.
182. Trams, E. G., and Lauter, C. J.: On the isolation and characterization of gangliosides. Biochim. Biophys. Acta, **60**, 350, 1962.
183. Trams, E. G., Guiffrida, L. E., and Karmen, A.: Gas chromatographic analysis of long chain fatty acids in gangliosides. Nature (London), **193**, 680, 1962.
184. Howard, R. E., and Burton, R. M.: Studies on the ganglioside micelle. Biochim. Biophys. Acta, **84**, 435, 1964.
185. Lowden, J. A., and Wolfe, L. S.: Studies on brain gangliosides. III. Evidence for the location of gangliosides specifically in neurones. Canad. J. Biochem., **42**, 1587, 1964.
186. Van Heyningen, W. E., and Miller, P. A.: The fixation of tetanus toxin by ganglioside. J. Gen. Microbiol., **24**, 107, 1961.
187. Mellanby, J., and Whittaker, V. P.: The fixation of tetanus toxin by synaptic membranes. J. Neurochem., **15**, 205, 1968.
188. Gielen, W.: Über die Funktion vom Gangliosiden. Die Verbreitung des Serotonin-Receptors. Z. Naturforsch. **23b**, 117, 1968.
189. Rapport, M. M., and Graf, L.: Immunochemical reaction of lipids. Progr. Allerg., **13**, 273, 1969.
190. Morrel, F., and Torres, F.: Electrophysiological analysis of a case of Tay-Sachs disease. Brain, **83**, 213, 1960.
191. Suzuki, K., and Korey, S. R.: Study on ganglioside metabolism. I. Incorporation of D-[U-^{14}C] glucose into individual gangliosides. J. Neurochem., **11**, 647, 1964.
192. Harzer, K., Jatzkewitz, H., and Sandhoff, K.: Incorporation of labelled glucose into the individual major gangliosides of the brain of young rats. J. Neurochem., **16**, 1279, 1969.
193. Maker, H. S., and Hauser, G.: Incorporation of glucose carbon into gangliosides and cerebrosides by slices of developing rat brain. J. Neurochem., **14**, 457, 1967.
194. Rubiolo de Maccioni, A. H., and Caputto, R.: Synthesis of gangliosides during development and its relation to the quantitative changes of subcellular particles of rat brain. J. Neurochem., **15**, 1257, 1968.
195. Brady, R. O., and Koval, G. J.: The enzymatic synthesis of sphingosine. J. Biol. Chem., **233**, 26, 1958.
196. Brady, R. O., Formica, J. V., and Koval, G. J.: The enzymatic synthesis of sphingosine. II. Further studies on the mechanism of the reaction. J. Biol. Chem., **233**, 1072, 1958.
197. Brady, R. O.: Sphingolipid metabolism in neural tissues, Neurosci. Res., **2**, 301, 1969.
198. Braun, P. E., and Snell, E. E.: Biosynthesis of sphingolipid bases. II. Keto intermediates in synthesis of sphingosine and dihydrosphingosine by cell-free extracts of *Hansenula ciferri.* J. Biol. Chem., **243**, 3775, 1968.
199. Braun, P. E., Morell, P., and Radin, N. S.: Synthesis of C_{18}- and C_{20}-dihydrosphingosines, ketodihydrosphingosines, and ceramides by microsomal preparations from mouse brain. J. Biol. Chem., **245**, 335, 1970.
200. Stoffel, W., Sticht, G., and Lekim, D.: Metabolism of sphingosine bases. VI. Synthesis and degradation of sphingosine bases in *Hansenula ciferrii.* Hoppe Seyler. Z. Physiol. Chem., **349**, 1149, 1968.
201. Fujino, Y., and Zabin, I.: The configuration of sphingosine synthesized in rat brain homogenates. J. Biol. Chem., **237**, 2069, 1962.
202. Fujino, Y.: Studies on conjugated lipids. XVIII. Enzymatic synthesis of the sphingosine base. Agr. Biol. Chem., **28**, 807, 1964.
203. Morell, P., and Radin, N. S.: Specificity in ceramide biosynthesis from long-chain bases and various fatty acyl coenzyme A's by brain microsomes. J. Biol. Chem., **245**, 342, 1970.
204. Basu, S., Kaufman, B., and Roseman, S.: Conversion of Tay-Sachs ganglioside to monosialoganglioside by brain uridine diphosphate D-galactose: glycolipid galactosyltransferase. J. Biol. Chem., **240**, PC4115, 1965.
205. Basu, S., and Kaufman, B.: Ganglioside synthesis in embryonic chicken brain. Fed. Proc., **24**, 479, 1965.
206. Kaufman, B., Basu, S., and Roseman, S.: Studies on the biosynthesis of gangliosides, in *Inborn Disorders of Sphingolipid Metabolism* (proceedings of the 3rd international symposium on the cerebral sphingolipidoses, 1965), edited by S. M. Aronson and B. W. Volk, p. 193. Pergamon, New York, 1967.
207. Basu, S.: Synthesis of glucosylceramide by an enzyme from embryonic chicken brain. Fed. Proc., **27**, 346, 1968.
208. Basu, S., Kaufman, B., and Roseman, S.: Enzymatic synthesis of ceramide-glucose and ceramide-lactose by glycosyltransferases from embryonic chicken brain. J. Biol. Chem., **243**, 5802, 1968.
209. Kaufman, B., Basu, S., and Roseman, S.: Enzymatic synthesis of disialogangliosides from monosialogangliosides by sialyltransferases from embryonic chicken brain. J. Biol. Chem., **243**, 5804, 1968.
210. Hauser, G.: The enzymatic synthesis of ceramide lactoside from ceramide glucoside and UDP-galactose. Biochem. Biophys. Res. Commun., **28**, 502, 1967.
211. Curtino, J. A., Calderon, R. O., and Caputto, R.: Enzymatic synthesis of gangliosides—the binding of glucose. Fed. Proc., **27**, 346, 1968.
212. Arce, A., Maccioni, H. F., and Caputto, R.: Enzymic binding of sialyl groups to ganglioside derivatives by preparations from the brain of young rat. Arch. Biochem., **116**, 52, 1966.
213. Kanfer, J. N., Blacklow, R. A., Warren, L., and Brady, R. O.: The enzymatic synthesis of gangliosides. Biochem. Biophys Res. Commun., **14**, 287, 1964.
214. Kanfer, J. N., and Richards, R. L.: Effect of puromycin on the incorporation of radioactive sugars into gangliosides in vivo. J. Neurochem., **14**, 513, 1967.
215. Gatt, S., and Rapport, M. M.: Enzymic hydrolysis of sphingolipids. Hydrolysis of ceramide lactoside by an enzyme from rat brain. Biochem. J., **101**, 680, 1966.
216. Gatt, S.: Comparison of four enzymes from brain which hydrolyze sphingolipids, in *Inborn Disorders of Sphingolipid Metabolism* (proceedings of the 3rd international symposium on the cerebral sphingolipidoses, 1965), edited by S. M. Aronson and B. W. Volk, p. 261. Pergamon, New York, 1967.
217. Gatt, S.: Enzymatic hydrolysis of sphingolipids. V. Hydrolysis of monosialoganglioside and hexosylceramides by rat brain -β-galactosidase. Biochim. Biophys. Acta, **137**, 192, 1967.
218. Sandhoff, K., Andreae, U., and Jatzkewitz, H.: Deficient hexosaminidase activity in an exceptional case of Tay-Sachs disease with additional storage of kidney globoside in visceral organs. Path. Europ., **3**, 278, 1968.
219. Sandhoff, K., and Jatzkewitz, H.: Preliminary note. A particle-bound sialyl lactosidoceramide splitting mammalian sialidase. Biochim. Biophys. Acta, **141**, 442, 1967.
220. Leibovitz, L., and Gatt, S.: Enzymatic hydrolysis of sphingolipids. VII. Hydrolysis of gangliosides by a neuraminidase from calf brain. Biochim. Biophys. Acta, **152**, 136, 1968.
221. Kolodny, E. H.: Studies on the metabolic defect in Tay-Sachs disease. Personal communication.
222. Gatt, S.: Enzymatic hydrolysis of sphingolipids. I. Hydrolysis and synthesis of ceramides by an enzyme from rat brain. J. Biol. Chem., **241**, 3724, 1966.
223. Yavin, E., and Gatt, S.: Enzymatic hydrolysis of sphingolipids. VII. Further purification and properties of rat brain ceramidase. Biochemistry, **8**, 1698, 1969.
224. Nilsson, A.: The presence of sphingomyelin- and ceramide-cleaving enzymes in the small intestinal tract. Biochim. Biophys. Acta, **176**, 339, 1969.
225. Stoffel, W., and Sticht, G.: Metabolism of sphingosine bases. 1. Degradation and incorporation of (3-^{14}C) erythro-DL-dihydrosphingosine and (7-$^{3}H_2$) erythro-DL-sphingosine into sphingolipids of rat liver. Hoppe Seyler. Z. Physiol. Chem., **348**, 941, 1967.
226. Stoffel, W., and Sticht, G.: Metabolism of sphingosine bases. II. Studies on the degradation and transformation of [3-^{14}C]erythro-DL-dihydrosphingosine, [7-^{3}H]erythro-DL-sphingosine, [5-^{3}H]threo-L-dihydrosphingosine and [3-^{14}C; 1-^{3}H]erythro-DL-dihydrosphingosine in rat liver. Hoppe Seyler. Z. Physiol. Chem., **348**, 1345, 1967.

227. Barenholz, Y., and Gatt, S.: Degradation of sphingosine, dihydrosphingosine, and phytosphingosine in rats. Biochemistry, **7**, 2603, 1968.
228. Gatt, S., and Barenholz, Y.: Degradation of sphingosine bases by cell-free preparations. α-Hydroxy palmitic acid, an intermediate of phytosphingosine degradation. Biochem. Biophys. Res. Commun., **32**, 588, 1958.
229. Keenan, R. W., and Okabe, K.: The degradation of tritiated dihydrosphingosine in the intact rat. Biochemistry, **7**, 2696, 1968.
230. Keenan, R. W., and Maxam, A.: The in vitro degradation of dihydrosphingosine. Biochim. Biophys. Acta, **176**, 348, 1969.
231. Keenan, R. W., and Haegelin, B.: The enzymatic phosphorylation of sphinganine. Biochem. Biophys. Res. Commun., **37**, 888, 1969.
232. Stoffel, W., Sticht, G., and LeKim, D.: Metabolism of sphingosine bases. X. Degradation of [1-^{14}C]dihydrosphingosine (sphinganine), [1-^{14}C]2-amino-1, 3-dihydroxyheptane and [1-^{14}C]dihydrosphingosine phosphate in rat liver. Hoppe Seyler. Z. Physiol. Chem., **350**, 63, 1969.
233. Stoffel, W., Sticht, G., and Lekim, D.: Metabolism of sphingosine bases. IX. Degradation in vitro of dihydrosphingosine and dihydrosphingosine phosphate to palmitaldehyde and ethanolamine phosphate. Hoppe Seyler. Z. Physiol. Chem., **349**, 1745, 1968.
234. Stoffel, W., Lekim, D., and Sticht, G.: Metabolism of sphingosine bases. XI. Distribution and properties of dihydrosphingosine-1-phosphate aldolase (sphinganine-1-phosphate alkanal-lyase). Hoppe Seyler. Z. Physiol. Chem., **350**, 1233, 1969.
235. Stoffel, W., Lekim, D., and Sticht, G.: Metabolism of sphingosine bases. IV. 2-Amino-1-hydroxyoctadecane-3-one(3-oxodihydrosphingosine), the common intermediate in the biosynthesis of dihydrosphingosine and sphingosine and in the degradation of dihydrosphingosine. Hoppe Seyler. Z. Physiol. Chem., **348**, 1570, 1967.
236. Batzdorf, U., Sarlieve, L. L., Gold, V. A., and Menkes, J. H.: Tay-Sachs Disease: demonstration of the stored ganglioside in cultured cells from brain biopsy. Arch. Neurol., **20**, 650, 1969.
237. Svennerholm, L., and Zettergren, L.: Infantile amaurotic idiocy. Acta Path. Microbiol. Scand., **41**, 127, 1957.
238. Wagner, A., Dain, I. D., and Schmidt, G.: Accumulation of an abnormal brain ganglioside in Tay-Sachs disease. Fed. Proc., **22**, 234, 1963.
239. Svennerholm, L.: Isolation of gangliosides. Acta Chem. Scand., **17**, 239, 1963.
240. Rouser, G., Galli, C., and Kritchevsky, G.: Lipid class composition of normal human brain and variations in metachromatic leucodystrophy, Tay-Sachs, Niemann-Pick, chronic Gaucher's and Alzheimer's diseases. J. Amer. Oil Chem. Soc., **42**, 404, 1965.
241. Wagner, A.: Über hirnganglioside bei Tay-Sachsscher Erkrankung. Klin. Wschr., **44**, 398, 1966.
242. Booth, D. A., Goodwin, H., and Cumings, J. N.: Abnormal gangliosides in Tay-Sachs disease, Niemann-Pick's disease and gargoylism. J. Lipid Res., **7**, 337, 1966.
243. Ledeen, R., Salsman, K., and Cabrera, M.: Structural studies of the Tay-Sachs ganglioside and its normal brain counterpart, in *Inborn Disorders of Sphingolipid Metabolism* (proceedings of the 3rd international symposium on the cerebral sphingolipidoses, 1965), edited by S. M. Aronson and B. W. Volk, p. 231. Pergamon, New York, 1967.
244. Dvorackova, I., and Michalec, C.: Two cases of Tay-Sachs disease and a case of atypical gargoylism. Path. Europ, **3**, 474, 1968.
245. Tamai, Y., and Yamakawa, T.: Study on glucoscerebroside in Tay-Sachs brain. Jap. J. Exp. Med., **39**, 85, 1969.
246. Suzuki, K., and Chen, G. C.: Brain ceramide hexosides in Tay-Sachs disease and generalized gangliosidosis (G_{M1}-gangliosidosis). J. Lipid Res., **8**, 105, 1967.
247. Sandhoff, K., Andreae, U., and Jatzkewitz, H.: Deficient hexosaminidase activity in an exceptional case of Tay-Sachs disease with additional storage of kidney globoside in visceral organs. Life Sci., **7**, 283, 1968.
248. Edgar. G. W. F.: Amino sugar in Tay-Sachs brain. Psychiat. Neurol. Neurochir., **70**, 141, 1967.
249. Bogoch, S., and Belval, P.: Brain proteins in the sphingolipidoses: Tay-Sachs disease protein, in *Inborn Disorders of Sphingolipid Metabolism* (proceedings of the 3rd international symposium on the cerebral sphingolipidoses, 1965), edited by S. M. Aronson and B. W. Volk, p. 273. Pergamon, New York, 1967.
250. Gregoire, P. E., Jonniaux, G., Loeb, H., Voet, W., and Capelle, R.: Étude biochimique des lipides cérébraux et hépatiques dans un cas de maladie de Tay-Sachs. Rev. Franc. Étud. Clin. Biol., **14**, 568, 1969.
251. Taketomi, T., and Kawamura, N.: Cerebral and visceral glycolipids in a case of Tay-Sachs disease. J. Biochem., **66**, 165, 1969.
252. Bernheimer, H.: Ganglioside im Liquor cerebrospinalis und Tay-Sachssche Erkrankung. Klin. Wschr., **46**, 258, 1968.
253. Suzuki, K., Suzuki, K., and Chen, G. C.: Membranous cytoplasmic bodies from Tay-Sachs disease G_{M1}-gangliosidosis (generalized gangliosidosis). J. Neuropath. Exp. Neurol., **27**, 142, 1968.
254. Edgar, G. W. F., Hooghwinkel, G. J. M., and Borri, P.: Erythrocyte lipids in amaurotic familial idiocy. Lancet, **2**, 693, 1965.
255. Rouser, G., Bauman, A. J., Nicolaides, N., and Heller, D.: Paper chromatography of lipids, methods, applications and interpretations. J. Amer. Oil Chem. Soc., **38**, 565, 1961.
256. Schneck, L.: The early electroencephalopathic and seizure characteristics of Tay-Sachs disease. Acta Neurol. Scand., **41**, 163, 1965.
257. Karacan, I., Schneck, L., Hinterbuchner, L. P., and Gross, K.: The sleep-dream pattern in Tay-Sachs disease (preliminary observations), in *Inborn Disorders of Sphingolipid Metabolism* (proceedings of the 3rd international symposium on the cerebral sphingolipidoses, 1965), edited by S. M. Aronson and B. W. Volk, p. 413. Pergamon, New York, 1967.
258. Balint, J. A., Spitzer, H. L., and Kyriakides, E. C.: Studies of red-cell stromal lipids in Tay-Sachs disease and other lipidoses. J. Clin. Invest., **42**, 1661, 1963.
259. Balint, J. A., Kyriakides, E. C., and Spitzer, H. L.: On the chemical changes in the red cell stroma in Tay-Sachs disease: their value as genetic tracers, in *Inborn Disorders of Sphingolipid Metabolism* (proceedings of the 3rd international symposium on the cerebral sphingolipidoses, 1965), edited by S. M. Aronson and B. W. Volk, p. 423. Pergamon, New York, 1967.
260. Balint, J. A., and Kyriakides, E. C.: Studies of red cell stromal proteins in Tay-Sachs disease. J. Clin. Invest., **47**, 1858, 1968.
261. Strouth, J. C., Zeman, W., and Merritt, A. D.: Leukocyte abnormalities in familial amaurotic idiocy. New Eng. J. Med., **274**, 36, 1966.
262. Rosner, F., Weisfogel, G., and Feinerman, A.: Infantile amaurotic familial idiocy. Leukocyte granulation and leukocyte alkaline phosphatase. J.A.M.A., **205**, 873, 1968.
263. Spiegel-Adolf, M., Baird, H. W., Coleman, H. S., and Szehely, G.: Vacuolized blood lymphocytes in the lipidoses and other central nervous system diseases with special reference to histochemical studies, in *Cerebral Sphingolipidoses, A Symposium on Tay-Sachs Disease and Allied Disorders,* edited by S. M. Aronson, and B. W. Volk, p. 129. Academic, New York, 1962.
264. Lazarus, S. S., Vethamany, V. G., Schneck, L., and Volk, W.: Fine structure and histochemistry of peripheral blood cells in Niemann-Pick disease. Lab. Invest., **17**, 155, 1967.
265. Aronson, S. M., Saifer, A., Kanof, A., and Volk, B. W.: Progression of amaurotic family idiocy as reflected by serum and cerebrospinal fluid changes. Amer. J. Med., **24**, 390, 1958.
266. Aronson, S. M., Perle, G., Saifer, A., and Volk, B. W.: Biochemical identification of the carrier state in Tay-Sachs disease. Proc. Soc. Exp. Biol. Med., **111**, 664, 1962.
267. Volk, B. W., Aronson, S. M., and Saifer, S. M.: Fructose-1-phosphate aldolase deficiency in Tay-Sachs disease. Amer. J. Med., **36**, 481, 1964.
268. Saifer, A., Schneck, L., Perle, C., and Volk, B. W.: Lactate dehydrogenase isoenzyme distribution in the cerebral sphingolipidoses and other neurological disorders. Neurology, **19**, 147, 1969.
269. Saifer, A., Volk, B. W., and Aronson, S. M.: Neuraminic (sialic) acid studies of biological fluids in amaurotic family idiocy and related disorders. A.M.A. J. Dis. Child., **97**, 745, 1959.
270. Spiegel-Adolf, M., Baird, H. W., and McCafferty, M.: Increased lysolecithin in serum extracts of lipidoses, particularly of Tay-Sachs patients. Confin. Neurol., **28**, 407, 1966.

271. Aronson, S. M., Saifer, A., Perle, G., and Volk, B. W.: Cerebrospinal fluid enzymes in central nervous system lipidoses. Proc. Soc. Exp. Biol. Med., **97,** 331, 1958.
272. Aronson, S. M., Saifer, A., and Volk, B. W.: Serial enzyme studies of serum and cerebrospinal fluid in amaurotic family idiocy. A.M.A. J. Dis. Child., **97,** 684, 1959.
273. Tourtellotte, W. W., Allen, R. J., and DeJong, R. N.: A study of lipids in cerebrospinal fluid (and serum). VII. In several sphingolipidoses (Tay-Sachs disease, metachromatic leucodystrophy, and Niemann-Pick disease), in *Cerebral Sphingolipidoses, A Symposium on Tay-Sachs Disease and Allied Disorders,* edited by S. M. Aronson and B. W. Volk, p. 317. Academic, New York, 1962.
274. Tourtellotte, W. W., Allen, R. J., Haerer, A. F., Kelly, S. A., Gustafson, K. A., Bryan, E. R., and DeJong, R. N.: A study of lipids in the cerebrospinal fluid. IX. Two new laboratory observations on the cerebrospinal fluid in Tay-Sachs disease. Trans. Amer. Neurol. Ass., **88,** 104, 1963.
275. Pascal, T. A., Saifer, A., and Gitlin, J.: Comparative studies of normal human and Tay-Sachs gangliosides—an immunochemical approach, in *Inborn Disorders of Sphingolipid Metabolism* (proceedings of the 3rd international symposium on the cerebral sphingolipidoses, 1965), edited by S. M. Aronson and B. W. Volk, p. 289. Pergamon, New York, 1967.
276. Pascal, T. A., and Saifer, A.: Immunochemical studies of isolated human brain ganglioside components. J. Neurochem., **16,** 301, 1969.
277. Kanfer, J. N.: Personal communication.
278. Robinson, D., and Sterling, J. L.: N-Acetyl-β-glucosaminidases in human spleen. Biochem. J., **107,** 321, 1968.
279. O'Brien, J. S., Okada, S., Chen, A., and Fillerup, D. L.: Tay-Sachs disease: detection of heterozygotes and homozygotes by serum hexosaminidase assay. New Eng. J. Med., **283,** 15, 1970.
279*a*. Friedland, J., Schneck, L., Saifer, A., Pourfar, M., and Volk, B. W.: Identification of Tay-Sachs disease carriers by acrylamide gel electrophoresis. Clin. Chim. Acta, **28,** 397, 1970.
280. O'Brien, J. S.: Diagnosis of Tay-Sachs. Nature (London), **224,** 1038, 1969.
281. Suzuki, Y., Berman, P. H., Hanson, P. A., and Suzuki, K.: Diagnosis of Tay-Sachs disease by cellulose acetate electrophoresis of hexosaminidase components. Abstract, p. 287. Society for Pediatric Research. Atlantic City, May, 1970.
282. Fredrickson, D. S.: Classification and features of the lipidoses affecting the nervous system. Path. Europ., **3,** 121, 1968.
283. Jatzkewitz, H., Pilz, H., and Sandhoff, K.: Quantitative Bestimmungen von Gangliosiden und ihren Neuraminsäurefreien Derivaten bei infantilen, juvenilen und adulten Formen der amaurotischen Idiotie und einer spätinfantilen biochemischen Sonderform. J. Neurochem., **12,** 135, 1965.
284. Suzuki, K.: The pattern of mammalian brain gangliosides. II. Evaluation of the extraction procedures, post mortem changes and the effect of formalin preservation. J. Neurochem., **12,** 629, 1965.
285. Kanof, A., Dunkell, S., and Abramson, I.: Principles and practices on a ward for children with Tay-Sachs disease, in *Cerebral Sphingolipidoses, A Symposium on Tay-Sachs Disease and Allied Disorders,* edited by S. M. Aronson and B. W. Volk, p. 413. Academic, New York, 1962.
286. Slome, D.: The genetic basis of amaurotic family idiocy. J. Genet., **27,** 363, 1934.
287. Ktenidès, M.: Au subjet de l'hérédité de l'idiotie amaurotique infantile (Tay-Sachs), thèse no. 2264, l'Université de Genève, 1954. Cited in S. M. Aronson, M. P. Valsamis, and B. W. Volk, Pediatrics, **26,** 229, 1960.
288. Kozinn, P. J., Weiner, H., and Cohen, P.: Infantile amaurotic family idiocy. J. Pediat., **51,** 58, 1957.
289. Goldschmidt, E., Lenz, R., Merin, S., Ronen, A., and Ronen, I.: Frequency of the Tay-Sachs gene in the Jewish communities of Israel. Abstract, 25th Annual Meeting of Genetics Society of America, Aug. 27, 1956. Cited in S. M. Aronson, M. P. Valsamis, and B. W. Volk. Pediatrics, **26,** 229, 1960.
290. Goldschmidt, E., Lenz, R., and Merin, S.: Tay-Sachs Disease, in *The Genetics of Migrant and Isolate Populations,* edited by E. Goldschmidt, p. 290. Williams & Wilkins, Baltimore, 1963.
291. Myrianthopoulos, N. C.: Some epidemiologic and genetic aspects of Tay-Sachs disease, in *Cerebral Sphingolipidoses, A Symposium on Tay-Sachs Disease and Allied Disorders,* edited by S. M. Aronson and B. W. Volk, p. 359. Academic, New York, 1962.
292. Myrianthopoulos, N. C., and Aronson, S. M.: Population dynamics of Tay-Sachs disease. I. Reproduction fitness and selection. Amer. J. Hum. Genet., **18,** 313, 1966.
293. Myrianthopoulos, N. C., and Aronson, S. M.: Reproductive fitness and selection in Tay-Sachs disease, in *Inborn Disorders of Sphingolipid Metabolism* (proceedings of the 3rd international symposium on the cerebral sphingolipidoses, 1965), edited by S. M. Aronson and B. W. Volk, p. 431. Pergamon, New York, 1967.
294. Knudson, A. G., Jr., and Kaplan, W. D.: Genetics of the sphingolipidoses, in *Cerebral Sphingolipidoses, A Symposium on Tay-Sachs Disease and Allied Disorders,* edited by S. M. Aronson and B. W. Volk, p. 395. Academic, New York, 1962.
295. Knudson, A. G., Jr.: Genetics and the lipidoses. J. Amer. Oil Chem. Soc., **44,** 623, 1967.
296. Shaw, R. F., and Smith, A. P.: Is Tay-Sachs disease increasing? Nature (London), **224,** 1214, 1969.
297. Abood, L. G., and Lipman, V. C.: Blood ceruloplasmin activity during human pregnancy with special reference to Tay-Sachs disease. Amer. J. Obstet. Gynec., **92,** 529, 1965.
298. Pilz, H., Muller, D., Sandhoff, K., and Meulen, V.: Tay-Sachssche Krankheit mit Hexosaminidase-Defekt. Deutsch. Med. Wschr., **93,** 1833, 1968.
299. O'Brien, J. S.: Five gangliosidoses. Lancet, **2,** 805, 1969.
300. Raine, D. N.: Tay, Sachs et al. Lancet, **2,** 959, 1959.
301. Suzuki, K., and Suzuki, Y.: Globoid cell leucodystrophy (Krabbes disease): deficiency of galactocerebroside β-galactosidase. Proc. Nat. Acad. Sci., **66,** 302, 1970.
302. Seitelberger, F., Sluga, E., and Bernheimer, H.: Studies on neuronal lipid dystrophies, in *Cerebral Lipidoses,* vol. 2, edited by A. Nuñes Vicente, P. Dustin, and A. Lowenthal, p. 116. Presses Académiques Européennes, Brussels, 1968.
303. Bernheimer, H., and Seitelberger, F.: Über das Verhalten der Ganglioside im Gehirn bei 2 Fällen von spätinfantiler amaurotischer Idiotie. Wien. Klin. Wschr., **80,** 163, 1968.
304. Volk, B. M., Adachi, M., Schneck, L., and Saifer, A.: Systemic late infantile amaurotic idiocy—monosialogangliosidosis. J. Neuropath. Exp. Neurol., **28,** 171, 1969.
305. Volk, B. W., Adachi, M., Schneck, L., Sanifer, A., and Kleinberg, W.: G_5-Ganglioside variant of systemic late infantile lipidosis: generalized gangliosidosis. Arch. Path., **87,** 393, 1969.
305*a*. Schneck, L., Friedland, J., Pourfar, M., Saifer, A., and Volk, B. W.: Hexosaminidase activities in a case of systemic G_{M2} gangliosidosis of late infantile type. Proc. Soc. Exp. Biol. Med., **133,** 997, 1970.
306. Klibansky, C., Saifer, A., Feldman, N. I., Schneck, L., and Volk, B. W.: Cerebral lipids in a case of systemic G_{M2}-gangliosidosis of a late infantile type. J. Neurochem., **17,** 339, 1970.
307. Suzuki, K., Kinuko, M. D., Rapin, I., Suzuki, Y., and Ishii, N.: Juvenile G_{M2}-gangliosidosis: clinical variant of Tay-Sachs disease or a new disease. Neurology, **20,** 190, 1970.
308. Pilz, H., Sandhoff, K., and Jatzkewitz, H.: Eine Gangliosidstoffwechselstörung mit Anhäufong von Ceramid-lactosid, Monosialo-ceramid-lactosid und Tay-Sachs-Gangliosid im Gehirn. J. Neurochem., **13,** 1273, 1966.
309. Jörgensen, .L., Blackstad, T. W., Harmark, W., and Steen, J. A.: Niemann-Pick's disease. Report of a case with histochemical evidence of neuronal storage of acid glycolipids. Acta Neuropath., **4,** 75, 1964.
310. Schneck, L., Wallace, B. J., Saifer, A., and Volk, B. W.: A clinical, biochemical and electron microscopic study of late infantile amaurotic family idiocy. Amer. J. Med., **39,** 285, 1965.

CHAPTER THIRTY

G_{M1} GANGLIOSIDOSES

John S. O'Brien

This chapter deals with two fatal inherited disorders involving cerebral storage of ganglioside G_{M1}; (1) *generalized gangliosidosis* (G_{M1} gangliosidosis Type 1), a rapidly progressive disorder with infantile onset and severe bony deformities; and (2) *juvenile G_{M1} gangliosidosis* (G_{M1} gangliosidosis Type 2), a more slowly progressive disorder with late infantile beginnings and mild bony deformities or absence of them. In both disorders mental and motor deterioration apparently results from the massive cerebral accumulation of ganglioside G_{M1} (Fig. 30-1).

Generalized gangliosidosis and juvenile G_{M1} gangliosidosis involve the visceral storage of mucopolysaccharides as well as gangliosides. The classification of both as gangliosidoses is imprecise; both could be classified as mucopolysaccharidoses with equal justification. However, although in both disorders mental and motor deterioration is severe, mucopolysacchariduria is not found by the usual assay methods, and bony deformities, though prominent in generalized gangliosidosis, are mild in juvenile G_{M1} gangliosidosis. It seems logical to direct attention to the nervous system manifestations of both diseases by classifying them as gangliosidoses.

G_{M1} GANGLIOSIDOSIS TYPE 1 (GENERALIZED GANGLIOSIDOSIS)

The first clinical description of generalized gangliosidosis was published by R. N. Norman et al. in 1959 under the title, "Tay-Sachs Disease with Visceral Involvement" [1]. Since then more than 25 patients with this disorder have been reported in the literature or are personally known to the author of this chapter [1–13]. The disease has been described by various terms (Table 30-1). The term *generalized gangliosidosis* was selected by Landing and O'Brien in 1965 [3], since (1) it is easy to pronounce, (2) no personal name is associated with it, (3) it emphasizes the neurovisceral storage, (4) it directs attention to the ganglioside storage, and (5) it delineates the disorder from the entities with which it is most easily confused—Tay-Sachs disease and Hurler's syndrome.

Generalized gangliosidosis presents as (1) severe progressive cerebral degeneration leading to death within the first 2 years of life, (2) the accumulation of a specific ganglioside in brain and viscera and of a mucopolysaccharide in viscera, and (3) bony deformities resembling those seen in Hurler's syndrome. Generalized gangliosidosis has been confused clinically with other storage diseases, including Tay-Sachs disease, Niemann-Pick disease, and the mucopolysaccharidoses (Types 1 to 3), since it resembles these disorders in some of its aspects. It is, however, phenotypically and genotypically distinct from them.

The enzyme defect responsible for the pathogenesis of generalized gangliosidosis has recently been uncovered [4]. A total of 10 years transpired between the first clinical description in 1959 and the elucidation of the fundamental enzymatic defect in 1969.

Phenotypic Aspects

Clinical Features

The psychomotor development of the infant with generalized gangliosidosis is retarded from birth. Appetite is poor, sucking is weak, and gain in weight is subnormal. Physical examination in the newborn period reveals a dull-looking, hypoactive, hypotonic infant with facial and peripheral edema (Figs. 30-2, 30-3). Facial abnormalities include frontal bossing, depressed nasal bridge, large low-set ears, increased distance between nose and upper lip, and downy hirsutism of the forehead and neck. These abnormalities may be present at birth (Fig. 30-3). The gums are hypertrophied, and slight to moderate macroglossia is present. The corneas have been clear in all but one patient. Cherry-red spots in the macular region, identical to those seen in Tay-Sachs disease, are present in one-half the patients.

Mental and motor development is severely retarded. The infant may hold his head up but does not crawl and can sit only with support. He may follow objects with his eyes and reach for them, but cannot grasp well because of weakness and incoordination. Arm movements are jerky and uncoordinated. He rarely smiles, has a feeble cry, is lethargic, and does not appear interested in the environment. He usually remains immobile throughout the day, sleeps often, and is said to be a "good baby."

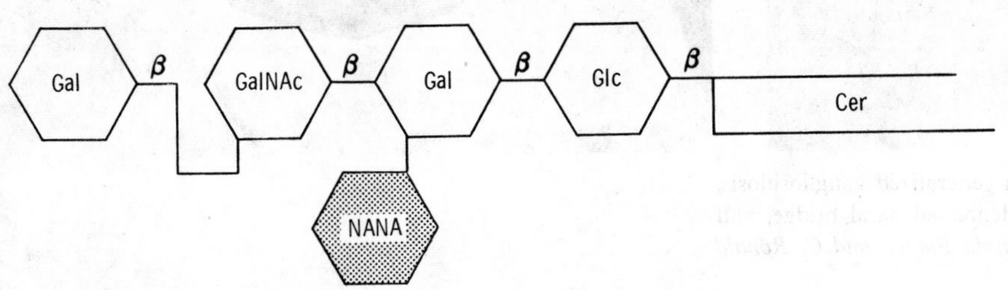

Figure 30-1. Ganglioside G_{M1}.

Table 30-1. NOMENCLATURE APPLIED TO GENERALIZED GANGLIOSIDOSIS

Term	Authors	Year
Tay-Sachs disease with visceral involvement	Norman et al. [1]	1959
Hurler's variant	Craig et al. [5]	1959
Pseudo-Hurler's disease	Landing and Rubinstein [14]	1962
A biochemically special form of infantile amaurotic idiocy*	Jatzkewitz and Sandhoff [15]	1963
Familial neurovisceral lipidosis	Landing et al. [2]	1964
Generalized gangliosidosis	O'Brien et al. [3]	1965
Late infantile systemic lipidosis	Gonatas and Gonatas [6]	1965
Idiotie amaurotic infantile avec surcharge viscérale	Farkas-Bargeton et al. [9]	1967
G_{M1} gangliosidosis	Suzuki et al. [16]	1968
La maladie de Landing	Sacrez et al. [7]	1967
Gangliosidose généralisée du type Norman-Landing, à G_{M1}	Seringe et al. [10]	1968
Cerebral G_{M1} gangliosidosis	Suzuki and Chen [17]	1967

* It is questionable whether this patient had the disease, since a clinical history was not available.

On physical examination internal strabismus and coarse lateral nystagmus may be found. Macrocephaly may develop but is neither as frequent nor as massive as that in Tay-Sachs disease. The heart and lungs are unremarkable early in the disease, but later bronchopneumonia frequently occurs. Hepatomegaly is invariably present after 6 months of age, and splenomegaly is present in 80 percent of the patients at this age. The liver extends 2 to 6 cm below the costal margin, and the edge is smooth, sharp, and nontender. Often only the tip of the spleen is palpable. Lymphadenopathy is of minor degree; it is much more prominent in Niemann-Pick disease and is somewhat more prominent in Gaucher's disease (Type 2).

Dorsolumbar kyphoscoliosis is usually present. The hands are often broad, and the fingers are short and stubby. Flexion contractures of the fingers, especially of the fifth finger, occur, and the interosseous muscles are atrophic, resulting in a "claw-hand" deformity. Hard, nontender enlargements

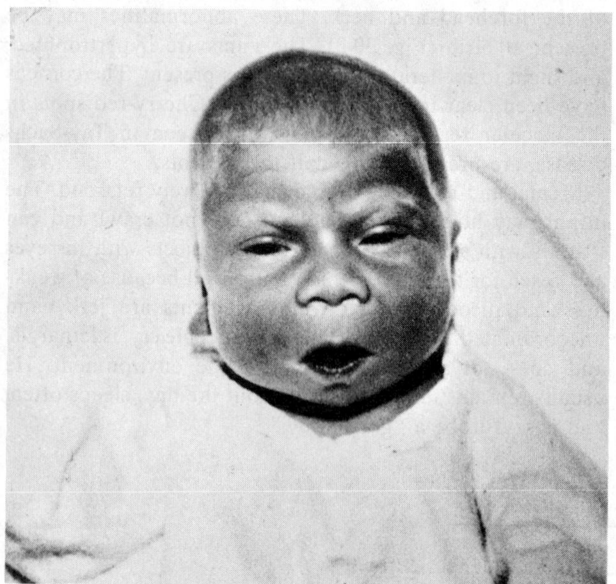

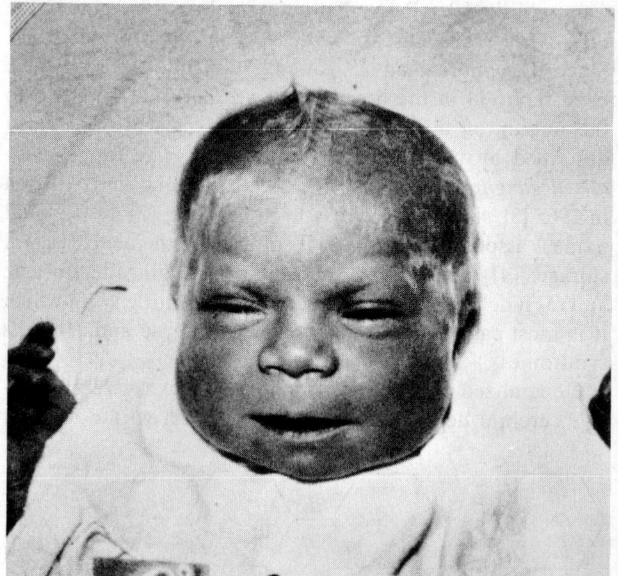

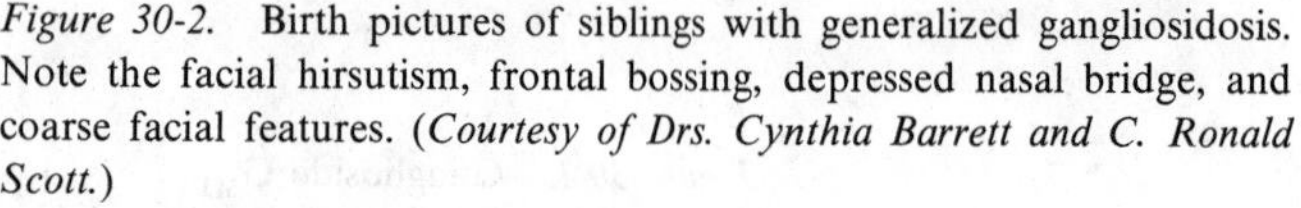

Figure 30-2. Birth pictures of siblings with generalized gangliosidosis. Note the facial hirsutism, frontal bossing, depressed nasal bridge, and coarse facial features. (*Courtesy of Drs. Cynthia Barrett and C. Ronald Scott.*)

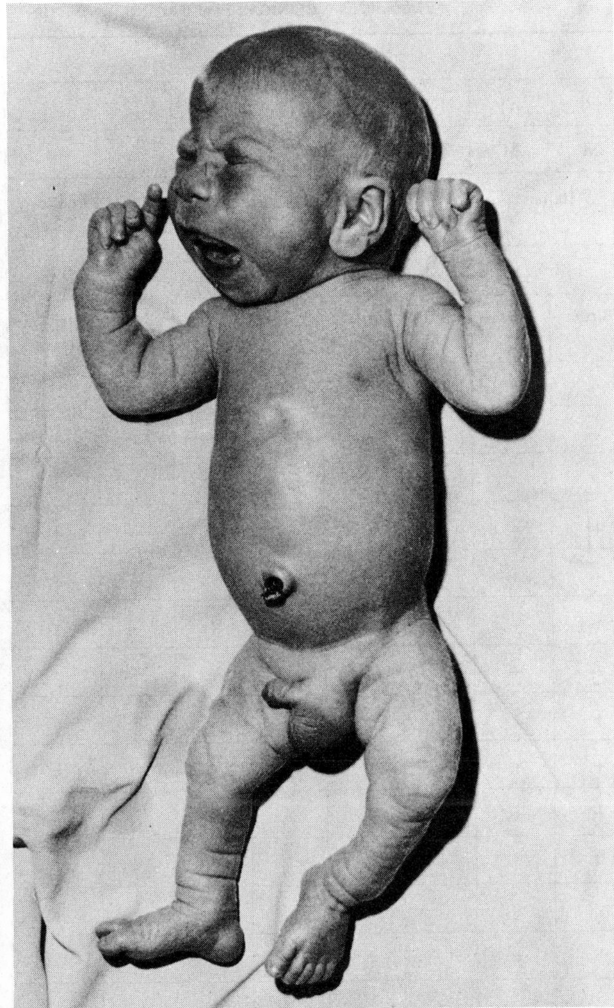

Figure 30-3. Patient with generalized gangliosidosis at 2 weeks of age. Note the frontal bossing, low-set ears, depressed nasal bridge, wide upper lip, maxillary hyperplasia, and prominent wrist and ankle joints. (*From Scott et al.* [8], *by permission of authors and publishers.*)

of epiphyseal joints, especially wrist and ankle joints, may be present (Fig. 30-2). Joints are stiff, and flexion contractures occur at elbows and knees.

Reflexes are hyperreactive. Muscle strength is poor, and generalized hypotonia is present. Hand and arm movements are poorly coordinated. Upon elevation of the trunk, a marked head lag occurs. The infant may demonstrate an exaggerated acousticomotor response (hyperacusis). The skin is often thick, hirsute, and rough. One patient had numerous telangiectasias over the abdomen [11].

After the first year of age deterioration is rapid. Clonic-tonic convulsions occur many times daily. Tube feeding is necessary because of ineffective swallowing. Respirations are labored and irregular. Recurrent bronchopneumonia is a major problem in medical management. Several patients have died suddenly at home; one had recurrent bouts of paroxysmal auricular tachycardia [2]. The sudden death of several patients raises suspicion as to the frequency of this complication.

If survival extends beyond 16 months of life the patient presents the picture of decerebrate rigidity. He is blind, deaf, and out of contact with his surroundings. There are extreme flexion contractures of the upper and lower extremities. The patient lies constantly in the "frog-leg" position and is unresponsive to stimuli. Death occurs by age 2 years and is usually due to bronchopneumonia.

A summary of 25 carefully studied cases is given in Table 30-2 [1–13].

Bony Deformities

The bony abnormalities in the newborn period differ from those seen later on (Figs. 30-4, 30-5). Abnormalities of the bodies of the lumbar vertebrae may be minimal in the first few months of life, and peripheral bony changes predominate. In the Syracuse patient (Patient 18) at 6 weeks of age, generalized symmetric periosteal new bone formation cloaked the shafts of all the long bones, including the ribs. Subepiphyseal transverse rarefactions and corner fractures of the metaphyses were present. These changes were reminiscent of those seen in congenital syphilis. By 7 months of age the periosteal lesions in the long bones had diminished and abnormalities of the vertebral bodies were prominent.

In the patients of Scott et al. [8] periosteal new bone formation surrounding the shaft of the long bones, most markedly in the humerus and femur, was a prominent lesion in the newborn period. The ribs were generally thickened, especially along the lateral margin, but the spine was normal at 1 week of age. At 3 months of age, thoracolumbar kyphosis appeared and vertebral body abnormalities became prominent. In these patients the severity of the peripheral skeletal lesions tended to diminish with time.

After 6 months of age the most important radiologic signs are in the spine and upper extremity [2]. There is generalized rarefaction of the cortex of most bones. One or more hypoplastic, beaked vertebral bodies are usually found at or near the site of a well-defined lumbar kyphosis (Fig. 30-4). The humeri and other long bones show a reversal of the usual contours; i.e., they are wider in the midshaft region, tapering both proximally and distally (Fig. 30-5). This uneven increase in the girth of the shafts may be the single most important diagnostic change in the skeleton. The radiologic changes at the cartilage-shaft junctions are minimal except for the tilting towards each other of the distal epiphyseal lines of the radius and ulna. The metacarpal bones become wedge-shaped, with a constriction proximally in the four lateral metacarpals. The fifth metacarpal is frequently the most expanded and deformed.

With increasing age the externally thickened cortical wall is removed by expansion of the medullary cavity, causing

Table 30-2. CLINICAL FEATURES OF 25 PATIENTS

Feature											
Reference	[1]	[5]	[2]	[2]	[2]	[2]	[2]	[2]	[2]	[3]	[6]
Sex	M	F	F	M	M	F	M	F	M	M	M
Ethnic origin	?	Ital.-French	N. Europ. Jewish	Italian		?	Jewish	Negro		Mexican	Puerto Rican +
Number of patients in sibship	3/8	1/2	1/1	2/5		1/3	?	2/2		1/1	1/4
Age at onset	?	Birth	7 days	Birth	Birth	Birth	Birth	?	?	Birth	Early infancy
Age at death, mo	17	3.5	16	4	?	4.5	10	15	21	8	25
Mental-motor retardation	+	+	+	+	+	+	+	+	+	+	+
Abnormal facies	+	+	. . .	. . .	+	+	. . .	. . .	+	+	+
Edema	. . .	+	+	+	+	?	. . .	. . .	. . .	+	+
X-ray changes, long bones	0	+	+	+	+	+	+	+	. . .	+	‡
Vertebrae	0	+	+	+	+	+	. . .	+	+	+	‡
Vacuolated lymphocytes	. . .	+	+	+	+	+	+	. . .	+	+	. . .
Foam cells in marrow	+	+	+	+	. . .	+	+	. . .	+	+	+
Hepatomegaly	+	+	+	+	+	+	+	. . .	+	+	+
Splenomegaly	0	+	+	+	+	. . .	+	+	. . .	. . .	0
Cherry-red spot	+	. . .	+	0	0	0	0	. . .	. . .	0	0
Macroglossia	+	. . .	+	. . .	. . .	+	. . .	. . .	+	. . .	0
Glomerular lesion	+	+	+	+	+	+	+	+	. . .	+	. . .
G_{M1} accumulation in:											
Brain	*	. . .	. . .	. . .	. . .	. . .	. . .	. . .	. . .	+	+
Viscera	. . .	. . .	. . .	. . .	. . .	. . .	. . .	. . .	. . .	+	. . .
Galactosidase deficiency	. . .	. . .	. . .	. . .			. . .			+	. . .
Mucopolysacchariduria	. . .	. . .	. . .	. . .	. . .	. . .	0	. . .	. . .	. . .	0
Mucopolysaccharide accumulation in viscera	. . .	. . .	. . .	. . .	. . .	. . .	. . .	. . .	. . .	+	. . .

* Found subsequently (R. M. Norman, personal communication).
† In urine and skin.
‡ Bony changes noted at autopsy but not reported on x-ray examination.
§ Mucopolysacchariduria early, which later disappeared.
Note: +, consanguineous parents. Blank indicates feature was not described.

a "reamed-out" appearance and resulting in a synchronous thinning of the cortical wall. In addition to the deformities of the long bones and vertebral bodies, other radiologic changes include a shallow, elongated pituitary fossa (shoe-shaped sella), widened spatulate ribs, and flared iliums [2].

The skeletal lesions of generalized gangliosidosis are not pathognomonic. Similar bony deformities occur in patients with mucopolysaccharidosis Type 1 or Hurler's syndrome [18], lipomucopolysaccharidosis [19], and I-cell disease [20]. Caffey's [21] careful descriptions of the prenatal and early postnatal bony abnormalities in patients with the mucopolysaccharidoses (probably including generalized gangliosidosis as well) provide an especially valuable source of reference.

Occasional patients have been reported in whom radiologic abnormalities were absent. In one of these bony de-

WITH GENERALIZED GANGLIOSIDOSIS

[7]	[8]	[8]	[9]	[10]	[13]	[13]	[13]	[11]	[13]	[13]	[12]	[12]	[12]	Frequency
F	M	F	M	F	M	M	M	F	M	F	F	F	M	
Algerian+	English-German		?+	French	Negro	Italian-Polish	?	?	Portuguese+	Maltese	Scandinavian+	Italian*	Maltese+	
1/3	2/3		1/2	1/1	1/4	1/1	1/1	1/2	1/1	?	1/1	1/1	1/1	
5 mo	Birth	Birth	15 days	Birth	Birth	Birth	Birth	Birth	6 mo	Early infancy	4 mo	1 mo	3 mo	
24	4	6	20	10	24	Alive	12	19	?	17	20	16	22	
+	+	+	+	+	+	+	+	+	+	+	+	+	+	25/25
+	+	+	...	+	...	+	+	+	+	...	+	+	+	18/18
±	...	...	+	+	...	...	+	+	0	...	...	+	+	12/13
...	+	+	+	...	+	+	+	+	+	+	+	+	+	21/22
+	+	...	+	+	+	+	+	+	+	+	+	+	+	22/23
+	+	...	0	+	+	+	0	+	+	...	+	+	+	18/20
...	±	...	...	...	+	+	+	+	+	...	+	+	+	17/18
+	0	...	+	+	+	+	+	+	+	+	+	+	+	22/23
+	0	...	...	+	+	+	+	+	+	+	+	+	+	17/20
+	0	...	...	+	+	...	+	+	+	+	0	+	+	11/19
+	±	±	...	...	...	...	+	...	+	...	...	...	+	10/11
...	+	+	...	+	+	...	...	...	...	...	+	+	+	16/16
+ +	... ...	... ...	+ ...	+ +	+ +	... ...	+ +	+ +	+ ...	+ ...	+ ...	+ ...	+ ...	14/14 6/6
+	...	...	...	+	+	+†	+	+	+	+				
0	0	...	+	0	...	...	±§	±	+	±	...	...	...	3/10
...	+	...	+	...	...	...	...	...	...	+	...	...	...	4/4

formities were found at autopsy [6], and in the other facial abnormalities were present [1]. The bony abnormalities may have been missed in these patients or may have been insufficiently developed for detection at the time roentgenograms were taken. At this writing it is my opinion that the diagnosis of generalized gangliosidosis cannot be made in the absence of deformities of the vertebral bodies or of the long bones if the patient is 6 months of age or older.

Genetics

Both sexes have been affected with about equal frequency (14 boys, 11 girls) (Table 30-2). Consanguinity has been present in 7 of 22 reported sibships. The ratio of affected to unaffected sibs is 0.51, higher than that expected for autosomal recessive inheritance (0.25), but if one corrects for incomplete ascertainment in 20 sibships there is close agreement between observation and expectation (Table 30-3). Unfortunately, the sample is too small to prove recessive inheritance, although the results are consistent with this mode of transmission. Fibroblasts cultured from the parents of one affected child contained metachromatic material, consistent with each having minimal abnormality detectable in this manner [12]. The cumulated evidence for autosomal recessive inheritance includes the high consanguinity rate, the pattern of familial occurrence, the equal sex ratio, the absence of signs of the disease in the parents, and the presence of cellular metachromasia in the fibroblasts of heterozygotes.

A severe deficiency of β-galactosidase activity occurs in leukocytes [53], urine [25] and cultured skin fibroblasts [27] from patients with generalized gangliosidosis. Leukocytes from parents of probands have enzyme activity intermediate to that in leukocytes from patients and controls [53], providing further evidence that the disease is autosomal recessive.

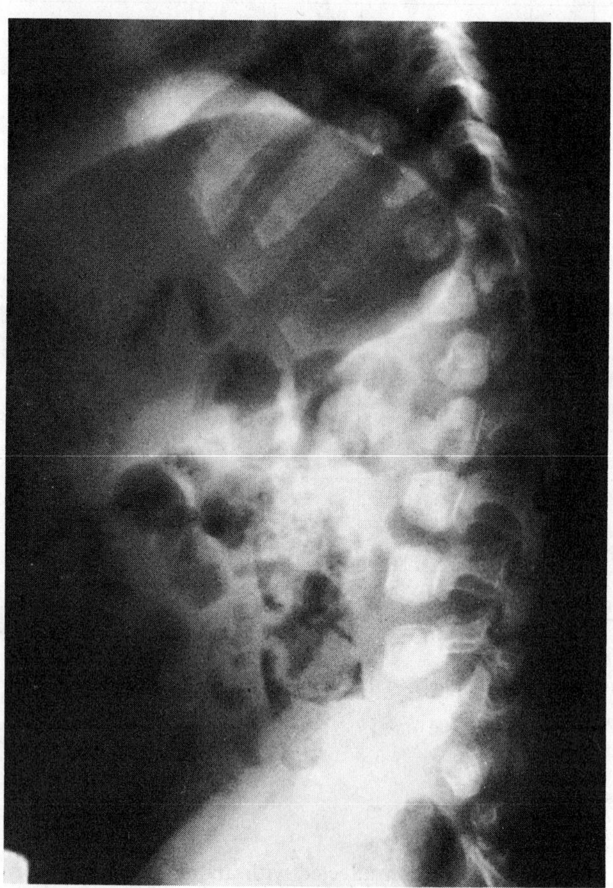

Figure 30-4. Spinal column deformities in generalized gangliosidosis at 7 months of age. Note the hypoplastic vertebral bodies, the beaking of L1 and L2, and the lumbar kyphosis. *(From G. Mitchell and A. Berne, Syracuse Memorial Hospital, Syracuse, N.Y., with their kind permission.)*

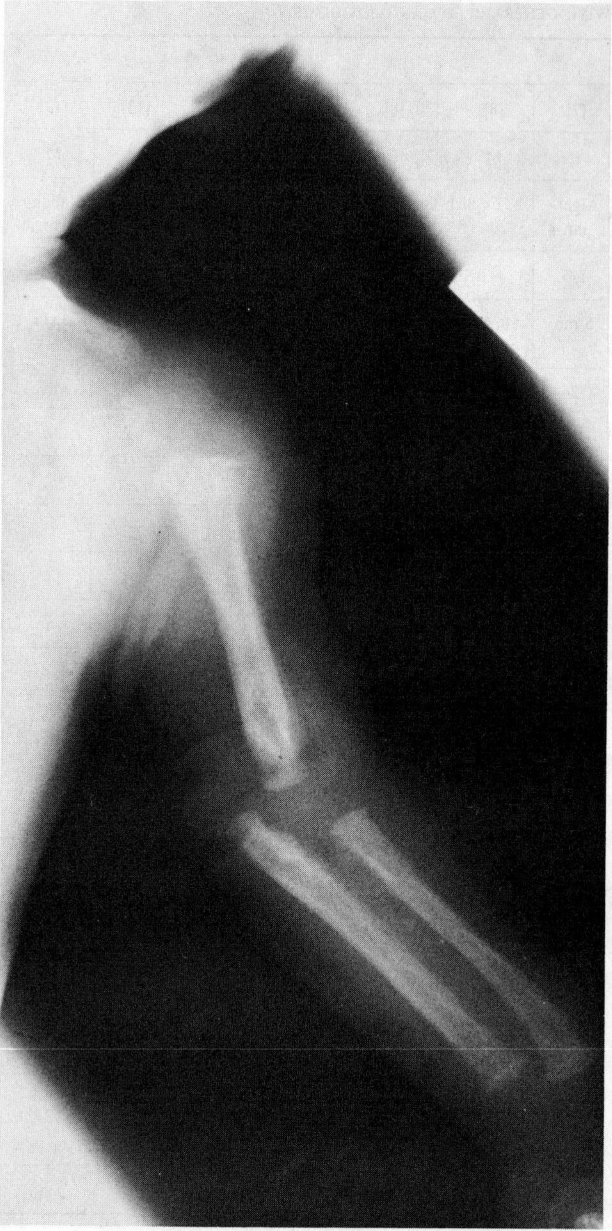

A

Figure 30-5. Upper extremity in generalized gangliosidosis. A. At 2 weeks of age. B. At 2 months. C. At 7 months. Note the hypoplastic appearance, the midshaft widening, the periosteal "cloaking," and the pinching-off of the ends of the humerus. *(From G. Mitchell and A. Berne, Syracuse Memorial Hospital, Syracuse, N.Y., with their permission.)*

No ethnic predilection has appeared. Patients of Italian-French, Jewish, Italian, Negro, Maltese, Mexican, Algerian, English-German, French, Italian-Polish, Portuguese, Japanese [22], and Puerto Rican origin have been reported. Two families out of 25 (Patients 22 and 25) trace their origin

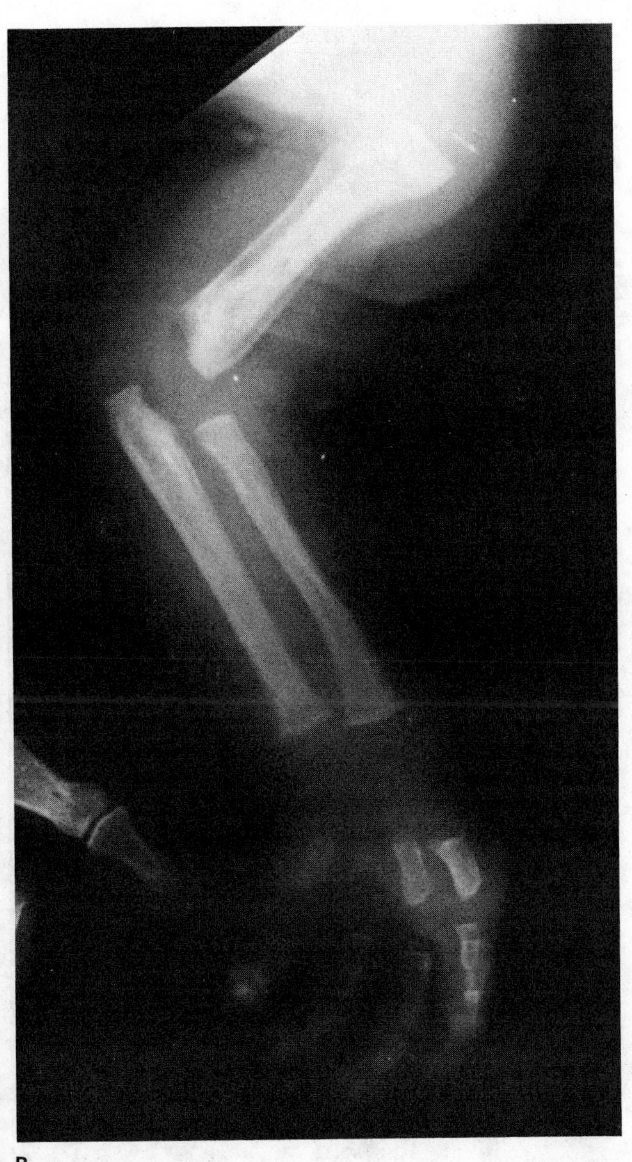

B

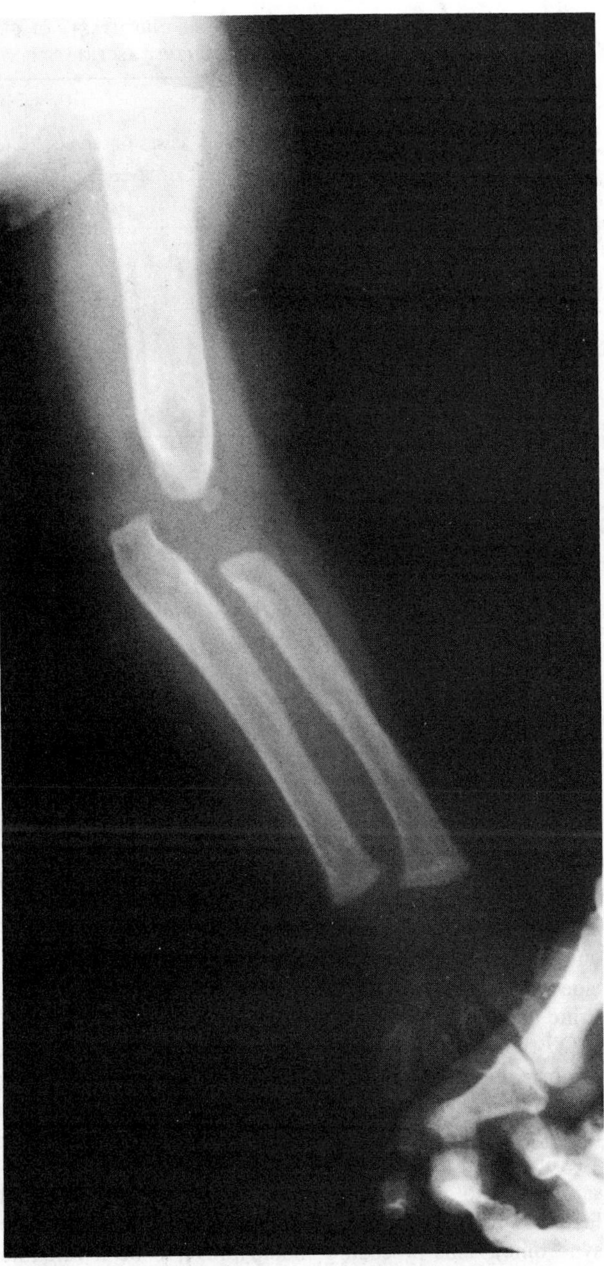

C

to Malta. This suggests an increase in the gene frequency for generalized gangliosidosis in that locale. The pan-ethnic nature of generalized gangliosidosis is in contrast to the situation in the other sphingolipidoses such as Tay-Sachs disease, Niemann-Pick disease, and "adult" Gaucher's disease (Type 1), which have an increased gene frequency in the Ashkenazi Jewish population [23].

The gene frequency of generalized gangliosidosis is unknown. With increased awareness of the disease, its frequency may be ascertained.

Table 30-3. A PRIORI TEST OF RECESSIVE INHERITANCE OF GENERALIZED GANGLIOSIDOSIS USING TRUNCATE ASCERTAINMENT

Size of sibship	No. of sibships of each size	No. of children	No. of cases observed	No. of cases expected
s	n_s	$t = sn_s$	r_s	C_s
1	9	9	9	9.00
2	4	8	5	4.56
3	3	9	4	3.87
4	2	8	2	2.88
5	1	5	2	1.65
8	1	8	3	2.24
	20	47	25	24.20

Laboratory Data

Lymphocytes in the peripheral blood smear are vacuolated; 10 to 80 percent of the lymphoctyes contain three or four vacuoles per cell. The vacuoles are not osmophilic and appear empty by electron microscopy [7]. Vacuolated histiocytes are present in fixed preparations of the bone marrow. The number of involved histiocytes is not as large as that in Niemann-Pick or Gaucher's disease.

Foamy mononuclear cells may be found in the urine sediment. The quantity of mucopolysaccharides in urine is usually normal or only slightly elevated as measured by the albumin turbidity test, the Berry-Spinanger spot test, or cetylpyridinium chloride precipitation. Patient 21 of Lowden excreted in urine twofold increased levels (15 to 20 mg per day) of a mucopolysaccharide which had a carbohydrate composition similar to that of keratan sulfate [24]. Gangliosides are not excreted, as determined by lipid extraction of urine samples and chromatography [3].

O'Brien found a reduction of β-galactosidase to 10 percent of normal in the urine of Patient 18. A more definitive study has been made by Thomas [25], who developed a urinary assay for β-galactosidase and β-N-acetylglucosaminidase and applied it to the urine of Patient 19. The ratio of glucosaminidase to galactosidase was over 100 in the patient and less than 20 in controls (including patients with Hurler's syndrome). This procedure should prove to be a valuable diagnostic test.

A deficiency of β-galactosidase has also been found in tissue obtained by skin biopsy [26]. Kaback and Howell [13] have reported a severe deficiency (0.5 percent of normal) of β-galactosidase in fibroblasts cultured from the skin of Patient 19, thereby demonstrating the defect in tissue culture. Similar findings have been published by Sloan et al. [27] using ganglioside G_{M1} as substrate (see Fig. 1-6).

Other laboratory procedures have revealed normal urine amino acid patterns [1, 3, 10], normal chromosomal karyotype [10], normal cytoarchitecture on skin biopsy with no evidence of mucopolysaccharide storage by the Haust-Landing stain [1], and slightly increased levels of serum α_2-globulin [9] and haptoglobin [10]. Serum fructose-1-phosphate aldolase levels have been in the normal range [10]. Lactose, galactose, and saccharose have been detected in the urine of one child [9].

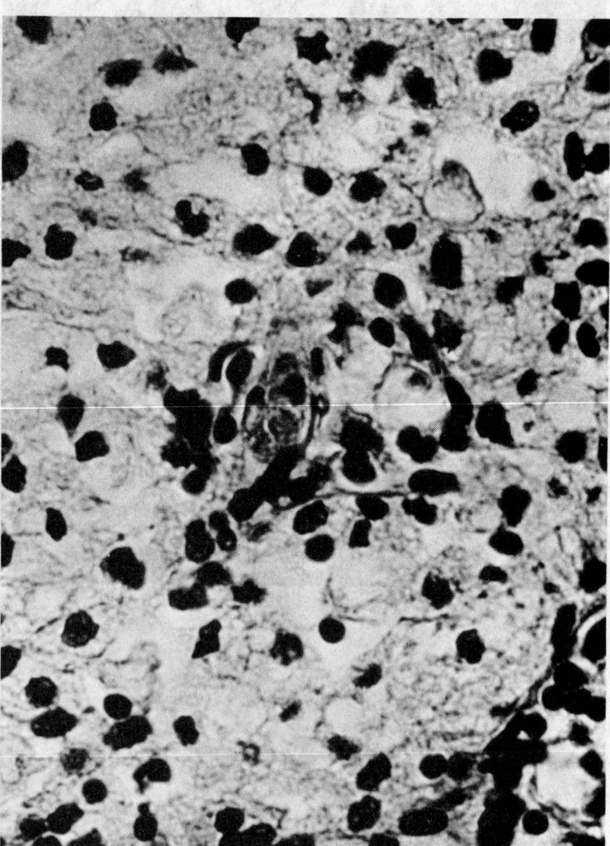

Figure 30-6. Vacuolation of splenic histiocytes in generalized gangliosidosis. (Hematoxylin and eosin, ×250.) (*Courtesy of B. H. Landing.*)

Pathologic Aspects

The most striking pathologic changes are (1) visceral histiocytosis, (2) neuronal lipidosis, and (3) cytoplasmic vacuolation of renal glomerular epithelium cells [1]. The inclusions in visceral histiocytes (Fig. 30-6) are periodic acid–Schiff (PAS)-positive, weakly metachromatic (pH 2), and weakly sudanophilic [2]. The Haust-Landing stain for acid mucopolysaccharides is negative [2]. The substance stored in visceral histiocytes is very soluble in aqueous fixatives.

Neuronal lipidosis occurs throughout the cortex, brain stem, and spinal cord as well as in Meissner's plexus. Rectal biopsy has been useful in demonstrating neurolipidosis for diagnostic purposes [2]. The neuronal cytoplasm is ballooned with storage material, displacing the nucleus to the periphery (Fig. 30-7). The storage substance appears as finely dispersed

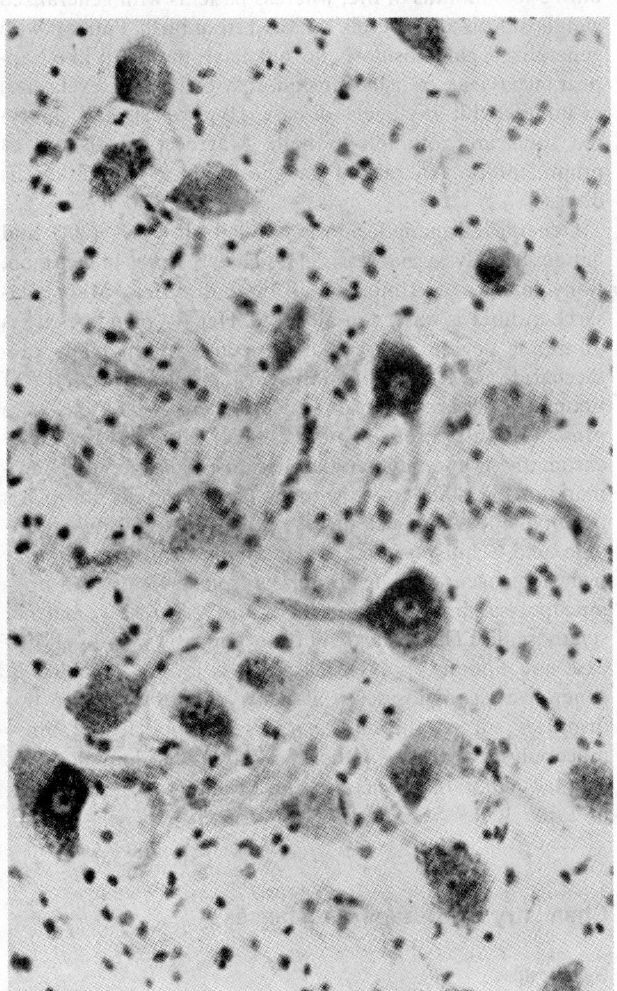

Figure 30-7. Cytoplasmic ballooning of neurons in cranial nerve nucleus in generalized gangliosidosis. (Acetic acid–cresyl violet, ×200.) (*From Landing et al.* [2], *by permission of authors and publishers.*)

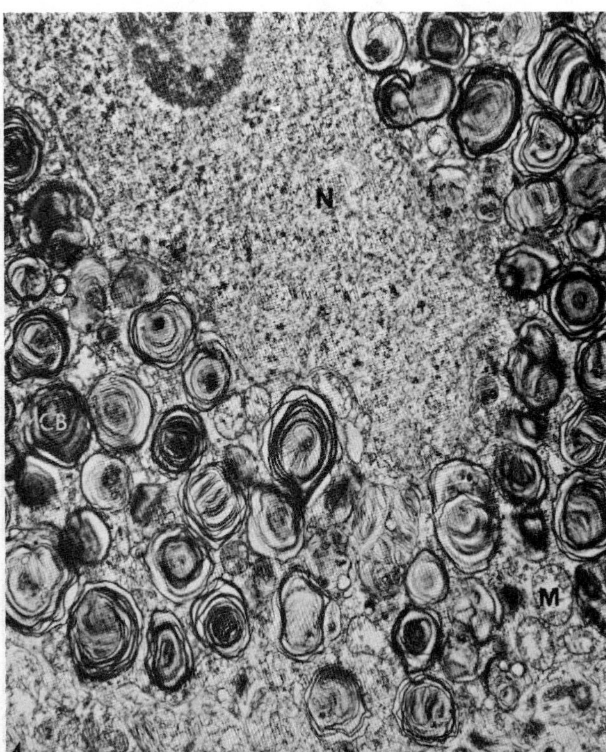

Figure 30-8. Cytoplasmic membranous bodies in neuronal cytoplasm in generalized gangliosidosis. (×8,000.) (*From N. K. Gonatas and J. Gonatas,* [6], *by permission of authors and publishers.*)

particles under the light microscope [2]. By electron microscopy (Fig. 30-8) cytoplasmic membranous inclusion bodies similar to those seen in Tay-Sachs disease [28] are seen. The inclusion bodies are comprised of spirally wound membranes enclosed within a limiting membrane [6, 7]. A single coiled membrane has a cross-sectional thickness of 60 Å [6].

The involvement of renal glomerular epithelial cells (Fig. 30-9) is a characteristic lesion not found in any other known lipidosis except Fabry's angiokeratoma corporis diffusum and juvenile G_{M1} gangliosidosis. The glomerular epithelial cells store large quantities of cytoplasmic material, giving the glomerulus a swollen appearance [1, 2]. The storage material is very soluble in aqueous fixatives; empty vacuoles remain after fixation for electron microscopy (Fig. 30-10) [7, 8]. Small amounts of osmophilic lamellated lipid-like material are also present. In splenic histiocytes the storage material appears as interwoven bundles of closely packed tubules approximately 200 Å in diameter [16].

Differential Diagnosis

Generalized gangliosidosis is most readily confused with Hurler's syndrome (mucopolysaccharidosis Type 1), Nie-

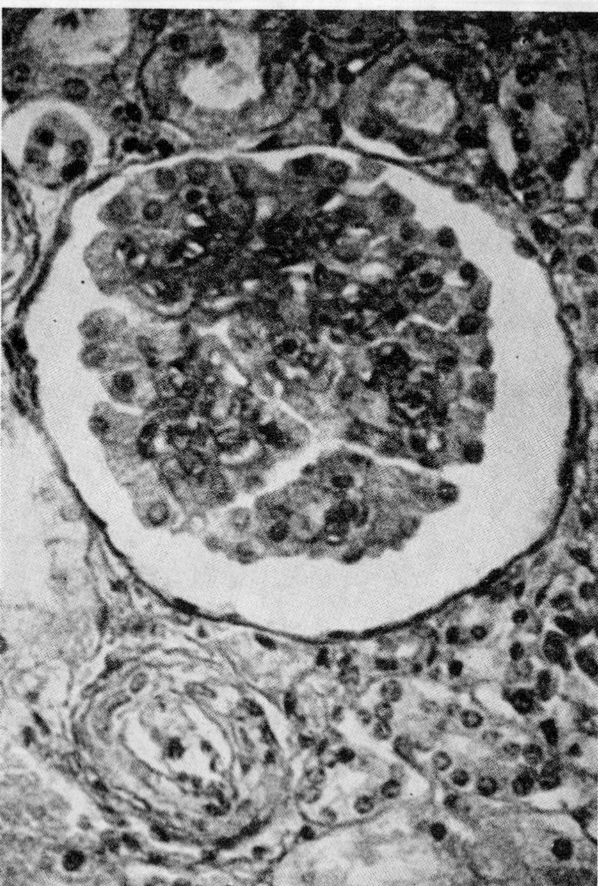

Figure 30-9. Cytoplasmic ballooning of renal glomerular epithelial cells in generalized gangliosidosis. (Periodic acid–Schiff stain, ×80.) (*From Landing et al.* [2], *by permission of authors and publishers.*)

mann-Pick disease, and Tay-Sachs disease. It can be differentiated from mucopolysaccharidosis Type 1 by a more rapid downhill course. Generalized gangliosidosis is fatal by 2 years; patients with Hurler's syndrome often survive beyond the first decade. Mental and motor retardation is much more severe in generalized gangliosidosis. Patients with Hurler's syndrome usually can walk and speak; patients with generalized gangliosidosis cannot. Radiologically, the two diseases mimic each other, although the bony lesions are somewhat more severe at an earlier age in generalized gangliosidosis. Cherry-red spots are found in one-half the patients with generalized gangliosidosis; they are absent in Hurler's syndrome. While corneal clouding is usually absent in generalized gangliosidosis and present in the Hurler's syndrome (mucopolysaccharidosis Type 1), slit-lamp examinations of the cornea have not been made in large enough numbers of patients to determine the frequency of small corneal opacities. Patients with generalized gangliosidosis excrete normal or only slightly elevated quantities of mucopolysaccharides in their urine; patients with the mucopolysaccharidoses excrete grossly elevated quantities. The renal glomerular epithelial ballooning seen in generalized gangliosidosis is absent in mucopolysaccharidoses.

Generalized gangliosidosis may be differentiated from infantile cerebral Niemann-Pick disease (Type A) by the bony deformities and facial abnormalities which are present in the former and absent in the latter. Hepatosplenomegaly is similar in both. Lymphadenopathy is greater in Niemann-Pick disease. Psychomotor retardation, progressive rapid deterioration, and cherry-red spots occur in both diseases. Visceral histiocytosis and neuronal lipidosis are common to both. Renal glomerular epithelial involvement is not found in Niemann-Pick disease.

Generalized gangliosidosis can be differentiated from Tay-Sachs disease by the presence of hepatosplenomegaly, the bony changes, and the renal lesion. Patients with Tay-Sachs disease do not exhibit severe psychomotor retardation until 3 to 6 months of life, whereas patients with generalized gangliosidosis are severely retarded from birth. Patients with generalized gangliosidosis do not have the "doll-like" appearance (clear, translucent skin, rosy color, long eyelashes) of infants with Tay-Sachs disease. Hyperacusis and cherry-red spots are common to both. Macrocephaly is not as prominent in generalized gangliosidosis as in Tay-Sachs disease.

Generalized gangliosidosis, "I-cell disease" [20], and "lipomucopolysaccharidosis" [19] have features in common. Bony changes are similar in all three disorders. Mucopolysacchariduria is absent in all three. Hepatosplenomegaly is of minor degree in I-cell disease and in lipomucopolysaccharidosis. Glycoproteinuria is a prominent feature of lipomucopolysaccharidosis. Lymphocyte inclusions are present in all three disorders; the inclusions are metachromatic in lipomucopolysaccharidosis, and nonmetachromatic in the other two disorders. Cultured skin fibroblasts from patients with I-cell disease contain PAS-positive (periodic acid–Schiff-positive), sudanophilic inclusions. Similar inclusions occur in skin fibroblasts from patients with lipomucopolysaccharidosis, and these are PAS-positive but not sudanophilic. The clinical course of patients with I-cell disease and lipomucopolysaccharidosis is longer than that in generalized gangliosidosis. Patients with the former two disorders survive beyond 2 years of age [19, 20], lipomucopolysaccharidosis patients surviving the longest.

A tabulation of the main points of differentiation is given in Table 30-4.

Chemistry of Storage Substances

Gangliosides

A discussion of ganglioside structure and metabolism is given in Chap. 29 of this volume. The ganglioside which accumulates in the brain and viscera in generalized gangliosidosis is ganglioside G_{M1}. The magnitude of the ganglioside G_{M1} accumulation is tenfold in gray matter [3, 6] (Fig. 30-11) and approximately twenty- to fiftyfold in liver [3, 17, 29] when compared to normal. The ganglioside has been isolated from the brain of affected patients; its sugar composition [3, 6], fatty acid composition [3], sugar sequence [30], and linkages of each sugar [31] are identical to those of the normal major monosialoganglioside G_{M1}, viz., {galactosyl-(1 → 3)-N-acetylgalactosaminyl-(1 → 4)-[(2 → 3)-N-acetylneuraminyl]-galactosyl-(1 → 4)-glucosyl-(1 → 1)-[2-N-acyl]-sphingosine}. (Fig. 30-1).

A structurally related glycolipid—a ceramide tetrahexoside—also accumulates in the brain in generalized gangliosidosis [17]. This compound, Gal-Gal (NAC)-Gal-Glc-Cer, is identical to ganglioside G_{M1} except that it lacks neuraminic acid.

The ganglioside stored in generalized gangliosidosis differs from ganglioside G_{M2}, which is stored in Tay-Sachs disease (see Chap. 29). Both generalized gangliosidosis and Tay-Sachs disease involve the massive cerebral accumulation of gangliosides which are normally present in the brain. Both may be classified as inborn errors of ganglioside metabolism. It is assumed that cerebral degeneration in generalized gangliosidosis and in Tay-Sachs disease is chiefly due to the

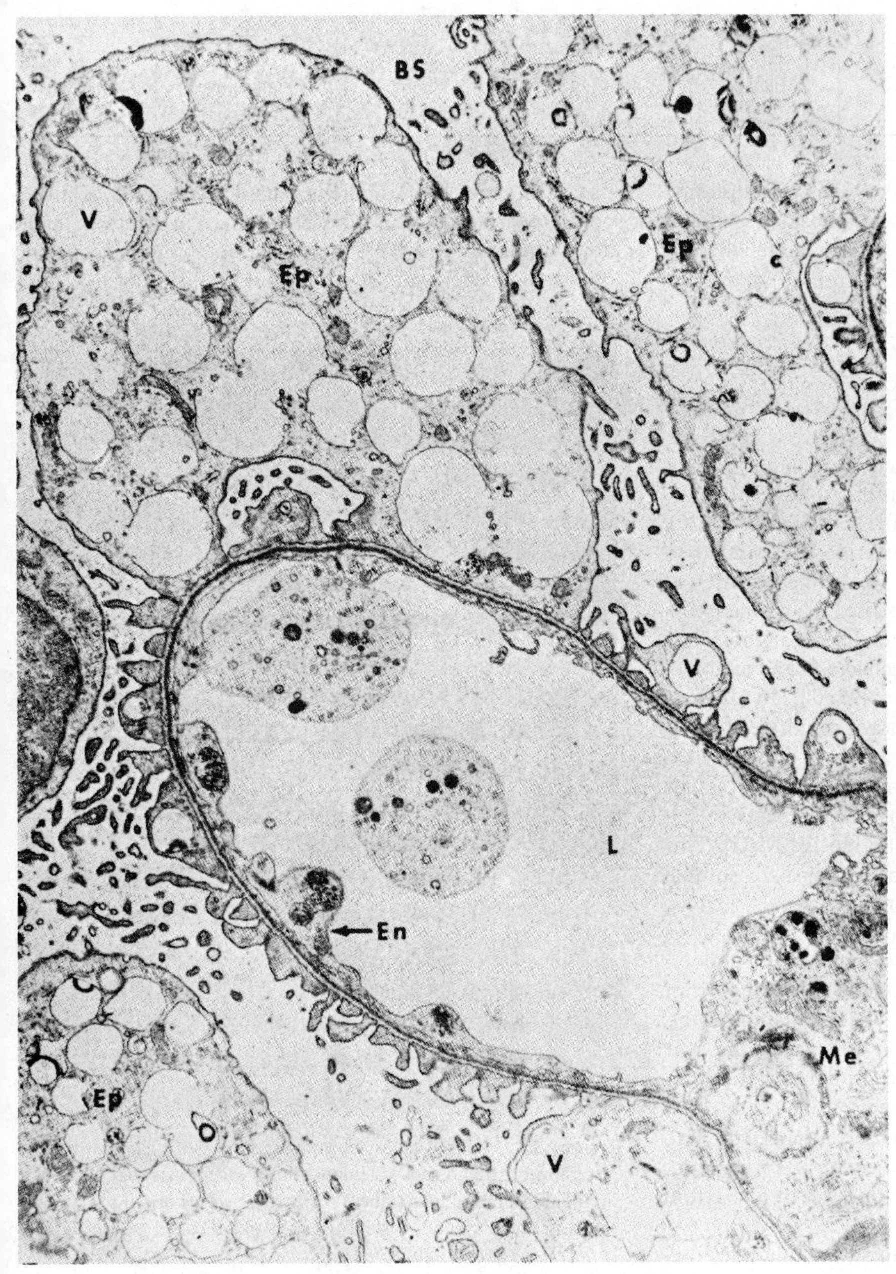

Figure 30-10. Cytoplasmic vacuolation of renal glomerular epithelial cells in generalized gangliosidosis. *BS,* Bowman's space, *L,* capillary lumen, *V,* vacuole. (×23,000.) (*From Scott et al.* [8], *by permission of authors and publishers.*)

Table 30-4. DIFFERENTIAL DIAGNOSTIC POINTS—GENERALIZED GANGLIOSIDOSIS

Feature	Generalized gangliosidosis	Tay-Sachs disease	Infantile cerebral Niemann-Pick disease	Mucopolysaccharidosis Type 1 [recessive]	Mucopolysaccharidosis Type 2 (X-linked)	Acute neuronopathic Gaucher's disease
Mental-motor retardation	Severe early	Severe after 6 mo	Severe early	Severe after several years	Severe after several years	Severe early
Cherry-red spot	+	+	+	−	−	+
Macrocephaly	±	+	−	+	+	−
Hepatosplenomegaly	+	−	+	+	+	+
Vacuolated lymphocytes	+	−	±	+	+	±
Bony abnormalities	+	−	−	+	+	−
Abnormal facies	+	−	−	+	+	−
Corneal clouding	±	−	−	+	−	−
Mucopolysacchariduria	±	−	−	+	+	−
Behavior	Apathetic	Placid	Apathetic	Placid	Aggressive	Apathetic
Lymphadenopathy	±	−	+	−	−	+

neuronal accumulation of gangliosides. This assumption is based on the belief that cytoplasmic gangliosidosis impairs neuronal function. Nonetheless, the precise metabolic and functional mechanisms responsible for cerebral impairment are unknown.

Mucopolysaccharides

Mucopolysaccharides are stored in the viscera in generalized gangliosidosis. This has been demonstrated by both morphologic [8, 29, 30] and analytic chemical studies [2, 30, 32]. The magnitude of the mucopolysaccharidosis is similar to that in mucopolysaccharidoses Types 1 to 3 [30], but different compounds accumulate in each disease. The mucopolysaccharide which accumulates in generalized gangliosidosis contains equimolar proportions of galactose and glucosamine, and is similar to keratan sulfate [29, 32]. In Hurler's syndrome, heparitin sulfate and chondroitin sulfate B accumulate [12].

A second polysaccharide, containing sialic acid residues as well as galactose and glucosamine, accumulates in the liver and spleen in generalized gangliosidosis [29, 32]. This sialomucopolysaccharide appears to be an unusually soluble compound, structurally similar to keratan sulfate.

The visceral histiocytosis in generalized gangliosidosis appears to be chiefly due to the storage of mucopolysaccharides rather than of ganglioside. Calculating from Suzuki's data [30], the ganglioside G_{M1} accumulation in the liver (his Patient 2) amounts to 0.02 percent of the wet weight, whereas the mucopolysaccharide accumulation (assuming the keratan sulfate structure) amounts to 0.80 percent and the sialomucopolysaccharide accumulation to 0.18 percent (assuming a sialic acid content of 20 percent). Thus, the amount of mucopolysaccharide stored is fiftyfold higher than that of ganglioside.

It is assumed that the polysaccharide accumulation gives rise to the bony abnormalities. The accumulation of mucopolysaccharide in connective tissue may interfere with the normal maturation of bone. The metabolic mechanisms involved in delayed mineralization and retarded bony maturation are unknown.

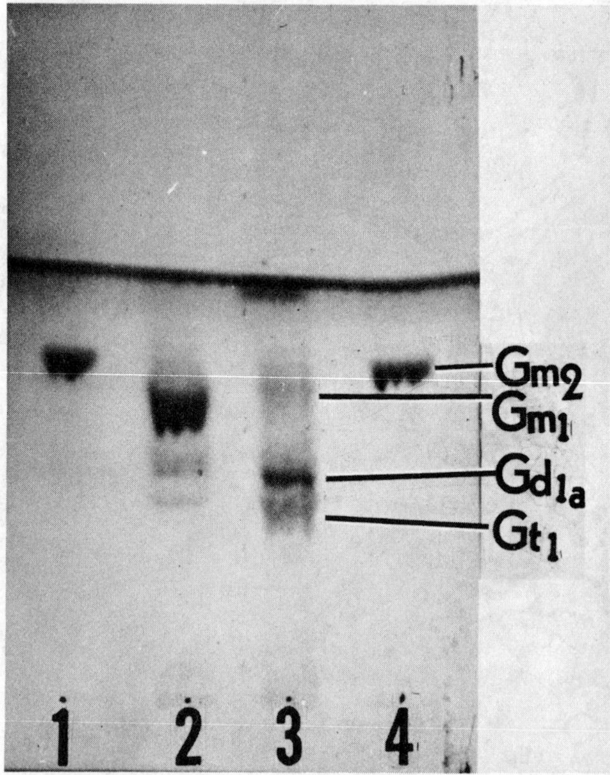

Figure 30-11. Thin-layer chromatography of gangliosides in generalized gangliosidosis demonstrating excess of ganglioside G_{M1} in patient's gray matter (lane 2) compared with normal gray matter (lane 3). Lanes 1 and 4 are Tay-Sachs ganglioside. (*From O'Brien et al.* [3], *by permission of the publishers.*)

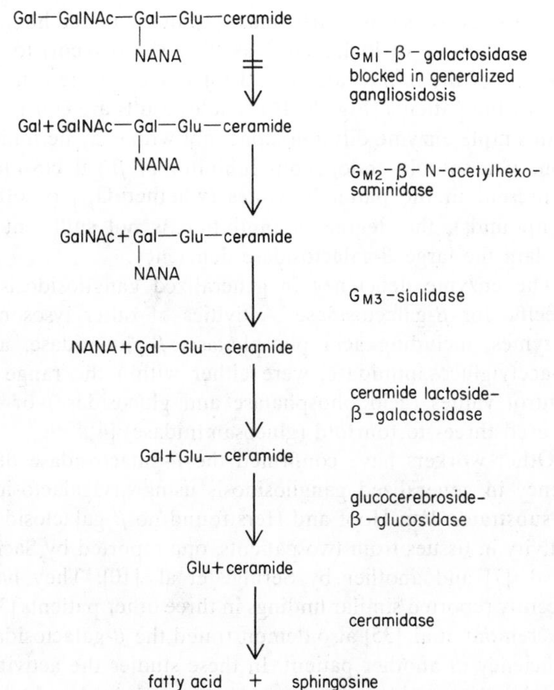

Figure 30-12. Scheme for ganglioside catabolism and metabolic block in generalized gangliosidosis. *Gal,* galactose; *glu,* glucose; *gal NAc,* N-acetylgalactosamine; *NANA,* N-acetylneuraminic acid.

Enzymatic Defect

Once the structure of the stored ganglioside was known, it was possible to think of mechanisms which could result in its accumulation. Obvious potential defects were (1) increased synthesis, (2) decreased degradation, or (3) a combination of both. The degradative pathway, involving sequential hydrolysis of sugar residues from ganglioside G_{M1} by lysosomal glycosidases, has been demonstrated in brain by Gatt and his coworkers [33] (Fig. 30-12). The first step is cleavage of the β-linked terminal galactose from ganglioside G_{M1}, a reaction carried out by a β-galactosidase localized in lysosomes. This defect appeared to be a likely one to test for in the disease.

One straightforward approach involved the assay of β-galactosidase activity using *p*-nitrophenyl-β-D-galactopyranoside as substrate. Activity for *p*-nitrophenylgalactoside and that for ganglioside G_{M1} are not directly equatable. Nonetheless, the *p*-nitrophenyl assay is easy to perform and was chosen for that reason.

β-Galactosidase Deficiency

Okada and O'Brien found a marked deficiency of β-galactosidase activity in the tissues of two patients with generalized gangliosidosis [4]. This study was performed on frozen tissue taken at autopsy; fortunately the enzyme is stable in the frozen state. The β-galactosidase activity in visceral organs (Table 30-5) was 2 to 5 percent of normal in generalized gangliosidosis, and the activity in brain was 10 percent of normal (Table 30-6).

β-Galactosidase activity was not depressed in other sphingolipid storage diseases in which the diagnosis was confirmed chemically; these diseases included Tay-Sachs disease, Niemann-Pick disease, metachromatic leukodystrophy, acute neuronopathic Gaucher's disease, and a variety of other disorders (Tables 30-5, 30-6) in which cerebral degeneration was present in patients of comparable age.

The low β-galactosidase activity was not due to the presence of soluble endogenous inhibitors [4]. This was demonstrated in two ways. First, ganglioside G_{M1} (which was soluble in the buffers used) was added to brain and liver homogenates from control subjects in amounts equivalent to those found stored in the patients' tissues (0.5 percent of the wet weight). A slight inhibition of β-galactosidase activity was found in the G_{M1}-enriched homogenates of control liver (Fig. 30-13), and a slightly larger inhibition (10 to 15 percent) was found in gray matter, but the degree of inhibition was small.

In another experiment liver homogenates from controls and patients were mixed in equal proportions and β-galactosidase activity was assayed under conditions in which the

Table 30-5. β-GALACTOSIDASE ACTIVITY OF VISCERAL ORGANS

Age	Diagnosis	Organ	Enzyme activity*
2 days	Meconium peritonitis	Liver	17.1
1 mo	Multiple congenital defects	Liver	18.0
3 mo	Gastroenteritis	Liver	16.7
11 mo	Lymphangioma	Liver	14.4
13 mo	Gastrointestinal hemorrhage	Liver	16.2
18 yr	Congenital renal disease	Liver	17.1
59 yr	Adenocarcinoma of lung	Liver	23.0
6 yr	Chronic granulomatous disease	Liver	20.4
10 yr	Niemann-Pick disease	Liver	23.9
5 yr	Niemann-Pick disease	Liver	13.6
8 mo	Generalized gangliosidosis	Liver	1.0
2 yr	Generalized gangliosidosis	Liver	0.8
2 mo	Maple syrup urine disease	Kidney	16.2
7 yr	Hereditary nephritis	Kidney	18.5
5 yr	Late infantile amaurotic idiocy	Kidney	15.3
59 yr	Adenocarcinoma of lung	Kidney	10.8
2 yr	Generalized gangliosidosis	Kidney	0.5
6 yr	Chronic granulomatous disease	Spleen	13.5
10 yr	Adult Gaucher's disease	Spleen	8.0
3 yr	Niemann-Pick disease	Spleen	13.0
5 yr	Late infantile amaurotic idiocy	Spleen	7.7
59 yr	Adenocarcinoma of lung	Spleen	5.5
8 mo	Generalized gangliosidosis	Spleen	0.3
2 yr	Generalized gangliosidosis	Spleen	0.7

* β-Galactosidase activity is expressed as nanomoles of *p*-nitrophenol released per milligram of wet tissue per hour. Assay conditions are given in [4].

Table 30-6. β-GALACTOSIDASE ACTIVITY OF CEREBRAL GRAY MATTER

Age	Diagnosis	Enzyme activity*
2 mo	Sudden-death syndrome	103
3 yr	Cardiac anomaly	146
6 yr	Auto accident	211
59 yr	Adenocarcinoma of lung	120
81 yr	Myocardial infarction	162
3 yr	Tay-Sachs disease	327
3 yr	Tay-Sachs disease	278
2 yr	Tay-Sachs disease	216
2 yr	Tay-Sachs disease	278
6 yr	Late infantile amaurotic idiocy	93
5 yr	Late infantile amaurotic idiocy	105
15 mo	Gaucher's disease (Type 2)	164
7 mo	Gaucher's disease (Type 2)	125
5 yr	Metachromatic leukodystrophy	151
11 yr	Metachromatic leukodystrophy	122
3 yr	Niemann-Pick disease	151
13 mo	Kinky-hair disease	169
11 yr	Cystic fibrosis	138
4 yr	Cerebellar hypoplasia	111
2 yr	Generalized gangliosidosis	18

* Enzyme units are in nanomoles of *p*-nitrophenol released per 100 mg of tissue per hour. Assay conditions given in [4]. In the first five assays, ganglioside G_{M1} was added to the homogenate in concentrations equivalent to those found in generalized gangliosidosis (0.5 percent of the wet weight).

rate of hydrolysis was nearly linear [4]. In the mixed homogenates, the rate of hydrolysis was close (85 percent) to the average of the initial rates found for tissues of the controls and of the patients (Fig. 30-14). These results are consistent with simple enzyme dilution alone, not with enzyme inhibition; if a soluble endogenous inhibitor of β-galactosidase is present in the patient's tissues (whether G_{M1} or other compounds), the degree of inhibition is not sufficient to explain the large β-galactosidase deficiency.

The enzyme deficiency in generalized gangliosidosis is specific for β-galactosidase. Activities of other lysosomal enzymes, including acid phosphatase, β-glucosidase, and N-acetylglucosaminidase, were either within the range of control values (acid phosphatase and glucosidase) or increased three- to fourfold (glucosaminidase) [4].

Other workers have confirmed the β-galactosidase deficiency in generalized gangliosidosis using arylgalactosides as substrates. Van Hoof and Hers found no β-galactosidase activity in tissues from two patients, one reported by Sacrez et al. [7] and another by Seringe et al. [10]. They have recently reported similar findings in three other patients [34]. Dacremont et al. [35] also demonstrated the β-galactosidase deficiency in another patient. In these studies the activities of related glycosidases such as α-galactosidase, N-acetyl-β-glucosaminidase, and α-mannosidase were increased four- to eightfold.

A number of β-galactosidases are known to occur in mammalian tissues. These β-galactosidases differ in their ability to cleave various galactose-containing substrates [36–38]. For example, a purified β-galactosidase from brain

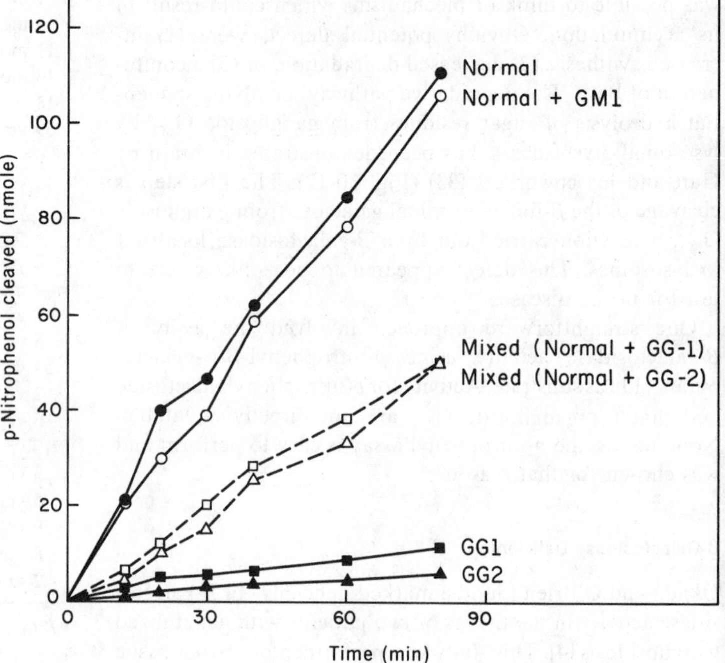

Figure 30-13. β-Galactosidase activity in liver in generalized gangliosidosis. *Normal,* liver tissue of a boy who died at 2 days of age from meconium peritonitis; *normal* + G_{M1}, ganglioside G_{M1} added to give a concentration of 0.5 percent of the wet weight; *GG-1,* 8-month-old patient with generalized gangliosidosis; *GG-2,* 2-year-old patient with generalized gangliosidosis; *mixed,* mixtures of equal proportions of normal and patients' homogenates. (*From S. Okada and J. S. O'Brien,* [4], *with permission of the publishers. Copyright, 1968, by the American Association for the Advancement of Science.*)

hydrolyzes *p*-nitrophenyl-β-D-galactopyranoside but does not catalyze the hydrolysis of glycosphingolipids [36, 37]. A purified β-galactosidase from liver hydrolyzes the *p*-nitrophenylgalactoside but not a galactose-containing glycoprotein; another β-galactosidase in this tissue hydrolyzes galactose from the glycoprotein but not from the *p*-nitrophenyl derivative [38]. Thus, β-galactosidase activity for synthetic galactosides may not accurately reflect activity for natural substrates, such as ganglioside G_{M1}.

GM_1-galactosidase Deficiency

In order to prove that the β-galactosidase deficiency is responsible for the ganglioside accumulation in generalized gangliosidosis, β-galactosidase activity had to be determined using ganglioside G_{M1} as the substrate. This was accomplished by Okada and O'Brien [4], who prepared ganglioside G_{M1}, exclusively labeled with ^{14}C in the terminal galactose, and used this compound as the substrate for β-galactosidase.

The rate of cleavage of galactose ^{14}C from G_{M1} was markedly lower in generalized gangliosidosis when partially purified preparations of β-galactosidase from liver (Fig. 30-14) or cerebral gray matter (Fig. 30-15) were used. When

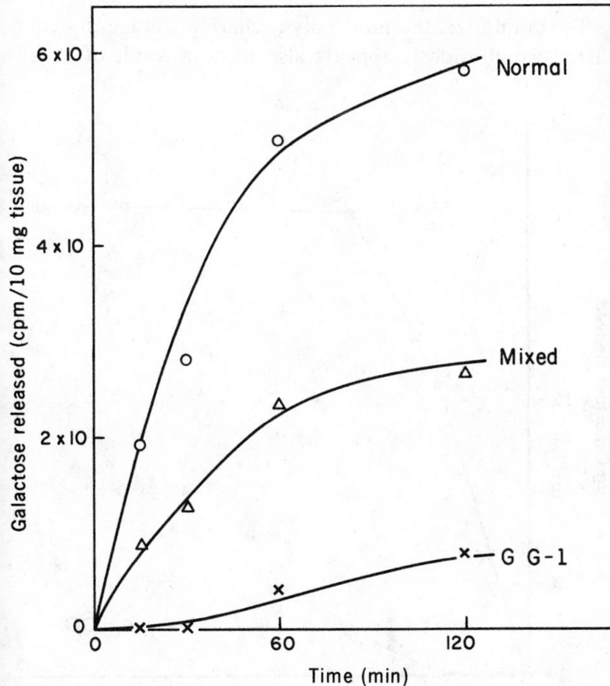

Figure 30-14. β-Galactosidase activity for ganglioside G_{M1} in liver in generalized gangliosidosis. *Normal,* 3-year-old boy who died from congenital heart disease; *GG-1,* 8-month-old patient with generalized gangliosidosis; *mixed,* mixture of equal proportions of the normal and patient's enzyme preparations. (*From S. Okada and J. S. O'Brien,* [4], *by permission of the publishers. Copyright,* 1968, *by the American Association for the Advancement of Science.*)

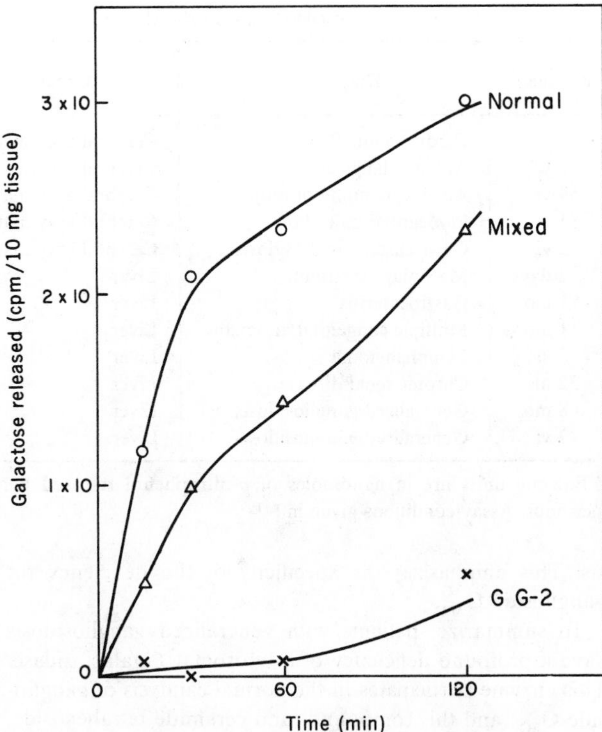

Figure 30-15. β-Galactosidase activity for ganglioside G_{M1} in brain in generalized gangliosidosis. *Normal,* 32-month-old boy who died from chronic renal disease; *GG-2,* 2-year-old patient with generalized gangliosidosis; *mixed,* mixture of equal proportions of the normal and patient's enzyme preparations. (*From S. Okada and J. S. O'Brien, et al.* [4], *by permission of the publishers. Copyright,* 1968, *by the American Association for the Advancement of Science.*)

preparations of β-galactosidase from control tissues and the tissues of the patient were mixed in equal proportions the rate of galactose hydrolysis was close to the average of the two initial rates, both in liver and in cerebral gray matter. This finding demonstrated that soluble endogenous inhibitors were not responsible for the lowered G_{M1}-β-galactosidase activity. Assays of β-galactosidase preparations from a number of control subjects demonstrated that activity directed against ganglioside G_{M1} in the patients with generalized gangliosidosis was diminished to 3 percent of normal in brain and to 3 to 6 percent of normal in liver (Table 30-7).

The degree of deficiency of β-galactosidase differs depending on the substrate used. Although the deficiency in liver is nearly the same for both the *p*-nitrophenyl derivative and the ganglioside, the deficiency in brain is threefold greater when ganglioside is used as the substrate. Recently, Brady and coworkers [52] have demonstrated that cerebral β-galactosidase activity for cerebroside (galactosyl ceramide), ceramide lactoside (galactosylglucosyl ceramide), and ceramide trihexoside (galactosylgalactosylglucosyl ceramide) is normal or increased in generalized gangliosido-

Table 30-7. GANGLIOSIDE G_{M1} β-GALACTOSIDASE ACTIVITY

Age	Diagnosis	Organ	Enzyme activity*
3 yr	Cardiac anomaly	Cerebral gray matter	46
10 yr	Ataxia-telangiectasia	Cerebral gray matter	23
59 yr	Adenocarcinoma of lung	Cerebral gray matter	25
81 yr	Myocardial infarction	Cerebral gray matter	36
2 yr	Generalized gangliosidosis	Cerebral gray matter	1
2 days	Meconium peritonitis	Liver	77
1 mo	Gastroenteritis	Liver	73
1 mo	Multiple congenital anomalies	Liver	52
2 yr	Lymphangioma	Liver	65
32 mo	Chronic renal disease	Liver	51
8 mo	Generalized gangliosidosis	Liver	4
2 yr	Generalized gangliosidosis	Liver	2

* Enzyme units are in nanomoles of *p*-nitrophenol released per 100 mg of tissue per hour. Assay conditions given in [4].

sis. This emphasizes the specificity of the deficiency for ganglioside G_{M1}.

To summarize, patients with generalized gangliosidosis have a profound deficiency of a lysosomal β-galactosidase. This enzyme participates in the normal catalysis of ganglioside G_{M1}; and this compound (and ceramide tetrahexoside, a structurally related lipid) accumulate as a result of a block in degradation. The reaction blocked is schematically represented in Fig. 30-12.

Impaired Cleavage of Mucopolysaccharides

The mucopolysaccharide which accumulates in the viscera contains galactose and glucosamine, probably linked in 1,4-β linkage [16, 17]. When galactose is terminal, this linkage should also be cleaved by a β-galactosidase. The accumulation of the mucopolysaccharide could also be explained by a block in degradation. In order to test this hypothesis, MacBrinn et al. [39] determined the rate of cleavage of galactose from the mucopolysaccharide which accumulates in generalized gangliosidosis.

The mucopolysaccharide was isolated from liver tissue of a patient with the disease. The mucopolysaccharide was then incubated in the presence of normal and generalized gangliosidosis liver tissue over an 18-hr time period, and galactose release was measured. The rate of cleavage of galactose from the stored mucopolysaccharide was 10 percent of normal in generalized gangliosidosis; 38.9 percent of the galactose was released by the enzyme prepared from normal liver, whereas 3.8 percent was released by the preparation from the patient's liver (Fig. 30-16) [39].

A similar experiment involved the cleavage of galactose from fetuin. This glycoprotein contains an oligosaccharide chain with a terminal galactose linked to hexosamine, and a sialic acid moiety linked to the galactose. Sialic acid–free fetuin was prepared by mild acid hydrolysis to give a glycoprotein with a free terminal galactose. When this glycoprotein was incubated with purified preparations of β-galactosidase from liver, normal tissue liberated 5.5 μg of galactose after 18 hr at 37°C. No detectable galactose was liberated by the enzyme prepared from the patient's liver [39].

To summarize, the mucopolysaccharide storage in generalized gangliosidosis appears also to be a result of a defi-

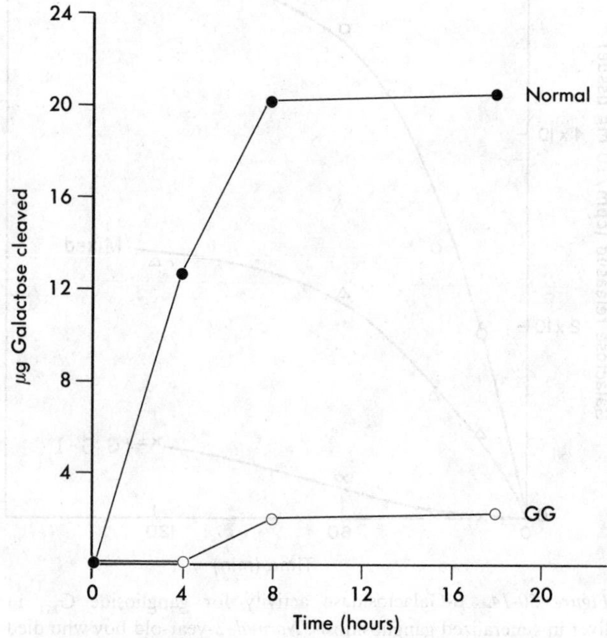

Figure 30-16. Cleavage of galactose from keratan sulfate by β-galactosidase prepared from equivalent amounts of normal (*N*) and generalized gangliosidosis (*GG*) liver tissue. (*From M. C. MacBrinn et al.* [39], *by permission of the publishers. Copyright,* 1968, *by the American Association for the Advancement of Science.*)

ciency of β-galactosidase, an enzyme which normally participates in its catabolism. Glycoprotein storage can be explained on the same basis.

Polymorphism of β-Galactosidases

A number of β-galactosidases with acid pH optimums (pH 3 to 5) occur in human liver. The pH activity curves of these β-galactosidases demonstrate two optimums—a major one at pH 4 to 5 and a minor one at pH 6.6. In generalized gangliosidosis, the peaks at pH 4 to 5 and 6.6 are both much diminished (Fig. 30-17) [40].

Ho and O'Brien [41] have separated liver β-galactosidase, by starch-gel electrophoresis, into three components, a fast-moving component (A) and two slower-moving ones (B and C). In generalized gangliosidosis, all three components are deficient (Fig. 30-18). At this writing it is not clear how a single gene mutation can lead to the deficiency of all three β-galactosidases. One possibility is that they share a common subunit which is structurally abnormal. Other possibilities, including operator-gene repression, could lead to the same result. It is also not clear which β-galactosidase component

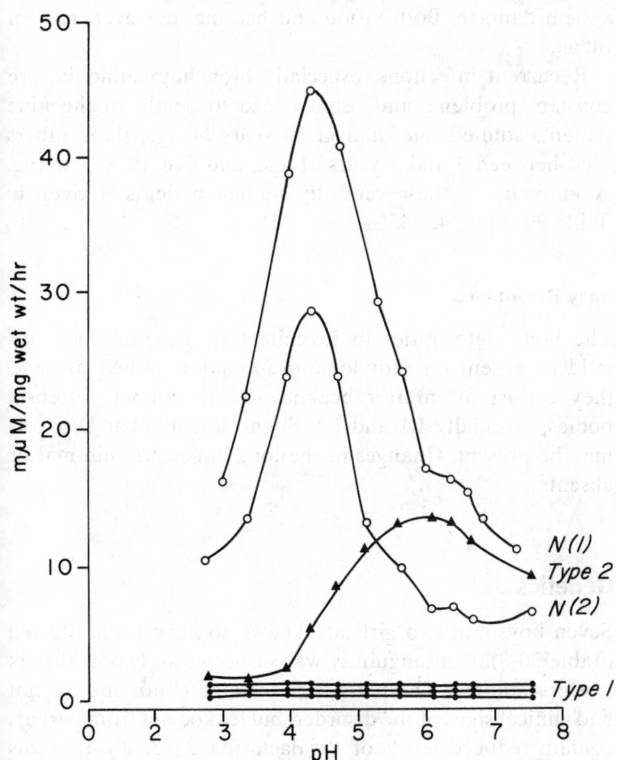

Figure 30-17. pH activity curves of human liver β-galactosidase from two control patients (*N1* and *N2*), three patients with generalized gangliosidosis (three lower curves designated Type 1), and one patient with juvenile G_{M1} gangliosidosis (Type 2). Activity was determined using 4-methylumbelliferyl-β-D-galactopyranoside as substrate according to Ho and O'Brien [41].

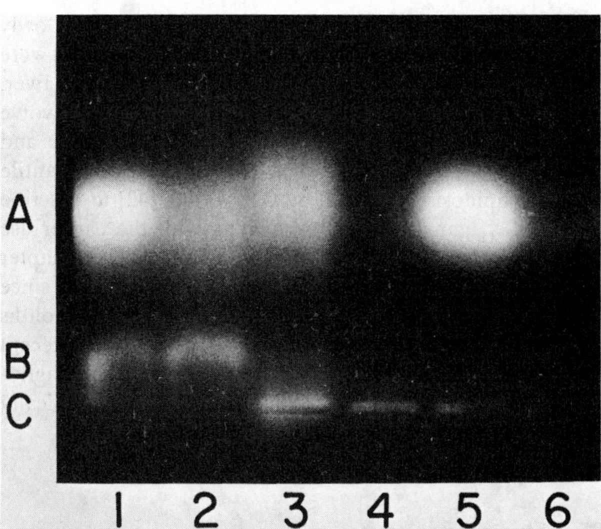

Figure 30-18. Starch-gel electrophoresis of liver β-galactosidase from two normal subjects (lanes 1 and 2), a patient with cystic fibrosis (lane 3), two patients with generalized gangliosidosis (lanes 4 and 6), and a patient with juvenile G_{M1} gangliosidosis (lane 5). Electrophoresis was carried out according to Ho and O'Brien [41] at pH 4.9. Note absence of β-galactosidase components A, B, and C in generalized gangliosidosis and preservation of component A in juvenile G_{M1} gangliosidosis.

(A, B, or C) possesses activity for ganglioside G_{M1}, mucopolysaccharides, or glycoproteins. Further work needs to be carried out to answer these questions.

Therapy

No specific therapy for generalized gangliosidosis is presently available. Supportive therapy includes prompt use of antibiotics to combat infections, attentive long-term bed care to prevent skin lesions and aspiration pneumonia, tube feeding to allay malnutrition, and anticonvulsants to suppress tonic-clonic convulsions. Even with careful management, patients with generalized gangliosidosis die by approximately 2 years of life.

Preventive approaches are discussed after the section on juvenile G_{M1} gangliosidosis.

G_{M1} GANGLIOSIDOSIS TYPE 2 (JUVENILE G_{M1} GANGLIOSIDOSIS)

In 1968, Derry et al. [42] reported two sibs of French-Canadian ancestry with the clinical picture of progressive mental and motor deterioration beginning at 1 year of age and progressing to death by age 4 to 5. Post-mortem examination disclosed ganglioside G_{M1} accumulated in the brain. Their patients differed from those with generalized gangliosidosis. The disorder had a later onset and a more slowly progressive course, visceromegaly and bony deformities were absent, and ganglioside G_{M1} was not stored in the liver. They suggested that there are two diseases which involve G_{M1} ganglioside storage, an infantile (Type 1) disease and a later-onset (Type 2) disease. The term "late infantile systemic lipidosis" was used by Derry et al. [42] to describe Type 2 G_{M1} gangliosidosis, in keeping with the earlier use of the term by Gonatas and Gonatas [6]. In this chapter the term "juvenile G_{M1} gangliosidosis" will be used, since the onset of symptoms has varied between 6 and 20 months of age and the age at death between 3 and 10 years. Recent enzyme studies support the belief that generalized gangliosidosis and juvenile G_{M1} gangliosidosis are genotypically distinct entities.

Phenotypic Aspects

Clinical Features

The mental and motor development of the child with juvenile G_{M1} gangliosidosis is usually normal for the first year of life. Appetite is good, weight gain is adequate, and the patient appears to be an active, thriving child. Developmental milestones are not delayed. He smiles, recognizes his parents, laughs, transfers objects from one hand to the other, sits up, crawls, stands with support, and walks at the usual times. By 1 year of age, he is usually able to say several words, and parents are not aware of mental or motor impairment.

The initial symptom, which appears after 1 year, is usually locomotor ataxia. Parents observe that the child is having difficulty walking; gait is awkward and unsteady, and the patient falls more frequently than normal. They may also observe a loss in coordinated manipulative hand movements at this time. Speech becomes difficult and subsequently is lost.

Examination at the time of initial neurologic symptoms reveals an alert, cooperative child in no apparent distress. Vision and hearing are intact. There are no facial deformities. Pupils are round, regular, and equal in size, and they react normally to light, both directly and consensually. Internal strabismus and unsustained bilateral nystagmus may be present. The corneas are clear. The retina is normal in appearance; there is a normal light reflex at the macula, and macular degeneration and retinal pigmentation do not occur. Neither the liver nor the spleen is palpable, and lymphadenopathy does not occur.

The gait is clumsy and wide-based. Ataxia occurs both while standing and while sitting. There are generalized moderate muscular weakness and hypotonia of both upper and lower extremities but no tremors or fasciculations, and muscle bulk is not reduced. Deep-tendon reflexes are hyperreactive, Babinski's reflex is usually plantar early and becomes flexor later on. Sensation appears to be intact.

Mental and motor deterioration may progress rapidly over the next few months. The child loses interest in his surroundings, seldom smiles, is lethargic, and does not socialize. He loses the ability to walk and can sit only with support. Spasticity of upper and lower extremities becomes apparent and, with time, progresses to spastic quadriplegia. Purposeless movements, facial grimacing, eye blinking, and an exaggerated acousticomotor response (hyperacusis) may be present.

After 16 months of age, seizures may develop. In several patients these began with an initial cry, followed by generalized stiffening and hyperextension of the head, upward rolling of the eyes, and spontaneous recovery after about 30 sec. Seizures may increase in severity and frequency; they were a major problem in the medical management of four of the patients in Table 30-8. Therapy with anticonvulsants may be effective in reducing the severity of the seizures to episodes of unresponsiveness and staring of a few seconds' duration.

After the second year of life mental deterioration increases, and the patient presents the clinical picture of decorticate rigidity, with the attendant problems in nursing and general care resulting from severe progressive nervous system damage. Both vision and hearing, however, remain intact.

Recurrent infections, especially bronchopneumonia, are constant problems and usually lead to death. In the nine patients studied one died at 10 years of age, three others died between 3 and 5 years of age, and five are still living. A summary of these carefully studied patients is given in Table 30-8 [25, 42, 45].

Bony Deformities

The bony deformities in juvenile G_{M1} gangliosidosis are mild or absent on radiologic examination. When present, they consist of inferior beaking of the lumbar vertebral bodies, especially L1 and L2. Slight dorsolumbar kyphosis may be present. Changes in the long bones are minimal or absent.

Genetics

Seven boys and two girls are known to have been affected (Table 30-8). Consanguinity was suspected in two of the six sibships studied. The parents of affected children have not had clinical signs of the disorder, but leukocytes from parents contain reduced levels of β-galactosidase [43, 46]. It seems probable that the disease is transmitted as an autosomal recessive trait.

Assays of cultured skin fibroblasts also demonstrate a profound deficiency of β-galactosidase [40, 43] persisting after many cellular generations. In two families we have studied [40], both parents have intermediate activity of β-galactosidase in skin biopsies and in cultured skin fibro-

Table 30-8. FEATURES OF NINE PATIENTS WITH JUVENILE G_{M1} GANGLIOSIDOSIS

Feature									
Reference	[42]	[42]	[16]	[43]	[43]	[44]	[44]	[45]	[45]
Sex	M	M	M	M	F	M	M	M	F
Ethnic origin	Fr.-Canad.	Fr.-Canad.	Irish	Mohawk Indian–Fr.-Canad.	Mohawk Indian–Fr.-Canad.	Eng.-Ger.	Eng.-Ger.	Flemish	Eng.-Jewish
Place of patient in sibship	2/6	2/6	1/3	2/5	2/5	3/4	3/4	1/2	2/5
Consanguinity	*	*	. . .	. . .	. . .	0	0	0	0
Age at onset, mo	11	13	6	12	10–12	18	20	13	14
Age at death, mo	56	48	37	10 (yr)	Alive at 3 yr	Alive	Alive	Alive	Alive at 7 yr
Mental-motor retardation	+	+	+	+	+	+	+	+	+
Abnormal facies	0	0	. . .	. . .	0	0	‡	Hypertelorism	0
Edema	0	0	. . .	. . .	0	0	0	0	±
Bony changes	0	. . .	0	. . .	0**	+	+	0	+
Seizures	0	0	. . .	+	+	+	+	0	+
Spasticity-ataxia	+	+	+	+	+	+	+	+	+
Vacuolated lymphs	. . .	. . .	. . .	. . .	. . .	. . .	. . .	0	+
Foam cells in marrow	+	. . .	+	. . .	0	+	+	0	+
Foam cells in viscera	+	. . .	+	. . .	. . .	+			
Hepatomegaly	0	0	†	. . .	0	0	0	0	0
Splenomegaly	0	0	0	. . .	0	0	0	0	0
Cherry-red spots	0	0	0	. . .	0	0	0	0	0
Corneal clouding	0	. . .	. . .	. . .	0	0	0	0	0
Other eye-ground changes	Pale disks	0	Pigmentation around disks	. . .	0	0	0	0	
Macroglossia	0	0	. . .	. . .	0	0	0	. . .	0
Glomerular lesion	+	. . .	+						
G_{M1} accumulation in brain	+	. . .	+	. . .	+	+	. . .	+	
G_{M1} accumulation in viscera	0 (Spleen)	. . .	0 (Liver)	. . .	. . .	0	. . .	0	
AMPS§ accumulation in urine	±	. . .	. . .	. . .	+	0	0	0	
AMPS§ accumulation in organs	. . .	. . .	+						
β-Galactosidase deficiency	. . .	. . .	. . .	. . .	+ Severe in brain & WBC	+	. . .	+ In WBC & liver	+

*Suspected.

†Liver enlarged 1 cm below costal margin.

‡Multiple minor congenital anomalies were present, including microcephaly, micrognathia, and epicanthal folds.

§AMPS = acid mucopolysaccharide.

**Mild bony abnormalities have subsequently been found in this patient (J. Spranger, personal communication.)

Note: Blank indicates feature was not described.

blasts. In one child, we made the diagnosis of juvenile G_{M1} gangliosidosis at 7 months of age, prior to the onset of clinical symptoms, by enzyme assay of cultured skin fibroblasts.

No ethnic predilection has appeared. Patients of French-Canadian, Irish, Mohawk-Indian, English, German, Flemish, and Jewish stock have been reported. The frequency of the disorder is unknown; nine cases have been collected in 2 years.

Laboratory Data

Vacuolated lymphocytes in the peripheral blood smear were found in one patient but not in another [45]. Foam cells appeared in the bone marrow in five patients but were not found in two others. Parenchymal cells in the liver were vacuolated in three patients in whom the liver was examined. The quantity of mucopolysaccharides in urine has been either normal or only slightly elevated. Leukocyte β-galactosidase was reduced to low levels in homozygotes and to intermediate levels in heterozygotes [43, 46]. Other laboratory findings include diffuse spike and slow-wave discharges by electroencephalography, cortical atrophy by pneumoencephalography, normal sural nerve conduction velocity time, normal karyotype, normal 24-hr urine amino acid pattern, normal 24-hr urinary protein, and normal serum fructose-1,6-phosphate aldolase [44]. In two patients, high levels of serum lactate dehydrogenase and glutamic-oxaloacetic acid transaminase were found; the lactate dehydrogenase isoenzyme pattern was indicative of extrahepatic origin [44].

Pathologic Aspects

The most striking pathologic changes are (1) foamy vacuolization of visceral parenchymal cells and histiocytes, (2) neuronal lipidosis, and (3) cytoplasmic vacuolization of renal glomerular epithelial cells. Neuronal lipidosis occurs throughout the cortex, brain stem, and spinal cord, as well as the neurons of Meissner's plexus [25, 42–45]. Rectal biopsy has been useful in demonstrating neuronal lipidosis as well as histiocytosis of the lamina propria [45]. The neuronal cytoplasm is ballooned with storage material, which displaces the nucleus to the periphery. The storage granules appear as finely dispersed particles under the light microscope. Electron microscopy reveals cytoplasmic membranous bodies similar to those seen in generalized gangliosidosis [16, 43, 44].

The involvement of renal glomerular epithelial cells is similar to that seen in generalized gangliosidosis (Fig. 30-9). The epithelial cells store large quantities of cytoplasmic material, giving the glomerulus a "choked" appearance [42]. Foamy vacuolization of the cytoplasm of histiocytes and parenchymal cells occurs in the liver and spleen [42, 44]. The histiocytosis appears less severe than that seen in generalized gangliosidosis. An electron microscopic study of the visceral lesions has not yet been reported in juvenile G_{M1} gangliosidosis.

Differential Diagnosis (Table 30-9)

The clinical picture of juvenile G_{M1} gangliosidosis is similar to that of late infantile amaurotic idiocy (Jansky-Bielschowsky disease) and metachromatic leukodystrophy.

Table 30-9. DIFFERENTIAL DIAGNOSTIC POINTS—JUVENILE G_{M1} GANGLIOSIDOSIS

Feature	Juvenile G_{M1} gangliosidosis	Jansky-Bielschowsky	Metachromatic leukodystrophy	Juvenile G_{M2} gangliosidosis
Onset	1–3 yr	1–3 yr	1–3 yr	1–3 yr
Blindness	Late	Early	Late	Late
X-ray changes of vertebrae	±	0	0	0
Retinal lesion	0	Macular degeneration	0	0
Foam cells in marrow	+	0	0	0
Peripheral nerve conduction	Normal	Normal	Slow	Normal
Convulsions	+	+	+	+
Spasticity	+	+	+	+
β-Galactosidase deficiency	+	0	0	0
Compound stored in brain	Ganglioside G_{M1}	Lipofuscin	Cerebroside sulfate	Ganglioside G_{M2}
Compound stored in viscera	Mucopoly-saccharide	. . .	Cerebroside sulfate	. . .

Mental and motor retardation progresses at about the same pace in all three disorders. Macular degeneration and early blindness occur in Jansky-Bielschowsky disease, not in the other two disorders. Foam cells are found in the bone marrow in juvenile G_{M1} gangliosidosis, not in the other disorders. Bony abnormalities of the lumbar vertebral bodies, although mild, are specific for juvenile G_{M1} gangliosidosis. Cortical neurons contain PAS-positive, nonautofluorescent, sudanophilic inclusion bodies in juvenile G_{M1} gangliosidosis; PAS-positive, sudanophilic, strongly autofluorescent inclusions in Jansky-Bielschowsky disease; and PAS-positive, nonautofluorescent, strongly metachromatic inclusions in metachromatic leukodystrophy. β-Galactosidase activity is normal in Jansky-Bielschowsky disease and metachromatic leukodystrophy; it is reduced in juvenile G_{M1} gangliosidosis. Urine, skin, and leukocytes from patients with metachromatic leukodystrophy are deficient in arylsulfatase A (see Chap. 32); the activity of this enzyme is normal in the other two disorders.

Another disorder which closely resembles juvenile G_{M1} gangliosidosis is juvenile or Type 3 G_{M2} gangliosidosis, a recently described slowly progressive disorder of late infantile or juvenile onset which involves the cerebral storage of ganglioside G_{M2} [47–49] (Chap. 29). Enzyme assays may aid in differentiating this disorder; hexosaminidase A activity has been found diminished in one patient with juvenile G_{M2} gangliosidosis, but β-galactosidase is not diminished [50].

Chemistry of the Storage Substances

Gangliosides

The ganglioside stored in juvenile G_{M1} gangliosidosis migrates on thin-layer chromatograms with an R_f identical to that of ganglioside G_{M1} [16, 42–45]. The magnitude of the cerebral storage of ganglioside G_{M1} in juvenile G_{M1} gangliosidosis is similar to that in generalized gangliosidosis [16, 43, 44], but in four patients studied G_{M1} ganglioside was not found to accumulate in the liver or spleen.

Mucopolysaccharides

The mucopolysaccharide stored in the viscera in juvenile G_{M1} gangliosidosis has been partially characterized as a keratan sulfate-like compound [43] similar to that in generalized gangliosidosis. It contains equimolar proportions of galactose and glucosamine. In addition, a second mucopolysaccharide containing sialic acid residues, as well as galactose and glucosamine, accumulates in the liver and spleen. It is quite likely that the polysaccharides accumulating in juvenile G_{M1} gangliosidosis are similar to those in generalized gangliosidosis, although further studies need to be carried out to decide this point. Both ganglioside G_{M1} and the keratan sulfate-like mucopolysaccharide have been demonstrated to accumulate in skin fibroblasts cultured from patients with juvenile G_{M1} gangliosidosis and generalized gangliosidosis [54].

Enzymatic Defect

The deficiency of β-galactosidase (assayed using synthetic substrates) in the brain in juvenile G_{M1} gangliosidosis is nearly as severe as that in generalized gangliosidosis. The deficiency of β-galactosidase in the liver of one patient studied by O'Brien was not as severe; the activity of this enzyme was ten times higher than that in generalized gangliosidosis (Table 30-10). As yet, no studies have been carried out using the ganglioside or the mucopolysaccharide which accumulate as substrate. It seems likely that these substrates will be found to be cleaved at a reduced rate in this disease; this would be similar to what happens in generalized gangliosidosis.

The pH activity curve of liver β-galactosidase in juvenile G_{M1} gangliosidosis differs from that in generalized gangliosidosis (Fig. 30-17) [40]. In both disorders there is a profound reduction of activity at pH 4. In generalized gangliosidosis, the activity at pH 6.6 is also much reduced, but in juvenile G_{M1} gangliosidosis the activity at this pH is nearly normal. Starch-gel electrophoresis of liver β-galactosidase reveals differences in the isoenzyme patterns in the two disorders [40]. In generalized gangliosidosis all three liver β-galactosidase isoenzymes (A, B, and C) are deficient (Fig. 30-18); in a patient with juvenile G_{M1} gangliosidosis, isoenzymes B and C are deficient but A is present at nearly normal levels. These differences in the pH activity curves and the isoenzyme patterns of β-galactosidase in the two disorders support the contention that they are genotypically distinct. Further studies need to be carried out in additional patients to determine whether the disturbances in β-galactosidase pattern are constant in all patients.

The activities of other lysosomal hydrolases, such as β-glucosidase and N-acetyl-β-D-glucosaminidase, are increased in the brain and liver of patients with juvenile G_{M1} gangliosidosis. This emphasizes the specificity of the β-galactosidase deficiency [44].

Therapy

No specific therapy for juvenile G_{M1} gangliosidosis is available. The clinical problems are those expected in a deteriorating neuropathic condition, and include special difficulty in the management of seizures. Enzyme replacement therapy in juvenile G_{M1} gangliosidosis and in generalized gangliosidosis has not been attempted. The need for a large supply of the enzyme in a highly purified state, the necessity of long-term systemic administration, and the danger of allergic reactions are obvious. The difficulty of getting a large protein molecule across the blood-brain barrier also reduces the possibility of success with this approach.

Table 30-10. GLYCOHYDROLASES IN JUVENILE G_{M1} GANGLIOSIDOSIS*

Subjects	β-Glucosidase	β-Galactosidase	β-N-Acetyl-glucosaminidase
		Cerebral Cortex	
Controls (9)	0.82 (0.42–1.32)	2.19 (1.87–2.56)	50.5 (30.7–78.6)
Generalized gangliosidosis			
J.C.	. . .	0.04	
J.Y.	8.6	0.07	105
M.B.	. . .	0.04	310
Juvenile G_{M1} gangliosidosis†	5.5	0.04	79
		Liver	
Controls (17)	5.8 (1.3–13.7)	30.3 (16.3–46.0)	323 (121–563)
Generalized gangliosidosis			
J.C.	14.0	0.3	467
J.Y.	4.5	0.6	640
M.B.	11.6	0.9	466
Juvenile G_{M1} gangliosidosis†	7.2	6.4	367

* Values are expressed as nanomoles of substrate cleaved per milligram of wet tissue per hour. Assayed according to MacBrinn et al [51] by Ho and O'Brien [40].
† Patient 6, Table 30-8; tissue obtained at surgery.

Prevention

Clinicians must be aware of the possibility of genetic disorders, such as generalized gangliosidosis and juvenile G_{M1} gangliosidosis, in their patients, and must be alert to their presence. Prompt recognition, early diagnosis, and immediate genetic counseling are the simplest and most effective means available for preventing the conception and birth of children who will die of these devastating diseases.

Homozygote detection is crucial in this effort and depends on the recognition of each phenotype by primary physicians, pediatricians, radiologists, geneticists, and pathologists. The diagnosis may be confirmed by biopsy and analytic lipid chemistry or by enzyme assay. Brain biopsy and ganglioside analysis have been used to make the diagnosis during life. Less traumatic and equally diagnostic are β-galactosidase assays of leukocytes, urine, and skin.

Prenatal detection of homozygotes in early pregnancy should be possible by amniocentesis followed by tissue culture of fetal cells and β-galactosidase assay. β-Galactosidase (pH 4.5) is present in normal fetal fibroblasts. Cultured fibroblasts from the skin of a patient with generalized gangliosidosis have a sharp reduction of this enzyme (Table 30-11) [50]. Thus this approach is feasible.

Several pregnancies have recently been monitored by amniocentesis [55]; each were in women who had previously delivered a child with generalized gangliosidosis. Enzyme assays of amniotic fluid cells after culture indicated that each of the fetuses was unaffected. Examination of each child after birth revealed no symptoms or signs of the disease [55].

Detection of homozygotes and heterozygotes for the genes for generalized gangliosidosis and juvenile G_{M1} gangliosidosis may be accomplished by assay of β-galactosidase in leukocytes, urine, skin biopsies, or cultured skin fibroblasts. Intermediate decreases in enzyme activity have been demonstrated in leukocytes [43, 53], skin biopsies [40] and cultured skin fibroblasts [40, 43] from heterozygotes for both diseases.

SUMMARY

1 Two phenotypically distinct childhood diseases involve the accumulation of ganglioside G_{M1}: generalized gangliosidosis (G_{M1} gangliosidosis Type 1) and juvenile G_{M1} gangliosidosis (G_{M1} gangliosidosis Type 2).
2 Generalized gangliosidosis is an acute infantile disorder characterized by psychomotor deterioration beginning at or near birth, severe bony deformities resembling those seen in the mucopolysaccharidoses, hepatosplenomegaly, visceral histiocytosis, neuronal lipidosis, and fatal outcome usually by 2 years of age.

Table 30-11. β-GALACTOSIDASE ACTIVITY IN FIBROBLASTS*

	N-Acetyl-β-D-glucosaminidase	β-D-galactosidase
Cultured skin fibroblasts:		
Control 1	7.61	0.83
Control 2	8.58	0.83
Control 3	8.09	0.73
Generalized gangliosidosis	9.60	0.02
Cultured amniotic cells:		
Control 1	1.18	0.16
Control 2	1.76	0.21

* Enzyme units are in nanomoles of substrate cleaved per microgram of protein per hour. The *p*-nitrophenyl derivatives of each sugar were incubated at pH 4.4 in 0.04*M* citrate-phosphate buffer at 37°C, and activity was assayed spectrophotometrically [51]. Amniotic cells were obtained by amniocentesis at 16 weeks of pregnancy.

3 Juvenile G_{M1} gangliosidosis is a more slowly progressive disorder characterized by the onset of psychomotor difficulties at about 1 year of age and progressing to spastic quadriplegia with a fatal outcome between 3 and 10 years. Hepatosplenomegaly is not present, and bony deformities, if present, are mild.

4 These diseases appear to be transmitted as autosomal recessive traits and have a pan-ethnic distribution. Ganglioside G_{M1} accumulates in the brain in both disorders; visceral accumulation of ganglioside G_{M1} has been found only in generalized gangliosidosis. A polysaccharide, structurally similar to keratan sulfate, accumulates in the viscera in both generalized gangliosidosis, and juvenile G_{M1} gangliosidosis.

5 A striking deficiency of β-galactosidase is present in both disorders. In generalized gangliosidosis, the enzyme deficiency has been demonstrated using both ganglioside G_{M1} and the "keratan sulfate-like" polysaccharide as substrates. Related hydrolases, including β-galactosidases, which cleave similar glycolipids (cerebroside, ceramide lactose, ceramide trihexoside) are not deficient. The storage of ganglioside G_{M1} and of polysaccharide appears to be due to a block in the catabolism of these galactose-containing macromolecules due to the profound β-galactosidase deficiency.

6 Three β-galactosidase components are separable from human liver. In generalized gangliosidosis, all three components are deficient; in juvenile G_{M1} gangliosidosis two of these are deficient, the other is not. These data, although preliminary, support the contention that generalized gangliosidosis and juvenile G_{M1} gangliosidosis are genotypically distinct.

7 Therapy for these diseases is palliative at present. Heterozygotes may be detected by β-galactosidase assay, and homozygotes may be detected prenatally by amniocentesis and enzyme assay. In this manner, family planning may reduce the number of children born with these fatal diseases.

BIBLIOGRAPHY

1. Norman, R. M., Urich, H., Tingey, A. H., and Goodbody, R. A.: Tay-Sachs disease with visceral involvement and its relationship to Niemann-Pick's disease. J. Path. Bact., **72**, 409, 1959.
2. Landing, B. H., Silverman, F. N., Craig, M. M., Jacoby, M. D., Lahey, M. E., and Chadwick, D. L.: Familial neurovisceral lipidosis. Amer. J. Dis. Child., **108**, 503, 1964.
3. O'Brien, J. S., Stern, M. B., Landing, B. H., O'Brien, J. K., and Donnell, G. N.: Generalized gangliosidosis. Amer. J. Dis. Child., **109**, 338, 1965.
4. Okada, S., and O'Brien, J. S.: Generalized gangliosidosis, β-galactosidase deficiency. Science, **160**, 1002, 1968.
5. Craig, J. M., Clarke, J. T., and Banker, B. Q.: Metabolic neurovisceral disorder with accumulation of an unidentified substance: variant of Hurler's syndrome? Amer. J. Dis. Child., **98**, 577, 1959.
6. Gonatas, N. K., and Gonatas, J.: Ultrastructural and biochemical observations on a case of systemic late infantile lipidosis and its relationship to Tay-Sachs disease and gargoylism. J. Neuropath. Exp. Neurol., **24**, 318, 1965.
7. Sacrez, R., Juif, J. G., Gigonnet, J. M., and Gruner, J. E.: La Maladie de Landing, ou idiote amaurotique infantile précoce avec gangliosidose généralisée. Pediatrie, **22**, 143, 1967.
8. Scott, C. R., Lagunoff, D., and Trump, B. F.: Familial neurovisceral lipidosis. J. Pediat., **71**, 357, 1967.
9. Attal, C., Farkas-Bargeton, E., Edgar, G. W. F., Pham-Huu-Trung, Girard, F., and Mozziconacci, P: Idiotie amaurotique infantile avec surcharge viscérale. Ann. Pediat. (Paris), **14**, 457, 1967.
10. Seringe, P., Plainfosse, B., Lautmann, F., Lorilloux, J., Calamy, G., Berry, J. P., and Watchi, J. M.: Gangliosidose généralisée du type Norman-Landing, à GM_1. Ann. Pediat. (Paris), **15**, 165, 1968.
11. Hooft, C., Senesael, L., Delbeke, M. J., Kint, J., and Dacremont, G.: The GM_1 gangliosidosis (Landing disease). Europ. Neurol., **2**, 225, 1969.
12. Grossman, H., and Danes, B. S.: Neurovisceral storage disease; roentgenographic features and mode of inheritance. Amer. J. Roentgen., **103**, 149, 1968.
13. Singer, L., Children's Hospital, Washington, D.C.; Mitchell, G., Syracuse Memorial Hospital; Kaback, M., and Howell, R. R., Johns Hopkins Hospital; and Lowden, J. A., Children's Hospital, Toronto, supplied data on Patients 18, 19, 21, and 22.
14. Landing, B. H., and Rubinstein, J. H.: Biopsy diagnosis of neurologic diseases in childhood with emphasis on lipidosis, in *Cerebral Sphingolipidosis: Symposium on Tay-Sachs Disease and Allied Disorders,* edited by S. M. Aronson and B. W. Volk, p. 14. Academic, New York, 1962.

15. Jatzkewitz, H., and Sandhoff, K.: On a biochemically special form of infantile amaurotic idiocy. Biochim. Biophys. Acta, **70,** 354, 1963.
16. Suzuki, K., Suzuki, K., and Chen, G. C.: Morphological and biochemical studies on a case of systemic late infantile lipidosis (generalized gangliosidosis). J. Neuropath. Exp. Neurol., **27,** 15, 1968.
17. Suzuki, K., and Chen, G. C.: Brain ceramide hexosides in Tay-Sachs disease and generalized gangliosidosis (GM_1-gangliosidosis). J. Lipid Res., **8,** 105, 1967.
18. McKusick, V. A.: *Heritable Disorders of Connective Tissue,* p. 325. Mosby, St. Louis, 1966.
19. Spranger, J., Wiedmann, H. R., Tolksdorf, J., Graucob, E., and Caesar, R.: Lipomucopolysaccharidose, eine neue Speicherkrankheit. Z. Kinderheilk., **103,** 285, 1968.
20. Leroy, J. G., DeMars, R. I., and Opitz, J. M.: 1-Cell disease. Birth Defects: Original Article Series, Vol. V, No. 4, edited by D. Bergsma, Natl. Foundation Publ., New York, 1969, p. 174.
21. Caffey, J.: Gargoylism: prenatal and neonatal bone lesions and their early postnatal evolution. Amer. J. Roentgen., **67,** 715, 1952.
22. Handa, S., and Yamakawa, T.: Personal communication.
23. Knudson, A.: *Genetics and Disease,* chap. 1. McGraw Hill, New York, 1965.
24. Lowden, A.: Personal communication, 1969.
25. Thomas, G. H.: β-Galactosidase in urine: deficiency in generalized gangliosidosis. J. Lab. Clin. Med., **74,** 125, 1969.
26. O'Brien, J. S.: Generalized gangliosidosis. J. Pediat., **75,** 167, 1969.
27. Sloan, H. R., Uhlendorf, B. W., Jacobson, C. B., and Fredrickson, D. S.: β-Galactosidase in tissue culture derived from human skin and bone marrow: enzyme in G_{M1} gangliosidosis. Pediat. Res., **3,** 532, 1969.
28. Terry, R. D., and Weiss, M.: Studies on Tay-Sachs disease. II. Ultrastructure of the cerebrum. J. Neuropath. Exp. Neurol., **22,** 18, 1963.
29. Suzuki, K., Suzuki, K., and Kamoshita, S.: Chemical pathology of GM_1 gangliosidosis (generalized gangliosidosis). J. Neuropath. Exp. Neurol., **28,** 25, 1969.
30. Suzuki, K.: Cerebral GM_1-gangliosidosis: chemical pathology of visceral organs. Science, **159,** 1471, 1968.
31. Ledeen, R., Salsman, K., Gonatas, J., and Taghavy, A.: Structure comparison of the major monosialogangliosides from brains of normal human, gargoylism and late infantile system lipidosis. J. Neuropath. Exp. Neurol., **24,** 341, 1965.
32. Farkas-Bargeton, E.: Idiotie amaurotique infantile avec surcharge viscérale. Proc. Fifth Int. Congr. Neuropath. Excerpta Med. Int., **100,** 135, 1965.
33. Gatt, S.: Enzymatic hydrolysis of sphingolipids. V. Hydrolysis of monosialoganglioside and hexosylceramides by rat brain β-galactosidase. Biochim. Biophys. Acta, **137,** 192, 1967.
34. Van Hoof, F., and Hers, H. G.: The abnormalities of lysosomal enzymes in the mucopolysaccharidoses. Europ. J. Biochem., **7,** 34, 1969.
35. Dacremont, G., and Kint, J. A.: GM_1-ganglioside accumulation and β-galactosidase deficiency in a case of GM_1 gangliosidosis (Landing disease). Clin. Chim. Acta, **21,** 421, 1968.
36. Hajra, A. K., Bowen, D. M., Kishimoto, Y., and Radin, N. S.: Cerebroside galactosidase of brain. J. Lipid Res., **7,** 379, 1966.
37. Jungalwala, F., and Robins, E.: Glycosidases in the nervous system. III. Separation, purification and substrate specificities of β-galactosidase and β-glucuronidase from brain. J. Biol. Chem., **243,** 4258, 1968.
38. Langley, T. J., and Jevons, F. R.: Action of beef liver enzymes on a glycoprotein substrate. Arch. Biochem. Biophys., **128,** 304, 1968.
39. MacBrinn, M. C., Okada, S., Ho, M. W., Hu, C. C., and O'Brien, J. S.: Generalized gangliosidosis: impaired cleavage of galactose from a mucopolysaccharide and a glycoprotein. Science, **163,** 946, 1969.
40. Ho, M. W., and O'Brien, J. S.: Unpublished results, 1969.
41. Ho, M. W., and O'Brien, J. S.: Hurler's syndrome: deficiency of a specific β-galactosidase isoenzyme. Science, **165,** 611, 1969.
42. Derry, D. M., Fawcett, J. S., Anderman, F., and Wolfe, L. S.: Late infantile systemic lipidosis: major monosialogangliosidosis, delineation of two types. Neurology, **18,** 340, 1968.
43. Wolfe, L. S., Callahan, J., Fawcett, J. S., Andermann, F., and Scriver, C.: GM_1 gangliosidosis without chondrodystrophy or visceromegaly: β-galactosidase deficiency with gangliosidosis and the excessive excretion of a keratan sulfate. Neurology, **20,** 23, 1970.
44. Opitz, J., ZuRhein, G., Ho, M. W., and O'Brien, J. S.: Juvenile GM_1 gangliosidosis: clinical, morphological and chemical analyses of two siblings., 1969 (in preparation).
45. Lowden, J. A., Children's Hospital, Toronto, and Hooft, C., Kindergeneeskunde, Rijksuniversiteit, Ghent, Belgium, for information on Patients 8 and 9, personal communication, 1969.
46. Kint, J. A., Dacremont, G., and Wlietinck, R.: Type II GM_1 gangliosidosis? Lancet, **2,** 108, 1969.
47. Bernheimer, H., and Seitelberger, F.: Über des Verhalten der Ganglioside im Gehirn bei 2 Fällen von spätinfantiler amaurotische Idiotie. Wien. Klin. Wschr., **80,** 163, 1968.
48. Volk, B. W., Adachi, M., Schneck, L., Saifer, A., and Kleinberg, W.: G-5 ganglioside variant of systemic late infantile lipidosis: generalized gangliosidosis. Arch. Path. (Chicago), **87,** 393, 1969.
49. Suzuki, K., Suzuki, K., Rapin, I., and Suzuki, Y.: A case of juvenile GM_2-gangliosidosis. Neurology, **19,** 304, 1969.
50. Okada, S., and O'Brien, J. S.: Unpublished data, 1969.
51. MacBrinn, M. C., Okada, S., Woollacott, M., Patel, V., Ho, M. W., Tappel, A. L., and O'Brien, J. S.: β-Galactosidase deficiency in the Hurler syndrome. New Eng. J. Med., **281,** 338, 1969.
52. Brady, R. O., O'Brien, J. S., Bradley, R. M., and Gal, A. E.: Sphingolipid hydrolases in brain tissue of patients with generalized gangliosidosis. Biochim. Biophys. Acta, **210,** 193, 1970.
53. Singer, H. S. and Schaffer, I. A.: White cell β-galactosidase activity. New Eng. J. Med., **282,** 571, 1970.
54. Callahan, J. W., Pinsky, L., and Wolfe, L. S.: G_{M1} gangliosidosis (type II); studies on a fibroblast cell strain. Biochem. Med., **4,** 295, 1970.
55. Sloan, H. R. and Kaback, M.: Personal Communication.

CHAPTER THIRTY-ONE

FABRY'S DISEASE: GLYCOSPHINGOLIPID LIPIDOSIS

Charles C. Sweeley, Bernard Klionsky, William Krivit, and Robert J. Desnick

Fabry's disease is a systemic disorder of glycosphingolipid metabolism transmitted by an X-linked gene and resulting from the progressive accumulation of galactosylgalactosylglucosyl ceramide (Gal-Gal-Glc-Cer) in most tissues of the body (Fig. 31-1). The metabolic abnormality is the absence of an α-galactosyl hydrolase required for the catabolism of the trihexosyl ceramide. The birefringent lipid is deposited in endothelial, perihelial, and smooth-muscle cells of blood vessels, in ganglion cells and perineural cells of the autonomic nervous system, in reticuloendothelial, myocardial, and connective tissue cells, and in epithelial cells of the cornea, kidney, and other tissues.

Clinically, the hemizygous males have a characteristic skin lesion which led to the descriptive name of *angiokeratoma corporis diffusum universale.* They also have corneal opacities, crises of fever and burning pain in the extremities, peripheral edema, and renal dysfunction. Death usually occurs in adult life from renal failure or from cardiac and cerebral complications of hypertension or of vascular disease. Heterozygous females, who may exhibit the disease in an attenuated form, are most likely to show the corneal opacities. Over 200 cases have been reported, most of them since 1961.

HISTORICAL ASPECTS

In 1898, Anderson [1], in England, and Fabry [2], in Germany, independently described patients with angiokeratoma corporis diffusum. Anderson designated his case as one of angiokeratoma. Fabry originally made a diagnosis of purpura nodularis but subsequently suggested the name *angiokeratoma corporis diffusum.* Anderson's original patient showed proteinuria, finger deformities, varicose veins, and edema of the legs. Because of the proteinuria, Anderson suspected that the disease might be a generalized disorder and suggested that abnormal vessels might be present in kidneys as well as in skin. The disease might, therefore, more properly be called Fabry-Anderson disease, but to minimize confusion in indexing, the term Fabry's disease has been retained.

Steiner and Voerner [3] and Gunther [4] described a patient with anhydrosis and intermittent peripheral pain aggravated by hot weather; the patient also had a diabetes insipidus-like syndrome, since he excreted daily 3 to 5.5 liters of urine of low specific gravity. A skin biopsy showed atrophy of the sweat glands as well as aneurysmal dilatation of the capillaries. The lesions involved not only the skin but the conjunctiva and the nasal mucosa as well. Weicksel [5] first described the corneal opacities and the vascular abnormalities in the conjunctiva and retina.

In 1947, Pompen et al. [6, 7] reported autopsies of two men who were known to have had the disease. The most significant observation was the presence of vacuoles in the media of abnormal blood vessels throughout the body. Similar vacuoles were found about the nuclei of hypertrophied myocardial fibers. Although special stains were negative for fat and glycogen in their paraffin-embedded material, they suggested the possibility of a generalized storage disease.

Scriba [8] definitely established the lipid nature of the storage material. He observed birefringent lipid crystals in frozen sections of blood vessels, glomerular and tubular epithelium, spleen, adrenal glands, lymph nodes, and ganglion cells of the brain and peripheral nervous system. On the basis of morphologic findings he concluded that the pattern of lipid storage was unlike that of the cerebrosides of Gaucher's disease. He also noticed that Formalin-fixed tissues contained a Best's carmine-stainable material, which he believed to be glycogen. This material was present in the liver, skeletal and cardiac muscle, the endothelium and smooth muscle of blood vessels, and the ganglion cells. Hornbostel and Scriba were the first to confirm the diagnosis histologically in a living patient by demonstrating a refractile lipid in vessels of a skin biopsy specimen [9].

Fessas et al. [10] demonstrated birefringent globules in the urinary sediment and found vacuolated cells in the bone marrow.

The first confirmation of the disease in a woman was reported by Wallace [11] and Colley et al. [12], who, following the death of the patient's son from this disorder, reviewed her autopsy material and demonstrated vacuolated glomerular epithelial cells. Subsequently, Burda and Winder [13] documented the occurrence and clinical features of the more limited disease which occurs in heterozygous females. Wise et al. [14] described 21 patients from eight families and presented the first definite evidence of corneal dystrophy in females whose other manifestations of disease were very slight. Stiles and Opitz [15] and Opitz [16] have studied a kindred with at least 21 carrier females and affected males. They have been able to make the diagnosis in childhood or, in severe cases, in infancy, and have offered confirmation of the X-linked transmission of the disorder.

Chemical analyses have confirmed the lipid nature of the storage material. Early and incomplete studies indicated that a phospholipid might be involved [8, 17, 18], but in 1963

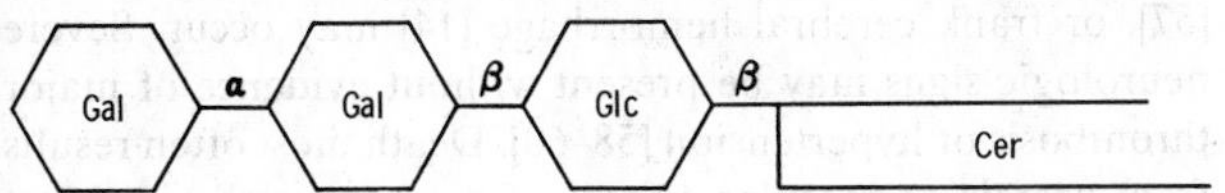

Figure 31-1. Galactosylgalactosylglucosyl ceramide (trihexosyl ceramide).

Sweeley and Klionsky [19] isolated and characterized two neutral glycosphingolipids—galactosylgalactosylglucosyl ceramide (Gal-Gal-Glc-Cer) and digalactosyl ceramide (Gal-Gal-Cer)—from a kidney of a Fabry hemizygote, obtained at autopsy [20, 21]. On the basis of these findings, they classified Fabry's disease as a sphingolipidosis. Chemical analyses of various Fabry tissues, including brain [22], plasma [23], urinary sediment [24–26], cultured skin fibroblasts [27], and most internal tissues [19, 22, 28–30], have demonstrated increased levels of Gal-Gal-Glc-Cer. Gal-Gal-Cer was found in the kidney [19, 22, 29–31], urinary sediment [24], and pancreas [29].

Brady et al. [32] demonstrated that the enzymatic defect in this inborn error of glycosphingolipid catabolism is the absence of enzymatic trihexosyl ceramide galactosyl hydrolase activity; this enzyme is required for the metabolism of Gal-Gal-Glc-Cer. Recently developed methods for the chemical determination of Gal-Gal-Glc-Cer levels in plasma [23], urinary sediment [24], and cultured skin fibroblasts [27, 33] have provided a biochemical means for the diagnostic confirmation of affected hemizygotes and the identification of heterozygotes, genetic variants, and affected hemizygotes before clinical onset of the disease [34].

Because many heterozygous females and hemizygous males do not have the classic skin lesion, the descriptive name angiokeratoma corporis diffusum universale seems inappropriate, as does the chemically imprecise term hereditary dystopic lipidosis [35]. In keeping with the terminology applied to other lipidoses and for the benefit of information retrieval, it would seem advisable to retain the commonly used eponym and to append the chemical nature of the storage lipid. Thus, an appropriate term is *tri- and dihexosyl ceramide lipidosis: Fabry's disease.* Recent comprehensive reviews are available [10, 14, 21, 36–40].

CLINICAL FEATURES

The Hemizygote

Clinical manifestations of Fabry's disease are the sequelae of the anatomic and physiologic alterations produced by deposits of glycosphingolipids in the tissues. The disease usually becomes quite evident and often severe during childhood and adolescence. It is characterized by periodic crises of fever and severe pain in the extremities; the appearance of vascular lesions of the skin, conjunctiva, and oral mucosa; and crystalline deposits in the conjunctiva.

Pain

Pain, which may be the initial symptom in childhood or adolescence [15], is often excruciating and has a burning or lightning quality. It is noted most often in the fingers and toes, where it may be accompanied by paresthesias, and it may extend into the palms and soles. It may be induced by changes in environmental temperature. Pain may be so severe that the patient may contemplate suicide [13, 28]. Because pain is often associated with fever and elevation of the erythrocyte sedimentation rate, the disease has been misdiagnosed as rheumatic fever [28, 39]. Attacks of abdominal or flank pain may simulate appendicitis or renal colic [35].

Skin Lesion

Telangiectases may be one of the earliest manifestations and may lead to diagnosis in childhood [15]. There is a progressive increase of cutaneous vascular lesions with age. Classically, the lesions develop slowly as clusters of individual punctate, dark-red angiectases in the superficial layers of the skin (Fig. 31-2). The lesions may be flat or slightly raised and do not blanch with pressure. The clusters of lesions are most dense between the umbilicus and the knees and have a tendency toward bilateral symmetry. The hips, back, thighs, buttocks, penis, and scrotum are most commonly involved, but there is a wide variation both in the pattern of distribution and in the density of the lesions. Involvement of the oral mucosa and conjunctiva are common, and other areas may also be involved. Recently, variants without the characteristic skin lesions have been reported [31, 41–50].

Renal Manifestations

Progressive accumulation of glycosphingolipids in the kidney results in proteinuria and other signs of renal impairment, with gradual deterioration of renal function and development of azotemia in middle age. Casts, red blood cells, and birefringent lipid globules within and outside the cells appear in the urine. The urine specific gravity becomes fixed in the range from 1.008 to 1.012. Polyuria and a syndrome similar to pitressin-resistant diabetes insipidus occasionally develop [51].

Vascular Lesions

Diffuse glycosphingolipid deposits in the vascular system and the heart may be associated with hypertension, cardiomegaly, myocardial ischemia, or infarction [8, 14, 52], and with cerebral vascular disease. Cerebral manifestations are common and often occur before the age of 25, at a time when hypertension and renal disease may not be prominent [14]. Thromboses [53], seizures [54], hemiplegia [49, 55], hemianesthesia [56], aphasia [11, 14], labyrinthine disorders [57], or frank cerebral hemorrhage [14] may occur. Severe neurologic signs may be present without evidence of major thrombosis or hypertension [58–60]. Death most often results from uremia or vascular disease of the heart or brain. Most patients die between ages 40 and 50, but occasionally a patient survives into his sixties [39, 61].

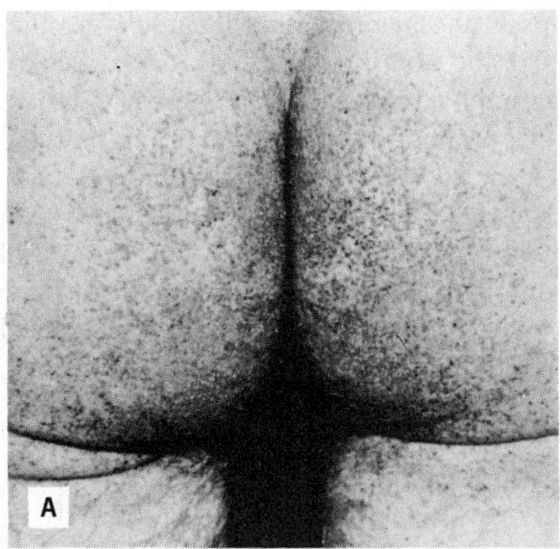

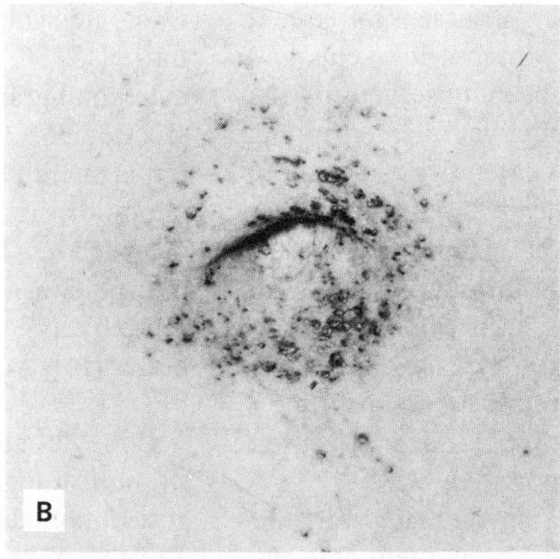

Figure 31-2. Clusters of dark-red skin lesions (telangiectases) of Fabry's disease on the buttocks (A) and in the umbilical area (B) of a hemizygote. (See also Plate II-1.)

Ocular Features

Although ocular lesions in Fabry's disease may be present in all elements of the eye, involvement is most prominent in the cornea and retina. Conjunctival and retinal vascular lesions may be present as part of the diffuse systemic involvement of vessels. These characteristically include aneurysmal dilatation of thin-walled venules and angulation and segmental, sausage-like dilatation of veins (Fig. 31-3). The vascular lesions in the conjunctiva and retina and the dystrophy of corneal epithelium do not impair vision. Edema of the lids is commonly observed [62]. As the disease progresses, with development of hypertension and uremia, retinal changes associated with these complications may be superimposed.

Corneal opacities are found in males with the disease and in many heterozygous females. They have been observed in a 6-month-old hemizygote [62]. The earliest lesion revealed by the slit lamp is a diffuse haziness in the epithelial layer. In more advanced cases many of the opacities appear as whorled streaks extending from the periphery toward the center of the cornea [14, 52].

Other Clinical Features

Because of the widespread distribution of the lipid deposits, signs and symptoms of this disorder arise in many other organs and systems. Several patients have had chronic bronchitis and wheezing respiration [14, 63] or dyspnea with

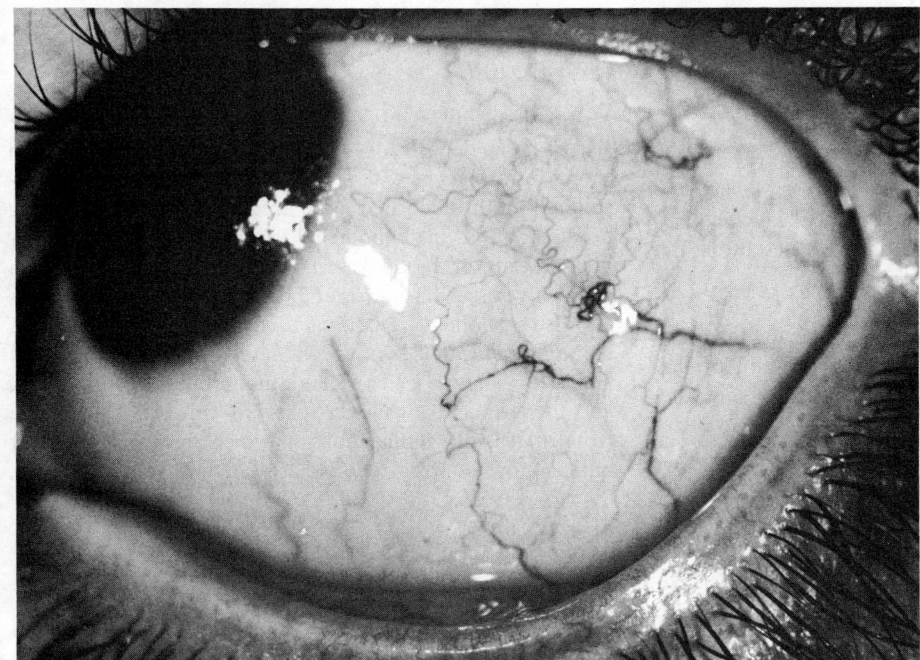

Figure 31-3. Typical conjunctival vessels in Fabry's disease. (*Courtesy of Dr. Philip Frost and George L. Spaeth, National Institutes of Health.*)

alveolar capillary block [51]. Pulmonary disease is a frequent cause of death. Many patients have varicose leg veins and hemorrhoids. Lipid deposits have been observed in the saphenous veins of a patient who underwent vein stripping for varices [64]. Edema of the legs is often present without hypoproteinemia, varices, or any clinically manifest vascular disease. Hypohidrosis is a common symptom. Nausea, vomiting, and diarrhea are common and may be related to deposition of glycosphingolipid in the autonomic ganglia of the bowel. Anemia is probably due to decreased red blood cell survival [28, 65]. A decreased serum iron concentration [66], normal red blood cell fragility [66], and an elevated reticulocyte count [52] have been reported.

Many patients have evidence of involvement of the musculoskeletal system. A characteristic permanent deformity arises from changes in the distal interphalangeal joint of the fingers [14, 39, 67, 68], causing limitation of extension of the terminal joint [14]. Avascular necrosis of the head of the femur [69] or talus [41] and multiple small infarct-like opacities in the femoral heads [70] and involvement of the metacarpals and metatarsals and temporal mandibular joint [62] have been reported. Local severe osteoporosis in a dorsal vertebra is recorded [53].

Many of the affected males seem to have retarded growth or delayed puberty [64, 71], sparse, fine facial [38] and body hair, and decreased fertility. In some kindreds an acromegalic-like appearance has been reported [38, 39, 41, 62, 72]. Affected individuals may complain of fatigue and weakness and may be incapacitated for prolonged periods of time [7, 73].

The Heterozygote

Heterozygous females are generally less severely affected than hemizygotic males [11–14, 35, 37, 39, 74–77]. The clinical manifestations in heterozygous females are usually limited and variable, however, and a few heterozygotes have been reported in which the expression was comparable to that seen in fully affected males [15]. Of over 45 heterozygotes reported in the literature, the corneal involvement is the most frequent and often singular manifestation [14, 36, 37, 42, 43, 46].

The skin lesions are generally less prominent in affected females than in males; often they are not clinically manifest [12, 36, 42, 44, 46]. The characteristic distribution of the lesions is present, but they may occasionally be seen on the uvula [14], tongue, and palms [37]. The lesions have been detected in a heterozygote as early as age 6 [78].

Other manifestations include intermittent pain of the extremities [13, 36–38, 46, 49, 79], sensitivity to changes in environmental temperature [38, 49], edema, particularly of the ankles [13, 14, 36, 46, 49], vascular lesions in the conjunctiva and retina [36–38, 43, 46, 49], and cardiovascular changes such as hypertension, abnormal electrocardiogram (ECG), and left ventricular hypertrophy [12–14, 36, 49]. Urologic symptoms in the heterozygotes include hyposthenuria [13, 36, 38, 49], the occurrence of erythrocytes, leukocytes, and granular and hyaline casts in the urinary sediment [12, 13, 36, 38, 49], proteinuria, and other signs of renal impairment [12–14, 36, 38, 46, 79]. Mucosal lesions [13, 38], hypohidrosis [35, 36, 38], and diarrhea [79, 80] have been recorded less frequently. Heterozygotes may develop a distal interphalangeal joint arthritis of the fingers, and they are more likely to develop urinary tract infections than affected males [16]. Autopsy findings have been reported [11, 13, 79, 81, 82].

Colley et al. [12] were the first to demonstrate lipid deposition histologically in the kidney of a 47-year-old heterozygote obtained at autopsy. Renal biopsy material of two living affected male relatives appeared histologically identical to that of the heterozygote. Subsequently, Rahman et al. [35] found a birefringent substance in the cytoplasm of epithelial cells from the glomerular tufts of a 17-year-old heterozygote. Renal biopsy of a 3-year-old heterozygote demonstrated the characteristic glomerular lesion by electron microscopy [83], and skin biopsies from two heterozygotes (8 and 35 years old) contained deposits of lipid in the endothelial and muscularis cells of clinically unaffected skin [38].

The clinical course and prognosis are better in heterozygotes than in affected hemizygotes. Heterozygotes experience little difficulty at ages at which hemizygous males are already severely affected [13]. Although the life expectancy is greater in affected women, most heterozygotes become more symptomatic as they grow older, and most of them die of the disease. Death usually results from renal and cardiac insufficiency [13], although two heterozygotes had central nervous system complications [12, 84].

PATHOLOGY

Morphologically, Fabry's disease is characterized by widespread tissue deposits of crystalline glycosphingolipid which shows birefringence with typical maltese crosses. The glycosphingolipid is deposited in all areas of the body, occurring predominantly in endothelial, perithelial, and smooth-muscle cells of blood vessels, and to a lesser degree in connective tissue histiocytic and reticular cells. Lipid deposits are also prominent in epithelial cells of the cornea and of glomeruli and tubules of the kidney, in muscle fibers of the heart, in ganglion cells of the autonomic nervous system, and in peripheral Schwann cells. Information is available from at least 20 publications in which findings of one or more autopsies were reported [6–8, 21, 29, 30, 35, 50, 52, 81, 82, 85–95].

Skin

The skin lesions (Fig. 31-4) are angiectases rather than angiomas. After a silent period, cumulative vascular damage

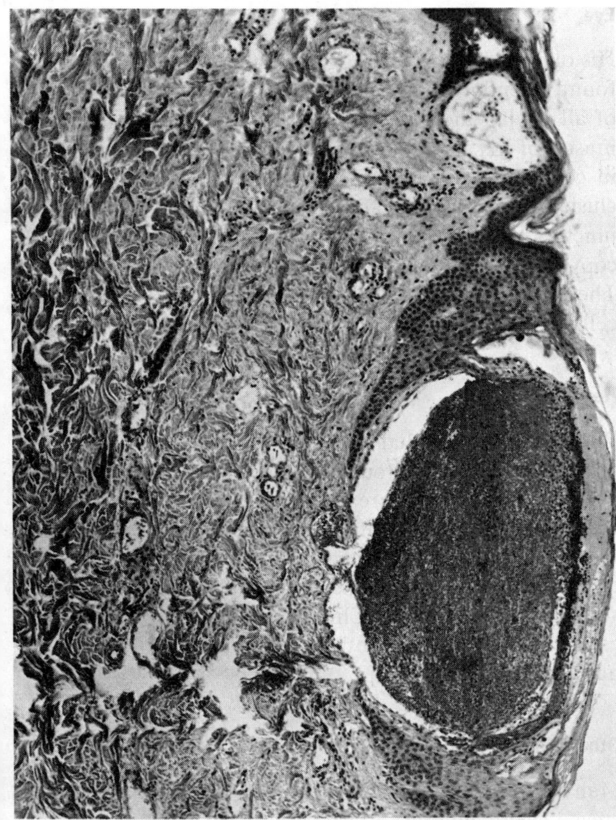

Figure 31-4. Photomicrographs of the skin lesions reveal dilated vascular channels of varying size in the upper dermis. The vessels may contain thrombi, and the overlying epithelium may be thinned or ulcerated.

leads eventually to clinically apparent progressive telangiectases. This pathogenetic sequence is suggested by the biopsy finding of lipid deposits in areas of clinically normal skin [96] or in patients with no skin lesions [97], and by recognition of patients who have visceral lesions but whose skin lesions either are of minimal consequence [31, 44, 98] or are delayed [99].

Capillaries, venules, and arterioles contain pathologic lipid stores in the endothelium, perithelium, or smooth muscle [64, 89, 96, 100]. Lipid stores have been noted in arrectores pilorum muscles [10, 37, 64, 67, 69, 89, 96, 101], sweat gland epithelium [67, 101], and perineural cells [67, 89, 101–104]. Atrophic [88] or scarce sweat and sebaceous glands have been reported.

The fully developed classic lesions are usually located in the upper dermis, where they may produce elevation and flattening of the epithelium. Thrombosis and organization may occur, as may erythema nodosum-like lesions [105]. There may be slight to moderate keratosis.

Clinical and pathologic details of diagnosis and differential diagnosis of skin lesions are available in reviews [96, 105–107].

Kidney

Accumulation of glycosphingolipids in the kidney is a progressive process, the earliest documentation of which was found in the examination of a 3-year-old heterozygote [83]. The earliest lesions are due to the accumulation of glycosphingolipid in endothelial and epithelial cells of the glomerulus and of Bowman's space (Fig. 31-5) and in the epithelium of the loops of Henle and of distal tubules (Fig. 31-6). In later stages, and to a lesser degree, proximal tubules [11, 108], interstitial histiocytes, and fibrocytes [109] may show lipid accumulation. Lipid-laden distal tubular epithelial cells desquamate (Fig. 31-6) and may be detected in the urinary sediment [24].

Concurrently renal blood vessels are also progressively involved, often extensively. Other histologic findings described in the kidney are the sequelae of nonspecific, severe end-stage renal disease with evidence of severe arteriolar sclerosis, glomerular atrophy and fibrosis, pseudotubular proliferation of residual glomerular epithelium, tubular atrophy, and diffuse interstitial fibrosis. Recent reviews of the renal involvement have been reported [98, 108, 110, 111].

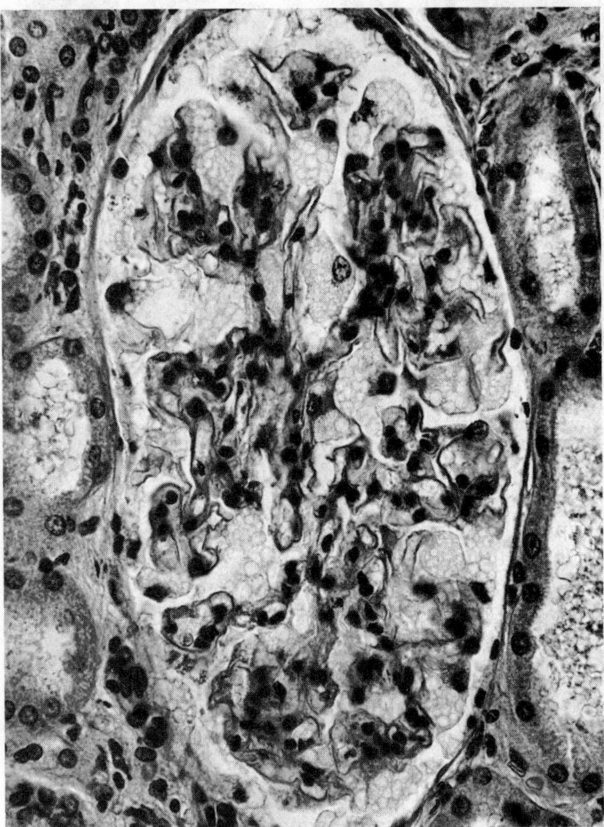

Figure 31-5. In this glomerulus the epithelial cells of the parietal and visceral layers of Bowman's capsule show the multiple vacuoles from which the lipid has been extracted. Zenker's fixation; paraffin embedding. (Hematoxylin and eosin, ×225.)

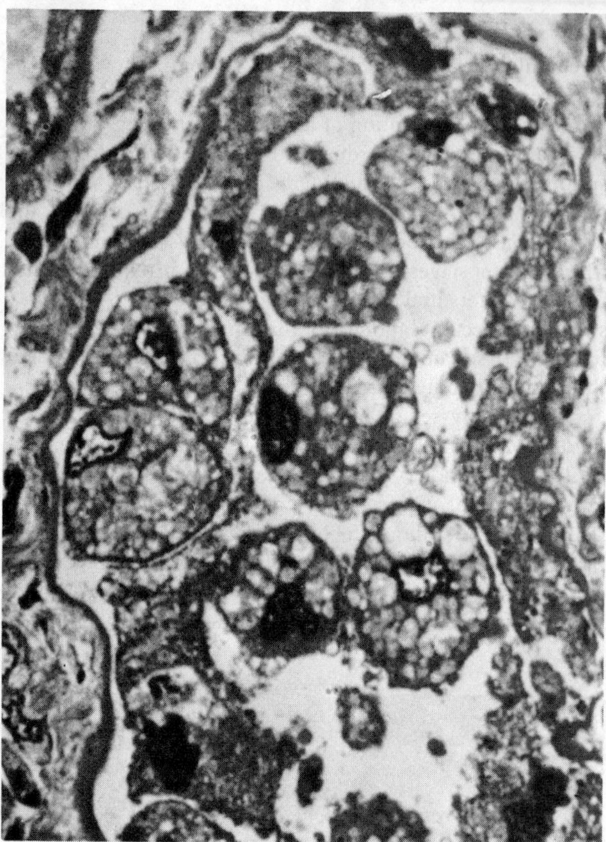

Figure 31-6. Lipid-laden cells in the lining and in the lumen of a renal tubule. Formalin fixation; postfixation in osmium tetroxide and embedding in Vestopal. "Thick" section, approximately 1 mm.

Nervous System

Vascular involvement is prominent in the nervous system, as it is elsewhere in the body [21, 31, 93]. In both heterozygotes and hemizygotes involvement of the nervous tissue appears to be limited to perineural or Schwann cells of peripheral nerves [21, 67, 89, 96, 101–103, 112], neurons of peripheral and central autonomic nervous system [8, 31, 81, 93, 113], and certain primary neurons of somatic afferent pathways [81]. Lipid-filled cells have been noted in peripheral ganglia of pancreas, intestine, prostate, and other viscera, in dorsal root ganglia, and in cells of the intermediolateral gray column of the spinal cord. Brain stem centers that are involved include the nuclei gracilis and cuneatus, the dorsal autonomic vagal nuclei, salivary nuclei, nucleus ambiguus, thalamus, reticular substance, mesencephalic nucleus of the fifth nerve, and the substantia nigra. Hemisphere involvement is noted in the amygdaloid, hypothalamic, and hippocampal nuclei [81]. The lipid storage in neuronal cells of the anterior and posterior lobes of the pituitary is described [101]. Detailed reviews of the neurologic findings are available [67, 93].

Eye

Histologically abnormal glycosphingolipid deposits are found in endothelial, perivascular, and smooth-muscle cells of all ocular and orbital vessels [101, 114, 115], in smooth muscle of iris and ciliary body [115], in perineural cells, and in connective tissue of the lens and cornea [101, 115]. Inclusions have been localized in the epithelium of the conjunctiva, cornea, and lens [101, 115], and, by electron microscopy, in the basal layer of conjunctival epithelial cells [114]. There may be hyperplasia and edema of corneal epithelial cells.

Heart

Within the myocardial cells, there is extensive deposition of Gal-Gal-Glc-Cer around the nucleus and between myofibrils. In addition there is involvement of vascular and connective tissue elements, as noted elsewhere in the body. Nonspecific findings frequently observed relate to the associated hypertension, cardiac hypertrophy, and vascular obstruction and infarction. Clinical and pathologic features of cardiac involvement in both hemizygotes and heterozygotes have been reviewed [82].

Other Tissues

Many other parenchymal organs, including the liver, pancreas, testis, thyroid, prostate, urinary bladder, adrenal glands, and gastrointestinal tract, show involvement of the blood vessels, smooth muscle, ganglia, and nerves. In addition, vacuoles or lipid stores have been demonstrated in epithelial cells [7, 21], in mucous glands [101], in smooth muscle of the bronchus [82], and in alveolar epithelial pneumocytes of type II [28]. Involvement of reticuloendothelial cells has been noted in the bone marrow [10, 21, 37, 49, 60, 73, 74, 91, 105] and in the liver, spleen, or lymph nodes [8, 10, 43, 49, 52, 58, 83, 88, 90, 116]. Foam cells containing birefringent lipid droplets are nearly always present in the urinary sediment (Fig. 31-7). Involvement of the interstitial cells of the testis has been noted [101]. No morphologic involvement of striated muscle has been documented. The finding of Gal-Gal-Glc-Cer in a thenar muscle [29] is probably attributed to microscopic involvement of blood vessels within the muscle [114]. Hyalinization and loss of cross striations in skeletal muscle have been observed, as have alterations in the electromyogram [117].

Histochemistry

Scriba [8] demonstrated that the accumulated lipid is birefringent in polarized light, that it can be stained in frozen sections with lipid-soluble dyes, and that it may be removed from the tissues by the process of dehydration and embedding in paraffin. He also reported Best's carmine–positive

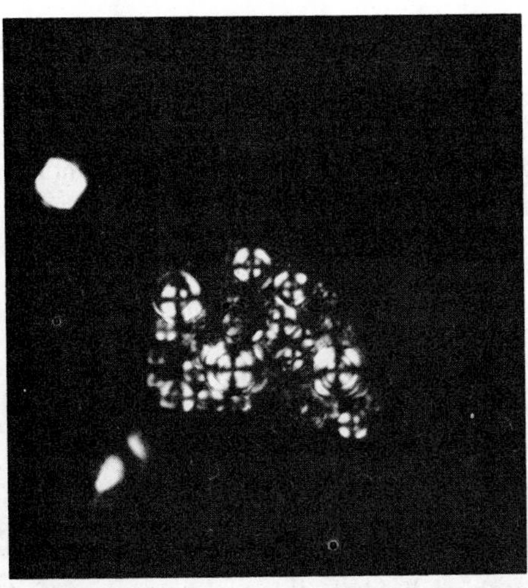

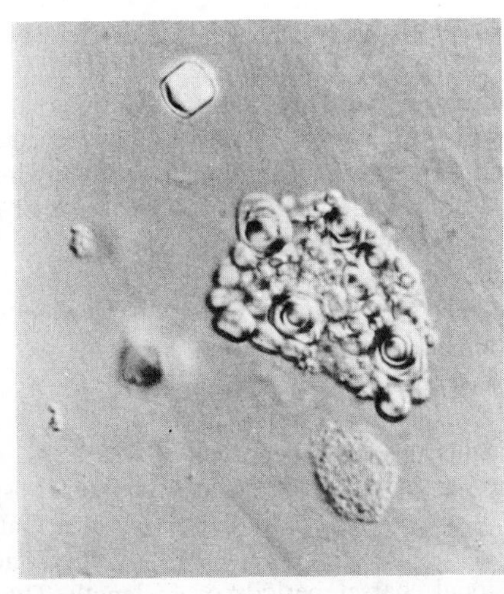

Figure 31-7. Photomicrographs of the urinary sediment from a heterozygote, showing lipid accumulation by polarized light microscopy (*left*) and interference-contrast microscopy (*right*). (×1,000.)

material in many of the same organs in which he found the lipid.

Studies with free-floating frozen sections and with blocks of Formalin-fixed tissues demonstrate that most of the lipid crystals are retained through alcohol dehydration, but are lost on exposure to xylene [21] or pyridine [100]. Ruiter [100] claimed that exposure of Formalin-fixed tissue for 1 week to 3 percent potassium chromate helped to preserve the lipid, and similar reports have been made for fixation in 1 percent calcium formol [64, 114]. Diastase digestion of Formalin-fixed frozen sections does not alter the subsequent staining of the lipids by the PAS (periodic acid–Schiff) procedure.

The significance of a residual Luxol blue material [21, 53, 94] after removal of the glycosphingolipid is uncertain, as is the significance of nonspecific staining by Luxol blue in general [118]. Caulet [94] described criteria of solubility and distribution to distinguish between a glycosphingolipid and a Luxol blue–positive material which he presumed to represent a phosphosphingolipid.

The presence of a phosphotungstic acid–positive matrix in electron micrographs [83] raises the question of mucopolysaccharide storage in the lesions, but other studies have indicated that the PAS-positive lipid [111] does not contain acid mucopolysaccharide [8, 21, 82, 114, 119], glycogen, phospholipid, sulfatide, or ganglioside [119, 120]. A modified PAS stain specific for neutral glycosphingolipids [119] and a positive test for sphingosine [120] have served to confirm the chemical identification of the storage lipid as a glycosphingolipid.

Ultrastructure

Additional details of the morphologic characteristics of the lesions and of the lipid inclusions have been revealed by electron microscopy in more than 30 published reports. These have dealt with skin [28, 50, 71, 81, 96, 99, 102–105, 107, 109, 114, 120–125], kidney [44, 67, 72–74, 83, 108, 109, 111, 121, 122, 126], bone marrow [114, 127], gastrointestinal tract [28, 114], lymph node [91, 94], liver [83, 122, 126], spleen [83, 126], heart [82], skeletal muscle [114], lungs [28], conjunctiva [114], peripheral nerve [102, 112], urinary sediment [127] (Fig. 31-8), and isolated trihexosyl ceramide [128]. The findings in the various tissues are similar.

The size and location of the lipid bodies suggest that enzyme-deficient lysosomes fail to hydrolyze Gal-Gal-Glc-Cer, which accumulates progressively and remains, following lysosomal rupture, as free intracytoplasmic bodies. Lipid subparticles, ranging from 0.1 to 0.5 microns in diameter [83, 114, 123], aggregate and fuse into larger masses, which may measure up to 10 microns in diameter. These are often limited by a single-unit membrane [71, 82, 83, 97, 99, 109], but when present in larger quantities they are usually free in the cytoplasm. A relationship to lysosomes is suggested by the prominence of pinocytic activity and multivesicular

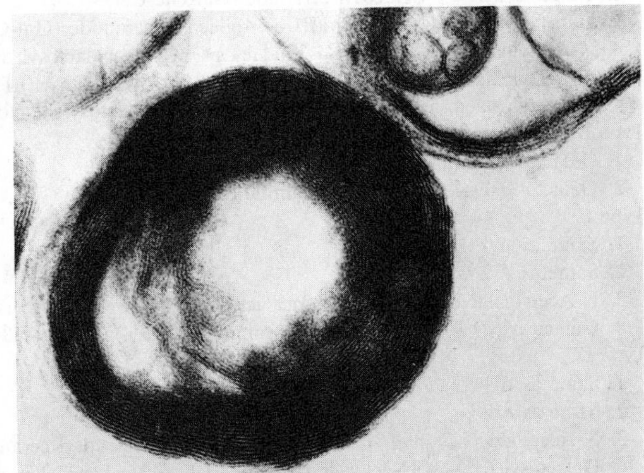

Figure 31-8. Electron photomicrograph of urinary sediment from a hemizygote with Fabry's disease. The lamellar arrangement has a periodicity of 50 to 60 Å. The bodies are also present in the urinary sediment of heterozygotes for this disorder. (×100,000.)

bodies [99, 103], by the demonstration of acid phosphatase within the inclusion-bearing bodies [97–99], and by analogy with the localization of other sphingolipid hydrolases [129].

Possible evidence against a lysosomal origin of the bodies includes the reported close relationship to mitochondria [28, 103], the presence of lipid inclusions within mitochondria [73, 82], the existence of a surrounding double membrane [28, 114], and the absence of acid phosphatase [114].

Although amorphous or pleomorphic lipid may be seen [114], well-preserved material examined at high resolution reveals a pattern of parallel, concentric, or interlacing lamellae with alternating light- and dark-staining bands (Fig. 31-8). The periodicity of these bands has been reported variably as 40 to 50 Å [81, 82, 91, 94, 97, 114, 127], 50 to 60 Å [28, 71, 96, 102, 104, 112], 60 to 65 Å [83, 103, 123], or as great as 98 Å [109]. The electron-dense component is 20 to 30 Å in thickness. Occasional coarser periods of 150 to 200 Å are noted [96, 104]. The tubular arrangement, which is observed with purified glucosyl ceramide, with trihexosyl ceramide [128], and in tissue deposits of lipids in Gaucher's disease [128, 130], is rarely found in the tissues in Fabry's disease [102, 114, 127].

CHEMISTRY OF NEUTRAL GLYCOSPHINGOLIPIDS

Neutral Glycosyl Ceramides

Structure

The glycolipids involved in Fabry's disease are members of a family of closely related neutral glycosphingolipids that are widely distributed in mammalian tissues. All of them have a common lipid structure called *ceramide,* to which various carbohydrate units are attached by a glycosidic bond between the reducing end of the carbohydrate and the terminal hydroxyl group of the ceramide. The ceramide moiety consists of a

$$\text{Carbohydrate—O—}CH_2CH(NH\text{—}CO(CH_2)_{22}CH_3)CH(OH)CH{=}CH(CH_2)_{12}CH_3$$

Ceramide

mixture of sphingosine and other related long-chain aliphatic amines that are joined in amide linkages with a mixture of fatty acids generally ranging from C_{16} to C_{26} in chain length. The glycosphingolipids in this category are neutral molecules, as contrasted with the gangliosides and sulfatides, which have acidic functional groups (N-acylneuraminic acid and sulfuric acid, respectively). The physical chemical behavior of neutral glycosphingolipids in solutions and in membranes is entirely due to the effects of the hydrophobic ceramide and hydrophilic carbohydrate portions of the molecule.

Carbohydrate Component

The neutral glycosphingolipids can be arranged in four groups with characteristic chemical similarities, as shown in Table 31-1. The compounds of Type A are closely related to one another, and all of them can be derived from globo-

Table 31-1. NEUTRAL GLYCOSPHINGOLIPIDS OF MAMMALIAN ORIGIN*

Type A:
1. Glucosyl ceramide (Glc-Cer)
2. Galactosyl(β1 → 4)glucosyl ceramide (Gal-Glc-Cer)
3. Galactosyl(α1 → 4)galactosyl(β1 → 4)glucosyl ceramide (Gal-Gal-Glc-Cer)
4. N-Acetylgalactosaminyl(β1 → 3)galactosyl(α1 → 4)galactosyl(β1 → 4)glucosyl ceramide (GalNAc-Gal-Gal-Glc-Cer)
   N-Acetylgalactosaminyl(α1 → 3)galactosyl(1 → 4)galactosyl(β1 → 4)glucosyl ceramide (GalNAc-Gal-Gal-Glc-Cer)
5. N-Acetylgalactosaminyl-N-acetylgalactosaminylgalactosylgalactosylglucosyl ceramide (GalNAc-GalNAc-Gal-Gal-Glc-Cer)

Type B:
1. Galactosyl ceramide (Gal-Cer)
2. Galactosyl(1 → 4)galactosyl ceramide (Gal-Gal-Cer)

Type C:
1. Same as A.1
2. Same as A.2
3. N-Acetylgalactosaminyl(β1 → 4)galactosyl(β1 → 4)glucosyl ceramide (GalNAc-Gal-Glc-Cer)
4. Galactosyl(β1 → 3)N-acetylgalactosaminyl(β1 → 4)galactosyl(β1 → 4)glucosyl ceramide (Gal-GalNAc-Gal-Glc-Cer)

Type D:
1. Same as A.1
2. Same as A.2
3. N-Acetylglucosaminyl(β1 → 3)galactosyl(β1 → 4)glucosyl ceramide (GlcNAc-Gal-Glc-Cer)
4. Galactosyl(β1 → 4)N-acetylglucosaminyl(β1 → 3)galactosyl(β1 → 4)glucosyl ceramide (Gal-GlcNAc-Gal-Glc-Cer)
   Galactosyl(β1 → 3)N-acetylglucosaminyl(β1 → 3)galactosyl(β1 → 4)glucosyl ceramide (Gal-GlcNAc-Gal-Glc-Cer)
5. Galactosyl(1 → 3)galactosyl(1 → 3)N-acetylglucosaminyl(1 → 3)galactosyl(1 → 4)glucosyl ceramide (Gal-Gal-GlcNAc-Gal-Glc-Cer)
   Galactosyl(β1 → 3)[fucosyl-(α1 → 4)]N-acetylglucosaminyl(1 → 3)galactosyl(1 → 4)glucosyl ceramide (Gal[Fuc]-GlcNAc-Gal-Glc-Cer)

*Stereochemical configurations of anomeric linkages are given unless unknown. When differences in the positions of anomeric linkages are known, both structures are shown.

Table 31-2. CONCENTRATIONS OF NEUTRAL GLYCOSPHINGOLIPIDS IN VARIOUS NORMAL HUMAN TISSUES, MG PER GM WET WEIGHT

Source	Reference	Glc-Cer	Gal-Glc-Cer (Gal-Gal-Cer)	Gal-Gal-Glc-Cer	GalNAc-Gal-Gal-Glc-Cer	Total
Kidney	Martensson [136]	0.10	0.16	0.37	0.64	1.27
	Snyder, Krivit, and Sweeley [230]	0.08	0.14	0.36	0.35	0.93
	Klionsky and Sweeley [231]	.....	.....	.....	.....	1.0
Spleen	Snyder, Krivit, and Sweeley [230]	0.098	0.16	0.072	0.107	0.44
	Suomi and Agranoff [153]	0.18	0.88			
	Klionsky and Sweeley [231]	.....	.....	.....	.....	0.8
Liver	Snyder, Krivit, and Sweeley [230]	0.041	0.10	0.045	0.035	0.20
	Klionsky and Sweeley [231]	.....	.....	.....	.....	0.4
Placenta	Svennerholm [232]	0.022	0.044	0.056	0.11	0.23
Erythrocytes	Vance [233]	0.004	0.014	0.015	0.09	0.124
Heart	Klionsky and Sweeley [231]	.....	.....	.....	.....	0.8
Lung	Klionsky and Sweeley [231]	.....	.....	.....	.....	3.4
Prostate	Klionsky and Sweeley [231]	.....	.....	.....	.....	0.6

side (A.4), a major constituent of many species of mammalian erythrocytes, by the addition or deletion of monomeric carbohydrate units. The simplest example of this class of lipids is glucosyl ceramide, or "glucocerebroside" (A.1); more complex oligosaccharide units are derived from the glucosyl ceramide by addition of Gal and GalNAc units in an order of arrangement that is maintained throughout the series. Normally glycosphingolipids of Type A are the predominant type in nonneural tissues and in blood, but the relative proportions of individual lipids in this class are quite dependent on the tissues from which they are obtained. In plasma, for example, Glc-Cer (A.1) is predominant, but in liver and spleen the concentration of lactosyl ceramide (A.2, Gal-Glc-Cer) is higher than that of Glc-Cer. In the erythrocytes and in kidney tetrahexosyl ceramides of Type A.4, GalNAc-Gal-Gal-Glc-Cer, are major substituents of the glycosphingolipid fraction [131]. Table 31-2 shows the relative distribution of these lipids in selected normal tissues.

The positions of glycosidic bonds and their stereochemical configurations are generally the same in all the glycosphingolipids of Type A, but variations are known to occur. In the globoside of erythrocyte membranes the GalNAc $(1 \rightarrow 3)$ Gal linkage is β [131, 132], whereas it is α in a globoside, called Forssman hapten [133], from kidney and other sources. Still another globoside, called cytolipin R, has been isolated from a lymphosarcoma of male Wistar rats [134]; this lipid has the same arrangement of hexose and hexosamine units, GalNAc-Gal-Gal-Glc-Cer, but it is immunochemically distinguishable from both red blood cell globoside and Forssman hapten. To what extent mixtures of these different globosides occur in various organs has not been established. The Gal-Gal linkage in human erythrocyte globoside and in trihexoside from human kidney and erythrocytes has recently been shown to have the α configuration [134a, 134b].

The pentahexosyl ceramide with two GalNAc units (A.5) has been isolated from canine intestine, where it is the major glycosphingolipid [135]; it has not been found in human tissues.

Glycosphingolipids of Type B are derived from galactosyl ceramide (B.1, Gal-Cer) instead of glucosyl ceramide. In the central nervous system Gal-Cer is the major neutral glycosphingolipid; it also occurs in substantial amounts in kidney [136] and in trace amounts in urine sediment cells [24]. Digalactosyl ceramide (B.2, Gal-Gal-Cer) has also been found in the kidney and in normal urine sediment [24, 136]. More complex glycolipids of Type B have not been reported but may be expected to occur in small amounts.

The same sugars are used as building blocks in both Type C and Type A, but the order in which they are arranged in the trihexosyl and tetrahexosyl ceramides is different. The GalNAc-Gal-Glc-Cer arrangement of C.3 is also a component of C.4 and is identical with part of the ganglioside structures from brain and several other tissues that have been examined [137]. They are generally referred to as asialo G_{M2} (C.3) and asialo G_{M1} (C.4) (see also Chap. 29). Ordinarily only small amounts of these neutral glycosphingolipids are found in the body, but large amounts may accumulate in certain glycosphingolipidoses (Chap. 29). Simpler glycolipids of Type C are identical with those of Type A, indicating the possibility of similar metabolic pathways.

Glycosphingolipids containing glucosamine (GlcN) rather than galactosamine (GalN) occur in some of the blood group active sphingolipids [138], in a Lewis^a-active glycosphingolipid from human adenocarcinoma [139, 140], and in gangliosides from spleen [138] and erythrocytes [131, 137, 141]. The glycosphingolipids of Types D.3 and D.4 are the asialo forms of the glucosamine-containing gangliosides. The pentahexosyl ceramide D.5, Gal-Gal-GlcNAc-Gal-Glc-Cer, has been found in erythrocytes of rabbits [142] but has not been isolated from human sources.

Sphingosine Base

The most common sphingolipid base in all the neutral glycosphingolipids is sphingosine, the chemistry of which is discussed in detail in Chap. 29. It accounts for 80 to 95 percent of the total "sphingosine" fraction in most lipids, and the remainder is usually dihydrosphingosine with the same C_{18} chain length. The glycosphingolipids of kidney are an unusual exception. Relatively high concentrations of phytosphingosine have been found in Glc-Cer and Gal-Cer from human kidney [143–146]. Other glycosphingolipids of kidney contained lesser amounts of phytosphingosine, but it was present in every fraction that was analyzed. Recent work has shown that phytosphingosine is also a component of the "sphingosine" fraction of bovine kidney gangliosides. [147]. In all these studies the level of phytosphingosine was highest in lipids rich in α-hydroxy fatty acids. The major long-chain base in Gal-Cer from brain is C_{18} sphingosine [148], but the ganglioside fraction of brain contains approximately equal amounts of C_{18} and C_{20} sphingosine [149]. On the basis of their long-chain base fraction, it is thus possible to differentiate glycosphingolipids of kidney origin from those synthesized in other nonneural organs and from those derived from brain and gangliosides.

Fatty Acid Components

The fatty acid compositions of neutral glycosphingolipids are similar to those of other sphingolipids. Gas chromatographic analyses have established that the glycosphingolipids have a characteristic mixture of components in which behenic (22:0), lignoceric (24:0), and nervonic (24:1) acids are usually predominant. Table 31-3 summarizes the fatty acid composition of selected human tissue glycosphingolipids.

The α-hydroxy fatty acids are either absent or present in trace amounts in most glycosphingolipids analyzed except kidney monohexosyl and dihexosyl ceramides [136] and galactosyl ceramide of brain [150], where they may be greater than 50 percent of the total fatty acids.

Variation in fatty acid composition by organ, species, and chain length of the oligosaccharide moiety has been reported. For example, in porcine erythrocytes the amounts of palmitic, stearic, and oleic acids were highest in glucosyl ceramide and decreased with increasing oligosaccharide chain length; the amounts of behenic, lignoceric, and nervonic acids increased with oligosaccharide chain length [151].

Isolation and Determination

The neutral glycosphingolipids can be isolated from tissues [19, 22, 29, 30, 152–155], formed elements of blood [156–158], plasma [22, 157, 159], fibroblasts [27, 160], and urinary sediment cells [24, 26] by extraction with chloroform-methanol (2:1, v/v), yielding a mixture of total lipids. Differential extraction of the glycosphingolipids after initial acetone or ethanol-ether precipitation is especially useful with large-scale isolations [135, 152, 161–163]. Polar glycerophosphatides are generally removed by alkali-catalyzed methanolysis of a lipid fraction containing glycosphingolipids, either before [22, 136, 154, 159, 160, 162] or after chromatographic purification [24, 135, 156, 157]. The individual glycosphingolipids can then be separated on silicic acid [30, 135, 136, 154, 158, 159, 162] or Florisil [29, 30, 136, 154–156, 160]. Subsequent chromatography on DEAE-cellulose has been used to remove acidic glycosphingolipids [135, 136, 155, 159, 164]. With samples of less than 10 gm of tissue or less than 50 ml of plasma or erythrocytes, these separations are carried out most conveniently by preparative thin-layer chromatography.

The quantitative estimation of the individual glycosphingolipids can be based on colorimetric and gas-chromatographic determinations of carbohydrate after acid hydrolysis or acid-catalyzed methanolysis of the lipids [165].

Table 31-3. FATTY ACID COMPOSITION OF THE NEUTRAL GLYCOSPHINGOLIPIDS FROM VARIOUS NORMAL HUMAN SOURCES*

	Monohexosyl ceramide		*Dihexosyl ceramide*				*Trihexosyl ceramide*				*Tetrahexosyl ceramide*		
Fatty acid	Kidney† [136]	Spleen [153]	Erythrocytes [234]	Leukocytes [156]	Kidney† [136]	Spleen [153]	Erythrocytes [235]	Kidney [136]	Liver [230]	Cultured skin fibroblasts [236]	Erythrocytes [234]	Kidney [136]	Spleen [230]
16:0	9.0	29.5	6.0	27.4	14.9	46.1	3.5	6.3	12.6	3.5	6.0	5.5	6.8
18:0	2.8	7.6	4.0	3.9	2.8	3.9	2.4	3.3	6.1	7.3	2.0	3.2	2.7
18:1	1.7	6.2	. . .	5.6	0.6	0.1	1.4	0.2	2.2	1.7	. . .	0.3	1.0
20:0	5.3	2.7	2.0	0.6	5.3	4.4	0.6	7.3	5.2	1.9	1.0	6.8	4.1
22:0	22.2	12.6	14.0	4.3	17.2	13.0	14.3	21.8	25.7	32.4	12.0	20.6	21.4
23:0	9.6	6.6	. . .	. . .	3.9	5.0	4.2	2.7	13.0	6.1	3.0	2.8	8.0
24:0	27.1	14.8	48.0	12.9	20.4	24.2	54.9	23.8	29.2	41.4	35.0	24.8	36.2
24:1	17.5	16.5	24.0	38.3	29.5	2.7	15.5	30.1	5.2	3.7	40.0	32.0	19.5
Other‡	4.8	3.5	2.0	7.0	5.4	0.6	3.2	4.5	0.8	2.	1.0	4.0	0.3

* Results are expressed as percentage of total fatty acids.
† Mixtures of glucosyl and galactosyl ceramides; digalactosyl and lactosyl ceramides.
‡ Small amounts of shorter- and longer-chain fatty acids were summed for convenience.

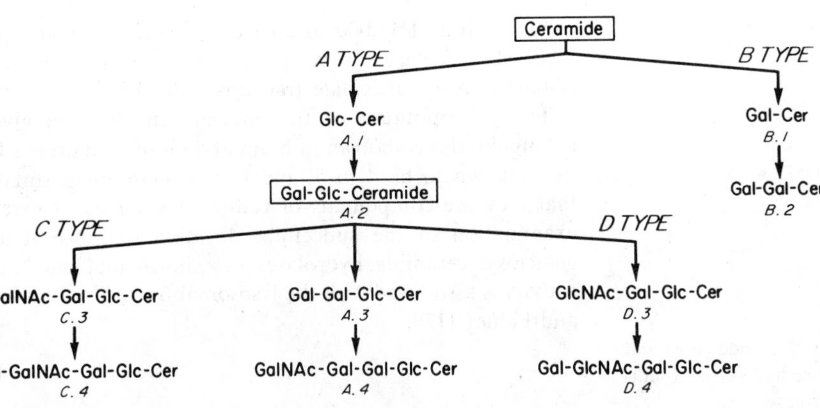

Figure 31-9. Steps in the biosynthesis of neutral glycosphingolipids from ceramide, involving sugar nucleotides and specific glycosyl transferases. The occurrence of enzymes involved in the formation of B.2, C.4, and D.4 has not yet been demonstrated, but these steps are included to show complete pathways.

Biosynthesis

The neutral glycosphingolipids are believed to be synthesized in all cells from ceramide by a multienzyme system of glycosyl transferases. Although only a few studies in vitro have been made with the glycolipids, there is a growing body of evidence in support of such a system from studies of ganglioside biosynthesis in cell-free preparations from embryonic chicken brain [166, 167]. The stepwise conversion of ceramide to Glc-Cer and Gal-Glc-Cer, as shown in Fig. 31-9, has been demonstrated with glucosyl transferase and galactosyl transferase from embryonic brain [167], and confirms earlier work on the biosynthesis of cerebrosides in the brain [167–170] and in other tissues such as spleen [171]. The conversion of Glc-Cer to Gal-Glc-Cer has also been observed with crude homogenates from rat spleen [172].

The scheme shown in Fig. 31-9 is tentative from Gal-Glc-Cer to globoside, Forssman hapten, and Gal-Gal-Cer, since the analogous steps in their synthesis have not been demonstrated with cell-free preparations.

There are two important points where the pathway divides to give three different families of glycosphingolipids. Ceramide itself can react with either of two sugar nucleotides, UDP-Glc or UDP-Gal, to form the Type A and Type B glycolipids, respectively. Lactosyl ceramide (Gal-Glc-Cer) is a key intermediate in the synthesis of the neutral tetrahexosyl ceramides such as red blood cell globoside and Forssman hapten, and it is also involved in the initiation of ganglioside biosynthesis by reaction with UDP-galactosamine to give GalNAc-Gal-Glc-Cer (C.3) [173] or with CMP-N-acetylneuraminic acid to give the simplest ganglioside, G_{M3} (NANA-Gal-Glc-Cer) [166].

It has been suggested that the glycosphingolipids are primarily associated with plasma membrane fractions of the cell in visceral organs, and it is probable that these glycosphingolipids are made by the cells where they are found. The recent observation of a striking degree of organ specificity in the nature and proportions of various glycolipids is compatible with these suggestions.

Erythrocyte glycosphingolipids such as Gal-Glc-Cer, Gal-Gal-Glc-Cer, and GalNAc-Gal-Gal-Glc-Cer (globoside) are probably synthesized in the bone marrow and incorporated there into the erythrocyte membrane. It has been shown, for example, that cultured bone marrow cells are capable of incorporating ^{14}C-glucosamine into acid-insoluble stromal components that are presumed to be gangliosides [174]. The kinetics of incorporation of ^{14}C-glucose into globoside and other glycosphingolipids of circulating porcine erythrocytes also supports this hypothesis [151, 201].

Plasma neutral glycosphingolipids are derived from at least two sources [151, 201]. Experiments using labeled glucose have shown that the plasma pools of glycosphingolipids are labeled in a manner comparable to the labeling of triglycerides and phospholipids after injection of fatty acids. This suggests that the glycolipids are also synthesized in the liver [151, 175, 201]. In an experiment in pigs, the plasma glycolipid pools were also found to be relabeled at a later time that corresponded both to the average life-span of the erythrocyte and to the time when labeled glycosphingolipid was lost from the erythrocyte pool [201]. This latter period of labeling accounted for approximately 80 percent of the total found in the pool of plasma glycosphingolipids during the 3 months of the study. This suggested that the glycolipids of senescent red blood cell membrane are lost directly into plasma and account for much of the circulating plasma glycosphingolipids.

METABOLISM

Glycosphingolipid catabolism has been studied in a number of laboratories, and a large number of relatively specific glycosyl hydrolases have been isolated [176–181]. It is apparent from these studies that a specific catabolic enzyme controls each step in the degradation of the glycosphingolipids by a pathway that is the reverse of biosynthesis, as shown in Fig. 31-10 for globoside. Preparations have been obtained from hog epididymis that contain a β-N-acetylgalactosaminyl hydrolase specific for hydrolysis of the terminal GalNAc residue of erythrocyte globoside [182]. The Forssman-active kidney globoside that contains a terminal N-acetylgalactosamine residue with an α glycosidic bond is not a substrate for this enzyme [133].

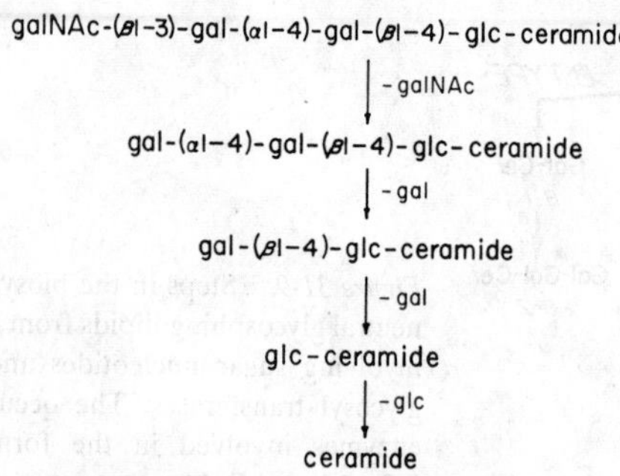

Figure 31-10. Pathway for the catabolism of globoside (top) and related glycosphingolipids, involving the stepwise hydrolysis of individual sugar residues by specific glycosyl hydrolases.

A galactosyl hydrolase that is specific for Gal-Gal-Glc-Cer has been found in particulate fractions from small intestine, spleen, kidney, brain, and liver [180]. It is inert toward glycosphingolipids such as Gal-Glc-Cer and Gal-Cer, both of which have β-galactosidic linkages. Recently, it has been shown that human and porcine plasma contain a protein fraction that is highly active in hydrolyzing the terminal Gal of this trihexosyl ceramide, and this enzymatic activity exhibited a bimodal pH optimum at 5.4 and 7.2. These findings suggest that there are two forms of the enzyme [183].

Enzymes that are capable of cleaving lactosyl ceramide (Gal-Glc-Cer) and Glc-Cer have been partially purified from brain [176, 184], small intestine [179], and spleen [185], and a β-galactosyl hydrolase that catalyzes the removal of galactose from Gal-Cer has also been studied [177, 179]. A glucosyl hydrolase that acts upon Glc-Cer has been found in leukocytes [186, 187]. The metabolism of neutral glycosphingolipids has been reviewed recently [151, 188, 189].

Ceramide is hydrolyzed by a ceramidase that has been isolated from rat brain [176]. Sphingosine formed by this reaction can be further degraded, through an intermediate phosphate and palmitaldehyde, to palmitic acid [190, 191], as shown in Fig. 31-11.

The subcellular distribution of several of the glycosyl hydrolases and ceramidase has been studied. The α-galactosyl hydrolase for Gal-Gal-Glc-Cer is contained in a particle that sediments between 700 and 12,000 × g [180]. The β-galactosyl and β-glucosyl hydrolases and ceramidase from brain are also associated with particles that sediment with

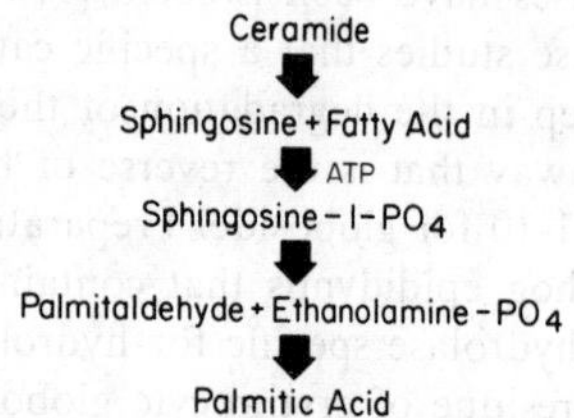

Figure 31-11. Metabolism of ceramide to fatty acid, with the intermediate formation of sphingosine-1-phosphate.

mitochondria at 15,000 to 20,000 × g [192]. Similarly, the glycosyl hydrolases from spleen and intestine were also obtained from particulate fractions [179, 185].

The pH optimum of the enzymes involved in glycosphingolipid metabolism in brain and peripheral organs has been shown to be 4 to 5, and it was therefore postulated that they are components of cellular lysosomes. A careful examination of the subcellular location of glucosyl and galactosyl ceramide hydrolases has shown that maximum activity is associated with the lysosomal fractions of rat liver and kidney [129].

CHEMICAL ABNORMALITIES IN FABRY'S DISEASE

The Nature of Accumulated Glycosphingolipids

Trihexosyl Ceramide

The enzymatic defect in Fabry's disease leads to widespread deposition of Gal-Gal-Glc-Cer, a trihexosyl ceramide of Type A.3. The complete chemical structure of this glycosphingolipid is illustrated in Fig. 31-12. The arrangement of the glucose and two galactose units in the Gal-Gal-Glc-Cer isolated from Fabry kidney [19, 22, 30], heart [22], and lymph nodes [30] was identical with that from normal kidney [136, 152], spleen [163], and serum [159]. The assignment of the positions of the linkages of glycosidic bonds was based on chemical analyses of material from kidney [19, 20, 30, 193] and lymph nodes [30] and agrees with the results obtained for material isolated from normal kidney [152], spleen [163], and serum [159].

The stereochemical configuration of the terminal Gal-Gal linkage of the trihexoside was more difficult to establish. Initially it was concluded that this linkage was β [193]. Enzymatic studies [206, 206a], however, suggested that the activity of an α-galactosidase was deficient in Fabry's disease. We have recently performed further nuclear magnetic resonance studies of sodium borohydride–reduced oligosaccharide purified from Fabry trihexosyl ceramide. These indicate that either the Gal-Gal or Gal-Glc linkage is α [193a], and identical results have been reported by Handa, Ariga, Miyatake, and Yamakawa [193b]. Li and Li have shown with highly specific glycosidases that the Gal-Gal linkage in the trihexoside is α and the Gal-Glc linkage is β [134b]. The same is true for trihexoside in normal human kidney [134b].

Digalactosyl Ceramide

Digalactosyl ceramide (Gal-Gal-Cer, Type B.2) was also found in abnormally high concentrations in kidneys from several patients with Fabry's disease [19–22, 30]. Abnormal amounts of this glycosphingolipid were also present in urine sediment cells [24] and in pancreas [29]. The Gal (1 → 4) Gal structure of the carbohydrate portion of the lipid in

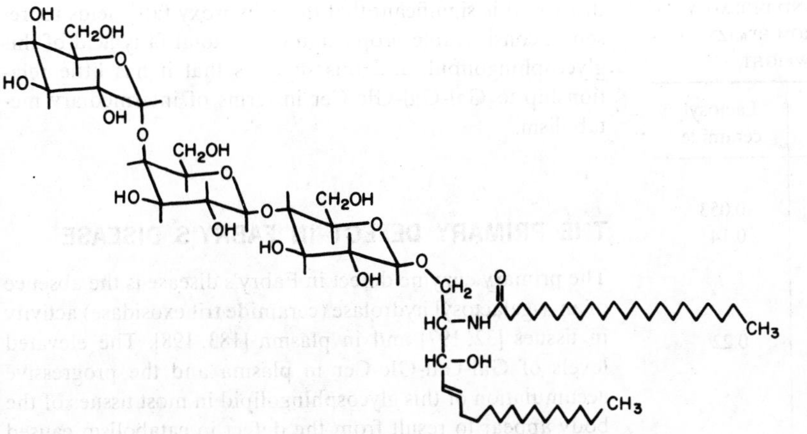

Figure 31-12. Complete chemical structure of the ceramide trihexoside that accumulates in tissues and fluids in Fabry's disease.

Fabry's tissues has been established by permethylation studies [21, 30] and is identical with results reported for a digalactosyl ceramide from mouse kidney [194] and rat kidney [195]. Small amounts of the same glycosphingolipid appear to be present in normal human kidney [136, 196], but chemical confirmation of the structure has not been made. Handa and colleagues have recently reported nuclear magnetic resonance studies indicating that the Gal-Gal linkage in the dihexoside accumulating in Fabry kidney also has the α configuration [193b].

Abnormal Distribution in Tissues

The distribution of glycosphingolipids in the organs and tissues of patients with Fabry's disease has been investigated in several laboratories [22, 29, 30]. Since increased concentrations of Gal-Gal-Glc-Cer were found in all the sources analyzed except erythrocytes, it appeared that most tissues are involved in the catabolism of glycosphingolipids of the globoside type. The level of Gal-Gal-Glc-Cer in erythrocytes was normal, and it is probable that globoside catabolism does not occur in these cells.

A summary is given in Table 31-4 of tissues in which increased concentrations of glycosphingolipids have been reported in patients with Fabry's disease. In one patient the magnitude of glycosphingolipid accumulation was thirty- to three-hundred-fold higher than normal levels [29]. The greatest accumulations of lipid were found in kidney, lymph node, vessels, prostate, and autonomic ganglia [22, 29, 30]. Lower concentrations of glycosphingolipids were found in cerebral cortex than in other parts of the brain [22, 29].

Table 31-5 contains a summary of the concentrations of Gal-Gal-Glc-Cer, Gal-Glc-Cer, and Gal-Gal-Cer found by several investigators for kidney, lymph node, and heart from patients with Fabry's disease. Thin-layer and gas chromatographic studies of isolated tissue glycosphingolipids show

Table 31-4. TISSUES AND ORGANS CONTAINING INCREASED CONCENTRATIONS OF NEUTRAL GLYCOSPHINGOLIPIDS FROM PATIENTS WITH FABRY'S DISEASE

Source	Reference
Nervous system:	
Autonomic ganglia	[29]
Brachial plexus	[231]
Brain	[231]
Brain stem	[29]
Cerebral cortex	[22, 29]
Corona radiata	[22]
Globus pallidus	[22]
Thalamus	[29]
Sympathetic nerve	[231]
Organs:	
Heart	[22, 29, 231]
Kidney	[22, 29, 30, 231]
Large intestine	[30]
Small intestine	[32]
Liver	[29, 30, 126, 231]
Lung	[28, 231]
Lymph node	[29, 30, 32, 205]
Pancreas	[29]
Prostate	[29, 30, 231]
Spleen	[29, 30, 231]
Tonsils	[205]
Vessels:	
Aorta	[30, 231]
Renal artery	[29]
Tissues:	
Smooth muscle	[29]
Striated muscle	[29]
Subcutaneous fat	[205]
Other sources:	
Cultured skin fibroblasts	[33]
Plasma or serum	[22, 23]
Urinary sediment	[24–26, 205]

Table 31-5. CONCENTRATIONS OF TRIHEXOSYL AND DIHEXOSYL CERAMIDES IN KIDNEY, LYMPH NODE, AND HEART FROM HEMIZYGOTES WITH FABRY'S DISEASE, MG PER GM WET WEIGHT

Source	Trihexosyl ceramide	Digalactosyl ceramide	Lactosyl ceramide
Kidney:			
Normal [136]	0.23	0.053	0.053
Normal [230]	0.36	.....	0.14
Fabry [19]	15.0		
Fabry [22]	3.0–23.0*		
Fabry [30]	28.0	16.0	
Fabry	1.80	0.69	0.22
Lymph node:			
Fabry [30]	30.0		
Fabry [205]	8.4–13.2*		
Heart:			
Fabry [22]	14.0		

* Range of three patients with Fabry's disease.

that Gal-Gal-Glc-Cer is the major glycosphingolipid in these and all other tissues that have been examined [22, 28–30]. No preferential accumulation of these glycosphingolipids was found in the renal cortex or papillary regions [29]. Table 31-6 compares the levels of Gal-Gal-Glc-Cer and other neutral glycosphingolipids in plasma, urinary sediment, and cultured skin fibroblasts from normal volunteers and patients.

Accumulation of Gal-Gal-Cer has been reported only in the kidney [19, 21, 22, 29, 30], pancreas [29], and urinary sediment [24]. The lipid precursor of Gal-Gal-Cer has not yet been identified, and the mechanism for the storage of this lipid is not clearly understood.

Table 31-7 contains a summary of the fatty acid compositions of Gal-Gal-Glc-Cer isolated from various sources in patients with Fabry's disease. Behenic, lignoceric, and nervonic acids were the major components, but there was considerable variation in the proportions of these fatty acids from tissue to tissue. Only small amounts of α-hydroxy fatty acids have been found in this glycosphingolipid. Table 31-8 compares the percentages of normal and α-hydroxy fatty acids in the dihexosyl ceramide (predominantly Gal-Gal-Cer) accumulated in the kidney of hemizygotes with Fabry's disease. It is significant that the α-hydroxy fatty acids represent a considerable proportion of the total fatty acid of this glycosphingolipid, and this suggests that it has little relationship to Gal-Gal-Glc-Cer in terms of intermediary metabolism.

THE PRIMARY DEFECT IN FABRY'S DISEASE

The primary enzyme defect in Fabry's disease is the absence of an α-galactosyl hydrolase (ceramide trihexosidase) activity in tissues [32, 197] and in plasma [183, 198]. The elevated levels of Gal-Gal-Glc-Cer in plasma and the progressive accumulation of this glycosphingolipid in most tissues of the body appear to result from the defect in catabolism caused by the absence of this enzyme activity (see Fig. 31-10).

Brady and colleagues [180] noted that the ceramide trihexosidase was not inhibited by many β-galactosides, and Kint [206] found that the leukocytes in Fabry's disease had normal activities of β-galactosidase. He then provided the first definite evidence that α-, not β-, galactosidase activity was severely deficient or absent. This has been confirmed by Romeo and Migeon using leukocytes and skin fibroblasts [206a] and by Handa and colleagues [193b] using Fabry kidney. In an elegant study Romeo and Migeon also used α-galactosidase assays to show that skin fibroblasts from female carriers of the disease have two distinct clonal populations of cells, one containing almost no α-galactosidase activity, the other normal activity. The activity of β-galactosidase was the same, and at normal levels, in both cell populations from the heterozygous females [206a]. Several artificial α- or β-galactosides were used as substrates for the above studies. The final proof of the configuration of the Gal-Gal bond, and, hence, of the enzymatic deficiency, awaits the synthesis of trihexoside and dihexoside having the terminal α linkage and their employment as substrates to test the enzymatic activities in normal and Fabry tissues. It now appears reasonably certain, however, that deficiency of an α-glycosidase is the basis for accumulation of both of the glycolipids accumulating in Fabry's disease.

Assays for enzymatic activity in a particulate fraction (presumably lysosomes) [125, 129] from biopsied kidney and

Table 31-6. CONCENTRATIONS OF NEUTRAL GLYCOSYL CERAMIDES IN VARIOUS TISSUES IN NORMAL SUBJECTS AND HEMIZYGOTES WITH FABRY'S DISEASE

Neutral glycosyl ceramides	*Plasma* [23], *μmoles/100 ml*		*Urinary sediment* [24], *μmoles/24-hr urine*		*Cultured skin fibroblasts* [27], *μmoles/gm dry wt*	
	Normal	Fabry	Normal	Fabry	Normal	Fabry
GL-1*	0.98	0.78	0.04	0.02–0.16	1.44	1.45
GL-2	0.55	0.47	0.04	0.02–0.40	0.34	0.22
GL-3	0.21	0.76	0.02	0.12–4.91	0.69	2.23
GL-4	0.28	0.31	0.02	0.03–0.64	0.31	0.33

*Denotes number of glycosyl residues.

Table 31-7. FATTY ACID COMPOSITION OF TRIHEXOSYL CERAMIDE IN VARIOUS SOURCES FROM HEMIZYGOTES WITH FABRY'S DISEASE*

Fatty acid	Kidney		Pancreas [94]	Heart		Lymph node [30]	Cultured skin fibroblasts [236]
	[30]	[19]		[29]	[22]		
16:0	8.5	2.6	9.0	4.1	2.4	13.6	7.8
16:1	. . .	. . .	1.4	0.8	. . .	. . .	1.4
17:0	. . .	. . .	0.3	tr	. . .	. . .	0.2
18:0	4.6	2.4	3.3	15.9	7.2	3.8	13 6
18:1	2.0		1.7	1.9	0.8	1.0	4.4
20:0	6.6	6.7	5.9	10.2	9.6	6.8	2.9
21:0	. . .	0.3	. . .	. . .	1.5	1.3	0.2
22:0	28.1	35.8	17.2	24.5	23.9	22.7	21.4
22:1	. . .	1.8	15.7	1.0			
23:0	6.2	4.7	5.1	9.3	2.5	8.6	5.0
24:0	27.8	33.5	23.4	10.3	19.2	30.5	37.9
24:1	16.2	13.1	14.6	20.8	25.5	11.7	4.8
Other†	. . .	. . .	1.9	1.4	7.4	. . .	0.4

* Results are expressed as percentage of total fatty acids.
† Shorter- and longer-chain fatty acids have been summed for convenience.

small-intestinal mucosal cells and in heparinized plasma are summarized in Table 31-9. There was no detectable enzymatic activity in any of the hemizygous male patients. Heterozygous females had intermediate levels of enzymatic activity, which can be associated with a less severe accumulation of Gal-Gal-Glc-Cer in the plasma and urinary sediment [23, 24].

Table 31-8. FATTY ACID COMPOSITION OF DIHEXOSYL CERAMIDE FROM HEMIZYGOTES WITH FABRY'S DISEASE*

Component	[193]	[29]†	[30]
16:0	2.0	16.0	0.8
h‡16:0	1.1	. . .	1.4
18:0	1.1	8.3	0.4
h18:0	0.7	. . .	0.6
18:1	0.3	13.1	
20:0	1.2	6.1	2.9
h20:0	1.5	. . .	2.3
22:0	3.0	18.8	8.3
h22:0	12.0	. . .	18.5
22:1	. . .	3.9	
23:0	0.4	2.0	2.1
h23:0	2.5	. . .	5.9
24:0	2.6	15.4	12.4
h24:0	15.4	. . .	39.9
24:1	1.4	9.5	2.0
h24:1	3.5	. . .	1.5
26:1	11.5		

* Results are expressed as percentage of total fatty acids.
† Analyses of hydroxy fatty acids were not reported by the authors.
‡ Signifies hydroxy acid.

The absence of ceramide trihexosidase in plasma and tissues has so far been restricted to patients with Fabry's disease. Normal levels of enzymatic activity were observed in particulate fractions from small intestine of abnormal control subjects such as patients with lymphoma, Hodgkin's disease, lymphosarcoma, and recurrent hypernephroma [32], and plasma levels of enzymatic activity were normal in patients with metachromatic leukodystrophy, Gaucher's disease (Type 1), and Tay-Sachs disease [199].

Normal plasma exhibited a bimodal curve of pH optimums with maximum ceramide trihexosidase activity at pH 5.4 and 7.2 [183]. The specific activity at pH 7.2 was about twice that at pH 5.4 (Table 31-9). It is not clear whether there are two forms of ceramide trihexosidase with different polypeptide chains or whether the two pH optimums are related to different arrangements of identical subunits. Both forms of the enzymatic activity were completely absent in blood from male patients with Fabry's disease. In the heterozygous females, on the other hand, the activity at pH 5.4 was diminished and that at pH 7.2 was absent. Studies of the purified proteins from hemizygous and heterozygous patients will probably provide an answer to the question about the relationship between the two forms of activity in plasma. The acidic form in plasma is presumed to be identical with that found in tissues, although the pH optimums are slightly different.

Enzyme Replacement

An attempt has been made to replace the deficient ceramide trihexosidase activity by infusion of normal plasma into patients with Fabry's disease [199]. Measurable levels of enzymatic activity were found in the plasma of these patients

Table 31-9. CERAMIDE TRIHEXOSIDASE ACTIVITIES IN PATIENTS WITH FABRY'S DISEASE AND CONTROL SUBJECTS*

Subject	Ceramide trihexosidase activity			
	Intestine [32], pH 5	Kidney [197], pH 5	Plasma [183, 198]	
			pH 5.4	pH 7.2
Controls	6.3 ± 0–9 (12)	4.6 (1)	7.8 ± 0.7 (20)	15.8 ± 1.8 (20)
Hemizygous males	<0.05 (2)	0 (1)	<0.7 (8)	<0.7 (8)
Heterozygous females	1.6 (1)		5.0 ± 0.9 (5)	<0.7 (5)

*Enzymatic activities with intestine and kidney are expressed as nanomoles of hexose liberated per milligram per hour; those with plasma are expressed as nanomoles of galactose liberated per milliliter per hour. Values in parentheses are the numbers of subjects.

after the infusion was completed, and the activity rose in 6 hr to maximum levels which were approximately 150 percent of the average found in normal plasma. Loss of ceramide trihexosidase from the plasma after the peak followed a complex curve which suggested a rapid turnover during the first day and a slower rate of loss for the following 6 days; after a week the activity could no longer be detected.

There was a gradual decrease in the concentration of Gal-Gal-Glc-Cer in the plasma following the infusion of normal plasma into the patients. Plasma enzyme replacement might therefore be used as a therapy for control of the glycosphingolipid levels in plasma and, possibly, to decrease the rate of accumulation of the lipid in tissues. Clinical examination after prolonged periods of intermittent plasma infusions will provide a test of this possibility.

PATHOPHYSIOLOGY

The majority of anatomic and physiologic abnormalities observed in Fabry's disease can be related directly to the cumulative deposition of glycosphingolipid in a variety of tissues. As the lipid deposition at a particular site reaches "threshold level," functional changes become manifest. Correlations have been reported between clinical severity and the level of glycosphingolipid deposition, on the basis of histochemistry [18, 200], chemical analysis [22], and electron microscopy [71]. Variations in glycosphingolipid deposition among affected individuals and families most likely depend on the residual activity of the deficient ceramide trihexosidase. It is known, for example, that heterozygotes having approximately 25 percent of normal enzymatic activity are only mildly affected [32, 183].

The pattern of accumulation of glycosphingolipids in Fabry's disease, particularly its predilection for blood vessels, is uniquely different from that seen in other sphingolipidoses. The difference may be explained mainly by the fact that globoside (GalNAc-Gal-Gal-Glc-Cer) is possibly released into the circulation from senescent erythrocytes [19, 201] and degraded there to trihexosyl ceramide. In Fabry's disease absence of trihexosyl ceramide α-galactosyl hydrolase [183] leads to an increased plasma level of Gal-Gal-Glc-Cer, which is presumably transported in a lipoprotein fraction. Globoside and other glycosphingolipids have been identified in both plasma high and low density lipoproteins, predominantly in the latter (personal communication from Sloan and Fredrickson). The Gal-Gal-Glc-Cer gains access to the endothelial and adjacent epithelial cells of the glomerulus and to endothelial cells and adjacent perithelial and smooth-muscle cells of blood vessels throughout the body, sites that are the most extensively involved areas of glycosphingolipid deposition. Deposits in other tissues may also be derived from diffusion of the globoside or Gal-Gal-Glc-Cer from the plasma and interstitial fluid. It is presumed that lysosomes in all cells are deficient in the acidic form of the enzyme, and fail to degrade glycosphingolipids of the globoside type, with resultant accumulation of the intermediate Gal-Gal-Glc-Cer. The latter is stored within extended multivesicular bodies or, in more advanced stages, as free intracytoplasmic masses which may lead to cellular dysfunction or degeneration. The metabolism of one other compound is also abnormal, as demonstrated by the presence of digalactosyl ceramide in the kidney [21, 22, 24, 29–31, 81] and pancreas [29]. The total amount of glycosphingolipids stored depends on time, the rate of accumulation, and possibilities for excretion.

That glycosphingolipid deposition is partly a function of time is illustrated by events after corneal biopsy. The regenerating corneal epithelium is initially clear but develops a golden haze within 3 months [202]. The rate of accumulation of lipid is probably determined by a number of factors. Perhaps the most important variable is the fractional activity of the mutant enzyme. Assuming that globoside from the erythrocyte membrane is a major precursor of accumulated Gal-Gal-Glc-Cer, factors affecting red blood cell survival and red blood cell mass may also be involved.

Excretion of glycosphingolipids from the kidney may be in the range of 0.1 to 6.0 mg per day [24]. There is little likelihood of appreciable excretion from other sites, although minor losses must occur by desquamation of corneal or bronchial epithelium.

The clinical signs and symptoms are best explained by consideration of the vascular lesions, the nervous system involvement, and the deposits of glycosphingolipid within kidney, myocardium, and other sites.

Vasculature

Narrowing, dilatation, motor unresponsiveness, and instability of blood vessels are major features of the altered physiology of Fabry's disease. The swollen endothelial cells, often accompanied by endothelial proliferation [29], encroach upon the lumen, with resultant focal increase of intraluminal pressure and peripheral ischemia. Such changes are frequently the precursors of thromboses and infarcts of the brain and other tissues. Muscle ischemia may contribute to pain or fatigue.

There may be progressive aneurysmal dilatation of the weakened vascular wall. This process is apparent in the transition from normality to telangiectasia and frank angiokeratoma in the skin, and in the progressive dilatation and microaneurysm formation of the retinal and conjunctival vessels [31].

Observed alterations of vasomotor control may reflect either the vascular lesions themselves or the extensive glycosphingolipid deposits in autonomic ganglia and perineural Schwann cells. The alteration of vasomotor response has been compared to that seen in patients with cold injury [35]. Both hemizygotes and heterozygotes with Fabry's disease demonstrate an impaired ability for vasoconstriction, and the more severely involved hemizygotes show, in addition, an inability of vasodilatation. Such a combined vascular and neural lesion may also explain the clinically observed temperature intolerance.

Nervous System

The peripheral neuropathy and involvement of peripheral and central autonomic nerve cells may be responsible for the paresthesias, pain, alteration of sweat production, such gastrointestinal symptoms as nausea and diarrhea, and a variety of vague neurologic signs and symptoms. The episodic fevers may be related to lesions of the hypothalamus [93].

Kidney

The observed disorders in renal function have their basis in lesions of the nephron and of renal vessels, and possibly in disorders of the posterior pituitary and hypothalamus. Early glycosphingolipid deposits antedate clinical signs and symptoms. During this early period, the lesions of the renal vasculature are less prominent than those of the nephron, and renal architecture is maintained [31]. The observed mild proteinuria may be explained by alteration of the glomerular epithelial cells and their foot processes [108] or by increased desquamation of lipid-laden tubular epithelial cells.

Loss of renal concentrating ability with polyuria [12, 111] and polydypsia [11, 37, 111] may occur well in advance of a significant decrease in glomerular filtration or evidence of renal failure. This diabetes insipidus-like syndrome, which is not related to faulty electrolyte transfer in distal tubules [111], may result from tubular insensitivity to antidiuretic hormone [111] or to combined dysfunction of the renal tubular cells and lesions of the glycosphingolipid-laden supraoptic nucleus, an antidiuretic center of the hypothalamus [38].

The later and more severe renal changes are the result of vascular lesions and of hypertension. The known immunologic properties of glycosphingolipids [203] have led to speculation that there may be an immune component in pathogenesis, particularly of the joint abnormalities and of certain nodose vascular lesions [114]. None of the electron microscopic observations of the glomerular basement membrane support such speculations for any immune type of glomerulonephritis.

Heart

Cardiac disorders seem to be related to the progressive infiltration of glycosphingolipid into myocardial cells and to the effects of hypertension and occlusive vascular lesions. Although infiltration of connective tissue of the valves has been observed [82], valvular lesions are infrequent.

Other Involvement

Pulmonary symptoms have been attributed to involvement of lung vasculature or bronchial and mucous gland epithelium. The dependent edema is not usually associated with hypoproteinemia or heart failure. Lymphatic obstruction or venous insufficiency with occasional frank varices may be responsible.

Reports of growth retardation, delayed puberty [46, 71], abnormal beard [38], or impaired fertility [80, 204] associated with a decrease of gonadotropins [63] may correlate with observations of testicular atrophy [205] or with glycosphingolipid storage in anterior and posterior lobes of the pituitary gland [101] or in the interstitial cells of the testis [81, 101]. No explanations have been offered for the frequently observed acromegaly-like appearance [38, 39, 41, 62, 72].

GENETICS

Mode of Inheritance

The genetics of Fabry's disease has been the subject of several recent reports [39, 46, 80, 204, 207, 208]. The disease is transmitted by an X-linked structural gene which is presumably responsible for the gene product, ceramide trihexosidase [32, 183]. Of the sphingolipidoses, only in Fabry's disease is the gene controlling the deficient hydrolytic enzyme on the X chromosome. As Brady [209] indicated, this is evidence that the entire sequence of genes for hydrolases involved in glycosphingolipid catabolism cannot be linked on the same chromosome, grouped in a particular operon.

The X-linked mode of inheritance is supported by the absence of male-to-male transmission, the absence of parental consanguinity, the occurrence of female-to-male transmission, and the measurable linkage between the loci for Fabry's disease and the Xg^a blood group antigen [46, 80, 208]. Further, the absence of any sign of the disease in more than 35 known sons of affected fathers, and the presence of three pedigrees in which two affected sons were born to the same mother by different fathers [14, 58, 207], clearly indicate the maternal transmission of this disease. Ten family pedigrees studied by Opitz [80] did not show a significant deviation from the 1:3 ratio of affected-to-normal sons expected in X-linked inheritance from all the daughters of known heterozygous grandmothers. Johnston et al. [46] identified an informative pedigree consistent with the Xg^a negative and deutan color-blindness genes being present on the same X chromosome of a male with Fabry's disease. The presence of these two well-established X-linked genes associated with Fabry's disease in this pedigree further supports the X-chromosomal locus of the Fabry gene. Chromosome studies of affected males demonstrated only normal karyotypes [31, 44, 46, 49, 210].

The disease is rare, and no estimate has been made of its frequency. Of over 200 reported cases, most of them have occurred in Caucasians. Latin American [66, 211, 212], Egyptian [213], and Oriental [87, 88, 214–216] patients have also been reported. No record of an affected Negro or Indian has been reported.

Penetrance and Variable Expressivity

The Fabry gene is highly penetrant in the hemizygote; no clinically normal sons of proved heterozygotes have had affected sons or carrier daughters. Clinical onset is variable, occurring usually during childhood, but may be delayed until the second or third decade [31, 46, 48, 49, 51, 99, 217–219].

Both intrafamilial and interfamilial variations in the clinical expression have been reported, the intrafamilial being less than the interfamilial variation [31, 39, 204]. It has been suggested [39] that modifying genes and environmental factors may be responsible for intrafamilial variations. Fabry variants have been reported without the classic skin lesions [31, 41, 43–50], and some without either skin lesions or corneal dystrophy [42].

On a molecular basis it is interesting to speculate that the interfamilial variation might be due to different intragenic mutations at the Fabry locus. These different structural mutations might alter the primary amino acid sequence of the Fabry enzyme and result in a quantitative heterogeneity of enzymatic activity among the families with the different Fabry alleles [220]. This is analogous to the findings in two other X-linked genes demonstrating variable expressivity: glucose-6-phosphate dehydrogenase [221] and hypoxanthine-guanine phosphoribosyl transferase [222]. Differing enzymatic activities might account for the Fabry genetic variants. Some mutant structural alleles may produce proteins with enough enzymatic activity so that glycosphingolipid deposition may not attain the threshold level necessary for certain clinical manifestations. Biochemical support for this speculation has already been reported. A Fabry hemizygote (W.R.), without the classic skin lesions, had the lowest levels of Gal-Gal-Glc-Cer in plasma [23] and urinary sediment [24] of the hemizygotes analyzed. Furthermore, Vance et al. [23] observed that the plasma glycosphingolipid profiles of four hemizygous sibs were similar to one another but were different from those of other families; they suggested a different mutation at the Fabry locus.

In heterozygous females penetrance is not complete, although the presence of the mutant gene may be demonstrated biochemically [23, 26, 34, 42]. Clinical expressivity in the heterozygote is variable. Proved heterozygotes may be completely asymptomatic throughout a normal life-span [80]. Franceschetti et al. [42] have identified clinically asymptomatic heterozygotes by their increased urinary Gal-Gal-Glc-Cer excretion. Approximately 20 percent of the heterozygotes have some skin lesions [80], a smaller percentage have the characteristic intermittent pain in the extremities [204], and about 80 percent have the whorl-like corneal dystrophy [42, 46]. Full clinical expression of the Fabry gene has been reported in a heterozygote who died at 47 years of age [13]. The variable expression in the heterozygote may be satisfactorily explained by Lyon's hypothesis [223]. At the cellular level, this hypothesis predicts that Fabry heterozygotes will have two populations of cells, one population with mutant enzyme and the other with normal enzyme activity [224]. The occurrence of two such cell populations in Fabry heterozygotes has been demonstrated in cultured skin fibroblasts [206a] as described above, but the intermediate level of trihexosyl ceramide galactosyl hydrolase activity assayed in a heterozygote [32] is consistent with Lyon's hypothesis.

Linkage Studies

The relative position of the Fabry locus on the X chromosome was first studied by Opitz et al. [80]. In an analysis of six families, these workers estimated that the loci for Fabry's disease and the X-linked blood group antigen, Xg^a, were linked by a distance of 27 centimorgans, with a recombination fraction of 0.27. Recently, Johnston et al. [208] pooled all available data on 10 families [46, 80] and reestimated the distance between these loci (Fabry and Xg^a). From the pooled data, the odds in favor of X linkage (as against autosomal linkage) were 6.4 to 1. A map interval of 24 centimorgans (with 95 percent confidence interval of 8 to 100 centimorgans) and a corresponding recombination fraction of 0.24 were calculated by a computer program for linkage analysis. An informative family provided data on the linkage relationship between the Fabry locus and the X-linked deutan color-blindness locus. These loci mapped with an interval of 17 centimorgans and a corresponding recombination fraction of 0.17 [208]. However, the confidence limits for the Fabry:deutan map interval were wide (1 to 156 centimorgans). This indicated weak linkage and the need for more data.

Genetic Counseling

Inheritance of the Fabry gene from hemizygotes and heterozygotes should be considered, since both genotypes transmit the gene. All sons of hemizygotes will be unaffected, but all daughters will be carriers of the gene. On the average, half the sons of heterozygotes will have the disease and half the daughters will be carriers. All possible carriers among close female relatives should be examined clinically and biochemically [23, 34, 225] for heterozygote identification. Fabry's disease has been detected antenatally from cultured fetal cells obtained by amniocentesis [226]. Genetic counseling should be made available to all families in which the diagnosis of Fabry's disease is made.

DIAGNOSIS

Many patients with Fabry's disease, both hemizygotes and heterozygotes, are discovered by deliberate investigation of the families of victims of the disease. The diagnosis in hemizygous males is most readily made clinically from the history and by observation of the characteristic skin lesions and corneal dystrophy. The diagnosis has been made in some boys during infancy [15]. The most common childhood manifestation before appearance of the lesions is recurrent fever in association with pain of the hands and feet. The disorder is often misdiagnosed as rheumatic fever [15, 66, 227, 228], neurosis, or erythromelalgia [229].

Presumptive diagnosis can be made by biopsy or from examination of the urinary sediment. Biopsy of the skin may reveal the characteristic refractile lipid in blood vessels. The presence of doubly refractile lipid bodies (Maltese crosses) in the urinary sediment confirms renal involvement, as does the demonstration in a renal biopsy of the characteristic renal lesions. The lipid-containing cells may occasionally be observed in aspirations of bone marrow [10]. The observation of dilated, tortuous retinal and conjunctival vessels and particularly the characteristic corneal dystrophy [43] may aid in the diagnosis.

The person suspected of being a heterozygote should be carefully examined for isolated skin lesions, particularly of the labia and posterolateral thighs. Detection may also be accomplished by careful ophthalmic examination [35, 37, 43], renal [35] and skin biopsies [38], or the finding of lipid-laden cells in the urinary sediment (Fig. 31-6) [62, 73].

Heterozygotes, hemizygous variants, and affected males can be identified biochemically even before the onset of clinical manifestations by the demonstration of increased levels of Gal-Gal-Glc-Cer in plasma [23], urinary sediment [24, 238], or cultured skin fibroblasts [33]. In addition the level of enzymatic activity can be assayed in biopsied intestinal mucosal cells [32] or, more easily, in plasma [183] leucocytes [206, 206a], or cultured skin fibroblasts [206a]. The diagnosis of Fabry's disease should be confirmed by biochemical analyses.

TREATMENT

In Fabry's disease the chronicity of the clinical events causes severe debilitation and incapacity that extends over years. Several therapeutic endeavors, based on the recent biochemical advances, are being actively investigated in an attempt to reduce this significant morbidity.

Enzyme replacement by infusion of normal plasma has been accomplished [199]. This offers the most immediate and direct approach. Enzymatic activity in hemizygous patients with Fabry's disease reached 150 percent of normal levels in plasma subsequent to infusion of normal plasma. This finding indicated that some form of enhancement had occurred, the mechanism of which is under active study. The enzymatic activity remained detectable in plasma for 7 days. During this period and subsequently, there was progressive decrease in the level in plasma of the substrate, Gal-Gal-Glc-Cer. The next approach will need to be prevention and control of glycosphingolipid deposition by administering plasma over a period of years to patients identified before clinical onset [24, 26]. More efficient replacement therapy may eventually be possible with purified enzyme from normal plasma.

Another approach to control of the levels of Gal-Gal-Glc-Cer by normal enzyme replacement conceivably could be renal transplantation. The active enzyme is present in normal renal tissues [197]; furthermore, renal transplantation would secondarily allow for direct treatment of overt or incipient azotemia.

Utilization of a Scribner shunt might provide a means for an ongoing glycosphingolipid substrate dialysis in which the coiled tubing [237] may act as a collector of the accumulated glycosphingolipid. If this latter method permits maintenance of sterility, an attachment of the arteriovenous shunt to a specific type of column packing devised to remove glycosphingolipids might also be feasible.

Further consideration ought to be given to methods for the reduction of the substrate load by decreasing the amount of the precursor, NAcGal-Gal-Gal-Glc-Cer. Since the major source of this glycosphingolipid presumably is the red blood cell membrane, a reduction of the erythrocyte population by phlebotomy would presumably decrease the amount of Gal-Gal-Glc-Cer in the plasma and its subsequent tissue deposition.

The crises of Fabry's disease are the most significant problem in morbidity. These painful, agonizing, and incapacitating days are of special importance to the patient and rank only behind azotemia in medical significance. Physiologic studies of patients in these crises indicate that electrolytes, pH, calcium, and phosphorus are normal [235]. The Gal-Gal-Glc-Cer level in plasma decreases during these crises (Desnick and Krivit et al., unpublished work), which may result from the precipitation of this compound into vascular endothelium, filtration into the nephron, or kidney epithelial deposition. During the crises, Seconal and Demerol have provided relief. Recently, prophylactic use of a low maintenance dose of diphenylhydantoin has been found to provide relief from the periodic crises of excruciating pain in hemizygotes and heterozygotes with Fabry's disease [239]. The results of a double blind triple cross-over study indicated that patients maintained on diphenylhydantoin had a striking remission of Fabry crises and discomfort, and that exacerbation of these episodes occurred when either an analgesic or placebo was substituted [239]. Symptomatic care of the patient with regard to cardiac, pulmonary, central nervous system, and renal symptoms otherwise remains nonspecific and empirical.

SUMMARY

1 Fabry's disease is an inborn error of glycosphingolipid catabolism characterized by the accumulation of a trihexosyl ceramide, Gal-Gal-Glc-Cer, in plasma and most tissues. Another glycolipid, Gal-Gal-Cer, is also elevated in kidney, pancreas, and urinary sediment. The trihexoside is a normal constituent of plasma and many tissues; the dihexoside has been isolated from normal kidney.

2 The specific biochemical defect is the absent enzymatic activity of trihexosyl ceramide galactosyl hydrolase (an α-galactosidase) in the lysosomes and plasma of hemizygous males. Heterozygotes have an intermediate level of enzymatic activity.

3 Hemizygous males have a characteristic skin lesion and extensive deposition of lipid in the endothelium, perithelium, and smooth muscle of blood vessels, in ganglion cells, in the heart, kidneys, eyes, and in most other tissues. The clinical sequelae include pain and paresthesias of the extremities, vessel ectasia in skin and mucous membrane, edema of the legs, hypohidrosis, albuminuria, and hyposthenuria. Severe renal impairment leads to hypertension and uremia. Death usually results from renal failure or from cardiac or cerebrovascular disease.

4 Heterozygous females may have an attenuated form of the disease, which includes most of the symptoms of the hemizygous males. Diagnosis has been confirmed by observation of a corneal epithelial dystrophy, demonstration of birefringent material in urinary sediment, demonstration of lipid deposition in skin and renal biopsies, biochemical assay of Gal-Gal-Glc-Cer levels from various sources, and enzymatic assay.

5 The disorder is transmitted by an X-linked gene. Intrafamilial and interfamilial variations occur. Genetic variants without the classic skin lesion have been described.

6 Confirmation of the clinical diagnosis in hemizygotes or heterozygotes should be made by chemical analyses for the stored lipids or by measurement of trihexoside ceramide hydrolase.

BIBLIOGRAPHY

1. Anderson, W.: A case of angiokeratoma. Brit. J. Derm., **10,** 113, 1898.
2. Fabry, J.: Ein Beitrag zur Kenntnis der Purpura haemorrhagica nodularis (Purpura papulosa hemorrhagica Hebrae). Arch. Derm. Syph., **43,** 187, 1898.
3. Steiner, L., and Voerner, H.: Angiomatosis miliaris: eine idiopathische Gefässerkrankung. Deutsch. Arch. Klin. Med., **96,** 105, 1909.
4. Gunther, H.: Anhidrosis und Diabetes insipidus. Z. Klin. Med., **78,** 53, 1913.
5. Weicksel, J.: Angiomatosis, bzw. Angiokeratosis universalis (eine sehr seltene Haut- und Gefässkrankheit). Deutsch. Med. Wschr., **51,** 898, 1925.
6. Ruiter, M., Pompen, A. W. M., and Wyers, H. J. G.: Über interne und pathologische-anatomische Befunde bei Angiokeratoma corporis diffusum (Fabry). Dermatologica (Basel), **94,** 1, 1947.
7. Pompen, A. W. M., Ruiter, M., and Wyers, H. J. G.: Angiokeratoma corporis diffusum (universale) Fabry, as a sign of an unknown internal disease: two autopsy reports. Acta Med. Scand., **128,** 234, 1947.
8. Scriba, K.: Zur Pathogenese des Angiokeratoma corporis diffusum Fabry mit cardio-vasorenalem Symptomenkomplex. Verh. Deutsch. Ges. Path., **34,** 221, 1950.
9. Hornbostel, H., and Scriba, K.: Zur Diagnostik des Angiokeratoma Fabry mit kardio-vasorenalem Symptomenkomplex als Phosphatid-speicherungskrankheit durch Probeexcision der Haut. Klin. Wschr., **31,** 68, 1953.
10. Fessas, P., Wintrobe, M. M., and Cartwright, G. E.: Angiokeratoma corporis diffusum universale (Fabry): first American report of a rare disorder. A.M.A. Arch. Intern. Med., **95,** 469, 1955.
11. Wallace, H. J.: Angiokeratoma corporis diffusum. Brit. J. Derm., **70,** 354, 1958.
12. Colley, J. R., Miller, D. L., Hutt, M. S. R., Wallace, H. J., and de Wardener, H. E.: The renal lesion in angiokeratoma corporis diffusum. Brit. Med. J., **1,** 1266, 1958.
13. Burda, C. D., and Winder, P. R.: Angiokeratoma corporis diffusum universale (Fabry's disease) in female subjects. Amer. J. Med., **42,** 293, 1967.
14. Wise, D., Wallace, H. J., and Jellinck, E. H.: Angiokeratoma corporis diffusum: a clinical study of eight affected families. Quart. J. Med., **31,** 177, 1962.
15. Stiles, F. D., and Opitz, J. M.: Diffuse angiokeratosis (Fabry's disease) in children (abstract). Meeting of the Midwest Society for Pediatric Research, Chicago, November, 1963.
16. Opitz, J.: Angiokeratoma corporis diffusum. Arch. Derm. (Chicago), **90,** 330, 1964.
17. Ruiter, M.: Das Angiokeratoma corporis diffusum Syndrom und seine Hauterscheinungen: Übersicht und eignene Erfahrungen der letzten zehn Jahre. Hautarzt, **9,** 15, 1958.
18. Ruiter, M.: Milestones in dermatology: angiokeratoma corporis diffusum. Excerpta Med., sect. XIII, 61, 1959.
19. Sweeley, C. C., and Klionsky, B.: Fabry's disease: classification as a sphingolipidosis and partial characterization of a novel glycolipid. J. Biol. Chem., **238,** 3148, 1963.

20. Sweeley, C. C., and Klionsky, B.: Fabry's disease: the isolation and characterization of a ceramide-trihexoside from kidney. Abstracts, Sixth International Congress of Biochemistry, New York, 1964.
21. Sweeley, C. C., and Klionsky, B.: Glycolipid lipidosis: Fabry's disease, in *The Metabolic Basis of Inherited Disease,* edited by J. B. Stanbury, J. B. Wyngaarden, and D. S. Fredrickson, 2d ed., p. 618. McGraw-Hill, New York, 1966.
22. Christenson-Lou, H. O.: A biochemical investigation of angiokeratoma corporis diffusum. Acta Path. Microbiol. Scand., **68,** 332, 1966.
23. Vance, D. E., Krivit, W., and Sweeley, C. C.: Concentrations of glycosyl ceramides in plasma and red cells in Fabry's disease: a glycolipid lipidosis. J. Lipid Res., **10,** 188, 1969.
24. Desnick, R. J., Sweeley, C. C., and Krivit, W.: A method for the quantitative determination of the neutral glycosphingolipids in urine sediment. J. Lipid Res., **11,** 31, 1970.
25. Kremer, G. J., and Denk, R.: Angiokeratoma corporis diffusum (Fabry). Lipoidchemische Untersuchungen des Harnsediments. Klin. Wschr., **46,** 24, 1968.
26. Philippart, M., Sarlieve, L., and Manacorda, A.: Urinary glycolipids in Fabry's disease: their examination in the detection of atypical variants and the presymptomatic state. Pediatrics, **43,** 201, 1969.
27. Matalon, R., Dorfman, A., Dawson, G., and Sweeley, C. C.: Glycolipid and mucopolysaccharide abnormality in fibroblasts of Fabry's disease. Science, **164,** 1522, 1969.
28. Bagdade, J. D., Parker, F., Ways, P. O., Morgan, T. E., Lagunoff, D., and Eidelman, S.: Fabry's disease: a correlative clinical, morphologic, and biochemical study. Lab. Invest., **18,** 681, 1968.
29. Schibanoff, J. M., Kamoshita, S., and O'Brien, J. S.: Tissue distribution of glycosphingolipids in a case of Fabry's disease. J. Lipid. Res., **10,** 515, 1969.
30. Miyatake, T.: A study on glycolipid in Fabry's disease. Jap. J. Exp. Med., **39,** 35, 1969.
31. Jensen, E.: On the pathology of angiokeratoma corporis diffusum (Fabry). Acta Path. Microbiol. Scand., **68,** 313, 1966.
32. Brady, R. O., Gal, A. E., Bradley, R. M., Martensson, E., Warshaw, A. L., and Laster, L.: Enzymatic defect in Fabry's disease: ceramide trihexosidase deficiency. New Eng. J. Med., **276,** 1163, 1967.
33. Dawson, G., Sweeley, C. C., Matalon, R., and Dorfman, A.: Chemical abnormalities of cultured skin fibroblasts in Fabry's disease. Fed. Proc., **28**(2), 540, 1969.
34. Desnick, R. J., and Krivit, W.: Fabry's disease: early detection and heterozygote identification by urine sediment glycolipid analyses. Presented before the American Society for Human Genetics, Austin, Texas, Oct.10, 1968.
35. Rahman, A. N., Simcone, F. A., Hackel, D. B., Hall, P. W., III, Hirsch, E. Z., and Harris, J. W.: Angiokeratoma corporis diffusum universale (hereditary dystopic lipidosis). Trans. Ass. Amer. Physicians, **74,** 366, 1961.
36. Colombi, A., Kostyal, A., Bracher, R., Gloor, F., Mazzi, R., and Tholen, H.: Angiokeratoma corporis diffusum—Fabry's disease. Helv. Med. Acta, **34,** 67, 1967.
37. von Gemmingen, G., Kierland, R. R., and Opitz, J. M.: Angiokeratoma corporis diffusum (Fabry's disease). Arch. Derm. (Chicago), **91,** 206, 1965.
38. de Groot, W. P.: Angiokeratoma corporis diffusum Fabry (thesaurismosis hereditaria Ruiter-Pompen-Wyers). Dermatologica (Basel), **128,** 321, 1964.
39. Johnston, A. W., Weller, S. D., and Warland, B. J.: Angiokeratoma corporis diffusum. Some clinical aspects. Arch. Dis. Child., **43,** 73, 1968.
40. Kahlke, W.: Angiokeratoma corporis diffusum (Fabry's disease), in *Lipids and Lipidoses,* edited by G. Schettler, p. 332. Springer, Berlin, 1967.
41. Fone, D. J., and King, W. E.: Angiokeratoma corporis diffusum (Fabry's syndrome). Aust. Ann. Med., **13,** 339, 1964.
42. Franceschetti, A. T., Philippart, M., and Franceschetti, A.: A study of Fabry's disease. I. Clinical examination of a family with cornea verticillata. Dermatologica (Basel), **138,** 209, 1969.
43. Francois, J., Snacken, J., and Stockmans, L.: Fabry's disease (glycolipid lipidosis). Path. Europ., **3,** 347, 1968.
44. Hamburger, J., Dormont, J., de Montera, H., and Hinglais, No.: Sur une singulière malformation familiale de l'épithélium renal. Schweiz. Med. Wschr., **94,** 871, 1964.
45. Johnston, A. W.: Fabry's disease without skin lesions. Lancet, **1,** 1277, 1967.
46. Johnston, A. W., Warland, B. J., and Weller, S. D. V.: Genetic aspects of angiokeratoma corporis diffusum. Ann. Hum. Genet., **30,** 25, 1966.
47. Kemp, G. L.: Fabry's disease involving the myocardium and coronary arteries. Vasc. Dis., **4,** 100, 1967.
48. Urbain, G., Peremans, J., and Philippart, M.: Fabry's disease without skin lesions? Lancet, **1,** 1111, 1967.
49. Wallace, R. D., and Cooper, W. J.: Angiokeratoma corporis diffusum universale (Fabry). Amer. J. Med., **39,** 656, 1965.
50. Wyers, H. J. F., Brugge, R. J., Pompe, C. A., and Pijpers, P. M.: Histologische Aspecten bij Ziekte van Fabry (angiokeratoma corporis diffusum). Nederl. T. Geneesk., **109,** 548, 1965.
51. Parkinson, J. E., and Sunshine, A.: Angiokeratoma corporis diffusum universale (Fabry) presenting as suspected myocardial infarction and pulmonary infarcts. Amer. J. Med., **31,** 951, 1961.
52. Falck, I., and Weicksel, A.: Angiokeratoma corporis diffusum Fabry mit vasorenalem Symptomenkomplex. Samml. Selt. Klin. Falle, **13,** 20, 1957.
53. Bethune, J. E., Landrigan, P. L., and Chipman, C. D.: Angiokeratoma corporis diffusum (Fabry's disease in two brothers). New Eng. J. Med., **264,** 1280, 1961.
54. Van Roey, A., and Wellens, W.: Angiokeratoma corporis diffusum van Fabry. Arch. Belg. Derm. Syph., **17,** 325, 1961.
55. Duperrat, B.: L'Angiokératome diffus de Fabry (angiokeratoma corporis diffusum). Presse Med., **67,** 1814, 1959.
56. Curry, H. B., and Fleisher, T. L.: Angiokeratoma corporis diffusum: a case report. J.A.M.A., **175,** 864, 1961.
57. Stoughton, R. B., and Clendenning, W. E.: Angiokeratoma corporis diffusum (Fabry). Arch. Derm. (Chicago), **79,** 601, 1959.
58. Brown, A., and Milne, J. A.: Diffuse angiokeratoma: report of two cases with diffuse skin changes, one with neurological symptoms and splenomegaly. Glasgow J. Med., **33,** 361, 1952.
59. Duperrat, B., and G. Pluvinage: Angiokératose diffuse de Fabry avec hémiplégie. Bull. Soc. Med. Hop. Paris, **72,** 748, 1956.
60. Hofmann, A., and Hauser, W.: Angiokeratoma corporis diffusum (Fabry) with cerebral manifestations. Deutsch. Z. Nervenheilk., **183,** 351, 1962.
61. Jacob, W., Gahlen, W., and Diekmann, H.: Zur differential-diagnosides Angiokeratoma Fabry und der Periarteriitis nodosa. Arz. Wschr., **8,** 551, 1953.
62. Spaeth, G. L., and Frost, P.: Fabry's disease: its ocular manifestations. Arch. Ophthal. (Chicago), **74,** 760, 1965.
63. Price, J. H.: Angiokeratoma corporis diffusum. Brit. J. Derm., **67,** 105, 1955.
64. Pittelkow, R. B., Kierland, R. R., and Montgomery, H.: Polariscopic and histochemical studies in angiokeratoma corporis diffusum. A.M.A. Arch. Derm., **76,** 59, 1957.
65. Krivit, W., Vance, D. E., Desnick, R., Whitecar, J. P., and Sweeley, C. C.: Red cell physiology in Fabry's disease. J. Lab. Clin. Invest., **12,** 906, 1968.
66. Karr, W. J., Jr.: Fabry's disease (angiokeratoma corporis diffusum universale): an unusual syndrome with multiple system involvement and unique skin manifestation. Amer. J. Med., **27,** 829, 1959.
67. Garcin, R., Hewitt, J., Godlewski, S., Laudat, P., De Montera, H., and Emile, J.: Les Aspects neurologiques de l'angiokératose de Fabry. À propos de deux cas. Presse Med., **75,** 435, 1967.
68. Lilis, M., Vulcan, P., and Peresecenschi, G.: Notes on a case of angiokeratoma corporis diffusum (Fabry's disease). Rum. Med. Rev., **20,** 29, 1966.
69. Pittelkow, R. B., Kierland, R. R., and Montgomery, H.: Angiokeratoma corporis diffusum. A.M.A. Arch. Derm., **72,** 556, 1955.
70. Lacroux, R.: Angiokératome diffus (angiokeratoma corporis diffusum) de Fabry. Bull. Soc. Franc. Derm. Syph., **67,** 474, 1960.
71. Ruiter, M., and Van Mullem, P. J.: Electron Microscopy Angiokeratoma corporis diffusum. Dermatologica (Basel), **138,** 346, 1969.

72. Dempsey, H., Hartley, M. W., Carroll, J., Balint, J., Miller, R. E., and Frommeyer, W. B.: Fabry's disease (angiokeratoma corporis diffusum): case report on a rare disease. Ann. Intern. Med., **63**, 1059, 1965.
73. Dubach, U. C., and F. Gloor: Fabry-Krankheit (Angiokeratoma corporis diffusum universale). Phosphatid-speicherkrankheit bei zwei Familien. Deutsch. Med. Wschr., **91**, 241, 1966.
74. Jeffries, J. L., and Barrett, J. C.: Medical grand rounds from the University of Alabama Medical Center. Southern Med. J., **56**, 518, 1963.
75. Rahman, A. N.: The ocular manifestations of hereditary dystopic lipidosis (angiokeratoma corporis diffusum universale). Arch. Ophthal. (Chicago), **69**, 708, 1963.
76. Siguier, F., Duperrat, B., Betourne, C., and Hanaut, A.: Angiokératose de Fabry, expression cutanée d'une maladie générale, nouvellement individualisée. Bull. Soc. Med. Hop. Paris, **72**, 291, 1956.
77. Wallace, H. J., and Colley, C.: Angiokeratoma corporis diffusum. Bull. Soc. Franc. Derm. Syph., **4**, 348, 1958.
78. Leng-Levy, Le Coulant, David-Chausse, Maleville, and Geniaux: Angiokératose familiale des membres inférieurs. Bull. Soc. Franc. Derm. Syph., **71**, 740, 1964.
79. Campbell, A. M. G., and Halford, M. E. H.: Syndrome of diarrhea and peripheral nerve changes due to generalized vascular disease. Brit. Med. J., **2**, 1509, 1964.
80. Opitz, J. M., Stiles, F. C., Wise, D., von Gemmingen, G., Race, R. R., Sander, R., Cross, E. G., and de Groot, W. P.: The genetics of angiokeratoma corporis diffusum (Fabry's disease), and its linkage with Xg (a) locus. Amer. J. Hum. Genet., **17**, 325, 1965.
81. Steward, V. W., and Hitchcock, C.: Fabry's disease (angiokeratoma corporis diffusum): a report of 5 cases with pain in the extremities as the chief symptom. Path. Europ., **3**, 377, 1968.
82. Ferrans, V. J., Hibbs, R. B., and Burda, C. D.: The heart in Fabry's disease: a histochemical and electron microscopic study. Amer. J. Cardiol., **24**, 95, 1969.
83. Tondeur, M., et al.: Fabry's disease in children: an electron microscopic study. Virchow. Arch. (Zellpath.), **2**, 239, 1969.
84. Leder, A. A., and Bosworth, W. C.: Angiokeratoma corporis diffusum universale (Fabry's disease) with mitral stenosis. Amer. J. Med., **38**, 814, 1965.
85. Ruiter, M., Pompen, A. W. M., and Wijers, H. J. G.: Angiokeratoma corporis diffusum (universale) als symptom van een onbekende en nog niet beschreven inwendige ziekte. Nederl. T. Geneesk., **90**, 1757, 1946.
86. Witschel, H., and Meyer, W.: Der Morbus Fabry als Beispiel einer erblichen Lipoidspeicherkrankheit. Klin. Wschr., **46**, 72, 1968.
87. Nakao, K., Mizuno, Y., Kano, S., Santo, H., Yano, Y., Mizoguchi, H., Uono, M., and Shibata, S.: A case of angiokeratoma corporis diffusum (Fabry's disease). J. Jap. Soc. Intern. Med., **56**, 369, 1967.
88. Uono, M.: Fabry's disease—from the standpoint of neuronal lipidosis. Jap. J. Clin. Med., **25**, 1587, 1967.
89. Ruiter, M.: Histological investigation of the skin in angiokeratoma corporis diffusum in particular with regard to the associated disturbance of phosphatid metabolism. Dermatologica (Basel), **109**, 273, 1954.
90. Hornbostel, H.: Das Angiokeratoma corporis diffusum universale mit kardio-vasorenalem Symptomenkomplex als neuartige Thesaurismoseform. Helv. Med. Acta, **19**, 388, 1952.
91. Germain, P., Caulet, T., Girard, P., Etienne, J. C., Adnet, J.-J., and Hopfner, C.: Angiokératose de Fabry familiale avec retentissement vasculaire et polyvisceral. Bull. Soc. Med. Hosp., **118**, 299, 1967.
92. Falck, I.: Angiokeratoma corporis diffusum Fabry mit vasorenalem Symptomenkomplex. Samml. Selt. Klin. Falle, **9**, 20, 1955.
93. Rahman, A. N., and Lindenberg, R.: The neuropathology of hereditary dystopic lipidosis. Arch. Neurol. (Chicago), **9**, 373, 1963.
94. Caulet, T., Germain, P., Adnet, J.-J., Hopfner, C., and Pluot, M.: Deux cas familiaux de maladie de Fabry: étude structurale et ultrastructurale. Ann. Anat. Path. (Paris), **12**, 49, 1967.
95. Raine, D. N.: Biochemical classification of the sphingolipidoses, in *Some Inherited Disorders of Brain and Muscle,* edited by J. D. Allan and D. N. Raine, p. 89. Livingston, Edinburgh, 1969.
96. Sagebiel, R. W., and Parker, F.: Cutaneous lesions of Fabry's disease: glycolipid lipidosis—light and electron microscopic findings. J. Invest Derm., **50**, 208, 1968.
97. Tarnowski, W. M., and Hashimoto, K.: New light microscopic skin findings in Fabry's disease. Acta Derm.-Venereol., **49**, 386, 1969.
98. Morel-Maroger, L., Ganter, P., Ardaillou, R., Cathelineau, G., and Richet, G.: Des rapports avec l'angiokératose de Fabry et la cytodystrophie rénale familiale. Bull. Soc. Med. Hop. Paris, **117**, 49, 1966
99. Hashimoto, K., B. G. Gross, and W. F. Lever: Angiokeratoma corporis diffusum (Fabry): histochemical and electron microscopic studies of the skin. J. Invest. Derm., **44**, 119, 1965.
100. Ruiter, M., Some further observations on angiokeratoma corporis diffusum. Brit. J. Derm., **69**, 137, 1957.
101. Witschel, H., and Meyer, W.: Fabry's disease: clinical and pathologic studies of a clinical case. Klin. Wschr., **46**, 305, 1968.
102. Bischoff, A., Fierz, U., Regli, G., and Ulrich, J.: Peripheral neurological disorders in Fabry's disease (angiokeratoma corporis diffusum universale): clinical and electron microscopic findings in a case. Klin. Wschr., **46**, 666, 1968.
103. Perrelet, A., Forssman, W. G., Franceschetti, A. T., and Rouiller, C. A.: A study of Fabry's disease. II. Light and electron microscopy. Dermatologica (Basel), **138**, 222, 1969.
104. Sagebiel, R., and Parker, F.: Electron microscopic observations relating Fabry's disease to other sphingolipidoses. Clin. Res., **14**, 273, 1966.
105. Frost, P., Spaeth, G. L., and Tanaka, Y.: Fabry's disease: glycolipid lipidosis. Skin manifestations. Arch. Intern. Med., **117**, 440, 1966.
106. Imperial, R., and Heliwig, E. B.: Angiokeratoma: a clinicopathological study. Arch. Derm. (Chicago), **95**, 166, 1967.
107. Van Mullem, P. J., and Ruiter, M.: Electron microscopic study of the skin in angiokeratoma corporis diffusum. Arch. Klin. Exp. Derm., **226**, 453, 1966.
108. McNary, W., and Lowenstein, L. M.: A morphological study of the renal lesion in angiokeratoma corporis diffusum universale (Fabry's disease). J. Urol., **93**, 641, 1965.
109. Rae, A. I., Lee, J. C., and Hopper, J.: Clinical and electron microscopic studies of a case of glycolipid lipidosis. J. Clin. Path., **20**, 21, 1967.
110. Funck-Brentano, J. L., Dormon, J., Mery, J. P., De Montera, H., and Moreira, M.: Les Lésions rénales de l'angiokératose de Fabry: á propos d'une observation. J. Urol. Nephrol., **70**, 826, 1964.
111. Henry, E. W., and Rally, C. R.: The renal lesion in angiokeratoma corporis diffusum (Fabry's disease). Canad. Med. Ass. J., **89**, 206, 1963.
112. Fierz, V., and Bischoff, A.: Angiokeratoma corporis diffusum. Dermatologica (Basel), **137**, 277, 1968.
113. Rahman, A. N.: The pathological basis of neurophysiological dysfunctions in hereditary dystopic lipidosis (angiokeratoma corporis diffusum universale). Clin. Res., **10**, 393, 1962.
114. Frost, P., Tanaka, Y., and Spaeth, G. L.: Fabry's disease—glycolipid lipidosis: histochemical and electron microscopic studies of two cases. Amer. J. Med., **40**, 618, 1966.
115. Witschel, H., and Mathyl, J.: Morphological elements of the specific ocular changes in Morbus Fabry. Klin. Mbl. Augenheilk., **154**, 599, 1969.
116. Knape, B. M., and Polman, H. A.: Fabry's disease diagnosed in childhood. Nederl. T. Geneesk., **113**, 1418, 1969.
117. Denk, R., and Sollberg, G.: Skelet Muskelbefunde beim Angiokeratoma corporis diffusum. Hautarzt, **17**, 248, 1966.
118. Adams, C. W. M.: *Neurohistochemistry.* Elsevier, Amsterdam, 1965.
119. Lehner, T., and Adams, C. W. M.: Lipid histochemistry of Fabry's disease. J. Path. Bact., **95**, 411, 1968.
120. Van Mullem, P. J., and Ruiter, M.: Histochemical studies on lipid metabolism in so-called Fabry's disease (angiokeratoma corporis diffusum). Arch. Klin. Exp. Derm., **232**, 148, 1968.
121. Hartley, M. W., and R. E. Miller: Renal and vascular changes in Fabry's disease, a dysphospholipidosis. J. Cell. Biol., **19**, 31A, 1963.
122. Hartley, M. W., Miller, R. E., and Lupton, C. H., Jr.: Dysphospholipidosis in Fabry's disease: a light and electron microscopic study. Alabama J. Med. Sci., **1**, 361, 1964.
123. Van Mullem, P. J., and Ruiter, M.: Electron microscopical investigation of the skin in angiokeratoma corporis diffusum. Dermatologica (Basel), **136**, 281, 1968.

124. Ruiter, M., and de Groot, W. P.: Methods of demonstration of lipid deposits in angiokeratoma corporis diffusum. Dermatologica (Basel), **135,** 75, 1967.
125. Tarnowski, W. M., and Hashimot, K.: Lysosomes in Fabry's disease. Acta Derm.-Venereol., **48,** 143, 1968.
126. Loeb, H., Jonniaux, G., Davis, P., Gregoire, P. E., and Wolff, P.: Étude clinique, biochimique et ultrastructurelle de la maladie de Fabry chez l'enfant. Helv. Paediat. Acta, **23,** 269, 1968.
127. Tanaka, Y., Frost, P., and Spaeth, G. L.: Figures myeliniques dans les cellules spumeuses de la maladie de Fabry. Nouv. Rev. Franc. Hemat., **5,** 425, 1965.
128. Lee, R. F., Balcerzak, S. P., and Westerman, M. P.: Gaucher's disease: a morphologic study and measurements of iron metabolism. Amer. J. Med., **42,** 891, 1967.
129. Weinreb, N. J., Brady, R. O., and Toppel, A. L.: The lysosomal localization of sphingolipid hydrolases. Biochim. Biophys. Acta, **159,** 141, 1968.
130. Jordan, S. W.: Electron microscopy of Gaucher cells. Exp. Molec. Path., **3,** 76, 1964.
131. Yamakawa, T., Nishimura, S., and Kamimura, M.: The chemistry of the lipids of posthemolytic residue or stroma of erythrocytes. XIII. Further studies on human red cell glycolipids. Japan J. Exp. Med., **35,** 201, 1965.
132. Ando, S., and Yamakawa, T.: On the oligosaccharide of Forssman-active sheep red-cell glycolipid, in *Chemistry and Metabolism of Glycosphingolipids,* edited by C. C. Sweeley, Chem. Phys. Lipids Suppl. North-Holland Publishing Company, Amsterdam, 1970, p. 91.
133. Makita, A., Suzuki, C., and Yosizawa, Z.: Biochemistry of organ glycolipid: chemical and immunological characterization of the Forssman hapten isolated from equine organs. J. Biochem. (Tokyo), **60,** 502, 1966.
134. Rapport, M. M., Schneider, H., and Graf, L., Cytolipin R: a pure lipid hapten isolated from rat lymphosarcoma. Biochim. Biophys. Acta, **137,** 409, 1967.
134a. Hakomori, S., Siddikui, B., Li, Y.-T., Li, S.-C., and Hellerquist, C. G.: Anomeric structures of globoside and ceramide trihexoside of human erythrocytes and hamster fibroblasts. J. Biol. Chem., **246,** 2271, 1971.
134b. Li, Y.-T., and Li, S.-C.: Anomeric configuration of galactose residues in ceramide trihexosides. J. Biol. Chem. In press.
135. Vance, W. R., Shook, C. P., III, and McKibbin, J. M.: The glycolipids of dog intestine. Biochemistry, **5,** 435, 1966.
136. Martensson, E.: Neutral glycolipid of human kidney. Isolation, identification, and fatty acid composition. Biochim. Biophys. Acta, **116,** 296, 1966.
137. Wiegandt, H.: The structure and the function of gangliosides. Angew. Chem. (Eng.), **7,** 87, 1968.
138. Hakomori, S. I., and Strycharz, G. D.: Investigations on cellular blood group substances. I. Isolation and chemical composition of blood group ABH and Le^b isoantigens of sphingoglycolipid nature. Biochemistry, **7,** 1279, 1968.
139. Hakomori, S. I., and Jeanloz, R. W.: Isolation of a glycolipid containing fucose, galactose, glucose and glucosamine from human cancerous tissue. J. Biol. Chem., **239,** PC3606, 1964.
140. Hakomori, S. I., Koscielak, J., Block, K. J., and Jeanloz, R. W.: Immunologic relationship between blood group substance and a fucose-containing glycolipid of adenocarcinoma. J. Immunol., **98,** 31, 1967.
141. Wiegandt, H.: Gangliosides of extra-neuronal tissue, in *Chemistry and Metabolism of Glycosphingolipids,* edited by C. C. Sweeley, Chem. Phys. Lipids Suppl. North-Holland Publishing Company, Amsterdam, 1970, p. 141.
142. Eto, T., Ichikawa, Y., Nishimura, K., Ando, S., and Yamakawa, T.: Occurrence of ceramide pentasaccharide in the membrane of erythrocytes and reticulocytes of rabbit. J. Biochem. (Tokyo), **64,** 205, 1968.
143. Carter, H. E., and Hirschberg, C. B.: Phytosphingosines and branched sphingosines in kidney. Biochemistry, **7,** 2296, 1968.
144. Karlsson, K. A.: Studies on sphingosines. VII. Existence of C_{18}- and C_{20}-phytosphingosines in animal tissues. Acta Chem. Scand., **18,** 2397, 1964.
145. Karlsson, K. A., and Martensson, E.: Studies on sphingosines. XIV. On the phytosphingosine content of the major human kidney glycolipids. Biochim. Biophys. Acta, **152,** 230, 1968.
146. Michalec, C., and Kolman, Z.: Biochemistry of sphingolipids. Chromatographic study of sphingolipids and sphingosine bases in normal human kidney. Clin. Chim. Acta, **13,** 525, 1966.
147. Puro, K., and Keranen, A.: Fatty acids and sphingosines of bovine-kidney gangliosides. Biochim. Biophys. Acta, **187,** 393, 1969.
148. Carter, H. E., Norris, W. P., Glick, F. S., Phillips, G. E., and Harris, R.: Biochemistry of the sphingolipides. II. Isolation of dihydrosphingosine from the cerebroside fractions of beef brain and spinal cord. J. Biol. Chem., **170,** 269, 1947.
149. Sambasivarao, K., and McCluer, R. H.: Lipid components of gangliosides. J. Lipid Res., **5,** 103, 1964.
150. Svennerholm, L., and Stallberg-Stenhagen, S.: Changes in the fatty acid composition of cerebrosides and sulfatides of human nervous tissue with age. J. Lipid Res., **9,** 215, 1968.
151. Sweeley, C. C., and Dawson, G.: Lipids of the erythrocyte, in *Red Cell Membrane Structure and Function,* edited by G. A. Jamieson and T. J. Greenwalt, p. 172. Lippincott, Philadelphia, 1970.
152. Makita, A.: Biochemistry of organ glycolipids. II. Isolation of human kidney glycolipids. J. Biochem. (Tokyo), **55,** 269, 1964.
153. Suomi, W. D., and Agranoff, B. W.: Lipids of the spleen in Gaucher's disease. J. Lipid Res., **6,** 211, 1965.
154. Gallai-Hatchard, J. J., and Gray, G. M.: The isolation and partial characterization of the glycolipids from pig lung. Biochim. Biophys. Acta, **116,** 532, 1966.
155. Philippart, M., Rosenstein, B., and Menkes, J. H.: Isolation and characterization of the main splenic glycolipids in the normal organ and in Gaucher's disease: evidence for the site of metabolic block. Biochem. Biophys. Res. Commun., **15,** 551, 1964.
156. Miras, C. J., Mantzos, J. D., and Levis, J. M.: The isolation and partial characterization of glycolipids of normal human leucocytes. Biochem. J., **98,** 782, 1966.
157. Vance, D. E., and Sweeley, C. C.: Quantitative determination of the neutral glycosyl ceramides in human blood. J. Lipid Res., **8,** 621, 1967.
158. Yamakawa, T., Irie, R., and Iwanaga, M.: The chemistry of lipid of posthemolytic residue or stroma of erythrocytes. IX. Silicic acid chromatography of mammalian stroma glycolipids. J. Biochem. (Tokyo), **48,** 490, 1960.
159. Svennerholm, E., and Svennerholm, L.: The separation of neutral blood-serum glycolipids by thin-layer chromatography. Biochim. Biophys. Acta, **70,** 441, 1963.
160. Hakomori, S., and Murakami, W. T.: Glycolipids of hamster fibroblasts and derived malignant-transformed cell lines. Proc. Nat. Acad. Sci. U.S.A., **59,** 254, 1968.
161. Carter, H. E., Rothfus, J. A., and Gigg, R.: Biochemistry of the sphingolipids. XII. Conversion of cerebrosides to ceramides and sphingosine: structure of Gaucher cerebroside. J. Lipid Res., **2,** 228, 1961.
162. Gray, J. M.: The isolation and partial characterization of the glycolipids of BP8/C3H ascites-sarcoma cells. Biochem. J., **94,** 91, 1965.
163. Makita, A., and Yamakawa, T.: Biochemistry of organ glycolipid. I. Ceramide—oligohexosides of human, equine, and bovine spleens. J. Biochem. (Tokyo), **51,** 124, 1962.
164. Rouser, G., Kritchevsky, G., and Yamamoto, A.: Column chromatographic and associated procedures for separation and determination of phosphatides and glycolipids, in *Lipid Chromatographic Analysis,* edited by G. V. Marinetti, p. 99. Marcel Dekker, Inc., New York, 1967.
165. Sweeley, C. C., and Vance, D. E.: Gas chromatographic estimation of carbohydrates in glycolipids, in *Lipid Chromatographic Analysis,* edited by G. V. Marinetti, p. 465. Marcel Dekker, Inc., New York, 1967.
166. Basu, S., Kaufman, B., and Roseman, S.: Conversion of Tay-Sachs ganglioside to monosialoganglioside by brain uridine diphosphate D-galactose: glycolipid galactosyl transferase. J. Biol. Chem., **240,** PC4115, 1965.
167. Basu, S., Kaufman, B., and Roseman, S.: Enzymatic synthesis of ceramide glucose and ceramide-lactose by glycosyltransferases from embryonic chicken brain. J. Biol. Chem., **243,** 5802, 1968.

168. Burton, R. M., Sodd, M. A., and Brady, R. O.: The incorporation of galactose in galactolipides. J. Biol. Chem., **233,** 1053, 1958.
169. Moser, H. W., and Karnovsky, M. L.: Studies on the biosynthesis of glycolipides and other lipides of the brain. J. Biol. Chem., **234,** 1990, 1959.
170. Nishimura, K., Ueta, N., and Yamakawa, T.: Incorporation of labeled hexose into brain cerebrosides. Jap. J. Exp. Med., **36,** 91, 1966.
171. Travis, E. G., and Brady, R. O.: Cerebroside synthesis in Gaucher's disease. J. Clin. Invest., **39,** 1546, 1960.
172. Hauser, G.: The enzymatic synthesis of ceramide lactoside from ceramide glucoside and UDP-galactose. Biochem. Biophys. Res. Commun., **28,** 502, 1967.
173. Burton, R. M.: Biochemistry of sphingosine containing lipids, in *Lipids and Lipidoses,* edited by G. Schettler, p. 134. Springer-Verlag, New York, 1967.
174. Dukes, P. P.: Erythropoietin-stimulated incorporation of 1-^{14}C-glucosamine into glycolipids of bone marrow cells in culture. Biochem. Biophys. Res. Commun., **31,** 345, 1968.
175. Baker, N.: The use of computers to study rates of lipid metabolism. J. Lipid Res., **10,** 1, 1969.
176. Gatt, S.: Enzymatic hydrolysis of sphingolipids. I. Hydrolysis and synthesis of ceramides by an enzyme from rat brain. J. Biol. Chem., **241,** 3724, 1966.
177. Gatt, S.: Enzymatic hydrolysis of sphingolipids. V. Hydrolysis of monosialoganglioside and hexosylceramides by rat brain β-galactosidase. Biochim. Biophys. Acta, **137,** 192, 1967.
178. Gatt, S., and Rapport, M. M.: Isolation of β-galactosidase and β-glucosidase from brain. Biochim. Biophys. Acta, **113,** 567, 1966.
179. Brady, R. O., Gal, A. E., Kanfer, J. N., and Bradley, R. M.: The metabolism of glucocerebrosides. III. Purification and properties of a glucosyl and galactosyl ceramide-cleaving enzyme from rat intestinal tissue. J. Biol. Chem., **240,** 3766, 1965.
180. Brady, R. O., Gal, A. E., Bradley, R. M., and Martensson, E.: The metabolism of ceramide trihexosides. I. Purification and properties of an enzyme that cleaves the terminal galactose molecule of galactosylgalactosylglucosyl-ceramide. J. Biol. Chem., **242,** 1021, 1967.
181. Frowein, Y., and Gatt, S.: Enzymatic hydrolysis of sphingolipids. VI. Hydrolysis of ceramide glycosides by calf brain β-N-acetylhexosaminidase. Biochemistry, **6,** 2783, 1967.
182. Miyatake, T., Handa, S., and Yamakawa, T.: Chemical structure of the main glycolipid of hog erythrocytes. Jap. J. Med., **38,** 135, 1968.
183. Mapes, C. A., Anderson, R. L., and Sweeley, C. C.: Trihexosyl ceramide: galactosyl hydrolase in normal human serum and plasma and its absence in patients with Fabry's disease. FEBS Letters, **7,** 180, 1970.
184. Gatt, S., and Rapport, M. M.: Hydrolysis of ceramide lactoside and ceramide glucoside by glycosidase from brain. Israel J. Med. Sci., **1,** 624, 1965.
185. Brady, R. O., Kanfer, J., and Shapiro, D.: Metabolism of glucocerebrosides. II. Evidence for an enzymatic deficiency in Gaucher's disease. Biochem. Biophys. Res. Commun., **18,** 221, 1965.
186. Kampine, J. P., Brady, R. O., Kanfer, J. N., Feld, M., and Shapiro, D.: Diagnosis of Gaucher's disease and Niemann-Pick disease with small samples of venous blood. Science, **155,** 86, 1967.
187. Kampine, J. P., Brady, R. O., Yankee, R. A., Kanfer, J. N., Shapiro, D., and Gal, A. E.: Sphingolipid metabolism in leukemic leukocytes, Cancer Res., **27,** 1312, 1967.
188. Brady, R. O.: Enzymatic defects in the sphingolipidoses, Advances Clin. Chem., **11,** 1, 1968.
189. Martensson, E.: *Progress in The Chemistry of Fats and Other Lipids,* edited by R. T. Holman. Pergamon, Oxford, 1969.
190. Stoffel, W., Sticht, G., and LeKim, D.: Degradation of (1-^{14}C) dihydrosphingosine (sphinganine), (1-^{14}C) 2-amino-1-3 dihydroxyheptane and (1-^{14}C) dihydrosphingosine phosphate in rat liver. Hoppe Seyler. Z. Physiol. Chem., **350,** 63, 1969.
191. Keenan, R. W., and Haegelin, B.: The enzymatic phosphorylation of sphinganine. Biochem. Biophys. Res. Commun., **37,** 888, 1969.
192. Gatt, S.: Comparison of four enzymes from brain which hydrolyze sphingolipids, in *Inborn Disorders of Sphingolipid Metabolism,* edited by S. M. Aronson and B. W. Volk, p. 261. Pergamon, New York, 1967.
193. Sweeley, C. C., Snyder, P. D., and Griffen, C. E.: Chemistry of glycosphingolipids in Fabry's disease. Chem. Phys. Lipids, **4,** 393, 1970.
193a. Sweeley, C. C. et al., in preparation.
193b. Handa, A., Ariga, T., Miyatake, T., and Yamakawa, T.: Presence of α-anomeric glycosidic configuration in the glycolipids accumulated in kidney with Fabry's disease. J. Biochem. (Tokyo), **69,** 625, 1971.
194. Adams, E. P., and Gray, G. M.: The carbohydrate structures of the neutral ceramide glycolipids in kidneys of different mouse strains with special reference to the ceramide dehexosides. Chem. Phys. Lipids, **2,** 147, 1968.
195. Kawanani, J.: Glycolipids from rat kidney. J. Biochem. (Tokyo), **64,** 625, 1968.
196. Makita, A., and Yamakawa, T.: Biochemistry of organ glycolipids. III. The structures of human kidney cerebroside sulfuric ester, ceramide dihexoside, and ceramide trihexoside. J. Biochem. (Tokyo), **55,** 365, 1964.
197. Dubach, U. C., Enderlin, F., and Mannhart, M.: Absent renal ceramide-trihexosidase activity in Fabry's disease. German Med. Monthly, **14,** 34, 1969.
198. Mapes, C. A., Anderson, R. L., and Sweeley, C. C.: Trihexosyl ceramide: galactosyl hydrolase in normal human serum and plasma and its absence in patients with Fabry's disease. Fed. Abstr., **29,** 409, 1970.
199. Mapes, C. A., Anderson, R. L., Sweeley, C. C., Desnick, R. J., and Krivit, W.: Enzyme replacement in Fabry's disease, and inborn error of metabolism. Science, **169,** 987, 1970.
200. Wachtel, H. L., and Mattei, I. R.: Angiokeratoma corporis diffusum universale. Arch. Intern. Med., **114,** 805, 1964.
201. Dawson, G., and Sweeley, C. C.: *In vivo* studies on glycosphingolipid metabolism in porcine blood. J. Biol. Chem., **245,** 410, 1970.
202. Dilorenzo, P. A., Kleinfeld, J., Tellman, W., and Nay, L.: Angiokeratoma corporis diffusum (Fabry's disease). Acta Dermatovener. (Stockholm), **49,** 319, 1969.
203. Rapport, M. M., and Graf, L.: Immunochemical reactions of lipids. Progr. Allerg., **13,** 273, 1969.
204. Wise, D.: Diffuse angiokeratoma (J. Fabry), in *Jadassohn's Handbuch des Haut- und Geschlechtskrankheiten,* vol. 7, sec. 743. Springer, Berlin, 1966.
205. Vogelberg, K. H., Solbach, H. G., and Gries, F. A.: Lipoidchemische Untersuchungen beim Angiokeratoma corporis diffusum (Fabry-syndrom). Klin. Wschr., **47,** 916, 1969.
206. Kint, J. A.: Fabry's disease, alpha-galactosidase deficiency. Science, **167,** 1268, 1970.
206a. Romeo, G., and Migeon, B. R.: Genetic inactivation of the α-galactosidase locus in carriers of Fabry's disease. Science, **170,** 180, 1970.
207. de Groot, W. P.: Genetic aspects of the thesaurismosis lipoidica hereditaria Ruiter-Pompen-Wyers (angiokeratoma corporis diffusum Fabry). Dermatologica (Basel), **129,** 281, 1964.
208. Johnston, A. W., Frost, P., Spaeth, G. L., and Renwick, J. H.: Linkage relationships of the angiokeratoma (Fabry) locus. Ann. Hum. Genet. (Lond.), **32,** 369, 1969.
209. Brady, R. O.: Genetics and the sphingolipidoses. Med. Clin. N. Amer., **53,** 327, 1969.
210. Yunis, J. J.: Human chromosomes in disease, in *Human Chromosome Methodology,* p. 234. Academic, New York, 1965.
211. Garza Toba, M.: Angioqueratoma corporis diffusum. Communicación de un caso clínico. Medicina (Mexico), **37,** 525, 1957.
212. Rodriquez, O.: Angioqueratomas. Communicación de un caso de angioqueratoma corporis diffusum. Dermatologica (Mexico), **1,** 309, 1957.
213. Madden, F. C.: Papilliform lesions (lymphangioma) of the scrotum. Associated with multiple petechial spots on the trunk and limbs. Brit. Med. J., **2,** 302, 1912.
214. Kuang-Yuan, Y.: Angiokeratoma corporis diffusum universale (Fabry): report of a case with lipoiduria. Chinese Med. J., **74,** 478, 1956.
215. Yeoh, S. A., and Asan, P.: Fabry's disease with renal tubular acidosis. Singapore Med. J., **8,** 275, 1967.
216. Yoshitoshi, Y., et al.: A case of Fabry's disease with special references

to changes in the skin, urinary albumin, anhydroses and kidney function. Naika, **15**, 555, 1965.

217. Calmettes, L., Deodati, F., Dupre, A., and Bec, P.: Manifestations oculaires du syndrome de Fabry. Bull. Soc. Ophthal. France, **72**, 513, 1959.
218. Rhodes, E. L.: Angiokeratoma corporis diffusum. Proc. Roy. Soc. Med. U.S.A., **57**, 43, 1964.
219. Zakon, S. J.: Angiokeratoma corporis diffusum (Mibelli). Arch. Derm. Syph. (Chicago), **51**, 155, 1945.
220. Childs, B., and Der Kalouslian, V. M.: Genetic heterogeneity. New Eng. J. Med., **279**, 1205, 1968.
221. Beutler, E., Mathai, C. K., and Smith, J. E.: Biochemical variants of glucose-6-phosphate dehydrogenase giving rise to congenital non-spherocytic hemolytic disease. Blood, **31**, 131, 1968.
222. Kelley, W. N., Rosenbloom, F. M., Henderson, J. F., and Seegmiller, J. E.: Specific enzyme defect in gout associated with overproduction of uric acid. Proc. Nat. Acad. Sci. U.S.A., **57**, 1735, 1967.
223. Lyon, M.: Gene action in the X-chromosome of the mouse (*Mus musculus* L.). Nature (London), **190**, 372, 1961.
224. Lyon, M.: Sex chromatin and gene action in the X-chromosome of mammals, in *The Sex Chromatin,* edited by K. L. Moore, p. 370. Saunders, Philadelphia, 1966.
225. Krivit, W., and Desnick, R. J.: Glycolipid analysis of urinary sediment in Fabry's and Gaucher's disease (abstract). J. Pediat., **72**, 571, 1968.
226. Brady, R. O., Uhlendorf, B. W., and Jacobson, C. B.: Antenatal detection of Fabry's disease. Science, in press.
227. Ende, M., and Peabody, C.: Angiokeratoma corporis diffusum universale (Fabry). Virginia Med. Monthly, **85**, 192, 1958.
228. Vineyard, W. R., and Kamin, E. J.: Angiokeratoma corporis diffusum. A. M. A. Arch. Derm., **82**, 817, 1960.
229. Cross, E. G.: The familial occurrence of erythromelalgia and nephritis. Canad. Med. Ass. J., **87**, 1, 1962.
230. Snyder, P. D., Krivit, W., and Sweeley, C. C.: Unpublished results.
231. Klionsky, B., and Sweeley, C. C.: Unpublished results.
232. Svennerholm, L.: Gangliosides and other glycolipids of human placenta. Acta Chem. Scand., **19**, 1506, 1965.
233. Vance, D. E.: The chemistry and metabolism of human blood glycolipids. Thesis, University of Pittsburgh, Pittsburgh, 1967.
234. Yamakawa, T.: Glycolipids of mammalian red blood cells, in *Lipoide,* edited by C. E. Schutte, p. 87. Springer-Verlag, New York, 1966.
235. Krivit, W., and Desnick, R. J.: Unpublished results.
236. Dawson, G., and Sweeley, C. C.: Unpublished results.
237. Folkman, M. J., and Mark, V. H.: Diffusion of anesthetics and other drugs through silicone rubber: therapeutic implications. Trans. N.Y. Acad. Sci., **30**, 1187, 1968.
238. Desnick, R. J., Dawson, G., Desnick, S. J., Sweeley, E. C., and Krivit, W.: Diagnosis of glycosphingolipidoses by urinary sediment analysis. New Engl. J. Med., **284**, 739, 1971.
239. Lockman, L. A., Krivit, W., and Desnick, R. J.: Relief of the painful crises of Fabry's disease by diphenylhydantoin. Presented at the annual meeting of the American Academy of Neurology, New York, New York, April 29-May 1. (Abst). Neurology, **21**, 423, 1971.

CHAPTER THIRTY-TWO

SULFATIDE LIPIDOSIS: METACHROMATIC LEUKODYSTROPHY *

Hugo W. Moser

Metachromatic leukodystrophy (MLD) represents several closely related disorders in which myelin degeneration is associated with accumulation of galactosyl (SO_4) ceramide or cerebroside sulfate (Fig. 32-1). At least two discrete forms appear to be due to deficient activity of a specific enzyme, cerebroside sulfatase. A rare form may be associated with decreased activity of more than one sulfatase. In addition to progressive and fatal central nervous system degeneration, there is in this disorder an accumulation of sulfatides in peripheral nerves, liver, and kidney.

Several types of leukodystrophy have been defined. Apart from metachromatic leukodystrophy, these include the globoid cell type of Krabbe (Chap. 34), spongy degeneration of the white matter [1, 2, 3], the leukodystrophy described by Pelizaeus and Merzbacher [4, 5, 6], sudanophilic leukodystrophy [7], and Alexander's disease [8, 9]. It is likely that all the leukodystrophies are genetically determined enzymatic defects. This has been shown to be the case for MLD and for the globoid cell type. The biochemical basis of the other leukodystrophies remains obscure.

The leukodystrophies must be distinguished from other disorders of the white matter which have distinct pathogenic mechanisms. The most common of these is multiple sclerosis, in which there is an inflammatory response and the nervous system is involved in an asymmetric fashion [10]. The pathogenesis of multiple sclerosis is unknown: an autoallergic or a viral cause has been proposed. It does not appear to be genetically determined [11].

For two other disorders which affect the white matter, a viral origin either has been established or appears likely. Subacute sclerosing panencephalitis is a progressive disorder of children which is due to a virus identical to or closely related to the measles virus [12]. Multifocal leukoencephalopathy, a white matter disorder which affects patients with leukemia or certain other debilitating disorders, is almost certainly due to a virus [13, 14].

There is one rare genetically determined disease entity in which there are cerebral lesions which closely resemble those of multiple sclerosis. This disorder is Addison-Schilder disease, or adrenocortical atrophy and diffuse cerebral sclerosis. It has an x-linked mode of inheritance [15, 16]. The basic defect is unknown. The distribution and appearance of the lesions in the white matter suggest that they do not represent a primary defect of brain metabolism. It seems probable that the brain lesions are secondary to another phenomenon such as the adrenal insufficiency.

* Supported in part by grant NB 0276 from the Public Health Service and by the Maternal and Child Health Service Project No. 906.

HISTORY

Metachromatic staining of the nervous system from a patient with diffuse sclerosis was first reported by Alzheimer in 1910 [17]. In 1921 Witte [18] briefly reported a similar patient with an accumulation of metachromatic material in the pituitary, liver, kidney, and testis. The detailed account of a familial progressive leukodystrophy of children by Scholz in 1925 [19] included histologic studies of celloidin- or paraffin-embedded blocks which had been dehydrated in alcohol. Most lipids would be removed by this procedure, and the metachromatic properties of the tissue were missed. The disease entity which Scholz described became known as *leukodystrophy, type Scholz,* and patients with similar conditions were reported later. Thirty years later Peiffer examined frozen sections of tissue from the original patients of Scholz and demonstrated a striking metachromasia [20]. Thus the report of Scholz is the first complete clinical and pathologic description of the metachromatic leukodystrophy briefly noted by Alzheimer.

A significant biochemical advance was made in 1958 when Jatzkewitz [21] and Austin [22] independently demonstrated a large excess of sulfatides in tissues from patients with metachromatic leukodystrophy. These observations have been confirmed, and it now seems appropriate to refer to this condition as *sulfatide lipidosis.* Since then, knowledge about MLD has increased rapidly. The most important advances are the demonstration of the enzymatic basis for the lipid accumulation, viz., deficiency of cerebroside sulfatase; the development of reliable diagnostic procedures based on assays of arylsulfatase A activity; the biochemical diagnosis of the heterozygote state; and, most recently, diagnosis of the disorder prenatally, so that this birth defect can be prevented. At this time there is no effective treatment.

SULFATIDES

Structure

The existence of sulfur in certain lipids was first reported by Thudichum [23] when he isolated a fraction containing

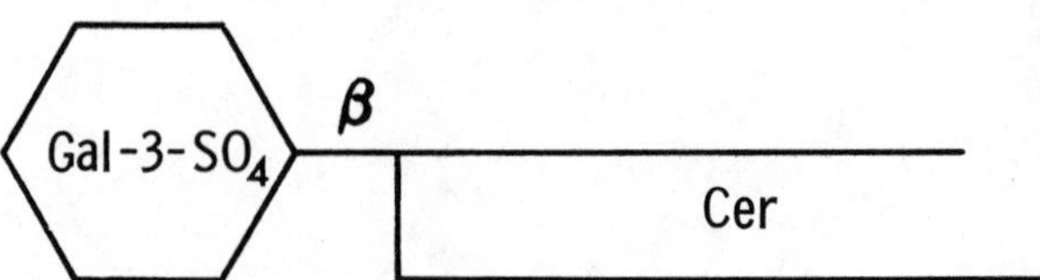

Figure 32-1. Galactosyl-3-sulfate ceramide.

both sulfur and phosphorus from protagon, a crude extract of brain soluble in hot ethanol but insoluble in acetone or ether. Blix, in 1933, isolated from brain protagon a sulfatide which contained approximately equimolar amounts of cerebronic acid, sphingosine, galactose, and sulfate, and which he presumed to be the sulfate ester of cerebroside [24]. All data accumulated since have confirmed this proposition. The demonstration of Lees that sulfatides contain no free amino or reducing group indicated that the constituent fatty acids and sphingosine are linked by an amide bond and that the galactose is attached by a glycosidic linkage [25]. The galactoside linkage has been shown to have the beta configuration [26]. Stoffyn et al. [27] treated sulfatides with dilute methanolic HCl and showed that they were converted in high yield to galactocerebrosides with the same properties and constituents as those which occur naturally. This result demonstrated that the sulfatides, indeed, are sulfate esters of the cerebrosides. As is true for cerebrosides, the sphingosine base of sulfatides consists almost exclusively of C_{18} sphingosine [26]. The structural formula of a sulfatide appears in Fig. 32-2.

In order to determine the location of the sulfate linkage Yamakawa et al. [28] and Stoffyn et al. [29] subjected sulfatides to methylation and subsequent methanolysis, and isolated the resulting methylated galactoside. With the conditions used in these studies all unsubstituted hydroxy groups of the galactose moiety of the sulfatide molecule are methylated. It is thus possible to define the position of the ester linkage by determining the structure of the isolated methylated galactoside. Both groups of investigators found that 2,4,6-trimethylgalactoside was the only methylated derivative present, and concluded that the sulfate ester linkage involves the hydroxy group of carbon-3. The hydroxy group of carbon-5 is not available for methylation because it is involved in the hemiacetal linkage. Prior to these studies it had been thought that the sulfate group was linked to carbon-6.

The fatty acid composition of sulfatides and cerebrosides is distinctive in that both compounds contain a high proportion of long-chain fatty acids, and of fatty acids which contain an α-hydroxy group. In fact, nearly all the α-hydroxy fatty acids found in brain lipids are constituents of these

```
                  H
                  |
CH3—(CH2)12— C = C — C — C — CH2 — O — C—H
             |       |    |               |
             H      OH   NH           H—C—OH
                          |               |        O
                         CO    HO-SO2-O-C-H
                          |               |
                        CHOH          HO—C—H
                          |               |
                        (CH2)21         H—C
                          |               |
                         CH3            CH2OH
```

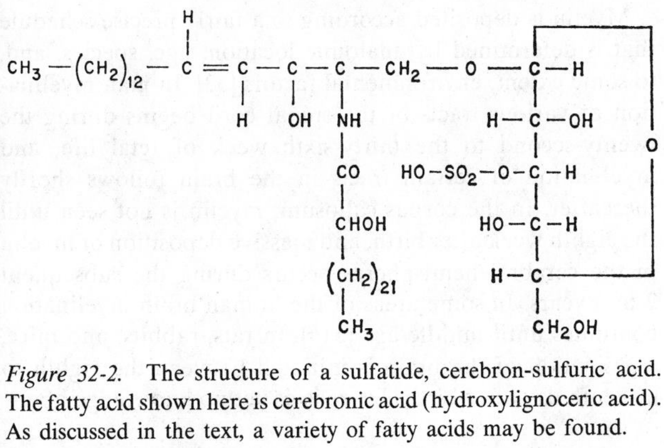

Figure 32-2. The structure of a sulfatide, cerebron-sulfuric acid. The fatty acid shown here is cerebronic acid (hydroxylignoceric acid). As discussed in the text, a variety of fatty acids may be found.

two glycolipids. With the advent of gas-liquid chromatography, detailed information concerning the fatty acid composition of these glycolipids has emerged. Consistent differences have been demonstrated between the sulfatide fatty acid pattern of adult and immature brain, and between the sulfatides of the nervous system and those in the kidney. In adult brain 20 to 25 percent of sulfatide fatty acids contain an α-hydroxy group. Among the nonhydroxy acids, nervonic acid (24:1) and lignoceric acid (24:0) predominate; the concentration of nervonic acid is approximately twice that of lignoceric. Cerebronic (24 H:O), oxynervonic (24 H:1), and the 22- and 23-carbon saturated fatty acids predominate among the α-hydroxy acids [30]. In fetal and immature brain medium-chain-length fatty acids (16:0, 18:0, and 18:1) predominate, and the proportion of hydroxy fatty acids is smaller than in mature brain tissue [31]; development of the pattern characteristic of adult brain coincides with myelination.

The fatty acid pattern of kidney sulfatides differs from that in the brain. The kidney sulfatides contain more than 10 times as much behenic acid (22:0) than do those in the brain. Kidney sulfatides also contain a higher proportion of lignoceric acid (24:0) than nervonic acid (24:1); in brain the reverse holds true [32, 33].

Ceramide-dihexoside Sulfate

In 1963 Martensson demonstrated a ceramide-dihexoside sulfuric acid ester fraction in human kidney [34]. The structure of this compound was determined by mild acid hydrolysis and by methylation studies. Hydrolysis with 0.05*N* HC1 removed the sulfate group and was shown to yield a compound with the same properties as ceramide-lactoside. Subsequent hydrolysis with 0.3*N* HCl yielded ceramide-glucose, thus demonstrating that the sequence in the ceramide-lactoside must have been ceramide-glucose-galactose [33]. Methylation studies, analogous to those carried out with sulfatides, showed that the sulfate ester linkage involved carbon-3 of the galactose [35]. Figure 32-3 shows the structure of ceramide-dihexoside sulfate. As is true for sulfatide, it contains mostly C_{18} sphingosine. The fatty acid composition of kidney ceramide-dihexoside sulfate resembles that of kidney sulfatide; nearly half the fatty acids contain an α-hydroxy group [33]. Normal human kidney contains 0.14 to 0.20 mg ceramide-dihexoside sulfate per gram of dry weight, slightly less than half the sulfatide level of 0.39 to 0.49 [33].

Isolation of Sulfatides

Prior to the development of chromatographic techniques, the isolation of sulfatides was difficult and most methods resulted in poor yields. To a considerable extent this is because most complex polar lipids are likely to enter into more or less stable associations with other substances, a

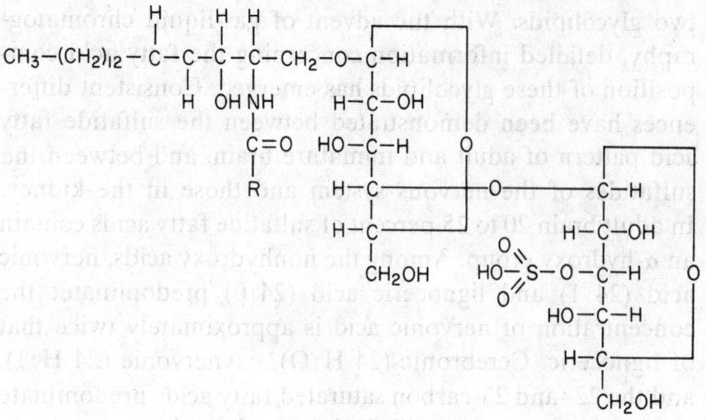

Figure 32-3. Structure of kidney ceramide-dihexoside sulfate.

feature which, as Stoffyn has emphasized, is probably essential to their function as membrane constituents in the living cell [26].

Modern isolation procedures depend on column and thin-layer chromatographic techniques; these are described in detail in several recent publications [36-38]. As the initial step, a total lipid extract is prepared [39]. This is then processed by column chromatography. To achieve purification, it is necessary to use different supports in succession. Several systems have been shown to provide a reasonably pure product in good yield. These include silicic acid followed by DEAE cellulose [40]; florisil (magnesium silicate) followed by DEAE cellulose and silicic acid [31]; DEAE cellulose followed by silicic acid or florisil [41], or charcoal-celite followed by florisil [32].

It is advantageous to combine column chromatography with thin-layer chromatography [36, 37]. This technique involves the use of silica gel in the form of thin layers on glass plates [37]. Particularly good separations are achieved with the two-dimensional techniques described by Rouser and his associates [37]. After the sulfatides have been purified by column or thin-layer chromatography or both, they can be quantitated by estimating the content of sulfate [42], galactose [43], or sphingosine [44], or, if sufficient material is available, by weighing the purified lipid.

Occurrence of Sulfatides

Sulfatides occur in highest concentration in adult brain white matter. Here they represent 0.8 to 0.9 percent of fresh weight and 2.5 to 4.1 percent of dry weight [41, 45, 46]. In adult gray matter they account for 0.1 to 0.15 percent of wet weight and 0.4 to 0.8 percent of dry weight. Next to nervous tissue, they occur in highest concentration in the kidney. Here sulfatide makes up 0.04 percent of dry weight. As already noted, the kidney also contains ceramide-dihexoside sulfate, which makes up 0.014 to 0.018 percent of dry weight. Lower levels of sulfatide also occur in other tissues, such as the spleen [46], liver [47], and plasma [48].

Brain sulfatide levels increase during maturation both in man and in experimental animals. For human tissue the most comprehensive data are those of Rouser and Yamamoto [49]; for the rat those of Wells and Dittmer [50], of Davison and Gregson [51], and of Hauser [51*a*] are the most complete. Figure 32-4 shows that in respect to sulfatide concentration, the maturational changes in these two species are in many respects comparable: at 3 days after birth the brain sulfatide levels in both rat and man are about 0.15 μmoles per gm fresh weight. The most rapid increases in sulfatide concentration coincide with the period of myelination—in man, the first 2 years of life; in the rat, between the tenth and fortieth days. Subsequent to this period, differences in rate of deposition exist between the two species. In man, brain sulfatide levels more than double between the second and the tenth years, and thereafter increase by another 40 percent until age 40, when the highest level is achieved. In their studies of rat brain sulfatide level, Davison and Gregson extended their observations to include rats up to 1,000 days old. They found that the sulfatide levels increased up to 120 days of age, and that, thereafter, they did not change significantly. Wells and Dittmer observed that the peak sulfatide level in 330-day-old rats was 30 percent in excess of that at 40 days, which marks the end of the period of rapid accumulation. Thus, in the rat most brain sulfatides are deposited during a relatively early stage of maturation, while in man sulfatide deposition continues until middle age. This finding is in agreement with the histologic observation that myelination of certain areas of the human brain is not completed until the fifth or sixth decade [51*b*]. The data cited so far refer to the sulfatide content of whole brain; it has been shown that the maturational increases are due mainly to increases in white matter sulfatide levels [46, 31].

The Formation of Myelin

Studies of brain sulfatide synthesis and metabolism have contributed significantly to the understanding of myelin formation. It is appropriate, therefore, that these two topics be considered together.

Myelin is deposited according to a fairly precise schedule that is determined by anatomic location, age, species, and, to some extent, environmental factors [52]. In man myelination of various tracts of the spinal cord begins during the twenty-second to the thirty-sixth week of fetal life, and myelination of certain tracts in the brain follows shortly thereafter. In the corpus callosum, myelin is not seen until the eighth week after birth, and massive deposition of myelin in the cerebral hemispheres occurs during the subsequent 2 to 3 years. In some areas of the human brain myelination continues until middle age [51*b*]. In rats, rabbits, and mice, myelination of the brain is initiated between the eighth to fifteenth day after birth. There is as yet no knowledge about

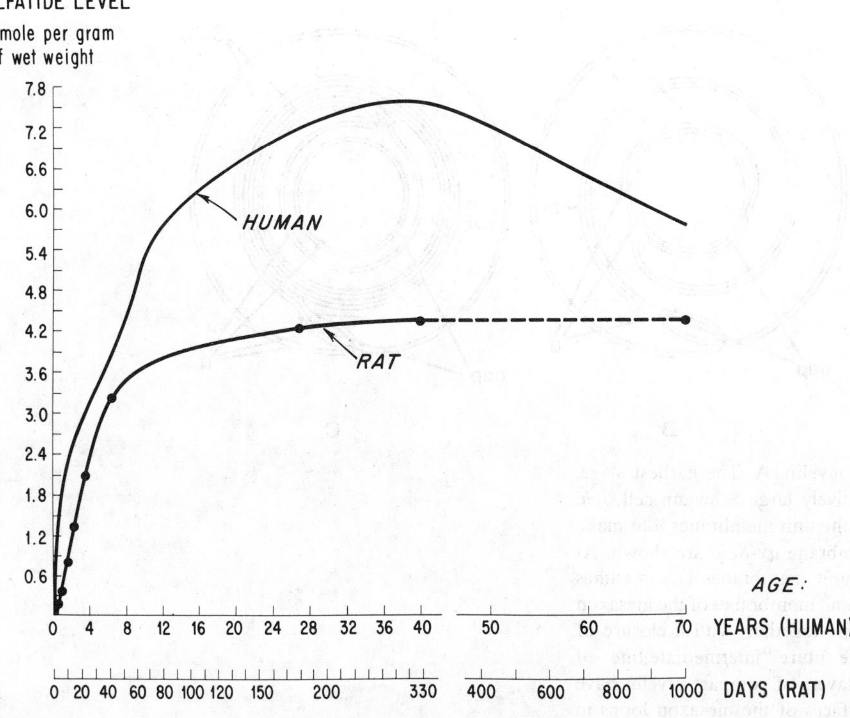

Figure 32-4. Brain sulfatides and maturation. The data for human brain tissue were calculated from equations developed by Rouser and Yamamoto to define the variation of sulfatide content with age. The calculated values did not deviate from measured values by more than 2 percent [49]. The data for rats up to 330 days old are those of Wells and Dittmer [50]. Davison and Gregson have shown that rat brain sulfatide levels remain constant between the ages of 300 and 1,000 days [51]. In all studies, including those of human material, sulfatide levels were measured in homogenates of whole brains.

the nature of the mechanisms which initiate the rapid assembly of myelin during maturation, and those which turn it "off" or "down" in adulthood.

Recent studies with the electron microscope have clarified the anatomic relationships between the myelin-forming cells and the myelin sheath. In the central nervous system myelin is formed by the oligodendrocyte [53], and in the peripheral nervous system by the Schwann cell [54]. During myelination the axon is surrounded by a process of the myelinating cell. This process is spiraled about the axon so that multiple layers are formed, and simultaneously or subsequently the membranes of the spiraling process come together in unusually close apposition. Together these steps are referred to as "ensheathment." Bunge describes this phenomenon in detail in a recent review [53]. The myelin sheath thus represents multiple compacted plasma membrane layers of the myelin-forming cell; the sheath is continuous with the plasma membrane of the myelin-forming cell, and it lies within the cytoplasm of this cell. These relationships are shown in Fig. 32-5.

Sulfatides as Myelin Constituents

Until the early 1960s knowledge about the composition of myelin was based on indirect evidence obtained from comparison between the composition of adult white and gray matter [55] and from studies of the changes in the chemical composition of the brain during maturation [56, 57, 50]. The latter approach proved particularly valuable since dramatic and reproducible changes in brain composition could be correlated with the deposition of myelin as judged by histologic criteria. On the basis of such correlations it was concluded that cholesterol, cerebrosides, sphingomyelins, acetal phosphatides, and proteolipid protein are components of the myelin sheath [56, 57]. Noting the rapid deposition of sulfatides occurring at the time of myelination, Davison and Gregson included them among the myelin lipids [51]. However, Wells and Dittmer noted that in rats, brain sulfatide concentration already increased before myelination began, and concluded that brain sulfatides are associated with both myelin and nonmyelin structures. [50].

Methods for the isolation of myelin were first described in 1960 to 1962 [58–60], and a variety of methods have been introduced since then [61, 62]. A popular technique is that developed by Autilio, Norton, and Terry in 1964 [63]. This is based on the fact that the myelin sheath has the highest lipid content and the lowest hydrated density of any subcellular particle of brain. As a result ultracentrifugation makes it possible to layer myelin-rich fractions between 0.32*m* and 0.656*m* sucrose solutions and to separate them from the denser cellular components which collect at the bottom of the tube. On the basis of their very low content of RNA and DNA, the absence of enzymes such as cytochrome oxidase, K^+-activated ATPase, and acid phosphatase [61], and on the basis of electron microscopic studies, carefully prepared myelin fractions have been judged to be 95 to 99 percent pure [63]. Fractions obtained by the technique

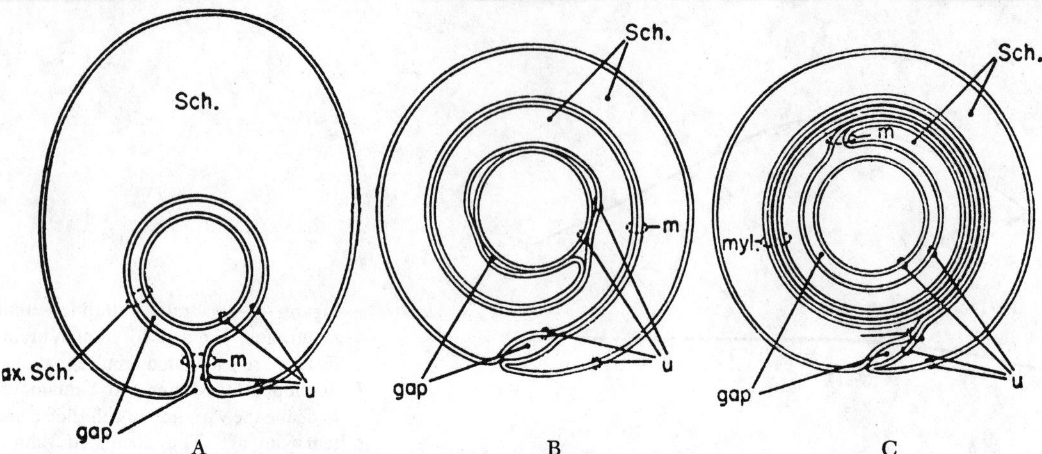

Figure 32-5. The development of nerve myelin. A. The earliest stage. Here a small axon is enveloped by a relatively large Schwann cell *Sch.* to make a protofiber. The combination of the unit membranes *u* to make a mesaxon *m* and the axon-Schwann membrane *ax-Sch.* are shown. At the earliest stages the gap between the unit membranes is sometimes present. B. An intermediate fiber. Here the unit membranes of the mesaxon and to some extent of the axon have come together, with a closure of most of the gap. Their line of contact is the future "intermediate line" of myelin. C. A later stage, in which a few layers of compact myelin have formed by contact of the cytoplasmic surfaces of the mesaxon loops to make the major lines of myelin. (*From Robertson* [79].)

Table 32-1. COMPOSITION OF BOVINE MYELIN*

Components	Molar percentage of total lipids	*Calculated percentage of total amount of each white matter constituent in:*	
		Myelin	Nonmyelin
Cholesterol	44.3	78	22
Total galactolipids	21.2	66	34
Minor galactolipids	0.7	72	28
Cerebrosides	18.3	69	31
Sulfatides	2.3	47	53
Total phospholipids	34.6	61	39
Ethanolamine phosphatides	14.6	83	17
Serine phosphatides	4.9	38	62
Phosphatidyl inositol	0.3	60	40
Lecithin	8.5	56	44
Sphingomyelin	5.8	71	29
Total plasmalogens	11.9	74	26
Phosphatidal ethanolamine	10.5		
Phosphatidal serine	0.2		
Phosphatidal choline	0.1		

* The molar percentage of lipids listed here represents the average of the values reported by Norton and Autilio [45] for "light" and "heavy" myelin. The partition of each white matter constituent between "myelin" and "nonmyelin" was calculated from its concentration within myelin, with the assumption that the total fraction represents 50 percent of white matter solids. Norton and Autilio have discussed the justification and limitations of this assumption. The actual value probably lies somewhere between 40 and 50 percent.

Source: Modified from Norton and Autilio [45].

of Autilio et al. [63] represent approximately 15 percent of the dry weight of mature white matter [45]. Since myelin is estimated to account for approximately 50 percent of the dry weight of mature white matter, the isolation procedures thus have approximately a yield of 30 percent. Myelin has also been isolated from intradural nerve roots [64], optic nerve [65], and peripheral nerves [66]. The results obtained by these several techniques in a variety of mammalian species are in rather close agreement. Table 32-1 summarizes the data of Norton and Autilio.

Myelin contains a high proportion of lipid. Whether or not a particular lipid is a "myelin lipid" can be judged by calculating the percentage of the substance associated with myelin, and comparing this with the percentage found in the white matter devoid of myelin. Table 32-1 outlines the procedure used and the results of these calculations. Since they involve certain assumptions, they represent approximations only. With this procedure cholesterol, cerebroside, ethanolamine phosphatides, sphingomyelin, and plasmalogens are classed as myelin lipids. These conclusions agree in most respects with those cited previously, which were derived from a study of data based on the changes of brain composition that accompany myelination. The studies of isolated myelin suggest that the distinction between a "myelin" and a "nonmyelin" lipid is not as absolute as had been thought. Thus, although cerebrosides are absent from brain tissue before myelination, and their deposition in brain matches the time of myelination as judged histologically, the calculations based on a study of isolated myelin suggest that a substantial proportion of white matter cerebroside (28 percent) is associated with structures other than myelin. In respect to sulfatide, the nonmyelin component appears to be even larger (53 percent). The composition of peripheral nerve myelin differs slightly, but consistently, from that of myelin in the central nervous system. Peripheral nerve myelin contains more sphingomyelin but less cholesterol, cerebroside, sulfatide, and phosphatidyl ethanolamine than does central myelin [66].

O'Brien and Sampson found that the composition of human myelin did not vary significantly between the ages of 10 months and 55 years [67, 30]. For the most part, therefore, the changes in brain composition during myelination reflect the quantity of myelin, not its composition. Myelin deposited at very early stages of development has a somewhat different composition from that in older animals. This has been shown in 14-day-old mice [68] and in 21- and 22-day-old rats [69, 70].

Determination of the composition of purified myelin will, no doubt, prove of great value in elucidating the structure of the myelin sheath at the molecular level. The available information on this point has recently been reviewed by Finean [71]. Figure 32-6 shows his proposed schematic structure of myelin. Vandenheuvel has constructed an ingenious model of the myelin membrane based on the most recent knowledge of the size and shape of the known myelin constituents [72, 73]. This is shown in Fig. 32-7. Korn has

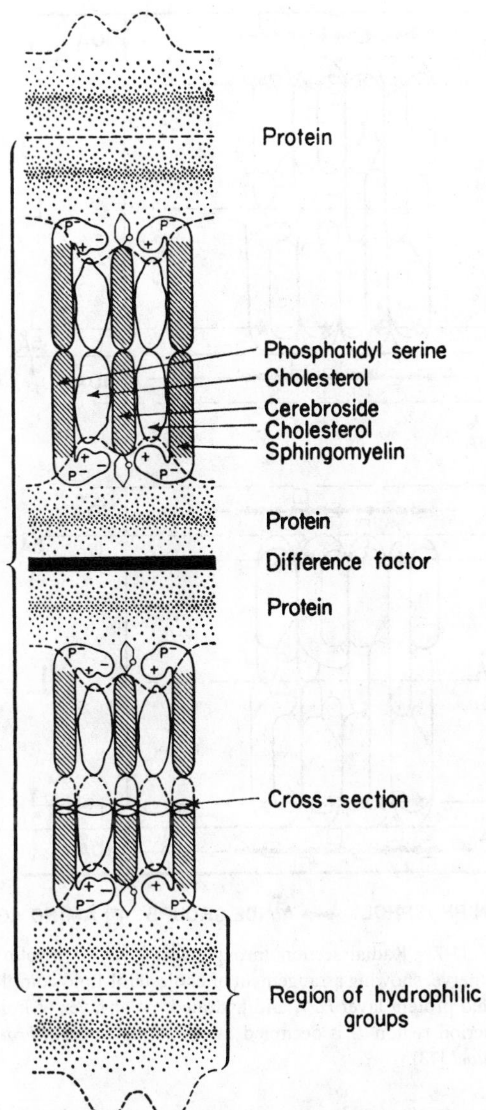

Figure 32-6. Finean's hypothesis of the arrangement of the lipid components in myelin. This scheme does not take into account the fact that normally approximately every fourth cerebroside molecule exists as a sulfate ester. (*From Finean* [71].)

presented a cogent critique of current concepts of membrane structure [74]; it must be emphasized that the structural models are hypothetical.

Sulfatides in White Matter Components Other than Myelin

Norton and Autilio, on the basis of their studies of purified myelin, calculated that 47 percent of white matter sulfatides forms part of the myelin sheath, and that 53 percent is part of other subcellular components [45]. This calculation is

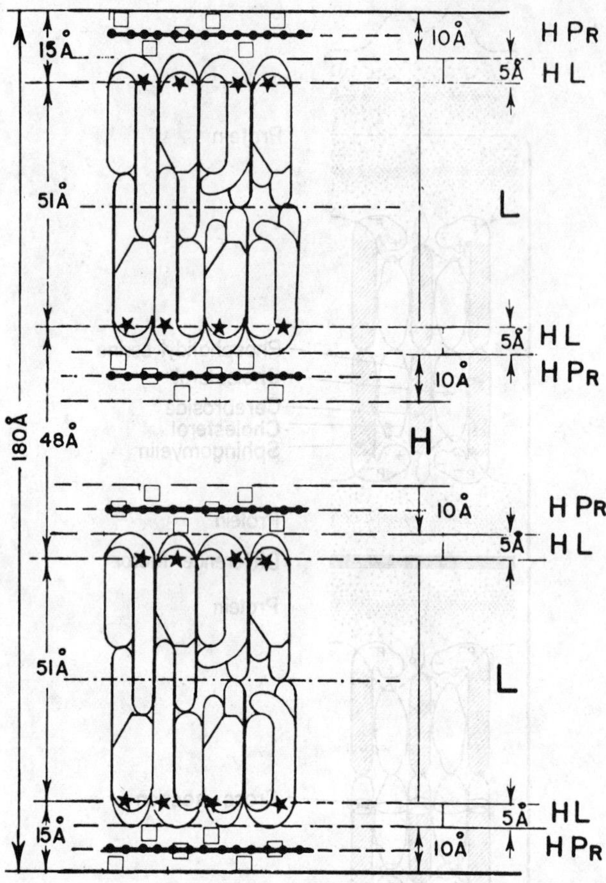

Figure 32-7. Radial section through unit layer of myelin of rat sciatic nerve, showing arrangement of cholesterol-lipid complexes *L*, hydrated protein layer *HPr*, and hydrated, polar layer of lipids *HL*. Intraperiod region *H* is occupied by water molecules. (*From Vandenheuvel* [73].)

based on the assumption that myelin comprises 50 percent of white matter dry weight. Were myelin in fact a larger fraction of white matter dry weight, the fraction of sulfatide in myelin would be proportionately larger. The subcellular localization of nonmyelin sulfatide is a matter of controversy. The sum of sulfatides that can be accounted for in nonmyelin structures, such as the microsomes, mitochondria, and the supernatant, appears to be less than the 53 percent of total sulfatides calculated by Norton and Autilio.

The largest portion of nonmyelin sulfatides is present in the microsomal fraction. Glycolipids make up a smaller fraction of lipids in the microsomes than in the myelin sheath. The molar ratios of cholesterol/phospholipid/glycolipid are 5:7:1 in the microsomes, compared with 2:2:1 for myelin [75]. Davison and Gregson recovered 15 percent of total white matter sulfatide in the microsomes. However, this is probably an overestimate, since their microsomal fraction was contaminated with myelin [51]. As will be discussed below, sulfatides are synthesized mainly within the microsomes [92, 95]. Microsomal sulfatides are metabolically active, and they turn over much more rapidly than those in the myelin sheath [97].

Most controversy exists in respect to the sulfatide content of brain mitochondria. Lovtrup and Svennerholm reported that glycolipids (cerebroside plus sulfatide) accounted for 18 percent of brain mitochondrial lipids [76]. This value is larger than that reported by other groups, and has been questioned [77]. Rouser and Yamamoto report the isolation of brain mitochondria free of cerebroside and sulfatide [38]. They found that the composition of bovine brain mitochondria was the same as that of bovine heart and liver mitochondria, and they take the position that the cerebrosides and sulfatides which others have isolated from brain mitochondria represent contamination by myelin fragments. Other authors report small but measurable amounts of cerebrosides and sulfatides in brain mitochondria, somewhat less than 1 percent of their total lipid content [78]. Metabolic studies also indicate that the mitochondrial sulfatides are not exclusively artifacts resulting from myelin contamination. Davison and Gregson injected ^{35}S methionine into 16-day-old rats, and then sacrificed them 334 days later. The myelin isolated from the brains of these animals contained significant and comparable levels of radioactivity in the sulfatide and proteolipid protein fractions, but only the mitochondrial sulfatide fraction contained radioactivity. Had the mitochondrial sulfatide represented myelin contamination only, comparable levels of radioactive myelin proteolipid protein would have been expected [51].

Herschkowitz and associates have isolated a sulfatide-containing lipoprotein in the $105{,}000 \times g$ supernatant fraction of rat brain [95]. This fraction, which accounts for only a very small proportion of white matter sulfatide, may represent the vehicle by which sulfatides are transported to the myelin sheath from their site of synthesis in the microsomes [95].

Sulfatides as Acidic Lipids

In addition to their importance as structural components of myelin, sulfatides may play a role in maintaining the electrolyte balance of the nervous system. They are acidic lipids and can combine with inorganic cations or organic bases to maintain electrical neutrality. Katzman, and Wilson [80] have calculated that 1 kg brain tissue containing half gray and half white matter would contain a total of 26 mEq of anionic sites attributable to lipids and that 8 mEq would be accounted for by sulfatides. The isolation by Blix of cerebron sulfuric acid as a potassium salt [24] is not necessarily of biologic significance, since Folch-Pi et al. [81] have shown that in the common lipid solvents various cations can displace one another from combination with the lipids. No information is available concerning the specific affinity of sulfatides for one or another of the physiologic cations in vivo. It is possible that the accumulation of sulfatides in brain tissue causes a quantitative disturbance of the normal electrolyte pattern; this in turn might affect the structure and properties of the myelin sheath.

Green et al. found that sulfatide increases the solubility of 5-hydroxytryptamine, acetylcholine, histamine, and norepinephrine in chloroform-methanol [82]. Although it is unlikely that sulfatides normally serve as the storage site for amines, it is of interest that the histologic studies of Dengler and Diezel [83] suggest an increase in catecholamines in metachromatic leukodystrophy.

Sulfatides as Metachromatic Lipids

The term *metachromasia* refers to the capacity of certain cationic dyes to shift their absorption spectrums toward shorter wavelengths in the presence of chemical substances with appropriately arranged anionic groups [84, 85]. Correspondingly, light of a longer wavelength is transmitted, and a dye such as toluidine blue will appear pink or red. Other dyes capable of undergoing this change include cresyl violet, methylene blue, and thionine. Biologic substances capable of inducing the color change (chromotropes) include heparin, chondroitin sulfate, sulfatides, and gangliosides [86]. These compounds are either high-molecular-weight polyelectrolytes or substances capable of polymerizing or aggregating. Metachromasia can be induced in artificial colloids by sulfate, phosphate, or carboxyl groups, the efficiency decreasing in the order cited. The phenomenon of metachromasia has been known since 1875, but its mechanism is still a matter of controversy. The most generally accepted theory is that the anionic group of the chromotrope must be arranged in such a manner that the bound dye molecules can interact with one another. The resulting additional resonance energy causes a shift in the absorption spectrum to a shorter wavelength.

Sulfatides fulfill the requirements for a chromotrope in that they are anionic lipids which are capable of aggregating into micelles under certain conditions. Metachromasia associated with an abnormally high sulfatide concentration in the tissue can be demonstrated only on frozen sections, since the lipid is usually lost during celloidin or paraffin embedding. Under appropriate conditions, purified sulfatide or tissue sections from patients with metachromatic leukodystrophy show a striking pink metachromasia when stained with toluidine blue. Cresyl violet in acetic acid also stains sulfatides in these tissues metachromatically, but the color is generally brown. This latter phenomenon is apparently specific for metachromatic leukodystrophy, and is useful for clinical diagnosis.

Sulfatide Biosynthesis

Formation of Active Sulfate

The mechanisms underlying the biologic activation of sulfate and its transfer to a variety of receptor compounds have been extensively studied.

Lipmann [87] and his coworkers have established that 3′-phosphoadenosine-5′-phosphosulfate (PAPS) is the active sulfate in all biologic reactions. Adenosine-5′-phosphosulfate (APS) is an intermediate in the formation of PAPS. The reactions appear to proceed as follows:

$$\text{ATP} + \text{sulfate} \longrightarrow \text{APS} + \text{pyrophosphate}$$
$$\text{APS} + \text{ATP} \longrightarrow \text{PAPS} + \text{ADP}$$

In the first reaction the enzyme ATP-sulfurylase catalyzes the formation of APS from ATP and inorganic sulfate, with the release of pyrophosphate. The equilibrium for this reaction is highly favorable for the formation of APS, but the reaction proceeds because the products are metabolized further. The pyrophosphate is broken down to inorganic phosphate by pyrophosphatase, and the APS participates in the second step of the sulfate activation. In this second reaction APS-kinase catalyzes the phosphorylation of the 3′-hydroxyl group of APS to form the active sulfate (PAPS). Several relatively specific sulfokinases catalyze the transfer of the sulfate from PAPS to the various acceptors, which include neutral cerebroside for sulfatide synthesis, glycosaminoglycans, and steroids.

Sulfation of Ceramide Galactose (Cerebroside) and Ceramide Lactose

Radin, Martin, and Brown [88] and Hauser [89] injected rats of various ages with ^{14}C-labeled glucose and measured the specific activities of brain cerebrosides and sulfatides. In both studies the specific activity of cerebrosides was several times that of sulfatides. These results were consistent with the hypothesis that cerebrosides are the precursors of sulfatides.

Studies in vitro by three groups of investigators have shown this hypothesis to be correct. Balasubramanian and Bachhawat [90] demonstrated that extracts of sheep brain catalyzed the formation of ^{35}S-labeled sulfatide from ^{35}S-labeled PAPS. The enzyme was prepared from the $18{,}500 \times g$ supernate of a white matter homogenate. The reaction was carried out at pH 7.4, and it was activated by EDTA (ethylenediaminetetraacetic acid) and sulfhydryl agents. The role of endogenous galactocerebroside as the sulfate acceptor was indicated by the observation that preincubation with galactose oxidase reduced sulfatide formation by 90 percent. Galactose oxidase is known to act on galactocerebroside but not on sulfatide. Addition of exogenous galactocerebroside did not stimulate sulfatide synthesis, nor did it restore the activity lost by preincubation with galactose oxidase. These latter observations indicated that galactocerebroside already present in the tissue was the sulfate acceptor. The acceptor appeared to be bound to the enzyme protein, as enzyme activity was retained after passage through a Sephadex column.

McKhann et al. [91] demonstrated sulfatide synthesis in vitro in the $100{,}000 \times g$ sediment, i.e., the microsomal fraction, from the brain of 16- to 18-day-old rats. The reaction was carried out at pH 8. They were able to solubilize the enzyme, at least in part, by sonication and treatment with deoxycholate. Under these circumstances sulfatide synthesis became dependent upon exogenous substrate, and this then made it possible to examine the specificity of the reaction. Natural or synthetic galactocerebrosides stimulated the reaction, and thus were presumed to act as ^{35}S-labeled PAPS acceptors. Glucocerebroside, in contrast, failed to stimulate ^{35}S-labeled sulfatide formation. In a later study Herschkowitz et al. [93] examined more closely the subcellular localization of sulfatide synthesis. They subdivided the microsomes into three fractions and found that the most rapid sulfatide synthesis took place in a fraction which consisted mainly of membranes and single ribosomes. The most rapid protein synthesis took place in a more dense microsomal fraction which consisted mainly of polyribosomes.

The most detailed studies concerning the sulfation of glycosphingolipids are those of Cumar et al. [92]. Preparations from the brain of young rats were found to contain enzymes which catalyze the transfer of ^{35}S from PAPS to galactose containing glycosphingolipids and to galactose and water-soluble galactosides. The enzymes were found in all the subcellular fractions as well as in the high-speed supernatant. The microsomal fraction had the highest specific activity, and the enzyme in this fraction could be solubilized by treatment with deoxycholate. By adding relevant substrates it was shown that galactosyl sphingosine (psychosine), lactosyl ceramide, and galactosyl ceramide could each act as acceptors. Gangliosides and glucocerebrosides were inactive. The apparent K_m for these three substrates varied between 3.3 and $8.5 \times 10^{-5}M$, and the pH optimum was 6.8 to 7.0. Studies with mixed acceptors carried out at concentrations above those required to saturate the system demonstrated that each of the three galactosphingolipids inhibited sulfation of the others. Addition of water-soluble galactosides had no effect. For this and other reasons, it seems likely that the glycosphingolipid sulfotransferase and the carbohydrate sulfotransferase are separate enzymes.

In all three enzymatic studies cited [90, 91, 92], synthesis of sulfatide in vitro required the presence of a PAPS-generating system. Thus, there is now sound evidence for the reaction:

$$\text{Galactocerebroside} + \text{PAPS} \longrightarrow \text{sulfatide} + \text{PAP}$$

Cumar et al. [92] have also demonstrated the following reaction:

$$\text{Lactosyl ceramide} + \text{PAPS} \longrightarrow \text{ceramide-dihexoside sulfate} + \text{PAP}$$

McKhann and Ho have isolated a galactocerebroside sulfotransferase from the microsomal fraction of rat kidney [94]. The kidney enzyme had the same pH optimum and substrate specificity as that in the brain. The difficulty of solubilizing sufficient quantities of sulfotransferase enzyme from either organ has hampered more detailed study; it is not known whether the brain and kidney cerebroside sulfotransferases are the same enzyme.

Cumar et al. have shown that galactosyl sphingosine (psychosine) can also act as a sulfate acceptor [92]. Thus, theoretically, sulfation could precede acylation in the biosynthesis of sulfatides. However, while the affinities of the sulfotransferase for psychosine and for galactocerebroside are approximately equal, the concentration of psychosine in brain tissue is much lower than that of cerebroside. It is unlikely, therefore, that the pathway psychosine → psychosine sulfate → sulfatide is quantitatively significant under ordinary circumstances.

Transport of Sulfatides to the Myelin Sheath

The mechanisms by which the constituents of the myelin sheath are transported and assembled into this highly organized structure have not been determined. Recent studies by Herschkowitz et al. have provided new data about the transport of brain sulfatides. They first demonstrated that the soluble proteins of brain homogenates contain lipoproteins which differ from those of serum in terms of lipid composition, density, and reaction to serum lipoprotein antibodies [96]. Newly synthesized ^{35}S-labeled sulfatide was found to be associated with certain specific proteins within this supernate fraction. Turnover studies showed that ^{35}S-labeled sulfate was *first* incorporated into microsomal sulfatides, *then* into those associated with supernate proteins, and *finally* into myelin [95] (Fig. 32-8). In another study they showed that the sulfatide and protein portions of the lipoprotein complex were synthesized in separate microsomal fractions, and that puromycin inhibited protein synthesis without altering sulfatide synthesis [93]. These findings suggested that the sulfatide became associated with carrier protein which had been previously formed.

The data of Herschkowitz et al. suggest that sulfatides synthesized within the microsomes become associated with more or less specific soluble proteins and that these then transport the sulfatides to the myelin sheath. The capacity of this proposed carrier system is undetermined; it is not known if it could transport the substantial amounts of sulfatides that must be incorporated during the period of most rapid myelination. It is also unknown if such a transport system would also be available for myelin lipids such as cerebrosides or cholesterol. As already described in other sections, there is sound evidence for the concept that the central nervous system myelin represents apposed plasma membranes of the oligodendrocyte. It is not known whether oligodendrocytes synthesize sulfatides, or whether this takes place in other brain cells as well. The proposed lipoprotein transport system might thus function for intracellular or extracellular transport or both.

Rates of Sulfatide Synthesis at Various Stages of Maturation

Sulfatide synthesis has been studied mainly in the brain and in the kidney, the organ which, next to the nervous system, contains the highest level of sulfatide. During maturation

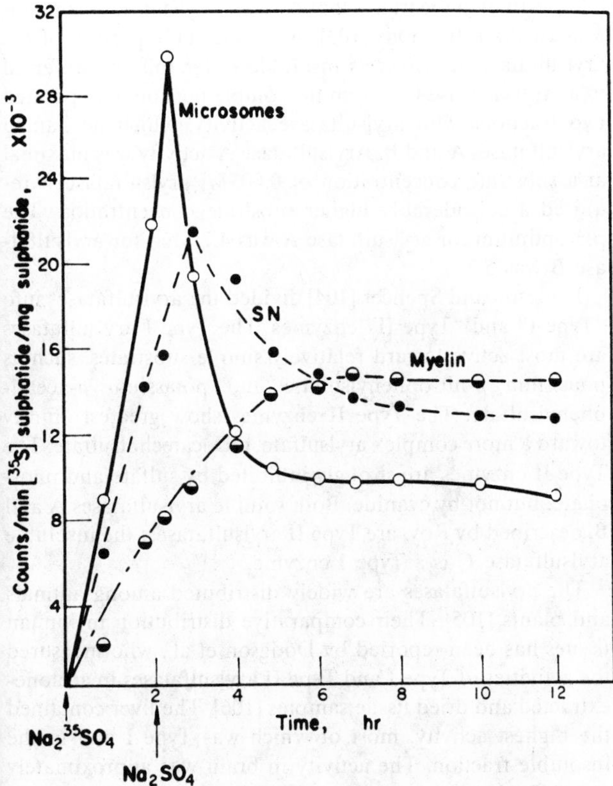

Figure 32-8. Turnover of ^{35}S-labeled sulfatide in subcellular fractions and supernatant. Animals received an intraperitoneal injection of 2 microcuries of ^{35}S Na_2SO_4 per gram of body weight and after 2 hr a second intraperitoneal injection of 0.5 ml of 7 percent Na_2SO_4. Animals were killed by decapitation at various times after the first injection. Specific activity of ^{35}S sulfatide was determined. High levels of specific activity are observed first in the microsomes, then in the supernatant (SN), and finally in the myelin. Zilversmit's criteria for a precursor-product relationship [274] were fulfilled in each instance. (*From McKhann et al.* [94].)

the activity of kidney cerebroside sulfotransferase increases at approximately the same rate as kidney weight [94], and the turnover time of kidney sulfatides appears to be independent of the animal's age [47]. In contrast, the rate of brain sulfatide synthesis varies greatly with age, presumably because myelination is discontinuous.

Maximum incorporation of ^{14}C-labeled glucose or of ^{35}S-labeled sulfate into sulfatides is observed in 15- to 22-day-old rats or mice [97, 51, 98, 99] (Fig. 32-9A). Davison and Gregson showed that brain slices from 19-day-old rats incorporated ^{35}S into sulfatides 5 to 12 times as rapidly as did those from adult animals [97]. McKhann and Ho found that rat brain galactocerebroside sulfotransferase was maximally active at 20 days after birth [94]. There was close correspondence between the variation with age of this brain enzyme (Fig. 32-9B) and the amount of label in brain sulfatide following the injection of a radioactive precursor (Fig. 32-9A). During maturation maximum capacity for brain

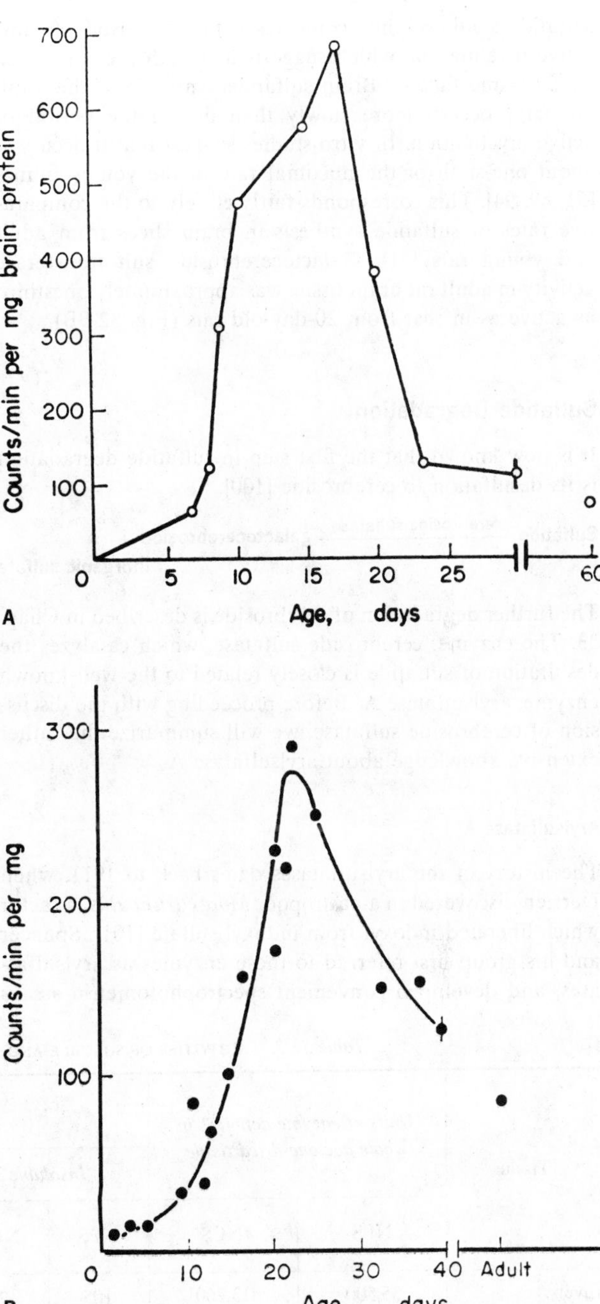

Figure 32-9. A. Incorporation of ^{35}S-labeled sulfate into the lipid extract of rat brain at various ages. Animals were killed 24 hr after injection of 0.3 microcurie of ^{35}S Na_2SO_4 per gm of body weight. Over 90 percent of the radioactivity could be accounted for in the sulfatide fraction. (*From McKhann and Ho* [94].) B. Incorporation of ^{35}S sulfate into sulfatide by a modified homogenate (750 × *g* supernatant). The incubation medium contained 100 micromoles tris buffer, pH 8; 10 micromoles ATP; 0.8 micromole K_2SO_4; 5 micromoles KCl; 50 microcuries ^{35}S-labeled Na_2SO_4; and 0.2 ml of a 750 × *g* supernatant. Incubation was for 2 hr at 37°C. Maximum incorporation was obtained in brain samples of 20-day-old rats. (*From McKhann and Ho* [94].)

sulfatide synthesis thus coincides with the period of most active myelination, which suggests that both are controlled by the same factors. Brain sulfatide synthesis in the adult animal proceeds more slowly than during the period of active myelination. In vitro studies suggest that it occurs at about one-sixth of the maximal rate in the young animal [51, 89, 94]. This corresponds fairly closely to the comparative rates of sulfatide synthesis in brain slices from adult and young rats [51]. Galactocerebroside sulfotransferase activity in adult rat brain tissue was approximately one-third as active as in that from 20-day-old rats (Fig. 32-9B).

Sulfatide Degradation

It is now known that the first step in sulfatide degradation is its desulfation to cerebroside [100].

$$\text{Sulfatide} \xrightarrow{\text{cerebroside sulfatase}} \text{galactocerebroside} + \text{inorganic sulfate}$$

The further degradation of cerebroside is described in Chap. 33. The enzyme, cerebroside sulfatase, which catalyzes the desulfation of sulfatide is closely related to the well-known enzyme, arylsulfatase A. Before proceeding with the discussion of cerebroside sulfatase, we will summarize the rather extensive knowledge about arylsulfatase A.

Arylsulfatase A

The history of the arylsulfatases dates back to 1911, when Derrien discovered in a gastropod, *Morex trunculus,* a factor which liberated indoxyl from indoxyl sulfate [101]. Spencer and his group first referred to these enzymes as arylsulfatases, and developed convenient spectrophotometric assays [102]. Roy demonstrated that ox liver arylsulfatase contains at least three fractions [103]. A considerable portion of the arylsulfatase activity was insoluble (later this was referred to as arylsulfatase C). From the soluble portion he separated two fractions with arylsulfatase activity, which he named arylsulfatases A and B. Arylsulfatase A activity was maximal at a substrate concentration of 0.003*M*; arylsulfatase B required a considerably higher substrate concentration. The pH optimum for arylsulfatase A was 4.7; that for arylsulfatase B was 5.7.

Dodgson and Spencer [104] divided the arylsulfatases into "Type I" and "Type II" enzymes. The Type I arylsulfatases are most active toward relatively simple substrates, such as potassium ρ-nitrophenylsulfate and potassium ρ-acetylphenylsulfate. The Type II enzymes show greatest affinity toward a more complex arylsulfate, nitrocatecholsulfate. The Type II enzymes are strongly inhibited by sulfate and phosphate, but not by cyanide. Both soluble arylsulfatases A and B, described by Roy, are Type II arylsulfatases; the insoluble arylsulfatase C is a Type I enzyme.

The arylsulfatases are widely distributed among animals and plants [105]. Their comparative distribution in human tissues has been reported by Dodgson et al., who measured the activities of Type I and Type II arylsulfatases in acetone-extracted and dried tissue samples [106]. The liver contained the highest activity, most of which was Type I and in the insoluble fraction. The activity in brain was approximately one-fifth that of liver, but in brain the soluble Type II enzymes predominate. The results of Dodgson et al. are summarized in Table 32-2.

Arylsulfatase A and B activities have also been demonstrated in urine [107–109] and in white blood cells [110, 111]. In white blood cells arylsulfatase activity resides mainly in the granulocyte series; cells of the lymphocytic series have

Table 32-2. ACTIVITIES OF SOLUBLE AND INSOLUBLE ARYLSULFATASES IN HUMAN TISSUES

Tissue	*Units of enzyme activity* in whole acetone-dried tissue*		*% of activity of whole tissue*				*Ratio of NPS to NCS*		
			"Insoluble"		*"Soluble"*				
	NPS	NCS	NPS	NCS	NPS	NCS	Whole tissue	Insoluble fraction	Soluble fraction
Liver	35,500	13,260	105	26	4	103	1:0.4	1:0.1	1:11
Pancreas	16,600	8,000	78	11	14	101	1:0.5	1:0.1	1:55
Kidney	13,700	22,750	96	13	4	108	1:1.6	1:0.2	1:49
Lung	1,150	4,780	97	16	13	123	1:3.4	1:0.6	1:34
Brain	510	2,900	73	19	133	120	1:4.1	1:0.9	1:176
Heart	100	2,100	77	22	18	123	1:22	1:6	1:150
Large intestine	950	390	94	15	7	98	1:2.3	1:0.4	1:30
Small intestine	2,500	4,200	56	28	14	116	1:1.7	1:0.3	1:14
Spleen	3,500	3,900							

*A unit of enzyme activity refers to the number of micrograms of phenol liberated after 1 hr of incubation at 37°C. For each fraction and tissue the activity arising from 1 gm acetone-dried tissue was measured.
NOTE: NPS, potassium ρ-nitrophenylsulfate; NCS, nitrocatecholsulfate.
Source: Modified from Dodgson et al. [106].

only little activity [110, 111]. Erythrocytes have none. Contrary to previous impressions, blood platelets have arylsulfatase activity. In the reported studies arylsulfatases A and B are not separated. The fact that optimal activity was achieved at pH 5 suggests that the platelet activity was, at least in part, activity of arylsulfatase A [112, 113]. Of considerable importance is the fact that arylsulfatase A activity can also be demonstrated in cultured skin fibroblasts [114] and in cells cultured from amniotic fluid [115]. Arylsulfatase A activity is located in the lysosomes [118]. This is true both in the liver [116] and in the brain [117]. Arylsulfatase C, in contrast, is a microsomal enzyme [117, 119].

The recent upsurge of interest in prenatal diagnosis has made it of crucial importance to determine the stage of fetal development at which arylsulfatase A activity normally develops. Precise information on this point is still lacking. Jatzkewitz reported that at birth rabbit brain has low levels of arylsulfatase A and cerebroside sulfatase activity; activity of both enzymes increases during myelination, and reaches maximal levels 24 weeks after birth [120]. Austin reported that in rat brain, arylsulfatase A activity is relatively low at birth and then increases during the next 20 days; rat kidney and liver arylsulfatase A activities are nearly fully developed by the first day after birth [121].

In recent years the arylsulfatase A from ox liver [122] and from ox brain [123] has been purified to such a degree that it may be nearly free of extraneous material. This represents an important advance in that it will permit knowledge of the structure of this enzyme and the mechanism of the reactions catalyzed by it. Furthermore, it is not inconceivable that such highly purified enzymes might have a place in therapy. Nichol and Roy achieved a 7,000-fold purification of arylsulfatase from ox liver, and they found this material to be homogeneous by ultracentrifugal analysis [122]. They found that it had a surprisingly high content of proline. At 0.10 ionic strength this enzyme exists as a monomer (molecular weight, 105,000) at pH 7.5, and as a tetramer (molecular weight, 411,000) at pH 5 [124]. They carried out several studies to determine the factors which control the aggregation of the monomer. At pH 5, the monomer has a smaller negative charge than at pH 7.5. They concluded that polymerization at pH 5 resulted from attractive hydrophobic intermolecular bonds which were sufficient to counteract the electrostatic repulsive forces at the lower pH. Treatment with detergent further broke up the monomer into enzymatically inactive subunits of approximately equal size (molecular weight, 24,000).

In studies with this purified ox liver arylsulfatase A, Jerfy and Roy showed that tyrosyl, and possibly histidyl, residues are essential for enzymatic activity [125]. They suggested that during arylsulfatase A-catalyzed desulfations, a tyrosyl residue at the active center of the enzyme is sulfated, and that subsequent desulfation of the enzyme-sulfate complex is aided by an adjacent histidyl residue [125].

Bleszynski et al. [126] achieved a 21,000-fold purification of ox brain arylsulfatase A, and a nearly comparable purification of ox brain arylsulfatase B. Detailed comparisons of the purified arylsulfatase A from brain and liver are not yet available. Allen and Roy have prepared small quantities of purified arylsulfatase B from ox liver [127]. They demonstrated that arylsulfatase B consists of at least two fractions—B-alpha and B-beta; both have molecular weights of 25,000 and, like arylsulfatase A, may aggregate into polymers. It is of interest that the molecular weight of the arylsulfatase B monomer (25,000) appears to be the same as that of the arylsulfatase A subunits (24,000) referred to previously. In view of the marked differences in the isoelectric points and certain other properties, Allen and Roy considered interconversion between arylsulfatase A and B to be highly improbable.

Recently, Goldstone, Konecny and Koenig have reported the effects of neuraminidase on a series of lysosomal hydrolases [275]. Neuraminidase converts hexosaminidase A into hexosaminidase B, and there is considerable evidence that this conversion is due to removal of neuraminic acid. These investigators also presented preliminary evidence that incubation with neuraminidase caused a partial conversion of arylsulfatase A to arylsulfatase B. They have presented the interesting hypothesis that the multiple forms of several lysosomal hydrolases differ from each other mainly in respect to the number of neuraminic acid residues. At first glance, this hypothesis appears at variance with the work of Allen and Roy [127] who considered the interconversions of arylsulfatases A and B to be unlikely. There is insufficient information to resolve this issue. Purified arylsulfatase A does contain amine sugars, but they have not yet been identified [122]. Neither the amino acid nor the carbohydrate components (if any) of arylsulfatase B have been determined [127].

Cerebroside Sulfatase

In 1964 Mehl and Jatzkewitz isolated a cerebroside sulfatase from pig kidney [100]. This enzyme was present in a mixed lysosome and mitochondrial fraction; additional fractionation suggested a lysosomal localization. A 6,000-fold purification of the enzyme was achieved. The final purification step involved high-voltage electrophoresis. The enzymatic activities of the fractions obtained by electrophoresis are shown in Fig. 32-10. Fractions 36 to 44 had arylsulfatase B activity but were essentially devoid of cerebroside sulfatase or arylsulfatase A activity. Fractions 12 to 16 were devoid of cerebroside sulfatase, arylsulfatase A, or arylsulfatase B activity. It is of great interest that combination of fractions 12 to 16 with fractions 16 to 28 brought about an eightfold stimulation of cerebroside sulfatase activity. Heating fractions 12 to 16 at 100°C for 20 min did not diminish this activation. Fractions 12 to 16 thus contained a heat-stable complementary factor for cerebroside sulfatase activity. The nature of this cofactor is under investigation and may prove of considerable importance. The complementary factor has no effect on arylsulfatase A activity.

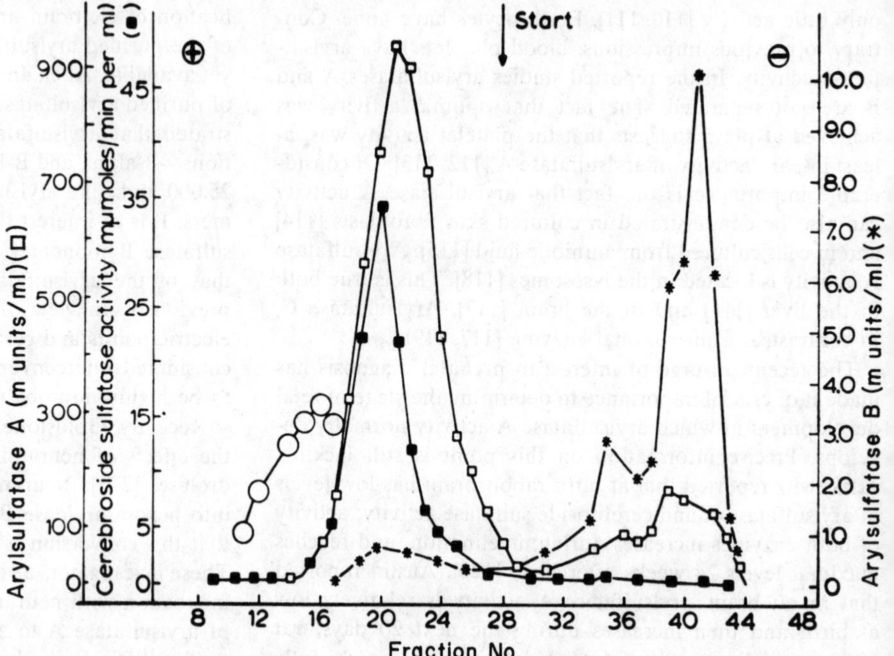

Figure 32-10. Sulfatase activities of pig kidney after fractionation by carrier-free electrophoresis at pH 5.1. (*From Mehl and Jatzkewitz* [129].)

□—□ Arylsulfatase A
■—■—■ Cerebroside sulfatase activity
○—○—○ Complementary fraction
* * Arylsulfatase B

Cerebroside sulfatase has a sharp pH optimum at 4.5. The K_m for kerasin sulfate is 1.05×10^{-4} mole per liter; for cerebron sulfate it is 2.9×10^{-4}. Highest activity was present in pig kidney; but even there, and under optimal conditions, its activity was only 40 to 70 mμmoles per kg per min. Corresponding values for spleen, lymph node, liver, and brain were 39 to 42, 20 to 29, and 7. In a later publication [128] these investigators reported comparable levels of activity in post-mortem human tissues, some of which had been stored in the frozen state for over 2 years.

Cerebroside sulfatase is active toward both natural and synthetic kerasin-3-sulfate and phrenosine-3-sulfate [the two major galactosyl (SO_4) ceramides]. Its specificity is indicated by the fact that it had slight activity with respect to galactose-3-sulfate but was inactive toward galactose-6-sulfate [129]. The cerebroside sulfatase was inactive against steroid sulfate or chondroitin sulfate. At all stages of purification, the enzyme was at least 30 times more active toward ρ-nitrocatecholsulfate than toward cerebroside sulfate. ρ-Nitrocatecholsulfate is the artificial substrate used to measure the activities of the enzymes arylsulfatase A and B.

While cerebroside sulfatase [galactosyl (SO_4) ceramide sulfatase] is clearly distinct from arylsulfatase B, there is considerable evidence that it bears a close relationship to arylsulfatase A. Thus, at all stages of purification cerebroside sulfatase and arylsulfatase A activities were found to reside in the same fractions [100]. Furthermore, in all instances mammalian arylsulfatase A, prepared by a variety of methods, showed cerebroside sulfatase activity provided that the complementary factor was added. Cerebroside sulfatase and arylsulfatase A are inhibited by the same compounds, viz., sulfate, sulfite, phosphate, pyrophosphate, and fluoride, but not by cyanide. Cerebroside sulfatase is inhibited by cerebroside; no data have been reported on the effect of cerebroside on arylsulfatase A activity. Sulfate liberation from cerebroside sulfate is reduced in the presence of ρ-nitrocatecholsulfate, and the sulfate liberation from ρ-nitrocatecholsulfate is reduced in the presence of cerebroside sulfate [129]. Finally, cerebroside sulfatase and arylsulfatase are both deficient in the tissues and body fluids of patients with MLD (see below). Present evidence suggests, therefore, that arylsulfatase A may be the same protein as the heat-labile component of cerebroside sulfatase (fractions 16 to 28, Fig. 32-10). Substantiation of this hypothesis must await preparation of sufficient quantities of this fraction so that it can be compared to highly purified arylsulfatase A.

Physiologic Role of the Arylsulfatases

The substrates which provide the most convenient measures of their activity are not found in biologic materials, and thus provide, at best, only indirect clues to the function of these enzymes. Arylsulfatases A and B are distinct from steroid sulfatases. They occur in different subcellular fractions, have a different pH optimum, and are inactive toward steroid sulfates [100]. Arylsulfatase C and steroid sulfatase are microsomal enzymes with alkaline pH optima. The fact that arylsulfatase C activity, but not dehydroepiandrosterone sulfatase activity, is present in human fetal tissues [130, 131], as well as certain other differences, suggests that these are separate enzymes. Probably a variety of mammalian polysaccharide sulfatases exists [132–134].

At present, study of patients with MLD provides the most significant clue to the physiologic role of arylsulfatase A. MLD is the only known disease in which there is a deficiency of arylsulfatase A, and accumulation of sulfatide is the most consistent and striking abnormality in this disease. The close relationship between arylsulfatase A and cerebroside sulfatase has already been discussed. Thus, it is likely that participation in the desulfation of sulfatides represents one of the physiologic functions of arylsulfatase A. It is possible that additional as yet unidentified physiologic roles may exist.

Previously, tyrosine-*o*-sulfate had been proposed as a possible physiologic substrate for arylsulfatase A [135]. This metabolite is normally present in mammalian urine [136] and bears a chemical resemblance to the artificial substrates used to test arylsulfatase activity. Furthermore, tyrosine-*o*-sulfate is known to be a constituent of fibrinopeptides B, fibrinogen, and gastrin II [136], and, as has already been discussed, it has been proposed as a constituent of arylsulfatase A itself [125]. However, arylsulfatase A has only slight activity against free tyrosine-*o*-sulfate, while arylsulfatases B and C are inactive [136]. Levels of tyrosine-*o*-sulfate have not been measured in patients with MLD.

The Turnover of Myelin Sulfatides

The question of whether there is turnover of the myelin sheath and its sulfatide components is of considerable general interest, and is of importance to a consideration of the pathogenesis of MLD. If myelin does not undergo turnover, i.e., remains *in situ* without renewal during the life of the individual, then a failure of myelin sulfatide degradation could not be the cause of the abnormal myelin composition characteristic of this disease (see below). As will be discussed here, there is now considerable evidence that myelin is not devoid of turnover. That myelin has a remarkable degree of metabolic stability has been established by the metabolic studies of Davison and others. They showed that radioactive precursors injected into chick embryos or suckling rats persisted in the myelin lipids in adult animals that had lived out a significant portion of their life-span [137]. In such studies the estimate of turnover depends on the slope of a curve obtained when the specific activity of the lipid under study is plotted as the ordinate, and the time interval between isotope injection and the sacrifice of the experimental animal as the abscissa. A steep negative slope indicates rapid turnover; a horizontal or slowly declining specific activity indicates slow or even absent turnover [97, 138]. Smith has demonstrated heterogeneity in the turnover rates of different myelin lipids. Some lipid components, even though they appeared to be part of the myelin sheath, had a relatively rapid turnover; this was true particularly for phosphatidyl inositol. For other substances, such as phosphatidyl ethanolamine, intermediate values were obtained. Sulfatides showed the slowest turnover (Fig. 32-11).

More recently the question of myelin turnover has been approached by studies in which the precursor is injected into adult animals. Such studies are technically more demanding, since a smaller fraction of the precursor is incorporated into the brain lipids of adult animals. It has now been clearly demonstrated that ^{35}S-labeled sulfate is incorporated into myelin sulfatides of adult rats injected with isotope at an age when net deposition of sulfatide has ceased [139, 94, 138]. The studies of Davison and Gregson [97] and those of Smith [139, 138] suggest that myelin deposition in the adult animal differs from that in the young animal. It appears that sulfatides synthesized in adult rats are incorporated into myelin within a few hours after injection, whereas those in the young animal are first incorporated into microsomes, and may not reach the myelin until after some days (possibly through the lipoprotein transport system described by Herschkowitz et al. [95, 96]). In addition, the myelin sulfatides synthesized in the adult animal appear to be assignable to at least two metabolic compartments. One is a small, "fast" pool that comprises 0.2 percent of myelin and has a half-life of 2.7 days. It is in slow equilibrium with the larger pool of myelin sulfatide, which either has a slow

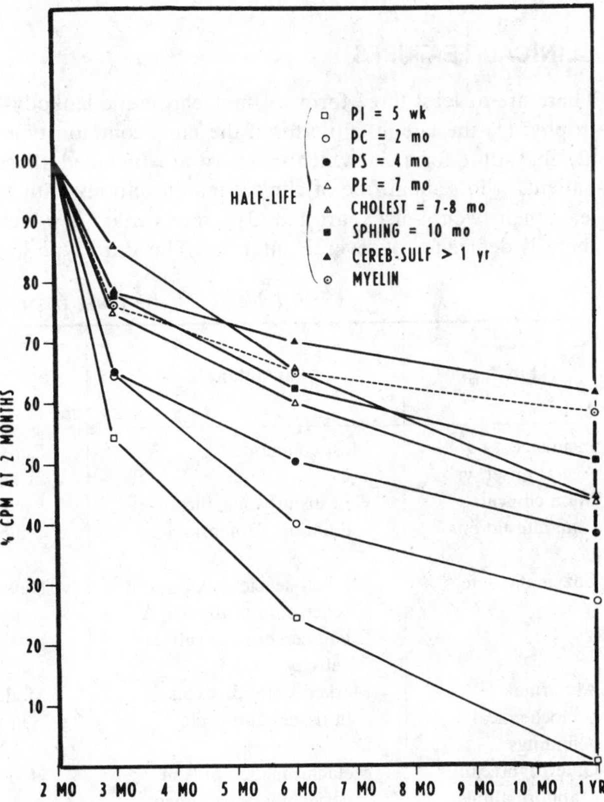

Figure 32-11. Specific activities of brain myelin lipids expressed as percentage of counts per minute at 2 months after injection. These values were corrected for dilution from newly synthesized myelin. (*From Smith* [138].) Abbreviations are: PI = phosphoinositide, PE = phosphatidyl ethanolamine, PS = phosphatidyl serine, PC = phosphatidyl choline, Cholest = cholesterol, Sphing = sphingomyelin, and Cereb. Sulf = sulfatide.

turnover or is metabolically stable. The anatomic localization of this "turnover myelin" is a matter of great interest. Hirano and Dembitzer approached this question by performing electron microscopic studies in rats subjected to a variety of experimental conditions which are known to be noxious to cerebral white matter. In this way they demonstrated clearly the presence of formed organelles and islands of cytoplasm among the myelin loops. They suggested that this myelin formation occurred at the inner and lateral myelin loops [140].

Jatzkewitz has demonstrated cerebroside sulfatase activity in human brain [128], and Bleszyński has prepared his highly purified arylsulfatase A from ox brain [123]. Clendenon and Allen have shown that the levels of arylsulfatase A activity in gray and white matter are approximately equal [118]. Finally, two histochemical studies suggest that arylsulfatase activity is located within or near the myelin sheath both in the central and in the peripheral nervous system [141, 142]. It seems plausible, therefore, that normal myelin sulfatide turnover results from the action of cerebroside sulfatase, the enzyme which is deficient in MLD.

CLINICAL FEATURES

There are at least three forms of metachromatic leukodystrophy: (1) the late infantile form, the most common type; (2) the adult form, in which category are included those patients who remain free of clinical manifestations until at least their twenty-first year; and (3) a rare variant in which there is deficiency of several sulfatases. The third type has been documented in only two unrelated patients (Table 32-3).

A juvenile form of MLD also exists in which the disease becomes apparent between the fourth and fifteenth years. Since in all other respects this form is similar to the late infantile form, it will not be described separately.

Late Infantile Form of MLD

The discussion of the clinical features of this entity is based mainly on the detailed descriptions of Hagberg [143–145], on a review of 42 cases described in the literature [146–163], and on five cases seen by Moser. Several additional clinical reports have appeared recently [164–169].

The late infantile form of MLD is a striking and distressing progressive neurologic disease. Early development is almost always normal. Thirty-seven of forty-two patients achieved locomotion and speech at the expected age. In 30 of the 42 patients symptoms first appeared between the ages of 12 and 18 months; the presenting symptom in almost all was a disturbance in locomotion or other motor activities.

Hagberg has subdivided the clinical course of the disease into four stages which are based on the degree of motor handicap [143].

CLINICAL STAGE I: This is the stage at which the disease first becomes evident. In most patients there are a flaccid weakness and hypotonia of both legs or of all four limbs. The deep tendon reflexes may be diminished or absent. Genu recurvation is often present. A common observation

Table 32-3. THE THREE FORMS OF METACHROMATIC LEUKODYSTROPHY*

Findings	Late infantile	Adult	MLD variant with multiple sulfatase deficiencies
Incidence	Most common	Rare (19 cases known)	Rare
Age at onset, yr	1–4	21 or more, by definition	1–3
Main clinical manifestations	Gait disturbance, incoordination, dementia	Psychosis and dementia; motor signs much later	Slow development, progressive psychomotor deterioration, deafness, skeletal changes, hepatomegaly
Enzymatic defect	Marked deficiency or absence of arylsulfatase A and cerebroside sulfatase activity	Deficient, but not absent, arylsulfatase A activity	Marked deficiency or absence of activity of arylsulfatase A and C and steroid sulfatase; reduced activity of arylsulfatase B
Abnormal biochemical findings	Marked sulfatide excess in tissues and urine	Moderate sulfatide excess in tissues and urine	Marked sulfatide excess in tissues and urine; polysaccharide excess in tissues (and usually in urine)
Other significant abnormalities	Metachromatic lipids in nerve biopsy specimen; progressive impairment of gallbladder function	None proved	Metachromatic lipids in nerve biopsy specimen; Alder-Reilly granules in leukocytes; usually increased urinary polysaccharides

*The classification of patients whose symptoms begin between the ages of 4 and 21 years is uncertain. They seem to fall into two categories: those whose symptoms begin between age 4 and the early teens (the juvenile group), and those in whom symptoms develop in late adolescence. Juvenile MLD probably is the same disorder as the late infantile form of MLD, while patients whose symptoms begin in late adolescence probably belong to the adult group.

is that a child who had already learned to walk becomes unsteady and requires support to stand or walk (Figs. 32-12A, and 32-13A). These features lead to the suspicion of a peripheral neuropathy, a myopathy, or Werdnig-Hoffmann disease.

Rarely, there is spastic paraplegia or diplegia, with increased muscular tone but without exaggerated deep tendon reflexes. Until the progressive nature of the disease becomes clear it may be diagnosed as "cerebral palsy" or brain injury secondary to hypoxia. Ataxia is present in some cases but is slight and not easily found unless specifically searched for. The mean duration of this stage is $1\frac{1}{4}$ years.

CLINICAL STAGE II: In this stage the patient can sit up but can no longer stand. Mental regression is obvious; speech deteriorates as a result of a combination of dysarthria and aphasia. Hypotonia may be replaced by hypertonicity, particularly in the legs. Ataxia is now clearly evident. Deep tendon reflexes continue to be diminished or absent. Hagberg has emphasized that intermittent pain in the arms and legs is a frequent feature in this stage of disease, and he believes that this is a manifestation of peripheral nerve or root involvement. This stage may be of short duration. Some patients appear to pass through it in only a few days; most commonly it is 3 to 6 months in duration.

CLINICAL STAGE III: At this stage the child is bedridden and quadriplegic. Muscle tone is variable. There may be decorticate, decerebrate, or dystonic postures (Fig. 32-13C), upon which hypertonic fits may be superimposed. There is difficulty in feeding and in maintaining the airway because of a combination of bulbar and pseudobulbar palsies. Six of nine patients observed by Hagberg had optic atrophy. The mental deficit is much more severe, and speech is no longer distinct, but the child may still be able to smile and respond to his parents. Deep tendon reflexes are nearly always absent. In Hagberg's series this stage lasted from $\frac{1}{4}$ to $3\frac{1}{2}$ years.

CLINICAL STAGE IV: In this final stage the patient appears to have lost all meaningful contact with his surroundings. He is blind, without speech, and without volitional movement. Usually he must be fed through a nasogastric or gastrostomy tube. This final stage may last for long periods. One of our patients, whose illness began at 9 years of age, remained in this vegetative state for 7 years, until her death at age 17.

Cogan et al. have described the ocular changes in five patients with MLD—four with the late infantile type and one with the variant in which there is a deficiency of multiple sulfatases [170, 171]. The most characteristic feature was grayness of the macula, with a red spot in the center. The macular changes resemble those in Tay-Sachs disease in that the accumulated material produces some opacification of the retina, but it results in a grayish discoloration rather than the conspicuous white opacification of the retina seen in Tay-Sachs disease. This is presumably because in MLD the glycolipid accumulation in the ganglion cells is less striking. The grayness was relatively indistinct and could escape casual examination, but was readily detected when looked for. In all five instances the change was present at clinical stage II, and in one instance the ophthalmologic finding represented the initial diagnostic clue.

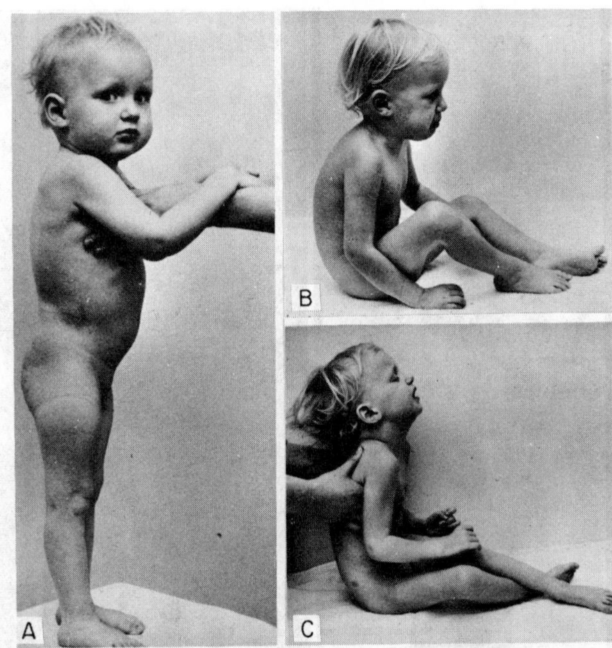

Figure 32-12. Late infantile MLD. A. Hagberg Stage One. B. Hagberg Stage Two (the child is no longer able to stand, even with support). C. Hagberg Stage Three. (*From Hagberg* [143].)

The juvenile type of MLD includes those cases in which illness first appears between 4 and 21 years of age, most commonly, between 5 and 10 years. The clinical course resembles that in the late infantile form, but in the juvenile form failure of schoolwork, emotional lability, and slight visual disturbances may be the initial or early symptoms. This was true of the original patients described by Scholz [19]. It is possible that the earlier prominence of mental and visual changes may be explained by their easier recognition in older children. The juvenile and late infantile types of MLD may occur within the same kinship. Austin reported a patient whose initial symptom began at age $5\frac{1}{2}$ years and who died at age 9 [172]. A maternal cousin of this patient died of MLD at age $3\frac{1}{4}$ years, following a 6-month illness. This observation, together with the clinical similarities, suggests that the late infantile and the juvenile type of MLD are the same clinical entity.

The Adult Type of MLD

The adult form of MLD is a rare disorder which is difficult to diagnose. It is listed here as a separate disease type because the clinical manifestations are relatively distinctive and because recent biochemical studies suggest differences from

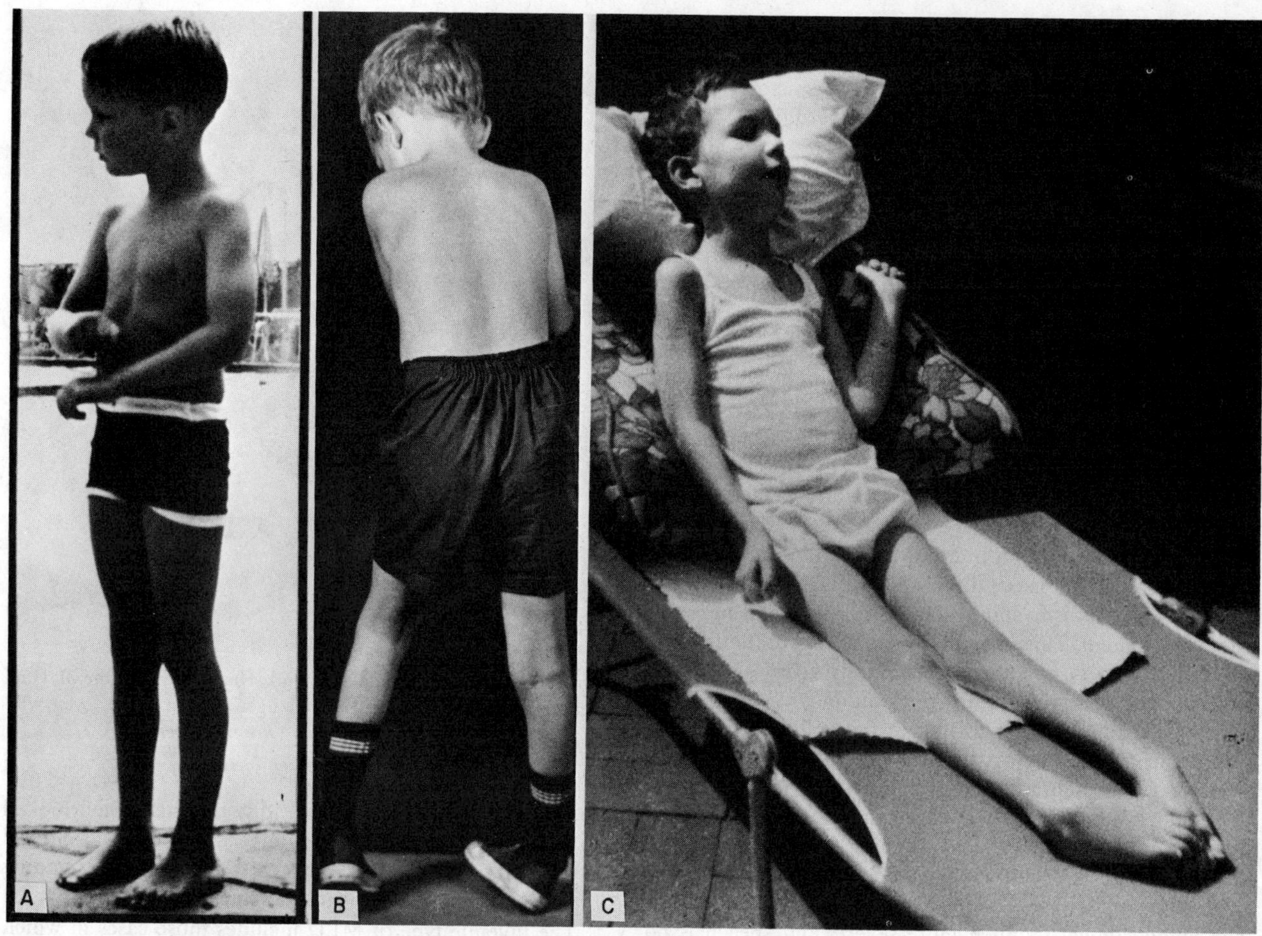

Figure 32-13. Juvenile MLD. A. Age $5\frac{1}{2}$ years, 1 year before onset of symptoms; the child is entirely normal. B. Age $6\frac{11}{12}$ years; the child has increasing gait difficulty and is unable to stand without support. C. Age $8\frac{10}{12}$ years; the patient is bedridden, has increasing difficulty in swallowing, and requires tube feeding. He is no longer able to speak, but recognizes family and displays pleasure when people pay attention to him.

the late infantile type of MLD. According to a recent compilation, 19 cases have been reported [173], including the cases of Alzheimer [17] and Witte [18] referred to in the introduction. In only two instances has the diagnosis been achieved during life [173, 174], and both of these patients were sibs of individuals in whom the diagnosis of adult MLD had been made by post-mortem studies.

The main clinical features have been summarized in a recent review [173]. Of 19 reported patients 5 were women and 13 men; in one the sex was not mentioned. Age at initial symptoms varied between 19 and 46 years. The patient whose disease began at 19 years of age died when she was 46 years old, and she has an affected brother and sister whose disease became symptomatic at ages 32 and 36. The illness may have an extremely protracted course. One patient died 44 years after the initial symptoms [175], and another patient was still alive 36 years after his first symptoms [174]. In a total of 7 patients clinical symptoms lasted more than 10 years; in 8 others the course of the illness was less than a decade, the shortest course being $1\frac{2}{12}$ years. Prior to the final stages of the disease the symptoms suggest schizophrenia or an organic dementia. This is illustrated by the patient reported by Van Bogaert and Dewulf, who when he was "21 years old began to drink heavily and developed ideas of grandeur. He thought he was going to be ambassador and gave himself honorary titles (although still working as a clerk); his writing became illegible and irregular; . . . he became childish, . . . proposed to passers-by that they box with him. He became unable to read newspapers and rested for hours in a chair immobile" [176]. It is not surprising that, faced with this type of history, the examining physician would fail to consider a leukodystrophy. However, since such symptoms have been reported in nearly all cases [174, 175, 177–183], it seems justified to attribute these mental and emotional changes to the leukodystrophy. Generalized seizures [183, 184], slight tremors or choreic movements [184], or other slight signs of motor incoordination are usually seen only in the later stages of the disease, at times not until several decades after the appearance of mental symptoms [174]. During the final stages of the illness the patient is in a severely deteriorated state, incontinent, mute, and subject to generalized seizures.

The term *adult MLD* here has been restricted arbitrarily to apply only to those patients who did not develop symptoms until they were at least 21 years old. Since the initial symptoms usually are in the mental and emotional sphere, and since they may, at first, be subtle, it is difficult to date their onset accurately. Austin et al. have tabulated 10 cases of MLD in which the illness began in late adolescence. The average age of the patients at the earliest symptoms was 17 years (range, 13 to 20 years) [174]. We have already referred to the patient of Müller et al., who became symptomatic at age 19 years but whose affected sibs did not develop symptoms until their mid-thirties [173]. There seems little doubt that at least some of the "late juvenile" cases should be classed with the adult type of MLD, but this cannot be proved until the biochemical and morphologic characteristics of the late infantile and the adult types have been more closely defined.

MLD Variant with Multiple Sulfatase Deficiencies

In 1963 and 1965 Austin described a brother and sister with MLD, members of the "M" family, who showed certain abnormalities beyond those which are usually associated with MLD [172, 185]. They did not achieve their early milestones at the appropriate age. The best performance at age 2 years included the ability to crawl but not to walk. The girl was then able to say "mommy" but lacked other words. As is true of other patients with MLD, she gradually lost these skills, a progressive quadriplegia, nystagmus, and brief seizures developed, and the patient and her brother died in a vegetative state when they were 11 and 12 years old. When the girl was 7 years old, it was first observed that her lower ribs flared and that the sternum was convex. The peripheral white blood cells contained large granules resembling the Alder-Reilly bodies seen in the mucopolysaccharidoses [186, 187]. The urine contained a large excess of mucopolysaccharides. At post-mortem examination the kidney was found to contain mucopolysaccharide levels comparable to those seen in the mucopolysaccharidoses [188]. In addition to the changes in the brain characteristic of MLD, there was lipid accumulation in the cortical neurons. The excess neuronal lipid appeared to consist of gangliosides rather than sulfatides. It is of great interest that the tissues of these patients were deficient in arylsulfatases A, B, and C, whereas in the usual form of MLD only arylsulfatase A is lacking [189].

Moser has studied another unrelated patient (G. L.), who bears a close resemblance to the affected members of the "M" family [190].

CASE REPORT. The patient, G. L. (MGH No. 113-72-55), was admitted to the Massachusetts General Hospital on three occasions in 1961 and 1962 for the study of his progressive neurologic disorder and for supportive medical therapy. He was the product of an unremarkable first pregnancy to unrelated parents of Canadian and French-Canadian descent. Three younger sibs, now ages 3 to 7, are normal.

As a neonate the patient had respiratory difficulties and a weak suck. Vomiting accompanied each feeding, and wheezing was frequent. Surgical repair of a pectus excavatum and a feeding gastrostomy were performed when he was 3 months old. When he was 5 months of age the mother suspected a developmental delay. At 12 months he was able to lift his head, crawl, and sit with support. At 18 months he could sit without support and walk a short distance independently. This last skill was retained only briefly. Speech never progressed beyond unintelligible sounds, and a progressive hearing loss was suspected at age 26 months.

At 26 months of age he appeared alert and effectively reached for objects in his immediate environment. He used a reflex hammer appropriately and exchanged toys from one hand to another. Body length and weight were normal; the head circumference was about the 90th percentile, and the head did not grow over the ensuing year (Fig. 32-14).

Other findings included thick, dry skin, labored respiration, generalized pulmonary rhonchi, 2- to 3-cm hepatomegaly, 2-cm splenomegaly, short and incurving fifth fingers, bilateral ptosis, a high myopia, lack of response to loud sounds, hyperactive deep tendon reflexes, resistance to passive movements, and generalized weakness. Sensation seemed intact to pinprick. There was a marked tremor of the upper extremities, aggravated by volitional movements. The corneae were clear, and extraocular movements were full.

X-ray examination showed broad humeri with thick cortices and thick, wide phalanges and metacarpals. The phalanges of the fifth fingers were hypoplastic. The second and fifth lumbar vertebrae protruded anteriorly. The cerebrospinal fluid was under normal pressure and only on the first of three occasions contained excessive protein (102 mg per 100 ml). An electroencephalogram performed during sedated sleep was normal; the lack of an arousal response to sound confirmed the prior impression of deafness. A bone marrow aspiration showed Alder-Reilly bodies [186, 187] in the white blood cell series, and later these were recognized in the peripheral blood. A screening test for excess urinary mucopolysaccharides was negative. Urinary polysaccharide uronic acid, measured as described by deFerrante's method [191], was 3 to 11 mg (average 7 mg) per 24 hr. This value is within normal limits for the age [192]. Urinary polysaccharides have not yet been fractionated.

By age 35 months, 9 months after initial evaluation, he could no longer follow visual stimuli, could not crawl or

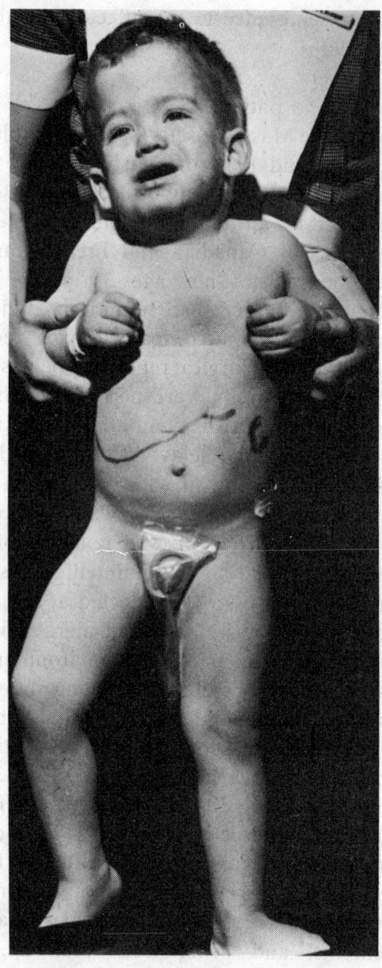

Figure 32-14. MLD variant with multiple sulfatase deficiencies. Patient G.L. at 26 months of age. Note enlarged head circumference, depressed bridge of nose, enlarged liver and spleen, pectus excavatum, and incurved little finger. (*From Murphy* [190].)

sit, and was unable to hold objects. Swallowing difficulties necessitated reinstitution of the feeding gastrostomy. He maintained a posture of flexion of his upper extremities and rigid extension of his lower extremities. Frequent and brief tonic seizures occurred, and were poorly controlled with Dilantin and phenobarbital.

At 40 months of age a gray hazy appearance about the maculae was first noted [171].

At that time the "fluff test" for urinary sulfatides [193] and a sural nerve biopsy were both positive for metachromatic leukodystrophy. Detailed metabolic studies were undertaken, including a therapeutic trial of a low-sulfur diet. The latter caused a reduction of urinary inorganic sulfate levels to less than 10 percent of control, but did not alter the clinical status, the urinary sulfatide level (approximately 5 mg per 24 hr), or the rate of incorporation of intravenously administered ^{35}S-labeled sulfate into urinary sulfatides. The patient died at the age of 3½ years.

Post-mortem examination was performed 3 hr after death. Recent bilateral tracheitis and pneumonitis were present. The free borders of the mitral valves contained nodular thickenings, 0.2 cm in greatest diameter. Microscopically these nodules were whorls of collagenous tissue. Except for this, the heart was normal. The liver weighed 900 gm (normal for age, 516 gm), and the spleen, 250 gm (normal for age, 39 gm). The hepatic Kupffer cells and the parenchymal cells were heavily vacuolated, as were the cells lining the splenic sinusoids. The gallbladder was normal. It did not contain the polypoid metachromatic deposits which are frequently present in classical MLD [216]. The kidneys weighed 130 gm (normal for age, 100 gm), and the renal collecting tubules stained metachromatically with acid cresyl violet.

The brain weighed 860 gm (normal for age, 1,140 gm). The meninges were thick, and there was marked cerebral and cerebellar atrophy. The number of cortical neurons was decreased. There was storage of PAS-positive but non-metachromatic material in all the remaining neurons. This stored material stained purple red with acid cresyl violet and pale pink with Scharlach red. The Purkinje cells contained storage material with similar histochemical properties and showed prominent dendritic enlargement. The white matter of the peripheral and central nervous systems showed striking brown metachromasia with acid cresyl violet, as in classical MLD. Similar metachromatic material was seen in the neurons of the dentate nucleus, inferior olives, brain stem nuclei, and motor nuclei of the spinal cord. Oligodendroglia, though reduced in number, were not as rare as in the usual case of metachromatic leukodystrophy. The only electron microscopic studies were done on the retina [171]. Here the ganglion cells contained single membrane-limited organelles with laminated inclusions which were thought to represent lysosomal storage.

In addition to sulfatide accumulation, certain of the visceral organs contained water-soluble metachromatic materials with properties similar to those of the tissue deposits found in the genetic mucopolysaccharidoses. These abnormal substances were present in the parenchymal and reticuloendothelial cells of the spleen and the liver and in the tubular epithelium of the kidney. Under the light microscope they appeared as small granules within the cell cytoplasm, and they showed alcohol-resistant metachromasia with toluidine blue.

As in the "M" family, Patient G. L. achieved delayed peak psychomotor development, at 2 years of age, and then showed progressive neurologic deterioration. He had a sternal abnormality (pectus excavatum), and the leukocytes showed Alder-Reilly granulations [186, 187]. Unlike the members of the "M" family, this child had hepatosplenomegaly. Though the urine did not contain excess mucopolysaccharide, the post-mortem tissues showed a mucopolysaccharide excess comparable to that in Hurler's syndrome. Neuropathologic examination showed the changes characteristic of MLD, but, again as in members of the "M" family, the cortical neurons were distended with nonmetachromatic lipids, probably gangliosides.

Enzymatic studies provide the most convincing evidence for placing Patient G. L. and the "M" family in the same category. Moser has had the opportunity to perform these assays on post-mortem liver tissue from one of the "M" family cases, and has compared the findings with those on post-mortem tissues of Patient G. L. and of patients with classical MLD. Both G. L. and the "M" family tissues showed deficiencies of arylsulfatases A, B, C, and of steroid sulfatases. Tissues from classical MLD patients showed a specific deficiency of arylsulfatase A; the activity of all four enzymes was either normal or increased in tissues from patients with Hurler's syndrome.

A combination of MLD with other disease entities has been reported in four additional patients from three separate kinships. Luthy et al. [194] reported a girl in whom MLD was combined with storage of nonmetachromatic lipids in the cortical neurons. Additional data about the pathologic and histochemical findings of this case have since been reported [195, 196]. Pilz and Jatzkewitz examined the gray matter lipids of formalin-fixed brain tissue from Luthy's case. Though they found a moderate increase in G_{M2} ganglioside, the main abnormality was an excess of ceramide-lactoside [196]. Mossakowski et al. reported similar findings in a French-Canadian family [197]. They concluded that the excess lipid in the cortical neurons of their patients was a ganglioside. In the patient of Thieffry et al., the skeletal, roentgenologic, and hematologic changes resembled those of Patient G. L., and, as in the "M" family, there was mucopolysacchariduria [198, 199]. Since post-mortem examination was not performed, there is no way to determine if there was also storage of nonmetachromatic lipids in the cortical neurons.

Table 32-4 shows the main features of the MLD variant. Patients G. L. and members of the "M" family show features of MLD, of a lipidosis, and of a mucopolysaccharidosis. Since deficiencies of arylsulfatases B and C and of steroid sulfatase have not been observed in any other known disorder of lipid or mucopolysaccharide metabolism, it is likely that this entity does not represent a random association of diseases, but rather that it is a new and separate disease. In view of the strong clinical and biochemical resemblance, we believe that the case of Thieffry et al. [198, 199] belongs in the same category. In respect to the patients of Mossakowski [197] et al. and of Luthy [194, 195], there is no information about mucopolysaccharide levels and no evidence that skeletal or roentgenologic abnormalities existed. Information is insufficient, therefore, to decide whether or not these cases should be assigned to this category.

Rampini et al. [276] have presented complete clinical data on three patients with this form of MLD. Pathologic features of one of these patients had been described previously [194, 195]. Urinary polysaccharides were increased in all

Table 32-4. FEATURES OF THE MLD VARIANT WITH MULTIPLE SULFATASE DEFICIENCIES

Feature	Murphy et al. [190], Patient G.L.	Austin et al. [172], Case CM	Mossakowski et al. [197]			Thieffry et al. [198, 199]	Luthy et al. [194, 195]
			Case 1	Case 2	Case 3		
Early development	Slow	Slow	Slow	Normal	Normal	Normal	N.M.
Best skill	Walked	Single words	Walked	Single words	Single words	Single words	N.M.
Age at start of deterioration	18 mo	24 mo	24 mo	14 mo	15 mo	15 mo	1 yr
Hearing	Deaf	Present	Deaf (?)	Deaf (?)	N.M.	Deaf	N.M.
Age at onset of seizures, yr	3	2	2	N.M.	N.M.	1½	N.M.
Age at death, yr	3½	12½	3	5	3	4	3
Skin	Thick, dry	Yellow, loose	N.M.	N.M.	N.M.	Ichthyosis	Ichthyosis
Head circumference, percentile	75th	Normal	Below 3d	N.M.	N.M.	10th	N.M.
Sternum	Pectus excavatum	Convex	N.M.	N.M.	N.M.	Protuberant	N.M.
Hepatosplenomegaly	Yes	No	No	N.M.	N.M.	No	Yes
Alder-Reilly bodies in WBCs	Yes	Yes	N.M.	N.M.	N.M.	Yes	Yes
Bone roentgenogram	Broad phalanges & humerus	Advanced age	N.M.	N.M.	N.M.	Broad metacarpals & carpals	N.M.
Urinary metachromasia	Yes	Yes	N.M.	N.M.	N.M.	Yes	Yes
Increased urinary mucopolysaccharides	No	Yes	N.M.	N.M.	N.M.	Yes	N.M.
CSF protein	40–102	N.M.	Normal	N.M.	N.M.	70	242
Positive nerve biopsy	Yes	N.M.	N.M.	N.M.	N.M.	Yes	Yes

three of these patients. One of them excreted equal amounts of heparan sulfate and dermatan sulfate. In the two other patients heparan sulfate accounted for 60.8 and 73 percent and dermatan sulfate for 39.2 and 27 percent of urinary polysaccharides. All patients showed Alder-Reilly granulations in leukocytes of peripheral blood and bone marrow. Urinary arylsulfatase A activity was deficient and nerve biopsy findings were similar to those in late infantile metachromatic leukodystrophy. The authors have proposed the designation "mucosulfatidosis" for this entity.

Other Atypical Forms of MLD

Bubis and Adlesberg [200] and Feigin [201] have reported cases of congenital metachromatic leukodystrophy. The patient described by Bubis and Adlesberg died 20 hr after birth. The neuronal cytoplasm in the cerebral cortex and basal ganglia was distended with acidophilic lipids. Numerous eosinophilic bodies up to 25 microns in diameter were disseminated throughout the white matter. The staining properties did not correspond exactly to those described for MLD, and there is no information about sulfatide levels or enzymatic activities. In our opinion there is insufficient evidence to assign this case to the MLD category.

Neimann et al. [202] described a 7-year-old patient in whom the main clinical abnormalities consisted of repeated convulsions and mental deterioration. They also described a 12-year-old patient with progressive external ophthalmoplegia, facial diplegia, progressive auditory impairment, impaired vision associated with retinitis pigmentosa, repeated convulsions, and, eventually, coma. The diagnosis of MLD was documented by sural nerve biopsy. Particularly for the 12-year-old patient, the clinical manifestations differ from those of any other cases known to me. The brief reports so far available do not allow full assessment of these patients.

PATHOLOGY

In metachromatic leukodystrophy the most severe damage occurs in the white matter of the central nervous system. In contrast to most other types of leukodystrophy, there is also a striking involvement of the peripheral nervous system, of certain groups of neurons, and of visceral organs. The diseased white matter is firmer than normal, has a gray or sometimes brown discoloration, and in severely affected regions may show cavitation. In most cases there is a relative sparing of the U fibers, the subcortical association fibers between adjacent convolutions.

Histopathology

The white matter shows a loss of normal myelin sheaths, a diminished number of interfascicular oligodendrocytes [146], and a striking accumulation of spherical granular masses of lipid material measuring 15 to 20 microns in diameter. These masses may be contained within macrophages which are prominent in perivascular spaces, or they may appear to lie free within the tissue [203]. They may also be found within oligodendrocytes in areas where the myelin sheaths are relatively spared [162]. These granules and inclusions are strikingly metachromatic, and this feature is responsible for the name assigned to this disorder. The most effective way to demonstrate this phenomenon is to stain frozen tissue sections with 1 percent cresyl violet adjusted to pH 3.6 with acetic acid, as described by Hirsch and Peiffer [205]. With this technique the white matter of MLD patients stains brown and stands in sharp contrast to the purple staining of the adjacent cerebral cortex. Dayan has shown that when sections of MLD tissues stained with cresyl violet are viewed by polarized light with the polarizer and analyzer 90° out of phase, the metachromatic granules show a specific lime-green to yellow-green dichroism [206]. Use of this device enhances the specificity of the cresyl violet staining reaction.

There is now ample evidence that the metachromatic staining reaction is due to sulfatide. The *in situ* staining characteristics are entirely consistent with this hypothesis. The material in the granules is extractable by solvents such as alcohol, pyridine, petroleum ether, and chloroform-methanol and is stained by Sudan black. It shows only a slight affinity for Sudan IV, which stains nonpolar lipids such as cholesteryl esters and neutral fats. An important and consistent observation is a strongly positive periodic acid–Schiff reaction (PAS). Preextraction of the tissue with lipid solvents results in the parallel disappearance of staining with PAS and Sudan black.

A positive PAS reaction which disappears upon extraction with lipid solvents generally indicates the presence of either an unsaturated fatty acid or a glycolipid. These can be distinguished by the fact that a positive PAS reaction due to a carbohydrate unit can be blocked by prior acetylation [207]. With this technique the material accumulated in MLD reacted like a glycolipid. Furthermore the metachromatic properties and the positive reaction with Alcian blue indicate that this glycolipid contains an acidic group. The two common acidic glycolipids in the nervous system are sulfatides and gangliosides. Gangliosides would appear to be ruled out by the fact that the lipids which accumulate in MLD fail to react with Bial's test for neuraminic acid [197], which is a characteristic component of these lipids. This indirect histochemical evidence thus points toward sulfatides as the cause of metachromasia.

The most conclusive evidence for the nature of the metachromatic material was provided by Suzuki et al. [208]. These investigators isolated the metachromatic bodies by ultracentrifugal and density-gradient techniques. Sulfatides accounted for 39 percent of the total lipid content of the metachromatic bodies. The preparation did not contain significant quantities of other acidic lipids or chromotropes.

It is characteristic of metachromatic leukodystrophy that, in addition to changes in the white matter, certain groups of neurons are also involved in the disease process. These are distended with metachromatic lipids which have histochemical reactions similar to those of the white matter. The dentate nucleus of the cerebellum is involved in all patients who have been adequately studied. In contrast to the observations in amaurotic familial idiocy, the Purkinje cells are spared.

Other groups of neurons which are frequently involved are the cranial nerve nuclei, hypothalamus, thalamus, basal ganglia, pons, anterior horn cells, and spinal root ganglion cells. The neurons in the cerebral cortex are normal, with the exception of the large Betz cells which sometimes contain metachromatic material. In contrast, in the MLD variant with multiple sulfatase deficiencies, the cortical neurons are distended with nonmetachromatic lipids.

The changes in peripheral nerves are similar to those in the central white matter, and this has permitted the utilization of peripheral nerve biopsy as a means of diagnosis (see below). Varying degrees of demyelination are seen, along with an accumulation of metachromatic granules within Schwann cells and phagocytes.

Dayan has reported that the peripheral nerve lesion in MLD is a segmental demyelination [209]. Webster had reached a similar conclusion on the basis of earlier electron microscopic studies [210]. The term "segment" here refers to that portion of the myelin sheath (and axon) situated between two adjacent nodes of Ranvier. Each myelin segment lies within the cytoplasm of one Schwann cell. Dayan studied post-mortem peripheral nerves of a 15-year-old patient with MLD. He had teased apart individual nerve fibers so that he could examine the changes in the myelin sheath segments of individual fibers. He then studied the pattern of demyelination in these fibers. If the primary lesion were within the anterior horn or dorsal ganglion cell, or if the nerve were damaged proximally, then all segments of that particular nerve fiber would be expected to show damage, while all segments of an adjacent uninvolved fiber might be intact. On the other hand, in segmental demyelination some segments may be demyelinated while other adjacent segments along the same nerve fiber remain intact. This was the case in the MLD nerves: Dayan found that 80 percent of all nerve fibers had some damage, but with the patchy distribution characteristic of segmental demyelination. The demonstration of this segmental pattern is of importance in considering the pathogenesis of MLD. As will be discussed, it directs attention to the importance of changes within the Schwann cells, and by implication, to those of the oligodendrocyte in the central nervous system.

A careful histologic study of the eyes has been reported by Cogan and Kuwabara [170, 171]. Metachromatic material was found in the ganglion cells of the retina. Even the large ganglion cells, which were preferentially affected, showed no distension. By contrast, in Tay-Sachs disease the small ganglion cells around the fovea are markedly distended with glycolipids which do not show the striking metachromasia seen in metachromatic leukodystrophy.

Involvement of visceral organs has been observed in all patients whose tissues have been carefully examined [214]. Metachromatic material is present in the epithelial cell cytoplasm of the convoluted tubules of the kidney and in the loops of Henle and collecting tubules, but not in the glomeruli. In one patient there were additional changes consistent with chronic nephritis [18], but in others there is only a swelling of the tubular epithelium corresponding to sites of accumulation of metachromatic material. In no patient has there been clinical evidence of impaired renal function. The gallbladder is small and fibrotic, and the mucosal cells and villi are distended with macrophages containing metachromatic material [148, 154]. Hagberg and Svennerholm have demonstrated a progressive inability of the gallbladder to concentrate dyes [215]. A moderate number of metachromatic granules are seen in the portal histiocytes, in the epithelial cells of intrahepatic bile ducts, and less frequently in Kupffer cells and parenchymal cells, particularly those in the peripheral zones of the lobule. Deposits of metachromatic lipids have been demonstrated occasionally in the islets of Langerhans [162, 144], the anterior pituitary [18], the adrenal cortex [162], and the testis [18]. The reticuloendothelial system is generally not involved.

Multiple large polypoid masses or papillomas project from the mucosa into the lumen of the gallbladder, and these masses contain abundant metachromatic material [216]. In another report multiple nonopaque calculi were demonstrated in the gallbladder of a $4\frac{1}{2}$-year-old boy with MLD [217].

Studies with the Electron Microscope

Studies with the electron microscope have demonstrated the presence of inclusion bodies, as well as structural changes in the myelin and mitochondria. Inclusions have been noted within neurons, glial cells, Schwann cells [204, 208, 210, 213, 218, 219], and retinal ganglion cells [171]. The inclusions vary in size. The small ones often are granular; the larger ones have a lamellar structure. The periodicity of the lamellar structure varied from 40 to 90 Å, with 60 Å the most common [208]. In the Schwann cell, inclusions are most frequently seen near the mitochondria and the node of Ranvier [210]. Inclusions also are noted within those Schwann cells which surround unmyelinated axons. Some of the inclusions form fusiform or saccular swellings along nerve fibers.

In addition to intraneuronal or intraglial inclusions, there are also large round masses of similar texture which are not clearly associated with any cellular element. These masses are probably the metachromatic bodies seen under the light microscope. Using a technique similar to that used for the isolation of the metachromatic bodies in Tay-Sachs disease, Suzuki et al. were able to isolate these bodies and have determined their chemical composition [208]. This important achievement establishes that the metachromatic bodies and

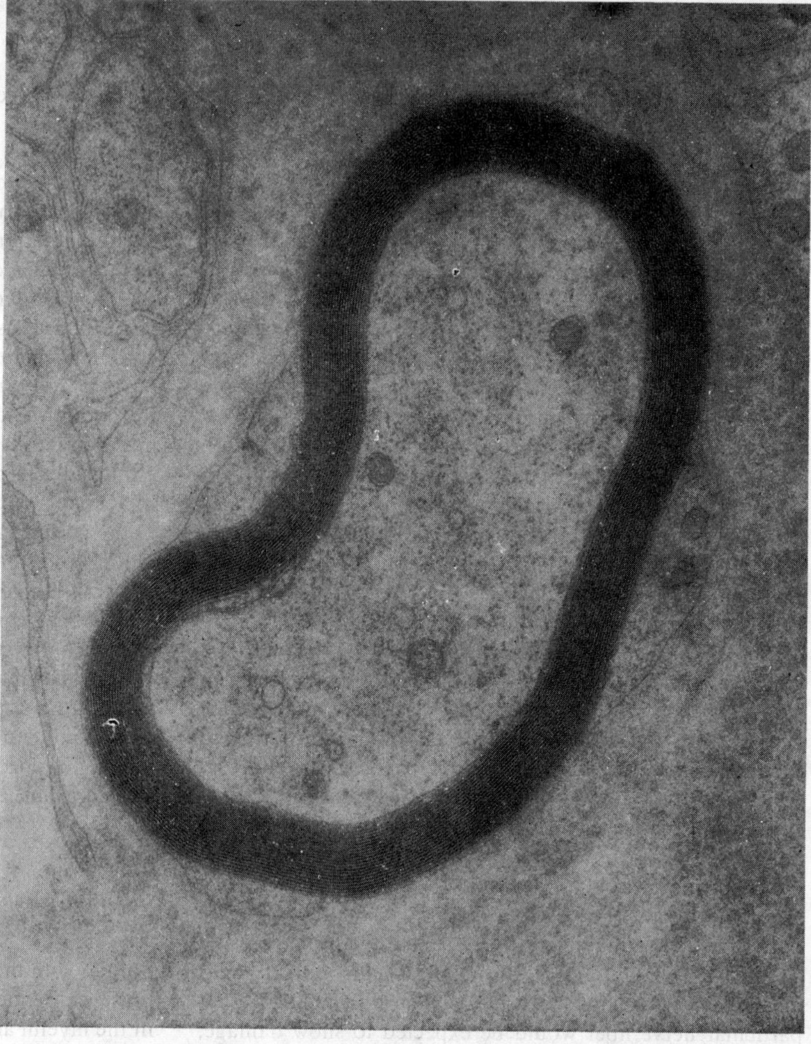

Figure 32-15. Cross section, normal human myelinated fiber. The myelin sheath, with its lamellar period of approximately 120 Å, lies within Schwann cell cytoplasm and surrounds the axon, containing filaments, mitochondria, and tubules of agranular endoplasmic reticulum. (×29,000.) (*From Webster* [210].)

inclusions are rich in sulfatide, and improves our understanding about the structure and formation of the inclusions. Résibois et al. [218] have shown that the less-structured inclusions are richest in acid phosphatase, and on the basis of this and other evidence, it appears likely that the sulfatide-containing granules and bodies are accumulated within lysosomes [220]. As has already been discussed, arylsulfatase A and cerebroside sulfatase activity are normally located within the lysosome.

Webster [210] and Cravioto et al. [213], in their studies with the electron microscope, have demonstrated abnormal myelin in MLD. In advanced lesions the myelin lamellas were almost totally disintegrated. In addition, they noted milder and earlier changes. Certain fibers showed a change in their lamellar pattern characterized by an overall increase in density and a decrease in the distance between dense lines. At times, this focal, bandlike change in the lamellar pattern occupied the entire circumference of the sheath (Figs. 32-15, 32-16). In the future it may be possible to correlate these alterations in the myelin lamellar pattern with the abnormal chemical composition of myelin isolated from MLD tissue by O'Brien [221], Suzuki [208], and Cumings [222]. Cravioto et al. have demonstrated greatly thickened cristae in the Schwann cell mitochondria [213].

Chemical Pathology

Sulfatide Accumulation

Jatzkewitz [21] and Austin [22] independently demonstrated an accumulation of sulfatides in the white matter of patients with MLD, and this observation has been confirmed in all instances where sulfatide analysis has been performed [46, 128, 149, 197, 209, 221, 223–228]. The data listed in Table 32-5 are representative. In the late infantile form of MLD white matter sulfatide levels are 3 to 10 times normal. The levels of the other myelin lipids such as cholesterol and sphingomyelin may be decreased by 30 to 50 percent, presumably secondary to the loss of myelin. Cerebroside levels are diminished out of proportion to those of the other myelin lipids. They vary between less than 10 percent and 50 percent of normal. As a result, the ratio of cerebroside to sulfatide is the most sensitive and consistent abnormality in MLD tissues. In normal white matter this ratio is approximately 4; in late infantile MLD it may be reduced to 0.25.

As has already been mentioned, an excess of sulfatide is also demonstrable in myelin prepared from MLD white matter. This was first shown by O'Brien [221] (Table 32-6), and has been confirmed by Suzuki [208] and Cumings [222].

The most striking accumulation of sulfatide is found in the kidney. Here sulfatide levels are 25 to 70 times normal [227]. There is also a marked increase of the ceramide-dihexoside sulfate level. This observation lends additional support to the suggestion that the same enzyme catalyzes the desulfation of both compounds [92, 94].

In the adult type of MLD, chemical abnormalities in the white matter are less severe than in the late infantile type. Expressed as a percentage of dry weight, the sulfatide level may be only moderately increased, or it may even be diminished. The cerebroside/sulfatide ratio has been abnormal in all the adult patients in whom it has been examined. The highest ratio has been 1.4, compared with the normal ratio of 4 [46, 226]. In the adult MLD patients the gray matter sulfatide levels may be increased to a greater extent than in the late infantile type [46]. This may be correlated with the observation that tissues from adult MLD patients may show accumulation of metachromatic lipids in cortical neurons [173]; this does not usually occur in the late infantile MLD.

Fibroblasts derived from skin biopsies of patients with MLD under ordinary circumstances do not accumulate sulfatides. However, Porter et al. have shown [277] that when sulfatides are added to the incubation medium, cells from MLD patients develop intracellular sulfatide accumulation, whereas this does not occur in cell lines from normal indi-

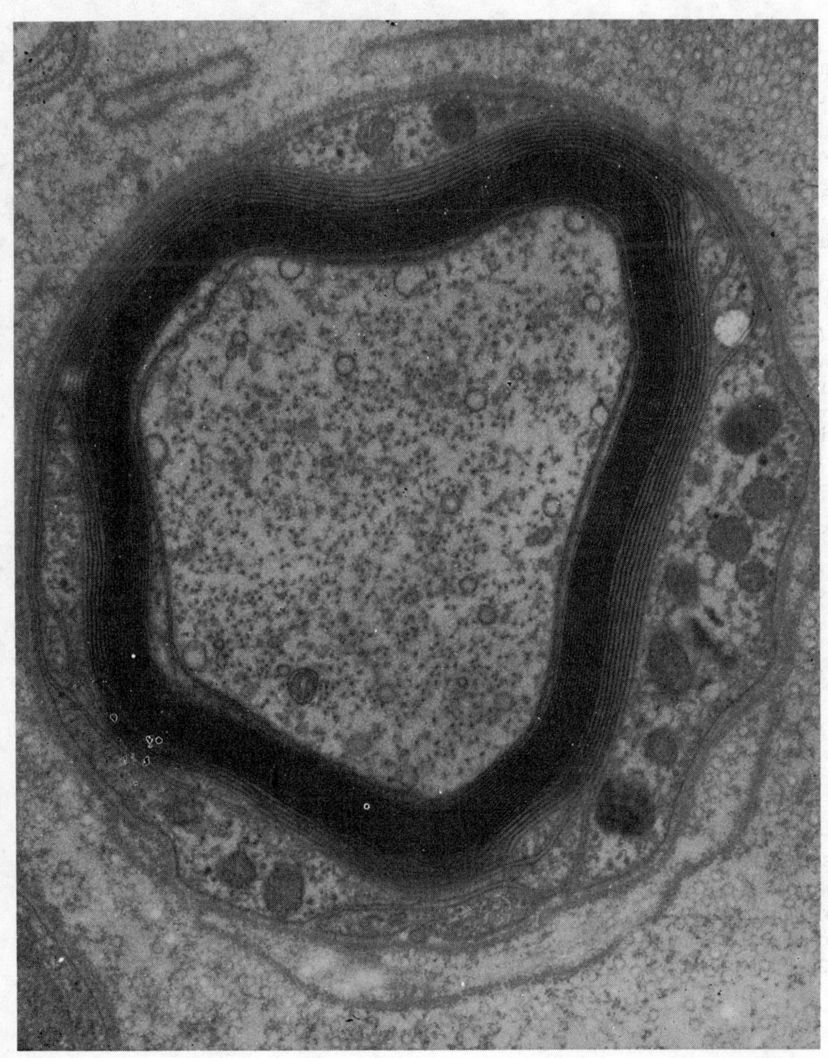

Figure 32-16. Cross section, myelinated fiber in metachromatic leukodystrophy. A circumferential band of compact myelin lamellas adjacent to the axon shows an increase in overall density. The spacing of lamellas external to this band is slightly increased (approximately 140 Å), and two small inclusions are present in the Schwann cell cytoplasm. (×29,000.) (*From Webster* [210].)

Table 32-5. COMPOSITION OF CEREBRAL WHITE MATTER AND KIDNEY IN METACHROMATIC LEUKODYSTROPHY, PERCENT OF DRY WEIGHT

Components	*Cerebral white matter*				*Kidney*		
	Normal, 6 subjects, age range 4–5 yr	Metachromatic leukodystrophy			Normal, 3 subjects, all 2 mo old	Metachromatic leukodystrophy, infantile	
		Infantile		Adult, age 29 yr			
		Age, 3¾ yr	Age, 4½ yr			Age, 3¾ yr	Age, 4½ yr
Total lipids	55.6–61.9	39.9	40.9	50.1	9.4–10.5	10.8	12.5
Cholesterol	12.2–15.7	8.1	7.8	13.5	1.3–1.7	1.7	1.6
Phospholipids	28.0–30.6	17.1	14.1	22.4	7.4–8.5	6.8	5.6
Cephalins	14.4–16.5	8.1	5.1	9.0	3.3–4.0	2.0	1.6
Lecithins	8.5–9.9	6.9	7.9	8.7	2.6–3.4	3.6	3.0
Sphingomyelin	4.1–5.2	2.5	2.2	4.7	1.0–1.22	1.1	1.0
Cerebrosides	10.3–13.8	2.8	3.2	7.8	0.41–0.45	1.21	0.71
Sulfatides	1.7–4.1	12.8	15.8	6.5	0.09–0.17	1.26	4.60
Lipid hexosamine	0.05	0.08	0.09	0.03			
Nonlipid hexosamine	0.23	0.7	0.65				

viduals. In similar studies with (^{35}S) sulfatides, fibroblast preparations from normal individuals degraded the sulfatide to inorganic (^{35}S) sulfate, which appeared in the medium. No demonstrable (^{35}S) inorganic sulfate was produced by cell lines from MLD patients. Such loading studies provide an interesting in vitro model of this disease, and may prove of value in screening possible therapeutic agents.

Table 32-6. MYELIN AND WHITE MATTER LIPIDS (PERCENTAGE OF TOTAL LIPID) IN A 6-YEAR-OLD BOY WHO HAD DIED OF METACHROMATIC LEUKODYSTROPHY

Component	Normal myelin*	MLD white matter	MLD myelin
Total lipid (% of dry weight)	78–81	47.7	76.0
Cholesterol	24.4	17.8	17.0
Total phospholipids	47.6	53.3	55.0
Ethanolamine GP	16.2	19.3	
Serine GP	6.0	7.5	
Choline GP	13.3	15.7	
Sphingomyelin	5.6	4.0	
Cerebroside	19.5	6.5	6.7
Cerebroside sulfate	5.6	20.4	20.2
Ceramide	1.3	2.0	
Uncharacterized†	6.5	6.8	

* Average of four human beings aged 10 months, 6 years, 9 years, and 55 years.
† Includes inositol glycerophosphatides as major components and smaller proportions of free fatty acids, gangliosides, and other phosphatides. Data from O'Brien and Sampson [221].
Note: GP, glycerophosphatides.
Source: From O'Brien [226].

Chemical Structure of Sulfatides Accumulated in MLD

All evidence indicates that the sulfatides which accumulate in MLD tissue have the same structure as in the normal subject. Malone et al. showed that galactose was the only carbohydrate component in sulfatides isolated from MLD white matter, and that, as in the normal, the sulfate group was located at the C-3 position of the galactopyranose moiety [229]. Taketomi et al. confirmed Malone's findings in respect to the galactose-sulfate linkage; they demonstrated also that, as in the normal, MLD sulfatide contained mostly C_{18} sphingosine [230]. The fatty acid composition of sulfatides from MLD brain tissue has been shown to be the same as in the normal subject [32, 226, 230]. Malone et al. showed that the kidney sulfatides from MLD patients have the same fatty acid composition as those in normal human kidney.

Abnormal Fatty Acid Composition in White Matter Sphingomyelin and Cerebrosides

O'Brien found that in patients with MLD the white matter sphingomyelin and cerebrosides have an abnormal fatty acid composition. The change is most striking for the cerebrosides. In MLD the fatty acids with 21 to 26 carbons make up 22 percent of the total unsubstituted group, compared to 78 percent in the normal subject (Table 32-7, [226]). A relative decrease in long-chain fatty acids also exists in white matter sphingomyelin. Ställberg-Stenhagen reported similar changes in the white matter sphingomyelin of MLD patients and also observed that changes of the same type were present in patients with globoid leukodystrophy and "subchronic leukoencephalitis" (subacute sclerosing panencephalitis) [231]. Malone and Stoffyn confirmed the diminution of long-chain fatty acids in brain white matter cerebrosides [32],

Table 32-7. FATTY ACIDS IN POST-MORTEM WHITE MATTER SPHINGOLIPIDS FROM TWO PATIENTS WITH METACHROMATIC LEUKODYSTROPHY, PERCENT OF TOTAL UNSUBSTITUTED FATTY ACIDS IN EACH LIPID

	Sphingomyelin			*Cerebroside*			*Cerebroside sulfate*		
Acid	Case 1	Case 2	Normal	Case 1	Case 2	Normal	Case 1	Case 2	Normal
14:0	3.0	1.0	7.8	0.7	0.8	0.8	0.1	1.2	4.6
16:1	0.8	0.3	0.5	1.5	2.2	tr	0.9	1.0	0.4
16:0	10.3	9.8	6.7	18.1	22.8	8.3	9.4	4.3	3.5
18:1	3.8	1.2	1.3	32.8	19.0	3.3	4.7	2.0	1.5
18:0	50.0	73.8	30.5	26.4	25.9	7.9	7.2	8.2	3.1
20:1	0.1	tr	tr	1.3	0.3	0.1	tr	. . .	tr
20:0	0.9	1.2	0.9	0.5	0.3	0.4	1.8	1.6	0.5
22:1	0.1	. . .	0.4	0.1	0.3	0.4	0.8	. . .	tr
22:0	0.9	0.8	1.4	0.3	0.6	1.8	2.7	3.3	1.8
23:1	0.1	tr	0.5	0.3	0.2	0.8	0.9	tr	0.6
23:0	1.0	0.6	1.6	0.8	0.7	3.1	3.2	4.0	3.3
24:1	16.5	7.2	25.2	6.8	7.3	40.0	27.3	27.3	38.7
24:0	3.4	1.7	6.5	1.9	6.2	11.3	17.9	19.2	16.1
25:1	2.5	0.8	3.2	1.1	2.2	7.0	6.6	7.6	9.0
25:0	1.5	tr	1.4	0.3	0.3	3.5	5.5	3.7	5.0
26:1	3.0	1.0	2.3	1.2	0.2	7.4	9.8	9.6	9.8
26:0	tr	tr	tr	tr	0.2	1.0	0.9	2.8	1.8
14–20	72.6	87.6	57.5	84.1	78.0	22.7	25.5	22.7	13.4
21–26	27.4	12.4	42.5	15.9	22.0	77.7	74.5	77.3	86.6

Source: From O'Brien and Sampson [221].

and Taketomi and Yabuucki confirmed the change in respect to sphingomyelin [225]. In spite of the altered fatty acid patterns in cerebroside and sphingomyelin, all authors agree that the fatty acid composition of sulfatides in the tissues of MLD patients is normal.

When the abnormality of white matter cerebroside fatty acids was first detected, O'Brien proposed as a working hypothesis that in MLD there is a deficiency of the fatty acid chain-elongation system, and that the resulting deficit in long-chain fatty acid compromises the stability of the myelin sheath [226]. The subsequent description of the cerebroside sulfatase deficiency and the demonstration of the normal pattern of sulfatide fatty acids have made this hypothesis unlikely. Instead, we favor the interpretation advanced by Ställberg-Stenhagen and Svennerholm, viz., that the diminished proportion of long-chain fatty acids reflects the loss of myelin [231]. As has already been mentioned, during the process of maturation, accumulation of long-chain fatty acids coincides with myelination. Loss of myelin would be expected, therefore, to be associated with return to the fatty acid pattern of immature white matter. This interpretation also accounts for the diminution of long-chain fatty acids which has been observed in other demyelinating disorders [231]. Proof of the Ställberg-Stenhagen–Svennerholm hypothesis would require demonstration of a normal fatty acid pattern in the myelin cerebrosides isolated from an MLD patient. To our knowledge such analyses have not been performed.

An Increase in White Matter Nonlipid Hexosamine

An increased level of white matter nonlipid hexosamine in MLD was first reported by Edgar, and he has recently summarized his studies on this topic [232]. The lipid hexosamine level probably reflects brain ganglioside content. The nonlipid hexosamines form part of a variety of compounds including mucopolysaccharides and glycoprotein. In normal white matter the lipid hexosamine represents 0.08 ± 0.01 percent of dry weight, while the nonlipid hexosamine level is 0.31 ± 0.04 percent. In nine patients with MLD, the corresponding values were 0.11 ± 0.01 percent and 0.53 ± 0.10 percent. Svennerholm has reported similar results ([46] and Table 32-5). The gray matter hexosamine levels are normal. The increase in white matter nonlipid hexosamine is roughly proportional to the increase of sulfated mucopolysaccharides which Yabuuchi et al. have reported in MLD white matter [225], and thus may reflect an increase in these constituents. Compared to the changes in sulfatide levels, the alterations in hexosamine content are of modest proportion. Furthermore, they are not specific, in that similar changes are observed in the white matter in Tay-Sachs disease.

Levels of Certain Other Tissue Constituents

The ganglioside levels in late infantile MLD have not been studied in detail. O'Brien reported no abnormality in the total ganglioside level [226], and as already noted the gray matter lipid hexosamine content is not increased [46]. Cumings et al., however, reported a small increase in the ganglioside content of a myelin fraction from MLD white matter [233]. Martensson reported that, though total kidney ganglioside levels in MLD were normal, the ganglioside pattern showed an increase of disialogangliosides and of an incompletely identified monosialoganglioside [227]. Austin and coworkers found that in late infantile MLD the acid polysaccharide levels of brain, kidney, and urine were within normal limits [188]. However, Yabuuchi et al. found an increase of sulfated acid mucopolysaccharide in white matter (0.449 γ-uronic acid per milligram of dry weight, compared to the normal value of 0.282 [225]). Such an increase would account approximately for the increase in the white matter nonlipid hexosamine level reported by Edgar [232] and Svennerholm [46]. Much greater increases in tissue polysaccharide levels are observed in the MLD variant, which will be discussed next.

Tissue Constituents in the MLD Variant Associated with Multiple Sulfatase Deficiencies

These have been studied in only two patients. As in late infantile MLD, the tissues contain the expected sulfatide excess. They differ from MLD in that there is also an increase of tissue polysaccharide levels. In his "M"-family patient, Austin demonstrated a fivefold excess in the kidney, a five- to tenfold excess in the urine, and approximately a twofold increase in brain. Most of the polysaccharide in kidney and urine belonged to the heparin or heparitin sulfate category [188]. Murphy et al. demonstrated a still larger excess of mucopolysaccharide in the liver of their patient, and histochemical studies indicated that this excess also existed in the spleen [190]. In addition, Murphy et al. reported the accumulation of cholesterol sulfate in the liver, kidney, plasma, and urine of their patient. Steroid sulfate accumulation has not been observed in the usual late infantile form of MLD, nor was it present in the liver of the "M"-family patients described by Austin. There is also suggestive evidence for an increased ganglioside level in the gray matter [172], and for an abnormality in the gray matter ganglioside pattern, which resembles that seen in Hurler's syndrome [190].

The Enzymatic Basis of Late Infantile MLD

The enzymatic basis of late infantile MLD is now firmly established, as a result of the work of Mehl and Jatzkewitz [234, 128] and that of Austin [189]. In the kidney, liver, and brain tissues of eight patients with MLD, activity of cerebroside sulfatase was at the limit of detection [128] (Fig. 32-17). Austin had shown previously that arylsulfatase A activity is absent or markedly reduced in the same tissues [189], and Mehl and Jatzkewitz showed that the small amount of arylsulfatase A activity which was detected in MLD kidney appeared to be due to an isoenzyme [234]. The relationship between arylsulfatase A and cerebroside sulfatase has already been discussed. In late infantile MLD the activities of other degradative enzymes, such as arylsulfatase B and C, acid phosphatase, and β-galactosidase, are normal [128, 189]. Steroid sulfatase activity is also normal [190].

The Enzymatic Basis of the Adult Type of MLD

Austin found diminished arylsulfatase A activity in the urine of an adult patient with MLD [174], but the activity appeared to be greater than that in patients with late infantile MLD.

Recently Stumpf and Austin considered this problem in more detail [235]. They compared the levels and certain of the properties of urinary arylsulfatase A in the juvenile or adult type of MLD with those in the late infantile type. In two sibs with the late infantile type the average morning urinary sulfatase A activity was 1.2 ± 0.4, compared with 17.3 ± 8.8 in three sibs with the juvenile form, and with 529 ± 233 in normal children. They also studied the effects of three types of inhibitors: (1) ρ-hydroxymercuribenzoate (PMB), a sulfhydryl group inhibitor; (2) diethyldithiocarbamic acid (DDCA); and (3) excess nitrocatecholsulfate, the substrate for the enzymatic reaction. Though PMB inhibited arylsulfatase A activity in normal subjects and in juvenile MLD patients, it did so only to a negligible extent in the late infantile patients. DDCA inhibited enzyme activity in juvenile MLD but not in normal samples. Excess nitrocatecholsulfate inhibited arylsulfatase A activity in normal urine but failed to do so in the samples from juvenile or adult MLD patients.

The differential effects of the inhibitors are difficult to interpret. They provide suggestive but as yet inconclusive evidence that the arylsulfatase A enzymes in the urine of normal, late infantile MLD, and juvenile or adult MLD patients are qualitatively different. The evidence for the existence of higher levels of arylsulfatase A activity in the urine of the older MLD patients is more convincing. To establish this point studies in additional patients will be required.

These studies suggest that in adult MLD the activity of arylsulfatase A, and, by implication, that of cerebroside sulfatase activity, is somewhat higher than in the late infantile form. Analogous findings have been reported in respect to glucocerebrosidase activity in individuals with the adult (Type 1) form of Gaucher's disease. It is of interest that in the normal human brain net accumulation of sulfatides continues until the fortieth year [49]. This, together with the demonstration of a small degree of myelin turnover in adult animals, indicates that the need for cerebroside sulfatase continues into adulthood. It is tempting to speculate that in the face of the slow normal turnover of sulfatide, the residual enzyme activity allows the accumulation of this

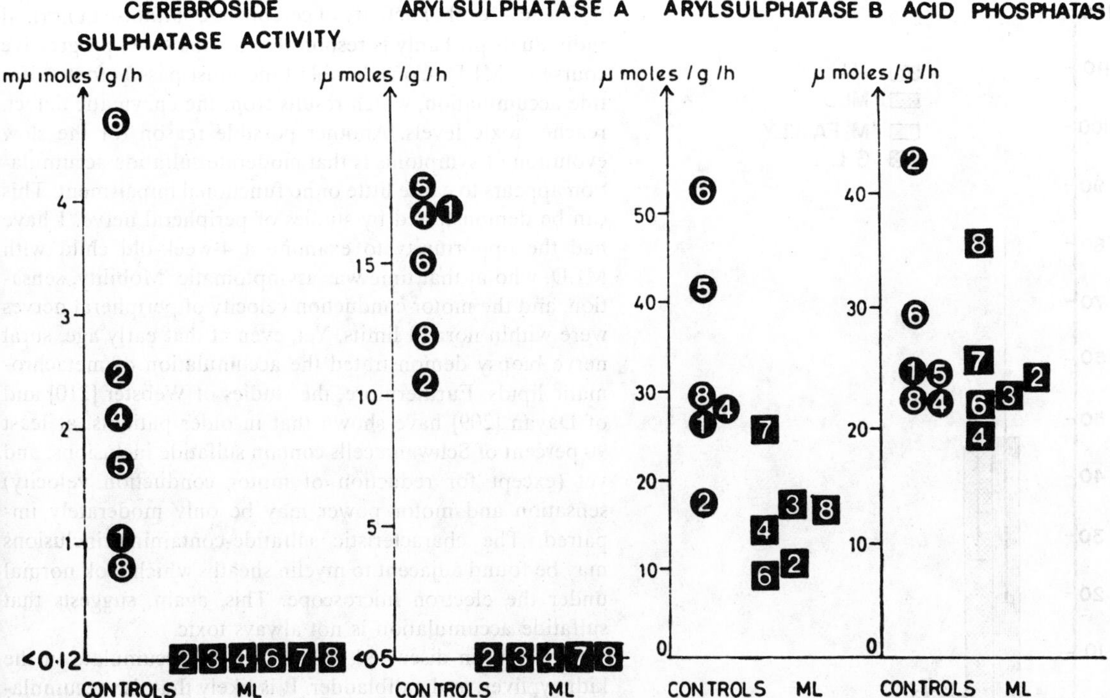

Figure 32-17. Deficiency of cerebroside sulfatase activity and arylsulfatase A activity in the renal cortex of eight patients with late infantile MLD. Circles represent the enzyme activities in control subjects, and the squares those in eight patients with late infantile MLD. (*From Jatzkewitz and Mehl* [128].)

substrate to occur at such a slow rate that toxic levels are not reached until adulthood.

The Enzymatic Basis of MLD with Multiple Sulfatase Deficiencies

Austin [189] and Murphy et al. [190] have demonstrated that in these individuals there is a deficiency of arylsulfatases A, B, and C in the kidney and brain, and of arylsulfatases A and C in the liver (Fig. 32-18). Liver arylsulfatase B activity appears to be diminished also, but it is not absent. Recently, Murphy et al. have shown that dehydroepiandrosterone sulfatase and cholesterol sulfatase activities also are reduced to the limit of detection ([190], Fig. 32-19). The activities of acid phosphatase, mannosidase, and fucosidase were normal or increased. Studies in vivo in one patient also demonstrated impaired degradation of mucopolysaccharides (Fig. 32-20). The biochemical basis for the impaired mucopolysaccharide degradation has not been determined, but it is tempting to speculate that it is due to impaired ability to desulfate either the mucopolysaccharides or the oligosaccharide sulfates which result from the action of other degradative enzymes.

The accumulation of sulfatide is almost certainly related to the arylsulfatase A deficiency, and the accumulation of cholesterol sulfate to the deficiency of cholesterol sulfatase. The metabolic consequences of the arylsulfatase B and arylsulfatase C deficiencies are not yet clear; indeed, the physiologic roles of these enzymes have not yet been defined. The mechanism by which a presumed single genetic defect can lead to a deficiency of five separate sulfatases is unknown.

MLD in Experimental Animals

Christensen et al. [236] have described a disorder in mink in which metachromatic lipids accumulate in the nervous system white matter as well as in the kidney and in the liver. In the affected animals myelination appeared to be incomplete or totally absent. Study of nervous system lipids by thin-layer chromatography indicated that the sulfatide levels were increased. The disorder first becomes clinically manifest when the kits are 40 to 120 days old. Tremor is the first symptom, and eventually paralysis occurs. The mode of inheritance was autosomal recessive. The relatively brief description available so far suggests that this disorder is related to human MLD. Enzymatic studies in these experimental animals have not been reported.

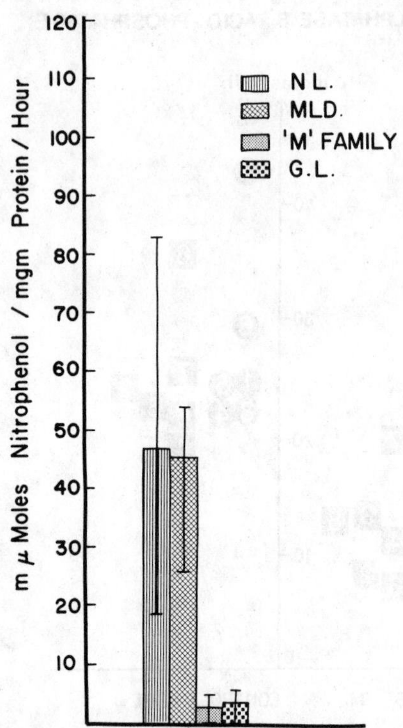

Figure 32-18. Hepatic arylsulfatase C activity. Arylsulfatase C was measured as described by Murphy et al. [190], with nitrophenylsulfate as the substrate. First bar, average level in post-mortem samples of eight age-matched controls; second bar, three patients with late infantile MLD and one patient with the juvenile form; third bar, liver from one of the patients of Austin's "M" family [172]; fourth bar, Patient G.L. ([190] and Fig. 32-14). The samples of the "M"-family patient and Patient G.L. showed the same degree of arylsulfatase A deficiency as those of late infantile MLD patients. Hepatic arylsulfatase B activity was diminished but not absent. However, in the kidney and brain of both patients arylsulfatase B activity was reduced to below the limits of detection.

THE PATHOGENESIS OF MLD

The basic biochemical disturbance in MLD is the impaired capacity to degrade sulfatides, which results from the deficiency of cerebroside sulfatase activity. The enzymatic defect is firmly established on the basis of carefully controlled studies in vitro. Moser et al. have confirmed this degradative defect with turnover studies in vivo ([237], Fig. 32-21). Compared to many other enzymes, cerebroside sulfatase has a rather low level of activity. Activity appears to be highest in the renal cortex [128]. Jatzkewitz has calculated that under optimal conditions, kidney cerebroside sulfatase can desulfate approximately 90 mg sulfatide per kilogram of kidney per 24 hr [100]. For children between 1 and 6 years of age this would mean that both kidneys desulfate 5 to 8 mg sulfatide per 24 hr. This value corresponds roughly to the daily turnover estimated from studies in vivo [237].

The low level of activity of cerebroside sulfatase in normal individuals probably is responsible for the slow, progressive course of MLD. Considerable time must pass before sulfatide accumulation, which results from the enzymatic defect, reaches toxic levels. Another possible reason for the slow evolution of symptoms is that moderate sulfatide accumulation appears to cause little or no functional impairment. This can be demonstrated by studies of peripheral nerve. I have had the opportunity to examine a 4-week-old child with MLD, who at that time was asymptomatic. Mobility, sensation, and the motor conduction velocity of peripheral nerves were within normal limits. Yet, even at that early age, sural nerve biopsy demonstrated the accumulation of metachromatic lipids. Furthermore, the studies of Webster [210] and of Dayan [209] have shown that in older patients, at least 90 percent of Schwann cells contain sulfatide inclusions, and yet (except for reduction of motor conduction velocity) sensation and motor power may be only moderately impaired. The characteristic sulfatide-containing inclusions may be found adjacent to myelin sheaths which look normal under the electron microscope. This, again, suggests that sulfatide accumulation is not always toxic.

As has been discussed, sulfatides also accumulate in the kidney, liver, and gallbladder. It is likely that the accumulation in the kidney results from the deficient degradation of sulfatides synthesized within that organ. It had previously been proposed that they represented breakdown products of the myelin sheath which had been transported to the kidney by phagocytes. This earlier concept appears untenable because the fatty acid pattern of sulfatides in MLD kidney differs from that in the brain [32]. Furthermore, the specific activity relationships during the in vivo turnover studies did not support the concept that brain sulfatides were the precursors of those in the kidney [237]. Hansson et al. have shown that sulfatides injected intracerebrally are transported to the kidney, provided that the site of intracerebral injection had been previously damaged by cold injury [238]. It is possible, therefore, that a relatively small fraction of kidney or urinary sulfatides does originate from the brain, but, for the reasons cited, it seems likely that the largest fraction originates in the kidney.

As far as is known, the sulfatide accumulation does not impair kidney or liver function. Though there is clear evidence that sulfatide accumulation interferes with gallbladder function [216, 215], this appears to be of much less clinical significance than the eventually devastating nervous system damage.

Even though, as has been pointed out, the sulfatide accumulation appears to be relatively well tolerated, eventually it leads to disruption of the myelin sheath and in this way causes the patient's death. In our opinion the most significant question in respect to the pathogenesis of MLD is the mechanism by which sulfatide accumulation causes the breakdown of myelin. In approaching this question, two facts appear of foremost importance: (1) the abnormal composition of myelin in patients who have died of MLD;

and (2) the observation that in the peripheral nerves the pattern of demyelination is segmental.

As already noted, O'Brien [221] was the first to demonstrate a large excess of sulfatide in the central nervous system myelin of a 6-year-old patient who had died of MLD. Table 32-6 shows that this abnormality was far from subtle. The cerebroside/sulfatide ratio was reduced to 0.25 from its normal value of 4. The degree to which the myelin composition deviated from normal is surprising, and raises the question of how long this abnormality had existed. Was the myelin already abnormal when it was first formed? If that is the case, many myelin lamellas must have functioned to some degree for several years. This would imply that the composition of the myelin sheath need not be as precisely fixed or invariable as had previously been thought. A priori, one would tend to believe that a sixteenfold increase in the sulfate groups of myelin would seriously compromise the stability of myelin. Several investigators have examined the effects of cations on isolated myelin in vitro [239–243], and their results suggest that such changes do affect its structure and function. An alternative hypothesis, which we consider more plausible, is that throughout the course of the patient's life there is a gradual increase in the sulfatide content of myelin. If myelin were completely stable, such a possibility would be precluded, but there is now considerable evidence that this substance does turn over.

Another important element in the pathogenesis of MLD consists of the "trophic" or "maintenance" functions of the oligodendrocyte in the central nervous system, and of the Schwann cell in the peripheral nervous system. The myelin sheath is continuous with the plasma membranes of these cells and lies within their cytoplasm. It is not known in what way these cells function in the maintenance of myelin, but it is highly probable that they are in some way required for its integrity. Of significance here is that in MLD the demyelination of the peripheral nerve follows a segmental pattern. The segmental distribution of demyelination thus suggests that the myelin breakdown was related to impaired function of the Schwann cell. Accumulation of sulfatides within Schwann cells has been demonstrated, and the altered appearance of the mitochondria may be of particular significance in this respect [213]. Analogous considerations may apply to the oligodendrocytes and the central nervous system, but here the complex anatomic relationships make it difficult to determine whether the demyelination follows a segmental pattern. Thus, the myelin breakdown in MLD

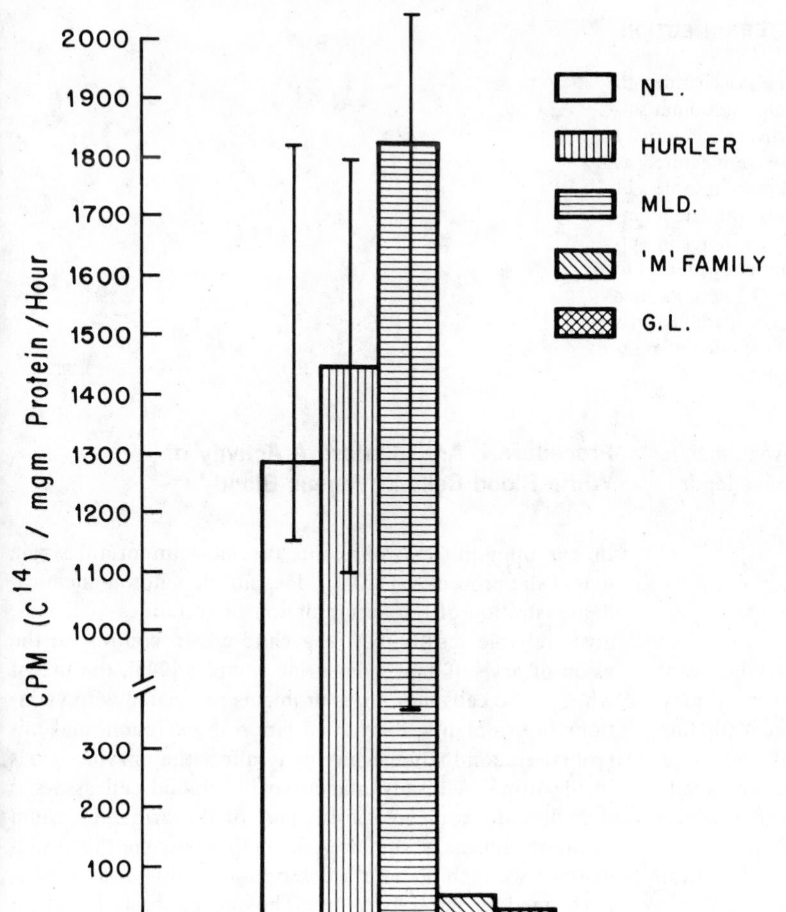

Figure 32-19. Hepatic dehydroepiandrosterone sulfatase activity. Steroid sulfatase in Patient G.L. and Austin's "M" family. Dehydroepiandrosterone sulfate was used as substrate. The assay was performed as described by Murphy et al. [190]. Cholesterol sulfatase activity also was found to be deficient in samples from Patient G.L. and Austin's "M" family [172].

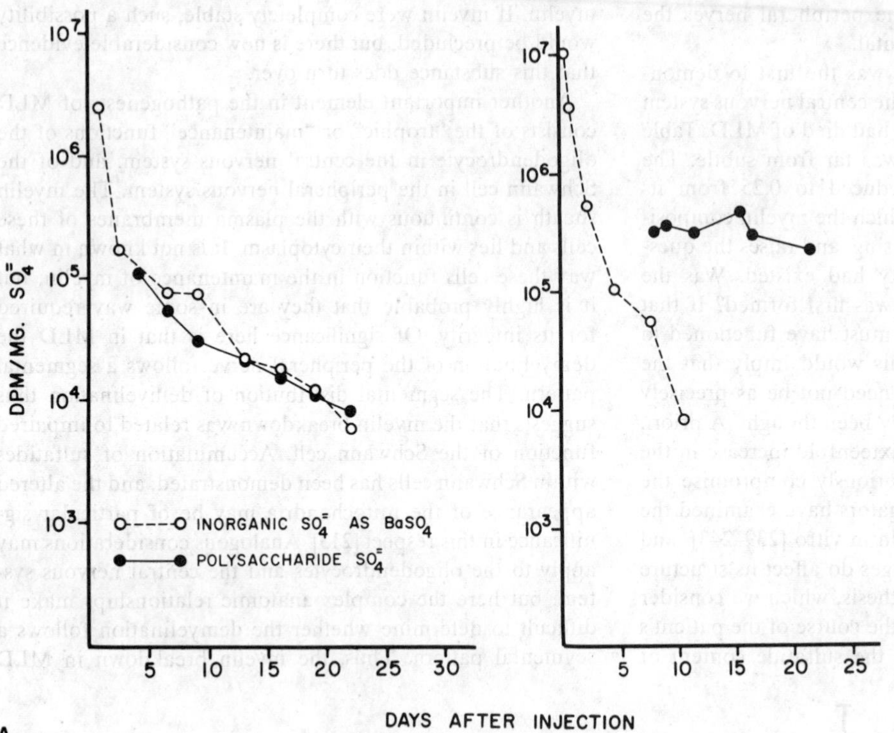

Figure 32-20. Incorporation of $^{35}SO_4^{--}$ into urinary polysaccharides. In these studies 25 to 50 microcuries of carrier-free ^{35}S-labeled sodium sulfate were injected intravenously and the specific activities of urinary inorganic sulfate and urinary polysaccharide sulfate were measured as described [237]. A. Findings in eight patients without known disorders of polysaccharide or sulfatide metabolism, in three patients with late infantile MLD, and in one patient with juvenile MLD. Urinary inorganic sulfate and polysaccharide sulfate reached isotopic equilibrium within 24 to 60 hrs after isotope injection. B. The results in Patient G.L. Radioactive polysaccharides persisted for an abnormally long time. Comparable levels of radioactivity were found in hepatic polysaccharides studied at postmortem examination 60 days following the isotope injection.

may be due to the abnormal composition of the myelin sheath, or impaired function of the Schwann cell or oligodendrocyte, or to a combination of these two factors.

LABORATORY DIAGNOSIS OF MLD

Many procedures are now available for the laboratory diagnosis of MLD. In some ways this very diversity may present a problem. The physician may be faced with this diagnostic possibility only relatively infrequently and is apt not to be fully informed about the tests that are now available. We list here the diagnostic tests in the order which reflects our own preferences. Procedures II, IV, and V are recommended for laboratories with limited biochemical resources.

Procedure I: Arylsulfatase A Activity of White Blood Cells in Venous Blood

In our opinion, this represents the most important single diagnostic procedure [110]. It does not depend on chemical demonstration of the accumulation of sulfatides and, thus, gives reliable results in young children. In contrast to the assay of arylsulfatase from urine samples [245], the use of white blood cells minimizes problems associated with variations in osmolality, diurnal variation in excretion, and microbial contamination which may affect the enzyme levels in the urine. A disadvantage of white blood cell assays is that they do not as yet form part of the armamentarium of many clinical laboratories. To help overcome this disadvantage we include here a description of this assay as it is performed in our laboratory. The procedure is based on those described by Percy and Brady [110], Snyder and Brady [111], and Bass et al. [246].

Assay of Leukocyte Arylsulfatase A Activity

Preparation of White Blood Cells

REAGENTS:

1. ACD (acid citrate dextrose) solution, consisting of 24.5 gm anhydrous dextrose, 22.0 gm anhydrous sodium citrate, 7.3 gm anhydrous citric acid per liter of 0.9 percent sodium chloride
2. 6 percent dextran type 200C (Sigma Chemical Co.) in 0.9 percent sodium chloride
3. 5 percent dextrose in 0.9 percent sodium chloride
4. 3.6 percent sodium chloride
5. 0.9 percent sodium chloride

To 10 ml venous blood add 10 ml of a solution prepared by mixing 1.5 ml ACD solution, 5.0 ml 6 percent dextran, and 3.5 ml 5 percent dextrose, and mix thoroughly. Cover with parafilm and let stand for 30 to 45 min at room temperature. Remove top layer, place in 12-ml centrifuge tube, and centrifuge for 15 min at 1,250 rpm in refrigerated centrifuge (4°C).

After centrifuging, discard supernatant, and to the pellet add 0.8 ml 0.9 percent NaCl and 2.4 ml double-distilled water. Cover tube with parafilm, mix vigorously, and then let stand 90 sec. Then add 0.8 ml 3.6 percent NaCl, and centrifuge at 1,250 rpm for 3 to 5 min. If pellet still has red blood cells in it, repeat above step; if after this the pellet still has a pink color add 1.5 ml double-distilled water, mix as before, then add 0.5 ml 3.6 percent NaCl, and centrifuge.

To the light-tan pellet add 1 ml 0.9 percent NaCl or 0.25*M* sucrose, mix to suspend white blood cells, and freeze. This preparation will keep about 6 months without substantial loss of activity.

Arylsulfatase A Assay

REAGENTS:

1. 0.5*M* sodium acetate–acetic acid buffer, pH 5, prepared by adding 0.5*M* acetic acid to 0.5*M* sodium acetate (3:7 v/v).
2. Substrate solution consisting of 0.01*M* *p*-nitrocatecholsulfate dipotassium salt, 0.0005*M* sodium pyrophosphate·$10H_2O$, 10 percent sodium chloride, sodium acetate–acetic acid buffer, prepared by weighing 155.7 mg *p*-nitrocatecholsulfate dipotassium salt, 11.2 mg sodium pyrophosphate, and 5 gm NaCl dissolved in 50 ml buffer.
3. Sodium hydroxide 1*N*.
4. 4-Nitrocatechol, a 0.01*M* solution containing 0.0005*M* sodium pyrophosphate, 10 percent sodium chloride in 0.5*M* buffer, pH 5.

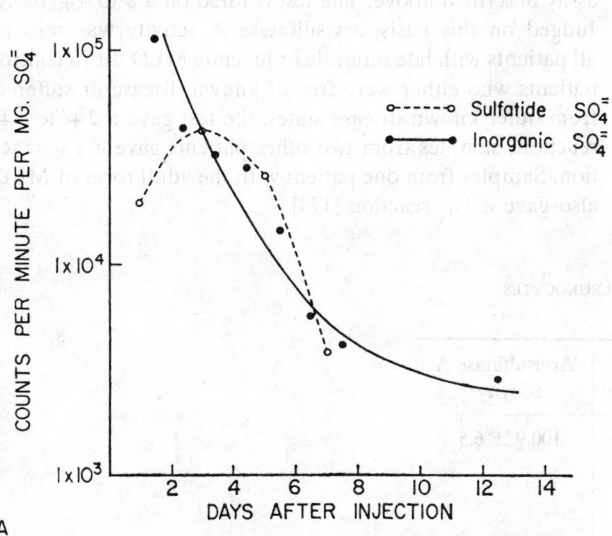

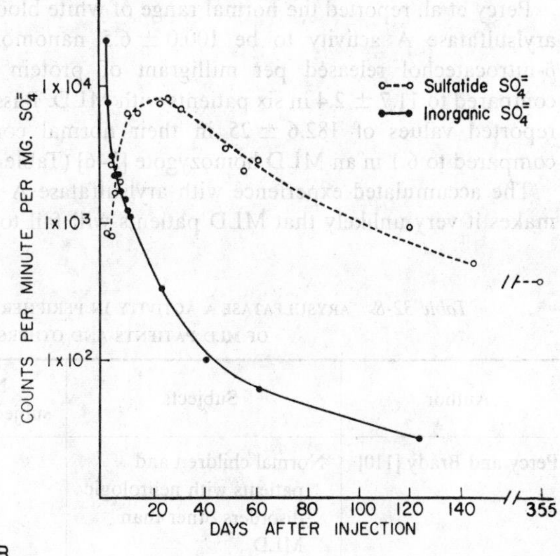

Figure 32-21. Specific activities of urinary sulfatides and inorganic sulfatide following administration of 250 microcuries of ^{35}S-labeled Na_2SO_4. A. Results in patients without known disorders of polysaccharide or sulfatide metabolism. B. Findings in five patients with MLD. Note difference in time scale. In the MLD patients radioactivity in urinary sulfatides persisted up to one year after isotope injection.

The frozen suspension of leukocytes is thawed and frozen (−75°C) six times, or sonicated for 5 min while in an ice bath. The 1-ml sample is then dialyzed overnight against 0.25*M* sucrose at 4°C. Following dialysis the leukocyte preparation is again made to the volume of 1 ml and is ready for analysis.

Two hundred microliters of substrate are transferred to a glass-stoppered test tube, followed immediately by the addition of 50 microliters of the enzyme preparation. The mixture is agitated on a vortex mixer and placed at 37°C for 1 hr. After incubation the reaction is terminated by the addition of 200 μl of 1*N* sodium hydroxide and centrifuged for 5 min at 2,000 rpm at 4°C. The supernatant is transferred to a fused quartz microcuvette, and the absorption at 515 mμ is measured against a water blank. Each sample is assayed in duplicate and is compared with a zero time control and the 4-nitrocatechol standard.

Aliquots of the leukocyte suspension are assayed for protein by the method of Lowry et al. [246*a*]. Leukocyte arylsulfatase A activity is expressed as nanomoles of 4-nitrocatechol released per hour per milligram of protein.

The initial parts of the procedure which deal with the preparation of a white blood cell suspension are applicable to other assays using leukocytes. Bass et al. list 22 inborn errors of metabolism which can be diagnosed by the study of white blood cell extracts [246]. Before undertaking the study of disease suspects, each laboratory must establish its own range of normal, and at least one control sample also should be assayed concurrently with a sample from the patient in whom the diagnosis of MLD is suspected.

Percy et al. reported the normal range of white blood cell arylsulfatase A activity to be 100.0 ± 6.5 nanomoles of ρ-nitrocatechol released per milligram of protein [110], compared to 11.7 ± 2.4 in six patients with MLD. Bass et al. reported values of 182.6 ± 25 in their normal controls, compared to 6.1 in an MLD homozygote [246] (Table 32-8).

The accumulated experience with arylsulfatase A assays makes it very unlikely that MLD patients will fail to show a deficiency of arylsulfatase A. Sources of technical error might be the use of an erroneously high pH and failure to include the phosphate inhibitor. Under such circumstances the assay might not distinguish the activities of arylsulfatase A and B, the activity of the latter enzyme being normal in the common form of MLD.

Are there disorders other than MLD which are associated with a deficiency of arylsulfatase A? None are known at this time, but the possibility cannot be excluded. Bass et al. [246] report that in MLD heterozygotes, white blood cell arylsulfatase A activity is intermediate between the normal and the MLD homozygote. Thus, in one MLD heterozygote the arylsulfatase A activity was only 23.7 nanomoles of ρ-nitrocatechol released per hour per milligram of protein. Confusion between the MLD heterozygote and homozygote might thus arise.

In view of the grave prognosis in the homozygous phenotype for MLD, it is advised that before this diagnosis is accepted at least one other laboratory test also yield a positive result. The most convenient confirmatory tests are the demonstration of excess sulfatide in the urine, or the demonstration of the characteristic brown metachromasia with acid cresyl violet in a sural nerve biopsy specimen.

Procedure II: Rapid Test for Sulfatase A Deficiency in the Urine

This important assay was developed by Austin et al. [245]. It is somewhat simpler to perform than the white blood cell assay described above. The test is rated on a 0 to 4+ basis. Judged on this basis, arylsulfatase A activity was zero in all patients with late infantile or juvenile MLD. In 70 control patients who either were free of known disease or suffered from other known disease states, the test gave a 2+ to 4+ reaction; samples from two other patients gave a 1+ reaction. Samples from one patient with the adult form of MLD also gave a 1+ reaction [174].

Table 32-8. ARYSULFATASE A ACTIVITY IN PERIPHERAL BLOOD LEUKOCYTES OF MLD PATIENTS AND OTHERS

Author	Subjects	No. of subjects studied	Arylsulfatase A activity*
Percy and Brady [110]	Normal children and patients with neurologic disorders other than MLD	16	100.9 ± 6.5
	MLD patients	6	11.7 ± 2.4
Bass et al. [246]	Normal controls	12	182.6 ± 25
	Presumably normal members of MLD pedigree	15	136.8 ± 15.8
	MLD heterozygotes	12	49.4 ± 6.6
	MLD patient	1	6.1

* Nanomoles ρ-nitrocatechol released per hour per milligram of protein.

Procedure III: Demonstration of Excess Sulfatide in the Urine

Urinary glycolipids can be quantitated by several more or less complex techniques, all of which utilize column and thin-layer chromatography [247, 237] and gas-liquid chromatography [248]. Excess of sulfatide in the urine of MLD patients can be readily demonstrated with all these techniques. The sulfatide levels in MLD urine are increased more than 100-fold over those in normal urine. In our experience patients with MLD excrete 1 to 5 mg sulfatide per 24 hr [237]. The quantitative assays noted above may be too time consuming for routine diagnosis; they also have the disadvantage that 24-hr urine collections are needed, and when column separations are used the result may not be available for at least several days.

For these reasons screening tests for excess urinary sulfatide are often used. One of these is the "fluff test" devised by Austin [193]. In this test a 24-hr urine sample is collected and refrigerated, the lipids of the sediment are extracted with 2:1 chloroform/methanol, and the extract is equilibrated with a large volume of water. The white fluff which collects at the interface is applied to filter paper and stained with 0.01 percent toluidine blue in 0.5 percent acetic acid. A strong metachromasia which persists at pH 2 is a positive test result (Fig. 32-22). Several investigators have questioned the specificity of this procedure, since they obtained false positive results in a variety of patients other than those with MLD [249, 250]. In our experience the test has proved of considerable value, provided that all samples that yield positive or borderline test results are examined by thin-layer chromatographic techniques. A useful solvent system is *n*-propanol/ammonia/water (12:1:2 v/v). The MLD urine samples show two spots with the same characteristics as brain sulfatides. Most frequently, a false positive metachromasia has been found attributable to steroid sulfates, which, in the solvent system mentioned here, move ahead of the sulfatides. Other investigators have summarized their experience with these tests [251, 252]. Hagberg and Svennerholm have described a semiquantitative assay for urine sulfatides [253, 254].

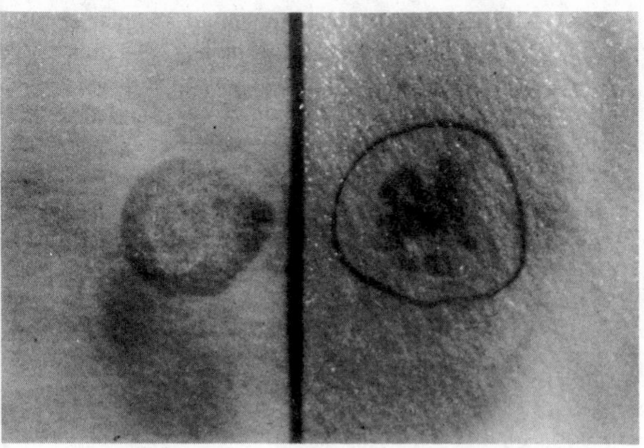

Figure 32-22. Lipids were extracted from the urine, spotted on filter paper, as described by Austin [255], and stained with 0.01 percent toluidine blue in 0.5 percent acetic acid. *Left,* a test of the urine from a patient with MLD; *right,* that from normal urine.

IV: Demonstration of Metachromatic Bodies in the Urine Sediment

This technique is the first diagnostic procedure described by Austin [255]. A freshly voided urine sample is centrifuged, and two drops of a 2 percent aqueous solution of toluidine blue are added to the sediment. The presence of various types of golden-brown bodies is characteristic of MLD. In practice, the urinary sediment may contain debris, including bacteria and phosphates, and these may be a source of confusion. Read has described a procedure to remove these contaminants [256]; this should improve the reliability of the test.

Lake [257] has described a modification of this procedure:

The urine, which must be fresh and preferably not an early morning specimen, is centrifuged at 2,000–3,000 rpm for 10 minutes. The supernatant is decanted, and 6 smears from the sediment are made on glass slides and then fixed in formalin vapour at 60°C. for one hour. The slides are washed in water and stained at room temperature for 10 minutes in a 1 percent aqueous solution of cresyl fast violet (E. Gurr, or Hopkins and Williams), the pH of which has been adjusted to 3.5–3.6 with acetic acid. The smears are washed in water and mounted in glycerine jelly.

A positive result is indicated by the presence of brown metachromatic-staining material in the cytoplasm of renal epithelial cells. These were observed in the urine of all 10 patients of MLD who were examined. A total of 128 control urine samples gave negative results.

Procedure V: Sural Nerve Biopsy

In 1959 Thieffry et al. introduced sural nerve biopsy as an aid to the diagnosis of MLD [258]. Olsson and Sourander have recently reviewed their experience with 8 patients who had MLD and 37 patients with other diseases. In all instances, the correct diagnosis was achieved [259]. Moser has had a similar experience with six other MLD patients, in one of whom the diagnostic changes were already present at 4 weeks of age. In MLD, frozen sections of the biopsy specimens show granules which exhibit brown metachromasia with cresyl violet in 1 percent acetic acid (Fig. 32-23) and which are extractable with 2:1 chloroform/methanol. The granules are located within phagocytes, which, singly or in clusters, surround the vasa nervorum or lie just under

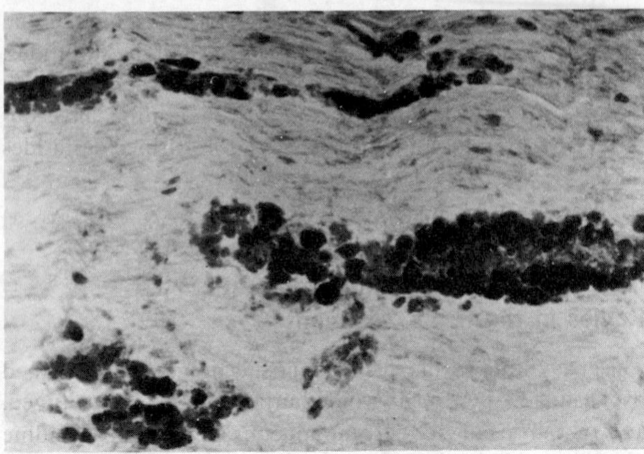

Figure 32-23. Sural nerve biopsy in MLD. A small portion of sural nerve obtained by biopsy was fixed in Formalin, and a frozen section was prepared and stained with cresyl violet in 1 percent acetic acid. Brown metachromatic granules are seen within Schwann cells and macrophages. These granules are also PAS-positive, and both reactions are abolished by prior treatment with fat solvents. The demonstration of brown metachromasia with this technique is diagnostic of MLD. See Plate II-2 for color version of this photomicrograph. (*From Olsson and Sourander* [259]. *Photomicrograph courtesy of Dr. Bengt Hagberg, Uppsala, Sweden.*)

the perineurium. The granules may also be seen within the Schwann cells or in the myelin sheath, or as apparently free-lying bodies between nerve fibers.

Other Laboratory Tests

Fullerton [260], Thieffry et al. [261], and Jacobs [262] have demonstrated a marked reduction in the conduction velocity of peripheral nerves in patients with MLD. This test is of limited diagnostic value, since such conduction is abnormal in peripheral neuropathy due to other causes. It should prove of particular utility in the evaluation of possible therapeutic agents.

Hagberg and Svennerholm have demonstrated that in patients with MLD there is progressive inability of the gallbladder to concentrate dyes [215]. Though this test is not without diagnostic value, we have found it difficult to carry out in the young children in whom the diagnosis is being considered.

The cerebrospinal fluid protein level is almost always elevated in patients with the late infantile form of MLD. Blom and Hagberg have described the electroencephalographic changes [263]. They found that the EEG was normal in the beginning of the disease but that in the more advanced stages, abnormal slow-wave activity appeared and that this was often mixed with paroxysmal or epileptogenic activity. The changes were nonspecific and did not contribute significantly to the differential diagnosis. Hultberg et al. [264] studied the urinary free amino acids in three patients with MLD, and demonstrated an increased excretion of serine and threonine.

TREATMENT

Three specific therapeutic approaches have been tried, but so far none has proved successful. Moser administered a specially prepared low-sulfur diet to the patient with MLD who had multiple sulfatase deficiencies [190]. Since a feeding gastrostomy had previously been inserted, the dietary intake could be monitored conveniently. During the 8-week period of the low-sulfur diet urinary inorganic sulfate excretion fell to less than 10 percent of normal, but urinary sulfatide excretion was unaltered, and there was no change in the rate of incorporation of intravenously administered ^{35}S-labeled sulfate into the urinary sulfatides.

Melchior and Clausen have reported on the effect of a diet low in vitamin A which was administered to a 3-year-old girl with advanced MLD for a 4-month period. During this period they noted a reduction in urinary glycolipid excretion, but there was no change in the clinical status [265]. Moser has followed the course of a boy with MLD, now 1½ years old, who has been maintained on a low-vitamin A diet since he was 4 weeks old. At that early stage he was asymptomatic, but since age 11 months he has become increasingly ataxic, has developed a strabismus, and has not yet learned to stand up. Motor conduction velocity was normal for age until he was 8 months old but has been below normal since then. No signs or symptoms of vitamin A deficiency have developed.

Greene et al. [266] administered arylsulfatase A to a 3½-year-old boy with advanced MLD. The enzyme had been prepared from brain and purified approximately 800-fold according to the method of Bleszynski and Dzialoszynski [267]. Prior to enzyme administration there was no demonstrable arylsulfatase A activity in the serum or in liver and brain biopsy specimens. High levels of arylsulfatase A activity were present in the liver 6 and 18 hr following intravenous administration of the enzyme, and this was accomplished without apparent ill effect. The patient also received one intrathecal injection of the enzyme. Up to 20 hr after this injection cerebrospinal fluid samples showed arylsulfatase A activity, but a brain biopsy speciman taken 8 hr after the intrathecal injection showed none. The fact that arylsulfatase A activity was demonstrable in the liver after intravenous injection holds out some hope of achieving the desulfation of sulfatide in visceral organs, but meaningful therapeutic results could be expected only if arylsulfatase A activity can be introduced into the appropriate tissues in the nervous system.

GENETICS

The author has reviewed the genetic data in 65 patients with MLD in 51 families [143–163, 225, 246, 268–271]. The sexes were found to be equally affected: 32 of the reported patients were males and 33 famales. Patients have been reported from England, Germany, Sweden, Denmark, France, Hungary, Japan, and from varying racial backgrounds in the

United States. One Negro child with the disease is known. There is no predilection for Jews. Involvement of a previous or subsequent generation has not been reported, but affliction of sibs has been frequently reported. Weinberg's "simple sib method" has been utilized to evaluate the mode of inheritance [272]. In this method the incidence of affected and unaffected sibs is compared, but the propositi are excluded from the calculation in order to avoid statistical bias. When this method was applied to 51 sibships, 20 sibs were found to be affected and 57 unaffected by the disease. Thus 26 percent of the sibs were affected, a number which is only slightly higher than the 25 percent that would be anticipated for an autosomal recessive mode of inheritance.

Parental consanguinity was reported in 7 of the 51 families. In two Japanese families the parents were first cousins [225, 270], and in another the maternal grandparents were cousins [272]. Bass et al. described four cases of MLD in four families which formed part of a large kindred living in an isolated community in southwest Virginia [246]. They were able to trace 110 members in 7 generations of this pedigree and found that there were many instances of consanguinity.

Recent enzymatic studies indicate that it is possible to detect the heterozygote state of MLD. Kaback and Howell, who studied arylsulfatase A activity in the cultured skin fibroblasts from four MLD families, showed that in samples from obligatory heterozygotes enzyme activity was significantly diminished ([115], Table 32-9). Leroy et al. reported similar observations in respect to the skin fibroblasts cultured from the parents of a patient with juvenile MLD [273]. Bass et al. also demonstrated diminished arylsulfatase A activity in leukocytes from the obligatory heterozygote members of their large MLD pedigree ([246], Table 32-8). Percy and Brady failed to demonstrate diminished arylsulfatase A activity in the white blood cells of the parents of three MLD patients [110], however, and it appears that the most promising method for the detection of the heterozygote state may be assay of arylsulfatase A activity in cultured skin fibroblasts.

Kaback and Howell have recently studied the arylsulfatase A activities of cultured amniotic fluid cells, obtained during amniocenteses performed during the seventeenth to twenty-fourth weeks of gestation ([115], Table 32-9). The enzyme specific activity of cultured amniotic fluid cells derived from normal subjects was only one-half to one-third as high as that of cultured fibroblasts from neonatal or adult skin, but still approximately ten times as high as in skin fibroblasts from MLD-affected patients. It is likely, therefore, that it will prove possible to detect prenatally a fetus that is homozygous for MLD. Before this can be accomplished with the required degree of certainty more data will be required concerning the range of arylsulfatase A activity in cultured amniotic fluid cells, with particular reference to cell lines obtained relatively early in the gestational period, and from fetuses subsequently shown to be heterozygous for this disorder.

SUMMARY

1 MLD is a familial disorder characterized pathologically by disintegration of myelin and accumulation of metachromatic lipids in the white matter of the central nervous system and in the peripheral nerves. Metachromatic lipids also accumulate within certain groups of neurons as well as in the kidney, the liver, and certain other visceral organs.

2 Clinically, the disease is characterized by progressive paralysis and dementia, which most commonly become apparent during the second year of life. The disease is usually fatal within 2 to 10 years. Two other rare forms of the disease have been defined. In the adult form psychic disorders and dementia may precede by decades the development of motor dysfunction. Changes resembling the mucopolysaccharidoses and the gangliosides are a feature of metachromatic leukodystrophy associated with multiple sulfatase deficiencies.

3 The main biochemical abnormality is the accumulation of sulfuric acid esters of cerebrosides. This is due to deficient activity of the degradative enzyme, cerebroside sulfatase [galactosyl (SO_4) ceramide sulfatase]. Optimal cerebroside

Table 32-9. ARYLSULFATASE A ACTIVITY IN FIBROBLASTS CULTURED FROM SKIN AND AMNIOTIC FLUID CELLS

Fibroblast source	No. studied	No. of determinations	*Arylsulfatase A activity**		
			Mean	S. D.	Range
MLD patients	3	16	16.6	6.3	7.5–26.8
Parents of MLD patients	7	34	117.8	58.5	54.1–265.0
Controls:					
Infant	8	26	414.0	181.0	286.2–727.1
Adult	6	20	635.2	270.0	320.4–982.5
Non-MLD	9	32	482.0	184.1	260.7–808.0
Amniotic fluid cells	4	12	187.9	66.9	106.8–295.2

* Expressed as millimicromoles nitrocatechol produced per hour per milligram of soluble fibroblast protein.
Source: From Kaback [115].

sulfatase activity requires both a heat-stable and a heat-labile factor. The heat-labile factor appears to be identical to the enzyme arylsulfatase A. A specific deficiency of arylsulfatase A is the basic biochemical defect in the late infantile and adult forms of MLD. In a rare additional variant form, there appear to be also deficiencies of arylsulfatases B and C and of steroid sulfatase.

4 MLD can be diagnosed by demonstration of arylsulfatase A deficiency in white blood cells, in urine, or in cultured skin fibroblasts; by the demonstration of excess sulfatides in the urine; and by demonstration of metachromatic lipids in biopsies of peripheral nerve or other tissues. It is likely that the disorder can be diagnosed prenatally by measuring the arylsulfatase A activity of fibroblasts cultivated from amniotic fluid samples.

5 The disorder is transmitted as an autosomal recessive trait. The heterozygote state can be identified by measuring arylsulfatase A activity in cultured skin fibroblasts.

BIBLIOGRAPHY

1. Van Bogaert, L., and Bertrand, I: Spongy degeneration of the brain in infancy. North-Holland Publishing Company, Amsterdam, 1970.
2. Banker, B. Q., Robertson, J. T., and Victor, M.: Spongy degeneration of the central nervous system in infancy. Neurology, **14**, 981, 1964.
3. Kamoshita, S., Rapin, I., Suzuki, K., and Suzuki, K.: Spongy degeneration of the brain: a chemical study of two cases including isolation and characterization of myelin. Neurology, **18**, 975, 1968.
4. Pelizaeus, F.: Ueber eine eigenthümliche Form spastischer Lähmung mit Cerebralerscheinungen auf hereditärer Grundlage (multiple Sclerose). Arch. Psychiat. Nervenkrankh., **16**, 698, 1885.
5. Merzbacher, L.: Eine eigenartige familiär-hereditäre Erkrankungsform (aplasia axialis extracorticalis congenita). Z. Ges. Neurol. Psychiat., **3**, 1, 1910.
6. Zeman, W., Demyer, W., and Falls, H. F.: Pelizaeus-Merzbacher disease: a study of nosology. J. Neuropath. Exp. Neurol., **23**, 334, 1964.
7. Norman, R. M., Tingey, A. H., Harvey, P. W., and Gregory, A. M.: Pelizaeus-Merzbacher disease: a form of sudanophil leucodystrophy. J. Neurol. Neurosurg. Psychiat., **29**, 521, 1966.
8. Alexander, W. S.: Progressive fibrinoid degeneration of fibrillary astrocytes associated with mental retardation in a hydrocephalic infant. Brain, **72**, 373, 1949.
9. Schochet, S. S., Lampert, P. W., and Earle, K. M.: Alexander's disease: a case report with electron microscopic observations. Neurology, **18**, 543, 1968.
10. Adams, R. D., and Kubik, C. S.: The morbid anatomy of the demyelinative disease. Amer. J. Med., **12**, 5, 510, 1952.
11. McAlpine, D., Lumsden, C. E., and Acheson, E. D.: Multiple sclerosis: a reappraisal. Williams & Wilkins, Baltimore, 1965.
12. Lehrich, J. R., Katz, M., Rorke, L. B., Barbanti-Brodano, G., and Koprowski, H.: Subacute sclerosing panencephalitis: encephalitis in hamsters produced by viral agents isolated from human brain cells. Arch. Neurol. (Chicago), **23**, 97, 1970.
13. Richardson, E. P.: Progressive multifocal leukoencephalopathy. New Eng. J. Med., **265**, 815, 1961.
14. ZuRhein, G. M., and Chou, S-M.: Particles resembling papova viruses in human cerebral demyelinating disease. Science, **148**, 1477, 1965.
15. Siemerling, E., and Creutzfeldt, H. G.: Bronzekrankheit und sklerosierende Encephalomyelitis (diffuse Sklerose). Arch. Psychiat. Nervenkr., **68**, 217, 1923.
16. Hoefnagel, D., Noort, S., Van Den, and Ingbar, S. H.: Diffuse cerebral sclerosis with endocrine abnormalities in young males, in *Brain,* edited by D. Williams, vol. 85, pp. 553–568. Macmillan, London, 1962.
17. Alzheimer, A.: Beiträge zur Kenntnis der pathologischen Neuroglia und ihrer Beziehung zu den Abbauvorgängen im Nervengewebe. Nissl-Alzheimer's Histol. Histopathol. Arb., **3**, 493, 1910.
18. Witte, F.: Ueber pathologische Abbauvorgänge im Zentralnervensystem. München. Med. Wschr., **68**, 69, 1921.
19. Scholz, W.: Klinische, pathologisch-anatomische und erbbiologische Untersuchungen bei familiärer, diffuser Hirnsklerose im Kindesalter. Z. Ges. Neurol. Psychiat., **99**, 42, 1925.
20. Peiffer, J.: Über die metachromatischen Leukodystrophien (Typ Scholz). Arch. Psychiat. Nervenkr., **199**, 386, 1959.
21. Jatzkewitz, H.: Zwei Typen von Cerebrosid-schwefelsäureestern als Sog. "Prälipoide" und Speichersubstanzen bei der Leukodystrophie, Typ Scholz (metachromatische Form der diffusen Sklerose). Z. Physiol. Chem., **311**, 279, 1958.
22. Austin, J. H.: Metachromatic sulfatides in cerebral white matter and kidney. Proc. Soc. Exp. Biol. Med., **100**, 361, 1959.
23. Thudichum, J. L. W.: Die chemische Konstitution des Gehirns des Menschen und der Tiere. Franz Pietzeker, Tübingen, 1901.
24. Blix, G.: Zur Kenntnis der schwefelhaltigen Lipid Stoffe des Gehirns: über cerebron Schwefelsäure. Z. Physiol. Chem., **219**, 82, 1933.
25. Lees, M., Folch, J., Sloane Stanley, G. H., and Carr, S.: A simple procedure for the preparation of brain sulphatides. J. Neurochem., **4**, 9, 1959.
26. Stoffyn, P. J.: The structure and chemistry of sulfatides. J. Amer. Oil Chem. Soc., **43**, 69, 1966.
27. Stoffyn, P., and Stoffyn, A.: Direct conversion of sulfatides into cerebrosides. Biochim. Biophys. Acta, **70**, 107, 1963.
28. Yamakawa, T., Kiso, N., Handa, S., Makita, A., and Yokoyama, S.: On the structure of brain cerebroside sulfuric ester and ceramide dihexoside of erythrocytes. J. Biochem., **52**, 226, 1962.
29. Stoffyn, P., and Stoffyn, A.: Structure of sulfatides. Biochim. Biophys. Acta, **70**, 218, 1963.
30. O'Brien, J. S., and Sampson, E. L.: Fatty acid and fatty aldehyde composition of the major brain lipids in normal human gray matter, white matter, and myelin. J. Lipid Res., **6**, 545, 1965.
31. Menkes, J. H., Philippart, M., and Concone, M. C.: Concentration and fatty acid composition of cerebrosides and sulfatides in mature and immature human brain. J. Lipid Res., **7**, 479, 1966.
32. Malone, M. J., and Stoffyn, P.: A comparative study of brain and kidney glycolipids in metachromatic leucodystrophy. J. Neurochem., **13**, 1037, 1966.
33. Martensson, E.: Sulfatides of human kidney isolation, identification, and fatty acid composition. Biochim. Biophys. Acta, **116**, 521, 1966.
34. Martensson, E.: On the sulfate containing lipids of human kidney. Acta Chem. Scand., **17** (4), 1174, 1963.
35. Stoffyn, A., Stoffyn, P., and Martensson, E.: Structure of kidney ceramide dihexoside sulfate. Biochim. Biophys. Acta, **152**, 353, 1968.
36. Rouser, G., Kritchevsky, G., Galli, C., and Heller, D.: Determination of polar lipids: quantitative column and thin-layer chromatography. J. Amer. Oil Chem. Soc., **42** (3), 215, 1965.
37. Rouser, G., Kritchevsky, G., and Yamamoto, A.: Column chromatographic and associated procedures for separation and determination of phosphatides and glycolipids, in *Lipid Chromatographic Analysis,* edited by G. V. Marinetti, p. 99. Marcel Dekker, Inc., New York, 1967.
38. Rouser, G., and Yamamoto, A.: Lipids of the nervous system, in *Handbook of Neurochemistry,* edited by A. Lajtha. Plenum, New York, 1969.
39. Folch, J., Lees, M., and Sloane Stanley, G. H.: Simple method for the isolation and purification of total lipides from animal tissues. J. Biol. Chem., **226**, 497, 1957.
40. Svennerholm, L., and Thorin, H.: Quantitative isolation of brain sulfatides. J. Lipid Res., **3**, 483, 1962.
41. O'Brien, J. S., and Sampson, E. L.: Lipid composition of the normal human brain: gray matter, white matter, and myelin. J. Lipid Res., **6**, 537, 1965.
42. Kean, E. L.: Rapid, sensitive spectrophotometric method for quantitative determination of sulfatides. J. Lipid Res., **9**, 319, 1968.
43. Sweeley, C. C., and Walker, B.: Determination of carbohydrates in glycolipides and gangliosides by gas chromatography. Anal. Chem., **36**, 1461, 1964.

44. Lauter, C. J., and Trams, E. G.: A spectrophotometric determination of sphingosine. J. Lipid Res., **3**, 136, 1962.
45. Norton, W. T., and Autilio, L. A.: The lipid composition of purified bovine brain myelin. J. Neurochem., **13**, 213, 1966.
46. Svennerholm, L.: Some aspects of the biochemical changes in leucodystrophy, in *Brain Lipids and Lipoproteins and the Leukodystrophies,* edited by J. Folch-Pi and H. Bauer, pp. 104–119. Elsevier, Amsterdam, 1963.
47. Green, J. P., and Robinson, J. D., Jr.: Cerebroside sulfate (sulfatide A) in some organs of the rat and in mast cell tumor. J. Biol. Chem., **235**, 1621, 1960.
48. Austin, J. H., and Maxwell, W. E.: Significance of plasma glycolipid levels in normals and in 3 disorders of brain glycolipids. Proc. Soc. Exp. Biol. Med., **107**, 197, May, 1961.
49. Rouser, G., and Yamamoto, A.: Curvilinear regression course of human brain lipid composition changes with age. Lipids, **3** (3), 284, 1968.
50. Wells, M. A., and Dittmer, J. C.: A comprehensive study of the postnatal changes in the concentration of the lipids of developing rat brain. Biochemistry, **6** (10), 3169, 1967.
51. Davison, A. N., and Gregson, N. A.: The physiological role of cerebron sulphuric acid (sulphatide) in the brain. Biochem. J., **85**, 558, 1962.
51*a*. Hauser, G.: Cerebroside and sulphatide levels in developing rat brain. J. Neurochem., **15**, 1237, 1968.
51*b*. Yakovlev, P. I.: Morphological criteria of growth and maturation of the nervous system in man, in *Mental Retardation,* vol. 39, pp. 1–46. Research Publications, A.R.N.M.D., 1962.
52. Davison, A. N., and Dobbing, J.: Myelination as a vulnerable period in brain development. Brit. Med. Bull., **22** (1), 40, 1966.
53. Bunge, R. P.: Glial cells and the central myelin sheath. Physiol. Rev., **48** (1), 197, 1968.
54. Geren, B. B.: The formation from the Schwann cell surface of myelin in the peripheral nerves of chick embryos. Exp. Cell Res., **7**, 558, 1954.
55. Brante, G.: Studies on lipids in the nervous system with special reference to quantitative chemical determination and topical distribution. Acta Physiol. Scand., **18**, suppl. 63, pp. 1–189, 1949.
56. Folch-Pi, J.: Composition of the brain in relation to maturation, in *Biochemistry of the Developing Nervous System,* edited by H. Waelsch, Academic Press, New York, 1955, pp. 121–135.
57. Folch-Pi, J.: Brain proteolipids in *Brain Lipids and Lipoproteins, and the Leucodystrophies,* edited by J. Folch-Pi and H. Bauer, pp. 18–30. Elsevier, Amsterdam, 1963.
58. Patterson, J. D. E., and Finean, J. B.: Ultracentrifugal fractionation of nerve tissue. J. Neurochem., **7**, 251, 1961.
59. August, C., Davison, A. N., and Maurice-Williams, F.: Phospholipid metabolism in nervous tissue. 4. Incorporation of ^{32}P into the lipids of subcellular fractions of the brain. Biochem. J., **81**, 8, 1961.
60. Laatsch, R. H., Kies, M. W., Gordon, S., and Alvord, E. C.: The encephalomyelitic activity of myelin isolated by ultracentrifugation. J. Exp. Med., **115**, 777, 1962.
61. Shapira, R., Binkley, F., Kibler, R. F., and Wundram, I. J.: Preparation of purified myelin of rabbit brain by sedimentation in a continuous sucrose gradient. Proc. Soc. Exp. Biol. Med., **133**, 238, 1970.
62. Thompson, E. J., Goodwin, H., and Cumings, J. N.: Caesium chloride in the preparation of membrane fractions from human cerebral tissue. Nature (London), **215**, 168, 1967.
63. Autilio, L. A., Norton, W. T., and Terry, R. D.: The preparation and some properties of purified myelin from the central nervous system. J. Neurochem., **11**, 17, 1964.
64. O'Brien, J. S., Sampson, E. L., and Stern, M. B.: Lipid composition of myelin from the peripheral nervous system: intradural spinal roots. J. Neurochem., **14**, 357, 1967.
65. MacBrinn, M. C., and O'Brien, J. S.: Lipid composition of optic nerve myelin. J. Neurochem., **16**, 7, 1969.
66. Horrocks, L. A.: Composition of myelin from peripheral and central nervous systems of the squirrel monkey. J. Lipid Res., **8**, 569, 1967.
67. O'Brien, J. S., and Sampson, E. L.: Lipid composition of the normal human brain: gray matter, white matter, and myelin. J. Lipid Res., **6**, 537, 1965.
68. Horrocks, L. A.: Composition of mouse brain myelin during development. J. Neurochem., **15**, 483, 1968.
69. Eng, L. F., and Noble, E. P.: The maturation of rat brain myelin. Lipids, **3**, 157, 1968.
70. Banik, N. L., and Davison, A. N.: Desmosterol in rat brain myelin. J. Neurochem., **14**, 594, 1967.
71. Finean, J. B.: The molecular organization of cell membranes. Progr. Biophys., **16**, 145, 1968.
72. Vandenheuvel, F. A.: Lipid-protein interactions and cohesional forces in the lipoproteins systems of membranes. J. Amer. Oil Chem. Soc., **43**, 258, 1966.
73. Vandenheuvel, F. A.: Structural studies of biological membranes: the structure of myelin. Ann. N.Y. Acad. Sci., **122**, 57, 1965.
74. Korn, E. D.: Current concepts of membrane structure and function. Fed. Proc., **28** (1), 6, 1969.
75. Cuzner, M., Louise, Davison, A. N., and Gregson, N. A.: The chemical composition of vertebrate myelin and microsomes. J. Neurochem., **12**, 469, 1965.
76. Lovtrup, S., and Svennerholm, L.: Chemical properties of brain mitochondria. Exp. Cell Res., **29**, 298, 1963.
77. Eichberg, J., Whittaker, V. P., and Dawson, R. M. C.: Distribution of lipids in subcellular particles of guinea-pig brain. Biochem. J., **92**, 91, 1964.
78. Parsons, P., and Basford, R. E.: Brain mitochondria. VI. The composition of bovine brain mitochondria. J. Neurochem., **14**, 823, 1967.
79. Robertson, J. D.: The molecular structure and contact relationships of cell membranes. Prog. Biophys., **10**, 343, 1960.
80. Katzman, R., and Wilson, C. E. J.: Extraction of lipid and lipid cation from frozen brain tissue. J. Neurochem., **7**, 113, 1961.
81. Folch-Pi, J., Lees, M., and Sloane Stanley, G. H.: The role of acidic lipids in the electrolyte balance of the nervous system of mammals, in *Metabolism of the Nervous System,* edited by D. Richter, p. 174. Pergamon, New York, 1957.
82. Green, J. P., Robinson, J. D., and Day, M.: Interaction between cerebroside sulfate and amines. J. Pharmacol. Exp. Therap., **131**, 12, 1961.
83. Dengler, H., and Diezel, P. B.: Speicherung eines Katecholamin-Lipoidkomplexes bei der degenerativen diffusen Sklerose vom Typus Scholz, Bielschowsky und Henneberg. Naturwissenschaften, **45**, 244, 1958.
84. Bergeron, J. A., and Singer, M.: Metachromasy: an experimental and theoretical reevaluation. J. Biophys. Biochem. Cytol., **4**, 433, 1958.
85. Schubert, M., and Hamerman, D.: Metachromasia: chemical theory and histochemical use. J. Histochem., **4**, 159, 1956.
86. Harris, A. F., and Saifer, A.: The metachromasy of strandin. J. Neurochem., **5**, 218, 1960.
87. Lipmann, F.: Biological sulfate activation and transfer. Science, **128**, 575, 1958.
88. Radin, N. S., Martin, F. B., and Brown, J. R.: Galactolipide metabolism. J. Biol. Chem., **224**, 499, 1957.
89. Hauser, G.: Labeling of cerebrosides and sulfatides in rat brain. Biochim. Biophys. Acta, **84**, 212, 1964.
90. Balasubramanian, A. S., and Bachhawat, B. K.: Formation of cerebroside sulphate from 3′-phosphoadenosine 5′-phosphosulphate in sheep brain. Biochim. Biophys. Acta, **106**, 218, 1965.
91. McKhann, G. M., Levy, R., and Ho, W.: Metabolism of sulfatides. I. The effect of galactocerebrosides on the synthesis of sulfatides. Biochem. Biophys. Res. Commun., **20**, 109, 1965.
92. Cumar, F. A., Barra, H. S., Maccioni, H. J., and Caputto, R.: Sulfation of glycosphingolipids and related carbohydrates by brain preparations from young rats. J. Biol. Chem., **243** (14), 3807, 1968.
93. Herschkowitz, N., McKhann, G. M., Saxena, S., Shooter, E. M., and Herndon, R.: Synthesis of sulphatide-containing lipoproteins in rat brain. J. Neurochem., **16**, 1049, 1969.
94. McKhann, G. M., and Ho, W.: The in vivo and in vitro synthesis of sulphatides during development. J. Neurochem., **14**, 717, 1967.
95. Herschkowitz, N., McKhann, G. M., Saxena, S., and Shooter, E. M.: Characterization of sulphatide-containing lipoproteins in rat brain. J. Neurochem., **15**, 1181, 1968.

96. Herschkowitz, N., McKhann, G. M., and Shooter, E. M.: Studies of water soluble lipoproteins in rat brain. J. Neurochem., **15,** 161, 1968.
97. Davison, A. N., and Gregson, N. A.: Metabolism of cellular membrane sulpholipids in the rat brain. Biochem. J., **98,** 915, 1966.
98. Burton, R. M., Sodd, M. A., and Brady, R. O.: The incorporation of galactose into galactolipids. J. Biol. Chem., **223,** 1053, 1958.
99. Moser, H. W., and Karnovsky, M. L.: Studies on the biosynthesis of glycolipides and other lipides of the brain. J. Biol. Chem., **234,** 1990, 1959.
100. Mehl, E., and Jatzkewitz, H.: Eine Cerebrosidsulfatase aus Schweineniere. Z. Physiol. Chem., **339,** 260, 1964.
101. Derrien, M.: Bull. Soc. Chim. Biol. (Paris), **9,** 110, 1911.
102. Robinson, D., Spencer, B., and Williams, R. T.: Spectrophotometric determination of phenolsulphatase (arylsulphatase). Biochem. J., **48,** XXVIII, 1951.
103. Roy, A. B.: The sulphatase of ox liver. 1. The complex nature of the enzyme. Biochem. J., **53,** 12, 1953.
104. Dodgson, K. S., and Spencer, B.: Assay of sulfatases. Meth. Biochem. Anal., **4,** 211, 1957.
105. Ney, K. H., and Ammon, R.: Die Verbreitung der Aryl- und Steroid-sulfatasen. Hoppe Seyler. Z. Physiol. Chem., **315,** 145, 1959.
106. Dodgson, K. S., Spencer, B., and Wynn, C. H.: Studies on sulphatases. 12. The arylsulphatases of human tissues. Biochem. J., **62,** 500, 1956.
107. Clausen, J., and Asboe-Hansen, G.: Urinary sulphatase activity in mastocytosis. Clin. Chim. Acta, **16** (1), 131, 1967.
108. Dodgson, K. S., and Spencer, B.: The occurrence of arylsulphatases A and B in human urine. Clin. Chim. Acta, **1,** 478, 1956.
109. Ammon, R., and Ney, K-H.: Arylsulfatase des menschlichen Harns. Arch. Biochem. Biophys., **69,** 178, 1957.
110. Percy, A. K., and Brady, R. O.: Metachromatic leukodystrophy: diagnosis with samples of venous blood. Science, **161,** 594, 1968.
111. Snyder, R. A., and Brady, R. O.: The use of white cells as a source of diagnostic material for lipid storage diseases. Clin. Chim. Acta, **25,** 331, 1969.
112. Polášek, J., and Rotrekl, B.: Arylsulphatases of human blood platelets. Nature (London), **214,** 187, 1967.
113. Rotrekl, B., and Polášek, J.: Nitrocatecholsulfatase in human blood platelets. Acta Haemat. (Basel), **39,** 129, 1968.
114. Porter, M. T., Fluharty, A. L., and Kihara, H.: Metachromatic leukodystrophy: arylsulfatase-A deficiency in skin fibroblast cultures. Proc. Nat. Acad. Sci. USA, **62,** 887, 1969.
115. Kaback, M. M., and Howell, R. R.: Infantile metachromatic leukodystrophy: heterozygote detection in skin fibroblasts and possible applications to intrauterine diagnosis. New Eng. J. Med., **282,** 1336, 1970.
116. DeDuve, C., and Wattiaux, R.: Functions of lysosomes. Ann. Rev. Physiol., **28,** 435, 1966.
117. Dodgson, K. S., Spencer, B., and Thomas, J.: Studies on sulphatases. 9. The arylsulphatases of mammalian livers. Biochem. J., **59,** 29, 1955.
118. Clendenon, N. R., and Allen, N.: Assay and subcellular localization of the arylsulphatases in rat brain. J. Neurochem., **17,** 865, 1970.
119. Milsom, D. W., Rose, F. A., and Dodgson, K. S.: Assay of a microsomal marker enzyme: rat liver arylsulphatase C. Biochem. J., **109,** 40P, 1968.
120. Jatzkewitz, H.: Zerebrale Sphingolipidosen als angeborene Stoffwechselstörungen. Deutsch. Med. Wschr., **16,** 131, 1970.
121. Austin, J., Armstrong, D., Fouch, S., Mitchell, C., Stumpf, D., Shearer, L., and Briner, O.: Metachromatic leukodystrophy (MLD). VIII. MLD in adults; diagnosis and pathogenesis. Arch. Neurol. (Chicago), **18,** 225, 1968.
122. Nichol, L. W., and Roy, A. B.: The sulfatase of ox liver. IX. The polymerization of sulfatase A. Biochemistry, **4,** 386, 1965.
123. Bleszyński, W.: Purification and separation of four soluble arylsulphatases from ox brain. Enzymologica, **32,** 169, 1967.
124. Nichol, L. W., and Roy, A. B.: The sulfatase of ox liver. X. Some observations on the intermolecular bonding in sulfatase A. Biochemistry, **5,** 1379, 1966.
125. Jerfy, A., and Roy, A. B.: The sulphatase of ox liver. XII. The effect of tyrosine and histidine reagents on the activity of sulphatase A. Biochim. Biophys. Acta, **175,** 355, 1969.
126. Bleszynski, W., Leznicki, A., and Lewosz, J.; Kinetic properties of three soluble arylsulphatases from ox brain, homogeneous in polyacrylamide gel electrophoresis. Enzymology, **37,** 314, 1969.
127. Allen, E., and Roy, A. B.: The sulphatase of ox liver. XI. The isoelectric focussing of a purified preparation of sulphatase B. Biochim. Biophys. Acta, **168,** 243, 1968.
128. Jatzkewitz, H., and Mehl, E.: Cerebroside-sulphatase and arylsulphatase A deficiency in metachromatic leukodystrophy (ML). J. Neurochem., **16,** 19, 1969.
129. Mehl, E., and Jatzkewitz, H.: Cerebroside 3-sulfate as a physiological substrate of arylsulfatase A. Biochim. Biophys. Acta, **151,** 619, 1968.
130. Pulkkinen, M. O.: Arylsulphatase and the hydrolysis of some steroid sulphates in developing organism and placenta. Acta Physiol. Scand., **52,** suppl. 180, 1961.
131. French, A. P., and Warren, J. C.: Properties of steroid sulphatase and arylsulphatase activities of human placenta. Biochem. J., **105,** 233, 1967.
132. Dietrich, C. P.: A heparin sulfamidase from mammalian lymphoid tissues. Canad. J. Biochem. (in press).
133. Tudball, N., and Davidson, E. A.: Isolation of a novel sulphatase from rat liver. Biochim. Biophys. Acta, **171,** 113, 1969.
134. Held, Von, E., and Buddecke, E.: Nachweis, Reinigung und Eigenschaften einer Chondroitin-4-Sulfatase[2] aus der Aorta des Rindes. Hoppe Seyler. Z. Physiol. Chem., **348,** S. 1047, 1967.
135. Dodgson, K. S., Rose, F. A., and Tudball, N.: Studies on sulphatases. 23. The enzymic desulphation of tyrosine O-sulphate. Biochem. J., **71,** 10, 1959.
136. John, R. A., Rose, F. A., Wusterman, F. S., and Dodgson, K. S.: The detection and determination of L-tyrosine O-sulphate in rabbit and other mammalian urine. Biochem. J., **100,** 278, 1966.
137. Davison, A. N., Dobbing, J., Morgan, R. S., and Wright, G. P.: Metabolism of myelin: the persistence of (4-^{14}C) cholesterol in the mammalian central nervous system. Lancet, **1,** 658, 1959.
138. Smith, M. E.: The metabolism of myelin lipids. Advances Lipid Res., **5,** 241, 1967.
139. Smith, M. E.: The turnover of myelin in the adult rat. Biochim. Biophys. Acta, **164,** 285, 1968.
140. Hirano, A., and Dembitzer, H. M.: A structural analysis of the myelin sheath in the central nervous system. J. Cell Biol., **34,** 555, 1967.
141. Mietkiewski, Von K., and Kozik, M.: Histotopochemische Untersuchungen über die Aktivität der Arylsulfatase im Nervensystem des Kaninchens. Acta Histochem., **25,** 205, 1966.
142. Kozik, M., and Wenclewski, A.: Histochemical localization of arylsulphate sulphydrolase (E.C. 3.1.6.1.) in the nervous system of guinea pigs. Acta Histochem., **21,** 135, 1965.
143. Hagberg, B.: Clinical symptoms, signs and tests in metachromatic leucodystrophy, in *Brain Lipids and Lipoproteins and the Leukodystrophies,* edited by J. Folch-Pi and H. Bauer, pp. 134–146. Elsevier, Amsterdam, 1963.
144. Hagberg, B., Sourander, P., and Svennerholm, L.: Sulfatide lipidosis in childhood. Amer. J. Dis. Child., **104,** 644, 1962.
145. Hagberg, B.: Sulfatid-Lipidosen im Kindesalter. Mschr. Kinderheilk., **115,** 250, 1967.
146. Greenfield, J. G.: A form of progressive cerebral sclerosis in infants associated with primary degeneration of the interfascicular glia. J. Neurol. Psychopath., **13,** 289, 1933.
147. Brandberg, O., and Sjovall, E.: Zur Kenntnis der diffusen Hirnsklerose (ein Fall von familiärem, Spätinfantilem Typus). Z. Ges Neurol. Psychiat., **170,** 131, 1940.
148. Norman, R. M.: Diffuse progressive metachromatic leucoencephalopathy: a form of Schilder's disease related to the lipoidoses. Brain, **70,** 234, 1947.
149. Norman, R. M., Urich, H., and Tingey, A. H.: Metachromatic leucoencephalopathy: a form of lipidosis. Brain, **83,** 369, 1960.
150. Brain, W. R., and Greenfield, J. G.: Late infantile metachromatic leucoencephalopathy, with primary degeneration of the interfascicular oligodendroglia. Brain, **73,** 291, 1950.
151. Leslie, D. A.: Diffuse progressive metachromatic leucoencephalopathy. J. Path. Bact., **64,** 841, 1954.

152. Hain, R. F., and LaVeck, G. D.: Metachromatic leuko-encephalopathy. Pediatrics, **22,** 1064, 1958.
153. Wohlwill, F. J., and Paine, R. S.: Progressive demyelinating leuko-encephalopathy. Neurology, **8,** 285, 1958.
154. Hagberg, B., Sourander, P., Svennerholm, L., and Voss, H.: Late infantile metachromatic leucodystrophy of the genetic type. Acta Paediat. Scand., **49,** 135, 1960.
155. Jervis, G. A.: Infantile metachromatic leukodystrophy (Greenfield's disease). J. Neuropath. Exp. Neurol., **19,** 323, 1960.
156. Ogawa, K.: Late infantile metachromatic leukodystrophy. Arch. Neurol. (Chicago), **4,** 418, 1961.
157. Allen, R. J., McCusker, J. J., and Tourtellotte, W. W.: Metachromatic leukodystrophy: clinical histochemical and cerebrospinal fluid abnormalities. Pediatrics, **30,** 629, 1962.
158. ZuRhein, G. M., and Chou, S.-M.: Particles resembling papova viruses in human cerebral demyelinating disease. Science, **148,** 1477, 1965.
159. Einarson, L., Neel, A. V., and Stromgren, E.: On the problem of diffuse brain sclerosis with special reference to the familial forms. Acta Jutlandica, **16,** 178, 1944.
160. Einarson, L., and Stromgren, E.: Diffuse progressive leucoencephalopathy (diffuse cerebral sclerosis) and its relationship to amaurotic idiocy, histological and clinical aspects. Acta Jutlandica, **10,** 40, 1961.
161. Tariska, S.: Über die sog. metachromatische Leukodystrophie. Psychiat. Neurol., **137,** 65, 1959.
162. Denny-Brown, D. E., Richardson, E. P., Jr., and Cohen, R. B.: Difficulty in walking and petit mal attacks in a child. New Eng. J. Med., **267,** 1198, 1962.
163. Hallervorden, J.: Die degenerative diffuse Sklerose, im *Handbuch der speziellen pathologischen Anatomie und Histologie,* edited by O. Lubarsch, p. 716. Springer, Berlin, 1957.
164. Yabuuchi, H., Okada, S., and Kamio, M.: Case of metachromatic leukodystrophy. Jap. J. Clin. Med., **24,** 1949, 1966.
165. Allegranza, A., D'Angelo, C., and Strada, G. P.: A case of metachromatic leucodystrophy. Acta Neurol. Napoli, **23,** 912, 1968.
166. Metz, H.: Sulfatide lipidosis, a review of 21 cases of metachromatic leucodystrophy (M.L.G.). Bull. Soc. Sci. Med. Luxemb., **102,** 351, 1965.
167. Schutta, H. S., Pratt, R. T., and Metz, H.: A family study of the late infantile and juvenile forms of metachromatic leucodystrophy. J. Med. Genet., **3,** 86, 1966.
168. Bryniarska, D., Guminska, M., and Pajak, B.: Pituitary disorders and some biochemical studies in two sisters suffering from metachromatic leukodystrophy. Bull. Pol. Med. Sci. Hist., **9,** 26, 1966.
169. Taori, G. M., Mathew, N. T., Bhaktaviziam, A., et al.: Metachromatic leucodystrophy sulphatide lipidoses. Juvenile type—case report. Indian J. Med. Res., **57,** 914, 1969.
170. Cogan, D. G., Kuwabara, T., Richardson, E. P., and Lyon, G.: Histochemistry of the eye in metachromatic leukoencephalopathy. A.M.A. Arch. Ophthal., **60,** 397, 1958.
171. Cogan, D. G., Kuwabara, T., and Moser, H.: Metachromatic leucodystrophy. Ophthalmology, **160,** 2, 1970.
172. Austin, J. H.: Mental retardation, metachromatic leucodystrophy (sulfatide lipidosis, metachromatic leucoencephalopathy), in *Medical Aspects of Mental Retardation,* edited by C. H. Carter, p. 768. Charles C Thomas,
173. Müller, D., Pilz, H., and Meulen, V. T.: Studies on adult metachromatic leukodystrophy. Part 1. Clinical, morphological and histochemical observations in two cases. J. Neurol. Sci., **9,** 567, 1969.
174. Austin, J., Armstrong, D., Fouch, S., Mitchell, C., Stumpf, D., Shearer, L., and Briner, O.: Metachromatic leukodystrophy (MLD) VIII. MLD in adults; diagnosis and pathogenesis. Arch. Neurol. (Chicago), **18,** 225, 1968.
175. Roizin, L., Scheinesson, G., and Eros, G.: Comparative histological and histochemical studies of infantile and adult metachromatic leucodystrophy. Path. Europ., **3** (2-3), 286, 1968.
176. Bogaert, L., van, and Dewulf, A.: Diffuse progressive leukodystrophy in the adult with production of metachromatic degenerative products (Alzheimer-Baroncini). A.M.A. Arch. Neurol. Psychiat., **42,** 1083, 1939.
177. Peiffer, J.: Über die metachromatischen Leukodystrophien (Typ Scholz). Arch. Psychiat., **199,** 386, 1959.
178. Stam, F. C.: New histochemical and colloid chemical aspects of leucodystrophy. Psychiat. Neurol. Neurochir., **63,** 237, 1960.
179. Helmstaedt, E. R.: Über eine Beobachtung von metachromatischer Leukodystrophie. Deutsch. Z. Nervenheilk., **184,** 213, 1963.
180. Holländer, H., and Pilz, H.: Über metachromatische Leukodystrophie, Part 1 (Kasuistische Mitteilung). Arch. Psychiat. Nervenkr., **205,** 293, 1964.
181. Ettinger, A.: Adult form of leukodystrophy of type Scholz-Beilschowsky-Henneberg, with metachromatic breakdown products, in a 55-year-old male (clinical-anatomical study). Psychiat. Neurol. (Basel), **149,** 225, 1965.
182. Segarra, J., Abramowicz, A., and Malone, M.: Metachromatic leucodystrophy in the elderly, in *Proceedings of the 8th International Congress of Neurology,* vol. 4, part 2, pp. 183–194. Excerpta Medica Foundation, Amsterdam, 1965.
183. Betts, T. A., Smith, W. T., and Kelly, R. E.: Adult metachromatic leukodystrophy (sulphatide lipidosis) simulating acute schizophrenia: report of a case. Neurology, **18,** 1140, 1968.
184. Sourander, P., and Svennerholm, L.: Sulphatide lipidosis in the adult with the clinical picture of progressive organic dementia with epileptic seizures. Acta Neuropath. (Berlin), **1,** 384, 1962.
185. Austin, J. H.: Recent studies in the metachromatic and globoid body forms of diffuse sclerosis, in *Brain Lipids and Lipoproteins, and the Leucodystrophies,* edited by J. Folch-Pi and H. Bauer, p. 120. Elsevier, Amsterdam, 1963.
186. Alder, A.: Über konstitutionell bedingte Granulations-veränderungen der Leukocyten. Deutsch. Arch. Klin. Med., **183,** 372, 1939.
187. Reilly, W. A.: The granules in the leukocytes in gargoylism. Amer. J. Dis. Child., **62,** 489, 1941.
188. Bischel, M., Austin, J., and Kemeny, M.: Metachromatic leukodystrophy (MLD). VII. Elevated sulfated acid polysaccharide levels in urine and postmortem tissues. Arch. Neurol. (Chicago), **15,** 13, 1966.
189. Austin, J., Armstrong, D., and Shearer, L.: Metachromatic form of diffuse cerebral sclerosis. V. The nature and significance of low sulfatase activity: a controlled study of brain, liver and kidney in four patients with metachromatic leukodystrophy (MLD). Arch. Neurol. (Chicago), **13,** 593, 1965.
190. Murphy, J. V., Wolfe, H. J., Balazs, E. A., and Moser, H. W.: A patient with deficiency of arylsulfatases A, B, C, and steroid sulfatase, associated with storage of sulfatide, cholesterol sulfate and glycosaminoglycans, in *Lipid Storage Diseases: Enzymatic Defects and Clinical Implications,* edited by J. Bernsohn and H. J. Grossman, Academic, New York, 1971, pp. 67–110.
191. DiFerrante, N. M.: The measurement of urinary mucopolysaccharides. Anal. Biochem., **21,** 98, 1967.
192. Teller, W. M., Burke, E. C., Rosevear, J. W., and McKenzie, B. F.: Urinary excretion of acid mucopolysaccharides in normal children and patients with gargoylism. J. Lab. Clin. Med., **59,** 95, 1962.
193. Austin, J. H.: Metachromatic form of diffuse cerebral sclerosis. 2. Diagnosis during life by isolation of metachromatic lipids from urine. Neurology, **7,** 716, 1957.
194. Luthy, F., Ulrich, J., Regli, F., and Isler, W.: Amaurotic idiocy with metachromatic change in the white matter? in *Proceedings of the Fifth International Congress* of Neuropathology, International Congress Series No. 100, p. 125. Excerpta Medica Foundation, Zurich, 1965.
195. Bischoff, A., and Ulrich, J.: Amaurotic idiocy connected with metachromatic leukodystrophy: transitional form or combination. Electron microscopic and histochemical finding. Acta Neuropath. (Berlin), **8,** 292, 1967.
196. Pilz, H., and Jatzkewitz, H.: Biochemical evaluation of a combined sulfatidosis and gangliosidosis (glycolipidosis) of the brain. Path. Europ., **3,** 409, 1968.
197. Mossakowski, M., Mathieson, G., and Cumings, J. N.: On the relationship of metachromatic leucodystrophy and amaurotic idiocy. Brain, **84,** 585, 1961.
198. Thieffry, S., Lyon, G., and Maroteaux, P.: Leucodystrophie métachromatique (sulfatidose) mucopolysaccharidose associées chez un même malade. Rev. Neurol. (Paris), **114,** 193, 1966.

199. Thieffry, S., Lyon, G., and Maroteaux, P.: Metabolic encephalopathy associating mucopolysaccharidosis and sulfatidosis. Arch. Franc. Pediat., **24**, 425, 1967.
200. Bubis, J. J., and Adlesberg, L.: Congenital metachromatic leukodystrophy: report of a case. Acta Neuropath. (Berlin), **6**, 298, 1966.
201. Feigin, I.: Diffuse cerebral sclerosis (metachromatic leuko-encephalopathy). Amer. J. Path., **30**, 715, 1954.
202. Neimann, N., Pierson, M., Tridon, P., Grignon, G., Marchal, C., Floquet, J., Vidailhet, M., and Humbel, R.: Les formes atypiques de la leucodystrophie métachromatique. Arch. Franc. Pediat., **25**, 957, 1968.
203. Greenfield, J. G.: Demyelinating diseases, in *Neuropathology,* chap. 7, p. 465. E. Arnold, London, 1958.
204. Liu, H. M.: Ultrastructure of central nervous system lesions in metachromatic leukodystrophy with special reference to morphogenesis. J. Neuropath. Exp. Neurol., **27**, 624, 1967.
205. Hirsch, T. V., and Peiffer, J.: Über histologische Methoden in der Differentialdiagnose von Leukodystrophien und Lipoidosen. Arch. Psychiat. Z. Neurol., **194**, 88, 1955.
206. Dayan, A. D.: Dichroism of cresyl violet–stained cerebroside sulfate ("sulfatide"). J. Histochem. Cytochem., **15**, 421, 1967.
207. McManus, J. F. A., and Cason, J. E.: Carbohydrate histochemistry studied by acetylation techniques. I. Periodic acid methods. J. Exp. Med., **91**, 651, 1950.
208. Suzuki, K., Suzuki, K., and Chen, G. C.: Isolation and chemical characterization of metachromatic granules from a brain with metachromatic leukodystrophy. J. Neuropath. Exp. Neurol., **26**, 537, 1967.
209. Dayan, A. D.: Peripheral neuropathy of metachromatic leucodystrophy: observations on segmental demyelination and remyelination and the intracellular distribution of sulphatide. J. Neurol. Neurosurg. Psychiat., **30**, 311, 1967.
210. Webster, H. deF.: Schwann cell alterations in metachromatic leukodystrophy: preliminary phase and electron microscope observations. J. Neuropath. Exp. Neurol., **21**, 534, 1962.
211. Yudell, A., Gomez, M. R., and Lambert, E. H.: The neuropathy of sulfatide lipidosis (metachromatic leukodystrophy). Neurology, **17**, 103, 1967.
212. Aziz, H., and Pearce, J.: Peripheral neuropathy in metachromatic leucodystrophy. Brit. Med. J., **4**, 300, 1968.
213. Cravioto, H., O'Brien, J. S., and Landing, B. H.: Ultrastructure of peripheral nerve in metachromatic leucodystrophy. Acta Neuropath. (Berlin), **7**, 111, 1966.
214. Wolfe, H. J., and Pietra, G. G.: The visceral lesions of metachromatic leukodystrophy. Amer. J. Path., **44**, 921, 1964.
215. Hagberg, B., and Svennerholm, L.: Metachromatic leucodystrophy—a generalized lipidosis: determination of sulfatides in urine, blood plasma and cerebrospinal fluid. Acta Paediat. Scand., **49**, 690, 1960.
216. Dische, M. R.: Metachromatic leucodystrophic polyposis of the gall bladder. J. Path., **97**, 388, 1969.
217. Dalinka, M. K., Rosen, R. A., Kurth, R. J., and Hemming, V. G.: Metachromatic leukodystrophy, A cause of cholelithiasis in childhood. Amer. J. Dig. Dis., **14** (8), 603, 1969.
218. Résibois, A.: Electron microscopic study of metachromatic leucodystrophy. III. Lysosomal nature of the inclusions. Acta Neuropath. (Berlin), **13**, 149, 1969.
219. Aurebeck, G., Osterberg, K., Blaw, M., Chov, S., and Nelson, E.: Electron microscopic observations on metachromatic leukodystrophy. Arch. Neurol. (Chicago), **11**, 273, 1964.
220. Hers, H. G., and Van Hoof, F.: The genetic pathology of lysosomes, in *Progress in Liver Disease,* vol. III, chap. 12, pp. 185–205. Grune & Stratton, New York, 1970.
221. O'Brien, J. S., and Sampson, E. L.: Myelin membrane: a molecular abnormality. Science, **150**, 1613, 1965.
222. Cumings, J. N.: The lipid composition of pure myelin in some demyelinating disorders. Neuropat. Pol., **7** (3), 255, 1969.
223. Jatzkewitz, H.: Cerebron- und Kerasin-schwefelsäureester als speicher Substanzen bei der Leukodystrophie, Typ Scholz (metachromatische Form der diffusen Sklerose). Z. Physiol. Chem., **320**, 134, 1960.
224. Tingey, A. H., and Edgar, G. W. F.: A contribution to the chemistry of the leukodystrophies. J. Neurochem., **10**, 817, 1963.
225. Yabuuchi, H., Okada, S., Honda, M., and Hanai, J.: Pathological and biochemical study of metachromatic leucodystrophy. Med. J. Osaka Univ., **18** (4), 361, 1968.
226. O'Brien, J. S.: A molecular defect of myelination. Biochem. Biophys. Res. Commun., **15** (5), 484, 1964.
227. Martensson, E., Percy, A., and Svennerholm, L.: Kidney glycolipids in late infantile metachromatic leucodystrophy. Acta Paediat. Scand., **55**, 1, 1966.
228. Pilz, H., and Müller, D.: Studies on adult metachromatic leukodystrophy. Part 2. Biochemical aspects of adult cases of metachromatic leukodystrophy. J. Neurol. Sci., **9**, 585, 1969.
229. Malone, M. J., Stoffyn, P., and Moser, H.: Structural studies on sulphatides in metachromatic leucodystrophy. J. Neurochem., **13**, 1033, 1966.
230. Taketomi, T., and Kawamura, N.: Cerebroside and sulfatide isolated from the cerebral frontal lobe of a patient with metachromatic leukodystrophy. Med. J. Shinshu Univ., **13** (2), 103, 1968.
231. Ställberg-Stenhagen, S., and Svennerholm, L.: Fatty acid composition of human brain sphingomyelins: normal variation with age and changes during myelin disorders. J. Lipid Res., **6**, 146, 1965.
232. Edgar, G. W. F.: Hexosamine in normal and pathological nerve tissue. Acta Neuropath. (Berlin), **13**, 182, 1969.
233. Cumings, J. N., Thompson, E. J., and Goodwin, H.: Sphingolipids and phospholipids in microsomes and myelin from normal and pathological brains. J. Neurochem., **15**, 243, 1968.
234. Mehl, E., and Jatzkewitz, H.: Evidence for the genetic block in metachromatic leucodystrophy (ML). Biochem. Biophys. Res. Commun., **19** (4), 407, 1965.
235. Stumpf, D., and Austin, J.: Metachromatic leukodystrophy (MLD) IX. Qualitative and quantitative differences in urinary arylsulfatase A in different forms of MLD. Arch. Neurol., **24**, 117, 1971.
236. Christensen, E., and Palludan, B.: Late infantile familial metachromatic leucodystrophy in minks. Acta Neuropath. (Berlin), **4**, 640, 1965.
237. Moser, H. W., Moser, A. B., and McKhann, G. M.: The dynamics of a lipidosis: turnover of sulfatide, steroid sulfate, and polysaccharide sulfate in metachromatic leukodystrophy. Arch. Neurol. (Chicago), **17**, 494, 1967.
238. Hansson, H-A., Olsson, Y., and Sourander, P.: Experimental studies on the pathogenesis of leucodystrophies. III. Cellular accumulation of injected sulphatides in brain, peripheral nerve and kidney. Acta Neuropath. (Berlin), **9**, 134, 1967.
239. Leitch, G. J., Horrocks, L. A., and Samorajski, T.: Effects of cations on isolated bovine optic nerve myelin. J. Neurochem., **16**, 1347, 1969.
240. Wolman, M.: Myelin breakdown in vitro. Biochim. Biophys. Acta, **102**, 261, 1965.
241. Wolman, M., and Wiener, H.: Structure of the myelin sheath as a function of concentration of ions. Biochim. Biophys. Acta, **102**, 269, 1965.
242. Meves, H.: Zur Wirkung hypertoner Lösungen auf die markhaltige Nervenfaser. Experientia, **20**, 31, 1964.
243. Webster, H. deF., and Ames, A., III: The effects of osmotic changes on the phase and electron microscopic appearance of nervous tissue. J. Neuropath. Exp. Neurol., **26**, 160, 1967.
244. Ledig, M.: Mise en évidence d'echangeurs de cations dans les membranes intracellulaires et dans les gaines de myéline. J. Physiol. (Paris) Comm., **59**, 254, 1967.
245. Austin, J., Armstrong, D., Shearer, L., and McAfee, D.: Metachromatic form of diffuse cerebral sclerosis. VI. A rapid test for the sulfatase A deficiency in metachromatic leukodystrophy (MLD) urine. Arch. Neurol. (Chicago), **14**, 259, 1966.
246. Bass, N. H., Witmer, E. J., and Dreifuss, F. E.: A pedigree study of metachromatic leukodystrophy: biochemical identification of the carrier state. Neurology, **20**, 52, 1970.

246*a*. Lowry, O. H., Rosenbrough, N. S., Farr, A. L., and Randall, R. J.: Protein measurement with the Folin phenol reagent. J. Biol. Chem., **193**, 265, 1951.

247. Wherrett, J. R.: Analysis of polar lipids in the urine sediment. Clin. Chim. Acta, **16** (1), 135, 1966.
248. Desnick, R. J., Sweeley, C. C., and Krivit, W.: A method for the quantitative determination of neutral glycosphingolipids in urine sediment. J. Lipid Res., **11**, 31, 1970.

249. Hagberg, B., Sourander, P., and Svennerholm, L.: Clinical and laboratory diagnosis of metachromatic leucodystrophy. Cerebral Palsy Bull., **3**, 438, 1961.
250. Helfant, M., Borjeson, M., and Hellström, B.: Value of urinary sediment examination as a screening method in suspected cases of metachromatic leukodystrophy. Acta Paediat. Scand., **51**, 49, 1962.
251. Brande, J. L., Van den Hooft, C., and Roose, A.: Metachromatic coloring matter in urinary sediment and cerebrospinal fluid and paper chromatography of the sulfatides: a comparative study in normal and centrally disturbed children. Maandschr. Kindergeneesk., **34**, 141, 1966.
252. Dacremont, G., Vandenbussche, P., Mortier, E., et al.: Study of urinary sulfatides by paper chromatography in a group of children with important psychomotor retardation. Rev. Franc. Etud. Clin. Biol., **14**, 297, 1969.
253. Hagberg, B., and Svennerholm, L.: Metachromatic leucodystrophy—a generalized lipidosis: determination of sulfatides in urine, blood plasma and cerebrospinal fluid. Acta Paediat. Scand., **49**, 690, 1960.
254. Svennerholm, L.: Chromatographic determination of sulfatides. Acta Chem. Scand., **17**, 1170, 1963.
255. Austin, J. H.: Metachromatic form of diffuse sclerosis. 1. Diagnosis during life by urine sediment examination. Neurology, **7**, 415, 1957.
256. Read, C. R.: Screening for metachromatic leucodystrophy. J. Clin. Path., **20**, 301, 1967.
257. Lake, B. D.: A reliable rapid screening test for sulphatide lipidosis. Arch. Dis. Child., **40**, 284, 1965.
258. Thieffry, S., and Lyon, G.: Diagnostic d'un cas de leucodystrophie métachromatique (type Scholz) par la biopsie d'un nerf périphérique. Rev. Neurol. (Paris), **100**, 452, 1959.
259. Olsson, Y., and Sourander, P.: The reliability of the diagnosis of metachromatic leucodystrophy by peripheral nerve biopsy. Acta Paediat. Scand., **58**, 15, 1969.
260. Fullerton, P. H.: Peripheral nerve conduction in metachromatic leucodystrophy (sulfatide lipidosis). J. Neurol., Neurosurg. Psychiat., **27**, 100, 1964.
261. Thieffry, S., Lyon, G., Aicardi, J., Chaumont, P., and Lerique, A.: L'Atteinte du système nerveux périphérique dans la leucodystrophie métachromatique. Signes cliniques et électriques. Rev. Neurol. (Paris), **110**, 508, 1964.
262. Jacobs, K., Radermecker, J., and Claes, C.: Caractères cliniques et électrophysiologiques des atteintes nerveuses périphériques dans la leucodystrophie métachromatique (7 cas). Rev. Neurol. (Paris), **118** (6), 545, 1968.
263. Blom, S., and Hagberg, B.: EEG findings in late infantile metachromatic and globoid cell leucodystrophy. Electroenceph. Clin. Neurophysiol., **22**, 253, 1967.
264. Hultberg, B., Ockerman, P-A., and Eriksson, O.: Urinary amino acids in storage disorders: mucopolysaccharidosis, Gaucher's disease and metachromatic leucodystrophy. Metabolism, **18** (8), 713, 1969.
265. Melchior, J. C., and Clausen, J.: Metachromatic leucodystrophy in early childhood: treatment with a diet deficient in vitamin A. Acta Paediat. Scand., **57**, 2, 1968.
266. Greene, H. L., Hug, G., and Schubert, W. K.: Metachromatic leukodystrophy: treatment with arylsulfatase-A. Arch. Neurol. (Chicago), **20**, 147, 1969.
267. Bleszynski, W., and Dzialoszynski, L. M.: Purification of soluble arylsulphatases from ox brain. Biochem. J., **97**, 360, 1965.
268. Omori, K., Masuda, M., Yogo, T., Matsuyama, H., and Watanabe, I.: An autopsied case of leucodystrophy. Shonika Shinryo, **25**, 1005, 1962.
269. Kamoshita, S., Matsubayashi, A., Suzuki, M., and Arima, M.: An autopsied case of leucodystrophy. Pediat. Univ. Tokyo, **8**, 43, 1963.
270. Kamoshita, S.: Studies on metachromatic leucodystrophy. Acta Paediat. Jap., **6**, 1, 1964.
271. Nishh, A.: An autopsied case of metachromatic leucodystrophy. Ann. Paediat. Jap., **11**, 467, 1965.
272. Stern, C.: In *Principles of Human Genetics,* 2d ed. Freeman, San Francisco, 1960.
273. Leroy, J. G.: Deficiency of arylsulphatase A in leucocytes and skin fibroblasts in juvenile metachromatic leucodystrophy. Nature (London), **226**, 553, 1970.
274. Zilversmit, D. B., Entenman, C., and Fishler, M. C.: On the calculation of "turnover time" and "turnover rate" from experiments involving the use of labeling agents. J. Gen. Physiol., **26**, 325, 1942.
275. Goldstone, A., Konecny, P., and Koenig, H.: Lysosomal hydrolases: Conversion of acidic to basic forms by neuraminidase. Federation of European Biochemical Societies, **13**, 68, 1971.
276. Rampini, S., Isler, W., Baerlocher, K., Bischoff, A., Ulrich, J., and Plüss, H. J.: Die Kombination von metachromatischer Leukodystrophie und Mukopolysaccharidose als selbständiges Krankheitsbild (Mukosulfatidose). Helv. Paediat. Acta, **25**, 436, 1970.
277. Porter, M. T., Fluharty, A. L., Harris, S. E., and Kihara, H.: The accumulation of cerebroside sulfates by fibroblasts in culture from patients with late infantile metachromatic leukodystrophy. Arch. Biochem., **138**, 646, 1970.

CHAPTER THIRTY-THREE

GLUCOSYL CERAMIDE LIPIDOSES: Gaucher's Disease

Donald S. Fredrickson and Howard R. Sloan

The name *Gaucher's disease* applies to two or more hereditary disorders in the metabolism of glucocerebrosides, compounds more accurately called *glucosyl ceramides* (and here abbreviated as Glc-Cer) (Fig. 33-1). The underlying defect appears to be deficient activity of a β-glucosidase that catalyzes the cleavage of glucose from glucosyl ceramide. Excess Glc-Cer accumulates in reticuloendothelial cells, which take on a characteristic appearance. Increasing masses of such "Gaucher cells" cause organs such as the spleen, liver, and lymph nodes to enlarge; they also frequently alter the structure and compromise the functions of the bones and lungs. In a majority of patients, the pathologic process proceeds slowly, the major manifestations being hypersplenism and bone pain and pathologic fractures. Patients so affected have chronic Gaucher's disease, sometimes called the adult form. In a smaller number of patients, the disorder is associated with obvious neurologic signs. Usually these cases progress rapidly and are fatal in infancy. Occasionally, neurologic manifestations occur later in childhood and death is delayed until the second decade. These several variants of Gaucher's disease seem to be due to different mutations affecting the same or similar genetic loci. They will be referred to here as Type 1 (chronic nonneuronopathic, adult), Type 2 (acute neuronopathic), and Type 3 (subacute neuronopathic, juvenile). A different order of types has been used previously [1, 2]; the present one is in accord with an earlier suggestion by Knudson and Kaplan [3] and has the advantage of considering the oldest known form as the first type and relegating the least certain to the last.

HISTORICAL ASPECTS

In the first report of this disease in 1882, Philippe Gaucher [4] described the chronic, progressive course with hepatosplenomegaly that is characteristic of Type 1 Gaucher's disease. It was early believed that the peculiar large cells in the spleen were evidence of a primary neoplasm [4] or connective tissue proliferation [5]. With discovery of more cases the concepts of causation gradually evolved through a theory of toxic origin [6] to one of a diffuse systemic disease of the lymphatic-hematopoietic system [5], to the suggestion that a "foreign" substance was being deposited in the reticulum cells [7], this substance being either carried there by the blood [8] or elaborated *in situ* [9].

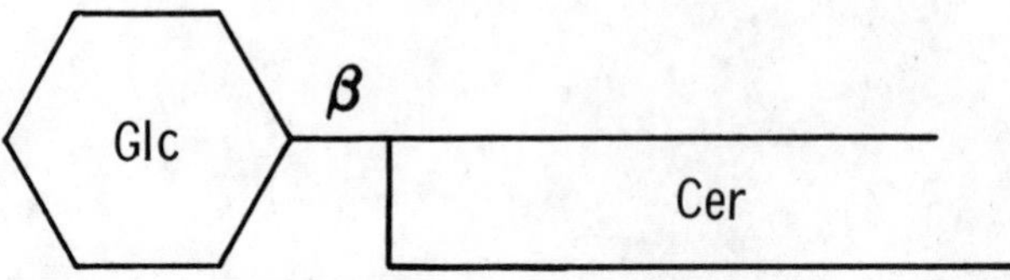

Figure 33-1. Glucosyl ceramide (glucocerebroside).

A number of investigations then indicated that the abnormal cells contained "lipoid" material. These early studies were thoroughly reviewed by Epstein [10], who, working with Lorenz [10, 11], found the "Gaucher spleen" to contain large amounts of an alcohol-soluble, acetone-insoluble material. In 1924, Lieb [12–14] isolated from this tissue large amounts of cerebrosides, compounds that had been isolated from brain 50 years earlier and given their name by Thudichum [15, 16]. Although Thudichum correctly described the general structure of cerebrosides, it is through the subsequent work of many other workers that the precise nature of their component sphingosine bases, fatty acids, and hexoses has become known [17].

Lieb [12–14] concluded that he had isolated from a Gaucher spleen the galactocerebroside containing lignoceric acid, which was also known by the trivial name of *kerasin*. Hence the name *kerasin lipidosis* was early given to Gaucher's disease. Klenk and Harle [18, 19] noted a few years later, however, that there was a difference in optical rotation between galactosyl ceramide and the cerebroside they had isolated from Gaucher tissue. The explanation of this discrepancy was discovered by Aghion, who reported in 1934 [20] that Glc-Cer, not Gal-Cer, accumulates in the Gaucher spleen. This was supported by Halliday et al. [21], established firmly by Rosenberg and Chargaff [22], and confirmed by others [23, 24].

Another major step forward was made in 1965, when deficiency of glucocerebrosidase activity in the spleens of patients with Gaucher's disease was first convincingly demonstrated by Brady, Kanfer, and Shapiro [25].

CLINICAL ASPECTS

Probably as many as a thousand patients with all types of Gaucher's disease have been reported. Most of these cases are examples of the chronic form (Type 1). No complete tabulation of children with neurologic involvement has appeared since the scholarly reviews of Giampalmo [26, 27], over 20 years ago. All available reports of the neuronopathic forms through 1969 have been reevaluated in this review. More than 70 patients have been described with typical neurologic manifestations that contributed to death before age 3. Most of them are compatible with a single disorder, the acute neuronopathic form (Type 2). From the 25 or more descriptions of patients dying later with neurologic deficits, the dual impressions are gained that there is a "juvenile" form of Gaucher's disease (Type 3), but that its clinical and chemical manifestations are heterogeneous; no satisfying classification of such intermediate cases is yet possible.

All forms of Gaucher's disease share certain common clinical features: hepatosplenomegaly, the presence of Gaucher cells in the bone marrow, and an elevated concentration of serum acid phosphatase. The three different forms all may begin in infancy, and phenotypic distinctions sometimes depend on the evolution of manifestations, the key one being evidence of neurologic involvement. As with many other heritable disorders, the best evidence for genotypic heterogeneity in Gaucher's disease is the repeated observation that affected relatives in the same kindred share a similar pattern of expression. There is also a marked difference in the frequency of the various types in one particular ethnic group, the Ashkenazi Jews.

Type 1: Chronic Nonneuronopathic (Adult) Gaucher's Disease

Freedom from signs of cerebral involvement is the *sine qua non* for classification of Type 1 Gaucher's disease. Although usually called the "adult" form, it often develops in childhood and may not have a benign indolent course. Death may occur early in life because of episodes of bleeding aggravated by thrombocytopenia or the conversion of intercurrent illnesses to fatal ones by the presence of severe anemia or pulmonary infiltration.

Perhaps someday there will emerge several forms of "chronic nonneuronopathic" Gaucher's disease, including some with symptomless, histologic evidence of neuronal involvement [28]. Certainly there is no single "typical" example of Type 1, and possibly case reports have tended to emphasize the more serious or spectacular manifestations. The following two examples illustrate the differences in severity that are possible.

PATIENT Z. K. This patient (NIH No. 02-62-62, also described previously [29]) was the second-born of two male children of Ashkenazi Jews. The mother came from Palestine; she has had one bone marrow examination which revealed no abnormality. The father, who came from Lithuania, died at a relatively young age of a coronary thrombosis. The patient's older sib is normal. Between the ages of 9 months and 1 year, the patient was taken to physicians because of a question of retarded growth and abdominal enlargement. When he was 4 years old, hepatosplenomegaly was established and Gaucher cells were discovered in the sternal marrow. When he was 7 years of age thrombocytopenia and discomfort led to removal of his greatly enlarged spleen. For the next 20 years he led a courageous, outwardly normal life. He was an excellent student and was admitted to the bar. Throughout his school life, however, he had repeated episodes of bone pain and fractures associated with minor trauma that eventually led to permanent deformities of the left hip and leg. He married and had two normal daughters.

The patient was first examined by us when he was 28 years of age. He had previously been reported by Thannhauser (Patient 48) [9]. He had not had bone pain or fractures for about 10 years; his liver was enormous, extending to the iliac crest. His skin was a rather sallow yellow, with a little duskiness over the tibias, and he had small, unimpressive pingueculae in both eyes. The pulmonic second sound was markedly accentuated, and this, in association with electrocardiograph evidence of right ventricular hypertrophy, suggested pulmonary hypertension. His serum acid phosphatase level was markedly elevated (3.08 Bessey-Lowry units, 0.15 being tartrate-inhibitable).

During the next 2½ years the patient had numerous bouts of severe chest pain, intermittent cardiac arrhythmia, and steadily increasing signs of pulmonary hypertension. At the age of 31 years he died shortly after admission to the hospital with severe congestive heart failure and hemopericardium. At post-mortem examination [30] a "raging diffuse hemorrhagic pericarditis" was found, but no Gaucher cells could be detected in the pericardium or heart. There was extensive infiltration of the pulmonary arteries, other changes indicative of pulmonary hypertension, and severe pulmonary artery atheromatosis. The liver weighed 8.1 kg and contained 86 mg per gm dry weight of glycolipids (normal, <10 mg per gm) (Fig. 33-8). There was evidence of extramedullary erythropoiesis in the liver, lung, lymph nodes, and adrenal glands, but not in the heart or pericardium.

At the opposite end of the spectrum from Patient Z. K. is the following patient.

PATIENT D. E. This patient (NIH No. 04-24-47) was an only child of Jewish parents. The mother was born in Lithuania and the father in Russia; there is no other known instance of Gaucher's disease in the family. The patient is married and the father of four apparently normal girls. He is a college graduate and has never had any neurologic abnormalities. At age 43 he noted a tendency to bruising or bleeding after mild trauma such as from shaving. Two years later hepatosplenomegaly was discovered, and at age 46 he was found to have leukopenia and thrombocytopenia; the edges of both liver and spleen were 4 cm below the costal margins, and there were definite Gaucher cells in several aspirates of sternal marrow. The serum acid phosphatase level was twice the normal (1.35 Bessey-Lowry units, the bulk being noninhibitable by tartrate). All other tests were negative. For about 10 years the patient continued to have a platelet count of about 50,000 and leukocytes in the range of 3,000 to 4,000. He had no detectable osseous lesions. His spleen was eventually removed at another hospital, and he continues to lead a normal and productive life.

Many reviews and case reports have dealt with the clinical features of Type 1 Gaucher's disease [29, 31, 35]. One of these reports [34] describes a series of 34 Israeli patients, many of whose cases have been followed for a number of years. Ethnic origin is not always identified in case reports, and there has been no complete tabulation of origins. Far more than half of all reported patients appear to have been Ashkenazi Jews; only two known cases have been described in Sephardic Jews [34].

Type 1 may manifest itself at any age. The earliest report is that of a post-mortem diagnosis made at 14 days of age in a child whose sib had definite Type 1 disease [36]. Many other cases have been detected in infancy, and probably a majority of patients have symptoms or signs before the age of 15 to 20 years. Some cases are not discovered until middle age, and at least one patient was an octogenarian before the diagnosis was made [37].

Although the clinical course of Type 1 can run rapidly downhill in childhood [38–40], the usual outlook is much more optimistic. For example, of 26 patients whose disease was detected at ages varying from 2 to 50 and was followed for at least 10 years, 4 had died at ages from 22 to 58 years [34]. One Australian patient with Type 1 was found to have splenomegaly at 61 years of age and reached the age of 82 [41]. Most affected children have reasonably normal development and survive into adulthood. If the disease first becomes evident in adulthood, normal life expectancy is possible.

Type 2: Acute Neuronopathic Gaucher's Disease

Of the many adjectives used for this form of Gaucher's disease, acute [42], infantile [43], cerebral [3], or malignant [44], the last is the single most descriptive. The commonly used term "infantile" is the least accurate and has often been misunderstood. We prefer the names malignant or acute neuronopathic and, for convenience, will usually refer to the condition here simply as Type 2. A reasonably typical description of Type 2 is provided by the following case history [29].

PATIENT W. M. C. This patient (NIH 04-29-10) was the second-born of young, healthy parents. One normal female sib was 3 years older. The mother, born in Central America, was of mixed Spanish, Italian, and Indian descent. The father was an American of Anglo-Saxon origin. Neither parent knew of Jewish ancestry. The patient developed normally until age 4 to 6 months, when he stopped gaining weight and was found to be anemic. By the time he was 8 months old, his motor development began to regress and abdominal protuberance was noted. At 10 months of age Gaucher cells were present in the bone marrow. When examined at age 12 months, he could no longer sit; the liver was 6 cm and the spleen 10 cm below the costal margins. There were left internal strabismus and some hypertonicity and "stiffness" of the extremities. The deep tendon reflexes were brisk, the plantar reflexes were flexor, and the ocular fundi were normal. He had microcytic anemia with evidence of iron deficiency, and his serum acid phosphatase level was markedly elevated to 30 King-Armstrong units, only 0.3 unit of which was tartrate-inhibitable. He soon developed trismus, laryngospasm, sustained retroflexion of the head, and increasing spasticity (Fig. 33-2). He also had a chronic cough and frequent unexplained fever. He died at 14 months of age after a brief severe intestinal infection associated with cyanosis, and severe thrombocytopenia.

There was massive infiltration of Gaucher cells in the liver (600 gm), spleen (420 gm), lymph nodes, Peyer's patches, thymus, and adrenal glands. There were scattered foci of similar cells in the lungs and adrenal cortices, and a few were also seen in the thyroid and other organs. The liver contained 17.1 μmoles of monohexosyl ceramide per gm wet weight [45] (normal 0.05 μmoles per gm [46]) (Fig. 33-8). The brain appeared grossly normal, and although no histologic abnormalities were initially reported by the pathologist [29], later review of PAS-stained paraffin-fixed sections revealed all the features described below as typical of the Type 2 brain, including some storage of glycolipid in neurons.

At least 67 patients with a reasonably similar story have been reported since Rusca's first description of a patient with the acute form of neuronopathic Gaucher's disease in 1921 [47]. These cases are summarized in Table 33-1. Omitted from this compilation are 21 other patients who also may have had Type 2 Gaucher's disease. Some, like the patients of Gerstl and Kraus [95, 96], Pick-Nauwerck [97], Kohn [98], Hoffman and Makler [99], Lindau [100], Findlay [101, 102], and Girgensohn [103], have been included in prior reviews. For each of these, however, and for others [36, 104–116] the

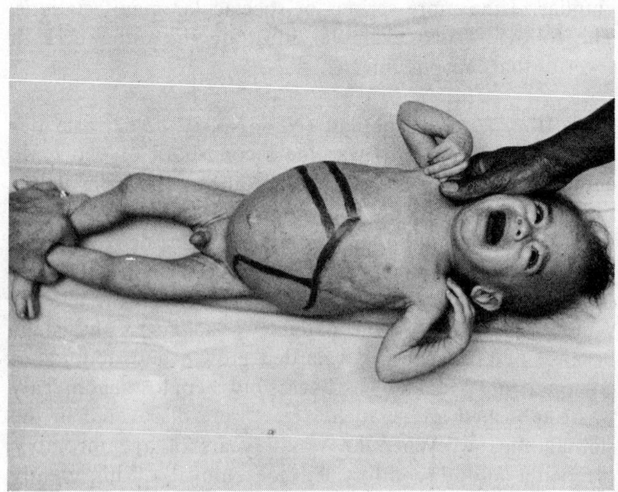

Figure 33-2. Acute neuronopathic Gaucher's disease (Type 2) in a 12-month-old child. The hyperextension of the head, position of the upper extremities, retraction of the lips, and strabismus, in association with hepatosplenomegaly, are characteristic of this form of the disease.

Table 33-1. REPORTED EXAMPLES OF ACUTE NEURONOPATHIC (TYPE 2) GAUCHER'S DISEASE

Patient	References	Year	Ethnic origin	Sibships		Sex	Age, mo		Confirmation of diagnosis	
				No. affected	Total live births		Onset	Death	Chemical	Neuro-pathologic
1	[47]	1921	Italian	1	?	M	6	12		
2	[48]	1924	....	2	3	M	5	8		
3	[48]	1924	....	2	3	F	6	7	...	+
4	[50]	1927	Non-Jewish	3	?	F	2	5	+	+
5	[51, 52]	1929	Non-Jewish	3	?	?	?	3		
6	[53]	1930	Non-Jewish	3	?	M	2	7		
7	[43]	1927	Non-Jewish	5	7	M	5	12		
8	[43]	1927	Non-Jewish	5	7	F	5	11	...	+
9	[43]	1927	Non-Jewish	5	7	F	1.5	11		
10	[43]	1927	Non-Jewish	5	7	M	0.8	1	...	+
11	[54, 55]	1934	Non-Jewish	5	7	F	3	7		
12	[56]	1927	....	2	2	?	?	3		
13	[56]	1927	....	2	2	F	2	5		
14	[57, 58]	1930	Non-Jewish	1	4	M	2.5	4	+	+
15	[59]	1932	French	1	1	F	6	8.5		
16	[60]	1934	Italian	1	?	M	6	7		
17	[61]	1938	Non-Jewish	1	1	F	0.3	4.5	+	
18	[62]	1939	Non-Jewish	1	?	M	3	8	+	+
19	[44]	1940	Non-Jewish	2	3	F	2	6	...	+
20	[44]	1940	Non-Jewish	2	3	M	1	4	...	+
21	[63]	1941	Cuban	1	?	F	3	Living		
22	[64]	1942	....	1	?	M	3	8	...	+
23	[65]	1942	....	1	?	F	6	8		
24	[66]	1943	....	1	2	F	2	6.5		
25	[67]	1945	Spanish	3	4	F	Birth	?		
26	[67]	1945	Spanish	3	4	M	Birth	8		
27	[67]	1945	Spanish	3	4	?	?	?		
28	[26]	1946	Italian	2	4	M	16	20	+	+
29	[27]	1949	Italian	2	4	F	0.3	1.5		
30	[68]	1948	....	1	?	M	4	?	+	+
31	[69]	1948	Jewish	1	?	M	1	7	+	+
32	[70]	1949	....	3	7	M	<5	9.5	...	+
33	[70]	1949	....	3	7	F	3	9	...	+
34	[70]	1949	....	3	7	M	0.3	10	...	+
35	[71]	1951	English-Dutch–	2	3	F	3.5	11	+	+
36	[72]	1953	Non-Jewish	2	3	M	2.5	10	+	+
37	[73]	1951	Non-Jewish	1	3	F	3	7	+	+
38	[74]	1951	....	1	3	M	0.3	6	...	+
39	[75]	1952	Non-Jewish	1	1	M	3	4.5	...	+
40	[76]	1956	....	1	2	M	2	14	...	+
41	[77]	1957	Negro	1	2	M	1	22	+	+
42	[78]	1961	German	1	?	F	<3	4	...	+
43	[79]	1961	Jewish	1	1	M	3	6	...	+
44	[80]	1961	Italian	1	2	F	12	>22		
45	[81]	1962	Jewish	2	3	M	<3	7	+	+
46	[81]	1962	Jewish	2	3	F	?	10		
47	[81]	1962	Non-Jewish	1	2	M	Birth	3	+	+
48	[81]	1962	Non-Jewish	1	4	F	6	16	+	+
49	[3]	1962	Mexican	3	4	M	?	5	...	+
50	[3]	1962	Mexican	3	4	M	?	5		
51	[3]	1962	Mexican	3	4	F	0.3	4.5		
52	[82]	1962	Nigerian	1	3	F	4	9		
53	[83]	1962	Italian	2	2	F	7	>13		
54	[83]	1962	Italian	2	2	F	?	20		
55	[84, 85]	1964	....	1	1	?	<1	8	...	+
56	[84, 85]	1964	....	1	?	M	4	18	...	+
57	[86, 87]	1964	....	2	3	M	<1	6.5		
58	[86, 87]	1964	....	2	3	F	4	8	...	+
59	[88]	1965	Slovak	1	?	F	9	16		
60	[29]	1966	English-Spanish-Italian	1	2	M	4	14	+	+
61	[89]	1966	Tunisian	1	?	M	2	24	...	+
62	[90]	1966	....	1	?	M	18	20	+	+
63	[91]	1967	Jewish	2	4	M	3	11	...	+
64	[91]	1967	Jewish	2	4	M	?	10		
65	[92]	1968	Italian	1	?	M	7.5	12	...	+
66	[93, 94]	1969	Negro	2	?	M	7	17	...	+
67	[93, 94]	1969	Negro	2	?	M	7	18	...	+

evidence of progressive central nervous system involvement consistent with Type 2 seems insufficient to add them to the compilation. Two "acute cerebral" cases reported by Makita et al. [115] and several cases mentioned by Svennerholm [116] were proved by chemical analyses to be Gaucher's disease, but the clinical descriptions were not complete enough to be tabulated. Also omitted from Table 33-1 are other patients who have been included in various reviews of the Type 2 form but whose case reports indicate that they had Type 1 [117–124] or probably did not have Gaucher's disease at all [125]. One of the most interesting omissions from Table 33-1 is the report of Girgensohn, Kellner, and Sudhof [103] of an infant who died 16 hr after birth with typical Gaucher cells throughout the body. There were also changes in ganglion cells, medial calcification in the great vessels, and good clinical evidence of erythroblastosis fetalis. We share the concern of the authors of the report [103] that the Gaucher cells and erythroblastosis may have been connected.

Onset and Survival

From the patients in Table 33-1 it is possible to construct a profile of Type 2. The child is usually born at term, after an uneventful pregnancy, and appears normal at birth. An average of 3 months passes before the earliest signs appear. These may be any combination of enlargement of the spleen, and usually of the liver, difficulty in feeding or swallowing, a chronic cough that ushers in progressive pulmonary infections, or simply a failure to thrive. About 10 percent of patients will be obviously abnormal at birth or within the first week of life; several patients have not been considered abnormal until 16 to 18 months old. Once the neurologic signs become evident, they usually progress rapidly. The average age at death is 9 months, and the range is from 1 month to 2 years. The principal immediate causes of death are anoxia and infection related to pulmonary involvement.

Neurologic Signs

By definition, every child with Type 2 Gaucher's disease has some evidence of progressive central nervous system dysfunction before death. Neurologic deficits are usually evident by 6 months of age. They tend to be highly stereotyped and feature cranial nerve and extrapyramidal tract involvement. Three findings that occur in 90 percent of cases at some time during the disease are strabismus, muscular hypertonicity or spasticity, and persistent retroflexion of the head (frequently and incorrectly termed "opisthotonos"). The next most common manifestations are rigidity of the neck, trismus, dysphagia, laryngeal stridor, and increased deep tendon reflexes. Babinski's sign and other pathologic reflexes may be present. A few patients will have seizures. Occasionally "sensory loss" or "paralysis" is mentioned. Many patients become hypotonic, and most of them become apathetic and mentally retarded near the end of the illness.

The appearance (Fig. 33-2) of a child with hepatosplenomegaly who also has ocular palsy, retracted lips, head held in severe hyperextension, and arms in a flexion posture is highly suggestive of Type 2 Gaucher's disease. Further corroboration is obtained by the finding of a high serum acid phosphatase level, and diagnosis is made reasonably certain with the demonstration of Gaucher cells in the bone marrow. The latter are almost always present by 6 months of age. It is reemphasized that children with other forms of Gaucher's disease may also have hepatosplenomegaly and Gaucher cells in the marrow in the first year of life.

Type 3: Subacute Neuronopathic (Juvenile) Gaucher's Disease

A "subacute neuronopathic" or a "juvenile" form of Gaucher's disease has been arbitrarily defined to include older children with hepatosplenomegaly, "Gaucher cells" in tissues, and neurologic abnormalities. The course is variable but more protracted than the malignant one seen in Type 2. Death usually occurs well after 2 years of age. No fewer than 25 patients have been reported who fit into this rough category. There is much doubt about inclusion of some of them, and inadequate chemical information for most of them. One can have little confidence that a single mutation or a unique disorder is represented. Because most of these patients have been cited one or more times as prototypic of a juvenile or subacute form of Gaucher's disease, each report is here briefly analyzed.

The report of Evans [126] involves a $3\frac{1}{2}$-year-old Jewish boy who very probably had Type 1 Gaucher's disease and a localized brain lesion, possibly due to hemorrhage. The pathologic studies of the brain (performed by Dr. Tilney) have apparently never been published. A patient of Howland and Rich was cited by Giampalmo [26] as having subacute Gaucher's disease. The only neurologic abnormalities were seizures that began at age 12, the year of his death, and the diagnosis of neuronopathic Gaucher's disease is most equivocal.

In 1931, Reiss and Kato described three Japanese children in a sibship of six [127]. Neurologic signs appeared in the two children who died at ages 6 and 7 years. The third sib had no such signs when he died at 2 years of age. Norman, Urich, and Lloyd [76] considered this sibship to include both "infantile" and "juvenile" variants; it is more likely that these cases represent a single mutation for a "juvenile" or Type 3 form. Tissue lipids were not analyzed. A girl described by Myers [128], sometimes considered as having Type 3 [76, 129], had hyperirritability and facial tics a year or so before she succumbed to an apparent pulmonary infection at the age of 9 years. The brain structure and tissue lipids were not examined.

A boy who died at 11 years reported by Bird [130] and another who died at 6 years described by Brain [131, 132] often are cited as having juvenile Gaucher's disease. This assignment has been both criticized [28, 133, 134] and defended [27, 76]. In the patient of Brain, Brante [134] was later unable to find any evidence of cerebroside accumulation in the spleen. No chemical data exist for Bird's case [130]. The equivocal data suggest that neither of these cases should continue to be used as examples of subacute neuronopathic Gaucher's disease.

One of the most extraordinary reports is that of Bernard and coworkers [109] of two French children who were born to the same mother but had different fathers. The first was a girl with chronic brain stem signs and choreoathetoid movements, hepatosplenomegaly, and Gaucher cells in the marrow. She was institutionalized for behavior problems before her death at 8 years of age. One of her five half-sibs, also a girl, died at the age of 14 months, with severe pulmonary involvement. Her story was a truncated version of the history of the other affected child, and the neuropathology, reported by Berard-Badier et al. [135], was compatible with that seen in Type 2 except perhaps for an unusual amount of neuronal lipid storage. The authors [109] considered that these cases demonstrated a dominant inheritance of Gaucher's disease. It seems more likely that the father of the first child may have carried one allele for the Type 1 form, whereas the mother and the father of the second bore alleles for Type 2. The implications of phenotypic modification are most interesting. No chemical analyses of tissues were made.

The patient of Maloney and Cumings [129] was a 9-year-old non-Jewish girl whose story is very similar to that of the Swedish families described below. They reported an increase in Glc-Cer in the spleen and brain, and an unusual amount of Gal-Cer in the spleen. These findings are atypical of other forms of Gaucher's disease. Jervis, Harris, and Menkes [136] reported an interesting case in a girl who died at age 4 years with neurologic signs very reminiscent of Type 2. The first signs of abnormality occurred at 18 months. "Gaucher cells" were present in the marrow and, at autopsy, in many other tissues. The chemical findings in the spleen [137] included a prominent rise in level of other neutral glycolipids in addition to Glc-Cer. Inose et al. [84, 85] studied a Japanese child who died at age 10. There were no neurologic signs except a stiff neck [84]. Striking fibrous proliferation of adventitial cells but few enlarged Gaucher type cells were seen in the brain. The brain, the only tissue examined chemically, had an increased content of dihexosyl ceramide in both gray and white matter. There was morphologic evidence of neuronal lipid storage in the brains of the first two patients, but very little in the patient of Inose.

Among other patients who may have had "juvenile" Gaucher's disease is a child mentioned by Philippart, Rosenstein, and Menkes [138] whose only possible neurologic abnormality at age 30 months was strabismus. An Italian girl with Gaucher's disease studied by Aronson and Carter [110] died at age 6 years. Her neurologic signs included strabismus, a stiff neck, and convulsions. The neuropathologic picture was suggestive of acute neuronopathic Gaucher's disease (Type 2). There was no ballooning of the neurons. A Spanish girl described by Sanchez-Villares and coworkers [111] was noted at 9 months of age to have psychomotor retardation, splenomegaly, and pulmonary infiltrates. When she was $2\frac{1}{2}$ years of age Gaucher cells were found in the marrow and spleen, and there were punctate areas of rarefaction in the skull. By 5 years of age, generalized hypertonia, hyperreflexia, and choreoathetoid movements were present. The electroencephalogram was diffusely abnormal. Attenuation of nervous manifestations and a late death (at 31 months of age) also occurred in a Turkish male described by Cura and Aksu [112]. Possibly both these patients had a protracted form of Type 2. A Polish boy, still living at age 14, who had Gaucher's disease with EEG changes and psychomotor retardation, has been reported by Klodnicka et al. [139]. Two other teen-age Belgian children, described by Claes and Carpentier [140], apparently had Gaucher's disease along with mental retardation and cerebellar and brain stem abnormalities. One also had hyperamino aciduria. Of this group of seven patients, tissues were submitted to chemical analyses only in the case of Philippart et al. [138]. In this patient there was an accumulation of both Glc-Cer and the dihexoside, Gal-Glc-Cer.

This leaves the largest single group of patients those with "juvenile" Gaucher's disease who come from four interrelated families from the province of Norrbotten in Northern Sweden and who have been described by Hillborg and coworkers [116, 141–144]. In all, there were 12 children, both boys and girls, who had Gaucher's disease. Six of them died between the ages of 1 and 3 years, all with splenomegaly and several with neurologic findings compatible with Type 2. Six other affected children, some of them sibs of the patients dying before 3 years of age, were studied at ages ranging from 6 to 20 years. All these last six appeared to be normal at birth, but each developed splenomegaly by 6 months to 1 year of age; this was followed by a slow increase in the size of the liver. Five of the 6 had anemia, leukopenia, and thrombocytopenia, and the spleen was removed from all six at ages ranging from $1\frac{1}{2}$ to 12 years. All the spleens contained typical Gaucher cells. At the time of splenectomy the patients were carefully examined and found to have no roentgenographic evidence of skeletal involvement. Within 4 years after splenectomy, all developed osseous lesions.

Careful neurologic assessment of the children was made when they were from 6 to 20 years of age. Five were mentally retarded, four of these and the child with normal intelligence had behavioral disturbances, two of them quite severe. Five of the six had other abnormalities, including hypertonicity or muscular stiffness, ticlike hyperkinesia, deficient coordination, strabismus, trismus, laryngeal stridor, or dysphagia. Half of them had epileptic seizures; all had EEG abnormalities. Svennerholm [116] has found no alterations in the glycolipid pattern in brain in the Swedish juvenile form (Type 3).

In summary, a group of children have been described who have central nervous system abnormalities and cells in nonneural tissues that have the histologic appearance of Gaucher cells. They usually survive longer than patients with Type 2, or if they die in infancy their clinical course has been subacute and other affected sibs have survived much longer. There has been inadequate evidence that most of these patients have the accumulation of Glc-Cer in extraneural tissues that is characteristic of other patients with Gaucher's disease. They undoubtedly represent a heterogeneous group, and though certain of their collective manifestations will be discussed further under the cover of "Type 3," no single certain disorder is implied.

CLINICOPATHOLOGIC CORRELATIONS

Several morphologic and functional alterations in Gaucher's disease merit elaboration: (1) the fine structure of the Gaucher cell itself, in which storage of Glc-Cer, apparently in lysosomes, is attended by unique cytoarchitectural distortions; (2) the disturbance in function of extraneural tissues that attends the gross anatomic changes; (3) the nature of the neuronal lesion, the poorly understood key to the phenotypic differences in Gaucher's disease.

The Gaucher Cell

Structure and Distribution

The storage cells in Gaucher's disease are mainly reticulum cells [5, 96, 145–149] or others, such as endothelial cells, with phagocytic potential. These storage cells undergo a remarkable change, while adjacent cells of other types may appear unaltered. The typical macrophages are especially abundant in lymphoid tissues, where they commonly occupy the area of the general reticulum outside the lymph sinuses [146]. Changes in lymph nodes are much more marked in the deep abdominal and thoracic nodes than in peripheral ones. The normal architecture of the spleen is sometimes replaced with sheets of "Gaucher cells"; this may also happen in sectors of the bone marrow. The Kupffer cells in the liver can become Gaucher cells, as may cells in the inner walls and adventitia of arterioles, veins, sinusoids, lymphatic vessels, and capillaries, especially the alveolar capillaries in the lung. Although osteoblasts and fibroblast-like spindle cells adjacent to spicules may be the source of Gaucher cells in the marrow [149, 150], some investigators have believed the endothelial cells of vessels to be primarily involved [151]. Many other organs may contain Gaucher cells, including the pancreas [152], thyroid [145], and adrenal cortex and medulla [153]. The distribution of abnormal cells is less than in the most severe forms of sphingomyelin lipidoses (Chap. 35) but wider than that in many other glycolipid storage diseases.

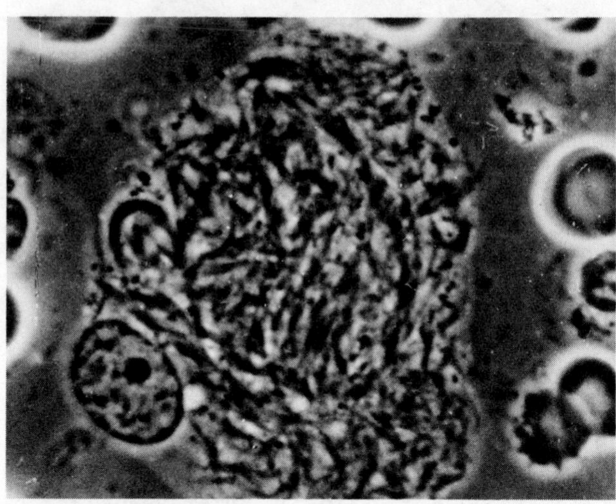

Figure 33-3. A Gaucher cell from bone marrow viewed without staining under the phase microscope. The size of the cell may be compared with that of the adjacent erythrocytes. (*Courtesy of Dr. George Brecher.*)

Light Microscopy

The appearance of the Gaucher cell is unique enough to permit an almost certain diagnosis when supravital preparations are viewed under the phase microscope (Fig. 33-3). The cells are usually between 20 and 100 microns in size, with a nucleus that is often eccentric. The cytoplasm appears to contain many fibrils of different lengths, giving the impression of "wrinkled tissue paper" or "crumpled silk" [150, 154]. This is in contrast to the foamy, particulate or mulberry appearance of storage cells in most of the other lipidoses (see Fig. 35-6, for example). The most appropriate stain for fixed preparations is the periodic acid–Schiff (PAS) reaction or PAS-leukofuchsin stain [155–157]. These tests remain positive after glycogen has been removed by diastase. Mallory's trichrome connective tissue stain is useful in bringing out the irregular cytoplasmic features. Cells that are easily distinguishable in supravital preparations may be less so when fixed and stained with Wright's or the Giemsa techniques. The histochemical reactions of Gaucher cells have been compared to those in other lipidoses by Wolman [158] and by Diezel [157]. The latter deduces from differential solubility of stored material that the cerebroside is "protein-bound" [159, 160], and also that several glycolipids, including gangliosides, are present in increased amounts. The cells are also strongly positive for acid phosphatase [161–163], and often contain ferritin [146, 154, 164, 165]; however, neither of these features is diagnostic.

Ultrastructure

Under the electron microscope the Gaucher cell is seen to contain characteristic cytoplasmic residual bodies or secondary lysosomes [91, 165–183]. These are illustrated in Fig.

33-4A and B from the studies of Lee, Balcerzak, and Westerman [177, 179]. The residual bodies appear to have a single limiting membrane surrounding a pale matrix, which is filled with tubular structures. The tubular diameters of 120 to 750 Å are fairly constant within each cell, but vary from cell to cell. The tubules are up to 5 microns in length. Each contains 10 to 12 fibrils twisted around the long axis of the tubule as a right-handed helix with a pitch of about 1,600 Å (Fig. 33-4B). The distance between the fibrils is about 80 Å, compared with the 40-Å length of a single molecule of glucosyl ceramide [177, 179]. Similar-appearing tubules can be formed in vitro from pure Glc-Cer [179]. Acid phosphatase is localized in the intertubular matrix of the lysosomes [183].

As summarized by Pennelli [182], three concepts of the origin of glucosyl ceramide in the Gaucher cells have arisen from study of electron micrographs. It was first assumed that the primary abnormality lay in the mitochondria. These sometimes appear abnormal [167, 168], but recent work suggests that the changes are nonspecific [173, 181, 182]. A second concept favors the heterophagous uptake of Glc-Cer, possibly in a "lipoprotein" form, by the Gaucher cells. Intense phagocytic and pinocytotic activity is suggested by numerous microvilli that appear at the cell borders of such

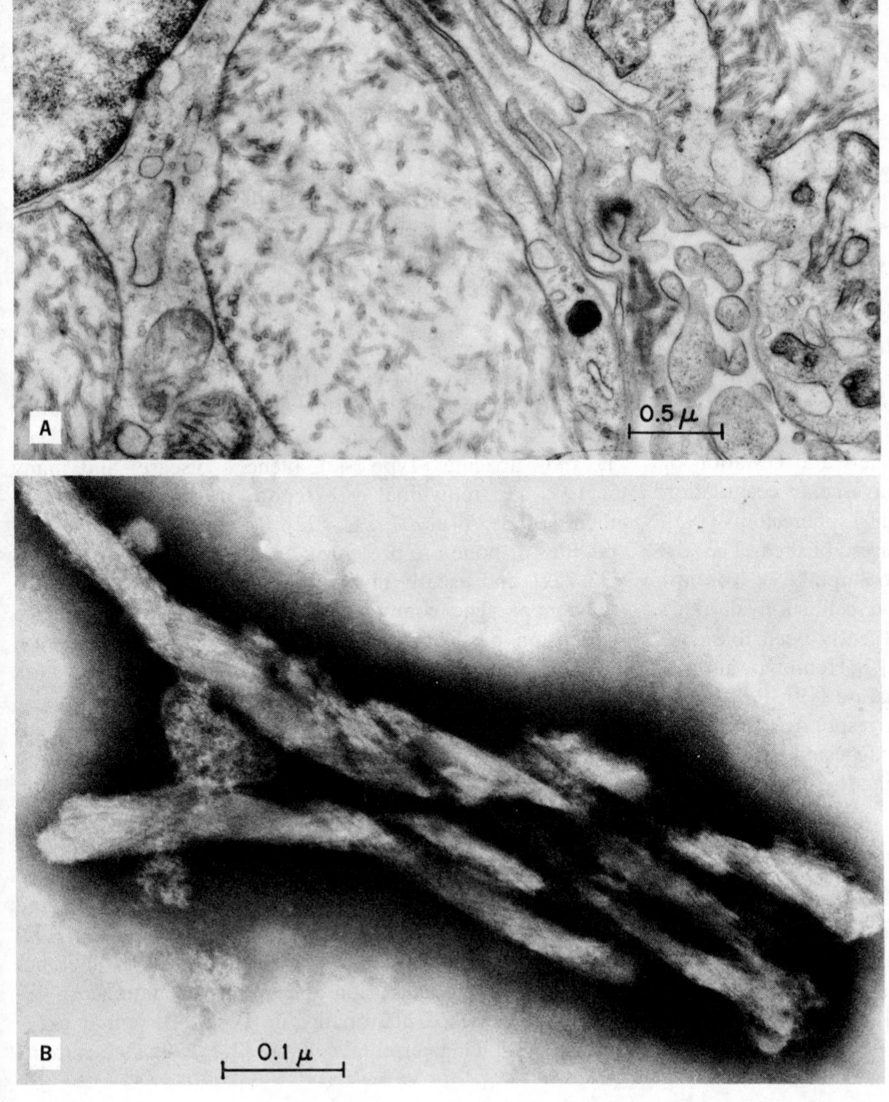

Figure 33-4. A. Portions of two Gaucher cells as seen with the electron microscope. Approximately ×36,000. Part of the nucleus of one is present, and within the cytoplasm of both are sacs containing typical tubules set in a pale matrix. B. Higher magnification of the strands, or tubules, of glucocerebroside present within the inclusion bodies seen in A. (*Courtesy of Dr. Robert E. Lee, University of Pittsburgh.*)

cells [166, 182]. The observation of partially digested erythrocytes, or "erythrophagosomes," at the cell border or within the cytoplasm suggests a third source of Glc-Cer within the cells [171, 176, 177, 179, 180, 182, 184]. There is also evidence that the tubular material (Glc-Cer) is often spilled into extracellular spaces, possibly from Gaucher cells undergoing lysis [182]. It is relevant to later discussions of pathogenesis and of the association of "Gaucher cells" with leukemia to note that electron micrographs have not shown conspicuous evidence of phagocytosis of leukocytes by Gaucher cells. The behavior of Gaucher cells in tissue culture has also been observed [184], the stages of their formation in tissues have been described [185], and similar cells have been produced by administration of cerebrosides [155, 186–190].

Clinical Consequences of Visceral Storage of Glc-Cer

Hypersplenism

The spleen is a primary focus of the disease. Splenomegaly is usually the earliest sign and, with rare exceptions [34, 37, 150, 185, 187, 191–194], is nearly always present. The enlarged spleen is usually painless but may cause distress. Hypersplenism eventually occurs in nearly all patients with Type 1 and Type 3 Gaucher's disease, and sometimes in those with the acute neuronopathic form (Type 2). Thrombocytopenia may be the only consequence, but it is usually accompanied by moderate leukopenia and mild microcytic anemia. Epistaxis, purpura, hemorrhagic infarcts, and other bleeding episodes eventually lead to splenectomy in well over half of patients. This is practically always followed by an immediate, sustained rise in platelets and cessation of bleeding phenomena. Increased intravascular coagulation noted in one patient was also corrected by splenectomy [195].

The cause of anemia has not been established. The absorption, plasma turnover, and marrow uptake of iron appear to be normal [177]. Red blood cell survival, once thought to be decreased [196], has recently been found to be normal or only slightly shortened [177]. Hemolytic anemia has been reported with Gaucher's disease [197, 198] but is not characteristic. The anemia often responds to removal of the spleen [199], and it has been suggested that splenomegaly may cause anemia by expanding the plasma volume [200].

Lymph Node Enlargement

In many children with the acute and subacute neuronopathic forms of Gaucher's disease, peripheral lymph nodes are enlarged and contain typical Gaucher cells. The thymus, Peyer's patches in the intestine [151], and the pharyngeal tonsils are frequently involved [31].

Hepatic and Renal Function

Groups of Gaucher cells frequently surround the central and hepatic veins and obstruct the liver capillaries [75, 175, 201, 202]. Lobular architecture is often destroyed, and fibrosis may be severe. Portal hypertension [203] and ascites [202, 204] may occur in all three types of the disease but are not characteristic. The enlarged liver may contain centers of extramedullary erythropoiesis. Although liver function test results are frequently abnormal, there are no characteristic changes [201, 205, 206]. Elevations in alkaline phosphatase level are more likely due to severe osseous lesions [207]. Jaundice is not a feature of Gaucher's disease. The kidney is occasionally involved, either in the glomeruli [208] or by scattered Gaucher cells throughout the cortex and medulla [152, 209]. Renal function is not characteristically disturbed.

Bone Lesions

Involvement of bone marrow was first reported in 1904 [210], and the striking anatomic changes in bone structure were appreciated somewhat later [8, 207]. The bone lesions are most likely due to interference with vascular supply by expanding masses of Gaucher cells within the marrow and enlargement of the vascular endothelial cells. True "invasion" of the periosteum, cartilage, or cortex is relatively rare [149, 152]. The possibility that acid hydrolases or other enzymes released from Gaucher cells contribute to destruction of bone and cartilage has not been excluded.

Aside from rare expansion of the marrow space or small osteolytic lesions visible on roentgenograms [77, 91, 109], bone lesions are not a feature of the acute neuronopathic (Type 2) variant. They are characteristic of chronic (Type 1) and subacute (Type 3) Gaucher's disease, and many reviews and individual case reports deal extensively with them [34, 39, 141, 207, 211–222]. Roentgenographic abnormalities of bone are present in 50 to 75 percent of patients [32, 222], and usually this is the only evidence of bone involvement. The commonest roentgenographic sign is an expansion of the cortex at the lower end of the femur, leaving radiolucence in the contour of an Erlenmeyer flask [39, 207, 213, 214, 218].

Bone pain and fracture are uncommon presenting signs of Gaucher's disease [34]. Pathologic fractures are most common in the acetabulum or head and neck of the femur, and hip lesions are frequently confused with Legg-Calvé-Perthes disease. The remainder of the pelvis, other long bones, phalanges, and ribs are more commonly involved than the skull, although lesions of both the calvarium and mandible have been noted. Destruction of the vertebral bodies often produces a thin, shortened cylinder, sometimes with complete spinal fusion and gibbus formation. An exceptional cause of neuropathy in Type 1 is spinal nerve damage following vertebral collapse [215, 220]. One extraordinary patient with a boot-shaped sella and acro-osteolysis has been reported [223]; he may have had a unique lipidosis.

Episodic Bone Pain

Bone involvement may proceed painlessly, but particularly in children and adolescents acute episodes of severe pain occur, often lasting days or weeks. These usually involve the end of a long bone and are believed to be due to vascular changes in the metaphysis attendant upon storage of glycolipid [218]. Pain is associated with local swelling, redness, tenderness, heat, and muscular spasm. Fever, leukocytosis, and increased sedimentation rate are common. Such "aseptic osteomyelitis" may initially be unaccompanied by roentgenographic changes; a few weeks later periosteal reaction is observed and, subsequently, often a pathologic fracture. Attacks usually subside spontaneously. They are not obviously made better by steroids [218] or radiation [224], but pain may be relieved by decompression [218]. Sinus tracts with Gaucher cells in the drainage [211] may form spontaneously or follow surgical intervention.

Relationship to Splenectomy

There has long been a debate about the possible association between splenectomy and the development of osseous lesions in Gaucher's disease [34, 141, 143, 218, 222, 225]. It has been suggested [222] that removal of the spleen takes away a reservoir for Glc-Cer storage and thus increases Gaucher cell development in the marrow. There is no proof for this, and it is possible that both hypersplenism and bone involvement are independent expressions of more severe illness [115]. The sum of the evidence suggests that splenectomy should be performed only when hypersplenism absolutely requires it; it is not an "elective" procedure in Gaucher's disease.

Pulmonary and Cardiovascular Abnormalities

Children affected with any form of Gaucher's disease often have a severe, productive cough, chest pain, and recurrent pneumonitis and respiratory distress. The reticular pattern of infiltration seen so often on roentgenograms in Niemann-Pick disease is rare [40, 109, 226]. Post-mortem examination, however, often reveals masses of typical Gaucher cells in the alveolar capillaries and lung lymphatic vessels [84, 128]. Occasionally Gaucher cells are also free in the alveoli [78, 108], and they have been seen in the sputum in a rare patient [227]. Very infrequently there has been massive consolidation due to Gaucher cells [40]. Some pulmonary distress and infection may also be related to enlarged mediastinal lymph nodes [128]. Patient Z. K. (above) had severe pulmonary hypertension in association with blockage of pulmonary capillaries (Fig. 33-5). His immediate cause of death [30] was a recurrent hemorrhagic pericarditis that

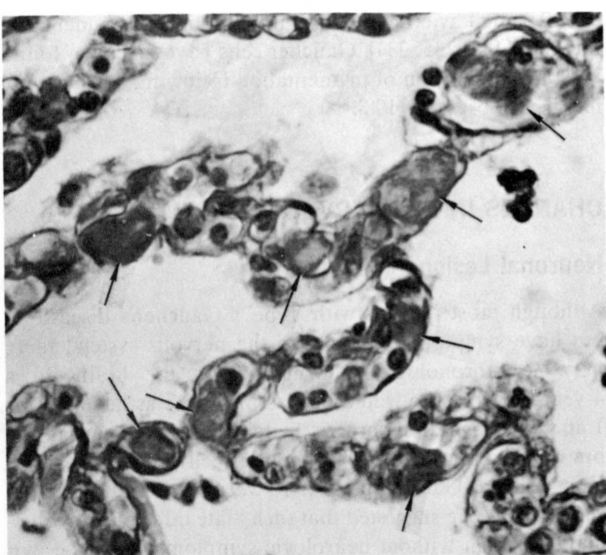

Figure 33-5. Pulmonary alveolar capillaries occluded by Gaucher cells (arrows). Periodic acid-Schiff stain. (×780.) (*Courtesy of Dr. William O. Roberts, National Heart and Lung Institute; reprinted from* [30] *with permission of Circulation.*)

has also been reported in several other patients [204, 228, 229]. Other than the presence of a few Gaucher cells in the myocardium, cardiac lesions have not been reported in any form of Gaucher's disease.

Eyes

The cherry-red spot seen in some other sphingolipid or mucopolysaccharide storage diseases does not occur in Gaucher's disease. Occasionally, macular lesions have been seen [230], but the fundus is usually normal. Corneal clouding has occurred in only one reported case [231]. There is a single report of the presence of Gaucher's cells in the choroid layer [232].

Yellow-brown, wedge-shaped lesions situated on the conjunctiva, their bases abutting on the cornea and the apices extending to the canthi, were described in Gaucher's disease as early as 1901 [233]. These pingueculae are usually seen only in the chronic form, and by no means universally so. It has been reported that small collections of Gaucher-like cells may occur in the pingueculae [234].

Skin

Some children and adults with Gaucher's disease have a peculiar yellow pallor that is not well correlated with the degree of anemia. Diffuse yellow-brown pigmentation also develops on the exposed surfaces in many older patients. It is sometimes localized or unilateral [9], symmetrically distributed over the lower part of the legs [235] or on the face. This pigmentation has not been explained, but it is accompanied by both increased iron-containing pigment and melanin [147, 235, 237]. Gaucher cells have not been found in skin. Diminution of pigmentation following splenectomy has been observed [198].

CHANGES IN THE NERVOUS SYSTEM

Neuronal Lesions in Type 1

Although most patients with Type 1 Gaucher's disease do not have symptoms referable to the nervous system, there may be morphologic abnormalities in the brain. In a 4-year-old boy who would be classified here as having Type 1 and who died after surgery, Seitelberger [87] found in the brain a striking degree of adventitial cell proliferation and an occasional Gaucher cell; there were no definite ganglion cell changes. He suggested that such "late infantile" involvement of brain without neurologic symptoms might be evidence of an obligatory involvement of the reticuloendothelial system in the brain. Diezel [28] described finding both perivascular cell storage and ganglion cell changes in the brain of a 61-year-old man, apparently with Type 1 Gaucher's disease. He believed that the storage of PAS-positive material in the neurons was nonspecific and that it possibly represented lipofuscin (ceroid) accumulation. Gaucher cells have been described in the hypophysis [238] and in the leptomeninges [152] in Type 1, as have lipid deposits in the axon and Schwann cells of the sural nerve [220]. There have also been a few adults with Gaucher's disease with clinical evidence of neurologic disorder [239, 240], but the symptoms were quite unlike those in the neuronopathic forms, and the neuropathologic change was nonspecific. A careful examination of the brain employing frozen sections and PAS stains is still indicated in autopsies of patients with Type 1 Gaucher's disease. It is not possible to ascertain from the literature how often the neurons or the reticuloendothelial cells in brain may show involvement without disturbance of function.

The Brain in Type 2

Practically all the examinations of the brain of patients dying with the acute neuronopathic form of Gaucher's disease have revealed abnormalities. These have been recurrently described in reports of neuropathologic changes in individual patients (Table 33-1), and in other articles [28, 87, 133, 136]. The reviews contained in the articles of Norman et al. [76], Banker et al. [81], Diezel [28, 157], and Seitelberger [87] are especially recommended.

The brain is usually not remarkable in gross appearance. Under light microscopy a fairly predictable pattern of involvement is seen. A striking feature, first described by Debré in 1951 [74], is the presence of *swollen periadventitial* cells that contain many PAS-positive fibrils (Fig. 33-6). This staining reaction is retained after paraffin fixation. Many of these cells are contiguous with the adventitia of small vessels, and sometimes the endothelial cells are also involved. Occasional "Gaucher cells" appear to be lying free in the brain tissue [81]. For unknown reasons the swollen adventitial cells are most frequent in the cortex or deep in the white matter and are less prominent in the brain stem, where neuronal damage is most pronounced.

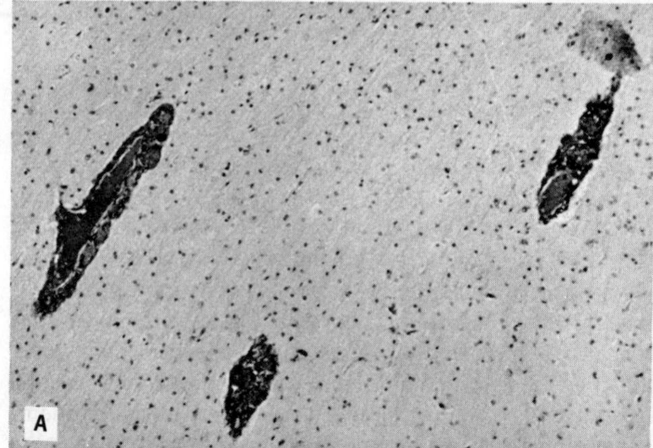

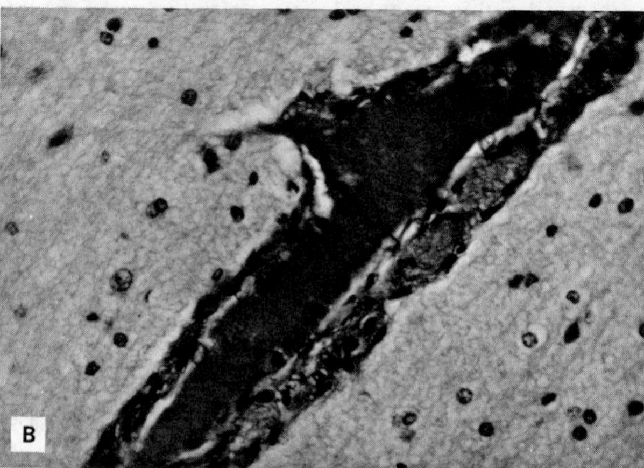

Figure 33-6. A. White matter of frontal lobe of brain from child with Type 2 Gaucher's disease. Three small arterioles are surrounded by periadventitial cells that contain many PAS-positive fibrils. B. Higher-power view of one of these arterioles. (*Courtesy of Dr. Ronald A. DeLellis, National Institutes of Health.*)

Examination also reveals scattered areas of *neuronal loss*. These occur in the pyramidal and ganglionic layers of cerebral cortex, thalamus, globus pallidus, subthalamus, hypothalamus, midbrain, pons, and medulla. Frequently depletion of the Purkinje cells in the cerebellum is especially marked. Many other neurons may be still visible but are obviously abnormal in regard to their irregular or crumpled outlines, chromatolysis, and loss of Nissl substance in the cytoplasm.

The issue of whether *neuronal cytoplasmic storage* occurs in acute neuropathic Gaucher's disease has been debated in the literature for years. The "classic" earliest descriptions of the brain in this phenotype by Oberling and Woringer [43], as well as other subsequent reports [64, 68, 69, 76, 81, 84], support its occurrence. It has been minimal or not observed in other patients described in Table 33-1. When it is observed, lipid storage is particularly evident in the neurons of the thalamus, basal ganglia, brain stem, spinal cord, nucleus dentatum, and some of the remaining Purkinje cells. The involved neurons are slightly distended and occasionally vacuolated [43, 69, 76, 81, 84, 111]. The nucleus and clumps of Nissl substance are pushed to the periphery. The cytoplasm is weakly sudanophilic, metachromatic, and PAS-positive, failing to react with Luxol fast blue. The staining is best observed with frozen sections [81], although some PAS reaction does survive fixation. Under the electron microscope [91], most of the affected neurons appear shrunken, with clumped cytoplasm. Other cells contain enlarged and anastomosing endoplasmic reticulum, as well as myelin figures or membranous cytosomes filled with flat parallel membranes. Some of these resemble the Zebra bodies seen in the mucopolysaccharidoses. The rodlike structures filled with tubules that are reminiscent of the cytoplasm of Gaucher cells are very rare. The neurons in the Type 2 brain are not ballooned to the degree seen in other neurolipidoses. Whether all the PAS-positive material represents gangliosides, Glc-Cer, or other glycolipids has not been completely resolved. The staining reactions are similar to those in Krabbe's disease [81], but the two diseases may be distinguished neuropathologically [28].

Neuronophagia is prominent in some areas of the brain, especially in the deeper layers of the cortex and in the nuclei of the basal ganglia and brain stem, areas correlating with much of the neurologic dysfunction in Type 2. This process is characterized by the presence of many microglia and histiocytes, representatives of the reticuloendothelial system of the brain that are mobilized as scavenger cells when acute nerve cell destruction is underway.

The degree of *demyelination* in the Type 2 brain is variable. It may not be obvious in the cortex [81], yet may be marked in other areas of the brain [93].

The Brain in Type 3

The children with neurologic deficits who have succumbed to "Gaucher's disease" after 3 years of age have usually had more conspicuous storage of PAS-positive material in the neurons than infants dying of the acute neuronopathic form. This may be accompanied by neuron loss, neuronophagia, and gliosis [84, 85, 129, 136]. No reports are available on the brain morphologic changes in the deceased members of the Swedish Type 3 families. Classifications of "acute" and "subacute" neuronal involvement in Gaucher's disease have been made [76, 87], the distinction resting mainly on the degree of neuronal cytoplasmic storage. More chemical evidence is needed to bolster such correlations and particularly to provide assurance that the patients involved all have a primary defect in catabolism of Glc-Cer.

In summary, correlation between clinical signs and neuropathologic changes in Gaucher's disease is mainly restricted to the acute neuronopathic form (Type 2). Here there is evidence of a swiftly destructive process. Some of the neurons are slightly swollen, and PAS-positive material is stored in the cytoplasm in a manner suggesting hasty and ineffective lysosomal function. Most of the affected neurons, however, appear shriveled and damaged. Often only crowds of scavenger cells attest to their prior destruction. Involvement is somewhat capricious. The large nuclear masses of the cranial nerves in the midbrain, pons, and medulla are usually heavily affected. This explains the near-universality of strabismus, dysphagia, trismus, and other brain stem abnormalities. Concomitant involvement of the basal ganglia, thalamus, cerebellum, and spinal cord is consonant with the hypertonicity, abnormal reflexes, and eventual total deterioration of motor functions.

In the brains of patients considered to have juvenile Gaucher's disease (Type 3), cytoplasmic storage in neurons manages to proceed further before cell death. There is still predilection for brain stem lesions, but seizures and behavior disorders, rather than severe demyelination and total failure of motor functions, are characteristic. Some of the patients with Type 1, or the nonneuronopathic form of Gaucher's disease, have also been found to have glycolipid storage in the reticuloendothelial elements of the brain.

THE CHEMISTRY OF CEREBROSIDES

Cerebroside is a generic name for the group of monohexosyl ceramides consisting of sphingosine base, fatty acid, and either glucose or galactose in a molar ratio of 1 :1 :1. The glucosyl ceramides (Fig. 33-7) are normally found outside the nervous system. The galactosyl ceramides are in largest concentration in the nervous system, where they are an important constituent of myelin and are found primarily in white matter.

Cerebroside Structure

Sphingosine Moiety

The chemistry and biochemistry of sphingosine are discussed in Chap. 29. The sphingosine moiety of neutral glycolipids

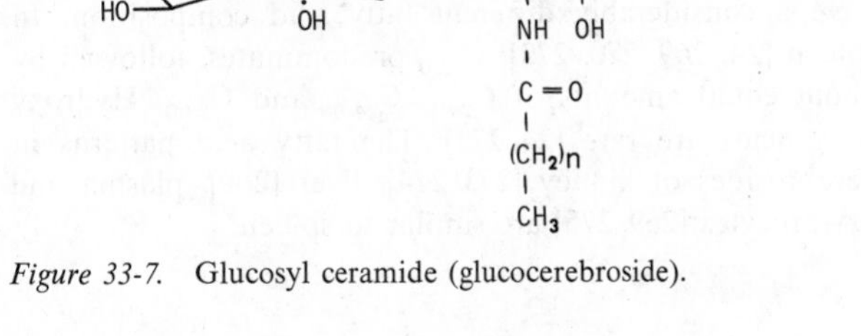

Figure 33-7. Glucosyl ceramide (glucocerebroside).

has been most studied in material isolated from the nervous system. Here the sphingosine in the monohexosyl ceramides is mainly the base common to other naturally occurring sphingolipids. It contains a double bond at C-4 and C-5, which is in the *trans* configuration [241, 242], and the substitutions at C-2 and C-3 are in the *erythro* configuration [243, 244]. Some of the cerebrosides contain the saturated base dihydrosphingosine [245] and small amounts of longer-chain congeners of sphingosine. Most of the studies of the visceral glucosyl ceramides have been made in connection with Gaucher's disease and indicate that the sphingosine moiety is the same as that in the galactosyl ceramides. Human kidney cerebrosides also contain significant amounts of 3,4-dihydroxysphingosine (phytosphingosine) [246, 247].

Hexose

The hexose in brain cerebrosides, called cerebrose by Thudichum, was later identified as D-galactose [248, 249], and many subsequent analyses have indicated that virtually all the myelin cerebrosides and cerebroside sulfates (see Chap. 32) contain this sugar [250–252]. Although brain cerebrosides contain small amounts of glucose [253, 254], the hexose in these compounds is not less than 99 percent galactose [255]. As already noted, the opposite is true for cerebrosides outside the nervous system. In both types of glycosyl ceramides the hexose is linked through its C-1 hydroxyl to the C-1 of sphingosine by a $(1 \rightarrow 4)$ β-glycosidic bond [22, 256, 257].

Fatty Acid

A number of different fatty acids are joined in amide linkage to sphingosine in cerebrosides [255, 258–263]. The neuronal galactosyl ceramides in the adult brain contain predominantly C_{24} monounsaturated acids and 2-hydroxy saturated acids [255, 264]. The total hydroxy fatty acid content is about double that of the total normal (straight-chain, unhydroxylated) fatty acids [255]. The infant human brain has a lower percentage of hydroxy, very long-chain (C_{22} to C_{26}), and monounsaturated fatty acids than does the child or adult [255]. This suggests that the activity of elongating [265, 266], hydroxylating, and unsaturating systems is enhanced after myelination is complete. Similar developmental changes in the fatty acid content of the brain have also been observed in the rat [267, 268].

The glucosyl ceramides found outside the nervous system have a considerably different fatty acid composition. In spleen [24, 269, 270, 271], $C_{16:0}$ predominates, followed by about equal amounts of $C_{24:1}$, $C_{24:0}$, and $C_{22:0}$. Hydroxy fatty acids are rare [24, 272]. The fatty acid patterns in cerebrosides of kidney [273, 274], liver [269], plasma and erythrocytes [269, 275] are similar to spleen.

Tissue Distribution of Cerebrosides

Glucosyl and galactosyl ceramides are the simplest members of a large family of oligohexosyl ceramides that are widely distributed in animal tissues. Their composition and distribution have been recently reviewed by Martensson [273], and one classification is discussed in Chap. 31. Monohexosyl ceramides have been demonstrated in each of the following organs outside the nervous system: aorta [276], erythrocytes [275], intestine [277, 278], kidney [274, 279], lens [280], leukocytes [281], liver [46, 269, 282], lung [283], placenta [284], plasma [269, 275, 285, 286], and spleen [24, 269, 270]. In these tissues, monohexosyl ceramides constitute about 25 percent of all neutral glycolipids and are primarily glucosyl ceramides. Nervous tissue is particularly rich in glycolipids, and the monohexosyl ceramide component is almost exclusively galactosyl ceramide [273]. The nature and distribution of other glycolipids are described in Chaps. 29 to 32 and 34.

THE BIOCHEMISTRY OF CEREBROSIDES

Biosynthesis of Glycosyl Ceramides

The immediate precursors of the glycosyl ceramides in vivo are fatty acids, carbohydrates, and sphingosines [287–290]. The biosynthesis of sphingosine and ceramide (N-acylsphingosine) has been described in Chap. 29.

Galactosyl Ceramide

Two possible pathways for the biosynthesis of galactosyl ceramide are known. One sequence proceeds through transfer of the galactose moiety of UDP-Gal to ceramide.

$$\text{Cer} + \text{UDP-Gal} \longrightarrow \text{Gal-Cer} + \text{UDP} \qquad (1)$$

Experiments employing UDP-Gal and young rat brain microsomes initially suggested the importance of this pathway [291]. Burton later reported [292] that exogenous ceramide enhanced the activity of the system, and this was unequivocally demonstrated by Fujino and Nakano [293]. There is evidence that this pathway is also active in rat and chicken liver [293] and in embryonic chicken brain [294]. In microsomes of young mouse brain, there is a similar system that requires ceramides containing hydroxy fatty acids as substrates; galactosyl ceramides containing hydroxy fatty acids are the products [295]. Kopaczyk and Radin [266], however, have noted that ceramide [N-stearoyl-(1-^{14}C) sphingosine] injected into the cerebrum of young rats is not incorporated into glucosyl ceramides, and certain evidence that ceramide is the precursor of Gal-Cer still needs to be obtained.

A second reaction sequence for the biosynthesis of cerebrosides involves the acylation of galactosyl sphingosine (psychosine). Cleland and Kennedy [296] observed the biosynthesis of galactosyl sphingosine from UDP-Gal and DL-erythrosphingosine (Reaction 2*a*).

$$\text{Sphingosine} + \text{UDP-Gal} \longrightarrow \text{Galactosyl sphingosine} + \text{UDP} \qquad (2a)$$

Brady demonstrated that rat brain microsomes can catalyze the acylation of the free amino group of galactosyl sphingosine [297].

$$\text{Galactosyl sphingosine} + \text{stearoyl CoA} \longrightarrow \text{Gal-Cer} + \text{CoA} \qquad (2b)$$

In the Jimpy mouse, a mutant in which there is a marked reduction of brain cerebrosides, the activity of the enzyme catalyzing Reaction 2*a* is significantly reduced [298]. This observation suggests that the second pathway is probably the major route for the biosynthesis of galactosyl ceramides containing normal fatty acids.

Glucosyl Ceramide

There appears to be general agreement that glucosyl ceramides are synthesized according to Reaction 3.

$$\text{Cer} + \text{UDP Glc} \longrightarrow \text{Glc-Cer} + \text{UDP} \qquad (3)$$

The enzyme catalyzing this reaction is present in microsomes of embryonic chicken brain [294, 299] and young rat brain [253, 300]. Reaction 3 may be the first step in ganglioside synthesis (see Chap. 29). It is also possible that a pathway analogous to Reactions 2*a* and 2*b* will be demonstrated for the synthesis of glucosyl ceramides.

Catabolism of Glycosyl Ceramides

By demonstrating the conversion of injected Gal-Cer to ceramide and galactose in rat brains, Kopaczyk and Radin showed that the initial step in the catabolism of glycosyl ceramides is a hydrolytic cleavage to a glycose (either glucose or galactose) and ceramide [266].

$$\text{Glycosyl ceramide} + H_2O \longrightarrow \text{glycose} + \text{ceramide}$$

Glycosidases that specifically catalyze the hydrolysis of Gal-Cer are present in rat brain [301–304], calf brain [301], pig brain [302], and rat spleen, lung, and kidney [302]. Glycosidases specific for glucosyl ceramides are present in rat, calf, and ox brain [301, 305, 306] and in rat and human spleen [307]. A glycosidase that cleaves both glucosyl and galactosyl ceramide has been demonstrated in rat small intestine [308]. The further catabolism of ceramide has been described in Chap. 29. Gatt [309] has suggested that the enzymes responsible for sphingoglycolipid catabolism are located together in particulate multienzyme systems; this hypothesis awaits further proof.

Intravenous injection of human erythrocyte stroma or sphingolipids into rats results in increased levels of hepatic glucosyl ceramide β-glucosidase [310]. Increased activity of the enzyme is also present in leukocytes from patients with acute and chronic myelogenous leukemia [311]. A marked deficiency of this enzymatic activity has been observed in tissues from patients with Gaucher's disease [25, 312–314].

CHEMICAL ABNORMALITIES IN GAUCHER'S DISEASE

Organs Other Than Brain

Glucosyl Ceramide Accumulation

It has been clearly established that visceral organs laden with Gaucher cells contain abnormally high amounts of monohexosyl ceramides. The organs most frequently analyzed are the liver and spleen. The increase is obvious in thin-layer chromatograms of the lipid extracted from these organs (Fig. 33-8). The concentration of monohexosyl ceramides in the liver (Table 33-2) and spleen (Table 33-3) may be more than

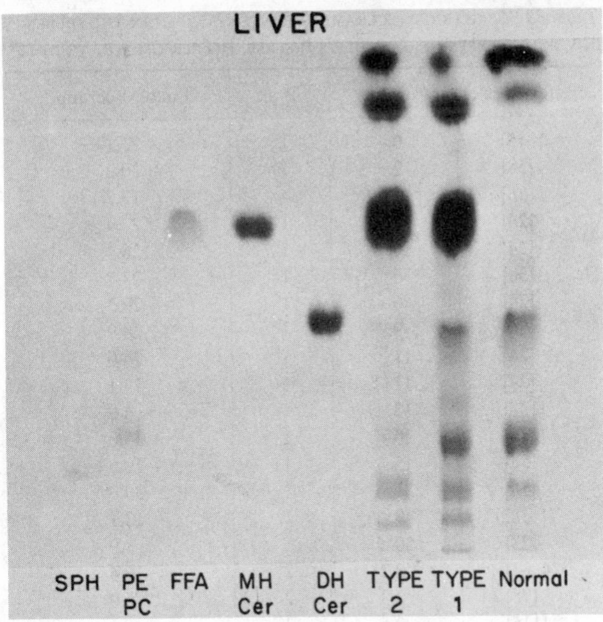

Figure 33-8. Thin-layer chromatogram comparing the lipid content of equal amounts of liver from patients with Type 1 and Type 2 Gaucher's disease and a normal subject. The massive increase in monohexosyl ceramides (MH Cer) in liver from either patient is apparent. The co-migrating free fatty acids (FFA) can easily be distinguished from MH Cer in other solvent systems and on the basis of different colors produced by anisaldehyde stain. Other abbreviations are: *SPH,* sphingomyelin; *PE,* phosphatidyl ethanolamine; *PC,* phosphatidyl choline; and *DH Cer,* dihexosyl ceramide. The solvent system used was chloroform:methanol:water (50:21:3).

Table 33-2. GLUCOSYL CERAMIDE CONCENTRATION IN THE LIVER IN VARIOUS TYPES OF GAUCHER'S DISEASE, MG PER GM WET WEIGHT*

References	Age, yr	Type	*Glucosyl ceramide*	
			Patient	Control
[38, 81]	0.8	1	16.3	2–6†
[29, 45]	1.2	2	13.7	0.05
[81]	0.2	2	15.0	2–6†
[81]	0.6	2	12.4	2–6†
[81]	1.3	2	12.9	2–6†
[110, 81]	6	3	6.4	2–6†

* Those concentrations originally reported on the basis of dry weight of tissue were arbitrarily divided by five to approximate the values at wet weight.

† These control values represent total water-insoluble glycolipid and are much higher than presently accepted values [45, 269, 273].

Table 33-3. GLUCOSYL CERAMIDE CONCENTRATION IN THE SPLEEN IN VARIOUS TYPES OF GAUCHER'S DISEASE, MG PER GM WET WEIGHT*

References	Age, yr	Type	Glucosyl ceramide
[315]	0.4	1	22.1
[58]	2	1†	30.2
[138]	2.5	1	13.2
[24]	3	1	22.4
[24]	4	1	26.4
[58]	6	1	23.8
[24]	6	1	20.3
[24]	9	1	28.9
[24]	11	1	24.0
[24]	11	1	13.1
[138]	13	1	4.9
[115]	14	1	15.0
[58]	15	1	10.6
[58]	31	1	39.0
[138]	49	1	13.1
[23]	50	1	8.9
[24, 81]	0.3	2	16.4
[78]	0.3	2	6.0
[115]	0.5	2	6.5
[24, 81]	0.6	2	14.4
[115]	1	2	12.2
[138]	2.5	3	40.5
[129]	9	3†	3.0
Normal	. . .	. . .	0.17

* Those concentrations originally reported on the basis of dry weight of tissue were arbitrarily divided by five to approximate the values at wet weight. The normal value represents the average of the data from three sources [24, 58, 115].

† Assignment of phenotype uncertain.

100 times normal. Monohexosyl ceramides have been increased in examples of all three types of Gaucher's disease.

Hexose Component

Previous editions of this book have dealt in detail with the history of the search for clarification of the hexose in the cerebrosides stored in the viscera in Gaucher's disease [29, 316]. The more recent studies [24, 58, 115, 138] have removed any doubts that glucosyl ceramides are being selectively stored. Unusual instances of associated galactosyl ceramide storage have been restricted to some possible examples of the juvenile, or Type 3, form [129, 137].

Fatty Acid and Sphingosine Moieties

The fatty acids of the Gaucher cerebrosides in the spleen resemble those in the Glc-Cer present in the normal organ. There may be a modest decrease in $C_{16:0}$ and $C_{24:1}$ acids and a higher proportion of saturated long-chain acids in the Gaucher cerebrosides [11, 115, 138, 317–319].

The usual erythro form [244] of the sphingosine base, containing 18 carbons and one double bond [22–24, 138, 317, 319] in the *trans* configuration [23], has been found in the Glc-Cer in extraneural tissues in Gaucher's disease. The C-20 base has been specifically excluded [24, 317, 319], and only a small percentage of dihydrosphingosine has been noted to be present [24, 319]. The hexose also appears to be joined to the C-1 hydroxyl of the sphingosine [23] and in a β-glucosidic linkage [24].

Other Neutral Glycolipids

Careful analyses of other glycolipids have been performed in relatively few organs from patients with Gaucher's disease. Normal amounts of dihexosyl ceramides have been found in spleens from patients representing clear-cut examples of Type 1 or Type 2 [24, 58, 115]. The Gal-Glc-Cer present in normal and Gaucher tissues has the same fatty acid pattern [24]. Increases in trihexosyl and tetrahexosyl ceramides (globosides) have been specifically excluded in several instances. Makita et al. isolated a "fast-moving cerebroside" from one spleen [115]. This proved to be a fatty acid ester of Glc-Cer. Similar esters of Gal-Cer have been isolated from normal brain [320–324]; the additional fatty acid is esterified either to the C_3-OH of sphingosine or to the hexose.

As described in the summary of patients who have been considered to have a juvenile form, tissue glycolipid patterns differing from those in other forms of Gaucher's disease have sometimes been present. Increases in galactosyl ceramides have accompanied a rise in Glc-Cer in some reports. Gal-Glc-Cer has also been increased [85, 138]. Such ceramide lactoside, however, does not accumulate in most patients with Gaucher's disease [24], at least one prior report of such accumulation [325] having recently been corrected by other investigators [58]. Of considerable importance for the establishment of juvenile examples as clearly representing a form of Gaucher's disease is the information supplied by Svennerholm in a personal communication [326] that Glc-Cer is definitely increased in the Swedish Type 3 patients.

Gangliosides

Gangliosides may also be increased, particularly ganglioside G_{M3} (hematoside) (Chap. 29), which is normally the predominant ganglioside in liver and spleen. Such an increase has been demonstrated in Type 1 [58, 115, 138] and Type 2 [115, 317] patients, as well as in two patients of uncertain phenotype described by Philippart et al. [138]. The hematoside in the Type 1 or 2 spleens has the same fatty acid pattern as that in the small amounts of ganglioside usually found in the spleen [115, 317]. Philippart and Menkes suggest that the hematoside may be a major precursor of Glc-Cer in the spleen [317].

Other Lipids

The concentrations of other major lipids such as total phospholipids, sphingomyelin, and sterol have repeatedly been demonstrated to be normal [9, 23, 24, 58, 143, 325]. Occasionally, elevated levels of sphingomyelin [128, 325] or "neutral lipids" [24] have been reported. Cholesteryl ester content may be elevated if the spleen has been infarcted [58].

The Brain

The chemical information about the brain in Gaucher's disease is inadequate, considering the number of patients who have come to autopsy. This paucity is related to difficulties in the interpretation of chemical analyses of nervous tissue. Adjustment is required for losses of either ganglion cells or white matter due to demyelination or for failure of normal myelination. A decrease in myelin depresses the content of cholesterol, monohexosyl ceramides, and sphingomyelins, and decrease in gray matter especially affects the content of gangliosides.

Glucosyl Ceramide Content

Svennerholm [116] has reported that the Glc-Cer content of brains of patients with "infantile" (Type 2) Gaucher's disease is increased. Other recent studies have failed to find an increase in Glc-Cer in the brain. One of these studies involved a child described by Espinas and Faris [93] (Table 33-1). French et al. found no increase in brain Glc-Cer even though the tissue extracted contained many of the perivascular "Gaucher cells" often seen in the Type 2 brain [94]. Similar failure to find increased Glc-Cer in a Type 2 brain was reported by Inose [85]. The brain of the child with an especially attenuated course for Type 2 examined by Philippart and coworkers [90] (Table 33-1) contained only a trace of glucose in the monohexosyl ceramides. The Gal-Cer present in the brain appeared to have its normal structure. There is often a decrease in total cerebroside (Gal-Cer) content, the degree being a function of the amount of decrease in myelin [81, 94, 327].

Interpretation of changes in the brain in "Type 3" patients is complicated by the possible heterogeneity of the presumed examples of this form. Menkes and Migeon believe that the major lipid accumulating may be Gal-Glc-Cer [328]. Inose et al. also found an increase of dihexosides but not of monohexosides [85]. Svennerholm has reported that he could find no Glc-Cer accumulation in the brain in "juvenile" Gaucher's disease [116]. In two cases of uncertain relationship to Gaucher's disease, Maloney and Cumings reported that the monohexosyl ceramides in brain contained more glucose than galactose [129]. No characteristic change in brain lipids was found by Jervis et al. [136].

In a 51-year-old patient with Type 1 Gaucher's disease who had a definite elevation in spleen Glc-Cer content, the cerebrosides and sulfatides of the brain contained only a trace of glucose, and the overall lipid content of gray and white matter was normal [90].

Gangliosides

Svennerholm [116] has provided the most provocative theory to explain the lesions in the brain from study of his cases of "infantile" (Type 2) Gaucher's disease. He has reported an increase in the ganglioside and Glc-Cer content of the brain. Moreover, the Glc-Cer present contained C_{20} sphingosine and a high content of C_{18} fatty acids, characteristic of brain gangliosides. He concluded that gangliosides, which contain Glc-Cer as a basic unit, are normally degraded to the latter through a predictable sequence of hydrolytic reactions. This is compatible with the findings of Gatt [309] as reviewed in detail in Chap. 29. A block in this pathway at the level of hydrolysis of Glc-Cer would cause the accumulation in the neuron of this compound and some of its precursors. The blockade in catabolism could also account for the overload of glycolipids in periadventitial cells and microglia within the brain. Inherent in Svennerholm's hypothesis is the conclusion that the excess Glc-Cer in brain arises there and is not transported from extraneural tissues. Confirmation of his important observations is awaited.

BLOOD ABNORMALITIES

Formed Elements

The glycolipid content of circulating leukocytes has not been reported in Gaucher's disease, but they do not contain distinctive vacuoles or inclusions. In one or two patients nonspecific changes in the erythrocyte phospholipid patterns have been reported [329], but these are not considered to be diagnostic.

Plasma Components

Glycolipids

The normal plasma content of neutral glycolipids is very low (Chap. 31). Thannhauser, using the methods developed by Svennerholm and Svennerholm [269], found 1.83 mg cerebroside per 100 ml plasma in a normal male, and 1.23 and 1.83 mg per 100 ml in two adults with Type 1 Gaucher's disease [9]. Hillborg, Svennerholm, and Herrlin, however, reported definite increases in plasma neutral glycolipids in six patients with the Swedish Type 3 form of the disease *after* splenectomy [142, 143]. The latter patients were 6 to 20 years of age. Polonovski and Petit [330, 331] have also reported increased plasma cerebrosides in three patients with Gaucher's disease. More precise definition of the plasma glycolipid content prior to splenectomy is still needed in all forms of Gaucher's disease. Cerebroside determinations in the cerebrospinal fluid have not been reported.

Acid Phosphatase

A characteristic of lysosomal storage diseases is increased tissue concentrations of acid hydrolase activities, including acid phosphatase [332]. Among all such diseases, however, Gaucher's disease is alone in the consistency with which plasma acid phosphatase activity is increased. This was first pointed out by Tuchman and coworkers [333, 334], who also noted that, in contrast to the prostatic enzyme [335], the enhanced phosphatase activity is not inhibited by L-tartrate. Neither is it inhibited significantly by copper ions or by formaldehyde, in contrast to normal erythrocyte phosphatase [335]. Isozymes of acid phosphatases in plasma, formed elements of the blood, and tissues have been partially characterized in Gaucher's disease [336–338]. The splenic and plasma enzymes may be the same, and the elevated plasma levels are possibly due to "spillage" from Gaucher cells [184]. It is not yet certain, however, that the enzyme in plasma arises from lysosomes. Kaulen and coworkers have reported that acid phosphatase activity in lysosomal membranes is inhibited by tartrate [338a]. Elevations occur in all three types of Gaucher's disease [144, 161]. The increase in acid phosphatase is helpful in making the diagnosis, but it is not specific. Elevations occur in some patients with Niemann-Pick disease (Chap. 35), in osteopetrosis [161, 339], multiple myeloma and other blood dyscrasias [337, 338], pregnancy, renal disease, thrombophlebitis, and embolic disease [340]. Increased activities of other acid hydrolases have been reported in the plasma of patients with Gaucher's disease [341].

Lipoproteins

Hypercholesterolemia has been reported in some patients with Gaucher's disease. In all three forms of the disease, the concentrations are usually not remarkably high. On the contrary, rather low levels of plasma lipids and lipoproteins are common in Gaucher's disease. Alpha- (high density) lipoproteins may be quite decreased in some patients, but this feature is not specific for Gaucher's disease [342].

Amino Acids

The plasma amino acid pattern has been described as normal [343]. Several instances of hyperamino aciduria have been reported [140, 344], including abnormal excretion of serine and threonine [344].

Other Plasma Proteins: Hyperglobulinemia

Plasma immunoglobulin levels are often abnormally high in adults with Type 1 Gaucher's disease. In younger patients several species of γ-globulin may be increased, while in older patients the elevated species usually appears to be monoclonal in origin [345]. The coincidence of multiple myeloma and Gaucher's disease (Type 1) has been reported [346].

Because Gaucher cells often are in contact with plasma cells [182, 345], it has been suggested that this association may provoke abnormal antibody formation and hence dysglobulinemia in Gaucher's disease [182]. Gaucher cells have themselves been examined for the presence of antigen-antibody reactions with α-globulin by immunofluorescent techniques. Fisher and Reidbord [168] found evidence supporting this; Lake [163] did not. Like many other lipids, Glc-Cer is a potent haptene [347], but circulating antibodies to Glc-Cer or other glycolipids have not yet been demonstrated in Gaucher's disease.

Gaucher Cells in Leukemia

Patients with leukemia often have cells in the bone marrow that, under both light and electron microscopy, appear similar to Gaucher cells [348–353]. There are some differences in the appearance of the stored material [354] (Fig. 33-9). Such cells have been observed in approximately 10 percent of three series of patients with chronic myelogenous leukemia [349, 350, 351, 352, 353]. These patients have not had known preexisting Gaucher's disease. Leukocytes in patients with leukemia have an increased glucocerebrosidase activity [311, 352]. It would appear that in leukemia a marked increase in turnover of leukocytes imposes a demand for glycolipid degradation that cannot be met even by induction of higher levels of the glucosidase. A result is Glc-Cer accumulation in reticuloendothelial cells. Plasma acid phosphatase activity also is increased in patients with chronic leukemia; it falls when remission is induced by treatment.

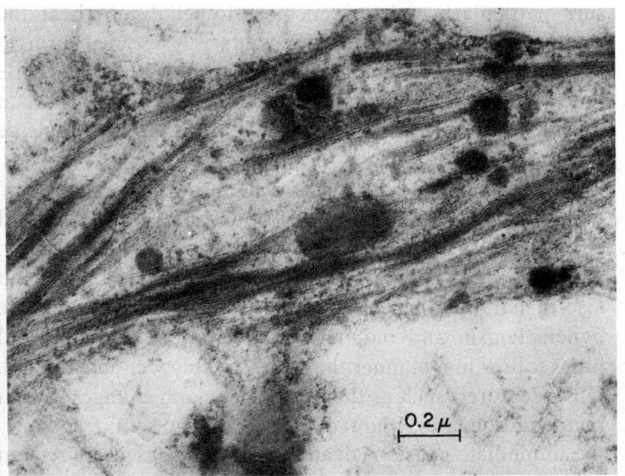

Figure 33-9. Electron micrograph of Gaucher-like cell from bone marrow of patient with chronic myelogenous leukemia. The glucocerebrosides have a membranous appearance and do not form tubules in the same fashion as do the glucocerebrosides seen in true Gaucher cells. ×72,000. (*Courtesy of Dr. Robert E. Lee and Dr. Lawrence D. Ellis, University of Pittsburgh.*)

The alternate possibility, that Gaucher's disease leads to leukemia, is not supported by available evidence. Several patients, however, are of interest in this regard. One reported child with acute lymphoblastic leukemia had a family history of Gaucher's disease [353]. Another man, who at age 37 had apparently typical Type 1 Gaucher's disease with bone lesions, developed "chronic lymphatic leukemia" at age 56 [219]. In the family reported by Strengers [70], three of seven sibs had Type 2 Gaucher's disease (Table 33-1). In a survey of the other family members, none of the Gaucher cells sometimes present in "heterozygotes" were seen in the marrow, but the father was discovered to have myelogenous leukemia. There are other reports of patients who have developed "leukoerythroblastic" reactions [152, 229, 356] long after splenectomy.

THE METABOLIC BASIS OF GAUCHER'S DISEASE

The metabolic defect that probably underlies all three types of Gaucher's disease is deficient activity of glucosyl ceramide β-glucosidase (glucocerebrosidase). Inadequate activity of this enzyme causes glucosyl ceramides to accumulate in many tissues.

Evidence of Glucocerebrosidase Deficiency

Types 1 and 2

A severe deficiency of glucocerebrosidase activity has been unequivocally demonstrated in patients with Gaucher's disease. Brady et al. found a marked deficiency in the activity of this enzyme in the spleens of 11 patients with Gaucher's disease [25, 313]. Patrick [312] observed decreased glucocerebrosidase activity in the spleens of four others. Brady and coworkers have also determined glucocerebrosidase activity in brain [314], leukocytes [314, 356, 357], and skin fibroblasts [357] from patients with Gaucher's disease. In each tissue the enzymatic activity was reduced. Employing an artificial substrate, Öckermann has demonstrated decreased β-glucosidase activity in liver and spleen of Gaucher patients [358, 359]. No clinical details accompanied any of the reports of these enzymatic studies. The majority of tissue samples clearly were obtained from patients with the Type 1 form; one or more "infantile" cases may have been examples of the Type 2 form. In the report of Espinas and Faris [93] of identical twins affected with Type 2, the glucocerebrosidase activity in liver was reduced to 6 percent of normal and in spleen was 17 percent of normal.

Type 3

Svennerholm [326] has observed reduced activity of brain glucocerebrosidase in several Swedish patients with Type 3 Gaucher's disease. Glucocerebrosidase activity in tissues from other Type 3 patients has not been reported.

Glucosyl Ceramide Precursors

The Glc-Cer that is the substrate for the deficient hydrolase may arise from several precursors that themselves are products of normal metabolic processes. Considered the steadiest and largest contributors are leukocytes and erythrocytes, whose degradation yields a number of gangliosides and neutral glycolipids, such as globoside (Chap. 31). Sequential removal from these compounds of sialic acids, galactosamine, and galactose eventually yields Glc-Cer, whose β-glucopyranoside linkage is attacked to release glucose and ceramide.

The overall pathways for glycolipid degradation have not been completely characterized, and their relative contributions to the Glc-Cer "pool" can be only crudely approximated. Estimates have been made by Kattlove et al. [352] that the release of Glc-Cer and its precursors from degraded leukocytes is 40 to 80 times larger than that contributed by the breakdown of erythrocytes. Assuming that the glycolipids released during degradation of both cell types find their way into the pool of Glc-Cer undergoing catabolism, the leukocytes are thus the more important source of this substrate. The chemical structure and turnover of glycolipids in formed elements of the blood are now subjects of intensive study; the available information is summarized in Chap. 31. It is noteworthy that the fatty acid composition of the neutral glycolipids in leukocytes is similar enough to that in the Glc-Cer stored in Gaucher's disease to permit a precursor-product relationship [281].

As already described, disorders leading to accelerated granulocyte destruction, such as leukemia, are associated with lysosomal accumulation of Glc-Cer in reticulum cells. The accumulation is even accompanied by induction of higher than normal glucosyl ceramide hydrolase activity [352] in leukemic cells. Presumably an increase in Glc-Cer formation from erythrocyte destruction does not reach the levels that can occur in leukemia. There are, however, rare cases of Gaucher's disease associated with hemolytic anemia [197, 198, 360].

Synthesis of Glc-Cer in Gaucher's Disease

Trams and Brady [361] incubated labeled glucose, galactose, and acetate with tissue slices of spleens from four children with Gaucher's disease, two with Niemann-Pick disease, and an adult with thrombocytopenia. The rates of incorporation of these substrates into cerebrosides appeared to be the same in all the spleens. Two other studies, however, have been interpreted as showing possible abnormalities in synthetic pathways in Gaucher tissues. Stein and Gardner [362] incubated fractions of splenic homogenates with labeled hexoses and concluded that the Gaucher spleen might be deficient in a heat-labile epimerase that theoretically converts Glc-Cer to Gal-Cer. Okada [363] concluded from similar experiments that epimerase activity, as well as conversion of Glc-Cer to dihexoside, might be defective. These studies are difficult to interpret, for there is little information about the normal occurrence of such reactions.

Accumulation of Other Glycolipids in Viscera

In contrast to other sphingolipidoses discussed in this book, Gaucher's disease is unusual in the paucity of data showing accumulation of more than one class of lipids. It is possible that Gal-Glc-Cer and gangliosides also accumulate more frequently than has been reported and that other related compounds do so as well. The tissue content of other compounds containing the Glc-Cer unit may increase from rate limitation in the hydrolysis of Glc-Cer. Accumulation of Glc-Cer could also inhibit other enzymes involved in glycolipid metabolism. Finally, the absolute specificity for Glc-Cer of the β-glucosidase, whose deficiency appears to be primary in Gaucher's disease, has not been established.

SPECULATION ABOUT PATHOPHYSIOLOGY

We may summarize the probable course of events in Gaucher's disease from the available evidence. The normal turnover of glycolipids from the formed elements of the blood and in many other tissues gives rise to compounds which are sequentially degraded to Glc-Cer. In Gaucher's disease, the β-glucosidase activity catalyzing the hydrolysis of Glc-Cer is deficient, and this relatively water-insoluble compound begins to accumulate. The spleen and other tissues particularly rich in reticuloendothelial cells bear the initial brunt of the disease. Secondary lysosomes form to sequester the Glc-Cer. The plasma level of Glc-Cer is little increased until after splenectomy, and removal of this organ may abruptly increase the load on reticulum cells outside the spleen.

In the chronic (Type 1) form of the disorder, much of the attendant difficulties can be ascribed to mechanical encroachment by masses of storage cells. The spleen, liver, and lymph nodes enlarge, not only to store glycolipids but also to maintain their other functions. The almost inevitable hypersplenism and the frequent disabilities in bones and lungs follow in a manner that is reasonably well understood. Other features, such as the pingueculae and changes in skin pigmentation, are without explanation at present; frequently the immediate cause of death is also only obscurely related to the visceral changes in the disease.

The pathologic changes in the central nervous system in Gaucher's disease are poorly understood. Perhaps the oldest theory to explain them is that of Tropp [364], who speculated that failure to transport preformed cerebroside to the brain hampered its development. Later awareness that the major cerebrosides within and outside the brain were different rendered this theory obsolete. The recent discovery of the catabolic defect in the periphery has not yet been completely explored as an explanation of the lesions in brain. There is no consistent observation of storage of Glc-Cer in brain. The evidence of Svennerholm [116] that Glc-Cer does accumulate and that it probably arises from a block in the normal catabolism of gangliosides offers an attractive explanation of the neuronal abnormalities in Gaucher's disease. There is enough evidence of neuronal storage in the brains of most children with Type 2 to support this thesis, especially if one acknowledges that relatively little storage of Glc-Cer in the young brain may carry with it severe consequences for the neuron. Not obvious now is a correlation between chemical, enzymatic, and morphologic changes that allow some children with brain involvement to survive longer. Better definition of the "juvenile form" (Type 3) may resolve this problem.

The fundamental question is why the brain escapes in one form of the disorder and is so seriously damaged in others. The answer may lie in a different alteration in the same enzyme in each of the forms of the disease. The activity of a single enzyme can be reduced to varying degrees by mutations at the same or different loci. Possibly the variations in phenotypes could be due to quantitative differences in glucocerebrosidase activity in the tissues. The level of activity in the brain may be particularly critical in determining whether or not neurologic abnormalities will be evident. The same level of reduced activity may result from several different mutations. Therefore the different phenotypes, grouped here as Types 1, 2, and 3, may themselves be heterogeneous and may each result from more than one mutation. The possibilities of polymorphism and other forms of heterogeneity in enzymes having glucocerebrosidase activity have yet to be clarified in the normal state as well as in Gaucher's disease.

TREATMENT

There is yet no rational basis for specific therapy of Gaucher's disease. Treatment is entirely supportive. The most common problem is the selection of the time for splenectomy. The basic disease process is not alleviated by removal of the spleen, and there are no arguments for splenectomy in advance of the time when either the hematologic effects of hypersplenism or serious mechanical distress provide definite indication. Patients may do well for years with a platelet count below 50,000; the decision is an individual one.

The bone lesions and especially the pain that accompanies them provide the most severe disability in chronic Gaucher's disease. There is no special form of therapy; steroids may be helpful. Replacement of the deficient enzyme is not yet practicable.

GENETICS

The second and third examples of Gaucher's disease, reported in 1895, were in sisters [365]. Ample evidence has since been obtained to indicate that the condition is inheritable. The genetics of the disease have been reviewed repeatedly [3, 9, 32, 38, 99, 366, 367], and several computations of familial incidence have been made from fairly large numbers of families [3, 366, 368]. At least three mutations are required to explain the different phenotypes that have been described.

Type 1

Extensive analyses of a few families, such as the five related Negro sibships studied by Herndon and Bender [38], indicate that Gaucher's disease without clinical evidence of neuronal involvement (Type 1, by present definition) can be inherited as an autosomal recessive trait. In 1962, Hsia, Naylor, and Bigler [366] collected 110 families from the literature affected with Gaucher's disease. In 85 families, they found no historical evidence of Gaucher's disease in either parent. In 79 of these sibships, assuming truncate ascertainment, they found the rate of occurrence most consistent with autosomal recessive inheritance. As they noted, however, about 10 percent of the sibships were representative of a neuronopathic form of the disease.

There are at least two families in which Gaucher's disease has been reported in successive generations, in one instance in father and son [366], and in the other, in mother and two daughters [369]. In two other families paternal uncles and their nephews unequivocally had Type 1 [39, 370]. In other families, one or more members had fairly clear-cut disease (Type 1) and first- or second-degree relatives had either splenomegaly or bone changes suggestive of Gaucher's disease [32, 34, 61, 185, 371–373]. Gaucher-like cells have also been found in the bone marrow of asymptomatic relatives of about 10 patients with Type 1 [32, 374–379]. Thus, one or more mutations may lead to development of Gaucher cells in the marrow and possibly lesser involvement of other tissues in the heterozygous state. As has been pointed out [366], a family has not yet been reported in which three successive generations have clearly been affected with Type 1. This event would lend needed support for the suggestion [380] that the disease may be produced by single dosage of an abnormal allele. The suggestions of Groen [380] of increased frequency of miscarriage and neonatal deaths among offspring of patients with Type 1 and that Gaucher's disease becomes increasingly severe in successive generations were not supported in the analyses of Hsia et al. [366].

The distribution of the gene or genes giving rise to Type 1 Gaucher's disease is very wide, and one or more cases have been reported in most ethnic groups. It has long been apparent that the prevalence is unusually high among Ashkenazi Jews [367, 380]. Estimates in Israel have varied from as high as one case per 2,000 to one per 20,000 Ashkenazi in that country [380–382]. The first known cases among Sephardic or Oriental Jews have recently been reported [34]. Most patients with Type 1 have been reported from Europe, the United States, or Israel. Many cases have also been reported from Latin America [63, 67, 121, 122, 230, 378, 383–385], Asia and India [84, 115, 120, 123, 124, 127, 319, 374, 375, 386, 387], and a few others from other Middle Eastern countries [112, 388–390, 391], Africa [82, 89, 203, 295], and Australia and New Zealand [41, 391, 392].

Type 2

Unequivocal examples of both Types 1 and 2 Gaucher's disease have never been reported in the same family. The 67 examples of Type 2 in Table 33-1 occurred in 46 families. Of the 62 patients for which sex was identified, 35 were males. An analysis of the 29 kindreds for which family history was available is presented in Table 33-4. The group of patients is slightly larger and somewhat different from that used for similar calculations by Knudson and Kaplan [3]. There is an excess of affected sibs over that expected for an autosomal recessive trait, whether single or truncate selection is used. None of the clinical abnormalities of Gaucher's disease have been reported in a parent of a Type 2 child. In several families [70, 72] Gaucher cells were specifically not found in the marrow of parents or unaffected sibs. Consanguinity has been noted in 2 of the 46 affected families [27, 78]. Of 31 families in which ethnic origin or religion was described, 4 were Jewish. The prevalence of Type 2 among Jews is thus relatively high, but it is far less striking than the extraordinary prevalence of Type 1 among

Table 33-4. GENETIC ANALYSIS OF FAMILIES AFFECTED WITH GAUCHER'S DISEASE, TYPE 2*

Family size	No. of sibships	Total no. of children	No. of children affected
1	5	5	5
2	8	16	10
3	8	24	13
4	6	24	11
7	2	14	8
Totals	29	83	47

* The data presented here are from 29 of the families in Table 33-1. The actual ratio of affected to total siblings is 0.57. The expected proportion calculated by single selection is 0.33 ± 0.06; by truncate selection it is 0.44 ± 0.11. The data were analyzed by Dr. Ntinos C. Myrianthopoulos.

Jews. The number of different ethnic groups affected is large (Table 33-1). In agreement with Knudson and Kaplan [3], it is concluded that the available data best support an autosomal recessive mode of inheritance for Type 2 Gaucher's disease.

Type 3

Of the number of possible cases of "juvenile" Gaucher's disease, roughly half are represented by the Norrbotten families in Sweden [141, 143]. In that group the consanguinity and mode of expression are most consistent with an autosomal recessive mode of inheritance. There have been no reasonably acceptable cases of the juvenile form involving Jews.

Heterozygote Detection

No evidence of clinical abnormality has been reported in a parent of a Type 2 child. The presence of Gaucher cells in asymptomatic parents and sibs of some patients with Type 1 has been discussed above. This examination frequently yields negative results, and it is not a reliable basis for detection of heterozygotes. Danes and Bearn [393] have reported that cultured skin fibroblasts from patients with Gaucher's disease and from heterozygous carriers stain metachromatically. This phenomenon is not limited to Gaucher's disease [394], and the clinical value of this test is therefore uncertain. At the present time the heterozygous state of Gaucher's disease has not been detected with certainty by enzymatic analyses. Evaluation of glucosidase activity in circulating leukocytes shows promise in this regard [394a]. Possible abnormalities in red blood cell lipids in patients [329] have not been observed in the erythrocytes of relatives. Plasma acid phosphatase levels have also not been elevated in the few sibs or parents of affected patients who have been examined [144, 161].

DIAGNOSIS

Gaucher's disease must always be considered in any patient with an enlarged spleen. In a child under 1 year of age who has retarded psychomotor development in addition to splenomegaly, the following diseases should be excluded (in approximate order of their prevalence): mucopolysaccharidoses (Types 1, 2, and 3); Niemann-Pick disease (Type A, Chap. 35); Gaucher's disease, Type 2; G_{M1} gangliosidosis with visceral involvement; and Wolman's disease. In these children the combination of hyperextended head, strabismus, and other signs of brain stem involvement, in the absence of corneal clouding, retinal abnormalities, bone deformities, or urinary excretion of metachromatic material, is most suggestive of Gaucher's disease. In a young child who has *only* hepatosplenomegaly with or without hypersplenism, Gaucher's disease (Type 1) may be confused with Niemann-Pick disease (Type B, Chap. 35).

In all suspected patients a thorough examination of the nervous system, careful roentgenographic survey of the lungs and bones, hemogram, plasma acid phosphatase, cholesterol and triglyceride determinations, and examination of a bone marrow aspirate are indicated. Usually the appearance of the Gaucher cells is typical enough to permit a satisfactory diagnosis. If there is doubt, liver biopsy is suggested. Sufficient liver (20 mg) can be procured by needle biopsy to permit a qualitative demonstration of increased cerebroside by thin-layer chromatography (Fig. 34-8). An open biopsy is preferable; 0.5 to 1.0 gm liver should be obtained. A small aliquot is used for histologic examination, including frozen and fixed preparations and electron microscopy. Most of the sample should be preserved *frozen*, in the absence of fixatives, to permit definitive chemical analyses and determination of enzymatic activities. If the spleen eventually requires removal, it should be handled in the same way. A thorough characterization of tissue glycolipid content is obligatory in all patients suspected of having the subacute or juvenile form (Type 3) of Gaucher's disease. Transmural rectal biopsy may also be helpful in determining the presence of nervous system involvement [395, 396].

Fucosidosis

A new glycolipid storage disease that must be differentiated from Gaucher's disease has recently been described [397, 398]. Its clinical manifestations include progressive neuromuscular degeneration leading to dementia, cardiovascular and respiratory disturbances, thick skin, abundant sweating, and hypoplasia and beaking of vertebral bodies. Tissues contain increased amounts of unusual glycolipids and mucopolysaccharides containing fucose. The defect is apparently due to deficiency of an α-fucosidase.

Lactosyl Ceramidosis

Dawson, Stein, and Matalon have recently described a new disease that they have termed lactosyl ceramidosis [399, 400], and Dr. Glynn Dawson, who has studied this patient extensively, has provided us with additional unpublished information about the clinical course and tissue analyses.

The patient was a negro female 3-½ years old. Her development was somewhat slow for the first two years of life and by 30 months of age psychomotor deterioration was obvious. Her eyes bulged and there was an oscillating nystagmus. Both the liver and spleen were enlarged and there was also generalized lymphadenopathy. She had tremors of the lower jaw and of all her extremities, marked truncal and limb ataxia, spasticity, hyperextension of the head, and bilateral Babinski responses. By 41 months of age the child was no longer able to hold objects or swallow food; there was almost total retinal degeneration and the maculae were slightly pink.

Clinopathological Correlations

Large mononuclear foam cells (30 to 40 μ in diameter) were found in bone marrow aspirates at 34 months of age; they contained clear lipid droplets, rather than the fibrillar material observed in Gaucher's disease. The serum acid phosphatase was elevated (28 I.U.) but not to the extent observed in Gaucher's disease.

The hepatic parenchymal cells and architecture were normal; the sinusoids, however, were focally dilated and contained large Kupffer cells with a pale foamy cytoplasm. The Kupffer cells did not stain with oil-red-O. Electron microscopy demonstrated the presence of abnormal organelles within the parenchymal cells.

A biopsy of the cerebral cortex contained slightly swollen neurons and greatly enlarged apical dendrites that contained inclusions of various sizes. Under electron microscopy these inclusions contained membranous, granular, and amorphous regions. The inclusions were readily differentiated from those seen in Tay-Sachs disease.

Chemical Abnormalities and Metabolic Defect

The concentration of lactosyl ceramide (galactosylglucosyl ceramide) was elevated in plasma, erythrocytes, urinary sediment, liver, cerebral cortex, and in fibroblasts derived from skin and bone marrow. Employing radioactively labeled galactosylglucosyl ceramide, Dawson et al. demonstrated a deficiency of galactosyl hydrolase activity in the liver and fibroblasts from their patient. It therefore appears that the accumulation of lactosyl ceramide in this disease is due to deficient activity of the enzyme that catalyzes the hydrolysis of the terminal galactose.

Relationship to Gaucher's Disease

It is possible that some of the patients with "Gaucher's disease, Type 3" described in this chapter were actually examples of lactosyl ceramidosis. Reference was made to apparent increase of lactosyl ceramide in the tissues of some of these patients.

SUMMARY

1. Gaucher's disease is a relatively common familial disease characterized by tissue accumulation of cerebrosides, specifically glucosyl ceramides. These compounds contain sphingosine, fatty acid, and glucose in equimolar amounts. The accumulation occurs in cells of the reticuloendothelial system, which take on a characteristic appearance and are called Gaucher cells. The proliferation of these cells in various tissues is responsible for most of the clinical abnormalities, which include hepatosplenomegaly, hypersplenism, and bone lesions.

2. The disease has been detected at all ages and occurs in two major clinical forms. The adult, or chronic, nonneuronopathic form (Type 1) may manifest itself any time from birth to old age. Hematologic abnormalities attributable to hypersplenism and bone lesions are the major manifestations. The acute neuronopathic, or malignant, form (Type 2) is usually apparent before 6 months of age and fatal by 2 years of age. The course of this form of the disease is rapidly progressive and associated with characteristic involvement of the cranial nerves and brain stem. The brain reveals minimal storage of lipid in ganglion cells, neuronal loss, neuronophagia, and prominent deposition of glycolipid in periadventitial cells. There is also a subacute neuronopathic, or juvenile, form (Type 3) in which the onset of cerebral abnormalities is delayed. Death may occur in infancy or as late as the third decade.

3. In all three types of the disease there is deficient activity of tissue glucosyl ceramide hydrolase (glucocerebrosidase). This enzyme normally cleaves glucose from glucosyl ceramides.

4. The observation of typical Gaucher cells in bone marrow or other tissues provides a tentative diagnosis. This should be confirmed by determination of tissue content of glycolipids and glucocerebrosidase activity. The level of plasma acid phosphatase (nontartrate-inhibitable) is elevated in nearly every case.

5. There is no specific treatment for the disease.

6. The three forms of the disease appear to be due to different mutations. All three forms are most likely an expression of a double dose of these different mutant autosomal alleles. Possibly some patients may have complex heterozygote conditions. An "incompletely dominant" inheritance of Type 1 in some families has not been excluded. Types 2 and 3 are much less common among Ashkenazi Jews than is Type 1. A reliable test for detection of heterozygotes is not yet available.

BIBLIOGRAPHY

1. Fredrickson, D. S.: Classification and features of the lipidoses affecting the nervous system. Path. Europ., **3**, 121, 1968.
2. Lowenthal, A., and Zeman, W.: Considerations on a classification of neurolipidoses. Path. Europ., **3**, 494, 1968.
3. Knudson, A. G., Jr., and Kaplan, W. D.: Genetics of the sphingolipidoses, in *Cerebral Sphingolipidoses,* edited by S. M. Aronson and B. W. Volk, p. 395. Academic, New York, 1962.
4. Gaucher, P.: De l'épithélioma primitif de la rate. Thèse de Paris, 1882.
5. Schlaugenhaufer, F.: Über meist familiar vorkommende, histologisch, characteristische Splenomegalien (Typus Gaucher). Arch. Path. Anat., **187,** 125, 1907.
6. Bovaird, D., Jr.: Primary splenomegaly. Amer. J. Med. Sci., **120,** 377, 1900.
7. Marchand, F.: Über sog. idiopathische Splenomegalie—Typus Gaucher. München. Med. Wschr., **54,** 1102, 1907.
8. Pick, L.: Zur pathologischen Anatomie des Morbus Gaucher. Med. Klin., **18,** 1408, 1922.
9. Thannhauser, S. J.: *Lipidoses, Diseases of the Intracellular Lipid Metabolism.* Grune & Stratton, New York, 1958.
10. Epstein, E.: Beitrag zur Chemie der Gaucherschen Krankheit. Biochem. Z., **145,** 3098, 1924.
11. Epstein, E., and Lorenz, K: Die Phosphatidzellverfettung der Milz bei Niemann-Pickschen Krankheit verglichen mit der Lipoidchemie des Morbus Gaucher und der Schüller-Christianschen Krankheit. Z. Physiol. Chem., **192,** 145, 1930.
12. Lieb, H.: Cerebrosidspeicherung bei Morbus Gaucher. Z. Physiol. Chem., **140,** 305, 1924.
13. Lieb, H.: Cerebrosidspeicherung bei Splenomegalie, Typus Gaucher. Z. Physiol. Chem., **170,** 60, 1927.
14. Lieb, H., and Mladenovic, M.: Cerebrosidspeicherung bei Morbus Gaucher. Z. Physiol. Chem., **181,** 208, 1929.
15. Thudichum, J. L. W.: *Die chemische Konstitution des Gehirns des Menschen und der Tiere.* Franz Pietzcker, Tübingen, 1901.
16. Drabkin, D. L.: *Thudichum, Chemist of the Brain,* University of Pennsylvania Press, Philadelphia, 1958.
17. Carter, H. E., Johnson, P., and Weber, E. J.: Glycolipids, in *Annual Review of Biochemistry,* edited by J. M. Juch and P. D. Boyer, vol. 34, pp. 109-142. Annual Reviews, Inc., Palo Alto, Calif., 1965.
18. Klenk, E., and Harle, R.: Teilsynthese des Kerasins und einige Bemerkungen über Nervon. Z. Physiol. Chem., **189,** 243, 1930.
19. Klenk, E.: Beitrage zur Chemie der Lipoidosen. Z. Physiol. Chem., **267,** 128, 1940.
20. Aghion, A.: *La Maladie de Gaucher dans l'enfance.* Thèse, Paris, 1934.
21. Halliday, N., Deuel, H., Jr., Tragerman, L. J., and Ward, W. E.: On isolation of glucose-containing cerebroside from spleen in a case of Gaucher's disease. J. Biol. Chem., **132,** 171, 1940.
22. Rosenberg, A., and Chargaff, E.: A reinvestigation of the cerebroside deposited in Gaucher's disease. J. Biol. Chem., **233,** 1323, 1958.
23. Marinetti, G. V., Ford, T., and Stotz, E.: The structure of cerebrosides in Gaucher's disease. J. Lipid Res., **1,** 203, 1960.
24. Suomi, W. D., and Agranoff, B. W.: Lipids of the spleen in Gaucher's disease. J. Lipid Res., **6,** 211, 1965.
25. Brady, R. O., Kanfer, J. N., and Shapiro, D.: Metabolism of glucocerebrosides. II. Evidence of an enzymatic deficiency in Gaucher's disease. Biochem. Biophys. Res. Commun., **18,** 221, 1965.
26. Giampalmo, A.: Stato attuale degli studi sull'anatomia pathologica e sulla patogenesi delle malattie di Niemann-Pick, di Gaucher e di v. Gierke. Arch. Maragliano Pat. Clin., **1,** 219, 1946.
27. Giampalmo, A.: Über die Pathologie der Gaucherschen Krankheit im fruhen Kindersalter (mit besonderer Berucksichtigung der neurologischen Form). Acta Paediat. Scand., **37,** 6, 1949.
28. Diezel, P. B.: Histochemische Untersuchungen an den Globoidszellen der familiaren infantilen diffusen Sklerose vom Typus Krabbe (Zugleich eine differentialdiagnostiche Betrachtung der zentralnervösen Veränderungen beim Morbus Gaucher). Virchow. Arch. [Path. Anat.], **327,** 206, 1955.
29. Fredrickson, D. S.: Cerebroside lipidosis: Gaucher's disease, in *The Metabolic Basis of Inherited Disease,* 2d ed., edited by J. B. Stanbury, J. B. Wyngaarden, and D. S. Fredrickson, p. 565. McGraw-Hill, New York, 1966.
30. Roberts, W. C., and Fredrickson, D. S.: Gaucher's disease of the lung causing severe pulmonary hypertension with associated acute recurrent pericarditis. Circulation, **35,** 783, 1967.
31. Reich, C., Siefe, M., and Kessler, B. J.: Gaucher's disease: a review and discussion of twenty cases. Medicine, **30,** 1, 1951.
32. Groen, J., and Garrer, A. H.: Adult Gaucher's disease with specific reference to the variations in its clinical course and the value of sternal puncture as an aid to its diagnosis. Blood, **3,** 1221, 1948.
33. Doss, M., and Matiar-Vahar, H.: Neurolipidosen und angeborene Entmarkungskrankheiten. Fortschr. Neurol. Psychiat., **33,** 617, 1965.
34. Matoth, Y., and Fried, K.: Chronic Gaucher's disease: clinical observations on 34 patients. Israel J. Med. Sci., **1,** 521, 1965.
35. Schettler, G., and Kahlke, W.: Gaucher's disease in *Lipids and Lipidoses,* edited by G. Schettler, pp. 260-287. Springer-Verlag, New York, 1967.
36. Bernstein, J., and Shelden, W. E.: A note on the development of Gaucher cells in a newborn infant. J. Pediat., **55,** 577, 1959.
37. Brinn, L., and Glabman, S.: Gaucher's disease without splenomegaly: oldest patient on record, with review. New York J. Med., **62,** 2346, 1962.
38. Herndon, C. N., and Bender, J. R.: Gaucher's disease; cases in 5 related Negro sibships. Amer. J. Hum. Genet., **2,** 49, 1949.
39. Levin, B.: Gaucher's disease: clinical and roentgenologic manifestations. Amer. J. Roentgen., **85,** 685, 1961.
40. Jackson, D. C., and Simon, G.: Unusual bone and lung changes in a case of Gaucher's disease. Brit. J. Radiol., **38,** 698, 1965.
41. McKelvie, I. J., and Edwards, L. R.: Gaucher's disease: report of a case. Med. J. Aust., **2,** 297, 1969.
42. Rowland, R. S.: Constitutional disturbances of lipid metabolism, in *Brennemann's Practice of Pediatrics,* vol. 3, chap. 23, p. 77. Prior, Hagerstown, Md., 1936.
43. Oberling, C., and Woringer, P.: La Maladie de Gaucher chez le nourrisson. Rev. Franc. Pediat., **3,** 475, 1927.
44. DeLange, C.: Über die maligne Form der Gaucherschen Krankheit. Acta Paediat. Scand., **27,** 34, 1940.
45. Kwiterovich, P. O., Jr., Sloan, H. R., and Fredrickson, D. S.: Unpublished data.
46. Kwiterovich, P. O., Jr., Sloan, H. R., and Fredrickson, D. S.: The glycolipids and other lipid constituents of normal human liver. J. Lipid Res., **11,** 322, 1970.
47. Rusca, C. L.: Sul morbo del Gaucher. Haematologica, **2,** 441, 1921.
48. Reber, M.: Gaucher's splenomegaly in infants. Jahrb. Kinderheilk., **105,** 277, 1924.
49. Jenny, E.: Beitrag zur Kenntnis der Varianten der Gaucherischen und Niemann-Pickschen Krankheit. Thesis, Basel, 1930.
50. Dienst, N., and Hamperl, H.: Ein Fall von lipoidzelliger Splenomegalie. Wien. Med. Wschr., **77,** 1597, 1927.
51. Dienst, G.: Über einen Fall von lipoidzelliger Splenohepatomegalie. J. Kinderheilk. Phys. Erziehung, **123,** 181, 1929.
52. Hamperl, H.: Über die pathologisch-anatomischen Veranderungen bei Morbus Gaucher im Säuglingsalter. Virchow. Arch. Path. Anat., **271,** 147, 1929.
53. Stransky, E.: Über grosszellige Splenohepatomegalie. Jahrb. Kinderheilk., **126,** 204, 1930.
54. Meyer, R.: Nouveau cas de syndrome pseudobulbaire du nourrisson (maladie du Gaucher du nourrisson). Rev. Neurol. (Paris), **2,** 612, 1934.
55. Meyer, R.: A proposito du un nuova caso di malattia di Gaucher nel lattante. Pediatria (Napoli), **45,** 434, 1937.
56. Corcan, P., Oberling, C., and Dienst, G.: La Maladie de Niemann-Pick. Rev. Franc. Pediat., **3,** 789, 1927.
57. Moncrieff, A.: Infantile type of Gaucher's disease. Arch. Dis. Child., **5,** 265, 1930.
58. Kennaway, N. G., and Woolf, L. I.: Splenic lipids in Gaucher's disease. J. Lipid Res., **9,** 755, 1968.
59. Meyer, R.: Syndrome neurologique et diagnostic clinique de la maladie du Gaucher du nourrisson. Rev. Franc. Pediat., **8,** 559, 1932.

60. De Sylla Robles: Bol. Soc. Ital. Pediat. (Torino), cited by A. Giampalmo, **3**, 181, 1934.
61. Aballi, A. J., and Kato, K.: Gaucher's disease in early infancy: review of literature and report of case with neurological symptoms. J. Pediat., **13**, 364, 1938.
62. Köhne, G.: Über Morbus Gaucher mit Hirnveranderungen. Z. Path. Anat., **102**, 512, 1939.
63. Tosco, M. A. F.: Enfermedad de Gaucher en un lactante. Bol. Soc. Cubana Pediat., **13**, 252, 1941.
64. Schairer, E.: Gaucher's disease. Virchow. Arch. [Path. Anat.], **309**, 726, 1942.
65. Ullrich, O.: Morbus Gaucher im Säuglingsalter. Kinderaerztl. Prax., **13**, 113, 1942.
66. Frisell, E.: Gaucher's disease in infants. Acta Paediat. Scand., **30**, 460, 1943.
67. Garrahan, J. P., Gambirassi, A. C., Albores, J. N., and Moran, J.: La Enfermedad de Gaucher en el lactante con motivo de una observación clinica. Arch. Argent. Pediat., **23**, 3, 1945.
68. Landolt, R. F., Zollinger, H. U., and Eugster, C. H.: Über die maligne, akut verlaufende Form des Morbus Gaucher. Helv. Paediat. Acta, **3**, 319, 1948.
69. Schairer, E.: Die Gehirnveranderungen beim Morbus Gaucher des Säuglings. Virchow. Arch. [Path. Anat.], **315**, 395, 1948.
70. Strengers, L.: Acute vorm van de ziekte van Gaucher bij drie kinderen uit één gezin. Maandschr. Kindergeneesk., **17**, 237, 1949.
71. Rodgers, C. L., and Jackson, S. H.: Acute infantile Gaucher's disease. Pediatrics, **7**, 53, 1951.
72. Geddes, A. K., and Moore, S.: Acute (infantile) Gaucher's disease: report of a case, the second in a family. J. Pediat., **43**, 61, 1953.
73. Seitz, H., and Stammler, A.: Morbus Gaucher beim Säugling. Zbl. Allg. Path., **87**, 336, 1951.
74. Debré, R., Bertrand, I., Grumbach, R., and Bargeton, G.: Maladie de Gaucher du nourrisson. Arch. Franc. Pediat., **8**, 38, 1951.
75. Kostitch-Yoksitch, S. A.: À Propos d'un cas de maladie de Gaucher. Le Sang. Biol. Path., **23**, 586, 1952.
76. Norman, R. M., Urich, J., and Lloyd, O. C.: The neuropathology of infantile Gaucher's disease. J. Path. Bact., **72**, 121, 1956.
77. Barlow, C. F.: Neuropathologic findings in a case of infantile Gaucher's disease. J. Neuropath. Exp. Neurol., **16**, 238, 1957.
78. Kubler, W.: Histologische und histochemische Untersuchungen an einem Fall von Gaucher-Krankheit bei einem Säugling. Frankfurt. Z. Path., **71**, 33, 1961.
79. Stein, M., and Gardner, L. I.: Acute infantile Gaucher's disease. Pediatrics, **27**, 491, 1961.
80. Pecorella, F.: Considerazioni su un case di malattia di Gaucher acuta nella infanzia. Riv. Clin. Pediat., **68**, 110, 1961.
81. Banker, B. Q., Miller, J. Q., and Crocker, A. C.: The cerebral pathology of infantile Gaucher's disease, in *Cerebral Sphingolipidoses,* edited by S. M. Aronson and B. W. Volk, p. 73. Academic, New York, 1962.
82. Ogunlesi, T. O.: Gaucher's disease in a Nigerian infant. J. Trop. Pediat., **8**, 45, 1962.
83. Bianchedi, S., and Vignolo, L.: La malattia di Gaucher nella prima infanzia. Minerva Pediat., **14**, 1349, 1962.
84. Inose, T., Inoue, K., Sawaizumi, S., and Matsuoka, T.: Beitrag zur Neuropathologie des Morbus Gaucher im Kindesalter. Acta Neuropath. (Berlin), **3**, 297, 1964.
85. Inose, T., Sakai, M., Tano, T., and Kaneko, Y.: Biochemische Analyse der Glycolipoide im Gehirn beim Morbus Gaucher. Yokohama Med. Bull., **18**, 215, 1967.
86. Rath, F.: Akuter Morbus Gaucher bei einem Säugling. Mschr. Kinderheilk., **112**, 355, 1964.
87. Seitelberger, F.: About the brain involvement in Gaucher's disease in children. Acta Psychiat. Nervenkrankh., **206**, 419, 1964.
88. Pavkovčeková, O., Jactna, J., and Tischler, V.: Infantilna forma Gaucherovej Choroby U 13 mesacneho dietata. Cesk. Pediat., **20**, 1092, 1965.
89. Jedidi, H., Hampa, B., and Chadley, A.: Maladie de Gaucher du nourrisson et manifestations neurologiques prédominates. Tunisie Med., **44**, 85, 1966.
90. Philippart, M., and Menkes, J. H.: Isolation and characterization of the principal cerebral glycolipids in the infantile and adult forms of Gaucher's disease, in *Inborn Disorders of Sphingolipid Metabolism,* Proceedings of the Third International Symposium on the Cerebral Sphingolipidoses, edited by S. M. Aronson and B. W. Volk, p. 389. Pergamon, New York, 1967.
91. Adachi, M., Wallace, B. J., Schneck, L., and Volk, B. W.: Fine structure of central nervous system in early infantile Gaucher's disease. Arch. Path. (Chicago), **83**, 513, 1967.
92. Scaravilli, F., and Tavolato, B.: Neuropathological aspects of the infantile form of Gaucher's disease. Acta Neurol. Belg., **68**, 674, 1968.
93. Espinas, O. E., and Faris, Amin A.: Acute infantile Gaucher's disease in identical twins: an account of clinical and neuropathologic observations. Neurology, **19**, 133, 1969.
94. French, J. H., Brotz, M., and Poser, C. M.: Lipid composition of the brain in infantile Gaucher's disease. Neurology, **19**, 81, 1969.
95. Kraus, E. J.: Zur Kenntnis der Splenomegalie Gaucher, insbesondere der Histogenese der grosszelligen Wucherung. Z. Angew. Anat., **7**, 186, 1920.
96. Gerstl, P.: Rachitischer Zwergwuchs und Splenomegalie Gaucher bei einer Fruhgeburt. Arch. Kinderheilk., **69**, 357, 1921.
97. Pick, L.: Über den Morbus Gaucher, seine Klinik pathologische Anatomie und histio-pathogenetische Umgrenzung, nebst Untersuchungen über den MG der Säuglinge und über die Beteiligung des Skelettsystems. Med. Klin., **20**, 1399, 1924.
98. Kohn: Cited by Aballi and Kato [61] and by Oberling and Woringer [43].
99. Hoffman, S. J., and Makler, M. I.: Gaucher's disease; a review of the literature and report of a case diagnosed from section of an inguinal lymph gland. Amer. J. Dis. Child., **38**, 775, 1929.
100. Lindau, A.: Neuere Auffassungen über die Pathogenese der familiaren amaurotischen Idiotie. Acta Psychiat. Neurol., **5**, 167, 1930.
101. Findlay, L.: Gaucher's disease verified by splenic puncture. Proc. Roy. Soc. Med., **24**, 848, 1931.
102. Findlay, L.: Microscopic sections from case of Gaucher's disease. Proc. Roy. Soc. Med., **24**, 1336, 1931.
103. Girgensohn, H., Kellner, H., and Sudhof, H.: Angeborener Morbus Gaucher bei Erythroblastose und Gefassverkalkung. Klin. Wschr., **32**, 57, 1954.
104. Frick, P., and Friedrich, G.: Morbus Gaucher in frühen Kindesalter. Arch. Kinderheilk., **90**, 1, 1930.
105. Winter, S. J.: Lipoid histiocytosis (Niemann-Pick type). Amer. J. Dis. Child., **43**, 1150, 1932.
106. Vickery, D.: A case of the infantile form of Gaucher's disease (Niemann-Pick's disease). Med. J. Aust., **2**, 546, 1934.
107. Acuna, M., and DeFilippi, F.: Enfermedad de Gaucher en un lactante esplenectomia. Semana Med. (Argentina), **42**, 735, 1935.
108. Donat, R.: Die Beteiligung der Lungen beim Morbus Gaucher. Zbl. Allg. Path. Anat., **78**, 273, 1941.
109. Bernard, R., Payan, H., and Albovy, E.: Maladie de Gaucher du nourrisson a manifestations cérébrales prédominantes, étude anatomo-clinique. Pediatrie, **16**, 285, 1961.
110. Aronson, S. M., and Carter, A. C.: Infantile form of Gaucher's disease, in *Clinicopathologic Conference,* edited by M. S. Bruno and W. B. Ober. New York State J. Med., **62**, 3599, 1962.
111. Sanchez-Villares, E., Crespo-Hernandez, M., and Gonzalez-Hernandez, P.: Enfermedad de Gaucher de forma juvenil. Rev. Esp. Pediat., **19**, 415, 1963.
112. Cura, S., and Aksu, O.: Akut Infantil Gaucher Vak'asi Dolayisi Ile. Ege Universitesi Tip Fakultesi Mecmuasi, **1**, 35, 1962.
113. Coutel, Y., Paugam, P., Guivarch, J., Morel, H., and Thomet, G.: Deux observations de maladie de Gaucher du nourrisson. Pediatrie, **19**, 957, 1964.
114. Andrada, Maria da Graça: Forma aguda de doença de Gaucher. Rev. Port. Pediat., **29**, 228, 1966.
115. Makita, A., Suzuki, C., and Yosizawa, Z.: Glycolipids isolated from the spleen of Gaucher's disease. Tohoku J. Exp. Med., **88**, 277, 1966.

116. Svennerholm, L.: Metabolism of gangliosides in cerebral lipidoses, in *Inborn Disorders of Sphingolipid Metabolism,* Proceedings of the Third International Symposium on the Cerebral Sphingolipidoses, edited by S. M. Aronson and B. W. Volk, p. 169. Pergamon, New York, 1967.
117. Fahr, T. H., and Stamm, M. C.: Kurtz Beitrage zur Frage der Splenomegalie Type Gaucher. Mschr. Kinderheilk., **26,** 169, 1923.
118. Harper, W. W.: Splenomegaly of the Gaucher type, with case report. Southern Med. J., **19,** 726, 1926.
119. Donovan, E. J.: Splenectomy in a child 11 months of age for Gaucher's disease. Surg. Clin. N. Amer., **11,** 517, 1931.
120. Nagao, N.: Über einen fall von Gaucherscher Krankheit. Nippon Byori Gakkai Kaishi, **24,** 464, 1934.
121. Macera, J., and Brachetto-Brain, D.: Enfermedad de Gaucher en un niño de 19 meses de edad. Cron. Med. (Lima, Peru), **54,** 256, 1937.
122. Aballi, A. J., Panicello, F. S., and Gispert, J. P.: La Enfermedad de Gaucher, primera observación en un niño Cubano. Bol. Soc. Cubana Pediat., **10,** 547, 1938.
123. Stransky, E., and Pecache, L. V.: Gaucher's disease in early infancy. Acta Med. Philipina, **2,** 21, 1940.
124. Wang, C. S., and Lin, K. S.: Gaucher's disease in a pair of twin girls. Acta Paediat. Sinica, **4,** 257, 1963.
125. Pounders, C. M.: The lipoid degenerative diseases. Discussion of infantile amaurotic family idiocy (Tay-Sachs' disease) and essential lipoid histiocytosis (Niemann-Pick's disease): report of a case of each type in Gentiles. J. Pediat., **2,** 216, 1933.
126. Evans, F. A.: Gaucher splenomegaly in a child. Proc. N. Y. Path. Soc., **16,** 114, 1916.
127. Reiss, O., and Kato, K.: Gaucher's disease: a clinical study, with special reference to the roentgenography of bones. Amer. J. Dis. Child., **43,** 365, 1932.
128. Myers, B.: Gaucher's disease of the lungs. Brit. Med. J., **2,** 8, 1937.
129. Maloney, A. F. J., and Cumings, J. N.: A case of juvenile Gaucher's disease with intraneuronal lipid storage. J. Neurol. Neurosurg. Psychiat., **23,** 207, 1960.
130. Bird, A.: Lipidoses and central nervous system. Brain, **71,** 434, 1948.
131. Brain, R.: The kerasin storage disorders, in *Fifth International Neurological Congress,* Lisbon, 7–12 Sept., 1953, vol. 1, p. 261.
132. Brain, R.: Les Affections dues à la thésaurismose de kérasine. Acta Neurol. Belg., **54,** 597, 1954.
133. Philippart, M., Rosenstein, B., and Menkes, J. H.: Isolation and characterization of the main splenic glycolipids in the normal organ and in Gaucher's disease: evidence for the site of metabolic block. J. Neuropath. Exp. Neurol., **24,** 290, 1965.
134. Brante, G.: Cerebral lipidoses: findings and aspects, in *Third International Neurochemistry Symposium,* Strasbourg, 1958, edited by Jordi Folch-Pi. Symposium Publications Division, Pergamon, New York, 1961.
135. Berard-Badier, M., Payan, H., and Edgar, G. W. F.: Étude histologique du système nerveux central d'un cas de maladie de Gaucher dans une fratrie, in *Proceedings of the IVth International Congress of Neuropathology,* edited by H. Jacob, p. 102. Georg Thieme Verlag, Stuttgart, 1962.
136. Jervis, G., Harris, R. C., and Menkes, J. H.: Cerebral lipidosis of unclear nature, in *Cerebral Sphingolipidoses,* edited by S. M. Aronson and B. W. Volk, p. 101. Academic, New York, 1962.
137. Rosenberg, A.: The sphingolipids from the spleen of a case of lipidosis, in *Cerebral Sphingolipidoses,* edited by S. M. Aronson and B. W. Volk, p. 119. Academic, New York, 1962.
138. Philippart, M., Rosenstein, B., and Menkes, J. H.: Isolation and characterization of the main splenic glycolipids in the normal organ and in Gaucher's disease: evidence for the site of metabolic block. J. Neuropath. Exp. Neurol., **24,** 290, 1965.
139. Klodnicka, J., Ograbek, E., and Kuberski, Z.: Report of Gaucher's disease with central nervous system abnormalities. Neurol. Neurochir. Pol., **1,** 267, 1967.
140. Claes, C., and Carpentier, G.: Sur la forme juvénile de la maladie de Gaucher. J. Neurol. Sci., **4,** 571, 1967.
141. Hillborg, P. O.: Morbus Gaucher i Norrbotten. Nord. Med., **61,** 303, 1959.
142. Hillborg, P. O., and Svennerholm, L.: Blood level of cerebrosides in Gaucher's disease. Acta Paediat. Scand., **49,** 707, 1960.
143. Herrlin, K. M., and Hillborg, P. O.: Neurological signs of a juvenile form of Gaucher's disease. Acta Paediat. Scand., **51,** 137, 1962.
144. Hillborg, P. O., and Estborn, B.: Acid phosphatase activity of serum thrombocytes and erythrocytes in a juvenile form of Gaucher's disease. Acta Paediat. Scand., **53,** 558, 1964.
145. Risel, W.: Uber die grosszellige Splenomegalie (Typus Gaucher) und über das endotheliale Sarkom der Milz. Beitr. Path. Anat., **46,** 241, 1909.
146. Mandlebaum, F. S., and Downey, H.: The histopathology and biology of Gaucher's disease (large cell splenomegaly). Folia Haemat. (Frankfurt), **20,** 139, 1916.
147. Bloom, W.: Splenomegaly (type Gaucher) and lipoid histiocytosis. Amer. J. Path., **1,** 595, 1925.
148. Oberling, C.: La maladie de Gaucher. Ann. Anat. Path. Anat. Normale Méd.-chir., **3,** 353, 1926.
149. Pick, L.: A classification of the diseases of lipoid metabolism and Gaucher's disease. Amer. J. Med. Sci., **185,** 453, 1933.
150. Block, M., and Jacobson, L. O.: The histogenesis and diagnosis of the osseous type of Gaucher's disease. Acta Haemat. (Basel), **1,** 165, 1948.
151. Mandlebaum, F. S.: A contribution to the pathology of primary splenomegaly (Gaucher type), with the report of an autopsy on a male child four and one half years of age. J. Exp. Med., **16,** 797, 1912.
152. Chang-Lo, M., Yam, L. T., and Rubenstone, A. I.: Gaucher's disease. Amer. J. Med. Sci., **254,** 303, 1967.
153. Case records of the Massachusetts General Hospital. New Eng. J. Med., **222,** 680, 1940.
154. Pittaluga, P. G., and Goyanes, J.: Contribution à l'étude de la cellule de Gaucher. Arch. Mal. Coeur, **26,** 65, 1933.
155. Morrison, R. W., and Hack, M. H.: Histochemical studies in Gaucher's disease. Amer. J. Path., **25,** 497, 1949.
156. Kovacs, K., Traut, A., and Horvath, E.: Cytochemistry of the Gaucher cell. Schweiz. Z. Allg. Path., **17,** 605, 1954.
157. Diezel, P. B.: Histochemische Untersuchungen an primaren Lipoidosen: amaurotische Idiotie, Gargoylismus, Niemann-Picksche Krankheit, Gauchersche Krankheit, mit besonderer Berucksichtigung des Zentralnervensystems. Arch. Path. Anat., **326,** 89, 1954.
158. Wolman, M.: II. The lipidoses, in *Handbook of Histochemistry,* vol. V, Lipides, 2d part, edited by W. Graumann and K. Neumann, p. 172. Gustav Fischer Verlag, Stuttgart, 1964.
159. Uzman, L. L.: The lipoprotein of Gaucher's disease. A.M.A. Arch. Path., **51,** 329, 1951.
160. Uzman, L. L.: Polycerebrosides in Gaucher's disease. I. Isolation, composition and physical properties, A.M.A. Arch. Path., **55,** 181, 1953.
161. Crocker, A. C., and Landing, B. H.: Phosphatase studies in Gaucher's disease. Metabolism, **9,** 341, 1960.
162. Pesce, V. D., and Ricco, R.: Comportamento istochimico del cerebroside delle cellule di Gaucher dopo solfatazione. Boll. Soc. Ital. Biol. Sper., **44,** 2135, 1968.
163. Lake, B. D.: A histochemical study of Gaucher's disease and Niemann-Pick's disease. J. Roy. Micr. Soc., **86,** 417, 1966.
164. Lorber, M.: The occurrence of intracellular iron in Gaucher's disease. Ann. Intern. Med., **53,** 293, 1960.
165. Lorber, M., and Nemes, J. L.: Identification of ferritin within Gaucher cells: an electron microscopic and immunofluorescent study. Acta Haemat. (Basel), **37,** 189, 1967.
166. DeMarsh, Q. B., and Kautz, J.: The submicroscopic morphology of Gaucher cells. Blood, **12,** 324, 1957.
167. Roos, B., Cottier, H., and Rossi, E.: Electron-optical observations in storage diseases. Experientia, **17,** 430, 1961.
168. Fisher, E. R., and Reidbord, H.: Gaucher's disease: pathogenetic considerations based on electron microscopic and histochemical observations. Amer. J. Path., **41,** 679, 1962.
169. Salomon, J. C., and Caroli, J.: À propos d'un cas de maladie de Gaucher: étude au microscope électronique d'un fragment de tissu hépatique. Rev. Int. Hepat., **12,** 281, 1962.
170. Tanaka, Y., Brecher, G., and Fredrickson, D. S.: Cellules de la maladie de Niemann-Pick et de quelques autres lipoidoses. (The storage cells of Niemann-Pick disease and some other lipidoses.) Nouv. Rev. Franc. Hemat., **3,** 5, 1963.

171. Jordan, S. W.: Electron microscopy of Gaucher cells. Exp. Molec. Path., **3**, 76, 1964.
172. Oliva, H., and Navarro, V.: Consideraciónes sobre la histopatología ultraestructural del higado: microscopia electronica de la localización hepática de la enfermedad de Gaucher. Rev. Esp. Enferm. Apar. Dig., **24**, 431, 1965.
173. Toujas, L., Cussac, Y., Juif, J. G., and Porte, A.: Traduction ultrastructurale des phénomènes de stockage de glycolipides dans la maladie de Gaucher. C. R. Soc. Biol. (Paris), **160**, 394, 1966.
174. Toujas, L., Juif, J. G., Cussac, Y., and Porte, A.: Sur les modifications ultrastructurales du foie dans un cas de maladie de Gaucher. Ann. Anat. Path. (Paris), **11**, 101, 1966.
175. Volk, B. W., and Wallace, B. J.: The liver in lipidosis: an electron microscopic and histochemical study. Amer. J. Path., **49**, 203, 1966.
176. Blicharski, J., Czyzewska-Wazewska, M., Pawlicki, R., and Urbanczyk, J.: Problems of ultrastructure and metabolism of Gaucher cells. Folia Histochem. Cytochem. (Krakow), **5**, 249, 1967.
177. Lee, R. E., Balcerzak, S. P., and Westerman, M. P.: Gaucher's disease: a morphologic study and measurements of iron metabolism. Amer. J. Med., **42**, 891, 1967.
178. Oliva, H., Navarro, V., and Forteza-Vila, J.: Submikroskopische Morphologie der Leber beim Morbus Gaucher. Frankfurt. Z. Path., **76**, 435, 1967.
179. Lee, R. E.: The fine structure of the cerebroside occurring in Gaucher's disease. Proc. Nat. Acad. Sci. U.S.A., **61**, 484, 1968.
180. Neimann, N., Grignon, G., Gentin, G., Guedenet, J.-C., and Vidailhet, M.: Étude de la cellule de Gaucher en microscopie électronique. Ann. Pediat. (Paris), **15**, 625, 1968.
181. Schafer, A., and Bassler, R.: Pathomorphogenese der Kerasinablagerung bei Morbus Gaucher: licht- und elektronenmikroskopische Untersuchungen der Leber und Milz. Frankfurt. Z. Path., **75**, 37, 1966.
182. Pennelli, N., Scaravilli, F., and Zacchello, F.: The morphogenesis of Gaucher cells investigated by electron microscopy. Blood, **34**, 331, 1969.
183. Hibbs, R. G., Ferrans, V. J., Cipriano, P. R., and Tardiff, K. J.: A histochemical and electron microscopic study of Gaucher cells. Arch. Path. (Chicago), **89**, 137, 1970.
184. Fraccaro, M., Magrini, U., Scappaticci, S., and Zacchello, F.: In vitro culture of spleen cells from a case of Gaucher's disease. Ann. Hum. Genet., **32**, 209, 1968.
185. Erf, A. E.: Studies of Gaucher cells by the supravital technique. Amer. J. Med. Sci., **195**, 144, 1938.
186. Pasternak, L., and Page, I. H.: Das Schicksal intravenös injizierter Phosphatide. Biochim. Z., **252**, 254, 1932.
187. Beumer, H., and Fasold, H.: Versuche einer Cerebrosidspeicherung. Z. Ges. Exp. Med., **90**, 661, 1933.
188. Kimmelstiel, P., and Laas, E.: Morphologische Studien zur Frage des Lipoid-antagonismus. Beitr. Path. Anat., **93**, 417, 1934.
189. Dworacek, E., and Pesta, H.: Über einen spektralanalytischen Nachweis des Kerasins und experimentelle Cerebrosidspeicherung im Sinne eines Morbus Gaucher. Wien. Klin. Wschr., **52**, 332, 1939.
190. Christianson, O. O.: Experimental lesions produced by cerebrosides. Arch. Path. (Chicago), **32**, 369, 1941.
191. Petit, J. V., and Schleicher, E. M.: "Atypical" Gaucher's disease. Amer. J. Clin. Path., **13**, 260, 1943.
192. Morgans, M. F.: Gaucher's disease without splenomegaly. Lancet, **2**, 576, 1947.
193. Harrison, W. E., Jr., and Louis, H. J.: Osseous Gaucher's disease in early childhood: report of case with extensive bone changes and pathological fractures without splenomegaly. J.A.M.A., **187**, 997, 1964.
194. Geerling, J.: Gaucher's disease without splenomegaly. Folia Med. Neerl., **9**, 43, 1966.
195. Vreeken, J., Meinders, A. E., Keeman, J. N., and Feltkamp, T. E. W.: A chronic clotting defect with some characteristics of excessive intravascular coagulation in a patient with Gaucher's disease. Folia Med. Neerl., **19**, 180, 1967.
196. Motulsky, A. G., Casserd, F., Giblett, E. R., Broun, G. O., and Finch, C. A.: Anemia and the spleen. New Eng. J. Med., **259**, 1164, 1958.
197. Carling, E. R., Carlill, H., and Pulvertaft, R. J.: Splenectomy in Gaucher's disease with haemoglobinuria. Proc. Roy. Soc. Med., **26**, 361, 1933.
198. Mandlebaum, H., Barber, L., Lederer, M., Sobel, A. E., and Kaye, I. A.: Gaucher's disease. Ann. Intern. Med., **16**, 438, 1942.
199. Bowdler, A. J.: Dilution anemia corrected by splenectomy in Gaucher's disease. Ann. Intern. Med., **58**, 664, 1963.
200. Prankerd, T. A. J.: The red cell and the spleen. Schweiz. Med. Wschr., **93**, 1485, 1963.
201. Edlin, P., Kepler, W. E., Jr., and Knabe, G. W.: Gaucher's disease. Gastroenterology, **28**, 120, 1955.
202. Morrison, A. N., and Lane, M.: Gaucher's disease with ascites; a case report with autopsy findings. Ann. Intern. Med., **42**, 1321, 1955.
203. Javett, S. N., Kew, M. C., and Liknaitsky, D.: Gaucher's disease with portal hypertension: case report. J. Pediat., **68**, 810, 1966.
204. Benbassat, J., Bassan, H., Milwidsky, H., Sacks, M., and Groen, J. J.: Constrictive pericarditis in Gaucher's disease. Amer. J. Med., **44**, 647, 1968.
205. Pachman, D. J.: Chronic Gaucher's disease. Amer. J. Dis. Child., **56**, 248, 1938.
206. Medoff, A. S., and Bayrd, E. D.: Gaucher's disease in 29 cases; hematologic complications and effect of splenectomy. Ann. Intern. Med., **40**, 481, 1954.
207. Junghägen, S.: Röntgenologische Skelettveranderungen bei Morbus Gaucher. Acta Radiol. (Stockholm), **5**, 506, 1926.
208. Ross, L.: Gaucher's cells in kidney glomeruli. Arch. Path. (Chicago), **87**, 164, 1969.
209. Horsley, J. S., Jr., Baker, J. P., and Apperly, F. L.: Gaucher's disease of late onset with kidney involvement and huge spleen. Amer. J. Med. Sci., **190**, 511, 1935.
210. Brill, N. E.: Large-cell splenomegaly (Gaucher's disease): a clinical and pathological study. Amer. J. Med. Sci., **146**, 863, 1913.
211. Gordon, G. L.: Osseous Gaucher's disease. Amer. J. Med., **8**, 332, 1950.
212. Davies, F. W. T.: Gaucher's disease. J. Bone Joint Surg. [Brit.], **34**, 454, 1954.
213. Tennent, W.: Gaucher's disease—the early radiological diagnosis. Brit. J. Radiol., **18**, 356, 1945.
214. Strickland, B.: Skeletal manifestations of Gaucher's disease with some unusual findings. Brit. J. Radiol., **31**, 246, 1958.
215. Raynor, R. R.: Spinal-cord compression secondary to Gaucher's disease. J. Neurosurg., **19**, 902, 1962.
216. Alberti, G. P., and Giannasi, F.: Lesioni ossee in corso di malattia di Gaucher. Cir. Org. Mov., **51**, 205, 1963.
217. Rourke, J. A., and Heslin, D. J.: Gaucher's disease: roentgenologic bone changes over 20 year interval. Amer. J. Roentgen., **94**, 621, 1965.
218. Yossipovitch, Z. H., Herman, G., and Makin, M.: Aseptic osteomyelitis in Gaucher's disease. Israel J. Med. Sci., **1**, 531, 1965.
219. Amstutz, H. C., and Carey, E. J.: Skeletal manifestations and treatment of Gaucher's disease: a review of twenty cases. J. Bone Joint Surg., **48**, 670, 1966.
220. Bischoff, A., Reutter, F. W., and Wegmann, T.: Erkrankung des peripheren Nervensystems beim Morbus Gaucher: neue Erkenntnisse auf Grund der Elektronenmikroskopie. Schweiz. Med. Wschr., **97**, 1139, 1967.
221. Katz, J. F.: Recurrent avascular necrosis of the proximal femoral epiphysis in the same hip in Gaucher's disease. J. Bone Joint Surg. [Amer.], **49**, 514, 1967.
222. Silverstein, M. N., and Kelly, P. J.: Osteoarticular manifestations of Gaucher's disease. Amer. J. Med. Sci., **253**, 569, 1967.
223. Taubman, J., and MacKeith, M.: Gaucher's disease with acroosteolysis. Proc. Roy. Soc. Med., **56**, 294, 1963.
224. Schettler, G.: Cerebrosidose, in *Handbuch der inneren medizin*, vol. 7, p. 665. Springer, Berlin, 1955.
225. Logan, V. H.: The results of splenectomy in Gaucher's disease. Surg. Gynec. Obstet., **72**, 807, 1941.
226. Habermann, P.: Pseudomiliares Lungenbild bei Morbus Gaucher. Arch. Kinderheilk., **144**, 268, 1952.
227. Merklen, P., Waitz, R., and Warter, J.: Un cas de maladie de Gaucher a determinations osseuses, avec cellules de Gaucher dans les crachats. Bull. Soc. Med. Hop. Paris, **49**, 36, 1933.
228. Brill, N. E., Mandlebaum, F. S., and Libman, E.: Primary splenomegaly—Gaucher type. Amer. J. Med. Sci., **129**, 491, 1905.

229. Zlotnick, A., and Groen, J. J.: Observations on a patient with Gaucher's disease. Amer. J. Med., **30**, 637, 1961.
230. Carbone, A. O., and Petrozzi, C.: Gaucher's disease: case report with stress on eye findings. Henry Ford Hosp. Med. J., **16**, 55, 1968.
231. Boudet, Ch., Costeau, J., and Raynaud, J. M.: Opacities cornéennes et maladie de Gaucher. Bull. Soc. Ophtal. Franc., **66**, 443, 1966.
232. Redslob, E., and Gery, L.: Localisations oculaires de la "maladie de Gaucher." Ann. Oculist. (Paris), **169**, 865, 1932.
233. Brill, N. E.: Primary splenomegaly. Amer. J. Med., **121**, 377, 1901.
234. East, T., and Savin, L. H.: A case of Gaucher's disease with biopsy of typical pingueculae. Brit. J. Ophth., **24**, 611, 1940.
235. Bloem, T. F., Groen, J., and Postma, C.: Gaucher's disease. Quart. J. Med., **5**, 517, 1936.
236. Wechsler, H. F., and Gustafson, E.: Gaucher's disease. New York J. Med., **40**, 133, 1940.
237. Baer, I., and Zimmermann, H. -B.: Morbus Gaucher beim Erwachsenen. Deutsch. Gesundh., **28**, 1297, 1967.
238. Teilum, G.: Die Gauchersche Krankheit; mit der Beschreibung eines Falles, der Veranderungen in der Hypophyse und im Hypothalamus zeigte. Acta Med. Scand., **116**, 170, 1944.
239. vanBogaert, L., and Fröhlich, A.: Un cas de maladie de Gaucher de l'adulte avec syndrome de Raynaud, pigmentation, et rigidité du type extra-pyramidal aux membres inférieurs. Ann. Med., **45**, 55, 1939.
240. Davison, C.: Disturbances in lipoid metabolism and the central nervous system. J. Mt. Sinai Hosp., **9**, 389, 1942.
241. Mislow, K.: The geometry of sphingosine. J. Amer. Chem. Soc., **74**, 5155, 1953.
242. Marinetti, G., and Stotz, E.: Studies on the structure of sphingomyelin. IV. Configuration of the double bond in sphingomyelin and related lipids and a study of their infrared spectra. J. Amer. Chem. Soc., **76**, 1347, 1954.
243. Carter, H. E., and Fujino, Y.: Biochemistry of the sphingolipides. IX. Configuration of the cerebrosides. J. Biol. Chem., **221**, 879, 1956.
244. Carter, H. E., Rothfus, J. A., and Gigg, R.: Biochemistry of the sphingolipids. XII. Conversion of cerebrosides to ceramides and sphingosine; structure of Gaucher cerebroside. J. Lipid Res., **2**, 228, 1961.
245. Carter, H. E., Norris, W. P., Glick, F. J., Phillips, G. E., and Harris, R.: Biochemistry of the sphingolipides. II. Isolation of dihydrosphingosine from the cerebroside fractions of beef brain and spinal cord. J. Biol. Chem., **170**, 269, 1947.
246. Carter, H. E., and Hirschberg, C. B.: Phytosphingosines and branched sphingosines in kidney. Biochemistry, **7**, 2296, 1968.
247. Karlsson, K. A., and Martensson, E.: Studies on sphingosines. XIV. On the phytosphingosine content of the major human kidney glycolipids. Biochim. Biophys. Acta, **152**, 230, 1968.
248. Thierfelder, H.: Ueber die Identität des Gehirnzuckers mit Galactose. Z. Physiol. Chem., **14**, 209, 1890.
249. Brown, H. T., and Morris, G. H.: VIII. Note on the identity of cerebrose and galactose. J. Chem. Soc., **57**, 57, 1890.
250. Klenk, E., and Rennkamp, F.: Über die Ganglioside und Cerebroside der Rindermilz. Z. Physiol. Chem., **273**, 253, 1942.
251. Brante, G.: Studies on the lipids in morbus Gaucher. I. Qualitative and quantitative determination of the hexose components in normal and Gaucher glycolipids. Acta Soc. Med. Upsal., **56**, 125, 1951.
252. Klenk, E.: The pathological chemistry of the developing brain, in *Biochemistry of the Developing Nervous System,* edited by E. Waelsch, p. 397. Academic, New York, 1955.
253. Nishimura, K., and Yamakawa, T.: Isolation of cerebroside containing glucose (glucosyl ceramide) and its possible significance in ganglioside synthesis. Lipids, **3**, 262, 1968.
254. Tamai, Y., and Yamakawa, T.: Glucocerebroside in brain of old patients. Jap. J. Exp. Med., **38**, 143, 1968.
255. Svennerholm, L., and Stallberg-Stenhagen, S.: Changes in the fatty acid composition of cerebrosides and sulfatides of human nervous tissue with age. J. Lipid Res., **9**, 215, 1968.
256. Nakayawa, T.: Studies on the conjugated lipids. I. On the configuration of cerebrosides. J. Biochem. (Japan), **37**, 309, 1950.
257. Carter, H. E., and Greenwood, F. L.: Biochemistry of the sphingolipides. VII. Structure of the cerebrosides. J. Biol. Chem., **199**, 283, 1952.
258. Radin, N. S., and Akahori, Y.: Fatty acids of human brain cerebrosides. J. Lipid Res., **2**, 335, 1961.
259. Bernhard, K., and Lesch, P.: Ein Beitrag zur Fettsäurezusammensetzung der Cerebroside, Sphingomyeline und Lecithine aus menschlichen Hirn. Helv. Chim. Acta, **46**, 1798, 1963.
260. Kishimoto, Y., and Radin, N. S.: Structures of the 2-hydroxy unsaturated fatty acids of pig brain sphingolipids. J. Lipid Res., **5**, 94, 1964.
261. Eng, L. F., Gerstl, B., Hayman, R. B., Lee, Y. L., Tietsort, R. W., and Smith, J. K.: The 2-hydroxy fatty acids in white matter of infant and adult brains. J. Lipid Res., **6**, 135, 1965.
262. O'Brien, J. S., and Sampson, E. L.: Fatty acid and fatty aldehyde composition of the major brain lipids in normal human gray matter, white matter and myelin. J. Lipid Res., **6**, 545, 1965.
263. Menkes, J. H., Philippart, M., and Concone, M. C.: Concentration and fatty acid composition of cerebrosides and sulfatides in mature and immature human brain. J. Lipid Res., **7**, 479, 1966.
264. Capella, P., Galli, C., and Fumagalli, R.: Hydroxy fatty acids from cerebrosides of the central nervous system: GLC determination and mass spectrometric identification. Lipids, **3**, 431, 1968.
265. Kishimoto, Y., and Radin, N. S.: Biosynthesis of nervonic acid and its homologues from carboxyl-labeled oleic acid. J. Lipid Res., **4**, 444, 1963.
266. Kopaczyk, K. C., and Radin, N. S.: In vivo conversions of cerebroside and ceramide in rat brain. J. Lipid Res., **6**, 140, 1965.
267. Kishimoto, Y., and Radin, N. S.: Composition of cerebroside acids as a function of age. J. Lipid Res., **1**, 79, 1959.
268. Kishimoto, Y., and Radin, N. S.: Isolation and detection methods for brain cerebrosides, hydroxy fatty acids and unsaturated fatty acids. J. Lipid Res., **1**, 72, 1959.
269. Svennerholm, E., and Svennerholm, L.: Neutral glycolipids of human blood serum, spleen and liver. Nature (London), **198**, 688, 1963.
270. Wagner, A.: Untersuchungen über Cerebroside aus menschlicher Milz. Clin. Chim. Acta, **10**, 175, 1964.
271. Makita, A., and Yamakawa, T.: Biochemistry of organ glycolipid. I. Ceramide oligo-hexosides of human, equine and bovine spleens, J. Biochem. (Japan), **51**, 124, 1962.
272. Kishimoto, Y., and Radin, N. S.: Occurrence of 2-hydroxy fatty acids in animal tissues. J. Lipid Res., **4**, 139, 1963.
273. Martensson, E.: Glycosphingolipids of animal tissue. Prog. Chem. Fats and Other Lipids, **10**, 365, 1969.
274. Martensson, E.: Neutral glycolipids of human kidney isolation, identification, and fatty acid composition. Biochim. Biophys. Acta, **116**, 296, 1966.
275. Vance, D. E., and Sweeley, C. C.: Quantitative determination of the neutral glycosyl ceramides in human blood. J. Lipid Res., **8**, 621, 1967.
276. Foote, J. L., and Coles, E.: Cerebrosides of human aorta: isolation, identification of the hexose, and fatty acid distribution. J. Lipid Res., **9**, 482, 1968.
277. Yurkowski, M., and Walker, B. L.: The carbohydrate moiety of rat mucosal cerebrosides. Biochim. Biophys. Acta, **158**, 299, 1968.
278. McKibbin, J. M.: The composition of the glycolipids in dog intestine. Biochemistry, **8**, 679, 1969.
279. Makita, A.: Biochemistry of organ glycolipids. II. Isolation of human kidney glycolipids. J. Biochem., **55**, 269, 1964.
280. Feldman, G. L., Feldman, L. S., and Rouser, G.: Occurrence of glycolipids in the lens of the human eye. J. Amer. Oil. Chem. Soc., **42**, 742, 1965.
281. Miras, C. J., Mantzos, J. D., and Levis, G. M.: The isolation and partial characterization of glycolipids of normal human leukocytes. Biochem. J., **98**, 782, 1966.
282. Dod, B. J., and Gray, G. M.: The localization of the neutral glycosphingolipids in rat liver cells. Biochem. J., **110**, 50P, 1968.
283. Gallai-Hatchand, J., and Gray, G. M.: The isolation and partial characterisation of the glycolipids from pig lung. Biochim. Biophys. Acta, **116**, 532, 1966.
284. Svennerholm, L.: Gangliosides and other glycolipids of human plasma. Acta Chem. Scand., **19**, 1506, 1965.
285. Svennerholm, E., and Svennerholm, L.: Isolation of blood serum glycolipids. Acta Chem. Scand., **16**, 1282, 1962.

286. Svennerholm, E., and Svennerholm, L.: The separation of neutral blood-serum glycolipids by thin layer chromatography. Biochim. Biophys. Acta, **70,** 432, 1963.
287. Moser, H. W., and Karnovsky, M. L.: Studies on the biosynthesis of glycolipides and other lipides of the brain. J. Biol. Chem., **234,** 1990, 1959.
288. Kishimoto, Y., and Radin, N. S.: Metabolism of brain glycolipid fatty acids. Lipids, **1,** 47, 1966.
289. Nishimura, K., Ueta, N., and Yamakawa, T.: Incorporation of labeled hexose into brain cerebrosides. Jap. J. Exp. Med., **36,** 91, 1966.
290. Maker, H. S., and Hauser, G.: Incorporation of glucose carbon into gangliosides and cerebrosides by slices of developing rat brain. J. Neurochem., **14,** 457, 1967.
291. Burton, R. M., Sodd, M. A., and Brady, R. O.: The incorporation of galactose into galactolipides. J. Biol. Chem., **233,** 1053, 1958.
292. Burton, R. M.: Biochemistry of sphingosine containing lipids, in *Lipids and Lipidoses,* edited by G. Schettler, p. 122. Springer-Verlag, New York, 1967.
293. Fujino, Y., and Nakano, Mo.: Enzymic synthesis of cerebroside from ceramide and uridine diphosphate galactose. Biochem. J., **113,** 573, 1969.
294. Basu, S., Kaufman, B., and Roseman, S.: Enzymatic synthesis of ceramide-glucose and ceramide-lactose by glycosyltransferases from embryonic chicken brain. J. Biol. Chem., **243,** 5802, 1968.
295. Morell, P., and Radin, N. S.: Synthesis of cerebroside by brain from uridine diphosphate galactose and ceramide containing hydroxy fatty acid. Biochemistry, **8,** 506, 1969.
296. Cleland, W. W., and Kennedy, E. P.: The enzymatic synthesis of psychosine. J. Biol. Chem., **235,** 45, 1960.
297. Brady, R. O.: Studies on the total enzymatic synthesis of cerebrosides. J. Biol. Chem., **237,** PC2416, 1962.
298. Neskovic, N. M., Nussbaum, J. L., and Mandel, P.: Enzymatic synthesis of psychosine in "jimpy" mice brain. FEBS Letters, **3,** 199, 1969.
299. Basu, S.: Synthesis of glucosylceramide by an enzyme from embryonic chicken brain. Fed. Proc., **27,** 346, 1968.
300. Curtino, J. A., Calderon, R. O., and Caputto, R.: Enzymatic synthesis of gangliosides—the binding of glucose. Fed. Proc., **27,** 346, 1968.
301. Gatt, S., and Rapport, M. M.: Isolation of β-galactosidase and β-glucosidase from brain. Biochim. Biophys. Acta, **113,** 567, 1966.
302. Hajra, A. K., Bowen, D. M., Kishimoto, Y., and Radin, N. S.: Cerebroside galactosidase of brain. J. Lipid Res., **7,** 379, 1966.
303. Bowen, D. M., and Radin, N. S.: Purification of cerebroside galactosidase from rat brain. Biochim. Biophys. Acta, **152,** 587, 1968.
304. Bowen, D. M., and Radin, N. S.: Properties of cerebroside galactosidase. Biochim. Biophys. Acta, **152,** 599, 1968.
305. Gatt, S., and Rapport, M. M.: Hydrolysis of ceramide lactoside and ceramide glucoside by glycosidases from brain. Israeli J. Med. Sci., **1,** 624, 1965.
306. Gatt, S.: Enzymic hydrolysis of sphingolipids: hydrolysis of ceramide glucoside by an enzyme from ox brain. Biochem. J., **101,** 687, 1966.
307. Brady, R. O., Kanfer, J., and Shapiro, D.: The metabolism of glucocerebrosides. I. Purification and properties of a glucocerebroside-cleaving enzyme from spleen tissue. J. Biol. Chem., **240,** 39, 1965.
308. Brady, R. O., Gal, A. E., Kanfer, J. N., and Bradley, R. M.: The metabolism of glucocerebrosides. III. Purification and properties of a glucosyl- and galactosylceramide-cleaving enzyme from rat intestinal tissue. J. Biol. Chem., **240,** 3766, 1965.
309. Gatt, S.: Comparison of four enzymes from brain which hydrolyze sphingolipids, in *Inborn Disorders of Sphingolipid Metabolism,* Proceedings of the Third International Symposium on the Cerebral Sphingolipidoses, edited by S. M. Aronson and B. W. Volk, p. 261. Pergamon, New York, 1967.
310. Kampine, J. P., Kanfer, J. N., Gal, A. E., Bradley, R. M., and Brady, R. O.: Response of sphingolipid hydrolases in spleen and liver to increased erythrocytorhexis. Biochim. Biophys. Acta, **137,** 135, 1967.
311. Kampine, J. P., Brady, R. O., Yankee, R. A., Kanfer, J. N., Shapiro, D., and Gal, A. E.: Sphingolipid metabolism in leukemic leukocytes. Cancer Res., **27,** 1312, 1967.
312. Patrick, A. D.: A deficiency of glucocerebrosidase in Gaucher's disease. Biochem. J., **97,** 17c, 1965.
313. Brady, R. O., Kanfer, J. N., Bradley, R. M., and Shapiro, D.: Demonstration of a deficiency of glucocerebroside-cleaving enzyme in Gaucher's disease. J. Clin. Invest., **45,** 1112, 1966.
314. Snyder, R. A., and Brady, R. O.: The use of white cells as a source of diagnostic material for lipid storage diseases. Clin. Chim. Acta, **25,** 331, 1969.
315. Rouser, G., Bauman, A. J., and Kritchevsky, G.: New methods for the separation and quantitative isolation of lipids: initial applications to the study of beef brain and spleen lipids in Gaucher's disease. Amer. J. Clin. Nutr., **9,** 112, 1961.
316. Fredrickson, D. S., and Hofmann, A. F.: Gaucher's disease, in *The Metabolic Basis of Inherited Disease,* 1st ed., edited by J. B. Stanbury, J. B. Wyngaarden, and D. S. Fredrickson, p. 603. McGraw-Hill, New York, 1960.
317. Philippart, M., and Menkes, J.: Isolation and characterization of the main splenic glycolipids in Gaucher's disease: evidence for the site of metabolic block. Biochem. Biophys. Res. Commun., **15,** 551, 1964.
318. Valdiguie, P., Douste-Blazy, L., Didier, A., and Soula, G.: Les Cérébrosides spléniques dans la maladie de Gaucher. Ann. Biol. Clin. (Paris), **23,** 857, 1965.
319. Taketomi, T., and Yamakawa, T.: Sphingomyelin and glucocerebroside of spleen in cases of Gaucher's and Niemann-Pick's diseases. Japan J. Exp. Med., **37,** 505, 1967.
320. Norton, W. T., and Brotz, M.: New galactolipids of brain: a monoalkyl-monoacyl-glyceryl galactoside and cerebroside fatty acid esters. Biochem. Biophys. Res. Commun., **12,** 198, 1963.
321. Klenk, E., and Doss, M.: Über das Vorkommen von Estercerebrosidin im Gehirn. Hoppe Seyler. Z. Physiol. Chem., **346,** 296, 1966.
322. Tamai, Y., Taketomi, T., and Yamakawa, T.: New glycolipids in bovine brain. Jap. J. Exp. Med., **37,** 79, 1967.
323. Klenk, E., and Lohr, J. P.: Über die Estercerebroside des Gehirns. Hoppe Seyler. Z. Physiol. Chem., **348,** 1712, 1967.
324. Kishimoto, Y., Wajda, M., and Radin, N. S.: 6-Acyl galactosyl ceramides of pig brain: structure and fatty acid composition. J. Lipid Res., **9,** 27, 1968.
325. Parke, D. V.: The occurrence of lactose in the spleen cerebrosides of Gaucher's disease. Clin. Sci., **22,** 119, 1962.
326. Svennerholm, L.: Personal communication.
327. Rouser, G., Galli, C., and Kritchevsky, G.: Lipid class composition of normal human brain and variations in metachromatic leucodystrophy, Tay-Sachs, Niemann-Pick, chronic Gaucher's and Alzheimer's diseases. J. Amer. Oil. Chem. Soc., **42,** 404, 1965.
328. Menkes, J. H., and Migeon, B. R.: Biochemical and genetic aspects of mental retardation. Ann. Rev. Med., **17,** 407, 1966.
329. Balint, J. A., Spitzer, H. L., and Kyriakides, E. C.: Studies of red-cell stromal lipids in Tay-Sachs disease and other lipidoses. J. Clin. Invest., **42,** 1661, 1963.
330. Polonovski, J., and Petit, M.: Determination of cerebrosides in the blood serum. Ann. Biol. Clin. (Paris), **21,** 583, 1963.
331. Polonovski, J., and Petit, M.: Osidolipides du sérum sanguin humain. Bull. Soc. Chim. Biol. (Paris), **45,** 111, 1963.
332. VanHoof, F., and Hers, H. G.: The abnormalities of lysosomal enzymes in mucopolysaccharidoses. Europ. J. Biochem., **7,** 34, 1968.
333. Tuchman, L. R., Suna, H., and Carr, J. J.: Elevation of serum acid phosphatase in Gaucher's disease. J. Mt. Sinai Hosp., **23,** 227, 1956.
334. Tuchman, L. R., Goldstein, G., and Clyman, M.: Studies on the nature of the increased serum acid phosphatase in Gaucher's disease. Amer. J. Med., **27,** 959, 1959.
335. Abul-F-Adl, M. A. M., and King, E. J.: Properties of the acid phosphatases of erythrocytes and human prostate gland. Biochem. J., **45,** 51, 1949.
336. Czitober, H., Grundig, E., and Schobel, B.: Histochemische und biochemische Untersuchungen bei Morbus Gaucher. Klin. Wschr., **42,** 1179, 1964.
337. Goldberg, A. F., Takakura, K., and Rosenthal, R. L.: Electrophoretic separation of serum acid phosphatase isoenzymes in Gaucher's disease, prostatic carcinoma and multiple myeloma. Nature (London), **211,** 41, 1966.
338. Ramot, B., and Streifler, C.: Serum and tissue acid α-naphthylphosphatase isozymes in various diseases. Israel J. Med. Sci., **3,** 505, 1967.

338a. Kaulen, H. D., Henning, R., and Stoffel, W.: Comparison of some enzymes of the lysosomal and the plasma membrane of the rat liver cell. Z. Physiol. Chem., **351,** 1555, 1970.

339. Kessel, A. W. L., and Signy, A. G.: Acid hyperphosphatasia in three families with osteogenesis imperfecta. Lancet, **2,** 1217, 1956.

340. Trimble, G. X.: Critique and cavil. J. Amer. Med. Ass., **195,** 379, 1966.

341. Öckerman, P. A., and Kohlin, P.: Acid hydrolases in plasma in Gaucher's disease. Clin. Chem., **15,** 61, 1969.

342. Fredrickson, D. S.: Sphingomyelin lipidosis: Niemann-Pick disease, in *The Metabolic Basis of Inherited Disease,* 2d ed., edited by J. B. Stanbury, J. B. Wyngaarden, and D. S. Fredrickson, chap. 28, p. 586. McGraw-Hill, New York, 1966.

343. Stacher, A., and Stockl, W.: Freie Aminosauren in Plasma and Milz von Patienten mit Morbus Gaucher. Wien. Klin. Wschr., **80,** 104, 1968.

344. Hultberg, B., Öckerman, P. A., and Eriksson, O.: Urinary amino acids in storage disorders: mucopolysaccharidosis, Gaucher's disease and metachromatic leucodystrophy. Metabolism, **18,** 713, 1969.

345. Pratt, P. W., Estren, S., and Kochwa, S.: Immunoglobulin abnormalities in Gaucher's disease: report of 16 cases. Blood, **31,** 633, 1968.

346. Pinkhas, J., Djaldetti, M., and Yaron, M.: Coincidence of multiple myeloma with Gaucher's disease. Israel J. Med. Sci., **1,** 537, 1965.

347. Rapport, M. M., and Graf, L.: Immunochemical reactions of lipids. Progr. Allerg., **13,** 274, 1969.

348. Gelfand, M. I., and Griboff, S. I.: Gaucher's disease and acute leukemia. J. Mt. Sinai Hosp., **28,** 278, 1961.

349. Albrecht, V. M.: "Gaucher-Zellen" bei chronisch myeloischer Leukamie. Blut, **13,** 169, 1966.

350. Smith, W. C., Kaneshiro, M. M., Goldstein, B. D., Parker, J. W., and Lukes, R. J.: Gaucher cells in chronic granulocytic leukemia. Lancet, **2,** 780, 1968.

351. Gerdes, J., Marathe, R. L., Bloodworth, J. M. B., and Mackinney, A. A., Jr.: Gaucher cells in chronic granulocytic leukemia. Arch. Path. (Chicago), **88,** 194, 1969.

352. Kattlove, H. E., Williams, J. C., Gaynor, E., Spivack, M., Bradley, R. M., and Brady, R. O.: Gaucher cells in chronic myelocytic leukemia: an acquired abnormality. Blood, **33,** 379, 1969.

353. Rosner, F., Dosik, H., Kaiser, S. S., Lee, S. L., and Morrison, A. N.: Gaucher cells in leukemia. J. A. M. A., **209,** 935, 1969.

354. Lee, R. E., and Lawrence, D. Ellis: "Gaucher cells" in chronic myelogenous leukemia, abstract, 67th Annual Meeting of the American Association of Pathologists and Bacteriologists, St. Louis, Mo., 1970 (to be published in American Journal of Pathology).

355. Melamed, S., and Chester, W.: Osseous form of Gaucher's disease. Arch. Intern. Med., **61,** 798, 1938.

356. Kampine, J. P., Brady, R. O., Kanfer, J. N., Feld, M., and Shapiro, D.: Diagnosis of Gaucher's disease and Niemann-Pick disease with small samples of venous blood. Science, **155,** 86, 1967.

357. Brady, R. O.: Genetics and the sphingolipidoses. Med. Clin. N. Amer., **53,** 827, 1969.

358. Öckerman, P. A.: Identity of β-glucosidase, β-xylosidase and one of the β-galactosidase activities in human liver when assayed with 4-methylumbelliferyl-beta-D-glycosides; studies in cases of Gaucher's disease. Biochim. Biophys. Acta, **165,** 59, 1968.

359. Öckerman, P. A., and Kohlin, P.: Tissue acid hydrolase activities in Gaucher's disease. Scand. J. Clin. Lab. Invest., **22,** 62, 1968.

360. Hayduk, K., Eggstein, M., Kaufmann, W., and Waller, H. D.: Morbus Gaucher mit Glutathionreduktase-Mangel in den Blutzellen. Deutsch. Med. Wschr., **93,** 1063, 1968.

361. Trams, E. G., and Brady, R. O.: Cerebroside synthesis in Gaucher's disease. J. Clin. Invest., **39,** 1546, 1960.

362. Stein, M. H., and Gardner, L. I.: Possible site of biochemical error in Gaucher's disease. Lancet, **2,** 1254, 1960.

363. Okada, M.: Gaucher's disease. Tokyo Med. Coll. J., **24,** 407, 1966.

364. Tropp, C.: Beitrag zur Pathogenese der Gaucherschen und Niemann-Pickschen Erkrankung. Klin. Wschr., **1,** 562, 1936.

365. Collier, W. A.: A case of enlarged spleen in a child aged six. Trans. Path. Soc. London, **46,** 148, 1895.

366. Hsia, D. Y., Naylor, J., and Bigler, J. A.: The genetic mechanism of Gaucher's disease, in *Cerebral Sphingolipidoses,* edited by S. M. Aronson and B. W. Volk, p. 327. Academic, New York, 1962.

367. Groen, J. J.: Gaucher's disease: hereditary transmission and racial distribution. Arch. Intern. Med., **113,** 543, 1964.

368. Hsia, D. Y., Naylor, J., and Bigler, J. A.: Gaucher's disease: report of two cases in father and son and review of the literature. New Eng. J. Med., **261,** 164, 1959.

369. Farber, S.: in *The Child in Health and Disease: A Textbook for Students and Practitioners of Medicine,* edited by C. G. Grulee, and R. C. Eley, 2d ed., p. 600. Williams & Wilkins, Baltimore, 1952.

370. Josephson, A.: Cited by D. Y. Hsia, J. Naylor, and J. A. Bigler, in *Cerebral Sphingolipidoses,* edited by S. M. Aronson and B. W. Volk, p. 327. Academic, New York, 1962.

371. Anderson, J. P.: Hereditary Gaucher's disease. J.A.M.A., **101,** 979, 1933.

372. Lowinger, S.: Die Bedeutung der Knochenmark- und Milzpunktion für die Diagnose des Morbus Gaucher. Folia Haemat. (Frankfurt), **53,** 126, 1935.

373. Gordon, W. H., and Kaufman, J. M.: Gaucher's disease; discussion and case presentation. J. Mich. State Med. Soc., **49,** 785, 1950.

374. Stransky, E., and Dauis-Lawas, D. F.: Heredity in the infantile type of Gaucher's disease. Amer. J. Dis. Child, **78,** 694, 1949.

375. Stransky, E., and Conchu, T. L.: Heredity in the infantile type of Gaucher's disease. Ann. Paediat. Fenn., **177,** 319, 1951.

376. Gerken, H., Graucob, E., and Wiedemann, H.-R.: Inheritance in Gaucher's disease. Brit. Med. J., 5424, 1594, 1964.

377. Wiedemann, H.-R., and Gerken, H.: Gaucher cells in healthy relatives of patients with Gaucher's disease. Lancet, **2,** 866, 1964.

378. Macario, A. J. L.: Enfermedad de Gaucher. Estudio hemático de una enferma y sus padres. Prensa Med. Argent., **52,** 245, 1965.

379. Gerken, V. A., and Wiedemann, H.-R.: Zur Frage des Erbganges und eines Heterozygotennachweises bei der Gaucherschen Krankheit. Deutsch. Med. Wschr., **91,** 1267, 1966.

380. Groen, J. J.: Present status of knowledge of Gaucher's disease. Israel J. Med. Sci., **1,** 507, 1965.

381. Fried, K.: Gaucher's disease among the Jews of Israel. Bull. Res. Council Israel, **7B,** 213, 1958.

382. Fried, K., Matoth, Y., and Goldschmidt, E.: Gaucher's disease—chronic adult type, in *The Genetics of Migrant and Isolate Populations,* edited by E. Goldschmidt, p. 292. Williams & Wilkins, Baltimore, 1963.

383. Notti, J., and Giunta, J. J.: Gaucher's disease. J. Dis. Child., **85,** 90, 1958.

384. Solidoro, A., Cabello, T., Orlandini, O., and Pasco, T.: Enfermedad de Gaucher: à propósito de tres casos. Acta Cancer, **4,** 24, 1965.

385. Lascano, R. J., and Barcia, J. M.: Enfermedad de Gaucher. Prensa Med. Argent., **53,** 1260, 1966.

386. Spackman, W. C., and Mackie, F. P.: Gaucher's type of splenomegaly in a Mahratta village, with a case treated by splenectomy. Indian Med. Gaz., Feb., p. 69, 1925.

387. Rao, K. S., Subramanyam, T. N., Gangadharan, D., and Reddy, S. S.: Gaucher's disease. J. Indian Med. Ass., **52,** 219, 1969.

388. Hashem, N.: Genetics of Gaucher's disease: clinico-pathological study of a case. J. Egypt. Med. Ass., **45,** 863, 1962.

389. Tümay, S. B., Bigler, M., and Ulukutlu, L.: Gaucher Hastalinginda Teshis Dayanaklani, Ist. Tip Fak. Mec., **28,** 327, 1965.

390. Ghandur-Mnaymneh, L., and Darbous, I.: Clinico-pathological conference. Lebanese Med. J., **19,** 263, 1966.

391. Berry, P. R.: Gaucher's disease: report of a New Zealand case. New Zeal. Med. J., **64,** 15, 1965.

392. Woodfield, D. G., and Rouse, J. E.: Gaucher's disease in a Maori. New Zeal. Med. J., **65,** 701, 1966.

393. Danes, B. S., and Bearn, A. G.: Gaucher's disease: a genetic disease detected in skin fibroblast cultures. Science, **161,** 1347, 1968.

394. Taysi, K., Kistenmacher, M. L., Punnett, H. H., and Mellman, W. J.: Limitations of metachromasia as a diagnostic aid in pediatrics. New Eng. J. Med., **281,** 1108, 1969.

394a. Beutler, E., and Kuhl, W.: Detection of the defect of Gaucher's disease and its carrier state in peripheral-blood leucocytes. Lancet, **1** (Mar. 21), 612, 1970.

395. Bodian, M., and Lake, B. D.: The rectal approach to neuropathology. Brit. J. Surg., **50,** 702, 1963.
396. Kamoshita, S., and Landing, B. H.: Distribution of lesions in myenteric plexus and gastrointestinal mucosa in lipidoses and other neurologic disorders of children. Amer. J. Clin. Path., **49,** 312, 1968.
397. Durand, P., Philippart, M., Borrone, C., Cella, G. D., and Bugiani, O.: Una nuova malattia da accumulo di glicolipidi. Minerva Pediat., **19,** 2187, 1967.
398. Durand, P., Borrone, C., and Della Cella, G.: Fucosidosis. J. Pediat., **75.** 665, 1969.
399. Dawson, G., and Stein, A. O.: Lactosyl ceramidosis: Catabolic enzyme defect of glycosphingolipid metabolism. Science, **170,** 556, 1970.
400. Dawson, G., and Matalon, R.: Lactosyl ceramidosis: Biochemical and genetic studies in cultured fibroblasts. J. Pediat. (in press).

CHAPTER THIRTY-FOUR

GALACTOSYL CERAMIDE LIPIDOSIS: GLOBOID CELL LEUCODYSTROPHY (KRABBE'S DISEASE)*

Kunihiko Suzuki and Yoshiyuki Suzuki

Globoid cell leucodystrophy, or Krabbe's disease, is an inherited metabolic disorder of the nervous system, generally becoming clinically evident during the first year of life. The majority of the patients show the first signs of the disease by age 3 to 6 months, with progressive retardation in development, prominent long-tract signs such as spastic quadriparesis, cortical blindness, optic atrophy, deafness, and pseudobulbar palsy. The clinical course is almost invariably rapidly progressive and patients rarely survive beyond the second year of life. Histopathologically, lesions are confined to the nervous system, particularly to the central nervous system. In the white matter, there is a paucity of myelin and oligodendroglia, severe astrocytic gliosis, and massive infiltration with unique multinucleated globoid cells. Gray matter is relatively preserved, but the peripheral nerves often show degenerative changes in the axons and the myelin sheath. The white matter shows a severe decrease of glycolipids, of both galactosyl ceramide and sulfatide.

The degree of sulfatide loss is disproportionately greater than that of cerebroside. The globoid cells are rich in galactosyl ceramide (Fig. 34-1), and intracerebrally injected galactosyl ceramide elicits a globoid cell reaction in a normal brain. Deficiencies of two enzymes, both directly related to galactosyl ceramide metabolism, have been reported. These are cerebroside-sulfatide sulfotransferase and galactosyl ceramide β-galactosidase. The more recently reported deficiency of galactosyl ceramide β-galactosidase appears to be the genetically determined primary enzymatic defect.

HISTORY

Krabbe described the clinical and histologic findings of two siblings who died of an "acute infantile familial diffuse sclerosis of the brain" in 1916 [1]. He noted familial occurrence, early onset of spasticity, and a rapidly progressive course to death. He gave a detailed description of the globoid cells, which are now considered the histological hallmark of the disease. A retrospective search of the neuropathological literature revealed two earlier descriptions of similar abnormal cells. Bullard and Southard [2] described multinucleated giant cells in the perivascular regions of the brain in a patient who developed an acutely progressive illness at age 6 years. Death occurred only 6 months after the clinical onset of the disease. The clinical features, as well as the distribution of lesions within the brain, were not typical of what is now known as Krabbe's globoid cell leucodystrophy, and the lack of illustrations makes it difficult to assess the exact histological nature of the case. In 1908, Beneke [3] also described similar large cells in the brain, which showed, in addition, areas of both diffuse sclerosis and patchy plaques of demyelination. In view of the uncertainties in these earlier reports, the first description of the disease is now credited to Krabbe. Collier and Greenfield [4] were the first to coin the term *globoid* to describe the numerous abnormal cells in the white matter. Although they called the disease *encephalitis periaxialis of Schilder,* they clearly described the morphological features of the disease now known as Krabbe's globoid cell leucodystrophy.

There was little progress in the understanding of the disease until the development of chemical and histochemical means of investigation. Hallervorden's earlier suggestion [5] that globoid cells might contain kerasin (a cerebroside) received the support of chemical [6, 7] and histochemical studies [8–10]. The experimental induction of the globoid reaction—demonstrated by Austin and coworkers [11, 12] and also by Olsson et al. [13]—by intracerebral injection of galactosyl ceramide, but not by any other lipids, further supported the notion of a close relationship between the globoid cells and cerebroside. Analytically, the most consistent abnormality in the white matter appeared to be the reduced ratio of sulfatide to cerebroside [14, 15]. In 1967, Austin and coworkers [16, 17] reported deficient activities of cerebroside-sulfatide sulfotransferase in the brains and kidneys of two patients, and concluded that this deficiency was probably responsible for the relative lack of sulfatide. Most recently profound deficiency of galactosyl ceramide β-galactosidase was demonstrated in the brain, liver, spleen, and kidney in eight patients [18, 19, 20]. The same deficiency was also found in peripheral leukocytes, serum, and cultured fibroblasts [21].

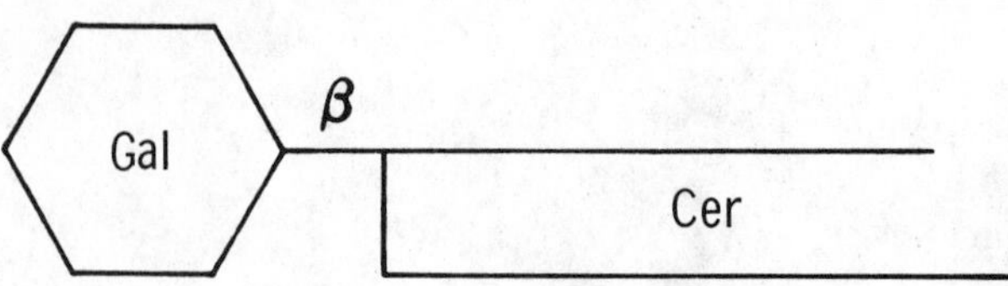

Figure 34-1. Galactosyl ceramide (galactocerebroside).

*Work carried out in the authors' laboratory was supported by research grants NS-08420 and NS-08075 from the Public Health Service, and the Inex J. Warriner Memorial Grant for Research on Multiple Sclerosis (670–A–1) from the National Multiple Sclerosis Society.
We thank Drs. Nicholas K. Gonatas and Kinuko Suzuki, Department of Pathology, Division of Neuropathology, University of Pennsylvania School of Medicine, for their advice regarding the section on morphology.

CLINICAL ASPECTS

Incidence and Heredity

Globoid cell leucodystrophy is a rare disease. Less than 100 cases have been recorded since the first description of Krabbe [1]. The incidence among the general population is not known. The geographical distribution is widespread. This disease has been reported in England, Germany, France, Italy, Switzerland, Sweden, the Netherlands, Poland, Russia, the United States, Canada, Denmark, and Japan. There seems to be no ethnic preponderance in incidence.

The disease occurs equally in both sexes. It is hereditary and in about half of the examples in the literature more than one member of the family has been involved. Krabbe himself reported two instances in sibs (Cases 1 and 2; 3 and 4). The consanguinity of parents has been reported in three families [22, 23]. The mode of inheritance is considered to be autosomal recessive. Involvement of more than one generation is not recorded.

Age of Onset

The clinical onset of the disease in most patients in the literature is during the period between 3 and 6 months after birth. Usually, the patient develops normally until this age, but patients may show clinical abnormalities soon after birth. The patient of Schochet et al. [24] was "stiff" from birth, and had a tendency to keep her fists clenched and her arms and legs extended. The patient of Hagberg et al. [25] vomited from the first week of life, which, together with malnutrition, prompted the parents to bring the baby to the hospital at age 2½ months. Some patients developed slowly for the first few months [7, 26, 27]. It is possible that more might have had earlier undetected symptoms.

Rarely, the disease occurs in late infancy [28]. Some of the patients with later onset, in childhood [2, 4, 23] or in adulthood [29–33], are often classified as having globoid cell leucodystrophy. The histological features are similar and they may well have been examples of this disease. All of these reports of atypical late cases appeared in 1954 or earlier, however, and the diagnoses merit reevaluation in the light of current clinical and histological diagnostic criteria.

Clinical Manifestations

Krabbe's original description [1] of five patients well represents what remains the typical clinical course and manifestations of the disease. It is steadily progressive. Hagberg [34] divided the entire course into three stages. Stage I is characterized by generalized hyperirritability, hyperaesthesia, episodic fever of unknown origin, and some stiffness of the limbs. The child, apparently normal for the first few months after birth, becomes hypersensitive to external stimuli, auditory, tactile, or visual, and begins to cry frequently without any apparent cause. Slight retardation or regression of psychomotor development, vomiting with feeding difficulty, and convulsive seizures may occur as initial clinical symptoms. The CSF protein is already increased. In stage II, rapid and severe motor and mental deterioration develop. There is marked hypertonicity, with extremely extended and crossed legs, flexed arms, and backward-bent head. Tendon reflexes are hyperactive. Minor tonic or clonic seizures occur. Optic atrophy and sluggish pupillary reactions to light may be observed. Stage III is the "burnt-out stage" which is attained often within a few weeks or months. The infant is decerebrate, blind, and has no contact with his surroundings. Deafness may appear. This final stage may last for many years, although the patient rarely survives for more than 2 years.

Head size is often small [35, 36, 37], but Yunis et al. [38] reported a patient with a large head suggesting macrocephaly at age 7½ months. It remained relatively large compared to body weight, with a large and open anterior fontanel at age 12 months. The head size of patient 2 in the report of Nelson et al. [28] was 50 cm at 1 year and 3 months, exceeding the 97th percentile.

The symptoms and signs are confined almost exclusively to those of the nervous system. The viscera are not enlarged. Vomiting is sometimes prominent, resulting in progressive loss of weight. Musty ammoniacal breath was present in one case [38], the origin of which was unknown.

Involvement of the peripheral nerves was considered uncommon in globoid cell leucodystrophy, in contrast to metachromatic leucodystrophy, in which it was first observed pathologically by Jacobi [39]. But since Matsuyama et al. [40] emphasized the pathological changes in peripheral nerves in globoid cell leucodystrophy, the peripheral nerve lesion has been intensively studied clinically and pathologically. Clinical examination does not always reveal neuropathy, especially in the early stages, because symptoms and signs of central nervous system involvement are overwhelming. Krabbe [1] pointed out originally that the knee jerks could not be elicited in any of his five patients, and that stiffness passed into a flaccid state toward the end of the disease. Since then several authors have reported absent or depressed tendon reflexes in a single examination [22, 35, 41–46] or disappearance of tendon reflexes in the course of the disease [36, 46, 47], although there are descriptions of patients with normal [28] or hyperactive [48] tendon reflexes at age 15 months. Dunn et al. [46] concluded that tendon reflexes are usually depressed after the first 6 months.

A Typical Clinical History [35]

The patient, a male, was born at 40-weeks of gestation with a birth weight of 7 lb 10 oz. The family history was noncontributory. Growth, development, and general health appeared to be unremarkable until age 4½ months, when he had a generalized seizure associated with fever. At 5 months definite motor and developmental retardation as well as marked irritability were observed. Head control was poor. A "clasp-knife" response was present in all extremities. In contrast the deep-tendon reflexes were decreased. Inspection of the fundi indicated loss of the foveal light reflex with equivocal pallor of the optic disc. Response to auditory stimuli was normal. An appropriate response to pain was demonstrated in all extremities. There was no enlargement of the viscera. Cerebral, muscle, and sural nerve biopsies at age 8 months established the diagnosis. At age 1 year the infant required tube feedings and responded poorly to environmental stimuli. Occasional myoclonic seizures were observed. Spastic quadriparesis, prominent initially, later gave way to flaccidity with diminished deep tendon reflexes. The head circumference at age 5 months was in the 25th percentile, and by age 9 months was below the 3rd percentile. The patient deteriorated steadily and died at age 14 months.

Atypical Cases

Some patients in the literature show atypical or misleading clinical histories. Wallace et al. [41] reported a patient who developed mental deterioration, apparently after mumps, at age 5 months. Convulsions started at age 7 months and the disease progressed. The clinical diagnosis was mumps encephalitis, and the final diagnosis was established only at autopsy. A patient with a rapid course (total of 3 months) reported by Osetowska et al. [42] was diagnosed as having "encephalitis." The symptoms in the patient of Nelson et al. [28] were apparently triggered by a fall at age 9 months and were further aggravated by a second fall at age 14 months. The patient of Bullard et al. [2], age 5½ years, who has been considered by many authors as a case of globoid cell leucodystrophy, started with "nervousness" and difficulty walking, after falling backward down the stairs without loss of consciousness.

Collier and Greenfield [4] described a 4½-year-old girl who developed a spastic and ataxic gait, with loss of vision, which gradually became worse during the following 6 months. Mentation was normal and she had no seizures. The CSF was normal. It was more than a year later that mental deterioration appeared. This patient was reported as having Schilder's disease, but numerous "globoid" cells were seen histologically. This report seems to be generally accepted as a case of globoid cell leucodystrophy.

A boy recorded by Blackwood and Cumings [7] had slight left hemiparesis at birth. This became worse following measles, when left hemiconvulsions occurred. He died at age 3 years and 2 months, and was diagnosed histologically as globoid cell leucodystrophy.

The morphological diagnosis of some patients with the so-called *adult type* of globoid cell leucodystrophy [29, 30] has been questioned by Poser and van Bogaert [49] and by Norman et al. [50].

Laboratory Findings

No specific abnormalities have been recorded in blood chemistry.

The CSF protein is usually high with a normal cell count. The CSF was reported to be normal in only a few cases in the literature [4, 22]. Hagberg et al. [25] stated that the electrophoretic pattern of CSF protein was of diagnostic help, in that albumin and α_2-globulin were elevated and β_1- and γ-globulins were decreased. This remained constant throughout the course of the disease, and the same pattern was found only in metachromatic leucodystrophy [51]. A marked increase of globulin in the CSF was reported by Dunn et al. [46].

Allen et al. [52] found much increased β-glucuronidase activity in the CSF in globoid cell leucodystrophy, as well as in diffuse meningeal dissemination of neoplasm and in acute necrotic myelopathy. The activity of this enzyme is normal in metachromatic leucodystrophy. They claimed that the increased β-glucuronidase activity is of diagnostic value in globoid cell leucodystrophy, if the clinical features are fully considered [53].

Radiological examinations usually reveal only diffuse and symmetrical cerebral atrophy. Rarely there is asymmetry demonstrated by pneumoencephalography or brain scan [38].

The EEG is normal in the initial stages, but gradually the cerebral rhythms become abnormal. Background activity becomes slow and disorganized [24, 28, 35, 37, 38, 48, 54–56], with changes that may be asymmetrical [38]. This is often accompanied by paroxysmal or epileptic discharges [24, 26, 28, 35, 37, 55–57]. One of two atypical patients with late onset [58] had three successive normal EEGs; in the other there was increasingly slow activity and a few focal spikes.

In accord with the clinical and pathological observations of peripheral neuropathy, various abnormal results have been obtained by electrophysiological procedures. Those include a mild increase in polyphasic motor unit potentials [37] and a few fibrillations [35, 37] in the routine EMG. Motor nerve conduction velocity seems to be more sensitive in the detection of peripheral neuropathy in globoid cell leucodystrophy, and all patients who have been examined show low conduction velocity [22, 24, 35, 37]. Even in one patient with a normal EMG, motor nerve conduction velocity was reduced, and this became more prominent as the disease progressed [46]. Distal sensory latency of the median nerve was also prolonged in one patient [37].

Clinical Diagnosis

Poser and van Bogaert [49] stated that it was almost impossible to make a clinical diagnosis of the leucodystrophies unless there was a well-documented family history. The statement, in its strictest sense, remains valid for globoid cell leucodystrophy. As already described, many patients have typical histories and clinical manifestations. Even though there are no pathognomonic signs, globoid cell leucodystrophy can be suspected clinically.

The disease can be differentiated from nonprogressive CNS disorders of congenital or perinatal origin on the basis of the history of normal development for the first few months after birth, proceeding to psychomotor deterioration. Rarely, the disease may first be considered to be of traumatic, inflammatory, or neoplastic origin in atypical cases, but careful evaluation of the clinical picture and appropriate laboratory investigation usually exclude these possibilities.

Differential diagnosis from other heredodegenerative diseases of infancy is often a major problem. *Metachromatic leucodystrophy* usually begins in the second year of life, with slowly progressive motor disturbance as the initial symptom. *Spongy degeneration of white matter* begins in early infancy and is characterized by enlarged head, initial hypotonia, and normal CSF protein. *Alexander's disease* includes megalencephaly as a characteristic symptom, but otherwise there are no specific clinical manifestations. *Pelizaeus-Merzbacher disease* may occur in the first year of life. This disease has a slowly progressive course, and abnormal involuntary eye movements, often described as nystagmus, are prominent and of diagnostic help. The CSF protein is normal. Inheritance is generally considered to be X-linked, recessive. *Tay-Sachs disease* (Chap. 29) becomes manifest in early infancy. The presence of cherry-red spots is characteristic. The initial clinical finding is sluggishness or apathy, rather than hyperirritability. *G_{M1}-gangliosidosis* (Chap. 30) is of early onset and more resembles Hurler's disease clinically and radiologically than it does Krabbe's disease. *Gaucher's disease* (Chap. 33) and *Niemann-Pick disease* (Chap. 35) can be differentiated by the enlarged viscera.

These clinical points are helpful in the differential diagnosis of globoid cell leucodystrophy, but in patients atypical with respect to age and certain symptoms, it may be almost impossible to make a clinical diagnosis. As will be described later assays of galactosyl ceramide β-galactosidase activity in serum or leukocytes now provide definitive antemortem diagnosis.

PATHOLOGY

All important pathological changes are confined to the nervous system. Austin found abnormal droplets in the renal tubular epithelial cells which stained bluish with toluidine blue [45, 59]. Although its significance is uncertain, this is a noteworthy finding because the kidney is the only extraneural organ that normally contains significant amounts of galactocerebroside [60, 61]. Multinucleated giant cells have been occasionally observed outside the nervous system, but they differ morphologically and can be distinguished from typical globoid cells [54, 62]. In only one patient have giant cells similar to the globoid cells in white matter been observed in lung, lymph nodes, and spleen [63].

Central Nervous System

Gross Anatomy

The brain is usually markedly and uniformly reduced in size, but otherwise the external appearance is normal except for shrunken gyri and widened sulci. On cut section the white matter is extremely deficient and has a whitish-gray appearance and a firm, rubberlike consistency. This is due to a widespread diffuse demyelination with severe astrocytic gliosis. White matter changes are often more severe posterosuperiorly within the cerebral hemispheres, and the subcortical arcuate fibers tend to be spared. Phylogenetically newer tracts are usually more severely involved. In contrast to the grossly abnormal appearance of the white matter, the gray matter appears relatively normal, except for reduced cortical thickness.

Histology

Histological involvement of the white matter is always much more severe than that of the gray matter. The major abnormalities are the presence of a large number of globoid cells, a severe lack of myelin, and astrocytic gliosis (Fig. 34-2).

Globoid Cells

Conventionally, the characteristic abnormal cells, abundantly present in the white matter of brains with globoid cell leucodystrophy, are divided into two categories, epithelioid cells (globoid cells) and globoid bodies [64, 65]. The epithelioid cells are medium-sized, round, or oval mononuclear cells. The globoid bodies are large, irregular, multinucleated cells, ranging from 20 to 50 microns in diameter, with as many as 15 to 20 nuclei located near the plasma membrane. In the past undue emphasis may have been placed on the differences between epithelioid cells and globoid bodies. But aside from the number of nuclei, these cells are identical in staining characteristics, and among them are always cells which could be considered transitional. Experimental evidence strongly indicates that these two types of cells have the same origin [11–13]. Therefore, the term *globoid cells* will be used in this chapter for both cell types, modified as *mononuclear* or *multinuclear* when it is necessary to differentiate between the two different types.

The mononuclear globoid cells are scattered in white matter, most typically as perivascular packets of 10 to 20 cells. These cells are more common in recently affected areas than in the old lesions in the deep white matter. These globoid cells are the dominant histological feature. It is estimated histologically that in some cases the globoid cells constitute 30 to 50 percent of the total white matter [66]. The globoid cells contain pale nuclei with prominent nucleoli. The cytoplasm is abundant and stains moderately positive with periodic acid–Schiff stain (PAS), and faintly

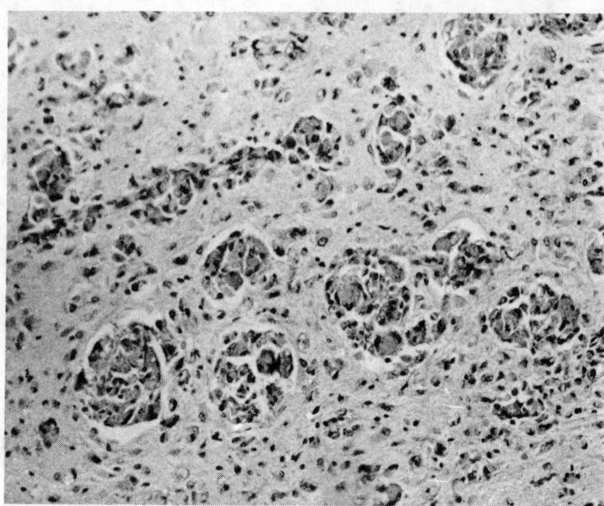

Figure 34-2. Typical light microscopic appearance of the white matter of globoid cell leucodystrophy. Conspicuous clusters of globoid cells occupy a considerable portion of whole white matter. Globoid cells are PAS-positive as shown here, and many contain multiple nuclei. The remainder of the tissue is mostly occupied by reactive astrocytes. PAS stain. Magnification ×120. (*Courtesy Dr. Kinuko Suzuki.*)

positive with Sudan Black B and Sudan IV. The cytoplasm is not metachromatic with the toluidine blue stain at acid pH. The globoid cells exhibit intense acid phosphatase activity [36, 41, 59]. The similarities in the morphological and histochemical characteristics between the globoid cells and the glucocerebroside-containing abnormal cells in Gaucher's disease have often been pointed out [5, 8].

A globoid cell reaction, virtually indistinguishable from the one in globoid cell leucodystrophy, can be produced experimentally in rats by intracerebral injection of solid galactocerebroside [11–13]. The experimental globoid cells are identical in appearance and staining properties to the globoid cells in Krabbe's disease. Their production is specifically confined to one type of injected lipid. Galactocerebroside appears to be the only compound capable of inducing the histological globoid cell reaction; and sulfatide, glucocerebroside, ceramide, psychosine, ceramide lactoside, ganglioside, and acid mucopolysaccharides are all ineffective. Similar multinucleated cells also have been produced in tissue culture of the retina by the addition of cerebroside to the media [67].

The origin of the globoid cells in Krabbe's disease has been the subject of considerable controversy. Collier and Greenfield thought that they might be of glial origin [4], and subsequent hypotheses in support of this have proposed that the originating species of glial cells were the microglia [7], the microglia and astrocytes [68], astrocytes and adventitial cells [69], and oligodendroglia [70]. Nevertheless, the experimental production of globoid cells by Austin and coworkers represented strong evidence that globoid cells originate in nonneural, mesodermal cells. No transition from oligodendroglial cells or astrocytes to globoid cells was observed. The predominantly perivascular localization of globoid cells is difficult to explain on the basis of oligodendrocytic or astrocytic origin. The fact that ultrastructural studies of affected human brains failed to demonstrate glial fibers in globoid cells has made it more likely that globoid cells derive from mesodermal cells, and that they are essentially macrophages. Although the globoid cells and most, if not all, microglia [71–73] now appear to be hematogenous in origin and histiocytic in nature, it does not follow, of course, that globoid cells necessarily arise through transformation of microglia. Globoid cells could possibly be derived from other cells of mesodermal origin.

Lack of Myelin

Myelin deficiency in the white matter of patients with globoid cell leucodystrophy is generally profound, but the subcortical U fibers tend to be spared, except in unusually severe cases in which practically no myelin can be demonstrated within the cerebral hemispheres. Among the various white matter systems, the phylogenetically newer areas tend to be more severely affected. Thus, fornix, hippocampus, mamillothalamic tract, or white matter of basal ganglia tend to be less involved than centrum semiovale or cerebellar white matter [50, 74, 75]. In the spinal cord, the pyramidal tracts are more severely affected than the dorsal columns. The areas with the most intense globoid cell infiltration are usually the areas with the least amount of preserved myelin, and vice versa. There is concomitant axonal degeneration, and generally no tendency to axonal preservation, such as that characteristically seen in multiple sclerosis. The oligodendroglial population is also severely diminished, and at the terminal state of some unusually severe cases they may be difficult to find. Generally, there are no inflammatory changes or deposits of amorphous sudanophilic material. Rarely, in the areas of recent acute myelin breakdown, there may be some indication of inflammation or a few sudanophilic droplets, but these findings are the exception rather than the rule in globoid cell leucodystrophy. Typically, the white matter is not spongy or edematous.

Astrocytic Gliosis

Aside from the globoid cells, the areas of white matter previously occupied by axons, myelin, and oligodendroglial cells are filled with dense fibrous astrocytic proliferation. The astrocytes contain faintly PAS-positive cytoplasm and large pleomorphic nuclei. Although unusually severe, this appears to be fundamentally the same reactive astrocytic gliosis found in many other pathological conditions.

Changes in Gray Matter

In contrast to the devastated white matter, the gray matter is generally much less affected. Neurons do not show the "ballooned-out" appearance as in many other lipid storage disorders. The case reported by de Vries [76] is exceptional in that there were severe degenerative changes in the cerebral cortex. Typically, changes in the gray matter are limited to mild focal or laminar degenerative changes in the cerebral cortex and regressive changes in neurons of the pons, dentate nuclei, thalamus, and other areas [7, 42, 68, 76].

Evolution of Morphological Changes

It is difficult to determine the chronological sequence of the various histological changes described above, because it is rarely possible to follow morphological changes in the same patient during the course of the illness. Even if this were possible, there are always great regional variations at any given moment. D'Agostino et al. [26] attempted to formulate the chronological evolution of the morphological changes based on a study of multiple sections from three cases. Utilizing the degree of demyelination, axonal loss, and glial response as criteria of chronicity, they divided the course into four stages: (1) early, (2) advanced, (3) late, and (4) final. The early lesions are characterized by "the presence of both intracellular and extracellular PAS-positive material, with subsequent formation of mononuclear globoid cells and only a slight decrease in the intensity of myelin staining." In the advanced stage, myelin and axons are decreased and astrocytic gliosis becomes prominent. The globoid cells are more numerous and tend to cluster around blood vessels, and many become multinucleated. In the late stage, the globoid cells become fewer in number and mostly clumped around blood vessels. Myelin and axons are markedly diminished at this stage. The final stage is characterized by predominant astrocytic gliosis, with remaining globoid cells and total loss of myelin and axons.

Ultrastructure

For many years the report by Nelson et al. [28] was the only electron microscopic study of globoid cell leucodystrophy. Then in 1969 to 1970, eight articles appeared in less than a year [24, 35, 38, 46, 77–80], describing the ultrastructure of both the central and peripheral nervous systems. These reports are essentially in agreement as to the ultrastructure of the central nervous system. At the ultrastructural level, mononuclear and multinucleated globoid cells appear similar, except for the number of nuclei. They are distinguished by numerous fine tortuous cytoplasmic processes (pseudopods), characteristic of macrophages, moderately electron-dense granular cytoplasm containing prominent rough endoplasmic reticulum, many free ribosomes, abundant fine filaments of approximately 90 to 100 Å, and scattered or clustered abnormal cytoplasmic inclusions (Fig. 34-3). The inclusions have moderately electron-dense straight or curved hollow tubular profiles in longitudinal sections and appear irregularly crystalloid in cross section (Figs. 34-4 and 34-5). Often they are freely scattered among

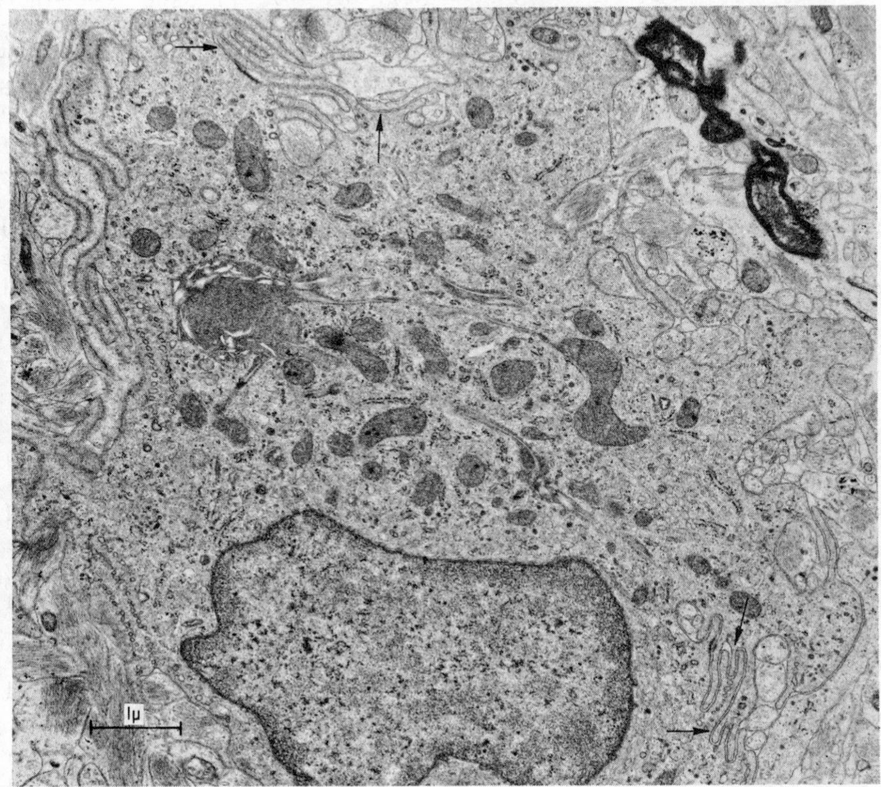

Figure 34-3. A low magnification electron micrograph showing a globoid cell. Only one nucleus is visible. There are numerous tortuous pseudopods (arrows) which characterize this cell as a macrophage. Within the cytoplasm, near the center of the picture, there are many abnormal tubular inclusions (for details, see Figs. 34-4 and 34-5). The line indicates a scale of 1 micron. (*Courtesy Dr. Kinuko Suzuki.*)

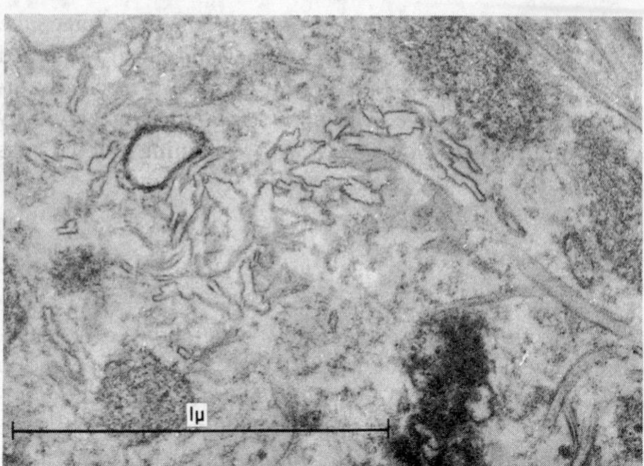

Figure 34-4. An electron micrograph showing the characteristic hollow, polygonal, or crystalloid cut sections of the abnormal inclusions in the cytoplasm of a globoid cell. Several longitudinal sections of tubules of the same type are seen on the right side of the picture. The line indicates a scale of 1 micron. (*Courtesy Dr. Kinuko Suzuki.*)

the normal cytoplasmic organelles, but sometimes they are packed in an electron-lucent space in the cytoplasm, with or without an outer limiting membrane. These tubules often have longitudinal striations of variable density, approximately 60 Å in width. Another type of abnormal tubular inclusion, described by Yunis and Lee [38], has the structure of twisted tubules with 40 to 50 Å longitudinal striations and rectangular or irregularly round cross sections (Fig. 34-6). This second type of tubule is similar to those in Gaucher's disease, but the first larger tubules, with irregular, polygonal, or crystalloid cross sections, seem to be unique to globoid cell leucodystrophy. Yunis and Lee [38] pointed out the morphological similarities of these abnormal inclusions to negatively stained pure brain galactocerebroside. Ultrastructural study of the experimental globoid cells produced

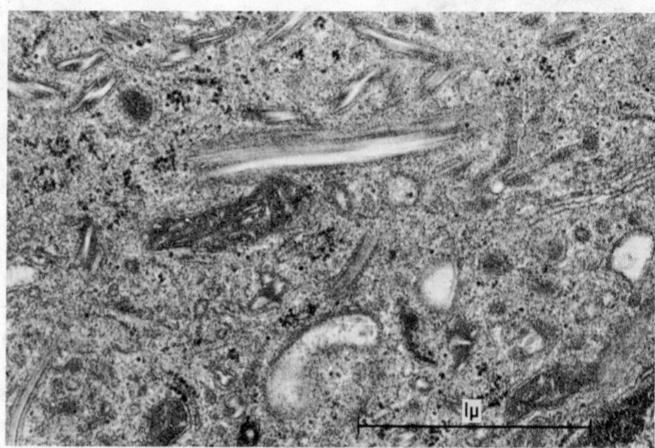

Figure 34-5. The abnormal hollow tubules show longitudinal striations, approximately 60 Å wide. The line indicates a scale of 1 micron.

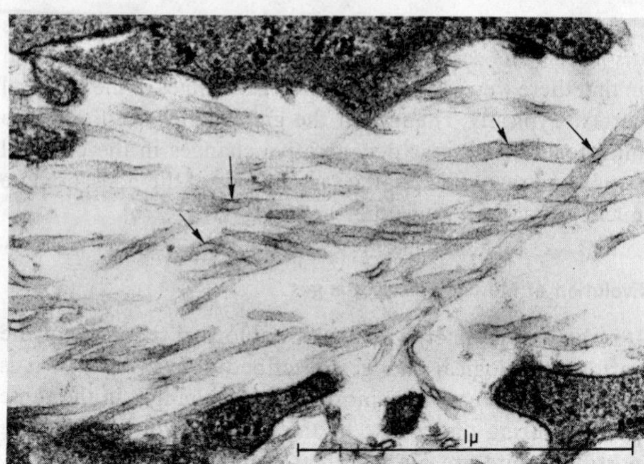

Figure 34-6. Another type of abnormal inclusions in globoid cells. They have the structure of twisted tubules with 40- to 50-Å striations (arrows). The line indicates a scale of 1 micron. (*Courtesy Dr. Eduardo J. Yunis.*)

by the intracerebral injection into rats of pure galactocerebroside, prepared from the brain of a patient with Krabbe's disease, showed both types of tubules. This further supported their close relationship to galactocerebroside [81]. In fact, the ultrastructure of the experimental globoid cells was essentially identical to that of human globoid cells (Figs. 34-7 and 34-8).

The ultrastructural appearance of human and experimental globoid cells, particularly the presence of numerous pseudopods, supports the view that these cells are macrophages. Astrocytes, identified by glial filaments, did not contain the abnormal tubular inclusions. The few remaining oligodendroglial cells, identifiable by the dense cytoplasm and microtubules, were also free of the tubules. On the other hand, endothelial and perithelial cells often contained cytoplasmic inclusions similar to those in globoid cells [35].

Degeneration of myelin, with or without associated axonal degeneration, is found in the white matter, but the remaining myelin has normal multilamellar configuration, with normal periodicity. Cortical neurons appear normal ultrastructurally.

Peripheral Nervous System

Peripheral nerves, including the cranial nerves, usually do not show gross abnormalities. The optic nerve is an exception, but it is actually a white matter tract of the central nervous system and not a peripheral nerve. It shares the same gross and histological abnormalities of CNS white matter.

Earlier, pathological changes in peripheral nerves had been reported rather sporadically [36, 45]. Some investigators, in fact, did not find morphological changes in peripheral nerves [10, 25, 47, 74]. More recent histological and ultrastructural studies have shown that the peripheral nervous system is commonly affected [35, 37, 40, 46, 79, 80, 82]. Dunn et al. [46] found peripheral nerve lesions in all of seven

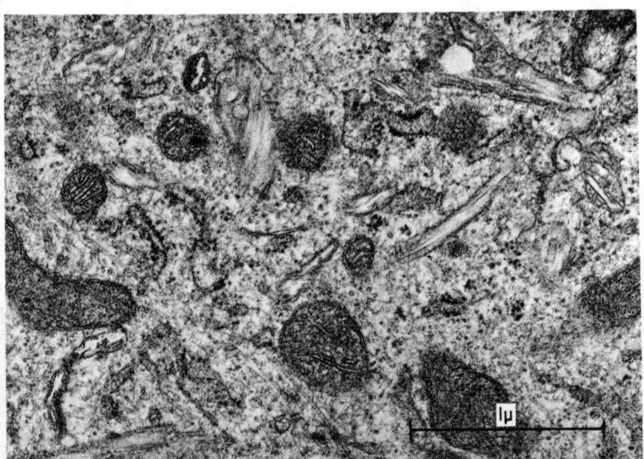

Figure 34-7. A high magnification electron micrograph of cytoplasm of a globoid cell, experimentally produced in rat brain by intracerebral injection of solid galactocerebroside. Abnormal hollow tubules, identical to those seen in human globoid cells (Figs. 34-4 and 34-5), are scattered within the cytoplasm. Note the similarities of the overall appearance to Fig. 34-5, which was taken from a human globoid cell. The line indicates a scale of 1 micron. (*Courtesy Dr. Kinuko Suzuki.*)

patients. Under light microscopy the peripheral nerve lesions consist of minimum to severe degenerative changes in axons and the myelin sheaths, associated with endoneurial fibrosis and the accumulation of foamy histiocytes around endoneurial blood vessels or trabeculae of the endoneurium. Segmental demyelination is common [35, 46, 79]. Typical globoid cells are not found in peripheral nerves. Ultrastructurally, straight or curved tubular inclusions, similar to those in globoid cells in the brain, are found scattered or clustered in the cytoplasm of histiocytes, in the proliferated endoneurial collagenous tissue, or around small blood vessels. Suzuki and Grover [35] did not find these abnormal inclusions within Schwann cells, but Bischoff and Ulrich found some in Schwann cells as well [80].

BIOCHEMISTRY OF GALACTOSYL CERAMIDE

Chemistry of Galactosyl Ceramide and Related Compounds

Galactocerebroside (galactosyl ceramide) belongs to the group of lipids generically called sphingoglycolipids. This name indicates that the molecule contains a long chain base, sphingosine, and a sugar moiety. Sphingosine is an unsaturated amino diol. The major sphingosine found in nature is C_{18}-sphingosine, having the structure D(+)*erythro*-1,3-dihydroxy-2-amino-4-*trans*-octadecene [83–86]. Besides this major form, C_{20}-sphingosine (icosisphingosine) occurs in smaller amounts [87–89]. Small portions of these sphingosines are also present in saturated (dihydro) forms [90, 91]. In the galactocerebroside and sulfatide of normal adult human brains, C_{18}-sphingosine constitutes 95 percent or more of the total sphingosine, the remainder being C_{18}-dihydrosphingosine and much smaller amounts of a shorter chain analogue, C_{16}-sphingosine. In immature human brains there are higher proportions of C_{18}-dihydrosphingosine, sometimes 10 percent of the total [92]. C_{20}-sphinogosine and its dihydro form do not appear to be components of brain galactocerebroside or sulfatide [91, 92].

Ceramide

The amino group of sphingosine is almost always acylated with a long-chain fatty acid, ranging from C_{14} to C_{26}. N-Acyl-sphingosine is generically called ceramide, the basic common building block of almost all sphingolipids. The fatty acid composition of galactocerebroside and sulfatide has been extensively studied both in normal adult brains and during development [93–97]. Generally, the fatty acids of galactocerebroside and sulfatide in the brain are characterized by the predominance of longer chain fatty acids (C_{20} to C_{26}), lack of polyunsaturated fatty acids, and the presence of α-hydroxy acids. Approximately two-thirds of the fatty acid in cerebrosides and one-third of those in sulfatides are α-hydroxy fatty acids. Alpha-hydroxy fatty acids are generally absent in other lipids of the brain, including glycerophospholipids, sphingomyelin, ceramide oligohexosides, and gangliosides. In galactocerebrosides and sulfatides, particularly those in white matter, 65 to 80 percent of the total unsubstituted fatty acids have chain lengths longer than 20 carbons. In the α-hydroxy fatty acids, the proportion of longer chain fatty acids is even greater. Except for the sphingomyelins of white matter and myelin, the predomi-

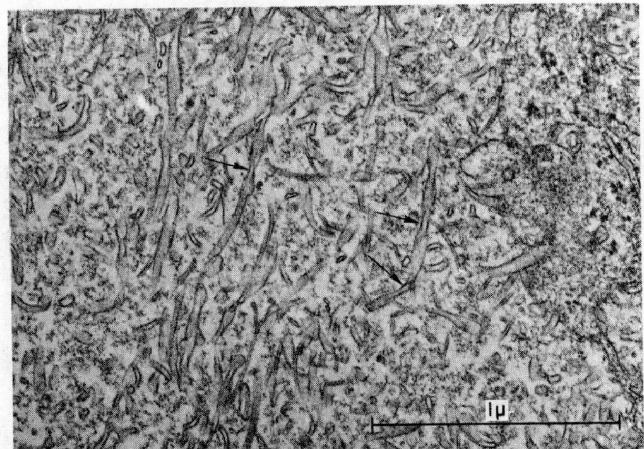

Figure 34-8. Numerous slender, twisted tubules that were produced within experimental globoid cells in rat brain by the intracerebral injection of galactocerebroside purified from the brain of a human patient with globoid cell leucodystrophy. The twisted configurations of the tubules are clearly seen (arrows). The ultrastructural appearance of these tubules is identical to those described by Yunis and Lee [38] in human globoid cell leucodystrophy (Fig. 34-6). The line indicates a scale of 1 micron. (*Courtesy Dr. Kinuko Suzuki.*)

nance of longer chain fatty acid is unique for brain galactocerebrosides and sulfatides. Stearic acid ($C_{18:0}$) is the predominant fatty acid in brain gangliosides [15, 89, 98–100] and a variety of ceramide oligohexosides in the brain [101]. Lack of fatty acids with more than one double bond is a characteristic shared by all sphingolipids in the brain.

Galactocerebrosides and Sulfatides

The hydroxyl group of C_1 of ceramide can be substituted for by a variety of compounds. Cerebroside is defined as a monohexosyl ceramide, the hexose being linked to the carbon-1 of ceramide by a glycosidic linkage. The hexose is either D-glucose or D-galactose. Depending on the nature of the hexose, cerebroside is named glucocerebroside (glucosyl ceramide) or galactocerebroside (galactosyl ceramide). Both the glucose and galactose are in β-configuration. Glucocerebrosides occur predominantly in systemic tissues other than the nervous system and are essentially absent in normal human brain after age 1 year. They are present in small amounts in the brains of normal human fetuses and newborns [102], and in the brains of older children with certain diseases, notably ganglioside storage disorders [101, 103].

In contrast, galactocerebroside is characteristically a lipid of the nervous system. As indicated by the preceding descriptions, it has the structure shown in Fig. 34-9.

Brain sulfatide is derived from galactocerebroside and it has an additional sulfate group, ester-linked to the C_3 of galactose [104, 105]. While the detailed structures of the individual moieties differ among these two groups of sphingolipids, for purposes of discussion the following simplified notations are convenient:

Sphingosine—galactose
|
Fatty acid
Galactosyl ceramide

Sphingosine—galactose-sulfate
|
Fatty acid
Sulfatide

A related compound, galactosyl-sphingosine (galactocerebroside minus fatty acid), is called psychosine. It is not present in the brain or in any systemic organs in measurable amounts, but the compound has potential importance when

```
              H       H  H
CH3(CH2)12—C=C—C—C—CH2—O—CH———————┐
              H    |  |          |         |
                  OH NH        HCOH        |
                      |          |         |
                     C=O       HOCH        O
                      |          |         |
                      R        HOCH        |
                                 |         |
                                HC—————————┘
                                 |
                                CH2OH
```

Figure 34-9. Structure of galactocerebroside (galactosyl ceramide). The molecule consists of sphingosine, fatty acid, and galactose. $R = -(CH_2)CH_3$.

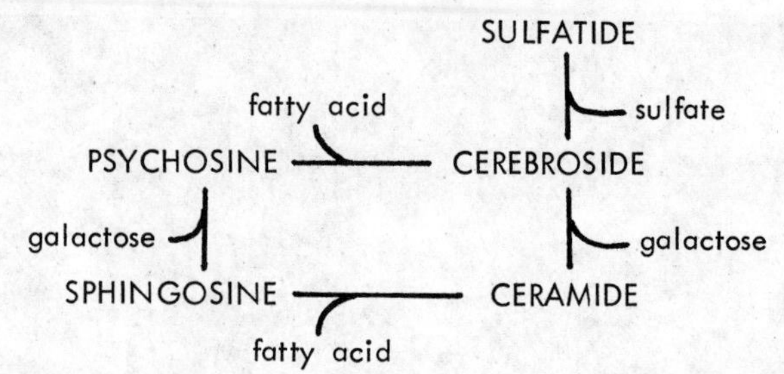

Figure 34-10. Chemical relationship of galactocerebroside and related compounds.

the dynamic behavior of galactocerebrosides is considered. The scheme in Fig. 34-10 summarizes the structural (but not necessarily metabolic) relationship of galactocerebrosides and related compounds.

Metabolism of Galactocerebroside

Two alternate pathways have been proposed for the biosynthesis of galactocerebroside. One is through psychosine, which is formed from sphingosine and UDP-galactose [106, 107]. Psychosine, in turn, may be acylated by acyl CoA to form galactocerebroside [108, 109]. More recent experimental data indicate that at least the galactocerebrosides containing α-hydroxy fatty acids are synthesized through ceramide rather than through psychosine [110]. It remains to be established whether or not galactocerebroside with unsubstituted fatty acids can also be synthesized from ceramide and UDP-galactose, and if so, which of the two alternative routes, either through psychosine or ceramide, is the major biosynthetic pathway of brain galactocerebroside. Biosynthesis of sulfatide occurs through cerebroside with the "active sulfate," 3′-phosphoadenosine 5′-phosphosulfate (PAPS), as sulfate donor [111–116]. The actual biosynthetic process of sulfatide appears to be complex, involving participation of an intermediate lipid-protein complex [116–118].

The initial step in degradation of sulfatide is removal of the sulfate group to convert it to galactocerebroside. This reaction is catalyzed by cerebroside sulfate sulfatase which is present in the arylsulfatase A fraction [119]. Deficiency of this enzyme characterizes another inherited leucodystrophy, metachromatic leucodystrophy, in which abnormal accumulation of sulfatide occurs [120, 121, also Chap. 32].

Galactocerebroside is degraded to ceramide and galactose by a lysosomal hydrolytic enzyme, galactocerebroside β-galactosidase.

Fatty acid
|
Sphingosine—galactose $\xrightarrow{\text{galactocerebroside } \beta\text{-galactosidase}}$
Cerebroside

Fatty acid
|
sphingosine + galactose
Ceramide

The nature of this enzyme in the brain has been extensively studied by Radin and coworkers [122–125]. Ultracentrifugal fractionation indicates that the enzyme is associated with the lysosomal fraction. Approximately 300-fold purification has been achieved by extraction with detergents, DEAE-Sephadex column chromatography, and differential precipitation at different pH's. The pH optimum of the enzyme is 4.5. Ceramide, sphingosine, ceramide lactoside, galactose, galactonolactone, and galactitol inhibit the enzyme in vitro. The enzyme is active on galactocerebroside with either unsubstituted or α-hydroxy fatty acids. The chain lengths of fatty acids do not affect the enzymatic activity; both cerebroside with stearic acid ($C_{18:0}$) and with lignoceric acid ($C_{24:0}$) are hydrolyzed. In rat brain, galactocerebroside β-galactosidase is present before myelination when little galactocerebroside is present in the brain (4 days), but the enzyme level then rises considerably (three to four times the 4-day level) during active cerebroside deposition and myelination. The activity remains high in mature animals. In man, galactocerebroside β-galactosidase activity in a 72-year-old brain was the same as that in a 21-year-old brain in gray matter, but was decreased to 60 percent of the activity of the young brain in white matter [18].

Galactocerebroside, Myelin, and Their Metabolism

The distribution of galactocerebrosides in mammalian organs is uniquely restricted. They are not found in any systemic organs except the kidneys, which contain normally appreciable amounts of galactocerebroside, although much less than the brain [60, 61]. The brain, particularly white matter, is rich in galactocerebroside and its sulfate ester, sulfatide. Gray matter contains much smaller amounts of these glycolipids. Galactocerebroside may be mostly, if not exclusively, localized in the myelin sheath and, probably, oligodendroglial cells, since the myelin sheath is a specialized extension of the oligodendroglial cell membrane. This contention is supported (but not proven) by the virtual absence of galactocerebroside in the brain before myelination [126–128], and similarly low cerebroside concentrations in pathological conditions where almost total loss of myelin occurs [129, 130]. The sum of cerebroside and sulfatide is the most sensitive biochemical indicator of the mass of myelin present in the brain [131]. Increase in the brain cerebroside content coincides with the active myelination period and, in fact, the amounts of total brain cerebroside correlate precisely with the amounts of myelin which can be isolated from the brain, whereas the other lipids do not [132].

Myelin of adult mammalian brains generally contains galactocerebroside at a concentration of 15 to 18 percent dry weight. The sum of galactocerebroside and sulfatide amounts to 20 percent of the dry weight of myelin. The content of galactocerebroside of myelin from the peripheral nerve is somewhat less than that of CNS myelin [133]. There are numerous original reports on the chemical composition of myelin isolated from mammalian brains and readers are referred to recent review articles on this subject [134–138]. In view of the unusually high concentration of galactocerebrosides and sulfatides in the myelin sheath, metabolic diseases involving these lipids would be expected to manifest themselves primarily in disturbances of white matter functions and peripheral neuropathy (globoid cell leucodystrophy and metachromatic leucodystrophy).

The metabolism of brain galactocerebroside is closely linked to the metabolism of myelin. This topic has been covered in a few recent review articles [139, 140]. The most significant metabolic feature of CNS myelin is its high rate of formation and turnover during the period of active myelination and its relative inertness in the adult. The period of most active myelination in man probably extends from the perinatal period to about age 18 months. Myelination is by no means stopped after this period. Histological study indicates that myelination in the human brain may not be complete until age 20 years [141]. The amount of cerebroside in the immature brain is very low, whereas cholesterol and phospholipids are present in reasonable concentrations. When measured by incorporation of labeled galactose administered in vivo, the rate of cerebroside synthesis in rat brain reaches a peak at 10 to 20 days, coinciding well with the most active period of myelination [106]. Synthesis of cerebroside occurs at a much lower rate in the adult. A series of long-term experiments by Davison and coworkers convincingly established the relative metabolic inertness of adult myelin. Their earlier studies, carried out on total white matter, were later confirmed by more refined experiments in which the incorporated labeled precursors were followed in isolated pure myelin fractions [142–144]. Smith and Eng [145] also studied the long-term turnover and the short-term formation of myelin lipids. There are still unresolved questions in regard to the metabolism of myelin, but there is general agreement that myelin is formed at a high rate during development and that once formed, it is very stable metabolically with a slow turnover rate. The half-life of cerebroside and sulfatide in the mature brain is 1 year or longer. At any developmental stage, myelin is metabolically the most stable component of the subcellular fractions of the brain.

Let us summarize a few key features of galactocerebroside metabolism, which will be crucial later in considering the pathophysiology of globoid cell leucodystrophy: (1) Galactocerebroside consists of a sphingosine, a fatty acid, and galactose. (2) Galactocerebroside is the precursor of sulfatide. (3) Both galactocerebroside and sulfatide are highly concentrated in the myelin sheath. (4) Sulfatide is normally degraded through galactocerebroside. (5) A lysosomal hydrolytic enzyme, galactocerebroside β-galactosidase, is responsible for the first step in normal degradation of cerebroside, in which galactocerebroside is cleaved to ceramide and galactose. (6) Biosynthesis of galactocerebroside in vivo reaches a peak, coincident with the maximum myelination period (during the first year and a half in humans). (7) Galactocerebroside β-galactosidase, present in low concentration before myelination, increases sharply during the active myelination period, when myelin is turning over relatively rapidly. (8) Once formed, adult myelin is unusually stable metabolically, although by no means completely inert. (9) The high level of galactocerebroside β-galactosidase, attained during the active myelination period, is retained in the adult brain.

CHEMICAL PATHOLOGY

Analytical Chemistry

Hallervorden was the first to point out the morphological similarities of the globoid cells to the storage cells in Gaucher's disease, and to suggest that the globoid cells also might contain cerebroside in excess [5]. Diezel, after careful histochemical examination of globoid cells and Gaucher cells, concluded that the stored material in both diseases was cerebroside, probably bound to protein [8, 9]. Stammler similarly interpreted his histochemical findings that the globoid cell contained cerebroside in a form that was almost insoluble in either aqueous or organic solvents [10]. The strong tetrazonium reaction within the cytoplasm of the globoid cell is consistent with the presence of a protein-cerebroside complex [62, 68, 146]. These histochemical findings were later substantiated by Austin [6], who obtained fractions enriched in globoid cells from seven patients with globoid cell leucodystrophy; he found that globoid cells contain unusually large amounts of galactocerebroside but little sulfatide.

Earlier, Blackwood and Cumings found an abnormally high cerebroside concentration in white matter in one case of globoid cell leucodystrophy [7]. They attributed this increased cerebroside to the abnormal material in globoid cells, but increased concentrations of cerebroside in the brains of patients with globoid cell leucodystrophy are now considered exceptional. More recent analyses almost invariably record both galactocerebrosides and sulfatides much lower than normal in white matter [9, 14, 15, 25, 44, 45, 48, 50, 147–155]. Pilz reported that α-hydroxy fatty acid–containing cerebroside was more decreased than that with unsubstituted fatty acids [155]. The most consistent, although not necessarily the most invariable, finding in white matter of globoid cell leucodystrophy is the increased ratio of cerebroside to sulfatide. In eight cases of globoid cell leucodystrophy, Austin [14, 147] found the cerebroside/sulfatide ratio to be between 5 to 10, whereas it is normally about 4. All of his patients had reduced total glycolipids in white matter. In that series patients who showed more globoid cells histologically tended to have higher absolute and relative cerebroside values. The increased cerebroside/sulfatide ratio was also pointed out by Svennerholm [15] in two cases. In a later study by Hagberg et al. [25], three of the four patients showed increased ratios of cerebroside to sulfatide in white matter, but a fourth patient had a normal ratio. Eto and Suzuki [151] also showed an almost normal cerebroside/sulfatide ratio. To evaluate whether an abnormal ratio was due to increase of cerebroside or decrease of sulfatide, Austin related the values of these lipids to those of cholesterol and found in six patients that the average increase of cerebroside was greater (plus 57 percent) than the average decrease of sulfatide (minus 30 percent) [65]. Suzuki et al. [18, 19] found that the sulfatide concentrations in white matter of globoid cell leucodystrophy were generally similar to those in the white matter of other devastating white matter diseases in which almost complete myelin loss also occurs, such as Schilder's disease [130] or spongy degeneration of white matter [129]. These authors concluded that the relative preservation of cerebroside is more impressive than the loss of sulfatide.

Beside the abnormalities of the major glycolipids of white matter, galactocerebrosides, and sulfatides, Menkes et al. [150] found an abnormal amount of a dihexosyl ceramide and possibly a trihexosyl ceramide. They identified the dihexosyl ceramide as glucosylgalactosyl ceramide, but Evans and McCluer [156] were unable to confirm this finding and found, instead, that the dihexosyl ceramide was galactosylglucosyl ceramide. Eto and Suzuki [151] studied the sphingoglycolipids of the brain of a patient with globoid cell leucodystrophy and also identified the dihexosyl ceramide as galactosylglucosyl ceramide, rather than glucosylgalactosyl ceramide. In addition, 16 percent of white matter cerebroside was glucocerebroside, and two other sphingoglycolipids, digalactosylglucosyl ceramide and globoside (N-acetylgalactosaminyldigalactosylglucosyl ceramide) were also present in significant amounts. These "visceral type" sphingoglycolipids in white matter were attributed to globoid cells, consistent with the idea that the globoid cells are of mesodermal origin, a secondary phenomenon rather than a direct result of the primary enzymatic defect (Table 34-1).

Earlier, isolated myelin from globoid cell leucodystrophy was reported to have a disproportionate lack of sulfatide [157], approximately half normal when expressed as a percentage of the total sphingosine. These experiments, however, did not refer the sulfatide content to either the content of protein, total lipids, or sphingolipids of the myelin fraction, and did not distinguish between a fraction with abnormally low sulfatide and normal cerebroside and one with abnormally high cerebroside and normal sulfatide. Moreover, the technique of myelin isolation used would not eliminate possible contamination of the myelin with subcellular components of lighter density. The abnormal tubular or polygonal inclusions found in globoid cells are lighter than myelin, and contain a high proportion of cerebroside but no sulfatide [158]. Therefore, the analytical values of the myelin fraction reported by these authors are likely to include the abnormal cerebroside-rich inclusions. In a more recent study [159], the abnormal tubular inclusions were present in even a larger amount than myelin. When they were carefully eliminated, the yield of myelin was, as ex-

Table 34-1. ANALYTICAL CHEMISTRY OF GLOBOID CELL LEUCODYSTROPHY

	Gray matter		*White matter*	
	Globoid	Normal	Globoid	Normal
Water content, % fresh wt	87.0	82.1	83.5	73.0
Chloroform-methanol insoluble residue	58.1	51.0	70.0	29.3
Total lipid	27.4	31.8	18.0	54.0
Proteolipid protein	0.7	3.2	0.5	8.6
Upper phase solids	13.6	14.0	11.5	8.0
Cholesterol	5.8	7.6	3.5	15.0
Phospholipid, total	21.4	22.1	12.9	23.9
Ethanolamine phospholipid	6.8	7.2	3.1	8.1
Lecithin	8.7	9.0	5.1	6.8
Sphingomyelin	2.5	1.8	2.3	4.3
Monophosphoinositide	0.8	0.7	0.5	0.4
Serine phospholipid	2.8	3.2	1.7	4.2
Glycolipids, total	0.44	0.92	1.6	14.6
Cerebroside*	0.25	0.50	0.99	12.5
Sulfatide	0.16	0.14	0.22	2.2
Ceramide dihexoside†	Trace	0.07	0.09	Trace
Ceramide trihexoside‡	.....	.....	0.04	
Globoside§			0.20	
Ceramide tetrahexoside¶	.....	Trace	0.04	

* Glucocerebroside constituted 32 and 13 percent of total cerebroside in gray and white matter, respectively, in globoid cell leucodystrophy, whereas only galactocerebroside was present in the normal brain. This patient is somewhat atypical in that the cerebroside sulfatide ratio in white matter is normal.

† Galactosylglucosyl ceramide.

‡ Visceral type trihexoside, i.e., digalactosylglucosyl ceramide.

§ N-Acetylgalactosaminyldigalactosylglucosyl ceramide.

¶ Asialo G_{M1} ganglioside.

Note: Expressed as percent dry weight except for the water content.
Source: Data from Eto and Suzuki [*151*].

pected from histological findings, only 0.4 percent of normal. The myelin had a normal ultrastructural configuration, and lipid composition was quite similar to normal myelin. Particularly, the amounts of glycolipids, cerebrosides, and sulfatides were normal. The cerebrosides were all galactocerebrosides and none of the ceramide oligohexosides found in the whole white matter were present in the myelin (Table 34-2). Thus, in globoid cell leucodystrophy the brain is apparently capable of forming myelin with normal morphological appearance and normal chemical composition. This finding is in contrast to metachromatic leucodystrophy, in which myelin is formed with an excess sulfatide content [157, 160, 161].

Besides these specific aspects of chemical abnormalities, white matter in globoid cell leucodystrophy typically shows increased water content, drastic reduction of proteolipid protein and total lipid, with consequent relative, but not absolute, increase of proteins. Cholesterol, lecithin, sphingomyelin, ethanolamine, and serine phospholipids are all reduced in similar degrees. These findings are primarily the reflection of the devastating myelin loss. As expected from the histological absence of sudanophilia, cholesterol ester is not present in white matter (Table 34-1).

The chemical content of the gray matter, in contrast to the white matter, may be normal or only slightly abnormal (Table 34-1). Glycolipids in gray matter may be moderately low [15, 25, 151, 152] or normal [7, 147]. The ratio of cerebroside to sulfatide is often increased.

Enzymatic Deficiency

Austin et al. [162] assayed brain, liver, and kidney tissues in Krabbe's disease for a number of enzymatic activities. They found normal activities of acid and alkaline phosphatase, UDPG-pyrophosphorylase, UDP-acetylglucosamine pyrophosphorylase, N-acetylglucosamine kinase, PAPS-degrading enzyme, and arylsulfatase. In the brain, the activities of two enzymes, UDPG-glycogen transglucosylase and glucosamine 6-P deaminase, were somewhat increased. In this study no enzyme was found to be deficient.

Cerebroside-sulfatide Sulfotransferase

In 1967, Austin and coworkers reported that the activity of cerebroside-sulfatide sulfotransferase was deficient in the gray and white matter, and in the kidneys of two patients with globoid cell leucodystrophy, compared to four matched control patients and one patient with metachromatic leucodystrophy [16, 17]. Cerebroside-sulfatide sulfotransferase is a synthetic enzyme which catalyzes the formation of sulfatide

Table 34-2. CHEMICAL COMPOSITION OF ISOLATED MYELIN

	Globoid cell leucodystrophy	Normal control*
Yield, mg/10 gm wet wt	3.8	1,000
Chloroform-methanol insoluble residue	25.7	12.4
Proteolipid protein	12.3	21.0
Total lipid	62.0	66.6
Cholesterol	12.2	15.6
Total phospholipid	30.3	30.1
Ethanolamine phospholipid	7.6	9.7
Lecithin	12.9	9.2
Sphingomyelin	5.0	5.1
Monophosphoinositide and serine phospholipid	4.2	5.8
Total galactolipid	17.0	17.4
Cerebroside	12.4	13.6
Sulfatide	4.6	3.8

* Average of two myelin preparations from normal brains, ages 2.5 and 5.5 years.

Note: Expressed as percent dry weight except for the yield.
Source: Data from Eto et al. [*159*].

from cerebroside and active sulfate, phosphoadenosine phosphosulfate (PAPS) [114–116].

$$\text{Cerebroside} + \text{PAPS} \xrightarrow[\text{sulfotransferase}]{\text{cerebroside-sulfatide}} \text{cerebroside sulfate (sulfatide)}$$

Deficiency of cerebroside-sulfatide sulfotransferase appeared to provide the enzymatic basis for the relative lack of sulfatide in white matter. A close examination of the morphological and chemical abnormalities in globoid cell leucodystrophy indicated that certain features were difficult to explain on the basis of the supposed sulfotransferase deficiency. As described earlier, the concentration of sulfatide is not particularly low for white matter that is almost totally devoid of myelin, and it is the relative preservation of galactocerebroside that characterizes the white matter of globoid cell leucodystrophy [18, 19]. The normal glycolipid composition of myelin was also out of keeping with a deficiency of sulfotransferase activity, for this should lead to formation of myelin relatively deficient in sulfatide. Both morphological and biochemical evidence of the storage of galactocerebroside in the globoid cells and the experimental production of globoid cells exclusively by intracerebral injection of galactocerebroside was also not obviously explained by sulfotransferase deficiency. If the degradative pathway of galactocerebroside were intact, abnormal storage would not be expected with a metabolic block in the synthetic pathway of cerebroside to sulfatide. One laboratory found it difficult to confirm the deficiency of sulfotransferase in two cases, one biopsy and another unfrozen postmortem specimen [163, 164]. The deficiency has been confirmed in additional cases by Austin [20]. Although consistent in gray and white matter, the deficiency was present, however, only in four of seven kidney samples studied. Thus, it now appears reasonable to assume that cerebroside-sulfatide sulfotransferase is often moderately decreased in globoid cell leucodystrophy, but this is probably not the primary genetic defect. The mechanism by which the reduction of sulfotransferase activity occurs is not known.

Deficiency of Galactocerebroside β-Galactosidase

Specific experimental production of the globoid reaction by galactocerebroside and the presence of galactocerebroside within the globoid cell, the most conspicuous and characteristic feature of globoid cell leucodystrophy, strongly suggested an abnormality in the degradative pathway of galactocerebroside. The first step of galactocerebroside degradation occurs normally by cleavage of the galactose moiety from the ceramide portion of cerebroside by the action of a specific enzyme, galactocerebroside β-galactosidase [122–125] (see diagram on page 768).

Profound deficiency of galactocerebroside β-galactosidase activity has now been demonstrated in the gray and white matter, liver, and spleen of three patients with globoid cell leucodystrophy [18, 19] (Table 34-3). The enzyme activity was assayed in tissue homogenates against the specific substrate, galactocerebroside. The labeled substrate was prepared from commercial bovine spinal cord galactocerebroside by oxidation with galactose oxidase and reduction by tritium-labeled sodium borohydride [165]. The label was located on C_6 of galactose, and the radioactivity of released galactose was determined as the measure of the enzyme activity. The activities of galactocerebroside β-galactosidase in these tissues were generally in the range of 5 to 10 percent of that in tissues from normal controls and patients with a variety of other diseases. Postmortem handling and storage of the tissues were adequately controlled. Four other lysosomal hydrolytic enzymes were assayed with appropriate *p*-nitrophenyl compounds, β-glucosidase, β-galactosidase, N-acetyl-β-glucosaminidase and N-acetyl-β-galactosaminidase. The high activities of these *p*-nitrophenyl glycosidases in globoid cell leucodystrophy further indicated satisfactory preservation of tissue. It is noteworthy that β-galactosidase was not deficient when assayed with the synthetic substrate, in spite of the profound deficiency of galactocerebroside β-galactosidase. This indicated that only this specific β-galactosidase was deficient. This was in clear contrast to G_{M1}-gangliosidosis in which galactocerebroside β-galactosidase is normal or even higher than normal,

Table 34-3. GALACTOCEREBROSIDE β-GALACTOSIDASE IN GLOBOID CELL LEUCODYSTROPHY

		Galactocerebroside β-galactosidase, mμmoles/hr/gm
Gray matter		
Krabbe's disease	1	12.1
	2	10.8
	3	5.7
Pathological controls ($n = 9$)*		123 ± 32
Normal controls ($n = 4$)		123 ± 17
White matter		
Krabbe's disease	1	17.7
	2	21.8
	3	7.5
Pathological controls ($n = 9$)*		197 ± 59
Normal controls ($n = 4$)		199 ± 55
Liver		
Krabbe's disease	3	6.4
Normal controls ($n = 2$)		125 and 113
Spleen		
Krabbe's disease	3	20.4
Normal controls ($n = 2$)		157 and 186

* Pathological controls included metachromatic leucodystrophy, Schilder's disease, early and late onset G_{M1} gangliosidosis, Tay-Sachs disease, G_{M2} gangliosidosis with total hexosaminidase deficiency, Hurler's syndrome, Gaucher's disease, and Niemann-Pick disease.

Note: Activities of four lysosomal *p*-nitrophenyl glycosidases were all normal in globoid cell leucodystrophy.

Source: Data from Suzuki and Suzuki [*18*].

whereas β-galactosidase assayed with *p*-nitrophenyl β-galactoside is extremely deficient [166, also Chap. 30].

The deficiency of galactocerebroside β-galactosidase was also not attributable to the extreme devastation of the white matter, because gray matter, much less involved histologically, and the histologically normal liver and spleen also showed the same deficiency. The galactocerebroside β-galactosidase activity was also normal in the white matter in Schilder's disease, in which there is almost complete loss of myelin and oligodendroglia. White matter in a patient with total hexosaminidase deficiency also exhibited severe loss of myelin, but no loss of galactocerebroside β-galactosidase. The presence of an inhibitor in the tissue of globoid cell leucodystrophy was ruled out by mixing experiments: there was no decrease of cerebroside cleavage by normal brain homogenates when homogenate of Krabbe's disease brain was added to the incubation (Fig. 34-11). The deficiency was also not due to a shift of the pH optimum of galactocerebroside β-galactosidase in Krabbe's disease. The activity was uniformly deficient throughout the pH range of 4.1 to 8.1, whereas there was an optimum around pH 4.5 for a normal brain, as reported previously for a rat brain [122] (Fig. 34-12).

Deficiency of galactocerebroside β-galactosidase activity has since been confirmed in the brain, liver, and kidney of five additional patients [20]. The average activity of galactocerebroside β-galactosidase was less than 5 percent of that of the controls in all organs examined. The highest activities

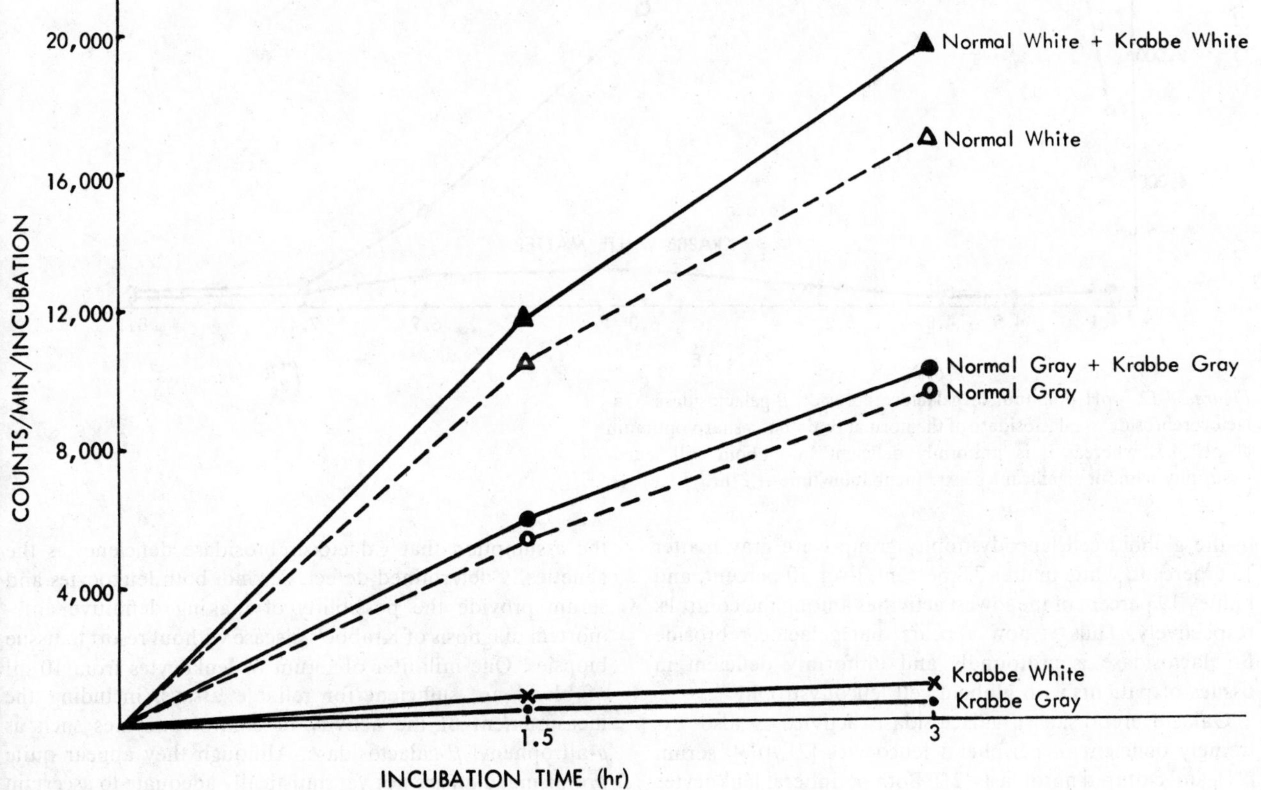

Figure 34-11. A mixing experiment for galactocerebroside β-galactosidase between globoid cell leucodystrophy and a normal control. The vertical scale indicates the radioactivity of the enzymatically liberated galactose. When incubated in the complete assay system, homogenates of either gray or white matter of globoid cell leucodystrophy exhibit little activity of galactocerebroside β-galactosidase (two solid lines at bottom). Both gray and white matter of a control brain show high enzyme activity (broken lines). Addition of homogenates of globoid cell leucodystrophy to normal control systems does not affect the high activities of normal gray and white matter (solid lines). This experiment excludes the possibility that either the presence of an inhibitor or the lack of a cofactor other than the enzyme is causing the apparent deficiency of galactocerebroside β-galactosidase in globoid cell leucodystrophy.

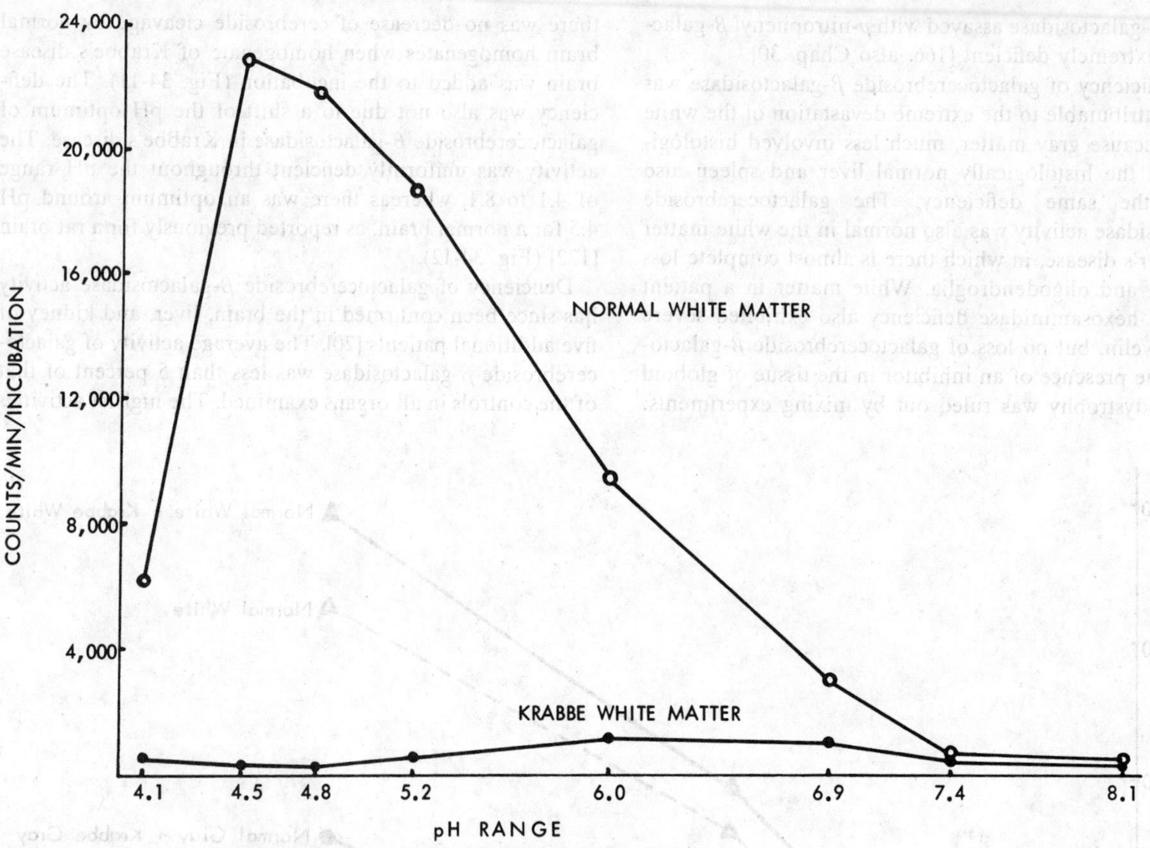

Figure 34-12. pH optimum of galactocerebroside β-galactosidase. Galactocerebroside β-galactosidase of the normal brain has a sharp optimum at pH 4.5, whereas it is uniformly deficient in globoid cell leucodystrophy without significant peaks. Incubation time = 3 hr.

in the globoid cell leucodystrophy group were gray matter 13.6 percent, white matter 7.8 percent, liver 30 percent, and kidney 19 percent of the lowest activities among the controls, respectively. Thus, it now appears that galactocerebroside β-galactosidase is profoundly and uniformly deficient in tissues of patients with globoid cell leucodystrophy.

Galactocerebroside β-galactosidase activity is also extremely deficient in peripheral leucocytes [21, 167], serum [21], and cultured fibroblasts [21]. Both peripheral leukocytes and serum from patients with globoid cell leucodystrophy had galactocerebrosidase activities that were only a few percent of those obtained in normal or pathological controls. Peripheral leukocytes and serum from parents of patients with Krabbe's disease, who are obligate heterozygous gene carriers, have galactocerebroside β-galactosidase activity that is intermediate between normal control individuals and patients. As in other organs, *p*-nitrophenyl β-galactosidase is normal in leukocytes and serum from patients with Krabbe's disease or their parents.

These findings are significant in two aspects, one fundamental and the other practical. First, the intermediate enzyme activities in heterozygous individuals strongly support the assumption that galactocerebrosidase deficiency is the genetically determined defect. Second, both leukocytes and serum provide the possibility of making definitive antemortem diagnosis of Krabbe's disease without resort to tissue biopsies. One milliliter of serum or leukocytes from 10 ml of blood are sufficient for reliable assays, including the measurement of the activity of control enzymes such as *p*-nitrophenyl β-galactosidase. Although they appear quite promising, data are not yet statistically adequate to ascertain whether or not heterozygous carriers can be detected reliably by assaying these materials for galactocerebroside β-galactosidase. In addition to peripheral leukocytes and serum, cultured skin fibroblasts from normal individuals had highly active galactocerebroside β-galactosidase, and this activity was severely deficient in cultured fibroblasts from a patient with Krabbe's disease [21].

PATHOPHYSIOLOGY

Available biochemical data strongly indicate that the deficiency of galactocerebroside β-galactosidase is most probably the genetically determined primary enzymatic defect in globoid cell leucodystrophy. If it is indeed the primary defect of the disease, then we should be able to explain the morphological and biochemical characteristics of the disease on the basis of this deficiency. Some of the major characteristics that have to be explained are (1) almost total loss of myelin and oligodendroglia; (2) normal chemical composition of remaining myelin [151]; (3) morphological evidence of decrease of the amount of myelin during the illness [26]; (4) massive infiltration by globoid cells; and (5) absence of excess accumulation of cerebroside in the brain despite a block in the degradative pathway.

A satisfactory hypothesis can be constructed based on the two apparently unique features of galactocerebroside. First, cerebroside is almost exclusively a constituent of myelin and oligodendroglia, as indicated by its virtual absence in the brain before myelination, and its almost complete loss in white matter of severely demyelinated brains [129, 130]. Second, galactocerebroside appears to be unique among sphingoglycolipids in its ability to elicit the globoid cell reaction when injected into normal rat brain [11–13].

This hypothesis is speculative, lacks the support of detailed experimental evidence, and is offered to be either proved or disproved by future investigations. But it does present a plausible explanation of the characteristics of the disease on the basis of the deficiency of galactocerebroside β-galactosidase. The following steps could occur in the brain of a patient with galactocerebroside β-galactosidase deficiency. Before myelination there is practically no cerebroside in the brain [126–128]. Therefore, lack of the enzyme is of little consequence, although it is normally present at low concentrations even at this premyelination stage [125]. As soon as myelination begins, just before birth in man, newly formed myelin begins to undergo normal turnover. This period coincides with a rapid rise of galactocerebroside β-galactosidase activity in a normal brain [125]. On the other hand, in the brain of patients with Krabbe's disease, galactocerebroside from the catabolized myelin cannot be disposed of because of lack of the enzyme. This undegraded cerebroside elicits globoid cell infiltration. While the globoid cell reaction in a normal brain in experimental conditions subsides as excess cerebroside is digested, the globoid cells in Krabbe's disease remain because galactocerebroside is not degraded. As myelination proceeds, more myelin is formed, and more myelin turns over to provide more free excess galactocerebroside. This in turn produces further globoid cell infiltration. However, myelination cannot proceed indefinitely, for ever-increasing globoid cells overwhelm the oligodendroglial cells, which soon die. When the stage of the massive death of oligodendroglial cells is reached, rapid myelin breakdown occurs. Because myelin is an extension of oligodendroglial cell membranes, myelin breakdown contributes more cerebrosides and these elicit further rapid increase of globoid cells. Finally, when all the oligodendroglial cells die and all the myelin is broken down, resulting in the maximum globoid cell infiltration, there will be no further production of myelin, nor of cerebrosides. Therefore, the total amount of cerebroside that can accumulate in the brain during the short life span of the patient is limited by the small amount of myelin produced before the death of all the oligodendroglial cells; and such total destruction usually takes place at what would have been normally a very early stage of myelination.

This hypothesis appears to explain the characteristic features of globoid cell leucodystrophy satisfactorily. The most crucial point of any hypothesis in regard to the pathophysiology of this disease is how to explain the lack of overt accumulation of galactocerebroside in the brain. As long as the deficient galactocerebroside β-galactosidase is assumed to be present in vivo, the only logical explanation is that, by some mechanism, production of galactocerebroside ceases at a certain stage of the disease when the total amount of cerebroside produced is still well below the concentration in a normal brain. The almost exclusive localization of galactocerebroside in myelin and oligodendroglia, coupled with the almost total loss of these neural components in the terminal stage of the disease, supports the above hypothesis. One recent preliminary report, however, indicates that axons isolated after myelination contain unexpectedly large amounts of galactocerebroside [168]. If these data are confirmed, the above hypothesis needs to be revised to include the disappearance of axons as an important aspect of the disease process. A competition between globoid cells and oligodendroglia is not the only possible mechanism of the death of oligodendroglia. The presence of excess cerebroside itself may be directly detrimental to the metabolism of the oligodendroglia and responsible for their disappearance. In metachromatic leucodystrophy, the amount of sulfatide becomes excessive in white matter as the result of faulty sulfatide degradation, but there is no globoid cell reaction or massive oligodendroglial cell death, and overt accumulation of sulfatide does occur (Chap. 32). Whatever the precise mechanism, either the globoid cell reaction or the excess of cerebrosides must be the key factor leading to the death of oligodendroglia.

There has been some controversy as to whether Krabbe's disease represents the early cessation of myelination or the rapid breakdown of already formed myelin. On the basis of the above hypothesis, both processes are involved, and both occur as the result of the death of the oligodendroglial cells. The destruction of myelin is not due to the formation of chemically abnormal myelin, as often previously postulated.

The low activity of sulfotransferase frequently found in tissues of patients with globoid cell leucodystrophy is difficult to explain. The possibility of two enzymatically distinct types of Krabbe's disease, one with galactocerebroside β-galactosidase deficiency and another with sulfotransferase deficiency, has been excluded; in several cases in which sulfotransferase had been found deficient, galactocerebrosidase was also profoundly deficient [20]. As indicated earlier, the deficiency of sulfotransferase may not be uniform, and some of the characteristic features of the disease are difficult to explain on the basis of sulfotransferase deficiency. It appears to be a secondary phenomenon.

Involvement of the peripheral nervous system is expected from the fact that the peripheral nerve myelin also contains galactocerebroside. Presumably the same disease process is operating in the peripheral nervous tissue as in the CNS. It is not clear why histiocytes in peripheral nerves, which contain abnormal inclusions similar to those in the brain, are not transformed to the typical multinucleated globoid cells. The absence of discernible morphological and functional abnormalities outside the nervous system is understandable, because, normally, galactosyl ceramide is practically absent in most nonneural tissues. The residual activity of galactocerebroside β-galactosidase in these organs may be sufficient to maintain the normal turnover of any minute amount of galactocerebroside present. It is possible that future investigations may reveal an increased concentration of galactocerebrosides in these organs. In most organs, an enormous increase over the normal concentration would be required before the increase in galactocerebrosides was sufficient to cause morphological or functional abnormalities. In this regard, intensive ultrastructural and biochemical examination of kidneys would be of interest, because the kidney is one of the few extraneural organs that normally contains measurable amounts of galactocerebroside [60, 61].

Krabbe's Disease As a Sphingolipidosis

Galactocerebroside β-galactosidase is a hydrolytic enzyme, normally localized in lysosomes. Therefore, the fundamental metabolic defect of Krabbe's disease corresponds with those in other inherited disorders of sphingolipid metabolism, in which lysosomal hydrolytic enzymes involved in the degradation of particular sphingolipids are genetically defective: Gaucher's disease, Niemann-Pick disease, various types of ganglioside storage diseases, metachromatic leucodystrophy, Fabry's disease, and possibly others. Of particular interest is the relationship of globoid cell leucodystrophy to Gaucher's disease. The sphingolipid involved in Gaucher's disease is glucocerebroside and the missing enzyme is glucocerebrosidase. Glucocerebroside and galactocerebroside differ only in the sugar moiety, one being glucose and the other galactose. The missing enzymes are those which cleave the sugar moieties of the respective cerebrosides. Therefore, the fundamental metabolic derangements in these diseases are quite similar. This probably explains the morphological similarities of the globoid cells of Krabbe's disease and the giant cells of Gaucher's disease. Nevertheless, the clinical and pathological features are entirely different. Such differences are expected because galactocerebroside is almost exclusively localized in the nervous system, whereas glucosyl ceramide (glucocerebroside) is primarily a nonneural cerebroside, normally present in visceral organs but nearly absent in the normal brain except in the early developmental stages. Krabbe's disease is unique among the sphingolipidoses in that there is no overt accumulation of galactocerebroside in spite of a metabolic block in its degradative pathway.

DIAGNOSIS AND TREATMENT

Brain biopsy had long been the final resort for the definitive antemortem diagnosis of globoid cell leucodystrophy since Blackwood and Cumings [7] emphasized the presence of the characteristic globoid cells. Due to the wide variations of morphological changes in different stages of the disease and in different areas of the brain, brain biopsy does not always establish the diagnosis. Giant cells, similar to globoid cells, may be encountered in other diseases such as "the syndrome of familial leucodystrophy, adrenal insufficiency and cutaneous melanosis," in which half of the cases showed globoid-like cells in cerebral white matter [169]. The diagnostic value of the peripheral nerve biopsy has not been fully explored, but, in view of consistent pathological changes, particularly on the ultrastructural level, it may prove useful.

Assays of galactocerebroside β-galactosidase activity in readily available materials, such as serum, peripheral leukocytes, or cultured fibroblasts, offer unquestionably the best and most reliable means for definitive antemortem diagnosis. So far, extremely low activities of this enzyme have been found only in globoid cell leucodystrophy. Specimens from normal individuals and from patients with varieties of pathological conditions other than globoid cell leucodystrophy invariably showed a high activity of galactocerebroside β-galactosidase.

Although larger numbers of samples are still needed for a strict statistical evaluation of the data, preliminary findings strongly indicate that an assay of white cells or serum for galactocerebroside β-galactosidase may also be used for reliable detection of heterozygotes. Furthermore, in view of recent developments in other inherited metabolic disorders, it is highly probable that an intrauterine diagnosis of affected children can be made by assaying cultured or uncultured amniotic fluid cells for the activity of this enzyme.

None of the other laboratory diagnostic procedures advocated earlier for the diagnosis of globoid cell leucodystrophy, such as the pattern of CSF protein [25] or the elevated β-glucuronidase activity in CSF [52], are specific, and their usefulness is limited.

There is no specific treatment for globoid cell leucodystrophy other than supportive care, nor is it expected that any effective specific treatment can be developed in the near future. One may hope with reasonable certainty that the day is not too far away when fewer patients will be born with globoid cell leucodystrophy through a combination of genetic counseling and preventive abortion, on the basis of prenatal enzymatic diagnosis of affected fetuses.

CANINE GLOBOID CELL LEUCODYSTROPHY

In 1963, Fankhauser et al. first reported that globoid cell leucodystrophy occurs in certain strains of dogs [170]. The strains in which the disease is known are West Highland and Cairn Terriers. The disease has been studied extensively from the clinical, morphological, and biochemical standpoints [171–178]. The disease appears to be transmitted as an autosomal recessive trait. The clinical picture is quite similar to the human disease. An example of a clinical history is given here [172].

This male West Highland White Terrier seemed normal until three months of age when he gradually developed increasing difficulty in walking down stairs and in running on paved surfaces. He showed knuckling of digits while standing and began to fall on his hind limbs with bilateral extension of hock and stifle. On examination at 9 months of age, there was paraplegia with loss of placing and hopping reactions, hypoactive to absent deep reflexes of the posterior limbs, loss of sensation of the tail, and urinary incontinence.

Morphologically, there are remarkable similarities between the human and the canine forms of globoid cell leucodystrophy. The most conspicuous changes are the massive infiltration of globoid cells in the white matter, with morphology, distribution pattern, and staining characteristics identical to human globoid cells. There is severe loss of myelin, oligodendroglia, and axons, with concomitant marked astrocytic gliosis. The ultrastructure of canine globoid cells is also quite similar to human globoid cells, containing the characteristic abnormal tubular inclusions. There are peripheral nerve lesions, again similar to human cases [179]. Information regarding the lipid composition of the brain is still limited, but in one report there was decreased total lipid, decreased sulfatide, and slightly increased cerebroside [174].

Suzuki et al. demonstrated that the canine globoid cell leucodystrophy is also characterized by deficient galactocerebroside β-galactosidase activity [180]. The enzyme was deficient in gray and white matter of the brain, liver, and kidney of two affected dogs. As in human patients, there was no deficiency of *p*-nitrophenyl β-galactosidase. Moreover, one apparently healthy litter mate of an affected dog had galactocerebrosidase activities intermediate between those of the affected dogs and another healthy litter mate. The latter healthy litter-mate dog had the same high enzyme activities as a healthy mixed-breed dog. Therefore, it is not unreasonable to consider that the litter-mate dog with intermediate enzyme values was a heterozygote. There was no cerebroside-sulfatide sulfotransferase deficiency in the affected dogs [180]. It appears certain that galactosyl ceramide β-galactosidase deficiency is the genetically determined primary enzymatic defect in canine globoid cell leucodystrophy (Table 34-4). It is, therefore, an authentic animal model, and not a mere facsimile, of the human disease.

SUMMARY

1 Krabbe's globoid cell leucodystrophy is a rapidly progressive, invariably fatal disease of infants. The onset of clinical symptoms is usually between age 3 to 6 months. The disease usually begins with ambiguous symptoms such as irritability or hypersensitivity to external stimuli, but soon progresses to severe mental and motor deterioration. Long-tract signs are prominent. There is hypertonicity with hyperactive reflexes in the early stages, but patients become flaccid and hypotonic later. Blindness and deafness are common. Patients rarely survive the second year. There are clinical and laboratory signs of peripheral neuropathy. Systemic manifestations are rare. The disease is transmitted as an autosomal recessive trait.

2 The presence of numerous characteristic globoid cells in the white matter is the morphological basis of diagnosis. The globoid cells are mesodermal in origin, essentially macrophages. They are either mononuclear or multinucleated and contain PAS-positive material which has characteristic ultrastructural features. The morphological evidence, as well as the experimental production of globoid reactions by intracerebral injection of galactocerebroside, indicates that

Table 34-4. GALACTOCEREBROSIDE β-GALACTOSIDASE IN CANINE GLOBOID CELL LEUCODYSTROPHY

		Gray matter mμmoles/hr/gm	White matter mμmoles/hr/gm	Liver mμmoles/hr/gm	Kidney mμmoles/hr/gm
Globoid cell leucodystrophy	1	14.1	13.0	16.7	12.3
	2	15.1	15.0	37.6	
Normal	1	127	.....	133	78.2
	2	120	169	138	91.7
Heterozygous?*		76.2	108	75.6	29.5

*This dog was an asymptomatic litter mate of the affected dog No. 1 and the normal dog No. 1.
Note: There was no significant difference in the activities of *p*-nitrophenyl β-galactosidase in all specimens.
Source: Data from Suzuki et al. [*180*].

these abnormal inclusions in globoid cells may be galactocerebroside. Severe myelin loss and astrocytic gliosis complete the pathological picture of the white matter. Morphological changes are also common in the peripheral nervous system.

3 White matter usually shows profound loss of all lipids, particularly glycolipids, as would be expected from the severe loss of myelin. Although much lower than normal, galactocerebroside is relatively preserved compared to sulfatide. Galactocerebroside is a sphingoglycolipid containing sphingosine, fatty acid, and galactose, and is highly concentrated in the myelin sheath.

4 Profound deficiency in the activity of galactocerebroside β-galactosidase, the enzyme which normally cleaves galactocerebroside to ceramide and galactose as the first step in degradation, appears to be the genetically determined enzymatic defect. The defect is generalized and affects brain, liver, spleen, kidneys, peripheral leukocytes, serum, and cultured fibroblasts. The features of the disease can be explained by this enzymatic defect when the two unique characteristics of galactocerebroside are taken into consideration: (1) its highly restricted localization in the myelin sheath and oligodendroglia, and (2) its capability to elicit the globoid cell reaction. The lack of overt accumulation of galactocerebroside, in spite of the block on its degradative pathway, can be explained as the result of the cessation of further galactocerebroside production because of almost complete loss of oligodendroglial cells. While there is no "storage" of galactocerebroside in whole tissue, the disease fundamentally belongs to the group of "lipid storage diseases" in which genetically determined deficiencies of lysosomal hydrolytic enzymes result in the accumulation of various lipids.

5 Galactocerebroside β-galactosidase assays on white cells or serum provide the means for definitive antemortem diagnosis of the disease.

6 There is no specific therapy for affected patients, but preventive measures may become available through genetic counseling and intrauterine diagnosis of affected individuals on the basis of galactocerebroside β-galactosidase assays on amniotic fluid cells.

7 Globoid cell leucodystrophy occurs in some strains of dogs with clinical and pathological features similar to the human disease. It is also characterized by deficient galactocerebroside β-galactosidase. The existence of this authentic animal model provides an invaluable tool for further investigation of globoid cell leucodystrophy.

BIBLIOGRAPHY

1. Krabbe, K.: A new familial, infantile form of diffuse brain sclerosis. Brain, **39,** 74, 1916.
2. Bullard, W. N., and Southard, E. E.: Diffuse gliosis of the cerebral white matter in a child. J. Nerv. Ment. Dis., **33,** 188, 1906.
3. Beneke, R.: Ein Fall hochgradigster ausgedehnter Sklerose des Centralnervensystems. Arch. Kinderheilk., **47,** 420, 1908.
4. Collier, J., and Greenfield, J. G.: The encephalitis periaxialis of Schilder: A clinical and pathological study with an account of two cases, one of which was diagnosed during life. Brain, **47,** 489, 1924.
5. Hallervorden, J.: Eine Speicherungshistiocytose des kindlichen Gehirns (Gauchersche Krankheit?). Verh. Deutsch. Ges. Pathol., **32,** 96, 1948.
6. Austin, J. H.: Studies in globoid (Krabbe) leukodystrophy. II. Controlled thin-layer chromatographic studies of globoid body fractions in seven patients. J. Neurochem., **10,** 921, 1963.
7. Blackwood, W., and Cumings, J. N.: A histochemical and chemical study of three cases of diffuse cerebral sclerosis. J. Neurol. Neurosurg. Psychiat., **17,** 33, 1954.
8. Diezel, P. B.: Histochemische Untersuchungen an den Globoidzellen der familiären infantilen diffusen Sklerose vom Typus Krabbe. Virchow Arch. Path. Anat., **327,** 206, 1955.
9. Diezel, P. B.: Histochemical investigations of degenerative diffuse sclerosis (leucodystrophy and diffuse sclerosis of the Krabbe type), in *Cerebral Lipidoses: A Symposium,* edited by J. N. Cumings and A. Lowenthal, p. 52. Charles C Thomas, Springfield, Ill., 1957.
10. Stammler, A.: Klinik, Pathologie und Histochemie der infantilen diffusen Sklerose vom Typus Krabbe. Deutsch. Z. Nervenheilk., **174,** 505, 1956.
11. Austin, J , Lehfeldt, D., and Maxwell, W.: Experimental "globoid bodies" in white matter and chemical analysis in Krabbe's disease. J. Neuropath. Exp. Neurol., **20,** 284, 1961.
12. Austin, J. H., and Lehfeldt, D.: Studies in globoid (Krabbe) leucodystrophy: III. Significance of experimentally produced globoid-like elements in rat white matter and spleen. J. Neuropath. Exp. Neurol., **24,** 265, 1965.
13. Olsson, R., Sourander, P., and Svennerholm, L.: Experimental studies on the pathogenesis of leucodystrophies. I. The effect of intracerebrally injected sphingolipids in the rat brain. Acta Neuropath. (Berlin), **6,** 153, 1966.
14. Austin, J. H.: Recent studies in the metachromatic and globoid body forms of diffuse sclerosis, in *Brain Lipids and Lipoproteins, and the Leucodystrophies,* edited by J. Folch-Pi and H. Bauer, p. 120. Elsevier, Amsterdam, 1963.
15. Svennerholm, L.: Some aspects of biochemical changes in leucodystrophy, in *Brain Lipids and Lipoproteins, and the Leucodystrophies,* edited by J. Folch-Pi and H. Bauer, p. 104. Elsevier, Amsterdam, 1963.
16. Bachhawat, B. K., Austin, J., and Armstrong, D.: A cerebroside sulphotransferase deficiency in a human disorder of myelin. Biochem. J., **104,** 15C, 1967.
17. Austin, J., Armstrong, D., Stumpf, D., Kretschmer, L., Mitchell, C., VanZee, B., and Bachhawat, B.: Defective sulfatide synthesis in Krabbe's disease (globoid leukodystrophy). Trans. Amer. Neurol. Ass., **175,** 179, 1967.
18. Suzuki, K., and Suzuki, Y.: Globoid cell leucodystrophy (Krabbe's disease): Deficiency of galactocerebroside β-galactosidase. Proc. Nat. Acad. Sci. USA., **66,** 302, 1970.
19. Suzuki, K., Suzuki, Y., and Eto, Y.: Deficiency of galactocerebroside β-galactosidase in Krabbe's globoid cell leucodystrophy, in *Lipid Storage Diseases: Enzymatic Defect and Clinical Implications,* edited by J. Bernsohn and H. J. Grossman, p. 396, Academic, New York, 1971.
20. Austin, J., Suzuki, K., Armstrong, D., Brady, R., Bachhawat, B. K., Schlenker, J., and Stumpf, D.: Studies in globoid (Krabbe) leukodystrophy (GLD). V. Controlled enzymic studies in ten human cases. Arch. Neurol. (Chicago), **23,** 502, 1970.
21. Suzuki, Y., and Suzuki, K.: Krabbe's globoid cell leukodystrophy: deficiency of galactocerebrosidase in serum, leukocytes, and fibroblasts. Science, **171,** 73, 1971.
22. Jervis, G. A.: Early infantile "diffuse sclerosis" of the brain (Krabbe's type): Report of two cases, with a review of the literature. Amer. J. Dis. Child., **64,** 1055, 1942.
23. Gehuchten, P. van: Sur l'origine des cellules globoides dans un cas de sclérose diffuse. Rev. Neurol. (Paris), **94,** 253, 1956.
24. Schochet, S. S., Jr., Hardman, J. M., Lampert, P. W., and Earle, K. M.: Krabbe's disease (globoid leukodystrophy): Electron microscopic observations. Arch. Path. (Chicago), **88,** 305, 1969.

25. Hagberg, B., Sourander, P., and Svennerholm, L.: Diagnosis of Krabbe's infantile leukodystrophy. J. Neurol. Neurosurg. Psychiat., **26,** 195, 1963.
26. D'Agostino, A. N., Sayre, G. P., and Hagles, A. B.: Krabbe's disease. Arch. Neurol. (Chicago), **8,** 82, 1963.
27. Globus, J. H., and Strauss, I.: Progressive degenerative subcortical encephalopathy. Arch. Neurol. Psychiat., **20,** 1190, 1928.
28. Nelson, E., Aurebeck, G., Osterberg, K., Berry, J., Jabbour, J. T., and Bornhofen, J.: Ultrastructural and chemical studies on Krabbe's disease. J. Neuropath. Exp. Neurol., **22,** 414, 1963.
29. Verhaart, W. J. C.: A case of multiple sclerosis with an Indian in the Dutch East Indies. Psychiat. Neurol. Bladen (Amst.), **35,** 511, 1931.
30. Guillain, G., Bertrand, I., and Gruner, J.: Sur un type anatomoclinique spécial de leucoencéphalite à nodules morulés gliogénes. Rev. Neurol. (Paris), **73,** 401, 1941.
31. Ferraro, A.: Familial form of encephalitis periaxialis diffusa. J. Nerv. Ment. Dis., **66,** 329, 1927.
32. Ferraro, A.: Familial form of encephalitis periaxialis diffusa. J. Nerv. Ment. Dis., **66,** 479, 1927.
33. Ferraro, A.: Familial form of encephalitis periaxialis diffusa. J. Nerv. Ment. Dis., **66,** 616, 1927.
34. Hagberg, B.: The clinical diagnosis of Krabbe's infantile leucodystrophy. Acta Paediat. Scand., **52,** 213, 1963.
35. Suzuki, K., and Grover, W. D.: Krabbe's leukodystrophy (globoid cell leukodystrophy): An ultrastructural study. Arch. Neurol. (Chicago), **22,** 385, 1970.
36. Allen, N., and de Veyra, E.: Microchemical and histochemical observations in a case of Krabbe's leukodystrophy. J. Neuropath. Exp. Neurol., **26,** 456, 1967.
37. Hogan, G. R., Gutmann, L., and Chou, S. M.: The peripheral neuropathy of Krabbe's (globoid) leukodystrophy. Neurology (Minneap.), **19,** 1093, 1969.
38. Yunis, E. J., and Lee, R. E.: The ultrastructure of globoid (Krabbe) leukodystrophy. Lab. Invest., **21,** 415, 1969.
39. Jacobi, M.: Über Leukodystrophie und Pelizaeus-Merzbachersche Krankheit. Virchow. Arch. Path. Anat., **314,** 460, 1947.
40. Matsuyama, H., Minoshima, I., and Watanabe, I.: An autopsy case of leucodystrophy of Krabbe type. Acta Path. Jap., **13,** 195, 1963.
41. Wallace, B. J., Aronson, S. M., and Volk, B. W.: Histochemical and biochemical studies of globoid cell leucodystrophy (Krabbe's disease). J. Neurochem., **11,** 367, 1963.
42. Osetowska, E., Gail, H., Lukasewicz, D., Karcher, D., and Wisniewski, H.: Leucodystrophie infantile précoce (Type Krabbe): (Remarques sur les proliférations gliales et les atrophies de système qui peuvent s'y observer). Rev. Neurol. (Paris), **102,** 463, 1960.
43. Kass, A.: Acute infantile sclerosis of the brain (Krabbe's disease). Acta Paediat., **42,** 70, 1953.
44. Bignami, A., Tingey, A. H., and Torre, C.: La sclerosi cerebrale diffusa tipo Krabbe. Riv. Neurol., **31,** 712, 1961.
45. Austin, J. H.: Recent studies in the metachromatic and globoid forms of diffuse sclerosis. Res. Publ. Ass. Res. Nerv. Ment. Dis., **40,** 189, 1962.
46. Dunn, H. G., Lake, B. D., Dolman, C. L., and Wilson, J.: The neuropathy of Krabbe's infantile cerebral sclerosis (globoid cell leucodystrophy). Brain, **92,** 329, 1969.
47. Sacrez, R., Levy, J. M., Gruner, J. E., Billuart, J., and Carlier, G.: La leucodystrophie de Krabbe. Arch. Franç. Pédiat., **22,** 641, 1965.
48. Cumings, J. N., and Rozdilsky, B.: The cerebral lipid composition of the brain in six cases of Krabbe's disease. Neurology (Minneap.), **15,** 177, 1965.
49. Poser, C. M., and van Bogaert, L.: Natural history and evolution of the concept of Schilder's diffuse sclerosis. Acta Psychiat. Scand., **31,** 285, 1956.
50. Norman, R. M., Oppenheimer, D. R., and Tingey, A. H.: Histological and chemical findings in Krabbe's leucodystrophy. J. Neurol. Neurosurg. Psychiat., **24,** 223, 1961.
51. Hagberg, B., and Svennerholm, L.: Metachromatic leucodystrophy—a generalized lipidosis: Determination of sulfatides in urine, blood plasma and cerebrospinal fluid. Acta Paediat., **49,** 690, 1960.
52. Allen, N., and Reagan, E.: Beta-glucuronidase activities in cerebrospinal fluid. Arch. Neurol. (Chicago), **11,** 144, 1964.
53. Allen, N. E., Shuttleworth, C., Clendenon, N. R., and Gordon, W. A.: Cerebrospinal fluid β-glucuronidase activity in the diagnosis of Krabbe's leucodystrophy. Int. Congr. Series No. 193, Excerpta Med., Amsterdam, p. 181, 1969.
54. Austin, J. H.: Some newer findings in Krabbe (globoid) leucodystrophy. Trans. Amer. Neurol. Ass., **87,** 66, 1962.
55. Blom, S., and Hagberg, B.: EEG findings in late infantile metachromatic and globoid cell leucodystrophy. Electroenceph. Clin. Neurophysiol., **22,** 253, 1967.
56. Kliemann, F. A., Harden, A., Pampiglione, G.: Some EEG observations in patients with Krabbe's disease. Develop. Med. Child. Neurol., **11,** 475, 1969.
57. Bugiani, O., Mastropaolo, C., and de Negri, M.: Association d'une leucodystrophie à cellules globoides d'une gliomatose et d'une abiotrophie. Acta Neurol. Belg., **68,** 799, 1968.
58. Christensen, E., Melchior, J. C., and Andersen, H.: Diffuse infantile familial sclerosis (Krabbe-type). Acta Psychiat. Neurol. Scand., **35,** 431, 1960.
59. Austin, J. H.: Histochemical and biochemical studies in diffuse cerebral sclerosis (metachromatic and globoid-body forms). *IVth Internat. Congr. Neuropath. Stuttgart,* Thieme, **1,** 35, 1962.
60. Makita, A.: Biochemistry of organ glycolipids. II. Isolation of human kidney glycolipids. J. Biochem. (Tokyo), **55,** 269, 1964.
61. Martensson, E.: Neutral glycolipids of human kidney: Isolation, identification and fatty acid composition. Biochim. Biophys. Acta, **116,** 296, 1966.
62. Diezel, P. B.: *Die Stoffwechselstörungen der Sphingolipoide.* Springer-Verlag, Berlin, 1957.
63. Hager, H., and Oehlert, W.: 1st die diffuse Hirnsklerose des Typ Krabbe eine entzündliche Allgemeinerkrankung? Z. Kinderheilk., **80,** 82, 1957.
64. Greenfield, J. G., and Norman, R. M.: Demyelinating Diseases, in *Greenfield's Neuropathology,* edited by W. Blackwood, W. H. McMenemy, A. Meyer, R. M. Norman, and D. S. Russel, 2d ed. p. 475. Williams and Wilkins, Baltimore, 1963.
65. Austin, J. H.: Globoid (Krabbe) leukodystrophy, in *Pathology of the Nervous System,* edited by J. Minkler, p. 843. McGraw-Hill, New York, 1968.
66. Suzuki, Kinuko: Personal communication.
67. Sourander, P., Hansson, H. A., Olsson, Y., and Svennerholm, L.: Experimental studies on the pathogenesis of leucodystrophies. II. The effect of sphingolipids on various cell types in cultures from the nervous system. Acta Neuropath. (Berlin), **9,** 231, 1966.
68. Pfeiffer, J.: Zur formalen Genese der Globoidzellen bei der diffusen Sklerose vom Typus Krabbe. Arch. Psychiat. Nervenkr., **195,** 446, 1957.
69. Einarson, L., and Strömgren, E.: Diffuse progressive leucoencephalopathy (diffuse cerebral sclerosis) and its relationship to amaurotic idiocy: Histological and clinical aspects. Acta Jutland, 33, 5, 1961.
70. Christensen, E., Melchior, J. C., and Negri, S.: A comparative study of 16 cases of diffuse sclerosis with special reference to the histopathological findings. Acta Neurol. Scand., **37,** 163, 1961.
71. Konigsmark, B. W., and Sidman, R. L.: The origin of brain macrophages in the mouse. J. Neuropath. Exp. Neurol., **22,** 643, 1963.
72. Huntington, H. W., and Terry, R. D.: The origin of the reactive cells in cerebral stab wounds. J. Neuropath. Exp. Neurol., **25,** 646, 1966.
73. Roesmann, U., and Friede, R. L.: Entry of labeled donor cells from the blood stream into the CNS. J. Neuropath. Exp. Neurol., **26,** 144, 1966.
74. Einarson, L., Neel, A. F., and Strömgren, E.: On the problem of diffuse brain sclerosis with special reference to the familial forms. Acta Jutland, **16,** 1, 1944.
75. Hallervorden, J.: Die degenerative diffuse Sklerose, in *Handbuch der speziellen pathologischen Anatomie und Histologie,* edited by H. Lubarsch and B. Rossle, XIII/1, p. 758. Springer-Verlag, Berlin, 1956.
76. de Vries, E.: Gliomatous polio- and leucodystrophy in a young child. J. Neuropath. Exp. Neurol., **17,** 501, 1958.

77. Andrews, J. M., and Cancilla, P.: Cytoplasmic inclusions in human globoid cell leukodystrophy. Arch. Path. (Chicago), **89,** 53, 1970.
78. Shaw, C.-M., and Carlson, C. B.: Crystalline structures in globoid-epithelioid cells: An electron microscopic study of globoid leukodystrophy (Krabbe's disease). J. Neuropath. Exp. Neurol., **29,** 306, 1970.
79. Lake, B. D.: Segmental demyelination of peripheral nerves in Krabbe's disease. Nature (London), **217,** 171, 1968.
80. Bischoff, A., and Ulrich, J.: Peripheral neuropathy in globoid cell leukodystrophy (Krabbe's disease): Ultrastructural and histochemical findings. Brain, **92,** 861, 1969.
81. Suzuki, K.: Ultrastructural study of experimental globoid cells. Lab. Invest., **23,** 612, 1970.
82. Sourander, P., and Olsson, Y.: Peripheral neuropathy in globoid cell leucodystrophy (Morbus Krabbe). Acta Neuropath. (Berlin), **11,** 69, 1968.
83. Carter, H. E., Glick, F. J., Norris, W. P., and Phillips, G. E.: Biochemistry of the sphingolipides. III. Structure of sphingosine. J. Biol. Chem., **170,** 285, 1947.
84. Carter, H. E.: Sphingolipids, in *Chemistry of Lipids as Related to Atherosclerosis,* edited by I. H. Page, p. 82. Charles C Thomas, Springfield, Ill., 1958.
85. Grob, C. A., and Gadient, F.: Die Synthese des Sphingosins und seiner Stereoisomeren. Helv. Chim. Acta, **40,** 1145, 1957.
86. Shapiro, D., Segel, H., and Flowers, H. M.: The total synthesis of sphingosine. J. Amer. Chem. Soc., **80,** 1194, 1958.
87. Prostenik, M., and Majhder-Orescanin, B.: Occurrence of a new sphingolipid base, C_{20}-sphingosine in horse and beef brain. Naturwissenschaften, **47,** 399, 1960.
88. Stanacev, N. Z., and Chargaff, E.: Icosisphingosine, a long chain base constituent of mucolipids. Biochim. Biophys. Acta, **59,** 733, 1963.
89. Sambasivarao, K., and McCluer, R. H.: Lipid components of gangliosides. J. Lipid Res., **5,** 103, 1965.
90. Sweeley, C. C., and Moscatelli, E. A.: Qualitative microanalysis and estimation of sphingolipid bases. J. Lipid Res., **1,** 40, 1959.
91. Moscatelli, E. A., and Mayes, J. R.: Sphingosine bases of normal human white matter. Biochemistry (Wash.), **4,** 1386, 1965.
92. Isaacson, E., and Moscatelli, E. A.: Sphingolipids of developing human central nervous tissue: Changes in composition of sphingosine bases. J. Neurochem., **17,** 365, 1970.
93. O'Brien, J. S., and Rouser, G.: The fatty acid composition of brain sphingolipids: Sphingomyelin, ceramide, cerebroside, and cerebroside sulfate. J. Lipid Res., **5,** 339, 1964.
94. Eng, L. F., Gerstl, B., Hayman, R. B., Lee, Y. L., Tietsort, R. W., and Smith, J. K.: The 2-hydroxy fatty acids in white matter of infant and adult brains. J. Lipid Res., **6,** 135, 1965.
95. Ställberg-Stenhagen, S., and Svennerholm, L.: Fatty acid composition of human brain sphingomyelins: Normal variation with age and changes during myelin disorders. J. Lipid Res., **6,** 146, 1965.
96. O'Brien, J. S., and Sampson, E. L.: Fatty acid and fatty aldehyde composition of the major brain lipids in normal human gray matter, white matter, and myelin. J. Lipid Res., **6,** 545, 1965.
97. Menkes, J. H., Philippart, M., and Concone, M. C.: Concentration and fatty acid composition of cerebrosides and sulfatides in mature and immature human brain. J. Lipid Res., **7,** 479, 1966.
98. Klenk, E., and Gielen, W.: Untersuchungen über die Konstitution der Ganglioside aus Menschengehirn und die Trennung des Gemisches in die Komponenten. Z. Physiol. Chem., **326,** 144, 1961.
99. Trams, E. G., Guiffrida, L. E., and Karmen, A.: Gas chromatographic analysis of long-chain fatty acids in gangliosides. Nature (London), **193,** 680, 1962.
100. Ledeen, R., Salsman, K., and Cabrera, M.: Gangliosides in subacute sclerosing leukoencephalitis: Isolation and fatty acid composition of nine fractions. J. Lipid Res., **9,** 129, 1968.
101. Suzuki, K., Suzuki, K., and Kamoshita, S.: Chemical pathology of G_{M1}-gangliosidosis (generalized gangliosidosis). J. Neuropath. Exp. Neurol., **28,** 25, 1969.
102. Svennerholm, L.: The distribution of lipids in the human nervous system. I. Analytical procedure: Lipids of foetal and newborn brain. J. Neurochem., **11,** 839, 1964.
103. Suzuki, Y., Jacob, J. C., Suzuki, K., and Suzuki, K.: G_{M2}-gangliosidosis with total hexosaminidase deficiency. Neurology (Minneap.) (in press).
104. Yamakawa, T., Kiso, N., Handa, S., Makita, A., and Yokoyama, S.: On the structure of brain cerebroside sulfuric ester and ceramide dihexoside of erythrocytes. J. Biochem. (Tokyo), **52,** 226, 1962.
105. Stoffyn, P., and Stoffyn, A.: Structure of sulfatides. Biochim. Biophys. Acta, **70,** 218, 1963.
106. Burton, R. M., Sodd, M. A., and Brady, R. O.: The incorporation of galactose into galactolipids. J. Biol. Chem., **233,** 1053, 1958.
107. Cleland, W. W., and Kennedy, E. P.: The enzymatic synthesis of psychosine. J. Biol. Chem., **235,** 45, 1960.
108. Brady, R. O.: Studies on the total enzymatic synthesis of cerebrosides. J. Biol. Chem., **237,** PC2416, 1962.
109. Brady, R. O.: Biosynthesis of glycolipids, in *Metabolism and Physiological Significance of Lipids,* edited by R. M. C. Dawson and D. N. Rhodes, p. 95. Wiley, London, 1964.
110. Morell, P., and Radin, N. S.: Synthesis of cerebroside by brain from uridine diphosphate galactose and ceramide containing hydroxy fatty acid. Biochemistry (Wash.), **8,** 506, 1969.
111. Goldberg, I. H.: The sulfolipids. J. Lipid Res., **2,** 103, 1961.
112. Radin, N. S., Martin, F. B., and Brown, J. R.: Galactolipide metabolism. J. Biol. Chem., **224,** 499, 1957.
113. Hauser, G.: Labelling of cerebroside and sulfatides in rat brain. Biochim. Biophys. Acta, **84,** 212, 1964.
114. McKhann, G., Lavy, R., and Ho, W.: Metabolism of sulfatides. I. The effect of galactocerebrosides on the synthesis of sulfatides. Biochem. Biophys. Res. Commun., **20,** 109, 1965.
115. Balasubramanian, A. S., and Bachhawat, B. K.: Studies on enzymic synthesis of cerebroside sulfate from 3′-phosphoadenosine-5′-phosphosulfate. Indian J. Biochem., **2,** 212, 1965.
116. Balasubramanian, A. S., and Bachhawat, B. K.: Formation of cerebroside sulfate from 3′-phosphoadenosine 5′-phosphosulfate in sheep brain. Biochim. Biophys. Acta, **106,** 218, 1965.
117. Herschkowitz, N., McKhann, G. M., Saxena, S., and Shooter, E. M.: Characterization of sulfatide-containing lipoproteins in rat brain. J. Neurochem., **15,** 1181, 1968.
118. Herschkowitz, N., McKhann, G. M., Saxena, S.: Synthesis of sulphatide-containing lipoproteins in rat brain. J. Neurochem., **16,** 1049, 1969.
119. Mehl, E., and Jatzkewitz, H.: Ein Cerebrosid Sulfatase aus Schweineniere. Z. Physiol. Chem., **339,** 260, 1964.
120. Austin, J. H., Armstrong, D., and Shearer, L.: Metachromatic form of diffuse cerebral sclerosis. V. The nature and significance of low sulfatase activity: A controlled study of brain, liver and kidney in four patients with metachromatic leucodystrophy (MLD). Arch. Neurol. (Chicago), **13,** 593, 1965.
121. Mehl, E., and Jatzkewitz, H.: Evidence for the genetic block in metachromatic leucodystrophy (ML). Biochem. Biophys. Res. Commun., **19,** 407, 1965.
122. Hajra, A. K., Bowen, D. M., Kishimoto, Y., and Radin, N. S.: Cerebroside galactosidase of brain. J. Lipid Res., **7,** 379, 1966.
123. Bowen, D. M., and Radin, N. S.: Purification of cerebroside galactosidase from rat brain. Biochim. Biophys. Acta, **152,** 587, 1968.
124. Bowen, D. M., and Radin, N. S.: Properties of cerebroside galactosidase. Biochim. Biophys. Acta, **152,** 599, 1968.
125. Bowen, D. M., and Radin, N. S.: Cerebroside galactosidase: A method for determination and a comparison with other lysosomal enzymes in developing rat brain. J. Neurochem., **16,** 501, 1969.
126. Folch-Pi, J.: Composition of the brain in relation to maturation, in *Biochemistry of the Developing Nervous System,* edited by H. Waelsch, p. 121. Academic, New York, 1955.
127. Cuzner, M. L., and Davison, A. N.: The lipid composition of rat brain myelin and subcellular fractions during development. Biochem. J., **106,** 29, 1968.
128. Wells, M. A., and Dittmer, J. C.: A comprehensive study of the postnatal changes in the concentration of the lipids of developing rat brain. Biochemistry (Wash.), **6,** 3169, 1967.
129. Kamoshita, S., Rapin, I., Suzuki, K., and Suzuki, K.: Spongy degeneration of the brain: A chemical study of two cases including isolation and characterization of myelin. Neurology (Minneap.), **18,** 975, 1968.

130. Suzuki, Y., Tucker, S. H., Rorke, L. B., and Suzuki, K.: Ultrastructural and biochemical studies of Schilder's disease. II. Biochemistry. J. Neuropath. Exp. Neurol. **29**, 405, 1970.
131. Bass, N. H., and Hess, H. H.: A comparison of cerebroside, proteolipid proteins and cholesterol as indices of myelin in the architecture of rat cerebrum. J. Neurochem., **16**, 731, 1969.
132. Norton, W. T.: Personal communication.
133. O'Brien, J. S., Sampson, E. L., and Stern, M. B.: Lipid composition of myelin from the peripheral nervous system. J. Neurochem., **14**, 357, 1967.
134. O'Brien, J. S.: Lipids and myelination, in *Developing Brain,* edited by H. E. Himwich and W. A. Himwich. Charles C Thomas, Springfield, Ill., 1968.
135. Dickerson, J. W. T.: The composition of nervous tissues, in *Applied Neurochemistry,* edited by A. N. Davison and J. Dobbing, p. 48. Davis, Philadelphia, Pa., 1968.
136. Eichberg, J., Hauser, G., and Karnovsky, M. L.: Lipids of nervous tissue, in *The Structure and Function of Nervous Tissue,* edited by G. H. Bourne, vol. III, p. 185. Academic, New York, 1969.
137. Mokrasch, L. C.: Myelin, in *Handbook of Neurochemistry,* edited by A. Lajtha, vol. 1, p. 171. Plenum, New York, 1969.
138. Norton, W. T.: The myelin sheath, in *The Cellular and Molecular Basis of Neurologic Disease,* edited by G. M. Shy, E. S. Goldensohn, and S. H. Appel, Lea and Febiger (in press).
139. Davison, A. N.: Myelin metabolism, in *Metabolism and Physiological Significance of Lipids,* edited by R. M. C. Dawson and D. N. Rhodes, p. 527. Wiley, London, 1964.
140. Smith, M. E.: The metabolism of myelin lipids, in *Advances in Lipid Research,* edited by R. Paoletti and D. Kritchevsky, vol. 5, p. 241. Academic, New York, 1967.
141. Yakovlev, P., and Lecours, A. R.: The myelogenetic cycles of regional maturation of the brain, in *Regional Development of the Brain in Early Life,* edited by A. Minkowski, p. 3. Blackwell, Oxford, 1967.
142. August, C., Davison, A. N., and Williams, F. M.: Phospholipid metabolism in nervous tissue. IV. Incorporation of ^{32}P into the lipids of subcellular fractions of the brain. Biochem. J., **81**, 8, 1961.
143. Cuzner, M. L., Davison, A. N., and Gregson, N. A.: Chemical and metabolic studies of rat myelin of the central nervous system. Ann. NY. Acad. Sci., **122**, 86, 1965.
144. Davison, A. N., and Gregson, N. A.: Metabolism of cellular membrane sulpholipids in the rat brain. Biochem. J., **98**, 915, 1966.
145. Smith, M. E., and Eng, L. F.: The turnover of the lipid contents of myelin. J. Amer. Oil Chem. Soc., **42**, 1013, 1965.
146. Rappay, G., and Posalaky, Z.: Beiträge zur Frage der Spezifität der Tetrazoniumreaktion. Acta Histochem. (Jena), **7**, 212, 1959.
147. Austin, J.: Studies in globoid (Krabbe) leukodystrophy. I. The significance of lipid abnormalities in white matter in 8 globoid and 13 control patients. Arch. Neurol. (Chicago), **9**, 207, 1963.
148. Tingey, A. H., and Edgar, G. W. F.: A contribution to the chemistry of the leucodystrophies. J. Neurochem., **10**, 817, 1963.
149. Jatzkewitz, H.: Die Leukodystrophie, Typ Scholz (metachromatische Form der diffusen Sklerose) als Sphingolipoidose (Cerebrosidschwefelsäureester-Speicherkrankheit). Z. Physiol. Chem., **318**, 265, 1960.
150. Menkes, J. H., Duncan, C., and Moossy, J.: Molecular composition of the major glycolipids in globoid cell leucodystrophy. Neurology (Minneap.), **16**, 581, 1966.
151. Eto, Y., and Suzuki, K.: Brain sphingoglycolipids in Krabbe's globoid cell leucodystrophy. J. Neurochem. (in press).
152. Lees, M. B.: The chemical pathology of lipidoses and leukodystrophies. Res. Publ. Ass. Res. Nerv. Ment. Dis., **40**, 222, 1962.
153. Lees, M. B., and Moser, H. W.: The chemical pathology of Krabbe's disease and metachromatic leucodystrophy, in *Cerebral Sphingolipidosis,* edited by S. M. Aronson and B. W. Volk, p. 179. Academic, New York, 1962.
154. Robinson, N., and Cumings, J. N.: Biochemical and histochemical observations on Krabbe's disease (globoid body diffuse sclerosis). Acta Neuropath. (Berlin), **9**, 280, 1967.
155. Pilz, H.: Die Sphingolipoidveränderungen bei der Leukodystrophie Typ Krabbe im Vergleich zum akuten und chronischen sudanophilen Markzerfall. Acta Neuropath. (Berlin), **4**, 16, 1964.
156. Evans, J. E., and McCluer, R. H.: The structure of brain dihexosylceramide in globoid cell leukodystrophy. J. Neurochem., **16**, 1393, 1969.
157. Cumings, J. N., Thompson, E. J., and Goodwin, H.: Sphingolipids and phospholipids in microsomes and myelin from normal and pathological brains. J. Neurochem., **15**, 243, 1968.
158. Eto, Y., and Suzuki, K.: Unpublished observations.
159. Eto, Y., Suzuki, K., and Suzuki, K.: Globoid cell leucodystrophy (Krabbe's disease): Isolation of myelin with normal glycolipid composition. J. Lipid Res., **11**, 473, 1970.
160. O'Brien, J. S., and Sampson, E. L.: Myelin membrane: A molecular abnormality. Science, **150**, 1613, 1965.
161. Norton, W. T., and Poduslo, S. E.: Metachromatic leucodystrophy: Chemically abnormal myelin and cerebral biopsy studies of three siblings, in *Variation in the Chemical Composition of the Nervous System,* edited by G. B. Ansell, p. 82. Pergamon, Oxford, 1966.
162. Austin, J. H., Balasubramanian, A. S., Pattabiraman, T. N., Saraswathi, S., Basu, D. K., and Bachhawat, B. K.: A controlled study of enzymic activities in three human disorders of glycolipid metabolism. J. Neurochem., **10**, 805, 1963.
163. Percy, A. K., and McKhann, G. M.: The biochemistry of myelin and the leukodystrophies, in *Handbook of Clinical Neurology,* North-Holland Pub. Co., Amsterdam (in press).
164. McKhann, G. M.: Personal communication.
165. Radin, N. S., Hof, L., Bradley, R. M., and Brady, R. O.: Lactosylceramide galactosidase: Comparison with other sphingolipid hydrolases in developing rat brain. Brain Res., **14**, 497, 1969.
166. Okada, S., and O'Brien, J. S.: Generalized gangliosidosis: Beta-galactosidase deficiency. Science, **160**, 1002, 1968.
167. Malone, M. J.: Deficiency in a degradative enzyme system in globoid leucodystrophy. Abstr. 1st Conf. Am. Soc. Neurochem., Albuquerque, N.M., p. 56, 1970.
168. Norton, W. T., and Turnbull, J. M.: The isolation and lipid composition of a myelin-free axon-enriched fraction. (Abstr.) Fed. Proc., **29**, 472, 1970.
169. Aguilar, M. J., O'Brien, J. S., and Taber, P.: The syndrome of familial leukodystrophy, adrenal insufficiency and cutaneous melanosis, in *Inborn Disorders of Sphingolipid Metabolism,* edited by S. M. Aronson and B. W. Volk, p. 149. Pergamon, Oxford, 1967.
170. Fankhauser, R., Luginbühl, H., and Hartley, W. J.: Leukodystrophie vom Typus Krabbe beim Hund. Schweiz. Arch. Tierheilk., **105**, 198, 1963.
171. Fletcher, T. F., Kurtz, H. J., and Low, D. G.: Globoid cell leukodystrophy (Krabbe type) in the dog. J. Amer. Vet. Med. Ass., **149**, 165, 1966.
172. Jortner, B. S., and Jonas, A. M.: The neuropathology of globoid cell leucodystrophy in the dog: A report of two cases. Acta Neuropath. (Berlin), **10**, 171, 1968.
173. Austin, J., Armstrong, D., and Margolis, G.: Studies of globoid leukodystrophy in dogs. Neurology (Minneap.), **18**, 300, 1968.
174. Austin, J., Armstrong, D., Margolis, G.: Canine globoid leukodystrophy: A model demyelinating disorder. Trans. Amer. Neurol. Ass., **93**, 181, 1968.
175. Fletcher, T.: Leukodystrophy in the dog. Minn. Veterin., **9**, 19, 1969.
176. Austin, J.: Recent studies in two inborn errors of glycolipid metabolism, in *The Future of the Brain Sciences,* edited by S. E. Bogoch, p. 397. Plenum, New York, 1969.
177. McGrath, J., Schutta, H., Yaseen, A., and Steinberg, A.: A morphologic and biochemical study of canine globoid leukodystrophy. J. Neuropath. Exp. Neurol., **28**, 171, 1969.
178. Hirth, R. S., and Nielsen, S. W.: A familial canine globoid cell leukodystrophy ("Krabbe type"). J. Small Anim. Pract., **8**, 569, 1967.
179. McGrath, J.: Personal communication.
180. Suzuki, Y., Austin, J., Suzuki, K., Armstrong, D., Schlenker, J., and Fletcher, T.: Studies in globoid leukodystrophy: enzymatic and lipid findings in the canine form. Exp. Neurol., **29**, 65, 1970.

Note Added in Proof

It has come to our attention that the patients reported in references 22 and 27 are generally considered by neuropathologists as having spongy degeneration of the brain, rather than globoid cell leucodystrophy.

The following articles, directly related to globoid cell leucodystrophy, were published after the manuscript of this chapter was completed.

Clinical and Genetic Aspects

181. Hagberg, B., Kollberg, H., Sourander, P., Åkesson, H. O.: Infantile globoid cell leucodystrophy (Krabbe's disease). A clinical and genetic study of 32 Swedish cases 1953–1967. Neuropädiatrie, **1**, 74, 1970.

182. Wilson, J., Lake, B. D., and Dunn, H. G.: Krabbe's leucodystrophy. Some clinical and pathogenetic considerations. J. Neurol. Sci., **10**, 563, 1970.

Morphology

183. Yunis, E. J., and Lee, R. E.: Tubules of globoid leukodystrophy: A right-handed helix. Science, **169**, 64, 1970.

184. Liu, H. M.: Ultrastructure of globoid leukodystrophy (Krabbe's disease) with reference to the origin of globoid cells. J. Neuropath. Exp. Neurol., **29**, 441, 1970.

185. Andrews, J. M., and Menkes, J. H.: Ultrastructure of experimentally produced globoid cells in the rat. Exp. Neurol., **29**, 483, 1970.

Animal Models

186. Kurtz, H. J., and Fletcher, T. F.: The peripheral neuropathy of canine globoid-cell leukodystrophy (Krabbe-type). Acta Neuropath. (Berlin), **16**, 226, 1970.

187. Fletcher, T. F.: Electroencephalographic features of leukodystrophic disease in the dog. J. Amer. Vet. Med. Assoc., **157**, 190, 1970.

188. Johnson, K. H.: Globoid leukodystrophy in the cat. J. Amer. Vet. Med. Assoc., **157**, 2057, 1970.

189. Fletcher, T. F., Lee, D. G., and Hammer, R. F.: Ultrastructural features of globoid cell leukodystrophy in the dog. Amer. J. Vet. Res., **32**, 177, 1971.

CHAPTER THIRTY-FIVE

SPHINGOMYELIN LIPIDOSES: NIEMANN-PICK DISEASE

Donald S. Fredrickson and Howard R. Sloan

The traditional picture of Niemann-Pick disease is that of a child dying before the age of 4 years with massive hepatosplenomegaly, foam cells in the bone marrow, and irreparable disordering of the nervous system. Postmortem examination reveals many cells in nearly every organ laden with lipids that react positively with stains for phospholipids and cholesterol. In more recent years, some of these features have been observed in other patients who live longer and may have no obvious abnormality of the nervous system.

Regardless of the ages of the patients and their clinical course, the definitive chemical abnormality found in tissues is an increase in the content of sphingomyelin. Sphingomyelin is the phosphorylcholine (PChol) ester of N-acylsphingosine or ceramide (Cer) (Fig. 35-1). There is usually also an increase in cholesterol which often overshadows that of the sphingomyelin on a molar basis. Such abnormalities are inheritable, and the heterogeneity of clinical and chemical changes indicates genotypic variation involving an uncertain number of mutants. Until the different phenotypes have been better resolved, the eponymic term *Niemann-Pick disease* remains a useful one for describing them collectively.

At present, there are at least four distinguishable forms of sphingomyelin lipidosis and a fifth group of indeterminate examples. They will be here referred to as types A to E. This classification is an adaptation of one proposed earlier by Crocker [1]. The types differ not only with respect to the age of onset, rate of progression, and degree of the nervous system involvement but also in regard to the relative excess of sphingomyelin and the activity of the enzyme, sphingomyelinase, present in the tissues. Moreover, these differences tend to be concordant in affected members of the same sibship. As in many other lipid storage diseases, the cells in Niemann-Pick disease contain dense bodies (lysosomes) when viewed under the electron microscope. These are filled with lipids that the cells have a severely limited capacity to degrade. The intracellular activity of acid hydrolases not specifically related to catabolism of the stored substance is often increased [2, 3]. Disorders having these last two characteristics have been referred to as *lysosomal diseases* [4].

A diagnosis of Niemann-Pick disease should not be made from morphologic or histochemical impressions alone. There are no stains absolutely specific for sphingomyelin. Chemical analyses are obligatory and enzymatic analyses are most useful in the establishment of a diagnosis.

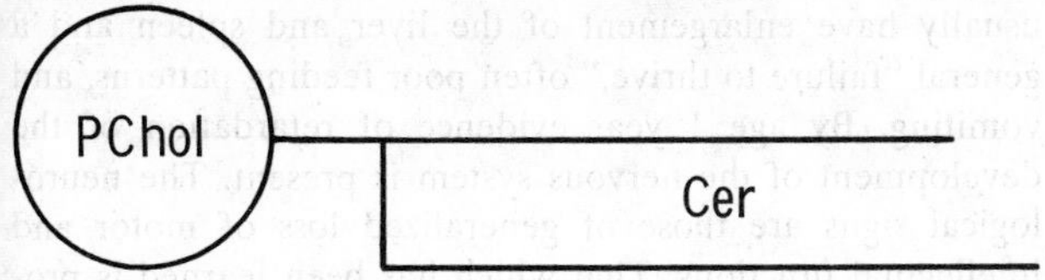

Figure 35-1. Sphingomyelin.

HISTORICAL ASPECTS

In 1914 Niemann, a Berlin pediatrician, observed a female infant who died at age 18 months after progressive deterioration associated with hepatosplenomegaly [5]. At autopsy the spleen, liver, and other organs had a striking yellow-white color. This proved to be due to the presence of large cells which Niemann thought were consistent with Gaucher's disease. He considered the early age of development and the rapid malignant course atypical of the available descriptions of Gaucher's disease and chose to report his case as *ein unbekanntes Krankheitsbild.*

Shortly thereafter several similar cases were reported as "Gaucher's disease" [6, 7], although not without dissent [8]. During the years 1922 to 1927, Pick correlated these into a single entity, distinct from Gaucher's disease on anatomic grounds, and called the new syndrome *lipoid cell splenomegaly* [9, 10]. It became more popularly known as Niemann-Pick disease as further reports appeared.

Over sixty examples which closely adhered to Niemann's description were reported before the same histochemical abnormalities were seen in an older patient. In 1946 Pfändler, in association with Dusendschon and Favarger, described typical pathologic and chemical changes found postmortem in two Swiss brothers who died at ages 29 and 33 years [11–13]. The disorder remains less common in adults, but a long-prevailing concept that the disease is virtually confined to Jewish female infants has been completely dispelled.

In the second and third patients reported [14], it was discovered that tissue phospholipids were increased, and this discovery was soon extended to other cases [15–21]. In 1934, Klenk made the important discovery that the predominant phospholipid accumulated is sphingomyelin [22, 23]. This observation was confirmed shortly thereafter by others [24–28], and an increased tissue content of sphingomyelin became the chemical hallmark of the disorder.

In 1966, Brady et al. reported the finding that sphingomyelinase activity was severely deficient in at least one form (type A) of sphingomyelin lipidosis [29]. Schneider and Kennedy confirmed this and reported measurements of the enzyme in other types [30]. Enzyme measurements have now been extended to tissue culture [31], and intrauterine diagnosis of one of the enzyme-deficient forms (type A) has recently been achieved [31a].

CLINICAL MANIFESTATIONS

In the preceding edition of this book, 165 patients with Niemann-Pick disease were tabulated from the world's literature [32]. Some of these cases were questionable, since chemical analyses were not made to confirm the diagnosis. This is unfortunately true for some cases reported subsequently. The present discussion of the disorder, including the citation of cases reported since 1966, will be confined mainly to examples of sphingomyelin storage proven by tissue analysis. There have been other extensive reviews of Niemann-Pick disease [33–37].

There is no generally agreed-upon classification of the sphingomyelin lipidoses. As suggested by Crocker [1] at least four different "phenotypes" can be defined clinically. We have added a fifth subgroup to include a few adult patients who do not obviously belong in one of the other four groups. It is not yet possible to use sphingomyelinase activity as an absolute basis of classification, for the assay has not been widely enough employed. It is anticipated that the mutants whose phenotypic expression has sphingomyelin storage as a common feature will be regrouped when they are better understood.

The Five Types

According to the present classification, the five types of sphingomyelin lipidoses are: type A (acute neuronopathic form; sphingomyelinase deficient); type B (chronic form without central nervous system involvement; sphingomyelinase deficient); type C (subacute form with central nervous system involvement; sphingomyelinase normal?); type D (Nova Scotia variant; sphingomyelinase normal); type E (indeterminate form in adults; sphingomyelinase normal?).

The definitions of these types that precede the general description of the features of sphingomyelin lipidoses include one or more illustrative case reports. More extensive biochemical data for these are included in Table 35-1.

Type A (Acute Neuronopathic Form)

Type A is characterized by the involvement of both viscera and nervous system in infancy, rapid and fatal progression, and severe deficiency of sphingomyelinase. It is the classical form first reported by Niemann [5] and called group A by Crocker [1]. Up to 1965, 121 examples of probable type A had been tabulated [32]. Fifty-one of these were familial [6, 7, 14, 17, 18, 22, 23, 32, 35, 38–60], and the remainder [5, 20, 32, 35, 49, 53, 60–116] not known to be familial. These constituted about 75 percent of all cases of Niemann-Pick disease in the literature by 1965 [32]. Among subsequent reports of type A patients are some with chemical confirmation of the diagnosis [117–119]. The following case report is typical of type A:

Patient P.W. (NIH No. 04-98-01); patient No. 71 in the previous review [32]. The patient, a male, was the third born of healthy Jewish parents of Northern European and Russian ancestry. Their first child, a girl, is now 11 years old and normal. Four other pregnancies ended in spontaneous abortions in the first trimester. Their second child, N. W. (patient No. 70 in [32]), also a girl, died at age 23 months of Niemann-Pick disease. P.W. was the product of a normal pregnancy and delivery. At birth his eyes, like his sister's (N.W.), were unusually prominent, his liver was slightly enlarged, and the occipital protuberance abnormally prominent. (The only other occurrence of this latter anomaly with Niemann-Pick disease was mentioned in a Russian child by Pashkova [104]). Cells from the amnion from this child were propagated in tissue culture; two subcultures contained 13.1 and 14.8 percent of the phospholipids as sphingomyelin, significantly higher than the mean of 7.4 percent in amnion cells from three controls. At 2 months of age the patient manifested a persistent fever and began to lose weight. At 10 weeks of age the liver was grossly enlarged, cherry-red spots were observed in both fundi, and foam cells were noted in the marrow. By 14 weeks extensive vacuolization of the circulating lymphocytes was noted. The patient then slowly regressed to an emaciated, vegetative state, without pathological reflexes. By 1 year of age diffuse reticular infiltration was present in both lungs and the SGOT and SGPT levels were markedly elevated.

The child expired at 23 months. At postmortem, 17 percent of the body weight of 5.8 kg was accounted for by the liver (750 gm) and spleen (210 gm). These organs, the lungs, and enlarged lymph nodes were reddish tan and mottled extensively with yellow infiltrations. Masses of foam cells virtually replaced the bone marrow, splenic pulp, lymph nodes, and adrenal medulla, and nearly filled the alveoli of the lungs. Similar cells were scattered throughout the testes and the lamina propria of the intestines and the subendocardium. Large numbers of foam cells were noted in the hepatic parenchyma. The brain weighed 1,100 gm. The cortex was abnormally firm and had a waxy appearance. Foamy macrophages were scattered throughout the cortical gray matter, and Purkinje cells were virtually absent from the cerebellum. Autonomic ganglion cells in the tongue, the plexi of Auerbach and Meissner, urinary bladder, and prostate were replaced by foam cells. The concentration of sphingomyelin in the spleen was increased more than twentyfold. The sphingomyelin-cleaving enzyme activity in the liver was 12 percent of normal.

Before they are 6 months of age, patients with type A usually have enlargement of the liver and spleen and a general "failure to thrive," often poor feeding patterns, and vomiting. By age 1 year evidence of retardation of the development of the nervous system is present. The neurological signs are those of generalized loss of motor and intellectual functions. That which has been learned is progressively lost and deterioration proceeds inexorably to

Table 35-1. TISSUE LIPID CONCENTRATIONS IN NIEMANN-PICK DISEASE

Reference number	Age, years	Type	*Liver, mg/gm dry wt*				*Spleen, mg/gm dry wt*				*Lymph node, mg/gm dry wt*			
			TL	PL	SPH	C	TL	PL	SPH	C	TL	PL	SPH	C
102	Fetus	A							30					
35	0.3	A	140	60	10	15	220	110	55	50			60	20
177	0.7			165	105	100								
59	0.7	A	180	115	25	55	305	185	85	105	290	180	70	95
119	0.9	A	470	320	225	70	510	345	265	100				
35	1.1	A	590	405	265	30	505	320	185	110	275	205	110	25
118	1.3	A					505	395	220	105				
118	1.5	A					410	320	210	85				
35, 151	1.5	A		370	260	70		425	330	65				
35, 151	1.9	A						515	370	180				
177	2.5	A		570	270	55	645	475	295	130				
177	2.6	A	520	420	260	100	490	360	255	100				
35, 60	2	B					615	410	280					
177	2.4	B		220	135	85								
177	4.7	B		550	335	140								
35, 120	9	B		585			550	330	250	40				
35, 120	21	B	170	145	30	15								
142	3.8	C		195	80			270	100					
144	5.5	C	245	145	45	25								
35	6.6	C	180	100	20	35					265	105	40	45
134	6.7	C	255	95	15	30	395	100	55	45				
141	6.8	C	325	130	15	45	495	155	100	70				
139	9.5	C							255					
133	13	C	260	130	30	15	365	100	65	50				
177	13	C		160	10	35		125	45	65				
141	22	C	300	105	15	15	455	105	25	50				
177	1.7	D		150	20	75								
177	9.5	D		180	10	35		165	55	85				
35, 60	19.1	D									175	70	20	20
			Upper limits of normal [178]											
			185	125	10	20	135	85	15	25	125	85	15	15

Note: TL, total lipid; PL, phospholipid; SPH, sphingomyelin; C, cholesterol.

death, nearly always by 4 years of age. The appearance of a patient early and late in the disease is shown in Fig. 35-2. Some children with type A have clearly been abnormal at birth or within age 1 month. Two probable fetal examples [102, 103] demonstrate that severe manifestations may develop in utero. In one instance, heavy infiltration of the placenta by foam cells may have led to abortion [103]. A child with type A may appear healthy for a year or more, however, and then rapidly develop signs of the disease [35, 94].

Type B (Chronic Form without Nervous System Involvement)

These patients may develop the visceral signs of the disease as early as type A and have a similar degree of sphingomyelin storage (Table 35-1); they are spared any obvious central nervous system (CNS) involvement. Sphingomyelinase activity is markedly decreased, although the deficiency is generally less severe than that in type A.

Patient A.S. (NIH No. 07-20-21), a male, is the firstborn of healthy Jewish parents of Northern European and Russian ancestry. The maternal great-grandparents were first cousins. The pregnancy and neonatal period and the patient's early development were unremarkable. At 4 years of age his spleen was enlarged. A year later the liver was also enlarged and an x-ray of the chest demonstrated a diffuse, reticular infiltration throughout both lungs. A bone marrow aspirate contained numerous foam cells which were strikingly birefringent. A liver biopsy was obtained at 5 years of age. The liver was butter-yellow and somewhat firm. Its architecture was normal and without fibrosis, but there were large collections of foamy macrophages primarily in the periportal regions. In frozen sections these stained heavily with the Smith-Dietrich and Schultz stains, suggesting excessive phospholipids and cholesterol, respectively. The concentration of sphingomyelin in the liver was increased thirty-five-fold. The sphingomyelin-cleaving enzyme activity of the

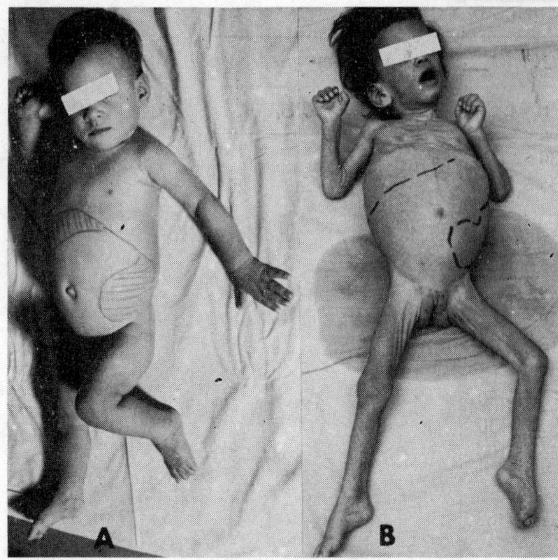

Figure 35-2. A. A patient with Niemann-Pick disease, type A, at the age of 11 months. B. Same patient at 22 months.

liver was 20 percent of normal and that of tissue culture cells derived from bone marrow and skin were each 6 percent of normal. The patient is now 9 years old and, except for marked hepatosplenomegaly, is in excellent health (Fig. 35-3). He is bright and alert. There are no neurological abnormalities and the fundi remain normal. Both the SGPT and SGOT are slightly elevated and the prothrombin time is somewhat prolonged; other liver functions are normal. A male sib is 7 years old and normal.

Patient A.S. is one of three similar examples of type B we are following. The oldest is 9 years of age. The first clear-cut descriptions of type B patients appeared in a review by Crocker and Farber in 1958 [35]; these and several others are also mentioned in later reports by Crocker [1, 120]. The literature contains other probable examples, including the patients of Chevrel [121], Fontan et al. (patients M.J.C. and M.F.C.) [111], Santelmann and Feyrter [122, 123], Forsythe and coworkers [124], Verger and coworkers [125], Lynn and Terry [126], a 21-year-old boy reported by Bourel and colleagues [127], and possibly several others [128–129]. Some adults with sphingomyelin lipidosis and no CNS symptoms, considered in this review to be the indeterminate or type E phenotype, may actually represent patients of type B who have survived to middle age or beyond. Examples include the adult sibs reported by Pfändler and Duscendschon [11–13], a man described by Terry et al. [131], and an elderly woman discovered at autopsy to have visceral sphingomyelin storage and low sphingomyelinase activity in the spleen [132]. Occasionally patients with Niemann-Pick disease who have low tissue sphingomyelinase activity survive into adulthood in spite of CNS changes. An example is a patient of ours (P.O., described earlier [32]), who is handicapped by cerebellar-ataxia but is otherwise in good health at age 29 years. Her liver sphingomyelin is modestly increased and the sphingomyelinase activity in skin fibroblasts is quite low. P.O. cannot readily be classified. Her CNS involvement excludes her from type B; and her sphingomyelinase activity is lower than the type C patients to be described presently.

Notwithstanding the uncertainties of phenotyping, there is a solid basis for encouragement concerning the outlook for patients who clearly fit the criteria for type B. This comes from patients "17" and "18" reported by Crocker and Farber [35]. Although each had hepatosplenomegaly between 6 and 24 months of age, neither had developed any neurological abnormalities by age 22 years (Crocker, personal communication). By 6 years of age both of the patients also had the diffuse x-ray evidence of the foam cell infiltration in the lungs that is frequently seen in Niemann-Pick disease. In type B patients, these severe roentgenologic changes may be accompanied by little functional impairment, but recurrent pulmonary infections are common and may possibly be fatal in childhood [125]. From the available information it is anticipated that patients of the type B phenotype may remain reasonably healthy and free from neurological abnormalities for at least 20 years. The outlook beyond this time is unknown.

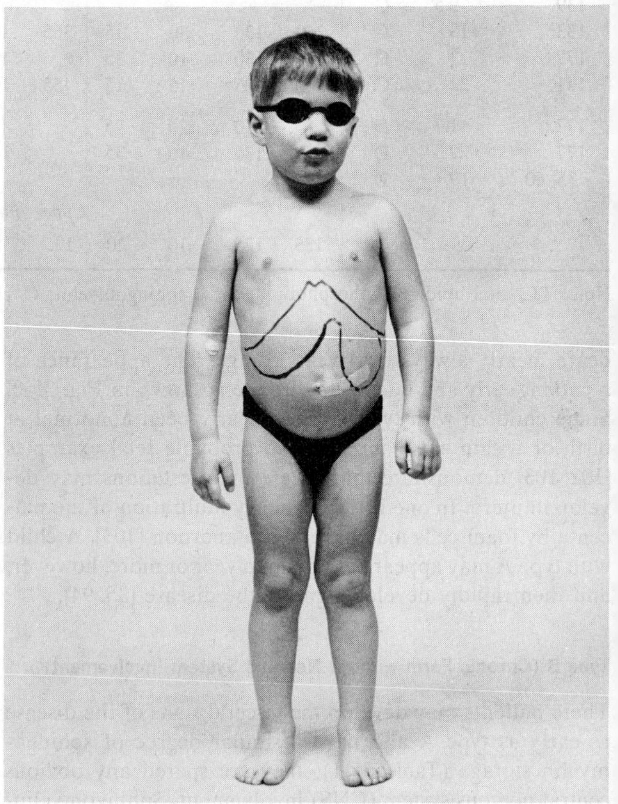

Figure 35-3. A patient with Niemann-Pick disease, type B, at 4.7 years of age.

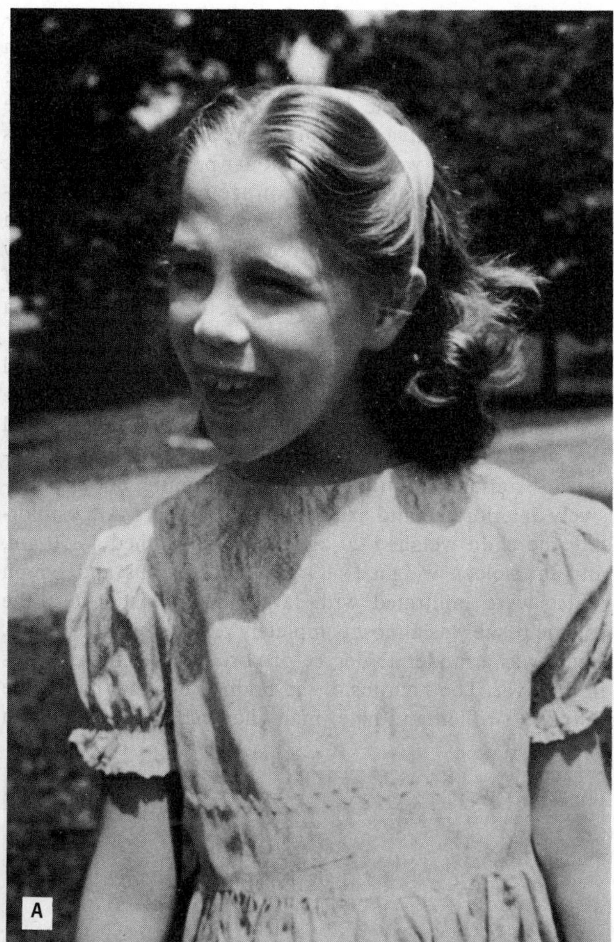

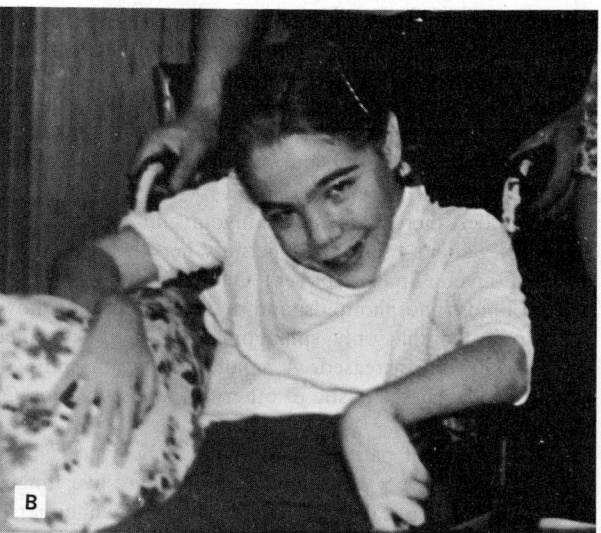

Figure 35-4. A patient with Niemann-Pick disease, type C, at 8 (A) and (B) at 10.5 years of age.

Type C

An increasing number of patients are being reported who have sphingomyelin lipidosis and CNS involvement, but a more prolonged course than type A. Usually appearing normal for 1 to 2 years and sometimes as long as 6 years [133], they eventually develop neurological abnormalities and usually die in childhood or adolescence. The presence of neurological involvement is the major clinical basis for assignment of patients with a chronic course to type C rather than to type B. Patients of type C further differ from both types A and B in that they have less obvious enlargement of liver and spleen, less increase in tissue sphingomyelin content [1], and normal or nearly normal tissue sphingomyelinase activity [30]. Patients classified as type C have sometimes been referred to as having *subacute* [134] or *juvenile* [133] Niemann-Pick disease.

Patients 2, 8, 11, and 12 described in the review of Crocker and Farber [35], many similar ones reported by others [1, 60, 133–145], and several not reported in detail by Crocker [1, 32, 120] comprise more than 20 known patients of probable type C. There are possible, but uncertain, additional examples of type C in the literature [34, 56, 136, 142, 132, 146–149]. Sphingomyelinase assays have been made on tissues from very few patients. We have followed one previously unreported patient with type C sphingomyelin lipidosis, whose history is representative of that type.

Patient L.B. (NIH No. 06-61-36), a female, was the third-born of healthy Protestant parents of Northern European ancestry. The pregnancy and neonatal periods were unremarkable. At her 6-week checkup, splenomegaly was found. At the age of 2 years, bone marrow aspiration was performed to exclude the possibility of leukemia. The slides obtained from this aspiration were reviewed 3 years later and many foamy macrophages were seen. Her development was entirely normal until the age of 5 years when she showed an abnormal gait and poor hand coordination. Her coordination deteriorated slowly and by age 9 years she could no longer care for herself. She never mastered the alphabet but could count from 1 to 20 with some dysarthria. By age 10 years, the patient began to deteriorate rapidly (Fig. 35-4). She was incontinent, unable to walk without falling, and her speech was significantly dysarthric although she understood most simple verbal commands. During the next 4 months the downhill course accelerated further; the patient could no longer walk, had frequent grand mal seizures, developed bilateral Babinski signs, was hypertonic and had lost nearly all coordination. Liver function studies and chest x-rays were normal throughout the course of her illness. The patient became totally helpless and died at 13 years of age.

At postmortem the liver was modestly enlarged (2,060 gm; normal 1,400 gm) and there was massive splenomegaly (750 gm). Foam cells were found in the lymph nodes, lungs, and spleen. The weight of the brain was somewhat less than normal. The cortical neurons were ballooned and the cytoplasm appeared foamy. The abnormal neurons (formalin-fixed tissues) did not stain strongly with either the Baker or Luxol fast blue reactions.

The sphingomyelin concentration in liver was normal; in the spleen it was threefold increased. The sphingomyelinase activity in the liver, spleen, and bone marrow fibroblasts was normal.

The modest increase in the sphingomyelin content of the spleen of Patient L.B. barely permits her classification as a sphingomyelin lipidosis patient. Qualitative analyses of all neutral lipids, phospholipids, and neutral glycolipids, however, indicated that only sphingomyelin and unesterified cholesterol were increased. A small increase in sphingomyelin is also characteristic of other examples of "type C" [1] (Table 35-1).

The majority of patients considered to be type C have died between ages 5 and 15 years. Some may live longer. For example, identical twins described by Oppenheimer et al. [141] were discovered at age 4 years to have enlarged spleens. Mental defectiveness was suspected between ages 10 to 15 years, and they started to have seizures at age 18 years. One twin died at age 22 years of infection.

It was noted by Crocker [120] that some patients considered to be type C apparently had a considerable decline in tissue accumulation of sphingomyelin between the analyses of tissue removed at biopsy or splenectomy in childhood and tissues obtained years later at autopsy. Possibly some induction of sphingomyelinase activity occurs as patients become older. The classification of patients with the clinical manifestations of "type C" will remain uncertain until both chemical and enzymatic assays have been correlated with age in many more patients.

Type D

At present the designation of type D is reserved for patients of Nova Scotian ancestry who otherwise have a course similar in many respects to type C. They will probably prove to be a distinct variant of the latter. Type D [1] was first described by Crocker and Farber (Patients 13, 14, 15, and 16 [35]). The following report of one sibship studied by us is given as an example of the Nova Scotia variant.

The sibship (Patients 67, 68, and 69, in [32]) consists of five children. The father's parents are French Canadian Catholics from near Yarmouth in Nova Scotia. Other paternal relatives are described who have had abdominal enlargement, seizures, and mental retardation. The mother's parents came from Italy, and in their extensive kindreds there are no suggestions of other instances of lipid storage disease. The firstborn of the couple is a 14-year-old girl who is healthy.

Patient D.D. (NIH No. 05-49-18 and Patient 67 in the previous review [32]), a female and the second-born, appeared to be normal at birth. Neonatal jaundice lingered for a few weeks but had disappeared before massive hepatosplenomegaly was detected at the age of 4 months. Foam cells were found in the biopsies of lymph nodes and spleen; none were seen in the liver, but there was considerable increase in connective tissue in the portal triads. A diagnosis of tissue lipidosis with the additional possibility of chronic hepatitis was made. At 3 years of age her mental development began to fall behind; and soon she developed an unsteady "tabetic" gait, poor coordination with increasingly frequent "seizures" or brief periods of falling, and lack of awareness of her surroundings, sometimes followed by a short postictal state.

By 8 years of age (Fig. 35-5), the patient had deteriorated further, could not talk coherently, and was unable to care for herself. The seizures gradually increased in severity and the patient was constantly obtunded and had profuse tracheal secretions requiring frequent suctioning. She progressively deteriorated and expired at age 9½ years. At postmortem the child weighed 20 kg; the liver weighed 1,350 gm, and the spleen weighed 580 gm. The thymus and lymph nodes were infiltrated with large foamy histiocytes; the splenic tissue was almost completely replaced by these cells. There was a moderate degree of portal and central fibrosis in the liver. The neurons of the brain and spinal cord were diffusely swollen and pale; many had eccentric nuclei with

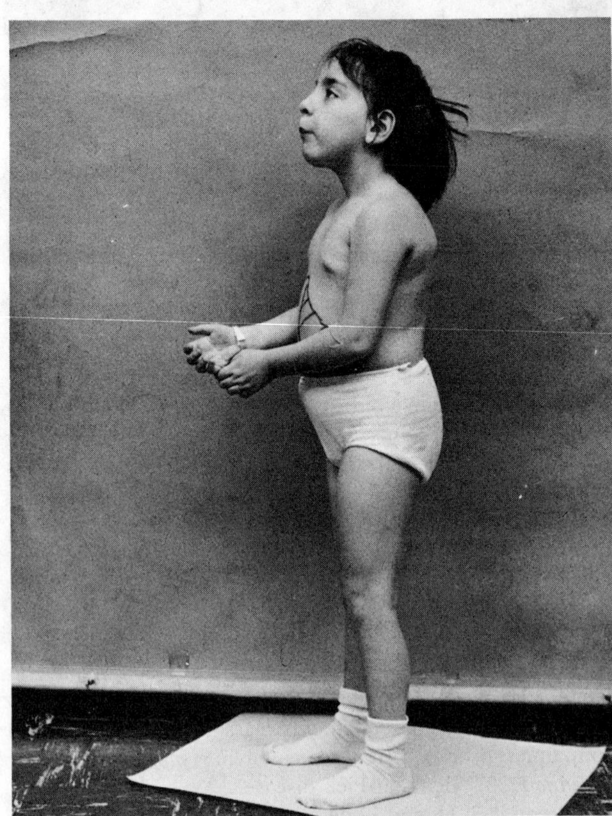

Figure 35-5. A patient with Niemann-Pick disease, type D, at 5 years of age.

extensive loss of Nissl substance. Purkinje cells were depleted in the cerebellum. The sphingomyelin content of the spleen was increased three- to fourfold, but that of the liver was normal. The sphingomyelin-cleaving enzyme activities in the liver and bone marrow fibroblasts were normal.

Patient J.D. (Patient No. 68 [32]), a male and the third-born, was icteric from shortly after birth until his death. At 2 months of age he had hepatosplenomegaly with elevated serum bilirubin and alkaline phosphatase levels. He developed ascites and died at age 6 months after a rapid downhill course. The liver contained swollen Kupffer cells with foamy cytoplasm, some fibrosis, chronic inflammation, and inspissation of bile in the small triad ducts. There were many foam cells in the spleen, lungs, lymph nodes, pancreas, and gastrointestinal tract. Lipid analyses were made on small sections of liver and spleen that had been in formalin for 3 years. The cholesterol content was definitely increased, and sphingomyelin apparently so.

The fourth child, a female, is now 8 years old and normal.

Patient R.D. (NIH No. 05-47-40 and Patient No. 69 [32]) was the last-born. He had moderate jaundice for a few days after birth, and then he was normal until age 7 weeks, when jaundice reappeared and enlargement of the liver and spleen became evident. The total serum bilirubin was 2.5 mg per 100 ml, half of which was conjugated; foam cells were found in the bone marrow. By age 5 months his jaundice had again completely disappeared. By 16 months of age his spleen was enormous and the liver was significantly enlarged, but his development seemed normal. At 3 years of age his mental development began to lag and he acquired an unsteady, broad-based gait. The liver was biopsied at 1.7 years and the sphingomyelin content was 20 mg per gm dry weight (normal 10). Microscopic examination of the biopsy revealed considerable fibrosis and alteration of the normal architecture; many Kupffer cells had become foam cells which stained positively for phospholipids. The sphingomyelin-cleaving enzyme activity of the liver was normal. The patient is now 7 years of age; the course of his illness has been quite similar to that described for his sister. The fundi are normal. The SGPT and SGOT are elevated and the prothrombin time is somewhat prolonged.

Patients considered to be of type D have all shared certain family names, common ancestry derived from one Nova Scotia community, and have a protracted course in which neurologic abnormalities slowly progress to severe disability and death. Early jaundice is a prominent feature of their disease. Rabinowicz and coworkers have reported a Swiss child whom they believe is an example of type D [145]. No chemical analyses or sphingomyelinase assays were performed and it is possible that this patient actually represents type C. A serious question exists as to whether type D is a sphingomyelin storage disease, considering the relatively minor increases in the concentration of this lipid in the liver and spleen and the proportionately greater increase in cholesterol (Table 35-1). Sphingomyelinase may be normal (Table 35-2) or perhaps decreased [30].

Type E

A few adults without neurological abnormalities have been discovered incidentally to have sphingomyelin accumulation in one or more tissues. Among the examples are two Swiss brothers who died in their thirties [11–13], a 53-year-old male [131, 150], and a patient briefly mentioned by Thannhauser [151]. As already noted, it is conceivable that some of these represent mild and long-surviving examples of type B. The following example [152], however, illustrates unsuspected visceral involvement in an otherwise healthy male whose tissue contained normal sphingomyelinase activity. If sphingomyelinase deficiency is to be used as a criterion for defining type B, then at least one other form of sphingomyelin lipidosis with neither CNS involvement nor enzyme deficiency must be recognized. The designation of type E is therefore employed here to encompass adults with visceral sphingomyelin storage and normal sphingomyelinase. With the possible exception of the two brothers mentioned above, "type E" is not known to be familial.

Patient R.S., a 27-year old male, had been in excellent health until age 25. At that time he sustained an injury to the left side of his chest and two ribs were fractured. His condition improved but he noted residual left upper quadrant distress that gradually increased in severity. An abdominal mass developed two to three weeks after the accident and his hemoglobin dropped from 15 to 12.5 gm percent. At laporatomy the spleen was found to be lacerated and was removed. The spleen contained many large foamy macrophages. The patient completely recovered. Unfortunately, the spleen was stored in formalin for several months before lipid analyses were performed. At that time the concentrations of sphingomyelin and cholesterol were 67 and 61 mg per gm dry weight, respectively. (See Table 35-1 for normal values). Several months following the splenectomy, a bone marrow biopsy and liver biopsy were performed. Lamellar membranous bodies were present in storage cells in the marrow and in liver parenchymal cells. The sphingomyelinase activity in cultured bone marrow fibroblasts was normal; the activity in skin fibroblasts, however, was depressed.

Summation of Case Reports

The preceding analysis of the various phenotypes of Niemann-Pick disease covers approximately 180 reported examples. Most of the reported cases have represented type A, the next most common being type C. The more recent literature contains a proportionately higher number of case

Table 35-2. SPHINGOMYELIN-CLEAVING ENZYME ACTIVITY IN HUMAN TISSUE PREPARATIONS

Reference number	Type	Liver*	Spleen†	Fibroblasts	
				Bone marrow‡	Skin‡
29	A	0.0			
29, 31	A	0.54		0.3	0.1
29	A	0.61			
29, 31	A	0.26		0	0
29, 31	A	0.46			0.1
29, 31	A	0.89		0	0.2
30	A		1.0		
30	A		1.4		
31	A			0.0	
31	A			0.0	
30	B		3.0		
30	B		7.6		
30	B		3.3		
31, 177	B	1.3		2.9	2.0
31, 177	B	0.9		3.5	1.8
31, 177	B§				1.3
31, 177	B	1.2			1.9
30	C		181		
30	C		88		
30	C		152		
30	C		254		
30	C		117		
177	C	8.8	3.2*	30.6	
30	D		36		
31, 177	D	6.7		30.1	
177	D	5.8			
Normal range		4.4–11.1	65–200	52 ± 10	35 ± 6

* Units per milligram of protein.
† Microinternational units per milligram of protein.
‡ Units per million cells.
§ This is patient P.O. of uncertain type who is described in the text under type B.

reports concerned with patients having a prolonged course. It is possible that the relative frequency of type A is diminishing, although it is more likely that the pattern of type A has become well enough established to discourage further case reporting. In addition to cases previously cited, the literature contains reference to at least 25 more cases of "Niemann-Pick disease." We believe seven of these are most probably Gaucher's disease or Wolman's disease [153–159]. The available information for the others [160–176] was not sufficiently detailed to allow us to attempt their classification.

CLINICOPATHOLOGIC CORRELATIONS

Involvement Outside the Nervous System

The Foam Cell

While the foam cell is often considered a histologic trademark of Niemann-Pick disease, it is not an exclusive feature. It should not be called a "Niemann-Pick cell" in the same sense that one refers to "Gaucher cells," for the latter have a distinctive appearance which is diagnostic of that disease.

The best way to distinguish Niemann-Pick foam cells from Gaucher cells is by phase microscopy of unstained preparations. As seen in Fig. 35-6, the cell found in sphingomyelin lipidoses is 20 to 90 microns in diameter. The cytoplasm is filled with many droplets or particles which usually, but not always, are fairly uniform in size and which give the cell a foamy, or "mulberry," appearance. There may be a single nucleus or many. In polarized light many of the droplets are birefringent, and in ultraviolet light they fluoresce a greenish-yellow color.

For histochemical examination under light microscopy, marrow smears and tissues should be prepared in *frozen sections* that are only briefly fixed in calcium-formalin or gluteraldehyde, as well as in the conventional paraffin blocks. The latter processing removes the lipid and leaves vacuoles in which only the margins may be stained. In frozen sections,

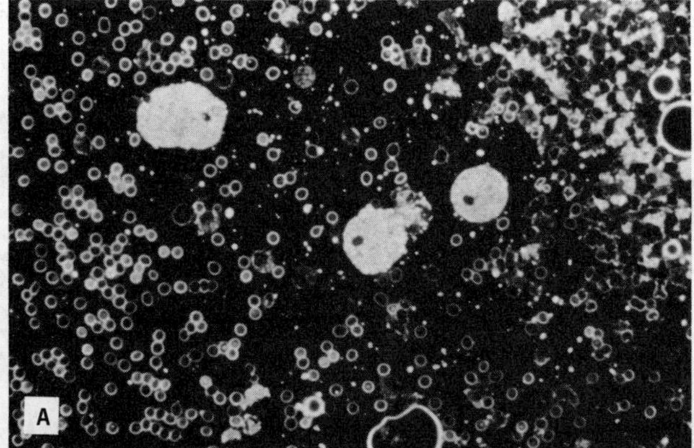

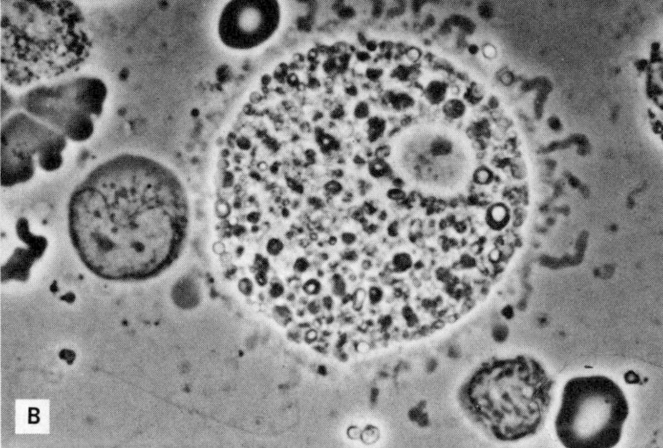

Figure 35-6. Foam cells in Niemann-Pick disease viewed in an unstained preparation with the phase microscope. A. Field magnified 25×. B. Magnified 430×.

the droplets in the foam cells usually stain blue-black with Smith-Dietrich, black with Sudan Black B, red with oil-red-O, blue-violet with Nile blue sulfate, violet with mercuric nitrate, blue-black with acid hematin, and negative or red with periodic acid–Schiff stain [179, 180]. Acid phosphatase activity is present [2]. Other papers [33, 35, 46, 126, 179, 180] may be consulted for a detailed discussion of the staining reactions of these cells.

Fine Structure

Foam cells in Niemann-Pick tissues have been studied extensively under the electron microscope [126, 181–183]. Scattered about the cytoplasm of these large cells are many round or oval residual bodies of 0.5 to 5 microns in diameter (Fig. 35-7). Some cells contain only a few large residual bodies; others, many small ones. Some of the bodies contain discrete myelin figures consisting of concentric osmophilic layers (considered to be phosphorylcholine). These alternate with clear, osmophobic layers having a width of about 27 Å [126], which is compatible with estimates of the length of the ceramide portion of sphingomyelin [184]. The periodicity of these concentric membranes is about 50 Å [126] (Fig. 35-7). This distance is probably indicative of the combination of sterol, sphingomyelin, and perhaps other lipids and protein to form bimolecular leaflets. It has not yet been resolved whether sphingomyelin lipidoses can be differentiated by electron microscopy from the other lipid storage disorders in which the cells contain similar appearing lysosomes [126, 183].

Origin

Foam cells arise through lipid accumulation mainly in reticulum cells in lymphoid tissue; but certain cells of the connective tissue, "perivascular embryonic cells and phagocytes all over the body," and some parenchymal cells also are involved [33]. In the advanced stages of the disease these alterations are nearly universally distributed, and it is rare to find any tissues without at least a few foam cells. The residual bodies in the foam cells are presently considered to represent secondary lysosomes and the lipid they contain to have arisen by endocytosis of extracellular lipid (heterophagy) or by autophagy of intracellular lipid.

Ceroid

Evidence of ceroid deposition can be seen in tissue of all patients with Niemann-Pick disease and is especially prominent in older patients (types B to E). The histochemical changes typical of ceroid or lipofuscin pigment include autofluorescence in ultraviolet light and a reddish reaction with the PAS stain. Ceroid is believed to be a resultant of lipid peroxidation [185]. Presumably phospholipids containing unsaturated fatty acids are among compounds particularly susceptible to this transformation. Peroxidation is associated with the formation of free radicals that can damage tissues to the same extent as radiation [186]. It is possible that some patients described as having "ceroid storage disease" [187–189] may have represented a sphingomyelin lipidosis. Ceroid deposition is found in other lipid storage diseases [190] and in atheromatous lesions, and may be associated with aging [191].

Spleen, Lymphoid Tissue, and Bone Marrow

No doubt because of their high content of reticulum cells, the most heavily involved organs, and, judging from the fetal studies, probably the earliest affected [102, 103], are the spleen, bone marrow, and other lymphoid tissues, such as nodes and thymus. The splenic pulp and lymph nodes may be completely replaced by masses of foam cells. They may also be present in the tonsils [144].

Although foam cells may eventually crowd out most visible hematopoietic cells in the marrow, dramatic changes in the hemogram appear only late in the disease. The first abnormality is usually a moderate microcytic anemia, which is sometimes responsive to iron administration. The leukocyte count is variable and may be moderately elevated.

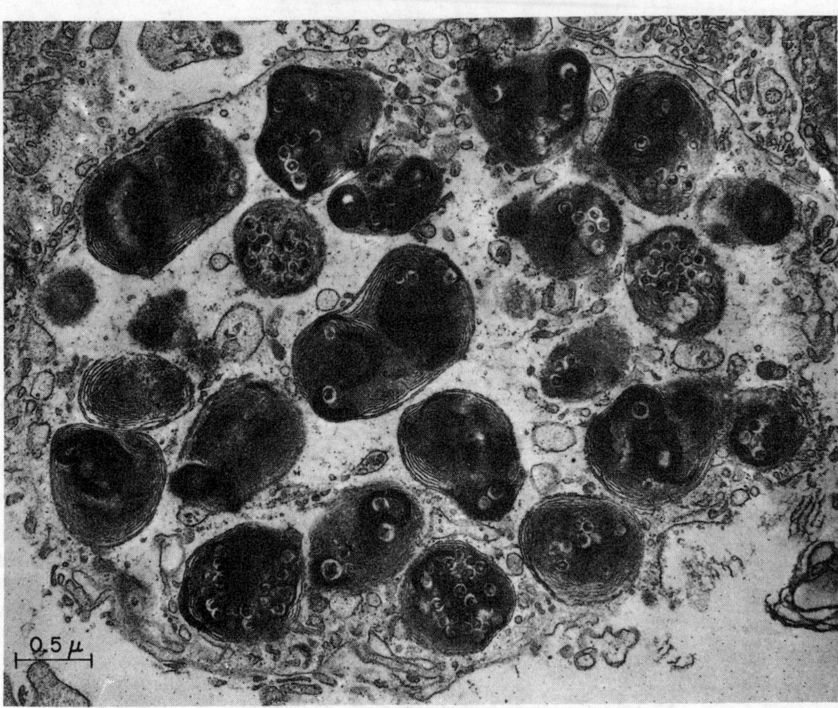

Figure 35-7. Electron micrograph of foam cell from lymph node of patient with Niemann-Pick disease. (*Courtesy of Dr. Robert Terry, Albert Einstein School of Medicine.*)

Thrombocytopenia occurs, and to a degree usually reflecting the severity and duration of splenomegaly. In many patients there are discrete vacuoles in lymphocytes and monocytes in smears of peripheral blood or bone marrow. These cells contain residual bodies similar to the foam cells [175, 192] (Fig. 35-8).

Lungs and Heart

The lungs are usually affected in patients of all ages. Infiltration is demonstrable by x-ray as a diffuse reticular or finely nodular pattern involving most of the lung fields (Fig. 35-9). The degree to which foam cells may fill the alveoli is hard to reconcile with the minimal or, in some cases, lack of respiratory embarrassment that may be evident. Pulmonary involvement may, however, lead to cyanosis, presumably by causing a diffusion block or arteriovenous shunting in the alveolar circulation [150]. Foam cells are found only rarely in the sputum. In the heart, foam cells are frequently seen adjacent to the myocardial fibers; cardiac dysfunction seems to have played a significant role in the death of at least one patient [11].

Liver and GI Tract

The enlarged liver usually contains "vacuolated" Kupffer and parenchymal cells that are distributed in spotty fashion throughout the organ. Persistent jaundice and a severe degree of disruption of hepatic architecture is common in the Nova Scotia variant (type D). These manifestations are unusual in other types of Niemann-Pick disease, although both have occurred in two Swedish sibs with type A [59]. At least one patient with type C has also had persistent jaundice [134]. Liver function test results and the serum proteins are usually normal in type A until the terminal stages. Children with type B, however, may early develop persistent elevations of alkaline phosphatase, SGOT, and SGPT. Ascites is uncommon. When it occurs, it is usually

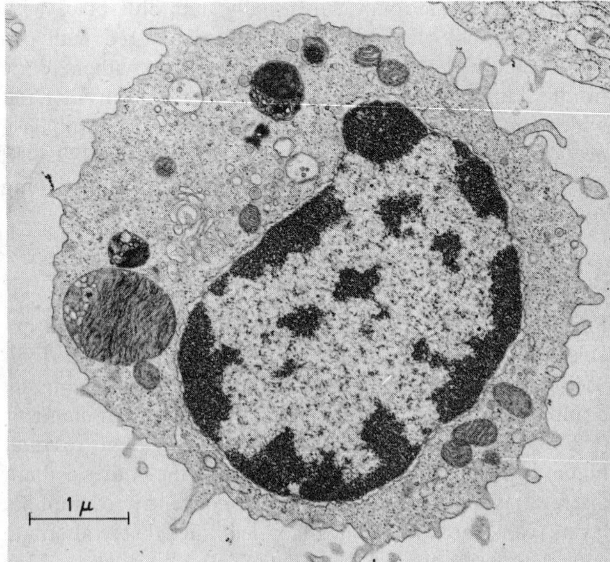

Figure 35-8. Electron micrograph of blood lymphocyte from patient with Niemann-Pick disease, type A. (*Courtesy of Dr. Bruno Volk, Isaac Albert Research Institute.*)

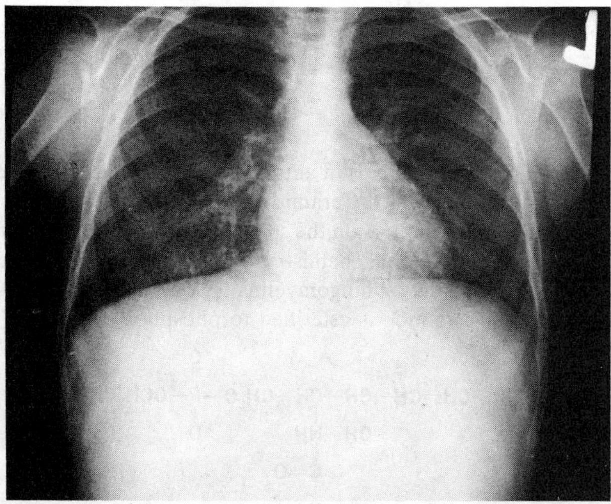

Figure 35-9. Chest x-ray of patient with Niemann-Pick disease, type B. Note the bilateral diffuse reticular infiltration.

attributable to venous obstruction by the greatly enlarged liver and spleen [59]. The lamina propria and smooth muscle cells of the intestine nearly always contain foam cells. These can be seen by rectal biopsy [2, 193].

Bones

The masses of foam cells in the marrow do not usually cause detectable changes in bones. Widened medullary cavities, occasionally seen at autopsy [77, 93], are rarely detected by x-rays [167], and the "Erlenmeyer flask deformities" often seen in Gaucher's disease are quite atypical. Osteoporosis, no doubt related to nutritional inadequacy and inactivity, is common in debilitated patients with type A. Bone age is usually normal. Serum calcium and phosphorous levels are normal.

Skin

Suppurative lesions about the face, associated with foam cell infiltration, and eruptive and infiltrative xanthomas, have been described [35]. Generalized thickening of the skin may occur [140]. Dark bluish Mongolian spots have been seen on the skin and oral mucosa [32, 35, 41, 43, 63], but their frequency and importance have perhaps been over-emphasized in earlier reviews. A peculiar brownish-yellow tint to the skin is common in type A and may also occur in type C [144]. *Café au lait* spots are rare [44].

Other Organs

Although lipid accumulation is present in many tissues not all the anatomic changes in epithelial and other cells express themselves in detectable abnormalities in function. Large yellow adrenal glands containing foam cells may be present without signs of adrenal insufficiency. Other endocrine organs, including the gonads, thyroid, and pituitary, and exocrine glands, such as the pancreas and salivary glands, may likewise be burdened with lipid without evident functional disability. Foam cells in the kidney glomeruli and swollen tubular epithelial cells are often present, but there are no definite abnormalities in renal function.

Nervous System

Survival of patients with all forms of Niemann-Pick disease is usually inversely correlated with the degree of nervous system involvement. Abnormalities may occur in both the central and peripheral portions of the nervous systems. The distribution of lesions is quite irregular. It has been suggested that the presence of ballooned ganglion cells in the plexi of Auerbach and Meissner might permit recognition of otherwise undetectable neuronal involvement [2] by rectal biopsy.

The ganglion cells are frequently swollen and have pale, vacuolated cytoplasm containing degenerated Nissl substance. The cytoplasm frequently fails to stain with lipophilic dyes; it usually has a weak periodic acid–Schiff reaction. Electron micrographs of the ballooned ganglion cells demonstrate residual bodies similar to the membranous cytoplasmic bodies described in Tay-Sachs disease [119, 171, 183] (Chap. 29). A severe loss of cells may occur in some areas of the cerebral or cerebellar cortex while adjacent areas appear to be unaffected. The white matter may appear to be normally myelinated or there may be a severe deficiency of myelin. Foam cells or lipid-laden glial cells are distributed about the leptomeninges, tela choroidea, and connective tissue in the perivascular spaces or endothelium of cerebral blood vessels [10, 73, 144, 169, 194, 195]. Proliferation of astrocytes or glial cells is also highly variable, but extensive gliosis is often seen in both gray and white matter. The cerebellum, basal ganglia, brain stem, spinal cord, and the spinal ganglia and roots, as well as the autonomic ganglia, may undergo morphologic changes similar to those in the cerebral cortex.

In patients with type A all areas of the brain may be affected, with a heavy emphasis on changes in the cerebellum, brain stem, and spinal cord [59, 102]. Frequently, the brain also shows considerable involvement of the cerebral cortex, the extensive fibrosis rendering it hard and leathery with gaping fissures [73]. The ventricles are usually not dilated and the weight of the brain is less than normal. It is difficult to correlate the degree of neurological dysfunction in type A with the evident changes in the brain. After the infant has passed some of the normal landmarks of motor and psychic development, there begins a complete regression to a vegetative state. Motor derangements are manifested mainly as hypotonia or flaccidity. Pathologic reflexes are often absent, as are "hyperacusis," common in Tay-Sachs disease, and the combination of brain stem signs and hypertonicity characteristic of neuronopathic Gaucher's disease.

In type C, neurological abnormalities usually appear between ages 2 to 4 years, but may come later. Spasticity and akinetic seizures, particularly myoclonic jerks, tend to be common [144]. Cerebellar involvement may vary from absent [35, 134] to quite conspicuous [133, 144]. Cerebral changes tend to be spotty and mental functioning deteriorates gradually. In some older children, difficulty in learning [141] or emotional lability and behavior problems [35] may be the first signs of CNS involvement. Philippart and coworkers [144] have given thoughtful consideration to possible differences in the brain changes in types A and C, but the available morphologic evidence does not permit a clear distinction between the pathologic processes.

There have not been enough well-studied patients with the type D variant to provide comparisons of neuronal damage and dysfunction with types A and C. Generally, the earliest manifestations in type D are ataxia and dyskinesia suggestive of cerebellar involvement. Severe retardation in mentation becomes evident in the early years of life. As the disease progresses, seizures become a serious problem.

In patients representing types A, C, and D, the cerebrospinal fluid pressure and contents have repeatedly been found to be normal. Electroencephalograms also do not show any specific changes.

Eyes

In keeping with the capricious distribution of lesions elsewhere in the nervous system, involvement of the retina may or may not be visible through the ophthalmoscope. When neurons in the macular area are destroyed, the dramatic result is the cherry-red spot. The detailed morphologic changes associated with it have been described by several observers [70, 196–198]. The cherry-red spot has been reported in about half of the patients with the type A disease [32]. It may also occur in type C and develop rather late in childhood. Sometimes only a grayish discoloration about the macula is evident.

SPHINGOMYELIN

Biochemistry

Sphingomyelin was first described by Thudichum late in the nineteenth century [193], but the general structure was not firmly established until much later [194–196]. The essential unit of the sphingolipids is sphingosine:

$$CH_3(CH_2)_{12}-CH{=}CH-\underset{OH}{CH}-\underset{NH_2}{CH}-CH_2OH$$

or one of its congeners. The N-acyl derivative of sphingosine is ceramide:

$$CH_3(CH_2)_{12}-CH{=}CH-\underset{OH}{CH}-\underset{NH-C(=O)-R}{CH}-CH_2OH$$

Most of the sphingolipids in animal tissues contain ceramide as a structural unit. Ceramide is abbreviated as Cer throughout the chapters on the sphingolipidoses. For further details on the general chemistry of the sphingolipids, see Chap. 29. In the sphingomyelins (Cer-PChol) the C_1-hydroxyl of ceramide is esterified to phosphorycholine:

$$CH_3(CH_2)_{12}-CH{=}CH-\underset{OH}{CH}-\underset{NH-C(=O)-R}{CH}-CH_2O-\underset{O^-}{\overset{O}{\overset{\|}{P}}}-OCH_2CH_2\overset{+}{N}(CH_3)_3$$

Sphingomyelin

The sphingosine base in sphingomyelins found in mammalian tissues and plasma is mainly the C_{18} monounsaturated base (2-amino-4-octadecene-1,3-diol) [202–205]. Smaller amounts of the saturated [203] and diunsaturated [204, 206] C_{18} bases and their shorter and longer-chain homologues [204, 207, 208], and of phytosphingosine (2-amino-octadecane-1,3,4-triol) [209, 210] are present. A branched-chain base has also been reported [209]. The sphingomyelins vary mainly in the structure of the long-chain fatty acids in their ceramide portions. As do most of the sphingolipid fatty acids [211], those in the sphingomyelins fall into two major groups. In sphingomyelins in cell cytoplasm and plasma, the fatty acids are primarily C_{16} and C_{18} in length. In cell membranes, there is a higher proportion of longer-chain acids such as C_{24}.

Svennerholm et al., examined the sphingomyelin fatty acids in plasma, red cells, spleen, placenta, lungs, and kidneys and found them to be relatively uniform [212]. Only eight acids appeared in quantities that were each greater than 1 percent of the total. The 16:0 and 24:1 acids were about equal in quantity and made up two-thirds of the total. The 22:0 acid was the next most common; it is the characteristic longer-chain acid of all extraneural sphingomyelin. These findings are in general accord with other reports [205, 213–219].

In the brain, the composition of the sphingomyelin fatty acids varies according to location and age [219–224]. Those in the gray matter have a higher proportion of C_{16} and C_{18} acids compared to those in the white matter, which tend to be of longer chain length. The brain of the newborn contains very little myelin, and as myelination takes place the relative content of $C_{24:1}$ acids in sphingomyelin rises markedly and the relative proportion of C_{16} and C_{18} acids declines [222–224]. In some tissues, the fatty acids of sphingomyelin are subject to rapid change. Examples are dietary-induced changes in sphingomyelin in the intestine [225], erythrocytes, and serum [226, 227].

Biosynthesis of Sphingomyelin

The biosynthesis of sphingosine and ceramide has been described in Chap. 29. Two possible pathways for the biosynthesis of sphingomyelin are presently known. One reaction sequence proceeds via the transfer of the phosphorylcholine moiety of cytidine diphosphate (CDP) choline to ceramide [228, 229].

Cer + **CDP-choline** ⟶ **Cer-P-choline** + **CMP** (1)
Ceramide **Sphingomyelin**

This reaction is catalyzed by the enzyme CDP-choline: ceramide choline phosphotransferase (EC 2.7.8.3). The enzyme has been found in both the mitochondria and the microsomes of chicken liver [228], and in homogenates of rat brain, kidney, and spleen [228]. Ceramide with either the *erythro* or *threo* conformation at carbons 2 and 3 can serve as the precursor in the biosynthesis of sphingomyelin [230, 231]. The enzyme catalyzing the reaction involving *erythro* ceramide is apparently located in the mitochondria.

A second reaction sequence involves the acylation of sphingosylphosphorylcholine [232, 233].

Sphingosine + **CDP-choline** ⟶
Sphingosylphosphorylcholine + **CMP** (*2a*)
Sphingosylphosphorylcholine + **fatty acyl CoA** ⟶
Cer-P-choline (*2b*)

The second reaction has been observed in mitochondria isolated from rat brain [233, 234], and either erythro- or threo-sphingosylphosphorylcholine can serve as the substrate [234]. It is believed that reaction (1) accounts for 95 percent of the sphingomyelin synthesized in the rodent brain (Brady, personal communication), but the more important biosynthetic route has not been established for all tissues.

Catabolism of Sphingomyelin

The initial step in the catabolism of sphingomyelin is a hydrolytic cleavage to phosphorylcholine and ceramide by an enzyme termed sphingomyelinase (phosphatidylcholine cholinephosphohydrolase, E.C.3.1.4.3) which is present in many tissues [30, 235–240].

Cer-P-choline ⟶ **Cer** + **P-choline**

In liver and kidney the enzymatic activity is primarily located in the lysosomes, but significant activity has also been found in the mitochondria [241]. Sphingomyelinase activity has also been measured in the intestinal epithelium [239] and in the arterial wall [240]. A deficiency of this enzyme in the tissues of patients with type A Niemann-Pick disease was first demonstrated by Brady et al. [29]. The further catabolism of ceramide has been described in Chap. 29. Schneider and Kennedy have demonstrated in the intact rat that dihydrosphingomyelin is probably catabolized according to the sequence dihydrosphingomyelin → dihydroceramide → dihydrosphingosine [242]. There is presently no evidence that sphingosylphosphorylcholine is an intermediate in the catabolism of sphingomyelin. In the studies just mentioned labeled dihydrosphingomyelin was injected intravenously as a micellar suspension. The largest part of the radioactivity was located in the liver [242].

Occurrence and Functions

The lipid phosphatides have in common certain properties derived from a general structure that incorporates both polar and nonpolar groups. They are therefore capable of both ionic associations with protein at aqueous interfaces and of interactions with less polar substances through forces deriving their strength from the close proximity of hydrophobic regions. Phospholipids thus play essential roles in the structure and function of lipoproteins and many tissue elements including membranes.

Differences in the constituent phospholipids undoubtedly bestow special properties on membranes and membranelike structures, but the specific functions served by the many different lipid phosphatides in tissues are poorly understood. Sphingomyelin differs considerably in structure from the more common glycerophosphatides. It is ubiquitous in distribution in animal tissues, usually making up 5 to 25 percent of the total lipid phosphatides (Table 35-3). The proportion represented by sphingomyelin in a given tissue, such as the erythrocyte [226, 243, 244] may vary considerably among different species. And at least in brain and the arterial wall [240], it also changes with age. In the liver (Table 35-4) sphingomyelin accounts for less than 10 percent of the total lipid phosphorus, a proportion that is retained in certain of the isolated liver cell components [245].

In the plasma, sphingomyelin comprises about 20 percent of the total phospholipids. The proportion varies among the different lipoprotein species [246-247], and a higher concen-

Table 35-3. APPROXIMATE CONCENTRATIONS OF TOTAL PHOSPHOLIPIDS (PL), SPHINGOMYELIN (SPH), AND CHOLESTEROL (C) IN VARIOUS HUMAN TISSUES

Tissue	PL, mg/gm dry wt	SPH, mg/gm dry wt	C, mg/gm dry wt	C/SPH, molar ratio wt
Cerebral gray*	230	20	60	6
Cerebral white*	295	45	145	6
Erythrocytes†	185	45	80	4
Liver‡	105	5	10	4
Kidney*	80	10	15	3
Spleen‡	65	8	16	4

* From Svennerholm [212]; brain data are means of frontal lobe analyses from six children, 4 to 5 years old; kidney data are from three infants, 2 months old.

† From combined data of Dodge et al. [243] and Ways and Hanahan [244].

‡ Analyses in the authors' laboratory of five livers and four spleens.

Table 35-4. PERCENTAGE DISTRIBUTION OF PHOSPHOLIPIDS IN NORMAL HUMAN LIVER

Phospholipid	Mean ± s.d.
Phosphatidyl choline	42.6 ± 4.3
Lysophosphatidyl choline	1.3 ± 0.7
Phosphatidyl ethanolamine	25.4 ± 2.0
Phosphatidyl inositol	6.9 ± 2.7
Phosphatidyl serine	7.5 ± 3.0
Sphingomyelin	7.0 ± 1.4
Cardiolipin	3.9 ± 1.2
Unidentified	5.5

Note: The mean total phospholipid content of normal human liver is approximately 100 mg/ml.
Source: Data from Kwiterovich et al. [178].

tration in lower density lipoproteins suggests that sphingomyelin is especially useful in the solubilization of triglycerides (see Chap. 26). The amount of net transport of sphingomyelin in plasma is not known.

CHANGES IN THE TISSUE LIPIDS IN NIEMANN-PICK DISEASE

Organs Outside the Central Nervous System

Chemical analyses of tissues obtained by biopsy, splenectomy, or at autopsy from patients with the several forms of sphingomyelin lipidosis are shown in Table 35-1.

Sphingomyelin Content

An increase in the sphingomyelin content of an organ such as the liver, spleen, lung, lymph node, or kidney is the primary basis for the diagnosis of a sphingomyelin lipidosis (Fig. 35-10). The concentration may rise from two- to over thirtyfold, and different organs in the same patient differ in the degree of abnormality. The greatest increases in sphingomyelin are found in patients with types A and B of the disorder. In some patients of type A the increase in total body content of sphingomyelin is of awesome proportions. Taking into account the great enlargement of the liver and spleen in one of our patients, we have estimated that sphingomyelin represented 2 to 5 percent of the total body weight. The increase in sphingomyelin is generally much less obvious in types C and D (Table 35-1). And the concentration in the liver may be normal in these latter patients.

Cholesterol

Tissue cholesterol is almost always increased in Niemann-Pick disease. On a molar basis, the excess of cholesterol often exceeds that of sphingomyelin (Table 35-1). The molar ratio between the two lipids also can vary markedly in different organs and there are differences between phenotypes in regard to this ratio (Table 35-1). The ratio of sphingomyelin to cholesterol in liver or spleen is high in types A and B, and low in types C and D, the relative increase in cholesterol being especially preponderant in type D tissues. Almost all the rise in tissue cholesterol is in the nonesterified form. One possible exception has been reported [20].

Other Lipids

The concentration of phospholipids other than sphingomyelin may also be elevated, but the changes are far less consistent and are probably nonspecific. Lecithins and "cephalins" (probably phosphatidylethanolamine and phosphatidylserine) may be increased [71, 131, 133, 134, 136, 141, 151, 248], but rarely to a greater extent than sphingomyelin [42, 43]. We have found [32], however, as have others [119, 141, 144, 249] that the major phospholipid classes other than sphingomyelin are often normal or lower than normal in tissues from type A patients. Rouser has recently reported the interesting finding of a greatly increased content of lysobisphosphatidic acid in the livers of three patients (probably of type A [249]). Normally present in only one-sixth the concentration of sphingomyelin, this phosphodiester may also be a substrate of sphingomyelinase [249]. In extraneural tissues there are no characteristic changes in glycerides, neutral glycolipids, or gangliosides.

Foam Cell Content

Comparison of lipids in the spleen of a type A patient and the foam cells isolated from it indicate that the increased

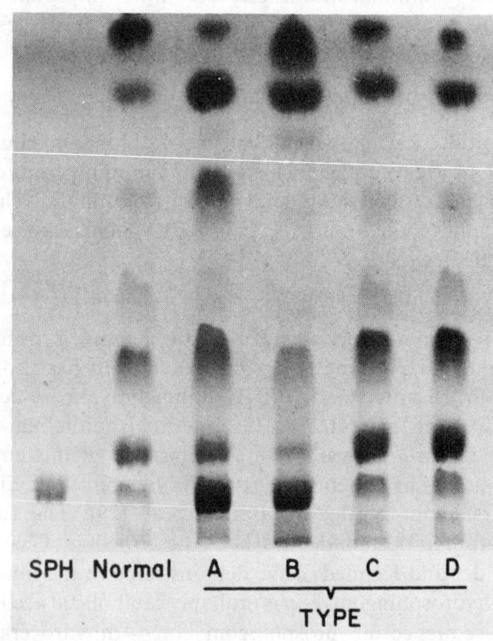

Figure 35-10. One-dimensional thin-layer chromatogram of liver lipids in four types of Niemann-Pick disease. SPH, sphingomyelin.

sphingomyelin and sterol are associated with the foam cells (Table 35-5). Residual bodies isolated from the organs of a patient with type A have also been found to have a lipid profile similar to that in the whole tissue [119].

Fibroblasts in Tissue Culture

Among the lipid storage diseases, the first demonstration of a chemical abnormality in tissues propagated in culture was obtained in patients with type A sphingomyelin lipidosis [250]. Diploid cells obtained from either skin, bone marrow, or amnion have two to three times the sphingomyelin and cholesterol content of normal fibroblasts. The defect persists through many passages and the cells are an excellent source of labeled sphingomyelin substrate for enzymatic analyses.

Lipid Content of the Nervous System

Analyses of brain lipids have been reported for a number of patients apparently of type A [1, 2, 23–25, 59, 92, 164, 220, 251–255], for a few patients apparently of type C [133, 134, 141, 142, 144], and one patient of type D [1]. The earlier studies usually involved extraction of whole brain; later ones have analyzed gray and white matter separately, and, most recently, Kamoshita and coworkers have analyzed residual bodies isolated from brain cells [119]. The quantitative results vary widely, in part because of the irregular loss of normal architecture in both the gray matter and myelin, the latter being a structure especially rich in sphingomyelin.

The concentrations of both sphingomyelin and cholesterol are increased in gray or white matter in most type A patients. Lesser increases or none at all are more characteristic of type C. Sphingomyelin in gray and white matter was reported as normal in the single type D patient, who was 19 years old at death [1]. The swollen neurons often fail to show histochemical evidence of either cholesterol or phospholipid storage, but the isolated residual bodies contain mainly cholesterol and sphingomyelin [119], and probably most of the excess lipid is stored in macrophages. In the type A brain, the sphingomyelin in the cortex contains the normal preponderance of C_{18} fatty acids and the sphingomyelin in white matter contains mainly its typical C_{24} fatty acids [220, 254]. In type C, abnormalities in the fatty acid components of both cerebral cerebrosides and sphingomyelin [144] have been suggested but not established.

Neutral glycolipids including glucosyl ceramides and lactosyl ceramides may be increased, especially in gray matter [133, 141, 144]. The concentration of gangliosides often is greater than usual in the brains of both type A [253] and type C patients. The excess mainly involves "fast moving" monosialogangliosides [117, 141, 142, 144, 170, 255], particularly gangliosides G_{M2} and G_{M3} (see Chap. 29) [141, 144]. Unusual gangliosides containing neither glucose nor hexosamine have also been found, but these are not specific for Niemann-Pick disease, being seen in other lipid and mucopolysaccharide storage disorders [170].

It has been pointed out [59, 144] that alterations in the normal profile of glycolipids and gangliosides in the brain probably are secondary to the disruption of both structure and function of neurons and myelin. The gangliosides in axons extending into the white matter will be relatively increased, for example, when the myelin sheath has disintegrated. Philippart and colleagues [144] have conjectured that the neuronal ballooning in the type C cortex may not be due to lipid storage, but to an accumulation of fluid. They interpret the frequent absence of any increase in brain sphingomyelin and the absence of a deficiency in (visceral) sphingomyelinase as possibly denoting different metabolic bases for CNS damage in type C compared to type A.

ANCILLARY CLINICAL FINDINGS

Plasma Lipids and Lipoproteins

Plasma cholesterol and total phospholipid concentrations are not consistently altered in patients with the several types of sphingomyelin lipidosis [32, 35]. Plasma sphingomyelin levels are not out of proportion to the total phospholipids [35, 151, 112]. Triglycerides and very low density lipoproteins tend to be abnormally high and high density lipoproteins tend to be low [32], but these changes are not specific for Niemann-Pick disease.

Other Plasma Components

An elevated plasma acid phosphatase is present in a few patients with the prolonged forms of Niemann-Pick disease. This was first observed by Hastrup and Videbaek [256], and we have noted it in type B. This enzyme is much more commonly elevated in Gaucher's disease. There are no *characteristic* changes in other plasma components. Absence of plasma α_2-globulins in one series of patients has been considered a nonspecific sign of hepatic failure [257].

Red Cells

A relative decrease in the proportion of noncholine containing phospholipids [112] and of sphingomyelin [113, 258, 259] in the erythrocytes has been described. These changes are difficult to interpret, particularly since similar ones have been reported in Tay-Sachs disease, Hurler's disease, and Gaucher's disease [259, 260]. Red cell fragility and life span have not been systematically studied in Niemann-Pick disease.

THE METABOLIC DEFECT IN THE SPHINGOMYELIN LIPIDOSES

Decreased Catabolism of Sphingomyelin

Types A and B

It appears that a widespread deficiency of sphingomyelinase is the primary defect in types A and B of the sphingomyelin lipidoses (Table 35-2). A marked decrease in hydrolysis of sphingomyelin was first observed in six livers and one kidney from patients with type A by Brady et al. [29]. Using a different assay system and the spleen as the enzyme source, Schneider and Kennedy [30] confirmed the finding in two other type A patients and extended it in three patients considered to be type B. The stability of the enzyme permitted the use of tissues kept for years in the frozen state. When the enzyme assays were extended to fibroblasts grown in tissue culture, cells derived from bone marrow aspirates or skin biopsies from patients of type A or type B were likewise found deficient in activity [31]. As was noted in solid tissues [30], the deficiency was more profound in fibroblasts from patients of type A. In each instance, when deficiency was apparent, care was taken to assure a great excess of labeled substrate in the assay employing fibroblasts [31], or correction was made for greater dilution by the endogenous substrate in solid tissues from affected subjects [29, 30]. No inhibitor has been found in experiments employing mixtures of control and either type A or B fibroblasts [31]. Representative enzyme assays are shown in Table 35-2. Kampine et al., have reported low sphingomyelinase activity in the peripheral white cells of patients with Niemann-Pick disease, some of whom almost certainly were of type A [261].

Other Types

Schneider and Kennedy [30] also measured sphingomyelinase activity in spleens from five patients classified by Dr. Allen Crocker as four type C's and one type D (Table 35-2).

Table 35-5. COMPARISON OF THE LIPID CONTENT OF WHOLE SPLEEN AND ITS ISOLATED FOAM CELLS IN TYPE A NIEMANN-PICK DISEASE

Lipid	Spleen, μmoles	Foam cells, μmoles
Phospholipids	100	100
Sphingomyelin	70	69
Lecithin	11	12
Other phospholipids	20	19
Cholesterol	55	62

Note: The lipids in each tissue are expressed on the basis of 100 μmoles of phospholipid. For conversion of normalized values to actual: spleen lipids × 4.8 = μmoles per gm dry tissue; foam cell lipids × 1.3 = μmoles per 10^7 cells. Cholesterol was 98 percent nonesterified in both whole spleen and cells.

In type C there was no obvious enzyme deficiency when compared to controls who had either Gaucher's disease or Hunter-Hurler syndrome. The activity in the spleen from the patient representing the Nova Scotia variant, type D, was appreciably lower than that of the controls but far above that in types A or B. In the patient, L.B., described above as an example of type C, we found the activity in the liver to be normal. In two sibs with type D (P.D. and R.D., described above), we found tissue culture sphingomyelinase to be normal. The patient R.S., cited as an example of type E, also had tissue culture levels of enzyme activity in the normal range. Obviously, more data are needed from well-classified patients. The available information indicates that type C and type D sphingomyelin lipidoses probably are not related to a sphingomyelinase deficiency in nonneural tissues. As defined in this chapter, type E does not include patients with sphingomyelinase deficiency. Studies of sphingomyelinase activity in the human brain are sorely needed in relation to Niemann-Pick disease. The level of activity of sphingomyelinase in visceral organs may not necessarily reflect that in the brain, and the nervous system damage in types A, C, and D cannot now be explained by a common mechanism.

Possible Increased Synthesis of Sphingomyelin

A few studies have been made of sphingomyelin synthesis in vivo [262–265], but not in patients with Niemann-Pick disease. Crocker and Mays have reported that the incorporation of labeled inorganic phosphate into sphingomyelin by liver and spleen slices or white cells from patients with Niemann-Pick disease does not appear to be greater than normal [120]. They used tissue samples freshly obtained at surgery from patients representing types B and C. Similar conclusions have been drawn from experiments involving sphingomyelin labeling in cultured fibroblasts from a type A patient and a control [266]. While there is no evidence that increased synthesis is the basis of sphingomyelin storage in types A, B, or C, technical problems in the reported experimentation did not permit complete exclusion of the possibility.

Possible Elaboration of Abnormal Sphingomyelin

It was earlier thought that the fatty acids in the sphingomyelins stored in Niemann-Pick disease might be unusual [23, 25, 267], but later examinations have not indicated any departure from normal patterns in the viscera of patients of types A and C [32, 59, 139, 142, 212]. The sphingomyelin fatty acid pattern in the isolated foam cells has also been found to be indistinguishable from that in the whole spleen [32]. Some possible alterations in brain sphingomyelin fatty acids have already been mentioned. There are no published data about sphingomyelin fatty acid composition in patients with types B, D, or E.

Other aspects of sphingomyelin structure, such as the configuration of the C_3-hydroxyl in the sphingosine, have not been thoroughly examined in Niemann-Pick tissues. We have obtained convincing evidence, however, that the sphingomyelin synthesized in type A cells is chemically normal. This was achieved by isolating labeled sphingomyelin from cultured fibroblasts. Although the sphingomyelinase activity in these cells was very low, the sphingomyelin proved to be an excellent substrate for the enzyme in both fibroblasts and solid tissues from normal subjects.

Chromosomal Abnormalities

Dr. B. W. Uhlendorf has examined the chromosome pattern in diploid cells carried in tissue culture from several patients with type A. There have been no detectable abnormalities.

PATHOPHYSIOLOGY AND PHENOTYPIC VARIATION

A general explanation for the sphingomyelin lipidoses is that sphingomyelin, a constituent of all cells and extracellular lipoproteins, accumulates in many cells with phagocytic potential because the demand for its catabolism exceeds the capacity of the degradative system. These cells become filled with secondary lysosomes [4] recognizable by their morphology and the increased activity of various nonspecific acid hydrolases. Organs containing a preponderance of these cells enlarge; perhaps they do so both to accommodate an undesired population of stuffed macrophages and to meet the minimum requirement for "working" cytoplasm necessary to carry out other essential functions. In organs outside the nervous system, the damage done by a steadily rising surplus of sphingomyelin is due mostly to physical destruction or inactivation of cellular organelles.

A metabolic disturbance involving one of its structural components is much less tolerable to the nervous system, however. The brain is confined in a rigid space and the spatial relationships of its components are critical. Neurons are also generally unable to regenerate damaged components. The events initiating and sustaining damage in the brain are not understood. The phagocytosis of lipid by glial cells and other macrophages is probably secondary to the defective metabolism of sphingomyelin within the neurons.

The pervasive nature of organ involvement in Niemann-Pick disease suggests that much of the accumulation of sphingomyelin comes locally from the turnover of an element of the cells themselves. Some organs may bear a heavier burden than others for the disposal of sphingomyelin derived from the circulating lipoproteins and blood cellular elements. There is no consistent increase in plasma sphingomyelin concentrations in Niemann-Pick disease and therefore no indication that an overflow of sphingomyelin is distributed from the liver and spleen to other tissues throughout the body.

Abnormal Hydrolases

Two forms of Niemann-Pick disease (types A and B) can be explained by gross failure of the normal capacity for sphingomyelin catabolism. In both forms the tissue activity of sphingomyelinase is low and the accumulation of sphingomyelin in extraneural tissues begins early in life, becoming massive and widely distributed. It appears that the degree of deficiency in sphingomyelinase activity in the liver or spleen is greater in type A than in type B (Table 35-2). Whether this is also true in the brain, and if it is, whether such a quantitative difference in activity could determine the presence or absence of clinically evident CNS involvement has not been ascertained. It has not been proved that the sphingomyelinases in brain and other tissues are the same. It is conceivable that different mutations at the same or different loci can differentially affect the activity of the same enzyme.

It has also not yet been excluded that a cofactor for sphingomyelinase may be differently affected by mutation. We have made preliminary studies of the effects of mixing sonicated normal and mutant fibroblasts that suggest that normal tissues cannot supply a missing cofactor to the abnormal cells and that the latter contain no transferable inhibitor affecting activity of the normal enzyme. Since types A and B appear to be caused by "leaky mutants"; i.e., some sphingomyelinase activity is present, there is hope of eventual purification and characterization of the possible mutant enzymes.

Defects Other than in Sphingomyelinase

Type C, at best an impure "phenotype" as now defined, includes examples in which sphingomyelinase activity in extraneural tissues is not clearly deficient. Thus at least part of those patients classified as type C have no demonstrated block in sphingomyelin catabolism. The same is true for one or two cases of type D in which sphingomyelinase activity has been assayed.

It is possible that some patients with type C and perhaps all of those with type D, the rare Nova Scotia variant, may be misplaced in their inclusion among the sphingomyelin lipidoses. The sphingomyelin storage is usually unimpressive and often overshadowed in degree by the cholesterol storage. There is inadequate published chemical data on the organs in both of these variants, but no other chemical or enzymatic abnormalities have been established.

Other Models of Sphingomyelin Storage

No explanation is available for the lipidosis in adults with visceral sphingomyelin storage and normal sphingomyelinase activity. They may represent sphingomyelin storage occurring under circumstances other than obvious genetic causes. Widespread accumulation of foam cells, containing a high concentration of sphingomyelin and sterol, have been associated with primary tumors of the liver [35, 268]. Secondary storage of lipid has been observed in animals after the injection of sphingomyelin suspensions [269–271]. Japanese workers have reported foam cells staining similarly to cells in Niemann-Pick disease in patients receiving large doses of polyvinylpyrrolidone parenterally [272].

Recently a group of patients has been collected under the name, "The Syndrome of the Sea Blue Histiocyte" [273]. The name is derived from large cells in the bone marrow that stain deep blue with Geimsa's or Wright's stain. The tissues in such patients have an increase of twofold or more in the concentration of sphingomyelin. The contents of certain unidentified neutral glycolipids are also increased. One of the patients described as representing this syndrome, first reported by Cogan and Federman [137], was found to have a marked increase in spleen sphingomyelin by Crocker [60]. She has splenomegaly, hyperteleorism, and macular lesions similar to cherry-red spots, but is otherwise healthy. We have found the sphingomyelin activity in skin fibroblasts from this patient to be low. Whether she represents a late stage of type B or C sphingomyelin lipidosis or a different syndrome is not clear.

A hereditary disease of mice, foam cell reticulosis [274], is associated with the accumulation of foam cells in the thymus and Peyer's patches. The content of sphingomyelin and cholesterol is greatly increased [275], but sphingomyelinase activity is normal. We have recently found that many glycolipids are also increased in these tissues. The disorder does not obviously resemble any particular human variant of Niemann-Pick disease.

Why Other Lipids Accumulate

It is characteristic of storage diseases that more than one chemical constituent is increased in the affected tissues. Sometimes this occurs because the altered enzyme acts upon several substrates. At other times compounds in pathways behind a metabolic block accumulate. These may also be degraded to derivatives rarely seen in the normal state. The concurrent piling up of compounds remote from any affected pathway is more difficult to explain. Such is the case for the invariable accumulation of unesterified cholesterol in the sphingomyelin lipidoses. It is possible that the accumulation of large amounts of sphingomyelin in lysosomes might interfere with the action of other acid hydrolyses, but there is no evidence that unesterified cholesterol is degraded by lysosomal enzymes. The possibility has been discussed [32, 59] that the simultaneous accumulation of cholesterol in Niemann-Pick disease facilitates the intracellular storage or "packing" of sphingomyelin. The spatial relationships and distribution of forces between these molecules relevant to this theory have been described by Vandenheuval [276]. Cholesterol metabolism has not been studied adequately in any of the sphingomyelin lipidoses.

DIAGNOSIS

The diagnosis of sphingomyelin lipidosis in a child is usually brought to mind because of hepatosplenomegaly coupled with abnormal psychomotor development. The earliest examination should include careful attention to neurological and mental development and examination of the eyes for cherry-red spots. X-rays should be taken of the lungs, of the bones to exclude changes typical of the mucopolysaccharidoses, and of the adrenals to exclude the calcification seen in Wolman's disease. The peripheral smear should be checked for vacuolation of leukocytes. A bone marrow aspirate should then be examined supravitally under the phase microscope for foam cells. Gaucher's disease may be differentiated from other lipidoses in this way. Whether other nonspecific foam cells are present or not, tissue biopsy is next considered. Open biopsy of a node or the liver is desirable for definitive diagnosis. Biopsy of the spleen is hazardous due to bleeding. Rectal biopsy does not permit a definitive diagnosis although otherwise undetectable neural involvement may be found upon examining the autonomic ganglion cells. Brain biopsy is an heroic diagnostic procedure.

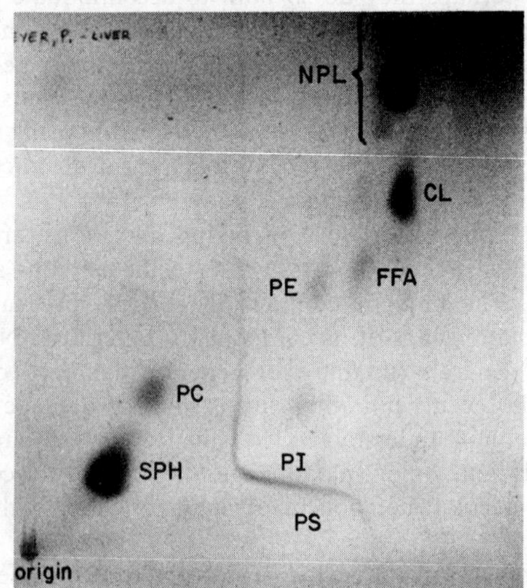

Figure 35-11. Two-dimensional thin-layer chromatogram of liver lipids in a patient with Niemann-Pick disease, type A. The sphingomyelin is about 20 times normal. Abbreviations: SPH, sphingomyelin; PC, phosphatidylcholine; PI, phosphatidyl inositol, PE, phosphatidyl ethanolamine; PS, phosphatidyl serine; CL, cardiolipin; FFA, free fatty acids; NPL, nonpolar lipids.

The 1.0 to 1.5 gm of liver usually obtained at biopsy should immediately be subdivided. A small aliquot is allotted for histological examination, including frozen and paraffin sections. Staining with oil-Red-O or other dyes for neutral lipids, and employing Baker hematoxylin (or Smith-Dietrich), periodic acid–Schiff (PAS), and Schultz techniques constitutes a minimum examination. The largest share of tissue, to be used for chemical and sphingomyelinase assays, is placed in several aliquots in sealed plastic bags and immediately frozen to at least −20°C. The diagnosis of sphingomyelin lipidosis can usually be made by qualitative thin-layer chromatography of phospholipids (Fig. 35-10), but quantitation is desirable (Fig. 35-11). Enzyme assays should be obtained if possible. *Failure to save frozen tissue for these purposes will usually expose the patient to the discomfort and risks of another biopsy to ascertain the diagnosis.*

Biopsy of the skin and bone marrow aspirates may be started in tissue culture and then stored for future analyses. It is now possible to use tissue culture instead of organ biopsy for diagnostic purposes. The same may eventually be true of peripheral leukocytes or lymphocyte cultures.

Differential Diagnosis

In children below 2 years, the sphingomyelin lipidoses may resemble many other storage diseases associated with the enlargement of the spleen and liver. These include especially Wolman's disease (Chap. 36), G_{M1}-gangliosidosis, (Chap. 30), and Gaucher's disease, type 2 (Chap. 33). Gaucher's disease, type 1, or glycogenosis may be confused with type B. In older children or adults with minimal hepatosplenomegaly and less striking neurological changes, Niemann-Pick disease may be confused with a variety of neurological or psychiatric disorders.

TREATMENT

Many medications have been tried without success in the treatment of sphingomyelin lipidoses [35]. Two possible treatments may be employed today. The first is splenectomy, when hypersplenism requires it. The second is the administration of antoxidants, at least to patients with the more chronic forms, in view of the likelihood of ceroid formation and the possibility of enhanced tissue damage due to free radical formation [186]. Antoxidants considered for long-term trial include vitamin C, vitamin E or α-tocopheral, and butylhydroxytoluene.

GENETICS

The tests for phenotypic ascertainment in the sphingomyelin lipidoses have only recently become both chemical and enzymatic, and extensive data to support many conclusions concerning genetics are not available. The majority of cases of all types have been reported in Caucausoids from the United States, Western Europe, and Scandinavia. They have also occurred in Orientals and Negroes. More is known about type A than any other form of Niemann-Pick disease.

Type A

The compilation of familial involvement in type A shown in Table 35-6 includes only families in which the diagnosis is unquestionable. The overall involvement of nearly 50 percent of sibs has been noted before [115] and is generally considered to be due to voluntary limitations on the size of affected families. There is an excess of affected males in Table 35-6. Two of the nine families were Jewish. We have also examined the case reports [32] of 110 "probable" type A patients dating from Niemann's first case. Of these 53 were males, 48 females, and for 9 the sex was not specified. Of those whose ethnic origin was identified, 46 percent were Jews. No vertical transmission of sphingomyelin lipidoses has been recorded in type A. The grandparents and father of one patient were noted to have splenomegaly [35].

Type A appears to be an autosomal recessive disease. The gene frequency is unusually high among Jews, particularly those of the Ashkenazim from Eastern Europe, but the distribution of the gene is panethnic.

Other Types

A group of 13 possible examples of type B, obtained by combining published reports [35, 111, 122–127] with our three patients with this variant, includes six males and seven females. Two sibs were affected in each of two families. Three of the affected families were described as Jewish.

A group of 21 possible examples of type C was obtained by combining published reports [32, 35, 60, 133–141, 143, 144] and adding the patient L.B. described here. Thirteen of these were females. A few patients were Jews, the majority Protestants or Catholics from the English-speaking world.

Table 35-6. FAMILIAL INCIDENCE IN TYPE A NIEMANN-PICK DISEASE

Number of families	Size of sibship	Total number of children	Number affected	Males among affected
3	2	6	4	2
3	3	9	4	3
2	4	8	4	4
1	5	5	1	1
9		28	13	10

Note: These data were compiled from a previous summation of cases [32]. They include only patients meeting the clinical criteria for type A, in whose families there were a known number of multiple births, and where chemical proof of the disorder in at least one sib was obtained.

Three sibs were affected in one family (patients 44, 45, 46 in [32]); two sibs in each of three others [134, 141, 143, 144], one pair being identical twins. It may be of interest that in two families [141, 143] the maternal line was Jewish, the father presumably was not, thereby raising the question of a genotype consisting of a mutant for type A and some other closely related mutant. A similar question may be raised concerning the D family, earlier presented as examples of type D. The Nova Scotia variant affects either sex.

At present the three phenotypes, types B, C, and D also appear to be the result of autosomal recessive inheritance. The father of one type C patient also had splenomegaly and vacuolated lymphocytes in the circulating blood [138, 139]. Nearly all of the other parents were reported as completely normal.

Detection of Heterozygotes

We have examined sphingomyelinase activity in fibroblasts from a few parents of children with either type A or type B. The resolution of these assays is not yet sufficient to employ them for heterozygote detection. It is probable that sensitive methods applicable either to cells in tissue culture or circulating leukocytes may someday be available for this purpose. There are presently no other reliable clinical findings or tests to permit the recognition of carriers.

SUMMARY

1 The sphingomyelin lipidoses (Niemann-Pick disease) are characterized by the presence of an increased tissue concentration of sphingomyelin (phosphorylcholine ceramide). The lipid is found particularly in secondary lysosomes in large foam cells. Many organs and cell types are affected. There is almost always hepatosplenomegaly, with foam cells in the bone marrow and pulmonary infiltration. The nervous system may be involved and to varying degrees. A cherry-red spot may be present in the retina.

2 In some forms of the disease, tissues are deficient in the activity of a lysosomal enzyme, sphingomyelinase (E.C. 3,1,4,3), that catalyzes the cleavage of phosphorylcholine from sphingomyelin.

3 At least four different phenotypes are recognizable. Type A develops in infancy and is always associated with severe CNS involvement that is fatal by 3 to 4 years of age. Sphingomyelinase is severely deficient. In type B visceral involvement may be as severe and is apparent in either infancy or childhood. The nervous system is spared, however, and patients may reach adulthood in reasonable health. Sphingomyelinase is also deficient in type B. Type C includes patients with neurovisceral involvement that follows a subacute or chronic course. It is usually fatal before age 20. Sphingomyelinase activity is normal or only slightly deficient. Type D is a variant similar to type C in patients of Nova Scotian ancestry. They have a slowly fatal course and their tissue sphingomyelinase activity is probably normal. Adults who are found incidentally to have tissue sphingomyelin accumulation without neurological involvement and with normal sphingomyelinase activity are classified here as a fifth form, type E.

4 Sphingomyelin storage is greatest in types A and B. It is usually much less in type C and least in type D. In all patients, unesterified cholesterol invariably accumulates with sphingomyelin.

5 Definitive diagnosis requires the chemical demonstration of sphingomyelin accumulation; histochemical techniques are not specific for this purpose. Sphingomyelinase assays are also useful in diagnosis and may be employed in frozen tissues or in fibroblasts grown in tissue culture.

6 Types A, B, C, and D, are considered to be inherited as autosomal recessive disorders. Ascertainment of the heterozygous phenotypes is not yet possible.

7 There is no specific therapy.

BIBLIOGRAPHY

1. Crocker, A. C.: The cerebral defect in Tay-Sachs disease and Niemann-Pick disease. J. Neurochem., **7,** 69, 1961.
2. Lake, B. D.: A histochemical study of Gaucher's disease and Niemann-Pick disease. J. Roy. Micr. Soc., **86,** 417, 1967.
3. Van Hoof, F., and Hers, H. G.: The abnormalities of lysosomal enzymes in mucopolysaccharidoses. Europ. J. Biochem., **7,** 34, 1968.
4. Hers, H. G.: Inborn lysosomal diseases. Gastroenterology, **48,** 625, 1965.
5. Niemann, A.: Ein unbekanntes Krankheitsbild. Jahrb. Kinderheilk. **79,** 1, 1914.
6. Knox, J. H. M., Jr., Wahl, H. R., and Schmeisser, H. C.: Gaucher's disease: A report of two cases in infants. Bull. Johns Hopkins Hosp., **27,** 1, 1916.
7. Siegmund, H.: Lipoidzellenhyperplasie der Milz und Splenomegalie Gaucher. Verh. Deutsch. Ges. Path., **18,** 59, 1921.
8. Mandlebaum, F. S., and Downey, H.: The cases of Gaucher's disease reported by Drs. Knox, Wahl, and Schmeisser. Bull. Johns Hopkins Hosp., **27,** 109, 1916.
9. Pick, L.: Uber die lipoidzellige splenohepatomegalie typus Niemann-Pick als Stoffwechselerkrankung. Med. Klin., **23,** 1483, 1927.
10. Pick, L.: II. Niemann-Pick's disease and other forms of so-called xanthomatoses. Amer. J. Med. Sci., **185,** 601, 1933.
11. Pfändler, U.: La maladie de Niemann-Pick dans le cadre des lipoidoses. Schweiz. Med. Wschr., **76,** 1128, 1946.
12. Dusendschon, A.: Deux cas familiaux de maladie de Niemann-Pick chez adulte. These, Faculte de medicine, Geneva, 1946.
13. Pfändler, U.: Nouvelles conceptions sur l'heredite et la pathogenie de la maladie de Niemann-Pick. Helv. Med. Acta, **20,** 216, 1953.
14. Wahl, H. R., and Richardson, M. L.: A study of lipid content of a case of Gaucher's disease in an infant. Arch. Intern. Med. (Chicago), **17,** 238, 1916.
15. Bloom, W., and Kern, R.: Spleens from Gaucher's disease and lipoid-histiocytosis; the chemical analysis. Arch. Intern. Med. (Chicago), **39,** 456, 1927.
16. Brahn, B., and Pick, L.: Zur chemischen Organalyse bei der lipoidzelligen Splenohepatomegalie typus Niemann-Pick. Klin. Wschr., **6,** 2367, 1927.
17. Corcan, P., Oberling, C., and Dienst, G.: La maladie de Niemann-Pick. Rev. Franc Pediat., **3,** 789, 1927.
18. McFate, R. P.: The chemical analysis of liver and spleen from a case of lipoid histiocytosis (Niemann-Pick's disease). Arch. Path. Lab. Med., **6,** 1054, 1928.

19. Epstein, E., and Lorenz, K.: Die Phosphatidzellverfettung in Gehirn, Leber and Milz bei Niemann-Pickschen Krankheit. Z. Physiol. Chem., **211,** 217, 1932.
20. Sobotka, H., Epstein, E. Z., and Lichtenstein, L.: The distribution of lipoid in a case of Niemann-Pick's disease associated with amaurotic family idiocy. Arch. Path. (Chicago), **10,** 677, 1930.
21. Sobotka, H., Glick, D., Reiner, M., and Tuchman, L. R.: The lipoids of spleen and liver in various types of lipoidoses. Biochem. J., **27,** 2031, 1933.
22. Klenk, E.: Uber die Natur der Phosphatide der Milz bei der Niemann-Pickschen Krankheit. Z. Physiol. Chem., **229,** 151, 1934.
23. Klenk, E.: Uber die Natur der Phosphatide und anderer lipoide des Gehirns und der Leber bei der Niemann-Pickschen Krankheit. Z. Physiol. Chem., **235,** 24, 1935.
24. Tropp, C., and Eckhardt, B.: Sphingomyelin bei Niemann-Pickschen Krankheit. Z. Physiol. Chem., **243,** 38, 1936.
25. Tropp, C., and Eckhardt, B.: Gehirn-sphingomyelin bei Niemann-Pickschen Krankheit. Z. Physiol. Chem., **245,** 1963, 1936.
26. Teunissen, P. H., and Den Ouden, A.: Nachtrag zu der Mitteilung: Beitrag zur Kenntnis der Chemie der Lipoidosis phosphatidica. Z. Chem., **252,** 271, 1938.
27. Thannhauser, S. J., Benotti, J., and Reinstein, H., cited by Thannhauser, S. J., in *Lipidoses: Diseases of the Intracellular Lipid Metabolism,* Grune & Stratton, New York, 1958.
28. Chargaff, E.: A study of the spleen in a case of Niemann-Pick disease. J. Biol. Chem., **130,** 503, 1939.
29. Brady, Roscoe O., Kanfer, Julian N., Mock, Michael B., and Fredrickson, Donald S.: The metabolism of sphingomyelin. II. Evidence of an enzymatic deficiency in Niemann-Pick disease. Proc. Nat. Acad. Sci. USA, **55,** 366, 1966.
30. Schneider, Peter B., and Kennedy, Eugene P.: Sphingomyelinase in normal human spleens and in spleens from subjects with Niemann-Pick disease. J. Lipid Res., **8,** 202, 1967.
31. Sloan, H. R., Uhlendorf, B. W., Kanfer, J. N., Brady, R. O., and Fredrickson, D. S.: Deficiency of sphingomyelin-cleaving enzyme activity in tissue cultures derived from patients with Niemann-Pick disease. Biochem. Biophys. Res. Commun., **34,** 582, 1969.
31a. Brady, R. O.: Personal Communication.
32. Fredrickson, D. S.: Sphingomyelin lipidosis: Niemann-Pick disease, in *The Metabolic Basis of Inherited Disease,* edited by J. B. Stanbury, J. B. Wyngaarden, and D. S. Fredrickson, 2d ed., p. 586. McGraw-Hill, New York, 1960.
33. Bloom, W.: The histogenesis of essential lipoid histicytosis (Niemann-Pick's disease). Arch. Path. (Chicago), **6,** 827, 1928.
34. Videback, A.: Niemann-Pick's disease: Acute and chronic type. Acta Paediat., **37,** 95, 1949.
35. Crocker, A. C., and Farber, S.: Niemann-Pick disease: A review of 18 patients. Medicine (Balt), **37,** 1, 1958.
36. Garmyn, F.: De ziekte van Niemann-Pick: Symptomatologie en evolutie. Maandschr. Kindergeneesk., **30,** 10, 1962.
37. Schettler, G., and Kahlke, W.: Niemann-Pick Disease in *Lipids and Lipidoses,* edited by G. Schettler, p. 289. Springer-Verlag, New York, 1967.
38. Hamburger, R.: Lipoidzellige splenohepatomegalie (Typus Niemann-Pick) in verbindung mit amaurotischer idiotie bei sinem 14 Monate alten Mädchen. Jahrb. Kinderheilk., **116,** 41, 1927.
39. Nordmann, J.: Les troubles oculaires dans les maladies de Gaucher et de Niemann-Pick. Bull. Soc. Opthal. Franc., **45,** 509, 1933.
40. Hess, J. H.: Niemann-Pick's disease. Amer. J. Dis. Child., **36,** 1068, 1928.
41. Kramer, B.: Lipoid-cell splenohepatomegaly, Niemann-Pick type: A clinical analysis of nine cases with a report of one additional case. Med. Clin. N. Amer., **11,** 905, 1928.
42. Lederer, M.: Lipoid cell splenohepatomegaly (Niemann). Arch. Path. (Chicago), **6,** 90, 1928.
43. Merksamer, D., and Kramer, B.: Niemann-Pick's disease: Report of three cases in one family. J. Pediat., **14,** 51, 1939.
44. Berman, S. L.: Lipoid histiocytosis (Niemann-Pick's disease). Amer. J. Dis. Child., **36,** 102, 1928.
45. Baty, J. M.: Lipoid histiocytosis (Niemann's disease). Amer. J. Dis. Child., **39,** 573, 1930.
46. Espinos, D., Uribes, M., and Vilaplana, E.: Contribucion al estudio de las histiocitomatosis por imoregnacion lipoidica (tipe Niemann-Pick). An. Med. Int., **5,** 307, 1936.
47. Freudenberg, E.: Klinische beobachtungen und untersuchungen an einem Zwillingspaar mit Niemann-Pickscher Krankheit (NPK). Z. Kinderheilk., **59,** 313, 1938.
48. Didion, H.: Vergleichend-histopathologische Untersuchungen an einem Zwillingspaar mit Niemann-Pickscher Krankheit. Frankfurt. Z. Path., **60,** 194, 1949.
49. Maurer, L. E.: Niemann-Pick's disease. Rocky Mountain Med. J., **38,** 460, 1941.
50. Kugelmass, I. N.: Case citation in *Blood Disorders in Children,* p. 777. Oxford Med. Pub., London, 1941.
51. Menten, M. L., and Welton, J. P.: Lipid analysis in a case of Niemann-Pick disease. Amer. J. Dis. Child., **72,** 720, 1946.
52. Driessen, O. A.: De l'identite de la maladie de Tay-Sachs et de Niemann-Pick. Acta Paediat. Belg., **42,** 447, 1953.
53. Denys, P., Therasse, Y., Malbrain, H., and Corbeel, L.: Contribution a l'etude de la lipidose de type Niemann-Pick. Acta Paediat. Belg., **9,** 233, 1955.
54. Jeune, M., Mouriquand, C., and Gilly, R.: Un cas de maladie de Niemann-Pick. Pediatrie, **11,** 457, 1956.
55. Jeune, M. D., Germain, R., Riedway, R., Hermier, M., and Sitnikow, M.: Sur les diagnotics de la maladie de Niemann-Pick, a propos de deux nouvelles observations. Pediatrie, **14,** 891, 1959.
56. Diaz-Rousselot, J., Valdez-Diaz, R., Salas-Danisello, F., Roque, A., and Pereiras, R.: Enfermedad de Niemann-Pick. Arch. Med. Infant. (Havana), **25,** 243, 1956.
57. Berek, B., Bogumil, M., and Sawicka, E.: A case of Niemann-Pick disease in a 4 months old infant. Pediat. Pol. **35,** 216, 1960.
58. McCusker, J. J., and Parsons, D. B.: Niemann-Pick disease: Report of two cases in siblings including the necropsy and histochemical findings in one. Arch. Path. (Chicago), **74,** 127, 1962.
59. Ivemark, B. I., Svennerholm, L., Thoren, C., and Tunnell, R.: Niemann-Pick disease in infancy: Report of two siblings with clinical, histologic and chemical studies. Acta Paediat., **52,** 391, 1963.
60. Crocker, A. C.: Personal communication, 1965.
61. Bloom, W.: Splenomegaly (type Gaucher) and lipoid-histiocytosis (type Niemann). Amer. J. Path., **1,** 595, 1925.
62. Henschen, F.: In comments on Klercker, K.: Contribution a l'etude de la maladie Gaucher. Acta Med. Scand., suppl. **16,** 590, 1926.
63. Schiff, E.: Im Leben diagnostizierte lipoidzellige Splenohepatomegalie (Typus Niemann-Pick) bei einem 17 monate alten Knaben. Jahrb. Kinderheilk., **112,** 1, 1926.
64. Abt, A. F., and Bloom, W.: Essential lipoid histiocytosis (type Niemann-Pick). JAMA, **90,** 2076, 1928.
65. Chwalibogowski, A., and Schusterowna, H.: O splenohepatomegalzi Niemann-Picka. Polska Gaz. Lek., **8,** 590, 1929.
66. Schmitz, J., and Thoenes, F.: Zum Problem der lipoidzelligen Splenohepatomegalie Niemann-Pick. Mschr. Kinderheilk., **43,** 341, 1929.
67. Jenny, E.: Beitrag zur Kenntnis der Varianten der Gaucherschen und Niemann-Pickschen Krankheit. Thesis, Basel, 1930, cited by Videback, ref. 34.
68. Kilchherr, H.: Beitrag zur Kenntnis der Niemann-Pick'schen Krankheit. Thesis. Zürich, 1930.
69. Smetana, H.: Ein Fall von Niemann-Pickscher Erkrankung. (Lipoidzellige Spleno-hepatomegalie). Arch. Path. Anat., **274,** 697, 1930.
70. Goldstein, I., and Wexler, D.: Niemann-Pick's disease with cherry-red spots in the macula. Arch. Ophthal. (Chicago), **5,** 704, 1931.
71. Wascowitz, B.: Niemann-Pick disease. Amer. J. Dis. Child., **42,** 356, 1931.
72. Poncher, H. G.: Lipoid histiocytosis. Amer. J. Dis. Child., **42,** 77, 1931.
73. Hassin, G. B.: Niemann-Pick's disease. Arch. Neurol. Psychiat., **24,** 61, 1930.
74. Schaferstein, S. J.: Die Pick-Niemann'sche Krankheit. Acta Paediat., **10,** 523, 1931.

75. Druss, J. G.: Pathologic changes in the ear in Niemann-Pick's disease. Arch. Otolaryng. (Chicago), **15**, 592, 1932.
76. Fisher, C. F.: Lipoid histiocytosis: Niemann-Pick's disease with leukemoid blood reaction. Arch. Pediat., **49**, 574, 1932.
77. Knox, R. A., and Ramsey, G. W.: Niemann-Pick's disease (essential lipoid histiocytosis). Ann. Intern. Med., **6**, 218, 1932.
78. Tow, A., and Wechsler, H. F.: Lipoid histiocytosis: Case report. New York J. Med., **33**, 203, 1933.
79. Van Bogaert, L.: L'idiotie amaurotique et les maladies du metabolisme lipidien. Bull. Acad. Roy. Med. Belg., **14**, 323, 1934.
80. Marin, P.: Splenomegalia lipoidocellulare tipo Niemann-Pick e suoi rapporti con il morbo di Gaucher. Minerva Med., **25**, 46, 1934.
81. Baumann, T., Klenk, E., and Scheidegger, S.: Die Niemann-Picksche Krankheit: eine kliniske, chemische und histopathologische Studie. Ergebn. Allg. Path., **30**, 183, 1936.
82. Guccione, F.: Su di una particolare forma di spleno-epatomegalie tipo N. Picl. Pediatria, **44**, 757, 1936.
83. Angel, E., and McConnell, J. S.: Niemann-Pick's disease. South. Med. Surg., **99**, 500, 1937.
84. Höra, J.: Ein Fall von Niemann-Pickscher Erkrankung mit benzonderer Beteiligung des Rückemmarkes. Beitr. Path. Anat., **99**, 16, 1937.
85. Tokugawa, H.: Über einen Sektions Fall der Niemann-Pickschen Krankheit. Nippon Byori Gakkai Kaishi, **27**, 114, 1937.
86. Kato, S.: A case of Niemann-Pick disease. Acta Paediat. Jap., **44**, 533, 1938; abstract, Amer. J. Dis. Child., **56**, 1364, 1938.
87. Lignac, G. D. E., and Teunissen, P. H.: Beitrag zur Kenntnis der Lipoidosis phosphatidica. Beitr. Path. Anat., **101**, 139, 1938.
88. Armand-Delille, M. P., Abricossof, M., and Joussemet, M.: Un cas de maladie de Niemann-Pick chez un enfant de 18 mois. Soc. Pediat. Paris, **37**, 464, 1939.
89. Ley, R. A.: Etude neuropathologique de la maladie de Niemann-Pick (splenohepatomegalie lipidienne). J. Belg. Neurol. Psychiat., **40**, 57, 1940.
90. Badanov, B. I.: A case of Niemann-Pick and Tay-Sachs disease. Pediat. (Russie) nr. 7/8, 76, 1940; abstract, Bormann, Zbl. Kinderheilk., **38**, 539, 1941.
91. Reeves, D. L., and Anderson, L. R.: Niemann-Pick's disease associated with amaurotic idiocy. Bull. Los Angeles Neurol. Soc., **6**, 177, 1941.
92. V. Cube, R., Schmitz, E., and Wienbeck, J.: Heichte bis mittelschwere Niemann-Picksche Krankheit. Arch. Path. Anat., **310**, 631, 1943.
93. Canmann, M. F.: Niemann-Pick disease (acute idiopathetic [sic] xanthomatosis, phosphatide lipidosis, lipoid cell splenomegaly—Niemann type). J. Pediat., **24**, 335, 1944.
94. Fakaçelli, N.: La maladie de Niemann-Pick (a propos d'un cas personnel). Ann. Pediat. (Paris), **162**, 218, 1944.
95. Giampalmo, A.: Sulla malattia di Niemann-Pick. Pathologica, **37**, 39, 1945.
96. Giampalmo, A.: State attuale degli studi sull'anatomia patologica e sulla patogenesi delle malattie di Niemann-Pick, di Gaucher e di v. Gierke. Arch E. Maragliano patologia e clin., **1**, 219, 1946.
97. Murray, H. A., and Bernstein, T. C.: Niemann-Pick's disease: Report of case. Arch. Pediat., **63**, 497, 1946.
98. Dina, M. A.: La malattia di Niemann-Pick: quadro endocrino ed interferenze con le splenoepatopatie fibrosclerotiche. Clin. Pediat. (Bologna), **32**, 329, 1950.
99. Haridas, G.: A case of Niemann-Pick disease. Med. J. Malaya, **4**, 285, 1950.
100. Chodkowska, S., and Lukaszewicz-Dancowa, D.: Przypadek choroby Niemann-Picka. Pediat. Pol., **26**, 422, 1951.
101. Crocco, G.: Su di un caso di malattia di Niemann-Pick: Osservasioni su talune particolarita della citomorfologia midollare. Pediatria (Napoli), **59**, 710, 1951.
102. Burne, J. C.: Niemann-Pick disease in a foetus. J. Path. Bact., **66**, 473, 1953.
103. Leal, A.: Niemann-Pick en un huevo de 5 meses: Aborto por desprendimiento placentario. Obstst. y. ginec. latino-am., **11**, 277, 1953.
104. Pashkova, T. F.: Lipoid-cellular genetic hepatosplenomegaly in child 1 year, 4 months. Pediatriaya, **2**, 57, 1953.
105. Malatesta, C.: Contributo alla conscenze della manifestazioni oculari nel morbo di Niemann-Pick. Boll. Oculist., **33**, 368, 1954.
106. Crosca, A., Recupero, C., and Blandino, G.: Il quadro ematomidollare, radiologico ed oculare nella lipoidosi fosfatidica di Niemann-Pick. Pediatria (Napoli), **54**, 797, 1956.
107. Bottura, C., and Buss, L.: Studio ematologico su di un caso di malattia di Niemann-Pick. Haemat. Arch., **43**, 73, 1958.
108. Chu, F. T.: Niemann-Pick Disease in *Practical Pediatrics,* vol. 2, p. 910. People's Medical Publishers, Peking, 1958.
109. Buckup, H. T., and Luisi, A.: Doenca de Nieman-Pick em crianca parda. Pediat. Prat., **30**, 1, 1959.
110. Sbraccia, C., and Varcasia, E.: Malattia di Nieman-Pick. Minerva Pediat., **11**, 87, 1959.
111. Fontan, A., Verger, P., Bentegeat, J., Leger, H., Kermarec, J., Channarond, J., and Lodeon, J.: Considerations sur les sphingolipidoses: Leurs caracteres histochimiques. Les formes a evolution prolongee de la maladie de Niemann-Pick. Ann. Pediat. (Paris), **8**, 475, 1961.
112. Balint, J. A., Nyhan, W. L., Lietman, P., and Turner, D. A.: Lipid patterns in Niemann-Pick disease. J. Lab. Clin. Med., **58**, 548, 1961.
113. Balint, J. A., and Spitzer, H. L.: Lipid metabolism in Niemann-Pick's disease. Clin. Res., **10**, 31, 1962.
114. Fakaçelli, N. M., and Araboglu, N.: Bir Niemann-Pick vak'asi münasebetiyle. Turk. Tip. Cem. Mec., **28**, 53, 1962.
115. Knudson, A. G., Jr., and Kaplan, W. D.: Genetics of the sphingolipidoses, in *Cerebral Sphingolipidoses: Symposium on Tay-Sachs Disease and Allied Disorders,* edited by S. M. Aronson and B. W. Volk, p. 395. Academic. New York, 1962.
116. Kao, Y. E., and Sui, S. L.: Niemann-Pick disease: Report of 2 cases in Chinese infants. China Med., **82**, 379, 1963.
117. Christensen-Lou, H. O., and Paerregaard, P.: Niemann-Pick's disease: A clinical and biochemical study. Danish Med. Bull., **14**, 62, 1967.
118. Fakatselli, N. M., Delta, B. G., Araboglu, N. S., and Hudaverdi, E. Y.: Niemann-Pick disease in two Moslem children. Clin. Pediat. (Bologna), **7**, 119, 1968.
119. Kamoshita, S., Aron, A. M., Suzuki, K., and Suzuki, K.: Infantile Niemann-Pick disease. A chemical study with isolation and characterization of membranous cytoplasmic bodies and myelin. Amer. J. Dis. Child., **117**, 379, 1969.
120. Crocker, A. C., and Mays, V. B.: Sphingomyelin synthesis in Niemann-Pick disease. Amer. J. Clin. Nutr., **9**, 63, 1961.
121. Chevrel, F., Chevrel-Bodin, M., Cormier, M., and Divet, H.: Maladie de Gaucher et maladie de Niemann-Pick. Ann. Anat. Path. (Paris), **14**, 297, 1937.
122. Santelmann, T.: Beitrag zur juvenillen Form der Niemann-Pickschen Krankheit. Mschr. Kinderheilk., **107**, 503, 1959.
123. Feyrter, F.: Uber die Unterschiedlichkeit der Speicherzellen beim Morbus Niemann-Pick. Frankfurt. Z. Path., **71**, 474, 1962.
124. Forsythe, W. I., McKeown, E. F., and Neill, D. W.: Three cases of Niemann Pick's disease in children. Arch. Dis. Child., **34**, 406, 1959.
125. Verger, P., Bentegeat, J., Kermarec, J., and Serville, F.: Maladie de Niemann-Pick chez un enfant de 4 ans sans manifestations nerveuses; importance remarquable des signes respiratoires pulmonaires. Arch. Franc. Pediat., **22**, 1109, 1965.
126. Lynn, R., and Terry, R. D.: Lipid histochemistry and electron microscopy in adult Niemann-Pick disease. Amer. J. Med., **37**, 987, 1964.
127. Bourel, M., Sabouraud, O., Chevrel, M.-L., Ferrand, B., Lenoir, P., Morel, H., and Badiche, A.: Maladie de Niemann-Pick de l'adulte a forme hepatospleno-pulmonaire. Sem. Hop. Paris, **44**, 1499, 1968.
128. Hollard, D., Revol, L., and Croizat, P.: Les dyslipoidoses d'evolution lente (Maladie de Gaucher et Niemann-Pick de L'adolescent et de l'adulte). Lyon Med., **33**, 217, 1961.
129. Hooft, C., Delbeke, M. J., Garmyn, F., and Vertruyen, H.: Lesions pulmonaires dans la maladie de Niemann-Pick. Ann. Pediat. (Paris), **10**, 385, 1963.
130. Olmer, J., Payan, H., Carcassonne, Y., Lallemand, M., Duc (Mlle): Dyslipoidose chez une malade de 24 ans, maladie de Niemann-Pick. Marseille Med., **100**, 607, 1963.
131. Terry, R., Sperry, W. M., and Brodoff, B.: Adult lipidosis resembling Niemann-Pick's disease. Amer. J. Path., **30**, 263, 1954.
132. Case records of the Massachusetts General Hospital, case 23. New Eng. J. Med., **278**, 1276, 1968.

133. Norman, R. M., Forrester, R. M., and Tingey, A. H.: The juvenile form of Niemann-Pick disease. Arch. Dis. Child., **42,** 91, 1967.
134. Norman, R. M., Tingey, A. H., and Fowler, M. C.: The subacute form of Niemann-Pick's disease, in *Proceedings of the Fifth International Congress of Neuropathology,* edited by F. Luthy and A. Bischoff, p. 143. Excerpta Medica Foundation, New York, 1966.
135. Bruton, O. C., Andrews, B. F., Searer, W. P., and Danoff, S. J.: Problems of the central nervous system simulating cerebral palsy. Clin. Proc. Child. Hosp. DC, **16,** 123, 1960.
136. Cumings, J. H.: Abnormalities in lipid metabolism in two members of a family with Niemann-Pick disease, in *Cerebral Sphingolipidoses: Symposium on Tay-Sachs Disease and Allied Disorders,* edited by S. M. Aronson and B. W. Volk, p. 171, Academic, New York, 1962.
137. Cogan, D. G., and Federman, D. D.: Retinal involvement with reticuloendotheliosis of unclassified type. Arch. Ophthal. (Chicago), **71,** 489, 1964.
138. Cap, J., Misikova, Z., Mezesova-Krajciova, V., and Porges, E.: Juvenilna forma Niemann-Pickovej choroby. Cesk. Pediat., **XXI,** 913, 1966.
139. Porges, E., Sojak, L., Solcaniova, E., and Cap, J.: Beitrag zum studium des milzsphingomyelin bei der Niemann-Pick'schen erkrankung. J. Neurochem., **13,** 879, 1966.
140. Galfi, I., Bata, G., and Imhof, S.: Niemann-Picksche krankheit bei en 11½ Jahre alten knaben. Acta Paediat. Acad. Sci. Hung., **8,** 355, 1966.
141. Oppenheimer, D. R., Norman, R. M., Tingey, A. H., and Aherne, W. A.: Histological and chemical findings in juvenile Niemann-Pick disease. J. Neurol. Sci., **5,** 575, 1967.
142. Lowden, J. A., LaRamee, M. A., and Wentworth, P.: The subacute form of Niemann-Pick disease. Arch. Neurol. (Chicago), **17,** 230, 1957.
143. Jansseune, H., Philippart, M., and Martin, J. J.: Sur deux observations de maladie de Niemann-Pick. Acta Paediat. Belg., **21,** 239, 1967.
144. Philippart, M., Martin, L., Martin, J. J., and Menkes, John H.: Niemann-Pick disease. Arch. Neurol. (Chicago), **20,** 227, 1969.
145. Rabinowicz, T., Klein, D., and Tchicaloff, M.: Juvenile form of Niemann-Pick disease. Path. Europ., **3,** 154, 1968.
146. Glanzmann, E.: Klinische demonstrationen, morbus Niemann-Pick. Schweiz. Med. Wschr., **73,** 1413, 1943.
147. Glanzmann, E.: Morbus Gaucher oder Niemann-Pick? in *Einführung in die Kinderheilkunde,* p. 293. Springer-Verlag, Vienna, 1949.
148. Chung, U-C., Lee, K. S., Chi, D. H., and Lee, U. S.: (A case of Niemann-Pick's disease). J. Korean M. A., **5,** 1590, 1962.
149. Videbaek, A.: Another case of Niemann-Pick's disease observed in Denmark. Acta Paediat., **41,** 355, 1952.
150. Fritts, H. W., Jr.: Clinical implications of cyanosis. Bull. NY Acad. Med., **37,** 291, 1961.
151. Thannhauser, S. J.: *Lipidoses: Diseases of the Intracellular Lipid Metabolism.* Grune & Stratton, New York, 1958.
152. Lee, R. E., Jr.: Personal communication.
153. Alexander, W. S.: Niemann-Pick disease: Report of a case showing calcification in the adrenal glands. New Zeal. Med. J., **45,** 43, 1946.
154. Fahr, T., and Stamm, C.: Kurzer Beitrag zur Frage der Splenomegalie Typ Gaucher. Mschr. Kinderheilk., **26,** 169, 1923.
155. Dienst, G.: Uber einen Fall von lipoidzellinger Splenohepatomegalie. Jahrb. Kinderheilk., **123,** 181, 1929.
156. Stransky, E.: Über groszellige Splenohepatomegalie. Jahrb. Kinderheilk., **126,** 204, 1930.
157. Pounders, C. M.: The lipoid degenerative diseases. J. Pediat., **2,** 216, 1933.
158. Winter, S. J.: Lipoid histiocytosis (Niemann-Pick type). Amer. J. Dis. Child., **43,** 1150, 1932.
159. Vickery, D.: A case of the infantile form of Gaucher's disease (Niemann-Pick's disease). Med. J. Aust., **2,** 546, 1934.
160. Chodkowska, S.: Roczurki proc mankowyck Arreszenia. Asylentow Universystatus Josef a Pilsudkiego, **1,** 1936.
161. Braithwaite, J. V., and Miller, J. H. D.: Hepatosplenomegaly resembling Niemann-Pick's disease: Recovery following liver therapy. Arch. Dis. Child., **15,** 61, 1940.
162. Sawitsky, A., Hyman, G. A., and Hyman, J. B.: An unidentified reticuloendothelial cell in bone marrow and spleen. Blood, **9,** 977, 1954.
163. Cumings, J. N.: The diagnostic value of lipid estimations in the cerebral lipidoses, in *Cerebral Lipidoses,* edited by J. N. Cumings and A. Lowenthal, p. 112. Blackwell, Oxford, 1957.
164. Bartsch, G.: The nature of the lipids in the brain in Niemann-Pick's disease, in *Cerebral Lipidoses,* edited by J. N. Cumings and A. Lowenthal, p. 159. Blackwell, Oxford, 1957.
165. Pansky, B., and Lee, R.: Niemann-Pick disease in a boy of 16 months: Electrophoretic study of blood serum proteins and lipoproteins following various types of therapy. J. Pediat., **51,** 290, 1957.
166. Mafalda-Rizzardini, V., Giorgio-Solimano, C., and Sergio-Oxman, V.: Enfermedad de Niemann-Pick. Pediatria (Santiago), **5,** 247, 1962.
167. Radiological notes, case no. 226. J. Mount Sinai Hosp. NY, **31,** 72, 1964.
168. Kyutoku, S.: Niemann-Pick disease: Report of a case. Jap. J. Pediat., **13,** 66, 1960.
169. Van Bogaert, L., Seitelberger, F., and Edgar, G. W. F.: Etudes neuropathologiques et neurochimiques sur un cas de Niemann-Pick chez un jeune enfant. Acta Neuropath., **3,** 57, 1963.
170. Booth, D. A., Goodwin, H., and Cumings, J. N.: Abnormal gangliosides in Tay-Sachs disease, Niemann-Pick's disease, and gargoylism. J. Lipid Res., **7,** 337, 1966.
171. Luse, S.: The fine structure of the brain and other organs in Niemann-Pick disease, in *Inborn Disorders of Sphingolipid Metabolism.* (*Proceedings of the Third International Symposium on the Cerebral Sphingolipidoses*), edited by S. M. Aronson and B. W. Volk, pp. 93–105. Pergamon, New York, 1967.
172. Van Hoof, F., and Hers, H. G.: L'Ultrastructure du foie dans certaines thesaurismoses. Rev. Int. Hepat, **17,** 815, 1967.
173. Taketomi, Tamotsu, and Yamakawa, Tamio: Sphingomyelin and glucocerebroside of spleen in cases of Gaucher's and Niemann-Pick's diseases. Jap. J. Exp. Med., **37,** 505, 1967.
174. Lampert, F., and Teller, W.: Niemann-Picksche Krankheit: Genetische, cytologische und biochemische Beobachtungen. Mschr. Kinderheilk., **115,** 439, 1967.
175. Lazarus, Sydney S., Vethamany, Victor G., Schneck, Larry, and Volk, Bruno W.: Fine structure and histochemistry of peripheral blood cells in Niemann-Pick disease. Lab. Invest., **17,** 155, 1967.
176. Hooghwinkel, G. J. M., and Borri, P. F.: Pathochemie van de sphingolipidosen. Chem. Weekbl., **60,** 578, 1964.
177. Unpublished data from the authors' laboratory.
178. Kwiterovich, P. O., Sloan, H. R., and Fredrickson, D. S.: The glycolipids and other lipid constituents of normal human liver. J. Lipid Res., **11,** 322, 1970.
179. Pearse, A. G. E.: *Histochemistry—Theoretical and Applied.* Little, Brown, Boston, 1960.
180. Wolman, M.: The Lipidoses, in *Handbook of Histochemistry,* edited by W. Graumann and K. Neumann, vol. V *Lipides,* 2d part, *Histochemistry of Lipids in Pathology,* p. 188. Gustav Fischer Verlag, Stuttgart, Germany, 1964.
181. Roos, B., Cottier, H., and Rossi, E.: Elektronenoptische Beobachtungen bei Speicherkrankheiten. Path. Microbiol. (Basel), **24,** 278, 1961.
182. Tanaka, Y., Brecher, G., and Fredrickson, D. S.: Cellules de la maladie de Niemann-Pick et de quelques autres lipoidoses. (The storage cells of Niemann-Pick disease and some other lipidoses). Nouv. Rev. Franc. Hemat., **3,** 5, 1963.
183. Wallace, Barbara J., Schneck, Larry, Kaplan, Harry, and Volk, Bruno W.: Fine structure of the cerebellum of children with lipidoses. Arch. Path. (Chicago), **80,** 466, 1965.
184. Stoekenius, W.: Osmium tetroxide fixation of lipids, in *Proceedings of the European Regional Conference on Electron Microscopy.* Nederlandsche Vereniging voor Electronen Microscope, Delft, 1960; cited by Lynn and Terry, ref. 126.
185. Chio, K. S., Reiss, U., Fletcher, B., and Tappel, A. L.: Peroxidation of subcellular organelles: Formation of lipofuscin-like fluorescent pigments. Science, **166,** 1535, 1969.
186. Tappel, A. L.: Free-radical lipid peroxidation damage and its inhibition by vitamin E and selenium. Fed. Proc., **24,** 73, 1965.
187. Oppenheimer, E. H., and Andrews, E. C., Jr.: Ceroid storage disease in childhood. Pediatrics, **23,** 1091, 1959.
188. Winkler, Helen H., Frame, Boy, Saeed, S. Mohammed, Spindler, A.

Curtis, and Brouillette, J. Nelson: Ceroid storage disease, complicated by rupture of the spleen. Amer. J. Med., **46**, 297, 1969.

189. Kristensson, K., and Sourander, P.: Occurrence of lipofuscin in inherited metabolic disorders affecting the nervous system. J. Neurol. Neurosurg. Psychiat., **29**, 113, 1966.
190. Levine, A. S., Lemieux, B., Brunning, R., White, J. G., Sharp, H. L., Stadlan, E., and Krivit, W.: Ceroid accumulation in a patient with progressive neurological disease. Pediatrics, **42**, 483, 1968.
191. Hartroft, W. S.: Pathogenesis and significance of hemoceroid and hyaloceroid, two types of ceroid-like pigment found in human atheromatous lesions. J. Geront. **8**, 158, 1953.
192. Lazarus, Sydney S., Vethamany, Victor G., and Volk, Bruno B.: Fine structure of phytohemagglutinin transformed lymphocytes. Arch. Path. (Chicago), **86**, 176, 1968.
193. Landing, B. H., and Rubinstein, J. H.: Biopsy diagnosis of neurologic diseases in children, with emphasis on lipidoses, in *Cerebral Sphingolipidoses: Symposium on Tay-Sachs Disease and Allied Disorders,* edited by S. M. Aronson and B. W. Volk, pp. 1–13. Academic, New York, 1962.
194. Pick, L., and Bielschowsky, M.: Über lipoidzellige Splenomegalie (Typus Niemann-Pick) und amaurotische Idiotie. Klin. Wschr., **6**, 1631, 1927.
195. Diezel, P. B.: Histochemical study of primary lipidoses, in *Cerebral Lipidoses,* edited by J. N. Cumings, and A. Lowenthal, p. 11. Blackwell, Oxford, 1957.
196. Rintelen, F.: Die Histopathologie der Augenhintergrunds veranderungen bei Niemann-Pickschen Lipoidose: Zugleich ein Beitrag zur Frage der Beziehungen zwischen Tay-Sachsscher Idiotie und Niemann-Pickschen Lipoidose. Arch. Augenh., **109**, 332, 1935.
197. Cogan, David G., and Kuwabara, Toichiro: The sphingolipidoses and the eye. Arch. Ophthal. (Chicago), **79**, 437, 1969.
198. Sebestyen, J., and Galfi, I.: Retinal functions in Niemann-Pick lipidosis: Ophthalmological aspects of the chronic form of sphyngomyelin lipidosis. Ophthalmologica (Basel), **157**, 349, 1969.
199. Thudichum, J. L. W.: *Die chemische Konstitution des Gehirns des Menschen und der Tiere.* Pietzcker, Tübingen, 1901.
200. Rouser, G., Berry, J. F., Marinetti, G. V., and Stotz, E.: Studies on the structure of sphingomyelin. I. Oxidation of products of partial hydrolysis. J. Amer. Chem. Soc., **75**, 310, 1953.
201. Marinetti, G., Berry, J. F., Rouser, G., and Stotz, E.: Studies on the structure of sphingomyelin. II. Performic and periodic acid oxidation studies. J. Amer. Chem. Soc., **75**, 313, 1953.
202. Carter, H. E., Johnson, P., and Weber, E. J.: Glycolipids. Ann. Rev. Biochem., **34**, 109, 1965.
203. Sweeley, C. C., and Moscatelli, E. A.: Qualitative microanalysis and estimation of sphingolipid bases. J. Lipid Res., **1**, 40, 1959.
204. Samuelsson, Bengt, and Samuelsson, Karin: Separation and identification of ceramides derived from human plasma sphingomyelins. J. Lipid Res., **10**, 47, 1969.
205. Hirvisalo, E. L., and Renkonen, O.: Composition of human serum sphingomyelin. J. Lipid Res., **11**, 54, 1970.
206. Karlsson, Karl-Anders: Studies on sphingosines. 16. The chemical structure of a dienic long chain base of human blood plasma sphingomyelins. Acta Chem. Scand., **21**, 2577, 1967. (Short communication).
207. Karlsson, K. A.: Studies on sphingosines 6. C_{16}- and C_{17}-sphingosines, hitherto unknown. Acta Chem. Scand., **18**, 2395, 1964.
208. Klenk, Ernst, and Huang, Richard T. C.: Zur Kenntnis der Gehirncer-amide und der darin vorkommenden Sphingosinbasen. Hoppe Seyler Z. Physiol. Chem., **349**, 451, 1968.
209. Carter, H. E., and Hirschberg, C. B.: Phytosphingosines and branched sphingosines in kidney. Biochemistry (Wash.), **7**, 2296, 1968.
210. Karlsson, Karl-Anders, and Steen, Goran O.: Studies on sphingosines. XIII. The existence of phytosphingosine in bovine kidney sphingomyelins. Biochim. Biophys. Acta, **152**, 798, 1968.
211. Svennerholm, L.: Some aspects of the biochemical changes in leucodystrophy, in *Brain Lipids and Lipoproteins and the Leucodystrophies,* edited by J. Folch-Pi, p. 104. Elsevier, Amsterdam, 1963.
212. Svennerholm, Elisabet, Stallberg-Stenhagen, S., and Svennerholm, Lars: Fatty acid composition of sphingomyelins in blood, spleen, placenta, liver, lung, and kidney. Biochim. Biophys. Acta, **125**, 60, 1966.
213. Hanahan, D. J., Watts, R. M., and Pappajohn, D.: Some chemical characteristics of the human and bovine erythrocytes and plasma. J. Lipid Res., **1**, 421, 1960.
214. Sweeley, Charles C.: Purification and partial characterization of sphingomyelin from human plasma. J. Lipid Res., **4**, 402, 1963.
215. O'Brien, John S., and Blankenhorn, David H.: Fatty acid composition of sphingomyelin and lecithin in normal human serum. Proc. Soc. Exp. Biol. Med., **119**, 862, 1965.
216. Williams, J. H., Kuchmak, M., and Witter, R. F.: Phospholipids of human serum. Lipids, **1**, 89, 1966.
217. Phillips, G. B., and Dodge, J. T.: Composition of phospholipids and of phospholipid fatty acids of human plasma. J. Lipid Res., **8**, 676, 1967.
218. Minari, Osamu, Tsubono, Hiroko, Akiyama, Masako, and Sakagami, Toshio: Sphingomyelins in human erythrocytes and plasma. J. Biochem. (Tokyo), **62**, 618, 1967.
219. Minari, Osamu, Tsubono, Hiroko, Akiyama, Masako, and Sakagami, Toshio: Distribution and metabolism of two sphingomyelins in rat tissues. J. Biochem. (Tokyo), **64**, 275, 1968.
220. Jatzkewitz, H., and Pilz, H.: Uber den Fettsaureanteil der Sphingomyeline im Grau und Weiss normaler und pathologischer Gehirne. Sonderdruck aus die Naturwissenschaften, **51**, 61, 1964.
221. O'Brien, John S., and Rouser, George: The fatty acid composition of brain sphingolipids: Sphingomyelin, ceramide, cerebroside, and cerebroside sulfate. J. Lipid Res., **5**, 339, 1964.
222. Svennerholm, L.: The distribution of lipids in the human nervous system. I. Analytical procedures, lipids of foetal and newborn brain. J. Neurochem. **11**, 839, 1964.
223. Stallberg-Stenhagen, S., and Svennerholm, L.: Fatty acid composition of human brain sphingomyelins: Normal variation with age and changes during myelin disorders. J. Lipid Res., **6**, 146, 1965.
224. Porges, Eduard, and Sojak, Ladislav: Sphingomyeline, Cerebroside und Sulphatide im Neugeborengehirn. J. Neurochem., **13**, 169, 1966.
225. Di Costanzo, G., and Clement, J.: Composition en acides gras des divers phospholipides de la muqueuse intestinale du rat a jeun et en periode d'absorption. Bull. Soc. Chim. Biol. (Paris), **45**, 137, 1963.
226. Van Deenen, L. L. M., De Gier, J., Houtsmuller, U. M. T., Montfoort, A., and Mulder, E.: Dietary effects on the lipid composition of biomembranes, in *Biochemical Problems of Lipids,* edited by A. C. Frazer, p. 404. Elsevier, Amsterdam, 1963.
227. Leat, W. M. F.: Serum phospholipids of pigs given different amounts of linoleic acid. 1. Fatty acid composition of the cephalin, lecithin, lysolecithin and sphingomyelin fractions. Biochem. J., **91**, 437, 1964.
228. Sribney, Michael, and Kennedy, Eugene: The enzymatic synthesis of sphingomyelin. J. Biol. Chem., **233**, 1315, 1958.
229. Kopaczyk, K. C., and Radin, N. S.: *In vivo* conversions of cerebroside and ceramide in rat. J. Lipid Res., **6**, 140, 1965.
230. Fujino, Y., Nakano, Mo., Negishi, T., and Ito, S.: Substrate specificity for ceramide in the enzymatic formation of sphingomyelin. J. Biol. Chem., **243**, 4650, 1968.
231. Sribney, Michael: Stimulation and inhibition of sphingomyelin synthetase. Arch. Biochem., **126**, 954, 1968.
232. Fujino, Y., Negishi, T., and Ito, S.: Enzymic synthesis of sphingosylphosphorylcholine. Biochem. J., **109**, 310, 1968.
233. Brady, R. O., Bradley, R. M., Young, O. M., and Kaller, Hans: An alternative pathway for the enzymatic synthesis of sphingomyelin (preliminary communication). J. Biol. Chem., **240**, PC 3693, 1965.
234. Fujino, Y., and Negishi, T.: Investigation of the enzymatic synthesis of sphingomyelin. Biochim. Biophys. Acta, **152**, 428, 1968.
235. Kanfer, Julian N., Young, Oscar M., Shapiro, David, and Brady, Roscoe O.: The metabolism of sphingomyelin. I. Purification and properties of a sphingomyelin-cleaving enzyme from rat liver tissue. J. Biol. Chem., **241**, 1081, 1966.
236. Heller, M., and Shapiro, B.: Enzymic hydrolysis of sphingomyelin by rat liver. Biochem. J., **98**, 763, 1966.
237. Barnholz, Y., Roitman, A., and Gatt, S.: Enzymatic hydrolysis of sphingolipids. II. Hydrolysis of sphingomyelin by an enzyme from rat brain. J. Biol. Chem., **241**, 3731, 1966.
238. Rachmilewitz, D., Eisenberg, S., Stein, Y., and Stein, D.: Phospholipases

in arterial tissue. I. Sphingomyelin choline phosphohydrolase activity in human, dog, guinea pig, rat and rabbit arteries. Biochim. Biophys. Acta, **144,** 624, 1967.

239. Nilsson, A.: The presence of sphingomyelin- and ceramide-cleaving enzymes in the small intestinal tract. Biochim. Biophys. Acta, **176,** 339, 1969.

240. Eisenberg, S., Stein, Y., and Stein, O.: Phospholipases in arterial tissue. III. Phosphatide acyl-hydrolase, and sphingomyelin choline phosphohydrolase in rat and rabbit aorta in different age groups. Biochim. Biophys. Acta, **176,** 557, 1969.

241. Weinreb, Neal J., Brady, Roscoe O., and Tappel, A. L.: The lysosomal localization of sphingolipid hydrolases. Biochim. Biophys. Acta, **159,** 141, 1968.

242. Schneider, Peter B., and Kennedy, Eugene P.: Metabolism of labeled dihydrosphingomyelin in vivo. J. Lipid Res., **9,** 58, 1968.

243. Dodge, J. T., Mitchell, C., and Hanahan, D. J.: The preparation and chemical characteristics of hemoglobin-free ghosts of human erythrocytes. Arch. Biochem., **100,** 119, 1963.

244. Ways, P., and Hanahan, D. J.: Characterization and quantification of red cell lipids in normal man. J. Lipid Res., **5,** 318, 1964.

245. Veerkamp, J. H., Mulder, I., and Van Deenen, L. L. M.: Comparative studies on the phosphatides of normal rat liver and primary hepatoma. Z. Krebsforsch., **64,** 137, 1961.

246. Phillips, G. B.: The phospholipid composition of human serum lipoprotein fractions separated by ultracentrifugation. J. Clin. Invest., **38,** 489, 1959.

247. Nye, W. H. R., Waterhouse, C., and Marinetti, G. V.: The phosphatides of human plasma. I. Normal values determined by paper and column chromatography. J. Clin. Invest., **40,** 1194, 1961.

248. Chargaff, E.: A study of the spleen in a case of Niemann-Pick disease. J. Biol. Chem., **130,** 503, 1939.

249. Rouser, G., Kritchevski, G., Yamamoto, A., Knudson, A. G., Jr., and Simon, G.: Accumulation of a glycerolphospholipid in classical Niemann-Pick disease. Lipids, **3,** 287, 1968.

250. Uhlendorf, B. W., Holtz, A. I., Mock, M. B., and Fredrickson, D. S.: Persistence of a metabolic defect in tissue cultures derived from patients with Niemann-Pick disease, in *Inborn Disorders of Sphingolipid Metabolism. (Proceedings of the Third International Symposium on the Cerebral Sphingolipidoses)*, edited by S. M. Aronson and B. W. Volk, pp. 443–453. Pergamon Press, New York, 1967.

251. Klenk, E.: Beiträge zur Chemie der Lipoidosen: Niemann-Pickschen Krankheit und amaurotische Idiotie. Z. Physiol. Chem., **262,** 128, 1939.

252. Klenk, E.: Beiträge zur Chemie der Lipoidosen. Z. Physiol. Chem., **267,** 128, 1940.

253. Klenk, E.: Uber die Verteilung der Neuraminsäure im Gehirn bei der familiären amaurotischen Idiotie und bei der Niemann-Pickschen Krankheit. Z. Physiol. Chem., **282,** 84, 1947.

254. Rouser, G., Galli, C., and Kritchevsky, G.: Lipid class composition of normal human brain and variations in metachromatic leucodystrophy, Tay-Sachs, Nieman-Pick, chronic Gaucher's and Alzheimer's diseases. J. Amer. Oil Chem. Soc., **42,** 404, 1965.

255. Wagner, A.: Biochemische Untersuchungen an den Gangliosiden eines Falles von Niemann-Pickschr Erkrankung. Verch. Deutsch. Ges. Inn. Med., **71,** 965, 1965.

256. Hastrup, B., and Videbaek, A.: Acid phosphatase in Niemann-Pick's disease and a therapeutic experiment with cortisone. Acta Med. Scand., **149,** 287, 1954.

257. Schneck, L., Saifer, A., Warshall, H. B., and Volk, B. W.: Absence of serum alpha-2 globulin in Nieman-Pick disease: A measure of hapatocellular involvement. Proc. Soc. Exp. Biol. Med. **122,** 1295, 1966.

258. Rouser, G., Bauman, A. J., Nicolaides, N., and Heller, D.: Paper chromatography of lipids: Methods, applications, and interpretations. J. Amer. Oil. Chem. Soc., **38,** 565, 1961.

259. Hooghwinkel, G. J. M., van Gelderen, H. H., and Staal, A.: Sphingomyelin of red blood cells in lipidosis and in dementia of unknown origin in children. Arch. Dis. Child., **44,** 197, 1969.

260. Balint, J. A., Spitzer, H. L., and Kyriakides, E. C.: Studies of red-cell stromal lipids in Tay-Sachs disease and other lipidoses. J. Clin. Invest., **42,** 1661, 1963.

261. Kampine, J. P., Brady, R. O., and Kanfer, J. N.: Diagnosis of Gaucher's disease and Niemann-Pick disease with small samples of venous blood. Science, **155,** 86, 1967.

262. Hunter, F. E., and Levy, S. R.: Occurrence and rate of turnover of sphingomyelin in tissues of normal and tumor-bearing rats. J. Biol. Chem., **146,** 577, 1942.

263. Zilversmit, D. B., Entenman, C., and Chaikoff, J. L.: The measurement of turnover of the various phospholipids in liver and plasma of the dog and its application to the mechanism of action of choline. J. Biol. Chem., **176,** 193, 1948.

264. Bieth, R., Rebel, G., and Mandel, P.: Methode de Separation Quantitative de sphingomyelines: Application a L'etude du Renouvellement de la splingomyeline in vivo. Bull. Soc. Chim. Biol. (Paris), 1959, 41, Nos. 7–8.

265. Kanfer, J., and Gal, A. E.: *In vivo* conversion of erythro and threo DL-sphingosine-^{3}H to ceramide and sphingomyelin. Biochem. Biophys. Res. Commun., **22,** 442, 1966.

266. Holtz, Albert I.: Quantitation of phospholipid analysis using P^{32} by a digital computer method in metabolic experiments on Niemann-Pick disease. J. Amer. Oil. Chem. Soc., **44,** 80, 1967.

267. O'Brien, J. S.: A molecular defect in myelination. Clin. Res., **12,** 276, 1964.

268. Wood, H.: Generalized essential xanthomatosis (type Niemann-Pick) associated with primary carcinoma of the liver in an infant. Arch. Path. (Chicago), **26,** 873, 1938.

269. Baumer, H., and Gruber, G.: Versuche zur experimentellen Erzengung der Niemann-Pickschen Krankheit. Jahrb. Kinderheilk., **146,** 125, 1936.

270. Ferraro, A., and Jervis, G. A.: Studies in experimental lipoidoses, I. Phosphatides. Arch. Path. (Chicago), **30,** 731, 1940.

271. Gochel, A.: Das Verhalten von Sphingomyelinen im Tiorkörper. Biochem. Z., **319,** 196, 1948.

272. Matsuda, N., Oba, Y., Yonehara, Y., Hirata, S., and Shibata, S.: Reticuloendothelial foam cells mistaken for Niemann-Pick's cells in the bone marrow, due to intravenous administration of polyvinylpyrrolidone. Med. Biol. (Tokyo), **73,** 3, 120, 1966.

273. Silverstein, M. N., Ellefson, R. D., and Ahern, E. J.: The syndrome of the Sea-Blue histiocyte. New Eng. J. Med., **282,** 1, 1970.

274. Lyon, M. F., Hulse, E. V., and Rowe, C. E.: Foam-cell reticulosis of mice, an inherited condition resembling Gaucher's and Niemann-Pick disease. J. Med. Genet., **2,** 99 (1965).

275. Fredrickson, D. S., Sloan, H. R., and Hansen, C. T.: Lipid abnormalities in foam cell reticulosis of mice, an analogue of human sphingomyelin lipidosis. J. Lipid Res., **10,** 288, 1969.

276. Vandenheuvel, A.: Study of biological structure at the molecular level with stereomodel projections. I. The lipids in the myelin sheath of nerve. J. Amer. Oil Chem. Soc., **40,** 455, 1963.

CHAPTER THIRTY-SIX

RARE FAMILIAL DISEASES WITH NEUTRAL LIPID STORAGE: Wolman's Disease, Cholesteryl Ester Storage Disease, and Cerebrotendinous Xanthomatosis

Howard R. Sloan and Donald S. Fredrickson

This chapter describes three diseases that are arbitrarily bound together by the thinnest of criteria: the tissue storage of large amounts of relatively nonpolar lipids. The first two, Wolman's disease and cholesteryl ester storage disease (CESD), have in common the accumulation of cholesteryl esters. In Wolman's disease, this is a generalized phenomenon and there is prominent tissue storage of triglycerides as well. In CESD, the stockpiling of cholesteryl esters reaches massive proportions in the liver but, except possibly for the intestine and bone marrow, does not occur elsewhere to a remarkable degree. The third disorder, cerebrotendinous xanthomatosis, is quite different. Here both cholesterol and cholestanol, the latter normally present in the body in very small amounts, are stored in sites that prominently include the tendons and nervous tissue. Deficient activity of a lysosomal hydrolase has been put forward as the cause of Wolman's disease. No enzyme defect has been demonstrated in the others. All three represent interesting, rare disorders about which a great deal remains to be discovered.

WOLMAN'S DISEASE

Wolman's disease is an abnormality of lipid metabolism that usually becomes clinically evident in the first weeks of life and is characterized by gastrointestinal symptoms, failure to thrive, hepatosplenomegaly, steatorrhea, and adrenal enlargement and calcification. It is invariably fatal, usually by the age of 6 months. Nearly every organ contains many cells loaded with neutral lipids, particularly cholesteryl esters and glycerides. The underlying defect appears to be deficient activity of one or more acid hydrolases that catalyze the catabolism of these neutral lipids. The morphologic changes and histochemical reactions in affected tissues are not specific, and a diagnosis of Wolman's disease should be made from chemical and enzymatic analyses. The presence of calcified adrenals associated with tissue lipid storage is, however, highly suggestive of Wolman's disease.

Historical Aspects

In 1956 Abramov, Schorr, and Wolman described an infant with abdominal distention, hepatosplenomegaly, and massive calcification of the adrenal glands [1]. The child died following a short illness at 2 months of age. In 1965 Wolman et al. reported two more affected sibs in this same family [2]. Since that time a number of very similar patients have been reported [3–21] (Table 36-1). Wolman [2] also suggested that two further examples may have been erroneously reported as Niemann-Pick disease [22–26]. In retrospect, it seems certain that one of these, the patient described by Alexander [26] may have represented the first reported case of Wolman's disease. It is more likely that the other, a patient of Dienst and Hamperl, died of Gaucher's disease, Type 2 (see Chap. 33); this assumption is supported by the fact that a sibling of this child also appeared to die of Gaucher's disease, Type 2 [27]. Henschen also described a 7-week-old infant with "Niemann's disease" whose adrenals were extensively involved [28]. Adrenal calcification was not mentioned, but it is possible that this was another instance of Wolman's disease.

In the initial case report, Wolman [1] and his colleagues noted the accumulation of both cholesterol and triglycerides in the liver, adrenal glands, spleen, and lymph nodes. The original patient was reported as a case of "generalized xanthomatosis with calcified adrenals." Wolman later modified this name to "primary familial xanthomatosis with adrenal calcification" [3, 17]. Later Crocker et al. [4] suggested the eponym *Wolman's disease.*

In 1961 Wolman et al. demonstrated that most of the accumulated cholesterol was in the esterified form [3]. Later studies have repeatedly confirmed these observations [8, 11, 18, 19, 21, 29]. In 1969 Patrick and Lake [29, 30] demonstrated that an acid hydrolase catalyzing the hydrolysis of both cholesteryl esters and triglycerides was severely deficient in the liver and spleen of patients with Wolman's disease. It has not yet been established whether the primary inherited defect in Wolman's disease is a defect in the metabolism of glycerides, cholesteryl esters, or both of these lipid classes.

Clinical Manifestations

With only two exceptions [18, 19], all of the patients with Wolman's disease (Table 36-1) have had a remarkably similar clinical course and died in the first few months of life.

Onset

Wolman's disease usually has its onset in the first weeks of life. In most cases, the abnormality first noticed by the parents is persistent and forceful vomiting associated with

Table 36-1. PATIENTS WITH WOLMAN'S DISEASE

Patient	Reference	Race or religion	*Sibships*			*Age*		*Clinical findings*					*Confirmation of diagnosis*	
			Total live births	Number affected	Sex	Onset, weeks	Death, months	Gastro-intestinal symptoms	Hepato-spleno-megaly	Adrenal calcifi-cation	Foam cells in marrow	Vacuolated lymphocytes	Chemical analyses	Pathological examination
1	[26]	–	–	–	M	0	3	+	+	+	–	–	–	+
2	[1]	Persian-Jew	3	3	F	7	2	+	+	+	–	–	–	+
3	[2]	Persian-Jew	3	3	F	1	3	+	+	+	+	–	+	+
4	[2]	Persian-Jew	3	3	F	3	2	+	+	+	–	–	+	+
5	[4, 6]	Rumanian-Irish	3	1	F	3	4	+	+	+	+	+	+	+
6	[4]	Ger.-Eng.	3	2	M	2	4	+	+	+	+	+	–	+
7	[4]	Ger.-Eng.	3	2*	M	–	4	+	+	+	–	–	–	–
8	[4, 9]	Ger.-Ir.-Eng.	4	3	F	3	5	+	+	+	+	+	+	+
9	[9]	Ger.-Ir.-Eng.	4	3	F	–	–	–	–	+	–	+	–	–
10	[7]	Ger.-Ir.-Eng.	4	3	M	–	–	–	–	+	–	+	–	–
11	[8]	Japanese	4	3	F	<2	5	+	+	+	+	+	+	+
12	[8]	Japanese	4	3*	–	–	4	+	+	–	–	–	–	–
13	[8]	Japanese	4	3*	–	–	4	+	+	–	–	–	–	–
14	[11, 12]	Dutch	3	1	M	0	4	+	+	–	+	+	+	+
15	[13]	Iraqi-Jew	2	1	M	0	3	+	+	+	+	0	–	+
16	[15, 21]	Greek	3	1	F	0.5	3.5	+	+	+	0	+	+	+
17	[18]	Irish	2	1	F	5	4	+	+	+	+	+	+	+
18	[18]	English	3	2	M	16	14	+	+	+	+	–	+	+
19	[18, 20, 29]	English	3	2	M	52	–	+	+	–	+	–	–	+
20	[19]	Japanese	–	1	F	20	9	+	+	+	–	–	+	+

Note: + = present; 0 = absent; – = not specifically mentioned; * = anamnestic case. Ger. = German; Eng. = English; Ir. = Irish.

marked abdominal distention. Several patients have also had frequent and watery stools in the first few weeks of life [15, 18, 21]. In a few patients, jaundice [2, 4, 8] or persistent low-grade fever has been observed [2, 4].

Anemia usually appears by the sixth week of life and becomes more severe as the disease progresses; the hemoglobin may fall to 6 gm per 100 ml. Although thrombocytopenia has not been observed, vacuolization of lymphocytes has been repeatedly observed [4, 8, 9, 11, 15, 18, 21]; the vacuoles are both intracytoplasmic and intranuclear. Lipid-laden histiocytes, or foam cells, have been observed in bone marrow aspirates as early as age 40 days. The marrow almost invariably contains large numbers of foam cells in the later stages of the illness. Similar cells have been observed in the peripheral blood [2]. Acanthocytosis has been reported in one patient [19]. Plasma lipids are usually normal, although one patient had hyperlipidemia [18] and another had hypolipoproteinemia [19].

Hepatosplenomegaly has been observed as early as the fourth day of life [21]. It is a constant feature of the disease and may be of massive proportions. The degree of abdominal distention is, however, greater than that which would be expected if hepatosplenomegaly were the only cause. In one patient [13], marked abdominal distention was associated with paralytic ileus caused by fibrinous adhesions.

The most striking feature of Wolman's disease is calcification of the adrenal glands (Fig. 36-1). This abnormality has been present in every patient. It has also been consistently demonstrated antemortem by roentgenographic examination, except in the extraordinary patient reported by Marshall et al. [18]. The adrenals are markedly and symmetrically enlarged (up to 3.5 × 2.5 cm); their normal pyramidal or semilunar shape is retained. They are extensively seeded with finely stippled or punctate calcific deposits. The enlarged adrenals may somewhat flatten the superior poles of the kidneys [4]; they do not, however, deform the calyceal system or interfere with renal function.

Specific symptoms related to the central nervous system are uncommon in Wolman's disease, but neurologic development is not normal. The infants are frequently bright and alert at age 5 to 6 weeks. By age 9 weeks, however, there is usually a marked reduction of activity. It is not clear whether this is due to the development of a neurologic deficit or to the severe vomiting, diarrhea, and malabsorption that dominate the clinical picture. In several case reports, mention has been made of the fact that the optic fundi were normal and that a cherry-red spot was not present. In one patient a Babinski sign was elicited [4]. Konno et al. described a patient who had exaggerated tendon reflexes, ankle clonus, and opisthotonus [8]. Paralysis and convulsions have not been observed.

Ancillary Clinical Findings

There are no specific laboratory observations that suggest the diagnosis. Liver function tests are frequently abnormal [2, 4, 8, 18]. Laboratory studies support the clinical observations of malabsorption and malnutrition. As determined by feeding ^{131}I-triolein [19] or unlabeled fats [21], there appears to be a significant impairment of fat absorption. ACTH-

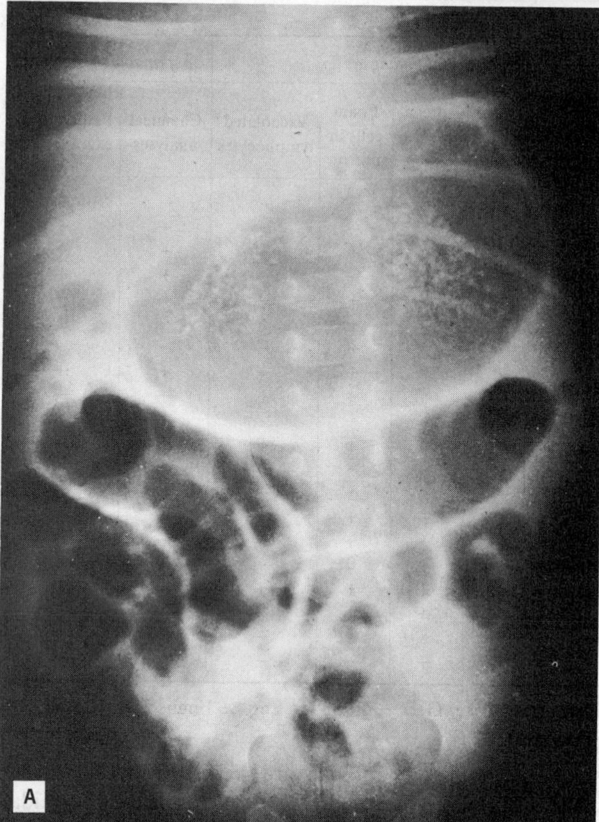

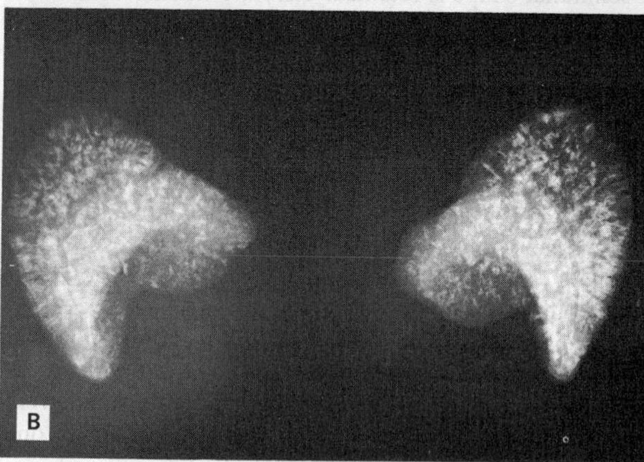

Figure 36-1. Roentgenograms showing the calcification of the enlarged adrenal glands in a patient with Wolman's disease. A. Patient in supine position. B. The adrenals after removal at autopsy. (*Photographs kindly supplied by Dr. Allen Crocker and reprinted from* [4] *with permission of the publishers.*)

stimulation studies have indicated depressed adrenal responsiveness [4, 21]. No gross abnormalities of the electroencephalogram have been observed in several patients [4, 8, 11, 19]. Chromosomal analyses in one patient were normal [8].

Course

Progressive vomiting and diarrhea, hepatosplenomegaly, abdominal distention, anemia, and inanition persist as the child's general condition progresses rapidly downhill. Death usually occurs by age 3 to 6 months.

Clinicopathological Correlations

Pathology

The Adrenal Glands

The adrenal glands are bright yellow and grossly and symmetrically enlarged; their configuration is, however, normal. Each gland may weigh as much as 13 gm compared with a normal weight of 5 gm. The adrenals are usually quite firm, contain flecks of gritty calcified tissue, and are difficult to cut. In cut section, the outer rim of cortex is intensely yellow, and the central zone is gray or white.

Under microscopic examination it can be seen that the architecture of the outer and part of the middle zone of the cortex, the zona glomerulosa, and zona fasciculata is relatively well preserved. Many of the cells, however, are swollen, vacuolated, and contain sudanophilic lipid [2,18]. The areas corresponding to the inner fasciculata and the entire zona reticularis (the innermost portion of the cortex) are replaced by a broad zone of haphazardly arranged large cells with a vacuolated, foamy cytoplasm. Many of the cells contain anisotropic crystals or large clefts in the shape of cholesterol crystals [21]. Other foam cells seem necrotic and their contents appear to have been released to form confluent lipid cysts. In the necrotic areas calcification may be quite prominent. Most of the calcium occurs in finely granular deposits, but there may be areas in which it is condensed into dense lumps [18]. There is frequently extensive fibrosis in the inner half of the cortex [2, 18]. The adrenal medulla is usually very narrow but normal in appearance.

Electron micrographs of the adrenals show that the histiocytes contain lipid in both the crystalline and droplet form [21]. In the severely affected portions of the cortex, histochemical techniques indicate the presence of large amounts of lipid with staining properties suggestive of cholesterol and triglyceride [2, 4, 13, 18, 21]. These include positive staining with oil-red-O, Sudan, and similar stains, as well as the Schultz stain for cholesterol. The histochemical findings in the large cells in the adrenal are also present in involved cells throughout other organs.

Liver

Hepatomegaly is a constant feature; the liver appears to increase in size throughout the course of the illness and by age 4 months may weigh 400 gm, or twice the normal weight [11]. The liver has a firm consistency and may be yellow.

The cut surface is yellow and greasy, and the normal hepatic pattern is replaced by a homogeneous appearance.

The normal architecture of the liver is so distorted that the portal spaces, even though infiltrated with lymphoid cells, provide the only readily recognizable landmarks [1, 2, 4, 18, 21]. The hepatic parenchymal cells are enlarged and vacuolated. Large numbers of foamy histiocytes are found in the portal and periportal areas and frequently in clusters between parenchymal cells. Grossly enlarged and vacuolated Kupffer cells are prominent. Portal and periportal fibrosis may be marked, and there may even be frank cirrhosis.

Under the electron microscope one sees that the organelles of the parenchymal cells have accumulated large osmiophilic lipid droplets. Some of these droplets are found adjacent to or apparently within lysosomes [21]. The smooth and rough endoplasmic reticulum may appear dilated and distended [21]. It is not certain from histochemical studies whether glycerides and cholesterol accumulate in both the Kupffer and the parenchymal cells [2, 4, 18, 21].

Spleen, Lymph Nodes, and Thymus

In Wolman's disease the spleen is always grossly enlarged and by age 3 months may weigh over 200 gm compared with the normal weight of 15 gm [2]. The spleen is firm, and the cut surface is red or reddish-yellow; the surface may be mottled with yellow or brown flecks. The normal follicular architecture is replaced by a homogeneous appearance. Microscopically, only a small number of follicles are present, and they are small and compressed. Most of the reticulum cells are transformed into large foam cells which make up the bulk of the organ. There is also swelling and vacuolization of the endothelial cells lining the sinusoids.

Lymph nodes throughout the body, particularly those in the mesentery, are enlarged, orange-yellow, firm, and elastic. Their cut surfaces are yellow and appear homogeneous. The microscopic and histochemical changes are quite similar to those found in the spleen. The bone marrow, thymus, and tonsils undergo changes that are almost identical to those in the spleen and lymph nodes.

Intestines

The colon is not significantly involved in the lipid storage process, although there may be some yellow zones in the mucosa. The small intestine is usually thickened and dilated, with a dull, opaque yellow serosa and a swollen yellow mucosa with thick, flattened, yellow villi. The changes are generally most marked in the proximal parts of the small intestine and least apparent in the terminal ileum. In the small intestine, and to some extent in the colon, the mucosa is infiltrated by foamy histiocytes. Some of the mucosal cells are also foamy. The infiltration of the mucosa by foam cells converts the villi into thick, club-shaped structures (Fig. 36-2). Some foam cells extend through the muscularis mucosa to form small clusters in the submucosa, and similar cells are also present in the lymphoid tissue. Some of the cells of the muscularis mucosa also stain positively for neutral lipids with Sudan stains. Sudanophilic staining may also be present in foamy endothelial cells within the intestinal adventitial layer.

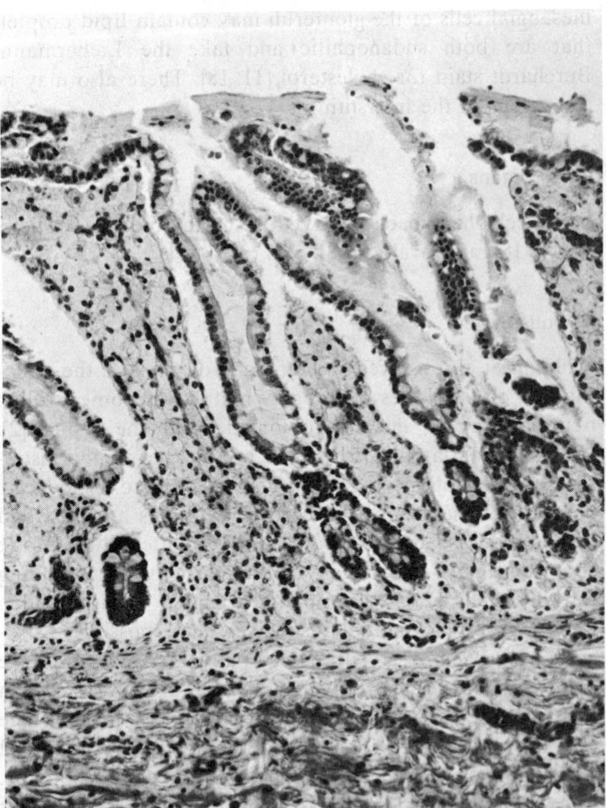

Figure 36-2. Photomicrograph of small intestine from a patient with Wolman's disease. The mucosa contains foamy histiocytes and the villi are thick and club-shaped. 160×. (*Kindly supplied by Dr. Allen Crocker.*)

Heart and Lungs

Upon gross examination the heart and lungs appear to be normal. Routine histological examination of the heart also reveals no abnormalities, but in frozen sections many sudanophilic droplets may be seen in the muscle fibers [11] and vascular endothelium [4, 11]. The lungs contain variable numbers [4, 11, 18] of foam cells in the alveoli and interstitial tissue.

Kidneys

There are no gross abnormalities in the renal parenchyma. Under the light microscope, the tubules appear normal, but mesangial cells of the glomeruli may contain lipid droplets that are both sudanophilic and take the Liebermann-Burchardt stain for cholesterol [11, 18]. There also may be foam cells in the interstitium.

Other Organs

Foam cells have been observed in the thyroid [11], testicles [4, 11, 18], and ovaries [18].

Nervous System

Wolman et al. observed sudanophilic droplets in the endothelium of capillaries of the gray matter and some swollen neurones in the medulla oblongata and the retina [2]. Crocker et al. later described the presence of foamy histiocytes in the leptomeninges [4]. They also noted a moderate decrease in the number of cortical neurones and retarded myelination. Foam cells also occur in the interstitium of the choroid plexus [8]. Lipid storage in neurons, including Purkinje cells [13], sudanophilic granules within swollen microglia, periadventitial histiocytes, and, possibly, astrocytes have been observed in some patients [13, 17, 18]. One of the most extensive studies of the central nervous system in Wolman's disease was made by Guazzi et al. [11, 12]. The autopsy was delayed for 2 days after death, however, and some of the reported changes may have been artefactual.

Kamoshita and Landing [14] first made the important observation that ganglion cells of both Auerbach's and Meissner's plexuses were packed with sudanophilic granules. These changes were found in the stomach, duodenum, and small intestine and have been repeatedly confirmed [11–13, 17, 18]. The storage of sudanophilic lipids in the sympathetic chain neurones has also been observed in one patient [13].

Lipid Abnormalities in Wolman's Disease

Organs outside the Central Nervous System

Chemical analyses of tissues from patients with Wolman's disease are shown in Table 36-2. An increase in the glyceride and cholesteryl ester content of an organ such as liver, spleen, or lymph node is the primary basis for the chemical diagnosis of Wolman's disease.

Glyceride Content

The triglyceride content of the liver may be 3 to 10 times the normal value. In the spleen, the triglycerides may be elevated from 8- to 100-fold. The triglyceride content of the adrenals has been reported in only one case [21] and was one-half the normal value. The concentrations of mono- and diglycerides were elevated five- to fifteenfold in the liver and spleen of the two patients in which they were measured [8, 21]; they were modestly, if at all, elevated in the adrenals of one patient [21].

The fatty acid composition of hepatic [8, 19] and splenic

Table 36-2. TISSUE LIPID CONCENTRATIONS IN WOLMAN'S DISEASE

Reference	Age, months	*Liver, mg/gm wet weight*				*Spleen, mg/gm wet weight*				*Adrenals, mg/gm wet weight*			
		TC	FC	CE	TG	TC	FC	CE	TG	TC	FC	CE	TG
[29]	?	170	9	161	61								
[29]	?	56	5	51	72								
[29]	?					35	8	27	99				
[8]	5	97	38	59	137	26	10	16	8				
[19]	9	13	6	7	208	8	4	4	29				
[11]	4	84	6	78	154								
[18]	4	21	2	19									
[18]	14	23	2	21									
[2]	3	65				37							
[2]	2	95				31				184			
[4]	4	46				18							
[4]	5	65				22							
[21]	4	49	23	26		20	5	15	9	185	15	170	23
Upper limits of normal [21, 31–33]		5*	4*	1*	20*	5†	4†	1†	<1†	33‡	10‡	23‡	41‡

* [31]
† [32, 33]
‡ [21]
Note: TC = total cholesterol; FC = free cholesterol; CE = cholesteryl esters; TG = triglycerides.

[8] triglycerides has been determined. The only striking observation was that linoleic acid could not be detected in splenic triglycerides.

Cholesteryl Ester Content

The total cholesterol concentration of liver, spleen, and adrenals has been elevated in every case of Wolman's disease (Table 36-2). Although the free cholesterol concentration has frequently been greater than normal, the bulk of the increase in total cholesterol is due to the accumulation of cholesteryl esters. The cholesteryl ester content of the liver may be 7 to 160 times the normal value; it was shown in one case [21] that cholesteryl esters were elevated eightfold in the adrenals.

The fatty acid composition of hepatic [8, 19] and splenic [8] cholesteryl esters has also been determined. Konno et al. [8] observed no alterations in the fatty acid content of hepatic cholesteryl esters. In the spleen there was a notable absence of linoleic acid in cholesteryl esters and an increase in palmitic acid content compared to the esters in the liver. Eto and Kitagawa [19] observed a marked increase in polyunsaturated 20-carbon fatty acids associated with a decreased content of oleic acid.

Other Lipids

The phospholipid and glycolipid contents of the liver and spleen are not remarkable. The free fatty acid content of the liver may be 9 to 16 times normal and that of the spleen may be 3 to 8 times the normal value [8, 29].

Lipid Content of the Nervous System

No consistent abnormalities have been detected in the neutral lipids, phospholipids, or glycolipids of the nervous system. The cholesterol and triglyceride concentrations of the brain have been found to be somewhat higher than normal in some patients [4, 18] and normal in others [11, 19]. There has been, however, no clear-cut increase in the concentration of any specific lipid class.

Plasma Lipids and Lipoproteins

Plasma cholesterol and triglyceride levels have been normal in most patients [2, 4, 8, 11, 13, 19, 21]. Marshall, however, described two patients with elevated triglycerides [18]. Triglycerides were directly determined in only one of these children. Marshall et al. showed that this patient had elevated serum levels of pre-β (very low density) lipoprotein [18]. The lipid composition of the plasma was consistent with Type IV hyperlipoproteinemia (Chap. 28). This pattern is nonspecific and is found as a secondary abnormality in individuals with many different disorders (Chap. 28). Eto and Kitagawa described one patient with low levels of both α- and β-lipoproteins and a somewhat depressed serum cholesterol level [19].

Cholesteryl Ester Metabolism

The reader is referred to excellent recent reviews of cholesterol [34–38] and cholesteryl ester [39–40] metabolism as a prelude to a brief summation of the biochemistry relevant to Wolman's disease and cholesteryl ester storage disease.

Cholesterol

Cholesterol (Δ_5-3β-cholesterol) is synthesized in practically all tissues of the body. The great bulk, however, is contributed by two organs, liver and intestine. The degradation of cholesterol involves alteration in both its side chain and ring structure. The major pathway of catabolism, conversion to bile acids, is limited to the liver.

Cholesteryl Esters

Esterified cholesterol may be derived from three major sources. An important contribution comes from the intestine in chylomicrons during the absorption of fat. This cholesterol is derived from the diet and from endogenous sterol coming from the bile, desquamated intestinal cells, and other secretions into the intestinal lumen. During digestion, cholesterol is converted to the free alcohol by action of pancreatic cholesteryl esterase. The cholesterol is then taken up into the intestinal mucosal cell where most of it is esterified and secreted into the lymph in chylomicrons and very low density lipoproteins (VLDL) (see Chap. 26). Upon entry into plasma, the cholesteryl esters are removed by many tissues, particularly the liver [39, 41]. All tissues receiving such cholesteryl esters appear to be capable of hydrolyzing them to cholesterol and fatty acid [39, 42]. It is known that in the liver uptake is not dependent upon hydrolysis [39].

In tissues, hydrolysis is catalyzed by cholesteryl ester hydrolase(s) that are found mainly in the supernatant fraction and usually have an acid pH optimum [39, 40]. Among tissues in which such hydrolytic activity has specifically been detected are liver, intestine, adrenal, spleen, kidney, muscle, lung, brain, pancreas, adipose tissue, and aorta [39, 40, 42]. The hydrolase in liver has been shown to act more rapidly upon the esters having a 9-*cis* unsaturated acyl group, a preference in keeping with the large amount of oleate and linoleate in plasma and tissue cholesteryl esters [43].

A second source of tissue cholesteryl esters is *in situ* esterification of cholesterol with a fatty acid. The cholesterol esterases that break down esters may also reversibly catalyze their synthesis, apparently without energy requirement. In certain tissues, however, there are more specific cholesterol esterifying enzymes. In the liver, and probably the adrenal, ester formation is mainly catalyzed by an acyl CoA cholesterol-O-acyl transferase that requires ATP [39, 40]. In the liver, transferase activity is exclusively particulate [39]. The pH optimum lies above 6.5, and the enzyme is markedly inhibited by fatty acids and conjugated bile acids.

A third major source of cholesteryl esters is limited to plasma. Here esterification is catalyzed mainly by lecithin-cholesterol acyl transferase (LCAT) (see Chap. 27). LCAT is believed to work in concert with plasma high density lipoproteins (HDL) to maintain stability of very low density lipoproteins as they are degraded and removed and, possibly, to mobilize cholesterol from tissues and transport it to the liver via high density lipoproteins for degradation. LCAT activity is apparently responsible for maintaining the balance between esterified and unesterified cholesterol in plasma.

The bulk of cholesterol in most tissues is unesterified. Only in the adrenals, as in the plasma, is most of the cholesterol esterified. There is very limited exchange of cholesteryl esters between plasma, red cells, and other tissues, and between different lipoprotein families, in contrast to the rapid equilibration of free cholesterol between plasma, red cells, and various extravascular pools. There is little evidence of direct uptake of cholesteryl esters by tissues, and the extent to which it occurs is not known. Normally, some esters in chylomicrons may be taken up by reticuloendothelial cells. On the other hand, the intestinal mucosa, for example, appears unable to take up cholesteryl esters; it is believed that only the free sterol is accepted across the boundary of these cells [39].

There is also inadequate knowledge to answer the corollary question of whether cholesteryl esters can pass from cells into extracellular fluid. Abnormal accumulation of cholesteryl esters is a characteristic of atheromas and probably also occurs in granulomas and other chronic lesions. Such progressive enrichment suggests that these lipids are among the most difficult for the cell to remove.

In summation, it appears most likely that in tissues other than liver, and perhaps the adrenal, cholesteryl esters arise mainly from intracellular esterification of cholesterol that has either been synthesized in the cell or has arrived there from plasma. Most cells contain cholesterol "esterases" or hydrolases that can hydrolyze esters, or acting reversibly, catalyze esterification. It is possible that the degradation of esterified cholesterol requires that it first be hydrolyzed to free cholesterol and then transported through the plasma to the liver, which has the sole capacity for conversion of cholesterol to bile acids. These acids, along with large quantities of cholesterol (all unesterified), are secreted in the bile.

Normally about 20 percent of cholesterol in liver is esterified. It is not known why esterification of the molecule is important in that organ [39]. It could be for purposes of storage prior to oxidation of the sterol to form bile acids. Conceivably, esterification might even be a facultative step in such a conversion. Cholesteryl esters are also important in the structure of plasma lipoproteins (Chap. 26), which the liver secretes. Esters probably also play some structural role in other cellular components involving lipid-protein interactions.

It is easy to surmise how failure of the capacity for hydrolysis of cholesteryl esters could seriously disturb the intracellular content of cholesterol. It is much less simple to determine both whether such failure is, in fact, responsible for cholesteryl ester storage when it occurs and the precise nature of metabolic disturbances that may attend upon such massive lipid accumulation.

Triglyceride Metabolism

The reader is referred to extensive reviews of triglyceride metabolism [44, 45] and to the discussion in Chap. 28. The action of pancreatic lipase and bile acids converts dietary triglycerides into monoglycerides and fatty acids which enter the intestinal mucosal cell and are immediately reesterified to triglycerides. The intestinal mucosal cells combine this triglyceride with cholesterol, phospholipid, and protein to form chylomicrons. The chylomicrons move out into the lymph channels and eventually enter the plasma via the thoracic duct (see Chap. 28 for a detailed description of triglyceride transport).

Chylomicrons are rapidly removed from the plasma. Recent experiments suggest that the first step in chylomicron metabolism occurs in extrahepatic tissue, particularly fat and muscle. Here most of the triglyceride is hydrolyzed by lipoprotein lipase (Chap. 28) to fatty acids that enter the tissue cells [46]. Removal of the triglycerides produces "remnants" rich in cholesteryl esters. These "remnants" contain small amounts of the triglyceride originally present in the chylomicrons and proceed to the liver for clearance [46]. The fatty acids that enter tissues are mainly incorporated into either triglycerides or other esterified lipids. It is not clear whether this reesterification occurs in the capillary endothelial cells or within parenchymal cells. Some of the fatty acids are completely metabolized to carbon dioxide.

Tissue triglyceride may arise not only from the diet but also from endogenous, or *de novo*, synthesis. The major pathway for the disposal of liver triglycerides appears to be their secretion into the plasma as constituents of very low density lipoproteins [44]. The sites and mechanisms for removal of VLDL triglyceride are likely similar to those involved in chylomicron glyceride metabolism, but this has not been well established [47].

The first step in tissue utilization of triglycerides for either energy production or biosynthetic processes is undoubtedly the removal of the fatty acid moieties. This hydrolysis *in situ* appears to be catalyzed by hydrolases other than lipoprotein lipase. It has been well documented that adipose tissue contains another "hormone-sensitive" triglyceride lipase [48–51] and that liver also contains a triglyceride lipase that is distinct from lipoprotein lipase [52]. Triglyceride lipases, definitely distinct from lipoprotein lipase, have not been adequately demonstrated in most other tissues.

Mahadevan and Tappel have demonstrated, however, the presence of acid lipases, active against triglycerides, in rat liver and kidney lysosomes [52*a*]. These lipases may account for the lipolysis of triglycerides entering lysosomes. The role of these enzymes in cellular physiology is unknown.

The Metabolic Defect in Wolman's Disease

The significant biochemical feature of Wolman's disease is the accumulation of both cholesteryl esters and triglycerides in many organs. The tissue concentrations of diglycerides, monoglycerides, and free fatty acids are also usually elevated. The lipids seem to collect in progressively increasing quantities. It is uncertain whether one lipid class may accumulate first, and others secondarily. Wolman [1, 13, 17] believes that the accumulation of triglyceride is of primary pathogenic importance and that the accumulations of cholesterol, cholesteryl esters, and free fatty acids are secondary phenomena. Crocker et al. [4] and Lough et al. [21] believe that storage of cholesteryl ester is the primary pathological process. Lough et al. [21] note that in the adrenal gland, an organ that is markedly affected in the disease, there is a striking accumulation of cholesteryl ester, but not of triglyceride (Table 36-2). Although their observation would strongly suggest the prominence of abnormal cholesterol metabolism in the pathogenesis, it is interesting that this is the only case report of adrenal lipid content in Wolman's disease. In most patients there seems to be an abnormality of both cholesteryl ester and triglyceride metabolism, and the work of Patrick and Lake [20, 29, 30] that will be cited later supports this possibility.

A key question is whether there is an increased synthesis of cholesteryl ester and triglyceride or whether these compounds accumulate because of a block in a normal pathway for their catabolism.

Possible Increased Synthesis of Cholesteryl Esters and Triglycerides

Sloviter et al. [7] have observed that red blood cell preparations from an infant with Wolman's disease incorporated ^{14}C-glycerol into triglyceride and ^{14}C-mevalonate into cholesterol and cholesteryl ester more rapidly than did those from control infants. Much more cholesteryl ester was formed than cholesterol. These experiments indicate an increase in the net synthesis of these lipids, but they did not provide any information about the rates of catabolism; a decreased rate of lipid degradation could also explain the results.

Possible Elaboration of Abnormal Lipids

The studies of Konno [8] and Eto [19] indicate that the fatty acid composition of the cholesteryl ester and triglyceride stored in Wolman's disease differs only slightly from that in normal tissue. Rosowsky et al. [6] employed gas chromatography to demonstrate that the sterol that accumulates is indeed cholesterol (Δ_5-3β-cholesterol) and that no significant amounts of any other sterol are present; Eto et al. have confirmed this result [19]. Konno [8] and Eto [19] have shown that the infrared spectrum of the cholesteryl ester that accumulates is quite similar to that of cholesteryl palmitate. Eto [19] has made a similar observation with respect to the stored triglyceride.

Acid Lipase Deficiency in Wolman's Disease

Patrick and Lake have demonstrated a total deficiency of acid lipase activity directed toward the hydrolysis of triglycerides and cholesteryl ester in the livers of two patients and the spleen of one patient [29, 30]. These patients had the characteristic lipid accumulation in tissues, but one had a quite atypical clinical course [18]. They suggest that the same enzyme may act on both lipid classes, but adequate attempts have not yet been made to separate or purify the enzymatic activities. No correction was made for dilution of substrate by the large amounts of endogenous substrate present in the tissues in Wolman's disease, and the possible presence of inhibitors was not excluded by experiments employing mixtures of control and affected tissue.

Lake and Patrick have further characterized the acid lipase deficiency in Wolman's disease by a histochemical technique [20]. Normal liver contains an acid lipase that hydrolyzes the artificial substrates, α-naphthyl-acetate and α-naphthyl-butyrate. In normal liver, this enzymatic activity is only partially inhibited by diethyl-*p*-nitrophenyl phosphate (E600). In liver in Wolman's disease, there is complete inhibition of residual acid lipase by E600. There is therefore either a deficiency of E600-resistant acid esterase in Wolman's disease, or the acid lipase that is present is abnormally sensitive to this inhibitor.

Pathophysiology

It now seems probable that the disease arises because the normal catabolism of cholesteryl ester and triglycerides is blocked at the step at which fatty acids are cleaved from the molecules. As a result, cholesteryl esters and triglycerides accumulate in many cells throughout the body. The consequences of such a metabolic block are not understood, and the lipid storage does not provide obvious explanations for all of the functional abnormalities.

The affected cells become filled with secondary lysosomes [53] recognizable by their morphology and the increased activity of various nonspecific acid hydrolases. Lake and Patrick [20] have shown by electron microscopy that, in the liver, lipid droplets are enclosed by a limiting membrane associated with acid phosphatase activity, a characteristic lysosomal enzyme. Lough et al. have made similar observations [21].

The lipid storage process apparently begins *in utero* and progresses steadily until the death of the patient. Hepatomegaly and adrenal calcification have been noted as early as the fifth day of life [21]. The pervasive nature of organ involvement in Wolman's disease and the fact that serum lipid levels are usually normal suggest that much of the lipid accumulation comes locally from the turnover of elements of the cells themselves. There is no clear explanation of why some organs, and particularly the adrenal glands, accumulate such large quantities of cholesteryl ester and triglycerides. Lough et al. suggest that lipids accumulate primarily in tissues that normally synthesize the largest amount of cholesteryl esters [21].

The striking involvement of the adrenal glands is possibly related to a normal involutionary process in these organs which takes place in infancy. Immediately after birth, dilated vascular channels, engorged with erythrocytes, appear in the wide fetal zone [54]. Within a few days, the cells of the fetal cortex degenerate and become necrotic; vascular engorgement may even take on the appearance of hemorrhage. By the fourth month of life, the fetal zone is 90 percent atrophic. Transient adrenal calcification is not rare in infants and may occur in the absence of obvious disease [55]. Konno et al. have suggested that adrenal calcification in Wolman's disease is a manifestation of an impairment of this process [8]. A probable cause of calcification is the precipitation of calcium soaps from free fatty acids released by the partial degradation of glycerides. Crocker et al. [4] and Abramov et al. [1] have drawn an analogy between the association of cholesterol deposition, necrosis, and calcification found in Wolman's disease with that also found in atheromas and sites of hemorrhage.

The persistent malabsorption that characterizes Wolman's disease is probably due to the structural distortions in the small intestine. Wolman has observed severe xanthomatous change in the neurons of a ganglion of the sympathetic chain in one patient and has suggested that the persistent abdominal distention may reflect disturbance in sympathetic tone in abdominal viscera [13, 17].

Why Other Lipids Accumulate

It is characteristic of storage diseases that more than one chemical constituent accumulates in the affected tissues. Patrick and Lake [29, 30] suggest that one lysosomal enzyme catalyzes the cleavage of both cholesteryl esters and triglycerides. It is possible that several enzymes are involved and that they are controlled by a single operon under faulty regulation, if an analogy may be drawn to bacterial genetics. These theories can be better tested when the metabolic role of acid hydrolases in the catabolism of cholesteryl esters and triglycerides is understood. It must be noted, however, that deficient hydrolase activity does not explain the accumulation of free fatty acids and free cholesterol that is occasionally found in Wolman's disease.

Diagnosis

Wolman's disease must be considered in any infant with hepatosplenomegaly, gastrointestinal symptoms, and failure to thrive. The earliest examination should include careful attention to neurological development. X-rays should be taken of the lungs and bones, and of the abdomen to observe the calcification of the adrenals that is almost invariably present.

Calcification of the adrenals may be observed in many other conditions such as Addison's disease [55], adrenal teratomas [55], hemorrhage [1, 15, 18], neuroblastoma, ganglioneuroma, adrenal cysts, cortical carcinoma, and pheochromocytoma [1, 15]. The presence of bilateral adrenal calcifications associated with hepatosplenomegaly and gastrointestinal symptoms strongly supports the diagnosis of Wolman's disease. It is noteworthy that in Niemann-Pick disease, type A, which sometimes resembles Wolman's disease, no adrenal calcification has ever been seen [5]. The decreased adrenal responsiveness that has been observed in some cases of Wolman's disease must be differentiated from the syndrome of familial leukodystrophy, adrenal insufficiency, and cutaneous melanosis [56]. The latter syndrome has a more protracted course, definite signs of central nervous system involvement, and the general clinical course is not easily confused with Wolman's disease.

The peripheral smear should be checked for vacuolization of lymphocytes. A bone marrow aspirate should then be obtained and unstained specimens examined by routine microscopy. Although no laboratory tests are diagnostic of Wolman's disease, liver function tests and a hemogram should be obtained.

Open biopsy of the liver is desirable for definitive diagnosis. The 1.0 to 1.5 gm of liver should immediately be subdivided for pathological, chemical, and enzymatic studies and processed as described in Chaps. 29, 33, and 35. A minimal lipid analysis of the liver includes the determination of cholesterol, cholesteryl ester, triglyceride, and phospholipid concentrations. Evaluation of acid lipase activities should also be obtained if possible.

Treatment

Many medications have been tried without success in the treatment of Wolman's disease. Antibiotics, cholestyramine [4], adrenal steroids [2, 4, 8, 15, 21], *d*-thyroxine [4], cyclophosphamide, and clofibrate [18] have not altered the progressive downhill course of the disease and treatment is entirely supportive.

Genetics

In the original family reported by Wolman and his colleagues [1, 2] three female infants died of the disease. Since that time, the disease has been observed in males and females with approximately equal frequency (Table 36-1). This, combined with the repeated occurrence in siblings with unaffected parents (Table 36-1), suggests that the mode of inheritance is probably autosomal recessive. Parental consanguinity has been noted only in the original family reported by Wolman [1, 2] and was specifically denied in several other cases [4, 11–13, 15, 18, 19, 21].

Heterozygote Detection

A technique for the detection of heterozygotes in the general population has not been developed. Spiegel-Adolf et al. [9] have observed vacuolized lymphocytes in the peripheral blood of parents, grandparents, and a sibling of three patients with Wolman's disease. The absence of vacuolized lymphocytes in the peripheral blood of one patient [13] and their presence in Niemann-Pick disease [9] suggest that this method is not sufficiently specific for use in the detection of heterozygotes.

CHOLESTERYL ESTER STORAGE DISEASE

Synonyms for this disease are *hepatic cholesteryl ester storage disease* and *polycorie cholestérolique.*

Cholesteryl ester storage disease (CESD) is a rare familial disease in which the liver is enlarged and contains a great excess of cholesteryl esters. Lipid also may accumulate in the lamina propria of the intestine, including the endothelial cells of the lacteals and vascular pericytes, and within bone marrow macrophages. Disability is minimal and life is not necessarily limited. The metabolic defect is not known.

History

Brief published mention of this disease was first made by Fredrickson in 1966 in reference to a child with marked hyperlipidemia, whose enlarged liver was found to contain 18 percent of its wet weight as cholesteryl esters. He called the disorder *hepatic cholesterol ester storage disease* [57, 58]. A detailed description of this patient, whose twin was also apparently affected, appears in this chapter. In 1967, Lageron et al. [59, 60] reported a 43-year-old man with apparently the same disease under the name *polycorie cholestérolique de l'adulte.* He had been known to have had hepatomegaly since age 14. At about the same time Schiff et al. reported a brother and sister with similar clinical, morphologic, and biochemical abnormalities [61]. Like the first patient, but in contrast to the second, the patients of Schiff et al. also had hyperlipidemia. Four of their five younger siblings also had hepatomegaly. Biopsy specimens of liver from three of these were interpreted as showing minimal morphologic abnormalities, suggesting a milder expression of the same inherited defect. These authors pointed out the presence of minimal cirrhosis in the liver in addition to the fat loading of all hepatocytes seen in the other cases. They also noted elevation of serum bile acids and a disproportion among the several bile acids present.

The following year Partin and Schubert [62] described detailed studies of jejunal and duodenal biopsy specimens in the two most severely affected children of the kindred of Schiff et al. [61]. The evidence they present of cholesterol storage in the intestine indicates that involvement in CESD extends beyond the liver. It is therefore suggested that the term *cholesterol* (or *cholesteryl*) *ester storage disease* used by Partin and Schubert is a more accurate name for the disorder until the responsible biochemical defect is uncovered.

It is possible that the three families thus far known to be affected are not representative of the same disease. It may also be that other reports of "fatty liver" or "congenital steatosis" in the older literature might include examples of CESD. In the main, however, these reports refer to glycogen storage disease with hepatic accumulation of both glycogen and glycerides (but not cholesteryl esters) [63–65].

Clinical Features

The history of the patient L.Mc. referred to by Fredrickson [58, 66] and of her twin sister, the latter providing the only autopsy report of a case of CESD, is as follows.

Patient L.Mc. (NIH 03-51-16) and a twin sister were the third and fourth children born to a woman, age 27, and her husband, age 25. The earlier born children, a brother and sister, now 23 and 29 years of age, were apparently normal. The gestation of the twins was considered normal and was terminated by induction at 8 months.

The twin sister (Patient 2, Table 36-3) weighed 3 lb 9 oz at birth. She expired of "respiratory distress" at the age of 24 days. At autopsy the body weighed 4 lb. The abdomen was distended and contained about 50 ml of yellow serous fluid. The spleen weighed 9 gm; the liver weighed 93 gm and was reported as "rather large and pale" and "tan or buff in color." The bile ducts were patent. The heart weighed 25 gm and the foramen ovale was open, but there were no congenital anomalies. The remainder of the gross examination was negative. The lungs were atelectatic. The cytoplasm of the hepatic cells was pale and granular and filled with fat vacuoles which were small to moderate in size. Microscopic examination of the thymus, spleen, kidneys, and adrenals was not remarkable.

The sib, L.Mc. (Patient 1, Table 36-3), remained in the hospital for 39 days and was discharged at 5 lb 4-½ oz in apparently good condition. At 16 months of age she was hospitalized for bronchopneumonia and "iron deficiency anemia." At 3 years of age she had a single episode of gross hematuria and at age 4 began to have recurrent epistaxes which continued for the next 10 to 11 years. Her appetite was considered poor from the postnatal period until her hospitalization for examination at the age of 8. A Grade II murmur at the base was heard and the liver was felt 6 cm below the right costal margin. The spleen was not palpable. There were several telangiectatic lesions—adjudged not to be spider angiomas—on the trunk. There was a slight microcytic, hypochromic anemia; platelets and coagulation studies were entirely normal. Alkaline phosphatase, thymol turbidity, cephalin flocculation and BSP were normal. The plasma cholesterol was 400 mg per 100 ml, 70 percent of which was esterified. Foam cells were seen in the marrow. A liver biopsy revealed an "enlarged, yellow and fibrotic appearing liver." Microscopic examination was interpreted as "fatty hepatosis"; no chemical analyses were made on the specimen.

By age 11 she weighed only 48 lb, had little appetite and her murmur and hepatic enlargement both seemed more prominent. She had moist rales at both bases and was digitalized and placed on strict bed rest for 3 months before she was admitted to the Clinical Center for the first time in April 1961.

At this time she was 49 in. tall and weighed 22 kg. The blood pressure was normal. A single telangiectatic lesion was present on an arm. The pharyngeal mucosa and tonsils appeared normal and there was no significant lymphadenopathy. Examination of the heart was consistent with aortic stenosis. The liver was nontender and a smooth edge was palpable 6 cm down from the costal margin. The spleen tip was palpable. The remaining examination, including a careful neurological survey, was within normal limits.

Urinalyses, hemograms, coagulation time, liver function tests, and 24-hr excretion of normetanephrine were normal. Plasma total cholesterol was 420, esterified cholesterol 275, and triglycerides 150 mg per 100 ml; postabsorptive free fatty acid concentrations were 0.5, 0.23, and 0.32 mEq per liter; and postheparin lipolytic activity was normal. Skull and other skeletal x-rays were negative.

Cardiac catheterization confirmed the diagnosis of aortic stenosis, probably congenital, with an aortic valve gradient of approximately 50 mm Hg. A bone marrow smear contained a few "foam cells" having irregular boundaries, eccentric, densely staining nuclei, and abundant cytoplasm containing doubly refractile droplets. Laparotomy was performed, at which the liver was markedly enlarged and had an extraordinary butter-yellow color. The chemical analyses of hepatic tissue are shown in Table 36-6, and the histological findings are summarized in the text. The liver content of glycogen, phosphorylase, and glucose-6-phosphatase activities were normal (H. Williams).

Skin and muscle biopsies were judged to be normal histologically, with the possible exception of oil-red-O positive droplets visible in the endothelium of arterioles seen in the muscle preparation.

In 1965, at age 15, she underwent successful correction of congenital supravalvular aortic stenosis (A. G. Morrow). Specimens of the aortic wall, left ventricular wall, thymus, and skin were carefully examined in frozen sections. Small amounts of oil-red-O staining material were present in the thymus, but less than that seen in Tangier disease (Chap. 26), for example. L.Mc. developed jaundice after the open-heart surgery, but recovered uneventfully.

She is now 22 and doing well. Her activity has been voluntarily restricted for 2 years, and she has been digitalized for vague attacks of breathlessness. Her stature is small but is similar to that of her mother, and her intelligence is normal.

In Table 36-3 are summarized some details concerning the five patients, four of them alive, who are here tentatively classified as having cholesteryl ester storage disease. If we assume that Patient 2 had the disease, it may be concluded that the abnormalities in the liver are obvious at birth. The principal and sometimes only sign, hepatomegaly, may be detected in early childhood and apparently becomes progressively greater with time. The spleen may be moderately enlarged but is not always palpable. Portal hypertension has not been obvious, although Patient 4 (Table 36-3) had esophageal varices visible by x-ray. Jaundice is not part of the disease, and liver function, as judged by conventional tests, is not obviously compromised. Gallstones were specifically not seen in direct examination of Patient 4 [61] or in cholecystograms of Patient 1. Perhaps significant is a possibly delayed puberty in 15-year-old male Patient 4. Patient 1 had recurrent epistaxes for years that were not obviously linked either to a few telangiectatic lesions seen on the skin or to

Table 36-3. PATIENTS WITH CHOLESTERYL ESTER STORAGE DISEASE

Patient	Initials	Reference	Sex	Age, years: Detection	Age, years: First biopsy	Hepatomegaly	Splenomegaly	Intestinal involvement
1	L. Mc.	[58, 66]	F	3	3	+	0	+
2	Mc.	[66]	F	1/12	1/12	+	+	−
3	Lem	[59, 60]	M	14	35	+	0	−
4	T. H.	[61, 62]	M	15	15	+	+	+
5	W. H. T.	[61, 62]	F	19	19	+	0	−

Note: + = present; 0 = absent; − = unknown.

her congenital heart disease. Patient 3 (Table 36-3) had severe rectal bleeding apparently due to benign rectal polyps. There is no obvious malabsorption or malnutrition, and no neurological abnormalities.

Clinical Laboratory Tests

Exclusive of the plasma lipids, there are no other definite abnormalities in routine laboratory tests. Patient 3 is said to have had an indirect bilirubin of 6 mg but no jaundice [59]. The hemogram and plasma protein electrophoresis are normal.

Several bone marrow aspirates in Patient 1 contained numerous large macrophages filled with droplets [66]. The only other recorded bone marrow examination, made in Patient 4, was normal [61].

Bile and Bile Acids

These have been examined only in Patients 4 and 5 and their relatives in the H. family of Schiff et al. [61]. Serum bile acids were quantified by gas chromatography in the patients, their five siblings, both parents, and an uncle and grandfather. The total bile acids were grossly elevated in Patient 4, probably normal in Patient 5, and elevated in all but three of the other relatives. The increased total bile acids reflected increases of deoxycholic, chenodeoxycholic, and cholic acids, but there appeared to be a disproportionate increase in chenodeoxycholic acid.

Bile was obtained from Patient 4 by both duodenal drainage and directly from the gall bladder. In both specimens the ratio of cholic acid to chenodeoxycholic acid was low. The total cholesterol content of bile was 0.17 mg per ml (normal 0.1 to 13 mg per ml) [61].

Plasma Lipids and Lipoproteins

Plasma lipids in the four living patients are shown in Table 36-4. The three younger ones clearly have hyperlipidemia, the cholesterol, phospholipids, and glycerides all being above the upper 5 percent of the population distribution for their ages. A normal proportion of the plasma cholesterol is esterified. In Patient 1 the lipoprotein pattern has repeatedly been consistent with Type II*b* (Chap. 28), or that characterized by a marked increase in low density lipoproteins (LDL) with some accompanying increase in very low density or pre-β-lipoproteins (Table 36-5). In qualitative terms, the electrophoretic patterns reported for Patients 4 and 5 are quite similar.

The LDL concentrations in Patient 1, expressed as cholesterol, have repeatedly been around 330 mg per 100 ml, somewhat above the average concentration of LDL seen in heterozygotes for familial Type II hyperlipoproteinemia. Neither of her parents, however, have a definite elevation of LDL (Table 36-5), a necessary genetic criterion for this condition (Chap. 28). The mother has hyperglyceridemia. The lipoprotein pattern in CESD should not yet be consigned to any of the major "types." The plasma phospholipids seem too high for conventional hyperbetalipoproteinemia and the high-density lipoproteins somewhat too low. Patient 1, for example, has had HDL concentrations in terms of cholesterol of 6, 17, 21, and 27 mg per 100 ml on different occasions (lower limits of normal, 35 mg per 100 ml) [66]. These are unusually low for familial Type II hyperlipoproteinemia and too high for Tangier disease (Chap. 26). Immunochemical tests indicate that HDL cross-reacting with antisera to normal HDL is present. The lipoproteins in CESD have not yet been characterized sufficiently well to exclude all significant abnormality.

Table 36-4. PLASMA LIPIDS IN CHOLESTERYL ESTER STORAGE DISEASE

Patient*	Reference	Age, years	TC	FC	PL	TG
			mg per 100 ml			
1	[66]	15	402	130	436	342
4	[61]	15	276	55	403	192
5	[61]	19	356	125	554	413
Normal limits†		1–19	120–230	...	155–265	10–140
3	[59–60]	35	270	...	220	140
Normal limits†		30–39	140–270	...	205–340	10–150

* As in Table 36-3.

† See Chap. 26, Table 26-10.

Note: TC = total cholesterol; FC = free cholesterol; PL = phospholipids; TG = triglycerides.

Pathology

Liver

The liver in CESD has an extraordinary orange or butter-yellow appearance. This has been viewed directly upon laparotomy in Patients 1, 2, 3, and 4 and in needle biopsy from Patient 5. The liver is smooth and soft in texture. With the light microscope, one views three major abnormalities: (1) Lipid droplets in all hepatic parenchymal cells which give the cytoplasm a lacework pattern. The vacuoles are of

Table 36-5. PLASMA LIPIDS AND LIPOPROTEINS IN Mc. KINDRED WITH CHOLESTERYL ESTER STORAGE DISEASE

Subject	Age when sampled	Cholesterol, mg per 100 ml				Triglycerides
		Total	VLDL	LDL	HDL	
Patient 1*	15	412	62	333	17	413
		378	30	327	21	293
		398	40	331	27	354
Brother	13	190	...	...	45	48
Upper limits of normal	1–19	230	25	170	70	140
Father	41	250	20	184	46	99
Mother	40	237	...	...	52	233
Upper limits of normal	40–49	310	35	190	80	160

* Repeated samples obtained several weeks apart in Patient 1 (Table 36-3) [66].
Note: VLDL = very low density lipoproteins; LDL = low density lipoproteins; HDL = high density lipoproteins.

different sizes and do not usually displace the nuclei. (2) A variable amount of septal fibrosis, considered to be early cirrhosis in the H. family (Patients 4 and 5) [61]. (3) A number of lymphocytes and some foamy macrophages in the portal areas, the latter presumably representing lipid-laden Kupffer cells.

The histological examination of liver has revealed similar findings in Patient 1 (as determined by P. T. Westlake and S. Spicer) [66], and Patients 3 [59], 4, and 5 [61]. Both frozen and paraffin-fixed tissues stained with hematoxylin and eosin give the appearance of nearly complete replacement of hepatocyte cytoplasm by droplets in the case of frozen sections or by vacuoles after paraffin-fixation.

In *frozen* sections, all cells stain intensely with the neutral lipid stains, oil-red-O, Sudan III, or Sudan Black; the Schultz stain for cholesterol or its esters is strongly positive at the edges of the hepatic cells, in small aggregates within some cells, and in the portal or septal areas. A comparison of the intensity of staining of hepatic cells by oil-red-O in CESD and in Niemann-Pick disease is shown in Fig. 36-3. The Baker hematoxylin (phospholipids) and dithioxamide (copper) stains are negative. The periodic acid–Schiff stain (vic-glycols) may be negative [66] or positive [59], the latter perhaps indicating some increase in glycogen. Nile blue stains the hepatocytes pink (neutral lipids) and the portal areas blue (acidic lipids). In the liver of Patient 4 [61], autofluorescence under ultraviolet light, believed typical of peroxidized lipid, was strong; there was none seen in the liver of Patient 1. Many needle-shaped crystals may be present under polarized light [61]. The staining reactions that are strikingly positive in frozen sections are negative in paraffin-fixed sections, indicating ready extractability of the reactants by lipid solvents.

Electron micrographs of the hepatocytes reveal normal mitochondria and many vacuoles or vesicles surrounded by a limiting membrane [59].

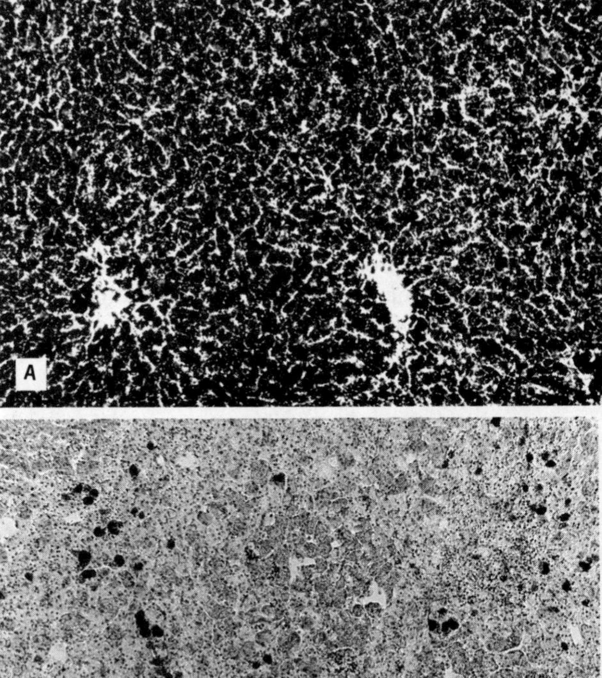

Figure 36-3. Frozen sections of liver stained with oil-red-O. A. Patient with cholesteryl ester storage disease (No. 1 in Table 36-3). B. Patient with Niemann-Pick disease, Type A (No. 70 in [67]), in which the hepatic cholesterol content was increased fivefold. Although oil-red-O staining of liver in Niemann-Pick disease is usually striking compared to normal, note the pale contrast with the staining in CESD. ×63.

Intestine

Partin and Schubert [62] have described in detail intestinal changes in CESD observed in peroral jejunal and duodenal biopsy specimens obtained in Patients 4 and 5. The mucosa has an orange color. The epithelium is normal. Beneath the epithelium in the region of the lacteals are collections of autofluorescent foam cells, especially densely packed in the villous tip. In frozen section, the foam cells stain intensely with oil-red-O, Sudan IV, or Sudan Black B. There is much extracellular lipid throughout the lamina propria that is crystalline, birefringent, and takes a stain similar to the fat in the foam cells. In contrast to the intracellular lipid, the extracellular lipid is more nonpolar. The Schultz reaction is weakly positive.

Electron microscopy of the lamina propria of the intestine of Patients 4 and 5 revealed several interesting features (Figs. 36-4 and 36-5). The lacteal endothelium was filled with round vacuoles that distended the smooth endoplasmic reticulum and looked as though they contained lipid taken up by pinocytosis. Many macrophages surrounded the lacteals with their irregular pseudopod extensions. The macrophages contained many vacuoles surrounded by limiting membranes. Similar nonosmophilic lipid droplets were present in adjacent smooth muscle cells, vascular pericytes, fibroblasts, and supporting cells of nerve fibers.

A rectal biopsy performed on Patient 1 at the age of 17 years revealed large, oil-red-O positive foam cells in the lamina propria. These were not as numerous as those seen in the biopsies from the other patients [62]. Scattered foam cells or mucus-laden macrophages occur in normal intestine,

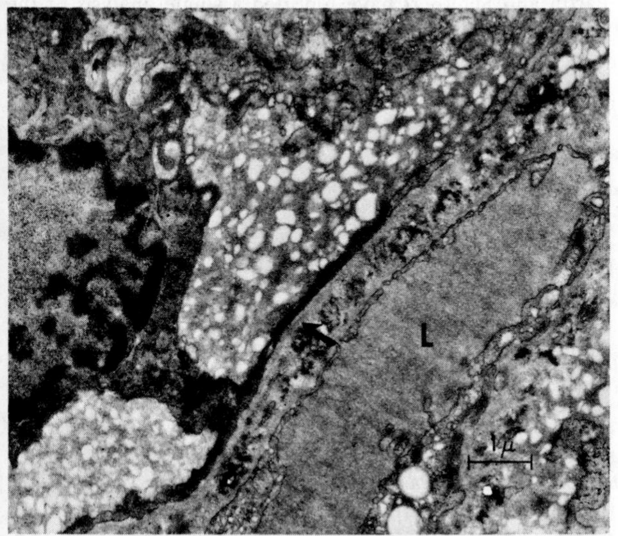

Figure 36-4. Electron micrograph of basement membrane region of small intestinal epithelium in patient (No. 4 in Table 36-3) with cholesteryl ester storage disease. Note the many angular droplets beyond the basement lamina (*arrow*). L = lumen of absorptive capillary. × 15,000. (*Kindly supplied by Dr. John C. Partin and reprinted from* [62] *with permission of the publishers.*)

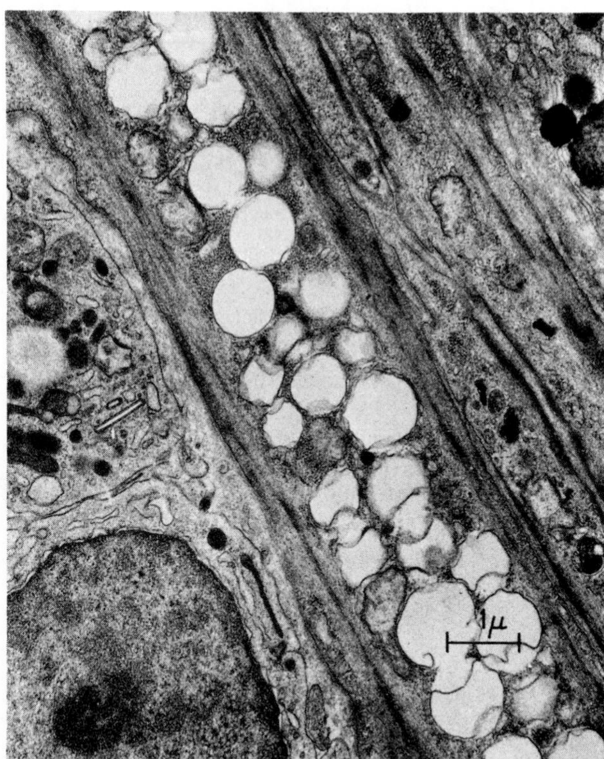

Figure 36-5. Electron micrograph of intestinal smooth muscle cell in patient with cholesteryl ester storage disease (No. 4 in Table 36-3). A portion of the cell is filled with large membrane-bound droplets, which were also birefringent. × 14,000. (*Kindly supplied by Dr. John C. Partin and reprinted from* [62] *with permission of the publishers.*)

and the pathologist was uncertain as to whether this lipid storage in the large intestine was indeed abnormal. Oil-red-O positive material was also present within and without large foam cells in the atrial appendage, skin, and thymus of Patient 1; its significance again was uncertain.

Bone Marrow

The large foam cells in the bone marrow of Patient 1 were birefringent. Under the phase microscope they could not be distinguished from the macrophages seen in Niemann-Pick disease (Chap. 35), Tangier disease (Chap. 26), or certain other lipidoses.

Tissue Chemistry

Lipids

Chemical abnormalities in tissues in CESD are thus far known to be present only in the liver and intestine. The analytical techniques employed by the three groups of investigators were not identical and there is a serious discrep-

Table 36-6. CONTENT OF LIVER IN CHOLESTERYL ESTER STORAGE DISEASE

Patient*	Reference	Lipids, mg/gm wet weight						CE fatty acids, percent						
		TL	TC	FC	CE	G	PL	14:0	16:0	16:1	18:0	18:1	18:2	<18
1	[66]	280	121	9	187	64	14	1	14	5	1	48	31	0
3	[60]	244	112	11	174	36	21	1	8	6	1	59	26	0
4	[62]	222	12	4	14	52	91	3	8	9	9	24	29	18
Controls	[31]	. . .	4	3	2	19	25							

*Numbered as in Table 36-3.
Note: TL = total lipid; TC = total cholesterol; FC = free cholesterol; CE = cholesteryl esters (cholesterol + fatty acid); G = glycerides; PL = phospholipids. Values are rounded to nearest milligram or percent.

ancy between the quantitative analyses of liver obtained in the first two families (Patients 1 and 3, Table 36-6) and those obtained in the third (Patient 4). From these data alone, one is not permitted to conclude that all three families represent the same disease. It has not been excluded, however, that experimental error accounts for the major differences.

Liver

Lipid analyses on three patients are displayed in Table 36-6. The major abnormality in Patients 1 and 3 was an increase in cholesteryl ester of such magnitude that 17 to 19 percent of the wet weight of the liver was due to this lipid alone. The concentration of sterol ester was more than 350 times normal. The sterol in Patient 1 was determined by the Liebermann-Burchardt reaction on a fraction prepared by silicic acid chromatography [66]. It was presumably a Δ_5-sterol, but absolute identification of cholesterol has not been made in any of the reported analyses.

It will be noted in Table 36-6 that in Patient 4 [62] the hepatic cholesteryl ester content appears to be far less than in the other patients, although the histochemical appearance of the liver and preliminary chromatographic evidence supported a very high content of neutral fats [61]. The sum of cholesterol, its esters, glycerides, and phospholipids accounts for 95 to 98 percent of the total lipid in Patients 1 and 3 but less than 75 percent in Patient 4. The difference in Patient 4 is reported as "carotene" [62], and in the extraordinary concentration of 52 mg per gm wet weight. This same abnormality was also reported in the intestinal mucosa of Patient 4 [62]. If it is correct, it may require segregation of the H. family (Patients 4 and 5) as a different disease. The great increase in hepatic phospholipids reported in the latter patients was also in contrast to low or normal values in Patients 1 and 3 (Table 36-6).

In Patient 1, 94 percent of the glyceride fraction was triglyceride, there being only small amounts of di- and monoglycerides as determined chromatographically [66]. The percentage distribution of hepatic phospholipids was phosphatidyl choline plus phosphatidyl inositol, 49; phosphatidyl ethanolamine, 31; sphingomyelin, 11.5; and lysophosphatidyl choline, 7 [66]. In Patient 3, it was considered that the liver sphingomyelin might be increased and the phosphatidyl ethanolamine decreased [60]. Liver glycolipids have not been studied adequately in any patient with CESD.

Intestine

Partin and Schubert have reported a single analysis of the lipid content of the small intestine in Patient 4 [62]. Cholesteryl ester content was more than twice normal, "carotene" three times normal, and phospholipids reduced. The contents of total lipids, unesterified cholesterol, triglycerides, monoglycerides, free fatty acids, and squalene were not obviously abnormal.

Cholesteryl Ester Fatty Acids

The acyl groups in the cholesteryl esters were predominantly oleic and linoleic acids [60, 61, 66], a pattern which is grossly similar to that seen in esters stored in Tangier disease, eosinophilic granuloma, or atheromas [68]. The fatty acid pattern shown for Patient 4 in Table 36-6 [61] is different

Table 36-7. PLASMA CHOLESTERYL ESTER FATTY ACIDS IN CHOLESTERYL ESTER STORAGE DISEASE

Patient	Reference	Percent							
		14:0	16:0	16:1	18:0	18:1	18:2	20:0	20:4
1	[66]	1	14	3	0	25	57	0	
3	[60]	10	26	6	5	37	15	0	2

from that described in a later report [62], where the predominant acids were C_{16} in length. The fatty acid composition of cholesteryl esters in the intestinal mucosa of Patient 4 did not differ remarkably from that in controls or from the liver [62]. The pattern of cholesteryl ester fatty acids in plasma is shown for two patients in Table 36-7. The methods used were not identical. The pattern in Patient 3 departs considerably from the preponderance of 18:2 fatty acids usually seen in plasma.

Other Lipid Analyses

The distribution of phospholipids in plasma in Patients 1 [66] and 3 [59] is not obviously abnormal. The same was true of one preliminary analysis of red cell phospholipids in Patient 1 [66].

Nonlipid Constituents

The liver glycogen content and several of the enzymes catalyzing glycogen metabolism were examined in Patient 1 (see case history above) and in Patient 3 [59, 60]. No abnormality was present. An increase in total bile acids in serum and a decrease in ratio of trihydroxy to dihydroxy bile acids in both bile and serum in Patients 4 and 5 [61] were mentioned earlier.

Biochemical Studies

Several studies of cholesteryl ester metabolism have been made in one or another patient with CESD. They have not been performed in any uniform way, and their value in interpreting the abnormal mechanism(s) responsible for this disorder (or these disorders) is limited.

In Vivo Studies

Experiments in which the plasma cholesterol in Patient 1 was labeled by two different means permit several conclusions about her disorder [66]. When she was fed a small amount of ^{14}C-cholesterol with fat, radioactive cholesterol appeared in the plasma within 15 min and reached its peak between 1 and 2 days later. The specific activity of esterified cholesterol exceeded that of nonesterified cholesterol until the fifth day when they became approximately the same. Thereafter, they declined at the same rate, the specific activity of the esterified sterol remaining only a little higher. The gross appearance of these curves differed from that obtained in similar studies in normal and hypercholesterolemic man [69]; normally, the specific activity of the esters lags slightly behind that of free sterol for almost 2 days after labeled cholesterol is ingested.

Patient 1 then received ^{14}C-mevalonic acid intravenously, and the plasma cholesterol was quickly labeled. The specific activity of plasma nonesterified cholesterol exceeded that of esterified cholesterol until the fourth day when the die-away curves were indistinguishable from those obtained when ^{14}C-cholesterol was fed. The experimental data in the mevalonic acid experiment were not dissimilar to those seen in hypercholesterolemic subjects by Nestel and Monger [70].

These labeling experiments indicate that there is little mixing of the esterified cholesterol in plasma, including that incoming in chylomicrons, with any significant part of the huge pool of esters in the liver. It also appears that the lecithin cholesterol acyl transferase system (Chap. 27), primarily responsible for the esterification of cholesterol in plasma, is operative. No direct measurement of plasma LCAT activity has been made in CESD.

Cholesteryl Esterase (Hydrolase) Activity

Specimens of liver from Patient 5 and a control were found to contain small but comparable amounts of cholesteryl ester hydrolase activity [61]. No measurements of acyl transferase activities that catalyze synthesis of cholesteryl esters in liver, intestine, or other tissues have been made in patients with CESD.

Lipid Synthesis

In Patient 3, Infante and colleagues report studies involving incorporation of different labeled substrates by liver slices [60]. The amounts of ^{14}C-tagged acetate, palmitate, and glucose that were incorporated into cholesteryl esters by the patient's liver exceeded that in the control by severalfold. The amounts of these substrates incorporated into glycerides, phospholipids, and cholesterol were considerably less than in the control. It is not possible to conclude from these studies alone whether there might be an accelerated synthesis of cholesteryl esters in the liver in vivo.

Pathophysiology

A section on cholesteryl ester metabolism earlier in this chapter is called to the reader's attention before he considers the possible defect in CESD. When first encountered in Patient 1, CESD seemed likely to be explicable on the basis of deficient activity of hepatic cholesterol esterase or hydrolase. One could conceive of cholesteryl esters arriving at the liver in chylomicrons and being sequestered in gradually enlarging stores, as they awaited the hydrolysis necessary for entry of the free sterol into its normal metabolic pathways.

Two pieces of information collected in the patients of Schiff et al. (Patients 4 and 5), however, were not consistent with this hypothesis. One was the evidence that cholesteryl esters were apparently also accumulating in the intestine. The second, and more important, was the finding in one biopsy specimen that liver cholesteryl ester hydrolase activity did not appear to be different from normal [61]. Reference has already been made to marked differences in the chemical content of tissues from different patients that may indicate (Table 36-6) that more than one disease has been collected under the descriptor CESD. It is quite possible that differences in techniques of lipid analyses account for this discrepancy.

If the hydrolase activity in CESD proves, on examination of more patients, to be normal, speculation must be directed to other possible defects. A more intimate examination of the plasma lipoproteins, both their total chemical content and, especially, the nature of the apolipoproteins, is in order. Recombination experiments (Chap. 26) indicate that phospholipids and cholesteryl esters may be the two most important lipids in determining the structure of lipoproteins. Conversely, the capacity of the lipoproteins to transport esters is probably a key factor in the regulation of tissue cholesterol concentrations. Excessive hepatic synthesis of cholesterol or of its esters, as suggested by experiments on tissue from Patient 3, cannot be excluded, although an error in degradative capacity is more probable. The examination of tissues other than liver, including fibroblasts grown in culture, for hydrolase activity and cholesteryl ester accumulation is also needed. It will also be necessary to follow up the peculiarities in bile acid distribution described in the patients of Schiff [61]. Although the type of bile acid present in intestinal lumen is quite important for proper emulsification and absorption of sterol [39], little else is known that might explain a relationship between the disparate hydroxylation of bile acids and a huge excess of hepatic cholesteryl esters.

Finally, it should be emphasized that, although the glyceride content of liver may also be somewhat high in CESD (Table 36-6), there is little to suggest that this disease and Wolman's disease are more than superficially similar. The death in early childhood of Patient 2 (Table 36-3) notwithstanding, it appears that the prognosis in CESD is far more benign and the tissue lipidosis much more localized.

Genetics

Of three known families affected with CESD, sibs were affected in two. Patients 1 and 2 (Table 36-3) were twins. The evidence for involvement of one, who survived only a few weeks, is entirely morphologic, but leaves little doubt that she also had the disease. The other two siblings appear to be normal. The father had a few foam cells in his bone marrow, but no other abnormalities.

The family of Schiff et al. [61] is more complicated. There were seven children, two of whom (Patients 4 and 5 in Table 36-3) are considered to have the full-blown syndrome. Four of the younger siblings, however, also had hepatomegaly and the abnormalities in plasma bile acid pattern found in Patients 4 and 5. The parents and three of four grandparents were examined. They had no hepatomegaly, but the father and paternal grandfather had an abnormal distribution within the plasma bile acids.

Biopsy specimens of the liver were obtained in three of the younger sibs with hepatomegaly. The tissue was grossly normal, but microscopic evidence of lipid storage, qualitatively similar to that seen in their two affected older siblings, was seen.

The identity of the disease in the three families has not yet been established. With regard to inheritance of the disorder(s) it is possible only to conclude that similar manifestations may appear in either sex. All of the three families described here were Caucasians.

Diagnosis

In a young child, the most likely disease to be confused with CESD is glycogen storage disease (see p. 155). In both disorders, marked hepatomegaly and hyperlipidemia without splenic enlargement may appear in a child whose mental and physical development is otherwise unremarkable. Provocative tests for adequacy of glycogenolysis should be performed and survey of glycogen content, glucose-6-phosphatase, phosphorylase and related enzymes should be made on liver removed by biopsy. The absence of jaundice in any patient with CESD thus far suggests that the disorder should not be confused with congenital biliary cirrhosis. A normal proportion of esters in the total cholesterol in plasma should help exclude biliary obstruction.

A child suspected of having CESD should have an examination of bone marrow for foam cells and, ideally, a biopsy of either rectal or intestinal mucosa to determine the presence of large cells reacting positively with the Schultz and oil-red-O stains. Liver biopsy will ultimately be necessary for diagnosis and the latter will depend upon a careful analysis of lipid content. A preponderant increase in cholesteryl esters—in the absence of the calcified adrenals and severe debilitation associated with Wolman's disease—provides a diagnosis. Liver and plasma should be retained frozen for more specific enzymatic and other analyses that may be developed in the future.

Treatment

There is no specific treatment for cholesteryl ester storage disease. Adequate trial of cholestyramine or other agents effective in decreasing cholesterol absorption has not been reported.

CEREBROTENDINOUS XANTHOMATOSIS

Cerebrotendinous xanthomatosis (CTX) is a rare disease that is characterized by xanthomas, cataracts, progressive cerebellar ataxia, and dementia [71]. Foam cells, myelin destruction, and gliosis are found in the brain stem and cerebellum. The large accumulations of cholesterol or cholesterol-like crystals in white matter and in xanthomas suggest an abnormality of cholesterol metabolism; the plasma cholesterol concentration, however, is usually normal.

A diagnosis of cerebrotendinous xanthomatosis was formerly based exclusively on clinical and pathological observations. Menkes et al., however, have recently demonstrated that 5α-cholestan-3β-ol (cholestanol; dihydrocholesterol) is stored within the nervous system [72]. Philippart and van Bogaert have confirmed this observation and have reported that cholestanol is also stored in tendon xanthomas [73].

The disease appears to be due to a double dose of a mutant autosomal allele. The basic inheritable metabolic defect is not yet known, and there is no specific therapy.

Historical Aspects

In 1936, Schneider described the finding of xanthomatous deposits in the nervous system of a mentally retarded and epileptic patient who died at 36 years of age [74]. Very little clinical information was provided, tendon xanthomas were not observed, and the published pathological data are insufficient to permit certain assignment of this patient as the first case of cerebrotendinous xanthomatosis. In 1937, van Bogaert et al. [71] provided a detailed clinical and pathological description of a patient with dementia, ataxia, cataracts, and xanthomas in tendons and in the nervous system. Van Bogaert observed similar symptoms in the paternal cousin of his first patient [71, 73, 75, 76]. In 1937, Epstein and Lorenz [77] and Epstein and Kreitner [78] described three patients with similar symptoms under the eponym *van Bogaert's disease.* Since that time about a dozen additional cases have been reported [72, 73, 75, 79–90]. In several of these patients, Van Bogaert et al. [71, 85] described massive deposits of "cholesterol" crystals in both white matter and in tendon xanthomas, observations that have been repeatedly confirmed. In 1968, Menkes et al. [72] made the important discovery that the cerebellum and cerebrum in two patients with CTX contained greatly increased concentrations of cholestanol.

Clinical Manifestations

Twelve well-documented patients with cerebrotendinous xanthomatosis have been reported [71–73, 75, 76, 79–86, 88–90]. Three other patients have been briefly alluded to in other reports [73, 87]. Table 36-8 contains a summary of the major clinical and pathological characteristics of 12 patients. From these data can be constructed a number of generalizations about the disease, but events are so variable that it is not possible to describe a typical case history.

Onset

The onset of CTX is insidious and unpredictable. Dementia has been observed as early as 10 years of age [71, 73], cataracts by age 15 [71], tendon xanthomas at 15 [80, 81], and ataxia by 18 years of age [77, 78].

Course

Van Bogaert et al. have suggested that the course may be divided into several arbitrary time phases [71]. The initial stage usually begins in childhood and is characterized by dementia. Mental retardation, mental deterioration, or borderline intelligence have been described repeatedly [71–73, 75–83, 85, 88–90]. In some of these patients, mental

Table 36-8. PATIENTS WITH CEREBROTENDINOUS XANTHOMATOSIS

Patient	Reference	Sex	Age, years		Clinical abnormalities							Confirmation of diagnosis	
					Mentality	Speech	Motor		Tendon xanthomas	Xanthelasma	Cataracts	Neuro-pathological	Chemical
			Onset*	Death			Paresis	Ataxia					
1	[71, 75]	M	<10	40	+	+	+	+	+	+	+	+	0
2	[71, 75, 73, 86]	F	10	55	+	+	+	+	0	+	+	+	+
3	[77, 78]	M	12	40	+	+	+	+	+	+	–	+	0
4	[77, 78]	F	44	–	+	–	+	+	+	0	–	0	0
5	[77, 78]	F	18	–	–	–	0	–	+	–	–	0	0
6	[79]	F	51	55	+	+	+	+	+	–	–	+	0
7	[80, 83]	F	15	–	+	–	–	–	+	–	+	0	0
8	[80, 83]	F	20	–	+	–	–	–	+	–	+	0	0
9	[84]	M	36	–	0	0	0	0	+	–	+	0	0
10	[86, 89, 72]	M	<10	60	+	+	+	+	+	0	+	+	+
11	[89, 72]	F	<24	–	+	–	–	+	+	+	+	0	0
12	[88, 90]	M	31	46	+	+	+	+	+	–	+	+	+

* = May indicate age at which patient was first seen.
+ = Present.
0 = Absent.
– = Not mentioned.

retardation or deterioration was present or began in childhood; in others, it is not possible to determine the age of onset. In one patient, mentation was normal at 41 years of age [84].

During adolescence and young adulthood there develops progressively severe spasticity, usually associated with ataxia. Juvenile cataracts and tendon xanthomas are also frequently observed in this second stage of the disease. Sometimes minimally present in childhood [71], spasticity typically becomes increasingly severe with advancing age [71, 75, 77, 78, 80, 81, 89] and may be incapacitating in the fourth and fifth decades [73, 75, 84]. Ataxia is usually associated with the spasticity, but it may be absent [71, 80, 84, 88, 90]. The juvenile cataracts are usually well developed by young adulthood and frequently require excision [71, 72, 75, 76, 80, 81, 88–90]. In some patients no mention was made of cataracts and presumably they are not always present [77–79].

Tendon xanthomas have been observed in the second decade [72, 77, 78, 80, 81, 89]; usually they are first noticed in the third or fourth decade [71, 75–78, 84, 88, 90]. The Achilles tendon is the most common site. They also may occur in the triceps [77, 78, 80, 81], tibial tuberosities [71, 77, 78, 84], and extensor tendons of the fingers [77, 78, 80, 81, 88, 90]. These lesions are superficially similar to those seen in Type II hyperlipoproteinemia (Chap. 28); they slowly increase in size but are not painful. Tendon xanthomas are not present in every case description [71, 73, 75, 79]. Xanthelasma (palpebral xanthomas) may also be present [71, 75, 77, 78, 89].

In the final stage of CTX, enlargement of xanthomas and neurological deterioration is severe. As spasticity and ataxia worsen, speech becomes difficult and tremors and muscular atrophy, particularly of the distal musculature, become quite noticeable [71, 75, 77–79, 84, 88–90]. Bilateral Babinski signs [71, 75, 79, 89] and loss of pain and vibratory sensations may be present [71, 75, 76].

The age at death, not always specified in case reports, has usually been between the fourth and sixth decades. A patient reported by Stein and Czuczwar [84] is noteworthy; at 44 years of age he had tendon xanthomas, cataracts, and a spastic gait but was otherwise apparently functioning normally.

Plasma Lipids

Van Bogaert's second patient had hypercholesterolemia [71, 75], the plasma cholesterol being over 400 mg per 100 ml on several occasions, although early in the course of the disease plasma lipids were normal. Only one other patient had a cholesterol concentration greater than 300 mg per 100 ml, but normal values were also obtained on several occasions [80, 81]. The plasma cholesterol in other patients has been normal [71, 84, 88–90]. Other plasma lipids and lipoproteins have not been well characterized.

Clinicopathological Correlations

The most striking pathologic changes in CTX occur in the tendons and in the nervous system.

Gross Pathology and Light Microscopy

Nervous System

Van Bogaert et al. have provided detailed descriptions of the pathological examination of the brain and spinal cord in CTX [71, 73, 75, 76]. The brain may be grossly normal or demonstrate minimal frontal atrophy.

CEREBELLUM: The most striking and consistent abnormalities within the nervous system occur in the cerebellum. The white matter of the lateral hemispheres usually contains yellowish granulomatous lesions that may be as large as 1.5 cm in diameter and replace most of the white matter [71, 73, 75, 77, 79, 88–90]. There may also be some atrophy of the adjacent folia [71, 89].

Microscopic examination reveals extensive demyelination of the cerebellar white matter lateral to the dentate nucleus and in the superior cerebellar peduncles; the white matter adjacent and medial to the dentate nucleus is spared [71, 75, 89]. The areas of extensive demyelination contain many cystic spaces and needle-shaped clefts (Fig. 36-6). Some of the cysts contain large mononuclear cells with a foamy, vacuolated cytoplasm [71, 78, 79, 89]. Similar macrophages and multinucleated giant cells may surround the clefts and cysts [71, 89]. When frozen sections of the cerebellum are stained with oil-red-O, neutral fat is evident around blood vessels and in the cystic spaces [71, 89]. The needle-shaped

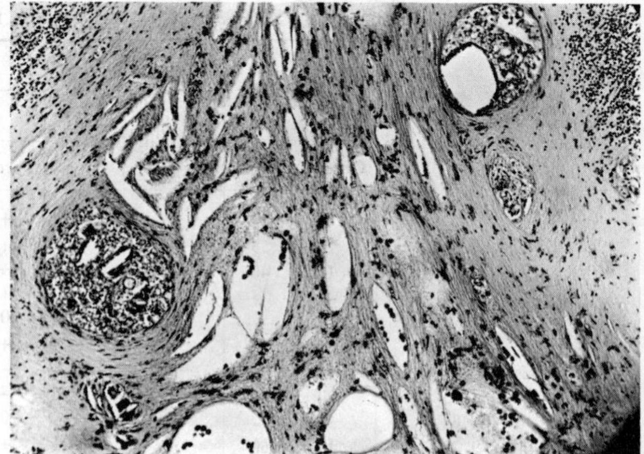

Figure 36-6. Section of cerebellum from patient with cerebrotendinous xanthomatosis. Clefts and cystic areas of necrosis are surrounded by macrophages with foamy cytoplasm and multinucleated giant cells. × 104. (*Kindly supplied by Dr. Phillip D. Swanson and reprinted from* [89] *with permission of the publishers.*)

clefts do not stain with oil-red-O but are birefringent [71, 89]. In the cerebellar cortex adjacent to the areas of extensive demyelination there is extensive loss of Purkinje and granule cells [71, 73, 89]. Philippart and van Bogaert noted almost complete destruction of the fastigial nuclei in one patient [73, 75]. Degeneration of the olivocerebellar fibers has also been observed [71, 75].

FOREBRAIN: Xanthomas have been observed in the globus pallidus and in the cerebral peduncles [71, 75]. Perivascular collections of large mononuclear cells with foamy cytoplasm may be found in the globus pallidus, the caudate nucleus, and the basal ganglia [71, 73, 75, 77, 89]. Scattered collections of foam cells have been observed in the thalamus [73] and in the white matter adjacent to the lateral ventricles [71, 75, 88, 90]. Extensive demyelination has been noted in the cerebral peduncles and in the fibers of the ansa lenticularis [71, 73, 89], and there may be areas of dense gliosis in the globus pallidus [71] and in the central part of the corona radiata [73]. Marked atrophy of the entire optic pathway has been observed [71, 79].

No abnormalities have been observed in the cerebral cortex. This is of interest in view of the marked dementia that has been noted in so many patients.

BRAIN STEM: Numerous lesions may be scattered throughout the brain stem, associated with gliosis and demyelination [71, 73, 75]. Van Bogaert et al. [71, 73, 75] have provided detailed descriptions of the pathological examination of the midbrain.

SPINAL CORD AND PERIPHERAL NERVES: As in other parts of the nervous system, perivascular cuffing by large mononuclear cells may occur in the spinal cord [71, 89]. There may be extensive demyelination of the posterior and lateral columns [71, 73, 75] and of the pyramidal tracts from the cerebral peduncles to the inferior extremes of the spinal cord [71, 73, 89]. No abnormalities of the peripheral nerves have been reported.

Other Tissues

TENDONS: As was noted above, tendon xanthomas are an almost constant feature of CTX. The gross appearance of the xanthomas is similar to that observed in patients with Type II hyperlipoproteinemia (see Fig. 28-17, Chap. 28). When viewed under the light microscope the xanthomas contain a dense accumulation of birefringent crystalline clefts surrounded by many multinucleated giant cells and large mononuclear cells with foamy cytoplasm [71, 77, 79, 89] (Fig. 36-7). Collections of free fat around blood vessels and throughout the granulomatous areas stain brightly with oil-red-O. Schimschock et al. [89] have observed that the crystalline clefts in tendon xanthomas are long and narrow, whereas those in the cerebellum are small and boxlike.

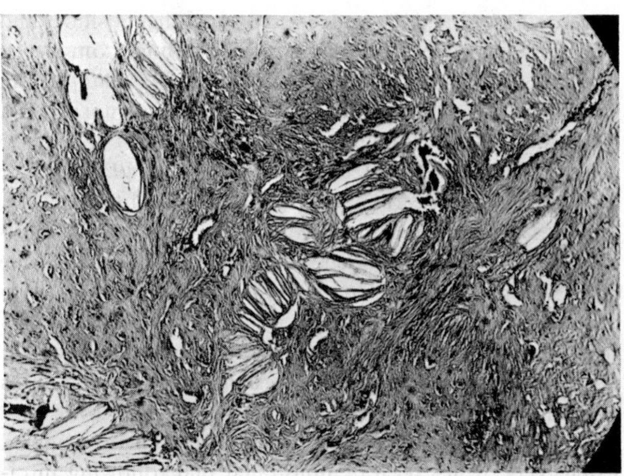

Figure 36-7. Section of Achilles tendon from patient with cerebrotendinous xanthomatosis. Large clefts are surrounded by evidence of cellular reaction including a few darkly staining multinucleated giant cells. × 104. (*Kindly supplied by Dr. Phillip D. Swanson and reprinted from* [89] *with permission of the publishers.*)

LUNG AND BONE: Granulomatous lesions containing needle-shaped birefringent crystalline clefts, multinucleated giant cells, and large foam cells have been observed in the lung [71, 89], in the femur [71, 75], and in the bodies of the lumbar vertebrae [71]. The lesions in the lung contained many extracellular deposits of lipid, particularly around the blood vessels [89].

CARDIOVASCULAR: Two patients with CTX have died following a myocardial infarction [88–90]. It is not known whether arteriosclerosis may be unusually common in this disease.

Chemistry of Cerebrotendinous Xanthomatosis

Cholestanol

The saturated sterol, 5α-cholestan-3β-ol or cholestanol (Fig. 36-8) appears to be associated with cholesterol in all mammalian tissues [91]. It differs from cholesterol by the absence of a double bond between carbon atoms 5 and 6. In the sterol 5α refers to the stereochemistry of the junction be-

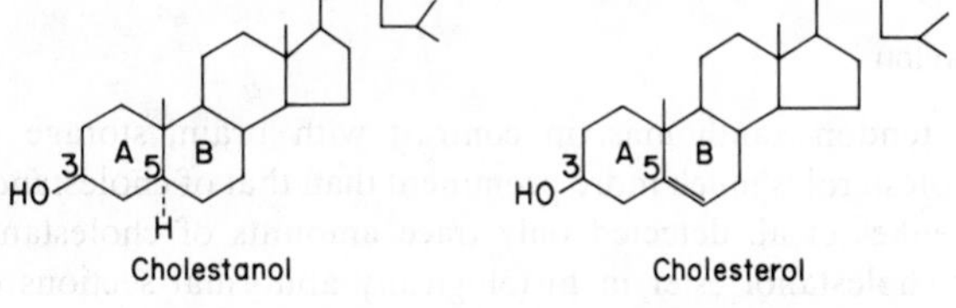

Cholestanol   Cholesterol

Figure 36-8. The structure of cholesterol and cholestanol.

tween rings A and B, and 3β refers to the position and configuration of the hydroxyl group at carbon atom 3.

Cholestanol is present in readily detectable quantities in liver, intestine, adrenals, gallstones, aorta, and serum [91, 92]. The biosynthesis of cholestanol from cholesterol appears to require the action of at least three enzymes [93, 94]. The hydroxyl group at carbon 3 is initially oxidized to a ketone, yielding cholest-5-ene-3-one. An enzyme-catalyzed isomerization converts cholest-5-ene-3-one to cholest-4-ene-3-one [93], which is then reduced by a specific reductase to 5α-cholest-3-one (or cholestanone) [94]. Cholestanone is then apparently reduced to cholestanol by another reductase [93, 94]. Like cholesterol, 5α-cholestan-3β-ol occurs both as free cholestanol and as the fatty acyl ester.

The catabolism of cholestanol has not been investigated extensively. It has been demonstrated that following intravenous injection or oral feeding, cholestanol is converted to several allocholanic bile acids that can be found in the feces [72, 95–97].

Chemical Abnormalities in Tissues

Brain

Only trace amounts of free or esterified cholestanol are normally found in brain. In 1968 Menkes et al. reported the presence of abnormally high concentrations of free and esterified cholestanol in the brain of one patient with CTX [72, 89]. Cholestanol comprised 25 percent of the total free sterols in histologically abnormal portions of cerebellum and about 20 percent of the total free sterols in normal-appearing gray and white matter samples of the cerebrum. Cholestanol esters accounted for 49 percent of the total esterified sterols in the histologically abnormal sections of cerebellum [72]. Philippart and van Bogaert then repeated these observations in the cerebellum of a second patient with CTX [73]. The brains in these two patients had been stored in formaldehyde prior to the analyses. Cholestanol storage has been recently confirmed, however, in brain that had been stored frozen from another patient with the disease [88, 90]. The presence of cholestanol has been determined by thin-layer and gas-liquid chromatography [73, 86, 89, 90], and recently by mass spectrometry [87].

The available data indicate that cerebral cholesterol is slightly increased, the augmentation being due almost entirely to selective increase in cholesteryl esters [72, 86].

Tendon

In tendon xanthomas, in contrast with brain, storage of cholesterol is much more prominent than that of cholestanol. Menkes et al. detected only trace amounts of cholestanol or cholestanol ester in histologically abnormal sections of tendon from two patients with CTX [72]. Philippart and van Bogaert, however, have demonstrated the accumulation of small amounts of free cholestanol (about 3 percent of total sterols) in tendon xanthomas of two patients with CTX [73]; one of these xanthomas was obtained from one of the two patients studied by Menkes et al. [72].

Plasma and Other Tissues

Although Menkes et al. were not able to detect abnormal concentrations of cholestanol in fasting or 2-hr postprandial plasma [72], Philippart and van Bogaert found that cholestanol accounted for 6 percent of total sterols (normal, < 1 percent) in the plasma of their patient with CTX [73]. In analyses of liver, lung, adrenal, and kidneys of one patient with CTX no cholestanol accumulation was found [72].

The Metabolic Defect in Cerebrotendinous Xanthomatosis

The metabolic defect in CTX has not been defined. The observation that cholestanol accumulates in the cerebrum, cerebellum, and possibly in tendon xanthomas suggests a basic derangement in cholestanol metabolism. Philippart and van Bogaert have proposed that, by analogy to other storage diseases, CTX may be due to a defect in the catabolism of cholestanol [73]. Menkes et al. have suggested that the metabolic abnormality in CTX is a defect in the transport of tissue cholesterol across the cell membrane, with the result that excess tissue cholesterol might be converted to cholestanol and stored as either the free sterol or the ester [72]. This theory has as one of its premises a marked limitation of capacity for removal of cholestanol from cells. This latter abnormality, or excessive conversion of cholesterol to cholestanol, could itself be the primary defect. One patient has been given labeled cholesterol intravenously. Three years later, labeled cholestanol was isolated from cerebral white matter [87].

Pathophysiology

The sequence of events by which cholestanol storage, if that is indeed the basic defect in CTX, causes the pathological abnormalities observed in the disease is not clear. Storage of cholestanol is gradual as indicated by the slow and progressive development of cataracts, tendon xanthomas, and neurological symptoms. The recent observation that plasma levels of cholestanol may be increased in CTX [73] suggests that the cholestanol stored in the nervous system and tendons may be derived from the blood, but intracellular conversion of cholesterol to cholestanol cannot be excluded.

Philippart and van Bogaert suggested that some of the cholesterol normally in myelin might be replaced by cholestanol [73], and Stahl et al [90] have demonstrated that unesterified cholestanol is present in myelin in this disease. Interestingly, this change in myelin composition was observed in the frontal lobe. This implies that, although the cerebral cortex does not usually contain either gross or microscopic lesions, the myelin nevertheless may be abnormal. This abnormality might in turn account for the severe changes in mentation that are typical of CTX.

If cholestanol storage is the primary defect in CTX, it is noteworthy that the tendon lesions [72, 73], and possibly the granulomas in lung [72], contain a good deal more cholesterol than cholestanol. There is no explanation for the apparent storage of both sterols. It should be mentioned here that there is inadequate information about possible cholestanol accumulation in other xanthomas or granulomatous diseases in which cholesterol storage is well documented.

Diagnosis

It is difficult to establish the diagnosis of CTX in the first decade of life. The disorder should be considered in any young adult with tendon xanthomas, juvenile cataracts, low or borderline intelligence, cerebellar abnormalities, and a normal plasma cholesterol. In a patient in whom the diagnosis is suspected, a thorough examination of the nervous system, x-ray of the lungs, and determination of fasting plasma cholesterol and triglyceride are indicated.

Until recently, a definitive diagnosis of CTX could not be made before death. Tissues obtained at biopsy or autopsy should be handled as described in Chaps. 29, 33, and 35. If the observation of Philippart and van Bogaert [73] is confirmed, it may be possible to diagnose CTX by determining the level of cholestanol in tendon xanthomas or in plasma.

Treatment

There is no specific therapy; cataract extraction may, however, relieve the visual symptoms. Stein et al. placed their patient on a low-cholesterol diet and repeated injections of heparin [84]; the results of this therapeutic trial have not been reported.

Genetics

Until recently, the diagnosis of CTX was based on clinical and pathological considerations and data are not available to support many conclusions concerning genetics. Twelve cases of CTX have been reported. The first and second examples of CTX were in paternal cousins [71, 73, 75, 76, 85] and the fourth and fifth cases were sisters [77, 78]. Two siblings have been affected in each of three families [72, 77, 78, 80, 81, 89] and possibly in a fourth [90]. Both sexes have been affected with the same frequency (see Table 36-8). The parents of the two patients reported by Schimschock et al. were first cousins [89]. These observations strongly support the conclusion that CTX is transmitted as an autosomal recessive disease.

Possibly Related Forms of Xanthomatosis

Several other diseases have been reported which resemble CTX and conceivably could be the same disorder. One of these was reported by Harlan and Still under the name *hereditary tendinous and tuberous xanthomatosis without hyperlipidemia* [98]. The patients were two black siblings. The younger, a 29-year-old male, had tendon and subcutaneous xanthomas and unspecified nodular densities in both lung fields. His 34-year-old sister had similar xanthomas and a cataract in one eye. No neurological symptoms or signs were present. Plasma lipids were normal in these patients. The xanthomas contained cholesterol clefts and numerous giant cells. Abundant cholesterol was present; no analyses for possible cholestanol were made. The authors classified these patients among the reticuloendothelioses. Subsequent debate about these cases [99] leaves unresolved their possible relationship to CTX.

A second disorder that is not clearly separated from CTX is so-called *spinal cholesterolosis.* In 1942 Thiebaut described a 34-year-old woman with progressive spastic paraplegia, bilateral Babinski signs, ankle and patellar clonus, and xanthomas of the Achilles and triceps tendons [100]. Her plasma cholesterol concentration was 250 mg per 100 ml; this value, we believe, has been erroneously interpreted as "2,050 mg per 100 ml" in several references to Thiebaut's report [89, 101]. Thiebaut attributed the symptoms to "cholesterolosis" of the spinal cord; there was, however, no pathological verification.

In 1962 van Bogaert reported a second case described as spinal cholesterolosis [101]. The 46-year-old woman had ataxia, bilateral Babinski signs, palmar and plantar xanthomas, and xanthelasmas. She also had hepatosplenomegaly, hyperlipemia, and a plasma cholesterol concentration of 630 mg per 100 ml. Postmortem examination revealed the presence of large numbers of cholesterol crystals and "free fatty granules" accompanied by severe demyelination in the lower medulla and upper spinal cord. Cataracts were not reported in either of these patients. Their clinical symptoms and the pathological observations in van Bogaert's patient indicate that these patients probably had a disease different from CTX.

Another patient, described by Ortiz de Zarate [102], cannot be classified with certainty as an example of CTX. This was a male who died at age 39 after a 12-year history of psychic abnormalities. There were no cerebellar symptoms, cataracts, or tendon xanthomas, and the only neurological sign was a bilateral increase in the patellar reflex with clonus. There were discrete areas of demyelination within the cerebrum and cholesterol crystals filled almost the entire head of the caudate nucleus and the adjacent internal capsule [102].

SUMMARY

1 Wolman's disease is a fatal familial disease characterized by tissue accumulation of large amounts of neutral lipids, particularly cholesteryl esters and glycerides. Gastrointestinal symptoms, hepatosplenomegaly, steatorrhea, adrenal calcification, and failure to thrive are usually observed in the first weeks of life; death usually occurs by 6 months of age. The biochemical basis remains to be firmly established; a marked deficiency of acid lipase activity that catalyzes hydrolysis of esterified lipids has been described. Wolman's disease is probably inherited as an autosomal recessive disorder. There is no specific therapy.

2 Cholesteryl ester storage disease is a rare familial disease in which the liver is enlarged and contains remarkably high concentrations of cholesteryl esters; lipid may also accumulate in the lamina propria of the intestine. The patients are usually asymptomatic and liver function is normal in spite of the marked hepatomegaly. Diagnosis is based on determination of the cholesteryl ester concentration of liver; the biochemical basis of the disease is not known. There is no known therapy.

3 Cerebrotendinous xanthomatosis (CTX) is a familial disease characterized by progressive cerebellar ataxia, dementia, cataracts, and tendon xanthomas. Cholesteryl esters and cholestanol (5α-cholestan-3β-ol) accumulate in the nervous system and possibly in the tendon xanthomas. Disability is progressive, although the patients may survive into the sixth decade. CTX is probably an autosomal recessive disorder, and its biochemical basis has not been established. There is no treatment for the disorder. Two additional diseases that resemble, and may be variants of, CTX are *hereditary tendinous and tuberous xanthomatosis without hyperlipidemia* and *spinal cholesterolosis.*

BIBLIOGRAPHY

1. Abramov, A., Schorr, S., and Wolman, M.: Generalized xanthomatosis with calcified adrenals. A.M.A. J. Dis. Child., **91**, 282, 1956.
2. Wolman, M., Sterk, V. V., Gatt, S., and Frenkel, M.: Primary familial xanthomatosis with involvement and calcification of the adrenals: Report of two more cases in siblings of a previously described infant. Pediatrics, **28**, 742, 1961.
3. Wolman, M.: Histochemistry of lipids in pathology, in *Handbuch der Histochemie,* edited by W. Graumann and K. Neumann, vol. V, pt 2, p. 228. Fischer Verlag, Stuttgart, 1964.
4. Crocker, A. C., Vawter, G. F., Neuhauser, E. B. D., and Rosowsky, A.: Wolman's disease: Three new patients with a recently described lipidosis. Pediatrics, **35**, 627, 1965.
5. Neuhauser, E. B. D., Kirkpatrick, J. A., and Wientraub, B.: Wolman's disease: A new lipidosis. Ann. Radiol. (Paris), **8** (numero special, Radiologie pediatrique), 175, 1965.
6. Rosowsky, A., Crocker, A. C., Trites, D. H., and Modest, E. J.: Gas-liquid chromatographic analysis of the tissue sterol fraction in Wolman's disease and related lipidoses. Biochim. Biophys. Acta, **98**, 617, 1965.
7. Sloviter, H. A., Janic, V., and Naiman, J. L.: Lipid synthesis by red blood cell preparations in Wolman's disease (a familial lipidosis). Clin. Chim. Acta, **20**, 423, 1968.
8. Konno, T., Fujii, M., Watanuki, T., and Koizumi, K.: Wolman's disease; the first case in Japan. Tohoku J. Exp. Med., **90**, 375, 1966.
9. Spiegel-Adolf, M., Baird, H. W., and McCafferty, M.: Hematologic studies in Niemann-Pick and Wolman's disease (cytology and electrophoresis). Confin. Neurol., **28**, 399, 1966.
10. Caffey, J., and Silverman, F. N.: *Pediatric x-ray diagnosis,* 5th ed. pp. 672–674. Year Book, Chicago, 1967.
11. Guazzi, G. C., Martin, J. J., Philippart, M., Roels, H., van der Eecken, H., Vrints, L., Delbeke, M. J., and Hooft, C.: Wolman's disease. Europ. Neurol., **1**, 334, 1968.
12. Guazzi, G. C., Martin, J. J., Philippart, M., Roels, H., Hooft, C., van der Eecken, H., Delbeke, M. J., and Vrints, L.: Wolman's disease: Distribution and significance of the central nervous system lesions. Path. Europ., **3**, 266, 1968.
13. Kahana, D., Berant, M., and Wolman, M.: Primary familial xanthomatosis with adrenal involvement (Wolman's disease): Report of a further case with nervous system involvement and pathogenetic considerations. Pediatrics, **42**, 70, 1968.
14. Kamoshita, S., and Landing, B. H.: Distribution of lesions in myenteric plexus and gastrointestinal mucosa in lipidoses and other neurological disorders of children. Amer. J. Clin. Path., **49**, 312, 1968.
15. Marks, M. J., and Marcus, A. J.: Wolman's disease. Canad. Med. Ass. J., **99**, 232, 1968.
16. Partin, J. C., Mereu, T. R., and Schubert, W. K.: Intestinal absorptive epithelium in Wolman's cholesterol lipidosis, in *Proc. 26th Ann. Meeting Electron Microscope Soc. Amer.,* edited by C. J. Arceneau, pp. 194–195. Claitor's Publishing Division, Baton Rouge, 1968.
17. Wolman, M.: Involvement of nervous tissue in primary familial xanthomatosis with adrenal calcification. Path. Europ., **3**, 259, 1968.
18. Marshall, W. C., Ockenden, B. G., Fosbrooke, A. S., and Cumings, J. N.: Wolman's disease: A rare lipidosis with adrenal calcification. Arch. Dis. Child., **44**, 331, 1969.
19. Eto, Y., and Kitagawa, T.: Wolman's disease with hypolipoproteinemia and acanthocytosis: Clinical and biochemical observations. J. Pediat., **77**, 862, 1970.
20. Lake, B. D., and Patrick, A. D.: Wolman's disease: Deficiency of E600-resistant acid esterase activity with storage of lipids in lysosomes. J. Pediat., **76**, 262, 1970.
21. Lough, J., Fawcett, J., and Wiegensberg, B.: Wolman's disease: An electron microscopic histochemical, and biochemical study. Arch. Path. (Chicago), **89**, 103, 1970.
22. Dienst, N., and Hamperl, H.: Über einen Fall von lipoidzelligen Splenohepatomegalie vom Typus Niemann-Pick. Wien. Klin. Wschr., **40**, 1432, 1927.
23. Dienst, N., and Hamperl, H.: Über einen Fall von lipoidzelliger Splenomegalie. Wien. Med. Wschr., **77**, 1597, 1927.
24. Dienst, N.: Über einen Fall von lipoidzelliger Splenohepatomegalie. J. Kinderheil. Physische Erziehung, **123**, 181, 1929.
25. Hamperl, H.: Über die pathologisch-anatomischen Veranderungen bei Morbus Gaucher im Sauglingsalter. Virchow. Arch. [Zellpath.], **271**, 147, 1929.
26. Alexander, W. S.: Niemann-Pick disease: Report of a case showing calcification in the adrenal glands. New. Zeal. Med. J., **45**, 43, 1946.
27. Stransky, E.: Über grosszellige Splenohepatomegalie. Jahrb. Kinderheilk., **126**, 204, 1930.
28. Henschen, F., in discussion of Klercker, O.: Contribution à l'étude de la maladie de Gaucher. Acta Med. Scand., suppl. **16**, 593, 1926.
29. Patrick, A. D., and Lake, B. D.: Deficiency of an acid lipase in Wolman's disease. Nature (London), **222**, 1067, 1969.
30. Patrick, A. D., and Lake, B. D.: An acid lipase deficiency in Wolman's disease. Biochem. J., **112**, 29P, 1969.
31. Kwiterovich, P. O., Sloan, H. R., and Fredrickson, D. S.: Glycolipids and other lipid constituents of normal human liver. J. Lipid Res., **11**, 322, 1970.
32. Suomi, W. D., and Agranoff, B. W.: Lipids of the spleen in Gaucher's disease. J. Lipid Res., **6**, 211, 1965.
33. Sloan, H. R.: Unpublished data.

34. Frantz, I. D., Jr., and Shroepfer, G. J., Jr.: Sterol biosynthesis. Ann. Rev. Biochem., **36,** 691, 1967.
35. Goodman, D. S., and Noble, R. P.: Turnover of plasma cholesterol in man. J. Clin. Invest., **47,** 231, 1968.
36. Grundy, S. M., and Ahrens, E. H., Jr.: Measurements of cholesterol turnover synthesis and absorption in man, carried out by isotope kinetic and sterol balance methods. J. Lipid Res., **10,** 91, 1969.
37. Nestel, P. J., Whyte, H. M., and Goodman, DeW. S.: Distribution and turnover of cholesterol in humans. J. Clin. Invest., **48,** 982, 1969.
38. Dietschy, J. M., and Wilson, J. D.: Regulation of cholesterol metabolism. New Eng. J. Med., **282,** 1128, 1179, 1241, 1970.
39. Goodman, DeW. S.: Cholesterol ester metabolism. Physiol. Rev., **45,** 747, 1965.
40. Vahouny, G. V., and Treadwell, C. R.: Enzymatic synthesis and hydrolysis of cholesterol esters. Meth. Biochem. Anal., **16,** 219, 1968.
41. Quarfordt, S. H., and Goodman, DeW. S.: Chylomicron cholesteryl ester metabolism in the perfused rat liver. Biochim. Biophys. Acta, **176,** 863, 1969.
42. Brot, N., Lossow, W. J., and Chaikoff, I. L.: *In vitro* uptake and hydrolysis, by rat tissues, of cholesterol esters of a very low density, chyle lipoprotein fraction. J. Lipid Res., **5,** 63, 1964.
43. Goller, H. J., Sgoutas, D. S., Ismail, I. A., and Gunstone, F. D.: Dependence of sterol ester hydrolase activity on the position of ethylenic bond in cholesteryl *cis*-octadecenoates. Biochemistry (Wash.), **9,** 3072, 1970.
44. Shapiro, B.: Lipid Metabolism. Ann. Rev. Biochem., **36,** 247, 1967.
45. Nikkila, E. A.: Control of plasma and liver triglyceride kinetics by carbohydrate metabolism and insulin, in *Advances in Lipid Research,* edited by R. Paoletti and D. Kritchevsky, vol. 7, p. 63. Academic, New York, 1969.
46. Redgrave, T. G.: Formation of cholesteryl ester-rich particulate lipid during metabolism of chylomicrons. J. Clin. Invest., **49,** 465, 1970.
47. Havel, R. J.: Metabolism of lipids in chylomicrons and very low density lipoproteins, in *Handbook of Physiology,* sec. 5, *Adipose Tissue,* edited by A. E. Renold and G. F. Cahill, Jr., chap. 50, p. 499. American Physiology Society, Wash., D.C., 1965.
48. Hollenberg, C. H.: Adipose tissue lipases II, in *Handbook of Physiology,* sec. 5, *Adipose Tissue,* edited by A. E. Renold and G. F. Cahill, Jr., chap. 29, p. 301. American Physiology Society, Wash., D.C., 1965.
49. Rizack, M. A.: Hormone-sensitive lipolytic activity of adipose tissue, in *Handbook of Physiology,* sec. 5, *Adipose Tissue,* edited by A. E. Renold and G. F. Cahill, Jr., chap. 30, p. 309. American Physiology Society, Wash., D.C., 1965.
50. Steinberg, D., and Vaughan, M.: Release of free fatty acids from adipose tissue *in vitro* in relation to rates of triglyceride synthesis and degradation, in *Handbook of Physiology,* sec. 5, *Adipose Tissue,* edited by A. E. Renold and G. F. Cahill, Jr., chap. 34, p. 335. American Physiology Society, Wash., D.C., 1965.
51. Vaughan, M., and Steinberg, D.: Glyceride biosynthesis, glyceride breakdown and glycogen breakdown in adipose tissue: Mechanisms and regulation, in *Handbook of Physiology,* sec. 5, *Adipose Tissue,* edited by A. E. Renold and G. F. Cahill, Jr., chap. 24, p. 239. American Physiology Society, Wash., D.C., 1965.
52. LaRosa, J. C., Levy, R. I., Windmueller, H. G., and Fredrickson, D. S.: Evidence for the heterogeneity of triglyceride lipases in post-heparin plasma. J. Clin. Invest., **49,** 55a, 1970.
52*a*. Mahadevan, S., and Tappel, A. L.: Lysosomal lipases of rat liver and kidney. Arch. Biochem., **126,** 945, 1968.
53. Hers, H. G.: Inborn lysosomal diseases. Gastroenterology, **48,** 625, 1965.
54. Bloodworth, J. M. B., Jr.: *Endocrine Pathology,* p. 224. Williams & Wilkins, Baltimore, 1968.
55. Meyers, M. A.: Diseases of the adrenal glands, in *Radiologic Diagnosis.* Charles C Thomas, Springfield, Ill., 1963.
56. Aguilar, M. J., O'Brien, J. S., and Taber, P.: The syndrome of familial leukodystrophy, adrenal insufficiency and cutaneous melanosis, in *Inborn Disorders of Sphingolipid Metabolism, Proc. Third Internat. Symp. Cerebral Sphingolipidoses,* edited by S. M. Aronson and B. W. Volk. Pergamon, New York, 1967.
57. Fredrickson, D. S.: Newly recognized disorders of cholesterol metabolism. Presented at the American College of Physicians Meeting, Denver, Colo., April 1–5, 1963.
58. Fredrickson, D. S.: Newly recognized disorders of cholesterol metabolism, in *The Metabolic Basis of Inherited Disease,* edited by J. B. Stanbury, J. B. Wyngaarden, and D. S. Fredrickson, 2d ed., chap. 23, p. 502. McGraw-Hill, New York, 1966.
59. Lageron, A., Caroli, J., Stralin, H., and Barbier, P.: Polycorie Cholestérolique de l'adulte. I. Étude clinique, électronique, histochimique. Presse Medicale (Paris), **75,** 2785, 1967.
60. Infante, R., Polonovski, J., and Caroli, J.: Polycorie Cholestérolique de l'adulte. II. Étude biochimique. Presse Medicale (Paris), **75,** 2829, 1967.
61. Schiff, L., Schubert, W. K., McAdams, A. J., Spiegel, E. L., and O'Donnell, J. F.: Hepatic cholesterol ester storage disease, a familial disorder. I. Clinical aspects. Amer. J. Med., **44,** 538, 1968.
62. Partin, J. C., and Schubert, W. K.: Small intestinal mucosa in cholesterol ester storage disease: A light and electron microscope study. Gastroenterology, **57,** 542, 1969.
63. Debré, R., Semelaigne, G., Nachmansohn, and Gilbrin: Les Hepatomegalies polycoriques. Bull. Soc. Med. Hop. Paris, **50,** 1023, 1934.
64. Van Creveld, S.: Glycogen disease. Medicine (Balt.), **18,** 1, 1939.
65. Tada, K., Katsushima, N., Hirono, H., and Arakawa, T.: Congenital steatosis of the liver: Biochemical approach to its pathogenesis. Tohoku J. Exp. Med., **77,** 317, 1962.
66. Fredrickson, D. S.: Unpublished data.
67. Fredrickson, D. S.: Sphingomyelin lipidosis: Niemann-Pick disease, in *The Metabolic Basis of Inherited Disease,* edited by J. B. Stanbury. J. B. Wyngaarden, and D. S. Fredrickson, 2d ed., p. 586. McGraw-Hill, New York, 1966.
68. Fredrickson, D. S.: Tangier disease, in *The Metabolic Basis of Inherited Disease,* edited by J. B. Stanbury, J. B. Wyngaarden, and D. S. Fredrickson, 2d ed., p. 486. McGraw-Hill, New York, 1966.
69. Hellman, L., Rosenfeld, R. S., Eidinoff, M. L., Fukushima, D. K., Gallagher, T. F., Wang, C. I., and Adlersberg, D.: Isotopic studies of plasma cholesterol of endogenous and exogenous origins. J. Clin. Invest., **34,** 48, 1955.
70. Nestel, P. J., and Monger, E. A.: Turnover of plasma esterified cholesterol in normocholesterolemic and hypercholesterolemic subjects and its relation to body build. J. Clin. Invest., **46,** 967, 1967.
71. van Bogaert, L., Scherer, H. J., and Epstein, E.: *Une Forme Cerebrale de la Cholestérinose Généralisée.* Masson et Cie, Paris, 1937.
72. Menkes, J. H., Schimschock, J. R., and Swanson, P. D.: Cerebrotendinous xanthomatosis: The storage of cholestanol within the nervous system. Arch. Neurol. (Chicago), **19,** 47, 1968.
73. Philippart, M., and van Bogaert, L.: Cholestanolosis (cerebrotendinous xanthomatosis): A follow-up study on the original family. Arch. Neurol. (Chicago), **21,** 603, 1969.
74. Schneider, C.: Über eine eigenartige Hirnerkrankung (vaskuläre Lipoidose). Allg. Zschr Psychiat., **104,** 144, 1936.
75. van Bogaert, L., Scherer, H. J., Froehlich, A., and Epstein, E.: Une deuxième observation de cholestérinose tendineuse symétrique avec symptômes cérébraux. Ann. Med., **42,** 69, 1937.
76. van Bogaert, L.: Les aspects neurologiques des cholestérinases généralisées. Progr. Med. (Paris), **22,** 785, 1938.
77. Epstein, E., and Lorenz, K.: Beitrag zur Pathologie und Pathochemie der cholesterinigen Lipoidose vom Typus van Bogaert-Scherer. Klin. Wschr., **16,** 1320, 1937.
78. Epstein, E., and Kreitner, H.: Beitrag zu einer vergleichenden Pathologie und Pathochemie der allgemeinen Cholesterinlipoidosen. Virchow. Arch. [Zellpath.], **306,** 53, 1940.
79. Guillain, G., Bertrand, I., and Godet-Guillain, M.: Étude anatomoclinique d'un cas de cholestérinose cerebrale. Rev. Neurol. (Paris), **74,** 249, 1942.
80. Giampalmo, A.: Über einen Fall von Cholesterinlipoidose vom Typus van Bogaert-Scherer. Verh. Deutsch Ges. Path., **34,** 227, 1950.
81. Vinditti, D.: Una Rara lipoidosi Di Interesse Ortopedico: Forma

Cerebro-Tendinea Della Colesterinosi Generalizzata. Chir. Organi Mov., **34,** 429, 1950.
82. Giampalmo, A.: Les Lipoidoses cholestériniques du système nerveux. Rev. Neurol. (Paris), **89,** 322, 1953.
83. Giampalmo, A.: Les lipidoses cholestériniques du système nerveux. Acta Neurol. Belg., **54,** 786, 1954.
84. Stein, W., and Czuczwar, S.: W sprawie cholesterozy mosgowoscieng-nowej v. Bogaerta-Scherera-Epsteina. Neurol. Neurochir. Pol., **9,** 599, 1959.
85. van Bogaert, L.: Le cadre des xanthomatoses et leurs differents types: Xanthomatoses secondaires. Rev. Med. (Liège), **17,** 433, 1962.
86. Menkes, J. H., and Philippart, M.: Cholestanol storage in the nervous system of two patients with cerebrotendinous xanthomatosis. Trans. Amer. Neurol. Ass., **93,** 66, 1968.
87. Mückenhausen, C., Derby, B. M., and Moses, H. W.: Conversion of ^{14}C-cholesterol to cholestanol in cerebrotendinous xanthomatosis. Fed. Proc., **28,** 882, 1968.
88. Naarden, A. L.: In discussion of ref. 86.
89. Schimschock, J. R., Alvord, E. C., Jr., and Swanson, P. D.: Cerebrotendinous xanthomatosis: Clinical and pathological studies. Arch. Neurol. (Chicago), **18,** 688, 1968.
90. Stahl, W. L., Sumi, S. M., and Swanson, P. D.: Subcellular distribution of cerebral cholestanol in cerebrotendinous xanthomatosis. J. Neurochem., in press.
91. Shefer, S., Milch, S., and Mosbach, E. H.: Biosynthesis of 5α-cholestan-3β-ol in the rabbit and guinea pig. J. Biol. Chem., **239,** 1731, 1964.
92. Werbin, H., Chaikoff, I. L., and Imada, M. R.: 5α-Cholestan 3β-ol: Its distribution in tissues and its synthesis from cholesterol in the guinea pig. J. Biol. Chem., **237,** 2072, 1962.
93. Werbin, H., Chaikoff, I. L., and Phillips, B. P.: Conversion of cholesterol to 5α-cholestan-3β-ol in germ free guinea pigs. Biochemistry (Wash.), **3,** 1558, 1964.
94. Shefer, S., Hauser, S., and Mosbach, E. H.: Studies on the biosynthesis of 5α-cholestan-3β-ol. I. Cholestenone 5α-reductase of rat liver. J. Biol. Chem., **241,** 946, 1966.
95. Harold, F. M., Chapman, D. D., and Chaikoff, I. L.: Metabolism of cholestanol. I. Fate of cholestanol-4-C^{14} in the rat. J. Biol. Chem., **224,** 609, 1957.
96. Gould, R. G., and Cook, R. P.: The metabolism of cholesterol and other sterols in the animal organism, in *Cholesterol: Pathology,* edited by R. P. Cook. Academic, New York, 1958.
97. Hofmann, A. F., Bokkenheuser, V., Hirsch, R. L., and Mosbach, E. H.: Experimental cholelithiasis in the rabbit induced by cholestanol feeding; effect of neomycin treatment on bile composition and gallstone formation. J. Lipid Res., **9,** 244, 1968.
98. Harlan, W. R., and Still, W. J. S.: Hereditary tendinous and tuberous xanthomatosis without hyperlipemia. New Eng. J. Med., **278,** 416, 1968.
99. Swanson, P. D., and Harlan, W. R., Jr.: Cerebrotendinous xanthomatosis: Letters to the editor. New Eng. J. Med., **278,** 857, 1968.
100. Thiebaut, F.: Paraplégie spasmodiques et xanthomes tendineux associés: Des rapports de ce syndrome avec la cholestérinose cérébrospinale. Rev. Neurol. (Paris), **74,** 313, 1942.
101. van Bogaert, L.: Spinal cholesterolosis. Brain, **88,** 687, 1965.
102. Ortiz de Zarate, J. C.: Colesterinos cristallina cerebral de Scherer, van Bogaert y Epstein. Rev. Neurol. Buenos Aires, **19,** 159, 1961.

CHAPTER THIRTY-SEVEN

PHYTANIC ACID STORAGE DISEASE: REFSUM'S SYNDROME

Daniel Steinberg

INTRODUCTION AND RÉSUMÉ

In 1946 Sigvald Refsum published his definitive monograph identifying a new familial neurologic syndrome which he designated *heredopathia atactica polyneuritiformis* [1]. The primary clinical features, almost all of them seen in Refsum's original cases, are listed in Table 37-1. Individually, none of the findings was unique but Refsum astutely concluded that the pattern in his five original cases, occurring in two inbred Norwegian families, could be distinguished from those seen in the many clinically related heredo-ataxic syndromes previously described. By 1960 there were 29 case reports in the literature [2] and the syndrome was widely accepted as a clinical entity, but there had been little progress toward defining the pathogenesis or the underlying biochemical lesion. Cammermeyer had called attention to lipid infiltration and, with Refsum, suggested a possible relation to the lipidoses (cited in Ref. 1) but the early postmortem findings were not completely consonant on this score [3].

The first direct evidence that the syndrome described by Refsum stemmed from a specific biochemical defect was published by Klenk and Kahlke in 1963 [4]. They anaylzed postmortem tissues from a 7-year-old girl diagnosed as an example of Refsum's syndrome by Richterich and coworkers in Berne [5]. Liver and kidney were grossly infiltrated with lipid, mostly neutral lipid, but no unusual complex lipids were detected. Gas chromatographic analysis revealed a large abnormal peak which accounted for over 50 percent of the total fatty acids in liver lipids. This component was isolated in pure form and fully characterized as phytanic acid, a 20-carbon branched-chain acid not previously reported in human tissues (Fig. 37-1). In plasma of patients with Refsum's syndrome, phytanic acid was found in amounts corresponding to 5 to 30 percent of the total fatty acids [6]. Normal human plasma contains traces of phytanic acid (less than 0.3 mg per 100 ml), amounts so small that they are generally undetectable in routine analyses [7, 8].

Two general hypotheses suggested themselves concerning the origin of the phytanic acid accumulating [9, 10]. The polyisoprenoid structure of phytanic acid suggested a biosynthetic origin by pathways related to that for sterol synthesis. However, studies in patients with Refsum's syndrome [11, 12] and in experimental animals [13] failed to demonstrate any endogenous synthesis. These results pointed to an exogenous origin for the accumulated phytanic acid and a defect in catabolism as the basis for its accumulation. Phytol (Fig. 37-1), a component of the chlorophyll molecule, was shown to be readily convertible to phytanic acid [11–17], and both phytol and phytanic acid itself were shown to be potential dietary sources since they accumulated when fed in large doses to experimental animals [14–16, 18, 19].

A series of studies by Steinberg and coworkers established the major pathway for phytanic acid oxidation in man and experimental animals (Fig. 37-2) [20–24]. It involves (1) an unusual initial α-oxidation to yield the $(n-1)$ fatty acid, pristanic acid; and (2) a series of successive β-oxidation steps for the further degradation of pristanic acid. Rates of phytanic acid oxidation in patients were shown to be less than 5 percent of normal [11, 12, 25, 26], and the defect was shown to persist in fibroblast cell cultures [27]. The latter finding greatly facilitated the further studies which led to identification of the site of the metabolic block. Evidence from clinical observations [26] and cell culture studies [27–29] indicated that the primary enzyme defect lies at the first step in the new metabolic pathway, i.e., in the conversion of phytanic acid to α-hydroxyphytanic acid. Results of

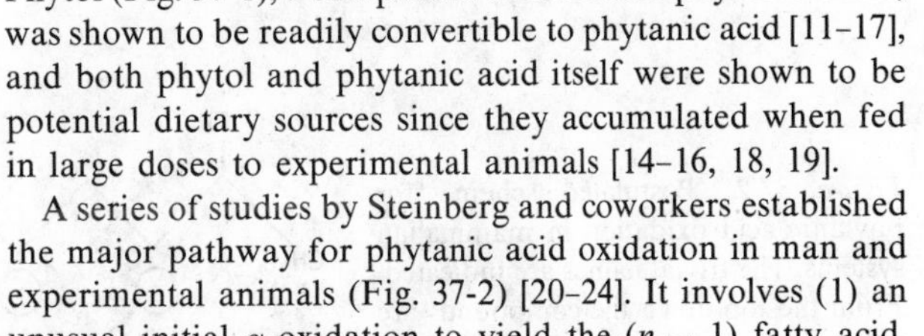

Table 37-1. CLINICAL FEATURES IN PHYTANIC ACID STORAGE DISEASE

Retinitis pigmentosa: failing night vision*; progressive constriction of visual fields; lenticular opacities (See Plate II-3)

Peripheral polyneuropathy: generally symmetrical; motor and sensory losses; absent or diminished deep tendon reflexes

Cerebellar ataxia: dyscoordination out of proportion to degree of peripheral neuropathy; unsteady gait; Romberg sign; intention tremor; nystagmus

Elevated cerebrospinal fluid protein level without pleocytosis

Familial incidence with autosomal recessive pattern of inheritance

Nerve deafness, anosmia, pupillary abnormalities

Nonspecific ECG changes

Ichthyosis-like changes: ranging from mild hyperkeratosis of palms and soles to florid ichthyosis on trunk

Epiphyseal dysplasia: short 4th metatarsal, syndactyly, hammer toe, pes cavus, osteochondritis dissecans

* Some authors have used the term *hemeralopia* to designate poor vision in dim light, whereas medical dictionaries define the term to mean "day blindness." We shall use the less ambiguous term "night blindness."

$$\mathrm{CH_3\text{-}CH(CH_3)\text{-}CH_2\text{-}CH_2\text{-}CH_2\text{-}CH(CH_3)\text{-}CH_2\text{-}CH_2\text{-}CH_2\text{-}CH(CH_3)\text{-}CH_2\text{-}CH_2\text{-}CH_2\text{-}C(CH_3){=}CH\text{-}CH_2\text{-}OH}$$

$$\mathrm{CH_3\text{-}CH(CH_3)\text{-}CH_2\text{-}CH_2\text{-}CH_2\text{-}CH(CH_3)\text{-}CH_2\text{-}CH_2\text{-}CH_2\text{-}CH(CH_3)\text{-}CH_2\text{-}CH_2\text{-}CH_2\text{-}CH(CH_3)\text{-}CH_2\text{-}COOH}$$

Figure 37-1. Structures of phytol (*top*) and phytanic acid (*bottom*). Note that the structures are identical, except for the presence of a double bond in the 2,3 position and the presence of an alcohol function rather than a carboxylic acid function at carbon 1 in phytol.

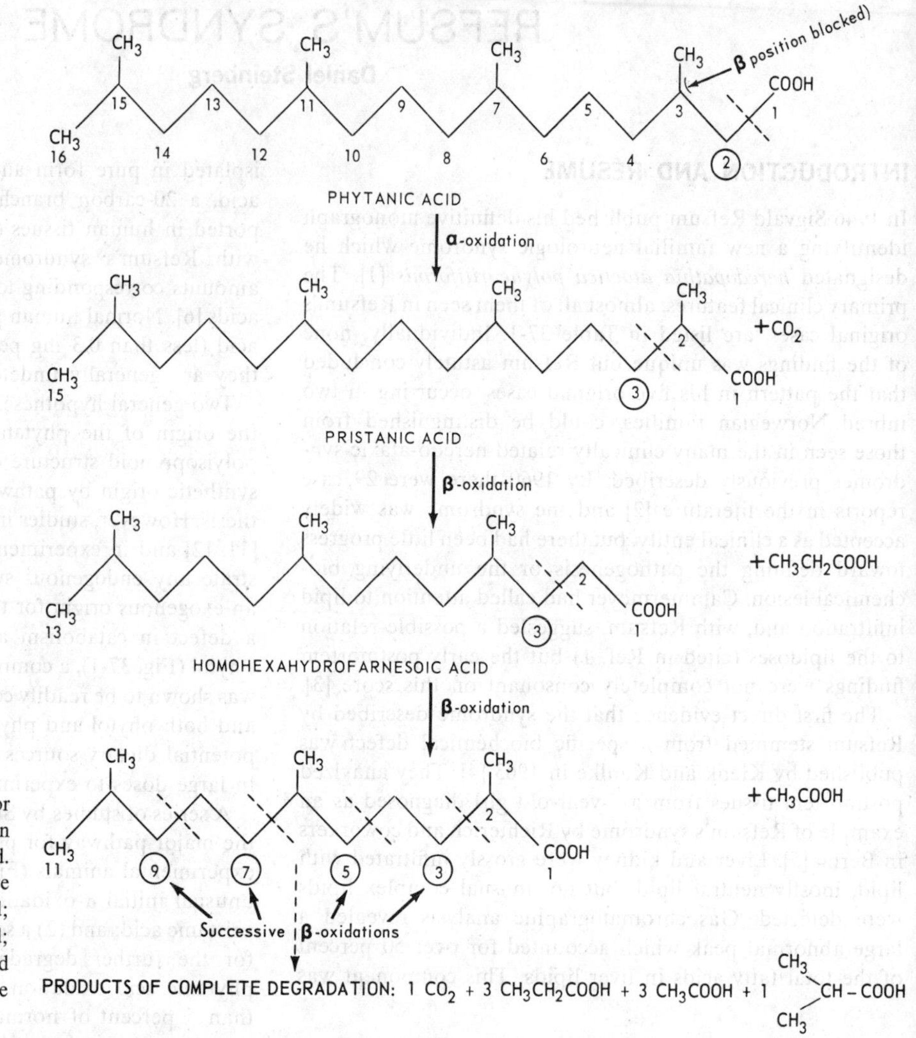

Figure 37-2. Postulated scheme for phytanic acid oxidation in mammalian systems. The trivial names are indicated. From the top down the compounds are 3,7,11,15-tetramethylhexadecanoic acid; 2,6,10,14-tetramethylpentadecanoic acid; 4,8,12-trimethyltridecanoic acid; and 2,6,10-trimethylundecanoic acid (see Fig. 37-7).

studies with model substrates structurally related to phytanic acid were compatible with this conclusion [30, 31].

As soon as it was established that phytanic acid had an exogenous origin, the possibility of therapeutic intervention by eliminating dietary sources of phytanate and its precursors was investigated. It has been clearly shown that dietary modification does indeed reduce plasma and tissue levels of phytanic acid [25, 32–34]. Changes in clinical progress are difficult to evaluate because of the irregularly fluctuating natural course of the disease. However, the limited experience available to date suggests that dietary treatment with reduction of phytanate levels may arrest progress and lead to partial remission [32–34].

Use of the cell culture technique has established that in presumed heterozygotes (parents of clinical cases) the rate of phytanate oxidation is reduced to about one-half the normal rate. Although parents of patients are symptom-free, elevation of plasma phytanic acid in presumed heterozygotes has been reported in a few instances, possibly because of a relative (and possibly intermittent) imbalance between their somewhat reduced oxidative capacity and their intake of phytanate or its precursors.

Thus, in the relatively short period of 6 years from the identification of phytanic acid by Klenk and Kahlke, it was possible (1) to establish that phytanic acid accumulates in Refsum's disease because of a defect in its removal; (2) to elucidate in some detail the novel α-oxidative pathway for its degradation; (3) to define narrowly the site of the metabolic block; (4) to demonstrate the carrier state biochemically; and (5) to propose and validate tentatively an approach to therapy through modification of the diet. The pace of these advances testifies to the power of modern tools for the study of metabolic disease, in this case including particularly gas-liquid chromatography, mass spectroscopy, and cell culture techniques. Phytanic acid storage disease is the first example of a genetic error in fatty acid oxidation. Complete deletion of straight-chain fatty acid oxidizing systems would probably represent a lethal mutation, but other nonlethal mutations affecting less vital systems (e.g., ω-oxidation or the α-oxidation system in nerve) will likely be detected. Incompletely expressed lesions may be found even in the key system for β-oxidation.

While the metabolic basis for phytanic acid accumulation is well established, the pathogenesis of the nerve degeneration remains uncertain. As discussed below, the fact that dietary treatment arrests progress and results in some amelioration of the neuropathy, coincident with reduction of plasma and tissue phytanate levels, supports a direct pathogenetic role for phytanate. Attempts to induce the disease in experimental animals by feeding phytol or phytanic acid have been negative [19, 36]. Further work is needed to explore the link between the well-defined biochemical abnormality and the poorly understood biological abnormality. Phytanic acid storage disease itself is relatively rare but many more common diseases with similar manifestations are known to the neurologist. In most cases, he is helpless to do more than classify. Perhaps closing the gap between biochemistry and biology in this demyelinating disease may open approaches to understanding others.

DEFINITIONS

Analysis of serum lipids, tissue biopsies, or postmortem tissues has revealed the presence of stored phytanic acid in almost every case diagnosed clinically as Refsum's syndrome, and normal (trace) levels have been found in a large number of related neurologic entities [25, 34, 37]. Concordance between clinical diagnosis and phytanic acid storage has been established in at least 34 cases thus far [38], but there are some exceptions. Two patients with clinical features difficult to distinguish from those typically found have been described in which there was no demonstrable accumulation of phytanate [34, 39]. Further work may clarify the relationship between pathogenesis in these cases *sine* phytanate and that of the more usual cases *cum* phytanate. At present it is preferable to designate as examples of *phytanic acid storage disease* only those patients with *both* (1) the typical clinical syndrome, *and* (2) demonstrated accumulation of phytanic acid *or* demonstrated reduction in capacity to oxidize phytanic acid. The latter stipulation is included since even patients with drastically reduced capacity to metabolize phytanate may, when kept on the appropriate diet, all but free themselves of the stored acid [33, 34]. Their capacity to oxidize phytanate, however, remains deficient [26].

Even narrower definition at the biochemical level can now be proposed. In 14 clinically typical patients studied in vivo or in cell culture, or both, the oxidation of pristanic acid, the α-oxidation product of phytanic acid, was normal. This established that the metabolic error is a phytanic acid α-oxidase deficiency [35]. In 3 of the 14 patients thus far tested, oxidation of α-hydroxyphytanate was also normal [26, 29]. Thus, these patients, and perhaps most or all others with phytanic acid storage disease, are examples of *phytanic acid α-hydroxylase deficiency.*

Presumed heterozygotes (parents or sibs of clinical cases) have occasionally shown phytanate accumulation without evidence of neurological involvement [40, 41]. Since heterozygotes have about a 50 percent reduction in capacity to oxidize phytanate [35], it is understandable that these individuals may tend to accumulate phytanic acid but to a much more limited extent than homozygotes. The normal level of oxidative capacity is far in excess of that needed to dissimulate the usual intake of phytanate and precursors in the diet. On the other hand, it is conceivable that under the appropriate circumstances (excessive dietary load or imposition of extrinsic factors accentuating the metabolic defect) these heterozygotes may store phytanic acid and possibly develop clinical disease. Thus, heterozygotes may be designated as examples of *phytanic acid storage trait.*

Several reviews are available that include extensive discussion of clinical aspects, differential diagnosis, and pathologic findings [1–3, 25, 37, 38, 42, 43]. The emphasis in this chapter is placed primarily on the metabolic pathway for phytanic acid oxidation, the nature of the enzymatic deficiency, genetic aspects, and pathogenesis.

CLINICAL FINDINGS AND DIFFERENTIAL DIAGNOSIS

The tetrad of retinitis pigmentosa, peripheral polyneuropathy, cerebellar ataxia, and a high CSF protein concentration in the absence of pleocytosis has been found in virtually every patient with phytanic acid storage disease. Additional clinical findings are listed in Table 37-1. As brought out below, the various clinical features may appear sequentially as the disease progresses; thus incomplete syndromes early in the course are to be expected and have been described in patients already showing storage of phytanic acid.

The onset of the disease has been detected in early childhood in some but not until the fifth decade in others. Most patients have clear-cut manifestations before age 20. Presenting complaints relate to failing vision and weakness in extremities or unsteadiness of gait. The earliest symptom is almost always night blindness, although it may require careful questioning to elicit this history and establish the true date of onset.

The course of the disease is one of gradually progressive deterioration, interrupted in over half of the patients by unexplained and sometimes lengthy periods of remission. Dramatic exacerbation associated with an ill-defined febrile illness, a surgical procedure, or pregnancy has been noted, as in Friedreich's ataxia. Gradual recovery of function following such episodes is the rule, but residual neurologic deficits remain.

A representative case history is that of patient J.S., reported first by Ashenhurst et al. [44] and later studied intensively from a clinical and biochemical point of view at the Clinical Center in Bethesda, Maryland [25, 33]:

Anosmia and night blindness were present from early childhood. The former caused no particular difficulty; the latter was sufficiently severe that at age 13 the patient was unable to make his way home from school in the dusk. However, medical advice was never sought for these problems. At age 21 he developed an influenza-like illness that persisted over a period of 2 weeks or so. Toward the end of this time an alarming weakness developed in all four extremities and he was admitted to the hospital. Examination at that time showed bilateral pes cavus, ataxia, marked muscular weakness, absence of all deep tendon reflexes, some generalized wasting in the upper and lower limbs, anosmia, constriction of visual fields with retinitis pigmentosa, and nystagmus. The diagnosis entertained at the time was Friedreich's ataxia. Over the next months there was progressive improvement and by 6 months motor power was almost fully restored. Previously absent reflexes were now elicited in the arms although knee jerks and ankle jerks were still unobtainable. Foot drop persisted bilaterally and was so severe as to require bilateral arthrodesis with considerable benefit to the patient. Lumbar puncture some 4 months after the acute attack revealed clear fluid with no increase in cell count, but a protein content of 450 mg per 100 ml, suggesting a diagnosis of acute idiopathic polyneuritis. Over the next few years there were two or three episodes of exacerbation of motor symptoms, each accompanied by a rise in CSF protein. A diagnosis of Refsum's syndrome was made. At the time of the first admission, opacities were noticed at the posterior pole of each lens. Eventually opacification became total and lenticular extraction was performed on the right, which restored some vision. Over these same years he developed tinnitus with progressive hearing loss. Ultimately, all hearing in both ears was totally lost.

When admitted to the Clinical Center at NIH in 1964 he showed mild scaling and thickening on palms and soles but no dermatologic changes elsewhere. Tendon reflexes were unobtainable and muscular weakness, particularly distally, was marked. In addition, there were clear-cut sensory losses, including decreases in light touch and pinprick in stocking-and-glove distribution to the knees and elbows. Vibration and position sense were almost absent in the toes and slightly diminished in the legs to the iliac crests. Shortly after admission he noted pain in the left eye and intraocular pressure was found to be elevated. A lenticular extraction was performed with relief of symptoms, but without significant improvement in visual acuity because of the underlying retinal degeneration. The diagnosis was confirmed by demonstration of phytanic acid as a major constituent of plasma fatty acids. Levels were initially about 100 mg per 100 ml. Blood urea nitrogen was slightly elevated (30 mg per 100 ml) and creatinine reduced but urine sediment was normal and there was no proteinuria. Lipid in the urine could not be demonstrated. Total urinary α-amino nitrogen was within normal limits. Plasma ceruloplasmin was within normal limits. Karyotype was normal. The electrocardiogram was interpreted as demonstrating left ventricular hypertrophy and strain.

Four of the eight deaths reported have occurred suddenly and without established cause. In view of the ECG changes that accompany the disease, nonspecific in most cases but including a few examples of impaired A-V conduction and bundle-branch block, a cardiac arrhythmia is suspected as the basis. Two deaths were attributed to respiratory paralysis and two to bacterial pneumonia, respiratory insufficiency not being mentioned explicitly as a factor.

Much increased levels of phytanic acid have been demonstrated in the serum of virtually every case of Refsum's syndrome examined for it. Conversely, no increases in phytanic acid level have been found in any of a wide variety of other neurologic syndromes, some of them closely related to Refsum's syndrome [25, 37, 38, 43]. Some of the more important negative results are those in Dejerine-Sottas hypertrophic peripheral neuropathy, Friedreich's ataxia, multiple sclerosis, retinitis pigmentosa of both the recessive and dominant types, a larger number of nonspecific heredoataxias, peroneal muscular atrophy (Charcot-Marie-Tooth syndrome), abetalipoproteinemia, high density lipoprotein deficiency (Tangier disease), amyotrophic lateral sclerosis, Sjögren-Larsson syndrome, Marinesco-Sjögren syndrome, Spielmeyer-Vogt disease, and Tay-Sachs disease.

METABOLIC BASIS FOR ACCUMULATION OF PHYTANATE

General Nature of the Metabolic Error

Both endogenous and exogenous origins of the stored phytanic acid have been considered. Thus far there is no evidence for any significant rate of endogenous synthesis from low molecular weight precursors. On the other hand, it has been shown that phytanic acid itself, phytol, and the side chain of vitamin $K_2(_{20})$ (phylloquinone) are potential dietary sources. The diet of patients has not been found to be unusual, i.e., there is no evidence for excessive intake of dietary precursors, nor do patients have any unusual capacity to absorb phytol either free or in chlorophyll-bound form. Clinical studies, as well as studies in isolated fibroblast cell cultures, establish directly a marked deficiency in the rate of phytanic acid oxidation in patients.

Evidence against Endogenous Synthesis

The polyisoprenoid structure of phytanic acid suggested that it might be endogenously synthesized by a pathway such as that outlined in Fig. 37-3. Geranylgeranyl pyrophosphate is a normal intermediate in carotene biosynthesis [45], and Nandi and Porter have reported its synthesis in pig-liver homogenates [46]. In plants, phytol is formed from mevalonic acid by such a pathway [47] and thus there is precedent for the reduction of double bonds in the polyisoprenoid series. The postulated conversion of the alcohol to a carboxylic acid would be analogous to the demonstrated oxidation of farnesol to farnesoic acid [48].

Attempts to demonstrate biosynthesis from 2-^{14}C-labeled mevalonic acid in a patient with phytanic acid storage dis-

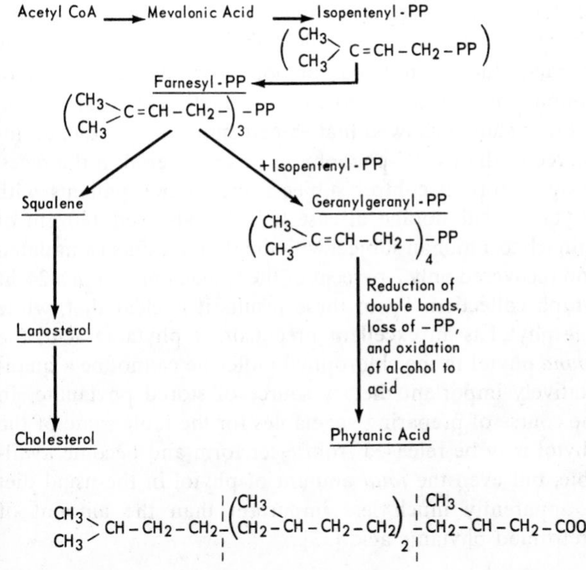

Figure 37-3. Postulated scheme for endogenous biosynthesis of phytanic acid by a pathway branching from that for sterol biosynthesis. No evidence for the operation of the pathway shown on the right has been obtained in animals or in man. While this pathway may operate in the biosynthetic pathway in plants and bacteria, it does not apparently operate at any significant rate in mammals.

ease were negative [11, 12], however, and neither labeled acetate nor mevalonate was incorporated into phytanate in experimental animals [13]. To rule out the possibility of a very slow rate of endogenous synthesis and to test for alternative pathways of biosynthesis from small molecules, clinical studies were carried out in two patients using D_2O as a precursor [12, 33]. Body water was held at a constant level of enrichment over 4 to 5 months. Plasma cholesterol showed the expected progressive enrichment in deuterium but plasma phytanate showed minimal enrichment, near the limits of detectability, corresponding to replacement of only two to four hydrogen atoms. Some enrichment would be expected as a result of the conversion of dietary phytol to phytanic acid. The results make it unlikely that there is any significant degree of endogenous *de novo* biosynthesis of phytanic acid in man or animals.

Origin from Dietary Phytanic Acid

Prior to the 1963 report of Klenk and Kahlke, phytanic acid had not been identified in plant or animal tissues. Hansen and Shorland had previously observed the presence in butterfat of a trace fatty acid component with 20 carbon atoms and properties indicating a branched-chain structure [49]. The first definitive proof of structure was published by Sonneveld et al. in 1962 [50]. They estimated that phytanic acid accounted for 0.05 percent of total fatty acids in butter.

Unusually large amounts of phytanic acid have been found in ruminant plasma lipids, accounting in some cases for up to 5 to 10 percent of total fatty acids [7, 51, 52]; trace amounts occur in other ruminant tissues, including the rumen [53–55]. Plasma of nonruminant animals and of normal man contains only traces (0.1 to 0.5 percent of total fatty acids) [7, 8].

A preliminary survey of some common foods revealed trace amounts of phytanic acid (e.g., in tomatoes and squash), but in most there was none detectable [25]. Marine lipids contain phytanic acid but again in only trace amounts [56–58]. A systematic survey of foods has yet to be carried out, but it appears that dairy products and ruminant fats may be the major sources.

Some measure of the daily intake of phytanic acid comes from analyses done of a typical American hospital diet [25]. Aliquots were taken of all foods consumed over a 7-day period and phytanate was determined in the saponified total lipid extract. The estimated daily intake was 56 mg. Similar analysis of the diet of a patient of Dr. I. A. M. Prior in New Zealand yielded an estimated daily intake of 89 mg [59].

In the rat, orally administered phytanic acid is well absorbed even when fed in large doses and most of the absorption occurs by way of the lymph [60]. Direct studies of phytanic acid absorption in man are not available. Since phytol absorption in man is similar to that in the rat [11, 15–17], it may be reasonable to assume that at least 50 to 75 percent of the small amounts of phytanic acid in the daily diet is in fact absorbed.

Origin from Dietary Phytol

Free Phytol

Phytol, differing in structure from phytanic acid only in having a Δ^2-double bond and an alcohol rather than a carboxylic acid function at carbon-1 (Fig. 37-1), is readily converted to phytanic acid [11–17]. Two pathways are possible, depending on the sequence in which the double-bond reduction and the oxidation of the alcohol function occurs (Fig. 37-4). Both the 2,3-unsaturated acid (phytenic acid; Δ^2-3,7,11,15-tetramethylhexadecenoic acid) and the saturated alcohol (dihydrophytol) can be converted to phytanic acid so that both pathways are potentially available [13, 16]. After administration of phytol to experimental animals, large amounts of phytenic acid are found but little or no dihydrophytol. This suggests that oxidation of the alcohol function is normally the initial step [13, 60]. But the possibility that there is a rapid turnover of dihydrophytol remains and further studies are needed before the alternative pathways can be properly evaluated.

Orally administered phytol is efficiently absorbed by normal human subjects (61 to 94 percent of a tracer dose) and similar values have been found in two patients with phytanic acid storage disease [12]. Studies in rats show that absorption is mainly by way of the thoracic duct [60] and in the course of absorption about 10 to 20 percent of the dose is converted to phytanic acid. Since similar values were found in a

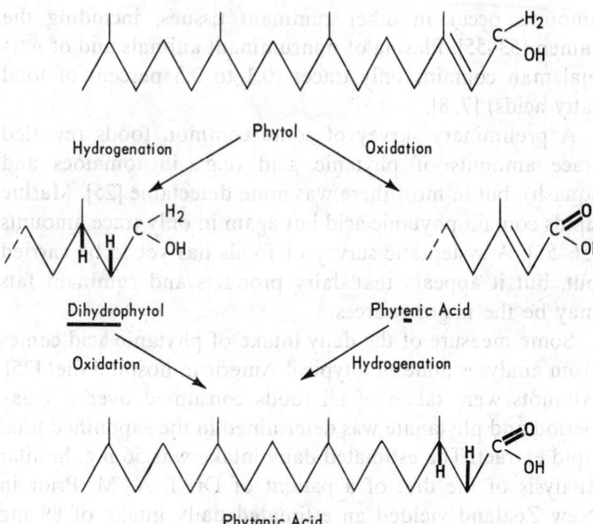

Figure 37-4. Two alternative pathways for the conversion of phytol to phytanic acid. The operation of the pathway shown on the right has been demonstrated. Conversion of dihydrophytol to phytanic acid has been demonstrated, but the overall pathway shown at the left has not been verified experimentally as yet.

germ-free rat it is unlikely that the intestinal flora play any major role in the phytol-phytanic acid conversion.

Klenk and Kremer on examining the liver fatty acids of phytol-fed rats noted the presence of three or four different isomeric forms of phytenic acid but these were not further characterized [16]. Baxter and Milne developed chromatographic methods that improved resolution of these isomers and made possible their individual isolation on a preparative scale [61]. They showed that the usual saponification procedures lead to isomerization but that transesterification under acid conditions does not. Five isomers were demonstrated in the lymph of phytol-fed rats: the *cis* and *trans* forms of Δ^2-phytenic acid, the *cis* and *trans* forms of Δ^3-phytenic acid, and the 3-methylene isomer. The *trans*-Δ^2 form predominated (70 percent of total phytenic acid). These findings are of interest in relation to the question of the mechanism of the phytol-phytanate conversion and may also be relevant to the question of the variable ratios of phytanic acid isomers found in different animal species and different patients with phytanic acid storage disease [62, 63].

Chlorophyll-bound Phytol

The ubiquitous presence of chlorophyll in green vegetables suggested that this might be an important dietary precursor since it contains 1 mole of phytol per mole bound in ester linkage to a propionic acid side chain of one of the pyrrole rings. Early balance studies, while imprecise, indicated that a significant fraction of chlorophyll phytol was lost from the tetrapyrrole nucleus during passage through the gastrointestinal tract [64, 65]. Reexamination of this question by Baxter and Steinberg using high-specific-activity ^{14}C-labeled pheophytin *a* (Mg^{++}-free chlorophyll *a*) showed that in the thoracic duct–cannulated rat not more than 2 percent of bound phytol was absorbed [66]. Baxter's careful clinical balance studies showed that 95 percent of the phytol administered orally as ^{14}C-pheophytin was recovered in the feces, both in normal control subjects and in two patients with phytanic acid storage disease [67]. He also fed 180 gm of spinach to a human subject with the thoracic duct cannulated and recovered only 2 percent of the spinach phytol in a 24-hr lymph collection. From these results it is clear that, while *free* phytol is an excellent precursor of phytanic acid, the *bound* phytol in the chlorophyll molecule cannot be a quantitatively important dietary source of stored phytanate. In the course of preparing vegetables for the table some of the phytol may be released from ester form and become available, but even the *total* amount of phytol in the usual diet is apparently much less important than the amount of preformed phytanic acid [33].

Other Precursors

Billeter et al. [68], studying the metabolism in pigeons of orally administered phylloquinone labeled both in the nucleus and in the phytyl side chain, found that the latter was split off by intestinal bacteria. The fate of the side chain was further studied using side chain-labeled phylloquinone. From breast muscle it was possible to isolate an acidic lipid with the properties of phytanic acid. Data are not available to assess the quantitative importance of this pathway.

It is possible that the intestinal flora contribute to the stored phytanate in patients. Some bacteria can synthesize phytanate itself and others may synthesize related isoprenoid compounds convertible to phytanate [69, 70]. If such synthesis occurs *de novo* in the bacteria (from acetate by way of mevalonate), the clinical studies with D_2O described above should have detected it since the total body water, including that in the intestine, was presumably at the same level of enrichment with deuterium. On the other hand, if the bacteria were to modify the structure of higher molecular weight branched-chain compounds in the diet, such structural modification might not necessarily entail incorporation of hydrogen from water and would go undetected. Additional evidence against a quantitatively important contribution by intestinal bacteria comes from clinical studies of phytanic acid excretion in feces. After 10 days on a phytanic acid–low formula diet, fecal excretion of phytanate fell to about 2 mg per day [33].

There is some reason to suspect that not all of the dietary precursors are known to us. The amounts of phytanic acid accumulated in the tissues of patients, as estimated from biopsies and postmortem analysis, are considerable. In the case reported by Hansen, for example, the liver alone contained over 50 gm and the kidneys about 10 gm [71]. Assuming a typical plasma concentration, the plasma accounts for another 2 to 3 gm. Adipose tissue, although it always contains a much lower percentage of phytanate (1 to 3 percent of total fatty acids), because of its enormous mass represents a large store (100 to 150 gm) and so does skeletal muscle. Thus, a reasonable estimate of total body phytanate in an adult patient might be 200 to 300 gm. Dietary intake of phytanate itself has been directly assessed in only two instances with values of about 50 to 100 mg per day [33, 59]. Even using the higher figure and assuming *complete* absorption and *no* degradation or excretion, it would take 6 to 9 years for dietary phytanate alone to account for the amounts stored. Since patients appear to have at least some limited capacity to oxidize and eliminate phytanic acid, the time needed to build up these stores may be even greater. There is no quantitative incompatibility in the case of adults such as Hansen's patient who died at age 33. However, the child studied by Klenk and Kahlke, who died at age 8 weighing 17 kg, may have had as much as 70 gm phytanate stored in the tissues [4]. On the basis of the same assumptions she would have had to take in and retain, on the average, 22 mg phytanate daily from birth. One liter of milk daily (4 percent fat and 0.05 percent of total fatty acids present as phytanic acid) would provide a daily intake of 20 mg phytanate. While again not quantitatively incompatible, the balance is so close that one must ask whether there are additional sources of phytanate. The possibility that there is endogenous biosynthesis in infants and children should be tested; other branched-chain dietary constituents should be considered as precursors, and production by unusual intestinal flora should be explored.

Defective Oxidation of Phytanic Acid

Normal Oxidative Capacity

A number of lines of evidence indicate that normal animals, including man, have a large capacity to dissimulate phytanic acid and prevent its accumulation even at high levels of intake. Phytanic acid-U-^{14}C injected intravenously into normal man as the albumin complex is converted to $^{14}CO_2$ at a rate comparable to that for palmitic acid-1-^{14}C [26]. This is so even though the initial rate of disappearance of the labeled free phytanic acid from the plasma is distinctly lower than that of palmitic acid. Orally administered phytol-U-^{14}C, which is probably oxidized to $^{14}CO_2$ in large part only after prior conversion to phytanic acid, is also efficiently oxidized—about 21 percent of the absorbed dose in the first 12 hr [12].

The capacity of experimental animals to oxidize and excrete phytanate can be exceeded, but this requires the addition of relatively large amounts of phytanic acid or phytol to the diet. In rats on a daily intake of 100 to 200 mg per day (over twice the estimated daily intake in man!) little accumulation occurs, phytanate accounting for less than 2 percent of the total fatty acids in liver and kidney [19]. At high levels of intake, 2 to 5 percent by weight in the diet, either phytol or phytanate can cause accumulation in the liver and serum to levels comparable to those seen in patients with phytanic acid storage disease [14–16, 18]. If after these high tissue levels have been reached the phytanic acid is removed from the diet, tissue phytanate is rapidly mobilized and eliminated, generally disappearing completely in a week or two. There are demonstrated species differences in oxidative capacity [72], so direct extrapolation of these results to man may not be justified. In man, Avigan reports that even after ingestion of 9.5 *gm* of phytol in a single dose by a normal subject, plasma phytanate at 18 hr had risen only to 2.4 mg per 100 ml [7]. In a heroic study this same volunteer ate 3.5 *kg* of boiled spinach over a 60-hr interval; his plasma phytanic acid level did not change perceptibly! Further evidence comes from studies showing that the fractional rate of oxidation of phytol to CO_2 in normal volunteers is the same whether only a tracer dose is given or whether a full 1-gm dose of carrier phytol is given with it [12].

Defective Oxidation in Patients

Clinical Studies

The first demonstration of the reduced capacity of patients to oxidize phytanic acid was with phytol-U-^{14}C as a precursor [11]. Animal studies had suggested that phytol is rapidly converted to phytanic acid and oxidized mostly or entirely subsequent to that conversion. Observed rates of $^{14}CO_2$ production in two patients were only about one-fifth those in normal volunteers. Subsequent studies in three additional cases using intravenously injected phytanic acid-U-^{14}C itself showed an even more striking deficit, initial rates of $^{14}CO_2$ production being less than 5 percent of those in control subjects [26]. The apparent difference in the degree of block suggested by the clinical studies using these two different precursors probably does not reflect basic differences in the degree of enzyme block in the patients studied. Later cell culture studies, using fibroblasts derived from skin biopsies, suggest that all five patients have comparably severe deficits, phytanic acid being oxidized at rates less than 5 percent of those observed with normal fibroblast cultures [35]. In retrospect, the results suggest the possibility that phytol can be oxidized to a significant degree by a pathway not involving phytanate as an intermediate.

After intravenous injection of labeled phytanic acid, less than 0.001 percent of the dose was recovered in the feces of either controls or patients, showing that biliary excretion or other mechanisms of excretion by way of the intestinal tract are quantitatively unimportant [26]. Less than 6 percent of the injected radioactivity appeared in the urine, 95 percent of it in nonlipid forms.

Eldjarn and coworkers have compared controls and patients with regard to oxidation of model compounds [73–75] but not phytanic acid itself. These model compounds (3,6-dimethyloctanoic acid and 3,14,14-trimethylpentadecanoic acid) resemble phytanate in having a methyl substituent on the 3-carbon and are thus not susceptible to ordinary β-oxidation. Moreover, the substituents at the omega ends of these molecules should prevent β-oxidation from that end also. The former compound, labeled in the ω-terminus (carbon-8), was oxidized to a limited extent by normal controls—2 to 3 percent in 10 hr—but in two patients with phytanic acid storage disease no $^{14}CO_2$ could be detected above background. One of these patients was restudied after plasma phytanate levels had been drastically reduced by dietary means [75]. At that time there was a small but significant yield of $^{14}CO_2$—0.5 to 1 percent of the administered dose. The oxidation of the other model compound, 3,14,14-trimethylpentadecanoic acid, which was labeled with tritium by catalytic exchange, was determined by measuring the release of tritium to body water. In control subjects, 31 to 37 percent of the dose was found in body water at the maximum but in two patients only 8 and 17 percent, respectively [75]. The metabolic pathway by which the trimethylpentadecanoic acid was degraded was not established and the cumulative yield of labeled metabolites in the urine was apparently no different in patients and controls. The other model compound, 3,6-dimethyloctanoic acid, is largely degraded by ω-oxidation, a small fraction undergoing α-oxidation as discussed below.

Fibroblast Cell Culture Studies

As in a growing list of inherited diseases of metabolism, the defect in phytanic acid storage disease persists in cultured fibroblasts [27]. Normal human fibroblasts derived from skin biopsies oxidize added phytanate at rates comparable to those for added palmitate. Cells derived from patients with phytanic acid storage disease, on the other hand, while oxidizing palmitate at a normal rate, oxidize phytanate at only about 1 percent of the normal rate. The low rate of phytanate oxidation is not due to a defect in uptake; the rate of incorporation of phytanate into cell lipids was in fact greater in the patients' cells than in the controls' cells but the *sum* of phytanate-^{14}C in cell lipids and in $^{14}CO_2$ was almost exactly the same. This indicated a normal uptake mechanism [29].

Another interpretation of the low observed rate of $^{14}CO_2$ production was that phytanate incorporated into ester linkages might be released at a low rate in the cells of patients and thus not be as readily available for subsequent oxidation. In other words, the defect might lie in a modified or deleted hydrolytic system(s) rather than in the oxidizing system per se. Direct studies of the rate of release of phytanate previously incorporated into cultured cells during incubation in unlabeled medium showed no difference in this regard between the cells of patients and control cells [29]. Laurell has shown that the phytanyl ester bonds in glyceryl triphytanate are extremely resistant to hydrolysis by lipoprotein lipase [76]. Since the plasma of patients contains diphytanyl and monophytanyl triglycerides but no detectable triphytanyl

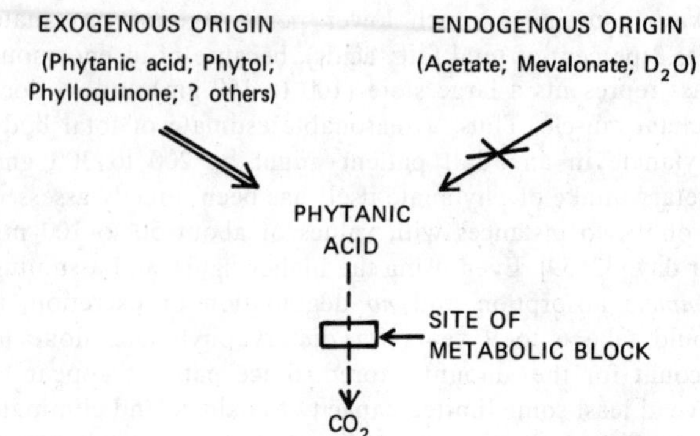

Figure 37-5.

triglycerides [77, 78], this finding leaves undecided the question of whether the phytanyl ester bonds in the naturally occurring mixed glycerides also are resistant to hydrolysis. Recent studies by Avigan and Steinberg, using the serum of a patient with phytanic acid storage disease or chyle from a phytanic acid-fed rat as substrate, indicate that even in mixed glycerides the phytanyl ester bond is resistant to the action of lipoprotein lipase [79]. Ellingboe, using synthetic mixed glycerides containing phytanate, has shown that the phytanyl ester bond is relatively resistant to hydrolysis by pancreatic lipase as well as by lipoprotein lipase from rat adipose tissue [80]. These findings may explain the fact that phytanic acid in the depot fat of patients or phytanic acid-fed rats accounts for a much lower percentage of the total than it does in the plasma. No difference has thus far been reported between control subjects and patients in their ability to hydrolyze phytanyl ester bonds. The studies in fibroblasts discussed above suggest that any such difference cannot be quantitatively important, but comparative studies of lipolytic specificity in other tissues have not been reported.

The studies summarized to this point establish that there is little or no endogenous biosynthesis of phytanic acid; that phytol and phytanic acid are potential dietary precursors (and perhaps other compounds); and that the metabolic error lies in a degradative pathway (Fig. 37-5).

Pathway for Phytanic Acid Oxidation in Relation to Previously Described Pathways for Fatty Acid Oxidation

Based on the present knowledge of fatty acid oxidizing mechanisms, the theoretically possible modes of initial attack on the phytanic acid molecule are indicated in Fig. 37-6 and each will be discussed in turn.

β-Oxidation [81]

This ubiquitous mitochondrial system for successive cleavage of two-carbon fragments from the carboxyl end of the chain is quantitatively the most important pathway for fatty acid

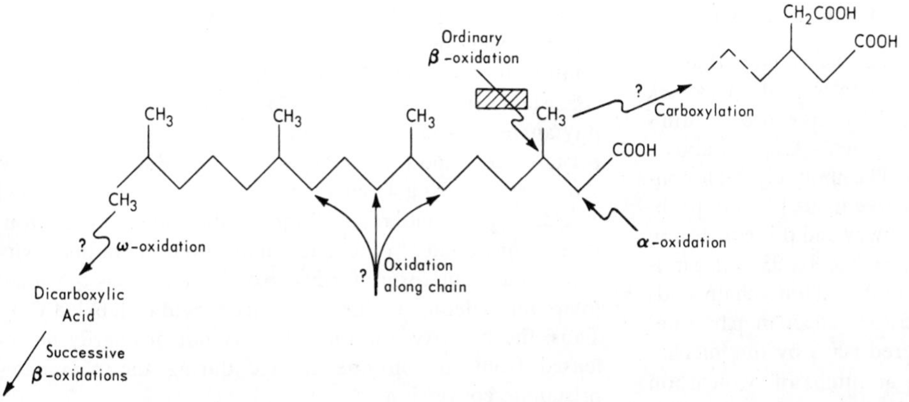

Figure 37-6. Schematic representation of the theoretically possible initial modes of oxidative attack on the phytanic acid molecule.

oxidation. Five basic steps, repeated in cyclic fashion, are involved:

Activation (acylthiokinase, long chain):

$$\mathrm{RCH_2CH_2COOH + CoASH + ATP \longrightarrow RCH_2CH_2COSCoA + AMP + PP_i} \quad (1)$$

Dehydrogenation (acyl CoA dehydrogenase):

$$\mathrm{RCH_2CH_2COSCoA + flavoprotein \longrightarrow RCH{=}CHCOSCoA + reduced\ flavoprotein:} \quad (2)$$

Hydration (enoyl hydrase):

$$\mathrm{RCH{=}CHCOSCoA + H_2O \longrightarrow RCHOHCH_2COSCoA} \quad (3)$$

Dehydrogenation (L(+)-β-hydroxyacyl-CoA dehydrogenase):

$$\mathrm{RCHOHCH_2COSCoA + NAD^+ \longrightarrow R\overset{O}{\overset{\|}{C}}CH_2COSCoA + NADH + H^+} \quad (4)$$

Thiolytic cleavage (β-ketoacyl-CoA thiolase):

$$\mathrm{R\overset{O}{\overset{\|}{C}}CH_2COSCoA + CoASH \longrightarrow R\overset{O}{\overset{\|}{C}}SCoA + CH_3\overset{O}{\overset{\|}{C}}SCoA} \quad (5)$$

Phytanic acid could undergo metabolism by way of this pathway only through step (3). Because of the 3-methyl substituent, it could not be dehydrogenated at this stage to yield the β-keto intermediate.

Fatty acids with 2-methyl substituents can be oxidized by the classical β-oxidation system. The reactions are presumably entirely analogous except that step (5) generates not acetyl CoA but rather propionyl CoA, as in the oxidation of α-methylbutyrate [82]:

$$\mathrm{CH_3\overset{O}{\overset{\|}{C}}{-}\overset{CH_3}{CH_2}\ COSCoA + CoASH \longrightarrow CH_3\overset{O}{\overset{\|}{C}}\ SCoA + CH_3CH_2\overset{O}{\overset{\|}{C}}\ SCoA} \quad (6)$$

There are two ways in which phytanate could be modified initially that would bring it under the jurisdiction of the β-oxidation system:

$$\mathrm{R\overset{CH_3}{\overset{|}{C}}HCH_2COOH \longrightarrow R\overset{CH_3}{\overset{|}{C}}HCOOH} \quad (7)$$

(Phytanate; 20 carbons) (Pristanate; 19 carbons)

This effectively converts a β-methyl fatty acid to an α-methyl fatty acid which, like α-methylbutyrate, could undergo the full cycle of β-oxidation steps. The first β-oxidation cycle would release propionyl CoA (see Eq. 6). A second cycle of β-oxidation would then yield acetyl CoA and an α-methyl fatty acid, whereupon the full cycle could repeat itself. As discussed below, this is in fact probably the major pathway after formation of the $(n-1)$ acid, pristanic acid.

$$\mathrm{\underline{\underline{CH_3}}\overset{CH_3}{\overset{|}{C}}HCH_2CH_2(CH_2\overset{CH_3}{\overset{|}{C}}HCH_2CH_2)_2CH_2\overset{CH_3}{\overset{|}{C}}HCH_2COOH \longrightarrow \underline{\underline{HOOC}}\underset{CH_3}{\underset{|}{C}}HCH_2CH_2(CH_2\underset{CH_3}{\underset{|}{C}}HCH_2CH_2)_2CH_2\underset{CH_3}{\underset{|}{C}}HCH_2COOH} \quad (8)$$

Note that at the ω-carboxyl end of the molecule the branch-methyl substituent is in the α position. Thus oxidation could, after activation, proceed from this end of the molecule by β-oxidation, yielding propionyl CoA and acetyl CoA alternatively.

α-Oxidation [83]

Straight-chain Fatty Acids—Plants

α-Oxidation of long-chain, straight-chain fatty acids, including the common fatty acids such as palmitate and stearate, appears to be an important pathway in plants. The mechanisms involved have been extensively studied in the laboratories of Stumpf [84–86] and of James [87–89]. At least two distinct systems appear to be operative. In germinating seeds (peanut cotyledon) Stumpf and coworkers describe a peroxide-dependent pathway involving the $(n-1)$ aldehyde as an intermediate, which is then oxidized to the acid by NAD. α-Hydroxy acids were not metabolized and if they are intermediates at all, it may be only in enzyme-bound form. In young pea leaves Hitchcock and James demonstrated the accumulation of α-hydroxy acids and the oxidation of added α-hydroxy acids [87–89], and, in the absence of NAD, accumulation of the $(n-1)$ aldehyde. This system does not require peroxide or a peroxidase.

Straight-chain Fatty Acids—Mammalian Nerve Tissue [83]

In mammalian systems, only brain and nerve have thus far been found to oxidize straight-chain fatty acids by attack at the α position, as shown by Mead's group and by Radin's group [90–98]. The longer-chain fatty acids, C_{20} and above, appear to be preferred substrates. The uniquely high concentrations of α-hydroxy acids in nerve tissue [92] are probably due to the operation of this pathway and this conclusion is supported by in vivo tracer studies [90, 91, 93, 94]. Similarly, the significant levels of odd-numbered long-chain acids (e.g., 21:0, 23:0, 25:0) in nerve tissue reflect in part one-carbon shortening of even-numbered acids by this mechanism while some may arise from additions of two-carbon units to propionate [93, 94]. The α-hydroxy and α-keto acids are believed to be intermediates, free or enzyme-bound. The overall sequence from even-numbered acid to $(n - 1)$ acid has been difficult to demonstrate in cell-free systems, particularly the initial α-hydroxylation. In any case, as discussed below, it appears that the system for α-oxidation of phytanate is *not* identical with the system for α-oxidation in nerve.

Phytanic Acid—Conversion to Pristanic Acid

Conversion of labeled phytanic acid to its $(n - 1)$ lower homologue, pristanic acid, was first demonstrated by Avigan and coworkers in 1966 [20]. The rate and extent of this conversion strongly suggested that this is the major normal pathway for phytanate oxidation and subsequent studies in vivo and in vitro have borne this out [21–24]. Unambiguous proof of direct conversion was provided by studies in which phytanic acid labeled with deuterium at the 2 and 3 positions was injected into rats. Pristanic acid was recovered from the liver and identified by mass spectrometry; one-half the deuterium was lost, as expected, as a result of oxidation of the 2-carbon, but the enrichment at position 3 was nearly the same as that of the injected phytanate [20]. This result also served to rule out the possibility that phytanate might first be dehydrogenated to phytenic acid (3,7,11,15-tetramethylhexadec-2-enoic acid) and then hydrated to form the α-hydroxy acid (see below).

Net accumulation of pristanic acid has been demonstrated in mice and in rats fed phytanic acid [21, 22, 100, 101], and trace amounts have been found in normal human tissues, including plasma [7], in butterfat [102], and in ruminant depot fat [103]. No systematic surveys of the relative capacities of different tissues to oxidize phytanate have been reported but it seems likely that the system will prove to be widely distributed. Attempts to demonstrate it in rat brain slices or after intracerebral injection in vivo have been negative [104].

Phytanic Acid—Role of α-Hydroxyphytanate as an Intermediate

α-Hydroxyphytanic acid was first isolated from incubations of phytanic acid with rat liver mitochondria, which contain all of the enzymes necessary for the complete oxidation of phytanic acid [23, 24]. That it is an obligatory intermediate was suggested by the following: (1) the rate of its formation relative to the rate of appearance of pristanic acid was consistent with such a role; (2) when labeled α-hydroxyphytanate was added as substrate it was converted to pristanic acid and further degradation products identical to those formed from labeled phytanate itself; (3) unlabeled α-hydroxyphytanate reduced the yield of labeled CO_2 from labeled phytanate. In the latter connection, the radioactivity recovered in the form of α-hydroxyphytanate was too small to account adequately for the reduced yield of labeled CO_2. Thus, the hydroxy intermediate may not ordinarily be released from the enzyme surface during the phytanate-pristanate conversion.

Studies on the mechanism of the hydroxylation in subcellular fractions of rat liver have shown that the activity is confined to the mitochondria [24]. The reaction is stimulated by NADPH and requires molecular oxygen. In these respects it resembles the several NADPH-dependent mixed function oxygenase reactions linked to the P_{450} system in liver microsomes, but the distinctly different subcellular localization distinguishes it clearly from them. Another unique property, not fully understood, is the marked stimulation due to the addition of fer*ric* iron whereas ferr*ous* iron inhibits. These properties further distinguish the phytanate oxidizing system in the liver from the straight-chain α-oxidation system in the brain. The latter is primarily microsomal and is *stimulated* by ferr*ous* iron [95, 98]. As noted above, the evidence for the conversion of long-chain, straight-chain fatty acids to the α-hydroxy form in subcellular preparations of mammalian brain is mostly indirect. The hydroxy acid may remain tightly bound as proposed for hydroxyphytanate; the latter, however, is to some extent dissociable and can be readily demonstrated as a major product.

Phytanic Acid—Further Oxidation of Pristanic Acid

The pathway for degradation beyond pristanic acid was first established by studies in mice fed phytanic acid [21]. This species, for reasons not fully understood, accumulates much larger quantities of pristanic acid when fed phytanic acid and, also, significant quantities of lower degradation products. The latter were clearly demonstrable by gas-liquid chromatography of liver fatty acids and could be completely characterized by the use of combined GLC-mass spectrometry [22]. Confirmation of their direct formation from phytanic acid was obtained by injecting U-^{14}C-phytanic acid and demonstrating the presence of radioactivity in the relevant GLC peaks. The structures of the products identified in this way are shown in Fig. 37-7. The products beyond pristanate obviously form the series that would be expected from successive β-oxidation of pristanic acid. Thus, β-oxidation of pristanic acid itself would yield 4,8,12-trimethyltridecanoic acid. This compound has been identified not only in mouse liver but also as a product of phytanate metabolism in rats in vivo [22], in rat liver mitochondria [23, 24], and in human fibroblast cell cultures [29]. Recently, Hansen has

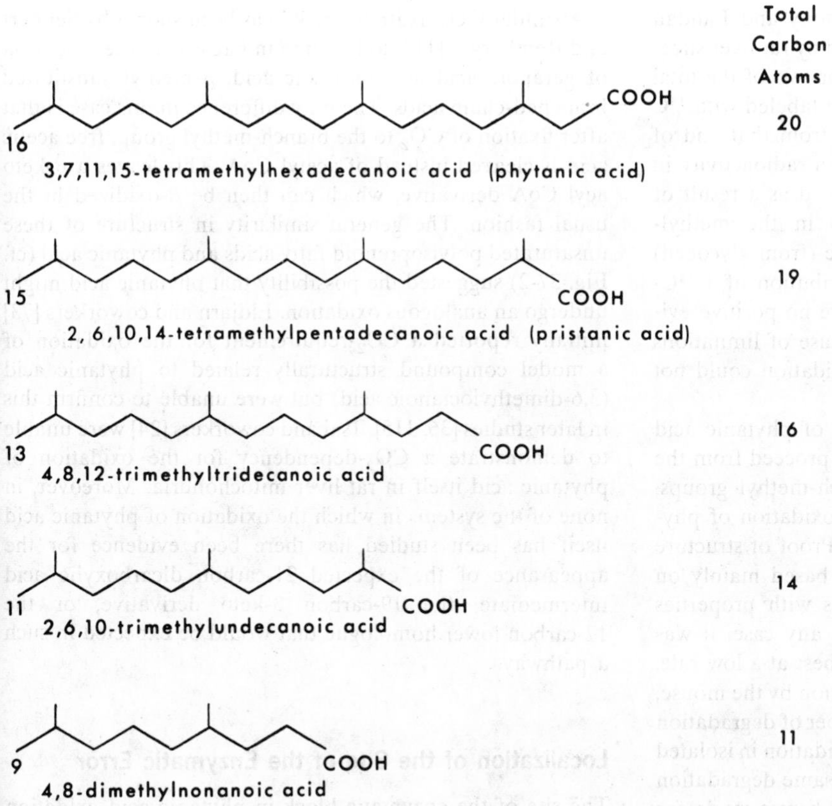

Compound	Total Carbon Atoms
16 ... COOH 3,7,11,15-tetramethylhexadecanoic acid (phytanic acid)	20
15 ... COOH 2,6,10,14-tetramethylpentadecanoic acid (pristanic acid)	19
13 ... COOH 4,8,12-trimethyltridecanoic acid	16
11 ... COOH 2,6,10-trimethylundecanoic acid	14
9 ... COOH 4,8-dimethylnonanoic acid	11

Figure 37-7. Intermediates in the oxidative degradation of phytanic acid identified by mass spectrometry or by demonstration of accumulation of the labeled compound, or both, after the administration of labeled phytanic acid.

shown that traces of this acid are present in butterfat and in ruminant fats [105, 106], which also contain phytanic acid and pristanic acid.

When labeled pristanic acid was incubated with rat liver mitochondria, a new component with a retention time on GLC greater than that of the starting material was detected. This was identified as the 2,3-unsaturated form of pristanic acid, Δ^2-pristenic acid [24]. This would be the expected dehydrogenation product in the classical β-oxidation sequence. Omission of NAD from the incubation mixture markedly increased the degree of accumulation of Δ^2-pristenic acid, but no evidence for accumulation of the corresponding β-hydroxy acid could be found. As discussed above, NAD is required for the dehydrogenation of the β-hydroxy acid in the classical β-oxidation sequence, i.e., it is required as a cofactor for the β-hydroxy acyl CoA dehydrogenase. If pristanic acid is oxidized by the same or by analogous enzymes, the result suggests that the equilibrium between Δ^2-pristenic acid and its hydrated β-hydroxy derivative lies in the direction favoring the unsaturated acid. In any case, the demonstrated formation of the α, β-unsaturated derivative supports the interpretation that further degradation of pristanic acid occurs by way of a β-oxidation pathway.

If the scheme shown in Fig. 37-2 is correct, 3 moles of propionic acid should be formed during the degradation of each mole of phytanic acid. Indirect evidence supporting this was obtained by the demonstration of an unusually large incorporation of radioactivity from phytanic acid into glucose in rats [20]. Completely satisfactory studies demonstrating the stoichiometric yield of propionic acid during phytanic acid oxidation have not yet been reported. The case for formation of propionic acid remains largely inferential, based on the structure of the degradation products.

ω-Oxidation

ω-Oxidation is initiated by oxygen attack at the ω-carbon or at the penultimate (ω-1) carbon of straight-chain fatty acids. As shown by Preiss and Bloch [107] and by Wakabayashi and Shimazono [108], the reaction requires NADPH and molecular oxygen and has the properties of a microsomal mixed function oxygenase. The major product is a dicarboxylic acid of the same number of carbon atoms as the substrate. While straight-chain fatty acids can readily be shown to undergo this form of oxidation in an isolated microsomal system, there is evidence that the mitochondrial β-oxidation system is quantitatively much more important, at least for the long-chain straight-chain fatty acids. When shorter-chain fatty acids are administered (C_6 to C_{10}), significant quantities of the dicarboxylic acid resulting from ω-oxidation are excreted in the urine. After injection of straight-chain, long-chain fatty acids (C_{16} to C_{18}), only traces of radioactivity appear in the urine. If oxidation from the carboxyl end is inhibited by dimethyl substitution at the α position, significant ω-oxidation takes place [109, 110].

Using a novel experimental design Antony and Landau have shown that ω-oxidation of stearic acid by rat liver slices cannot account for more than a percent or two of the total oxidized [110]. They incubated stearic acid labeled with ^{14}C in the 18-carbon so that acetate derived from that end of the molecule by ω-oxidation would contain radioactivity in the carboxyl-carbon whereas acetate derived as a result of β-oxidation would contain radioactivity in the methyl-carbon. The distribution of ^{14}C in glucose (from glycogen) allowed an estimate of the relative contribution of 1-^{14}C-acetate and 2-^{14}C-acetate. The results gave no positive evidence for any ω-oxidation although, because of limitations in methodology, a small amount of ω-oxidation could not be completely ruled out.

As discussed above, initial ω-oxidation of phytanic acid would make it possible for β-oxidation to proceed from the ω end without interference by the branch-methyl groups. Try has presented evidence suggesting ω-oxidation of phytanic acid in rat liver homogenates [111]. Proof of structure was not presented, the conclusion being based mainly on the finding of radioactivity in fatty acids with properties similar to those of dicarboxylic acids. In any case, it was concluded that ω-oxidation proceeded at best at a low rate. In the course of studies of phytanate oxidation by the mouse, which allowed the isolation of a large number of degradation products, and in studies of phytanic acid oxidation in isolated rat liver mitochondria, where many of the same degradation products could be identified, careful search was made for the formation of dicarboxylic acids but none was found [22, 24]. While some degree of oxidation by this pathway cannot be ruled out, the evidence available suggests that it must be at most a minor pathway.

Removal of Methyl Groups after Fixation of CO_2

A β-substituted fatty acid (β-methylbutyric acid) is formed in the course of the oxidative degradation of leucine. This fatty acid (as the acyl CoA) could undergo the second and third steps of the usual β-oxidation cycle, namely, α,β-dehydrogenation and hydration to form the β-hydroxy acyl CoA derivative (see subsection on β-Oxidation above). The second dehydrogenation to form the β-keto acid would be blocked. Degradation depends upon fixation of CO_2 to the β-methyl group of the α, β-unsaturated acid. Hydration yields hydroxymethyl glutaryl CoA which is cleaved to yield acetoacetic acid and acetyl CoA [112, 113].

Leucine

$$(CH_3)_2CHCH_2\overset{O}{\overset{\|}{C}}SCoA \xrightarrow[+CO_2]{-2H} HOOCCH_2(CH_3)C{=}CH\overset{O}{\overset{\|}{C}}SCoA \xrightarrow{+H_2O}$$

$$HOOCCH_2(CH_3)\overset{OH}{\overset{|}{C}}{-}CH_2\overset{O}{\overset{\|}{C}}SCoA \longrightarrow CH_3\overset{O}{\overset{\|}{C}}{-}CH_2COOH + CH_3COSCoA$$

A similar CO_2-fixation "trick" has been shown by Seubert and Remberger [114] to function in bacteria in the oxidation of geranoic acid and farnesoic acid, β-methyl substituted branched-chain acids. The only difference in this case is that after fixation of CO_2 to the branch-methyl group, free acetic acid is cleaved instead of acetyl CoA. This leaves a β-keto acyl CoA derivative, which can then be β-oxidized in the usual fashion. The general similarity in structure of these unsaturated polyisoprenoid fatty acids and phytanic acid (cf. Fig. 37-2) suggested the possibility that phytanic acid might undergo an analogous oxidation. Eldjarn and coworkers [73] initially reported a CO_2-requirement for the oxidation of a model compound structurally related to phytanic acid (3,6-dimethyloctanoic acid) but were unable to confirm this in later studies [36, 115]. Tsai and coworkers [24] were unable to demonstrate a CO_2-dependency for the oxidation of phytanic acid itself in rat liver mitochondria. Moreover, in none of the systems in which the oxidation of phytanic acid itself has been studied has there been evidence for the appearance of the expected 21-carbon dicarboxylic acid intermediate, the 19-carbon 3-keto derivative, or the 17-carbon lower homologue that would be expected in such a pathway.

Localization of the Site of the Enzymatic Error

The site of the enzymatic block in phytanic acid oxidation in the patients has been localized to the initial α-oxidation, probably in the α-hydroxylation step itself. This conclusion is based on studies of the rates of oxidation of phytanic acid and of its degradation products in cell cultures and is supported by studies in vivo in patients. The evidence can be summarized as follows:

1 While the rate of phytanic acid oxidation in cell cultures derived from patients is only 1 percent of that seen in control cell cultures, the rates of oxidation of labeled pristanic acid (Fig. 37-8) are comparable to the rates in control cells [27–29, 35]. A normal rate of oxidation of pristanic acid has been demonstrated in cultures derived from a total of 14 different clinically diagnosed cases of phytanic acid storage disease. This suggests that all patients have their metabolic error at the same biochemical site. The oxidation of α-hydroxyphytanic acid has only been studied in cultures derived from three patients and, consequently, the generalization that the metabolic block always lies in the hydroxylation step is less firmly established.

2 The rate of oxidation of intravenously injected phytanic acid is depressed in patients, but the rate of oxidation of pristanic acid or of α-hydroxyphytanic acid is comparable to that seen in normal subjects (Fig. 37-9) [25, 26].

3 After incubation of normal fibroblasts with labeled phytanic acid the cell lipids can be shown to contain labeled α-hydroxyphytanic acid and labeled pristanic acid as well as labeled 4,8,12-trimethyltridecanoic acid [29]. In contrast,

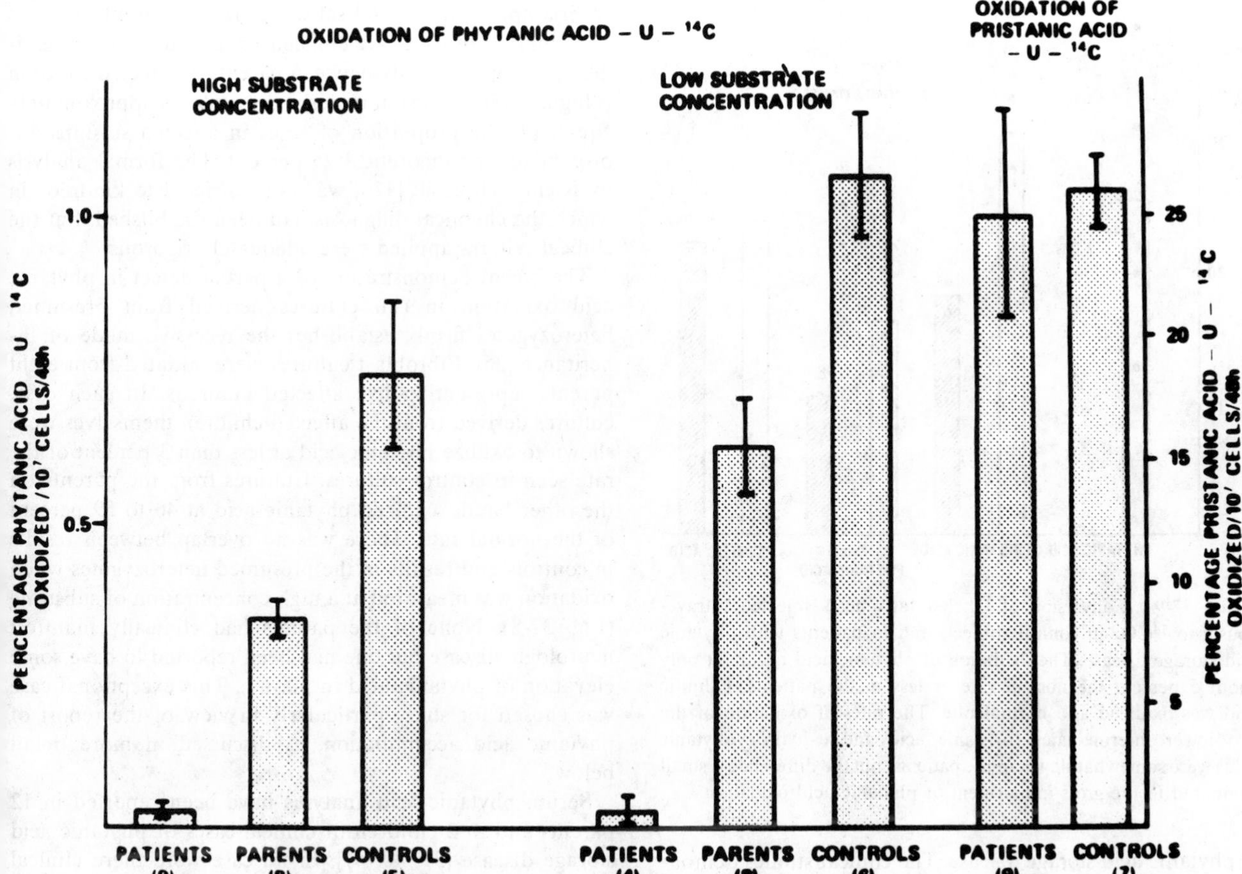

Figure 37-8. Rates of phytanic acid and pristanic acid oxidation in fibroblast cell cultures. The almost complete deletion of the phytanic acid oxidizing activity in homozygous patients is shown, as well as the normal rates of pristanic acid oxidation in patients. The rates of oxidation of phytanic acid in the presumed heterozygotes (parents) is approximately 50 percent of control values.

the cell lipids in fibroblasts derived from patients contain only labeled phytanic acid and no demonstrable radioactivity corresponding to any of the identified degradation products.

4 Careful study of serum and tissue lipids from patients with phytanic acid storage disease and of postmortem tissues has failed to reveal the accumulation of any branched-chain congeners other than phytanic acid itself. Were the metabolic block at some lower point in the degradation pathway one might expect to find at least some concentrations of accumulated intermediates [25].

5 After administration to normal subjects of a branched-chain model compound related to phytanic acid in having a β-methyl substitution (3,6-dimethyloctanoic acid-8-^{14}C), a small fraction of the administered dose of radioactivity is recovered in the urine in the form of the α-oxidation product (2,5-dimethylheptanoic acid) [74]. In contrast, patients failed to show any α-oxidation product in the urine. Normal subjects oxidized a small percentage of the administered radioactivity to CO_2 but patients oxidized none [73, 74]. If it is assumed that the model compound is metabolized by the same systems that oxidize phytanic acid itself, which is supported by the results in patients, these results support the conclusion that there is a defect in α-oxidation.

On the basis of indirect evidence obtained by using model compounds, it was proposed that the accumulation of phytanic acid reflected a defect in ω-oxidation [116]. However, studies showed that other compounds subject to ω-oxidation were handled normally [117], and even the oxidation of the model compound used originally (tricaprin) returned toward normal in the patients after they had been maintained on a phytanate-low diet [118]. Possibly the stores of phytanate secondarily affect some ω-oxidation systems. As discussed above, there is no evidence for a major role of ω-oxidation in the metabolism of phytanic acid itself.

The cell culture technique played a pivotal role in the studies leading to the characterization of the metabolic error

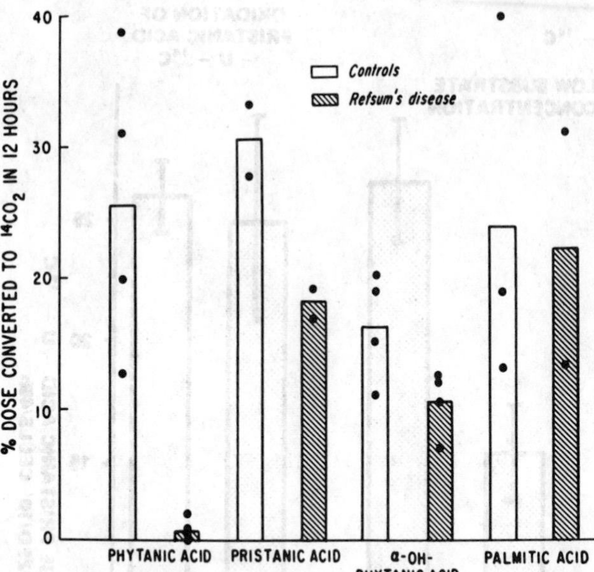

Figure 37-9. Conversion of labeled fatty acids injected intravenously to $^{14}CO_2$ in control subjects and in patients with phytanic acid storage disease. The oxidation of phytanic acid occurs at only about 5 percent the normal rate or less in the patients. Palmitic acid was oxidized at a normal rate. The rates of oxidation of the two lower intermediates (pristanic acid and α-hydroxyphytanic acid) were somewhat slower in the patients, but the difference is small compared to the gross impairment of phytanic acid oxidation.

in phytanic acid storage disease. The clinical studies demonstrating a low rate of $^{14}CO_2$ formation from ^{14}C-labeled phytanic acid presented an interpretational problem commonly encountered in the study of storage diseases. The patients, of course, have large stores of the metabolite under investigation (in this case, phytanic acid). A low yield of $^{14}CO_2$ might be attributable entirely or at least in part to dilution of the administered radioactivity in the large store of unlabeled material. The cell culture studies were free of this ambiguity because the cells in culture contained no stores of phytanic acid. Also, because of the rarity of this disease, it would have been difficult to extend the studies to any large series of cases at the clinical level. On the other hand, it proved perfectly feasible to take skin biopsies and ship them to the home laboratory by air express and there initiate the cultures [35]. Sterile biopsies were shipped refrigerated in small vials of Eagle's medium from Europe; cultures were initiated successfully in all cases, even when there were 2- and 3-day delays in transit. Both for diagnostic purposes and research purposes, the value of this approach becomes increasingly evident.

GENETICS

The observed inheritance pattern is that expected for autosomal recessive transmission [1, 2, 119, 120]. The classical criteria appear to be well satisfied, viz., (1) parents of cases and children of cases are clinically unaffected; (2) the incidence of consanguinity between parents of affected children is high; (3) incidence in males and females is approximately equal; (4) the proportion of cases in affected sibships approximates the theoretical 25 percent. The formal analysis by Richterich et al. [120] was not restricted to kindreds in which the chemical diagnosis had been established, but the clinical criteria applied were adequately rigorous.

The recent demonstration of a partial defect in phytanic acid oxidation in cell cultures derived from presumed heterozygotes firmly establishes the recessive mode of inheritance [35]. Fibroblast cultures were initiated from eight parents representing five affected kindreds. In each case, cultures derived from the affected children themselves were shown to oxidize phytanic acid at less than 3 percent of the rate seen in control cultures. Cultures from the parents on the other hand, oxidized phytanic acid at 46 to 59 percent of the normal rate. There was no overlap between results in controls and results in the presumed heterozygotes when oxidation was measured at a high concentration of substrate (Fig. 37-8). None of the parents had clinically manifest neurologic disease but one had been reported to have some elevation of phytanic acid in plasma. This exceptional case was chosen for study particularly in view of the report of phytanic acid accumulation, as discussed in more detail below.

Serum phytanic acid analyses have been reported in 12 parents and in 2 children of clinical cases of phytanic acid storage disease [37, 40, 41]. In no case were there clinical stigmata of Refsum's syndrome and, with the two exceptions just mentioned, phytanic acid levels were within normal limits. Thus, it appears that one-half the normal capacity for oxidation of phytanic acid is ordinarily adequate to prevent significant accumulation on ordinary diets. One of the exceptional parents was the mother of patient E.H., and was originally reported by Richterich [40] to have a phytanate level fully as high as that of her clinically affected son. A serum sample obtained from this same patient in 1967 showed only the usual normal trace levels of phytanate (Herndon and Steinberg, unpublished results). Unless the single analysis originally reported represents analytical error, one has to conclude that this presumed heterozygote accumulated phytanic acid transiently. The second exception is the mother of cases E.S. and J.S. reported by Nevin et al. in 1967 [41]. Her plasma phytanate accounted for 2.6 percent of total fatty acids. The fact that she was herself symptom-free seems to rule against her being homozygous. The cell culture results classify her as a heterozygote rather unambiguously. With a 50 percent reduction in capacity to oxidize phytanate, it is conceivable that under some conditions (e.g. changes in diet or alterations in the expression of the enzyme defect) heterozygotes may accumulate phytanate. While there are no recorded examples of established heterozygotes with clinical disease, such a possibility should probably not be ruled out. Prior et al. [59] have encountered a puzzling case, diagnosed clinically as Refsum's syndrome, in which phytanic acid was demonstrated in the plasma about two years prior to the patient's death, but in whom *no* phytanate was demonstrable in postmortem tissues.

For purposes of genetic counseling, especially helpful in the case of clinically unaffected individuals in affected sibships, the carrier state can be diagnosed using the fibroblast cell culture method. Now that it is established that there *is* a partial defect, it may prove possible to design a simpler and more direct clinical "loading" test. However, the cell culture method is becoming increasingly accessible. Normal amniotic cells have been shown to have the capacity to oxidize phytanic acid [121], and so it should be possible to make a diagnosis of the homozygous or heterozygous state ante partum.

The biochemical evidence available is compatible with the postulate of a single mutation leading to the loss of a functional phytanic acid hydroxylase (Fig. 37-10). The enzyme has not been purified, and demonstration of the functional defect is still limited to studies using intact cells. Thus, the primary defect might lie in a system necessary for phytanic acid hydroxylation (e.g., a cofactor regenerating system), but not in the phytanic acid α-hydroxylase itself. The possibility of multiple gene defects is always difficult to rule out but thus far no biochemical errors have been established beyond the defect in phytanic acid α-oxidation.

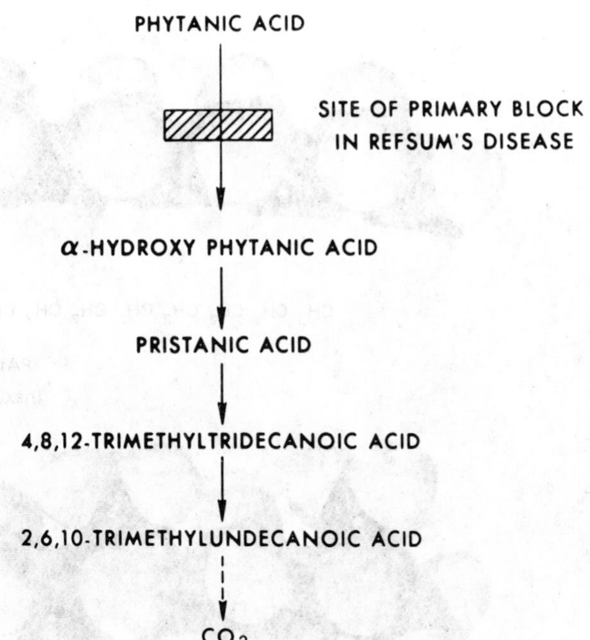

Figure 37-10. Major pathway for oxidation of phytanic acid in mammalian systems, indicating the probable site of the primary metabolic error.

PATHOGENESIS

While a great deal of insight has been gained into the biochemical basis for phytanic acid accumulation, it remains to be established how the accumulation of phytanic acid leads to the clinical manifestations of the disease. Indeed, it is not firmly established whether or not phytanic acid accumulation per se is the necessary and sufficient basis for all of the clinical signs and symptoms of Refsum's syndrome.

Molecular Distortion Hypothesis

The simplest hypothesis remains that the incorporation of the multiple-branched, "thorny" phytanic acid molecule into tissue lipids in place of the normal straight-chain fatty acids interferes with function of myelin or at least increases its susceptibility to damage [25; Fig. 37-11]. The cross-sectional area of the phytanic acid molecule is a good 50 percent greater than that of the straight-chain fatty acids [122] and the binding forces at close range would be considerably less than in the case of straight-chain fatty acids. Thus, in highly ordered structures, like that of myelin or membrane lipids generally, the displacement of straight-chain acids by phytanic acid might in itself lay the basis for evolution of the clinical disease. If this is the case, then elimination of phytanic acid and its precursors from the diet should prevent the development of lesions in very young patients and might arrest the progress or even lead to some reversal of symptoms in older patients. As discussed in the next section in more detail, four cases have been followed on phytanic acid–low diets for periods up to 4 years. None of them has had a relapse while on the special diet, and three have had modest but statistically significant improvement in some objective measures of neurologic status [32–34]. Plasma phytanate levels and levels in adipose tissue biopsies fell during treatment but there is as yet no evidence that the nerve content of phytanic acid was influenced. If further experience with low–phytanic acid diets confirms the therapeutic benefit indicated by these preliminary studies, that will constitute the best evidence favoring a simple cause-and-effect relationship between phytanic acid accumulation and clinical manifestations.

The corollary approach of trying to produce the disease in animals by feeding large amounts of phytanic acid or its precursors has been tried with negative results [14–16, 18, 19, 22, 36]. In the five species studied (rat, rabbit, chinchilla, mouse, and polecat), it has been possible to increase the phytanic acid levels in serum and in most tissues to values similar to those reported in postmortem tissues of patients with phytanic acid storage disease. The levels reached in nerve and brain have been low relative to those reported in the human disease. Consequently, the negative experimental results do not militate strongly against the hypothesis that phytanic acid storage in the nervous system is pathogenetic. Higher levels could not be attained because increasing the levels of intake still further caused serious

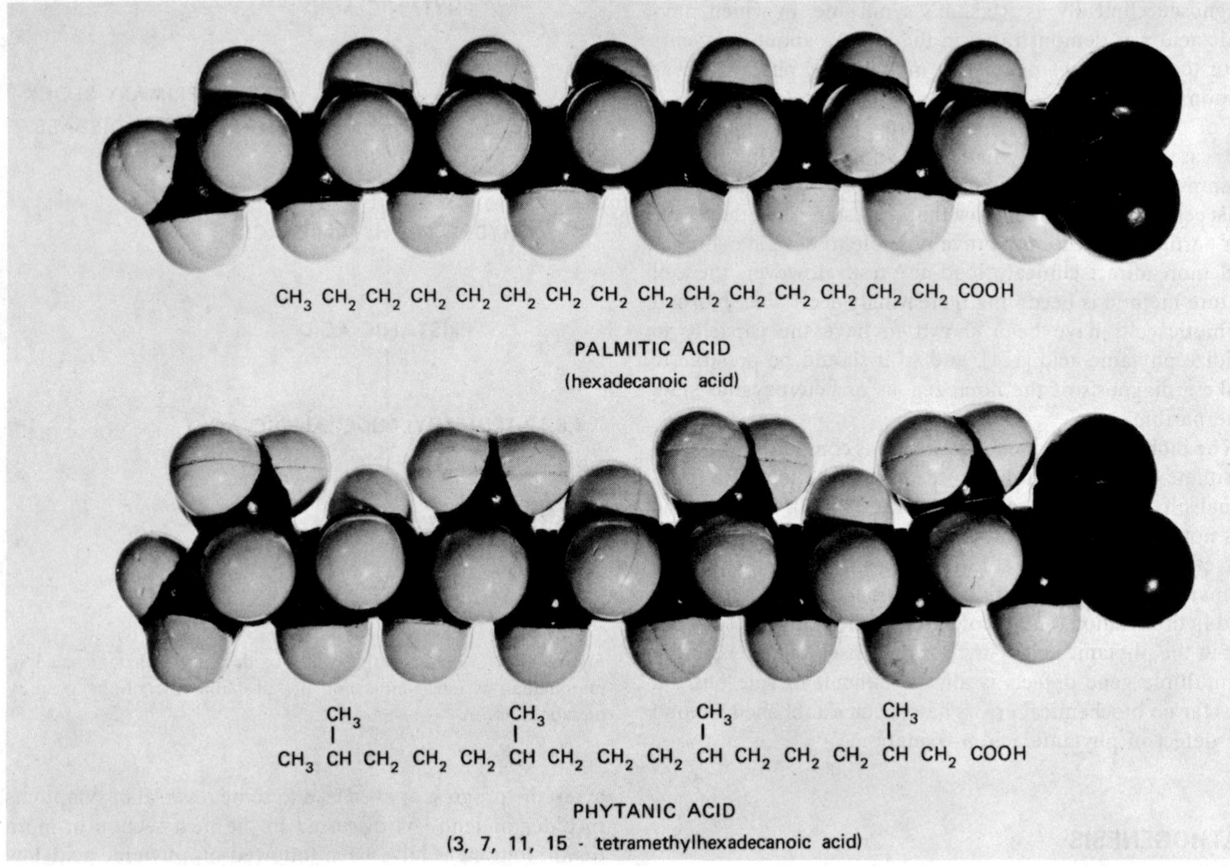

Figure 37-11. Molecular models indicating the space-occupying branch-methyl substituents as they influence the configuration of the phytanic acid molecule.

toxic effects, including the arrest of growth and the death of the test animals. The mechanism of this marked toxicity of phytol or phytanic acid remains unknown. The administration of large doses of fat-soluble vitamins and polyunsaturated fats afforded no protection [19, and unpublished results].

Any satisfactory hypothesis with regard to pathogenesis must account for the sometimes dramatic acute exacerbations and gradual remissions of symptoms seen in the natural course of the disease. From what we know about the sources and metabolism of phytanic acid in these patients, it seems highly unlikely that these rapid fluctuations in clinical expression could be accompanied by similarly rapid changes in tissue phytanate levels. More probably, the clinical expression is conditioned by intercurrent factors in the environment superimposed upon a basically defective nervous tissue structure. Mention has been made of the association between intercurrent infections, for example, or other physiologic stresses and the development of acute relapses. Recently, a preliminary report has appeared suggesting that rats maintained on a phytanic acid diet may be more susceptible to damage from experimental allergic encephalitis [123].

Antimetabolite Hypothesis

The close structural similarity between phytanic acid and the isoprenoid side chains of the fat-soluble vitamins, particularly vitamins E and K, led to the suggestion that phytanic acid might be toxic by interfering with the function of these fat-soluble vitamins. The arrest in the growth of rats or mice fed large doses of phytanate was not prevented by the simultaneous administration of large doses of fat-soluble vitamins [19]. But these negative results do not completely rule out the hypothesis. Phytanic acid might be competing successfully, even noncompetitively, at the site of vitamin function. One reason this hypothesis has received attention follows from the resemblance between some of the clinical features of abetalipoproteinemia (in which fat-soluble vitamin transport may be deficient) and the clinical features of phytanic acid storage disease. Other possibilities, such as interference with the function of coenzyme Q or other polyisoprenoid compounds can be mentioned speculatively, but no relevant data are as yet available.

"Double-function" Hypothesis

It could be proposed that the α-oxidation system necessary for the metabolism of phytanic acid (and deleted in patients) plays a physiologically important role in one or more other biochemical pathways. One specific hypothesis along these lines, one that seemed particularly attractive before the biochemical details of phytanic acid α-oxidation were further developed, related to the possibility of a generalized deficiency in α-hydroxylation. α-Hydroxylation of fatty acids in animals has only been observed in nerve tissue, as discussed above (subsection on α-Oxidation); thus, a deficiency in this system might understandably manifest itself primarily in nervous system disease. More recent studies on the properties of the phytanic acid oxidizing system show clearly that it is distinct from the long-chain, straight-chain fatty acid α-oxidation system. Moreover, analyses of postmortem tissues failed to show any abnormality in concentration or composition of the straight-chain α-hydroxy fatty acids in brain or nerve [124, 125]. Analyses of skin biopsies in two cases showed an α-hydroxy fatty acid concentration at the lower limits of normal and with a normal distribution [126]. Finally, rats fed a phytanic acid-rich diet have shown no abnormality in α-hydroxy fatty acid concentration or composition in brain. Thus, there is no evidence that patients with phytanic acid storage disease have any difficulty in making α-hydroxy acids in the straight-chain fatty acid series.

Until it has been shown that the inability to oxidize phytanic acid is the result of a simple deletion, one cannot rule out the possibility that the primary defect involves, for example, a cofactor generating system and thus influences other metabolic pathways in addition to the one for phytanic acid oxidation.

Multiple-gene Defects

Thus far there is no unambiguous evidence of a defect in any other biochemical pathway. The karyotype, when reported, has been normal. Nevertheless, the possibility of still undiscovered biochemical defects always remains open. One can ask whether the clinical features reported are all reasonably attributed to nerve damage or in some other way to phytanic acid accumulation. Certainly most of the clinical features are readily attributed to nerve damage, but not all. The electrocardiographic abnormalities may be on the basis of damage to the conduction system but there are reports also of myocardial fibrosis. Patients have been reported to have shortening of the metatarsal bones, pes cavus, epiphyseal dysplasia, and ichthyosis. These are not readily attributable to nerve damage. They may be due to incorporation of phytanic acid into and distortion of other cell membranes.

It may be hoped that this still elusive question of the pathogenesis of phytanic acid storage disease will be actively pursued. If, through the successful development of an animal model or an in vitro model, it can be shown how the molecular disorganization due to the presence of phytanic acid leads to demyelination in this disease, the insights gained may be valuable in understanding the many other neurologic disorders associated with demyelination.

TREATMENT

Four patients have been studied on phytanic acid–low diets for periods of from 2 to 4 years [25, 32, 33, 34]. The diets were originally drawn up to exclude dairy fats and ruminant fat (i.e., sources of phytanic acid itself) and also chlorophyll, which has one mole of phytol esterified to a propionic substituent of the porphyrin ring. Subsequent studies showed that the total amounts of phytol in the diet (free and chlorophyll-bound) are small relative to the amounts of phytanic acid [33] and, furthermore, that the phytol esterified in the chlorophyll molecule is largely unavailable [66, 67]. Consequently, the rigorous exclusion of vegetable products may not really be necessary. Specific details of a suitable diet have been published elsewhere [33].

All four patients studied showed highly significant decreases in plasma phytanic acid levels. The fall did not begin for as much as 3 months after the initiation of the diet but was then progressive. Levels one-third or more below the original level were reached in all cases and even normal levels in some. Adipose tissue biopsies were taken in two cases and both showed a decrease in phytanic acid content. No data are available with regard to possible changes in phytanic acid level in nerve tissue.

Two patients (J.S., whose history is given above, and his sister, K.S. [25, 44]) were intensively studied under carefully controlled hospital conditions for a period of approximately 15 months. Neurologic status was evaluated during a 4-½-month control period and then periodically through a year on a phytanic acid–low diet. Both patients showed definite improvement in a number of parameters. Perhaps the most convincing change was in the objective measurement of ulnar nerve conduction velocity. Using the variance of the measurements made during the control period and during the special diet period, it was shown that the difference in the mean values for the two periods was statistically significant, although the conduction values still did not approach normal (Table 37-2). In addition, there were a number of other objective signs of improvement, including increases in objective measures of muscle strength and coordination, return of previously unobtainable tendon reflexes,

Table 37-2. SUMMARY OF NEUROLOGIC CHANGES ON LOW PHYTANATE DIET

	J.S.	K.S.
Muscle strength	Increased	Increased
Reflexes	Biceps, triceps and patellar: 0 → +	Triceps and finger jerks: 0→ +
Light touch	Deficit to elbows → normal Deficit to knees → mid-calf	Mild deficit below mid-forearms → normal Mild deficit to mid-calf → normal
Ulnar nerve conduction velocity	20.3 ± 0.9 → 25.6 ± 0.9 $p < .001$	16.6 ± 1.2 → 24.9 ± 0.7 $p < .001$
Objective tests of coordination	Improvement in most (? learning component)	Improvement in all
Functional activity tests	±	±

No improvement in: cranial nerve function, vibratory sense, rapid alternating movements, finger-nose, and heel-knee-shin tests

amelioration of sensory deficits in the extremities, and reversion of the electrocardiogram to a normal pattern. At the end of this study the patients returned to Ireland with appropriate dietary instructions but dietary adherence was poor, as shown by a progressive rise in plasma phytanate levels. Coincident with this rise in phytanate levels, both patients underwent a definite relapse. When they were readmitted to the Clinical Center, both were found to have undergone a sharp decrease in ulnar nerve conduction velocity and showed deterioration in other neurologic parameters. They were then placed on a special liquid-formula diet containing only approximately 2 mg of phytanic acid daily. On this they showed a dramatic drop in plasma phytanate and an equally remarkable rise in ulnar nerve conduction velocity over a period of just a few months. The cycle of improvement, relapse and improvement again on diet in both of these patients occurring in parallel constitutes strongly suggestive evidence for the therapeutic value of the diet [33].

Of the two patients studied jointly by the Oslo group and the Bethesda group [12, 32, 34], one showed only minimal neurologic changes initially and did not change importantly with diet treatment. The other showed moderately impressive clinical improvement during the first year on the diet and an increase in ulnar nerve conduction velocity from 7 m per sec initially to 19 m per sec after 1 year. His clinical status then reached a plateau but when he was placed on a still more restricted diet in 1967, plasma phytanate levels fell still further and his ulnar nerve conduction velocity has increased still further over the past year (S. Refsum, personal communication).

Evaluation in diseases characterized by spontaneous relapses and remissions is difficult. More patients will have to be studied and over a longer period of time before a final statement can be made regarding the value of the diet treatment. Nevertheless, the evidence available is strong enough to indicate that any patient with phytanic acid storage deserves an intensive trial on dietary treatment. The rapidity of the chemical response depends on how completely phytanic acid is eliminated from the diet. By turning to a synthetic liquid-formula diet that contained less than 2 mg of phytanic acid daily, it was possible to bring the plasma levels of phytanic acid down much more rapidly. This diet is, of course, difficult for patients to adhere to for long periods of time. When more complete data are available concerning the phytanic acid content of foodstuffs, it should be possible to design more acceptable diets with appropriately low phytanic acid content.

Finally, it is reasonable to expect that any therapeutic benefits will be more significant if treatment is initiated early in the course of the disease. Once demyelination is extensive and connective tissue reaction has progressed to the stage of hypertrophy, restoration of function can probably not be achieved even if further progression is arrested.

SUMMARY

1 Phytanic acid storage disease, or Refsum's syndrome, is a rare inherited disorder of lipid metabolism characterized clinically by peripheral neuropathy and ataxia, retinitis pigmentosa, and changes in the skin and bones.

2 The disorder is accompanied by accumulation in the tissues, especially in the liver and kidney, of a 20-carbon branched-chain acid, phytanic acid. This lipid may comprise as much as 30 percent of the total fatty acids of the plasma. Only traces of this component are normally found in the plasma.

3 The origin of the phytanic acid in these patients is both dietary phytanic acid and phytol, a component of the chlorophyll molecule which is readily converted to phytanic acid. Normally phytanic acid is oxidized through an initial α-oxidation to pristanic acid, and then further by successive β-oxidation steps.

4 The primary defect is failure of the conversion of phytanic acid to α-hydroxyphytanic acid, the inital step in conversion to pristanic acid. This step is catalyzed by phytanic acid α-hydroxylase and activity of this enzyme is absent in the disease.

5 The defect has been demonstrated in fibroblast cultures from patients, and there is evidence for a partial defect in obligate heterozygotes. Inheritance follows a simple autosomal recessive pattern.

6 Significant improvement in clinical manifestations has accompanied prolonged dietary management.

BIBLIOGRAPHY

1. Refsum, S.: Heredopathia atactica polyneuritiformis. Acta Psychiat. Scand., suppl. **38,** 9, 1946.
2. Refsum, S.: Heredopathia atactica polyneuritiformis reconsideracion. World Neurol., **1,** 334, 1960.
3. Cammermeyer, J.: Neuropathological changes in hereditary neuropathies: Manifestation of the syndrome heredopathia atactica polyneuritiformis in the presence of interstitial hypertrophic polyneuropathy. J. Neuropath. Exp. Neurol., **15,** 340, 1956.
4. Klenk, E., and Kahlke, W.: Über das Vorkommen der 3,7,11,15-Tetramethylhexadecansäure (Phytansäure) in den Cholesterinestern und anderen Lipoidfraktionen der Organe bei einem Krankheitsfall unbekannter Genese (Verdacht auf Heredopathia atactica polyneuritiformis (Refsum's syndrome)). Hoppe Seyler Z. Physiol. Chem., **333,** 133, 1963.
5. Richterich, R., van Mechelen, P., and Rossi, E.: Refsum's disease (heredopathia atactica polyneuritiformis): An inborn error of lipid metabolism with storage of 3,7,11,15-tetramethylhexadecanoic acid. Amer. J. Med., **39,** 230, 1965.
6. Kahlke, W.: Refsum-Syndrom—Lipoidchemische Untersuchungen bei 9 Fällen. Klin. Wschr., **42,** 1011, 1964.
7. Avigan, J.: The presence of phytanic acid in normal human and animal plasma. Biochim. Biophys. Acta, **116,** 391, 1966.
8. Kremer, G. J.: Über das Vorkommen der 3,7,11,15-Tetramethylhexadecansäure in den Lipoiden von Normalseren. Klin. Wschr., **43,** 517, 1965.
9. Steinberg, D.: Remarks on the biochemical basis of Refsum's disease. Nord. Med., **73,** 570, 1965.
10. Eldjarn, L.: Biokjemiske synspunkter på phytansaurens opprinnelse. Nord. Med., **73,** 569, 1965.
11. Steinberg, D., Avigan, J., Mize, C., Eldjarn, L., Try, K., and Refsum, S.: Conversion of U-C^{14}-phytol to phytanic acid and its oxidation in heredopathia atactica polyneuritiformis. Biochem. Biophys. Res. Comm., **19,** 783, 1965.
12. Steinberg, D., Mize, C. E., Avigan, J., Fales, H. M., Eldjarn, L., Try, K., Stokke, O., and Refsum, S.: Studies on the metabolic error in Refsum's disease. J. Clin. Invest., **45,** 1076, 1966; **46,** 313, 1967.
13. Mize, C. E., Avigan, J., Baxter, J. H., Fales, H. M., and Steinberg, D.: Metabolism of phytol-U-^{14}C and phytanic acid-U-^{14}C in the rat. J. Lipid Res., **7,** 692, 1966.
14. Steinberg, D., Avigan, J., Mize, C., and Baxter, J. H.: Phytanic acid formation and accumulation in phytol-fed rats. Fed. Proc., **24,** 290, 1965.
15. Steinberg, D., Avigan, J., Mize, C., and Baxter, J.: Phytanic acid formation and accumulation in phytol-fed rats. Biochem. Biophys. Res. Comm., **19,** 412, 1965.
16. Klenk, E., and Kremer, G. J.: Untersuchungen zum Stoffwechsel des Phytols, Dihydrophytols und der Phytansäure. Hoppe Seyler Z. Physiol. Chem., **343,** 39, 1965.
17. Stoffel, W., and Kahlke, W.: The transformation of phytol into 3,7,11,15-tetramethylhexadecanoic (phytanic) acid in heredopathia atactica polyneuritiformis (Refsum's syndrome). Biochem. Biophys. Res. Comm., **19,** 33, 1965.
18. Hansen, R. P., Shorland, F. B., and Prior, I. A. M.: The fate of phytanic acid when administered to rats. Biochim. Biophys. Acta, **116,** 178, 1966.
19. Steinberg, D., Avigan, J., Mize, C. E., Baxter, J. H., Cammermeyer, J., Fales, H. M., and Highet, P. F.: Effects of dietary phytol and phytanic acid in animals. J. Lipid Res., **7,** 684, 1966.
20. Avigan, J., Steinberg, D., Gutman, A., Mize, C. E., and Milne, G. W. A.: Alpha-decarboxylation, an important pathway for degradation of phytanic acid in animals. Biochem. Biophys. Res. Comm., **24,** 838, 1966.
21. Mize, C. E., Steinberg, D., Avigan, J., and Fales, H. M.: A pathway for oxidative degradation of phytanic acid in mammals. Biochem. Biophys. Res. Comm., **25,** 359, 1966.
22. Mize, C. E., Avigan, J., Steinberg, D., Pittman, R. C., Fales, H. M., and Milne, G. W. A.: A major pathway for the mammalian oxidative degradation of phytanic acid. Biochim. Biophys. Acta, **176,** 720, 1969.
23. Tsai, S.-C., Herndon, J. H., Jr., Uhlendorf, B. W., Fales, H. M., and Mize, C. E.: The formation of alpha-hydroxyphytanic acid from phytanic acid in mammalian tissues. Biochem. Biophys. Res. Comm., **28,** 571, 1967.
24. Tsai, S.-C., Avigan, J., and Steinberg, D.: Studies on the alpha-oxidation of phytanic acid by rat liver mitochondria. J. Biol. Chem., **244,** 2682, 1969.
25. Steinberg, D., Vroom, F. Q., Engel, W. K., Cammermeyer, J., Mize, C. E., and Avigan, J.: Refsum's disease—a recently characterized lipidosis involving the nervous system. Ann. Intern. Med., **66,** 365, 1967.
26. Mize, C. E., Herndon, J. H., Jr., Blass, J. P., Milne, G. W. A., Follansbee, C., Laudat, P., and Steinberg, D.: Localization of the oxidative defect in phytanic acid degradation in patients with Refsum's disease. J. Clin. Invest., **48,** 1033, 1969.
27. Steinberg, D., Herndon, J. H., Jr., Uhlendorf, B. W., Mize, C. E., Avigan, J., and Milne, G. W. A.: Refsum's disease: Nature of the enzyme defect. Science, **156,** 1740, 1967.
28. Steinberg, D., Avigan, J., Mize, C. E., Herndon, J. H., Jr., Fales, H. M., and Milne, G. W. A. The nature of the metabolic defect in Refsum's disease. Path. Europ., **3,** 450, 1968.
29. Herndon, J. H., Jr., Steinberg, D., Uhlendorf, B. W., and Fales, H. M.: Refsum's disease: Characterization of the enzyme defect in cell culture. J. Clin. Invest., **48,** 1017, 1969.
30. Eldjarn, L., Stokke, O., and Try, K.: Alpha-oxidation of branched-chain fatty acids in man and its failure in patients with Refsum's disease showing phytanic acid accumulation. Scand. J. Clin. Lab. Invest., **18,** 694, 1966.
31. Stokke, O., Try, K., and Eldjarn, L.: Alpha-oxidation as an alternative pathway for the degradation of branched-chain fatty acids in man, and its failure in patients with Refsum's disease. Biochim. Biophys. Acta, **144,** 271, 1967.
32. Eldjarn, L., Try, K., Stokke, O., Munthe-Kaas, A. W., Refsum, S., Steinberg, D., Avigan, J., and Mize, C.: Dietary effects on serum-phytanic-acid levels and on clinical manifestations in heredopathia atactica polyneuritiformis. Lancet, **1,** 691, 1966.
33. Steinberg, D., Mize, C. E., Herndon, J. H., Jr., Fales, H. M., Engel, W. K., and Vroom, F. Q.: Phytanic acid in patients with Refsum's syndrome and response to dietary treatment. Arch. Intern. Med. (Chicago), **125,** 75, 1970.
34. Refsum, S., and Eldjarn, L.: Heredopathia atactica polyneuritiformis—an inborn defect in the metabolism of branched-chain fatty acids, in *Future of Neurology,* edited by H. G. Bammer, p. 36. Thieme, Stuttgart, 1967.
35. Herndon, J. H., Steinberg, D., and Uhlendorf, B. W.: Refsum's disease:

Defective oxidation of phytanic acid in tissue cultures derived from homozygotes and heterozygotes. New Eng. J. Med., **281,** 1034, 1969.
36. Stokke, O.: Alpha-oxidation of fatty acids in various mammals, and a phytanic acid feeding experiment in an animal with a low alpha-oxidation capacity. Scand. J. Clin. Lab. Invest., **20,** 305, 1967.
37. Try, K.: Heredopathia atactica polyneuritiformis (Refsum's disease), the diagnostic value of phytanic acid determination in serum lipids. Europ. Neurol., **2,** 1, 1969.
38. Steinberg, D., and Herndon, J. H., Jr.: Refsum's disease: Phytanic acid storage disease, in *The Cellular and Molecular Basis of Neurologic Disease,* edited by G. M. Shy, E. S. Goldensohn, and S. H. Appel. Lea and Febiger, Philadelphia, 1971. (In press.)
39. Kolodny, E. H., Hass, W. K., Lane, B., and Drucker, W. D.: Refsum's syndrome: Report of a case including electron microscopic studies of the liver. Arch. Neurol. (Chicago), **12,** 583, 1965.
40. Kahlke, W., and Richterich, R.: Refsum's disease (heredopathia atactica polyneuritiformis), an inborn error of lipid metabolism with storage of 3,7,11,15-tetramethyl hexadecanoic acid. II. Isolation and identification of the storage product. Amer. J. Med., **39,** 237, 1965.
41. Nevin, N. C., Cumings, J. N., and McKeown, F.: Refsum's syndrome, heredopathia atactica polyneuritiformis. Brain, **90,** 419, 1967.
42. Kahlke, W.: Heredopathia atactica polyneuritiformis (Refsum's disease), in *Lipids and Lipidoses,* edited by G. Schettler, Springer-Verlag, New York, 1967.
43. Refsum, S.: Diagnose und Differentialdiagnose der Heredopathia atactica polyneuritiformis. Dtsch. A. Nervenheik, **195,** 257, 1969.
44. Ashenhurst, E. M., Millar, J. H. D., and Milliken, T. G.: Refsum's syndrome affecting a brother and two sisters. Brit. Med. J., **2,** 415, 1958.
45. Grob, E. C., Kirschner, K., and Lynen, F.: Neues über die Biosynthese der Carotinoide. Chimia, **15,** 308, 1961.
46. Nandi, D. L., and Porter, J. W.: The enzymatic synthesis of geranyl-geranyl pyrophosphate by enzymes of carrot root and pig liver. Arch. Biochem., **105,** 7, 1964.
47. Fischer, F. G., Märkl, G., Hönel, H., and Rüdiger, W.: Einbau von Essigsäure und Mevalonsäure-(2-^{14}C) in Chlorophyll, Sterine und Carotinoide von Gerstenkeimlingen. Liebig. Ann. Chem., **657,** 199, 1962.
48. Christophe, J., and Popják, G.: Studies on the biosynthesis of cholesterol: XIV. The origin of prenoic acids from allyl pyrophosphates in liver enzyme systems. J. Lipid Res., **2,** 244, 1961.
49. Hansen, R. P., and Shorland, F. B.: The branched-chain fatty acids of butterfat. 3. Further investigations on a multibranched C_{20} saturated fatty acid fraction. Biochem. J., **52,** 662, 1953.
50. Sonneveld, W., Begemann, P. H., van Beers, G. J., Keuning, R., and Schogt, J. C. M.: 3,7,11,15-Tetramethylhexadecanoic acid, a constituent of butterfat. J. Lipid Res., **3,** 351, 1962.
51. Duncan, W. R. H., and Garton, G. A.: Blood lipids. 3. Plasma lipids of the cow during pregnancy and lactation. Biochem. J., **89,** 414, 1963.
52. Lough, A. K.: Blood lipids. 4. The isolation of 3,7,11,15-tetramethyl-hexadecanoic acid (phytanic acid) from ox-plasma lipids. Biochem. J., **91,** 584, 1964.
53. Hansen, R. P.: 3,7,11,15-Tetramethylhexadecanoic acid: Its occurrence in sheep fat. New Zeal. J. Sci., **8,** 158, 1965.
54. Hansen, R. P.: Occurrence of 3,7,11,15-tetramethylhexadecanoic acid in ox perinephric fat. Chem. Industr., **303,** 1965.
55. Patton, S., and Benson, A. A.: Phytol metabolism in the bovine. Biochim. Biophys. Acta, **125,** 22, 1966.
56. Ackman, R. G., and Sipos, J. C.: Isolation of the saturated fatty acids and branched-chain fatty acids. Comp. Biochem. Physiol., **15,** 445, 1965.
57. Peters, H., and Wieske, Th.: Detection of traces of polybranched fatty acids. Fette, Seifen, Anstrichmittel, **68,** 947, 1966.
58. Sen Gupta, A. K., and Peters, H.: Isolation and structure determination of polybranched-chain fatty acids from fish oil. Fette, Seifen, Anstrichmittel, **68,** 349, 1966.
59. Prior, I. A. M., Alexander, W. S., Steinberg, D., Mize, C. E., and Herndon, J. H., Jr.: Unpublished results.
60. Baxter, J. H., Steinberg, D., Mize, C. E., and Avigan, J.: Absorption and metabolism of uniformly ^{14}C-labeled phytol and phytanic acid by the intestine of the rat studied with thoracic duct cannulation. Biochim. Biophys. Acta, **137,** 277, 1967.
61. Baxter, J. H., and Milne, G. W. A.: Phytenic acid: Identification of five isomers in chemical and biological products of phytol. Biochim. Biophys. Acta, **176,** 265, 1969.
62. Ackman, R. G., and Hansen, R. P.: The occurrence of diastereomers of phytanic and pristanic acids and their determination by gas-liquid chromatography. Lipids, **2,** 357, 1967.
63. Eldjarn, L., and Try, K.: Different ratios of the LDD and DDD diastereoisomers of phytanic acid in patients with Refsum's disease. Biochim. Biophys. Acta, **164,** 94, 1968.
64. Fischer, H., and Hendschel, A.: Gewinnung von Chlorophyllderivaten aus Elefanten und Menschenexkrementen. Z. Physiol. Chem., **216,** 57, 1933.
65. Brugsch, J. T., and Sheard, C.: Determination and quantitative estimation of the decomposition of chlorophyll in the human body. J. Lab. Clin. Med., **24,** 230, 1938.
66. Baxter, J. H., and Steinberg, D.: Absorption of phytol from dietary chlorophyll in the rat. J. Lipid Res., **8,** 615, 1967.
67. Baxter, J. H.: Absorption of chlorophyll phytol in normal man and in patients with Refsum's disease. J. Lipid Res., **9,** 636, 1968.
68. Billeter, M., Bolliger, W., and Martius, C.: Untersuchungen über die Umwandlung von verfütterten K-Vitaminen durch Austausch der Seitenkette und die Rolle der Darmbakterien hierbei. Biochem. Z., **340,** 290, 1964.
69. Velick, S. F., and Anderson, R. J.: The chemistry of phytomonas tumefaciens. III. Phytomonic acid, a new branched-chain fatty acid. J. Biol. Chem., **152,** 523, 1944.
70. Kates, M., Yengoyan, L. W., and Sastry, P. S.: A diether analog of phosphatidyl glycerophosphate in *Halobacterium cutirubrum.* Biochim. Biophys. Acta, **98,** 252, 1965.
71. Hansen, R. P.: 3,7,11,15-Tetramethylhexadecanoic acid: Its occurrence in the tissues of humans afflicted with Refsum's syndrome. Biochim. Biophys. Acta, **106,** 304, 1965.
72. Stokke, O.: Alpha-oxidation of fatty acids in various mammals, and a phytanic acid feeding experiment in an animal with a low alpha-oxidation capacity. Scand. J. Clin. Lab. Invest., **20,** 305, 1967.
73. Eldjarn, L., Try, K., and Stokke, O.: The existence of an alternative pathway for the degradation of branched-chain fatty acids, and its failure in heredopathia atactica polyneuritiformis (Refsum's disease). Biochim. Biophys. Acta, **116,** 395, 1966.
74. Stokke, O., Try, K., and Eldjarn, L.: α-Oxidation as an alternative pathway for the degradation of branched-chain fatty acids in man, and its failure in patients with Refsum's disease. Biochim. Biophys. Acta, **144,** 271, 1967.
75. Try, K.: Indications of only a partial defect in the alpha-oxidation mechanism in Refsum's disease. Scand. J. Clin. Lab. Invest., **20,** 255, 1967.
76. Laurell, S.: The action of lipoprotein lipase on glyceryl triphytanate. Biochim. Biophys. Acta, **152,** 80, 1968.
77. Karlsson, K-A., Norrby, A., and Samuelsson, B.: Use of thin-layer chromatography for the preliminary diagnosis of Refsum's disease (heredopathia atactica polyneuritiformis). Biochim. Biophys. Acta, **144,** 162, 1967.
78. Laudat, P., and Wolf, L.-M.: Répartition des esters phytaniques parmi les triglycérides plasmatiques de cinq patients atteints de maladie de Refsum. Étude par chromatographie en couche mince. Biochim. Biophys. Acta, **176,** 425, 1969.
79. Avigan, J., and Steinberg, D.: Unpublished results.
80. Ellingboe, J.: Personal communication.
81. Green, D. E., and Allmann, D. W.: Fatty acid oxidation, in *Metabolic Pathways,* edited by D. M. Greenberg, vol. II, p. 1. Academic, New York, 1968.
82. Robinson, W. G., Bachhawat, B. K., and Coon, M. J.: Tiglyl coenzyme A and α-methylacetoacetyl coenzyme A, intermediates in the enzymatic degradation of isoleucine. J. Biol. Chem., **218,** 391, 1956.
83. Bowen, D. M., and Radin, N. S.: Hydroxy fatty acid metabolism in brain. Advances Lipid Res., **6,** 255, 1968.
84. Castelfranco, P., Stumpf, P. K., and Contopolon, R.: Fat metabolism in higher plants. V. A soluble palmitate oxidase requiring glycolic acid as activator. J. Biol. Chem., **214,** 567, 1955.

85. Stumpf, P. K.: Fat metabolism in higher plants. J. Biol. Chem., **223,** 643, 1956.
86. Martin, R. O., and Stumpf, P. K.: Fat metabolism in higher plants. XII. α-Oxidation of long chain fatty acids. J. Biol. Chem., **234,** 2548, 1959.
87. Hitchcock, C., and James, A. T.: Oxidation of unsaturated fatty acids by leaf tissue. J. Lipid Res., **5,** 593, 1964.
88. Hitchcock, C., and James, A. T.: The mechanism of α-oxidation in leaves. Biochim. Biophys. Acta, **116,** 413, 1966.
89. Hitchcock, C., Morris, L. J., and James, A. T.: The stereochemistry of α-oxidation of fatty acids in plants. Isotopic competition experiments. Europ. J. Biochem., **3,** 419, 1968.
90. Fulco, A. J., and Mead, J. F.: The biosynthesis of lignoceric, cerebronic, and nervonic acids. J. Biol. Chem., **236,** 2416, 1961.
91. Hajra, A. K., and Radin, N. S.: Isotopic studies of the biosynthesis of the cerebroside fatty acids in rats; in vivo conversion of labeled fatty acids to the sphingolipid fatty acids in rat brain. J. Lipid Res., **4,** 448, 1963.
92. Kishimoto, Y., and Radin, N. S.: Occurrence of 2-hydroxy fatty acids in animal tissues. J. Lipid Res., **4,** 139, 1963.
93. Hajra, A. K., and Radin, N. S.: Biosynthesis of odd- and even-numbered cerebroside fatty acids: Evidence for two routes. Biochim. Biophys. Acta, **70,** 97, 1963.
94. Mead, J. F., and Levis, G. M.: A 1 carbon degradation of long chain fatty acids of brain sphingolipids. J. Biol. Chem., **238,** 1634, 1963.
95. Levis, G. M., and Mead, J. F.: An α-hydroxy acid decarboxylase in brain microsomes. J. Biol. Chem., **239,** 77, 1964.
96. Levis, G. M.: The possible role of ascorbic acid in the α-hydroxyacid decarboxylase of brain microsomes. Biochim. Biophys. Acta, **99,** 194, 1965.
97. Macdonald, R. C., and Mead, J. F.: The *alpha*-oxidation system of brain microsomes: Cofactors for *alpha*-hydroxy acid decarboxylation. Lipids, **3,** 275, 1966.
98. Davies, W. E., Hajra, A. K., Parmar, S. S., Radin, N. S., and Mead, J. F.: Decarboxylation of 2-keto fatty acids by brain. J. Lipid Res., **7,** 270, 1966.
99. Lippel, K., and Mead, J. F.: Alpha-oxidation of 2-hydroxystearic acid *in vitro.* Biochim. Biophys. Acta, **152,** 669, 1968.
100. Shorland, F. B., Hansen, R. P., and Prior, I. A. M.: The effect of phytanic acid on the fatty acid composition of the lipids of the rat with further observations on its metabolism, in *Proceedings of the Seventh International Congress of Nutrition,* vol. 5, p. 399. Verlag Friedr. Vieweg & Sohn GmbH, West Germany, 1966.
101. Hansen, R. P., Shorland, F. B., and Prior, I. A. M.: The occurrence of 4,8,12-trimethyltridecanoic acid in the tissues of rats fed high levels of phytanic acid. Biochim. Biophys. Acta, **152,** 642, 1968.
102. Hansen, R. P., and Morrison, J. D.: The isolation and identification of 2,6,10,14-tetramethylpentadecanoic acid from butterfat. Biochem. J., **93,** 225, 1964.
103. Hansen, R. P.: Occurrence of 2,6,10,14-tetramethylpentadecanoic acid in sheep fat. Chem. Industr., p. 1258, 1965.
104. Blass, J. P., Avigan, J., and Tsai, S.-C.: Unpublished results (cited in ref. 126).
105. Hansen, R. P.: 4,8,12-Trimethyltridecanoic acid: Its isolation and identification from sheep perinephric fat. Biochim. Biophys. Acta, **164,** 550, 1968.
106. Hansen, R. P.: The isolation and identification of 4,8,12-trimethyltridecanoic acid from butterfat. J. Dairy Res., **36,** 77, 1969.
107. Preiss, B., and Bloch, K.: Omega-oxidation of long chain fatty acids in rat liver. J. Biol. Chem., **239,** 85, 1964.
108. Wakabayashi, K., and Shimazono, N.: Studies on omega-oxidation of fatty acids *in vitro.* I. Overall reaction and intermediate. Biochim. Biophys. Acta, **70,** 132, 1963.
109. Bergström, S., Borgström, B., Tryding, N., and Westöö, G.: Intestinal absorption and metabolism of 2,2-dimethylstearic acid in the rat. Biochem. J., **58,** 604, 1954.
110. Antony, G. J., and Landau, B. R.: Relative contributions of alpha, beta and omega-oxidative pathways to in vitro fatty acid oxidation in rat liver. J. Lipid Res., **9,** 267, 1968.
111. Try, K.: The in vitro omega-oxidation of phytanic acid and other branched chain fatty acids by mammalian liver. Scand. J. Clin. Lab. Invest., **22,** 224, 1968.
112. Bachhawat, B. K., Robinson, W. G., and Coon, M. S.: Enzymatic carboxylation of β-hydroxyisovaleryl coenzyme A. J. Biol. Chem., **219,** 539, 1956.
113. Bachhawat, B. K., Robinson, W. G., and Coon, M. J.: The enzymatic cleavage of β-hydroxy-β-methylglutaryl coenzyme A to acetoacetate and acetyl coenzyme A. J. Biol. Chem., **216,** 727, 1955.
114. Seubert, W., and Remberger, U.: Untersuchungen über den bakteriellen Abbau von Isoprenoiden. II. Die Rolle der Kohlensäure. Biochem. Z., **338,** 245, 1963.
115. Stokke, O.: Evidence against a CO_2-fixation mechanism in the degradation of a beta-methyl-substituted fatty acid in mammals. Biochim. Biophys. Acta, 176, 230, 1969.
116. Eldjarn, L.: Heredopathia atactica polyneuritiformis (Refsum's disease)—a defect in the omega-oxidation mechanism of fatty acids. Scand. J. Clin. Lab. Invest., **17,** 178, 1965.
117. Eldjarn, L., Try, K., and Stokke, O.: The ability of patients with heredopathia atactica polyneuritiformis to omega-oxidize and degrade several isoprenoid branch-chained fatty structures. Scand. J. Clin. Lab. Invest., **18,** 141, 1966.
118. Try, K., and Eldjarn, L.: Normalization of the tricaprin test for omega-oxidation in Refsum's disease upon lowering of serum phytanic acid. Scand. J. Clin. Lab. Invest., **20,** 294, 1967.
119. Refsum, S.: Heredopathia atactica polyneuritiformis. Acta Genet. (Basel), **7,** 344, 1957.
120. Richterich, R., Rosin, S., and Rossi, E.: Refsum's disease (heredopathia atactica polyneuritiformis): An inborn error of lipid metabolism with storage of 3,7,11,15-tetramethyl hexadecanoic acid. Formal Genetics. Humangenetik, **1,** 333, 1965.
121. Uhlendorf, B. W., Jacobson, C. B., Sloan, H. R., Mudd, S. H., Herndon, J. H., Brady, R. O., Seegmiller, J. E., and Fujimoto, W.: Cell cultures derived from human amniotic fluid: The possible application in the intra-uterine diagnosis of heritable metabolic disease. In Vitro, **4,** 158, 1969.
122. O'Brien, J. D.: Cell membranes—composition, structure, function. J. Theor. Biol., **15,** 307, 1967.
123. Blass, J. P., Avigan, J., and Clark, R. G.: Effects of phytol feeding and experimental allergic encephalomyelitis on myelin synthesis. (Abstract), Fed. Proc., **28,** 838, 1969.
124. MacBrinn, M. C., and O'Brien, J. S.: Lipid composition of the nervous system in Refsum's disease. J. Lipid Res., **9,** 552, 1968.
125. Kishimoto, Y., Radin, N. S., and Steinberg, D.: Cited in ref. 83.
126. Blass, J. P., Avigan, J., and Steinberg, D.: α-Hydroxy fatty acids in hereditary ataxic polyneuritis (Refsum's disease). Biochim. Biophys. Acta, **187,** 36, 1969.

PART FIVE

DISORDERS OF STEROID METABOLISM

CHAPTER THIRTY-EIGHT

DISORDERS OF ADRENOCORTICAL STEROID BIOGENESIS

(The Adrenogenital Syndrome Associated with Congenital Adrenal Hyperplasia)

Alfred M. Bongiovanni

The appellation *adrenogenital syndrome* to designate a disease of man probably stems from the coincidence of gross adrenal disease (usually hyperplasia) and disorders of the genitalia which are often congenital. It is advisable to discard the generic terminology "congenital *virilizing* adrenocortical hyperplasia" since there are now several recognized categories within this theme which do not display virilization, and in some forms the normal masculine embryogenesis of the genotypic male fetus is wanting. The adrenogenital syndrome associated with adrenocortical hyperplasia is a genetic disorder in the biosynthesis of adrenal corticoids (primarily cortisol and at times aldosterone) stemming from a deficiency of one of several enzymatic systems required for "complete" steroidal biogenesis.[1]

The first forms of the adrenogenital syndrome to be recognized were characterized by clinical virilization and attributed to an excessive production of androgens by the disordered adrenal cortex. This was eventually found to be the result of defective cortisol formation and the diversion of certain crucial intermediary metabolites into other pathways, leading to the production of testosterone. Later, different loci of enzymatic deficiency were shown to exclude the pathways to androgens. Hence virilization is not a common clinical denominator in all forms. Nonetheless, the more common varieties involve those enzymes which permit excessive androgen secretion and thus represent the more frequent types.

The first unmistakable and thorough description of the adrenogenital syndrome is that of de Crecchio [1] in 1865. The author was an anatomist who dissected the cadaver of an apparent male of some 40 years, with bilateral cryptorchidism and partial hypospadias. The penis had normal corpora cavernosa and there were ejaculatory ducts, a well-developed prostate and Cowper's glands. On further examination the cadaver revealed a vagina, uterus, fallopian tubes, ovaries, and extremely large adrenal glands. It is interesting that the subject of this study was said to have had frequent diarrhea and vomiting and that he died during such an episode. In "his" last illness, "he became reduced in a very few days to a state of extreme weakness and exhaustion." Might this have been an addisonian crisis? Finally the author describes his investigations into the subject's psychosexual orientation. There were some doubts of the gender until 4 years of age, at which time he was declared a male, and thereafter conducted himself in all arenas, including sexual intercourse, as a man. This description is a classic for the virilizing form of the disease, sufficiently extreme to masculinize the external genitalia of a genotypic female, so that she was believed to be of the male sex.

CLINICAL FEATURES

The clinical expression of the disordered adrenocortical metabolism depends upon the inadequate secretion of active critical hormones, primarily cortisol and aldosterone, and the excessive production of certain precursors which may directly affect the organism (e.g., deoxycorticosterone) or be diverted in large amounts into pathways producing androgens. In the event that the biochemical defect occurs early in the normal pathway, virtually no hormonally active substances will be produced, including those fetal steroids required for normal male organogenesis of the lower genital tract. Under the latter circumstance, there can be no viriliza-

[1] The following trivial names are used here: *Aldosterone:* 11β,21-dihydroxypregn-4-en-3,20-dion-18-al; *tetrahydro aldosterone:* 3α,11β,21-trihydroxy-5β-pregnane-3,20-dione-18-al; *androstenedione:* androst-4-ene-3,17-dione; *11β-hydroxyandrostenedione:* 11β-hydroxyandrost-4-ene-3,17-dione; *cholesterol:* cholest-5-en-3β-ol; *corticosterone, compound B:* 11β,21-dihydroxypregn-4-ene-3,20-dione; *18-hydroxycorticosterone (B):* 11β,18,21-trihydroxypregn-4-ene-3,20-dione; *cortisol, compound F:* 11β,17α,21-trihydroxypregn-4-ene-3,20-dione; *dehydroepiandrosterone:* 3β-hydroxyandrost-5-en-17-one; *16α-hydroxydehydroepiandrosterone:* 3β,16α-dihydroxyandrost-5-en-17-one; *deoxycorticosterone, DOC:* 21-hydroxypregn-4-ene-3,20-dione; *20α-dihydroprogesterone:* 20α-hydroxypregn-4-en-3-one; *20β-dihydroprogesterone:* 20β-hydroxypregn-4-en-3-one; *pregnanediol:* 5β-pregnane-3α,20α-diol; *pregnenolone:* 3β-hydroxypregn-5-en-20-one; *17-hydroxypregnenolone:* 3β,17α-dihydroxypregn-5-en-20-one; *progesterone:* pregn-4-ene-3,20-dione; *16α-hydroxyprogesterone:* 16α-hydroxypregn-4-ene-3,20-dione; *17-hydroxyprogesterone:* 17α-hydroxypregn-4-ene-3,20-dione; *17-hydroxypregnanolone:* 3α,17α,5β-pregnane-20-one; *testosterone:* 17β-hydroxyandrost-4-en-3-one; *cortisone, compound E:* 17α,21-dihydroxypregn-4-ene-3,11,20-trione; *21-deoxy-F:* 11β,17α-dihydroxypregn-4-ene-3,20-dione; *substance S:* 17α,21-dihydroxypregn-4-ene-3,20-dione; *pregnanetriol:* 5β-pregnane-3α,17α,20α-triol; *pregnanetriolone:* 3α,17α,20α-trihydroxy-5β-pregnane-11-one; *androsterone:* 3α-hydroxy-5α-androstan-17-one; *etiocholanolone:* 3α-hydroxy-5β-androstan-17-one; *THS, tetrahydro S:* 3α,17α,21-trihydroxy-5β-pregnan-20-one; *THE, tetrahydro E:* 3α,17α,21-trihydroxy-5β-pregnane-11,20-dione; *THF, tetrahydro F:* 3α,11β,17α,21-tetrahydroxy-5β-pregnan-20-one; *THDOC, tetrahydro DOC:* 3α,21-dihydroxy-5β-pregnan-20-one; *THB, tetrahydro B:* 3α,11β,21-trihydroxy-5β-pregnan-20-one; *tetrahydro-18-hydroxycorticosterone:* 3α,11β,11,18-tetrahydroxy-β-pregnan-20-one.

tion and there is profound expression of adrenocortical deficiency. Since there is evidence for varying degrees of defective metabolism at several enzymatic steps, the clinical manifestations may vary.

In those forms (most common) with excessive androgen secretion, virilization is usually apparent at birth in the female and within the first 2 to 3 years of life in the male. Since adrenocortical activity begins in the fetus prior to complete development of the external genitalia, the affected female is exposed to excessive androgens from her own adrenal and the external genitalia are masculinized to a variable degree. At birth there is hypertrophy of the clitoris associated with its ventral binding, as in chordee, and variable fusion of the labioscrotal folds conceal the introitus (Fig. 38-1). The internal female duct structures and gonads remain unaltered, although as noted in the classical case of de Crecchio, certain caudal male structures, such as the prostate, may become prominent. The external appearance is similar to that of a male with bilateral cryptochidism and hypospadias, from which the adrenogenital syndrome in a female may not be differentiated by inspection alone. The labioscrotal folds are bulbous and rugated, and resemble a scrotum [2]. In a small percentage the labioscrotal fusion may be so extensive that the urethra traverses the phallus. A penile urethra has been described in a number of females with the adrenogenital syndrome [3, 4, 5, 6, 7, 8, 9, 10]. These

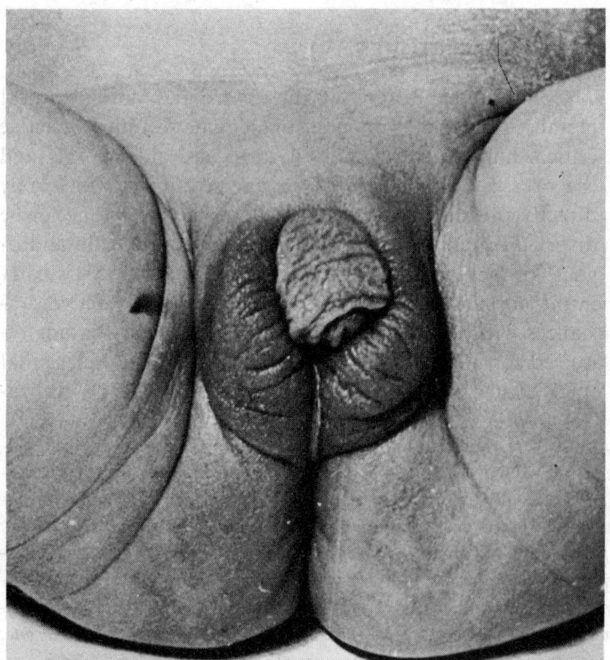

Figure 38-1. External genitalia of female infant with congenital adrenal hyperplasia (21-hydroxylase defect) demonstrating the usual malformation. The labia majora are almost completely fused and scrotal in appearance, the clitoris is enlarged and somewhat bound by chordee, and there is a single small orifice (not visible) at its base. (*From Bongiovanni et al.* [160].)

subjects resemble males with cryptorchidism and are often reared as boys. Under these circumstances, clinical sexual differentiation becomes extremely difficult and the error in sex assignment is common. Weldon et al. [11] reviewed several such errors.

Similar alterations in the human female fetus are produced by administration of androgenic substances to the mother early in gestation or by maternal androgen-secreting tumors. This condition has been termed female pseudohermaphroditism. In a few cases the fusion is slight or rarely absent. The virilization may become evident for the first time in such females in later infancy, adolescence, or adulthood with the appearance of extreme hirsutism, seborrhea, clitoral enlargement and deepening of the voice. Decourt, Jayle, and Baulieu [12], Jayle et al. [13], Lipsett and Riter [14], Mahesh et al. [15], and Brooks [16] have described older girls with virilization in later life and the biochemical findings typical of the adrenogenital syndrome. An occasional male has been described, as that of Guenel at al. [17], with the disorder appearing in later life. Whether these are acquired forms of the disease or the later pictures of mild congenital forms, with few signs in early life, cannot be ascertained. In all such instances it is important to rule out an adrenal tumor, since neoplasm rather than the adrenogenital syndrome due to hyperplasia explains most instances of acquired virilization. Marie et al. [18] report what they consider to have been the adrenogenital syndrome in a female infant with normal genitalia, but with the early acquisition of pubic hair and progressive virilization in very early life. They suggest that although the condition was congenital, the excessive androgens may not have been secreted until after the fifth fetal month when development of the external genitalia was complete.

The untreated female grows rapidly during the first years of life with relentless progessive virilism. At puberty there is, almost always, failure of normal female sexual development and menstruation. In both sexes rapid somatic maturation is displayed by extreme advance of epiphyseal ossification. As a result there is the paradox of a dwarfed adult in a previously abnormally tall child [2]. Many of the signs of virilization, such as beard, are difficult to reverse, hence the importance of early replacement therapy, particularly in girls.

In the absence of complications, i.e., saltwater loss, the condition is usually not recognized in the male at birth. In the commonest types, there has been no disturbance of normal male embryogenesis and the sexual organs appear normal. There is early and excessive development of the penis and appearance of the secondary sexual characteristics (Fig. 38-2). Rapid growth, early acne, deepening of the voice, frequent erections and excessive muscular development occur within the first few years of life. This condition has been termed macrogenitosomia precox or pseudosexual precocity. The testes usually remain infantile in size despite the rapid development, and this finding excludes constitutional sexual precocity.

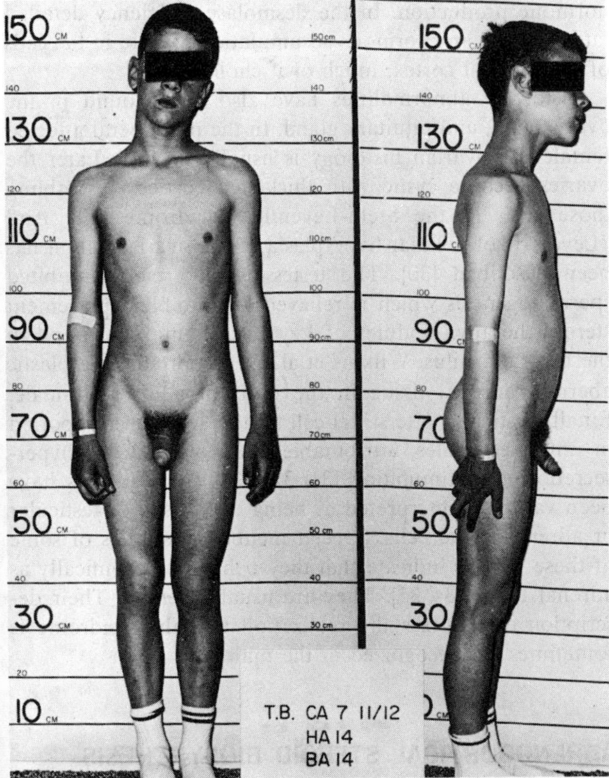

Figure 38-2. Male of 7 years with congenital adrenal hyperplasia (21-hydroxylase defect) demonstrating the usual appearance. Both the height age (HA) and bone age (BA) are advanced but the testes are infantile in size and are not visible in the photograph. (*From Bongiovanni et al.* [160].)

Generally the gonads fail to develop so that the affected individual may be expected to be infertile without therapy. The additional disadvantage in the female resides in the absence of normal feminine sexual development, which is perhaps due to both lack of ovarian hormones and excessive adrenal androgens. It is thought that the "abnormal" adrenal products suppress the secretion of gonadotropins.

Rare varieties of the disease due to different but well-defined enzymatic defects are known in which the male does not achieve normal masculine embryogenesis of the external genitalia. There may be hypospadias or indeed complete failure of masculine development. At times both males and females with these forms resemble one another. They may both have female external genitalia or there may be a partial masculinization of the genitalia which is equal in both sexes. The latter may be explained by the production of androgens, in type and amount, enough to virilize mildly the female fetus, but insufficient to bring about full male development in the opposite sex. Generally these types are characterized by defective enzymatic systems shared by both adrenals and gonads.

In some patients with the adrenogenital syndrome, vomiting and dehydration resembling addisonian crisis develop within a few weeks of birth. The first cases of this complication were recorded by Phillips in 1888 [19]. Four of seven sibs with the adrenogenital syndrome died under such circumstances. It was not until 1939, when Butler et al. [20] reported a case, that the electrolyte disturbance was clarified as resembling that seen in adrenal insufficiency, and the beneficial response to the administration of sodium chloride was described. Wilkins et al. [21], soon thereafter, reported similar findings. The basis for this manifestation is not as yet clear and is discussed below. It is not strictly associated with only one type of the recognized biochemical defects. This so-called "salt-losing" form of the disease is reported to occur in from as few as 30 percent to as many as 65 percent of all cases according to Marks et al. [22].

EMBRYOLOGY

In the human embryo between the fifth and sixth fetal week the gonadal anlagen are recognized as genital ridges on either side of the dorsal mesentery. At this time, the primitive gonad consists of approximately equal cortical (ovarian) and medullary (testicular) components. They are bipotential and capable of developing into either structure. Testicular differentiation occurs in this ambiguous structure at about the seventh fetal week with proliferation of the primary sex cords and invasion by the coelemic epithelium carrying the germ cells. The interstitial cells become abundant by the eighth week and their secretion plays an important role in male sexual differentiation. On the other hand, ovarian differentiation begins about 2 weeks later with proliferation of the cortex and migration of the secondary sex cords into the interior, at the expense of the medulla. Between the third and fourth fetal month, the cortex undergoes further proliferation with further contraction of the medulla.

The human fetus of 7 weeks contains the primordial anlage of both the male and female genital ducts. The müllerian ducts represent the forerunners of the uterus and fallopian tubes whereas the wolffian ducts become the epididymis, vas deferens, seminal vesicles, and ejaculatory ducts of the male. One predominates by the third month as the other involutes. So too, the external genitalia remain identical at the eighth week, consisting of a urogenital slit, surrounded by urethral folds and the labioscrotal folds. The genital tubercle is present consisting of corpora cavernosa and the glans. These structures may remain patent to form the labia majora and the introitus (female) or they may fuse in the midline to form the scrotum and penile urethra. Normally the differentiation of genital ducts and the external genitalia will conform to the chromosomal and the gonadal sex, either testis or ovary.

Alfred Jost [23, 24] has demonstrated in a series of brilliant experiments that the secretions of the fetal testis play a critical role in the differentiation of these structures. There are probably two different hormonal products of the testis. One, apparently a polypeptide, which inhibits the müllerian elements and stimulates the wolffian ducts produces male internal sex differentiation. The fetal ovary is passive, so that even in its absence equally good development of the uterus, tubes, and external genitalia will occur. The testis produces a second secretion, almost certainly testosterone or a closely related androgenic steroid, which causes fusion of the urogenital slit and growth of the genital tubercle. The administration of androgens experimentally brings about variable male differentiation of the external genitalia in the female fetus, depending upon the dosage and the stage of development.

Thus, errors in steroidogenesis may influence sexual embryonogenesis, but only of the external structures. The internal differentiation depends upon a separate secretory product and is therefore not subject to disturbances in steroid hormone production. The female fetus exposed to androgens at an early stage of embryonic development, as occurs in disorders of steroid hormone production with inordinate adrenocortical activity, will develop variable virilization of the external structures whereas the uterus and tubes remain intact. Or in certain types of steroidal disorders with an enzymatic defect shared by the gonads, the adrenal may not be engaged in large androgen production, but the defect will impair the secretion of testosterone by the fetal testis, leading to a failure of appropriate male development of the external genitalia. At times the picture is not so clear-cut. Certain disorders of steroidogenesis may lead to the high secretion of steroids having modest virilizing action on the fetus, so that the female fetus develops mildly masculinized external genitalia and the male is incompletely formed, as in hypospadias.

These considerations are important since the genetic disorders in steroid hormone production express themselves early in fetal life and thus influence differentiation of the caudal sexual structures. But since the steroids play no role in the differentiation of the internal structures, these coincide with the chromosomal and gonadal sex.

ANATOMIC PATHOLOGY

Blackman [25] described progressive hyperplasia of the zona reticularia in the adrenal cortex of patients with congenital adrenal hyperplasia. He concluded that this was the source of the excessive androgens. There was a variable amount of poorly developed zona glomerulosa and attempts were made to correlate this with the "salt-losing" form. Tonutti [26] believed the zona fasciculata to be hyperplastic and Seelen [27] found both zones enlarged in material obtained upon adrenalectomy or biopsy.

Symington [28] demonstrated that in normal adrenal glands, adrenocorticotropin stimulation causes the "clear" cells of the zona fasciculata to become indistinguishable from those of the reticularis. He proposes that the two zones function as a single unit, the fasciculata as a storage area for steroidal precursors and the reticularis as the site of hormone production. In the desmolase deficiency detailed later, there is an enormous accumulation of lipid in the cells of the adrenal cortex, much of it cholesterol.

Histologic abnormalities have also been found in the ovary, testis, and pituitary gland. In the prepuberal affected female the ovarian histology is usually normal. Later the ovaries become cystic with thickened cortices resembling those seen in the Stein-Leventhal syndrome [29]. And "Leydig-like" cellular hyperplasia of the ovarian hilum has been described [30]. The testes usually reveal inhibited spermatogenesis which is relieved by suitable replacement steroid therapy. Nodules of Leydig cells may be found in the testicular hilus. Wilkins et al. [21] reported hyperplastic aberrant adrenal tissue in the testis of a diseased male. Finally testicular interstitial cell tumors have been reported in untreated males, attributable to chronic ACTH hypersecretion and stimulation [31, 32, 33]. These tumors have been variously interpreted as being comprised of testicular or adrenocortical cells. Special incubation studies of some of these tumors indicate that they behave biochemically as adrenal tissue [34, 35]. They are usually benign. Their description emphasizes the realization that the syndrome is sometimes not recognized in the male.

ADRENOCORTICAL STEROID BIOSYNTHESIS

The primary steroidal secretory products of the adrenal cortex are C_{21} compounds with a cyclopentanophenanthrene nucleus, two angular methyl groups, and a two-carbon side chain at C-17 (Fig. 38-3). These are generated from cholesterol. Cholesterol is formed from acetate by way of β-hydroxy-β-methylglutaric acid, mevalonic acid, isopentyl pyrosphosphate, geranyl pyrophosphate, and farnesyl pyrophosphate. Squalene forms by the condensation of two molecules of farnesyl pyrophosphate, which cyclizes to lanosterol, and which is then converted to cholesterol

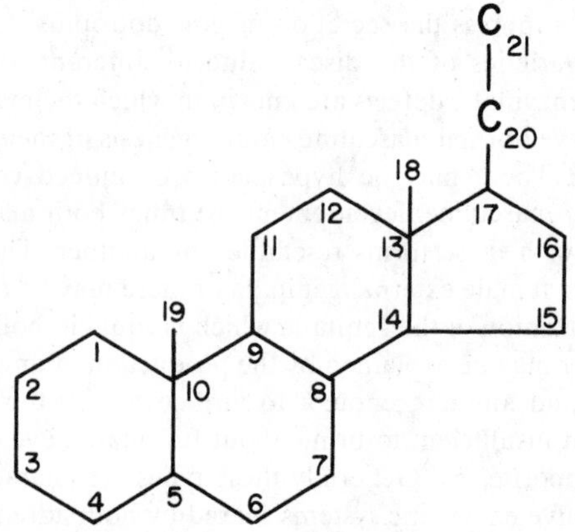

Figure 38-3. The dimethyl cyclopentanophenanthrene nucleus with side chain, also designated as the pregnane skeleton, with carbon atoms numbered according to convention.

[36–44]. It is possible that the C_{21} steroids (corticoids) may arise in some small measure from acetate without passage through the cholesterol.

Cleavage of cholesterol to pregnenolone has been reasonably well established. Solomons et al. [45] first suggested that 20α-hydroxycholesterol was a possible intermediate and subsequently 20α, 22ξ-dihydroxycholesterol was demonstrated as a further intermediate (Fig. 38-4). The side chain of cholesterol is cleaved as isocaproaldehyde, which is oxidized to isocaproic acid [46]. The enzyme complex for the cleavage of cholesterol is not highly specific and demonstrates an affinity for a number of sterols with variations in the nucleus as well as the side chain. Normally all of the enzymes involved in the process ("desmolase") are present in the cell as an organized complex, and the overall rate of conversion to pregnenolone is determined by the first reaction, i.e., the formation of 20α-hydroxycholesterol [47]. NADPH is a required cofactor. It is to be noted that pregnenolone retains the 3β-hydroxyl function and the 5-6 unsaturation of cholesterol. Thereafter a series of oxidations occur on the pregnenolone molecule as outlined below.

Steroid Hydroxylations in Steroidogenesis

The principal biochemical reactions in the conversion of cholesterol into active adrenocortical steroids require a series of hydroxylations which have the same general requirements. The hydroxylation of deoxycorticosterone at carbon-11β was first studied in some detail, It was found that NADPH was required and the reaction was facilitated by certain Krebs' cycle intermediates [48, 49]. Furthermore, molecular oxygen was incorporated from the atmosphere [50]. It became apparent that the system conformed to a mixed function oxidase, one atom of molecular oxygen being incorporated into the substrate and the other being reduced to water. This may be represented as follows where RH is the steroid substrate and H_2X, reduced nicotinamide-adenine dinucleotide phosphate (NADPH):

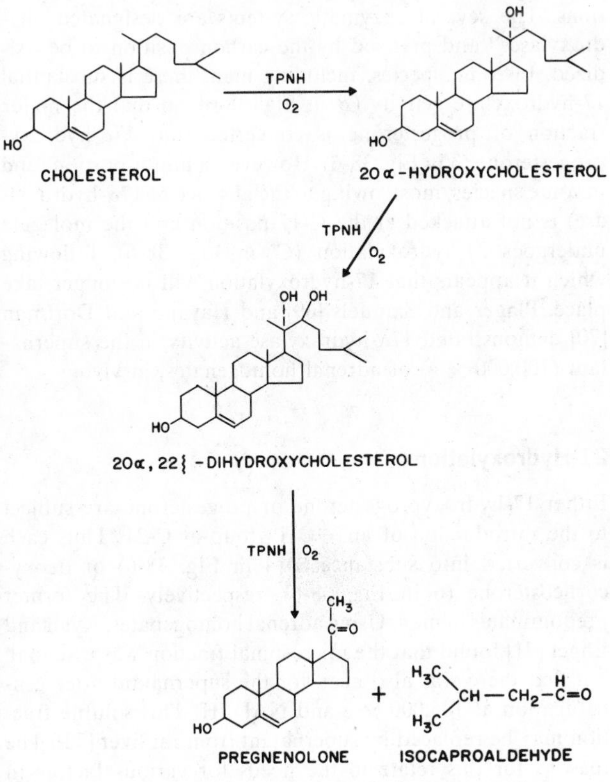

$$\text{RH} + O_2 + H_2X \longrightarrow \text{R-OH} + X + H_2O$$

Tomkins et al. [51] indicated the need for several components, and Omura [52] and Kimura [53] resolved the 11β-hydroxylase system into three components. Harding et al. [54, 55] reported a cytochrome of the P-450 type serving as the terminal oxidase. Cooper et al. [56] assigned cytochrome P-450, the carbon monoxide binding pigment of adrenal mitochondria, as the oxygen-activating enzyme. This type of hemoprotein was first found by Garfinkel in liver [57] and, subsequently, in adrenal microsomes by Ryan and Engel [58].

Estabrook's group, studying C-21 hydroxylation [59], and Harding's group [60], examining 11β-hydroxylation, further implicated the following components in steroidal hydroxylation: NADPH; a flavoprotein dehydrogenase (FP), also known as adrenodoxin reductase specific for NADPH; adrenodoxin, a nonheme iron containing pigment (NHI-P), and cytochrome P-450. The flow of electrons through this system is shown in Fig. 38-5. NADPH transfers electrons to cytochrome P-450. The reduced P-450 forms an activated complex with the steroidal substrate and molecular oxygen. In the process P-450-Fe(++) is oxidized to Fe(+++). Note that NADPH is also directly involved in the steroid hydroxylation by generating the hydroperoxo complex. This has been reviewed by Sih [61].

There may exist a number of pathways for this flow of electrons as stressed by Harding et al. [60], who find that ascorbate may serve as a potential donor under suitable conditions.

These pathways may prove applicable to the several recognized hydroxylations in steroidal biogenesis: 20α, 22ξ, 17α, 21, 11β, and 18. The first two are required to cleave the cholesterol side chain producing the 21-carbon steroid molecule. The remainder provide further embellishments toward the formation of cortisol, aldosterone, and, ultimately, the sex hormones. Four are present in adrenocortical mitochondria (20α, 22ξ, 18, and 11β) and the remaining two in microsomes. Although "zonation" will not be emphasized herein, it is important to recognize the localization of certain hydroxylases in a single region of the gland. For example, 18-hydroxylase predominates in the zona glomerulosa. This implies certain complexities of substrate migration from one part of the organ to another.

CHOLESTEROL → (TPNH, O_2) → 20α-HYDROXYCHOLESTEROL → (TPNH, O_2) → 20α, 22ξ-DIHYDROXYCHOLESTEROL → (TPNH, O_2) → PREGNENOLONE + ISOCAPROALDEHYDE

Figure 38-4. The conversion of cholesterol to pregnenolone.

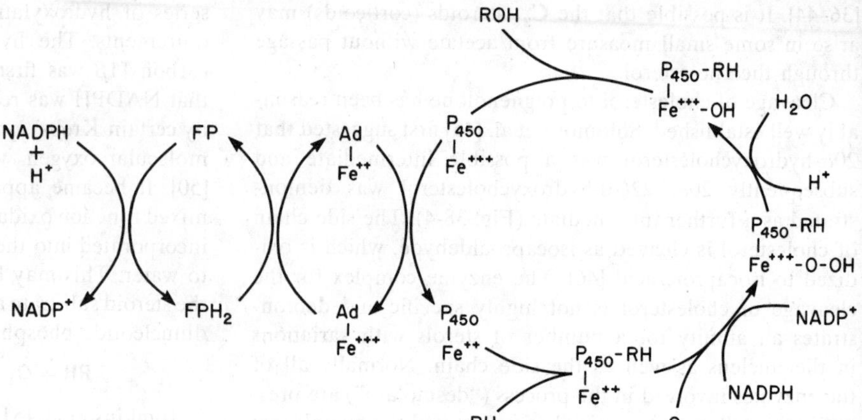

Figure 38-5. The several components for the flow of electrons in the hydroxylation of the steroid (R) molecule.

Conversion of Pregnenolone to Progesterone

Pregnenolone (1 in Fig. 38-6) is the "earliest" C_{21} precursor in the synthesis of cortisol and aldosterone. It is required that the molecule assume the ring A-B structure of these active corticoids through oxidation of the 3β-hydroxyl group and isomerization from Δ^5 to Δ^4. The former process is accomplished by an enzymatic system designated 3 β-hydroxysteroid dehydrogenase (*A* in Fig. 38-6) which catalyzes the oxidation of the —OH group at C-3 to a ketonic function. This enzyme was first recognized by Samuels et al. [62] in testicular tissue and in both adrenal and gonadal tissues it would seem to be required for active hormone synthesis, whether sex hormone or adrenocortical steroid. Samuels et al. [62], as well as Beyer and Samuels [63], have demonstrated this activity in ovarian, testicular, adrenal, and placental tissue, with the major activity in the microsomal fraction. It is NADH dependent. A specific isomerase may also be necessary for this conversion, and such an enzyme has been demonstrated in *Pseudomonas testosteroni.* This isomerase has also been demonstrated in mammalian tissues, but the mechanism appears to be different. Whereas the bacterial enzyme causes a direct transfer of the 4β-H to C-6β, most of the labeled 4β-H was "lost" in the mammalian system. Fukushima et al. [64] and Bradlow et al. [65] demonstrated this peculiarity in man in vivo and in vitro with beef adrenal microsomes and rat liver 100,000 $\times$ *g* supernatant. Werbin and Chaikoff [66] had observed this difference in mammals in their studies of cholesterol metabolism. In spite of the evidence for this isomerase, it should be noted that certain chemical oxidations, such as the Oppenauer, not only oxidize the 3β-ol to a ketone but effect a rearrangement from Δ^5 to Δ^4. Thus, cholesterol on treatment with aluminum isopropoxide and cyclohexanone is converted to Δ^4-cholestene-3-one.

It does not appear that the reorganization of rings A-B in this fashion is obligatory at this point. There is evidence that 17-hydroxypregnenolone (8 in Fig. 38-6) may serve as a substrate for cortisol in certain in vitro studies [67, 68]. And in the rare disease associated with a deficiency of 3β-hydroxysteroid dehydrogenase, steroidal products have been isolated, thereby demonstrating that subsequent hydroxylations had taken place on the pregnenolone molecule without 3-oxidation or isomerization. Furthermore, the entire sequence of cortisol biosynthesis is apparently not obliged to adhere to the usual order of events as presented.

17-Hydroxylation

In order to achieve the formation of cortisol, progesterone (2 in Fig. 38-6) is hydroxylated at the 17, 21, and 11β positions. The several enzymatic systems are designated "hydroxylases" and prefixed by the carbon position to be oxidized. In some species, including man, there is substantial 17-hydroxylase activity (*B* in Fig. 38-6), so that the major fraction of progesterone is converted into 17α-hydroxyprogesterone (3 in Fig. 38-6). However, a minor portion (and in some species, most, owing to the absence of 17α-hydroxylase) is not attacked at the C-17 position and the molecule undergoes 21-hydroxylation (*C′* in Fig. 38-6), following which it appears that 17-hydroxylation will no longer take place. Plager and Samuels [69] and Hayano and Dorfman [70] demonstrated 17α-hydroxylase activity in the supernatant (100,000 $\times$ *g*) of adrenal homogenates, in vivo.

21-Hydroxylation

Either 17-hydroxyprogesterone or progesterone are subject to the introduction of an —OH group at C-21. Thus each is converted into substance S (4 in Fig. 38-6) or deoxycorticosterone (6 in Fig. 38-6), respectively. The former predominates in man. Using adrenal homogenates, Ryan and Engel [71] found that the microsomal fraction was essential, but that there was also need for the supernatant after centrifugation at 105,000 $\times$ *g* and NADPH. This soluble fraction may be replaced by supernatant from rat liver [72]. The reasons for this relate to the needs for various factors in the chain of electron transfer described above.

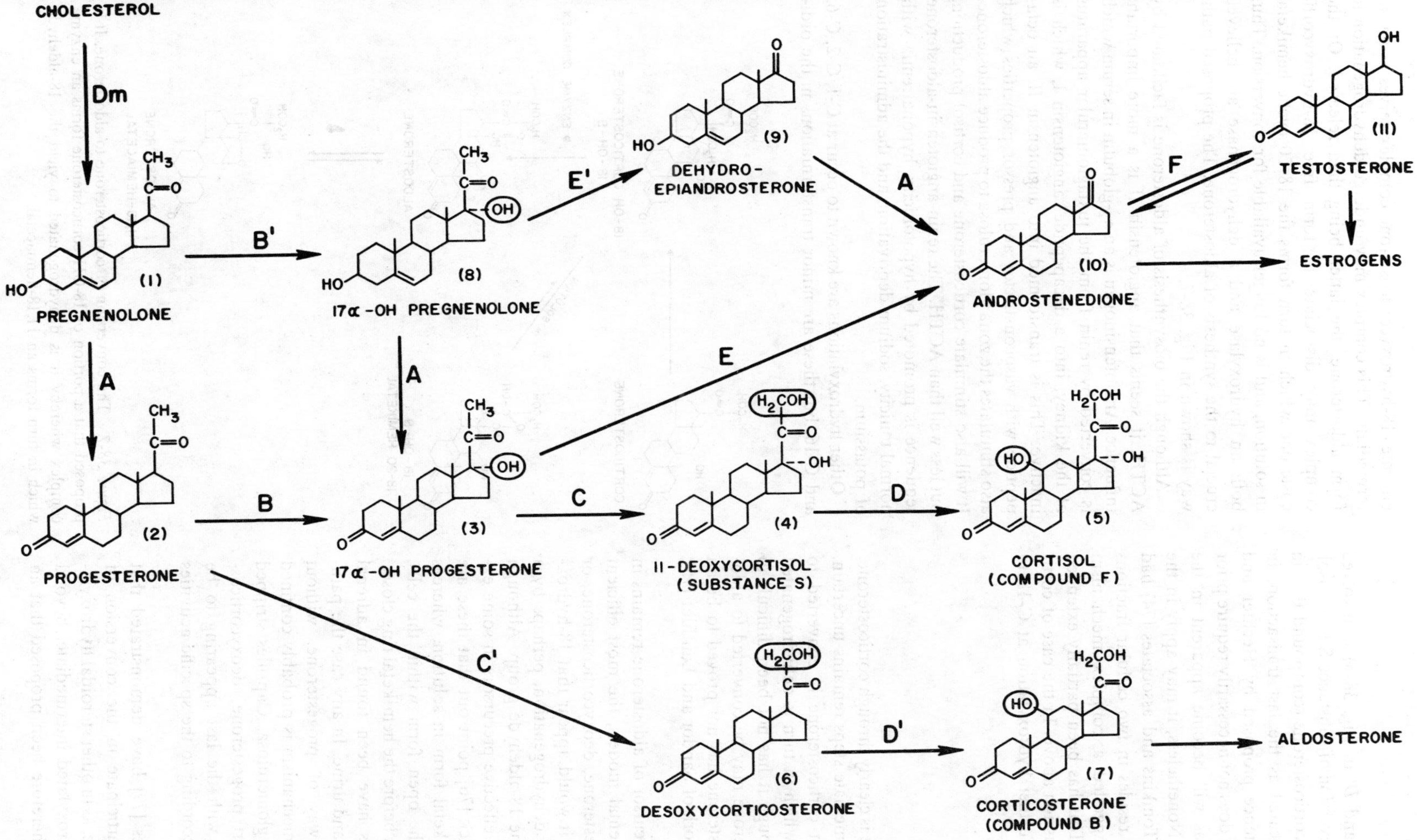

CHOLESTEROL

Dm

PREGNENOLONE (1)

B′

17α-OH PREGNENOLONE (8)

E′

DEHYDRO-EPIANDROSTERONE (9)

A

ANDROSTENEDIONE (10)

F

TESTOSTERONE (11)

ESTROGENS

A

PROGESTERONE (2)

B

17α-OH PROGESTERONE (3)

E

C

11-DEOXYCORTISOL (SUBSTANCE S) (4)

D

CORTISOL (COMPOUND F) (5)

C′

DESOXYCORTICOSTERONE (6)

D′

CORTICOSTERONE (COMPOUND B) (7)

ALDOSTERONE

Figure 38.6. The biosynthetic pathways to cortisol and other steroids including the sex hormones. The enzyme systems include Dm (cholesterol desmolase), *A* (3β-hydroxysteroid dehydrogenase and Δ^5-Δ^4-isomerase), *B,B′* (17-hydroxylase), *C,C′* (21-hydroxylase), *D,D′* (11-hydroxylase), *E,E′* (17-hydroxycorticoid cleaving enzyme), and *F* (17-hydroxysteroid dehydrogenase). In man the major pathway normally proceeds through *B* to cortisol while a smaller amount of progesterone is first hydroxylated at C-21 through *C′* to yield corticosterone and aldosterone. Most of the enzymes are present in both adrenocortical and gonadal tissue, but *C,C′* and *D,D′* are probably confined to the adrenal.

11β-Hydroxylation

The 11β-hydroxylase (*D* and *D′* in Fig. 38-6) is involved in the final step for the conversion of substance S to cortisol, or deoxycorticosterone to corticosterone (compound B, 7 in Fig. 38-6). Although indicated as the last transaction, in accordance with the sequence proposed by Hechter and Pincus [73], this occurrence does not necessarily require prior 17- or 21-hydroxylation, as will become apparent in the examination of disorders. Nonetheless, it may apply in the normal course of events. Tomkins and associates [74] had indicated that the activity resides in two cellular fractions of adrenal cortex and suggested a complex mechanism requiring several factors. This has been partially extended and elucidated in the discussion above. In the case of corticosterone, there may be further hydroxylation at C-18 to produce aldosterone.

18-Hydroxylation

The pathway to aldosterone is clearly through corticosterone, but the matter of the intermediate steps remains uncertain. It has been proposed that corticosterone is converted to 18-hydroxycorticosterone, which in turn is dehydrogenated to form aldosterone. Although it has not been difficult to demonstrate that corticosterone may be converted to aldosterone, 18-hydroxycorticosterone has not proved to be an efficient precursor in the work of Sandor and Lanthier [75], and many others.

Thus, the immediate precursor of aldosterone remains in doubt. In various experimental models, the most efficient intermediate may be progesterone, deoxycorticosterone, or corticosterone. In any case it would appear that 18-hydroxylation occurs followed by dehydrogenation, perhaps by a specific enzyme, to form the 18-aldehyde group. Although 18-hydroxysteroids are less effective precursors in some experiments, Nicolis and Ulick [76] point out that these are present as the 18–20 hemiketal form in solution, whereas they may be present as the open form within the cells, capable of dehydrogenation before the hemiketal ring closes. In fact, 18-hydroxysteroids have been found in adrenal tissue, adrenal vein blood, and urine. In any case the pathway would proceed by way of progesterone, without 17-hydroxylation, and the mechanism is probably confined to the region of the zona glomerulosa. Capsules stripped from beef adrenals convert progesterone, deoxycorticosterone and corticosterone, with the last appearing to be the immediate precursor according to the specific activities encountered [77, 78].

Greengard and associates [79] have demonstrated that cytochrome P-450 does participate in the conversion of corticosterone to aldosterone, as in other steroidal hydroxylations. This suggests an hydroxylated intermediate, beyond corticosterone, and it has therefore been proposed that an enzyme · 18-hydroxycorticosterone complex serves as an intermediate. This complex may undergo dehydrogenation to form aldosterone, the latter being then released. Or the complex may dissociate to form free 18-hydroxycorticosterone which in turn forms the 18–20 cyclic hemiketal in solution, and is no longer available for conversion. Thus both an hydroxylase and a dehydrogenase are believed crucial to the synthesis of aldosterone. The proposed pathway is shown in Fig. 38-7.

Although the biosynthesis of aldosterone is facilitated by ACTH, it seems that angiotensin II is a more important influence. Angiotensinogen is an α_2-globulin in serum which is converted by renin from the juxtaglomerular apparatus of the kidney, into a decapeptide, angiotensin I, which is inactive. This is transformed into angiotensin II, an octapeptide with vasoconstrictor and pressor properties which also stimulates the zona glomerulosa to produce aldosterone. It will also stimulate corticosterone and cortisol production, but less well than ACTH. The renin-angiotensin-aldosterone sequence is promoted by hypotonicity, hyponatremia with normal tonicity, sodium deprivation, and the administration of potassium.

Other hydroxylations are known to occur at C-1, C-2, C-6, and C-16, but these are minor transformations in the ordi-

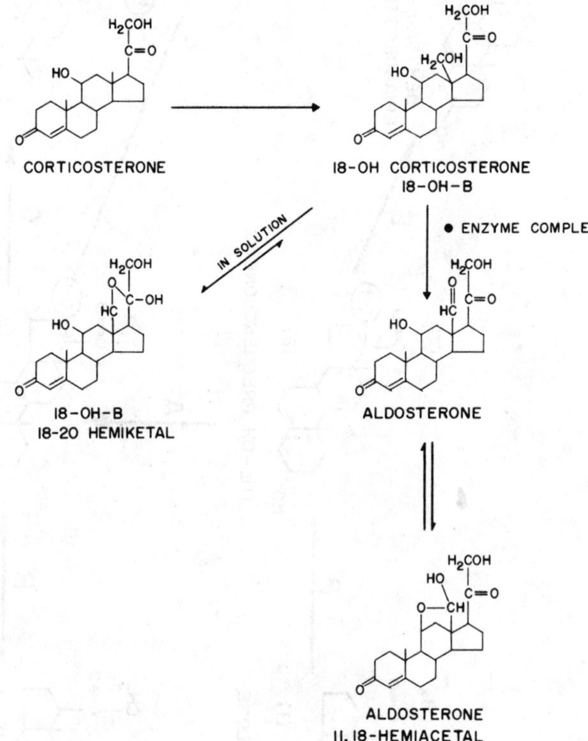

Figure 38-7. The conversion of corticosterone to aldosterone. It is proposed that a portion of 18-OH corticosterone forms an enzyme complex whereby it is dehydrogenated to yield the 18-aldehyde which in turn forms an 11,18-hemiacetal.

nary course of events and require no detailing in this discussion. Under special circumstances relating to age or drug administration, certain of these become more significant.

ADRENAL ANDROGENS

Slaunwhite and Samuels [80] demonstrated the pathway to Δ^4-androstenedione in the testis by way of progesterone → 17α-hydroxyprogesterone, and this may apply to the adrenal gland as well (3 to 10 to 11 in Fig. 38-6). In addition to the detection of these steroids in adrenal tissue, Bloch et al. [81] isolated radioactive Δ^4-androstenedione and its 11β-hydroxy derivative from beef adrenal glands perfused with tagged cholesterol and acetate. The pathway may also proceed (8 to 9 to 10 in Fig. 38-6) through 17α-hydroxypregnenolone, dehydroepiandrosterone, and Δ^4-androstenedione [82]. The mechanism for the removal of the side chain is not entirely clear but the supposed enzymatic system has been designated a desmolase by some. Ichii provided evidence for the reduced 20α-hydroxy derivative of 17-hydroxyprogesterone as the immediate precursor of Δ^5-androstenedione in the adrenal but not in the testis [83]. Thereafter, in some tissues, Δ^4-androstenedione is converted to testosterone through NADH-dependent 17β-hydroxysteroid dehydrogenase (*F* in Fig. 38-6). Horton and Tait [84] have found that androstenedione is the major adrenal product in this sequence, with peripheral conversion to testosterone at least in female subjects. The possible genesis of testosterone from cholesterol and 17-hydroxypregnene derivatives seems unquestioned but the role of acetate as a precursor through other channels remains unclear. The human disorder to be described, 17α-hydroxylase deficiency, provides evidence against the latter as an important pathway in man.

The urinary 17-ketosteroids thus arise from partial reduction of the aforementioned C_{19} or C_{21} steroids, including cortisol. These aspects are summarized in Fig. 38-8.

ESTROGEN

The early precursors of estrogens appear to be the same as for testosterone. The important proximal intermediate is Δ^5-androstenedione. This undergoes hydroxylation at the C-19 position, probably according to the general rules for such reactions as described, and finally removal of the C-19 grouping with aromatization of ring A. Although Ryan [85] has been able to show that microsomes prepared from human placenta catalyze these events, it has been extremely difficult to prove the case in the adrenal. There are instances of human disease, including rare adrenocortical tumors, associated with elevated estrogen production. There are enzymes in the adrenal which can hydroxylate estrogens, but these may have little to do with the provision of so-called natural major hormones.

ADRENOCORTICOTROPIN (ACTH)

A pituitary-adrenocortical homeostatic mechanism controls the secretion of adrenal steroids so that relatively constant tissue levels are maintained. The hypothalamus contains an ACTH-releasing factor which provokes the release of ACTH from the anterior pituitary, and the hypothalamic center is sensitive both to tissue levels of glucocorticoids and to stress. In the latter event, more ACTH and hence more adrenocortical steroid is secreted and released than under normal conditions.

ACTH produces both adrenocortical growth and increased steroidogenesis. The major site of action involves the conversion of cholesterol into pregnenolone. In various studies in vitro, the hormone does not increase the conversion of pregnenolone or progesterone to cortisol [86]. It has been postulated that the rate limitation on steroidogenesis is related to the availability of NADPH. Other NADPH-requiring enzymes in steroidogenesis, including those required for the synthesis of cholesterol from acetate and several hydroxylases, are present. Why then does the site of action appear to be limited to a specified locus? Are there variable loci within subcellular particles with separation of units? Since this theory invokes the role of 3′,5′-AMP, it should be noted that under special conditions Creange and Roberts found that high levels stimulated 11- and 18-hydroxylation of progesterone added to adrenal homogenates [87]. Haynes [88] demonstrated that ACTH increases the concentration of 3′,5′-adenosine monophosphate (3′,5′-AMP) in adrenal tissue, which in turn activates phosphorylase, providing more glucose-6-phosphate (G6P) and thus giving rise to increased NADPH from the active pentose shunt. This mechanism parallels the action of other peptide hormones on their respective target organs. The increased production of 3′,5′-AMP may be the result of the activation of adenyl cyclase by ACTH.

McKerns proposes a direct ACTH-induced conformational change in glucose-6-phosphate dehydrogenase [89]. In addition it has been shown that cyclic AMP in other tissues activates phosphofructokinase as well, and this should lead to a chain of events including a decrease in G6P and further entry of glucose [90].

A reaction similar to that of insulin has been proposed on the basis that optimal ACTH stimulation depends upon glucose in the medium and that there is an increase in the aminoisobutyrate, mannitol, and D-xylose space in adrenal slices [91, 92].

Cyclic AMP causes mitochondrial swelling with increased permeability [88], and in some experiments ACTH seems to facilitate the passage of specific steroid substrates required for pregnenolone synthesis [93]. Further, Harding [60] speculates that there may be an activation of ascorbate transport into the mitochondria. Finally, he suggests that ACTH may produce a "pull"-type stimulus near the termination of steroid hydroxylation by increasing the transport of substrate

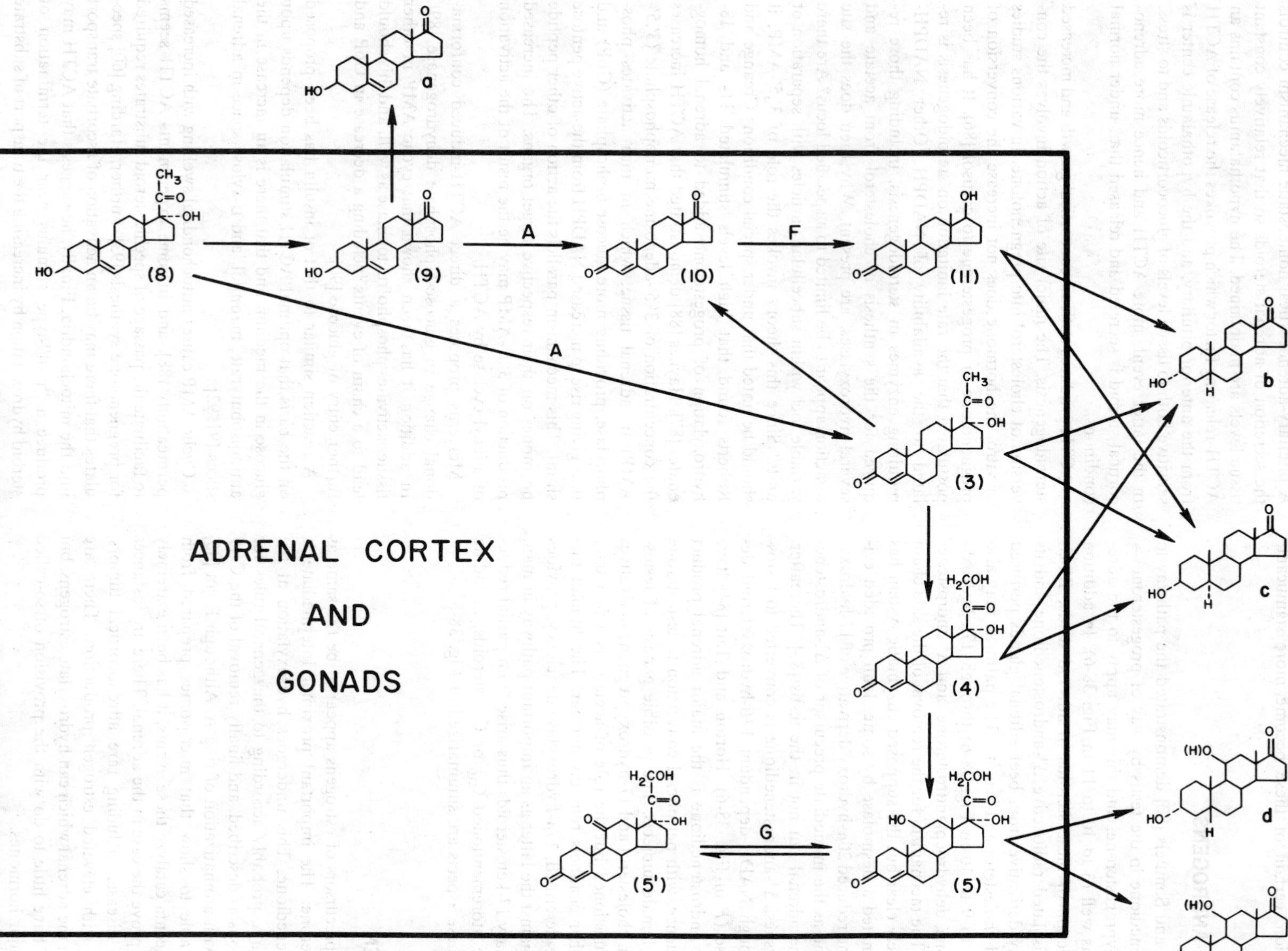
ADRENAL CORTEX
AND
GONADS
URINARY C-19 STEROIDS
(8)
(9)
(10)
(11)
(3)
(4)
(5)
(5')
a
b
c
d
e
A
F
G

to cytochrome P-450 through various mechanisms. This last is supported by the observations of Chance et al. [94], who demonstrate rapid oxidation of adrenal cortical pyridine nucleotides under the influence of ACTH. There is a possibility that several of these mechanisms work in consonance to account for the effects of ACTH on the adrenal cortex.

ACTH also regulates the DNA-directed regulation of RNA and of protein synthesis in the adrenal cortex. Whether this is an effect, primary or secondary to steroidogenesis, is uncertain. This matter has been reviewed by McKerns who proposes that the pentose phosphate shunt increases phosphorylated ribose sugar, with the stimulation of protein synthesis [95].

STEROID BIOTRANSFORMATION

As the principal steroidal products are released from the adrenal they undergo a series of reductions and conjugation prior to excretion, primarily through the urine. This is well reviewed by Rosenfeld et al. [96]. The recognition of these products and their precursors permits conclusions concerning adrenocortical steroidogenesis employing either classical isolation and measurement of products as such or secretion rates. The transformation of C_{21} steroids is shown in Fig. 38-9.

There is a reversible oxidation of cortisol (11—OH) to cortisone (11=O) the latter having about two-thirds the biological activity of cortisol. Reduction of ring A occurs predominantly in the liver, and may occur in one of two directions. Reduction to a 5α-steroid is catalyzed by a particulate enzyme which is NADPH dependent. The 5β-reduction, also NADPH dependent, involves a soluble protein and this reaction predominates. Further reduction of ring A to the "tetrahydro derivatives" (IV, V, VI, VII, XIII, and XIV in Fig. 38-9) requires a dehydrogenase with dual nucleotide requirement, and in man the 3α-hydroxy compounds predominate so that the 3β-derivatives are not indicated. Although these tetrahydro derivatives may now be conjugated, principally with glucuronic acid, and excreted, and while they do represent the major urinary components, there is nonetheless some further reduction at C-20 to the respective 20α- and 20β-cortols and cortolones (XI and XII in Fig. 38-9).

Discussion of cortisol as the prototype for C_{21} ketonic corticoids is applicable to the transformations of deoxycorticosterone, corticosterone, and substance S with certain minor exceptions. Corticosterone undergoes a similar reversible oxidation at C-11 to compound A, but reduction at C-20 may be the first major reaction, and corticosterone yields a greater percentage of fully reduced urinary products. In addition there is a greater reduction to the 5α-steroid with corticosterone. The ratio of 5β:5α products with cortisol is 4:1, but with corticosterone it is approximately unity. Deoxycorticosterone and substance S closely resemble cortisol in their disposition.

The C-21 deoxy compounds, such as 17-hydroxyprogesterone, are in a great measure reduced to the 3α,20α-dihydroxy-5β-pregnane derivatives, although small amounts of the allo- (5α) and 20β-OH metabolites may be found. Under pathologic conditions where large amounts of this group may be released from the adrenal, transformation may be somewhat suppressed. Thus a large fraction of 17-hydroxypregnanolone (III in Fig. 38-9) and 3α-hydroxy-5 β-pregnane-20-one (II in Fig. 38-9) appear in the urine. Or its precursors, the 3β-hydroxy-Δ^5-pregnenes (XV and XVI in Fig. 38-9), may be excreted as such, with variable reduction at C-20, and predominantly as sulfate conjugates.

Figure 38-8. The origin of the major urinary 17-ketosteroids is illustrated and certain derivatives theoretically arise from adrenal and gonadal secretions (*a, b,* and *c*), whereas others are restricted to adrenal sources (*d, e*). The designations are the same as for Fig. 38-7 except for the interconversion between cortisol (5) and cortisone (5′) through an 11-dehydrogenase (*G*). The common urinary 17-ketosteroids are dehydroepiandrosterone (*a*), etiocholanolone (*b*), androsterone (*c*), 11-hydroxy or 11-keto etiocholanolone (*d*), and 11-hydroxy or 11-keto androsterone (*e*). Other products reduced at C-17 or dehydrogenated at C-3, and with additional hydroxyl groupings in other positions, may occur in small quantities or may abound under abnormal conditions.

THE BIOCHEMICAL BASIS OF THE ADRENOGENITAL SYNDROME

The adrenogenital syndrome is divided into several categories:

- I. Virilizing
  - A. 21-hydroxylase deficiency
    1. Compensated
    2. Salt losing
  - B. 11-Hydroxylase deficiency
    1. Hypertensive
    2. Nonhypertensive (?)
- II. Mixed
  - A. 3β-Hydroxysteroid dehydrogenase deficiency (usually salt losing)
- III. Nonvirilizing
  - A. 17-Hydroxylase deficiency (hypertensive)
  - B. Desmolase deficiency (salt losing)

In the earlier observations, studies were apparently confined to the 21-hydroxylase deficiency wherein virilization, rapid somatic development, and high urinary 17-ketosteroids (androgens) were the rule. Independently, Bartter et al. [97] and Wilkins et al. [98] noted that the administration of exogenous cortisone led to a diminution of the urinary 17-ketosteroids. At first the significance of this observation was not clear and was believed by some to represent merely

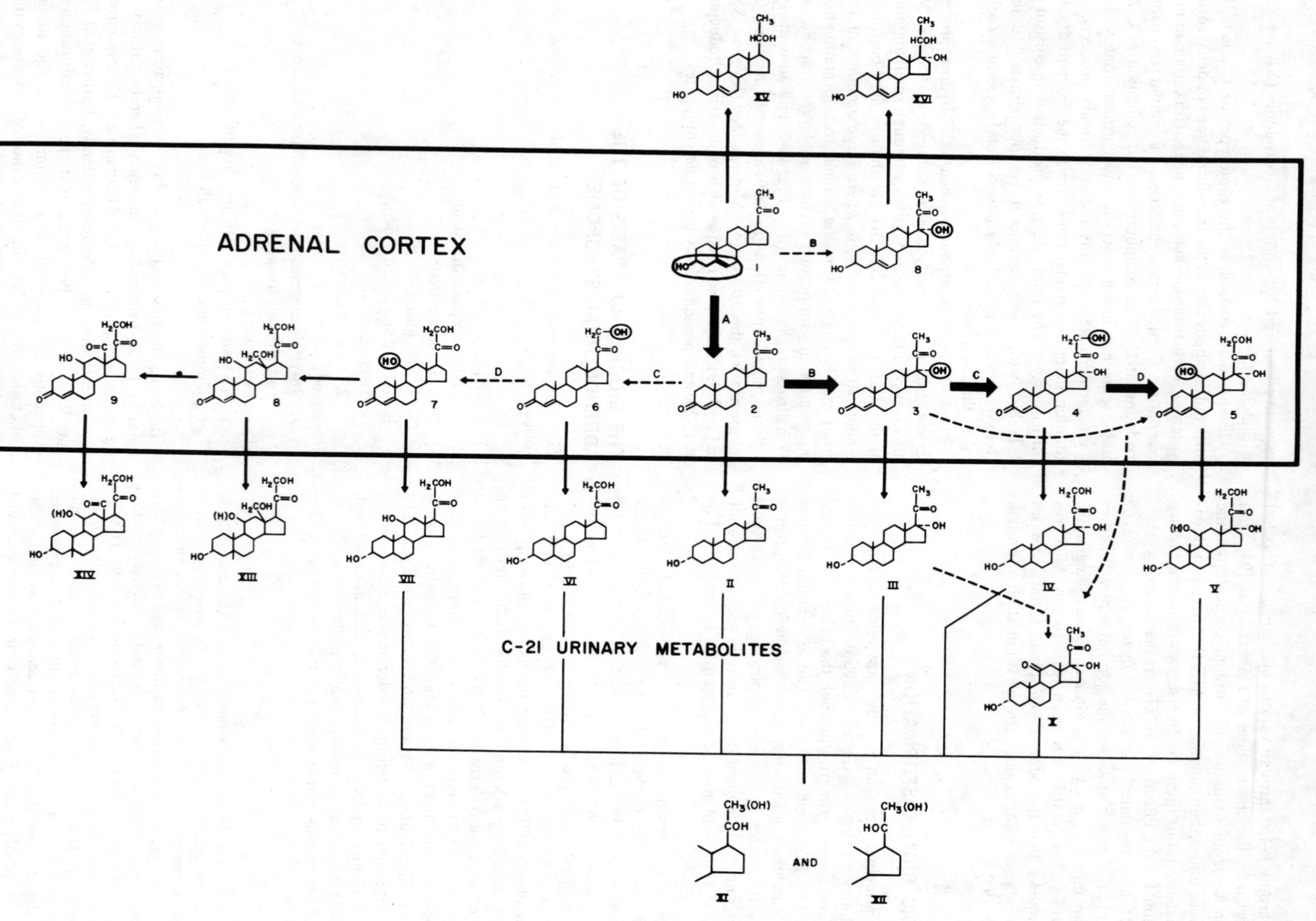
ADRENAL CORTEX
C-21 URINARY METABOLITES
AND
URINARY METABOLITES

the well-accepted adrenocortical suppression which occurs generally upon administration of corticoids. In 1951, Bartter et al. [99] studied the urinary reducing corticoids of individuals with the adrenogenital syndrome. There was no rise in response to the administration of ACTH, nor were the other expected responses observed, including salt retention, negative nitrogen balance, or eosinopenia. It was suggested that the basic defect was one of decreased production of glucocorticoids, a compensatory increase in ACTH secretion causing an excessive androgen production. Earlier, Lewis and Wilkins [100] reported on the failure to produce the expected potassium loss and sodium retention in affected subjects. Thus it appeared that a basic defect in steroidogenesis was the cause, rather than an aimless independent adrenocortical hyperplasia with androgen excess. These basic realizations remained valid upon further scrutiny of the disease and the revelation of precise foci of disturbances. However, the pattern of urinary and blood steroids, including the elevated urinary 17-ketosteroids, varied from one form to another.

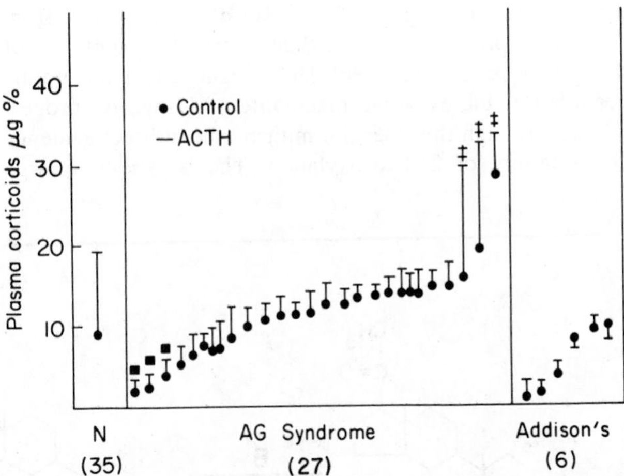

Figure 38-10. Serum cortisol measured by the Porter-Silber reaction before (•) and 4 hr after intramuscular ACTH 25 units per square meter (—). All instances of congenital adrenal hyperplasia (AG syndrome) are of the 21-hydroxylase variety except for three with 11-hydroxylase deficiency (‡). The initial levels may be low or within the normal limits, but the response to ACTH is always insignificant in the 21-hydroxylase deficiency. Three salt losers are included (solid boxes).

21-Hydroxylase Deficiency

This represents the commonest form of the adrenogenital syndrome, accounting for perhaps more than 90 percent of all the cases currently recognized. It is associated with congenital virilization and elevation of the urinary 17-ketosteroids. It was within this form that further support for the earlier theses was found by studying the serum levels of cortisol. These were often normal, occasionally low, and did not respond to the administration of ACTH to the same degree as control subjects (Fig. 38-10). Although this particular feature can be generally applied to all the other forms presently delineated, a word of caution is needed, since it is not applicable to the 11-hydroxylase deficiency when using the more commonly employed techniques for the measurement of steroids in blood or urine.

In order to present the evolution of discoveries culminating in the localization of the defect, it is necessary to return to the era of pioneering extraction, separation, and identification of adrenal steroids in biologic fluids. Very often, urine from patients with peculiar syndromes were selected for such excursions. In 1937 Butler and Marrian [101] and again in 1945 Mason and Kepler [102] isolated 5β-pregnane-3α,17α,20α-triol (pregnanetriol) from the urine of several virilized adults, most of whom had the adrenogenital syndrome, although one was believed to have an adrenal tumor. In 1953 [103] it became possible to demonstrate that large amounts of this "abnormal" steroid were present in virtually all cases of the disease studied at that time and that indeed small amounts were to be found normally. This corresponded to Jailer's [104] theory of a block between 17-hydroxyprogesterone and cortisol, based on the assumption that the former was a potent androgen.

In 1945 Lieberman and Dobriner [105] had reported large amounts of 3α,17α-dihydroxypregnane-20-one in the urine of a patient. This is another C-21 deoxy steroid, and its presence accords with defective 21-hydroxylation. For some years it has been recognized that pregnanediol in the urine is also elevated above normal in this disease [106, 107], although to a lesser extent than pregnanetriol. It is likely that some "back-up" occurs in the chain of events even though the major defect is farther along.

Strott et al. [108] reported an increased blood level of progesterone as well as increased production rates, but in their studies there was a considerably higher urine and plasma level and a higher production rate (112 mg per day) of 17-hydroxyprogesterone.

Although it has been amply demonstrated that pregnanetriol arises from 17-hydroxyprogesterone and is its reduced

Figure 38-9. The C_{21} adrenal steroids (within box) and their urinary C_{21} metabolites (roman numerals). Variable amounts of early precursors with the Δ^5-3β-hydroxy configuration may be excreted (XV and XVI), and these are predominantly conjugated as sulfates. Later intermediates undergo reduction of ring A and of the 3-keto group (primarily to 3α-hydroxy steroids) and appear predominantly as conjugates of glucosiduronic acid. Although the C-20 ketonic metabolites are the ones usually measured by standard techniques, there is a variable and further reduction at this position (XI and XIII). The designations are the same as in Fig. 38-6. Included are 18-hydroxy corticosterone (8) and aldosterone (9). The reduced urinary derivatives (II to XIV) are commonly named as the "tetrahydro" derivatives of their parent compounds. One urinary derivative, 11-ketopregnanetriol (*X*) indicates 17- and 11-hydroxylation of progesterone without the "normal" 21-hydroxylation between these two steps.

urinary product (Fig. 38-11), it also derives, in part, from 17-hydroxypregnenolone without the intervention of 17-hydroxyprogesterone [96]. Thus pregnanetriol may not be regarded as the exclusive metabolite of 17-hydroxyprogesterone although this does not mitigate the indirect evidence for a failure of 21-hydroxylation. The isolation of large amounts of $3\alpha,17\alpha,20\alpha$-pregnanetriol-11-one (pregnanetriolone X1X, Fig. 38-11) by Finkelstein et al. [109] from the urine of subjects with this form of the disease indicates the efficiency of 11-hydroxylation, while further supporting the lack of 21-hydroxylation. So too, the presence of large amounts of 11-oxygenated 17-ketosteroids in the urine of

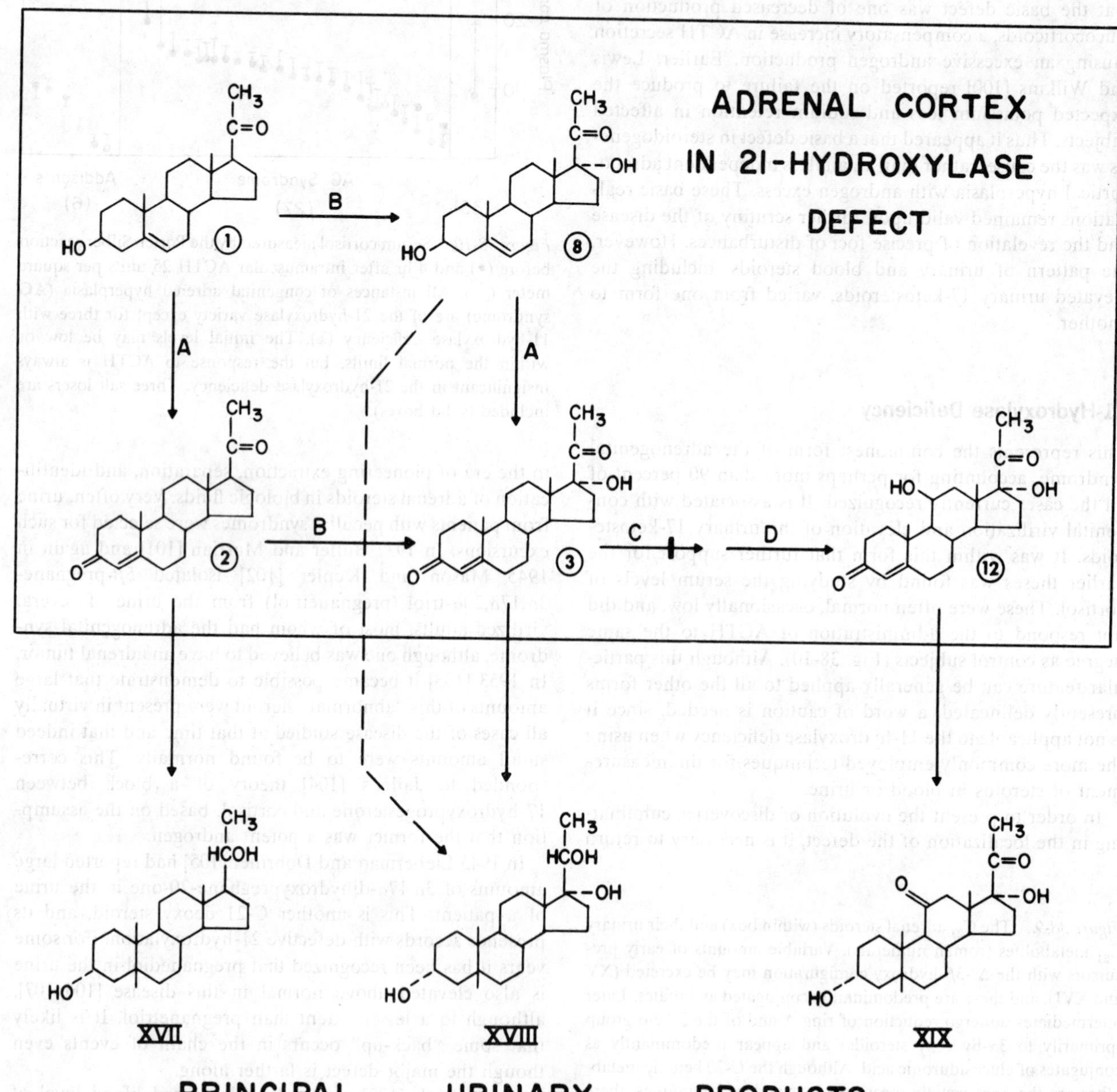

Figure 38-11. The intermediary steroidal metabolites which accumulate in the adrenal cortex in the 21-hydroxylase deficiency (2, 3, and 12) with their urinary metabolites: pregnanediol (XVII), pregnanetriol (XVIII), and 11-ketopregnanetriol (XIX). The enzymes are designated as in Fig. 38-6, and the deficient 21-hydroxylation (*C*) does not preclude 11-hydroxylation (*D*).

these subjects attests to the integrity of 11-hydroxylation and supports this commonest type as representing a single enzymatic defect in 21-hydroxylation.

The evidence which points to defective cortisol biogenesis with a specific defect at 21-hydroxylation may be summarized as follows:

1 The blood levels of cortisol and the urinary excretion of metabolites of cortisol [110–114], as well as cortisol secretion rates [115, 116], may be low, and although more often within the low normal range are incapable of increasing normally upon stimulation with ACTH.

2 It has been demonstrated on several occasions that the serum level of ACTH is elevated in this condition, as it is in Addison's disease, and that it falls upon the administration of small replacement doses of corticoids [117]. Binoux et al. [118] examined the blood levels of ACTH by bioassay from 24 children with congenital adrenal hyperplasia, 23 due to 21-hydroxylase deficiency. The values while extremely variable were all high, with an average of 2.5 times normal. There was no correlation with the blood cortisol levels or the degree of virilization, and the circadian rhythm of ACTH and cortisol occurred as in normal subjects. The ACTH in blood fell with replacement steroid therapy.

3 Not only is the urinary excretion of pregnanetriol and pregnanetriolone elevated well above normal, but a large assortment of C-21 methylated steroids (lacking C-21-OH) are to be found (Table 38-1) which are either absent or present in minute amounts in normal subjects. While there are several specific methods for the measurement of certain of these compounds, convenient group reaction will detect most of them by a single determination [114]. Borohydride reduction of suitable urinary extracts followed by periodate oxidation will yield acetaldehyde, mole for mole, for all 17-hydroxy C-21 methylated steroids. With this technique the "defective" C-21 deoxy steroids are greatly elevated in urine (Figs. 38-12 and 38-13).

4 The secretion rate of 17-hydroxyprogesterone is greatly elevated in this disease. It has been estimated as 240 to 280 mg per day by Fukushima et al. [119] and 111 to 112 mg per day by Strott et al. [108], as compared to normal values of 1.7 to 3.0 mg per day.

5 The blood levels of 17-hydroxyprogesterone have been shown to be elevated in this disorder after the administration of ACTH, 12.0 μg per 100 ml versus 0.09 μg per 100 ml normally [108]. And 21-deoxy-F (the steroidal product which resembles cortisol in all respects except for the absence of C-21-OH) has been found in the blood of affected subjects [120]. Although this substance is not regarded as a usual intermediate in cortisol biogenesis, its presence once more attests to the occasional exceptions to the "rules."

6 The adrenal glands of several affected individuals have been extracted and found to contain diminished quantities of cortisol but greatly elevated amounts of 17-hydroxyprogesterone [121, 122].

7 Finally, in a few limited experiments, Bongiovanni [121] and Axelrod and Goldzieher [123] found that fresh adrenal tissue from afflicted individuals was unable to perform 21-hydroxylation of suitable substrates, although other activities were intact. Unfortunately, in spite of diligent efforts to demonstrate 21-hydroxylation by red blood cells, white blood cells, serum, and cultured fibroblasts from normal individuals, little was found [124]. Thus these more simple approaches to detecting enzymatic defects in other disorders have little promise in the adrenogenital syndrome due to the 21-hydroxylase deficiency.

Table 38-1. URINARY C_{21} STEROIDS IN 21-HYDROXYLASE DEFICIENCY

5β-Pregnane-3α,20α-diol (pregnanediol)
3α-Hydroxy-5β-pregnane-20-one (pregnanolone)
3α,17α-Dihydroxy-5β-pregnane-20-one (17-hydroxypregnanolone)
3α,17α-Dihydroxy-5α-pregnane-20-one
3β,16α-Dihydroxy-5α-pregnane-20-one
3α,20α-Dihydroxy-5β-pregnane-11-one
5β-Pregnane-3α,17α,20α-triol (pregnanetriol)
5α-Pregnane-3α,17α,20α-triol
5α-Pregnane-3α,17α,20β-triol
3α,17α,20α-Trihydroxy-5β-pregnane-11-one (pregnanetriolone)
5β-Pregnane-3α,11β,17α,20α-tetrol
Pregn-5-ene-3β,20α-diol
3α-Hydroxy-5β-pregnane-11,20-dione
5β-Pregnane-3,20-dione
5β-pregnane-3β,20α-diol
5α-Pregnane-3α,20α-diol
3α,16α-Dihydroxy-5β-pregnane-20-one
3β,16α-Dihydroxy-5β-pregnane-20-one
3α,16α-Dihydroxy-5α-pregnane-20-one
3β,16α-Dihydroxy-5α-pregnane-20-one'
3α,17α-Dihydroxy-5β-pregnane-11,20-dione

In Fig. 38-11, 21-hydroxylase is designated as *C*. The metabolites of the immediate precursor accumulate, but as discussed do not entirely escape other hydroxylations beyond the defect.

The urine contains large quantities of adrenocortical steroids, the result of compensatory hyperactivity of the biosynthetic pathway with the production of excessive steroidal intermediates. Some of these intermediates are variously reduced, conjugated, and excreted. A portion may be diverted into the pathways for androgen and estrogen synthesis. The total urinary 17-ketosteroids are elevated. Mizutami et al. [125] find androsterone to be the most abundant C_{19} steroid, with less etiocholanolone. Of the 11-oxygenated 17-ketosteroids, 11β-hydroxyandrosterone predominates and there is a large amount of 11-ketoetiocholanolone as well. Dehydroepiandrosterone is generally within normal range in 21-hydroxylase deficiency. Of the C_{21} steroids, pregnanetriol and 17-hydroxypregnanolone predominate. A large number of C_{21} methyl compounds are also present (Table 38-1). The reduced products of cortisol secretion, tetrahydrocortisol and tetrahydrocortisone, are present in normal or

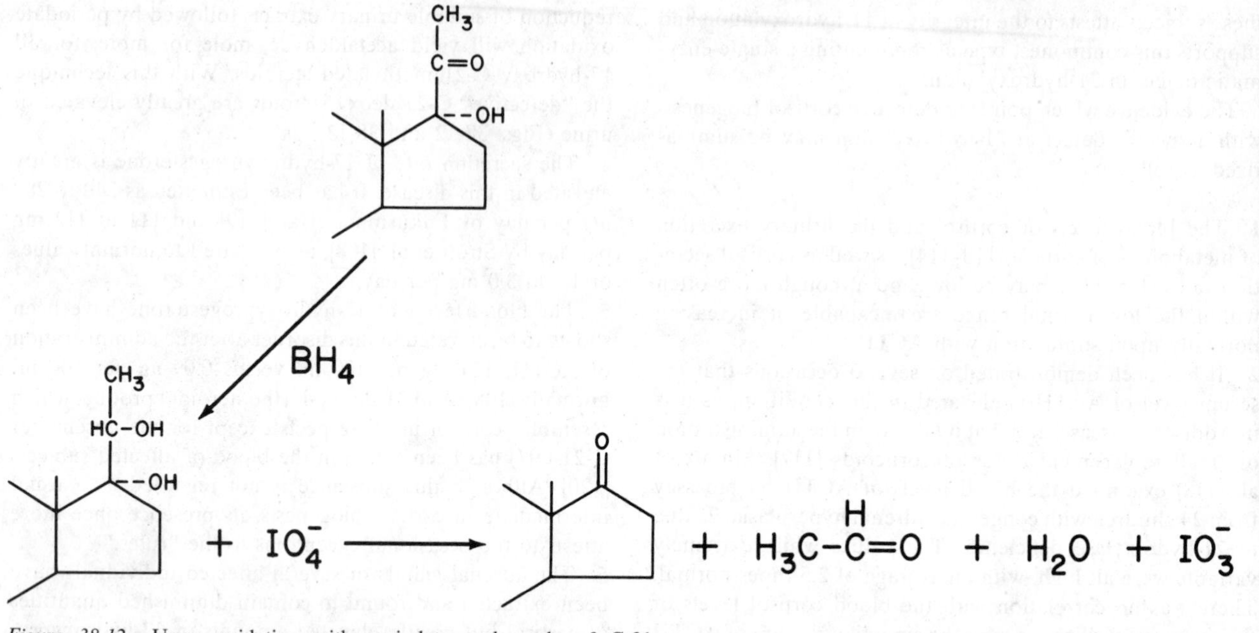

Figure 38-12. Upon oxidation with periodate each mole of C-21 methylated steroid (reduced at C-20) yields a mole of acetaldehyde. Prior treatment of urinary extracts with borohydride (BH_4) will include C-21 methylated compounds with a C-20 ketonic function, thereby reducing them. This convenient group reaction is valuable in revealing the 21-hydroxylase defect.

diminished quantities [125, 126]. The C_{19} steroids are probably derived in great measure from the C_{21} methyl steroids after cleavage of the side chain and reduction.

The production of cortisol itself may be limited, but in most instances normal amounts are produced, as indicated above. Eberlein and Bongiovanni [126] compared the ratio of pregnanetriol to cortisol metabolites as an index of the large quantities of 21-deoxy intermediates secreted in order to achieve normal cortisol production. This was much elevated in the adrenogenital syndrome, but the absolute quantity of the latter was often normal in the disease. This has come to be regarded as the "compensatory" form of the disease, whereby vigorous metabolic activity producing large amounts of "abnormal" intermediates nonetheless achieves normal levels of cortisol and the clinical manifestations of cortisol deficiency do not appear. They also demonstrated that in the salt-losing form the urinary metabolites of cortisol are so extremely low that virtually a complete block is indicated. In addition, subjects were found who were intermediate in their ability to compensate and demonstrated clinical adrenal insufficiency only under stress. Migeon and Kenny [116] measured cortisol production rates after the administration of trace quantities of labeled steroid. When compared with controls matched by age, the cortisol production rates were normal, except in the salt-losing form, where they were much reduced. Thus the enzymatic deficiency is apparent by indirect methods, but it is often incomplete and may be overcome by increased metabolic activity within the adrenal gland and the accumulation of excessive intermediary steroids. The defect is "complete" in the salt-losing form, but this particular matter merits further discussion below.

The clinical virilization, typical of this form of the disorder, is to be attributed to excess production of testosterone. Several investigators have described elevated levels of testosterone in the peripheral and adrenal blood or urine. As with the urinary 17-ketosteroids, these fall to normal values after the administration of glucocorticoids in replacement dosages [127–131]. The blood levels of androstenedione are also elevated. More refined studies by Horton [132] and Rivarola et al. [133] point to an increased secretion of androstenedione by the disordered adrenal, with peripheral conversion of this steroid to testosterone. It is likely that the excessive 17-hydroxyprogesterone produced is diverted in some increased measure to the synthesis of androstenedione (3 to 10 in Fig. 38-6). More recently, Frasier et al. [134] have shown that this also applies to that form of the disease caused by 11-hydroxylase deficiency, as described below.

It might be supposed that the compensatory adrenocortical hyperactivity is the result of a fundamentally normal ability to secrete cortisol with an abnormal enzymatic dehydroxylation at carbon-21 and the production of large amounts of C-21 methyl steroids. Fukushima and Gallagher [135] ruled out this hypothesis by demonstrating normal metabolism of cortisol administered to a diseased person. They also demonstrated a deficient secretion of cortisol by isotopic techniques.

Although pregnanetriol, among the C_{21} compounds excreted in excess, appears to predominate, the picture is somewhat different in the early months of life in this disorder. Bergstrand et al. [136] and Bongiovanni et al. [137] have shown a preponderance of 11-ketopregnanetriol during infancy, and certain Δ^5-16-hydroxy-21-methyl pregnene derivatives are present [138].

The elevated 17-ketosteroids probably arise in large measure from C_{21} precursors such as 17-hydroxyprogesterone, and not from C_{21} compounds lacking the 17-OH. Some C_{19} compounds may arise differently. Bloch et al. [81] have incubated labeled acetate with adrenal tissue from an affected subject and found radioactive dehydroepiandrosterone, androstenedione, and 11β-hydroxyandrostenedione, with very little 17-hydroxyprogesterone. Others have isolated these same compounds from human adrenal vein blood [139–142]. Bradlow and Gallagher [143] found 11β-hydroxyandrosterone to be the principal metabolite of tagged 11β-hydroxyandrostenedione. The large amounts of 11-hydroxylated 17-ketosteroids suggest an increased adrenocortical 11-hydroxylase in the 21-hydroxylase defect, probably the consequence of increased ACTH. However, it is not entirely clear that these C_{19} steroids may not be shunted through 17-hydroxy C_{21} compounds. Cohn and Mulrow [144] studied the metabolism of 17-hydroxypregnenolone by human adrenal slices and found it to be converted to dehydroepiandrosterone, androstenedione, and 11β-hydroxyandrostenedione. Perhaps the 11-hydroxylation occurs on a C_{19} substrate, but the large amounts of 11-ketopregnanetriol in the urine indicate that it may occur on C_{21} steroids. Perhaps both occur.

Migeon and Gardner [145] have studied urinary estrogens in this form of the disease and have found them to be elevated. Since they diminish upon the administration of corticoids they are probably of adrenal origin.

11-Hydroxylase Deficiency

In 1956 Eberlein and Bongiovanni [146] described a female pseudohermaphrodite with the usual clinical characteristics of congenital adrenal hyperplasia but associated with severe hypertension. At first the urine and blood appeared to contain excessive amounts of cortisol by the usual chemical methods for measuring this steroid. On further analysis the predominant compound in the blood was found to be substance S (4 in Fig. 38-6) and in the urine tetrahydro S (IV in Fig. 38-9). These findings indicated a defect in 11-hydroxylation (*D* and *D′* in Fig. 38-6). Blood cortisol and its urinary metabolites were in fact diminished. The second most abundant urinary C_{21} steroid was tetrahydro DOC (VI in Fig. 38-9), an intermediate in the alternate pathway to corticosterone. It was derived from the adrenal secretion of large amounts of deoxycorticosterone (6 in Figs. 38-6, 38-9) and probably accounted for the hypertension. Administration of replacement doses of cortisol suppressed the secretion of these compounds, the hypertension remitted and the virilization was suppressed. The urine contained only modestly elevated pregnanetriol. The urinary 17-ketosteroids were elevated as in the 21-hydroxylase deficiency, but etiocholanolone (*b* in Fig. 39-9) comprised 75 percent of the total and there were no 11-oxy-17-ketosteroids which are generally elevated in the usual form. Substance S is known to be converted in great measure to etiocholanolone rather than androsterone. Blunck [147] has reported a similar urinary steroidal pattern in two patients with increased substance S, tetrahydro S, and tetrahydro DOC. They found androsterone to predominate among the 17-ketosteroids and that the 11-oxy-17-ketosteroids were diminished.

Other patients of this type have been described with a similar steroidal pattern, providing indirect evidence for the 11-hydroxylase defect. But hypertension is not always present [147, 148–150] and the defect is sometimes partial, as indicated by variable cortisol production. Whether the hypertension is related to the duration of the abnormal secretions, the degree of the defect or variations in salt intake is not clear. Studies are needed, as in the 21-hydroxylase defect, to assess better the severity of the enzymatic defect in an attempt to correlate this with the hypertension. Indeed, in one patient without hypertension, Gandy et al. [149] found 11-oxygenated 17-ketosteroids, which were absent in the first case reported, in spite of an overall steroidal pattern consistent with this form of the disorder. They consider that this may have reflected a partial enzymatic deficiency. Nevertheless, virilization occurs in all patients.

That there may be milder forms has been established by Dyrenfurth [151] and Gabrilove [152]. They have described a condition in adult women simulating the Stein-Levinthal syndrome, sometimes with hypertension. The basic urinary pattern may coincide with that described but often is not distinctive until after the administration of ACTH. It is believed to be the result of a partial enzymatic deficiency, mild enough to elicit no clinical disturbance in early life but becoming more and more apparent with advancing age.

Kowarski et al. [153] studied aldosterone secretion in four subjects with the syndrome due to the 11-hydroxylation defect. In all, the production of aldosterone was very low and remained so even after sodium restriction. In two subjects who had been on suppressive steroid treatment for long periods, the production was somewhat higher and responded moderately to sodium deprivation. In a fourth patient, following initiation of therapy, while on a low sodium diet, there was sodium loss and the aldosterone remained low on the sixth day of treatment. One could speculate that the excessive deoxycorticosterone secretion in this disorder suppressed aldosterone, and that the latter was unable to restore itself in the early phase of therapy. Even so, the persistence of low aldosterone production after prolonged treatment is a reflection of the specific enzymatic defect which affects aldosterone as well as cortisol synthesis.

17-Hydroxylase Deficiency

Biglieri [154] and subsequently others [155, 156] have described four genotypic female adults with apparent hypogonadism, no secondary sexual characteristics, hypokalemic alkalosis, and hypertension. The cortisol secretion, as well as blood levels and cortisol urinary metabolites, was virtually zero. The major secretory product was corticosterone (7 in Fig. 38-6) but deoxycorticosterone (6 in Fig. 38-6) was also well above normal. Urinary 17-ketosteroids and estrogens were absent. This spectrum of findings places the defect at 17-hydroxylation (*B* and *B′* in Fig. 38-6) and suggests that in man, 17-hydroxylation is crucial in the formation of C_{19} and C_{18} steroids, androgens, and estrogens, as indicated in the schema. Although the aldosterone secretion was at first low in some, probably secondary to excessive deoxycorticosterone production and saltwater retention, this returned to normal after suppressive doses of glucocorticoids. Thus, there is not an accompanying defect in aldosterone biogenesis which does not require 17-hydroxylation. The data in some of these cases suggest a partial defect of the enzyme, but in all amenorrhea, absent sexual hair and hypertension were common clinical manifestations. One would not expect that an inability to produce sex hormones would affect female sexual differentiation during the embryonic development, although secondary sexual development would not occur. On the other hand, if this syndrome were to occur in a male it would be anticipated that the fetal testis would be impaired in its induction of distal masculine sexual differentiation.

Such now appears to be the case. New [157] has described a genotypic male adolescent with congenitally ambiguous genitalia. The labia had failed to fuse, and there was a rudimentary penis with complete hypospadias and a shallow vagina. One testis was partially and the other fully descended into the labioscrotal folds. There was no sexual hair and mild hypertension without hypokalemia. The pattern of steroidal secretion was similar to the cases described in females and pointed to a 17-hydroxylase deficiency. The administration of testosterone produced sexual hair, hitherto absent, and growth of the phallus. The karyotype and gonadal tissues were appropriate to a male. The testosterone secretion in this patient was below normal and responded neither to ACTH nor to gonadotropins. The plasma dehydroepiandrosterone level was also depressed. This case once again points to the absence of a similar enzymatic mechanism in both the adrenal and gonad, both probably associated with a single gene. It is, in part, a clinical example of Jost's experiments indicating the important role of fetal testicular function in producing a steroidal androgen for complete male embryogenesis.

3β-Hydroxysteroid Dehydrogenase Deficiency

A rare form of defective cortisol biogenesis has been described in several infants by Bongiovanni [158, 159]. The urinary steroids consisted almost entirely of compounds with the Δ^5-3β-OH configuration. The major compounds isolated and identified are indicated in Table 38-2. This then represents a block at *A* in Figure 38-6. Clinically, an exception to the usual appearance of severe virilization is to be found, as also in the 17-hydroxylase and desmolase deficiency. Male infants are usually incompletely developed, having varying degrees of hypospadias or complete failure of masculinization with a vagina. In addition, in most cases described there has been marked salt and water wasting. Failure to thrive in spite of apparently adequate replacement therapy is common and the outcome is often fatal in the first months of life. Female infants may be moderately virilized at birth but the extent is often less than with other varieties. It is as if the steroidal compounds produced were "intermediate" in androgenic potency, producing a neuter gender with respect to the external genitalia in both sexes. It has been possible to demonstrate the absence of the enzyme 3β-hydroxysteroid dehydrogenase in the tissues [160]. It is absent from both the adrenal cortex and the gonads. Its lack in the fetal testis explains the incomplete masculine development. Migeon and Blizzard [161] have described a patient who appeared to have only a partial enzymatic deficiency. They showed that the plasma testosterone and androstenedione levels were not elevated as in instances of 21-hydroxylase deficiency [133]. Thus the deficiency of this enzyme interferes both with the biogenesis of testosterone as well as cortisol. Kogut [162] has also described a patient with severe salt and water loss who had a fatal outcome. It is probable that a single gene accounts for this enzyme in both the adrenal and gonadal tissues.

Table 38-2. URINARY STEROIDS IN 3β-HYDROXYSTEROID DEHYDROGENASE DEFICIENCY

Δ^5-Pregnene-3β,17α,20α-triol
3β,17α-Dihydroxy-Δ^5-pregnen-20-one
Δ^5-Pregnene-3β,20α-diol
Δ^5-Pregnene-3β,17α,20β,21-tetrol
3β,16α-Dihydroxy-Δ^5-pregnen-20-one
3β,16α-Dihydroxy-Δ^5-androsten-17-one
3β-Hydroxy-Δ^5-androsten-17-one

As indicated earlier, the rearrangement of rings A-B at the locus where the deficiency occurs (*A* in Fig. 38-6) requires two enzymes, the second an isomerase known to be present in adrenal tissue. The direct evidence for lack of the dehydrogenase in the tissues seems clear, but there is no information on the activity of this second enzyme in this disorder. It is of interest to note that certain hydroxylations occur on this molecule (Table 38-2) even with persistence of the Δ^5-3β-OH configuration.

However, recently several cases of this form of the disease have been described with more prolonged survival and some appear to be partial deficiencies [162*a*–*d*]. A notable feature about the steroidal pattern after the first few months of life is the appearance of respectable amounts of pregnanetriol while at the same time the Δ5-3β-hydroxysteroids remain prominent. This had been noted earlier in a single case and was at that time attributed to a possible double enzyme defect, to include the 21-hydroxylase. This no longer seems probable. It is likely that there is some conversion of pregnenetriol to pregnanetriol with the maturation of hepatic enzymes with 3β-hydroxysteroid dehydrogenase activity. This peripheral conversion may render the urinary pattern confusing. Presumably the hepatic enzyme is different and is under separate control from that in the adrenal cortex and the gonads.

Desmolase Deficiency (Lipoid Adrenal Hyperplasia)

Prader and his colleagues [163, 164] have described a form of congenital adrenal hyperplasia wherein there are virtually no detectable urinary 17-ketosteroids. As in the previous form, males are not masculinized during fetal life and all subjects have feminine external genitalia. This again is testimony to the role of a single enzyme in both adrenal and gonadal tissues. The adrenal glands are much enlarged and contain tremendous quantities of cholesterol and other lipids. There is usually salt and water loss. Camacho et al. [165] studied an affected genotypic male with incomplete external sexual development. They were able to demonstrate low secretion rates of cortisol and aldosterone. There were virtually no detectable steroids in the urine. The subject died and was found to have large lipid-filled adrenals, testes, and male internal ducts. These authors have suggested that there is a deficiency prior to pregnenolone (1 in Fig. 38-6), possibly of the enzymatic system responsible for the cleavage of the side chain of cholesterol (Dm in Fig. 38-6). As detailed earlier, although this has been designated as "desmolase deficiency," there are several steps in this transaction. More precise delineation of this defect awaits further investigation. A deficiency at this locus is a reasonable conjecture and such has been demonstrated in the adrenal gland following the administration of aminoglutethimide, which inhibits the desmolase system [166]. This experimental condition resembles lipoid adrenal hyperplasia.

Coupled Defects

It has already been indicated that in the 21-hydroxylase defect, although the 17-hydroxy C-21 methyl steroids predominate in urine, pregnanediol is also significantly increased. Does this mean that in this type there is also a relative deficiency of 17-hydroxylase? This may be an expression of product inhibition or the deficiency of enzyme or cofactor common to two hydroxylations. Or perhaps a "normal" preceding enzyme system is unable to cope with the excessive substrate precursors presented to it.

It has been noted in the 11-hydroxylase deficiency that pregnanetriol is elevated although there are more 21-hydroxy-11-deoxy steroids [167, 168]. Stempfel [169] studied a patient with partial 11-hydroxylase deficiency who had elevated urinary pregnanetriol as well. Upon administration of an 11-hydroxylase inhibitor metyrapone [2-methyl-1,2-bis(3-pyridyl)-1-propanone] there was a fall in the urinary cortisol metabolites and a further rise in the production of substance S. The pregnanetriol also fell. Stempfel reasoned that were the pregnanetriol merely related to an accumulation of 17-hydroxyprogesterone, the result of product inhibition arising from the 11-hydroxylase defect, the pregnanetriol should have risen under these circumstances and that therefore a milder 21-hydroxylase deficiency was present as well.

Bongiovanni [159], in his description of the 3β-hydroxysteroid dehydrogenase defect, reported one patient in whom there was a deficiency of 21-hydroxylated steroids as well. Perhaps this was a coupled genetic defect also involving 21-hydroxylase. Although this was originally interpreted as a coupled genetic defect also involving 21-hydroxylase, this no longer appears likely. Several such cases have been reported as described above.

The Electrolyte and Water Disturbance

This aspect of the disease merits further discussion. Although the propensity to lose salt and water is not confined to a single form of this disease, most available studies have been conducted in subjects with the 21-hydroxylase deficiency. Attention has logically been directed toward the production of aldosterone in attempting to elucidate this problem. Although some aspects seem indisputable, others remain controversial.

Various propositions have been set forth and are not necessarily mutually exclusive. These may be summarized as follows:

1 In the salt-losing form of the disorder there is a deficiency of aldosterone as well as cortisol. On this point there is general agreement, although the deficiency of aldosterone was not revealed in some earlier studies due to technical deficiencies. With more recent methods [170–175] it is apparent that aldosterone is truly deficient in the salt-losing form of congenital adrenal hyperplasia, whether determined by secretion rates or measurement of urinary metabolites of aldosterone. The "salt losers" secrete little aldosterone under all conditions including the deficiency of sodium, excessive potassium, and hypovolemia. In the compensated form, aldosterone secretion is not suppressed and it rises with sodium deprivation. But the problem has become complicated since Bartter et al. [176] reported aldosterone hypersecretion in the untreated compensated, "non-salt-losing" form of the disease, with extraordinary rises following sodium deprivation. Such high values have not been found in some other studies although occasional modest elevations are reported. Nonetheless, there is agreement that in the salt losers, aldosterone production is poor.

2 There are degrees of defect in 21-hydroxylase, a single enzyme, which when most severe not only reduces cortisol production sharply, but interferes with aldosterone synthesis as well. In the studies of Eberlein and Bongiovanni [177] such a thesis was proposed and in all of their patients the salt losers had the lowest levels of urinary cortisol metabolites. In addition they were able to demonstrate in one [178] a permissive action of cortisol on the response to aldosterone, so that in the virtual absence of the former, the latter was without effect. Most other studies, employing various techniques, support the greater defect in cortisol production in salt losers but do not all agree with the thesis of a single genotype for both forms, i.e., a single gene abnormality with variable expression. Childs et al. [179] and Prader et al. [180] found one form or the other (salt loser or non-salt loser) within individual families and proposed separate genotypes. On the other hand, Rosenbloom et al. [181] described salt losers and non-salt losers within sibships. They suggest that there are not necessarily two different genetic defects and that the varying expression might be due to environmental factors such as stress and salt intake. A single genotype is attractive because it is unlikely that a double defect of this nature would occur in so high a percentage of cases.

3 There are two different 21-hydroxylases, one specific for 17-hydroxyprogesterone (the precursor of cortisol), the other for progesterone (the precursor of aldosterone). Sharma and Dorfman [182] have described the kinetics of 21-hydroxylation with mammalian adrenal tissue, which differ significantly between the two substrates. Bartter [176] supports this view, which is strengthened by the high aldosterone production in the compensated form, which nonetheless reveals relative deficiencies in cortisol production. Furthermore, Degenhart et al. [115] report that in the compensated form of the disease there are in fact differences in the ability to produce cortisol and aldosterone which clearly point to two different mechanisms. Their evidence is based upon a more brisk rise of aldosterone upon salt deprivation than of cortisol following ACTH administration in the compensated form of the disease. Their study is meritorious in its presentation of data on both aldosterone and cortisol secretion rates in nine subjects. The additional aspects are in agreement with the isolated studies of others: there is a relative defect in cortisol synthesis in the compensated form that appears to be severest in most salt losers; aldosterone secretion is very low in salt losers and does not respond to stimulation.

4 Among the unusual secretory products in congenital adrenal hyperplasia is a salt-excreting factor. Kowarski [172] and Klein [183] have supported this thesis. It is favored by Bartter [176] and others [184], who have observed hyperaldosteronism in the compensated form. Bartter reasons that the elevated aldosterone, which does not produce the expected chemical or clinical consequences, represents a compensatory mechanism for the overproduction of salt-excreting steroids. But he does not rule out other possibilities. The salt losers, who in addition have a defect in the "second" hydroxylase required to produce aldosterone, suffer the consequences of the salt-excreting factor. Visser and Degenhart [185] have described an infant with 21-hydroxylase deficiency who in spite of normal aldosterone production was unable to retain sodium effectively. This they attributed to the hypothetical salt-wasting substance. On the other hand, if Bartter's findings apply, this patient should have had a high aldosterone production and must be regarded as somewhat handicapped in aldosterone synthesis.

Even so, there has been no firm demonstration of such a factor to date. The administration of ACTH has been said to cause salt loss in this syndrome, an argument favoring the production of such a hormone. And from time to time, progesterone or other steroids have been incriminated. Coppage et al. [186], by careful studies, have discredited these previous claims concerning ACTH and steroid-induced water and salt loss. Nevertheless, a salt-losing factor cannot be excluded at present.

The subtle details of the salt-losing complication of the adrenogenital syndrome remain to be resolved. Godard et al. [187] and Imai et al. [188] have studied the plasma renin in this disease. Godard et al. measured aldosterone secretion as well. The renin values were greatly elevated in salt losers, only slightly so in the compensated form, and low in a single patient with 11-hydroxylase deficiency. The normal values for children were 19 ± 16 mμg per liter per min. In the compensated 21-hydroxylase disorder, values were 26 to 39 mμg and in three salt losers 115, 249, and 1,250 mμg per liter min. The significant finding of interest was the sharp rise in plasma renin on a low salt diet, much more than in normal subjects; however, the aldosterone rise was modest. Because of this Godard et al. [187] suggest a partial defect in aldosterone synthesis in all forms of the disease. Imai [188] also finds a high renin level in salt losers and suggests that angiotensin may be the salt-excreting factor.

Further studies relative to the question of aldosterone metabolism in congenital adrenal hyperplasia should be mentioned. Ulick [189] described the excessive production of 18-hydroxycorticosterone relative to aldosterone in congenital adrenal hyperplasia. The ratio was higher in the salt losers than in the non-salt losers. His demonstration was based on the levels of urinary 18-hydroxytetrahydro-A (3α,18,21-trihydroxy-5β-pregnane-11,20-dione) (XIII in Fig. 38-9) which is the major metabolite of 18-hydroxycorticosterone. As in other studies, the absolute quantities of urinary metabolites of the aldosterone itself were much lower in the salt losers. While this pattern of excessive aldosterone precursors is abnormal, its precise significance is unknown. Ulick then took up the question of 21-deoxyaldosterone metabolites in subjects with congenital adrenal hyperplasia with 21-hydroxylase deficiency [190]. This substance conforms to aldosterone itself with the exception that C-21 is not hydroxylated. Ulick demonstrated first that it could be converted into aldosterone by the adrenal tissue of the bullfrog although he did not indicate that this was necessarily a major pathway. He then compared the urinary levels of 21-deoxyaldosterone, aldosterone, and tetrahydroaldosterone in the urine of affected children with the urinary levels of normal subjects. Two of seven children with congenital adrenal hyperplasia had somewhat more 21-deoxyaldosterone than three normal adults, but he did not consider his overall results as evidence of overproduction of 21-deoxyaldosterone. Unfortunately, the urinary excretion of these three substances is generally so low in this condition, particularly in the salt losers, that it is difficult to interpret. In none of these studies were any of the metabolites greatly elevated, as might be expected in the non-salt losers in accordance with the hyperaldosteronism described by Bartter.

Throughout this discussion little emphasis has been placed on the different adrenal zones. It has been mentioned that aldosterone formation occurs primarily in the zona glomerulosa and cortisol in the fasciculata. These different sites for certain crucial transactions may be important and may account for some differences in the secretion of individual steroids. It may be speculated that a specific enzyme defect in one zone is not applicable to another.

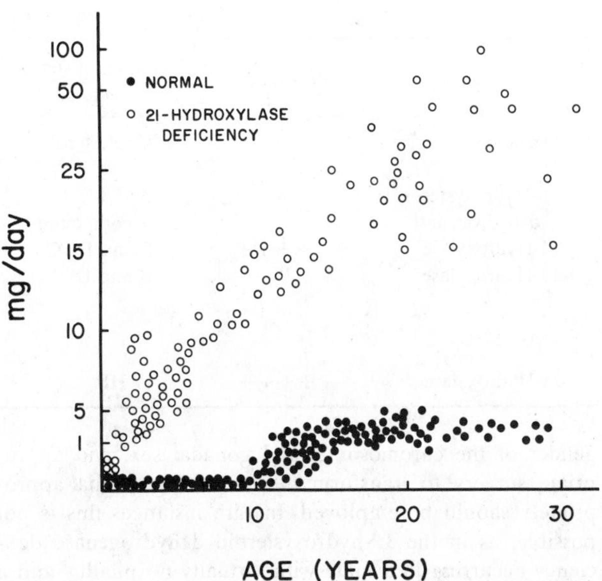

Figure 38-13. Urinary C-21 methyl steroid levels by measurement of acetaldehyde after periodate oxidation in normal subjects and those with the 21-hydroxylase defect. The quantities in this disorder greatly exceed the normal values, except in the first few days of life.

ADRENAL TUMORS

Adrenal neoplasms, as distinguished from the hereditary disorders herein discussed, sometimes simulate the various forms of the adrenogenital syndrome. They usually occasion little difficulty in differential diagnosis since they become manifest well after the neonatal period.

It has long been appreciated that many virilizing adrenal tumors secrete large quantities of Δ^5-3β-OH steroids which may be easily determined by such group tests as those used for the Pettenkofer or Allen chromogens. Thus dehydroepiandrosterone is likely to be the predominant 17-ketosteroid in the presence of such tumors. The total 17-ketosteroids in the urine are often extremely elevated beyond the levels seen in the adrenogenital syndrome [191]. Tumors may reveal peculiar enzymatic characteristics, and it has been shown that the neoplastic tissue may be deficient in 3β-hydroxysteroid dehydrogenase [192].

Other tumors appear to be deficient in 11-hydroxylase. Thus Touchstone et al. [193] and Rosselet et al. [194] have found tetrahydro-S to be the principal steroid in the urine of subjects with an adrenal tumor and hypertension. Although an increased secretion of deoxycorticosterone was not described in these cases, it is a likely accompaniment and suggests deficient 11β-hydroxylase. Fraser et al. [195] have described a corticosterone-secreting tumor which was probably deficient in 17-hydroxylase.

The administration of replacement doses of cortisol will always suppress the abnormal steroids in congenital adrenal hyperplasia, but usually will have little or no effect on their levels when the source is a tumor.

DIAGNOSIS AND TREATMENT

Ambiguous external genitalia at birth always suggest a diagnosis of the adrenogenital syndrome. In the most common form due to 21-hydroxylase deficiency, it is the genotypic female who displays abnormalities of the external genitalia. But as has been stressed, in certain of the less common types the male may also have such ambiguity. These external malformations or transitional states are limited, and there is usually no alteration of the internal duct system or the gonads. These will conform to the chromosomal sex. Thus a buccal smear or karyotyping is helpful in determining the "basic" sex. Injection of radiopaque dye into the external genital orifice is usually helpful in defining the internal structures. Thus in the common instance of the female with 21-hydroxylase deficiency and ambiguous external genitalia, a vagina, uterus, and sometimes fallopian tubes may be demonstrated.

The urinary steroidal pattern will usually establish the diagnosis. Generally the total 17-ketosteroids will be elevated and in the most frequent type of the disease, the total C-21 methyl compounds will be elevated. These may be determined by specific techniques for the measurement of pregnanetriol or pregnanetriolone, or by group reactions for total C-21 deoxy compounds, as by periodate oxidation and the determination of acetaldehyde (Fig. 38-13). The other forms are less common, and often have distinctive steroidal patterns (Table 38-3). It is essential that the diagnosis be established as soon as possible, in order that suitable replacement therapy with cortisol or its analogues may be started. Treatment not only suppresses the abnormal steroidal pattern, and hence the relentless virilization of most forms, but it avoids the possible consequences of cortisol deficiency. In the salt-losing forms it is also necessary to administer mineralocorticoids such as deoxycorticosterone or 9α-fluorohydrocortisone.

Insofar as possible, the patient should be reared in the

Table 38-3. FORMS OF CONGENITAL ADRENAL HYPERPLASIA

Deficiency	Virilization	Dominant steroid secreted	Urinary 17 KS	Salt loss	Miscellaneous
Desmolase	0	Cholesterol?	Low	Usually	Rare; males have female external genitalia
3β-Hydroxysteroid dehydrogenase	+	Δ^5-3β-OH compounds	Elevated	Usually	Rare; males have female external genitalia
11-Hydroxylase	+++++	S and DOC	Elevated	No	Usually hypertensive
17-Hydroxylase	0	B and DOC	Low	No	No sex hormones; males have ambiguous genitalia; no 2° sex dev.; hypertensive
21-Hydroxylase	+++++	17 HP	Elevated	Often	Most common type

gender of the chromosomal and gonadal sex, and appropriate surgery to transform the external genitalia appropriately should be employed. In rare instances this is not possible, as in the 3β-hydroxysteroid dehydrogenase deficiency occurring in a male with virtually no phallus and a suitable vagina. Such an individual should be reared as a female. These decisions must be made as quickly as possible.

Medical treatment with cortisol or its analogues not only arrests the rapid virilization, but also prevents the precipitous somatic maturation including epiphyseal advancement. The advantages are illustrated in Fig. 38-14. Furthermore, the suppression of the abnormal urinary steroidal pattern by treatment represents further confirmation of the diagnosis. Approximately 25 mg cortisol per m^2 or equivalent doses of other related compounds are replacement dosages. The

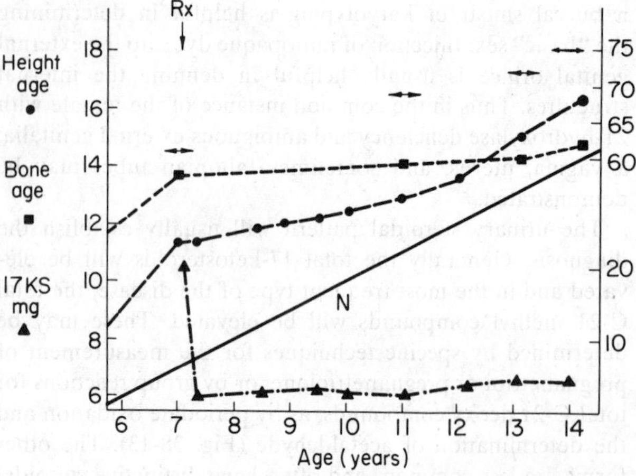

Figure 38-14. The clinical response with respect to an abnormally rapid somatic maturation in a boy with congenital adrenal hyperplasia after the administration of hydrocortisone. The urinary 17-ketosteroids (17 KS) have fallen and the abnormally rapid rate of growth and epiphyseal maturation are arrested. In this manner the limitation of ultimate stature is avoided. At several points are shown the estimates for final height (↔) according to the Bayley prediction tables were the epiphyseal maturation to continue at the same pace. In the fourteenth year of life he has already exceeded the original prediction.

exact requirement varies depending upon the route of administration and from one patient to another. Thus the therapy must be determined by the response of each individual: the clinical response, and the suppression of urinary 17-ketosteroids and pregnanetriol (in 21-hydroxylase deficiency) or of other steroids peculiar to each type as described.

GENETICS

The exact genetic basis for defective steroidal synthesis is unknown. It may be assumed that a structural gene is at fault, but it is possible that the graded reductions in a single enzyme, such as appears to occur in congenital adrenocortical hyperplasia, is attributable to control genes. Jacob and Monod [196] have shown that mutation of control genes has a variety of effects on structural genes, leading to decreased production of a specific protein in microorganisms. The variations in the commonest form of congenital adrenocortical hyperplasia, due to a 21-hydroxylase deficiency, could be explained by variable mutations in control genes. Whatever the exact "gene disorder," the human disease behaves as a Mendelian autosomal recessive.

Most of the genetic information has been gathered among cases of 21-hydroxylase deficiency. Bentinck [197] in a study of 33 affected families finds an average incidence of 60 percent, but this becomes closer to the expected 25 percent when he includes only sibships of seven or more. The gene frequency for this disease varies among different human populations. In Switzerland, Prader [180] reports the gene frequency as 0.014 with the heterozygous state as $1/_{35}$ and the homozygous, $1/_{5,000}$. In the United States (Maryland) Childs et al. [179] report a gene frequency of 0.004, heterozygosity $1/_{128}$ and homozygosity $1/_{67,000}$. The figures for Eskimos are unusually high as reported by Hirschfeld and Fleshman [198]. For the total Alaskan natives these are 0.026, $1/_{20}$, and $1/_{1,481}$; for the Yupik Eskimos alone, these become 0.045, $1/_{11}$, and $1/_{490}$ with a very high incidence of the salt-losing state. In this last group it may be that the frequency is even higher, based on the supposition that non-salt losers, especially males, are not being well detected. Indeed the majority of the cases reported among the Eskimos are female.

Although some series would indicate a predominance of females, the sex incidence is probably equal. Clinical attention is more often drawn to the female because of the congenital abnormalities of the external genitalia. At one time it was believed that the condition was associated with subnormal intellectual development, a supposition based on the consequence of inadequate treatment of salt losers and repeated circulatory collapse. This is not the case. Money and Lewis [199] reported somewhat superior intelligence, although the difference from control subjects was barely significant.

There have been several studies directed to the prenatal diagnosis of congenital adrenal hyperplasia due to 21-hydroxylase deficiency. Jeffcoate [199*a*] detected high 17-ketosteroids and pregnanetriol in the amniotic fluid toward the end of gestation, and the infant proved to have the disorder. Nichols [199*b, c*] found an elevated pregnanetriol level in amniotic fluid collected at delivery of an affected infant. He also found elevation of pregnanetriol in another instance when amniotic fluid was obtained between 273 and 278 days from conception. Thereafter, upon the injection of cortisol into the amnion, the level gradually fell. Cathro et al. [199*d*] studied maternal urines for their estrogen levels during the 26th, 29th, and 34th weeks of gestation. These levels were significantly higher during a pregnancy which produced an affected infant. This finding may represent evidence for accelerated steroid biosynthesis in the fetal adrenal gland. On the other hand, Merkatz et al. [199*e*] were unable to detect any abnormalities in amniotic fluid collected between the 23rd and 42nd week of gestation. They believe that these procedures were of no value in distinguishing between affected and unaffected infants.

PSYCHOLOGICAL ASPECTS

Certain experiments in rodents indicate that during fetal or neonatal life, sex hormones play a crucial role in the sexually undifferentiated neural tissues. Specifically, androgens appear to organize the male pattern of gonadotropin secretion and later sexual behavior. The absence of androgen (as in castrated males) at certain early crucial periods leads to behavioral and physiological feminization with cyclic patterns of gonadotropin secretion. In addition, exposure of the young female to androgens diminishes normal feminine receptivity in adulthood. For a review see Levine [200]. Since in certain common forms of the adrenogenital syndrome, the fetus and newborn are exposed to high androgen levels, might there not occur problems in psychosexual orientation?

It is generally agreed among clinicians that the female with congenital adrenal hyperplasia who is recognized early in life should be reared as a female and have appropriate surgical and medical treatment. Under these circumstances she will almost always undergo female sexual maturation, with the potential for complete realization of her gender, including motherhood. In the classic studies of these patients, by Money and the Hampsons [201–205] the environment, hence the sex of rearing, appears as the most important determinant of psychosexual orientation. The firm ascertainment of the gender role becomes ingrained in the first few years of life and can rarely be reversed with impunity. More recently, Money et al. [206, 207] have described masculine behavior and fantasy in such women, which is more marked when medical treatment was not instituted soon after birth. This was interpreted in the light of the experiments in rodents briefly outlined above. It is difficult to translate these experiments from animals to man. To be sure, the majority of affected girls, unlike certain experiments in rodents, achieve cyclic gonadotropin secretion with normal menses and ovulation. Thus the physiologic pattern does not appear to be reversed as in other species. Furthermore, it is difficult to assess the role of the environment which is chosen for indoctrination of gender in the young child. This is especially difficult for parents confronted with an infant of ambiguous sex.

These considerations emphasize the necessity for early recognition of disorders of sex, including the adrenogenital syndrome, early administration of medical therapy which inhibits adrenocortical androgen production, and early forthright sex assignment. Even in Money's more recent observations certain subtle differences which he detected in affected women treated early did not exclude appropriate romance, marriage, and motherhood.

EXPERIMENTAL ADRENOGENITAL SYNDROME

There are no spontaneous animal models of the syndrome which are known to correspond precisely to the human disorder. For this reason there have been attempts to induce its occurrence by the employment of relatively specific enzyme inhibitors.

There has already been allusion to the virilization of female fetuses induced by androgen administration to the pregnant animal at the crucial time for genital formation. The question remains, particularly in regard to the 3β-hydroxysteroid dehydrogenase deficiency in females wherein testosterone would not be expected to be formed in sufficient amount, and yet in fact moderate virilization occurs. Here the predominant 17-ketosteroid is dehydroepiandrosterone. Goldman [208] has recently shown that a similar malformation may be produced in female rat fetuses by the administration of this steroid to the mother. Hence there seems to be reason to attribute the changes in this form of the disease to this substance.

It has been possible to reproduce the 3β-hydroxysteroid dehydrogenase in rats by employing a synthetic inhibitor, 2α-cyano-4,4,17α-trimethyl-17β-hydroxyandrost-5-en-3-one. By direct analysis of tissues, Goldman et al. [209] have demonstrated inhibition of long duration in both adrenal and testicular tissue. The adrenal glands are much enlarged, there is increased activity of glucose-6-phosphate dehydrogenase (the consequence of increased ACTH), and the clinical features are duplicated in the newborn rat when the inhibitor is administered on the fifteenth to sixteenth day of gestation. The inhibitor is an analogue of the usual substrate and is of an unusual irreversible, stoichiometric type. Large doses of 17β-estradiol produce an identical type of inhibition and clinical picture in rats [210].

In like fashion, Goldman [211] has reproduced the clinical features of 11β-hydroxylase in newborn rats by the administration of metyrapone to pregnant rats during days 15 to 20 of gestation. It was shown that 11β-hydroxylation had in fact been inhibited in the tissues of the treated animals.

SUMMARY

1 The disorders of adrenocortical steroidal biogenesis leading to congenital adrenal hyperplasia in man have been resolved into several different and specific enzymatic deficiencies. The clinical manifestations vary and depend upon the particular intermediate compounds which accumulate and their specific actions.

2 In all forms there is a detectable, if sometimes subtle, limitation of cortisol and, on occasion, of aldosterone, production. There are a number of hydroxylating enzymatic systems required for the conversion of cholesterol to cortisol. Cholesterol requires both C-20 and C-22 hydroxylation for conversion to pregnenolone. Both 3β-hydroxy steroid dehydrogenase and Δ^5-Δ^4-isomerase act to produce progesterone. Thereafter 17α-, 11β, and 21-hydroxylating systems convert progesterone to cortisol. A minor portion of progesterone normally escapes 17-hydroxylation in man and becomes corticosterone. This in turn is hydroxylated at C-18 and dehydrogenated at this same position to yield aldosterone. Most of these systems require a flow of electrons through NADPH, adrenodoxin reductase (flavoprotein reductase), a nonheme iron containing pigment and cytochrome P-450.

3 The most common form of the disease is the result of 21-hydroxylase deficiency. Its frequency varies among populations and is especially high in certain Eskimos. The disorder is transmitted as a simple autosomal recessive trait. Virilization is usual in this form and is accompanied by elevated urinary 17-ketosteroids as well as pregnanetriol and a large assortment of C-21 deoxy steroids which attest indirectly to the locus of the defect. A few direct studies of enzymatic activity in adrenal tissue confirm the deficiency of 21-hydroxylase. The virilization appears to be the consequence of large amounts of androstenedione which are generated from excessive 17-hydroxyprogesterone, the precursor for the defective enzyme through cleavage of its side chains. The androstenedione is then, in large measure, converted to testosterone in peripheral tissue.

4 The 21-hydroxylase defect is variable. In most affected individuals, the disturbance is compensated so that virtually normal amounts of cortisol are produced at the cost of the accumulation of intermediary metabolites in large quantity. In other instances, the defect is almost complete so that little or no cortisol is produced, and under these circumstances there is salt and water loss as well. Aldosterone production also varies, and, while often normal, in the presence of a complete 21-hydroxylase deficiency it is low. Serum renin levels may then be elevated; nevertheless, there is a poor response to further aldosterone secretion.

5 The 11β-hydroxylase defect is also accompanied by virilization and elevated urinary 17-ketosteroids. The urinary pattern reveals the defect by the abundance of 11-deoxy compounds. The typical C_{21} steroid which predominates is 11-deoxycortisol (substance S) and its reduced metabolites in urine, and there is also evidence for a lesser rise in deoxycorticosterone secretion. Thus hypertension is usually present in the complete form of the disease. As with the 21-hydroxylase defect there are indications that excessive testosterone production accounts for the virilization.

6 In the other three recognized varieties of the disorder steroidal biogenesis virilization is not prominent. The "desmolase" deficiency reflects an inability to convert cholesterol to pregnenolone, and the urine is devoid of detectable steroids. When 3β-hydroxy steroid dehydrogenase is deficient, its activity has been undetectable in either gonads or adrenal glands. Male subjects are not fully developed at birth, having hypospadias or complete failure to fuse the labioscrotal folds. Females, on the other hand, may be slightly virilized. The urine contains large amounts of several steroids retaining the Δ^5-3β-hydroxy configuration. When 17-hydroxylase is deficient, the major secretory product is corticosterone, but deoxycorticosterone is also produced in excessive quantity so that hypertension is common. There are almost no 17-ketosteroids or estrogens in the urine and adult female subjects are eunuchoid. This last form indicates that C_{19} steroids and estrogens in man arise from C_{21} precursors.

7 The latter three forms of this disorder indicate that the same gene controls the synthesis of an enzyme common to the gonads and the adrenal glands.

8 The salt-losing complication has been best studied in the 21-hydroxylase deficiency, although it may occur in other forms. This aspect of the disease is not yet resolved. Although there is general agreement that in the presence of this complication cortisol secretion and aldosterone secretion are sharply limited, there are conflicting results in the compensated form and conflicting theories of etiology. While many investigators find aldosterone secretion to be normal in the compensated variety, others find a hypersecretion without the expected consequence of hyperaldosteronism. This could be explained by the additional production of an unidentified salt-losing steroid which evokes compensatory aldosterone production. Under these conditions it has been proposed that there are two 21-hydroxylases, one concerned with cortisol and the other with aldosterone synthesis.

Therefore in the salt loser a defect of both enzymes is proposed. Other investigators prefer the theory that there is a single enzyme, which when completely defective interrupts both cortisol and aldosterone synthesis, with consequent salt and water loss.

9 The administration of cortisol or its analogues usually corrects the disordered steroidal secretory pattern and leads to remission of the clinical manifestations. The abnormal pattern of rapid somatic maturation and virilization is arrested, and in the 11β- and 17α-hydroxylase deficiencies the hypertension subsides. Aside from appropriate surgical correction of the genitalia, replacement doses of steroids are all that is required. In the less common forms when an enzymatic defect is shared by the gonads, normal sex hormone secretion will not take place. Therefore sex hormones must also be administered at the appropriate age. The sooner the diagnosis is established and treatment initiated the better will be controlled the apparent clinical manifestations and the psychosexual development of the patient.

BIBLIOGRAPHY

1. de Crecchio, L.: Sopra un caso di apparenze virili in una donna. Il Morgagni, **7,** 151, 1865.
2. Wilkins, L.: *The Diagnosis and Treatment of Endocrine Disorders in Childhood and Adolescence,* 2d ed., 556 pp. Thomas, Springfield, Ill, 1957.
3. Ainger, L. E., Zapata, G. C., Ely, R. S., and Kelley, V. C.: Female pseudohermaphroditism with penile urethra: Report of unusual case of congenital adrenal hyperplasia. J. Dis. Child., **95,** 410, 1958.
4. Bentinck, R. C., Lisser, H., and Reilly, W. A.: Female pseudohermaphrodism with penile urethra, masquerading as precocious puberty and cryptorchidism: Case report. J. Clin. Endocr., **16,** 412, 1956.
5. Matheson, W. J., and Ward, E. M.: Hormone sex reversal in female. Arch. Dis. Child., **29,** 22, 1954.
6. Perloff, W. H., Conger, K. B., and Levy, L. M.: Female pseudohermaphrodism: Description of 2 unusual cases. J. Clin. Endocr., **13,** 783, 1953.
7. Reilly, W. A., Hinman, F., Jr., Pickering, D. E., and Crane, J. T.: Phallic urethra in female pseudohermaphroditism. J. Dis. Child., **95,** 9, 1958.
8. Jeune, M., and Bertrand, J.: Pseudo-hermaphrodisme féminin avec virilisation totale (urèthre pénien) par hyperplasie surrénale: A propos d'un cas. Sem. Hop. Paris, **35,** 2131, 1959.
9. Prader, A. Vollkommen männliche äussere Genitalentwicklung und Salzverlustsyndrom bei Mädchen mit kongenitalem adrenogenitalem Syndrom. Helv. Paediat. Acta, **13,** 5, 1958.
10. Peris, L. A.: Congenital adrenal hyperplasia producing female hermaphroditism with phallic urethra. Obstet. Gynec., **16,** 156, 1960.
11. Weldon, V. V., Blizzard, R. M., and Migeon, C. J.: Newborn girls misdiagnosed as bilaterally cryptorchid males. New Eng. J. Med., **274,** 829, 1966.
12. Decourt, J., Jayle, M. F., and Baulieu, E.: Virilisme cliniquement tardif avec excrétion de prégnanetriol et insuffisance de la production du cortisol. Ann. Endocr. (Paris), **18,** 416, 1957.
13. Jayle, M. F., Weinmann, S. H., Baulieu, E. E., and Vallin, Y.: Virilisme postpubertaire discret par deficience de l'hydroxylation en C_{21}. Acta Endocr., (Kobenhavn), **29,** 513, 1958.
14. Lipsett, M. B., and Riter, B. D.: Urinary steroids in post-natal adrenal hyperplasia with virilism. Acta endocr. (Kobenhavn), **38,** 481, 1961.
15. Mahesh, V. B., Greenblatt, R. B., and Coniff, R. F.: Adrenal hyperplasia—a case report of delayed onset of the congenital form or an acquired form. J. Clin. Endocr., **28,** 619, 1968.
16. Brooks, R. V., Mattingly, D., Mills, I. H., and Prunty, F. T. G.: Postpubertal adrenal virilism with biochemical disturbance of congenital type of adrenal hyperplasia. Brit. Med. J., **I,** 1294, 1960.
17. Guenel, J., Bureau, L., and Orieux, J.: Deficit en 21-hydroxylase tardivement chez un homme a l'occasion d'un asthenie chronique. Ann. Endocr. (Paris), **28,** 71, 1967.
18. Marie, J., Kostich-Jaksitch, S., Bricaire, H., Salet, J., See, G., and Leveque, B.: Hyperplasie congenitale des surrenales ne comportant pas de sinus urogenital et s'accompagnant de developpement premature des siens. Sem. Hop. Paris, **33,** 1594, 1957.
19. Phillips, J.: Four cases of spurious hermaphroditism in one family. Trans. Obstet. Soc., London, **28,** 158, 1888.
20. Butler, A. M., Ross, R. A., and Talbot, N. B.: Probable adrenal insufficiency in infant: Report of case. J. Pediat., **15,** 831, 1939.
21. Wilkins, L., Fleischmann, W., and Howard, J. E.: Macrogenitosomia praecox associated with hyperplasia of androgenic tissue of adrenal and death from cortico-adrenal insufficiency: Case report. Endocrinology, **26,** 385, 1940.
22. Marks, J. F., and Fink, C. W.: Incidence of the salt-losing form of congenital hyperplasia. Pediatrics, **43,** 636, 1969.
23. Jost, A.: Embryonic sexual differentiation: Morphology, physiology, abnormalities, in *Hermaphroditism, Genital Anomalies and Related Disorders,* edited by H. W. Jones and W. W. Scott, p. 15. Williams and Wilkins, Baltimore, 1958.
24. Jost. A.: Problems of fetal endocrinology: The gonadal and hypophyseal hormones. Recent Progr. Hormone Res., **8,** 379, 1953.
25. Blackman, S. S., Jr.: Concerning function and origin of reticular zone of adrenal cortex: Hyperplasia in adrenogenital syndrome. Bull. Johns Hopkins Hosp., **78,** 180, 1946.
26. Tonutti, E., Bayer, J. M., and Spiegelhoff, W.: Beitrag zur Kenntnis der Struktur der Nebennierenrinde beim connatalen adrenogenitalen Syndrom. Endokrinologie, **40,** 310, 1961.
27. Seelen, J. C.: Pathological anatomical findings in adrenal cortex in two cases of congenital adrenocortical hyperplasia. Acta Endocr. (Kobenhavn), **34,** 457, 1960.
28. Symington, T.: Morphology and secretory cytology of human adrenal cortex. Brit. Med. Bull., **18,** 117, 1962.
29. Codaccioni, J. L., and Ruf, H.: L'état des ovaries dans le hyper et les dyscorticismes. Sem. Hop. Paris, **37,** 3661, 1961.
30. Landing, B. H.: Hilar-cell proliferation in adrenogenital syndrome. J. Clin. Endocr., **14,** 245, 1954.
31. Earll, J. M., Newman, S. G., and DiRaimondo, V. C.: Bilateral testicular tumors in untreated congenital adrenocortical hyperplasia. JAMA, **209,** 937, 1969.
32. Schoen, E. J., DiRaimondo, V. C., and Dominguez, O. V.: Bilateral testicular tumors complicating congenital adrenocortical hyperplasia. J. Clin. Endocr., **21,** 518, 1961.
33. Miller, E. C., and Murray, H. L.: Congenital adrenocortical hyperplasia: Case previously reported as bilateral interstitial cell tumor of the testicle. J. Clin. Endocr., **22,** 655, 1962.
34. Besch, P.: In vitro biosynthesis studies of endocrine tumors. III. Cortisol production by a testicular tumor. J. Clin. Endocr., **24,** 1339, 1964.
35. Engel, L. L., Lanman, G., Scully, R. E., and Villee, D. B.: Studies on an interstitial cell tumor of the testes: Formation of cortisol-^{14}C from acetate-1-^{14}C. J. Clin. Endocr., **26,** 381, 1966.
36. Bloch, K.: The biological synthesis of cholesterol. Recent Progr. Hormone Res., **6,** 111, 1951.
37. Würsch, J., Huang, R. L., and Bloch, K.: The origin of the isooctyl side-chain of cholesterol. J. Biol. Chem., **195,** 439, 1952.
38. Cornforth, J. W., Hunter, G. D., and Popjak, G.: Studies of cholesterol biosynthesis. 1. Biochem. J., **54,** 590, 1953.
39. Cornforth, J. W., Hunter, G. D., and Popjak, G.: Studies of cholesterol biosynthesis. 2. Biochem. J., **54,** 597, 1953.
40. Cornforth, J. W., Gore, I. Y., and Popjak, G.: Studies on the biosynthesis of cholesterol. 4. Biochem. J., **65,** 94, 1957.
41. Bloch, K.: Über die Herkunft des Kohlenstoff-atoms 7 in Cholestrin: Ein Beitrag zur Kenntnis der Biosynthese der Steroide. Helvet. Chim. Acta, **36,** 1611, 1953.

42. Little, H. N., and Bloch, K.: Studies on the utilization of acetic acid for the biological synthesis of cholesterol. J. Biol. Chem., **183,** 33, 1950.
43. Srere, P. A., Chaikoff, I. L., Treitman, S. S., and Burkstein, L. S.: The extrahepatic synthesis of cholesterol. J. Biol. Chem., **182,** 629, 1950.
44. Srere, P. A., Chaikoff, I. L., and Dauben, W. G.: The in vitro synthesis of cholesterol from acetate by surviving adrenal cortical tissue. J. Biol. Chem., **176,** 829, 1948.
45. Solomons, S., Levitan, P., and Lieberman, S.: Possible intermediates between cholesterol and pregnenolone in corticoidogenesis. Canad. Rev. Biol., **15,** 282, 1956.
46. Staple, E., Lynn, W. S., and Gurin, S.: An enzymatic cleavage of the cholesterol side chain. J. Biol. Chem., **219,** 845, 1956.
47. Shimizu, K., Hayano, M., Gut, M., and Dorfman, R. I.: The transformation of 20α-hydroxycholesterol to isocaproic acid and C21 steroids. J. Biol. Chem., **236,** 695, 1961.
48. Sweat, M. L., and Lipscomb, M. D.: A transdehydrogenase and reduced diphosphopyridine nucleotide involved in the oxidation of desoxycorticosterone to corticosterone by adrenal tissue. J. Amer. Chem. Soc., **77,** 5185, 1955.
49. Grant, J. K., and Brownie, A. C.: The role of fumarate and TPN in steroid enzymatic 11β-hydroxylation. Biochim. Biophys. Acta, **18,** 433, 1955.
50. Hayano, M., Lindberg, M. C., Dorfman, R. I., Hancock, J. E. H., and Doering, W. V. E.: Mechanisms of the C-11β-hydroxylation of steroids. Arch. Biochem., **59,** 529, 1955.
51. Tomkins, G. M., Curran, J. F., and Michael, P. J.: Further studies on enzymatic adrenal 11β-hydroxylation. Biochim. Biophys. Acta, **28,** 449, 1958.
52. Omura, T., Sanders, E., Estabrook, R. W., Cooper, D. Y., and Rosenthal, O.: Isolation from adrenal cortex of a non-heme iron protein and a flavoprotein functional as a reduced NADPH-cytochrome P-450 reductase. Arch. Biochem., **117,** 660, 1966.
53. Kimura, T., and Suzuki, K.: Components of the electron transport system in adrenal steroid hydroxylase: Isolation and properties of non-heme iron protein. J. Biol. Chem., **242,** 485, 1966.
54. Harding, B. W., Wong, S. H., and Nelson, D. H.: Carbon monoxide-combining substances in rat adrenal. Biochim. Biophys. Acta, **92,** 415, 1964.
55. Harding, B. W., and Nelson, D. H.: Electron carriers of the bovine adrenal cortical respiratory chain and hydroxylating pathways. J. Biol. Chem., **241,** 2212, 1966.
56. Cooper, D. Y., Novack, B., Foroff, O., Slade, A., Saunders, E., Narasimhulu, S., and Rosenthal, O.: Photochemical action spectrum of reconstituted steroid 11-β hydroxylase of bovine adrenocortical mitochondria. Fed. Proc., **26,** 341, 1967.
57. Garfinkel, D.: Studies on pig liver microsomes. I. Enzymatic and pigment composition of different microsomal fractions. Arch. Biochem., **77,** 493, 1958.
58. Ryan, K., and Engel, L.: Hydroxylation of steroids at carbon 21. J. Biol. Chem., **225,** 103, 1957.
59. Estabrook, R. W., Cooper, D. Y., and Rosenthal, O.: The light reversible carbon monoxide inhibition of the steroid C-21 hydroxylase system of the adrenal cortex. Biochem. Z., **338,** 741, 1963.
60. Harding, B. W., Bell, J. J., Oldham, S. B., and Wilson, L. D.: Corticosteroid biosynthesis in adrenal cortical mitochondria, in *Functions of the Adrenal Cortex,* edited by K. W. McKerns. Appleton-Century-Crofts, New York, 1968.
61. Sih, C. J.: Enzymatic mechanism of steroid hydroxylation. Science, **163,** 1297, 1969.
62. Samuels, L. T., Helmreich, M. L., Lasater, M. B., and Reich, H.: Enzyme in endocrine tissues which oxidizes Δ^5-3 hydroxy steroids to α,β unsaturated ketones. Science, **113,** 490, 1951.
63. Beyer, K. F., and Samuels, L. T.: Distribution of steroid-3β-ol-dehydrogenase in cellular structures of adrenal gland. J. Biol. Chem., **219,** 69, 1956.
64. Fukushima, D. K., Bradlow, H. L., Yamauchi, T., Yagi, A., and Koerner, D.: Fate of 48-hydrogen in Δ^5-androstene-3,17-dione on isomerization with mammalian enzyme preparations. Steroids, **11,** 541, 1968.
65. Bradlow, H. L., Fukushima, D. K., Zumoff, B., and Hellman, L.: Metabolism of dehydroepiandrosterone-4-^{14}C-4β-^{3}H in man. Steroids, **11,** 273, 1968.
66. Werbin, H., and Chaikoff, I. L.: Fate of the 4-beta-hydrogen of cholesterol during its conversion of steroid hormones. Biochem. Biophys. Acta, **82,** 581, 1964.
67. Mulrow, P. J., Cohn, G. L., and Kuljian, A.: Conversion of 17-hydroxypregnanolone to cortisol by normal and hyperplastic human adrenal slices. J. Clin. Invest., **41,** 1584, 1962.
68. Welike, I., and Engel, L. L.: 17-Hydroxypregnenolone as a precursor for cortisol. Fed. Proc., **20,** 179, 1961.
69. Plager, J. E., and Samuels, L. T.: Conversion of progesterone to 17-hydroxy-11-desoxycorticosterone by fractionated beef adrenal homogenates. J. Biol. Chem., **211,** 21, 1954.
70. Hayano, M., and Dorfman, R. I.: Enzymatic C-11β-hydroxylation of steroids. J. Biol. Chem., **201,** 175, 1953.
71. Ryan, K. J., and Engel, L. L.: Hydroxylation of steroids at carbon 21. J. Biol. Chem., **225,** 103, 1957.
72. Ryan, K. J.: Steroid 21-hydroxylation by adrenal cell fractions. Fed. Proc., **15,** 344, 1956.
73. Hechter, O., and Pincus, G.: Genesis of adrenocortical secretion. Physiol. Rev., **34,** 459, 1954.
74. Tomkins, G. M., Michael, P. J., and Curran, J. F.: Studies on nature of steroid 11-β-hydroxylation. Biochim. Biophys. Acta, **23,** 655, 1957.
75. Sandor, T. J., and Lanthier, A.: The in vitro biosynthesis of 18-hydroxycorticosterone-4-^{14}C by slices of zona glomerulosa of beef adrenals and by human adrenals. Acta Endocr. (Kobenhavn), **42,** 355, 1963.
76. Nicolis, G. L., and Ulick, S.: Role of 18-hydroxylation in the biosynthesis of aldosterone. Endocrinology, **76,** 514, 1965.
77. Ayres, P. J., Pearlman, W. H., Tait, J. F., and Tait, S. A. S.: Biosynthetic preparation of aldosterone and corticosterone. Biochem. J., **70,** 230, 1958.
78. Stachenko, J., and Giroud, C. P. J.: Some aspects of steroidogenesis in the zona glomerulosa, in *The Human Adrenal Cortex,* edited by A. R. Curie, T. Symington, and J. K. Grant. Livingstone, Edinburgh, 1962.
79. Greengard, P., Psychoyoss, H., Tallan, H. H., Cooper, D. Y., Rosenthal, O., and Estabrook, R. W.: Aldosterone synthesis by adrenal mitochondria. 3. Participation of cytochrome P-450. Arch. Biochem., **121,** 298, 1967.
80. Slaunwhite, W. R., Jr., and Samuels, L. T.: Progesterone as a precursor of testicular androgens. J. Biol. Chem., **220,** 441, 1956.
81. Bloch, E., Dorfman, R., and Pincus, G.: The conversion of acetate to C19 steroids by human adrenal gland slices. J. Biol. Chem., **224,** 737, 1957.
82. Cohn, G. L., and Mulrow, P. J.: Androgen release and synthesis in vivo by human adult adrenal glands. J. Clin. Invest., **42,** 64, 1963.
83. Ichii, S., Kobayashi, S., and Matsuba, M.: Studies on the sidechain cleavage of C21 steroids. Steroids, **5,** 123, 1965.
84. Horton, R., and Tait, J. F.: Androstenedione production and interconversion rates measured in peripheral blood and studies on the possible site of its conversion to testosterone. J. Clin. Invest., **45,** 301, 1966.
85. Ryan, K. J.: Biological aromatization of steroids. J. Biol. Chem., **234,** 268, 1959.
86. Stone, D., and Hechter, O.: Studies on ACTH action in perfused bovine adrenals: The site of action of ACTH in corticosteroidogenesis. Arch. Biochem., **51,** 457, 1954.
87. Creange, J. E., and Roberts, S.: Stimulation of steroid C-11β and C-18 hydroxylations in rat adrenal homogenates by adenosine 3′,5′-phosphate via a mechanism not requiring endogenous precursor, glycogen phosphorylation or NADPH generation. Steroids, suppl. II, 13, 1965.
88. Haynes, R. C. Jr.,: The activation of adrenal phosphorylase by the adrenocorticotropic hormone. J. Biol. Chem., **233,** 1220, 1958.
89. McKerns, K. W.: Mechanism of action of adrenocorticotropic hormone through activation of glucose-6-phosphate dehydrogenase. Biochim. Biophys. Acta, **90,** 357, 1964.
90. Lowry, O. H., and Passonneau, J. V.: The relationship between substrates and enzymes of glycolysis in brain. J. Biol. Chem., **239,** 31, 1964.
91. Schonbaum, E., Birmingham, M. K., and Saffran, M.: Metabolism of glucose and steroid formation by rat adrenals in vitro. J. Biochem., **34,** 527, 1956.
92. Hechter, O., and Lester, G.: Cell permeability and hormone action. Recent Progr. Hormone Res., **16,** 139, 1960.

93. Hirshfield, I. N., and Koritz, S. B.: The stimulation of pregnenolone synthesis in the large particles from the adrenals of rats administered adrenocorticotropin in vivo. Biochim. Biophys. Acta, **111,** 313, 1965.
94. Chance, B., Schoener, B., and Ferguson, J. J.: In vivo induced oxidation by adrenocorticotropic hormone of reduced pyridine nucleotides in adrenal cortex of hypophysectomized rats. Nature (London), **195,** 776, 1962.
95. McKerns, K. W.: Mechanisms of ACTH regulation of the adrenal cortex, in *Functions of the Adrenal Cortex.* Appleton-Century-Crofts, New York, 1968.
96. Rosenfeld, R. S., Fukushima, D. K., and Gallagher, T. F.: Metabolism of adrenal cortical hormones, in *The Adrenal Cortex,* edited by A. B. Eisenstein, p. 103, Little, Brown, Boston, 1967.
97. Bartter, F. C., Forbes, A. P., and Leaf, A.: Congenital adrenal hyperplasia associated with the adrenogenital syndrome: An attempt to correct its disordered hormonal pattern. J. Clin. Invest., **29,** 797, 1950.
98. Wilkins, L., Lewis, R. A., Klein, K., and Rosenberg, E.: Suppression of androgen secretion by cortisone in case of congenital adrenal hyperplasia: Preliminary report. Bull. Johns Hopkins Hosp., **86,** 249, 1950.
99. Bartter, F. C., Albright, F., Forbes, A. P., Leaf, A., Dempsey, E., and Carroll, E.: The effects of adrenocorticotropic hormone and cortisone in the adrenogenital syndrome associated with congenital adrenal hyperplasia: An attempt to explain and correct its disordered hormonal pattern. J. Clin. Invest., **30,** 237, 1951.
100. Lewis, R. A., and Wilkins, L.: The effect of adrenocorticotropic hormone in congenital adrenal hyperplasia with virilism and in Cushing's syndrome treated with methyl testosterone. J. Clin. Invest., **28,** 394, 1949.
101. Butler, G. C., and Marrian, G. F.: Isolation of pregnane-3,17,20-triol from urine of women showing adrenogenital syndrome. J. Biol. Chem., **119,** 565, 1937.
102. Mason, H. L., and Kepler, E. J.: Isolation of steroids from urine of patients with adrenal cortical tumors and adrenal cortical hyperplasia: New 17-ketosteroid, androstane-3(α), 11-diol-17-one. J. Biol. Chem., **161,** 235, 1945.
103. Bongiovanni, A. M.: Detection of pregnandiol and pregnantriol in urine of patients with adrenal hyperplasia: Suppression with cortisone: Preliminary report. Bull. Johns Hopkins Hosp., **92,** 244, 1953.
104. Jailer, J. W.: Virilism. Bull. N. Y. Acad. Med., **29,** 377, 1953.
105. Lieberman, S., and Dobriner, K.: Isolation of pregnanediol-3α,17-one-20 from human urine. J. Biol. Chem., **161,** 269, 1945.
106. Fukushima, D. K., and Gallagher, T. F.: Steroid isolation studies in congenital adrenal hyperplasia. J. Biol. Chem., **229,** 85, 1957.
107. Bergstrand, C. G., and Gemzell, C. A.: Pregnanediol excretion in normal children and in children with various endocrine disorders, including congenital adrenal hyperplasia. J. Clin. Endocr., **17,** 870, 1957.
108. Strott, C. A., Yoshimi, T., Bardin, C. W., and Lipsett, M. B.: Blood progesterone and 17-hydroxyprogesterone levels and production rates in a boy with virilizing congenital adrenal hyperplasia. J. Clin. Endocr., **28,** 1085, 1968.
109. Finkelstein, M., von Euw, J., and Reichstein, T.: Isolierung von 3α,17,20α,-trioxy-pregnanon-11 aus pathologischen menschlichen Harn. Helv. Chim. Acta, **36,** 1266, 1953.
110. Kelley, V. C., Ely, R. S., and Raile, R. B.: Metabolic studies in patients with congenital adrenal hyperplasia: Effects of cortisone therapy. J. Clin. Endocr., **12,** 1140, 1952.
111. Kelley, V. C., Ely, R. S., and Raile, R. B.: Hormone patterns with congenital adrenal hyperplasia. Pediatrics, **12,** 541, 1953.
112. Bongiovanni, A. M., Eberlein, W. R., and Cara, J.: Studies on metabolism of adrenal steroids in adrenogenital syndrome. J. Clin. Endocr., **14,** 409, 1954.
113. Christy, N. P., Wallace, E. Z., and Jailer, J. W.: Effect of intravenously-administered ACTH on plasma 17,21-dihydroxy-20-ketosteroids in normal individuals and in patients with disorders of adrenal cortex. J. Clin. Invest., **34,** 899, 1955.
114. Eberlein, W. R., and Bongiovanni, A. M.: Partial characterization of urinary adrenocortical steroids in adrenal hyperplasia. J. Clin. Invest., **34,** 1337, 1955.
115. Degenhart, H. J., Visser, H. K., Wilmink, A., and Croughs, W.: Aldosterone and cortisol secretion rates in infants and children with congenital adrenal hyperplasia suggesting different 21-hydroxylase defects. Acta Endocr. (Kobenhavn), **48,** 587, 1965.
116. Migeon, C. J., and Kenny, F. M.: Cortisol production rate. V. Congenital virilizing adrenal hyperplasia. J. Pediat., **69,** 779, 1966.
117. Sydnor, K. L., Kelley, V. C., Raile, R. B., Ely, R. S., and Sayers, G.: Blood adrenocorticotrophin in children with congenital adrenal hyperplasia. Proc. Soc. Exp. Biol. Med., **82,** 695, 1953.
118. Binoux, M., Girard, F., Pham-Huu-Trung, M. T., Canlorbe, P., and Mozziconacci, P.: La Regulation Hypophyso-Surrenale dans L'Hyperplasie Congenitale des Surrenales. Arch. Franc. Pediat., **24,** 369, 1967.
119. Fukushima, D. K., Bradlow, H. L., Hellman, L., Zumoff, B., and Gallagher, T. F.: Study of 17-hydroxyprogesterone-4-C^{14} in man. J. Clin. Endocr., **21,** 765, 1961.
120. Wieland, R. G., Maynard, D. E., Tiley, T. R., and Hamsi, G. J.: Detection of 21-deoxycortisol in blood from a patient with congenital adrenal hyperplasia. Metabolism, **14,** 1276, 1965.
121. Bongiovanni, A. M.: In vitro hydroxylation of steroids by whole adrenal homogenates of beef, normal man, and patients with adrenogenital syndrome. J. Clin. Invest., **37,** 1342, 1958.
122. Zander, J.: Nachweis von Progesteron und 17α-Hydroxyprogesteron in hyperplastichen Nebennieron bei adrenogenitalem Syndrom. Klin. Wschr., **38,** 5, 1960.
123. Axelrod, F., and Goldzieher, J. W.: Steroid biosynthesis by adrenal and ovarian tissue in congenital adrenal hyperplasia. Acta Endocr. (Kobenhavn), **56,** 453, 1967.
124. Bongiovanni, A. M.: Unpublished data.
125. Mizutami, S., Kusunoki, T., Matsumoto, K., and Seki, T.: Urinary steroids in fifteen cases of congenital adrenal hyperplasia. Endocr. Jap., **14,** 148, 1967.
126. Eberlein, W. R., and Bongiovanni, A. M.: Defective steroidal biogenesis in congenital adrenal hyperplasia. Pediatrics, **21,** 661, 1958.
127. Gandy, H. M., Moody, C. B., and Peterson, R. E.: Androgen levels in ovarian and adrenal venous plasma, in *Proceedings VI Pan-American Congress of Endocrinology,* p. 223. Excerpta Medica, New York, 1966.
128. Camacho, A. M., and Migeon, C. J.: Testosterone excretion and production rate in normal adults and patients with congenital adrenal hyperplasia. J. Clin. Endocr., **26,** 893, 1966.
129. Rosner, J. M., Conte, N. F., Briggs, J. H., Chao, P. Y., Sudman, E. M., and Forsham, P.: Determination of urinary testosterone by chromatography and colorimetry. J. Clin. Endocr., **25,** 95, 1965.
130. Lim, N. Y., and Dingman, J. F.: Measurement of testosterone excretion and production rate by glass chromatography. J. Clin. Endocr., **25,** 563, 1965.
131. Butenandt, O., and Knorr, D.: Die Testosteroneausscheidung im Urin beim kongenitalen adrenogenitalen Syndrom. Z. Kinderheilk., **100,** 20, 1967.
132. Horton, R., and Frasier, S. D.: Androstenedione and its conversion to plasma testosterone in congenital adrenal hyperplasia. J. Clin. Invest., **46,** 1003, 1967.
133. Rivarola, M. A., Saez, J. M., and Migeon, C. J.: Studies of androgens in patients with congenital adrenal hyperplasia. J. Clin. Endocr., **27,** 624, 1967.
134. Frasier, S. D., Horton, R., and Ulstrom, R. A.: Androgens in 11β-hydroxylase deficiency adrenal hyperplasia. Pediatrics, **44,** 209, 1969.
135. Fukushima, D. K., and Gallagher, T. F.: Absence of 21-hydroxylation in congenital adrenal hyperplasia. J. Clin. Endocr., **18,** 694, 1958.
136. Bergstrand, C. G., Birke, G., and Plantin, L.: The corticosteroid excretion pattern in infants and children with the adrenogenital syndrome. Acta Endocr. (Kobenhavn), **30,** 500, 1959.
137. Bongiovanni, A. M., Eberlein, W. R., Smith, J. D., and McPadden, A. J.: The urinary excretion of three C-21 methyl corticosteroids in the adrenogenital syndrome. J. Clin. Endocr., **19,** 1608, 1959.
138. Reynolds, J. W.: Isolation of 16-OH-pregnenolone from urine of newborn infants. Proc. Soc. Exp. Biol. Med., **113,** 980, 1963.
139. Bush, I. E., and Mahesh, V. B.: Adrenocortical hyperfunction with sudden onset of hirsutism. J. Endocr., **18,** 1, 1959.
140. Romanoff, E. B., Hudson, P., and Pincus, G.: Isolation of hydrocortisone and corticosterone from human adrenal vein blood. J. Clin. Endocr., **13,** 1546, 1953.

141. Lombardo, M. E., McMorris, C., and Hudson, P. B.: The isolation of steroidal substances from human adrenal vein blood. Endocrinology, **65**, 426, 1959.
142. Hirschmann, H., DeCourcy, C., Levy, R. P., and Miller, K. L.: Adrenal precursors of urinary 17-ketosteroids. J. Biol. Chem., **235**, PC48, 1960.
143. Bradlow, H. L., and Gallagher, T. F.: Metabolism of 11β-hydroxy-Δ^4androstene-3,17-dione in congenital adrenal hyperplasia. J. Clin. Endocr., **19**, 1575, 1959.
144. Cohn, G. L., and Mulrow, P. J.: Androgen release and synthesis in vitro by human adult adrenal glands. J. Clin. Invest., **42**, 64, 1963.
145. Migeon, C. J., and Gardner, L. I.: Urinary estrogens (measured fluorometrically and biologically) in hyperadrenocorticism: Influence of cortisone, compound F, compound B, and ACTH. J. Clin. Endocr., **12**, 1513, 1957.
146. Eberlein, W. R., and Bongiovanni, A. M.: Plasma and urinary corticosteroids in hypertensive form of congenital adrenal hyperplasia. J. Biol. Chem., **223**, 85, 1956.
147. Blunck, W.: Die alpha-ketolischen Cortisol und Corticosteron-metaboliten sowie die 11-Oxy-und 11-Desoxy-17-ketosteroide im Urin von Kindern, Acta Endocr. (Kobenhavn), **59**, suppl. 134, 1968.
148. Chaptal, J., Jean, R., Cristol, P., and Bonnet, H.: Augmentation des 17-hydroxycorticoides plasmatiques et urinaires dans un cas d'hyperplasie congenitale es surrenales sans hypertension arterielle. Ann. Endocr. (Paris), **20**, 323, 1959.
149. Gandy, H. M., Keutmann, E. H., and Izzo, A. J.: Characterization of urinary steroids in adrenal hyperplasia: Isolation of the metabolites of cortisol, Compound S and desoxycorticosterone from normotensive patient with adrenogenital syndrome. J. Clin. Invest., **39**, 364, 1960.
150. Green, O. D., Migeon, C. J., and Wilkins, L.: Urinary steroids in hypertensive form of congenital adrenal hyperplasia. J. Clin. Endocr., **20**, 929, 1960.
151. Dyrenfurth, I., Sybulski, S., Notchev, V., Beck, J. C., and Venning, E. H.: Urinary corticosteroid excretion patterns in patients with adrenocortical dysfunction. J. Clin. Endocr., **18**, 391, 1958.
152. Gabrilove, J. L., Sharma, E. C., and Dorfman, R. I.: Adrenocortical 11-beta-hydroxylase deficiency and virilism first manifest in the adult women. New Eng. J. Med., **272**, 1189, 1965.
153. Kowarski, A., Russell, A., and Migeon, C. J.: Aldosterone secretion rate in the hypertensive form of congenital adrenal hyperplasia. J. Clin. Endocr., **28**, 1445, 1968.
154. Biglieri, E. G., Herron, M. A., and Brust, N.: 17-Hydroxylation deficiency in man. J. Clin. Invest., **45**, 1946, 1966.
155. Goldsmith, O., Solomon, D. H., and Horton, R.: Hypogonadism and mineralocorticoid excess: The 17-hydroxylase deficiency syndrome. New Eng. J. Med., **277**, 673, 1967.
156. Mallin, S. R.: Congenital adrenal hyperplasia secondary to 17-hydroxylase deficiency. Ann. Intern. Med., **70**, 69, 1969.
157. New, M.: Male pseudohermaphroditism due to 17α-hydroxylase deficiency. J. Clin. Invest., **49**, 1930, 1970.
158. Bongiovanni, A. M.: Unusual steroid pattern in congenital adrenal hyperplasia: Deficiency of 3β-hydroxy dehydrogenase. J. Clin. Endocr., **21**, 860, 1961.
159. Bongiovanni, A. M.: Adrenogenital syndrome with deficiency of 3β-hydroxysteroid dehydrogenase. J. Clin. Invest., **41**, 2086, 1962.
160. Bongiovanni, A. M., Eberlein, W. R., Goldman, A. S., and New, M.: Disorders of adrenal steroid biogenesis. Recent Progr. Hormone Res., **23**, 375, 1967.
161. Migeon, C. J., and Blizzard, R. M.: Personal communication, 1962.
162. Kogut, M. D.: Adrenogenital syndrome associated with 3β-hydroxysteroid dehydrogenase deficiency. Amer. J. Dis. Child., **110**, 562, 1965.
162*a*. Jänne, O., Perheentupee, J., and Vikho, R.: Plasma and urinary steroids in an eight-year-old boy with 3β-hydroxysteroid dehydrogenase deficiency. J. Clin. Endocr., **531**, 162, 1970.
162*b*. Zachman, M., Vollmin, J. A., Murset, G., Curtius, H. Ch., and Prader A.: Unusual type of adrenal hyperplasia probably due to deficiency of 3β-hydroxysteroid dehydrogenase. J. Clin. Endocr., **30**, 719, 1970.
162*c*. Kenny, F. M., Reynolds, J. W., and Green, O. C.: Partial 3β-hydroxy steroid dehydrogenase and 21-hydroxylase deficiency in a family with congenital adrenal hyperplasia with evidence for increasing 3β-hydroxysteroid dehydrogenase activities with age. Program Abstracts, 40th Annual Meeting, Society for Pediatric Research, p. 62, 1970.
162*d*. Parks, G. A., New, M. I., Bermudez, J. A., Anast, C. S., and Bongiovanni, A. M.: A pubertal boy with the 3β-hydroxysteroid dehydrogenase defect. J. Clin. Endocr. In press.
163. Prader, A., and Gurtner, H. P.: Das Syndrom des Pseudo-hermaphroditismus masculinus bei kongenitaler Nebennierenrinden Hyperplasie ohne Androgenüberproduktion. Helv. Paediat. Acta, **10**, 397, 1955.
164. Prader, A., and Siebermann, R. E.: Nebenniereninsuffizienz bei kongenitaler Lipoidhyperplasie der Nebennieren. Helv. Paediat. Acta, **12**, 509, 1957.
165. Camacho, A. M., Kowarski, A., Migeon, C. J., and Brough, A. J. Congenital adrenal hyperplasia due to a deficiency of one of the enzymes involved in the biosynthesis of pregnenolone. J. Clin. Endocr., **28**, 153, 1968.
166. Cash, R., Brough, A. J., Cohen, M. N. P., and Satch, P. S.: Aminoglutethimide as an inhibitor of adrenal steroidogenesis: Mechanism of action and therapeutic trial. J. Clin. Endocr., **27**, 1239, 1967.
167. Green, O. C., Migeon, C. J., and Wilkins, L.: Urinary steroids in the hypertensive form of congenital adrenal hyperplasia. J. Clin. Endocr., **20**, 929, 1960.
168. Stempfel, R. S., Jr.: Familial variations in adrenocorticosteroid excretion in hypertensive congenital adrenal hyperplasia. Southern Med. J., **53**, 1584, 1960.
169. Stempfel, R. S., Jr., and Billings, R. B.: Relatively deficient 21-hydroxylation vs. precursor "pile-up" in hypertensive congenital adrenal hyperplasia. Proc. Soc. Pediatric Res., Atlantic City, 1963.
170. Blizzard, R. M., Liddle, G. W., Migeon, C. J., and Wilkins, L.: Aldosterone excretion in virilizing adrenal hyperplasia. J. Clin. Invest., **38**, 1442, 1959.
171. Bryan, G. T., Kliman, B., and Bartter, F. C.: Impaired aldosterone production in "salt-losing" congenital adrenal hyperplasia. J. Clin. Invest., **44**, 957, 1965.
172. Kowarski, A., Finkelstein, J. W., Spaulding, J. S., Holman, G. H., and Migeon, C. J.: Aldosterone secretion rate in congenital adrenal hyperplasia: A discussion of the theories on the pathogenesis of the salt-losing form of the syndrome. J. Clin. Invest., **44**, 1505, 1965.
173. Lieberman, A. H., and Luetscher, J. A.: Some effects of abnormalities of pituitary, adrenal or thyroid function on excretion of aldosterone and the response to corticotropin or sodium deprivation. J. Clin. Endocr., **20**, 1004, 1960.
174. Mattox, V. R., and Lewbart, M. L.: The determination of aldosterone in urine. J. Clin. Endocr., **19**, 1151, 1959.
175. New, M. I., Miller, B., and Peterson, R. E.: Aldosterone excretion in normal children and children with adrenal hyperplasia. J. Clin. Invest., **45**, 412, 1966.
176. Bartter, F. C., Henkin, R. I., and Bryan, G. T.: Aldosterone hypersecretion in "non-salt-losing" congenital adrenal hyperplasia. J. Clin. Invest., **47**, 1742, 1968.
177. Eberlein, W. R., and Bongiovanni, A. M.: Defective steroidal biogenesis in congenital adrenal hyperplasia. Pediatrics, **21**, 661, 1958.
178. Eberlein, W. R., and Bongiovanni, A. M.: Steroid metabolism in the "salt-losing" form of congenital adrenal hyperplasia. J. Clin. Invest. **37**, 889, 1958.
179. Childs, B., Grumbach, M. M., and VanWyk, J. J.: Virilizing adrenal hyperplasia: A genetic and hormonal study. J. Clin. Invest., **35**, 213, 1956.
180. Prader, A.: Die Haufigkeit des Kongenitalen Adrenogenitalen Syndromes. Helv. Paediat. Acta, **13**, 426, 1958.
181. Rosenbloom, A. L., and Smith, D. W.: Varying expression for salt-losing in related patients with congenital adrenal hyperplasia. Pediatrics, **38**, 215, 1966.
182. Sharma, D. C., and Dorfman, R. I.: Studies on in vivo C-21 hydroxylation of progesterone and 17α-hydroxyprogesterone. Fed. Proc., **22**, 530, 1963.

183. Klein, R.: Evidence for and against existence of salt-losing hormone. J. Pediat., **57**, 452, 1960.
184. Hall, K., and Hökfelt, B.: Clinical and steroid metabolic studies in four siblings with congenital virilizing adrenal hyperplasia. Acta Endocr. (Kobenhavn), **52**, 535, 1966.
185. Visser, H. K. A., and Degenhart, H. J.: Salt-losing in an infant with congenital adrenal hyperplasia and normal aldosterone production. Acta Paediat. Scand., **56**, 216, 1967.
186. Coppage, W. C., Jr., and Liddle, G. W.: Metabolic studies with a steroid isolated from the urine of patients with "salt-losing" congenital adrenal hyperplasia. J. Clin. Endocr., **20**, 729, 1960.
187. Godard, C., Riondell, A. M., Veyrat, R., Megevand, A., and Miller, A. F.: Plasma renin activity and aldosterone secretion in congenital adrenal hyperplasia, Pediatrics, **41**, 883, 1968.
188. Imai, M., Igarashi, Y., and Sokabe, H.: Plasma renin activity in congenital virilizing adrenal hyperplasia. Pediatrics, **41**, 897, 1968.
189. Ulick, S.: Aldosterone biosynthesis in congenital adrenal hyperplasia. Program of the 49th Meeting of the Endocrine Society, p. 31, 1967.
190. Ulick, S.: The metabolism and secretion of 21-deoxy-aldosterone. In press.
191. Kepler, E. J., and Mason, H. L.: Relation of urinary steroids to diagnosis of adrenal cortical tumors and adrenal cortical hyperplasia: Quantitative and isolation studies. J. Clin. Endocr., **7**, 343, 1947.
192. Goldman, A. S., Bongiovanni, A. M., Yakovac, W. C., and Prader, A.: Study of Δ^5-3β-hydroxysteroid dehydrogenase in normal, hyperplastic, and neoplastic adrenal cortical tissue. J. Clin. Endocr., **24**, 894, 1964.
193. Touchstone, J. C., Bulaschenko, H., Richardson, E. M., and Dohan, F. C.: Excretion of pregnane-3α,17α,21-triol-20-one in normal and pathologic urine. J. Clin. Endocr., **17**, 250, 1957.
194. Rosselet, J. P., Overland, I., Jailer, J. W., and Lieberman, S.: Die Isolierung von 3α,17α,21-trioxy-pregnanon-(20) aus menschlichem Harn. Helv. Chim. Acta, **37**, 1933, 1954.
195. Fraser, R., James, V. H. T., Landon, J., Peart, W. S., Rawson, A., Giles, C. A., and McKay, A. M.: Clinical and biochemical studies of a patient with a corticosterone secreting adrenocortical tumor. Lancet, **2**, 1116, 1968.
196. Jacob, F., and Monod, J.: Genetic regulatory mechanisms in the synthesis of proteins. J. Molec. Biol., **3**, 318, 1961.
197. Bentinck, R. C., Hinman, F., Lisser, H., and Traut, H. F.: Familial congenital adrenal syndrome: Report of two cases and review of literature. Postgrad. Med., **11**, 301, 1952.
198. Hirschfeld, A. J., and Fleshman, J. K.: An unusually high incidence of salt-losing congenital adrenal hyperplasia in the Alaskan Eskimo. J. Pediat., **75**, 492, 1969.
199. Money, J., and Lewis, V.: I.Q., genetics and accelerated growth; adrenogenital syndrome. Bull. Johns Hopkins Hosp., **118**, 365, 1966.
199*a*. Jeffcoate, T. N. A., Fliegner, J. R. H., Russell, S. H., Davis, J. C., and Wade, A. P.: Diagnosis of the adrenogenital syndrome before birth. Lancet, **2**, 553, 1965.
199*b*. Nichols, John: Antenatal diagnosis of adrenocortical hyperplasia. Lancet, **1**, 1151, 1969.
199*c*. Nichols, John: Antenatal diagnosis and treatment of the adrenogenital syndrome. Lancet, **1**, 83, 1970.
199*d*. Cathro, D. M., Coyle, M. G., and Bertrand, J.: Antenatal diagnosis of adrenocortical hyperplasia. Lancet, **1**, 732, 1969.
199*e*. Merkatz, I. R., New, M. I., Peterson, R. E., and Seaman, M. P.: Prenatal diagnosis of adrenogenital syndrome by amniocentesis. J. Ped., **75**, 977, 1969.
200. Levine, S.: Endocrines and the central nervous system: Hormones in infancy and adult behavior, in *Malnutrition, Learning and Behavior,* edited by N. S. Scrimshaw and J. E. Gordon, p. 151. M.I.T., Cambridge, Mass., 1968.
201. Hampson, J. G.: Hermaphroditic genital appearance, rearing and eroticism in hyperadrenocorticism. Bull. Johns Hopkins Hosp., **96**, 265, 1955.
202. Hampson, J. G., Money, J., and Hampson J. L.: Hermaphrodism: Recommendations concerning case management. J. Clin. Endocr., **16**, 547, 1956.
203. Money, J.: Hermaphroditism, gender and precocity in hyperadrenocorticism: Psychologic findings. Bull. Johns Hopkins Hosp., **96**, 253, 1955.
204. Money, J., Hampson, J. G., and Hampson, J. L.: Hermaphroditism: Recommendations concerning assignment of sex, change of sex and psychologic management. Bull. Johns Hopkins Hosp., **97**, 284, 1955.
205. Money J., Hampson, J. G., and Hampson, J. L.: Sexual incongruities and psychopathology: Evidence of human hermaphroditism. Bull. Johns Hopkins Hosp., **98**, 43, 1956.
206. Ehrhardt, A. A., Epstein, R., and Money, J.: Influence of androgen and some aspects of sexually dimorphic behavior in women with the late-treated adrenogenital syndrome. Bull. Johns Hopkins Hosp., **122**, 160, 1968.
207. Ehrhardt, A. A., Evers, K., and Money, J.: Fetal androgens and female gender identity in early-treated women with the adrenogenital syndrome. Johns Hopkins Med. J., **123**, 115, 1968.
208. Goldman, A. S.: Virilization of the external genitalia of the female rat fetus by dehydroepiandrosterone. Endocrinology (in press).
209. Goldman, A. S.: Maternal and fetal effects of two inhibitors of 3β-hydroxysteroid dehydrogenase and Δ^5,3-ketosteroid isomerase in the rat. Endocrinology, **85**, 325, 1969.
210. Goldman, A. S.: Production of congenital adrenocortical hyperplasia in rats by estradiol-17β and inhibition of 3β-hydroxysteroid dehydrogenase. J. Clin. Endocr., **28**, 231, 1969.
211. Goldman, A. S.: Experimental model of congenital adrenal cortical hyperplasia produced in utero with an inhibitor of 11β-steroid hydroxylase. J. Clin. Endocr., **27**, 1390, 1967.

PART SIX

DISORDERS OF PURINE AND PYRIMIDINE METABOLISM

CHAPTER THIRTY-NINE

GOUT

James B. Wyngaarden and William N. Kelley

Gout is a clinical disorder found exclusively in man. The disease chiefly affects the joints and produces a characteristic type of acute and chronic arthritis, related to the presence of crystals of sodium urate. The cardinal biochemical feature is hyperuricemia. In *primary gout,* of which there are several biochemically distinct forms, the hyperuricemia is attributable to an inborn error of metabolism. In *secondary gout,* of which there are many varieties, the hyperuricemia occurs as a complication of an acquired disorder or of the use of certain drugs. A classification of gout is presented in Table 39-1.

In primary gout the hyperuricemia is initially asymptomatic. In some affected individuals it may remain so throughout their lifetimes. In others the disorder becomes clinically manifest by recurrent attacks of acute gouty arthritis or renal lithiasis, or both. In time the arthritis may become chronic because of the destructive effects of tissue deposits of urate, called *tophi,* which are prone to form in and around the joints of the extremities and in cartilaginous structures. Most gouty subjects develop renal disease involving particularly the tubular and interstitial tissue, which may contain deposits of crystalline urate; glomerular and renal vascular changes and hypertension are also common. The renal disease is generally only slowly progressive and is often without noticeable effect upon life expectancy.

Secondary gout may also evolve through the stages of asymptomatic hyperuricemia, recurrent acute gouty arthritis or renal lithiasis, and chronic gouty arthritis. The acute attacks are indistinguishable from those of primary gout. In secondary gout, complicating myeloproliferative disease, the interval phases between acute attacks tend to be shorter than in primary gout, and chronic gouty arthritis and tophi occur earlier in the course of the disease and are often more severe.

This chapter deals chiefly with primary gout. A large portion of the inquiry is directed toward the pathophysiology of hyperuricemia.

HISTORY

The clinical descriptions of gout can be traced to ancient medical literature. Early Greek and Roman physicians possessed an intimate knowledge of its varied features. In the fifth century B.C., Hippocrates described gout as podagra,

Table 39-1. CLASSIFICATION OF HYPERURICEMIA AND GOUT

Type	Metabolic Disturbance	Inheritance
Primary		
Idiopathic		
Normal excretion (75 to 80% of primary gout)	Overproduction of uric acid and/or underexcretion of uric acid (specific defects undefined)	Polygenic Autosomal dominant forms?
Overexcretion (20 to 25% of primary gout)	Overproduction of uric acid (specific defects undefined)	
Associated with specific enzyme defects		
Glucose-6-phosphatase: deficiency or absence	Overproduction plus underexcretion of uric acid; glycogen storage disease, Type I (von Giercke)	Autosomal recessive
Hypoxanthine-guanine phosphoribosyltransferase: deficiency, partial or "virtually complete" (Lesch-Nyhan syndrome)	Overproduction of uric acid	X linked
Glutamine-PP-ribose-P-amidotransferase: feedback resistance	Overproduction of uric acid	Unknown
Glutathione reductase variant: increased activity	Overproduction of uric acid suspected, but undetermined	Autosomal dominant
Secondary		
Associated with increased nucleic acid turnover	Overproduction of uric acid	
Associated with decreased renal excretion of uric acid	Reduced renal functional mass Inhibited tubular secretion of uric acid Enhanced tubular reabsorption of uric acid	

cheiagra, or gonagra, depending on whether the big toe, wrist, or knee was involved. Tophi were first described by Galen (A.D. 131 to 200) [1]. The term *gout,* introduced in the thirteenth century, is derived from the Latin *gutta,* a drop, and reflects an early belief that the disease was caused by a *noxa,* a poison, falling drop by drop into the joint [2].

Colchicine was known to Byzantine physicians as early as the fifth century A.D. under the name of *hermodactyl* (finger of Hermes). A drug probably identical with colchicine was described in the Ebers papyrus (1500 B.C.). *Colchicum autumnale* (or meadow saffron) was introduced into Europe in 1763 by Baron Anton von Storch, physician to Empress Maria Theresa [3], and subsequently into this country by Benjamin Franklin [4]. The term *colchicum* probably originates from an ancient district in Asia Minor called Colchis.

The modern clinical history of gout began with Thomas Sydenham, whose unsurpassed description of the disease, drawn from 34 years of personal affliction, first clearly differentiated gout from other articular disorders [5]. The chemical history of gout began a century after Sydenham, when in 1776 Scheele [6] discovered uric acid as a constituent of a kidney stone. Shortly thereafter Wollaston (1797) and Pearson (1798) demonstrated urate in the tophi of patients with gout [7, 8]. Another 50 years later, Garrod performed his historic experiments in which he demonstrated first by the murexide test [9] and later by his famous "thread" test (1854) [10] an increased amount of uric acid in the blood of gouty subjects.

At this time the structure of uric acid was unknown. With the establishment by Fischer [11] in 1898 that uric acid was a purine compound, its potential relationship to the nucleic acid constituents adenine and guanine was appreciated, and a key role of purine metabolism in the pathophysiology of gout was recognized. With the introduction of a reliable method for the determination of uric acid in the blood by Folin and Denis in 1913 [12], clinical and metabolic studies of gout were greatly facilitated. The pathways of enzymatic synthesis of purine compounds were elucidated by Buchanan, Greenberg, and others during the 1950s. The first specific enzymatic defect responsible for one subtype of adult primary gout was discovered by Seegmiller and associates in 1967.

Through the centuries, gout has enjoyed a royal patronage, and victims of gout have been favored subjects of caricatures, novels, and biographies. Many writers have compiled rosters of distinguished personages in history who have had gout. The list includes men of such diverse claims to fame as the Medici, Isaac Newton, Charles Darwin, Martin Luther, John Calvin, Benjamin Franklin, Ben Jonson, William Pitt, Samuel Johnson [13], Cotton Mather [14], and George IV of England [15]. Several illuminating articles on the history of gout have appeared in recent years, chiefly by Hartung [2], Rodnan and Benedek [14, 16–18], and Bywaters [15].

CLINICAL FEATURES OF GOUT

Asymptomatic Hyperuricemia

Asymptomatic hyperuricemia is that stage at which the serum urate level is raised but arthritic symptoms, tophi or uric acid stones, have not yet appeared. This stage begins at puberty in the male at risk from the common form of gout but may be delayed until the menopause in the female [19, 20]. In patients with hyperuricemia secondary to a specific enzyme deficiency, this trait is present from birth. Renal calculi composed partially or wholly of uric acid may occur at any stage of gout; their significance in the prearticular stage is often overlooked. Rarely, tophi may antedate the development of articular gout. Very rarely, renal injury due to hyperuricemia may occur in otherwise asymptomatic persons.

Acute Gouty Arthritis

It is difficult to improve on Sydenham's [21] description of the acute attack:

The victim goes to bed and sleeps in good health. About two o'clock in the morning he is awakened by a severe pain in the great toe; more rarely in the heel, ankle or instep. This pain is like that of a dislocation, and yet the parts feel as if cold water were poured over them. Then follow chills and shivers, and a little fever. The pain, which was at first moderate, becomes more intense. With its intensity the chills and shivers increase. After a time this comes to its height, accommodating itself to the bones and ligaments of the tarsus and metatarsus. Now it is a violent stretching and tearing of the ligaments—now it is a gnawing pain and now a pressure and tightening. So exquisite and lively meanwhile is the feeling of the part affected, that it cannot bear the weight of the bedclothes nor the jar of a person walking in the room. The night is passed in torture, sleeplessness, turning of the part affected, and perpetual change of posture; the tossing about of the body being as incessant as the pain of the tortured joint, and being worse as the fit comes on. Hence the vain effort, by change of posture, both in the body and the limb affected, to obtain an abatement of the pain.

The attack usually subsides spontaneously in a few days to a few weeks, and recovery following the initial episode is generally complete. About 50 percent of initial attacks involve the great toe (podagra), and occasionally the initial attack is bilateral [22]. Ninety percent of gouty patients experience attacks in the great toe at some time during the course of their disease. Next in order of frequency as sites of initial involvement are the instep, ankle, heel, knee, and wrist. Any joint in the body may be involved. Hench [23] has emphasized that the more distal the site of involvement, the more typical is the character of the attack.

Prevalence and Incidence

The prevalence of gout varies widely in different parts of the world. A figure of 0.3 percent in Europe was recorded by Lawrence [24]. In the United States it has been estimated to be some 275 per 100,000 (0.27 percent) [25]. In the Heart Disease Epidemiology Study conducted in Framingham, Massachusetts, a prevalence of gouty arthritis of 0.2 percent was found in a population of 5,127 subjects (2,283 men and 2,844 women) aged 30 to 59 years (mean age 44). Fourteen years later the prevalence had increased to 1.5 percent of this population (mean age 58), 2.8 percent in men, 0.4 percent in women [26]. Prevalence appears to be even higher among Filipino males in Northwestern North America [27, 28], and very much higher among the Chamorros and the Carolinians in the Mariana Islands [29] and in the Maori of New Zealand [30, 31]. In the last group the prevalence in males is 10 percent [31]! The relationship of prevalence to the serum urate level is shown in Table 39-2, which summarizes the situation in the Framingham population admitted at mean age 44 and followed for 14 years.

During World Wars I and II acute gouty arthritis was uncommon in Europe. When protein again became plentiful, the prevalence returned to prewar levels [32, 33]. In Japan, where protein intake per capita has doubled since World War II, gout is becoming increasingly prevalent. These and other observations underscore the importance of dietary and environmental influences in determining whether the genetic factor or factors are expressed in subjects at risk. Gout has long been considered a disease of middle and upper social classes. A study in Manchester, England, documented this belief [34], and a similar correlation noted in Pittsburgh led to the studies cited below on the distribution of serum urate values among members of various social and educational classes [35, 36]. Nevertheless, the disease is widely distributed and involves all nationalities and all social classes. It is said to be rare in African nationals [37], but it is common in the American Negro [38, 39].

Acute gout is preeminently a disease of the adult male. Since the time of Hippocrates it has been known that gout is uncommon in women. In large series, only 3 to 7 percent of the cases of primary gout are found in women, and these are chiefly in the postmenopausal group [40–44]. In limited series, higher percentages of women are occasionally noted [38, 45]. These series may include cases of secondary gout complicating hypertension, renal disease, or the use of diuretics.

Gout in women may be more severe and more destructive than in men. When gout is inherited from the mother, its onset may be at an earlier age, and it may be more severe than usual. Gout is very rare in prepubertal children and, when it occurs, it may represent a form of gout associated with a specific enzymatic deficiency leading to the overproduction of urate [46, 47].

The usual form of primary gout is uncommon before the third decade, and its peak incidence in various series is in the thirties [3], forties [38], or fifties [48]. In general, the higher the serum urate level, the earlier the onset of gouty arthritis [26]. In the population study in Framingham, Massachusetts, the cumulative incidence of gouty arthritis in men appeared to be approaching a plateau at mean age 58 years. This occurred in spite of the fact that only one-third of the men with urate levels of 8 mg per 100 ml or more had experienced an attack of gout [26]. The age factor may explain the low fraction of 21 patients with gout among 5,400 cases of arthritis (0.4 percent) in one United States Army Arthritis Center during World War II [49, 50], compared with the usual frequency of 4 or 5 percent of gouty patients among all arthritic patients in civilian clinic populations in this country [51, 52].

Plasma and Urinary Uric Acid

There are no characteristic changes of plasma urate levels that precede, accompany, or follow an acute attack of gouty arthritis. There may be an elevation of urinary uric acid excretion values during the acute attack [53, 54], perhaps mediated by the uricosuric action of corticosteroids [55] secreted during the stress of gouty inflammation. Such a uricosuric effect would normally be anticipated to reduce the serum urate level, and perhaps this explains some of

Table 39-2. PREVALENCE OF GOUTY ARTHRITIS BY MAXIMUM URATE LEVEL IN A POPULATION OF MEAN AGE 58

Serum urate concentration, mg/100 ml	*Men*		*Women*	
	Fraction with gout	Percent with gout	Fraction with gout	Percent with gout
<6	8/1,281	0.6	2/2,665	0.08
6.0–6.9	15/790	1.9	5/151	3.3
7.0–7.9	27/162	16.7	4/23	17.4
8.0–8.9	10/40	25.0	0/4	0
9+	9/10	90.0	0/1	0
Total	65/2,283	2.8	11/2,844	0.4

Source: Hall et al. [26].

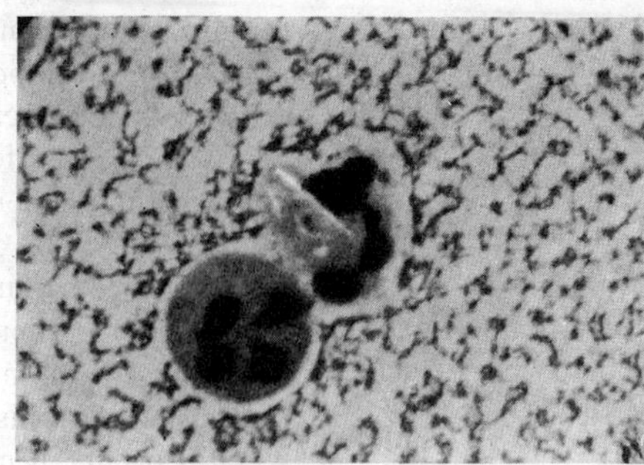
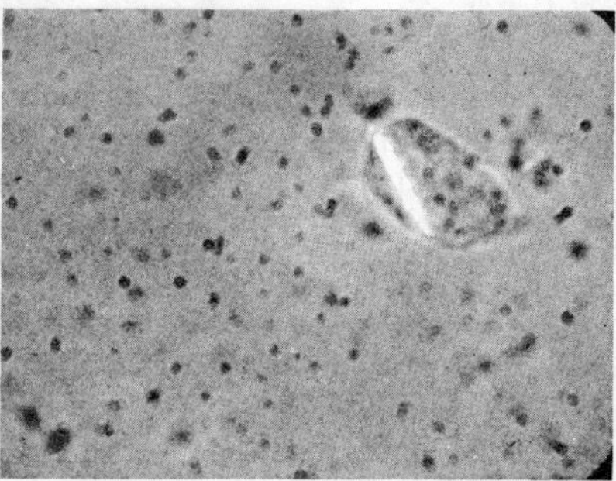

Figure 39-1. Crystals of sodium urate monohydrate in leukocytes of synovial fluid in acute gouty arthritis, as seen under polarized light. (*Courtesy of Dr. Daniel J. McCarty, Jr.*)

the normal values observed during acute attacks. In general, however, the values do not fall, and an increased production of uric acid, a consequence of leukocytosis, enhanced leukocyte turnover, and increased nucleic acid production, has been postulated as offsetting the effects of uricosuria. Intravenously administered deoxyribonuclease increases uric acid excretion in symptomatic gouty subjects (as well as in nongouty subjects with inflammatory disease) but not in gouty subjects in the asymptomatic phase [56], and these observations support the concept described above [54]. An increase in urinary 7-methyl-8-hydroxyguanine and a decrease in urinary 6-succinoaminopurine have been reported during the acute attack [57, 58].

Mechanism of the Acute Attack

Garrod [59] proposed in 1876 that the acute gouty paroxysm was triggered by precipitation of sodium urate crystals in the joint or neighboring tissues. In 1899, Freudweiler [60] reproduced acute gouty attacks by the injection of microcrystals of sodium urate, and also of other crystals such as those of hypoxanthine, or xanthine [61]. The subcutaneous injection of urate crystals was followed by the evolution of a histologically characteristic tophus [62]. Freudweiler also proposed a central role for the urate crystal in the genesis of the acute gouty attack.

These observations were lost sight of, and when the measurement of serum and urinary uric acid revealed no characteristic changes during the acute attack and infusions of urate solutions [63, 64] or injections of them near, or even into, the joints of gouty subjects evoked no inflammatory response [65], the concept of a direct role of urate in the pathogenesis of the acute attack fell into disfavor. Theories of a primary vascular disturbance [66], metabolic abnormalities [58], endocrine imbalance [67, 68], or allergy to food or bacterial products [69, 70] were then proposed.

A study of joint fluid by McCarty and Hollander [71] led to a renewed interest in crystals of sodium urate in gouty effusions [72], and particularly in the diagnostic value of large numbers of negatively birefringent crystals within synovial fluid leukocytes during the acute attack as demonstrated with the use of polarized light [73] (Fig. 39-1). With the use of a first-order red compensator, the urate crystal may be recognized by its yellow color when oriented in parallel with the axis of the compensator and its blue color when oriented perpendicularly to it [74]. Intracellular urate crystals are virtually constant in acute gouty arthritis [75, 76] and are a more reliable diagnostic criterion than the presence of crystals in the synovial membrane, which are only inconsistently observed in tissue obtained by needle biopsy [70, 77, 78] (Fig. 39-2).

Following the recognition of crystals in gouty effusions (a confirmation of the *gutta-noxa* theory!) Faires and McCarty [79] and Seegmiller, et al. [80–82] rediscovered the capacity of microcrystals of sodium urate to evoke an inflammatory response in the skin, subcutaneous tissues, and joints of animals and man. In man, both normouricemic and gouty, the inflammatory response strikingly resembles the acute gouty attack. It may be successfully treated with [83] or prevented by [84] colchicine. The response is not limited to crystals of sodium urate but may also be evoked by calcium oxalate [79], sodium orotate [80], and certain steroids [79] (see Pseudogout below).

The mechanism by which crystals induce inflammation

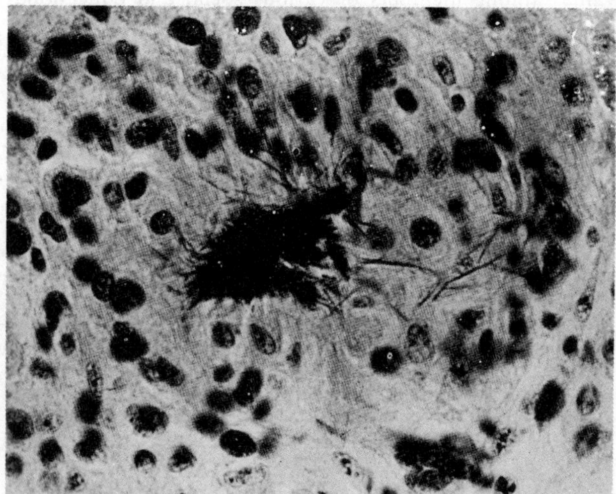

Figure 39-2. Acute gouty synovitis. The tissue has been fixed in absolute alcohol and the section stained by the method of de Galantha. Individual and aggregated needle-like crystals have deposited in incipient tophus formation. This lesion has been included in The Pathology Teaching Collection of Lantern Slides. (*By permission of the Arthritis Foundation, and of Dr. Leon Sokoloff.*)

is complex and imperfectly understood. It has been suggested that ingested crystals cause *mechanical damage* to cells by the release of intracellular substances, e.g., lysosomal enzymes, into the synovial tissues and fluid that then lead to the characteristic finding of inflammation [85, 86]. It has also been proposed that urate crystals initiate *chemical reactions* in the synovial fluid resulting in the development of inflammatory mediators. Kellermeyer [87] proposes that the negatively charged urate crystals activate the Hageman factor, which in turn initiates a series of reactions resulting in the development of permeability enhancing activity, perhaps PF/dil (permeability factor/diluted serum), kallikrein, or kinins. These factors can induce vasodilatation, increased vascular permeability, and leukocyte emigration through the vessel wall. It is further proposed that urate crystals may activate still another series of reactions in the synovium resulting in the activation of chemotactic factors from complement components, which could then direct the movement of leukocytes to the urate crystals. Release of lysosomal proteolytic and hydrolytic enzymes from the accumulated leukocytes may enhance and prolong the inflammatory process. Thus acute gouty arthritis can be viewed as the end result of several reaction sequences, each responsible for a phase of the inflammatory process.

This hypothesis is supported by considerable data [87]: (1) the Hageman factor is activated in vitro by urate crystals [88]; (2) the Hageman factor is present in normal synovial fluid [89]; (3) permeability enhancing factors are found in normal human synovial fluid exposed to urate crystals in vitro [90]; (4) the permeability enhancing factors are not activated in normal human synovial fluid if the Hageman factor is inactivated by a specific antibody [90]; (5) kinins are present in synovial fluid exudates from individuals with acute gout [91]; and (6) the chicken, which lacks the Hageman factor, does not develop an acute inflammatory response following the intraarticular injection of monosodium urate crystals [87].

In dogs, the inflammatory response to sodium urate shows an absolute requirement for leukocytes. The response is markedly suppressed in dogs rendered leukopenic with vinblastin [92] or with antipolymorphonuclear leukocyte serum [93], unless the leukocyte count is restored by cross circulation from a normal donor dog [92] or time for recovery is allowed [93]. Following the intraarticular injection of microcrystalline urate into a canine joint the pressure increases, and the pH of the synovial fluid falls slightly as a consequence of a rise in the concentration of lactic acid, produced by the metabolic activity of the leukocytes [94]. The maximal pH drop is only 0.5 unit however [95], probably inconsequential in terms of its effect upon urate solubility [96] though perhaps significant in activating proteins of the inflammatory process [87]. The ingested crystals are either destroyed by the verdoperoxidases of the leukocytes [97] or released if the leukocyte ruptures and may then be reingested by other leukocytes [94]. The concentration of kinin-like peptides in synovial fluid may rise as much as fiftyfold during crystal-induced attacks in man, as it does during spontaneous attacks of gout and in other inflammatory states such as rheumatoid arthritis [91], but bradykinin is not thought to be the mediator of inflammation [98]. Complement is depleted in human serum by urate crystals [99], and chemotactic activity develops [100, 101]. A formulation of the role of the urate crystal in acute gout is presented in Fig. 39-3.

The effect of colchicine upon the leukocyte and the possible relation of this action to its specific anti-inflammatory effect in gout is reviewed below.

Pseudogout (Chondrocalcinosis Articularis)

The renewed interest in the examination of synovial fluids from patients with acute arthritis led to the recognition of a second type of crystal-induced synovitis which is rather like gout but which must be differentiated from it. The first patients were suffering from attacks of apparently typical gout, but their synovial fluids disclosed nonurate crystals, and they were often not hyperuricemic [102]. The crystals were established by x-ray diffraction studies to be calcium pyrophosphate dihydrate [103]. Injection of the isolated calcium pyrophosphate crystals into the normal joints of experimental animals provoked an acute arthritis [104], and calcium pyrophosphate crystals were recovered from the synovial fluid of these joints. McCarty et al. [105] regard this sequence of events to be the fulfillment of Koch's postulates in a new context.

The acute episodes tend to affect middle-aged or elderly people [106–108]. Often they are precipitated by trauma. Gout and pseudogout may affect the same patient [109–111], so that both types of crystal appear in the same sample of joint fluid [111]. The larger joints are affected more often than the smaller ones. What the great toe is to gout the knee is to pseudogout [102, 107, 111]. Recurrent attacks, separated by normal intervals, may progress through longer subacute attacks to a chronic degenerative arthropathy, with or without exacerbations. The disease may be polyarticular and lead to deformities including bony ankylosis [110]. Familial examples have been described but no conclusions about genetic transmission have been formed [110–112]. Calcification of joint cartilage is seen on x-ray in nearly all cases. In hyaline articular cartilage this appears as a thin, dense band separate from, and parallel to, the bone cortex. The cartilage of the menisci is almost always affected, as is the pubic symphysis [106, 108, 111, 113]. Urinary excretion and plasma and synovial fluid levels of pyrophosphate are normal [114, 115], but the pyrophosphate hydrolase activity of synovial fluid may be low [116]. Chondrocalcinosis and arthropathy are frequent findings in hemochromatosis [117]. Salicylates, phenylbutazone, and indomethacin [118] control the acute attacks of pseudogout, but colchicine yields inconsistent results [106].

Acute inflammatory episodes rather like gout may also be associated with periarticular calcific deposits in tendons, joint capsules, and ligaments [119, 120]. The deposit may

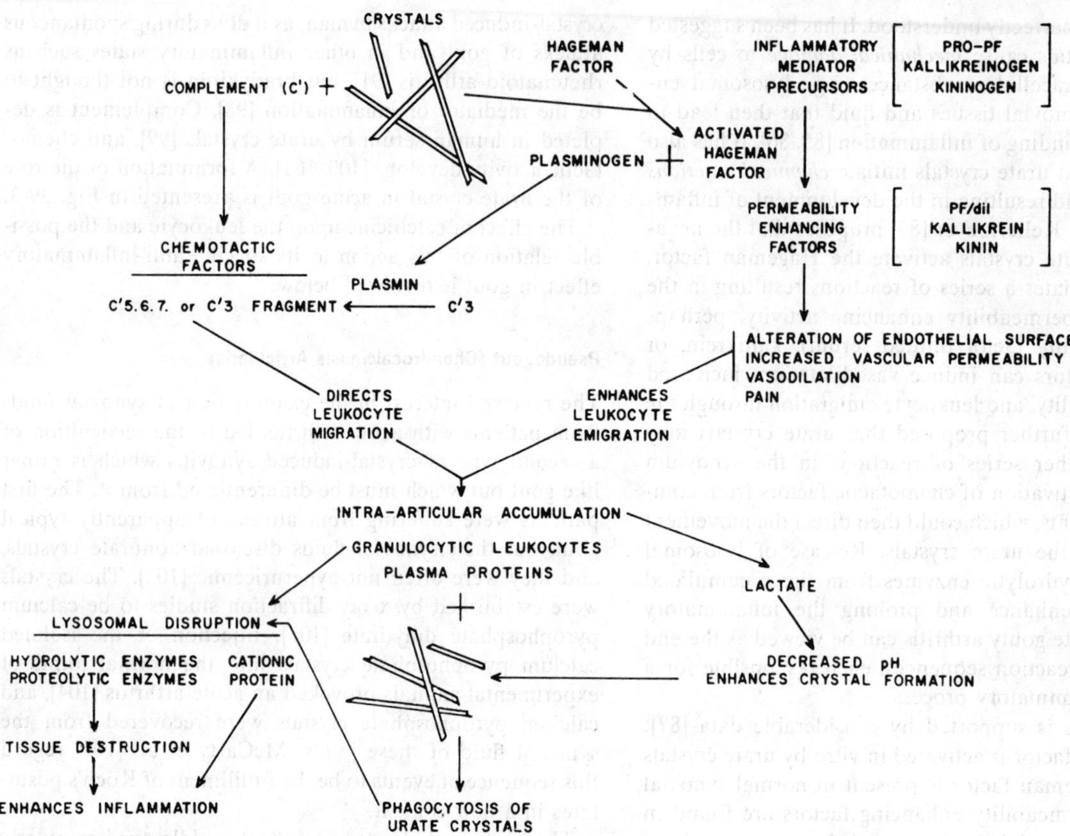

Figure 39-3. Hypothesis of the roles of urate crystals in the pathogenesis of acute gouty inflammatory reaction. Crystal surfaces are postulated to activate Hageman factor; ingestion of crystals by leukocytes is postulated to lead to lysosomal disruption. (*From R. W. Kellermeyer* [87] *with permission of Arthritis and Rheumatism.*)

disappear after the acute phase [121] but attacks may be recurrent [120]. Attacks occur more often in women than in men, are commonest around the shoulder, but may involve the big toe, hip, finger, wrist, or knee. The material in the deposit is amorphorus hydroxyapatite [119, 120]. The pain usually responds to phenylbutazone or indomethacin [118] but may require injections of a local anesthetic or of hydrocortisone. Rather similar episodes of acute localized soft-tissue inflammation may arise in uremic patients maintained by periodic hemodialysis, associated also with hydroxyapatite deposits [122–124]. Attacks of inflammation may be induced at these sites by raising the uric acid concentration of the dialysis bath and, hence, also of the patient's serum [122, 123].

Interval Gout

Following the initial acute attack, the gouty subject enters an asymptomatic interval phase which may last from a few weeks to many years. Generally in 6 months to 2 years the patient will suffer another episode in the same or another joint, and the events of the initial attack will be repeated, unless modified by therapy. In the natural history of the disease acute attacks recur with increasing frequency. Later attacks are often polyarticular, more severe, longer, and perhaps febrile. Roentgenographic changes may develop, and the attacks may abate more gradually than before, but the joints may nevertheless recover complete symptomless function.

Chronic Gouty Arthritis

The duration of time from the initial attack to the beginning of chronic symptoms or visible tophaceous involvement is highly variable, ranging in one large series from 3 to 42 years, with an average of 11.6 years [23]. Chronic gouty arthritis may develop as the residue of an acute attack, or it may develop insidiously in a previously uninvolved joint. Acute attacks may be superimposed on the chronically affected joints, although late in the chronic phase they may

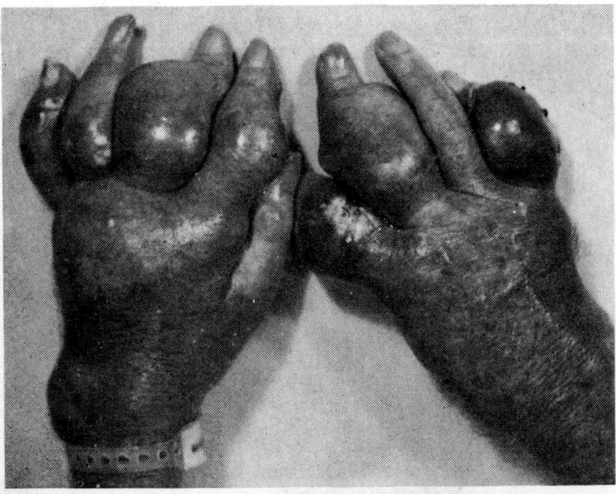

Figure 39-4. Chronic tophaceous gout of severe degree (see Plate I-6, facing page 114). (*Courtesy of Dr. R. Wayne Rundles.*)

disappear altogether. Chronic gouty arthritis is generally polyarticular and may be destructive, grotesquely deforming, and totally disabling (Fig. 39-4). Tophi may ulcerate and drain chalky material, although they are usually relatively painless. Tophi may produce a marked limitation of joint movement by the direct involvement either of the joint structure or of tendons serving the joint. Any joint may be involved, although those of the lower extremity are chiefly affected. Spinal joints do not escape urate deposition, but acute gouty spondylitis almost never occurs. Tophaceous involvement of the sacroiliac joint was found in 7 of 95 gouty patients on a routine x-ray examination [124*a*]. Aseptic necrosis of the hip has been reported as a manifestation of gout [125, 126].

Prior to the advent of uricosuric agents, 50 to 60 percent of gouty patients developed visible tophi, permanent joint changes (Figs. 39-5 and 39-6), or chronicity of symptoms [127, 128]. In a more recent series, the incidence of tophi has ranged from 13 to 25 percent [129, 130]. The development of tophi is correlated with the height of the serum urate concentration, the severity of renal involvement, and the duration of the disease [131], occurring primarily in subjects who have had gout for 6 to 10 years or more [23, 132].

Pathology

The specific pathologic changes in gout depend upon the deposition of urate in tissues and the associated inflammatory reaction and degenerative changes. The one pathognomonic lesion of gout is the tophus, a urate deposit surrounded by tissue exhibiting inflammatory and foreign body reaction. Because urate crystals are water soluble, nonaqueous fixatives are necessary to preserve urate deposits in histologic sections. Urate crystals, if preserved in bulk, are brilliantly anisotropic when viewed with polarized light under the microscope. A useful staining technique is that of de Galantha, in which tissue is fixed in absolute alcohol and subsequently stained with silver [133]. Urate crystals are stained brown-black by this method. However, provided the initial fixation is done with absolute alcohol, staining with hematoxylin and eosin is also usually successful, even though the bulk of the crystals may have been dissolved out.

Two general categories of mechanisms have been proposed regarding the deposition of urate in gout. Borrowing some terms from concepts of pathologic calcification, Sokoloff [77] has grouped these as follows: (1) metastatic, implying that urate is deposited in tissues because excessive quantities are

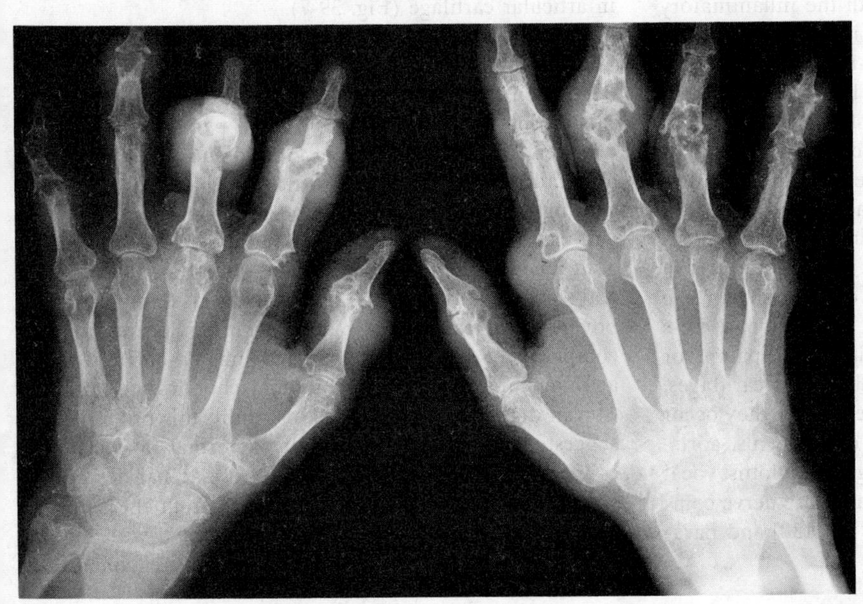

Figure 39-5. Chronic gouty arthritis of the hands. Note the extensive destruction of bone by urate deposits and the large soft-tissue tophi.

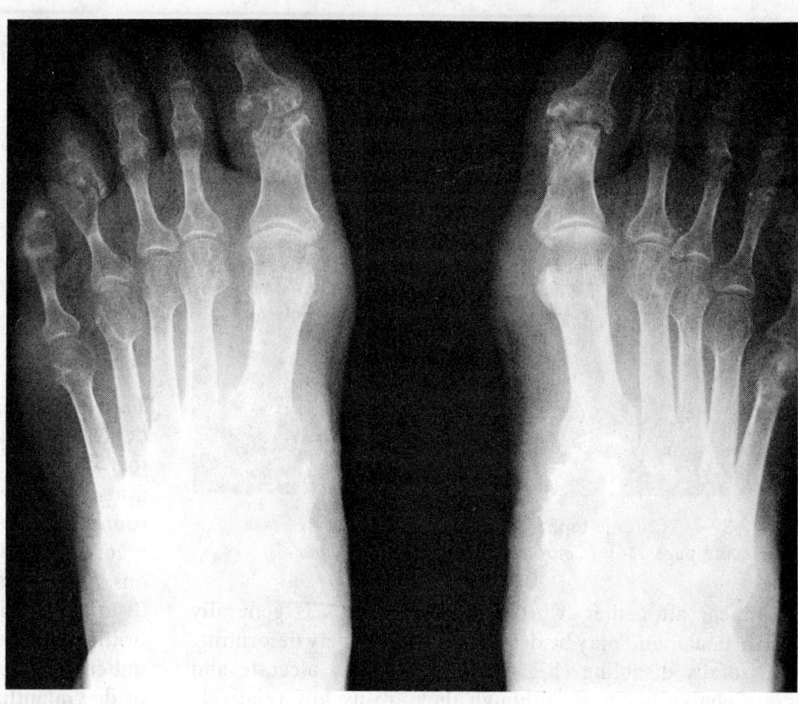

Figure 39-6. Chronic gouty arthritis of the feet of the patient shown in Fig. 39-5.

presented to them by circulating blood; and (2) dystrophic, implying that urate is deposited in tissues because the latter have undergone some primary pathologic alteration rendering them susceptible to urate deposition. These two categories are not mutually exclusive. In gout, urates tend to deposit in cartilage, epiphyseal bone, periarticular structures, and kidneys. The deposits produce local necrosis and (unless the tissue is avascular) an ensuing foreign body reaction with proliferation of fibrous tissue. The characteristic tophaceous nodule consists of the multicentric deposit of urate crystals and intercrystalline matrix, together with the inflammatory reaction and foreign body granuloma it has evoked. The crystals, which have been proved by x-ray crystallography to be monosodium urate monohydrate [134, 135], are acicular and arranged radially in small clusters. Granular and amorphous deposits have also been described. Calcific material deposited in the matrix may render the tophus radiopaque, and rarely this process may reach the proportions of heterotopic ossification [136]. Protein, lipid, and polysaccharide components are also found in the tophus [77].

Tophi commonly occur in the helix or antihelix of the ear, the olecranon and patellar bursae, and tendons. Less commonly, they occur in the skin of fingertips, palms, or soles, the tarsal plates of the eyelids, the nasal cartilages, or the cornea or sclerotic coats of the eye. Rarely they occur in the corpus cavernosum and prepuce of the penis, aorta, myocardium, aortic or mitral valves, tongue, epiglottis, vocal cords, and arytenoid cartilages. Tophi may cause nerve compressions, the carpal tunnel syndrome, [137, 138] and paraplegia [139].

In the joint, cartilaginous degeneration, synovial proliferation, destruction of subchondral bone, proliferation of marginal bone, often synovial pannus, and sometimes fibrous or bony ankylosis may develop [140, 141]. In vertebral bodies, urate deposits are found in the marrow spaces adjacent to intervertebral disks, as well as in disk tissue itself. The punched-out lesions of bones commonly seen in the roentgenograms of gouty patients represent marrow tophus deposits, which in most instances communicate with the urate crust on the articular surface through erosions and defects in articular cartilage (Fig. 39-7).

Urates tend to deposit in relatively avascular tissue [2]. Sokoloff [77] has pointed out that several sites of urate deposition in gout—articular and other cartilages, synovial tissues, interstitial tissue of the renal pyramid, and sclerae and heart valves—are rich in ground substance containing acid mucopolysaccharide. Cartilage has an affinity for absorbing urates in vitro [143], and the tarsal bones of swine will cause the precipitation of needles such as are seen in gout when suspended in saturated solutions of urate [72]. Katz and Schubert [144] have identified substances from bovine nasal cartilage, which are protein polysaccharides composed of protein and chondroitin sulfate and which augment urate solubility. Unbound chondroitin sulfate or trypsin digested material fails to exhibit this property. It is suggested that when, as a result of normal or accelerated connective tissue turnover, protein polysaccharides are destroyed, urate crystals may precipitate from the saturated tissue fluids. This concept may be integrated with the role of lysosomes in joint disease [85, 86]. Lysosomes contain acid

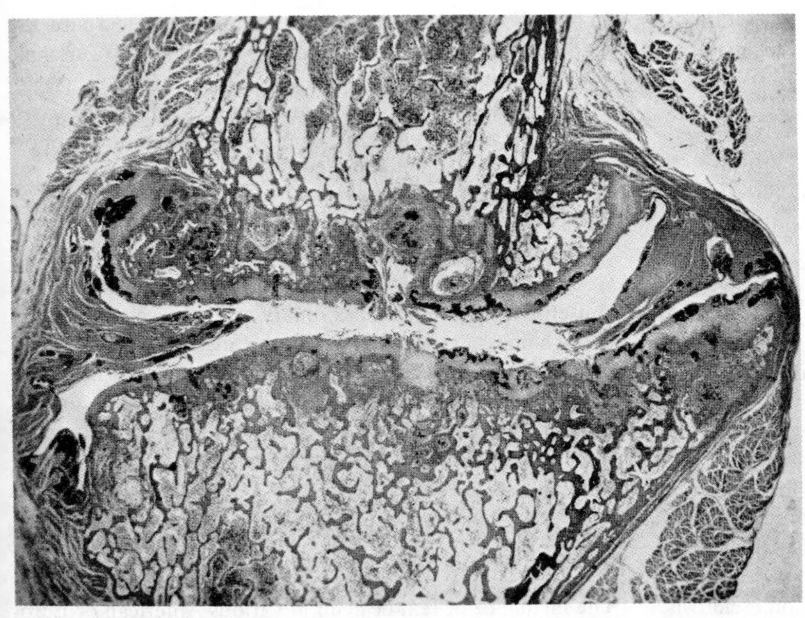

Figure 39-7. Chronic gouty arthritis. Urate crystals in the synovial membrane, articular cartilages, and subchondral bone appear black. Advanced osteoarthritic changes with marginal osteophyte formation are seen. (*From L. Sokoloff and I. O. Gleason* [142], *with permission of the Amer. J. Clin. Path.*)

proteases capable of breaking down the protein polysaccharides of cartilage matrix. One may now envision a link between hyperuricemia, recurrent acute attacks, and chronic tophaceous gout. Injury may result in damage to the lysosomes, release of cathepsins, degradation of cartilage matrix, and, in the case of hyperuricemic individuals, perturbation of the equilibrium between solubilized and soluble urate, with the resultant crystal formation leading to the triggering of acute attacks, deposition in tophi, or both.

Crystals have been recovered from the sputum of gouty subjects, but they apparently do not occur in the central nervous system. The concentration of uric acid is very low in spinal fluid [145], ranging in normal and gouty subjects from 0.25 to 1.0 mg per 100 ml. The low concentration has been attributed to selective impermeability of the blood-brain barrier to urates. Values are said to be slightly higher in children (0.3 to 1.5 mg per 100 ml) and to be increased in all forms of meningitis. The low levels of uric acid in spinal fluid probably explain the absence of tophaceous deposits in the central nervous system even in advance cases of gout.

Renal Disease in Primary Gout

Renal disease is the most frequent complication of gout apart from arthritis [146–148]. Ordinarily the process is only slowly progressive and does not materially reduce life expectancy [149, 150]. The incidence of proteinuria varies from 20 to 40 percent. It may be intermittent or persistent; only rarely is the quantity heavy. Hypertension is approximately as common as albuminuria. Usually it is benign [147].

Renal Hemodynamics

Inulin Clearance

The majority of inulin clearance values in gouty subjects are within the low-normal range; about one-third fall below 90 ml per min [131, 151]. The mean values fall somewhat below those of nongouty subjects of an equivalent age [152]. The lowest values are found in patients of advanced age or those with hypertension or coronary artery disease [131].

C_{PAH}

The mean value in 110 gouty subjects was 414 ± 90 ml per min per 1.73 m^2 (range 208 to 722 ml) [131]. A comparison with the distribution in nongouty subjects of an equivalent age [152] indicated a moderate but significant reduction in the effective renal plasma flow ($p < 0.01$ in all age groups) in patients with gout. The reduction in C_{PAH} was disproportionate to the minimal reduction of inulin clearances, especially in the older patients, and as a consequence the filtration fraction tended to rise with age from 0.19 to 0.25. Arterial hypertension was present in about half of the subjects with a statistically significant increase in filtration fractions [131].

Tm_{PAH}

The mean value in 14 patients was 62.3 ± 10.4 mg per min per 1.73 m^2 [131], compared with a mean normal value of 77.2 ± 15.0 [153]. In only three patients were the values below 60.0 mg per min. The mean C_{inulin}/Tm_{PAH} was

1.58 ± 0.35, a normal value. The mean ratio C_{PAH}/Tm_{PAH} was 6.63 ± 1.49. The normal mean value in males is 8.44 ± 2.45 [153].

Pathology

The only distinctive histologic feature of the gouty kidney is the presence of urate crystals in the medulla [154] or pyramids [77] and surrounding giant cell reaction. These may be associated with pyelonephritic or vascular changes, or both. In a review of 191 patients with gout, on whom clinical information and postmortem renal tissue permitted adequate evaluation, Talbott and Terplan [147] found only 3 that revealed neither urate crystals nor pyelonephritic or vascular changes. In all others these features were present in variable proportions. There was a strong correlation between the clinical severity of gout and the severity of the histologic lesions in the kidney, in the case of both predominantly pyelonephritic changes and predominantly vascular changes. The pyelonephritic changes were both acute and chronic; the vascular changes included arterial and arteriolar sclerosis, and in 11 instances the changes were those of malignant renal hypertension. A total of 30 patients revealed well-developed vascular changes and pyelonephritis with extensive structural alterations from urate deposits.

A few notable exceptions in the correlation between severity of clinical symptoms and of renal disease were also found. Some patients with advanced tophaceous gout showed only minimal clinical evidence of renal insufficiency; conversely, some patients with severe renal disease had suffered only minimal articular distress. The extreme degree of the latter phenomenon may be represented by reports of fatal "gout nephrosis" occurring without clinical evidence of gout. In four patients purported to represent this syndrome [154–156] no uric acid analyses had been performed during life. The concept of hyperuricemic nephropathy has been applied by Duncan and Dixon [157] to an English family in which eight members had hyperuricemia and six showed evidence of renal disease, while only two reported articular gout. A similar family has been reported by Rosenbloom et al. [158].

The traditional view has been that the renal lesions stem from the deposition of urates in collecting tubules, with resultant obstruction, atrophy of the more proximal tubules, and secondary necrosis and fibrosis [154, 159, 160]. The associated interstitial inflammatory process has been attributed to complicating pyelonephritis [154, 161]. More recent studies have shown that the earliest structural abnormality in the kidney is tubular damage associated with interstitial reaction [162]. There is a distinctive glomerulosclerosis, with uniform fibrillar thickening of glomerular capillary basement membranes, different from that of nephrosclerosis or diabetic glomerulosclerosis. The Henle loops show early atrophy and dilatation, occasionally associated with brown pigment degeneration of the epithelium. The interstitial reaction is maximal in the region near the changes in the Henle loops. In kidneys without tophi this reaction tends to spare the medulla and juxtamedullary cortex. The changes of chronic pyelonephritis may, therefore, not be of infectious origin. The vessels, both arteries and arterioles, show increased basophilia and degenerative changes that are out of proportion to the parenchymal changes [163].

Renal failure is the eventual cause of death in from 22 to 25 percent of gouty subjects [147, 164]. The majority of gouty patients die of cardiac or cerebral vascular disease [165]. In the epidemiological study in Framingham, Massachusetts, the incidence of coronary artery disease was twice as high in gouty subjects as in the male population with normal serum urate values but was not increased in hyperuricemic subjects without clinical gout [166]. In Tecumseh, Michigan, the serum urate levels of patients with coronary disease were not significantly different from the mean of the population [167].

Urolithiasis in Gout

The incidence of renal calculi in various American or European series of gout is 5 to 33 percent [130, 168]. In the experience of Yü and Gutman [169], the incidence was 22 percent in 1,258 patients with primary gout and 42 percent in 59 patients with secondary gout, or at least 1,000 times that of the general population. In 40 percent of the cases of primary gout, lithiasis antedated acute arthritis, occasionally by more than 20 years. Uric acid nephrolithiasis may rather frequently be associated with hyperuricemia without acute arthritis. About one-third of such patients give a family history of gout. Over 80 percent of calculi in gouty subjects are composed of uric acid [169]. Occasionally they may be mixed, or have only a central nidus of uric acid [170], or contain only calcium oxalate or phosphate [169].

Factors which predispose toward uric acid nephrolithiasis in gout include undue acidity of the urine, increased urinary excretion of uric acid, increased urinary concentration, and perhaps qualitative or quantitative abnormalities of urinary constituents which affect the solubility of uric acid [168].

Gouty patients have a tendency toward unusually acid urine both in fasting morning specimens and throughout the day [169, 171–174] and a substandard rise of urinary pH in response to oral alkali. There is no correlation between urine pH and urinary uric acid excretion [169]. In the three-fourths of gouty subjects whose urinary uric acid values fall within the normal range, the high incidence of renal stones is probably in part related to low urinary pH. This in turn is a reflection of a low NH_4^+/titratable acidity ratio attributed by some to a subnormal ammonium excretion at a given acid load or pH [173, 175–177] and by others to high values of titratable acidity [174, 178–180]. The deficit of ammonium excretion, when present, has been assigned to the effects of occult or measurable renal damage [179, 181], aging [182], or high purine intake [183] by some authors, but is regarded as an intrinsic defect in the production of ammonia, presumably from glutamine, by Gutman and Yu [177, 184, 185].

The pK_{a_1} and pK_{a_2} of uric acid are 5.75 and 10.3, respectively [186]. Therefore at urinary pH values of 4.5 to 5 the predominant form is uric acid, not sodium urate. X-ray crystallographic studies have shown that the stones are uric acid [135, 170]. The solubility of uric acid is only one-seventeenth that of sodium urate in water at 37°C.

The prevalence of renal stones rises with increasing plasma urate levels in the general population (see Table 39-3) and approximates 50 percent when serum urate levels exceed 12 mg per 100 ml in patients with gout [169]. The influence of hyperuricemia is probably chiefly significant as it affects urinary uric acid excretion. The prevalence of urolithiasis increases from 11 percent in patients with excretion values under 300 mg per day to 50 percent in patients with values over 1,100 mg per day [169].

According to Dulce [187] and Boshamer [188], uric acid stones are formed only when supersaturation prevails and when there is a crystallation nucleus of organic matrix. Sperling and De Vries [96, 189] conclude that urine is invariably supersaturated with uric acid if the pH is below 5.5 or 5.7. Uric acid stone formers have normal urinary uric acid solubility and a normal capacity to form supersaturated urine.

The significance of highly concentrated urine is illustrated by an incidence of uric acid nephrolithiasis of 75 percent in gouty subjects in Israel [168].

Uric Acid Nephrolithiasis in Nonhyperuricemic Subjects

Only about 20 percent of patients without clinical gout who form uric acid stones are hyperuricemic [130, 190]. In *idiopathic* uric acid nephrolithiasis, by definition occurring in patients with normal plasma and urinary uric acid values, a consistent finding, as in gouty and in otherwise asymptomatic hyperuricemic subjects, is a tendency toward a low urine pH. Henneman et al. [175], Woeber et al. [175], and Rapoport et al. [191] have reported reduced ammonium excretion and normal or increased titratable acidity in such patients, whereas Metcalfe-Gibson and associates [179] found normal ammonium excretion in relation to pH, except in patients with overt renal damage. Ammonium excretion per nephron was normal.

A familial form of uric acid lithiasis is found in Israel, in which patients are normouricemic but may have unusually acid urines, in the absence of other abnormalities of renal function. Frank et al. [178] and Barzel et al. [180] found normal rates of ammonium excretion and elevated values for titratable acidity in these subjects. The excretion of ammonium, with or without administration of an acid load, was not lower than in control subjects of equivalent age [182]. There is no apparent deficiency of urinary "solubilizers" of uric acid [192]. This disorder appears to be an inherited disease distinct from gout with an autosomal dominant mode of inheritance and high penetrance in both sexes [171].

The risk of uric acid stones is also increased in patients with ileostomies [193–195] who exhibit increased renal conservation of sodium, a decreased urinary Na/K ratio, increased urinary acid excretion, and low urinary pH values [195].

Uric acid stones may at times be dissolved with protracted fluid and alkali therapy [168, 196] but allopurinol is the treatment of choice (see below).

Association of Gout with Other Metabolic Disorders

Obesity

Many gouty subjects are moderately obese. Studies and reviews of gouty patients show body weights above ideal values for age and height in a large number of subjects (see for example, Table 39-4). Serum urate values are positively correlated with weight and surface area [65, 197–199]. In obese patients with gout, urinary uric acid values are often normal when factored by body weight [199, 200].

Diabetes Mellitus

The possible association of gout and diabetes mellitus continues to be a complex issue. Hyperuricemia has been reported in 2 to 50 percent of patients with diabetes [201], whereas gouty arthritis has been reported in from less than 0.1 to 9.0 percent of diabetic subjects [201]. Abnormal glucose tolerance tests have been noted in 7 to 74 percent of patients with gout [201–205] depending, in part, on the criteria used; when overt clinical diabetes is present in such patients it tends to be mild. Despite this apparently high incidence of hyperuricemia in diabetes, and of glucose intolerance in gout, several epidemiologic studies have failed

Table 39-3. PREVALENCE OF URINARY CALCULI BY MAXIMUM URATE CATEGORY IN A POPULATION OF MEAN AGE 58

Serum urate concentration, mg/100 ml	*Men*		*Women*	
	Number	Percent with stones	Number	Percent with stones
7.0+	212	12.7	28	7.1
8.0+	50	22.0	5	0
9.0+	10	40.0	1	0

Source: Hall et al. [26].

to find an association of serum urate and blood glucose concentrations [167, 201, 206]. In such studies the mean serum urate concentration was actually lower in patients with overt diabetes. This has been attributed to the apparent uricosuric effect of glucose [207–209].

The frequent occurrence of hyperuricemia in diabetic ketoacidosis is undisputed. This is most likely due to the inhibitory effect of acetoacetate and β-hydroxybutyrate on the renal tubular secretion of uric acid [210], although depletion of extracellular fluid volume probably also plays a role. Hyperuricemia in this situation is usually transient and of little clinical significance.

Relationship to Hyperlipoproteinemia and Atherosclerosis

A representative study of hyperlipoproteinemia in primary gout [211] is summarized in Table 39-4. Hypertriglyceridemia has been reported in 75 to 84 percent of patients with gout [204, 211–214] and hyperuricemia in 82 percent of patients with hypertriglyceridemia [214]. A rank order correlation of serum urate and serum triglyceride values has been described [214]. An α_1,α_2-globulin has been reported to bind urate [215] but also reported to be *reduced* in quantity in many gouty subjects [216]. Treatment with clofibrate (Atromid-S) results in the reduction of both serum triglyceride and urate values [204], possibly by different mechanisms, as clofibrate is a uricosuric agent [217]. Although many gouty subjects are hypercholesterolemic [218, 219], many studies have failed to show a correlation between serum urate and cholesterol values [212–214, 220, 221], which perhaps would obtain if the binding of urate by β-lipoprotein, reported by Alvsaker [215], was of quantitative importance. Although earlier studies suggested a relationship between hyperuricemia and atherosclerosis [222–227], this association has been seriously challenged by a number of excellent epidemiologic studies [166, 167].

Role of Ethanol

In his classic review on gout published in 1863, A. B. Garrod [228] wrote: "There is no truth in medicine better established than the fact that the use of fermented liquors is the most powerful of all the predisposing causes of gout; nay, so powerful, that it may be a question whether gout would ever have been known to mankind had such beverages not been indulged in."

The centuries-old belief that the acute gouty paroxysm may be associated with overindulgence in drink has at long last acquired a physiologic explanation. Hyperuricemia is common in inebriated subjects [229], and infusions of ethanol result in hyperuricemia [230]. As ethanol is metabolized by alcohol dehydrogenase, NAD is reduced, and this may account in part for the excessive conversion of pyruvate to lactate. The levels of hyperlacticacidemia achieved [230] are adequate to suppress the renal excretion of uric acid (see below) and to induce hyperuricemia [231], thus increasing the probability of crystal formation.

More recently, MacLachlan and Rodnan [232] have observed that the combination of ethanol ingestion and fasting may be additive or synergistic with respect to the effects of each of these factors on uric acid metabolism. Several epidemiologic studies have reported a correlation between serum urate levels and habitual alcohol intake [233, 234]. The daily ingestion of alcohol in significant but tolerated

Table 39-4. SERUM LIPOPROTEIN LEVELS IN HEALTHY, ATHEROSCLEROTIC, AND GOUTY SUBJECTS

	Healthy		*Atherosclerotic*		*Gouty*	
	Male	Female	Male	Female	Male	Female
Total numbers	70	70	80	30	44	9
Mean age, years	52 ± 7	50 ± 6	55 ± 8	58 ± 10	57 ± 10	61 ± 17
Mean body-weight deviation from ideal, lb	+11	+4	+11	−4	+20	+23
Number with diabetes mellitus	0	0	2	2	3	2
Diastolic B.P. > 100 mm Hg, %	Not recorded		30	23	45	44
Total cholesterol, mg/100 ml	184 ± 32	190 ± 32	258 ± 52	259 ± 45	231 ± 49	255 ± 82
β-Lipoprotein cholesterol, mg/100 ml	144 ± 27	146 ± 31	215 ± 51	211 ± 40	189 ± 46	212 ± 72
α-Lipoprotein cholesterol, mg/100 ml	38 ± 8	45 ± 9	38 ± 5	43 ± 5	38 ± 4	39 ± 9
Triglycerides, mg/100 ml	103 ± 48	90 ± 38	176 ± 70	141 ± 67	199 ± 139	270 ± 316
Urate, mg/100 ml	5.1 ± 0.8	4.1 ± 0.7	5.2 ± 1.2	4.4 ± 1.3	8.2 ± 1.0	8.7 ± 2.2

Values are: Mean ± s.d.
Source: Barlow [211].

amounts, e.g., 100 ml per 24 hr, may be associated with hyperuricemia and *increased* urinary excretion of uric acid, both of which may return toward or to normal during protracted periods (days) of abstinence and normal diet. These cycles are not explained by reduced urinary clearance of uric acid. An effect upon purine synthesis has been postulated [235]. The possible role of lead, a frequent contaminant of unbonded whiskey, in producing a chronic nephritis with secondary hyperuricemia and gout is discussed below.

HYPERURICEMIA

Methods

Standard colorimetric methods for the measurement of uric acid, such as those of Folin [236] or Archibald [237] depend upon the ability of urate to reduce phosphotungstic acid solutions. Some urate is lost during protein precipitation; also some nonurate reducing substances may be detected. The errors thus introduced are partially compensating ones. Current autoanalyzer methods [238–240] appear to overestimate true urate by an average of about 0.4 mg per 100 ml [240]. A minimal protein binding of urate may retard the diffusion of urate and offset a tendency toward even higher readings based on nonspecificity of the colorimetric method. The nonurate chromogens are labile and disappear on storage of samples for 3 weeks [241] or at 60°C for 1 hr [242].

A variety of compounds accumulating in serum or urine may interfere with the chemical determination of uric acid. These include caffeine, theophylline, theobromine, and their metabolites [243], salicylates and metabolites [244, 245], homogentisic acid [246], L-dopa [247], high glucose levels [248], and certain chromogens retained in renal failure. Accuracy of determinations is increased by the analysis of differences in concentrations of chromogen following the incubation of plasma or urine samples with uricase [240, 249, 250].

The most accurate values are obtained with the enzymatic spectrophotometric method of Kalckar [251] and Praetorius [252], in which the change in the absorbency of serum or urine at 292 mμ, the absorbency peak of uric acid at pH 8.2, is measured after treatment with purified uricase. This method is sensitive, accurate, and specific. It avoids errors inherent in colorimetric methods requiring the precipitation of protein or involving some degree of nonspecificity in color development. The modification of Liddle et al. [253] facilitates the handling of numbers of samples with reasonable efficiency. It is currently the method of choice for research determinations. Autoanalyzer methods appear to have less variability than manual methods and are recommended for routine use [254]. Table 39-5 summarizes several population studies of serum urate values employing the enzymatic spectrophotometric method.

Normal Values

In plasma at pH 7.4, about 98 percent of uric acid exists as the monoalkali salt [261]. Human serum values vary with age and sex. In children there is normally no sex difference in serum urate levels, which are lower than in adults, averaging about 3.6 mg per 100 ml [262]. After puberty the levels rise in both sexes, but more so in males. These differences have been attributed to higher renal clearances of urate in children than in adults and, among adults, in women than in men [263, 264].

Sex-age-specific mean serum urate values in nearly 6,000 members of a healthy population in Tecumseh, Michigan [260], are shown in Fig. 39-8. Values in males reach a plateau in the early twenties and are essentially stable thereafter. Values in females are constant from age 20 to about age 40. With the menopause, the values rise further and approach [256, 260] or equal [20, 34] values in males.

The sex difference in urate levels in adults is found with all methods. The ratio of values in males to those in females averaged 1.19 in 11 published studies [65, 260, 265]. Figure 39-9 presents a good example of the distribution of serum urate values in the two sexes in a large healthy population. The values are distributed in bell-shaped curves with skewing toward higher levels. The curves are not bimodal, that is, the curves for each sex do not separate the population into two distinct groups, one normal and one hyperuricemic. The serum urate concentration value is a continuous variable, much like height or blood pressure. Statistically, hyperuricemia can be defined exactly. The upper limit of normal, defined as the mean value + 2 s.d., is 7.3 mg per 100 ml in postpubertal males and 5.9 mg per 100 ml in postpubertal females [26] for a colorimetric method involving a protein precipitation step [236, 266]. With the enzymatic and spectrophotometric method, it ranges from 6.9 to 7.5 mg per 100 ml in males and 5.7 to 6.6 in females in the United States and most of Europe (Table 39-5).

Ethnic Variations

The mean serum urate value is similar for American and European Caucasian men [34, 256, 257, 259, 260], North American Indians (Pima and Blackfeet of Arizona [198] and the Haida of British Columbia [267]), North American Negroes [268], Australians of European origin [269], full-blooded Hawaiians and national groups of Japanese, Chinese, Portuguese, and Caucasians living in Hawaii [270], and Filipinos living in the Philippines [271].

By contrast, studies of other indigenous Pacific peoples have disclosed populations with mean serum urate concentrations significantly higher than in Caucasian populations. These have included the Maoris of New Zealand [31, 272] and other Polynesians living in Rarotonga and Pukapuka in the Cook Islands [234, 273] and in American Samoa [274],

Table 39-5. SERUM URATE CONCENTRATION VALUES

Population, Class or Group	Males			Females			References
	No.	Mean	s.d.	No.	Mean	s.d.	
Population							
Tecumseh, Mich.	2,987	4.9	1.4	3,013	4.2	1.2	[260]
Framingham, Mass.*	2,283	5.12	1.11	2,844	4.00	0.94	[26]
U.S.A.	22	5.32	0.93	18	4.32	0.81	[258]
U.S. Army inductees	817	5.06	0.94	—	—	—	[257]
U.S. prisoners (Caucasian)	90	5.01	1.11	—	—	—	[27]
Denmark	150	5.10	1.19	150	4.00	0.94	[256]
Wensleydale, England	436	4.46	—	475	3.70	—	[34]
West Germany	265	4.86	1.32	119	4.05	1.29	[259]
Australia (Caucasian)*	100	5.56	0.95	100	4.52	0.70	[269]
Social class							
Pittsburgh executives	339	5.73	1.21	—	—	—	[36]
ORNL Ph.D. scientists	76	5.34	1.23	—	—	—	[36]
U.S. craftsmen†	532	4.77	1.13	—	—	—	[36]
U.S. high school students	138	5.16	—	—	—	—	[35]
Univ. of Mich. professors	113	5.66	1.17	—	—	—	[286]
Edinburgh executives	100	6.00	0.88	—	—	—	[285]
Ethnic group							
American Negro	154	5.17	—	—	—	—	[268]
North American Indians							
Pima	949‡	4.89	1.19	—	—	—	[198]
Blackfeet	1,018‡	4.22	1.19	—	—	—	[198]
Haida	237	4.41	0.99	—	—	—	[267]
Filipinos, in Seattle	118	6.29	1.29	—	—	—	[27, 271]
Subgroup I	92	5.80	0.89	—	—	—	[27, 271]
Subgroup II	26	8.07	0.89	—	—	—	[27, 271]
Filipinos in Hawaii	60	6.1	1.3	—	—	—	[271]
Filipinos in Philippines	483	5.2	1.3	—	—	—	[270]
Hawaiians (full bloods)	49	5.4	1.1	—	—	—	[281]
Mariana Islanders							
Chamorros (>40 yr.)	160	6.23	1.51	175	5.10	1.41	[29]
Carolinians (>40 yr.)	26	7.27	1.67	29	5.70	1.01	[29]
Polynesians							
Maori (New Zealand)	366	7.06	1.54	381	5.77	1.55	[273]
Rarotongans	243	6.96	1.39	228	5.97	1.20	[273]
Pukapukans	188	7.04	1.10	191	6.18	1.09	[273]
Australian Aborigines (Aurukun)	82	6.03	1.25	135	4.78	1.23	[279]

* Colorimetric methods. All other values determined by enzymatic spectrophotometric methods.
† Pittsburgh and ORNL (Oak Ridge National Laboratories).
‡ Males and females about equally distributed in each group.

two Micronesian groups in the Mariana Islands (the Chamorros and Carolinians) [29], Filipinos living in Hawaii, Alaska, and other parts of the United States [27, 271, 275, 276], and some groups of Chinese [277] or Malaysians [278]. In addition, mean serum urate values are higher in Australian aborigines [279] and in Xavante Indians of Brazil [274] than in Caucasians in the same regions.

No racial differences in serum urate values were observed between healthy Caucasians and Indians in India and Indonesia, but the mean values in both groups were lower than in most other studies, perhaps owing to the use of a colorimetric method [280].

Selected examples of ethnic variations in mean serum urate values are included in Table 39-5.

Association of Serum Urate Values with Other Variables

The positive correlation of serum urate values with weight and with surface area, commented on above, is true of peoples of widely differing races and cultures throughout the world [234], but exceptions exist among Hawaiians [281], Brazilian recruits [199], and a tribe of Australian aborigines,

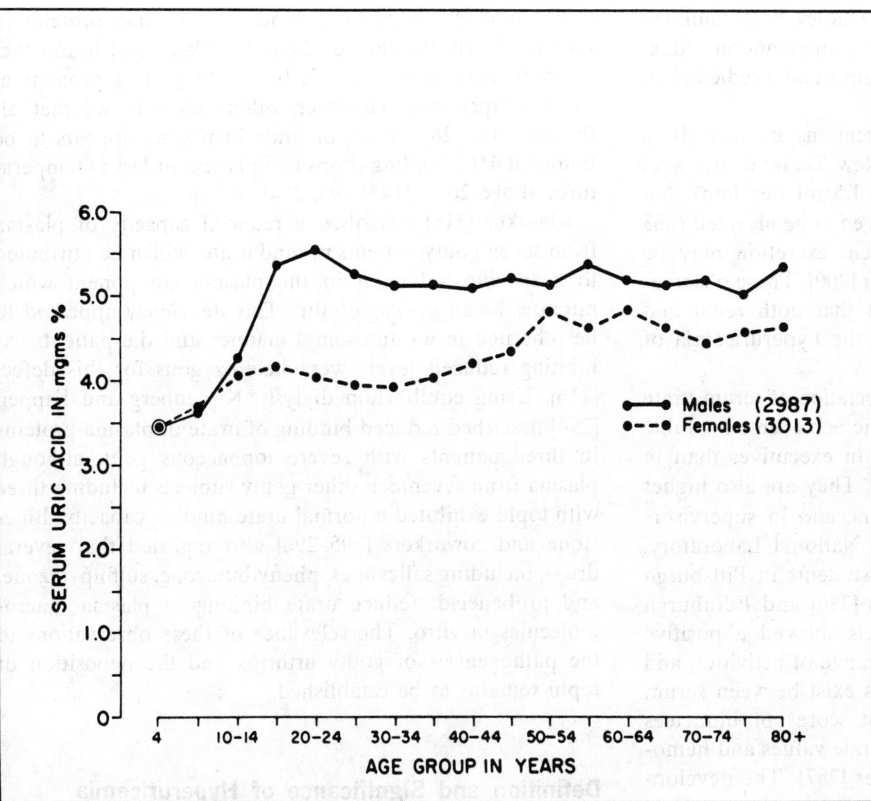

Figure 39-8. Sex–age-specific mean serum urate values in the population of Tecumseh, Michigan, 1959 to 1960, determined with ultraviolet differential spectrophotometric (uricase) method. (*From Mikkelsen et al.* [260], *with permission of Amer. J. Med.*)

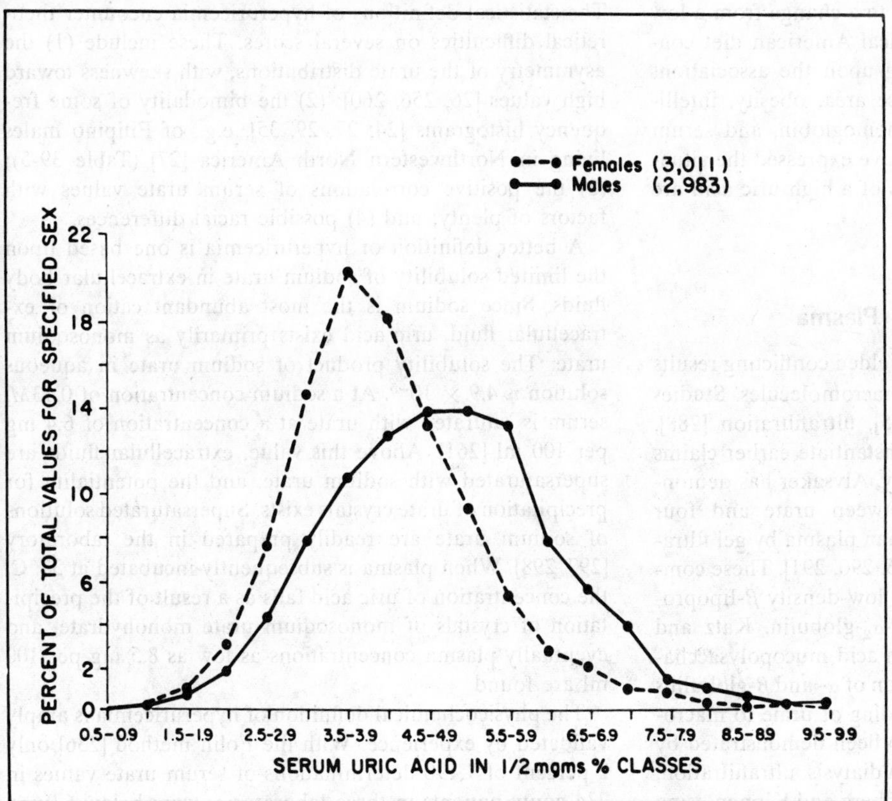

Figure 39-9. Distributions of serum urate values in the male and female population of Tecumseh, Michigan, 1959 to 1960. Note skewness toward high values in both sexes. (*From Mikkelsen et al.* [260], *with permission of Amer. J. Med.*)

the Aurukun [279]. In epidemiologic studies, body bulk (as estimated by body weight, surface area, or ponderal index) has proved to be one of the most important predictors of hyperuricemia [282].

The nature of this relationship remains unclear. In a population of 25 obese Maoris in New Zealand uric acid clearance was somewhat low (5.0 ± 1.5 ml per min), but the daily excretion of uric acid appeared to be elevated (663 mg) [283]. In obese subjects uric acid excretion may be normal when factored by body weight [200]. These observations, although fragmentary, suggest that both renal and metabolic factors may contribute to the hyperuricemia of obesity.

In the United States there is an association of serum urate values with "social class" or academic achievement (Table 39-5). Mean urate levels are higher in executives than in craftsmen [35, 36, 273, 274, 284, 285]. They are also higher in Ph.D. scientists than in supervisors, and in supervisors than in craftsmen, at the Oak Ridge National Laboratory, and in medical than in high school students in Pittsburgh [35, 36]. Among university professors [286] and Edinburgh business executives [285], urate levels showed a positive correlation with drive, achievement, range of activities, and leadership. Also, positive correlations exist between serum urate levels and Army aptitude test scores of inductees ($p = 0.03$) [257], as well as between urate values and hemoglobin [197] and serum protein values [287]. The development of hyperuricemia in some Filipinos upon moving to the United States has been ascribed to a change from a low purine, low protein diet to the typical American diet containing more meat. In commenting upon the associations of urate values with weight, surface area, obesity, intelligence, social status, achievement, hemoglobin, and serum proteins, Acheson and Chan [282] have expressed the situation well by stating, "The associates of a high uric acid are the associates of plenty."

The Physical State of Urate in Plasma

Studies over the past 30 years have yielded conflicting results on the binding of urate to plasma macromolecules. Studies employing equilibrium dialysis [145], ultrafiltration [288], and electrophoresis [70] failed to substantiate earlier claims of substantial binding [289]. Recently, Alvsaker has demonstrated a reversible interaction between urate and four macromolecular components in human plasma by gel filtration and immunoelectrophoresis [215, 290, 291]. These components were identified as albumin, low-density β-lipoprotein, β_2-macroglobulins, and an α_1-α_2-globulin. Katz and Ehrlich [292] have identified a serum acid mucopolysaccharide component migrating in the region of α- and β-globulins which increases urate solubility. Binding of urate to macromolecules in human plasma has also been demonstrated by Skeikh and Moller using equilibrium dialysis, ultrafiltration, and gel filtration [293], and by Klinenberg and Kippen using a modified equilibrium dialysis procedure [294].

The importance of urate binding to plasma proteins in vivo has been questioned [293]. Alvsaker [215] found that 25 to 30 percent of urate is bound to plasma proteins at room temperature. However, others have found that although 20 to 26 percent of urate in plasma appears to be bound at 4°C, binding drops to 5 percent or less at temperatures above 20°C [145, 293, 294].

Alvsaker [215] described a reduced capacity of plasma from seven gouty patients to bind urate, which he attributed to a specific reduction in the plasma component which migrates as an α_1-α_2-globulin. This deficiency appeared to be inherited in an autosomal manner and the patients exhibiting reduced levels were heterozygous for this defect [216]. Using equilibrium dialysis, Klinenberg and Kippen [294] described reduced binding of urate in plasma proteins in three patients with severe tophaceous gout, although plasma from seventeen other gouty subjects including three with tophi exhibited a normal urate binding capacity. Bluestone and coworkers [295, 296] also reported that several drugs, including salicylates, phenylbutazone, sulfinpyrazone, and probenecid, reduce urate binding to plasma macromolecules in vitro. The relevance of these observations to the pathogenesis of gouty arthritis and the deposition of tophi remains to be established.

Definition and Significance of Hyperuricemia

The statistical definitions of hyperuricemia encounter theoretical difficulties on several scores. These include (1) the asymmetry of the urate distributions, with skewness toward high values [26, 256, 260]; (2) the bimodality of some frequency histograms [24, 27, 29, 35], e.g., of Filipino males living in Northwestern North America [27] (Table 39-5); (3) the positive correlations of serum urate values with factors of plenty; and (4) possible racial differences.

A better definition of hyperuricemia is one based upon the limited solubility of sodium urate in extracellular body fluids. Since sodium is the most abundant cation of extracellular fluid, uric acid exists primarily as monosodium urate. The solubility product of sodium urate in aqueous solution is 4.9×10^{-5}. At a sodium concentration of $0.13M$, serum is saturated with urate at a concentration of 6.4 mg per 100 ml [261]. Above this value, extracellular fluids are supersaturated with sodium urate, and the potentiality for precipitation of urate crystals exists. Supersaturated solutions of sodium urate are readily prepared in the laboratory [297, 298]. When plasma is subsequently incubated at 37°C, the concentration of uric acid falls as a result of the precipitation of crystals of monosodium urate monohydrate, and eventually plasma concentrations as low as 8.5 mg per 100 ml are found.

The physicochemical definition of hyperuricemia is amply validated by experience. With the Folin method [236] only 2 percent of 1,190 determinations of serum urate values in 234 gouty patients in three laboratories were below 6.0 mg per 100 ml [266, 299, 300]. Ninety-four percent of 177 serum analyses in 21 gouty patients exceeded 7.0 mg per 100 ml [266]. The prevalence of gout is high in ethnic groups whose mean serum uric acid values are above the American mean [27–31].

The study of Seegmiller et al. [76] of the distribution of serum urate values for 940 nongouty males and 60 gouty males (Fig. 39-10) employing the enzymatic spectrophotometric method [253] shows an appreciable overlap of the distributions of values in nongouty and gouty subjects in the region of 6.0 to 7.5 mg per 100 ml. Nine percent of gouty patients at times showed serum values below 7.0 mg per 100 ml. With the enzymatic method, 21 percent of 3,000 males in Tecumseh, Michigan, had serum levels above 6.0 mg per 100 ml [260], and in three studies from 3 to 7.4 percent of males had values above 7.0 mg per 100 ml [26, 76, 260]. For purposes of population surveys, arbitrary normal limits of 7.0 mg per 100 ml for males and 6.0 mg per 100 ml for females have been suggested for the spectrophotometric method [32]. For such purposes these are probably acceptable limits for the normal range with this method, but the upper reaches of this range in males may well represent supersaturation values of monosodium urate in serum. A 9 percent incidence of values of less than 7.0 mg per 100 ml in gouty subjects suggests that this is the case.

In population studies the prevalences of gout, and of renal stones, are correlated with the height of the serum urate value in both males and females (Tables 39-2 and 39-3). In subjects with serum urate values above 9 mg per 100 ml at mean age 58, the prevalence of gout was 90 percent and of renal stones was 40 percent. The figures on the prevalence

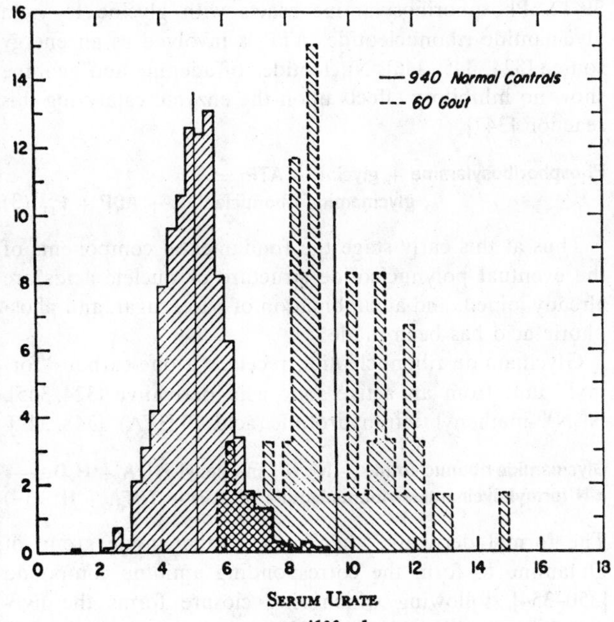

Figure 39-10. Distribution of serum uric acid concentration in a normal and gouty population. (*Reproduced from Seegmiller et al.* [76], *with permission of the New Eng. J. Med.*)

of stones at various serum urate levels in this population agree well with the prevalence values of stones in a large series of patients with gout in a referral practice [169].

Potential Pathophysiologic Mechanisms of Hyperuricemia

In theory, hyperuricemia could result from increased absorption of precursor purines or from increased plasma protein binding, increased production, decreased excretion, or decreased destruction of uric acid, or from some combination of these abnormalities.

A purine-free diet results in an average reduction of the serum urate level of 1 to 1.2 mg per 100 ml in gouty subjects [65, 301] but, with rare exceptions [302], does not correct hyperuricemia. Feeding of 4 gm yeast RNA per day for 4 days results in comparable elevations of serum urate levels in nongouty [303, 304] and gouty subjects [305]. Clearly hyperuricemia cannot be attributed to abnormal absorption of precursor purines.

There is considerable evidence that both increased production of uric acid and reduced renal excretion of uric acid play important roles in the pathogenesis of hyperuricemia in primary gout. This evidence will be considered in detail below.

Such uricolysis as occurs in man [306] can be accounted for almost entirely by the action of intestinal flora upon uric acid entering the gastrointestinal tract in gastric, biliary, pancreatic, and intestinal secretions [307, 308]. There is no evidence that extrarenal disposal of uric acid is diminished in gout, whereas, on the contrary, in gouty patients with reduced renal excretion of uric acid extrarenal disposal may constitute the chief route of disposal of urate [309]. The topic of uricolysis will also be considered below, but first we will review the normal processes of synthesis and excretion of uric acid, and studies of these processes in patients with primary gout.

BIOCHEMISTRY OF PURINE COMPOUNDS

Biosynthesis of the Purine Ring

Early work concerned with the biosynthesis and metabolism of purine compounds in animals and man has been reviewed elsewhere [64, 310–312]. Because of structural similarities, urea [313], arginine, and histidine [314] were at one time proposed as precursors of purines. When experiments were performed with these substances in labeled form [315, 316] and no labeling of tissue purines resulted, these theories were discarded. In 1943, Barnes and Schoenheimer [315] fed ammonium citrate containing ^{15}N to pigeons and rats and demonstrated that the purines of internal organs and the uric acid of the avian excreta contained appreciable ^{15}N in the ring structure and substituent amino groups.

Following these early studies, the use of labeled substrates

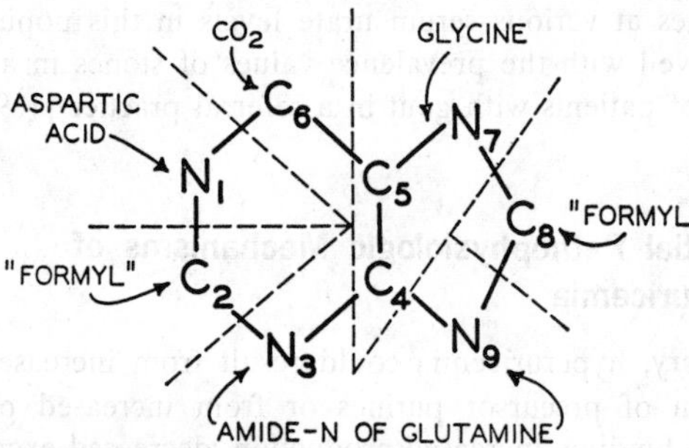

Figure 39-11. Origins of the atoms of the purine ring.

in bacterial, avian, and mammalian systems soon defined the origin of the individual atoms of the purine ring (Fig. 39-11). Glycine contributes carbon atoms 4 and 5, and nitrogen atom 7 [317–319]. Carbon atoms 2 and 8 come from formate [319, 320], carbon atom 6 comes from CO_2 [318, 321], nitrogen atoms 3 and 9 come from the amide-N of glutamine [322–324], and nitrogen atom 1 comes from aspartic acid [323].

A key intermediate in the synthesis of purines is 5-phosphoribosyl-1-pyrophosphate (PP-ribose-P). This high-energy compound is involved in purine synthesis in two types of reactions: in one it is a substrate, together with L-glutamine, in the first specific reaction of purine synthesis *de novo*]325]; in the other it participates with purine bases in the direct synthesis of purine ribonucleotides by a condensation reaction with liberation of inorganic pyrophosphate [326, 327]. PP-ribose-P is formed by transfer of the terminal pyrophosphate group of ATP to the carbon-1 of ribose-5-phosphate [328, 329].

$$\textbf{Ribose-5-phosphate + ATP} \longrightarrow \textbf{PP-ribose-P + AMP} \quad (1)$$

Ribose-5-phosphate has three possible pathways of origin: it may arise as an intermediate in the 6-phosphogluconic acid oxidation pathway of glucose; as a product of nonoxidative cleavage of fructose-6-phosphate; or as a late product of the metabolism of glucose-1-phosphate via the uronic acid cycle. The 6-phosphogluconic acid pathway is probably the major source of ribose esters in tissues with an active oxidative pathway of glucose catabolism, such as liver [330] and bone marrow [331]. The fructose cleavage pathway is demonstrable in tissues which catabolize glucose chiefly by the glycolytic pathway, such as skeletal muscle [330]. Both pathways appear to be operative in man [332]. The uronic acid cycle is thought to be of minor quantitative importance as a source of ribose-5-phosphate [333].

The first specific reaction of purine synthesis *de novo* is that in which 5β-phosphoribosyl-1-amine is generated [324, 325]. In this reaction, the pyrophosphate group of PP-ribose-P is displaced by the amide group of glutamine, and there is an inversion of the substituents to yield the β linkage characteristic of the glycosidic bond of all known ribonucleotides [325] (Fig. 39-12).

$$\alpha\textbf{-PP-ribose-P} + \textbf{glutamine} + H_2O \xrightarrow{Mg^{++}} \beta\textbf{-phosphoribosylamine} + \textbf{glutamic acid} + PP_i \quad (2)$$

The reaction generating phosphoribosylamine is the first irreversible reaction dealing specifically with the synthesis of purines *de novo,* and it thus becomes a potentially important reaction in control of purine synthesis. The enzyme catalyzing this reaction, glutamine phosphoribosylpyrophosphate amidotransferase, is the site of a synergistic feedback control by adenine and guanine ribonucleotides [336–338]. The regulation of purine biosynthesis will be discussed more fully below.

An alternative pathway for the synthesis of phosphoribosylamine by the direct reaction of ammonia with ribose-5-phosphate was described in bacterial extracts by Nierlich and Magasanik [339] and later shown to have occurred nonenzymatically at high ammonium chloride concentrations. Suggestive evidence for such a pathway in bacteria was provided by Le Gal et al. [340], in Ehrlich ascites cells by Herscovics and Johnstone [341], and in pigeon liver extracts by Reem [342]. The assays were indirect, and performed in crude extracts. Feedback effects were similar to those described for the amidotransferase, which is known to accept ammonium as a substrate in vitro in the absence of glutamine [343]. Westby and Gots [344] have now described bacterial mutants which lack any activity of glutamine-PP-ribose-P-amidotransferase (*pur* F mutants) and show complete dependence upon exogenous purines for growth. The conclusion that there is a second enzyme which catalyzes the formation of phosphoribosylamine is presently unwarranted.

The stepwise synthesis of the purine ring is shown in Fig. 39-12. Phosphoribosylamine reacts with glycine to yield glycinamide ribonucleotide. ATP is involved as an energy source [324, 345, 346]. Nucleotides of adenine and guanine show no inhibitory effects upon the enzyme catalyzing this reaction [347].

$$\textbf{Phosphoribosylamine} + \textbf{glycine} + \textbf{ATP} \rightleftharpoons \textbf{glycinamide ribonucleotide} + \textbf{ADP} + P_i \quad (3)$$

Thus at this early stage the fundamental components of the eventual polynucleotide structure of nucleic acids are already joined, and a combination of base, sugar, and phosphoric acid has been made.

Glycinamide ribonucleotide receives a one-carbon "formyl" unit from an active folic acid derivative [324, 345], N^5,N^{10}-methenyl tetrahydrofolic acid (THFA) [348, 349].

$$\textbf{Glycinamide ribonucleotide} + N^5,N^{10}\textbf{-methenyl-THFA} + H_2O \longrightarrow \alpha\textbf{-N-formylglycinamide ribonucleotide (FGAR)} + \textbf{THFA} + H^+ \quad (4)$$

The formyl derivative then receives the amide group of glutamine to form the corresponding amidine compound [350–354], following which ring closure forms the five-membered imidazole ring [355], one of two fused heterocyclic rings comprising the eventual purine structure. Each of these reactions requires ATP as an energy source.

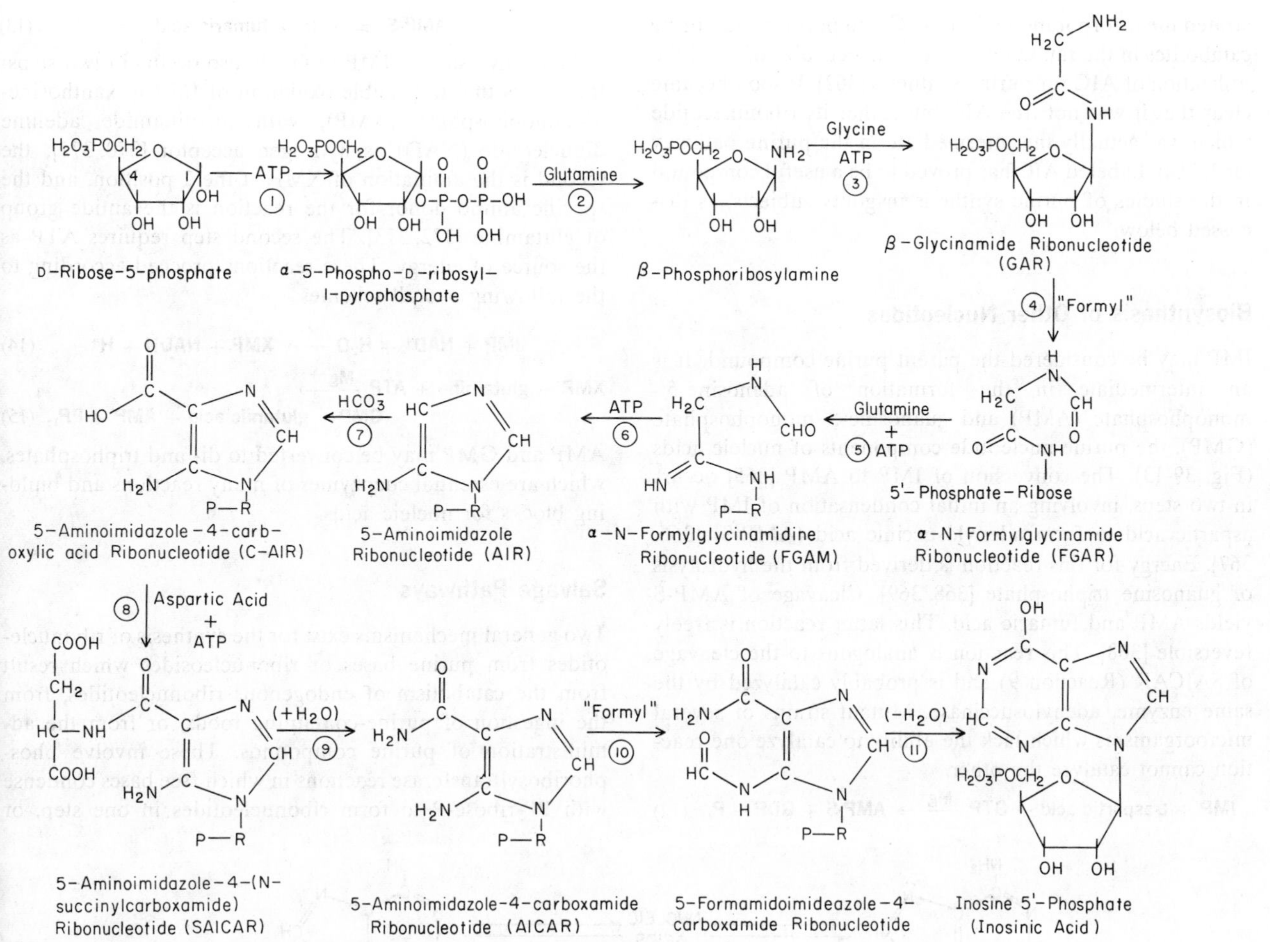

Figure 39-12. Biosynthesis of the purine ring. The encircled numbers in this figure and in Fig. 39-13 refer to numbered reactions in the text.

$$\text{FGAR} + \text{glutamine} + \text{ATP} + H_2O \xrightarrow{Mg^{++}} \alpha\text{-N-formylglycinamidine ribonucleotide (FGAM)} + \text{glutamic acid} + \text{ADP} + P_i \quad (5)$$

$$\text{FGAM} + \text{ATP} \xrightarrow{Mg^{++},\,K^{+}} \text{5-aminoimidazole ribonucleotide} + \text{ADP} + P_i \quad (6)$$

5-Aminoimidazole ribonucleotide (AIR) now receives a carboxyl group at C-4 by a CO_2-fixation reaction which requires a high concentration of bicarbonate [356]. The carboxyl serves as a point for the condensation of this intermediate with aspartic acid through an amide linkage involving another ATP as the source of energy [356]. Hydrolysis of the intermediate yields 5-aminoimidazole-4-carboxamide ribonucleotide, a compound lacking only carbon atom 2 of a complete purine ribonucleotide.

$$\text{AIR} + CO_2 \rightleftharpoons \text{5-aminoimidazole-4-carboxylic acid ribonucleotide (C-AIR)} \quad (7)$$

$$\text{C-AIR} + \text{aspartic acid} + \text{ATP} \xrightleftharpoons{Mg^{++}} \text{5-aminoimidazole-4-N-succinocarboxamide ribonucleotide (SAICAR)} + \text{ADP} + P_i \quad (8)$$

$$\text{SAICAR} \rightleftharpoons \text{fumaric acid} + \text{5-aminoimidazole-4-carboxamide ribonucleotide (AICAR)} \quad (9)$$

AIC-ribonucleotide receives a second formyl group from a tetrahydrofolic acid derivative [357, 358], and ring closure completes the biosynthesis of the purine structure by forming inosine-5′-monophosphate (IMP) [358].

$$\text{AICAR} + N^{10}\text{-formyl-THFA} \xrightarrow{K^{+}} \text{5-formamidoimidazole-4-carboxamide ribonucleotide} + \text{THFA} \quad (10)$$

$$\text{5-Formamidoimidazole-4-carboxamide ribonucleotide} \rightleftharpoons \text{IMP} + H_2O \quad (11)$$

One intermediate in the synthesis of IMP deserves special comment, viz., 5-aminoimidazole-4-carboxamide ribonucleotide. Its free base, 4(5)-aminoimidazole-5(4)-carboxamide (AIC), was first isolated in 1945 by Stetten and Fox [359] from cultures of *Escherichia coli* grown in the presence of sulfonamide. The elucidation of its structure by Shive and coworkers [360] stimulated considerable interest, since it was immediately recognized as a potential purine precursor. This postulate was confirmed when Miller et al. [361] demonstrated the incorporation of AIC-^{14}C into purines and purine catabolites in the rat. Other studies further substantiated the utilization of AIC for purine synthesis [362]. It soon became clear that it was not free AIC but rather its ribonucleotide which was actually the intermediate in the purine pathway [363, 364]. Labeled AIC has proved to be a useful compound in the studies of purine synthesis in gouty subjects, as discussed below.

Biosynthesis of Other Nucleotides

IMP may be considered the parent purine compound. It is an intermediate in the formation of adenosine-5′-monophosphate (AMP) and guanosine-5′-monophosphate (GMP), the purine nucleotide components of nucleic acids (Fig. 39-13). The conversion of IMP to AMP [365] occurs in two steps, involving an initial condensation of IMP with aspartic acid to form adenylosuccinic acid (AMP-S) [366, 367]. Energy for this reaction is derived from the hydrolysis of guanosine triphosphate [368, 369]. Cleavage of AMP-S yields AMP and fumaric acid. This latter reaction is freely reversible [368]. This reaction is analogous to the cleavage of SAICAR (Reaction 9) and is probably catalyzed by the same enzyme, adenylosuccinase. Mutant strains of several microorganisms which lack the ability to catalyze one reaction cannot catalyze the other.

$$\text{IMP} + \text{L-aspartic acid} + \text{GTP} \xrightarrow{Mg^{++}} \text{AMP-S} + \text{GDP} + P_i \quad (12)$$

$$\text{AMP-S} \rightleftharpoons \text{AMP} + \text{fumaric acid} \quad (13)$$

The conversion of IMP to GMP also occurs in two steps: the first is the irreversible oxidation of IMP to xanthosine-5′-monophosphate (XMP), with nicotinamide adenine dinucleotide (NAD) as hydrogen acceptor [370, 371]; the second is the amination of XMP at the 2 position, and the specific amino donor for the reaction is the amide group of glutamine [372, 373]. The second step requires ATP as the source of energy. These reactions proceed according to the following overall schemes:

$$\text{IMP} + \text{NAD}^+ + H_2O \xrightarrow{K^+} \text{XMP} + \text{NADH} + H^+ \quad (14)$$

$$\text{XMP} + \text{glutamine} + \text{ATP} \xrightarrow{Mg^{++}} \text{GMP} + \text{glutamic acid} + \text{AMP} + PP_i \quad (15)$$

AMP and GMP may be converted to di- and triphosphates, which are essential coenzymes of many reactions and building blocks for nucleic acids.

Salvage Pathways

Two general mechanisms exist for the synthesis of ribonucleotides from purine bases or ribonucleosides which result from the catabolism of endogenous ribonucleotides, from the ingestion of purine-containing foods, or from the administration of purine compounds. These involve phosphoribosyltransferase reactions in which free bases condense with PP-ribose-P to form ribonucleotides in one step, or

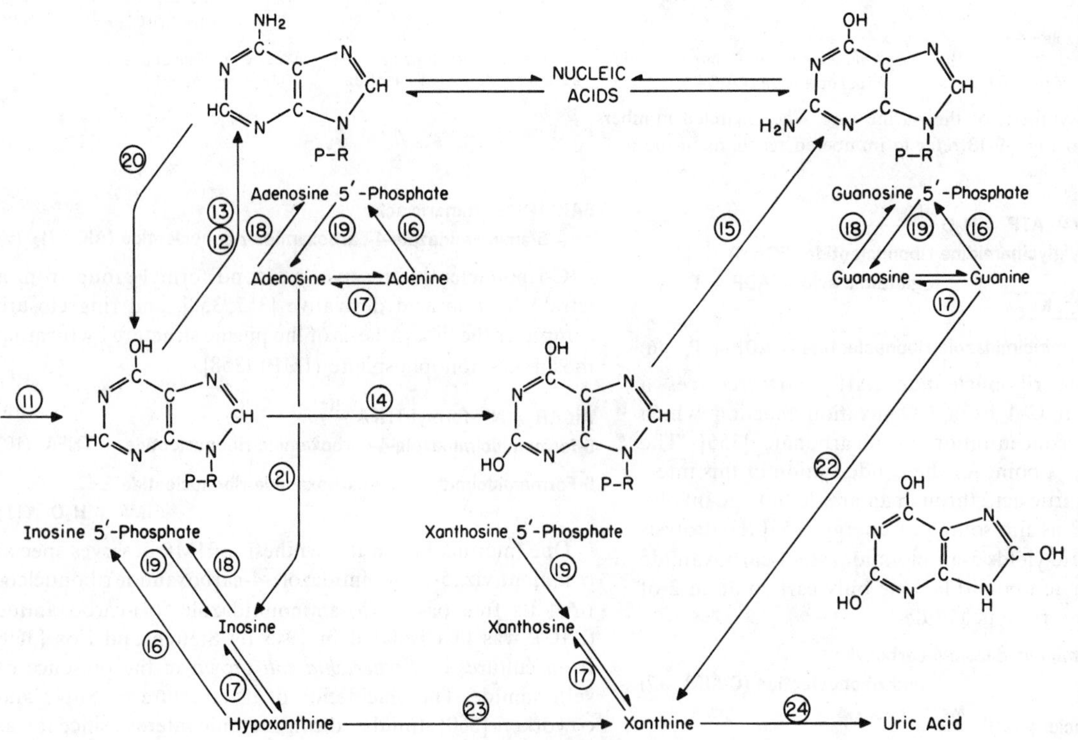

Figure 39-13. Biosynthesis of purine ribonucleotides, ribonucleosides, and bases.

phosphorylase reactions in which free bases react with ribose-1-phosphate to form ribonucleosides, operating in conjunction with kinase reactions in which ribonucleosides are phosphorylated to form ribonucleotides.

The phosphoribosyltransferase reaction has the following form:

$$\text{Base} + \text{PP-ribose-P} \rightleftharpoons \text{base-ribose-phosphate} + PP_i \quad (16)$$

This general reaction is responsible for the conversion of purines [326, 327], pyrimidines [374], nicotinamide [375], and certain other nitrogenous bases to their respective ribonucleotides. Two different purine phosphoribosyltransferases (formerly termed ribonucleotide pyrophosphorylases) have been identified, one acting upon AIC and adenine [326, 376], the other upon hypoxanthine and guanine [327, 375]. Adenine phosphoribosyltransferase (A-PRT) will also accept adenine analogues such as 2,6-diaminopurine and 8-azadenine.

Hypoxanthine-guanine phosphoribosyltransferase (PRT, or occasionally H-G-PRT) will catalyze the conversion of xanthine to XMP, but at only about 0.3 percent of the rate of the reaction with hypoxanthine or guanine [377]. PRT will also catalyze the conversion of 6-thiopurine [327], 6-thioguanine, 8-azaguanine, allopurinol [378], and probably oxipurinol to their respective ribonucleotides. These enzymes have been studied in yeast [364], beef liver [326, 327], ascites cells [376], and human erythrocytes [375, 379, 380]. In man, PRT activity is widely distributed and is especially rich in brain, where activity is greatest in basal ganglia [200]. Activity is low in muscle and bone marrow [200]. The K_{eq} of both phosphoribosyltransferases is far toward the ribonucleotide; a value of 290 has been estimated for A-PRT [376]. Both phosphoribosyltransferases are inhibited by purine ribonucleoside monophosphates. The regulation of phosphoribosyltransferase activities, and the role of these enzymes in maintaining the homeostasis of intracellular nucleotide concentrations, will be discussed below.

The two-step pathway has the following form:

$$\text{Base} + \text{ribose-1-phosphate} \rightleftharpoons \text{base-ribose} + P_i \quad (17)$$
$$\text{Base} - \text{ribose} + \text{ATP} \longrightarrow \text{base-ribose-phosphate} + \text{ADP} \quad (18)$$

Purine nucleoside phosphorylase is widely distributed in mammalian tissue and active with guanine, hypoxanthine, and, to a lesser extent, xanthine, but not with adenine [381–383]. In the case of hypoxanthine, the equilibrium point is far toward the ribonucleoside. The phosphorylase has been extensively studied in human erythrocytes [383, 384].

Present indications are that the phosphoribosyltransferases are responsible for a much more extensive recycling of purine bases back into nucleotide pools than was initially appreciated. By contrast, studies in subjects who lack activity of H-G-phosphoribosyltransferase, and of their cells in culture, indicate that recycling of hypoxanthine and guanine via the nucleoside phosphorylase–nucleoside kinase route is not very active. Kinases capable of phosphorylating inosine or guanosine have been described in animal tissues [385], and labeled inosine is incorporated into adenine and guanine nucleotides in liver of both normal and PRT-deficient subjects [386]. However, these kinases appear to be absent in human fibroblasts [387]. Normally the action of purine nucleoside phosphorylase upon inosine or guanosine is probably largely degradative. The situation with adenosine is quite different. Adenosine is converted to acid-soluble nucleotides by dog heart muscle even more actively than adenine [388]. Also, AIC-ribonucleoside is readily utilized by rabbit erythrocytes for the synthesis of ATP and GTP [389]. Adenosine kinase is a well-known, active enzyme with an extensive distribution among mammalian tissues [390, 391].

By either of these salvage pathways only one high-energy bond, in the form of PP-ribose-P or ATP, is expended in the synthesis of a ribonucleotide, whereas synthesis of AMP or GMP *de novo* from glutamine and PP-ribose-P requires the expenditure of a minimum of six high-energy bonds.

Economy of Purine Biosynthesis in the Mammal

Purine biosynthesis *de novo* is especially active in liver. All enzymes of purine biosynthesis, nucleotide interconversion, degradation, and base salvage are found in the soluble portion of the cell, except for uricase which when present is particulate, and is found in lysosomes. Uricase is not present in birds, higher apes, and man. There is evidence that the enzymes of purine biosynthesis *de novo* are not in free solution, circulating within the cytosol at random, but rather that they exist in a macromolecular aggregate of molecular weight well in excess of 1 million, capable of conducting the complete synthesis of inosinic acid [392].

Such nonhepatic tissues as have been studied appear capable of only limited synthesis of purines *de novo.* The mature erythrocyte actively synthesizes PP-ribose-P, and purine ribonucleotides from free bases via phosphoribosyltransferase reactions, but it cannot synthesize phosphoribosylamine [393]. Therefore, it is incapable of purine synthesis *de novo.* Reactions beyond AIC-ribonucleotide are active in the erythrocyte, including those of nucleotide interconversion [389].

Data of Lajtha and Vane [394] suggest that nonhepatic tissues, for example bone marrow, are dependent upon an advanced purine precursor originating in liver for their sources of nucleic acid purine bases. On the basis of studies of turnover of purine nucleotides in various tissues of the rat, Henderson and LePage [395] suggested that erythrocytes may transport an auxiliary supply of purines. Mager and associates [396] have assigned this function to ATP synthesized in liver and delivered to distant tissues by the erythrocyte. The critical role of phosphoribosyltransferase pathways in nonhepatic tissues is thus clear. In the presence of a limited capacity for purine synthesis *de novo,* and partial dependence upon purine imports, recovery of purine bases generated by catabolic reactions becomes a function of major importance to the cell. Because of the restricted distribution in man of catabolic enzymes capable of acting upon free purines, those bases generated in nonhepatic or nonintestinal tissue are largely protected from catabolism and available for recycling, unless lost from the cell and transported to the liver.

Nucleic Acid Catabolism

Enzymatic hydrolysis of the polynucleotide chains of nucleic acids occurs through the action of various nucleases [397]. The major products released by ribonuclease *a* and *b* and by deoxyribonuclease I and II are oligonucleotides. The oligonucleotides are further cleaved by phosphodiesterases to yield 5′- and 3′-mononucleotides.

The mononucleotides are split by group-specific nucleoside-5′-phosphatases [398], as well as by a variety of nonspecific phosphatases]399], to yield the corresponding purine or pyrimidine nucleoside and orthophosphate. The purine nucleoside is then split by purine nucleoside phosphorylase [381] to yield the free purine base and ribose-1-phosphate, or deoxyribose-1-phosphate [381, 400].

$$\text{Purine mononucleotide} \longrightarrow \text{purine nucleoside} + P_i \quad (19)$$

$$\text{Purine nucleoside} + P_i \rightleftharpoons \text{purine base} + \text{ribose-1-}PO_4 \quad (17)$$

In addition to these general reactions, AMP and adenosine are acted upon by specific deaminating enzymes. AMP is converted to IMP by adenylic deaminase (Reaction 20, Fig. 39-13) [401] and adenosine to inosine by adenosine deaminase (Reaction 21, Fig. 39-13) [402].

A number of purine bases other than adenine and guanine occur as minor constituents of nucleic acids. The mononucleotides derived from certain bacterial and bacteriophage DNAs contain small quantities of 6-methylaminopurine [403]. Ribosomal and transfer RNAs of bacterial and mammalian cells contain small amounts of hypoxanthine, as well as of several methylated purine bases, including 1-methylguanine, N^2-methylguanine, N^2-dimethylguanine, 7-methylguanine, 2-methyladenine, N^6-methyladenine, N^6-dimethyladenine, 1-methyladenine, and 1-methylhypoxanthine [404]. tRNAs contain approximately four times as many methyl groups as rRNAs. The 16S species of ribosomal RNA contains approximately 20 percent more methyl groups than the 23S. Methylations occur at the polynucleotide level [405–407] and a number of different methylating enzymes have been identified which will methylate specific purine sites in DNA [408], rRNA [409], or methyl-deficient tRNA [404]. In all known instances the methyl donor is S-adenosylmethionine. Most of the methylated bases listed above have been identified in human urine in small quantities.

Catabolism of Ingested Nucleoproteins

Nucleic acids of dietary nucleoproteins are liberated in the intestinal canal by the action of proteolytic enzymes. Nucleic acids are degraded in turn to nucleotides by nucleases and phosphodiesterases secreted by the pancreas. The nucleotides are chiefly hydrolyzed to nucleosides by various nucleotidases and phosphatases, and the nucleosides may be absorbed intact, or they may be cleaved phosphorolytically to yield the free base. The small intestinal mucosa of man is rich in nucleoside phosphorylase and xanthine oxidase, and ingested nucleoprotein purines may potentially be converted to uric acid in the gastrointestinal mucosa. The uric acid may be further catabolized by intestinal bacteria or may be absorbed. From experiments in which normal and gouty subjects ingested ^{15}N-labeled nucleic acid [410], it appeared that the purine moieties were converted to uric acid largely by direct routes without prior incorporation into body nucleic acids. However, small quantities of dietary nucleosides and even nucleotides may also be utilized directly for the synthesis of nucleic acids [411].

Formation of Uric Acid

The free purine bases that result from nucleoside cleavage are adenine, guanine, hypoxanthine, and xanthine. Since purine nucleoside phosphorylase acts most readily upon inosine and guanosine [381, 412, 413], the major bases generated are very likely hypoxanthine and guanine. In mammalian tissue free adenine is not deaminated as it is in certain bacterial systems [399], so that adenine does not give rise directly to hypoxanthine. If it is not reconverted to its nucleoside or nucleotide, it may be excreted unchanged, and normal human subjects excrete adenine in small quantities in urine [414]. By contrast, the other purine bases are readily converted to uric acid. Guanine is deaminated by guanase to yield xanthine (Reaction 22, Fig. 39-11). Hypoxanthine is oxidized by xanthine oxidase to yield xanthine (Reaction 23), which in turn is further oxidized by the same enzyme to yield uric acid (Reaction 24) [415]. It will be noted from Fig. 39-11 that, whereas adenine, hypoxanthine, and guanine appear to be derived exclusively by cleavage of the corresponding nucleoside, xanthine has at least three direct precursors, namely, its nucleoside (xanthosine or deoxyxanthosine), free hypoxanthine, and guanine.

In man, xanthine oxidase is found in high activity only in liver and small intestinal mucosa [416, 417]. Traces of activity are found in heart and skeletal muscle, kidney and spleen, none in leukocytes, erythrocytes, stratum cornium, or fibroblasts in tissue culture [417]. Activity may be present inconstantly in bone marrow [418]. The enzyme is a flavoprotein containing iron and molybdenum, capable of oxidizing a wide variety of purines, aldehydes, and pteridines.

Because of the restricted distribution of xanthine oxidase and its great activity in liver, uric acid synthesis appears largely to be a hepatic process in man. Presumably purine degradation products of other tissues are transported to the liver for further oxidation. Plasma contains small quantities of xanthine and hypoxanthine, together amounting to about 0.1 to 0.3 mg per 100 ml [419, 420], but no other uric acid precursors have been detected in normal plasma, with the possible exception of IMP following anoxic muscle injury [421].

Uric Acid Ribonucleoside

Since the discovery of uric acid ribonucleoside in beef erythrocytes [422] and liver [423], the possibility has been entertained that this nucleoside is an intermediate of an alternative pathway of uric acid synthesis. Its existence in human erythrocytes has been claimed [424] and denied [425, 426]. Although Falconer and Gulland [423] originally concluded that the beef compound was a 9-N-ribosyl derivative, more recent spectral studies [427] indicate that the ribosyl group is attached to the N-3 position of uric acid [426]. This structure has been confirmed by synthesis [428, 429]. The ribonucleoside is cleaved to uric acid and ribose-1-phosphate by a specific phosphorylase found in several species and purified extensively from dog small intestinal mucosa [430]. The phosphorylase is inhibited by colchicine ($K_i = 1.2 \times 10^{-3}M$) and phenylbutazone ($K_i = 1.8 \times 10^{-3}M$) but not probenecid, pyrazinamide, or certain other alkaloids [431]. It is now known that the ribonucleoside is formed by the action of phosphatase or 5′-nucleotidase upon uric acid ribonucleotide [(3-N-ribosyluric acid)-5′-phosphate], which is formed by a direct condensation of uric acid and PP-ribose-P [432, 433]. Therefore, the pathway does not result in net synthesis of uric acid. Small amounts of the ribonucleotide exist in beef erythrocytes [434].

The enzyme catalyzing synthesis of the ribonucleotide has been purified over 5,000-fold from beef erythrocytes. It also catalyzes reaction with xanthine, uracil, orotic acid, and thymine [433, 435]. With xanthine and uric acid the products are both 3-N-ribosephosphate derivatives [434] (see Fig. 39-16, later). The K_m values for the pyrimidine substrates are lower than for uric acid or xanthine. For this reason the enzyme is considered to be a 2, 4-diketo pyrimidine phosphoribosyltransferase with overlapping specificity towards purines, with a 2, 6-diketo construction and unsubstituted nitrogen atoms. Competition experiments indicate that the enzyme is identical with orotate phosphoribosyltransferase [436]. In addition, a phosphoribosyltransferase derived from *Lactobacillus plantarus* forms a 9-N-ribosephosphate derivative of uric acid [437], but it is not known whether such a compound is formed by mammalian enzymes.

REGULATION OF PURINE BIOSYNTHESIS

Rate-limiting Step

Although the reaction rates of the individual steps of the pathway of purine biosynthesis have not been measured under steady state conditions, a number of arguments collectively suggest that the first committed reaction, that in which L-glutamine and 5-phosphoribosyl-1-pyrophosphate form 5-phosphoribosyl-1-amine, is rate limiting for the entire sequence: (1) Phosphoribosylamine is the first specific purine precursor, and no branching of the succeeding pathway occurs prior to the synthesis of inosinic acid. (2) No intermediates of the *de novo* pathway accumulate unless a genetic or chemical block of a reaction is introduced, e.g., in bacteria [438] or in tissue culture of surviving mammalian cells [439, 440]. (3) The activity of the first enzyme is regulated by purine ribonucleotides [336–338], but that of the second enzyme is not [347], and no functional inhibition is observed in the portion of the sequence from GAR to IMP [393]. Although inhibition of the amidation of FGAR to FGAM by AMP and GMP can be demonstrated with the isolated enzyme, the required concentrations of inhibitor ribonucleotides are unphysiologically high [441]. (4) Bacterial purine auxotrophs grown on limiting concentrations of purines show derepression of synthesis of the first enzyme as well as of five others concerned with purine synthesis *de novo* [442, 443]. (5) Measures which raise intracellular concentrations of PP-ribose-P accelerate purine biosynthesis; measures which lower PP-ribose-P concentrations reduce the rate of purine biosynthesis [444–446]. (6) The availability of glutamine can be rate limiting for purine synthesis under certain circumstances [447].

The regulation of the rate of formation of phosphoribosylamine may therefore be the single most important factor in the control of purine synthesis *de novo.* The chief influences upon the rate of its synthesis are the concentrations of the substrates of the first reaction and the activity of the enzyme catalyzing it. The activity is determined by the intrinsic properties of the enzyme and the effects of inhibitors or activators upon it.

Substrates

α5-Phosphoribosyl-1-Pyrophosphate

The biosynthesis of PP-ribose-P from ribose-5-phosphate and ATP has been discussed above. Only a small fraction of pentose phosphate is converted to PP-ribose-P [448]. Accordingly, control of its synthesis by one or more end products has been investigated. The activity of bacterial PP-ribose-P-synthetase is regulated by both purine and pyrimidine ribonucleotides, most strongly by ADP, GTP, CTP, and ATP, and also by tryptophan, but not by histidine alone or in combination with other inhibitors, nor by pyridine nucleotides [449]. PP-ribose-P-synthetase from Ehrlich ascites tumor cells is inhibited by a large number of nucleoside mono-, di-, and triphosphates [450]. The enzyme from human erythrocytes appears to be strongly inhibited by ADP and GDP [451, 452].

Atkinson and Fall [453, 454] postulate that the activity of a biosynthetic reaction is controlled by the "energy charge" of the cell, as well as by cumulative feedback inhibition:

$$\text{“Energy charge”} = \frac{\text{ATP} + \frac{1}{2}\,\text{ADP}}{\text{ATP} + \text{ADP} + \text{AMP}}$$

This concept predicts that the synthesis of PP-ribose-P will be inhibited by nucleoside diphosphates and monophosphates, irrespective of specific feedback effects, which appears to be true in bacteria [449] and mammalian cells [450, 452]. The experiments of Klungsøyr et al. [455] suggest an interaction between the energy charge modulation and cumulative product inhibition in control of the activity of bacterial PP-ribose-P-synthetase.

Normal levels of PP-ribose-P range from 1 to 5 $\times 10^{-6}M$ in erythrocytes; and perhaps as high as $1.3 \times 10^{-5}M$ in fibroblasts in tissue culture [456]. These values are below the Michaelis constants for the PP-ribose-P-amidotransferases of bacteria [338], avian liver [337, 457], and mammalian adenocarcinoma cells [458], which range from 6×10^{-5} to $4.7 \times 10^{-4}M$.

Methylene blue will raise the intracellular concentration of PP-ribose-P in Ehrlich ascites cells in vitro [444], in human fibroblasts in tissue culture [445], and in human erythrocytes in vitro [446], presumably by accelerating the regeneration of NADP in the oxidative pathway of glucose metabolism and thereby stimulating the rate of production of ribose-5-phosphate. Purine biosynthesis *de novo* is enhanced. PP-ribose-P synthesis is also stimulated in vitro by glucose, fructose, and mannose [444, 445]. Ingestion of fructose [459–463] or galactose, or rapid infusions of fructose, mannose, or glucose [461], lead to hyperuricemia and increased uric aciduria in man and animal. Patients with essential fructosuria due to fructokinase deficiency do not show this effect, but children with hereditary fructose intolerance associated with phosphofructaldolase deficiency and fructose-1-phosphate accumulation show marked responses following fructose ingestion or infusion [459]. In vivo, fructose induced hyperuricemia appears to result, at least in part, from rapid degradation of adenyl nucleotides [460], and effects the PP-ribose-P synthesis remain to be documented.

PP-ribose-P concentration values are elevated in cells with deficient hypoxanthine-guanine phosphoribosyltransferase activity [464]. PRT-deficient fibroblasts show accelerated rates of purine biosynthesis [464]. Intracellular PP-ribose-P concentrations may be reduced by stimulating PP-ribose-P consumption with allopurinol [465], orotic acid [466], adenine [445], or 2, 6-diaminopurine [445]. Such measures reduce the rate of purine biosynthesis *de novo,* except in PRT-deficient cells which have a surfeit of PP-ribose-P [446].

L-Glutamine

This compound is often regarded as a storage form of ammonia-N:

$$\alpha\text{-Ketoglutarate} + NH_3 + NADH + H^+ \rightleftharpoons \text{L-glutamate} + H_2O + NAD^+$$

$$\text{L-Glutamate} + NH_3 + ATP \longrightarrow \text{L-glutamine} + H_2O + P_i + ADP$$

The reversible fixation of ammonia by α-ketoglutarate is catalyzed by glutamic acid dehydrogenase, an enzyme subject to complex regulation by purine ribonucleotides and certain steroids. Frieden [467] has discussed the possibility that the inhibition of glutamic acid dehydrogenase, which catalyzes a reaction usually operating to convert glutamic acid to α-ketoglutaric acid, may indirectly influence the rate of glutamine synthesis and, therefore, of purine synthesis.

The reaction of L-glutamate, NH_3, and ATP is catalyzed by glutamine synthetase, an enzyme found in high activity in liver [468], cerebral cortex [469], and rat kidney [470], but apparently absent from dog kidney [470, 471]. Glutamine synthetase of *E. coli* is a polymeric enzyme which requires adenylylation by ATP for conversion from an inactive to an active state [472]. The active enzyme is subject to cumulative end-product inhibition: each of eight end products of pathways entered by glutamine contributes a fractional inhibition of residual enzyme activity; all eight end products are required in saturating concentrations for complete inhibition. These include glycine, alanine, histidine, tryptophan, glucosamine-6-phosphate, carbamylphosphate, and CTP, as well as AMP an end product of the purine biosynthetic pathway [473]. Glutamine synthetase is also inhibited both in vivo and in vitro by the phosphorylated derivative of methionine sulfoximine [474, 475].

Liver, brain, and kidney of all species studied are rich in glutamine [476]. L-Glutamine of plasma is the immediate precursor of perhaps 80 percent of urinary ammonia [477, 478]. Two glutaminases are present in the kidney and liver [479, 480]. One, designated as glutaminase I, is activated (or stabilized) by phosphate [471, 481, 482] and splits off the amide nitrogen of glutamine to form glutamic acid and ammonia. Its pH optimum is 8; it is found in the mitochondria. The other, designated as glutaminase II, is in reality a glutamine-transaminase-ω-deamidase system and is activated by α-keto acids. Alpha-ketoglutaramide is the hypothetical direct precursor of ammonia [483]. The pH optimum of this enzyme is about 9, and it is found in the soluble fraction of the cell.

Normal human fibroblasts grown in a glutamine-free medium for 1 or 2 days show a roughly linear increase in purine synthesis with increasing glutamine concentrations, the maximal stimulation being five to tenfold [447]. The stimulation of purine biosynthesis *de novo* by a high protein diet in both normal and gouty man [484] may operate by providing additional glutamine. The K_m of glutamine in the first reaction is $5.4 \times 10^{-4}M$ with rat liver enzyme [337] and 7.5×10^{-4} to $1.1 \times 10^{-3}M$ with pigeon liver enzyme [337, 457, 485]. The plasma level of glutamine in both normal and gouty man is about $7 \times 10^{-4}M$ [419].

Glutamine Phosphoribosylpyrophosphate Amidotransferase

Properties of the Enzyme

The enzyme has been studied in bacteria [338], yeast [486], pigeon, chicken, and rat liver [337, 457, 485], Ehrlich ascites cells [487, 488], and adenocarcinoma 755 cells [458]. The avian enzyme has a molecular weight of about 200,000, and dissociates into electrophoretically identical subunits of 50,000 mol. wt. There is nothing unusual about the amino acid composition. The enzyme is activated by PP-ribose-P and Mg^{++}, which are required for the subsequent binding of glutamine. A plot of velocity versus substrate concentration is sigmoidal with respect to PP-ribose-P, linear with respect to glutamine. With the most highly purified enzyme from pigeon liver the K_m value of PP-ribose-P is $6 \times 10^{-5}M$, of Mg^{++} is $3 \times 10^{-4}M$, and of glutamine is $7.5 \times 10^{-4}M$ [457]. Optimal pH is about 8. The enzyme contains 12 atoms of nonheme iron per 200,000 mol. wt.

End-product Inhibition

The enzyme is inhibited by purine-5′-ribonucleotides, but not by purine deoxyribonucleotides, 2′, 3′ ribonucleotides, ribonucleosides, or bases, or by pyrimidine compounds [336]. The K_i values for various ribonucleotide inhibitors range from 10^{-5} to $10^{-3}M$ (Table 39-6). The enzyme may be desensitized to its inhibitors without loss of catalytic activity. The enzyme has two inhibitor-binding sites, one for 6-aminopurine and one for 6-hydroxypurine ribonucleotides, and both sites appear to be distinct from either substrate site. Some of the iron atoms are concerned with inhibitor binding, others appear to be involved in maintaining the tetramer structure [457]. The sigmoidal kinetics observed with the variation of PP-ribose-P concentrations are greatly accentuated in the presence of ribonucleotide inhibitors [485]. The inhibitory effects of AMP and GMP acting in concert are more than additive. These results define a cooperative end-product control of purine biosynthesis, which is maximal when the two types of negative effectors are present in optimal concentration and ratio [337, 338, 488]. The cooperative nature of the inhibition permits a more effective curtailment of the first reaction when both types of inhibitor are present in abundance, but allows for a more moderate control when only one kind is in excess.

Enzyme Derepression

Bacteria which require purines for growth will show remarkable increases in the activity of several of the purine biosynthetic enzymes, including the amidotransferase, when grown in limiting amounts of purines [442, 443]. There are indications that derepression of enzymes of purine synthesis may also occur in mammalian cells growing in tissue culture on marginal concentrations of purines [489]. In general, however, the changes in enzyme activity that can be attributed to different nutritional or metabolic conditions are small compared with those observed in bacteria [490]. Swiss mice infected with Friend leukemia virus show a marked increase in the activity of splenic glutamine-PP-ribose-P-amidotransferase, which shows a preference for NH_4Cl as a substrate and exhibits greater sensitivity to 6-amino than to 6-hydroxypurine ribonucleotide inhibitors [491, 492].

Nucleotide Regulators

The intracellular concentration of purine nucleotides tend to fall as nucleotides are removed by conversion into macromolecules of RNA and DNA, by consumption in other

Table 39-6. MICHAELIS CONSTANTS FOR GLUTAMINE PP-RIBOSE-P AMIDOTRANSFERASE

		References
Substrate	K_m*, M	
Glutamine	7.5×10^{-4} to 1.1×10^{-3}	[325, 336, 337, 338, 338*a*, 457, 458, 485]
PP-ribose-P	6.0×10^{-5} to 2.4×10^{-4}	
Mg^{++}	3.0×10^{-4}	
Inhibitor	K_i*, M	
AMP	9.2×10^{-5} to 2.5×10^{-3}	[336, 337]
ADP	3.8×10^{-5} to 6.4×10^{-4}	
IMP	1.8×10^{-4} to 3.5×10^{-3}	
GMP	8.6×10^{-5} to 3.5×10^{-3}	
GDP	3.8×10^{-4} to 5.4×10^{-3}	
6-Mercaptopurine-ribonucleoside monophosphate (RP)†	4.2 to 8.5×10^{-5}	
6-Thioguanine-RP†	1.7 to 2.0×10^{-4}	[378]
8-Azaguanine-RP†	5.4×10^{-4}	
Allopurinol-RP†	6×10^{-4}	

* Values vary with source of enzyme and stage of purification.

† These K_i values were obtained with an enzyme preparation with which AMP gave a value of $1 \times 10^{-3}M$.

biosynthetic reactions, or by degradative processes. Nucleotide concentrations are maintained within physiological levels by the salvage of purine bases and their reconversion to ribonucleotides, by such additional biosynthesis *de novo* as is required, and by interconversion of purine ribonucleotide base forms. Low concentrations of adenyl or guanyl ribonucleotides, or an unfavorable ratio between them, release glutamine-PP-ribose-P-amidotransferase from end-product inhibition and allow synthesis *de novo* to proceed. There are in addition complex regulatory mechanisms for maintaining the optimal distribution of various purine nucleotide forms, and for coordinating the activities of purine and pyrimidine biosynthetic pathways.

Regulation of Synthesis of AMP and GMP from IMP

The synthesis of AMP from IMP involves a two-step reaction sequence, the first of which is irreversible and requires GTP as a source of energy [368]. This reaction is inhibited by AMP [493]. The synthesis of GMP from IMP also involves two reaction steps. The first is irreversible and is inhibited by GMP [494]. The second requires ATP as an energy source. The combined influences of "forward" control, based on the availability of GTP and ATP [495], each of which is concerned with the synthesis of the other nucleotide, and of feedback inhibition, by which AMP and GMP each controls its own biosynthesis, may regulate the intracellular level of adenyl and guanyl nucleotides. AMP may be converted to IMP by adenylic deaminase and thus potentially serve as a source of guanyl ribonucleotides. Adenylic deaminase is stimulated by ATP and strongly inhibited by GTP [496]. Free guanine may be deaminated and reduced to hypoxanthine in mammalian tissue [497], and GMP may be converted to IMP in bacteria [494]. Thus guanine compounds may potentially serve as sources of adenyl ribonucleotides.

Regulation of Phosphoribosyltransferases

Adenine phosphoribosyltransferase is inhibited by AMP [376]. Hypoxanthine-guanine phosphoribosyltransferase is inhibited by IMP and GMP whether the substrate is hypoxanthine or guanine [379]. The inhibitions are formally competitive against PP-ribose-P, and appear to involve product inhibition at the substrate site [379].

Regulation of Ribonucleotide Reductase

Formation of deoxyribonucleotides involves reduction of the ribose moiety at the 2 position. This occurs only in nucleotide linkage. In *Leishamania,* reduction occurs at the nucleoside triphosphate level [498]. In *E. coli,* Novikoff hepatoma and rat embryo reduction occur at the nucleoside diphosphate level [499–502]. Ribonucleoside diphosphate reductases are subject to complex regulation. Reduction of ADP to dADP is inhibited by dATP, but stimulated by dGTP. Reduction of GDP to dGDP is inhibited by dGTP but stimulated by ATP. Both purine ribonucleoside diphosphate reductions are stimulated by thymidine triphosphate (TTP). By contrast, reductions of pyrimidine ribonucleoside diphosphates are inhibited by all deoxyribonucleoside triphosphates and stimulated by ATP [501].

Integration of Controls

These relationships illustrate the existence of a complex coordination of purine and pyrimidine deoxyribonucleotide biosynthesis in both bacterial and mammalian cells. Reciprocal controls also operate at the initial reaction of pyrimidine synthesis. In *E. coli,* aspartate transcarbamylase, the enzyme catalyzing the initial reaction of pyrimidine biosynthesis, is inhibited by CTP. The inhibition is blocked and the enzyme stimulated by ATP [503]. Mammalian aspartate transcarbamylase is insensitive to pyrimidine or purine ribonucleotides, and control of pyrimidine biosynthesis appears to operate at the prior step, that of the synthesis of carbamyl phosphate (see Chap. 42). Extramitochondrial carbamyl phosphate synthetase, which is thought to be concerned with pyrimidine rather than urea synthesis, is inhibited by pyrimidine ribonucleotides [379].

The major known regulatory mechanisms for coordinating purine biosynthesis *de novo,* purine base salvage, nucleotide interconversions, and the removal of nucleotides into macromolecules are shown in Fig. 39-14. The reader should bear in mind that certain of the regulations have been demonstrated with bacterial enzymes and have not yet been studied in animal systems.

Pharmacologic Control of Purine Biosynthesis

Inhibition

Purine biosynthesis *de novo* can be inhibited by compounds which compete for PP-ribose-P in phosphoribosyltransferase reactions. Included in this group are orotic acid [466, 504], allopurinol [465, 505], adenine [480], and 2,6-diamino purine [481], all of which have been shown to reduce intracellular PP-ribose-P levels in erythrocytes in vivo and in cultured fibroblasts in vitro. The glutamine analogues, aza-L-serine [506–509] and 6-diazo-5-oxo-L-norleucine (DON) [506, 510], inhibit the three steps of purine synthesis in which L-glutamine serves as substrate. The enzyme which catalyzes the conversion of FGAR to FGAM is a 100-fold more sensitive to azaserine than is glutamine-PP-ribose-P-amidotransferase [506]. Azaserine blocks the formation of a γ-glutamyl-enzyme complex through the formation of a stable compound with a sulfhydryl group on the enzyme surface [353, 354]. As a result FGAR accumulates in intact cells

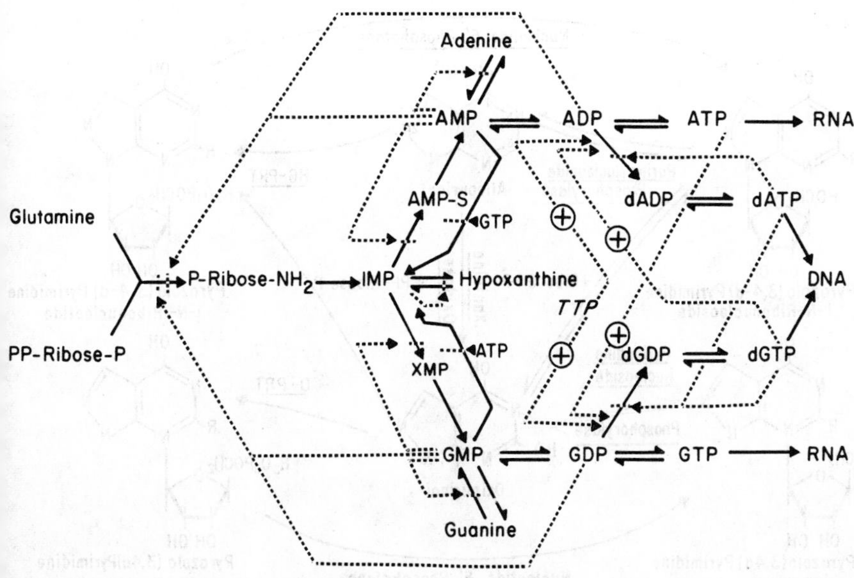

Figure 39-14. Summary of feedback controls operating upon reactions of purine biosynthesis and utilization. Reactions are shown by heavy solid arrows. Controls are shown by dotted lines and bars. All controls are negative (inhibitory), except those of ATP, dGTP, and TTP indicated by ⊕ symbol.

[440, 487], or in tissue cultures [505] treated with azaserine. In studies with such cells, the incorporation of labeled precursor into the accumulated FGAR provides an index of purine synthesis *de novo.* Both azaserine [511] and DON [512] have been shown to inhibit purine synthesis in man, but they are too toxic for therapeutic use.

The purine analogues, 6-mercaptopurine, 6-thioguanine, 8-azaguanine, allopurinol, and 6-methylmercaptopurine ribonucleoside, inhibit the accumulation of FGAR in azaserine-treated tissues [439, 440, 513, 514] and the accumulation of AICAR in a bacterial purine auxotroph [515]. The inhibitions depend upon prior conversion of the base to ribonucleotide. Cultured fibroblasts deficient in PRT activity are resistant to the lethal action of 6-mercaptopurine, 8-azaguanine, and 6-thioguanine, all of which require PRT activity for conversion to their nucleotide form [439, 514]. The ribonucleotide derivatives of these bases and of allopurinol act as pseudofeedback inhibitors of glutamine phosphoribosylpyrophosphate amidotransferase [378, 514]. Approximate K_i values of these inhibitors are shown in Table 39-6.

5-Aminoimidazole-4-carboxamide (AIC) [516], adenine [517], 6-thiopurine [518], and azathioprine [519, 520] inhibit purine synthesis *de novo* when administered in large doses in man. The effects of azathioprine (6-imidazolylthiopurine) in inhibiting purine synthesis *de novo* are probably dependent upon its hydrolysis to 6-mercaptopurine and conversion of the latter substance to ribonucleotide form. Azathioprine does not inhibit purine synthesis in patients who are deficient in PRT activity [520, 521]. Adenine exhibits its effect even in PRT-deficient fibroblasts in culture, which have very high levels of PP-ribose-P and are resistant to the inhibition of purine biosynthesis by agents such as orotic acid which also compete with glutamine for this substrate [522]. Accordingly, the inhibition of purine synthesis *de novo* by AIC and adenine probably represents the activation of endogenous feedback control mechanisms by normal nucleotides derived from these bases, rather than competition for PP-ribose-P. AIC, adenine, 6-thiopurine, and azathioprine are themselves catabolized in part to uric acid, so that the net change in serum urate concentration is often quite small in spite of the fact that they inhibit purine synthesis [516, 517, 519]. Hence, even if these drugs were nontoxic, their potential use as hypouricemic agents would be quite limited.

Methotrexate (4-amino-N^{10}-methylpteroylglutamic acid) inhibits the incorporation of single carbon fragments into positions 2 and 8 of the purine ring [362, 528] and thereby reduces purine synthesis in man [524]. Hadacidine (N-formyl hydroxyaminoacetic acid), an analogue of L-aspartate, inhibits the conversion of IMP to AMP-S [525, 526], in concentrations which appear to have little effect upon the conversion of C-AIR to SAICAR, a reaction in which aspartate also participates. Both methotrexate and hadacidine are too toxic for use as hypouricemic agents in man.

Xanthine Oxidase Inhibitors

Many inhibitors of xanthine oxidase are known, including 6-pteridylaldehyde [527] and various purine analogues such as adenine [528], 2,6-diaminopurine [528], 6-thiopurine [529, 530], 6-chloropurine [531], 4-diazoimidazole-5-carboxamide [532], symmetrical triazines [533], allopurinol [4-hydroxypyrazolo-(3,4-d)pyrimidine], and oxipurinol [2,4-dihydroxypyrazolo-(3,4-d)pyrimidine].

Allopurinol is an analogue of hypoxanthine in which the positions of N-7 and C-8 are reversed [534] (Fig. 39-15). It is a potent inhibitor of xanthine oxidase [535–537] and an agent of considerable importance in the control of hyperuricemia and uric acid calculus formation in man (see below). Allopurinol is metabolized to oxipurinol by xanthine

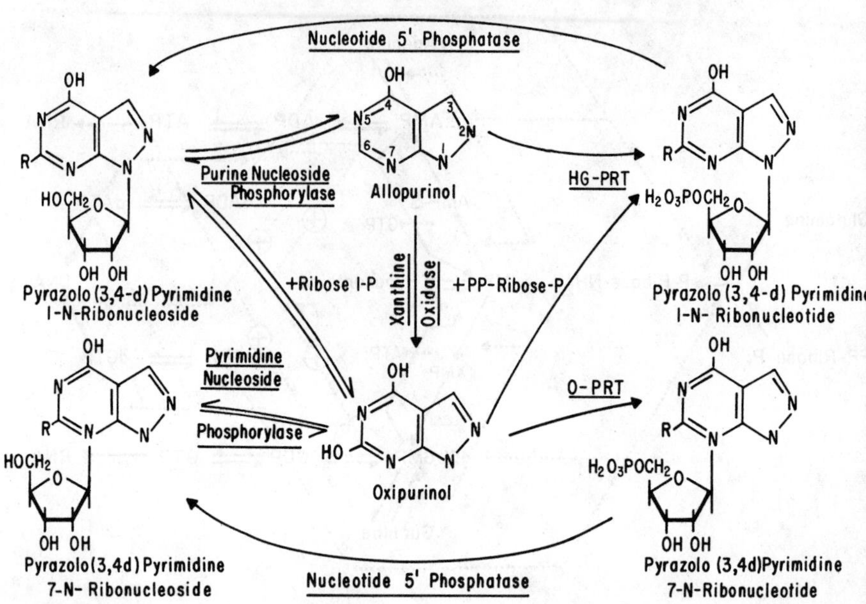

Figure 39-15. Reactions of allopurinol and of its oxidation product oxipurinol. Enzymes are underlined. R = H-(allopurinol) or HO-(oxipurinol).

oxidase [536]. Oxipurinol is also an inhibitor of xanthine oxidase. The Michaelis constant of allopurinol is some 15- to 200-fold lower than that of xanthine, whereas that of oxipurinol is comparable to that of xanthine [536] (Table 39-7). Allopurinol may show substrate-competitive kinetics. Both allopurinol and oxipurinol produce pseudoirreversible inactivation of xanthine oxidase: Inactivation occurs when allopurinol and the enzyme are incubated in the absence of substrate, but enzyme activity can be restored by prolonged dialysis. Oxipurinol has no effect on the enzyme alone, but inactivates it in the presence of xanthine [536, 536a, 537].

In man, there is no evidence for irreversible inactivation of xanthine oxidase, nor, for that matter, of enzyme induction. The maximum depression of the serum urate level is reached within a few days after beginning therapy, and remains relatively constant over prolonged periods [538, 539]. Withdrawal usually results in a return to pretreatment serum urate levels. Allopurinol has a very short biological half-life of only 2 to 3 hr [540]. Three to ten percent of an administered dose is excreted with a clearance rate approximately equal to the GFR [540]. The majority of allopurinol (45 to 65 percent) is rapidly oxidized to oxipurinol in vivo, with a portion being converted to 1-N-allopurinol ribonucleoside [541] and probably allopurinol-1-ribonucleotide [465]. Most of the oxipurinol formed is excreted unchanged by

Table 39-7. MICHAELIS CONSTANTS FOR XANTHINE OXIDASE

	Source of xanthine oxidase				Reference
	Human liver		Bovine cream		
	pH 7.4	pH 8.6	pH 7.4	pH 8.26	
Substrate (K_m, *M*)					
Hypoxanthine	—	—	—	8.4×10^{-6}	[528]
Xanthine	3.0×10^{-6}	4.1×10^{-5}	4.0×10^{-6}	—	[536]
		1.6×10^{-5}*	—	—	[417]
				5.4×10^{-6}	[528, 530]
6-Mercaptopurine	—	—	—	1.7×10^{-5}	[530]
Adenine	—	—	—	1.2×10^{-5}	[528]
Inhibitor (K_i, *M*)					
Adenine	—	—	—	1.1×10^{-5}	[528]
2,6-Diaminopurine	—	—	—	7.4×10^{-6}	[528]
6-Mercaptopurine	—	—	—	1.8×10^{-6}	[528]
Allopurinol	1.9×10^{-7}	2.0×10^{-7}	7.0×10^{-7}	—	[536]
Oxipurinol	1.1×10^{-6}	3.6×10^{-6}	6.3×10^{-6}	—	[536]

* Human intestinal xanthine oxidase (pH 8.3) [417].

the kidney with a relatively long half-life (28 hr) [540], although a small portion is metabolized to 7-N-ribosyloxipurinol (oxipurinol ribonucleoside) and perhaps to 1-N-ribosyloxipurinol [542] (Fig. 39-15). Factors which affect uric acid excretion generally alter oxipurinol excretion in a similar manner [542]. It has been suggested that oxipurinol rather than allopurinol, is primarily responsible for xanthine oxidase inhibition in vivo [536], but a direct comparison of the two drugs indicated that allopurinol was probably the more effective [543].

Allopurinol has a number of additional effects. Through its action upon xanthine oxidase it inhibits tryptophan pyrrolase [544], probably by limiting the availability of H_2O_2 for use by the latter enzyme [545, 546]. In vitro, allopurinol also inhibits purine nucleoside phosphorylase [383, 541] and pyrimidine deoxyribosyltransferase [547]. It activates, and at higher concentration inhibits, urate oxidase [548]. In ribonucleotide linkage, allopurinol inhibits early enzymes of both purine and pyrimidine biosynthesis. Its inhibition of glutamine phosphoribosylpyrophosphate amidotransferase was described above. The increased urinary excretion of orotic acid and orotidine in patients receiving allopurinol [549–551] has been traced to the inhibition of orotidylic decarboxylase by allopurinol ribonucleotide [550]. The action occurs also in PRT-deficient subjects [552]. Furthermore, high concentrations of both allopurinol and oxipurinol inhibit purine biosynthesis *de novo* in azaserine-treated PRT-deficient fibroblasts in culture [505]; they also inhibit the orotidylic decarboxylase of PRT-deficient cells [550]. It now appears that these actions are also dependent upon the presence of PP-ribose-P and upon the activity of another enzyme, orotate phosphoribosyltransferase, which converts oxipurinol to oxipurinol-7-N-ribonucleotide [436], analogous to the purine-3-N-ribonucleotides described above (Fig. 39-14).

Allopurinol therapy results in an eightfold increase in activity of both the orotate phosphoribosyltransferase and the orotidylic decarboxylase of erythrocytes, apparently through an activation mechanism rather than as an effect upon enzyme synthesis or turnover [552*a*].

Thiopurinol (mercapto pyrazolo-pyrimidine), although developed for use as a xanthine oxidase inhibitor, apparently reduces uric acid synthesis without a concomitant increase in oxypurine excretion [553]. This effect has also been postulated to reflect inhibition of purine biosynthesis *de novo,* although this hypothesis remains to be documented. Further discussion of the clinical use of allopurinol, and of its modified effects in PRT-deficient subjects are presented below. K_i values for a number of xanthine oxidase inhibitors are shown in Table 39-6.

Stimulation

2-Ethylamino-1, 3, 4-thiadiazole (EAT) has been found to cause marked hyperuricemia and hyperuricaciduria in man [554], by stimulation of purine synthesis *de novo* [555]. The effects of EAT are countermanded by the simultaneous administration of nicotinamide [555] or nicotinic acid [556]. In mice, EAT causes an enhanced incorporation of formate or glycine into acid-soluble adenine of liver [557]. In human beings receiving EAT, the incorporation of glycine into urinary uric acid resembles that found in gouty subjects with unequivocal overproduction of uric acid [556, 558]. The mechanism of the action of EAT remains unknown. Its action does not depend upon PRT activity, for children deficient in PRT treated with EAT show an even further acceleration of purine biosynthesis [559]. EAT does not alter the enzymatic activity of the purine sequence *de novo,* nor does it block the inhibition of amidotransferase by adenine ribonucleotides [560].

The effects of methylene blue, and of hexoses in stimulating uric acid synthesis have been discussed above.

PRODUCTION OF URIC ACID IN GOUT

Chemical Balance

In theory, the rate of purine synthesis may be assessed from the difference between purine intake and excretion in the dynamic steady state. In practice this approach fails because the urinary excretion of uric acid represents a variable fraction of total purine turnover, and there are no convenient methods for the measurement of extrarenal excretion of urate. Purine intake may be reduced to levels of less than 3 mg purine-N per day by severe dietary purine restriction. The average urinary uric acid value then becomes a minimal estimate of purine production. Values in normal adult males show a very wide range. Frequency histograms show skewness toward high values without evidence for bimodality. The normal range of urinary uric acid excretion has been defined on a statistical basis as representing the range, mean $\pm$ 2 s.d., of nongouty subjects studied under standard conditions of activity and dietary intake. Such values in normal adult males range from 278 to 558 mg per day (mean 418 $\pm$ 70 mg) [131], or from 264 to 588 mg per day (mean 426 $\pm$ 81 mg) [301].

The distribution of urinary uric acid values in males with primary gout extends from values of 150 mg per day or less to values of 1,500 mg per day or more. Low values are found in patients with overt renal damage. From 21 to 28 percent of subjects with primary gout consistently excrete quantities of urate exceeding the mean + 2 s.d. [131, 301]. Such patients have arbitrarily been classified as *overexcretors* of uric acid. The theoretical possibility that an increased urinary excretion is secondary to a decreased extrarenal disposal of urate has been excluded by normal urinary recoveries of injected labeled uric acid in the majority of overexcretor patients [301]. Therefore, sustained overexcretion of uric acid is evidence for excessive synthesis of purines *de novo.* However, a normal urinary excretion of uric acid does not exclude overproduction of uric acid in gouty subjects, for in the hyperuricemic subject with reduced renal urate excretion, the disposal of urate by extrarenal processes may be much increased, occasionally accounting for over 80 percent of the urate turnover [301].

In the past two decades the mechanisms and rates of uric acid production have been under intensive study by means of two general types of biochemical techniques: (1) the turnover study, employing principles of isotope dilution; and (2) precursor administration, with evaluation of the rate and extent of conversion of the administered substance into uric acid. More recently, studies of purine metabolism in gout have been amplified by direct enzyme assays in human tissue and by the use of cell culture techniques.

The Miscible Pool of Uric Acid and Its Turnover

The isotope dilution technique for the measurement of the miscible pool of uric acid and the rate of its turnover was introduced by Benedict et al. [561] in 1949. Isotopic uric acid is injected intravenously and permitted to mix intimately with uric acid in the body. Urinary uric acid is isolated serially for several days, and the isotope concentration of each sample is determined. Values are plotted on semilogarithmic coordinates, and the theoretical concentration of isotope in the body at the moment of mixing (I_0) is obtained by extrapolation of the decay curve to zero time. The *miscible pool* of uric acid is defined as the quantity of uric acid in the body of the recipient by which the injected uric acid is promptly diluted. The quantity of uric acid present in the miscible pool (A) may be readily calculated from knowledge of the amount of uric acid injected (a), of the concentration of isotope in it (I_i), and of the concentration of isotope in the uric acid of the body at the moment of mixing (I_0):

$$A = a\left(\frac{I_i}{I_0} - 1\right)$$

After mixing has occurred, a further progressive decline in the concentration of isotope in uric acid occurs because of the continuous dilution of the labeled uric acid pool by newly synthesized nonisotopic uric acid molecules. From the rate of this decline in isotope concentration, the rate of addition of unlabeled uric acid may be calculated [561]. In the normal subject, this addition may be presumed to represent newly synthesized uric acid. The majority of studies have employed the original technique of determining the isotope concentration of uric acid isolated from urine. Sorensen [307, 309] has injected uric acid-^{14}C intravenously and has calculated the specific activity of uric acid from the radioactivity value and uric acid content of a volume of serum, on the reasonable assumption (in man) that all ^{14}C in serum is in the form of uric acid.

In about 25 normal male subjects [301, 306, 307, 561–567, 579], the rapidly miscible pool was an average of 1,200 mg uric acid, with values ranging from 866 to 1,587 mg. In three normal females, the pool ranged from 541 to 687 mg [567, 579]. These values confirmed earlier analytic values of Gudzent [69].

From the rate of decline in concentration of ^{15}N or ^{14}C in urinary uric acid, it was calculated that from 45 to 85 percent of the uric acid of the miscible pool was normally replaced each day by newly formed, nonisotopic uric acid. The turnover of uric acid averaged 695 mg per day, with values ranging from 513 to 1,108 mg per day. In each case, the quantity of uric acid entering the pool exceeded the amount leaving it in urine by 100 to 260 mg uric acid per day [307, 561]. The significance of this surplus will be discussed below.

In gouty subjects, the miscible pool is generally enlarged to 2,000 to 4,000 mg in patients without tophi [301, 561, 564, 566] and may reach 18,000 to 31,000 mg in patients with severe tophaceous gout [562]. Even so, the value of the miscible pool may represent only a small fraction of the total urate in the body, for only the peripheral layers of tophi are readily exchangeable with urate in solution in body fluids [562]. In one patient, the amount of uric acid in the tophaceous compartment participating in a slow exchange with the soluble uric acid was estimated by Sorensen [309] to be 300 times the size of the rapidly miscible pool.

Because of the possibility of exchange of labeled urate of the miscible pool with unlabeled urate of the solid phase, the rate of change of isotope concentration of the soluble phase may not be a dependable measure of the synthesis of new urate in subjects with tophaceous gout. Even so, the derived value for turnover of urate often agrees very well with another calculation of rate of synthesis [200, 301], viz.,

$$\frac{\text{Basal urinary uric acid, mg per day}}{\text{Urinary recovery of injected isotopic uric acid, fraction of administered dose}}$$

In gouty patients whose miscible pool is within, or just above, the normal range it is sometimes possible to calculate that all the urate measured in the miscible pool is in solution. In two patients meeting these criteria, Sorensen [307] found excessive turnover of uric acid. However, in five patients also meeting these criteria, Seegmiller et al. [301] found a normal turnover of uric acid, and these five patients also showed normal incorporations of isotopic glycine into uric acid (see below).

Incorporation of Labeled Precursors into Uric Acid

The rate of generation of uric acid has been studied in both normal and gouty subjects by observing the rate at which isotope appears in uric acid when a labeled precursor is administered. Studies of this type have been performed with glycine-^{15}N, glycine-1-^{14}C, glycine-2-^{14}C, ammonium-^{15}N, formate-^{14}C, 4-aminoimidazole-5-carboxamide-4-^{13}C and -4-^{14}C, hypoxanthine-8-^{14}C, and adenine-8-^{14}C and -8-^{13}C.

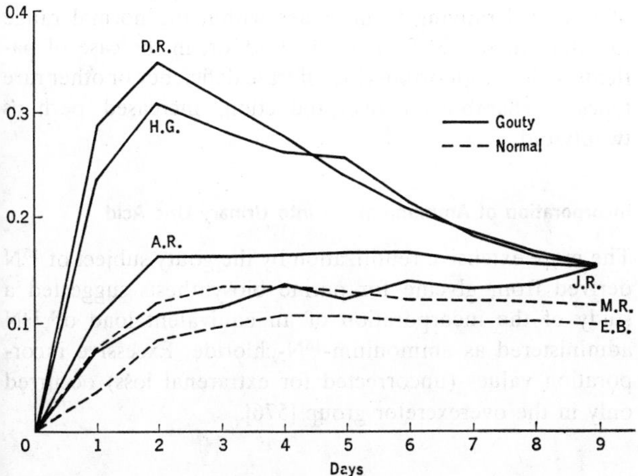

Figure 39-16. Concentration of ^{15}N in urinary uric acid following ingestion of glycine-^{15}N by normal and gouty subjects. (*From J. D. Benedict et al.* [554], *with permission of the J. Clin. Invest.*)

Incorporation of Labeled Glycine into Urinary Uric Acid

A large number of studies of the incorporation of labeled glycine into urinary uric acid have been performed since the technique was introduced by Benedict and associates in 1952 [568, 569] (Fig. 39-16). The following discussion is based on studies of the incorporation of glycine-1-^{14}C, glycine-U-^{14}C, and glycine-^{15}N under standardized experimental conditions. The few studies in which glycine-2-^{14}C was administered orally [570], or in which glycine-^{15}N was given in small amounts [571] will be omitted, since they are not strictly comparable.

Labeled glycine is given orally with a light breakfast [568], or injected intravenously [309] after the subject has been prepared with a very low purine diet for about 5 days. The labeled glycine will be diluted with glycine of dietary origin and by glycine of various intracellular and extracellular pools. Variations in the amount of diluting unlabeled glycine and in the size and turnover of the hepatic glycine pool will influence the specific activity of uric acid, quite apart from differences in the rates of purine synthesis. In addition, differences in the sizes of the pools of intermediates of purine synthesis and of uric acid will be reflected in corresponding influences upon the specific activity of uric acid. Because many of these variables are beyond the ability of the investigator to control or to assess in a quantitative manner, the significance of small differences in results found in nongouty and certain gouty subjects is difficult to evaluate.

Glycine-1-^{14}C can be given in tracer doses of a few milligrams, whereas with glycine-^{15}N doses of 0.1 gm per kg are required. The latter quantity of glycine-^{15}N is approximately equal to that of the free glycine pool in man, which is 80 to 90 mg per kg [570, 572]. Since glycine enters the purine sequence beyond the rate-limiting step of purine synthesis, one would anticipate that approximately one-half as much isotope would be incorporated into uric acid when such a glycine load is given as when a tracer dose is given. Average incorporation values for ^{14}C and ^{15}N in control and gouty subjects (Fig. 39-16) as well as a direct appraisal of this question in four control subjects given glycine-1-^{14}C with and without carrier glycine [570] confirm this prediction.

The studies of Benedict et al. [568, 569] established that the incorporation of glycine-^{15}N into urinary uric acid was excessive in gouty subjects with abnormally large excretions of urate but normal or only slightly elevated in those subjects with normal excretion values. Subsequent studies with glycine-^{15}N and with glycine-1-^{14}C have confirmed and extended these observations. Figure 39-17 summarizes the majority of published incorporation values observed in studies in which glycine-1-^{14}C or -U-^{14}C was administered. Those in which glycine-^{15}N were employed have been summarized elsewhere [570]. In gouty subjects with uric acid

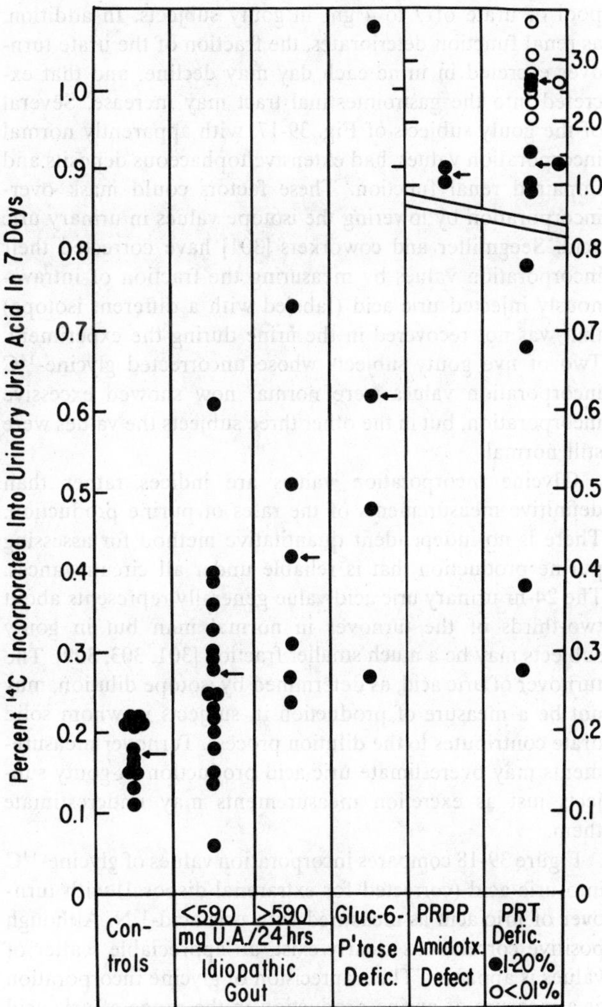

Figure 39-17. Summary of incorporations of glycine-1-^{14}C and glycine U-^{14}C into urinary uric acid. Values represent data from published studies [200, 301, 512, 568–581] in which glycine was administered to subjects on purine-restricted diets.

excretions of less than 590 mg per day, the cumulative incorporation of ^{15}N is normal in six of seven instances, whereas that of ^{14}C is excessive in one-half to two-thirds of the cases. In subjects with excretions of more than 590 mg per day, both tracers are incorporated excessively. The plots of specific activity, or of cumulative incorporation against time, show a considerable heterogeneity in both control and gouty subjects. The values plotted represent incorporations during the 7 days following the administration of isotope, although the incorporations are by no means linear for this period in most subjects. However, the conclusions would not be materially altered by plotting values representing 1- or 2-day incorporations.

Incorporation of Labeled Glycine into Total Body Uric Acid

Newly synthesized isotopic urate will mix with a miscible pool of urate of 2 to 4 gm in gouty subjects. In addition, as renal function deteriorates, the fraction of the urate turnover excreted in urine each day may decline, and that excreted into the gastrointestinal tract may increase. Several of the gouty subjects of Fig. 39-17, with apparently normal incorporation values, had extensive tophaceous deposits and impaired renal function. These factors could mask overincorporation by lowering the isotope values in urinary uric acid. Seegmiller and coworkers [301] have corrected their incorporation values by measuring the fraction of intravenously injected uric acid (labeled with a different isotope) that was not recovered in the urine during the experiment. Two of five gouty subjects whose uncorrected glycine-^{14}C incorporation values were normal now showed excessive incorporation, but in the other three subjects the values were still normal.

Glycine incorporation values are indices rather than definitive measurements of the rates of purine production. There is no independent quantitative method for assessing purine production that is reliable under all circumstances. The 24-hr urinary uric acid value generally represents about two-thirds of the turnover in normal man but in gouty subjects may be a much smaller fraction [301, 303, 309]. The turnover of uric acid, as determined by isotope dilution, may not be a measure of production in subjects in whom solid urate contributes to the dilution process. Turnover measurements may overestimate uric acid production in gouty subjects just as excretion measurements may underestimate them.

Figure 39-18 compares incorporation values of glycine-^{14}C into uric acid (corrected for extrarenal disposal) with turnover of uric acid as measured with uric acid-^{15}N. Although positive correlations clearly exist, an appreciable scatter of values is apparent. The imprecision of glycine incorporation as a measure of purine production in the range of uric acid turnover of 500 to 1,200 mg per day, in which the turnovers of the majority of gouty subjects fall, is clear. Taken altogether, the glycine incorporation studies suggest that subjects with primary gout show a spectrum of rates of production of uric acid ranging from values within the normal range to values increased four- or fivefold, or, in the case of patients with phosphoribosyltransferase deficiency or other rare types of flamboyant overproduction, increased perhaps twentyfold.

Incorporation of Ammonium-^{15}N into Urinary Uric Acid

The more extensive reutilization by the gouty subject of ^{15}N derived from glycine for purine biosynthesis suggested a study of the incorporation of an equivalent load of ^{15}N administered as ammonium-^{15}N-chloride. Excessive incorporation values (uncorrected for extrarenal loss) occurred only in the overexcretor group [576].

Incorporation of Formate-^{14}C into Urinary Uric Acid

The incorporation of formate-^{14}C into urinary uric acid is excessive in gouty patients with excessive excretion values of uric acid and is normal in patients with normal urinary excretion values [70, 583, 584]. Erratic results, bearing no relationship to urinary urate values, have been reported in patients in whom experimental conditions were not standardized [567].

Incorporation of Glycine, 5-Aminoimidazole-4-Carboxamide, Hypoxanthine, or Adenine into Urinary Uric Acid and Purine Bases

In both nongouty and gouty subjects, 5-aminoimidazole-4-carboxamide (AIC) [516, 586] and adenine [517] are rapidly converted to uric acid. The pathways of utilization involve initial conversion to ribonucleotide forms [326] (Reaction 16). Seegmiller, et al. found that in normal man

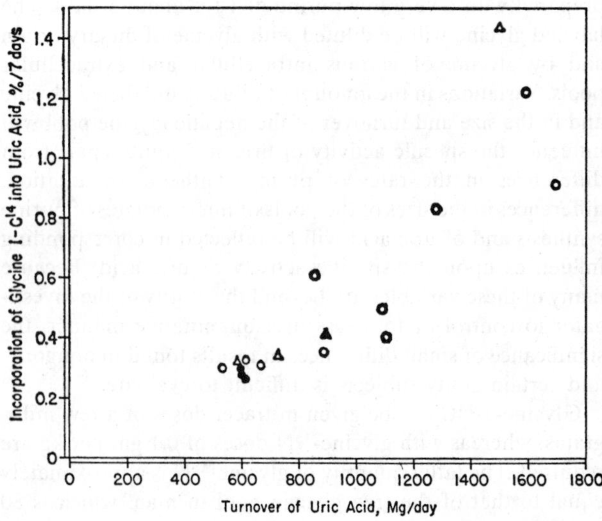

Figure 39-18. Comparison of incorporation of glycine-1-^{14}C into uric acid and turnover of uric acid. The incorporation values have been corrected for extrarenal disposal. (*Replotted from Seegmiller et al.* [301].)

approximately 20 percent of administered AIC-^{13}C was excreted in urine as uric acid in 14 days [516]. There was a biphasic incorporation, consisting of a prompt and extensive conversion of ingested AIC-^{13}C into uric acid, followed by a slower, less direct conversion process. In all of five gouty subjects studied [586], incorporation of AIC into uric acid was somewhat greater than normal irrespective of urinary urate excretion. The degree of abnormality was magnified when appropriate corrections were made for dilution factors within the urate pool and for uricolysis, on the basis of simultaneous studies with uric acid-^{14}C.

In a similar study with adenine-8-^{13}C, Seegmiller et al. [517] found a prompt incorporation of ^{13}C into urinary uric acid, with maximal labeling on the first or second day, and a first-order decline in isotope abundance thereafter. Three gouty subjects, who were known overproducers of uric acid and overincorporators of glycine-^{15}N, incorporated twice as much ^{13}C into urate as did two controls.

When AIC or adenine was administered together with glycine-^{15}N a marked and comparable suppression of the incorporation of ^{15}N into urinary uric acid was observed in normal and gouty subjects [516, 517]. This probably resulted from the activation of feedback inhibition of purine synthesis by nucleotides derived from AIC or adenine, rather than from the diversion of PP-ribose-P from the pathway of purine synthesis *de novo,* for reasons discussed below.

Further indications of the complexity of pathways between IMP and uric acid came from studies of the incorporation of labeled glycine or labeled purine bases into urinary purine bases in nongouty and gouty subjects [587–589]. Following the administration of glycine-1-^{14}C, there is a prompt and

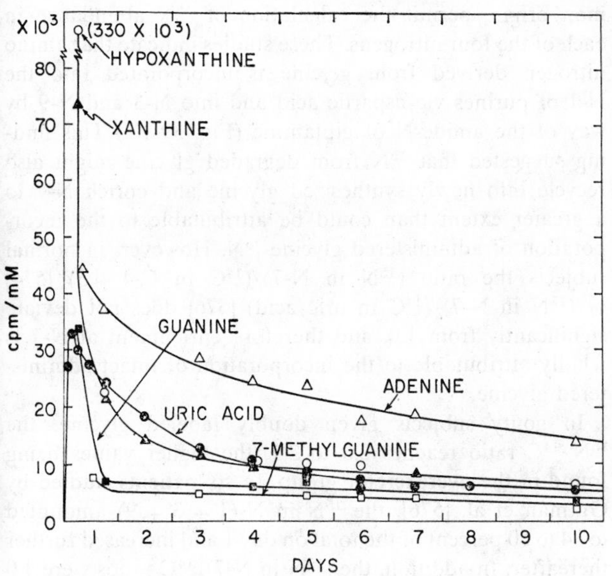

Figure 39-19. Specific activity values of urinary purines in a patient with chronic myelogenous leukemia following the intravenous administration of AIC-4-^{14}C. (*From J. B. Wyngaarden* [589], *with permission of Metabolism.*)

striking labeling of urinary hypoxanthine, indicative of the operation of an IMP cleavage pathway. Early labeling of adenine and 7-methylguanine suggest that other nucleotides are also subject to cleavage shortly after formation. Early labeling of 7-methylguanine, now known to be a constituent of DNA, and soluble and ribosomal RNAs [404] was particularly impressive in gouty subjects [587]. Labeled hypoxanthine administered intravenously is promptly converted to uric acid. Labeled adenine in tracer dose is only slowly and sparingly converted to uric acid [588], in contrast to larger doses which are converted to uric acid more promptly [517]. Labeled AIC gives rise to extensive labeling of all urinary purine bases, in particular hypoxanthine and xanthine [588] (Fig. 39-19). These findings strengthen the concept that IMP cleavage contributes to the rapid synthesis of uric acid in normal and gouty man. The findings that urinary-7-methylguanine is labeled promptly in gouty subjects and that excretion of 5-ribosyluracil (pseudouridine) (an important constituent of soluble and ribosomal RNA [403, 405]) may be increased in gouty subjects [590, 591] suggest that certain species of RNA may also turn over sufficiently rapidly to contribute to the hyperuricemia of gout.

Overproduction of Uric Acid in Gout

All the tracer studies discussed thus far involve the isolation of uric acid from urine and the determination of its isotopic enrichment, following the administration of labeled uric acid or some labeled precursor of uric acid. These studies have demonstrated the overproduction of uric acid in a substantial percentage of gouty subjects, but have not disclosed the mechanism.

Present concepts of control of purine synthesis *de novo* suggest three general categories of abnormalities which may potentially lead to overproduction of uric acid [592]. These are (1) metabolic defects, remote or proximate, which increase the *substrate levels* of L-glutamine or phosphoribosylpyrophosphate; (2) defects which increase the *amount* or intrinsic *activity* of the first enzyme of the pathway of purine synthesis; or (3) defects which reduce the concentrations of one or more *negative effectors* (nucleotide inhibitors) of the first enzyme.

Studies of mechanisms of hyperuricemia in primary gout of idiopathic varieties will be presented first. Information on hyperuricemia and gout occurring as a consequence of known specific enzyme defects will be presented below.

The Role of L-Glutamine in Gout

Amino Acids and Urinary Ammonia Production in Gout

Plasma glutamine values are normal in gout, and range from 7 to 10 mg per 100 ml, or 0.5 to 0.7 μmoles per ml [419, 593–595]. Concentration values of total amino acids in plasma, exclusive of proline and aspartic acid, are about 2.7

μmoles per ml in both nongouty [594, 596] and gouty subjects [593–595]. One report of hyperaminoacidemia in gout (2.6 μmoles per ml) is probably attributable to low values in the control groups (2.02 μmoles per ml) which included a large number of hospitalized subjects recovering from acute infectious illnesses [593]. Reported elevations of individual plasma amino acid values in gout largely disappear when protein intakes are standardized in the two groups [594]. An exception is glutamic acid, which remain higher than in controls [594, 595] even after casein loading of both groups [595]. Values in gouty subjects average 68 or 72 μmoles per ml compared with 45 or 51 μmoles per ml in controls [594, 595]. Plasma glycine values are distinctly lower in gouty subjects than in controls, and serine values are slightly so [594].

Renal clearances of several amino acids are less in gouty subjects than in controls [594, 597]. Deficits of some degree persisted for glutamine, serine, and threonine even after protein restriction. By far the most conspicuous deficit found in the gouty subjects was in the urinary excretion and clearance of glutamine. Following glutamine loading, plasma glutamine levels rose and fell indistinguishably in gouty and control subjects, but the differences in glutamine excretion and clearance persisted [594].

Gutman and Yü [184] have reported that when glycine-^{15}N is administered to gouty normal and overexcretor subjects, the first-day and cumulative ammonium-^{15}N values are less than found in control subjects with equivalently acid urines. In three subjects in each category, the average cumulative values in 7 days were 3.38 percent of administered ^{15}N in controls, 2.54 percent in gouty normal excretors, and 1.61 percent in gouty overexcretors. The enrichment values were the same in all groups: 2.61 to 2.72 atom percent excess ^{15}N. The deficit was attributed to a decrease in the quantity of ammonia produced in the gouty subjects. The ammonium/creatinine ratios were found to average 0.27 ± 0.09 in 77 gouty subjects as compared to 0.41 ± 0.10 in 17 nongouty subjects with comparable urinary pH values [184]. In 83 gouty subjects [177] with a urinary pH <5.7 the mean net deficit in the elimination of ammonia was 8 μEq per min in comparison with 46 nongouty controls excreting urine of the same pH. Yü et al. [177] have suggested that the increased tubular reabsorption of glutamine, and reduced urinary excretion of ammonia in primary gout (overexcretors and normoexcretors alike) are related in some way (see Glutaminase Hypothesis, below).

Plante et al. [183] noted that the apparent defect in ammonium excretion in gouty subjects was not present in patients on a low purine diet, but they did not control their studies with reexaminations of the same patients on normal or high purine diets. Metcalfe-Gibson et al. [179] found no abnormally low values of ammonium excretion in hyperuricemic subjects with creatinine clearance values above 65 ml per min. A low ammonium/titratable acidity ratio has been a well-known consequence of renal disease since the studies of Henderson and Palmer [598]. Tubular ammonia production also declines with age [599]. In gouty patients the earliest recognizable renal changes, as observed by both light and electron microscopy, involve the tubules [163]. Thus, even a normal glomerular filtration rate in gouty subjects may not exclude an acquired deficit in tubular function. Furthermore, values of ammonia production in gouty subjects show a very extensive overlap with normal values, even though mean values are different [177]. The significance of the deficit in urinary excretion of ammonium with respect to uric acid production and hyperuricemia in gouty subjects remains conjectural.

Intramolecular Distribution of ^{14}C or ^{15}N in Urinary Uric Acid

Glycine-1-^{14}C serves as a specific label of C-4 of the purine ring. No significant recycling of isotope from the degradation products of glycine into other carbon atoms of uric acid is detected in normal [570, 574] or gouty subjects [570]. When glycine-1-^{14}C, α-^{15}N is administered, the $^{15}N/^{14}C$ ratio in urinary uric acid is significantly above 1.0 in both nongouty and gouty subjects, indicating a greater incorporation of ^{15}N than can be attributed to the entry of the intact glycine molecule into the eventual purine structure [570, 574].

When the urate molecule is degraded into fractions representing N-7 and N-(1 + 3 + 9), the latter fraction is found to contain 23 to 34 percent of the total ^{15}N on day 1 and as much as 39 to 50 percent by day 7 in normal subjects [317, 574, 576]. Additional dissections of the molecule into fractions representing N-(1 + 3) and N-(7 + 9) [184] or N-(1 + 7) [574], and the assumption that the isotopic abundances of N-3 and N-9 are identical in view of their common origin, permit the calculation of ^{15}N abundance in each of the four nitrogens. These studies indicate that amino nitrogen derived from glycine is incorporated into the N-1 of purines via aspartic acid and into N-3 and N-9 by way of the amide-N of glutamine (Fig. 39-10.) This finding suggested that ^{15}N from degraded glycine might also recycle into newly synthesized glycine and enrich N-7 to a greater extent than could be attributable to the incorporation of administered glycine-^{15}N. However, in normal subjects the ratio (^{15}N in N-7)/(^{14}C in C-4 + 5) [574] or (^{15}N in N-7)/(^{14}C in uric acid) [576] does not deviate significantly from 1.0, and therefore enrichment at N-7 is wholly attributable to the incorporation of intact administered glycine.

In gouty subjects given doubly labeled glycine, the $^{15}N/^{14}C$ ratio reaches 2.0 to 2.9, the higher values being found in the overexcretor group. In six patients studied by Gutman et al. [576], the ^{15}N in N-(1 + 3 + 9) amounted to 34 to 50 percent of the total on day 1 and increased further thereafter. In addition, the (^{15}N in N-7)/^{14}C ratios were 1.0 to 1.3 in a normal excretor and 1.2 to 1.6 in two overexcretors, signifying the recycling of reconstituted glycine back into purine biosynthesis in these gouty subjects.

Hypothesis of Abnormal Glutamine Metabolism in Primary Gout

Further dissection of the urate molecule by Gutman and Yü [184] disclosed that the increase in percentage of ^{15}N in the N-(1 + 3 + 9) fraction in gouty subjects was accounted for by an increase in the percentage of ^{15}N in N-(3 + 9), relative to values observed in their control subjects. Representative values in three control subjects, three gouty normal excretors, and three gouty overexcretors are shown in Table 39-8. The percentage of the dose of glycine-^{15}N excreted as ammonium-^{15}N (see above) was found to be reduced in the gouty subjects of this study. This finding was attributed to a reduced rate of urinary ammonia excretion in the presence of normal or increased titratable acidity and normal or low urinary pH in gouty subjects. The preferential increase of labeling of N-(3 + 9) and the reduced excretion of ammonia in these gouty subjects (see above) suggested to Gutman and Yü [184] that there was a deviation of the amide nitrogen of glutamine from ammonia production into purine synthesis *de novo* in gout.

THE GLUTAMINASE HYPOTHESIS: On the basis of these findings a block of glutaminase I was proposed [176, 184]. This hypothesis, as originally stated, has now been disproved by the finding of normal activities of phosphate-activated glutaminase (glutaminase I), pyruvate-activated glutaminase (glutaminase II), and nonactivated glutaminase in renal biopsy tissue from four gouty subjects by Pollak and Mattenheimer [600]. In rebuttal, Yü and Gutman have called attention to the scatter of enzyme assay results on tissue obtained by biopsy and have cited the need for a functional assay of glutaminase I in vivo, by measurement of transrenal glutamine differences at various urinary pH values in nongouty and gouty subjects [177].

THE GLUTAMIC ACID DEHYDROGENASE HYPOTHESIS: The reaction catalyzed by glutamic acid dehydrogenase appears to operate chiefly in the direction of synthesis of α-ketoglutaric acid. Pagliari and Goodman [595] have confirmed an earlier observation [594] that plasma levels of glutamic acid are elevated in gout and have considered this finding, and those of Gutman and Yü cited above, in support of a suggestion first made by Frieden [467] that faulty control or reduced activity of glutamic acid dehydrogenase could result in the diversion of glutamic acid toward glutamine and purine biosynthesis.

Table 39-8. INTRAMOLECULAR DISTRIBUTION OF URIC ACID ^{15}N

Subjects	Atom percent excess			
	Uric acid-^{15}N	^{15}N-7	^{15}N-1	^{15}N-(3 + 9)
Controls (3)	0.063 (100)*	0.172 (68)	0.067 (26)	0.009 (6)
Gout normal excretors (3)	0.099 (100)	0.247 (61)	0.090 (22)	0.034 (17)
Gout over excretors (3)	0.308 (100)	0.699 (53)	0.286 (24)	0.141 (23)

* Numbers in parentheses below percentages are the percent of total.
Source: Day 2 values from Gutman and Yü [184].

The Kinetic Hypothesis

Studies have been conducted in three normouricemic controls and four gouty subjects in whom the transfer of ^{15}N, administered as glycine-^{15}N, has been traced with time into urinary hippuric acid, phenylacetylglutamine (both amide and amino nitrogens), and ammonia, and the values compared with the enrichment at each of the nitrogen atoms of the uric acid molecule [601]. The gouty subjects included one modest overexcretor with a minimal increase of glycine incorporation into urinary urate classified as having idiopathic gout, and three substantial overproducers with specific subtypes of gout: one was PRT deficient, one appeared to have a mutant amidotransferase of low sensitivity to regulatory end-products [602], and one was subsequently shown to overproduce PP-ribose-P because of a mutant PP-ribose-P synthetase and to excrete 2,400 mg of uric acid per day. No significant differences in enrichment of urinary hippurate were noted in control and gouty subjects. These results confirm those of others [301], which disclose normal enrichment and turnover kinetics of urinary glycine or hippurate in gout. Similarly, no abnormalities in enrichment or turnover kinetics of either the amide-N or amino-N of phenylacetylglutamine were noted among any of the four gouty subjects. These findings exclude a gross defect of nitrogen metabolism resulting in the excessive transfer of ammonia or amino nitrogen into glutamic acid or glutamine in gout.

In the three control subjects, the enrichment of N-(3 + 9) ranged from 9 to 17 percent of total uric acid ^{15}N on the first day and from 14 to 23 percent on the third day (see Table 39-8). The values for N-(3 + 9) from the first through the twenty-eighth day were higher than those found by Gutman and Yü [184] in their controls and overlapped 13 of 14 values reported by them in normoexcretor gouty subjects. Percentage enrichments of N-(3 + 9) were within or just above the normal range in the patient with minimal overexcretion of uric acid, somewhat higher in the PRT-deficient subject, and well above the normal range in the two overproducers with normal PRT activities. In the latter two subjects, 25 to 34 percent of the ^{15}N in urinary uric acid was in N-(3 + 9) in eight samples obtained throughout the first 24 hr after glycine administration. The enrichment values observed in phenylacetylglutamine indicate, however, that the increased percentage of ^{15}N found in N-(3 + 9) of uric acid in overproducers cannot be attributed to a greater enrichment of precursor glutamine in gouty than in nongouty subjects.

In tracer studies, the more rapid the rate of conversion of precursor to product, the more closely the isotopic enrichment of the product resembles that of the precursor. When glycine-^{15}N is administered orally the glycine pool is maximally labeled in 1 hr [603]. Free ammonia is more highly labeled within the first hour than either nitrogen atom of phenylacetylglutamine, both of which pass through their maximum enrichments between 2 and 4 hr following glycine ingestion, by which time the enrichments of glycine [603], hippurate, and ammonia are falling rapidly. The isotope abundances in all these substances, as sampled in urine, exhibit typical polyexponential die-away curves [601]. In the experiments referred to above, the greater the peak enrichment of uric acid, the earlier the peak enrichment occurred in both N-7 (maximal in a 2 to 4 hr urate sample and in N-(3 + 9) (maximal in a 4 to 7 hr sample). The maximal enrichment of N-7 was about one-eighth of the hippurate maximum, whereas the maximum enrichment of N-(3 + 9) was one-third that of the maximum of the amide-N of glutamine. The lag between the enrichment peaks of hippurate and N-7, and of glutamine and N-(3 + 9) was about 2 hr in each case. Clearly, when purine biosynthesis is accelerated, the enrichment of N atoms of the purine ring assumes the character of a pulse-labeling experiment: nitrogen atoms drawn from precursor pools at a time when they are highly enriched dominate the distribution pattern of ^{15}N in the purine ring.

The observation that an increase in the ratio (^{15}N in N-3 + N-9)/(^{15}N in uric acid) was found in the gouty overproducer with PRT deficiency as well as in those with normal PRT activity (see also [517]) suggests that the shift of percentage enrichment toward N-(3 + 9) in overproducers is a consequence of the complex kinetics of enrichment of precursor pools, following the administration of ^{15}N-glycine. One possible explanation is that in the overproducer a larger amount of purine is synthesized during that period of a few hours when the isotope abundance is already falling in glycine but still rising in glutamine. This relationship would tend to result in a greater percentage enrichment of N-(3 + 9) in the uric acid of accelerated producers, especially in samples obtained early, assuming a route of synthesis that largely bypasses the more slowly turning over nucleic acid pools. When $^{15}NH_4Cl$ rather than ^{15}N-glycine is the labeled precursor [576], isotope distribution among N atoms of the purine ring is indistinguishable between normal subjects and overproducers, as one would predict from the kinetic hypothesis on the expectation that precursor pools of glycine and glutamine would be simultaneously rather than sequentially labeled.

The postulate of a defect of glutamine metabolism in primary gout rests chiefly upon isotope data that are subject to more than one interpretation. In our view, the observed deviations from normal of isotope distribution patterns in overproducers following the administration of ^{15}N-glycine are related to the complex interrelationships of the kinetics of ^{15}N transfer from glycine to glutamine, and from these precursors to the purine ring. One does not need to invoke a defect in glutamine metabolism in order to explain the data. The observation that the distribution abnormalities are also present in PRT-deficient overproducers weakens the arguments for the glutamine hypothesis in other gouty subjects and favors the kinetic hypothesis advanced above.

The Role of Phosphoribosylpyrophosphate in Gout

Concentration values of PP-ribose-P are normal in the erythrocytes and fibroblasts of most gouty subjects with normal phosphoribosyltransferase activity and are not correlated with plasma or urinary uric acid values [445, 456]. In patients who are deficient in PRT activity, there is a gross underutilization of PP-ribose-P in purine salvage with resultant accumulation of PP-ribose-P (Table 39-9). The maxi-

Table 39-9. PP-RIBOSE-P CONCENTRATION VALUES IN HUMAN ERYTHROCYTES

	Number	PP-Ribose-P nmoles/ml	References
Controls	28	2.6 ± 0.7*	[465]
	12	4.4 ± 1.8	[456]
	10	3.1 ± 0.5	[445]
Gout—normal PRT activity	28	2.6 ± 0.7*	[465]
	14	2.7 ± 0.5	[445]
Gout—PRT partial deficiency (hemizygote)	3	4.6 ± 1.3	[445]
Lesch-Nyhan (hemizygote)	7	38.8 ± 4.0	[445]
Lesch-Nyhan (hemizygote)	3	35.3 (21–50)	[456]
Lesch-Nyhan (heterozygote)	3	4.2 (1.5–6.5)	[456]
A-PRT deficiency (heterozygote)	1	2.6	[456]
O-PRT deficiency (homozygote)	1	2.7	[456]
O-PRT deficiency (heterozygote)	2	3.4, 5.1	[456]
Glycogen storage disease, Type I	2	2.2, 2.4	[445]

* These controls and gouty subjects had similar values of PP-Ribose-P. Mean and Standard Deviations refer to data on all 56 subjects.

mal rates of synthesis of PP-ribose-P are not increased in PRT-deficient cells [464]. Erythrocyte levels of PP-ribose-P were normal in one patient with partial deficiency of A-PRT [456]. They were also normal in one patient with orotic aciduria [456], a disorder in which there is an absence of activity of orotic acid phosphoribosyltransferase (O-PRT) [604], which catalyzes another reaction in which PP-ribose-P is consumed. In erythrocytes and fibroblasts, the maximal rate of the reaction catalyzed by O-PRT is only about 0.2 percent of the maximum of the PRT reaction [456]. One subject with decreased enzymatic activities of O-PRT and orotidylic decarboxylase, thought possibly heterozygous for the defect of orotic aciduria, was found to be hyperuricemic [605]. However, other subjects with this pattern of enzyme deficiencies have not been hyperuricemic, nor have gouty subjects shown these enzyme deficiencies [605].

Hershko et al. [606] have reported that erythrocytes from at least 2 of 19 gouty patients exhibited an increased capacity for the synthesis of nucleotides from preformed purines as well as an increased rate of PP-ribose-P formation. They suggested that increased PP-ribose-P synthesis was related to the increased availability of ribose-5-phosphate.

Glutathione Reductase Variants and Gout

In addition a highly significant association of hyperuricemia and gout with *increased* enzymatic activity of a mutant glutathione reductase has been provisionally attributed to an increased rate of operation of the hexose monophosphate shunt, and of synthesis of ribose-5-phosphate and PP-ribose-P. Twenty-three of twenty-eight Negro patients with gout were found to have the glutathione reductase variant. The fast variant is 28 percent more active than the normal enzyme [607]. Elevated activity of erythrocyte glutathione reductase has also been observed in a group of Caucasians with untreated primary gout [608]. A similar consequence is envisioned in glycogen storage disease Type I (glucose-6-phosphatase deficiency) because of the diversion of hexose phosphate toward pentose-phosphate synthesis [609]. Fructose ingestion leads to a greater and more prolonged rise in serum urate levels in gouty patients, and in children of gouty patients, than in normal controls [462]. As discussed, above, elevated hexose levels lead to increased intracellular PP-ribose-P levels in vitro.

Phosphoribosylpyrophosphate Turnover in Gout

An additional approach to the question of the mechanism of overproduction of purines in gout has been the assessment of the rate of turnover of PP-ribose-P by determination of the specific activity of the ribose moiety of PP-ribose-P in control and gouty subjects following the administration of labeled glucose [610]. Current evidence suggests that net flux of carbon is from glucose-6-phosphate to ribose-5-phosphate, via the oxidative limb of the hexose monophosphate shunt, rather than from fructose-6-phosphate to pentose via the nonoxidative limb [448]. Apparently only a small fraction, perhaps one-sixth, of ribose-5-phosphate is normally converted to PP-ribose-P [448]. However, as pointed out above, measures which increase the production of ribose-5-P may be reflected in an increased synthesis of PP-ribose-P and of purines. A small increase in production and turnover of PP-ribose-P from ribose-5-P would not necessarily be reflected in an increase in the specific activity of PP-ribose-P, if the turnover of the pool of PP-ribose-P was normally rapid compared with that of the pool of ribose-5-P. However, a gross acceleration of production of ribose-5-P from labeled glucose, or of PP-ribose-P from ribose-5-P could be reflected in an increased specific activity of PP-ribose-P. This should be true whether this occurs as a "primary" or idiopathic overproduction of PP-ribose-P, or as a "secondary" or compensatory overproduction because of the increased utilization of PP-ribose-P in accelerated purine biosynthesis. "Aliquots" of the PP-ribose-P pool can be obtained by the administration of imidazoleacetic acid and the isolation of its ribonucleoside derivative from the urine [611]. The reactions occur in liver [612] and are as follows:

$$\text{Imidazoleacetic acid} + \text{ATP} + \text{PP-ribose-P} \longrightarrow \text{IAA-ribose-P} + \text{ADP} + \text{PP}_i + \text{P}_i$$

$$\text{IAA-ribose-P} \longrightarrow \text{IAA-ribose} + \text{P}_i$$

This study has been performed on seven control and nine gouty subjects, including three overexcretors and six normal excretors of uric acid [610]. Specific activity values in the ribose moiety of IAA-ribonucleoside isolated from the 0- to 10-hr urine samples are shown in Fig. 39-20. The values in the three gouty subjects who excreted more than 600 mg uric acid per day are clearly excessive. Those of the six gouty

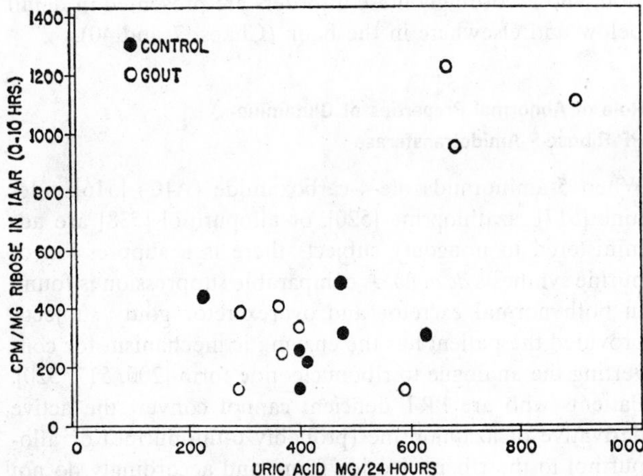

Figure 39-20. Specific activity of the ribose moiety of imidazoleacetic acid ribonucleoside in control and gouty subjects. Values obtained during the 10-hr period after administration of imidazoleacetic acid and glucose-U-^{14}C are plotted against uric acid excretion values. (*Reproduced from Jones et al.* [610], *with permission of the J. Clin. Invest.*)

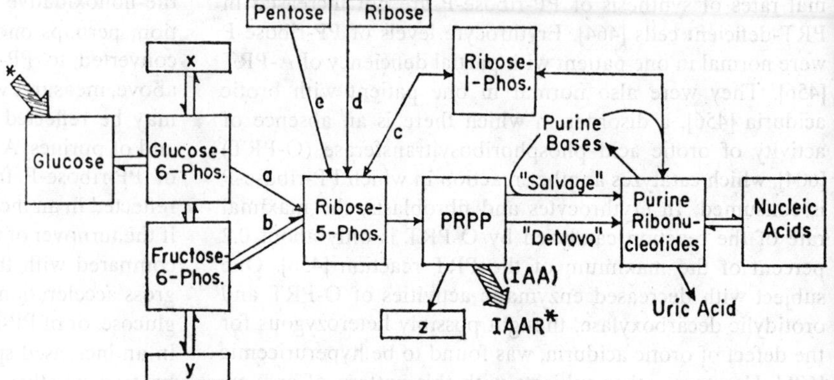

Figure 39-21. Model of hypothetical metabolic pools and known biochemical reactions which may influence isotopic labeling of ribose. (*Reproduced from Jones et al.* [610], *with permission of the J. Clin. Invest.*)

subjects who excreted normal amounts of uric acid are indistinguishable from those of the controls.

It would appear that the postulate of an increase in turnover of PP-ribose-P is substantiated in these gouty overexcretors. It is not known whether there was a primary overproduction of PP-ribose-P, or a secondary increase in its rate of renewal from labeled glucose because of some other cause of accelerated purine biosynthesis. No studies of erythrocyte PRT activity were performed. The results in the gouty normoexcretor do not rigorously exclude an increase in turnover of PP-ribose-P in this group, for an enhancement of rate of renewal of PP-ribose-P could take place at the expense of labeled glucose and unlabeled precursors equally, such that the specific activity of the precursor ribose-5-phosphate pool would remain unchanged (see Fig. 39-21).

The mechanisms of hyperuricemia in Type I glycogen storage disease (glucose-6-phosphatase deficiency) and phosphoribosyltransferase deficiency warrant extensive discussion, and accordingly these disorders are presented in detail below and elsewhere in the book (Chaps. 7 and 40).

Role of Abnormal Properties of Glutamine-PP-Ribose-P-Amidotransferase

When 5-aminoimidazole-4-carboxamide (AIC) [516], adenine [517], azathioprine [520], or allopurinol [538] are administered to nongouty subjects there is a suppression of purine synthesis *de novo.* A comparable suppression is found in both normal excretor and overexcretor gouty subjects, provided the patient has the enzymatic mechanism for converting the analogue to ribonucleotide form [200, 517, 520]. Patients who are PRT deficient cannot convert the active derivative of azathioprine (probably 6-thiopurine) or allopurinol to the ribonucleotide form, and accordingly do not respond to these agents with suppression in purine production [200, 520, 521]. They do respond normally to adenine [517], which is converted to adenylic acid by A-PRT, and (in tissue culture) to 6-methylmercaptopurine ribonucleoside [464], which is converted to its ribonucleotide by adenosine kinase [613, 614] and then behaves as an analogue of inosinic acid [514]. Thus in these gouty subjects, including those who are PRT deficient, it appears that both the 6-amino and 6-hydroxyribonucleotide control sites of the amidotransferase are intact.

The possibility that these inhibitions of purine synthesis *de novo* occur because of depletion of PP-ribose-P appears unlikely for two reasons: (1) Adenine is inhibitory in PRT-deficient cells in spite of elevated concentrations of PP-ribose-P [464], whereas orotic acid does not inhibit purine synthesis *de novo* in PRT-deficient cells [466], even though it lowers intracellular PP-ribose-P levels as effectively as does adenine [445]. The products of the phosphoribosyltransferase reactions are AMP, a known inhibitor of this enzyme, and orotidylic acid, which has no effect upon PP-ribose-P-amidotransferase [336]. (2) 6-Methylmercaptopurine ribonucleoside is converted to its ribonucleotide stage without consumption of PP-ribose-P [514].

Henderson and associates [602] found that purine biosynthesis *de novo* in fibroblasts cultured from two patients with extraordinary overexcretion and overproduction of uric acid and normal PRT activity appeared to be abnormally resistant to feedback inhibition by both 6-amino and 6-hydroxypurine compounds (Table 39-10). These results suggest the presence of a mutation which has altered the regulatory properties of glutamine-PP-ribose-P-amidotransferase. Many bacterial mutants are known in which a biosynthetic enzyme has become resistant to feedback control, presumably through structural alterations of the protein affecting only the inhibitor site. An Ehrlich ascites cell tumor appears to be resistant to 6-methylmercaptopurine ribonucleoside because of decreased feedback sensitivity to 6-hydroxypurine compounds [615]. A mutant strain of *Schizosaccharomyces pombe,* which shows a tenfold reduction in sensitivity of its PP-ribose-P amidotransferase to 6-hydroxypurine ribonucleotides, overproduces purines and excretes hypoxanthine and inosine into the medium [486]. Since the regulatory sites of the amidotransferase are distinct from its substrate sites [337, 338], loss of regulatory control is a theoretical explanation for excessive purine production in gout.

The situation in these two patients is unclear, however. PP-ribose-P levels were somewhat above normal in fibro-

Table 39-10. REDUCED SENSITIVITY OF PURINE BIOSYNTHESIS TO INHIBITION BY PURINE COMPOUNDS IN FIBROBLASTS OF TWO GOUTY SUBJECTS

Addition	Conc., *M*	Normal cells, %	Gout B.P., %	Gout T.B., %
None	0	100	100	100
Adenine	10^{-5}	95	—	—
	10^{-4}	25	70	63
	10^{-3}	18	49	39
Hypoxanthine	10^{-4}	47	83	88
	10^{-3}	37	56	68
6-Methyl-mercapto-purine ribonucleoside	10^{-7}	78	—	—
	10^{-6}	65	—	—
	10^{-5}	24	—	—
	10^{-4}	20	79	65
	10^{-3}	19	37	41

Values represent synthesis of FGAR (α-N-formylglycinamide ribonucleotide) in fibroblasts in presence of azaserine, expressed as percent of control value of each cell line. Control values were: Normal cells, 1,740 cpm (range 1380–1980); B.P., 6,470 cpm; T.B., 6,320 cpm.
Source: Henderson et al. [602].

blasts [602], a result unanticipated on the basis of altered feedback properties of the enzyme. Furthermore, ^{14}C-glycine incorporation into urinary urate was normally inhibited in response to administered adenine [517] or azathioprine [520]. Also allopurinol inhibited total purine production in both subjects [200]. The question of altered responsiveness to feedback inhibitors can only be resolved by kinetic or inhibitor-binding studies of partially purified enzyme, the technical requirements of which have not yet been solved in human tissue.

Increased Levels of Glutamine-PP-Ribose-P-Amidotransferase

There is a precedent for an increase in the quantity and activity of a specific enzyme in an inherited human "over-production" disease, namely, acute intermittent porphyria, in which a sevenfold increase in the activity of δ-amino-levulinic acid synthetase has been found in liver [616]. Derepression (induction) of enzymes of purine biosynthesis can be brought about in bacteria [442, 443] and in mammalian cells [489] growing on marginal concentrations of purines. There is at present no evidence for or against this concept in hyperuricemic subjects, for current techniques do not permit the direct assay of amidotransferase activity in accessible tissue in man.

The Role of Inhibitor Ribonucleotides in Gout

Disturbances of control of purine biosynthesis could result from alterations of the concentrations of active feedback inhibitors at the surface of glutamine-PP-ribose-P-amidotransferase. In normally growing or neoplastic cells, presumably it is the removal of nucleotides into nucleic acids, or into other products, which reduces the inhibitory constraints upon the amidotransferase and allows synthesis of purines *de novo* to proceed. An abnormally rapid degradation of nucleotides might have the same effect. There are a few clues that the latter mechanism may operate in specific hyperuricemic patients. In one overproducer gouty subject studied by Seegmiller et al. the rate constant for the turnover of labeled adenine was twice that of two other gouty subjects and two controls [517]. In addition, fibroblasts cultured from a patient with familial gout associated with normal uric acid production showed a twentyfold increase in the rate of deamination of adenylic acid to inosinic acid [602], which was thought possibly to correlate with an abnormally rapid rate of breakdown of azathioprine to uric acid in this patient *in vivo* [520].

Patients with PRT deficiency show an inability to convert hypoxanthine and guanine to their respective ribonucleotides (see below). They show extraordinary degrees of acceleration of purine synthesis *de novo*. One potential explanation is that the deficiency of PRT activity results in an inability to maintain normal intracellular concentrations of nucleotides. The only direct measurements of cellular nucleotide content in this disease are in fibroblasts in culture where the total concentrations of adenyl and guanyl ribonucleotides appeared to fall within normal limits [464].

The discovery of the synergistic feedback control of the amidotransferase effected by adenyl and guanyl ribonucleotides raises an additional possibility that relaxation of control may result from a nonoptimal balance between 6-amino- and 6-hydroxypurine ribonucleotides. Regulatory defects of the AMP and GMP pathways will need to be considered. Weissmann and Gutman [57] suggested a nucleotide imbalance in explanation of the increased excretion of 7-methyl-8-hydroxyguanine and decreased excretion of 6-succinoaminopurine in acute gout. Gouty patients given glycine-1-^{14}C show enhanced labeling of urinary-7-methylguanine, but not of urinary adenine [587]. No definite conclusions can be drawn from these observations at the present time.

Xanthine Oxidase Activity in Gout

Carcassi et al. [617] have reported elevated values of xanthine oxidase activity in liver biopsy specimens obtained from eight overexcretor gouty subjects. Mean values were fourfold greater than in controls. It is not known whether the increase in xanthine oxidase activity is primary, or secondary to another metabolic lesion. PRT activity was not assayed in these subjects, nor have assays been published from patients with secondary hyperuricemia, e.g., associated with polycythemia vera. As discussed in Chap. 41, xanthine oxidase is an inducible enzyme [618]. In any case, increased xanthine oxidase activity would be expected to augment the conversion of hypoxanthine and xanthine to uric acid, and to reduce their reconversion to ribonucleotides in the PRT reaction, at least in liver. It is possible that this shift in the balance of competition for hypoxanthine results in a reduction of intracellular nucleotide levels, with the relaxation of end product inhibition of glutamine-PP-ribose-P-amidotransferase.

EXCRETION OF URIC ACID IN GOUT

Renal Mechanisms of Uric Acid Excretion in Normal Man

The current view is that virtually all urate in plasma is freely filterable at the glomerulus, that all but a small fraction of filtered urate is reabsorbed in the tubule, and that the major fraction of excreted urate enters the tubule by a secretory process [619, 620].

Evidence that plasma urate is freely filterable has been reviewed above. Studies leading to the concept of tubular secretion of urate in man have been reviewed in detail elsewhere [621, 622]. Tubular secretion of uric acid, once thought to be restricted to birds and certain reptiles, has now been demonstrated in the rabbit [623], guinea pig [624], dog [625–627], Cebus monkey [628], man [629–631], and chimpanzee [632]. Tubular secretion of urate in the dog occurs in the proximal [633, 634] and perhaps also the distal segment [625, 626, 635]. The chimpanzee kidney is probably the closest model of the human with respect to urate mechanisms [632].

The first indication of this process in man was found by Praetorius and Kirk [629] in a young male with hypouricemia (plasma urate values of 0.2 to 0.6 mg per 100 ml), who showed urate clearances 28 to 46 percent above simultaneous inulin clearances. These findings were explained by postulating an absence of tubular reabsorption of filtered urate and the presence of substantial tubular secretion of urate. Supporting arguments came from the analysis of the biphasic response of urate excretion to uricosuric agents by Gutman et al. [619, 630]. At low doses, salicylates [636], phenylbutazone and sulfinpyrazone [637, 638], and probenecid [639] caused a reduction in the C_{urate}/C_{inulin} ratio; at higher doses all of these agents increased this ratio and were uricosuric [636–640]. These results have been explained by postulating an inhibition of urate secretion at low drug concentrations, and in addition an inhibition of tubular reabsorption at higher drug concentrations [636]. Finally, confirmatory data on tubular secretion were obtained from urate clearance values in normal man as much as 23 percent greater than the glomerular filtration rate under experimental conditions that were considerably altered from the normal [630]. Attempts to localize the site of urate secretion within the nephron in man have suggested that this process occurs in the proximal tubule [631].

The evaluation of the relative roles of filtration, reabsorption, and tubular secretion depends upon the use of a technique that allows specific analysis of each component of the bidirectional transport system for urate [620, 641]. Pyrazinamide is a potent inhibitor of uric acid excretion [642, 643] which has little or no effect on glomerular filtration rate [644]. In man, large doses of pyrazinamide or pyrazinoic acid will reduce uric acid excretion almost to the vanishing point [642]. On the basis of animal studies, the drug is presumed to inhibit the tubular secretion of urate [635, 644]. Uric acid which appears in urine in subjects given full doses of pyrazinamide is presumed to represent filtered urate that has escaped reabsorption.

In the normal kidney, the excreted quantity ranges from 1.2 to 1.6 percent of filtered urate. This value is constant over a wide range of plasma urate values [620, 641]. It represents a *maximal* figure. The normal value could be lower, perhaps even zero. Apparent excretion of a small fraction of filtered urate could represent (1) incomplete inhibition of tubular secretion of urate by pyrazinamide; or (2) complete inhibition of secretion plus some inhibition of urate reabsorption. The latter effect of pyrazinamide has been demonstrated in the rat and dog. Conclusions based on the use of the pyrazinamide test, described below, should be considered tentative at present.

In spite of the constancy of the fraction of filtered urate that is reabsorbed in the normal renal tubule, the C_{urate}/C_{inulin} ratio increases as plasma urate levels are raised [303–305, 645, 646]. The constancy and near completeness of fractional reabsorption of filtered urate suggest that the increase in clearance ratio results from increased tubular secretion of urate. A plot of the rate of uric acid excretion at various plasma levels shows that the increase in rate is more than proportional to the increment in plasma urate concentration and that there is a sharp augmentation of the rate of excretion in normal man at plasma urate concentrations of 9 or 10 mg per 100 ml [647]. A study of this phenomenon with the use of pyrazinamide suppression confirms that the augmented excretion of uric acid at high plasma levels is attributable entirely to the increased tubular secretion of urate [305, 620, 641].

Reduced Nephron Population

In the chronically diseased kidney, urate secretion is markedly reduced in association with a striking increase in the fractional excretion of filtered urate. When renal disease is severe, as much as 45 percent of filtered urate may escape reabsorption and be excreted. Thus although substrate-regulated tubular secretion is the principle homeostatic mechanism for urate excretion in normal and moderately diseased kidneys, glomerular filtration assumes this role in far advanced renal disease [648].

Renal Mechanisms of Uric Acid Excretion in Gout

It is also assumed that virtually all urate in the plasma of gouty man is freely filterable at the glomerulus. The binding of urate by plasma proteins, still a controversial subject, would account for only about 4 percent of plasma urate at 37°C, and a deficiency of a urate binding α_1-α_2-globulin in gout, as reported by Alvsaker [215], would result in more nearly complete filtration.

The C_{urate}/C_{inulin} ratio tends to be lower in gouty subjects than in normal controls at any specified serum urate level [131, 303, 304, 649–651]. This ratio increases in gouty subjects as the plasma urate level is raised, as it does in normal controls, but higher plasma urate values are required in gouty than in normal subjects to achieve a given clearance ratio (Fig. 39-22) [647, 652].

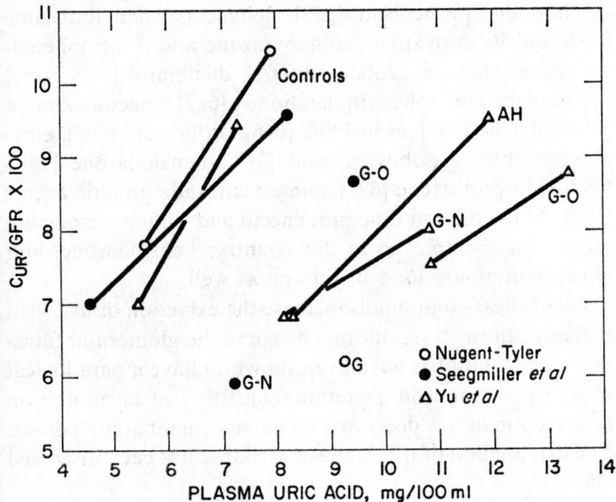

Figure 39-22. Renal clearance of uric acid in nongouty and gouty subjects, plotted against plasma urate concentrations. In the pairs of points connected by lines, the right-hand member represents the value observed after the serum urate concentration was raised by feeding of RNA. G = gouty subject; AH = asymptomatic hyperuricemic; N = normal excretor; O = overexcretor. (*Data of Nugent and Tyler* [303]; *Seegmiller et al.* [304]; *Yü et al.* [305]. *Reproduced from J. B. Wyngaarden* [647], *with permission of Academic, New York.*)

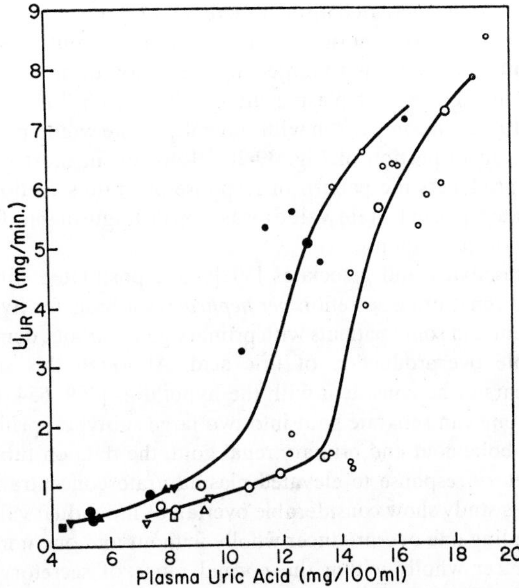

Figure 39-23. Rate of uric acid excretion at various plasma urate levels in nongouty (solid symbols) and gouty (open symbols) subjects. Large symbols represent mean values; small symbols represent individual data of a few mean values selected to illustrate the degree of scatter within groups. Studies were conducted under basal conditions, after RNA feeding, and after infusions of lithium urate. (▲, △, *Nugent and Tyler* [303]; ▼, ▽, *Seegmiller et al.* [304]; ●, ○, *Yü et al.* [305]; ■, □, *Lathem and Rodnan* [645]. *Reproduced from J. B. Wyngaarden* [647], *with permission of Academic, New York.*)

When the data of these studies are plotted as rates of uric acid excretion at various serum urate levels, it appears that the curve of excretion rates has the same form in gouty subjects as in nongouty controls, and that the *capacity* of the excretory mechanism for uric acid is not reduced in gout (Fig. 39-23). However, the excretion curve is shifted such that gouty subjects require serum values 2 or 3 mg per 100 ml higher than controls in order to achieve equivalent uric acid excretion rates. The sharp augmentation of rate of urate excretion occurs at approximately 13 mg per 100 ml rather than at 9 or 10 mg per 100 ml as in normal man.

The data plotted in Fig. 39-23 are from control and gouty subjects with normal renal mass, i.e., all subjects have a glomerular filtration rate of 100 ml per min or greater. The displacement of the curve in gouty subjects is not a consequence of sustained hyperuricemia, for in leukemic subjects the rates of uric acid excretion are generally normal or increased in relation to the titration curve in nongouty subjects [646, 653].

Application of the pyrazinamide suppression test to the study of uric acid excretion in gouty subjects shows that a normal fraction of filtered urate escapes reabsorption in both normal producers and overproducers, both at basal and increased filtered urate loads [302, 641]. The augmented excretion of uric acid at high plasma urate levels is attributable to the increased tubular secretion of urate in the gouty subjects, as it is in normal man [302]. In most gouty normal producers, there was a blunted augmentation of urate secretion in the range of plasma urate values from 7 to 13 mg per 100 ml in comparison with controls, as one would predict from an inspection of Fig. 39-20. However, in most gouty overproducers the pattern of response of urate secretion to elevated plasma urate values was not distinguishable from the normal response.

Rieselbach and associates [302] have postulated diminished renal urate secretion *per nephron* as a basis for hyperuricemia in some patients with primary gout without demonstrable overproduction of uric acid. Although this study appears to be consistent with the hypothesis [309, 654, 655] that one can separate gout into two large subtypes, primary metabolic gout and primary renal gout, the data on tubular secretory response to elevated plasma urate concentrations in this study show considerable overlap of individual values, including one overproducer wholly without and one normal producer wholly within the normal range of secretory response. These observations, together with others showing low C_{urate}/C_{inulin} ratios in relation to plasma urate concentrations in certain overproducers [131, 304], suggest that it may not be appropriate to separate patients with idiopathic primary gout so sharply into two groups on the basis of mean responses. Some gouty subjects appear to be simultaneous overproducers and underexcretors [656]. However, overproducers in the specific subgroup with partial or complete PRT deficiency have no demonstrable impairment of renal handling of urate apart from the effects of renal disease and reduced functional mass [200, 304].

The explanation of the shift of the velocity-substrate curve of the tubular secretion of uric acid toward higher plasma urate values in a large fraction of patients with gout is unknown. It does not appear that this finding can be attributed to hemodynamic changes. Tubular blood flow may be reduced in gout but not enough to explain these findings [131]. There is an active transport system for uric acid in erythrocytes [657], but little is known about the mechanism of the transfer of urate from renal cells into the tubular lumen.

Excretion of Purine Bases in Gout

Normal urine contains about 30 mg per day of purines other than uric acid. These include xanthine, hypoxanthine, 1-methylhypoxanthine, guanine, 1-methylguanine, 7-methylguanine, ^{2}N-methylguanine, 7-methyl-8-hydroxyguanine, adenine, and 6-succinoaminopurine [57, 414, 587, 658]. Their normal excretion values are given in Table 39-11. The origins of adenine, guanine, hypoxanthine, xanthine, and of the methylated adenines and guanines have been discussed. Succinoadenine is the aglycone of adenylosuccinic acid [366], the intermediate in the conversion of IMP to AMP.

Table 39-11. URINARY EXCRETION OF PURINE BASES IN NORMAL SUBJECTS, MG/DAY

Purine base	Range	Mean
Hypoxanthine	5.9–13.2	9.7
Xanthine	5.1–8.6	6.1
Adenine	1.1–1.7	1.4
Guanine	0.2–0.6	0.4
1-Methylhypoxanthine	0.2–0.7	0.4
6-Succinoaminopurine	0.8–1.5	1.2
1 + 7-Methylguanine	5.5–7.8	6.5
N^2-Methylguanine	0.4–0.6	0.5
7-Methyl-8-hydroxyguanine	1.1–2.0	1.6

Source: B. Weissmann and A. B. Gutman [57], and Weissmann et al. [401].

7-Methyl-8-hydroxyguanine arises from 7-methylguanine by action of human liver xanthine oxidase [684]; bovine milk xanthine oxidase will not catalyze this reaction [587].

The quantities of these bases found in the urine of gouty subjects do not differ significantly from those of normal subjects [57, 58].

Pharmacologic Control of Uric Acid Excretion in Man

Uricosuric Drugs

This category of compounds includes salicylates [636], cinchophen, probenecid [639], longacid, phenylbutazone [659] and its derivatives, sulfinpyrazone and *p*-nitrophenylbutazone [660], zoxazolamine [661], dicumarol [662], ethyl biscoumacetate, phenylindandione [663], acetoheximide [664], glycine [665], azauridine [666], orotic acid [667], ethyl *p*-chlorophenoxyisobutyric acid [217], benziodarone [668–670], chlorprothixene [671], and certain radiographic agents [672]. At the present time probenecid and sulfinpyrazone are most widely employed in this country; benziodarone, and zoxazolamine are used in Europe as well.

All of these compounds increase the excretion of uric acid without causing a significant change in the glomerular filtration rate. A number have been shown to have a paradoxical effect upon uric acid excretion, consisting of an inhibition of excretion at low doses and an enhancement at high doses. The explanation of this biphasic response has been discussed above.

Striking reductions of the miscible pool of uric acid have been demonstrated after the administration of adequate doses of salicylates [562], probenecid [639, 673], phenylbutazone [567, 659], and cortisone [564]. These are probably accounted for entirely by the increment in urate excretion. At least in the case of phenylbutazone, an increase in uricolysis or excretion by a nonrenal pathway has been excluded. No significant increase in the synthesis of uric acid was demonstrable when phenylbutazone was given for a few days [639], but in the case of one of two normal subjects given this drug for a longer time and in two hyperuricemic patients given probenecid [659] the increment in uric acid excretion exceeded the measured decrement in the miscible pool of uric acid. This suggests either mobilization of uric acid not measured within the pool or a concomitant or subsequent increase in the rate of synthesis. In the case of corticotropin, there is good evidence for increased uric acid production [564, 674, 675] in addition to the uricosuric effect.

The uricosuric actions of probenecid, sulfinpyrazone, and zoxazolamine are suppressed by salicylates in man, in part because of a countermanding of the inhibition of tubular reabsorption of uric acid produced by uricosuric drugs. The mechanism is complex, however, and also involves effects upon the tubular secretion of uric acid by salicylates and competition between salicylates and sulfinpyrazone for binding sites on transporting plasma proteins and perhaps elsewhere [676]. Probenecid, phenylbutazone, and salicylates are reported to reduce urate binding to protein [295]. Sulfinpyrazone may have a similar though less striking effect [296]. Such an action could at best account for only a fraction of their uricosuric effects.

Drugs and Metabolites Which Inhibit Urate Secretion Selectively

Pyrazinoic acid and pyrazinamide have been discussed above.

In normal man the uric acid/inulin clearance ratio (C_{ur}/C_{in}) is markedly reduced by the infusion of sodium lactate [231], as well as in clinical conditions in which arterial lactate levels are raised. These include preeclampsia [677], severe muscular exercise [678], acute alcohol ingestion [229, 230], and glycogen storage disease Type I [609]. Uric acid clearance is also reduced by infusions of β-hydroxybutyric acid [206, 679], as well as in ketoacidosis complicating starvation [679, 680] or uncontrolled diabetes [681]. During starvation-induced acidosis, hyperuricemia may reach 15 to 25 mg per 100 ml [680, 682]. These effects are most logically explained by postulating the suppression of urate secretion by lactate and β-hydroxybutyrate.

Extrarenal Disposal of Uric Acid in Gout

Uricolysis in Normal Man

Urinary recoveries of injected uric acid are incomplete in normal subjects. Forty years ago Folin et al. [64] and Koehler [683] reported recoveries that ranged from 28 to 91 percent, and averaged about 50 percent. Recoveries ranging from 55 to 95 percent of uric acid-^{15}N or uric acid-2^{14}-C have been reported [307, 308, 563, 565, 567]. The average of 14 studies with uric acid-^{15}N was 75.6 percent.

Studies of the turnover of uric acid in normal man have uniformly shown that the quantity of uric acid synthesized per day is greater than the quantity appearing in urine. In studies with uric acid-^{15}N [567] or uric acid-^{14}C [308], the fraction of the turnover appearing in urine is essentially the same as the fraction of injected uric acid recovered in urine. Thus a significant quantity of uric acid is disposed of by routes other than the kidney.

In initial studies with uric acid-^{15}N, small but significant concentrations of ^{15}N were found in urinary urea and ammonia [561]. Subsequently, when a relatively large quantity of uric acid-1, 3-^{15}N was administered intravenously to a normal subject [306, 685], about 25 percent of the isotope was found in urinary allantoin, urea, and ammonia and fecal nitrogen. In studies with uric acid-2-^{14}C, a comparable percentage of administered isotope was recovered in respiratory CO_2, urinary area, allantoin and allantoic acid, and feces [307]. In patients with biliary catheters given uric acid-^{15}N, labeled products were recovered in bile. These results suggested that uricolysis occurred in the intestinal tract.

Sites of Uricolysis

When labeled uric acid was administered orally to normal subjects, only 9 to 11 percent was absorbed and excreted unchanged in urine [307, 564]. With uric acid-^{15}N, 47 percent of the ^{15}N was recovered in urinary urea in 3 days [564]. With uric acid-2-^{14}C, only 2.4 percent appeared in urea, but 55 percent of the ^{14}C was excreted as respiratory CO_2 [307]. An additional 16.3 percent was recovered in feces, 83 to 91 percent of this amount being found within the intestinal bacteria themselves.

To verify the role of the intestinal flora in uricolysis in man, the degradation of intravenously administered uric acid was studied in a normal subject before and after an effective bacteriostasis was achieved with concomitant sulfonamide, streptomycin, and neomycin [307]. The quantity of ^{14}C recovered in various degradation products was reduced from 22.5 to 3.0 percent during drug treatment (Table 39-12). A variety of intestinal organisms have the capacity to destroy uric acid [306].

Sorensen [307] estimated that 100 mg of uric acid or more enters the alimentary tract in saliva, gastric juice, and bile. An equal quantity may enter in pancreatic and intestinal juices. These quantities of uric acid are larger than previously estimated [686, 687] and are adequate to account for the degradation of one-third of the uric acid normally turned over each day.

A trivial amount of uricolysis may occur within the tissues of man. Two enzyme systems of human tissues can destroy uric acid in vitro at physiologic pH. These are, verdoperoxidase [688] and cytochrome–cytochrome oxidase [689]. Bien and Zucker [690] showed that leukocytes and erythrocytes of normal subjects will destroy uric acid during prolonged incubations, and Villa et al. [70] demonstrated uricolytic properties of leukocyte extracts. This activity resides primarily

Table 39-12. RECOVERY OF INTRAVENOUSLY ADMINISTERED URIC ACID-2-^{14}C IN EXCRETORY PRODUCTS (5 TO 10 DAYS) BEFORE AND AFTER ESTABLISHMENT OF EFFECTIVE BACTERIOSTASIS OF THE INTESTINAL TRACT

Excretory product	*Recovery of ^{14}C, percent of dose*	
	Before bacteriostasis	During bacteriostasis
Urinary uric acid	69.0 (10 days)	55.7 (5 days)
Urinary allantoin	2.1	1.8
Urinary allantoic acid	0.2	
Urinary urea	2.2	0.7
Expired carbon dioxide	10.9	0.5
Fecal products	7.1	0.0
Total recovery in degradation products	22.5	3.0

Source: L. B. Sorensen [297].

in cells of the myeloid series [691], which are known to contain verdoperoxidase [692]. Uric acid crystals are degraded by leukocytes with the release of CO_2 from the 6 position [693]. The mechanism of the peroxidative reaction appears to be a two-electron–one-proton oxidation, which yields allantoin and CO_2 as the initial products [694]. Canellakis et al. [695] have shown that the products of the peroxidative destruction of uric acid in phosphate buffer are chiefly allantoin and urea.

Uricolysis in Gout

Decreased uricolysis has been proposed as a cause of hyperuricemia in gout [64, 70]. However, recoveries of injected unlabeled uric acid have ranged from 15 to 94 percent in the urine of gouty subjects [64, 683]. Recoveries of injected uric acid-^{14}N [684] or uric acid-^{14}C [307] have ranged from 35 to 54 percent in urine. All these values are lower, on the average, than those found in nongouty subjects. In gouty subjects, the fraction of the daily turnover of uric acid recovered in urine is smaller than in normal subjects. Other studies suggest that extrarenal disposal of uric acid is greater than normal in gouty subjects [307]. Uricolysis should be accentuated in hyperuricemic individuals, in whom larger than normal quantities of uric acid enter the intestinal tract. Pollycove et al. [695] have reported an increased yield of $^{14}CO_2$ from injected uric acid-^{14}C in hyperuricemic subjects.

The maximal uricolysis attributable to the tissues of man is 2 to 4 percent of the uric acid turnover [25]. No substantial evidence exists to implicate failure of tissue or intestinal uricolysis in the hyperuricemia of gout. On the contrary, emphasis should be placed upon enhanced enteral uricolysis as a compensatory factor in gout, tending to lessen hyperuricemia and constituting the major process of disposal of uric acid in certain patients with severe renal insufficiency [309, 654].

GOUT ASSOCIATED WITH SPECIFIC ENZYMATIC DEFECTS

Glucose-6-Phosphatase Deficiency in Gout

Patients with glycogen storage disease Type I (glucose-6-phosphatase deficiency) have hyperuricemia from infancy, and may develop gouty arthritis by the end of the first decade of life, sometimes of disabling severity [696–701]. Chronic tophaceous gout and gouty nephropathy may be responsible for a major portion of the morbidity in these patients as they become adults. Over 40 cases of glycogen storage disease and gout have been recorded [702]. In addition, in some cases of "primary juvenile gout," the clinical history and physical findings are suggestive of underlying glycogen storage disease [703].

Hyperuricemia in glycogen storage disease Type I is rather marked, often in the range of 10 to 16 mg per 100 ml of plasma [609, 701]. Two and perhaps three distinct pathophysiologic mechanisms contribute to the hyperuricemia of this disorder. They are reduced excretion of uric acid because of the presence of marked hyperlacticacidemia and ketonemia; increased production of uric acid *de novo,* possibly a consequence of increased synthesis of phosphoribosylpyrophosphate; and perhaps increased binding of urate in plasma by lipoproteins which are present in increased amounts.

Patients with glucose-6-phosphatase deficiency are unable to produce free glucose from phosphorylated carbohydrates. Recurrent hypoglycemia acts as a stimulus both to glycogenolysis and gluconeogenesis. One consequence is hyperlactic acidemia [609, 704, 705]. Blood lactate levels may be 50 mg per 100 ml or more (normal 5 to 18 mg per 100 ml). Recurrent hypoglycemia also results in ketonemia and elevated blood levels of β-hydroxybutyrate [609]. Both lactate and β-hydroxybutyrate are thought to suppress tubular urate secretion [231, 682]. Renal clearances of uric acid are low in Type I glycogen storage disease [609].

The hyperuricemia of Type I glycogen storage disease is also associated with an excessive uric acid production. Uric acid excretion values are high when expressed in terms of body weight [579]. The urinary uric acid/creatinine ratio may be >0.75 [706]. By tracer methods, both the turnover of the urate pool [579] and glycine-1-^{14}C incorporation into urinary urate may be excessive [579, 697, 707] (Table 39-13). The pattern of increased purine production is that of accelerated biosynthesis *de novo.* This finding has been attributed to the postulated overproduction of phosphoribosylpyrophosphate [579, 697]. The intracellular surfeit of carbohydrate intermediates that cannot be released as free glucose may lead to an excessive production of phosphorylated ribose compounds, including PP-ribose-P. The active operation of the oxidative pathway of glucose-6-phosphate catabolism has been demonstrated in liver in this disease [609]. However, an increased synthesis of PP-ribose-P, or increased

Table 39-13. TURNOVER AND SYNTHESIS OF URIC ACID IN GLYCOGEN STORAGE DISEASE, TYPE I

Subject	Sex	Age, yr	Serum urate, mg/100 ml	Pool size, mg	Turnover rate, pool/day	Turnover uric acid, mg/day	Excretion uric acid, mg/day	Turnover excreted, %	Recovery of isotope in urinary uric acid in 7 days		
									Administered uric acid, %	Administered glycine	
										Uncorrected, %	Corrected, %
Normal control subjects*	6 M 2 F	26 (19–38)	4.3 (2.9–5.5)	978 (541–1,290)	0.62 (0.46–0.80)	590 (431–729)	429 (357–536)	73 (65–82)	73 (63–82)	0.24 (0.16–0.29)	0.32 (0.27–0.37)
Patients with Type I glycogen storage disease	M*	14	10.9	1,380	0.85	1,176	528	45	54	1.09	2.02
	M*	17	16.4	2,843	0.48	1,365	569	42	39	0.61	1.56
	F*	19	14.7	1,917	0.61	1,175	343	29	35	0.48	1.37
	M†	34	15.0	1,920	0.42	807	362	45	42	0.26	0.62
	M‡	18	17.0	2,251	0.39	884	318	36	32	0.11	0.34

* Ref. [579]
† Ref. [578]
‡ Ref. [707]

intercellular levels of this compound, have not yet been documented. Greene and Seegmiller [445] found normal levels of PP-ribose-P in erythrocytes and cultured fibroblasts in two patients with this disorder. This result was perhaps to be expected, since erythrocytes from these tissues do not contain glucose-6-phosphatase activity even in normal subjects. The critical organ for study will be the liver.

The hyperlipoproteinemia of glycogen storage disease may be very marked, and may include elevations of triglycerides, phospholipids, and cholesterol [609]. Lipoprotein electrophoresis discloses a Type IV pattern. There is a rank order correlation between plasma levels of triglycerides and urate [214]. The possibility that lipoproteins may bind urate in this and other disorders requires further study.

Hyperuricemia has also been described in an undefined type of glycogen storage disease with normal hepatic glucose-6-phosphatase activity [708]. In this instance, renal retention of urate appeared to be related, at least in part, to hyperlactic acidemia.

Hypoxanthine-Guanine Phosphoribosyltransferase Deficiency in Gout

One of the major advances in the study of the mechanisms of hyperuricemia was the discovery by Seegmiller and associates of a deficiency of hypoxanthine-guanine phosphoribosyltransferase (PRT) in certain patients with flamboyant overproduction of uric acid. Complete or virtually complete deficiency of this enzyme activity is associated with a syndrome of choreoathetoses, spasticity, mental retardation, and a bizarre compulsive self-mutilation, known as the Lesch-Nyhan syndrome [709]. There is prodigious overproduction and overexcretion of uric acid, and renal stones and secondary renal damage are common. In a few patients, a severe gouty arthritis has occurred. All the patients are males, and the disorder is X-linked. The Lesch-Nyhan syndrome is sufficiently distinct to warrant a full description apart from its brief inclusion here. Accordingly, it is considered *in extenso* in Chap. 40.

Among adult patients with marked overproduction of uric acid, a portion has been found to have a high-grade, but partial, deficiency of PRT activity [710]. The incidence of this enzyme defect in the gouty population is not yet known. Six affected individuals, three of them in one family, were found among 110 gouty patients admitted for special study at the Clinical Center of the National Institutes of Health over a 14-year period. A total of 18 patients were described in a general review of the topic written in September, 1968 [200]. Included in this group were several patients who had been reported earlier as examples of juvenile gout associated with marked hyperexcretion of uric acid or with neurological abnormalities [309, 600, 711, 712]. Sperling et al. [713] found only 1 subject with a partial deficiency of PRT activity among 52 adult male gouty overproducers of urate. About 24 cases had been published throughout the world by the end of 1970 [200, 580, 713, 714].

Presenting symptoms in patients with partial PRT deficiency may be typical acute gouty arthritis, renal stones, crystalluria, or neurological dysfunction. Gouty arthritis usually presents in the second or third decade. Three-quarters of known patients have formed renal stones; half of these occurred before age 10. In 20 percent of patients there have been neurological manifestations, including mental retardation, mild spastic quadriplegia, dysarthria, cerebellar ataxia, and seizure. These suggest that there may be a relationship to the debilitating disease found in patients with complete PRT deficiency. Neurological findings have occurred in patients with 0.5 percent or less of normal PRT activity in erythrocyte lysates with guanine as substrate [714]. As little as 1 percent of normal enzyme activity in hemolysates is associated with no discernible neurological involvement [580]. A few patients have had a mild macrocytic anemia [200].

Gouty subjects with PRT deficiency tend to have rather high serum urate values. Most of them have been above 10 mg per 100 ml. Urinary uric acid excretion is elevated unless renal failure is present, often being well above 1,000 mg per day (Fig. 39-24). Patient TS of Fig. 39-24, whose uric acid excretion falls within the normal range, had a glomerular filtration rate of only 10 ml per min. Turnover studies of Patient TS disclosed a urate production of 1,693 mg per day of which only 34 percent was disposed of in the urine. The elevated excretion of uric acid in PRT-deficient subjects is reflected in a uric acid/creatinine ratio above 0.75 (normal, 0.15 to 0.75) [706]. In most patients with gout and normal PRT activity, the values are within the normal range.

Turnover studies with labeled uric acid have disclosed enlarged urate pools and increased urate turnovers in all of five patients studied [200]. Glycine-1-^{14}C incorporation into urinary uric acid is excessive, particularly after correction for extrarenal disposal. Values in five patients ranged from 0.88 to 3.94 percent of administered glycine in 7 days. These values are somewhat less than may be found in patients with complete PRT deficiency (4.3 to 6.1 percent) but very much greater than in normal subjects (0.1 to 0.3 percent). There is an overlap with values found in gouty overproducers with normal PRT activity (0.4 to 1.9 percent). In patients with PRT deficiency given glycine-1-^{14}C, the peak specific activity values in urinary uric acid occur earlier than in normal individuals. These results indicate that excessive purine production in these patients is the result of increased purine synthesis *de novo,* rather than an increased turnover of nucleic acids (compare Fig. 39-16 with Fig. 39-28 below).

PRT Assays

The clue to the discovery of PRT deficiency in the Lesch-Nyhan syndrome [709] was the unresponsiveness of purine biosynthesis and uric acid levels to administered azathioprine in children with this disorder [519]. Suppression of purine

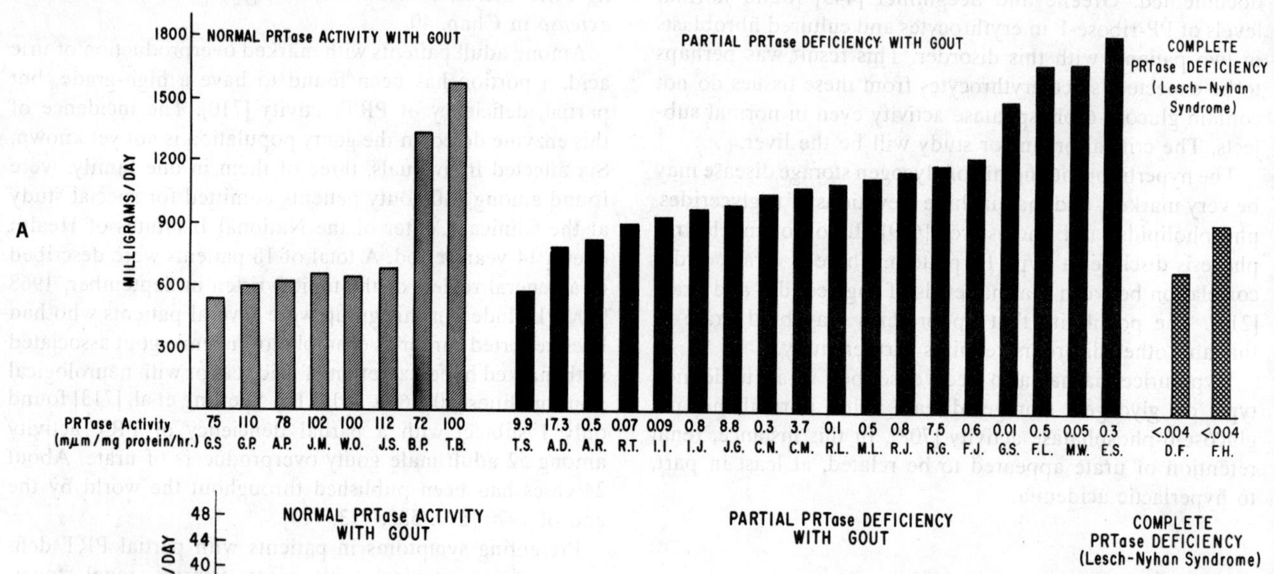

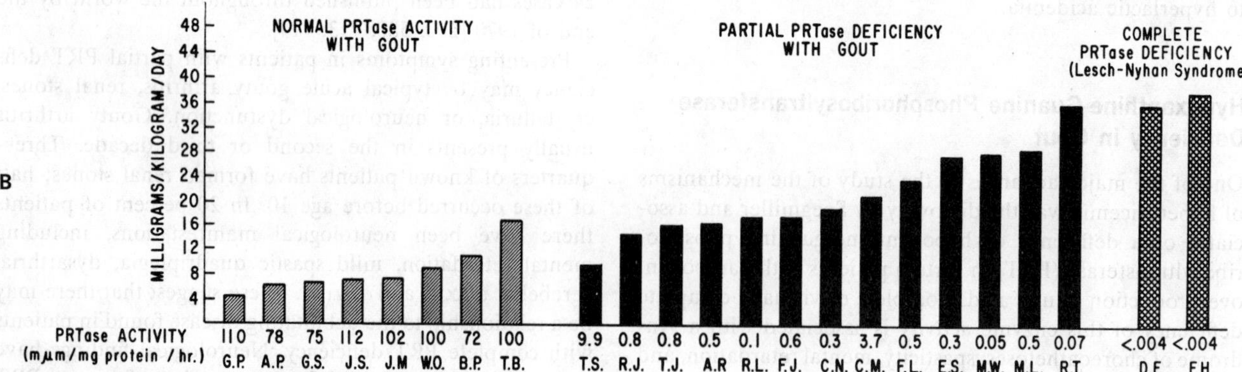

Figure 39-24. Daily uric acid excretions in patients producing excessive quantities of uric acid. Comparison of patients with normal, partially deficient, and "virtually completely" deficient hypoxanthine-guanine phosphoribosyltransferase (PRT) activity. A. Excretion values in milligrams per day (upper limit of normal is 590 mg per day). B. Excretion values in milligrams per killigram per day (upper limit of normal is 6 to 7 mg per kg per day). Source: Kelley et al. [300].

Table 39-14. SPECIFIC ACTIVITY OF PHOSPHORIBOSYLTRANSFERASES IN ERYTHROCYTES IN HYPERURICEMIC SUBJECTS

Subject	Number	*PRT activity, nmoles/mg protein/hr (mean ± s.d.)* Hypoxanthine	Guanine	Adenine
Normal controls	32	103 ± 18	103 ± 21	31.1 ± 6.0
Gout				
Normal uric acid production	6	99 ± 13	106 ± 10	31.2 ± 6.9
Excessive uric acid production				
Normal PRT activity	10	103 ± 18	104 ± 22	30.4 ± 5.3
Partial deficiency	24	0.03–12.2	0.009–17.3	26–74
Lesch-Nyhan syndrome	9	<0.01	<0.004	39–94

Source: Kelley et al. [200], except that data of Kogut et al. [580], Emmerson and Wyngaarden [582], and Sperling et al. [713], on patients with partial PRT deficiency, have been added, with corrections for differences in control values. Activity with hypoxanthine and guanine was reduced in parallel in patients with partial PRT deficiency, except in the L. family of Kelley et al. in which activity with hypoxanthine as substrate was 20-fold greater than with guanine.

biosynthesis by azathioprine requires prior conversion of this compound, or one of its metabolites, to a ribonucleotide form [514], in a reaction catalyzed by PRT [378]. Extension of the study of PRT activity to adult gouty subjects disclosed a partial deficiency in a limited number of overexcretors [710].

Activity values in dialyzed hemolysates have ranged from 0.01 to 17 percent of normal, with guanine as substrate (lowest activity detectable = 0.004 percent of normal) (Table 39-14). The amount of activity with either hypoxanthine or guanine as substrate varied greatly from one family to another, but was about the same among members of the same family. Further evidence of heterogeneity among the mutant enzymes was obtained in studies of heat stability and electrophoretic migration of the protein. In one family, the mutant enzyme was less stable than normal; in another, it was more stable; and in a third, it exhibited normal thermolability (Fig. 39-25) [200].

Leukocytes and fibroblasts of patients with partial PRT deficiency also show low activity values, indicating that this deficiency is not confined to a single cell line.

A-PRT Activity

An increase in the activity of the closely related enzyme, A-PRT, has been a consistent observation in hemolysates of patients with complete PRT deficiency [200], and was also observed in about one-half of patients with partial deficiency [200, 712, 713] (see Table 39-14). A-PRT activity values are normal in fibroblasts of PRT-deficient patients [715]. The elevated activity values of A-PRT in erythrocytes have been attributed to stabilization of the enzyme by the very high concentrations of phosphoribosylpyrophosphate in the erythrocytes of PRT-deficient subjects [716]. It is unlikely that the increase of activity values plays a role in the accelerated purine biosynthesis of PRT-deficient subjects, for reasons detailed elsewhere [200]. Also, it is pertinent to note that partial deficiencies of A-PRT activities, with values of approximately 20 percent [717], or 8 percent [718], of normal, are not associated with detectable abnormalities of purine metabolism. The gene for A-PRT is autosomal, rather than X-linked [717, 719].

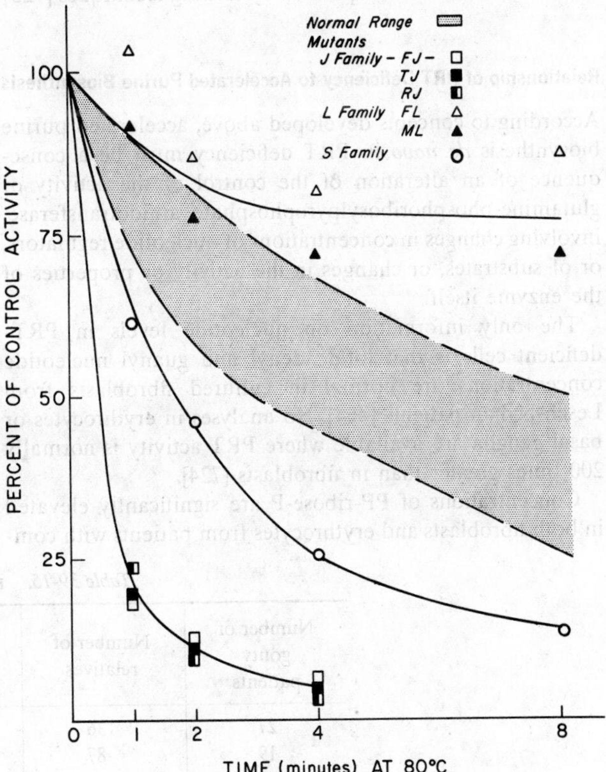

Figure 39-25. Inactivation of normal and mutant hypoxanthine-guanine phosphoribosyltransferase when heated at 80°C for the time indicated. (*Reproduced from Kelley et al.* [200], *with permission of Ann. Intern. Med.*)

Purine Metabolism in Heterozygotes

All mothers of PRT-deficient patients are obligate heterozygotes, except in the case of new mutations. In most instances heterozygotes have been clinically normal, without hyperuricemia or hyperuricaciduria [200, 580, 713]. However, three of nine heterozygotes studied by Kelley et al. [200] and two of three by Emmerson and Wyngaarden [714] were hyperuricemic. Only one of nine heterozygotes of the first series and one of three of the second showed reduced PRT activity values in erythrocytes, intermediate between those of hemizygotes and normal controls. Increased urinary uric acid, enlarged urate pools, increased urate turnover, and enhanced glycine incorporation into urinary urate have been reported in several obligate heterozygotes [714].

The fibroblasts of heterozygotes are mosaic, consisting of some cells having normal activity and some having no activity [720]. The proportion varies from 60 percent to virtually 100 percent of normal cells depending on the degree of cell contact in cultures. Demonstration of PRT-deficient cells may be enhanced by the use of selective growth conditions, in which an antimetabolite is employed to kill PRT-competent cells. At the present time, this is probably the simplest relatively dependable method available for the identification of heterozygotes [721, 722]. The two cell populations have also been separated by cloning techniques [723].

Relationship of PRT Deficiency to Accelerated Purine Biosynthesis

According to concepts developed above, accelerated purine biosynthesis *de novo* in PRT deficiency must be a consequence of an alteration of the control of the activity of glutamine-phosphoribosylpyrophosphate amidotransferase, involving changes in concentrations of nucleotide regulators, or of substrates, or changes in the activity or properties of the enzyme itself.

The only information on nucleotide levels in PRT-deficient cells is that total adenyl and guanyl nucleotide concentrations are normal in cultured fibroblasts from Lesch-Nyhan patients [464]. No analyses in erythrocytes or basal ganglia are available where PRT activity is normally 200 times greater than in fibroblasts [724].

Concentrations of PP-ribose-P are significantly elevated in both fibroblasts and erythrocytes from patients with complete or partial PRT deficiency [445, 464]. Representative values are shown in Table 39-9. Presumably these elevations reflect a reduced consumption of PP-ribose-P in the deficient PRT reaction. These values are sufficiently high that modest reductions induced by orotic acid or adenine, through consumption of PP-ribose-P in other phosphoribosyltransferase reactions, do not suppress purine biosynthesis *de novo* in vitro [466].

The activity and properties of glutamine-PP-ribose-P-amidotransferase have been approached indirectly. The rate of synthesis of formylglycinamide ribonucleotide is accelerated in fibroblasts from PRT-deficient subjects, but this may be a reflection of the elevated levels of substrate PP-ribose-P. Such fibroblasts appear to be at least normally susceptible to the inhibition of purine biosynthesis by derivatives of adenine or 6-methylmercaptopurine ribonucleoside, an adenosine analogue [464].

Relationship of PRT Deficiency to Neurological Dysfunction

Available information on this topic is presented in the chapter on the Lesch-Nyhan syndrome (Chap. 40).

HEREDITY

Familial Incidence of Gout

The familial nature of gout has been recognized since antiquity. Galen ascribed gout to "debauchery, intemperance and an hereditary trait." English observers have reported a familial incidence of gout of 38 to 81 percent in their cases [725]. In series reported from the United States the familial incidence has generally been from 6 to 18 percent [726, 727], but the true familial incidence may be higher as reflected in figures ranging up to 75 percent [728], obtained after persistent questioning.

Among hyperuricemic relatives of gouty subjects, the incidence of gout averaged 20 percent in five series reviewed by Smyth [265] (Table 39-15). In a population study in selected rural and urban populations in England a relatively high incidence of hyperuricemia was found in both localities, but no cases of clinical gout were found in the rural group and only two in the urban sample. The hyperuricemia was

Table 39-15. HYPERURICEMIA IN RELATIVES OF GOUTY PATIENTS

Number of gouty patients	Number of relatives	Number of gouty relatives	Number of hyperuricemic relatives	Percent hyperuricemic	Reference
27	136	3	34	25	[729]
19	87	3	21	24	[19]
44	136	0	16	11	[732]
3	29	11	21	72	[730]
32	261	16	71	27	[256]

Source: C. J. Smyth [265].

familial in 8 of 33 instances, but clinical gout was seen only in relatives where the proband was already suffering from gout. It was suggested that the inheritance of familial hyperuricemia does not necessarily determine the inheritance of clinical gout and that other factors, especially diet, may be concerned [34].

Asymptomatic Hyperuricemia in Families of Gouty Patients

The first recorded observation of asymptomatic hyperuricemia in a man in whose family gout occurred was by Folin and Lyman in 1913 [731]. In 1937 Jacobson found hyperuricemia in a son of each of two men with gout, and a brother of a third [266]. The first extensive study was by Talbott [729], who reported in 1940 that 25 percent of 136 asymptomatic blood relatives of 27 gouty persons had hyperuricemia. Smyth et al. [19] in the United States and Hauge and Harvald [256] in Denmark found similar prevalences (24 and 27 percent) in groups of 87 and 261 relatives, respectively. In other studies, prevalences ranging from 11 percent [289] to as high as 72 percent [730] have been recorded.

Hypothesis of an Autosomal Dominant Gene

The first studies of hyperuricemia in families of gouty subjects led to the conclusion that hyperuricemia was determined by an autosomal dominant gene whose penetrance was low, especially in women. Smyth et al. [19] found that a frequency diagram of serum urate values among relatives of gouty patients was bimodal for both males and females, with nadirs of 6.0 and 5.0 mg per 100 ml, respectively. Using these critical levels, they classified 10 of 48 male relatives and 11 of 39 females as hyperuricemic. The distribution of hyperuricemic individuals in 19 pedigrees conformed rather closely with expectations if such kindreds were segregated according to the presence or absence of a dominant autosomal gene for hyperuricemia. If this is the mode of inheritance, the ratio of hyperuricemic to normal offspring of matings in which only one patient is hyperuricemic should be 1:1. There were no hyperuricemic sons among 14 below the age of 16 years. However, when sons above age 16 years were considered, the ratio was six hyperuricemic to seven normal sons. Thus the data on male relatives were in agreement with the hypothesis of dominant autosomal inheritance if one assumed that the metabolic change resulting in hyperuricemia is not manifested in males until the age of puberty. Among daughters of the same matings, two of six below age 16 years and two of four above 16 years were hyperuricemic. These data in females do not fit an autosomal dominant pattern of inheritance. However, in females hyperuricemia frequently does not develop until after the menopause.

Stecher et al. [732] have published data which permit similar analyses. A frequency distribution of serum urate values of 137 relatives of gouty persons (excluding spouses) was shifted toward high values in comparison with a similar plot of 1,024 determinations on individuals from the general hospital population. It was also suggestively bimodal, the nadir being 6.0 to 6.4 mg per 100 ml, and 23 of 147 determinations on 137 relatives fell above this range. Among relatives, they observed hyperuricemia in 15 to 21 percent of mothers, brothers, sisters, and sons, but in none of 45 daughters of index cases. These workers also tentatively concluded that hyperuricemia was an autosomal dominant trait with low penetrance in both sexes, but considerably lower in females than in males. When this conclusion was put to numerical test for male offspring only, a correction being applied for small family size, the expected number of hyperuricemic individuals was 31. Actually 26 were found among 51 men. These figures were regarded as showing satisfactory conformity with the expected 1:1 ratio. The data were then used to estimate penetrance. Since 26 hyperuricemic sons were observed where 31 were expected, the penetrance was estimated at about 84 percent in heterozygote males. And since there were only 8 hyperuricemic females compared with 54 hyperuricemic males, despite the nearly equal sex distribution of the 203 individuals of the study, the penetrance was estimated to be about one-seventh as high in women as in men, or about 14 percent. Since not a single daughter of a gouty patient was found to be hyperuricemic, among 45 tested, no critical analysis could be applied in the case of female offspring. Both groups excluded sex-linked inheritance on the basis of male-to-male transmission patterns. Also a recessive genetic transmission pattern was excluded by Stecher et al. [732] on the basis of a probability analysis. In neither of these studies was a rigorous statistical analysis performed to exclude a unimodal distribution with skewness toward high values.

Hypothesis of Multifactorial Inheritance

The hypothesis of an autosomal dominant genetic control of hyperuricemia was questioned by Hauge and Harvald [256] following their study of 261 siblings of 32 gouty subjects. These writers came to the conclusion that hyperuricemia was a polygenic trait. Plots of serum uric acid values in both controls and relatives fitted unimodal distributions. No clear separation could be made between normal and abnormal uric acid values, although the mean values for both male and female relatives of gouty patients were higher than the mean values of their respective control groups. The data on male sibs conformed satisfactorily to the sum of two normal distributions, but those on female relatives did not. The writers therefore excluded inheritance due to a single autosomal dominant gene and concluded that to the extent that the higher uric acid values observed in these sibs as compared with the control group were genetically determined, multifactorial inheritance was responsible.

In 1965, Neel and associates [733] restudied 271 members

of 19 families first studied 18 years earlier by Smyth et al. [19] because of a gouty propositus. The new results showed a significant skewing to the right and the evidence for bimodality was less convincing than earlier. The hypothesis of multifactorial inheritance was considered at least as tenable as the "one-gene hyperuricemia" hypothesis.

Hyperuricemia in Population Studies

A study of 2,000 Blackfoot and Pima Indians showed an association of hyperuricemia with obesity and surface area, but in addition there were strong hereditary determinants of serum urate levels, which appeared to be polygenic. Transmission patterns suggested that some of the genes were autosomal dominants and others possibly sex-linked dominants [29]. The studies of Mikkelsen et al. [260, 734] of 6,000 residents of Tecumseh, Michigan, and of Hall et al. [26] of 5,000 residents of Framingham, Massachusetts, also favored multifactorial inheritance. The frequency histograms showed skewness toward high values without evidence of bimodality.

In contrast, the population studies of Lawrence et al. [24] in England, of Cobb and associates [35, 36] of Pittsburgh executives and medical students, of Decker et al. [27] of Filipino males living in Northwestern North America, and of Burch et al. [29] of the Chamorros and Carolinians of the Mariana Islands all showed bimodal distributions of serum uric acid values. Accordingly, these studies appear to support the dominant gene hypothesis.

When all available data are considered, they suggest a possible synthesis of views. In the species at large, the serum uric acid concentration is controlled by multiple genes. The probability of selecting out an apparently dominant genetic factor increases when the basis of selection is racial, when the group is an isolate, or when the study concerns several generations of families in which gout occurs, as in the studies of Smyth et al. [19] and Stecher et al. [732]. Evidence for polygenic control will be more prominent when the population is heterogeneous or when only sibs of gouty subjects are studied, as in the investigations of Hauge and Harvald [256].

Further progress in understanding the heredity of hyperuricemia will require a definition of the precise biochemical mechanism of hyperuricemia in each isolate or family, and study of the transmission of that trait. It is doubtful that additional population studies will contribute further to our understanding of hereditary mechanisms.

Genetic Control of Uric Acid Excretion

The renal excretion of uric acid is almost certainly under the control of both genetic and nongenetic factors. In the Dalmatian coach dog, failure of tubular reabsorption of urate [735, 736] is a recessive trait associated with spottedness. In man the hypouricemia of the Fanconi syndrome and Wilson's disease [737, 738] arise as a consequence of inherited metabolic defects.

In a study of uric acid excretion in 37 patients with primary gout and 96 of their first-degree relatives, Scott and Pollard [739] found a graded correlation between clearance values of patients and relatives, closer in the case of male than of female relatives. These observations suggest that the concept of multifactorial influences regulating urate levels in plasma may apply to the renal handling as well as the production of urate.

X-linked Hyperuricemia—Complete and Partial PRT Deficiencies

As pointed out above and in Chap. 40, hypoxanthine-guanine phosphoribosyltransferase deficiency is an X-linked condition, clinically manifest in fully expressed form only in the hemizygous male. A representative pedigree of complete deficiency (Lesch-Nyhan syndrome) is shown in Fig. 40-9, and one of partial deficiency in Fig. 39-26. Examples of complete [577] or partial [200] deficiencies among half-brothers are known. In both instances the half-brothers were related through their mothers. No examples of male-to-male transmission of PRT deficiency have been identified [200, 577].

Heterozygous subjects may be mildly hyperuricemic, may show abnormalities of kinetics of uric acid synthesis or turnover, and may show values of erythrocyte PRT activity intermediate between normal values and values in deficient subjects [200, 714]. However, in most obligate heterozygotes, erythrocyte phosphoribosyltransferase activity values are normal [200, 580, 713]. A selective growth or survival advantage of PRT-competent erythrocytes in competition with PRT-deficient cells appears to be a likely explanation. The mature erythrocyte cannot synthesize purine ribonucleotides *de novo.* It is possible that even normal or increased activity of A-PRT in PRT-deficient erythrocytes may not enable the cell to maintain normal nucleotide levels. An alternative explanation is that there is selective inactivation of the X chromosome which codes for the mutant PRT enzyme in erythropoietic cells.

Subjects who are heterozygous for PRT deficiency are mosaic: their fibroblasts grown in tissue culture show two populations of cells, one capable, the other incapable of utilizing hypoxanthine [720]. These results are consistent with the Lyon hypothesis [740] of early random irreversible inactivation of one of the X chromosomes in the cells of female subjects. When fibroblasts in tissue culture are grown to confluence the majority of cells may appear normal in their ability to utilize hypoxanthine or guanine. This phenomenon may reflect metabolic cooperation [741], a process in which some product of a competent cell is transferred to an incompetent cell. In this instance, the transfer apparently

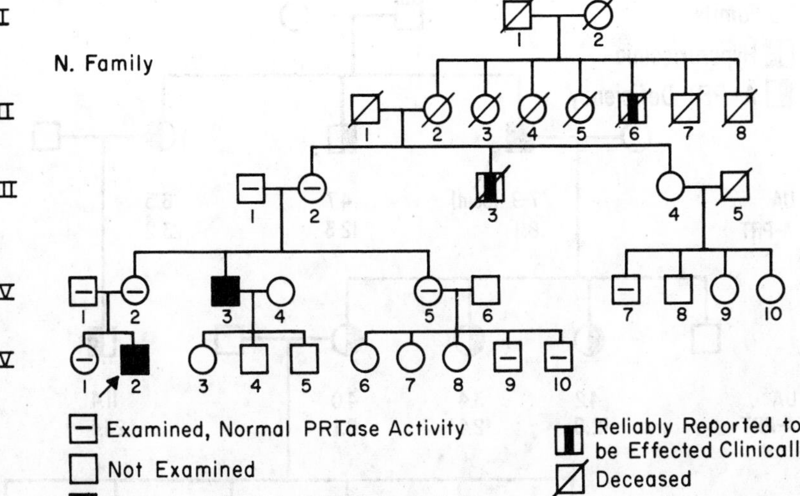

Figure 39-26 Pedigree of a family with partial PRT deficiency, gout, and spinocerebellar ataxia. (*Reproduced from Kelley et al.* [200], *with permission of Ann. Intern. Med.*)

involves the labeled nucleotide or one of its products synthesized in the PRT-competent cell with which the PRT-deficient cell is in contact [742].

A mouse fibroblast line, deficient in PRT activity, has been successfully transformed with competent mouse DNA by Szibalska and Szibalski [743].

Hyperuricemia in Autosomally Inherited Conditions

Glucose-6-Phosphatase Deficiency

The occurrence of hyperuricemia and gout in this condition was discussed above and in Chap. 7. The transmission of this disorder as an autosomal recessive trait is well established.

Glutathione Reductase Variant

During a survey of 1,473 Negro male outpatients for variants of erythrocyte glucose-6-phosphate dehydrogenase, an electrophoretically fast variant of glutathione reductase was detected [607]. In a subgroup of 196 consecutive samples there was no association between the common G-6-PD variants and the glutathione reductase variant. The gene frequency of the variant was 0.133 and of the usual form of the enzymes it was 0.867. A subsequent study of 125 presumably healthy Negroes, 79 males and 46 females, selected at random from the population, showed a gene frequency of 0.132 for the glutathione reductase variant, almost identical with that of the outpatient hospital population. Studies of nine Negro families [607] are consistent with the assumption of an autosomal mode of inheritance of the enzyme variant. The striking frequency of the fast variant among 28 gout patients (1.9 percent of the 1,473 subjects) compared with the predicted random distribution of the trait, and the findings in the last 196 general medical patients of the G-6-PD study (all Negro males), are shown in Table 39-16.

In a subsequent study [268] of 522 Negro volunteers, 10 phenotypes of glutathione reductase were detected by acrylamide-gel electrophoresis of plasma. These were judged to be the products of five alleles at the same autosomal gene locus. Gene frequencies were 0.2644 for type 1, 0.6322 for type 2, 0.0086 for type 4, 0.0431 for type 5, and 0.0517 for type 6. Mean plasma urate levels were higher for those who were heterozygous or homozygous for type 1 and type 6 variants than for those homozygous for the usual form of the enzyme, type 2 (type 2, 5.17 mg per 100 ml; type 1, 7.24 mg per 100 ml; type 6, 6.48 mg per 100 ml). Red cells with type 1 or 6 enzyme show greater glutathione reductase activity and less activation by FAD than those with type 2 or 5.

A-PRT Deficiency

Two families with partial A-PRT deficiency are known. In one, values about 20 percent of normal were found in four

Table 39-16. FREQUENCY OF GLUTATHIONE REDUCTASE PHENOTYPES IN GENERAL NEGRO POPULATION AND IN NEGRO MALES WITH GOUT OR OTHER MEDICAL ILLNESSES

GSSG-R phenotype	General Negro population, percent	*Negro male patients*	
		Gout	Other illnesses
S	75.16	5	150
FS	23.06	15	40
F	1.78	8	6

Source: W. K. Long [607].

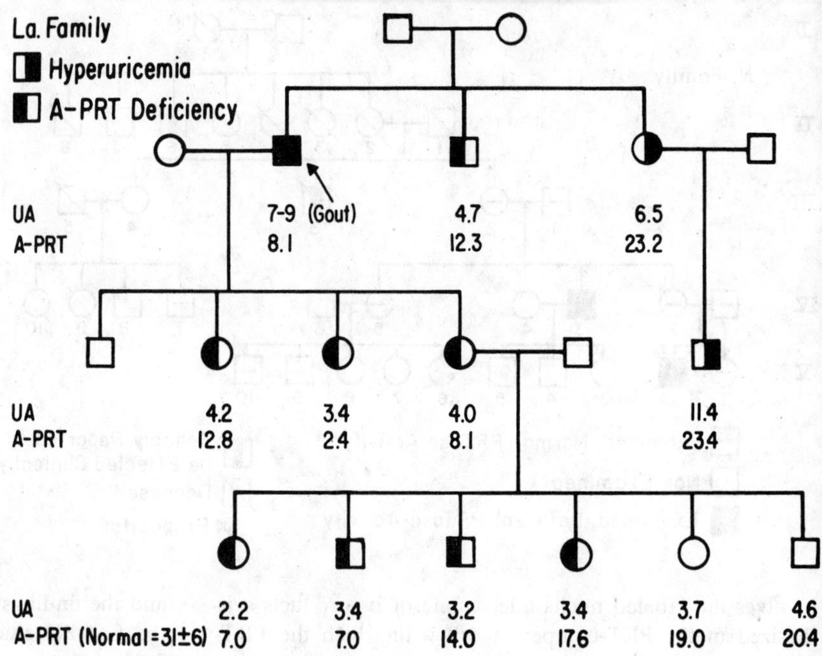

Figure 39-27. Pedigree of a family with partial adenine phosphoribosyltransferase (A-PRT) deficiency and hyperuricemia. Note lack of concordance of the two traits.

members of three generations. The transmission of the trait from father to two daughters but not to a third established the autosomal location of the gene for A-PRT [717, 719]. A novel mechanism of the association of mutant and normal A-PRT polypeptide strands in a hypothetical polymeric structure was proposed as a potential explanation of activity values appreciably lower than one-half of normal. The propositus of this pedigree was hyperlipoproteinemia. None of the A-PRT-deficient subjects was hyperuricemic.

In the second family, A-PRT deficiency was more variable. Activity values ranged from 8 to 60 percent of normal in erythrocytes. The propositus was hyperuricemic. Family study disclosed discordance of the two traits, with examples of all four possible combinations of findings [718]. (Fig. 39-27).

It is likely that a complete or high-grade deficiency of A-PRT would require a double dose of abnormal allele and be inherited as an autosomal recessive condition. No such patient has yet been identified, and it is therefore not presently possible to comment on the potential effect of total A-PRT deficiency upon purine metabolism, or health.

Hyperuricemia and Types III, IV, and V Hyperlipoproteinemia

This association [747] is discussed more fully in Chap. 28. The common denominator with reference to hyperuricemia is probably the presence of hypertriglyceridemia in each of these types of hyperlipoproteinemia. The mode of inheritance of these hyperlipoproteinemias is not yet certain. Type IV hyperlipoproteinemia may coexist with partial PRT deficiency [200] or glucose-6-phosphatase deficiency [609].

Idiopathic Familial Uric Acid Nephrolithiasis

This condition has been described among Israeli subjects with normal serum and urinary uric acid values. The defect appears to be one leading to undue acidity of the urine [178], as discussed above. It is reported to be a disorder distinct from gout and inherited as an autosomal dominant condition [171].

SECONDARY HYPERURICEMIA AND GOUT

A few decades ago it was widely held that all gout was hereditary [127]. The coexistence of gout and of polycythemia vera, for example, was viewed as the chance concurrence of primary gout with a second relatively common disease. Additional clinical observations and new insights into the mechanism of the acute attack of gout have altered these views. It is now recognized that acquired hyperuricemia is common, and that the potential for development of gout exists in all hyperuricemic subjects.

In one large series, 13.2 percent of hospitalized males were hyperuricemic, and in 70 percent of this group hyperuricemia was attributable to a specific nongenetic cause [748]. Gouty arthritis occurs relatively frequently in patients with polycythemia vera, myeloid metaplasia, or chronic lead intoxication, in whom hyperuricemia is usually quite severe and long standing. By contrast, gouty arthritis appears to be unusual in patients with hyperuricemia due to renal failure. In general, secondary hyperuricemia is caused by either the increased turnover of nucleic acid purines or the impaired renal excretion of uric acid. Thus in secondary gout, as in primary gout, hyperuricemia appears to have a dual pathogenesis. The differentiation of secondary metabolic gout from secondary renal gout [309] is often valid, although these categories are not mutually exclusive (Table 39-17).

Hematologic Disorders

Hyperuricemia and secondary gout occur in lymphoproliferative and myeloproliferative disorders [749–752], multiple myeloma [753], secondary polycythemia [754, 755], certain hemoglobinopathies, thalassemia, and pernicious anemia. All of these conditions are associated with chronically increased marrow activity.

In one large series of patients with leukemia, myeloid metaplasia, polycythemia vera, and multiple myeloma, hyperuricemia was noted in 66 percent of 113 male patients and 69 percent of 73 female patients, although only 10 patients had a history of gouty arthritis [756]. Gouty arthritis occurred most commonly in patients with myeloid metaplasia (6 of 22 patients). In other series, gouty arthritis has occurred in 2 to 14 percent (mean 6 percent) of patients with polycythemia vera, but 84 percent of the gouty patients have been males. Hyperuricemia probably occurs with increased frequency in all types of leukemia, with the possible exception of chronic lymphocytic leukemia, and in general the degree of hyperuricemia is correlated with bone marrow proliferation [756]. The serum urate concentration tends to be higher in these patients than in patients with primary hyperuricemia [43, 749]. Exacerbations of hyperuricemia and gout are commonly related to radiation or chemotherapy.

Table 39-17. SECONDARY (ACQUIRED) HYPERURICEMIA

Increased production of uric acid
- Associated with increased nucleic acid turnover
  - Myeloproliferative disorders
  - Lymphoproliferative disorders
  - Chronic hemolytic anemias
  - Psoriasis
- Associated with increased synthesis *de novo;* induced by:
  - 2-Ethylamino-1,3,4-thiadiazole
  - Fructose ingestion or infusion

Decreased renal excretion of uric acid
- Reduced renal functional mass
  - Chronic renal disease of various types
  - Reduced renal perfusion, e.g., myxedema
- Inhibited tubular secretion of uric acid
  - Condition associated with hyperlactic acidemia, e.g., acute ethanolism, toxemia of pregnancy, sarcoidosis
  - Condition associated with β-hydroxybutyric and acetoacetic acidemia, e.g., starvation, diabetic ketoacidosis
  - Induced by drugs
    - Pyrazinamide
    - Salicylates in low dosage
  - Lead nephropathy (plus reduced functional mass)
- Enhanced tubular reabsorption of uric acid
  - Conditions associated with intraarterial volume contraction
    - Natriuretic agents, especially thiazides and thiazide derivatives
    - Others, e.g., hepatorenal syndrome

Not established
- Hyperlipoproteinemias, types III, IV, and V
- Down's syndrome
- Obesity

Sandberg et al. [757] found that increased uric acid excretion was common in acute leukemias and in all chronic leukemias, except the lymphocytic variety. In 15 patients with acute leukemia and in 2 patients with chronic myelocytic leukemia. Rieselback et al. found that the uric acid excretion rate ranged from 0.92 to 10.3 mg per min per 1.73 M^2 compared with a mean control value of 0.71 $\pm$ 0.22 mg per min per 1.73 M^2 [653]. Gutman and Yü [43] found a mean urinary uric acid excretion value of 634 mg per 24 hr in 27 cases of secondary gout complicating hematologic disorders, as compared to a mean value of 497 mg per 24 hr in their control group. The fractional urate clearance, $C_{\text{uric acid}}$/GFR, is generally normal or increased [646, 653]. These patients tend to show normal or low values of hypoxanthine, xanthine, and 1 + 7-methylguanines, and normal or high values of adenine, guanine, 7-methyl-8-hydroxyguanine, pseudouridine, and succinoadenine in the urine [758]. In addition, increases of urinary inosine and guanosine and of certain other purine and pyrimidine compounds have been noted in leukemic subjects [759].

The miscible pool of uric acid and its turnover are increased in patients with myelogenous leukemia or polycythemia vera [564]. The incorporation of glycine-^{15}N [414, 760], glycine-1-^{14}C, and 5-aminoimidazole-4-carboxamide-4-^{14}C [588, 589] into urinary purine bases and uric acid has revealed striking labeling of the bases during the first day followed by secondary maxima in bases and uric acid between 7 and 12 days (Fig. 39-28). Cumulative incorporation of isotope into uric acid is approximately normal during the first few days but greatly exceeds the normal after 1 to 2 weeks [588]. All these data indicate an exaggerated turnover of nucleic acid purines as the cause of hyperuricemia in these subjects.

Hyperuricemia has been described in 11 of 12 males and 5 of 8 females with infectious mononucleosis [761]. The increase in plasma urate values was maximal within the first 2 weeks of the disease and tended to parallel the presence of abnormal lymphocytosis.

In sickle cell disease, 6 of 13 patients were found to have a serum urate concentration greater than 6.0 mg per 100 ml [762]. Two patients had a history strongly suggestive of gouty arthritis. One patient with SS disease and gout showed both overproduction of uric acid and diminished excretion due to diminished nephron mass [763]. Hyperuricemia has also been described in about one-third of patients with SC disease but gouty arthritis has occurred infrequently [764]. Gouty arthritis may also complicate β-thalassemia and other chronic hemolytic anemias [765, 766].

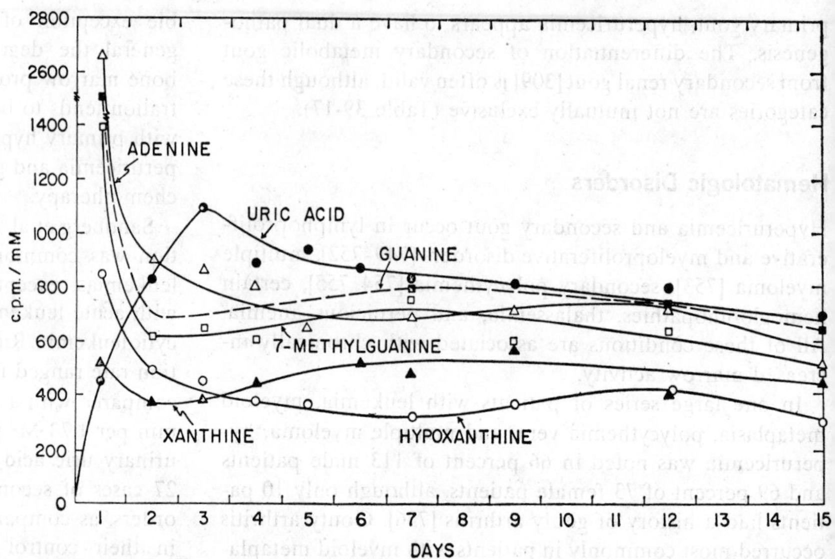

Figure 39-28. Specific activity values of urinary purines in a patient with myeloid metaplasia, following the oral administration of glycine-1-^{14}C. (*From J. B. Wyngaarden* [589], *with permission of Metabolism.*)

Drug-induced Hyperuricemia

This has become an important category in clinical medicine. Drug-induced hyperuricemia is a frequent antecedent of acute and chronic gouty arthritis. The list of drugs which lead to hyperuricemia includes the potent diuretics, alcohol, pyrazinamide, and salicylates in low doses. All of these agents, except the diuretics, have been discussed elsewhere in this chapter. Drug-induced gout has become increasingly important since the advent of the potent thiazide diuretics [767, 768].

Diuretics

In a study of hyperuricemic men admitted to a Veterans Administration hospital, diuretics were considered the causative factor in 20 percent [769]. Of the new cases of gout in Framingham, Massachusetts, 50 percent have developed in subjects taking thiazides or ethacrynic acid [274]. The mean urate level for this group prior to diuretic therapy was 5.8 mg per 100 ml, which is higher than the mean of 5.1 mg per 100 ml for men. Hyperuricemia has been noted in up to 75 percent of patients treated with diuretics [770], but it may not be appropriate to place sole responsibility for induction of hyperuricemia or of gout upon the drug.

There are several mechanisms by which potent diuretic agents may produce hyperuricemia [771]. The work of Steele and Oppenheimer [772, 773] suggests that a prerequisite is sufficient salt and water loss to produce volume contraction. Following the administration of furosemide or ethacrynic acid, tubular reabsorption of filtered urate is increased. In addition, in several studies inhibition of tubular secretion of urate seems likely. Neither effect appears to represent a direct action of the diuretic agent upon tubular transport of urate, for urate excretion values remained near control values when volume depletion was prevented by replacement of urinary salt and water losses with intravenous saline. Replacement studies also led Suki et al. [774] to postulate that thiazide-induced hyperuricemia was a byproduct of extracellular fluid volume contraction. These observations suggest that any diuretic sufficiently effective to produce volume contraction may produce hyperuricemia. Acetazolamide [775] and chlorthalidone [776] are also in this class.

Secondary extrarenal influences upon the kidney may be responsible for the hyperuricemia. Volume contraction leads to a generalized increase in solute reabsorption, perhaps mediated by changes in oncotic pressure [777–779]. In addition, furosemide induces hyperlacticacidemia sufficient to suppress tubular secretion of urate [780]. This is also true for diazoxide, a nondiuretic thiazide which promotes muscle glycolysis and leads to hyperlacticacidemia [781]. Thiazide-induced hyperuricemia is corrected by KCl or NH_4Cl, apparently in part by causing a uricosuria and in part by causing a redistribution of urate among body compartments [782]. Neither organomercurials nor xanthine diuretics appear to have been studied in detail with respect to hyperuricemia. Organomercurials are listed as capable of producing hyperuricemia by Beyer and Baer [783]. It is doubtful that xanthine diuretics are sufficiently potent by themselves to produce volume contraction and hyperuricemia. Their biotransformation into uric acid is not an issue. There is also little information on the production of hyperuricemia by diuretics which affect primarily the distal tubular sodium exchange site, such as spironolactone or triamterene, which tend to be rather weak natriuretic agents, unlikely by themselves to lead to volume contraction.

Hypertension

In untreated hypertensive patients without discernible renal disease the incidence of hyperuricemia ranges from 22 to

27 percent [784, 785]. When therapy and renal disease are not excluded, the incidence increases to 47 to 67 percent [784–787]. Hyperuricemia is equally common in essential and renovascular hypertension [784]. Values of 59 to 67 percent were recorded in patients in whom the disease was severe enough to warrant sympathectomy [786, 787] or adrenalectomy [788]. Gout was observed in 11 of 105 such patients. The overall incidence of gout in hypertension has been variably reported as 2 to 12 percent [784, 785].

In most hypertensive patients, hyperuricemia appears to be related to the reduced renal excretion of uric acid, attributed to a lower $C_{\text{uric acid}}$/GFR ratio than in nonhyperuricemic hypertensives [789]. The suggestion has been made that tubular dysfunction may be a consequence of vascular disease, tissue hypoxia, and local lactic acid excess, but attempts to relate hyperuricemia to hyperlacticacidemia have been controversial [784, 788].

Hyperuricemia is present in 24 to 52 percent of patients with myocardial infarction [223, 790]; it is also present in increased incidence in patients with moderate or severe peripheral vascular disease [791]. Multiple factors, including hypertension, renal disease, hyperlipoproteinemia, diuretic agents, anoxia, and hyperlacticacidemia, and occasionally primary gout, need to be considered in explanation of the hyperuricemia.

Chronic Renal Insufficiency

Hyperuricemia is common in the presence of renal insufficiency although it has not been possible to correlate the serum urate value or endogenous uric acid clearance with the degree of renal insufficiency [792]. This lack of correlation is at least partly attributable to the relative augmentation of fractional uric acid excretion which occurs with decreasing GFR [648, 793].

In spite of very high serum urate concentrations in some patients, gouty arthritis occurs only rarely. In a study of 496 patients with chronic renal insufficiency, Sarre [794] found 6 with gout, in 4 of whom the disease appeared to be primary. Several examples have also been reported by others [309, 795]. The paucity of gouty arthritis in these patients has been attributed to (1) a shortened life span; and (2) a decreased ability to respond to an inflammatory stimulus [796].

Recurrent attacks of acute arthritis may occur in patients with chronic renal failure treated with periodic hemodialysis. The clinical features of the acute inflammatory episodes, their response to colchicine, and the tendency for their frequency to vary directly with the plasma urate level have led to the diagnosis of acute gouty arthritis [122, 123]. However, examination of the synovial fluid frequently reveals the presence of calcium phosphate crystals rather than monosodium urate crystals [124]. Similarly the crystals in muscle have also been identified as calcium phosphate, not urate [124].

It is not yet clear whether prolonged hyperuricemia in renal insufficiency can lead to the deposition of monosodium urate within the kidney. Although several studies suggest this possibility, the crystals noted have not been positively identified. [797]

Saturnine Gout

The association of gout with chronic lead poisoning led many years ago to the concept of saturnine gout, in which gout was regarded as a complication of the chronic nephritis of plumbism [798]. A relatively high incidence of this type of gout appears still to exist in Queensland, Australia [799], and in France [800] where patients were exposed to leaded paint in childhood. When compared to primary gout, this group of patients has a higher incidence of renal disease prior to the first episode of arthritis, females are more frequently affected, the arthritis is milder, the mean age of onset is younger, there is a lower incidence of renal calculi, and they are less likely to have a family history of gout [801]. In the United States, saturnine gout is most often related to the habitual consumption of moonshine alcohol with an appreciable lead content. In a recent study at a southern Veterans Administration hospital, 37 of 43 cases of gout were found to be associated with chronic lead intoxication [802, 803].

The observation that 70 of 450 patients with gouty arthritis in Spain had a history of direct and prolonged contact with leaded gasoline suggests that subclinical lead intoxication from another source may also be important [804]. The hyperuricemia in chronic lead intoxication is due to decreased uric acid excretion [803, 805].

Sarcoid and Chronic Beryllium Disease

Hyperuricemia has been reported in 36 to 50 percent of patients with sarcoidosis [806–809] and in 40 percent of patients with chronic beryllium disease [810]. In the latter group of patients, the elevated serum urate concentration was due to a diminished fractional renal clearance of uric acid. Interestingly, uric acid retention occurred almost exclusively in those patients exhibiting a reduced carbon monoxide diffusing capacity [810], and was associated with hyperlacticacidemia quantitatively similar to that observed in eclampsia and following ethanol ingestion.

Starvation

Total caloric restriction is known to result in extreme degrees of hyperuricemia [811–814] attributable in part to a reduced renal clearance of uric acid [680] and in part to the overproduction of uric acid [812]. The retention of uric acid is correlated best with ketosis and with the serum concentration of β-hydroxybutyrate [210, 679, 682]. Refeeding of carbohydrate results in correction of ketosis, temporarily excessive excretion of uric acid, and reduction in serum urate levels.

Attacks of gouty arthritis may occur during periods of starvation [815], but are unusual except in patients with a prior history of gout [232].

Hyperparathyroidism

There is a high incidence of hyperuricemia in hyperparathyroidism [816–818]. Scott et al. [818] noted hyperuricemia in 11 of 12 patients, in 5 of whom they obtained a history consistent with gout. They postulated that the hyperuricemia is renal in origin, possibly related to nephrocalcinosis.

Most studies have failed to demonstrate any relationship between urate excretion and the plasma concentration, or urinary excretion of calcium or phosphate [819, 820] and the infusion of parathyroid hormone [821]. Synovial fluid examination is essential to the diagnosis of gout in these patients and must disclose urate rather than calcium pyrophosphate crystals, for pseudogout may also occur in this setting [822].

Down's Syndrome

The serum urate concentration is significantly higher in patients with Down's syndrome than in mentally retarded controls from the same institutions [823–826]. This appears to be due to a decreased fractional clearance of uric acid [825, 827]. The turnover of uric acid is not increased [828]. In one small series no significant difference in serum urate levels was noted in the trisomic and translocation forms of Down's syndrome [829]. There is currently no evidence to suggest an increased incidence of gouty arthritis in these patients.

Psoriasis

Hyperuricemia occurs in 30 to 50 percent of patients with psoriasis and tends to correlate with the extent of skin involvement [830]. The pattern of enrichment of urinary uric acid in hyperuricemic patients with psoriasis given glycine-1-^{14}C shows peak values intermediate in time between those of primary gout and those of secondary gout due to myeloproliferative disease. This has been interpreted as indicating increased nucleotide and nucleic acid turnover in the psoriatic lesions as probable pathogenetic factors in the hyperuricemia [830]. The association of sarcoidosis, psoriasis, and gout has been reported and regarded as a syndrome by some [808], as chance concurrence by others [807], or possibly as sarcoid arthritis in a hyperuricemic subject with psoriasis but without true gout [831].

THERAPY

The objectives of therapy differ in acute gouty arthritis, interval gout, and chronic tophaceous gout. Current concepts and practices in the treatment of primary and secondary gout are presented in detail elsewhere [832–835]. This discussion will be limited to the mechanisms of the actions of drugs which have specific effects in gout or upon purine metabolism.

Acute Gout

The acute gouty attack may be treated with colchicine, phenylbutazone, oxyphenbutazone, indomethacin, ACTH, or corticoids. The possible mechanism of action of colchicine will be discussed below.

Colchicine

The response of the inflammatory reaction of acute gouty arthritis to colchicine has long been considered specific, but this time-honored axiom has been questioned in reports of responses of acutely inflamed joints of serum sickness [836], experimental arthritis [837], sarcoid arthritis [838], rheumatoid arthritis [839], and the inflammation associated with hydroxyapatite calcific tendinitis [119]. Some of the disagreement results from the varying criteria for an adequate colchicine response. Using rigid criteria, Wallace et al. [840] noted a typical response to oral colchicine in 75 percent of 58 patients with gout, and in only 4 of 37 patients with a variety of other articular disorders. Response to colchicine given intravenously may be more specific for gouty arthritis [841].

The nature of the anti-inflammatory action of colchicine in gout has been one of the mysteries of medicine. Following its intravenous infusion colchicine rapidly enters cells [842, 843] where it is bound in a noncovalent complex to a subunit protein of microtubules [844–847]. These microtubules, which are ordinarily demonstrable in human polymorphonuclear leukocytes, are no longer visible in the presence of colchicine [844]. These observations led Malawista to suggest that colchicine may interfere with the locomotion of the leukocyte, a process which requires rapid, reversible sol-gel transformations within the cell [844–847]. Studies of leukocyte function in the presence of colchicine indicate that it inhibits a variety of functions including leukocyte adhesiveness [848], amoeboid motility [849], mobilization [850], chemotaxis [851], random motility under the influence of urate [852], degranulation of lysosomes [853, 854], and leukocyte metabolism during phagocytosis [854–856]. In addition, colchicine blocks kinin release from plasma under the influence of leukocytes [857]. The most potent inhibitory effects of colchicine are on the motility of leukocytes [852] and the development of chemotactic activity after phagocytosis of urate crystals [851]. It remains to be proven whether the effects of colchicine in the treatment of acute gouty arthritis are related to its actions upon the leukocyte [83, 97]. This drug does not alter serum concentration or renal excretion of uric acid [130], nor does it have any significant effect upon the miscible pool of uric acid or the rate of its turnover [562, 565]. It inhibits uric acid ribonucleoside phosphorylase, as do a number of other agents [431].

Colchicine Prophylaxis

The practice of giving small daily doses of colchicine as prophylaxis against acute attacks of gout was introduced by Cohen in 1936 [725] and advocated by Talbott and Coombs in 1938 [299]. In 1952 Gutman and Yü [858] reported that 18 of 31 patients who ingested colchicine daily for 18 months or more experienced a conspicuous reduction in the frequency of acute attacks. This program enabled restoration of full employment in 13 patients who had been virtually incapacitated because of frequent episodes of gout. Subsequently, Yü and Gutman [859] reported a series of 208 gouty subjects who had received 0.5 to 2.0 mg colchicine daily for from 2 to 10 years (mean 5.4 years) selected because of a prior history of frequent and disabling attacks of acute gouty arthritis. Of these, 119 received colchicine alone, and 89 tophaceous patients received colchicine and uricosuric agents concomitantly. In 74 percent, the results of prophylaxis were considered excellent, in 20 percent satisfactory, and in 6 percent unsatisfactory.

A number of physicians have recorded experiences in agreement with those above [728, 860, 861], whereas others have not been impressed with the value of maintenance colchicine [862–864] and have cited progressive development of chronic gouty arthritis in spite of its use [865].

Two children whose father had been taking colchicine prophylactically at the time of conception have been born with Down's syndrome [866]. Lymphocytes cultured from gouty patients treated with colchicine showed an increase of cells with abnormal numbers of chromosomes, including an increased frequency of cells with 47 chromosomes [866]. Large doses of colchicine given as a single intravenous injection have been reported to induce a chromosomal alteration [867]. However, Yü and Gutman did not observe an increased incidence of congenital abnormalities in the progeny of 34 patients treated with prophylactic colchicine [859]. Walker reported 200 patients with Down's syndrome, none of whom had been born to a parent known to be taking colchicine [868].

Colchicine at doses of 2.6 to 3.9 mg per day has produced a reversible malabsorption syndrome with an increase in fecal fat, a decreased absorption of *d*-xylose and B_{12}, and a decreased serum cholesterol value [869–871]. A rare manifestation of chronic colchicine toxicity is myopathy [872].

Regulation of Serum Urate Level

Four approaches have been employed in attempts to reduce serum urate levels in hyperuricemic subjects. These include (1) reduction of uric acid synthesis by dietary means—restriction of purine, protein, ethanol, or caloric intake; (2) promotion of increased uric acid excretion by the administration of uricosuric agents; (3) destruction of urate within the body by the administration of uricase; (4) inhibition of uric acid synthesis by the administration of agents which either inhibit xanthine oxidase or purine synthesis *de novo,* or both.

The efficacy of dietary measures has been touched upon elsewhere in this chapter. Influences upon both rates of production of purines and excretion of uric acid have been cited, but the full scope of these complex interrelationships is not yet known. In addition to the obvious effect of the restriction of purine intake upon the production of uric acid, protein restriction in and of itself reduces the rate of purine synthesis *de novo* in both normal and gouty man [484]. However, the advent of well-tolerated hypouricemic agents has rendered severe dietary measures unnecessary in most gouty patients.

This section will deal with the pharmacologic therapy of hyperuricemia or uricaciduria. Indications for therapy include recurrent attacks of acute gouty arthritis or of uric acid nephrolithiasis, or demonstrable accumulations of monosodium urate as visible or radiographically detectable tophi. Asymptomatic hyperuricemia is not an indication for therapy with drugs, unless serum urate levels are in a range where acute gouty attacks, early tophaceous gout, uric acid nephrolithiasis, or hyperuricemic nephropathy become statistically likely. From data presented elsewhere in this chapter, a critical value of 9 mg per 100 ml or above is suggested. In other hyperuricemic subjects, one can afford to wait for an attack of acute gout or of uric acid stone before instituting therapy. Evidence is scant that mild hyperuricemia in itself is associated with a more rapid decline of renal function than occurs in nonhyperuricemic subjects of equivalent age [873, 874].

When it is decided that administration of a hypouricemic drug is indicated, the objective of treatment is to reduce the serum urate level to 6 mg per 100 ml or lower and to maintain it in this range indefinitely. No resolution of tophi occurs unless the serum level is brought below 7 mg per 100 ml [875], but if lower levels are achieved, striking reductions in the size of visible tophi and regeneration and recalcification of bone matrix may take place [128, 864, 875]. The shift of the uric acid balance in tissues from positive to negative occurs as a consequence of the lowering of serum uric acid levels to values sufficiently undersaturated to permit the dissolution of tophi. In addition, the frequency of attacks of acute gout may eventually be considerably reduced in patients by the adequate control of hyperuricemia, although shortly after the institution of therapy acute attacks may be frequent [128].

Uricosuric Agents

The mechanisms of action of these drugs has been discussed above. An extensive clinical experience attests to the dramatic success of such agents as probenecid [875] and sulfinpyrazone [876] in the control of hyperuricemia and the prevention and resolution of tophi in a large segment of the gouty population. Nevertheless, in spite of careful management, a significant percentage of patients is not brought under ideal control. In one large clinic, 27 percent of the patients receiving probenecid failed to achieve serum urate levels of less than 7 mg per 100 ml [875]. In another study with various agents, only half of 64 patients achieved levels of 6 mg per 100 ml [877]. Leading causes of failure were drug intolerance, concomitant salicylate ingestion, and renal impairment. In the experience of de Seze et al. [878] and Kuzell et al. [876], about one-third of patients eventually became intolerant of probenecid. Tolerance for sulfinpyrazone is reported to be better than for probenecid. At times, combinations of uricosuric drugs prove superior to the use of one drug along [879].

The use of uricosuric agents adds to the risk of urinary stone formation and does not result in the improvement of impaired renal function, though further progression of renal damage may be arrested [880].

Inhibition of Uric Acid Synthesis

Agents which inhibit synthesis of purine compounds have been identified and their mechanisms of action discussed earlier in this chapter. The only agent in general clinical use in this country is allopurinol. Oxipurinol and occasionally orotic acid are also used in Europe.

Allopurinol

Allopurinol was first synthesized for trial as a chemotherapeutic agent, but by itself had little or no effect upon experimental tumors [881, 882]. It was found to be an inhibitor of xanthine oxidase [535] and to inhibit the conversion of 6-thiopurine to 6-thiouric acid in mouse and man [883]. It was first introduced clinically as an adjunct therapy for patients receiving 6-thiopurine for leukemia [538]. Patients given allopurinol showed a pronounced reduction in both serum and urinary uric acid values. These observations suggested a trial of the agent in gout [538, 884]. Allopurinol is now established as a standard form of therapy in gout [539, 885–889].

The administration of allopurinol to subjects with normal renal function is followed by a prompt decrease in the serum and urinary uric acid values occurring within 24 to 48 hr, reaching a maximum in 4 days to 2 weeks and remaining relatively constant over prolonged periods of time [887, 889]. With the inhibition of urate production by allopurinol, increased amounts of the precursors, hypoxanthine and xanthine, appear in the urine, usually within 4 to 6 hr [890]

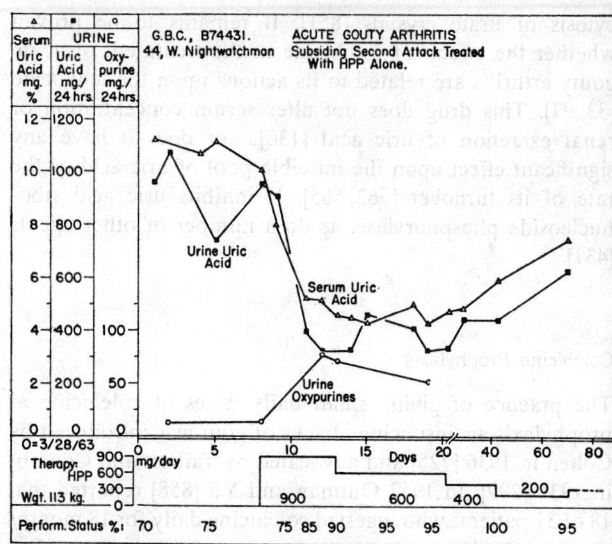

Figure 39-29. Effect of allopurinol on serum concentration of uric acid and on urinary excretion of uric acid and of oxypurines in a gouty subject. (*Reproduced from Rundles et al.* [538], *with permission of the Association of American Physicians.*)

(Fig. 39-29). Only trivial changes occur in the excretion of other urinary purine bases [551]. The combined increase in hypoxanthine and xanthine, though striking, usually falls far short of balancing the decrement in uric acid (see below). Withdrawal of allopurinol results in a return to pretreatment serum urate levels within a few days and the exceptional more prolonged effects are clearly associated with the delayed excretion of oxipurinol [537].

The concomitant administration of uricosuric agents usually results in appreciable increases of urinary uric acid excretion and a further decline in serum urate level [889]. The uricosuric response is accompanied by an increase in the clearance of oxipurinol [540, 542] and a decrease in the excretion of oxypurines [542]. Goldfinger et al. [891] cite evidence that hypoxanthine and xanthine are secreted by the renal tubules in man and that this process is inhibited by uricosuric agents.

Normal uricemic values can be achieved in all but a few patients. The doses required to reduce the elevated levels to normal average 200 to 300 mg per day for patients with mild disease and 400 to 600 mg per day for those with moderately severe tophaceous disease; rarely, doses of 700 to 1,000 mg per day have been required.

By the selection of the appropriate dose of allopurinol it is possible to reduce the serum urate level to normal or, if desired, to hold it as low as 2 or 3 mg per 100 ml indefinitely, unless renal function is markedly limited. Even then, appreciable reduction of serum urate values can be achieved with allopurinol.

When allopurinol is given, serum oxypurine levels rise only slightly, reaching 0.5 to 1.0 mg per 100 ml [538, 886] or, rarely, 2.0 mg per 100 ml [539] because of the high renal clearance of oxypurines. As Klinenberg and colleagues point out [886], the oxypurine levels achieved are well below the solubility limits of hypoxanthine or xanthine in serum.

THERAPEUTIC EFFECTS: In the early experience at Duke Hospital [538, 887, 889] the incidence of acute attacks did not change for 3 to 6 months, but thereafter their frequency and severity declined. Others have found the frequency of gouty attacks relatively high on initiation of therapy [539]. Typical attacks have occurred with serum urate levels as low as 2 mg per 100 ml and comparably low urinary urate excretions. It is recommended that daily colchicine be given during the first months of therapy of gout with allopurinol.

An extensive clinical experience attests to the usefulness of allopurinol as a hypouricemic agent in gout [539, 885–889]. Resolution of tophi occurs gradually with the maintenance of normal serum urate levels and is frequently extensive by 6 to 12 months. Slower improvement can be anticipated in patients with renal insufficiency [892]. Destructive arthritis improves. There is a corresponding improvement in functional status. The progression of gouty nephropathy appears to halt in most patients [889, 893–898].

Formation of uric acid stones can be virtually abolished with allopurinol. The drug has found wide utility in the treatment of idiopathic uric acid nephrolithiasis [899, 900], as it has in management of nephrolithiasis in otherwise asymptomatic hyperuricemia [901] and in frankly gouty subjects [169, 889]. In addition, it has proved very useful in controlling the marked hyperuricemia and hyperuricaciduria and urinary crystalluria that may accompany aggressive therapy of lymphoma or leukemia [653, 902–904]. A variety of forms of secondary gout have been effectively treated with allopurinol [537, 905].

TOXIC EFFECTS: More than one-half of the urinary oxypurine increase observed with allopurinol therapy consists of xanthine, a sparingly soluble compound in acid and neutral urine [886]. The levels attained with full doses of allopurinol equal those which in xanthinuria subjects (who lack xanthine oxidase activity as an inborn error of metabolism) have caused the formation of urinary calculi composed of xanthine (see Chap. 41). Thus far, the development of xanthine crystalluria or lithiasis has not been observed in any patient given allopurinol for treatment of gout or uric acid stones. Three instances of xanthine stone formation, induced by allopurinol therapy, have been reported in other circumstances. Two occurred in children with the Lesch-Nyhan syndrome [906, 907] and the third in an adult patient with lymphosarcoma [908]. All three excreted approximately 1,500 mg uric acid per day. One child, who received 9 mg allopurinol per kg, excreted as much as 800 mg xanthine per day while on therapy [906, 909]. It appears that allopurinol should be given cautiously and in minimal doses to patients with extraordinarily great uric acid excretion values, particularly those with an inability to reutilize hypoxanthine and xanthine because of PRT deficiency [909].

Serious complications of allopurinol therapy appear to have been rare during its initial 6 years of general use. A small percentage of patients (perhaps 5 percent) find it necessary to discontinue the drug [910]. Allopurinol may lead to the development of gastrointestinal intolerance [539], skin rashes, sometimes with fever [886], leukopenia, thrombocytopenia, hepatitis, and vasculitis [911]. The incidence of side effects of all kinds may be about 20 percent [910]. It is not clear whether these are related to hypersensitivity or to a toxic effect of the drug. These complications tend to occur more often in the presence of renal insufficiency. Despite earlier reports to the contrary, allopurinol has no effect on iron absorption, storage, or utilization [537].

EFFECT OF ALLOPURINOL ON PURINE SYNTHESIS *De Novo:* In most patients, the replacement of urinary uric acid by oxypurines is less than stoichiometric [538, 888, 889, 912]. The deficit ranges from 10 to 60 percent and is roughly proportional to the pretreatment level of uric acid excretion [912]. The deficit may amount to several hundred milligrams of purines per day [538, 539] (Fig. 39-30). In addition, the reduction in total purine excretion is associated with a decreased incorporation of isotopic glycine into urinary uric acid [913]. This effect of allopurinol requires the presence of hypoxanthine-guanine phosphoribosyltransferase [200, 914] and may be due to a combination of factors, including an increased conversion of hypoxanthine to IMP [889], the inhibitory action of purine ribonucleotides derived from IMP, or of allopurinol ribonucleotide, upon glutamine-PP-ribose-P-amidotransferase [337, 378], and the depletion of PP-ribose-P, an essential substrate for this enzyme [465].

The administration of allopurinol leads to a substantial reduction of erythrocyte PP-ribose-P content within 3 to 5 hr [465]. This effect in the erythrocyte is due to the consumption of PP-ribose-P resulting from the conversion of allopurinol to its ribonucleotide. It is probably not attributable to the increased reutilization of hypoxanthine and xanthine, since erythrocytes do not contain xanthine oxidase activity. PP-ribose-P levels do not fall after oxipurinol administration [465]. Nevertheless, it has been shown that the reutilization of hypoxanthine [915] and xanthine [916] for nucleic acid synthesis is markedly enhanced when their oxidation is inhibited by allopurinol in the intact rat.

EFFECT OF ALLOPURINOL ON PYRIMIDINE SYNTHESIS *De Novo:* The administration of allopurinol and oxipurinol in man is accompanied by a moderate increase in the excretion of orotidine and orotic acid [549–551] (Table 39-18). Studies in vivo and in cell culture demonstrate that this effect results from the inhibition of orotidylic decarboxylase which catalyzes a step in the conversion of orotic acid to uridine-5′-monophosphate (UMP). Allopurinol-1-N-ribonucleotide and xanthine ribonucleotide, which can be formed by action of the HG-PRT, and oxipurinol-7-N-ribosylphosphate,

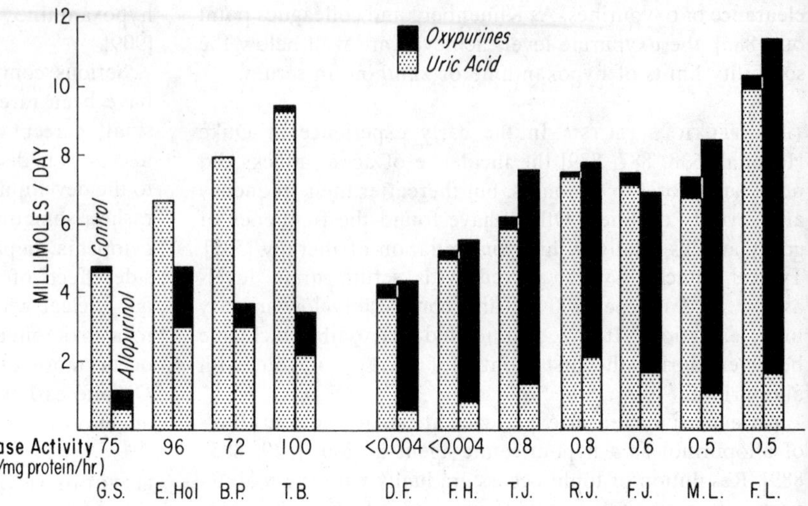

Figure 39-30. Effects of allopurinol on total purine excretion in patients who produce excessive quantities of uric acid. Comparison in patients with normal, virtually completely deficient, and partially deficient hypoxanthine-guanine phosphoribosyltransferase (PRT) activity. The height of each bar represents total purine excretion, oxypurines plus uric acid. (*Reprinted from Kelley et al.* [200], *with permission of Ann. Intern. Med.*)

which can be formed by action of O-PRT, are potent inhibitors of orotidylic decarboxylase [550].

EFFECTS OF ALLOPURINOL IN PATIENTS DEFICIENT IN HYPOXANTHINE-GUANINE PHOSPHORIBOSYLTRANSFERASE ACTIVITY: Allopurinol exerts its predicted effect upon xanthine oxidase in PRT-deficient subjects. Uric acid levels in blood and urine are reduced and urinary oxypurines are increased. However, in contrast to results in other subjects, there is a stoichiometric replacement of urinary uric acid by hypoxanthine and xanthine in PRT-deficient subjects [200, 522, 914]. (Fig. 39-27). Similarly, no reduction of total purine excretion occurs in response to azathioprine [520] (Table 39-19). These anomalous responses are attributed to the PRT deficiency itself, as inhibition of purine synthesis *de novo* requires prior conversion of these analogue bases to ribonucleotide form [378, 440, 514]. No reduction of intracellular PP-ribose-P content occurs on incubation of PRT-deficient erythrocytes with allopurinol [465].

In spite of the PRT deficiency, allopurinol does result in orotidinuria in children with the Lesch-Nyhan syndrome [552]. Furthermore, in PRT-deficient fibroblasts studied in vitro, high concentrations of both allopurinol and oxipurinol inhibit an early step of purine synthesis *de novo,* probably glutamine-PP-ribose-P-amidotransferase [505]. These effects probably involve the formation of oxipurinol-7-N-ribonucleotide, which is an analogue of the purine-3-N-ribonucleotides, and whose formation is also catalyzed by orotate phosphoribosyltransferase [436] (Fig. 39-15).

Orotic Acid

Orotic acid in doses ranging from 2 to 6 gm per day produces a modest reduction in serum urate concentration [667, 918]. This is related to its uricosuric effect [667] and to inhibition of purine biosynthesis *de novo* [466, 677]. Orotic acid is a normal intermediate of pyrimidine biosynthesis and reacts with PP-ribose-P to form orotidine-5′-monophosphate (OMP), a precursor of uridine and cytidine nucleotides [374]. Several studies suggest that this compound inhibits purine biosynthesis by competing with L-glutamine for the available PP-ribose-P [504]. Following the administration of orotic acid, erythrocyte PP-ribose-P levels fall and the incorporation of isotope glycine into urinary uric acid is reduced [667]. Although short-term therapy with orotic acid in man was not associated with the development of a fatty liver [667], as it is in the rat [918, 919], this agent does not appear to offer any therapeutic advantage over other hypouricemic drugs currently in use.

Table 39-18. EFFECTS OF ALLOPURINOL ON PYRIMIDINE EXCRETION

Subject	Number	Orotic acid excretion		Orotidine excretion	
		Basal, mg/24 hr	After allopurinol, mg/24 hr	Basal, mg/24 hr	After allopurinol, mg/24 hr
Normal	6	<2.0	—	<2.0	—
Gout (normal PRT activity)	12	<2.0	14.5 (5.8–29.8)	8.0 (3.2–10.2)	45.6 (24–121)
Lesch-Nyhan	2	<1.5	<1.5	<1.6	18.1, 24.3

Source: Kelley and Beardmore [550], and Beardmore et al. [552].

Table 39-19. EFFECTS OF AZATHIOPRINE ON PURINE SYNTHESIS IN PATIENTS PRODUCING EXCESSIVE QUANTITIES OF URIC ACID

Subject*	Serum urate, mg/100 ml	*Urinary uric acid, mg/24 hr*		Percent of control	Cumulative incorporation of glycine-^{14}C into urinary uric acid, percent of administered dose	Percent of control
		Uncorrected	Corrected			
Normal PRT activity						
B. P.						
Control	9.7	1,529			1.24	
Azathioprine	6.9	922	865	57	0.22	18
T. B.						
Control	10.5	1,241			1.11	
Azathioprine	6.8	740	701	56	0.28	25
Partial PRT deficiency						
M. L.						
Control	10.4	1,127			2.62	
Azathioprine	11.1	1,139	...	101	2.95	113
F. L.						
Control	15.0	1,693			2.74	
Azathioprine	15.6	1,762	...	104	2.88	105
Complete PRT deficiency						
D. F.						
Control	12.4	659			2.49	
Azathioprine	11.8	719	...	100	2.70	108
F. H.						
Control	10.0	828			3.16	
Azathioprine	10.9	926		100	3.15	100

* PRT = hypoxanthine-guanine phosphoribosyltransferase.
Source: Kelley et al. [200].

Increased Uric Acid Destruction

The infusion of highly purified uricase has been shown to bring about a transient reduction in the serum urate level [920–923]. An increased clearance of uric acid appears to be at least partly responsible for the effects observed [922]. Rapid development of antibodies to the enzyme is associated with diminished effectiveness.

SUMMARY

1 Gout is a clinical disorder manifested by hyperuricemia, recurrent attacks of acute arthritis ordinarily responsive to colchicine, and in some instances, eventually by tophaceous deposits of monosodium urate. The arthritis may become chronic and disabling. Rarely it is grotesquely deforming. Nephropathy is a frequent complication in gout. Nephrolithiasis is also common and often antedates articular gout.

2 Primary gout is a form of the disease that is attributable to an inborn error of metabolism. The category is biochemically and genetically heterogeneous. The largest subgroup consists of patients in whom the biochemical defect is as yet undefined. Most patients in this group can be shown to produce uric acid excessively, when studied by techniques for assessment of turnover of uric acid or of rate of incorporation of labeled precursors into uric acid. In many subjects there is a reduction in renal urate secretion per nephron. In addition to genetic factors, dietary excesses of caloric and alcohol ingestion often appear to be important.

3 Overproduction of uric acid in patients with idiopathic primary gout has been discussed in terms of the availability of L-glutamine and 5-phosphoribosyl-1-pyrophosphate (PP-ribose-P), the substrates of the initial and rate-limiting reaction of purine biosynthesis; and in terms of the regulation of the enzyme which catalyzes this reaction.

4 The best defined enzymatic defect leading to overproduction of uric acid and gout is the partial deficiency of hypoxanthine-guanine phosphoribosyltransferase (PRT). The flamboyant overproduction of purines observed in this disorder is at least partially attributable to elevated intracellular levels of PP-ribose-P that result from underutilization of this compound in the blocked salvage pathway.

5 Three other enzymatic derangements have been identified which may lead to accelerated purine biosynthesis and be responsible for the disease in a small fraction of gouty overproducers of uric acid. Glucose-6-phosphatase deficiency and a glutathione reductase variant with increased activity are both postulated to lead to excessive production of PP-ribose-P. A mutant glutamine phosphoribosylpyrophosphate amidotransferase with reduced sensitivity to inhibitory ribonucleotides has been associated with markedly accelerated purine production in two patients.

6 Reduction of renal secretion of urate per nephron is most readily demonstrable in gouty patients when serum urate concentration values are artificially raised. The defect is most prominent in those patients who show minimal evidence of excessive purine production. Some patients appear to exhibit this defect as the major or even the sole basis of hyperuricemia. This defect is present in some overproducers of uric acid, although not in patients with PRT deficiency.

7 The acute gouty attack is thought to be triggered by the formation of crystals of monosodium urate, which may initiate an inflammatory reaction by activation of Hageman factor and production of leukotactic and other factors involved in the reaction. Colchicine is thought to interrupt the attack by suppressing the activity of the leukocyte.

8 It is postulated that development of tophi may be initiated when breakdown of urate-solubilizing mucoproteins of relatively avascular tissue is accelerated following injury to lysosomes. This accelerated breakdown leads to local supersaturation with monosodium urate and crystal formation.

9 Solutions of the electrolyte composition of extracellular fluid are saturated with monosodium urate at a concentration of about 6.4 mg per 100 ml. Perhaps an additional 5 percent (i.e., 0.3 to 0.4 mg per 100 ml) is normally bound to nondiffusible elements of plasma. The most logical definition of hyperuricemia is one based not upon the statistical distribution of serum urate values in a population, but rather upon the limits of solubility of monosodium urate in body fluids.

10 There is significant variability of mean plasma urate values among certain racial groups, especially in the Pacific islands. For example, among adult male Maori, mean serum urate values are over 7 mg per 100 ml, and the prevalence of gout is 10 percent. In most populations, serum urate values are positively correlated with surface area and body weight.

11 In population studies hyperuricemia appears to be multifactorial, and attributable to a combination of genetic and nongenetic factors. Genetic factors may include both cumulative gene action and single-gene effects. In studies of families or isolates the latter sometimes suggest autosomal dominant factors, sometimes sex-linked factors. Known enzymatic abnormalities associated with hyperuricemia are of several genetic types. PRT deficiency is X-linked. Glucose-6-phosphatase deficiency is an autosomal recessive trait. The glutathione reductase variant is an autosomal factor demonstrable in both single and double gene dosage.

12 The prevalences of articular gout and of nephrolithiasis are strongly correlated with the height of the serum urate concentration value. In one population study the prevalences were 90 percent and 40 percent, respectively, in males with serum urate values of 9 mg per 100 ml or greater at mean age 58 years. The incidence of renal lithiasis in gout is 1,000 times that found in the general population. An important factor favoring stone formation in gouty subjects is a tendency toward excretion of persistently acid urine.

13 Secondary gout may occur as a complication of any acquired form of hyperuricemia. Gout occurs in a small percentage of patients with myeloproliferative diseases or chronic hemolytic anemias characterized by increased nucleic acid turnover and increased uric acid production. Gout also occurs secondary to drug-induced hyperuricemia, chiefly that caused by thiazide diuretics, and in certain other conditions leading to reduced renal uric acid excretion. Although the fraction of patients using diuretic agents who develop gout is small, the total is large enough to constitute an appreciable fraction of all new patients with gout in a general population.

BIBLIOGRAPHY

1. Neuwirth, E.: Milestones in the diagnosis and treatment of gout. Arch. Int. Med. (Chicago), **72**, 377, 1943.
2. Hartung, E. F.: Historical considerations. Metabolism, **6**, 196, 1957.
3. von Storch, A.: An essay on the use and effects of the root of the *Colchicum autumnale,* or meadow saffron, translated from the Latin. T. Becket and P. A. de Honet, 1764.
4. Schnitker, M. A., and Richter, A. B.: Nephritis in gout. Amer. J. Med. Sci., **192,** 241, 1936.
5. Sydenham, T.: Tractatus de podagra et hydrope. G. Kettilby, London, 1683.
6. Scheele, K. W.: Examen chemicum calculi urinarii. *Opuscula,* vol. 2, p. 73, 1776.
7. Wollaston, W. H.: On gouty and urinary concretions. Phil. Trans. London, **87,** 386, 1797.
8. Pearson, G.: Experiments and observations, tending to show the composition and properties of urinary concretions. Phil. Trans. London, **88,** 15, 1798.
9. Garrod, A. B.: Observations on certain pathological conditions of the blood and urine in gout, rheumatism and Bright's disease. Trans. M.-Chir. Soc. Edinburgh, **31,** 83, 1848.
10. Garrod, A. B.: On the blood and effused fluids in gout, rheumatism and Bright's disease. Trans. M.-Chir. Soc. Edinburgh, **37,** 49, 1854.
11. Fischer, E.: *Untersuchungen in der Puringruppe.* Springer, Berlin, 1907.
12. Folin, O., and Denis, W.: A new (colorimetric) method for the determination of uric acid in blood. J. Biol. Chem., **13,** 469, 1912–1913.
13. Stetten, D., Jr.: Gout and metabolism. Sci. Amer., **198,** 73, 1958.
14. Rodman, G. P., and Benedek, T. G: Cotton Mather and the gout. Arthritis Rheum., **6,** 789, 1963.
15. Bywaters, E. G. L.: Gout in the time and person of George IV: A case history. Ann. Rheum. Dis., **21,** 325, 1962.
16. Rodnan, G. P.: A gallery of gout. Arthritis Rheum., **4,** 27, 176, 1961.
17. Rodnan, G. P., and Benedek, T. G.: Ancient therapeutic arts and the gout. Arthritis Rheum., **6,** 317, 1963.
18. Benedek, T. G., and Rodnan, G. P.: Petrarch on medicine and the gout. Bull. Hist. Med., **37,** 397, 1963.
19. Smyth, C. J., Cotterman, C. W., and Freyberg, R. H.: The genetics of gout and hyperuricemia: An analysis of nineteen families. J. Clin. Invest., **27,** 749, 1948.
20. Smyth, C. J., Stecher, R. M., and Wolfson, W. Q.: Genetic and endocrine determinants of the plasma urate level. Science, **108,** 514, 1948.
21. Sydenham, T.: *The Works of Thomas Sydenham,* trans. by R. G. Latham, vol. II, p. 214. Sydenham Society, London, 1850.

22. Bauer, W., and Calkins, E.: Gout, in *Diseases of Metabolism,* edited by E. Duncan, 4th ed., p. 643. Saunders, Philadelphia, 1959.
23. Hench, P. S.: The diagnosis of gout and gouty arthritis. J. Lab. Clin. Med., **220,** 48, 1936.
24. Lawrence, J. S.: Heritable disorders of connective tissue. Proc. Roy. Soc. Med., **53,** 522, 1960.
25. Wyngaarden, J. B.: Gout, in *Metabolic Basis of Inherited Disease,* 1st ed., edited by J. B. Stanbury, J. B. Wyngaarden, and D. S. Fredrickson, p. 679. McGraw-Hill, New York, 1960.
26. Hall, A. P., Barry, P. E., Dawber, T. R., and McNamara, P. M.: Epidemiology of gout and hyperuricemia: A long-term population study. Amer. J. Med., **42,** 27, 1967.
27. Decker, J. L., Lane, J. J., Jr., and Reynolds, W. E.: Hyperuricemia in a Filipino population. Arthritis Rheum., **5,** 144, 1962.
28. Decker, J. L., and Lane, J. J., Jr.: Gouty arthritis in Filipinos. New Eng. J. Med., **261,** 805, 1959.
29. Burch, T. A., O'Brien, W. M., Need, R., and Kurland, L. T.: Hyperuricemia and gout in Mariana Islands. Ann. Rheum. Dis., **25,** 144, 1966.
30. Lennane, G. A. Q., Rose, B. S., and Isdale, I. C.: Gout in Maori. Ann. Rheum. Dis., **19,** 120, 1960.
31. Prior, I. A. M., and Rose, B. S.: Uric acid, gout and public health in the South Pacific. New Zeal. Med. J., **65,** 295, 1966.
32. Brochner-Mortensen, K.: Review of diagnostic criteria and known etiological factors in gout, in *Epidemiology of Chronic Rheumatism,* vol. 1, p. 140. Davis, Philadelphia, 1963.
33. Zollner, N.: Moderne Gichtprobleme Ätiologie, Pathogenese. Klin. Ergbn. inn. Med. Kinderheilk., **14,** 321, 1960.
34. Popert, A. J., and Hewitt, J. V.: Gout and hyperuricemia in rural and urban populations. Ann. Rheum. Dis., **20,** 154, 1962.
35. Cobb, S.: Hyperuricemia in executives, in *The Epidemiology of Chronic Rheumatism,* vol. 1, p. 182. Davis, Philadelphia, 1963.
36. Dunn, J. P., Brooks, G. W., Mausner, J., Rodnan, G. P., and Cobb, S.: Social class gradient of serum uric acid levels in man. JAMA, **185,** 431, 1963.
37. Sheperd-Wilson, W., and Gelfand, M.: Gout in the African: Report of a case. *Cent. Afr. J. Med.,* **8,** 181, 1962.
38. Turner, R. E., Frank, M. J., Van Ausdal, D., and Bollet, A. J.: Some aspects of the epidemiology of gout. Arch. Intern. Med. (Chicago), **106,** 400, 1960.
39. Nathan, L. A., Kubota, C. K., and Turnbull, G. C.: Relative incidence of gout in Negro and white males at Cook County Hospital (1944–1952). J. Lab. Clin. Med., **42,** 927, 1953.
40. Bartels, E. C.: Gout as a complication of surgery. Surg. Clin. N. Amer., **38,** 847, 1957.
41. Hoffman, W. S.: Some unsolved problems of gout. Med. Clin. N. Amer., **43,** 595, 1959.
42. McCracken, J. H.: Gout: An analysis of fifty cases. Bull. New Eng. Med. Center, **3,** 249, 1941.
43. Gutman, A. B., and Yü, T.-F.: Secondary gout. Ann. Intern. Med., **56,** 675, 1962.
44. Yü, T.-F., and Gutman, A. B.: Uric acid nephrolithiasis in gout: Predisposing factors. Ann. Intern. Med., **67,** 1133, 1967.
45. Delbarre, F., Braun, S., and Saint-Georges-Chaumet, F.: La Goutte Feminine (Analyse de quarante observations). Sem. Hop. Paris **43,** 19, 1967.
46. Kolb, F. O., de Lalla, O. F., and Gofman, J. W.: The hyperlipemias in disorders of carbohydrate metabolism: Serial lipoprotein studies in diabetic acidosis with xanthomatosis and in glycogen storage disease. Metabolism, **4,** 310, 1955.
47. Lesch, M., and Nyhan, W. L.: A familial disorder of uric acid metabolism and central nervous system function. Amer. J. Med., **36,** 561, 1964.
48. Harth, M., and Robinson, C. E. G.: Gouty arthritis in a D.V.A. hospital, a retrospective study. Med. Serv. J. Canada, **18,** 671, 1962.
49. Hollander, J. L.: Cited in ref. 50.
50. Smyth, C. J.: Gout, in *Arthritis,* edited by J. L. Hollander, 6th ed., p. 859. Lea & Febiger, Philadelphia, 1960.
51. Lockie, L. M., and Cooper, R. G.: Gout, the rediscovered disease. Geriatrics, **15,** 497, 1960.
52. Smyth, C. J., and Huffman, E. R.: Gouty arthritis, diagnosis and treatment. Rocky Mountain Med. J., **52,** 513, 1955.
53. Brochner-Mortensen, K.: Diagnosis of gout. Acta Med. Scand., **99,** 538, 1939.
54. Ayvazian, J. H., and Ayvazian, L. F.: Changes in serum and urinary uric acid with the development of symptomatic gout. J. Clin. Invest., **42,** 1835, 1963.
55. Ingbar, S. H., Kass, E. H., Burnett, C. H., Relman, A. S., Burrows, B. A., and Sisson, J. H.: The effects of ACTH and cortisone on the renal tubular transport of uric acid, phosphorus, and electrolytes in patients with normal renal and adrenal function. J. Lab. Clin. Med., **38,** 533, 1951.
56. Ayvazian, J. H., and Ayvazian, L. F.: Effect of intravenous administration of crystalline pancreatic desoxyribonuclease in patients with gout. New Eng. J. Med., **263,** 999, 1960.
57. Weissmann, B., and Gutman, A. B.: The identification of 6-succinoaminopurine and of 8-hydroxy-7-methylguanine as normal human urinary constituents. J. Biol. Chem., **229,** 239, 1957.
58. Gutman, A. B., Yü, T.-F., and Weissmann, B.: The concept of secondary gout: Relation to purine metabolism in polycythemia and myeloid metaplasia. Trans. Ass. Amer. Physicians, **69,** 229, 1956.
59. Garrod, A. B.: *A Treatise on Gout and Rheumatic Gout* (*Rheumatoid Arthritis*), 3d ed. Longmans, London, 1876.
60. Freudweiler, M.: Experimentelle untersuchungen uber das Wesen der Gichtknoten. Deutsch. Arch. Klin. Med., **63,** 286, 1899.
61. Freudweiler, M.: Experimentelle untersuchungen über die Entstehung der Gichtknoten. Deutsch. Arch. Klin. Med., **69,** 155, 1901.
62. His, W. J.: Schicksal und Wirkungen des sauren harnsauren Natrons in Bauch-und Gelenkhöhle des Kaninchens. Deutsch. Arch. Klin. Med., **67,** 81, 1900.
63. Berliner, R. W., Hilton, J. G., Yü, T.-F., and Kennedy, T. J., Jr.: The renal mechanism for urate excretion in man. J. Clin. Invest., **29,** 396, 1950.
64. Folin, O., Berglund, H., and Derick, C.: The uric acid problem: An experimental study on animals and man, including gouty subjects. J. Biol. Chem., **60,** 361, 1924.
65. Gutman, A. B., and Yü, T.-F: Gout, a derangement of purine metabolism. Advances Intern. Med., **5,** 27, 1952.
66. Mugler, A.: Le Traitement de la goutte aigue. *Congrès international de la goutte et de la lithiasis urique,* Evian, Sept. 4–6, 1964, p. 283.
67. Robinson, W. D., Conn, J. W., Block, W. D., and Louis, L. H.: Role of the adrenal cortex in urate metabolism and in gout. J. Lab. Clin. Med., **33,** 1473, 1948.
68. Hellman, L.: Production of acute gouty arthritis by adrenocorticotrophin. Science, **109,** 280, 1949.
69. Gudzent, F.: *Gicht und Rheumatismus.* Springer, Berlin, 1928.
70. Villa, L., Robecchi, A., and Ballabio, C. B.: Physiopathology, clinical manifestations, and treatment of gout. Part I. Ann. Rheum. Dis., **17,** 9, 1958.
71. McCarty, D. J., Jr., and Hollander, J. L.: Identification of urate crystals in gouty synovial fluid. Ann. Intern. Med., **54,** 452, 1961.
72. Roberts, W.: The Croonian lectures. On the chemistry and therapeutics of uric acid gravel and gout. Brit. Med. J., **2,** 61, 1892.
73. McCarty, D. J., Jr.: Phagocytosis of urate crystals in gouty synovial fluid. Arthritis Rheum., **4,** 425, 1961.
74. Phelps, P., Steele, A. D., and McCarty, J. D., Jr.: Compensated polarized light microscopy. JAMA, **203,** 508, 1968.
75. Zwaifler, N. J., and Pekin, T. J.: Significance of urate crystals in synovial fluids. Arch. Intern. Med. (Chicago), **111,** 99, 1963.
76. Seegmiller, J. E., Laster, L., and Howell, R. R.: Biochemistry of uric acid and its relation to gout. New Eng. J. Med., **268,** 712, 1963.
77. Sokoloff, L.: The pathology of gout. Metabolism, **6,** 230, 1957.
78. Zeveley, H. A., French, A. J., Mikkelsen, W. M., and Duff, I. F.: Synovial specimens obtained by knee joint punch biopsy. Amer. J. Med., **20,** 510, 1956.
79. Faires, J. S., and McCarty, D. J., Jr.: Acute synovitis in normal joints of man and dog produced by injections of microcrystalline sodium urate, calcium oxalate and corticosteroid esters. Arthritis Rheum., **5,** 295, 1962.

80. Malawista, S. E., Howell, R. R., and Seegmiller, J. E.: Factors modifying the inflammatory response to injected microcrystalline sodium urate. Arthritis Rheum., **5,** 307, 1962.
81. Seegmiller, J. E., and Howell, R. R.: The old and new concepts of acute gouty arthritis. Arthritis Rheum., **5,** 616, 1962.
82. Seegmiller, J. E., Howell, R. R., and Malawista, S. E.: Inflammatory reaction to sodium urate: Its possible relationship to genesis of acute gouty arthritis. JAMA, **180,** 469, 1962.
83. Seegmiller, J. E., Howell, R. R., and Malawista, S. E.: A mechanism of action of colchicine in acute gouty arthritis. J. Clin. Invest., **41,** 1399, 1962.
84. Malawista, S. E., and Seegmiller, J. E.: The effect of pretreatment with colchicine on the inflammatory response to injected microcrystalline monosodium urate: A model for gouty inflammation. Ann. Intern. Med., **62,** 648, 1965.
85. Weissmann, G.: Lysosomes and joint disease. Arthritis Rheum., **9,** 834, 1966.
86. Rajan, K. T.: Lysosomes and gout. Nature (London), **210,** 959, 1966.
87. Kellermeyer, R. W.: Hageman factor and acute gouty arthritis. Arthritis Rheum., **11,** 452, 1968.
88. Kellermeyer, R. W., and Breckenridge, R. T.: The inflammatory process in acute gouty arthritis. I. Activation of Hageman factor by sodium urate crystals. J. Lab. Clin. Med., **65,** 307, 1965.
89. Kellermeyer, R. W., and Breckenridge, R. T.: The inflammatory process in acute gouty arthritis. II. The presence of Hageman factor and plasma thromboplastin antecedent in synovial fluid. J. Lab. Clin. Med., **67,** 455, 1966.
90. Kellermeyer, R. W.: The inflammatory process in acute gouty arthritis. III. Vascular permeability enhancing activity in normal human synovial fluid; induction by Hageman factor activators and inhibition by Hageman factor activators and inhibition by Hageman factor antiserum. J. Lab. Clin. Med., **70,** 372, 1967.
91. Melmon, K., Webster, M. E., Goldfinger, S. E., and Seegmiller, J. E.: The presence of a kinin in inflammatory synovial effusion from arthritides of varying etiologies. Arthritis Rheum., **10,** 13, 1967.
92. Phelps, P., and McCarty, D. J., Jr.: Crystal induced inflammation in canine joints. II. Importance of polymorphonuclear leukocytes. J. Exp. Med., **124,** 115, 1966.
93. Chang, Y.-H., and Gralla, E. J.: Suppression of urate crystal-induced canine joint inflammation by heterologous anti-polymorphonuclear leukocyte serum. Arthritis Rheum., **11,** 145, 1968.
94. McCarty, D. J.: Pathophysiologie de la goutte. *Congrès international de la goutte et de la lithiasis urique,* Evian, Sept. 4–6, 1964, p. 161.
95. Howell, D. S.: Preliminary observations on local pH in gouty tophi and synovial fluid. Arthritis Rheum., **8,** 736, 1965.
96. Sperling, O., Kedem, O., and De Vries, A.: Étiologie de la lithiase urique. I. Solubilité de l'acide urique et de l'urate de sodium en solution tampon. Rev. Franc. Etud. Clin. Biol., **11,** 40, 1966.
97. Howell, R. R., and Seegmiller, J. E.: A mechanism of action of colchicine. Arthritis Rheum., **5,** 303, 1962.
98. Phelps, P., Prokop, D. J., and McCarty, D. D.: Crystal induced inflammation in canine joints. III. Evidence against bradykinin as a mediator of inflammation. J. Lab. Clin. Med., **68,** 433, 1966.
99. Naff, G. B., and Byers, P. H.: Possible implication of complement in acute gout. J. Clin. Invest., **46,** 1099, 1967.
100. Phelps, P.: Polymorphonuclear leukocyte motility in vitro. III. Possible release of a chemotactic substance after phagocytosis of urate crystals by polymorphonuclear leukocytes. Arthritis Rheum., **12,** 197, 1969.
101. Phelps, P.: Appearance of chemotactic activity following intraarticular injection of monosodium urate crystals: Effect of colchicine. J. Lab. Clin. Med., **76,** 622, 1970.
102. McCarty, D. J., Kohn, N. N., and Faires, J. S.: The significance of calcium phosphate crystals in the synovial fluid of arthritic patients: The "pseudo-gout syndrome." I. Clinical aspects. Ann. Intern. Med., **56,** 711, 1962.
103. Kohn, N. N., Hughes, R. E., McCarty, D. J., and Faires, J. S.: The significance of calcium phosphate crystals in the synovial fluid of arthritic patients: "Pseudogout syndrome." II. Identification of crystals. Ann. Intern. Med., **56,** 738, 1962.
104. McCarty, D. J., and Gatter, R. A.: Pseudogout syndrome. Bull. Rheum. Dis., **64,** 1964.
105. McCarty, D. J., Jr., Gatter, R. A., and Hughes, R. E.: Pseudogout syndrome. IV. Early (perilacunar) and "mature" cartilaginous deposits of monoclinic and triclinic crystals of calcium pyrophosphate dihydrate; Koch's postulates and possible pathogenesis. Arthritis Rheum., **6,** 287, 1963.
106. McCarty, D. J., Jr.: Crystal-induced inflammation; syndromes of gout and pseudogout. Geriatrics, **18,** 467, 1963.
107. Zitnan, D., and Sit'aj, S.: Chondrocalcinosis articularis. Section I. Clinical and radiological study. Ann. Rheum. Dis., **22,** 142, 1963.
108. Gatter, R. A., and McCarty, D. J., Jr.: Pseudogout syndrome. V. A clinical analysis of 30 cases. Arthritis Rheum., **6,** 271, 1963.
109. Dodds, W. J., and Steinbach, H. L.: Gout associated with calcification of cartilage. New Eng. J. Med., **275,** 745, 1966.
110. Reginato, M. A., Valenzuela, R. F., Martinez, C. V., Passano, G., and Daza, K. S.: Polyarticular and familial chondrocalcinosis. Arthritis Rheum., **13,** 197, 1970.
111. Skinner, M., and Cohen, A. S.: Calcium pyrophosphate dihydrate crystal deposition disease. Arch. Intern. Med. (Chicago), **123,** 636, 1969.
112. Moscowitz, R. W., and Katz, D.: Chondrocalcinosis (pseudogout syndrome): A family study. JAMA, **188,** 867, 1964.
113. Moskowitz, R. W., and Katz, D.: Chondrocalcinosis and chondrocalsynovitis (pseudogout syndrome): Analysis of 24 cases. Amer. J. Med., **43,** 322, 1967.
114. Pflug, M., McCarty, D., and Kawahara, F.: Basal urinary pyrophosphate excretion in pseudogout. Arthritis Rheum., **12,** 228, 1969.
115. Russell, R. G. G., Fleisch, S. B. H., Currey, H. L. F., Rubinstein, H. M., Dietz, A. A., Boussina, I., Micheli, A., and Fallet, G.: Inorganic pyrophosphate in plasma, urine, and synovial fluid of patients with pyrophosphate arthropathy (chondrocalcinosis or pseudogout). Lancet, **2,** 899, 1970.
116. Good, A. E., and Starkweather, W. H.: Synovial fluid pyrophosphate phosphohydrolase (PPPH) in pseudogout, gout and rheumatoid arthritis. Arthritis Rheum., **12,** 298, 1969.
117. Atkins, C. J., McIvor, J., Smith, P. M., Hamilton, E., and Williams, R.: Chondrocalcinosis and arthropathy: Studies in haemochromatosis and in idiopathic chondrocalcinosis. Quart. J. Med., **153,** 71, 1970.
118. Emmerson, B. T.: Regimen of indomethacin therapy in acute gouty arthritis. Brit. Med. J., **2,** 272, 1967.
119. Thompson, G. R., Ming Ting, Y., Riggs, G. A., Fenn, M. E., and Denning, R. M.: Calcific tendinitis and soft-tissue calcification resembling gout. JAMA, **203,** 464, 1968.
120. Swannell, A. J., Underwood, F. A., and Dixon, A. St. J.: Periarticular calcific deposits mimicking acute arthritis. Ann. Rheum. Dis., **29,** 380, 1970.
121. Sandstrom, C.: Peritendinitis calcarea. Amer. J. Roentgen., **40,** 1, 1938.
122. Caner, J. E. Z., Hegstrom, R. H., and Decker, J. L.: Gout-like arthritis in patients with chronic renal failure treated with periodic hemodialysis. Arthritis Rheum., **5,** 287, 1962.
123. Caner, J. E. Z., and Decker, J. L.: Recurrent acute (?gouty) arthritis in patients with chronic renal failure treated with periodic hemodialysis. Amer. J. Med., **36,** 571, 1964.
124. Moskowitz, R. W., Vertes, V., Schwartz, A., Marshall, G., and Friedman, B.: Crystal-induced inflammation associated with chronic renal failure treated with periodic hemodialysis. Amer. J. Med., **47,** 450, 1969.
124*a*. Malawista, S. E., Seegmiller, J. E., Hathaway, E., and Sokoloff, L.: Sacroiliac gout. JAMA, **194,** 954, 1965.
125. Hunder, G. G., Worthington, J. W., and Bickel, W. H.: Avascular necrosis of the femoral head in a patient with gout. JAMA, **203,** 47, 1968.
126. McCollum, D. E., Mathews, R. S., and O'Neil, M. T.: Aseptic necrosis of the femoral head: Associated diseases and evaluation of treatment. Southern Med. J., **63,** 241, 1970.
127. Bauer, W., and Klemperer, F.: Gout, in *Diseases of Metabolism,* edited by G. G. Duncan, 2d ed. Saunders, Philadelphia, 1947.
128. Bartels, E. C., and Matossian, G. S.: Gout: Six year follow-up on probenecid (Benemid) therapy. Arthritis Rheum., **2,** 193, 1959.
129. Bartels, E. C.: Gout. Postgrad. Med., **15,** 254, 1954.
130. Talbott, J. H.: *Gout.* Grune & Stratton, New York, 1957.

131. Gutman, A. B., and Yü, T.-F.: Renal function in gout with a commentary on the renal regulation of urate excretion, and the role of the kidney in the pathogenesis of gout. Amer. J. Med., **23**, 600, 1957.
132. Talbott, J. H.: *Gout,* 2d ed. Grune & Stratton, New York, 1964.
133. de Galantha, E.: Technic for preservation and microscopic demonstration of nodules in gout. Amer. J. Clin. Path., **5**, 165, 1935.
134. Brandenberger, E., De Quervain, F., and Schinz, H. R.: The nature of the deposits in gout. Helv. Med. Acta, **118**, 195, 1947.
135. Howell, R. R., Eanes, E. D., and Seegmiller, J. E.: X-ray diffraction studies on the tophaceous deposits in gout. Arthritis Rheum., **6**, 97, 1963.
136. Lichtenstein, L., Scott, H. W., and Levin, M. H.: Pathologic changes in gout: Survey of eleven necropsied cases. Amer. J. Path., **32**, 871, 1956.
137. Ward, L. E., Bickel, W. H., and Corbin, K. B.: Median neuritis (carpal tunnel syndrome) caused by gouty tophi. JAMA, **167**, 844, 1958.
138. O'Hara, L. J., and Levin, M.: Carpal tunnel syndrome and gout. Arch. Intern. Med. (Chicago), **120**, 180, 1967.
139. Koskoff, Y. D., Morris, L. E., and Lubic, L. G.: Paraplegia as a complication of gout. JAMA, **152**, 37, 1953.
140. Ludwig, A. P., Bennett, G. A., and Bauer, W.: Rare manifestation of gout: Widespread ankylosis simulating rheumatoid arthritis. Ann. Intern. Med., **11**, 1248, 1938.
141. Hughes, G. R., Barnes, C. G., and Mason, R. M.: Bony ankylosis in gout. Ann. Rheum. Dis., **27**, 67, 1968.
142. Sokoloff, L., and Gleason, I. O.: The sternoclavicular articulation in rheumatic diseases. Amer. J. Clin. Path., **24**, 406, 1954.
143. Brugsch, T., and Citron, J.: Ueber die Absorption der Harnsaure durch Knorpel. Z. Exp. Path. Therap., **5**, 401, 1908.
144. Katz, W. A., and Schubert, M.: The interaction of monosodium urate with connective tissue components. J. Clin. Invest., **49**, 1783, 1970.
145. Wyngaarden, J. B.: Uric acid, in *The Cyclopedia of Medicine, Surgery, Specialties,* edited by G. M. Piersol, p. 341. Davis, Philadelphia, 1955.
146. Wyngaarden, J. B.: The role of the kidney in the pathogenesis and treatment of gout. Arthritis Rheum., **1**, 191, 1958.
147. Talbott, J. H., and Terplan, K. L.: The kidney in gout. Medicine, **39**, 405, 1960.
148. Barlow, K. A., and Beilin, L. J.: Renal disease in primary gout. Quart. J. Med., **37**, 79, 1968.
149. Ungerleider, H. E.: The internist and life insurance. Ann. Intern. Med., **41**, 124, 1954.
150. Talbott, J. H., and Lilienfeld, A.: Longevity in gout. Geriatrics, **14**, 409, 1959.
151. Coombs, F. S., Pecora, L. J., Thorogood, E., Consolazio, W. V., and Talbott, J. H.: Renal function in patients with gout. J. Clin. Invest., **19**, 525, 1940.
152. Davies, D. F., and Shock, N. W.: Age changes in glomerular filtration rate, effective renal plasma flow, and tubular excretory capacity in adult males. J. Clin. Invest., **29**, 496, 1950.
153. Smith, H. W.: *The Kidney.* Oxford University Press, Fair Lawn, N.J., 1951.
154. Brown, J., and Mallory, G. K.: Renal changes in gout. New Eng. J. Med., **243**, 325, 1950.
155. Ebstein, W.: *Die Natur und Behandlung der Gicht.* Bergmann, Wiesbaden, 1906.
156. Umber, F.: *Ernahrung und Stoffwechselkrankheiten.* Corban und Schwarzenberg, Vienna, 1914.
157. Duncan, H., and Dixon, A. St. J.: Gout, familial hyperuricemia, and renal disease, Quart. J. Med., **29**, 127, 1960.
158. Rosenbloom, F. M., Kelley, W. N., Carr, A. A., and Seegmiller, J. E.: Familial nephropathy and gout in a kindred. Clin. Res., **15**, 270, 1967.
159. Minkowski, O.: *Die Gicht.* Holder, Vienna, 1903.
160. Modern, F. W. S., and Meister, L.: The kidney of gout, a clinical entity. Med. Clin. N. Amer., **36**, 941, 1952.
161. Fineberg, S. K., and Altschul, A.: The nephropathy of gout. Ann. Intern. Med., **44**, 1182, 1956.
162. Greenbaum, D., Ross, J. H. and Steinberg, V. L.: Renal biopsy in gout. Brit. Med. J., **1**, 1502, 1961.
163. Gonick, H. C., Rubini, M. E., Gleason, I. O., and Sommers, S. C.: The renal lesion in gout. Ann. Intern. Med., **62**, 667, 1965.
164. Mayne, J. G.: Pathological study of the renal lesions found in 27 patients with gout. Ann. Rheum. Dis., **15**, 61, 1965.
165. Rakic, M. T., Valkenburg, H. A., Davidson, R. T., Engels, J. P., Mikkelsen, W. M., Neel, J. V., and Duff, I. F.: Observations on the natural history of hyperuricemia and gout. I. An eighteen year follow-up of nineteen gouty families. Amer. J. Med., **37**, 862, 1964.
166. Hall, A. P.: Correlations among hyperuricemia, hypercholesterolemia, coronary disease and hypertension. Arthritis Rheum., **8**, 846, 1965.
167. Myers, A., Epstein, F. H., Dodge, H. J., and Mikkelsen, W. M.: The relationship of serum uric acid to risk factors in coronary heart disease. Amer. J. Med., **45**, 520, 1968.
168. Atsmon, A., de Vries, A., and Frank, M.: *Uric Acid Lithiasis.* Elsevier, Amsterdam, 1963.
169. Yü, T-F., and Gutman, A. B.: Uric acid nephrolithiasis in gout. Ann. Intern. Med., **67**, 1133, 1967.
170. Prien, E. L., and Prien, E. L., Jr.: Composition and structure of urinary stone. Amer. J. Med., **45**, 654, 1968.
171. de Vries, A., Frank, M., and Atsmon, A.: Inherited uric acid lithiasis. Amer. J. Med., **33**, 880, 1962.
172. Sérane, J., and Lederer, J.: Contribution a l'étude du rein des goutteux. Presse Med., **63**, 335, 1955.
173. Woeber, K. A., Ricca, L., and Hills, A. G.: Pathogenesis of uric acid urolithiasis. Clin. Res., **10**, 45, 1962.
174. Delbarre, F., Auscher, C., and DuLac, Y.: Documents pour l'étude du rein goutteux. IV. Documents sur le pH urinaire et ses variations. Rein Foie, **6**, 53, 1964.
175. Henneman, P. H., Wallach, S., and Dempsey, E. F.: The metabolic defect responsible for uric acid stone formation. J. Clin. Invest., **41**, 537, 1962.
176. Gutman, A. B., and Yü, T.-F.: On the nature of the inborn metabolic error(s) of primary gout. Trans. Ass. Amer. Physicians, **76**, 141, 1963.
177. Gutman, A. B., and Yü, T.-F.: Urinary ammonium excretion in primary gout. J. Clin. Invest., **44**, 1474, 1965.
178. Frank, M., de Vries, A., Atsmon, A., and Kochwa, S.: Urinary pH, ammonia and calcium excretion in renal uric acid stone patients. Israel Med. J., **12**, 299, 1960.
179. Metcalfe-Gibson, A., McCallum, F. M., Morrison, R.B.I., and Wrong, O.: Urinary excretion of hydrogen ion in patients with uric acid calculi. Clin. Sci., **28**, 325, 1965.
180. Barzel, U. S., Sperling, O., Frank, M., and de Vries, A.: Renal ammonium excretion and urinary pH in idiopathic uric acid lithiasis. J. Urol., **92**, 1, 1964.
181. Pak Poy, R. K.: Urinary pH in gout. Aust. Ann. Med., **14**, 35, 1965.
182. Sperling, O., Frank, M., and de Vries, A.: L'excretion d'ammoniac au cours de la goutte. Rev. Franc. Etud. Clin. Biol., **11**, 401, 1966.
183. Plante, G. E., Durivage, J., and Lemieux, G.: Renal excretion of hydrogen in primary gout. Metabolism, **17**, 377, 1968.
184. Gutman, A. B., and Yü, T.-F.: An abnormality of glutamine metabolism in primary gout. Amer. J. Med., **35**, 820, 1963.
185. Gutman, A. B., and Yü, T.-F.: Uric acid nephrolithiasis. Amer. J. Med., **45**, 756, 1968.
186. Bergmann, F., and Dikstein, S.: The relationship between spectral shifts and structural changes in uric acids and related compounds. J. Amer. Chem. Soc., **77**, 691, 1955.
187. Dulce, H. J.: Biochemie der harnsteinbildung. Urol. Int., **7**, 137, 1958.
188. Boshamer, K.: Morphologie und genese der Harnsteine, in *Handbuch der Urologie, vol.* X, *Die Steinerkrankungen.* Springer, Berlin, 1961.
189. Sperling, O., and de Vries, A.: Studies on the etiology of uric acid lithiasis. Part 2. Solubility of uric acid in urine specimens from normal subjects and patients with idiopathic uric acid lithiasis. J. Urol., **92**, 331, 1964.
190. Armstrong, W. A., and Greene, L. F.: Uric acid calculi with particular reference to determinations of uric acid content of blood. J. Urol., **70**, 545, 1953.
191. Rapoport, A., Crassweller, P. O., Husdan, H., From, G. L. A., Zweig, M., and Johnson, M. D.: The renal excretion of hydrogen ion in uric acid stone formers. Metabolism, **16**, 176, 1967.
192. Sperling, O., de Vries, A., and Kedem, O.: Studies on the etiology of uric acid lithiasis. IV. Urinary non-dialyzable substances in idiopathic uric acid lithiasis. J. Urol., **94**, 286, 1965.
193. Deren, J. J., Porush, J. G., Levitt, M. F., and Khilnani, M. T.: Nephro-

lithiasis as a complication of ulcerative colitis and regional enteritis. Ann. Intern. Med., **56,** 843, 1962.

194. Bennett, R. C., and Jepson, R. P.: Uric acid stone formation following ileostomy. Aust. New Zeal. J. Surg., **36,** 153, 1966.
195. Clarke, A. M., and McKenzie, R. G.: Ileostomy and the risk of urinary uric acid stones. Lancet, **2,** 395, 1969.
196. Atsmon, A., de Vries, A., Lazebnik, J., and Salinger, H.: Dissolution of renal uric acid stones by oral alkalinization and large fluid intake in a patient suffering from gout. Amer. J. Med., **27,** 167, 1959.
197. Acheson, R. M., and O'Brien, W. M.: Dependence of serum uric acid on haemoglobin and other factors in the general population. Lancet, **2,** 777, 1966.
198. O'Brien, W. M., Burch, T. A., and Bunim, J. J.: Genetics of hyperuricemia in Blackfeet and Pima Indians. Ann. Rheum. Dis., **25,** 117, 1966.
199. Acheson, R. M., and Florey, C. du V.: Body-weight, ABO blood-groups, and altitude of domicile as determinants of serum-uric-acid in military recruits in four countries. Lancet, **2,** 391, 1969.
200. Kelley, W. N., Greene, M. L., Rosenbloom, F. M., Henderson, J. F., and Seegmiller, J. E.: Hypoxanthine-guanine phosphoribosyl-transferase deficiency in gout. Ann. Intern. Med., **70,** 155, 1969.
201. Mikkelsen, W. M.: The possible association of hyperuricemia and/or gout with diabetes mellitus. Arthritis Rheum., **8,** 853, 1965.
202. Denis, G., and Launay, M. P.: Carbohydrate intolerance in gout. Metabolism, **18,** 770, 1969.
203. Bernheim, C., Ott, H., Zahnd, G., and Martin, E.: Goutte et diabète. 1. La goutte et ses relations avec le diabète. Schweiz. Med. Wschr., **98,** 33, 1968.
204. Berkowitz, D.: Gout, hyperlipidemia and diabetes interrelationships. JAMA, **197,** 117, 1966.
205. McKechnie, J. K.: Gout, hyperuricemia and carbohydrate metabolism. S. Afr. Med. J., **38,** 182, 1964.
206. Herman, J. B., Mount, F. W., Medalie, J. H., Groen, J. J., Dublin, T. D., Neufeld, N. H., and Riss, E.: Diabetes prevalence and serum uric acid: Observations among 10,000 men in a survey of ischemic heart disease in Israel. Diabetes, **16,** 858, 1967.
207. Padova, J., Patchefsky, A., Onesti, G., Faludi, G., and Bendersky, G.: The effect of glucose loads on renal uric acid excretion in diabetic patients. Metabolism, **13,** 507, 1964.
208. Herman, J. B., and Keynan, A.: Hyperglycemia and uric acid. Israel J. Med. Sci., **5,** 1048, 1969.
209. Skeith, M. D., Healey, L. A., and Cutler, R. E.: Urate excretion during mannitol and glucose diuresis. J. Lab. Clin. Med., **70,** 213, 1967.
210. Goldfinger, S., Klinenberg, J. R., and Seegmiller, J. E.: Renal retention of uric acid induced by infusion of beta-hydroxybutyrate and aceto-acetate. New Eng. J. Med., **272,** 351, 1965.
211. Barlow, K. A.: Hyperlipidemia in primary gout. Metabolism, **17,** 289, 1968.
212. Feldman, E. B., and Wallace, S. L.: Hypertriglyceridemia in gout. Circulation, **29,** 508, 1964.
213. Benedek, T. G.: Correlations of serum uric acid and lipid concentrations in normal, gouty, and atherosclerotic men. Ann. Intern, Med., **66,** 851, 1967.
214. Berkowitz, D.: Blood lipid and uric acid interrelationships. JAMA, **190,** 856, 1964.
215. Alvsaker, J. O.: Uric acid in human plasma. V. Isolation and identification of plasma proteins interacting with urate. Scand. J. Clin. Lab. Invest., **18,** 227, 1966.
216. Alvsaker, J. O.: Genetic studies in primary gout: Investigations on the plasma levels of the urate-binding α_1-α_2 globulin in individuals from two gouty kindreds. J. Clin. Invest., **47,** 1254, 1968.
217. Trevaks, G., and Lovell, R. R. H.: Effect of atromid and its components on uric acid excretion and on gout. Ann. Rheum. Dis., **24,** 572, 1965.
218. Harris-Jones, J. N.: Hyperuricemia and essential hypercholesterolemia. Lancet, **1,** 857, 1957.
219. Salvini, L., and Verdi, G.: Statistical study on correlation between blood level of cholesterol beta/alpha lipoprotein ratio and uric acid of normal and arteriosclerotic subjects. Gerontologia (Basel), **3,** 327, 1959.
220. Kornerup, V.: Blood-uric-acid levels in familial hypercholesterolemia. Lancet, **1,** 298, 1966.
221. Strejček, J., and Kučerová, L.: Idiopathic hyperlipemia and gout. Acta Rheum. Scand., **14,** 95, 1968.
222. Upmark-Ask, E., and Adner, L.: Coronary infarction and gout. Acta Med. Scand., **139,** 1, 1950.
223. Gertler, M. M., Garn, S. M., and Levine, S. A.: Serum uric acid in relation to age and physique in health and in coronary artery disease. Ann. Intern. Med., **34,** 1421, 1951.
224. Kramer, D. W., Perilstein, P. K., and De Medeiros, A.: Metabolic influences in vascular disorders with particular reference to cholesterol determinations in comparison with uric acid levels. Angiology, **9,** 162, 1958.
225. Dreyfuss, F.: The role of hyperuricemia in coronary heart disease. Dis. Chest, **38,** 332, 1960.
226. Eidlitz, M.: Uric acid and arteriosclerosis. Lancet, **2,** 1046, 1961.
227. Hansen, O. E.: Hyperuricemia, gout and atherosclerosis. Amer. Heart J., **72,** 570, 1966.
228. Garrod, A. B.: *The Nature and Treatment of Gout and Rheumatic Gout,* p. 251, Walton and Maberly, London, 1863.
229. Lieber, C. S., and Davidson, C. S.: Some metabolic effects of ethyl alcohol. Amer. J. Med., **33,** 319, 1962.
230. Lieber, C. S., Jones, D. P., Losowsky, M. S., and Davidson, C. S.: Interrelation of uric acid and ethanol metabolism in man. J. Clin. Invest., **41,** 1863, 1962.
231. Yü, T.-F., Sirota, J. H., Berger, L., Halpern, M., and Gutman, A. B.: Effect of sodium lactate infusion on urate clearance in man. Proc. Soc. Exp. Biol. Med., **96,** 809, 1957.
232. MacLachlan, M. J., and Rodnan, G. P.: Effects of food, fast and alcohol on serum uric acid and acute attacks of gout. Amer. J. Med., **42,** 38, 1967.
233. Saker, B. M., Tofler, O. B., Burvill, M. J., and Reilly, K. A.: Alcohol consumption and gout. Med. J. Aust., **1,** 1212, 1967.
234. Evans, J. G., Prior, I. A. M., and Harvey, H. P. B.: Relation of serum uric acid to body bulk, haemoglobin, and alcohol intake in two South Pacific Polynesian populations. Ann. Rheum. Dis., **27,** 319, 1968.
235. Delbarre, F., Auscher, C., Brouihlet, H., and de Géry, A.: Action de l'éthanol dans la goutte et sur le métabolisme de l'acide urique. Sem. Hop. Paris, **43,** 659, 1967.
236. Folin, O.: Standardized methods for determination of uric acid in unlaked blood and urine. J. Biol. Chem., **101,** 111, 1933.
237. Archibald, R. M.: Colorimetric measurement of uric acid. Clin. Chem., **3,** 102, 1957.
238. Nishi, H. H.: Determination of uric acid: Adaptation of the Archibald method on the autoanalyzer. Clin. Chem., **13,** 12, 1967.
239. Wheat, J. L.: Determination of uric acid. Clin. Chem., **14,** 630, 1968.
240. Crowley, L. V., and Alton, F. I.: Automated analysis of uric acid. Amer. J. Clin. Path., **49,** 285, 1968.
241. Buchanan, M. J., Isdale, E. C., and Rose, B. S.: Serum uric acid estimation. Ann. Rheum. Dis., **24,** 285, 1965.
242. Isdale, I. C., Buchanan, M. J., and Rose, B. S.: Serum uric acid estimation. Ann. Rheum. Dis., **25,** 184, 1966.
243. Buchanan, O. H., Christman, A. A., and Block, W. D.: Metabolism of methylated purines. II. Uric acid excretion following ingestion of caffeine, theophylline, and theobromine. J. Biol. Chem., **157,** 189, 1945.
244. Yü, T.-F., and Gutman, A. B.: Interference of gentisic acid in determination of urinary uric acid after administration of salicylates. Fed. Proc., **8,** 267, 1949.
245. Grayzel, A. I., Liddle, L., and Seegmiller, J. E.: Diagnostic significance of hyperuricemia in arthritis. New Eng. J. Med., **265,** 763, 1961.
246. Indenbaum, S., Ward, L. E., and Tauxe, W. N.: Spuriously increased urate values in alkaptonuria. Mayo Clin. Proc., **40,** 127, 1965.
247. Cawein, M. J., and Hewins, J.: False rise in serum uric acid after L-dopa. New Eng. J. Med., **281,** 1489, 1969.
248. Bien, E. J., and Troll, W.: Interference by glucose in quantitative determination of uric acid. Proc. Soc. Exp. Biol. Med., **73,** 370, 1950.
249. Caraway, W. T., and Marable, H.: Comparison of carbonate and uricase carbonate methods for the determination of uric acid in serum. Clin. Chem., **12,** 18, 1966.
250. Yü, T.-F., and Gutman, A. B.: Quantitative analysis of uric acid in blood and urine: Methods and interpretation. Bull. Rheum. Dis. Diag. Proc. (suppl.), **7,** 5, 1957.

251. Kalckar, H. M.: Differential spectrophotometry of purine compounds by means of specific enzymes. I. Determination of hydroxypurine compounds. J. Biol. Chem., **167**, 429, 1947.
252. Praetorius, E.: An enzymatic method for the determination of uric acid by ultraviolet spectrophotometry. Scand. J. Clin. Lab. Invest., **1**, 222, 1949.
253. Liddle, L., Seegmiller, J. E., and Laster, L.: Enzymatic spectrophotometric method for determination of uric acid. J. Lab. Clin. Med., **54**, 903, 1959.
254. Bywaters, E. G. L., and Holloway, V. P.: Measurement of serum uric acid in Great Britain in 1963. Ann. Rheum. Dis., **23**, 236, 1964.
255. Gjorup, S., Poulsen, H., and Praetorius, E.: The uric acid concentration in serum determined by enzymatic spectrophotometry. Scand. J. Clin. Lab. Invest, **7**, 201, 1955.
256. Hauge, M., and Harvald, B.: Heredity in gout and hyperuricemia. Acta Med. Scand., **152**, 247, 1955.
257. Stetten, DeW., Jr., and Hearon, J. Z.: Intellectual level measured by Army classification battery and serum uric acid concentration. Science, **129**, 1737, 1959.
258. Grayzel, A. I., Liddle, L., and Seegmiller, J. E.: Diagnostic significance of hyperuricemia in arthritis. New Eng. J. Med., **265**, 763, 1961.
259. Zollner, N.: Eine einfache Modifikation der enzymatischen Harnsaurebestimmung: Normalwerte der deutschen Bevolkerung. Z. Klin. Chem., **6**, 178, 1963.
260. Mikkelsen, W. M., Dodge, H. J., and Valkenburg, H.: The distribution of serum uric acid values in a population unselected as to gout or hyperuricemia: Tecumseh, Michigan 1959–1960. Amer. J. Med., **39**, 242, 1965.
261. Peters, J. P., and Van Slyke, K. K.: *Quantitative Clinical Chemistry,* 2d ed., vol. l, p. 937. Williams & Wilkins, Baltimore, 1946.
262. Harkness, R. A., and Nicol, A. D.: Plasma uric acid levels in children. Arch. Dis. Child., **44**, 773–778, 1969.
263. Wolfson, W. Q., Krevshy, D., Levine, R., Kadota, K., and Cohn, C.: Endocrine factors in gout: The significance of differences in childhood and adult urate metabolism. J. Clin. Endocr., **9**, 666, 1949.
264. Wolfson, W. Q., Hunt, H. D., Levine, R., Guterman, H. S., Cohn, C., Rosenberg, E. F., Huddlestun, B., and Kadota, K.: The transport and excretion of uric acid in man. V. A sex difference in urate metabolism: With a note on clinical and laboratory findings on gouty women. J. Clin. Endocr., **9**, 749, 1949.
265. Smyth, C. J.: Hereditary factors in gout: A review of recent literature. Metabolism, **6**, 218, 1957.
266. Jacobson, B. M.: The uric acid in the serum of gouty and non-gouty individuals: Its determination by Folin's recent method and its significance in the diagnosis of gout. Ann. Intern. Med., **11**, 1277, 1937.
267. Ford, D. K., and DeMos, A. M.: Serum uric acid levels of healthy Caucasian, Chinese and Haide Indian males in British Columbia. Canad. Med. Ass. J., **90**, 1295, 1964.
268. Long, W. K.: Association between glutathione reductase variants and plasma uric acid concentration in a Negro population. Program abstracts, Amer. Soc. Human Genetics, October, 1970, p. 14a.
269. Emmerson, B. T., and Sandilands, P.: The normal range of plasma urate levels. Aust. Ann. Med., **12**, 46, 1963.
270. Healey, L. A., Caner, J. E. Z., and Decker, J. L.: Ethnic variations in serum uric acid. I. Filipino hyperuricemia in a controlled environment. Arthritis Rheum., **9**, 288, 1966.
271. Healey, L. A., Skeith, M. D., Decker, J. L., and Banyani-Sioson, P. S.: Hyperuricemia in Filipinos: Interaction of heredity and environment. Amer. J. Hum. Genet., **19**, 81, 1967.
272. Prior, I. A. M., Rose, B. S., and Davidson, F.: Metabolic abnormalities in New Zealand Maoris. Brit. Med. J., **1**, 1065, 1964.
273. Prior, I. A. M., Rose, B. S., Harvey, H. P. B., and Davidson, F.: Hyperuricaemia, gout, and diabetic abnormality in Polynesian people. Lancet, **1**, 333, 1966.
274. Healy, L. A., and Hall, A. P.: The epidemiology of hyperuricemia. Bull. Rheum. Dis., **20**, 600, 1970.
275. Steuermann, N., and Farias, A. H.: Hyperuricemia in Filipinos. Hawaii Med. J., **20**, 151, 1960.
276. Steuermann, N.: Hyperuricemia in the Filipino population of the Puna district on the island of Hawaii, in *The Epidemiology of Chronic Rheumatism,* vol. 1, p. 170. Davis, Philadelphia, 1963.
277. T'sung-Po, K: Gout in tropical Taiwan. J. Formosan Med. Ass., **63**, 415, 1964.
278. Burns-Cox, C. J.: Thirty-three cases of acute arthritis in Sabah. Med. J. Malaya, **19**, 25, 1964.
279. Emmerson, B. T., Douglass, W., Doherty, R. L., and Feigl, P.: Serum urate concentrations in the Australian aboriginal. Ann. Rheum. Dis., **28**, 150, 1969.
280. Saha, N., and Banerjee, B.: Genetic influences on serum-uric-acid. Lancet, **2**, 911, 1969.
281. Healey, L. A., Caner, J. E. Z., Bassett, D. R., and Decker, J. L.: Serum uric acid and obesity in Hawaiians. JAMA, **196**, 364, 1966.
282. Acheson, R. M., and Chan, Y. K.: The prediction of serum uric acid in a general population. J. Chronic Dis., **21**, 543, 1969.
283. Wallace, M. R., and James, K. R.: Renal function in obese hyperuricaemic Maoris. New Zeal. Med. J., **70**, 84, 1969.
284. Montoye, H. J., Faulkner, J. A., Dodge, H. J., Mikkelsen, W. M., Willis, P. W., and Block, W. D.: Serum uric acid concentration among business executives. Ann. Intern. Med., **66**, 838, 1967.
285. Anumonye, A., Dobson, J. W., Oppenheim, S., and Sutherland, J. S.: Plasma uric acid concentrations among Edinburgh business executives. JAMA, **208**, 1141, 1969.
286. Brooks, G. W., and Mueller, E.: Serum urate concentrations among university professors. JAMA, **195**, 415, 1966.
287. Acheson, R. M., Chan, Y. K., and Payne, M.: The interrelationships between morning stiffness, nocturnal pain and swelling of the joints: New Haven survey of joint diseases. J. Chronic Dis., **21**, 533, 1969.
288. Yü, T.-F., and Gutman, A. B.: Ultrafilterability of plasma urate in man. Proc. Soc. Exp. Biol. Med., **84**, 21, 1953.
289. Adlersberg, D., Grishman, E., and Sobotka, H.: Uric acid partition in gout and hepatic disease. Arch. Intern. Med. (Chicago), **70**, 101, 1942.
290. Alvsaker, J. O.: Uric acid in human plasma. III. Investigations on the interaction between the urate ion and human albumin. Scand. J. Clin. Lab. Invest., **17**, 467, 1965.
291. Alvsaker, J. O.: Uric acid in human plasma. IV. Investigations on the interactions between urate and the macromolecular fraction in plasma from healthy individuals and patients with diseases associated with hyperuricemia. Scand. J. Clin. Lab. Invest., **17**, 476, 1965.
292. Katz, W. A., and Ehrlich, G. E.: The solubility of monosodium urate in serum and connective tissue fractions. Arthritis Rheum., **11**, 492, 1968.
293. Skeikh, M. I., and Moller, J. V.: Binding of urate to proteins of human and rabbit plasma. Biochim. Biophys. Acta, **158**, 456, 1968.
294. Klinenberg, J. R., and Kippen, I.: The binding of urate to plasma proteins determined by means of equilibrium dialysis. J. Lab. Clin. Med., **75**, 503, 1970.
295. Bluestone, R., Kippen, I., and Klinenberg, J. R.: Effect of drugs on urate binding to plasma proteins. Brit. Med. J., **4**, 590, 1969.
296. Bluestone, R., Kippen, I., Klinenberg, J. R., and Whitehouse, M. W.: Effect of some uricosuric and antiinflammatory drugs on the binding of uric acid to human serum albumin in vitro. J. Lab. Clin. Med., **76**, 85, 1970.
297. Bechold, H., and Ziegler, J.: Vorstudien uber Gicht. III. Biochem. Z., **64**, 471, 1914.
298. Klinenberg, J. R., Goldfinger, S., Miller, J., and Seegmiller, J. E.: The effectiveness of a xanthine oxidase inhibitor in the treatment of gout. Arthritis Rheum., **6**, 779, 1963.
299. Talbott, J. H., and Coombs, F. S.: Metabolic studies on patients with gout, JAMA, **110**, 1977, 1938.
300. Goldthwait, J. C., Butler, C. F., and Stillman, J. S.: The diagnosis of gout: Significance of an elevated serum uric acid value. New Eng. J. Med., **259**, 1095, 1958.
301. Seegmiller, J. E., Grayzel, A. I., Laster, L., and Liddle, L.: Uric acid production in gout. J. Clin. Invest., **40**, 1304, 1961.
302. Rieselback, R. E., Sorensen, L. B., Shelp, W. D., and Steele, T. H.: Diminished renal urate secretion per nephron as a basis for primary gout. Ann. Intern. Med., **73**, 359, 1970.
303. Nugent, C. A., and Tyler, F. H.: The renal excretion of uric acid in

patients with gout and in nongouty subjects. J. Clin. Invest., **38,** 1890, 1959.

304. Seegmiller, J. E., Grayzel, A. I., Howell, R. R., and Plato, C.: The renal excretion of uric acid in gout. J. Clin. Invest., **41,** 1094, 1962.
305. Yü, T.-F., Berger, L., and Gutman, A. B.: Renal function in gout. II. Effect of uric acid loading on renal excretion of uric acid. Amer. J. Med., **33,** 829, 1962.
306. Wyngaarden, J. B., and Stetten, D., Jr.: Uricolysis in normal man. J. Biol. Chem., **203,** 9, 1953.
307. Sorensen, L. B.: Degradation of uric acid in man. Metabolism, **8,** 687, 1959.
308. Sorensen, L. B.: The elimination of uric acid in man studied by means of C^{14}-labeled uric acid. Scand. J. Clin. Lab. Invest., **12,** suppl. 54, 1960.
309. Sorensen, L. B.: The pathogenesis of gout. Arch. Intern. Med. (Chicago), **109,** 379, 1962.
310. Rose, W. C.: Purine metabolism. Physiol. Rev., **3,** 544, 1923.
311. Christman, A. A.: Purine and pyrimidine metabolism. Physiol. Rev., **32,** 303, 1952.
312. Bishop, C., and Talbott, J. H.: Uric acid: Its role in biological processes and the influence upon it of physiological, pathological, and pharmacological agents. Pharmacol. Rev., **5,** 231, 1953.
313. Wiener, H.: Uber synthetische Bildung der Harnsaure im Tierkorper. Beitr. Chem. Physiol. Path., **2,** 42, 1902.
314. Ackroyd, H., and Hopkins, F. G.: Feeding experiments with deficiencies in the amino acid supply: Arginine and histidine as possible precursors of purines. Biochem. J., **10,** 551, 1916.
315. Barnes, F. W., and Schoenheimer, R.: On biological synthesis of purines and pyrimidines. J. Biol. Chem., **151,** 123, 1943.
316. Tesar, C., and Rittenberg, D.: The metabolism of L-histidine. J. Biol. Chem., **170,** 35, 1947.
317. Shemin, D., and Rittenberg, D.: On the utilization of glycine for uric acid synthesis in man. J. Biol. Chem., **167,** 875, 1947.
318. Buchanan, J. M., Sonne, J. C., and Delluva, A. M.: Biologic precursors of uric acid. II. The role of lactate, glycine, and carbon dioxide as precursors of the carbon chain and nitrogen atom 7 of uric acid. J. Biol. Chem., **173,** 81, 1948.
319. Karlson, J. L., and Barker, H. A.: Biosynthesis of uric acid labeled with radioactive carbon. J. Biol. Chem., **177,** 597, 1949.
320. Sonne, J. C., Buchanan, J. M., and Delluva, A. M.: Biological precursors of uric acid. I. The role of lactate, acetate and formate in synthesis of the ureido groups of uric acid. J. Biol. Chem., **173,** 69, 1948.
321. Heinrich, M. R., and Wilson, D. W.: Biosynthesis of nucleic acid components studied with C^{14}. I. Purines and pyrimidines in the rat. J. Biol. Chem., **186,** 447, 1950.
322. Sonne, J. C., Lin, I., and Buchanan, J. M.: Biosynthesis of the purines. IX. Precursors of the nitrogen atoms of the purine ring. J. Biol. Chem., **220,** 369, 1956.
323. Levenberg, B., Hartman, S. C., and Buchanan, J. M: Biosynthesis of the purines. X. Further studies in vitro on the metabolic origin of nitrogen atoms 1 and 3 of the purine ring. J. Biol. Chem., **220,** 379, 1956.
324. Goldthwait, D. A., Peabody, R. A., and Greenberg, G. R.: On the mechanism of synthesis of glycinamideribotide and its formyl derivative. J. Biol. Chem., **221,** 569, 1956.
325. Hartman, S. C., and Buchanan, J. M.: Biosynthesis of the purines. XXI. 5-Phosphoribosylpyrophosphate amidotransferase. J. Biol. Chem., **233,** 451, 1958.
326. Flaks, J. G., Erwin, M. J., and Buchanan, J. M.: Biosynthesis of the purines. XVI. The synthesis of adenosine 5′-phosphate and 5′-amino-4-imidazolecarboxamide ribotide by a nucleotide pyrophosphorylase. J. Biol. Chem., **228,** 201, 1957.
327. Lukens, L. N., and Herrington, K. A.: Enzymic formation of 6-mercaptopurine ribotide. Biochim. Biophys. Acta, **24,** 432, 1957.
328. Kornberg, A., Lieberman, I., and Simms, E. S.: Enzymatic synthesis and properties of 5-phosphoribosylpyrophosphate. J. Biol. Chem., **215,** 389, 1955.
329. Remy, C. N., Remy, W. T., and Buchanan, J. M.: Biosynthesis of the purines. VIII. Enzymatic synthesis and utilization of 5-phosphoribosylpyrophosphate. J. Biol. Chem., **217,** 885, 1955.
330. Bloom, B., and Stetten, D., Jr.: Pathways of glucose catabolism. J. Amer. Chem. Soc., **75,** 5446, 1953.
331. Bloom, B.: Catabolism of glucose by mammalian tissues. Proc. Soc. Exp. Biol. Med., **88,** 307, 1955.
332. Hiatt, H. H.: Studies of ribose metabolism. VI. Pathways of ribose synthesis in man. J. Clin. Invest., **37,** 1461, 1958.
333. Hiatt, H. H., and Lareau, J.: Studies of ribose metabolism. VII. An assessment of ribose biosynthesis from hexose by way of the C-6 oxidation pathway. J. Biol. Chem., **233,** 1023, 1958.
334. Goldthwait, D. A., Greenberg, G. R., and Peabody, R. A.: The involvement of 5-phosphoribosylamine in the biosynthesis of glycinamide ribotide. Biochim. Biophys. Acta, **18,** 148, 1955.
335. Goldthwait, D. A.: 5-Phosphoribosylamine, a precursor of glycinamide ribotide. J. Biol. Chem., **222,** 1051, 1956.
336. Wyngaarden, J. B., and Ashton, D. M.: The regulation of activity of phosphoribosylpyrophosphate amidotransferase by purine ribonucleotides: A potential feedback control of purine biosynthesis. J. Biol. Chem., **234,** 1492, 1959.
337. Caskey, C. T., Ashton, D. M., and Wyngaarden, J. B.: The enzymology of feedback inhibition of glutamine phosphoribosylpyrophosphate amidotransferase by purine ribonucleotides. J. Biol. Chem., **239,** 2570, 1964.
338. Nierlich, D. P., and Magasanik, B.: Regulation of purine ribonucleotide synthesis by end product inhibition. J. Biol. Chem., **240,** 358, 1965.
338*a*. Rottman, F., and Guarino, A. J.: The inhibition of phosphoribosylpyrophosphate amidotransferase activity by cordecepin monophosphate. Biochim. Biophys. Acta, **89,** 465, 1964.
339. Nierlich, D. P., and Magasanik, B.: Alternative first steps of purine biosynthesis. J. Biol. Chem., **236,** 32, 1961.
340. Le Gal, M.-L., Le Gal, Y., Roche, J., and Hedegaard, J: Purine biosynthesis: Enzymatic formation of ribosylamine-5-phosphate from ribose-5-phosphate and ammonia. Biochem. Biophys. Res. Commun., **27,** 618, 1967.
341. Herscovics, A., and Johnstone, R. M.: ^{14}C-Formate utilization in cell-free extracts of Ehrlich ascites cells. Biochim. Biophys. Acta, **93,** 251, 1964.
342. Reem, G.: Enzymatic synthesis of 5′-phosphoribosylamine from ribose-5-phosphate and ammonia, alternative first step in purine biosynthesis. J. Biol. Chem., **243,** 5695, 1968.
343. Hartman, S. C.: Phosphoribosylpyrophosphate amidotransferase: Purification and general catalytic properties. J. Biol. Chem., **238,** 3024, 1963.
344. Westby, C. A., and Gots, J. S.: Genetic blocks and unique features in the biosynthesis of 5′-phosphoribosyl-N-formylglycinamide in *Salmonella typhimurium.* J. Biol. Chem., **244,** 2095, 1969.
345. Hartman, S. C., Levenberg, B., and Buchanan, J. M.: Biosynthesis of the purines. XI. Structure, enzymatic synthesis, and metabolism of glycinamide ribotide and (α-N-formyl)-glycinamide ribotide, J. Biol. Chem., **221,** 1057, 1956.
346. Hartman, S. C., and Buchanan, J. M.: Biosynthesis of the purines. XXII. 2-Amino-N-ribosylacetamide-5′-phosphate kinosynthetase. J. Biol. Chem., **233,** 456, 1958.
347. Nierlich, D. P., and Magasanik, B.: Phosphoribosylglycinamide synthetase of *Aerobacter aerogenes.* J. Biol. Chem., **240,** 366, 1965.
348. Warren, L., and Buchanan, J. M.: Biosynthesis of the purines. XIX. 2-Amino-N-ribosylacetamide-5′-phosphate (glycinamide ribotide) transformylase. J. Biol. Chem., **229,** 613, 1957.
349. Warren, L., Flaks, J. G., and Buchanan, J. M.: Biosynthesis of the purines. XX. Integration of enzymatic transformylation reactions. J. Biol. Chem., **229,** 627, 1957.
350. Levenberg, B., and Buchanan, J. M.: Biosynthesis of the purine. XIII. Structure, enzymatic synthesis and metabolism of (α-N-formyl)-glycinamidine ribotide. J. Biol. Chem., **224,** 1019, 1957.
351. Melnick, I., and Buchanan, J. M.: Biosynthesis of the purines. XIV. Conversion of (α-N-formyl)-glycinamide ribotide to (α-N-formyl)-glycinamide ribotide; purification and requirements of the enzyme system. J. Biol. Chem., **225,** 157, 1957.
352. Mizobuchi, K., and Buchanan, J. M.: Biosynthesis of the purines: Purification and properties of formylglycinamide ribonucleotide amidotransferase from chicken liver. J. Biol. Chem., **243,** 4842, 1968.
353. Mizobuchi, K., and Buchanan, J. M.: Biosynthesis of the purines:

Isolation and characterization of formylglycinamide ribonucleotide amidotransferase-glutamyl complex J. Biol. Chem., **243,** 4853, 1968.
354. Mizobuchi, K., Kenyon, G. L., and Buchanan, J. M.: Binding of formylglycinamide ribonucleotide and adenosine triphosphate to formylglycinamide ribonucleotide, amidotransferase. J. Biol. Chem., **243,** 4863, 1968.
355. Levenberg, B., and Buchanan, J. M.: Biosynthesis of the purines. XII. Structure, enzymatic synthesis, and metabolism of 5-aminoimidazole ribotide. J. Biol. Chem., **224,** 1005, 1957.
356. Lukens, L. N., and Buchannan, J. B.: Further intermediates in the biosynthesis of inosinic acid *de novo.* J. Amer. Chem. Soc., **79,** 1511, 1957.
357. Flaks, J. G., Warren, L., and Buchanan, J. M.: Biosynthesis of the purines. XVII. Further studies of the inosinic acid transformylase system. J. Biol. Chem., **228,** 215, 1957.
358. Flaks, J. G., Erwin, M. J., and Buchanan, J. M.: Biosynthesis of the purines. XVIII. 5-Amino-1-ribosyl-4-imidazolecarboxamide 5′-phosphate transformylase and inosinicase. J. Biol. Chem., **229,** 603, 1957.
359. Stetten, M. R., and Fox, C. L., Jr.: An amine formed by bacteria during sulfonamide bacteriostasis. J. Biol. Chem., **161,** 333, 1945.
360. Shive, W., Ackermann, W. W., Gordon, M., Getzendaner, M. E., and Eakin, R. E.: 5(4)-amino-4(5)-imidazolecarboxamide, a precursor of purines. J. Amer. Chem. Soc., **69,** 725, 1947.
361. Miller, C. S., Gurin, S., and Wilson, D. W.: C^{14}-Labeled 4(5)-amino-5(4)-imidazolecarboxamide in the biosynthesis of purines. Science, **112,** 654, 1950.
362. Schulman, M. P., and Buchanan, U. M.: Biosynthesis of the purines. II. Metabolism of 4-amino-5-imidazolecarboxamide in pigeon liver. J. Biol. Chem., **196,** 513, 1952.
363. Buchanan, J. M., and Schulman, M. P.: Biosynthesis of the purines. III. Reactions of formate and inosinic acid and an effect of the citrovorum factor. J. Biol. Chem., **202,** 241, 1953.
364. Williams, W. J., and Buchanan, J. M: Biosynthesis of the purine. IV. The metabolism of 4-amino-5-imidazolecarboxamide in yeast. J. Biol. Chem., **202** 253, 1953.
365. Abrams, R., and Bentley, M.: Transformation of inosinic acid to adenylic and guanylic acids in a soluble enzyme system. J. Amer. Chem. Soc., **77,** 4179, 1955.
366. Carter, C. E., and Cohen, C. H.: The preparation and properties of adenylosuccinase and adenylosuccinic acid. J. Biol. Chem., **222,** 17, 1956.
367. Joklik, W. K.: Adenine succinic acid and adenylsuccinic acid from mammalian liver: Isolation and identification. Biochem. J., **66,** 333, 1957.
368. Lieberman, I.: Enzymatic synthesis of adenosine 5′-phosphate from inosine 5′-phosphate. J. Biol. Chem., **223,** 327, 1956.
369. Fromm, H. J.: On the equilibrium and mechanism of adenylosuccinic acid synthesis. Biochim. Biophys. Acta, **29,** 255, 1958.
370. Magasanik, B., Moyed, H. S., and Gehring, L. B.: Enzymes essential for the biosynthesis of nucleic acid guanine: Inosine 5′-phosphate dehydrogenase of *Aerobacter aerogenes.* J. Biol. Chem., **226,** 379, 1957.
371. Lagerkvist, U.: Biosynthesis of guanosine 5′-phosphate. I. Xanthosine 5′-phosphate as an intermediate. J. Biol. Chem., **233,** 138, 1958.
372. Lagerkvist, U.: Biosynthesis of guanosine 5′-phosphate. II. Amination of xanthosine 5′-phosphate by purified enzymes from pigion liver. J. Biol. Chem., **233,** 143, 1958.
373. Abrams, R., and Bentley, M.: Biosynthesis of nucleic acid purines. III. Guanosine 5′-phosphate formation from xanthosine 5′-phosphate and L-glutamine. Arch. Biochem., **79,** 91, 1959.
374. Lieberman, I., Kornberg, A., and Simms, E. S.: Enzymatic synthesis of pyrimidine nucleotides: Orotidine-5′-phosphate and uridine-5′-phosphate. J. Biol. Chem., **215,** 403, 1955.
375. Preiss, J., and Handler, P.: Enzymatic synthesis of nicotinamide mononucleotide. J. Biol. Chem., **222,** 759, 1957.
376. Hori, M., and Henderson, J. F.: Kinetic studies of adenine phosphoribosyltransferase. J. Biol. Chem., **241,** 3404, 1966.
377. Kelley, W. N., Rosenbloom, F. M., Henderson, J. F., and Seegmiller, J. E.: Xanthine phosphoribosyltransferase in man: Relationship to hypoxanthine-guanine phosphoribosyltransferase. Biochem. Biophys. Res. Commun., **28,** 345, 1967.
378. McCollister, R. J., Gilbert, W. R., Jr., Ashton, D. M., and Wyngaarden, J. B.: Pseudofeedback inhibition of purine synthesis by 6-mercaptopurine ribonucleotide and other purine analogues. J. Biol. Chem., **239,** 1560, 1964.
379. Henderson, J. F., Brox, L. W., Kelley, W. N., Rosenbloom, F. M., and Seegmiller, J. E.: Kinetic studies of hypoxanthine-guanine phosphoribosyltransferase. J. Biol. Chem., **243,** 2514, 1968.
380. Craft, J. A., Dean, B. M., Watts, R. W. E., and Westwick, W. J.: Studies on human erythrocyte IMP: Pyrophosphate phosphoribosyl transferase. Europ. J. Biochem., **15,** 367, 1970.
381. Kalckar, H. M.: The enzymatic synthesis of purine ribosides. J. Biol. Chem., **167,** 477, 1947.
382. Friedkin, M., and Kalckar, H.: Nucleoside phosphorylases, in *The Enzymes,* edited by P. D. Boyer, H. Lardy, and K. Myrback, vol. 5, p. 237. Academic, New York, 1961.
383. Krenitsky, T. A., Elion, G. B., Henderson, A. M., and Hitchings, G. H.: Inhibition of human purine nucleoside phosphorylase: Studies with intact erythrocytes and the purified enzyme. J. Biol. Chem., **243,** 2876, 1968.
384. Sandberg, A. A., Lee, G. R., Cartwright, G. E.,•and Wintrobe, M. D.: Purine nucleoside phosphorylase activity of blood. I. Erythrocytes. J. Clin. Invest., **12,** 1823, 1955.
385. Pierre, K. J., and Le Page, G. A.: Formation of inosine-5′-monophosphate by a kinase in cell-free extracts of Ehrlich ascites cells *in vitro.* Proc. Soc. Exp. Biol. Med., **127,** 432, 1968.
386. Wada, Y., Arakawa, T., and Koizumi, K.: Lesch-Nyhan syndrome: Autopsy findings and in vitro study of incorporation of ^{14}C-8-inosine into uric acid, guanosine-monophosphate and adenosine-monophosphate in the liver. Tohoku J. Exp. Med., **95,** 253, 1968.
387. Friedmann, T., Seegmiller, J. E., and Subak-Sharpe, J. H.: Evidence against the existence of guanosine and inosine kinases in human fibroblasts in tissue culture. Exp. Cell Res., **56,** 425, 1969.
388. Goldthwait, D.: Mechanisms of synthesis of purine nucleotides in heart muscle extracts. J. Clin. Invest., **36,** 1572, 1957.
389. Lowy, B. A., Williams, M. K., and London, I. M.: Enzymatic deficiencies of purine nucleotide synthesis in the human erythrocyte. J. Biol. Chem., **237,** 1622, 1962.
390. Caputto, R.: The enzymatic synthesis of adenylic acid: Adenosinekinase. J. Biol. Chem., **189,** 801, 1951.
391. Kornberg, A., and Pricer, W. E., Jr.: Enzymatic phosphorylation of adenosine and 2,6-diaminopurine riboside. J. Biol. Chem., **193,** 481, 1951.
392. Wyngaarden, J. B., Appel, S. H., and Rowe, P. B.: Control of biosynthetic pathways by regulatory enzymes, in *Exploitable Molecular Mechanisms and Neoplasia,* p. 415. Williams & Wilkins, Baltimore, 1969.
393. Wyngaarden, J. B., Silberman, H. R., and Sadler, J. H.: Feedback mechanisms influencing purine ribotide synthesis. Ann. NY Acad. Sci., **75,** 45, 1958.
394. Lajtha, L. G., and Vane, J. R.: Dependence of bone marrow cells on the liver for purine supply. Nature (London), **182,** 191, 1958.
395. Henderson, J. F., and Le Page, G. A.: Utilization of host purines by transplanted tumors. Cancer Res., **19,** 67, 1959.
396. Mager, J., Hershko, A., Zeitlin-Beck, R., Shoshami, T., and Razin, A.: Turnover of purine nucleotides in rabbit erythrocytes. I. Studies in vivo. Biochim. Biophys. Acta, **149,** 50, 1967.
397. Heppel, L. A., and Rabinowitz, J. C.: Enzymology of nucleic acids, purines, and pyrimidines. Ann. Rev. Biochem., **27,** 613, 1958.
398. Heppel, L. A., and Hilmoe, R. J.: Purification and properties of 5-nucleotidase. J. Biol. Chem., **188,** 665, 1951.
399. Schmidt, G.: Nucleases and enzymes attacking nucleic acid components, in *The Nucleic Acids,* edited by E. Chargaff and J. N. Davidson, vol. 1. Academic, New York, 1955.
400. Friedkin, M.: Enzymatic synthesis of desoxyxanthosine by the action of xanthosine phosphorylase in mammalian tissue. J. Amer. Chem. Soc., **74,** 112, 1952.
401. Nikiforuk, G., and Colowick, S. P.: The purification and properties of 5-adenylic acid deaminase from muscle. J. Biol. Chem., **219,** 119, 1956.
402. Kalckar, H. M.: Differential spectrophotometry of purine compounds by means of specific enzymes. III. Studies of the enzymes of purine metabolism. J. Biol. Chem., **167,** 461, 1947.

403. Dunn, D. B., and Smith, J. D.: The occurrence of 6-methylaminopurine in deoxyribonucleic acids. Biochem. J., **68,** 627, 1958.
404. Borek, E., and Srinivasan, P. R.: The methylation of nucleic acids. Ann. Rev. Biochem., **35,** 275, 1966.
405. Cantoni, G. L., Gelboin, H. V., Luborsky, S. W., Richards, H. H., and Singer, M. F.: Studies on soluble ribonucleic acid of rabbit liver. III. Preparation and properties of rabbit-liver soluble RNA. Biochim. Biophys. Acta, **61,** 354, 1962.
406. Magee, P. N., and Farber, E.: Toxic liver injury and carcinogenesis: Methylation of rat-liver nucleic acids by dimethylnitrosamine in vivo. Biochem. J., **83,** 114, 1962.
407. Fleissner, E., and Borek, E.: A new enzyme of RNA synthesis: RNA methylase. Proc. Nat. Acad. Sci. USA, **48,** 1199, 1962.
408. Gold, M., and Hurwitz, J.: The enzymatic methylation of ribonucleic acid and deoxyribonucleic acid. V. Purification and properties of the deoxyribonucleic acid–methylating activity of *Escherichia coli.* J. Biol. Chem., **239,** 3858, 1964.
409. Hurwitz, J., Anders, M., Gold, M., and Smith, I.: The enzymatic methylation of ribonucleic acid and deoxyribonucleic acid. VII. The methylation of ribosomal ribonucleic acid. J. Biol. Chem., **240,** 1256, 1965.
410. Wilson, D., Beyer, A., Bishop, C., and Talbott, J. H.: Urinary uric acid excretion after the ingestion of isotopic yeast nucleic acid in the normal and gouty human. J. Biol. Chem., **209,** 227, 1954.
411. Roll, P. M., Brown, G. B., DeCarlo, F. J., and Schultz, A. S.: The metabolism of yeast nucleic acid in the rat. J. Biol. Chem., **180,** 333, 1949.
412. Korn, E. D., and Buchanan, J. M.: Biosynthesis of the purines. VI. Purification of liver nucleoside phosphorylase and demonstration of nucleoside synthesis from 4-amino-5-imidazolecarboxamide, adenine, and 2,6-diaminopurine. J. Biol. Chem., **217,** 183, 1955.
413. Huennekens, F. M., Nurk, E., and Gabrio, B. W.: Erythrocyte metabolism. I. Purine nucleoside phosphorylase. J. Biol. Chem., **221,** 971, 1956.
414. Weissmann, B., Bromberg, P. A., and Gutman, G. B.: The purine bases of human urine. II. Semiquantitative estimation and isotope incorporation. J. Biol. Chem., **224,** 423, 1957.
415. Bergmann, F., and Dikstein, S.: Studies on uric acid and related compounds. III. Observations on the specificity of mammalian xanthine oxidase. J. Biol. Chem., **223.** 765, 1956.
416. Engelman, K., Watts, R. W. E., Klinenberg, J. R., Sjoerdsma, A., and Seegmiller, J. E.: Clinical physiological and biochemical studies of a patient with xanthinuria and pheochromocytoma. Amer. J. Med., **37,** 839, 1964.
417. Watts, R. W. E., Watts, J. E. M., Seegmiller, J. E.: Xanthine oxidase activity in human tissues and its inhibition by allopurinol (4-hydroxypyrazolo (3,4-d) pyrimidine). J. Lab. Clin. Med., **66,** 688–697, 1965.
418. Dunn, J., and Wyngaarden, J. B.: Unpublished results.
419. Segal, S., and Wyngaarden, J. B.: Plasma glutamine and oxypurine content in patients with gout. Proc. Soc. Exp. Biol. Med., **88,** 342, 1955.
420. Jorgensen, S., and Poulsen, H. E.: Enzymic determination of hypoxanthine and xanthine in human plasma and urine. Acta Pharmacol. (Kobenhavn), **11,** 223, 1955.
421. Hoffman, G. T., Rottino, A., and Albaum, H. G.: Levels of nucleotide in the blood during shock. Science, **114,** 188, 1951.
422. Davis, A. R., Newton, E. B., and Benedict, S. R.: The combined uric acid in beef blood. J. Biol. Chem., **54,** 595, 1922.
423. Falconer, R., and Gulland, J. M.: The constitution of purine nucleosides. VIII. Uric acid riboside. J. Chem. Soc. [Org.], 1939, p. 1369.
424. Newton, E. B., and Davis, A. R.: Combined uric acid in human, horse, sheep, pig, dog, and chicken blood. J. Biol. Chem., **54,** 603, 1922.
425. Overgaard-Hansen, K., and Nielsen, A. T.: Does human blood contain uric acid riboside? Scand. J. Clin. Lab. Invest., **9,** 194, 1957.
426. Forrest, H. S., Hatfield, D., and Lagowski, J. M.: Uric acid riboside. Part I. Isolation and reinvestigation of the structure. J. Chem. Soc. [Org.], 1961, p. 963.
427. Carter, C. E., and Potter, J. L.: Distribution and properties of uric acid riboside. Fed. Proc., **11,** 195, 1952.
428. Birkofer, L., Ritter, A., and Kuhlthan, H. P.: Uric acid-3-ribofuranoside and uric acid-3-glucopyranoside. Angew Chem. [Eng.], **2,** 155, 1963.
429. Lohrman, R., Lagowski, J. M., and Forrest, H. S.: 3-Ribosyluric acid. Part III. Unambiguous synthesis of 3-ribosyluric acid and related compounds. J. Chem. Soc. [Org.], 1964, p. 451.
430. Laster, L., and Blair, A.: An intestinal phosphorylase for uric acid ribonucleoside. J. Biol. Chem., **238,** 3348, 1963.
431. Laster, L., and Blair, A.: Uric acid riboside phosphorylase in human tissues: Inhibition by colchicine, and other properties. J. Clin. Invest., **37,** 909, 1958.
432. Hatfield, D., and Forrest, H. S.: Biosynthesis of 3-ribosyluric acid (uric acid riboside). Biochim. Biophys. Acta, **62,** 185, 1962.
433. Hatfield, D., and Wyngaarden, J. B.: 3-ribosylpurines. II. Studies on (3-ribosylxanthine)5′-phosphate and on ribonucleotide derivatives of certain uracil analogues. J. Biol. Chem., **239,** 2587, 1964.
434. Hatfield, D., Rinehart, R. R., and Forrest, H. S.: 3-Ribosyluric acid. Part II. Isolation of the corresponding nucleotide from beef blood. J. Chem. Soc. [Org.], 1963, p. 899.
435. Hatfield, D., and Wyngaarden, J. B.: 3-Ribosylpurines. I. Synthesis of (3-ribosyluric acid)5′-phosphate and (3-ribosylxanthine)5′-phosphate by a pyrimidine ribonucleotide pyrophosphorylase of beef erythrocytes. J. Biol. Chem., **239,** 2580, 1964.
436. Beardmore, T. D., and Kelley, W. N.: Studies on the mechanism of allopurinol-induced inhibition of pyrimidine metabolism. Clin. Res., **19,** 27, 1971.
437. Hatfield, D., Greenland, R. A., Stewart, H. L., and Wyngaarden, J. B.: Biosynthesis of a new uric acid ribonucleotide. Biochim. Biophys. Acta, **91,** 163, 1964.
438. Gots, J. S., and Goldstein, J.: Specific action of adenine as a feedback inhibitor of purine biosynthesis. Science, **130,** 622, 1959.
439. Brockman, R. W., and Anderson, E. P.: Biochemistry of cancer (metabolic aspects). Ann. Rev. Biochem., **32,** 463, 1963.
440. Brockman, R. W., and Chumley, S. W.: Inhibition of formylglycinamide ribonucleotide synthesis in neoplastic cells by purines and analogs. Biochim. Biophys. Acta, **95,** 365, 1965.
441. Howard, W. J., and Appel, S. H.: Control of purine biosynthesis: FGAR amidotransferase. Clin. Res., **16,** 344, 1968.
422. Nierlich, D. P., and Magasanik, B.: Control by repression of purine biosynthetic enzymes in aerogenes. Fed. Proc., **22,** 476, 1963.
443. Momose, H., Nishikawa, H., and Shus, L.: Regulation of purine nucleotide synthesis in *Bacillus subtilis.* J. Biol. Chem., **59,** 325, 1966.
444. Henderson, J. F., and Khoo, M. K. Y.: Synthesis of 5-phosphoribosyl-1-pyrophosphate from glucose in Ehrlich ascites tumor cells in vitro. J. Biol. Chem., **240,** 2349, 1965.
445. Greene, M. L., and Seegmiller, J. E.: Elevated erythrocyte phosphoribosylpyrophosphate in X-linked uric aciduria: Importance of PRPP concentration in the regulation of human purine biosynthesis. J. Clin. Invest., **48,** 32a, 1969.
446. Kelley, W. N., Fox. I. H., and Wyngaarden, J. B.: Essential role of phosphoribosylpyrophosphate (PRPP) in regulation of purine biosynthesis in cultured human fibroblasts. Clin. Res., **18,** 457, 1970.
447. Raivio, K. O., and Seegmiller, J. E.: Role of glutamine in purine synthesis and interconversion. Clin. Res., **19,** 161, 1971.
448. Katz, J., and Rognstad, R.: The labeling of pentose phosphate from glucose-^{14}C and estimation of the rates of transaldolase, transketolase, the contribution of the pentose cycle, and ribosephosphate synthesis. Biochemistry (Wash.), **6,** 2227, 1967.
449. Switzer, R. L.: End-product inhibition of phosphoribosylpyrophosphate synthetase. Fed. Proc., **26,** 560, 1967.
450. Wong, P. C. L., and Murray, A. W.: 5-Phosphoribosyl pyrophosphate synthetase from Ehrlich ascites tumor cells. Biochemistry (Wash.), **8,** 1608, 1969.
451. Hershko, A., Razin, A., and Mager, J.: Relation of the synthesis of 5-phosphoribosyl-1-pyrophosphate in intact red blood cells and in cell free preparations Biochim. Biophys. Acta, **184,** 64, 1969.
452. Fox, I., and Kelley, W. N.: Human erythrocyte phosphoribosylpyrophosphate synthetase: Conformational changes and regulation. Fed. Proc., **30,** 1255, 1971.
453. Atkinson, D. E., and Fall, L.: Adenosine triphosphate conservation in biosynthetic regulation: *Escherichia coli* phosphoribosylpyrophosphate synthetase. J. Biol. Chem., **242,** 3241, 1967.
454. Atkinson, D. E.: The energy charge of the adenylate pool as a regulatory

parameter: Interaction with feedback modifiers. Biochemistry (Wash.), **7,** 4030, 1968.

455. Klungsoyr, L., Hageman, J. H., Fall, L., and Atkinson, D. E.: Interaction between energy charge and product feedback in the regulation of biosynthetic enzymes: Aspartokinase, phosphoribosyladenosine triphosphate synthetase, and phosphoribosyl pyrophosphate synthetase. Biochemistry (Wash.), **7,** 4035, 1968.
456. Fox, I., and Kelley, W. N.: Phosphoribosylpyrophosphate in man: Biochemical and clinical significance. Ann. Intern. Med., **74,** 424, 1971.
457. Rowe, P. B., and Wyngaarden, J. B.: Glutamine phosphoribosylpyrophosphate amidotransferase: Purification, substructure, amino acid composition and absorption spectra. J. Biol. Chem., **243,** 6373, 1968.
458. Hill, D. L., and Bennett, L. L., Jr.: Purification and properties of 5-phosphoribosyl pyrophosphate amidotransferase from adenocarcinoma 755 cells. Biochemistry (Wash.), **8,** 122, 1969.
459. Perheentupa, J., and Raivio, K.: Fructose-induced hyperuricemia. Lancet, **2,** 528, 1967.
460. Maenpaa, P. H., Raivio, K. O., and Kekomaki, M. P.: Liver adenine nucleotides: Fructose-induced depletion and its effect on protein synthesis. Science, **161,** 1253, 1968.
461. Simkin, P. A.: Hexose-induced hyperuricemia and uricosuria in cebus monkeys. Arthritis Rheum., **12,** 332, 1969.
462. Stirpe, F., Corte, E. D., Bonetti, E., Abbondanza, A., Abbati, A., and de Stefano, F.: Fructose-induced hyperuricaemia. Lancet, **2,** 1310, 1970.
463. Forster, H., Meyer, E., and Ziege, M.: Erhohung von serumharnsaure und serumbilirubin nach hochdosierten infusionen von sorbit, xylit und fructose. Klin. Wschr., **48,** 14, 1970.
464. Rosenbloom, F. M., Henderson, J. F., Caldwell, I. C., Kelley, W. N., and Seegmiller, J. E.: Biochemical bases of accelerated purine biosynthesis *de novo* in human fibroblasts lacking hypoxanthine-guanine phosphoribosyltransferase. J. Biol. Chem., **243,** 1166, 1968.
465. Fox, I. H., Wyngaarden, J. B., and Kelley, W. N.: Depletion of erythrocyte phosphoribosylpyrophosphate in man, a newly observed effect of allopurinol. New Eng. J. Med., **283,** 1177, 1970.
466. Kelley, W. N., Fox, I. H., and Wyngaarden, J. B.: Regulation of purine biosynthesis in cultured human cells. I. Effects of orotic acid. Biochim. Biophys. Acta, **215,** 512, 1970.
467. Frieden, C.: Glutamate dehydrogenase. V. The relation of enzyme structure to the catalytic function. J. Biol. Chem., **238,** 3286, 1963.
468. Speck, J. F.: The synthesis of glutamine in pigeon liver dispersions. J. Biol. Chem., **179,** 1387, 1949.
469. Sellinger, O. Z., and Verster, F. de B.: Glutamine synthetase of rat cerebral cortex: Intracellular distribution and structural latency. J. Biol. Chem., **237,** 2836, 1962.
470. Rector, F. C., Jr., and Orloff, J.: The effect of the administration of sodium bicarbonate and ammonium chloride on the excretion of ammonia: The absence of alterations in the activity of renal ammonia-producing enzymes in the dog. J. Clin. Invest., **38,** 366, 1959.
471. Krebs, H. A.: Metabolism of amino-acids. IV. The synthesis of glutamine from glutamic acid and ammonia, and the enzymic hydrolysis of glutamine in animal tissues. Biochem. J., **29,** 1951, 1935.
472. Kingdon, H. S., Shapiro, B. M., and Stadtman, E. R.: Regulation of glutamine synthetase. VIII. ATP: glutamine synthetase adenyltransferase, an enzyme that catalyzes alterations in the regulatory properties of glutamine synthetase. Proc. Nat. Acad. Sci. USA, **58,** 1703, 1967.
473. Shapiro, B. M., and Stadtman, E. R.: The regulation of glutamine synthesis in microorganisms. Ann. Rev. Microbiol., **24,** 501, 1970.
474. Ronzio, R., Rowe, W. B., and Meister, A.: Studies on the mechanism of inhibition of glutamine synthetase by methionine sulfoximine. Biochemistry (Wash.), **8,** 1066, 1969.
475. Rowe, W. B., Ronzio, R. A., and Meister, A.: Inhibition of glutamine synthetase by methionine sulfoximine: Studies on methionine sulfoximine phosphate. Biochemistry (Wash.), **8,** 2674, 1969.
476. Waelsch, H.: Glutamic acid and cerebral function. Advances Protein Chem., **6,** 299, 1951.
477. Owen, E. E., and Robinson, R. R.: Amino acid extraction and ammonia metabolism by the human kidney during the prolonged administration of ammonium chloride. J. Clin. Invest., **42,** 263, 1963.
478. Pitts, R. F.: Renal production and excretion of ammonia. Amer. J. Med., **36,** 720, 1964.
479. Errera, M.: Liver glutaminases. J. Biol. Chem., **187,** 483, 1949.
480. Errera, M., and Greenstein, J. P.: Phosphate-activated glutaminase in kidney and other tissues. J. Biol. Chem., **187,** 495, 1949.
481. Sayre, F. W., and Roberts, E.: Preparation and some properties of a phosphate-activated glutaminase from kidneys. J. Biol. Chem., **233,** 1128, 1958.
482. Klingman, J. D., and Handler, P.: Partial purification and properties of renal glutaminase. J. Biol. Chem., **232,** 369, 1958.
483. Meister, A.: *Biochemistry of the amino acids.* Academic, New York, 1957.
484. Bien, E. J., Yü, T.-F., Benedict, J. D., Gutman, A. B., and Stetten, D., Jr.: The relation of dietary nitrogen consumption to the rate of uric acid synthesis in normal and gouty man. J. Clin. Invest., **32,** 778, 1953.
485. Rowe, P. B., Coleman, M. D., and Wyngaarden, J. B.: Glutamine phosphoribosylpyrophosphate amidotransferase: Catalytic and conformational heterogeneity of the pigeon liver enzyme. Biochemistry (Wash.), **9,** 1498, 1970.
486. Nagy, M.: Regulation of the biosynthesis of purine nucleotides in *Schizosaccharomyces pombe.* I. Properties of the phosphoribosylpyrophosphate glutamine amidotransferase of the wild strain and of a mutant desensitized towards feedback modifiers. Biochim. Biophys. Acta, **198,** 471, 1970.
487. Henderson, J. F.: Feedback inhibition of purine biosynthesis in ascites tumor cells. J. Biol. Chem., **237,** 2631, 1962.
488. Henderson, J. F., and Khoo, Mary K. Y.: On the mechanism of feedback inhibition of purine biosynthesis *de novo* in Ehrlich ascites tumor cells in vitro. J. Biol. Chem., **240,** 3104, 1965.
489. McFall, E., and Magasanik, B.: The control of purine biosynthesis in cultured mammalian cells. J. Biol. Chem., **235,** 2103, 1960.
490. Wyngaarden, J. B.: Genetic control of enzyme activity in higher organisms. Biochem. Genet., **4,** 105, 1970.
491. Reem, G. H., and Friend, C.: Phosphoribosylamidotransferase: Regulation of activity in virus-induced murine leukemia by purine nucleotides. Science, **157,** 1203, 1967.
492. Reem, G. H., and Friend, C.: Characteristics of phosphoribosylamidotransferase in experimental leukemia. J. Clin. Invest., **47,** 83a, 1968.
493. Wyngaarden, J. B., and Greenland, R. A.: The inhibition of succinoadenylate kinosynthetase of *Escherichia coli* by adenosine and guanosine 5′-monophosphates. J. Biol. Chem., **238,** 1054, 1963.
494. Mager, J., and Magasanik, B.: Guanosine 5′-phosphate reductase and its role in the interconversion of purine nucleotides. J. Biol. Chem., **235,** 1474, 1960.
495. Stetten, D., Jr.: Current status of purine biosynthesis: An interim report. Ann. Rheum. Dis., **15,** 404, 1956.
496. Setlow, B., Burger, R., and Lowenstein, J. M.: Adenylate deaminase. I. The effects of adenosine and guanosine triphosphate on activity and the organ distribution of the regulated enzyme. J. Biol. Chem., **241,** 1244, 1966.
497. Biswas, B. B., and Abrams, R.: Formation of hypoxanthine from guanine in rat liver extracts. Arch. Biochem., **92,** 507, 1961.
498. Beck, W. S.: Regulation of cobamide-dependent ribonucleotide reductase by allosteric effectors and divalent cations. J. Biol. Chem., **242,** 3148, 1967.
499. Larsson, A., and Reichard P.: Enzymatic synthesis of deoxyribonucleotides. IX. Allosteric effects in the reduction of pyrimidine ribonucleotides by the ribonucleoside diphosphate reductase system of *Escherichia coli.* J. Biol. Chem., **241,** 2540, 1966.
500. Larsson, A., and Reichard, P.: Enzymatic synthesis of deoxyribonucleotides. X. Reduction of purine ribonucleotides: Allosteric behaviour and substrate specificity of the enzyme system from *Escherichia coli* B. J. Biol. Chem., **241,** 2540, 1966.
501. Moore, E. C., and Hurlbert, R. B.: Regulation of mammalian deoxyribonucleotide biosynthesis by nucleotides as activators and inhibitors. J. Biol. Chem., **241,** 4802, 1966.
502. Murphree, S., Moore, E. C., and Beall, P. T.: Regulation by nucleotides of the activity of partially purified ribonucleotide reductase from rat embryos. Cancer Res., **28,** 860, 1968.

503. Blakley, R. L., and Vitols, E.: Control of nucleotide biosynthesis. Ann. Rev. Biochem., **37**, 201, 1968.

504. Higgins, J. T., Ashton, D. M., Speas, M., and Wyngaarden, J. B.: An evaluation of relative roles of substrate diversion and feedback inhibition in the control of purine synthesis. Clin. Res., **9**, 181, 1961.

505. Kelley, W. N., and Wyngaarden, J. B.: Effects of allopurinol and oxipurinol on purine synthesis in cultured human cells. J. Clin. Invest., **49**, 602, 1970.

506. Levenberg, B., Melnick, I., and Buchanan, J. M.: Biosynthesis of the purines. IV. The effect of aza-L-serine and 6-diazo-5-oxo-L-norleucine on inosinic acid biosynthesis de novo. J. Biol. Chem., **225**, 163, 1957.

507. French, T. C., Dawid, I. B., Day, R. A., and Buchanan, J. M.: Azaserine-reactive sulfhydryl group of 2-formamido-N-ribosylacetamide 5′-phosphate: L-Glutamine amido-ligase (adenosine diphosphate). I. Purification and properties of the enzyme from *Salmonella typhimurium* and the synthesis of L-azaserine-C^{14}. J. Biol. Chem., **238**, 2171, 1963.

508. Dawid, I. B., French, T. C., and Buchanan, J. M.: Azaserine-reactive sulfhydryl group of 2-formamido-N-ribosylacetamide 5′-phosphate: L-Glutamine amido-ligase (adenosine diphosphate). II. Degradation of azaserine-C^{14}-labeled enzyme. J. Biol. Chem., **238**, 2178, 1963.

509. French, T. C., Dawid, I. B., and Buchanan, J. M.: Azaserine-reactive sulfhydryl groups of 2-formamido-N-ribosylacetamide 5′-phosphate: L-Glutamine amido-ligase (adenosine diphosphate). III. Comparison of degradation products with synthetic compounds. J. Biol. Chem., **238**, 2186, 1963.

510. Hartman, S. C.: The interaction of 6-diazo-5-oxo-L-norleucine with phosphoribosyl pyrophosphate amidotransferase. J. Biol. Chem., **238**, 3036, 1963.

511. Zuckerman, R., Drell, W., and Levin, M. H.: Urinary purines in gout: Effect of azaserine. Arthritis Rheum., **2**, 46, 1959.

512. Grayzel, A. I., and Seegmiller, J. E.: Suppression of uric acid synthesis in the gouty human by the use of 6-diazo-5-oxo-L-norleucine (DON). J. Clin. Invest., **39**, 447, 1960.

513. Le Page, G. A., and Jones, M.: Purinethiols as feedback inhibitors of purine synthesis in ascites tumor cells. Cancer Res., **21**, 642, 1961.

514. Brockman, R. W.: Metabolism and mechanisms of action of purine analogues, in *Exploitable Molecular Mechanisms and Neoplasia,* pp. 435–464. Williams & Wilkins, Baltimore, 1969.

515. Gots J. S., and Gollub, E. G.: Purine analogs as feedback inhibitors. Proc. Soc. Exp. Biol. Med., **101**, 641, 1959.

516. Seegmiller, J. E., Laster, L., and Stetten, D., Jr.: Incorporation of 4-amino-5-imidazolecarboxamide-4-C^{13} into uric acid in the normal human. J. Biol. Chem., **216**, 653, 1955.

517. Seegmiller, J. E., Klinenberg, J. R., Miller, J., and Watts, R. W. E.: Suppression of glycine-N^{15} incorporation into urinary uric acid by adenine-8-C^{13} in normal and gouty subjects. J. Clin. Invest., **47**, 1193–1203, 1968.

518. Sorensen, L. B.: Mechanism of excessive purine biosynthesis in hypoxanthine-guanine phosphoribosyltransferase deficiency. J. Clin. Invest., **49**, 968, 1970.

519. Sorensen, L. B.: Suppression of the shunt pathway in primary gout by azathioprine. Proc. Nat. Acad. Sci. USA, **55**, 571, 1966.

520. Kelley, W. N., Rosenbloom, F. M., and Seegmiller, J. E.: The effect of azathioprine (Imuran) on purine synthesis in clinical disorders of purine metabolism. J. Clin. Invest., **46**, 1518, 1967.

521. Nyhan, W. L., Sweetman, L., Carpenter, D. G., Carter, C. H., and Hoefnagel, D.: Effects of azathioprine in a disorder of uric acid metabolism and cerebral function. J. Pediat., **72**, 111, 1968.

522. Sorensen, L. B., Kawahara, F., Chow, D., Benke, P. J., and Coben, L.: Excessive purine synthesis and neurologic dysfunction in children. Arthritis Rheum., **13**, 835, 1970.

523. Goldthwait, D. A., Peabody, R. A., and Greenberg, G. R.: Glycine ribotide intermediates in the *de novo* synthesis of inosinic acid. J. Amer. Chem. Soc., **76**, 5258, 1954.

524. Krakoff, I. H., Balis, M. E., Magill, J. W., and Nary, D.: Studies of purine metabolism in neoplastic diseases. Med. Clin. N. Amer., **45**, 521, 1961.

525. Shigeura, H. T., and Gordon, C. N.: Hadacidin, a new inhibitor of purine biosynthesis. J. Biol. Chem., **237**, 1932, 1963.

526. Shigeura, H. T., and Gordon, C. N.: The mechanism of action of hadacidin. J. Biol. Chem., **237**, 1937, 1963.

527. Kalckar, H. M., Kjeldgaard, N. O., and Klenow, H.: Inhibition of xanthine oxidase and related enzymes by 6-pteridyl aldehyde. J. Biol. Chem., **174**, 771, 1948.

528. Wyngaarden, J. B.: 2,6-Diaminopurine as substrate and inhibitor of xanthine oxidase. J. Biol. Chem., **224**, 453, 1957.

529. Bergmann, F., and Ungar, H.: The enzymatic oxidation of 6-mercaptopurine to 6-thiouric acid. J. Amer. Chem. Soc., **82**, 3957, 1960.

530. Silberman, H. R., and Wyngaarden, J. B.: 6-Mercaptopurine as substrate and inhibitor of xanthine oxidase. Biochim. Biophys. Acta, **47**, 178, 1961.

531. Duggan, D. E., and Titus, E.: 6-Chloropurine and 6-chlorouric acid as substrates and inhibitors of purine-oxidizing enzymes. J. Biol. Chem., **234**, 2100, 1959.

532. Iwata, H., Yamamoto, I., and Muraki, K.: Potent xanthine oxidase inhibitors-4(or 5)-diazo-imidazole-5(or 4)-carboxamide and two related compounds. Biochem. Pharmacol., **15**, 955, 1969.

533. Fridovich, I.: A new class of xanthine oxidase inhibitors isolated from guanidinium salts. Biochemistry (Wash.), **4**, 1098, 1965.

534. Robins, R. K.: Potential purine antagonists. I. Synthesis of some 4,6-substituted pyrazolo 3,4-d pyrimidines. J. Amer. Chem. Soc., **78**, 784, 1956.

535. Feigelson, P., Davidson, J. D., and Robins, P. K.: Pyrazolopyrimidines as inhibitors and substrates of xanthine oxidase. J. Biol. Chem., **226**, 993, 1957.

536. Elion, G. B.: Enzymatic and metabolic studies with allopurinol. Ann. Rheum. Dis., **25**, 608, 1966.

536*a*. Massey, V., Komai, H., Palmer, G., and Elion, G.: On the mechanism of inactivation of xanthine oxidase by allopurinol and other pyrazolo (3,4-d) pyrimidines. J. Biol. Chem., **245**, 2837, 1970.

537. Rundles, R. W., Wyngaarden, J. B., Hitchings, G. H., and Elion, G. B.: Drugs and uric acid. Ann. Rev. Pharmacol., **9**, 345, 1969.

538. Rundles, R. W., Wyngaarden, J. B., Hitchings, G. H. Elion, G. B., and Silberman, H. R.: Effects of a xanthine oxidase inhibitor on thiopurine metabolism, hyperuricemia and gout. Trans. Ass. Amer. Physicians, **76**, 126, 1963.

539. Yü, T.-F., and Gutman, A. B.: Effects of allopurinol [4-hydroxypyrazolo (3,4-d) pyrimidine] on serum and urinary uric acid in primary and secondary gout. Amer. J. Med., **37**, 885, 1964.

540. Elion, G. B., Kovensky, A., Hitchings, G. H., Metz, E., and Rundles, R. W.: Metabolic studies of allopurinol, an inhibitor of xanthine oxidase. Biochem. Pharmacol., **15**, 863, 1966.

541. Krenitsky, T. A., Elion, G. B., Strelitz, R. A., and Hitchings, G. H.: Ribonucleosides of allopurinol and oxoallopurinol. J. Biol. Chem., **242**, 2675, 1967.

542. Elion, G. B., Yü, T.-F., Gutman, A. B., and Hitchings, G. H.: Renal clearance of oxipurinol, the chief metabolite of allopurinol. Amer. J. Med., **45**, 69, 1968.

543. Chalmers, R. A., Kromer, H., Scott, J. T., and Watts, R. W. E.: A comparative study of the xanthine oxidase inhibitors, allopurinol and oxipurinol in man. Clin. Sci., **35**, 353, 1968.

544. Chytil, F.: Activation of liver tryptophan oxygenase by adenosine 3′,5′-phosphate and by other purine derivatives. J. Biol. Chem., **243**, 893, 1968.

545. Julian, J., and Chytil, F.: Participation of xanthine oxidase in the activation of liver tryptophan pyrrolase. J. Biol. Chem., **245**, 1161, 1970.

546. Ghosh, D., and Forrest, H. S.: Inhibition of tryptophan pyrrolase by some naturally occurring pteridines. Arch. Biochem., **120**, 578, 1967.

547. Gallo, R. D., Perry, S., and Breitman, T. R.: Inhibition of human leukocyte pyrimidine deoxynucleoside synthesis by allopurinol and 6-mercaptopurine. Biochem. Pharmacol., **17**, 2185, 1968.

548. Truseve, R., and Williams, V.: The effect of allopurinol on urate oxidase activity. Biochem. Pharmacol., **17**, 165, 1968.

549. Fox, R. M., Royse-Smith D., and O'Sullivan, W. J.: Orotidinuria induced by allopurinol. Science, **168**, 861, 1970.

550. Kelley, W. N., and Beardmore, T. D.: Allopurinol: alteration in pyrimidine metabolism in man. Science, **169**, 388, 1970.

551. Kelley, W. N., and Wyngaarden, J. B.: The effect of dietary purine

restriction, allopurinol and oxipurinol on the urinary excretion of ultraviolet absorbing compounds. Clin. Chem., **16,** 707, 1970.

552. Beardmore, T. D., Fox, I. H., and Kelley, W. N.: Effect of allopurinol on pyrimidine metabolism in the Lesch-Nyhan syndrome. Lancet, **2,** 830, 1970.

552*a*. Beardmore, T. D., and Kelley, W. N.: Increase of 2 essential enzymes in pyrimidine biosynthesis resulting from allopurinol therapy. Clin. Res. **19,** 27, 1971.

553. Delbarre, F., Auscher, C., DeGery, A., Brouilhet, H., and Olivier, J. L.: Le traitement de la dyspurinie goutteuse par la mercaptopyrazolopyrimidine (MPP: Thiopurinol). Presse Med., **76,** 2329, 1968.

554. Krakoff, I. H., and Magill, G. B.: Effects of 2-ethylamino-1,3,4 thiadiazole HC1 on uric acid production in man. Proc. Soc. Exp. Biol. Med., **91,** 470, 1956.

555. Krakoff, I. H., and Balis, M. E.: Studies on the uricogenic effect of 2-substituted thiadiazoles in man. J. Clin. Invest., **38,** 907, 1959.

556. Seegmiller, J. E., Grayzel, A. I., and Liddle, L.: Excessive uric acid production in the human induced by 2-ethylamino-1,3,4-thiadiazole. Nature (London), **183,** 1463, 1959.

557. Shuster, L., and Goldin, A.: Some biochemical effects of 2-ethylamino-1-3,4-thiadiazole. Biochem. Pharmacol., **2,** 17, 1959.

558. Seegmiller, J. E., Grayzel, A. I., Liddle, L., and Wyngaarden, J. B.: The effect of 2-ethylamino-1,3,4-thiadiazole on the incorporation of glycine into urinary purines and uric acid in man. Metabolism, **12,** 507, 1963.

559. Nyhan, W. L., Sweetman, L., and Lesch, M.: Effects of the uricogenic agent, 2-ethylamino-1,3,4-thiadiazole in hypoxanthine-guanine phosphoribosyl transferase deficiency. Metabolism, **17,** 846, 1968.

560. Bauman, N., and Wyngaarden, J. B.: Regulation of purine biosynthesis in the mouse. Fed. Proc., **23,** 324, 1964.

561. Benedict, J. D., Forsham, P. H., and Stetten, DeW., Jr.: The metabolism of uric acid in the normal and gouty human studied with the aid of isotopic uric acid. J. Biol. Chem., **181,** 183, 1949.

562. Benedict, J. D., Forsham, P. H., Roche, M., Soloway, S., and Stetten, DeW., Jr.: The effect of salicylates and adrenocorticotropic hormone upon the miscible pool of uric acid in gout. J. Clin. Invest., **29,** 1104, 1950.

563. Geren, W., Bendich, A., Bodansky, O., and Brown, G. B.: Fate of uric acid in man. J. Biol. Chem., **183,** 21, 1950.

564. Bishop, C., Garner, W., and Talbott, J. H.: Pool size, turnover rate, and rapidity of equilibration of injected isotopic uric acid in normal and pathological subjects. J. Clin. Invest., **30,** 879, 1951.

565. Buzard, J., Bishop, C., and Talbott, J. H.: Recovery in humans of intravenously injected isotopic uric acid. J. Biol. Chem., **196,** 179, 1952.

566. Scott, J. T., Holloway, V. P., Glass, H. I., and Arnot, R. N.: Studies of uric acid pool size and turnover rate. Ann. Rheum. Dis., **28,** 366, 1969.

567. Wyngaarden, J. B.: The effect of phenylbutazone on uric acid metabolism in two normal subjects. J. Clin. Invest., **34,** 256, 1955.

568. Benedict, J. D., Roche, M., Yü, T.-F., Bien, E. J., Gutman, A. B., and Stetten, DeW., Jr.: Incorporation of glycine nitrogen into uric acid in normal and gouty man. Metabolism, **1,** 3, 1952.

569. Benedict, J. D., Yü, T.-F., Bien, E. J., Gutman, A. B., and Stetten, DeW., Jr.: A further study of the utilization of dietary glycine nitrogen for uric acid synthesis in gout. J. Clin. Invest., **32,** 775, 1953.

570. Gutman, A. B., Yü, T.-F., Black, H., Yalow, R. S., and Berson, S. A.: Incorporation of glycine 1-C^{14}, glycine 2-C^{14} and glycine-N^{15} into uric acid in normal and gouty subjects. Amer. J. Med., **25,** 917, 1958.

571. Bishop, C., Rand, R., and Talbott, J. H.: Rate of conversion of isotopic glycine to uric acid in the normal and gouty humans and how this is affected by vitamin E and folic acid. Metabolism, **4,** 174, 1955.

572. Watts, R. W. E., and Crawhall, J. C.: The first glycine metabolic pool in man. Biochem. J., **73,** 277, 1959.

572*a*. Wyngaarden, J. B.: Gout, in *Metabolic Basis of Inherited Disease,* edited by J. B. Stanbury, J. B. Wyngaarden, and D. S. Fredrickson, 2d ed. McGraw-Hill, New York, 1966.

572*b*. Muller, A. F., and Bauer, W.: Uric acid production in normal and gouty subjects, determined by N^{15} labeled glycine. Proc. Soc. Exp. Biol. Med., **82,** 47, 1953.

572*c*. Wyngaarden, J. B.: Normal glycine-C^{14} incorporation into uric acid in primary gout. Metabolism, **7,** 374, 1958.

573. Seegmiller, J. E., Laster, L., and Liddle, L. V.: Failure to detect consistent over-incorporation of glycine 1-C^{14} into uric acid in primary gout. Metabolism, **7,** 376, 1958.

574. Howell, R. R., Speas, M., and Wyngaarden, J. B.: A quantitative study of recycling of isotope from glycine-1-C^{14}, α-N^{15} into various subunits of the uric acid molecule in a normal subject. J. Clin. Invest., **40,** 2076, 1961.

575. Wyngaarden, J. B., and Jones, O. W.: The pathogenesis of gout. Med. Clin. N. Amer., **45,** 1241, 1961.

576. Gutman, A. B., Yü, T.-F., Adler, M., and Javitt, N. B.: Intramolecular distribution of uric acid-N^{15} after administration of glycine-N^{15} and ammonium N^{15} chloride to gouty and nongouty subjects. J. Clin. Invest., **41,** 623, 1962.

577. Lesch, M., and Nyhan, W. L.: A familial disorder of uric acid metabolism and central nervous function. Amer. J. Med., **36,** 561, 1964.

578. Alepa, F. P., Howell, R. R., Klinenberg, J. R., and Seegmiller, J. E.: Relationships between glycogen storage disease and tophaceous gout. Amer. J. Med., **42,** 58, 1967.

579. Kelley, W. N., Rosenbloom, F. M., Seegmiller, J. E., and Howell, R. R.: Excessive production of uric acid in type 1 glycogen storage disease. J. Pediat., **72,** 488, 1968.

580. Kogut, M. D., Donnell, G. N., Nyhan, W. L., and Sweetman, L.: Disorder of purine metabolism due to partial deficiency of hypoxanthine-guanine phosphoribosyltransferase: A study of a family. Amer. J. Med., **48,** 148, 1970.

581. Kelley, W. N., Green, M. L., Fox, I. H., Rosenbloom, F. M., Levy, R. L., and Seegmiller, J. E.: The effects of orotic acid on purine and lipoprotein metabolism in man. Metabolism, **19,** 1025, 1970.

582. Emmerson, B., and Wyngaarden, J. B.: Variant of the Lesch-Nyhan syndrome associated with partial deficiency of hypoxanthine-guanine phosphoribosyltransferase deficiency and gout. (In preparation.)

583. Spilman, E. L.: Uric acid synthesis in the nongouty and gouty human. Fed. Proc., **13,** 302, 1954.

584. Spilman, E. L.: Personal communication.

585. Buchanan, D. L., and Rollins, J. M.: Lack of correlation between gout and the incorporation of isotopic formate into uric acid. Yale J. Biol. Med., **34,** 31, 1961.

586. Seegmiller, J. E., Laster, L., and Stetten, D., Jr.: Uric acid formation in patients with gout: The incorporation of 4-amino-5-imidazolecarboxamide-C^{13} into uric acid. *Ninth Int. Congr. Rheum. Dis.,* Toronto, Canada, June 23–28, 1957, vol. 2, p. 207.

587. Wyngaarden, J. B., Blair, A. E., and Hilley, L.: On the mechanism of overproduction of uric acid in patients with primary gout. J. Clin. Invest., **37,** 579, 1958.

588. Wyngaarden, J. B., Seegmiller, J. E., Laster, I., and Blair, A. E.: The utilization of hypoxanthine, adenine and 4-amino-5-imidazolecarboxamide for uric acid synthesis in man. Metabolism, **8,** 455, 1959.

589. Wyngaarden, J. B.: Intermediary purine metabolism and the metabolic defects of gout. Metabolism, **6,** 244, 1957.

590. Adler, M., and Gutman, A. B.: Uridine isomers (5-ribosyluracil) in human urine. Science, **130,** 862, 1962.

591. Weissman, S., Eisen, A. Z., and Karen, M.: Pseudouridine metabolism. II. Urinary excretion in gout, psoriasis, leukemia, heterozygous orotic aciduria. J. Lab. Clin. Med., **59,** 852, 1962.

592. Wyngaarden, J. B.: Pathophysiology of hyperuricemia in primary gout. Trans. Amer. Clin. Climat. Ass., **81,** 161, 1969.

593. Kaplan, D., Bernstein, D., Wallace, S. L., and Halberstam, D.: Serum and urinary amino acids in normouricemic and hyperuricemic subjects. Ann. Intern. Med., **62,** 658, 1965.

594. Yü, T.-F., Adler, M., Bobrow, E., and Gutman, A. B.: Plasma and urinary amino acids in primary gout, with special reference to glutamine. J. Clin. Invest., **48,** 885, 1969.

595. Pagliara, A. S., and Goodman, A. D.: Elevation of plasma glutamate in gout, its possible role in the pathogenesis of hyperuricemia. New Eng. J. Med., **281,** 767, 1969.

596. Swendseid, M. E., Tuttle, S. G., Figueroa, W. S., Mulcare, D., Clark, A. J., and Massey, F. J.: Plasma amino acid levels in men fed diets

differing in protein content. Some observations with valine deficient diets. J. Nutr., **88,** 239, 1966.

597. Kaplan, D., Diamond, H., Wallace, S. L., and Halberstam, D.: Amino acid excretion in primary hyperuricaemia. Ann. Rheum. Dis., **28,** 180, 1969.
598. Henderson, L. J., and Palmer, W. W.: On the several factors of acid excretion in nephritis. J. Biol. Chem., **21,** 37, 1915.
599. Hilton, J. G., Goodbody, M. F., Jr., and Kruesi, O. R.: The effect of prolonged administration of ammonium chloride on the blood acid-base equilibrium of geriatric subjects. J. Amer. Geriat. Soc., **3,** 697, 1955.
600. Pollak, V. E., and Mattenheimer, H.: Glutaminase activity in the kidney in gout. J. Lab. Clin. Med., **66,** 564, 1965.
601. Sperling, O., and Wyngaarden, J. B.: The effect of kinetic acceleration of purine biosynthesis on incorporation of glutamine amide-N into uric acid in man. (In preparation.)
602. Henderson, J. F., Rosenbloom, F. M., Kelley, W. N., and Seegmiller, J. E.: Variations in purine metabolism of cultured skin fibroblasts from patients with gout. J. Clin. Invest., **47,** 1511, 1968.
603. Wu, H., and Bishop, C. W.: Pattern of N^{15}-excretion in man following administration of N^{15}-labeled glycine. J. Appl. Physiol., **14,** 1, 1959.
604. Pinsky, L., and Krooth, R. S.: Studies on the control of pyrimidine biosynthesis in human diploid cell strains. I. Effect of 6-azauridine on cellular phenotype. Proc. Nat. Acad. Sci. USA, **57,** 925, 1967.
605. Smith, L. H., Jr., Sullivan, M., and Huguley, C. M., Jr.: Pyrimidine metabolism in man. IV. The enzymatic defect of orotic aciduria. J. Clin. Invest., **40,** 656, 1961.
606. Hershko, A., Hershko, C., and Mager, J.: Increased formation of 5-phosphoribosyl-1-pyrophosphate in red blood cells of some gouty patients. Israel Med. J., **4,** 939, 1968.
607. Long, W. K.: Glutathione reductase in red blood cells: Variant associated with gout. Science, **155,** 712, 1967.
608. Long, W. K.: Red blood cell glutathione reductase in gout. Science, **138,** 991, 1962.
609. Howell, R. R., Ashton, D. M., and Wyngaarden, J. B.: Glucose-6-phosphatase deficiency glycogen storage disease: Studies on the interrelationships of carbohydrate, lipid, and purine abnormalities. Pediatrics, **29,** 553, 1962.
610. Jones, O. W., Jr., Ashton, D. M., and Wyngaarden, J. B.: Accelerated turnover of phosphoribosylpyrophosphate, a purine nucleotide precursor, in certain gouty subjects. J. Clin. Invest., **41,** 1805, 1962.
611. Hiatt, H. H.: Studies of ribose metabolism. II. A method for the study of ribose synthesis in vivo. J. Biol. Chem., **229,** 725, 1957.
612. Crowley, G. M.: The enzymatic synthesis of 5′-phosphoribosylimidazoleacetic acid. J. Biol. Chem., **239,** 2593, 1964.
613. Caldwell, I. C., Henderson, J. F., and Paterson, A. R. P.: The enzymic formation of 6-(methylmercapto) purine ribonucleoside 5′-phosphate. Canad. J. Biochem., **44,** 229, 1966.
614. Allan, P. W., Schnebli, H. P., and Bennett, L. L., Jr.: Conversion of 6-mercaptopurine and 6-mercaptopurine ribonucleoside to 6-methylmercaptopurine ribonucleotide in human epidermoid carcinoma No. 2 cells in culture. Biochim. Biophys. Acta., **114,** 647, 1966.
615. Henderson, J. F., Caldwell, I. C., and Paterson, A. R. P.: Decreased feedback inhibition in a 6-methylmercaptopurine ribonucleoside resistant tumor. Cancer Res., **27,** 1773, 1927.
616. Tschudy, D. P., Perlroth, M. G., Marver, H. S., Collins, A., Hunter, G., Jr., and Rechceigl, M., Jr.: Acute intermittent porphyria: The first "over-production disease" localized to a specific enzyme. Proc. Nat. Acad. Sci. USA, **53,** 841, 1965.
617. Carcassi, A., Marcolongo, R., Jr., Marinello, E., Riario-Sforza, G., and Boggiano, C.: Liver xanthine oxidase in gouty patients. Arthritis Rheum., **12,** 17, 1969.
618. Rowe, P. B., and Wyngaarden, J. B.: The mechanism of dietary alterations in rat hepatic xanthine oxidase levels. J. Biol. Chem., **241,** 5571, 1966.
619. Gutman, A. B., Yü, T.-F.: A three-component system for regulation of renal excretion of uric acid in man. Trans. Ass. Amer. Physicians, **74,** 353, 1961.
620. Steele, T. H., and Rieselbach, R. E.: The renal mechanism for urate homeostasis in normal man. Amer. J. Med., **43,** 868, 1967.
621. Steele, T. H.: Control of uric acid excretion. New Eng. J. Med., **284,** 1193, 1971.
622. Milne, M. D.: Urate excretion. Proc. Roy. Soc. Med., **59,** 308, 1966.
623. Poulsen, H., and Praetorius, E.: Tubular excretion of uric acid in rabbits. Acta Pharmacol. (Kobenhavn), **10,** 371, 1954.
624. Mudge, G. H., McAlary, B., and Berndt, W. O.: Renal transport of uric acid in the guinea pig. Amer. J. Physiol., **214,** 875, 1968.
625. Kessler, R. H., Hierholzer, K., and Gurd, R. S.: Localization of urate transport in the nephron of mongrel and dalmatian dog kidney. Amer. J. Physiol., **197,** 601, 1959.
626. Yü, T.-F. Berger, L., Kupfer, S., and Gutman, A. B.: Tubular secretion of urate in the dog. Amer. J. Physiol., **199,** 1199, 1960.
627. Lathem, W., Davis, B. B., and Rodnan, G. P.: Renal tubular secretion of uric acid in the mongrel dog. Amer. J. Physiol., **199,** 9, 1960.
628. Fanelli, G. M., Jr., Bohn, D., and Stafford, S.: Functional characteristics of renal urate transport in the *Cebus* monkey. Amer. J. Physiol., **218,** 627, 1970.
629. Praetorius, E., and Kirk, J. E.: Hypouricemia: With evidence for tubular elimination of uric acid. J. Lab. Clin. Med., **35,** 865, 1950.
630. Gutman, A. B., Yü, T.-F., and Berger, L.: Tubular secretion of urate in man. J. Clin. Invest., **38,** 1778, 1959.
631. Podevin, R., Ardaillou, R., Paillar, F., Fontanelle, J., and Richet, G.: Etude chez l'homme de la cinetique d'apparition dans l'urine de l'acide urique 2 ^{14}C. Nephron, **5,** 134, 1968.
632. Fanelli, G. M., Jr., Bohn, D. L., and Reilly, S. S.: Renal urate transport in the chimpanzee. Amer. J. Physiol., **220,** 613, 1971.
633. Mudge, G. H., Cucchi, J., Platts, M., O'Connell, J. M. B., and Berndt, W. O.: Renal excretion of uric acid in the dog. Amer. J. Physiol., **215,** 404, 1968.
634. Zins, G. R., and I. M. Weiner.: Bidirectional urate transport limited to the proximal tubule in dogs. Amer. J. Physiol., **215,** 411, 1968.
635. Davis, B. B., Field, J. B., Rodnan, G. P., and Kedes, L. H.: Localization and pyrazinamide inhibition of distal transtubular movement of uric acid-2-^{14}C with a modified stop-flow technique. J. Clin. Invest., **44,** 716, 1965.
636. Yü, T.-F., and Gutman, A. B.: Study of the paradoxical effects of salicylate in low, intermediate and high dosage on the renal mechanisms for excretion of urate in man. J. Clin. Invest., **38,** 1293, 1959.
637. Yü, T.-F., and Gutman, A. B.: Paradoxical retention of uric acid by uricosuric drugs in low dosage. Proc. Soc. Exp. Biol. Med., **90,** 542, 1955.
638. Burns, J. J., Yü, T.-F., Ritterband, A., Perel, J. M., Gutman, A. B., and Brodie, B. B.: A potent new uricosuric agent, the sulfoxide metabolite of the phenylbutazone analogue, G-25671. J. Pharmacol. Exp. Ther., **119,** 418, 1957.
639. Sirota, J. H., Yü, T.-F., and Gutman, A. B.: Effect of Benemid [*p*-(di-*n*-propylsulfamyl)-benzoic acid] on urate clearance and other discrete renal functions in gouty subjects. J. Clin. Invest., **31,** 692, 1952.
640. Marson, F. G. W.: Studies in gout, with particular reference to the value of sodium salicylate in treatment. Quart. J. Med., **22,** 331, 1953.
641. Gutman, A., Yü, T.-F., and Berger, L.: Renal function in gout. III. Estimation of tubular secretion and reabsorption of uric acid by use of pyrazinamide (pyrazinoic acid). Amer. J. Med., **45,** 575, 1969.
642. Yü, T.-F., Berger, L., Stone, D. J., Wolf, J., and Gutman, A. B.: Effects of pyrazinamide and pyrazinoic acid on urate clearance and other discrete renal functions. Proc. Soc. Exp. Biol. Med., **96,** 542, 1955.
643. Cullen, J. H., LeVine, M., and Fiore, J. M.: Studies of hyperuricemia produced by pyrazinamide. Amer. J. Med., **23,** 587, 1957.
644. Yü, T.-F., Berger, L., and Gutman, A. B.: Suppression of tubular secretion of urate by pyrazinamide in the dog. Proc. Soc. Exp. Biol. Med., **107,** 905, 1961.
645. Lathem, W., and Rodnan, G. P.: Impairment of uric acid excretion in gout. J. Clin. Invest., **41,** 1955, 1962.
646. Nugent, C. A., MacDiarmid, W. D., and Tyler, F. H.: Renal excretion of uric acid in leukemia and gout. Arch. Intern. Med. (Chicago), **109,** 54, 1962.
647. Wyngaarden, J. B.: Gout. Advances Metab. Dis., **2,** 2, 1965.
648. Steele, T. H., and Rieselback, R. E.: The contribution of residual

nephrons within the chronically diseased kidney to urate homeostasis in man. Amer. J. Med., **43**, 876, 1967.
649. Mugler, A., Pernet, A., and Friedrich, S.: Le pouvoir d'epuration du rein pour l'acide urique chez l'hyperuricemique d'apres l'etude de 400 clearances, in *Contemporary Rheumatology,* edited by J. Goslings and H. Van Swaay, p. 574. Elsevier, Amsterdam, 1956.
650. Sala, G., Ballabio, C. B., Amira, A., Ratti, G., and Cirla, E.: Renal mechanism for urate excretion in normal and gouty subjects, in *Contemporary Rheumatology,* edited by J. Goslings and H. Van Swaay, p. 581. Elsevier, Amsterdam, 1956.
651. Houpt, J. B., and Ogryzlo, M. A.: Persistence of impaired uric acid excretion in gout during reduced synthesis with allopurinol. Arthritis Rheum., **7**, 316, 1964.
652. Nugent, C. A., MacDiarmid, W. D., and Tyler, F. H.: Renal excretion of urate in patients with gout. Arch. Intern. Med. (Chicago), **113**, 165, 1964.
653. Rieselbach, R. E., Bentzel, C. J., Cotlove, E., Frei, E., III, and Freireich, E. J.: Uric acid excretion and renal function in the acute hyperuricemia of leukemia: Pathogenesis and therapy of uric acid nephropathy. Amer. J. Med., **37**, 872, 1964.
654. Sorensen, L. B.: Current concepts of gout and its treatment. Med. Clin. N. Amer., **47**, 169, 1963.
655. Sorensen, L. B.: Hyperuricemia and gout. Advances Intern. Med., **15**, 177, 1969.
656. Wyngaarden, J. B.: On the dual etiology of hyperuricemia in primary gout. Arthritis Rheum., **3**, 414, 1960.
657. Lassen, U. K.: Kinetics of uric acid transport in human erythrocytes. Biochim. Biophys. Acta, **53**, 557, 1961.
658. Weissmann, B., Bromberg, P. A., and Gutman, A. B.: The purine bases of human urine. I. Separation and identification. J. Biol. Chem., **224**, 407, 1957.
659. Yü, T.-F., Sirota, J. H., and Gutman, A. B.: Effect of phenylbutazone (3,5-dioxo-1,2-diphenyl-4-N-butylpyrazolidine) on renal clearance of urate and other discrete renal functions in gouty subjects. J. Clin. Invest., **32**, 1121, 1953.
660. Von Rechenberg, H. K.: *Phenylbutazone,* p. 48. Arnold, London, 1962.
661. Burns, J. J., Yü, T.-F., Berger, L., and Gutman, A. B.: Zoxazolamine: Physiological disposition, uricosuric properties. Amer. J. Med., **25**, 401, 1958.
662. Hansen, O. E., and Holten, C.: Uricosuric effect of dicumarol. Lancet, **1**, 1047, 1958.
663. Sougin-Mibashin, R., and Horwitz, M.: The uricosuric action of ethyl bis-coumacetate (Tromexan). Lancet, **1**, 1191, 1955.
664. Yü, T.-F., Berger, L., and Gutman, A. B.: Hypoglycemic and uricosuric properties of acetohexamide and hydroxyhexamide. Metabolism, **17**, 309, 1968.
665. Yü, T.-F., Kaung, C., and Gutman, A. B.: Effect of glycine loading on plasma and urinary uric acid and amino acids in normal and gouty subjects. Amer. J. Med., **49**, 352, 1970.
666. Fallon, H. J., Frei, E., III, Block, J., and Seegmiller, J. E.: The uricosuria and orotic aciduria induced by 6-azauridine. J. Clin. Invest., **40**, 1906, 1961.
667. Kelley, W. N., Greene, M. L., Fox, I. H., Rosenbloom, F. M., Levy, R. I., and Seegmiller, J. E.: Effects of orotic acid on purine and lipoprotein metabolism in man. Metabolism, **19**, 1025, 1970.
668. Ryckewaert, A., Kuntz, D., Henrard, J.-C., Puel, M., et de Seze, S.: Basic treatment of gout using Benziodarone. Presse Med., **77**, 1157, 1969.
669. Delbarre, F., Auscher, C., Olivier, J. L., and Rose, A.: Traitement des hyperuricémies et de la goutte par des dérivés du benzofuranne. Sem. Hop. Paris, **43**, 1127, 1967.
670. Zollner, N., Stern, G., Gröbner, W., and Dofel, W.: Lowering of uric acid level by action of benzbromarone. Klin. Wschr., **46**, 1318, 1968.
671. Healey, L. A., Harrison, M., and Decker, J. L.: Uricosuric effect of chlorprothixene. New Eng. J. Med., **272**, 526, 1956.
672. Postlethwaite, A. E., and Kelley, W. N.: Uricosuric effect of some commonly used radiocontrast agents in man. Ann. Intern. Med. In press.
673. Bishop, C., Rand, R., and Talbott, J. H.: The effect of Benemid [*p*-(di-*n*-propylsulfamyl)-benzoic acid] on uric acid metabolism in one normal and one gouty subject. J. Clin. Invest., **30**, 889, 1951.
674. Forsham, P. H., Thorn, G. W., Prunty, F. T. G., and Hills, A. G.: Clinical studies with pituitary adrenocorticotropin. J. Clin. Endocr., **8**, 15, 1948.
675. Fajans, S. S., Conn., J. W., Johnson, D., and Christman, A. A.: ACTH-induced changes in purine and carbohydrate metabolism in Dalmatian and mongrel dogs. Endocrinology, **49**, 225, 1951.
676. Yü, T.-F., Dayton, P. G., and Gutman, A. B.: Mutual suppression of the uricosuric effects of sulfinpyrazone and salicylate: A study in interactions between drugs. J. Clin. Invest., **42**, 1330, 1963.
677. Handler, J. S.: Role of lactic acid in reduced excretion of uric acid in toxemia of pregnancy. J. Clin. Invest., **39**, 1526, 1960.
678. Quick, A. J.: The effect of exercise on the excretion of uric acid, with a note on the influence of benzoic acid on uric acid elimination in liver diseases. J. Biol. Chem., **110**, 107, 1935.
679. Healey, A. A.: The effect of fasting and ketosis on uric acid excretion. Arthritis Rheum., **7**, 313, 1964.
680. Lennox, W. G.: A study of the retention of uric acid during fasting. J. Biol. Chem., **66**, 521, 1925.
681. Padova, J., and Bendersky, G.: Hyperuricemia in diabetic ketoacidosis. New Eng. J. Med., **267**, 530, 1962.
682. Shapiro, J. R., Klinenberg, J. R., Peck, W., Goldfinger, S. E., and Seegmiller, J. E.: Hyperuricemia associated with obesity and intensified by caloric restriction. Arthritis Rheum., **7**, 343, 1964.
683. Koehler, A. E.: Uric acid excretion. J. Biol. Chem., **60**, 621, 1924.
684. Skupp, S., and Ayvazian, J. H.: Oxidation of 7-methylguanine by human xanthine oxidase. J. Lab. Clin. Med., **73**, 909, 1969.
685. Buzard, J., Bishop, C., and Talbott, J., II: The fate of uric acid in the normal and gouty human. J. Chronic Dis., **2**, 42, 1955.
686. Lucke, H.: Das Harnsaureproblem und seine klinische Bedeutung. Ergebn. Inn. Med. Kinderheilk., **44**, 499, 1932.
687. Kurti, L.: Untersuchungen uber den Harnsaurestoffwechsel bei Nierenkranken. Z. Klin. Med., **122**, 585, 1932.
688. Canellakis, E. S., Tuttle, A. L., and Cohen, P. P.: A comparative study of the end products of uric acid oxidation by peroxidases. J. Biol. Chem., **213**, 397, 1955.
689. Griffiths, M.: Oxidation of uric acid catalyzed by copper and by the cytochrome-cytochrome oxidase system. J. Biol. Chem., **197**, 399, 1952.
690. Bien, E. J., and Zucker, H.: Uricolysis in normal and gouty individuals. Ann. Rheum. Dis., **14**, 409, 1955.
691. Ratti, G.: Sull esistenza di una attivita, uricolitica nell'uomo. Reumatiso, **10**, suppl. **2**, 33, 1958.
692. Agner, K.: Crystalline myeloperoxidase. Acta Chem. Scand., **12**, 89, 1958.
693. Howell, R. R., and Seegmiller, J. E.: Uricolysis by human leukocytes. Nature (London), **196**, 482, 1962.
694. Howell, R. R., and Wyngaarden, J. B.: On the mechanism of peroxidation of uric acids by hemoproteins. J. Biol. Chem., **225**, 3544, 1960.
695. Pollycove, M., Tolbert, B. M., Lawrence, J. H., and Harman, D.: Uric acid metabolism: The oxidation of uric acid in normal subjects and patients with gout, polycythemia and leukemia. Clin. Res. Proc., **5**, 38, 1957.
696. Jeune, M., Charrat, A., and Bertrand, J.: Polycorie hepatique, hyperuricemic et goutte. Arch. Franc. Pediat., **14**, 897, 1957.
697. Howell, R. R.: The interrelationship of glycogen storage disease and gout. Arthritis Rheum., **8**, 780, 1965.
698. Holling, H. E.: Gout and glycogen storage disease. Ann. Intern. Med., **58**, 654, 1963.
699. Fine, R. N., Strauss, J., and Donnell, G. N.: Hyperuricemia in glycogen storage disease Type I. Amer. J. Dis. Child., **112**, 572, 1966.
700. Von Hogningen-Huene, C. B. G.: Gout and glycogen storage disease in preadolescent brothers. Arch. Intern. Med. (Chicago), **118**, 471, 1966.
701. Kelley, W. N., Rosenbloom, F. M., Seegmiller, J. E., and Howell, R. R.: Excessive production of uric acid in Type I glycogen storage disease. J. Pediat., **72**, 488, 1968.
702. Seegmiller, J. E.: Diseases of purine and pyrimidine metabolism, in *Duncan's Diseases of Metabolism,* edited by P. K. Bondy, p. 516. Saunders, Philadephia, 1969.
703. Smythe, C. M., and Cutchin, J. H.: Primary juvenile gout. Amer. J. Med., **32**, 799, 1962.
704. Jeandet, J., and Lestradet, H.: L'hyperlactacidemie cause probable de

l'hyperuricemie dans la glycogenose hepatique. Rev. Franc. Etud. Clin. Biol., **6,** 71, 1961.

705. Alepa, F. P., Howell, R. R., and Seegmiller, J. E.: The occurrence of glycogen storage disease with tophaceous gout. Arthritis Rheum., **5,** 634, 1962.
706. Kaufman, J. M., Greene, M. L., and Seegmiller, J. E.: Urine uric acid to creatinine ratio: A screening test for inherited disorders of purine metabolism. J. Pediat., **73,** 583, 1968.
707. Jakovcic, S., and Sorensen, L. B.: Studies of uric acid metabolism in glycogen storage disease associated with gouty arthritis. Arthritis Rheum., **10,** 129, 1967.
708. Briggs, J. M., and Haworth, J. C.: Liver glycogen disease. (Report of a case of hyperuricemia, renal calculi and no demonstrable enzyme defect.) Amer. J. Med., **36,** 443, 1964.
709. Seegmiller, J. E., Rosenbloom, F. M., and Kelley, W. N.: An enzyme defect associated with a sex-linked human neurological disorder and excessive purine synthesis. Science, **155,** 1682, 1967.
710. Kelley, W. N., Rosenbloom, F. M., Henderson, J. F., and Seegmiller, J. E.: A specific enzyme defect in gout associated with overproduction of uric acid. Proc. Nat. Acad. Sci. USA, **57,** 1735, 1967.
711. Decker, J. L., and Vanderman, P. R.: Renal calculi preceding gouty arthritis in a child. Amer. J. Med., **32,** 805, 1962.
712. Rosenthal, I. M., Gaballah, S., and Rafelson, M. E., Jr.: Gout in infancy manifested by renal failure. Pediatrics, **33,** 251, 1964.
713. Sperling, O., Frank, M., Ophir, R., Liberman, U. A., Adam, A., and DeVries, A.: Partial deficiency of hypoxanthine-guanine phosphoribosyltransferase associated with gout and uric acid lithiasis. Rev. Europ. Etud. Clin. Biol., **15,** 942, 1970.
714. Emmerson, B. T., and Wyngaarden, J. B.: Purine metabolism in heterozygous carriers of hypoxanthine guanine phosphoribosyltransferase deficiency. Science, **166,** 1533, 1969.
715. Kelley, W. N., and Wyngaarden, J. B.: Studies on the purine phosphoribosyltransferase enzymes in fibroblasts from patients with the Lesch-Nyhan syndrome. Clin. Res., **18,** 394, 1970.
716. Green, M. L., Boyles, J. R., and Seegmiller, J. E.: Substrate stabilization: Genetically controlled reciprocal relationship of two human enzymes. Science, **167,** 887, 1970.
717. Kelley, W. N., Levy, R. I., Rosenbloom, R. M., Henderson, J. F., and Seegmiller, J. E.: Adenine phosphoribosyltransferase deficiency: A previously undescribed genetic defect in man. J. Clin. Invest., **47,** 2281, 1968.
718. Kelley, W. N., Fox, I. H., and Wyngaarden, J. B.: Further evaluation of adenine phosphoribosyltransferase deficiency in man: Occurrence in a patient with gout. Clin. Res., **18,** 53, 1970.
719. Henderson, J. F., Kelley, W. N., Rosenbloom, F. M., and Seegmiller, J. E.: Inheritance of purine phosphoribosyltransferases in man. Amer. J. Hum. Genet., **21,** 61, 1969.
720. Rosenbloom, F. M., Kelley, W. N., Henderson, J. F., and Seegmiller, J. E.: Lyon hypothesis and x-linked disease. Lancet, **2,** 305, 1967.
721. Migeon, B. R.: X-linked hypoxanthine-guanine phosphoribosyl transferase deficiency: Detection of heterozygotes by selective medium. Biochem. Genet., **4,** 377, 1970.
722. Felix, J. S., and DeMars, R.: Detection of female heterozygous for the Lesch-Nyhan mutation by 8-azaguanine resistant growth of cultured fibroblasts. J. Lab. Clin. Med., **77,** 596, 1971.
723. Migeon, B. R., Der Kaloustian, V. M., Nyhan, W. L., Young, W. J., and Childs, B.: X-linked HG-PRTase deficiency: Heterozygote has two clonal populations. Science, **160,** 425, 1968.
724. Kelley, W. N., and Meade, J. C.: Studies on hypoxanthine-guanine phosphoribosyltransferase in fibroblasts from patients with the Lesch-Nyhan syndrome: Evidence for genetic heterogeneity. J. Biol. Chem., **246,** 2953, 1971.
725. Cohen, H.: Gout, in *Textbook of the Rheumatic Diseases,* edited by W. S. C. Copeman, p. 361. Livingston, Edinburgh, 1955.
726. Neel, J. V.: The clinical detection of the genetic carriers of inherited disease. Medicine (Balt.), **26,** 115, 1947.
727. Rosenberg, E. F.: Gout and male hermaphroditism: Report of a case. Ann. Rheum. Dis., **2,** 273, 1941.
728. Talbott, J. H.: Gout. J. Chronic Dis., **1,** 338, 1955.
729. Talbott, J. H.: Serum urate in relatives of gouty patients. J. Clin. Invest., **27,** 749, 1940.
730. Wilson, D., Collins, D. H., and Marson, R. M.: Gout: Discussion, Proc. Roy. Soc. Med., **44,** 285, 1951.
731. Folin, O., and Lyman, H.: On the influence of phenylquinolin carbonic acid (Atophan) on uric acid elimination. J. Pharmacol., **4,** 539, 1913.
732. Stecher, R. M., Hersh, A. H., and Solomon, W. M.: The heredity of gout and its relationship to familial hyperuricemia. Ann. Intern. Med., **31,** 595, 1949.
733. Neel, J. V., Rakic, M. T., Davidson, R. I., Valkenburg, H. A., and Mikkelsen, W. M.: Studies on hyperuricemia. II. A reconsideration of the distribution of serum uric acid values in the families of Smyth, Cotterman, and Freyberg. Amer. J. Hum. Genet., **17,** 14, 1965.
734. French, J. G., Dodge, H. J., Kjelsberg, M. O., Mikkelsen, W. M., and Schull, W. J.: A study of familial aggregation of serum uric acid levels in the population of Tecumseh, Michigan. Amer. J. Epidem., **86,** 214, 1967.
735. Friedman, M., and Byers, S. O.: Observations concerning the causes of excess excretion of uric acid in the Dalmation dog. J. Biol. Chem., **175,** 127, 1948.
736. Harvey, A. H., and Christensen, H. N.: Uric acid transport system: Apparent absence in erythrocytes of the Dalmation coach hound. Science, **145,** 826, 1964.
737. Bishop, C., Zimdahl, W. T., and Talbott, J. H.: Uric acid in two patients with Wilson's disease (hepatolenticular degeneration). Proc. Soc. Exp. Biol. Med., **86,** 440, 1954.
738. Sorensen, L. B., Reilly, R., and Kappas, A.: Uric acid metabolism in Wilson's disease. Arthritis Rheum., **7,** 347, 1964.
739. Scott, J. T., and Pollard, A. C.: Uric acid excretion in relatives of patients with gout. Ann. Rheum. Dis., **29,** 397, 1970.
740. Lyon, M. F.: Gene action in the X-chromosome of the mouse. Nature (London), **190,** 372, 1961.
741. Fujimoto, W. Y., and Seegmiller, J. R.: Hypoxanthine-guanine phosphoribosyltransferase deficiency: Activity in normal, mutant and heterozygote-cultured human skin fibroblasts. Proc. Nat. Acad. Sci. USA, **65,** 577, 1970.
742. Cox, R. P., Krauss, M. R., Balis, M. E., and Dancis, J.: Evidence for transfer of enzyme product as the basis of metabolic cooperation between tissue culture fibroblasts of Lesch-Nyhan disease and normal cells. Proc. Nat. Acad. Sci. USA, **67,** 1573, 1970.
743. Szybalska, E. H., and Szybalski, W.: Genetics of human cell lines. IV. DNA-mediated heritable transformation of a biochemical trait. Proc. Nat. Acad. Sci. USA, **48,** 2026, 1962.
744. Meloni, C. R., and Canary, J. J.: Cystinuria with hyperuricemia. JAMA, **200,** 257, 1967.
745. Stanton, King J., and Wainer, A.: Cystinuria with hyperuricemia and methioninuria. Amer. J. Med., **43,** 125, 1967.
746. Schulman, J. D., Lustberg, T. J., and Seegmiller, J. E.: Hyperuricemia in branched chain ketoaciduria (maple syrup urine disease). Arthritis Rheum., **13,** 347, 1970.
747. Khachadurian, A. K.: Migratory polyarteritis in familial hypercholesterolemia (Type II hyperlipoproteinemia). Arthritis Rheum., **11,** 385, 1968.
748. Paulus, H. E., Coutts, A., Calabro, J. J., and Klinenberg, J. R.: Clinical significance of hyperuricemia in routinely screened hospitalized men. JAMA, **211,** 277, 1970.
749. Gutman, A. B.: Primary and secondary gout. Ann. Intern. Med., **39,** 1062, 1953.
750. Hickling, R. A.: Gout, leukemia, and polycythaemia. Lancet, **1,** 57, 1953.
751. Talbott, J. H.: Gout and blood dyscrasias. Medicine (Balt.), **38,** 173, 1959.
752. Yü, T.-F: Secondary gout associated with myeloproliferative diseases. Arthritis Rheum., **8,** 765, 1965.
753. Bronsky, D., and Bernstein, A.: Acute gout secondary to multiple myeloma, a case report. Ann. Intern. Med., **41,** 820, 1954.
754. Yü, T.-F., Wasserman, L. R., Benedict, J. D., Bien, E. J., Gutman, A. B., and Stetten, D., Jr.: A simultaneous study of glycine-N^{15} incorpo-

ration into uric acid and heme, and of Fe utilization in a case of gout associated with polycythemia secondary to congenital heart disease. Amer. J. Med., **15,** 845, 1953.

755. Sommerville, J.: Gout in cyanotic congenital heart disease. Brit. Heart J., **23,** 31, 1961.
756. Lynch, E. C.: Uric acid metabolism in proliferative diseases of the marrow. Arch. Intern. Med. (Chicago), **109,** 639, 1962.
757. Sandberg, A. A., Cartwright, G. E., and Wintrobe, M. D.: Studies on leukemia. I. Uric acid excretion. Blood, **11,** 154, 1956.
758. Yü, T.-F., Weissmann, B., Sharney, L., Kupfer, S., and Gutman, A. B.: On the biosynthesis of uric acid from glycine-N^{15} in primary and secondary polycythemia. Amer. J. Med., **21,** 901, 1956.
759. Adams, W. S., Skoog, W. A., and Davis, F. W.: An investigation of purine and pyrimidine excretion in normal and leukemic subjects utilizing ion exchange column and paper chromatographic techniques. J. Clin. Invest., **37,** 875, 1958.
760. Laster, L., and Muller, A. F.: Uric acid production in a case of myeloid metaplasia associated with gouty arthritis, studied with N^{15}-labeled glycine. Amer. J. Med., **15,** 857, 1953.
761. Cowdrey, S. C.: Hyperuricemia in infectious mononucleosis. JAMA, **196,** 319, 1966.
762. Gold, M. S., Williams, J. C., Spivack, M., and Guann, V.: Sickle cell anemia and hyperuricemia. JAMA, **206,** 1572, 1968.
763. Ball, G. V., and Sorensen, L. B.: The pathogenesis of hyperuricemia and gout in sickle cell anemia. Arthritis Rheum., **13,** 846, 1970.
764. River, G. L., Robbins, A. A., and Schwartz, S. O.: S-C hemoglobin: A clinical study. Blood, **18,** 385, 1961.
765. March, H. W., Schlyen, S. M., and Schwartz, S. E.: Mediterranean hemopathic syndromes (Cooley's anemia) in adults. Amer. J. Med., **13,** 46, 1952.
766. Paik, C. H., Alavi, I., Dunea, G., and Weiner, L.: Thalassemia and gouty arthritis. JAMA, **213,** 296, 1970.
767. Aronoff, A.,: Acute gouty arthritis precipitated by chlorothiazide. New Eng. J. Med., **262,** 767, 1960.
768. Naimark, A., and Fyles, T. W.: Gout as a complication of chlorothiazide therapy. Canad. Med. Ass. J., **83,** 819, 1960.
769. Paulus, H. E., Coutts, A., Calabro, J. J., and Klinenberg, J. R.: Clinical significance of hyperuricemia in routinely screened hospitalized men. JAMA, **211,** 277, 1970.
770. Demartini, F. E., Wheaton, E. A., Healey, L. A., and Laragh, J. H.: Effect of chlorothiazide on the renal excretion of uric acid. Amer. J. Med., **32,** 572, 1962.
771. Wyngaarden, J. B.: Diuretics and hyperuricemia. New Eng. J. Med., **283,** 1170, 1970.
772. Steele, T. H.: Evidence for altered renal urate reabsorption during changes in volume of the extracellular fluid. J. Lab. Clin. Med., **74,** 288, 1969.
773. Steele, T. H., and Oppenheimer, S.: Factors affecting urate excretion following diuretic administration in man. Amer. J. Med., **47,** 564, 1969.
774. Suki, W. N., Hull, A. R., Rector, F. C., Jr., and Seldin, D. W.: Mechanism of the effect of thiazide diuretics on calcium and uric acid. J. Clin. Invest., **46,** 1121, 1967.
775. Ayvazian, J. H., and Ayvazian, L. F.: A study of the hyperuricemia induced by hydrochlorothiazide and acetazolamide separately and in combination. J. Clin. Invest., **40,** 1961, 1961.
776. Bryant, J. M., Yü, T.-F., Berger, L., Schvartz, N., Torosdag, S., Fletcher, L., Jr., Fertig, H., Schwartz, M. S., and Quan, R. B. F.: Hyperuricemia induced by administration of chlorthalidone and other sulfonamide diuretics. Amer. J. Med., **33,** 408, 1962.
777. Rector, F. C., Jr., Sellman, J. C., Martinez-Maldonado, M., and Seldin, D. W.: The mechanism of suppression of proximal tubular reabsorption by saline infusions. J. Clin. Invest., **46,** 47, 1967.
778. Clapp, J. R., Nakajima, K., Nottebohm, G. A., and Robinson, R. R.: Volume-mediated regulation of furosemide. Clin. Res., **17,** 426, 1969.
779. Cannon, P. J., Svahn, D. S., and Demartini, F. E.: The influence of hypertonic saline infusions upon the fractional reabsorption of urate and other ions in normal and hypertensive man. Circulation, **41,** 97, 1970.
780. Schirmeister, J., Man, N. K., and Hallauer, W.: Study on renal and extrarenal factors involved in the hyperuricemia induced by furosemide, in *Progress in Nephrology,* edited by G. Peters and F. Roch-Ramel, p. 59. Springer-Verlag, Berlin-Heidelberg-New York, 1969.
781. Schultz, G., Gesaft, G., Losert, W., and Sitt, R.: Biochemische Grundlagen der Diazoxide Hyperglykamic. Naunyn Schmiedeberg. Arch. Pharm., **255,** 372, 1966.
782. Zweifler, A. J., and Thompson, G. R.: Correction of thiazide hyperuricemia by potassium chloride and ammonium chloride. Arthritis Rheum., **8,** 1134, 1965.
783. Beyer, K. H., and Baer, J. E.: Physiological basis for the action of newer diuretic agents. Pharmacol. Rev., **13,** 517, 1961.
784. Cannon, P. J., Stason, W. B., Demartini, F. E., Sommers, S. C., and Laragh, J. H.: Hyperuricemia in primary and renal hypertension. New Eng. J. Med., **275,** 457, 1966.
785. Breckenridge, A.: Hypertension and hyperuricemia. Lancet, **1,** 15, 1966.
786. Dollery, C. T., Duncan, H., and Schumer, B.: Hyperuricemia related to treatment of hypertension. Brit. Med. J., **2,** 832, 1960.
787. Kinsey, D.: Gout and hyperuricemia in hypertensive patients 15–35 years following lumbodorsal splanchnicectomy. Arthritis Rheum., **6,** 778, 1963.
788. Itskovitz, H. D., and Sellers, A. M.: Gout and hyperuricemia after adrenalectomy for hypertension. New Eng. J. Med., **268,** 1105, 1963.
789. Simon, N. M., Smucker, J. E., O'Conor, J., Jr., and Del Gueco, F.: Differential uric acid excretion in essential and renal hypertension. Circulation, **39,** 121, 1969.
790. Kohn, P. M., and Prozan, G. B.: Hyperuricemia: Relationship to hypercholesteremia and acute myocardial infarction. JAMA, **170,** 1909, 1959.
791. Schrade, W., Boehl, E., and Biegler, R.: Humoral changes in arteriosclerosis: Investigations on lipids, fatty acids, ketone bodies, pyruvic acid, lactic acid, and glucose in blood. Lancet, **2,** 1409, 1960.
792. Kasanen, A., Kallio, V., and Markkanen, T.: On serum uric acid and endogenic uric acid clearance in renal failure. Acta Med. Scand., **160,** 503, 1958.
793. McPhaul, J., Jr.: Hyperuricemia and urate excretion in chronic renal disease. Metabolism, **17,** 430, 1968.
794. Sarre, H.: Goutte secondaire a une insuffisance rénale. *Congres international de la goutte et de la lithiase urique,* Evian, Sept. 4–6, 1964, p. 245.
795. Richet, G., Ardaillon, R., De Montera, H., Slama, R., and Bougault, Th.: Etude de 31 cas de nephropathic associee a la goutte. J. Urol. Nephrol. (Paris), **67,** 1, 1961.
796. Buchanan, W. W., Klinenberg, J. R., and Seegmiller, J. E.: The inflammatory response to injected microcrystalline monosodium urate in normal, hyperuricemic, gouty, and uremic subjects. Arthritis Rheum., **8,** 361, 1965.
797. Ostberg, Y.: Renal urate deposits in chronic renal insufficiency. Acta Med. Scand., **183,** 197, 1968.
798. Ludwig, G. D.: Saturnine gout: A secondary type of gout. A.M.A. Arch. Intern. Med., **100,** 802, 1957.
799. Emmerson, B. T.: Chronic lead nephropathy: The diagnostic use of calcium EDTA and the association with gout. Aust. Ann. Med., **12,** 310, 1963.
800. Richet, G., Albahary, C., Ardaillou, R., Sultan, C., and Morel-Maroger, A.: Le rein du saturnisme chronique. Rev. Franc. Etud. Clin. Biol., **9,** 188, 1964.
801. Emmerson, B. T.: The clinical differentiation of lead gout from primary gout. Arthritis Rheum., **11,** 623, 1968.
802. Ball, G. V., and Morgan, J. M.: Chronic lead ingestion and gout. Southern Med. J., **61,** 21, 1968.
803. Ball, G. V., and Sorensen, L. B.: Pathogenesis of hyperuricemia in saturnine gout. New Eng. J. Med., **280,** 1199, 1969.
804. Rapado, A.: Gout and saturnism. New Eng. J. Med., **281,** 851, 1969.
805. Emmerson, B. T.: The renal excretion of urate in chronic lead nephropathy. Aust. Ann. Med., **14,** 295, 1965.
806. Bunim, J. J., Kimberg, D. V., Thomas, L. B., Van Scott, E. J., and Klatskin, G.: The syndrome of sarcoidosis, psoriasis, and gout. Ann. Intern. Med., **57,** 1018, 1962.
807. Zimmer, J. G., and Demis, D. J.: Associations between gout, psoriasis,

and sarcoidosis (with consideration of their pathogenic significance). Ann. Intern. Med., **64,** 786, 1966.

808. Kaplan, H., and Klatskin, G.: Sarcoidosis, psoriasis, and gout: Syndrome or coincidence? Yale J. Biol. Med., **32,** 335, 1960.
809. Chetrick, A.: Co-existent sarcoidosis, erythema nodosum, and gout. JAMA, **186,** 950, 1963.
810. Kelley, W. N., Goldfinger, S. E., and Hardy, H. L.: Hyperuricemia in chronic beryllium disease. Ann. Intern. Med., **70,** 977, 1969.
811. Lennox, W. G.: Increase of uric acid in the blood during prolonged starvation. JAMA, **82,** 602, 1924.
812. Pablico, R. C., Canfield, C. J., and Barry, K. G.: The effects of acute total caloric starvation on uric acid metabolism in obese human subjects. Clin. Res., **13,** 45, 1965.
813. Drenick, E. J., Swenseid, M. E., Blahd, W. H., and Tuttle, S. G.: Prolonged starvation as treatment for severe obesity. JAMA, **187,** 100, 1964.
814. Cristofori, F. C., and Duncan, G. G.: Uric acid excretion in obese subjects during periods of total fasting. Metabolism, **13,** 303, 1964.
815. Runcie, J., and Thomson, T. J.: Total fasting, hyperuricemia and gout. Postgrad. Med. J., **45,** 251, 1969.
816. Mintz, D. H., Canary, J. J., Carreon, G., and Kyle, L. H.: Hyperuricemia in hyperparathyroidism. New Eng. J. Med., **265,** 112, 1961.
817. Bywaters, E. C. L., Dixon, A. St. J., and Scott, J. T.: Gout lesions of hyperparathyroidism. Ann. Rheum. Dis., **22,** 171, 1963.
818. Scott, J. T., Dixon, A. St. J., and Bywaters, E. G. L.: Association of hyperuricemia and gout with hyperparathyroidism. Brit. Med. J., **5390,** 1070, 1964.
819. Duarte, C. G., and Bland, J. H.: Uric acid, calcium and phosphorous clearances in normal subjects on a low calcium, low phosphorous diet: Uric acid, calcium and phosphorous clearances after calcium infusion in normal and gouty patients. Metabolism, **14,** 203, 1965.
820. Garrod, P. R., McSwiney, R. R., and Bold, A. M.: Investigation of renal excretion of phosphate and urate. Clin. Sci., **31,** 9, 1966.
821. Shelp, W. D., Steel, T. H., and Rieselbach, R. E.: Comparison of urinary phosphate, urate and magnesium excretion following parathyroid hormone administration to normal man. Metabolism, **18,** 63, 1969.
822. Jackson, W. P. U., and Harris, F.: Gout with hyperparathyroidism: Report of a case with examination of synovial fluid. Brit. Med. J., **2,** 211, 1965.
823. Fuller, R. W., Luce, M. W., and Mertz, E. T.: Serum uric acid in mongolism. Science, **137,** 868, 1962.
824. Kaufman, J. M., and O'Brien, W. M.: Hyperuricemia in mongolism. New Eng. J. Med., **276,** 953, 1967.
825. Goodman, H. O., Lofland, H. B., and Thomas, J. J.: Serum uric acid levels in mongolism. Amer. J. Ment. Defic., **71,** 437, 1966.
826. Appleton, M. D., Haab, W., Burti, U., and Orsulak, P. J.: Plasma urate levels in mongolism. Amer. J. Ment. Defic., **74,** 196, 1969.
827. Coburn, S. P., Seidenberg, M., and Mertz, E. T.: Clearance of uric acid, urea, and creatinine in Down's syndrome. J. Appl. Physiol., **23,** 579, 1967.
828. Coburn, S. P., Sirlin, E. M., and Mertz, E. T.: Metabolism of N^{15} labeled uric acid in Down's syndrome. Metabolism, **17,** 560, 1968.
829. Rosner, F., Ong, B. H., Paine, R. S., and Mahanand, D.: Biochemical differentiation of trisomic Down's syndrome (mongolism) from that due to translocation. New Eng. J. Med., **273,** 1356, 1965.
830. Eisen, A. Z., and Seegmiller, J. E.: Uric acid metabolism in psoriasis. J. Clin. Invest., **40,** 1486, 1961.
831. Bunim, J. J., Kimberg, D. V., Thomas, L. B., Van Scott, E. J., and Klatskin, G.: The syndrome of sarcoidosis, psoriasis, and gout: Combined clinical staff conference at the National Institutes of Health. Ann. Intern. Med., **57,** 1018, 1962.
832. Kersley, G. D.: Pharmaceutical treatment of gout. Ann. Phys. Med., **8,** 199, 1966.
833. Krakoff, I. H.: Clinical pharmacology of drugs which influence uric acid production and excretion. Clin. Pharmacol. Ther., **8,** 124, 1967.
834. Gutman, A. B.: Recent developments in the therapy of gout. J. Amer. Geriat. Soc., **16,** 499, 1968.
835. Wyngaarden, J. B.: Gout and other disorders of uric acid metabolism, in *Principles of Internal Medicine,* edited by T. R. Harrison, R. D. Adams, I. L. Bennett, W. H. Resnik, G. W. Thorn, and M. M. Wintrobe, 6th ed., pp. 597–606. McGraw-Hill, New York, 1970.
836. Mugler, A.: Action de la colchicine dans les accidents allergiques. Ann. Med. Paris, **51,** 495, 1950.
837. Hoppe, D.: Uber die Verwendung von Colchysat in der Therapie chronisch rheumatischer Erkrankunger ausser bei Gicht. Deutsch. Gesundh., **12,** 896, 1957.
838. Kaplan, H.: Further experience with colchicine in the treatment of sarcoid arthritis. New Eng. J. Med., **268,** 761, 1963.
839. Zuckner, J.: Colchicine therapeutic trial responses in rheumatoid arthritis. Arthritis Rheum., **5,** 329, 1962.
840. Wallace, S. L., Bernstein, D., and Diamond, H.: Diagnostic value of the colchicine therapeutic trial. JAMA, **199,** 525, 1967.
841. Kantor, T. G., and Brown, R.: Test of non-specific anti-inflammatory activity of colchicine. Arthritis Rheum., **9,** 862, 1966.
842. Levine, M: The action of colchicine on cell division in human cancer animal and plant tissues. Ann. NY Acad. Sci., **51,** 1406, 1951.
843. Wallace, S. L., Omokoku, B., and Ertel, N. H.: Colchicine plasma levels: Implications as to pharmacology and mechanism of action. Amer. J. Med., **48,** 443, 1970.
844. Borisy, G. G., and Taylor, E. W.: The mechanism of action of colchicine: Binding of colchicine-^{3}H to cellular protein. J. Cell Biol., **34,** 525, 1967.
845. Shelanski, M. L., and Taylor, E. W.: Isolation of a protein subunit from microtubules. J. Cell. Biol., **34,** 549, 1967.
846. Malawista, S. E.: Colchicine: A common mechanism for its anti-inflammatory and anti-mitotic effects. Arthritis Rheum., **11,** 191, 1968.
847. Weisenberg, R. C., Borisy, G. G., and Taylor, E. W.: The colchicine-binding protein of mammalian brain and its relation to microtubules. Biochemistry (Wash.), **7,** 4466, 1968.
848. Malawista, S. E.: Sols, gels, and colchicine: A common formulation for the effects of colchicine in gouty inflammation and on cell devision. Arthritis Rheum., **7,** 325, 1964.
849. Malawista, S. E.: The action of colchicine in acute gout. Arthritis Rheum., **8,** 752, 1965.
850. Fruhman, G. J.: Inhibition of neutrophil mobilization by colchicine. Proc. Soc. Exp. Biol. Med., **104,** 284, 1960.
851. Phelps, P.: Polymorphonuclear leukocyte motility in vitro. IV. Colchicine inhibition of chemotactic activity formation after phagocytosis of urate crystals. Arthritis Rheum., **13,** 1, 1970.
852. Phelps, P.: Polymorphonuclear leukocyte motility in vitro. II. Stimulatory effect of monosodium urate crystals and urate in solution; partial inhibition by colchicine and indomethacin. Arthritis Rheum., **12,** 189, 1969.
853. Malawista, S. E., and Bodel, P. T.: The dissociation by colchicine of phagocytosis from increased oxygen consumption in human leukocytes. J. Clin. Invest., **46,** 786, 1967.
854. Rajan, K. T.: Lysosomes and gout. Nature, (London), **210,** 959, 1966.
855. Wechsler, R., Wallace, S. L., Gerber, D., and Scherrer, J.: Colchicine and trimethylcolchicinic acid: A comparison of their effects on human white blood cells in vitro. Arthritis Rheum., **8,** 1104, 1965.
856. Goldfinger, S. E., Howell, R. R., and Seegmiller, J. E.: Suppression of metabolic accompaniments of phagocytosis by colchicine. Arthritis Rheum., **8,** 1112, 1965.
857. Melmon, K. L., and Cline, M. J.: The interaction of leukocytes and the kinin system. Biochem. Pharmacol., **17,** 271, 1968.
858. Gutman, A. B., and Yü, T.-F: Current principles of management in gout. Amer. J. Med., **13,** 744, 1952.
859. Yü, T.-F., and Gutman, A. B.: Efficacy of colchicine prophylaxis in gout. Ann. Intern. Med., **55,** 179, 196.
860. Bauer, W.: Panel discussion on rheumatic diseases. J. Amer. Geriat. Soc., **4,** 572, 1956.
861. Robinson, W. D.: Current status of the treatment of gout. JAMA, **164,** 1670, 1957.
862. Rosenberg, E. F.: Gout: A summary of recent developments in therapy. J. Amer. Geriat. Soc., **2,** 229, 1954.
863. Smyth, C. J., Huffman, E. R., and Wilson, G. M.: Treatment of gout. A.M.A. Arch. Intern. Med., **97,** 783, 1956.
864. Bartels, E. C.: Treatment of gout. Metabolism, **6,** 297, 1957.

865. Smyth, C. J., and Huffman, E. R.: Gouty arthritis: Diagnosis and treatment. Med. Clin. N. Amer., **39**, 543, 1955.

866. Ferreira, M. L., and Buoniconti, A.: Trisomy after colchicine therapy. Lancet, **2**, 1304, 1968.

867. Hansteen, I. L.: Colchicine and chromosome aberrations. Lancet, **2**, 744, 1969.

868. Walker, F. A.: Trisomy after colchicine therapy. Lancet, **1**, 257, 1969.

869. Wallace, S. L., and Ertel, N. H.: Colchicine: Current problems. Bull. Rheum. Dis., **20**, 582, 1969.

870. Faloon, W. W., Webb, D. I., and Race, T. F.: Cholesterol lowering effect of colchicine. Ann. Intern. Med., **66**, 1058, 1966.

871. Webb, D. I., Chodos, R. B., Mahar, C. Q., and Faloon, W. W.: Mechanism of vitamin B_{12} malabsorption in patients receiving colchicine. New Eng. J. Med., **279**, 845, 1968.

872. Kontos, H. A.: Myopathy associated with chronic colchicine toxicity. New Eng. J. Med., **266**, 38, 1962.

873. Colton, R. S., Ward, L. E., Maher, F. I., and Ferguson, R. H.: Occult renal impairment in gouty and hyperuricemic individuals. Amer. J. Med. Sci., **252**, 575, 1966.

874. Klinenberg, J. R., Dornfield, L. P., and Gonick, H. C.: Renal function in patients with asymptomatic hyperuricemia. Arthritis Rheum., **12**, 307, 1969.

875. Gutman, A. B., and Yü, T.-F.: Protracted uricosuric therapy in tophaccous gout. Lancet, **2**, 1258, 1957.

876. Kuzell, W., Glover, R., Gibbs, J., and Blau, R.: Effect of anturane on serum uric acid and cholesterol in gout: A long-term study. Acta. Rheum. Scand., suppl. **8**, 31, 1964.

877. Thompson, G. R., Dull, I. F., Robinson, W. D., Mikkelsen, W. M., and Falindez, H.: Long term uricosuric therapy in gout. Arthritis Rheum., **5**, 384, 1962.

878. De Seze, S., Ryckewaert, A., Caroit, M., Kahn, M. F., and D'Anglejan, G.: Le traitement uricosurique de la goutte. *Congres International de la goutte et de la lithiase urique,* Evian, Sept. 4–6, 1964, p. 297.

879. Seegmiller, J. E., and Grayzel, A. I.: Use of the newer uricosuric agents in the management of gout. JAMA, **173**, 1076, 1960.

880. Robinson, W. D.: The present status of colchicine and uricosuric agents in management of primary gout. Arthritis Rheum., **8**, 865, 1965.

881. White, F. R.: 4-Aminopyrazolo (3,4-d) pyrimidine and three derivatives. Cancer Chemother. Rep., **3**, 26, 1959.

882. Shaw, R. K., Shulman, R. N., Davidson, J. D., Rall, D. P., and Frei, Emil, III: Studies with the experimental antitumor agent 4-aminopyrazolo (3,4-d) pyrimidine. Cancer, **13**, 482, 1960.

883. Elion, G. B., Callahan, S., Nathan, H. Bieber, S., Rundles, R. W., and Hitchings, G. H.: Potentiation by inhibition of drug degradation: 6-Substituted purines and xanthine oxidase. Biochem. Pharmacol., **12**, 85, 1963.

884. Wyngaarden, J. B., Rundles, R. W., Silberman, H. R., and Hunter, S.: Control of hyperuricemia with hydroxypyrazolopyrimidine, a purine analogue which inhibits uric acid synthesis. Arthritis Rheum., **6**, 306, 1963.

885. Rundles, R. W., Silberman, H. R., Hitchings, G. H., and Elion, G. B.: Effects of xanthine oxidase inhibitor on clinical manifestations and purine metabolism in gout. Ann. Intern. Med., **60**, 717, 1964.

886. Klinenberg, J. R., Goldfinger, S. E., and Seegmiller, J. E.: The effectiveness of the xanthine oxidase inhibitor allopurinol in the treatment of gout. Ann. Intern. Med., **62**, 639, 1965.

887. Wyngaarden, J. B., Rundles, R. W., and Metz, E. N.: Allopurinol in the treatment of gout. Ann. Intern. Med., **62**, 842, 1965.

888. Delbarre, F., Amor, B., Auscher, C., and DeGery, A.: Treatment of gout with allopurinol, a study of 106 cases. Ann. Rheum. Dis., **25**, 627, 1966.

889. Rundles, R. W., Metz, E. N., and Silberman, H. R.: Allopurinol in the treatment of gout. Ann. Intern. Med., **64**, 229, 1966.

890. Elion, G. B., Kovensky, A., and Hitchings, G.: Metabolic studies of allopurinol: An inhibitor of xanthine oxidase. Biochem. Pharmacol., **15**, 863, 1966.

891. Goldfinger, S., Klinenberg, J. R., and Seegmiller, J. E.: The renal excretion of oxypurines. J. Clin. Invest., **44**, 623, 1965.

892. Delbarre, F., Lagrue, G., Frugier, J-C., and Aignan, M.: Le traitement, par L'allopurinol, de la Goutte avec insuffisance rénale. Sem. Hop. Paris, **43**, 644, 1967.

893. Emmerson, B. T.: The use of the xanthine oxidase inhibitor, allopurinol, in the control of hyperuricemia, gout and uric acid calculi. Aust. Ann. Med., **16**, 205, 1967.

894. Levin, N. W., and Abrahams, O. L.: Allopurinol in patients with impaired renal function. Ann. Rheum. Dis., **25**, 681, 1966.

895. Ogryzlo, M. A., Urowitz, M., Weber, H. M., and Haupt, J. B.: Effects of allopurinol on gouty and nongouty uric acid nephropathy. Ann. Rheum. Dis., **25**, 673, 1966.

896. Stoberg, K.-H.: Allopurinol therapy of gout with renal complications. Ann. Rheum. Dis., **25**, 688, 1966.

897. Rundles, R. W.: Allopurinol in gouty nephropathy and renal dialysis. Ann. Rheum. Dis., **25**, 694, 1966.

898. Wilson, J. D., Simmonds, H. A., and North, J. D. K.: Allopurinol in the treatment of uremic patients with gout. Ann. Rheum. Dis., **26**, 136, 1967.

899. De Vries, A., Frank, M., Liberman, U. A., and Sperling, O.: Allopurinol in the prophylaxis of uric acid stones. Ann. Rheum. Dis., **25**, 691, 1966.

900. Alexander, S., and Brendler, H.: Treatment of uric acid urolithiasis with allopurinol, a xanthine oxidase inhibitor, J. Urol., **97**, 340, 1967.

901. Anderson, E. E., Rundles, R. W., Silberman, H. R., and Metz, E. N.: Allopurinol control of hyperuricosuria: A new concept in the prevention of uric acid stones. J. Urol., **97**, 344, 1967.

902. Krakoff, I. H.: Xanthine oxidase inhibition in the management of hyperuricemia in leukemias and lymphomas. Arthritis Rheum., **8**, 896, 1965.

903. Vogler, W. R., Bain, J. A., Huguley, C. M., Jr., Palmer, H. B., Jr., and Lowrey, M. E.: Metabolic and therapeutic effects of allopurinol in patients with leukemia and gout. Amer. J. Med., **40**, 548, 1966.

904. Watts, R. W. E., Watkins, P. J., Matthias, J. Q., and Gibbs, D. A.: Allopurinol and acute uric acid nephropathy. Brit. Med. J., **1**, 205, 1966.

905. Scott, J. T.: Symposium on allopurinol. Ann. Rheum. Dis., **25**, 599, 1966.

906. Sorensen, L., and Seegmiller, J. R.: Seminars on the Lesch-Nyhan syndrome: Management and treatment, discussion. Fed. Proc., **27**, 1097, 1968.

907. Greene, M. L., Fujimoto, W. Y., and Seegmiller, J. E.: Urinary xanthine stones—a rare complication of allopurinol therapy. New Eng. J. Med., **280**, 426, 1969.

908. Band, P. R., Silverberg, D. S., Henderson, J. F., Ulan, R. A., Wensel, R. H., Banerjee, T. K., and Little, A. S.: Xanthine nephropathy in a patient with lymphosarcoma treated with allopurinol. New Eng. J. Med., **283**, 354, 1970.

909. Wyngaarden, J. B.: Allopurinol and xanthine nephropathy. New Eng. J. Med., **283**, 371, 1970.

910. Kuzell, W. C., Seebach, L. M., Glover, R. P., and Jackman, A. E.: Treatment of gout with allopurinol and sulphinpyrazone in combination and with allopurinol alone. Ann. Rheum. Dis., **25**, 634, 1966.

911. Jarzobski, J., Ferry, J., Wombolt, D., Fitch, D. M., and Egan, J. D.: Vasculitis with allopurinol therapy. Amer. Heart J., **79**, 116, 1970.

912. Hitchings, G. H.: Effects of allopurinol in relation to purine biosynthesis. Ann. Rheum. Dis., **25**, 601, 1966.

913. Emmerson, B. T.: Discussion: Symposium on allopurinol. Ann. Rheum. Dis., **25**, 622, 1966.

914. Kelley, W. N., Rosenbloom, F. M., Miller, J., and Seegmiller, J. E.: An enzymatic basis for variation in response to allopurinol. New Eng. J. Med., **278**, 287, 1968.

915. Pomales, R., Bieber, S., Friedman, R., and Hitchings, G. H.: Augmentation of the incorporation of hypoxanthine into nucleic acids by the administration of an inhibitor of xanthine oxidase. Biochim. Biophys. Acta, **72**, 119, 1963.

916. Pomales, R., Elion, G. B., and Hitchings, G. H.: Xanthine as a precursor of nucleic acid purines in the mouse. Biochim. Biophys. Acta, **95**, 505, 1965.

917. Delbarre, F., and Auscher, C.: Traitement de la goutte par l'acide uracil-6-carboxylique et ses derives. Presse Med., **71**, 1765, 1963.

918. Standerfer, S. B., and Handler, P.: Fatty liver induced by orotic acid feeding. Proc. Soc. Exp. Biol. Med., **90**, 270, 1959.

919. Creasey, W. A., Hankin, L., and Handschumacher, R. E.: Fatty livers induced by orotic acid. I. Accumulation and metabolism of lipids. J. Biol. Chem., **236**, 2064, 1961.

920. Altman, K. I., Smull, K., and Guzman-Barron, E. S.: A new method for the preparation of uricase and the effect of uricase on the blood uric acid levels of the chicken. Arch. Biochem., **21**, 158, 1949.

921. London, M., and Hudson, P. B.: Uricolytic activity of purified uricase in two human beings. Science, **125**, 937, 1957.

922. Royer, R., Vindel, J., Lamarche, M., and Kissel, P.: Modalities d'élimination des purines au cours du traitement enzymatique de la goutte et des états hyperuricémiques par une urate-oxydase. Presse Med., **76**, 2325, 1968.

923. Kissel, P., Lamarche, M., and Royer, R.: Modification of uricemia and the excretion of uric acid nitrogen by an enzyme of fungal origin. Nature (London), **217**, 72, 1968.

CHAPTER FORTY

THE LESCH-NYHAN SYNDROME

William N. Kelley
James B. Wyngaarden

The Lesch-Nyhan syndrome is an inherited disorder associated with a virtually complete deficiency of an enzyme of purine metabolism, hypoxanthine-guanine phosphoribosyl transferase. The disease affects only males. It is characterized clinically by hyperuricemia, excessive production of uric acid, and certain characteristic neurologic features, including self-mutilation, choreoathetosis, spasticity, and mental retardation.

CLINICAL FEATURES

Central Nervous System Function

Patients with the Lesch-Nyhan syndrome generally appear normal at birth. Although hypotonia, recurrent vomiting, and difficulty with secretions occur in some patients during the first 3 months of life [1], the earliest consistent abnormality is a delay in motor development which appears by 3 to 4 months of age (Table 40-1). Between 8 months and 1 year, extrapyramidal signs develop. These signs are characterized by fine athetoid movements of the hands and feet, dystonia, and chorea. The athetosis, which is similar to that associated with asphyxia, birth injury, and hyperbilirubinemia, accounts at least in part for the dysarthria which appears later in life [2]. At about 1 year signs of pyramidal tract involvement, such as hyperreflexia, sustained ankle clonus, extensor plantar responses, and scissoring of the legs, also develop. These findings preclude ambulation in the older patient.

The most striking neurologic feature of the Lesch-Nyhan syndrome is compulsive self-destructive behavior (Fig. 40-1). At 2 or 3 years of age affected children begin to bite their fingers, lips, and buccal mucosa. This compulsion for self-mutilation becomes so extreme that it is necessary to keep the elbows in extension with splints and hands wrapped with gauze or restrained in some other manner. In several patients mutilation of lips could only be controlled by extraction of teeth.

The compulsive urge to inflict painful wounds appears to grip the patient irresistibly. Often he will appear to be content until one begins to remove an arm splint. At this point a communicative patient will plead that the restraints be left alone. If one continues in freeing the arm, the patient will become extremely agitated and upset. Finally, when completely unrestrained, he will begin to put his fingers into his mouth. An older patient will plead for help, and if one then takes hold of the arm which has previously been freed, the patient will show obvious relief. If help is not forthcoming, a painful and often severe injury may be inflicted. The apparent urge to bite fingers is often not symmetrical. In several patients it has been possible to leave one arm unrestrained without concern even though freeing the other would result in an immediate attempt at self-mutilation.

Retarded children with a variety of other disorders will also often exhibit finger biting as well as other types of self-destructive behavior, but lip biting seems to be almost unique to the Lesch-Nyhan syndrome. Severe self-biting also occurs in a number of neurologic disorders characterized by loss of pain sensation [3], but detailed study of patients with the Lesch-Nyhan syndrome has failed to reveal any sensory abnormalities.

These patients also attempt to injure themselves by banging their heads against inanimate objects or by placing their extremities in dangerous places such as the spokes of a wheelchair. If the hands are unrestrained, their mutilation becomes the patient's main concern, and effort to inflict injury in some other manner seems to be sublimated.

Patients with this syndrome also exhibit unusual aggressiveness directed at others. They will strike out at those around them including children, nurses, physicians, relatives, and friends. A typical maneuver is a swing at the physician in an apparent attempt to knock his glasses off. This is done in a peculiarly jovial but extremely aggressive manner and is usually followed by an apology. In addition, patients will spit and use abusive language, often apologizing while doing so.

The degree to which self-mutilation and aggressiveness occur is quite variable. One patient had no apparent evidence of any behavioral abnormality other than mental deficiency until the age of 16, when he first developed self-mutilation. On the other hand, many patients have tended to improve as they became older. Behavior may also improve with prolonged hospitalization. The degree of mutilation and aggressiveness varies from day to day depending at least in part on surrounding events.

These patients respond to stressful situations by increased agitation, episodes of opisthotonic posturing, and increasing attempts at self-mutilation. Menkes has compared the aggressiveness which they direct toward others upon being disturbed to "sham rage" [4]. In the older patient the internal struggle between the desire to inflict injury and the attempt to control this urge can be quite overt.

Most patients with the Lesch-Nyhan syndrome appear to be mentally deficient. IQ testing by routine methods usually gives values ranging from 30 to 65. Their poor performance on formal testing is in part related to dysarthria and choreoathetosis, which make communication difficult. One patient was found to have normal intelligence when testing was designed to minimize these factors [5].

Approximately 50 percent of patients reported in the literature have had seizures. In several instances this has

Table 40-1. CLINICAL FEATURES IN PATIENTS WITH THE LESCH-NYHAN SYNDROME

Family	Date of birth	*Onset of symptoms*		Family history	Serum urate (mg/100 ml)	Urinary uric acid (mg/kg/24 hr)	Other features	Reference
		Age	Type					
1*	1956			+	9.9–15.5	38.9		[19]
2	1951	12 mo	Slow development		10.6	44.2	Anemia	[17]
3*a*		3 mo	Slow development	+	8.9–16.8	46.8	Renal calculi	[1]
3*b*		5 mo	Slow development		9.9–11.2	43.7		[13]
4*a*		6 mo	Slow motor development	+	10.5–12.4	32.4–55.6	Renal calculi	[13]
4*b*		1 year	Slow motor development	+	12.3		Renal calculi	[23]
5*a*			Abnormal posturing	+		37.8–53.0	Crystalluria	
5*b*		6 mo	Slow motor development		8.6–9.4	37.8–53.0		
6	1961	4 mo	Urethral obstruction	–	13.3–25.1	57.5	Imperforate anus	
7		2 mo	Hypotonia, dysphagia	+	7.2		Crystalluria tophi	[16]
8	1961	birth	Delayed development		9.5	37–58		[78]
9					6.6–14.7			[14]
10	1960		Delayed development	?	10.4			[113]
11	1963	6 mo	Delayed development	+	7.0–12.5	35.0–60.0	Renal calculi	[114]
12	1957	5½ mo	"Jerking spell"	–	8.1	66.5		[13]
13	1960	2 mo	Diarrhea and vomiting	–	9.3–13.2	24.5		[13]
14	1955	birth	Irritable	–	8.0	29.3		[13]
15		4 mo	Delayed motor development	–	7.4–9.9	36.4–56.5		[79] [79]
16		birth	Listless		11.7			
17	1948	birth	Choreoathetosis, psychomotor retardation	–	12.6–14.0	25.0–30.0	Macrocytic anemia, tophi	[20]
18	1963			+	5.8–22.0	55	Megaloblastic anemia	[21]
19	1956			–	7.9–8.6	30.6–46.4	Megaloblastic anemia	[21]
20*a*	1962	10 mo	Slow motor development	+	6.1–16.9	81.1	Anemia	[15]
20*b*		16 mo	Slow motor development	+	4.9–14.9	36.8	Hirschsprung's disease, anemia	
21*a**	1967	4 mo	Spasticity	+	9.1	143		[15]
21*b*	1963	7 mo	Poor development, vomiting		18.6	79.0	Anemia	
22	1965	Not stated	Not stated	+	8.6–9.0	47–62	Anemia	[18]
23*a*	1956						Megaloblastic anemia	[22]
23*b*	1959			+	14.5–18.5	40.3–44.9	Megaloblastic anemia	
23*c*	1966				11.3	49	Megaloblastic anemia	
24	1966	3½ mo	Delayed motor development	+	8.0–18.9	93.6	Hypocalcemia	[6]
25	1958	7 wk	Vomiting, delayed development	–	8.3–11.0	45		[4]
26	1963	3 mo	Delayed motor development	+	7.5–9.6		Ur. UA/Cr 2.55–3.20	[9]

Table 40-1. CLINICAL FEATURES IN PATIENTS WITH THE LESCH-NYHAN SYNDROME (*continued*)

Family	Date of birth	Onset of symptoms		Family history	Serum urate (mg/100 ml)	Urinary uric acid (mg/kg/24 hr)	Other features	Reference
		Age	Type					
27	1961	7 mo	Delayed motor development	+	8.0–10.4		Ur. UA/Cr 2.07–4.68	[9]
28	1962	8 mo	Seizures	−	7.6–9.0		Ur. UA/Cr 2.40–3.10	[9]
29	1963	2½ mo	Spastic torticollis	−	6.3–9.2		Ur. UA/Cr 2.48–2.56	[9]
30†	1963	Not stated	Delayed development	+	8.1	Not stated		[5]

*No self mutilation. All patients in this table exhibited self-mutilation, choreoathetosis, and spasticity with developmental and mental retardation, except where indicated.
† Normal intelligence.

been attributed to some apparently unrelated event such as hypocalcemia [6] or hypoglycemia [7]. The seizures in some patients have been interpreted as decerebrate cerebellar fits [8].

Routine studies of cerebrospinal fluid are uniformly normal. Electromyograms and nerve conduction velocities are also normal [9]. Electroencephalograms may be normal or may reveal diffuse slowing.

Hyperuricemia and Overproduction of Uric Acid

All patients with the Lesch-Nyhan syndrome exhibit excessive production of uric acid. This is reflected in an increased excretion of uric acid in the urine. Although the daily excretion of uric acid may not be in excess of that seen in normal adults, the values are extremely high when one considers the small size of these patients. As can be seen in Table

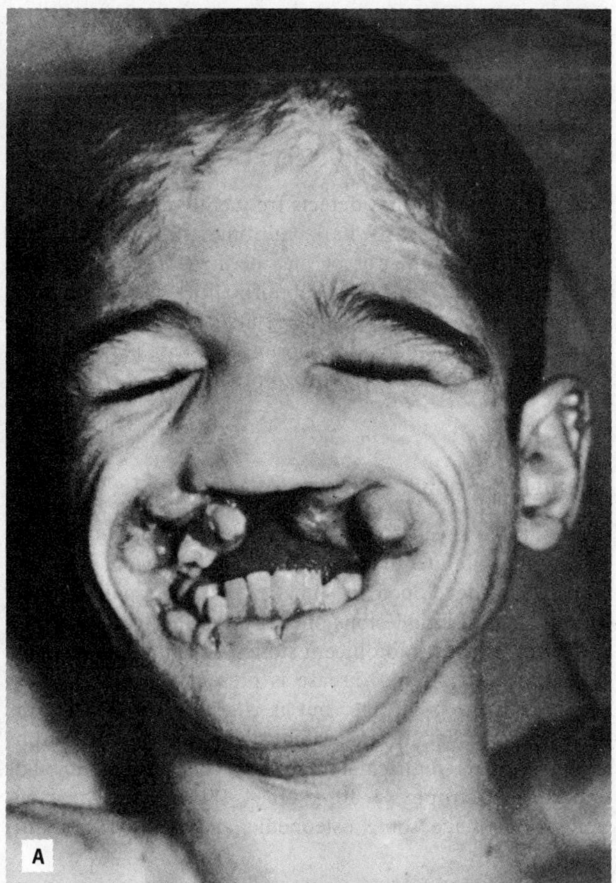

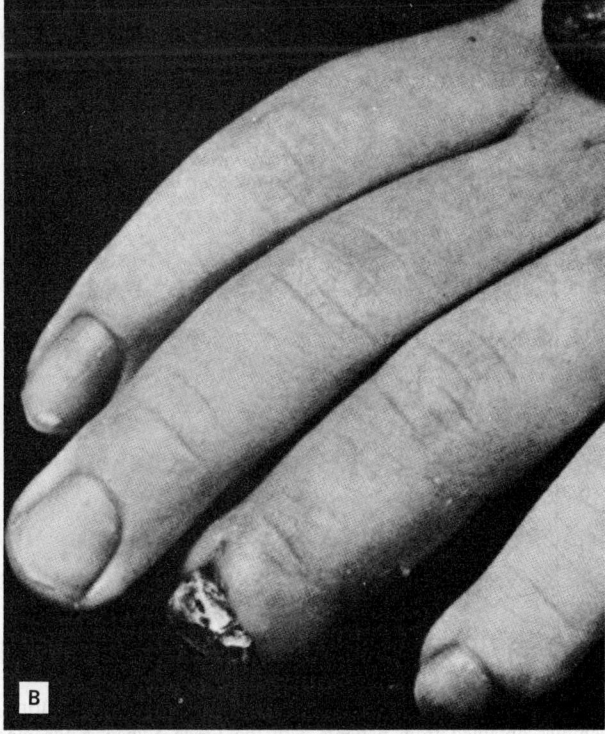

Figure 40-1A and B. Evidence of severe mutilation of lips and fingers in a patient with the Lesch-Nyhan syndrome. (*From Nyhan, W. L., Fed. Proc.,* **27,** 1027, 1968.)

40-1, the excretion of uric acid, when expressed on the basis of body weight, ranges from 25 to 143 mg per kg per day [10, 11] compared to an upper limit of normal in children of 18 mg per kg per day [10]. The excretion of uric acid can also be expressed in relation to creatinine excretion, another measure of body mass. As indicated in Fig. 40-2, the ratio of uric acid to creatinine concentration in urine samples obtained from patients with the Lesch-Nyhan syndrome is uniformly larger than in age-matched controls. The consistency of this elevated ratio, the ease of collecting random urine samples, and the simplicity of the chemical determinations make the uric acid/creatinine ratio in urine an excellent, although nonspecific, screening test for this disorder [12]. Although false negative results are unusual, several other disorders also associated with excessive uric acid production, such as Type I glycogen storage disease and certain lymphoproliferative disorders, will cause an occasional false positive test result.

The increased quantity of uric acid excreted in the urine leads to the development of uric acid crystalluria in most patients at some time. The finding of orange crystals on a diaper during the first few weeks of life has occasionally been the first sign observed by the mother [13]. Unfortunately, this is rarely brought to the attention of the physician, and even when recognized, these crystals are easily mistaken for some other urinary constituent such as cystine. Many patients progress to symptomatic uric acid nephrolithiasis, and this may lead to obstructive uropathy with severe and unrelenting azotemia. Such a course has been a common cause of death during the first decade of life in untreated patients with this syndrome. Hematuria and colicky abdominal pain often occur, but the radiolucency of uric acid stones delays clinical recognition.

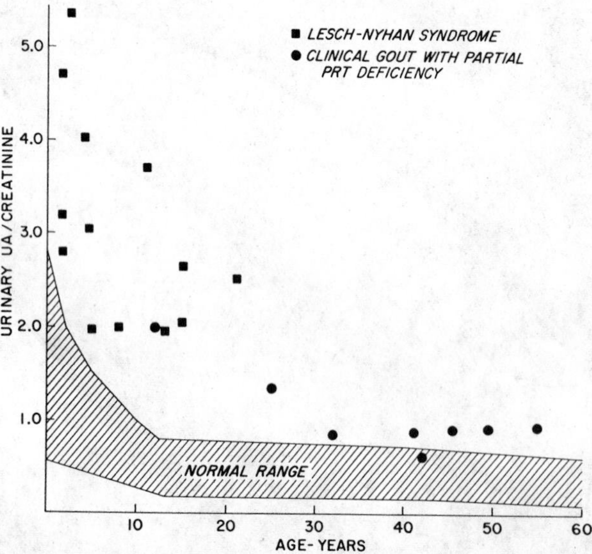

Figure 40-2. Ratio of uric acid to creatinine concentration in urine samples obtained from patients with the Lesch-Nyhan syndrome (complete PRT deficiency) and those with gout and a partial deficiency of PRT. The normal range represents the mean ± 2 s. d. in a total of 284 control subjects of various ages. (*From Kaufman, J. M., et al., J. Pediat.,* **73**, 583, 1968.)

The excessive production of uric acid leads to hyperuricemia. The serum urate concentration usually ranges from 7 to 10 mg per 100 ml in the absence of renal insufficiency, but in an occasional patient a random value will fall within the normal range [14, 15, 9]. The serum urate concentration may provide an initial clue to the diagnosis, but because of its variability, it is not an infallible screening test. An occasional patient has developed classical gouty arthritis and tophaceous deposits of monosodium urate [16, 17]. These symptoms rarely occur before the age of 12 or 13, even when the serum urate has been elevated since birth.

Hematologic Abnormalities

At least 10 of the reported patients were anemic prior to the occurrence of renal insufficiency [11, 15, 17, 18–22]. Catel and Schmidt described the anemia in their patient as megaloblastic in character [19]. More recently a number of investigators have confirmed the presence of macrocytic erythrocytes in the peripheral blood and megaloblastic changes in the bone marrow [20–22]. These changes may be present even in the absence of overt anemia. Possible mechanisms for these morphologic changes and approaches to therapy will be considered later.

Associated Congenital Defects

Some of the congenital defects frequently observed in children with the Lesch-Nyhan syndrome, such as bilaterally dislocated hips and clubfeet, may be the result of the severe spasticity. Other congenital abnormalities have also been seen which are not necessarily related to the basic disease process. These include Hirschsprung's disease [15], imperforate anus [23], and bilateral cryptorchidism [24, 7].

Roentgenographic Findings

There are no specific x-ray findings in this syndrome. Most patients have bilaterally dislocated hips. Tophaceous deposits which have developed in some of the older patients may be apparent as lytic lesions on x-ray. An intravenous pyelogram may suggest radiolucent stones, or small kidneys with poor function if renal disease is present. There is usually some delay in bone age, but it is not as marked as the retardation in height and weight. Pneumoencephalography usually reveals ventricular dilatation consistent with bilateral cortical atrophy [1, 10, 11, 16, 4, 18]. Finally, these patients often have some osteopenia and bone demineralization.

Pathology

At least eight patients dying with the Lesch-Nyhan syndrome have been autopsied [13, 15, 16, 24, 25, 26, 27]. In addition to the evidence of growth retardation and self-mutilation, a consistent finding has been bilaterally shrunken kidneys with striking deposits of monosodium urate and uric acid.

Distinctive changes in the central nervous system have not been apparent. The findings described by Sass et al., which included demyelinative and vascular lesions of the cerebral and cerebellar white matter, degeneration of the granules in Purkinje cells, multiple small chronic infarcts, and the presence of De Galantha staining material, can probably be attributed to the severe uremia preceeding death [16]. Partington and Hennen noted occasional perivascular birefringent crystals which were not uric acid in the alcohol-fixed brain of one patient [15]. One of the two original patients reported by Lesch and Nyhan was autopsied at the National Institutes of Health in 1966. Gross examination disclosed a brownish pigmentation over the cerebral cortex, but this could not be detected histologically in either formalin- or alcohol-fixed tissue [25]. The patient originally described by Riley was found at autopsy to have thinning of the cerebellar cortex and loss of cells in the granular layer [24]. Autopsies on four additional cases have failed to reveal any significant changes in the central nervous system [13, 26, 27].

BIOCHEMICAL FEATURES

Regulation of Purine Metabolism in Man

The mechanism of purine synthesis and its regulation have been considered in detail in the previous chapter and will only be summarized here.

The purine nucleotides, guanylic acid (GMP) and adenylic acid (AMP), can be synthesized by several mechanisms (Fig. 40-3). The free purine bases can be converted directly to their respective ribonucleotides by the appropriate purine phosphoribosyl transferase in the presence of PP-ribose-P [28, 29]. In addition, GMP and AMP can be synthesized *de novo* from smaller precursors including PP-ribose-P, glutamine, glycine, asparate, formate, and bicarbonate through a common intermediate, inosinic acid (IMP) [30–32].

Data obtained in bacterial [33], avian [34, 35], and mammalian [36] systems indicate that AMP and GMP inhibit PP-ribose-P amidotransferase, the initial and rate-limiting step of *de novo* purine biosynthesis, by interacting at separate sites on the enzyme, termed the *6-amino* and *6-hydroxy sites,* respectively. AMP and GMP are also effective inhibitors of formylglycinamide ribonucleotide (FGAR) amidotransferase, although the importance of this feedback site to the control of the rate of purine synthesis *de novo* is not established [37]. Each nucleotide further regulates its own *de novo* formation by inhibiting the appropriate nucleotide interconversion; GMP inhibits inosinic dehydrogenase that catalyzes the formation of xanthylic acid, XMP, from IMP [38, 39]; AMP inhibits the formation of adenylosuccinic acid (AMP-S) from IMP that is catalyzed by adenylosuccinate synthetase [40]. Finally, AMP and GMP also inhibit their respective purine phosphoribosyl transferases, A-PRT and G-PRT, and thereby regulate their synthesis from the free purine bases [41, 42].

Regulation of purine biosynthesis and purine interconversions by end product repression of enzyme synthesis has been shown to be important in bacterial systems [43, 44], but in man this mechanism has not been conclusively shown to play a significant role in the regulation of purine synthesis or metabolism.

Enzyme Defect

In 1967, Seegmiller, Rosenbloom, and Kelley described a virtually complete deficiency of an enzyme of purine metabolism, hypoxanthine-guanine phosphoribosyl transferase, in erythrocyte lysates from three patients and in cultured skin fibroblasts from another patient with this disorder [45]. The enzyme defect was subsequently confirmed in other tissues including liver, brain, and leukocytes as well as cultured skin fibroblasts and erythrocytes from many similarly affected patients [46, 47] (Tables 40-2, 40-3, 40-4).

Hypoxanthine-guanine phosphoribosyl transferase catalyzes the conversion of hypoxanthine to inosinic acid and

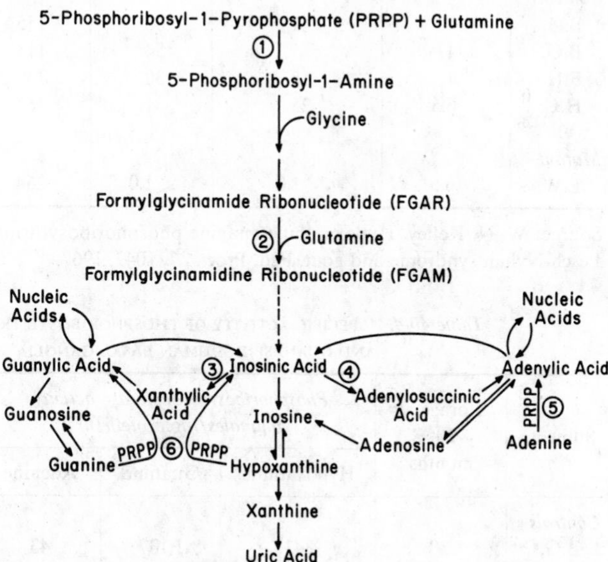

Figure 40-3. Regulation of purine metabolism in man. Enzymes subject to feedback inhibition by adenylic acid (AMP) or guanylic acid (GMP) are indicated as follows: (1) 5-phosphoribosyl-1-pyrophosphate amidotransferase, (2) α-N-formylglycinamide ribonucleotide amidotransferase, (3) inosinate dehydrogenase, (4) adenylosuccinate synthetase, (5) adenine phosphoribosyl transferase, and (6) hypoxanthine-guanine phosphoribosyl transferase.

Table 40-2. SPECIFIC ACTIVITY OF PHOSPHORIBOSYL TRANSFERASE OF ERYTHROCYTE HEMOLYSATES FROM SUBJECTS WITH LESCH-NYHAN SYNDROME

Subjects	*Phosphoribosyl transferase activity mμmoles/mg protein/hr*		
	Hypoxanthine, mean ± s.d.	Guanine, mean ± s.d.	Adenine, mean ± s.d.
Normal [32]*	103 ± 18	103 ± 21	31 ± 6
Lesch-Nyhan syndrome			
J.W.	<0.01	<0.004	58
T.S.	<0.01	<0.004	39
D.F.	<0.01	<0.004	53
B.M.	<0.01	<0.004	49
M.B.	<0.01	<0.004	56
S.M.	<0.01	<0.004	51
F.H.	<0.01	<0.004	94
M.W.	<0.01	<0.004	65
J.S.	<0.01	<0.004	71

* Number of subjects studied.

Source: W. N. Kelley, Hypoxanthine-guanine phosphoribosyl transferase deficiency in the Lesch-Nyhan syndrome and gout, Fed. Proc., **27**, 1047, 1967.

Table 40-3. SPECIFIC ACTIVITY OF PHOSPHORIBOSYL TRANSFERASE AND GUANASE IN HUMAN LIVER

Subject	Storage at −20°C, months	*Phosphoribosyl transferase activity, mμmoles/mg protein/hr*			Guanase activity, mμmoles/mg protein/hr
		Hypoxanthine	Guanine	Adenine	
Controls					
B.G.	0	41	66	155	1,439
B.G.	1		54	118	1,497
F.H.	1	18	30	139	2,372
H.C.	6.5	25	31	163	917
Mutant					
E.W.	6.5	<1.0	<1.0	264	1,546

Source: W. N. Kelley, Hypoxanthine-guanine phosphoribosyl transferase deficiency in the Lesch-Nyhan syndrome and gout, Fed. Proc., **27**, 1047, 1967.

Table 40-4. SPECIFIC ACTIVITY OF PHOSPHORIBOSYL TRANSFERASE AND GUANASE IN HUMAN BASAL GANGLIA

Subject	Storage at −20°C, months	*Phosphoribosyl transferase activity, mμmoles/mg protein/hr*			Guanase activity, mμmoles/mg protein/hr
		Hypoxathine	Guanine	Adenine	
Controls					
B.G.	0	843	1,137	43	3,786
B.G.	1	685	715	37	5,027
F.H.	1	315	413	27	2,662
Mutant					
E.W.	6.5	<4	<4	71	6,839

Source: W. N. Kelley, Hypoxanthine-guanine phosphoribosyl transferase deficiency in the Lesch-Nyhan syndrome and gout, Fed. Proc., **27**, 1047, 1967.

Hypoxanthine + PRPP (5-phosphoribosyl-1-pyrophosphate) ⟶ Inosinic Acid + P–P

Figure 40-4. The reaction catalyzed by hypoxanthine-guanine phosphoribosyl transferase illustrated with hypoxanthine as substrate.

guanine to guanylic acid in the presence of PP-ribose-P [28, 29] (Fig. 40-4). The natural purine base, xanthine, is also converted to its nucleotide by this enzyme, although at only about 1 percent of the rate found with hypoxanthine or guanine [48, 42]. Several purine analogues, including 6-mercaptopurine, allopurinol, 8-azaguanine, and 6-thioguanine, are also substrates for the enzyme [42, 49] (Fig. 40-5). Significantly, azathioprine, adenine, uric acid, and uracil are not substrates [42]. The enzyme is activated by magnesium ions and is inhibited by the end products of the reaction. Guanylic acid and its di- and triphosphates are much stronger inhibitors than inosinic or xanthylic acid [42].

Erythrocytes are generally used as a source of this enzyme in clinical assays. The level of enzyme activity in erythrocytes is ordinarily higher than in any other tissue except the central nervous system [46] (Table 40-5). In addition, other enzymes such as xanthine oxidase, guanase, 5′-nucleotidase, and adenylosuccinic acid synthetase, which would compete for substrates or products of the hypoxanthine-guanine phosphoribosyl transferase reaction, are either absent or present in relatively low activities in erythrocytes [50]. The relatively low activity of these interfering enzymes allows one to assay for very low activities of hypoxanthine-guanine phosphoribosyl transferase in erythrocyte lysates, whereas this is not possible with crude homogenates from other tissues. When hemolysates obtained from patients with the Lesch-Nyhan syndrome were assayed for hypoxanthine-guanine phosphoribosyl transferase activity, until recently no trace of

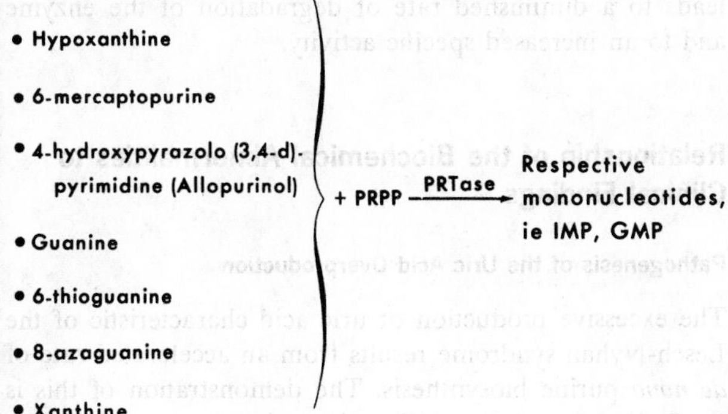

Figure 40-5. Purine substrates for hypoxanthine-guanine phosphoribosyl transferase.

Table 40-5. SPECIFIC ACTIVITY OF PHOSPHORIBOSYL TRANSFERASE IN HUMAN NECROPSY TISSUE

Tissue	Phosphoribosyl transferase		
	Hypoxanthine	Guanine	Adenine
Brain			
Frontal lobe	497	736	12
Basal ganglia	843	1137	43
Spinal cord	42	57	4
Cerebellum	463	660	68
Liver	41	66	155
Spleen	36	60	50
Kidney	28	48	11
Muscle	0.1	5	15
Ovary	143	194	46
Pancreas	42	41	5
Jejunum	18	27	9
Adrenal	35	58	31
Erythrocytes	103	103	31
Leukocytes	128	183	221

Source: W. N. Kelley, M. L. Greene, F. M. Rosenbloom, J. F. Henderson, and J. E. Seegmiller. Hypoxanthine-guanine phosphoribosyl transferase deficiency in gout, Ann. Intern. Med., **70**, 155, 1969.

activity could be demonstrated. McDonald and Kelley [50a] have now described a patient with all the classical features of the Lesch-Nyhan syndrome in whom erythrocyte hypoxanthine-guanine phosphoribosyl transferase appeared to be inactive under usual assay conditions. However, when the concentrations of both guanine and PP-ribose-P were increased to 10 times those ordinarily used for the assay, the enzyme exhibited nearly normal activity. Further evaluation of the mutant enzyme from this patient indicated that it had markedly altered Michaelis constants for both substrates (Fig. 40-6).

The major disadvantage of erythrocytes as the source for any enzyme is that the enzymes must be relatively stable, since synthesis of new protein does not occur once the erythrocyte has matured. A mutation leading to synthesis of a labile enzyme protein might well result in failure to detect that enzyme in erythrocytes, even though significant quantities might be present in other tissues. The use of tissue obtained at the time of autopsy is subject to the same limitation in that a labile enzyme might be more susceptible to post-mortem degradation.

Several lines of evidence have suggested that low levels of hypoxanthine-guanine phosphoribosyl transferase activity may be present in cultured skin fibroblasts from patients with the Lesch-Nyhan syndrome. (1) Mutant cells cultured in the presence of hypoxanthine-^3H occasionally incorporate large enough quantities of this isotope into nucleic acids for detection by radioautography [51]. (2) Hypoxanthine and guanine in relatively high concentrations appear to inhibit the early steps of *de novo* purine synthesis in these cells, an effect usually considered to require prior synthesis of

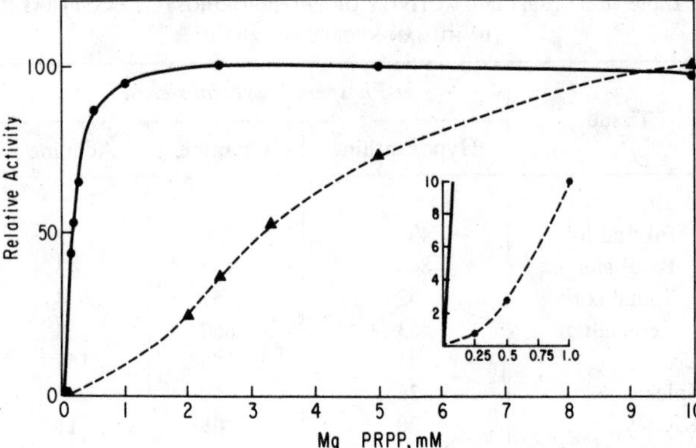

Figure 40-6. Effect of MgPP-ribose-P concentration on GMP synthesis by normal and mutant PRT enzymes. The data are expressed as relative activity (v/v × 100) using the GMP formed at 2.5 × $10^{-3}M$ and 1 × $10^{-2}M$ MgPP-ribose-P as V for the normal (70.2 mμmoles/mg prot/hr) and mutant (6.1 mμmoles/mg prot/hr) enzyme, respectively. Virtually identical results were obtained with hypoxanthine as the fixed substrate. Normal enzyme, .——.; mutant enzyme, — — —. (*From McDonald, J. A., and Kelley, W. N.* [50a]).

inosinic and guanylic acids by hypoxanthine-guanine phosphoribosyl transferase [52]. Fujimoto and Seegmiller [53] and Kelley and Meade [53*a*] have recently reported that low levels of hypoxanthine-guanine phosphoribosyl transferase activity can be demonstrated in extracts of fibroblasts derived from these patients when thymidine triphosphate is added to inhibit the extremely high level of 5′-nucleotidase activity which normally interferes with the assay.

In the four mutant strains studied by Fujimoto and Seegmiller, the hypoxanthine-guanine phosphoribosyl transferase present appeared to be relatively heat labile when compared to the normal enzyme [53]. Kelley and Meade also found that this enzyme from eight of nine mutant strains studied exhibited relative thermolability [53*a*]. However, they also noted that the enzyme from one mutant strain was not subject to product inhibition by IMP and GMP as would be expected. These studies provide evidence that the genetic alteration responsible for the deficiency of hypoxanthine-guanine phosphoribosyl transferase usually (if not always) resides on the structural gene coding for this enzyme. In addition, the latter study provides evidence of substantial heterogeneity of the mutations leading to a deficiency of hypoxanthine-guanine phosphoribosyl transferase (Table 40-6) in the Lesch-Nyhan syndrome.

Table 40-6. GENETIC HETEROGENEITY OF HYPOXANTHINE-GUANINE PHOSPHORIBOSYL TRANSFERASE DEFICIENCY IN FIBROBLASTS DERIVED FROM PATIENTS WITH THE LESCH-NYHAN SYNDROME*

Type	Product inhibition*	Thermal stability*	Prototype (cell strain)
1	+	+	193
2	+	−	182, 197, 198, 199
3	−	−	121

* +, normal; −, abnormal

Source: Kelley, W. N., and Meade, J. C. [53*a*].

Alterations in Adenine Phosphoribosyl Transferase Activity

In addition to the deficiency of hypoxanthine-guanine phosphoribosyl transferase, a substantial increase in the activity of adenine phosphoribosyl transferase has been a constant finding in nearly all patients with the "complete" enzyme defect and the Lesch-Nyhan syndrome [45, 47] (Table 40-3). There has been much interest in the molecular nature of this association, since the two enzymes, although functionally and kinetically similar, appear to represent different proteins which are coded by structural genes from different chromosomes [54, 55]. The increased adenine phosphoribosyl transferase activity in erythrocytes is associated with an increased resistance to thermal inactivation [54]. More recently it has become apparent that although adenine phosphoribosyl transferase activity is elevated in erythrocytes, it is either normal or only slightly elevated in other tissues such as cultured skin fibroblasts from these patients [54, 46, 56]. This suggests that the increased activity is not the result of a genetic alteration but more likely reflects a change in the environment of the erythrocyte.

Balis et al. have recently shown that the half-life of adenine phosphoribosyl transferase is prolonged in erythrocytes obtained from several patients with hypoxanthine-guanine phosphoribosyl transferase deficiency [57]. They suggest that this prolonged half-life accounts for the increased activity. Such a mechanism is consistent with the observation that when the enzyme is increased in activity, it is also more thermostable [54]. Greene et al. have recently demonstrated that PP-ribose-P stabilizes purified adenine phosphoribosyl transferase in vitro and that free PP-ribose-P levels are increased in erythrocytes from patients with increased erythrocyte adenine phosphoribosyl transferase activity [58]. They suggest that increased PP-ribose-P levels stabilize the adenine phosphoribosyl transferase enzyme in vivo and that this leads to a diminished rate of degradation of the enzyme and to an increased specific activity.

Relationship of the Biochemical Abnormalities to Clinical Findings

Pathogenesis of the Uric Acid Overproduction

The excessive production of uric acid characteristic of the Lesch-Nyhan syndrome results from an accelerated rate of *de novo* purine biosynthesis. The demonstration of this is the finding that glycine-^{14}C, an isotopic precursor of *de novo* purine synthesis, is rapidly incorporated into uric acid in these patients (Fig. 40-7) and that the cumulative incorpo-

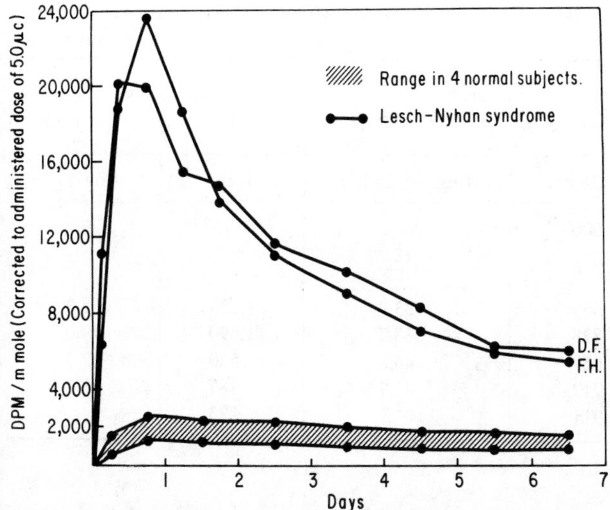

Figure 40-7. A comparison of the incorporation of orally administered glycine-1-^{14}C into urinary uric acid in two patients with the Lesch-Nyhan syndrome and four normal subjects. (*Adapted from Kelley, W. N., et al., Ann. Intern. Med.,* **73**, 583, 1969.)

ration into urinary uric acid over a 7-day period may be as much as 20 times normal (Table 40-6) [1, 23, 59]. The striking increased turnover rate of uric acid which also occurs in these patients is a reflection of this increased uric acid synthesis (Table 40-7).

Hypoxanthine and xanthine, the immediate precursors of uric acid, are readily converted to uric acid by the ample quantities of xanthine oxidase in the liver, so that only a moderate increase in the total urinary excretion of these compounds is observed. In normal persons xanthine is usually excreted in excess of hypoxanthine because of reutilization of hypoxanthine into inosinic acid. In patients with the Lesch-Nyhan syndrome the absence of hypoxanthine-guanine phosphoribosyl transferase is associated with an inability to convert hypoxanthine to inosinic acid and a substantial increase in the excretion of hypoxanthine relative to that of xanthine [60, 61] (Table 40-8).

Increased urinary excretion of another purine derivative, 4-amino imidazole-5-carboxamide, has also been reported in a patient with this syndrome [62]. The exact significance of this finding is difficult to evaluate, since this compound is also elevated in the urine from patients depleted of folic acid [63], and patients with the Lesch-Nyhan syndrome may be deficient in this vitamin [54].

The tissues responsible for excessive production of uric acid are unknown. Although most studies on purine synthesis and its regulation have involved the liver, it is clear that certain other tissues, including human fibroblasts in culture [64], can also synthesize purines *de novo.* In fact, fibroblasts cultured in vitro from patients deficient in hypoxanthine-guanine phosphoribosyl transferase activity exhibit an accelerated rate of *de novo* purine synthesis similar to the observations in vivo [64, 65] (Table 40-9). Although this finding was important in establishing the value of these mutant fibroblasts for studying the regulation of purine synthesis in vitro, there is no evidence that these cells contribute significantly to the excessive purine synthesis observed in vivo.

The capability for *de novo* purine synthesis exists in the central nervous system [66], and indirect evidence suggests that excessive purine synthesis may occur in the brain in patients with the Lesch-Nyhan syndrome. The concentration of hypoxanthine and xanthine in cerebrospinal fluid is four times higher than that observed in normouricemic control patients [46, 67]. In addition, the concentration of these oxypurines in CSF is nearly three times higher than the simultaneous plasma concentration, whereas the normal CSF/plasma ratio is 0.33 [46] (Table 40-10). Although the elevated concentration of oxypurines in the cerebrospinal fluid could be the result of transport from the plasma against a concentration gradient [68, 69], the alternative possibility exists that their increased concentration reflects an accelerated production of purines within the central nervous system. The central nervous system lacks xanthine oxidase activity, so that hypoxanthine and xanthine are not further oxidized to uric acid within this tissue. The concentration of uric acid in the CSF is consistently normal in patients with this syndrome [46].

There are several possible mechanisms by which a deficiency of hypoxanthine-guanine phosphoribosyl transferase could result in excessive purine synthesis. The deficiency of this enzyme, which catalyzes the conversion of guanine to GMP and hypoxanthine to IMP, might accomplish this by virtue of a decreased synthesis of either IMP or GMP, since these nucleotides are normally important inhibitors of *de novo* purine biosynthesis. Attempts to measure intracellular levels of GMP and IMP have been of only limited value, partly because of the very low intracellular concentration of these compounds under normal conditions [64].

An elevated concentration of intracellular PP-ribose-P has been demonstrated in erythrocytes [58, 58a] and in cultured fibroblasts [64] from patients with the Lesch-Nyhan syndrome (Table 40-11). The elevated concentration in fibroblasts has been further shown to be due to decreased utilization of the compound rather than to increased synthesis [64]. An increased concentration of PP-ribose-P could increase *de novo* purine biosynthesis by providing more substrate for the enzyme of the limiting step of this pathway, PP-ribose-P amidotransferase. The increased synthesis of purines observed in patients with Type 1 glycogen storage disease due to a deficiency of glucose-6-phosphatase, has also been attributed on theoretical grounds to an increased concentration of PP-ribose-P [70–72]. In order for an increased concentration of PP-ribose-P to increase purine synthesis *de novo* in either of these conditions, the normal concentration of PP-ribose-P would need to be substantially less than that required for saturation of the enzyme. The intracellular concentration of PP-ribose-P in normal human erythrocytes ranges from 1 to 5 $\times$ $10^{-6}M$ whereas in cultured fibroblasts

Table 40-7. INCORPORATION OF ISOTOPICALLY LABELED URIC ACID AND LESCH-NYHAN

Subject	Reference	Serum urate (mg/100 ml)	*Urinary uric acid*		*Urate pool size*	
			(mg/24 hr)	(mg/kg/24 hr)	(mg)	(mg/kg)
Normal adults	[115]*	<7.0	<600		866–1587	
Normal children	[1, 10]*	3.6 ± 1.2		<18		
Lesch-Nyhan syndrome						
D.F.	[59]	12.4	659	33.9	1,130	58.3
F.H.	[59]	10.0	828	38.7	1,690	79.0
M.W.	[1]	9.9	669	46.8	530	37.1
E.W.	[1]	8.9	712	43.7	787	48.3
S.M.	[116]	7.2	911		833	

* See also Chap. 39.

concentrations as high as $1.3 \times 10^{-5} M$ have been observed [72a]. These values are substantially less than the K_m for the PP-ribose-P amidotransferase in mammalian adenocarcinoma cells [73] (2.3 to $4.7 \times 10^{-4} M$). The Michaelis constants for this enzyme in normal human tissue are not known, and the intracellular concentration of PP-ribose-P in tissues other than the mature erythrocyte and fibroblast has not been established. Recent studies in cultured human fibroblasts as well as in man in vivo have demonstrated that the intracellular concentration of PP-ribose-P has a critical role in the regulation of purine biosynthesis *de novo* (73a, 73b). Therefore, it appears that increased levels of PP-ribose-P are at least partly responsible for the increased rate of purine biosynthesis observed in the Lesch-Nyhan syndrome.

The free bases, hypoxanthine and guanine, produce a modest increase in the rate of *de novo* purine biosynthesis in cultured fibroblasts which lack hypoxanthine-guanine phosphoribosyl transferase [64, 56]. Although the mechanism of this apparent stimulatory effect in the mutant cells has not been elucidated, the stimulation produced is not of sufficient magnitude alone to account for the excessive purine synthesis observed in these mutant fibroblasts.

Table 40-8. OXYPURINE EXCRETION* IN PATIENTS WITH THE LESCH-NYHAN SYNDROME

		Uric acid	Hypoxanthine	Xanthine	H/X
Controls					
Adults (5)	mean	370	1.5	30	0.05
	range	(270–580)	(0.4–3.5)	(13–45)	
Children (4)	mean	670	6	21	0.3
	range	(475–880)	(3.5–9)	(10–33)	
Lesch-Nyhan syndrome					
C.W.		2,500	78	38	2.0
R.K.		2,700	70	28	2.5
V.A.		2,600	90	38	2.4
D.C.		2,800	100	43	2.3

* Values are expressed as mg/gm creatinine. (Adapted from M. E. Balis, I. H. Krakoff, P. H. Berman, and J. Dancis, *Science*, **156**, 1122, 1967.)

Pathogenesis of Central Nervous System Disease

Patients with the Lesch-Nyhan syndrome share certain devastating neurologic and behavioral abnormalities which are almost unique. Patients with a partial deficiency of the same enzyme, however, have only mild, if any, neurologic involvement [54]. These findings suggest that this characteristic neurologic syndrome is somehow related to the severe deficiency of hypoxanthine-guanine phosphoribosyl transferase.

Early studies suggested that the disease might be directly related to the presence of hyperuricemia. This is clearly not the case since (1) these children are not always hyperuricemic and (2) hyperuricemia observed in other conditions is not associated with neurologic findings. The concentration of uric acid has been repeatedly normal in the cerebrospinal fluid of these patients.

The finding of a high concentration of the oxypurines,

GLYCINE INTO URINARY URIC ACID IN PATIENTS WITH THE SYNDROME

Turnover rate (pools/day)	Turnover		Turnover excreted	7-day recovery of isotope into urinary uric acid		
				Administered uric acid	*Administered glycine*	
	(mg/day)	(mg/kg/day)			(uncorrected)	(corrected)
0.45–0.85	513–1108		55–76	57–77	<0.22 <0.15	<0.30
1.02	1,150	59.4	58	61	2.49	4.29
0.98	1,650	77.1	50	54	3.16	6.08
2.06	1,090	76.2	61		2.37	3.89
1.61	1,270	77.9	56		2.05	3.66
1.55	1,294		70	71	3.67	5.19

hypoxanthine and xanthine, seemed particularly pertinent, since the administration of caffeine, a methylated xanthine, will lead to self-mutilation in rats [74]. The finding of a similarly elevated concentration of oxypurines in four patients with a partial deficiency of hypoxanthine-guanine phosphoribosyl transferase, including two with no evidence of central nervous system disease, suggests that these compounds themselves are not the cause of the central nervous system disease [54].

Observations in man [46] and in the Rhesus monkey [75] that hypoxanthine-guanine phosphoribosyl transferase activity is normally higher in the central nervous system than in any other tissue and that the activity of PP-ribose-P amidotransferase, the rate-limiting step in the *de novo* pathway, is normally lower in this tissue [66], suggest that the brain may be unusually dependent on this salvage pathway for the synthesis of IMP and GMP. The possibility exists, therefore, that in the absence of hypoxanthine-guanine phosphoribosyl transferase, the central nervous system may be unable to maintain an intracellular concentration of GMP or IMP necessary for normal function. The necessity for synthesis of these purine nucleotides entirely from the *de novo* pathway in the absence of hypoxanthine-guanine phosphoribosyl transferase may lead to depletion of certain cofactors such as ATP or folic acid which could also limit normal function. The suggestion has also been made that there may be deficiencies of amino acids, particularly of glutamine, secondary to increased utilization in purine biosynthesis and poor protein intake [74a]. There are no data currently available which would allow further consideration of these possibilities.

Table 40-9. PURINE BIOSYNTHESIS DE NOVO IN FIBROBLASTS LACKING HYPOXANTHINE-GUANINE PHOSPHORIBOSYL TRANSFERASE ACTIVITY

Cells	*Source*		FGAR* (cpm)
	Sex	Age (years)	
Normal			
R.S.	Male	23	1,710
G.C.	Male	21	1,980
W.M.	Male	17	1,870
G.R.	Female	15	1,380
Hypoxanthine-guanine phosphoribosyl transferase deficient			
D.F.	Male	15	7,320
F.H.	Male	15	8,060
M.W.	Male	8	7,100
J.S.	Male	3	7,310

*Formylglycinamide ribonucleotide. See Fig. 40-3.

Note: Fibroblasts (8 mg, wet weight) derived from four normal individuals and from four patients lacking hypoxanthine-guanine phosphoribosyl transferase activity were incubated in Krebs'-Ringer-phosphate medium, pH 7.4, in an air atmosphere for 1 hr at 37°C with 4 mM glycine, 20 mM L-glutamine, 5.5 mM glucose, 0.3 mM azaserine, and 1.52 mM formate-^{14}C.

Source: F. M. Rosenbloom et al. [64].

Megaloblastic Anemia

Several patients with megaloblastic changes in the bone marrow and macrocytic erythrocytes have had a low serum folate concentration [54]. It has been demonstrated in fibroblasts derived from similar individuals that there is an increased growth requirement for adenine which can be overcome by high concentrations of folic acid [76]. These findings suggest that the accelerated rate of *de novo* purine synthesis leads to an increased utilization of folate, an essential cofactor at two sites in the *de novo* pathway. Adenine is readily converted to AMP and then to IMP. These purine nucleotides inhibit PP-ribose-P amidotransferase and thereby reduce the rate of *de novo* synthesis, and presumably the rate of folate utilization. It is not known whether the deficiency of folate observed *in vivo* is due to its increased utilization or in fact is even related to the anemia. The

Table 40-10. OXYPURINE AND URIC ACID CONCENTRATION IN PLASMA AND CEREBROSPINAL FLUID (mg/100 ml)

Subject*	Uric acid			Oxypurines†		
	CSF	Plasma	CSF/plasma	CSF	Plasma	CSF/plasma
Control (7)	0.29	4.3	0.07	0.13	0.18	0.72
Complete PRT deficiency (5)	0.32	8.2	0.04	0.55	0.20	2.75
Partial PRT deficiency (4)						
F.L.	1.25	14.1	0.09	0.32	0.12	2.56
M.L.	0.39	9.8	0.04	0.45	0.15	3.02
T.J.	0.72	7.5	0.10	0.44	0.19	2.32
C.M.	1.25	10.9	0.11	0.23	—	—

* PRT, hypoxanthine-guanine phosphoribosyl transferase.
† Hypoxanthine and xanthine.
Source: W. N. Kelley et al. Hypoxanthine-guanine phosphoribosyl transferase deficiency in gout, Ann. Intern. Med., **70,** 155, 1969.

finding by Van Der Zee et al. that the megaloblastic anemia in their patient failed to respond to exogenous folate but did respond to adenine indicates that additional factors may be important in vivo [77] (Fig. 40-8).

GENETICS

The familial nature of this syndrome was recognized in the original report by Lesch and Nyhan [1]. The patients have not had any particular ethnic background. Although most patients are Caucasian, the disease has been described in at least five Oriental and two Negro families.

Major clinical manifestations only occur in affected males, and transmission is through carrier females. In all large pedigrees the pattern of inheritance has been consistent with either an X-linked or sex-limited mode of transmission [78, 79] (Figs. 40-9 and 40-10). The absence of male-to-male transmission, a critical test of X-linked inheritance, cannot be evaluated because patients with the Lesch-Nyhan syndrome do not reproduce. The finding of patients with a partial deficiency of the same enzyme was particularly valuable in this regard, since they have a milder disease and do reproduce. No male-to-male transmission of the defect has been observed in this latter group [54], and this is consistent with the enzyme being coded by DNA on the X chromosome. X-linked inheritance would also account for the absence of parental consanguinity in spite of the rarity of the disease.

It has been possible, using fibroblasts in culture, to demonstrate that obligate heterozygotes for the severe enzyme defect are mosaics in terms of hypoxanthine-guanine phosphoribosyl transferase activity. Using an autoradiographic technique, 60 percent of the cells from an obligate heterozygote appeared to have normal activity, whereas the remaining 40 percent had no detectable activity [80] (Figs. 40-11 and 40-12). The two cell populations have also been separated by cloning techniques and selective chemical treatment [81, 82, 82a]. These findings provide substantial support for the X-linked mode of inheritance and are consistent with the Lyon hypothesis [83].

Several observations indicate that heterozygotes for a deficiency of hypoxanthine-guanine phosphoribosyl transferase exhibit certain subtle biochemical abnormalities in vivo, although they are generally asymptomatic clinically. An elevated serum urate concentration has been detected in at least three such patients [54], and one patient has had recurrent monoarticular arthritis thought clinically to be gout. In addition, several obligate heterozygotes have excreted greater than normal quantities of uric acid in their urine [13, 78]. Bland et al. have reported three obligate heterozygotes with histories of renal calculi. The chemical nature of the stones was not known [84]. It has been suggested that the increased excretion of uric acid may be a reflection of a higher than normal conversion of dietary

Table 40-11. PP-RIBOSE-P CONCENTRATIONS IN NORMAL FIBROBLASTS AND FIBROBLASTS DEFICIENT IN HYPOXANTHINE-GUANINE PHOSPHORIBOSYL TRANSFERASE

	A. PP-Ribose-P, mμmoles/gm	*B.* Adenine nucleotide synthesis, mμmoles/gm
Normal	0.85	4.02
Deficient in hypoxanthine-guanine phosphoribosyl transferase	3.59	4.16

Note: Normal fibroblasts and fibroblasts deficient in hypoxanthine-guanine phosphoribosyl transferase were incubated with 5.5 mM glucose (Part *A*), or with 5.5 mM glucose and 0.5 mM adenine-^{3}H (Part *B*). Fibroblasts of 16 mg wet weight were used.
Source: F. M. Rosenbloom et al. [64].

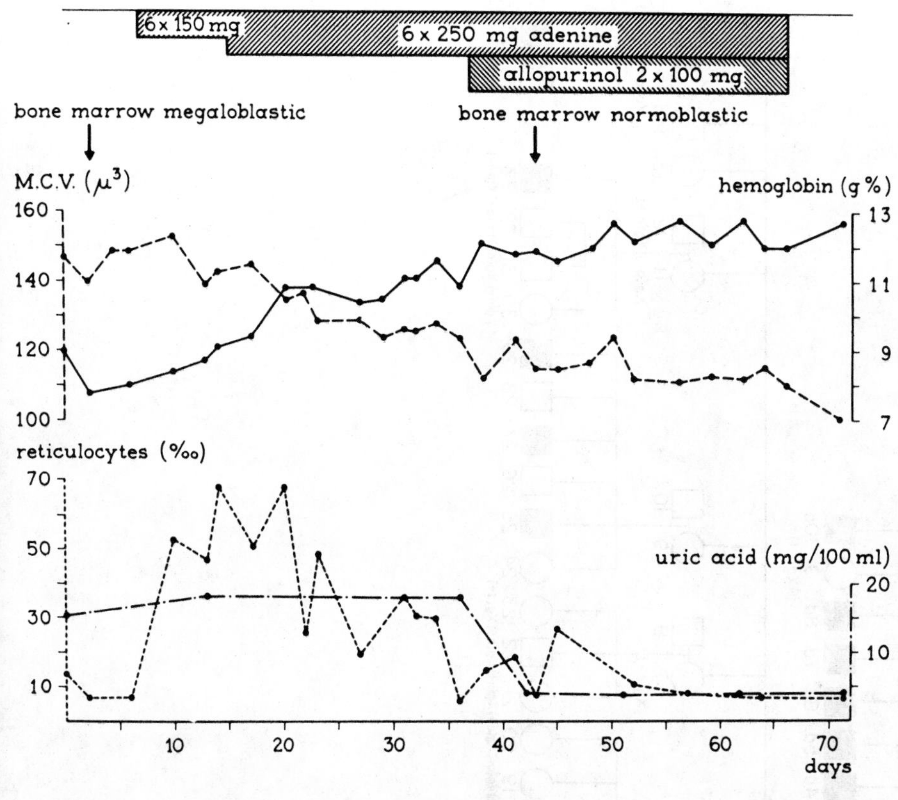

Figure 40-8. Response of megaloblastic anemia and serum urate concentration to the administration of adenine and allopurinol. (*From Van Der Zee, S. P. M., et al., Lancet,* **1,** 1427, 1968.)

purines to uric acid [79]. While this may be true, studies on the incorporation of glycine-1-^{14}C into uric acid in five heterozygous individuals have demonstrated that there is also a moderate increase in the rate of *de novo* purine synthesis [54, 85].

Obligate heterozygotes cannot be reliably detected by assay of the enzyme in erythrocyte lysates, since in most cases enzyme activity has been within the normal range [47, 85, 86] (Table 40-12). In addition, several studies have shown both indirectly [86a] and directly [86b] that the mutant enzyme is not present in circulating erythrocytes from proven heterozygotes. This suggests that either the X chromosome coding for the mutant enzyme in erythropoietic precursors is preferentially inactivated or that the erythropoietic cells lacking the enzyme are unable to proliferate. Efforts to detect mosaicism in circulating lymphocytes have also been unsuccessful [86].

At the present time cultured fibroblasts seem to provide the most reliable method for detection of mutants heterozygous for this enzyme defect. Tissue for culture can be readily obtained by skin biopsy or even by amniocentesis. The culture of cells obtained from amniotic fluid has allowed the heterozygous as well as the hemizygous state to be diagnosed in utero [87, 88]. Although this technique is not suitable for routine screening, it should prove useful for genetic counseling in specific circumstances. Assay of hair follicles provides a promising new approach to the detection of heterozygotes for this enzyme defect [88*a*].

Since hypoxanthine-guanine phosphoribosyl transferase is coded by DNA on the X chromosome, this marker provides another locus which might prove useful in mapping the X chromosome in man. Initial studies suggested that the PRT locus might be relatively close to the Xga locus, but recent data involving a large number of patients have failed to demonstrate measurable linkage [54]. So far, no families of patients with the Lesch-Nyhan syndrome with multiple marker alleles at another locus on the X chromosome have been studied in detail.

Pharmocogenetics

In addition to the naturally occurring substrates for hypoxanthine-guanine phosphoribosyl transferase, including hypoxanthine, guanine, and xanthine, a number of purine analogues are converted to their nucleotide derivatives by this enzyme. Several of these analogues, 6-mercaptopurine and its nitroimidazole derivative, azathioprine, 8-azaguanine, and allopurinol, are used clinically. The deficiency of hypoxanthine-guanine phosphoribosyl transferase in patients with the Lesch-Nyhan syndrome is associated with an altered response to certain effects of these drugs both in vivo and in vitro.

The administration of azathioprine to patients with normal hypoxanthine-guanine phosphoribosyl transferase activity leads to a striking reduction in *de novo* purine synthesis that

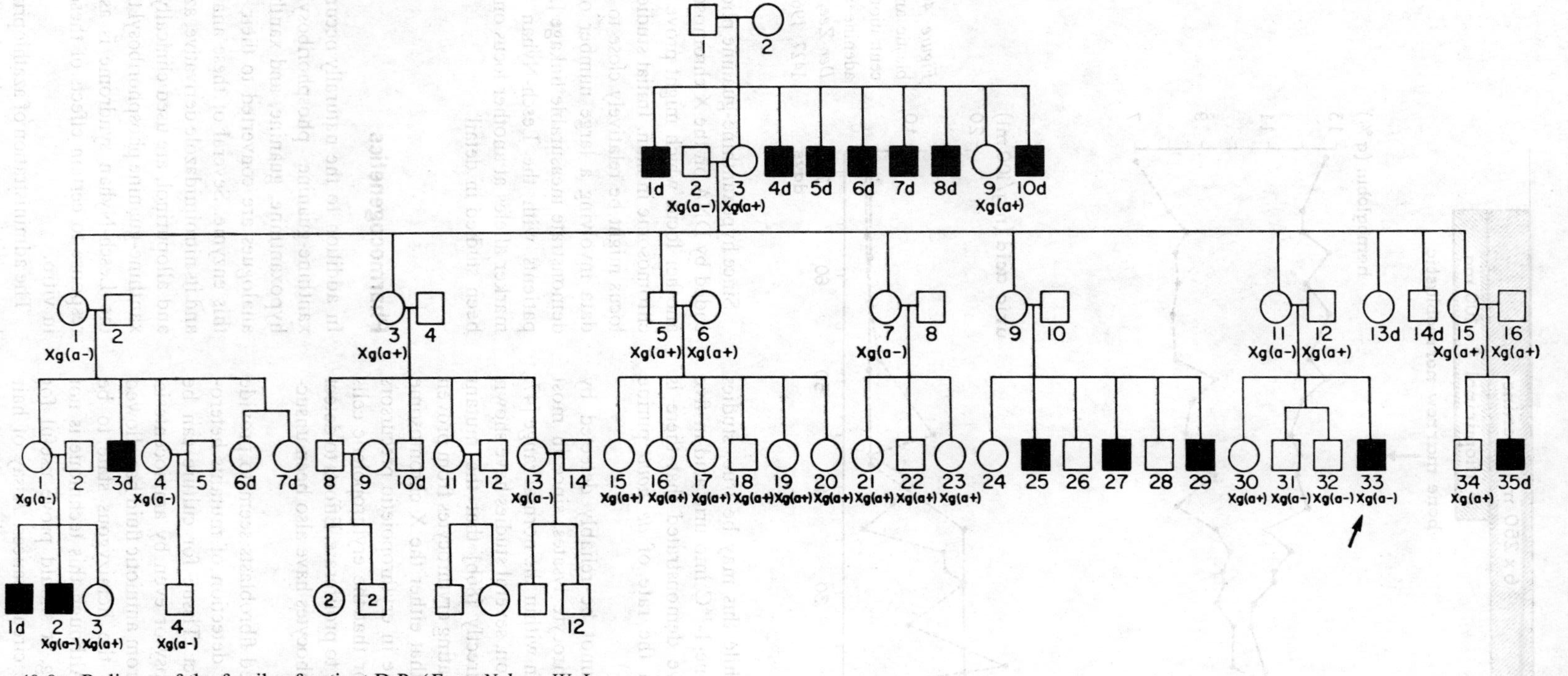

Figure 40-9. Pedigree of the family of patient D.B. (*From Nyhan, W. L., Fed. Proc.,* **27**, 1091, 1968.)

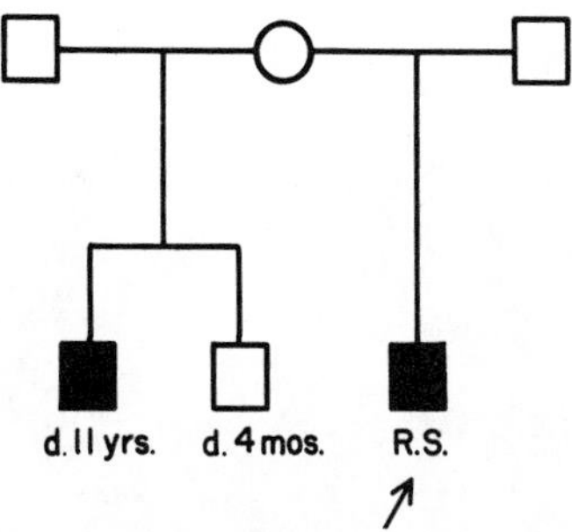

Figure 40-10. Pedigree of the family of patient R.S. suggesting X-linked inheritance. (*From Nyhan, W. L., Fed. Proc.,* **27,** 1091, 1968.)

is often accompanied by a decrease in both the serum and urinary uric acid (Fig. 40-13). This is presumably due to the conversion of azathioprine to 6-mercaptopurine, which is then converted to its ribonucleotide by hypoxanthine-guanine phosphoribosyl transferase. The ribonucleotide derivative of 6-mercaptopurine, but not the free base, is a

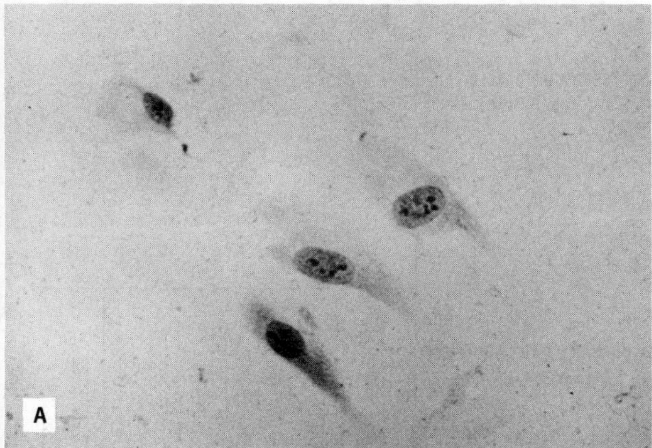

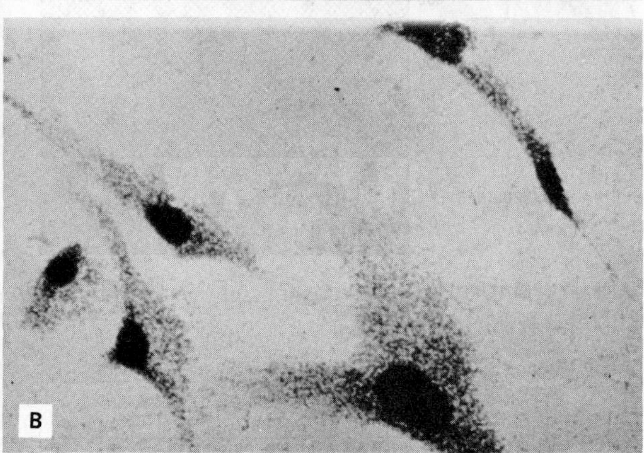

Figure 40-11. Radioautographs of fibroblasts from an affected child incubated with (A) ^{3}H-hypoxanthine and (B) ^{3}H-adenine. Black granules throughout the nucleus and cytoplasm show distribution of tritiated purine base incorporated into trichloroacetic acid precipitable RNA. (*Courtesy of Dr. F. M. Rosenbloom.*)

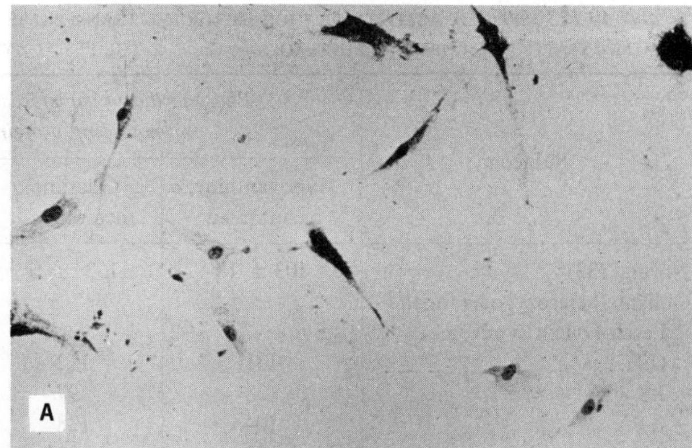

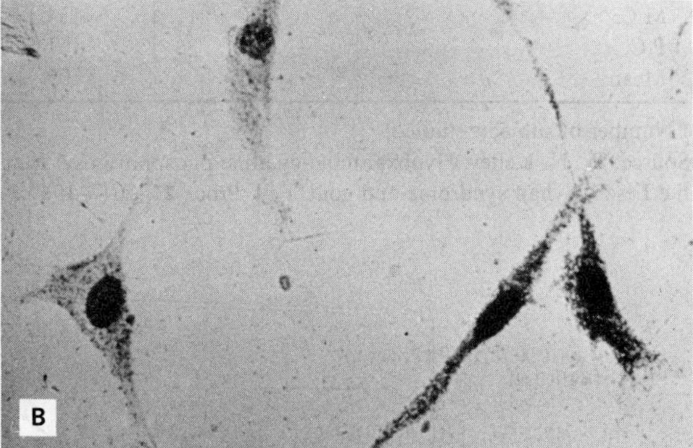

Figure 40-12. Radioautographs of fibroblasts from an obligate heterozygote incubated with ^{3}H-hypoxanthine, demonstrating the presence of two cell populations. (A) $\times 160$. (B) $\times 400$. (*Courtesy of Dr. F. M. Rosenbloom.*)

potent inhibitor of PP-ribose-P amidotransferase, the rate-limiting step in the *de novo* pathway [89]. In patients lacking hypoxanthine-guanine phosphoribosyl transferase, azathioprine has no effect on the *de novo* synthesis of purines [59, 90, 91] (Fig. 40-14). In addition, absence of this enzyme in lymphocytes obtained from these patients is associated with a loss of the ability of azathioprine to suppress phytohemagglutinin-induced transformation of these cells as measured by incorporation of tritiated thymidine into DNA [92]. Resistance to the potential inhibitory effects of 6-mercaptopurine on *de novo* purine synthesis has also been demonstrated in cultured fibroblasts derived from these patients [45].

The effects of administration of allopurinol to patients lacking hypoxanthine-guanine phosphoribosyl transferase differ in several distinctive ways from its effects in normal subjects. In patients with the Lesch-Nyhan syndrome, (1) allopurinol does not have its usual inhibitory effect on purine biosynthesis *de novo* [93–95], (2) allopurinol does not deplete erythrocyte PP-ribose-P (95a), (3) a normally occurring ribonucleoside derivative of allopurinol does not appear in the urine [67]; and (4) the drug appears to produce an even more striking inhibitory effect on xanthine oxidase [54]. All

Table 40-12. SPECIFIC ACTIVITY OF PHOSPHORIBOSYL TRANSFERASE OF ERYTHROCYTE HEMOLYSATES FROM OBLIGATE HETEROZYGOTES FOR THE LESCH-NYHAN SYNDROME

Subjects	*Phosphoribosyl transferase activity, mμmoles/mg protein/hr*		
	Hypoxanthine, mean ± s.d.	Guanine, mean ± s.d.	Adenine, mean ± s.d.
Normal (32)*	103 ± 18	103 ± 21	31 ± 6
Obligate heterozygotes for the Lesch-Nyhan syndrome			
O.H.	131	112	46
J.S.	58	97	35
L.F.	104	128	25
S.G.	71	82	19
M.C.	130	134	54
P.C.	110	101	48
Mean	101	109	38

* Number of subjects studied.
Source: W. N. Kelley, Hypoxanthine-guanine phosphoribosyl transferase deficiency in the Lesch-Nyhan syndrome and gout, Fed. Proc., **27**, 1047, 1967.

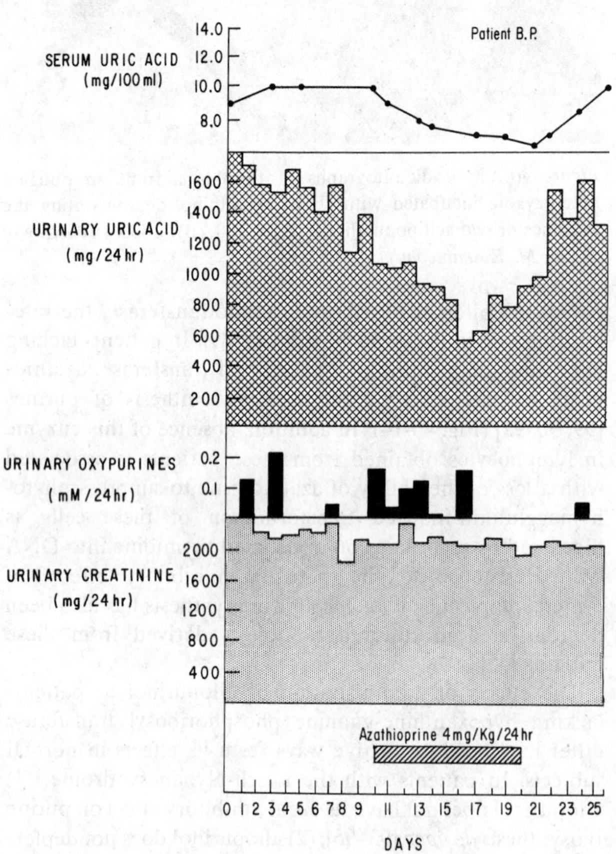

Figure 40-13. The effect of azathioprine treatment on the serum urate and 24-hr urinary uric acid excretion of a gouty patient who produces excessive quantities of uric acid. (*From Kelley, W. N., et al., J. Clin. Invest.,* **46,** 1518, 1967.)

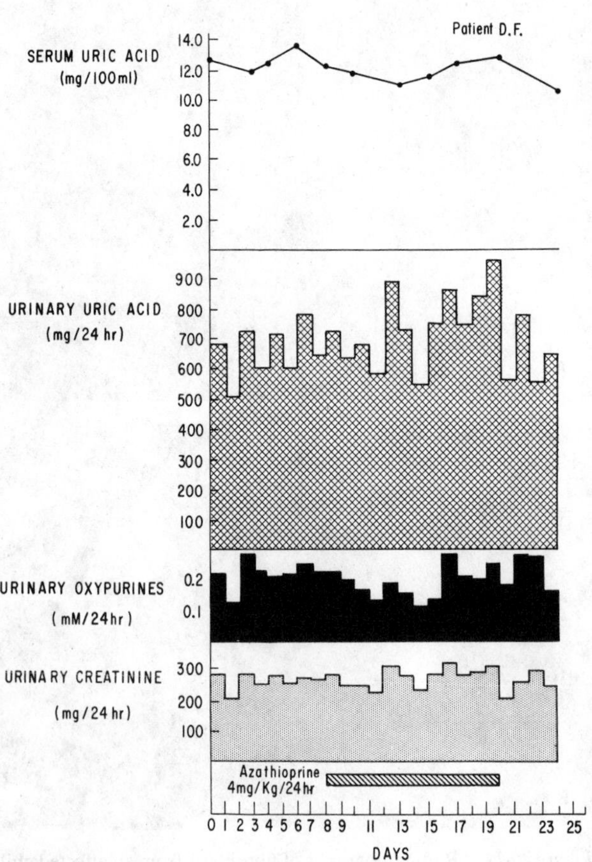

Figure 40-14. The effect of azathioprine treatment on the serum urate and 24-hr urinary uric acid excretion of a patient with the Lesch-Nyhan syndrome. (*From Kelley, W. N., et al., J. Clin. Invest.,* **46,** 1518, 1967.)

these observations can readily be attributed to the deficiency of hypoxanthine-guanine phosphoribosyl transferase.

In most patients the decrease in uric acid excretion produced by allopurinol is not accompanied by a stoichiometric increase in the excretion of the immediate precursors of uric acid, hypoxanthine, and xanthine. This decrease in total purine excretion is due to a decrease in the rate of purine synthesis [96]. Although the exact mechanism of this effect is not clear, several possibilities have been considered. These include (1) an increased conversion of hypoxanthine to IMP as an indirect result of the inhibition of xanthine oxidase, (2) the conversion of allopurinol to its ribonucleotide, or (3) a depletion of intracellular PP-ribose-P as a result of either mechanism 1 or 2 (Fig. 40-15). Both IMP and allopurinol ribonucleotide are inhibitors of PP-ribose-P amidotransferase, whereas the free bases are not; therefore, an increase in their formation would lead to a decrease in *de novo* purine biosynthesis. In addition, PP-ribose-P is an essential and rate-limiting substrate for this reaction: a decrease in its concentration would also decrease purine synthesis (95a). Since each of these possible inhibitory mechanisms depends on the presence of hypoxanthine-guanine phosphoribosyl transferase, it is logical that allopurinol has no inhibitory effect on the *de novo* synthesis of purines in patients lacking this enzyme. The failure of allopurinol to inhibit *de novo* purine synthesis in these patients results in a striking increase in the excretion of hypoxanthine and xanthine which roughly equals the decrease in uric acid formation. Although hypoxanthine usually predominates in the urine under these conditions, the excretion of xanthine can be high enough to exceed solubility levels. In fact, two of the three patients who have been reported to have developed xanthine stones while on allopurinol have been patients with this enzyme defect [97, 98].

The major catabolic products of allopurinol found in urine of normal subjects are oxipurinol and allopurinol ribonucleoside [99, 100] (Fig. 39-15). Allopurinol is rapidly converted to oxipurinol by xanthine oxidase [99], although some of the latter compound may be formed in vivo by another mechanism [101]. The origin of allopurinol ribonucleoside in the urine is less clear. This compound may result from the conversion of allopurinol to its ribonucleotide by hypoxanthine-guanine phosphoribosyl transferase, with subsequent degradation to the ribonucleoside derivative by an enzyme with nucleotidase activity. This ribonucleoside derivative would be able to cross cell membranes and, therefore, appear in the urine, whereas this would probably not be the case for a ribonucleotide derivative. The observation that patients lacking hypoxanthine-guanine phosphoribosyl transferase do not excrete the ribonucleoside derivative in their urine when given allopurinol is consistent with the hypothesis that this compound is derived from the ribonucleotide. The ribonucleoside derivative may also be formed directly from allopurinol by the action of a purine ribonucleoside phosphorylase [102]. If this were an important source of the ribonucleoside in man, however, its absence in the urine from hypoxanthine-guanine phosphoribosyl transferase–deficient individuals would have to be attributed to some less-direct mechanism, such as saturation of the phosphorylase enzyme by the higher levels of hypoxanthine.

Patients lacking hypoxanthine-guanine phosphoribosyl transferase appear to be somewhat more sensitive to the inhibitory effect of allopurinol on xanthine oxidase than is the normal person [54] (Fig. 40-16). This may be because of failure of allopurinol to be catabolized to its ribonucleoside derivative, leaving more of the free bases allopurinol and oxipurinol to inhibit xanthine oxidase. The serum urate concentration also tends to drop faster once xanthine

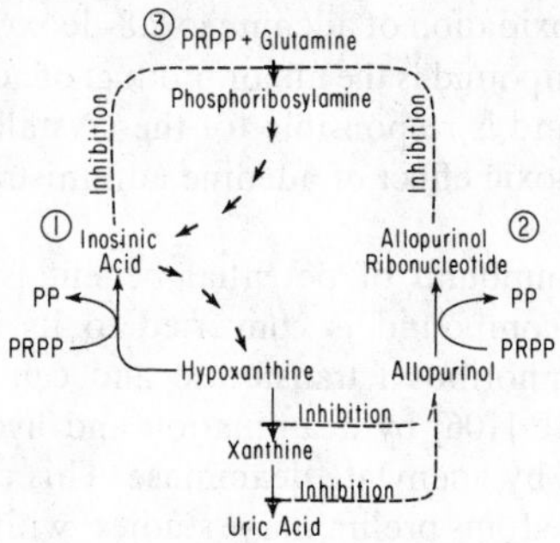

Figure 40-15. Possible mechanisms to account for the inhibitory effect of allopurinol on *de novo* purine synthesis. These include (1) an increased conversion of hypoxanthine to inosinic acid, (2) a direct conversion of allopurinol to its ribonucleotide, and (3) a depletion of intracellular P-ribose-PP.

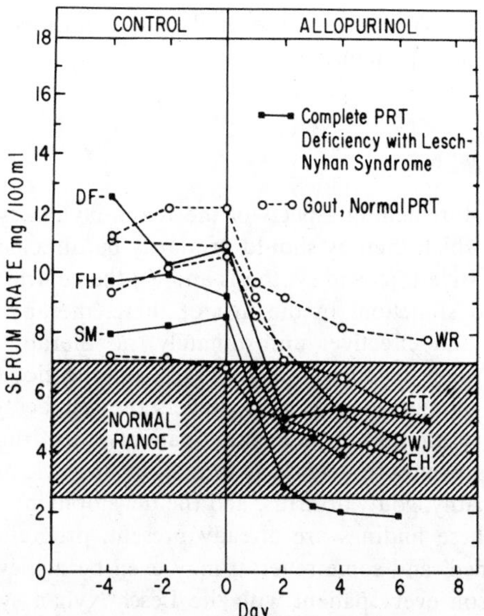

Figure. 40-16. The effect of allopurinol administration on the concentration of urate in serum of hyperuricemic patients. Comparison of effects in patients with the Lesch-Nyhan syndrome and patients with normal hypoxanthine-guanine phosphoribosyl transferase activity. (*Adapted from Kelley, W. N., et al., Ann. Intern. Med.,* **70,** 155, 1969.)

oxidase is inhibited because of the rapid turnover of uric acid in these patients.

TREATMENT

The life-threatening aspects of the Lesch-Nyhan syndrome toward which therapy should primarily be directed are (1) the excessive uric acid synthesis and (2) the central nervous system dysfunction. In the first of these, therapy is well-defined and effective; unfortunately, no therapy has yet proved to be beneficial for the latter complication.

Since allopurinol effectively lowers the uric acid content of both serum and urine in these patients, this drug can be used to prevent uric acid stone formation, uric acid and urate nephropathy, gouty arthritis, and the development of tophi. When these findings are already present, progression can be stopped, and some reversal may even be achieved. For this reason every patient with the Lesch-Nyhan syndrome should be treated with allopurinol. Uricosuric therapy probably should not be used unless allopurinol is also being administered because of the extremely large load of uric acid already being presented to the kidney. In most patients without tophi, allopurinol alone will be adequate to maintain a normal serum urate concentration, and uricosurics will not be needed. The possibility of xanthine stone formation during allopurinol treatment exists but can be minimized by increasing urine flow. This potential complication should not deter the use of allopurinol in this disease. Allopurinol has not been shown to affect the progression of central nervous system dysfunction in either a beneficial or detrimental manner, although only a few patients with this syndrome have been treated with allopurinol from birth.

Approaches toward prevention or correction of the central nervous system dysfunction remain experimental. Since these children have no apparent abnormalities in central nervous system function at birth and because no distinctive pathologic changes are noted at post-mortem examination, it seems possible that this aspect of the disease may be preventable or treatable. Several major problems continue to plague this area of investigation. First, the pathogenesis of the disease remains unclear. Secondly, there are few dependable and objective methods of evaluating subtle changes in neurologic function in these patients. Finally, the patients seem to improve generally when they begin to receive the care and attention associated with hospitalization. This is particularly true when they are transferred from the environment of a large institution to a clinical research facility. Evaluation of the results of therapy should consider these latter two factors before conclusions are drawn.

A major experimental approach in treating the central nervous system dysfunction has been directed toward replacing the presumed but undocumented deficiency of either GMP or IMP. The administration of GMP or AMP has been tried without evidence of clinical improvement [11]. This might be anticipated, since these purine nucleotides cross cell membranes poorly if at all. Guanosine has been tried with the hope that it would be converted to GMP by guanosine kinase [54]. Failure to find evidence of an inhibitory effect of guanosine on *de novo* purine biosynthesis in one patient with this disorder provides indirect evidence that significant quantities of GMP were not formed. The patient did not improve clinically. In one patient, the oral administration of inosine (20 to 40 mg per kg per day) produced no change in uric acid excretion [9]. Since inosine is converted to uric acid, this finding suggests that the compound must have inhibited *de novo* purine synthesis to some degree. Since inosine itself is not an effective inhibitor of purine synthesis but requires conversion to IMP in order to effect inhibition, this observation implies that inosine somehow increased the intracellular concentration of IMP. No clinical improvement was described in this patient during the course of these studies. The free bases hypoxanthine or guanine would not be effective, since they cannot be converted to their nucleotides in the absence of hypoxanthine-guanine phosphoribosyl transferase.

Adenine may be a reasonable therapeutic agent for several reasons. Adenine is readily converted to AMP by adenine phosphoribosyl transferase, and might then increase IMP or GMP levels by (1) its direct conversion to IMP and GMP through the purine interconversion pathway or (2) by inhibiting the 5′nucleotidase responsible for the catabolism of IMP and GMP. In addition, the formation of AMP itself should lead to inhibition of *de novo* purine synthesis. Because of these theoretical considerations and the observation that exogenous adenine is required for the normal growth of fibroblasts derived from patients deficient in hypoxanthine-guanine phosphoribosyl transferase, several patients have been treated from birth with adenine [103, 104]. It is too early at this time to state with certainty what the outcome of these studies will be. One 9-year-old patient was treated with 1,500 mg adenine daily for nearly 2 months [77]; although this produced a striking improvement in his megaloblastic anemia, no changes in neurological behavior were noted [104*a*]. The potential beneficial effects of adenine might even be enhanced with allopurinol, since xanthine oxidase catalyzes the oxidation of adenine to 2,8-deoxyadenine [105]. This latter compound is the major product of adenine catabolism in man and is responsible for the crystalluria observed as the major toxic effect of adenine administration in lower animals.

Another compound of potential benefit is 2,6-diaminopurine. This compound is converted to its nucleotide by adenine phosphoribosyl transferase and can then be converted to GMP [106] by deamination and hydroxylation at the 6 position by adenylate deaminase. This compound has also been used in preliminary studies without apparent benefit [9].

Since several patients have been depleted of folate and since the apparent adenine requirement of cultured fibroblasts can be replaced with high concentrations of folate, it seems reasonable to determine whether folic acid is of any benefit in vivo. Several patients are now being treated in this way, but it is not yet possible to determine what beneficial effects, if any, this treatment has had [103].

In one instance, low plasma levels of glutamine were observed, and were returned to normal on a regimen of glutamate supplementation which led to improved appetite and increased protein intake. The suggestion was made that behavior improved on this regimen, but additional studies are needed to determine whether improvement was attributable to nutritional factors or to supportive measures, such as padding and restraining of hands and exemplary nursing care [75a].

Approaches to therapy have so far been directed almost entirely at correcting possible consequences of the enzyme defect. It may be possible in the future to design means for increasing the in vivo levels of enzyme activity. The discovery, in a patient with the Lesch-Nyhan syndrome, of a mutant form of hypoxanthine-guanine phosphoribosyl transferase which exhibits normal activity at high concentrations of substrates PP-ribose-P and hypoxanthine suggests that attempts to elevate the intracellular levels of these compounds might be beneficial in some patients (50a). Since patients with low levels of functioning enzyme in vivo have little if any neurologic disease, one might reason that such an approach would be helpful in preventing the neurologic dysfunction even if only minimal enzymatic activity could be achieved in vivo. Initial studies are now proceeding in a number of laboratories using cultured fibroblasts as a model system to test possibilities which might be of therapeutic benefit. These possibilities include induction or stabilization of the mutant enzyme by chemical agents or even by viral transformation. Perhaps fibroblasts themselves could be used as a source of enzyme if conditions were such that they could survive in vivo.

VARIANTS AND PHENOCOPIES

A number of patients have been described who are hyperuricemic and produce excessive quantities of uric acid but have a low level of hypoxanthine-guanine phosphoribosyl transferase activity at usual concentrations of substrates rather than a complete deficiency of the enzyme in their erythrocytes [107, 54] (see Chap. 39). These patients usually have gouty arthritis or uric acid calculi but do not have the devastating neurologic and behavioral features characteristic of the Lesch-Nyhan syndrome. Several of the patients with the partial enzyme defect have had some findings related to the central nervous system which suggest a *forme fruste* relationship to the classic Lesch-Nyhan syndrome. These include choreoathetosis, mental retardation, and spasticity. Several of the patients with the incomplete Lesch-Nyhan syndrome reported in the literature probably have the partial rather than the complete enzyme defect. It will be important to assay hypoxanthine-guanine phosphoribosyl transferase activity and to determine kinetic constants in all patients suspected of being deficient in the enzyme. The finding of a low level of enzyme activity with normal kinetic constants in erythrocytes may be of significant prognostic value, especially in the young patient.

Nyhan et al. have recently reported a 3-year-old boy who exhibited excessive purine synthesis and hyperuricemia in addition to mental retardation, dysplastic teeth, absence of tears on crying, absence of speech, and unusual autistic behavior [108]. This patient did not appear to have the Lesch-Nyhan syndrome, because erythrocyte hypoxanthine-guanine phosphoribosyl transferase activity was normal and there was no self-mutilation or choreoathetosis. If the kinetic constants for the hypoxanthine-guanine phosphoribosyl transferase from this patient are normal then he may represent another inborn error of purine metabolism associated with abnormal behavior. Perhaps the increased level of erythrocyte adenine phosphoribosyl transferase activity in this patient will provide some insight into the possible molecular abnormality.

Hooft et al. have studied a young girl with delayed psychomotor development, mutilation of fingers and buccal mucosa, choreoathetosis, episodes of opisthotonos, and generalized spasticity [109]. In spite of a repeatedly normal serum urate concentration (3.5 to 5.0 mg per 100 ml) excessive purine synthesis was clearly present, as evident in the excretion of 35.0 to 45.0 mg uric acid per kg body weight and the incorporation of 1.7 percent of an intravenously administered dose of glycine-^{14}C into urinary uric acid in 7 days. Both parents were normal clinically. This patient therefore has most of the classic features of the Lesch-Nyhan syndrome, except that by both clinical and chromosomal analysis she is female. Several other less striking differences are also apparent. These include (1) the occurrence of parental consanguinity, (2) a relatively delayed peak in the incorporation of isotopic glycine into urinary uric acid, (3) marked improvement with allopurinol therapy to the point that she was able to walk, and (4) persistent normouricemia in absence of hypouricemic agents. Speculation on the nature and significance of the findings in this exciting patient must await additional biochemical information, such as the determination of hypoxanthine-guanine phosphoribosyl transferase activity.

Bazelon et al. have recently described three females with hyperuricemia, mental retardation, and mutilation of the lips and hands [110]. These patients differ significantly from patients with the Lesch-Nyhan syndrome in that the urinary excretion of uric acid is normal, erythrocyte hypoxanthine-guanine phosphoribosyl transferase activity is normal, and there is no choreoathetosis, spasticity, or severe growth retardation.

It is not surprising that other patients are being described who exhibit some degree of neurologic disease and hyperuricemia [111], since the latter finding occurs with a relatively high frequency in the general population [112]. An increased excretion of uric acid will no doubt prove to be a much more significant finding than an elevated serum urate concentration when associated with one of the types of neurologic or behavioral disorders described here.

SUMMARY

1 The Lesch-Nyhan syndrome is an inherited disorder associated with a deficiency of an enzyme of purine metabolism, hypoxanthine-guanine phosphoribosyl transferase. The disease is characterized by the excessive production of uric acid and certain characteristic neurologic features, including self-mutilation, choreoathetosis, spasticity, and mental retardation.

2 The abnormalities of purine metabolism are present at birth and may lead to hyperuricemia, uric acid crystalluria, and stone formation early in life. Other direct complications of the purine overproduction and hyperuricemia, such as gouty arthritis, tophaceous deposits, and monosodium urate deposits within the kidney, may not develop for many years.

3 At birth the patients generally have no apparent central nervous system dysfunction. Beginning at about 3 to 4 months of age, developmental retardation is usually apparent, and by the age of 2 years, they usually have the other neurologic manifestations of the syndrome. No characteristic pathologic changes have been noted in the central nervous system at the time of autopsy.

4 Deficiency of hypoxanthine-guanine phosphoribosyl transferase is generalized to all tissues in patients with this syndrome. Although in most patients no trace of enzyme activity has been detected in erythrocytes, in one patient a mutant enzyme has been described which is active at high substrate concentrations and which has quantitatively and qualitatively altered kinetic properties. Despite the "complete" absence of detectable enzyme activity in erythrocytes in most patients, fibroblasts cultured from these patients have low levels of activity. Further evaluation of the hypoxanthine-guanine phosphoribosyl transferase enzyme in these mutant cells indicates that the mutations leading to the enzyme defect are on the structural gene coding for the enzyme and that there is considerable genetic heterogeneity within the Lesch-Nyhan syndrome.

5 The deficiency of hypoxanthine-guanine phosphoribosyl transferase is associated with an increased intracellular concentration of PP-ribose-P. The increased concentration of this compound is probably at least partly responsible for both the increased rate of *de novo* purine biosynthesis and the increased amounts of the enzyme adenine phosphoribosyl transferase found in erythrocytes from these patients.

6 The mechanism by which the deficiency of hypoxanthine-guanine phosphoribosyl transferase produces the central nervous system disorder characteristic of this disease remains unknown.

7 Hypoxanthine-guanine phosphoribosyl transferase is coded by DNA in the X chromosome in man. Hemizygous males are affected with the disease, which is transmitted through heterozygous females. Heterozygotes may exhibit biochemical evidence of excessive purine synthesis and hyperuricemia, although generally they remain asymptomatic. Detection of the heterozygous state has only been successful in cultured fibroblasts; hypoxanthine-guanine phosphoribosyl transferase activity is usually normal in erythrocytes obtained from heterozygotes.

8 Patients lacking hypoxanthine-guanine phosphoribosyl transferase activity exhibit several distinctive pharmacogenetic features. They are resistant to the effect of allopurinol and certain other purine analogues on *de novo* purine synthesis, but they are slightly more sensitive to the inhibitory effects of allopurinol on xanthine oxidase.

9 Allopurinol should be used to prevent or reverse the consequences of the excessive uric acid synthesis. No therapy has been successful so far in treating the devastating central nervous system dysfunction characteristic of this disease.

BIBLIOGRAPHY

1. Lesch, M., and Nyhan, W. L.: A familial disorder of uric acid metabolism and central nervous system function. Amer. J. Med., **36,** 561, 1964.
2. Dreifuss, F. E., Newcombe, D. S., Shapiro, S. L., and Sheppard, G. L.: X-linked primary hyperuricemia (Hypoxanthine-guanine phosphoribosyltransferase deficiency encephalopathy). J. Ment. Defic. Res., **12,** 100, 1968.
3. Gillespie, J. B., and Perucca, L. G.: Congenital generalized indifference to pain (Congenital analgia). Amer. J. Dis. Child., **100,** 124, 1960.
4. Munsat, T. L., Klinenberg, J., Carrel, R. E., and Menkes, J.: Defects in purine metabolism and neurologic disease. Bull. Los Angeles Neurol. Soc., **33,** 101, 1968.
5. Scherzer, A. L., and Ilson, J. B.: Normal intelligence in the Lesch-Nyhan syndrome. *Pediatrics,* **44,** 116, 1969.
6. Marks, J. F., Baum, J., Kelle, D. K., Kay, J. L., and Mac Farlen, A.: Lesch-Nyhan syndrome treated from the early neonatal period. Pediatrics, **42,** 357, 1968.
7. Smith, M. G., Bland, J. H., Kelley, W. N., and Seegmiller, J. E.: Unpublished observations.
8. Hoefnagel, D.: Seminars on the Lesch-Nyhan syndrome: Discussion. Fed. Proc., **27,** 1045, 1967.
9. Berman, P. H., Balis, M. E., and Dancis, J.: Congenital hyperuricemia, an inborn error of purine metabolism associated with psychomotor retardation, athetosis, and self-mutilation. Arch. Neurol., **20,** 44, 1969.
10. Michener, W. M.: Hyperuricemia and mental retardation with athetosis and self-mutilation. Amer. J. Dis. Child., **113,** 195, 1967.
11. Rosenberg, D., Monnet, P., Mamelle, J. L., Colombel, M., Salle, B., and Bovier-Lapierre, M.: Encephalopathie avec troubles du metabolisme des purines. Presse Med., **76,** 2333, 1968.
12. Kaufman, J. M., Greene, M. L., and Seegmiller, J. E.: Urine uric acid to creatinine ratio: screening test for disorders of purine metabolism. J. Pediat., **73,** 583, 1968.
13. Hoefnagel, D., Andrew, E. D., Mireault, N. G., Berndt, W. O.: Hereditary choreoathetosis, self mutilation, and hyperuricemia in young males. New Eng. J. Med., **273,** 130, 1965.
14. Van Bogaert, L., Damme, J. V., Verschueren, M.: Sur un syndrome professif d'hypertonie extrapyramidale avec osteoarthropathies goutteuses chez duex freres. Rev. Neurol., **114,** 15, 1966.
15. Partington, M. W., and Hennen, B. K. E.: The Lesch-Nyhan syndrome: Self-destructive biting, mental retardation, neurological disorder and hyperuricemia. Develop. Med. Child. Neurol., **9,** 563, 1967.
16. Sass, J. K., Itabashi, H. H., and Dexter, R. A.: Juvenile gout with brain involvement. *Arch. Neurol.,* **13,** 639, 1965.
17. Riley, J. D.: Gout and cerebral palsy in three-year-old boy. Arch. Dis. Child., **35,** 293, 1960.

18. Labrune, B., Cartier, M., Hamet, M. M., Bonnenfant, F., Velin, J., Ribierre, M., and Mallet, R.: Encephalopathie familiale avec hyperuricemie. Presse Med., **76**, 2337, 1968.
19. Catel, W., and Schmidt, J.: Uber familiare gichtische Diathese in Verdundung mit zerebralen and renalen Symptomen bei einem Kleinkind. Deutsch Med. Wschr., **84**, 2145, 1959.
20. Marie, J., Royer, P., and Rappaport, R.: Hyperuricemie congenitale avec troubles neurologiques, renaux et sanguinis. Arch. Franc. Pediat., **24**, 501, 1967.
21. Manzke, H.: Hyperuricamie mit cerebralparese Syndrom eines hereditaren Purenstoffwechselleidens. Helv. Paediat. Acta, **22**, 258, 1967.
22. Van Der Zee, S. P. M., Monnens, L. A. H., and Schretlen, E. D. A. M.: Hereditary disorder of purine metabolism with cerebral affection and megaloblastic anemia. Nederl. T. Geneesk., **112**, 1475, 1968.
23. Nyhan, W. L., Oliver, W. J., Lesch, M.: A familial disorder of uric acid metabolism and central nervous system function. II., J. Pediat., **67**, 257, 1965.
24. Seegmiller, J. E.: Summary. Pathology and pathologic physiology. Fed. Proc., **27**, 1042, 1968.
25. Rosenblum, W. I., Rosenbloom, F. M., and Seegmiller, J. E.: Unpublished results.
26. Renuart, A. W.: Personal communication.
27. Crussi, F. G., Robertson, D. M., Hiscox, J. L.: The pathological condition of the Lesch-Nyhan syndrome. Amer. J. Dis. Child., **118**, 501, 1969.
28. Kornberg, A., Lieberman, I., Sims, E. S.: Enzymatic synthesis of purine nucleotides. J. Biol. Chem., **215**, 417, 1955.
29. Korn, E. D., Remy, C. N., Wasileyko, H. C., Buchanan, J. M.: Biosynthesis of nucleotides from bases by partially purified enzymes. J. Biol. Chem., **217**, 875, 1955.
30. Buchanan, J. M., Hartman, S. C.: Enzymatic reactions in synthesis of the purines. Advances Enzym., **21**, 199, 1959.
31. Buchanan, J. M.: The enzymatic synthesis of the purine nucleotides. Harvey Lect., **54**, 104, 1960.
32. Gutman, A. B., Yu, T. F.: Uric acid metabolism in normal man and in primary gout. New Eng. J. Med., **273**, 252, 313–321, 1965.
33. Nierlich, D. P. Magasanik, B.: Regulation of purine ribonucleotide synthesis by end product inhibition. The effect of adenine and guanine ribonucleotides on the 5′-phosphoribosylpyrophosphate amidotransferase of *Aerobacter aerogenes.* J. Biol. Chem., **240**, 358, 1965.
34. Wyngaarden, J. B., Ashton, D. M.: The regulation of activity of phosphoribosylpyrophosphate amidotransferase by purine ribonucleotides; a potential feedback control of purine biosynthesis. J. Biol. Chem., **234**, 1492, 1959.
35. Caskey, C. T., Ashton, D. M., and Wyngaarden, J. B.: The enzymology of feedback inhibition of glutamine phosphoribosylpyrophosphate amidotransferase by purine ribonucleotides. J. Biol. Chem., **239**, 2570, 1964.
36. Henderson, J. F.: Feedback inhibition of purine biosynthesis in ascites tumor cells. J. Biol. Chem., **237**, 2631, 1962.
37. Howard, W. J., and Appel, S. H.: Control of purine biosynthesis: FGAR amidotransferase (abstract). Clin. Res., **16**, 344, 1968.
38. Magasanik, B., and Karibian, D.: Purine nucleotide cycles and their metabolic role. J. Biol. Chem., **235**, 2672, 1960.
39. Mager, J., and Magasanik, B.: Guanosine 5′-phosphate reductase and its role in the interconversion of purine nucleotides. J. Biol. Chem., **235**, 1474, 1960.
40. Wyngaarden, J. B., and Greenland, R. A.: The inhibition of succinadenylate kinosynthetase of *Escherichia coli* by adenosine and guanosine 5′-monophosphates. J. Biol. Chem., **238**, 1054, 1963.
41. Henderson, J. F.: Kinetic properties of hypoxanthine-guanine and adenine phosphoribosyltransferase. Fed. Proc., **27**, 1053, 1968.
42. Krenitsky, T. A., Papaioannou, R., and Elion, G. B.: Human hypoxanthine phosphoribosyltransferase I. Purification, properties and specificity. J. Biol. Chem., **244**, 1263, 1969.
43. Nierlich, D. P., and Magasanik, B.: Control by repression of purine biosynthetic enzymes in *Aerobacter aerogenes.* Fed. Proc., **22**, 476, 1963.
44. Momose, H., Nishikawa, H., and Katsuya, N.: Genetic and biochemical studies of 5′ nucleotide fermentation. II. Repression of enzyme formation in purine nucleotide biosynthesis in Bacillus subtilis and derivation of derepressed mutants. J. Gen. Appl. Microbiol., **11**, 211, 1965.
45. Seegmiller, J. E., Rosenbloom, F. M., and Kelley, W. N.: An enzyme defect associated with a sex-linked human neurological disorder and excessive purine synthesis. Science, **155**, 1682, 1967.
46. Rosenbloom, F. M., Kelley, W. N., Miller, J., Henderson, J. F., and Seegmiller, J. E.: Inherited disorder of purine metabolism: correlation between central nervous system dysfunction and biochemical defects. JAMA, **202**, 175, 1967.
47. Kelley, W. N.: Hypoxanthine-guanine phosphoribosyltransferase deficiency in the Lesch-Nyhan syndrome and gout. Fed. Proc., **27**, 1047, 1968.
48. Kelley, W. N., Rosenbloom, F. M., Henderson, J. F., and Seegmiller, J. E.: Xanthine phosphoribosyltransferase in man: relationship to hypoxanthine-guanine phosphoribosyltransferase. Biochem. Biophys. Res. Comm., **28**, 340, 1967.
49. Brockman, R. W.: Resistance to purine antagonists in experimental leukemia systems. Can. Res., **25**, 1596, 1965.
50. Lowy, B. A., Williams, M. K., and London, I. M.: Enzymatic deficiencies of purine nucleotide synthesis in the human erythrocyte. J. Biol. Chem., **237**, 1622, 1962.
50*a*. McDonald, J. A., and Kelley, W. N.: Lesch-Nyhan syndrome: altered kinetic properties of mutant enzyme. Science, **171**, 689, 1971.
51. Fujimoto, W. Y., and Seegmiller, J. E.: Personal communication, 1969.
52. Kelley, W. N., and Wyngaarden, J. B.: The effect of allopurinol and oxipurinol on purine synthesis in cultured human cells. J. Clin. Invest., **49**, 602, 1970.
53. Fujimoto, W. Y., and Seegmiller, J. E.: Hypoxanthine-guanine phosphoribosyltransferase deficiency activity in normal mutant and heterozygote cultured human skin fibroblasts. Proc. Nat. Acad. Sci., **65**, 577, 1970.
53*a*. Kelley, W. N., and Meade, J. C.: Studies on hypoxanthine-guanine phosphoribosyltransferase in fibroblasts from patients with the Lesch-Nyhan syndrome: Evidence for genetic heterogeneity. J. Biol. Chem., **246**, 2953, 1971.
54. Kelley, W. N., Greene, M. L., Rosenbloom, F. M., Henderson, J. F., and Seegmiller, J. E.: Hypoxanthine-guanine phosphoribosyltransferase deficiency in gout. Ann. Intern. Med., **70**, 155, 1969.
55. Henderson, J. F., Kelley, W. N., Rosenbloom, F. M., and Seegmiller, J. E.: Inheritance of purine phosphoribosyltransferase in man. Amer. J. Hum. Genet., **21**, 61, 1969.
56. Kelley, W. N.: Studies on the adenine phosphoribosyltransferase enzyme in human fibroblasts lacking hypoxanthine-guanine phosphoribosyltransferase. J. Lab. Clin. Med., **77**, 33, 1971.
57. Rubin, C. S., Balis, M. E., Piomelli, S., Berman, P. H., and Dancis, J.: Elevated AMP pyrophosphorylase activity in congenital IMP pyrophosphorylase deficiency (Lesch-Nyhan disease). J. Lab. Clin. Med., **74**, 732, 1969.
58. Greene, M. L., Bayles, J. R., and Seegmiller, J. E.: Substrate stabilization: genetically controlled reciprocal relationship of two human enzymes. Science, **167**, 887, 1970.
58*a*. Fox, I. H., and Kelley, W. N.: Phosphoribosylpyrophosphate in man: biochemical and clinical significance. Ann. Intern. Med., **74**, 424, 1971.
59. Kelley, W. N., Rosenbloom, F. M., and Seegmiller, J. E.: The effects of azathioprine (imuran) on purine synthesis in clinical disorders of purine metabolism. J. Clin. Invest., **46**, 1518, 1967.
60. Balis, M. E., Krakoff, I. H., Berman, P. H., and Dancis, J.: Urinary metabolites in congenital hyperuricosuria. Science, **156**, 1122, 1967.
61. Balis, M. E.: Aspects of purine metabolism. Fed. Proc., **27**, 1067, 1968.
62. Newcombe, D. S., Lapes, M., Thomson, C., and Wright, E. Y.: Urinary excretion of 4-amino-5-imidazolecarboxamide in X-linked primary hyperuricemia. Clin. Res., **15**, 45, 1967.
63. Herbert, V., Streiff, R. R., Sullivan, L. W., and McGeer, P. L.: Deranged purine metabolism manifested by aminoimidazolecarboxamide excretion in megaloblastic anemias, hemolytic anemia, and liver disease. *Lancet,* **2**, 45, 1964.
64. Rosenbloom, F. M., Henderson, J. F., Caldwell, I. C., Kelley, W. N., and Seegmiller, J. E.: Biochemical bases of accelerated purine biosyn-

thesis *de novo* in human fibroblasts lacking hypoxanthine-guanine phosphoribosyltransferase. J. Biol. Chem., **243**, 1166, 1968.

65. Rosenbloom, F. M., Henderson, J. F., Kelley, W. N., and Seegmiller, J. E.: Accelerated purine biosynthesis *de novo* in skin fibroblasts deficient in hypoxanthine-guanine phosphoribosyltransferase. Biochim. Biophys. Acta, **166**, 258, 1968.
66. Howard, W. J., Kerson, L. A., and Appel, S. H.: Synthesis *de novo* of purines in slices of rat brain and liver. J. Neurochem., **17**, 121, 1970.
67. Sweetman, L.: Urinary and cerebrospinal fluid oxypurine levels and allopurinol metabolism in the Lesch-Nyhan syndrome. Fed. Proc., **27**, 1055, 1967.
68. Lassen, U. V.: Hypoxanthine transport in human erythrocytes. Biochim. Biophys. Acta, **135**, 146, 1967.
69. Berlin, R. D.: Purines: Active transport by isolated choroid plexus. Science, **163**, 1194, 1969.
70. Alepa, F. P., Howell, R. R., Klinenberg, J. R., and Seegmiller, J. E.: Relationships between glycogen storage disease and tophaceous gout. Amer. J. Med., **42**, 58, 1967.
71. Jakovcic, S., and Sorensen, L. B.: Studies of uric acid metabolism in glycogen storage disease associated with gouty arthritis. Arthritis Rheum., **10**, 129–134, 1967.
72. Kelley, W. N., Rosenbloom, F. M., Seegmiller, J. E., and Howell, R. R.: Excessive uric acid production in type I glycogen storage disease. J. Pediat., **72**, 488, 1968.

72*a*. Kelley, W. N., Fox, I. H., and Wyngaarden, J. B.: Essential role of phosphoribosylpyrophosphate in regulation of purine biosynthesis in cultured human fibroblasts. Clin. Res., **18**, 457, 1970 (abstract).

73. Hill, D. L., and Bennett, L. L.: Purification and properties of 5-phosphoribosylpyrophosphate amidotransferase from adenocarcinoma 755 cells. Biochemistry, **8**, 122, 1969.

73*a*. Kelley, W. N., Fox, I. H., and Wyngaarden, J. B.: Regulation of purine biosynthesis in cultured human cells. Biochim. Biophys. Acta, **215**, 512, 1970.

73*b*. Kelley, W. N., Green, M. L., Fox, I. H., Rosenbloom, F. M., Levy, R. I., and Seegmiller, J. E.: Effects of orotic acid on purine and lipoprotein metabolism in man. Metabolism, **19**, 1025, 1970.

74. Boyd, E. M., Dolman, M., Knight, L. M., and Sheppard, E. P.: The chronic oral toxicity of caffeine. Canad. J. Physiol. Pharmacol., **43**, 995, 1965.
75. Krenitsky, T. A.: Tissue distribution of purine ribosyl- and phosphoribosyltransferase in the Rhesus monkey. Biochim. Biophys. Acta, **179**, 506, 1969.

75*a*. Ghadimi, H., Bhalla, C. K., and Kirchenbaum, D. M.: The significance of the deficiency state in Lesch-Nyhan disease. Acta Paediat. Scand., **59**, 233, 1970.

76. Felix, J. S., and DeMars, R.: Purine requirement of cells cultured from humans affected with Lesch-Nyhan syndrome (Hypoxanthine-guanine phosphoribosyltransferase deficiency). Proc. Nat. Acad. Sci., **62**, 536, 1969.
77. Van Der Zee, S. P. M., Schretlen, E. D. A. M., and Monnens, L. A. H.: Megaloblastic anemia in the Lesch-Nyhan syndrome. Lancet, **1**, 1427, 1968.
78. Shapiro, S. L., Sheppard, G. L., Jr., Dreifuss, F. E., and Newcombe, D. S.: X-linked recessive inheritance of a syndrome of mental retardation with hyperuricemia. Proc. Soc. Exp. Biol. Med., **122**, 609, 1966.
79. Nyhan, W. L., Pesek, J., Sweetman, L., Carpenter, D. G., and Carter, C. H.: Genetics of an X-linked disorder of uric acid metabolism and cerebral function. Pediat. Res., **1**, 5, 1967.
80. Rosenbloom, F. M., Kelley, W. N., Henderson, J. F., and Seegmiller, J. E.: Lyon hypothesis and X-linked disease. Lancet, **2**, 305, 1967.
81. Migeon, B. R., Der Kaloustian, V. M., Nyhan, W. L., Young, W. J., and Childs, B.: X-linked hypoxanthine-guanine phosphoribosyltransferase deficiency: Heterozygote has two clonal populations. Science, **160**, 425, 1968.
82. Salzmann, J., DeMars, R., and Benke, P.: Single allele expression at an X-linked hyperuricemia locus in heterozygous human cells. Proc. Nat. Acad. Sci., **60**, 545, 1968.

82*a*. Migeon, B. R.: X-linked hypoxanthine-guanine phosphoribosyltransferase deficiency: detection of heterozygotes by selective medium. Biochem. Genetics, **4**, 377, 1970.

83. Lyon, M. F.: Gene action in the X-chromosome of the mouse (Mus musculus L.). Nature (London), **190**, 372, 1961.
84. Bland, J. H.: Discussion of epidemiology and genetic implications. Fed. Proc., **27**, 1091, 1968.
85. Emmerson, B. T., and Wyngaarden, J. B.: Purine metabolism in heterozygous carriers of hypoxanthine-guanine phosphoribosyltransferase deficiency. Science, **166**, 1533, 1969.
86. Dancis, J., Berman, P. H., Jansen, V., and Balis, M. E.: Absence of mosaicism in the lymphocyte in X-linked congenital hyperuricosuria. Life Sciences, **7**, 587, 1968.

86*a*. Nyhan, W. L., Bakay, B., Connor, J. D., Marks, J. F., and Keele, D. K.: Hemizygous expression of glucose-6-phosphate dehydrogenase in erythrocytes of heterozygotes for the Lesch-Nyhan syndrome. Proc. Nat. Acad. Sci. USA, **65**, 214, 1970.

86*b*. McDonald, J. A., and Kelley, W. N. (in preparation).

87. Fujimoto, W. Y., Seegmiller, J. E., Uhlendarf, B. W., and Jacobson, C. B.: Biochemical diagnosis of an X-linked disease in utero. Lancet, **2**, 511, 1968.
88. DeMars, R., Sarto, G., Felix, J. S., and Benke, P.: Lesch-Nyhan mutation: Prenatal detection with amniotic fluid cells. Science, **164**, 1303, 1969.

88*a*. Gartler, S. M., Scott, R. C., Goldstein, J. L., Campbell, B., and Sparkes, R.: Lesch-Nyhan syndrome: Rapid detection of heterozygotes by the use of hair follicles. Science, **172**, 572, 1971.

89. McCollister, R. J., Gilbert, W. R., Jr., Ashton, D. M., and Wyngaarden, J. B.: Pseudofeedback inhibition of purine synthesis by 6-mercaptopurine ribonucleotide and other purine analogues. J. Biol. Chem., **239**, 1560, 1964.
90. Sorensen, L. B., and Benke, P. J.: Biochemical evidence for a distinct type of primary gout. Nature (London), **213**, 1122, 1967.
91. Nyhan, W. L., Sweetman, L., Carpenter, D. G., Carter, C. H., and Hoefnagel, D.: Effects of azathioprine in a disorder of uric acid metabolism and cerebral function. J. Pediat., **72**, 111, 1968.
92. Brown, R. S., Kelley, W. N., Seegmiller, J. E., and Carbone, P. P.: The action of thiopurines in lymphocytes lacking hypoxanthine guanine phosphoribosyltransferase. J. Clin. Invest., **47**, 12*a*, 1968. (Abstract.)
93. Newcombe, D. S., Shapiro, S. L., Sheppard, G. L., and Dreifuss, F. E.: Treatment of X-linked primary hyperuricemia with allopurinol. JAMA, **198**, 315, 1966.
94. Sweetman, L., and Nyhan, W. L.: Excretion of hypoxanthine and xanthine in genetic disease of purine metabolism. Nature (London), **215**, 859, 1967.
95. Kelley, W. N., Rosenbloom, F. M., Miller, J., and Seegmiller, J. E.: An enzymatic basis for variation in response to allopurinol. New Eng. J. Med., **278**, 287, 1968.

95*a*. Fox, I. H., Wyngaarden, J. B., and Kelley, W. N.: Depletion of erythrocyte phosphoribosylpyrophosphate in man: a newly observed effect of allopurinol. N. Eng. J. Med., **283**, 1177, 1970.

96. Emmerson, B. T.: Discussion. Session I. Biochemistry and metabolism. Symposium on allopurinol. Ann. Rheum. Dis., **25 (Suppl. 6)**, 621, 1966.
97. Greene, M. L., Fujimoto, W. Y., and Seegmiller, J. E.: Urinary xanthine stones: A rare complication of allopurinol therapy. New Eng. J. Med., **280**, 426, 1969.
98. Sorensen, L. B.: In Proceedings of the Seminars on the Lesch-Nyhan syndrome. Fed. Proc., **27**, 1099, 1968.
99. Elion, G. B., Kovensky, A., Hitchings, G. H., Metz, E., and Rundles, R. W.: Metabolic studies of allopurinol, an inhibitor of xanthine oxidase. Biochem. Pharmacol., **15**, 863, 1966.
100. Simmonds, H. A.: Urinary excretion of purines, pyrimidines and pyrazolopyrimidines in patients treated with allopurinol or oxipurinol. Clin. Chim. Acta, **23**, 353, 1969.
101. Chalmers, R. A., Parker, R., Simmonds, H. A., Snedden, W., and Watts, R. W. E.: The conversion of 4-hydroxypyrazolo [3,4-d] pyrimidine (allopurinol) into 4,6-dihydroxypyrazolo [3,4-d] pyrimidine (oxipurinol) *in vivo* in the absence of xanthine oxidase. Biochem. J., **112**, 527, 1969.
102. Krenitsky, T. A., Elion, G. A., Sterlitz, R. A., and Hitchings, G. H.:

Ribonucleosides of allopurinol and oxoallopurinol. Isolation from human urine, enzymatic synthesis, and characterization. J. Biol. Chem., **242**, 2675, 1967.

103. Benke, P. J., and Anderson, J.: Use of folic acid, adenine, and bicarbonate in newborn twins with the Lesch-Nyhan syndrome. Pediat. Res., **3**, 356, 1969 (abstract).
104. Seegmiller, J. E.: Personal communication.
104*a*. Van Der Zee, S. P. M., Lommen, E. J. P., Frijbels, J. M. P., and Schretten, E. D. A. M.: The influence of adenine on the clinical features and purine metabolism in the Lesch-Nyhan syndrome. Acta Paediat. Scand., **59**, 259, 1970.
105. Klenow, H.: The enzymic oxidation and assay of adenine. Biochem. J., **50**, 404, 1952.
106. Hamilton, L.: Utilization of purines for nucleic acid synthesis in man. Nature (London), **172**, 457, 1953.
107. Kelley, W. N., Rosenbloom, F. M., Henderson, J. F., and Seegmiller, J. E.: A specific enzyme defect in gout associated with overproduction of uric acid. Proc. Nat. Acad. Sci., **57**, 1735, 1967.
108. Nyhan, W. L., James, J. A., Seberg, A. J., Sweetman, L., and Nelson, L. G.: A new disorder of purine metabolism with behavioral manifestations. J. Pediat., **74**, 20, 1969.
109. Hooft, C., Van Nevel, C., and De Schaepdryver, A. F.: Hyperuricosuric encephalopathy without hyperuricemia. Arch. Dis. Child., **43**, 734, 1968.
110. Bazelon, M., Stevens, H., Davis, M., Seegmiller, J. E., and Greene, M.: Mental retardation, self-mutilation and hyperuricemia in females. Trans. Amer. Neurol. Ass., **93**, 187, 1968.
111. Rosenberg, A. L., and Bartholomew, B. A.: Hyperuricemia and neurologic deficits: A family study. Arthritis Rheum., **17**, 837, 1968 (abstract).
112. Wyngaarden, J. B.: Gout, in *The Metabolic Basis of Inherited Disease*, 2nd ed., edited by J. B. Stanbury, J. B. Wyngaarden, and D. S. Fredrickson, pp. 667–728, McGraw-Hill, New York, 1966.
113. Reed, W. B., and Fish, C. H.: Hyperuricemia with self-mutilation and choreoathetosis. Lesch-Nyhan syndrome. Arch. Derm., **94**, 194, 1966.
114. Jeune, M., Hernier, M., and Rosenberg, D.: Encephalopathie familiale avec hyperuricemie. A propos d'une observation. Pediatrie, **21**, 663, 1966.
115. Seegmiller, J. E., Grayzel, A. I., Laster, L., and Liddle, L.: Uric acid production in gout. J. Clin. Invest., **40**, 1304, 1961.
116. Greene, M. L., and Seegmiller, J. E.: Unpublished observations, 1969.

CHAPTER FORTY-ONE

XANTHINURIA

James B. Wyngaarden

Xanthinuria is a rare hereditary disorder characterized by a gross deficiency of xanthine oxidase activity in the tissues, by the resultant excretion of xanthine and hypoxanthine as the chief end products of purine metabolism, and by low concentration values of uric acid in serum and urine. Nine well-documented patients have been reported [1–10]. Three have presented with xanthine calculi of the urinary tract [1, 6, 7]. Two have had a unique type of myopathy associated with crystalline deposits of xanthine and hypoxanthine in the skeletal muscles [2, 9, 11]. The disorder is probably transmitted as an autosomal recessive condition.

About 40 additional cases of xanthine stones have been recorded since they were first identified by Marcet [12] in 1817. In some patients, chiefly adults, serum or urinary uric acid values were normal, and xanthine was only a minor component of the calculus. At least seven xanthine stones occurred in subjects under age 15 who may have had hereditary xanthinuria, but since xanthine excretion studies were not performed, the relationship is uncertain [13–24].

CLINICAL FEATURES

Case 1. In 1954 Dent and Philpot [1] described a 4½-year-old girl with hematuria and urinary frequency who passed a smooth oval calculus weighing 0.9 gm. It was nonopaque to x-rays, contained only traces of calcium and magnesium, and was almost ash-free. In the murexide test it gave a reddish-brown color quite unlike that of uric acid. Extracts of the stone, analyzed by paper chromatography in the presence of various purine markers, matched xanthine exactly. Xanthine excretion was 176 mg per day, or 607 mg per gm creatinine. By a nonspecific chemical method uric acid excretion was 30 mg per day, and plasma uric acid was 0.5 mg per 100 ml.

This patient was restudied at age 9 by Dickinson and Smellie [2]. She had had no further calculi but had developed clubbing of the calyces of the left kidney. By specific enzymatic methods plasma oxypurines were 0.75 mg per 100 ml, and plasma uric acid was 0.2 mg per 100 ml. The renal clearance of oxypurines was 94 ml per min per 1.73 m^2 body surface area, a value equivalent to 82 percent of the simultaneous endogenous creatinine clearance (normal = 10 to 20 percent). When the patient was given a low-purine diet, fresh urine and plasma contained no detectable uric acid but contained hypoxanthine equivalent to 10 to 20 percent of xanthine. Larger quantities of both hypoxanthine and uric acid were found in stored urine specimens.

At age 14 a pyelogram showed some persistent clubbing of the left renal calyces, with reduction of size of the left kidney (10.5 cm) compared with the right (14 cm). At age 19 she was normotensive and in good health [25].

Case 2. In 1964 Engleman and colleagues [3, 4] described a 23-year-old Negro woman suffering from pheochromocytoma and heart failure who was found to have a very low serum uric acid value. In addition, she had mental retardation, with an IQ of 53, congenital skeletal abnormalities, and on a later admission, glucose-6-phosphate dehydrogenase deficiency [25]. There was no clinical or radiologic evidence of urinary calculi. Further study disclosed diminished amounts of uric acid and increased quantities of oxypurines in both serum and urine. The renal clearance of oxypurines was 87 percent of the endogenous creatinine clearance. The increased excretion of uric acid which normally follows the ingestion of 5-amino-4-imidazole carboxamide was replaced by an approximately equivalent increase in the urinary excretion of xanthine [4]. Activity of xanthine oxidase in homogenates of liver and jejunal mucosa was determined (1) by measurement of conversion of hypoxanthine-8-^{14}C to xanthine as separated by paper electrophoresis, (2) by conversion of xanthine-6-^{14}C to $^{14}CO_2$ in the presence of uricase, and (3) by spectrophotofluorometric measurement of conversion of xanthopterin to leukopterin. With each of these assays xanthine oxidase activities of jejunal mucosa and liver corresponded to no more than 0.1 percent of activities found in specimens from control subjects. Normal activities of lactic dehydrogenase and guanase activities indicated that the tissue was metabolically active. No evidence was found for an inhibitor of xanthine oxidase in intestinal mucosa or blood [3, 4]. By age 27 she had developed muscle cramps in her legs following walking or strenuous exercise. A muscle biopsy contained numerous crystals which were identified as xanthine and hypoxanthine by Chalmers et al. [11] and by Parker, Snedden, and Watts [26].

Case 3. The third patient, described by Ayvazian [5], was a 47-year-old man of Irish ancestry with hemochromatosis and serum uric acid values of 0.2 and 0.6 mg per 100 ml. On a low-purine diet, the values fell to 0.04 to 0.1 mg per 100 ml. Plasma oxypurine levels were 0.2 to 0.5 mg per 100 ml. Urinary uric acid excretion values ranged up to 42 mg per 24 hr on a standard diet, but fell to undetectable levels when dietary purines were restricted. When urine was incubated with xanthine oxidase, the uric acid values increased to 408 to 620 mg per 24 hr. In fresh urine almost all the oxypurine was xanthine, but in an 8-day-old specimen xanthine accounted for only about 80 percent of the total. A liver biopsy specimen was found to contain xanthine oxidase activity of "less than 10 percent of normal."

Cases 4 and 5. Cifuentes Delatte and Castro-Mendoza [6] have described an interesting family in which two brothers excreted abnormal amounts of oxypurines in urine, ranging from 462 to 566 mg per day, and almost no uric acid. One suffered severe recurrent stone formation from the age of 6, leading to a nephrectomy at age 12 and cystotomy for a bladder stone at age 13; the other, who excreted comparable amounts of oxypurines, never formed stones. In both patients 90 to 95 percent of the oxypurines was xanthine. A 24-year-old sister excreted 60 to 83 mg oxypurines per day, in addition to 371 to 421 mg uric acid. Clearly, she had significant activity of xanthine oxidase and differed metabolically from her two brothers.

Case 6. The sixth patient, described by Frézal and associates [7], was a 20-month-old Negro male who developed urinary symptoms, and later passed a stone measuring 1 cm in its greatest dimension. The stone gave a positive murexide test for xanthine, and more precise analysis by x-ray diffraction, ultraviolet absorption spectra, and chromatography established its identity. The serum contained 0.3 to 1.6 mg uric acid per 100 ml; the urine contained an average of 60 mg uric acid per day, and quantities of oxypurines estimated to be more than 10 times normal. By various studies xanthine appeared to be present in somewhat larger amounts than hypoxanthine. X-ray examination 2 months later disclosed a nonopaque stone in the left ureter. It eventually produced hydronephrosis, and 3 months later was removed surgically. Hepatic tissue obtained at the time of surgery showed no xanthine oxidase activity in an assay that gave $20\text{–}50 \times 10^{-6}$ μmoles of substrate oxidized per mg protein per hour with normal intestinal mucosa.

Case 7. Bradford et al. [8] have described a seventh patient, a 62-year-old Puerto Rican woman, with a 30-year history of mild psoriasis, who entered Bellevue Hospital because of acute monoarticular arthritis. This became migratory and polyartricular, affecting ankles, knees, elbows, wrists, and hands over a 6-week period, with fever to 104°F. The etiology of the arthritis was not established, but the finding of a serum uric acid of 0.8 to 1.1 mg per 100 ml prompted study of xanthinuria. On a low-purine diet urinary uric acid ranged from 0 to 38.5 mg per day, urinary total oxypurines from 212 to 399 mg (of xanthine equivalents) per day, urinary xanthine from 125 to 325 mg per day, and urinary hypoxanthine from 27 to 76 mg per day.

Case 8. In 1969, Chalmers et al. [9] reported a 31-year-old Negro male from Guyana who had been an active athlete until 3 years earlier, when he developed "tight sensations" and a feeling of "distension" at the back of both thighs and calves, often aggravated by exertion. He lost 7 kg in weight over the next 30 months but remained otherwise well. Examination disclosed no vascular abnormalities, and the neurologic findings were normal except for universally sluggish reflexes and absent ankle jerks. Muscle strength was normal, no muscle tenderness was found at rest or following exertion, and there was no myotonia, but the calves felt firmer than normal. The finding of a very low serum uric acid value led to further investigation in the hospital, where the mean of four determinations was 0.78 mg per 100 ml. Plasma oxypurines, calculated as xanthine, were 0.29 mg per 100 ml. Urinary excretion values were: uric acid, 12 to 52 mg; xanthine 245 mg; and hypoxanthine, 19 mg per 24 hr. No xanthine oxidase activity was demonstrated by histochemical techniques in a jejunal biopsy. Electromyographic studies were in keeping with a diffuse myopathic process. Four muscle biopsies were performed over a period of 12 months. A striking feature was the unusually high average diameter of muscle fibers, which also showed increased numbers of centrally placed muscle nuclei. A few of the fibers contained intensely staining rodlike inclusions, which on electron microscopy consisted of aggregations of electron-dense material, much of which was crystalline in appearance. By polarized light, phase-contrast, and interference microscopy, the optical properties of the crystals were compatible with their being hypoxanthine and xanthine [11]. Identification was subsequently accomplished by high-resolution mass spectrometry [26] both with crystals from this patient and from Case 2.

Case 9. Sperling and coworkers [10] recently reported a 32-year-old Iranian-born housewife who suffered from attacks of palpitation and dizziness. There was no history of renal stone or muscle disorder. Physical examination disclosed aortic and mitral insufficiency and systolic hypertension. Tests for pheochromocytoma and hemochromatosis were negative. Routine examinations of blood and urine were normal except for the consistent findings of hypouricema. By enzymatic methods plasma urate was 0.20 and 0.42 mg per 100 ml; plasma oxypurines, 0.30 mg per 100 ml; urinary uric acid, 9 and 23 mg per 24 hr; xanthine, 346 and 359 mg per 24 hr; and hypoxanthine, 44 and 138 mg per 24 hr. Urinary xanthine thus accounted for 70 to 88 percent of oxypurines. Xanthine oxidase activity of jejunal mucosa obtained by peroral biopsy was about 5 percent of that of a control tissue. The assay involved conversion of 8-^{14}C hypoxanthine to uric acid, followed by thin-layer chromatographic separation of purine bases. Plasma urate values in a sister and two brothers ranged from 4.8 to 6.0 mg per 100 ml.

Clinical Summary

Data on the nine reported patients with xanthinuria and on the sister of the two Spanish subjects are summarized in Table 41-1.

In the majority of patients, xanthinuria appears to be a relatively benign disorder, first suggested by the finding of a very low serum uric acid value during investigation of presumably unrelated medical problems. In three of the nine

Table 41-1. CLINICAL AND CHEMICAL DATA ON REPORTED CASES OF PRIMARY XANTHINURIA

Patient	Age	Sex	Serum		Urine		Percent xanthine	Stones	Xanthine oxidase		Reference
			Uric acid mg/100 ml	Oxypurines mg/100 ml	Uric acid mg/day	Oxypurines mg/day			Assay	Tissue	
1	4½, 9	F	0.2–0.5	0.75	30	176	80–90	+		—	[1, 2]
2	23	F	0.3–0.5	0.4–0.9	2–12	100–358	70	0	<0.1% of normal	liver and jejunum	[3, 4]
3	47	M	0.2–0.6	0.2–0.5	<42	408–620*	80	0	<10% of normal	liver	[5]
4	17	M	<0.05	0.3–0.6	2.4–4.9	473–542	90	+		—	[6]
5	21	M	<0.05	0.4–0.6	3.5–5.1	462–566	95	0			[6]
6	1½	M	0.3–1.6	—	~60	>160	">50"	+	"no activity"	liver	[7]
7	62	F	0.8–1.1	—	0–38.5	X = 125–325 Hx = 27–76	83	0	"no activity" "traces"	liver jejunum	[8]
8	31	M	0.8	0.29	12–52	X = 245 Hx = 19	94	0	"no activity"	jejunum	[9]
9	32	F	0.2–0.4	0.30	9–29	X = 346, 359 Hx = 49, 138	72–88	0	5.7% of normal	jejunum	[10]

* Uric acid equivalents.

subjects, xanthine calculi of the urinary tract developed; in one it led to mild calyceal clubbing and in another, to hydronephrosis and eventual nephrectomy. In two patients a myopathy was present, associated with crystalline deposits of xanthine and hypoxanthine. One patient presented with recurrent polyarthritis, which Seegmiller has suggested may have represented a crystal-induced synovitis [27].

The association of pheochromocytoma and xanthinuria in Case 2 is probably fortuitous. Plasma from eight other patients with pheochromocytoma studied by Engleman et al. [4] contained normal amounts of uric acid, and urine from the xanthinuric patient of Dent and Philpot contained normal amounts of catecholamines and their metabolites [1]. In the patient of Frézal et al. [7] urinary excretion of vanillomandelic acid was normal. The association of xanthinuria and hemochromatosis in Case 3 is also probably coincidental. In 4 of 11 patients with proved hemochromatosis in whom serum uric acid values were available, the values were normal [5]. The patient with xanthinuria described by Engleman and associates [4] developed iron deficiency anemia and hypoferremia that responded promptly to iron administered orally. Seegmiller and associates [27] later found a normal absorption of ^{59}Fe and a normal incorporation of absorbed iron into erythrocytes of this patient.

XANTHINE OXIDASE

Xanthine oxidase catalyzes the oxidation of hypoxanthine to xanthine and of xanthine to uric acid (Fig. 41-1). It functions both as an oxidase with molecular oxygen, and as a dehydrogenase with a variety of other electron acceptors, including methylene blue, cytochrome, ferricyanide, nitrate, and in some species NAD. Its relative activity as an oxidase or dehydrogenase varies from species to species. In man the enzyme of liver is substantially more active in vitro when functioning as a dehydrogenase with methylene blue than with oxygen as acceptor [25]. Both activities are inhibited by 6-pteridylaldehyde, and both are virtually absent in tissue from xanthinuric subjects. Accordingly, it is concluded that a single protein is capable of functioning both aerobically and anaerobically.

Xanthine oxidase is not a highly discriminating enzyme. It attacks a variety of substrates including aldehydes, pteridines, and purines other than hypoxanthine and xanthine. Adenine is oxidized to 2,8-dihydroxyadenine [28] by way of 2-hydroxy and 8-hydroxyadenine intermediates [29]. 2,6-Diaminopurine [30], 2-azadenine, 2-azahypoxanthine [31], 6-mercaptopurine [32], and several other substituted purines are also substrates. The enzyme does not attack methylxanthines other than the 1-methyl compound [33]. Table 41-2 gives data on relative rates of oxidation of purine derivatives by bovine milk and human liver xanthine oxidases functioning aerobically [34].

Xanthine Oxidase Inhibitors

Many purine compounds, including particularly those that are not substrates, act as competitive inhibitors of xanthine oxidase [30, 32, 35]. In addition, two classes of purine analogues are inhibitors of the enzyme. Fridovich has described

Hypoxanthine → Xanthine → Uric Acid

Figure 41-1. Conversion of hypoxanthine to xanthine, and of xanthine to uric acid by xanthine oxidase. Structures are shown in their lactim forms.

Table 41-2. RELATIVE RATES OF OXIDATION OF PURINE DERIVATIVES BY BOVINE MILK AND HUMAN LIVER XANTHINE OXIDASES

Substrate	Product	Oxidative pathway†	Relative rate with	
			Bovine milk xanthine oxidase	Human liver xanthine oxidase
Xanthine*	Uric acid	....	1.0	1.0
1-Methylxanthine	1-Methyluric acid	....	0.45	1.0
6,8-Dioxypurine	Uric acid	....	1.0	1.1
Hypoxanthine	Xanthine, uric acid (6,8-dioxypurine?)	→ 2,6 → 2,6,8	0.7	0.7
Purine	Uric acid	→ 6 → 2,6 → 2,6,8	0.2	0.15
2-Oxypurine	2,8-Dioxypurine	→ 2,8 → 2,6,8	0.16	0.04
8-Oxypurine	2,8-Dioxypurine	→ 2,8 → 2,6,8	0.015	0.002
8-Oxypurine	Uric acid	....	0.002	0.0005
2,8-Dioxypurine	Uric acid	....	0.002	0.0005

* Xanthine served as reference compound.
† Indicates order in which the oxidizable compounds were attacked by the enzyme.
Source: Bergmann and Dikstein [34].

competitive inhibition of xanthine oxidase by symmetrical triazines and compounds of guanidine [36]. More important from the clinical point of view are the pyrazolopyrimidines, which are used therapeutically to control production of uric acid from hypoxanthine and xanthine. Allopurinol (4-hydroxypyrazolo-[3,4-*d*] pyrimidine) is both a powerful inhibitor and substrate of the enzyme [37–39]. It is oxidized to oxipurinol (4,6-dihydroxypyrazolo-[3,4-*d*] pyrimidine) which is also an inhibitor of xanthine oxidase [38, 39] and useful in patients sensitive to allopurinol. Among the pteridines, xanthopterin [40] and 6-pteridyl aldehyde [41] are xanthine oxidase inhibitors.

Xanthine Oxidase as an Aldehyde Oxidase

All aldehydes which have been tested are oxidized to the corresponding acids by xanthine oxidase, although at variable rates [42]. Aldehyde oxidases distinct from xanthine oxidase are known. One, purified extensively from rabbit liver, has properties similar to xanthine oxidase but also important differences, such as its content of coenzyme Q_{10} [43]. The extent to which xanthine oxidase functions as an aldehyde oxidase in vivo is unknown. For example, glyoxylic acid is oxidized to oxalic acid by xanthine oxidase in vitro [42], but oxalate excretion in hyperoxaluric subjects is unaffected by treatment with allopurinol [44]. The pteridines xanthopterin and 2-amino-4-hydroxy pteridine are oxidized to their 8-hydroxy derivatives (leukopterin and isoxanthopterin) by xanthine oxidase.

Molecular Weight and Cofactors

The molecular weight of the enzyme from milk is 275,000 [45, 45*a*] to 300,000 [46], from pig liver 288,000 [47], and from chicken liver 300,000 [48]. The bovine milk enzyme can be dissociated into subunits of 150,000 MW in guanidine or acid [46]. Amino acid analysis of purified milk enzyme discloses no unusual percentage composition [49].

Bovine milk xanthine oxidase contains two gm atoms molybdenum, two FAD residues, eight gm atoms of nonheme iron, and eight moles of labile sulfide per 300,000 MW [50]. Different Mo/FAD/Fe ratios have been reported for the enzyme obtained from mammalian intestine and liver and from avian liver [51], but these values may reflect inadvertent removal of cofactors during purification. The molybdenum-free enzyme is nonfunctional [52]. Flavin-free enzyme is devoid of xanthine oxygen reductase activity and can be reconstituted by a short incubation with FAD [53].

Mechanism of Action

The complexity of xanthine oxidase approaches that of enzyme systems with multiple intermediates, such as the respiratory chain. Studies employing circular dichroism, electron paramagnetic resonance spectroscopy (EPR), and optical rotatory dispersion have shown that electron flow during purine oxidation is first to molybdenum, which is reduced from valence to 6+ to 5+, from molybdenum to FAD, and terminally from iron to oxygen or anaerobically to methylene blue, cytochrome c, or other receptor [52–55]. Under anaerobic conditions lower valence states of molybdenum are detected by EPR [50]. Uncertainty exists whether one iron atom is interposed between Mo and FAD. The inhibitory action of allopurinol and oxipurinol apparently involves complex formation with enzyme-bound molybdenum in the Mo^{4+} state and is dependent upon prior reduction of enzyme by substrate. Binding studies with ^{14}C-oxipurinol suggest that 1 mole of purine is bound per molybdenum, and therefore that there are two active sites per molecule of enzyme [39]. This accords with the observation that the enzyme can be dissociated into halves [46].

The two-step dehydrogenation of hypoxanthine to uric acid involves release of intermediate xanthine from the enzyme surface and reorientation of xanthine on rebinding, possibly to different active centers. Bergmann and Dikstein [34] have suggested that hypoxanthine is bound at N1, N3, and N7, whereas xanthine is bound at N3, N7, and N9. The rate of the first dehydrogenation step is 0.7 [34] to 0.8 [56] that of the second. A small but detectable steady state concentration of xanthine exists during hypoxanthine oxidation, greater than can be accounted for by the amount of intermediate xanthine bound to the enzyme surface.

Distribution

The distribution of xanthine oxidase in mammalian and avian tissues varies from species to species [57]. In most mammals, liver and small intestinal mucosa are rich sources. In man these are the only tissues that normally show abundant xanthine oxidase activity, although significant traces of activity exist in kidney, spleen, and skeletal and heart muscle [58]. Activity has been detected inconstantly in marrow of leukemic children [59]. Although activity is undetectable in serum of normal persons, individuals with acute infectious hepatitis and jaundice may have striking levels of activity in serum [60]. Xanthine oxidase is also regularly present in human milk [61].

Enzyme Induction and Repression

Hepatic xanthine oxidase levels can be altered tenfold by changes in dietary protein intake [62]. Rats maintained on an 8 percent protein diet show a decrease of xanthine oxidase activity to about 10 percent of control values in 10 days. Thereafter the values remain constant. Return to a 23 percent protein diet results in a fivefold increase in activity within 12 hr. This increase is inhibited completely by actinomycin D, 5-fluorouracil, and puromycin and indicate that both ribonucleic acid and protein synthesis are involved in the repletion. Administration of ^{14}C-leucine resulted in identical specific activities in hepatic xanthine oxidase in control and protein-depleted animals, in spite of a tenfold difference in activity levels. These results show that the fractional turnover rates are the same in the two groups of rats and suggest that the rate of xanthine oxidase synthesis was reduced tenfold in the depleted rats. Hepatic guanase and uricase activities are also markedly reduced during protein restriction [63], but in spite of the marked reduction in activities of these hepatic enzymes, allantoin excretion is unchanged [62]. Reductions in hepatic xanthine oxidase activity also result from induced dietary deficiencies of iron or molybdenum in experimental animals [64].

Activity of xanthine oxidase in hepatic tissue has been reported elevated fourfold in certain subjects with gout who excrete large quantities of uric acid [65], but it is not yet established whether this represents induction of enzyme by the surfeit of purine precursors or a primary disturbance.

METABOLIC DEFECTS IN XANTHINURIA

Xanthine Oxidase Activity

The findings of Dent and Philpot [1] that xanthine had replaced uric acid as the chief end product of purine metabolism in their patients and of Dickinson and Smellie [2] that the plasma level of oxypurines was elevated pointed toward a deficiency of xanthine oxidase activity in xanthinuria. Watts, Engleman, and associates [3] subsequently demonstrated less than 0.1 percent of normal activity in jejunal mucosa and liver biopsy material from their patient. Activity was deficient using xanthine, hypoxanthine, or xanthopterin as substrate and was not restored by addition of FAD, molybdenum, or ferric iron. Xanthine dehydrogenase activity measured with addition of methylene blue as electron acceptor was also missing. Residual activity was abolished by heating the homogenate to 100°C for several minutes and by the inhibitors allopurinol and pteridylaldehyde.

Deficiency of xanthine oxidase activity has been reported in five additional patients. Ayvazian [5] found less than 10 percent of normal activity in the liver of his patient. Frézal and colleagues [7] reported no measurable activity in liver in their patient. Bradford et al. [8] detected traces of activity in small intestine but no demonstrable activity in hepatic tissue in biopsy material from their patient. Chalmers et al. [9] were unable to detect xanthine oxidase activity by a histochemical technique in intestinal mucosa from their patient. Sperling et al. [10] reported about 5 percent of normal activity in jejunal mucosa from their patient.

Assay methods differed in the various laboratories, and limits of accuracy and sensitivity were not given. Accordingly, it is not yet known whether the apparent variation in levels of residual activity represents methodologic limitations or heterogeneity of the genetic and molecular defect.

Muscle Hypoxanthine and Xanthine Content in Xanthinuria

Concentrations of hypoxanthine and xanthine in skeletal muscle of Cases 2 and 8 have been determined by Parker, Snedden, and Watts [66] using quantitative high-resolution mass spectrometry. The results are given in Table 41-3. The values are much too high to be accounted for by oxypurines uniformly distributed in total muscle water or extracellular water at the concentrations that prevail in plasma. They therefore lend quantitative support to the view that hypo-

Table 41-3. CONCENTRATION OF HYPOXANTHINE AND XANTHINE IN SKELETAL MUSCLE FROM XANTHINURIC AND CONTROL SUBJECTS

	Hypoxanthine (ng/mg dry wt)	Xanthine (ng/mg dry wt)
Case 8	350 ± 40	315 ± 30
Control	22 ± 3	<50
Case 2	240 ± 30	450 ± 40
Control	29 ± 3	<50

Source: Parker, Snedden, and Watts [66].

xanthine and xanthine accumulate locally in muscle tissue in xanthinuria [11, 26].

Plasma Purine Concentration Values in Xanthinuria

Plasma normally contains from 0.1 to 0.3 mg oxypurines per 100 mg [67, 68], of which hypoxanthine appears to be the major component. Both hypoxanthine and xanthine accumulate in the plasma of shed blood [69] and may increase 100-fold during standing at room temperature for 48 hr, presumably from catabolism of erythrocyte purine compounds. From 10 to 30 percent of the increment may be due to xanthine [70].

Plasma oxypurine concentration values have been recorded in seven of nine reported xanthinuric patients, and have ranged from 0.2 to 0.9 mg per 100 ml. Borderline or elevated concentration values were found in all seven at one time or another; in four patients values were sometimes within the normal range. Serum uric acid concentration values ranged from 0.05 to 1.6 mg per 100 ml. On a purine-restricted diet virtually all values were less than 1.0 mg per 100 ml (Table 41-1).

Purine Excretion in Xanthinuria

Urinary excretion of xanthine normally ranges from 5.1 to 8.6 mg (average 6.1) per day, and of hypoxanthine, from 5.9 to 13.2 mg (average 9.7) per day [71]. In the nine reported cases of xanthinuria, the excretion of hypoxanthine plus xanthine ranged from 100 to over 500 mg per day, and of uric acid, from 0 to 60 mg per day. The urinary uric acid is at least in part of endogenous origin, for in the patient of Engleman et al. ^{14}C-xanthine given intravenously was converted to ^{14}C-uric acid found in serum and urine. It was calculated that the low level of xanthine oxidase activity detected in liver and intestinal mucosa was sufficient to account for the small amounts of uric acid excreted, 2 to 12 mg per day [4].

In all patients the urinary excretion of xanthine has greatly exceeded that of hypoxanthine (average 84 percent xanthine, range ">50" to 95 percent). The ratio of xanthine to hypoxanthine may be changed in the xanthinuric subject given allopurinol [4]. This suggests that the preponderance of xanthine is in part attributable to the low level of residual activity of xanthine oxidase.

An additional and perhaps more important explanation for the preponderance of urinary xanthine has emerged from isotope dilution studies of the size of the miscible pools of hypoxanthine and xanthine, and of the rates of their turnovers in two xanthinuric subjects. Based on the decline of specific activity in plasma, Engleman et al. [4] calculated an immediate xanthine pool of 144 mg with a turnover of 264 mg per day. Because of the rapidity of turnover of hypoxanthine in plasma, pool values of hypoxanthine could not be calculated. Their patient excreted 126 mg xanthine and only 52 mg hypoxanthine. In more detailed studies of a second patient (Table 41-4), Bradford et al. [8] showed that the initial pool of xanthine was 73 mg and of hypoxanthine, 118 mg. Daily turnovers of these pools were calculated to be 276 and 960 mg, respectively. Of these quantities 79 percent of the xanthine turnover (219 mg) was excreted in urine, compared with only 5.7 percent of the hypoxanthine turnover (54 mg). Qualitatively similar results were obtained by Ayvazian and Skupp [72], who found utilization of administered purines greatest with adenine, intermediate with hypoxanthine, and least with xanthine.

These data disclose a very considerable reutilization, or "salvage," of hypoxanthine, but very little of xanthine in the tissues of man. Although the same phosphoribosyltransferase which efficiently catalyzes the conversion of hypoxanthine and guanine to their respective ribonucleotides also catalyzes the reutilization of xanthine, it does so at less than 1 percent of the rate of the reaction with hypoxanthine [73]. Accordingly, a much larger percentage of the xanthine produced each day is permanently lost from the purine nucleotide pool, and in the absence (or severe deficiency) of xanthine oxidase activity is excreted unchanged. There is nevertheless evidence of some reutilization of xanthine in both mouse [74] and man [75].

Table 41-4. DIMENSIONS AND TURNOVER OF PURINE POOLS IN A XANTHINURIC PATIENT

Purine	Miscible pool, mg	Turnover, mg/day	Urinary excretions, mg/day	% of turnover excreted/day
Hypoxanthine	118	960	54.5	5.7
Xanthine	72.5	276	219	79
Uric Acid	19	11	6.5	61

Source: Bradford et al. [8].

Renal Handling of Xanthine

Dent and Philpot [1] originally suggested that gross xanthinuria with very low levels of uric acid in both plasma and urine might be a consequence either of a block in oxidation of xanthine to uric acid or of a "deviation" mechanism by which xanthine is excreted in urine too rapidly to allow much of it to be oxidized to uric acid.

The finding that plasma oxypurine levels are higher than normal in xanthinuria [2, 4] excluded the renal deviation mechanism as the sole basis of this condition. Moreover, the direct evidence that xanthine oxidase activity is grossly deficient provided a satisfying confirmation of the suspected enzymatic lesion.

Studies showing a renal clearance of oxypurines approaching that of the glomerular filtration rate in the original patient of Dent and Philpot suggested to Dickinson and Smellie [2] that there were two metabolic defects, one of xanthine oxidase function and another of the renal tubular reabsorptive mechanism for xanthine. A high renal clearance of oxypurines was also found in the patient of Engleman and associates [4]. However, when serum oxypurine levels were raised in normal subjects to those found in xanthinuria, either by administration of a xanthine oxidase inhibitor [76] or by infusion of xanthine [4], the clearance of oxypurines rose from normal values of 0.1 to 0.2 of the filtered load to 0.7 to 1.9 times the endogenous creatinine clearance. The high clearances found in xanthinuria may therefore be regarded as normal responses to the elevated serum levels of oxypurines.

Available information about the normal renal handling of xanthine relates in actuality to "oxypurines" composed of hypoxanthine and xanthine in unknown proportions. The normal clearance of oxypurines ranges from 15 to 40 ml per min in man and is therefore three to five times the urate clearance [77]. Xanthine plus hypoxanthine excretion is not influenced by probenecid in man [77]. The accumulation of *p*-aminohippurate by surviving slices of rabbit kidney cortex is inhibited by uric acid, but not by xanthine or hypoxanthine [78]. These results suggest that oxypurine bases are reabsorbed in the renal tubules by a mechanism distinct from that responsible for urate reabsorption.

OTHER CASES OF HYPOURICEMIA

Hypouricemia also occurs in association with certain other inborn errors of metabolism, but except in patients with xanthinuria, it appears to be attributable to failure of renal tubular reabsorption of uric acid. The classic prototype of such a defect is the Dalmatian coach dog, in which clearance of urate equals [79] or exceeds [80, 81] that of inulin. In man hypouricemia occurs in the Fanconi syndrome (Chap. 7) and in Wilson's disease (Chap. 43) as one manifestation of the renal tubular defects of these disorders. Hypouricemia has also been reported in association with carcinoma of the lung in one patient [82].

Praetorius and Kirk [83] discovered an interesting instance of hypouricemia: he was a healthy young man with a plasma uric acid value ranging from 0.2 to 0.6 mg per 100 ml and a urinary output of uric acid of 690 mg per day. Uric acid clearances ranged from 162 to 284 ml per min (normal = 7 to 10 ml per min) and averaged 46 percent greater than simultaneous inulin clearances. The defect appears to be an extraordinarily high uric acid clearance, best explained as total failure of tubular reabsorption plus persistence of normal tubular secretion (Chap. 39). The original report also described an elevated level of "oxypurine" in the plasma of the patient, and in that of his father and son, both of whom had normal plasma uric acid levels. Subsequently the high oxypurine levels were attributed by other authors [68] to breakdown of red cell nucleotides occurring before the plasma was separated from erythrocytes.

A report [84] that serum oxypurine levels are elevated in gout has not been confirmed [67].

IDENTIFICATION OF XANTHINE STONES

Xanthine stones are rare. Hsieh and Hsu [24] found 1 pure xanthine calculus in 760 cases of urinary calculi. Herring [85] found 4 stones containing xanthine among 10,000 urinary calculi. One was pure xanthine (possibly the one obtained from Hsieh and Hsu), and three contained 5 to 19 percent xanthine.

The majority of xanthine stones have been described as brownish or brown-yellow, smooth, round or oval, friable, easily cut with a razor, and white and laminated inside. A few have been irregular in shape. They have ranged in size from a few millimeters in diameter to the size of a hen's egg [13] and in weight from "a few grains" to 3 gm [13] or more [20]. Xanthine stones are nonopaque to x-rays unless calcium is trapped within the stone.

A variety of methods has been used for identification of xanthine in the stone. Most of these leave much to be desired, and identification should be based upon the highly sensitive and specific methods now available, including differential spectrophotometry, paper and column chromatography, and x-ray crystallography [24]. Methods for detection of xanthine in stones are given elsewhere [86]. A detailed description of the two types of crystal structure found in xanthine stones is given by Hsieh and Hsu [24].

Other Cases of Xanthine Stones

Xanthine stones have been found in patients ranging from 2 to 72 years of age [13–24]. Three-quarters of the subjects have been males. Two-thirds of the xanthine stones have been "pure" and one-third, "mixed." The mixed stones have frequently contained uric acid, or calcium oxalate or phosphate in addition to xanthine.

Except in the patients of Dent and Philpot [1], Cifuentes Delatte [6], and Frézal et al. [7], urinary excretion of xanthine has not been measured, nor has hypouricemia been reported in any other patient with xanthine stones. The level of blood or serum uric acid has been normal [14, 20, 23] or even somewhat high [19] in the few cases studied, all adults. In two Duke Hospital patients who had passed mixed xanthine–uric acid stones, excretions of xanthine and of other urinary purines [87] were normal, and serum uric acid levels were not low. A third subject, a woman who had passed stones since early childhood, had pure xanthine stones at age 28 (1947). No uric acid analyses were performed, and she has since been lost to follow-up.

It is clear that not all patients who form xanthine stones have a deficiency of xanthine oxidase activity. Among the patients with xanthine stones are several about whom a strong suspicion exists that xanthine excretion may have been elevated.

Taylor and Taylor [20] reported a 60-year-old male who had xanthine stones weighing 12 gm. If xanthine excretion was normal in this subject (6 mg per day), these stones would represent quantitative precipitation and retention of the cumulative urinary xanthine excretion of 6 years. In addition, seven cases of xanthine stone formation have involved children under age 15, an age group in which the suspicion of an underlying metabolic defect is high. For example, the 2-year-old Taiwanese girl from whom surgeons removed a pure xanthine stone weighing 0.2 gm [24] may very well have xanthinuria. Unfortunately the critical studies required to establish the presence or absence of xanthinuria have not been performed in these subjects.

Ichikawa [22] reported a 44-year-old male who had a left nephrectomy after a lengthy history of hematuria and negative study for urinary calculi. The kidney was grossly normal but on palpation was studded with numerous small nodules. The cut surface disclosed many small holes with brownish granular concrements, which were round or oval, smooth, and friable. Chemical tests showed these to be xanthine, and some tubules contained xanthine casts.

XANTHINURIA INDUCED BY XANTHINE OXIDASE INHIBITORS

When allopurinol or oxipurinol is administered, a portion of urinary uric acid is replaced by xanthine and hypoxanthine. In patients with normal phosphoribosyl transferase activity, the increment of excretion of hypoxanthine plus xanthine is about two-thirds of the decrement of excretion of uric acid [88–90]. Total purine production has been reduced. In this circumstance the excretion of xanthine exceeds considerably that of hypoxanthine, presumably because of the salvage of hypoxanthine discussed above. By contrast, in patients with gross deficiencies of phosphoribosyl transferase activity the decrement of uric acid excretion is matched exactly by the increment of oxypurine excretion [91], and the quantity of hypoxanthine may exceed the quantity of xanthine by a ratio of 1.5 or 3 to 1 [92].

The quantities of xanthine excreted in urine during allopurinol therapy may reach levels comparable to those of patients with hereditary xanthinuria. In spite of the large numbers of patients with gout or urate stones treated with allopurinol, in only two instances has induced xanthine crystal formation been reported. Both were in patients with the Lesch-Nyhan syndrome in whom the basal excretion of uric acid was prodigious, and in whom urinary oxypurine excretion under therapy reached 1,500 to 1,800 mg per day, 42 percent of which was xanthine [92, 93]. In addition, one patient with lymphosarcoma who received allopurinol for control of hyperuricemia showed renal xanthine stones and parenchymal xanthine deposits at post-mortem examination [94].

GENETICS

Of the nine known patients with xanthinuria, four have been females and five males. Six patients have been Caucasian and three, Negro. Thirteen relatives of the xanthinuric subject examined by Dent and Philpot [1] showed no abnormal excretion of xanthine and had normal urinary values of uric acid. These included an only sister, both parents, and three surviving grandparents. None gave a history of renal stone, and the parents were not related. The paternal aunts and the three children of the patient of Ayvazian [5] had ample uric acid in urine; urinary oxypurines were not measured. The mother of the patient of Engleman and associates had normal uric acid and oxypurine levels in plasma and urine and normal xanthine oxidase activity in jejunal mucosa [4]. The patient has no sibs, and the father was not available for study. All three sibs of the patient of Sperling et al. [10] had normal plasma urate values.

The family reported by Cifuentes Delatte and Castro-Mendoza [6] included two brothers with near total replacement of urinary uric acid by xanthine and a sister who excreted 60 to 83 mg of oxypurines per day in addition to 371 to 421 mg of uric acid per day. Seegmiller [25] has suggested that she may be heterozygous for the defect found in its homozygous state in the brothers.

All known data are consistent with the interpretation that xanthinuria is an autosomal recessive disorder. No abnormalities have been detected in any of several presumed obligate heterozygotes. If the young woman cited above is a heterozygote, heterogeneity of the genetic and molecular defect is probable.

A *Drosophila* mutant (rosy^2) seems to lack xanthine oxidase and accumulates hypoxanthine and 2-amino-4-hydroxypteridine [95]. It contains no isoxanthopterin and fails to make red eye pigment [96].

TREATMENT

Prevention of xanthine stone formation in predisposed individuals depends upon recognition of the low solubility of xanthine in acid solutions. The pK_{a_1} of xanthine is 7.7; and

Table 41-5. SOLUBILITY OF PURINES IN BODY FLUIDS

	pH	Uric acid, mg/100 ml	Xanthine, mg/100 ml	Hypoxanthine, mg/100 ml
Serum	7.4	7	10	115
Urine	5	15	5	140
Urine	7	200	13	150

Source: Klinenberg et al. [89].

the pK_{a_2} is 10.6 [97]. Dent and Philpot [1] found that 100 ml normal urine at 26°C dissolved 6.7, 6.5, and 16.5 mg xanthine at a pH of 5.8, 7.0, and 8.1, respectively.

A high fluid intake and maintenance of a large urinary volume would appear to be indicated, as in all instances of stone formation. Oral alkali may be useful in specific instances, but the hazards of continuous alkali therapy must be borne in mind. Furthermore, alkalinization produces only a modest increase in the solubility of xanthine compared with its effect upon uric acid (Table 41-5) [89]. Dietary regulation of purine intake is not indicated in the patient with a normal xanthine output, for xanthine excretion is independent of diet in such patients [87]. On the other hand, in a patient with a block in xanthine oxidation, dietary purines would no doubt add to the burden of xanthine excretion and should be limited. Allopurinol therapy in high doses reversed the xanthine/hypoxanthine ratio in one patient [4] and might be useful in xanthinuric subjects with xanthine stones and residual xanthine oxidase activity. The potential advantage of substitution of the more soluble hypoxanthine for a portion of xanthine is clear from Table 41-3. Methylxanthines, such as caffeine and theophylline, are very much more soluble than xanthine and are not metabolized by xanthine oxidase. It is unnecessary to prohibit their use in xanthinuric subjects.

SUMMARY

1 Xanthinuria is a rare disorder characterized by the replacement of uric acid by xanthine and hypoxanthine in urine. When dietary purines are restricted, there is a virtual absence of uric acid in serum and urine. Nine well-documented cases have been reported. In five the metabolic defect was an incidental finding. In two patients a myopathy was associated with crystalline deposits of hypoxanthine and xanthine in muscle, and in three patients, urinary xanthine stones developed.

2 There is a gross deficiency of xanthine oxidase activity in xanthinuria. Jejunal and hepatic biopsy material show absent or extremely low enzyme activity toward hypoxanthine, xanthine, and xanthopterin.

3 Several additional patients have formed xanthine stones in childhood and may have had xanthinuria. Many of the adults who have formed xanthine stones have clearly not had a defect in xanthine oxidase activity, for in several instances normal or elevated serum uric acid levels were found. Circumstantial evidence, such as the finding of xanthine deposits in the renal parenchyma in one case, suggests that xanthine excretion may have been excessive in a few, but this is unproved.

4 All available data on genetic factors are consistent with an autosomal recessive pattern of inheritance, but in only one family have sibs been involved, and none of the presumed obligate heterozygotes has shown hypouricemia or abnormality of purine excretion.

BIBLIOGRAPHY

1. Dent, C. E., and Philpot, G. R.: Xanthinuria, an inborn error (or deviation) of metabolism. Lancet, **1,** 182, 1954.
2. Dickinson, C. J., and Smellie, J. M.: Xanthinuria. Brit. Med. J., **2,** 1217, 1959.
3. Watts, R. W. E., Engleman, K., Klinenberg, J. R., Seegmiller, J. E., and Sjoerdsma, A.: The enzyme defect in a case of xanthinuria. Biochem. J., **90,** 4P, 1964.
4. Engleman, K., Watts, R. W. E., Klinenberg, J. R., Sjoerdsma, A., and Seegmiller, J. E.: Clinical, physiological and biochemical studies of a patient with xanthinuria and pheochromocytoma. Amer. J. Med., **37,** 839, 1964.
5. Ayvazian, J. H.: Xanthinuria and hemochromatosis. New Eng. J. Med., **270,** 18, 1964.
6. Cifuentes Delatte, L., and Castro-Mendoza, H.: Xanthinuria familiar. Rev. Clin. Esp., **107,** 244, 1967.
7. Frézal, J., Malassenet, R., Cartier, P., Fessard, C., Roy, C., Rey, J., and Lamy, M.: Sur un cas de xanthinurie. Arch. Franç. Pediat., **24,** 129, 1967.
8. Bradford, M. J., Krakoff, I. H., Leeper, R., and Balis, M. E.: Study of purine metabolism in a xanthinuric female. J. Clin. Invest., **47,** 1325, 1968.
9. Chalmers, R. A., Johnson, M., Pallis, C., and Watts, R. W. E.: Xanthinuria with myopathy. Quart. J. Med., New Series, **38,** 493, 1969.
10. Sperling, O., Liberman, U. A., Frank, M., and DeVries, A.: Xanthinuria. An additional case with demonstration of xanthine oxidase deficiency. Am. J. Clin. Path., **55,** 351, 1971.
11. Chalmers, R. A., Watts, R. W. E., Bitensky, L., and Chayen, J.: Microscopic studies on crystals in skeletal muscle from two cases of xanthinuria. J. Path., **99,** 45, 1969.
12. Marcet, A.: *An Essay on the Chemical History and Medical Treatment of Calculous Disorders.* London, 1817.
13. Kretschmer, H. L.: Xanthin calculi: Report of a case and a review of the literature. J. Urol., **38,** 183, 1937.
14. Ratner, M., and Strasberg, A.: A case of xanthine calculosis. Can. Med. Ass. J., **40,** 350, 1939.
15. Hyman, A., and Leiter, H. E.: A case of xanthine calculi. J. Mount Sinai Hosp. NY, **8,** 84, 1941.
16. Butt, A. J., and Holliman, H. E., Jr.: Xanthine calculus: A case report. J. Urol., **52,** 89, 1944.
17. Gersh, I. J., and Meltzer, H. L.: Xanthine urinary calculi: Two cases. J. Urol., **55,** 169, 1946.
18. Berman, L. S.: Twenty-second case of xanthine urinary calculus. J. Urol., **60,** 420, 1948.
19. Pearlman, C. K.: Xanthine urinary calculus. J. Urol., **64,** 799, 1950.
20. Taylor, W. N., and Taylor, J. N.: Xanthine calculus: Case report. J. Urol., **68,** 659, 1952.
21. Mackey, J. F., Jr.: Xanthine calculus. Missouri Med., **50,** 617, 1953.
22. Ichikawa, T.: Xanthine calculi of kidney. J. Urol., **72,** 770, 1954.
23. Jordan, H.: Multiple Xanthinsteinbildung. Bericht über einen Fall. Deutsch. Z. Verdau., **15,** 143, 1955.
24. Hsieh, Y. F., and Hsu, T. C.: Xanthine calculus: a case report. J. Formosan Med. Ass., **62,** 83, 1963.

25. Seegmiller, J. E.: Hereditary xanthinuria, in *Duncan's diseases of Metabolism. Sixth edition. Genetics and Metabolism,* edited by P. K. Bondy and L. E. Rosenberg, pp. 581–599, Saunders, Philadelphia, 1969.
26. Parker, R., Snedden, W., and Watts, R. W. E.: The mass-spectrometric identification of hypoxanthine and xanthine ("oxypurines") in skeletal muscle from two patients with congenital xanthine oxidase deficiency (xanthinuria). Biochem. J., **115,** 103, 1969.
27. Seegmiller, J. E., Engleman, K., Klinenberg, J. R., Watts, R. W. E., and Sjoerdsma, A.: Xanthine oxidase and iron. New Eng. J. Med., **270,** 534, 1964.
28. Klenow, H.: Adenine oxidase. Biochem. J., **50,** 404, 1951–1952.
29. Wyngaarden, J. B., and Dunn, J. T.: 8-Hydroxyadenine as the intermediate in the oxidation of adenine to 2,8-dihydroxyadenine by xanthine oxidase. Arch. Biochem., **70,** 150, 1957.
30. Wyngaarden, J. B.: 2,6-Diaminopurine as substrate and inhibitor of xanthine oxidase. J. Biol. Chem., **224,** 453, 1957.
31. Shaw, E., and Wooley, D. W.: Imidazo-1,2,3-triazines as substrates and inhibitors for xanthine oxidase. J. Biol. Chem., **194,** 641, 1952.
32. Silberman, H. R., and Wyngaarden, J. B.: 6-Mercaptopurine as substrate and inhibitor of xanthine oxidase. Biochim. Biophys. Acta, **47,** 178, 1961.
33. De Renzo, E. C.: Chemistry and biochemistry of xanthine oxidase. Advances Enzym., **17,** 293, 1956.
34. Bergmann, F., and Dikstein, S.: Studies on uric acid and related compounds. III. Observations on the specificity on mammalian xanthine oxidases. J. Biol. Chem., **223,** 765, 1956.
35. Coombs, H. I.: Studies on xanthine oxidase. IX. The specificity of the system. II. Biochem. J., **21,** 1259, 1927.
36. Fridovich, I.: A new class of xanthine oxidase inhibitors isolated from guanidinium salts. Biochemistry, **4,** 1098, 1965.
37. Feigelson, P., Davidson, J. D., and Robins, R. K.: Pyrazolopyrimidines as inhibitors and substrates of xanthine oxidase. J. Biol. Chem., **226,** 993, 1957.
38. Elion, G. B.: Enzymatic and metabolic studies with allopurinol. Ann. Rheum. Dis., **25,** 608, 1966.
39. Massey, V., Komai, H., Palmer, G., and Elion, G. B.: On the mechanism of inactivation of xanthine oxidase by allopurinol and other pyrazolo [3,4-d] pyrimidines. J. Biol. Chem., **245,** 2837, 1970.
40. Krebs, E. G., and Norris, E. R.: The competitive inhibition of xanthine oxidation by xanthopterin. Arch. Biochem., **24,** 49, 1949.
41. Kalckar, H. M., Kjeldgaarde, N. O., and Klenow, H.: Inhibition of xanthine oxidase and related enzymes by 6-pteridyl aldehyde. J. Biol. Chem., **174,** 771, 1948.
42. Booth, V. H.: The specificity of xanthine oxidase. Biochem. J., **32,** 494, 1938.
43. Rajagopalan, K. V., Fridovich, I., and Handler, P.: Hepatic aldehyde oxidase. I. Purification and properties. J. Biol. Chem., **237,** 922, 1962.
44. Gibbs, D. A., and Watts, R. W. E.: Biochemical studies on the treatment of primary hyperoxaluria. Arch. Dis. Child., **42,** 505, 1967.
45. Andrews, P., Bray, R. C., Edwards, P., and Shooter, K. V.: The chemistry of xanthine oxidase. II. Ultracentrifuge and gel-filtration studies on the milk enzyme. Biochem. J., **93,** 627, 1964.
45*a*. Hart, L. I., McGartoll, M. A., Chapman, H. R., and R. C. Bray.: The composition of milk xanthine oxidase. Biochem. J., **116,** 851, 1970.
46. Nelson, C. A., and Handler, P.: Preparation of bovine xanthine oxidase and the subunit structures of some iron flavoproteins. J. Biol. Chem., **243,** 5368, 1968.
47. Brumby, P. E.: Ph.D. Thesis. University of Sheffield, 1963.
48. Rajagopalan, K. V., and Handler, P.: Purification and properties of chicken liver xanthine dehydrogenase. J. Biol. Chem., **242,** 4097, 1967.
49. Bray, R. C., and Malmstrom, B. G.: The chemistry of xanthine oxidase. 12. The amino acid composition. Biochem. J., **93,** 633, 1964.
50. Massey, V., Brumby, P. E., Komai, H., and Palmer, G.: Studies on milk xanthine oxidase. Some spectral and kinetic properties. J. Biol. Chem., **244,** 1682, 1969.
51. Mehler, A. H.: *Introduction to Enzymology,* p. 178. Academic, New York, 1957.
52. Bray, R. C., Chisholm, J., Hart, L. I., Meriwether, L. S., and Watts, D. C.: Studies on the composition and mechanism of action of milk xanthine, in *Flavines and Flavoproteins,* edited by E. C. Slater, p. 117, Elsevier, Amsterdam, 1966.
53. Komai, H., Massey, V., and Palmer, G.: The preparation and properties of deflavo xanthine oxidase. J. Biol. Chem., **244,** 1692, 1969.
54. Bray, R. C., Palmer, G., and Beinert, H.: Direct studies on the electron transfer sequence in xanthine oxidase by electron paramagnetic resonance spectroscopy. II. Kinetic studies employing rapid freezing. J. Biol. Chem., **239,** 2667, 1964.
54*a*. Palmer, G., and Massey, V.: Electron paramagnetic resonance and circular dichroism studies on milk xanthine oxidase. J. Biol. Chem., **244,** 2614, 1969.
55. Handler, P., Rajagopalan, K. V., and Aleman, V.: Structure and function of iron-flavoproteins. Fed. Proc., **23,** 30, 1964.
56. Mackler, B., Mahler, H. R., and Green, D. E.: Studies on metalloflavoproteins. I. Xanthine oxidase, a molybdoflavoprotein. J. Biol. Chem., **210,** 149, 1954.
57. Al-Khalidi, U. A. S., and Chaglassian, T. H.: The species distribution of xanthine oxidase. Biochem. J., **97,** 318, 1965.
58. Watts, R. W. E., Watts, J. E. M., and Seegmiller, L. E.: Xanthine oxidase activity in human tissues and its inhibition by allopurinol (4-hydroxypyrazolo [3,4-d] pyrimidine). J. Lab. Clin. Med., **66,** 688, 1965.
59. Dunn, J. T., and Wyngaarden, J. B.: Unpublished data.
60. Shamma'a, M. H., Masrallah, S., Chaglassian, T., Kachadurian, A. K., and Al-Khalidi, U. A. S.: Serum xanthine oxidase: A sensitive test of acute liver injury. Gastroenterology, **48,** 226, 1965.
61. Morgan, E. J.: The distribution of xanthine oxidase. I. Biochem. J., **20,** 1282, 1926.
62. Rowe, P. B., and Wyngaarden, J. B.: The mechanism of dietary alterations in rat hepatic xanthine oxidase levels. J. Biol. Chem., **241,** 5571, 1966.
63. Rowe, P. B., and Wyngaarden, J. B.: Unpublished data.
64. Bray, R. C.: Xanthine oxidase, in *The Enzymes,* edited by P. Boyer, H. Lardy, and K. Myrbäch p. 533, vol. 7, 2nd ed., Academic, New York, 1963.
65. Carcassi, A., Marcolongo, R., Jr., Marinello, E., Riario-Sforza, G., and Boggiano, C.: Liver xanthine oxidase in gouty patients. Arthritis Rheum., **12,** 17, 1969.
66. Parker, R., Snedden, W., and Watts, R. W. E.: The quantitative determination of hypoxanthine and xanthine ("oxypurines") in skeletal muscle from two patients with congenital xanthine oxidase deficiency (xanthinuria). Biochem. J., **116,** 317, 1970.
67. Segal, S., and Wyngaarden, J. B.: Plasma glutamine and oxypurine content in patients with gout. Proc. Soc. Exp. Biol. Med., **88,** 342, 1955.
68. Jorgensen, S., and Poulsen, H. E.: Enzymic determination of hypoxanthine and xanthine in human plasma and urine. Acta Pharmacol. Toxicol., **11,** 223, 1955.
69. Jorgensen, S.: Hypoxanthine and xanthine accumulated in stored human blood: Determination of relative amounts by spectrophotometry. Acta Pharmacol. Toxicol., **11,** 265, 1955.
70. Jorgensen, S.: Xanthine formation from guanine, guanosine or xanthosine in human blood. Acta Pharmacol. Toxicol., **12,** 303, 1956.
71. Weissmann, B., Bromberg, P. A., and Gutman, A. B.: The purine bases of human urine. II. Semiquantitative estimation and isotope incorporation. J. Biol. Chem., **224,** 423, 1957.
72. Ayvazian, J. H., and Skupp, S.: Purine utilization and excretion in xanthinuria. J. Clin. Invest., **44,** 1248, 1965.
73. Kelley, W. N., Rosenbloom, F. M., Henderson, J. F., and Seegmiller, J. E.: Xanthine phosphoribosyltransferase in man: relationship to hypoxanthine-guanine phosphoribosyltransferase. Biochem. Biophys. Res. Commun., **28,** 340, 1967.
74. Pomales, R., Elion, G. B., and Hitchings, G. H.: Xanthine as a precursor of nucleic acid purines in the mouse. Biochim. Biophys. Acta, **95,** 505, 1965.
75. Kelley, W. N., and Wyngaarden, J. B.: Effects of allopurinol and oxipurinol on purine synthesis in cultured human cells. J. Clin. Invest., **49,** 602, 1970.
76. Klinenberg, J. R., Goldfinger, S., Miller, J., and Seegmiller, J. E.: The effectiveness of a xanthine oxidase inhibitor in the treatment of gout. Arthritis Rheum., **6,** 779, 1963.

77. Gjorup, S., and Poulsen, H.: Effects of probenecid cinchophen and colchicine on the plasma concentrations and renal excretion of oxypurine in patients with gout. Acta Pharmacol. Toxicol., **11**, 343, 1955.
78. Despopoulos, A.: Renal excretory transport of organic acids: Inhibition by oxypurines. Amer. J. Physiol., **197**, 1107, 1959.
79. Friedman, M., and Byers, S. O.: Observations concerning the causes of excess excretion of uric acid in the Dalmatian dog. J. Biol. Chem., **175**, 127, 1948.
80. Kessler, R. H., Hierholzer, K., and Gurd, R. S.: Localization of urate transport in the nephron of mongrel and Dalmatian dog kidney. Amer. J. Physiol., **197**, 601, 1959.
81. Yu, T. F., Berger, L., Kupfer, S., and Gutman, A. B.: Tubular secretion of urate in the dog. Amer. J. Physiol., **199**, 1199, 1960.
82. Weinstein, I. B., Irreverre, F., and Watkin, D.: Lung carcinoma, hypouricemia and aminoaciduria. Amer. J. Med., **39**, 520, 1965.
83. Praetorius, E., and Kirk, J. E.: Hypouricemia: With evidence for tubular elimination of uric acid. J. Lab. Clin. Med., **35**, 865, 1950.
84. Orstrom, A., and Orstrom, M.: The role of glutamine in metabolism, with special regard to the formation of uric acid in gout. Acta Med. Scand., **138**, 108, 1950.
85. Herring, L. C.: Observations on the analysis of 10,000 urinary calculi. J. Urol., **88**, 545, 1962.
86. Wyngaarden, J. B.: Xanthinuria, in *Metabolic Basis of Inherited Disease,* 1st ed., p. 761, edited by J. B. Stanbury, J. B. Wyngaarden, and D. S. Fredrickson, McGraw-Hill, New York, 1960.
87. Weissmann, B., Bromberg, P. A., and Gutman, A. B.: The purine bases of human urine. I. Separation and identification. J. Biol. Chem., **224**, 407, 1957.
88. Rundles, R. W., Wyngaarden, J. B., Hitchings, G. H., Elion, G. B., and Silberman, H. R.: Effects of a xanthine oxidase inhibitor on thiopurine metabolism, hyperuricemia and gout. Trans. Ass. Amer. Physicians, **76**, 126, 1963.
89. Klinenberg, J. R., Goldfinger, S., Miller, J., and Seegmiller, J. E.: The effectiveness of a xanthine oxidase inhibitor on the treatment of gout. Ann. Intern. Med., **62**, 639, 1965.
90. Rundles, R. W., Wyngaarden, J. B., Hitchings, G. H., and Elion, G. B.: Drugs and uric acid. Ann. Rev. Pharmacol. **9**, 345, 1969.
91. Kelley, W. N., Greene, M. L., Rosenbloom, F. M., Henderson, J. J., and Seegmiller, J. E.: Hypoxanthine guanine phosphoribosyltransferase deficiency in gout. Ann. Intern. Med., **70**, 155, 1969.
92. Greene, M. J., Fujimoto, W. Y., and Seegmiller, J. E.: Urinary xanthine stones—a rare complication of allopurinol therapy. New Eng. J. Med., **280**, 426, 1969.
93. Sorensen, L., and Seegmiller, J. E.: Seminars on the Lesch-Nyhan syndrome: Management and treatment, discussion. Fed. Proc., **27**, 1097, 1968.
94. Band, P. R., Silverberg, M. D., Henderson, J. H., Ulan, R. A., Wensel, R. H., Banerjee, T. K., and Little, A. S.: Xanthine nephropathy in a patient with lymphosarcoma treated with allopurinol. New Eng. J. Med., **283**, 354, 1970.
95. Morita, T.: Purine catabolism in Drosophila melanogaster. Science, **128**, 1135, 1958.
96. Hadorn, E., and Schwinck, I.: A mutant of *Drosophila* without isoxanthopterine which is non-autonomous for the red eye pigments. Nature, **177**, 940, 1956.
97. Bergmann, F., and Dikstein, S.: The relationship between spectral shifts and structural changes in uric acids and related compounds. J. Amer. Chem. Soc., **77**, 691, 1955.

CHAPTER FORTY-TWO

HEREDITARY OROTIC ACIDURIA

Lloyd H. Smith, Jr., Charles M. Huguley, Jr., and James A. Bain

Hereditary orotic aciduria represents two rare genetic disorders of pyrimidine metabolism characterized usually by retarded growth and development, hypochromic anemia associated with a megaloblastic marrow unresponsive to usual hematinic therapy, and excessive urinary excretion of orotic acid [1–4]. Replacement therapy with pyrimidine nucleotides or uridine leads to a clinical and hematologic remission and to a reduction in the excretion of orotic acid. Studies of hemic cells, liver homogenates, and of fibroblasts grown in tissue culture have demonstrated reduced activities of both orotidylic pyrophosphorylase and orotidylic decarboxylase, sequential enzymes which catalyze the conversion of orotic acid to uridine-5′-phosphate [5, 6, 7]. More recently a single patient with isolated deficiency of orotidylic decarboxylase activity has been discovered, indistinguishable clinically from the prototype disorder [2]. In this discussion *hereditary orotic aciduria* will be used as a general description, with the specific disorders designated as Type I (double enzyme defect) and Type II (isolated deficiency of orotidylic decarboxylase).

Hereditary orotic aciduria has several features which lend added importance to its investigation [8]: (1) it represents the only specific disorder of pyrimidine nucleotide synthesis so far elucidated in man or in any nonmicrobial organism; (2) the phenotype can be partially simulated by the use of a pharmacologic agent; (3) it is pyrimidine auxotrophism in man, perhaps the clearest example of auxotrophism in a multicellular organism; (4) the "pyrimidine starvation" of hereditary orotic aciduria illustrates intracellular metabolic control mechanisms previously described in microorganisms; and (5) the presence of a double enzyme defect in the Type I disorder suggests a mutation in a regulatory gene, although this possibility has not been established.

CLINICAL FEATURES

Only eight cases of hereditary orotic aciduria are known to the authors. Their case reports will be summarized briefly.

Patient J.R. [1]. This white male infant, the product of a normal delivery at full term, weighed 8 lb, 9 oz at birth and appeared to be in good health until the age of 3 months. He was then observed to be pale, lethargic, and somnolent and was subject to repeated respiratory infections and chronic diarrhea, with large, pale, foul-smelling stools. His hemoglobin was 6 gm per 100 ml. This anemia failed to respond to iron, ascorbic acid, folic acid, vitamin B_{12}, or crude liver concentrate.

When first studied at age 9 months, the patient was pale and weak but well developed and well nourished. The scleras appeared blue, and the edge of the liver and tip of the spleen were palpable. There was no atrophy of his tongue. There was outward torsion of the left tibia but no other skeletal abnormalities. No neurologic abnormalities were found. Laboratory studies revealed a severe hypochromic anemia (hemoglobin 6.7 gm; erythrocytes 2.8 million per mm^3), with striking anisocytosis and poikilocytosis (Fig. 42-1). There was leukopenia (leukocytes 2,050 per mm^3) with monocytosis, but a normal platelet count. The bone marrow was hypercellular, and there were striking abnormalities of the megaloblastic type in cells of both the granulocytic and erythrocytic series. Urinalysis was normal except for a moderate number of crystals which were later proved to be orotic acid.

The clinical course of patient J.R. has been presented in detail elsewhere [1]. Appropriate diagnostic studies, including failure of therapeutic response, excluded deficiency of vitamin B_{12}, folic acid, pyridoxine, or iron as contributing to his anemia. Studies for hemoglobin abnormalities, thalassemia, and erythremic myelosis (DiGuglielmo's syndrome) were also negative. There was a partial hematologic remission during glucocorticoid therapy without reversal of the bone marrow abnormalities. Throughout his course large numbers of crystals would precipitate from the urine on standing or, occasionally, within the urinary tract. On several occasions urethral obstruction, and on one occasion right ureteral obstruction, occurred. These crystals were identified as orotic acid by a series of tests described elsewhere [1]. Orotic acid excretion was variable but usually was in the range of 800 to 1,400 mg per 24 hr. When the child was treated with a yeast extract containing a mixture of pyrimidine nucleotides, there was a prompt reticulocytosis, rise of hemoglobin to normal, disappearance of marrow megaloblasts, and a striking reduction in urinary orotic acid (Fig. 42-2). The prompt improvement in his general health was equally as marked. He gained weight for the first time in 18 months and recovered from an apparent retardation in walking, talking, and general activity. After approximately 3 months nucleotide therapy was discontinued because it was poorly tolerated. It was planned to reinstitute treatment with other preparations, but there was a prompt relapse. Death occurred shortly thereafter secondary to varicella (Fig. 42-2). Autopsy showed only generalized varicella.

The patient's three sibs and his parents exhibited no

This work was supported in part by Research Grant AM-09406, National Institute of Arthritis and Metabolic Diseases, U.S. Public Health Service.

The authors express their gratitude to Drs. S. H. Appel, D. M. O. Becroft, R. M. Fox, M. E. Haggard, R. S. Krooth, A. Y. Najean, F. S. Porter, and G. M. Tomkins for suggestions and for allowing the use of unpublished data in the preparation of this chapter.

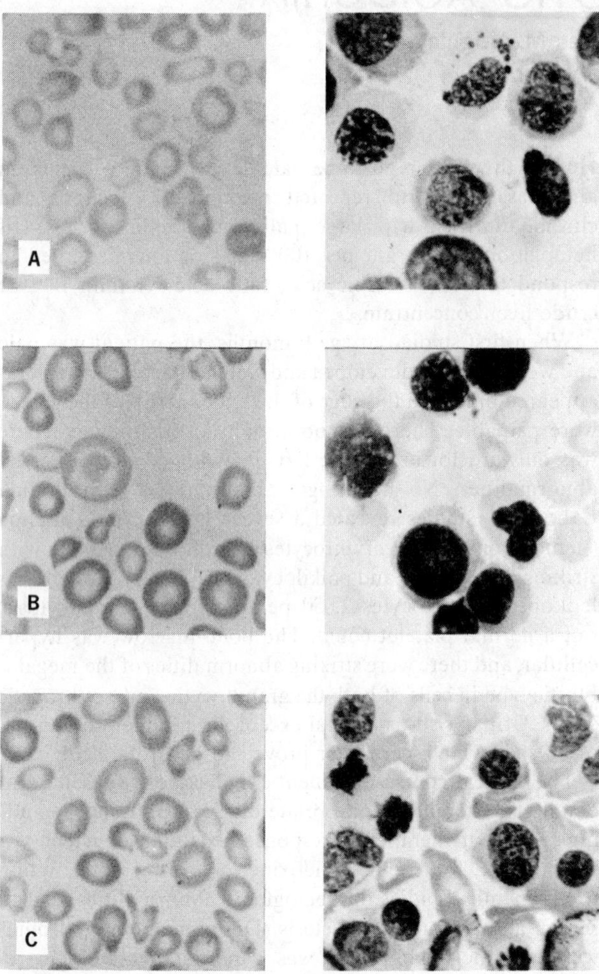

Figure 42-1. Peripheral blood (*left*) and bone marrow preparations (*right*) from three patients with untreated hereditary orotic aciduria. A. Patient J.R. B. Patient D.G. C. Patient J.P.

clinical or hematologic abnormalities. Studies on the R. family are presented in the sections on Pathogenesis and Genetics.

Patient D.G. [9, 10]. This male infant, a quarter-caste Maori in New Zealand, weighed 9 lb, 2 oz at birth and seemed to grow and develop normally for the first 2 to 3 months. Beginning at about age 3 months he appeared pale and apathetic, and was retarded in motor development. At age 13 months, at which time he could not sit unsupported, he received a short course of treatment with chloramphenicol for bronchopneumonia. He was discovered to be severely anemic (hemoglobin 4.6 gm per 100 ml) and leukopenic (leukocytes 2,400 per mm^3). Further investigation revealed a megaloblastic marrow and a low serum iron (11 μg per 100 ml), but there was no hematologic response to iron, folic acid, vitamin B_{12}, pyridoxine, or thyroxine. Additional studies seemed to exclude blood loss, malabsorption, hepatic disease, or renal disease as contributing causes of his illness.

When examined at age 17 months at the Auckland Hospital he was found to be a pale, lethargic child with an alternating strabismus, weighing 21½ lb (<3rd percentile). Although there were no specific neurologic abnormalities, his general physical and mental development appeared to be retarded. He was unable to sit up alone but could maintain a sitting position. There was sparse growth of short, fine hair, and it was noted that his fingernails had failed to grow over a period of several months. The spleen tip was palpable. There was no glossitis. The initial hemoglobin was 8.0 gm per 100 ml, and the smear showed hypochromic cells with marked anisocytosis and poikilocytosis (Fig. 42-1). The presence of megaloblastic changes in the bone marrow was confirmed. There was histamine-fast achlorhydria. Serum levels of vitamin B_{12} and folic acid were normal. A urine specimen on standing developed a heavy, flocculent precipitate of fine, needle-shaped crystals (Fig. 42-3) with the ultraviolet absorption spectrum of orotic acid. The excretion of orotic acid averaged 1.15 gm daily. Absence of orotidylic pyrophosphorylase and orotidylic decarboxylase activities was demonstrated in frozen erythrocytes (see below). A brief trial of cytidylic acid therapy was given, following which the patient was treated with oral uridine (Fig. 42-4). There was a rapid hematologic response to uridine, most marked when the initial dose of 0.75 gm was increased to 1.5 gm daily. One month after the beginning of uridine therapy the hemoglobin was 13.7 gm per 100 ml, hematocrit 44 percent, and the bone marrow was normoblastic. Orotic acid excretion decreased to approximately 0.2 to 0.3 gm per 24 hr. There was an accompanying improvement in general health, with weight gain, increased strength and activity, and renewed growth of hair and nails. Treatment has now continued until age 7 at a dose of approximately 150 mg uridine per kg body weight in divided doses. At last report [10] he was at the 75th percentile for height and weight. Although there was initial rapid improvement in intellectual skills on uridine, his IQ using the Wechsler Scale at age 7 was in the range of 73–81. Slight alternating convergent strabismus continues, and there are small areas of scleral pigmentation. On uridine his hemoglobin, platelets, and leukocytes have been normal, and orotic acid excretion has stabilized in the range of 0.4 to 0.6 gm per day. No renal complications have resulted from this level of excretion in spite of crystalluria.

Extensive family studies have not as yet been carried out. The father, of Irish descent, has reduced levels of orotidylic pyrophosphorylase and orotidylic decarboxylase in his erythrocytes (see below). A hydrocephalic sib died of a subdural hematoma. No orotic acid was found in his urine. At the time of writing no studies have been carried out on the patient's mother, who is three-fourths Maori, or on an older male sib, who is reported to be in good health.

Patient J.P. [11]. This white male infant, the product of a 35-week gestation, weighed only 4 lb at birth but was thought

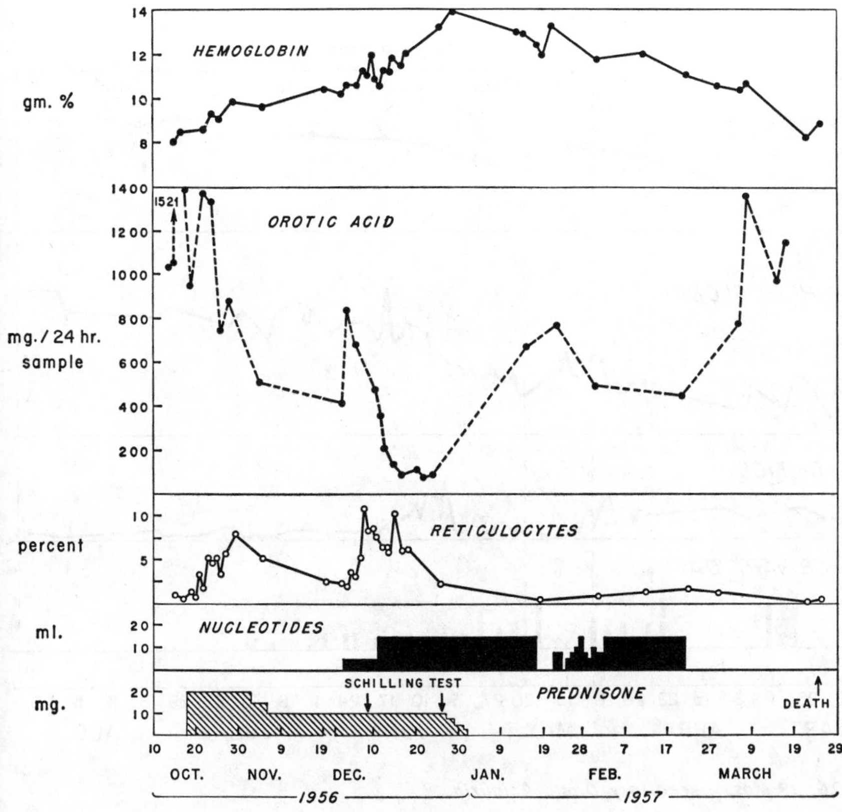

Figure 42-2. Changes in hemoglobin, reticulocytes, and urinary orotic acid in patient J.R. during treatment with prednisone and a mixture of nucleotides (uridylic acid, 115 mg per ml; cytidylic acid, 269 mg per ml).

to grow and develop normally for the first few months. At age 7 months, he appeared pale and listless, and his hematocrit was 22 percent. Iron therapy was ineffective, and he was sent at age 10 months to the Children's Hospital, Galveston, Texas, for further investigation. Physical examination revealed a pale, blond infant, 68 cm in length, weighing 19 lb, 11 oz (25th percentile). There was an alternating esotropia

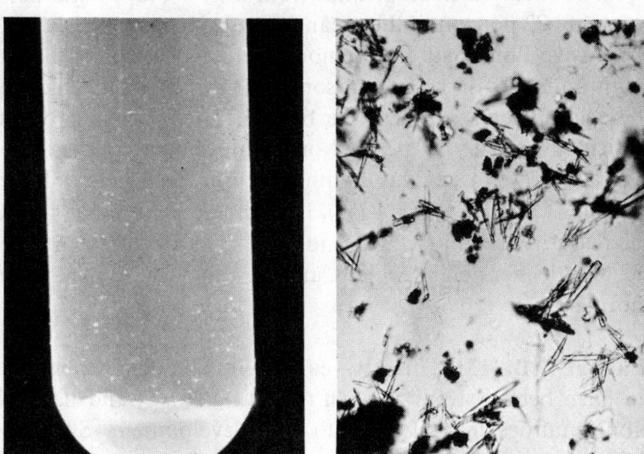

Figure 42-3. Sediment of crystalline orotic acid in the urine of patient D.G.

but no glossitis or specific neurologic abnormalities.

Laboratory studies revealed a severe anemia (hemoglobin 4.8 gm per 100 ml) and leukopenia (leukocytes 1,500 per mm^3). The peripheral blood smear demonstrated hypochromic erythrocytes with marked anisocytosis and poikilocytosis (Fig. 42-1), and repeated bone marrow aspirations showed a megaloblastic pattern. Serum folic acid and vitamin B_{12}, hemoglobin electrophoresis, red cell osmotic fragility, formiminoglutamic acid excretion (after histidine loading), serum iron, and gastric acidity were normal. There was no response to therapeutic trials with folic or folinic acids, vitamin B_{12}, crude liver extract, pyridoxine, or α-tocopherol. Immunoelectrophoresis demonstrated absence of γA- and γD-globulins. At age 13½ months his performance by Gesell testing was at the 9-month level. On prednisone therapy (30 mg per day in divided doses) there was a reticulocytosis to 6.4 percent with a rise of hemoglobin to 10.2 gm per 100 ml and reversal of leukopenia, but with no change in the marrow megaloblastosis. Hematologic relapse followed withdrawal of prednisone, with a second partial remission when it was reinstituted. At age 19 months, while on prednisone therapy, the child developed partial ureteral obstruction associated with marked crystalluria. Urinary orotic acid was found to be 930 mg per day, and orotidylic decarboxylase activity was absent from his erythrocytes. Uridine therapy (250 mg orally six times per day) was begun at age 22

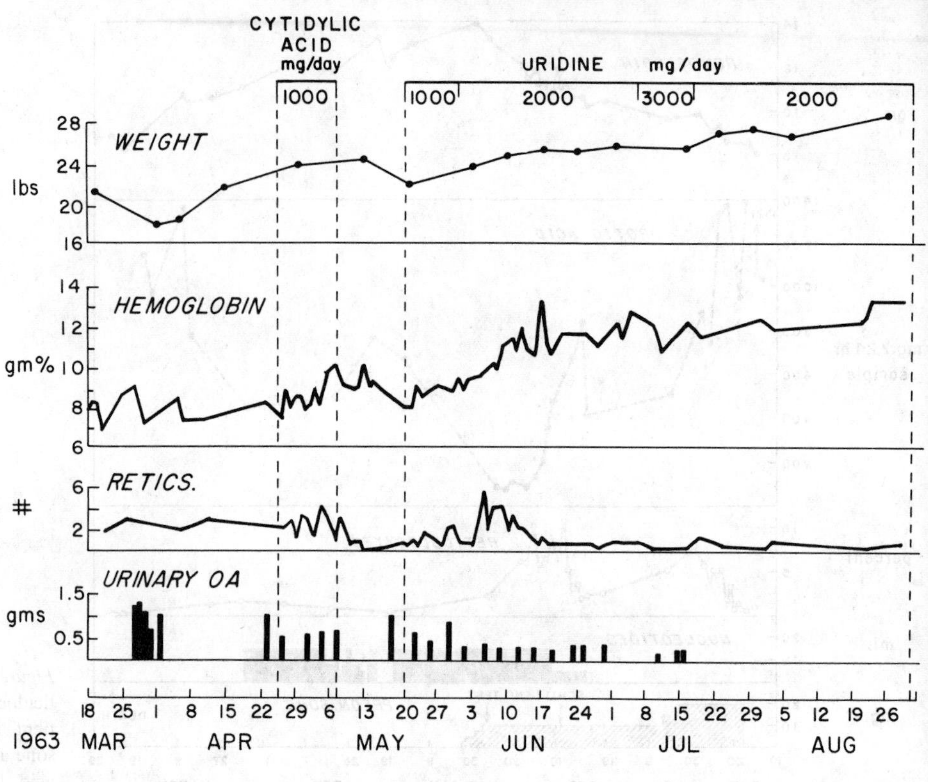

Figure 42-4. Changes in weight, hemoglobin, reticulocytes, and urinary orotic acid in patient D.G. during treatment with cytidylic acid and with uridine.

months. There was a prompt reticulocytosis (17.2 percent), with rise of hemoglobin to 12.1 gm and reversion of his bone marrow to a normal cytologic pattern. Orotic acid excretion was reduced to 147 mg per day. At age 7½ years the patient is still being maintained on uridine, 1.5 gm orally daily, and has normal growth and development. His hematologic remission has been maintained, but his IQ is only 80–84 [12]. His parents and male sib have normal hemograms but reduced activities of erythrocyte orotidylic decarboxylase.

Patient T. H. [6]. This white female, the product of a normal pregnancy, weighed 6 lb, 7¾ oz at birth, and was considered to have normal development until age 2 months when anemia (7.7 gm per 100 ml) was noted. Because of failure to respond to oral iron and vitamin C, she was referred to the North Carolina Baptist Hospital, Winston-Salem, for further studies. Physical examination revealed pallor, bilateral strabismus, and a harsh precordial systolic murmur (subsequently interpreted as a probable interventricular septal defect). No other neurologic abnormality was noted, and there was no hepatosplenomegaly. The infant's weight was 7.4 kg (50th percentile) and her length was 68 cm (90th percentile).

Laboratory studies revealed anemia (hemoglobin 7.8 gm per 100 ml; hematocrit 28 percent; erythrocytes 2.9 million per mm^3), leukopenia (3,300 per mm^3), and a megaloblastic marrow with erythroid hyperplasia. The peripheral blood smear showed moderately hypochromic cells with anisocytosis, poikilocytosis, and hypersegmentation of granulocytes. There was no response to folic acid or vitamin B_{12}. Several months later crystalluria was noted and orotic acid was identified. Orotic acid excretion was 1.11 to 3.57 gm per gm creatinine (while receiving 0.75 gm oral uridine daily). The conversion of orotic acid to uridylic acid was markedly reduced in hemolysates of the infant's erythrocytes, and orotidylic pyrophosphorylase and orotidylic decarboxylase were reduced in homogenates from a liver biopsy (1.5 percent and 22 percent of the mean control values, respectively). Extensive family studies demonstrated a pattern consistent with transmission as an autosomal trait with partial enzyme defects in heterozygotes (see below). There was a prompt reticulocytosis to 14 percent on institution of oral uridine therapy (1.5 gm per day), with a return of all hematologic findings to normal (Fig. 42-5). In addition there was a rapid increase in growth (weight and length) and activity. At age 52 months her height, weight, and mental development were normal.

Patient D.B. [13]. This 7½-year-old female child appeared to have been normal at birth (weight 2.95 kg) and had no abnormalities in early growth and development. She had been observed to be somewhat pale and for perhaps a year had fatigued easily and had complained of backache and flank pain. Following an episode of gross hematuria she was

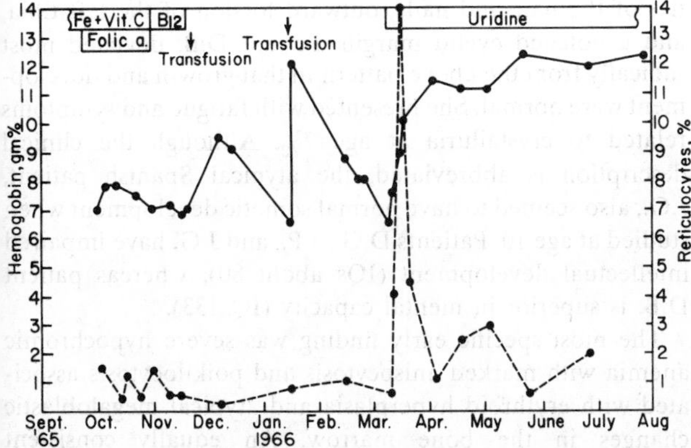

Figure 42-5. Hemoglobin and reticulocyte response in patient T.H. following uridine administration. Lack of response to treatment with iron, vitamin C, vitamin B_{12}, and folic acid is demonstrated. (*From Pediatrics,* **42,** 415, 1968, *with permission of the publishers.*)

found to be anemic and was admitted to the University of Michigan Medical Center. Physical examination revealed a pale but alert girl of height 122 cm (25th percentile) and weight 25 kg (50th percentile). The only abnormalities were a small notch with absence of lashes in the margin of the right upper eyelid and a soft systolic murmur heard over the pulmonic area.

Laboratory studies revealed anemia (hemoglobin 7.4 gm per 100 ml; hematocrit 27 percent; erythrocytes 3.39 million per mm^3) and leukopenia (3,200 per mm^3). The peripheral blood smear showed moderate hypochromia with marked anisocytosis and poikilocytosis without hypersegmentation of the neutrophils. The bone marrow aspirate revealed erythroid hyperplasia with megaloblastic changes and giant metamyelocytes in the granulocytic series. Normal studies included serum iron, serum folate, serum B_{12}, a Schilling's test, gastric acidity, serum protein electrophoresis, and the direct Coombs test. The creatine clearance and intravenous pyelogram were normal. At 7½ years the patient had an IQ of 133 (Stanford-Binet), with a mental age of 10.0 years. Performance on nonverbal tasks was less proficient than on verbal tasks, and there was "a relative lag in numerical concepts and integrative capabilities" [13]. Crystals from her urine were identified by ultraviolet absorption spectroscopy as orotic acid (650 mg per day while receiving uridine, 20 mg per kg per day). Markedly deficient activities of orotidylic pyrophosphorylase and orotidylic decarboxylase were demonstrated in erythrocyte hemolysates and in a diploid cell strain established in tissue culture from a skin biopsy. There was a prompt response of the erythrocytic abnormalities to oral uridine, 100 mg per kg per day. Leukopenia, however, was reversed only at a dose of 150 mg per kg per day. During subsequent months the hematologic remission has persisted, and there have been no further urinary tract symptoms (attributed to crystalluria) or unusual fatigue. No change in growth pattern occurred during the 40 weeks of observation on uridine. The mother of the patient exhibited a heterozygous pattern of enzyme deficiencies in erythrocyte hemolysate preparations. Her father was not available for examination.

Patient C.P. [2] This male infant of Greek parentage was born after 32 weeks gestation with numerous deformities and weight 3 lb, 5 oz. At age 3 months he was admitted to the Royal Alexandra Hospital for Children (Sydney, Australia) because of failure to thrive. Physical examination revealed generalized hypertonicity, kyphoscoliosis, and a scaphoid skull. There were umbilical and bilateral inguinal hernias and "herniation of lung into the supraclavicular regions."

Laboratory studies revealed anemia (hemoglobin 6.3 gm per 100 ml) and leukopenia (2,600 per mm^3). The peripheral blood smear was hypochromic with anisocytosis, and the bone marrow aspirate was megaloblastic with increased iron stores. Serum B_{12} was 1,000 pg per ml and serum folic acid 0.4 ng per ml. There was no hematologic response to iron, folic acid, or vitamin B_{12}. Heavy crystalluria was noted, leading at one time to urethral obstruction. The crystals were identified as orotic acid by ultraviolet absorption spectroscopy. Low levels of orotidylic pyrophosphorylase and orotidylic decarboxylase were found in hemolysates of the patient's erythrocytes. Levels of these enzyme activities in his parents' hemolysates were not low as compared to a control subject, but the reliability of these absolute values is diminished by a 6-months' storage period (−25°C) prior to analysis. There was an initial hematologic response to uridine replacement therapy (150 mg per kg per day orally), but the child was removed from the hospital against advice by his parents and died soon afterwards from meningitis and pneumonia.

Patient P.M. [2, 3] This male infant was born at full term with a birth weight of 7 lb. There was a family history of mental retardation with possible consanguinity as well. The patient is thought to be the product of a brother-sister mating. At 5½ months of age he was admitted to the Royal Alexandra Hospital for Children because of failure to thrive. Physical examination at that time revealed retarded motor development, mild seborrheic dermatitis, and fine, dry hair. Laboratory studies showed anemia (7.4 gm per 100 ml). The leukocyte count was not reported. The bone marrow aspirate was megaloblastic. Serum B_{12} was 548 pg per ml and serum folic acid 6.4 ng per ml. There was no response to oral iron or folic acid or to parenteral vitamin B_{12}. Profuse crystalluria was noted with identification of orotic acid by ultraviolet spectrophotometry. Orotidine excretion was elevated also (about 50 to 100 mg per day). Studies on erythrocyte hemolysates revealed virtual absence of orotidylic decarboxylase activity. In contrast to all previous patients with hereditary orotic aciduria, the activity of orotidylic pyrophosphorylase was elevated rather than reduced. This patient is therefore the propositus of Type II hereditary orotic aciduria. The patient's mother has exhibited a partial enzyme defect in her erythrocytes and excretes excessive orotic acid and orotidine. By urinary screening techniques P.M.'s brother and probable father-uncle exhibit excretion patterns of orotic acid consistent with heterozygosity. Oral uridine therapy was begun (150 mg per kg per day) with a prompt hematologic response. After almost 2 years of therapy, his hemoglobin was 11.1 gm per 100 ml, leukocytes 12,900, and platelets normal. His seborrheic dermatitis remained symptomatic and he has continued to be retarded in mental development [3].

Patient J.G. [14, 15]. This Spanish boy (residing in France), who had severe anemia beginning at age 3 months and requiring 10 transfusions, was studied at 5 years of age [14] and more recently at age 10 [15]. His somatic growth and development have been normal despite anemia, and no urinary symptoms from crystalluria were reported. At age 10 he is unable to read or write and has an IQ of about 80. He was found to have megaloblastic anemia (Hb 8.5 gm) without leukopenia or thrombocytopenia. There was no response to treatment with pyridoxine or B_{12}. There was a partial response to folic acid and folinic acid (2.5 mg per day), with a rise of hemoglobin and a marrow remission. The patient has continued to be anemic over the past few years but has required no further transfusions while on folic acid. Crystals were observed in the urine and were identified as orotic acid by melting point, spectroscopy, and chromatographic characteristics. The amount excreted was not quantified; it was stated that no orotidine was found in the urine. Trials of uridine, thymine, thymidine, and cytidine orally have been ineffective [15]. Studies of marrow preparations in vitro were interpreted to show decreased decarboxylation of ^{14}C-aspartate and increased recovery of the label in orotic acid. The parents and three other sibs appear to be normal and have no excess urinary orotic acid by a survey method [15]. A 9-month-old sister, however, has severe macrocytic megaloblastic anemia which has already required 15 transfusions. She also has no leukopenia or thrombocytopenia and has been similarly resistant to treatment with even less response to folic acid. So far no excess orotic acid has been found in her urine, although orotic aciduria persists in patient J.G. These patients probably represent a different genetic disorder, as will be commented upon later.

Some of the clinical and laboratory findings in the 8 reported patients with hereditary orotic aciduria have been summarized in Table 42-1. Six have been male and two female. With the exception of C.P., the patients appeared to be normal at birth. Typically, poor growth and development were evident during the first few months of life with lassitude, pallor, and nonspecific "failure to thrive." No characteristic neurologic picture was found although three of the seven patients were noted to have strabismus (D.G., J.P., T.H.). Splenomegaly was noted in two patients. Other abnormalities seen in single patients were kyphoscoliosis, hernias, presumed interventricular septal defect, abnormalities of the hair and nails, outward torsion of the left tibia, and a notched eyelid margin. Patient D.B. deviated most radically from the above pattern in that growth and development were normal. She presented with fatigue and symptoms related to crystalluria at age 7½. Although the clinical description is abbreviated, the atypical Spanish patient, J.G., also seemed to have normal somatic development when studied at age 10. Patients D.G., J.P., and J.G. have impaired intellectual development (IQs about 80), whereas patient D.B. is superior in mental capacity (IQ 133).

The most specific early finding was severe hypochromic anemia with marked anisocytosis and poikilocytosis associated with erythroid hyperplasia and atypical megaloblastic changes in the bone marrow. An equally consistent finding was leukopenia (except in J.G.), but thrombocytopenia was not observed (Table 42-1). In each patient the hematologic abnormalities failed to respond to an array of hematinic agents. In patients J. R. and J. P. glucocortical therapy improved the anemia significantly without reversing the megaloblastic changes in the marrow. This form of treatment was not tried on the other six patients. In each patient the degree of orotic aciduria was sufficient to result in its spontaneous crystallization in urine specimens (Fig. 42-3) and in three cases (J.R., J.P., and D.B.) evidence of partial obstruction of the urinary tract occurred. The response to uridine replacement therapy was prompt. There was reticulocytosis, rise of hemoglobin, reversal of megaloblastosis, and improvement in general health, growth, and development (except in patient D.B. where no blunting of growth and development had occurred). Leukopenia also was reversed but was noted to require larger doses of uridine for effective therapy in one patient. As noted in patient J.G. a partial hematologic remission was obtained with folic or folinic acid. When measured quantitatively, the urinary excretion of orotic acid was found to decrease but not to disappear (Figs. 42-2 and 42-4). As an exception, no reduction of urinary orotic acid was noted in patient T.H. during therapy. In only one family (J.G.) has the clinical disorder appeared more than once. The atypical disease in these sibs is probably different from hereditary orotic aciduria. The inheritance of hereditary orotic aciduria will be considered in detail in the section on Genetics.

METABOLISM OF OROTIC ACID

The detection of orotic acid in the urine was the key observation leading to the discovery of this first demonstrated disorder of pyrimidine metabolism. The metabolism of orotic acid will be briefly reviewed.

Absorption

The normal dietary content of orotic acid is not known. Very low levels are present in animal tissue. Even on diets con-

Table 42-1. CLINICAL FINDINGS IN PATIENTS WITH HEREDITARY OROTIC ACIDURIA

Patient; sex	Onset of symptoms	Age at diagnosis	Clinical features	Physical examination	Urine and urinary tract	Hb	WBC	Platelets	Response to treatment
J.R.; M [1]	3 mo	1 yr	Weakness, lethargy, diarrhea, repeated infections. Mental and motor development appeared normal	Pallor, splenomegaly, outward torsion of left tibia	Gross crystalluria. Ureteral and urethral obstruction	6.7	2,050	260,400	Partial response to glucocorticoids. Early response to pyrimidines. Died of varicella off treatment.
D.G.; M [9, 10]	3 mo	1½ yr	Failure to thrive, retarded in motor development, alternating strabismus	Splenomegaly, strabismus, weakness, fine short hair	Heavy crystalluria	4.6	2,400	220,000	Good response to uridine, 1,500 mg/day orally.
J.P.; M [11]	7 mo	1½ yr	Failure to thrive, strabismus, slow motor development—at age 1½ yr, tested at 9-mo level (Gesell)	Pallor and strabismus	Crystalluria with partial ureteral obstruction	4.8	1,500	213,000	Partial response to glucocorticoids. Good response to uridine, 1,500 mg/day.
T.H.; F [6]	2 mo	10 mo	Weakness, bilateral strabismus, normal size	Heart murmur of interventricular septal defect. Strabismus	Crystalluria	7.8	3,300	570,000	Good response to uridine, 1,500 mg/day orally.
D.B.; F [13]	6½ yr	7½ yr	Fatigue, back and flank pain. Normal mental and physical development	Small notch at margin of right upper eyelid. Soft systolic murmur over pulmonic area	Crystalluria and hematuria. Symptoms probably related to crystalluria	7.4	3,200	300,000	Response to uridine, 150 mg/kg/day. Leukopenia responded last.
C.P.; M [2]	Birth	4 mo	Failure to thrive with generalized hypertonicity	Kyphoscoliosis, hernias, scaphoid skull	Crystalluria	6.3	2,600	364,000	Early response to uridine, 150 mg/kg/day. Death from meningitis and pneumonia.
P.M.; M [2, 3]	5½ mo	6–7 mo	Failure to thrive with retarded motor development	Seborrheic dermatitis and fine, dry hair	Crystalluria	7.4	?	?	Response to uridine, 150/kg/day orally.
J.G.; M [14, 15]	3 mo	5 yr	Anemia, normal growth and development	Not described	Crystalluria	8.5	10,000	270,000	Partial response to folic and folinic acids.

taining 1 percent orotic acid by weight, the free compound cannot be demonstrated in rat liver [16]. Orotic acid was first discovered in milk 60 years ago [17], and recent measurements confirm its presence in cow's milk, human milk [18], and especially in food milk powders [19]. Its content in other dietary constituents is not known. As a highly insoluble pyrimidine, orotic acid is not readily absorbed. In rats from 2 to 59 percent of the radioactivity recovered after the oral administration of ^{14}C-orotate was found in the feces [16]. No data are available on the absorption of orotic acid in man. Some is absorbed, as indicated by the partial efficacy of large oral doses of orotic acid (3 to 6 gm per day) in the treatment of pernicious anemia [20]. Active transport of other pyrimidine bases occurs in the small intestine, with considerable structural specificity required [21]. There is no evidence that dietary orotic acid is a quantitatively important source of pyrimidines.

Excretion

The normal adult excretes approximately 1.4 mg orotic acid in the urine per 24 hr (Fig. 42-6) [22]. Orotic acid in bile and gastrointestinal secretions has not been studied, although the relatively high content in milk has been noted. Orotic acid is actively secreted by the avian renal tubule, and this secretory mechanism is inhibited by probenecid [23]. No orotic acid was detectable in plasma by a sensitive isotope-dilution technique [24] or by an enzymatic spectrophotometric method [25]. This has prevented direct renal

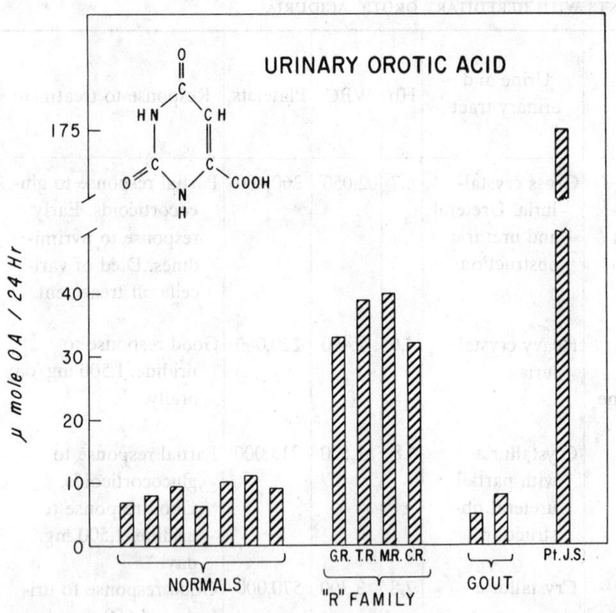

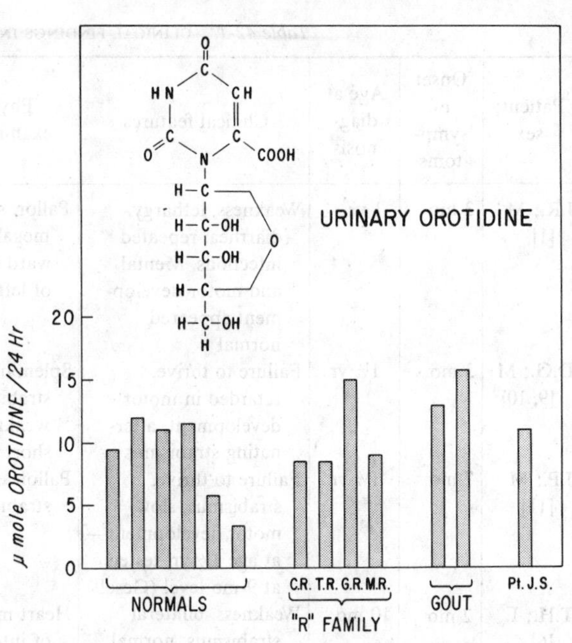

Figure 42-6. Urinary excretion of orotic acid and orotidine in normal subjects, presumed heterozygotes of hereditary orotic aciduria, and two patients with gout. (*From Nature, London,* **197**, 194, 1963, *with permission of the publishers.*)

clearance studies in man in the absence of induced orotic aciduria. During infusion of ring-labeled ^{14}C-orotic acid, the clearance of radioactivity approached that of creatinine clearance [26]. During drug-induced orotic aciduria (see below), the clearance of orotic acid exceeds glomerular filtration. If the normal excretion of orotic acid (1.4 mg) is derived from glomerular filtrate without tubular reabsorption, the plasma concentration would be approximately 0.8 μg per 100 ml. The same assumptions indicate a plasma level in hereditary orotic aciduria of $>$ 1.0 mg per 100 ml. No measurement of plasma orotic acid in hereditary orotic aciduria has been attempted. Infused orotic acid increases the clearance of uric acid, presumably by competing for a renal transport mechanism [27]. Excretion of orotic acid may increase more than 1,000-fold in hereditary orotic aciduria. Presumably this is due to an increased plasma concentration. A primary renal tubular defect in the reabsorption of orotic acid seems unlikely in hereditary orotic aciduria in view of the enzyme defects to be described.

Biosynthesis

Increased urinary excretion of orotic acid might result from overproduction through increased synthesis of a rate-limiting enzyme or through some other abnormality of intracellular metabolic regulatory mechanisms. The pathway for the *de novo* synthesis of orotic acid (Fig. 42-7), first demonstrated in bacteria [28, 29], has subsequently been confirmed as valid in man [24]. The individual enzymes concerned will be described.

Carbamyl Phosphate Synthase

Carbamyl phosphate (CAP) is an unstable, high-energy intermediate which serves as the donor of the carbamyl moiety in the synthesis of citrulline and carbamylaspartate. In aqueous solution at physiologic pH, carbamyl phosphate is in equilibrium with phosphate and cyanate. Its enzymatically governed carbamylation reactions with amino groups are analogous to chemical reactions of cyanate to yield the same products.

Although evidence is not yet complete, it seems probable that in animal systems there are two separate carbamyl phosphate synthase enzymes with different physiologic functions and control [30, 31].

$$2\ ATP + NH_4^+ + HCO_3^- + \xrightarrow[Mg^{++}]{acetylglutamate} CAP + 2\ AMP + P_i$$

This CAP synthase is a hepatic mitochondrial enzyme which utilizes ammonia as a nitrogen donor and requires N-acetylglutamate, or one of its analogues [32], as a cofactor. It seems to be linked primarily to citrulline synthesis as part of the urea cycle [33]. This enzyme has been demonstrated to appear at the stage of metamorphosis during which the ammonotelic tadpole becomes a ureotelic frog [34]. Genetic studies in *Neurospora crassa* have also suggested the functional separation of CAP synthesis for the two main pathways of carbamylation [35].

$$2\ ATP + glutamine + HCO_3^- + H_2O \xrightarrow[Mg^{++}]{K^+} CAP + 2\ ADP + P_i + glutamate$$

This carbamyl phosphate synthetase, originally described in mushrooms [36], has now been demonstrated in microorganisms [37], yeasts [38], plants [39], and animal tissues [40–42]. It is a soluble enzyme with greatest affinity for glutamine as a nitrogen donor, although NH_4^+ may also serve as a substrate. The glutamine-dependent enzyme appears to function primarily as the source of CAP for the pyrimidine biosynthetic pathway. Evidence will be presented later concerning its role as a site of metabolic regulation.

Carbamyl phosphate can also be formed by the phosphorolytic cleavage of citrulline [43]. Carbamate kinase catalyzes the interconversion of carbamate and CAP in microorganisms, but this reaction does not appear to be an important source of CAP [44, 45]:

$$NH_2COO^- + ATP \rightleftharpoons CAP + ADP$$

It has not been established whether CAP is synthesized *de novo* in all mammalian tissues. Because of the very low activities of carbamyl phosphate synthase found, it is possible that "carbamyl carriers" may exist, such as citrulline or, by analogy with bacterial studies, creatine, allantoin, and urea [46].

Aspartate Transcarbamylase

This enzyme catalyzes the first reaction unique to pyrimidine biosynthesis, the irreversible carbamylation of L-aspartate by carbamyl phosphate to form carbamylaspartate (Fig. 42-7). In contrast to carbamyl phosphate synthase this enzyme is widely distributed in mammalian tissues. Highest activities are found in the testis, spleen, intestine, bone marrow, and liver [47]. The crystalline enzyme from *Escherichia coli* has been extensively studied in several laboratories as a model system for allosteric interactions [48, 49, 50]. It is composed of two catalytic and four regulatory subunits of molecular weight 2.7×10^4 and 1×10^5, respectively. Other studies have suggested six catalytic and six regulatory units [51]. It is available in gram quantities and can readily be dissociated into these separable catalytic and regulatory units. Activity

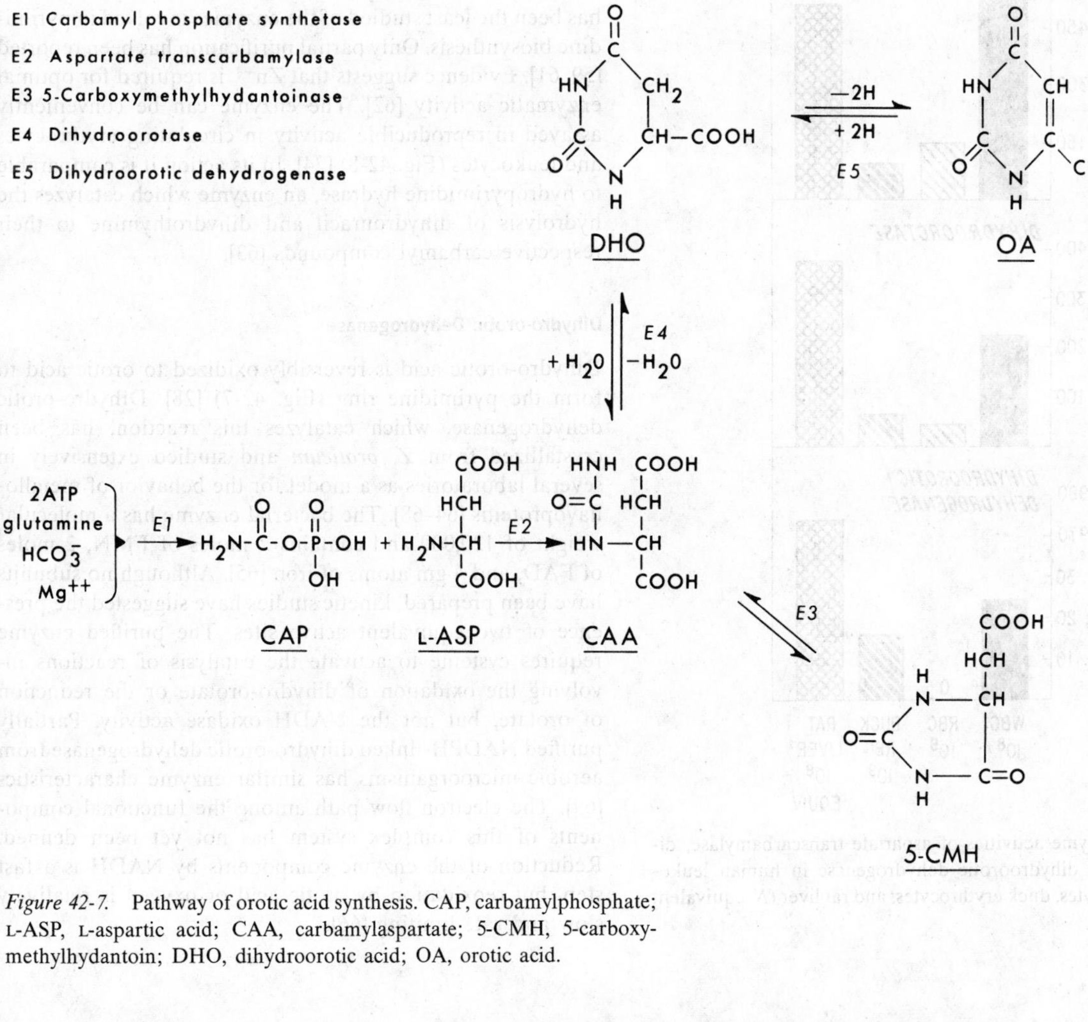

E1 Carbamyl phosphate synthetase
E2 Aspartate transcarbamylase
E3 5-Carboxymethylhydantoinase
E4 Dihydroorotase
E5 Dihydroorotic dehydrogenase

2ATP, glutamine, HCO_3^-, Mg^{++} —E1→ $H_2N\text{-}C(=O)\text{-}O\text{-}P(=O)(OH)\text{-}OH$ (CAP) + $H_2N\text{-}CH(COOH)\text{-}CH_2\text{-}COOH$ (L-ASP) —E2→ CAA

CAA ⇌ (E3) 5-CMH

CAA ⇌ (E4; $+H_2O$ / $-H_2O$) DHO

DHO ⇌ ($-2H$ / $+2H$; E5) OA

Figure 42-7. Pathway of orotic acid synthesis. CAP, carbamylphosphate; L-ASP, L-aspartic acid; CAA, carbamylaspartate; 5-CMH, 5-carboxymethylhydantoin; DHO, dihydroorotic acid; OA, orotic acid.

is reduced by sulfhydryl-reactive agents and also is inhibited by certain inorganic anions [52]. Aspartate transcarbamylase has been studied in bacteria, fungi, higher plants [53], birds, Ehrlich ascites cells [54], rat, and man [24].

The mammalian enzyme, partially purified from rat liver, differs significantly from *E. coli* aspartate transcarbamylase in pH optimum, stability, sensitivity to metals, and insensitivity to allosteric inhibition [55, 56]. The presence or absence of subunits in the mammalian enzyme has not been determined. Enzyme preparations from human erythrocytes resemble bacterial preparations in the high concentrations of L-aspartate (1 to $1.6 \times 10^{-2}M$) and carbamyl phosphate (3 to $5 \times 10^{-3}M$) required for enzyme saturation [24]. Aspartate transcarbamylase is present as a soluble enzyme in circulating mature erythrocytes and in the particulate fraction of leukocytes, in which its activity approximates that found in rat liver (Fig. 42-8) [24]. In rat liver, activity is highest in the microsomal fraction [57]. The role of this enzyme in the control of pyrimidine nucleotide synthesis will be considered below.

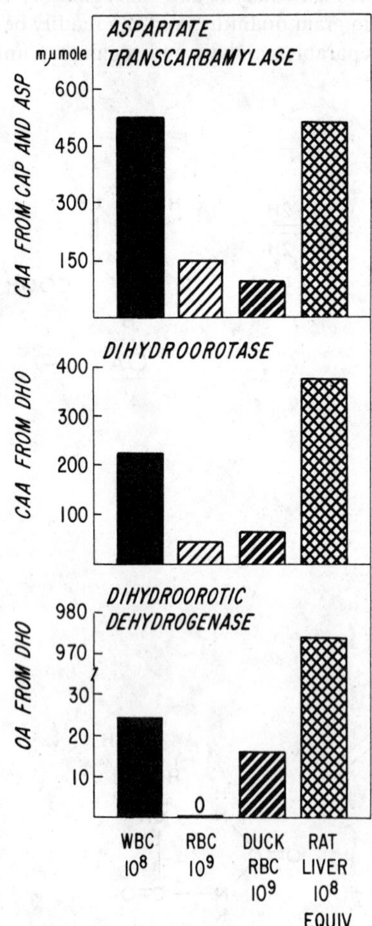

Figure 42-8. Enzyme activities of aspartate transcarbamylase, dihydroorotase, and dihydroorotic dehydrogenase in human leukocytes and erythrocytes, duck erythrocytes, and rat liver (*N* equivalent to 10^8 WBC) [24].

5-Carboxymethylhydantoinase

This enzyme catalyzes the reversible ring closure of carbamylaspartate to form the corresponding hydantoin (Fig. 42-7). It was described first in *Zymobacterium oroticum* [29]. It has limited distribution in bacteria and is absent in rat liver and human leukocytes and erythrocytes [24]. There is no current evidence to support its participation in mammalian pyrimidine metabolism.

Dihydro-orotase

The major fate of carbamylaspartate is ring closure to form dihydro-orotic acid, a reaction catalyzed by dihydro-orotase (Fig. 42-7). This reaction, originally described in bacteria [29], has been confirmed in rat liver [58], Novikoff ascites hepatoma cells [59], human hemic cells [24], fibroblast cultures [7], and gut mucosa [60]. The K_m for carbamylaspartate is $2.8 \times 10^{-4}M$ and at equilibrium there is a ratio of carbamylaspartate to dihydro-orotate of 1.9. Dihydro-orotase has been the least studied of the enzymes involved in pyrimidine biosynthesis. Only partial purification has been reported [59, 61]. Evidence suggests that Zn^{++} is required for optimal enzymatic activity [62]. The enzyme can be conveniently assayed in reproducible activity in circulating erythrocytes and leukocytes (Fig. 42-8) [24]. In its action it is comparable to hydropyrimidine hydrase, an enzyme which catalyzes the hydrolysis of dihydrouracil and dihydrothymine to their respective carbamyl compounds [63].

Dihydro-orotic Dehydrogenase

Dihydro-orotic acid is reversibly oxidized to orotic acid to form the pyrimidine ring (Fig. 42-7) [28]. Dihydro-orotic dehydrogenase, which catalyzes this reaction, has been crystallized from *Z. oroticum* and studied extensively in several laboratories as a model for the behavior of metalloflavoproteins [64–68]. The bacterial enzyme has a molecular weight of 120,000 and contains 2 moles of FMN, 2 moles of FAD, and 4 gm atoms of iron [65]. Although no subunits have been prepared, kinetic studies have suggested the presence of two equivalent active sites. The purified enzyme requires cysteine to activate the catalysis of reactions involving the oxidation of dihydro-orotate or the reduction of orotate, but not the NADH oxidase activity. Partially purified NADPH-linked dihydro-orotic dehydrogenase from aerobic microorganisms has similar enzyme characteristics [69]. The electron flow path among the functional components of this complex system has not yet been defined. Reduction of the enzyme components by NADH is a fast step, but reoxidation by orotic acid or oxygen is relatively slow and rate limiting [66].

Dihydro-orotic dehydrogenase has not been highly purified from mammalian sources. It is present in circulating human leukocytes [24], gut mucosa [60], and fibroblasts grown in vitro [70]. The enzyme is absent from mature erythrocytes but present in nucleated avian erythrocytes and in reticulocytes (Fig. 42-8) [24, 71]. No requirement for NAD or NADP could be found in leukocyte preparations. Dihydro-5-azaorotic acid has been recently described as a specific inhibitor of the enzyme [72]. The absence of dihydro-orotic dehydrogenase activity in the mature human erythrocyte, and its presence in reticulocytes suggest that the enzyme is lost during cell maturation with a resulting block in *de novo* pyrimidine synthesis at the stage of orotic acid formation [71].

Fate of Orotic Acid

Orotic acid has not been detected in normal tissue, and only 1.2 to 1.8 mg is normally excreted in the urine [22]. Nevertheless, pyrimidine base turnover in man is approximately 0.6 gm per 24 hr [26]. Orotic acid has only two known pathways of metabolism. By a reversal of reactions described above it may be reduced to dihydro-orotic acid and subsequently hydrolyzed to carbamylaspartate [Fig. 42-7]. The carbamylaspartate may be irreversibly converted to aspartate, carbon dioxide, and ammonia by ureidosuccinase (carbamylaspartase), a reaction which has been studied only in bacteria [73]. Carbamylaspartate may also undergo decarboxylation to form carbamyl-β-alanine [74], which in turn is irreversibly decarbamylated [75]. Through the operation of this degradative pathway orotic acid is converted to an amino acid (aspartate or β-alanine), carbon dioxide, and ammonia. Evidence reviewed elsewhere suggests that this degradative pathway is not quantitatively important [16, 76]. Most of the orotic acid is converted to uridine-5′-phosphate, with intermediate formation of orotidine-5′-phosphate (Fig. 42-9). The ultimate degradative pathway of orotic acid is therefore that of uracil—which is catabolized through dihydrouracil and carbamyl-β-alanine to carbon dioxide, ammonia, and β-alanine [77].

Orotidine-5′-phosphate Pyrophosphorylase

This enzyme catalyzes the formation of orotidine-5′-phosphate (O5P) from orotic acid and 5-phosphoribosylpyrophosphate (PRPP) in the presence of Mg^{++} (Fig. 42-9). This reaction, a reversible pyrophosphorolysis analogous to the formation of purine nucleotides from free purine bases, has been studied most rigorously using a partially purified enzyme from yeast [78, 79] and from calf thymus [80]. It has also been demonstrated in rat liver homogenates [81], human erythrocytes [5] and fibroblasts [7], and cow brain [82]. The K_m values for orotic acid and 5-phosphoribosylpyrophosphate were found to be 3.2×10^{-5} and $2.1 \times 10^{-5} M$, respectively, with the calf thymus enzyme [80] in good agreement with earlier studies of the yeast enzyme [78, 79]. Orotidine-5′-phosphate inhibits the forward reaction [78], which can also be inhibited by several structural analogues of orotate [79] as well as certain inorganic anions [83]. The enzyme catalyzes the conversion of 5-fluoro-orotic acid to its corresponding nucleotide [84], but otherwise exhibits specificity for orotate. Reproducible activities of this enzyme have been found in mature human erythrocytes, but activities in leukocytes have been low and variable in sonicated cell preparations. This enzyme activity was not separable from that of orotidine-5′-phosphate decarboxylase during a 600-fold purification from cow brain [82], but was separated by starch gel electrophoresis in the calf thymus preparation [80]. This reaction is the only known pathway for orotidine-5′-phosphate synthesis, a small amount of which is irreversibly dephosphorylated to orotidine. The normal urinary

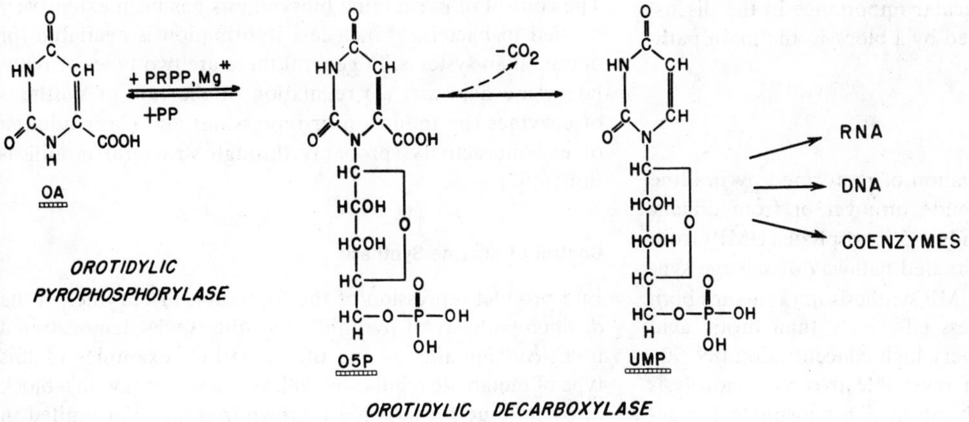

Figure 42-9. Pathway of conversion of orotic acid to pyrimidine nucleotides. OA, orotic acid; O5P, orotidine-5′-phosphate; UMP, uridine-5′-phosphate; PRPP, 5-phosphoribosylpyrophosphate.

excretion of orotidine is about 2.5 mg per 24 hr (Fig. 42-6) [22].

Orotidine-5′-phosphate Decarboxylase

Orotidine-5′-phosphate decarboxylase catalyzes the irreversible decarboxylation of orotidine-5′-phosphate to uridine-5′-phosphate (Fig. 42-9). The enzyme was first demonstrated in extracts of yeast [78], but has also been studied in higher plants [85], rat liver [81, 86], calf thymus [80], cow brain [82], and human hemic cells [5] and fibroblast cultures [7]. No cofactors have been demonstrated. Rat liver preparations differ from those of yeast in not being susceptible to sulfhydryl inhibitors. In human erythrocytes the apparent K_m for orotidine-5′-phosphate is $1.1 \times 10^{-5}M$ [5]. The K_m in the cow brain preparation was $3 \times 10^{-6}M$ [82]. Although irreversible, this reaction is subject to end product inhibition by uridine-5′-phosphate and is also competitively inhibited by a number of other pyrimidine and purine nucleotides, in decreasing order: CMP, AMP, GMP, CDP, UDP, and CTP [82]. 6-Azauridine is converted to 6-azauridylic acid in vivo and serves as a specific inhibitor of the decarboxylase [87]. Reproducible activities of O5P decarboxylase are found in preparations of human erythrocytes [5] and leukocytes [88]. The close association of O5P pyrophosphorylase and decarboxylase activities during purification has been noted above. The possibility that both activities may be catalyzed by the same protein will be discussed further in the consideration of the pathogenesis of hereditary orotic aciduria.

Alternate Pathways of Pyrimidine Nucleotide Synthesis

There are two general types of alternate pathways for pyrimidine nucleotide synthesis: (1) "salvage synthesis" and (2) *de novo* synthesis by a pathway exclusive of orotic acid. These pathways are of particular importance in the discussion of a disease characterized by a block in the main pathway of pyrimidine synthesis.

Salvage Synthesis

This term refers to the utilization of preformed pyrimidine bases available from nucleotide turnover or from dietary sources. The formation of uridine-5′-phosphate (UMP) from uracil is the most carefully studied pathway of salvage synthesis. Uracil is utilized for UMP synthesis in rat tissues both in vivo and in vitro, but less effectively than orotic acid except under conditions of very high concentration [89, 90]. UMP may be formed by a reversible pyrophosphorolysis between uracil and 5-phosphoribosylpyrophosphate, a reaction analogous to that catalyzed by orotidine-5′-phosphate pyrophosphorylase [83, 91, 92]. In mammalian tissue the most important pathway appears to involve the prior formation of uridine (catalyzed by uridine phosphorylase), which is then phosphorylated by uridine kinase [90]. The importance of these pathways in man cannot be assessed at present. Uracil in large doses (15 to 30 gm per 24 hr) has produced a partial and temporary remission in certain megaloblastic anemias [93]. A relatively short-term trial of uracil (2.5 gm per day for 10 days) failed to produce a reticulocytosis in patient J.R., although later there was a prompt response to oral nucleotides (Fig. 42-4) [1]. Uracil was similarly ineffective in patient D.G. [10]. Uridine has demonstrated its continued effectiveness in the treatment of hereditary orotic aciduria (see below), presumably being converted to uridine-5′-phosphate by uridine kinase. If salvage synthesis from pyrimidine bases is of importance in man, it might be exaggerated in the pyrimidine starvation of hereditary orotic aciduria. This warrants further investigation.

Alternate de novo Synthetic Pathways

Uracil undergoes a series of degradative reactions in mammalian systems to form β-alanine, carbon dioxide, and ammonia. In theory, by reversal of these steps, uracil might be formed *de novo* from simple precursors by a pathway not involving orotic acid. Evidence is reviewed elsewhere that this pathway does not normally operate in mammalian tissues [94]. It would be of interest to determine whether such a "shunt" synthesis could be demonstrated in tissue culture of hereditary orotic aciduria fibroblasts, although this seems unlikely, since certain bacterial mutants which require uracil cannot grow on dihydrouracil or carbamyl-β-alanine [95]. In a preliminary report a high rate of incorporation of carbamyl-β-alanine ribonucleotide and dihydrouridylic acid into ribonucleic acid of avian liver was found [96]. This possible alternate pathway remains to be confirmed.

Control of Pyrimidine Nucleotide Synthesis

The control of pyrimidine biosynthesis has been extensively studied in bacteria. Much less information is available for mammalian systems. In general there are two types of regulatory mechanisms: (1) regulation of the rate of synthesis of enzymes (by induction or repression) and (2) regulation of enzyme activity (probably through structural modifications) [97].

Control of Enzyme Synthesis

End product repression of the formation of enzymes in the *de novo* pathway of pyrimidine synthesis was demonstrated in *E. coli* mutants as one of the earliest examples of this type of metabolic regulation [98]. When mutants with a block in pyrimidine formation are grown in a medium limited in pyrimidines ("pyrimidine starvation"), there is a release of end product repression (derepression). This results in a compensatory increased production of enzymes which catalyze pyrimidine synthesis (Fig. 42-10) [98, 99]. Conversely, the

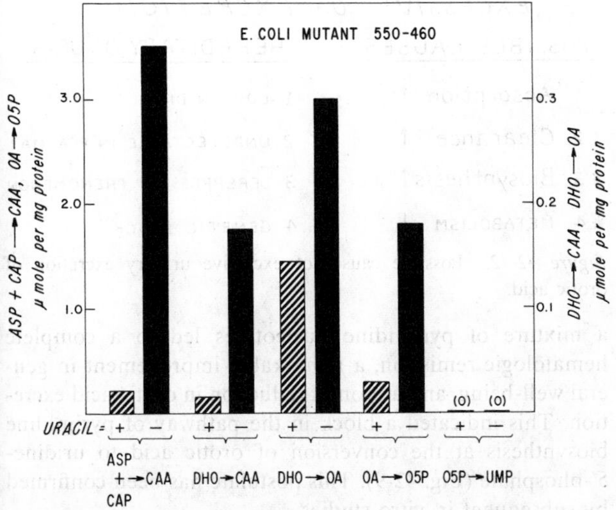

Figure 42-10. Enzyme activities in an *E. coli* mutant during control periods (uracil +) and during pyrimidine starvation (uracil −). The increase of enzyme activities during growth in media limited in uracil (solid bars) represents release of end product repression. ASP + CAP ⟶ CAA, aspartate transcarbamylase; DHO ⟶ CAA, dihydroorotase; DHO ⟶ OA, dihydroorotic dehydrogenase; OA ⟶ O5P, orotidylic pyrophosphorylase; O5P ⟶ UMP, orotidylic decarboxylase.

addition of end products of the pathway, derived from uracil, inhibits enzyme synthesis. Evidence has been presented for the existence of a common repressor in *E. coli* for all five enzymes catalyzing the formation of uridine-5′-phosphate [100]. Less rigorous evidence for derepression of pyrimidine synthesis in mammalian cells has been reported in pernicious anemia [101] and sarcoma-180 cells [102].

The study of induction and repression of enzyme activity in bacteria has led to the hypothesis of a system of genetic control schematically shown in Fig. 42-11 [103]. A cluster of structural genes may be under the control of a single adjacent operator, constituting a genetic unit of transcription termed an *operon.* The operator in turn is controlled by a product of a regulatory gene, called a *repressor.* Enzyme synthesis is induced by a release of the operator from repression by inactivation of the repressor. This allows expression of all the structural genes within the operon to be proportionately coinduced. Conversely, enzyme repression results from activation of the repressor of the operon. Evidence for the operon hypothesis as it relates to genetic regulatory mechanisms in microorganisms has been reviewed elsewhere [103]. Data have been particularly confirmatory in elegant series of studies on the lac operon of *E. coli* [104–106]. It has not been established that the operon hypothesis is applicable to the eucaryotic cells of higher organisms. It has been postulated, in contrast, that in higher organisms there is posttranscriptional regulation of enzyme synthesis [107]. At the present time there is no firm evidence for the mechanisms of repression and derepression of the synthesis of enzymes in the pyrimidine biosynthetic sequence in mammalian systems. The relationship of the enzyme alterations in hereditary orotic aciduria will be discussed below.

Control of Enzyme Activity

There are a number of ways in which the activity of an enzyme may be altered. These include changes in its primary structure, changes in its association-dissociation into subunits, or changes in conformation [97, 108, 109]. Feedback inhibition of the first step unique to a biosynthetic sequence by one of the end products is one of the most widespread metabolic control mechanisms. In microbial systems it has been demonstrated that cytidine triphosphate (CTP) is a powerful competitive inhibitor and adenosine triphosphate (ATP) is an activator of aspartate transcarbamylase, the first enzyme unique to pyrimidine biosynthesis [109]. Evidence indicates that the inhibition occurs because of CTP binding at an allosteric site, which presumably reduces the enzymatic activity through a change in configuration [109, 110]. *Escherichia coli* aspartate transcarbamylase has four regulatory subunits which can be physically separated from the catalytic subunits [48–50]. Because of its availability and relative simplicity, this enzyme has been used as a model for the study of allosteric control mechanisms [111, 112]. Aspartate transcarbamylase partially purified from rat liver does not exhibit specificity for CTP or such a high degree of sensitivity to feedback inhibition. It is equally inhibited by uridine or cytidine derivatives and maximally inhibited by deoxyribonucleosides (thymidine) [55]. It is also inhibited by purine deoxyribonucleosides and deoxyribonucleotides [113]. Aspartate transcarbamylase has also been found to be resistent to nucleotide inhibition in human leukocytes [114], rabbit erythrocytes [115], and mouse spleen [40].

As noted earlier there are two separate carbamyl phosphate synthases in mammalian cells. One is mitochondrial, uses ammonia as a nitrogen donor, and requires N-acetylglutamate as a cofactor. It appears to function primarily in citrulline synthesis. The second CAP synthase is soluble, uses glutamine as a nitrogen donor, and appears to be linked to pyrimidine biosynthesis. In the mouse spleen this latter enzyme is inhibited by UTP [40]. Similarly in *E. coli* the

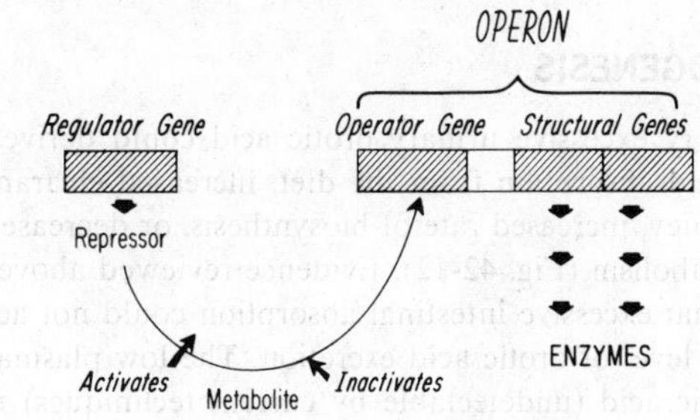

Figure 42-11. Theoretical scheme for the genetic control of enzyme synthesis, as proposed by Jacob and Monod [103]. (*From Tr. Ass. Amer. Physicians,* **76,** 214, 1963, *with permission of the publishers.*)

glutamine requiring CAP synthase is inhibited by pyrimidine nucleotides and stimulated by purine nucleotides [116]. Comparison of relative activities indicates that CAP synthase rather than aspartate transcarbamylase is rate-limiting in pyrimidine synthesis in Ehrlich ascites carcinoma [42], avian and fetal rat liver [117], and the frog egg [30]. At this time it appears that the most important site of feedback inhibition of pyrimidine synthesis in mammalian systems is at the level of the soluble CAP synthase [118].

Feedback inhibition of mammalian dihydro-orotase is exhibited by a number of pyrimidines and purines [59]. Product inhibitions of orotidylic pyrophosphorylase by orotidine-5′-phosphate and of orotidylic decarboxylase by uridine-5′-phosphate have been discussed above. The coordination of these various metabolic control mechanisms in vivo in mammalian systems is not clear. Hereditary orotic aciduria represents "pyrimidine starvation" in man and exhibits marked alterations in rate control of pyrimidine synthesis, as will be discussed below.

PHARMACOLOGY OF OROTIC ACID

Large oral doses of orotic acid induce a partial remission in patients with pernicious anemia, but relapse occurs after some months of maintenance therapy [20]. The mechanism of this response is unknown. A diet high in orotic acid leads to severe fatty liver in the rat associated with a block in the synthesis and release of beta lipoproteins [119–121]. There is an accompanying increase in the hepatic content of uridine nucleotides (two- to fourfold increase) associated with a decrease in adenine nucleotides [16, 122]. Adenine prevents or reverses fat accumulation in the liver induced by orotic acid. It has been reported that a diet containing 1 percent orotic acid increases rather than represses hepatic aspartate transcarbamylase and dihydro-orotase in spite of high levels of free pyrimidine nucleotides [123]. Orotic acid increases the clearance of uric acid [27] and has been reported to reduce uric acid formation in gouty patients [124]. There is a large and uncritical literature suggesting that oral therapy with orotic acid is beneficial in a variety of hepatic, gastrointestinal, and hematologic disorders.

PATHOGENESIS

In theory excessive urinary orotic acid could derive from increased absorption from the diet, increased clearance by the kidney, increased rate of biosynthesis, or decreased rate of metabolism (Fig. 42-12). Evidence reviewed above indicates that excessive intestinal absorption could not account for the level of orotic acid excretion. The low plasma level of orotic acid (undetectable by current techniques) makes it unlikely that a renal tubular defect contributes to its excessive urinary excretion. In the initial clinical studies of the first patient with orotic aciduria the administration of

EXCESSIVE OA EXCRETION

POSSIBLE CAUSES	HEREDITARY OA'URIA
1 Absorption ↑	1 LOW IN DIET
2 Clearance ↑	2 UNDETECTABLE IN PLASMA
* 3 Biosynthesis ↑	3 DEREPRESSION PHENOMENON
* 4 METABOLISM ↓	4 GENETIC BLOCK

Figure 42-12. Possible causes of excessive urinary excretion of orotic acid.

a mixture of pyrimidine nucleotides led to a complete hematologic remission, a remarkable improvement in general well-being, and a prompt reduction in orotic acid excretion. This indicated a block in the pathway of pyrimidine biosynthesis at the conversion of orotic acid to uridine-5′-phosphate (Fig. 42-9). This postulate has been confirmed by subsequent in vitro studies.

Enzymatic Defect in Hemic Cells

Studies have been carried out on enzymes involved in orotic acid synthesis and metabolism in preparations from circulating hemic cells.

Orotidine-5′-phosphate Pyrophosphorylase

Erythrocytes from the parents and two of the three sibs of the propositus of orotic aciduria (R. family) had reduced activities of pyrophosphorylase (Fig. 42-13). Erythrocytes

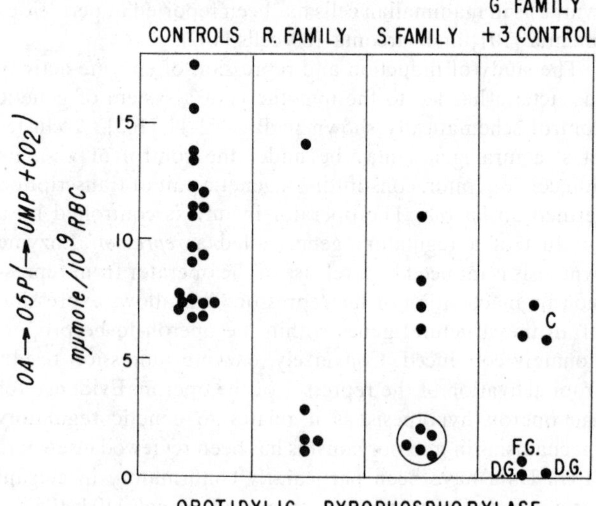

Figure 42-13. Activity of orotidylic pyrophosphorylase in erythrocyte preparations from control subjects and members of the R. family, S. family, and G. family. The circle encloses five determinations over a period of 1 year in a presumed heterozygote in the S. family. *C,* controls obtained in New Zealand; D.G., 2 determinations on patient D.G.: F.G., father of D.G.

from the third sib had values in the normal range. In the course of these studies a subject (J.S.), chosen as an apparently normal control, was found to have consistently low levels of enzyme activity on repeated determinations over a period of several months. Studies of the parents and two brothers of J.S. (the S. family) revealed a tendency toward reduced activity of O5P pyrophosphorylase, but no single value in the range found for other presumed heterozygotes (Fig. 42-13). In frozen erythrocytes from another patient with homozygous hereditary orotic aciduria (D.G.), no enzyme activity was found in one preparation and < 0.2 mμmole per 10^9 RBC in a second preparation. His father's erythrocytes had an enzyme activity of 0.35 mμmole per 10^9 RBC (Fig. 42-13). The quantitative significance of these values is uncertain because of the instability of O5P pyrophosphorylase in frozen erythrocytes, as indicated by the low values of control specimens obtained in New Zealand at the same time as those of the patient (C in Fig. 42-13). Erythrocyte orotidine-5′-phosphate pyrophosphorylase was also markedly reduced in patient D.B., who had survived untreated to age 8 without any abnormality in growth and development [13]. The pyrophosphorylase activity was < 1 percent of the control value in D.B.'s erythrocytes and approximately 12 percent of control in her mother's erythrocytes. In patient T.H. the overall conversion of orotic acid to uridine-5′-phosphate was markedly depressed (0.2 mμ $^{14}CO_2$ per 10^9 RBC per hr) with a normal control range of 2.4 to 14.9 [6]. Both parents had values of < 1.0. The pyrophosphorylase was not specifically measured. Similarly low levels of activity were found in patient C.P., but his parents had minimal reductions in pyrophosphorylase activity as noted in the S. family [2]. No studies of pyrophosphorylase were conducted in patients J.P. and J.G.

In contrast to all other patients and presumed heterozygotes studied, patient P.M. was found to have elevation of orotidine-5′-phosphate pyrophosphorylase (approximately two- to threefold) expressed per 10^8 RBC [2]. The patient was treated with uridine, and enzyme activity returned to normal levels. Reproducible values for O5P pyrophosphorylase activity have not been obtained in leukocyte preparations by current assay techniques.

Orotidine-5′-phosphate Decarboxylase

O5P decarboxylase activity was also studied in erythrocyte preparations (Fig. 42-14). A pattern of reduced enzyme activity similar to that of O5P pyrophosphorylase was observed in four of the five surviving members of the R. family and in subject J.S. In two erythrocyte preparations from patient D.G. there was no detectable orotidylic decarboxylase activity, and erythrocytes from his father exhibited an intermediate value (2.5 mμmoles per 10^9 RBC) consistent with those of other presumed heterozygotes. In erythrocytes from patient J.P. there was also less than 1 percent of the normal orotidine-5′-phosphate decarboxylase activity, and his parents also had activities in the range of 5 to 10 percent

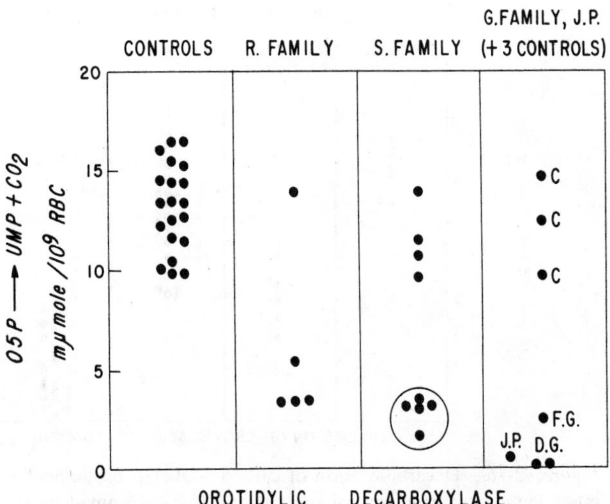

Figure 42-14. Activity of orotidylic decarboxylase in erythrocyte preparations from control subjects and members of the R. family, S. family, G. family, and patient J.P. Abbreviations are as in Figure 42-13.

of control values. Similarly low activities of O5P decarboxylase were found in patient D.B. and her mother [13] and in patients C.P. and P.M. [2]. The parents of patient C.P. failed to exhibit significant reductions of decarboxylase activity. Orotidine-5′-phosphate decarboxylase is stable in frozen erythrocyte preparations, and the activity of this enzyme is a convenient means of detecting heterozygotes [125, 126].

Orotidylic decarboxylase activity was also reduced in leukocytes from the R. family and subject J.S. (Fig. 42-15). The block in the overall metabolism of orotic acid was shown by using an assay of the decarboxylation of orotic acid by intact leukocytes, which reflects the sequential activities of

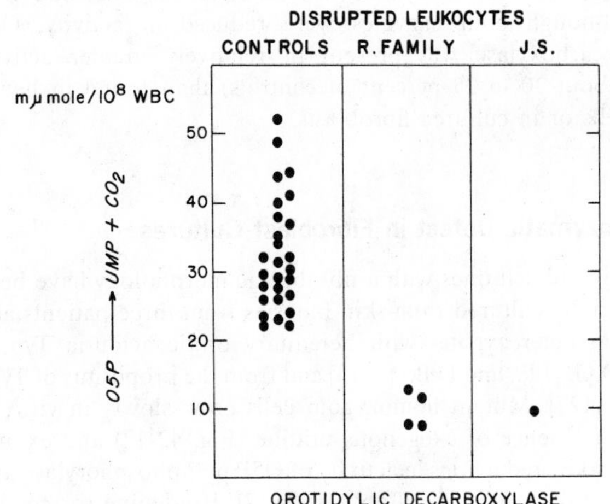

Figure 42-15. Activity of orotidylic decarboxylase in disrupted leukocyte preparations from control subjects and from presumed heterozygotes in the R. family and subject J.S. (*From Blood,* **20,** 700, 1962, *with permission of the publishers.*)

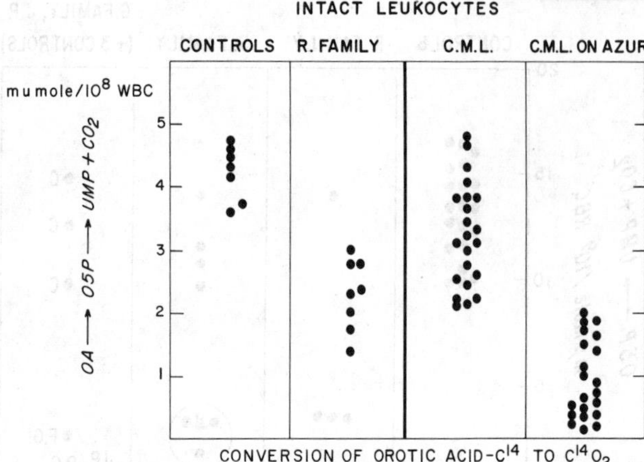

Figure 42-16. Decarboxylation of carboxyl-labeled orotic acid by intact leukocytes from control subjects and from presumed heterozygotes of hereditary orotic aciduria in the R. family. These values are compared with those of leukocytes from patients with untreated chronic myelocytic leukemia (CML) or from patients during the secondary orotic aciduria induced by therapy with 6-azauridine (AZUR). (*From Blood,* **20**, 700, 1962, *with permission of the publishers.*)

both orotidylic pyrophosphorylase and orotidylic decarboxylase (Fig. 42-16) [88].

Enzymatic Defect in Liver

Assays of the activities of orotidine-5′-phosphate pyrophosphorylase and decarboxylase have been reported on patient T.H. in preparations from a percutaneous liver biopsy [6]. The values obtained were: O5P pyrophosphorylase, 0.02 mμmoles CO_2 per 5 mg liver per hr (controls 0.79 and 1.90); and O5P decarboxylase, 0.96 (controls 5.4, 4.1, and 3.6). Although both enzymes were reduced in activity, O5P decarboxylase was present in relatively greater activity (about 20 to 25 percent of controls) than found in hemic cells or in cultured fibroblasts.

Enzymatic Defect in Fibroblast Cultures

Diploid cell lines with a fibroblastic morphology have been serially cultured from skin biopsies from three patients and two heterozygotes with hereditary orotic aciduria Type I (D.G., J.P., and D.B.) [7, 13] and from the propositus of Type II [127]. Mutant homozygous cells grow slowly in vitro in the absence of exogenous uridine (Fig. 42-17) and exhibit marked reductions in activity of O5P pyrophosphorylase and O5P decarboxylase (Table 42-2) [7]. If adenine (or certain purine nucleosides) is added to the medium, activities of the affected enzymes are further depressed, and mutant homozygous cells develop an absolute nutritional requirement for uridine [128]. As shown in Table 42-2, homozygous hereditary orotic aciduria cells retain about 0.2 percent of the normal activity of O5P pyrophosphorylase and about 0.5 percent of O5P decarboxylase activity. Heterozygous cells exhibit a partial defect in both enzymes, but not so striking as that found in erythrocytes. No abnormality in either the number or structure of the chromosomes was found in karyotypes of the cultured cells.

The development of these cell lines by Krooth and his colleagues has provided an important tool for the study of the mechanism of the double enzyme defect in hereditary orotic aciduria and the control of pyrimidine biosynthesis in human diploid cells. Growth of the mutant homozygous cells in the presence of certain inhibitors of pyrimidine biosynthesis, 6-azauridine, 5-azaorotic acid, and barbituric acid (which inhibit respectively the activities of O5P decarboxylase, O5P pyrophosphorylase, and dihydro-orotic dehydrogenase), leads to an increase in the activities of both O5P pyrophosphorylase and O5P decarboxylase [129, 130]. Enzyme levels have been produced comparable to those found in normal cell lines. This occurs in the presence of added cytidine, suggesting that this increase is not secondary to derepression because of further pyrimidine starvation. Based on these observations, it has been postulated that one or more earlier intermediates in the pyrimidine biosynthetic sequence, most likely dihydro-orotic acid, are necessary for the normal induction of the two enzymes at fault in hereditary orotic aciduria, O5P pyrophosphorylase and O5P decarboxylase [130]. This will be commented upon later.

Urinary Excretion Data

The patients studied have excreted approximately 600 to 1,500 mg orotic acid per day. If normal values obtained in adults (Fig. 42-6) [22] are applicable in relationship to surface area in childhood, this is an increase of approximately 3,000- to 5,000-fold in urinary orotic acid. Orotidine, dihydro-orotic acid, and carbamylaspartic acid have been found elevated in the urines of patients J.P. and D.G. during relapse [131]. In patients J.P. and D.G. urinary orotidine was 15.8 and 18.4 mg per 24 hr, respectively. This represents an increase of approximately twenty- to fortyfold and is consistent with some residual orotidylic pyrophosphorylase activity. On the other hand the relatively small degree of orotidinuria, in spite of the rise of precursor orotic acid, is further evidence for the double enzyme defect, since selective inhibition of orotidylic decarboxylase using 6-azauridine produces comparable degrees of orotic aciduria and orotidinuria [132]. Urinary orotidine should be markedly elevated in patient P.M., with a selective defect of O5P decarboxylase. No measurements have as yet been reported.

Studies of the incorporation of ring-labeled orotic acid into urinary pseudouridine (5-ribosyluracil) have suggested that the *de novo* synthesis of pyrimidine bases is approximately 0.6 gm per 24 hr in adults [26]. This value is similar to that of purine turnover, estimated from the rate of uric

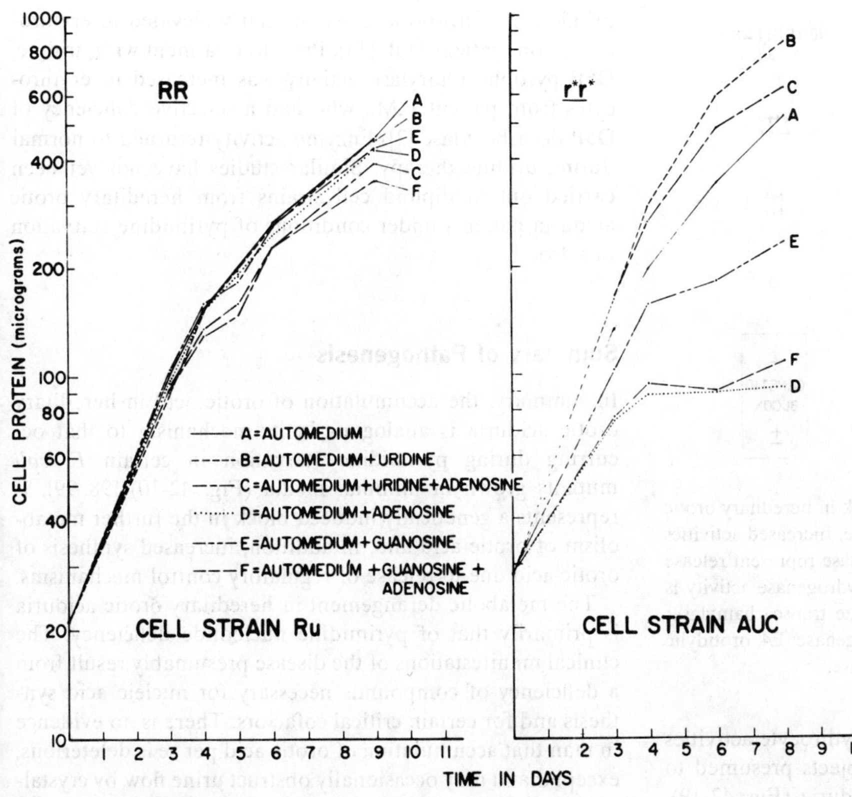

Figure 42-17. Growth of the homozygous mutant and normal cells in various nucleoside supplements. (*From Cold Spring Harbor Symp. Quant. Biol.* 29, **189**, 1964, *with permission of the publishers.*)

acid synthesis [133]. In patients with untreated hereditary orotic aciduria, excretion of orotic acid has varied from 0.5 to 1.5 gm per 24 hr (up to 8 gm per 24 hr per 1.73 m^2). This suggests a marked increase in the rate of orotic acid synthesis in these small children. With a single exception [6], in all patients studied there was a reduction in the rate

Table 42-2. SPECIFIC OROTIDINE-5′-MONOPHOSPHATE PYROPHOSPHORYLASE AND DECARBOXYLASE ACTIVITIES IN DIPLOID CELL STRAINS FROM CONTROLS, THREE PATIENTS WITH HEREDITARY OROTIC ACIDURIA AND ONE HETEROZYGOTE

Cell strain	Presumed genotype*	Specific OMP pyrophosphorylase activity†	Specific OMP decarboxylase activity‡
CR	RR	4.154	0.3350
PD	RR	4.833	0.3240
DB [13]	rr	0.173	0.0094
DG [9, 10]	rr	0.068	0.0028
JP [11]	rr	0.072	0.0022
OR [1, 5]	Rr	2.580	0.1020

* r denotes the mutant gene for orotic aciduria, and R denotes its normal allele.

† mμmoles of orotidine-5′-monophosphate produced per hour of incubation per milligram of cell protein.

‡ mμmoles of orotidine-5′-monophosphate decarboxylated per hour of incubation per milligram of cell protein.

Source: From the Amer. J. Dis. Child. [13] with permission of the publishers.

of orotic acid excretion (from 0.7 to 1.5 gm to 0.1 to 0.2 gm per 24 hr) during the clinical and hematologic remission produced by oral pyrimidine replacement therapy.

Derepression of Orotic Acid Synthesis

The studies carried out in hemic cells, in liver, and in tissue culture have demonstrated a block in two consecutive enzymes which catalyze the conversion of orotic acid to uridine-5′-phosphate (Fig. 42-18). This double enzyme defect leads to a deficiency of pyrimidine nucleotides which can be rectified in vivo by oral replacement therapy using uridine [9] or in vitro by the inclusion of uridine or cytidine in the tissue culture medium (Fig. 42-17) [127]. Since the enzyme defects remain unchanged, this must represent a reduced rate of orotic acid synthesis. This reduction in orotic acid synthesis and excretion may be attributable to the operation of both types of metabolic regulatory mechanisms discussed above: end product repression of enzyme synthesis and negative feedback control in which the pyrimidine nucleotides suppress the activity of one or more enzymes acting early in pyrimidine synthesis, especially carbamyl phosphate synthase.

In an attempt to show increased enzymatic activities prior to the site of the block, as an example of enzyme control by repression-derepression, studies were carried out on aspartate transcarbamylase and dihydro-orotase in erythro-

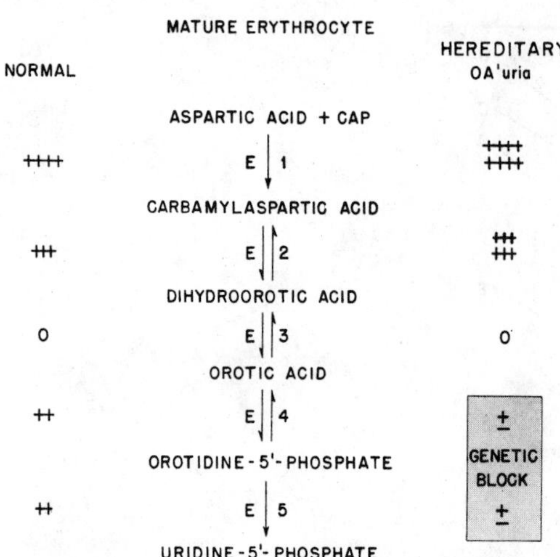

Figure 42-18. Site of the double enzyme block in hereditary orotic aciduria, as measured in the mature erythrocyte. Increased activities of aspartate transcarbamylase and dihydroorotase represent release of end product repression. Dihydroorotic dehydrogenase activity is absent in the mature erythrocyte. E1, aspartate transcarbamylase; E2, dihydroorotase; E3, dihydroorotic dehydrogenase; E4, orotidylic pyrophosphorylase; E5, orotidylic decarboxylase.

cytes. With a possible single exception, erythrocyte activities of these enzymes were normal in all subjects presumed to be heterozygous for hereditary orotic aciduria (Fig. 42-19). This would be anticipated in subjects without clinical or laboratory evidence of pyrimidine deficiency, although presumed heterozygotes did excrete a small excess of orotic acid in the urine (Fig. 42-6). In patient D.G. both enzymes were greatly increased in activity in circulating erythrocytes (Fig. 42-19) and returned to normal on treatment with

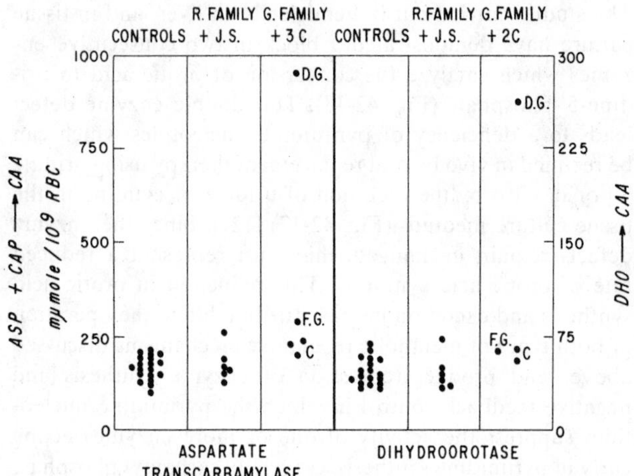

Figure 42-19. Activities of aspartate transcarbamylase and dihydroorotase in erythrocyte preparations from control subjects, from presumed heterozygotes from the R., S., and G. families, and from patient D.G. The elevated activities in D.G. returned to normal levels during uridine treatment (Fig. 42-4).

uridine. Dihydro-orotase was similarly elevated in erythrocytes from patient D.B. [13]. Prior to treatment with uridine, O5P pyrophosphorylase activity was increased in erythrocytes from patient P.M., who had a selective deficiency of O5P decarboxylase [2]. Enzyme activity returned to normal during uridine therapy. Similar studies have not yet been carried out in diploid cell strains from hereditary orotic aciduria patients under conditions of pyrimidine starvation in vitro.

Summary of Pathogenesis

In summary, the accumulation of orotic acid in hereditary orotic aciduria is analogous in its mechanism to that occurring during pyrimidine starvation in certain *E. coli* mutants grown in minimal media (Fig. 42-10) [98, 99]. It represents a genetically induced block in the further metabolism of orotic acid and, in addition, increased synthesis of orotic acid due to release of regulatory control mechanisms.

The metabolic derangement in hereditary orotic aciduria is primarily that of pyrimidine nucleotide deficiency. The clinical manifestations of the disease presumably result from a deficiency of compounds necessary for nucleic acid synthesis and for certain critical cofactors. There is no evidence in man that accumulation of orotic acid per se is deleterious, except that it may occasionally obstruct urine flow by crystalline deposits. The pharmacologic properties of orotic acid have been reviewed above. It is presumed that the toxic properties of this pyrimidine are in some way related to its further metabolism and resulting nucleotide imbalance [134, 135]. The enzymatic block in the conversion of orotic acid to uridine-5′-phosphate is presumably protective against this mode of toxicity in hereditary orotic aciduria.

The most striking clinical feature has been megaloblastosis, which is associated with hypochromia of the erythrocytes. A critical discussion of megaloblastosis is beyond the scope of this chapter. It has been suggested that megaloblastosis results from a selective defect in DNA synthesis which interferes with mitosis [136]. It is a provocative finding, therefore, that hereditary orotic aciduria is associated with megaloblastosis, since the genetic block occurs at a position in the pyrimidine biosynthetic sequence which should result equally in deficient formation of both RNA and DNA. Possibly limited amounts of pyrimidine nucleotides are more efficiently used for RNA than for DNA synthesis. The megaloblasts in hereditary orotic aciduria are not as large as those found in pernicious anemia or folic acid deficiency, and the cellular abnormalities are considerably more striking in the more mature red cell precursors. The degree of microcytosis and hypochromia in circulating erythrocytes (Fig. 42-1) also differs from that usually found in other megaloblastic anemias. These differing structural abnormalities may reflect the coexistence of deficient RNA production and therefore reduced protein synthesis in these patients, with a block in the common pathway of pyrimidine nucleotide synthesis. This speculation is not yet supported by experimental evidence.

OTHER CAUSES OF OROTIC ACIDURIA

A disorder of pyrimidine metabolism somewhat analogous to genetically induced orotic aciduria is produced in man by the administration of the antineoplastic agent 6-azauridine [132]. This substance, following its enzymatic conversion to 6-azauridylic acid, is a specific competitive inhibitor of the decarboxylation of orotidine-5′-phosphate to form uridine-5′-phosphate (Fig. 42-9) [87]. When it is used in therapeutic doses, there is a prompt urinary excretion of both orotic acid (up to 12 gm per 24 hr) and orotidine (up to 10 gm per 24 hr) (Fig. 42-20). 6-Azauridine therapy decreases orotic acid decarboxylation in the intact subject [76] or in leukocytes isolated from the patient under treatment [88]. Although administration of 6-azauridine simulates many of the features of the genetic disease, a major point of dissimilarity lies in the absence of marked orotidinuria in hereditary orotic aciduria. This is probably the result of the additional block of the enzyme catalyzing the conversion of orotic acid to orotidine-5′-phosphate in the genetic disease. Prolonged administration of 6-azauridine to patients without hematologic disease has produced a mild anemia and often, but not invariably, a megaloblastic bone marrow. This has not simulated closely the hypochromic, megaloblastic anemia of hereditary orotic aciduria, perhaps because severe anemia has not been produced. Quite recently it has been shown that the administration of allopurinol in the usual therapeutic doses leads to orotic aciduria and orotidinuria of moderate degree [137, 138]. Allopurinol ribonucleotide has been found to be a competitive inhibitor of orotidylic decarboxylase comparable to 6-azauridylic acid. In patients receiving allopurinol, erythrocyte levels of orotidylic decarboxylase and orotidylic pyrophosphorylase activities are increased, perhaps representing derepression secondary to partial interference with the synthesis of uridine-5′-phosphate. A comparison of hereditary and drug-induced orotic aciduria is discussed more fully elsewhere [88].

Increased excretion of orotic acid, uracil, and uridine has

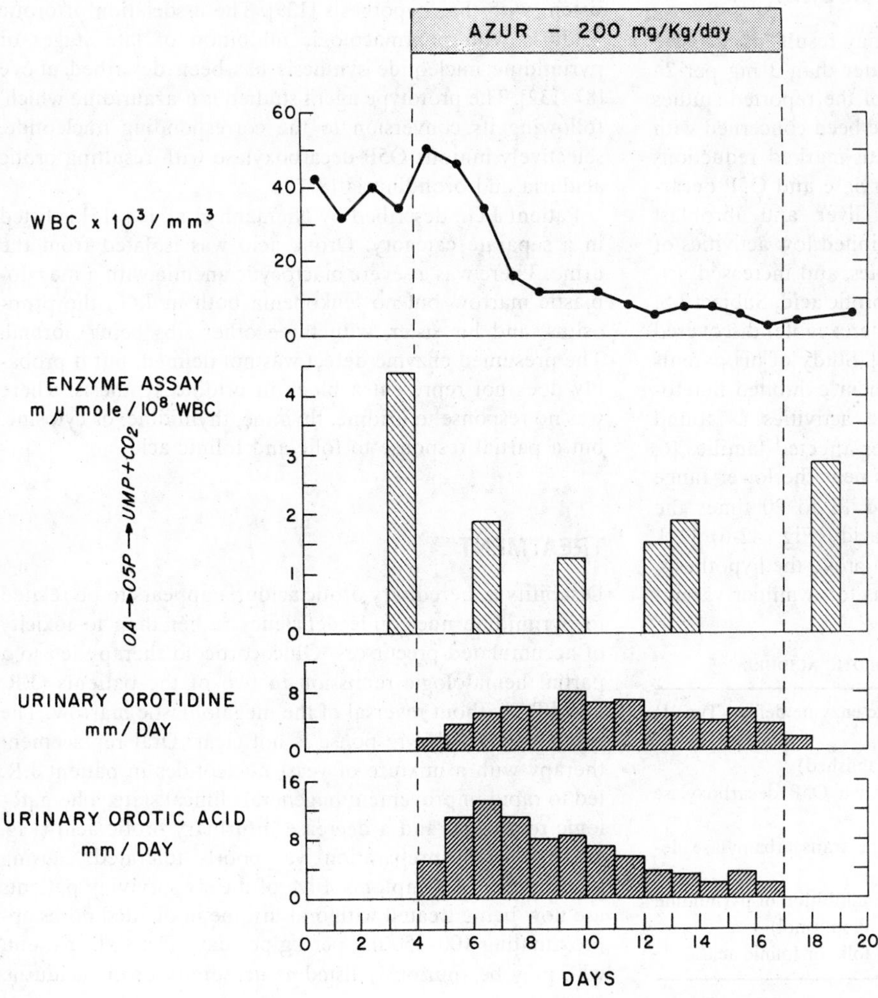

Figure 42-20. Effect of 6-azauridine treatment of a patient with chronic myelocytic leukemia. There was a prompt, coincident orotic aciduria and orotidinuria and a block in the metabolism of orotic acid by isolated leukocytes. (*From Blood,* **20,** 700, 1962, *with permission of the publishers.*)

been reported in two children with ornithine transcarbamylase deficiency [139]. In one patient urinary orotic acid was 240 mg per 100 ml while on a normal protein diet, falling to undetectable levels on a very low-protein diet. It was postulated that carbamyl phosphate might accumulate in this disorder secondary to the partial block in citrulline synthesis resulting in a secondary increase in pyrimidine synthesis by way of aspartate transcarbamylase [139]:

$$\text{CAP} \begin{cases} + \text{ ornithine} \xrightarrow{\text{block}} \text{citrulline} \\ + \text{ aspartate} \longrightarrow \text{carbamylaspartate} \end{cases}$$

The presence of orotic aciduria in hyperammonemia secondary to ornithine transcarbamylase deficiency has been recently confirmed [140]. Evidence was reviewed earlier that separate enzymes catalyze the synthesis of CAP destined for the urea cycle and for pyrimidine synthesis. The compartmentalization of these two CAP pools in mitochondria and in cytosol, respectively, may not be complete.

CLASSIFICATION OF OROTIC ACIDURIA

There are several conditions which may result in excessive urinary excretion of orotic acid (greater than 3 mg per 24 hr), as outlined in Table 42-3. Most of the reported studies and the discussion in this chapter have been concerned with hereditary orotic aciduria Type I with marked reductions in activity of both O5P pyrophosphorylase and O5P decarboxylase in erythrocytes, leukocytes, liver, and fibroblast cultures. Heterozygotes have also exhibited low activities of both enzymes, especially in erythrocytes, and increased urinary excretion (three- to fourfold) of orotic acid. Subject J.S. has been previously reported as a heterozygote, discovered by chance in a small control series [5]. Study of his parents indicated, however, that neither of them exhibited heterozygote levels of erythrocyte enzyme activities as found consistently in genetic studies of other affected families [6, 125, 126]. Both had enzyme activities near the lower range of normal. Subject J.S. also excreted 18 to 20 times the normal amount of urinary orotic acid (Fig. 42-6) [22]. Although the data are not sufficient to prove the hypothesis, it seems likely that J.S. is homozygous for a milder variant of Type I hereditary orotic aciduria. This would be somewhat analogous to the Duarte variant of galactosemia [141]. More extensive studies of the S. family including the children of the propositus might lend further support to this hypothesis.

Table 42-3. CLASSIFICATION OF OROTIC ACIDURIA

I. Hereditary orotic aciduria with double enzyme defect (Type I)
   A. Symptomatic
   B. S. family variant (not clearly established)
II. Hereditary orotic aciduria with selective O5P decarboxylase deficiency (Type II)
III. Orotic aciduria secondary to ornithine transcarbamylase deficiency
IV. Orotic aciduria secondary to analogue inhibition of pyrimidine nucleotide biosynthesis (6-azauridine, allopurinol)
V. Orotic aciduria partially responsive to folic or folinic acid

In Type II hereditary orotic aciduria there is a selective deficiency of activity of O5P decarboxylase [2, 3]. Orotidine-5′-phosphate pyrophosphorylase activity was increased in the propositus during "pyrimidine starvation" and presumed derepression, returning to normal levels during uridine replacement therapy. At this time a single case has been discovered, with demonstration of intermediate enzyme activity or urinary orotic acid excretion values, presumptive of heterozygosity in the patient's mother, brother, and probable father [3].

Orotic aciduria associated with ornithine transcarbamylase deficiency was described above [139]. It is presumed that elevated levels of intracellular carbamyl phosphate behind the block in citrulline synthesis (urea cycle) accelerated pyrimidine biosynthesis, since CAP is beyond the probable major site of feedback control in mammalian systems. This remains to be demonstrated directly, but the marked reduction in orotic acid excretion on a low-protein diet is consistent with that hypothesis [139]. The association of orotic aciduria with pharmacologic inhibition of late stages of pyrimidine nucleotide synthesis has been described above [87, 132]. The prototype agent studied is 6-azauridine which, following its conversion to the corresponding nucleotide, selectively inhibits O5P decarboxylase with resulting orotic aciduria and orotidinuria [87].

Patient J.G., described by Niemann et al. [14, 15] is listed in a separate category. Orotic acid was isolated from the urine. There was a severe macrocytic anemia with a megaloblastic marrow but no leukopenia both in J.G., the propositus, and his sister, with three other sibs being normal. The presumed enzyme defect was not defined, but it probably does not represent a block in uridine synthesis. There was no response to uridine, thymine, thymidine, or cytosine, but a partial response to folic and folinic acid.

TREATMENT

Disability in hereditary orotic aciduria appears to be related to pyrimidine nucleotide deficiency rather than to toxicity of accumulated precursors. Glucocorticoid therapy led to a partial hematologic remission in two of the patients (J.R. and J.P.) without reversal of the megaloblastic marrow. The mechanism of this response is not clear. Oral replacement therapy with a mixture of yeast nucleotides in patient J.R. led to rapid improvement in general clinical state, a hematologic remission, and a decrease in urinary orotic acid (Fig. 42-2) [1]. This preparation was poorly tolerated, causing gastrointestinal symptoms. Five of the six surviving patients are now being treated with oral uridine in divided doses approximating 100–150 mg per kg per day. The sixth patient, who may be spuriously listed as hereditary orotic aciduria, was treated with folic and folinic acids [14, 15]. The details of therapy and response have been summarized in the case reports earlier in the chapter and are summarized for patient D.G. in Fig. 42-4 and patient T.H. in Fig. 42-5. Attempts at maintenance therapy with uracil were unsuccessful when tried in two patients [1, 10]. In general, hematologic abnormalities have responded promptly and completely to full doses of uridine, as have growth and development. In spite of normal growth, two of the patients still have mental deficiency (D.G. and J.P.). T.H. is stated to have normal intelligence, and D.B. was reported to have an IQ of 133. The severe illness which may occur (patient C.P.) and the residual impairment of mental function noted indicate the importance of early diagnosis and treatment.

Seegmiller has suggested that in families in which this disorder has been discovered, prenatal diagnosis might be attempted in order to allow pyrimidine therapy from birth or possibly termination of the pregnancy [4, 142]. It is possible that uridine treatment of the mother might prevent or reduce the occurrence of congenital abnormalities (such as those noted in Table 42-1) although the ability of uridine to cross the placental barrier has not been established.

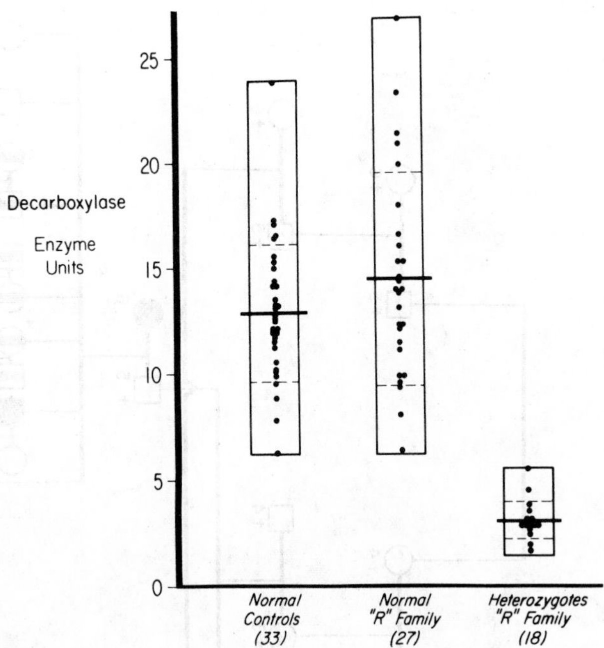

Figure 42-21. Activities of orotidylic decarboxylase in erythrocytes from control subjects and from members of the R. family. (*From Tr. Ass. Amer. Physicians,* **76,** 214, 1963, *with permission of the publishers.*)

GENETICS

The existence of a partial enzyme defect in presumed heterozygotes with hereditary orotic aciduria Type I (Figs. 42-13 and 42-14) has allowed a convenient means of determining its mode of inheritance. A survey was made of the available members of the R. family (that of the proband), using the activity of orotidylic decarboxylase in erythrocytes as a marker [125, 126]. The range and mean values of the enzyme studies performed on a normal control group and on 63 members of the affected family are summarized in Fig. 42-21. The 18 family members with low enzyme levels were provisionally considered heterozygous for hereditary orotic aciduria. It is assumed that the deceased proband was homozygous, although his enzyme levels were not determined. Both parents and two of the three sibs of this original case were heterozygous. The transmission of the defect was apparent through four generations, as shown in the pedigree (Fig. 42-22). The minor degree of consanguinity of the parents appeared to be irrelevant. No increased incidence of abortions, neonatal death, or anemia could be established in the family. Two other pedigrees have been subsequently published with similar patterns of transmission of the trait [6]. Family studies carried out on hereditary orotic aciduria Type II similarly suggest autosomal recessive transmission [3]. The different pattern found in the parents of subject J.S. was discussed in the section on classification.

From these studies it can be concluded that orotic aciduria is transmitted as an autosomal recessive disease. Heterozygotes exhibit decreased activities of orotidylic pyrophosphorylase and orotidylic decarboxylase and excrete a slightly increased amount of orotic acid in the urine. They are not deficient in pyrimidine nucleotide production, as is indicated by absence of symptoms, of anemia, and of the pattern of "pyrimidine starvation" in their pyrimidine biosynthetic pathway.

The frequency of the heterozygous trait of hereditary orotic aciduria in the general population has not been established. In the initial study of the enzyme defect subject J.S. was discovered in a series of about 40 controls [2]. The question of whether he represents a heterozygote or a homozygote of a milder variant has been discussed above. In a subsequent study of approximately 200 specimens from donors at a blood bank, no heterozygotes were discovered by the erythrocyte O5P decarboxylase assay [143]. In studies of the family of T.H., a new heterozygote was discovered in an unrelated in-law [6]. Three other presumed heterozygotes were then found in this "I family." A simplified urinary screening test has been introduced in the survey for heterozygotes which gave only two false positives in 100 random urines screened [144]. Although some patients have undoubtedly escaped detection, homozygous hereditary orotic aciduria must be very rare, in that resistant megaloblastic anemia of infancy is rare. The rarity of this disease suggests that a homozygous defect in the *de novo* pathway of pyrimidine biosynthesis may usually be lethal. In analogy, mutants of *E. coli* are known which have "hereditary orotic aciduria" in that they exhibit a block at orotidylic pyrophosphorylase or orotidylic decarboxylase and accumulate orotic acid in the medium [99, 100]. These organisms fail to grow in the absence of an exogenous source of pyrimi-

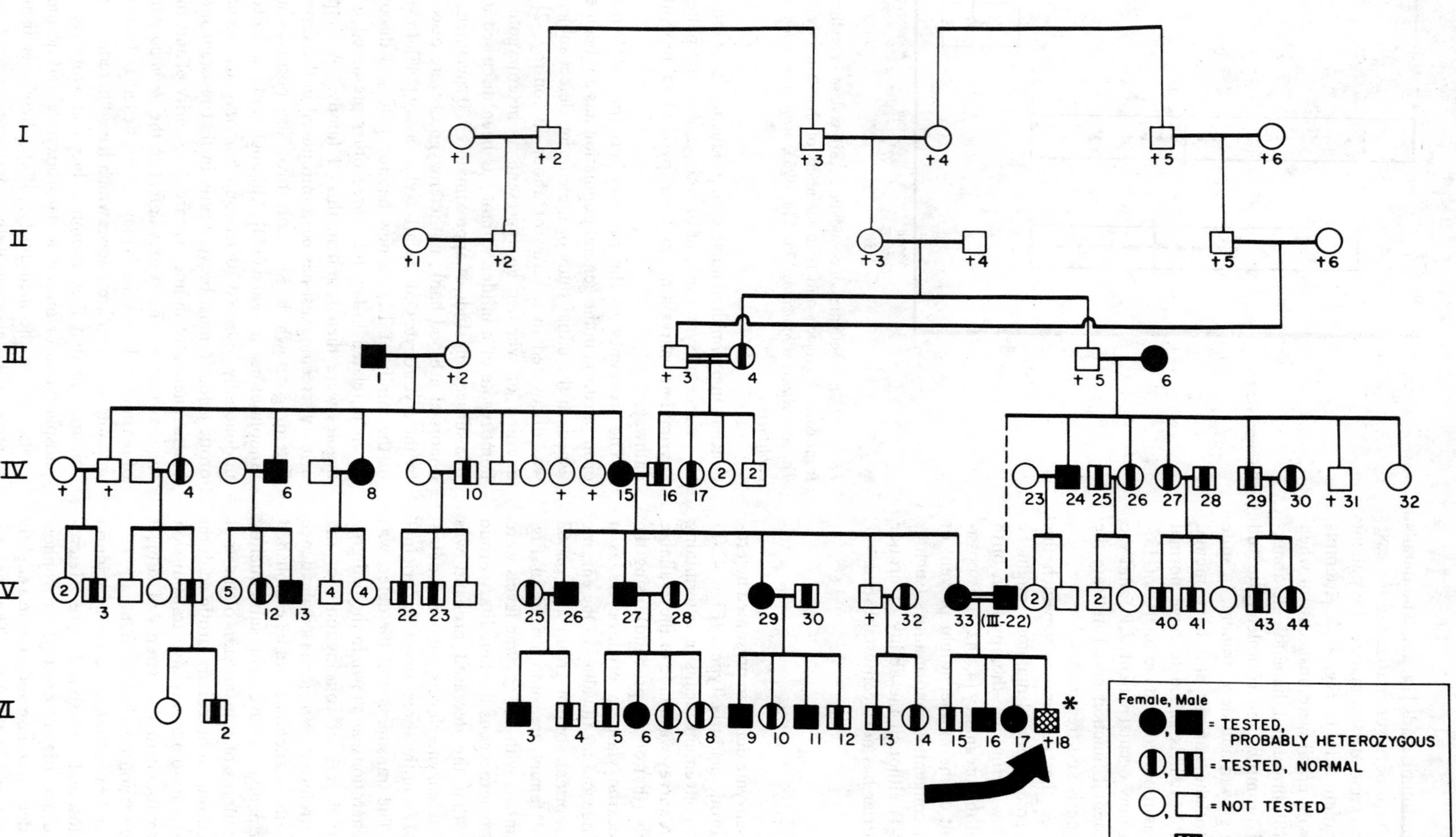

Figure 42-22. Pedigree of the R. family. The proband, patient J.R., is marked by an arrow. Presumed heterozygotes were identified in members of all four surviving generations. (*From. Tr. Ass. Amer. Physicians,* **76**, 214, 1963, *with permission of the publishers.*)

dines. It should be noted that orotidine-5′-phosphate pyrophosphorylase and decarboxylase activities are not absent in diploid cell lines from these patients [7, 13, 127]. Activities have approximated 0.4 to 2.0 percent of those of control cell lines. In the face of accumulation of substrate it is presumably this residual activity which allows the marginal survival of an occasional homozygous case of hereditary orotic aciduria. The role of salvage synthesis of pyrimidine nucleotides from pyrimidine bases or nucleosides present in the diet or released during catabolism has not been investigated in these patients.

Hereditary orotic aciduria is unique as an "involuted genetic disorder" in that it is a genetic defect in the production of genetic material. Also it is the only genetic disease so far found in man in which two sequential enzymes are involved. Evidence has been presented that maple syrup urine disease may be secondary to separate enzymes which in parallel catalyze the decarboxylations of the branched chain keto acids [145]. There are several possible interpretations of this double enzyme defect:

1 Are both biochemical steps carried out by the same enzyme in man? Orotidylic pyrophosphorylase and orotidylic decarboxylase activities have been clearly separated in partially purified preparations from yeast [78], rat liver [86], and calf thymus [80]. In the latter study O5P pyrophosphorylase and decarboxylase were closely associated through successive stages of purification, complete separation being finally attained only by starch gel electrophoresis [80]. During a 600-fold purification of O5P decarboxylase from cow brain no separation from O5P pyrophosphorylase was obtained [82]. There was greater lability of pyrophosphorylase activity, as has been noted in human erythrocyte preparations [5]. There is loss of pyrophosphorylase activity and retention of decarboxylase activity on storage at $-20°C$. The selective inhibition of O5P decarboxylase which occurs during 6-azauridine therapy results in excretion of both orotic acid and orotidine in contrast to the genetic disorder. Finally, the recent discovery of hereditary orotic aciduria Type II with loss of decarboxylase activity associated with elevation of O5P pyrophosphorylase suggests different proteins [2]. None of this evidence is definitive since there could be functionally separate catalytic sites on the same protein. In the opinion of the authors it seems unlikely that these two activities are associated with the same enzyme. It remains a possibility, however, until physical separation of the enzyme activities is achieved in human preparations. For example, recent studies in *Neurospora* have shown three separate steps in the histidine pathway to be catalyzed by a single protein species [146]. It might also be speculated that O5P decarboxylase and pyrophosphorylase are separate proteins which share a common polypeptide. The defect in Type I disease with both enzyme activities affected might reflect a mutation in the structural gene for this subunit. Type II disease might then represent a mutation in the gene for the polypeptide unique to O5P decarboxylase [147].

2 Does a primary genetic defect of one enzyme produce a secondary "nongenetic" decreased activity of the adjacent enzyme? The genotype is only one of many factors affecting the cellular level of either constitutive or inducible enzymes [97, 107]. This is a difficult possibility to exclude in studies on man. In bacteria a selective genetic block of either orotidylic pyrophosphorylase or orotidylic decarboxylase is associated with an increased activity of the other enzyme during periods of pyrimidine starvation, as would be anticipated by release of repression (Fig. 42-10) [99]. As noted above, pharmacologic block of orotidylic decarboxylase with 6-azauridine in man must similarly be associated with increased activity of orotidylic pyrophosphorylase in that there is overproduction of orotidine-5′-phosphate (as reflected in urinary orotidine). The pattern of pyrimidine starvation is seen in aspartate transcarbamylase and dihydro-orotase activities in homozygous hereditary orotic aciduria (Fig. 42-19), in analogy to more rigorous studies in bacterial mutants. It could be speculated that the two enzyme activities are in separate but interacting proteins in which the decarboxylase protein stabilizes the pyrophosphorylase protein [147]. As noted, the mammalian enzymes are very difficult to separate during purification and when separated the pyrophosphorylase activity is extremely unstable [80]. Protection against the inactivation of O5P decarboxylase activity during purification protects against the inactivation of pyrophosphorylase activity [82]. It might therefore be speculated that orotic aciduria Type I is the result of a single structural gene mutation which results in an abnormal polypeptide with impaired decarboxylase activity and impaired ability to stabilize the pyrophosphorylase polypeptide [147]. The presence of increased activity of O5P pyrophosphorylase in Type II disease with O5P decarboxylase deficiency is not consistent with this hypothesis, although the active enzymatic site and the postulated stabilization configuration might represent different parts of the molecule. In addition the remarkable increases in both enzyme activities in tissue culture with 6-azauridine, 5-azaorotic acid, barbituric acid, and even dihydro-orotic acid do not suggest a simple structural gene mutation [129, 130].

3 Does hereditary orotic aciduria result from coincidental mutations of two structural genes (Fig. 42-11)? This possibility cannot be excluded. Genetic studies in *E. coli* show that the four loci determining the structure of dihydro-orotase, dihydro-orotic dehydrogenase, orotidylic pyrophosphorylase, and orotidylic decarboxylase are closely linked [100]. No such genetic mapping is available in man. In an extensive study of enzyme activities in more than sixty pyrimidine-requiring bacterial mutants, none was found which lacked more than one enzyme [100]. The enzyme pattern of hereditary orotic aciduria is compared with that of certain mutants in Fig. 42-23. As will be noted, hereditary orotic aciduria Type II is analogous to *E. coli* mutant 550-460 and *Neurospora crassa* 36601. If the loci of structural genes determining the synthesis of orotidylic pyrophosphorylase and orotidylic decarboxylase are adjacent on the human

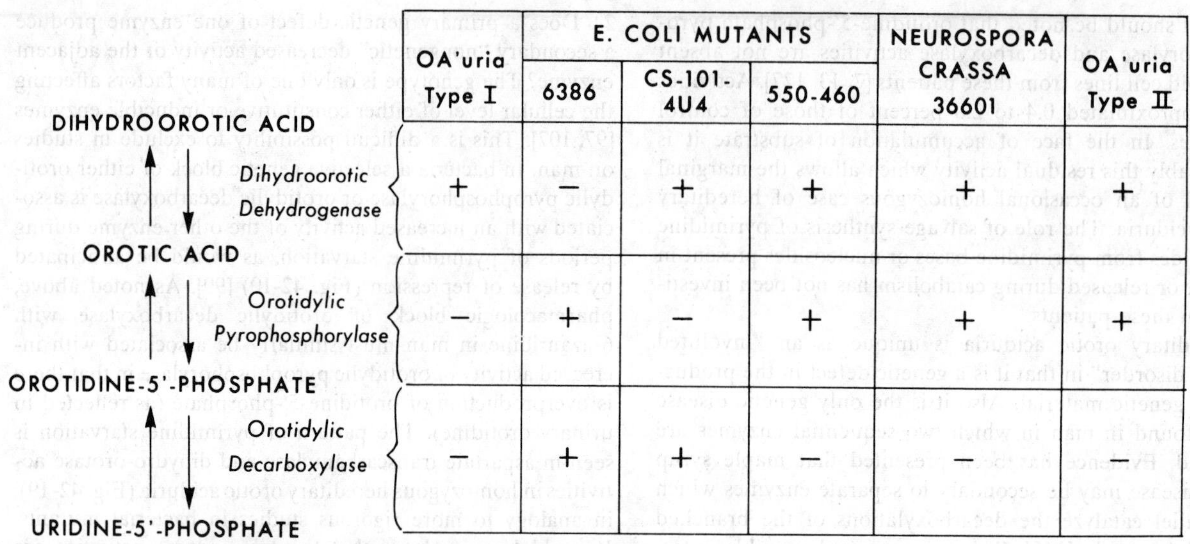

	OA'uria Type I	E. COLI MUTANTS 6386	CS-101-4U4	550-460	NEUROSPORA CRASSA 36601	OA'uria Type II
DIHYDROOROTIC ACID ↓ Dihydroorotic Dehydrogenase	+	−	+	+	+	+
OROTIC ACID ↓ Orotidylic Pyrophosphorylase	−	+	−	+	+	+
OROTIDINE-5'-PHOSPHATE ↓ Orotidylic Decarboxylase	−	+	+	−	−	
URIDINE-5'-PHOSPHATE						

Figure 42-23. Comparison of the enzyme defects in hereditary orotic aciduria with those found in *E. coli* mutants 6386, CS-101-4U4, and 550-460 and in *Neurospora crassa* mutant 36601.

chromosome, a single, possibly extensive genetic defect might overlap both coding sites. This speculation is not open to experimental confirmation. The presence of the double enzyme defect in all but one subject so far studied makes such a fortuitously situated defect unlikely. Also the rise of activities to normal levels in tissue culture during growth on 6-azauridine has been noted.

4 Is hereditary orotic aciduria Type I produced by a mutation in a gene affecting a regulatory mechanism controlling the synthesis of two sequential enzymes in pyrimidine biosynthesis? A brief discussion of controlling mechanisms for the pyrimidine pathway was presented earlier in the chapter. It was emphasized that there is no direct evidence that the Jacob and Monod model (Fig. 42-11), which is based on microbial studies, is applicable to the cells of a metazoan organism [107]. In such organisms the control of the expression of genetic information may in fact be posttranscriptional [107]. Concurrent loss of adjacent enzyme activities in orotic aciduria Type I is consistent with a defect in a controlling mechanism. Earlier enzymes in pyrimidine biosynthesis are unaffected or increased in activity (measured in erythrocytes and fibroblasts) and uridine alone constitutes effective replacement therapy (evidence against undetected enzymatic defects in the further metabolism of pyrimidine nucleotides). The ability of the structural genes to code for normal activities of both enzymes in fibroblast cultures grown in the presence of certain inhibitors of pyrimidine biosynthesis would be more consistent with a regulatory defect, although these important observations do not establish what the regulatory mechanism may be [129, 130]. Evidence has been obtained in yeast [148] and in diploid cell lines from patients with homozygous orotic aciduria Type I [130] which suggests that levels of enzymes in pyrimidine biosynthesis are sequentially induced by certain intermediates, especially dihydro-orotic acid.

Krooth has suggested that the primary defect in hereditary orotic aciduria may be an inappropriate excretion of (or inability to concentrate) orotic acid or other precursors by cells with resultant failure of induction or stabilization of the subsequent two enzymes [149]. This interesting hypothesis is open to experimental verification.

SUMMARY

1 Hereditary orotic aciduria Type I is a rare genetic disorder usually characterized by failure of normal growth and development, hypochromic anemia associated with a megaloblastic marrow resistant to the usual hematinic agents, and excessive urinary excretion of orotic acid. A second form of the disease (Type II) has been recently described which is indistinguishable clinically but which exhibits a different enzymatic defect.

2 The excessive excretion of orotic acid in the homozygous Type I patient is secondary to a block in its further metabolism because of deficient activities of orotidine-5′-phosphate pyrophosphorylase and orotidine-5′-phosphate decarboxylase. There is also overproduction of orotic acid because of release of metabolic control mechanisms. In hereditary orotic aciduria Type II orotidine-5′-phosphate decarboxylase is deficient, but pyrophosphorylase is increased in activity.

3 The pattern of pyrimidine metabolism in hereditary orotic aciduria resembles that of "pyrimidine starvation" studied in bacterial mutants. It can also be partially simulated in man by use of the antineoplastic agent 6-azauridine.

4 The patient with hereditary orotic aciduria is a "pyrimidine auxotroph," requiring pyrimidine replacement therapy for survival. Uridine alone results in a hematologic remission, marked improvement in growth and development, and a decrease in urinary orotic acid. Glucocorticoid therapy is partially effective, but the mechanism of this response is obscure.

5 Hereditary orotic aciduria Type I is transmitted as an autosomal trait. Heterozygotes have partial enzyme deficiencies of orotidine-5′-phosphate pyrophosphorylase and orotidine-5′-phosphate decarboxylase and excrete increased amounts of orotic acid in the urine, but are asymptomatic. No family studies have been reported concerning the single patient so far seen with hereditary orotic aciduria Type II.

6 The loss of two adjacent enzyme activities in hereditary orotic aciduria Type I is consistent with a defect in a genetic control mechanism. Both enzyme activities return toward normal levels in homozygous diploid cell lines grown in the presence of certain inhibitors of pyrimidine biosynthesis. Current evidence does not allow definition of the postulated control mechanism at fault in this genetic disease.

BIBLIOGRAPHY

1. Huguley, C. M., Jr., Bain, J. A., Rivers, S., and Scoggins, R.: Refractory megaloblastic anemia associated with excretion of orotic acid. Blood, **14**, 615, 1959.
2. Fox, R. M., O'Sullivan, W. J., and Firkin, B. G.: Orotic aciduria. Differing enzyme patterns. Amer. J. Med., **47**, 332, 1969.
3. Fox, R. M.: Personal communication.
4. Seegmiller, J. E.: Hereditary orotic aciduria, in *Duncan's Diseases of Metabolism,* edited by P. K. Bondy, p. 570, Saunders, Philadelphia, 1969.
5. Smith, L. H., Jr., Sullivan, M., and Huguley, C. M., Jr.: Pyrimidine metabolism in man. IV. The enzymatic defect of orotic aciduria. J. Clin. Invest., **40**, 656, 1961.
6. Rogers, L. E., Warford, L. R., Patterson, R. B., and Porter, F. S.: Hereditary orotic aciduria. I. A new case with family studies. Pediatrics, **42**, 415, 1968.
7. Howell, R. R., Klinenberg, J. R., and Krooth, R. S.: Enzyme studies on diploid cell strains developed from patients with hereditary orotic aciduria. Johns Hopkins Med. J., **120**, 81, 1967.
8. Smith, L. H., Jr.: Hereditary orotic aciduria—pyrimidine auxotrophism in man. Amer. J. Med., **38**, 1, 1965.
9. Becroft, D. M. O., and Phillips, L. I.: Hereditary orotic aciduria and megaloblastic anaemia: a second case, with response to uridine. Brit. Med. J., **1**, 547, 1965.
10. Becroft, D. M. O., Phillips, L. I., and Simmonds, A.: Hereditary orotic aciduria: Long-term therapy with uridine and a trial of uracil. J. Pediat., **75**, 885, 1969.
11. Haggard, M. E., and Lockhart, L. H.: Megaloblastic anemia with orotic aciduria. Amer. J. Dis. Child., **113**, 733, 1967.
12. Haggard, M. E.: Personal communication.
13. Tubergen, D. G., Krooth, R. S., and Heyn, R. M.: Hereditary orotic aciduria with normal growth and development. Amer. J. Dis. Child., **118**, 864, 1969.
14. Neimann, N., Najean, Y., Scialom, C., Boulard, M., Pierson, M., and Bernard, J.: Étude d'un cas d'anémie mégaloblastique de l'enfant avec excrétion anormale d'àcide orotique. Nouv. Rev. Franç. Hémat., **5**, 445, 1965.
15. Najean, A. Y.: Personal communication.
16. Von Euler, L. H., Rubin, R. J., and Handschumacher, R. E.: Fatty livers induced by orotic acid. II. Changes in nucleotide metabolism. J. Biol. Chem., **238**, 2464, 1963.
17. Biscaro, G., and Belloni, E.: Über die Orotsäure. Ann. Soc. Chim. Milano, **11**, 1, 2, 1905. Chem. Zentralbl., **2**, 64, 1905.
18. Kobata, A., Suzuoki, J., and Kida, M.: Acid-soluble nucleotides of milk. I. Quantitative and qualitative differences of nucleotide constituents in human and cow milk. J. Biochem. (Tokyo), **51**, 277, 1962.
19. Okonkovo, P. O., and Kinsella, J. E.: Orotic acid in food milk powders. Amer. J. Clin. Nutr., **22**, 532, 1969.
20. Rundles, R. W., and Brewer, S. S., Jr.: Hematologic responses in pernicious anemia to orotic acid. Blood, **13**, 99, 1958.
21. Schanker, L. S., and Jeffrey, J. J.: Structural specificity of the pyrimidine transport process of the small intestine. Biochem. Pharmacol., **11**, 961, 1962.
22. Lotz, M., Fallon, H. J., and Smith, L. H., Jr.: Excretion of orotic acid and orotidine in heterozygotes of congenital orotic aciduria. Nature (London), **197**, 194, 1963.
23. Volle, R. L., Green, R. E., Peters, L., Handschumacher, R. E., and Welch, A. D.: Renal tubular excretion studies with pyrimidine derivatives and analogues. J. Pharmacol. Exp. Therap., **136**. 353, 1962.
24. Smith, L. H., Jr., and Baker, F. A.: Pyrimidine metabolism in man. I. The biosynthesis of orotic acid. J. Clin. Invest., **38**, 798, 1959.
25. Rosenbloom, F. M., and Seegmiller, J. E.: An enzymatic spectrophotometric method for determination of orotic acid. J. Lab. Clin. Med., **63**, 492, 1964.
26. Weissman, S. M., Eisen, A. Z., Fallon, H., Lewis, M., and Karon, M.: The metabolism of ring-labeled orotic acid in man. J. Clin. Invest., **41**, 1546, 1962.
27. Fallon, H. J., Frei, E., III, Block, J., and Seegmiller, J. E.: The uricosuria and orotic aciduria induced by 6-azauridine. J. Clin. Invest., **40**, 1906, 1961.
28. Lieberman, I., and Kornberg, A.: Enzymatic synthesis and breakdown of a pyrimidine, orotic acid. I. Dihydro-orotic dehydrogenase. Biochim. Biophys. Acta, **12**, 223, 1953.
29. Lieberman, I., and Kornberg, A.: Enzymatic synthesis and breakdown of a pyrimidine, orotic acid. II. Dihydroorotic acid, ureidosuccinic acid, and 5-carboxymethylhydantoin. J. Biol. Chem., **207**, 911, 1954.
30. Lan, S. J., Sallach, H. J., and Cohen, P. P.: The enzymatic steps of pyrimidine biosynthesis in the unfertilized frog egg. Biochemistry, **8**, 3673, 1969.
31. Kerson, L. A., and Appel, S. H.: Kinetic studies on rat liver carbamyl phosphate synthetase. J. Biol. Chem., **243**, 4279, 1968.
32. Schooler, J. M., Fahien, L. A., and Cohen, P. P.: 2-Acetoxyglutarate as an activator of carbamyl phosphate synthetase. J. Biol. Chem., **238**, 1909, 1963.
33. Cohen, P. P.: Biochemical aspects of metamorphosis: transition from ammonotelism to ureotelism. Harvey Lect., **60**, 119, 1966.
34. Metzenberg, R. L., Marshall, M., Paik, W. K., and Cohen, P. P.: The synthesis of carbamyl phosphate synthetase in thyroxin-treated tadpoles. J. Biol. Chem., **236**, 162, 1961.
35. Davis, R. H.: Carbamyl phosphate synthesis in *Neurospora crassa.* II. Genetics, metabolic position, and regulation of arginine-specific carbamyl phosphokinase. Biochim. Biophys. Acta, **107**, 54, 1965.
36. Levenberg, B.: Role of L-glutamine as donor of carbamyl nitrogen for the enzymatic synthesis of citrulline in *Agaricus bisporus.* J. Biol. Chem., **237**, 2590, 1962.
37. Piérard, A., and Wiame, J. M.: Regulation and mutation affecting a glutamine dependent formation of carbamyl phosphate in *Escherichia coli.* Biochem. Biophys. Res. Commun., **15**, 76, 1964.
38. Lacroute, F., Piérard, A., Grenson, M., and Wiame, J. M.: The biosynthesis of carbamoyl phosphate in *Saccharomyces cerevisiae.* J. Gen. Microbiol., **40**, 127, 1965.
39. O'Neal, D., and Naylor, A. W.: Purine and pyrimidine nucleotide inhibition of carbamyl phosphate synthetase from pea seedlings. Biochem. Biophys. Res. Commun., **31**, 322, 1968.
40. Titibana, M., and Ito, K.: Carbamyl phosphate synthetase of the hematopoietic mouse spleen and the control of pyrimidine biosynthesis. Biochem. Biophys. Res. Commun., **26**, 221, 1967.
41. Titibana, M., and Ito, K.: Control of pyrimidine biosynthesis in mammalian tissues. I. Partial purification and characterization of glutamine-

utilizing carbamyl phosphate synthesis of mouse spleen and its tissue distribution. J. Biol. Chem., **244,** 5403, 1969.

42. Hager, S. E., and Jones, M. E.: Initial steps in pyrimidine synthesis in Ehrlich ascites carcinoma *in vitro.* II. The synthesis of carbamyl phosphate by a soluble, glutamine-dependent carbamyl phosphate synthetase. J. Biol. Chem., **242,** 5667, 1967.
43. Smith, L. H., Jr., and Reichard, P.: Enzymic synthesis of carbamyl-aspartate from citrulline in extracts from rat liver mitochondria. Acta Chem. Scand., **10,** 1024, 1956.
44. Piérard, A., Glansdorff, N., Mergeay, M., and Wiame, J. M.: Control of the biosynthesis of carbamoyl phosphate in *Escherichia coli.* J. Molec. Biol., **14,** 23, 1965.
45. Marshall, M., and Cohen, P. P.: A kinetic study of the mechanism of crystalline carbamate kinase. J. Biol. Chem., **241,** 4197, 1966.
46. Jones, M. E.: Carbamyl phosphate. Science, **140,** 1373, 1963.
47. Young, J. E., Proger, M. D., and Atkins, I. C.: Comparative activities of aspartate transcarbamylase in various tissues of the rat. Proc. Soc. Exp. Biol. Med., **125,** 860, 1967.
48. Yates, R. A., and Pardee, A. B.: Control of pyrimidine biosynthesis in Escherichia coli by a feed-back mechanism. J. Biol. Chem., **221,** 757, 1956.
49. Changeux, J.-P., Gerhart, J. C., and Schachman, H. K.: Allosteric interactions in aspartate transcarbamylase. I. Binding of specific ligands to the native enzyme and its isolated subunits. Biochemistry, **7,** 531, 1968.
50. Hervé, G. L., and Stark, G. R.: Aspartate transcarbamylase. Amino-terminal analyses and peptide maps of the subunits. Biochemistry, **6,** 3743, 1967.
51. Weber, K.: New structural model of E. coli aspartate transcarbamylase and the amino acid sequence of the regulatory polypeptide chain. Nature (London), **218,** 1116, 1968.
52. Kleppe, K.: Aspartate transcarbamylase from *Escherichia coli.* I. Inhibition by inorganic anions. Biochim. Biophys. Acta, **122,** 450, 1966.
53. Stein, L. I., and Cohen, P. P.: Correlation of growth and aspartate transcarbamylase activity in higher plants. Arch. Biochem., **109,** 429, 1965.
54. Bresnick, E., and Hitchings, G. H.: Feedback control in Ehrlich ascites cells. Cancer Res., **21,** 105, 1961.
55. Bresnick, E.: Inhibition by pyrimidines of aspartate transcarbamylase partially purified from rat liver. Biochim. Biophys. Acta, **67,** 425, 1963.
56. Weitzman, P. D. J., and Wilson, I. B.: Studies on aspartate transcarbamylase and its allosteric interaction. J. Biol. Chem., **241,** 5481, 1966.
57. Bottomley, R. H., and Lovig, C. A.: Subcellular distribution of rat aspartate carbamoyltransferase. Biochim. Biophys. Acta, **148,** 588, 1967.
58. Cooper, C., Wu, R., and Wilson, D. W.: Studies of some precursors of pyrimidines. J. Biol. Chem., **216,** 37, 1955.
59. Bresnick, E., and Blatchford, K.: Inhibition of dihydroorotase by purines and pyrimidines. Biochim. Biophys. Acta, **81,** 150, 1964.
60. Shafritz, D. A., and Senior, J. R.: Synthesis of pyrimidine nucleotide precursors in human and rat small intestinal mucosa. Biochim. Biophys. Acta, **141,** 332, 1967.
61. Sander, E. G.: *Studies on Dihydroorotate.* Ph. D. Thesis, Cornell Univ., 1965. University Microfilms, Ann Arbor, 66-4502.
62. Sander, E. G., Wright, L. D., and McCormick, D. B.: Evidence for function of a metal ion in the activity of dihydroorotase from *Zymobacterium oroticum.* J. Biol. Chem., **240,** 3628, 1965.
63. Wallach, D. P., and Grisolia, S.: The purification and properties of hydropyrimidine hydrase. J. Biol. Chem., **226,** 277, 1957.
64. Friedmann, H. C., and Vennesland, B.: Crystalline dihydroorotic dehydrogenase. J. Biol. Chem., **235,** 1526, 1960.
65. Aleman, V., and Handler, P.: Dihydroorotate dehydrogenase. I. General properties. J. Biol. Chem., **242,** 4087, 1967.
66. Aleman, V., Handler, P., Palmer, G., and Beinert, H.: Studies on dihydroorotate dehydrogenase by electron paramagnetic resonance spectroscopy. II. Electron paramagnetic resonance and optical spectra and titrations. J. Biol. Chem., **243,** 2560, 1968; III. Kinetic studies by rapid freezing. J. Biol. Chem., **243,** 2569, 1968.
67. Miller, R. W., and Kerr, C. T.: Dihydroorotate dehydrogenase. III. Interactions with substrates, inhibitors, artificial electron acceptors, and cytochrome *c.* J. Biol. Chem., **241,** 5597, 1966.
68. Eakin, R. T., and Mitchell, H. K.: A mitochondrial dihydroorotate oxidase system in *Neurospora crassa.* Arch. Biochem. Biophys., **134,** 160, 1969.
69. Udaka, S., and Vennesland, B.: Properties of triphosphopyridine nucleotide-linked dihydroorotic dehydrogenase. J. Biol. Chem., **237,** 2018, 1962.
70. Wuu, K.-D., and Krooth, R. S.: Dihydroorotic acid dehydrogenase activity of human diploid cell strains. Science, **160,** 539, 1968.
71. Lotz, M., and Smith, L. H., Jr.: The effect of reticulocytosis in the rabbit on the activities of enzymes in pyrimidine biosynthesis. Blood, **19,** 593, 1962.
72. Santilli, V., Škoda, J., Gut, J., and Šorm, F.: Dihydro-5-azaorotic acid, the first specific inhibitor of dihydro-orotate dehydrogenase. Biochim. Biophys. Acta, **155,** 623, 1968.
73. Lieberman, I., and Kornberg, A.: Enzymatic synthesis and breakdown of a pyrimidine, orotic acid. III. Ureidosuccinase. J. Biol. Chem., **212,** 909, 1955.
74. Grisolia, S., Caravaca, J., Cardoso, S., and Wallach, D. P.: Metabolism of dihydropyrimidines and related compounds. Fed. Proc., **16,** 189, 1957.
75. Caravaca, J., and Grisolia, S.: Enzymatic decarbamylation of carbamyl β-alanine and carbamyl β-aminoisobutyric acid. J. Biol. Chem., **231,** 357, 1958.
76. Rabkin, M. T., Frederick, E. W., Lotz, M., and Smith, L. H., Jr.: Pyrimidine metabolism in man. V. The measurement *in vivo* of the biochemical effect of antineoplastic agents in animal and human subjects. J. Clin. Invest., **41,** 871, 1962.
77. Canellakis, E. S.: Pyrimidine metabolism. I. Enzymatic pathways of uracil and thymine degradation. J. Biol. Chem., **221,** 315, 1956.
78. Lieberman, I., Kornberg, A., and Simms, E. S.: Enzymatic synthesis of pyrimidine nucleotides: orotidine-5′-phosphate and uridine-5′-phosphate. J. Biol. Chem., **215,** 403, 1955.
79. Holmes, W. L.: Studies on the mode of action of analogues of orotic acid: 6-uracilsulfonic acid, 6-uracilsulfonamide, and 6-uracil methyl sulfone. J. Biol. Chem., **223,** 677, 1956.
80. Kasbekar, D. K., Nagabhushanam, A., and Greenberg, D. M.: Purification and properties of orotic acid-decarboxylating enzymes from calf thymus. J. Biol. Chem., **239,** 4245, 1964.
81. Blair, D. G. R., Stone, J. E., and Potter, V. R.: Formation of orotidine-5′-phosphate by enzymes from rat liver. J. Biol. Chem., **235,** 2379, 1960.
82. Appel, S. H.: Purification and kinetic properties of brain orotidine 5′-phosphate decarboxylase. J. Biol. Chem., **243,** 3924, 1968.
83. Canellakis, E. S.: Pyrimidine metabolism. II. Enzymatic pathways of uracil anabolism. J. Biol. Chem., **227,** 329, 1957.
84. Dahl, J. L., Way, J. L., and Parks, R. E., Jr.: The enzymatic synthesis of 5-fluorouridine 5′-phosphate. J. Biol. Chem., **234,** 2998, 1959.
85. Wolcott, J. H., and Ross, C.: Orotidine 5′-phosphate decarboxylase from higher plants. Biochim. Biophys. Acta, **122,** 532, 1966.
86. Creasey, W. A., and Handschumacher, R. E.: Purification and properties of orotidylate decarboxylases from yeast and rat liver. J. Biol. Chem., **236,** 2058, 1961.
87. Handschumacher, R. E.: Orotidylic acid decarboxylase: inhibition studies with azauridine 5′-phosphate. J. Biol. Chem., **235,** 2917, 1960.
88. Fallon, H. J., Lotz, M., and Smith, L. H., Jr.: Congenital orotic aciduria: demonstration of an enzyme defect in leukocytes and comparison with drug-induced orotic aciduria. Blood, **20,** 700, 1962.
89. Canellakis, E. S.: Pyrimidine metabolism. III. The interaction of the catabolic and anabolic pathways of uracil metabolism. J. Biol. Chem., **227,** 701, 1957.
90. Sköld, O.: Enzymes of uracil metabolism in tissues with different growth characteristics. Biochim. Biophys. Acta, **44,** 1, 1960.
91. Goldberg, A. R., Machledt, J. H., and Pardee, A. B.: On the action of fluorouracil on leukemia cells. Cancer Res., **26,** 1611, 1966.
92. Reyes, P.: The synthesis of 5-fluorouridine 5′-phosphate by a pyrimidine phosphoribosyltransferase of mammalian origin. I. Some properties of the enzyme from P1534J mouse leukemia cells. Biochemistry, **8,** 2057, 1969.
93. Vilter, R. W., Horrigan, D., Mueller, J. F., Jarrold, T., Vilter, C. F., Hawkins, V., and Seaman, A.: Studies on relationships of vitamin B_{12}, folic acid, thymine, uracil, and methyl group donors in persons with pernicious anemia and related megaloblastic anemias. Blood, **5,** 695, 1950.

94. Reichard, P.: The enzymatic synthesis of pyrimidines. Advances Enzymol., **21**, 263, 1959.
95. Wright, L. D., Miller, C. S., and Driscoll, C. A.: Inactivity of dihydrouracil and β-ureidoproprionic acid as pyrimidine precursors for lactic acid bacteria. Proc. Soc. Exp. Biol. Med., **86**, 215, 1954.
96. Mokrasch, L. C., and Grisolia, S.: Incorporation of hydropyrimidine derivatives in ribonucleic acid with liver preparations. Biochim. Biophys. Acta, **27**, 226, 1958.
97. Pardee, A. B., and Wilson, A. C.: Control of enzyme activity in higher animals. Cancer Res., **23**, 1483, 1963.
98. Yates, R. A., and Pardee, A. B.: Control by uracil of formation of enzymes required for orotate synthesis. J. Biol. Chem., **227**, 677, 1957.
99. Smith, L. H., Jr., and Lotz, M.: Studies on congenital orotic aciduria: comparison of orotic acid metabolism in microorganisms. J. Lab. Clin. Med., **61**, 211, 1963.
100. Beckwith, J. R., Pardee, A. B., Austrian, R., and Jacob, F.: Coordination of the synthesis of the enzymes in the pyrimidine pathway of *E. coli.* J. Molec. Biol., **5**, 618, 1962.
101. Smith, L. H., Jr., and Baker, F. A.: Pyrimidine metabolism in man. III. Studies on the leukocytes and erythrocytes in pernicious anemia. J. Clin. Invest., **39**, 15, 1960.
102. Ennis, H. L., and Lubin, M.: Capacity for synthesis of a pyrimidine biosynthetic enzyme in mammalian cells. Biochim. Biophys. Acta, **68**, 78, 1963.
103. Jacob, F., and Monod, J.: Genetic regulatory mechanisms in the synthesis of proteins. J. Molec. Biol., **3**, 318, 1961.
104. Ptashne, M.: Specific binding of the λ phage repressor by λ DNA. Nature (London), **214**, 232, 1967.
105. Gilbert, W., and Müller-Hill, B.: Isolation of the lac repressor. Proc. Nat. Acad. Sci. USA, **56**, 1891, 1966.
106. Gilbert, W., and Müller-Hill, B.: The lac operator is DNA. Proc. Nat. Acad. Sci. USA, **58**, 2415, 1967.
107. Tomkins, G. M., Gelehrter, T. D., Granner, D., Martin, D., Jr., Samuels, H. H., and Thompson, E. B.: Control of specific gene expression in higher organisms. Science, **166**, 1474, 1969.
108. Stadtman, E. R.: Allosteric regulation of enzyme activity. Advances Enzymol., **28**, 41, 1966.
109. Gerhart, J. C., and Pardee, A. B.: The enzymology of control by feedback inhibition. J. Biol. Chem., **237**, 891, 1962.
110. Monod, J., Changeux, J.-P., and Jacob, F.: Allosteric proteins and cellular control systems. J. Molec. Biol., **6**, 306, 1963.
111. McClintock, D. K., and Markus, G.: Conformational changes in aspartate transcarbamylase. I. Proteolysis of the intact enzyme. J. Biol. Chem., **243**, 2855, 1968.
112. Dratz, E. A., and Calvin, M.: Substrate- and inhibitor-induced changes in the optical rotatory dispersion of aspartate transcarbamylase. Nature (London), **211**, 497, 1966.
113. Bresnick, E.: Feedback inhibition of aspartate transcarbamylase in liver and in hepatoma. Cancer Res., **22**, 1246, 1962.
114. Proger, M. D., Young, J. E., and Atkins, I. C.: A study of the possible role of feedback inhibition of aspartate transcarbamylase in regulation of pyrimidine synthesis in human leukocytes. J. Lab. Clin. Med., **70**, 768, 1967.
115. Curci, M. R., and Donachie, W. D.: An attempt to find pyrimidine inhibitors of a mammalian aspartate carbamoyl-transferase. Biochim. Biophys. Acta, **85**, 338, 1964.
116. Anderson, P. M., and Meister, A.: Control of *Escherichia coli* carbamyl phosphate synthetase by purine and pyrimidine nucleotides. Biochemistry, **5**, 3164, 1966.
117. Hager, S. E., and Jones, M. E.: A glutamine-dependent enzyme for the synthesis of carbamyl phosphate for pyrimidine biosynthesis in fetal rat liver. J. Biol. Chem., **242**, 5674, 1967.
118. Blakley, R. L., and Vitols, E.: Control of nucleotide biosynthesis. Ann. Rev. Biochem., **37**, 201, 1968.
119. Standerfer, S. B., and Handler, P.: Fatty liver induced by orotic acid feeding. Proc. Soc. Exp. Biol. Med., **90**, 270, 1955.
120. Creasey, W. A., Hankin, L., and Handschumacher, R. E.: Fatty livers induced by orotic acid. I. Accumulation and metabolism of lipids. J. Biol. Chem., **236**, 2064, 1961.
121. Windmueller, H. G., and Levy, R. I.: Total inhibition of hepatic betalipoprotein production in the rat by orotic acid. J. Biol. Chem., **242**, 2246, 1967.
122. Marchetti, M., Puddu, P., and Caldarera, C. M.: Liver acid soluble nucleotides in orotic acid-fed rats. Biochim. Biophys. Acta, **61**, 826, 1962.
123. Bresnick, E., Mayfield, E. D., and Mosse, H.: Increased activity of enzymes for *de novo* pyrimidine biosynthesis after orotic acid administration. Molec. Pharmacol., **4**, 173, 1968.
124. Delbarre, F., and Auscher, C.: Traitement de la goutte par l'acide uracil-6-carboxylique et ses dérives. Presse Méd., **71**, 1765, 1963.
125. Fallon, H. J., Smith, L. H., Jr., Lotz, M., Graham, J. B., and Burnett, C. H.: Hereditary orotic aciduria. Tr. Ass. Amer. Physicians, **76**, 214, 1963.
126. Fallon, H. J., Smith, L. H., Jr., Graham, J. B., and Burnett, C. H.: A genetic study of hereditary orotic aciduria. New Eng. J. Med., **270**, 878, 1964.
127. Krooth, R. S.: Personal communication.
128. Krooth, R. S.: Properties of diploid cell strains developed from patients with an inherited abnormality of uridine biosynthesis. Cold Spring Harbor Symp. Quant. Biol., **29**, 189, 1964.
129. Pinsky, L., and Krooth, R. S.: Studies on the control of pyrimidine biosynthesis in human diploid cell strains. I. Effect of 6-azauridine on cellular phenotype. Proc. Nat. Acad. Sci. USA, **57**, 925, 1967.
130. Pinsky, L., and Krooth, R. S.: Studies on the control of pyrimidine biosynthesis in human diploid cell strains. II. Effects of 5-azaorotic acid, barbituric acid, and pyrimidine precursors on cellular phenotype. Proc. Nat. Acad. Sci. USA, **57**, 1267, 1967.
131. Bain, J. A., and Huguley, C. M., Jr.: Unpublished observations.
132. Cardoso, S. S., Calabresi, P., and Handschumacher, R. E.: Alterations in human pyrimidine metabolism as a result of therapy with 6-azauridine. Cancer Res., **21**, 1551, 1961.
133. Seegmiller, J. E., Grayzel, A. I., Laster, L., and Liddle, L.: Uric acid production in gout. J. Clin. Invest., **40**, 1304, 1961.
134. Rajalakshmi, S., and Handschumacher, R. E.: Control of purine biosynthesis *de novo* by orotic acid *in vivo* and *in vitro.* Biochim. Biophys. Acta, **155**, 317, 1968.
135. Bloomfield, R. A., Letter, A. A., and Wilson, R. P.: Effect of orotic acid on the lipid and acid-soluble nucleotide concentrations in avian liver. Biochim. Biophys. Acta, **187**, 266, 1969.
136. Thorell, B.: Studies on the formation of cellular substances during blood cell production. Acta Med. Scand., **Suppl. 200**, 1, 1947.
137. Fox, R. M., Royse-Smith, D., and O'Sullivan, W. J.: Orotidinuria induced by allopurinol. Science, **168**, 861, 1970.
138. Kelley, W. N., and Beardmore, T. D.: Allopurinol: alteration in pyrimidine metabolism in man. Science, **169**, 388, 1970.
139. Levin, B., Abraham, J. M., Oberholzer, V. G., and Burgess, E. A.: Hyperammonaemia: a deficiency of liver ornithine transcarbamylase. Arch. Dis. Child., **44**, 152, 1969.
140. Williams, H. E.: Unpublished observations.
141. Beutler, E., Baluda, M. C., Sturgeon, P., and Day, R.: A new genetic abnormality resulting in galactose-1-phosphate uridyltransferase deficiency. Lancet, **1**, 353, 1965.
142. Nadler, H. L.: Prenatal detection of genetic defects. J. Pediat., **74**, 132, 1969.
143. Howard, B., and Smith, L. H., Jr.: Unpublished observations.
144. Rogers, L. E., and Porter, F. S.: Hereditary orotic aciduria. II. A urinary screening test. Pediatrics, **42**, 423, 1968.
145. Goedde, H. W., and Keller, W.: Metabolic pathways in maple syrup urine disease, in *Amino Acid Metabolism and Genetic Variation,* edited by W. L. Nyhan, p. 191, McGraw-Hill, New York, 1967.
146. Minson, A. C., and Creaser, E. H.: Purification of a trifunctional enzyme, catalyzing three steps of the histidine pathway, from *Neurospora crassa.* Biochem. J., **114**, 49, 1969.
147. Appel, S. H.: Personal communication.
148. Lacroute, F.: Regulation of pyrimidine biosynthesis in *Saccharomyces cerevisiae.* J. Bact., **95**, 824, 1968.
149. Krooth, R. S.: Studies on the regulation of UMP synthesis in human diploid cells, in *Control Mechanisms in Expression of Cellular Phenotype,* edited by H. Padykula, Academic, New York, 1970, In press.

PART SEVEN

DISEASES MANIFEST PRIMARILY AS ABNORMALITIES OF METAL METABOLISM

CHAPTER FORTY-THREE

WILSON'S DISEASE

Alexander G. Bearn

Wilson's disease (hepatolenticular degeneration) is a rare autosomal recessively inherited disease characterized by degenerative changes in the brain, particularly the basal ganglia, and cirrhosis of the liver. The greenish-brown Kayser-Fleischer rings at the limbus of the cornea are pathognomonic of the disease (Fig. 43-1).

CLINICAL FEATURES

In 1912 Wilson published his monograph entitled "Progressive Lenticular Degeneration: A Familial Nervous Disease Associated with Cirrhosis of the Liver" [1]. While still a young man, Wilson had under his care a patient who died after a long illness characterized by muscular rigidity, tremor, and forced grimacing. Cirrhosis of the liver and gross degenerative changes in the lenticular nucleus of the brain were found at autopsy. On searching the literature, Wilson found other cases which were clinically similar. Six years earlier Gowers, in a paper entitled "On Tetanoid Chorea and Its Association with Cirrhosis of the Liver," described two patients whose symptoms were similar to those of Wilson's patient [2]. A review of the literature at that time disclosed that the disease has been seen sporadically in the past but had escaped systematic study. The first case of recognized Wilson's disease was probably described by Frerichs in his classic monograph on liver disease in 1861 [3]. The patient, a young boy, suffered from severe liver disease associated with violent tremors and convulsions and died at the age of 10. An autopsy revealed cirrhosis of the liver. The age of the patient and the nature of his symptoms make the diagnosis of Wilson's disease highly likely.

The clinical features of Wilson's disease may be so characteristic that the diagnosis is not in doubt. Unfortunately, the number of classic cases is relatively decreasing as recognition of the various clinical manifestations of the disease improves.

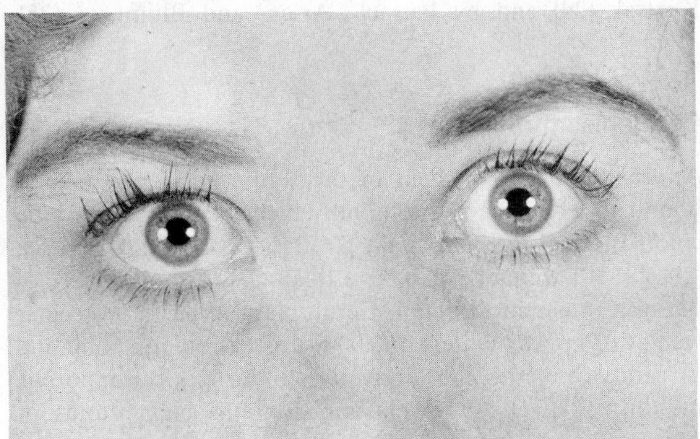

Figure 43-1. Typical Kayser-Fleischer ring in a patient with Wilson's disease.

Lenticular Degeneration

This form of the disease was the one seen by Wilson and overemphasized by subsequent observers. Classic lenticular degeneration is a severe but relatively uncommon form of the disease that occurs predominantly in young adults. Spasticity, rigidity, dysarthria, and dysphagia are the common presenting symptoms. Tremor is usually less pronounced, and clinical evidence of hepatic disease is minimal or absent, although, as in all varieties of Wilson's disease, pathologic evidence of cirrhosis is invariable. Acute unexplained febrile episodes were recognized by Wilson in some of his patients and may usher in the terminal phase of the disease.

Pseudosclerosis

Unnecessary and frequently acrimonious nosologic debate obscured the existence of this variety of hepatolenticular degeneration during the early part of this century. It is now clear that what has been known as pseudosclerosis of Westphal [4] is a form of Wilson's disease in which flapping tremor of the wrists and shoulders are usually the major disabling symptom, and rigidity and spasticity are less marked. Symptoms referable to hepatic dysfunction are uncommon, but pathologic evidence of cirrhosis can invariably be found, and slight impairment of bromsulfalein excretion can be demonstrated frequently. Other biochemical evidence of disturbed liver function is surprisingly minimal [5].

Kayser-Fleischer Ring

Despite the brilliance of Wilson's clinical acumen, the only pathognomonic sign of the disease escaped his notice. Ten years before the publication of Wilson's paper Kayser had observed a greenish ring at the limbus of the cornea in a patient diagnosed as having multiple sclerosis. A year later Fleischer reported a corneal ring as an integral part of a neurologic disease associated with cirrhosis of the liver. In a series of papers [6–8] Fleischer proposed the concept that the changes in the eye, brain, and liver were all due to a common metabolic cause. The Kayser-Fleischer ring is still rightly regarded as the single most important diagnostic sign of the disease. The ring is not always complete and is usually most marked at the superior and inferior aspects of the cornea. Although with experience most Kayser-Fleischer rings can be seen with the naked eye, its presence can be definitely excluded only by a slit-lamp examination. Kayser-Fleischer rings are almost invariably present in patients with overt neurologic disease. In young children, in whom hepatic disease is particularly liable to predominate, the Kayser-Fleischer ring may be absent when the patient is first seen [8, 9]. The finding of Kayser-Fleischer rings under the age of 7 is exceptional [10]. In a very few patients careful examination of the eye will reveal a *Sonnenblumenkatarakt*. Similar cataracts are known to follow the intraocular localization of a foreign body containing copper. Kayser-Fleischer rings may be expected to fade or disappear in 30 to 60 percent of the patients who have received adequate treatment with penicillamine [11, 12].

Cirrhosis of the Liver

The hepatic form of Wilson's disease, in which there is evidence of liver disease with minor or absent neurologic signs, has been recognized as a clinical variant for many years [13, 14] and is particularly common in children under the age of 10. Its frequency and significance have recently become increasingly appreciated [14, 15]. In a series of 32 cases collected at the Rockefeller University, 8 (25 percent) could be classified as belonging to this group. Similarly Walshe [16] in a series of 25 cases reported that 11 presented with jaundice in childhood or obscure hepatosplenomegaly. Hypersplenism with thrombocytopenia may occur early [17]. No patient with juvenile cirrhosis can be said to have been examined satisfactorily until the presence of Kayser-Fleischer rings has been sought for diligently, and the biochemical tests necessary for the diagnosis of Wilson's disease have been performed. The cirrhosis is similar pathologically to that seen in the pseudosclerotic variety of the disease but is generally more severe. Signs of portal hypertension can frequently be demonstrated. In some patients with Wilson's disease the presenting symptom is massive hemorrhage due to rupture of esophageal varices. Hepatic coma is uncommon but may usher in the terminal phase. Ascites rarely occurs and then only in the late stages of hepatic decompensation.

Other Clinical Variants

A sizable proportion of patients with Wilson's disease may present with symptoms suggesting schizophrenia; others may develop less pronounced abnormalities in behavior or personality. In one series of patients with Wilson's disease approximately 60 percent had significant psychiatric manifestations as the first clinical indication of the disease [18]. Tragic ignorance of this form of the disease has resulted in needless shock therapy and unnecessary detention in psychiatric hospitals. Occasionally patients may develop epileptic seizures, usually of the Jacksonian type. Hemiplegia is not so rare as is commonly supposed. A curious comatose state may persist for several weeks and does not necessarily herald an immediate fatal outcome.

An acute hemolytic anemia [17, 19] may occur during the course of the disease and may antedate other manifestations of the disease. The hemolytic episodes are thought to be due to a sudden release of copper from the tissues [19]. A similar hemolytic anemia has been seen in acute copper toxicity and in sheep with chronic copper intoxication [20]. Azure lunulae [21], unusual pigmentation of the lower extremities, spontaneous fractures, and bone lesions [22, 23] may be early manifestations of the disease.

Etiology

The primary abnormality in Wilson's disease is unknown. Numerous hypotheses have been constructed over the past decade, none of which has stood the test of time. It seems certain, however, that the signs and symptoms of the disease are best explained by the slow relentless abnormal accumulation of copper in the body.

NORMAL METABOLISM OF COPPER

Copper is a ubiquitous element. Under normal circumstances the average individual consumes between 2.5 and 5.0 mg copper per day. Foods with high copper content include liver, shellfish, nuts, and chocolate. Cow's milk usually contains only a small amount of copper and has been used successfully to induce copper deficiency in certain animals. In most foodstuffs copper is bound principally to proteins and amino acids. Copper may be present in significant quantities in drinking water, particularly if the pipes are copper-lined. Although small quantities of copper are excreted in the urine, the bile is the principal route of excretion of the metal. Extensive and valuable reviews of copper metabolism have recently been published by Sass-Kortsak [24] and by Peisach, Aisen, and Blumberg [25].

Ceruloplasmin Copper

Approximately 98 percent of the serum copper in man is bound to a specific α_2-globulin, which, because of its blue color, is called *ceruloplasmin* [26, 27]. Kasper and Deutsch [28, 29, 30] were the first investigators to examine ceruloplasmin in chemical detail. Ceruloplasmin has a molecular weight of approximately 160,000; it is extremely labile and is readily converted into derivatives of faster electrophoretic mobility [27, 31]. Ceruloplasmin contains eight atoms of copper per molecule, of which half are in the cupric form. Electron spin resonance studies on the state of copper in the ceruloplasmin molecule [32] confirm the chemical findings. Acid-base and spectrophotometric studies indicate that histidyl and either lysyl or tyrosyl residues are probably concerned with the binding of copper. Ceruloplasmin contains approximately 7.5 percent carbohydrate and has valine as the principal amino-terminal amino acid [28]. The observed heterogeneity of ceruloplasmin [31, 33] must be evaluated in the light of its known instability and its liability to form polymers [30, 34]. Under certain conditions ceruloplasmin can be cleaved to form nonidentical subunits. The subunits do not recombine to form the native ceruloplasmin [34]. Simons and Bearn have recently investigated the polypeptide-chain structure of human ceruloplasmin. Two different polypeptide chains, alpha and beta, have been isolated. The alpha chain has a molecular weight of 15,900, with valine as its N-terminal amino acid. It is antigenically distinct from the beta chains which are heterogeneous. Both beta chains have lysine as their N-terminal amino acid; the molecular weight of the beta chain is 58,900 [35]. Despite much chemical progress, more data will be required before an exact model for the polypeptide structure of ceruloplasmin can be formulated. Radioactive studies [36] indicate that human ceruloplasmin from which the sialic acid residues have been cleaved by neuraminidase disappears from the circulation of the rabbit within minutes, whereas native ceruloplasmin has been shown to have a half-life of 56 hr. If the galactosyl residue exposed by the neuraminidase is removed by galactosidase, the half-life of ceruloplasmin returns to normal. These studies have raised the possibility that in Wilson's disease there may be a genetic defect in the enzyme system which catalyzes the transfer of sialic acid to the ceruloplasmin molecule [36]. Ceruloplasmin exhibits oxidase activity toward certain polyphenols and polyamines including epinephrine and serotonin. The greatest oxidase activity has been demonstrated using paraphenylenediamine as substrate. Ceruloplasmin has been considered an ascorbic acid oxidase, but the evidence for this is highly controversial [37].

Procedures designed to dissociate copper from ceruloplasmin have resulted in loss of enzymatic activity. Under appropriate conditions half of the eight copper atoms of each ceruloplasmin molecule can exchange with ionic copper [38]. Exchange of copper absorbed from the intestinal tract with ceruloplasmin has not been convincingly demonstrated. It is possible that ceruloplasmin functions as a storage protein. A greatly decreased concentration of ceruloplasmin may occur in some healthy carriers of the abnormal gene of hepatolenticular degeneration.

The results of a number of important investigations have recently appeared, among which is one by Deutsch and his colleagues on the structure and immunologic properties of ceruloplasmin. Using immunologic methods, they demonstrated apoceruloplasmin in human serum. This relatively low copper-containing protein constitutes between 10 and 20 percent of the total serum ceruloplasmin in normal serum [136]. The level of apoceruloplasmin in patients with Wilson's disease did not differ in quantity or quality from that found in normal subjects [137]. An apoceruloplasmin has been found in rats raised on a copper-free diet in whom the serum ceruloplasmin concentration was undetectable. Holtzman and Gaumnitz have also identified an apoceruloplasmin in copper-deficient rats and performed turnover studies [138, 139]. Ceruloplasmin activity is restored to normal when copper-depleted rats are returned to a copper-rich diet [138]. Recent studies by the same investigators suggest that erythrocuprein, hepatocuprein, and cerebrocuprein are identical [140] (see below). All three proteins have been shown to contain zinc as well as copper [141].

Chemical and physical studies on ceruloplasmin have also been described by Morell and his colleagues [142–144]. The observation that asialoceruloplasmin disappears more rapidly from the serum than native ceruloplasmin has raised the possibility that a defective enzyme system, which normally catalyzes the transfer of sialic acid to ceruloplasmin, may be present in patients with Wilson's disease [145]. Additional evidence from Scheinberg and his colleagues indicates that degradation of ceruloplasmin takes place in the hepatocyte after removal of two of the terminal sialic acid residues. Cleavage of sialic acid and galactosyl residues probably occurs within hepatic lysosomes [146]. The suggestion that ceruloplasmin may function as a controller of cytochrome oxidase activity was raised by Shokeir and Shreffler, who reported a correlation between the depression of serum ceruloplasmin and a decreased leukocyte cytochrome oxidase [147].

Ceruloplasmin Determination

Serum ceruloplasmin can be measured in a variety of ways. Holmberg and Laurell originally demonstrated a positive correlation between the copper concentration of the serum and its oxidase activity. The latter can be measured directly in a Warburg apparatus and recorded in terms of micromoles of O_2 uptake per milliliter per hour [26]. Alternatively, the oxidase activity can be measured colorimetrically [39, 40]. Most colorimetric methods using a purified preparation of ceruloplasmin as a standard indicate that the normal ceruloplasmin concentration is approximately 36.0 ± 5.6 mg per 100 ml serum for males and 40.9 ± 6.8 per 100 ml for females. Other methods for estimating this protein depend upon the loss of the blue color. Ceruloplasmin can also be measured immunologically [41]. This, of course, is dependent upon the availability of a pure preparation of ceruloplasmin which can be used as an antigen. Broman [32] first reported the existence of multiple ceruloplasmins in normal plasma with similar enzymatic properties. The main component accounts for approximately 80 percent of the total ceruloplasmin. This heterogeneity has been confirmed by several investigators [31, 35, 42–45]. Walshe claims that purified ceruloplasmin is inhibited in its oxidase activity more by the serum of

Wilson's disease patients than by normal serum [46]. This interesting observation awaits further confirmation.

Nonceruloplasmin Copper

It can be shown by salt fractionation and, more precisely, by electrophoretic techniques, that the nonceruloplasmin copper is bound to serum albumin [47]. The physical and chemical characteristics of the copper-albumin complex have been studied extensively [48]. In general, it may be stated that the main copper-binding sites of the albumin molecule are the imidazole groups, but some weaker binding also occurs at the carboxyl groups. The extent of the binding depends on the pH and the competitive effect of other anions in solution. Heating to approximately 100°C does not disturb the ability of protein to form complexes with copper, in contrast to its effect on protein-anion complexes. The essential requirements for binding appear to be the presence of appropriate residues and favorable electrostatic conditions of the molecule [48].

Ionic copper reacts with diethyldithiocarbamate to form a characteristic yellow color. Copper in ceruloplasmin will not react with this reagent unless the copper is first released from the ceruloplasmin. Copper which is bound to albumin reacts directly and permits the detection and quantitation of the albumin-bound copper. This fraction was designated the *direct-reacting copper* by Gubler and his associates [49]. Measurement of the direct-reacting copper is extremely inaccurate. Recent studies on the direct-reacting copper have been performed by Neumann and Sass-Kortsak [50] and by Walshe [46, 51]. Neumann and Sass-Kortsak [52, 53] and Silverberg and coworkers [54] emphasize the importance of the small amount of copper in normal serum which is bound to histidine and certain other amino acids. Their studies suggest that copper can be transported across metabolically inert membranes and that this process is closely allied to amino acid transport. It seems probable that although the amount of albumin copper does not normally greatly exceed 5 percent of the total serum copper, it performs the essential task of transporting copper from the intestinal tract to the various tissues of the body and is metabolically the most active fraction of the serum copper. The copper amino acid complexes are probably also important in the transport of copper in the body.

Erythrocuprein

Copper is a normal component of adult red cells, where its function is unknown. At least 80 percent of the copper in erythrocytes is present in the form of erythrocuprein, a nearly colorless protein isolated from human red cells by Kimmel et al. [55] and by Markowitz and his colleagues [56]. A comparison of some of the physical properties of erythrocuprein and ceruloplasmin is shown in Table 43-1.

In copper-deficient animals a severe anemia develops which is morphologically similar to the anemia of iron deficiency. The erythrocytes of the copper-deficient pig have a shortened survival time but when transfused into a normal pig, they have an approximately normal life-span. Erythrocytes transfused from a normal to a copper-deficient pig also survive normally. Such evidence suggests that the shortened survival time of erythrocytes in copper-deficient animals is not due to an extracorpuscular abnormality other than the low serum copper and that rapid exchange can take place between the serum copper and the red cell copper. Such exchange has been shown both in vivo and in vitro.

Tissue Copper

It is hardly surprising that copper is widely distributed in all body tissues. The body of a normal adult contains approximately 150 mg copper [24]. The liver, central nervous system, and kidney have the highest copper content. Appropriately enough, the highest concentration of copper occurs in the locus ceruleus in the brain stem [57]. The muscles and bones, because of their total mass, contain over 50 percent of the total body copper. Curiously, the fetal liver contains about 10 times the amount of copper found in an adult liver, where it is stored as a 2 percent copper containing "mitochondroprotein" [58]. The copper content of the liver of a child reaches the level found in a young adult by the age of 10.

Several copper proteins have been isolated from the liver. Mann and Keilin isolated a colorless copper protein from the liver of an ox [59]. This protein was not crystallized and accounted for only a part of the total copper present in the liver. Mohamed and Greenberg isolated an apparently crystalline copper protein from horse liver. The protein was blue, contained 0.30 to 0.40 percent copper, had an estimated molecular weight of 30,000 to 40,000, and has been named *hepatocuprein.* Unlike ceruloplasmin, it does not exhibit any oxidase activity [60]. The protein containing most of the copper in normal human liver has been isolated and purified by Morell and coworkers [61]. The protein, which contains a large number of sulfhydryl groups, has also been isolated from the livers of patients with Wilson's disease.

Table 43-1. COMPARISON OF THE PHYSICAL AND CHEMICAL PROPERTIES OF ERYTHROCUPREIN AND CERULOPLASMIN

Property	Erythrocuprein	Ceruloplasmin
Color	Nearly colorless	Blue
Absorption maxima	655,265 mμ	605,280 mμ
Molecular weight	33,000	160,000
Percentage of copper	0.32–0.36	0.32–0.34
Atoms of copper per molecule	2	8
Isoelectric point	5.3	4.4

Source: Modified from Kimmel et al. [55] and Markowitz et al. [56].

The nature of the copper proteins of normal brain (cerebrocuprein) has been extensively studied by Porter [58, 62–64]. Thus far, three copper-containing fractions of normal brain have been isolated and their properties described. Fraction I is extracted with acetate buffer at pH 4.5; fraction II is obtained by extraction of the residue from fraction I with water at pH 3.5 at very low ionic strength; the final residue fraction is designated fraction III. From fraction I a green copper-containing protein has been isolated, named *cerebrocuprein I.* This protein contains 0.30 percent copper and appears 85 percent homogeneous by ultracentrifugal and electrophoretic techniques. It has a molecular weight of approximately 34,000. Cerebrocuprein I exhibits a singular property; copper is not released from it by dialysis at pH 4.5. Copper proteins in the subcellular soluble fraction of normal human brain and normal liver account for 60 percent of the total tissue copper. It seems possible that cerebrocuprein I and hepatocuprein may represent the same protein isolated from different tissues [58]. Copper is widely distributed in all parts of the brain. The selective deposition of copper in the basal ganglia has been unduly stressed. Vogel [65] has demonstrated an increased copper content of the brain of goldfish when reared in an environment in which the ionic copper is experimentally increased.

Ceruloplasmin in trace amounts has been found in the liver and the kidney [66]. The physiologic significance of these observations, if any, is uncertain.

Secretions

Copper is present in small amounts in most of the body fluids, including saliva, milk, tears, and sweat and bile. The urine, in the absence of significant proteinuria, contains only small amounts of copper. The daily 24-hr urine excretion rarely exceeds 0.1 mg per day. The form in which copper is present in normal urine is uncertain; only part is freely dialyzable.

Physiologic Variations in Copper Metabolism

The significance of the alterations in copper metabolism in Wilson's disease cannot be appreciated unless the normal physiologic variations are understood.

Ceruloplasmin increases under a variety of physiologic conditions. It may be increased in pregnancy, infections, thyrotoxicosis, cancer, and cirrhosis of the liver, particularly of the biliary type. It is frequently decreased in the newborn, and in sprue, nephrosis, anemia (in infants), and malnutrition (in infants). It is almost invariably decreased in Wilson's disease. The administration of estrogens to normal subjects increases the ceruloplasmin level [67, 68]. Increased levels are also found in women who take oral contraceptives.

ABNORMALITIES OF COPPER METABOLISM IN WILSON'S DISEASE

A number of early German workers implicated various heavy metals, including copper, as possible etiologic agents in Wilson's disease. In 1913, only 2 years after Wilson's classic paper, Rumpel reported an increased silver and copper content of the liver and kidneys of patients who had died from pseudosclerosis [69]. In retrospect, it appears that these patients were almost certainly suffering from unrecognized Wilson's disease. Nine years later, Siemerling and Oloff, on the basis of the similarity of the eye cataracts in Wilson's disease to those following injury from a copper-containing foreign body, made the bold suggestion that copper might be deposited in the liver and brain in this disease, as well as in the eye, and might be directly responsible for the disease [70]. Recent chemical studies have shown unequivocally that copper is deposited in Descemet's membrane in patients with Wilson's disease and is responsible for the characteristic Kayser-Fleischer ring.

Because of technical difficulties the possible role of heavy metals in the etiology of the disease remained confused until 1930, when Haurowitz convincingly demonstrated an increased copper content of the liver and brain [71]. In spite of this unequivocal clue the subject lay dormant until 1945, when Glazebrook reported a patient with Wilson's disease whose liver and brain at autopsy contained an increased copper concentration and whose serum copper was considered elevated [72]. In view of subsequent findings, the increased serum copper reported may possibly have been in error. The observations of Glazebrook proved to have catalytic consequences, and a bewildering spate of papers on copper metabolism ensued. The next major event was the chance finding by Mandelbrote and his coworkers [73] that a patient suffering from Wilson's disease excreted an increased quantity of copper in the urine. Numerous observers have now amply confirmed both the increased tissue copper and the high urinary copper excretion. Considerable additional disagreement has developed in regard to the serum copper concentration in Wilson's disease. Although initial observers reported both normal and elevated levels, it was subsequently shown that the levels were almost invariably decreased [74]. Recently, the wheel has turned full circle, and at least 14 patients with unequivocal Wilson's disease have now been reported in whom the serum copper is unquestionably normal. This subject has recently been reviewed by Scheinberg and Sternlieb [75] and by Sherlock [14].

Serum Ceruloplasmin

Almost simultaneously in different laboratories and with different methods diminished ceruloplasmin levels were found in patients with Wilson's disease. The first method used was based on its enzymatic activity [74], as described by Holmberg and Laurell, and the second, more elegant, was based on quantitative immunologic procedures in which antiserum had been prepared against crystalline ceruloplasmin [41].

Although the majority of patients with Wilson's disease have a diminished serum ceruloplasmin level, <20 mg per 100 ml, the degree of depression varies. In some essentially no ceruloplasmin can be detected. In others the level is depressed to about 25 percent of normal (Fig. 43-2). Several sibships with Wilson's disease have been reported in which the ceruloplasmin levels are within the normal range. Several investigators have emphasized that those cases of Wilson's disease in which a normal level of ceruloplasmin has been reported have severe liver disease. Approximately 5 percent of patients with Wilson's disease have a serum ceruloplasmin concentration in the normal range. Most of these patients are children with severe liver disease, and in many of the reported cases the patients have died in hepatic coma. The problem is complicated from a diagnostic viewpoint because Walshe [76] has reported low levels of ceruloplasmin in severe liver disease not due to Wilson's disease, but this appears to be exceptional.

In some patients with Wilson's disease, as in normal subjects, an increase in the ceruloplasmin concentration can be achieved by the administration of estrogens. This effect is most marked in those in whom the ceruloplasmin level is least depressed. As might be anticipated, in those patients in whom little or no ceruloplasmin can be detected, no measurable increase in the ceruloplasmin level occurs. In a few patients a poorly sustained cupruresis may follow the administration of estrogens [68].

Serum Copper

Early in the course of investigations of Wilson's disease it was found that the serum copper level was higher than would have been expected from the ceruloplasmin levels observed. Since there was no evidence that ceruloplasmin in Wilson's disease contained more copper per molecule, it seemed

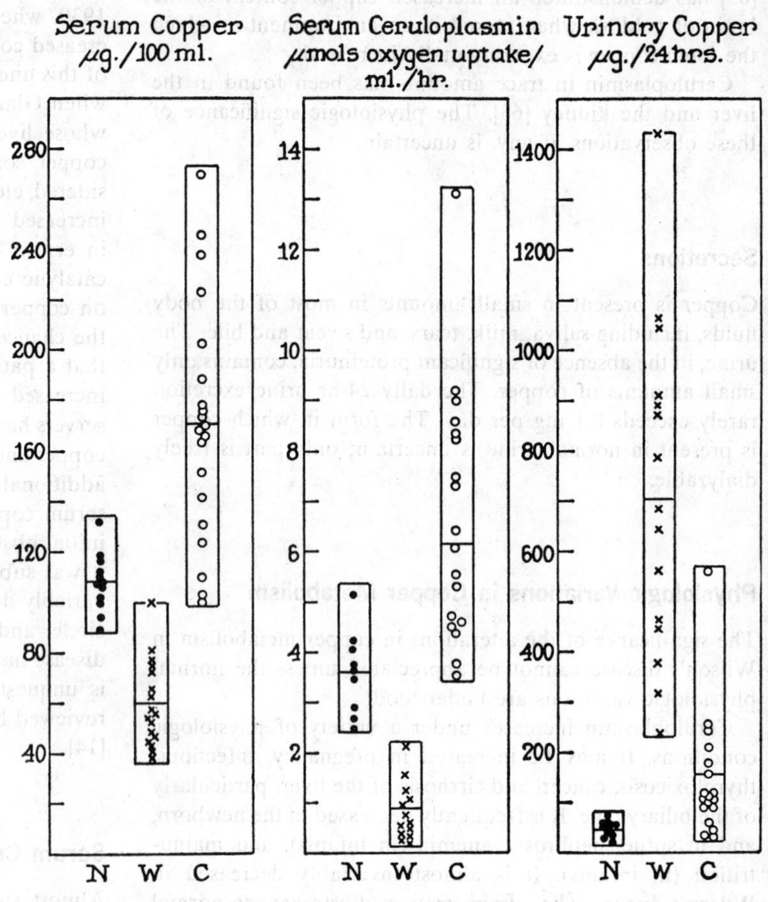

Figure 43-2. Comparison of amounts of serum copper, serum ceruloplasmin, and urinary copper in normal subjects, cirrhotic patients, and patients with Wilson's disease. Horizontal lines represent mean values. Note the one patient with Wilson's disease in whom a normal ceruloplasmin level occurred. (*Reproduced from A. G. Bearn* [102].)

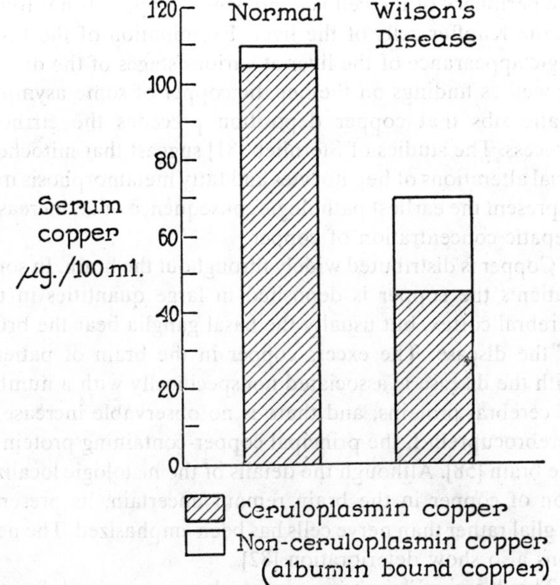

Figure 43-3. Note (1) decrease in total serum copper; (2) decrease in serum ceruloplasmin; (3) increase in direct-reacting copper (albumin-bound copper) in Wilson's disease.

probable that the nonceruloplasmin copper was increased. Observations by Cartwright established that the direct-reacting copper is elevated in Wilson's disease (Fig. 43-3). It is possible that the increased concentration of the direct-reacting copper reflects the mechanism by which excess copper is deposited in the tissue.

Urinary Copper

Although an increased copper excretion is usually considered to be one of the cardinal biochemical abnormalities in Wilson's disease, it should be appreciated that a moderate increase in urinary copper excretion can occur in cirrhosis of the liver particularly of the biliary type [77]. Urinary copper excretion estimations are, therefore, unreliable in excluding Wilson's disease as a cause for juvenile cirrhosis. Fortunately, this important clinical differential diagnosis can usually be settled by a determination of the level of serum ceruloplasmin (Fig. 43-2).

The extent of the increased urinary copper excretion in Wilson's disease varies considerably. In general, those individuals with the shortest duration of clinical disease tend to have the more nearly normal levels; those in whom the disease has been present for a long time may excrete as much as 1.5 mg copper daily. In untreated patients it is usually possible to observe a slow but progressive increase in the urinary excretion of copper over a period of years. Thus far, no untreated patient with clear clinical evidence of Wilson's disease has been seen in whom the urinary copper excretion was completely normal (<100 μg per 24 hr).

Under standard dietary conditions, day-to-day fluctuations in the urinary excretion of copper are relatively slight and are largely independent of the urinary volume and the dietary copper intake [77]. In contrast to the insensitivity of the urinary excretion of copper to a twenty-five-fold increase in copper intake, a tenfold increase in the dietary protein intake results in an approximately twofold increase in the urinary excretion of copper. In normal subjects trivial and inconsistant increases in copper excretion are observed following a similar increase in protein intake. The increased copper excretion which follows augmented protein intake is paralleled by increased amino acid excretion [77]. It is tempting to ascribe part of the increased copper excretion to the capacity of many amino acids to chelate copper. Quantitative considerations compel one to qualify such an interpretation, for chelation implies a necessary molar relationship between the quantity of amino acids and the quantity of copper excreted.

Tissue Copper

The intrahepatic distribution of copper in Wilson's disease was first investigated by Uzman [78] and has recently been extensively studied by Schaffner and coworkers [79]. Glycogen degeneration of hepatic cell nuclei accompanied by cytoplasmic fat droplets is frequently observed and may occur in the early stages of the disease [79, 80] (Fig. 43-4). Although these and other structural abnormalities have been observed in ultrastructural studies on the hepatocytes in Wilson's disease, none is specific. Recent studies have focused on mitochondrial abnormalities. An increased electron opacity of the mitochondrial matrix has been the most consistent finding, although other mitochondrial abnormalities may be present. Of particular interest has been the observation that these mitochondrial changes may occur in asymptomatic patients with the disease. Although it cannot be considered proved, it seems likely that these changes are caused by the increased concentrations of hepatic copper. In two asymptomatic sibs in whom hepatic copper was not elevated mitochondrial changes were absent [81]. Rubeanic acid forms a black precipitate with copper, possibly because of the formation of the imido internal salt of rubianic acid. Under neutral or slightly alkaline conditions this reaction has a reported sensitivity of 0.006 μg copper. The original method using rubeanic acid was grossly unreliable. Recent modifications have resulted in significant improvement, although attention to detail is still imperative if reproducible results are to be obtained [79]. A marked variation in the copper content of various liver lobules occurs.

The accumulation of intracellular hepatic copper occurs in successive stages. At first a fine diffuse distribution of copper is present throughout the cytoplasm of the liver cell. Later the copper is concentrated around one pole of the nucleus. In heavily involved lobules, the granular copper deposits near the nucleus are coarse but become finer as

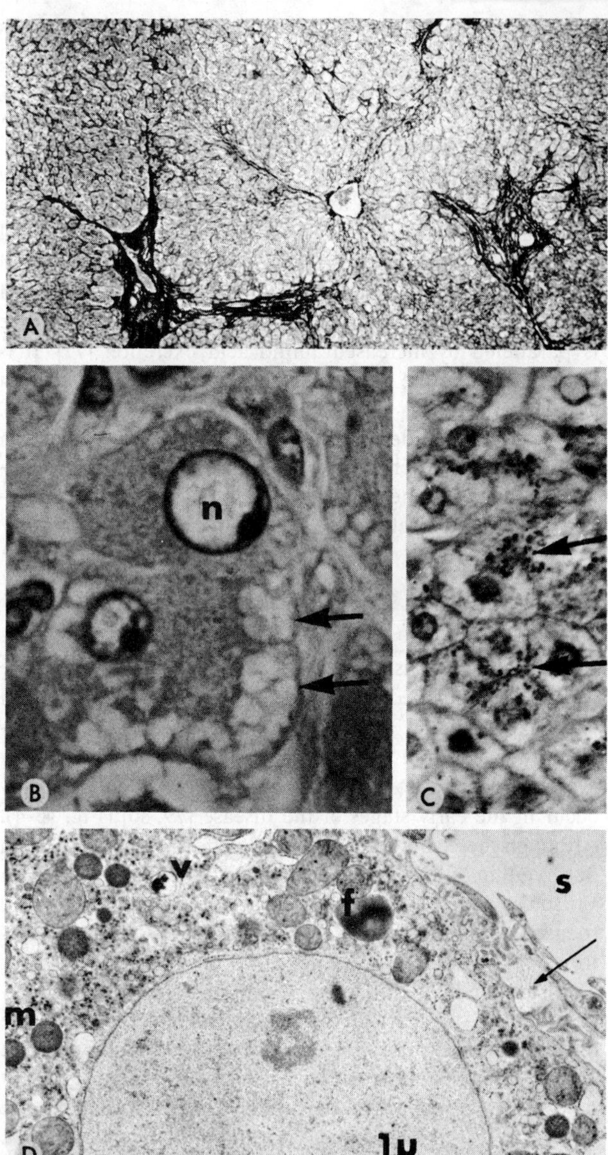

Figure 43-4. A. Stellate portal and central fibrosis, not yet cirrhosis, in the liver in Wilson's disease. The compression of the portal vein in fibrotic portal tracts, four of which are seen here around a central vein, may cause presinusoidal portal hypertension. (Gomori silver impregnation ×30.) B. Small droplets of fat along sinusoidal borders of hepatocytes (arrows) and glycogen degeneration of hepatocellular nuclei (n) with displacement of chromatin and nucleolus to the periphery. These are nonspecific cytologic changes found in all instances of Wilson's disease. (Hematoxylin and eosin ×875.) C. Granules of copper-containing pigment near bile canaliculi (arrows) in hepatocytes (Timm's ammonium sulfide—silver nitrate stain ×225.) D. Electron micrograph of a portion of liver cell in Wilson's disease with a large fiber bundle (arrow) beneath an endothelial cell lining the sinusoid(s), a small fat droplet (f), a vacuole (v) containing dense material, and numerous dense microbodies (m). (Lead citrate ×4,200.) (*Photomicrographs prepared by Dr. Fenton Schaffner, Mt. Sinai Hospital, New York.*)

the periphery of the cell is approached. Copper is not found in the Kupffer cells of the liver. Examination of the histologic appearance of the liver at various stages of the disease as well as findings on the hepatic copper of some asymptomatic sibs that copper deposition precedes the cirrhotic process. The studies of Sternlieb [81] suggest that mitochondrial alterations of hepatocytes and fatty metamorphosis may represent the earliest pathologic consequence of an increased hepatic concentration of copper.

Copper is distributed widely throughout the brain. In some patients the copper is deposited in large quantities in the cerebral cortex, but usually the basal ganglia bear the brunt of the disease. The excess copper in the brain of patients with the disease is associated nonspecifically with a number of cerebral proteins, and there is no observable increase in cerebrocuprein I, the principal copper-containing protein of the brain [58]. Although the details of the histologic localization of copper in the brain remain uncertain, its presence in glial rather than nerve cells has been emphasized. The neurons also show deterioration [82].

The Kayser-Fleischer ring has been examined for the presence of heavy metals ever since the early studies of Siemerling and Oloff. The histochemical and electron microscopic studies of Uzman first clarified a rather confused subject [83]. It has now been demonstrated by two groups of workers that the copper content of the substantia propria may be increased without causing any cloudiness of the cornea or any noticeable color change. The copper in the substantia propria is alcohol-insoluble but easily removed by dilute acids or chelating agents such as Versene. In Descemet's membrane, on the other hand, the copper is localized as a fine granular deposit arranged in two parallel zones to the endothelial surface of the membrane. The precise chemical form in which copper is deposited in the cornea is still unknown. The characteristic brown or gray-green color of the Kayser-Fleischer ring is not directly due to the deposition of copper in Descemet's membrane. The presence of dense layers of copper depositions separated by intervening clear zones provides an ideal physical system for the scattering and reflection of incident light on the cornea and gives rise to the characteristic appearance of the Kayser-Fleischer ring.

Dynamic Aspects of Copper Metabolism

Thus far, this account of the abnormalities of copper metabolism in Wilson's disease has been entirely restricted to the realm of descriptive biology; it seems appropriate now to consider some of its dynamic aspects. This problem has been clarified by the use of radioactive isotopes. ^{64}Cu has a half-life of only 12.88 hr, which limits the time during which studies on man can be performed. Another isotope of copper ^{67}Cu, with a half-life of 61.8 hr, has enabled more prolonged studies to be carried out (Fig. 43-5).

A characteristic and reproducible series of curves is ob-

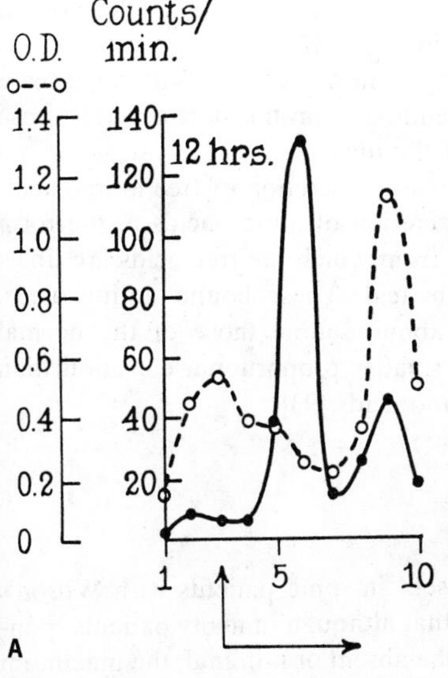

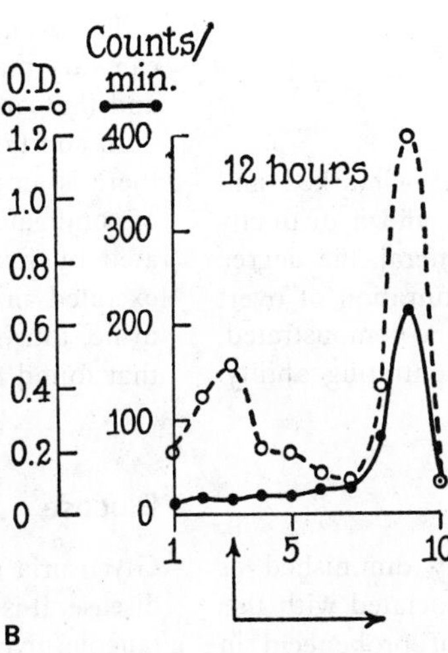

Figure 43-5. Distribution of radioactive copper in the electrophoretically separated fractions of the serum of control subjects (A) and a patient with Wilson's disease (B) 12 hr following oral administration of Cu^{64}. (*Adapted from A. G. Bearn and H. G. Kunkel* [47].)

tained after the intravenous administration of radioactive copper to normal subjects [84, 85]. An initial rapid fall in labeled serum copper is followed by a rise. This is succeeded by a decline of radioactivity, which is slower than in normal subjects, and has no observable secondary rise. Electrophoretic separation of serum and salt fractionation at various intervals after administration of the isotope has shown that immediately following the administration of ^{64}Cu the radioactivity is bound to serum albumin and possibly to amino acids; no radioactivity is detected in any of the other serum fractions. During the normal secondary rise the radioactivity is associated with the ceruloplasmin, and little or no labeled copper is found in association with the albumin. In patients with Wilson's disease, as in normal subjects, the ^{64}Cu is first associated with serum albumin, but it remains bound to albumin at a time when in normal persons the ^{64}Cu is associated with ceruloplasmin. Interestingly, the failure of the patient to incorporate copper into ceruloplasmin occurs even in those rare patients in whom the serum copper concentration is not greatly decreased.

The tentative explanation of these findings is that in both normal subjects and patients with Wilson's disease, copper is transported, attached to serum albumin, to various parts of the body. Some copper is transported to the site of ceruloplasmin synthesis, where provided the capacity to synthesize ceruloplasmin is normal, it becomes incorporated into newly synthesized ceruloplasmin. Since impaired ceruloplasmin synthesis is a usual feature of Wilson's disease, the copper transported to the liver is not utilized in this way; it is deposited at various tissue sites and remains bound to the albumin in quantities greater than in normal subjects. The copper-albumin complex is a relatively loose bond; the copper can easily be dissociated from the protein moiety. The increased quantity of copper in the urine in Wilson's disease is no longer anomalous, for although the total circulating copper is diminished, the copper bound to serum albumin is increased and copper is excreted in the urine, probably bound to amino acids. Asymptomatic normal sibs, in whom ceruloplasmin is deficient, handle intravenous ^{64}Cu in a fashion similar to patients with clinical Wilson's disease.

Since the total body copper is increased in Wilson's disease and because the urinary excretion is elevated, it is clear either that an increased quantity of dietary copper must be absorbed through the intestinal tract or that there must be a decreased biliary excretion of copper. Despite more than two decades of work, this issue is not yet firmly resolved. The copper content of bile in Wilson's disease is reported to be lower than normal. This is in contrast with observations using radioactive ^{64}Cu in mice where an increase in absorption of copper is accompanied by an increase in biliary excretion [86]. These experiments suggest that the increase in tissue copper in Wilson's disease may be, at least in part, due to a defect in biliary excretion. Balance studies have tended to indicate that increased absorption does indeed occur, as does a decreased excretion of copper through the intestinal tract. The use of radioactive copper has enabled the increased absorption of copper to be demonstrated clearly [84, 87, 88].

Uptake of ^{64}Cu by erythrocytes (in erythrocuprein) of patients with Wilson's disease is similar to that of normal subjects and emphasizes the rather specific nature of the ceruloplasmin defect in this condition.

RENAL ABNORMALITIES IN WILSON'S DISEASE

In 1948 Uzman and Denny-Brown reported an increased amino aciduria in patients with Wilson's disease [89]. Dent in the previous year had also observed an increased excretion of amino acids in Wilson's disease [90]. In the succeeding years it has become clear that the renal lesion in Wilson's disease is extremely diffuse and affects many aspects of renal function [91, 92].

Renal Hemodynamics

In most cases of Wilson's disease there is a marked and consistent reduction of renal plasma flow and a distinctly decreased glomerular filtration rate. In general, the degree of impairment parallels the severity and duration of overt disease. In most instances albuminuria can be demonstrated. There may be impairment in urine-concentrating ability.

Tubular Reabsorptive Mechanisms

The tubular secretory capacity is usually diminished as judged by impairment of the Tm_{PAH}. Associated with this defective function, a diminished effect of probenecid in eliciting a further reduction of Tm_{PAH} can be demonstrated.

Amino Acids

Impairment of renal tubular reabsorptive activities in Wilson's disease has been thoroughly demonstrated. The excessive amino aciduria can be attributed to defective renal reabsorption, since the amino acids in the serum are not elevated. It is known that the various amino acids are not reabsorbed in the tubules by a common process; thus it is of interest to examine the distribution of the amino acids excreted in the urine in patients with Wilson's disease. It should be emphasized that increased amino aciduria is not a constant feature of the disease and is usually present only in those patients in whom the disease is of long standing. In general, it appears that the largest excretion relative to normal subjects occurs with threonine and cystine, excretion of which may be elevated twentyfold [93]. Indeed, the excretion of cystine in Wilson's disease may exceed that found in patients with cystinuria. It is of interest that patients with Wilson's disease usually do not form cystine stones. The excretion of other amino acids, in relation to the normal excretion, is illustrated in Table 43-2.

The urinary excretion of amino acids in Wilson's disease can vary markedly depending upon the state of the disease and the composition of the diet.

In addition to an increased excretion of free amino acids there is an increased excretion of amino acids in the form of conjugated linkages, from which the free acids are liberated by hydrolysis with acid. These bound amino acids, excreted in quantities about double those of the normal urine, thus represent a smaller proportional elevation than that found for free amino acids [93].

Glucose

Glycosuria may be present in some patients with Wilson's disease. It is significant that although in many patients spontaneous glycosuria may be absent or minimal, the maximum tubular capacity to reabsorb glucose is reduced frequently and substantially [91]. These observations emphasize that a failure to find an increased excretion of glucose does not preclude a considerable defect in the capacity of the renal tubules to transport glucose across the tubular epithelium.

Bicarbonate

A tendency to excrete an alkaline urine in patients with Wilson's disease has been described and is associated with the renal excretion of bicarbonate at plasma levels that would ordinarily demand complete reabsorption of bicarbonate by the renal tubules. In addition many patients fail to acidify their urine in response to an ammonium chloride load [91, 92].

Uric Acid

In 1954 Bishop and coworkers reported a low serum uric acid associated with an increased uric acid excretion in a

Table 43-2. URINARY AMINO ACID EXCRETION IN WILSON'S DISEASE

Diminished	Normal	Increased (× normal) 2–4	Increased (× normal) 5–10	Increased (× normal) >10	Excretion of amino acids not found in normal urine
Taurine 1-Methyl histidine 3-Methyl histidine	Aminoadipic acid Methionine Isoleucine Leucine Arginine	Histidine Ornithine Phenylalanine	Serine Glycine Asparagine Glutamine Valine Tyrosine Lysine	Threonine Cystine	Proline Citrulline

Source: W. H. Stein et al. [93].

brother and sister with Wilson's disease [94]. Subsequent investigators have confirmed these findings, and renal clearance studies have demonstrated that, as originally postulated, the diminished reabsorption of filtered urate accounts for both the increased urinary excretion and the low serum urate levels observed. The capacity of probenecid further to increase the ratio C_{urate} to C_{inulin} diminished as the tubular transport systems for urate deteriorated with progression of the disease [91]. The low serum uric acid level is so constant a feature of Wilson's disease that a serum uric acid determination should be performed in all cases of cirrhosis of unexplained origin and in all obscure diseases of the central nervous system in which disturbances of the function of the basal ganglia are prominent.

Phosphate

A low serum inorganic phosphate level occurs in a high proportion of patients with Wilson's disease [91]. Renal clearance studies have revealed an even higher proportion of patients in whom the C_{PO_4} is increased. Thus, a failure of normal tubular transport of phosphate is a common feature of the disease and may be in part responsible for the occasional appearance of clinical osteomalacia and spontaneous fractures (Fig. 43-6) [22, 23].

Calcium

Radioactive studies using calcium 47 indicate that hyperabsorption of calcium can be demonstrated in many patients with Wilson's disease. Moreover, the hypercalciuria was decreased in response to a low calcium diet. Hypercalciuria occurs in many patients with Wilson's disease and is also related in part to the duration of the overt disease [95, 96].

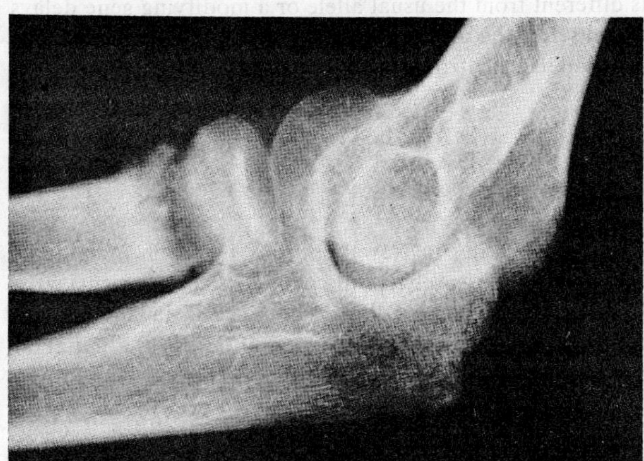

Figure 43-6. Radiograph illustrating fracture of the head of the right radius with no evidence of bone union. (*Reproduced from A. G. Bearn* [116].)

THE PATHOGENESIS OF WILSON'S DISEASE

Although the pathogenesis of the clinical syndromes of Wilson's disease has been clarified greatly during the past decade, the primary genetic abnormality remains obscure. Because a decreased serum ceruloplasmin has been such a constant biochemical abnormality in most patients with the disease, it has been tempting to assume that the primary defect is an inability to synthesize ceruloplasmin. This hypothesis, in its simplest form, is incompatible with a number of well-verified observations. (1) There is no correlation between the depression of ceruloplasmin synthesis and the amount of copper deposited in the tissues. (2) Certain patients with Wilson's disease have a normal serum concentration of ceruloplasmin. (3) Following treatment with penicillamine, the serum ceruloplasmin may decrease in the face of marked clinical improvement. (4) Individuals heterozygous for the Wilson's disease gene may have greatly decreased serum ceruloplasmin levels and yet never develop symptoms of the disease. The possibility has been raised that ceruloplasmin in Wilson's disease is structurally abnormal as well as being decreased in concentration. Holtzman et al. [97] isolated ceruloplasmin from a patient with Wilson's disease and using the techniques of peptide mapping, could not detect any difference from ceruloplasmin isolated from normal adult serum. Recently, however, Simons and Gahmberg [98] examined the K_m of normal ceruloplasmin and ceruloplasmin from Wilson's disease and found a marked decrease in the K_m value for N,N-dimethyl-*p*-phenylene-diamine in the serum from patients with Wilson's disease and in normal cord serum. These results, if confirmed, suggest that the conversion of ceruloplasmin with a low K_m value in cord serum to ceruloplasmin with a normal value in adult serum does not occur in individuals homozygous for the abnormal gene. Two other hypotheses have been advanced recently which deserve brief mention. Sass-Kortsak [24] raises the possibility that there may be a disturbance in copper transport in the liver cell. As a consequence, copper accumulates in the liver and prevents copper excretion from the cell into the bile and interferes with the availability of copper for ceruloplasmin synthesis. Walshe also emphasizes the decreased biliary excretion of copper in this disease [99], a view substantiated by the observation that less radioactive copper can be recovered in stools from patients with Wilson's disease than in normal subjects.

An alternative hypothesis was postulated by Uzman and outlined by him in a series of papers [100, 101]. This hypothesis ascribes the primary effects of the abnormal gene to an abnormal protein which has an increased capacity for binding ionic copper. This hypothetical protein is present in the liver and presumably in every tissue in which the copper is increased. The increased affinity of copper for certain tissues blocks the formation of ceruloplasmin; thus, the diminished ceruloplasmin level is a secondary phenomenon and is due to the diversion of copper to the tissues. Except for the postulation of a specific abnormal copper-binding protein in the serum, this hypothesis bears a superficial similarity to those advanced by Sass-Kortsak [24] and Walshe [99]. However Uzman also postulated an abnormality of protein metabolism in the liver which gave rise to specific oligopeptides which competed with amino acids and uric acid for reabsorption in the proximal renal tubule, causing amino aciduria and uricosuria. No evidence has emerged which supports this view, and it must be concluded that Uzman's hypothesis is untenable. Although it must be concluded that the primary genetic abnormality in Wilson's disease is unknown, a plausible narrative for the development of the signs and symptoms of the disease can be written [99]. Children who are homozygous for the gene causing Wilson's disease have at birth a normal content of copper in their tissues. The serum concentration of copper and ceruloplasmin is normally low at birth, and thus examination of the serum for a depressed ceruloplasmin would not yield useful diagnostic information. Although symptoms of the disease do not usually appear during the first 6 years of life, copper accumulates inexorably in the tissues from the time of birth. Initially the liver bears the brunt of the disease and copper is deposited in the hepatic cells. In the earliest stages, although no abnormality in liver function can be detected, minimal changes in the electron microscopic appearance of the liver cells may be apparent, and an estimation of the hepatic copper concentration indicates that it is above normal. As the binding sites for copper become saturated, the copper becomes deposited in other tissues of the body. Interestingly, the hepatic copper concentration is frequently higher in asymptomatic sibs than in patients with neurologic disease. That increasing accumulation of copper in the tissues results in disordered function is proved by the observation that elimination of the excess copper from the body by effective therapy reverses the signs and symptoms of the disease. The functions of the liver, brain, and kidney can be objectively studied and improvement documented. If this account of the natural history is correct, it is clearly imperative to treat all patients who are homozygous for the Wilson's disease gene before the accumulation of copper gives rise to clinical symptoms of disease.

GENETICS

In his original monograph Wilson pointed out that familial incidence is one of the striking features of the disease. Although he considered the possibility that the disease was inherited, the familial incidence was attributed to environmental rather than genetic causes [1].

Study of a large number of patients with Wilson's disease has permitted a genetic analysis [102, 103]. Inspection of the pedigrees immediately confirmed the familial concentration observed by Wilson and, in addition, disclosed that many of those afflicted were the offspring of consanguine unions (Table 43-3).

Table 43-3. THE CONSANGUINITY RATE IN 30 FAMILIES WITH WILSON'S DISEASE

No. of sibships	*Consanguinity rate in parents of patients with Wilson's disease*					
	First cousins		*Second cousins*		*Unrelated*	
	No.	Percentage	No.	Percentage	No.	Percentage
30	11	36.7	3	10.0	16	53.3

Source: Adapted from A. G. Bearn [103].

This remarkably high consanguinity rate is good evidence that the disease is inherited in an autosomal recessive fashion (Table 43-4). Calculations based on the incidence of Wilson's disease in sibs with unaffected parents are in accord with this hypothesis [103]. The method of calculation used is variously known as *Hogben's factorial method* or the *a priori method of Bernstein.*

Sex Incidence

The disease may be slightly more common in males than in females. Most series of cases show a slight excess in males which, because of the small numbers, is statistically insignificant. In the author's series, 21 of 32 patients were male.

Age of Onset

The age of onset of Wilson's disease is variable and does not differ in the two sexes (Table 43-4). The apparent excess of Jewish males when the disease has a late onset raises the problem of genetic heterogeneity. The possibility exists that either the allele causing disease in this group of patients is different from the usual allele or a modifying gene delays the onset of the disease in these patients. There is no clear-cut evidence that the disease is caused by more than one gene.

Racial Incidence

Of the 30 families in New York City in whom individuals with Wilson's disease were discovered, 13 (43 percent) were Jewish and came from the border of Russia and Poland within a radius of approximately 100 miles. If a mutation occurred in this population, breeding structure would favor the formation of many homozygotes. Seven of the thirty families (23 percent) were Italians who came from Sicily and the southernmost tip of Italy. The breeding structure in this isolated area would tend also to produce individuals homozygous for the abnormal gene. Nearly all the remainder

Table 43-4. THE ESTIMATED AGE OF ONSET AND GEOGRAPHIC ORIGIN OF 32 PATIENTS WITH WILSON'S DISEASE

Age of onset, years	Consanguinity	Sex		Geographic origin				Total
		Male	Female	Eastern European (Jewish)	Mediterranean	Negro	Other	
10–24	R	5	3	3*	3	0	2	8
	U	5	3	1	2*	1	4	8
	T	10	6	4	5	1	6	16
25–39	R	4	4	6	1	1	0	8
	U	7	1	4	2	0	2	8
	T	11	5	10	3	1	2	16

* Includes one sibling pair.
Note: R = related; U = unrelated; T = total.
Source: Adapted from A. G. Bearn [103].

of the patients of this series came from various parts of Europe. In interpreting these data it must be recalled that these patients were largely collected from New York City and that their racial distribution reflects to some extent the geographic origins of the population of New York.

Patients with Wilson's disease continue to be reported from all parts of the world. Recent studies from India by Dastur and his colleagues have indicated that the disease affects all racial and religious groups [148, 149].

Gene Frequency

Estimations of gene frequency are hazardous. One of the essential assumptions, namely, that the disease is genetically homogeneous, may be unjustified. Another difficulty encountered, if the method devised by Dahlberg [104] is used, is the uncertainty of the estimate of the frequency of first-cousin marriage in the population from which the sample is drawn. Few precise data are available concerning the estimate of the first-cousin consanguinity rate in the populations of Eastern Poland or Sicily 50 years ago. To be sure, the figure of 0.0006 estimated by Bell [105] for England is far too low and would give too low an estimate of the gene frequency. If accurate data on the consanguinity rate were known, it would be possible to give a rough estimate of the gene frequency in the original populations of Eastern Poland and Sicily. If we assume that in these countries 50 years ago the consanguinity rate was 0.1, then the gene frequency can be calculated to be approximately 0.0006, the disease incidence 0.001, a carrier frequency of 0.002 [106]. Although recent estimates of the gene frequency in Japan yield results of a similar order of magnitude [107], a population on the Japanese island of Mikura, recently studied by Arima, suggests that the carrier frequency may be as high as 0.01 [107–109].

Diagnosis of the Disease and Detection of Carriers

The recognition of asymptomatic carriers of deleterious genetic traits is being attempted in many heritable disorders. Related to this problem, but frequently more difficult to demonstrate, is the important question of whether the heterozygote possesses any increased biologic fitness over either homozygote [110]. Unfortunately, with a disease as rare as Wilson's disease it would be virtually impossible to demonstrate any heterozygous advantage.

If the gene product were known with certainty, then the three genotypes—homozygous normal, homozygous affected, and heterozygous carrier—could be distinguished. A decreased ceruloplasmin level, a relatively constant biochemical abnormality in patients with Wilson's disease, has been found in some heterozygotes and not in others [102, 111–116]. In addition, some asymptomatic adult sibs without Kayser-Fleischer rings have had low levels of ceruloplasmin and were found to be unable to incorporate ^{64}Cu into ceruloplasmin [117]. A method for distinguishing heterozygotes without the need for liver biopsy has been proposed by Sternlieb and coworkers [114]. It depends on the ratio of incorporation of ^{64}Cu into ceruloplasmin at 48 hr to the level reached at 1 to 2 hr after oral ingestion of ^{64}Cu. A ratio of ^{64}Cu at 48 hr to ^{64}Cu at 1 to 2 hr of less than 0.559 was considered to indicate a heterozygote with 99 percent confidence limits, whereas a ratio of greater than 1.253 was considered homozygote normal with similar confidence. Unfortunately the ratio in control subjects appears to be correlated with age. When this correlation is borne in mind, accurate discrimination of heterozygotes becomes less certain. Similar studies reviewed by Walshe [99] did not enable a distinction to be drawn between control subjects and heterozygous carriers, and is in conformity with results from the author's laboratory. The finding of a low serum ceruloplasmin in an asymptomatic sib of a patient with Wilson's

Table 43-5. SERUM CERULOPLASMIN CONCENTRATION AND HEPATIC COPPER CONCENTRATION IN PATIENTS WITH WILSON'S DISEASE, HETEROZYGOUS CARRIERS, AND CONTROL SUBJECTS

Group	*Serum Ceruloplasmin*			*Hepatic Copper Concentration*		
	No. of Patients	Range (mg/100 ml)	Mean ± s.d. (mg/100 ml)	No. of Patients	Range (μg/gm dry weight)	Mean ± s.d. (μg/gm dry weight)
Wilson's disease						
Asymptomatic	31	0–19.5	3.6 ± 5.3	36	152–1,828	983.5 ± 368
Symptomatic	84	0–43.0	5.9 ± 7.1	33	94–1,360	588.3 ± 304
Heterozygous carriers	95*	1–50.1	28.4 ± 8.5	14	39–213	117.0 ± 51
Normal subjects	180	18.5–65.9	30.7 ± 3.5	16	20–45	31.5 ± 6.8

* 71 parents of patients with Wilson's disease and 24 children, each of whom had 1 parent with Wilson's disease.
Source: Adapted from I. Sternlieb and I. H. Scheinberg [115].

disease in the face of a normal level of hepatic copper is strongly suggestive of the heterozygous state (Table 43-5).

There is evidence that the disease in certain families conforms to a distinctive clinical and biochemical pattern. In any one sibship, the age of onset, the predominant clinical symptoms, and the biochemical abnormalities may be remarkably similar. In some families only the hepatic form of the disease is present; in others the liver injury is minimal, and neurologic symptoms are prominent. Unfortunately, there are many exceptions to this rule, and sibs may have different types of disease. Thus, the possibility that variations in the disease are due to different alleles, which may not be at the same locus, cannot be presently substantiated [103].

TREATMENT

Since treatment is designed to reduce the tissue stores of copper, the copper content of the diet should be kept as low as possible. Although it is not possible to decrease the copper intake below 1 mg per day without severe caloric restriction, avoidance of high copper-containing foods (liver, nuts, mushrooms, chocolate, certain shellfish) should be encouraged. The ingestion of potassium sulfide with meals has been advocated to reduce copper absorption.

In addition to diminishing the copper intake, efforts should be made to achieve a large and persistent increase in urinary copper excretion. A variety of agents which chelate copper has been used with success. BAL, introduced simultaneously by Denny-Brown and Porter [118] and by Cumings [119], has proved a valuable agent in increasing the urinary excretion of copper. It suffers from the disadvantage that it must be administered intramuscularly. Local induration or abscesses may occur at the site of injection. Moreover, toxic reactions to BAL, including high fever, faintness, nausea, and vomiting are not uncommon.

The introduction of penicillamine (β,β-dimethylcysteine) in 1956 by Walshe was a spectacular landmark in the treatment of Wilson's disease [120]. The beneficial results of penicillamine have been amply documented [121, 122, 123] over the intervening years. In 1968 [57] Walshe reviewed his extensive experience with penicillamine over a 10-year period. This compound, which can be given by mouth, is a much more effective cupruric agent than BAL, and its administration is not accompanied by so many side reactions. Nevertheless toxic reactions also occur with penicillamine [124]. In about 30 percent of patients minor skin eruptions, fever, and lymphadenopathy may occur within the first 2 weeks of initiating treatment. If the drug is withdrawn for a few days, gradual reinstitution of therapy, beginning with 50 mg penicillamine, can frequently be undertaken [125]. Thrombocytopenia and leukopenia may appear during the course of therapy but almost never lead to serious depression of the bone marrow. The most serious complication is nephrosis, which may follow the administration of both *d*- and *dl*-penicillamine [126, 127]. Fortunately, this complication is rare. Regular examination of the urine for protein is advisable, since the nephrotic syndrome is promptly reversed on discontinuation of therapy. Other complications include optic neuritis, reversible by pyridoxine [128], a decrease in taste perception [129], and skin lesions characterized by the eruption of purpuric lesions on the elbows, knees, and shoulders. The lesions may appear hemorrhagic without any abnormality in coagulation. The lesions are characteristically covered by small pearly white milia [125, 130]. Although D-penicillamine is unquestionably the treatment of choice, in those very few patients in whom penicillamine is not tolerated, or who continue to deteriorate after adequate amounts of therapy, a trial with BAL is indicated. Penicillamine should be given indefinitely in a dose of 1 to 2 gm (orally) depending on body weight. D-Penicillamine is the isomer of choice. L-Penicillamine, in addition to decreasing the growth rate of rats fed on a choline-deficient diet, acts as a pyridoxine antimetabolite.

The natural course of the disease is downhill all the way. Dramatic improvement, particularly in the neurologic manifestations, frequently follows the use of penicillamine. Patients with predominantly hepatic forms of the disease may also show considerable improvement [131, 132]. In some instances improvement may be delayed for over 6 months.

Not uncommonly a period of deterioration may follow the initial therapy. Patients in whom gross pathologic changes in the brain have already occurred cannot be expected to respond favorably.

In many instances a presumptive diagnosis of Wilson's disease can be made before the onset of symptoms. The recognition of a deficiency or absence of ceruloplasmin (less than 20 mg per 100 ml) associated with an elevated hepatic copper (greater than 100 μg per gm dry weight), as judged by liver biopsy in a sib of an affected individual, is an indication to begin therapy [133, 134], for without therapy symptoms of the disease will eventually develop. In newborn infants the decision to start therapy should be delayed for 6 months, since low ceruloplasmin levels and elevated hepatic copper occur normally. Persistent low levels of ceruloplasmin and an elevated hepatic copper concentration indicate that therapy should be initiated.

Penicillamine reduces the serum ceruloplasmin concentration and appears to act by releasing copper from ceruloplasmin and albumin and permitting its excretion by way of the kidneys [132, 135]. A decrease in hepatic copper can be monitored by serial hepatic biopsies, although this is not usually indicated. It has been suggested that the sulfhydryl group in penicillamine exerts a therapeutic effect in addition to that of chelating copper.

The passage of time has strengthened the evidence that, provided Wilson's disease can be detected in the asymptomatic stage, symptoms of the disease can be prevented. The effectiveness of penicillamine in the treatment of overt cases is now well established. Toxic effects of penicillamine continue to be reported. The induction of a lupus-like syndrome may be a rare complication of penicillamine therapy. Walshe [150] has described the use of a new chelating agent, triethyl tetramine dihydrochloride, in the treatment of the disease. This agent may prove to be useful for those few patients who develop the nephrotic syndrome while on penicillamine or in whom other serious toxic manifestations arise.

SUMMARY

1 Wilson's disease (hepatolenticular degeneration) is a rare inherited disease which usually occurs in young people. Pathologically it is characterized by cirrhosis of the liver and degenerative changes in the brain, particularly in the basal ganglia. Kayser-Fleischer corneal rings are pathognomonic of the disease. An increased deposition of copper in the tissues can be demonstrated. The increased copper in the body is localized primarily in the liver, brain, kidneys, and cornea.

2 Clinical manifestations rarely occur before the age of 6 years and may be delayed until the fifth decade. Approximately 40 percent of patients develop symptoms of hepatic disease as their presenting symptom, and 40 percent develop symptoms referable to the nervous system. The hepatic form of the disease is common in childhood and must be distinguished from other forms of juvenile cirrhosis. In approximately 20 percent the initial symptoms are psychiatric or behavioral.

3 Biochemical abnormalities in Wilson's disease are multiple. Low serum copper concentration and decreased serum ceruloplasmin levels are observed in the majority of patients with the disease and are associated with an increased excretion of copper. The plasma levels of amino acids and glucose are usually normal or slightly decreased. The serum phosphate level is often decreased and the serum uric acid usually decreased.

4 Abnormalities in renal function are demonstrable; they consist primarily of a progressive failure of tubular transfer mechanisms for amino acids, glucose, uric acid, calcium, and phosphate. A decrease in the normal capacity of the kidney to acidify the urine also occurs.

5 Family studies indicate that the disease is inherited in an autosomal recessive fashion. A decreased serum copper and, more particularly, a decreased serum ceruloplasmin is found in a small proportion of clinically normal heterozygotes.

6 The pathogenesis of the disease is obscure. The primary genetic defect is not known with certainty. A decreased synthesis of structurally normal serum ceruloplasmin is closely related to the primary action of the gene. The possibility that the small amount of ceruloplasmin synthesized by most patients with Wilson's disease is structurally abnormal has not yet been excluded.

7 D-Penicillamine is the treatment of choice and usually results in striking clinical improvement, particularly when given in the early stages of the disease. Treatment is indicated in asymptomatic sibs who demonstrate a consistently low serum ceruloplasmin level and an increased hepatic copper.

BIBLIOGRAPHY

1. Wilson, S. A. K.: Progressive lenticular degeneration: a familial nervous disease associated with cirrhosis of the liver. Brain, **34**, 295, 1912.
2. Gowers, W. R.: On tetanoid chorea and its association with cirrhosis of the liver. Rev. Neurol. Psychiat., **9**, 249, 1906.
3. Frerichs, F. T.: *Pathologisch-anatomischer Atlas zur Klinik der Leberkrankheiten,* vol. 2, p. 62. Vieweg, Brunswick, Germany, 1861.
4. Westphal, C.: Über eine dem Bilde der cerebrospinalen grauen Degeneration ähnliche Erkrankung des centralen Nervensystems ohne anatomischen Befund, nebst einigen Bemerkungen uber paradoxe Contraction. Arch. Psychiat., **14**, 87, 1883.
5. Franklin, E. C., and Bauman, A.: Liver dysfunction in hepatolenticular degeneration: a review of eleven cases. Amer. J. Med., **15**, 450, 1953.
6. Fleischer, B.: Zwei weitere Fälle von grünlicher Verfärbung der Kornea. Klin. Mbl. Augenheilk., **41**, 489, 1903.
7. Fleischer, B.: Die periphere braungrünliche Hornhautverfärbung als Symptom einer eigenartigen Allgemeinerkrankung. München. Med. Wschr., **56**, 1120, 1909.
8. Fleischer, B.: Über einer der "Pseudoklerose" nahestehende bisher unbekannte Krankheit (gekennzeichnet durch Tremor, psychische Störungen, bräunliche Pigmentierung bestimmter Gewebe, insbesondere auch der Hornhautperipherie, Lebencirrhose). Deutsch Z. Nervenheilk., **44**, 179, 1912.

9. Sternlieb, I.: The Kayser-Fleischer ring. Med. Radiogr. Photogr., **42,** 14, 1966.
10. Arima, M., and Kurumada, T.: Genetical studies of Wilson's disease in childhood. I. Ped. Univ., Tokyo, **7,** 1, 1962.
11. Sternlieb, I. Penicillamine therapy for hepatolenticular degeneration. J. A. M. A., **189,** 749, 1964.
12. Lange, L.: Long-term therapy of Wilson's disease with D-penicillamine, in Wilson's Disease. Birth Defects Original Article Series, **4,** 130, 1968.
13. Kehrer, F.: Zur Ätiologie und Nosologie der Pseudosklerose Westphal-Wilson. Z. Neurol. Psychiat., **129,** 488, 1930.
14. Sherlock, S.: *Diseases of the Liver and Biliary System,* 4th ed., Blackwell, Oxford, 1968.
15. Chalmers, T. C., Iber, F. L., and Uzman, L. L.: Hepatolenticular degeneration (Wilson's disease) as a form of idiopathic cirrhosis. New Eng. J. Med., **256,** 235, 1957.
16. Walshe, J. M.: Wilson's disease. Arch. Dis. Child., **37,** 253, 1962.
17. Scheinberg, I. H., and Sternlieb, I.: The liver in Wilson's disease. Gastroenterology, **37,** 550, 1959.
18. Scheinberg, I. H., Sternlieb, I., and Richman, J.: Psychiatric manifestations in patients with Wilson's disease, in Birth Defects Original Article Series, **4,** 85, 1968.
19. McIntyre, N., Clink, H. M., Leir, H. J., Cumings, J. W., and Sherlock, S.: Hemolytic anemia in Wilson's disease. New Eng. J. Med., **276,** 439, 1967.
20. Holtzman, N. A., Elliott, D. A., and Heller, R. H.: Copper intoxication. Report of a case with observations on ceruloplasmin. New Eng. J. Med., **275,** 347, 1966.
21. Bearn, A. G., and McKusick, V. A.: Azure lunulae: an unusual change in the fingernails in two patients with hepatolenticular degeneration (Wilson's disease). J. A. M. A., **166,** 903, 1958.
22. Finby, N., and Bearn, A. G.: Roentgenographic abnormalities of the skeletal system in Wilson's disease (hepatolenticular degeneration). Am. J. Roentgen., **79,** 603, 1958.
23. Warnock, C. G.: Hepatolenticular degeneration (Wilson's disease): a report of five cases, with commentary, Ulster Med. J., **21,** 155, 1952.
24. Sass-Kortsak, A.: Copper metabolism, Advances Clin. Chem., **8,** 1, 1965.
25. Peisach, J., Aisen, P., and Blumberg, W. E.: *The Biochemistry of Copper,* Academic, New York, 1966.
26. Holmberg, C. G., and Laurell, C. B.: Investigations in serum copper. II. Isolation of the copper containing protein, and a description of some of its properties. Acta Chem. Scand., **2,** 550, 1948.
27. Curzon, G.: Studies on the oxidase properties of caeruloplasmin, in *Wilson's Disease: Some Current Concepts,* edited by J. M. Walshe and J. N. Cumings, Blackwell, Oxford, 1961.
28. Kasper, C. B., and Deutsch, H. F.: Physicochemical studies of human ceruloplasmin. J. Biol. Chem., **238,** 2325, 1963.
29. Kasper, C. B., and Deutsch, H. F.: Studies on the state of copper in native and modified human ceruloplasmin. J. Biol. Chem., **238,** 2338, 1963.
30. Kasper, C. B., and Deutsch, H. F.: Immunochemical studies of crystalline human ceruloplasmin and derivatives. J. Biol. Chem., **238,** 2343, 1963.
31. Poulik, M. D., and Bearn, A. G.: Heterogeneity of human ceruloplasmin. Clin. Chim. Acta, **7,** 374, 1962.
32. Broman, L., Malmström, B. G., Aasa, R., and Vanngard, T.: Quantitative electron spin resonance studies on native and denatured ceruloplasmin and lactase. J. Molec. Biol., **5,** 301, 1962.
33. Broman, L.: Separation and characterization of two caeruloplasmins from human serum. Nature (London), **182,** 1655, 1958.
34. Poulik, M. D.: Heterogeneity and structural subunits of human ceruloplasmin, in *Protides of Biological Fluids,* edited by H. Peeters, vol. 10, p. 170, Elsevier, Amsterdam, 1963.
35. Simons, K., and Bearn, A. G.: Isolation and partial characterization of the polypeptide chains in human ceruloplasmin. Biochim. Biophys. Acta, **175,** 260, 1969.
36. Morell, A. G., Irvine, R. A., Sternlieb, I., and Scheinberg, I. H.: Physical and chemical studies on ceruloplasmin. V. Metabolic studies on sialic acid-free ceruloplasmin in vivo. J. Biol. Chem., **243,** 155, 1968.
37. Morell, A. G., Aisen, P., and Scheinberg, I. H.: Is ceruloplasmin an ascorbic acid oxidase? J. Biol. Chem., **237,** 3455, 1962.
38. Morell, A. G., and Scheinberg, I. H.: Preparation of an apoprotein from ceruloplasmin by reversible dissociation of copper. Science, **127,** 588, 1958.
39. Ravin, H. A.: Rapid test for hepatolenticular degeneration. Lancet, 1, 726, 1956.
40. Aisen, P., Schorr, J. B., Morell, A. G., Gold, R. Z., and Scheinberg, I. H.: A rapid screening test for deficiency of plasma ceruloplasmin and its value in the diagnosis of Wilson's disease. Amer. J. Med., **28,** 550, 1960.
41. Scheinberg, I. H., and Gitlin, D.: Deficiency of ceruloplasmin in patients with hepatolenticular degeneration (Wilson's disease). Science, **116,** 484, 1952.
42. Morell, A. G., and Scheinberg, I. H.: Heterogeneity of human ceruloplasmin. Science, **131,** 930, 1960.
43. Sass-Kortsak, A., Jackson, S. J., and Charles, A. F.: Studies on ceruloplasmin. Vox Sang., **5,** 87, 1960.
44. Hirschmann, S. Z., Morell, A. G., and Scheinberg, I. H.: The heterogeneity of the copper-containing protein of human plasma, ceruloplasmin. Ann. N.Y. Acad. Sci., **94,** 960, 1961.
45. McAllister, R., Martin, S. M., and Benditt, E. P.: Evidence for multiple ceruloplasmin components in human serum. Nature (London), **190,** 927, 1961.
46. Walshe, J. M.: Studies on the oxidase properties of ceruloplasmin: factors in normal and Wilson's disease serum affecting oxidase activity. J. Clin. Invest., **42,** 1048, 1963.
47. Bearn, A. G., and Kunkel, H. G.: Localization of Cu^{64} in serum fractions following oral administration: an alteration in Wilson's disease. Proc. Soc. Exp. Biol. Med., **85,** 44, 1954.
48. Fiess, H. A., and Klotz, I. M.: The thermodynamics of metalloprotein combinations: comparison of copper complexes with natural proteins. J. Amer. Chem. Soc., **74,** 887, 1952.
49. Gubler, C. J., Lahey, M. E., Cartwright, G. E., and Wintrobe, M. M.: Studies on copper metabolism. X. The transportation of copper in blood. J. Clin. Invest., **32,** 405, 1953.
50. Neumann, P. Z., and Sass-Kortsak, A.: Binding of copper by serum proteins. Vox Sang., **8,** 111, 1963.
51. Walshe, J. M.: Filterable and non-filterable serum copper. I. The action of penicillamine. Clin. Sci., **25,** 405, 1963.
52. Neumann, P. Z., and Sass-Kortsak, A. The state of copper in human serum: Evidence for an amino acid bound fraction. J. Clin. Invest., **46,** 646, 1967.
53. Harris, D. I. M., and Sass-Kortsak, A. The influence of amino acids on copper uptake by rat liver slices. J. Clin. Invest., **46,** 659, 1967.
54. Silverberg, M., Neumann, P. Z., and Rotenberg, A. D.: The role of amino acids in the physiologic and pathologic copper transport: In vitro and in vivo studies in Wilson's disease. Birth Defects Original Article Series, **4,** 8, 1968.
55. Kimmel, J. R., Markowitz, H., and Brown, D. M.: Some chemical and physical properties of erythrocuprein. J. Biol. Chem., **234,** 46, 1959.
56. Markowitz, H., Cartwright, G. E., and Wintrobe, M. M.: Studies on copper metabolism. XXVII. The isolation and properties of an erythrocyte cuproprotein (erythrocuprein). J. Biol. Chem., **234,** 40, 1959.
57. Walshe, J. M.: The physiology of copper in man and its relation to Wilson's disease. Brain, **90,** 149, 1967.
58. Porter, H. Copper proteins in brain and liver in normal subjects and in cases of Wilson's disease, in Wilson's Disease. Birth Defects Original Article Series, **4,** 23, 1969.
59. Mann, T., and Keilin, D.: Haemocuprein and hepatocuprein, copper-protein compounds of blood and liver in mammals. Proc. Roy. Soc. [Biol], **126,** 303, 1938.
60. Mohamed, M. S., and Greenberg, D. M.: Isolation of purified copper protein from horse liver. J. Gen. Physiol., **37,** 433, 1954.
61. Morell, A. G., Shapiro, J. R., and Scheinberg, I. H.: Copper binding protein from human liver, in *Wilson's Disease: Some Current Concepts,* edited by J. M. Walshe and J. N. Cumings, Blackwell, Oxford, 1961.
62. Porter, H., and Folch, J.: Brain copper-protein fractions in the normal and in Wilson's disease. A.M.A. Arch. Neurol. Psychiat., **77,** 8, 1957.
63. Porter, H., and Ainsworth, S.: Reaction of brain copper proteins with

sodium diethyldithiocarbamate in normal and in hepatolenticular degeneration. Proc. Soc. Exp. Biol. Med., **98,** 277, 1958.
64. Porter, H.: Copper protein combinations in the brain in Wilson's disease, in *Wilson's Disease: Some Current Concepts,* edited by J. M. Walshe and J. N. Cumings, Blackwell, Oxford, 1961.
65. Vogel, F. S.: The deposition of exogenous copper under experimental conditions with observations on its neurotoxic and nephrotoxic properties in relation to Wilson's disease. J. Exp. Med., **110,** 801, 1959.
66. Cartwright, G. E., Hodges, R. E., Gubler, C. J., Mahoney, J. P., Daum, K., Wintrobe, M. M., and Bean, W. B.: Studies on copper metabolism. XIII. Hepatolenticular degeneration. J. Clin. Invest., **33,** 1487, 1954.
67. Russ, E. M., and Raymunt, J.: Influence of estrogens on total serum copper and caeruloplasmin. Proc. Soc. Exp. Biol. Med., **92,** 465, 1956.
68. German, J. L., and Bearn, A. G.: Effect of estrogens on copper metabolism in Wilson's disease. J. Clin. Invest., **40,** 445, 1961.
69. Rumpel, A.: Über das Wesen und die Bedeutung der Leberveranderungen und der Pigmentierungen bei den damit verbunden Fällen von Pseudosklerose zugleich ein Beitrag zur Lehre von der Pseudosklerose (Westphal-Strümpell). Deutsch. Z. Nervenheilk., **49,** 54, 1913.
70. Siemerling, E., and Oloff, H.: Pseudosklerose (Westphal-Strümpell) mit Corneal-ring (Kayser-Fleischer) und doppelseitiger Scheinkatarakt, die nur bei seitlicher Beleuchtung sichtbar ist und die der nach Verletzung durch Kupfersplitter entstehenden Katarakt ähnlich ist. Klin. Wschr., **1,** 1087, 1922.
71. Haurowitz, F.: Über eine Anomalie des Kupferstoffwechsels. Z. Physiol. Chem., **190,** 72, 1930.
72. Glazebrook, A. J.: Wilson's disease. Edinburgh Med. J., **52,** 83, 1945.
73. Mandelbrote, B. M., Stanier, M. W., Thompson, R. H. S., and Thruston, M. N.: Studies on copper metabolism in demyelinating diseases of the central nervous system. Brain, **71,** 212, 1948.
74. Bearn, A. G., and Kunkel, H. G.: Biochemical abnormalities in Wilson's disease. J. Clin. Invest., **31,** 616, 1952.
75. Scheinberg, I. H., and Sternlieb, I.: Wilson's disease and the concentration of ceruloplasmin in serum. Lancet, **2,** 1420, 1963.
76. Walshe, J. M., and Briggs, J.: Ceruloplasmin in liver disease: a diagnostic pitfall. Lancet, **1,** 263, 1962.
77. Bearn, A. G., and Kunkel, H. G.: Abnormalities of copper metabolism in Wilson's disease and their relationship to the aminoaciduria. J. Clin. Invest., **33,** 400, 1954.
78. Uzman, L. L.: Histochemical localization of copper with rubeanic acid. Lab. Invest., **5,** 299, 1956.
79. Schaffner, F., Sternlieb, I., Banka, T., and Popper, H.: Hepatocellular changes in Wilson's disease. Amer. J. Path., **41,** 315, 1962.
80. Scheinberg, I. H., and Sternlieb, I.: The liver in Wilson's disease. Gastroenterology, **37,** 550, 1959.
81. Sternlieb, I.: Mitochondrial and fatty changes in hepatocytes of patients with Wilson's disease. Gastroenterology, **55,** 354, 1968.
82. Uzman, L. L.: in *Proceedings of the Third International Neurochemistry Symposium, Strasbourg, 1958.* Pergamon, New York, 1961.
83. Uzman, L. L., and Jakus, M. A.: The Kayser-Fleischer ring: a histochemical and electron microscope study. Neurology, **7,** 341, 1957.
84. Bearn, A. G., and Kunkel, H. G.: Metabolic studies in Wilson's disease using Cu^{64}. J. Lab. Clin. Med., **45,** 623, 1955.
85. Bush, J. A., Mahoney, J. P., Marfkowitz, H., Gubler, C. J., Cartwright, G. E., and Wintrobe, M. M.: Studies on copper metabolism. XIV. Radioactive copper studies in normal subjects and in patients with hepatolenticular degeneration. J. Clin. Invest., **34,** 1766, 1955.
86. Gitlin, D., Hughes, W. L., Janeway, C. A.: Absorption and excretion of copper in mice. Nature (London), **188,** 150, 1960.
87. Sternlieb, I., Morell, A. G., Tucker, W. D., Greene, M. W., and Scheinberg, I. H. The incorporation of copper into ceruloplasmin in vivo; studies with Cu^{64} and Cu^{67}. J. Clin. Invest., **40,** 1834. 1961.
88. Scheinberg, I. H., and Sternlieb, I.: Wilson's disease. Ann. Rev. Med., **16,** 119, 1965.
89. Uzman, L. L., and Denny-Brown, D.: Aminoaciduria in hepatolenticular degeneration (Wilson's disease). Amer. J. Med. Sci., **215,** 599, 1948.
90. Dent, C. E.: Chromatography studies, in liver injury, *Transactions of the 6th Conference on Liver Injury, May 1–2, 1947,* pp. 53–62. Josiah Macy, Jr. Foundation, New York, 1948.
91. Bearn, A. G., Yu, T. F., and Gutman, A. B.: Renal function in Wilson's disease. J. Clin. Invest., **36,** 1107, 1957.
92. Reynolds, E. S., Tannen, R. L., and Tyler, H. R.: The renal lesion in Wilson's disease. Amer. J. Med., **40,** 518, 1966.
93. Stein, W. H., Bearn, A. G., and Moore, S.: The amino acid content of the blood and urine in Wilson's disease. J. Clin. Invest., **33,** 410, 1954.
94. Bishop, C., Zimdahl, W. T., and Talbott, J. H.: Uric acid in two patients with Wilson's disease (hepatolenticular degeneration). Proc. Soc. Exp. Biol. Med., **86,** 440, 1954.
95. Litin, R. B., Randall, R. V., Goldstein, N. P., Power, N. H., and Diessner, G. R.: Hypercalcuria in hepatolenticular degeneration (Wilson's disease). Amer. J. Med. Sci., **238,** 614, 1959.
96. Kinney, V. R., Randall, R. V., Rosevear, J. W., Tauxe, W. N., and Goldstein, N. P. Calcium studies in Wilson's disease, in Birth Defects Original Series, **4,** 109, 1968.
97. Holtzman, N. A., Naughton, M. A., Iber, F. L., and Gaumnitz, B. M.: Ceruloplasmin in Wilson's disease. J. Clin. Invest., **46,** 993, 1967.
98. Simons, K., and Gahmberg, C. G.: Ceruloplasmin in serum from newborn infants and patients with Wilson's disease. Unpublished.
99. Osborn, S. B., and Walshe, J. M.: Studies with radioactive copper (^{64}Cu and ^{67}Cu) in relation to the natural history of Wilson's disease. Lancet, **1,** 346, 1967.
100. Uzman, L. L., Iber, F. L., and Chalmers, T. C.: Mechanism of copper deposition in the liver in hepatolenticular degeneration (Wilson's disease). Amer. J. Med. Sci., **231,** 511, 1956.
101. Iber, F. L., Chalmers, T. C., and Uzman, L. L.: Studies of protein metabolism in hepatolenticular degeneration. Metabolism, **6,** 388, 1957.
102. Bearn, A. G.: Genetic and biochemical aspects of Wilson's disease. Amer. J. Med., **15,** 442, 1953.
103. Bearn, A. G.: A genetical analysis of thirty families with Wilson's disease (hepatolenticular degeneration). Ann. Hum. Genet., **24,** 33, 1960.
104. Dahlberg, G.: Biometric evaluation of findings, in *Clinical Genetics,* edited by A. Sorsby, pp. 83–100. Butterworth, London, 1953.
105. Bell, J.: A determination of the consanguinity rate in the general hospital population of England and Wales. Ann. Eugen., **10,** 370, 1940.
106. Bearn, A. G.: Genetic considerations in Wilson's disease, in *Wilson's Disease: Some Current Concepts,* edited by J. M. Walshe and J. N. Cumings. Blackwell, Oxford, 1961.
107. Arima, M., and Kurumada, T.: Genetical studies of Wilson's disease in childhood. Paediat. Univ. Tokyo, **7,** 7, 1963.
108. Arima, M., and Sano, I.: Genetic studies of Wilson's disease in Japan, in Birth Defects Original Series, **4,** 54, 1968.
109. Arima, M., Kamoshita, S., Komiya, H., and Murokawa, H.: Genetical studies of Wilson's disease. 3. Genetical and epidemiological studies of Wilson's disease in Mikura Island. Paediat. Univ. Toyko, **10,** 5, 1964.
110. Penrose, L. S.: Quelques principes sur la frequence des genes et sa stabilité dans les populations humaines. J. Gen. Hum., **3,** 159, 1954.
111. Bickel, H., Neale, F. C., and Hall, G.: A clinical and biochemical study of hepatolenticular degeneration (Wilson's disease). Quart J. Med., **26,** 527, 1957.
112. Neale, F. C., and Fischer-Williams, M.: Copper metabolism in normal adults and in clinically normal relatives of patients with Wilson's disease. J. Clin. Path., **2,** 441, 1958.
113. Sass-Kortsak, A., Glatt, B. S., Cherniak, M., and Cederlund, I.: Observations on copper metabolism in homozygotes and heterozygotes of Wilson's disease, in *Wilson's Disease: Some Current Concepts,* edited by J. M. Walshe and J. N. Cumings. Blackwell, Oxford, 1961.
114. Sternlieb, I., Morell, A. G., Bauer, C. D., Combes, B., Sternberg, S. De B., and Scheinberg, I. H.: Detection of the heterozygous carrier of the Wilson's disease gene. J. Clin. Invest., **40,** 707, 1961.
115. Sternlieb, I., and Scheinberg, I. H.: Prevention of Wilson's disease in asymptomatic patients. New Eng. J. Med., **278,** 352, 1968.
116. Bearn, A. G.: Wilson's disease: an inborn error of metabolism with multiple manifestations. Amer. J. Med., **22,** 747, 1957.
117. Bearn, A. G.: Wilson's disease (hepatolenticular degeneration). Postgrad. Med. J., **32,** 477, 1956.

118. Denny-Brown, D., and Porter, H.: The effect of BAL (2,3-dimercaptopropanol) on hepatolenticular degeneration (Wilson's disease). New Eng. J. Med., **245,** 917, 1951.
119. Cumings, J. N.: The effect of BAL in hepatolenticular degeneration. Brain, **74,** 10, 1951.
120. Walshe, J. M.: Penicillamine, a new oral therapy for Wilson's disease. Amer. J. Med., **21,** 487, 1956.
121. Richard, J., Rosenoer, V. M., Tompsett, S. L., Draper, I., and Simpson, J. A. Hepatolenticular degeneration (Wilson's disease) treated by penicillamine. Brain, **87,** 619, 1964.
122. Hsia, Y. E., Combs, J. T., Hook, L., and Brandt, I. K.: Hepatolenticular degeneration: Comparative effectiveness of D-penicillamine, potassium sulfide and diethyldithiocarbamate as decoppering agents. J. Pediat., **68,** 921, 1966.
123. Sternlieb, I., and Scheinberg, I. H.: Penicillamine therapy for hepatolenticular degeneration. J.A.M.A., **189,** 748, 1964.
124. Supplement: Postgraduate Medical Journal, October, 1968.
125. Scheinberg, I. H.: Toxicity of penicillamine, Suppl. Postgrad. Med. J., p. 11, Oct., 1968.
126. Hirschman, S. Z., Isselbacher, K. J.: The nephrotic syndrome as a complication of penicillamine therapy for hepatolenticular degeneration. Ann. Intern. Med., **62,** 1297, 1965.
127. Sternlieb, I.: Penicillamine and the nephrotic syndrome. J.A.M.A., **198,** 1311, 1966.
128. Tu, J. B., Blackwell, R. W., and Lee, P. F.: DL-penicillamine as a cause of optic axial neuritis. J.A.M.A., **85,** 83, 1963.
129. Henkin, R. I., Keisen, H. R., Jaffe, I. A., Sternlieb, I., and Scheinberg, I. H.: Decrease taste sensitivity after dl-penicillamine reversed by copper administration. Lancet, **ii,** 1268, 1967.
130. Kueppers, F., and Daniels, F.: Penicillamine induced skin lesions in patients with Wilson's disease. Cutis, **5,** 35, 1969.
131. Sherlock, S.: Hepatic aspects of Wilson's disease, in *Wilson's Disease: Some Current Concepts,* edited by J. M. Walshe and J. N. Cumings. Blackwell, Oxford, 1961.
132. Walshe, J. M.: Penicillamine. Practitioner, **191,** 789, 1963.
133. Sternlieb, I., and Scheinberg, I. H.: The diagnosis of Wilson's disease in asymptomatic patients. J.A.M.A., **183,** 747, 1963.
134. Walshe, J. M.: The movement of copper through membranes, in *Wilson's Disease: Some Current Concepts,* edited by J. M. Walshe and J. N. Cumings. Blackwell, Oxford, 1961.
135. Walshe, J. M.: The liver in hepatolenticular degeneration, in *Diseases of the Liver,* edited by L. Schiff. Lippincott, Philadelphia, 1968.
136. Carrico, R. J., Deutsch, H. F., Beinert, H., and Orme-Johnson, W. H.: Some properties of an apoceruloplasmin-like protein in human serum. J. Biol. Chem., **244,** 4141, 1969.
137. Carrico, R. J., and Deutsch, H. F.: Some properties of ceruloplasmin from patients with Wilson's disease. Biochem. Med., **3,** 117, 1969.
138. Holtzman, N. A., and Gaumnitz, B. M.: Identification of an apoceruloplasmin-like substance in the plasma of copper-deficient rats. J. Biol. Chem., **245,** 2350, 1970.
139. Holtzman, N. A., and Gaumnitz, B. M.: Studies on the rate of release and turnover of ceruloplasmin and apoceruloplasmin in rat plasma. J. Biol. Chem., **245,** 2354, 1970.
140. Carrico, R. J., and Deutsch, H. F.: Isolation of human hepatocuprein and cerebrocuprein. Their identity with erythrocuprein. J. Biol. Chem., **244,** 6087, 1969.
141. Carrico, R. J., and Deutsch, H. F.: The presence of zinc in human cytocuprein and some properties of the apoprotein. J. Biol. Chem., **245,** 723, 1970.
142. Morell, A. G., Van Den Hamer, C. J. A., and Scheinberg, I. H.: Physical and chemical studies on ceruloplasmin. IV. Preparation of radioactive, sialic acid-free ceruloplasmin labeled with tritium on terminal D-galactose residues. J. Biol. Chem., **241,** 3745, 1966.
143. Van Den Hamer, C. J. A., Morell, A. G., and Scheinberg, I. H.: Physical and chemical studies on ceruloplasmin. IX. The role of galactosyl residues in the clearance of ceruloplasmin from the circulation. J. Biol. Chem., **245,** 4397, 1970.
144. Morell, A. G., Van Den Hamer, C. J. A., and Scheinberg, I. H.: Physical and chemical studies on ceruloplasmin. VI. Preparation of human ceruloplasmin crystals. J. Biol. Chem., **244,** 3494, 1969.
145. Morell, A. G., Irvine, R. A., Sternlieb, I., and Scheinberg, I. H.: Physical and chemical studies on ceruloplasmin. V. Metabolic studies on sialic acid-free ceruloplasmin in vivo. J. Biol. Chem., **243,** 155, 1968.
146. Gregoriadis, G., Morell, A. G., Sternlieb, I., and Scheinberg, I. H.: Catabolism of desialylated ceruloplasmin in the liver. J. Biol. Chem., **245,** 5833, 1970.
147. Shokeir, M. H. K., and Schreffler, D. C.: Cytochrome oxidase deficiency in Wilson's disease: a suggested ceruloplasmin function. Proc. Nat. Acad. Sci., **62,** 867, 1969.
148. Dastur, D. K., Manghani, D. K., and Wadia, N. H.: Wilson's disease in India. I. Geographic, genetic, and clinical aspects in 16 families. Neurology, **18,** 21, 1968.
149. Manghani, D. K., and Dastur, D. K.: Wilson's disease in India. II. Biochemical and pathogenic considerations in patients, parents, and siblings. Neurology, **18,** 117, 1968.
150. Walshe, J. M.: Management of penicillamine nephropathy in Wilson's disease: A new chelating agent. Lancet, **2,** 1401, 1969.

CHAPTER FORTY-FOUR
HEMOCHROMATOSIS*

Myron Pollycove

A diagnosis of primary, or endogenous, hemochromatosis is based classically on the clinical triad of pigment (hemosiderin) cirrhosis, darkening of the skin to a bronze or slate-gray color, and diabetes. Probably Trousseau [1] first described a patient with this disease in 1865 during a lecture on diabetes. His patient had a peculiar color of the liver, with cirrhosis, "bronzing" of the skin, and glycosuria. Troisier first recognized primary hemochromatosis as a disease entity in 1871, designating it as *la cirrhose pigmentaire dans le diabète sucré* [2]. In 1889 von Recklinghausen [3] introduced the term *hemochromatosis.* He thought the excessive tissue pigment was the result of hemoglobin decomposition following hemorrhage. Subsequently, the term *bronze diabetes* was also used to describe this entity. Sheldon in 1927 [4] was the first to suggest that primary hemochromatosis is an inherited metabolic disorder, and in his classic monograph of 1935 [5], which included over 300 cases from the literature, he reported reliable data establishing the familial incidence of the disease. Finch and Finch in 1955 reviewed over 1,000 cases from the literature and 80 of their own in the light of current knowledge of iron metabolism [6]. They emphasized that primary hemochromatosis is an iron storage disease in which massive iron deposition is the result of increased gastrointestinal absorption of iron. Clarification of the pathogenesis of primary hemochromatosis and its differentiation from other iron storage diseases with iron overload require an understanding of iron metabolism.

THE METABOLISM OF IRON

Function, Distribution, and Properties of the Iron Compounds in Man

The most important function of iron in the human body is to combine with protoporphyrin to form the pigment heme (ferrous protoporphyrin). Heme combines with various protein moieties to form heme compounds (hemoglobin and myoglobin), which bind oxygen reversibly, and heme enzymes (cytochromes, catalase, and peroxidase), which make oxygen available for intracellular oxidation. Unicellular organisms contain heme enzymes. More complex organisms cannot obtain oxygen directly by diffusion from the environment but must obtain it through specialized organs such as gills or lungs. Hemoglobin in erythrocytes transports oxygen from these organs to all cells. The iron in heme is thus pivotally involved in the basic energy-exchange reactions of cellular metabolism.

*Personal investigations cited were supported by the United States Atomic Energy Commission and National Institutes of Health Grant CA 01440–14.

A normal adult requires 3 to 5 gm elemental iron for transporting oxygen from the lung and carbon dioxide from the tissues, storing oxygen in muscle, utilizing oxygen in cellular oxidation, and maintaining an adequate iron storage reserve. This iron is distributed as follows (Fig. 44-1): 65 percent in red blood cell hemoglobin, 3 percent in myoglobin (muscle hemoglobin), 25 percent in storage iron almost equally divided between ferritin and hemosiderin, and less than 1 percent in plasma and extracellular fluid attached to transferrin (siderophilin) and heme enzymes. Approximately 6 percent of the total body iron is unaccounted for; this may represent unknown constituents or errors in determinations [7, 8].

The Heme Compounds (Fig. 44-1)

Human hemoglobin, a protein with a molecular weight of 66,700, is composed of four molecules of heme bound to four amino acid chains comprising one molecule of globin. Ferrous iron is bound in six coordinate linkages. Four of these bind each of the four nitrogen atoms of protoporphyrin, one binds to a nitrogen atom of globin, and the remaining linkages bind oxygen reversibly. Each gram of hemoglobin contains 3.4 mg iron.

Myoglobin

This is a small protein with a molecular weight of approximately 17,000. It is composed of one heme molecule bound to one protein molecule. It, too, binds oxygen reversibly and rapidly, thereby providing a labile reserve supply of oxygen to muscle cells during peak or intermittent muscular activity. The very large content of myoglobin in marine animals such as the whale and the seal enables these mammals to exert themselves under water for long periods [9].

The intracellular heme enzymes contain only a few tenths of 1 percent of the total body iron and yet are absolutely essential for all cellular life. Cytochrome b, cytochrome c_1, cytochrome c, and cytochrome a successively accept and release electrons in the oxidation chain leading from the substrates of the dehydrogenating systems to cytochrome oxidase (cytochrome a). Cytochrome oxidase is the terminal member of the cytochrome chain, inasmuch as it is the only member capable of reducing oxygen. Peroxidases and catalase employ hydrogen peroxide as substrate in oxidative reactions. Peroxidative reactions result in oxidation of many types of compounds. Catalytic splitting of H_2O_2 to H_2O and O represents a special case of the peroxidatic reaction in which H_2O_2 serves as substrate and acceptor.

The heme molecule alone can carry out the varied functions of these compounds, but at a markedly lower level of efficiency. It is the specific combination with a particular

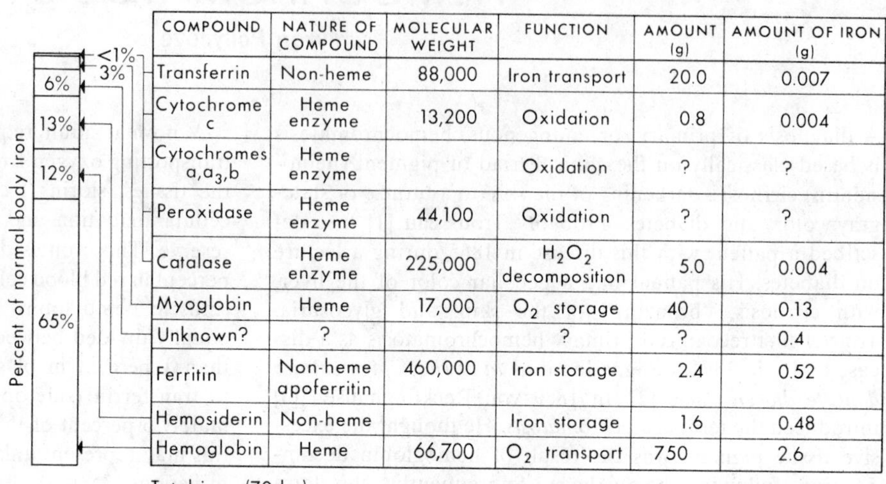

COMPOUND	NATURE OF COMPOUND	MOLECULAR WEIGHT	FUNCTION	AMOUNT (g)	AMOUNT OF IRON (g)
Transferrin	Non-heme	88,000	Iron transport	20.0	0.007
Cytochrome c	Heme enzyme	13,200	Oxidation	0.8	0.004
Cytochromes a, a_3, b	Heme enzyme		Oxidation	?	?
Peroxidase	Heme enzyme	44,100	Oxidation	?	?
Catalase	Heme enzyme	225,000	H_2O_2 decomposition	5.0	0.004
Myoglobin	Heme	17,000	O_2 storage	40	0.13
Unknown?	?		?	?	0.4
Ferritin	Non-heme apoferritin	460,000	Iron storage	2.4	0.52
Hemosiderin	Non-heme		Iron storage	1.6	0.48
Hemoglobin	Heme	66,700	O_2 transport	750	2.6
Total iron (70 kg)					4 grams

Figure 44-1. Distribution and functions of the iron compounds in normal man.

protein that enhances and differentiates the various functions of heme.

The Nonheme Iron Compound (Fig. 44-1)

Ferritin

This compound is composed of apoferritin, a protein of molecular weight 460,000, in which are held ferric hydroxide micelles (clusters) to the extent that 20 to 24 percent of crystallized ferritin is iron. It is colorless and usually is so finely dispersed in tissue that it cannot be detected microscopically except diffusely after staining for iron; it may aggregate into microscopically visible siderotic granules, which normally are present in immature red blood cells. Ferritin is the primary and most readily available iron storage protein of the body. It may also participate in the regulation of iron movement at various body barriers [7]. When sufficient concentrations of iron are presented to the cells of the marrow erythroid series, intestinal mucosa, renal tubules, or placental villi, newly formed or increased ferritin can be demonstrated at these sites [10–15]. Recent studies in the rat suggest that this increased synthesis of ferritin in response to iron is the result of increased formation of messenger RNA, i.e., that ferritin synthesis is under gene transcriptional control and is not controlled at a later stage of the biosynthetic pathway [16]. Ferritin also may possibly inhibit the vasoconstrictor action of epinephrine and may be involved in the phenomena of irreversible shock, hypotension, and antidiuresis [17].

Hemosiderin

This compound normally comprises almost one-half the total body storage iron [18–20]. The difference between hemosiderin and ferritin is that an increased percentage of iron is associated with apoferritin denaturation, and the hemosiderin iron-protein complex is insoluble in water [21]. The iron content of hemosiderin varies between 25 and 36 percent; ferritin contains 20 to 24 percent iron [22, 23]. Very old deposits in hematoxylin-eosin-azure-stained tissue usually appear as a golden crystalline substance which is coarse enough to be seen with the light microscope and takes an iron stain. More recent deposits may appear yellow, green, blue-green, or blue in order of decreasing age [24]. Tissues in which a moderate amount of hemosiderin is present also have a high concentration of ferritin. Ferritin appears to be the precursor of hemosiderin that is formed when the rate of iron deposition exceeds the rate of apoferritin formation. Hemosiderin aggregates into particles large enough to be visible microscopically as blue granules after staining with Prussian blue.

The pattern of hemosiderin distribution in bone marrow varies in accordance with the functional state of red blood cell production and destruction [25–27]. Hemosiderin iron also is available for hemoglobin formation but is more slowly mobilized than is ferritin iron, the oldest deposits being mobilized most slowly. Normally, about one-third of the body irons stores is found in the liver, another third is contained in the bone marrow, and the balance is contained in the spleen, muscle, and elsewhere [28–33].

Transferrin

Also called *siderophilin,* this compound is a plasma protein (found in Cohn's plasma fraction IV-7) with the electrophoretic mobility of a β_1-globulin. It is probably a real carrier of iron, just as hemoglobin is the carrier of oxygen. Various genetically determined transferrins of slightly different electrophoretic mobilities but similar iron-binding capacity have been demonstrated [34, 35]. Transferrin has a molecular weight of 88,000 and can bind two ferric atoms per molecule. When ferrous or ferric ions are added to this protein at physiologic pH in the presence of carbon dioxide,

Table 44-1. HUMAN DAILY BODY REQUIREMENTS FOR IRON

Individual status (development, function, sex)	Total daily requirement for Fe, mg	Daily requirement of Fe, mg				
		Excretion 1	Normal menses 0.8	Rapid growth 1	Pregnancy 2.7	Lactation 0.8
Adult normal male, 70 kg	1	1				
Adult menstruating female, 70 kg	1.8	1	0.8			
Adult postmenopausal female	1	1				
Infant male or female, 12 kg	1.2	0.2	...	1		
Adolescent male in puberty	2	1	...	1		
Adolescent female in puberty	2.8	1	0.8	1		
Normal pregnancy	3.7	1	...	..	2.7	
Adult lactating female without menses	1.8	1	...	..	...	0.8
Adult lactating female with menses	2.6	1	0.8	..	...	0.8

a tightly bound ferric chelate is formed. The 8 gm (0.27 gm per 100 ml) transferrin which is present normally in the plasma carries about 3.5 mg iron at a concentration of 120 μg per 100 ml. This is approximately one-third the maximum amount of iron that it is capable of carrying, so that there remains a latent iron-binding capacity of 230 μg per 100 ml [36, 37]. This iron is probably randomly distributed so that each transferrin molecule has either two atoms or one atom of iron or none. Iron attached at one of the binding sites may be more readily available to the cells than iron attached at the other [38]. Approximately another 8 gm transferrin containing 3.5 mg bound iron is in the extracellular fluid in equilibrium with the plasma transferrin [39, 40]. Transferrin molecules with one or two iron atoms are rapidly attached to immature red blood cells. With random iron binding of transferrin to a normal saturation level of 33 percent, four-ninths of the transferrin molecules would have no iron atoms, four-ninths would have one iron atom, and one-ninth of the molecules would have two atoms of iron. There is preferential erythron[1] binding of transferrin binding two iron atoms, as well as rapid transfer of iron from transferrin to erythron low-molecular-weight iron, ferritin, and hemoglobin [11, 12, 41], and detachment of transferrin and replacement by saturated transferrin. Jandl and Katz have found that reticulocytes may bind 50,000 molecules of transferrin per cell and that these may occupy approximately 2 percent of the cell surface, with a 5:1 binding ratio of saturated to unsaturated transferrin [42, 43]. Transferrin binding and iron transfer to hepatic cells (storage exchange) occur much more slowly, and iron transfer becomes considerable only when there is a high degree of saturation of transferrin [42–44].

[1] *Erythron,* as used in this chapter, signifies red blood cells at any stage of maturity, from the proerythroblast (rubriblast) to the senescent erythrocyte. In this sense it is synonymous with *red blood cells,* although the latter term has usually been associated with the erythrocyte, the mature red blood cell. The term erythron, in addition to being succinct, possesses a general meaning that emphasizes the various stages of red blood cell development. This definition differs from previous use of the term, which, in addition to erythroid elements of the marrow and circulating red corpuscles, included all other bone marrow elements and plasma.

Total Body Requirements for Iron (Table 44-1)

The normal adult male requires approximately 1 mg iron per day to remain in balance, provided there is no abnormal blood loss. The excretion of iron in the urine amounts to about 0.1 mg per day, and urinary loss is not significantly increased except in patients with hematuria, hemoglobinuria, or hemosiderinuria. Desquamation of skin and sweat formation comprise a loss of approximately 0.2 mg per day. Iron lost by shedding of intestinal mucosa and biliary excretion constitute another 0.2 mg per day [45]. The remaining daily iron loss of 0.5 mg per day is the result of normal gastrointestinal bleeding of approximately 1 ml per day [45–52].

In other physiologic conditions the daily requirement for iron may be sharply increased. Thus, the additional iron requirement for maximal growth during infancy and puberty is about 1 mg per day [53]. Approximately 0.8 mg per day is required to balance the iron lost in the average menstrual blood flow of 50 ml per month [54, 55]. During the last two trimesters of pregnancy, an additional 2.7 mg per day is required to meet the fetal demand for iron and to compensate for blood loss at parturition [49, 56, 57]. Following pregnancy 0.8 mg per day is needed to balance the iron lost in lactation [49, 58]. Human requirements for iron vary between 1 and 4 mg per day, depending on the development, function, and sex of the individual. The total daily requirements for iron in man under various circumstances are listed in Table 44-1.

Absorption of Iron

The total iron loss normally is approximately 1 mg per day and remains within relatively narrow limits (0.7 to 2.4 mg per day) in spite of iron depletion or excess [45, 48, 59]. Total body iron is regulated physiologically by the rate at which iron is absorbed from the intestine. Balance studies performed on normal adult males indicate that the daily iron requirement (approximately 1 mg per day to meet fixed excretion) is met by a dietary iron intake of 12 to 15 mg per day [46, 49]. Thus absorption of iron amounts to 7 to 8 percent of intake. Normal absorption of 4 mg ferrous iron varies from 3 to 22 percent and is well correlated with the reticulocyte count [60]; the amount of iron absorbed from a single dose increases approximately sevenfold with a tenfold increase of ingested iron [61].

Absorption of food iron is increased up to 40 percent [62] in a variety of circumstances, as indicated in Fig. 44-2. Absorption is increased in the following conditions in which body or plasma iron is low: in childhood, in adolescence, in the latter half of pregnancy, in menstruating women, following acute blood loss, and in iron deficiency anemia [62–68]. It is also increased in conditions in which the blood hemoglobin concentration is low without reduction of body or plasma iron: pernicious anemia, hypoplastic anemia, refractory anemias with erythroid hyperplasia, and hemolytic anemias [64, 69–72]. Increased iron absorption also occurs in patients with polycythemia or compensated hemolysis in which there is no significant decrease of blood hemoglobin concentration, plasma iron concentration, or storage iron. Other observations also indicate that increased erythropoiesis, per se, increases iron abosorption [65, 69, 70, 73–77]. Conversely, markedly decreased erythropoiesis occurring in persons or animals acclimatized to high altitude when taken to sea level is associated with a virtual cessation of iron absorption [76–78]. Hypoxia, per se, increases iron absorption [73]. For unknown reasons iron absorption is increased in patients with primary hemochromatosis, even though plasma and storage iron are increased and erythropoiesis and hemoglobin concentration are normal [6, 63, 79–81]. Whether absorption of iron is increased or decreased during infection is not clear [46].

Iron is absorbed from the intestine as ferrous ions, or when hemoglobin is ingested, as heme. Virtually all food iron is in the ferric state. Ferric hydroxide and the tightly bound ferric-organic chelates in food decompose to ferric ions and loose ferric chelates when the pH of the stomach content is less than 4. This ionic iron can react with suitable ligands such as fructose, ascorbic acid, and citric acid or with an iron-binding fraction of human gastric juice, gastroferrin [82–90]. Initial characterization of gastroferrin showed it to be a glycoprotein, with a molecular weight of 260,000, consisting of approximately 85 percent carbohydrate and 15 percent protein [87]. The formation of soluble iron complexes at acid pH normally found in the stomach maintains the solubility of iron during the subsequent rise of pH in the duodenum which approaches neutrality in the jejunum [91]. Saltman and colleagues have emphasized the importance of iron chelates for the transportation and absorption of iron [82, 83]. If the soluble complexes of iron are not formed at low pH, then neutralization results in the polymerization and precipitation of iron as unabsorbable ferric hydroxide [88, 89]. In collaboration with Saltman and Freeman we have compared iron absorption of ferric fructose (100:1 molar fructose:iron) with ferrous sulfate in each of 10 normal subjects. Fifteen doses of each compound con-

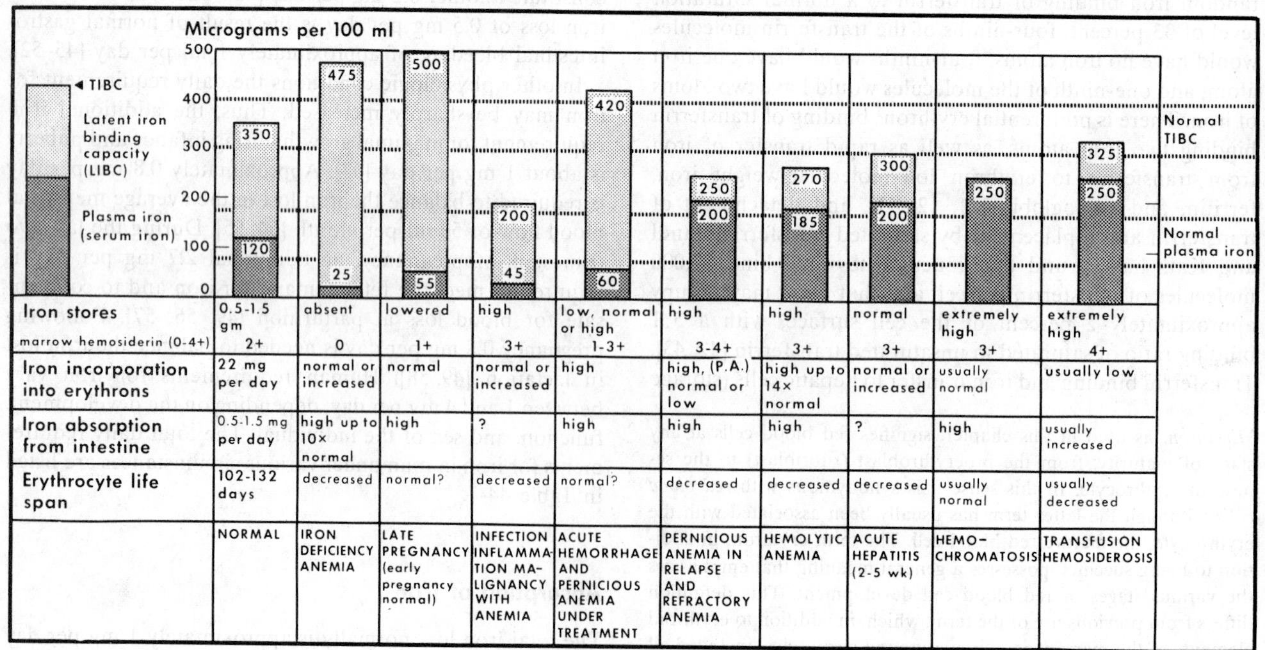

	NORMAL	IRON DEFICIENCY ANEMIA	LATE PREGNANCY (early pregnancy normal)	INFECTION INFLAMMATION MALIGNANCY WITH ANEMIA	ACUTE HEMORRHAGE AND PERNICIOUS ANEMIA UNDER TREATMENT	PERNICIOUS ANEMIA IN RELAPSE AND REFRACTORY ANEMIA	HEMOLYTIC ANEMIA	ACUTE HEPATITIS (2-5 wk)	HEMO-CHROMATOSIS	TRANSFUSION HEMOSIDEROSIS
Iron stores	0.5-1.5 gm	absent	lowered	high	low, normal or high	high	high	normal	extremely high	extremely high
marrow hemosiderin (0-4+)	2+	0	1+	3+	1-3+	3-4+	3+	3+	3+	4+
Iron incorporation into erythrons	22 mg per day	normal or increased	normal	normal or increased	high	high, (P.A.) normal or low	high up to 14× normal	normal or increased	usually normal	usually low
Iron absorption from intestine	0.5-1.5 mg per day	high up to 10× normal	high	?	high	high	high	?	high	usually increased
Erythrocyte life span	102-132 days	decreased	normal?	decreased	normal?	decreased	decreased	decreased	usually normal	usually decreased

Figure 44-2. Iron metabolism in man under various conditions.

taining 50 mg iron were ingested over a 10-day period. Red cell ^{55}Fe and ^{59}Fe and whole body ^{59}Fe were measured 2 weeks after the tenth day of daily alternation of ^{55}Fe-ferric fructose (50 mg Fe tid) and ^{59}Fe ferrous sulfate (50 mg Fe tid). Iron absorption of ferric fructose was 1.8 times greater than iron absorption of ferrous sulfate [83*a*]. Conflicting evidence has not yet resolved the question of whether binding of iron by gastroferrin decreases or increases iron absorption [89, 92]. In collaboration with Davis and Saltman we recently demonstrated that the ingestion of 4 mg Fe^{++} together with 200 mg human gastroferrin increased iron absorption by a factor of 1.5 [87*a*]. There is also a current unresolved controversy concerning the possible existence of an undefined gastric factor that promotes iron absorption [93–99]. The iron of ingested hemoglobin does not become ionic, but after peptic digestion remains in solution and enters mucosal cells as heme [100–103]. Ionic iron and heme are absorbed chiefly in the duodenum and proximal jejunum; gastric absorption is negligible [104–109]. Increasing alkalinity of the small intestine, pancreatic secretions, and the lapse of time permit the formation of unabsorbable ferric complexes so that only a small amount of iron is absorbed distal to the jejunum (see Fig. 44-3) [110–117]. Adequate dietary protein and amino acids facilitate the absorption of iron [118–120], probably through the fomation of iron-amino complexes [121–124]. Food phosphates and phytates greatly impair iron absorption by forming undissociated complexes. Food low in phosphates and high in iron and protein, such as liver, fish, and beef muscle, are excellent sources of dietary iron. Foods containing large amounts of phosphate, such as eggs, milk, and cheese, are relatively poor sources of available iron, although they may be relatively high in iron content [62, 63, 125].

The mechanisms of absorption of iron from human duodenal and jejunal mucosa have been partially clarified by animal and human experimentation. The mucosal cells of the guinea pig duodenum absorb ferrous iron, a part of which may become attached to the apoferritin to form ferritin [126]. In dog and man the ingestion of a sufficient dose of iron decreases the absorption of any iron subsequently fed for 6 to 24 hr [23, 127, 128]. The period of time during which absorption of iron is "blocked" corresponds well to the time sequence of appearance and disappearance of ferritin in the duodenal mucosa of the guinea pig. It has been proposed that when iron enters the mucosal cell, a portion forms a nonprotein complex and is transferred rapidly into the plasma while the remainder is oxidized to ferric hydroxide and unites with apoferritin in the cell to form ferritin [13, 129]. The iron stored in mucosal cells as ferritin is subsequently largely lost to the body by sloughing of the cells within 7 to 10 days [130]. Absorbed heme derived from digested hemoglobin is split within the mucosal cell, thereby freeing the iron so that it may also either be transferred into the plasma or remain bound as ferritin. When absorption is increased, almost all the mucosal iron is rapidly transferred to the plasma, with minimal ferritin formation. Conversely, when absorption is decreased, most of the mucosal iron is trapped in ferritin and lost as the mucosal cells exfoliate [103, 131].

The rapid phase of iron transfer from mucosal cell to plasma occurs within the first 4 hr after iron ingestion. The slow phase requires a few days. Usually more than half the total iron transfer to plasma occurs during the rapid phase [107, 132–134]. The iron of ferritin is bound to apoferritin, so that as more ferritin is formed by the transfer of intraluminal iron, the apoferritin of the cell tends to become saturated, with inhibition of further transfer of iron from the intestinal lumen (Fig. 44-3). Thus mucosal cells may become "blocked" within a few hours by the presence of high concentrations of intraluminal iron. The "mucosal block" may be considered a protective mechanism preventing the harmful accumulation of excessive iron, such as occurs in hemochromatosis [135].

Mucosal cells of the rat may also be similarly conditioned to absorb small and limited amounts of iron by incorporation of circulating transport iron while they are developing in the villous crypts of Lieberkühn in the presence of highly saturated transferrin. Parenteral iron saturation of transferrin does not decrease gastrointestinal absorption until a few days later, when the conditioned gastrointestinal crypt cells have migrated into functional positions along the villi [13, 136–138]. Consequently, although acute complete iron saturation of transferrin does not immediately decrease iron absorption in man, chronic high levels of transferrin saturation in equilibrium with body iron stores sharply reduce iron absorption. In both circumstances, most of the absorbed iron is not attached to transferrin and is immediately removed from the portal circulation by deposition in the liver prior to entrance into the systemic circulation [65, 81, 139, 140]. Conversely, iron absorption is increased when plasma iron concentration is reduced and the latent plasma iron-binding capacity (concentration of total transferrin plasma iron-binding capacity minus plasma iron concentration) is increased [141]. This was first suggested by Laurell in 1947 [36] and was clearly demonstrated in man by Hallberg and Solvell [132]. With the simultaneous use of ^{55}Fe and ^{59}Fe they have shown that intravenous administration of transferrin increases iron absorption. In this way the plasma iron-transferrin transport system may participate in the regulation of gastrointestinal iron absorption in accordance with requirements for iron.

Increased absorption of iron occurs in hypoxia and anemic states even if body and plasma iron are not decreased or erythropoiesis increased [64, 69, 72, 73]. Since the intestinal mucosa has an active aerobic metabolism, it seems plausible that decrease in oxygen supply, brought about by a low content of hemoglobin in the blood, leads to a greater reducing tendency in these cells. This could facilitate the reduction of the ferric iron to ferrous iron and its passage into the blood. Low oxygen supply may similarly facilitate delivery of ferrous iron to the plasma from other tissues which store iron as ferritin. This kind of regulatory mecha-

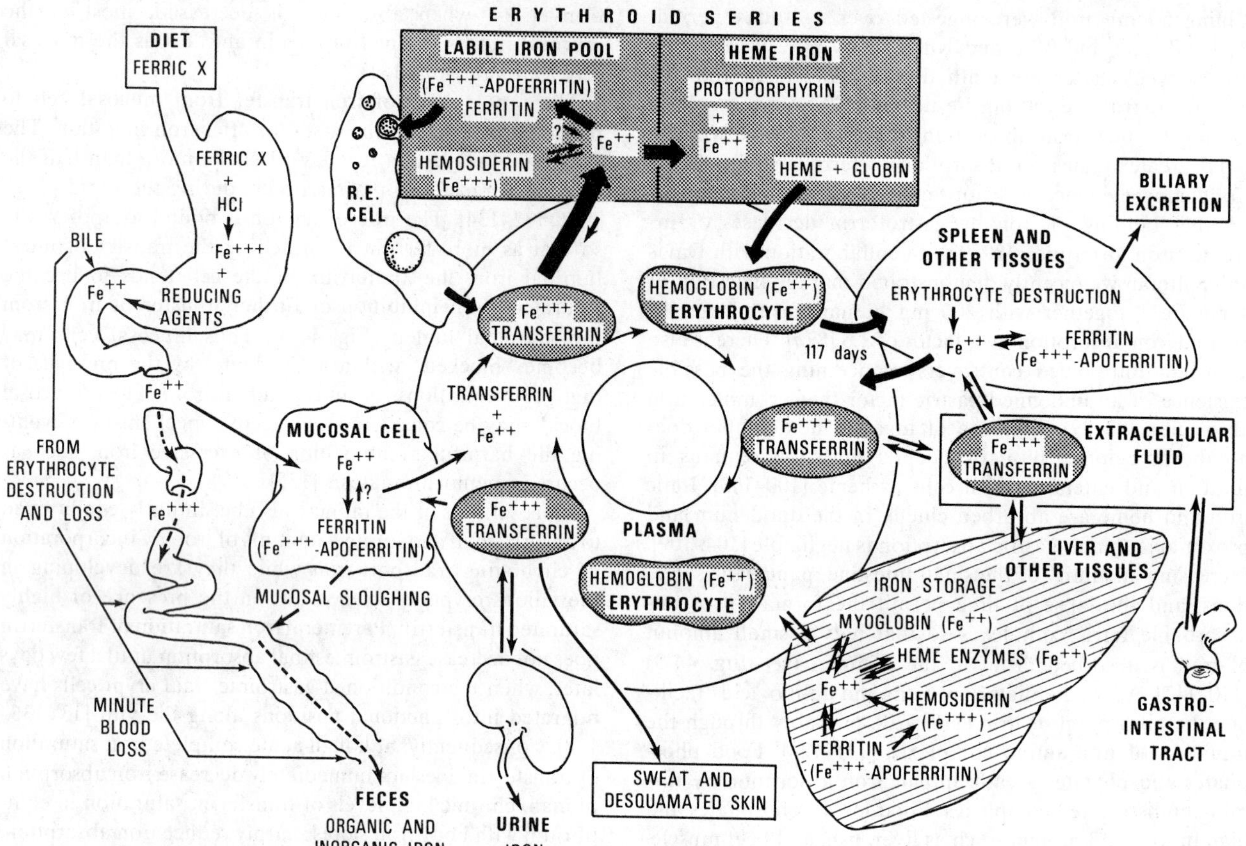

Figure 44-3. Iron metabolism. Ingested organic chelates, subjected to the action of hydrochloric acid (low pH) and reducing agents, are broken down in the stomach with the formation of ferric ions, which are then reduced to ferrous ions. Iron is absorbed only in the ferrous state and chiefly by the mucosal cells of the duodenum and proximal jejunum, where ferritin is formed. Ferrous ions leave the mucosal cell to enter the plasma, where they are bound tightly in the ferric state to the β_1-globulin transferrin. Iron leaves the plasma very largely by entering the labile iron pool of the erythroid series, from which there is a large feedback of iron into the plasma. Within the developing erythroid cells of the bone marrow ferrous ions combine with protoporphyrin to form the porphyrin heme, which in turn combines with globin to form hemoglobin. Hemoglobin is released within circulating erythrocytes that have an average life-span of 117 days. These cells at the time of their disintegration are removed from the circulation by the spleen and other reticuloendothelial tissues with excretion of the split porphyrin as bilirubin in the bile and conservation of almost all the iron, which reenters the plasma and is bound once more to transferrin. These phagocytic reticuloendothelial cells are normally the chief source of iron entering the plasma. Approximately two-thirds of normal total-body iron loss (1.0 mg per day) occurs as the result of the gastrointestinal blood loss of 1.2 ml per day (0.6 mg Fe per day). Approximately 10 percent of the iron leaving and entering the plasma does so in equilibration with extracellular fluid transferrin, the formation and breakdown of myoglobin and the heme enzymes, iron absorption, and iron storage.

nism does not explain other conditions already mentioned in which iron absorption is increased without any demonstrable reduction of oxygen supply to the intestinal mucosa. It must be concluded that though oxygen supply and ferritin production in the mucosa are important factors influencing iron absorption, these mechanisms do not provide a complete description of how iron absorption is regulated. Some evidence suggests the possible existence of humoral factor(s) [142–146].

Plasma Iron Equilibria (Figs. 44-2, 44-3)

The amount of iron in the plasma is determined by a dynamic equilibrium. Thus iron flows into plasma from reticulum cells after erythrophagocytosis of senescent or damaged cells, from plasma to bone marrow for hemoglobin synthesis in erythroblasts and reticulocytes, into plasma from the intestinal mucosa, to and from the erythropoietic labile iron pool (chiefly in bone marrow), and to and from tissue iron stores. In addition, the amount of plasma iron is affected by the rate of formation, entry, and removal of the β_1-globulin transferrin (Fig. 44-3) [147]. The balance established by these movements of iron results in a normal mean plasma iron level of about 120 μg per 100 ml (70 to 170 μg per 100 ml) bound to transferrin and a residual latent transferrin iron-binding capacity of about 230 μg per 100 ml (Fig. 44-2). Women have a mean plasma iron level about 10 μg per 100 ml lower than that of men [36, 148–150]. There is a diurnal variation in plasma iron [151–155]. The evening level is about 30 μg per 100 ml lower than the morning level in day workers; for night workers the rhythm is reversed.

It is apparent that if the rate at which iron leaves the plasma exceeds its rate of entry, the plasma iron level will fall, and if this is reversed, the level will rise. The amount of iron leaving the plasma daily and transferred to the bone marrow is approximately nine times the total iron content of the plasma. Thus if erythropoiesis is rapidly increased several-fold in response to severe hemorrhage, for example, the corresponding increase of iron transferred to marrow cannot be met by mere depletion of plasma iron. Rather, the additional plasma iron utilized by the bone marrow for increased hemoglobin synthesis is supplied by a correspondingly increased entry of iron into plasma, largely from iron stores, and relatively little increased entry from the intestine in response to the decreased iron saturation of transferrin.

The equilibrium of iron between storage (ferritin and hemosiderin) and plasma (Fe^{3+}-transferrin) is strongly affected by the degree of transferrin saturation. Low plasma iron concentration with reduced transferrin saturation shifts the equilibrium so as to favor the transfer of iron from stores to plasma, while an elevated plasma concentration of iron with a high degree of transferrin saturation increases the transfer of iron from plasma to stores [44, 156]. Plasma iron appears to be deposited as storage iron first in ferritin, with subsequent transformation of ferritin into hemosiderin [21, 157, 158]. The removal of more iron from plasma by an increased number of immature red blood cells initially decreases the plasma iron and lowers transferrin saturation. Consequently the net transfer of iron from stores to plasma increases as transferrin saturation falls, until the rate of transfer of iron from stores to plasma compensates for the increased rate of marrow removal of iron from plasma. At this point plasma iron concentration and transferrin saturation stabilize at a lower level. As increased erythropoiesis lessens the severity of the anemia, erythropoietin stimulation of the marrow becomes less intense, and the erythroid hyperplasia and associated marrow removal of plasma iron diminish. The excess of iron entry from stores increases the saturation, thereby diminishing the transfer of iron from storage to plasma, so that the supply of iron to plasma is again equated to the marrow demand. After repair of the anemia the major resultant effect of the hemorrhage on iron metabolism is a transfer of iron from stores into circulating erythrocytes to compensate for the lost erythrocyte iron. This depletion of storage iron is, in turn, during the period of hemoglobin normalization only partially compensated by an increased absorption of dietary iron that occurs in response to two stimuli: increased erythropoiesis and decreased transferrin saturation. During a period of a year or more, a persistent slight increase of iron absorption will gradually restore iron stores to normal [59].

The transfer of iron from storage Fe^{3+}-ferritin to plasma involves the reduction of iron to the ferrous state, so that it can be bound to transferrin and circulate in the plasma. Storage iron is significantly increased in the liver of rats given allopurinol, a potent xanthine oxidase inhibitor [159]. Mazur and his associates have demonstrated that liver xanthine oxidase may be involved in the reduction of Fe^{3+}-ferritin to Fe^{++}-ferritin and with the oxidation of hypoxanthine and xanthine to uric acid, as shown in Fig. 44-4. In rat liver slices [160] and in rabbits, guinea pigs, and dogs, in vivo [161], xanthine oxidase was found to function as an enzyme required for the release of iron from liver ferritin. Induced hypoxia was associated with an increase of xanthine and

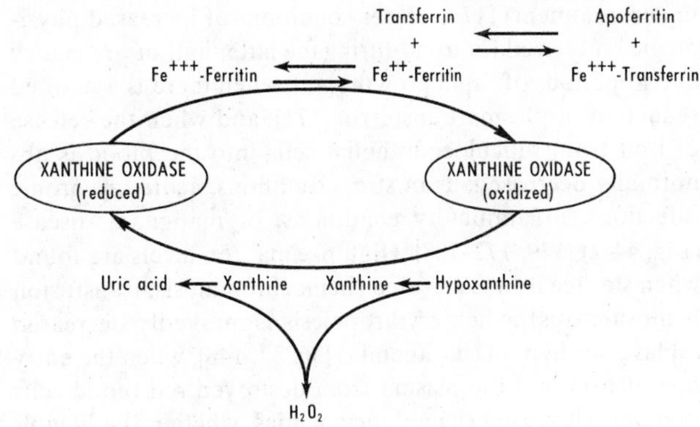

Figure 44-4. Xanthine oxidase mediation of the coupled reduction of ferric-ferritin and oxidation of hypoxanthine and xanthine.

hypoxanthine in the liver. In the presence of ferritin and under anaerobic conditions, hypoxanthine and xanthine were oxidized to uric acid by the dehydrogenase activity of xanthine oxidase. Ferric ferritin acts as an electron acceptor, thereby oxidizing xanthine oxidase, and the iron is reduced to the ferrous state. The ferrous iron can then be removed by transferrin, leaving the iron-free protein apoferritin. Whether xanthine oxidase is absolutely needed in the process is doubtful. Pigeon liver lacks xanthine oxidase. Also in xanthinuria, in which xanthine oxidase activity is low or absent, iron metabolism may be normal [162]. Xanthine oxidase may also be involved in the mucosal transfer of iron to plasma. Hemoglobin and myoglobin ingested in meat and chicken are excellent sources of iron. Normal subjects absorb as much iron from hemoglobin as from inorganic ferrous iron [102]. Iron is not released from heme in the intestinal lumen but is absorbed into mucosal cells as a stable heme complex. Recent evidence suggests that the xanthine oxidase present in canine epithelial cells of the small intestine facilitates opening of the heme ring by the generation of peroxides (Fig. 44-4) which oxidize the α-methene bridge of heme, thereby forming biliverdin and releasing iron [131]. Feeding of allopurinol did not decrease heme absorption in the rat or dog, nor did it decrease ferrous iron absorption in man [131, 163, 164]. In spite of suggestive data obtained in some animals, there is still no evidence that in man xanthine oxidase is an essential factor in the mobilization of storage iron or mucosal transport of iron.

The ferrous oxidase activity of ceruloplasmin may facilitate the mobilization of iron from hepatic parenchymal cells, intestinal mucosal cells, and reticuloendothelial cells by catalyzing the oxidation of ferrous iron so that it may be bound to transferrin in the ferric state [165, 166]. Though observations in copper-deficient swine with low ceruloplasmin level support this concept [167], similar changes have not been observed in patients with Wilson's disease and congenital deficiency of ceruloplasmin [168].

Plasma iron level is low in many circumstances. It is low when storage iron is low or absent (iron deficiency anemia) [36, 169, 170], when erythropoiesis is increased without corresponding hemolysis (acute hemorrhage, pernicious anemia under treatment) [171], under conditions of increased physiologic body need for iron (during the latter half of pregnancy and in periods of rapid growth) [49], when there is a marked reduction of plasma transferrin [171], and when the release of iron from reticuloendothelial cells into the blood is abnormally decreased, as in stress situations, acute or chronic infections, inflammatory conditions, or malignant disease (Fig. 44-2) [149, 172–188]. High plasma iron levels are found when storage iron is elevated (hemochromatosis, transfusion hemosiderosis), when erythropoiesis is markedly decreased (aplastic or hypoplastic anemia) [36, 37, 148], when the entry rate of iron into the plasma from destroyed red blood cells is greatly increased (hemolytic anemias, whether the hemolysis occurs after cell release from the marrow into the circulation or during cell maturation within the marrow, as in pernicious anemia) [37, 148, 189], and when rapid hepatocellular damage occurs (acute hepatitis with release of storage iron from injured cells to plasma) (Fig. 44-2) [190–195].

Whenever the plasma iron level is low, the total iron-binding capacity (TIBC) of the plasma tends to be high, and, accordingly, the percentage saturation is low [(plasma iron/TIBC) $\times$ 100]. This reciprocal action is so sensitive in iron deficiency states that an abnormally low percentage saturation occurs before the concentration of iron in the plasma is decreased unequivocally below the normal range. Conversely, high plasma iron levels are associated with low total iron-binding capacities and a high percentage saturation (Fig. 44-2). The most notable exception to this correlation occurs in patients with infection, inflammation, or malignant disease when both the plasma iron concentration and the total iron-binding capacity are reduced. The percentage saturation in these conditions is usually reduced but not to the same extent as in iron depletion, in which the total iron-binding capacity is increased [36, 149]. Elevated total iron-binding capacity associated with an increase in plasma iron concentration occurs in women using oral contraceptives [196].

Iron Kinetics

Normal Pattern

The total plasma iron of a normal man weighing 70 kg is about 3.5 mg and normally remains fairly constant from day to day except for diurnal variations and moderate post-absorptive increases. Of the normal mean plasma iron turnover of 35 mg per day, approximately 21 mg is utilized daily by the bone marrow for hemoglobin synthesis within immature erythrons. More than five times the total plasma iron enters the plasma daily from the catabolism of erythrocytes within reticuloendothelial cells, while approximately only one-eighth of this amount enters the plasma from the intestine, tissue stores, and extracellular fluid combined (Fig. 44-5). The use of radioactive iron has made it possible to measure this and other aspects of iron movement using the general iron-kinetics model shown in Fig. 44-8 [158, 166, 197–204]. After intravenous injection of a tracer amount of transferrin-bound radioactive iron (^{59}Fe), the amounts of radioactive iron in plasma, red blood cells, sacral bone marrow, liver, and spleen are determined at intervals. Study of normal subjects in this way leads to the following observations (Fig. 44-5).

Virtually all administered tracer radioactive iron initially moves rapidly from plasma to bone marrow, remaining there approximately 1 day. There is a small shunt of plasma transferrin through the liver and thoracic duct lymph, which contains approximately 2 percent of the plasma iron and turns over every half-hour (Fig. 44-6) [147, 201]. This shunt may be of special significance with respect to hepatic heme enzyme synthesis and breakdown, as well as storage iron

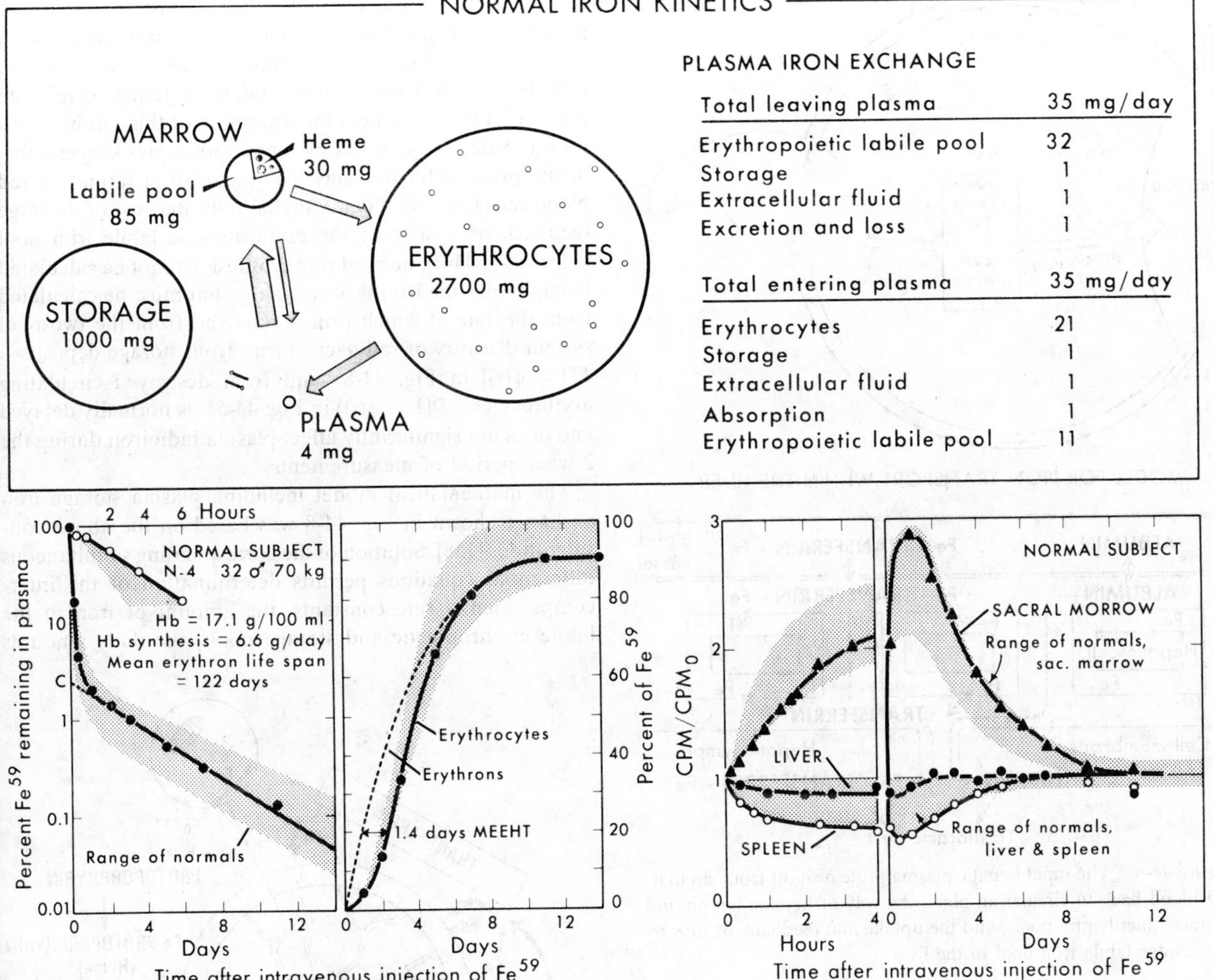

Figure 44-5. Quantitative aspects of normal iron kinetics, with distribution of iron in various compartments and measurements of radioiron in the plasma and erythrocytes and surface radioactivity, in a normal subject. The interrupted curve, showing cumulative fixation of radioiron in the erythrons, and the mean effective erythron hemoglobinization time (MEEHT) are calculated.

deposition and mobilization. During the next 5 to 7 days radioiron leaves the marrow and appears in circulating erythrocytes. After 4 to 8 hr, the initial rapid exponential rate of decrease of plasma radioiron diminishes progressively.

After approximately 2 days, a second, much slower exponential rate of radioiron decrease is established, which persists for the next 8 to 12 days (Fig. 44-5). This pattern indicates continuous feedback of radioactive iron from and equilibration with at least one other iron pool, and continuous removal of iron from both these pools.

Since virtually all plasma radioiron transfers to marrow, it seems plausible that feedback of radioactivity occurs from the marrow. This pool is designated "labile," in contrast to the relatively fixed iron stores. The existence of a labile pool is confirmed by several observations. Thus, measurements of canine marrow and rabbit and human reticulocytes demonstrated labile nonheme iron associated with the stroma of immature erythrons [44, 158, 201, 205, 206]. Electron microscopic observations have shown ferritin in normal human immature erythrons [207, 208], and microspectrographic studies of individual salamander erythrons showed that the ratio of nonheme iron (probably Fe^{++}) to hemoglobin iron exceeded 20 in the youngest cells but was approximately 2 from the time hemoglobin synthesis was one-third complete until maturity [209]. Recent studies by Zail, Charlton, Terrance, and Bothwell as well as by Primosigh and Thomas utilizing in vivo and in vitro studies of hu-

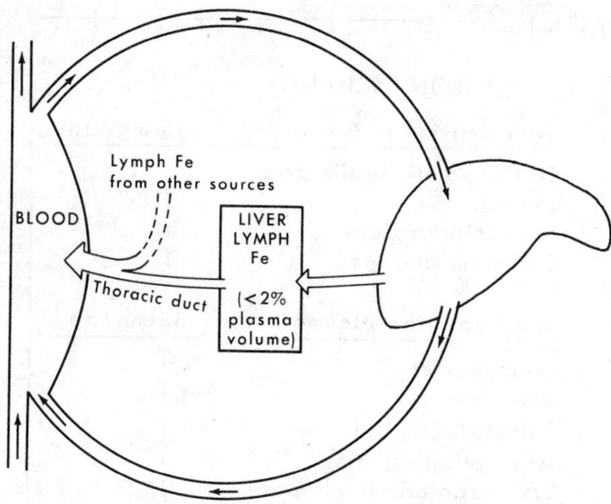

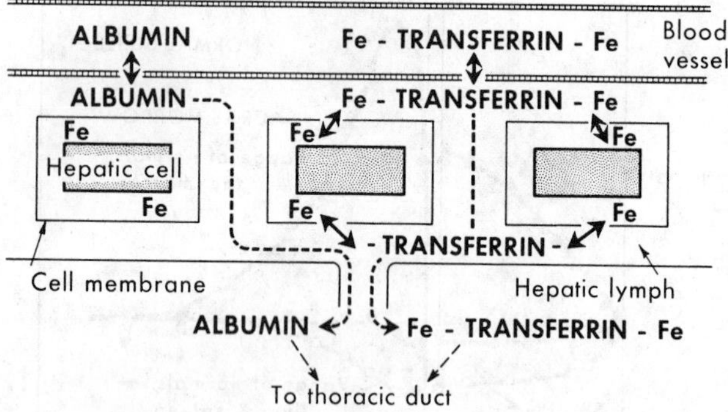

Figure 44-6. The rapid hepatic plasma protein shunt from circulating blood back to circulating blood, by way of hepatic lymph and thoracic duct lymph pools, and the uptake and feedback of iron by the storage labile iron pool in the liver.

man, canine, and rat marrow strongly suggest that erythron iron not required for hemoglobin synthesis is incorporated into ferritin [11, 12]. No evidence was obtained that erythron ferritin iron is a significant precursor of hemoglobin, as previously suggested by Mazur and Carleton on the assumption that ferritin was uniformly labeled with ^{59}Fe [41]. This was a questionable assumption, since iron-poor ferritin molecules incorporate transferrin-bound iron to a greater extent than iron-rich ferritin molecules [210]. Zail et al. demonstrated with incubation of human marrow that approximately one-quarter of the radioiron was incorporated into ferritin [11]. Since labeled ferritin could not be identified in the circulating red blood cells of a splenectomized human subject or splenectomized rat, it appears probable that ferritin normally leaves the cell during its maturation in the marrow, rather than in the spleen. This is consistent with the electron microscopic observations that ferritin can move freely between immature red blood cells and reticuloendothelial cells [207, 208]. Although Bessis originally suggested that the movement of ferritin was from reticuloendothelial cell to nucleated red blood cell, the validity of this interpretation is highly questionable [11]. Recent findings by Deiss and Cartwright have demonstrated the excretion of soluble ferritin from porcine siderotic reticulocytes into plasma [211]. Subsequent incorporation of this soluble ferritin into siderotic granules by blood monocytes suggests that in the marrow ferritin may also move from immature red blood cells into reticuloendothelial cells. Because of the large feedback of iron from the erythropoietic labile iron pool (Figs. 44-5, 44-7), hemoglobin synthesis cannot be calculated from the plasma iron turnover alone but must be calculated from the rate at which iron is removed from the two-pool system. Reentry of radioactive iron from storage deposits—$E[1 - \psi(t)]$ in Fig. 44-8—and from destroyed circulating erythrocytes—$D[1 - \phi(t)]$ in Fig. 44-5—is normally delayed and does not significantly affect plasma radioiron during the 2-week period of measurements.

The mathematical model including plasma storage iron exchange shown in Fig. 44-8 was based on the above considerations [158]. Solution of the corresponding simultaneous differential equations permits determination of the intercompartmental rate constants, the amount of iron in the labile erythropoietic and storage pools, the daily amounts

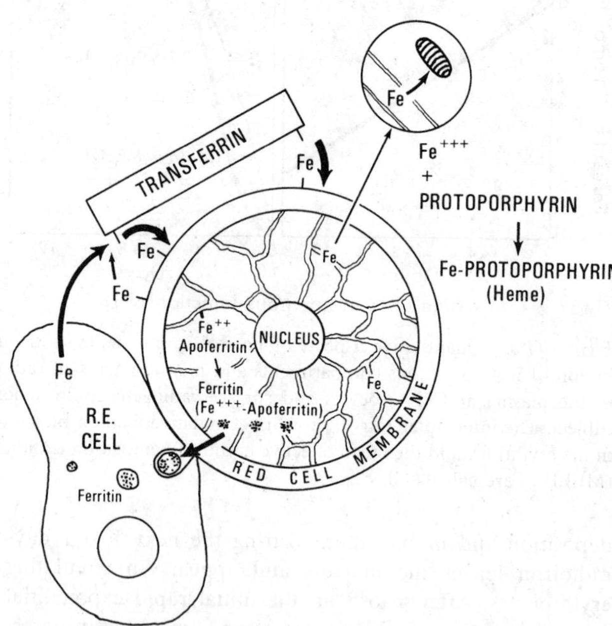

Figure 44-7. The erythropoietic labile iron pool in the stroma of immature erythrons. Transfer of iron is shown from and to transferrin, as well as irreversible incorporation of iron into heme after movement from the stroma into the cell interior. Iron not utilized for heme synthesis combines with apoferritin to form ferritin, which subsequently enters an adjacent reticuloendothelial cell from which the iron returns to transferrin. This feedback to transferrin of iron not utilized for hemoglobin synthesis occurs predominantly in the marrow. For some red cells, however, this feedback of "excess" iron to transferrin is completed by splenic RE cells after release as reticulocytes into the circulation.

of iron leaving the plasma and returning to plasma from the labile erythropoietic and storage pools, and the iron fixed in maturing erythrons for hemoglobin synthesis. Since nonhemoglobin iron in normal erythrocytes is negligible and 1 gm hemoglobin contains 3.4 mg iron, hemoglobin synthesis is readily calculated. Mean erythron life-span is calculated by relating daily hemoglobin synthesis to total body hemoglobin, as measured with ^{51}Cr- or ^{32}P-labeled red blood cells at the beginning and end of the 2-week period of study.

Movement of iron after it leaves the plasma is traced by measuring gamma-ray emission of radioiron over the sacrum (marrow), liver (representing tissue iron stores), and spleen. Data so obtained appear in Fig. 44-5. The surface radioactivity at any time is plotted as a ratio to extrapolated zero-time radioactivity, when all radioiron is in the plasma. The spleen and liver counting rates decrease as the marrow accumulates iron. Active uptake of iron persists beyond 4 hr. This decrease in spleen and liver counting ratios below unity signifies that their uptake of radioiron is less than the initial amount of radioiron contained in the relatively small volumes of plasma in these organs. It is apparent that the marrow is the principal accumulator of plasma iron. Subsequently, radioiron remains in the marrow near its peak level for approximately 1 day and then during the next 5 days rapidly leaves the marrow. During this period of radioiron decrease in the marrow, the simultaneous increases in splenic and hepatic radioactivity toward their initial levels indicate reappearance of radioiron circulating through these organs, but now in erythrocytes. It should be noted that this increase in splenic radioactivity is not greater than its preceding decrease. An increase in splenic radioactivity exceeding the previous decrease ($cpm/cpm_o > 1$) would indicate splenic sequestration and destruction of erythrocytes, characteristic of hemolytic anemia [198, 200, 202, 203]. Extramedullary erythropoiesis is present whenever the pattern of accumulation and release of radioiron characteristic of marrow occurs in spleen or liver [200, 202, 203].

As radioiron leaves the marrow, it reappears simultaneously in the blood within red blood cells. Figure 45-5 includes the curve obtained when the percentage of ^{59}Fe present in the total red blood cell mass is plotted as a function of time for a period of 2 weeks. Within the first week, when most of the radioiron has left the marrow, tracer iron is almost completely incorporated into circulating erythrocytes. Normally 85 to 100 percent of the removed plasma iron is incorporated into circulating erythrocytes. The rate of irreversible incorporation of radioiron into marrow erythrons, as calculated from analysis of plasma radioiron disappearance, is shown by the dotted line. The lag between irreversible incorporation of radioiron into marrow erythrons and its appearance within circulating erythrocytes is designated as *the mean effective erythron "hemoglobinization" time.* Normally, this period varies from 1.0 to 1.8 days; in this subject it is 1.4 days.

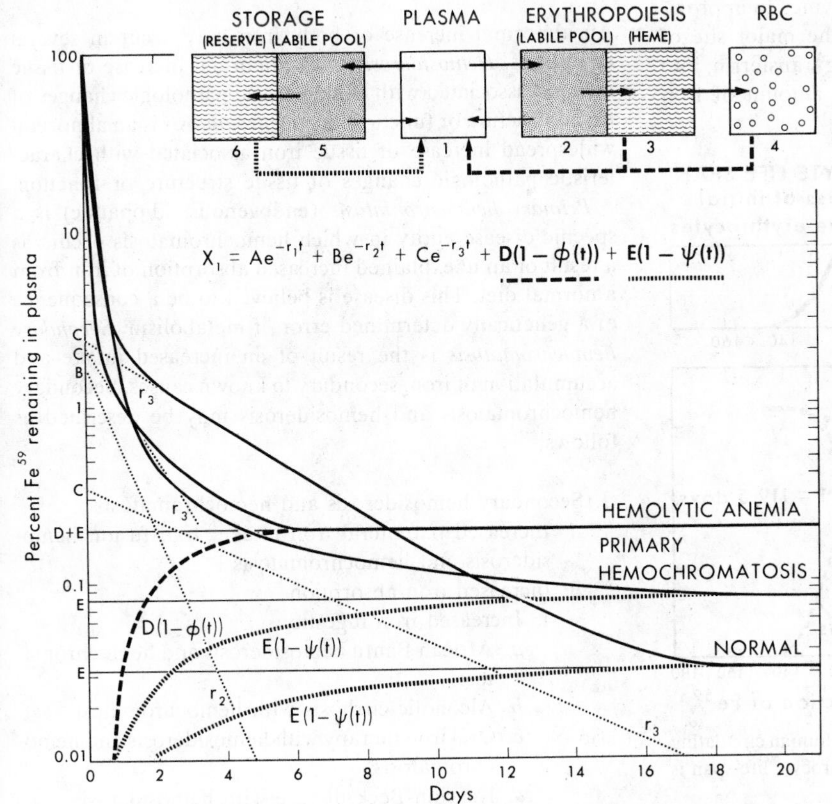

Figure 44-8. General iron-kinetics model. In normal subjects plasma radioiron equilibrates at a constant level after approximately 2 weeks as a result of the slow feedback of radioiron to the plasma from the reserve miscible storage iron pool, $E[1 - \psi(t)]$; patients with primary hemochromatosis similarly feed back radioiron from storage reserve, but to a greater degree, with a resultant higher level of radioiron equilibration. In patients with hemolytic anemia, however, plasma radioiron equilibrates relatively rapidly at a still higher level, this being a result of the hemolysis of maturing erythrons of circulating erythrocytes, $D[1 - \phi(t)]$. When plasma-to-storage iron exchange is greatly increased, as in patients with endogenous hemochromatosis or hypoplastic anemia, the intermediate exponential component (r_2, with intercept B) is markedly prolonged and must be used when applying the model.

After 7 to 10 days, the amount of erythrocyte radioiron remains constant for approximately 100 days (Fig. 44-9). Subsequently, as erythrocyte death occurs, erythrocyte radioiron decreases slowly. Because of reincorporation, erythrocyte radioiron, after reaching a minimum (in this subject at 122.5 days), increases to near its original value at 140 days. The amount of radioiron in circulating erythrocytes can be calculated from a normal distribution curve of erythrocyte longevity, assuming that after a given delay period reincorporation of radioiron proceeds as measured initially [212]. In this subject, the *calculated* amount of radioiron in erythrocytes (heavy line) is derived from the normal distribution curve shown in Fig. 44-9. In this way, the erythrocyte life-span *distribution* of this subject is determined, in addition to the mean life-span of 115.5 days.

The main pathways of normal iron transit and amounts of iron involved in various components of plasma iron exchange shown in Fig. 44-5 are based on many observations similar to those described above [158]. The main flow of iron is from plasma to marrow to erythrocytes and then, following death of the erythrocyte, back to plasma. Approximately 32 mg per day leaves the plasma for the marrow. Of this amount, 21 mg is fixed in red blood cells, while 11 mg returns to the plasma [158]. Plasma iron exchange from intestinal absorption and excretion in bile, urine, sweat, and from cell desquamation amounts to approximately 1 mg per day [45–47, 50, 63, 125], that from storage exchange approximately 1 mg per day [158], and from exchange with extracellular fluid, myoglobin, and heme enzymes to approximately 1 mg per day [158]. The liver is the major site of rapid shunting of plasma proteins, including transferrin, into thoracic duct lymph [147, 201]. The daily amount of iron

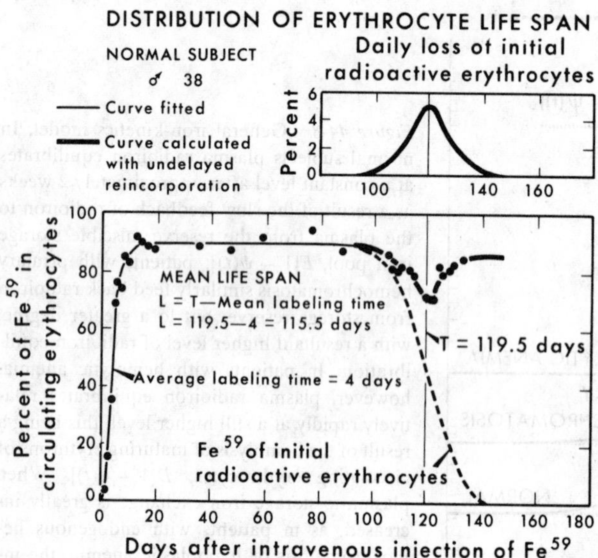

Figure 44-9. Net incorporation of ^{59}Fe in normal human circulating erythrocytes, from which the distribution of erythrocyte life-span is obtained.

involved in all these exchanges is approximately 10 percent of the mean daily amount of iron going to marrow (Fig. 44-5).

Although normally quite small, storage iron exchange is included in Fig. 44-5, since it may, in pathologic conditions, constitute a larger or even major fraction of plasma iron exchange. Though over 90 percent of iron leaving plasma enters erythropoietic marrow, only two-thirds of this is used in hemoglobin formation. The remainder reenters the plasma [158]. In Fig. 44-5 the area of each compartment corresponds to the amount of iron contained in it. Plasma iron exchange is not proportional to the amount of iron in the compartment involved. Storage iron reserve of 1,000 mg is approximately 25 percent of total iron, but storage iron exchange is less than 5 percent of total iron exchange. The erythropoietic labile pool, containing only 85 mg of iron, receives 90 percent of the iron leaving the plasma [158].

Whole-body counter measurements [213] have shown that 1 to 2 percent of iron leaving plasma becomes "fixed" in a compartment from which iron is removed slowly at a fractional rate of only 0.0046 per day. This corresponds to a half-time of approximately 150 days. This fixation and slow turnover occur even in the presence of iron deficiency anemia (Fig. 44-10). This suggests that this compartment may represent iron in myoglobin.

CLASSIFICATION AND DEFINITIONS

An abnormal increase of body iron may occur in several conditions. *Hemosiderosis* is an abnormal increase of tissue iron not associated with characteristic pathologic changes of tissue structure or function. *Hemochromatosis* is an abnormal widespread increase of tissue iron associated with characteristic pathologic changes of tissue structure or function.

Primary hemochromatosis (endogenous, idiopathic) is a specific disease entity in which hemochromatosis occurs as a result of an unexplained increased absorption of iron from a normal diet. This disease is believed to be a consequence of a genetically determined error of metabolism. *Secondary hemochromatosis* is the result of an increased intake and accumulation of iron, secondary to known causes. Secondary hemochromatosis and hemosiderosis may be described as follows:

I. Secondary hemosiderosis and hemochromatosis
   A. Increased parenteral iron intake: transfusion hemosiderosis and hemochromatosis
   B. Increased iron absorption
      1. Increased iron ingestion
         a. African Bantu hemosiderosis and hemochromatosis
         b. Alcoholic cirrhosis with hemochromatosis
         c. Oral iron therapy with hemosiderosis and hemochromatosis
         d. Kaschin-Beck disease with hemosiderosis

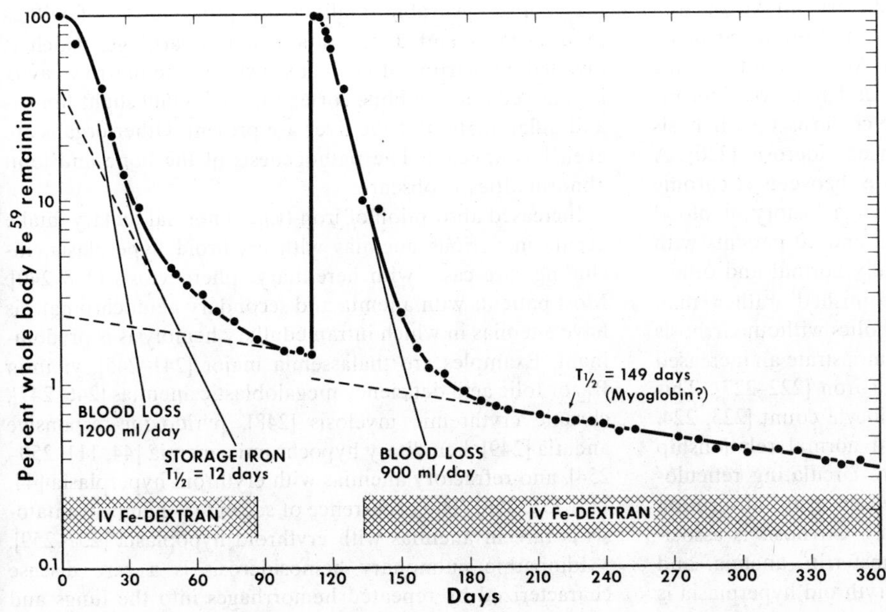

Figure 44-10. Fixation and slow turnover of iron derived from plasma transferrin in a nonhemoglobin, nonstorage compartment.

2. Increased iron absorption from a normal amount of dietary iron: anemia with erythroid hyperplasia

II. Focal hemosiderosis
  A. Idiopathic pulmonary hemosiderosis
  B. Renal hemosiderosis

Congenital and familial iron overload is a condition characterized by the intrauterine accumulation of excessive hepatic iron, as recently reported by Vitale and colleagues [214]. The abnormal amounts of hemosiderin in the liver were associated with very high serum iron concentration and saturation of transferrin; hemolysis, anemia, and unusual iron intake were absent. The iron overload present in these two neonatal sibs was also associated with hypotonia and minor congenital anomalies.

SECONDARY HEMOCHROMATOSIS AND HEMOSIDEROSIS

Transfusion therapy may add a considerable burden of iron to the body. Some patients with transfusion hemosiderosis develop hemochromatosis that may differ from primary hemochromatosis only in that hepatic damage is slight or absent [215–217]. Included in this group are patients with erythroid hypoplasia who have had more than 100 blood transfusions. These patients have received more than 25 gm parenteral iron, an amount comparable to that present in a patient with primary hemochromatosis, as hemoglobin. The iron absorbed from the gastrointestinal tract of such a patient probably constitutes only a small fraction of body iron [61, 178]. The transfusion iron overload initially is distributed predominantly in reticuloendothelial cells as a result of phagocytosis of nonviable transfused erythrocytes. This deposition appears to be relatively innocuous. In time, a variable degree of redistribution into parenchymal cells occurs which seems to determine the extent of supervening tissue damage.

Prolonged increased absorption of iron from the gastrointestinal tract results in an iron excess which is distributed predominantly in parenchymal cells. Secondary hemosiderosis and secondary hemochromatosis are relatively frequent in the adult African Bantu population as a result of a high daily dietary intake of iron. This often exceeds 100 mg per day, or approximately seven times the normal dietary requirement [61]. Most of this intake is obtained from the iron utensils they employ in cooking and in the preparation of alcoholic beverages, chiefly Kaffir beer. A similar distribution of iron develops in the relatively small number of Bantu who accumulate amounts of iron comparable to that found in primary hemochromatosis. These patients give a history of excessive alcohol intake and show decreased plasma transferrin concentrations with high transferrin saturations; in contrast are Bantu with hemosiderosis but no cirrhosis, in whom transferrin concentration is increased so that the percentage saturation is normal or only moderately raised in spite of a high plasma iron concentration [179, 218]. Tissue studies in vitro have shown that high saturation of transferrin increases the tissue uptake of iron [156], so that this mechanism may be involved in the widespread deposition of iron in epithelial cells of cirrhotic subjects. The anemia of cirrhosis with erythroid hyperplasia and associated increased iron absorption and turnover of reticuloendothelial iron may also be an important etiologic factor.

The relatively high incidence of hemochromatosis in subjects with alcoholic cirrhosis has been reemphasized during the last decade [219, 220]. Wines produced in Europe or the United States contain from 5 to 22 mg iron per liter

[219]. Cirrhosis and an increased dietary intake of iron probably occur in hemochromatosis with alcoholic cirrhosis, as well as in hemochromatosis of the African Bantu. In the Bantu much more iron is ingested, and massive siderosis precedes cirrhosis [179]; in alcoholic cirrhosis the cirrhosis precedes the development of advanced siderosis [220]. A recent comparison of hepatic iron stores between 41 chronic abusers of alcohol without cirrhosis or a history of blood loss, transfusions, or iron medication, and 20 patients with gallbladder disease but hematologically normal and otherwise healthy, indicated slightly diminished, rather than increased, iron stores in chronic alcoholics without cirrhosis [221]. Many patients with cirrhosis demonstrate an increased absorption of a standard oral dose of iron [222–227]. This increase is proportional to the reticulocyte count [223, 224, 228] and lies within the extrapolated normal relationship existing between iron absorption and circulating reticulocytes, as contrasted with the increased iron absorption observed in primary hemochromatosis. Cirrhosis is associated with inadequate circulating transferrin, anemia, and erythroid hyperplasia. Anemia with erythroid hyperplasia is associated with increased absorption of iron and widespread deposition of iron in epithelial cells, while insufficient transferrin to maintain adequate plasma latent iron-binding capacity also is associated with an increased epithelial deposition of iron [179]. These factors as well as increased dietary iron may be involved in the development of hemochromatosis secondary to alcoholic cirrhosis. A small fraction of cirrhotic patients who had undergone end-to-side portacaval anastomosis have subsequently developed marked hemosiderosis. Gastrointestinal absorption of iron has not been increased above preoperative levels [227, 229, 230]. The development of advanced hepatic siderosis appears to be largely the result of body iron redistribution. Why this occurs specifically in a few such patients is unknown. Possible explanations for such enhanced hepatic iron deposition include (1) decreased transferrin production with increased percentage saturation of transferrin, and (2) increased oxygenation of the liver consequent to exclusively arterial blood supply. Both these factors promote hepatic iron deposition.

Prolonged oral iron therapy in patients with anemia not secondary to iron deficiency may result in hemochromatosis [231–236]. It is apparent that the administration of iron to anemic patients with normal or increased stores of iron is needless and, if prolonged, may be harmful.

Kaschin-Beck disease is localized to several regions of Asia, especially in Manchuria, where the water and food have a high iron content (0.3 to 10 mg per liter) [237]. Although extensive deposition of iron pigment is found in all organs, supervening pathologic changes characteristic of hemochromatosis, such as cirrhosis or diabetes, have not been observed. The disease is characterized by recurrent attacks of polyarthritis in adolescence with symmetric joint deformities and shortness of stature. The small joints, especially the interphalangeal, are most seriously affected. The long bones may be symmetrically shortened but are not otherwise deformed as in rickets or chondrodystrophy. The major histologic abnormalities are proliferation of villous joint surfaces and degeneration of the cartilage, which is invaded by marrow of normal structure. The marrow cavity is enlarged and the bone cortex thinned. Only slight fibrosis and inflammation of the liver are present. Other organs are even less affected. The pathogenesis of the bone and joint abnormalities is obscure.

Increased absorption of iron from a normal dietary intake occurs in various anemias with erythroid hyperplasia, including rare cases with hereditary spherocytosis [238–240]. Most patients with anemia and secondary hemochromatosis have anemias in which intramedullary hemolysis is predominant. Examples are thalassemia major [241–245], vitamin B_{12} or folic acid deficiency megaloblastic anemias [246, 247], chronic erythremic myelosis [248], pyridoxine-responsive anemia [249], hereditary hypochromic anemia [44, 111, 250–254], and refractory anemias with erythroid hyperplasia [44, 111, 255, 256]. The occurrence of secondary hemochromatosis is rare in anemias with erythroid hypoplasia [257–259].

Idiopathic pulmonary hemosiderosis is a rare disease characterized by repeated hemorrhages into the lungs and hemosiderosis localized to the lungs [260, 261]. The pulmonary vessels are frequently defective in elastic fibers, but not in cases with recent onset [260, 262]. The frequent occurrence of glomerular nephritis and, in addition, occasionally associated eosinophilia, reticuloendothelial hyperplasia, mast cells, cold agglutinins, hemolysins, and necrotizing pulmonary arteritis suggest that the vascular lesions in the lung are frequently the consequence of antigen-antibody reactions that result in the rupture of small pulmonary blood vessels [263–275]. Massive amounts of hemosiderin are found in alveolar and interstitial macrophages. Several grams of iron localized in the lungs may exceed the normal amount of total body iron. By contrast, iron deposits are absent from all other organs. Iron-kinetics studies have demonstrated that the anemia, which frequently is severe during bouts of pulmonary hemorrhage, is the result of iron deficiency and hemorrhage, i.e., chronic and acute blood loss [276]. Hemolysis and splenic destruction of erythrocytes are absent. As shown in Fig. 44-11, much, if not all, of the erythrocyte iron extravasated into the lungs is fixed as hemosiderin in pulmonary tissue macrophages and is unavailable to transferrin for transport to the marrow for hemoglobin synthesis.

Renal hemosiderosis occurs whenever there is persistent glomerular filtration of free hemoglobin. This is usually the result of an intravascular hemolysis which releases hemoglobin into the blood at a rate which exceeds the binding capacity of circulating haptoglobin and albumin. The tubular reabsorption of hemoglobin from the glomerular filtrate is accompanied by degradation of hemoglobin and storage of the iron as ferritin in the tubular cells. Persistence of this process results in tubular deposition of hemosiderin, which may be found in the desquamated tubular cells of the urinary sediment. Thus persistent intravascular hemolysis associated with various anemias, such as paroxysmal nocturnal hemoglobinuria, acquired hemolytic anemias (idiopathic, autoimmune, or isoimmune), and occasionally pernicious

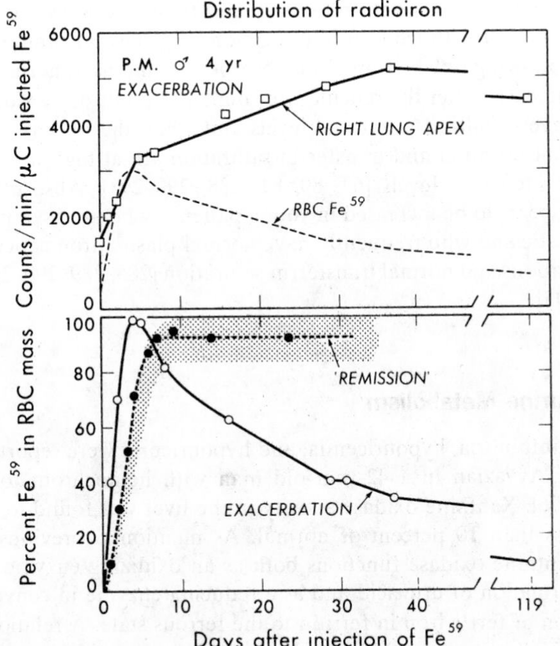

Figure 44-11. Distribution of iron removed from plasma during exacerbation (and remission) in a patient with idiopathic pulmonary hemosiderosis. Increasing pulmonary radioactivity while radioactivity in the blood decreases suggests continuing pulmonary hemorrhage, which comprised at least two-thirds of the blood volume within the month.

anemia, will result in hemoglobinemia, hemoglobinuria, and hemosiderinuria [277, 278]. Persistence of intense renal siderosis does not impair renal function. This lack of damage may be ascribed to the normal rapid turnover of tubular cells. As shown in Fig. 44-12, renal radioactivity derived from ^{59}Fe-erythrocytes reaches a maximum in approximately 18 days, with a half-time of 6 days. This indicates a tubular cell functional life-span of approximately 9 days.

In patients with porphyria cutanea tarda a curious association exists between mild iron overload, storage iron increased to approximately 1.5 to 7.0 gm with a mean of 3.5 gm (normal, 0.5 to 1.5 gm), and the manifestations of skin fragility and blister formation in sun-exposed areas, hirsutism, hyperpigmentation, sclerodermoid changes, and excretion of large amounts of uroporphyrin in the urine and stool. After the removal of 1 to 7 gm (mean, 2 gm) of iron by venesection, urinary uroporphyrin excretion fell below 1 mg per day, and all the above-mentioned manifestations disappeared within several months after treatment was discontinued [279–282]. Although porphyria cutanea tarda is frequently associated with alcoholism [283], in many cases alcoholism is absent [281]. Since these patients are not anemic, the mild increase of iron stores is not readily explained in the nonalcoholic patients. Possibly an increased retention and consequent abnormal deposition of iron in the liver are related to the defective hepatic metabolism, which produces excessive uroporphyrin in the liver. The mechanism of the beneficial effect of phlebotomy is not clear, but the therapeutic results suggest that the accumulation of iron together with porphyrins in the liver cells may exacerbate the underlying cellular biochemical defect (see Chap. 45).

PRIMARY HEMOCHROMATOSIS

Iron Metabolism

Patients with primary hemochromatosis may accumulate 20 to 60 gm iron during a 50-year period [6]. Most of the iron is deposited in tissues as hemosiderin. As excessive tissue

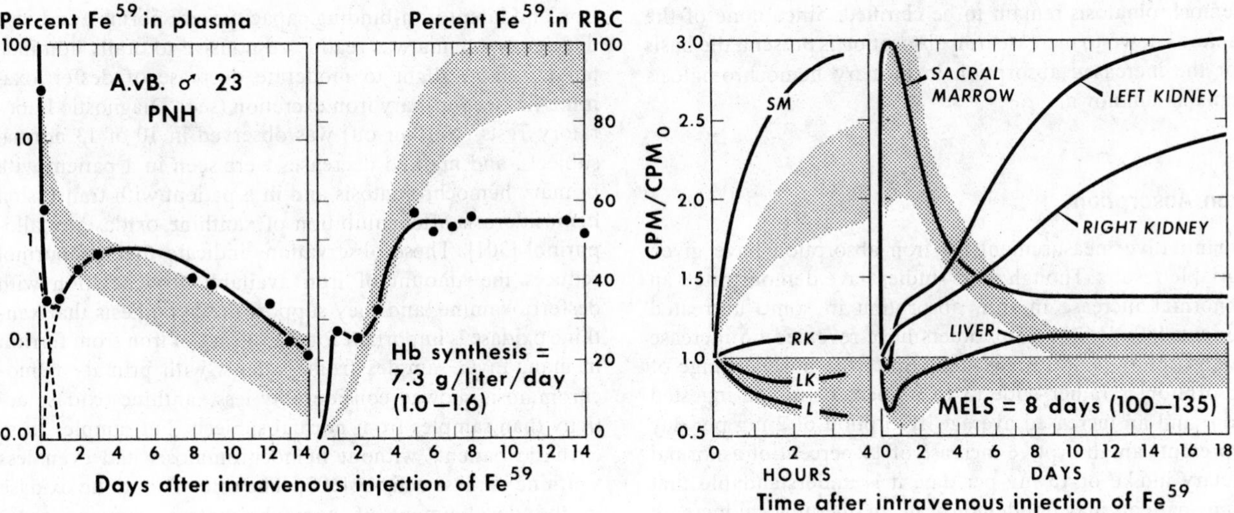

Figure 44-12. Distribution of iron removed from plasma in a patient with paroxysmal nocturnal hemoglobinuria.

iron accumulates, there is a progressive increase in the proportion of hemosiderin. The normal ratio of hemosiderin to ferritin iron is approximately 0.9; in primary or secondary hemochromatosis this ratio is increased to between 4 and 11 [15, 23]. In order to accumulate this massive amount of iron it is evident that a positive iron balance of approximately 2 mg per day must have been present for several decades. This implies that iron absorption is increased to an average of approximately 4.0 mg per day, since iron loss in patients with primary hemochromatosis is increased to approximately 2.0 mg per day. Dietary intake of iron is usually normal [6, 283]. Anemia, increased erythropoiesis, and hypoxia are usually absent. Pancreatic function is normal [6, 283]. Plasma iron-binding capacity is not increased. On the contrary and characteristically, total iron-binding capacity is decreased; also the latent iron-binding capacity is much reduced or absent, and plasma iron concentration is abnormally high, i.e., greater than 170 μg per 100 ml (Fig. 44-3). A glycoprotein in gastric juice was detected by Davis and colleagues and designated by them as gastroferrin [86, 87]. Using their method of in vitro assay of gastric juice, they found a striking reduction of gastroferrin in patients with iron deficiency anemia and primary hemochromatosis [92, 92*a* and *b*], which indicated that gastroferrin inhibits iron absorption by producing a poorly absorbed iron chelate, and suggested that defective production of gastroferrin is the basic genetic defect in patients with primary hemochromatosis. Wynter and Williams, however, were not able to confirm these observations, finding no significant difference between the gastroferrin concentration in gastric juice of control subjects and in that of patients with primary hemochromatosis [92*c* and *d*]. Employing an improved assay method and simultaneous whole-body counter measurement of iron absorption in collaboration with Davis and Saltman, we, too, have been unable to confirm the observations of Davis and colleagues [44]. The function of gastroferrin in iron absorption and its possible significance in primary hemochromatosis remain to be clarified. Since none of the factors known to increase iron absorption is present, the basis for the increased absorption in primary hemochromatosis remains unknown.

Iron Absorption

Quantitative measurements of iron absorption have given variable results. Though most studies have demonstrated an abnormal increase in iron absorption in some untreated patients [80, 81, 284–286], others have revealed no increase in absorption [63, 223, 287–289]. Since the normal range of absorption is rather wide (3 to 22 percent of the ingested iron) and an increased average absorption of 2 mg per day represents an absorptive increase of 13 percent of a normal dietary intake of 15 mg per day, it is understandable that many patients may not demonstrate an unequivocal increase of iron absorption. It also appears that in the later stages of the disease, when transferrin and the mucosa are highly saturated with iron, iron absorption is somewhat inhibited. Following phlebotomy, iron absorption remains abnormally increased after the reticulocyte count and erythrocyte values have stabilized at normal levels and when the plasma iron concentration and transferrin saturation are at high normal or increased levels [63, 80, 81, 288, 290–293]. Absorption appears to be increased in young patients, who are asymptomatic and who frequently have normal plasma iron concentrations and normal transferrin saturation [285, 289, 290, 294, 295].

Purine Metabolism

Xanthinuria, hypouricemia, and hypouricuria were reported by Ayvazian in a 42-year-old man with hemochromatosis [296]. Xanthine oxidase activity in the liver was found to be less than 10 percent of normal. As mentioned previously, xanthine oxidase functions both as an oxidizing enzyme in formation of uric acid and as a reducing enzyme in conversion of ferric iron in ferritin to the ferrous state. A relationship between xanthine oxidase insufficiency and excessive iron storage was postulated by the author. Such a relationship, even if causal in this case, is apparently not general. Uric acid values have been normal in all other reported patients [296], and two other known patients with xanthinuria have not shown abnormalities of iron metabolism. The lack of evidence of hemochromatosis in the 4-year-old girl of Dent and Philpot [297], even when restudied at age 9 [298], is not necessarily compelling evidence against an association of xanthinuria and hemochromatosis, in view of the absence of clinically demonstrable hemochromatosis below the age of 20. A similar argument may be applied in the instance of the 29-year-old woman with xanthinuria reported by Watts et al. [299, 300], in view of the rarity of hemochromatosis in premenopausal women. In this patient serum iron and latent iron-binding capacity were normal, and iron deficiency anemia was readily responsive to orally administered iron. A slight to moderate decrease of desferrioxamine-induced urinary iron excretion (see "Diagnostic Laboratory Tests," further on) was observed in 10 of 13 normal subjects, and marked decreases were seen in a patient with primary hemochromatosis and in a patient with transfusion hemosiderosis after inhibition of xanthine oxidase by allopurinol [301]. These observations indicate that allopurinol reduces the amount of iron available for chelation with desferrioxamine, and they support the hypothesis that xanthine oxidase is important for the release of iron from ferritin in man. Liver samples from patients with primary hemochromatosis showed considerably less xanthine oxidase activity than samples from normal subjects, but samples from cirrhotic patients without hemochromatosis had even less xanthine oxidase activity [302]. The role of xanthine oxidase in the development of hemochromatosis remains questionable.

Iron Overload

Whether iron, per se, in sufficient amount will produce hemochromatosis is unsettled. Massive iron overload alone in animals has not resulted in the production of tissue damage resembling that seen in primary hemochromatosis. These studies have been of short duration (1 to 4 years), compared to the decades required for the development of primary hemochromatosis in man. In rats fed a lipotrope-deficient diet with excessive iron which produced fatty livers with cirrhosis, a pattern of iron distribution resembling that in hemochromatosis developed within several months. Administration of choline or folic acid prevented or slowed the development of cirrhosis and limited the presence of excess iron to liver cells [303, 304]. Although hemochromatosis secondary to multiple transfusions occurs in some patients, many others receiving a greater number of transfusions have no evidence of tissue damage. Tissue damage appears to be correlated with the location of iron in cells other than those of the reticuloendothelial system [6]. Iron within reticuloendothelial cells appears to be innocuous. Though the capacity of the reticuloendothelial system is great, a combination of massive iron accumulation for a long period of time and a marked decrease of plasma latent iron-binding capacity, i.e., transferrin saturation, leads to deposition of iron in other tissues, and results in cellular damage.

Iron Kinetics

Iron kinetics in patients with primary hemochromatosis is characterized by a much increased plasma-to-storage iron exchange. Iron kinetics of a nonanemic patient with primary hemochromatosis is shown in Fig. 44-13.

The slow feedback of radioiron from storage reserve—$E[1 - \psi(t)]$ from compartment 6, Fig. 44-8—is shown as a dashed curve increasing toward its asymptote. The plasma radioiron curve can be resolved into three distinct exponentials, which indicate considerable plasma-to-storage iron exchange. Measurement of the three slopes and the zero-time intercepts permits quantitation of the iron kinetics. Hemoglobin synthesis (6 gm per day) and mean erythron life-span (110 days) are normal in this patient. Measurements in vivo show an initial accumulation of radioiron in the liver as well as in the marrow (Fig. 44-13). Subsequently, liver accumulation continues and finally remains constant at a high level. These findings indicate increased plasma-to-storage iron exchange. The incorporation of radioiron into circulating erythrocytes is correspondingly low.

The Kinetics Abnormality

The main pathways of iron transit and the compartments and rates of iron transfer in patients with primary hemochromatosis appear in Fig. 44-13. The principal abnormal finding is a ten-to twentyfold increase in the movement of iron from plasma to storage, i.e., 20 mg per day. This metabolic abnormality is associated with a thirtyfold increase in storage iron, to about 40,000 mg. The increase in plasma-to-storage iron exchange is not merely a passive consequence of the size of the storage pool but is largely the result of an active affinity of storage cells for iron. This is suggested by the iron-kinetics studies of patients with primary hemochromatosis and postphlebotomy iron deficiency anemia. Four such studies have been performed, and in all four patients findings were similar to the following: In a male patient with primary hemochromatosis and iron deficiency anemia resulting from systematic venesection therapy [305], a sixfold increase in the movement of iron from plasma to storage (6 mg per day) was measured (Fig. 44-14). Body-surface measurements in this patient disclosed a rapid net hepatic uptake and release of plasma radioiron (not observed previously in patients with iron deficiency anemia or non-hemochromatotic patients with cirrhosis and iron deficiency, as shown in Figs. 44-15, 44-16) at a rate corresponding closely to the rate constant ($\alpha_{51} = 11.4$ per day, $t\frac{1}{2} = 1.46$ hr) of feedback from the storage labile iron pool ($X_5 = 0.52$ mg) to the plasma ($X_1 = 1.06$ mg). These values were derived by mathematic analysis of plasma radioiron measurements; the calculated rate of storage feedback corresponds closely to the measured release of hepatic radioiron (Fig 44-14). It is remarkable that the hepatic cells in this patient were able to remove iron from the plasma at six times the normal rate in spite of a slightly increased marrow uptake of plasma iron (36 mg per day) and in spite of complete absence of storage iron deposits, a low plasma iron concentration of 38 μg per 100 ml, and transferrin saturation of only 10 percent. This abnormal tissue avidity for iron may be an inherited disorder which results in increased absorption of iron in persons with primary hemochromatosis. These findings would be compatible with impaired release of iron from ferric ferritin to plasma transferrin.

The storage iron which equilibrates with plasma iron within a month is probably in the form of ferritin and comprises approximately one-eighth of total storage iron (Fig. 44-13). The storage labile iron pool is a small fraction of the stores (16 mg); yet it contains more than twice the iron in the plasma (7 mg). Increases in the plasma and erythrocyte labile iron (110 mg) pools produce only slight changes in the iron kinetics involved in erythropoiesis. Patients with superimposed hemolysis associated with congestive splenomegaly secondary to cirrhosis show splenic sequestration together with destruction of red blood cells and compensatory increases in erythropoiesis (Fig. 44-17).

Clinical Features

Primary hemochromatosis is a rare disorder of worldwide distribution which tends to be rarer in areas where iron deficiency is common. It is diagnosed once in approximately

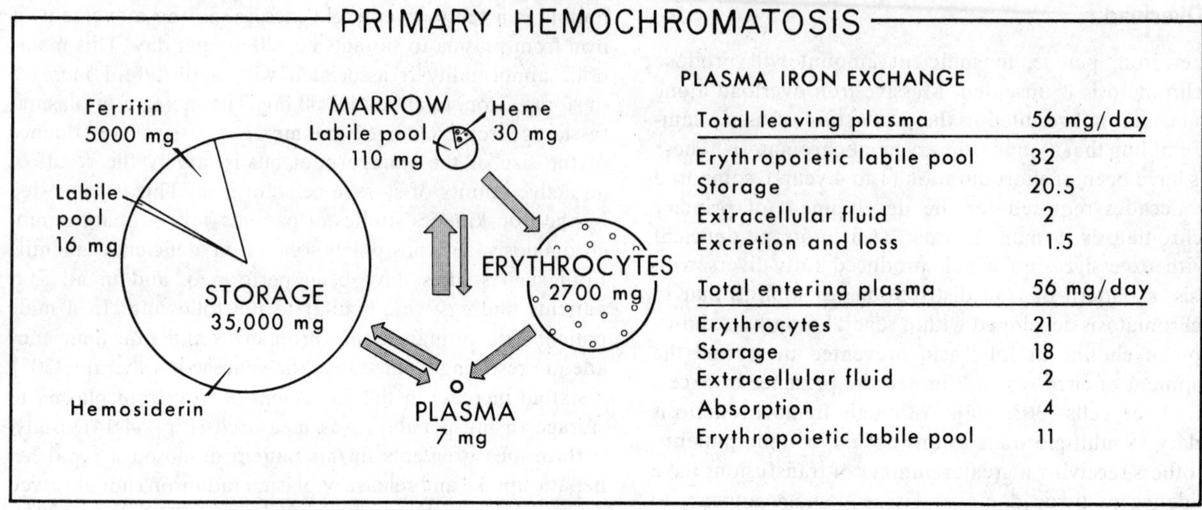

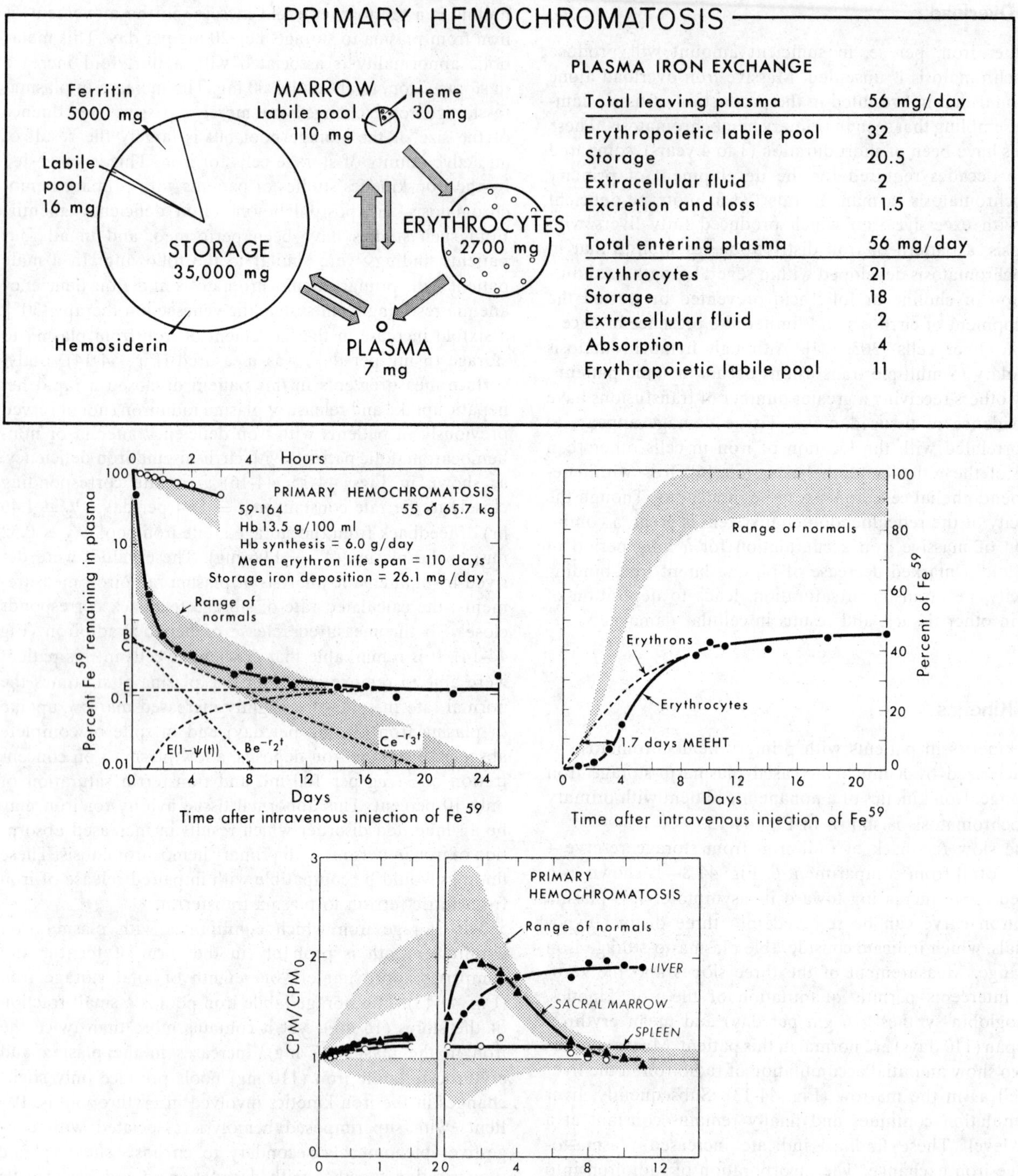

Figure 44-13. Quantitative aspects of iron kinetics in patients with primary hemochromatosis, with distribution of iron in various compartments. Radioiron in the plasma, erythrocytes, and surface radioactivity are shown in a patient with primary hemochromatosis. The interrupted curve, showing cumulative fixation of radioiron in the erythrons, and the mean effective erythron hemoglobinization time (MEEHT) are calculated.

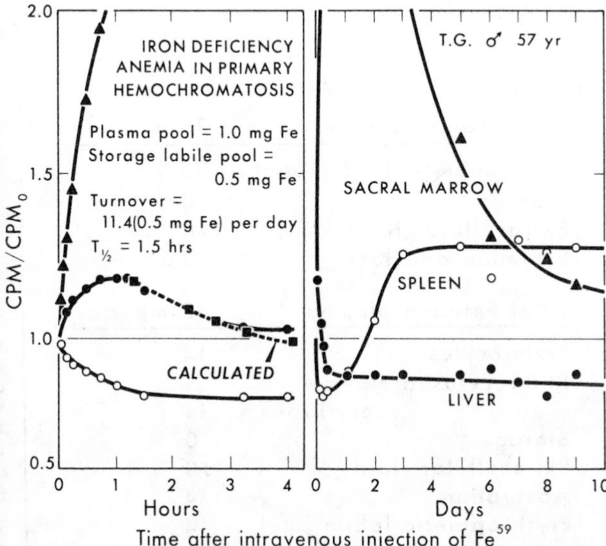

Figure 44-14. Body surface radioactivity in a patient with primary hemochromatosis and iron deficiency anemia (therapeutically induced). The interrupted hepatic curve shown between 1 and 4 hr (almost completely superimposed upon the measured hepatic curve) is a plot of the storage labile iron pool ($X_5 = 0.5$ mg) washout rate ($\alpha_{51} = 11.4$ per day) calculated from analysis of plasma radioiron data ($\alpha_{56} = X_6 = 0$).

7,000 hospital deaths [306–308] and once in approximately 20,000 hospital admissions [307, 309, 310]. These figures suggest that in the United States there are approximately 20,000 persons with primary hemochromatosis, and most of them are in the asymptomatic period during which the gradual accumulation of body iron occurs. This prehemochromatotic phase is rarely recognized, since physical findings are normal and the only laboratory abnormalities are increased tissue iron demonstrated by biopsy, increased absorption of radioiron, and possibly an elevation of plasma iron concentration.

The clinical aspects of primary hemochromatosis have been described in detail by Sheldon [5], von Heilmeyer [286], Finch and Finch [6], and others [283, 309, 311].

Clinical Course

Most patients with primary hemochromatosis become symptomatic between the ages of 40 and 60 years (80 percent after the age of 40). Unequivocal cases below the age of 13 have not been reported. This prolonged asymptomatic prelude to hemochromatosis is understandable in terms of the many years required to accumulate 20 to 60 gm iron by absorption from a normal dietary intake of 15 mg per day. Since the average woman loses approximately 10 to 35 gm iron during her lifetime as the result of menstruation, pregnancy, and lactation, it is understandable that hemochromatosis is 10 to 20 times more common in men than in women and that its onset is delayed in women. Approximately 50 percent of all women with this disorder give a history of scanty or absent menses. Onset of hemochromatosis between the ages of 20 and 30 years occurs in approximately 4 percent of reported patients. Without proper venesection therapy (discussed later), patients in this small group have a fulminating course and an average survival of 1 to 2 years, as compared with an average survival of approximately 5 years when symptoms begin between the ages of 30 and 60 years [61, 312].

Initial Symptoms

These are usually related to the classic triad of cirrhosis, skin pigmentation, and diabetes. The most frequent initial complaints are weight loss, weakness, lassitude and malaise, and loss of libido, in order of decreasing frequency of occurrence. These complaints are usually related to the presence of diabetes, hypopituitarism, or cirrhosis. One or more of these symptoms are present in virtually all patients. Skin pigmentation increases gradually. The distribution is similar to that of sunlight pigmentation, so that it is unnoticed by the majority of patients. Ascites is reported infrequently as a late complication of cirrhosis. Dyspnea and edema resulting from cardiac failure are also infrequent initial symptoms but carry a grave prognosis and appear in approximately half the relatively small number of patients (20 percent) between ages 20 and 40 years. Cardiac symptoms frequently develop rapidly in a few days and may progress to extreme degrees of congestion and peripheral edema that frequently are resistant to cardiotherapeutic measures [313].

Physical Signs

Hepatomegaly and increased skin pigmentation are the earliest signs to develop and are almost invariably present in symptomatic patients. Hepatic enlargement usually exists for many years prior to the development of laboratory evidence or symptoms of liver dysfunction and fibrosis. The liver is usually firm, smooth, and nontender. Portal hypertension is usually only slight or moderate, so that esophageal varices and ascites are much less common complications of primary hemochromatosis than of Laennec's cirrhosis. Palpable splenomegaly of moderate degree occurs in approximately half the symptomatic patients.

Gynecomastia, loss of body hair, fine hair with female distribution, soft and atrophic skin that is frequently dry and finely desquamating, and palmar erythema and spider angiomas may all be related to hepatic impairment. Testicular atrophy (resulting in loss of libido, loss of body hair, and weakness) may be the result of liver disease or, more probably, of pituitary hypofunction, rather than of the slight deposition of hemosiderin in the testes.

The pigmentation in naturally light-skinned patients is usually a peculiar grayish metallic or dark tan. The tan bronzing is largely the result of increased melanin deposition in

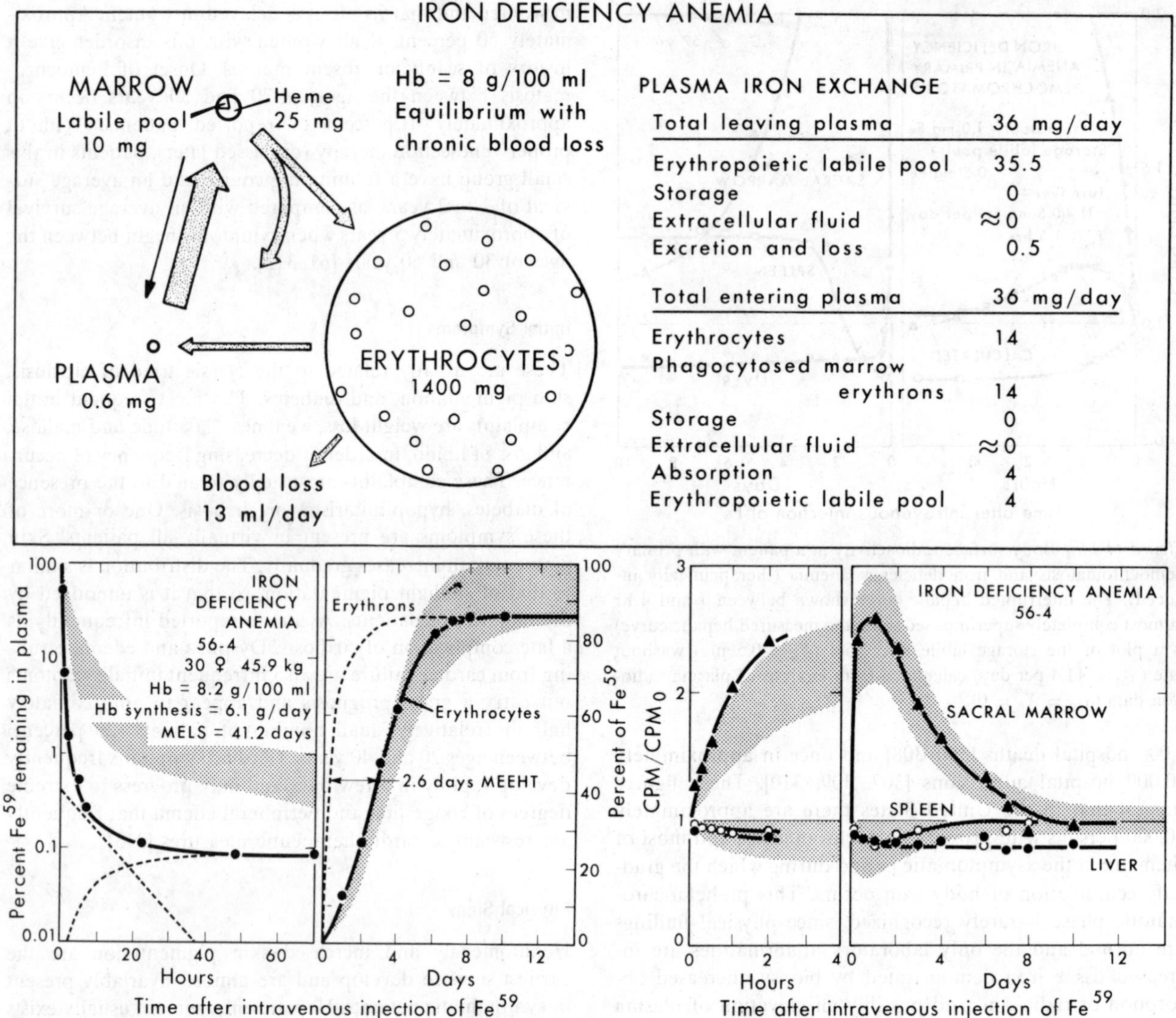

Figure 44-15. Quantitative aspects of iron kinetics in patients with iron deficiency anemia, with distribution of iron in various compartments. Radioiron in the plasma, erythrocytes, and surface radioactivity are shown in a patient with iron deficiency anemia. The interrupted curve, showing cumulative fixation of radioiron in the erythrons, and the mean effective erythron hemoglobinization time (MEEHT) are calculated.

the skin, not iron; but increased iron deposition may also occur with an associated metallic gray. "Slate gray" and "bronze" are terms frequently used to describe the peculiar sheen and hue of the skin. The pigment, although generalized, is usually darker on the face and neck, dorsum of the forearms and hands, lower part of the legs, genital and axillary regions, nipples, and in scars.

Roentgenographic Examinations

Occasionally these may demonstrate an increased radiographic density of the liver because of its high iron content and, to a greater extent, nonfatty increase of mass. The hepatic opacity may be sufficient to produce a sharp line appearing just below the shadow of the right side of the diaphragm.

Heart Findings

Congestive failure and cardiac arrhythmias may develop as a result of damage from the progressive myocardial hemosiderosis. In congestive failure both ventricles are dilated. The roentgenographic shadow of the heart is globular and resembles that observed with pericardial effusion. The rate of deposition of hemosiderin may be an important factor in determining the degree of cardiac damage, since heart

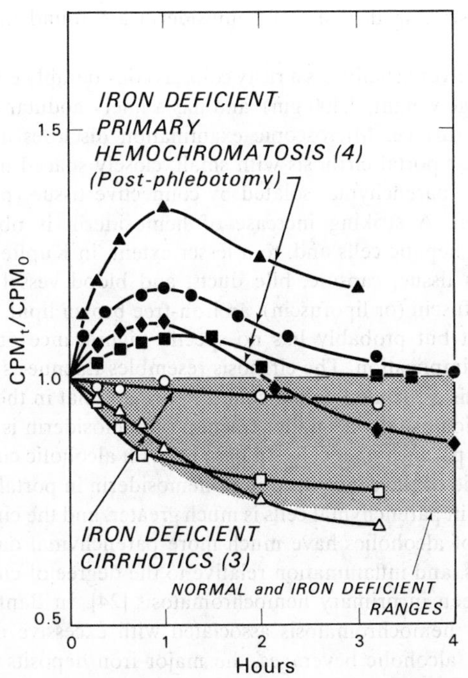

Figure 44-16. Hepatic iron kinetics after administration of radioiron to four patients with iron-deficient primary hemochromatosis and to three patients with cirrhosis and iron deficiency.

disease is common in younger subjects in whom symptoms may develop suddenly. Cardiac arrhythmia is an ominous sign. Ventricular extrasystoles or paroxysmal auricular tachycardia are the most common disturbances. Response to cardiac therapy is usually only transient. Since the use of insulin, cardiac failure has become the leading single cause of death. Approximately one-third of the patients die in congestive heart failure.

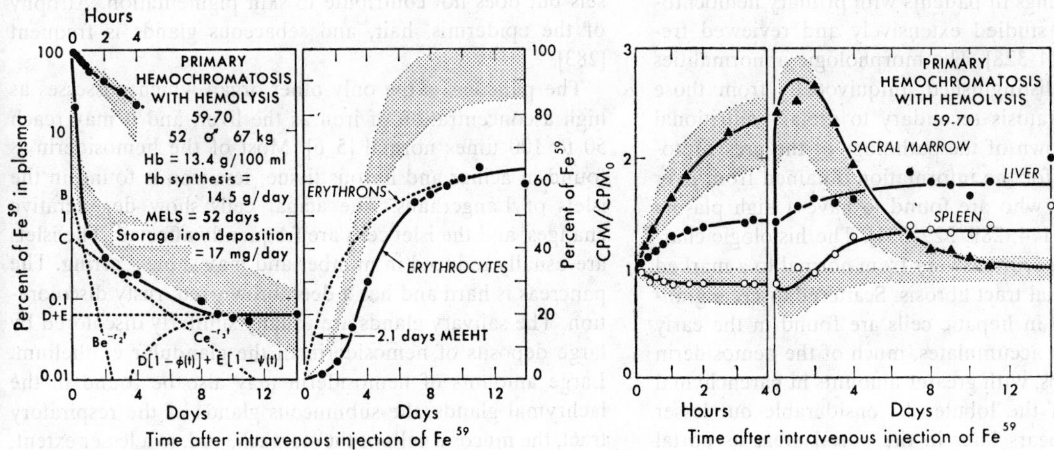

Figure 44-17. Radioiron in plasma and erythrocytes, and surface radioactivity in a patient with primary hemochromatosis and mild hemolysis. Plasma radioiron stabilizes at a constant level within 9 days as a result of the hemolytic component $D[1 - \phi(t)]$ superimposed upon the more gradual storage feedback component $E[1 - \psi(t)]$.

Pituitary Function

The characteristic symptoms of weakness, lassitude, and loss of libido encountered in patients with primary hemochromatosis are also characteristically present in panhypopituitarism. Although occasional reports of pituitary deficiency in primary hemochromatosis have appeared since 1933 [314–318], only recently has pituitary function been investigated in an unselected group of 15 patients. Stocks and Martin have reported that only 6 of the 15 patients had no evidence of pituitary dysfunction as determined by the measurement of urinary gonadotropins, plasma luteinizing hormones, the responses of plasma cortisol and plasma human growth hormone to hypoglycemic stress, plasma protein-bound iodine and response to TSH (thyroid-stimulating hormone), plasma testosterone, and 24-hr total urinary estrogens. Pituitary growth hormone and ACTH (adrenocorticotropic hormone) responses were abnormal in 9 and 6 patients, respectively. Six patients had absent or low gonadotropins, and two had TSH deficiency with hypothyroidism. Four patients had severe hypopituitarism with the typical clinical features and demonstrable failure of three trophic hormones [319]. These findings suggest that hypopituitarism is a frequent complication of primary hemochromatosis.

Arthropathy

The occurrence of a specific arthropathy was first suggested in 1964 by Schumacher, on the basis of his studies of two patients with hemochromatosis [320]. Subsequent systematic joint studies in unselected patients with primary hemochromatosis [321, 322] reveal a characteristic arthropathy in approximately half the 60 patients investigated. There was progressive polyarthritis, usually beginning in the metacarpophalangeal joints, with severe pain and disability. Approximately half the arthritic patients had acute episodes of inflammatory arthritis, apparently associated with the liberation into the joint fluid of calcium pyrophosphate crystals. These crystals were also responsible for the frequent radiographic finding of articular chondrocalcinosis, occurring most often in the menisci of the knee, the articular hyaline cartilage of the pubis, symphysis and the triangular ligament of the wrist. In general, patients with hemochromatosis who develop arthritis are older and have had the disease longer than those without arthritis. Although hemosiderin may be present in synovium and, less commonly, in articular cartilage [5, 320, 323], it may be absent in venesected patients with progressive arthropathy. The precise relationship of the arthritis to excessive iron deposition is obscure. Unfortunately, venesection therapy does not result in improvement of arthritis. In some patients arthritis develops after excess iron has been removed, possibly the irreversible consequence of previously induced damage to articular cartilage.

Other Systems

Pain in the extremities, cutaneous hyperesthesia, muscle tenderness, and leg cramps occur as late complications. Muscular weakness and atrophy and diminished tendon reflexes may be present. These findings are not infrequently attributable to diabetic neuritis. Psychic disturbances may appear and may be related to the deposition of iron in various areas of the brain.

Hematologic, renal, biliary, and gastric functions are usually normal.

Pathology

The pathologic findings in patients with primary hemochromatosis have been studied extensively and reviewed frequently [5, 6, 61, 324–328]. The morphologic abnormalities cannot always be distinguished uniquivocally from those seen in hemochromatosis secondary to dietary nutritional disease. Little is known of the pathology of the presymptomatic stages except for the information obtained from liver biopsies of relatives who are found to have a high plasma iron concentration [174, 289, 329–331]. The histologic characteristics of these specimens vary from normal to a marked iron excess with portal tract fibrosis. Scattered discrete granules of hemosiderin in hepatic cells are found in the early stages. As more iron accumulates, much of the hemosiderin coalesces into clumps, with greater amounts in parenchymal cells at the edge of the lobule. A considerable but lesser amount of iron appears later in the portal areas as portal tract fibrosis develops. Characteristic fully developed portal cirrhosis occurs only in association with symptomatic disease. During the earlier stages of the disease almost all the excess iron is localized to the liver, in contrast to the late stages, when striking deposits of hemosiderin are found in many organs.

The liver usually has a rusty color, is considerably enlarged (average weight, 2,400 gm), and has a finely nodular ("hobnail") surface. Microscopic examination discloses a finely granular portal cirrhosis with small, closely spaced nodules of liver parenchyma isolated by connective tissue (pseudolobules). A striking increase of hemosiderin is observed within hepatic cells and, to a lesser extent, in Kupffer cells, fibrous tissue, capsule, bile ducts, and blood vessel walls. Hemofuscin (or lipofuscin), an iron-free brown lipid, is also present but probably has no specific significance or diagnostic implication. The cirrhosis resembles Laennec's portal cirrhosis associated with alcoholism, except that in the latter condition usually a smaller fraction of hemosiderin is found within parenchymal cells. In patients with alcoholic cirrhosis the ratio of the concentration of hemosiderin in portal tissue to that in parenchymal cells is much greater, and the cirrhotic livers of alcoholics have much more parenchymal damage, fibrosis, and inflammation relative to the degree of cirrhosis than seen in primary hemochromatosis [24]. In Bantu secondary hemochromatosis associated with excessive dietary iron in alcoholic beverages, the major iron deposits are in Kupffer cells and portal tract phagocytes, not in parenchymal cells [332]. Primary hepatoma is found three times more frequently (approximately one patient in seven) than in Laennec's cirrhosis; cholangiomas have been observed rarely [326].

The skin usually contains increased deposits of melanin in the deepest layers of the epidermis and in the Malpighian cells of the corium. To a lesser degree hemosiderin also frequently contributes to the grossly observable increase in pigmentation (approximately 50 percent of cases) [283]. Hemosiderin is most prominent in the corium near or within the sweat gland cells. The hemofuscin is present in small amounts in the corium and in the walls of blood vessels but does not contribute to skin pigmentation. Atrophy of the epidermis, hair, and sebaceous glands is frequent [283].

The pancreas is the only other organ which possesses as high a concentration of iron as the liver, and it may reach 50 to 100 times normal [5, 6]. Most of the hemosiderin is found in acinar and fibrous tissue; less iron is found in the islets of Langerhans. The acinar cells show degenerative changes, and the islet cells are frequently affected. The islets are usually reduced in number and may show scarring. The pancreas is hard and has a deep brown-red, rusty discoloration. The salivary glands are usually similarly discolored by large deposits of hemosiderin in the glandular epithelium. Large amounts of hemosiderin may also be found in the lachrymal glands, the submucous glands of the respiratory tract, the mucosal cells of the stomach, and, to a lesser extent, the proximal duodenum.

The heart usually is a deep brown. The hemosiderin deposition (roughly 10 to 15 times normal) is confined to the myocardium and is most marked in the perinuclear area of the cells. Fatty degeneration and fibrosis of the muscle fibers are present in varying degrees. Hemosiderin and accompanying tissue damage are found in the atrioventricular node in association with arrhythmias. The sinus node is selectively spared [333].

The spleen is usually only slightly enlarged and often shows the fibrocongestive changes secondary to portal hypertension. Hemosiderin deposits are only approximately five times normal and are located chiefly in the trabeculae, blood vessel walls, and capsule. These findings are in contrast to the greater degree of splenomegaly and much increased iron content of the spleen, kidney, and bone marrow observed in transfusion hemosiderosis or hemochromatosis.

The pituitary, thyroid, and parathyroid glands usually show a brown discoloration resulting from increased (approximately 25 times normal) deposits of hemosiderin in epithelial cells. In the pituitary gland hemosiderin is limited to the anterior lobe. Hemosiderin deposition in the adrenal gland is approximately 10 to 15 times normal and is localized to the cortex, usually the outer zona glomerulosa. A correlation between the amount of iron deposited in the zona glomerulosa and the degree of melanin pigmentation has been found [334]. In one case of primary hemochromatosis with minimal pigmentation no hemosiderin was found in the zona glomerulosa [335]. Deposition of hemosiderin in the testes is usually small and is usually in the blood vessel walls and interstitial connective tissue. The frequently observed atrophy of the testicular germinal epithelium is probably related to pituitary hypofunction or advanced liver disease. The ovaries usually do not contain increased quantities of hemosiderin.

The kidneys show a relatively small increase of iron (roughly five times normal). The hemosiderin is found in the epithelial cells of the convoluted tubules. The iron may be demonstrable in the desquamated epithelial cells of the urinary sediment. Intercapillary glomerulosclerosis is relatively infrequent in the diabetes associated with hemochromatosis [336, 337].

A moderate increase of hemosiderin is usually observed within the reticulum cells of the bone marrow. Bone marrow hemosiderin is strikingly less than the amount of hemosiderin observed in liver biopsy specimens. By contrast, patients with transfusion hemosiderosis or hemochromatosis show a decided increase of marrow hemosiderin, comparable to the high concentration of hemosiderin observed in the liver.

Iron may be found in many other tissues unaccompanied by demonstrable pathologic changes. In the central nervous system small amounts of iron may be found in the choroid plexus, extrapyramidal areas, and the pineal gland. Iron may also be found in the peritoneum, synovial tissue, cartilage of joints and the tracheobronchial tree, and striated muscle. Considerable deposits of hemosiderin may be found in the lymph nodes draining areas containing high concentrations of iron.

Diagnostic Laboratory Tests

Determination of the plasma iron concentration and latent iron-binding capacity is probably the most useful initial diagnostic test in the evaluation of a patient in whom primary hemochromatosis is suspected. In the absence of infection, inflammation, neoplasia, or recent blood loss, the plasma iron concentration of symptomatic patients with hemochromatosis will be high, usually in the range of 175 to 275 μg per 100 ml. The plasma iron concentration in uncomplicated Laennec's cirrhosis is within the normal range [192]. The total iron-binding capacity is usually decreased below 300 μg per 100 ml, and the latent iron-binding capacity is less than 50 μg per 100 ml. In patients with transfusion hemochromatosis or hemosiderosis the plasma iron concentration is similarly elevated, but the total iron-binding capacity usually remains above 300 μg per 100 ml, and the latent iron-binding capacity is higher. Iron staining of aspirated marrow smears or sections reveals high-normal to moderately increased hemosiderin deposits. These are located in the reticuloendothelial cells. Marrow hemosiderin is strikingly less than hepatic hemosiderin. Patients with transfusion hemosiderosis or hemochromatosis have considerably greater deposits of iron in the marrow reticuloendothelial cells, comparable in amount to that present in the liver. When the plasma iron concentration and marrow hemosiderin deposits are compatible with a diagnosis of primary hemochromatosis, then a needle biopsy of the liver (in the presence of normal blood coagulation test values) is indicated.

The characteristic findings of primary hemochromatosis may be demonstrated by liver biopsy but cannot always be definitely distinguished from those of Laennec's cirrhosis with secondary hemosiderosis. The latter usually shows more hemosiderin in the periportal areas and less in the parenchymal (polygonal) cells.

A skin biopsy may be confirmatory, but a negative finding does not rule out primary hemochromatosis. The Rous [6, 338] test for hemosiderinuria within epithelial cells is helpful. This test will be positive in primary hemochromatosis and other conditions with iron overload if a sufficient number of overnight urine specimens is examined. Hemosiderinuria is also demonstrable in patients with various types of hemoglobinemia and hemoglobinuria and in pernicious anemia. If iron deficiency fails to develop in spite of weekly venesection of 500 ml blood for several months, then one may assume an abnormally increased iron store. A more rapid and useful test for iron overload involves measurement of the increase in urinary iron excretion during 24-hr periods before and after intravenous or intramuscular injections of a chelating agent, desferrioxamine (see below). The slow intravenous administration of 8.3 or 10 mg desferrioxamine per kg body weight according to the method of Hallberg and Hedenberg or Fielding results in good reproducibility in a given individual and facilitates comparisons between individuals [301, 339, 340]. Urinary iron excretion in the absence of renal failure is highly correlated with hepatic iron and, more specifically, with parenchymal rather than periportal or reticuloendothelial liver iron [341, 342]. This test is useful then not only in screening for iron overload, but also in determining the degree of iron overload and differentiation between iron overload associated with alcoholic cirrhosis and that stemming from primary hemochromatosis [301, 342–344].

Treatment

The removal of excess body iron is the only effective therapy of primary hemochromatosis. The most effective and convenient method is by a systematic program of phlebotomy. Venesection of 500 ml blood once or twice a week will remove 10 to 20 gm iron annually. Care is taken to maintain the hemoglobin concentration at a level of 11 gm per 100 ml or higher (hematocrit = 34 percent). Patients without complications such as infection, inflammation, hepatoma, and other malignant tumors are able to increase erythropoiesis and maintain it at three- to fivefold normal for a year or more. Venesection should be maintained at the maximal steady rate that will permit maintenance of hemoglobin concentration. Usually after removal of 20 to 40 gm iron in 1 to 4 years, a rapid decrease in the frequency of compensatable phlebotomies will occur. Unless some complication has supervened, this indicates exhaustion or near-exhaustion of storage iron. If after a 2-month suspension of venesection erythrocyte values remain depressed, measurements of plasma iron concentration and binding capacity are indicated. If these determinations indicate iron deficiency, then a liver biopsy serves to confirm the reduction or absence of storage iron. This biopsy may contrast strikingly with the base-line liver biopsy obtained before initiation of venesection therapy. Subsequent reaccumulation of excess iron is prevented by annual reinstitution of the venesection program until a mild iron deficiency anemia again appears.

Several years of intensive phlebotomy may be required for removal of the abnormal accumulation of iron, but distinct clinical improvement usually occurs within 3 months after starting the venesection program. Patients feel much more energetic and have a sense of well-being. During therapy insulin requirements may be reduced, pigmentation is decreased, and there may be improvement of hepatic and cardiac function [44, 61, 312, 345].

The recent availability of desferrioxamine B provides for the first time an effective chelating agent which can remove considerable amounts of iron. Intramuscular injections of 1,000 mg per day (500 mg twice daily) will usually result in the urinary excretion of 5 to 18 gm iron per year. Occasional patients may not respond [346–350]. Rapid clinical improvement similar to that seen with venesection therapy has been observed within a month or two after initiation of desferrioxamine therapy. No side effects have been noted when desferrioxamine is administered intramuscularly. It may also be administered slowly intravenously; rapid infusion may result in flushing and faintness. One patient had a fatal pontine hemorrhage following intravenous use of desferrioxamine [346], but the relationship of the severe thrombocytopenia and hemorrhage to the use of desferrioxamine in this patient is not clear, since no other instance of thrombocytopenia associated with desferrioxamine therapy has been reported. Cataracts develop in dogs after administration of desferrioxamine for many months. While desferrioxamine therapy may be fairly effective, the disadvantages of expense, inconvenience, possible complications, and occasional lack of response all favor venesection as the safest, most convenient, and most satisfactory method of therapy. Rarely, a concurrent anemia of sufficient degree may indicate the use of desferrioxamine.

Chelation therapy with desferrioxamine is of value and importance in the treatment of various forms of secondary hemochromatosis and hemosiderosis. It may be of benefit in transfusion hemochromatosis (or siderosis) associated with erythroid hypoplasia (or aplasia) and in hemochromatosis associated with various types of refractory anemia with intramedullary hemolysis (i.e., marked erythroid hyperplasia without corresponding reticulocytosis such as thalassemia major, severe hereditary hypochromic hypersideremic anemia, chronic erythremic myelosis, and primary hyperplastic refractory anemia). Secondary hemochromatosis occurs rather frequently in the above categories and constitutes the most important indication for the clinical use of chelation therapy. Patients with secondary hemochromatosis and hemolytic anemia with distinct reticulocytosis tolerate venesection therapy well, even at hemoglobin levels of 7 to 9 gm per 100 ml, since the red blood cells removed by phlebotomy each week constitute a small fraction of the red blood cells released from the marrow into the circulation.

Genetics

A number of family studies have demonstrated hemochromatosis, or iron overload, or both in a highly significant fraction of the relatives of patients with the disease [5, 289, 295, 329, 331, 351–375]. The fully developed clinical disease appears 10 times more commonly in males than in females. Clinical manifestations of primary hemochromatosis occur with a frequency as high as 50 percent in sibs, but the florid disease has rarely been observed in successive generations. It is difficult for an investigator to follow this disorder through two generations because of the long time required for the complications of primary hemochromatosis to develop and become clinically apparent. In order to investigate the genetics of hemochromatosis various measurements have been made to detect abnormalities of iron metabolism characteristic of primary hemochromatosis before the organic changes become symptomatic.

Measurements of plasma iron concentration and iron-binding capacity have been performed in several hundred sibs or children of nearly a hundred patients with primary hemochromatosis [44, 355, 357, 376–378]. The largest series is that of Dreyfus and Schapira [379]. One hundred and sixty-one children (80 females and 81 males) of 40 patients with hemochromatosis have been studied [379]. The average serum iron concentration of the patients with hemochromatosis was 250 μg per 100 ml, whereas it was 140 μg per 100 ml in 38 normal controls. All the daughters and all the sons below age 15 years averaged approximately 140 μg per 100 ml, while 40 sons above age 15 years averaged 195 μg per 100 ml. Of the latter, approximately 40 percent had values above those of the control group.

Liver biopsies of relatives of patients with hemochromatosis demonstrate a high incidence of increased hepatic deposition of iron. The most extensive investigation demonstrated histologically detectable iron (grades 1+ to 4+) in 28 (61 percent) of 46 relatives of 17 patients [79, 380]. Though Zimmerman et al. were able to detect iron in only 13 percent of autopsied patients [381], Pechet et al. were able to detect iron in 55 to 77 percent of their 601 patients autopsied in San Francisco, Boston, South Africa, and Israel [382]. If grades 2+ and above are considered to indicate increased iron storage, then 13 (28 percent) of the relatives were abnormal. The mean plasma iron concentration of this group (2+ to 4+) was 180 μg per 100 ml.

Oral iron absorption studies, using the double-isotope technique of measurement of erythrocyte ^{55}Fe and ^{59}Fe radioactivity after oral administration of ^{55}Fe and intravenous injection of ^{59}Fe have been done in one group of 29 relatives of patients with primary hemochromatosis without iron deficiency or previous venesection therapy. Increased absorption was found in 16 of the relatives (55 percent) and normal absorption in the others [295], in spite of the erroneously low absorption values obtained with this method in patients with high levels of transferrin saturation [140].

In another series using a whole-body counter, iron absorption was measured in 29 relatives of 10 patients with primary hemochromatosis. Only five were older than 15 years, and all had normal plasma iron concentration [294]. As shown in Fig. 44-18 and Table 44-2, increased absorption was found in seven relatives, or 24 percent of those tested. Twenty-seven percent of the male relatives and 21 percent of the female relatives showed increased absorption of iron. Most patients with primary hemochromatosis demonstrated

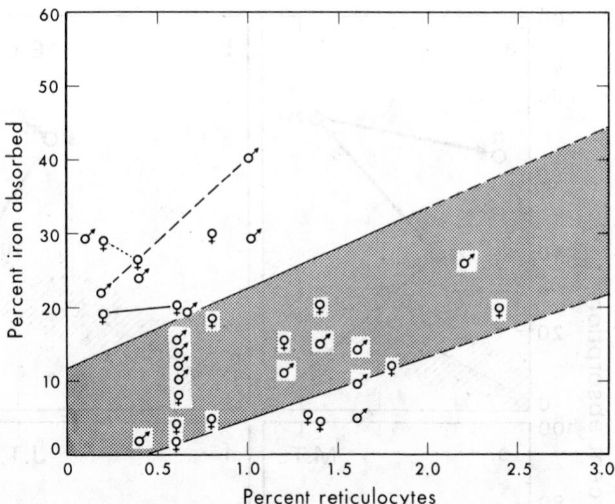

Figure 44-18. Iron absorption of 4 mg ingested Fe^{++} (as ferrous sulfate) related to reticulocyte count of relatives of patients with primary hemochromatosis.

normal iron absorption before venesection, but absorption was always abnormally increased after venesection, usually even when plasma iron concentration and reticulocyte counts returned to normal (Fig. 44-19) [81]. Iron-kinetics studies may also be used to detect metabolic abnormalities in asymptomatic relatives of patients with primary hemochromatosis. Increased plasma-to-storage iron exchange may be demonstrated by this means in patients with normal plasma iron concentration [158] or with normal iron deposits in the liver biopsy specimen (Fig. 44-20) [383].

These investigations constitute strong evidence in support of the hypothesis that the metabolic abnormality resulting in primary hemochromatosis is inherited. The occurrence of the metabolic abnormality in males of successive generations and in females is sufficiently frequent to suggest that the genetic defect is not X-linked.

The data are insufficient to determine whether (1) autosomal homozygosity is required for development of symptomatic primary hemochromatosis and heterozygous individuals merely manifest abnormalities of iron metabolism that are not of sufficient magnitude to lead to primary hemochromatosis, (2) heterozygosity is associated with variable degrees of manifestations of the genetic defect which results

Table 44-2. INCIDENCE OF INCREASED IRON ABSORPTION IN 29 RELATIVES OF 10 PATIENTS WITH PRIMARY HEMOCHROMATOSIS

	Sibling	Children	Niece or nephew	Grandniece or grandnephew	Male	Female	Average age of nonsiblings, years
Test positive	0	3	1	3	4	3	14.6
Test negative	3	10	5	4	11	11	19.0
Percent positive	0%	23%	17%	43%	27%	21%	

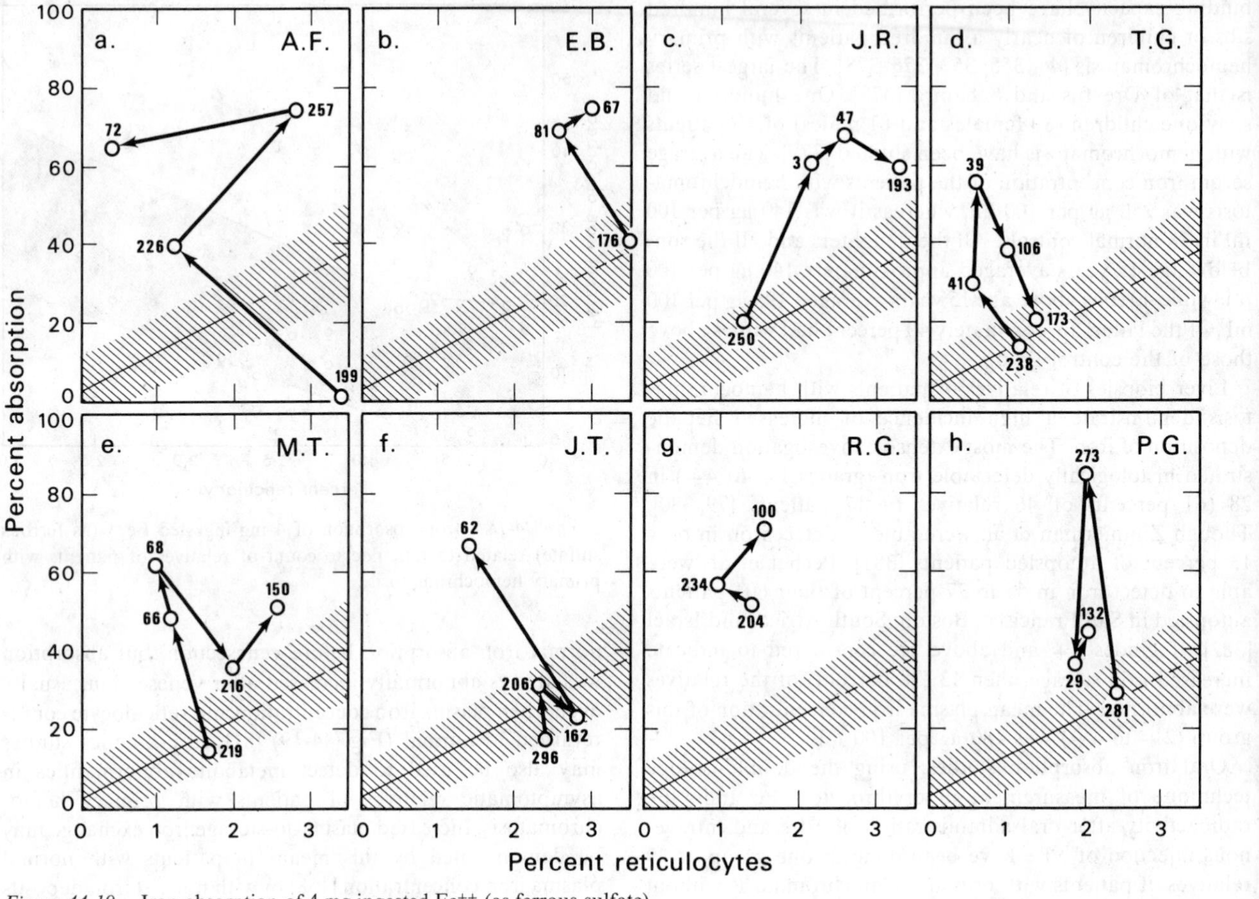

Figure 44-19. Iron absorption of 4 mg ingested Fe^{++} (as ferrous sulfate) related to reticulocyte count and plasma iron concentration (μg/100 ml) of patients with primary hemochromatosis before and after iron depletion.

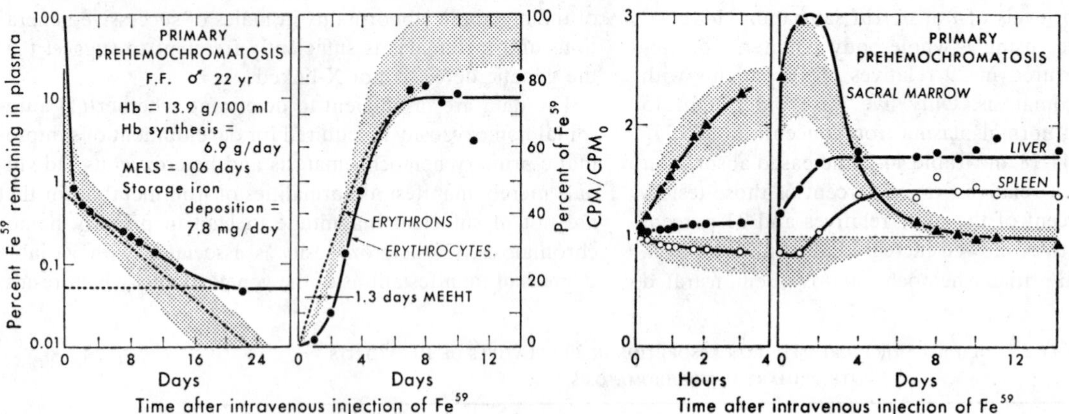

Figure 44-20. Radioiron in plasma and erythrocytes, and surface radioactivity in an asymptomatic son of a father with primary hemochromatosis. Two uncles also had primary hemochromatosis. Liver biopsy demonstrated increased deposition of hemosiderin, and iron absorption was increased, while plasma iron concentration was normal, 140 μg per 100 ml. Plasma-storage iron exchange is increased to 7.8 mg per day (normal range, 0.2 to 2 mg per day).

in primary hemochromatosis, or (3) the metabolic defect and the extent of its manifestations are determined by the cumulative action of several genes (polymerism) such that the patient with primary hemochromatosis suffers from a cumulative gene defect.

SUMMARY

1 Primary hemochromatosis is a genetically determined disorder of iron metabolism characterized by massive widespread accumulation of iron as hemosiderin, with associated impairment of hepatic, pancreatic, and cardiac structure and function. Pigmentation, hepatic cirrhosis, and diabetes mellitus form the classic triad of this disease.

It differs from other iron overload diseases in that the excess iron, accumulated as a result of persistently increased intestinal absorption of iron, is unassociated with known causes of excessive iron absorption such as iron deficiency anemia, excessive dietary iron, and increased erythropoiesis, especially that associated with intramedullary hemolysis.

2 The excessive absorption of iron is 2 to 3 mg per day, and several decades are usually required in order to accumulate the 20 to 60 gm iron present in the body at the time the disease becomes clinically apparent. As a result, 80 percent of patients with primary hemochromatosis become symptomatic only after the age of 40. The iron loss in females associated with menstruation, pregnancy, and lactation is partially protective, so that the clinical disease occurs 10 times more frequently in men than in women.

3 Deposits of hemosiderin appear in liver, pancreas, heart, pituitary, adrenals, and other organs. The increase in hepatic hemosiderin, primarily parenchymal in distribution, is much greater than that in the marrow. The characteristic metallic-slate to bronze-tan pigmentation of skin occurs primarily as a result of increased melanin deposition in the skin and atrophy of the epidermis. Hemosiderin deposition in the corium may also contribute to the pigmentation to a variable degree. The signs and symptoms of the disease arise from organ damage occurring as a tissue reaction to the hemosiderin deposits.

4 Plasma iron concentration is elevated, while plasma transferrin is decreased and characteristically is nearly completely saturated with iron. The exchange of iron between plasma and storage depots is increased, while plasma-erythropoiesis iron exchange is usually normal. Hemosiderinuria is present.

5 Differentiation from several types of secondary hemochromatosis may be difficult. The most reliable finding in a patient with clinically suggestive features is an elevation of the degree of saturation of plasma transferrin with iron. Hemosiderinuria, if present, is helpful. Occasionally the diagnosis must be established from a careful history or functional measurements, such as iron-kinetics study, urinary iron excretion in response to a chelating agent, or the response to systematic phlebotomy.

6 Treatment by systematic venesection of 500 to 1,000 ml whole blood per week will usually arrest development of the disease and result in striking symptomatic improvement and decreased insulin requirements. Phlebotomy should be continued until mild iron deficiency anemia results and then reinstituted annually. Characteristically postphlebotomy iron absorption measurements remain abnormally elevated for many months or years after reticulocyte and erythrocyte values and serum iron concentration and transferrin saturation have become normal or elevated.

7 Family studies indicate that the metabolic abnormality that results in primary hemochromatosis is inherited, but the mode of inheritance has not been established.

BIBLIOGRAPHY

1. Trousseau, A.: *Clinique médicale de l'Hôtel-Dieu de Paris,* 2d ed., p. 672. Baillière, Paris, 1865.
2. Troisier, M.: Diabète, sucré. Bull. Soc. Anat. Paris, **16,** 231, 1871.
3. von Recklinghausen, F. D.: Über Hämochromatose. Tagebl. Versamml. Natur. Arzte, Heidelberg, **62,** 324, 1889.
4. Sheldon, J. H.: The iron content of the tissues in hemochromatosis, with special reference to the brain. Quart. J. Med., **21,** 123, 1927.
5. Sheldon, J. H. *Hemochromatosis.* Humphrey Milford, London, 1935.
6. Finch, S. C., and Finch, C. A.: Idiopathic hemochromatosis, an iron storage disease. Medicine, **34,** 381, 1955.
7. Granick, S.: Iron metabolism. Bull. N.Y. Acad. Med., **30,** 81, 1954.
8. Drabkin, D. L.: Metabolism of the hemin chromoproteins. Physiol. Rev., **31,** 345, 1951.
9. Kendrew, J. C., Parrish, R. G., Marrack, J. R., and Orlans, E. S.: The species specificity of myoglobin. Nature (London), **174,** 946, 1954.
10. Granick, S.: Increase of protein apoferritin in gastrointestinal mucosa as direct response to iron feeding. J. Biol. Chem., **164,** 737, 1946.
11. Zail, S. S., Charlton, R. W., Torrance, J. D., and Bothwell, T. H. Studies on the formation of ferritin in red cell precursors. J. Clin. Invest., **43,** 670, 1964.
12. Primosigh, J. V., and Thomas, E. D.: Studies on the partition of iron in bone marrow cells. J. Clin. Invest., **47,** 1473, 1968.
13. Charlton, R. W., Jacobs, P., Torrance, J. D., and Bothwell, T. H.: The role of the intestinal mucosa in iron absorption. J. Clin. Invest., **44,** 543, 1965.
14. Hamilton, J. K., and Mayerson, H. S.: Hemoglobin iron as stimulus for production of ferritin by the kidney. Amer. J. Physiol., **160,** 1, 1950.
15. Tecce, Di G., and Tecce, T.: Presenza di ferritina nella placenta umana a termine di gravidanza. Quad. Nutr., **11,** 42, 1950.
16. Yoshino, Y., Manis, J., and Schachter, D.: Regulation of ferritin synthesis in rat liver. J. Biol. Chem., **243,** 2911, 1968.
17. Mazur, A., Litt, I., and Shorr, E.: Chemical properties of ferritin and their relation to its vasodepressor activity. J. Biol. Chem., **187,** 473, 1950.
18. Kaldor, I.: Studies of intermediary iron metabolism. XII. Measurement of the iron derived from water soluble and water insoluble non-haem compounds (ferritin and haemosiderin iron) in liver and spleen. Aust. J. Exp. Biol. Med. Sci., **36,** 173, 1958.
19. Shoden, A., Gabrio, B. W., and Finch, C. A.: The relationship between ferritin and hemosiderin in rabbits and man. J. Biol. Chem., **204,** 823, 1953.
20. Weinfeld, A.: Storage iron in man. Acta Med. Scand., suppl. **427,** 1965.
21. Sturgeon, P., and Shoden, A.: Mechanisms of iron storage, in *Iron Metabolism,* edited by F. Gross, p. 121. Springer-Verlag, Berlin, 1964.
22. Heilmeyer, L., and Weissbecker, L.: Funktion und Stoffwechsel der Schwermetalle, in *Handbuch der allgemeine Pathologie,* edited by F. Buchner, E. Letterer, and F. Roulet, vol. 4, part 2, p. 1. Springer-Verlag, Berlin, 1957.

23. Heilmeyer L.: Ferritin, in *Iron in Clinical Medicine,* edited by R. O. Wallerstein, p. 24. University of California Press, Berkeley, 1958.
24. Block, M., Moore, G., Wasi, P., and Haiby, G.: Histogenesis of the hepatic lesion in primary hemochromatosis: with consideration of the pseudo-iron deficient state produced by phlebotomies. Amer. J. Path., **47,** 89, 1965.
25. Wallerstein, R. O., and Pollycove, M.: Bone marrow hemosiderin and ferrokinetics patterns in anemia. A.M.A. Arch. Intern. Med., **101,** 418, 1958.
26. Nixon, R. K., and Olson, J. P.: Diagnostic value of marrow hemosiderin patterns. Ann. Intern. Med., **69,** 1249, 1968.
27. Kariyone, S., and Miyake, T.: Reticuloendothelial cell in the bone marrow and its relationship to iron metabolism. Tohoku J. Exp. Med., **89,** 213, 1966.
28. Hallgren, B.: Hemoglobin formation and storage iron in protein deficiency. Acta Soc. Med., Upsal. **59,** 81, 1954.
29. Butt, E. M., Nusbaum, R. E., Gilmour T. C., and Didio, S. L.: Trace metal patterns in diseased states. I. Hemochromatosis and refractory anemia. Amer. J. Clin. Path., **26,** 225, 1956.
30. Gross, H., Sandberg, M., and Holly, O. M.: Changes in copper and iron retention in chronic diseases accompanied by secondary anemia: changes in liver, spleen, and stomach. Amer. J. Med. Sci., **204,** 201, 1942.
31. Mazur, A., and Shorr, E.: A quantitative immunochemical study of ferritin and its relation to the hepatic vasodepressor material. J. Biol. Chem., **182,** 607, 1950.
32. Roth, O., Jasinski, B., and van Bidder, H.: Das Gewebeeisen beim Menschen bei normalen und pathologischen Zuständen. Helv. Med. Acta, **18,** 159, 1951.
33. Gale, E., Torrance, J., and Bothwell, T.: The quantitative estimation of total iron stores in human bone marrow. J. Clin. Invest., **42**(2), 1076, 1963.
34. Barnicott, N. A.: Haptoglobins and transferrins, in *Genetical Variation in Human Populations,* edited by G. A. Harrison, p. 41. Pergamon, New York, 1961.
35. Turnbull, A., and Giblett, E. R.: The binding and transport of iron by transferrin variants. J. Lab. Clin. Med., **57,** 450, 1961.
36. Laurell, C. B.: Studies in the transportation and metabolism of iron in the body. Acta Physiol. Scand., suppl. **46,** 1, 1947.
37. Laurell, C. B.: Plasma iron and the transport of iron in the organism. Pharmacol. Rev., **4,** 371, 1952.
38. Fletcher, J.: Variation in the availability of transferrin-bound iron for uptake by immature red cells. Clin. Sci., **37,** 273, 1969.
39. Gitlin, D., Janeway, C. A., and Farr, L. E.: Studies on metabolism of plasma proteins in nephrotic syndrome: albumin, γ-globulin and iron-binding globulin. J. Clin. Invest., **35,** 44, 1956.
40. Katz, J. H.: Iron and protein kinetics studied by means of doubly labeled human crystalline transferrin. J. Clin. Invest., **40,** 2143, 1961.
41. Mazur, A., and Carleton, A.: Relation of ferritin to heme synthesis. J. Biol. Chem., **238,** 1817, 1963.
42. Jandl, J. H., and Katz, J. H.: The plasma to cell cycle of transferrin in iron utilization. Trans. Ass. Amer. Physicians, **74,** 72, 1961.
43. Jandl, J. H., and Katz, J. H.: The plasma to cell cycle of transferrin. J. Clin. Invest., **42,** 314, 1963.
44. Pollycove, M.: Unpublished data.
45. Green, R., Charlton, R., Seftel, H., Bothwell, T., Mayet, F., Adams, B., Finch, C., and Layrisse, M.: Body iron excretion in man. Amer. J. Med., **45,** 336, 1968.
46. Josephs, H. W.: Iron metabolism and the hypochromic anemia of infancy. Medicine, **32,** 125, 1953.
47. Josephs, H. W.: Absorption of iron as a problem in human physiology: a critical review. Blood, **13,** 1, 1958.
48. Saito, H., Sargent, T., III, Parker, H., and Lawrence, J. H.: Whole-body iron loss in normal man measured with a gamma spectrometer. Univ. Calif. Rad. Lab. 11387 Semiann. Rep. Biol. Med., p. 96, Spring, 1964. J. Nucl. Med., **5,** 571, 1964. Cited in *Iron Metabolism,* edited by F. Gross, p. 462. Springer-Verlag, Berlin, 1964.
49. Moore, C. V.: Iron nutrition, in *Iron Metabolism,* edited by F. Gross, p. 241. Springer-Verlag, Berlin, 1964.
50. Dubach, R., Moore, C. V., and Callender, S.: Studies in iron transportation and metabolism. IX. The excretion of iron as measured by the isotope technique. J. Lab. Clin. Med., **45,** 599, 1955.
51. Man, Y. K., and Wadsworth, G. R.: Urinary loss of iron and the influence on it of dietary levels of iron. Clin. Sci., **36,** 479, 1969.
52. Cavill, I., Jacobs, A., Beamish, M., and Owen, G.: Iron turnover in the skin. Nature (London), **222,** 167, 1969.
53. Heath, C. W., and Patek, A. J.: Anemia of iron deficiency. Medicine, **16,** 267, 1937.
54. Frenchman, R., and Johnston, F. A.: Relation of menstrual losses to iron requirement. J. Amer. Diet. Ass., **25,** 217, 1949.
55. Millis, J.: Iron losses in healthy women during consecutive menstrual cycles. Med. J. Aust., **2,** 874, 1951.
56. Hynes, M.: Iron metabolism. J. Clin. Path., **1,** 57, 1948.
57. Widdowson, E. M., and Spray, C. M.: Chemical development in utero. Arch. Dis. Child., **26,** 205, 1951.
58. Feuillen, Y. M., and Plumier, M.: Iron metabolisms in infants: the intake of iron in breast feeding, and artificial feeding (milk and milk foods). Acta Paediat., (Scand.), **41,** 138, 1952.
59. Finch, C. A.: Physiopathologic mechanisms of iron excretion, in *Iron Metabolism,* edited by F. Gross, p. 452, Springer-Verlag, Berlin, 1964.
60. Saito, H., Sargent, T., Parker, H. G., and Lawrence, J. H.: Whole-body iron loss in normal man measured with a gamma spectrometer. J. Nucl. Med., **5,** 571, 1964.
61. Bothwell, T. H., and Finch, C. A.: *Iron Metabolism.* Little, Brown, Boston, 1962.
62. Layrisse, M., Cook, J. D., Martinez, C., Roche, M., Kuhn, I. N., Walker, R. B., and Finch, C. A.: Food iron absorption: a comparison of vegetable and animal foods. Blood, **33,** 430, 1969.
63. Chodos, R. B., Ross, J. F., Apt, L., Halkett, J., and Pollycove, M.: The absorption of food iron and inorganic iron by normal, iron-deficient, and hemochromatotic subjects. Clin. Res. Proc., **2,** 53, 1955; J. Clin. Invest., **36,** 314, 1957.
64. Dubach, R., Callender, S. T. E., and Moore, C. V.: Absorption of radioactive iron in patients with fever and anemias of various etiology. Blood, **3,** 526, 1948.
65. Bothwell, T. H., Pirzio-Biroli, G., and Finch, C. A.: Iron absorption. I. Factors influencing absorption. J. Lab. Clin. Med., **51,** 24, 1958.
66. Hahn, P. F., Bale, W. F., Ross, J. F., Balfour, W. M., and Whipple, G. H.: Radioactive iron absorption by gastrointestinal tract: influence of anemia, anoxia, and antecedent feeding: distribution in growing dogs. J. Exp. Med., **78,** 169, 1943.
67. Monsen, E. R., Kuhn, I. N., and Finch, C. A.: Iron states of menstruating women. Amer. J. Clin. Nutr., **20,** 842, 1967.
68. Kuhn, I. N., Monsen, E. R., Cook, J. D., and Finch, C. A.: Iron absorption in man. J. Lab. Clin. Med., **71,** 715, 1968.
69. Mendel, G. A., Weiler, R. J., and Mangalik, A.: Studies on iron absorption. II. The absorption of iron in experimental anemias of diverse etiology. Blood, **22,** 450, 1963.
70. Ley, A.: The relationship of erythropoiesis to iron absorption. J. Clin. Invest., **39,** 1006, 1960.
71. Erlandson, M. E., Walden, B., Stern, G., Hilgartner, M. W., Wuhman, J., and Smith, C. H.: Studies of congenital hemolytic syndromes. IV. Gastrointestinal absorption of iron. Blood, **19,** 359, 1962.
72. Schiffer, L. M., Price, D. C., and Chronkite, E. P.: Iron absorption and anemia. J. Lab. Clin. Med., **65,** 316, 1965.
73. Mendel, G. A.: Studies of iron absorption. I. The relationship between the rate of erythropoiesis, hypoxia and iron absorption. Blood, **18,** 727, 1961.
74. Krantz, S., Goldwasser, E., and Jacobson, L. O.: Studies on erythropoiesis. XIV. The relationship of humoral stimulation to iron absorption. Blood, **14,** 654, 1959.
75. Stewart, W. B., Vassar, P. S., and Stone, R. S.: Iron absorption in dogs during anemia due to acetylphenylhydrazine. J. Clin. Invest., **32,** 1225, 1953.

76. Weintraub, L. R., Conrad, M. E., and Crosby, W. H.: Regulation of the intestinal absorption of iron by the rate of erythropoiesis. Brit. J. Haemat., **11**, 432, 1965.
77. Sauer, J. P., Chapman, C. W., and Gallagher, N. I.: Effects of altered erythropoiesis on iron absorption. Lab. Invest., **20**, 558, 1969.
78. Reynafarje, C., and Ramos, J.: Influence of altitude changes on intestinal iron absorption. J. Lab. Clin. Med., **57**, 848, 1961.
79. Sherlock, S.: Introduction to the general discussion of iron overload, in *Iron Metabolism,* edited by F. Gross, p. 392. Springer-Verlag, Berlin, 1964.
80. Smith, P. M., Godrey, B. E., and Williams, R.: Iron absorption in idiopathic haemochromatosis and its measurement using a whole-body counter. Clin. Sci., **37**, 519, 1969.
81. Sargent, T. W., Saito, H., and Winchell, H. S.: Iron absorption in hemochromatosis before and after phlebotomy therapy. Donner Laboratory Semiannual Report UCRL, **19420**, p. 30, Fall, 1969. J. Nucl. Med. August, 1971.
82. Saltman, P.: The role of chelation in iron metabolism. J. Chem. Educ., **42**, 682, 1965.
83. Helbock, H., and Saltman, P.: The transport of iron by rat intestine. Biochim. Biophys. Acta, **135**, 979, 1967.
83*a*. Pollycove, M., Saltman, P., Freeman, L., Newman, R., and Tono, M.: Unpublished data.
84. Davis, P. S., and Deller, D. J.: Prediction and demonstration of iron chelating ability of sugars. Nature (London), **212**, 404, 1966.
85. Conrad, M. E., and Schade, S. G.: Ascorbic acid chelates in iron absorption: a role for hydrochloric acid and bile. Gastroenterology, **55**, 35, 1968.
86. Davis, P. S., Luke, C. G., Deller, D. J.: Gastric iron binding protein in iron chelation by gastric juice. Nature (London), **214**, 1126, 1967.
87. Davis, P. S., Multani, J. S., Cepurneek, C. P., and Saltman, P.: Isolation of gastroferrin from human gastric juice. Biochem. Biophys. Res. Commun., **37**, 532, 1969.
87*a*. Pollycove, M. Davis, P. S., Saltman, P., Newman, R., and Tono, M.: Unpublished data.
88. Jacobs, A., and Miles, P. M.: Intraluminal transport of iron from stomach to small-intestinal mucosa. Brit. Med. J., **4**, 778, 1969.
89. Jacobs, A., and Miles, P. M.: The iron-binding properties of gastric juice. Clin. Chim. Acta, **24**, 87, 1969.
90. Jacobs, A., and Miles, P. M.: Role of gastric secretion in iron absorption. Gut, **10**, 226, 1969.
91. Jacobs, P., Bothwell, T., and Charlton, R. W.: Role of hydrochloric acid in iron absorption. J. Appl. Physiol., **19**(2), 187, 1964.
92. Luke, C. G., Davis, P. S., and Deller, D. J.: Change in gastric iron-binding protein (gastroferrin) during iron-deficiency anaemia. Lancet, **1**, 926, 1967.
92*a*. Luke, C. G., Davis, P. S., and Deller, D. J.: Gastric iron binding in haemochromatosis, secondary iron overload, cirrhosis, and diabetes. Lancet, **2**, 844, 1968.
92*b*. Luke, C. G., Davis, P. S., and Deller, D. J.: Gastric iron-binding in haemochromatosis (letter to editor). Lancet, **2**, 1392, 1968.
92*c*. Wynter, C. V. A., and Williams, R.: Iron-binding properties of gastric juice in idiopathic haemochromatosis. Lancet, **2**, 534, 1968.
92*d*. Wynter, C. V. A., and Williams, R.: Gastric iron binding in haemochromatosis (letter to editor). Lancet, **2**, 1243, 1968.
93. Koepke, J. A., and Stewart, W. B.: Role of gastric secretion in iron absorption (29081). Proc. Soc. Exp. Biol. Med., **115**, 927, 1964.
94. Mignon, M., Russell, M. C., Semb, L. S., Morgan, E. H., Finch, C. A., and Nyhus, L. M.: The effect of gastric juice on the absorption of iron. Surg. Forum, **16**, 319, 1965.
95. Jacobs, A., Rhodes, J., and Eakins, J. D.: Gastric factors influencing iron absorption in anemic patients. Scand. J. Haemat., **4**, 105, 1967.
96. Murray, M. J., and Stein, N.: A gastric factor promoting iron absorption. Lancet, **1**, 614, 1968.
97. Murray, M. J., and Stein, N.: The effects on iron absorption of gastro-intestinal secretions from patients with iron-deficiency anaemia and haemochromatosis. Brit. J. Haemat., **15**, 87, 1968.
98. Turnberg, L. A.: Gastric factor in iron absorption. Lancet, **1**, 921, 1968.
99. Smith, P., and Williams, R.: Gastric factor in iron absorption. Lancet, **1**, 824, 1968.
100. Turnbull, A., Cleton, F., and Finch, C. A.: Iron absorption. IV. The absorption of hemoglobin iron. J. Clin. Invest., **41**, 1897, 1962.
101. Hwang, Y., and Brown, E.: Studies of the effect of desferrioxamine on human absorption and excretion. J. Lab. Clin. Med., **62**, 885, 1963.
102. Hallberg, L., and Solvell, L.: Absorption of hemoglobin iron in man. Acta Med. Scand., **181**, 335, 1967.
103. Weintraub, L. R., Weinstein, M. B., Huser, H. J., and Rafal, S.: Absorption of hemoglobin iron: the role of a heme-splitting substance in the intestinal mucosa. J. Clin. Invest., **47**, 531, 1968.
104. Moore, C. V., and Dubach, R.: Iron, in *Mineral Metabolism: An Advanced Treatise,* p. 287. Academic, New York, 1962.
105. Callender, S. T.: Digestive absorption of iron, in *Iron Metabolism,* edited by F. Gross, p. 89. Springer-Verlag, Berlin, 1964.
106. Duthie, H. L.: The relative importance of the duodenum in the intestinal absorption of iron. Brit. J. Haemat., **10**, 59, 1964.
107. Fawwaz, R. A., Winchell, H. S., Pollycove, M., Sargent, T., Anger, H., and Lawrence, J. H.: Intestinal iron absorption studies using iron-52 and Anger positron camera, J. Nucl. Med., **7**, 569, 1966.
108. Dagg, J. H., Kuhn, I. N., Templeton, F. E., and Finch, C. A.: Gastric absorption of iron. Gastroenterology, **53**, 918, 1967.
109. Wheby, M. S.: Site of iron absorption in man. Scand. J. Haemat., **7**, 56, 1970.
110. Davis, A. E., and Badenoch, J.: Iron absorption in pancreatic disease. Lancet, **2**, 6, 1962.
111. Taylor, J., Stiven, D., and Reid, E. W.: Experimental and idiopathic siderosis in cats. J. Path. Bact., **41**, 397, 1935.
112. Taylor, J., Stiven, D., and Reid, E. W.: Haemochromatosis in a depancreatised cat. J. Path. Bact., **34**, 793, 1931.
113. Kaufman, N., Klavins, J. V., and Kinney, T. D.: Excessive iron absorption in rats fed low-protein, high-fat diets. Lab. Invest., **7**, 369, 1958.
114. Kinney, T. D., Kaufman, N., and Klavins, J.: Effect of ethionine induced pancreatic damage on iron absorption. J. Exp. Med., **102**, 151, 1955.
115. Andersen, D. H.: Cystic fibrosis of the pancreas and its relation to celiac disease: a clinical and pathologic study. Amer. J. Dis. Child., **56**, 344, 1938.
116. Murray, M. J., and Stein, N.: Does the pancreas influence iron absorption? A critical review of information to date. Gastroenterology, **51**, 694, 1966.
117. Davis, A. E., and Biggs, J. C.: The pancreas and iron absorption: current views. Amer. J. Dig. Dis., **12**, 293, 1967.
118. Klavins, J. V., Kinney, T. D., and Kaufman, N.: Iron absorption in rats fed a protein-free diet. Amer. J. Path., **35**, 690, 1959.
119. Klavins, J. V., Kinney, T. D., and Kaufman, N.: The influence of dietary protein on iron absorption. Brit. J. Exp. Path., **43**, 172, 1962.
120. Kroe, D., Kinney, T. D., Kaufman, N., and Klavins, J. V.: The influence of amino acids on iron absorption. Blood, **21**, 546, 1963.
121. Brown, E. B., and Rother, M.: Studies of the process of intestinal iron absorption in rats. Blood, **18**, 780, 1961.
122. Brown, E. B., and Rother, M.: Studies of the mechanism of intestinal iron absorption. Presented at IX Cong. Int. Hemat. Soc., Mexico City, 1962.
123. Kroe, D. J., Kaufman, N., Klavins, J. V., and Kinney, T. D.: Interrelation of amino acids and pH on intestinal iron absorption. Amer. J. Physiol., **211**, 414, 1966.
124. Van Campen, D., and Gross, E.: Effects of histidine and certain other amino acids on the absorption of iron-59 by rats. J. Nutr., **99**, 68, 1969.
125. Moore, C. V.: The importance of nutritional factors in the pathogenesis of iron deficiency anemia. Amer. J. Clin. Nutri., **3**, 3, 1955.
126. Granick, S.: Ferritin: its properties and significance for iron metabolism. Chem. Rev., **38**, 379, 1946.
127. Brown, E. B., Jr., Dubach, R., and Moore, C. V.: Studies in iron transportation and metabolism. XI. Critical analysis of mucosal block by large dose of inorganic iron in human subjects. J. Lab. Clin. Med., **52**, 335, 1958.

128. Stewart, W. B., Yuile, C. L., Claiborne, H. A., Snowman, R. T., and Whipple, G. H.: Radioiron absorption in anemic dogs. J. Exp. Med., **92,** 375, 1950.
129. Hartman, R. S., Conrad, M. E., Jr., Hartman, R. E., Joy, J. T. R., and Crosby, W. H.: Ferritin-containing bodies in human small intestinal epithelium. Blood, **22,** 397, 1963.
130. Conrad, M. E., Jr., and Crosby, W. H.: Intestinal mucosal mechanisms. Blood, **22,** 406, 1963.
131. Dawson, R. B., Rafal, S., and Weintraub, L. R.: Absorption of hemoglobin iron: the role of xanthine oxidase in the intestinal heme-splitting reaction. Blood, **35,** 94, 1970.
132. Hallberg, L., and Solvell, L.: Iron absorption studies. Acta Med. Scand., **168,** suppl. 358, 1960.
133. Stewart, W. B., and Gambino, S. R.: Kinetics of iron absorption in normal dogs. Amer. J. Physiol., **201,** 67, 1961.
134. Wheby, M. S., and Crosby, W. H.: The gastrointestinal tract and iron absorption. Blood, **22,** 416, 1963.
135. Granick, S.: Structure and physiologic functions of ferritin. Physiol. Rev., **31,** 489, 1951.
136. Conrad, M. E., Jr., and Crosby, W. H.: Intestinal mucosal mechanisms controlling iron absorption. Blood, **22,** 406, 1963.
137. Conrad, M. E., Weintraub, L. R., and Crosby, W. H.: The role of the intestine in iron kinetics. J. Clin. Invest., **43,** 963, 1964.
138. Greenberger, N. J., Balcerzak, S. P., and Ackerman, G. A.: Iron uptake by isolated intestinal brush borders: changes induced by alterations in iron stores. J. Lab. Clin. Med., **73,** 711, 1969.
139. Wheby, M. S., and Umpierre, G.: Effect of transferrin saturation on iron absorption in man. New Eng. J. Med., **271,** 1391, 1964.
140. Fawwaz, R. A., Winchell, H. S., Pollycove, M., and Sargent, T.: Hepatic iron deposition in humans. I. First-pass hepatic deposition of intestinally absorbed iron in patients with low plasma latent iron-binding capacity. Blood, **30,** 417, 1967.
141. Taylor, M. R. H., and Gatenby, P. B. B.: Iron absorption in relation to transferrin saturation. Brit. J. Haemat., **12,** 747, 1966.
142. Moore, C. V.: Iron metabolism and nutrition. Harvey Lect., **55,** 67, 1959.
143. Krantz, S., Goldwasser, E., and Jacobson, L. O.: Studies on erythropoiesis. XIV. The relationship of humoral stimulation to iron absorption. Blood, **14,** 654, 1959.
144. Beutler, E., and Buttenweiser, E.: The regulation of iron absorption. I. A search for humoral factors. J. Lab Clin. Med., **55,** 274, 1960.
145. Fischer, D. S., and Price, D. C.: A possible humoral regulator of iron absorption. Proc. Soc. Exp. Biol. Med., **112,** 228, 1963.
146. MacDermott, R. P., and Greenberger, N. J.: Evidence for a humoral factor influencing iron absorption. Gastroenterology, **57,** 117, 1969.
147. Winchell, H. S., Pollycove, M., Kusubov, N., and Fawwaz, R.: Kinetics of ^{125}I-albumin and ^{131}I-transferrin in lymph, in *Preparation and Biomedical Application of Labeled Molecules,* edited by J. Sirchis. Euratom, Brussels, 1964.
148. Cartwright, G. E., Huguley, C. M., Jr., Ashenbrucker, H., Fay, J., and Wintrobe, M. M.: Studies on free erythrocyte protoporphyrin, plasma iron and plasma copper in normal and anemic subjects. Blood, **3,** 501, 1948.
149. Cartwright, G. E., and Wintrobe, M. M.: The anemia of infection: studies of the iron binding capacity of serum. J. Clin. Invest., **28,** 86, 1949.
150. Powell, J. F.: Serum iron in health and disease. Quart. J. Med., **13,** 19, 1944.
151. Hamilton, L. B., Gubler, C. J., Cartwright, G. E., and Wintrobe, M. M.: Diurnal variations in the plasma iron level of man. Proc. Soc. Exp. Biol. Med., **75,** 65, 1950.
152. Vahlquist, B. C.: Das Serumeisen, eine pädisatrischklinische und experimentelle Studie. Acta Paediat. Scand., **28,** suppl. 5, 1941.
153. Waldenstrom, J.: Incidence of "iron deficiency" (sideropenia) in some rural and urban populations. Acta Med. Scand., suppl. **170,** 252, 1946.
154. Hemmeler, G.: Nouvelles recherches sur le métabolisme du fer: les oscillations du fer sérique dans la journée. Helv. Med. Acta, **11,** 201, 1944.
155. Johnston, F. A.: Serum iron levels in adolescent girls. Amer. J. Dis. Child., **74,** 716, 1947.
156. Jandl, J. H., Inman, J. K., Simmons, R. L., and Allen, D. W.: Transfer of iron from serum iron binding protein to human reticulocytes. J. Clin. Invest., **38,** 161, 1959.
157. Shoden, A., and Sturgeon, P.: On the formation of haemosiderin and its relation to ferritin. II. A radioisotopic study. Brit. J. Haemat., **9,** 513, 1963.
158. Pollycove, M., and Mortimer, R.: The quantitative determination of iron kinetics and hemoglobin synthesis in human subjects. Clin. Res. Proc., **4,** 51, 1956; J. Clin. Invest., **40,** 753, 1961.
159. Powell, L. W., and Emmerson, B. T.: Haemosiderosis associated with xanthine oxidase inhibition. Lancet, **1,** 239, 1966.
160. Green, S., and Mazur, A.: Relation of uric acid metabolism to release of iron from hepatic ferritin. J. Biol. Chem., **227,** 653, 1957.
161. Mazur, A., Green, S., Saha, A., and Carleton, A.: Mechanism of release of ferritin iron *in vivo* by xanthine oxidase. J. Clin. Invest., **37,** 1809, 1958.
162. Seegmiller, J. E., Engleman, K., Klineberg, J. R., Watts, R. W. E., and Sjoerdsma, A.: Xanthine oxidase and iron. New Eng. J. Med., **270,** 534, 1964.
163. Davis, P. S., and Deller, D. J.: Effect of a xanthine oxidase inhibitor (allopurinol) on radioiron absorption in man. Lancet, **2,** 470, 1966.
164. Awai, M., and Brown, E. B.: Examination of the role of xanthine oxidase in iron absorption by the rat. J. Lab. Clin. Med., **73,** 366, 1969.
165. Osaki, S., Johnson, D. A., and Frieden, E.: The possible significance of the ferrous oxidase activity of ceruloplasmin in normal human serum. J. Biol. Chem., **241,** 2746, 1966.
166. Osaki, S., and Johnson, D. A.: Mobilization of liver iron by ferroxidase (ceruloplasmin). J. Biol. Chem, **244,** 5757, 1969.
167. Lee, G. R., Nacht, S., Lukens, J. N., and Cartwright, G. E.: Iron metabolism in copper-deficient swine. J. Clin. Invest., **47,** 2058, 1968.
168. O'Reilly, S., Pollycove, M., and Bank, W. J.: Iron metabolism in Wilson's disease. Neurology, **18,** 634, 1968.
169. Coleman, D. H., Stevens, A. R., Jr., and Finch, C. A.: The treatment of iron deficiency anemia. Blood, **10,** 567, 1955.
170. Verloop, M. C., Meeuwissen, J. E. Th., and Blokhuis, E. W. M.: Comparison of the "iron absorption test" with the determination of the iron binding capacity of serum in the diagnosis of iron deficiency. Brit. J. Haemat., **4,** 70, 1958.
171. Heilmeyer, L.: Human hyposideraemia, in *Iron Metabolism,* edited by F. Gross, p. 201. Springer-Verlag, Berlin, 1964.
172. Freireich, E. J., Miller, A., Emerson, C. P., and Ross, J. F.: The effect of inflammation on the utilization of erythrocyte and transferrin-bound iron for red cell production. Blood, **12,** 972, 1957.
173. Schaefer, K. H.: Neuro-endocrine control of iron metabolism, in *Iron Metabolism,* edited by F. Gross, p. 280. Springer-Verlag, Berlin, 1964.
174. Freireich, E. J., Ross, J. F., Bayles, T. B., Emerson, C. P., and Finch, S. C.: Radioactive iron metabolism and erythrocyte survival studies of the mechanism of the anemia associated with rheumatoid arthritis. J. Clin. Invest., **36,** 1043, 1957.
175. Cartwright, G. E., Lauritsen, M., Jones, P., Merrill, I., and Wintrobe, M. M.: Anemia of infection. II. Experimental production of hypoferremia and anemia in dogs. J. Clin. Invest., **25,** 81, 1946.
176. Heilmeyer, L., and Plotner, K.: *Das Serumeisen und die Eisenmangelkrankheit.* Fischer, Jena, 1937.
177. Jasinski, B.: Eisenresorption und Infektion erkennung des Eisenmangels bei Infektions Krankheiten durch Blastungsversuch: Pathogenese der Infektanämie. Acta Haemat. (Basel), **3,** 17, 1950.
178. Cleton, F. J., and Blok, A. P. R.: Post-transfusional haemosiderosis, in *Iron Metabolism,* edited by F. Gross, p. 347. Springer-Verlag, Berlin, 1964.
179. Bothwell, T. H.: Iron overload in the Bantu, in *Iron Metabolism,* edited by F. Gross, p. 362. Springer-Verlag, Berlin, 1964.
180. Miller, A., Chodos, R. B., Emerson, C. P., and Ross, J. F.: Studies of the anemia and iron metabolism in cancer. J. Clin. Invest., **35,** 1248, 1956.
181. Bothwell, T. H., Kramer, S., Keeley, K. J., Seftel, H., and Bradlow, B.: Iron metabolism in scurvy. South African J. Med. Sci., **24,** 144, 1959.
182. Brendstrup, P.: Serum copper, serum iron and total iron-binding capacity

of serum in patients with chronic rheumatoid arthritis. Acta Med. Scand., **146,** 384, 1953.
183. Bronte-Stewart, B.: The anaemia of adult scurvy. Quart. J. Med., **22,** 309, 1953.
184. Nylander, G.: Iron metabolism in fractures. Acta Endocr. (Kobenhavn), **20,** 148, 1955.
185. Rath, C. E., and Finch, C. A.: Chemical, clinical and immunological studies of the products of human plasma fractionation. XXXVIII. Serum iron transport: measurement of iron-binding capacity of serum in man. J. Clin. Invest., **28,** 79, 1949.
186. Haurani, F. I., Burke, W., and Martinez, E. J.: Defective reutilization of iron in the anemia of inflammation. J. Lab. Clin. Med., **65,** 560, 1965.
187. Quastel, M. R., and Ross, J. F.: The effect of acute inflammation on the utilization and distribution of transferrin-bound and erythrocyte radioiron. Blood, **28,** 738, 1966.
188. Mowat, A. G., and Hothersall, T. E.: Nature of anaemia in rheumatoid arthritis. VIII. Iron content of synovial tissue in patients with rheumatoid arthritis and in normal individuals. Ann. Rheum. Dis., **27,** 345, 1968.
189. Smith, C. H., Schulman, I., and Morgenthau, J. E.: Iron metabolism in infants and children: serum iron and iron-binding protein; diagnostic and therapeutic implications. *Advances in Pediatrics,* vol. 5, pp. 195–231. Year Book Medical Publishers, Inc., Chicago, 1952.
190. Reissman, K. R., Boley, J., Christianson, J. F., and Delp, M. H.: The serum iron in experimental hepatocellular necrosis. J. Lab. Clin. Med., **43,** 572, 1954.
191. Rechenberger, J.: Die Bestimmung des Serumeisens und Serunkupfers in der Diagnostik der Erkrankungen des Leberparenchyms und der Gellenwege: Serumeisen und Serumkupfer bei der Hepatitis epidemica und beim Verschlussikterus. Deutsch. Z. Verdau., **15,** 70, 1955.
192. Peterson, R. E.: The serum iron in acute hepatitis. J. Lab. Clin. Med., **39,** 225, 1952.
193. Reissman, K. R., and Dietrich, M. R.: On the presence of ferritin in the peripheral blood of patients with hepatocellular disease. J. Clin. Invest., **35,** 588, 1956.
194. Rumball, J. M., Stone, C. M., Jr., and Hassett, C.: The behavior of serum iron in acute hepatitis. Gastroenterology, **36,** 219, 1959.
195. Stone, C. M., Jr., Rumball, J. M., and Hassett, C. P.: An evaluation of the serum iron in liver disease. Ann. Intern. Med., **43,** 229, 1955.
196. Burton, J. L.: Effect of oral contraceptives on haemoglobin, packed-cell volume, serum-iron, and total iron-binding capacity in healthy women. Lancet, **1,** 978, 1967.
197. Pollycove, M.: Iron kinetics, in *Iron in Clinical Medicine,* edited by R. O. Wallerstein, p. 43. University of California Press, Berkeley, 1958.
198. Pollycove, M.: Ferrokinetics: techniques, in *Eisenstoffwechsel,* edited by W. Keiderling, p. 20. Thieme, Stuttgart, 1959.
199. Huff, R. L., Hennessy, T. G., Austin, R. E., Garcia, J. F., Roberts, B. M., and Lawrence, J. H.: Plasma and red cell iron turnover in normal subjects and in patients having various hematopoietic disorders. J. Clin.
200. Huff, R. L., Elmlinger, P. J., Garcia, J. F., Oeda, J. M., Cockrell, M. C., and Lawrence, J. H.: Ferrokinetics in normal persons and in patients having various erythropoietic disorders. J. Clin. Invest., **30,** 1512, 1951.
201. Pollycove, M.: Iron kinetics, in *Iron Metabolism,* edited by F. Gross, p. 148. Springer-Verlag, Berlin, 1964.
202. Pollycove, M.: *Iron Metabolism:* Thannhauser's Textbook of Metabolism and Metabolic Disorders, vol. II, 2d ed., revised, edited by N. Zollner and S. Estren, p. 809. Grune & Stratton, New York, 1964.
203. Pollycove, M.: Iron metabolism and kinetics. Seminars Hemat., **3,** 235, 1966.
204. Pollycove, M., Winchell, H. S., and Lawrence, J. H.: Classification and evolution of patterns of erythropoiesis in polycythemia vera as studied by iron kinetics. Blood, **28,** 807, 1966.
205. Pollycove, M., and Maqsood, M.: Existence of an erythropoietic labile iron pool in animals. Nature (London), **194,** 152, 1961.
206. Morgan, E. H., and Laurell, C. B.: Studies on the exchange of iron between transferrin and reticulocytes. Brit. J. Haemat., **9,** 471, 1963.
207. Bessis, M.: Étude au microscope électronique du rôle de la ferritine dans le cycle hémoglobinique du fer, in *Eisenstoffweschsel,* edited by W. Keiderling, p. 11. Thieme, Stuttgart, 1959.
208. Bessis, M.: Erythropoiesis as seen with the electron microscope, in *Kinetics of Cellular Proliferation,* edited by F. Stohlman, Jr., p. 22. Grune & Stratton, New York, 1959.
209. Sondhaus, G. A., and Thorell, B.: Microspectrophotometric determinations of nonheme iron in maturing erythroblasts and its relationship to the endocellular hemoglobin formation. Blood, **16,** 1285, 1960.
210. Mazur, A., Green, S., and Carleton, A.: Mechanism of plasma iron incorporation into hepatic ferritin. J. Biol. Chem., **235,** 595, 1960.
211. Deiss, A., and Cartwright, G. E.: Ferritin metabolism in reticulated siderocytes. J. Clin. Invest., **49,** 517, 1970.
212. Pollycove, M., Elmlinger, P. J., Sarkes, L. A., Apt, L., and Ross, J. F.: Radioiron determination of human erythrocyte lifespan distribution. Clin. Res. Proc., **4,** 79, 1956.
213. Sargent, T., Pollycove, M., Carpe, L., and Lawrence, J. H.: Dynamics of total body iron: gastrointestinal blood, storage and "fixed" components. Clin. Res., **10,** 78, 1962.
214. Vitale, L., Opitz, J. M., and Shahidi, N. T.: Congenital and familial iron overload. New Eng. J. Med., **280,** 642, 1969.
215. Schwartz, S. O., and Blumenthal., S. A.: Exogenous hemochromatosis resulting from blood transfusions. Blood, **3,** 617, 1948.
216. Bothwell, T. H.: The relationship of transfusional haemosiderosis to idiopathic haemochromatosis. South African J. Clin. Sci., **4,** 53, 1953.
217. Oliver, R. A.: Siderosis following transfusions of blood. J. Path. Bact., **77,** 171, 1959.
218. Seftel, H. C., Keeley, K. J., Isaacson, C., and Bothwell, T. H.: Siderosis in the Bantu: the clinical incidence of haemochromatosis in diabetic subjects. J. Clin. Med., **58,** 837, 1961.
219. MacDonald, R. A.: *Hemochromatosis and Hemosiderosis.* Charles C Thomas, Springfield, Ill., 1964.
220. Caroli, J., and André, J.: Surcharge ferrique dans les cirrhosis (à l'exclusion de l'hémochromatose idiopathique), in *Iron Metabolism,* edited by F. Gross, p. 326. Springer-Verlag, Berlin, 1964.
221. Lundvall, O., Weinfeld, A., and Lundin, P.: Iron stores in alcohol abusers. Acta Med. Scand., **185,** 259, 1969.
222. Callender, S. T., and Malpas, J. S.: Absorption of iron in cirrhosis of liver. Brit. Med. J., **2,** 1516, 1963.
223. Greenberg, M. S., Strohmeyer, G., Hine, G. J., Keene, W. R., Curtis G., and Chalmers, T. C.: Body radioactivity measurements in patients with liver disease. Gastroenterology, **46,** 651, 1964.
224. Linscheer, W. G., Greenberg, M. S., Moore, E. W., and Chalmers, T. C.: Absorption in the proximal small intestine in patients with cirrhosis. Gastroenterology, **46,** 682, 1964.
225. Murray, J., and Stein, N.: The case for increased iron absorption in liver disease. Medicine, **45,** 507, 1966.
226. Friedman, B. I., Schaefer, J. W., and Schiff, L.: Increased iron-59 absorption in patients with hepatic cirrhosis. J. Nucl. Med., **7,** 594, 1966.
227. Williams, R., Williams, H. S., Scheuer, P. J., Pitcher, C. S., Loiseau, E., and Sherlock, S.: Iron absorption and siderosis in chronic liver disease. Quart. J. Med., **36,** 151, 1967.
228. Sargent, T. W.: Personal communication.
229. Grace, N. D., and Balint, J. A.: Hemochromatosis associated with end-to-side portacaval anastomosis. Amer. J. Digest. Dis., **11,** 351, 1966.
230. Ecker, J. A., Gray, P. A., McKittrick, J. E., and Dickson, D. R.: The development of postshunt hemochromatosis—parenchymal siderosis in patients with cirrhosis occuring after portasystemic shunt surgery. Amer. J. Gastroent., **50,** 13, 1968.
231. Castleman, B., and Towne, V. W.: Case records of the Massachusetts General Hospital: Case no. 38512. New Eng. J. Med., **247,** 992, 1952.
232. Castleman, B., and Towne, V. W.: Case records of the Massachusetts General Hospital: Case no. 39472. New Eng. J. Med., **249,** 859, 1953.
233. Wallerstein, R. O., and Robbins, S. L.: Hemochromatosis after prolonged oral iron therapy in a patient with chronic hemolytic anemia. Amer. J. Med., **14,** 256, 1953.
234. Turnberg, L. A.: Excessive oral iron therapy causing haemochromatosis. Brit. Med. J., **1,** 1360, 1965.
235. Bannerman, R. M., Keusch, G., Kreimer-Birnbaum, M., Vance, V. K.,

and Vaughn, S.: Thalassemia intermedia, with iron overload, cardiac failure, diabetes mellitus, hypopituitarism and porphyrinuria. Amer. J. Med., **42,** 476, 1967.

236. Johnson, B. F.: Hemochromatosis resulting from prolonged oral iron therapy. New Eng. J. Med., **278,** 1100, 1968.
237. Hiyeda, K.: The cause of Kaschin-Beck's disease. Jap. J. Med. Sci., **4,** 91, 1939.
238. Kent, G., and Popper, H.: Secondary hemochromatosis: its association with anemia. Arch. Path. (Chicago), **70,** 623, 1960.
239. Wilson, J. D., Scott, P. J., and North, J. D. K.: Hemochromatosis in association with hereditary spherocytosis. Arch. Intern. Med., **120,** 701, 1967.
240. Barry, M., Scheuer, P. J., Sherlock, S., Ross, C. F., and Williams, R.: Hereditary spherocytosis with secondary hemochromatosis. Lancet, **2,** 481, 1968.
241. Frumin, A. M., Waldman, S., and Morris, P.: Exogenous hemochromatosis in Mediterranean anemia. Pediatrics, **9,** 290, 1952.
242. Howell, J., and Wyatt, J. P.: Development of pigmentary cirrhosis in Cooley's anemia. A.M.A. Arch. Path., **55,** 423, 1953.
243. Ellis, J. I., Schulman, I., and Smith, C. F.: Generalized siderosis with fibrosis of liver and pancreas in Cooley's (Mediterranean) anemia, with observations on the pathogenesis of siderosis and fibrosis. Amer. J. Path., **30,** 287, 1954.
244. Currin, J. F.: Occurrence of secondary hemochromatosis in patient with thalassemia major. A.M.A. Arch. Intern. Med., **93,** 781, 1954.
245. Engle, M. A.: Cardiac involvement in Cooley's anemia. Ann. N.Y. Acad. Sci., **119,** 694, 1964.
246. Koszewski, B. J.: Occurrence of megaloblastic erythropoiesis in patients with hemochromatosis. Blood, **7,** 1182, 1952.
247. Granville, N., and Dameshek, W.: Hemochromatosis with megaloblastic anemia responding to folic acid: report of a case. New Eng. J. Med., **258,** 586, 1958.
248. Dickerman, R. C., Rom, J., and Kobernick, S. D.: Chronic erythremic myelosis with exogenous hemochromatosis. Amer. J. Clin. Path., **27,** 56, 1957.
249. Maier, C.: Megaloblastare Vitamin B_6 Mangelanämie bei Hämochromatose. Schweiz. Med. Wschr., **87,** 1234, 1957.
250. Goldish, R. J., and Aufderheide, A. C.: Secondary hemochromatosis. II. Report of a case not attributable to blood transfusion. Blood, **8,** 837, 1953.
251. Caroli, J., Bessis, M., Combrisson, A., Malassenet, R., and Breton, J.: Hémochromatose avec anémie hypochrome et absence d'hémoglobine anormal. Presse Med., **65,** 1991, 1957.
252. Von Lukl, P., Widermann, B., and Barborik, M.: Hereditare Leptocyten-Anämie bie Mannern mit Hämochromatose. Folia Haemat. (Frankfurt Am Main), **3,** 17, 1958.
253. Byrd, R. B., and Cooper, T.: Hereditary iron loading anemia with secondary hemochromatosis. Ann. Intern. Med., **55,** 103, 1961.
254. Gelpi, A. P., and Ende, M.: An hereditary anemia with hemochromatosis: studies of the unusual hemopathic syndrome resembling thalassemia. Amer. J. Med., **25,** 303, 1958.
255. Block, M.: Hemosiderosis and hemochromatosis, in *Iron in Clinical Medicine,* edited by R. O. Wallerstein and S. R. Mettier, p. 115. University of California Press, Berkeley, 1958.
256. Recant, L., and Lacy, P. (editors): Hemosiderosis versus hemochromatosis: refractory anemia, hepatic dysfunction, diabetes and increased tissue iron deposits, in Clinicopathologic Conference. Amer. J. Med., **38,** 450, 1965.
257. Houston, J. C.: Hemochromatosis and refractory anemia. Guy's Hosp. Rep., **100,** 355, 1951.
258. Norris, R. P., and McEven, F. J.: Exogenous hemochromatosis following multiple blood transfusions. J.A.M.A., **143,** 740, 1950.
259. Morningstar, W. A.: Exogenous hemochromatosis: a report of 3 cases, A.M.A. Arch. Path., **59,** 355, 1955.
260. Ceelen, W.: Die Kreislaufstoerungen der Lungen in Henke-Lubarsch, in *Handbuch der speziellen pathologischen Anatomie und Histologie,* vol. III, part 3, p. 20. Springer-Verlag, Berlin, 1931.
261. Soergel, K. H., and Sommers, S. C.: Idiopathic pulmonary hemosiderosis and related syndromes. Amer. J. Med., **32,** 499, 1962.
262. Waldenström, J.: Relapsing, diffuse, pulmonary bleedings or haemosiderosis pulmonum: new clinical diagnosis. Acta Radiol. [Diagn.] (Stockholm), **25,** 149, 1944.
263. Bruwer, A. J., Kennedy, R. L. J., and Edwards, J. E.: Recurrent pulmonary hemorrhage with hemosiderosis: so-called idiopathic pulmonary hemosiderosis. Amer. J. Roentgen., **76,** 98, 1956.
264. MacGregor, C. S., Johnson, R. S., and Turk, K. A. D.: Fatal nephritis complicating idiopathic pulmonary haemosiderosis in young adults. Thorax, **15,** 198, 1960.
265. Heptinstall, R. H., and Salmon, M. V.: Pulmonary haemorrhage with extensive glomerular disease of the kidney. J. Clin. Path., **12,** 272, 1959.
266. Parkin, T. W., Rusted, I. E., Burchell, H. B., and Edwards, J. E.: Hemorrhagic and interstitial pneumonitis with nephritis. Amer. J. Med., **18,** 220, 1955.
267. Sande, E.: Essential pulmonary haemosiderosis: Account of 2 cases, 1 treated experimentally with ACTH. Danish Med. Bull., **1,** 175, 1954.
268. Hanssen, P.: Haemosiderosis pulmonum. Acta Pediat. Scand., **34,** 103, 1947.
269. Gluck, E.: Idiopathic pulmonary haemosiderosis: report of a case with special regard to the pathogenesis. Acta Path. Microbiol. Scand., **37,** 241, 1955.
270. Wiesmann, W., Wolvius, D., and Verloop, M. C.: Idiopathic pulmonary hemosiderosis. Acta Med. Scand., **146,** 341, 1953.
271. Wyllie, W. G., Sheldon, W., Bodian, M., and Barlow, A.: Idiopathic pulmonary haemosiderosis (essential brown induration of the lungs). Quart. J. Med., **17,** 25, 1948.
272. Anspach, W. E.: Pulmonary hemosiderosis. Amer. J. Roentgen., **41,** 592, 1939.
273. Edwards, J. W., Parkin, T. W., and Burchell, H. B.: Recurrent hemoptysis and necrotizing pulmonary alveolitis in a patient with acute glomerulonephritis and periarteritis nodosa. Proc. Staff Meet. Mayo Clin., **29,** 193, 1954.
274. Schuler, D., and Flesch, I.: Über die Ätiologie und Pathogenese der essentiellen Lungenhämosiderose. Ann. Pediat. (Basel), **185,** 96, 1955.
275. Steiner, B.: Essential pulmonary haemosiderosis as an immunohaematological problem. Arch. Dis. Child., **29,** 391, 1954.
276. Apt, L., Pollycove, M., and Ross, J. F.: Idiopathic pulmonary hemosiderosis: a study of the anemia and iron distribution using radioiron and radiochromium. J. Clin. Invest., **36,** 1150, 1957.
277. Crosby, W. H.: Paroxysmal nocturnal hemoglobinuria: relation of the clinical manifestations to underlying pathogenic mechanisms. Blood, **8,** 769, 1953.
278. Wintrobe, M. M.: Hemolytic anemias, in *Clinical Hematology,* chap. 12, p. 598. Lea & Febiger, Philadelphia, 1961.
279. Ippen, H.: Entstehung und Behandlung der Porphyria cutanea tarda. Klin. Wschr., **38,** 89, 1960.
280. Ippen, H.: Beobachtungen bei der Aderlassbehandlung der Porphyria cutanea tarda. Arch. Klin. Exp. Derm., **213,** 863, 1961.
281. Lundvall, O., and Weinfeld, A.: Studies of the clinical and metabolic effects of phlebotomy treatment in porphyria cutanea tarda. Acta Med. Scand., **184,** 191, 1968.
282. Epstein, J. H., and Redeker, A. G.: Porphyria cutanea tarda: a study of the effect of phlebotomy. New Eng. J. Med., **279,** 1301, 1968.
283. Althausen, T. L., Doig, R. K., Weiden, S., Motteram, R., Turner, C. N., and Moore, A.: Hemochromatosis: investigation of 23 cases, with special references to etiology, nutrition, iron metabolism, and studies of hepatic and pancreatic functions. A.M.A. Arch. Intern. Med., **88,** 553, 1951.
284. Alper, T., Savage, D. V., and Bothwell, T. H.: Radioiron studies in a case of hemochromatosis. J. Lab. Clin. Med., **37,** 665, 1951.
285. Peterson, R. E., and Ettinger, R. H.: Radioactive iron absorption in siderosis (hemochromatosis) of the liver. Amer. J. Med., **15,** 518, 1953.
286. Heilmeyer, L., von: Die Hämochromatose: Klinik, Eisenstoffwechsel und Pathogenese. Acta Haemat. (Basel), **11,** 137, 1954.
287. Balfour, W., Hahn, P. F., Bale, W. F., Pommerenke, W. T., and Whipple, G. H.: Radioactive iron absorption in clinical conditions: normal, pregnancy, anemia, and hemochromatosis. J. Exp. Med., **76,** 15, 1942.
288. Williams, R., Manenti, F., Williams, H. S., and Pitcher, C. S.: Iron absorption in idiopathic haemochromatosis before, during, and after venesection therapy. Brit. Med. J., **2,** 78, 1966.

289. Balcerzak, S. P., Westerman, M. P., Lee, R. E., and Doyle, A. P.: Idiopathic hemochromatosis. Amer. J. Med., **40,** 857, 1966.
290. Pirzio-Biroli, G., Bothwell, T. H., and Finch, C. A.: Iron absorption. II. The absorption of radioiron administered with a standard meal in man. J. Lab. Clin. Med., **51,** 37, 1958.
291. Bothwell, T. H., Elliz, B. C., Van Doorn-Wittkampf, H., and Abraham, O. L.: Radioiron studies in hemochromatosis: the effects of repeated phlebotomies. J. Lab. Clin. Med., **45,** 167, 1955.
292. Deller, D. J.: Iron-59 absorption measurements by whole body counting: studies in alcoholic cirrhosis, hemochromatosis, and pancreatis. Amer. J. Dig. Dis., **10,** 249, 1965.
293. Boender, C. A., and Verloop, M. C.: Iron absorption, iron loss and iron retention in man: studies after oral administration of a tracer dose of $^{59}FeSO_4$ and $^{131}BaSO_4$. Brit. J. Haemat., **17,** 45, 1969.
294. Sargent, T.: Increased iron absorption in relatives of patients with endogenous hemochromatosis. Presented at Tenth Congr. Int. Soc. Hemat., Stockholm, 1964.
295. Williams, R., Pitcher, C. S., Parsonson, A., and Williams, H. S.: Iron absorption in the relatives of patients with idiopathic hemochromatosis. Lancet, **1,** 1243, 1965.
296. Ayvazian, J. H.: Xanthinuria and hemochromatosis. New Eng. J. Med., **270,** 18, 1964.
297. Dent, C. E., and Philpot, G. R.: Xanthinuria, inborn error (or deviation) of metabolism. Lancet, **1,** 182, 1954.
298. Dickinson, C. J., and Smellie, J. M.: Xanthinuria. Brit. Med. J., **2,** 1217, 1959.
299. Watts, R. W. E., Engleman, K., Klinenberg, J. R., Seegmiller, J. E., and Sjoerdsma, A.: The enzyme defect in a case of xanthinuria. Biochem. J., **90,** 4P, 1964.
300. Engleman, K., Watts, R. W. E., Klinenberg, J. R., Sjoerdsma, A., and Seegmiller, J. E.: Clinical, physiological and biochemical studies of a patient with xanthinuria and pheochromocytoma. Amer. J. Med., **37,** 839, 1964.
301. Hedenberg, L.: Studies on iron metabolism with desferrioxamine in man. Scand. J. Haemat., suppl. **6,** 1969.
302. Mazur, A., and Sackler, M.: Hemochromatosis and hepatic xanthine oxidase. Lancet, **1,** 254, 1967.
303. MacDonald, R. A., Jones, R. S., and Pechet, G. S.: Folic acid deficiency and hemochromatosis. Arch. Path. (Chicago), **80,** 153, 1965.
304. MacDonald, R. A., Endo, H., and Pechet, G. S.: Studies of experimental hemochromatosis. Arch. Path. (Chicago), **85,** 366, 1968.
305. Pollycove, M., Fawwaz, R. A., and Winchell, H. S.: Transient hepatic deposition of iron in primary hemochromatosis with iron deficiency following venesection. J. Nucl. Med., **12,** 28, 1971.
306. Guye, P.: La Cirrhose pigmentaire. À propos de cas de cette affection examinés a l'Institut Pathologique de Genève, au cours de 30 années. Helv. Med. Acta, **4,** 209, 1937.
307. Lisa, J. R., and Hart, J. F.: Pigment cirrhosis: rate of occurrence and difficulties in diagnosis. New York J. Med., **39,** 521, 1939.
308. Vogt, J. H.: Hemochromatosis. Acta Path. Microbiol. Scand., **21,** 461, 1944.
309. Butt, H. R., and Wilder, R. N.: Hemochromatosis: report of 30 cases in which the diagnosis was made during life. Arch. Path. (Chicago), **20,** 262, 1938.
310. King, W. E., and Downie, E.: Hemochromatosis: observations on the incidence and on the value of liver biopsy in diagnosis. Quart. J. Med., **17,** 247, 1948.
311. Kleckner, M. S., Kark, R. M., Baker, L. A., Chapman, A. Z., Kaplan, E., and Moore, T. J.: Clinical features, pathology, and therapy of hemochromatosis. J.A.M.A., **157,** 1471, 1955.
312. Williams, R., Smith, P. M., Spicer, E. J. F., Barry, M., and Sherlock, S.: Venesection therapy in idiopathic haemochromatosis. Quart. J. Med., **38,** 1, 1969.
313. Charlton, R. W., Abrahams, C., and Bothwell, T. H.: Idiopathic hemochromatosis in young subjects. Arch. Path. (Chicago), **83,** 132, 1967.
314. Althausen, T. L., and Kerr, W. J.: Haemochromatosis. II. A report of 3 cases with endocrine disturbances and notes on a previously reported case. Discussion and etiology. Endocrinology, **17,** 621, 1933.
315. Clinicopathological Conference: Haemochromatosis versus Addison's disease. Amer. J. Med., **9,** 383, 1950.
316. deGennes, C.: Le Syndrome endocrinien des cirrhoses bronzées. Acta Gastroent., Belg., **15,** 208, 1952.
317. Azérad, E., and Lubetzki, J.: Évolution particuliére de l'insuffisance endocrinienne et syndrome de Sheehan terminal dans une hémochromatose idiopathique. Bull. Soc. Med. Hop. Paris, **144,** 777, 1963.
318. Kent, J. R., Aronow, W. S., and Meister, L.: Hypogonadotrophic hypogonadism in hemochromatosis. Calif. Med. **3,** 450, 1969.
319. Stocks, A. E., and Martin, F. I. R.: Pituitary function in haemochromatosis. Amer. J. Med., **45,** 839, 1968.
320. Schumacher, H. R.: Hemochromatosis and arthritis. Arthritis Rheum., **7,** 41, 1964.
321. Hamilton, E., Williams, R., Barlow, K. A., and Smith, P. M.: The arthropathy of idiopathic haemochromatosis. Quart. J. Med., **37,** 171, 1968.
322. Wardle, E. N., and Patton, J. T.: Bone and joint changes in haemochromatosis. Ann. Rheum. Dis., **28,** 15, 1969.
323. Kra, S. J., Hollingsworth, J. W., and Finch, S. C.: Arthritis with synovial iron deposition in a patient with hemochromatosis. New Eng. J. Med., **272,** 1268, 1965.
324. Aufderheide, A. C., Horns, H. L., and Goldish, R. J.: Secondary hemochromatosis. I. Transfusion (exogenous) hemochromatosis. Blood, **8,** 824, 1953.
325. Kleckner, M. S., Baggenstoss, A. H., and Weir, J. F.: Hemochromatosis and transfusional hemosiderosis: a clinical and pathologic study. Amer. J. Med., **16,** 682, 1954.
326. Dubin, I. N.: Idiopathic hemochromatosis and transfusion siderosis. Amer. J. Clin. Path., **25,** 514, 1955.
327. Wyatt, J. P.: Patterns of pathological iron storage. A.M.A. Arch. Path., **61,** 42, 1956.
328. Hedinger, C.: Zur Pathologie der Hämochromatose: Hämochromatose als Syndrom. Helv. Med. Acta (suppl. 32), **20,** 1, 1953.
329. Brick, I. B.: Liver histology in 6 asymptomatic siblings in family with hemochromatosis: genetic implications. Gastroenterology, **40,** 210, 1961.
330. Pirart, J., and Carpent, G.: Aspects dynamiques de l'hémochromatose. Acta Gastroent. Belg., **18,** 7, 1955.
331. Powell, L. W.: Iron storage in relatives of patients with haemochromatosis and in relatives of patients with alcoholic cirrhosis and haemosiderosis. Quart. J. Med., **34,** 427, 1965.
332. Bothwell, T. H., Abrahams, C., Bradlow, B. A., and Charlton, R. W.: Idiopathic and Bantu hemochromatosis. Arch. Path. (Chicago), **79,** 163, 1965.
333. James, T. N.: Pathology of the cardiac conduction system in hemochromatosis. New Eng. J. Med., **271,** 92, 1964.
334. Hellier, F. F.: The nature and causation of the skin pigmentation in hemochromatosis. Brit. J. Derm. Syph., **47,** 1, 1935.
335. Holmes, N. E.: A case of hemochromatosis with almost complete absence of skin pigment, and with fatal rupture of an esophageal varix. Ann. Intern. Med., **13,** 1075, 1939.
336. Lonergan, P., and Robbins, S. L.: Absence of intercapillary glomerulosclerosis in the diabetic patient with hemochromatosis. New Eng. J. Med., **260,** 366, 1959.
337. Becker, D., and Miller, M.: Presence of diabetic glomerulosclerosis in patients with hemochromatosis. New Eng. J. Med., **263,** 367, 1960.
338. Rous, P.: Urinary siderosis: haemosiderin granules in the urine as an aid in the diagnosis of pernicious anaemia, haemochromatosis, and other diseases causing siderosis of the kidney. J. Exp. Med., **28,** 645, 1918.
339. Hallberg, L., and Hedenberg, L.: The effect of desferrioxamine on iron metabolism in man. Scand. J. Haemat., **2,** 67, 1965.
340. Fielding, J.: Differential ferrioxamine test for measuring chelatable body iron. J. Clin. Path., **18,** 88, 1965.
341. Hallberg, L., Hedenberg, L., and Weinfeld, A.: Liver iron and desferrioxamine-induced urinary iron excretion. Scand. J. Haemat., **3,** 85, 1966.
342. Harker, L. A., Funk, D. D., and Finch, C. A.: Evaluation of storage iron by chelates. Amer. J. Med., **45,** 105, 1968.
343. Fielding, J., O'Shaughnessy, M. C., Brunstrom, G. M.: Differential ferrioxamine test in idiopathic haemochromatosis and transfusional haemosiderosis. J. Clin. Path., **19,** 159, 1966.

344. Smith, P. M., Studley, F., Williams, R.: Assessment of body-iron stores in cirrhosis and hemochromatosis with the differential ferrioxamine test. Lancet, **1**, 133, 1967.
345. Knauer, C. M., Gamble, C. N., and Monroe, L. S.: The reversal of hemochromatotic cirrhosis by multiple phlebotomies. Gastroenterology, **49**, 667, 1965.
346. Moeschlin, S. (moderator): Erfahrungen mit Desferrioxamin bei pathologischen Eisenablagerungen. Schweiz. Med. Wschr., **92**, 1295, 1962.
347. Heilmeyer, L., and Wohler, F.: Moderne Hämochromatose Probleme mit besonderer Berucksichtigung Desferrioxaminbehandlung. Deutsch. Med. Wschr., **87**, 2661, 1962.
348. Wohler, F.: The treatment of haemochromatosis with desferrioxamine. Acta Haemat. (Basel), **30**, 65, 1963; and in *Iron Metabolism,* edited by F. Gross, p. 551. Springer-Verlag, Berlin, 1964.
349. Moeschlin, S., and Schnider, U.: Treatment of primary and secondary haemochromatosis and acute iron poisoning with a new, potent, iron-eliminating agent (desferrioxamine B), in *Iron Metabolism,* edited by F. Gross, p. 525. Springer-Verlag, Berlin, 1964.
350. Albahary, C.: Introduction to the general discussion of the therapeutic effects of desferrioxamine and calcium—D.T.P.A., in *Iron Metabolism,* edited by F. Gross, p. 580. Springer-Verlag, Berlin, 1964.
351. Frisch, A. V.: Über familiäre Hämochromatose. Wien. Arch. Inn. Med., **4**, 149, 1922.
352. Boland, B. F., and Curran, L. G.: Hemochromatosis: two atypical cases occurring in brothers. J.A.M.A., **97**, 379, 1931.
353. Rogers, W. F., Jr.: Familial hemochromatosis: with comments on adrenal function in hemochromatosis. Amer. J. Med. Sci., **220**, 530, 1960.
354. Lesieur, A.: À propos d'un cas familial de cirrhose bronzée. Arch. Mal. App. Digest., **39**, 960, 1950.
355. Lohr, K., and Reinwein, H.: Konkordantes Aufreten von Lebercirrhose und Diabetes mellitus (Hämochromatose) bei eineiigen Zwillingen. Deutsch. Arch. Klin. Med., **200**, 53, 1952.
356. Boulin, R., and Bamberger, J.: L'Hémochromatose familiale. Sem. Hop. Paris, **29**, 3153, 1953.
357. Nussbaumer, T., Plattner, H. C., and Rywlin, A.: Hémochromatose juvénile chez trois soeurs et un frère avec consanguinité des parents: étude anatomoclinique et génétique due syndroms endocrino-hépatomyocardinique. J. Genet. Hum., **1**, 53, 1953.
358. Houston, J. C., and Zilkha, K. J.: Hemochromatosis in a family. Guy. Hosp. Rep., **104**, 262, 1955.
359. Darnis, F.: L'Hémochromatose idiopathique familiale. Rev. Prat., **8**, 2985, 1958.
360. Conte, J., Ristelhueber, J., and Malvezin, J. C.: Les Hémochromatoses familiales et héréditaires. Bull. Soc. Med. Hop. Paris, **74**, 267, 1958.
361. Pirart, J., and Gatz, P.: L'Étiologie de l'hémochromatose nontransfusionelle; révue de la question; étude de l'hérédité dans 21 familles. Sem. Hop. Paris, **34**, 1044, 1958.
362. Bothwell, T. H., Cohen, I., Abrams, O. L., and Perold, S. M.: A familial study in idiopathic hemochromatosis. Amer. J. Med., **27**, 730, 1959.
363. Dillingham, C. H.: Familial occurrence of hemochromatosis. New Eng. J. Med., **262**, 1128, 1960.
364. Brick, I. B., and Rath, C. E.: Familial hemochromatosis: comparison and diagnostic procedures in 7 siblings with liver biopsy findings. Clin. Res., **8**, 199, 1960.
365. Davison, R. H.: Inheritance of haemochromatosis. Brit. Med. J., **2**, 1262, 1961.
366. Morgan, E. H.: Idiopathic haemochromatosis: a family study. Aust. Ann. Med., **10**, 114, 1961.
367. Frey, W. C., Milne, J., Johnson, G. B., and Ebaugh, F. G.: Management of familial hemochromatosis. New Eng. J. Med., **265**, 7, 1961.
368. Brunner, H. E., Frick, P. G., and Hitzig, W. H.: Familiar Hämochromatosen nachweis der Stoffwechselstorung in der Fruphase mit Fe^{59}. Schweiz. Med. Wschr., **92**, 343, 1962.
369. Johnson, G. B., and Frey, W. G.: Familial aspects of idiopathic hemochromatosis. J.A.M.A., **179**, 747, 1962.
370. Lloyd, H. M., Powell, L. W., and Thomas M. J.: Idiopathic hemochromatosis in menstruating women. Lancet, **2**, 555, 1964.
371. Ploem, J. E., Otten, K., Huizinga, J., and Verloop, M. C.: Idiopathic haemosiderosis. Scand. J. Haemat., **2**, 3, 1965.
372. Perkins, K. W., McInnes, I. W. S., Blackburn, C. R. B., and Beal, R. W.: Idiopathic haemochromatosis in children. Amer. J. Med., **39**, 118, 1965.
373. Turner, P. P.: Idiopathic hemochromatosis in a family. Lancet, **2**, 72, 1966.
374. Felts, J. H., Nelson, J. R., Herndon, C. N., and Spurr, C. L.: Hemochromatosis in two young sisters. Ann. Intern. Med., **67**, 117, 1967.
375. Charlton, R. W., and Bothwell, T. H.: Hemochromatosis: dietary and genetic aspects. Progr. Hemat., **5**, 298, 1966.
376. Risola, A.: Su un cas di emochromatosi ad impronta familliare. Rass. Giuliana Med., **6**, 66, 1950.
377. Debré R., Dreyfus, J., Frezal, J., Labie, D., Lamy, M., Maroteaux, P., Schapira, F., and Schapira, G.: Genetics of haemochromatosis. Ann. Hum. Genet., **23**, 16, 1958.
378. Sinniah, R.: Environmental and genetic factors in idiopathic hemochromatosis. Arch. Intern. Med., **124**, 455, 1969.
379. Dreyfus, J. C., and Schapira, G.: The metabolism of iron in hemochromatosis, in *Iron Metabolism,* edited by F. Gross, p. 296. Springer-Verlag, Berlin, 1964.
380. Williams, R., Scheuer, P. J., and Sherlock, S.: The inheritance of idiopathic haemochromatosis: a clinical and liver biopsy study of 16 families. Quart. J. Med., **31**, 249, 1962.
381. Zimmerman, H. J., Chomet, B., Kulesh, M. H., and McWhorter, C. A.: Hepatic hemosiderin deposits; incidence in 558 biopsies from patients with and without intrinsic hepatic disease. Arch. Intern. Med., **107**, 494, 1961.
382. Pechet, G. S., French, S., Levy, J., and Mac Donald, R. A.: Stainable tissue iron: significance for hemochromatosis. Lab. Invest., **13**, 948, 1964.
383. Frick, P.: Discussion of the metabolism of iron in primary hemochromatosis, in *Iron Metabolism,* edited by F. Gross, p. 343. Springer-Verlag, Berlin, 1964.

PART EIGHT

DISEASES OF PORPHYRIN AND HEME METABOLISM

CHAPTER FORTY-FIVE

THE PORPHYRIAS *

Harvey S. Marver† and Rudi Schmid

Since the end of the nineteenth century porphyria has aroused the curiosity and interest of clinicians and investigators alike and has received widespread attention in spite of its relatively infrequent occurrence. A continuing interest in disorders of porphyrin metabolism is largely due to three factors: (1) the unusual variety of clinical manifestations of these disturbances, (2) the relative ease with which very small amounts of porphyrins can be identified and estimated because of their unique spectroscopic and fluorescent properties, and (3) the fundamental importance of porphyria as a model of genetic defects in enzyme regulation.

Porphyria has been the subject of innumerable clinical reports and of many biochemical investigations, but only relatively recently has information been accumulated regarding the nature and location of the metabolic defects which appear to be responsible for the occurrence of this group of diseases. In the last 20 years, with the advent of tracer techniques, impressive progress has been made, and much of the biosynthetic pathway by which porphyrins and heme are formed has been clarified. This better understanding of the normal pathway of metabolism has provided an indispensable basis for the elucidation of the biochemical defects involved in the various types of porphyria.

HISTORY

The first authentic case of porphyria recorded in the literature was reported by Schultz [1] and by Baumstark [2] under the diagnosis of "pemphigus leprosus." The patient was a 33-year-old craftsman with a lifelong history of photosensitivity and excretion of wine-red urine; the presence of splenomegaly and slight chronic icterus suggested the possibility of a hemolytic anemia. From his urine Baumstark [2] isolated two pigments, "urorubrohaematin" and "urofuscohaematin," the former of which unmistakably exhibited the spectroscopic and solubility properties of the compound now designated as uroporphyrin.

A few years later, MacMunn [3] reported five patients suffering from "subacute rheumatism," or "idiopathic pericarditis," whose urine contained a red pigment which he named "urohaematin." Although "urohaematin" undoubtedly was a porphyrin, it is questionable whether MacMunn was actually describing uroporphyrin. Its solubility in chloroform and its spectroscopic properties, which differed slightly from those of Baumstark's "urorubrohaematin" [2], suggest that MacMunn may have been dealing with the pigment which today is known as *coproporphyrin.* In spite of the recognized slight spectroscopic differences, Salkowski [4], Hammersten [5], Garrod [6], Stokvis [7], Saillet [8], Anderson [9], Nebelthau [10], and others regarded these pigments as identical with hematoporphyrin,* which Hoppe-Seyler [11] and Nencki and Sieber [12] had prepared by exposing hemoglobin to concentrated sulfuric acid. Garrod [6] discovered "haematoporphyrin or allied pigments" in the urine of 76 out of a group of 126 patients of a mixed hospital population. His conclusion that "haematoporphyrin" was an "almost constant constituent of urine in health and disease" reached far ahead into modern concepts of porphyrin metabolism. During the next two decades massive "hematoporphyrinuria" was observed in a large number of patients with such diverse manifestations as photodermatitis, colicky abdominal pain, bizarre involvement of the nervous system, or psychic disturbances [13].

PROPOSED CLASSIFICATIONS

Günther [14] was the first in attempting to arrange the reported cases according to certain recurrent clinical patterns. His classification distinguished between *haematoporphyria congenita* and *haematoporphyria acuta:* the latter included idiopathic and toxic forms. In addition, he designated a few cases as *haematoporphyria chronica,* which he originally considered as a separate entity but later tended to regard as mild and late forms of porphyria congenita [15]. In such patients the photosensitivity and the excretion of red urine are indeed characteristic of what is now termed congenital (erythropoietic) porphyria; yet these two conditions differ strikingly in their clinical course, particularly in the time of onset of the first symptoms. In 1937 Waldenström [16] proposed substituting the term *porphyria cutanea tarda* for Günther's original "chronic porphyria." In recent years the fundamental difference between congenital photosensitive porphyria as a defect in the *erythropoietic system* and porphyria cutanea tarda as a disturbance in *liver metabolism* has become well recognized [13, 17, 19].

Under the term *acute porphyria* Waldenström [16] included a variety of clinical subforms with different manifestations, such as abdominal colic, peripheral neuropathy and paralysis, psychosis, and coma. In addition, patients who excreted abnormal amounts and types of porphyrins, including

*This work was supported in part by National Institutes of Health grants AM-11275 and AM-11296, and Career Development Award K04 AM-14301-01.

†Deceased.

*Hematoporphyrin is not found in nature but can be prepared from hemoglobin in vitro. In the earlier literature, *hematoporphyrin* was used as a generic term to designate all naturally occurring porphyrins as well as those which can be derived from hemoglobin in vitro. *Hematoporphyria, hematoporphyrinuria,* and *porphyria* were terms employed interchangeably.

porphobilinogen, but in whom clinical manifestations of porphyria were lacking, were classified as having *latent porphyria* [16, 19–21]. Such persons, many of whom were blood relatives of patients with manifest porphyria, were believed to exhibit the inherited metabolic abnormality, but for unknown reasons they remained free of symptoms. It was recognized, however, that in such asymptomatic individuals acute clinical manifestations could at times be precipitated by ingestion of relatively small amounts of sedatives such as barbiturates and sulfonal [16, 22, 23]. In these instances the drug undoubtedly converted a genetically determined latent porphyria into an acute form [16].

On the other hand, "acute porphyria" was reported with increasing frequency in individuals who were addicted to sedatives but in whom no evidence of preexisting porphyria or familial occurrence of the disease could be elucidated [15, 24–26]. Soon after 1888, the year of the introduction of ethyl sulfones into clinical medicine [27], massive "haematoporphyria" was observed in two patients with chronic sulfonal poisoning [28]. By 1900, Taylor and Sailer [29] were able to collect from the literature 31 cases of fatal sulfonal poisoning: most of these patients showed a marked increase in "haematoporphyrin" excretion in the urine. Particularly striking was a patient with fatal porphyria described by Duesberg [26], who over a period of many years had ingested very large amounts of Sedormid (allylisopropylacetyl carbamide) and other sedatives. His urine exhibited high concentrations of uroporphyrin, and at autopsy intense porphyrin fluorescence was demonstrable in the liver, gallbladder, and bile ducts [30].

The concept that in previously normal individuals sedatives of the sulfonal group could produce a porphyria-like syndrome gained strong support from animal experiments. In rabbits it was observed that sulfonal poisoning regularly produced marked "haematoporphyrinuria" [7, 27, 31–33]. With more refined analytic methods, Fischer and Duesberg [34] demonstrated uroporphyrin in the urine of such rabbits, but a few years later Waldenström and Wendt [35] failed to confirm these observations. The problem remained undecided until 1952, when it was discovered that an experimental form of porphyria, similar to human hepatic porphyria, could be produced by the sedative Sedormid [36]. In relation to their body weight, rabbits [36, 37] and rats [37, 38] poisoned with this compound excreted more porphobilinogen and porphyrins than porphyric patients in relapse. It was recognized, however, that Sedormid-induced porphyria in experimental animals differed in some respects from the hereditary forms of the human disorder [39]. For example, Sedormid leads to a profound reduction in liver catalase activity [38], which is not observed in human hepatic porphyria [40, 41].

In recent years, four chemically unrelated groups of compounds have been found to produce porphyria in laboratory animals [13, 42–44] and in primary tissue culture [45]. These include dialkyl-substituted acetamides, acetyl carbamides, and barbiturates [37, 46, 47]; 3,5-diethoxycarbonyl-1,4-dihydro-2,4,6-trimethylpyridine [48]; hexachlorobenzene [43]; and the antibiotic griseofulvin [42]. Granick and Urata [49], Granick [45], and Marver et al. [50] demonstrated that these structurally dissimilar chemicals share the biologic property of inducing formation of hepatic δ-aminolevulinic acid synthetase (ALA synthetase). Later, in a series of elegant experiments, Granick [45] and Granick and Kappas [51] discovered that in addition to compounds that induce ALA synthetase in *intact* animals, a number of substances stimulate this enzyme in cell culture; these include the naturally occurring 5β-reduced steroids, such as etiocholanolone.

The ease with which experimental porphyria could be produced in animals lent credence to the belief that some forms of human porphyria may have a similar toxic, rather than a hereditary, cause. It was recognized that because of species differences in the susceptibility to these porphyrinogenic compounds, observations made in laboratory animals could not simply be applied to human physiology. With noted, for instance, that chronic abuse of allyl-allyl-substituted barbiturates known to produce porphyria in animals [43] usually did not result in increased urinary porphyrin excretion in man [52]. Similarly, Sedormid readily induced porphyria in rats, rabbits, mice, and chickens [43], but dogs and guinea pigs were found to be too sensitive to its hypnotic effect to permit administration in doses sufficient to induce porphyria [41].

Direct evidence for the occurrence in man of an *acquired porphyric syndrome* mimicking hereditary porphyria was obtained through an accidental large-scale intoxication with hexachlorobenzene [53–55]; this is discussed in detail further on in this chapter.

On the basis of these and other considerations, the classification presented in Table 45-1 appears to be most useful. General considerations of porphyrin metabolism may be found in reviews by Watson [56, 57], Rimington [58], Waldenström [19], Vannotti [59], Bénard [60], Goldberg and Rimington [13], With [61], Tschudy [62], Lascelles [63], and

Table 45-1. CLASSIFICATION OF THE PORPHYRIAS*

1. Erythropoietic porphyria
   a. Congenital erythropoietic porphyria (congenital photosensitive, Günther's disease)
   b. Erythropoietic porphyria in animals, including cattle
2. Hepatic porphyria
   a. Acute intermittent porphyria (acute porphyria, pyrroloporphyria, Swedish type)
   b. Variegate porphyria (mixed hepatic porphyria, cutanea tarda hereditaria, South African type)
   c. Coproporphyria
   d. Porphyria cutanea tarda (symptomatic, acquired porphyria, cutanea tarda symptomatica, constitutional or idiosyncratic, Bantu porphyria)
   e. Toxic porphyria, including experimental porphyria in animals
3. Protoporphyria (erythropoietic protoporphyria, erythrohepatic protoporphyria)

* Synonyms are given in parentheses.

Burnham [64], and in the proceedings of recent symposia on porphyrin metabolism and porphyria in London (1955) [65], Saclay (1962) [66], Perugia (1962) [67], Cape Town (1963) [68], and London (1968) [69].

RELATIONSHIP OF PORPHYRINS TO HEMOPROTEINS

The name porphyrin appeared for the first time in the literature in 1871, when Hoppe-Seyler [11] prepared "haematoporphyrin" from hemoglobin. A few years later Nencki and Sieber [12] identified hematoporphyrin as a derivative of hemin, the prosthetic group of hemoglobin. Although a number of investigators [3, 4, 6, 8, 33] recognized the slight spectroscopic differences between hematoporphyrin and the porphyrins excreted in the urine, these pigments were considered identical for practical purposes. This led to the widely accepted but erroneous belief that the urinary porphyrins are derived from breakdown of hemoglobin [3, 7, 15, 59, 70–72], although several observers, including Kast and Weiss [33], Garrod [6], and later Liebig [73], raised doubts as to the validity of this concept. It was not until 1925 that direct proof became available for the independence of porphyrin excretion from hemoglobin breakdown. (Catabolism of hemoglobin results in formation of bile pigments, not porphyrins, as discussed in the following chapter.) Fischer and his coworkers [74] found significant structural differences between hematoporphyrin prepared from red blood cells and the porphyrins present in the urine. Of more importance was the finding that the urinary porphyrins belong in part to an isomeric series different from that of hemoglobin protoporphyrin (Fig. 45-1).* These and other observations led Fischer to suggest that in developing erythroid cells of the bone marrow, small amounts of porphyrins of the type I isomer are synthesized along with, and parallel to, formation of the isomer type III porphyrins, which are the precursors of hemoglobin [74]. This concept is to a large extent in agreement with more recent investigations.

Although as a result of these observations it was generally accepted that porphyrins are formed along with hemoglobin in the bone marrow, it soon became apparent that this hypothesis was not applicable to patients with acute porphyria or porphyria cutanea tarda. On the basis of extensive clinical and necropsy studies, Waldenström [75] came to the conclusion that there must exist a fundamental difference in the pathogenesis of the various forms of porphyria. He reasoned that ". . . the porphyrin must either be an anomalous product on the way to hemoglobin, which is then excreted . . . (or) the other possibility is to try to find another source from which porphyrin might appear."

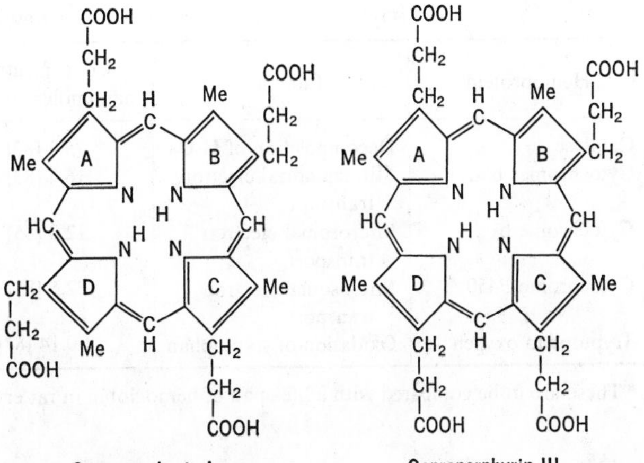

From biopsies [76] and autopsy studies [30, 40, 59, 76–80] and from animal experiments [38] it soon became clear that not only the erythropoietic system but also other organs, particularly the liver, may be important sites of porphyrin formation. This is not surprising, because most mammalian cells can synthesize the porphyrin required for formation of their essential heme-containing enzymes such as cytochromes, catalase, and peroxidase [81]. Although the amount of these heme proteins in the organism is quite small compared with hemoglobin, they have a more rapid rate of turnover than hemoglobin; approximate turnover rates for hemoproteins in the liver are given in Table 45-2. Synthesis of these hepatic hemoproteins requires appreciable quantities of the intermediates in heme biosynthesis [90]. Thus, although abnormalities resulting in excessive formation and liberation of porphyrins and of precursors may occur in any tissue of the body, the liver appears to be of particular importance as the site of such disturbances. Indeed, the liver probably is the major site of the metabolic derangement in most forms of human porphyria other than the erythropoietic type, and in experimentally produced porphyria in laboratory animals. This has led to the proposal that these disturbances be classified under the group name of *hepatic porphyria* [76, 91] (Table 45-1).

Of particular relevance to the hepatic porphyrias is the intracellular hemoprotein, cytochrome P450. Microsomal oxidation of many drugs and steroids depends on the antecedent combination of this unique cytochrome with oxygen. This heme protein derives its name from the fact that it

Coproporphyrin I   Coproporphyrin III

Figure 45-1. Coproporphyrin of type I and type III isomer series. In porphyrins of type III isomer, the sequence of the side chains in the β positions of pyrrole ring D is reversed. *Me,* methyl.

*The classification of porphyrin isomers is based on the four synthetically prepared isomers of etioporphyrin, designated as I, II, III, and IV. Only porphyrins belonging to the isomer series I and III have been identified in nature. The protoporphyrin of hemoglobin and of other heme proteins has the basic structure of a porphyrin type III isomer. However, since the β positions of the pyrrole rings are substituted by three different side chains (Fig. 45-3), the total number of possible isomers for protoporphyrin is 15. The protoporphyrin occurring in all known heme proteins is designated as isomer IXα and corresponds in its basic structure to etioporphyrin III.

Table 45-2. RELATIVE TURNOVER RATES OF HEMOPROTEINS IN RAT LIVER*

Hemoprotein	Function	Concentration, nanomoles/gm liver	Turnover (T ½)
Catalase	Decomposition of H_2O_2	5.3 [82]	29 hr [82]
Cytochromes b, c	Mitochondrial electron transport	16.4 [83]	5.5, 6.1 days [84]
Cytochrome b_5	Microsomal electron transport	12.0 [85]	2.3 days [84] or 45 hr [617]
Cytochrome P450	Microsomal electron transport	22.5 [85]	Biphasic: 7–10 hr and 24–48 hr [86, 618]
Tryptophan oxygenase	Oxidation of tryptophan	0.14 [87]	2.2 hr [88]

* These are to be compared with a life-span of hemoglobin in rat erythrocytes of 60 days [89].

combines with carbon monoxide to produce an intense absorption peak at 450 μm. Measurements of the turnover of cytochrome P450 suggest a biphasic curve with apparent half-lives of 8 and 40 hr (Table 45-2) [86]. This has been interpreted as indicating two forms of the hemoprotein; in particular, synthesis of the cytochrome with the shorter half-life would be expected to require considerable quantities of heme and its precursors.

BIOSYNTHESIS OF PORPHYRINS AND OF HEME

Prior to 1946 little was known about the chemical building blocks from which the body synthesizes porphyrins and heme. In that year Shemin and Rittenberg [92, 93] observed that after administration of isotopically labeled glycine, the concentration of the label in the circulating hemoglobin heme rose rapidly, remained more or less steady for about 100 days, and then rapidly declined (Fig. 45-2). The disappearance of the label from the circulating heme was accompanied by a marked though temporary increase in the fecal excretion of labeled urobilinogen [95, 96]. These observations permitted the conclusions that (1) glycine is a specific precursor of heme protoporphyrin; (2) hemoglobin of the circulating erythrocytes remains outside the general metabolic pool of protein interchange; (3) most of the normal red blood cells have a mean life-span of about 120 days; (4) a large fraction of the fecal urobilinogen is derived from the breakdown of circulating red blood cells; and (5) the metabolites of heme protoporphyrin are not reutilized for the synthesis of hemoglobin in newly formed erythrocytes.

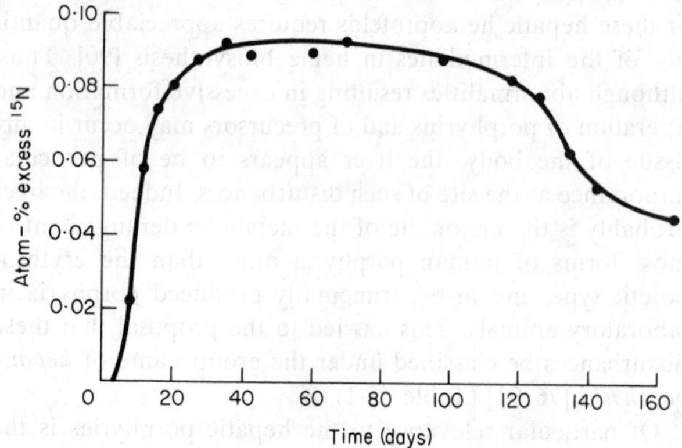

Figure 45-2. Concentration of ^{15}N in hemoglobin heme of a normal subject, given 12 gm glycine-^{15}N (31.65 atom-percent excess ^{15}N) during the first 4 days of the experiment. (*By permission of C. H. Gray* [94].)

Additional studies carried out in various laboratories showed that blood from ducks and chickens which contains nucleated erythrocytes [97, 98] and blood from rabbits which had been made anemic to produce a high percentage of reticulocytes [99] are able to synthesize labeled heme from glycine-^{14}C in vitro. The availability of these systems greatly facilitated subsequent studies, which revealed that all four nitrogen atoms [92, 100, 101] and eight carbon atoms of the protoporphyrin molecule are derived from glycine [101–103] (Fig. 45-3). Four of the carbon atoms are still attached to the nitrogen atoms of glycine; the four which are not form the methyne bridges which link the four pyrrole rings to make up the porphyrin ring (Fig. 45-3). All eight carbon atoms are derived from the α-carbon atom of glycine, while the carboxyl carbon of glycine is not utilized for any of the carbon atoms of porphyrin [103, 104].

The remaining 26 carbon atoms of protoporphyrin arise from intermediates of the tricarboxylic acid cycle [101, 105]. Acetate, labeled either in the methyl or in the carboxyl group, α-ketoglutarate-5-^{14}C, α-ketoglutarate-1,2-^{14}C, or citrate-1,5-^{14}C lead to characteristic and predictable labeling patterns, which strongly suggests that the same four-carbon chain is utilized in the formation of both sides of all four pyrrole rings [101, 106]. With methyl-labeled acetate, for example, highest labeling of heme protoporphyrin is observed in the carbon atoms 6 and 9 (Fig. 45-4); less activity is present in positions 4, 8, 5, and 3 [107]. Moreover, there is equal labeling each to each, in the position pairs 6 and 9, 4 and 8, 5 and 3 [107]. The labeling pattern obtained in protoporphyrin synthesized from succinate-1,4-^{14}C is pictured in Fig. 45-4.

These results indicate that the biosynthesis of the proto-

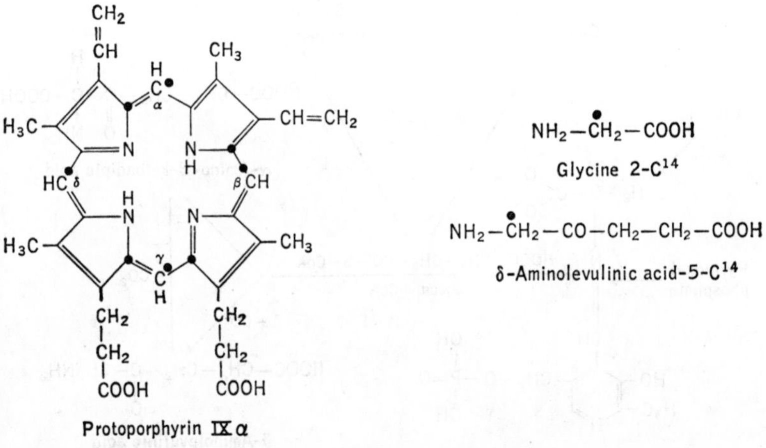

NH_2-CH_2-COOH

Glycine 2-C[14]

$NH_2-CH_2-CO-CH_2-CH_2-COOH$

δ-Aminolevulinic acid-5-C[14]

Protoporphyrin IX α

Figure 45-3. The carbon atoms of protoporphyrin IXα derived from the α-carbon of glycine and the δ-carbon of δ-aminolevulinic acid (ALA). (*By permission of D. Shemin* [101].)

porphyrin molecule requires 8 moles of glycine and 8 moles of a four-carbon intermediate of the tricarboxylic acid cycle, presumably succinate [101]. The finding that the α-carbon atom of glycine is always utilized equally for both the pyrrole ring and the methyne bridge carbon atoms limits the possible ways by which succinate and glycine could combine to form a pyrrole unit [101, 108].

These and other observations led Shemin and Russell [101, 109] to suggest that the intermediate, which is formed by condensation of glycine and succinate, is the five-carbon amino ketone δ-aminolevulinic acid (ALA) (Fig. 45-5). With the use of ALA-5-^{14}C in a system of hemolyzed duck red blood cells, the position of this amino ketone as a true intermediate in porphyrin biosynthesis has been well documented [110–112]. Not only was the labeling pattern of the δ-carbon atom of ALA identical with that of the α-carbon atom of glycine [101, 110] (Fig. 45-3), but the heme synthesized from an equimolar amount of ALA-5-^{14}C was about 65 times more radioactive than heme synthesized from glycine-2-^{14}C [101]. From these observations Shemin [109] postulated a metabolic pathway by which "active" succinate can be condensed with glycine to form ALA and subsequently the pyrrole precursor, porphobilinogen (PBG).

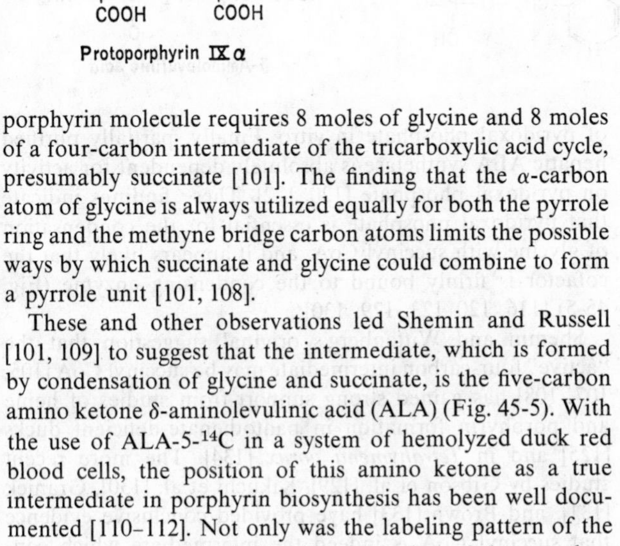

Quantitatively, the principal pathway for utilization of ALA is the formation of PBG (i.e., heme biosynthesis) [90]. However, Nemeth et al. demonstrated that (δ-^{14}C)-ALA labeled not only PBG and porphyrins but also the ureido group of guanine, uric acid, and formate [110, 113]; the remainder of the ALA molecule was reconverted into succinate. This indicated that the δ-carbon atom of ALA functioned as a "one-carbon" unit. Similar findings were obtained using the aldehyde analogue of ALA, γ,δ-dioxovaleric acid [114]. Thus, it has been suggested that ALA undergoes transamination to γ,δ-dioxovaleric acid with subsequent loss of a "one-carbon" fragment upon conversion to succinate. That this pathway occurs in the intact organism is suggested by the observation of Dowdle et al. that in man (δ-^{14}C)-ALA labels the 2 and 8 carbon atoms of uric acid [115]. It is apparent that in mammals this so-called succinate-glycine cycle [101, 110, 113] is quantitatively unimportant, as shown by studies with liver preparations [90] and in the intact animal. Indeed, it has been postulated that the equilibrium of the transamination reaction is toward ALA formation and, thus, that this may represent an alternate mechanism for ALA biosynthesis [114].

$+ 6CO_2$ from positions 7 and 10

Figure 45-4. The labeling pattern obtained in protoporphyrin IXα synthesized from succinate-1,4-^{14}C. Carbon 7, which gives rise to the CO_2, is the carbon of the original carboxyl group attached to carbon 6. (*By permission of D. Shemin* [101].)

Biosynthesis of δ-Aminolevulinic Acid (ALA)

Condensation of glycine with succinyl coenzyme A to form ALA in vitro has been demonstrated in systems containing particulate matter which is present in nucleated avian red blood cells and in mammalian reticulocytes, liver, and kidney [49, 101, 109, 110, 116–118] but is absent from mature mammalian erythrocytes [99]. The enzyme responsible for catalyzing this reaction is ALA synthetase. In the intact

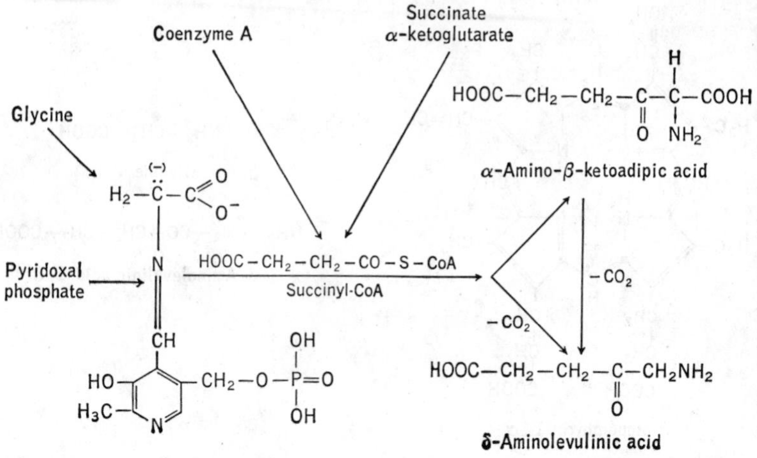

Figure 45-5. Condensation of succinyl CoA with glycine in the presence of pyridoxal phosphate. (*Adapted from Kikuchi et al.* [130].)

mammalian cell, ALA can be formed only within mitochondria [49, 116, 118], since this organelle is uniquely endowed with the capacity to generate succinyl coenzyme A and contains the major fraction of intracellular ALA synthetase [49, 119, 120]. Recently, McKay et al. have further localized ALA synthetase in the matrix of the mitochondrion [121]. ALA also has been identified in the cytosol of the liver [49, 119, 120], where it is not functional but appears to be in transit to mitochondria [119, 120]. The enzyme has been partially purified from rat liver cytosol [119, 120, 122] and from *Rhodopseudomonas spheroides.* Both in bacterial and in animal cells [123, 124] ALA synthetase activity is regulated; this regulation plays a critical role in determining intracellular heme levels. For example, ALA synthetase partially purified from *R. spheroides* [124] or from porphyric rat liver [120, 122] is subject to end product inhibition by heme. Certain aspects of these control mechanisms will be discussed under "Regulation of Heme and Hemoprotein Biosynthesis."

All enzyme preparations require pyridoxal phosphate as cofactor. The requirement for pyridoxal was demonstrated along four different lines of evidence. In blood of pyridoxine-deficient ducklings, Schulman and Richert [125] observed reduced heme synthesis from glycine-^{14}C, a defect that could be corrected by the addition of pyridoxal phosphate. Similarly, in a patient with acute intermittent porphyria, urinary excretion of ALA and porphobilinogen was diminished following induction of pyridoxine deficiency, and was greatly enhanced by subsequent pyridoxine loading [126]. These findings are in line with earlier observations by Wintrobe [127] that pigs deficient in vitamin B_6 produced small, pale red blood cells with a low content of hemoglobin and free protoporphyrin. Compounds known to inhibit enzymes which contain pyridoxal phosphate [90, 128] have been shown to reduce formation of ALA [116, 129, 130] and of porphyrins [131, 132] in vitro. Marked inhibition was obtained with L-penicillamine and isonicotinic acid hydrazide. Biosynthesis of ALA [116, 129, 130, 133] and of porphyrin [131, 125, 134] was found to be enhanced by the addition of pyridoxal phosphate in vitro. Finally, partially purified hepatic ALA synthetase is absolutely dependent for activity on pyridoxal phosphate [120, 122]. These findings indicate that pyridoxal phosphate is essential for the condensation of glycine with succinyl CoA, and it appears likely that the cofactor is firmly bound to the condensing enzyme (Fig. 45-5) [116, 120–123, 129, 130].

Shemin and Wittenberg's original suggestion that the "active" four-carbon intermediate may be succinyl CoA [105, 107, 108] has gained strong support from studies of heme and porphyrin formation in pantothenate-deficient ducks [125] and in *Tetrahymena vorax* [134]. The more recent studies by Gibson et al. [129], Kikuchi et al. [130], Granick [131], and Brown [133] have provided conclusive evidence that succinyl CoA is indeed the intermediate which condenses with glycine. The succinyl CoA can be derived from α-ketoglutarate by the action of α-ketoglutaric dehydrogenase [116, 129], or it may be formed from succinate by succinyl CoA synthetase in the presence of ATP or GTP [49, 119, 120, 124, 129, 130].

Although it had initially been expected that α-amino-β-ketoadipic acid (Fig. 45-5) would be the primary product obtained on condensation of succinyl CoA with glycine [101, 109, 111], the lability of this compound [129] has prevented verification of this hypothesis. Indeed, it has been suggested that decarboxylation of the pyridoxal phosphate derivative of glycine and condensation with succinyl CoA may be simultaneous reactions (Fig. 45-5) [123, 130].

The condensation of glycine with succinyl CoA may be the prototype of a more general reaction involving glycine metabolism [101, 123]. Distinct mitochondrial enzymes appear to catalyze the condensation of glycine with other acyl CoA substrates, such as acetyl CoA and propionyl CoA, forming aminoacetone and other amino ketones [135].

The biosynthetic pathway of ALA formation is summarized in Fig. 45-6. The substrates involved in this reaction are succinyl CoA, which is generated by the tricarboxylic acid cycle, and glycine. An enzyme functional in mitochondria, ALA synthetase, which requires pyridoxal phosphate

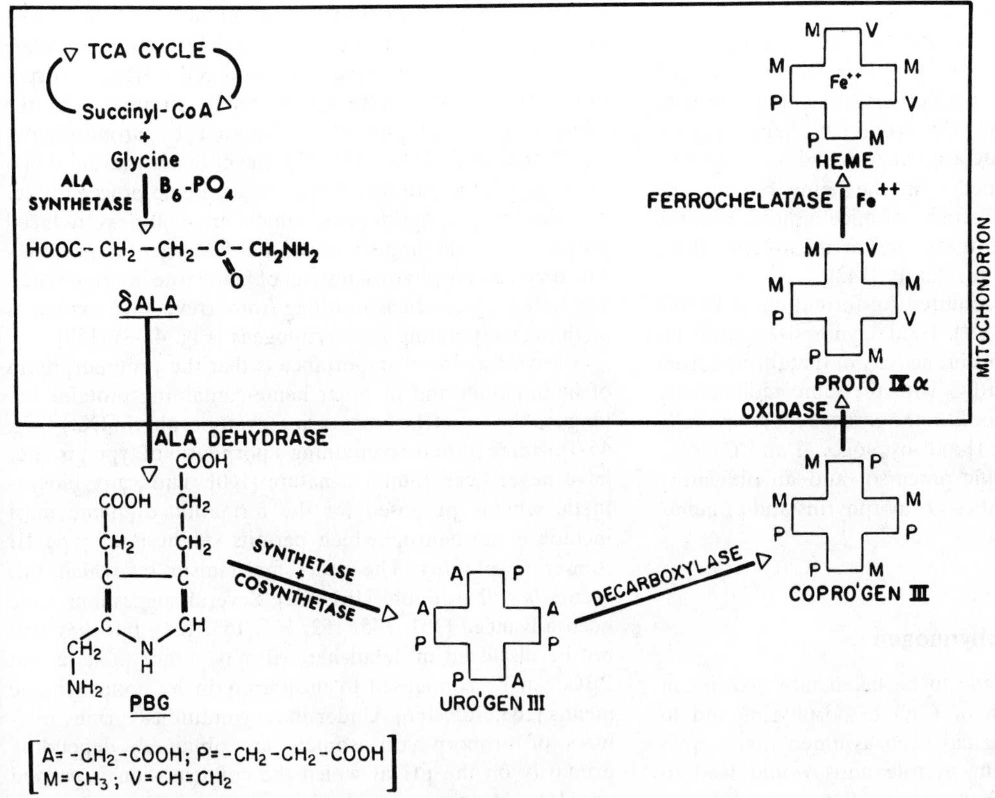

Figure 45-6. Outline of heme biosynthesis. The boxed area represents intramitochondrial reactions; below are reactions occurring in the cytosol.

as a cofactor, catalyzes the condensation of succinyl CoA with glycine to form ALA. The initial reaction of this pathway requires a functioning tricarboxylic acid cycle and thus is oxygen-dependent; the condensing enzyme system is operative under anaerobic conditions. The lack of mitochondria in mature mammalian erythrocytes precludes formation of succinyl CoA and, hence, of ALA.

Biosynthesis of Porphobilinogen (PBG)

With the establishment of ALA as an obligatory intermediate in porphyrin and heme biosynthesis, studies of the subsequent enzymatic steps were greatly facilitated. ALA dehydrase was found to catalyze condensation of 2 moles of ALA to form a precursor pyrrole [136, 137] (Fig. 45-7). The theoretical formulation of the structure of this pyrrole [109] yielded the same structure as PBG, a chromogen excreted in the urine of patients with acute porphyria [16], first isolated by Westall [138]. The soluble enzyme ALA dehydrase has been purified from a number of sources, including *R. spheroides* [124, 139], duck erythrocytes [137], chicken erythrocytes [140], ox liver [137], mouse liver and spleen [141, 142], and spinach leaves [143]. Reduced glutathione is required for activation of the enzyme system [137, 144, 145]. SH-group inhibitors such as iodoacetamide and *p*-chloromercuribenzoate have an inhibitory effect [137], which can be overcome by the addition of reduced glutathione [137]. In addition, marked inhibition of ALA dehydrase from most mammalian sources [145] has been noted with the chelating agent, ethylenediaminetetraacetic acid, a finding which originally suggested that a metal, possibly copper [146], may be essential for this enzymatic step. Subsequent studies have yielded enzyme preparations which were fully active in the absence of copper [147] or iron [123].

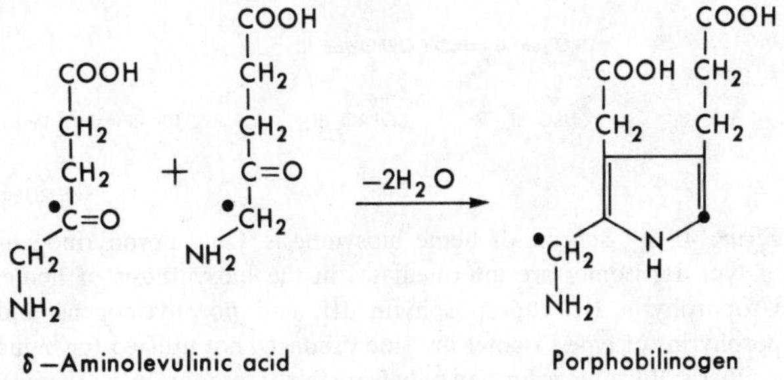

δ−Aminolevulinic acid + δ−Aminolevulinic acid $\xrightarrow{-2H_2O}$ Porphobilinogen

Figure 45-7. Condensation of 2 moles δ-aminolevulinic acid to form 1 mole porphobilinogen. The carbon atoms bearing the label are the original α-carbon atoms of glycine. (*By permission of D. Shemin* [101].)

The partially purified enzyme from *R. spheroides* has an apparent molecular weight of 250,000 and is allosterically activated by potassium ions [139]. The protein is composed of six subunits [148, 149]. These observations, together with the strong inhibition of ALA dehydrase by heme, suggest that, similar to ALA synthetase, ALA dehydrase may perform some regulatory function in the heme biosynthetic pathway. Studies in inbred strains of mice indicate that the enzyme in the liver is under the control of at least two alleles [150], which are probably regulatory [142].

Two moles of ALA are required for formation of 1 mole of PBG [101, 136] (Fig. 45-7). Heme synthesized from labeled ALA has twice the specific activity of that formed from an equimolar amount of PBG with the same radioactivity [101, 144]. These findings confirm the earlier reports by Falk, Dresel, and Rimington [151] and by Bogorad and Granick [152] that PBG is a specific precursor and an obligatory intermediate in the biosynthesis of porphyrins and of heme.

Biosynthesis of Uroporphyrinogen

Two important findings have to be taken into account in considering the conversion of PBG to porphyrins and to heme. In earlier studies it had been assumed that simple linear condensation of four pyrrole units would lead to formation of the next metabolic intermediate, uroporphyrin. The latter would then undergo stepwise decarboxylation to yield protoporphyrin. It was soon discovered that this simple scheme was not correct. In a variety of systems capable of converting PBG to heme or to porphyrins with less than eight carboxyl groups, uroporphyrin was ineffective as a substrate and could not replace PBG (Fig. 45-8) [101, 153, 154]. These observations suggested that the true intermediate

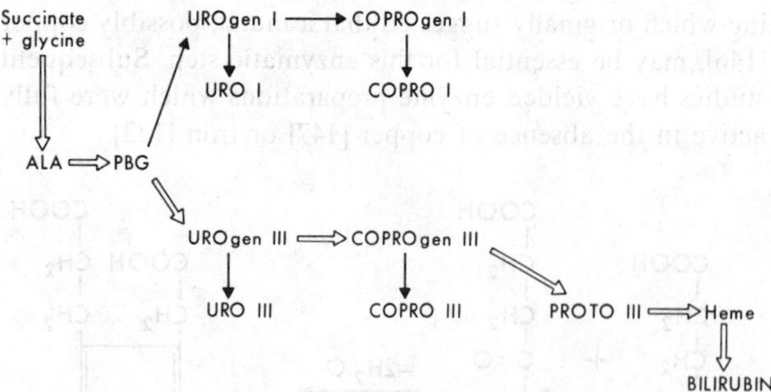

Figure 45-8. Scheme of heme biosynthesis. Only porphyrinogens of type III isomer are intermediates in the biosynthesis of heme. Uroporphyrin III, coproporphyrin III, and porphyrinogens and porphyrins of type I isomer are side products, not utilized for heme synthesis. Bilirubin is formed only from ferroprotoporphyrin (heme), not from porphyrins. *PBG*, porphobilinogen; *UROgen, COPROgen, PROTOgen,* uroporphyrinogen, coproporphyrinogen, protoporphyrinogen; *URO, COPRO, PROTO,* uroporphyrin, coproporphyrin, protoporphyrin.

formed from PBG is not uroporphyrin but its reduced form, uroporphyrinogen. Indeed, Neve and his coworkers [155] found that in a hemolyzed red blood cell system, incorporation of ^{59}Fe into heme was markedly stimulated by the addition of uroporphyrinogen but not by uroporphyrin. Additional studies [143, 156, 157] have clearly indicated that the biosynthetic pathway from PBG to heme proceeds over a series of porphyrinogens, which are colorless reduced porphyrins containing six additional hydrogen atoms [158]. The oxidized porphyrins, instead of being true intermediates, are merely by-products resulting from irreversible oxidation of the corresponding porphyrinogens (Fig. 45-8) [159].

A second point of importance is that the protoporphyrin of hemoglobin and of other heme-containing proteins belongs to the type III isomer series (protoporphyrin IXα) (Fig. 45-3). Heme proteins containing a porphyrin of type I isomer have never been found in nature [160]. Thus, any biosynthetic scheme proposed for the formation of heme must include a mechanism which permits synthesis of type III isomer porphyrins. The exact mechanism by which this occurs is still in doubt [161, 162]. Several suggestions have been advanced [101, 145, 152, 161, 163, 164], but they will not be discussed in detail here. It may suffice to state that PBG can be condensed to uroporphyrin by nonenzymatic means [163, 165, 166]. Under these conditions various mixtures of uroporphyrin isomers are obtained, depending primarily on the pH at which the condensation is carried out [166]. Moreover, porphyrinogens may undergo isomerization in hot acid [167].

Although knowledge regarding the precise mechanism and the nature of some of the intermediates involved in the formation of porphyrins of type III isomer is as yet incomplete, sufficient information is available to formulate a reasonable working hypothesis [13, 156, 161, 162, 168, 169] (Figs. 45-8, 45-9). Incubation of PBG with an enzyme system obtained from Chlorella [152], *R. spheroides* [170], red blood cell hemolyzates [171–175], or mouse spleen [168, 169] results in formation of porphyrins of type III isomer. If such a system is heated to 60°C, it is altered in such a way that only porphyrins of type I isomer are formed [161, 171]. This finding suggests that the enzyme "porphobilinogenase" may have more than one component. Indeed, from plants and bacteria, Bogorad [173, 174] and Hoare and Heath [176] succeeded in preparing two separate enzyme fractions, uroporphyrinogen I synthetase, which is relatively heat-stable, and uroporphyrinogen III cosynthetase, which is heat-labile. More recently, Levin [169] separated and purified the cosynthetase from hematopoietically active mouse spleen. It appears that one of the actions of uroporphyrinogen I synthetase is to remove the amino group of PBG and to condense individual monopyrroles to form polypyrrylmethanes (Fig. 45-9) [145, 174, 168, 169]. The enzyme, when acting alone, converts PBG to the symmetric uroporphyrinogen I [173]. Uroporphyrinogen I synthetase is inhibited by silver and mercuric ions, *p*-chloromercurobenzoate [173], opsopyrroledicarboxylic acid [177], isoporphobilinogen [178],

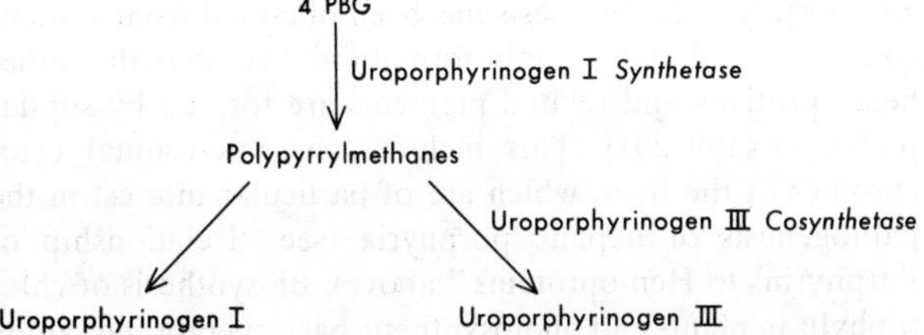

Figure 45-9. Enzymatic condensation of 4 moles porphobilinogen (PBG) to 1 mole uroporphyrinogen. Uroporphyrinogen III cosynthetase acts on postulated intermediary polypyrrylmethanes to form uroporphyrinogen III.

ammonium ions [161], and formaldehyde [173]. On the basis of studies with inhibitors, Stevens et al. [613] suggested that uroporphyrinogen I synthetase (porphobilinogen deaminase) may contain at least two identifiable enzyme activities: one converting PBG to some as yet unidentified intermediate and the other transforming this intermediate to uroporphyrinogen I. More recently, this intermediate has tentatively been identified as 5-aminomethyl-4,3′-di(carboxymethyl)-3, 4′-di(2-carboxyethyl)dipyrrylmethane [614]; the cyclic uroporphyrinogen I appears to be formed by successive addition of PBG residues to this dipyrrylmethane intermediate.

If uroporphyrinogen III cosynthetase is added to a system containing PBG and uroporphyrinogen I synthetase, the reaction product is uroporphyrinogen III [174] (Fig. 45-9). Since by itself uroporphyrinogen III cosynthetase reacts with neither PBG nor uroporphyrinogen I [156, 174], it is clear that its enzymatic function is dependent on some effect of uroporphyrinogen I synthetase on PBG. It seems reasonable to assume that uroporphyrinogen I synthetase catalyzes the formation of a noncyclized intermediate, probably a dipyrrylmethane [145, 174] (Fig. 45-9). Uroporphyrinogen III cosynthetase then permits isomerization of this intermediate, which results in a "flip-over" of one of the pyrrole rings, producing the unsymmetric uroporphyrinogen III (Fig. 45-9). This concept is supported by the findings that only four molecules of PBG are required for formation of uroporphyrinogen III [145, 173, 174, 179], that formaldehyde is neither produced nor incorporated in this reaction [175, 179], and that dipyrrylmethenes do not participate as reactants.

Metabolism of Uroporphyrinogen

The further metabolism of uroporphyrinogen can proceed along one of two separate lines: it may undergo either a stepwise oxidation to uroporphyrin or a stepwise enzymatic decarboxylation to porphyrinogens with less than eight carboxyl groups [155–157, 171, 176] (Figs. 45-6, 45-8). The oxidative process leads to uroporphyrin, which is a side product and does not serve as a substrate for the enzyme uroporphyrinogen decarboxylase. Nonenzymatic oxidation of uroporphyrinogen can occur by photocatalytic auto-oxidation, a process activated by the product, uroporphyrin [145]. Photo-oxidation is partially inhibited by glutathione, 2-mercaptoethylamine, cysteine, or sodium sulfite and is markedly reduced under strictly anaerobic conditions or by exclusion of light [145, 173]. On the other hand, ferric ion at acid pH catalyzes the photo-oxidative process [145, 176]. Mauzerall and Granick [156] have suggested that the conversion of uroporphyrinogen to uroporphyrin proceeds stepwise with the cyclized tetrapyrroles porphomethene and porphodimethene as intermediates; the former has two and the latter four hydrogen atoms less than uroporphyrinogen. Since the amount of uroporphyrin normally excreted in the urine is exceedingly small compared with the magnitude of heme synthesis, the fraction of uroporphyrinogen that is oxidized and escapes from the biosynthetic path must be insignificant. It appears likely that the exclusion of light and the presence in the cells of antioxidants such as glutathione and cysteine are of importance in keeping most of the tetrapyrroles in a reduced state [156].

The major fraction of the uroporphyrinogen is enzymatically decarboxylated to porphyrinogens with less than eight carboxyl groups [140, 156, 157, 171, 176] (Figs. 45-6, 45-8). Uroporphyrinogen decarboxylase activity has been demonstrated in erythrocytes of man [171, 172], ducks [155], and chickens [180–183], in rabbit reticulocytes [156], in Chlorella [152], and in *R. spheroides* [176]. With enzyme preparations obtained from rabbit reticulocytes [156], or Chlorella [152], anaerobic incubation of uroporphyrinogen resulted in formation of coproporphyrinogen exhibiting four carboxyl groups. The enzyme has a high degree of specificity; ALA, PBG, and uroporphyrin cannot replace uroporphyrinogen as substrates [156, 157]. Mercury, copper, manganese, and oxygen strongly inhibit the reaction [156, 157], the last probably by enhancing auto-oxidation of the substrate to uroporphyrin. On the other hand, reduced glutathione and cysteine greatly increase the yield of coproporphyrinogen. Uroporphyrinogen decarboxylase is active with all uroporphyrinogen isomers, but the rate of decarboxylation is highest with the type III isomer [156, 157, 184].

The removal of the four acetic acid side chains of uroporphyrinogen probably occurs stepwise and randomly, so that intermediate porphyrinogens with seven, six, and five carboxyl groups are formed [143, 156, 159, 182–184]. Since the decarboxylating enzyme appears to have a low Michaelis constant and a high turnover number [156], the concentration of these intermediate porphyrinogens at any one time is very low, and the reaction is rapidly carried through to coproporphyrinogen. It is not known whether the successive removal of carboxyl groups of uroporphyrinogen to form, ultimately, coproporphyrinogen is catalyzed by a single enzyme system or by several closely related enzyme systems [156]. For convenience, the term *uroporphyrinogen decarboxylase* is used, although the enzyme as defined can react with porphyrinogens which exhibit fewer carboxyl groups than uroporphyrinogen [156, 615].

Biosynthesis of Protoporphyrin and Protoheme

With uroporphyrinogen I as substrate, coproporphyrinogen I or its oxidation product, coproporphyrin I, is the end product, since further decarboxylation of the type I isomer series does not occur [13, 156, 157, 159, 185]. Protoporphyrin or heme corresponding to type I isomer has never been demonstrated in nature [13, 160] (Fig. 45-8). On the other hand, coproporphyrinogen III is readily converted to protoporphyrin IXα, an enzymatic process which requires oxygen. The conversion involves decarboxylation and oxidation of the propionate groups at positions 2 and 4, yielding two vinyl groups; the resulting protoporphyrinogen IXα is then converted to protoporphyrin IXα by removal of six hydrogens [185, 186]. The enzyme coproporphyrinogen (oxidative) decarboxylase is a mitochondrial enzyme that has been prepared from chicken red blood cells [187], *Euglena* [188], and beef liver [185]. Enzymatic activity is highest in tissues which have a rapid rate of heme turnover [185], such as bone marrow and liver. The reaction is highly substrate-specific for coproporphyrinogen III; neither coproporphyrinogen I nor coproporphyrin III serve as substrates [185] (Fig. 45-8). It is not clear whether coproporphyrinogen decarboxylase is a single enzyme responsible for the entire conversion of coproporphyrinogen III to protoporphyrin IXα. The most attractive hypothesis is that the first step, requiring molecular oxygen, involves formation of 2,4-bis (β-hydroxypropionic acid) deuteroporphyrinogen IX [190]. This intermediate then is decarboxylated and dehydrated to protoporphyrinogen IXα, a reaction that may proceed under anaerobic conditions [190]. It is most likely that the conversion of protoporphyrinogen to protoporphyrin occurs simultaneously with the decarboxylation, but it is unknown whether this also is an enzymatic process or whether it may occur spontaneously in the presence of oxygen [185, 186, 190] (Fig. 45-6).

The final step in heme biosynthesis is the incorporation of iron into the protoporphyrin ring (Fig. 45-6). This can be accomplished nonenzymatically by various chemical manipulations [191, 192]. On the other hand, Krueger et al. [193], Goldberg et al. [194], Lochhead et al. [195], Labbe et al. [196], and others have presented convincing evidence that in vivo the incorporation of iron to form protoheme is regulated enzymatically. The presence of an iron-incorporating enzyme system (ferro-protoporphyrin chelatase) [196] was demonstrated in mitochondrial preparations obtained from liver, bone marrow, duck erythrocytes, and rabbit reticulocytes [195–199, 202]. Enzymatic activity is dependent on the presence of reducing substances such as ascorbic acid, cysteine, or glutathione [195], and the enzyme appears to be substrate-specific for porphyrins with free carboxyl groups on the propionic acid side chains in positions 6 and 7 [196]. Copro- and uroporphyrin are not attacked by the enzyme, presumably because of steric effects which interfere with enzyme-substrate interaction [197, 198].

Though most of this evidence for the mechanism of heme and porphyrin biosynthesis has been obtained from systems concerned with hemoglobin formation, it is likely that other heme proteins and related pigments are formed by similar pathways [199–201]. This includes the microsomal cytochromes of the liver, which are of particular interest in the pathogenesis of hepatic porphyria (see "Relationship of Porphyrins to Hemoproteins," above). Biosynthesis of chlorophylls in plants and photosynthetic bacteria proceeds along comparable lines [63, 199, 200], and ALA and PBG are specific precursors for the formation of vitamin B_{12} [201], which has a structure closely related to that of uroporphyrin III.

Recapitulation

The nearly complete elucidation of the pathway by which glycine and succinate are used for the biosynthesis of porphyrins and heme provides an impressive example of the biochemical progress made during the last two decades. There can be little doubt that the few remaining regions of uncertainty and ignorance will soon be explored and clarified. This applies particularly to the enzymatic mechanism which catalyzes the condensation of 4 moles of PBG to form the asymmetric uroporphyrinogen III, and also to the steps involved in the oxidative decarboxylation of coproporphyrinogen III to protoporphyrin IXα.

Some aspects of the biosynthetic pathway in the intact organism which are believed to be of particular importance with regard to porphyria are summarized below.

1 ALA and PBG are obligatory intermediates in the biosynthesis of porphyrins and of heme.

2 The following cofactors are essential: pantothenate for the formation of succinyl CoA, and pyridoxal phosphate and possibly biotin for the condensation of succinyl CoA with glycine.

3 Though most of the individual biosynthetic steps proceed in the absence of oxygen, three reactions require aerobic conditions: (*a*) the formation of succinyl coenzyme A, which is dependent on a functioning tricarboxylic acid cycle; (*b*) the oxidative decarboxylation of coproporphyrinogen III to protoporphyrinogen IXα, which is catalyzed by the mitochondrial enzyme coproporphyrinogen decarboxylase; and (*c*) the oxidation of protoporphyrinogen IXα, which may be a spontaneous process that occurs simultaneously with the decarboxylation.

4 These reactions are catalyzed by enzyme systems which are bound to mitochondria and which are inoperative in mature nonnucleated erythrocytes. On the other hand, the steps from ALA to coproporphyrinogen III are catalyzed by soluble enzymes present both in nucleated cells and in mature mammalian erythrocytes.

5 Porphyrinogens and porphyrins of the type I isomer series are by-products of heme synthesis without known physiologic function. In vivo, the biosynthetic pathway is conditioned in such a way that formation of porphyrins of type I isomer is insignificant in comparison with the amount of protoheme IXα formed.

6 With the exception of protoporphyrin IXα, porphyrins of the type III isomer series are not intermediates in heme biosynthesis but are by-products resulting from *irreversible* oxidation of the respective porphyrinogens. The *true intermediates* are porphyrinogens of the type III isomer, which are reduced porphyrins containing an additional six hydrogen atoms. They may be converted to the corresponding porphyrins by photocatalytic auto-oxidation. Oxidation of porphyrinogens to porphyrins in vivo is minimized by the exclusion of light and by the presence of antioxidants in the cell.

7 The dynamics of the uroporphyrinogen decarboxylase system favors the formation of porphyrins with eight carboxyl groups (uroporphyrin) and with four carboxyl groups (coproporphyrin), but smaller amounts of porphyrins with seven, six, five, and three carboxyl groups are also formed.

8 Catabolism of heme and heme proteins does not lead to porphyrins but results in formation of bile pigments (see the following chapter).

9 The control and regulation of porphyrin and heme biosynthesis are of fundamental importance for the pathogenesis of porphyria. This will be considered in detail in a following section.

FORMATION OF PORPHYRINS AND PORPHYRIN PRECURSORS IN THE INTACT ORGANISM

The bone marrow of an adult individual forms approximately 300 mg heme per day. This amount is needed for hemoglobin formation to compensate for the physiologic decay of aged erythrocytes [203]. Additional heme is synthesized for the formation of other heme proteins, but the lack of precise information regarding the rate of turnover of these compounds (Table 45-2) precludes exact estimation of the total daily heme production. Undoubtedly it is considerably larger than the 300 mg required for hemoglobin synthesis in the bone marrow, since heme-containing compounds, which are believed to be synthesized *in loco,* are present in almost all aerobic cells [81]. In relation to this rate of heme formation, the excretion of porphyrins and of porphyrin precursors in urine and bile is very small. If one visualizes the excreted compounds as the sum of all porphyrins and porphyrin precursors which "escape" during heme formation, it becomes obvious that heme biosynthesis proceeds with a remarkable degree of efficiency. It is not known how much individual organs contribute to the "pool" of excreted porphyrins and porphyrin precursors, but it is apparent that the bone marrow and the liver are major contributors.

δ-Aminolevulinic Acid and Porphobilinogen

In man, approximately 2 mg ALA is excreted in the urine per day [21, 204–206]. No data are available for its excretion in bile, but it is believed to be negligible [207–209] (Table 45-3). Significant elevation of ALA excretion in the urine is observed in lead poisoning [210].

Injection or oral administration of labeled ALA to man and to animals results in the excretion of a large portion of the unaltered compound in the urine [207]. Smaller fractions are converted to PBG, to protoporphyrin, and to stercobilin, the first being excreted in the urine, the latter two in the bile [207–209]. All three compounds are believed to be formed outside the hematopoietic system, probably largely in the liver [207, 208]. In addition, ALA-1,4-^{14}C gives rise to labeled CO_2 in the breath [201]. A small fraction of the injected ALA is used for heme biosynthesis in immature red blood cells [101, 207, 208], but in contrast to the observations with glycine-2-^{14}C, isotopically labeled ALA is much more efficiently incorporated into hepatic heme than into hemoglobin of circulating erythrocytes (see Chap. 46, Hyperbilirubinemia). This probably is largely because of the relative impermeability of the red blood cell membrane for ALA [207, 208, 211].

In healthy individuals daily excretion of PBG in the urine is approximately 1.0 to 1.5 mg [21, 204–206] (Table 45-3). At the low concentrations which exist in normal urine, the conventional test for its detection [212, 213] is inadequate and gives negative results [214]. Increased urinary excretion of PBG is at times observed in patients with hepatic, malignant, or infectious diseases [215], and it is frequently present in lead poisoning [210, 216]. In animals poisoned with Sedormid [36] or related compounds [37, 43], large amounts of PBG are excreted in the urine and are present in the

Table 45-3. RANGE OF NORMAL VALUES FOR THE EXCRETION OF PORPHYRINS AND PORPHYRIN PRECURSORS*

	Urine, μg/24 hr	Feces, μg/gm dry wt	Erythrocytes, μg/100 ml cells
ALA	Trace–2,000		
PBG	Trace–1,500		
Uroporphyrin	10–40	Trace	Trace
Coproporphyrin	100–250	Trace–50	0.5–1.5
Protoporphyrin	0	Trace–120	25–75

* Ranges used in the laboratory of H. S. Marver and R. Schmid.

liver but not in the bone marrow or circulating erythrocytes [39].

If injected parenterally, PBG is rapidly excreted in the urine [217]; fecal excretion or conversion of PBG to porphyrins is insignificant [209, 217]. Since in animals injected PBG cannot be demonstrated in the liver [217], it may not pass the liver cell membrane. Similar findings have been reported for fowl erythrocytes in vitro [218]. It is evident, nevertheless, that the impermeability of the cell membrane is only relative, since in instances where endogenous PBG production is increased it *does* escape from the cells and gain access to the urine. Thus, in acute porphyria of man and in Sedormid porphyria of animals, large amounts of PBG are derived from the liver and excreted in the urine [39, 76, 217].

Porphyrins

Normal human urine contains small amounts of porphyrins. The predominant one is coproporphyrin, which is excreted at a daily rate of 100 to 300 μg [219–222], the values being somewhat smaller in the female [219]. Both type I and type III isomers are present, but the ratio is subject to considerable variation [223, 224]. In a variety of conditions, such as hemolytic anemia, liver disease, and lead poisoning, a slight to moderate increase in urinary coproporphyrin excretion is observed [221], and changes in isomer ratio have been reported [20]. Coproporphyrin is also present in the bile, where the daily excretion rate is estimated to be 400 to 1,000 μg [221]. Thus, elevated values for urinary coproporphyrin excretion may result not only from increased porphyrin production but also from liver damage leading to diversion of excretion from the biliary to the urinary route [20]. For example, Hoffbauer et al. [225] and Sano and Rimington [226] have found that in rats, injected coproporphyrin III is almost entirely eliminated in the bile unless the bile ducts are occluded or the liver is damaged by carbon tetrachloride. By contrast, injected coproporphyrinogen normally is in part excreted by the kidneys [226]. This is of physiologic importance, because a significant fraction of what ultimately is measured in the urine as coproporphyrin is excreted in the form of coproporphyrinogen [227] (Table 45-3).

Other porphyrins present in normal human urine include uroporphyrin [220, 221, 228, 229] and traces of porphyrins with seven, six, five, and three carboxyl groups [223, 230]. Most of the uroporphyrin appears to be of type I isomer, with only trace amounts of uroporphyrin III [228].

Protoporphyrin is normally absent from the urine [20, 221, 226] but is present in bile and feces [20, 231]. Even in Sedormid poisoning, where very large amounts of protoporphyrin are excreted by way of the bile, this porphyrin could not be demonstrated in the urine [36]. As a general rule, it may be said that ALA, PBG, and uroporphyrin are mainly excreted in the urine, while coproporphyrin is preferentially and protoporphyrin exclusively eliminated through the bile.

A large fraction of the porphyrins present in normal urine is excreted in the form of precursors, which are converted to porphyrins by exposure to light and air or, more efficiently, by oxidation with dilute iodine [226, 227, 232, 233]. These precursors probably include porphyrinogens and PBG, and possibly ALA, all of which can be converted nonenzymatically to porphyrins [137, 215, 234]. It appears likely that the quantity and isomer types of porphyrins formed from precursors in the urine depend to some extent on environmental factors, such as pH of the urine and type of oxidizing agent employed [235].

Significant amounts of porphyrins are excreted in the feces [9, 231]; they may represent pigments or precursors which have reached the intestinal tract with the bile, or they may be derived from chlorophyll and heme proteins of ingested food or intestinal hemorrhages. In part, they may be formed by the intestinal microorganisms [236, 237]. It is not yet known how much these potential sources contribute to the total fecal porphyrin excretion. It appears likely that most of the coproporphyrin and much of the protoporphyrin in the stool represents pigment that has reached the intestinal tract with the bile. On the other hand, fecal deutero-, meso-, and pemptoporphyrins may be largely of exogenous origin, or they may be formed by the colonic flora [236–238].

Under these conditions, it is not surprising that fecal porphyrin excretion is highly variable in normal individuals. Expressed per gram of dried fecal material, coproporphyrin concentration ranges from 0 to approximately 40 μg, and protoporphyrin from 0 to about 100 μg [19, 220, 237, 239] (Table 45-3). Calculated on the basis of excretion per 24 hr, mean values of 422 μg coproporphyrin and 955 μg protoporphyrin have been reported [236]. Total porphyrin concentrations of up to 200 μg per gm dry fecal material probably do occur in normal individuals and therefore, in the absence of other evidence, should not be considered as indicative of porphyria [240].

Except for circulating erythrocytes, information is scant regarding the concentration of free porphyrins in normal human tissues. Erythrocytes contain approximately 15 to 60 μg protoporphyrin, and 1 to 2 μg coproporphyrin per 100 ml of cells [221, 241]. These values may be greatly increased in iron deficiency, hemolytic anemia, lead poisoning, and other disorders of erythropoiesis [20, 56, 221, 242].

Because of differences in methodology and because of nutritional, ethnic, and geographic variations, it is difficult to define generally applicable ranges for normal prophyrin excretion. The values listed in Table 45-3 have been found to be of practical usefulness in our laboratory.

PHARMACOLOGIC ACTION OF PORPHYRINS AND OF PORPHYRIN PRECURSORS

Photosensitivity

The photosensitizing activity of porphyrins is well known and has been the subject of many studies [243–250]. It is probably related to the intense fluorescence of porphyrins

[250], since both properties are most effectively produced by long-wave ultraviolet light of about 400-mμ wavelength. This corresponds to the peak absorption of porphyrins in the ultraviolet region of the spectrum [251–253]. In the famous self-experiment of Meyer-Betz [246], 200 mg hematoporphyrin was injected intravenously; this resulted in marked erythema and edema of the exposed parts of the body. Similar observations have been reported by Schwartz [254]. The photodynamic effect in the skin may be mediated by release of histamine [225].

In spite of the recognized relation between porphyrins and photosensitivity, the pathogenesis of hydroa aestivale, the vesicular eruption occurring on exposed parts of patients who suffer from photosensitive porphyria, is not fully understood. Blum and his coworkers [248], Watson [23], and Gray [256] failed to produce the characteristic vesicles by exposing areas of skin of porphyric patients to ultraviolet radiation, although the wavelength of the emitted light corresponded to the absorption maximum of porphyrins. These negative results may be ascribed to the use of light sources emitting inadequate radiant energy in the 400-mμ band. Indeed, in more recent investigations, Magnus et al. were able to reproduce experimentally the skin lesions typical of cutaneous porphyria by employing a powerful monochromator and a 70-amp d-c Xenon arc lamp [251, 252]. Predictably, the action spectrum was found to be a small waveband in the 400-mμ region (cf. Fig. 45-20). During or immediately after the exposure to light, the patients experienced the sensations of pricking, itching, or burning associated with strictly localized erythema. Two to three hours later, more extensive erythema and edema formation occurred. This was reminiscent of common sunburn, except that the latter normally is provoked by ultraviolet light in the 300-mμ band. Occasionally in the irradiated sites ecchymosis or blisters developed, followed in 2 to 3 weeks by cutaneous atrophy. It is likely that these skin manifestations are mediated by substances produced by photochemical reactions which are initiated by the radiant energy absorbed by the porphyrins. It is probable that release of lysosomal enzymes plays a major role in this process [257]. Individual porphyrins, such as protoporphyrin or uroporphyrin, may produce quantitatively different photocutaneous reactions; these differences probably are related to the physicochemical characteristics of the porphyrin, such as solubility properties, interaction with proteins, and subcellular distribution in the skin. The presence of significant porphyrin concentrations in the skin of porphyric patients has repeatedly been demonstrated [253, 258, 259]. The beneficial effect of chloroquine on the photosensitivity of patients with porphyria cutanea tarda has been shown to be due to formation of a water-soluble chloroquine-porphyrin complex in the liver [260]. This complex is readily excreted in the urine, thereby ridding the body of excess uroporphyrin.

Administration of ALA to man has resulted in marked but transient hypersensitivity to sunlight [208]. In rats, injection of ALA followed by exposure to radiation from a carbon arc lamp has produced marked photosensitivity [261]. Injection of PBG had no such effect. This difference is believed to be related in part to the rate at which these compounds can enter epidermal cells [261]. Fluorescence microscopic examination of skin obtained from animals injected with ALA suggests that ultraviolet radiation may enhance the intracellular conversion of ALA to uroporphyrin [261]. This is reminiscent of the photocatalytic auto-oxidation of porphyrinogens to porphyrins in vitro, a process which is sensitized by the product, porphyrin [145]. In vivo, Pimenta de Mello [262, 263] observed that in rabbits poisoned with lead acetate or injected with the photosensitizing dye rose Bengal, ultraviolet irradiation resulted in a marked increase in urinary coproporphyrin excretion. A similar elevation of fecal and urinary porphyrins has been reported in patients with cutaneous porphyria who were exposed to sunlight [259]. It is not known whether this enhanced pigment excretion is attributable to photocatalytic conversion of precursors [264] or to light-induced release of preformed porphyrin from the skin [253, 259]. On the other hand, it is noteworthy that most patients with acute intermittent porphyria are free from photosensitivity [18, 57], although large amounts of porphyrin precursors are present in the liver [76] and are excreted in the urine. High concentration of protoporphyrin in erythrocytes greatly enhances their photohemolysis. Thus, red blood cells of patients with erythropoietic protoporphyria are rapidly hemolyzed by exposure to near-ultraviolet radiation [265–267].

Other Pharmacologic Effects

In addition to their photosensitizing properties, porphyrins have been said to produce a variety of toxic effects, including vascular and intestinal spasm and neuropathologic changes [59, 268, 269]. Reinvestigations of the pharmacologic action of naturally occurring porphyrins have failed to produce convincing evidence of demonstrable effects of these compounds on smooth muscle or on the nervous system [13, 261, 270–272]. Further, neither injection of hematoporphyrin [246] nor the excessive production of endogenous uroporphyrin which occurs in congenital erythropoietic porphyria give rise to intestinal or neurologic symptoms, nor are such symptoms produced by injection of PBG or ALA in man or in animals [208, 261, 270, 271, 273]. In vitro these compounds are without effect on the smooth muscle of rat intestine [261, 270], but recent findings suggest a possible inhibitory effect of PBG and of its oxidation product, porphobilin, on the neuromuscular junction [274, 619]. PBG and porphobilin have been shown in vitro to inhibit potassium-augmentation of miniature end-plate potential frequencies [619]. The results suggest that these pyrroles reduce the release of acetylcholine that normally follows ionic depolarization. It is of note that PBG and porphobilin exert these effects at concentrations of the same order of magnitude as can be found in the sera of patients with the genetically transmitted hepatic porphyrias. A preliminary report has provided data suggesting that ALA may inhibit brain tissue (sodium + potassium)-dependent ATPase [620]. Thus, in spite of earlier failures to demonstrate that intermediates in heme biosynthesis are neurotoxic in vivo, a pharmacologic basis for such toxicity may be forthcoming.

REGULATION OF HEME AND HEMOPROTEIN BIOSYNTHESIS

The human porphyrias and their animal prototypes are a diverse collection of conditions that have in common derangements in the regulation of heme and hemoprotein biosynthesis. These may lead to distinctive patterns of excessive levels of intermediates of this pathway which accumulate in the involved tissues and subsequently are excreted. The understanding of many of the factors that influence regulatory phenomena in microbes and in higher organisms advanced remarkably during the past several years, and therefore it is now feasible to define more clearly the logical alternatives that may account for the regulatory aberrations present in the porphyrias. This section will deal with the mechanisms that are known to influence the regulation of heme biosynthesis in higher organisms. Additional factors governing tetrapyrrole biosynthesis in bacteria, particularly in organisms capable of photosynthesis, will not be discussed here, but this fascinating subject is described in detail in recent treatises by Lascelles [63] and by Burnham [64].

Regulation of a sequence of metabolic events leading from precursor A to an end product Z that is several steps removed is a function of a number of factors that include (1) the activities and quantities of the enzymes involved (Fig. 45-6). In this regard, of particular importance is regulation of the enzymatic effectiveness of the rate-controlling enzyme in the pathway. In general, this enzyme initiates the pathway and utilizes a high-energy intermediate as substrate. In heme biosynthesis, ALA synthetase fulfills these criteria (Figs. 45-6, 45-10). (2) The availability of the initial substrates and the subsequent intermediates. (3) The ultrastructural interrelationships of the enzymes in the pathway. (4) The efficiency of the system in terms of intercellular and intracellular retention of intermediates and the availability of alternative mechanisms for the utilization of these intermediates.

In eukaryotic cells enzymatic function can be influenced by the following regulatory processes: (1) Alterations of enzyme activity by modifications of preexisting protein without changing the actual quantity of enzyme present. For example, pepsinogen is activated to pepsin by hydrogen ions [275]. Alternatively, enzyme activity may be diminished by substances which are generally termed *inhibitors.* (2) Enzyme levels may be regulated by changes in the rates of degradation. Since a "dynamic state" [276] of proteins exhibiting differing rates of turnover is a general feature of animal cells, enzyme levels may be increased by factors which diminish the rate of protein degradation [88, 277] or they may be decreased by enhanced catabolism. Thus, either of the above processes (1) or (2) provides a mechanism for altering an enzymatic pathway *without* actually changing the rates of protein synthesis; these regulatory mechanisms therefore are little affected by inhibitors of protein synthesis such as cycloheximide or puromycin. (3) Enzyme levels may also be regulated by changes in the rate of protein synthesis. "Induction" implies an increase in the rate of enzyme synthesis, thereby leading to more enzyme; conversely, "repression" indicates interference with enzyme synthesis.

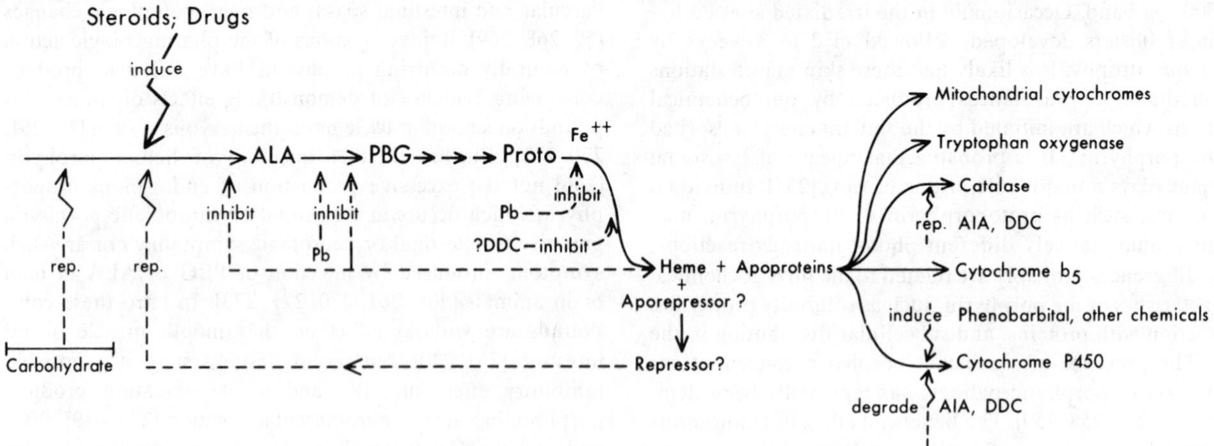

Figure 45-10. Specific sites and mechanisms of action of substances known to influence hepatic heme and hemoprotein biosynthesis. As discussed in the text, it is uncertain whether the action of a drug at one site in the pathway is responsible for activity at another point. For example, does the action of AIA (allylisopropylacetamide) on cytochrome P450 result in the capacity of the latter to induce ALA (δ-aminolevulinic acid) synthetase? (*PBG,* porphobilinogen; *PROTO,* protoporphyrin IXα; *DDC,* 3,5-dicarbethoxy-1,4-dihydrocollidine; *rep,* repress.)

Obviously, new protein synthesis also influences enzymatic effectiveness at the level of activation or degradation, or in the formation of new proteins with similar enzymatic specificities but with different functional capacities. The regulation of protein synthesis, particularly in eukaryotic cells, is complex [277–282] and may involve control at almost any level of protein synthesis from the transcription of DNA into RNA to translation of messenger RNA into protein on ribosomes.

Enzymatic Regulation of Heme Biosynthesis

Inhibition and possibly activation may play a role in regulating the activity of the enzymes in heme and hemoprotein biosynthesis. Of some importance is the negative feedback inhibition exercised by heme. Though this effect previously had been documented in bacteria [124], only recently have similar phenomena been observed in eukaryotic cells [120, 122]. As seen in Fig. 45-10, heme inhibits ALA synthetase [120, 122] and ALA dehydrase [124, 142]; ferrochelatase (not shown in Fig. 45-10) probably also is inhibited by heme [283]. This inhibition can be markedly impeded by a variety of proteins that interact with heme and may be present within the cell [120]. Thus, it is often impossible to demonstrate inhibition with cruder enzyme preparations that contain significant quantities of protein contaminants [45, 120, 284]. Therefore, it is difficult to assess the physiologic importance of this type of negative feedback effect that is demonstrable only with purified enzyme systems [120]. Moreover, heme has been shown to inhibit at least one enzyme not directly involved in heme biosynthesis, ribonuclease [285]. This observation raises interesting speculations regarding the possibility that heme inhibits enzyme systems not directly involved in its formation.

Negative feedback systems commonly are characterized by the fact that the enzyme under control is the first one leading exclusively to a particular end product so that the end product governs its own rate of synthesis by interacting with the first enzyme in the pathway [286, 287]. The effect of heme deviates from this general principle in that heme also inhibits the activity of ALA dehydrase (Fig. 45-10) [124, 142] and, additionally, of ferrochelatase [283]. Another feature of such a negative feedback system is that it involves an enzymatic site topologically distinct from the site of catalysis (allostery) and undergoes reversible inhibition [288–290]. Though data related to allosteric effects are scant, reversibility has been observed in all cases in which it has been examined [120, 122, 124, 142].

Pyridoxal-5-phosphate is a cofactor absolutely required for the synthesis of ALA [122, 125, 127], but under physiologic conditions and even in experimental porphyria it does not appear to assume an important regulatory role [90, 291]. Recently, divalent and monovalent cations have been shown to activate ALA synthetase [122] and ALA dehydrase [124, 139, 148, 149], but these ions appear to play no major homeostatic role, because their concentrations required for influencing enzyme activity lie outside the limits compatible with life.

Lead inhibits the activities of at least two enzymes in the heme biosynthetic pathway (ALA dehydrase and ferrochelatase) in erythrocytes [203, 210, 216, 292, 293] and probably in other tissues. At least with ALA dehydrase, the presumed mechanism of action is combination with sulfhydryl groups essential for enzymatic activity [292, 293]. Characteristic manifestations of these metabolic blocks in heme biosynthesis (see Fig. 45-10) are seen in chronic lead poisoning and include hypochromic anemia, increased free erythrocyte protoporphyrin, and excessive urinary excretion of ALA and coproporphyrin with near normal levels of porphobilinogen. This latter pattern of urinary metabolites is almost pathognomonic of lead intoxication.

Tschudy and Collins have reported that in sufficient concentration the herbicide 3-amino-1,2,4-triazole partially inhibits ALA dehydrase [294]. Although there is conflicting evidence as to whether the degree of inhibition effected by this compound can alter overall heme synthesis [45, 295], a recent report suggests that aminotriazole can interfere with the synthesis of cytochrome P450 [295].

As shown in Fig. 45-10, alterations in the turnover of protein have been identified as significant regulatory events in heme biosynthesis only in relationship to enhancement of cytochrome P450 degradation by certain porphyria-inducing drugs [296–300]. The possible relevance of this observation to the pathogenesis of porphyria will be discussed in the subsequent sections.

Although control of metabolic activity can be exercised at the level of enzyme activity or turnover, a more efficient system is effected by control of *enzyme synthesis.* Control by enzyme "repression" permits the cell to regulate a metabolic pathway more economically by avoiding the unnecessary formation of new protein. According to the model of Jacob and Monod [301] proposed on the basis of bacterial studies, the last small molecule in a biosynthetic sequence reacts with an aporepressor substance to form a repressor. In turn, the repressor impedes synthesis of the messenger RNA coding for certain enzymes in the metabolic pathway. While dramatic discoveries of the past few years have indeed demonstrated the existence of the postulated repressor molecules involved in the β-galactosidase system [302, 303] and in replication of lambda phage [304, 305], it is not certain that a similar series of events accounts for feedback repression in animal cells.

Repression by heme of drug-mediated induction of ALA synthetase appears to have been demonstrated in a number of laboratories. That is, administration of heme to intact animals [306–308], or addition of this metalloporphyrin [45, 309, 310] or of ALA [311] (which is converted largely to heme) to cultured hepatocytes, interferes with induction of ALA synthetase. As already indicated, heme does not interfere with ALA synthetase activity when added directly to crude liver homogenates containing the enzyme even if the heme concentrations far exceed those which repress ALA synthetase induction [45, 284]. The possibility cannot be excluded of course that heme could localize specifically at the appropriate enzyme sites within the intact cell, thereby reaching effective inhibitory concentrations, but the available data do not favor this possibility. It should be noted that the biologic half-life of hepatic ALA synthetase is approximately 72 min [50, 312], which is short in comparison with other liver proteins. Therefore, primary regulation of this enzyme at the level of its synthesis provides a relatively sensitive control mechanism. If heme does indeed influence the rate of synthesis of ALA-synthetase, the site of this action is still uncertain; i.e., the effect could be on transcription, translation, or an alternative mechanism that modifies the formation of the active enzyme. Recent indirect data have been interpreted as indicating that heme regulates the hepatic concentration of ALA-synthetase at the level of translation [621].

Granick and Urata first demonstrated that following administration of certain drugs to experimental animals the increased hepatic content of porphyrins and their precursors was an ultimate consequence of drug-mediated induction of hepatic ALA synthetase (Fig. 45-10). These observations have been extended and confirmed in a number of laboratories [50, 119, 120, 306, 307, 313]. More recently, Granick introduced the elegant technique of quantitating induction of ALA synthetase by determination of porphyrin fluorescence in primary cultures of avian hepatocytes [45]. Many compounds of diverse structure are inducers [45, 51, 310, 314]. A few representative substances are illustrated in Fig. 45-11. There is considerable variation in the inductive potency of these agents. Moreover, in rodents the less-active compounds produce only a transient increase in ALA synthetase, which fails to provide the persistent and sustained overproduction of porphyrins and their precursors typical of the chemically induced forms of porphyria in animals and in certain forms of human hepatic porphyria. The more active porphyria-inducing compounds (i.e., allylisopropylacetamide and the trimethylpyridine derivatives) appear unique in this regard. Though the relatively slow rates of detoxification of these agents may account for some of these differences [315], they do not appear to explain the entire phenomenon, since equivalent differences in potency are observed in cell culture in which detoxification plays only a minor role [45, 311].

Drugs such as phenobarbital induce cytochrome P450 (Figs. 45-10, 45-11) as part of an adaptive response of the liver to enhance its capacity for detoxification of phenobarbital and of a host of other chemicals [316, 317]. It has been postulated that this induction of a heme protein would necessitate increased availability of heme and, hence, call

INDUCTION OF HEPATIC ALA-SYNTHETASE

AGENTS	RODENTS	CULTURED AVIAN HEPATOCYTES	PATIENTS WITH IAP
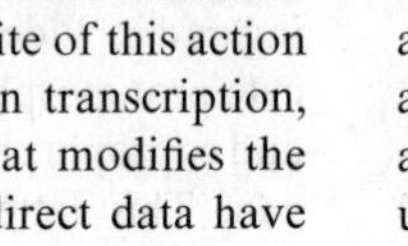 Diethyl-1, 4-dihydro-2,4,6-trimethylpyridine 3, 5-dicarboxylate	++++[a]	++++[b]	Not tested
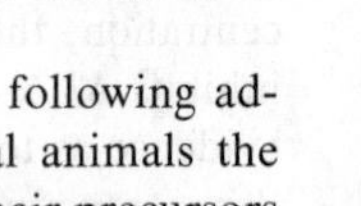 Allylisopropylacetamide	++++[c]	++++[b]	Not tested
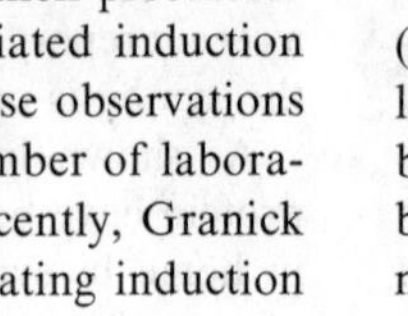 Phenobarbital	+[d]	+[b]	Active[e]
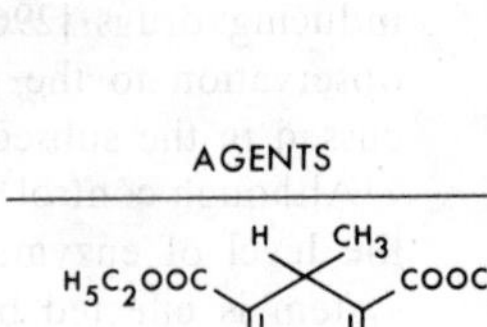 Etiocholanolone-17β	0 – +[a]	++++[f]	?

Figure 45-11. Structures of several representative compounds known to induce hepatic ALA (δ-aminolevulinic acid) synthetase in the species and under the conditions listed. The marked diversity in the structure of these compounds and their potency in different systems are to be noted. (References: *a* [49]; *b* [45]; *c* [50]; *d* [306]; *e* [19, 20]; *f* [328].)

Table 45-4. δ-AMINOLEVULINIC ACID (ALA) UTILIZED IN THE BIOSYNTHESIS OF HEPATIC HEME ENZYMES*

Enzyme	ALA utilized, nanomoles/gm/hr
Catalase	3.5
Cytochromes b, c_1, c, a, a^3	1.3
Mitochondrial cytochrome b_5	0.2
Microsomal cytochrome b_5	1.4
Cytochrome P450	14.4
	0.7
Tryptophan oxygenase	0.3
Total	21.8

* Calculations based on the data in Table 45-2.

for induction of ALA synthetase [317, 318, 319]. A number of experimental studies provide tentative support for this hypothesis [295, 300, 306, 318, 320] (Table 45-4).

The mechanism accounting for the excessive induction of ALA synthetase by allylisopropylacetamide and similar compounds is not readily explained. A review of recent reports indicates that these compounds have the unique capacity of promoting degradation of cytochrome P450 [296–300]. It has been postulated, therefore, that this chemically mediated acceleration of cytochrome P450 turnover tends to remove heme from its role as a repressor, thereby magnifying and prolonging induction of ALA synthetase.

Indeed, reciprocal control mechanisms between ALA synthetase and the hemoprotein tryptophan oxygenase (Fig. 45-10) have been observed [284]. Thus, diversion of heme from its participation in enzyme repression and, possibly, enzyme inhibition by the selective increase of one or more hemoproteins may constitute a more general mechanism for the regulation of coordinate synthesis of heme and apoproteins.

An alternative mechanism for the inductive effect of dicarbethoxydihydrocollidine on ALA synthetase may involve inhibition of the enzymatic formation of heme from protoporphyrin and iron [321] (Figs. 45-10, 45-11); this would reduce heme synthesis, thereby derepressing ALA synthetase. Such an inhibitory effect of DDC has been found by some [322] but not all investigators [300]. Moreover, the magnitude of the effect described may be insufficient to account for the profound inducing capacity of this agent and its analogues.

Stein et al. have recently reported that chelated iron, in the form of ferric citrate, but not nonchelated iron salts, such as ferric chloride, exerts a marked synergistic effect on the chemical induction of ALA synthetase [323]. Chelated iron compounds are ineffective as inducers when administered alone. The mechanism of this effect is unknown, but because of the absence of ionic charge, passage of iron chelates across membranes is facilitated, as shown, for example, by their ready entrance into liver [324] and into mitochondria in vitro [325]. Moreover, this synergistic effect of ferric citrate and inducers of chemical porphyria suggests that these agents induce ALA synthetase by different mechanisms. This study may be relevant to the pathogenesis of porphyria cutanea tarda (Table 45-1), since, as will be discussed in the appropriate section, iron appears to have a unique effect in this disorder.

Kappas, Granick, and coworkers have recently described an important group of physiologic substances that at least in avian liver are potent inducers of ALA synthetase [45, 51, 326, 327]. These substances are reduced steroids (Fig. 45-11) containing alcohol or ketone substituents at the C-3, C-17, C-20, and possibly C-11 positions. Reportedly such steroids with the beta configuration (i.e., in which the A:B ring function is highly angular) are significantly more active than steroids of the more planar alpha configuration. C-21 hydroxylated steroids such as cortisol and aldosterone do not appear to possess inducing activity [51, 326]. It is of interest that steroids that are potent inducers of the hepatic enzyme both in primary cultures of avian liver and in the liver of intact chick embryos have only a slight and transient effect in rodent liver in vivo [328]. Recent studies by Necheles and Rai [329], Gorshein and Gardner [330], and Gordon et al. [331] demonstrated that, unlike other active chemicals, steroids which induce ALA synthetase in avian liver stimulate heme biosynthesis in mammalian marrow. A similar effect on erythroid cell formation has also been described in the chick blastoderm [332]. The factors accounting for the unusual properties of this group of steroids and their peculiar species and tissue specificity are not easily understood, particularly as the "classical" porphyria-inducing drugs are all ineffective in erythroid cells while displaying complete additivity with these steroids in cultured hepatocytes.

Tschudy and coworkers [333, 334], and subsequently De Matteis reported that ingestion of relatively large amounts of carbohydrate or protein, but not of fat, reduced the excretion of porphyrin precursors in chemically induced experimental porphyria in rodents and in patients with acute intermittent porphyria [335]. This effect was shown to be mediated through hepatic ALA synthetase. Chemical induction of ALA synthetase is enhanced by fasting but is significantly suppressed by feeding [45, 50, 118]. It also is likely that the physiologic activity of ALA synthetase in the liver is lowered by administration of large quantities of carbohydrate or protein, but may be modestly increased by fasting [328]. Experimental alterations of carbohydrate concentrations fail to affect directly hepatic ALA synthetase activity in in vitro assays [90]. This suggests that this "glucose effect" involves alterations in the rate of synthesis of ALA synthetase. Nevertheless in experimental porphyria, the "glucose effect" is clearly synergistic with the porphyria-inducing compounds [50, 118], so that it most probably influences the induction of ALA synthetase by a distinct mechanism.

Despite extensive studies and obvious therapeutic implications, the "glucose effect" on ALA synthetase remains mechanistically unexplained. The effect is unique, in that it cannot be reproduced in primary culture of hepatocytes

[45]; moreover, in contrast to similar effects of carbohydrate on other enzyme systems [336, 337], glucagon neither induces ALA synthetase nor reverses its repression [50].

Although ALA synthetase appears to be rate-limiting in heme biosynthesis [45, 49, 90, 118], this enzyme has a relatively high requirement (Michaelis constant, K_m) for one of its two substrates, glycine [122, 124]. This implies that within the narrow limits set by the quantity of enzyme present, the amount of ALA and of subsequent intermediates in heme biosynthesis may be modified by the intracellular availability of glycine [122]. It should be emphasized that under ordinary conditions, a mere increase in the amount of glycine available would not augment the rate of ALA production sufficiently to account for the development of experimental or human genetic porphyria. Indeed, a number of studies have failed to provide conclusive evidence for abnormalities of glycine metabolism either in human [338] or in chemically induced, experimental porphyria [339].

In general, under conditions of maximum substrate availability, the overall velocity of a multienzyme system is limited by the enzymatic step with the least activity [340]. When substrate concentrations are *not* saturating for certain enzymes in the pathway, then the overall velocity of the pathway will be regulated by both substrate *and* enzyme concentrations. The degree to which each of these influences the overall pathway is, of course, highly variable. Indeed, unlike the role of glycine in the formation of ALA, substrate concentrations may assume a dominant role. The relevance of this point for the genetically transmitted porphyrias will be discussed in subsequent sections.

The ultrastructural interrelationships of the enzymes in heme biosynthesis may play an additional regulatory role in the overall pathway. For example, compartmentalization of enzymes between the cytosol and mitochondria may provide regulation by alteration of mitochondrial permeability. The proximity of ALA synthetase and of ferrochelatase in the matrix and on the inner membrane of the mitochondrion respectively [121] may subject ALA synthetase to high local concentrations of heme, and thereby exert an inhibitory effect [120]. Findings suggesting that ALA synthetase is formed on the endoplasmic reticulum and then transported into the mitochondrion [119, 120] provide an additional potential site of control. The role of these and similar factors in the regulation of heme biosynthesis has not been sufficiently evaluated to permit definitive conclusions.

As a final point, it should be noted that retention of intermediates within the cell, utilization of intermediates by alternate pathways, and preservation of porphyrinogens in their reduced form, essential for their role as biochemical intermediates, may also function as controlling factors of heme biosynthesis. Little information is available regarding the first and last possibilities. The alternative utilization of ALA has been discussed already in the section dealing with this intermediate.

Recapitulation

The principal factors known to control the heme biosynthetic pathway are outlined in Figs. 45-6 and 45-10. These include (1) inhibition of enzyme activity; (2) repression of enzyme synthesis; and (3) enzyme induction. Of particular relevance is the regulation of ALA synthetase, since this is the first and rate-limiting enzyme of the pathway.

1 Heme inhibits the activity of ALA synthetase, ALA dehydrase, and ferrochelatase. The physiologic significance of these inhibitory effects is uncertain, since high concentrations of heme are required for enzyme inhibition in crude systems. Lead is a potent inhibitor of ALA dehydrase and ferrochelatase; this accounts for the effects of lead poisoning on the metabolism of porphyrins and porphyrin precursors.

2 Relatively low concentrations of heme administered to intact rodents or to cultured hepatocytes repress the synthesis of ALA synthetase.

3 ALA synthetase is induced by diverse drugs and steroids. Some of these compounds, such as allylisopropylacetamide, are particularly potent inducers; they produce an experimental porphyria in rodents. They also share the property of enhancing the catabolism of cytochrome P450. It is uncertain whether these two effects are causally related. Chemically mediated induction of ALA synthetase is repressed by administration of heme. Also, ingestion of carbohydrate or protein represses the induction of ALA synthetase, while fasting augments enzyme synthesis. This phenomenon, termed the *glucose effect,* appears to act at a site distinct from that responsible for the chemical induction of ALA synthetase.

CONGENITAL ERYTHROPOIETIC PORPHYRIA

Incidence and Clinical Manifestations

Erythropoietic porphyria (Günther's disease) is a rare congenital disease which occurs much less frequently than other forms of porphyria. The prominence of photosensitivity and of massive porphyrinuria has often caused it to be confused with the hepatic types of cutaneous porphyria [15], although it differs fundamentally in its pathogenesis from the latter disorders [76]. In the earlier literature [15, 341], many of the reported cases clearly had features of the hepatic forms, while in other instances the data were insufficient to permit distinction [17]. A reexamination of the cases of so-called congenital photosensitive porphyria reported up to 1954 permitted the diagnosis of erythropoietic porphyria beyond doubt in a total of 34 cases [17]. An additional 26 cases reported up to 1964 are included in Table 45-5, which summarizes the essential features of these 60 patients. During the last few years at least 10 more cases have come to our attention [377, 402, 408–414], but because of incomplete reporting it is often difficult to be sure that these patients have not been described previously [377, 378, 388, 393, 394, 402, 404, 407–409, 411, 413, 414]. Of the 60 patients listed in Table 45-5, 28 were female and 32 male. In the earlier literature it was generally held that congenital porphyria was more common in males, but this was undoubtedly caused by confusion with porphyria cutanea tarda, which is more frequent in males [415, 416]. As shown in Table 45-5, the disease has a wide racial distribution and has been observed in children of parents of Japanese, Bantu, Sudanese, Aleutian Indian, and Bengali-Hindu extraction.

The first sign suggesting the presence of erythropoietic porphyria is usually the excretion of red urine containing much uroporphyrin but no increase in PBG. This may be noted at birth or during infancy, only rarely later in life [377]. Although porphyrinuria is probably present at all times, the amounts of porphyrins excreted, and hence the red color of the urine, may show considerable daily or seasonal fluctuation [9, 76, 354, 405]. In some instances, the color of the urine was light except during periods of active photodermatitis occurring in the summer months [9, 76, 226]. In others, large and relatively constant amounts of uroporphyrin were excreted over long periods of time [15].

Photosensitivity is frequently absent in the neonatal period, but it may become apparent during the first years of life as exposure to sunlight increases. A vesicular or bullous eruption appears on the face, the back of the hands, and other exposed parts of the body. This is commonly referred to as hydroa aestivale, the adjective indicating the seasonal recurrence of the lesions. The vesicles contain a serous fluid which may exhibit red fluorescence, heal slowly, and leave depressed pigmented scars. Infected bullae often ulcerate, causing marked scarring and deformity, particularly of the tips of the fingers, the ears, the nose, and the eyelids. After years of repeated attacks severe mutilation may ensue, with contractions of the face and loss of parts of digits and ears [15]. In other cases the cutaneous manifestations may be relatively mild, leaving little if any scarring. In several patients a definite decrease in photosensitivity and a reduction in urinary porphyrin excretion followed splenectomy [76, 354, 360, 369, 373, 387, 390, 392, 402, 405]. In one of these children [354], removal of the spleen resulted in virtual loss of photosensitivity, but porphyrin-containing vesicles were observed on those parts of the hands which became infested with scabies [41].

Hypertrichosis is a frequent finding in these patients [15, 23]. Blond, downy hair resembling lanugo may cover the face and extremities [15, 23, 343, 356, 369]. Deciduous and permanent teeth may show a red or brownish discoloration (erythrodontia) [15, 258, 393], but in some cases this has been inconspicuous [20, 406]. Under the ultraviolet light the teeth always exhibit marked red fluorescence. Deposition of porphyrin in the developing teeth and in bones is believed to be due to its physical affinity for calcium phosphate [20]. The presence of porphyrin in the deciduous teeth suggests that the metabolic disorder was present during fetal life [342, 406].

Splenomegaly is an almost constant feature of the disease (Table 45-5). It may remain undetected during the neonatal period and appear only as the patient grows older [17]. In one patient the spleen was enlarged in early childhood but could no longer be palpated 10 years later [344]. In five patients splenomegaly was absent; at times this was correlated with normal erythrocyte survival and absence of hemolytic anemia at the time of study [372, 373, 384, 400, 402]. Hypertension and abdominal or neurologic symptoms so frequently observed in other forms of porphyria are not found in erythropoietic porphyria.

Hematologic Findings

In the majority of the reported cases, increased hemolytic activity was present, as indicated by the following findings: normochromic anemia, associated with elevated reticulocyte levels and circulating normoblasts; normoblastic hyperplasia of the bone marrow; and increased excretion of fecal urobilinogen [17]. In most patients the reduction in hemoglobin concentration was only slight and the hemolysis was largely compensated by increased red blood cell production. Only rarely was the anemia severe, requiring multiple transfusion [389, 406] or leading to early death [347]. It was stated that the famous patient Petry [258] at the time of his death suffered from pernicious anemia in addition to congenital porphyria, but Aldrich et al. [354] raised justified doubts of this interpretation of the autopsy findings and suggested that Petry may have had an unrecognized hemolytic anemia with splenomegaly. In another patient, originally reported by Ashby [348] and later by Garrod [344], outspoken hemolytic anemia was repeatedly demonstrated [349]. At the time of her death at age 27, she was found to have a coarse-nodular cirrhosis of the liver, and the bone marrow showed "extensive myeloid hyperplasia and no significant erythroid haemopoiesis" [349]. The available information is inadequate to permit speculation as to the possible factors which could have led to this marrow failure [17].

Erythrocyte life-span has been directly estimated in most of the patients reported more recently [94, 363, 367, 369, 372, 377, 402, 403, 405, 417, 418]; most of them had hematologic findings suggestive of hemolytic anemia. A decreased survival of autologous erythrocytes was demonstrated by the glycine-^{15}N method in the two patients studied, the first by Grinstein et al. [417], the second by Watson et al. [367]. In the former patient splenectomy resulted in remarkable improvement in hemoglobin concentration, porphyrin excretion, and photosensitivity [354]. In the case reported by London et al. [363], the average life-span of the erythrocytes appeared to be normal, but the reticulocyte count was elevated, and the marrow showed erythroid hyperplasia. In a study reported by Rosenthal et al. [369], erythrocytes of

Table 45-5. CASES OF CONGENITAL ERYTHROPOIETIC PORPHYRIA REPORTED IN THE LITERATURE UP TO 1964

Reference	Year	*Essential features of patient*								Remarks
		Sex	Racial background	Age at onset of symptoms	Anemia	Splenomegaly	Erythrodontia	Parental consanguinity		
[1]	1874	M	German	3 mo	0	+	0	0		Also studied by Baumstark [2].
[9]	1898	M	English	4 yr	0	0	0	–		Sister believed to have died with porphyria. 4 normal sibs. Birth order: 3, 4, 5 [342].
[9]	1898	M	English	3 yr	0	0	0	–		
[343]	1914	M	Italian	3 yr	+	+	0	0		No sibs.
[342, 344]	1922	M	English	Birth	Hemolytic	+	+	–		Splenectomy; died, 1952, in uremia [345]; 3 normal and 1(?) normal elder sibs.
[344, 346]	1924	F	English	5 yr	Hemolytic	+	+	+		6 normal sibs. Birth order: 3.
[347]	1926	M	Japanese	Birth	Hypochromic	+	+	–		2 sibs died with similar symptoms. 4 normal sibs. Birth order: 4, 6, 7.
[344, 348]	1926	F	English	Birth	Hemolytic	+	+	–		Died 1949 in hepatic coma after delivery of second child [349]. No sibs.
[350]	1926	F	German	2 yr	Hemolytic	+	0	0		Splenectomy discussed but not performed.
[351]	1927	F	Japanese	Birth	Hemolytic	+	0	0		2 normal sibs. Second patient's time of onset of first symptoms not clearly stated.
[352]	1928	M	Japanese	16 yr (?)	Hemolytic	+	0	0		
[352]	1928	F	Japanese	3 yr	Hemolytic	+	+	+		No sibs.
[353]	1929	M	Italian	Birth	+	+	+	–		1 normal younger sib.
[258]	1929	M	German	Birth	+	+	+	0		Patient Petry; anemia believed to be pernicious but may have been hemolytic [354]; 2 offspring aborted but found to be normal [355].
[356]	1931	M	Italian	5 yr	Hemolytic	+	+	0		Studied again in 1948 [357] and 1962 [358]; 2 normal elder sibs.
[359]	1933	M	White	1 yr	+	+	0	0		Type of anemia not stated.
[360]	1934	F	Argentine	5 yr	Hemolytic	+	0	0		Splenectomy with partial remission of photosensitivity.
[361]	1938	F	Spanish	1 yr	0	0	0	+		Sibs. Hydroa aestivale, red urine, hypertrichosis.
[361]	1938	F	Spanish	1 yr	0	0	0	+		
[361]	1938	F	Spanish	Early in life	0	0	0	0		Sibs
[361]	1938	F	Spanish	Early in life	0	0	0	0		1 additional sib, normal (?).
[361]	1938	M	Spanish	Early in life	0	0	0	0		
[362]	1938	F	White	Birth	Hemolytic	+	+	0		Later studied by London et al. [363]. Delivered normal infant [364, 365]. 1 normal elder sib.
[366]	1938	F	White	3 yr	+	+	+	0		Splenectomized, 1957, with remission of hemolytic anemia [367].
[368]	1947	F	White	Birth	–	+	+	–		Increased hemolysis; splenectomy, 1953 [369]. 1 sib possibly affected.
[370, 371]	1948	M	French	Birth	–	–	+	–		6 normal sibs. 2 of the 3 patients had normal survival of chromated erythrocytes [372]; all 3 were splenectomized in 1960 [373]. Birth order: 5, 6, 9.
[370, 371]	1948	F	French	Birth	–	–	+	–		
[370, 371]	1948	M	French	Birth	Hemolytic	+	+	–		
[374]	1948	M	Italian	3–4 yr	+	0	0	–		11 healthy sibs.
[375, 376]	1950	F	Bantu	11 mo	Hemolytic	+	+	+		Delivered normal infant [377, 378]. No sibs.
[354]	1951	F	Norwegian	2 mo	Hemolytic	+	+	0		Splenectomy with remission of photosensitivity. 3 normal elder sibs.

Table 45-5. CASES OF CONGENITAL ERYTHROPOIETIC PORPHYRIA REPORTED IN THE LITERATURE UP TO 1964 (*continued*)

Reference	Year	*Essential features of patient*							Remarks
		Sex	Racial background	Age at onset of symptoms	Anemia	Splenomegaly	Erythrodontia	Parental consanguinity	
[379, 380]	1951	F	White	1 yr	Hemolytic	+	+	0	Splenectomy with partial remission of photosensitivity.
[381]	1953	F	Italian	Birth	Hemolytic	+	+	0	Severe photodermatitis with scarring.
[17, 76]	1954	F	English	3 yr	Hemolytic	+	+	0	Splenectomy with partial remission of photosensitivity.
[382]	1954	F	Polish	1 yr	Hemolytic	+	+	0	Eldest and youngest of 4 sibs.
[382]	1954	F	Polish	Birth	Hemolytic	+	+	0	
[383]	1956	M	Indian	6 mo	Hemolytic	+	+	+	3 normal sibs. Birth order: 1, 5.
[383]	1956	M	Indian	1 yr	Hemolytic	+	+	+	Second case splenectomized.
[376, 384]	1957	M	Sudanese	9 mo	–	–	+	–	2 normal younger sibs. Parents had common tribal background.
[376, 384]	1957	F	Sudanese	7 mo	Hemolytic	+	+	–	First patient had normoblastic hyperplasia of bone marrow.
[385]	1957	M	Brazilian	4 mo	Hemolytic	+	+	–	Patients said to have another affected sister and 5 normal sibs [386].
[385]	1957	M	Brazilian	10 mo	Hemolytic	+	+	–	
[385]	1957	M	Brazilian	10 mo	Hemolytic	+	+	–	
[387]	1958	F	Bantu	Birth	Hemolytic	+	+	0	Splenectomy with partial remission of photosensitivity. 5 normal sibs [388].
[389]	1958	M	German	Birth	Hemolytic	+	+	0	Splenectomy for severe hemolytic anemia.
[390]	1958	F	English	Birth	Hemolytic	+	+	0	Splenectomy partially beneficial. 1 normal younger sib [393, 394].
[391]	1958	M	Indian	3 mo	+	+	+	–	2 normal sibs. Birth order: 2, 4.
[391]	1958	M	Indian	3 mo	Hemolytic	+	0	–	
[392]	1960	M	Sardinian	0	Hemolytic	+	+	0	Splenectomy without benefit.
[395, 396]	1960	F	Italian	1 mo	Hemolytic	+	+	0	3 normal sibs. Studied again in 1962 [397].
[395, 396]	1960	M	Italian	1 mo	Hemolytic	+	+	0	
[398]	1960	M	French	3 yr	+	+	+	0	Onset of first symptoms not clearly stated.
[399]	1961	F	Indian Hindu	Birth	Hemolytic	+	+	+	Clinical and hematologic improvements on steroids. 2 normal sibs.
[400]	1962	M	Bengali Hindu	Few months	–	–	+	–	Clinical and laboratory improvement on steroids. 4 normal sibs. Birth order: 4.
[400]	1962	M	Bengali Hindu	Birth	Hemolytic	+	+	+	4 normal younger sibs.
[401, 402]	1963	F	Aleutian Indian	3 mo	Hemolytic	–	+	–	3 normal elder sibs.
[403, 404]	1963	F	French	1 yr	–	+	+	0	Normal survival of chromated erythrocytes; reticulocytosis.
[405]	1963	M	German	Birth	–	+	+	+	Increased hemolysis; laboratory improvement after splenectomy. 5 normal sibs; 1 died in infancy. Heterozygotes detected.
[405]	1963	M	German	4 yr	–	+	+	–	Reticulocyte count 2%; 3 normal sibs. Heterozygotes detected.
[406, 407]	1964	M	Irish	7 mo	Hemolytic	+	+	0	Splenectomy without benefit. 4 normal sibs. Birth order: 3.

Key: + = present; – = absent; 0 = no statement. Braces indicate sibs.

a patient with erythropoietic porphyria were infused into a recipient with ulcerative colitis, and the disappearance of the donor's cells from the recipient's circulation was followed by differential agglutination. Although the analysis of the results was complicated by the fact that the recipient was bleeding, the findings suggested a more rapid rate of removal of the porphyric cells than occurred with cells from a normal donor. Splenectomy in this patient resulted in only temporary improvement, although 4 years after the operation survival of chromated erythrocytes was almost normal [419]. A similar normalization of red blood cell survival following splenectomy was observed by Heilmeyer et al. [405]. On the other hand, in the patient reported by Gajdos et al. [403, 404] and in two of the three sibs studied by May et al. [370] and Canivet et al. [372] red blood cell survival as estimated by the ^{51}Cr method appeared to be normal, and there was no evidence of hemolytic anemia as judged by normal hemoglobin concentration, reticulocyte counts, fecal urobilinogen excretion, and absence of erythroid hyperplasia of the bone marrow. One of the latter two patients subsequently developed splenomegaly, and all three sibs were splenectomized [373].

A possible explanation for these seemingly contradictory results may be found in the observation that a hemolytic component may be present during one phase of the disease but absent at other times. Thus, in a patient in whom hemolytic anemia had repeatedly been demonstrated [342, 344] over the course of 25 years, Gray et al. [94, 418] found that approximately half the erythrocytes appeared to have a mean life-span of less than 20 days while other red blood cell fractions survived for periods of 40 to 70 days and for 110 to 120 days, respectively. At the time of this study, the patient was believed to have a hemolytic crisis, as suggested by the presence of anemia, reticulocytosis, normoblasts in the peripheral blood, and increased excretion of fecal urobilinogen. At a later date, when the reticulocyte count had returned to normal, a second study of erythrocyte survival suggested that at least 80 percent of the cells appeared to have a normal life-span while only a minor fraction appeared to be removed between the thirtieth and the eightieth days. All these values were calculated on the basis of data obtained by following the ^{15}N content of circulating hemoglobin heme after administration of ^{15}N-labeled glycine (Fig. 45-2) [94, 418]. The limitations of this method for determining the apparent life-span of circulating erythrocytes must be kept in mind.

The above findings suggest that increased hemolysis, although present in the majority of cases, may be intermittent in nature and at times may be so slight as to make detection difficult. It is interesting that the porphyric brother of the two patients with normal erythrocyte survival reported by Canivet et al. [372] exhibited marked hemolytic anemia [370, 371]. Furthermore, of the two Sudanese sibs studied by Townsend-Coles and Barnes [376, 384], one had severe hemolytic anemia, whereas the other had a normal hemoglobin concentration, erythrocyte count, and reticulocyte count, although the bone marrow showed normoblastic hyperplasia.

The mechanism responsible for the hemolytic process is not understood. Osmotic resistance of the erythrocytes was normal in all instances in which it was tested [13]. The absence of a positive Coombs' test and the finding of decreased survival of porphyric cells in a normal recipient [369] are suggestive of an intracorpuscular defect. It is possible that increased porphyrin concentrations predispose erythrocytes to hemolysis and that the life-span of porphyrin-containing cells may be further shortened by exposure of the patients to sunlight [265]. An alternative explanation was provided by Hausmann's observation [420] that hematoporphyrin sensitizes normal red blood cells to hemolysis by light in vitro. This suggested that the presence of porphyrins in the circulating plasma may exert a hemolytic effect in vivo [418]. It should be noted that none of these explanations is based on concrete experimental evidence.

Studies of unstained bone marrow preparations in the fluorescence microscope show intense porphyrin fluorescence in nucleated red blood cells, and to a lesser degree in reticulocytes [17, 76, 367, 390, 397, 402, 403, 405, 406] (Fig. 45-12). In normoblasts most of the porphyrin appears to be present either inside or at the surface of the cell nucleus [17, 390, 397] (Fig. 45-12). A portion of the normoblasts in all developmental stages and some of the reticulocytes in the peripheral blood fail to exhibit red fluorescence [17, 390, 397, 405]. Furthermore, many fluorescing normoblasts exhibit morphologic abnormalities in nuclear structure, consisting of single or at times multiple inclusions (Fig. 45-13) that stain dark with benzidine (Fig. 45-14) and show strong absorption

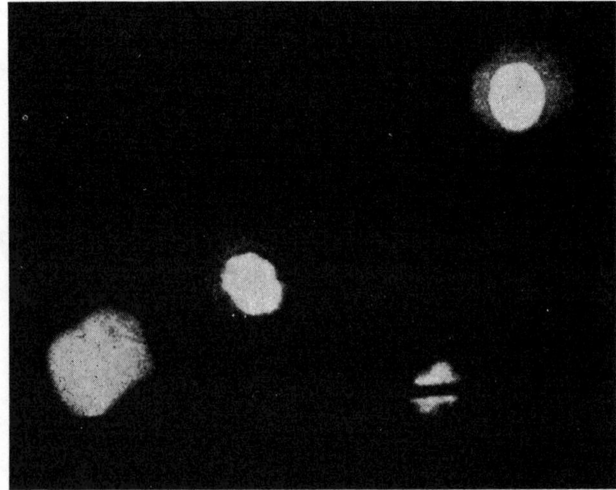

Figure 45-12. Unstained bone marrow smear of a patient with erythropoietic porphyria, photographed in the fluorescence microscope (×800.) Red fluorescence (reproduced in white) is particularly intense in the normoblastic nuclei. The polychromatophilic erythrocyte in the left lower corner exhibits a lesser degree of porphyrin fluorescence. (*By permission of R. Schmid et al.* [76].)

in the 400-mμ band [17, 390, 397, 405]. This nuclear abnormality does not seem to be present in normoblasts which lack porphyrin fluorescence. On electron microscopy, a striking difference in nuclear structure was observed between these two forms of normoblasts [407]. In addition, the cytoplasm of fluorescing normoblasts frequently shows clumping, vacuolization, and basophilic stippling [390, 397], and many of these cells contain iron granules [390]. In some of these normoblasts and in occasional erythrocytes, Varadi [390] has detected fine, needle-like structures which may have been porphyrin crystals. It is interesting to note that similar observations have been reported in the bone marrow of porphyric cattle [367].

These observations gave rise to the suggestion that there may be two different types of erythropoietic cells, only one of which exhibits a detectable defect in porphyrin metabolism [17]. The concept of two types of red blood cell precursors is difficult to reconcile with the genetics of erythropoietic porphyria (see below). Unless one makes the unlikely assumption that these types represent two colonies of cells under separate genetic control, it is hard to explain why a defect present in all cells manifests itself in only a portion of them. Experimental manipulations, including stress [421, 422] or partial suppression [364, 423] of the erythroid apparatus, failed to yield clarification, so that the problem at present remains unsolved.

In patients in whom increased hemolysis was demonstrable, the excretion of fecal urobilinogen was elevated [17, 76, 354, 369, 390, 418]. More important was the observation that a major fraction of the excreted bile pigment was not derived from breakdown of hemoglobin of mature circulating erythrocytes [94, 96, 363, 417]. Although in normal subjects 80 to 90 percent of the fecal urobilinogen originates from destruction of red blood cells which have reached the end of their physiologic life-span [94, 424], this does not apply

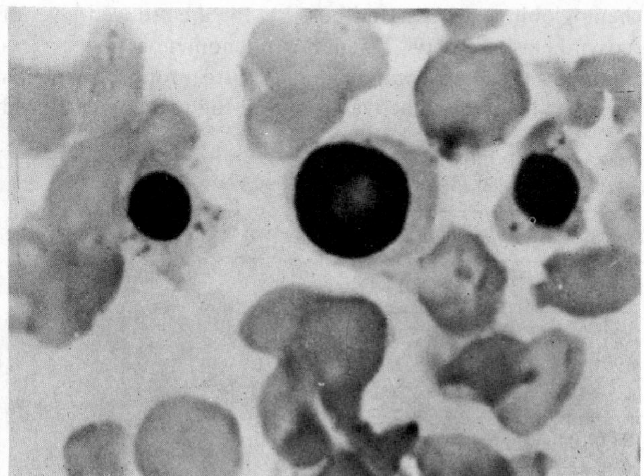

Figure 45-13. Bone marrow smear from a patient with erythropoietic porphyria stained with Wright's stain. The nucleus of the large normoblast shows a central inclusion. (*By permission of R. Schmid et al., Acta Haemat. (Basel)*, **10,** 153, 1953.)

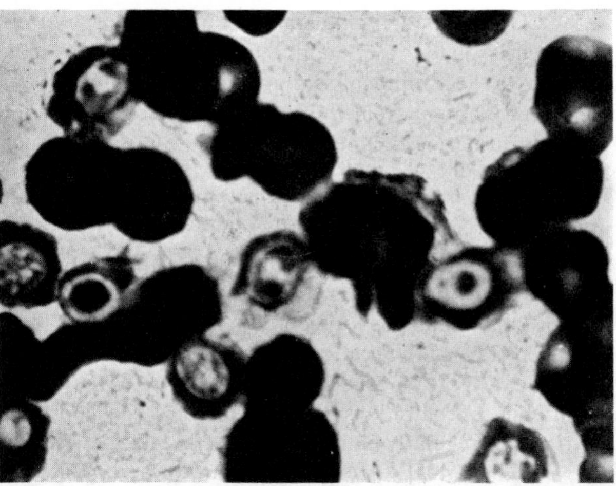

Figure 45-14. Bone marrow smear from a patient with erythropoietic porphyria, stained with benzidine. Abnormal normoblasts contain dark-staining nuclear inclusions. Nuclei of normal immature normoblasts appear granular (*left border*); those of normal mature normoblasts appear white (*left lower corner*). Hemoglobin-containing erythrocytes stain dark. (*By permission of R. Schmid et al.* [17].)

in erythropoietic porphyria [94, 96, 363]. At least 31 percent, and in one patient as much as 80 percent, of the excreted urobilinogen appeared to be derived from sources other than circulating hemoglobin; most of this urobilinogen fraction was excreted during the first 20 days after the administration of labeled glycine.

The various potential sources of this "early-labeled" bile pigment fraction are discussed in the following chapter. In congenital erythropoietic porphyria, this fraction most likely is derived from maturing erythroid cells which have undergone destruction in the bone marrow before being released into the circulation (ineffective erythropoiesis). It is also possible that part of the bile pigment fraction originates from porphyrin-laden erythrocytes which have a very short circulating life-span.

Chemical Findings

The color of the urine of patients with erythropoietic porphyria may vary from a faint pink to a Burgundy red to a dark reddish brown, depending on the concentration of porphyrins. The amounts of uroporphyrin excreted are always increased, and daily excretion of as much as 500 mg has been reported [15, 390, 405]. In addition, the urine contains large amounts of coproporphyrin, but the concentration is usually less than that of uroporphyrin [76, 354, 390, 405, 425]. Smaller amounts of porphyrins with seven, six, five, and three carboxyl groups have also been demonstrated [372, 389, 405, 425]. Most of the urinary porphyrins are of the type I isomer [56, 74], but small fractions of uroporphyrin III have been identified [425, 426]. For coproporphyrin, the type I to type III isomer ratio may be as high as 99:1 [354], although small amounts of coproporphyrin III have been isolated in crystalline form [354]. PBG as identified by the conventional semiquantitative method [212] is consistently absent from the urine. With chromatographic methods, urinary excretion of ALA and PBG is within normal limits [389, 396, 405].

The feces regularly contain large amounts of coproporphyrin [17, 349, 354, 367, 376, 390, 396, 405, 418]; the amount of uroporphyrin is usually smaller [354, 367, 396, 405]. Most of the coproporphyrin is of type I isomer, although small amounts of coproporphyrin III have been identified [349, 354]. Fecal excretion of protoporphyrin IXα, although variable, is usually not significantly elevated.

Variable concentrations of uroporphyrin I and coproporphyrin I are regularly demonstrable in the plasma [76, 354, 367, 369, 396, 405]. Circulating erythrocytes contain high concentrations of uroporphyrin I [76, 354, 367, 369, 389, 390, 396, 405] and somewhat lower concentrations of coproporphyrin I; the values for protoporphyrin are usually not higher than those found in other hemolytic conditions [427]. Typical values in a patient studied before and after splenectomy are given in Table 45-6. Highest concentrations of these porphyrins are present in the bone marrow, where the ratio of uroporphyrin I to coproporphyrin I is about the same as in the peripheral blood [76, 367, 389, 405]. Uroporphyrin I in crystalline form has been isolated from bone marrow obtained by needle aspiration [76].

Large amounts of uroporphyrin I are also present in the spleen [76, 258, 354, 369, 389]. On fluorescence microscopic examination, fine dustlike granules of porphyrin are visible in the red pulp but not in the Malpighian corpuscles [76, 258, 405]. In contrast to the marrow, splenic cells do not exhibit nuclear fluorescence [76]. In the liver, red fluorescence is minimal, but considerable amounts of uroporphyrin I are demonstrable on extraction [76, 258, 367, 369].

Watson et al. [422] and other investigators [16, 397] have reported that while uroporphyrin I exceeds by far the type III isomer (which proportionally is very small indeed), the actual amount of uroporphyrin III present in the blood or excreted in the urine is often increased above normal values. In view of the enormous excretion of uroporphyrin I, it may, of course, be difficult to exclude the possibility of contamination during isomer analysis which would result in an apparent increase in the uroporphyrin III fraction. Nonetheless, this observation may have a direct bearing on the pathogenetic mechanism involved in the disease.

Nature of the Metabolic Defect

Evaluation of the nature of the metabolic defect in this disease must include consideration of the unique chemical findings and of the numerous observations that overall hemoglobin synthesis appears to be normal, or increased in response to hemolysis.

The earlier indirect evidence of Booij and Rimington [171] and the recent biochemical studies by Levin [428] and by Romeo and Levin [429] have demonstrated a marked decrease of uroporphyrinogen III cosynthetase activity in the erythrocytes both of cattle and of human patients homozygous for erythropoietic porphyria. These important observations suggest a finite number of testable alternatives which could account for the aberrations in porphyrin metabolism in this disorder.

1 There may be a primary overproduction of uroporphyrinogen I as a consequence of increased activity either of uroporphyrinogen I synthetase or of ALA synthetase (Fig. 45-9). Consequently, production of the intermediate which is the substrate for the uroporphyrinogen III cosynthetase would exceed the amount that can be handled by the enzyme, so that the ratio of the uroporphyrinogen I isomer to the type III isomer would increase [422]. This hypothesis not only would explain the massive formation of uroporphyrin I, but also would account for the additional overall increase in the type III isomer, for the normal capacity for hemoglobin synthesis, and possibly for the reduced level of cosynthetase activity. This latter phenomenon may be explained by the observation that in vitro uroporphyrinogen III cosynthetase is inactivated during the reaction catalyzed

Table 45-6. PORPHYRIN CONCENTRATIONS IN ERYTHROCYTES, BONE MARROW, AND URINE OF A 6-YEAR-OLD GIRL WITH ERYTHROPOIETIC PORPHYRIA

Date	*Erythrocytes, μg/100 ml*			*Bone marrow, μg/100 ml*			*Urine, μg/24 hr*	
	URO	COPRO	PROTO	URO	COPRO	PROTO	URO	COPRO
11/9/50	11.0	5.6	55	2,635	302	124	8,450	2,280
4/2/51	377	91	44	2,492	614	190	21,500	3,450
6/21/51	440	150	105	.....	...	...	52,300	2,800
6/21/51	Splenectomy; spleen contained 3,400 μg URO/100 gm							
7/3/51	.....	.....	.....	.....	.....	...	1,200	400
10/6/51	122	20	60	176	84	284	6,970	2,310

Note: URO, COPRO, PROTO = uroporphyrin, coproporphyrin, protoporphyrin, respectively.
Source: R. Schmid et al. [76].

by uroporphyrinogen I synthetase [169, 429]. However, Smith and Kaneko [430] have provided suggestive evidence of a defect in heme biosynthesis, in that formation of isotopically labeled heme from 2-^{14}C-glycine was less with bovine porphyric blood than with normal blood per 10^{10} reticulocytes. In addition, these investigators reported that the maturation time of porphyric reticulocytes was prolonged.
2 A second possibility, which may be more attractive, is that the genetic defect results in a primary deficiency of uroporphyrinogen III cosynthetase [174, 428, 429, 431, 432] (Fig. 45-9). Since this enzyme usually is present in large excess compared with uroporphyrinogen I synthetase [168, 169], hemoglobin synthesis could proceed unimpaired even though the ratio of the type I to the type III isomer is markedly increased. The apparent net increase in uroporphyrinogen III would remain unexplained unless it were assumed to be a systematic artifact occurring in the course of the isomer analysis. Alternatively, a decrease in cosynthetase activity might interfere with heme synthesis to a degree sufficient to enhance ALA synthetase so that, eventually, an increased amount of substrate is available for the cosynthetase. This latter possibility, of course, would depend on the K_m's of uroporphyrinogen synthetase and cosynthetase and on the amount of substrate normally available. This concept will be discussed further on in this chapter, under Introduction to the Hepatic Porphyrias and Acute Intermittent Porphyria.

Further evidence supporting the concept that a defect in uroporphyrinogen III cosynthetase is the primary inherited trait leading to congenital porphyria is provided by the following observations: (1) cosynthetase activity is lower in the hemolyzates from carriers of the disease than in hemolyzates from normal subjects [432], and (2) cultured skin fibroblasts from patients with erythropoietic porphyria display less cosynthetase activity than similar cells from normal persons [431]. This latter observation also provides evidence that the lesions in heme biosynthesis in at least some of the porphyrias may not necessarily be restricted to the tissue overtly expressing the defect. That is, modifying factors in different cells may limit the manifestations of the abnormality. Further aspects of this question are discussed further on in this chapter, under Protoporphyria.

Genetic Considerations*

It has been possible in many hereditary metabolic disorders, to obtain strong support for an autosomal recessive mode of inheritance (i.e., one in which the disease results from a double dose of a mutant gene) by direct measurements of enzyme levels in cells from heterozygous and homozygous individuals. Except for the families described by Heilmeyer et al. [405] and for the very recent report by Romeo et al. [432], biochemical studies of this type have not been performed in erythropoietic porphyria, and it has been necessary to rely upon examination and statistical analysis of pedigree data to derive evidence favoring this type of inheritance. The pertinent genetic data are summarized in Tables 45-5 and 45-7.

Estimates of the fraction of affected individuals (p) within sibships were made from the data on the 27 sibships suitable for analysis (Table 45-7). In these calculations, all persons with probable cases were considered to be affected. Correction for ascertainment bias was made by the single (simple sib) and the truncate (complete) ascertainment methods [433, 434], and the values of p obtained were (p_0) 0.159 ($\sigma p_0 = 0.036$) and (p_1) 0.242 ($\sigma p_1 = 0.046$), respectively. The value theoretically to be expected in autosomal recessive inheritance is 0.25. In practice, the single ascertainment method, which depends on discarding all propositi from the calculations, usually underestimates p, while the truncate method often results in an overestimate. Therefore, the following test has been suggested to determine whether the estimates obtained by these two methods are compatible with the theoretical expectation: $p_1 + \sigma p_1 > 0.25 > p_0 + \sigma p_0$ [433]. The estimates of p obtained from the data on erythropoietic porphyria clearly meet this test. The fact that p_1 is virtually identical with the theoretical value suggests either that truncate ascertainment (i.e., ascertainment of *all* sibships containing affected individuals) was completely operative, or that not all affected individuals within families were detected or reported. The latter explanation would appear to be more reasonable, especially since a few persons who were considered as normal in the calculations may well have been affected.

From the available information, maximal and minimal estimates of the frequency of consanguine marriages among the parents of affected individuals can be made. In the 20 families for whom specific data are given, consanguinity (varying in degree from first to second cousins) occurred in six, giving a maximal estimate of 30 percent consanguinity.

Table 45-7. DISTRIBUTION WITHIN SIBSHIPS OF INDIVIDUALS WITH CONGENITAL ERYTHROPOIETIC PORPHYRIA

Size of sibship	No. of sibships	Total no. of sibs	Total no. of affected individuals
2	4	8	4
3	2	6	2
4	8	32	14
5	5	25	7
6	2	12	2
7	3	21	7
9	2	18	7
12	1	12	1
Total	27	134	44

*Prepared by Dr. Charles J. Epstein, Department of Pediatrics, University of California, San Francisco, Calif.

If it is assumed that no consanguinity exists in the other 26 reported families, a minimal estimate of 13 percent is obtained. Both estimates appear to be considerably greater than would be expected from the general population and conform to the increase in consanguinity expected in recessively inherited disease.

Vertical transmission of erythropoietic porphyria has not been observed. Parents of patients have never been affected, and the four live-born [349, 364, 377, 378] and two spontaneously aborted offspring [355] of porphyric individuals have been found to be normal. Of the 60 patients listed in Table 45-5, 28 are female and 32 are male, resulting in a sex ratio close to 1:1. An analysis of birth order was carried out for the 19 sibships for whom sufficient data were available, and no significant birth order effect could be detected [435]; i.e., the chance of being affected was not related to an individual's position in his sibship.

Thus, all formal genetic data on erythropoietic porphyria, including estimates of the proportion of sibs who are affected and of the frequency of consanguineous marriages among their parents, the absence of vertical transmission and of a birth order effect, and the sex ratio are consistent with an autosomal recessive mode of inheritance. Chromosomal abnormalities have not been detected [405, 406].

Direct biochemical evidence relating to the inheritance of erythropoietic porphyria has been reported by Heilmeyer et al. and Romeo et al. [405, 432]. In an investigation of two families, the parents and some of the sibs of two porphyric patients were found to have slightly elevated levels of erythrocyte uroporphyrin and, in some instances, of coproporphyrin and protoporphyrin. In one of these families, the patient's grandmothers also had slight elevations of erythrocyte porphyrins [405]. It is possible, therefore, that some of the heterozygous "carriers" of the gene for erythropoietic porphyria may be identified by measurement of erythrocyte porphyrins. Levin's group [432] observed that in presumed heterozygous carriers of the disease, uroporphyrinogen III cosynthetase activity of circulating red blood cells was intermediate between normal controls and affected homozygous patients. This is consistent, of course, with an autosomal recessive mode of inheritance.

Congenital Porphyria in other Mammals

Cattle

Congenital porphyria has been observed in cattle in South Africa, Denmark, England, and the United States [13, 367, 436–442]. In all instances the disease was inherited as a simple Mendelian recessive character. Heterozygous animals are clinically and biochemically normal [13, 367, 438, 439]. Porphyric calves were obtained by breeding animals which were known to be heterozygous for the trait [13, 367, 440].

Afflicted animals exhibit photosensitivity of those areas of the skin which are not pigmented or covered with dark hair [13, 367]. The first case of bovine porphyria recognized in Denmark was discovered because "the cow was not getting on at pasture but did well in the stable." When the animals are slaughtered, bones and teeth are found to be dark and to contain large amounts of porphyrin [13, 367, 436, 438, 440, 443].

Bovine congenital porphyria appears to have distinct similarities to the human form of erythropoietic porphyria [422]. Anemia, reticulocytosis, and splenomegaly may be present [367, 444], but splenectomy performed in one porphyric cow failed to result in significant improvement [367]; the spleen contained much porphyrin, mostly uroporphyrin I. Isotopic studies revealed a marked reduction in median erythrocyte survival time and a greatly increased iron turnover [444], and these abnormalities were present even in the absence of significant anemia [444]. Porphyrin concentrations in the liver were insignificant [13, 367, 439, 443]. As in the human disease, highest porphyrin concentrations were found in the bone marrow [367], and on fluorescence microscopic examinations unstained bone marrow preparations exhibited intense red fluorescence, which was most prominent in normoblastic nuclei. On staining, these cells exhibited abnormalities of nuclear structure similar to those described in congenital erythropoietic porphyria in man (Figs. 45-13, 45-14). In contrast to the human disease, circulating erythrocytes contained relatively little uroporphyrin but much protoporphyrin [13, 367, 443]. Plasma porphyrins comprised mostly uro- and coproporphyrin [13, 443]. Nearly all the porphyrins in bone marrow, red blood cells, and plasma were of the type I isomer [13, 367, 440, 443].

The urine of porphyric cattle contained mainly uro- and coproporphyrin I [13, 367, 438–440, 443], but smaller amounts of hepta- and hexa-, pentacarboxylic porphyrins were also identified [13, 443]; a significant fraction of these porphyrins was excreted in the form of the reduced porphyrinogens [440]. PBG was not increased in the urine [13, 367, 440], nor could it be detected in the liver of afflicted animals [13, 367, 439]. Coproporphyrin I was greatly increased in the feces [13, 367, 440].

It is apparent that bovine erythropoietic porphyria, like its human counterpart, is characterized by overproduction of porphyrins of type I isomer in cells of the erythroid series [422]. The observation by Rimington and Booij [445] that incubation of ALA or PBG with hemolyzed erythrocytes from porphyric cattle resulted in formation of both uroporphyrinogen I and uroporphyrinogen III, suggested that the metabolic defects in the bovine and the human form of the disease may be similar. This is further supported by Levin's recent demonstration [428] that in erythrocytes of porphyric cattle, uroporphyrinogen III cosynthetase is greatly reduced.

Pigs

Congenital porphyria is also observed in pigs [438, 440, 446, 447]. In contrast to the human and bovine forms, the porcine disease is probably inherited as a Mendelian dominant trait [438, 440, 447], although further studies on the precise mode of inheritance are necessary. Porphyric pigs excrete in the urine large amounts of uroporphyrin and smaller quantities of coproporphyrin and of porphyrins with seven, six, and five carboxyl groups. The feces contain mostly coproporphyrin [446]. Almost all the excreted porphyrins belong to the type I isomer series [440, 447], and porphobilinogen is not demonstrable [438]. Affected pigs do not exhibit photosensitivity, and the diagnosis rests mainly on the discovery of red fluorescence in bones and teeth. Teeth of newborn pigs with porphyria contain considerable amounts of uroporphyrin I [440, 447], a finding which serves as a convenient mode of diagnosis during the lifetime of the animal [438].

Little is known of the biochemical nature and the anatomic site of the metabolic defect. It remains to be shown whether the overproduction of porphyrins of the type I isomer occurs in erythroid cells, as in the human and bovine forms of the disease, or whether the pigments are derived from other sites. Chemical and microscopic studies of bone marrow have not yet been reported, but Joergensen, With, et al. [440, 447] observed high concentrations of porphyrins in the spleen and much smaller amounts in liver, kidneys, and blood. Pigs affected with the disease appear to show a considerable degree of fluctuation in the amounts of porphyrins produced [440, 447]. In some instances where high concentrations of uroporphyrin were demonstrated in the teeth at birth, no evidence of a disturbance in porphyrin metabolism was detectable a few months later at autopsy [440, 447]. This has been taken to indicate that the porcine form of porphyria may show a high degree of latency, a factor which renders genetic studies most difficult.

Cats

Congenital porphyria recently was reported in a black domestic short-haired cat and two of her kittens [448]. Litters with affected kittens were obtained by breeding the proposita with nonrelated, nonaffected males, which is consistent with a single dominant inheritance [449]. Uro- and coproporphyrin were excreted in excessive quantities, but photosensitivity was lacking. The diagnosis can be readily made on the basis of the brownish pigmentation of the deciduous teeth, which exhibit intense pinkish fluorescence under ultraviolet light [449].

Other Species

Finally, it should be noted that in at least two species, the fox squirrel (*Sciurus niger*) and the touraco bird (*Musophagidae*), uroporphyrin is a physiologic end product of metabolism [450–453]. The metabolic origin of the pigment in these species is not known.

HEPATIC PORPHYRIAS

The hepatic porphyrias are a group of disorders characterized by excessive levels of porphyrins and porphyrin precursors formed in the liver. They may be distinguished on the basis of their clinical manifestations, but the main discriminant in classification is the unique pattern of porphyrin and porphyrin precursor excretion in the urine and feces in each disorder (Table 45-1; Fig. 45-15). The defects responsible for most of these disorders are genetically transmitted as autosomal dominant traits [13, 19, 421, 454–457]; the only exception is porphyria cutanea tarda, which generally is believed to be acquired [458, 459], with genetic factors playing an uncertain role [19, 421, 454].

The three genetically transmitted porphyrias (acute intermittent porphyria, variegate porphyria, and hereditary coproporphyria) have certain features in common [13, 19, 310, 421, 459, 460]: (1) The acute phase of each of these diseases is associated with increased urinary excretion of ALA and PBG (Fig. 45-15). This increase is due, at least in part, to enhanced activity of ALA synthetase [310, 460–463]. (2) In all three disorders, exacerbations may be precipitated by therapeutic doses of certain drugs, most of which induce ALA synthetase in avian hepatocyte culture [44, 45, 51, 310, 314] and often in the liver of intact animals [49, 50, 306, 307, 313, 318]. (3) Clinical exacerbations are associated with the same neurologic syndrome. (4) Frequently the initial clinical and biochemical manifestations occur during late puberty. These features will be discussed in more detail in the sections dealing with the individual diseases.

In the following discussion we consider the logical alternatives that may account for the common occurrence of the features listed above [62, 310, 421, 460, 461]. In arriving at these alternatives, it is essential to recall that (1) heme participates in the end product repression of ALA synthetase [45, 306–310], and (2) the unique patterns of porphyrin and porphyrin precursor excretion that distinguish the hepatic porphyrias are reported to run generally "true to form" even in heterogeneous populations [19, 57, 421, 458].

First, in all forms of hepatic porphyria, a primary defect (genetically determined or acquired) may result in increased activity of ALA synthetase. For example, Watson et al. [422], Granick [45], and others [461, 464] have suggested the possibility that a defect similar to an operator constitutive mutation in bacteria [301] might account for excessive production of ALA synthetase, inappropriate responsiveness to chemical inducers, and a dominant mode of inheritance. While such a hypothesis may explain one form of hepatic porphyria (i.e., variegate porphyria), in order to encompass *all* forms the additional assumption must be made that constitutional differences involving the activity of enzymes beyond ALA synthetase determine the unique patterns of porphyrin and porphyrin precursor excretion that characterize each individual disorder. Such a postulated modification of a single mutation appears unlikely in view of the observation that, in general, the excretory pattern remains "true to form" in families with individual types of hepatic porphyria. In other words, if a mutation leading to increased ALA synthesis were to explain *all* these disorders, this defect would have to be combined with additional mutations, which statistically is highly improbable.

A second possibility is that each of the hepatic porphyrias

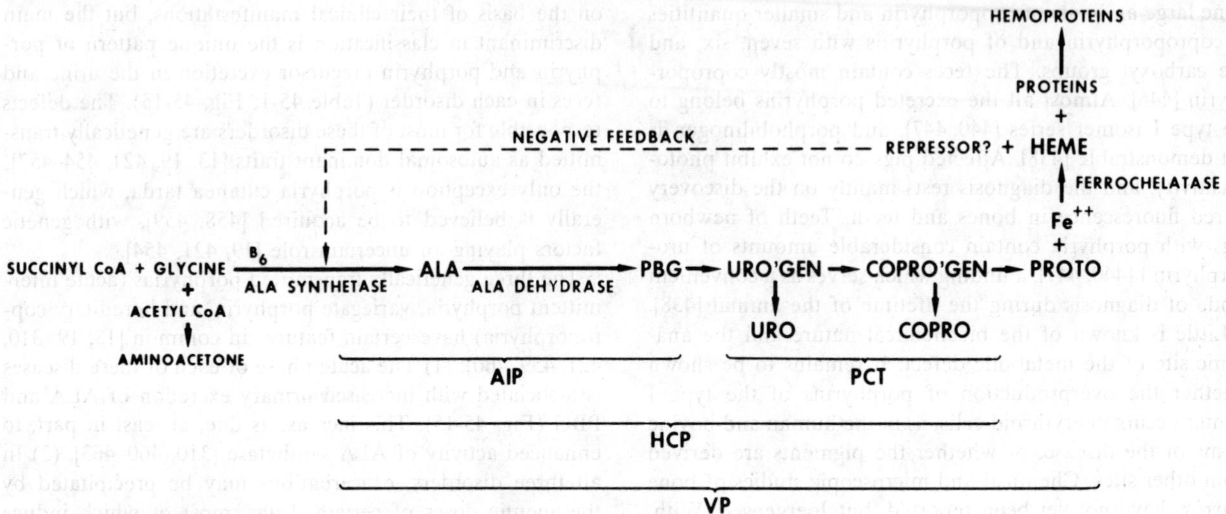

Figure 45-15. Outline of heme biosynthesis and its regulation. Intermediates of the pathway excessively excreted during the acute phase of each of the hepatic porphyrias are within the respective brackets. The porphyrinogens are reduced hexahydroporphyrins and are the true intermediates in heme biosynthesis. (*ALA*, δ-aminolevulinic acid; *PBG*, porphobilinogen; *URO'GEN*, uroporphyrinogen; *COPRO'GEN*, coproporphyrinogen; *PROTO*, protoporphyrin; *AIP*, acute intermittent porphyria; *PCT*, porphyria cutanea tarda; *HCP*, hereditary coproporphyria; *VP*, variegate porphyria.) (*By permission of L. Kaufman and H. S. Marver* [460].)

is the primary result of a partial block in heme biosynthesis such as (1) diminished activity of enzymes involved at specific steps in the pathway; (2) loss of intermediates due to alterations in membrane permeability of the hepatocyte; or (3) excessive, irreversible conversion of reduced porphyrinogens to oxidized porphyrins (Figs. 45-6, 45-8). Such defects would be expected to dampen the end product repression exerted by heme on ALA synthetase; this would result in increased production of ALA synthetase, accentuation of its sensitivity to inducers, and accumulation of intermediates prior to the "block" [310, 460]. If the unaffected allele is incapable of adaptive response, the defect in the involved allele would be expressed dominantly. Moreover, if the effectiveness of the involved step normally is subject to regulation by substrate availability (because the concentration of substrate is below the K_m), then the accumulation of precursor may totally, or partially, overcome the enzyme deficiency, and consequently the net production of heme may be essentially undiminished [310]. Observations consistent with this alternative have been mentioned under Congenital Erythropoietic Porphyria, and a further discussion will be included under Acute Intermittent Porphyria.

A third possible alternative is that the primary defect consists of the diversion of heme from its participation in the feedback control of ALA synthetase. As discussed previously under Regulation of Heme and Hemoprotein Biosynthesis, chemically induced hepatic porphyria in rodents is associated with enhanced degradation of cytochrome P450 (Fig. 45-10) [284, 296–300, 322], which in turn may divert heme from its participation in the repression of ALA synthetase. If a similar mechanism were postulated for all the genetic, hepatic porphyrias, one would have to make additional assumptions comparable to those discussed in relation to the first alternative.

The onset of the hepatic porphyrias during puberty may be related to the capacity of certain naturally occurring steroids to induce ALA synthetase [45, 51, 326, 327]. This may suggest that in addition to a genetic lesion porphyria may become overt only in the presence of certain endogenous or exogenous compounds that are inducers of ALA synthetase.

The neurologic syndrome associated with the acute phase of all three genetically transmitted hepatic porphyrias is difficult to interpret because of the paucity of relevant information. If the primary defect indeed involves a mutation in the heme biosynthetic pathway, then one would predict the neuropathy to be related to overproduction of porphyrin precursors. Although neurotoxicity of these compounds has not yet been demonstrated experimentally, they are the only known substances that are excreted in excess in the acute phase of all three forms of hepatic porphyria (Fig. 45-15). Alternatively, one may postulate a defect in heme biosynthesis in the nervous system itself which would interfere with proper formation of hemoproteins essential for cell function.

Acute Intermittent Porphyria

The most extensive study of this type of familial porphyria was undertaken by Waldenström in 1937 [16], although many similar cases had been reported previously [14, 15]. The condition has been described as acute porphyria [15, 16], acute intermittent porphyria [20], or pyrroloporphyria [19, 458]. A synonym is Swedish type of porphyria.

Clinical Manifestations

Abdominal pain of moderate to severe degree and often colicky in nature is the initial and frequently the most prominent symptom [465]. The pain may be generalized or localized, but the abdomen is usually soft, and tenderness is not marked. Rebound tenderness is lacking. X-ray examination frequently reveals areas of intestinal distension proximal to areas of spasm [466, 467]. Constipation is usually marked and may give rise to confusion with bowel obstruction [468, 469]. Distension of the stomach and pernicious vomiting are at times outspoken. These manifestations are characteristically intermittent in nature. Acute attacks may last from several days to several months. Between acute episodes, periods of remission occur during which symptoms may be slight or even absent [13, 20, 467]. The gastrointestinal manifestations frequently lead to weight loss and occasionally to severe emaciation, while prolonged vomiting may cause oliguria and azotemia. Although death normally occurs from respiratory paralysis, uremia and cachexia may be contributing factors.

Neurologic manifestations are extremely variable. They may involve peripheral nerves, autonomic nervous system, brain stem, cranial nerves, or cerebral function. Extensive reviews of the neurologic, mental, and neuropathologic findings have recently been published [19, 20, 22, 273, 467, 470–473]. As noted earlier, the role of porphyrins and porphyrin precursors in the pathogenesis of the abdominal and neurologic manifestations is not clear. It is noteworthy that at autopsy the brain and the spinal cord of patients with porphyria usually fail to exhibit PBG or increased concentrations of porphyrins [76, 273, 474].

Many patients have hypertension, but this is not always present, and at times the blood pressure may actually be low [465, 475]. During acute attacks, sinus tachycardia is frequently observed [476], and the pulse rate has been found to be a good index for judging the activity of the disease [467]. Photosensitivity and increased mechanical fragility of the skin are conspicuously absent, although Watson has pointed out that exceptions to this rule may occur [57].

In some of the patients acute episodes may be associated with slight fever and leukocytosis, but these are by no means constant findings [19, 56, 467].

In many instances the metabolic defect is present in a latent form, so that afflicted persons are entirely free of symptoms or exhibit only vague complaints such as dyspepsia or nervousness [13, 16, 19, 467]. In latent porphyria, chromatographic analysis of the urine frequently [465] but not invariably [61] reveals increased excretion of ALA or PBG or both [13, 57, 213, 477]. With the conventional qualitative test for PBG [212, 213], negative results are not uncommon [19, 21, 56, 61, 213, 467, 477]. Latent porphyria may never become clinically manifest, or acute attacks may occur at a later date [16, 467]. Such attacks may be precipitated by administration of various drugs, notably barbiturates, sulfonamides, griseofulvin, and estrogens [16, 20, 22, 68, 273, 467, 470, 471, 478], but this is not an invariable sequence [465, 479, 480]; we have repeatedly observed patients with latent porphyria who underwent major surgical procedures under barbiturate anesthesia without developing symptoms of porphyria.

It is generally recognized that porphyric manifestations usually begin at puberty or shortly thereafter [19, 56, 467] (Fig. 45-16); in fact manifest porphyria is exceedingly rare before puberty [19, 21, 56, 482–485]. In children of afflicted kinships even the presence of latent porphyria is often difficult to detect before adolescence [21, 61, 481]. Furthermore, symptomatic manifestations are most pronounced during the early part of the reproductive period, and the death rate for porphyria is highest in young adults [19, 467].

The effect of pregnancy on porphyria is unpredictable.

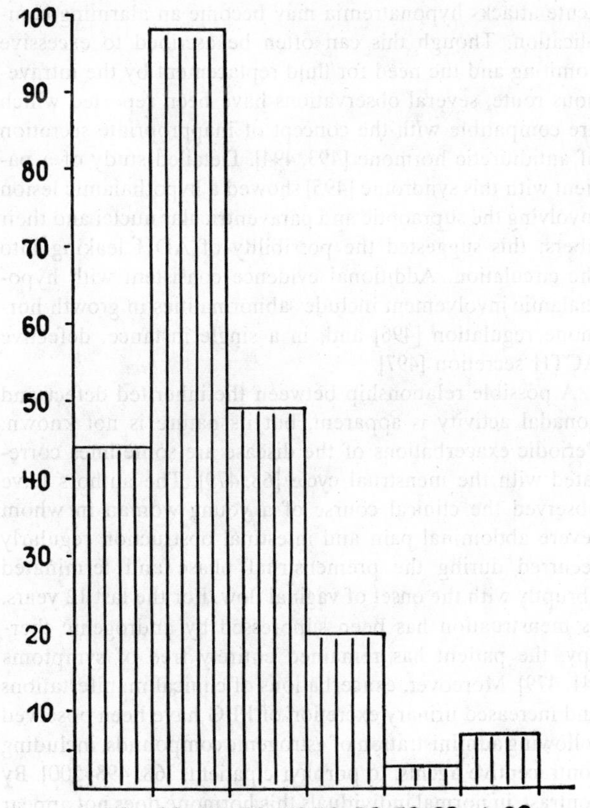

Figure 45-16. Age at first clinical manifestations of acute intermittent porphyria. (*By permission of J. Waldenström* [19].)

Acute manifestations may occur during the latter part of gestation [486–489] or during, or shortly after, delivery [20, 56], but this is not a constant feature [490]. In a recent study [465] in 72 out of 74 instances pregnancy did not affect the course of the porphyria. Infants of porphyric mothers frequently excrete porphyrin precursors and porphyrins during the first few days of life [490].

Acute attacks, unless fatally terminated, frequently are followed by periods of latency, which may last from weeks to years [467]. During a 5-year-observation period of 50 patients with acute intermittent porphyria, Goldberg [467] reported an overall mortality of 24 percent. The death rate was highest during the third decade of life [19, 467]. In a recent study only four deaths attributable to porphyria were encountered in a series of 46 patients with acute intermittent porphyria [465]; this improved prognosis may reflect better recognition of latent cases and avoidance of drugs that precipitate attacks.

Acute intermittent porphyria, particularly during an acute attack, frequently is associated with a variety of metabolic and endocrine abnormalities which are difficult to relate pathogenetically to the underlying disease. Plasma protein-bound iodine and thyroxine-binding globulin often are increased, and the biologic half-life of thyroxine is prolonged, but the patients are eumetabolic [491, 492]. During acute attacks hyponatremia may become an alarming complication. Though this can often be ascribed to excessive vomiting and the need for fluid replacement by the intravenous route, several observations have been reported which are compatible with the concept of inappropriate secretion of antidiuretic hormone [493, 494]. Detailed study of a patient with this syndrome [495] showed a hypothalamic lesion involving the supraoptic and paraventricular nuclei and their fibers; this suggested the possibility of ADH leaking into the circulation. Additional evidence consistent with hypothalamic involvement includes abnormalities in growth hormone regulation [496] and, in a single instance, defective ACTH secretion [497].

A possible relationship between the inherited defect and gonadal activity is apparent, but its nature is not known. Periodic exacerbations of the disease are sometimes correlated with the menstrual cycle [68, 479]. The authors have observed the clinical course of a young woman in whom severe abdominal pain and intestinal obstruction regularly recurred during the premenstrual phase and terminated abruptly with the onset of vaginal flow. For the last 12 years, as menstruation has been suppressed by androgenic therapy, the patient has remained entirely free of symptoms [41, 479]. Moreover, exacerbations of clinical manifestations and increased urinary excretion of PBG have been observed following administration of estrogenic compounds, including contraceptive agents, to porphyric patients [68, 498–500]. By contrast, in normal individuals this hormone does not appear to effect the excretion of porphyrin precursors and porphyrins [498].

Abnormalities in glucose tolerance and hypercholesterolemia are frequently encountered [465]. Conventional liver function tests usually are normal, except for frequently increased retention of Bromsulphalein [76, 465]. The striking effect of a high-carbohydrate intake on the excretion of ALA and PBG ("glucose effect") was discussed earlier. In 13 out of 16 symptomatic patients in a recent series [465], carbohydrate administration resulted in a sharp fall in PBG excretion and in significant clinical improvement.

Chemical Findings

The most characteristic finding in this type of porphyria is the urinary excretion of large amounts of PBG [16, 165, 501]. As discussed earlier, PBG is an obligatory intermediate in the biosynthesis of porphyrins and heme (Figs. 45-6, 45-8), and small amounts of it are normally excreted in the urine. It is a colorless monopyrrolic chromogen (Fig. 45-7), giving an intense red color with Ehrlich's aldehyde (*p*-dimethylaminobenzaldehyde). The red aldehyde complex has a strong absorption band at 560 mμ and a weaker one at 525 mμ [165, 213]. In contrast to the red products obtained with urobilinogen and other chromogens, the Ehrlich's aldehyde-PBG complex is not extractable with chloroform [165] or butanol [213]. The concentration of PBG present in normal urine is too small to be detected with the conventional method [214] described by Watson and Schwartz [212]. During acute attacks of porphyria the test is strongly positive, and a positive result is frequently, but not invariably, obtained during latency [61, 212, 213]. Estimation of PBG excretion during acute manifestations has yielded values ranging from less than 30 to several hundred milligrams per liter of urine or per day [61, 204, 205, 458, 465, 477, 502]. Although in individual patients there is a rough correlation between severity of clinical manifestations and PBG excretion, the amount of chromogen in the urine of different patients shows wide variations [61, 502]. During periods of latency, urinary PBG excretion may be much lower and, indeed, may approach normal values [13, 21, 61, 205, 213, 265, 502].

In addition to PBG, the urine usually contains large quantities of ALA, another obligatory intermediate in the biosynthesis of heme (Figs. 45-6, 45-8). During an acute episode the urine may contain as much as 180 mg ALA per day [61, 204, 205, 477, 502]; during remission the values may be much lower [61, 502]. In individual patients the amounts of ALA and PBG excreted in the urine usually fluctuate in a roughly parallel manner [465, 502].

Although the urinary excretion of large amounts of these two compounds is a typical feature of this form of porphyria, the urine may also contain other porphyrin precursors, which give a negative Ehrlich's reaction [56, 227, 232, 233, 503]. Some of these chromogens are undoubtedly porphyrinogens or their partially oxidized derivatives, porphomethene and porphodimethene. In the urine, most of these porphyrin precursors, including PBG and possibly ALA, can be converted to porphyrins [160, 215, 234], but the extent of this process and the nature of the porphyrins obtained depend largely on external factors such as pH, exposure to light and air, and the presence of oxidizing substances [13, 160, 163, 215, 504]. Freshly voided urine of patients with acute porphyria may contain little if any increase in uroporphyrin concentration [163]; porphyrins are formed only on standing or during the extraction procedure. This is probably why freshly passed urine frequently is of normal color but darkens on standing in light and air [165]. It should be noted that the color is not all due to porphyrins but in part reflects formation of porphobilin, a brown amorphous oxidation product of PBG [165].

The many extensive studies that have been undertaken in an attempt to define more clearly the nature of the porphyrins present, or formed on standing, in the urine of patients with acute porphyria [16, 40, 78, 79, 163, 234, 504–508] have yielded seemingly contradictory results. One can probably reconcile these different findings by realizing that most of the isolated porphyrins are actually formed after the urine has been passed and thus are largely artifactual [160, 163]. There is little doubt that uroporphyrin of both isomer types is present, but the isomer ratio appears to be influenced by the conditions under which precursors are converted to porphyrins. A curious and as yet unexplained finding is that most of the porphyrins in the urine seem to be present as metal complex, the metal probably being zinc [20, 509]. On the other hand it has been reported that total zinc excretion is not increased [510].

In addition to these porphyrin precursors and porphyrins, the urine of patients with acute intermittent porphyria may contain increased amounts of amino acids [511] and indolic compounds [213, 512]. Some of the latter may give a positive Ehrlich's reaction which can mimic that produced by PBG [213, 512]. Contrary to earlier reports, urinary aminoacetone excretion appears to be normal [513].

A slight to moderate elevation in fecal porphyrin excretion may be observed [13, 56, 57, 61, 79, 205, 239, 458, 477, 481]. In some of the patients uroporphyrin has been isolated from stool [56, 76, 79, 514], and fecal copro- and protoporphyrin concentrations have been found to be slightly increased [205, 239, 477]. Small increases may be found in peptide-conjugated porphyrins, but the values are usually much lower than in variegate porphyria [515]. It is evident that, in contrast to other forms of porphyria, in acute intermittent porphyria fecal elimination of pyrrolic compounds is of minor significance.

With the exception of the liver, tissues obtained at autopsy usually failed to reveal increased porphyrin concentrations [13, 16, 20, 30, 76–79, 467]. In some cases uroporphyrin or coproporphyrin or both have been identified and isolated from hepatic tissue [59, 76, 79], but this was not possible in all instances [75]. More important was the demonstration that the liver regularly contained large amounts of PBG [40, 76, 78, 467, 516], while this precursor has not been detected in other organs such as the spleen or in muscle or bone marrow [40, 76]. Biopsy studies performed on a larger group of patients with acute or latent porphyria showed that fresh liver tissue contained only insignificant amounts of porphyrins but that a marked increase in uroporphyrin concentration could be obtained by converting precursors to porphyrin [76].

These findings indicate that in acute intermittent porphyria the principal metabolic abnormality is the presence and excretion not of porphyrins but of porphyrin precursors. The large amounts of ALA and PBG excreted in the urine are probably derived from the liver, since this is the only organ in which they regularly are present in detectable quantities. It appears unlikely that these compounds could have reached the liver from other sites of formation, because in experimental animals injection of ALA and PBG failed to result in their accumulation in the liver [217].

Nature of the Metabolic Defect

A number of laboratories have demonstrated a profound increase in hepatic ALA synthetase in this disorder [310, 460–464]. This "enzyme overproduction" [461] surely contributes to the excessive excretion of porphyrin precursors in acute porphyria. As already discussed, it has been suggested that this disease is a consequence of a genetic defect akin to an operator constitutive mutation in microorganisms [45, 422, 461]. However, the pattern of excessive porphyrin *precursor* excretion with little, if any, increase in porphyrin excretion (Fig. 45-15) is distinctly atypical for experimentally induced porphyria in rodents [7, 36, 44] and differs from the findings in a few normal subjects following the oral ingestion of a "loading dose" of ALA [115]. In the latter two conditions, levels of urinary coproporphyrin and 2- and 4-carboxyl fecal porphyrins are much elevated. This difference in the excretory pattern has suggested alternatively that the primary metabolic defect in acute intermittent porphyria may be a consequence of the diminished enzymatic conversion of PBG to uroporphyrinogen (uroporphyrinogen I synthetase) [19, 421, 460]. Heilmeyer and Clotten already had reported reduced formation of porphyrins from ALA in the liver of a patient with acute intermittent porphyria [517]. On the other hand, Nakao et al. observed that in porphyric liver ALA disappeared at a rate similar to that in control preparations [462].

Recent findings in the liver of three patients with acute intermittent porphyria revealed that in addition to major elevations of ALA synthetase, uroporphyrinogen I synthetase activity was reduced more than 50 percent as compared with the values obtained in 12 nonporphyric subjects and in patients with other forms of hepatic porphyria [310, 622]. This observation is entirely consistent with the finding that patients with this disease excrete excessive amounts of porphyrin precursors, rather than of porphyrins. It remains to be determined, of course, whether this reduction in hepatic uroporphyrinogen I synthetase activity reflects familial or ethnic factors which may modulate inappropriate overproduction of ALA, or whether it is the result of a primary mutation unique to patients with acute intermittent porphyria. At present, the latter alternative appears more plausible for the following reasons: (1) acute intermittent porphyria is characterized by a unique pattern of porphyrin precursor excretion which in heterogeneous populations is said generally to run "true to form" [19, 57, 421, 454]; (2) on the basis of the patients studied [310, 517, 622] it would appear that the hepatic conversion of PBG to porphyrins in acute intermittent porphyria is far below that of non-porphyric controls. It is evident that these preliminary findings require further validation by sampling of larger population groups.

Since patients with acute intermittent porphyria are presumed to be heterozygous for the underlying metabolic defect, an apparent decrease of uroporphyrinogen I synthetase of greater than 50 per cent is puzzling. This apparent inconsistency may be a consequence of technical difficulties with the enzyme assay or of the small sample size so far studied; or it may indicate that the defect is a consequence of an abnormality in the regulation of the activity or the synthesis of uroporphyrinogen I synthetase [310, 622].

On the basis of limited studies, erythrocytes from patients with acute intermittent porphyria appear to exhibit a diminished enzymatic capacity to convert PBG to porphyrins [623]. If correct, these data suggest that the metabolic abnormality in acute intermittent porphyria may be present but unexpressed in tissues other than liver.

If the above finding should prove to be correct, then the increased activity of the ALA synthetase in the liver of these patients most likely would be a consequence of the diminished enzymatic conversion of PBG to porphyrins. The two phenomena can easily be reconciled because a partial defect in the conversion of PBG to uroporphyrinogen would be expected to interfere with the formation of heme, which in turn has been shown both to inhibit [120, 122] and to repress [45, 284, 306–311] ALA synthetase. By necessity, such a defect can be only partial, since complete absence of the enzymatic activity would be incompatible with life. On the basis of indirect evidence obtained in the study of a patient with acute intermittent porphyria, Dowdle et al. suggested that the rate of hepatic heme synthesis may be unimpaired [115]. This is not inconsistent with a partial defect in the conversion of PBG to porphyrins, since the K_m of uroporphyrinogen I synthetase appears to be higher than the normal concentration of PBG in the liver. This is suggested by the observation that PBG cannot be found in normal liver even with the use of a method that can detect it at concentrations of 10^{-6} M [310]; the latter figure is the approximate K_m of uroporphyrinogen I synthetase [168, 310]. Thus, by inducing ALA synthetase, the hepatic concentration of PBG may be increased sufficiently to compensate, in part or in whole, for the enzymatic defect in heme synthesis [310, 622].

As indicated earlier, acute intermittent porphyria is associated with a multitude of clinical abnormalities. The information currently available is insufficient to allow speculation about their relationship to the nature of the metabolic defect beyond the aspects discussed in the introductory paragraph under Hepatic Porphyrias, earlier in this chapter.

Heredity and Incidence

Genetic studies are rendered difficult by the frequency with which the disturbance remains asymptomatic and by the fact that even genetically true carriers may fail to exhibit an easily detectable increase in PBG excretion [21, 61, 481]. Waldenström's extensive studies in Sweden [16, 19, 518] showed that a positive family history could definitely be established for 242 of 321 proved cases of porphyria. One hundred and thirty-seven patients belonged to a single family. The three next largest families contained 14, 12, and 9 porphyric members, respectively. A representative pedigree from the Swedish study is given in Fig. 45-17. The youngest generation, comprised largely of children, cannot be adequately evaluated, because quantitative determinations of PBG and ALA excretion have not yet been reported [19, 21]. On the basis of these findings it has been assumed that affected individuals are heterozygous for a rare, autosomal gene [16, 19, 481, 518].

Familial occurrence of acute porphyria has been reported by other investigators [473, 481, 512, 519]. Watson [56] studied 97 cases, and Markovitz [471] collected from the literature 69 cases of acute porphyria, many with a positive family history. Acute attacks of porphyria were observed in two pairs of identical twins [19, 520]. In earlier studies, strong predilection for the female sex was reported [16]. Later reports, based on a larger amount of case material, yielded an approximate female/male ratio of 3:2 [19, 56, 471, 477]. Latent porphyria, on the other hand, appeared to be more frequent in males [56, 473], although exceptions to this rule have been described [512]. Most of the reported observations are consistent with the concept that acute intermittent porphyria is due to a single dose of a rare autosomal gene and that this hereditary defect leads to clinical manifestations most frequently in young adults of the female sex.

The incidence of the disease is obviously influenced by its occurrence in large families. For Lapland, for example, Waldenström [19] has calculated an incidence of 1:1,000, largely because a single family with no less than 137 known porphyric persons lives in this Northern region. On the other hand, for Sweden proper, the incidence is about 1.5:100,000. Comparable values have been reported for Denmark [61], Ireland [521], and Western Australia [522]. Judging from the number of reported cases in the literature, it would appear that the disease is more frequent in individuals of Scandinavian or English ancestry; in Negroes its occurrence is extremely rare [523–525].

Recapitulation

Acute intermittent porphyria is characterized by abdominal and neurologic manifestations which are frequently intermittent in nature. Photosensitivity is lacking. The abnormality is believed to be due to a single dose of a rare

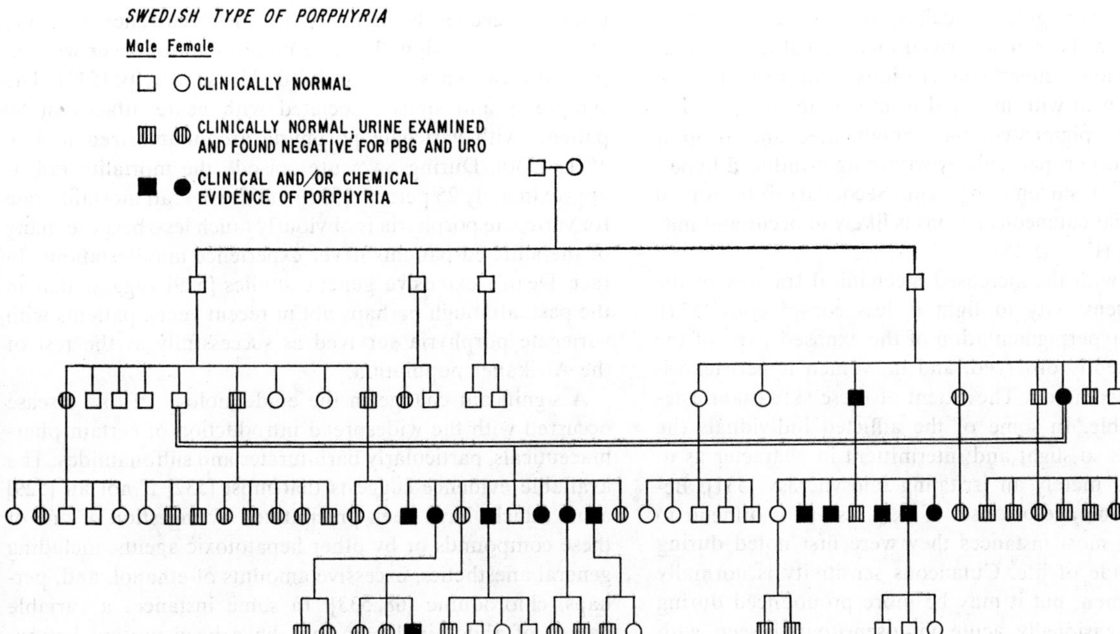

Figure 45-17. Pedigree of a family with acute intermittent porphyria. Urine of clinically normal individuals was examined with the semiquantitative method for porphobilinogen. It is probable that with the advent of refined methods for estimation of urinary porphobilinogen and δ-aminolevulinic acid, more cases of latent porphyria will be discovered. This applies particularly to the fifth generation, which is comprised largely of children [21]. (*By permission of J. Waldenström* [19].)

autosomal gene, but afflicted individuals frequently remain free of symptoms. Qualitative methods of investigation may fail to reveal the metabolic derangement in asymptomatic persons who are genetically sure carriers.

The defect involves overproduction of the porphyrin precursor ALA in the liver, which results in increased excretion of ALA and PBG in the urine. Alternative genetic mechanisms have been discussed which may account for this metabolic abnormality in the liver.

It has been pointed out [19, 205] that "acute porphyria" and "intermittent acute porphyria" are misnomers for this condition, for the disease is based on a genetically controlled metabolic disorder of chronic nature. Furthermore, the primary disturbance probably does not involve porphyrin metabolism but occurs at the level of pyrrole biosynthesis which is interrelated with the tricarboxylic acid cycle.

Variegate Porphyria

This disorder is also called South African genetic porphyria or protocoproporphyria hereditaria.

Clinical Manifestations

In the years between 1951 and 1955, Dean and Barnes [526–528] reported a large group of porphyric individuals in the white population of South Africa. In 13 families a total of 236 patients with porphyria were discovered, all of whom could be traced back to a pair of early settlers who migrated from Holland and married at the Cape of Good Hope in 1688 [526, 529]. Over the last few years many more cases from this genetic line have been reported [529, 530]; the overall incidence of the disease in the Afrikaners of the Republic of South Africa is estimated at 3 per 1,000 [529].

The type of hepatic porphyria which occurs in this population group differs significantly from acute intermittent porphyria [205, 477]. Its main features are:

1 A positive family history of chronic skin involvement and, at times, of acute abdominal and neurologic manifestations
2 Increased sensitivity of the exposed skin to minor mechanical trauma and to light
3 Occasional occurrence of transient episodes (usually precipitated by ingestion of drugs, particularly barbiturates) of acute abdominal and neurologic manifestations, associated with porphobilinogenuria
4 Continuous excretion of greatly increased amounts of proto- and coproporphyrin, and of peptide conjugates of dicarboxylic porphyrins in the feces

The cutaneous manifestations are of chronic nature and usually are limited to those parts of the body which normally are exposed to sunlight, particularly the face and the back of the hands. In these areas, trivial mechanical trauma may lead to abrasions, superficial erosions, and formation of bullae which heal with minimal to moderate scarring. The scars are often pigmented, but depigmented and atrophic scarring may occur, particularly within light-induced hyperpigmentation of surrounding skin. Secondary infection of these superficial cutaneous lesions is likely to occur and may delay healing (Fig. 45-18).

Compared with the increased mechanical fragility of the skin, direct sensitivity to light is less conspicuous [531]. Generalized hyperpigmentation of the exposed parts of the body is frequently observed, and in women hypertrichosis of the face is common. The extent of these skin manifestations is variable. In some of the afflicted individuals the abnormality is so slight and intermittent in character as to be considered merely an irritating idiosyncrasy [531]. Because of this the age of onset of skin lesions is difficult to determine; in most instances they were first noted during the third decade of life. Cutaneous sensitivity is normally milder in women, but it may be more pronounced during pregnancy. Occasionally, acute photosensitivity is seen, with exposure to sunlight resulting in pruritus, erythema, and edema [530, 531]. This variability may be related to the concentration of porphyrins in the skin or plasma. Magnus et al. [251, 252] have shown that the action spectrum for producing cutaneous lesions lies in the 400-mμ band, corresponding to the maximal spectral absorption of porphyrins (Fig. 45-20).

Although skin lesions are the only manifestations of porphyria in almost half the affected individuals, episodes of acute abdominal pain and neuropathy similar to those in acute intermittent porphyria are not uncommon [205, 477, 526, 528, 531]. Chronic cutaneous involvement usually precedes by many years the occurrence of acute attacks, but occasionally acute manifestations occur without previous awareness of increased skin sensitivity [532]. The symptoms and signs associated with acute attacks in 80 patients with variegate porphyria are summarized in Fig. 45-18 [530]. During an acute episode the mortality rate is approximately 25 percent [532], but the overall mortality rate for variegate porphyria is obviously much less, because many of the afflicted patients never experience manifestations. In fact, Dean's extensive genetic studies [529] suggest that in the past, although perhaps not in recent years, patients with variegate porphyria survived as successfully as the rest of the Afrikaner population.

A significant change in the epidemiology of this disease occurred with the widespread introduction of certain pharmaceuticals, particularly barbiturates and sulfonamides. The available evidence suggests that most [532] if not all [529] acute attacks have been precipitated by ingestion of one of these compounds or by other hepatotoxic agents, including general anesthetics, excessive amounts of ethanol, and, perhaps, chloroquine [68, 533]. In some instances a variable degree of abdominal pain may have been present beforehand, but drug administration appeared to be responsible for its aggravation as well as for the initial development of neurologic lesions [532]. Acute attacks frequently are associated with prerenal azotemia, hypochloremia, hyponatremia, and hypokalemia [531], probably because of excessive vomiting and sweating. Unless they terminate fatally, acute attacks usually resolve completely, but neuropathic changes may persist long after the subsidence of the initial acute episode. Necropsy examinations have failed to reveal major anatomic abnormalities [534], and histologic and laboratory evidence of significant hepatic dysfunction is lacking [530, 532].

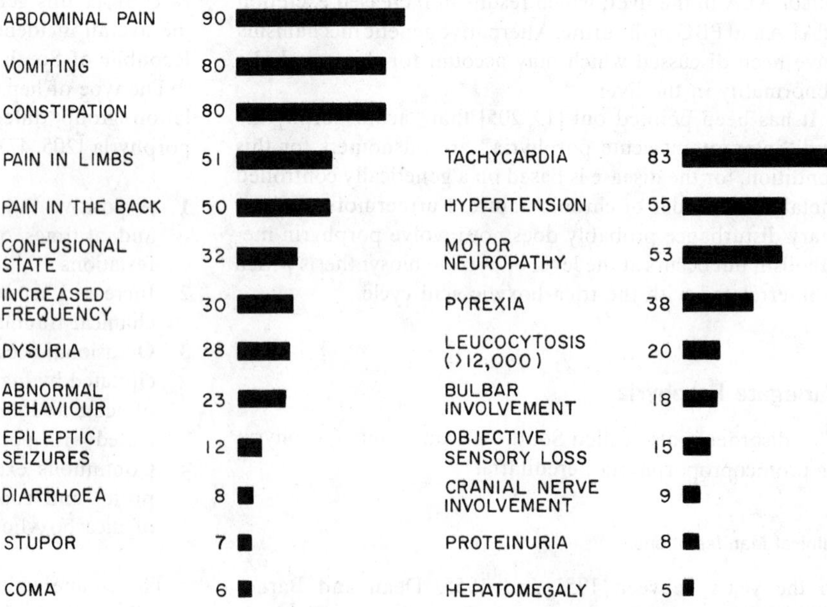

Figure 45-18. Acute attack in variegate porphyria. Percentage frequency of symptoms and signs in 80 patients. (*By permission of L. Eales* [530].)

Table 45-8. URINARY ALA AND PBG EXCRETION AND FECAL PORPHYRIN EXCRETION IN VARIEGATE PORPHYRIA

Sex	Age, yr	Clinical status	Urine			Stool (dry)	
			PBG qualitative [205]	PBG, mg/l	ALA, mg/l	COPRO, μg/gm	PROTO, μg/gm
M	28	Acute attack	+++	194	219	890	1,400
F	47	Acute attack	+++	99	45	520	574
M	29	Acute attack	++	40	41	805	810
F	35	Acute attack	++	138	81	623	805
M	29	Acute attack	++	31	30	670	785
F	43	Mild attack	+	25	26	620	1,240
F	42	Recent attack	+	20	8	345	568
F	35	Recent attack	Neg.	6	7	623	392
M	29	Recent attack	Trace	24	81	580	890
M	28	Recent attack	Neg.	2	7	270	508
M	52	Mild pain	Neg.	3	3	363	266
F	39	Mild pain	Neg.	8	5	477	930
M	23	Mild pain	Neg.	6	11	630	760
F	35	Cutaneous	Neg.	2	2	1,220	1,310
M	54	Cutaneous	Neg.	1	5	106	186
F		Cutaneous	Neg.	0	1	70	165
M	29	Cutaneous	Neg.	2	3	414	490
F	33	Cutaneous	Neg.	1	1	743	2,000
M	49	Cutaneous	Neg.	1	2	159	131

Note: COPRO, PROTO = coproporphyrin, protoporphyrin, respectively.
Source: G. Dean and H. D. Barnes [205].

Since the original description of variegate porphyria in South Africa, many similar cases, occurring individually or in family groups, have been reported. In retrospect, it is likely that some of the patients and families described as having chronic porphyria [14, 15, 535], mixed porphyria [56, 76, 536], porphyria cutanea tarda [18, 19, 415, 537] or protocoproporphyria hereditaria [458, 477] had genetically determined metabolic abnormalities similar to, or indeed identical with, those which have been described in variegate porphyria in the Afrikaners of South Africa. Large families with variegate porphyria have been studied in Sweden [538], Holland [537], Great Britain [539], and the United States [536]. It has been claimed that variegate porphyria occurred in the Royal Houses of Stuart, Hanover, and Prussia, and indeed, that George III suffered from the disease [540]; validation of these claims is difficult because of the almost complete lack of supporting laboratory data.

Chemical Findings

In this form of porphyria the characteristic chemical finding is the continuous excretion of large amounts of protoporphyrin and coproporphyrin in the feces. In normal persons the upper limits of fecal porphyrin concentration are assumed to be 30 to 40 μg for coproporphyrin and approximately 100 μg for protoporphyrin, all expressed per gram of dry stool [18, 220, 237, 239] (Table 45-3). As shown in Table 45-8, in patients with variegate porphyria the concentration of these porphyrins in the feces is greatly increased [205, 376, 529–531, 541], even when clinical manifestations are minimal [205, 531, 539, 542]. Furthermore, increased porphyrin concentration in the stool is demonstrable in asymptomatic children of patients with porphyria [376] (Table 45-9). Fourteen of thirty-five such children under the age of 18 were found to have elevated values. It is assumed that these children have "latent porphyria" which may become manifest during adult life [376]. Recent reports indicate that patients with variegate porphyria excrete in the feces

Table 45-9. PORPHYRIN CONCENTRATION IN THE FECES OF ASYMPTOMATIC CHILDREN OF PARENTS WITH VARIEGATE PORPHYRIA

Group	No. of children	Stool (dry weight)			
		COPRO, μg/gm		PROTO, μg/gm	
		Mean	Range	Mean	Range
Normal	23	7.5	0–14	23	5–51
Abnormal, but asymptomatic	14	52	16–158	116	51–212
Control: normal Bantu	13	5	1–11	10	3–27

Note: COPRO, PROTO = coproporphyrin, protoporphyrin, respectively.
Source: H. D. Barnes [376].

hitherto unrecognized peptide-conjugated dicarboxylic porphyrins that normally are present in only very small amounts [515].

In patients exhibiting only cutaneous manifestations at the time of examination, whether or not they have experienced acute episodes in the past, urinary excretion of porphyrins and porphyrin precursors is either normal or only moderately increased (Table 45-8) [205, 530, 541]. In a recent series of 45 cases [530] the following average values were obtained in milligrams per liter (range in parentheses): ALA, 4.3 (0.3 to 27.8); PBG, 1.7 (0 to 13.8); uroporphyrin, 0.240 (0 to 1.4); coproporphyrin, 0.630 (0.017 to 5.1). During acute attacks, on the other hand, much larger amounts of ALA, PBG, and porphyrins appear in the urine (Table 45-8) [205, 526, 529, 530, 541]. Urinary ALA and PBG concentrations may reach values comparable to those in patients with acute intermittent porphyria in relapse. Concomitantly, fecal porphyrin concentrations usually are higher than they are during periods of remission when only cutaneous manifestations are present (Table 45-8) [205, 530, 541], and the stool may contain significant amounts of uroporphyrin and of uro-type porphyrins with five to seven carboxyl groups [541].

These observations indicate that the clinical and biochemical aspects of acute attacks are remarkably similar in variegate and in acute intermittent porphyria, except for significantly higher fecal porphyrin concentrations in the variegate form.

Nature of the Metabolic Defect

In several patients with variegate porphyria hepatic ALA synthetase activity has been shown to be increased [310, 463]; this, of course, is similar to the situation in acute intermittent porphyria and may account in part, or entirely, for the increased excretion of porphyrin precursors and of porphyrins (Fig. 45-15) that is characteristic of this disorder. Moreover, Dowdle et al. [115] have demonstrated that in nonporphyric subjects administration of large amounts of ALA resulted in an excretory pattern of porphyrin precursors and porphyrins that was similar to that found in patients with variegate porphyria [421, 458]. In view of these observations, the primary metabolic defect in porphyrin metabolism most probably results in an exaggerated responsiveness of hepatic ALA synthetase. The studies of Dowdle et al. [115] and the characteristic excretory pattern appear to exclude a partial block in heme biosynthesis, at least at a step prior to ferrochelatase. An alternative, albeit unlikely, pathogenetic mechanism is that heme may be diverted from its participation in ALA synthetase repression in a manner similar to what appears to occur in chemically induced, experimental porphyria [296–300] (see also, Regulation of Heme and Hemoprotein Biosynthesis, earlier in this chapter).

Inheritance

The impressive investigations by Dean and Barnes [526, 529, 543] in South Africa and in other parts of the world [536–539] clearly indicate the hereditary nature of variegate porphyria. By tracing the disease back through 10 to 12 generations, Dean has accumulated records of over 1,400 porphyric individuals in 118 family groups, all with a common ancestry. Afflicted individuals appear to be heterozygous for a gene which, at least in the Afrikaner population, is not uncommon. It is not known whether inheritance of a double dose of this gene is compatible with life. The relative frequency of this genetic abnormality in this population group should offer a reasonable probability for the marriage of two heterozygotes, which eventually should provide an answer to this question [543].

A representative family tree is given in Fig. 45-19 [526]. The progenitor of this family was born in 1814 and had 478 descendants, many of whom could be traced and were still alive at the time of this study. As shown in Table 45-10, there were 62 porphyric patients among the 125 descendants with a porphyric parent, excluding children under 18 years of age in the sixth generation. In all cases only one parent had porphyria. In the second generation, 5 of the 10 members had porphyria; in the third generation, 16 out of 37; in the fourth generation, 32 out of 59; in the fifth generation, 9 out of the 19 descendants who were over 18 years of age had porphyria. Thus, 50 percent of the adults with one porphyric parent inherited the disturbance, 25 males and 37 females. At the time of the original study [526], all descendants in the sixth generation were under 18 years of age; in more recent investigations, 12 of the 32 children were found to have increased fecal porphyrin excretion [376, 529]. In the other 117 family groups studied a similar pattern of inheritance was demonstrated [529].

Hereditary Coproporphyria

Clinical and Chemical Manifestations

Hereditary coproporphyria resembles variegate porphyria clinically, but the unique pattern of porphyrin excretion in this condition appears to justify its consideration as a separate entity. The first family study carried out with modern investigative techniques was reported in 1955 by Berger and Goldberg [544]. It is probable that the patient described by Dobriner in 1936 [545] and the two patients reported by Watson and coworkers in 1949 [546] represented individual instances of this condition.

Hereditary coproporphyria undoubtedly occurs more frequently than was initially assumed. In 1967, Goldberg et al. [547] reported 10 new cases and summarized the 20 recorded in the literature. These included 14 male and 16 female patients, ranging in age from 7 to 75 years. Additional reports have appeared more recently [548–551].

Many of the subjects with this disease are asymptomatic, or they have mild, intermittent, and generally ill-defined abdominal, neurologic, or psychiatric manifestations. Photosensitivity appears to be infrequent [551, 552]. Acute

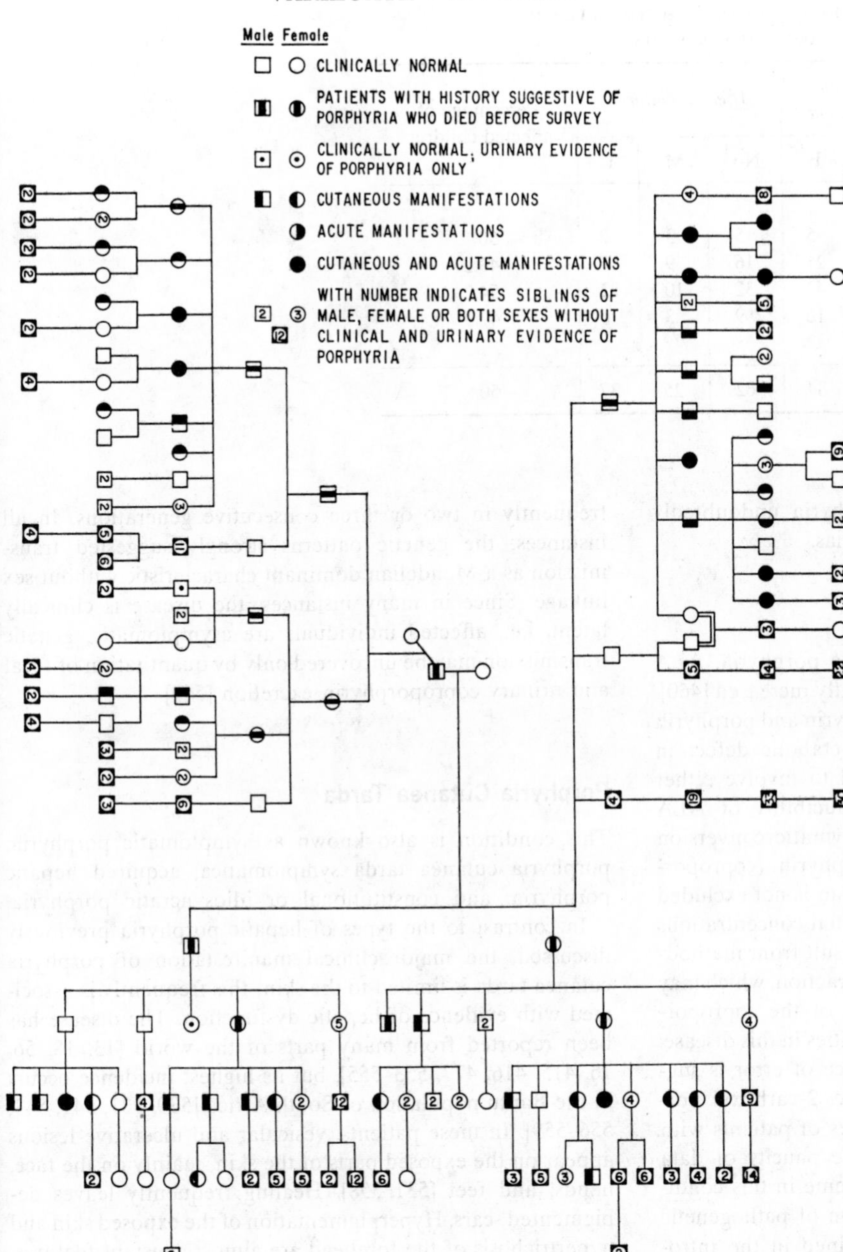

Figure 45-19. Pedigree of a family with variegate porphyria. The diagnosis was established on the basis of clinical manifestations and urinary analysis, but fecal examinations for porphyrins have not yet been reported for this family. The last generation is comprised largely of children under 18 years of age, many of whom may exhibit increased porphyrin excretion in the feces [376]. (*By permission of G. Dean and H. D. Barnes* [526].)

attacks similar to those seen in acute intermittent or in variegate porphyria may occur spontaneously or, more often, are precipitated by drugs such as barbiturates, anticonvulsants, or tranquilizers [547, 548]. This may happen at any age, including childhood and adolescence.

The most striking biochemical abnormality in hereditary coproporphyria is the unremitting excretion of large amounts of coproporphyrin III in the feces. Values of several milligrams coproporphyrin per gram dry feces have been reported [547–549]. Fecal protoporphyrin excretion is usually much less impressive, although it may be above the normal range. The hydrophilic "X porphyrin," characteristic of variegate porphyria [515], is not found in hereditary coproporphyria [547, 548]. Coproporphyrin excretion also is frequently increased in the urine, particularly during acute attacks, but it may return to normal values during clinical remissions. ALA and PBG concentrations in the urine are commonly elevated, and during acute attacks these values may approach those seen in acute intermittent porphyria. A fragment of liver tissue obtained from a patient exhibited intense red fluorescence [547], but no increase in porphyrins was demonstrable in bone marrow and in circulating red

Table 45-10. NUMBER OF MEMBERS IN EACH GENERATION, TOTAL ADULT CHILDREN OF AFFECTED PARENTS, AND NUMBER AND PERCENTAGE OF AFFECTED CHILDREN IN A FAMILY WITH VARIEGATE PORPHYRIA

Generation	Total members	*Adult children of affected parent*			*Affected children*			Percentage of affected children
		No.	M	F	No.	M	F	
I	1							
II	10	10	5	5	5	3	2	50
III	62	37	16	21	16	9	7	43.2
IV	173	59	17	42	32	10	22	54.2
V	201	19	3	16	9	3	6	47.5
VI	32							
Total	479	125	41	84	62	25	37	50

Source: G. Dean and H. D. Barnes [526].

blood cells. Thus hereditary coproporphyria undoubtedly belongs in the group of hepatic porphyrias.

Nature of the Metabolic Defect

As in acute intermittent and in variegate porphyria, ALA synthetase activity in the liver is significantly increased [460]. In view of this and of the pattern of porphyrin and porphyrin precursor excretion (Fig. 45-15), the metabolic defect in porphyrin biosynthesis may be expected to involve either a primary genetic alteration in the inducibility of ALA synthetase or a partial block in the enzymatic conversion of coproporphyrinogen III to protoporphyrin (coproporphyrinogen oxidase). This latter mechanism is not excluded by occasional reports of greater than normal concentrations of fecal protoporphyrin, since this may result from methodologic errors in measuring this porphyrin fraction, which may be contaminated by a small percentage of the coproporphyrin that is excreted in such large quantities in this disease. That this indeed may be a possible source of error is suggested by the absence of the hydrophilic, 2-carboxyl porphyrins ("X-type" porphyrins) in the feces of patients with hereditary coproporphyria [547, 548]. The paucity of data relating to the biosynthetic pathway of heme in this condition precludes a more extensive discussion of pathogenetic mechanisms. The general approach outlined in the introductory material under Hepatic Porphyrias above seems applicable.

Genetic Considerations

The original description of coproporphyria [544] emphasized the genetic nature of the disease, in that the propositus was the offspring of consanguine parents, both of whom exhibited elevated coproporphyrin excretion. Of the 30 cases collected by Goldberg et al. [547], 24 had a positive family history. Most of the patients reported subsequently [548, 549, 551, 552] also exhibited familial occurrence of the disease, frequently in two or three consecutive generations. In all instances, the genetic patterns strongly suggested transmission as a Mendelian dominant characteristic without sex linkage. Since in many instances, the disease is clinically latent, i.e., affected individuals are asymptomatic, genetic transmission may be uncovered only by quantitation of fecal and urinary coproporphyrin excretion [549].

Porphyria Cutanea Tarda

This condition is also known as symptomatic porphyria, porphyria cutanea tarda symptomatica, acquired hepatic porphyria, and constitutional or idiosyncratic porphyria.

In contrast to the types of hepatic porphyria previously discussed, the major clinical manifestation of porphyria cutanea tarda is limited to the skin; this frequently is associated with evidence of hepatic dysfunction. The disease has been reported from many parts of the world [13, 18, 56, 76, 415, 416, 477, 553–555], but its highest incidence occurs in the Bantu population of South Africa [530, 531, 541, 543, 556–559]. In these patients, vesicular and ulcerative lesions appear on the exposed parts of the skin, mainly on the face, hands, and feet [531, 558]. Healing frequently leaves depigmented scars. Hyperpigmentation of the exposed skin and hypertrichosis of the forehead are almost constant features. Virtually all patients have hepatomegaly and exhibit laboratory and histologic evidence of liver disease [528], but acute attacks with abdominal and neurologic manifestations do not occur. The onset of these symptoms is usually insidious and occurs most often in middle age [458, 558]. Although in most instances a recent increase in facial pigmentation and intermittent excretion of red urine has been noticed, tle skin lesions attributable to porphyria frequently are not the primary reason for seeking medical attention. Many of these patients suffer from other unrelated diseases, including tuberculosis, leprosy, intestinal infections, and pellagra, and the discovery of coexistent porphyria is incidental [558].

Chemically, this type of porphyria is characterized by increased urinary excretion of uroporphyrin and of other ether-insoluble porphyrins [530, 531, 541, 556, 558] (Fig. 45-15). In contrast to variegate porphyria, fecal porphyrin concentrations are highly variable, ranging from normal to distinctly increased [376, 421, 519, 530, 531, 558]; elevated urinary excretion of ALA and PBG is uncommon [530, 558, 559]. Hepatic tissue shows intense red fluorescence and greatly increased porphyrin concentrations [541, 558].

Because evidence for a hereditary transmission of this disease is lacking [458, 530, 558], it is generally assumed to be an acquired abnormality (symptomatic porphyria [530]; porphyria cutanea tarda symptomatica [19, 458]). Most of these patients have a high consumption of alcohol, consisting mainly of a variety of home-brewed concoctions with a high iron content [558, 560]. Although the siderosis which is prevalent in this population group [560, 561] does not appear to be causally related to the porphyria [558], there is strong but indirect evidence that alcoholism may be an important etiologic factor [19, 458, 477, 558]. It should be noted that though alcohol consumption is widespread among the Bantus of South Africa [558], the incidence of porphyria is much lower. Among the patients attending the out-patient department of the Baragwanath Hospital in Johannesburg, 13 per 1,000 had porphyria, and in ward patients the ratio was 5:1,000 [562]. This leaves open the possibility of an underlying but occult genetic abnormality which is activated by superimposed liver injury such as that produced by alcohol.

The anamnestic, clinical, and laboratory patterns of patients with porphyria cutanea tarda reported from other parts of the world are similar [13, 18, 76, 415, 416, 421, 477, 519, 553–555]. Photosensitivity characterized by blisters, increased mechanical fragility, and hyperpigmentation of the exposed parts of the skin, is the outstanding feature [563]. Uro- and coproporphyrin excretion in the urine frequently is sufficiently high to produce a pink or brownish color; in other instances, the urine color may be normal but increased porphyrin excretion is evident from the red or pink fluorescence of the acidified urine under ultraviolet light [76, 421, 519, 541]. The liver contains high porphyrin concentrations [76], whereas in red blood cells the values invariably are normal.

Varying degrees of hepatic injury, frequently of ethanolic nature, are common in these patients [76, 421]. This has led to the belief [13] that the liver disease is the primary disorder and the disturbance in porphyrin metabolism is only a secondary manifestation; accordingly, the term *porphyria cutanea tarda symptomatica* has been proposed [19]. It is evident however that only a small minority of chronic alcoholics with liver disease develop porphyria cutanea tarda. Among 360 patients with cirrhosis of alcoholic type [564], only 7 instances of porphyria could be detected [519]. Moreover, in these seven porphyric patients the extent of the hepatic dysfunction was relatively slight. It seems reasonable to assume, therefore, that these patients have a genetically determined but normally undetectable predisposition for porphyria [43, 57, 421, 477, 519]. In accord with this concept is the observation by Waldenström and Haeger-Aronsen that it occasionally is possible to detect increased porphyrin excretion in relatives of patients with porphyria cutanea tarda [477, 519].

The pathogenesis of this condition is unclear. A current hypothesis holds that the primary defect is overproduction of ALA, as is assumed to be the case in the other forms of hepatic porphyria. This seemed to be supported by the finding of increased ALA synthetase activity in the liver [565–568]. It should be noted that in these studies the small amount of liver obtained by needle biopsy prevented the quantitative separation of the formed ALA from aminoacetone (which also gives a positive Ehrlich reaction). Indeed, with a new and highly specific assay method for ALA synthetase, studies in five patients with porphyria cutanea tarda demonstrated hepatic enzyme activity within the *normal* range [310, 460]. This, of course, is in accord with the observation that urinary excretion of ALA and PBG usually is not elevated [530, 558, 559]. Moreover, patients with porphyria cutanea tarda do not exhibit the exquisite sensitivity to barbiturates characteristic of most other types of hepatic porphyria [421]. Rimington [569] postulated that increased formation of porphyrins in the liver and their excretion in the urine may result from excessive oxidation of porphyrinogens, leading to irreversible diversion of these intermediates from hepatic heme biosynthesis (Fig. 45-8), but experimental support for this concept is not available.

Several other observations tend to characterize porphyria cutanea tarda as a distinct clinical entity. In several instances first manifestations of the disease appear to have followed therapeutic administration of estrogens, e.g., for carcinoma of the prostate or for postmenopausal disturbances [421, 569–571]. Repeated phlebotomy has been established as an effective means of treatment [554, 572, 573]. This beneficial effect is probably related to removal of excessive iron from the liver [574], but it should be noted that "spontaneous" remissions of the disease do occur, particularly after abstinence from ethanol. Finally, patients with porphyria cutanea tarda respond in a unique way to chloroquine [575–578]. On administration of this drug in therapeutic doses there is evidence of transitory liver injury associated with nausea, vomiting, and fever; this is accompanied by an almost explosive efflux of porphyrin in the urine. Felsher and Redeker [576] suggested that the chloroquine may bind uroporphyrin in the liver. This has now been substantiated by demonstrating formation of a water-soluble chloroquine-uroporphyrin complex that is readily excreted in the urine [260]. This "purging" process is associated with selective destruction of hepatic mitochondria [260]. In a group of patients, the coexistence of porphyria cutanea tarda and lupus erythematosus has been reported [616]. Although occurring more frequently than would be expected on the basis of chance alone, the cause for this association of two distinct diseases, both exhibiting photosensitivity, is unclear.

Toxic Acquired Porphyria

An almost explosive outbreak of porphyria involving several thousand individuals was reported in 1956 from three southeastern provinces of Turkey [54, 55]. The syndrome was characterized by hepatomegaly, marked porphyrinuria, photosensitivity, pigmentation, and hypertrichosis. The patients belonged to several ethnic groups living in this region, including Turks, Kurds, and Armenians; children and adolescents, particularly of the male sex, appeared to be affected more frequently and more severely [55]. In four representative patients, urine uroporphyrin excretion ranged from 3 to 12 mg per day, with corresponding coproporphyrin values between 0.5 and 2 mg [41]. Fecal excretion in two patients was as follows: coproporphyrin, 30 and 430, and protoporphyrin, 8.8 and 50 μg per gm dry weight [41]. Qualitative tests for porphobilinogen gave negative results.

This disturbance in porphyrin metabolism could be traced to chronic ingestion of hexachlorobenzene, which was used as a fungicidal agent in wheat [54, 55] distributed in these three provinces by the Turkish government. When this practice was discontinued in 1959 new cases of porphyria ceased to occur, and the syndrome gradually disappeared [55]. On the basis of this epidemiologic information and confirmative animal experiments [579], it was evident that hexachlorobenzene-induced porphyria represented an acquired derangement of porphyrin metabolism, occurring without a genetic predisposition to porphyria.

An interesting case of seemingly acquired cutaneous porphyria was reported by Tio et al. [580]. Photosensitivity and marked porphyrinuria had gradually developed in an 80-year-old woman over the course of a year, when she was discovered to have a large benign liver cell adenoma. On resection this was found to contain large amounts of proto-, copro-, and uroporphyrin. The surrounding liver tissue was normal. Following the operation the cutaneous manifestations disappeared and porphyrin excretion returned to normal. This seemed to indicate that the defect in porphyrin metabolism was limited to the hepatic tumor.

PROTOPORPHYRIA

Synomyns for this disorder are erythropoietic protoporphyria and erythrohepatic protoporphyria.

Incidence and Clinical Manifestation

In 1961, Magnus and his coworkers [581] described a hitherto unrecognized type of congenital and probably inherited photosensitive porphyria which differs fundamentally from classic erythropoietic porphyria. In retrospect, it is likely that the first case of this condition had been reported by Sir Archibald Gray [346, 582], and Kosenow and Treibs [583] appear to have observed patients with this condition without fully recognizing the separate disease entity with which they were dealing. In the short period of 9 years since its first comprehensive description, protoporphyria has been recorded with considerable frequency [252, 265, 584–600]. The reason for the belated and almost accidental discovery of this malady lies in the fact that it fails to exhibit some of the major manifestations commonly associated with congenital porphyria: there is no increase in urinary porphyrin excretion, and erythrodontia, hirsutism, and hyperpigmentation are absent. Moreover, exposed parts of the skin show neither the abnormal mechanical fragility nor the chronic bullous eruptions which are so characteristic of the other forms of photosensitive porphyria.

Instead, the skin lesions appear in the form of solar urticaria [581] or solar eczema [584, 601]. In the majority of patients a few minutes of exposure to sunlight results in intense pruritus, erythema, and edema [581, 587]. These manifestations commonly begin during or immediately after the period of exposure, involve the uncovered areas of the body, and subside in the course of 12 to 24 hr. As a rule, healing occurs without leaving significant scarring, atrophy, or pigmentation [595]. Magnus et al. [252, 581, 601] have been able to demonstrate conclusively that the photodermatitic lesions are produced by a narrow band of near-ultraviolet light in the 400-mμ region (Fig. 45-20). The position of this action spectrum is identical with that of the maximal spectral absorption of porphyrins (Soret's band).

In a few patients cutaneous manifestations occurred only after prolonged exposure to sunlight [584, 585, 588, 590, 601]; in others, the initial skin lesions progressed to a chronic

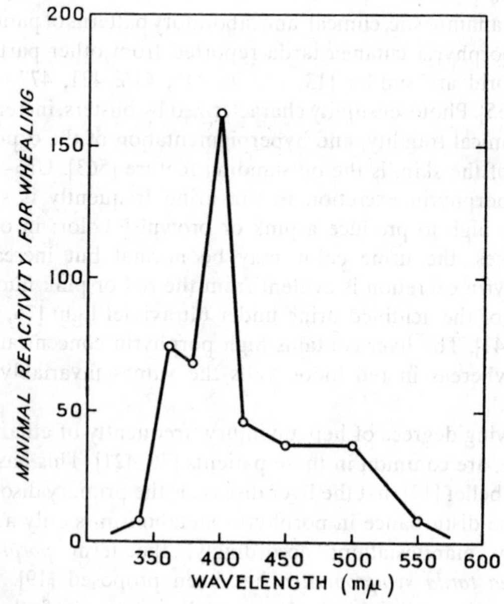

Figure 45-20. Action spectrum for cutaneous edema (whealing) in erythropoietic protoporphyria. (The ordinate scale—minimal reactivity for whealing—is the reciprocal of the minimal dose required to produce whealing. This dose of radiation is expressed in arbitrary units—i.e., t [time in seconds] $\times$ I [intensity].) Intensity was measured with a galvanometer and linear vacuum thermopile with quartz window. (*By permission of I. A. Magnus* [581].)

eczematous phase, which persisted for several weeks and healed with scar formation [584, 585, 590, 596]. In individual patients skin sensitivity exhibits considerable fluctuation [581, 591], and seasonal variations in susceptibility are frequently observed [581, 585, 587, 591]. In most cases, the cutaneous manifestations of the disease are first noted during childhood or adolescence and persist throughout life. In other instances cutaneous lesions are inconspicuous or absent and the disease in its latent form is uncovered by fecal or erythrocyte porphyrin analysis in the course of a family survey [594, 597, 600].

The clinical manifestations of protoporphyria are limited almost entirely to the skin, except for disturbances of the hepatobiliary apparatus. The disease appears to be associated frequently with cholelithiasis, the gallstones consisting in part of precipitated protoporphyrin [599]. Focal intrahepatic deposits of precipitated protoporphyrin have been reported [599], and in one instance these concretions were so extensive as to result in a veritable cholestasis [602]. Hemolytic anemia is only rarely seen in this condition [588, 589, 602]; when it occurs, it appears to respond favorably to splenectomy [588].

Laboratory Findings

Except for the rare patient with hemolytic anemia, the formed elements of the blood and bone marrow appear morphologically normal. Reticulocyte counts, red blood cell survival, and iron kinetics are within normal limits [581, 590, 597, 598]. Conventional liver function tests usually give normal results, and the urine is unremarkable. Urinary excretion of ALA, PBG, and porphyrins is within, or close to, the normal range [581, 584–588, 598].

The most striking findings are present in the red blood cells and in the feces. The concentration of free protoporphyrin in circulating erythrocytes is increased five- to thirtyfold [581, 584–588, 590, 597, 598] (Table 45-11), and the pigment has the structure of isomer type IXα protoporphyrin [581, 589]. In the fluorescence microscope, up to half the erythrocytes in the blood and bone marrow exhibit intense red fluorescence [603, 604] which fades rapidly on ultraviolet illumination [581, 587, 588, 590, 605]. Normoblasts also contain fluorescing porphyrins [581, 587, 588], but in contrast to congenital erythropoietic porphyria, the red fluorescence is limited to the cytoplasm [587]. Protoporphyrin concentration appears to be normal in the red blood cell population that fails to exhibit red fluorescence [603]. On exposure to light of 400-mμ wavelength, porphyrin-containing erythrocytes are readily hemolyzed; subsequently, nonfluorescing red blood cells also undergo hemolysis, presumably because of sensitization by protoporphyrin released into the suspending solution [603]. The erythrocyte coproporphyrin concentration may also be slightly increased [594, 598]. Protoporphyrin concentrations frequently are elevated also in the plasma [581, 582, 585, 586, 588]. This appears to be accentuated by fasting ("glucose effect") [606].

Large amounts of protoporphyrin usually are excreted in the stool (Table 45-11) [581, 582, 584–591, 594, 597, 598], and at times coproporphyrin values are also increased. Fecal porphyrin concentration often is high enough to produce red fluorescence on direct illumination with ultraviolet light. No increase in uroporphyrin concentrations has been detected in the excreta or tissues. In several instances liver tissue exhibited red fluorescence, presumably due to protoporphyrin [607], whereas in another case no increase in hepatic porphyrin was demonstrable [588]. In a porphyric patient with associated hemolytic anemia, liver tissue removed prior to splenectomy contained increased porphyrin concentrations, but 2 years after surgery a liver biopsy failed to reveal porphyrin fluorescence or abnormal pigmentation [588].

In several patients skin biopsies revealed variable degrees of red fluorescence [591, 607]. It is likely, although not proved, that the porphyrin in the skin is derived from the elevated protoporphyrin level in the plasma. The cutaneous lesions of these patients are probably the result of photochemical reactions produced by light that is absorbed by porphyrins present in the skin [252, 595, 601].

Table 45-11. PORPHYRINS IN PROTOPORPHYRIA

Case	Manifestations	*Stool, μg per 100 gm wet weight*		Plasma, μg per 100 ml, PROTO	Erythrocytes, μg per 100 ml, PROTO
		COPRO	PROTO		
Twin son	Photosensitivity	140	1,078	8.7	873
		589	10,610	....	1,510
Twin son	Photosensitivity	160	1,040	18.0	758
		495	2,700	....	653
Father	Normal	450	303	....	55
Mother	Asymptomatic	875	2,940	....	47
		462	3,067	0	50
Daughter	Normal	222	206	....	64
Daughter	Normal	75	132	....	176

Note: COPRO, PROTO = coproporphyrin, protoporphyrin, respectively.
Source: Adapted from A. G. Redeker and R. S. Bronow [585].

Site and Nature of the Metabolic Defect

Protoporphyrin-laden erythrocytes exhibiting intense red fluorescence under ultraviolet light have become accepted as the hallmark of protoporphyria. This has led to the assumption that defective heme biosynthesis in the maturing red blood cells is the source of the excessive protoporphyrin. Several more recent observations are difficult to reconcile with the concept of a genetic abnormality that is expressed metabolically solely in the erythroid apparatus.

1 In a number of instances, marked discrepancies were noted between erythrocyte concentration and fecal excretion of protoporphyrin [597, 598]; the quantity excreted daily in the feces exceeded by as much as 50 times the total amount of protoporphyrin in the circulating red blood cell mass. Since most of these patients exhibited a normal erythrocyte life-span, it is apparent that only a small portion of their fecal protoporphyrin could have been derived from senescent red blood cells. Significant "leakage" of protoporphyrin from intact circulating erythrocytes into the plasmas has been ruled out by direct experimental observation [607]. Furthermore, no increase in fecal porphyrin excretion is demonstrable in lead intoxication and in iron deficiency [608], both of which are associated with high levels of free red blood cell protoporphyrin [608–610].

2 Investigation of kinships with the disease revealed several affected individuals with elevated fecal porphyrin excretion who failed to exhibit a concomitant increase in red blood cell protoporphyrin [587, 611].

3 In a patient with protoporphyria studied with ^{15}N-glycine, Gray et al. [582] noted that the specific isotope concentration of erythrocyte protoporphyrin could not readily account for the isotope values of the porphyrin in the feces.

In a recent study employing simultaneous pulse labeling of protoporphyrin with ^{14}C-glycine and ^{3}H-ALA in vivo, additional evidence was obtained that the excessive excretion of protoporphyrin is a consequence of disordered heme synthesis in *several* tissues [612]. In this particular study, the liver and the maturing erythrocytes appeared to be the most important sources of protoporphyrin, with the liver providing the major fraction. Aside from kinetic considerations, a dominant role of the liver in protoporphyrin overproduction appears plausible, because (1) it is a well-known site of active porphyrin and heme biosynthesis, and (2) protoporphyria exhibits a reciprocal relationship between caloric intake and porphyrin excretion, similar to the "glucose effect" [465, 606] in the hepatic porphyrias.

The concept of protoporphyria as a disorder of heme biosynthesis that involves more than one organ raises the question of whether in other forms of porphyria the metabolic defect may appear also in more than one cell type but may become manifest only when the "milieu" of a particular cell renders the involved step rate-limiting [310, 431]. This could result from quantitative differences between various cell types in the relative activity of enzymes in heme biosynthesis [310, 431], in membrane permeability properties, or in inducer concentrations.

The nature of the metabolic defect in heme biosynthesis in protoporphyria is unknown. In a study of tissues from two patients with an atypical form of protoporphyria associated with hemolytic anemia, Porter [588, 589] failed to uncover a specific lesion. This single report does not rule out, of course, a possible defect in ferrochelatase, but the paucity of available data does not permit a more detailed consideration of the pathogenicity.

Genetic Considerations

In over half the cases reported to date, the disease occurred in more than one member of a family [582, 585–588, 594, 596, 597, 600, 601]. The patient studied by Gray et al. [582] had a twin sister and a daughter with porphyria. The mother of the twin boys reported by Redeker and Bronow [585] was found to have elevated fecal protoporphyrin concentrations (Table 45-11) but was clinically normal. Haeger-Aronsen described a family with affected members in three generations [587] (Fig. 45-21), but only the father and his two daughters suffered from photosensitivity; two other members were clinically normal but exhibited slightly increased red blood cell protoporphyrin concentrations. Four out of nine sibs in Langhof's family had the disease [591], and Redeker and Bryan have recently studied a family with affected members in four successive generations [611].

These observations indicate that protoporphyria is a hereditary disease occurring in both sexes. The available data suggest that the disturbance in porphyrin metabolism is due to a single dose of a rare gene, i.e., that the disease is

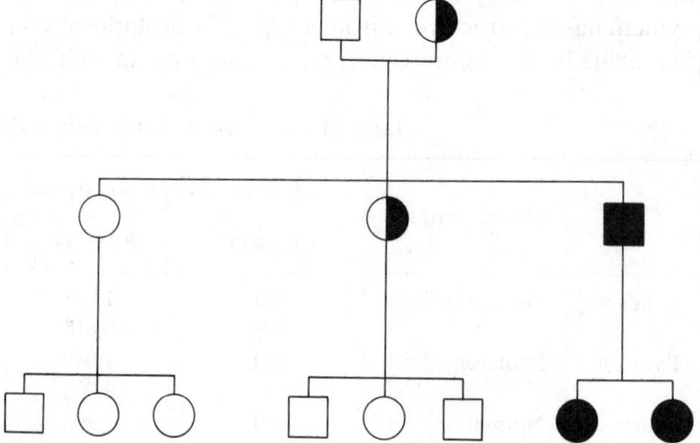

Figure 45-21. Pedigree of a family with erythropoietic protoporphyria. Squares indicate males; circles, females. Solid black indicates clinically manifest disease; black and white, latent cases, recognized by increased erythrocyte or stool protoporphyrin; white, unaffected family members. (*By permission of B. Haeger-Aronsen* [587].)

transmitted as an autosomal dominant trait. It is evident that a significant percentage of individuals carrying this genetic abnormality remains clinically asymptomatic, and in such patients repeated determinations of erythrocyte *and* fecal protoporphyrin concentrations may be the only means of detecting the genetic defect.

SUMMARY

1 Among the various forms of inherited disorders of porphyrin metabolism, *congenital erythropoietic porphyria* (Günther's disease) stands out as a well-defined and easily recognizable disease (Table 45-1). To date, a total of approximately 70 proved cases has been reported. The metabolic defect is located in the maturing erythroid cells of the bone marrow and leads to overproduction of porphyrins of the isomer type I series. This results in chronic cutaneous photosensitivity and severe porphyrinuria, usually associated with hemolytic anemia. Affected individuals have a double dose of a rare autosomal gene; clinically latent cases are not observed. A single dose of the abnormal gene *rarely* produces demonstrable defects in porphyrin metabolism, but the genetic defect may be uncovered by enzyme studies.

2 *Acute intermittent porphyria* is the only inherited disturbance of porphyrin metabolism not associated with cutaneous sensitivity. The major clinical manifestations include abdominal colic, hypertension, peripheral and central neuropathy, mainly of the motor system, and psychosis. These characteristically are intermittent in nature and occur to a highly variable extent; clinically latent cases are frequently observed. Acute attacks or exacerbations of symptoms may be precipitated by a variety of drugs. Death may occur during an acute attack, usually as the result of respiratory paralysis. The metabolic defect is located in the liver and leads to overproduction of δ-aminolevulinic acid (ALA), resulting in urinary excretion of greatly increased amounts of this porphyrin precursor and of porphobilinogen (PBG). Affected individuals have a single dose of an abnormal autosomal gene.

3 *Variegate porphyria* is a hepatic type of inherited porphyria. Its clinical manifestations are highly variable in nature and in extent. The major symptom is chronic skin sensitivity to light and to mechanical trauma. Acute attacks, similar to those in acute intermittent porphyria, do occur and are usually precipitated by drugs or other hepatotoxins. The biochemical abnormality consists of greatly increased excretion of fecal proto- and coproporphyrin; these pigments are derived from the liver. During acute attacks, urinary excretion of ALA, PBG, and porphyrins is increased. Affected individuals have a single dose of an abnormal autosomal gene, which, at least in some population groups, appears to be relatively frequent.

4 *Hereditary coproporphyria* resembles variegate porphyria clinically. Photosensitivity and abdominal manifestations are usually mild, and latent cases are frequent. Acute attacks, often precipitated by ingestion of drugs, are similar to those occurring in acute intermittent and in variegate porphyria. The biochemical characteristic is the unremitting excretion of large amounts of coproporphyrin in the feces and, to a lesser extent, in the urine; the pigment originates in the liver.

5 In *porphyria cutanea tarda,* the role of genetic factors is unclear. Many cases appear to be acquired, usually in association with hepatic injury. Photosensitivity is the only noteworthy clinical manifestation. Chemically, large amounts of uroporphyrin, derived from the liver, are excreted in the urine. Acute attacks do not occur, and urinary excretion of ALA and PBG is normal. The disease clinically may resemble congenital erythropoietic porphyria, but the two conditions are entirely different in their pathogenesis, pathology, genetic transmission, and age of onset.

6 *Toxic acquired porphyria* has occurred in several thousand individuals accidentally exposed to hexachlorobenzene. This and other agents regularly induce experimental forms of hepatic porphyria in laboratory animals.

7 *Protoporphyria,* formerly called erythropoietic protoporphyria, is a relatively mild disorder, characterized by acute solar urticaria or more chronic solar eczema. The extent of the cutaneous manifestations is highly variable, and clinically latent cases appear to be frequent. The metabolic defect consists of overproduction of protoporphyrin IXα in the liver and in the erythroid cells, leading to greatly increased fecal excretion of this pigment. Affected individuals have a single dose of an abnormal autosomal gene.

BIBLIOGRAPHY

1. Schultz, J. H.: Ein Fall von Pemphigus leprosus, complicirt durch *Lepra visceralis* (thesis). Greifswald, 1874.
2. Baumstark, F.: Zwei pathologische Harnfarbstoffe. Arch. Ges. Physiol., **9**, 568, 1874.
3. MacMunn, C. A.: Observations on the colouring matters of the so-called bile of invertebrates, on those of the bile of vertebrates, and on some unusual urine pigments. Proc. Roy. Soc. London, **35**, 370, 1883.
4. Salkowski, E.: Ueber Vorkommen und Nachweis des Haematoporphyrins im Harn. Z. Physiol. Chem., **15**, 286, 1891.
5. Hammersten, O.: Ueber Haematoporphyrin in Harn. Skand. Arch. Physiol., **3**, 319, 1892.
6. Garrod, A. E.: On haematoporphyrin as a urinary pigment in disease. J. Path. Bact., **1**, 187, 1893.
7. Stokvis, B. J.: Zur Pathogenese der Haematoporphyrie. Z. Klin. Med., **28**, 1, 1895.
8. Saillet: De l'urospectrine (ou urohématoporphyrine normale) et de sa transformation en hémochromogène sans fer. Rev. Med. Paris, **16**, 542, 1896.
9. Anderson, M. T.: Hydroa aestivale in two brothers, complicated with the presence of haematoporphyrin in the urine. Brit. J. Derm., **10**, 1, 1898.
10. Nebelthau, E.: Beitrag zur Lehre von Haematoporphyrin des Harnes. Z. Physiol. Chem., **27**, 324, 1899.
11. Hoppe-Seyler, F.: *Medizin.-chem.: Untersuchungen.* Tübingen, 1871.
12. Nencki, M., and Sieber, N.: Ueber das Haematoporphyrin. Arch. Exp. Path. Pharmakol., **24**, 430, 1888.
13. Goldberg, A., and Rimington, C.: *Diseases of Porphyrin Metabolism.* Charles C Thomas, Springfield, Ill., 1962.

14. Günther, H.: Die Haematoporphyria. Deutsch. Arch. Klin. Med., **105,** 89, 1911.
15. Günther, H.: In *Handbuch der Krankheiten des Blutes und der blutbildenden Organe,* edited by A. Schittenhelm, vol. 2. Springer-Verlag, Berlin, 1925.
16. Waldenström, J.: Studien ueber Porphyrie. Acta. Med. Scand., suppl. **82,** 1937.
17. Schmid, R., Schwartz, S., and Sundberg, D.: Erythropoietic (congenital) porphyria: a rare abnormality of the normoblasts. Blood, **10,** 416, 1955.
18. Holti, G., Rimington, C., Tate, B. C., and Thomas, G.: An investigation of "porphyria cutanea tarda." Quart. J. Med., **27,** 1, 1958.
19. Waldenström, J.: The porphyrias as inborn errors of metabolism. Amer. J. Med., **22,** 758, 1957.
20. Watson, C. J.: In *Diseases of Metabolism,* 3d ed. Saunders, Philadelphia, 1953.
21. Haeger, B.: Urinary δ-aminolaevulinic acid and porphobilinogen in different types of porphyria. Lancet, **2,** 606, 1958.
22. Waldenström, J.: Neurological symptoms caused by so-called acute porphyria. Acta Psychiat. Neurol., **14,** 375, 1939.
23. Watson, C. J.: In *Oxford Medicine,* vol. IV, chap. 9-A, p. 251. Oxford, New York, 1951.
24. Ellinger, A., and Riesser, O.: Zur Kenntnis des im Harn nach Trionalvergiftung auftretenden Porphyrins. Z. Physiol. Chem., **48,** 1, 1916.
25. Micheli, F., and Dominici, G.: Ueber zwei Fälle von familiärer Porphyrie mit letalem Ausgang. Deutsch. Arch. Klin. Med., **171,** 154, 1931.
26. Duesberg, R.: Toxische Porphyrie. München. Med. Wschr., **79,** 1821, 1932.
27. Nakarai: Ueber Haematoporphyrie. Deutsch. Arch. Klin. Med., **58,** 165, 1897.
28. Stokvis, B. J.: Cited in A. E. Garrod, *Inborn Errors of Metabolism,* 2d ed. Oxford, London, 1923.
29. Taylor, A. E., and Sailer, J.: A fatal case of sulphonal poisoning. Contribution, Pennsylvania University William Pepper Laboratory, 1900.
30. Emminger, E.: Fluoreszenz-mikroskopische Untersuchungen bei einem Fall von Schlafmittelvergiftung. Klin. Wschr., **12,** 1840, 1933.
31. Neubauer, O.: Haematoporphyrin und Sulfonalvergiftung. Arch. Exp. Path., **43,** 456, 1900.
32. Perutz, A.: Ueber Hydroa aestivale und vacciniforme. Arch. Derm. Syph., **124,** 531, 1917.
33. Kast, A., and Weiss, Th.: Zur Kenntnis der Haematoporphyrinurie. Berlin. Klin. Wschr., **33,** 621, 1896.
34. Fischer, H., and Duesberg, R.: Ueber Porphyrine bei klinischer und experimenteller Porphyrie. Arch. Exp. Path. Pharmakol., **166,** 95, 1932.
35. Waldenström, J., and Wendt, S.: Tierexperimentelle Studien ueber den Porphyrinstoffwechsel. Z. Physiol. Chem., **259,** 157, 1939.
36. Schmid, R., and Schwartz, S.: Experimental porphyria. III. Hepatic type produced by Sedormid. Proc. Soc. Exp. Biol. Med., **81,** 685, 1952.
37. Goldberg, A., and Rimington, C.: Experimentally produced porphyria in animals. Proc. Roy. Soc. London, ser. B, **143,** 257, 1955.
38. Schmid, R., Figen, J. F., and Schwartz, S.: Experimental porphyria. IV. Studies of liver catalase and other heme enzymes in Sedormid porphyria. J. Biol. Chem., **217,** 263, 1955.
39. Schmid, R., and Schwartz, S.: Studies of some liver heme proteins and porphyrins in experimental Sedormid porphyria, in *Porphyrin Biosynthesis and Metabolism,* Ciba Foundation. Churchill, London, 1955.
40. Gray, C. H.: Acute porphyria. A.M.A. Arch. Intern. Med., **85,** 459, 1950.
41. Schmid, R.: Unpublished observations.
42. De Matteis, F., and Rimington, C.: Disturbance of porphyrin metabolism caused by griseofulvin in mice. Brit. J. Derm., **75,** 91, 1963.
43. Schmid, R.: Hepatotoxic drugs causing porphyria in man and animals. South African J. Lab. Clin. Med., **9,** 212, 1963.
44. De Matteis, F.: Disturbances of liver porphyrin metabolism caused by drugs. Pharmacol. Rev., **19,** 523, 1967.
45. Granick, S.: The induction in vitro of the synthesis of δ-aminolevulinic acid synthetase in chemical porphyria: a response to certain drugs, sex hormones and foreign chemicals. J. Biol. Chem., **241,** 1359, 1966.
46. Hirsch, G. H., Bubbar, G. L., and Marks, G. S.: Studies of the relationship between chemical structure and porphyria-inducing activity, III. Biochem. Pharmacol., **16,** 1455, 1967.
47. Talman, E. L., Labbe, R. F., and Aldrich, R. A.: Porphyrin metabolism IV. Molecular structure of acetamide derivatives affecting porphyrin metabolism. Arch. Biochem. Biophys., **66,** 289, 1957.
48. Solomon, H. M., and Figge, F. H. J.: Disturbance in porphyrin metabolism caused by feeding diethyl-1,4-dihydro-2,4,6-trimethylpyridine-3,5-dicarboxylate. Proc. Soc. Exp. Biol. Med., **100,** 583, 1959.
49. Granick, S., and Urata, G.: Increase in activity of δ-aminolevulinic acid synthetase in liver mitochondria induced by feeding of 3,5-dicarbethoxy-1,4-dihydrocollidine. J. Biol. Chem., **238,** 821, 1963.
50. Marver, H. S., Collins, A., Tschudy, D. P., and Rechcigl, M., Jr.: δ-Aminolevulinic acid synthetase. II. Induction in rat liver. J. Biol. Chem., **241,** 4323, 1966.
51. Granick, S., and Kappas, A.: Steroid induction of porphyrin synthesis in liver cell culture. I. Structural basis and possible physiological role. J. Biol. Chem., **242,** 4587, 1967.
52. With, T. K.: Porphyrin metabolism and barbiturate poisoning: observations on cases of acute and chronic poisoning. J. Clin. Path., **10,** 165, 1957.
53. Cam, C.: Cutaneous porphyria, related to intoxication. Dirim (Istanbul), **34,** 11, 1959.
54. Schmid, R.: Cutaneous porphyria in Turkey. New Eng. J. Med., **263,** 397, 1960.
55. Cam, C., and Nigogoysan, G.: Acquired toxic porphyria cutanea tarda due to hexachlorobenzene. J.A.M.A., **183,** 88, 1963.
56. Watson, C. J.: The porphyrias. Advances Intern. Med., **6,** 2, 1954.
57. Watson, C. J.: The problem of porphyria—some facts and questions. New Eng. J. Med., **263,** 1205, 1960.
58. Rimington, C.: Haem pigments and porphyrins. Ann. Rev. Biochem., **26,** 561, 1957.
59. Vannotti, A.: *Porphyrins: Their Biological and Chemical Importance.* Hilger and Watts, Ltd., London, 1954.
60. Bénard, H.: *Hémoglobine et pigments apparentés.* Masson et Cie, Paris, 1949.
61. With, T. K.: Acute intermittent porphyria: family studies on the excretion of PBG and delta-ALA with ion exchange chromatography. Z. Klin. Chem., **1,** 134, 1963.
62. Tschudy, D. P.: Biochemical lesions in porphyria. J.A.M.A., **191,** 718, 1965.
63. Lascelles, J.: *Tetrapyrrole Biosynthesis and Its Regulation.* W. A. Benjamin, Inc., New York, 1964.
64. Burnham, B. F.: Metabolism of porphyrins and corrinoids, in *Metabolic Pathways,* 3d ed., edited by David M. Greenberg, vol. 3, chap. 18. Academic, New York, 1969.
65. Wolstenholme, G. E. W., and Millar, E. C. P. (editors): *Porphyrin Biosynthesis and Metabolism,* Ciba Foundation. Churchill, London, 1955.
66. *Les Maladies du métabolisme des porphyrines,* 2ᵉ Colloque international de biologie de Saclay. Presses Universitaires de France, Paris, 1962.
67. Symposium on the normal and pathological metabolism of porphyrins. Panminerva Med., **4,** 305, 368, 1962.
68. Proceedings of the International Conference on the Porphyrias. South Afr. J. Lab. Clin. Med., **9,** 143, 1963.
69. Goodwin, T. W. (editor): *Porphyrins and Related Compounds,* Biochem. Soc. Symp. No. 28. Academic, New York, 1968.
70. Zoja, L.: Sur quelques pigments de certaines urines, et specialement sur la présence, dans celles-ci, de l'hématoporphyrine et de l'uroérythrine. Arch. Ital. Biol., **19,** 425, 1893.
71. Robitschek, W.: Haematoporphyria congenita. Z. Klin. Med., **101,** 540, 1925.
72. Hegler, C., Fraenkel, E., and Schumm, O.: Zur Lehre von der Haematoporphyria congenita. Deutsch. Med. Wschr., **39,** 842, 1913.
73. Liebig, H.: Ueber die experimentelle Bleihaematoporphyrie. Arch. Exp. Path. Pharmakol., **125,** 16, 1927.
74. Fischer, H., Hilmer, H., Lindner, F., and Puetzer, B.: Zur Kenntnis der natuerlichen Porphyrine: chemische Befunde bei einem Fall von Porphyrinurie (Petry). Z. Physiol. Chem., **150,** 44, 1925.
75. Waldenström, J.: Some observations on acute porphyria and other conditions with a change in the excretion of porphyrins. Acta Med. Scand., **83,** 281, 1934.
76. Schmid, R., Schwartz, S., and Watson, C. J.: Porphyrin content of bone

marrow and liver in the various forms of porphyria. A.M.A. Arch. Intern. Med., **93**, 167, 1954.

77. Derrien, E., and Benôit, C.: Notes et observations sur les urines et sur quelques organes d'une femme morte en crise de porphyrie aigue. Arch. Soc. Sci. Med. Biol. Montpellier et Languedoc, **10**, 456, 1929.
78. Prunty, F. T. G.: Acute porphyria: investigations on pathology of porphyrins and identification of excretion of uroporphyrin I. A.M.A. Arch. Intern. Med., **77**, 623, 1946.
79. Watson, C. J., Schwartz, S., and Hawkinson, V.: Studies of the uroporphyrins. II. Further studies of the porphyrins of the urine, feces, bile and liver in cases of porphyria with particular reference to a Waldenström-type porphyrin behaving as an entity on the Tswett column. J. Biol. Chem., **157**, 345, 1945.
80. MacGregor, A. G., Nicholas, R. E. H., and Rimington, C.: Porphyria cutanea tarda. A.M.A. Arch. Intern. Med., **90**, 483, 1952.
81. Drabkin, D. L.: Independent biosynthesis of different heme chromoproteins: cytochrome C in various tissues. Proc. Soc. Exp. Biol. Med., **76**, 527, 1951.
82. Price, V. E., Sterling, W. R., Tarantola, V. A., Hartley, R. W., Jr., and Rechcigl, M., Jr.: The kinetics of catalase synthesis and destruction in vivo. J. Biol. Chem., **237**, 3468, 1962.
83. Williams, J. N., Jr.: A method for the simultaneous quantitative estimation of cytochromes a, b, c_1, and c in mitochondria. Arch. Biochem. Biophys., **107**, 537, 1964.
84. Druyan, R., DeBerndard, B., and Rabinowitz, M.: Turnover of cytochromes labeled with δ-aminolevulinic acid-^{3}H in rat liver. J. Biol. Chem., **244**, 5874, 1969.
85. Omura, T., and Sato, R.: The carbon monoxide-binding pigment of liver microsomes. I. Evidence for its hemoprotein nature. J. Biol. Chem., **239**, 2370, 1964.
86. Levin, N., and Kuntzman, R.: Biphasic decrease of radioactive hemoprotein from liver microsomal CO-binding particles. J. Biol. Chem., **244**, 3671, 1969.
87. Schimke, R. T., Sweeney, E. W., and Berlin, C. M.: Studies of the stability in vivo and in vitro of rat liver tryptophan pyrrolase. J. Biol. Chem., **240**, 4609, 1965.
88. Schimke, R. T., Sweeney, E. W., and Berlin, C. M.: The roles of synthesis and degradation in the control of rat liver tryptophan pyrrolase. J. Biol. Chem., **240**, 322, 1965.
89. Prankerd, T. A. J.: *The Red Cell.* Blackwell Scientific Publications, Ltd., Oxford, 1961.
90. Marver, H. S., Tschundy, D. P., Perlroth, M. G., and Collins, A.: δ-Aminolevulinic acid synthetase. I. Studies in liver homogenates. J. Biol. Chem., **241**, 2803, 1966.
91. Watson, C. J., Lowry, P. T., Schmid, R., Hawkinson, V. E., and Schwartz, S.: The manifestations of the different forms of porphyria in relation to chemical findings. Trans. Ass. Amer. Physicians, **64**, 345, 1951.
92. Shemin, D., and Rittenberg, D.: The biological utilization of glycine for the synthesis of the protoporphyrin of hemoglobin. J. Biol. Chem., **166**, 621, 1946.
93. Shemin, D., and Rittenberg, D.: The life span of the human red blood cell. J. Biol. Chem., **166**, 627, 1946.
94. Gray, C. H.: Isotope studies in porphyria. Brit. Med. Bull., **8**, 229, 1952.
95. London, I. M., Shemin, D., West, R., and Rittenberg, D.: Heme synthesis and red blood cell dynamics in normal humans and in subjects with polycythemia vera, sickle-cell anemia, and pernicious anemia. J. Biol. Chem., **179**, 463, 1949.
96. Gray, C. H., Neuberger, A., and Sneath, P. H. A.: Studies in congenital porphyria. 2. Incorporation of ^{15}N in the stercobilin in the normal and in the porphyric. Biochem. J., **47**, 87, 1950.
97. Shemin, D., London, I. M., and Rittenberg, D.: The in vitro synthesis of heme from glycine by the nucleated red blood cell. J. Biol. Chem., **173**, 799, 1948.
98. Dresel, E. I. B., and Falk, J. E.: Studies on the biosynthesis of blood pigments. 1. Haem synthesis in haemolyzed erythrocytes of chicken blood. Biochem. J., **56**, 156, 1954.
99. London, I. M., Shemin, D., and Rittenberg, D.: Synthesis of heme in vitro by the immature non-nucleated mammalian erythrocyte. J. Biol. Chem., **183**, 749, 1950.
100. Muir, H. M., and Neuberger, A.: The biogenesis of porphyrins: the distribution of ^{15}N in the ring system. Biochem. J., **45**, 163, 1949.
101. Shemin, D.: The succinate-glycine cycle: the role of δ-aminolevulinic acid in porphyrin synthesis, in *Porphyrin Biosynthesis and Metabolism,* Ciba Foundation. Churchill, London, 1955.
102. Muir, H. M., and Neuberger, A.: The biogenesis of porphyrins. 2. The origin of the methene carbon atoms. Biochem. J., **47**, 97, 1950.
103. Radin, N. S., Rittenberg, D., and Shemin, D.: The role of glycine in the biosynthesis of heme. J. Biol. Chem., **184**, 745, 1950.
104. Grinstein, M., Kamen, M. D., and Moore, C. V.: Observation on the utilization of glycine in the biosynthesis of hemoglobin. J. Biol. Chem., **174**, 767, 1948.
105. Shemin, D., and Kumin, S.: The mechanism of porphyrin formation: the formation of a succinyl intermediate from succinate. J. Biol. Chem., **198**, 827, 1952.
106. Wriston, J. C., Jr., Lack, L., and Shemin, D.: The mechanism of porphyrin formation: further evidence on the relationship of the citric acid cycle and porphyrin formation. J. Biol. Chem., **215**, 603, 1955.
107. Shemin, D., and Wittenberg, J.: The mechanisms of porphyrin formation: the role of the tricarboxylic acid cycle. J. Biol. Chem. **192**, 315, 1951.
108. Wittenberg, J., and Shemin, D.: The location in protoporphyrin of the carbon atoms derived from the α-carbon atom of glycine. J. Biol. Chem., **185**, 103, 1950.
109. Shemin, D., and Russell, C. S.: Delta-aminolevulinic acid, its role in the biosynthesis of porphyrins and purines. J. Amer. Chem. Soc., **75**, 4873, 1953.
110. Shemin, D., Russell, C. S., and Abramsky, T.: The succinate-glycine cycle. I. The mechanism of pyrrole synthesis. J. Biol. Chem., **215**, 613, 1955.
111. Neuberger, A., and Scott, J. J.: Aminolaevulic acid and porphyrin biosynthesis. Nature (London), **172**, 1093, 1953.
112. Dresel, E. I. B., and Falk, J. E.: Conversion of δ-aminolaevulic acid to porphobilinogen in a tissue system. Nature (London), **172**, 1185, 1953.
113. Nemeth, A. M., Russell, C. S., and Shemin, D.: The succinate-glycine cycle. II. Metabolism of δ-aminolevulinic acid. J. Biol. Chem., **229**, 415, 1957.
114. Tait, G. H.: General aspects of haem synthesis, in *Porphyrins and Related Compounds,* edited by T. W. Goodwin, pp. 19–34. Academic, New York, 1968.
115. Dowdle, E., Mustard, P., Spong, N., and Eales, L.: The metabolism of [5-^{14}C] δ-aminolevulinic acid in normal and porphyric human subjects. Clin. Sci., **34**, 233, 1968.
116. Laver, W. G., Neuberger, A., and Udenfriend, S.: Initial stages in the biosynthesis of porphyrins. 1. The formation of δ-aminolaevulic acid by particles obtained from chicken erythrocytes. Biochem. J., **70**, 4, 1958.
117. Miyakoshi, T., and Kikuchi, G.: Studies on experimental porphyria. Report I. Increased synthesis of δ-aminolevulinic acid in allylisopropylacetamide-induced porphyria rat. Tohoku J. Exp. Med., **79**, 199, 1963.
118. Tschudy, D. P., Welland, F. H., Collins, A., and Hunter, G. W., Jr.: The effect of carbohydrate feeding on the induction of δ-aminolevulinic acid synthetase. Metabolism, **13**, 396, 1964.
119. Hayashi, N., Yoda, B., and Kikuchi, G.: Mechanisms of allylisopropylacetamide-induced increase of δ-aminolevulinate synthetase in liver mitochondria. IV. Accumulation of the enzyme in the soluble fraction of rat liver. Arch. Biochem. Biophys., **131**, 83, 1969.
120. Scholnick, P. L., Hammaker, L. E., and Marver, H. S.: Soluble hepatic δ-aminolevulinic acid synthetase: end-product inhibition of the partially purified enzyme. Proc. Nat. Acad. Sci. U.S.A., **63**, 65, 1969.
121. McKay, R., Druyan, R., Getz, G. S., and Rabinowitz, M.: Intramitochondrial localization of δ-aminolaevulinate synthetase and ferrochelatase in rat liver. Biochem. J., **114**, 455, 1969.
122. Scholnick, P. L., Hammaker, L. E., and Marver, H. S.: Regulation of the activity of purified hepatic δ-aminolevulinic acid synthetase (abstract). Fed. Proc., **29**, 542, 1970.
123. Shemin, D., Kikuchi, G., and Abramsky, T.: Enzymatic studies of the synthesis of some intermediates in porphyrin biogenesis, in *Les Maladies du métabolisme des porphyrines.* Presses Universitaires de France, Paris, 1962.

124. Burnham, B. F., and Lascelles, J.: Control of porphyrin biosynthesis through a negative feedback mechanism. Biochem. J., **87,** 462, 1963.
125. Schulman, J. P., and Richert, D. A.: Heme synthesis in vitamin B_6 and pantothenic acid deficiencies. J. Biol. Chem., **226,** 181, 1957.
126. Elder, T. D., and Mengel, C. E.: Effect of pyridoxine deficiency on porphyrin precursor excretion in acute intermittent porphyria. Amer. J. Med., **41,** 369, 1966.
127. Wintrobe, M. M.: Factors and mechanisms in the production of red corpuscles. Harvey Lect., **45,** 87, 1949–1950.
128. du Vigneaud, V., Kuchinskas, E. J., and Horvath, A.: L-Penicillamine and rat liver transaminase activity. Arch. Biochem. Biophys., **69,** 130, 1957.
129. Gibson, K. D., Laver, W. G., and Neuberger, A.: Initial stages in the biosynthesis of porphyrins. 2. The formation of δ-aminolaevulic acid from glycine and succinyl-coenzyme A by particles from chicken erythrocytes. Biochem. J., **70,** 71, 1958.
130. Kikuchi, G., Kuman, A., Talmage, P., and Shemin, D.: The enzymatic synthesis of δ-aminolevulinic acid. J. Biol. Chem., **233,** 1214, 1958.
131. Granick, S.: Porphyrin biosynthesis in erythrocytes. I. Formation of δ-aminolevulinic acid in erythrocytes. J. Biol. Chem., **232,** 1101, 1958.
132. Larsen, E. G., and Orten, J. M.: Studies of porphyrin biosynthesis in the nucleated avian erythrocyte. Abstract 69C, American Chemical Society 128th Meeting, Minneapolis, September, 1955.
133. Brown, E. G.: The relationship of the tricarboxylic acid cycle to the synthesis of δ-aminolaevulic acid in avian erythrocyte preparations. Biochem. J., **70,** 313, 1958.
134. Lascelles, J.: Synthesis of porphyrins by cell suspensions of *Tetrahymena vorax:* effect of members of the vitamin B group. Biochem. J., **66,** 65, 1957.
135. Urata, G., and Granick, S.: Biosynthesis of α-aminoketones and the metabolism of aminoacetone. J. Biol. Chem., **238,** 811, 1963.
136. Granick, S.: Enzymatic conversion of δ-aminolevulinic acid to porphobilinogen. Science, **120,** 1105, 1954.
137. Gibson, K. D.: Some properties of δ-aminolaevulinic acid dehydrase, in *Porphyrin Biosynthesis and Metabolism,* Ciba Foundation. Churchill, London, 1955.
138. Westall, R. G.: Isolation of porphobilinogen from the urine of a patient with acute porphyria. Nature (London), **170,** 614, 1952.
139. Nandi, D. L., France Baker-Cohen, K., and Shemin, D.: δ-Aminolevulinic acid dehydratase of *Rhodopseudomonas spheroides.* I. Isolation and properties. J. Biol. Chem., **243,** 1224, 1968.
140. Dresel, E. I. B., and Falk, J. E.: Studies on the biosynthesis of blood pigments. 3. Haem and porphyrin formation from δ-aminolaevulinic acid and from porphobilinogen in haemolyzed chicken erythrocytes. Biochem. J., **63,** 80, 1956.
141. Coleman, D. L.: Purification and properties of δ-aminolevulinate dehydratase from tissues of two strains of mice. J. Biol. Chem., **241,** 5511, 1966.
142. Doyle, D., and Schimke, R. T.: The genetic and developmental regulation of hepatic δ-aminolevulinate dehydratase in mice. J. Biol. Chem., **244,** 5449, 1969.
143. Bogorad, L.: Intermediates in the biosynthesis of porphyrins from porphobilinogen. Science, **121,** 878, 1955.
144. Schmid, R., and Shemin, D.: The enzymatic formation of porphobilinogen from δ-aminolevulinic acid and its conversion to protoporphyrin. J. Amer. Chem. Soc., **77,** 506, 1955.
145. Granick, S., and Mauzerall, D.: Porphyrin biosynthesis in erythrocytes. II. Enzymes converting δ-aminolevulinic acid to coproporphyrinogen. J. Biol. Chem., **232,** 1119, 1958.
146. Iodice, A. A., Richert, D. A., and Schulman, M. P.: Copper content of purified δ-aminolevulinic acid dehydrase. Fed. Proc., **17,** 248, 1958.
147. Wilson, M. L., Iodice, A. A., Schulman, M. P., and Richert, D. A.: Studies on liver δ-aminolevulinic acid dehydrase. Fed. Proc., **18,** 352, 1959.
148. van Heyningen, S., and Shemin, D.: Quaternary structure of δ-aminolevulinate dehydratase. Fed. Proc., **29,** 937, 1970.
149. Shemin, D.: On the synthesis of heme. Naturwissenschaften, **57,** 185, 1970.
150. Russell, R. L., and Coleman, D. L.: Genetic control of hepatic δ-aminolevulinate dehydratase in mice. Genetics, **48,** 1033, 1963.
151. Falk, J. E., Dresel, E. I. B., and Rimington, C.: Porphobilinogen as a porphyrin precursor, and interconversion of porphyrins in a tissue system. Nature (London), **172,** 292, 1953.
152. Bogorad, L., and Granick, S.: The enzymatic synthesis of porphyrins from porphobilinogen. Proc. Nat. Acad. Sci. U.S.A., **39,** 1176, 1953.
153. Schwartz, S.: Porphyrins and porphyrin precursors in human and experimental porphyria. Fed. Proc., **14,** 717, 1955.
154. Dresel, E. I. B.: The role of some porphyrins and porphyrin precursors in the biosynthesis of haeme, in *Porphyrin Biosynthesis and Metabolism,* Ciba Foundation. Churchill, London, 1955.
155. Neve, R. A., Labbe, R. F., and Aldrich, R. A.: Reduced uroporphyrin III in the biosynthesis of heme. J. Amer. Chem. Soc., **78,** 691, 1956.
156. Mauzerall, D., and Granick, S.: Porphyrin biosynthesis in erythrocytes. III. Uroporphyrinogen and its decarboxylase. J. Biol. Chem., **232,** 1141, 1958.
157. Bogorad, L.: The enzymatic synthesis of porphyrins from porphobilinogen. III. Uroporphyrinogens as intermediates. J. Biol. Chem., **233,** 516, 1958.
158. Fischer, H., and Orth, H.: *Die Chemie des Pyrrols.* Akademische Verlagsgesellschaft m.f.H., Leipzig, 1937.
159. Rimington, C.: The biosynthesis of haemoglobin. Brit. Med. J., **2,** 189, 1956.
160. Gray, C. H.: In *Biochemical Disorders in Human Disease.* Academic, New York, 1957.
161. Bogorad, L.: Enzymatic mechanisms in porphyrin synthesis: possible enzymatic blocks in porphyria. Ann. N.Y. Acad. Sci., **104,** 676, 1963.
162. Mauzerall, D.: Normal porphyrin metabolism. J. Pediat., **64,** 5, 1964.
163. Cookson, G. H., and Rimington, C.: Porphobilinogen. Biochem. J., **57,** 476, 1954.
164. Bullock, E., Johnson, A. W., Markham, E., and Shaw, K. B.: Formation of I- and III-type porphyrins by the polymerization of pyrroles. Nature (London), **185,** 607, 1960.
165. Waldenström, J., and Vahlquist, B.: Studien ueber die Entstehung der roten Harnpigmente (Uroporphyrin and Porphobilin) bei der akuten Porphyrie aus ihrer farblosen Vorstufe (Porphobilinogen). Z. Physiol. Chem., **260,** 189, 1939.
166. Mauzerall, D.: The condensation of porphobilinogen to uroporphyrinogen. J. Amer. Chem. Soc., **82,** 2605, 1960.
167. Mauzerall, D.: The thermodynamic stability of porphyrinogen. J. Amer. Chem. Soc., **82,** 2601, 1960.
168. Levin, E. Y., and Coleman, D. L.: The enzymatic conversion of porphobilinogen to uroporphyrinogen catalyzed by extracts of hematopoietic mouse spleen. J. Biol. Chem., **242,** 4248, 1967.
169. Levin, E. Y.: Uroporphyrinogen III cosynthetase from mouse spleen. Biochemistry, **7,** 3781, 1968.
170. Heath, H., and Hoare, D. S.: The biosynthesis of porphyrins from porphobilinogen by *Rhodopseudomonas spheroides.* Biochem. J., **72,** 13, 1959.
171. Booij, H. L., and Rimington, C.: Effect of preheating on porphyrin synthesis by red cells. Biochem. J., **65,** 4P, 1957.
172. Lockwood, W. H., and Rimington, C.: Purification of an enzyme converting porphobilinogen to uroporphyrin. Biochem. J., **67,** 8P, 1957.
173. Bogorad, L.: The enzymatic synthesis of porphyrins from porphobilinogen. I. Uroporphyrinogen I. J. Biol. Chem., **233,** 501, 1958.
174. Bogorad, L.: The enzymatic synthesis of porphyrins from porphobilinogen. II. Uroporphyrin III. J. Biol. Chem., **233,** 510, 1958.
175. Bogorad, L., and Marks, G.: The enzymatic synthesis of uroporphyrins from porphobilinogen. IV. Investigations on the participation of formaldehyde. J. Biol. Chem., **235,** 2127, 1960.
176. Hoare, D. S., and Heath, H.: Intermediates in the biosynthesis of porphyrins from porphobilinogen by *Rhodopseudomonas spheroides.* Nature (London), **181,** 1592, 1958.
177. Carpenter, A. T., and Scott, J. J.: The relationship of opsopyrroledicarboxylic acid to the biosynthesis of porphyrins. Biochem. J., **71,** 325, 1959.
178. Carpenter, A. T., and Scott, J. J.: The inhibition of porphobilinogen deaminase by isoporphobilinogen. Biochim. Biophys. Acta, **52,** 195, 1961.
179. Lockwood, W. H., and Benson, A.: The enzymatic condensation of porphobilinogen to porphyrins. Biochem. J., **75,** 372, 1960.

180. Shemin, D., Abramsky, T., and Russell, C. S.: The synthesis of protoporphyrin from δ-aminolevulinic acid in a cell-free extract. J. Amer. Chem. Soc., **76,** 1204, 1954.
181. Dresel, E. I. B., and Falk, J. E.: Studies on the biosynthesis of blood pigments. 5. Intermediates in haem biosynthesis. Biochem. J., **63,** 388, 1956.
182. Batlle, A. M., del C., and Grinstein, M.: Porphyrin biosynthesis. Phyriaporphyrinogen III, a normal intermediate in the biosynthesis of protoporphyrin IX. Biochim. Biophys. Acta, **62,** 197, 1962.
183. San Mártin de Viale, L. C., and Grinstein, M.: Porphyrin biosynthesis. IV. 5- and 6-COOH porphyrinogens (type III) as normal intermediates in haem biosynthesis. Biochim. Biophys. Acta, **158,** 79, 1968.
184. Cornford, P.: Transformation of porphobilinogen into porphyrins by preparations from human erythrocytes. Biochem. J., **91,** 66, 1964.
185. Sano, S., and Granick, S.: Mitochondrial coproporphyrinogen oxidase and protoporphyrin formation. J. Biol. Chem., **236,** 1173, 1961.
186. Batlle, A. M., del C., Benson, A. M., and Rimington, C.: Purification and properties of coproporphyrinogenase. Biochem. J., **97,** 731, 1965.
187. Granick, S., and Mauzerall, D.: Enzymes of porphyrin synthesis in red blood cells. Ann. N.Y. Acad. Sci., **75,** 115, 1958.
188. Granick, S., and Mauzerall, D.: Enzymic formation of protoporphyrin from coproporphyrinogen III. Fed. Proc., **17,** 233, 1958.
189. Schwartz, S., and Cardinal, R.: Incorporation of ALA-C^{14} into dog tissue hemes. Fed. Proc., **24,** 485, 1965.
190. Sano, S.: 2,4- Bis(β-hydroxypropionic acid) deuteroporphyrinogen IX, a possible intermediate between coproporphyrinogen III and protoporphyrin IX. J. Biol. Chem., **241,** 5276, 1966.
191. Heikel, T., Lockwood, W. H., and Rimington, C.: Formation of non-enzymic haem. Nature (London), **182,** 313, 1958.
192. Sano, S., and Tanaka, K.: Recombination of protoporphyrinogen with cytochrome c apoproteins. J. Biol. Chem., **239,** PC 3109, 1964.
193. Krueger, R. C., Melnick, I., and Klein, J. R.: Formation of heme by broken-cell preparations of duck erythrocytes. Arch. Biochem. Biophys., **64,** 302, 1956.
194. Goldberg, A., Ashenbrucker, H., Cartwright, G. E., and Wintrobe, M. M.: Studies on the biosynthesis of heme in vitro by avian erythrocytes. Blood, **11,** 821, 1956.
195. Lochhead, A. C., Kramer, S., and Goldberg, A.: Quantitative measurement of the iron-incorporating enzyme in relation to marrow cells and liver tissue in the rabbit. Brit. J. Haemat., **9,** 39, 1963.
196. Labbe, R. F., Hubbard, N., and Caughey, W. S.: Porphyrin specificity of ferro: protoporphyrin chelatase from rat liver. Biochemistry, **2,** 372, 1963.
197. Oyama, H., Sugita, Y., Yoneyama, Y., and Yoshikawa, H.: Stoichiometry of heme synthesis by partially purified enzyme preparation from duck erythrocytes. Biochim. Biophys. Acta, **47,** 413, 1961.
198. Yoneyama, Y., Oyama, H., Sugita, Y., and Yoshikawa, H.: Iron-chelating enzyme from duck erythrocytes. Biochim. Biophys. Acta, **62,** 261, 1962.
199. Granick, S.: Porphyrin and chlorophyll biosynthesis in *Chlorella,* in *Porphyrin Biosynthesis and Metabolism,* Ciba Foundation. Churchill, London, 1955.
200. Lascelles, J.: Synthesis of tetrapyrroles by micro-organisms. Physiol. Rev., **41,** 417, 1961.
201. Bray, R. C., and Shemin, D.: On the biosynthesis of vitamin B_{12}, J. Biol. Chem., **238,** 1501, 1963.
202. Porra, R. T., and Jones, O. T. G.: Studies on ferrochelatase. I. Assay and properties of ferrochelatase from a pig-liver mitochondrial extract. Biochem. J., **87,** 181, 1963.
203. Harris, J. W.: *The Red Cell, Production, Metabolism, Destruction: Normal and Abnormal.* Harvard, Cambridge, Mass., 1963.
204. Mauzerall, D., and Granick, S.: The occurrence and determination of δ-aminolevulinic acid and porphobilinogen in urine. J. Biol. Chem., **219,** 435, 1956.
205. Dean, G., and Barnes, H. D.: Porphyria in Sweden and South Africa. South Afr. Med. J., **33,** 274, 1959.
206. Malooly, D. A., and Hightower, N. C., Jr.: Quantitative determination of porphobilinogen and delta-aminolevulinic acid in the urine. J. Lab. Clin. Med., **59,** 568, 1962.
207. Berlin, N. I., Neuberger, A., and Scott, J. J.: The metabolism of δ-aminolaevulic acid. 2. Normal pathways, studied with the aid of ^{14}C. Biochem. J., **64,** 90, 1956.
208. Berlin, N. I., Neuberger, A., and Scott, J. J.: The metabolism of δ-aminolaevulic acid. 1. Normal pathways, studied with the aid of ^{15}N. Biochem. J., **64,** 80, 1956.
209. Granick, S., and Van den Schrieck, H. G.: Porphobilinogen and δ-aminolevulinic acid in acute porphyria. Proc. Soc. Exp. Biol. Med., **88,** 270, 1955.
210. Haeger-Aronsen, B.: Studies on urinary excretion of δ-aminolaevulic acid and other haem precursors in lead workers and lead-intoxicated rabbits. Scand. J. Clin. Lab. Invest., **12,** suppl. 47, 1960.
211. Robinson, S. H., Tsong, M., Brown, B. W., and Schmid, R.: The sources of bile pigment in the rat: studies of the "early labeled" fraction. J. Clin. Invest., **45,** 1569, 1966.
212. Watson, C. J., and Schwartz, S.: A simple test for urinary porphobilinogen. Proc. Soc. Exp. Biol. Med., **47,** 393, 1941.
213. Watson, C. J., Bossenmaier, I., and Cardinal, R.: Acute intermittent porphyria: urinary porphobilinogen and other Ehrlich reactors in diagnosis. J.A.M.A., **175,** 1087, 1961.
214. Hammond, R. L., and Welcker, M. L.: Porphobilinogen tests on a thousand miscellaneous patients in a search for false positive reactions. J. Lab. Clin. Med., **33,** 1254, 1948.
215. Watson, C. J.: Some studies of nature and clinical significance of porphobilinogen. A.M.A. Arch. Intern. Med., **93,** 643, 1954.
216. Schwartz, S., Keprios, M., and Schmid, R.: Experimental porphyria. II. Type produced by lead, phenylhydrazine, and light. Proc. Soc. Exp. Biol. Med., **79,** 463, 1952.
217. Goldberg, A.: Fate of porphobilinogen, administered enterally or parenterally, in the rat. Biochem. J., **59,** 37, 1955.
218. Dresel, E. I. B., and Falk, J. E.: Studies on the biosynthesis of blood pigments. 2. Haem and porphyrin formation in intact chicken erythrocytes. Biochem. J., **63,** 72, 1956.
219. Zieve, L., Hill, E., Schwartz, S., and Watson, C. J.: Normal limits of urinary coproporphyrin excretion determined by an improved method. J. Lab. Clin. Med., **41,** 663, 1953.
220. Eales, L., and Saunders, S. J.: The diagnostic importance of faecal porphyrins in the differentiation of the porphyrias. I. Values in normal subjects and in patients with non-porphyric disorders. South Afr. J. Lab. Clin. Med., **8,** 127, 1963.
221. Schwartz, S., Berg, M. H., Bossenmaier, I., and Dinsmore, H.: Determination of porphyrins in biological materials, in *Methods of Biochemical Analysis,* edited by D. Glick, vol. VIII. Interscience, New York, 1960.
222. Goldberg, A., Smith, J. A., and Lochhead, A. C.: Treatment of lead-poisoning with oral penicillamine. Brit. Med. J., **1,** 1270, 1963.
223. Comfort, A., Moore, H., and Weatherall, M.: Normal human urinary porphyrins. Biochem. J., **58,** 177, 1954.
224. Watson, C. J., Hawkinson, V., Schwartz, S., and Sutherland, D.: Studies of coproporphyrin. I. The per diem excretion and isomer distribution of coproporphyrin in normal human urine. J. Clin. Invest., **28,** 447, 1949.
225. Hoffbauer, F. W., Watson, C. J., and Schwartz, S.: Urinary and fecal coproporphyrin excretion in rats. III. Excretion of injected coproporphyrin. Proc. Soc. Exp. Biol. Med., **83,** 238, 1953.
226. Sano, S., and Rimington, C.: Excretion of various porphyrins and their corresponding porphyrinogens by rabbits after intravenous injection. Biochem. J., **86,** 203, 1963.
227. Watson, C. J., Pimenta de Mello, R., Schwartz, S., Hawkinson, V. E., and Bossenmaier, I.: Porphyrin chromogens or precursors in urine, blood, bile and feces. J. Lab. Clin. Med., **37,** 831, 1951.
228. Lockwood, W. H., and Bloomfield, B.: Uroporphyrins. III. Crystalline uroporphyrin from normal human urine. Aust. J. Exp. Biol. Med. Sci., **32,** 733, 1954.
229. With, T. K., and Petersen, H. C. A.: Symptomatic uroporphyrinuria. Lancet, **2,** 1148, 1954.
230. Nicholas, R. E. H., and Rimington, C.: Qualitative analysis of the porphyrins by partition chromatography. Scand. J. Clin. Lab. Invest., **1,** 12, 1949.
231. Watson, C. J.: Concerning the naturally occurring porphyrins. V. Porphyrins of the feces. J. Clin. Invest., **16,** 383, 1937.

232. Herbert, F. K.: The coproporphyrin precursor of human urine, and another pigment formed from a chromogen. Biochem. J., **69**, 10P, 1958.
233. Comfort, A., and Weatherall, M.: Urinary porphyrins in lead-treated rabbits. Biochem. J., **54**, 247, 1953.
234. Brockman, P. E., and Gray, C. H.: Studies on porphobilinogen. Biochem. J., **54**, 22, 1953.
235. Cookson, G. H., and Rimington, C.: Porphobilinogen. Biochem. J., **57**, 476, 1954.
236. England, M. T., Cotton, V., and French, J. M.: Faecal porphyrin excretion in normal subjects and in patients with the "malabsorption syndrome." Clin. Sci., **22**, 447, 1962.
237. Barnes, H. D.: Counter-current analysis of ether-soluble stool porphyrins. South Afr. J. Lab. Clin. Med., **9**, 177, 1963.
238. French, J. M., England, M. T., Lines, J., and Thonger, E.: Separation of ether-extractable fecal porphyrins by counter-current distribution. Arch. Biochem. Biophys., **107**, 404, 1964.
239. Haeger-Aronsen, B.: Fecal porphyrins in porphyria acuta intermittens, porphyria cutanea tarda and intoxicatio plumbi. Scand. J. Clin. Lab. Invest., **14**, 397, 1962.
240. Barnes, H.: In Conference discussion. South Afr. J. Lab. Clin. Med., **9**, 302, 1963.
241. Schwartz, S., and Wikoff, H. M.: The relation of erythrocyte coproporphyrin and protoporphyrin to erythropoiesis. J. Biol. Chem., **194**, 563, 1952.
242. Schmid, R., Schwartz, S., and Watson, C. J.: Porphyrins in the bone marrow and circulating erythrocytes in experimental anemia. Proc. Soc. Exp. Biol. Med., **75**, 705, 1950.
243. Dobriner, K., and Rhoads, C. P.: The porphyrins in health and disease. Physiol. Rev., **20**, 416, 1940.
244. Hausmann, W., and Haxthausen, H.: *Die Lichterkrankungen der Haut.* Urban & Schwarzenberg, Berlin, 1929.
245. Fischer, H., and Zerweck, W.: Ueber den Harnfarbstoff bei normalen und pathologischen Verhaeltnissen und seine lichtschuetzende Wirkung: zugleich einige Beitraege zur Kenntnis der Porphyrinurie. Z. Physiol. Chem., **137**, 176, 1924.
246. Meyer-Betz, F.: Untersuchungen ueber die biologische (photodynamische) Wirkung des Haematoporphyrins und anderer Derivate des Blut- und Gallenfarbstoffes. Deutsch. Arch. Klin. Med., **62**, 476, 1913.
247. Strauch, C. B.: Photosensitivation. Amer. J. Dis. Child., **40**, 800, 1930.
248. Blum, H. F., and Hardgrave, L. E.: Spectral region of photosensitivity in hydroa aestivale seu vacciniforme with porphyrinuria. Proc. Soc. Exp. Biol. Med., **34**, 613, 1936.
249. Blum, H. F., and Pace, N.: Studies of photosensitization by porphyrins. Brit. J. Derm. Syph., **49**, 465, 1937.
250. Fischer, H.: Ueber die Giftigkeit, die sensibilisierende Wirkung, das spektroskopische Verhalten der natürlichen Porphyrine. Z. Physiol. Chem., **97**, 109, 1916.
251. Magnus, I. A., Porter, A. D., and Rimington, C.: Action spectrum for skin lesions in porphyria cutanea tarda. Lancet, **1**, 912, 1959.
252. Magnus, I. A.: Action spectrum and other studies on patients with porphyria. South Afr. J. Lab. Clin. Med., **9**, 238, 1963.
253. Runge, W., and Watson, C. J.: Experimental production of skin lesions in human cutaneous porphyria. Proc. Soc. Exp. Biol. Med., **109**, 809, 1962.
254. Schwartz, S.: In discussion of J. J. Scott [65].
255. Feldberg, W., and Talesnik, J.: Reduction of tissue histamine by compound 48/80. J. Physiol., **120**, 550, 1953.
256. Gray, C. H.: In discussion of J. J. Scott [65].
257. Rimington, C., Magnus, I. A., Ryan, E. A., and Cripps, D. J.: Porphyria and photosensitivity. Quart. J. Med., **36**, 29, 1967.
258. Borst, M., and Koenigsdoerffer, H.: Untersuchungen ueber Porphyrie mit besonderer Beruecksichtigung der Porphyria congenita. S. Hirzel, Leipzig, 1929.
259. Burnett, J. W., and Pathak, M. A.: Pathogenesis of cutaneous photosensitivity in porphyria. New Eng. J. Med., **268**, 1203, 1963.
260. Scholnick, P., and Marver, H. S.: The molecular basis of chloroquine responsiveness in porphyria cutanea tarda. Clin. Res., **16**, 258, 1968.
261. Jarrett, A., Rimington, C., and Willoughby, D. A.: δ-Aminolaevulic acid and porphyria. Lancet, **1**, 125, 1956.
262. Pimenta de Mello, R.: Effect of rose Bengal and ultraviolet light on porphyrin excretion in rabbits. Proc. Soc. Exp. Biol. Med., **72**, 292, 1949.
263. Pimenta de Mello, R.: Effect of light on urinary coproporphyrin excretion in lead-poisoned rabbits. Proc. Soc. Exp. Biol. Med., **76**, 823, 1951.
264. Weatherall, M.: Drugs and porphyrin metabolism. Pharmacol. Rev., **6**, 133, 1954.
265. Harber, L. C., Fleischer, A. S., and Baer, R. L.: Erythropoietic protoporphyria and photohemolysis. J.A.M.A., **189**, 191, 1964.
266. Peterka, E. S., Runge, W. J., and Fusaro, R. M.: Erythropoietic protoporphyria. III. Photohemolysis. Arch. Derm. (Chicago), **94**, 282, 1966.
267. Fleischer, A. S., Haber, L. C., Cook, J. S., and Baer, R. L.: Mechanism of in vitro photohemolysis in erythropoietic protoporphyria (EPP). J. Invest. Derm., **46**, 505, 1966.
268. Schreus, H. T., and Carrié, C.: Untersuchungen zum Gallenfarbstoffwechsel. Klin. Wschr., **13**, 1670, 1934.
269. Reitlinger, K., and Klee, P.: Zur biologischen Wirkung der Porphyrine. Arch. Exp. Path. Pharmakol., **127**, 277, 1928.
270. Goldberg, A., Paton, W. D. M., and Thompson, J. W.: Pharmacology of the porphyrins and porphobilinogen. Brit. J. Pharmacol., **9**, 91, 1954.
271. Goldberg, A., and Rimington, C.: Fate of porphobilinogen in the rat: relation to acute porphyria in man. Lancet, **2**, 172, 1954.
272. Bingel, A.: Die Bedeutung der Porphyrine fur die Pathogenese gewisser neurologischer Krankheitsbilder. Z. Ges. Neurol. Psychiat., **158**, 79, 1937.
273. Gibson, J. B., and Goldberg, A.: The neuropathology of acute porphyria. J. Path. Bact., **71**, 495, 1956.
274. Feldman, D. S., Levere, R. D., Lieberman, J. S., Cardinal, R. A., and Watson, C. J.: Inhibition of the neuromuscular junction by porphobilinogen and porphobilin as compared with uroporphyrins I and III (abstract). J. Clin. Invest., **49**, 28*a*, 1970.
275. Herriot, R. M.: Kinetics of the formation of pepsin from swine pepsinogen and identification of an intermediate compound. J. Gen. Physiol., **22**, 65, 1938.
276. Schoenheimer, R.: *The Dynamic State of Body Constituents.* Harvard, Cambridge, Mass., 1942.
277. Schimke, R. T., Ganschow, R., Doyle, D., and Arias, I. M.: Regulation of protein turnover in mammalian tissues. Fed. Proc., **27**, 1223, 1968.
278. Tomkins, G., and Ames, B. N.: The operon concept in bacteria and in higher organisms. Nat. Cancer Inst. Monogr., **27**, 221, 1967.
279. Tomkins, G. M., Gelehrter, T. D., Granner, D., Martin, D., Jr., Samuels, H. H., and Thompson, E. B.: Control of specific gene expression in higher organisms. Science, **166**, 1474, 1969.
280. Harris, H.: Nuclear ribonucleic acid, in *Progress in Nucleic Acid Research,* edited by J. N. Davidson and W. E. Cohn, vol. 2, p. 19. Academic, New York, 1963.
281. Scherrer, K., Marcaud, L., Zajdela, F., London, I., and Gros, F.: Patterns of RNA metabolism in a differentiated cell: a rapidly labelled, unstable 60S RNA with messenger properties in duck erythroblasts. Proc. Nat. Acad. Sci. U.S.A., **56**, 1571, 1966.
282. Shearer, R., and McCarthy, B.: Evidence of ribonucleic acid molecules restricted to the cell nucleus. Biochemistry, **6**, 283, 1967.
283. Jones, O. T. G.: Personal communication.
284. Marver, H. S., Tschudy, D. P., Perlroth, M. G., and Collins, A.: Coordinate synthesis of heme and apoenzyme in the formation of tryptophan pyrrolase. Science, **154**, 501, 1966.
285. Burka, E. R.: Hemin: an inhibitor of erythroid cell ribonuclease. Science, **162**, 1287, 1968.
286. Umbarger, H. E.: Feedback control by endproduct inhibition, in Cellular Regulatory Mechanisms. Sympos. Quant. Biol., **26**, 301, 1961.
287. Moyed, Harris, S., and Umbarger, H. E.: Regulation of biosynthetic pathways. Physiol. Rev., **42**, 444, 1962.
288. Gerhart, J. C., and Pardee, A. B.: The enzymology of control by feedback inhibition. J. Biol. Chem., **237**, 891, 1962.
289. Monod, J., Changeux, J.-P., and Jacob, F.: On the nature of allosteric transitions: a plausible model. J. Molec. Biol., **12**, 88, 1965.
290. Koshland, D. E., Jr., and Neet, K. E.: The catalytic and regulatory properties of enzymes. Ann. Rev. Biochem., **37**, 359, 1968.

291. Chabner, B. A., Stein, J. A., and Tschudy, D. P.: Effect of dietary pyridoxine deficiency on experimental porphyria. Metabolism, **19**, 189, 1970.
292. Lichtman, H. C., and Feldman, F.: In vitro pyrrole and porphyrin synthesis in lead poisoning and iron deficiency. J. Clin. Invest., **42**, 830, 1963.
293. Goldberg, A.: Lead poisoning as a disorder of heme synthesis. Seminars Hemat., **5**, 424, 1968.
294. Tschudy, D. P., and Collins, A.: Effect of 3-amino-1,2,4-triazole on δ-aminolevulinic acid dehydrase activity. Science, **126**, 168, 1957.
295. Baron, J., and Tephly, T. R.: Effect of 3-amino-1,2,4-triazole on the stimulation of hepatic microsomal heme synthesis and induction of hepatic microsomal oxidases produced by phenobarbital. Molec. Pharmacol., **5**, 10, 1969.
296. Marver, H., Kaufman, L., and Manning, J.: Enhanced heme degradation in experimental porphyria. Fed. Proc., **27**, 774, 1968.
297. Wada, O.: Pathogenesis of hepatic porphyria. Jap. J. Med., **7**, 93, 1968.
298. Waterfield, M. D., Del Favero, A., and Gray, C. H.: Effect of 1,4-dihydro-3,5-dicarbethoxycollidine on hepatic microsomal haem, cytochrome b_5 and cytochrome P450 in rabbits and mice. Biochim. Biophys. Acta, **184**, 470, 1969.
299. De Matteis, F.: Rapid loss of cytochrome P-450 and haem caused in the liver microsomes by the porphyrogenic agent 2-allyl-2-isopropylacetamide. FEBS Letters, **6**, 343, 1970.
300. Meyer, U. A., and Marver, H. S.: Hepatic porphyria: inappropriate induction of δ-aminolevulinic acid synthetase by enhanced hemoprotein turnover. J. Clin. Invest., **49**, 66*a*, 1970.
301. Jacob, F., and Monod, J.: On the regulation of gene activity, in Cellular Regulatory Mechanisms. Sympos. Quant. Biol., **26**, 193, 1961.
302. Gilbert, W., and Müller-Hill, B.: Isolation of the Lac repressor. Proc. Nat. Acad. Sci. U.S.A., **56**, 1891, 1966.
303. Gilbert, W., and Müller-Hill, B.: The Lac operator is DNA. Proc. Nat. Acad. Sci. U.S.A., **58**, 2415, 1967.
304. Ptashne, M.: Isolation of the λ phage repressor. Proc. Nat. Acad. Sci. U.S.A., **57**, 306, 1967.
305. Ptashne, M.: Specific binding of the λ phage repressor to λ DNA. Nature (London), **214**, 232, 1967.
306. Marver, H. S.: The role of heme in the synthesis and repression of microsomal protein, in *Microsomes and Drug Oxidations,* edited by J. R. Gillete, A. H. Conney, G. J. Cosmides, R. W. Estabrook, J. R. Fouts, and G. J. Mannerning, p. 495. Academic, New York, 1969.
307. Marver, H. S., Schmid, R., and Schutzel, H.: Heme and methemoglobin: naturally occurring repressors of microsomal protein. Biochem. Biophys. Res. Commun., **33**, 969, 1968.
308. Waxman, A. D., Collins, A., and Tschudy, D. P.: Oscillations of hepatic δ-aminolevulinic acid synthetase produced in vivo by heme. Biochem. Biophys. Res. Commun., **24**, 675, 1966.
309. Kappas, A., and Granick, S.: Steroid induction of porphyrin synthesis in liver cell culture. II. The effects of heme, uridine diphosphate glucuronic acid, and inhibitors of nucleic acid and protein synthesis on the induction process. J. Biol. Chem., **243**, 346, 1968.
310. Strand, L. J., Felsher, B. W., Redeker, A. G., and Marver, H. S.: Enzymatic abnormalities in heme biosynthesis in intermittent acute porphyria: decreased hepatic conversion of porphobilinogen to porphyrins and increased δ-aminolevulinic acid synthetase activity. Proc. Nat. Acad. Sci. U.S.A., **67**, 1315, 1970.
311. Marver, H. S., and Manning, J.: In preparation.
312. Tschudy, D. P., Marver, H. S., and Collins, A.: A model for calculating messenger RNA half-life: short-lived messenger RNA in the induction of mammalian δ-aminolevulinic acid synthetase. Biochem. Biophys. Res. Commun., **21**, 480, 1965.
313. Narisawa, K., and Kikuchi, G.: Mechanism of allyl-isopropylacetamide-induced increase of δ-aminolevulinate synthetase in rat-liver mitochondria. Biochim. Biophys. Acta, **123**, 596, 1966.
314. Marks, G. S., Hunter, E. G., Terner, U. K., and Schneck, D.: Studies on the relationship between chemical structure and porphyria-inducing activity. Biochem. Pharmacol., **14**, 1077, 1965.
315. Kaufman, L., Swanson, A. L., and Marver, H. S.: Chemically induced porphyria: prevention by pretreatment with phenobarbital. Science, **170**, 320, 1970.
316. Remmer, H., and Merker, H. J.: Effect of drugs on the formation of smooth endoplasmic reticulum and drug metabolizing enzymes. Ann. N.Y. Acad. Sci., **123**, 79, 1965.
317. Conney, A. H.: Pharmacological implications of microsomal enzyme induction. Pharmacol. Rev., **19**, 317, 1967.
318. Marver, H. S.: Experimental and acute intermittent porphyria: a suggested role of disordered drug metabolism (abstract). J. Lab. Clin. Med., **68**, 996, 1966.
319. Marver, H. S., and Schmid, R.: Biotransformation in the liver: implications for human disease. Gastroenterology, **55**, 282, 1968.
320. Baron, J., and Tephly, T. R.: The role of heme synthesis during the induction of hepatic microsomal cytochrome P-450 and drug metabolism produced by benzpyrene. Biochem. Biophys. Res. Commun., **36**, 526, 1969.
321. Onisawa, J., and Labbe, R. F.: Effects of diethyl-1,4-dihydro-2,4,6-trimethylpyridine-3,5-dicarboxylate on the metabolism of porphyrins and iron. J. Biol. Chem., **238**, 724, 1963.
322. Wada, O., Yano, Y., Urata, G., and Nakao, K.: Behavior of hepatic microsomal cytochromes after treatment of mice with drugs known to disturb porphyrin metabolism in liver. Biochem. Pharmacol., **17**, 595, 1968.
323. Stein, J. A., Tschudy, D. P., Corcoran, P. L., and Collins, A.: δ-Aminolevulinic acid synthetase. III. Synergistic effect of chelated iron on induction. J. Biol. Chem., **245**, 2213, 1970.
324. Charley, P., Rosenstein, M., Shore, E., and Saltman, P.: The role of chelation and binding equilibria in iron metabolism. Arch. Biochem. Biophys., **88**, 222, 1960.
325. Strickland, E. H., and Daris, B. C.: Fe^{3+} uptake by rat-liver mitochondria. Biochim. Biophys. Acta, **104**, 596, 1965.
326. Granick, S., and Kappas, A.: Steroid control of porphyrin and heme biosynthesis: a new biological function of steroid hormone metabolites. Proc. Nat. Acad. Sci. U.S.A., **57**, 1463, 1967.
327. Kappas, A., Song, C. S., and Sachson, R. A., Levere, R. D., and Granick, S.: Induction of δ-aminolevulinic acid synthetase in vivo in chick embryo liver by natural steroids. Proc. Nat. Acad. Sci. U.S.A., **61**, 509, 1968.
328. Marver, H. S., and Manning, J.: Unpublished observations.
329. Necheles, T. F., and Rai, U. S.: Studies on the control of hemoglobin synthesis: the in vitro stimulating effect of a 5β-H steroid metabolite on heme formation in human bone marrow cells. Blood, **34**, 380, 1969.
330. Gorshein, D., and Gardner, F. H.: Erythropoietic activity of steroid metabolites in mice. Proc. Nat. Acad. Sci. U.S.A., **65**, 564, 1970.
331. Gordon, A. S., Zanjani, E. D., Levere, R. D., and Kappas, A.: Stimulation of mammalian erythropoiesis by 5β-H steroid metabolites. Proc. Nat. Acad. Sci. U.S.A., **65**, 919, 1970.
332. Levere, R. D., Kappas, A., and Granick, S.: Stimulation of hemoglobin synthesis in chick blastoderms by certain 5β androstane and 5β pregnane steroids. Proc. Nat. Acad. Sci. U.S.A., **58**, 985, 1967.
333. Rose, J. A., Hellman, E. S., and Tschudy, D. P.: Effect of diet on the induction of experimental porphyria. Metabolism, **10**, 514, 1961.
334. Welland, F. H., Hellman, E. S., Gaddis, E. M., Collins, A., Hunter, G. W., Jr., and Tschudy, D. P.: Factors affecting the excretion of porphyrin precursors by patients with acute intermittent porphyria. I. The effects of diet. Metabolism, **13**, 232, 1964.
335. De Matteis, F.: Increased synthesis of L-ascorbic acid caused by drugs which induce porphyria. Biochim. Biophys. Acta, **82**, 641, 1964.
336. Peraino, C., and Pitot, H. C.: Studies on the induction and repression of enzymes in rat liver. II. Carbohydrate repression of dietary and hormonal induction of threonine dehydrase and ornithine δ-transaminase. J. Biol. Chem., **239**, 4308, 1964.
337. Csányi, V., Greengard, O., and Knox, W. E.: The inductions of tyrosine aminotransferase by glucagon and hydrocortisone. J. Biol. Chem., **242**, 2688, 1967.
338. Richards, F. F., and Scott, J. J.: Glycine metabolism in acute porphyria. Clin. Sci., **20**, 387, 1961.
339. Tschudy, D. P., Rose, J., Hellman, E., Collins, A., and Rechcigl, M.,

Jr.: Biochemical studies of experimental porphyria. Metabolism, **11**, 1287, 1962.
340. Dixon, M., and Webb, E. C.: *Enzymes,* pp. 550–554. Academic, New York, 1964.
341. Turner, W. J., and Obermayer, M. E.: Studies on porphyria. II. A case of porphyria with epidermolysis bullosa, hypertrichosis and melanosis. Arch. Derm. Syph., **37**, 549, 1938.
342. Mackey, L., and Garrod, A. E.: On congenital porphyrinuria associated with hydroa aestivale and pink teeth. Quart. J. Med., **15**, 319, 1922.
343. Cappelli, J.: Caso singolare di hydroa vacciniforme con ematoporfirinuria ed ipertricosi. Gior. Ital. Mal. Vener., **55**, 481, 1914.
344. Garrod, A. E.: Congenital porphyria, a postscript. Quart. J. Med., n.s., **5**, 473, 1936.
345. Gray, C. H., and Neuberger, A.: Effect of splenectomy in a case of congenital porphyria. Lancet, **1**, 851, 1952.
346. Gray, A. M. H.: Haematoporphyria congenita with hydroa vacciniforme and hirsuties. Quart. J. Med., **19**, 381, 1926.
347. Sato, A., and Takahasi, N.: A new form of congenital hematoporphyria: oligochromemia, porphyrinuria (megalosplenica congenita). Amer. J. Dis. Child., **32**, 325, 1926.
348. Ashby, H. T.: Haematoporphyria congenita: its association with hydroa vacciniforme and pigmentation of the teeth. Quart. J. Med., **19**, 375, 1926.
349. Kench, J. D., Langley, F. A., and Wilkinson, J. F.: Biochemical and pathological studies of congenital porphyria. Quart. J. Med., n.s., **22**, 285, 1955.
350. Schmidt-La Baume, F.: Hydroa aestivale. Klin. Wschr., **6**, 827, 1926.
351. Kitagawa, K.: Ueber Haematoporphyria congenita "Hans Günther" und ihre experimentelle Untersuchung. Jap. J. Derm. Urol., **27**, 43, 1927.
352. Matsuoka, K.: Ueber Haematoporphyria congenita. Jap. J. Derm. Urol., **28**, 38, 1928.
353. Marcozzi, A.: Epidermolisi bullosa distrofica con ematoporfirinuria ed alterazione endocrino-simpatica (eritrodontia). Arch. Ital. Derm. Sif., **4**, 555, 1929.
354. Aldrich, R. A., Hawkinson, V., Grinstein, M., and Watson, C. J.: Photosensitive or congenital porphyria with hemolytic anemia. I. Clinical and fundamental studies before and after splenectomy. Blood, **6**, 685, 1951.
355. Fraenkel, E.: Experimentelles ueber Haematoporphyrie. Arch. Path. Anat., **248**, 125, 1924.
356. Meineri, A.: Sindrome cutanea a tipo di epidermolisi bullosa, a di idroa vacciniforme con porfiria. Dermosifilografo, **6**, 389, 1931.
357. Ottolenghi-Lodigiani, F., and Serhi, G.: Le porfirine ed il loro metabolismo nella porfiria congenita. Gior. Ital. Derm. Sif., **89**, 187, 1948.
358. Panconesi, E., Giannotti, B., and Zampi, G. C.: Preliminary note on the alterations revealed in a post-mortem case of porphyria congenita. Panminerva Med., **4**, 382, 1962.
359. Taussig, L. R.: Hypersensitivity of the skin to light. Calif. West. Med., **39**, 301, 1933.
360. De Marval, L., and Pons, R.: Concomitancía entre una porfirinuria congénita en ictericia hemolitica: esplanectomia. Arch. Argent. Pediat., **5**, 220, 1934.
361. Hernando, T.: La Porphyrie: ces manifestations digestives, cutanées et oculaires. Biol. Med., **36**, 293, 1938.
362. Peachey, C. H., Dobriner, K., and Strain, W. H.: Hydroa estivale in congenital porphyria. New York J. Med., **38**, 1, 1938.
363. London, I. M., West, R., Shemin, D., and Rittenberg, D.: Porphyrin formation and hemoglobin metabolism in congenital porphyria. J. Biol. Chem., **184**, 365, 1950.
364. Haining, R. G., Labbe, R. F., and Cowger, M-L.: Hypertransfusion in congenital erythropoietic porphyria. Clin. Res., **15**, 131, 1967.
365. Thiede, H., and Swisher, S. N.: Personal communication.
366. Dobriner, K., Strain, W. H., Guild, H., and Localio, S. A.: The excretion of porphyrins in congenital porphyria. J. Clin. Invest., **17**, 761, 1938.
367. Watson, C. J., Perman, V., Spurrell, F. A., Hoyt, H. H., and Schwartz, S.: Some studies of the comparative biology of human and bovine porphyria erythropoietica. Trans. Ass. Amer. Physicians, **71**, 196, 1958.
368. Dunsky, I., Freeman, S., and Gibson, S.: Porphyria and porphyrinuria: report of a case; review of porphyrin metabolism with a study of congenital porphyria. Amer. J. Dis. Child., **74**, 305, 1947.
369. Rosenthal, I. M., Lipton, E. L., and Asrow, G.: Effect of splenectomy on porphyria erythropoietica. Pediatrics, **15**, 663, 1955.
370. May, E., Bloch-Michel, H., Poncet-Guaret, and Tournier, P.: Porphyrie familiale (maladie de Gunther). Bull. Soc. Med. Hop. Paris, **64**, 340, 1948.
371. Bolgert, M., Canivet, J., and Le Sourd, L.: Trois cas de porphyrie cutanée congenitale (maladie de Gunther) dans la même fratrie. Bull. Soc. Franc. Derm. Syph., **59**, 233, 1952.
372. Canivet, J., and Pelhard-Considere, M.: Étude de l'hémolyse dans deux cas de porphyrie congénitale. Rev. Franc. Etud. Clin. Biol., **3**, 27, 1958.
373. Cordier, G., Canivet, J., and Barbier: Splénectomie dans trois cas de porphyrie congénitale. Mem. Acad. Chir. (Paris), **86**, 554, 1960.
374. Caletti, A.: Luciti a tippo epidermolisi bullosa con porfiria. Gior. Ital. Derm. Sif., **89**, 187, 1948.
375. Findlay, G. H., and Barnes, H. D.: Congenital porphyria, hydroa aestivale and hypertrichosis in a South African Bantu. Lancet, **2**, 846, 1950.
376. Barnes, H. D.: Porphyria in South Africa: the faecal excretion of porphyrin. South Afr. Med. J., **32**, 680, 1958.
377. Kramer, S., Viljoen, E., Meyer, A. M., and Metz, J.: The anaemia of erythropoietic porphyria with the first description of the disease in an elderly patient. Brit. J. Haemat., **11**, 666, 1965.
378. Zail, S. S., Krawitz, P., Viljoen, E., and Kramer, S.: The anaemia of erythropoietic porphyria II. Studies of some red cell intermediates. Brit. J. Haemat., **13**, 60, 1967.
379. Menagh, F., and Reyner, C. E.: Hydroa aestivale: congenital porphyria. A.M.A. Arch. Derm., **63**, 518, 1951.
380. Zuelzer, W. W., and Kaplan, E.: Personal communication.
381. Pozzan, M.: Porfiria congenita con iperemolisi. Acta Paediat. Latina, Parm., **6**, 995, 1953.
382. Weremowicz, I.: Congenital porphyria with erythrodontia, splenomegaly, and anemia in two sisters. Pol. Tyg. Lek., **9**, 550, 585, 1954.
383. Taneja, P. N., and Seth, R. K.: Congenital porphyria: case reports and review. Indian J. Child Health, **5**, 707, 1956.
384. Townsend-Coles, W. F., and Barnes, H. D.: Erythropoietic (congenital) porphyria: two cases in Sudanese siblings. Lancet, **2**, 271, 1957.
385. Guimaraes, N. A., Monteira, A. B., Lisboa, A., and da Costa Pereira, C. G.: Congenital porphyria. Hospital (Rio), **51**, 51, 1957.
386. Drabkin, D. L.: Some historical highlights in knowledge of porphyrins and porphyrias. Ann. N.Y. Acad. Sci., **104**, 658, 1963.
387. Baxter, B.: Erythropoietic (congenital) porphyria. Cent. Afr. J. Med., **4**, 148, 1958.
388. Leary, P. M.: Erythropoietic porphyria. South Afr. Med. J., **41**, 11, 1967.
389. Stich, W.: Die kongenitale Porphyrie, eine erythropathische haemolytische Anämie (Porphyrocytose). Schweiz. Med. Wschr., **41**, 1012, 1958.
390. Varadi, S.: Haematological aspects in a case of erythropoietic porphyria. Brit. J. Haemat., **4**, 270, 1958.
391. Chaudhuri, A., Chaudhuri, J. N., and Chaudhuri, C. C.: Congenital porphyria in siblings, with a brief review of congenital and hereditary porphyrias. Indian J. Pediat., **25**, 157, 1958.
392. Bisogno, E. M., and Rossetti, S. R.: La Milza nella porfiria congenita (studio istologico). Rass. Med. Sarda., **62**, 921, 1960.
393. Rayne, J.: Porphyria erythropoietica. Brit. J. Oral Surg., **5**, 68, 1967.
394. Kaufman, B. M., Vickers, H. R., Rayne, J., and Ryan, T. J.: Congenital erythropoietic porphyria. Brit. J. Derm., **79**, 210, 1967.
395. Caruso, P., and Previti, A.: Contributo allo studio della porfiria eritropoietica: due casi con anemia emolitica, splenomegalia, ipofunzionalitá surrenalica. Minerva Pediat., **12**, 250, 1960.
396. Ventura, S., Caruso, P., and Aresu, G.: La porfiria eritropoietica. Nota. I. Il comportamento del ricambio porfirinico. Haematologica, **44**, 993, 1959.
397. Larriza, P.: The problem of erythropoietic porphyria in the light of the latest advances in biochemistry and morphology. Panminerva Med., **4**, 315, 1962.
398. Teodoresco, St., Badanoiu, A., Atanasiu, M., and Balta, E.: Quelques remarques à propos d'un cas de porphyrie congénitale mutilante. Bull. Soc. Franc. Derm. Syph., **67**, 266, 1960.
399. Mandal, J. N.: Porphyria congenita. Bull. Calcutta Sch. Trop. Med., **9**, 141, 1961.
400. Chatterji, A. K., and Chatterjea, J. B.: Porphyria erythropoietica: review

of Indian literature and report of two new cases. J. Indian Med. Ass., **39,** 526, 1962.
401. Shurtleff, D. B., et al.: Personal communication.
402. Haining, R. G., Cowger, M. L., Shurtleff, D. B., and Labbe, R. F.: Congenital erythropoietic porphyria. I. Case report, special studies and therapy. Amer. J. Med., **45,** 624, 1968.
403. Gajdos, A., Gajdos-Török, M., Hartleyb, H., and Lausecker, C.: Un cas de porphyrie congénitale traitée par l'acide adénosine-5-monophosphorique. Presse Med., **71,** 1294, 1963.
404. Lausecker, C., Hartleyb, H., Gajdos, A., Gajdos-Török, M., and Fischer, D.: Porphyrie essentielle de l'enfant. À propos d'un cas de maladie de Guenther traité par l'acide adénosine-5-monophosphorique. Arch. Franc. Pediat., **22,** 137, 1965.
405. Heilmeyer, L. E., Clotten, R., Kerp, L., Merker, H., Parra, C. A., and Wetzel, H. P.: Porphyria erythropoietica congenita Günther: Bericht über zwei Familien mit Erfassung der Merkmalsträger. Deutsch. Med. Wschr., **88,** 2449, 1963.
406. Gross, S.: Hematologic studies on erythropoietic porphyria: a new case with severe hemolysis, chronic thrombocytopenia, and folic acid deficiency. Blood, **23,** 762, 1964.
407. Gross, S., Schoenberg, M. D., and Mumaw, V. R.: Electron microscopy of the red cells in erythropoietic porphyria. Blood, **25,** 49, 1965.
408. Handa, F.: Congenital porphyria. Arch. Derm. (Chicago), **91,** 130, 1965.
409. Chatterjea, J. B.: Erythropoietic porphyria. Blood, **24,** 806, 1964.
410. El-Mofty, A. M.: Cutaneous porphyria in Egyptians. Brit. J. Derm., **76,** 268, 1964.
411. Pecorella, F.: Su un nuovo caso di porfiria eritropoietica congenita (malattia di Ghünther). Riv. Clin. Pediat., **71,** 1226, 1963.
412. Hamaguchi, T., Kotani, Y., and Ishibuchi, M.: A case of porphyria congenita. Acta Derm. (Kyoto), **59,** 163, 1964.
413. Baldini, G., Bartalena, R., and Cipolloni, C.: Rilievi su di un caso di porfiria erithropoietica in lattante. Riv. Clin. Pediat., **77,** 113, 1966.
414. Mullick, D. N., Chawla, G. B. S., Sarin, G. S., and Ghai, O. P.: Porphyria erythropoietica. Indian J. Pediat., **30,** 327, 1963.
415. Brunsting, L. A.: Observations on porphyria cutanea tarda. Arch. Derm. Syph., **70,** 551, 1954.
416. Bolgert, M., Canivet, J., and LeSourd, M.: La Porphyrie cutanée de l'adulte: étude de neuf cas et description. Sem. Hop. Paris, **29,** 1587, 1953.
417. Grinstein, M., Aldrich, R. A., Hawkinson, V., and Watson, C. J.: An isotopic study of porphyrin and hemoglobin metabolism in a case of porphyria. J. Biol. Chem., **179,** 983, 1949.
418. Gray, C. H., Muir, H., and Neuberger, A.: Studies in congenital porphyria. 3. The incorporation of ^{15}N into the haem and glycine of haemoglobin. Biochem. J., **47,** 542, 1950.
419. Rosenthal, I. M.: Personal communication.
420. Hausmann, W.: Die sensibilisierende Wirkung des Haematoporphyrins. Biochem. Z., **30,** 276, 1910.
421. Taddeini, L., and Watson, C. J.: The clinical porphyrias. Seminars Hemat., **5,** 335, 1968.
422. Watson, C. J., Runge, W., Taddeini, L., Bossenmaier, I., and Cardinal, R.: A suggested control gene mechanism for the excessive production of types I and III porphyrins in congenital erythropoietic porphyria. Proc. Nat. Acad. Sci. U.S.A., **52,** 478, 1964.
423. Rosenthal, I. M., and Schmid, R.: Unpublished observations.
424. London, I. M., West, R., Shemin, D., and Rittenberg, D.: On the origin of bile pigment in normal man. J. Biol. Chem., **184,** 351, 1950.
425. Rimington, C., and Miles, P. A.: A study of the porphyrins excreted in the urine by a case of congenital porphyria. Biochem. J., **50,** 202, 1951.
426. Fischer, H., and Hofmann, H. J.: Ueber die Konstitution des Uro- und Muschelschalenporphyrins. Z. Physiol. Chem., **246,** 15, 1937.
427. Watson, C. J.: Porphyrin metabolism in the anemias. A.M.A. Arch. Intern. Med., **99,** 323, 1957.
428. Levin, E. Y.: Uroporphyrinogen III cosynthetase in bovine erythropoietic porphyria. Science, **161,** 907, 1968.
429. Romeo, G., and Levin, E. Y.: Uroporphyrinogen III cosynthetase in human congenital, erythropoietic porphyria. Proc. Nat. Acad. Sci. U.S.A., **63,** 856, 1969.
430. Smith, J. E., and Kaneko, J. J.: Rate of heme and porphyrin synthesis by bovine reticulocytes *in vitro.* Amer. J. Vet. Res., **27,** 931, 1966.
431. Romeo, G., Kaback, M. M., and Levin, E. Y.: Uroporphyrinogen III cosynthetase in fibroblasts from patients with congenital erythropoietic porphyria. Biochem. Genet., **4,** 659, 1970.
432. Romeo, G., Glenn, B. L., and Levin, E. Y.: Uroporphyrinogen III cosynthetase in asymptomatic carriers of congenital erythropoietic porphyria. Biochem. Genet., **4,** 719, 1970.
433. Steinberg, A. G.: Methodology in human genetics. J. Med. Educ., **34,** 315, 1959.
434. Finney, D. J.: The truncated binominal distribution. Ann. Eugen., **14,** 319, 1949.
435. Haldane, J. B. S., and Smith, C. A. B.: A simple exact test for birth order effect. Ann. Eugen., **14,** 117, 1948.
436. Fourie, P. J. J.: The occurrence of congenital porphyrinuria (pink tooth) in cattle in South Africa (Swaziland). Onderstepoort J. Vet. Res., **2,** 535, 1936.
437. Rimington, C.: Some cases of congenital porphyrinuria in cattle: chemical studies upon the living animals and post-mortem material. Onderstepoort J. Vet. Res., **7,** 567, 1936.
438. Joergensen, S. K., and With, T. K.: Congenital porphyria in swine and cattle in Denmark. Nature (London), **176,** 156, 1955.
439. Amoroso, E. C., Loosmore, R. M., Rimington, C., and Tooth, B. E.: Congenital porphyria in bovines: first living cases in Britain. Nature (London), **180,** 230, 1957.
440. Joergensen, S. K., and With, T. K.: Porphyria in domestic animals: Danish observations in pigs and cattle and comparison with human porphyria. Ann. N.Y. Acad. Sci., **104,** 701, 1963.
441. Rhode, E. A., and Cornelius, C. E.: Congenital porphyria (pink tooth) in Holstein-Friesian calves in California. J. Amer. Vet. Med. Ass., **132,** 122, 1958.
442. Nestel, B. L.: Bovine congenital porphyria (pink tooth), with a note on five cases observed in Jamaica. Cornell Vet., **48,** 430, 1958.
443. Chu, T. C., and Chu, E. J.-H.: Porphyrins from congenitally porphyric (pink tooth) cattle. Biochem. J., **83,** 318, 1962.
444. Kaneko, J. J.: Erythrokinetics and iron metabolism in bovine porphyria erythropoietica. Ann. N.Y. Acad. Sci., **104,** 689, 1963.
445. Rimington, C., and Booij, H. L.: Porphyrin biosynthesis in human red cells. Biochem. J., **65,** 3P, 1958.
446. Clare, N. Y., and Stephens, E. H.: Congenital porphyria in pigs. Nature (London), **153,** 252, 1944.
447. With, T. K., Clausen, H., and Hojgaard-Olson, N. J.: Undersogelser over kongenit porfyri hos svin. Beretn. forsogslaboratoriet, Copenhagen, **310,** 1959.
448. Tobias, G.: Congenital porphyria in a cat. J. Amer. Vet. Med. Ass., **145,** 462, 1964.
449. Glenn, B. L., Glenn, H. G., and Omtvedt, I. T.: Congenital porphyria in the domestic cat (*Felis catus*): preliminary investigations on inheritance pattern. Amer. J. Vet. Res., **29,** 1653, 1968.
450. Turner, W. J.: Studies on porphyria. I. Observations on the fox squirrel (*Sciurus niger*). J. Biol. Chem., **118,** 519, 1937.
451. Rimington, C.: A reinvestigation of turacin, the copper porphyrin pigment of certain birds belonging to the Musophagidae. Proc. Roy. Soc. London, s.B., **127,** 106, 1939.
452. Watson, C. J., and Berg, M.: Studies of the uroporphyrins. IV. Reexamination of a crucial Waldenström porphyrin. J. Biol. Chem., **214,** 537, 1955.
453. With, T. K.: Pure unequivocal uroporphyrin. III. Simplified method of preparation from turaco feathers. Scand. J. Clin. Lab. Invest., **9,** 398, 1957.
454. Waldenström, J., and Haeger-Aronsen, B.: The porphyrias: a genetic problem. Progr. Med. Genet., **5,** 58, 1967.
455. Dean, G.: *The Porphyrias: A Story of Inheritance and Environment.* Pitman Medical Publishing Co., London, 1963.
456. Dean, G.: The prevalence of the porphyrias. S. Afr. J. Lab. Clin. Med., **9,** 145, 1963.
457. Goldberg, A., Rimington, C., and Lochhead, A. C.: Hereditary coproporphyria. Lancet, **1,** 632, 1967.
458. Eales, L.: The porphyrins and the porphyrias. Ann. Rev. Med., **12,** 251, 1961.

459. Schmid, R.: Porphyria, in *Textbook of Medicine,* edited by P. B. Beeson, and W. McDermott, 12th ed., p. 1233. Saunders, Philadelphia, 1967.
460. Kaufman, L., and Marver, H. S.: The biochemical defects in two types of human hepatic porphyria. New Eng. J. Med., **283**, 954, 1970.
461. Tschudy, D. P., Perlroth, M. G., Marver, H. S., Collins, A., Hunter, G., Jr., and Rechcigl, M., Jr.: Acute intermittent porphyria: the first "overproduction disease" localized to a specific enzyme. Proc. Nat. Acad. Sci. U.S.A., **53**, 841, 1965.
462. Nakao, K., Wada, O., Kitamura, T., Uono, K., and Urata, G.: Activity of aminolevulinic acid synthetase in normal and porphyric human livers. Nature (London), **210**, 838, 1966.
463. Dowdle, E. B., Mustard, P., and Eales, L.: δ-Aminolevulinic acid synthetase activity in normal and porphyric human livers. S. Afr. Med. J., **41**, 1093, 1967.
464. Perlroth, M. G., Tschudy, D. P., Marver, H. S., Berard, C. W., Ziegel, R. F., Rechcigl, M., Jr., and Collins, A.: Acute intermittent porphyria: new morphologic and biochemical findings. Amer. J. Med., **41**, 149, 1966.
465. Stein, J. A., and Tschudy, D. P.: Acute intermittent porphyria: a clinical and biochemical study of 46 patients. Medicine, **49**, 1, 1970.
466. Mason, V. R., Courville, C., and Ziskind, E.: The porphyrins in human disease. Medicine, **12**, 355, 1933.
467. Goldberg, A.: Acute intermittent porphyria. Quart. J. Med., n.s., **28**, 183, 1959.
468. Calvy, G. L.: Porphyria: a consideration in surgical diagnosis. Surg. Gynec. Obstet., **90**, 716, 1950.
469. Watson, C. J., Varco, R. L., and Schmid, R.: An unusual case of acute porphyria with volvulus and gangrene of the cecum. Amer. J. Med., **22**, 980, 1957.
470. Denny-Brown, D., and Sciarra, D.: Changes in the nervous system in acute porphyria. Brain, **68**, 1, 1945.
471. Markovitz, M.: Acute intermittent porphyria: a report of five cases and a review of the literature. Ann. Intern. Med., **41**, 1170, 1954.
472. Ten Eyck, F. W., Martin, W. J., and Kernohan, J. W.: Acute porphyria: necropsy studies in nine cases. Proc. Staff Meet. Mayo Clin., **36**, 409, 1961.
473. Wetterberg, L.: *A Neuropsychiatric and Genetical Investigation of Acute Intermittent Porphyria.* Scandinavian University Books, Svenska Bskförlaget, Norstedts, 1967.
474. Kleuver, H.: In *Cerebral Mechanism in Behavior.* Wiley, New York, 1951.
475. Nesbitt, S.: Acute porphyria. J.A.M.A., **124**, 286, 1944.
476. Ridley, A., Hierons, R., and Cavanagh, J. B.: Tachycardia and the neuropathy of porphyria. Lancet, **2**, 708, 1968.
477. Waldenström, J., and Haeger-Aronsen, B.: Different patterns of human porphyria. Brit. Med. J., **2**, 272, 1963.
478. Redeker, A. G., Sterling, R. E., and Bronow, R. S.: Effect of Griesofulvin in acute intermittent porphyria. J.A.M.A., **188**, 466, 1964.
479. Perlroth, M. G., Marver, H. S., and Tschudy, D. P.: Oral contraceptive agents and the management of acute intermittent porphyria. J.A.M.A., **194**, 1037, 1965.
480. Tschudy, D. P.: Recent progress in the hepatic porphyrias. Prog. Liver Dis., **3**, 13, 1970.
481. Curnow, D. H., Morgan, S. H., and Sarfaty, G. A.: Acute intermittent porphyria: a family study. Aust. Ann. Med., **8**, 267, 1959.
482. Aldrich, R. A., Labbe, R. F., and Talman, E. L.: A review of porphyrin metabolism with special reference to childhood. Amer. J. Med. Sci., **230**, 675, 1955.
483. Lysaught, J. N., and McCleery, J. M.: Acute intermittent porphyria: report of a case in an infant aged eight months, with discussion of porphyrin metabolism. J. Pediat., **46**, 552, 1955.
484. Bleifer, S. B., and Alphas, S. J.: Acute intermittent porphyria: report of a case associated with porphobilinogen in the urine of four of five children. New Eng. J. Med., **260**, 978, 1959.
485. Basltrop, D.: Acute intermittent porphyria in a child with a note on the glycine loading test. Pediatrics, **34**, 696, 1964.
486. Vine, S., Shaffer, H. M., Pauler, G., and Margolis, E. J.: A review of the relationship between pregnancy and porphyria and presentation of a case. Ann. Intern. Med., **47**, 834, 1957.
487. Neilson, D. R., and Neilson, R. P.: Porphyria, complicated by pregnancy. Western J. Surg., **66**, 133, 1958.
488. Gould, S., Allison, H. M., and Bellew, L. N.: Acute porphyria, complicated by pregnancy: report of a case. Obstet. Gynec., **17**, 109, 1961.
489. Petrie, S. J., and Mooney, J. P.: Porphyria with the complication of pregnancy. Amer. J. Obstet. Gynec., **83**, 264, 1962.
490. James, G. W., III, Rudolph, S. G., and Abbott, L. D.: Delta-aminolevulinic acid, porphobilinogen, and porphyrin excretion throughout pregnancy in a patient with acute intermittent porphyria with "passive porphyria" in the infant. J. Lab. Clin. Med., **58**, 437, 1961.
491. Hellman, E. S., Tschudy, D. P., Robbins, J., and Rall, J. E.: Elevation of the serum protein-bound iodine in acute intermittent porphyria. J. Clin. Endocr., **23**, 1185, 1963.
492. Hollander, C. S., Scott, R. L., Tschudy, D. P., Perlroth, M., Waxman, A., and Sterling, K.: Increased protein-bound iodine and thyroxine-binding globulin in acute intermittent porphyria. New Eng. J. Med., **277**, 995, 1967.
493. Hellman, E. S., Tschudy, D. P., and Bartter, F. C.: Abnormal electrolyte and water metabolism in acute intermittent porphyria. Amer. J. Med., **32**, 734, 1962.
494. Ludwig, G. D., and Goldberg, M.: Hyponatremia in acute intermittent porphyria probably resulting from inappropriate secretion of antidiuretic hormone. Ann. N.Y. Acad. Sci., **104**, 710, 1963.
495. Perlroth, M. G., Tschudy, D. P., Marver, H. S., Berard, C. W., Ziegel, R. F., Rechcigl, M., Jr., and Collins, A.: Acute intermittent porphyria: new morphologic and biochemical findings. Amer. J. Med., **41**, 149, 1966.
496. Perlroth, M. G., Tschudy, D. P., Waxman, A., and Odell, W. D.: Abnormalities of growth hormone regulation in acute intermittent porphyria. Metabolism, **16**, 87, 1967.
497. Waxman, A. D., Berk, P. D., Schalch, D., and Tschudy, D. P.: Isolated ACTH deficiency in acute intermittent porphyria. Ann. Intern. Med., **70**, 317, 1969.
498. Watson, C. J., Runge, W., and Bossenmaier, I.: Increased urinary porphobilinogen and uroporphyrin after administration of stilbesterol in a case of latent porphyria. Metabolism, **11**, 1129, 1962.
499. Wetterberg, L.: Oral contraceptives and acute intermittent porphyria. Lancet, **2**, 1178, 1964.
500. Rimington, C., and DeMatteis, F.: Oral contraceptives and acute intermittent porphyria. Lancet, **1**, 270, 1965.
501. Sachs, P.: Ein Fall von akuter Porphyrie mit hochgradiger Muskelatrophie. Klin. Wschr., **10**, 1123, 1931.
502. Ackner, B., Cooper, J. E., Gray, C. H., Kelly, M., and Nicholson, D. C.: Excretion of porphobilinogen and δ-aminolaevulinic acid in acute porphyria. Lancet, **1**, 1256, 1961.
503. Taddeini, L., Kay, I. T., and Watson, C. J.: Inhibition of the Ehrlich's reaction of porphobilinogen by indican and related compounds. Clin. Chim. Acta, **7**, 890, 1962.
504. Gibson, Q. H., and Harrison, D. C.: A note on the urinary uroporphyrin in acute porphyria. Biochem. J., **46**, 154, 1950.
505. Grinstein, M., Schwartz, S., and Watson, C. J.: Studies of the uroporphyrins. I. The purification of uroporphyrin I and the nature of Waldenström's uroporphyrin, as isolated from porphyria material. J. Biol. Chem., **157**, 323, 1945.
506. Nicholas, R. E. H., and Rimington, C.: Studies on the "Waldenström porphyrin" of acute porphyria urines. Biochem. J., **55**, 109, 1953.
507. With, T. K.: Preparation of crystalline porphyrin esters from porphyria urines and normal human urine. Scand. J. Clin. Lab. Invest., **10**, 297, 1958.
508. Fischer, H., and Libowitzky, K.: Auftreten von Uro-bzw. Koproporphyrin I bei akuter Porphyrie. Z. Physiol. Chem., **241**, 220, 1936.
509. Lemberg, R., and Legge, J. W.: *Hematin Compounds and Bile Pigments.* Interscience, New York, 1949.
510. Olsson, R. A., and Ticktin, H. E.: Zinc metabolism in acute intermittent porphyria. J. Lab. Clin. Med., **60**, 48, 1962.
511. Mellincoff, S. M., Halpern, R. M., Frankland, M., and Greipel, M.: Abnormal urinary amino acid patterns in acute intermittent porphyria. J. Lab. Clin. Med., **53**, 358, 1959.
512. Ludwig, G. D., and Epstein, I. S.: A genetic study of two families having the acute intermittent type of porphyria. Ann. Intern. Med., **55**, 81, 1961.
513. Druyan, R., and Haeger-Aronsen, B.: Aminoacetone excretion in por-

phyrias and in chronic lead intoxication. Scand. J. Clin. Lab. Invest., **16,** 498, 1964.
514. Fischer, H.: Ueber das Kotporphyrin. Z. Physiol. Chem., **97,** 148, 1916.
515. Rimington, C., Lockwood, W. H., and Belcher, R. V.: The excretion of porphyrin-peptide conjugates in porphyria variegata. Clin. Sci., **35,** 211, 1968.
516. Smith, S. G.: The porphobilinogen in fresh postmortem tissues from a case of acute intermittent porphyria. Arch. Path. (Chicago), **70,** 361, 1960.
517. Heilmeyer, L., and Clotten, R.: Zur biochemischen Pathogenese der Porphyria acuta intermittens. Klin. Wschr., **47,** 71, 1969.
518. Waldenström, J.: Studies on the incidence and heredity of acute porphyria in Sweden. Acta Genet., **6,** 122, 1956.
519. Waldenström, J., and Haeger-Aronsen, B.: The porphyrias: a genetic problem. Progr. Med. Genet., **5,** 58, 1967.
520. Kehoe, E. L., Rudensky, H., and Reynolds, W. W.: Acute intermittent porphyria in identical twins. Ann. Intern. Med., **47,** 131, 1957.
521. Fennelly, J. J., Fitzgerald, O., and Hingerty, D. J.: Observations on porphyria with special reference to Ireland. Irish. J. Med. Sci., **411,** 130, 1960.
522. Saint, E. G., and Curnow, D. H.: Porphyria in Western Australia. Lancet, **1,** 133, 1962.
523. Curtis, V. J., and Giliberti, J. J.: Acute porphyria in a Negro. New York J. Med., **50,** 1966, 1950.
524. Wiggins, C. A.: Fatal case of acute porphyria in a Negro. Brit. Med. J., **2,** 866, 1950.
525. Lyon, L. J.: Acute porphyria in American Negro. New York J. Med., **68,** 2441, 1968.
526. Dean, G., and Barnes, H. D.: The inheritance of porphyria. Brit. Med. J., **2,** 89, 1955.
527. Barnes, H. D.: Further South African cases of porphyrinuria. South Afr. J. Clin. Sci., **2,** 117, 1951.
528. Dean, G.: Porphyria. Brit. Med. J., **2,** 1291, 1953.
529. Dean, G.: *The Porphyrias: A Story of Inheritance and Environment.* Pitman Medical Publishing Co., London, 1963.
530. Eales, L.: Porphyria as seen in Cape Town: a survey of 250 patients and some recent studies. South. Afr. J. Lab. Clin. Med., **9,** 151, 1963.
531. Eales, L.: Cutaneous porphyria: observations on 111 cases in three racial groups. South Afr. J. Lab. Clin. Med., **6,** 63, 1960.
532. Eales, L., and Linder, G. C.: Porphyria—the acute attack. South Afr. Med. J., **36,** 284, 1962.
533. Cripps, D. J., and Curtis, A. C.: Toxic effect of chloroquine on porphyria hepatica. Arch. Derm. (Chicago), **86,** 575, 1962.
534. Campbell, J. A. H.: The pathology of South African genetic porphyria. South Afr. J. Lab. Clin. Med., **9,** 197, 1963.
535. Gray, C. H., Rimington, C., and Thomson, S.: A case of chronic porphyria associated with recurrent jaundice. Quart. J. Med., **17,** 123, 1948.
536. Calvy, G. L., Jaruszewski, E. J., and Carroll, H. H.: Porphyria: clinical observations and a family vignette. Ann. Intern. Med., **34,** 767, 1951.
537. Tio, T. H.: Beschouwingen over de Porphyria cutanea tarda. Thesis, University of Amsterdam, 1956.
538. Hamnström, B., Haeger-Aronsen, B., Waldenström, J., Hysing, B., and Molander, J.: Three Swedish families with porphyria variegata. Brit. Med. J., **4,** 449, 1967.
539. Cochrane, A. L., and Goldberg, A.: A study of faecal porphyrin levels in a large family. Ann. Hum. Genet., **32,** 195, 1968.
540. Macalpine, I., Hunter, R., and Rimington, C.: Porphyria in the Royal Houses of Stuart, Hanover and Prussia. A followup study of George III illness. Brit. Med. J., **1,** 7, 1968.
541. Sweeney, G. D.: Patterns of porphyrin excretion in South African porphyric patients. South Afr. J. Lab. Clin. Med., **9,** 182, 1963.
542. Wetterberg, L., Haeger-Aronsen, B., and Stathers, G.: Faecal porphyrins as a diagnostic index between acute intermittent porphyria and porphyria variegata. Scand. J. Clin. Lab. Invest., **22,** 131, 1968.
543. Dean, G.: The prevalence of the porphyrias. South Afr. J. Lab. Clin. Med., **9,** 145, 1963.
544. Berger, H., and Goldberg, A.: Hereditary coproporphyria. Brit. Med. J., **2,** 85, 1955.
545. Dobriner, K.: Simultaneous excretion of coproporphyrin I and III in a case of chronic porphyria. Proc. Soc. Exp. Biol. Med., **35,** 175, 1936.
546. Watson, C. J., Schwartz, S., Schulze, W., Jacobson, L. O., and Zagaria, R.: Studies of coproporphyrin. III. Idiopathic coproporphyrinuria; a hitherto unrecognized form characterized by lack of symptoms in spite of the excretion of large amounts of coproporphyrin. J. Clin. Invest., **28,** 465, 1949.
547. Goldberg, A., Rimington, C., and Lochhead, A.: Hereditary coproporphyria. Lancet, **1,** 632, 1967.
548. Haeger-Aronsen, B., Stathers, G., and Swahn, G.: Hereditary coproporphyria: study of a Swedish family. Ann. Intern. Med., **69,** 221, 1968.
549. Lomholt, J. C., and With, T. K.: Hereditary coproporphyria: a family with unusually few and mild symptoms. Acta Med. Scand., **186,** 83, 1969.
550. Dean, G., Kramer, S., and Lamb, P.: Coproporphyria. S. Afr. Tydskrif Geneesk., Feb. 8, 1969, p. 138.
551. Connon, J. J., and Turkington, V.: Hereditary coproporphyria. Lancet, **2,** 263, 1968.
552. Langhof, H., Franken, E., and Kluge, K.: Kombinierte hereditäre Porphyria hepatica (hereditäre Koproporphyrie). Hautarzt, **16,** 101, 1965.
553. Tappeiner, S., and Tirschek, H.: Das Syndrom der aktinischtraumatischen bulloesen Porphyrindermatose. Arch. Derm. Syph., **196,** 65, 1953.
554. Ippen, H.: Porphyrin metabolism in porphyria cutanea tarda. Panminerva Med., **4,** 381, 1962.
555. Ventura, S.: La porfiria epatica. Minerva Med., **50,** 2381, 1959.
556. Barnes, H. D.: Porphyria in the Bantu races on the Witwatersrand. South Afr. Med. J., **29,** 781, 1955.
557. Eales, L., Dowdle, E. B., Saunders, S. J., and Sweeney, G. D.: The diagnostic importance of faecal porphyrins in the differentiation of the porphyrias. II. Values in the cutaneous porphyrias. South Afr. J. Lab. Clin. Med., **9,** 126, 1963.
558. Lamont, N. M., Hathorn, M., and Joubert, S. M.: Porphyria in the African. Quart. J. Med., n.s., **30,** 373, 1961.
559. Barnes, H. D.: The excretion of porphyrins and porphyrin precursors by Bantu cases of porphyria. South African Med. J., **33,** 274, 1959.
560. Bothwell, T. H., Seftel, H., Jacobs, P., Torrance, J. D., and Baumslag, N.: Iron overload in Bantu subjects: studies on the availability of iron in Bantu beer. Amer. J. Clin. Nutr., **14,** 47, 1964.
561. Hathorn, M., Gillman, T., Canham, P. A. S., and Lamont, N. M.: Plasma iron and iron-binding capacity in African males with siderosis. Clin. Sci., **19,** 35, 1960.
562. Keeley, K. J.: In Discussion. South Afr. J. Lab. Clin. Med., **9,** 162, 1963.
563. Magnus, I. A.: The cutaneous porphyrias. Seminars Hemat., **5,** 380, 1968.
564. Hällén, J., and Krook, H.: Follow-up studies on an unselected ten-year material of 360 patients with liver cirrhosis in one community. Acta Med. Scand., **173,** 479, 1963.
565. Dowdle, E. B., Mustard, P., and Eales, L.: δ-Aminolevulinic acid synthetase activity in normal and porphyric human liver. South Afr. Med., J., **41,** 1093, 1967.
566. Masuya, T.: Pathophysiological observations on porphyrias. Acta Haemat. Jap., **32,** 465, 1969.
567. Levere, R. D.: Stilbesterol-induced porphyria: increase in hepatic δ-aminolevulinic acid synthetase. Blood, **28,** 569, 1966.
568. Zail, S. S., and Joubert, S. M.: Hepatic δ-aminolaevulic acid synthetase activity in symptomatic porphyria. Brit. J. Haemat., **15,** 123, 1968.
569. Rimington, C.: Types of porphyria: some thoughts about biochemical mechanisms involved. Ann. N.Y. Acad. Sci., **104,** 658, 1963.
570. Becker, F. T.: Porphyria cutanea tarda induced by estrogens. Arch. Derm. (Chicago), **92,** 252, 1965.
571. Vail, J. T.: Porphyria cutanea tarda and estrogens. J.A.M.A., **20,** 671, 1967.
572. Hickman, R., Saunders, S. J., and Eales, L.: Treatment of symptomatic porphyria by venesection. South Afr. Med. J., **41,** 456, 1967.
573. Epstein, J. H., and Redeker, A. G.: Porphyria cutanea tarda: a study of the effect of phlebotomy. New Eng. J. Med., **279,** 1301, 1968.
574. Kramer, S.: Iron metabolism in the porphyrias. South Afr. J. Lab. Clin. Med., **9,** 283, 1963.
575. Cripps, D. J., and Curtis, A. C.: Toxic effect of chloroquine on porphyria hepatica. Arch. Derm. (Chicago), **86,** 575, 1962.

576. Felsher, B. F., and Redeker, A. G.: Effect of chloroquine on hepatic uroporphyrin metabolism in patients with porphyria cutanea tarda. Medicine, **45**, 575, 1966.
577. Sweeney, G. D., Saunders, S. J., Dowdle, E. B., and Eales, L.: Effects of chloroquine on patients with cutaneous porphyria of the "symptomatic" type. Brit. Med. J., **1**, 1281, 1965.
578. Saltzer, E. I., Redeker, A. G., and Wilson, J. W.: Porphyria cutanea tarda: remission following chloroquine administration without adverse effects. Arch. Derm. (Chicago), **98**, 496, 1968.
579. Ockner, R. K., and Schmid, R.: Acquired porphyria in man and rat due to hexachlorobenzene intoxication. Nature (London), **189**, 449, 1961.
580. Tio, T. H., Leijnse, B., Jarrett, A., and Rimington, C.: Acquired porphyria from a liver tumor. Clin. Sci., **16**, 517, 1957.
581. Magnus, I. A., Jarrett, A., Prankerd, T. A. J., and Rimington, C.: Erythropoietic protoporphyria: a new porphyria syndrome with solar urticaria due to protoporphyrinaemia. Lancet, **2**, 448, 1961.
582. Gray, C. H., Kulczycka, A., Nicholson, D. C., Magnus, I. A., and Rimington, C.: Isotope studies on a case of erythropoietic protoporphyria. Clin. Sci., **26**, 7, 1964.
583. Kosenow, W., and Treibs, A.: Lichtüberempfindlichkeit und Porphyrinämie. Z. Kinderheilk., **73**, 82, 1953.
584. Redeker, A. G., and Berke, M.: Erythropoietic protoporphyria with eczema solare: report of a case. Arch. Derm. (Chicago), **86**, 569, 1962.
585. Redeker, A. G., and Bronow, R. S.: Erythropoietic protoporphyria presenting as hydroa aestivale. Arch. Derm. (Chicago), **89**, 104, 1964.
586. Holti, G., Magnus, I. A., and Rimington, C.: Erythropoietic protoporphyria in sisters. Brit. J. Derm., **75**, 225, 1963.
587. Haeger-Aronsen, B.: Erythropoietic porphyria: a new type of inborn error of metabolism. Amer. J. Med., **35**, 450, 1963.
588. Porter, S., and Lowe, B. A.: Congenital erythropoietic protoporphyria. I. Case reports, clinical studies and porphyrin analyses in two brothers. Blood, **22**, 521, 1963.
589. Porter, S.: Congenital erythropoietic protoporphyria. II. An experimental study. Blood, **22**, 532, 1963.
590. Sweeney, G. D., Dowdle, E. B., Saunders, S. J., and Eales, L.: Erythropoietic protoporphyria. South Afr. J. Lab. Clin. Med., **9**, 247, 1963.
591. Langhof, H., Müller, H., and Rietschel, L.: Studies on familial protoporphyrinemic light urticaria. Arch. Klin. Exp. Derm., **212**, 506, 1961.
592. Gajdos, A., Gajdos-Török, M., Mantz, I. M., and Schirardin, H.: Protoporphyrie érythropoiétique: traitement par l'inosine. Presse Med., **73**, 119, 1965.
593. Baer, R. L., Miles, W. J., Rorsman, H., and Harber, L. C.: Erythropoietic protoporphyria. Dermatologica (Basel), **135**, 5, 1967.
594. Donaldson, E. M., Donaldson, A. D., and Rimington, C.: Erythropoietic protoporphyria: a family study. Brit. Med. J., **1**, 659, 1967.
595. Ryan, E. A.: Histochemistry of the skin in erythropoietic protoporphyria. Brit. J. Derm., **78**, 501, 1966.
596. Cripps, D. J.: Erythropoietic protoporphyria (Antea lipoid proteinosis) in sisters. Arch. Derm. (Chicago), **94**, 682, 1966.
597. Haeger-Aronsen, B., and Krook, G.: Erythropoietic protoporphyria. Acta Med. Scand., suppl. **445**, 48, 1966.
598. Peterka, E. S., Fusaro, R. M., Runge, W. J., Jaffe, M. O., and Watson, C. J.: Erythropoietic protoporphyria. J.A.M.A., **193**, 1036, 1965.
599. Cripps, D. J., and Scheuer, P. J.: Hepatobiliary changes in erythropoietic protoporphyria. Arch. Path. (Chicago), **80**, 500, 1965.
600. Wuepper, K. D., and Epstein, J. H.: Erythrocyte fluorescence in relatives of patients with erythropoietic protoporphyria. J.A.M.A., **200**, 70, 1967.
601. Magnus, I. A.: The cutaneous porphyrias. Seminars Hemat., **5**, 380, 1968.
602. Kniffen, J. C.: Protoporphyrin removal in intrahepatic porphyrastasis. Program of the 71st Meeting of the American Gastroenterology Association, p. A110, Boston, 1970.
603. Kaplowitz, N., Javitt, N., and Harber, L. C.: Isolation of erythrocytes with normal protoporphyrin levels in erythropoietic protoporphyria. New Eng. J. Med., **278**, 1077, 1968.
604. Cripps, D. J., Hawgood, R. S., and Magnus, I. A.: Iodine tungsten fluorescence microscopy for porphyrin fluorescence. Arch. Derm. (Chicago), **93**, 129, 1966.
605. Rimington, C., and Cripps, D. J.: Biochemical and fluorescence-microscopy screening-tests for erythropoietic protoporphyria. Lancet, **1**, 624, 1965.
606. Redeker, A. G., and Sterling, R. E.: The "glucose effect" in erythropoietic protoporphyria. Arch. Intern. Med., **121**, 446, 1968.
607. Redeker, A. G., Bronow, R. S., and Sterling, R. E.: Erythropoietic protoporphyria. South Afr. J. Lab. Clin. Med., **9**, 235, 1963.
608. Watson, C. J.: The erythrocyte coproporphyrin: variation in respect to erythrocyte protoporphyrin and reticulocytes in certain anemias. Arch. Intern. Med., **86**, 797, 1950.
609. Watson, R. J., Decker, E., and Lichtman, H.: Hematologic studies of children with lead poisoning. Pediatrics, **21**, 40, 1958.
610. Dagg, J. H., Goldberg, A., and Lochhead, A.: Value of erythrocyte protoporphyrin in the diagnosis of latent iron deficiency (sideropenia). Brit. J. Haemat., **12**, 326, 1966.
611. Redeker, A. G., and Bryan, H. G.: Erythropoietic protoporphyria. Lancet, **1**, 912, 1964.
612. Scholnick, P., Marver, H. S., and Schmid, R.: Erythropoietic protoporphyria: evidence for multiple sites of excess protoporphyrin formation. J. Clin. Invest., **50**, 203, 1971.
613. Stevens, E., Frydman, R. B., and Frydman, B.: Separation of porphobilinogen deaminase and uroporphyrinogen III cosynthetase from human erythrocytes. Biochim. Biophys. Acta, **158**, 496, 1968.
614. Pluscec, J., and Bogorad, L.: A dipyrrylmethane intermediate in the enzymatic synthesis of uroporphyrinogen. Biochemistry, **9**, 4736, 1970.
615. Tomio, J. M., Garcia, R. C., San Martin de Viale, L. C., and Grinstein, M.: Porphyrin biosynthesis. VII. Porphyrinogen carboxy-lyase from avian erythrocytes. Purification and properties. Biochem. Biophys. Acta, **198**, 353, 1970.
616. Hetherington, G. W., Jetton, R. L., and Knox, J. M.: The association of lupus erythematosus and porphyria. Brit. J. Derm., **82**, 118, 1970.
617. Griem, H., Schenkman, J. B., Klotzbücher, M., and Remmer, H.: The influence of phenobarbital on the turnover of hepatic microsomal cytochrome b_5 and cytochrome P-450 hemes in the rat. Biochim. Biophys. Acta, **201**, 20, 1970.
618. Meyer, U. A., and Marver, H. S.: Chemically induced porphyria: increased microsomal heme turnover after treatment with allylisopropylacetamide. Science, **171**, 64, 1971.
619. Feldman, D. S., Levere, R. D., Lieberman, J. S., Cardinal, R. A., and Watson, C. J.: Presynaptic neuromuscular inhibition by porphobilinogen and porphobilin. Proc. Nat. Acad. Sci. U.S.A., **67**, 1315, 1970.
620. Kramer, S., Becker, D. M., and Viljoen, D.: A possible mechanism for the development of the neurological disturbance in porphyria. So. Afr. J. Lab. Clin. Med., 1971 (in press).
621. Sassa, S., and Granick, S.: Induction of δ-aminolevulinic acid synthetase in chick embryo liver cells in culture. Proc. Nat. Acad. Sci. U.S.A., **67**, 517, 1970.
622. Strand, L. J., Manning, J., and Marver, H. S.: Acute intermittent porphyria: studies of the enzymatic basis of disordered heme biosynthesis. So. Afr. J. Lab. Clin. Med., 1971 (in press).
623. Strand, L. J., Felsher, B. F., Redeker, A. G., and Marver, H. S.: Intermittent acute porphyria: new evidence for a basic defect in uroporphyrinogen synthetase. J. Clin. Invest., **50**, 89a, 1971.

CHAPTER FORTY-SIX

HYPERBILIRUBINEMIA

Rudi Schmid*

Jaundice as a manifestation of liver disease has been known for centuries. Its diagnostic and prognostic aspects were discussed by Hippocrates [1], and its association with the presence of gallstones in the biliary tract was recognized by Galen [2].

The concept that bile pigment is derived from blood pigment is probably very old, but the first clear and experimentally supported indication was provided by Virchow [3], who observed and isolated bilirubin crystals from old blood extravasations. Through many classic experiments conducted over the ensuing years, unmistakable evidence accumulated that bilirubin is derived from the prosthetic group of hemoglobin [4–9]. The final proof was obtained much later when Fischer and his school elucidated the chemical constitution of heme and of bilirubin and demonstrated that both have a closely related tetrapyrrolic structure [10].

For a long time the anatomic site of bilirubin formation in the organism was a matter of much controversy. On the basis of the findings of Minkowski and Naunyn [11] that in hepatectomized geese induced hemolysis failed to produce jaundice, it was thought that the liver was the only organ capable of converting hemoglobin to bilirubin. This was an unfortunate interpretation of a correct observation, which was later clarified by the finding that in the goose virtually all reticuloendothelial cells are located in the liver. In mammals, McNee [6], Mann et al. [8], Rich [4], and others obtained conclusive evidence that formation of bilirubin occurs following total hepatectomy. As a result of these findings it became generally accepted that hemoglobin may be converted to bilirubin in a variety of organs and that this process is a function primarily of the reticuloendothelial system. Experimental proof for this concept was obtained recently with the demonstration that many tissues, including liver, spleen, kidney, bone marrow, and isolated macrophages, contain an enzyme system that converts hemoglobin to bilirubin in vitro [12, 13].

Quantitative studies of bile pigment metabolism were greatly facilitated when van den Bergh introduced Ehrlich's diazo reaction for estimation of bilirubin in biologic specimens [14]. When icteric sera were studied with this method, it became recognized that bilirubin appeared to be present in two different forms: one gave a direct reaction when diazotized sulfanilic acid was added to icteric serum, whereas the other coupled with the diazo reagent only after alcohol was also added to the reaction mixture (indirect reaction). Separate determination of these two pigment fractions was found to be of clinical usefulness in the differential diagnosis of jaundice [15]. For many years the basic reason for this difference in reaction type was unknown, and numerous explanations and hypotheses were offered [16]. The discovery that bilirubin is esterified by the liver and excreted largely as the glucuronide conjugate provided an answer to this problem [17–19]. Aqueous solutions of conjugated bilirubin react *directly* with diazotized sulfanilic acid (direct van den Bergh reaction), whereas native bilirubin requires the addition of alcohol in order for the reaction to occur (*indirect* van den Bergh reaction).

As the result of work performed during the past several years, it has become possible to characterize the manner in which bilirubin is handled by the liver. The individual steps of this process may be visualized as follows:

1 Transfer of bilirubin from the plasma into the liver cell
2 Conjugation of bilirubin by the microsomal enzyme system
3 Transport of conjugated bilirubin from the hepatic cell into the bile canalicular system

A defect in the first two steps results in decreased formation of conjugated bilirubin and, hence, in retention of unconjugated bilirubin in the plasma. A disturbance of the third step leads to impaired excretion of conjugated bilirubin and results in its "regurgitation" into the plasma. In practice it is often difficult to identify the cause of hyperbilirubinemia and to characterize it in terms of this simplified scheme. This is partly because the mechanisms involved in these three steps are functionally interrelated and, therefore, are difficult to analyze individually. Thus, the net transfer of bilirubin from the plasma into the liver cell (hepatic uptake) depends critically on the rate of pigment conjugation; in turn, the latter determines the upper limit at which conjugated bilirubin is secreted into the bile. Moreover, in hepatic injury, most, if not all, metabolic and excretory functions of the liver may be impaired to variable degrees, so that hyperbilirubinemia frequently is caused by a combination of defects.

In the following discussion, a number of syndromes will be considered in which icterus appears to be due to one or a combination of defects that have been shown to be or are suspected of being, genetically determined. Recent reviews containing more general discussions of bilirubin metabolism have been published by Arias [20], Beck [21], Bouchier and Billing [22], Lester and Troxler [23], and With [24].

*I wish to thank Dr. Roger Lester for his invaluable help and criticism in writing this review.

FORMATION OF BILIRUBIN

Chemistry of Bilirubin

Structure

Bilirubin is a compound which consists of four pyrrole rings

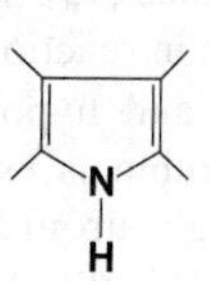

and associated subgroups, with a molecular weight of approximately 585 (Fig. 46-1) [25]. The rings are linked by three carbon bridges, of which two are unsaturated (outside) and one is saturated (central). A total of eight side chains is located on the pyrrole carbons farthest from the nitrogens. The order of these eight side chains in bilirubin is the same as that found in protoporphyrin IX. According to standard nomenclature, bilirubin is designated IXα, since it is formed by the oxidation of the α-carbon bridge of the protoporphyrin IX in heme. Although bilirubin is usually represented and referred to as a "linear tetrapyrrole," the ring-shaped structure shown in Fig. 46-1 is a more accurate representation. Free rotation is possible around the central saturated bridge carbon, but the outer unsaturated bridges confer a marked degree of steric rigidity to each half of the molecule.

Oxygen atoms are located on carbons of the outer pyrrole rings. It has been suggested that these structures are best represented as ketoamides rather than as enolimines [26]. Lemberg recognized the possibility of ketoenolization, and on the basis of deductions from indirect evidence [27], as well as from nuclear magnetic resonance (NMR) spectroscopy [28], it appears that in chloroform the enolimine form is predominant.

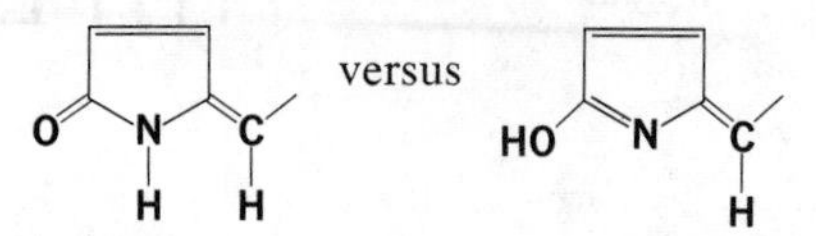

Bilirubin structure is further characterized by the presence of intramolecular hydrogen bonding. This possibility was first suggested by Fog [29] and later elaborated upon by others [30]. The original formulation probably was incorrect, in that it was proposed that hydrogen bonding exists between the propionic acid side chains and the pyrrole ring nitrogens. Although it can be shown with molecular models that such bonding is possible, recent studies with infrared and NMR spectroscopy suggest that hydrogen bonding occurs as an interaction between the two propionic acid side chains [28]. This "dimer" formation between the two propionic acid groups promotes additional hydrogen bonding between the two outer-ring hydroxyls, which tends to fix the molecule in the enolimine configuration.

Physical and Chemical Properties

Bilirubin is moderately soluble in chloroform and is most easily crystallized by displacement of chloroform with boiling methanol [31]. Bilirubin is minimally soluble in pure aqueous solution at physiologic pH, but can be "salted into solution" by adding electrolyte [32, 33]. The propionic acid side chains which ionize with a single pK at a pH between 7 and 8 confer weakly acidic properties on the molecule. Ionized species of the molecule are water-soluble, and bilirubin is therefore freely soluble in base. Basic solutions are unstable, however, especially when exposed to light and heat [31]. The "chromophore" (see below) of at least some of

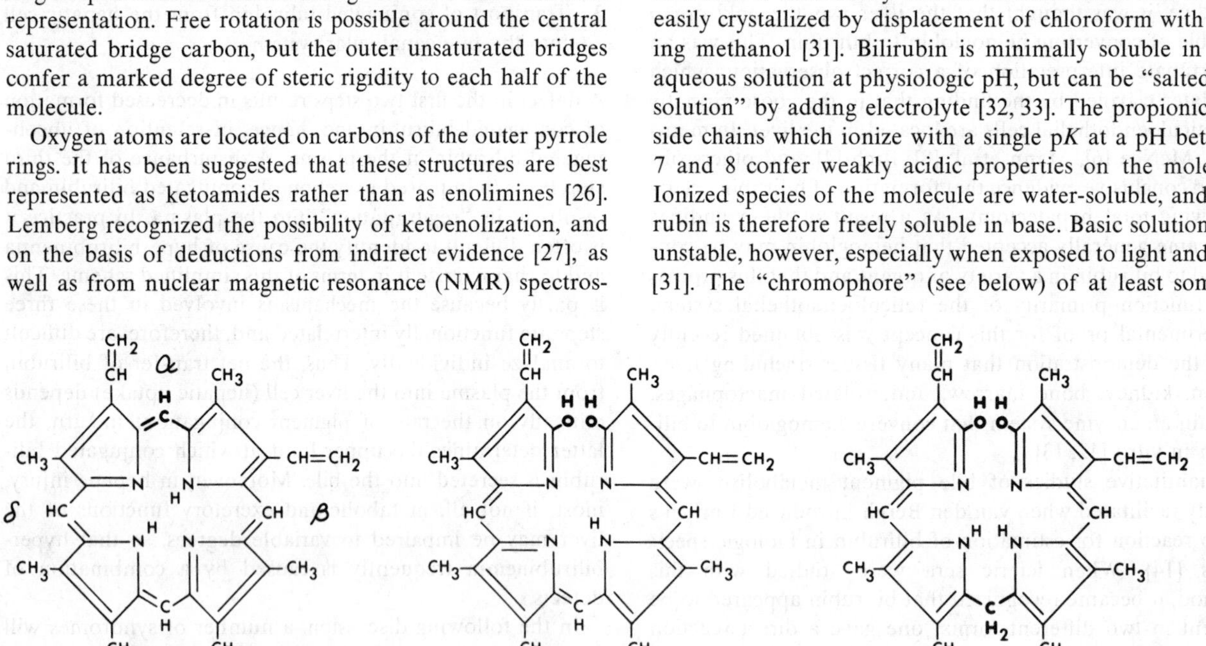

Protoporphyrin IX   Biliverdin IX α   Bilirubin IX α

Figure 46-1. Structural relationship of protoporphyrin, biliverdin, and bilirubin. Structural differences are represented in heavy print. The bridge carbons are designated as α, β, γ, and δ. (*Adapted from R. Lester and R. F. Troxler* [23].)

the tetrapyrroles has weakly basic characteristics by virtue of the free nitrogen positions of the ring structures [34].

Bilirubin is red orange in the solid crystalline form and yellow when in dilute solution. The color is conferred by the resonance of the two systems of five conjugated double bonds (alternating single and double bonds, —CH═CH—CH═CH—) which are separated by the central saturated bridge (—CH_2—), and which are referred to as the "chromophore" of the molecule [2]. Peak absorption in the visible range is at 450 mμ in nonpolar solvents such as chloroform, and 420 to 430 mμ in water. A second peak of absorption in the ultraviolet range at approximately 250 mμ is also observed. The fact that protein-bound bilirubin in aqueous solution absorbs light maximally at 450 mμ suggests that bilirubin is bound to a site on the protein molecule which provides a nonpolar milieu.

Bilirubin gives characteristic color reactions with oxidizing reagents. When exposed to nitric acid containing traces of nitrous acid, green, blue, violet, red, orange, and yellow derivatives appear in sequence (Gmelin's reaction) [2]. These colored derivatives are the result of a series of successive dehydrogenations and oxidations of the ring and bridge structures. The reaction is characteristic, but not specific for bilirubin, and is useful for qualitative, rather than for quantitative, analysis.

The purple diazo derivative formed by the reaction of bilirubin with diazotized sulfanilic acid is widely used for pigment quantitation ("diazo reaction," van den Bergh's reaction). The reaction involves the splitting of bilirubin into dipyrrolic halves, and the subsequent coupling of diazotized sulfanilic acid to each half-bilirubin moiety [26]. The most commonly used technique, originally devised by Malloy and Evelyn, is performed in acid media and involves quantitation by reading optical density at 540 mμ [35]. Modifications have been proposed in which alkaline media are employed and the solution is read at 600 mμ, but these are less commonly used in the United States [36]. Bilirubin reacts with diazotized sulfanilic acid only after the addition of "accelerator" substances such as methanol ("indirect reaction"), whereas conjugated bilirubin reacts immediately and without the addition of accelerators ("direct reaction"). Explanation of this phenomenon in terms of the difference in water solubility between unconjugated and conjugated bilirubin is inadequate, since unconjugated bilirubin maintained in aqueous solution by addition of bile salt gives in part an indirect reaction. Fog has suggested that hydrogen bonding between the propionic acid side chains and the ring nitrogens prevents interaction between the diazotized sulfanilic acid and bilirubin by steric interference [29]. Since bilirubin is conjugated by esterification of the propionic acids with glucuronic acid, this would cause disruption of the postulated hydrogen bonds and permit nucleophilic attack of the diazotized sulfanilic acid on the central carbon bridge. As noted above, this explanation must be modified in view of the probable hydrogen bonding between the two propionic acid residues and between the outer-ring enols [28]. As a modified interpretation which might explain the direct diazo reaction, one might postulate that disruption of the propionic acid dimer by glucuronic acid conjugation results in an alteration of hydrogen bonding of the outer-ring enols, which in turn leads to an electron shift in the bilirubin chromophore so as to open the central carbon bridge to nucleophilic attack. This entire area will remain obscure until purified conjugated bilirubin becomes available for study. Whatever the mechanism of the direct diazo reaction ultimately proves to be, for practical purposes direct-reacting bilirubin in the plasma approximates conjugated bilirubin. A partition method has been devised for more accurate determination of conjugated bilirubin concentration [37], but for clinical use the Malloy-Evelyn technique usually is adequate.

Isotopic Labeling

Bile pigments were initially labeled biosynthetically with ^{15}N [38, 39], but this method was never widely employed for metabolic studies. Stable isotope assay is relatively insensitive, and it requires access to a mass spectrometer. Subsequently, methods were devised for ^{14}C and ^{3}H labeling of bilirubin and its derivatives. Ostrow, Hammaker, and Schmid prepared ^{14}C-labeled bilirubin through the administration of ^{14}C-glycine to rats made anemic by induced hemolysis and phlebotomy [31]. Under these conditions "early-labeled bilirubin" (see "Formation of Bilirubin from Sources Other than Senescent Erythrocytes," further on) is markedly increased, and the labeled precursor is rapidly incorporated into pigment. Bilirubin-^{14}C of relatively high specific activity and of proved radiochemical purity was crystallized from bile samples obtained through an external biliary fistula. Although variants of the method were suggested subsequently, a notable advance was introduced by the substitution of δ-aminolevulinic acid-^{14}C(ALA-^{14}C) as pigment precursor [40]. ALA is the first specific precursor in the porphyrin-bile pigment series, and its fractional incorporation into bile pigment is much greater than that of labeled glycine. Moreover, in vivo it is incorporated almost exclusively into bile pigment derived from nonerythroid sources, and therefore the need for anemic animals is eliminated.

Methods for tritiating bilirubin in vitro were first devised by Grodsky et al. [41]. Unlabeled bilirubin was exposed to tritium gas under drastic conditions by Wilzbach's technique [42]. The major fraction of unlabeled bilirubin is destroyed in this process, but the residual intact bilirubin bearing the label can be extracted and purified chromatographically. Exchangeable tritium may be removed by standard methods and through interaction of the pigment with albumin. The labeling process is inexpensive, the specific activities achieved are very high, and the preparative process is extremely simple. On the other hand, labeling is nonspecific and the relative proportions of label at any one site in the molecule are unpredictable. Theoretically, the procedure may produce minor changes in the labile bilirubin molecule which may be difficult to detect, and which in turn may autocatalyze their own formation, thereby complicating purification procedures [42]. Use of this labeling procedure requires careful chemical technique and rigorous purification.

An alternative method was devised in which bilirubin was tritiated biosynthetically [43]. ALA-3,5-^3H was prepared by a process of enolization exchange, which is inexpensive and easily performed. The site of tritium labeling in the ALA molecule was evaluated by metabolic methods, and directly by NMR spectroscopy. ALA-3,5-^3H was then administered to rats and the labeled pigment recovered from bile. The resulting bilirubin-^3H is not as highly labeled as that prepared by the Wilzbach technique, but specific activities up to 10 millicuries per millimole have been obtained, which are adequate for most investigative purposes. Moreover, the labeling is at specific sites in the bilirubin molecule, and the possibility of significant contamination with closely related radioactive compounds is virtually eliminated. More recently, an alternate biosynthetic method for tritiating bilirubin has been introduced, in which ALA-2,3-^3H is employed as the labeled precursor [44]. Preparation of ALA-2,3-^3H is an arduous procedure, but this material is commercially available.

Catabolism of Hemoglobin

The average life-span of the normal human erythrocyte is approximately 120 days [45]. At the end of this period, the cell is removed from the circulation, and its hemoglobin is degraded. Sequestration of senescent red blood cells and hemoglobin catabolism take place primarily in the reticuloendothelial cells of the spleen, but other tissues, including the liver and bone marrow, may share this function [45, 46]. In hemolytic states and after splenectomy, these secondary sites may assume the major role in hemoglobin catabolism and bilirubin formation [46]. Hemoglobin, released by intravascular hemolysis or administered intravenously, is degraded predominantly in the liver, kidney, and bone marrow [47], whereas the liver is probably the sole site of conversion of methemalbumin [48]. Finally, bilirubin is formed in subcutaneous hematomas [3] and in other blood extravasations [49], and this suggests that tissue or circulating macrophages have the capacity to convert heme to bile pigment [89].

It is not known how much hemoglobin can be converted to bile pigment by the intact organism, but clinical and experimental observations suggest that the maximum capacity, whether constitutive or adaptive, is far in excess of the physiologic turnover of hemoglobin and other hemoproteins. Thus, relatively large amounts of dissolved hemoglobin [50] or antibody-coated erythrocytes [46, 50] infused into experimental animals are efficiently converted to bile pigment. In hemolytic anemia unconjugated hyperbilirubinemia is frequently observed, but significant hemoglobinemia or methemalbuminemia is unusual. This indicates that the rate of release of heme rarely exceeds the rate of heme degradation, but the rate of heme degradation may exceed the maximum rate of bilirubin removal by the liver. The older literature relating to red blood cell destruction and bilirubin formation was reviewed by Lepehne [51], With [24], and Watson [15].

Of the three hemoglobin constituents, iron is almost completely reutilized for formation of new iron-containing compounds [52]. The globin is degraded and returned to the amino acid pool [45]. The protoporphyrin moiety is not preserved; the porphyrin ring is cleaved at its α-methene bridge and yields equimolar amounts of bile pigment and carbon monoxide [10, 53, 54] (Figs. 46-1 and 46-2). Originally, it was postulated that the physiologic breakdown of hemoglobin was brought about by a coupled oxidation with ascorbate and molecular oxygen which led to formation of a series of green bile pigment iron-globin complexes (choleglobin, verdohemoglobin), and upon treatment with acetic acid these yielded biliverdin and free iron [25, 55]. Although choleglobin-like pigments were tentatively identified in stored human red blood cells [56] and in erythrocytes of rabbits treated with phenylhydrazine [57–59], the possibility was not excluded that these green pigments simply represented artifacts [60–63].

Though Lemberg and his school considered this catabolic system to be nonenzymatic, Nakajima and coworkers claimed to have characterized and partially purified a soluble enzyme system that converted heme to a possible precursor of biliverdin. The enzyme, which they called heme α-methenyl oxygenase, was obtained from liver and kidney homogenate; as cofactors, it required NADPH, ferrous iron, and an activator extracted from liver cell nuclei by boiling water [64]. The system was unusual in its substrate specificity in that it acted only on pyridine hemochromogen, hemoglobin-haptoglobin complex, and myoglobin [65], whereas it was inactive with hematin, oxyhemoglobin, and methe-

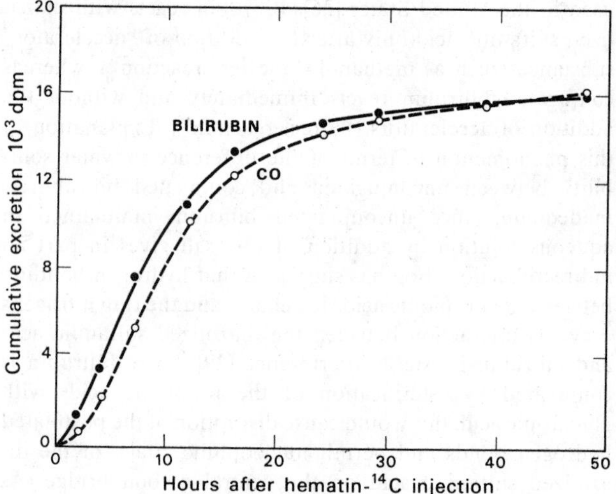

Figure 46-2. Cumulative production of ^{14}C-bilirubin and ^{14}CO in a rat with an external bile fistula injected with ^{14}C-hematin in a single pulse at a time zero. (*By permission of S. A. Landaw et al.* [54].)

moglobin. Moreover, spleen and bone marrow, both tissues presumably active in hemoglobin degradation, were relatively low in enzymatic activity. Subsequent reports failed to confirm the existence of a soluble heme α-methenyl oxygenase system. Levin [66] and Murphy and coworkers [67] showed that Nakajima's findings could be ascribed to a dialyzable and heat-stable factor of low molecular weight functioning as a reducing agent. Furthermore, Nichol and Morell [68] demonstrated that with this nonenzymatic system, mixtures of biliverdin isomers are obtained, whereas in vivo only the α isomer of the bile pigment is produced [10]. These findings argue strongly against a physiologic role of coupled oxidation or of "heme α-methenyl oxygenase" in the degradation of heme compounds in vivo. Compelling evidence that the activity of Nakajima's system is due to coupled oxidation with ascorbate was recently published by Colleran and O'Carra [385].

In preliminary communications, Wise and Drabkin described a light-mitochondrial system obtained from the hemophagous organ of the dog placenta that converted hemoglobin to biliverdin [69, 70]. This enzyme system resembled the microsomal heme oxygenase system discussed below [12] in being particulate in nature, but differed from it by requiring NAD and ATP. Moreover, because of its localization in an esoteric organ of unknown function, long known to contain biliverdin [71], the relevance of this system to the physiologic mechanism of bile pigment formation in the intact organism was not established.

A series of recent observations strongly support the concept originally proposed by Watson [15] that hematin is the first intermediate formed on hemoglobin degradation. According to this scheme, the initial catabolic step consists in the splitting of the iron-protoporphyrin complex from the globin [2, 15, 72, 73]. Green and Kench [74] and Bunn and Jandl [75] demonstrated that the ferriprotoporphyrin ring of methemoglobin may readily be dissociated from the globin; the separated hematin then is transferred to albumin, forming methemalbumin, or to hemopexin [384]. In conditions associated with intravascular hemolysis [76] and in some instances of severe liver disease [15, 77], the plasma may contain hematin bound to albumin (methemalbumin). Under physiologic conditions, hematin cannot be demonstrated in the blood, presumably because the breakdown of red blood cells occurs primarily inside the reticuloendothelial cells.

Conversion of hematin to bile pigments has been demonstrated in vivo [8, 79–81], and recent experiments in rats injected with ^{14}C-hematin revealed almost quantitative excretion of the label in the form of conjugated bilirubin [48]. Moreover, in the intact organism, hematin [48] and hemoglobin [50] are converted to bilirubin by similar kinetics; both are taken up preferentially by the liver [48], whereas sequestration of senescent erythrocytes normally occurs primarily in the spleen. The earlier belief that free protoporphyrin may represent an intermediate step in the catabolism of hematin [83] was shown to be erroneous, in that the presence of a central divalent or trivalent metal was found to be essential for the cleavage of the heme ring in vivo [12, 80]. Studies demonstrating the conversion of a small fraction of labeled protoporphyrin to bilirubin do not contradict this concept, since they suggest that a small fraction of the administered protoporphyrin was converted to heme which then was broken down to bile pigment [82]. It is well established that protoporphyrin may form heme by spontaneous coordination with ferrous iron [84, 85] or by serving as substrate for the enzyme ferrochelatase [86].

The conversion of hematin to bilirubin occurs in two steps (Fig. 46-3). The first involves the cleavage of the porphyrin

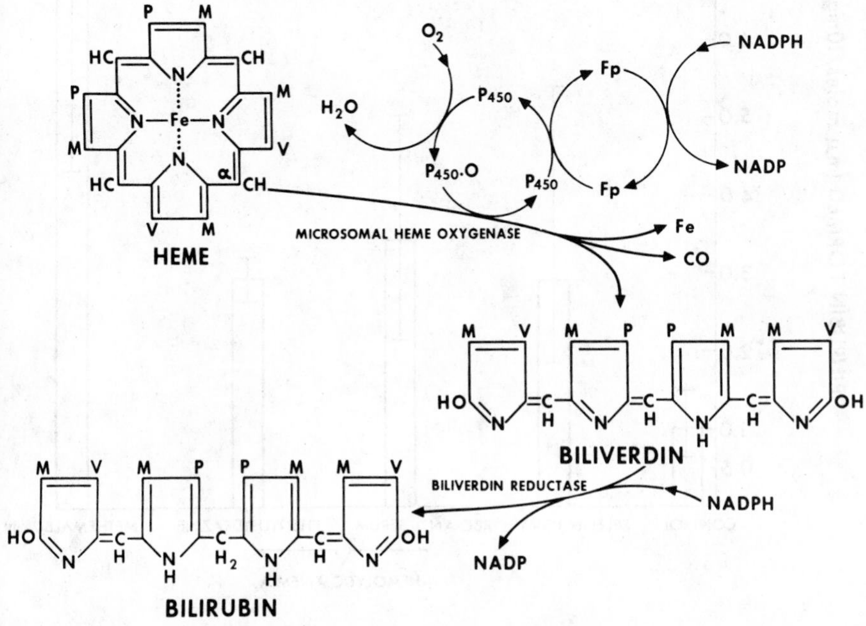

Figure 46-3. Enzymatic conversion of heme to bilirubin by microsomal heme oxygenase and soluble biliverdin reductase. (*By permission of R. Tenhunen et al., Trans. Ass. Amer. Physicians,* **8**, 1969.)

ring at the α-methene bridge by the microsomal enzyme heme oxygenase [12]. The resulting biliverdin IXα is then reduced to bilirubin IXα by soluble biliverdin reductase, which is closely coupled with the microsomal heme oxygenase system [87]. The heme oxygenase is rate-limiting, whereas the soluble biliverdin reductase is present in great excess.

Heme oxygenase activity was detected in several tissues, most of which contain cells with reticuloendothelial function [88]. Highest enzyme activity per gram of tissue protein was found in spleen, followed by bone marrow, liver, brain, kidney, and lung [88]. Heme oxygenase activity also is present in isolated macrophages, particularly after their exposure to hematin or hemoglobin [89]. The measured enzyme activity in the rat spleen is in good agreement with the kinetic requirements for red blood cell hemoglobin turnover in the intact animal [13]. After splenectomy hepatic heme oxygenase activity is greatly increased (Fig. 46-4), indicating the potential of the liver to substitute for the spleen as a major site of red blood cell destruction [88]. Experimentally induced hemolysis also results in a significant increase in hepatic heme oxygenase activity (Fig. 46-4). This points up the major role of this organ in the removal of damaged erythrocytes. Finally, parenteral administration of hemoglobin or hematin, both of which are converted to bilirubin predominantly in the liver [47, 48, 50], greatly enhances hepatic enzyme activity [88]. These findings leave little doubt that in individual tissues the level of heme oxygenase activity is regulated by the amount of heme that is being offered for catabolism. The exact mechanism of this enzyme stimulation is unknown, but recent findings in the kidney of rats made hemoglobinuric suggest that substrate-mediated enzyme induction is involved [90].

Heme oxygenase is a microsomal enzyme that catalyzes the mixed-function oxidation of heme by a mechanism similar to that involved in the oxidation of many drugs and endogenous steroids. The system utilizes cytochrome P450 as the terminal oxidase and requires NADPH and molecular oxygen [12, 13]; carbon monoxide inhibits the reaction. Methemalbumin, methemoglobin, isolated α and β chains of hemoglobin, and hemopexin-bound hemin readily serve as substrates [12]. In these hemoproteins, the heme group is easily dissociated from the protein moiety [74, 75]. By contrast, with oxyhemoglobin, carboxyhemoglobin, myoglobin, and haptoglobin-bound hemoglobin in which the heme group is more firmly bound, the enzyme system was nearly inactive [12]. Free porphyrins lacking a central iron atom, are not attacked by heme oxygenase.

Hematin is converted stoichiometrically to 1 mole of the α isomer of biliverdin and 1 mole of CO by purified micro-

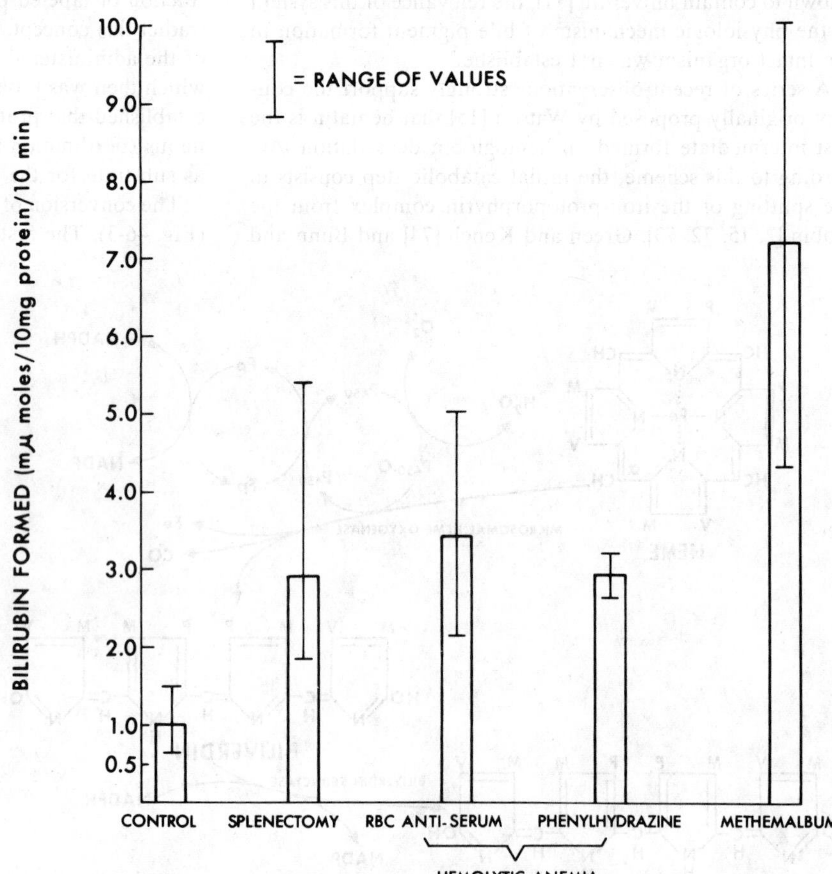

Figure 46-4. Enhancement of heme oxygenase activity in rat liver after splenectomy, after treatment with rat erythrocyte antiserum or phenylhydrazine, or after methemalbumin injection. (*By permission of R. Tenhunen et al., Trans. Ass. Amer. Physicians,* **8,** 1969.)

somal heme oxygenase [12] (Figs. 46-2 and 46-3). As already stated, the biliverdin IXα is rapidly reduced by biliverdin reductase to bilirubin IXα [87]. Biliverdin reductase is a soluble enzyme with an absolute requirement for NADPH (Fig. 46-3). Although biliverdin reductase is functionally coupled with the heme oxygenase system, its tissue distribution is wider than that of the latter, and it is not rate-limiting in the overall conversion of heme to bilirubin [12, 13, 87]. This explains why in vivo, even in severe hemolytic anemia, biliverdin rarely is detectable in plasma [91].

These recent observations clearly indicate that the metabolic conversion of hemoglobin to bilirubin is an enzymatic process in which microsomal heme oxygenase plays an essential role. The enzyme system is operational in a variety of tissues, including liver, spleen, kidney, brain, and macrophages. This explains the observation originally recorded by Virchow [3] that bilirubin may be formed in subcutaneous and pleural blood extravasations. Moreover, this enzymatic apparatus is capable of regulatory adaptation in response to substrate loads, thereby providing a mechanism for the efficient catabolism of relatively large amounts of hemoglobin that may be delivered in hemolytic or hemorrhagic states. Finally the product of the catabolic process is bilirubin IXα derived from cleavage of the ferriprotoporphyrin ring at the α-methene bridge (Figs. 46-1 and 46-3); the α-carbon is converted quantitatively to CO (Figs. 46-2 and 46-3).

Although there is little doubt that in vivo the bulk of the hemoglobin and probably most other hemoproteins are catabolized by this enzymatic route, there is strong evidence that even under normal conditions small amounts of heme are converted to metabolites other than bilirubin [54]. This is suggested by the frequent observation of significant discrepancies between estimated rates of hemoglobin turnover and the amounts of bile pigment recovered in the stool [16, 92–94]. In rats injected with ^{14}C-labeled antibody-sensitized red blood cells, only 63 to 81 percent of the sequestered heme pigment appeared in the bile as ^{14}C-labeled bilirubin [50]. When small amounts of ^{14}C-labeled hematin were administered, 50 to 68 percent of the isotope appeared in ^{14}C-bilirubin in the bile, and an equimolar amount of ^{14}CO was eliminated in the breath [54]; an additional 20 to 25 percent of the label was excreted in the bile in the form of unidentified metabolites. It is likely that in these experiments the hemoglobin or hematin not accounted for by labeled bilirubin in the bile was converted to di- or monopyrrolic derivatives, but, because of methodologic difficulties, isolation and identification of these metabolites in the bile have not been possible.

The heme of Heinz bodies, which consist of oxidatively denatured and precipitated hemoglobin [95], is broken down in vivo to diazo-negative and water-soluble metabolites [96] which are excreted in the bile; bilirubin is neither an intermediate nor an end product in this process. Moreover, in rats treated with the porphyrinogenic compound allylisopropylacetamide, exogenously administered hematin or heme formed in the liver is converted largely to metabolites other than bilirubin [54]. It is tempting to assume that these examples reflect instances of heme breakdown by alternate and presumably nonenzymatic routes. It remains to be determined whether these alternate pathways are unique for these specific situations or whether they simply represent an exaggeration of alternate routes of heme degradation that are functional under normal conditions. The metabolic pathways by which heme is degraded may be determined by the nature of the initial attack on the ferroprotoporphyrin ring; while enzymatic attack by heme oxygenase leads to bilirubin, chemical modification of the heme ring (e.g., by peroxides or related redox compounds) may result in formation of other pyrrolic derivatives [54].

Dipyrrolic compounds belonging to the group of bilifuscin, mesobilifuscin, and pentdyopent have been identified and isolated in the feces of healthy individuals [97–99], and pentdyopent has occasionally been found in the urine of jaundiced patients [100, 101]. The metabolic origin of these substances has not yet been established. On the basis of earlier investigations they were regarded as catabolites derived from breakdown of bilirubin in the intestine [97, 98], but more recent findings obtained with isotopic techniques do not support this concept [99, 102]. Dark pigments belonging to the mesobilifuscin group are excreted in the urine of patients with a rare congenital syndrome in which increased hemolysis is associated with the presence of erythrocyte inclusion bodies [103]. Similar dipyrrolic pigments are said to be detectable in the urine of patients with certain hemoglobinopathies [104]. In these instances the urinary pigments are believed to be derived from the abnormal red blood cells, but the nature of the metabolic defect in the erythrocytes is not yet known.

Formation of Bilirubin from Sources Other than Senescent Erythrocytes

At a relatively early date it was appreciated that not all bilirubin is derived from the breakdown of senescent erythrocytes [38, 39]. When glycine-^{15}N was administered to human subjects and experimental animals, most of the ^{15}N label recovered in fecal bile pigment was found, as expected, in a peak of isotope roughly 120 days after administration (Fig. 46-5). From 10 to 20 percent of the ^{15}N label was recovered from fecal bile pigment excreted in an early peak of isotope before maximum heme labeling of the circulating red blood cells. Glycine is incorporated into heme only in newly formed red blood cells. The "early-labeled peak" might be produced, therefore, by the rapid formation and degradation of hemoglobin *within* immature red blood cells [39], or by the loss of cytoplasmic hemoglobin in association with normoblast nuclear extrusion [105]. It appeared more probable, however, that early-labeled bilirubin (ELB) is derived from the heme of a unique population of red blood cells with an extremely short survival, or from nonerythroid heme sources. In subsequent studies several major technical refinements were em-

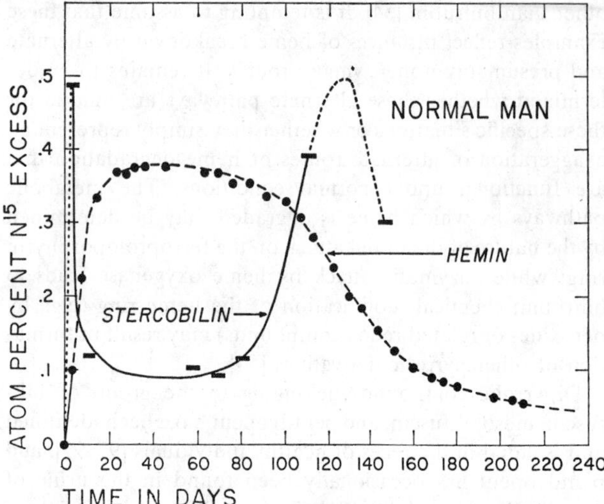

Figure 46-5. Formation of bile pigment in normal man. When glycine-^{15}N is administered to normal man, hemin of circulating hemoglobin shows a rapid increase in isotope content. Fecal stercobilin exhibits two separate peaks of high isotope concentration; a first maximum is reached during the first week, while the second maximum coincides with the period of maximal breakdown of labeled erythrocytes. (*By permission of I. M. London et al.* [38].)

ployed: radioactive labeling was substituted for the more cumbersome heavy-isotope labeling; bile or serum bilirubin was examined directly rather than the pigment derivatives recovered from the feces; and estimates of the rate of bilirubin production were substituted for the earlier expression of results in terms of the amount of pigment excreted [106–108]. These studies established that ELB production begins within *minutes* of labeled precursor administration, and reaches peak rates within 1 to 3 hr (Fig. 46-6) [109, 110]. The amount of label incorporated depends on the species investigated and on the precursor employed. Less than 1 percent of intravenously injected glycine-2-^{14}C is recovered as ELB, while fractional incorporation of the more specific porphyrin precursor δ-aminolevulinic acid-^{14}C (ALA-^{14}C) is much higher. Moreover, ALA-^{14}C penetrates red blood cells poorly so that fractional incorporation into hemoglobin in vivo is minimal, while labeling of nonhemoglobin heme and ELB is high [109–111].

The source or sources of ELB have been a matter of considerable controversy. On several occasions the possibility has been raised that ELB might be formed by the linear assembly of pyrrolic subunits without intermediary porphyrin or heme formation [38, 39]. It was suggested that ELB may include isomers other than the IXα isomer of bilirubin, which, in turn, would indicate that not all pigment in this fraction is derived from the oxidation of heme at its α-carbon bridge [112]. The possibility might, therefore, be raised that this non-IXα bilirubin might be formed through direct assembly of monopyrrolic subunits ("shunt bilirubin") rather than by way of heme formation and oxidation. It should be noted that the methods employed for the study of tetrapyrrole isomeric structure are far from quantitative. If the formation of non-IXα isomers in vivo is confirmed, these findings may be explained plausibly by the occurrence of limited heme oxidation at the β-, γ-, or δ-carbon bridges [112]. Under normal conditions, there is, in fact, an excellent molar relationship between bile pigment production and carbon monoxide formation (Fig. 46-2), which suggests strongly that bile pigment is formed by the oxidation of heme bridge carbons through a mechanism which yields 1 mole of carbon monoxide per mole of bilirubin formed [113]. Even in phylogenetically primitive unicellular organisms, "straight-chain" tetrapyrroles similar to bilirubin are formed from porphyrin intermediates [114] by a mechanism which causes the liberation of stoichiometric quantities of carbon monoxide [115]. Bile pigment formation through cleavage of a porphyrin ring is, therefore, a primal mechanism, and it appears highly improbable that there is a pathway for biosynthesis of shunt bilirubin that bypasses a porphyrin-metal complex as an intermediary.

Another possible origin of ELB that has been mentioned is myoglobin heme [116], but its rate of turnover is so slow as to make it a highly improbable candidate [116, 117]. On the other hand, two sources that deserve serious consideration include heme contained in, or synthesized for, cytochromes and other hemoprotein enzymes, and hemoglobin-heme of maturing red blood cells with a very short life-span.

ALA-^{14}C, which, as noted above, labels primarily nonerythroid heme, was found to label sequentially, first, hepatic "freely extractable heme" (i.e., unbound or loosely bound heme), and then bilirubin [118]. Isolated rat liver perfused with mature red blood cells or with plasma produced bilirubin-^{14}C from both glycine-^{14}C and ALA-^{14}C [119]. In this system no precursor was incorporated into hemoglobin, since no hemoglobin was newly synthesized, and the bilirubin-^{14}C excreted could be derived only from nonerythroid hepatic sources. Of interest was the finding that the amount of bilirubin-^{14}C formed by the isolated perfused rat liver was similar to the amount produced over a comparable period when labeled precursor was administered intravenously to an intact rat. This suggested that nonerythroid heme synthesized and located in the liver is the major source of ELB. The microsomal cytochrome P450, which is part of the drug-metabolizing apparatus of the liver, may be a source of nonerythroid ELB [120], but a major fraction appears to be derived from hepatic "free-tissue heme," (i.e. heme which is not bound to an apoprotein) [121].

Israels was the first to point out that ELB formation is diphasic or multiphasic [106]. He attributed the initial component of the early-labeled peak to nonerythroid sources, and the later component(s) to rapid turnover of red blood cell precursors. This view has, in part, been substantiated. In clinical states associated with a rapid turnover of red blood cell precursors ("ineffective erythropoiesis"), ELB is markedly increased. Thus in congenital erythropoietic porphyria [39, 122], pernicious anemia [123], and thalassemia

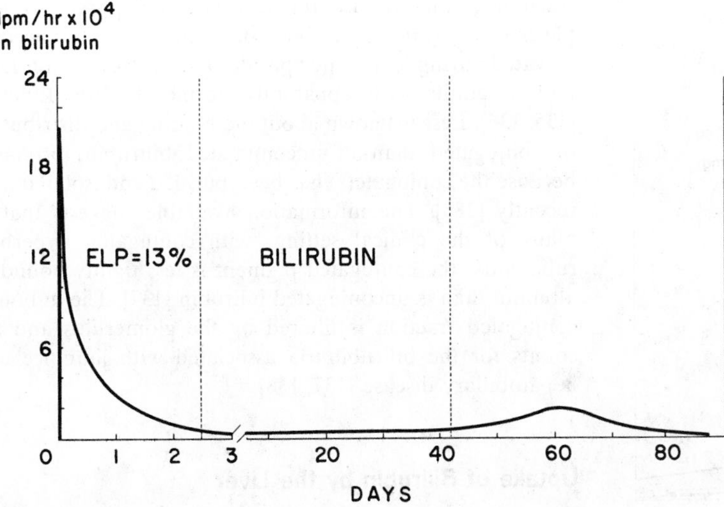

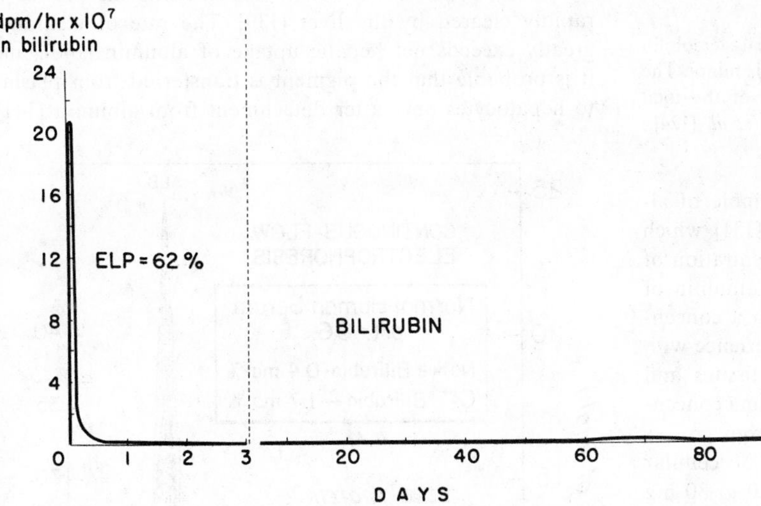

Figure 46-6. Formation of ^{14}C-bilirubin after the administration of glycine-2-^{14}C (*top*) or δ-amino-levulinic acid-4-^{14}C (*bottom*) to Gunn rats. *ELP,* early-labeled peak, expressed in percentage of the *total* production of labeled bile pigment. With glycine-2-^{14}C, a late-labeled peak containing the major fraction of radio-labeled bilirubin is evident. This reflects catabolism of labeled hemoglobin in senescent erythrocytes. The ELP formed with δ-amino-levulinic acid-4-^{14}C is sharper and contains the major fraction of radio-labeled bilirubin. (*By permission of S. H. Robinson et al.* [109].)

minor [124], from 30 to 80 percent of the fecal bile pigment may originate from sources other than mature red blood cells (Fig. 46-7). When erythropoiesis was altered under relatively well-controlled clinical conditions, there appeared to be little effect on the initial component of ELB, but the later component(s) was markedly influenced [121, 125]. Moreover, it has been shown that reticulocytes produced under conditions in which the bone marrow is stressed may show limited survival [126, 127]. These observations may suggest that, normally, prematurely destroyed red blood cell precursors contribute to the formation of ELB. On the other hand, at least in the rat, complete suppression of erythropoiesis by hypertransfusion failed to alter the shape of both the early and the late components of the early-labeled peak [109]. This disparate finding may be the result of species differences or may represent relative insensitivity of the methods for measuring bile pigment formation.

Thus, in brief, it is clear that the initial component of ELB is largely hepatic in origin. The relative contribution of erythroid and of nonerythroid elements to the later phases of ELB formation under normal conditions remains controversial [128].

TRANSPORT, CONJUGATION, AND EXCRETION OF BILIRUBIN

Transport of Bilirubin in the Plasma

Bilirubin is sparingly soluble in aqueous solution at physiologic pH and ionic strength [32, 33]. It has been known for many years that in plasma it is bound to protein. The vast and often contradictory older literature on the subject has been reviewed by With [16]. The best evidence suggests that bilirubin is bound exclusively to albumin (Fig. 46-8) and that the equilibrium

$$[\text{Bilirubin}] + [\text{Albumin}] = [\text{Bilirubin} - \text{Albumin}]$$

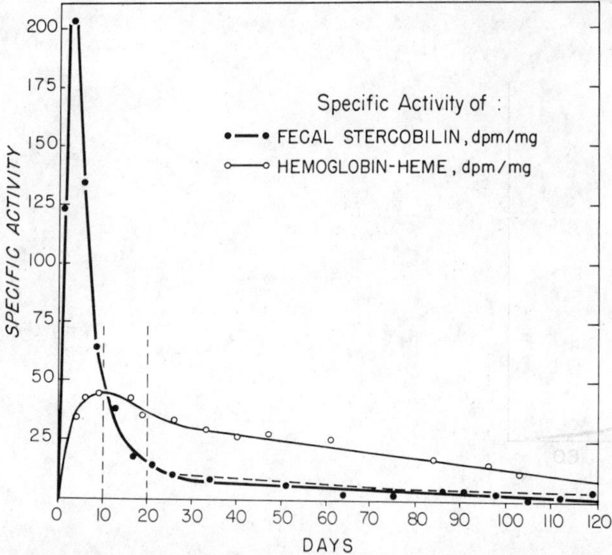

Figure 46-7. Incorporation of glycine-2-^{14}C into fecal stercobilin and into hemoglobin-heme in a patient with thalassemia minor. The early-labeled fraction comprises at least 75 percent of the total stercobilin output. (*By permission of S. H. Robinson et al.* [124].)

is preponderantly to the right [129–131]. One mole of albumin can maximally bind 2 moles of bilirubin [131], which would mean, assuming a plasma albumin concentration of 4 gm per 100 ml and a molecular weight for albumin of 68,000, that bilirubin in plasma is bound up to a concentration of about 70 mg per 100 ml. Clinical experience with kernicterus suggests that bilirubin penetrates tissues and produces evidence of toxicity at much lower plasma concentrations [132]. Presumably only unbound bilirubin crosses cellular membranes, and the clinical finding of cellular toxicity at plasma bilirubin concentrations of 20 to 30 mg per 100 ml suggests that the second mole of bilirubin is bound to albumin less tightly than the first [129, 130]. In addition, other factors such as plasma pH, the presence of organic anions which compete for albumin binding, and differences in the ease with which bilirubin penetrates membranes and is bound to intracellular constituents, may all influence the distribution and toxic effects of bilirubin (see "Neonatal Hyperbilirubinemia," further on in this chapter).

In healthy persons the total serum bilirubin concentration ranges from 0.1 to 0.8 mg per 100 ml [133]. Many animals such as rats, mice, dogs, and cats, consistently have low values [16]; in horses the bilirubin concentration is higher than in man. This variability may in part reflect species differences in the degree of albumin-bilirubin binding [134].

Less than 10 percent of bilirubin in the plasma of normal individuals gives a direct van den Bergh reaction [133]. Whether this small fraction really represents conjugated bilirubin or is an artifact is uncertain. In hepatocellular and obstructive disease both the unconjugated and conjugated fractions commonly rise. It is less generally appreciated that plasma *conjugated* bilirubin concentrations may become elevated during hemolytic episodes both in newborn infants and in adults with apparently normal hepatic function [135, 136]. Less is known about the binding and distribution of conjugated than of unconjugated bilirubin, primarily because the conjugate(s) has been purified and isolated only recently [386]. The information available suggests that in many of the clinical settings with conjugated hyperbilirubinemia, the conjugated pigment is less tightly bound to albumin than is unconjugated bilirubin [137]. The unbound conjugated fraction is filtered by the glomerulus and accounts for the bilirubinuria associated with jaundice and hepatobiliary disease [137, 138].

Uptake of Bilirubin by the Liver

Bilirubin formed in the tissues and entering the plasma is rapidly cleared by the liver [139]. The rate of clearance greatly exceeds net hepatic uptake of albumin [140], and it is probable that the pigment is transferred from plasma to hepatocytes only after detachment from albumin [141].

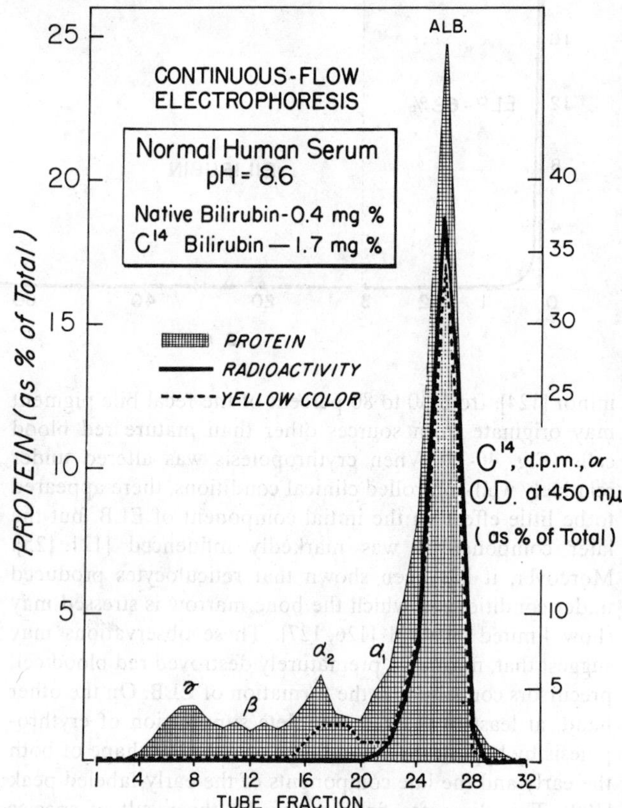

Figure 46-8. Continuous-flow electrophoresis of human serum, containing 1.7 mg percent ^{14}C-bilirubin. All radioactive pigment is bound to albumin. (*By permission of J. D. Ostrow et al.* [131].)

Competitive inhibition of bilirubin uptake has been demonstrated [142–144], and presumably uptake is carrier-mediated. Reversible movement of labeled bilirubin into and out of liver cells has been demonstrated [144], and similarly, kinetic analyses of plasma bilirubin disappearance curves [145, 146] are compatible with the concept of bidirectional fluxes across the sinusoidal surface of the liver cell. Under normal conditions, and especially in the face of a bilirubin load, net movement is into the liver.

Little is known about bilirubin transport within the hepatic cell. An intrahepatic storage space for bilirubin comparable to that for Bromsulphalein (BSP) has been described [147]. After intravenous injection of radioactive bilirubin relatively small quantities of label are associated with hepatocellular organelles [141, 148]. Of this small portion, a disproportionately large amount is associated with microsomes, which may indicate pigment binding to smooth endoplasmic reticulum during the process of conjugation. The great proportion of intrahepatic radioactive bilirubin is found in the soluble fraction of the liver cell. Recent studies suggest that bilirubin in liver cells is bound to specific soluble proteins of low molecular weight designated Y and Z [150]. Binding is saturable, and other organic anions secreted by the liver (e.g., BSP) also are bound by these proteins and compete with bilirubin for binding. Both proteins have been identified in the liver of man and other mammals, but only small quantities are found in brain, kidney, and other organs. The precise role of Y and Z in the hepatic uptake and intracellular transport of bilirubin has not yet been defined. Attempts have been made to correlate concentration of intrahepatic binding proteins with changes in hepatic bilirubin uptake that may be associated with maturation of the fetus and newborn. These studies suggest that Y may play a greater role than Z in the intracellular pigment binding in vivo [151]. In order to establish conclusively the functional role of these soluble protein fractions, it will be necessary to demonstrate that hepatic pigment uptake critically depends on their presence.

Conjugation of Bilirubin

Glucuronyl Transferase

In the liver cell synthesis of conjugated bilirubin is enzymatically catalyzed [17–19], and glucuronic acid is transferred from the nucleotide uridine diphosphate glucuronic acid (UDPGA) to the carboxyl groups of the pigment; the resulting product is an alkali-labile ester-glucuronide (Fig. 46-9). UDPGA is derived from glucose-1-phosphate through the formation of uridine diphosphate glucose (UDP-glucose), which is oxidized by a soluble dehydrogenase reaction [17, 18, 152, 153] (Fig. 46-10). The transferring enzyme, glucuronyl transferase, is associated with the microsomal fraction of the liver [154, 155], but it appears probable that several related but distinct microsomal enzymes catalyze the synthesis of the various ester and ether glucuronides [156–158] formed by the liver [159]. Biosynthesis of bilirubin glucuronide has been demonstrated with slices [160], homogenates [160–162], and microsomal preparations [153] of mammalian liver.

Most of the bilirubin excreted in the bile of man [17–19], cat [163], rat [164], guinea pig [165], dog [18], and sheep [166] is present as the diglucuronide, but a minor pigment fraction exhibits properties conforming to a "monoglucuronide" structure [167]. It is possible that this minor fraction is a labile equimolar complex of bilirubin and bilirubin diglucuronide [36, 168, 169]. Rats congenitally deficient in glucuronyl transferase ("Gunn Rat," further on), although unable to conjugate and excrete bilirubin, can transfer relatively large amounts of unconjugated pigment into bile if given an intravenous infusion of bilirubin glucuronide [170].

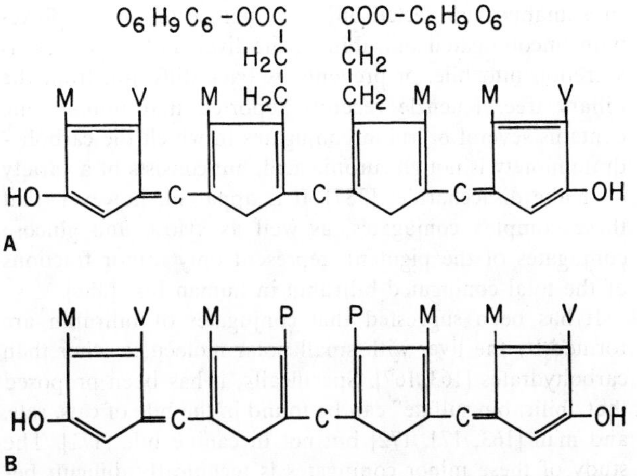

Figure 46-9. A. Conjugated bilirubin ("direct-reacting"). B. Free bilirubin ("indirect-reacting"). In conjugated bilirubin, glucuronic acid is attached to the two propionic acid groups to form an acyl-glucuronide.

UDPG + 2 DPN⁺ —UDPG-dehydrogenase (liver extract)→ UDPGA + 2DPNH + 2H⁺

2 UDPGA + BILIRUBIN —GA-transferase (liver microsomes)→ BILIRUBIN DIGLUCURONIDE + 2UDP

Figure 46-10. Enzymatic formation of bilirubin diglucuronide. Glucuronic acid is transferred from the nucleotide uridine diphosphate glucuronic acid (UDPGA) to bilirubin. UDPGA is formed by dehydrogenation of uridine diphosphate glucose (UDP-glucose).

Presumably the injected bilirubin diglucuronide complexes with unconjugated bilirubin in the liver and facilitates its secretion into bile, or prevents its back diffusion from the biliary tree. Kuenzle recently reported that human bile contains several bilirubin conjugates in which the carbohydrate moiety is not glucuronic acid, but consists of a variety of acidic disaccharides [387]. It is apparent, however, that these complex conjugates, as well as xylose and glucose conjugates of the pigment, represent only minor fractions of the total conjugated bilirubin in human bile [388].

It has been suggested that conjugates of bilirubin are formed by the liver with small polar molecules other than carbohydrates [163, 167]. Specifically, it has been proposed that "bilirubin sulfate" can be found in the bile of cats, rats, and man [163, 171, 172] but not in canine bile [171]. The study of these minor conjugates is technically difficult because of the small amounts of material available, the lability of the conjugates in biologic materials, the technical problems encountered in chromatographing pigments and their derivatives, and the lack of purified bilirubin glucuronide or adequately pure synthetic standards of the postulated derivates. The azo derivative of bilirubin sulfate found by one group migrated chromatographically with an R_f identical to that of bilirubin glucuronide [163]; the azo derivative obtained by another group migrated with an R_f different from that of bilirubin glucuronide but identical to that of a synthetic bilirubin sulfate [172]. Even if it is established that such minor conjugates exist, it appears improbable that conjugation of bilirubin by mechanisms other than glucuronide formation is of functional significance. In instances of congenital defects in glucuronide synthesis, compensatory increases in the formation of other pigment conjugates are not observed [134].

Attempts to estimate the capacity of the liver for conjugation of bilirubin have met with considerable difficulty. Because separate quantitation of conjugated and unconjugated pigment in tissue preparations is inaccurate, most investigators have assayed the rate of glucuronide synthesis by using other aglycones as substrates. This may not be justified, since investigations with solubilized purified enzyme preparations [158] and studies in vivo [173–175] have suggested the presence of two or more transferase enzymes, the activities of which may vary independently. Using available techniques it has been shown that pretreatment of animals with a variety of compounds leads to enhanced activity of microsomal enzyme systems in general [176] and of glucuronide synthesis in particular [177]. Similarly, a number of compounds added in vitro have been found to stimulate [178, 179] or inhibit [180–182] glucuronide synthesis, but it is not known whether this is because of a direct effect on the transferring enzyme or whether this represents structural alterations produced within or at the surface of the microsomal particles. Of particular interest is the finding that in homogenates of Gunn rat liver, which normally form little *o*-aminophenol glucuronide, this limited capacity is increased twentyfold upon addition of diethylnitrosamine [183]. Clearly, therefore, the conditions of study greatly influence the in vitro assay of glucuronyl transferase, and care is required in drawing conclusions about the *functional amounts* of this enzyme based on *in vitro activity* [184–186].

Physiologic Implications of Conjugation

In the formation of bilirubin diglucuronide, bilirubin is changed from a weakly charged, chloroform-soluble molecule (molecular weight, 585) to a larger, hydroxylated, water-soluble conjugate (molecular weight, approximately 941). Unconjugated bilirubin, as described above, is sparingly soluble in water at physiologic pH, but high concentrations can be maintained in aqueous solutions containing conjugated bile salts. Under many conditions such solutions are unstable, and it is, therefore, not surprising that an association between elevated levels of unconjugated bilirubin in the bile and pigment gallstone formation has been postulated [187, 188]. Pigment stones are commonly seen in association with biliary tree infection in Japan, and it has been suggested that bacterial β-glucuronidase in the bile liberates unconjugated bilirubin, which may then form a calcium salt and precipitate. Similarly, pigment stones seen in patients with chronic hemolysis may be due to the increased amounts of unconjugated bilirubin found in bile in association with high rates of bilirubin glucuronide excretion [170]. It would therefore appear that, under normal conditions, stable solubilization of pigment in bile is a direct result of glucuronide formation.

As noted above in the section on the chemistry of bilirubin, the molecular structure and physicochemical characteristics of the bilirubin molecule are much affected by the unsaturated bridges connecting the pyrrole rings, and by intramolecular hydrogen bonding involving the propionic acid side chains [28, 29]. Esterification of the acid side chains with glucuronic acid should alter intramolecular hydrogen bonding in bilirubin, and thus influence molecular configuration and charge distribution in the molecule. It is of interest, therefore, that tetrapyrroles closely resembling bilirubin, but with the outer carbon bridges saturated, are excreted by the liver *without* glucuronide conjugation [189]. Though alternative explanations are possible, one might speculate that the configurational changes conferred by saturation of the carbon bridges influence the "fit" of tetrapyrroles to the hepatic secretory "carrier." Tetrapyrroles with saturated carbon bridges might fit the secretory carrier directly, whereas bilirubin with its unsaturated bridges might require glucuronide conjugation before an adequate fit is achieved. Glucuronide formation may, therefore, represent an adaptive mechanism to permit more efficient secretion of bilirubin into the canaliculus [189].

Because of its solubility characteristics, bilirubin diffuses across lipoid surfaces, whereas bilirubin glucuronide does not. Thus, as discussed in several sections of this review, unconjugated, but not conjugated, bilirubin is absorbed from the intestine [190, 191] and the gallbladder [192], crosses the placenta [193–196], and penetrates the blood-brain barrier [197]. It may be concluded, therefore, that glucuronide formation prevents the transfer of bile pigment across biologic membranes, and by limiting cellular and organelle penetration, serves as an effective detoxification mechanism. Similarly, conjugation may increase the efficacy of the excretory process by preventing back-diffusion from the biliary tree and the intestine.

Secretion of Bilirubin into Bile

The excretion of bilirubin occurs by a poorly understood mechanism which may be shared by a diverse group of endogenous and exogenous organic anions that are secreted into bile. Some but not all of these molecules are conjugated, as bilirubin is, with small polar metabolites during the excretory process, and most of the excreted molecules have polar-nonpolar configuration. Biliary secretion proceeds against large concentration gradients, competitive inhibition has been demonstrated, and the mechanism is saturable [147]. It is reasonable, therefore, to conclude that the secretion of bilirubin glucuronide, and of other comparable organic anions, is carrier-mediated and is, directly or indirectly, associated with energy-consuming processes [198].

Of additional interest is the dissociation between the excretion of bile salts and that of other organic anions. Hepatic transport of the organic anion series is greatly reduced in mutant Corriedale sheep with a disorder similar to Dubin-Johnson syndrome [199]; in these sheep taurocholate secretion is maintained at normal rates [200]. Similarly, although the secretion of bilirubin and bilirubin glucuronide is defective in the primate fetus [193, 195, 196], cholate and taurocholate are efficiently secreted [201]. Thus both genetic and developmental evidence suggests that the secretion of bilirubin and that of bile salt are distinct.

Fate of Bilirubin in the Gastrointestinal Tract

Bile pigment reaches the intestine in the form of bilirubin glucuronide. As noted above, because of its molecular size and solubility characteristics, bilirubin glucuronide is not appreciably reabsorbed as such [190, 191]. The conjugate probably remains intact during transit through the human small intestine, although some hydrolysis occurs in the small intestine of the rat [190]. There is, therefore, no appreciable "enterohepatic circulation" of bilirubin in man. Bilirubin glucuronide is hydrolyzed in the terminal ileum and large intestine by bacterial β-glucuronidase, while at the same time bilirubin is reduced to a complex series of colorless tetrapyrrolic compounds, collectively termed the *urobilinogens* [26, 102]. It is not known whether reduction of bilirubin to urobilinogen precedes or follows glucuronide hydrolysis. It has been suggested that urobilinogen glucuronide may be formed from bilirubin glucuronide [203], but urobilinogen glucuronide would be expected to be rapidly hydrolyzed in the large intestine. Conversion of bilirubin to urobilinogen has been demonstrated by isolated cultures of clostridia [202] and by cultures of mixed fecal flora [203]. When performed in vitro, the conversion occurs only under anaerobic conditions, requires soluble cofactors, and appears to be mediated by an enzyme bound to bacterial membranes [204].

The urobilinogens are sparingly absorbed from the terminal ileum and large intestine, and then are excreted predominantly by the liver through the anionic transport mechanism described above for bilirubin [189, 205–207]. Under normal conditions, and especially in the presence of excessive bile pigment formation or liver disease, urobilinogen also is excreted by the kidney through a mechanism which includes glomerular filtration, tubular reabsorption, and probably tubular secretion [208, 209]. Urine urobilinogen excretion is affected, therefore, not only by the amount of urobilinogen produced, the fraction of this amount absorbed, and hepatic function, but also by renal function, urine volume, and urine pH.

PATHOPHYSIOLOGY OF HYPERBILIRUBINEMIA

Hyperbilirubinemia occurs as the result of two distinct, but at times associated, phenomena. Overproduction of pigment, inadequate hepatic uptake, or failure of the conjugating mechanism may lead to plasma "retention" of unconjugated bilirubin. "Regurgitation" into the plasma of bilirubin glucuronide may result from functional cholestasis, disruption of the hepatic architecture, or extrahepatic biliary obstruction.

In patients with overt hemolysis, the accelerated red blood cell destruction may lead to overproduction of bilirubin at rates far in excess of the physiologic pigment formation. Similar pigment overproduction may occur in disorders of red blood cell formation associated with high degrees of "ineffective erythropoiesis" [124, 210]. Since the normal human liver is believed to have a large functional reserve for the handling of bilirubin, it may be difficult to understand why these patients exhibit unconjugated hyperbilirubinemia. For this reason the coexistence of additional hepatic defects was postulated [211], involving perhaps the uptake or the conjugating mechanism. It should be noted that in rats with constant pigment infusions, the plasma bilirubin level rises at infusion rates far below what has been considered the maximal excretory rate for bilirubin in this species [144, 212, 213]. Thus in the more severe forms of hemolytic anemia or ineffective erythropoiesis, the pigment load may be sufficiently large to cause significant retention of unconjugated bilirubin in the plasma without the coexistence of a hepatic defect.

The syndromes associated with unconjugated hyperbilirubinemia in the absence of increased pigment production will be discussed in detail in subsequent sections.

In most instances of jaundice due to primary liver disease, the plasma exhibits elevated concentrations of both conjugated and unconjugated bilirubin, but the relative proportion of the two pigment types is highly variable. Elevation of the unconjugated bilirubin may be due to shortened erythrocyte life-span sometimes seen in association with liver disease [214], or may be related to reduction of the capacity of the liver to take up or to conjugate the pigment. The mechanisms which lead to raised plasma levels of bilirubin glucuronide in the absence of overt mechanical obstruction are equally unclear. It is possible that the defect involves primarily the secretory apparatus of the hepatic cells in a manner that results in regurgitation of conjugated pigment into the circulation. As an alternative, it might be postulated that the injury directly affects the endothelial lining of the bile ductules [215], permitting leakage of the secreted conjugated bilirubin into the plasma. Finally, some forms of liver injury, while sparing the major bile ducts, may block flow in the fine radicles of the biliary tree and thereby produce an obstructive jaundice. Structural derangements consistent with each concept have been observed on electron microscopy; they suggest that intrahepatic cholestasis may be the result of several, perhaps unrelated, disburbances.

UNCONJUGATED HYPERBILIRUBINEMIA

Bilirubin is normally cleared from the plasma at a sufficient rate to keep concentrations below 1.0 mg per 100 ml. Even in the face of low-grade hemolysis, the hepatic excretory capacity usually is adequate to maintain normal plasma concentrations in most (but not in all [216]) individuals. Unconjugated hyperbilirubinemia frequently develops in patients with more severe acute or chronic hemolysis or with severe "ineffective" erythropoiesis. Presumably in these circumstances the raised plasma bilirubin concentration enhances the flow of bilirubin from the plasma into the liver cell, thereby increasing the rate of conjugation and biliary excretion of the pigment. When excretion balances production, a new plasma bilirubin level is reached which is maintained as long as the overproduction persists.

A transient elevation of plasma unconjugated bilirubin due to a hepatic deficiency in one or more of the steps necessary to achieve conjugation is observed during the first few days of life (neonatal hyperbilirubinemia). Chronic intermittent or persistent unconjugated hyperbilirubinemia occurs in man and in animals in association with hepatic defects that have been shown to be or are suspected of being genetically determined.

Neonatal Hyperbilirubinemia

Transient jaundice in apparently healthy newborn infants is a well-recognized pediatric syndrome. In some premature babies plasma unconjugated bilirubin concentrations exceed 20 mg per 100 ml, and exchange transfusion may become necessary in order to prevent the development of neurologic damage. Low-grade elevation of plasma bilirubin concentration is a benign condition which occurs in virtually all newborn infants, usually reaches peak levels within 7 days, and returns to normal by 2 weeks of age [217, 218].

This so-called physiologic jaundice results from inadequate hepatic function in the near-term fetus and newborn infant. Studies performed in utero with isotopically labeled bilirubin have established that the monkey fetus depends primarily on placental transfer for bilirubin elimination [193, 195, 196]. Bilirubin excretion by the monkey fetal liver is minimal, and little bilirubin glucuronide is present in fetal bile. The bile merely contains some pyrrole pigment derivatives of unidentified structure [196]. It should be noted that marked species differences exist. Bilirubin excretion in the fetal guinea pig resembles that in the monkey [194], but the liver of the fetal dog has considerable capacity to conjugate and excrete bilirubin, and only minimal amounts of bilirubin are transferred intact across the dog placenta [196] (Fig. 46-11).

Since in monkeys and presumably in man fetal bilirubin excretion depends on placental transfer, hyperbilirubinemia develops as this excretory site is lost at birth, and it usually persists until the liver has sufficiently "matured" to provide adequate excretory function. The precise nature of the defect in the fetus and newborn has been the subject of extensive investigation. Bile formation, bile salt secretion, and the transfer of bile from the liver to the gallbladder and intestine are all intact [201, 219]. The failure to excrete bilirubin, therefore, is not due to a complete failure of hepatic excretory function, or to an anatomic block preventing the formation or excretion of bile. Fetal hepatic glucuronide formation, as measured in vitro, is reduced in man [220],

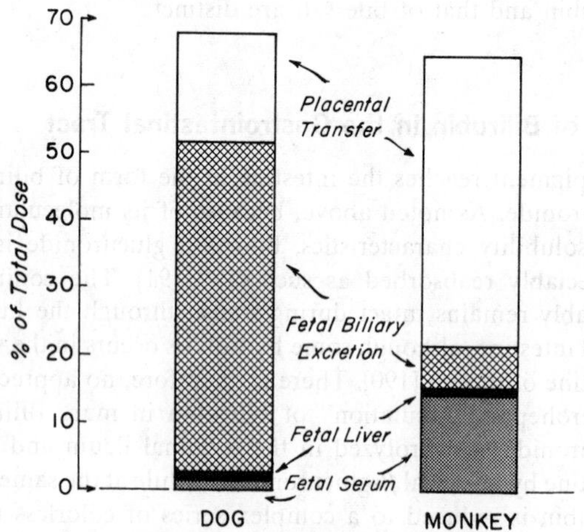

Figure 46-11. Distribution of radioactive label 10 hr after the intravenous administration of bilirubin-^{3}H to representative monkey and dog fetuses *in situ.* Total recovery of label averaged 60 to 70 percent of the administered dose. (*By permission of R. B. Bernstein et al.* [196].)

monkeys [218], and certain rodents [165, 221, 222]; the reduction may involve both the synthesis of UDPGA and the activity of glucuronyl transferase. Enzymatic activity increases slowly toward the end of gestation and reaches adult levels within a few days to 2 weeks after birth [165, 222, 223] (Fig. 46-12). A deficiency of the conjugating apparatus in the fetus and newborn, therefore, provides at least a partial explanation for the development of "physiologic jaundice."

In addition to deficient conjugation other factors appear to play a contributory role. BSP clearance is delayed in premature and full-term newborn infants [224, 225]. The secondary phase of clearance is slower than that observed in adults, which suggests that the biliary secretion of BSP is defective in the newborn. Even more striking is the virtual absence of an initial rapid phase of BSP clearance in 1-day-old infants. In adults, the initial phase of clearance is thought to reflect hepatic uptake, so that the altered BSP clearance curves observed in infants may indicate either incomplete vascularization of the newborn liver or "immaturity" of the postulated hepatic plasma membrane mechanism for BSP uptake, or both [224]. This abnormal BSP clearance, in turn, might suggest that hepatic uptake and biliary secretion of bilirubin may also be defective in the newborn. Recently it has been shown that the hepatic dye-binding protein, designated Y (see "Uptake of Bilirubin by the Liver," earlier in this chapter), is deficient in the fetal and neonatal guinea pig liver and that it only gradually increases to 75 percent of the adult level as the young guinea pig reaches a weight in excess of 200 gm [151]. If, as discussed above, Y protein plays an essential role in bilirubin uptake or intracellular

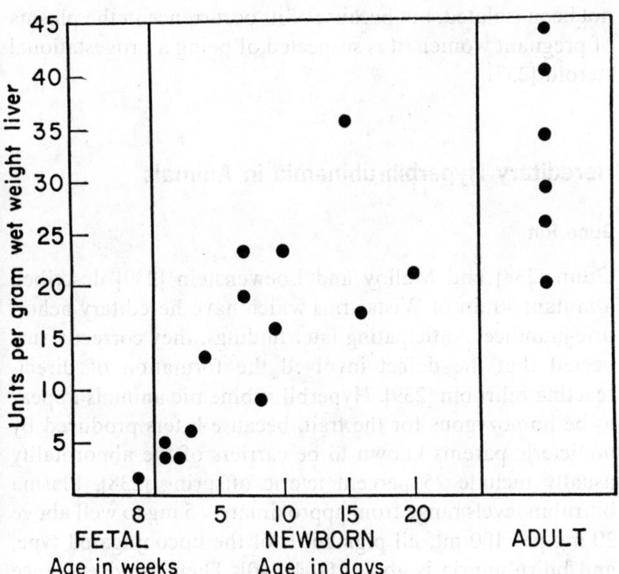

Figure 46-12. Glucuronide formation in fetal, newborn, and adult guinea pigs. Similar results were obtained with liver homogenate of other mammals. (*By permission of A. K. Brown and W. W. Zuelzer* [165].)

transport, or both, and if a comparable deficiency exists in the human neonatal liver, this might contribute to the inadequate excretion of bilirubin in newborn infants. Finally, it has been shown that labeled conjugated bilirubin administered intravenously to fetal guinea pigs or monkeys is minimally excreted in fetal bile [194, 195]. This clearly establishes that inadequate conjugation is not the sole factor limiting bilirubin excretion in the fetus. Taken together, these observations suggest that several components of the excretory mechanism are defective in the fetal and neonatal liver. The relative contributions of intrinsic hepatic "immaturity" and of the hormonal and metabolic environment of the fetus and newborn are uncertain. Similarly, it is not known whether hepatic "maturation" occurs in response to the accumulation of bilirubin in the newborn after interruption of the placental excretory mechanism. Nevertheless, it is apparent that multiple defective excretory mechanisms mature during the early postnatal period and that over the first several weeks of life the liver of the newborn infant develops adult excretory function.

When plasma unconjugated bilirubin concentrations rise toward 20 mg per 100 ml in the newborn infant, the threat of neurologic damage arises. In its extreme form (kernicterus), bilirubin toxicity in the brain results in ataxia, convulsions, and death. It has been suggested that low-grade neurologic damage may result from moderately elevated bilirubin concentrations [226].

As discussed already, there is an equilibrium between albumin-bound and unbound unconjugated bilirubin in plasma. Unbound pigment molecules can diffuse across the blood-brain barrier and enter the central nervous system [197]. The concentration of unbound bilirubin can be increased if hypoalbuminemia develops (Fig. 46-13), if endogenous metabolites (e.g., fatty acids) or drugs (e.g., salicylates) compete for binding, or if the plasma pH decreases. Therefore, several factors commonly operative in premature and debilitated infants substantially increase the risk of penetration of bilirubin into the brain.

Bilirubin neurotoxicity is usually (but not invariably [227]) limited to infants. Unbound bilirubin may penetrate the brain of adult rats, and it appears improbable that infants are more susceptible to bilirubin toxicity because of altered permeability properties of the blood-brain barrier [197]. The congruence of adverse physiologic phenomena described in the preceding paragraph may be less common in adults. Moreover, in most adults with severe jaundice the major fraction of bilirubin is conjugated. It has been shown that conjugated bilirubin does not cross the blood-brain barrier [197]. Furthermore, it is conceivable that bilirubin diglucuronide in the plasma exerts a protective effect by forming mixed molecular "monoglucuronide" complexes with unconjugated bilirubin (see "Conjugation of Bilirubin," earlier in this chapter) and thus prevents entry of the pigment into the brain. Neonatal central nervous tissue may be more susceptible to the toxic effects of bilirubin, but this has not been established.

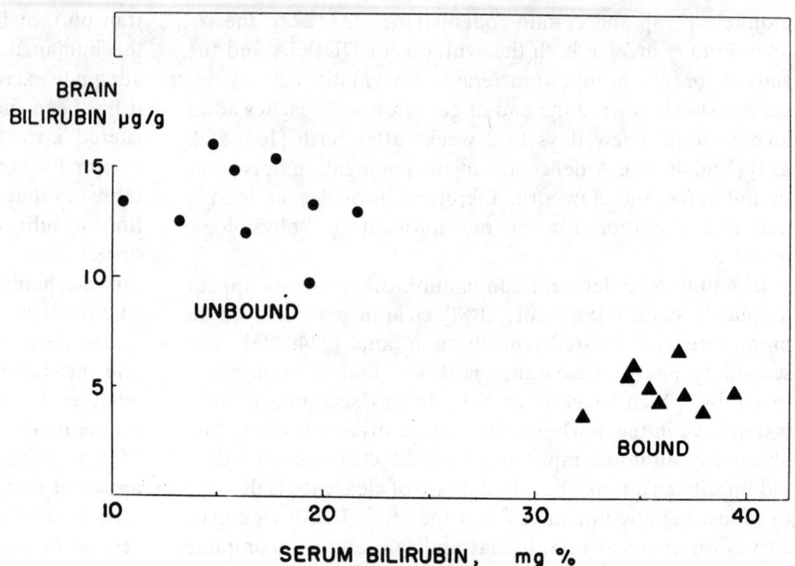

Figure 46-13. Brain and plasma concentrations of bilirubin in newborn guinea pigs infused for 1 hr at a constant rate with unbound or with albumin-bound ^{14}C-bilirubin. (*Adapted from I. Diamond and R. Schmid* [197].)

The precise mechanism by which bilirubin produces nerve cell damage is also in doubt. The concept that neural injury is the result of uncoupled oxidative phosphorylation has gained wide acceptance [228–230], but excessive amounts of unbound bilirubin were used in these studies [197]. When oxygen consumption and inorganic phosphorus utilization were measured in mitochondria obtained from the brain of guinea pigs with experimental kernicterus, no inhibition of oxidative phosphorylation was observed [231, 232]. Brain mitochondria incubated with bilirubin concentrations equal to those found in the brain of animals with experimental kernicterus yielded similarly negative results. Further investigation will be necessary, therefore, to clarify the mechanism of bilirubin neurotoxicity.

Kernicterus used to be observed most commonly in subjects with erythroblastosis fetalis. This disease can now be prevented by administration of anti-Rh-containing γ-globulin to Rh-negative mothers [233]. A major decline in the incidence of erythroblastosis can, therefore, be anticipated. In the future the most common threat of kernicterus probably will occur in premature sick infants, especially in those with associated hemolysis due to ABO incompatibility or with infection.

Prolonged unconjugated hyperbilirubinemia is not infrequently observed in association with breast feeding [234]. Jaundice, often seen in successive breast-fed sibs, becomes maximal during the first 10 to 20 days post partum, and disappears within 1 to 2 months of birth despite continued breast feeding. Development of hyperbilirubinemia is believed to be due to the presence of pregnane-3α,20β-diol in the milk of mothers of affected infants [235] (but for a contrary view see [236]). This and other steroid metabolites inhibit glucuronyl transferase activity in vitro [184]. Jaundice associated with this syndrome is mild and readily reversible if breast feeding is discontinued, and it is, therefore, usually not associated with kernicterus.

Several women have been described who gave birth to more than one infant with transient severe neonatal hyperbilirubinemia which was not attributable to hepatic dysfunction or overproduction of pigment [237]. Maximal plasma bilirubin concentrations ranged from 9 to 65 mg per 100 ml, and 4 out of 16 infants, unlike those with breast milk jaundice, developed kernicterus. An inhibitor of glucuronyl transferase assayed in vitro was present in the serum of the affected infants and their mothers. The inhibitor has not been isolated, but because of its occurrence in the plasma of pregnant women, it is suspected of being a progestational steroid [237].

Hereditary Hyperbilirubinemia in Animals

Gunn Rat

Gunn [238] and Malloy and Loewenstein [239] described a mutant strain of Wistar rats which have hereditary acholuric jaundice. Anticipating later findings, they correctly suspected that the defect involved the formation of direct-reacting bilirubin [239]. Hyperbilirubinemic animals appear to be homozygous for the trait, because litters produced by nonicteric parents known to be carriers of the abnormality usually include 25 percent icteric offspring [238]. Plasma bilirubin levels range from approximately 5 mg to well above 20 mg per 100 ml; all pigment is of the unconjugated type, and bilirubinuria is absent [164, 240]. There is no evidence of increased hemolysis [239], and, except for minor structural modifications of the endoplasmic reticulum [241], liver structure is normal [164].

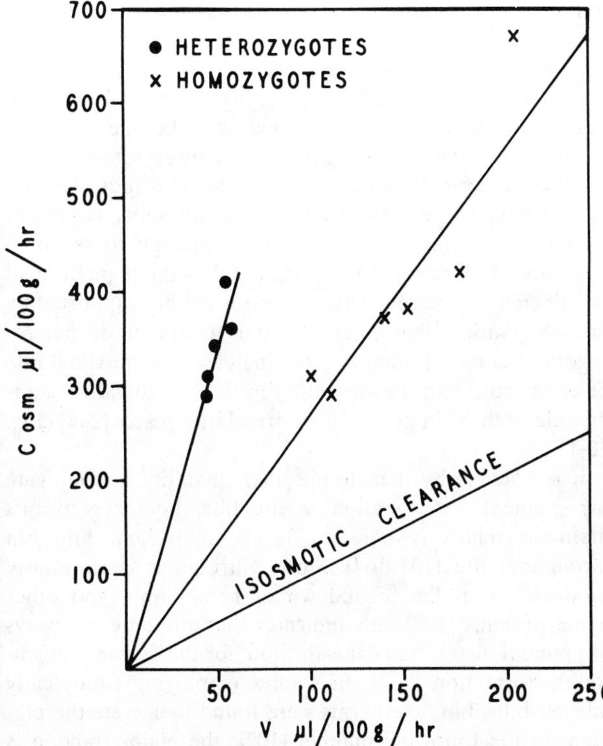

Figure 46-14. Relationship between osmolal clearance and urinary flow rates in control heterozygous and in homozygous jaundiced Gunn rats. Regression lines were drawn by inspection. (*By permission of G. B. Odell et al.* [244].)

In rats with bilirubin levels exceeding 12 to 15 mg per 100 ml, functional impairment and morphologic alterations of the central nervous system which resemble kernicterus frequently occur [242]. In homozygous jaundiced rats, slight diffuse yellow staining of the brain, that later becomes localized in the cerebellum and basal ganglia, is observed during the first days of life [243]. In ataxic animals the cerebellum is smaller than in normal and in heterozygous rats [243], and the cerebellum and basal ganglia contain significantly higher bilirubin concentrations than other parts of the central nervous system [197]. Striking morphologic abnormalities are seen in the Purkinje cells, which exhibit bizarre membranous bodies and altered mitochondria [243]; the degree of clinically discernible ataxia appears to be related to the severity and extent of these morphologic changes [243].

Adult jaundiced rats exhibit a striking polyuria and with water deprivation are subject to rapid dehydration and weight loss [244]. The bilirubin concentration in the renal papilla is much higher than in the cortical region of the kidney [164, 244]. These changes, which are less pronounced in young animals [245], are believed to reflect interference of bilirubin with sodium and urea transport in the renal medulla, and to result in a significant concentrating defect (Fig. 46-14). The hereditary hydronephrosis with cystic changes of the kidney which occurs in Gunn rats as an autosomal dominant trait appears to be entirely unrelated to the hereditary defect causing jaundice [246].

The biliary excretory system is patent, as demonstrated by the rapid appearance in the bile of injected radiopaque contrast medium (Cholografin), BSP [164], and urobilinogen and urobilin [189, 190]. The excretory rate for injected *conjugated* bilirubin is similar in icteric and in normal rats [164, 247]. In icteric rats, intravenous administration of *unconjugated* bilirubin fails to result in significant biliary excretion of the pigment [164, 247, 248]; in normal rats comparable pigment loads may lead to a 100-fold increase of the conjugated bilirubin concentration in the bile [164] (Fig. 46-15). The bile of icteric animals is devoid of conjugated bilirubin [102, 164], but it contains other bilirubin derivatives whose structure has not been clearly defined [102, 249, 250], and small amounts of unconjugated bilirubin [102, 170, 251, 252]. Unconjugated bilirubin excretion in the bile is greatly enhanced by the administration and excretion of exogenous conjugated bilirubin [170, 252]; this suggests that conjugated and unconjugated bilirubin form a complex with the characteristics of a "monoglucuronide" as discussed above under "Conjugation of Bilirubin" [170]. Fecal urobilinogen excretion is greatly reduced as compared with that in normal rats [164]. These observations indicate that the unconjugated hyperbilirubinemia observed in Gunn rats is due specifically to a defect in the conjugation of bilirubin, which in turn interferes with its elimination in bile.

Total urinary excretion of glucuronic acid and glucuronides in icteric rats is approximately half that in control animals [164]. After administration of menthol or *o*-aminobenzoate, icteric rats excrete much smaller fractions of these

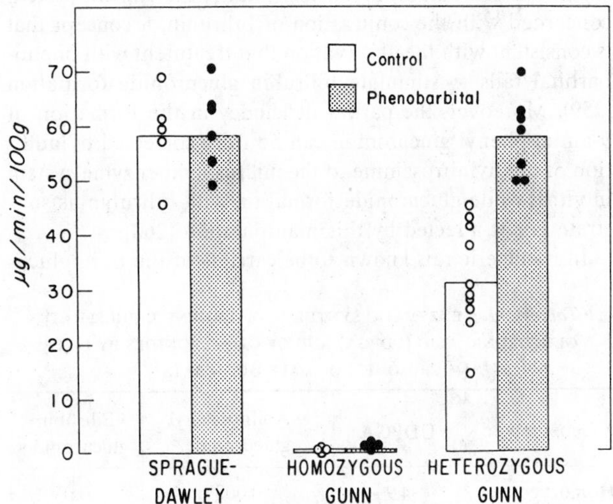

Figure 46-15. Maximum excretion of bilirubin in the bile of phenobarbital-treated rats and their controls. All animals received bilirubin infusions at constant rate. Height of the bars indicates mean value of each group; dots reflect individual values. (*By permission of S. H. Robinson* [248].)

compounds as glucuronides [164]. Similarly, after injection of benzoate, icteric rats form less benzoyl glucuronide and more hippurate than normal Wistar rats [164]. With other aglycones, including those forming N-linked glucuronides [173], similar differences are not observed [253].

Glucuronide formation in the liver of icteric rats was studied in vitro by incubating slices [160, 162, 173], homogenates [160, 254], and microsomal preparations [164, 255, 256]. With bilirubin as substrate, formation of bilirubin glucuronide cannot be detected [160, 162, 254], whereas with *o*-aminophenol, the glucuronide is formed, but at a greatly reduced rate [160, 162, 164] (Table 46-1). On the other hand, synthesis of aniline glucuronide [173] and of tetrahydrocortisone glucuronide [256] proceeds at normal rates; with *p*-nitrophenol as substrate controversial results were obtained [174, 256, 257]. Variations in the observed ability to conjugate aglycones other than bilirubin may reflect crossbreeding of the mutant rats with genetically distinct domestic and foreign strains [258]. The activity of UDP-glucose dehydrogenase is comparable to that in the liver of normal animals [164] (Table 46-1).

These findings indicate that the primary defect involves the glucuronyl transferase system of the liver microsomes. It is not clear why this enzymatic abnormality appears to result in complete abolition of glucuronide formation with bilirubin while with other aglycones the rate of synthesis is only reduced or remains unaffected. Though it has been suggested that bilirubin may be unsuccessful in competing with other aglycones for the deficient glucuronide-forming system [255], a more likely explanation is that there are two or more transferase enzymes, which may be under separate genetic control [253, 257]. The hereditary defect in Gunn rats presumably involves primarily the enzyme system concerned with the conjugation of bilirubin, a concept that is consistent with the observation that treatment with phenobarbital fails to stimulate bilirubin glucuronide formation [259]. Moreover, the partial deficiency in the formation of *o*-aminophenyl glucuronide can be fully corrected by addition of diethylnitrosamine to the microsomal enzyme system in vitro, while glucuronide formation with bilirubin as substrate is not affected by this manipulation [260].

In nonicteric rats known to be carriers of the trait, glucuronide formation in vivo and in vitro (Table 46-1) is reduced, as compared with that in genetically normal littermates, but it is greater than that in icteric rats [162, 164]. Similarly, after intravenous administration, unconjugated bilirubin disappears from the plasma, and it appears in the bile [248, 261] of the heterozygotes at significantly slower rates than in genetically normal animals (Fig. 46-15). This indicates that in heterozygous rats, the enzymatic abnormality is present to a lesser degree and is not severe enough to result in retention of bilirubin in the plasma unless the pigment load is artificially increased. This concept is further supported by the observation that phenobarbital treatment of heterozygotes, but not of homozygotes, increases the maximal rate of conjugated bilirubin excretion in the bile to values comparable to those in genetically normal littermates [248] (Fig. 46-15).

It is noteworthy that despite their inability to conjugate the pigment for excretion in the bile, homozygous rats maintain relatively constant levels of plasma bilirubin throughout life [102, 164]. Since bilirubin is continuously produced from the breakdown of hemoglobin and other heme proteins [109], this indicates that alternate pathways of pigment disposition can substitute for the deficient glucuronide formation [102]. In studies employing isotopically labeled bilirubin, icteric rats were found to excrete the pigment in the following manner [102]: the major fraction is broken down to polar, mostly diazo-negative derivatives of bilirubin which are excreted in the bile and, to a much smaller extent, in the urine [109]; some unconjugated bilirubin is transferred directly from the plasma across the intestinal mucosa into the intestine; a minute amount of the pigment appears as unconjugated bilirubin in the bile (Fig. 46-16). These combined excretory rates balance the rate of bilirubin formation, a steady state in pigment turnover is reached, and a constant level of plasma unconjugated bilirubin is maintained [102, 109]. The fractional turnover of

Table 46-1. ENZYMATIC SYNTHESIS OF URIDINE DIPHOSPHATE GLUCURONIC ACID (UDPGA) AND OF GLUCURONIDES BY LIVER (MICROSOMES) OF MALE GUNN RATS*

Genetic type	UDPGA	*o*-Aminophenyl glucuronide	Bilirubin glucuronide
Homozygous jaundiced	4.9	0.008	0.0
Heterozygous	4.3	0.034	0.011–0.039
Homozygous normal	5.8	0.061	0.056–0.089

* Results are expressed in micromoles per gram of liver.
Source: Adapted from Schmid et al. [164] and from Arias [162].

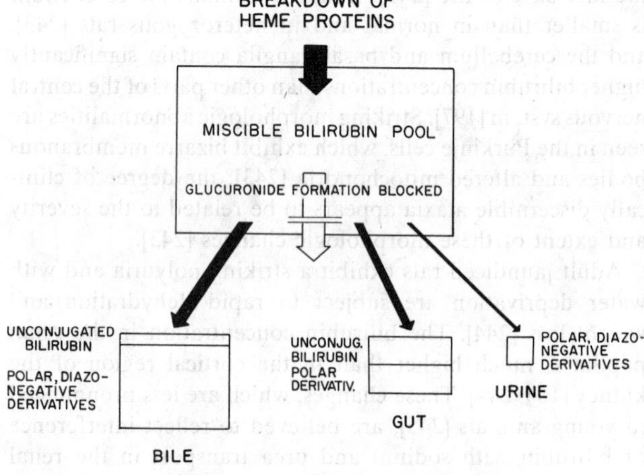

Figure 46-16. Schematic representation of alternate pathways of bilirubin disposition in icteric Gunn rats with defective glucuronide formation. (*From R. Schmid and L. Hammaker* [102].)

Table 46-2. POOL SIZE, BIOLOGIC HALF-LIFE, AND TURNOVER OF BILIRUBIN IN ICTERIC GUNN RATS

Weight, gm	200	275	355
Initial serum bilirubin level, mg per 100 ml	6.0	9.2	8.0
Biologic half-life of ^{14}C-bilirubin, hr	33	62	41
Bilirubin plasma pool, μg	360	763	845
Total miscible bilirubin pool, μg	3,520	5,470	4,000
Fractional turnover, per 24 hr	0.49	0.27	0.40

Source: Adapted from Schmid and Hammaker [102].

the total miscible pigment pool is inversely proportional to the bilirubin concentration in the blood (Table 46-2), but the plasma contains only approximately one-sixth of the total pigment pool [102]; the remainder is present in the extravascular compartments, primarily in the liver, kidneys, skin, and adipose tissue [102]. This large extravascular pigment space appears to reflect the relatively weak interaction of bilirubin with rat albumin as compared to human albumin [102, 262]. When homozygous Gunn rats were infused with *human* albumin, pigment was transferred from tissues, including the liver [144] and the brain [197], into the plasma (Fig. 46-17). Conversely, a marked reduction of the pigment level could be achieved by oral administration of cholestyramine [263, 264]. This polystyrene resin enhances pigment elimination with the feces and, in turn, reduces the pigment pool in the body by trapping bilirubin that has been transferred across the intestinal wall into the intestinal lumen.

These icteric rats provide an unusual opportunity for the study of bilirubin metabolism, and they are an excellent

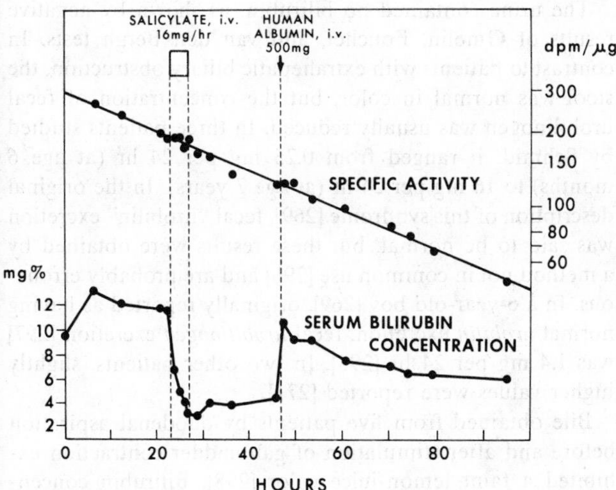

Figure 46-17. Effect of salicylate and of human albumin on the plasma bilirubin level of an icteric Gunn rat. The specific activity of the ^{14}C-bilirubin declined at a single exponential rate, indicating that the total miscible pigment pool remained unaltered despite the reversible shift of bilirubin from the plasma into the tissues. (*Adapted from R. Schmid et al.* [262].)

experimental tool for investigations into the pathogenesis and prevention of kernicterus [197, 240, 244, 249].

Southdown Mutant Sheep

Congenital hyperbilirubinemia associated with photosensitivity in a mutant line of Southdown sheep was first reported from New Zealand in 1962 [265]. The condition is inherited as a single autosomal recessive trait [266]. Plasma levels of unconjugated bilirubin range from 0.5 to 1.9 mg per 100 ml, while comparable values in normal sheep are less than 0.2 mg per 100 ml [267]. Animals homozygous for the defect have chronic facial eczema which is due to photosensitization by phylloerythrin, an intestinal breakdown product of chlorophyll that is absorbed into the portal blood and normally is excreted in the bile.

The recent discovery in California of a limited number of photosensitive Southdown sheep with a similar hepatic defect has permitted additional pathogenetic studies [267]. Animals homozygous for the defect exhibit delayed plasma disappearance but normal metabolism and secretion of a number of organic anions, including bilirubin, BSP, rose bengal, indocyanine green, and phylloerythrin [267]. The architecture and subcellular structure of the liver appear to be normal, and a number of other laboratory investigations failed to show significant abnormalities. These findings are most compatible with a defect in the hepatic uptake of selected organic anions [267]. Preliminary findings suggest that a similar defect may be present in the renal excretory apparatus [267].

Unconjugated Hyperbilirubinemia in Man

After the neonatal period, a wide spectrum of conditions is associated with chronic unconjugated hyperbilirubinemia without overt signs of hemolysis. This spectrum ranges from the frequently occurring *mild* and fluctuating hyperbilirubinemia commonly referred to as Gilbert's syndrome [268] to the rarely seen, *severe,* and often fatal syndrome first described by Crigler and Najjar [269]. Between these two extremes, occasional patients are seen with unconjugated hyperbilirubinemia of *intermediate* degree, often exhibiting considerable spontaneous fluctuation of the plasma pigment concentration [216, 270-277]. At present it is difficult to separate these forms of hyperbilirubinemia into clearly defined syndromes or distinct genetic or pathogenetic entities [24]. The reasons for this include the facts that hepatic bilirubin transport has not been fully characterized [23], that existing methods for the assay of bilirubin conjugation are inadequate, that minor degrees of hemolysis or ineffective erythropoiesis are difficult to recognize [278], and that only a rough correlation exists between demonstrable defects of conjugation and the degree of hyperbilirubinemia [216, 271]. Despite these difficulties, three patterns of unconjugated hyperbilirubinemia emerge which may be distinguished primarily on the basis of the bilirubin level in the plasma and the presence or absence of conjugated bilirubin in the bile [279]. The following syndromes will be considered: (1) Severe, lifelong unconjugated hyperbilirubinemia with no conjugated bilirubin in the bile: this condition usually is referred to as the Crigler-Najjar syndrome, and is believed to be a genetic defect in bilirubin conjugation, similar to that found in homozygous Gunn rats. (2) Chronic hyperbilirubinemia of intermediate degree, usually lifelong, but at times detected only in childhood or adolescence: the fact that the bile usually contains bilirubin glucuronide suggests that the enzymatic defect in conjugation may be only partial. (3) Mild asymptomatic fluctuating hyperbilirubinemia, generally known as Gilbert's syndrome or constitutional hepatic dysfunction: This may be a heterogeneous group including syndromes with widely differing pathogenesis [216, 279].

Severe Icterus Due to Defective Conjugation of Bilirubin (Crigler-Najjar Syndrome; Congenital Nonhemolytic Jaundice)

Clinical Findings

A familial form of severe nonhemolytic jaundice associated with disturbances of the central nervous system was described in 1952 by Crigler and Najjar [269]. In three related families six infants were observed in whom severe icterus appeared on the first to third day after birth and persisted throughout life. There was no evidence of increased hemolysis or of blood group incompatibilities. The serum bilirubin was virtually all of the indirect-reacting type, and bilirubinuria was absent. Liver histology and conventional liver function tests were normal.

All but one of these icteric infants developed a neurologic syndrome resembling kernicterus, and all five died during the first 15 months of life. In the one instance in which the brain was examined at autopsy, the cerebral cortex and the basal ganglia showed intense staining with bile pigment. The sixth icteric child of this family group initially escaped detectable neurologic damage [280, 281] and remained well except for persistent jaundice. At the age of 15½ years and without apparent precipitating cause, this boy developed signs and symptoms resembling kernicterus which were progressive and led to his death 6 months later [282]. At autopsy, the brain showed striking neuronal loss and gliosis of the thalamus and more moderate changes in the basal ganglia [283]. A similar but unrelated patient remained neurologically normal until age 3, when he developed severe ataxia, and eventually died at age 12 [284]; permission for autopsy was not obtained. It is unknown why despite lifelong severe hyperbilirubinemia, these patients developed encephalopathy only after puberty, although a partial explanation may be deduced from recent findings in animals with experimental bilirubin encephalopathy [197], as noted under "Neonatal Hyperbilirubinemia," above.

An additional patient belonging to the original family group described by Crigler and Najjar was discovered in 1956 [280]. This girl, who is now 15 years old (1970) and is a double first cousin of the other patients, became jaundiced on the first or second day of life. Plasma bilirubin concentrations of approximately 25 mg per 100 ml have persisted since birth, but in contrast to the patients described above she has shown no neurologic disturbances thus far.

Since the original description of this syndrome, approximately twenty additional patients have been studied and reported in adequate detail [102, 270, 271, 284–293]. Most of them died as a direct or indirect result of central nervous system damage; a few appear to have survived in spite of neurologic damage. At the time of this writing, only four patients are known to be alive and neurologically normal; two of them are in their teens [102, 280].

Laboratory Examinations

In none of these patients was there evidence of hemolytic anemia: all had normal hemoglobin concentration, low reticulocyte counts, normal bone marrow structure, and absence of splenomegaly. The liver was not enlarged, and on histologic examination the only abnormality found was the occasional presence of bile thrombi in some of the hepatic canaliculi [269]. On electron microscopy minor changes may be seen at the sinusoidal pole of the hepatocytes, but otherwise the subcellular structure is normal; the smooth endoplasmic reticulum tends to be prominent [294, 295]. Conventional liver function tests, including clearance of BSP, yielded uniformly normal results. Patency of the extrahepatic bile ducts was established by normal cholangiographic findings or by direct inspection at laparotomy or autopsy.

The urine contained no bilirubin, as shown by negative results of Gmelin, Fouchet, and van den Bergh tests. In contrast to patients with extrahepatic biliary obstruction, the stool was normal in color, but the concentration of fecal urobilinogen was usually reduced. In three patients studied by Schmid, it ranged from 0.23 mg per 24 hr (at age 6 months) to 16 mg per 24 hr (at age 7 years). In the original description of this syndrome [269], fecal "urobilin" excretion was said to be normal, but these results were obtained by a method not in common use [296] and are probably erroneous. In a 6-year-old boy [269], originally reported as having normal *urobilin* excretion, fecal *urobilinogen* excretion [297] was 1.4 mg per 24 hr [298]. In two other patients, slightly higher values were reported [271].

Bile obtained from five patients by duodenal aspiration before and after stimulation of gallbladder contraction exhibited a faint lemon-juice color [298]. Bilirubin concentrations ranged from 0.1 to 1.5 mg per 100 ml [299]; azo derivatives of conjugated pigment could not be detected on paper chromatography [300]. In other patients, aspirated bile failed to "show any pigment of type II and only minute amounts of pigment type I" [286], or was described as "pale grass-green . . . containing 5 mg per 100 ml bilirubin giving

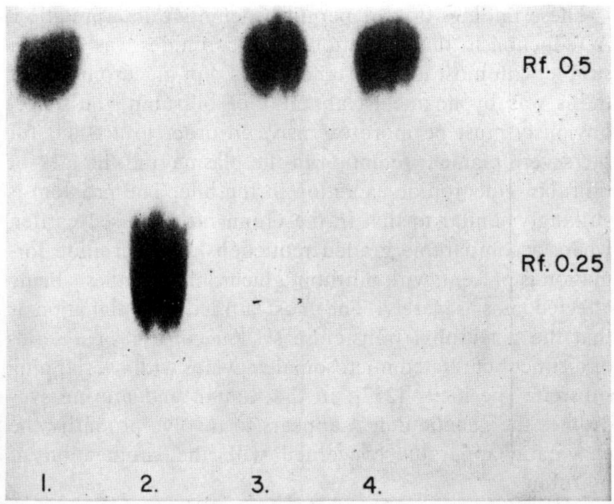

Figure 46-18. Bilirubin in serum of patients with congenital nonhemolytic jaundice (Crigler-Najjar syndrome). Ascending paper chromatogram of the azo derivatives of serum bilirubin from three patients with congenital nonhemolytic jaundice. All three sera contained only unconjugated bilirubin (R_f 0.5). The azo derivative of bilirubin diglucuronide has an R_f of 0.25. (1) Case J. D., male [284]. (2) Control, bilirubin diglucuronide. (3) Case J. H., female [285]. (4) Case J. D. H., male [280]. (*From R. Schmid* [299].)

a protracted direct reaction" [289] or as "virtually colorless, containing only a trace of unconjugated bilirubin" [271]. In a few instances, higher pigment concentrations were observed in gallbladder bile at laparotomy or at autopsy [287, 289], but chromatographic analysis of these specimens was not reported. The presence in bile of conjugated pigment would indicate that the defect in bilirubin glucuronide formation may be only partial [271], as discussed further on under "Formation of Glucuronides in Vivo and in Vitro."

In all patients studied, the plasma was deeply icteric. With one exception, bilirubin concentrations ranged from approximately 15 to 48 mg per 100 ml, and virtually all pigment gave an indirect van den Bergh reaction. In a 2½-year-old girl with severe brain damage [270], pigment concentrations during the first month of life exceeded 20 mg per 100 ml but later fell progressively to levels below 10 mg per 100 ml. This was ascribed to prolonged exposure to sunlight [270]. Although similar light-induced reductions of hyperbilirubinemia have been observed in other cases [291, 292], the data reported for this patient do not permit evaluation of this explanation [270]. Fluctuation of plasma bilirubin concentration was observed in individual patients, with a tendency to higher values during incidental illnesses [102]. It was established, by paper chromatographic analysis [299] (Fig. 46-18) and by crystallization [102, 269], that plasma bilirubin was unconjugated.

Bilirubin metabolism was investigated with isotopic techniques in a 4½-year-old boy with plasma bilirubin levels, ranging from 25 to 27 mg per 100 ml [102]. The biologic half-life of the pigment was 156 hr (Fig. 46-19); the daily bilirubin turnover of 60 mg closely approximated the anticipated value calculated on the basis of estimated hemoglobin degradation. The total miscible bilirubin pool was 568 mg (28 mg per kg body weight) and required approximately 30 hr for equilibration with the injected tracer (Fig. 46-19). Half the miscible pigment pool of the body was contained in the vascular compartment, and all the circulating bilirubin was bound to serum albumin [131]. It is of interest that the bilirubin distribution in this patient closely paralleled the estimated albumin space. The distribution of the miscible pigment pool between intra- and extravascular spaces differed significantly from that in the icteric Gunn rats described above. In the latter, approximately five-sixths of the total bilirubin pool was contained in the extravascular compartments, and the pigment levels in the plasma were much lower [102]. This difference between man and rat may be due to species differences in the degree of albumin-pigment interaction [262].

In the patient less than one-third of the daily bilirubin turnover was recovered as fecal urobilinogen; the remainder of the isotope was present in the form of a water-soluble derivative(s) of bilirubin which appeared in the feces and, to a much smaller extent, in the urine. This derivative(s) was not mesobilifuscin (a dipyrrole normally found in small quantities in stool), since mesobilifuscin isolated from the stool contained insignificant amounts of label [102]. The results of this study show that in the absence of a functioning conjugating apparatus, bilirubin is degraded by alternate metabolic pathways which establish a steady state between pigment formation and elimination at greatly increased plasma bilirubin concentrations.

Similar isotopic studies using ^{14}C-bilirubin were carried out in a 1½-year-old boy with bilirubin levels ranging from 17 to 39 mg per 100 ml [293]. On two separate occasions, the total miscible bilirubin pool was found to be 200 and

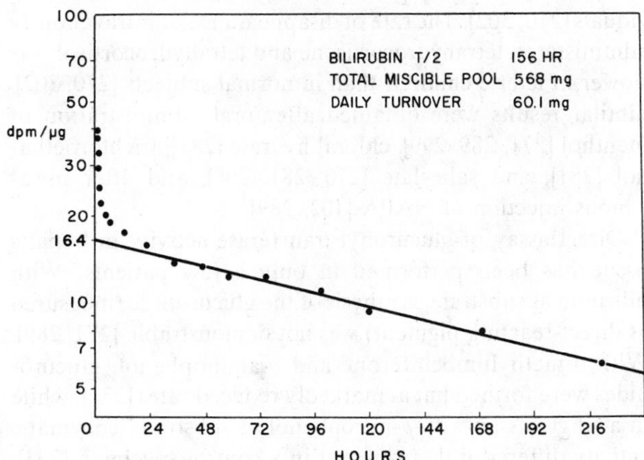

Figure 46-19. Specific activity of plasma bilirubin in a 4½-year-old boy with congenital nonhemolytic jaundice (Crigler-Najjar syndrome). At time zero, 4.3 microcuries ^{14}C-bilirubin was injected. (*From R. Schmid and L. Hammaker* [102].)

184 mg (25 and 23 mg per kg body weight), with 83 and 96 mg respectively in the vascular compartment. Studies with glycine-2-^{14}C and ALA-3,5-^{3}H [110] showed that the relative magnitude and kinetics of the early-labeled bile pigment fraction were similar to those demonstrated in the rat [109]. Although in these two patients studied with tracer techniques only a little more than half the total miscible bilirubin pool appeared to be contained in extravascular compartments, in the patient who died from kernicterus at the age of 15½ years [282] the apparent extravascular pool size was much larger. It is not known whether this was because of the unusually long duration of the disease in this patient or whether the tracer studies by which the "miscible pool" was measured caused an underestimation of the total pool size.

Formation of Glucuronides in Vivo and in Vitro

The above findings suggest that the metabolic defect in these patients involves the conversion of bilirubin to its water-soluble glucuronide [255, 271, 299]. Direct demonstration of this disturbance in vivo is technically difficult, but it was found that, in addition to impaired formation of bilirubin glucuronide, formation of other glucuronides is also reduced [255]. This was demonstrated with a variety of compounds which ordinarily are excreted in part as glucuronides. After oral administration of N-acetyl-*p*-aminophenol (NAPA), the concentration of NAPA glucuronide in the plasma was lower in an icteric child than in a normal subject of the same age and sex [255]. Plasma disappearance of cortisol[1] was normal [270, 281, 302], but the metabolites of tetrahydrocortisol conjugated with glucuronic acid appeared in the plasma at a slower rate than in normal subjects [281, 302]. Following infusion of cortisone-^{14}C recovery of labeled metabolites in the urine of icteric patients was quantitatively comparable to that in normal subjects, but the fraction of glucuronic acid–conjugated metabolites was much smaller, and the fraction of other conjugates was larger than in normal individuals [270, 302]. The rate of disappearance of intravenously administered tetrahydrocortisone and tetrahydrocortisol was slower in icteric children than in normal subjects [270, 302]. Similar results were obtained after oral administration of menthol [271, 289, 299], chloral hydrate [281], trichloroethanol [281], and salicylate [270, 281, 298], and after intravenous injection of NAPA [102, 289].

Direct assay of glucuronyl transferase activity in hepatic tissue has been performed in only a few patients. With bilirubin as substrate, synthesis of the glucuronide (measured as direct-reacting pigment) was not demonstrable [271, 289]. With 4-methylumbelliferone and *o*-aminophenol, glucuronides were formed but at markedly reduced rates [271], while in a single assay with *p*-nitrophenol as substrate, enzymatic activity differed little from that in a control specimen [293].

[1]Cortisol, in contrast to its derivative, tetrahydrocortisol, does not form a glucuronide, because it lacks the 3α-ol function in ring A [301].

These findings do not permit a definitive interpretation. A reduction in the formation of glucuronides was demonstrable with most test substances used, but glucuronide synthesis was by no means absent. For bilirubin, the defect obviously must be more extensive in order to account for the severe pigment retention in the plasma and the lack of bilirubin glucuronide excretion in the bile. The problem is strikingly similar to that in the Gunn rat discussed earlier, where a comparable graded reduction in glucuronide formation is present, with bilirubin glucuronide synthesis being affected most severely. The most attractive explanation is that the glucuronyl transferase system consists of a series of distinct but related microsomal enzymes with overlapping substrate specificity [257]; in the human and murine syndromes the genetic defect appears to involve primarily the enzymatic apparatus concerned with the conjugation of bilirubin.

Genetic Considerations

Familial occurrence of this syndrome was clearly demonstrated in the original report [269]. Six cases occurred in three related families, and later an additional case was discovered in a blood relative (M.E.H.) [281] (Fig. 46-20). The patients observed by Klingberg [285] and by Szabó et al. [289] were sibs, and a double cousin of the patient reported by Rosenthal et al. [284] died in infancy with severe unexplained jaundice. Lelong et al. [288] described a family of six sibs, three of whom were normal; in addition to the Patient F.L.L., two other sibs exhibited severe jaundice and brain damage and died at 21 days and 18 months, respectively. Finally, two of the five patients reported by Arias et al. [271] had affected sibs who died with kernicterus; the serum bilirubin level was normal in 16 other family members studied. Although the number of affected cases is too small

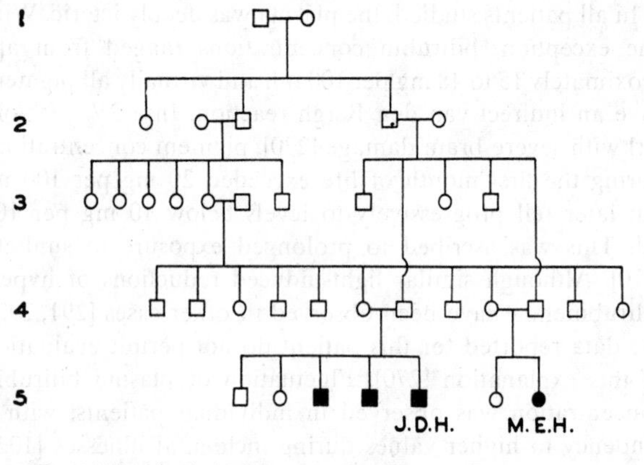

Figure 46-20. Pedigree of a family with congenital nonhemolytic jaundice (Crigler-Najjar syndrome). This family is part of an interrelated family group exhibiting a total of seven recognized cases of jaundice. (*By permission of B. Childs et al.* [281].)

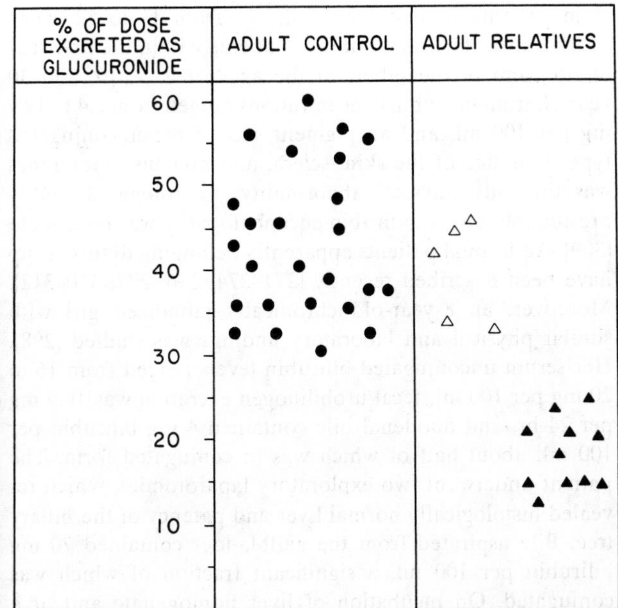

Figure 46-21. Urinary menthol glucuronide excretion in normal adults and in adult relatives of two sibs with congenital nonhemolytic jaundice (Crigler-Najjar syndrome). All urine was collected for 5 hr following oral administration of 2 gm menthol. Designation of a relative as homozygous normal or heterozygous was made on the basis of the response to this test. (*By permission of L. Szabó and P. Ebrey* [303].)

for statistical analysis, these observations leave little doubt that the defect is genetically determined. They are consistent with the concept that the disease is the result of a double dose of a rare, non-X-linked allele [271, 281, 303].

This mode of inheritance is supported by the findings in the nonicteric parents and sibs of some of these patients [271, 281, 303]. In the adult sibs, parents, and grandparents of three of Childs' patients [281], oral administration of salicylate resulted in significantly reduced excretion of salicyl glucuronide as compared with normal controls. Similarly, 11 of 16 relatives of Szabó's two patients exhibited reduced formation of menthol glucuronide [303] (Fig. 46-21). The abnormality was present in both parents and three grandparents of the jaundiced sibs (Fig. 46-22). Following intravenous injection of NAPA, the parents of Patient J.D. excreted slightly reduced amounts of NAPA glucuronide [298], but normal values were found in the parents of Patient J.d'E. [102]. In two of the five families studied by Arias et al. [271] parental consanguinity was acknowledged, and each of five parents examined exhibited reduced excretion of menthol glucuronide. These observations indicate that in the majority of relatives presumed to be heterozygous for the trait a minor defect in glucuronide formation is demonstrable. Since none of these individuals exhibited increased serum bilirubin concentrations [102, 271, 281, 284, 288, 303], the enzymatic abnormality does not appear to be of sufficient severity to interfere with pigment excretion. It should be noted, however, that the father of Patient F.L.L. [288] and a paternal uncle of Patient J.d'E. [102] had a mild unconjugated hyperbilirubinemia; in the latter the magnitude of glucuronide formation was estimated with NAPA [304] and was normal.

Treatment

Treatment of this condition obviously is aimed at a sustained reduction of the circulating bilirubin level, in the hope of preventing the development of bilirubin encephalopathy [197]. This would seem to be of particular importance in those patients who survived infancy without detectable neurologic damage [282, 284]. Therapeutic approaches were made along two different lines. The first was an attempt to enhance formation of bilirubin glucuronide in the liver by administration of drugs, notably phenobarbital, that stimulate the smooth endoplasmic reticulum [305]. As expected, this was without effect in those patients who are presumed to be homozygous for the defect in the glucuronyl transferase system [271, 282, 291, 292]. As discussed earlier, homozygous icteric Gunn rats also do not respond to phenobarbital administration, whereas the drug readily enhances pigment excretion in animals that are heterozygous for the defect [248, 259]. Thus, the lack of a therapeutic response to phenobarbital has been advocated as a means of identifying patients whose enzymatic defect appears to be complete, as contrasted with individuals who *do* respond and therefore are believed to be only partially deficient in the enzyme [271]. It is apparent, however, that this criterion needs further evaluation, particularly in relation to clinical findings and genetic aspects [271, 293].

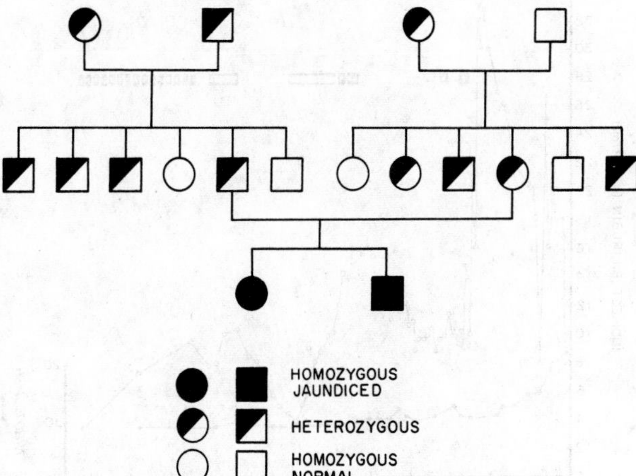

Figure 46-22. Pedigree of a family with congenital nonhemolytic jaundice (Crigler-Najjar syndrome). Two sibs were homozygous-jaundiced; 11 nonicteric relatives were identified as heterozygous for the trait by the menthol test (see Fig. 46-21). (*By permission of L. Szabó and P. Ebrey* [303].)

A second and more promising therapeutic approach to severe unconjugated hyperbilirubinemia is phototherapy. On exposure to visible light, bilirubin decomposes to breakdown products that are diazo-negative and are more polar [31, 250] and potentially less toxic than the parent compound [306]. These breakdown products formed in vitro resemble the bilirubin derivatives that are excreted normally in the bile of icteric Gunn rats [102, 249]. On the basis of these observations, Cremer et al. [307] first suggested exposure to sunlight as a possible treatment for neonatal hyperbilirubinemia. Subsequently, phototherapy was shown also to be successful in patients with congenital hyperbilirubinemia who had failed to respond to treatment with phenobarbital [291, 292] (Fig. 46-23). In these instances a sustained fall in the plasma bilirubin level from approximately 30 to 10 mg per 100 ml could be achieved provided that the patients were exposed continuously to an artificial light source for about 12 hr each day on a regular schedule. Isotopic studies carried out during illumination indicated that part of the bilirubin in the plasma or in a compartment in rapid exchange with plasma bilirubin (probably the skin) was degraded to water-soluble derivatives that were rapidly excreted in the bile and to a lesser extent in the urine [308]. It should be realized, of course, that this therapeutic approach is awkward to use in ambulatory patients, and its efficacy on a long-term basis remains to be evaluated.

Hyperbilirubinemia of Intermediate Degree Presumably Due to Partial Defects in Bilirubin Conjugation

A form of unconjugated hyperbilirubinemia, probably related to the Crigler-Najjar syndrome but clinically and chemically less severe, was described by Arias [216]. The eight patients studied ranged in age from 14 to 52 years. Jaundice was first noted in four patients within the first year of life, and in the others at the ages of 2, 7, 10, and 30 years. Serum bilirubin concentrations ranged from 6.4 to 19.9 mg per 100 ml, and all pigment was of the unconjugated type. Jaundice of the skin, sclera, and mucous membranes was the only physical abnormality; neurologic disability presumably due to bilirubin encephalopathy was infrequent [309]. Additional patients apparently belonging to this group have been described recently [271–274, 276, 277, 310–312]. Moreover, an 8-year-old chronically jaundiced girl with similar physical and laboratory findings was studied [298]. Her serum unconjugated bilirubin levels ranged from 16 to 20 mg per 100 ml, fecal urobilinogen excretion was 16.9 mg per 24 hr, and duodenal bile contained 4 mg bilirubin per 100 ml, about half of which was in conjugated form. The patient underwent two exploratory laparotomies, which revealed histologically normal liver and patency of the biliary tree. Bile aspirated from the gallbladder contained 70 mg bilirubin per 100 ml, a significant fraction of which was conjugated. On incubation of liver homogenate and of a microsomal preparation with bilirubin or *o*-aminophenol, no direct-reacting bilirubin was formed, but the microsomes synthesized *o*-aminophenol glucuronide at a rate which was approximately half that observed with similar preparations obtained from male rat liver.

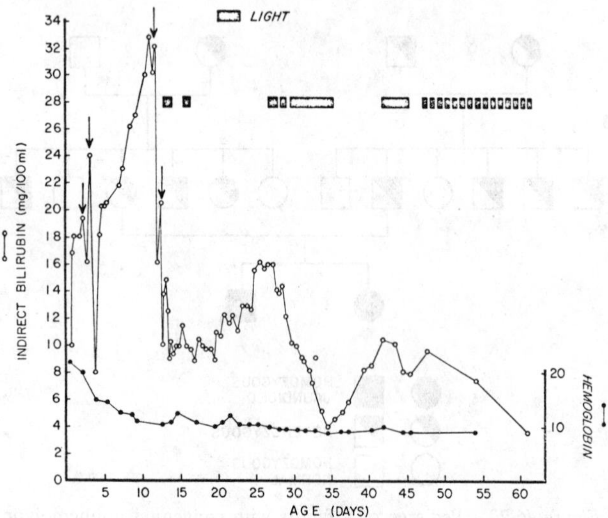

Figure 46-23. Phototherapy in an infant with severe unconjugated hyperbilirubinemia (Crigler-Najjar syndrome). The plasma bilirubin level promptly responded to illumination. Arrows indicate exchange transfusions. (*By permission of M. Karon et al.* [291].)

In these patients erythrocyte survival was normal, extrahepatic bile ducts were patent, and the histologic appearance of the liver failed to exhibit significant abnormalities. Evidence of bilirubin encephalopathy was less frequently encountered than in the more severe form of hyperbilirubinemia (Crigler-Najjar syndrome), but kernicterus was reported in occasional instances [270, 272, 287, 293, 309, 311]. One of these patients died at the age of 44 after having spent the last 20 years of her life in a mental institution [309]. At 6 months of age she had been diagnosed as having "Little's disease with idiocy and jaundice," and on her admission to the mental institution severe icterus, muscle rigidity, dystonia, partial deafness, and mental deficiency were noted. These manifestations did not progress, and the bilirubin level remained between 16 and 22 mg per 100 ml. At autopsy, the liver was found to be grossly and histologically normal, but the brain was reduced in weight and, on histologic examination, showed degenerative changes consistent with kernicterus [309].

In this syndrome plasma bilirubin levels range from approximately 6 to 25 mg per 100 ml. The direct-reacting pigment fraction invariably is normal. In some instances the icterus was not detected until later in life [271], whereas in others the bilirubin level appeared to peak shortly after birth and then fell progressively during infancy and childhood [270, 277]. No bilirubin was excreted in the urine.

The bile obtained by duodenal aspiration or at laparotomy invariably contained ample bilirubin, a significant fraction of which was conjugated with glucuronic acid [216, 270, 271, 274, 276, 286, 287]. The amount of fecal urobilinogen was

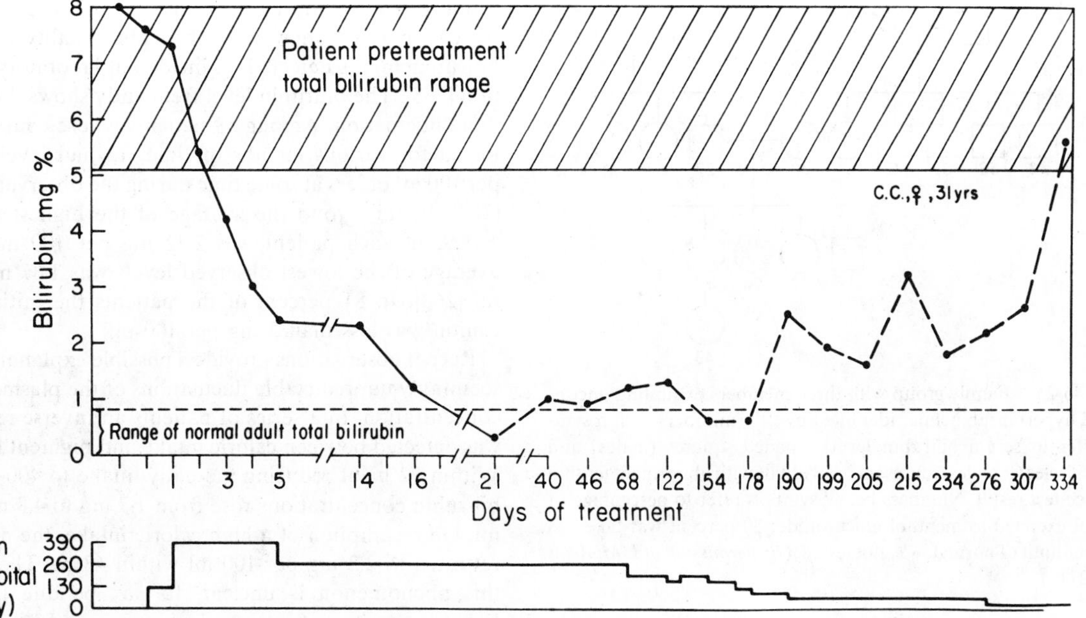

Figure 46-24. Effect of phenobarbital treatment in a patient with moderate unconjugated hyperbilirubinemia presumably due to a partial defect in bilirubin conjugation. (*Adapted from M. J. Kreek and M. H. Sleisenger*) [274].)

slightly to moderately decreased in the majority of these patients.

Studies with menthol or salicylamide in vivo suggested reduced glucuronide formation in most [216, 271, 273, 274, 310] but not in all cases [276]. Similarly, in vitro, liver tissue exhibited reduced glucuronide synthesis with *o*-aminophenol, 4-methylumbelliferone, and *p*-nitrophenol [216, 271, 274, 298]; with bilirubin as the substrate, significant formation of direct-reacting pigment was not demonstrable [216, 271, 274, 298].

In 1966, Yaffe and coworkers [273] and Crigler and Gold [293] reported a dramatic response of patients with this type of hyperbilirubinemia to treatment with relatively large amounts of phenobarbital. This was subsequently confirmed in a number of additional patients [271, 274, 275]. On daily administration of 60 to 180 mg phenobarbital in divided doses, the bilirubin concentration fell progressively over an interval of 2 to 3 weeks to near-normal levels; on withdrawal of the drug, the pigment level gradually returned to pretreatment values (Fig. 46-24). Similar results were obtained with oral administration of dichlorodiphenyl trichloroethane (pp'—D.D.T.) [310]. Treatment with these drugs also tended to increase the percentage of menthol and salicylamide excreted in the urine as glucuronides [271, 273, 310], but this was not a constant finding [274, 276]. It is tempting to speculate that this beneficial effect of phenobarbital and related drugs is related to their inductive properties for many microsomal enzymes in the liver, including glucuronyl transferase [313], but conclusive evidence in support of this hypothesis is not available [274]. On the basis of the reported information, the impressive improvement in jaundice cannot be ascribed solely to enhanced formation of bilirubin glucuronide [276], as other factors appear to play important roles [274, 314]. Nonetheless, the drug-mediated reduction of the bilirubin levels lends force to the argument that hyperbilirubinemia of intermediate degree results from a partial deficiency of glucuronyl transferase, which may be distinguished from the absolute enzyme deficiency characteristic of the Crigler-Najjar syndrome and of the homozygous Gunn rat.

The occurrence of this syndrome in families suggests that it is genetically determined, but the exact pattern of inheritance is difficult to determine; autosomal dominant transmission with incomplete penetrance and varied expressivity has been suggested as the most likely possibility (Fig. 46-25) [271]. The problem of genetic classification is related to the difficulty of identifying carriers of the trait who lack hyperbilirubinemia. The oral menthol tolerance test, though widely used, fails to discriminate between icteric patients and anicteric family members suspected of carrying the abnormal gene (Fig. 46-25) [216, 271]. On the other hand, frankly jaundiced patients may show normal menthol glucuronide excretion, as did the paternal grandfather in Fig. 46-25. It also should be remembered that the test result is abnormal in anicteric individuals presumed to be heterozygous for the Crigler-Najjar defect (Fig. 46-21). This lack of discriminatory power severely limits the diagnostic usefulness of the menthol tolerance test. The noted discrep-

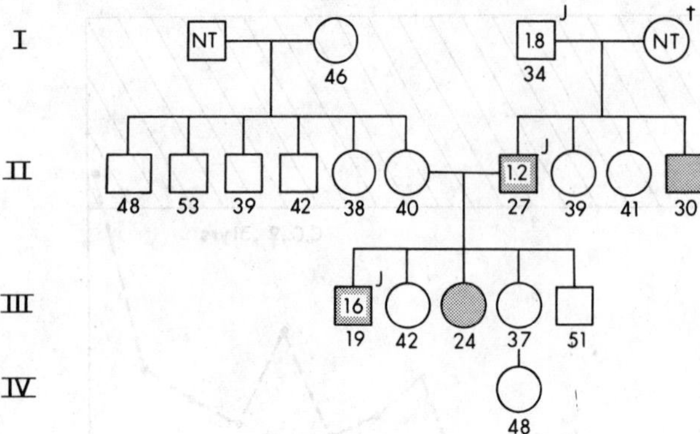

Figure 46-25. Family group with three members exhibiting unconjugated hyperbilirubinemia, identified by "J" (numbers within symbols refer to serum bilirubin level). Shaded squares (males) and shaded circles (females) represent individuals with abnormal menthol tolerance test result. Numbers below symbols refer to percentage of menthol excreted as menthol glucuronide; 30 percent was taken as the lower limit of normal. *NT,* not tested. (*By permission of I. M. Arias et al.* [271].)

ancies between the apparent rates of glucuronide formation with menthol and with bilirubin may not be surprising in view of the probable multiplicity of enzymes that catalyze glucuronide synthesis [257].

The findings in these patients are consistent with the concept that the chronic hyperbilirubinemia is the result of an enzymatic abnormality similar to that in the Crigler-Najjar syndrome but that the defect is functionally less severe. This is supported by the generally lower pigment levels in the plasma, the presence of conjugated bilirubin in the bile, and the positive response to phenobarbital. It should be realized that the difference between the two syndromes may be so subtle that a clear distinction is presently impossible. Similarly, the separation between unconjugated hyperbilirubinemia of intermediate degree and the mild chronic hyperbilirubinemia (Gilbert's syndrome) to be discussed in the following section is relative rather than absolute.

Low-grade Chronic Hyperbilirubinemia (Gilbert's Syndrome; Constitutional Hepatic Dysfunction)

Since the original report by Gilbert [315], patients with unexplained mild and chronic elevation of indirect-reacting serum bilirubin have been reported with increasing frequency [268, 316]. The condition has variously been referred to as icterus intermittens juvenilis [317], hereditary nonhemolytic bilirubinemia [318], familial nonhemolytic jaundice [319], and constitutional hepatic dysfunction [320]. None of these terms is adequate, but any is perhaps preferable to the frequently employed Gilbert's syndrome, since most of Gilbert's cases probably suffered from what is now recognized as a compensated hemolytic state.

Mild icterus may be detected shortly after birth but usually is not recognized until puberty or later in life [268, 317]. The patients may be unaware of their abnormality until hyperbilirubinemia is detected on incidental laboratory examination [268]. The bilirubin level frequently shows considerable daily fluctuation. Among 58 patients whose course was followed for various lengths of time, 13 had levels of 1 mg per 100 ml or less at some time during the observation period [268]. In this group the average of the highest values observed in each patient was 2.72 mg per 100 ml, and the average of the lowest observed levels was 1.67 mg per 100 ml [268]. In 81 percent of the patients the initial concentration was less than 3 mg per 100 ml.

Recent observations provide a possible explanation for the seemingly unpredictable fluctuations of the plasma bilirubin concentration. In a series of patients an inverse relationship was detected between caloric intake and pigment level [321]. Within 72 hr of reducing the daily intake to 400 cal., mean bilirubin concentrations rose from 1.7 mg to 4.8 mg per 100 ml. On resumption of a high caloric intake, the mean value returned to 2.2 mg per 100 ml within 48 hr. The nature of this phenomenon is unclear. It may be due to reduced hepatic excretory function during fasting, similar to that reported for BSP [322], or it may reflect increased pigment production in the liver analogous to the starvation effect in hepatic porphyria [314, 389].

Virtually all the serum bilirubin gives an indirect van den Bergh reaction [268], and on paper chromatographic analysis no conjugated bilirubin is detectable. Bilirubinuria is absent, liver and spleen are usually not enlarged, and conventional liver function tests give normal results, except for occasional increased BSP retention [304, 323]. The fecal excretion of urobilinogen is usually normal, but it may be slightly decreased [216, 319]. Histologic examination of the liver reveals no significant abnormalities [268], but recent electron microscopic studies suggest the presence of minor alterations in the liver cell membrane adjacent to the sinusoidal lumen [324] and occasional intracellular pigment granules similar to those seen in the Dubin-Johnson syndrome [325–327].

It is often stated that the hyperbilirubinemia is associated with subjective symptoms, such as fatigue, asthenia, weariness, and dyspepsia [317, 318, 328]. The multiplicity of complaints and the failure to elicit any common pattern of symptoms suggest that these manifestations are unrelated to the disorder in pigment metabolism [268]. Indeed, it seems likely that many of these symptoms develop after the patient has become aware of his icterus and that they are related to anxiety rather than to organic disease.

The pathogenesis of this syndrome is unresolved, but there is much evidence to suggest that persistent mild hyperbilirubinemia may be the result of several unrelated disturbances [216, 279]. In some patients studies of erythrocyte survival suggested a mild and compensated hemolytic state [216, 268, 278, 329], but it is not clear whether this relatively slight increase in pigment production is the sole cause of the hyperbilirubinemia or whether associated abnormalities in the liver may be present [278, 316]. It should be noted in this connection that in rats significant retention of unconjugated bilirubin in the plasma occurs on constant pigment infusion at rates that are far below those usually considered to be the maximal excretory capacity of the liver [139, 247, 330]. Scattered reports suggest that chronic mild icterus may be a late and inconsequential manifestation of infectious hepatitis [216, 328], but some of these cases may simply represent instances of hepatitis occurring in individuals with Gilbert's syndrome [279]. Also, it may be predicted that a fixed percentage of measured plasma bilirubin concentrations will lie outside the statistical confidence limits of the accepted range of "normal" and thus appear to be abnormal.

The remaining patients with unexplained unconjugated hyperbilirubinemia usually fulfill the following criteria for the diagnosis of Gilbert's syndrome [316]: chronic mild unconjugated hyperbilirubinemia with normal values for direct-reacting bilirubin; normal erythropoiesis and red blood cell survival; and absence of histologic or functional abnormalities of the liver and biliary tree. In these patients the retention of unconjugated bilirubin in the plasma most probably results from abnormalities either in hepatic uptake or in the hepatic conjugating mechanism. Incomplete understanding of the nature of these steps makes a definitive evaluation of the underlying defects difficult.

Attempts to demonstrate impairment of glucuronide formation in vivo generally have been unsuccessful [216, 268, 304, 332]. Incubation of liver biopsy material with bilirubin, *o*-aminophenol, or 4-methylumbelliferone in vitro yielded controversial results; some investigators reported levels of glucuronyl transferase activity comparable to that in normal liver [216, 333], whereas others found slightly to moderately reduced enzyme activity [334, 335]. The significance of these findings is difficult to assess, since, with the methods employed, even the reduced values (expressed as μmoles of bilirubin per gram of liver) are more than 10 times higher than the calculated hepatic enzyme activity required to conjugate the amount of bilirubin that is produced in vivo. This may render it doubtful that the mild hyperbilirubinemia of these patients is due primarily to an enzymatic abnormality. It should be noted that a few individuals genetically related to deeply jaundiced patients with established conjugating defects (Crigler-Najjar syndrome) have been found to exhibit *low-grade* unconjugated hyperbilirubinemia that is indistinguishable from Gilbert's syndrome [216, 271, 288, 298]. Although in two instances defective glucuronide formation could not be demonstrated with the available methods in vivo [216, 298], the possibility of a genetically determined but undetected conjugation defect obviously could not be ruled out with certainty [216].

As an alternate explanation it has been postulated that the uptake or extraction of the pigment by the liver may be impaired [304]. The underlying defect may lie in the carrier responsible for the transport of organic anions from the plasma into the liver, as had been postulated for the mutant Southdown sheep [267]. Another highly speculative possibility is that patients with Gilbert's syndrome have excessive plasma levels of an undetected anion normally excreted by the liver. Competitive inhibition of bilirubin uptake would then result in unconjugated hyperbilirubinemia comparable to that produced by flavaspidic acid [144, 336]. Indirect support for either of these mechanisms has been obtained by analysis of plasma bilirubin disappearance curves observed in patients with Gilbert's syndrome [337–340], but this approach is not sufficiently discriminatory to exclude other pathogenic mechanisms. Finally, the possibility should be considered that patients with Gilbert's syndrome may produce increased amounts of bilirubin from nonhemoglobin sources in the liver, as has been demonstrated in starved rats treated with phenobarbital [120]. To date, none of these experimental models has been able to explain fully the hyperbilirubinemia of this syndrome.

The occurrence of unexplained mild unconjugated hyperbilirubinemia in more than one member of a family has been reported repeatedly [268, 317–319, 341–345]. Dameshek and Singer [319] described two families with three and seven icteric members, and among 58 patients with unexplained hyperbilirubinemia studied by Foulk et al. [268], 8 had a positive family history for jaundice. In the group of 15 patients reported by Alwall et al. [345], 55 percent of the sibs and 26 percent of the parents of the probands had bilirubin levels above 1.3 mg per 100 ml. The pedigree of a family studied by Baroody and Shugart [341] is reproduced in Fig. 46-26. In another recent family study of 42 patients with Gilbert's syndrome, 27 percent of the examined sibs and 16 percent of the parents were found to have elevated bilirubin levels [316]; no affected relatives were discovered in the families of 25 of the 42 patients. It may be expected that a higher incidence of hyperbilirubinemia in relatives may be found if plasma bilirubin levels are determined repeatedly [268] and if the subjects are fasted for 48 hr [321].

These observations suggest that in many instances, mild chronic unconjugated hyperbilirubinemia may be genetically transmitted. Although the available data are insufficient to

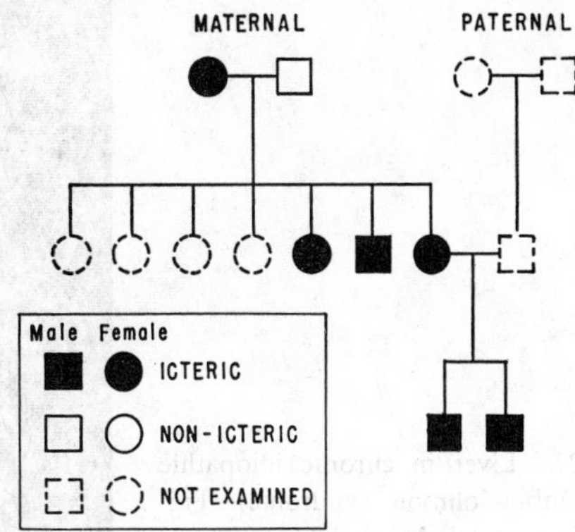

Figure 46-26. Pedigree of a family with constitutional hepatic dysfunction (Gilbert's syndrome). (*By permission of W. G. Baroody et al.* [341].)

establish the precise mode of inheritance, an autosomal dominant type of inheritance appears most probable [316, 319, 345].

Conjugated Hyperbilirubinemia

Chronic Idiopathic Jaundice (Dubin-Johnson Syndrome)

In 1954, Dubin and Johnson [346] and Sprinz and Nelson [347] described a previously unrecognized syndrome characterized by chronic icterus and an unidentified pigment in the liver cells. Since the original description, numerous cases of a similar nature have been observed and reported [348–351].

The presence of mild and often asymptomatic icterus may be detected in childhood or during adult life [348]. Hyperbilirubinemia usually is slight in degree and exhibits marked fluctuation in intensity [347, 348]. Characteristically the plasma contains a significant fraction of bilirubin, which gives a direct van den Bergh reaction [348, 352], and conjugated bilirubin can be demonstrated on paper chromatography. Bile pigment is detectable in the urine in the majority of patients [348, 352].

The hyperbilirubinemia may be entirely asymptomatic, or it may be associated with weakness, increased fatigability, and diverse gastrointestinal manifestations [348]. Enlargement and tenderness of the liver are occasionally observed [348]. The results of conventional liver function tests may be either normal or moderately impaired [348, 352]. After intravenous injection of Bromsulphalein, hepatic removal and storage of the dye are often unimpaired, but biliary excretion usually is greatly delayed [353, 354]; this may result in the appearance of conjugated BSP in the plasma and in its subsequent excretion in the urine [353, 355]. Oral cholecystography frequently fails to display the gallbladder [348] or shows it only faintly [352]. Intravenous administration of contrast medium may yield a higher percentage of visualization [348]. Glucuronide formation in vivo [355] and in vitro [356] is unimpaired.

Except for the presence of dark pigmentation, the gross appearance of the liver is usually normal [348]. The tissue core obtained by needle biopsy has been described as "green-black" or "dark-gray" [348, 352]. A slight degree of fibrosis or fatty infiltration may be detectable [348] on histologic examination of the liver, but the most striking finding is the presence of intracellular coarsely granular brown pigment, which is particularly conspicuous in cells of the centrolobular area (Fig. 46-27). The pigment tends to be confined to parenchymal cells [347] but is present to a lesser degree in Kupffer cells [348, 352]. On electron microscopy the granular material is recognizable as dense bodies located primarily in the pericanalicular region [241], and it has been suggested that these bodies are pigment-laden lysosomes [241, 357]. The nature of this pigment is unknown. Histochemically it differs from bile pigments, hemosiderin, and hematin [347, 348, 352]. Some investigators have assumed that the pigment belongs to the ill-defined group of lipofuscins [346, 347, 358, 359], but histochemical, spectroscopic, and physicochemical analyses suggest similarities with melanin [360, 361].

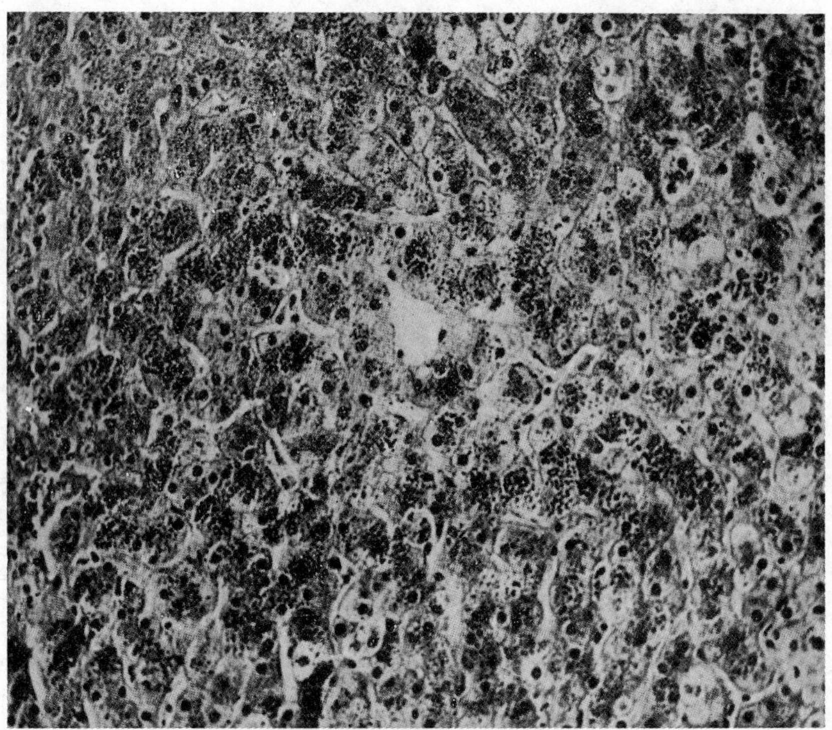

Figure 46-27. Liver in chronic idiopathic jaundice (Dubin-Johnson syndrome). Pigmentation is particularly marked in parenchymal liver cells of the centrolobular area. (*By permission of I. N. Dubin and F. B. Johnson* [346].)

The degree of hepatic pigmentation shows wide individual variations. In two families with 10 icteric members (Fig. 46-28) histologic examination of the liver revealed two instances with large amounts of pigment, four with a slight degree of pigmentation, and two with only minimal pigment deposition. In the last group the pigment differed little in character and quantity from the centrolobular pigment often found in parenchymal cells of normal livers [352]. In another family, two of three icteric members studied had marked hepatic pigmentation, whereas the liver of the third was histologically normal in spite of conjugated hyperbilirubinemia and of increased BSP retention [356]. Twenty-nine of 38 family members in whom a liver biopsy was performed in a recent study had variable degrees of hepatic pigmentation [349]. Not all these had hyperbilirubinemia, and in others significant pigmentation was lacking despite slight icterus.

These observations may indicate that the primary defect involves the biliary secretory mechanism of the liver. It is postulated that the organic anion series discussed elsewhere in this chapter is secreted abnormally, and this has been demonstrated for conjugated bilirubin [348], BSP [353–355], rose bengal dye [352], indocyanine green [355], and contrast media employed for cholecystography [348]. It has been suggested that the hepatic pigmentation may be due to a similar secretory defect [362]. On the other hand, taurocholate secretion is unimpaired, and organic cations, such as procaine amide ethobromide, are secreted normally [200]. The absence of pruritus in these patients is consistent with normal bile acid metabolism.

The syndrome occurs in both sexes and has been observed in widely varying ethnic groups, including Negroes, Persian Jews, and Caucasians [348]. A positive family history of icterus is obtained in a significant number of patients [348, 352, 353, 355, 356, 363–365], but a definite familial incidence can be established only by methodical performance of liver biopsies on family groups [352, 366]. The pedigree of a Puerto Rican family studied by Wolf et al. [352] is given in Fig. 46-28. One parent and 7 of 10 sibs had hyperbilirubinemia, and liver biopsy performed in all but two of these patients revealed a variable degree of pigmentation. This observation and similar ones [353, 356, 363, 364] suggest that the defect is genetically controlled and may be the heterozygous expression of a rare allele.

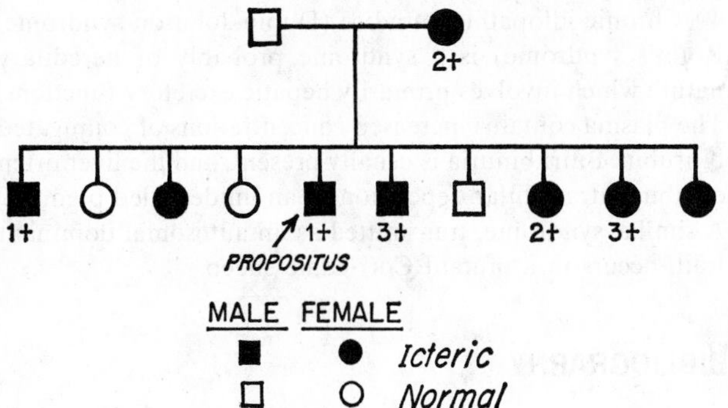

Figure 46-28. Pedigree of a family with chronic idiopathic jaundice. The degree of hepatic pigmentation is indicated on an arbitrary scale of 1+ to 3+. In two patients, liver biopsies were not performed. (*By permission of R. L. Wolf et al.* [352].)

In 1948, Rotor and his associates [367] described a Philippine family with several icteric members, three of whom were studied in detail. Mild and fluctuating icterus, discovered shortly after birth or during childhood, persisted throughout life. Serum bilirubin concentrations were slightly to moderately increased, and the van den Bergh reaction was predominantly direct, but bilirubinuria was not noted. There was intermittent epigastric discomfort, with occasional frank abdominal pain and fever. There was nothing to suggest cholelithiasis or increased hemolysis. Cholecystographic examination and estimation of erythrocyte life-span or fecal urobilinogen excretion were not reported. The only significant abnormality was marked retention of BSP. Liver biopsy performed in one patient showed no significant histologic abnormalities and no pigmentation. The pedigree of this family indicated the presence of jaundice in a total of eight members in three generations [368]. An additional two members gave a history of jaundice, although at the time of examination they were not icteric. Unfortunately, only three patients were reported in detail [367, 368].

More recently, a number of similar observations has been reported [369–376], and in several instances, familial occurrence of this syndrome has been well documented [369–374]. Studies of the original family [367, 368] and of those described by Haverback and Wirtschafter [374] and by Peck et al. [373] suggest that the defect is genetically controlled, affected members being heterozygous for the abnormal gene. In other families characterization of the genetic pattern is more difficult [377, 378].

The clinical and laboratory findings are suggestive of a hepatic excretory defect similar to that in the Dubin-Johnson syndrome, but pigmentation of the liver is lacking. As additional points of distinction, it is claimed that patients with hepatic pigmentation generally exhibit less severe BSP retention in the plasma and less frequently show cholecystographic visualization of the gallbladder [379], but these apparent differences are at best quantitative. The only indisputable justification for separation of the two syndromes would be the presence or absence of melanin-like pigment in the liver cells, but this argument loses much force with the recent demonstration that in the Dubin-Johnson syndrome the degree of hepatic pigmentation is variable and, indeed, may be minimal [349, 352, 356]. Moreover, accumulation of pigment granules in hepatic cells appears to be unspecific, in that it has been reported in the liver of patients with chronic unconjugated hyperbilirubinemia [325, 349, 359] and in others with reduced red blood cell survival [377]. These observations suggest that pathogenetic or clinical separation of the syndromes described by Dubin and Johnson and by Rotor may be arbitrary and that both conditions may be due to the same metabolic defect.

Mutant Corriedale Sheep with Conjugated Hyperbilirubinemia

In 1965, Cornelius et al. [380] discovered a photosensitive syndrome in mutant Corriedale sheep that resembled the icteric syndrome described by Dubin and Johnson in man [348]. Affected sheep have mild conjugated hyperbilirubinemia [380], and biliary secretion of conjugated bilirubin, BSP, rose bengal, indocyanine green, and iodopanoic acid is greatly reduced [361, 381]. On the other hand, hepatic transport of taurocholate and of the organic cation procaine amide ethobromide is unimpaired [361]. The facial photosensitivity results from retention in the plasma of phylloerythrin, a porphyrin which is formed in the rumen by bacterial degradation of chlorophyll [382]. This bovine disorder appears to be transmitted with the genetic characteristics of an autosomal dominant trait.

Morphologically the liver appears black from the accumulation of a brown-black pigment that is localized primarily in the centrolobular parenchymal cells; no other histologic abnormalities are detectable in the liver. The pigment granules are contained in hepatic organelles that by electron microscopy, histochemistry, and ultracentrifugation are recognized as lysosomes [361]. Isolated pigment has physicochemical properties that resemble melanin. Although mammalian liver lacks the enzymatic apparatus to synthesize true melanins, the hepatic cells readily excrete metabolites of tyrosine, tryptophan, and phenylalanine which, if oxidized, polymerize to form aggregates of the melanin type. Thus it was postulated that the hepatic pigmentation may result from a chronic defect in the biliary excretion of one or more of these metabolites [361]. This concept gained support from the observation that no pigment was detectable in the liver of newborn mutant sheep for the first 6 months of life in spite of the functional impairment in biliary excretion.

Experimental studies with radioactive epinephrine, which in the sheep is converted to the single metabolite metanephrine glucuronide, confirmed the presence of defective biliary excretion of organic amines [383]. In mutant Corriedale sheep, only 1 percent of the injected tracer dose appeared in the bile; in normal animals up to 20 percent of the isotope was excreted in the bile in the form of labeled metanephrine glucuronide. Moreover, radioactivity was incorporated into the hepatic pigment within 3 days of the tracer injection, and the pigment remained labeled for at least 3 weeks. This suggested a slow metabolic turnover.

These findings provide strong indirect evidence that the hepatic pigment belongs to the melanin group. The functional, morphologic, and genetic similarities between the condition in the mutant Corriedale sheep and the human Dubin-Johnson syndrome are so striking as to suggest that both may be due to the same inherited metabolic defect.

SUMMARY

1 Several syndromes characterized clinically by chronic nonhemolytic icterus have been shown to be or are suspected of being due to genetically controlled abnormalities of the liver. These may be divided into two major groups, depending on whether the principal defect involves the conversion of bilirubin to its conjugates or the excretion of conjugated pigment in the bile. The first group is comprised of congenital familial nonhemolytic jaundice (Crigler-Najjar syndrome and related conditions) and of constitutional hepatic dysfunction (Gilbert's syndrome). The second group includes chronic idiopathic jaundice (Dubin-Johnson syndrome) and related syndromes. (Congenital abnormalities in the development of intrahepatic bile ducts are not discussed here.)

2 Congenital nonhemolytic jaundice (Crigler-Najjar syndrome) is a rare familial and probably inherited disorder characterized by high concentrations of unconjugated bilirubin in the plasma and frequently associated with irreversible brain damage resembling kernicterus. The underlying defect involves failure of the enzymatic formation of bilirubin glucuronide, which impairs the proper excretion of pigment in the bile. Alternate metabolic pathways are operative for elimination of bilirubin which permit establishment of relatively constant levels of hyperbilirubinemia even though there is continuous pigment production from hemoglobin breakdown.

Patients with less-severe unconjugated hyperbilirubinemia appear to have a partial deficiency of bilirubin conjugation. The defect is probably genetically determined, but the mode of inheritance is unclear. Bilirubin encephalopathy occurs much less frequently. Dramatic lowering of the plasma bilirubin level may follow treatment with drugs that stimulate the microsomal drug-metabolizing enzyme system of the liver.

3 Patients with constitutional hepatic dysfunction (Gilbert's syndrome) usually have a much milder degree of chronic hyperbilirubinemia. The level of unconjugated bilirubin in the plasma fluctuates, and bilirubinuria is absent. Mild and intermittent icterus may be the only significant manifestation of the syndrome. It probably represents a heterogeneous group of benign metabolic abnormalities of unknown causes. Since several members of a family may be affected, at least in some instances the defect may be genetically controlled.

4 Chronic idiopathic jaundice (Dubin-Johnson syndrome, Rotor's syndrome) is a syndrome probably of hereditary nature which involves primarily hepatic excretory functions. The plasma contains increased concentrations of conjugated bilirubin. Bilirubinuria is usually present, and the liver often exhibits intracellular deposition of an unidentified pigment. A similar syndrome, transmitted as an autosomal dominant trait, occurs in a mutant Corriedale sheep.

BIBLIOGRAPHY

1. Adams, F.: *The Genuine Works of Hippocrates.* Williams & Wilkins. Baltimore, 1939.
2. Gray, C. H.: *The Bile Pigments.* Methuen, London, 1953.
3. Virchow, R.: Die pathologischen Pigmente. Arch. Path. Anat., **1**, 379, 1847.
4. Rich, A. R.: The formation of bile pigment. Physiol. Rev., **5**, 182, 1925.

5. Aschoff, L.: Das reticulo-endotheliale System und seine Beziehungen zur Gallenfarbstoffbildung. München. Med. Wschr., **69,** 1352, 1922.
6. McNee, J. W.: Jaundice: a review of recent work. Quart J. Med., **16,** 390, 1923.
7. Whipple, G. H., and Hooper, C. W.: Bile pigment output influenced by hemoglobin injections, anemia and blood regeneration. Amer. J. Physiol., **43,** 258, 1917.
8. Mann, F. C., Sheard, C., Bollman, J. L., and Blades, E. J.: The formation of bile pigment from hemoglobin. Amer. J. Physiol., **76,** 306, 1926.
9. Tarchanoff, J. F.: Ueber die Bildung von Gallenpigment aus Blutfarbstoff im Thierkoerper. Arch. Ges. Physiol., **9,** 53, 1874.
10. Fischer, H., and Orth, H.: *Die Chemie des Pyrrols.* Akademische Verlagsgesellschaft m.b.H., Leipzig, 1937.
11. Minkowski, O., and Naunyn, B.: Beitraege zur Pathologie der Leber und des Icterus. 2. Ueber den Icterus durch Polycholie und die Vorgaenge in der Leber bei demselben. Arch. Exp. Path. Pharmakol., **21,** 1, 1886.
12. Tenhunen, R., Marver, H. S., and Schmid, R.: Microsomal heme oxygenase: characterization of the enzyme. J. Biol. Chem., **244,** 6388, 1969.
13. Tenhunen, R., Marver, H. S., and Schmid, R.: The enzymatic conversion of heme to bilirubin by microsomal heme oxygenase. Proc. Nat. Acad. Sci. U.S.A., **61,** 748, 1968.
14. Hijmans van den Bergh, A. A., and Mueller, P.: Ueber eine direkte und indirekte Diazoreaktion auf Bilirubin. Biochem. Z., **77,** 90, 1916.
15. Watson, C. J.: The pyrrol pigments, with particular reference to normal and pathological hemoglobin metabolism, in *Handbook of Hematology,* edited by Hal Downey. Hamilton, London, 1938.
16. With, T. K.: *Biology of Bile Pigments.* Arne Forst-Hansen, Copenhagen, 1954.
17. Billing, B. H., Cole, P. G., and Lathe, G. H.: The excretion of bilirubin as a diglucuronide giving the direct van den Bergh reaction. Biochem. J., **65,** 774, 1957.
18. Talafant, E.: Properties and composition of the bile pigment giving a direct diazo reaction. Nature (London), **2,** 312, 1956.
19. Schmid, R.: Direct-reacting bilirubin, bilirubin glucuronide in serum, bile and urine. Science, **124,** 76, 1956.
20. Arias, I. M.: Formation of bile pigment, in *Handbook of Physiology,* sec. 6, vol. 5, chap. 110. American Physiological Society, Washington, D.C., 1968.
21. Beck, K.: *Ikterus.* International Symposium, Oct. 27–29, 1967. Freiburg i. Br., F. K. Schattauer, Stuttgart and New York, 1968.
22. Bouchier, I. A. D., and Billing, B. H.: *Bilirubin Metabolism.* Blackwell Scientific Publications, Oxford, 1967.
23. Lester, R., and Troxler, R. F.: Recent advances in bile pigment metabolism. Gastroenterology, **56,** 143, 1969.
24. With, T. K.: *Bile Pigments: Chemical, Biological and Clinical Aspects.* Academic, New York, 1968.
25. Lemberg, R., and Legge, J. W.: *Haematin Compounds and Bile Pigments.* Interscience, New York, 1949.
26. Gray, C. H.: *Bile Pigments in Health and Disease.* Charles C Thomas, Springfield, Ill., 1961.
27. Ó Carra, P.: Zinc complex salt formation by bilirubin and mesobilirubin. Nature (London), **195,** 899, 1962.
28. Nichol, A. W., and Morell, D. B.: Tautomerism and hydrogen bonding in bilirubin and biliverdin. Biochem. Biophys. Acta, **177,** 599, 1969.
29. Fog, J., and Jellum, E.: Structure of bilirubin. Nature (London), **198,** 88, 1963.
30. Brodersen, R., Flodgaard, H., and Hansen, J. K.: Intramolecular hydrogen bonding in bilirubin. Acta Chem. Scand., **21,** 2284, 1967.
31. Ostrow, J. D., Hammaker, L., and Schmid, R.: The preparation of crystalline bilirubin-C^{14}. J. Clin. Invest., **40,** 1442, 1961.
32. Overbeek, J.T.G., Vink, C. L. J., and Deenstra, H.: The solubility of bilirubin. Rec. Trav. Chim. Pays-Bas, **74,** 81, 1955.
33. Burnstine, R. C., and Schmid, R.: Solubility of bilirubin in aqueous solutions. Proc. Soc. Exp. Biol. Med., **109,** 356, 1962.
34. Gray, C. H., Kulczycka, A., and Nicholson, D. C.: The chemistry of the bile pigments. IV. Spectrophotometric titration of the bile pigments. J. Chem. Soc. [Org.], **2,** 2776, 1961.
35. Malloy, H. T., and Evelyn, K. A.: The determination of bilirubin with the photoelectric colorimeter. J. Biol. Chem., **119,** 481, 1937.
36. Nosslin, B.: The direct diazo reaction of bile pigments in serum: experimental and clinical studies. Scand. J. Clin. Lab. Invest., suppl. **49,** 1960.
37. Weber, A. P., and Schalm, L.: Quantitative separation and determination of bilirubin and conjugated bilirubin in human serum. Clin. Chim. Acta, **7,** 805, 1962.
38. London, I. M., West, R., Shemin, D., and Rittenberg, D.: On the origin of bile pigment in normal man. J. Biol. Chem., **184,** 351, 1950.
39. Gray, C. H., Neuberger, A., and Sneath, P. H. A.: Incorporation of N^{15} in the stercobilin in the normal and the porphyric. Biochem. J., **47,** 87, 1950.
40. Barrett, P. V. D., Mullins, F. X., and Berlin, N. I.: Studies on the biosynthetic production of bilirubin-C^{14}: an improved method utilizing δ-aminolevulinic acid-4-C^{14} in dogs. J. Lab. Clin. Med., **68,** 905, 1966.
41. Grodsky, G. M., Carbone, J. V., Fanska, R., and Peng, C. T.: Tritiated bilirubin: preparation and physiological studies. Amer. J. Physiol., **203,** 532, 1962.
42. Wilzbach, K. E.: Tritium gas exposure labeling, in *Advances in Tracer Methodology,* edited by S. Rothchild, vol. I., Plenum, New York, 1963.
43. Lester, R., and Klein, P. D.: Biosynthesis of tritiated bilirubin and studies of its excretion in the rat. J. Lab. Clin. Med., **67,** 1000, 1966.
44. Howe, R. B., Berk, P. D., Bloomer, J. R., and Berlin, N. I.: Preparation and properties of specifically labeled radiochemically stable ^{3}H-bilirubin. J. Lab. Clin. Med., **75,** 499, 1970.
45. Harris, J. W.: *The Red Cell: Production, Metabolism, Destruction: Normal and Abnormal.* Harvard, Cambridge, Mass., 1963.
46. Jandl, J. H., Jones, A. R., and Castle, W. B.: The destruction of red cells by antibodies in man. I. Observations on the sequestration and lysis of red cells altered by immune mechanisms. J. Clin. Invest., **36,** 1428, 1957.
47. Keene, W. R., and Jandl, J. H.: The sites of hemoglobin catabolism. Blood, **26,** 705, 1965.
48. Snyder, A. L., and Schmid, R.: The conversion of hematin to bile pigments in the rat. J. Lab. Clin. Med., **65,** 817, 1965.
49. Langhaus, Th.: Beobachtungen ueber Resorption der Extravasate und Pigmentbildung in denselben. Arch. Path. Anat. Physiol., **49,** 66, 1870.
50. Ostrow, J. D., Jandl, J. H., and Schmid, R.: The formation of bilirubin from hemoglobin in vivo. J. Clin. Invest., **41,** 1628, 1962.
51. Lepehne, G.: Das Problem der Gallenfarbstoffbildung Innerhalb und Ausserhalb der Leber. Folia Haemat., **39,** 277, 1930.
52. Moore, C. V., and Dubach, R.: Metabolism and requirements of iron in man. J.A.M.A., **162,** 197, 1958.
53. Sjöstrand, T.: The formation of carbon monoxide by the decomposition of haemoglobin in vivo. Acta Physiol. Scand., **26,** 338, 1952.
54. Landaw, S. A., Callahan, E. W., and Schmid, R.: Catabolism of heme in vivo: comparison of the simultaneous production of bilirubin and carbon monoxide. J. Clin. Invest., **49** (5), 914, 1970.
55. Lemberg, R.: The chemical mechanism of bile pigment formation. Rev. Pure Appl. Chem., **6,** 1, 1956.
56. Gajdos, A., and Tiprez, G.: La signification biologique des corpuscules de Heinz. C. R. Soc. Biol. (Paris), **139,** 545, 1945.
57. Mills, G. C., and Randall, H. P.: Hemoglobin catabolism. II. The protection of hemoglobin from oxidative breakdown in the intact erythrocyte. J. Biol. Chem., **232,** 589, 1958.
58. Kaziro, K., Kikuchi, G., and Hanaoka, C.: Verdohemoglobin, an immediate precursor of biliverdin in the model reaction of hemoglobin in vitro. J. Biochem., **42,** 423, 1955.
59. Kiese, M., and Seipelt, L.: Bildung und Elimination von Verdoglobin. Arch. Exp. Path., **200,** 648, 1943.
60. Kench, J. E., Gardikas, C., and Wilkinson, J. F.: Bile pigment formation in vitro from haematin and other haem derivatives. Biochem. J., **47,** 129, 1950.
61. Lemberg, R.: Bile pigments from normal erythrocytes. Nature (London), **163,** 97, 1949.
62. Gardikas, C., Kench, J. E., and Wilkinson, J. F.: Choleglobin formation in the erythrocyte. Nature (London), **161,** 607, 1948.
63. Gardikas, C., Kench, J. E., and Wilkinson, J. F.: Bile pigment precursors in normal human erythrocytes. Biochem. J., **46,** 85, 1950.
64. Nakajima, H.: Studies on heme α-methenyl oxygenase. II. The isolation

and characterization of the final reaction product, a possible precursor of biliverdin. J. Biol. Chem., **238,** 3797, 1963.

65. Nakajima, H., Takemura, T., Nakajima, O., and Yamaoka, K: Studies on heme α-methenyl oxygenase. I. The enzymatic conversion of pyridine hemichromogen and hemoglobin-haptoglobin into a possible precursor of biliverdin. J. Biol. Chem., **238,** 3784, 1963.
66. Levin, E. Y.: The conversion of protohemochrome to verdohemochrome with liver homogenate. Biochim. Biophys. Acta, **136,** 155, 1967.
67. Murphy, R. F., O'hEocha, C., and O'Carra, P.: The formation of verdohemochrome from pyridine protohemochrome by extracts of red algae and of liver. Biochem. J., **104,** 6c, 1967.
68. Nichol, A. W., and Morell, D. B.: Studies on the isomeric composition of biliverdin and bilirubin by mass spectrometry. Biochim. Biophys. Acta, **184,** 173, 1969.
69. Wise, C. D., and Drabkin, D. L.: Degradation of hemoglobin and hemin to biliverdin by a new cell-free enzyme system obtained from the hemophagous organ of dog placenta. Fed. Proc., **23,** 223, 1964.
70. Wise, C. D., and Drabkin, D. L.: Enzymatic degradation of hemoglobin and hemin to biliverdin and carbon monoxide. Fed. Proc., **24,** 222, 1965.
71. Lemberg, R., Barcroft, J., and Keilin, D.: Uteroverdin. Nature (London), **128,** 967, 1931.
72. Nencki, M., and Zaleski, J.: Untersuchungen ueber den Blutfarbstoff. Z. Physiol. Chem., **30,** 384, 1900.
73. Eppinger, H.: *Die Hepato-lienalen Erkrankungen.* Springer-Verlag, Berlin, 1920.
74. Green, M., and Kench, J. E.: A study of the transfer of haem from haemoglobin to serum albumin. S. Afr. Med. J., **41,** 895, 1967.
75. Bunn, H. F., and Jandl, J. H.: Exchange of heme among hemoglobins and between hemoglobin and albumin. J. Biol. Chem., **243,** 465, 1968.
76. Bingold, K.: Haemolyse, Blutfarbstoffabbau, Haematinaemie und Ikterus. Arch. Klin. Med., **97,** 257, 1923.
77. Schumm, O.: Haematin als pathologischer Bestandteil des Blutes. Z. Physiol. Chem., **97,** 32, 1916.
78. Fairley, N. H.: Methaemalbumin: clinical aspects. Quart. J. Med., **10,** 95, 1941.
79. Brugsch, T., and Retzlaff, K.: Blutzerfall, Galle und Urobilin. Z. Exp. Path., **11,** 508, 1912.
80. Pass, I. J., Schwartz, S., and Watson, C. J.: The conversion of hematin to bilirubin following intravenous administration in human subjects. J. Clin. Invest., **24,** 283, 1945.
81. London, I. M.: The conversion of hematin to bile pigment. J. Biol. Chem., **184,** 373, 1950.
82. Ibrahim, G. W., Schwartz, S., and Watson, C. J.: The conversion of protoporphyrin-C^{14} to heme compounds and bilirubin in dogs. Metabolism, **15,** 1120, 1966.
83. London, I. M., Yamasaki, M., and Sabella, A. G.: Conversion of protoporphyrin to bile pigment. Fed. Proc., **10,** 217, 1951.
84. Heikel, T., Lockwood, W. H., and Rimington, C.: Formation of nonenzymatic haem. Nature (London), **182,** 313, 1958.
85. Mauzerall, D., and Granick, S.: Porphyrin biosynthesis in erythrocytes. III. Uroporphyrinogen and its decarboxylase. J. Biol. Chem., **232,** 1141, 1958.
86. Nishida, G., and Labbe, R. F.: Heme biosynthesis: on the incorporation of iron into protoporphyrin. Biochim. Biophys. Acta, **31,** 520, 1959.
87. Tenhunen, R., Ross, M. E., Marver, H. S., and Schmid, R.: Reduced nicotinamide-adenine dinucleotide phosphate dependent biliverdin reductase: partial purification and characterization. Biochemistry, **9,** 298, 1970.
88. Tenhunen, R., Marver, H. S., and Schmid, R.: The enzymatic catabolism of hemoglobin: stimulation of microsomal heme oxygenase by hemin. J. Lab. Clin. Med., **75,** 410, 1970.
89. Pimstone, N. R., Tenhunen, R., Seitz, P. T., Marver, H. S., and Schmid, R.: The enzymatic degradation of hemoglobin to bile pigments by macrophages. J. Exp. Med., 1971, in press.
90. Pimstone, N. R., Engel, P., Tenhunen, R., Seitz, P. T., Marver, H. S., and Schmid, R.: Inducible heme oxygenase in the kidney: a model for the homeostatic control of hemoglobin catabolism. J. Clin. Invest., 1971, in press.
91. Rosen, H., and Sears, D. A.: Spectral properties of hemopexin-heme: the Schumm test. J. Lab. Clin. Med., **74,** 941, 1969.
92. Ottenberg, R.: Bilirubin and bile salts in jaundice. J. Mt. Sinai Hosp., **9,** 937, 1943.
93. With, T. K.: The bilirubin production of the human organism and its significance to the pathogenesis of jaundice. Acta Med. Scand., **123,** 166, 1946.
94. Deenstra, H.: L'excrétion des pigments biliaires par les reins. Ann. Med., **51,** 685, 1950.
95. Jandl, J. H.: The Heinz body hemolytic anemias. Ann. Intern. Med., **58,** 702, 1963.
96. Goldstein, G. W., Hammaker, L., and Schmid, R.: Catabolism of Heinz bodies: experimental model demonstrating conversion to nonbilirubin catabolites. Blood, **31,** 388, 1968.
97. Siedel, W., v. Poelnitz, W., and Eisenreich, F.: Bilifuscin und Mesobilifuscin als natuerliche Abbauprodukte des Blutfarbstoffes; ueber Vorkommen und Bildung. Naturwissenschaften, **34,** 314, 1947.
98. Siedel, W., Stich, W., and Eisenreich, F.: Promesobilifuscin (Mesobilileukan), ein neues physiologisches Abbauprodukt des Blutfarbstoffes. Naturwissenschaften, **35,** 316, 1948.
99. Gilbertsen, A. S., Lowry, P. T., Hawkinson, V., and Watson, C. J.: Studies of dipyrrylmethene ("fuscin") pigments. I. The anabolic significance of the fecal mesobilifuscin. J. Clin. Invest., **38,** 1166, 1959.
100. Bingold, K.: Eigenschaften und physiologische Bedeutung des Pentdyopents. Klin. Wschr., **17,** 289, 1938.
101. Hulst, L. A., and Grotepass, W.: Ueber das Pentdyopent von Bingold. Klin. Wschr., **15,** 201, 1936.
102. Schmid, R., and Hammaker, L.: Metabolism and disposition of C^{14}-bilirubin in congenital nonhemolytic jaundice. J. Clin. Invest., **42,** 1720, 1963.
103. Schmid, R.: Anémie hémolytique familiale avec inclusions érythrocytaires et trouble du métabolisme pigmentaire: un nouveau syndrome. Nouv. Rev. Franc. Hemat., **1,** 801, 1961.
104. Kreimer-Birnbaum, M., Pinkerton, P. H., and Bannerman, R. M.: Dipyrrolic urinary pigments in congenital Heinz-body anaemia due to Hb Koln and in thalassemia. Brit. Med. J., **2,** 396, 1966.
105. Bessis, M., Breton-Gorius, J., and Thiery, J. P.: Rôle possible de l'hémoglobine accompagnant le noyau des érythroblastes dans l'origine de la stercobiline éliminée précocement. C. R. Acad. Sci., **252,** 2300, 1961.
106. Israels, L. G., Yamamoto, T., Skanderberg, J., and Zipursky, A.: Shunt bilirubin; evidence for two components. Science, **139,** 1054, 1963.
107. Robinson, S. H., and Schmid, R.: The relation of erythropoiesis to bile pigment formation. Medicine, **43,** 667, 1964.
108. Yamamoto, T., Skanderberg, J., Zipursky, A., and Israels, L. G.: The early appearing bilirubin: evidence for two components. J. Clin. Invest., **44,** 31, 1965.
109. Robinson, S. H., Tsong, M., Brown, B. W., and Schmid, R.: The sources of bile pigment in the rat: studies of the "early-labeled" fraction. J. Clin. Invest., **45,** 1569, 1966.
110. Robinson, S. H., Lester, R., Crigler, J. F., and Tsong, M.: Early-labeled peak of bile pigment in man. Studies with glycine-C^{14} and δ-aminolevulinic acid-H^3. New Eng. J. Med., **277,** 1323, 1967.
111. Ibrahim, G. W., Schwartz, S., and Watson, C. J.: Early labeling of bilirubin from glycine and δ-aminolevulinic acid in bile fistula dogs, with special reference to stimulated versus suppressed erythropoiesis. Metabolism, **15,** 1129, 1966.
112. Petryka, Z. J.: Identification of isomers differing from 9α, in the early labeled bilirubin of the bile. Proc. Soc. Exp. Biol. Med., **123,** 464, 1966.
113. Coburn, R. F., Blakemore, W. S., and Forster, R. S.: Endogenous carbon monoxide production in man. J. Clin. Invest., **42,** 1172, 1963.
114. Troxler, R. F., and Lester, R.: Biosynthesis of phycocyanobilin. Biochemistry, **6,** 3840, 1967.
115. Troxler, R. F., Brown, A., Lester, R., and White, P.: Bile pigment formation in plants. Science, **167,** 192, 1970.
116. Daly, J. S. F., Little, J. M., Troxler, R. F., and Lester, R.: Metabolism of ^{3}H-myoglobin. Nature (London), **216,** 1030, 1967.
117. Åkeson, Å., Ehrenstein, G., Hevesy, G., and Theorell, H.: Life span of myoglobin. Arch. Biochim. Biophys., **91,** 310, 1960.

118. Schwartz, S., Ibrahim, G., and Watson, C. J.: The contribution of nonhemoglobin hemes to the early labeling of bile bilirubin (abstract). J. Lab. Clin. Med., **64,** 1003, 1964.
119. Robinson, S. H., Owen, C. A., Flock, E. V., and Schmid, R.: Bilirubin formation in the liver from nonhemoglobin sources: experiments with isolated, perfused rat liver. Blood, **26,** 823, 1965.
120. Schmid, R., Marver, H. S., and Hammaker, L.: Enhanced formation of rapidly labeled bilirubin by phenobarbital: hepatic microsomal cytochromes as a possible source. Biochem. Biophys. Res. Commun., **24,** 319, 1966.
121. Levitt, M., Schacter, B. A., Zipursky, A., and Israels, L. G.: The nonerythropoietic component of early bilirubin. J. Clin. Invest., **47,** 1281, 1968.
122. London, I. M., West, R., Shemin, D., and Rittenberg, D.: Porphyrin formation and hemoglobin metabolism in congenital porphyria. J. Biol. Chem., **184,** 365, 1950.
123. London, I. M., and West, R.: The formation of bile pigment in pernicious anemia. J. Biol. Chem., **184,** 359, 1950.
124. Robinson, S. H., Vanier, T., Desforges, J. F., and Schmid, R.: Jaundice in thalassemia minor: a consequence of "ineffective erythropoiesis." New Eng. J. Med., **267,** 523, 1962.
125. Israels, L. G., Skanderbeg, J., Guyda, H., Zingg, W., and Zipursky, A.: A study of the early-labeled fraction of bile pigment: the effect of altering erythropoiesis on the incorporation of $(2-{}^{14}C)$ glycine into haem and bilirubin. Brit. J. Haemat., **9,** 50, 1963.
126. Robinson, S. H.: Reticulocyte death: a source of early labeled bile pigment. J. Clin. Invest. (abstract), **46,** 1109, 1967.
127. Nagai, K., and Kakishita, E.: Destruction of immature erythrocytes measured by bilirubin excretion. Blood, **33,** 717, 1969.
128. Robinson, S. H.: The origins of bilirubin. New Eng. J. Med., **279,** 143, 1968.
129. Odell, G. B.: Studies in kernicterus. I. The protein binding of bilirubin. J. Clin. Invest., **38,** 823, 1959.
130. Odell, G. B.: The dissociation of bilirubin from albumin and its clinical implications. J. Pediat., **55,** 268, 1959.
131. Ostrow, J. D., and Schmid, R.: The protein-binding of C^{14}-bilirubin in human and murine serum. J. Clin. Invest., **42,** 1286, 1963.
132. Sass-Kortsak, A.: *Kernicterus:* report based on a symposium held at the IXth International Congress of Paediatrics, Montreal, July, 1959. University of Toronto Press, Toronto, 1961.
133. Powell, L. W., Hemingway, E., Billing, B. H., and Sherlock, S.: Idiopathic unconjugated hyperbilirubinemia (Gilbert's syndrome): a study of 42 families. New Eng. J. Med., **277,** 1108, 1967.
134. Schmid, R., and Hammaker, L.: Metabolism and disposition of C^{14}-bilirubin in congenital nonhemolytic jaundice. J. Clin. Invest., **42,** 1720, 1963.
135. Hsia, D. Y., Patterson, P., Allen, F. H., Diamond, L. K., and Gellis, S. S.: Prolonged obstructive jaundice in infancy. I. General survey of 156 cases. Pediatrics, **10,** 243, 1952.
136. Schalm, L., and Weber, A. Ph.: Jaundice with conjugated bilirubin in hyperhaemolysis. Acta Med. Scand., **176,** 549, 1964.
137. Fulop, M., Sandson, J., and Brazeau, P.: Dialyzability, protein binding, and renal excretion of plasma conjugated bilirubin. J. Clin. Invest., **44,** 666, 1965.
138. Schenker, S., and McCandless, D. W.: Renal disposition of conjugated bilirubin in aglomerular fish. Nature (London), **202,** 1344, 1964.
139. Weinbren, K., and Billing, B. H.: Hepatic clearance of bilirubin as an index of cellular function in the regenerating rat liver. Brit. J. Exp. Path., **37,** 199, 1956.
140. Katz, J. S., Rosenfeld, S., and Sellers, A. L.: Sites of plasma albumin catabolism in the rat. Amer. J. Physiol., **200,** 1301, 1961.
141. Bernstein, L. H., Ezzer, J. B., Gartner, L., and Arias, I. M.: Hepatic intracellular distribution of tritium-labeled unconjugated and conjugated bilirubin in normal and Gunn rats. J. Clin. Invest., **45,** 1194, 1966.
142. Hunton, D. B., Bollman, J. L., and Hoffman, H. N.: The plasma removal of indocyanine green and sulfobromophthalein: effect of dosage and blocking agents. J. Clin. Invest., **40,** 1648, 1961.
143. Berthelot, P., and Billing, B. H.: Effect of bunamiodyl on hepatic uptake of sulfobromophthalein in the rat. Amer. J. Physiol., **211,** 395, 1966.
144. Hammaker, L., and Schmid, R.: Interference with bile pigment uptake in the liver by flavaspidic acid. Gastroenterology, **53,** 31, 1967.
145. Billing, B. H., Williams, R., and Richards, T. G.: Defects in hepatic transport of bilirubin in congenital hyperbilirubinaemia: an analysis of plasma bilirubin disappearance curves. Clin. Sci., **27,** 245, 1964.
146. Berk, P. D., Howe, R. B., Bloomer, J. R., and Berlin, N. I.: Studies of bilirubin kinetics in normal adults. J. Clin. Invest., **48,** 2176, 1969.
147. Goresky, C. A.: The hepatic uptake and excretion of sulfobromophthalein and bilirubin. Canad. Med. Ass. J., **92,** 851, 1965.
148. Brown, W. R., Grodsky, G. M., and Carbone, J. V.: Intracellular distribution of tritiated bilirubin during hepatic uptake and excretion. Amer. J. Physiol., **207,** 1237, 1964.
149. Grodsky, G. M.: Studies in the uptake and intrahepatic transport of (^3H) bilirubin, in *Bilirubin Metabolism,* edited by I. A. D. Bouchier and B. H. Billing, p. 159. Blackwell Scientific Publications, Oxford, 1967.
150. Levi, A. J., Gatmaitan, Z., and Arias, I. M.: Two hepatic cytoplasmic protein fractions, Y and Z, and their possible role in the hepatic uptake of bilirubin, sulfobromophthalein and other anions. J. Clin. Invest., **48,** 2156, 1969.
151. Levi, A. J., Gatmaitan, Z., and Arias, I. M.: Deficiency of hepatic organic anion-binding protein as a possible cause of non-haemolytic unconjugated hyperbilirubinaemia in the newborn. Lancet, **2,** 139, 1969.
152. Schachter, D.: Nature of the glucuronide in direct-reacting bilirubin. Science, **126,** 507, 1957.
153. Schmid, R., Hammaker, L., and Axelrod, J.: The enzymatic formation of bilirubin glucuronide. Arch. Biochem., **70,** 285, 1957.
154. Dutton, G. J., and Storey, I. D. E.: Uridine compounds in glucuronic acid metabolism. I. The formation of glucuronides in liver suspensions. Biochem. J., **57,** 275, 1954.
155. Strominger, J. L., Kalckar, H. M., Axelrod, J., and Maxwell, E. S.: Enzymatic oxidation of uridine diphosphate glucose to uridine diphosphate glucuronic acid. J. Amer. Chem. Soc., **76,** 6411, 1954.
156. Axelrod, J., Inscoe, J. K., and Tomkins, G. M.: Enzymatic synthesis of N-glucosyluronic acid conjugates. J. Biol. Chem., **232,** 835, 1958.
157. Dutton, G. J.: *Glucuronide Conjugation,* Proceedings, First International Pharmacological Meeting, vol. 6, p. 39. Pergamon, New York, 1962.
158. Isselbacher, K. J., Chrabas, M. F., and Quinn, R. C.: The solubilization and partial purification of a glucuronyl transferase from rabbit liver microsomes, J. Biol. Chem., **237,** 3033, 1962.
159. Williams, R. T.: *Detoxication Mechanisms.* Wiley, New York, 1959.
160. Lathe, G. H., and Walker, M.: The synthesis of bilirubin glucuronide in animal and human liver. Biochem. J., **70,** 705, 1958.
161. Grodsky, G. M., and Carbone, J. V.: Synthesis of bilirubin glucuronide by tissue homogenates. J. Biol. Chem., **226,** 449, 1957.
162. Arias, I. M.: A defect in microsomal function in nonhemolytic acholuric jaundice. J. Histochem., **7,** 250, 1969.
163. Isselbacher, K. J., and McCarthy, E. A.: Studies on bilirubin sulfate and other nonglucuronide conjugates of bilirubin. J. Clin. Invest., **38,** 645, 1959.
164. Schmid, R., Axelrod, J., Hammaker, L., and Swarm, R. L.: Congenital jaundice in rats, due to a defect in glucuronide formation. J. Clin. Invest., **37,** 1123, 1958.
165. Brown, A. K., and Zuelzer, W. W.: Studies on the neonatal development of the glucuronide conjugating system. J. Clin. Invest., **37,** 332, 1958.
166. Schmid, R.: Unpublished observations.
167. Billing, B. H., and Lathe, G. H.: Bilirubin metabolism in jaundice. Amer. J. Med., **24,** 111, 1958.
168. Weber, A. Ph., Schalm, L., and Witmans, G.: Bilirubin monoglucuronide (pigment I): a complex. Acta Med. Scand., **173,** 19, 1963.
169. Gregory, C. H.: Studies of conjugated bilirubin. III. Pigment I, a complex of conjugated and free bilirubin. J. Lab. Clin. Med., **61,** 917, 1963.
170. Callahan, E. W., Jr., and Schmid, R.: Excretion of unconjugated bilirubin in the bile of Gunn rats. Gastroenterology, **57,** 134, 1969.
171. Gregory, C. H., and Watson, C. J.: Studies of conjugated bilirubin. II. Problems of sulfates of bilirubin in vivo and in vitro. J. Lab. Clin. Med., **60,** 17, 1962.
172. Noir, B. A., De Walz, A. T., and Rodriguez-Garay, E.: Studies on bilirubin sulphate in human bile, in *Bilirubin Metabolism,* edited by

I. A. D. Bouchier and B. H. Billing, p. 99. Blackwell Scientific Publications, Oxford, 1967.
173. Arias, I. M.: Ethereal and N-linked glucuronide formation by normal and Gunn rats in vitro and in vivo. Biochem. Biophys. Res. Commun., **6,** 81, 1961.
174. van Leusden, H. A. I. M., Bakkeren, J. A. J. M., Zilliken, F., and Stolte, L. A. M.: *p*-Nitrophenylglucuronide formation by homozygous adult Gunn rats. Biochem. Biophys. Res. Commun., **7,** 67, 1962.
175. Javitt, N. B.: In vivo studies of glucuronide formation (abstract). Gastroenterology, **46,** 299, 1964.
176. Remmer, H., and Merker, H. J.: Drug-induced changes in the liver endoplasmic reticulum: association with drug-metabolizing enzymes. Science, **142,** 1657, 1963.
177. Inscoe, J. K., and Axelrod, J.: Some factors affecting glucuronide formation in vitro. J. Pharmacol. Exp. Ther., **129,** 128, 1960.
178. Pogell, B. M., and Leloir, L. F.: Nucleotide activation of liver microsomal glucuronidation. J. Biol. Chem., **236,** 293, 1961.
179. Stevenson, I. H., and Dutton, G. J.: Mechanism of glucuronide synthesis in skin. Biochem. J., **77,** 19P, 1960.
180. Hargreaves, T., and Holton, J. B.: Jaundice of the newborn due to novobiocin. Lancet, **1,** 839, 1962.
181. Waters, W. J., Dunham, R., and Bowen, W. R.: Inhibition of bilirubin conjugation in vitro. Proc. Soc. Exp. Biol. Med., **99,** 175, 1958.
182. Lathe, G. H., and Walker, M.: Inhibition of bilirubin conjugation in rat liver slices by human pregnancy and neonatal serum and steroids. Quart. J. Exp. Physiol., **43,** 257, 1958.
183. Stevenson, I., Greenwood, D., and McEwen, J.: Hepatic UDP-glucuronyl-transferase in Wistar and Gunn rats—*in vitro* activation by diethylnitrosamine. Biochem. Biophys. Res. Commun., **32,** 866, 1968.
184. Lester, R., and Schmid, R.: Bilirubin metabolism. New Eng. J. Med., **270,** 779, 1964.
185. Lathe, G. H.: Disorders of bilirubin metabolism. The Warner-Chilcott Lecture. Clin. Chem., **11,** 309, 1965.
186. Boerth, R. C., Blatt, A. H., and Spratt, J. L.: Limitations in the determination of in vitro bilirubin glucuronide formation. J. Lab. Clin. Med., **65,** 475, 1965.
187. Maki, T., Sato, T., Yamaguchi, I., and Saito, Y.: Autopsy incidence of gallstones in Japan. Tohoku J. Exp. Med., **84,** 37, 1964.
188. Maki, T.: Pathogenesis of calcium bilirubinate gallstone: role of *E. coli, β*-glucuronidase and coagulation by inorganic ions, polyelectrolytes, and agitation. Ann. Surg., **164,** 90, 1966.
189. Lester, R., and Klein, P. D.: Bile pigment excretion: a comparison of the biliary excretion of bilirubin and bilirubin derivatives. J. Clin. Invest., **45,** 1839, 1966.
190. Lester, R., and Schmid, R.: Intestinal absorption of bile pigments. I. The enterohepatic circulation of bilirubin in the rat. J. Clin. Invest., **42,** 736, 1963.
191. Lester, R., and Schmid, R.: Intestinal absorption of bile pigments. II. Bilirubin absorption in man. New Eng. J. Med., **269,** 178, 1963.
192. Ostrow, J. D.: Absorption of bile pigments by the gallbladder. J. Clin. Invest., **46,** 2035, 1967.
193. Lester, R., Behrman, R. E., and Lucey, J. F.: Transfer of bilirubin-C^{14} across monkey placenta. Pediatrics, **32,** 416, 1963.
194. Schenker, S., Dawber, N. H., and Schmid, R.: Bilirubin metabolism in the fetus. J. Clin. Invest., **43,** 32, 1964.
195. Schenker, S., Bashore, R. A., and Smith, F.: Bilirubin disposition in foetal monkeys, in *Bilirubin Metabolism,* edited by I. A. D. Bouchier and B. H. Billing, p. 199. Blackwell Scientific Publications, Oxford, 1967.
196. Bernstein, R. B., Novy, M. J., Piasecki, G. J., Lester, R., and Jackson, B. T.: Bilirubin metabolism in the fetus. J. Clin. Invest., **48,** 1678, 1969.
197. Diamond, I., and Schmid, R.: Experimental bilirubin encephalopathy: the mode of entry of bilirubin-^{14}C into the central nervous system. J. Clin. Invest., **45,** 678, 1966.
198. Schanker, L. S.: Passage of drugs across body membranes. Pharmacol. Rev., **14,** 501, 1962.
199. Arias, I., Bernstein, L., Toffler, R., Cornelius, C., Novikoff, A. B., and Essner, E.: Black liver disease in Corriedale sheep: a new mutation affecting hepatic excretory function. J. Clin. Invest., **43,** 1249, 1964.
200. Arias, I. M.: The excretion of conjugated bilirubin by the liver cell. Medicine, **45,** 513, 1966.
201. Smallwood, R. A., Lester, R., Piasecki, G. J., Little, J. M., and Jackson, B. T.: Bile salt metabolism in the fetal monkey (abstract). Gastroenterology, **58,** 300, 1970.
202. Watson, C. J.: Recent studies of the urobilin problem. J. Clin. Path., **16,** 1, 1963.
203. Watson, C. J., Campbell, M., and Lowry, P. T.: Preferential reduction of conjugated bilirubin to urobilinogen by normal fecal flora. Proc. Soc. Exp. Biol. Med., **98,** 707, 1958.
204. Troxler, R. F., Dawber, N. H., and Lester, R.: Synthesis of urobilinogen by broken cell preparations of intestinal bacteria. Gastroenterology, **54,** 568, 1968.
205. Lester, R., Schumer, W., and Schmid, R.: Intestinal absorption of bile pigments. III. The enterohepatic circulation of urobilinogen in the rat. J. Clin. Invest., **44,** 722, 1965.
206. Lester, R., Schumer, W., and Schmid, R.: Intestinal absorption of bile pigments. IV. Urobilinogen absorption in man. New Eng. J. Med., **272,** 939, 1965.
207. Stumpf, W. E., and Lester, R.: Secretion and absorption of mesobilirubinogen-H^3 studied by autoradiography. Lab. Invest., **15,** 1156, 1966.
208. Bourke, E., Milne, M. D., and Stokes, G. S.: Mechanisms of renal excretion of urobilinogen. Brit. Med. J., **2,** 1510, 1965.
209. Levy, M., Lester, R., and Levinsky, N. G.: Renal excretion of urobilinogen in the dog. J. Clin. Invest., **47,** 2117, 1968.
210. Israels, L. G., Suderman, H. J., and Ritzman, S. E.: Hyperbilirubinemia due to alternate path of bilirubin production. Amer. J. Med., **27,** 693, 1959.
211. Arias, I. M.: The transport of bilirubin in the liver, in *Progress in Liver Disease,* edited by H. Popper and F. Schaffner. Grune & Stratton, New York, 1961.
212. Snyder, A. L., Satterlee, W., Robinson, S. H., and Schmid, R.: Conjugated plasma bilirubin in jaundice caused by pigment overload. Nature (London), **213,** 93, 1967.
213. Billing, B. H., Maggiore, Q., and Cartter, M. A.: Hepatic transport of bilirubin. Ann. N.Y. Acad. Sci., **111,** 319, 1963.
214. Jandl, J. H.: Anemia of liver disease: observations on its mechanism. J. Clin. Invest., **34,** 390, 1955.
215. Popper, H., and Schaffner, F.: Fine structural changes of the liver. Ann. Intern. Med., **59,** 674, 1963.
216. Arias, I. M.: Chronic unconjugated hyperbilirubinemia without overt signs of hemolysis in adolescents and adults. J. Clin. Invest., **41,** 2233, 1962.
217. Weech, A. A.: The genesis of physiologic hyperbilirubinemia. Advances Pediat., **2,** 346, 1947.
218. Lucey, J. F., Behrman, R. E., and Warshaw, A. L.: "Physiologic" jaundice in newborn rhesus monkeys. Amer. J. Dis. Child., **106,** 350, 1963.
219. Smallwood, R. A., Lester, R., Piasecki, G. J., Rauschecker, H. F. J., and Jackson, B. T.: Metabolism of bile salt in the fetal dog (abstract). J. Clin. Invest., **48,** 78a, 1969.
220. Lathe, G. H., and Walker, M.: The synthesis of bilirubin glucuronide in animal and human liver. Biochem. J., **70,** 705, 1958.
221. Karunairatnam, M. C., Kerr, L. M. H., and Levvy, G. A.: Glucuronide-synthesizing system in mouse and its relationship to β-glucuronidase. Biochem. J., **45,** 496, 1949.
222. Hartiala, K. H. V., and Pulkkinen, M.: Studies on detoxification mechanisms. IV. Glucuronide synthesis in the fetal rabbit. Ann. Med. Exp. Biol. Fenn., **33,** 246, 1955.
223. Dutton, G. J.: Glucuronide synthesis in foetal liver and other tissues. Biochem. J., **71,** 141, 1959.
224. Obrinsky, W., Denley, M. L., and Brauer, R. W.: Sulfobromophthalein sodium excretion test as a measure of liver function in premature infants. Pediatrics, **9,** 421, 1952.
225. Sussman, S., Carbone, J. V., Grodsky, G., Hjelte, V., and Miller, P.: Sulfobromophthalein sodium metabolism in newborn infants. Pediatrics, **29,** 899, 1962.
226. Boggs, T. R., Jr., Hardy, J. B., and Frazier, T. M.: Correlation of neonatal serum total bilirubin concentrations and developmental status at age eight months. J. Pediat., **71,** 553, 1967.

227. Blumenschein, S. D., Kallen, R. J., Storey, B., Natzschka, J. C., Odell, G. B., and Childs, B.: Familial nonhemolytic jaundice with late onset of neurological damage. Pediatrics, **42,** 786, 1968.
228. Ernster, L., Herlin, L., and Zetterstrom, R.: Experimental studies on the pathogenesis of kernicterus. Pediatrics, **20,** 647, 1957.
229. Menken, M., Waggoner, J. G., and Berlin, N. I.: The influence of bilirubin on oxidative phosphorylation and related reactions in brain and liver mitochondria: effects of protein-binding. J. Neurochem., **13,** 1241, 1966.
230. Schenker, S., McCandless, D. W., and Zollman, P. E.: Studies of cellular toxicity of unconjugated bilirubin in kernicteric brain. J. Clin. Invest., **45,** 1213, 1966.
231. Diamond, I., and Schmid, R.: Oxidative phosphorylation in experimental bilirubin encephalopathy. Science, **155,** 1288, 1967.
232. Menken, M., and Weinbach, E. C.: Oxidative phosphorylation and respiratory control of brain mitochondria isolated from kernicteric rats. J. Neurochem., **14,** 189, 1967.
233. Freda, V. J., Gorman, J. G., and Pollack, W.: Suppression of the primary Rh immune response with passive Rh IgG immunoglobulin. New Eng. J. Med., **277,** 1022, 1967.
234. Arias, I. M., Gartner, L. M., Seifter, S., and Furman, M.: Prolonged neonatal unconjugated hyperbilirubinemia associated with breast feeding and a steroid, pregnane-3 (alpha) 20 (beta)-diol, in maternal milk that inhibits glucuronide formation *in vitro.* J. Clin. Invest., **43,** 2037, 1964.
235. Gartner, L. M., and Arias, I. M.: Studies of prolonged neonatal jaundice in the breast-fed infant. J. Pediat., **68,** 54, 1966.
236. Ramos, A., Silverberg, M., and Stern, L.: Pregnanediols and neonatal hyperbilirubinemia. Amer. J. Dis. Child., **111,** 353, 1966.
237. Arias, I. M., Wolfson, S., Lucey, J. F., and McKay, R. J., Jr.: Transient familial neonatal hyperbilirubinemia. J. Clin. Invest., **44,** 1442, 1965.
238. Gunn, C. K.: Hereditary acholuric jaundice. J. Hered., **29,** 137, 1938.
239. Malloy, H. T., and Loewenstein, L.: Hereditary jaundice in the rat. Canad. Med. Ass. J., **42,** 122, 1940.
240. Johnson, L., Sarmiento, F., Blanc, W. A., and Day, R.: Kernicterus in rats with an inherited deficiency in glucuronyl transferase. A.M.A.J. Dis. Child., **99,** 591, 1959.
241. Novikoff, A. B., and Essner, E.: The liver cell. Amer. J. Med., **29,** 102, 1960.
242. Blanc, W. A., and Johnson, L.: Studies on kernicterus. J. Neuropath. Exp. Neurol., **18,** 165, 1959.
243. Schutta, H. S., and Johnson, L.: Bilirubin encephalopathy in the Gunn rat: a fine structure study of the cerebellar cortex. J. Neuropath. Exp. Neurol., **26,** 377, 1967.
244. Odell, G. B., Natzschka, J. C., and Storey, G. N. B.: Bilirubin nephropathy in the Gunn strain of rat. Amer. J. Physiol., **212,** 931, 1967.
245. Odell, G. B.: The response of jaundice and non-jaundiced weanling rats to thirsting. Pediat. Res., **2,** 237, 1968.
246. Lozzio, B. B., Chernoff, A. I., Machado, E. R., and Lozzio, C. B.: Hereditary renal disease in a mutant strain of rats. Science, **156,** 1742, 1967.
247. Arias, I. M., Johnson, L., and Wolfson, S.: Biliary excretion of injected conjugated and unconjugated bilirubin by normal Gunn rats. Amer. J. Physiol., **200,** 1091, 1961.
248. Robinson, S. H.: Increased bilirubin conjugation in heterozygous Gunn rats treated with phenobarbital. Nature (London), **222,** 990, 1969.
249. Ostrow, J. D.: Mechanism of the phototherapy of jaundice. Gastroenterology, **56,** 400, 1969.
250. Ostrow, J. D.: in *Bilirubin Metabolism,* edited by I. A. D. Bouchier and B. H. Billing, p. 117. Blackwell Scientific Publications, Oxford, 1967.
251. Berthelot, P., and Fauvert, R.: L'Excrétion de bilirubine non-conjugée dans la bile du rat: modification de cette excrétion par la novobiocine. Rev. Franc. Etud. Clin. Biol., **12,** 702, 1967.
252. Ostrow, J. D.: Mechanism for the appearance of unconjugated bilirubin in bile. Gastroenterology, **52,** 321, 1967.
253. Javitt, N. B.: Ethereal and acyl glucuronide formation in the homozygous Gunn rat. Amer. J. Physiol., **211,** 424, 1966.
254. Carbone, J. V., and Grodsky, G. M.: Constitutional nonhemolytic hyperbilirubinemia in the rat: defect of bilirubin conjugation. Proc. Soc. Exp. Biol. Med., **94,** 461, 1957.
255. Axelrod, J., Schmid, R., and Hammaker, L.: A biochemical lesion in congenital non-obstructive non-hemolytic jaundice. Nature (London), **180,** 1426, 1957.
256. Drucker, W. D.: Glucuronic acid conjugation of tetrahydrocortisone and *p*-nitrophenol in the homozygous Gunn rat. Proc. Soc. Exp. Biol. Med., **129,** 308, 1968.
257. Dutton, G. J.: in *Glucuronic Acid, Free and Combined,* edited by G. J. Dutton, pp. 222, 230. Academic, New York, 1966.
258. Boucher, I. A. D., and Billing, B.: *Bilirubin Metabolism,* edited by I. A. D. Bouchier & B. H. Billing, p. 188. Blackwell Scientific Publications, Oxford, 1967.
259. DeLeon, A., Gartner, L. M., and Arias, I. M.: The effect of phenobarbital on hyperbilirubinemia in glucuronyl transferase deficient rats. J. Lab. Clin. Med., **70,** 273, 1967.
260. Stevenson, I., Greenwood, D., and McEwen, J.: Hepatic UDP-glucuronyl-transferase in Wistar and Gunn rats—in vitro activation by diethylnitrosamine. Biochem. Biophys. Res. Commun., **32,** 866, 1968.
261. Arias, I. M., and Johnson, I.: Studies of bilirubin excretion in normal and Gunn rats. Clin. Res., **7,** 291, 1959.
262. Schmid, R., Diamond, I., Hammaker, L., and Gundersen, C. B.: The interaction of bilirubin with albumin. Nature (London), **206,** 1041, 1965.
263. Lester, R., Hammaker, L., and Schmid, R.: A new therapeutic approach to unconjugated hyperbilirubinaemia. Lancet, **2,** 1257, 1962.
264. Housett, E., Etienne, J. P., Petite, J. P., Oudéa, P., and Oudéa, M. C.: Le Rat Gunn, animal d'expérience privilégié. Path. Biol. (Paris), **15,** 546, 1967.
265. Cunningham, I. J., Hopkirk, C. S. M., and Filmer, J. F.: Photosensitivity diseases in New Zealand. I. Facial eczema: its clinical, pathological and biochemical characteristics. New Zeal. J. Sci. Tech., **24A,** 185, 1942.
266. Hancock, J.: Congenital photosensitivity in Southdown sheep. A new sub-lethal factor in sheep. New Zeal. J. Sci. Tech., **32A,** 16, 1950.
267. Cornelius, C. E., and Gronwall, R. R.: Congenital photosensitivity and hyperbilirubinemia in Southdown sheep in the United States. Amer. J. Vet. Res., **29,** 291, 1968.
268. Foulk, W. T., Butt, H. R., Owen, C. A., Whitcomb, F. F., and Mason, H. L.: Constitutional hepatic dysfunction (Gilbert's disease): its natural history and related syndromes. Medicine, **38,** 25, 1959.
269. Crigler, J. F., and Najjar, V. A.: Congenital familial nonhemolytic jaundice with kernicterus. Pediatrics, **10,** 169, 1952.
270. François, R., Bertholon, M. A., Bertrand, J., and Quincy, Cl.: La Maladie de Crigler-Najjar. Rev. Int. Hepat., **12,** 753, 1962.
271. Arias, I. M., Gartner, L. M., Cohen, M., Ezzer, J. B., and Levi, A. J.: Chronic nonhemolytic unconjugated hyperbilirubinemia with glucuronyl transferase deficiency. Amer. J. Med., **47,** 395, 1969.
272. Billing, B. H., Gray, C. H., Kulczycka, A., Manfield, P., and Nicholson, D. C.: The metabolism of ^{14}C-bilirubin in congenital non-hemolytic hyperbilirubinemia. Clin. Sci., **27,** 163, 1964.
273. Yaffe, S. J., Levy, G., Matsuzawa, T., and Baliah, T.: Enhancement of glucuronide-conjugating capacity in a hyperbilirubinemic infant due to apparent enzyme induction by phenobarbital. New Eng. J. Med., **275,** 1461, 1966.
274. Kreek, M. J., and Sleisenger, M. H.: Reduction of serum unconjugated bilirubin with phenobarbitone in adult congenital non-haemolytic unconjugated hyperbilirubinaemia. Lancet, **1,** 73, 1968.
275. Smith, P. M., Middleton, J. E., and Williams, R.: Studies on the familial incidence and clinical history of patients with chronic unconjugated hyperbilirubinaemia. Gut, **8,** 449, 1967.
276. Whelton, M. H., Krustev, L. P., and Billing, B. H.: Reduction in serum bilirubin by phenobarbital in adult unconjugated hyperbilirubinemia. Is enzyme induction responsible? Amer. J. Med., **45,** 160, 1968.
277. Wranne, L.: Congenital nonhaemolytic jaundice. Acta Paediat. Scand., **56,** 552, 1967.
278. Powell, L. W., Billing, B. H., and Williams, H. S.: An assessment of red cell survival in idiopathic unconjugated hyperbilirubinaemia (Gilbert's syndrome) by the use of radioactive diisopropylfluorophosphate and chromium. Aust. Ann. Med., **16,** 221, 1967.

279. Powell, L. W.: Bilirubin metabolism and jaundice with special reference to unconjugated hyperbilirubinaemia. Aust. Ann. Med., **16**, 343, 1967.
280. Childs, B., and Najjar, V. A.: Familial nonhemolytic jaundice with kernicterus: report of two cases without neurologic disease. Pediatrics, **18**, 369, 1956.
281. Childs, B., Sidbury, J. B., and Migeon, C. J.: Glucuronic acid conjugation by patients with familial non-hemolytic jaundice and their relatives. Pediatrics, **23**, 903, 1959.
282. Blumenschein, S. D., Kallen, R. J., Storey, B., Natzschka, J. C., Odell, G. B., and Childs, B.: Familial nonhemolytic jaundice with late onset of neurological damage. Pediatrics, **42**, 786, 1968.
283. Gardner, W. A., and Koningsmark, B. W.: Familial nonhemolytic jaundice: bilirubinosis and encephalopathy. Pediatrics, **43**, 365, 1969.
284. Rosenthal, I. M., Zimmerman, H. J., and Hardy, N.: Congenital nonhemolytic jaundice with disease of central nervous system. Pediatrics, **18**, 378, 1956.
285. Klingberg, W. G.: Personal communication.
286. Suger, P.: Familial nonhemolytic jaundice, congenital, with kernicterus. Arch. Intern. Med., **108**, 2, 1961.
287. Whitington, G. L.: Congenital nonhemolytic icterus with damage to the central nervous system: report of a case in a negro child. Pediatrics, **25**, 437, 1960.
288. Lelong, M., Colin, J., Alagille, D., Gentil, C., Bretagne, J., and Houllemare, L.: Ictére familial non-hémolytique avec ictére nucléaire (maladie de Crigler-Najjar). Arch. Franc. Pediat., **18**, 272, 1961.
289. Szabó, L., Kovács, Z., and Ebrey, P. B.: Crigler-Najjar syndrome. Acta Paediat. Hung., **3**, 49, 1962.
290. Moggi, P., and Mori, S.: Su un caso di ittero congenito anemolitico con kernicterus da difetto di glicuronil-transferasi. Riv. Clin. Pediat., **69**, 305, 1962.
291. Karon, M., Imach, D., and Schwartz, A.: Phototherapy in congenital nonobstructive, nonhemolytic jaundice. New. Eng. J. Med., **282**, 377, 1970.
292. Gorodischer, R., Levy, G., Krasner, J., and Yaffe, S. J.: Congenital nonobstructive nonhemolytic jaundice: effect of phototherapy. New. Eng. J. Med., **282**, 375, 1970.
293. Crigler, J. F., Jr., and Gold, N. I.: Effect of sodium phenobarbital on bilirubin metabolism in an infant with congenital nonhemolytic unconjugated hyperbilirubinemia and kernicterus. J. Clin. Invest., **48**, 42, 1969.
294. De Brito, T., Borges, M. A., and Da Silva, L. C.: Electron microscopy of the liver in nonhemolytic acholuric jaundice with kernicterus (Crigler-Najjar) and in idiopathic conjugated hyperbilirubinemia (Rotor). Gastroenterologia, **106**, 325, 1966.
295. Minio-Paluello, F., Gautier, A., and Magnenat, P.: L'Ultrastructure de foie humain dans un cas de Crigler-Najjar. Acta Hepatosplen. (Stuttgart), **15**, 65, 1968.
296. Josephs, H. W.: Urobilin excretion in infancy and childhood: relation to blood destruction and formation. Bull. Johns Hopkins Hosp., **55**, 154, 1934.
297. Schwartz, S., Sborov, V., and Watson, C. J.: Studies of urobilinogen. IV. The quantitative determination of urobilinogen by means of the Evelyn photoelectric colorimeter. Amer. J. Clin. Path., **14**, 598, 1944.
298. Schmid, R.: Unpublished observations.
299. Schmid, R.: Congenital defects in bilirubin metabolism, in *Liver Function,* Publication 4, p. 549. American Institute of Biological Sciences, Washington, 1958.
300. Schmid, R.: The identification of "direct-reacting" bilirubin as bilirubin glucuronide. J. Biol. Chem., **229**, 881, 1957.
301. Isselbacher, K. J., and Axelrod, J.: Enzymatic formation of corticosteroid glucuronide. J. Amer. Chem. Soc., **77**, 1070, 1955.
302. Peterson, R. E., and Schmid, R.: A clinical syndrome associated with a defect in steroid glucuronide formation. J. Clin. Endocr., **17**, 1485, 1957.
303. Szabó, L., and Ebrey, P.: Studies on the inheritance of Crigler-Najjar's syndrome by the menthol test. Acta Paediat. Hung., **4**, 153, 1963.
304. Schmid, R., and Hammaker, L.: Glucuronide formation in patients with constitutional hepatic dysfunction (Gilbert's disease). New Eng. J. Med., **260**, 1310, 1959.
305. Zeidenberg, P., Orrenius, S., and Ernster, L.: Increase in levels of glucuronylating enzymes and associated rise in activities of mitochondrial oxidative enzymes upon phenobarbital administration in the rat. J. Cell Biol., **32**, 528, 1967.
306. Diamond, I., and Schmid, R.: Neonatal hyperbilirubinemia and kernicterus: experimental support for treatment by exposure to visible light. Arch. Neurol. (Chicago), **18**, 699, 1968.
307. Cremer, R. J., Perryman, P. W., and Richards, D. H.: Influence of light on hyperbilirubinaemia of infants. Lancet, **l**, 1094, 1958.
308. Callahan, E. W., Thaler, M. M., Karon, M., Bauer, K., and Schmid, R.: Phototherapy in congenital nonhemolytic jaundice: kinetics of bilirubin metabolism and disposition of labeled degradation products (abstract). Gastroenterology, **58**, 305, 1970.
309. Jervis, G. A.: Constitutional nonhemolytic hyperbilirubinemia with findings resembling kernicterus. A.M.A. Arch. Neurol. Psychiat., **81**, 55, 1959.
310. Thompson, R. P. H., Stathers, G. M., Pilcher, C. W. T., McLean, A. E. M., Robinson, J., and Williams, R.: Treatment of unconjugated jaundice with dicophane. Lancet, **l**, 4, 1969.
311. Aziz, M. A., and Siddiqui, A. R.: Congenital familial nonhemolytic hyperbilirubinemia in an adult with central nervous system derangement. Gastroenterology, **52**, 254, 1967.
312. Newton, W. A., and Irtel, I. J.: Phenobarbital in the treatment of hyperbilirubinemia in the Crigler-Najjar syndrome. J. Pediat., **70**, 586, 1968.
313. Remmer, H.: The fate of drugs in the organism. Rev. Pharmacol., **5**, 405, 1965.
314. Marver, H. S., and Schmid, R.: Biotransformation in the liver: implications for human disease. Gastroenterology, **55**, 282, 1968.
315. Gilbert, A., Lereboullet, P., and Herscher, M.: Les trois cholémies congénitales. Bull. Soc. Med. Hop. Paris, **24**, 1203, 1907.
316. Powell, L. W., Hemingway, E., Billing, B. H., and Sherlock, S.: Idiopathic unconjugated hyperbilirubinemia (Gilbert's syndrome): a study of 42 families. New Eng. J. Med., **277**, 1108, 1967.
317. Meulengracht, E.: Icterus intermittens juvenilis (chronischer intermittierender juveniler Subicterus). Klin. Wschr., **18**, 118, 1939.
318. Alwall, N.: On hereditary nonhemolytic bilirubinemia. Acta Med. Scand., **123**, 560, 1946.
319. Dameshek, W., and Singer, K.: Familial nonhemolytic jaundice: constitutional hepatic dysfunction with indirect van den Bergh reaction. A.M.A. Arch. Intern. Med., **67**, 259, 1941.
320. Comfort, M. W.: Constitutional hepatic dysfunction. Proc. Staff Meet. Mayo Clin., **10**, 57, 1935.
321. Redeker, A. G., Rickard, D., and Felsher, B. F.: The reciprocal relationship between caloric intake and degree of hyperbilirubinemia in Gilbert's syndrome. Gastroenterology, **58**, 303, 1970.
322. Combes, B.: The importance of conjugation with glutathione for sulfobromophthalein sodium (BSP) transfer from blood to bile. J. Clin. Invest., **44**, 1214, 1965.
323. Rosendaal, H. M., Comfort, M. W., and Snell, A. M.: Slight and latent jaundice: significance of elevated concentrations of bilirubin giving indirect van den Bergh reactions. J.A.M.A., **104**, 374, 1935.
324. Simon, G., and Varonier, H. S.: Étude au microscope électronique du foie de deux cas d'ictère non-hémolytique congénital de type Gilbert. Schweiz. Med. Wschr., **93**, 459, 1963.
325. Sagild, U., Dalgaard, O. Z., and Tygstrup, N.: Constitutional hyperbilirubinemia with unconjugated bilirubin in the serum and lipochrome-like pigment granules in the liver. Ann. Intern. Med., **56**, 308, 1962.
326. Herman, J. D., Cooper, E. B., Takeuchi, A., and Sprinz, H.: Constitutional hyperbilirubinemia with unconjugated bilirubin in the serum and pigment deposition in the liver. Amer. J. Dig. Dis., **9**, 160, 1964.
327. Feldmann, G., Oudéa, P., Domart-Oudéa, M. C., Molas, G., and Fauvert, R.: L'Ultrastructure hépatique au cours de la maladie de Gilbert. Path. Biol., **16**, 943, 1968.
328. Hult, H.: "Cholémie simple familiale" (Gilbert) and posthepatic states without fibrosis of liver. Acta Med. Scand., **138**, Suppl. 244, l, 1950.
329. Kalk, H., and Wildhirt, E.: Die posthepatitische Hyperbilirubinaemie

(der sog. erworbene haemolytische Ikterus nach Hepatitis). Z. Klin. Med., **153,** 354, 1955.

330. Snyder, A. L., Satterlee, W., Robinson, S. H., and Schmid, R.: Conjugated plasma bilirubin in jaundice caused by pigment overload. Nature (London), **213,** 93, 1967.
331. Volwiler, W., and Elliott, J. A., Jr.: Late manifestations of epidemic infectious hepatitis. Gastroenterology, **10,** 349, 1948.
332. Barniville, H. T. F., and Misk, R.: Urinary glucuronic acid excretion in liver disease and the effect of a salicylamide load. Brit. Med. J., **1,** 337, 1959.
333. Wakisaka, G., et al.: Clinical and enzymological observations on cases with Gilbert's disease. Jap. Arch. Intern. Med., **8,** 634, 1961.
334. Metge, W. R., Owen, C. A., Foulk, W. T., and Hoffman, N. H.: Bilirubin glucuronyl transferase activity in liver disease. J. Lab. Clin. Med., **64,** 89, 1964.
335. Black, M., and Billing, B. H.: Hepatic bilirubin UDP-glucuronyl transferase activity in liver disease and Gilbert's syndrome. New Eng. J. Med., **280,** 1266, 1969.
336. Nosslin, B.: Bromsulphalein retention and jaundice due to unconjugated bilirubin following treatment with male fern extract. Scand. J. Clin. Lab. Invest., **15,** suppl. 69, 206, 1963.
337. Galambos, J. T., and McLaren, G. R.: Hepatic uptake defect in patients with "Gilbert's disease." Arch. Intern. Med., **111,** 214, 1963.
338. Billing, B. H., Williams, R., and Richards, T. G.: Defects in hepatic transport of bilirubin in congenital hyperbilirubinaemia: an analysis of plasma bilirubin disappearance curves. Clin. Sci., **27,** 245, 1964.
339. Barrett, P. V. D., Beck, P. D., Menken, M., and Berlin, N. I.: Bilirubin turnover studies in normal and pathologic states using bilirubin-C^{14}. Ann. Intern. Med., **68,** 355, 1968.
340. Nixon, J. C., and Monahan, G. J.: Gilbert's disease and the bilirubin tolerance test. Canad. Med. Assoc. J., **96,** 370, 1967.
341. Baroody, W. G., and Shugart, R. T.: Familial nonhemolytic icterus. Amer. J. Med., **20,** 314, 1956.
342. Carithers, H. A., Jr.: Non-hemolytic familial jaundice. J. Pediat., **19,** 817, 1941.
343. Manson, J. S.: Hereditary icterus or familial acholuric jaundice. Brit. Med. J., **1,** 131, 1928.
344. Tecon, R. M.: A propos d'ictères chroniques. Helv. Med. Acta, **5,** 671, 1938.
345. Alwall, N., Laurell, C. B., and Nilsby, I.: Studies on heredity in cases of "non-hemolytic bilirubinemia without direct van den Bergh reaction" (hereditary, non-hemolytic bilirubinemia). Acta Med. Scand., **124,** 114, 1946.
346. Dubin, I. N., and Johnson, F. B.: Chronic idiopathic jaundice with unidentified pigment in liver cells: new clinico-pathologic entity with report of 12 cases. Medicine, **33,** 155, 1954.
347. Sprinz, H., and Nelson, R. S.: Persistent nonhemolytic hyperbilirubinemia associated with lipochrome-like pigment in liver cells: report of 4 cases. Ann. Intern. Med., **41,** 952, 1954.
348. Dubin, I. N.: Chronic idiopathic jaundice: a review of 50 cases. Amer. J. Med., **24,** 268, 1958.
349. Butt, H. R., Anderson, V. E., Foulk, W. T., Baggenstoss, A. H., Schoenfield, L. J., and Dickson, E. R.: Studies of chronic idiopathic jaundice (Dubin-Johnson syndrome). II. Evaluation of a large family with the trait. Gastroenterology, **51,** 619, 1966.
350. Blanck, C., Dahlgren, S., Gullmar-Willcocks, M., and DeHevesy, S.: Chronic idiopathic jaundice (Dubin-Johnson's syndrome) in three sisters. Acta Paediat. Scand., **55,** 329, 1966.
351. Knoke, M., Guertler, H., and Markert, J.: Die chronisch-idiopathische Hyperbilirubinaemie mit Pigmentablagerungen in der Leber. Deutsch. Med. Wschr., **92,** 832, 1967.
352. Wolf, R. L., Pizette, M., Richman, A., Dreiling, D. A., Jacobs, W., Fernandez, O., and Popper, H.: Chronic idiopathic jaundice: a study of two afflicted families. Amer. J. Med., **28,** 32, 1960.
353. Mandema, E., de Fraiture, W. H., Niewig, H. O., and Arends, A.: Familial chronic idiopathic jaundice (Dubin-Sprinz disease), with a note on bromsulphalein metabolism in this disease. Amer. J. Med., **28,** 42, 1960.
354. Wheeler, H. O., Meltzer, J. I., and Bradley, S. E.: Biliary transport and hepatic storage of sulfobromophthalein sodium in the unanesthetized dog, in normal man, and in patients with hepatic disease. J. Clin. Invest., **39,** 1131, 1960.
355. Schoenfield, L. J., McGill, D. B., Hunton, D. B., Foulk, W. F., and Butt, H. R.: Studies of chronic idiopathic jaundice (Dubin-Johnson syndrome). I. Demonstration of hepatic excretory defect. Gastroenterology, **44,** 101, 1963.
356. Arias, I. M.: Studies of chronic familial non-hemolytic jaundice with conjugated bilirubin in the serum with and without an unidentified pigment in the liver cells. Amer. J. Med., **31,** 510, 1961.
357. Muscatello, U., Mussini, I., and Agnolucci, M. T.: The Dubin-Johnson syndrome: an electronmicroscopic study of the liver cell. Acta Hepat. splen. (Stuttgart), **14,** 162, 1967.
358. Brown, N. L., and Shnitka, T. K.: Constitutional non-hemolytic jaundice with "lipochrome" hepatosis (Dubin-Sprinz disease). Amer. J. Med., **21,** 292, 1956.
359. Hamperl, H.: Chronischer nichthaemolytischer Ikterus mit Ablagerung eines eigentuemlichen Pigmentes in der Leber. Klin. Wschr., **35,** 177, 1957.
360. Wegman, R., Rangier, M., Etève, J., Charbonnier, A., and Caroli, J.: Mélanose hépato-splénique avec ictère chronique à bilirubine directe. Sem. Hop. Paris, **36,** 1761, 1960.
361. Arias, I. M.: Chronic idiopathic jaundice, in *Ikterus,* edited by K. Beck. F. K. Schattauer, Stuttgart, 1968.
362. Post, J., Benton, J. G., and Breakstone, R.: Observations on a cytoplasmic hepatic cell pigment in man. A.M.A. Arch. Path., **52,** 69, 1951.
363. Beker, S., and Read, A. E.: Familial Dubin-Johnson syndrome. Gastroenterology, **35,** 387, 1958.
364. John, G. G., and Knudtson, K. P.: Chronic idiopathic jaundice: two cases occurring in siblings, with histochemical studies. Amer. J. Med., **21,** 138, 1956.
365. Warmoes, F., DeDeurwaerder, R. J., and Van den Eynde, P.: Un cas d'ictère de Dubin-Johnson. Acta Gastroent. Belg., **20,** 525, 1957.
366. Burka, E. R., Brick, I. B., and Wolfe, H. R.: "Lipochrome" hepatosis without jaundice: a variant of the Dubin-Johnson syndrome. Amer. J. Med. Sci., **240,** 746, 1961.
367. Rotor, A. B., Manahan, L., and Florentin, A.: Familial non-hemolytic jaundice with direct van den Bergh reaction. Acta Med. Philippina, **5,** 37, 1948.
368. Stransky, E.: Ueber kongenitalen, familiaeren, nichthaemolytischen Ikterus. Ann. Paediat. (Basel), **175,** 301, 1950.
369. Dagnini, G., and Moreschi, E.: Ittero familiare epatogeno. Recent. Progr. Med. (Roma), **23,** 47, 1957.
370. Canali, G.: Ittero congenito familiare "epatico." Recent. Progr. Med. (Roma), **23,** 69, 1957.
371. Cinotti, G. A., Fabiani, F., and Pericoli, F.: Ittero anemolitico familiare a bilirubinemia diretta e splenomegalia. Policlinico [Prat.], **64,** 1573, 1957.
372. Schiff, L., Billing, B. H., and Oikawa, Y.: Familial nonhemolytic jaundice with conjugated bilirubin in the serum. New Eng. J. Med., **260,** 1315, 1959.
373. Peck, O. C., Rey, D. F., and Snell, A. M.: Familial jaundice with free and conjugated bilirubin in the serum and without liver pigmentation. Gastroenterology, **39,** 625, 1960.
374. Haverback, B. J., and Wirtschafter, S. K.: Familial nonhemolytic jaundice with normal liver histology and conjugated bilirubin. New Eng. J. Med., **262,** 113, 1960.
375. Vest, M. F., Kaufmann, H. J., and Fritz, E.: Chronic non-haemolytic jaundice with conjugated bilirubin in the serum and normal liver histology: a case study. Arch. Dis. Child., **35,** 600, 1960.
376. Porush, J. G., Delman, A. J., and Feuer, M. M.: Chronic idiopathic jaundice with normal liver. Arch. Intern. Med., **109,** 302, 1962.
377. Dollinger, M. R., Brandborg, L. L., Sartor, V. E., and Bernstein, J. M.: Chronic familial hyperbilirubinemia: hepatic defect(s) associated with occult hemolysis. Gastroenterology, **52,** 875, 1967.
378. Lima, J. E. P., Utz, E., and Roisenberg, S. B.: Hereditary nonhemolytic conjugated hyperbilirubinemia without abnormal liver cell pigmentation: a family study. Amer. J. Med., **40,** 628, 1966.
379. Dubin, I. N.: Rotor's syndrome and chronic idiopathic jaundice. Arch. Intern. Med., **110,** 823, 1962.

380. Cornelius, C. E., Arias, I. M., and Osburn, B. I.: Hepatic pigmentation with photosensitivity: a syndrome in Corriedale sheep resembling Dubin-Johnson syndrome in man. J. Amer. Vet. Ass., **146**, 709, 1965.
381. Arias, I., Bernstein, L., Toffler, R., Cornelius, C., Novikoff, A. B., and Essner, E.: Black liver disease in Corriedale sheep: a new mutation affecting hepatic excretory function. J. Clin. Invest., **43**, 1249, 1964.
382. Goldberg, A., and Rimington, C: *Diseases of Porphyrin Metabolism.* Charles C Thomas, Springfield, Ill., 1962.
383. Arias, I. M., Bernstein, L., Toffler, R., and Ben-Ezzer, J.: Black liver disease in Corriedale sheep: metabolism of tritiated epinephrine and incorporation of isotope into the hepatic pigment in vivo (abstract). J. Clin. Invest., **44**, 1026, 1965.
384. Muller-Eberhard, U., Liem, H. H., Hanstein, A., and Saarinen, P. A.: Studies on the disposal of intravascular heme in the rabbit. J. Lab. Clin. Med., **73**, 210, 1969.
385. Colleran, E., and O'Carra, P.: Non-enzymic nature of the pyridine haemochrome-clearing activity of mammalian tissue extracts ("Haem α-methenyl oxygenase"). Biochem. J., **119**, 905, 1970.
386. Ostrow, J. D., and Murphy, N. H.: Isolation and properties of conjugated bilirubin from bile. Biochem. J., **120**, 311, 1970.
387. Kuenzle, C. C.: Bilirubin conjugates of human bile. The excretion of bilirubin as the acyl glycosides of aldobiouronic acid, with a branched-chain hexuronic acid as one of the components of the hexuronosylhexuronide. Biochem. J., **119**, 411, 1970.
388. Fevery, J., Degroot, J., Compernoble, F., and Heirwegh, K. P. M.: Xylose and glucose conjugates of bilirubin in man and animal: detection in bile and formation in vitro. Gastroenterology, **60**, 660, 1971.
389. Bakken, A. F., Thaler, M. M., Pimstone, N. R., and Schmid, R.: Stimulation of hepatic heme oxygenase activity by fasting and by hormones. Gastroenterology, **60**, 177, 1971.

PART NINE

DISEASES PRIMARILY OF CONNECTIVE TISSUE, MUSCLE, AND BONE

CHAPTER FORTY-SEVEN

THE PERIODIC PARALYSES

Carl M. Pearson and Krishna Kalyanaraman

The syndrome of periodic paralysis is characterized by episodic attacks of weakness and flaccid paralysis of skeletal muscles due to intermittent failure of muscle excitation and contractility, the pathogenesis of which is still unclear. These attacks often involve the extremities asymmetrically and only rarely involve the bulbar and cranial musculature. Spontaneous remissions are common, and sensory and sphincter involvement is virtually unknown. There is usually a family history of the attacks.

Alterations in serum potassium during attacks has led to recognition of three specific types of primary periodic paralysis, namely, hypokalemic, hyperkalemic, and normokalemic varieties. Also included is the syndrome of paramyotonia congenita, which is characterized by episodic attacks of massive paralysis on exposure to cold, in addition to its myotonic features. While myotonia occurs very rarely in the hypokalemic form, it is on occasion quite prominent in the hyperkalemic variety.

The following classification of periodic paralysis is useful for clinical purposes:

I. *Primary periodic paralysis*
   A. Hypokalemic (familial) periodic paralysis, in which there is a fall in serum potassium during attacks
   B. Hyperkalemic periodic paralysis with or without myotonia, characterized by a rise in serum potassium during attacks
   C. Normokalemic periodic paralysis, in which there is no significant alteration of serum potassium levels during attacks and which responds to sodium administration
   D. Paramyotonia congenita with myotonia and massive weakness on exposure to cold

II. *Secondary periodic paralysis*
   A. Paralysis in endocrine dysfunction, e.g., thyrotoxicosis and primary aldosteronism
   B. Paralysis secondary to disorders affecting potassium metabolism, e.g., renal tubular acidosis, diabetic acidosis, and ureterosigmoidostomy
   C. Licorice intoxication

In this chapter the emphasis will be on the three types of primary periodic paralysis associated with disturbance of serum potassium. Thyrotoxic periodic paralysis is clinically and biochemically indistinguishable from the hypokalemic type, except for its nonfamilial occurrence, its association with hyperthyroidism, and a predominant occurrence in the Orient, especially Japan. Brief mention will be made about paramyotonia congenita and myotonic periodic paralysis, and the many overlapping features of these symdromes with the periodic paralyses, especially the hyperkalemic type, will be pointed out.

HYPOKALEMIC PERIODIC PARALYSIS

Historical Background and Development of Knowledge

The first convincing description of periodic paralysis was by Musgrave in 1727 [1]. However, doubts about the organic origin of this disease were expressed [2]. Similar cases were rarely commented upon during the next 150 years until a report by Shakhnovitch in 1884 described a 44-year-old man with a classical picture of periodic paralysis, whose father had died of a similar illness at age 54 years [3]. Although Shakhnovitch in proposing the term *paraplegia spinalis intermittens nervosa* possibly thought that his patient had neurosis, yet his clinical description clearly points to a diagnosis of classical familial periodic paralysis. This report was soon followed by a description of similar cases by Westphal in 1885 [4]. The latter was the first to describe the complete loss of muscular contractility on electrical stimulation during attacks.

Goldflam in 1890 described some of the clinical features of hypokalemic periodic paralysis, emphasizing the frequent occurrence of attacks, the severe thirst during paralysis, and the tendency for the attacks to become less frequent with advancing age [5]. He was also the first to describe the pathologic changes in the muscle, pointing out "The ramifications beginning between the myofibrils in the muscle fibers, splitting of Cohnheim's fields and vacuolation," findings which have stood until now [6].

The turn of this century saw a few empirical discoveries such as mention of the efficacy of potassium salts in the therapy of periodic paralysis [7–9]. In 1908, Kramer discovered that a high-carbohydrate diet was capable of precipitating attacks [10]. This observation was confirmed later by Shinosaki, who was the first to use glucose for the experimental induction of paralysis [11].

The forerunner of the many metabolic and electrolyte studies was the report of Biemond and Daniels in 1934 of a patient with familial periodic paralysis who had a low serum potassium concentration during an attack [12]. They did not seem to grasp the significance of this finding, though they made the very important observation that permanent muscular wasting and weakness occurred in this patient. They were soon followed by many others. Aitken et al. (1937), Allott and McArdle (1938), Gammon et al. (1939), and Ferrebee et al. (1941) were among those who confirmed the relationship between attacks of paralysis and a low level of serum potassium [13–16]. These authors, basing their conclusions on balance studies, pointed out that the fall in serum potassium was not accompanied by any significant increase in urinary excretion of potassium, thereby discounting the possibility of negative potassium balance. Talbott, in a classical review in 1941, summarized clinical features of this syndrome [17].

The modern era in the study of periodic paralysis began in 1957 with the studies of Grob et al. [18], as well as those of Zierler and Andres [19], who further evaluated the role of potassium in this syndrome. Shy et al. [20], in 1961, made a thorough and classical study of hypokalemic periodic paralysis. In addition to investigating the role of potassium, they also described the electron microscopic features and speculated on the pathogenesis. The most recent thorough review of this subject was by Streeten [21], in 1966.

Conn et al. [22], in 1957, suggested that the primary defect in periodic paralysis might be due to intermittent hypersecretion of adrenal cortical hormones, especially aldosterone. However, other workers, namely Rowley and Kliman [23] and Vaughan Jones et al., [24], were unable to show a consistent relationship between sodium retention and the onset of paralysis, nor could increased aldosterone secretion be shown preceding an attack.

The last decade has seen determined efforts by workers scattered all over the world to solve the riddle of periodic paralysis. McArdle [25] and Satayoshi [26] have pointed to the possibility of an abnormality of carbohydrate metabolism. Histopathologic features have been well reviewed by Pearson [6] and others [27], who pointed to the occurrence of permanent myopathic weakness in this syndrome and reviewed the pathology in its entirety.

In addition to refined neurophysiologic and metabolic studies of this syndrome, recent workers have concentrated on the ultrastructure of the muscle in patients with and without permanent muscle weakness [28–30]. It is hoped that studies in this direction will be helpful if not conclusive in unraveling the pathogenesis of this interesting syndrome.

Clinical Features

Inheritance and Sex

Hypokalemic periodic paralysis is considered to be inherited as an autosomal dominant and affecting males far more often than females [31–34]. Although sporadic cases have been recorded, there is a considerable excess of familial over sporadic cases, e.g., a ratio of 34:6 in Denmark, as pointed out by Helweg-Larsen et al. [35]. Most pedigrees show regular autosomal dominance, and Meyer found that in those pedigrees in which all children had been recorded, 50 percent of males and 45 percent of females were affected [36]. But there are two or three males to one female in published studies, for instance, Bickerstaff's [33], with six males affected in three generations. In a survey of all cases in Denmark, where the prevalence was 0.8 per 100,000, Helweg-Larsen et al. [35] found that of all living patients 31 were male and only 3 were female. In their six pedigrees, about 50 percent of sons but only about 5 percent of daughters of affected males and females were themselves affected, suggesting sex limitation with frequent failure of manifestation of disease in females. Previous studies have also pointed out that the disease tends to be milder when it occurs in females [37, 38]. Pratt [31] concluded that most familial cases are probably dominant, completely so in some pedigrees and with frequent failure of manifestation in females in other pedigrees.

There is one pedigree with possible X-linked recessive inheritance reported from India [39]. McKusick [40] considers this pedigree to be a purely fortuitous occurrence due to the strong predilection of the disease for males. He cites the review of Sagild [41] in 1959, in which he found that of the 627 reported cases reviewed, 411 were men. Furthermore, 99 of the 109 probands were men. Among 52 cases of the disease in Denmark only 4 were females, a sex ratio of 12:1 in favor of males. Despite some evidence for X-linked recessive inheritance, numerous instances of male-to-male transmission have been recorded. Sagild [41], therefore, concluded that hypokalemic periodic paralysis is an autosomal dominant with marked reduction in penetrance and in expressivity in females.

Chen [42] has reported the occurrence of periodic paralysis in Taiwan, with rare familial incidence and disproportionately higher involvement of males.

Geographic and Racial Distribution

In spite of its rarity, the disease has been found in many parts of the world. There have been reports of patients from Russia, Japan, India, and Brazil. The disease was once thought to be unknown among the Chinese, but the already noted report by Chen [42] from Taiwan in 1965 cites the occurrence of 28 cases, 18 being mainland Chinese and the rest Taiwan Chinese. Almost all the reported cases from North America have been Caucasians, except for a single study by Glynn et al. [43] of members of a Negro family in which six individuals were affected. There has also been no report of cases from Africa, except for a single family from South Africa [44]. Dalinghaus [45] had drawn attention to the nearly complete absence of recognition of the condition in the tropics.

Age Incidence

Streeten [21] in his excellent review in 1966 pointed to the wide variation in the age of onset, the majority of attacks beginning between the ages of 7 and 21 years. He has also noted the similarity in ages of onset in familial and sporadic cases of periodic paralysis. In general, as McArdle [25] observed, the first episode commonly occurs in the second decade, and with increasing age the attacks tend to become less frequent and often to cease. The peak of severity is usually in the third decade [46]. The age of onset of paralysis tends to be similar among the members of an affected family, e.g., 7 to 8 years in the family of Biemond and Daniels [12], 12 to 16 years in one of Mankowsky's families [47], and 17 to 19 years in MacLachlan's [32]. Even though attacks frequently disappear between age 30 and 70 years [48], in some patients the course is not so benign, and severe attacks may continue into middle life and even into old age [5].

Duration and Frequency of Attacks

McArdle [25, 46, 49] has given an excellent and precise description of the attacks, on which the following account is based. They usually commence during the night or early morning and consist of flaccid paralysis of the limbs and trunk. The facial, respiratory, and pharyngeal muscles are usually spared, except in the most severe cases. Sweating, a feeling of heaviness of the extremities, and paresthesia may herald onset of an attack. The paralysis usually lasts about 6 to 24 hr. The severity often varies; a single muscle group may be affected for only a few minutes or massive paralysis may last several days.

The distribution of the paralysis is predominantly proximal and the muscles fail to respond to direct mechanical or electrical stimulation. The deep stretch reflexes are usually absent. The girth of the limb muscles may increase measurably during paralysis, and the muscles may have a firm rubbery consistency. No loss of any sensory modality or impairment of mental faculties or consciousness occurs in even the severest of attacks. The attacks may be associated with thirst and water retention during the early phases, and with diuresis and sweating on recovery [17, 50–52]. Positive water balance was found by Talbott [17].

The most important predisposing factors are prolonged rest after vigorous exercise [2], a heavy meal shortly beforehand [3, 5, 11, 14, 53, 54], anxiety [37, 50, 55], and cold [2]. A large carbohydrate meal [3, 5, 7, 14, 35, 53, 54] seems especially likely to be followed by paralysis. The administration of frequent doses of glucose, or preferably of glucose and insulin, is the most certain method of inducing an attack [11].

Associated Disorders

Migraine has been found to be associated in several reports in patients as well as relatives [9, 12, 47, 48, 53]. In Japan, thyrotoxicosis occurs commonly with periodic paralysis, usually among patients whose condition is nonfamilial; the combination seems to have a predilection for the Japanese [71].

Though myotonia of the tongue or extremities has not been reported, three patients of Resnick and Engel [72] showed a myotonic lid lag. One of these patients occasionally also showed percussion myotonia of thenar and extensor forearm muscles.

During the attack the electrocardiogram (ECG) shows the changes characteristic of hypokalemia [18, 33, 51, 56–59]. Grob et al. [18] have pointed out that the hypokalemic changes in the ECG are more severe than in normal persons at the same level of serum potassium. Klein et al. [60], described what they called a variant of familial periodic paralysis, characterized by premature ectopic heartbeats of varying locus and frequency, and most commonly manifested by bigeminy. In some of the earlier reports, like the one of Oppenheim [61], a description of transient bradycardia and cardiac dilatation, with the appearance of an apical systolic murmur, was given, which has since been confirmed by other workers. Coppen and Reynolds [62] reported that one of their six patients had mild hypertension, cardiac enlargement, auricular fibrillation, and widespread inversion of T waves on the electrocardiogram. Interestingly enough this patient also developed a proximal myopathy, giving rise to the intriguing possibility that he had a cardiomyopathy.

Laboratory Examinations, Excluding Electrolytes

Routine laboratory examination generally reveals no changes in urinalysis or hemogram. Occasional patients may have mild proteinuria, glycosuria, acetonuria, and cylindruria. Streeten [21] also has cited references to reports of neutrophilic leukocytosis and eosinopenia occurring during attacks, followed by lymphocytosis and eosinophilia after the attack. The cerebrospinal fluid has only rarely been examined, and on those occasions it has been essentially normal. The CSF potassium, as pointed out by Pudenz et al. [63], in 1938, has shown only a slight drop compared to serum levels during attacks. This was confirmed in another study by Gass et al. [64] in 1948. Rarely, it has been found to be quite low during an attack of paralysis [65].

The electroencephalogram, as noted by Jung [66] in 1939, was not different during the attack, when compared to attack-free periods. Hammes [67], in 1951, confirmed this finding, and Saunders [68], in 1954, found only minimal differences in the EEGs taken during and between the attacks.

The serum enzymes have generally been reported to be normal in periodic paralysis, although an increase of glutamic oxaloacetic transaminase and aldolase has been described in the occasional patient with paramyotonia congenita [69]. Even in a case with permanent myopathy, the serum enzymes were normal [6].

Electromyographic Changes

Between attacks, the biphasic muscle action potentials have been reported as normal in duration and shape [70]. Rapid faradic stimulation, however, caused rhythmic fluctuations in the amplitude of the action potentials, which were more pronounced than in the normal controls, suggesting that the muscle was abnormal even in the nonparalyzed state. During the process of recovery, the abnormalities in the electromyogram were still present when the serum potassium had returned to normal or elevated levels, and these abnormalities vanished only after further delay. In induced attacks with glucose and insulin, the onset of paralysis was heralded by progressive widening of the action potentials to twice or thrice their normal duration, with lengthening of the latent period between the stimulus and the response. Also, widening of the action potentials appeared before the onset of the motor response to indirect faradic stimulation. With the onset of complete paralysis, the action potentials, which had become progressively prolonged in duration and reduced in amplitude, were no longer elicited.

Fudema et al. [73], in 1962, reported on the electromyographic findings in cases of familial periodic paralysis. They found that electrophysiologic studies during induced attacks revealed no changes in nerve conduction velocity. Motor unit voltages were markedly decreased and lengthened. Increases in rheobase and chronaxie were noted, and marked shifts in strength–duration curves occurred. These electrophysiologic changes were comparable to those seen in denervated muscle [43].

Engel et al. [74] made detailed electromyographic studies on a patient with hypokalemic periodic paralysis on several occasions over several years. When weakness began, induced by oral administration of 100 gm glucose, the voluntary motor unit potentials decreased in amplitude and duration, whereas the proportion of polyphasic motor unit potentials increased. As weakness continued, there was a progressive reduction in the number of motor units that could be activated voluntarily, and drop-off in the response of the muscle fibers to stimulus by the needle electrode. No spontaneous activity was observed. The conduction velocity of the ulnar nerve was not appreciably different in the paralyzed and nonparalyzed states and was within normal limits. However, the amplitude of the action potential evoked by supramaximal stimulation of the ulnar nerve was appreciably higher in the nonparalyzed state than in the paralyzed state.

Niall and Pak Poy [75] did extensive electromyographic sampling of muscles in upper and lower extremities in a patient during attacks and found large areas of electrical silence on attempted voluntary contraction. In some areas, spontaneous repetitive motor units were seen to be firing, but overall there was no indication of a normal interference pattern. No typical fibrillations, positive sharp waves, or giant action potentials were seen. Motor conduction velocities were normal. During symptom-free periods the electromyogram was essentially normal.

Metabolic Alterations

Potassium

SERUM POTASSIUM CONCENTRATION: The importance of potassium in this disease was first clearly defined by Aitken et al. [13] in 1937, who demonstrated that the serum level of potassium declined in both spontaneous and induced attacks. During attacks the level of plasma potassium falls coincidentally with the development of the paralysis, with weakness usually becoming apparent at about 3 mEq per liter and becoming marked at 2 to 2.5 mEq per liter. However, in many cases the onset of weakness has been at levels only slightly below the normal range [49]. There is therefore an undue susceptibility to a fall in serum potassium among afflicted persons, since normal subjects do not become significantly weak until the level falls to about 2 to 2.5 mEq per liter or lower. The serum potassium remains low during paralysis and rises during recovery. Measures used to provoke attacks result in a greater and more long-lasting fall in serum potassium in patients than in normal subjects. Shy et al. [20] and Engel et al. [74] sometimes found normal serum potassium levels during attacks.

According to Streeten [21] the serum potassium concentration is normal between attacks in some patients and low in others. It repeatedly dropped below normal between attacks in patients described by Talbott [17] and by Gass et al. [64].

It has since been shown that there is a positive balance of potassium in the body during the attacks [14, 63, 76], and that potassium moves into the muscle during the development of an attack and is slowly released during recovery [18, 19]. The same release of potassium occurs during recovery following ingestion of potassium chloride, although in normal persons potassium chloride causes a shift of potassium into muscles. Agents like glucose, insulin, epinephrine, deoxycorticosterone acetate, adrenocorticotropic hormone, and 9α-fluorohydrocortisone would appear to precipitate attacks by virtue of their effect in lowering the serum potassium level [18]. Also, a low level of potassium in the diet, especially in association with a high carbohydrate intake, precipitates attacks, whereas the converse prevents them or reduces their number [79].

That the urinary excretion of potassium declines simultaneously with the fall in serum potassium during induced attacks of paralysis was shown by Streeten [21]. In spontaneous attacks of paralysis, too, the reduction in urinary potassium output accompanied, but never preceded, the fall in serum potassium. It was Streeten's conclusion that the reduced urinary excretion of potassium was secondary to the fall in the serum potassium. After the end of the attacks, the potassium diuresis usually continues for 1 or 2 days. Engel et al. [74] also observed a progressive decrease of urinary concentrations of sodium and chloride, in addition to potassium, from the onset of the attack to complete paralysis. They found that the reduction of urinary electrolyte excretion preceded changes in the patient's strength, while the major decrease in the patient's handgrip preceded the maximal decline in serum potassium concentration. It is possible that, in the later stages of attack, the low serum potassium level may have contributed to a decreased distal renal tubular secretion of potassium ions, and the decrease in the amount of sodium presented to the distal tubules may have reduced the amount of potassium secreted in exchange for sodium [78, 79]. A decreased renal plasma flow might also be the cause of reduced potassium excretion during attacks [80].

DeGraeff and Lameijer [81] found in one of their patients that the excretion of potassium and phosphate in the urine began to decrease in the days preceding a spontaneous attack. The quantity of potassium and phosphate in the urine decreased in both their patients during spontaneous or induced attacks, almost simultaneously with the decline in the levels in serum. Exchangeable body potassium levels have been found to be low normal [82] or low [83]. Talso et al. [84] confirmed these results in their patients during the nonparalyzed state, with findings of low normal levels of exchangeable body potassium levels. Coppen and Reynolds [62] recently also found a low total body potassium in their patients between attacks.

Sodium

SODIUM RETENTION: According to Streeten [21] severe attacks of paralysis, either spontaneous or induced, are usually preceded by sodium retention, resulting in a positive balance. A negative sodium balance usually occurs for 1 or 2 days after the end of the attacks and is sometimes of considerable magnitude. Sodium retention has also been noted in earlier reports by Pudenz et al. [63] and Ferrebee et al. [16], as well as by Danowski et al. [76]. Recently, Talso et al. [84], in a study of patients in a nonparalytic state, found total exchangeable body sodium to be increased, as mentioned in earlier reports. However, Coppen and Reynolds [62] in a recent study were unable to confirm these findings and found normal values of exchangeable and intracellular sodium in six patients between attacks of paralysis. DeGraeff and Lameijer [81] also found that on a diet containing salt, sodium retention indeed occurred. However, it should be noted that retention of sodium and chloride is not an essential part of the metabolic pattern of paralysis [24].

SERUM SODIUM LEVELS: The serum sodium shows a slight rise shortly before or during the onset of attacks [21]. This is probably of little consequence in affecting muscle power, but might contribute to the thirst and oliguria.

Chloride

Changes in the urinary chloride excretion parallel the changes in urinary output of sodium. There is reduced urinary excretion before and during attacks and diuresis at the end of the attack [16, 21, 24, 85].

Water

TOTAL BODY WATER: There are reports that spontaneous and induced attacks of paralysis may be preceded by gain in body weight [2]. However, this has not been the experience of other authors [16, 17, 76]. Poor correlation between the magnitude of the weight change and the severity of the attacks suggests that an increase in total body water is of little or no importance in the genesis of attacks. Coppen and Reynolds [62] found normal results, as pointed out earlier by Talso [84]. However, these studies were made between attacks. Engel et al. [74] studied their patient in the course of an acute attack and found data compatible with an increase of total body water content and a shift of water from the extracellular into the intracellular fluid compartment, even though the venous hematocrit did not reflect such a shift.

CHANGES IN INTERNAL DISTRIBUTION OF BODY WATER: Even though there are conflicting reports in the literature regarding changes in the fluid compartments in familial periodic paralysis, recent reports only tend to confirm these discrepancies [62, 75]. In summary, the present available evidence is inadequate to establish that any real and significant changes occur in the fluid compartments of the body.

Hormonal Alterations

Conn and Streeten [83] were the first to systematically study the changes in steroid excretion in periodic paralysis. They found a definite increase of output of 17-hydroxycorticoids in the most severe spontaneous attack, as well as in attacks induced by glucose and insulin [21]. Mild attacks, either spontaneous or induced, were unaccompanied by increased 17-hydroxycorticoid excretion.

The urinary 17-ketosteroids were also increased in two severe attacks [83], and even mild attacks were always associated with an increased output of 17-ketosteroids preceding and during attacks [21]. Cerny and Katzenstein-Sutro [86] had previously recorded the increase in urinary 17-ketosteroids during attacks in 1952.

A striking change in urinary aldosterone excretion was found by Conn and Streeten [83] in 1960. They found that a large increase in output of this hormone occurred on the day before five spontaneous attacks, and it usually remained increased throughout the paralysis. Smaller increases were observed during induced attacks. However, other workers were unable to confirm these results and to establish the occurrence of intermittent hypersecretion of aldosterone in their patients [20, 23, 24]. Less important, but worth mentioning, is the report of increased urinary excretion of a follicle-stimulating hormone during attacks in a patient with familial periodic paralysis [86]. Thyroid function has been normal in patients with sporadic periodic paralysis who had no clinical evidence of thyrotoxicosis [21]. The syndrome of periodic paralysis associated with thyrotoxicosis, though clinically and biochemically indistinguishable from familial periodic paralysis, has its own distinguishing features, e.g., its predominant occurrence in the Orient, especially Japan, and lack of familial occurrence [71]. Engel [87] found, in a classic case of familial periodic paralysis, that muscle weakness developed only after stopping the administration of triiodothyronine and of thyrotropin. This led him to the conclusion that metabolic abnormalities in familial periodic paralysis and thyrotoxic periodic paralysis are probably different.

Miscellaneous Findings

Alterations in the metabolism of a number of other substances have been reported, but only two seem likely to be directly relevant. The serum inorganic phosphate level falls during attacks and, in general, tends to follow the changes in serum potassium [14]. The blood pyruvate and lactate have been found to be increased both in spontaneous and induced attacks [25]. Satoyoshi et al. [26] found the fasting blood pyruvate level to be higher than normal, but the main and consistent abnormality was the markedly increased pyruvate and lactate levels during paralysis. Also the mean level of cocarboxylase in blood in 12 patients was significantly lower than controls [26]. Engel et al. [74] found an excessive accumulation of lactic and pyruvic acids in the blood after a standard work load.

Changes in Muscle

Chemical Composition

Biochemical analysis of muscle obtained by biopsy has been of considerable value in confirming the concepts of potassium shifts in periodic paralysis. Jantz [88] reported that the concentration of potassium in muscle was increased at the height of an attack of paralysis to 182 mEq per kg and returned to normal within ½ hr of recovery of normal muscle function. Vastola and Bertrand [89] found that the onset of paralysis was associated with the intracellular movement of 129 mEq potassium per kg muscle solids, together with an increase of the water content, especially in the extracellular fluid phase (i.e., the chloride space), of the muscle. The change in water content neutralized the effect of the potassium shift on the concentration of potassium in the sample of wet muscle, which was unchanged by the occurrence of the paralysis.

More recent determinations [21] of the electrolyte composition in muscle in periodic paralysis confirm the results of Jantz [88]. Between attacks of paralysis, the concentration of potassium in the muscle is low, probably indicating a chronic potassium deficiency state. The sodium concentration is considerably elevated, as is common in chronic potassium deficiency [90]. Paralyzed or weakened muscle consistently shows higher potassium concentrations than muscle sampled between the attacks, suggesting that an acute shift of potassium into muscle may have taken place during the attack of paralysis [18, 88, 89]. Conn and Streeten [83] showed the increased concentration of sodium and the decreased concentration of potassium in muscle between the attacks. Talso et al. [84], in an analysis of muscle, found that in the nonparalytic state the distribution of extracellular and intracellular water did not differ significantly from normal skeletal muscle. However, intracellular sodium concentration was strikingly increased. With induction of paralysis, the apparent mass of extracellular phase (chloride space) increased markedly, while the intracellular phase remained unchanged. Concomitantly, while the extracellular potassium concentration decreased, intracellular potassium increased. Moreover, paralysis was characterized by a decrease in intracellular sodium concentration [84]. Engel et al. [74] found that a fully paralyzed muscle and a muscle only somewhat weakened were similar in their electrolyte and water content, except for the higher calcium and magnesium content of the weaker muscle. Both muscles had chloride spaces and water levels which were higher than most normal values; sodium, chloride, and magnesium levels were higher than normal, and the potassium level was lower than most normal values. The chloride space values were too high to be a measure of the extracellular space and could not be used for calculating intracellular electrolyte concentrations [74].

Studies of Muscle In Vitro

Quite recently Hofmann and Smith [91] have conducted a series of unique studies on single isolated and resected muscle fibers from three patients with hypokalemic paralytic attacks. Their conclusions, upon comparison with studies on muscle fibers from normal subjects and by an analysis of membrane potentials, electrical excitability, neuromuscular transmission, inulin space, and intrafiber water, sodium, and potassium, were as follows:

1 All the diseased specimens were significantly depolarized in vitro, irrespective of the patient's clinical condition, or normality, at the time of biopsy. The muscle fibers from patients with hypokalemic periodic paralysis appeared unusually sensitive to isolation techniques.

2 When insulin was added to the fluid bathing the isolated muscle fibers, it further depolarized the diseased fibers when the potassium in bathing fluid was normal, but strongly repolarized the fibers when the extracellular potassium was reduced to near zero. Normal fibers, in zero potassium concentrations, were also repolarized by insulin.

3 The removal of 90 percent of the sodium caused the resting membrane potential of diseased fibers to return to normal but this maneuver did not restore the excitability of the fibers.

4 Insulin repolarization in hypokalemic periodic paralysis did not appear to be the result of chloride entry alone.

5 Substitution of nitrate ion for chloride caused repolarization, which is most conveniently explained by reduced sodium permeability.

6 Five times normal potassium concentration depolarized both normal and diseased fibers, but less than expected from the concentrations of intracellular potassium and sodium.

7 Exposure of diseased fibers to procaine partially restored the resting membrane potential and their ability to contract.

8 The diseased fibers appeared to contain too much sodium and too little potassium.

9 Manipulations in vitro were followed by vacuole formation only in the diseased fibers.

Hofmann and Smith [91] have speculated extensively concerning some of the observations that have been made in this rather unique series of experiments. It is quite obvious from recent findings that water may exist in skeletal muscle in two phases [92] and that at least potassium ion may be adsorbed within muscle fibers and other cells [93]. Therefore, a great deal of additional information will probably be forthcoming concerning sodium, potassium, magnesium, and other electrolyte shifts, and the movement of water into and out of muscle in the various forms of periodic paralysis.

Miscellaneous Findings

Engel [94] found reduced levels of AMP deaminase activity in the muscle of a patient with hypokalemic periodic paralysis. Very little is known presently of the physiologic function of AMP deaminase in muscle, and its relationship, if any, to the pathogenesis of this disorder is far from being settled.

Histopathologic Changes

Light-microscopic Observations

Goldflam [5, 95] was the first to describe characteristic and completely identical muscular changes. Cross sections of the muscle fibers showed that these were rather thick and of uniform size, and that the myofibrils were exceptionally distinct. In numerous fibers, vacuoles were demonstrable, and they were usually located in or near the center. They were found to be round or oval and to contain a transparent, nonstainable substance, which in rare cases was seen to be granulated. Most of the vacuoles were rather small, although some might occupy up to one-third of the diameter of the fibers concerned; fine vacuoles might be present in the cross section of a fiber, giving it an appearance of a multiloculated cyst.

In longitudinal section, Goldflam noted that the vacuoles appeared as cavities or slits of varying lengths and diameters, arranged parallel with the longitudinal axis. Transverse as well as longitudinal striations were normal, and no reactive changes were observed. Figure 47-1 is reproduced from Goldflam's historic paper published in 1890 [5].

Although autopsies or muscle biopsies were infrequently performed in the subsequent 50 years, a number of authors commented upon the histological normalcy of their cases [48, 96]. Others, such as Biemond and Daniels [12], considered Goldflam's beautiful demonstrations to be merely artifacts of tissue fixation or processing, even though they observed some mild muscle fiber vacuolation in their own material. Bekeny and associates, in 1961, pointed to the finding of muscle fiber vacuolation in their patients [97–99]. These findings were confirmed by Adams et al. [100], in 1962, in their classical study of the pathology of muscle diseases.

Impressive examples of vacuolar and other changes have been given more recently by many authors [6, 27–29, 101].

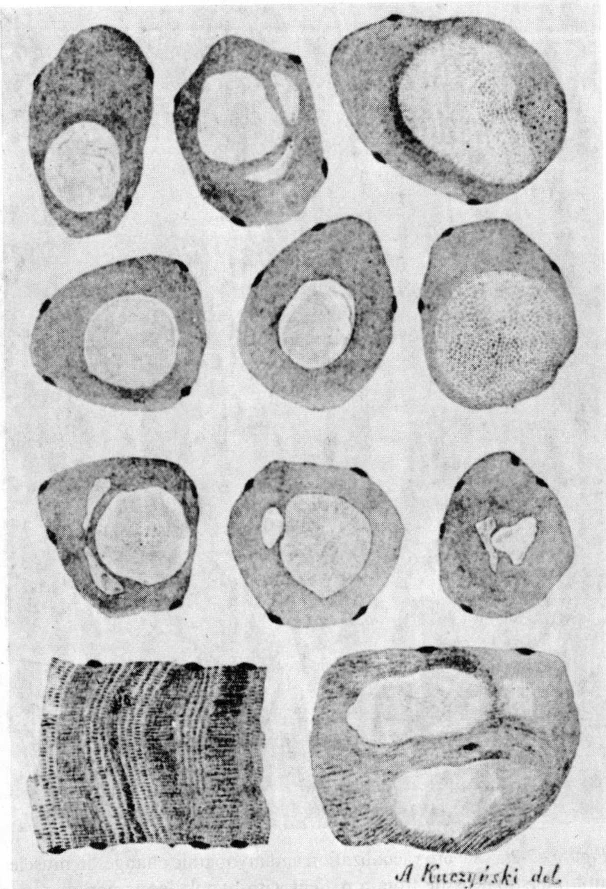

Figure 47-1. Reproduction of the 1890 drawings of vacuoles in muscle fibers. (*From S. Goldflam* [5].)

All these authors have noted the formation of large and small watery cisterns in muscle fibers (Figs. 47-2 and 47-3). These were in general longitudinal in orientation. They seemed to be larger during the peak of an attack in patients of Shy [20], but were more lasting between attacks in the others. Diffuse granular material within some of the cisterns was PAS-positive and was removable by diastase digestion, implying that it was glycogen or a glycogen complex.

Pearson [6] observed that the vacuolar changes may, after several years of intermittent paralytic attacks, become permanent anatomic features, which unquestionably contribute to the progressive clinical weakness that accompanies these findings. He also felt that the histologic picture was quite unlike that seen in any other human myopathic state, with the possible exception of some resemblance to certain cases of glycogen storage disease of muscle [102].

Generally, the vacuoles have been found to be empty or to contain some transparent, nonspecific substance. Zabriskie and Frantz [51] as far back as 1932 demonstrated the presence in the vacuoles of some nondescript granules which they said reacted negatively for glycogen straining. Olivarius and Christensen [27] found vacuoles in biopsies from three

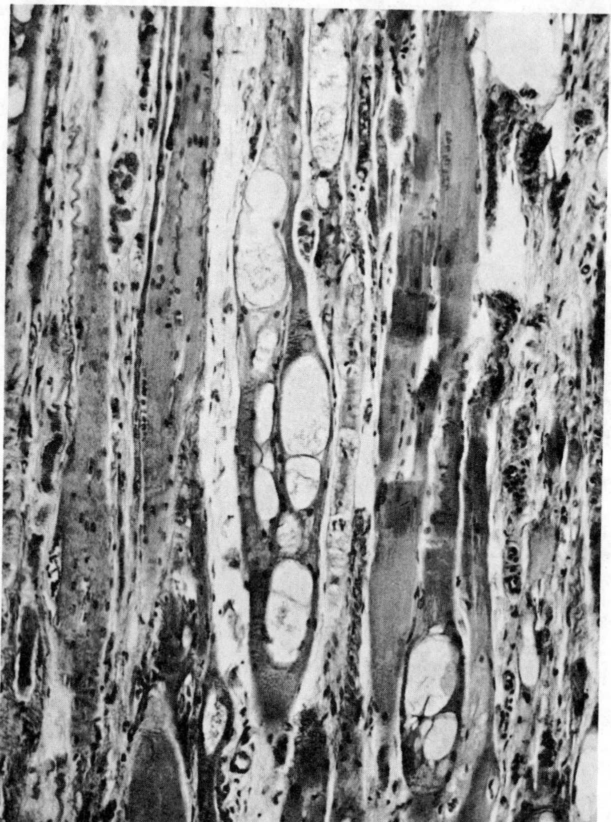

Figure 47-2. Severe vacuolization and myopathic changes in muscle and interstitial tissue from a patient with hypokalemic periodic paralysis and permanent myopathic weakness. (H and E, ×162.) (*From C. M. Pearson* [6], *with permission.*)

of their five patients. They also found that two of the patients without vacuolar changes in muscle were symptom-free for long periods, suggesting a correlation between frequency of attacks and vacuolation of muscle. Others, however, have shown large accumulations of PAS-positive glycogen granules in many fibers [6] (Fig. 47-4).

Engel et al. [74] studied a patient with hypokalemic periodic paralysis in whom multiple end-plates were innervated by collateral branches of a single terminal axon and in whom there was enlargement of some of the motor end-plates. These abnormalities may possibly explain the electromyographic signs of denervation, which are occasionally encountered in this disease.

Electron-microscopic Observations

Shy et al. [20] observed that the smallest vesicles appearing in the abnormal muscle fibers were membrane-limited and that larger cisterns evolved from vesicles adjacent to the Z line, as well as from longitudinally oriented tubules. They also found that the longitudinal channels of the sarcoplasmic (or endoplasmic) reticulum were irregularly dilated, sometimes over several sarcomeres in length, especially opposite the Z disks. Some of these dilatations apparently initiated the vacuole formation. Gruner and Porte [101] in an ultrastructural study noted vesiculation of lysosomes, focal degeneration of the sarcoplasm, and lysis of myofilaments.

Howes et al. [28] studied a patient with permanent muscle weakness between attacks. The smallest vacuoles that they found in the muscle fibers were thought to arise by dilatation of the lateral cisterns of the sarcoplasmic reticulum (Fig. 47-5A), while the larger ones were thought to evolve by further enlargement and fusion of the smaller ones (Fig. 47-5B). Glycogen was present in excessive amounts between the muscle fibers. Some of the degenerating fibers showed loss of A bands but persistence of randomly scattered and at times thickened Z lines and attached I-band filaments ("Z line degenerating units"). In some places the myofilaments formed tangles, were precipitated, or appeared to be finely particulate. Abnormally small, odd-shaped mitochondria with fewer than normal cristae were seen in degenerating fibers. Some fibers had lost most of their organelles and contained only a few myelin figures and glycogen granules.

Engel [29] was in essential agreement with Howes et al. [28] as to the origin and evolution of the vacuoles, the

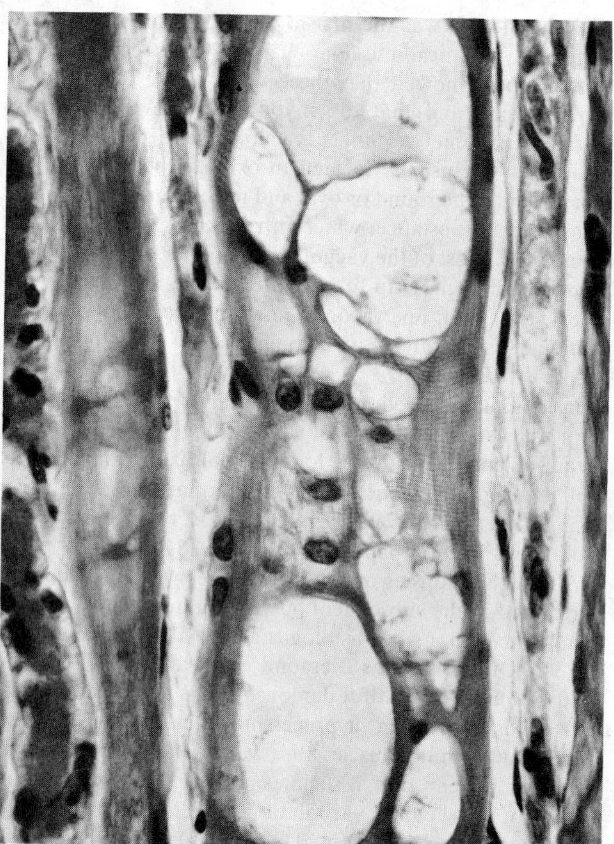

Figure 47-3. High magnification of multiloculated vacuoles and entrapped sarcolemmal nuclei in the patient described in Fig. 47-2. (H and E, ×650.) (*From C. M. Pearson* [6], *with permission.*)

persistence of large vacuoles in some muscle fibers between attacks, and the appearance of degenerative changes in organelles other than the sarcoplasmic reticulum as well. Engel [29, 182] concluded that the degenerative changes seen by him and by Howes et al. [28] were a consequence of the repeated distentions and distortions of the sarcoplasmic reticulum, with associated disruption of the normal architecture of the muscle fiber. These changes formed the morphologic basis of the permanent weakness that supervened after repeated attacks of paralysis. Recently Engel [182] found that most vacuoles communicate with the extracellular fluid via T tubules and the T system.

Odor et al. [30], in their ultrastructural studies of a patient with familial periodic paralysis and permanent weakness, considered the most interesting findings to be the presence of aggregates of tubules, approximately 73 mμ in diameter, which occurred in both subsarcolemmal and interfibrillar regions of the muscle fibers. The origin of these aggregates is unknown, but they could arise either from proliferation of tubules or from accumulations occurring after the breakdown of the myofibrils in these areas. They believed that these were derived from sarcoplasmic reticulum. Engel [103] noted the focal dilatations of the longitudinal elements of the sarcoplasmic reticulum at the point of contact with the transverse system in three different types of hypokalemic periodic paralysis. Longitudinally oriented cisterns appeared to result from a coalescence and rupture of the vesicles. Only in the hypokalemic type was "proliferation of sarcotubules" noted. Others have made similar observations [104, 105].

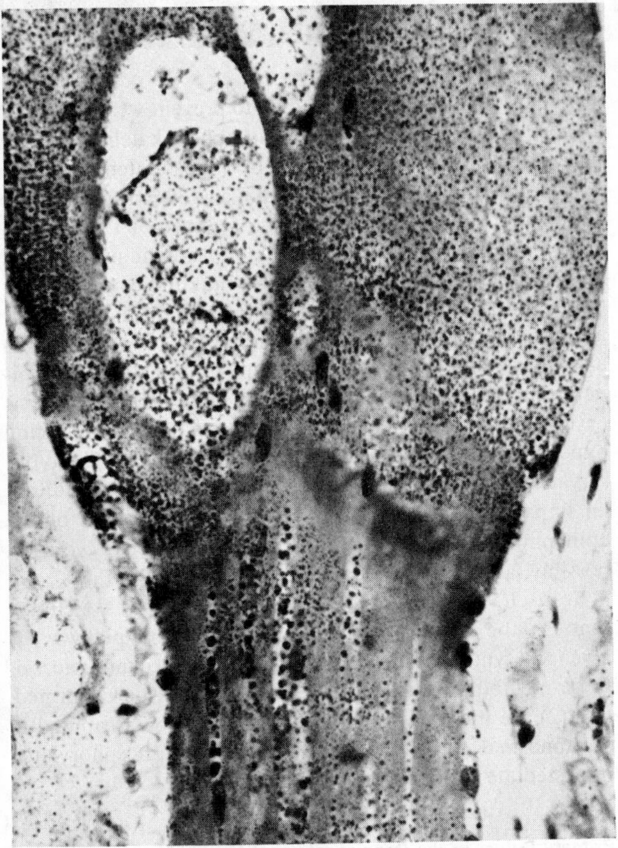

Figure 47-4. Massive deposition of glycogen droplets within vacuoles and overlying myofibrils in the patient described in Fig. 47-2. The droplets could be removed by prior digestion with diastase. (PAS stain, ×650.) (*From C. M. Pearson* [6], *with permission.*)

Abnormal and swollen mitochondria are frequently described as a nonspecific change in muscle fibers in hypokalemic periodic paralysis [20, 103]. A much less common alteration in skeletal muscle is the presence of subsarcolemmal mitochondrial aggregations, as observed by Engel [106] with histochemical methods in two cases of hypokalemic periodic paralysis and one case of congenital myotonia. Although this was confirmed by Odor et al. [30], such a change is probably nonspecific since similar changes have been found in other myopathies [103].

Pathogenesis

There has been no spectacular advance in solving the riddle of the pathogenesis of paralytic attacks in hypokalemic periodic paralysis, although several additional observations have been made in the last few years. The various theories regarding causation center primarily around (1) disturbances of adrenocortical hypersecretion; (2) disturbed carbohydrate metabolism in muscle, (3) a primary defect in the depolarization of muscle membrane, (4) a defect in the cellular organelles of the fiber, i.e., mitochondria, sarcoplasmic reticulum, T system, etc., and (5) a loss of integrity of higher neuronal function, i.e., in the area of the diencephalon.

Adrenocortical Hypersecretion

Streeten [21], in his comprehensive review, summarized the evidence for the participation of intermittent adrenocortical hypersecretion in the pathogenesis of the attacks. He argued that many of the precipitating factors of attacks, such as infection, stressful situations, and glucose and insulin administration, are known to be associated with, or followed by, adrenocortical overactivity. He also cited the increase in urinary excretion of 17-hydroxycorticoids and 17-ketosteroids in several attacks of paralysis as attributable to adrenocortical hyperactivity. Even though Conn and Streeten in 1960 [83] marshalled evidence in favor of their theory of intermittent hyperaldosteronism as a pathogenic factor, it has since been shown that no consistent relationship exists between sodium retention and onset of paralysis and that increased aldosterone excretion does not precede attacks of paralysis [23, 24]. Streeten [21] commented in his review that present evidence in the literature rules out intermittent hypersecretion of aldosterone as a pathogenic factor in hypokalemic periodic paralysis.

He did point out, however, that paralytic attacks consistently follow the administration of ACTH [109] and all other

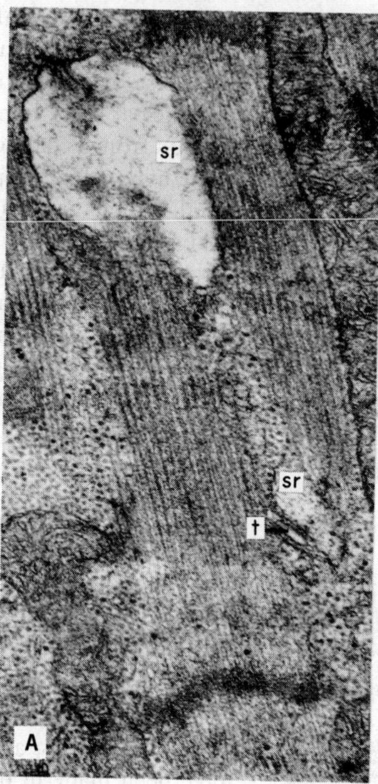

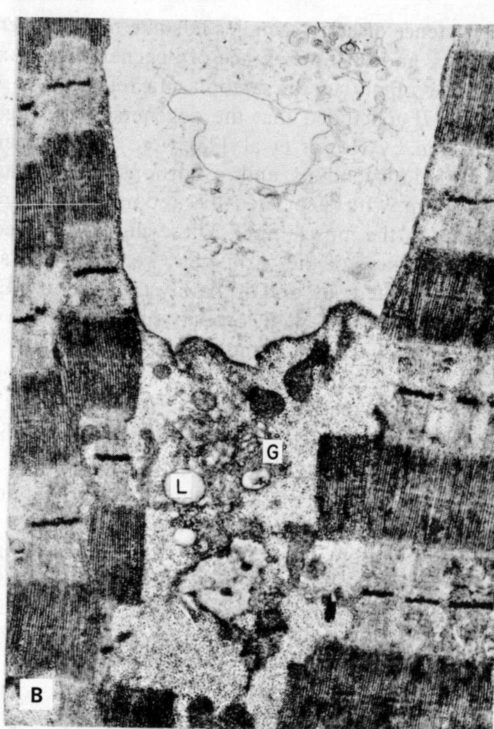

Figure 47-5. (A) Dilatation of the longitudinal component of the sarcoplasmic reticulum (*sr*), particularly the lateral cisterns. (EM, ×48,000.) (B) Large confluent vacuole spanning several sarcomeres and forcing apart the myofibrils. The vacuole contains granular material and some membrane forms. A Golgi apparatus (*G*) and a lipid droplet (*L*) are identified. (EM, ×12,000.) (*From E. L. Howes et al.* [28], *with permission.*)

potent mineralocorticoid substances, except aldosterone. Conn, in a presidential address [108], observed that hypokalemic muscle weakness may occur in primary aldosteronism, probably from the effects of chronic mineralocorticoid excess and not from any separate muscle membrane defect [108], in licorice intoxication [109, 110], and in dogs injected with DOCA [111]. He concluded that the paralytic attacks could be due to increased adrenal activity resulting in the release of a mineralocorticoid, not necessarily aldosterone. The protection of spontaneous and induced attacks by inhibitors of adrenal steroid synthesis (especially SU 9055) and by spironolactone adds support [108].

Disturbed Carbohydrate Metabolism as Cause of Attacks

Theories have been proposed at various times based on the long-known association of attacks and factors influencing carbohydrate metabolism. To explain the parallel movements of potassium and phosphate into cells, it was suggested that a defect in carbohydrate metabolism might be present at or about the hexose phosphate level [14, 26]. Shy et al. [20] were impressed by the relationship between the production of attacks and glycogen synthesis in muscle, and linked this with the appearance of numerous vacuoles within the muscle fibers. The vacuoles appeared to be predominantly fluid but contained some granules staining histochemically for glycogen. They postulated a metabolic defect in the synthetic pathway between glucose-1-phosphate and glycogen, giving rise to an accumulation of nondiffusible, anionic, subpolymerized glycogen molecules, causing by osmosis the influx of electrolytes and water into muscle. The administration of thiamine has been noted to prevent weakness after glucose administration in the primary hypokalemic form of periodic paralysis [26], and it has been postulated that there may be an impairment of metabolism of pyruvic acid or within the Krebs' cycle itself. The findings of Engel et al. [74] of excessive accumulation of lactic acid and pyruvic acid in blood after a standard workload may indicate a greater than normal release of these metabolites from muscle or an impaired metabolism by muscle, or both. These authors also found that small doses of epinephrine (not norepinephrine) administered intraarterially induced rapid paralysis of the muscles of the perfused forearm without inducing hypokalemia or hyperglycemia in arterial blood. These observations led them to conclude [112] that this may indicate an impairment of the assimilation of the products of the epinephrine-induced glycolysis into the Krebs' cycle or, possibly, a partial block of one or more steps in the Krebs' cycle itself. Based on biochemical studies, they concluded that (1) the hypothesis that a defect in the pathway of glycogen synthesis exists and leads to the accumulation of these metabolites during paralysis could not be confirmed, and (2) the mechanism of paralysis cannot be attributed to an abnormal accumulation of an anionic, phosphorylated intermediate of glycolysis in muscle.

Primary Defect in the Depolarization of Muscle Membrane

Electrophysiologic studies have led to a theory offering a rational explanation of the paralytic attacks. This hypothesis [113] predicts, and is dependent upon, the presence of hyperpolarization of the membrane. Actual measurements of the resting membrane potentials by Shy et al. [20], Creutzfeldt et al. [114], and more recently by others [115, 116], as well as the refined studies by Hofmann and Smith [91], have placed the theory under a cloud, as membrane potentials did not rise during paralysis. In fact, most of these investigators have observed significant depolarization of the muscle membrane in each of the several types of periodic paralysis [91, 114, 115]. Nonetheless, the theory focuses attention on the excitable membrane around and within the muscle cells as a possible site for the elusive biochemical lesion. Conduction of electrical impulses along these membranes requires active transport of sodium and potassium [117], which is dependent on energy and on carriers within the membrane [118, 119, 120]. Speculations about the hypoexcitable membrane during paralysis are very shaky because of our lack of knowledge of the basic disease process. Hofmann and Smith [91] have presented the current theories on this subject.

Changes in the Cellular Organelles as Cause of Attacks

Coppen and Reynolds [62] point to recent work, reviewed in 1964 by Adrian [121], which has focused attention on the peculiar properties of the sarcoplasmic reticulum with regard to its permeability to potassium. Hodgkin and Horowicz [122] have shown that at varying external potassium concentrations the potassium permeability in muscle is small for outward potassium movement but large for inward potassium movement. This "anomalous rectification" has puzzled physiologists, because these differing permeabilities for movement of potassium in opposite directions appear to be the reverse of those necessary to explain the recovery and loss of potassium during an impulse. Adrian presents evidence to suggest that the walls of the T-system component of the sarcoplasmic reticulum are the site of this anomalous permeability to potassium. He further suggests that this property is intimately concerned in the process of excitation-contraction coupling and that, following excitation, the failure of outward potassium movement across the T-system walls allows the inward movement of a negatively charged calcium ion complex which initiates contraction. If this hypothesis is correct, it can be seen that any disturbance in the permeability to potassium across the T system is likely to seriously interfere with muscle contraction. The problem of intracellular potassium ion adsorption to structural components is also just being explored [93]. Abnormalities to permeability of potassium in the membrane at that site may well be responsible for the paralysis of both the hypo- and hyperkalemic types of periodic paralysis. In this connection, it is significant that the most conspicuous structural changes in electron-microscopic studies have been dilatation of sarcoplasmic reticulum [20, 28–30, 105, 106].

Engel and Lambert [123] studied the effects of calcium on isolated muscle fibers in hypokalemic periodic paralysis and found that myofilaments of paralyzed fibers responded normally to calcium. Therefore, it appears that the block in excitation-contraction coupling resides in the membranous components of the fiber, either the surface membrane, the T system, the sarcoplasmic reticulum, or all three. Since sarcoplasmic reticulum of paralyzed muscle fibers could concentrate calcium from the myofilament space in a manner comparable to the sarcoplasmic reticulum of normal muscle, if the sarcoplasmic reticulum were affected in the paralyzed state, the abnormality would be one that affects the release but not the uptake of calcium.

Hypothetical Diencephalic Factors in Pathogenesis

Solomon [124] in a provocative discussion drew attention to the various similarities between periodic paralysis and the narcolepsy-cataplexy syndrome. He pointed out that except for the duration of the ictal episodes, which is very brief in narcolepsy-cataplexic attacks, they shared many other features. Of interest is the fact that there are isolated reports in the literature of hypopotassemic weakness, associated with hypothalamic obesity [125], adiposogenital dystrophy [126], and following meningoencephalitis [127]. Such reports suggest that disturbance of potassium metabolism may result from alteration in the hypothalamic electrolyte-regulating centers. As had already been pointed out, if Streeten's [21] assumption is correct, that hypersecretion of some mineralocorticoid other than aldosterone is the cause of the attacks, a defect in the diencephalic electrolyte-regulating center would still be appropriate.

In conclusion, it should be said that a strong case *does not* exist for considering periodic paralysis a neurohumoral disorder with disturbance of the hypothalamus, as suggested by Valso [128].

Treatment

Potassium salts were administered empirically from the turn of this century, even before the relationship of hypokalemia to attacks had been established [8, 9, 96]. Once it has been established that the paralysis is of the hypokalemic type, the attack is best treated by giving about 10 gm of potassium chloride orally in water, depending on the age of the patient and the muscle mass (Table 47-1) [49]. In severe attacks this may be insufficient and a further 5 gm may be required if there has been no improvement within 1 to 2 hr. When attacks are frequent and are not controlled by a high-potassium, restricted carbohydrate and sodium diet, a prophylactic dose of potassium, often best given at night, should be tried. Poskanzer and Kerr [129] found spironolactone helpful in one case and Okinaka et al. [130] have confirmed this.

A prophylactic dose of about 5 gm of potassium chloride (or its equivalent in organic potassium salts) given at night [46] often decreases the frequency of attacks. Streeten [21] has reviewed the literature regarding inefficacy of prophylactic potassium administration and the occurrence of more frequent attacks during maintenance therapy with potassium chloride. Conn and Streeten [83] have advised the use of diuretics, given to promote sodium loss, to stop attacks.

Table 47-1. DISTINGUISHING FEATURES OF THE THREE TYPES OF PERIODIC PARALYSIS

	Hypokalemic type	Hyperkalemic type (adynamia episodica hereditaria)	Normokalemic type
Age of onset	7 to 21 years	First decade	First decade
Duration of attacks	1 hr to 4 days (usually several hours)	Less than 1 hr	2 days to 3 weeks
Serum potassium during attack	Low	High	Normal or slightly low
Factors which induce attacks	Rest after exertion, large high-carbohydrate meals, cold, infections, trauma, mental tension, alcohol	Rest after exertion, cold and damp, hunger	Rest after exertion, sleeping late, alcohol, cold and damp, mental stress
Iatrogenic induction	Glucose and insulin, ACTH, DCA, fluorohydro-cortisone, epinephrine	Potassium chloride	Potassium chloride
Severity	Frequently complete paralysis, sparing face and respiratory muscles	Usually mild weakness, often localized	Often complete paralysis, including jaw and cough reflex
Time of onset	Awaken paralyzed	Usually during the day	Awaken paralyzed
Sex differences	More severe in males	More severe in males	Similar in both sexes
Sensory changes	None	May have paresthesias	Peripheral hypesthesia
Metabolic changes	Potassium and, usually, sodium retention	No retention of sodium or potassium	Potassium retention
Prophylaxis	Spironolactone, very low sodium diet and diuretics, acetazolea-mide	Gentle exercise after exertion; carbohydrate feedings, acetazolea-mide, hydrochlorthiazide	Gentle exercise after exertion; fluorohydro-cortisone and acetazola-mide
Treatment of attacks	Potassium salts	Calcium gluconate	Sodium chloride

Source: Modified from Poskanzer and Kerr [129].

Okinaka et al. [130], like Poskanzer and Kerr before them, also found aldosterone antagonists useful. The usual dose of spironolactone (Aldactone) is 100 to 200 mg daily in divided portions. Continuous administration of the drug for several years may cause androgenic effects in females and gynecomastia in males [21].

DeGraeff and Lameijer [81] found that administration of cortisone in sufficient dosage greatly diminished the frequency of paralytic attacks for a prolonged period of time in one of their two patients. This has not been confirmed by other workers, although Grob et al. [18] earlier found this form of therapy of value in protecting against glucose- and insulin-induced attacks.

The most recent development in the drug therapy of hypokalemic periodic paralysis is the 1968 report of Resnick et al. [131] on the prophylactic use of acetazolamide. They found striking improvement in three of the five patients on whom they tried this form of prophylactic therapy.

Prognosis

Talbott [17] in his review of the literature found a mortality of 10 percent during attacks. High mortality was the feature of families reported by Holtzapple [96]. Causes of death, as summarized by Streeten [21], have been respiratory paralysis, respiratory infections, inhalation pneumonia, cardiac failure, shock, and excessive therapeutic venesections.

McArdle [49] points to the fact that the attacks are at their worst in early adult life. They later become less severe and, especially in females, may disappear entirely. The outlook is less satisfactory for those who develop a permanent weakness, though the progression is very slow.

HYPERKALEMIC PERIODIC PARALYSIS

In the half-century or more during which extensive studies were done on hypokalemic periodic paralysis, it became standard treatment to administer adequate doses of potassium chloride. However, it gradually became clear that there were a number of families in which the paralysis not only failed to respond to oral potassium therapy but, in fact, worsened. In such cases, the serum potassium did not fall during attacks, and sometimes it even rose. Tyler et al. [133], in 1951, carefully studied such a family and suggested that the cases that they were reporting formed a distinct and separate entity. The situation was not further clarified until 1956, when Gamstorp [134] presented her extensive studies on two families with periodic paralysis in which the serum potassium almost invariably rose during the attacks. In total, she studied 139 cases. In addition to elevated potassium levels in the serum during paralytic episodes, she also noted that muscular weakness was precipitated by the oral ingestion of potassium salts, instead of being relieved as in the hypokalemic form of the disease. Gamstorp gave the condition the name *adynamia episodica hereditaria,* which in general has now been replaced by *hyperkalemic periodic paralysis.*

There appears to be a close relationship between this condition and a cold-susceptible form of myotonia described first in 1886 by Eulenberg [135] as *paramyotonia congenita.* A link with hyperkalemic periodic paralysis and paramyotonia was provided when French and Kilpatrick [136], in 1957, studied a patient with paramyotonia who was subject to attacks of generalized weakness. In that patient, an oral dose of potassium chloride induced an attack of weakness without a fall in the serum potassium level.

Since the original Scandanavian papers, approximately 30 reports of hyperkalemic periodic paralysis have appeared in the literature. The great majority of these describe myotonia, either on physical examination or by electromyography [137–153]. In none of the others was myotonia completely excluded [151]. It thus appears that hyperkalemic periodic paralysis without myotonic features is indeed rare.

The presence of myotonia would seem to link this condition with paramyotonia congenita, although myotonia in the latter condition develops primarily in response to cold. For many years, paramyotonia was considered by many investigators to be a variant of myotonia congenita [132]. However, more recently, discussions have concerned its relationship to hyperkalemic periodic paralysis. Drager et al. [154], in 1958, maintained that the two conditions were manifestations of the same disease, and there is much to be said for this view. It is the approach that many later workers such as Layzer et al. [151] have supported. Nevertheless, at the present time it appears best to preserve an open mind about either the pathogenic identity or dissimilarity of these two conditions, until more is known about the underlying biochemical and electrical or membrane abnormalities in these conditions.

Clinical Features

Paralytic Attacks

A typical severe attack of hyperkalemic periodic paralysis [142] occurs when the patient is relaxing after unusually energetic exertion. If the exercise has been strenous, resting for 30 min is often sufficient to induce an episode. Weakness is usually first noticed in the lower back, next in the thighs and calves, and then in the hands and arms. As the attack progresses the neck muscles become affected, and finally in severe attacks, significant difficulty may occur in coughing and swallowing. An early symptom of an attack, and one by which the family recognizes the infants that are affected, is an increased liability for the eyes to become temporarily "staring," as first pointed out by McArdle [142]. Thus, during the episodes of staring, the conjunctivae show above the corneae on looking down, after first looking up. In addition, transient blurring of vision from simple relaxation of accomodation or convergence may occur, as in looking up from a book to gaze out the window.

The development of paralysis is usually rapid, the peak in a severe attack being reached within 30 or 40 min or less. The attack then abates with equal rapidity. It is unusual for severe attacks to last for more than 1 to 2 hr or for moderate attacks to continue for longer than 1 hr. However, some patients have been described whose paralysis may last for 12 hr or more [6]. Mild weakness may persist much longer, the duration depending upon the level of activity. Thus, it is nearly always possible to prevent or abort an attack by exercise, though this usually results only in postponement until the exercise has ceased. If the attack is already at its peak or on the wane, its disappearance can be hastened by exercise without the likelihood of an immediate recurrence of the weakness on resting. In general, it takes from 2 to 10 min, depending upon the severity of the attack, for exercise to relieve the weakness. Even then it may not be wholly successful. Repeated postponement or abortion of mild attacks may sometimes result in painful, hard, tender lumps, involving the whole or part of one or both calves and persisting for hours or days.

Other factors which, in many patients, seem to predispose to attacks include excitement, emotion, generalized exposure to cold or chilling, hunger, infections, and general anesthesia. Other symptoms which have been described in some patients include aching in the muscles, occasional circumoral tingling, and indefinite paresthesia in the extremities, which are oftentimes experienced early in an attack. In addition, some patients experience a tingling sensation in the epigastrium at the onset of an attack [6], and others yawn regularly during the early stages of a spontaneous attack [142]. During the development of a severe or moderate attack, most patients have noticed an urgent need to urinate and that if they are able to do so the attack is likely to subside more quickly.

In hyperkalemic periodic paralysis, attacks occur frequently in many patients, but there is a great variation from one patient or one family to another. Most patients have brief, daytime attacks, varying from several every day to one a year, at different times of day in different patients. Some patients regularly experience their attacks nocturnally. In general, the daytime attacks are brief, while the nocturnal attacks are more prolonged and often more severe. During the diurnal attacks, where the onset could be observed, most patients described a similar pattern of onset and development.

Physical Signs

It is possible to assess accurately the power of muscles *between attacks* only by repeated examination, since minor transient weakness of one or more groups of muscles is commonly present, even at times of relative freedom from paralysis. However, nearly all patients show some degree of permanent weakness, although this may be slight. The distribution of permanent weakness is usually the same, there being weakness of the abdominal muscles and the hip flexors and, to a lesser extent, of the triceps muscles. Less frequently involved muscles include hip extensors and shoulder abductors. Most patients, even between attacks, have significant difficulty in arising from a deep knee bend. When the weakness becomes quite marked, as has been described in a number of patients [6, 152, 153], it is largely proximal in distribution, involving the shoulder and pelvic girdles, and is of a typical "myopathic" variety. In nearly all patients, even those with significant permanent weakness, neither wasting nor hypertrophy are unequivocal. Between attacks, the deep tendon reflexes are almost invariably preserved, although perhaps they might be somewhat diminished. Sometimes percussion myotonia may be observed in characteristic muscles such as in the tongue or the orbicularis oculi; myotonia in the latter causes the characteristic "squinting" after forceful closing of the eyes.

During *mild* attacks there is usually intensification of the preexisting weakness. In *severe attacks,* the paralysis is usually much more marked in the trunk and the proximal limb muscles, while the neck muscles and especially those of the face are rarely involved. As described previously, there may be a shallowness of breathing and a partial weakness of the intercostal muscles, as well as weakness of the bulbar pharyngeal muscles, often to the point of interference with swallowing of tablets, solids, or even liquids. During very severe attacks, the deep tendon reflexes have been found either much diminished or absent.

Inheritance and Sex Distribution

In nearly all the families so far described, inheritance is by an autosomal dominant pattern [134, 142, 144, 150, 151]. Only two sporadic cases have been described; in one [147], other family members were not examined, while in the other [155] paralysis was apparently sporadic, but "severe muscle cramps" occurred in a clearly autosomal dominant pattern. Certain other cases have been thought to be sporadic ones until relatives have been examined and found to demonstrate myotonia by electromyography.

Both sexes are equally affected in most reports. In the report by Layzer et al. [151], 15 males and 20 females were affected and all three asymptomatic but affected individuals were females. In McArdle's reports [46, 49, 142], an unduly small proportion of the children of affected males were themselves affected; this seems to be a rarity since it is not observed in other pedigrees.

Almost every affected individual in published pedigrees has had an affected parent, and as far back as the grandparents of the youngest affected generation only four examples of a skipped generation have been recorded. These individuals in question were apparently not examined.

In families in which paramyotonia congenita has been reported, there is also an autosomal dominant pattern with complete penetrance.

Age of Onset

In most patients, the earliest symptoms (myotonia or weakness) were noticed between 4 and 18 years of age. The initial appearance of these symptoms, however, has been noticed in infancy within the first few weeks of life [6], and only occasionally beyond the twentieth year [156]. The majority of patients have the onset of their initial symptoms in the second decade in some series [151], whereas Gamstorp [134], in her initial report stated that 90 percent of the patients she studied had attacks of weakness before age 10 years.

Laboratory and Metabolic Studies

Establishing a diagnosis of hyperkalemic periodic paralysis seldom should be difficult. The rise in serum potassium is usually modest and generally parallels the degree of paralysis. In some instances, however, the serum potassium may rise to a level of 8 mEq per liter, at which time cardiac irritability and significant ECG evidence of hyperkalemia may be seen. In a few patients, little or no rise in serum potassium has been demonstrated, even during severe paralysis. Also, sometimes in the same individual there may be a few episodes in which the potassium does not rise above the normal limits, and occasionally it may even fall [6, 49].

Levels of serum sodium, chloride, bicarbonate, calcium, and phosphorus are not consistently altered in any pattern during an attack [159]. Urinary excretion of potassium during paralysis usually parallels the serum level or remains unchanged. The latter observation tends to exclude control of potassium by the kidneys as a factor in the disorder.

Routine blood and urine examinations reveal no evidence of abnormality between attacks. Serum enzymes have been found to rise following some attacks in a few patients [160].

Electromyographic and Membrane Potential Studies

The most characteristic electromyographic findings in hyperkalemic periodic paralysis are focal evidences of insertional activity in the form of myotonic discharges [157, 158]. Such discharges, of a mild and brief character, are frequently provoked by needle movement and muscle percussion. Motor unit activity is, on the other hand, not significantly abnormal. No abnormality other than myotonia is usually detected by electromyography. Nerve conduction rates and terminal latencies in various peripheral nerves are almost invariably normal. When an extremity to be examined is cooled, myotonic discharges are frequently increased in number and magnitude.

In advanced myopathic weakness, which usually follows late in the course of hyperkalemic periodic paralysis, the electromyogram may disclose some myopathic electrical activity.

Muscle membrane potentials have now been recorded from a number of patients, both during attacks and in attack-free intervals [114, 153, 157]. These studies have in general revealed the following: (1) Measurements in vivo during an attack-free interval show the membrane potentials to be significantly lower than normal, that is −68.5 mv versus −87.4 mv in a normal subject [114]; (2) during either a spontaneous attack or one induced by potassium administration, the membrane potentials drop from −46 to −51.5 mv, therefore indicating major depolarization of the muscle cell membrane.

It thus appears that the paralytic episodes of hyperkalemic periodic paralysis are due to a reversible depolarization of the muscle fibers. There are reasons to suggest that this depolarization may not occur as a consequence of a disorder of membrane permeability, since, so far, no such change has been demonstrated. However, this point is clearly debatable, since Creutzfeldt et al. [114] postulated that the depolarization is due to an increased membrane permeability to sodium. They reached this conclusion when it appeared to be impossible to explain the degree of fall of the resting membrane potential as a consequence of a rise in the intracellular potassium concentration. Brooks speculated [157] that there may be an abnormality of the sodium-potassium pump mechanism as the primary disturbance in this condition, and he presented evidence to support this view.

Other Etiologic Findings

There is evidence that potassium may leak from muscle during the development of weakness [142], and Carson and Pearson [149] found low muscle potassium and high sodium content during a severe attack. Between attacks the muscle potassium and total exchangeable potassium have been normal or low; on the other hand, Liljestrand [161] and Gamstorp [134] found the muscle potassium lowered and the sodium and chloride increased. Hypocalcemia has been noted in some attacks [151], but the serum calcium has otherwise always been found to be normal.

A very interesting possibility has been raised that a humoral factor may be involved in the production of myotonia in hyperkalemic periodic paralysis. This was advanced in some interesting studies by Krull et al. [162], who closely observed one patient with venous occlusion (100 mm Hg) of a forearm. When this was accompanied by repeated contraction of the occluded hand for 15 min, it resulted in striking *generalized* and long-lasting myotonia on release of the occluded cuff; the duration of myotonic discharges increased progressively during the period of venous occlusion. The myotonia did not appear to be due to potassium. Upon release of the cuff, several hundred cubic centimeters of blood were removed from the antecubital vein of the arm that had been exercised. It was later reinjected into the same patient after a period of storage. The reinjection blood seemed to induce generalized myotonia in the patient. Serum taken from the blood removed during the compression period and injected intravenously into rabbits and rats was said to result in myotonic discharges on tapping the muscle. The nature of the humoral substance and how it acts is so far unknown.

Pathologic Studies

Light Microscopy

Comparisons of stained tissue sections from paralyzed and nonparalyzed muscle from a variety of patients have now been reported many times in the literature [104, 153, 163]. There are minimal histologic differences between the paralyzed and nonparalyzed state. Sections have exhibited scattered and isolated atrophic or degenerative muscle fibers, without any increase in fibrous connective tissue or accumulations of inflammatory cells. The usual polygonal configuration of the muscle fibers is preserved, except in the actual atrophic or degenerative ones. The latter sometimes become rounded and smaller in diameter and show a relative increase in sarcolemmal nuclei with a centralization of these nuclei. Sometimes a distinguishing feature in the paralyzed muscle is the vacuolization of the perinuclear area (Fig. 47-6), which is usually seen deep within the muscle fiber. Many of these vacuolated areas appear to be membrane-limited and to contain PAS-positive material. The vacuolizations are rarely seen in the nonparalyzed muscle. The massive central vacuolization changes, frequently described in hypokalemic periodic paralysis, are not usually seen. Bradley [153] described occasional vacuolated fibers and an increased amount of sarcoplasmic glycogen collections into subsarcolemmal blebs, as well as nonspecific myopathic changes of central nuclei and hyaline fibers. No grossly vacuolated fibers were noted in the material from his patients.

Electron Microscopy

In ultrastructural studies from nonparalyzed muscle, the sarcolemma was normal and the sarcolemmal nuclei were frequently crenated [104]. The mitochondria were elongated and smooth, and the cristae were at right angles to the outer membrane and parallel to one another. The sarcoplasmic reticulum was seen as a tubular system, and occasionally beneath the sarcolemma there was dilatation of the system.

In the paralyzed muscle of some patients, striking differences were noted [163]. The sarcoplasmic reticulum showed cisternal dilatations, most frequently in the perinuclear and subsarcolemmal areas, although they were present also within the substance of the muscle cell. The dilated sarcoplasmic reticulum was membrane-limited and in it were seen ribosome-like bodies. Within the lumina was an amorphous material with scattered discrete particles resembling ribosomes. The mitochondria appeared to be swollen, with distortion of the outer membrane and of the internal cristae.

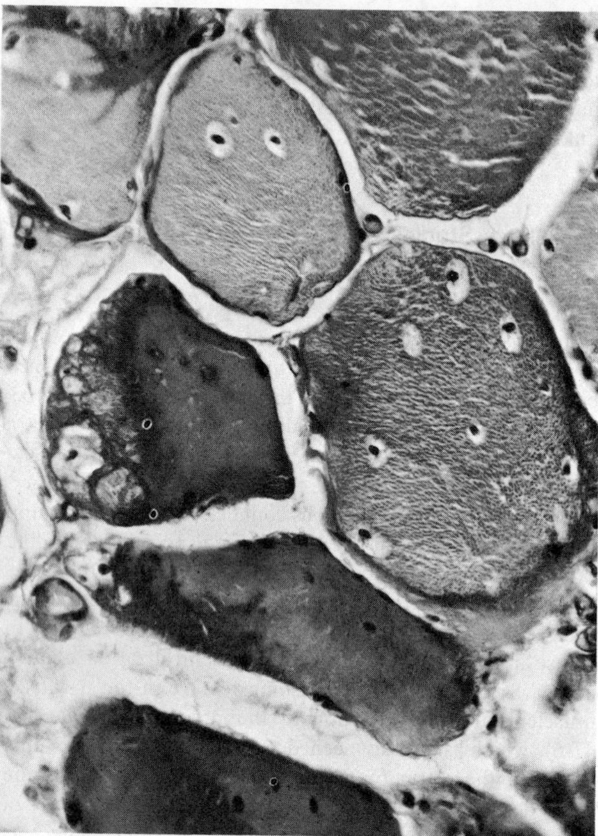

Figure 47-6. Biopsy from a patient with hyperkalemic periodic paralysis during an attack. The fibers reveal modest perinuclear vacuolation and other sparse myopathic changes. These represent the usual extent of the changes that are seen in this condition. (H and E, ×390.) (*From C. M. Pearson* [6], *with permission.*)

The dilated sarcoplasmic reticulum appeared to distort and displace the mitochondria from their normal distribution about the myofibrils. The modestly dilated sarcoplasmic reticulum is very similar to that seen in some of the milder examples of cistern formation found in hypokalemic periodic paralysis and demonstrated in Fig. 47-5A. In some biopsies, an increase in muscle glycogen has been noted in the regions of the I band of the myofibrils [104]. It was thought that these glycogen accumulations were probably secondary and compensatory. Bradley [164] has mentioned that the ultrastructure in the three forms of periodic paralysis (including the normokalemic type) cannot be distinguished at present, suggesting that the dilatation of the longitudinal elements of the sarcoplasmic reticulum, with consequent disruption of the excitation-contraction couplings, may play a major role in the production of paralysis in all three conditions, although the exact underlying defect in each case must presumably be somewhat different.

Relationship of Hyperkalemic Periodic Paralysis to Paramyotonia Congenita

Since the original report by Eulenberg [135], there has been a tendency to define paramyotonia as a form of myotonia which is present only, or primarily, in the cold [132, 165]. Magee [166] has shown that in a patient with classical paramyotonic symptoms, the myotonia could be induced at any temperature, although somewhat more readily in the cold. Moreover, cold also magnifies the difficulty in relaxation in two other conditions, namely mytonia congenita and myotonic muscular dystrophy [165]. What appears to be unique to paramyotonia is that *weakness* is brought about either by cold or, occasionally, spontaneously. It is the weakness which suggests a close relationship between paramyotonia and periodic paralysis.

In the families described by Layzer [151] there was strong evidence that paramyotonia and hyperkalemic periodic paralysis are one and the same. In some of the individuals in that study the clinical features of myotonia predominated, while in others, often in the same family, episodes of periodic paralysis were most evident. There was clear-cut evidence of myotonia in all affected individuals, and thus in those families myotonia appeared to be the minimal expression of the genetic trait. The presence or absence of associated hyperkalemic periodic paralysis and the severity of either myotonia or periodic paralysis, appeared to be independently variable. Presumably the paralytic episodes, Layzer thought, were the result of other modifying factors. He also pointed out that such a large variability in the expression of a genetic trait is well known in other disorders with an autosomal dominant inheritance, as exemplified by the variable characteristics which are seen in facioscapulohumeral dystrophy or myotonic dystrophy.

Some families have been described with a more homogeneous clinical syndrome of "pure" paramyotonia congenita [146, 166, 167]. On the other hand, hyperkalemic periodic paralysis has also been described without myotonia [168], but it is not clear in the latter series whether myotonia was specifically excluded by electromyographic and other studies. In order to demonstrate that paramyotonia is not the same disease as hyperkalemic paralysis it would be absolutely necessary to show that patients with "paramyotonia" were *not* made weak by feeding of potassium salts. There have been only two attempts of this type. In the original description of hyperkalemic periodic paralysis, by Gamstorp [134], weakness was induced by doses of KCl of less than 5 gm; however, one patient who received only 4 gm did not become weak. Gamstorp [146] later described a family with paramyotonia congenita in whom none of the five patients became weak after receiving 4 to 6 gm KCl, although the myotonia increased in some of these persons. Similarly, Magee [167] gave 6 gm KCl daily in divided doses to patients with paramyotonia without inducing weakness. Although larger amounts were not given by either investigator, it was implied that patients with paramyotonia were resistant to paralysis by potassium. However, considerable variation in susceptibility to weakness or paralysis after administration of potassium has been demonstrated by the patients described in the family studied by Layzer [151].

The sodium content of the diet also may influence the ease with which the attacks can be induced by either potassium or exercise. In some cases a high-sodium diet is protective while a low-sodium diet has an adverse effect [147, 169]. Therefore, unless a standard diet is used, the amount of potassium required to produce paralysis may not be a reliable diagnostic criterion. The studies of Layzer [151] suggest that the identity of paramyotonia with hyperkalemic periodic paralysis can be confirmed when a patient becomes weak after a potassium load of *any magnitude* if the serum potassium rises but remains below the level at which otherwise normal individuals may become weak. This level may, on some occasions, be as high as 8 mEq/liter [142]. It should be pointed out, however, that some individuals have not been paralyzed despite still higher blood levels [137], while others become weak with serum potassium levels as low as 7.2 mEq/liter [170]. It is difficult in practice to know exactly at what level one should challenge patients before deciding when to stop for fear of producing serious cardiac side effects. In practice it appears that single oral doses greater than 10 gm KCl are not likely to be required.

In summary, the evidence to date suggests that paramyotonia congenita and hyperkalemic periodic paralysis are one and the same disease. Proof, however, requires identification of the inherited metabolic abnormality.

Relation between Hyperkalemic Periodic Paralysis and Myotonia Congenita

It has been reported on many occasions that some individuals in families with classical periodic paralysis suffer from only myotonic symptoms—no attacks of paralysis are recorded. These persons resemble those with myotonia congenita. On the other hand, in most families who have clear-cut myotonia congenita, there are no attacks of paralysis. In one patient from a family with myotonia congenita that was studied by Layzer [151] doses up to 7 gm of KCl were followed by an increase in serum potassium to 5.0 mEq/liter, with aggravation of myotonia but no weakness. Since not enough patients have been studied, additional evidence will be required before it can be concluded that myotonia congenita is an entirely separate disorder, although upon present evidence this appears likely. Therefore, the term *myotonia congenita* should be restricted to families with pure myotonia (without attacks of weakness even in one family member), while at the same time it should be recognized that a thorough family study may be necessary to exclude the existence of individuals with occasional attacks of episodic weakness.

Pathogenesis

In a discussion concerning the etiologic or pathogenetic factors in hyperkalemic periodic paralysis, the reader is referred to the lengthy discussion concerning the pathogenetic mechanisms in *hypo*kalemic periodic paralysis, since much of the discussion of that section is perhaps relevant to the hyperkalemic disorder. It has been observed by many workers that during an attack of weakness in hyperkalemic periodic paralysis the myotonic phenomena often initially become more pronounced in some muscles than in others. It appears, therefore, that whatever changes take place during an attack seem to effect both myotonia and weakness. It is this reasoning that draws one to the conclusion that the mechanisms of myotonia and periodic paralysis are probably intimately related.

Local cooling in water to about 12°C can induce a much greater and long-lasting weakness or paralysis than is found in normal individuals [142]. Electromyography during weakness shows changes in the action potentials indicating functional loss of both individual muscle fibers and whole motor units. The remaining fibers often show hyperirritability of a myotonic type [114, 171]. Since it was also shown that muscles had a lowered threshold of motor response to injected acetylcholine, Buchthal and associates [171] suggested that the paralysis was due to an abnormally low resting membrane potential. This suggestion, which would account satisfactorily for all the main findings, was substantiated by Creutzfeldt et al. [114], as well as more recently by other workers [116, 157], who, using intracellular electrodes, found the membrane potential abnormally low between attacks, with a further fall during paralysis. All of these authors have pointed out that the potassium changes observed in plasma and muscle could not adequately explain the low membrane potential between the attacks, nor the extent of the fall during paralysis. Therefore they postulated that an abnormally increased membrane permeability to sodium existed. An alternative hypothesis had been advanced previously by Buchthal and associates [171], who attributed the low membrane potential to an increased permeability to chloride.

In hyperkalemic periodic paralysis there have been only a few measurements of the tissue electrolyte and water concentrations, but the results are compatible with a shift of potassium out of the muscle and into the extracellular fluid [159]. In this condition, however, these shifts of potassium cannot be clearly and unequivocally related to a well-defined metabolic abnormality. Moreover, there is no absolutely consistent relationship between the level of serum potassium and the severity of paralysis. It is not quite clear why diuretic (kaluretic) drugs should be beneficial in hyperkalemic periodic paralysis, as will be discussed. These findings have been noted in the absence of a striking reduction of serum potassium levels, and therefore the suggestion has been made [114] that these drugs may have a direct effect on muscle ion fluxes or even more specifically upon the muscle membrane or the sarcoplasmic reticulum. The latter appears to be a very likely possibility. The findings of increased sodium and lowered potassium content of muscle [139, 149], and of excessive potassium efflux following exercise [142], also suggest a defect in the permeability properties of the muscle membrane. We have observed that myotonia, as demonstrated both electromyographically and clinically, has appeared in some of our patients with hyperkalemic periodic paralysis within 30 min after the administration of a diuretic such as hydrochlorthiazide, before any demonstrable change in serum potassium or urinary excretion of potassium had occurred. Therefore it seems quite likely that such compounds have an effect upon the muscle membrane or on the membrane of the sarcoplasmic reticulum. The abnormality in hyperkalemic periodic paralysis might be magnified by these drugs, which allow myotonia to develop but protect against weakness. A defect in the membrane in the opposite direction could likewise, under some conditions, stimulate myotonia and initiate weakness because of depolarization, with a subsequent failure of the spike mechanisms of the membrane.

Treatment

Reference is made to Table 47-1 in which is outlined prophylactic treatment of hyperkalemic periodic paralysis, as well as treatment of attacks. Since 1962, when McArdle [142] first described the beneficial effects of various diuretics or kaluretics in patients with this condition, many authors have confirmed this finding. McArdle obtained considerable relief with acetazolamide in all six patients he treated with either this compound or with another carbonic anhydrase inhibitor, namely dichlorphenamide. In the series of Layzer (151) acetazolamide was symptomatically beneficial in four of five patients, but complete elimination of attacks was achieved in only two of the four. Two patients treated with chlorthiazide were similarly improved in Layzer's series, but a third developed a marked increase in myotonic symptoms after 2 days on chlorthiazide, 1.0 gm daily. Samaha [150] noted considerable improvement in seven patients treated with chlorthiazide, in none of whom were there any side effects. Carson and Pearson [149] treated three patients successfully with acetazolamide, chlorthiazide, or hydrochlorthiazide. However, one patient experienced increasing weakness while taking acetazolamide, 500 mg daily, but subsequently improved on that medication after the simultaneous administration of potassium. When the same patient was given hydrochlorthiazide, 100 mg daily, moderate symptomatic myotonia appeared and she required occasional supplements of potassium in order to counteract the persistent weakness that developed.

It is generally recommended that for prophylactic treatment of hyperkalemic periodic paralysis the individual should avoid vigorous exercise, that he should take a fairly sizable amount of carbohydrate in the diet, and that he should be treated with a diuretic such as acetazolamide in a dosage of approximately 500 mg a day, hydrochlorthiazide, 100 mg a day (50 mg twice daily), or chlorthiazide in a total dose of 1.0 gm daily. It has been stated that acute attacks of hyperkalemic periodic paralysis may be partially aborted or prematurely improved with the use of intravenous calcium gluconate, although clear-cut evidence for this last effect has not been documented in the literature. Obviously potassium salts or a high potassium diet should be avoided, unless the patient is also on one of the diuretics.

From the results that have so far accumulated in the literature it appears that the effectiveness of the carbonic anhydrase inhibitors or the thiazide diuretics varies from one patient to another. Although usually beneficial, it has been noted by some [149] that increased weakness, myotonic symptoms, or both may occur with either class of drug. It does appear that the magnified weakness in this situation may respond to supplemental potassium administration. At first glance, this may appear to be surprising, but there is now evidence for an intracellular deficit of muscle potassium in hyperkalemic periodic paralysis which may be aggravated by diuretic agents. Although still somewhat hypothetical, it seems reasonable to predict that the beneficial action of the diuretic drugs is probably not related to renal excretion of electrolytes but rather to a direct effect on the muscle membrane.

NORMOKALEMIC PERIODIC PARALYSIS

In 1961 Poskanzer and Kerr [129] described what they called a third type of hereditary periodic paralysis. It bears a close resemblance to hyperkalemic periodic paralysis except that the serum potassium was not raised, even during the most severe attacks. They named the condition normokalemic periodic paralysis. The attacks were often prolonged, lasting days or even weeks. Also they were usually more severe than those described in the hyperkalemic variety, and they occurred mainly at night.

The family that Poskanzer and Kerr studied comprised 45 family members, 21 of whom had suffered periodic episodes of paralysis. The illness started in the first decade, and was characterized by episodes of paralysis at intervals of 1 to 3 months. Each attack lasted from 2 days to 3 weeks, often with a severe degree of weakness including quadriplegia and weakness of the muscles of mastication but excluding any dysfunction of facial expression, bladder or bowel, or respiration. The pattern of inheritance of this condition was said to be autosomal dominant.

The characteristics of this disorder are summarized in Table 47-1. In essence, episodes were provoked by rest after physical exertion, prolonged inactivity such as sleeping late in the morning, or sitting or standing in one place for several hours. Alcoholic intake, cold and dampness, and mental stress also appeared to predispose to attacks. The serum potassium level was *normal* during all attacks. Administration of KCl could precipitate attacks and the attacks were improved by the use of large doses of NaCl. No attacks occurred while patients were given a combination of 250 mg acetazolamide and 0.1 mg 9α-fluorohydrocortisone daily over 3 months, despite attempts to provoke paralysis.

Muscle biopsy specimens obtained during an attack demonstrated mild vacuolation of muscle fibers in focal areas, with muscle fiber degeneration. Myotonia apparently did not exist in these patients, or at least it was not reported from the electromyographic studies of one patient who was investigated during two episodes of severe paralysis.

The disease appeared to have many features in common with classical hypokalemic periodic paralysis as well as with hyperkalemic periodic paralysis. However, in this carefully studied family the authors felt that there were sufficient dissimilarities to justify the description of a third syndrome. So far as is known, no additional similar families or patients have been studied in the intervening years.

PERIODIC PARALYSIS IN HYPERTHYROIDISM

Periodic paralysis of the hypokalemic type is a well-recognized complication of thyrotoxicosis. In 1961 Engel [87] was able to uncover 228 cases in the literature in which paralytic episodes were associated with overactive thyroid function. Almost an equal number have been reported since that time [71, 172, 173, 174]. Although there appears to be little or no relationship between thyroid function and the typical cases of familial hypokalemic periodic paralysis, the paralytic attacks in both the familial and the thyrotoxic varieties are similar in that (1) they can be induced by increased carbohydrate metabolism, (2) they follow excessive physical exertion, and (3) they are diminished or prevented by administration of potassium.

There appears to be a remarkable predeliction for periodic paralysis to occur in conjunction with hyperthyroidism in the Japanese [71, 175] and perhaps in other Asian races [172, 173]. Furthermore there is predominance of thyrotoxic periodic paralysis in males, the incidence being about 15 times that in women. Satoyoshi and his associates [71] reviewed the histories of 432 patients with hyperthyroidism in several hospitals in Tokyo, Japan, and found that 38 of these suffered from fairly representative attacks of thyrotoxic periodic paralysis. Although the large majority of cases of pure hyperthyroidism were in females, nevertheless they found that 30 percent of the males admitted for hyperthyroidism suffered from attacks of periodic paralysis, whereas only 2 percent of thyrotoxic females were so afflicted. At least half their patients suffered from initial attacks of paralysis between the ages of 21 and 30 years.

There are also many interesting similarities between thyrotoxic periodic paralysis and familial hypokalemic periodic paralysis. In both there is a preponderance in males, the factors which induce attacks are the same, and if the manifestations of thyrotoxicosis are excluded the clinical picture during attacks is identical. The biochemical changes are similar in both conditions. There appears generally to be a retention of water and sodium without alteration in the serum sodium concentration. There is invariably a fall in serum potassium concentration to levels of 2.0 to 3.0 mEq/liter, associated with a proportional reduction in the amount of potassium excreted in the urine. There is no evidence of excessive loss of potassium in the stools. Careful studies [176] have demonstrated that during the onset of an attack there is a constant positive arteriovenous difference of potassium. These findings indicate that during the onset of attacks there is intracellular migration of potassium from the extracellular space. On the other hand, the total body exchangeable potassium is within normal limits in thyrotoxic periodic paralysis [177] while direct measurements of the intracellular and extracellular contents of potassium in muscle tissue before and during attacks of paralysis demonstrated that the K_i/K_o ratio increases roughly parallel to the severity of the induced paralysis [178].

The response of attacks of paralysis to treatment in thyrotoxic periodic paralysis is similar to that in the familial variety. Potassium salts and aldosterone antagonists are prophylactically effective in a proportion of persons. Paralytic episodes could be completely reversed by treatment of the thyrotoxic condition. Furthermore, after the patient reaches normal thyroid function, an attack of paralysis can no longer be induced, even when hypokalemia is produced by priming with 9-α-fluorohydrocortisone [172].

There are some differences between thyrotoxic periodic paralysis and the familial form. In the thyrotoxic condition there is *never* a family history of the disease and the age of onset is usually somewhat later, corresponding to the age incidence of thyrotoxicosis. Furthermore, the occurrence of attacks of paralysis is not generally related to the duration or the severity of the thyrotoxicosis, and by no available thyroid function test could a distinction be made between those with and those without paralysis.

Careful assessment of the anatomic alterations in muscle fibers between and during attacks of thyrotoxic periodic paralysis has not shown any significant or specific alterations. Schutta and Armitage [179, 180] have seen minimal evidence of structural damage, with distention of the sarcoplasmic reticulum, especially the terminal sacs. These vacuolar distentions were filled with granular material which they suggested may represent excessive calcium accumulation within the sarcoplasmic reticulum. They also found vacuoles within muscle fibers which were not dilatations of the sarcoplasmic reticulum but which they felt may represent sequestered areas of focal myofiber necrosis. Also changes such as alterations in mitochondria, lipid droplets, and other nonspecific changes were observed. Others [174, 181] have observed minor vacuolar and other changes in muscle fibers in thyrotoxic periodic paralysis. Usually light microscopy will fail to reveal changes, even when the biopsy is taken during an attack of paralysis.

SUMMARY

1 Periodic paralysis is a syndrome characterized by attacks of flaccid paralysis. The paralysis rarely involves the bulbar and cranial musculature, and there are no sensory or sphincter changes. Three varieties of the disorder are recognized, one with reduced plasma concentrations of potassium during attacks, another with increased concentrations, and a third with normal plasma potassium. All are inherited as autosomal dominant traits. Periodic paralysis may also occur secondary to thyrotoxicosis and other metabolic disorders.

2 Hypokalemic periodic paralysis occurs more frequently and severely in males than in females. Attacks occur on rest after exertion, after a high-carbohydrate diet, or on exposure to cold or other stress. They may be induced by insulin with glucose, ACTH, adrenal cortical steroids, and epinephrine. Characteristic vacuoles appear within the myofibrils. During attacks the plasma potassium falls but there is a net positive balance of potassium before the attack commences. Sodium is retained as well. The muscle membranes are depolarized during attacks. The pathogenesis of the disease remains undetermined.

3 Hyperkalemic periodic paralysis is also more severe in males. Attacks are precipitated by rest after exertion, by cold and hunger, and may be induced by administration of potassium. During seizures the muscle content of potassium falls. The pathogenesis of this disorder is likewise unknown. Paramyotonia congenita is a related syndrome.

4 Normokalemic periodic paralysis has been described in a single large kindred. Duration of paralytic attacks is much longer than in the other two types. Muscle biopsy findings are indistinguishable from the other types.

5 Periodic paralysis which occurs in association with thyrotoxicosis is not familial. This disorder has been seen mostly but not exclusively in Japanese. It disappears with correction of the thyrotoxicosis. The clinical pattern is not distinguishable from that of hypokalemic periodic paralysis.

Preparation of this review was greatly aided by a grant from the Muscular Dystrophy Associations of America and by Grant GM-15759 from the U.S. Public Health Service.

BIBLIOGRAPHY

1. Musgrave, W.: A periodical palsy. The Philosophical Transactions and Collections to the end of the year 1700. London, **2,** 33, 1727.
2. Seiler: Periodische Lahmung. Arch. Med. Erfahr., **1,** 117, 1815. Cited by Talbott [17].
3. Shakhnovitch: On a case of intermittent paraplegia. Russk. Vrach., **32,** 537, 1882; abstracted in London Med. Rec., **12,** 130, 1884.
4. Westphal, C.: Ueber einen merkwurdigen Fall von periodischer Lahmung aller vier Extremitaten mit gleichzeitigem Erloschen der elektrischen Erregbarkeit wahrend der Lahmung. Berlin. klin. Wschr., **22,** 489, 509, 1885.
5. Goldflam, S.: Ueber eine Eigenthümliche Form von periodischer, familiarer, wahrscheinlich autointoxicatorischer Paralyse. Wien. Med. Presse, **31,** 1418, 1457, 1500, 1536, 1890.
6. Pearson, C. M.: The periodic paralyses: Differential features and pathological observations in permanent myopathic weakness. Brain, **87,** 341, 1964.
7. Buzzard, E. F.: Three cases of family periodic paralysis with a consideration of the pathology of the disease. Lancet, **2:** 1564, 1901.
8. Singer, H. D., and Goodbody, F. W.: A case of family periodic paralysis with a critical digest of the literature. Brain, **24,** 257, 1901.
9. Mitchell, J. K., Flexner, S., and Edsall, D. L.: A brief report of the clinical, physiological and chemical study of three cases of family periodic paralysis. Brain, **25,** 109, 1902.
10. Kramer, W. W.: Zur Frage der periodischen Paralyse der Extremitaten. Russ. Med. Rundschau, **6,** 453, 517, 1908.
11. Shinosaki, T.: Klinische Studien uber die periodische Extremitatenlahmung. Z. Ges. Neurol. Psychiat., **100,** 564, 1926.
12. Biemond, A., and Daniels, A. P.: Familial periodic paralysis and its transition into spinal muscular atrophy. Brain, **57,** 91, 1934.
13. Aitken, R. S., Allott, E. N., Castleden, L.I.M., and Walker, M.: Observations on a case of familial periodic paralysis. Clin. Sci., **3,** 47, 1937.
14. Allott, E. N., and McArdle, B.: Further observations on familial periodic paralysis. Clin. Sci., **3,** 229, 1938.
15. Gammon, G. D., Austin, J. H., Blithe, M. D., and Reid, C. G.: The relation of potassium to periodic family paralysis. Amer. J. Med. Sci., **197,** 326, 1939.
16. Ferrebee, J. W., Gerity, M. K., Atchley, D. W., and Loeb, R. F.: Behavior of electrolytes in familial periodic paralysis. Arch. Neurol. Psychiat., **44,** 830, 1940.
17. Talbott, J. H.: Periodic paralysis: A clinical syndrome. Medicine (Balt.), **20,** 85, 1941.
18. Grob, D., Johns, R. J., and Liljestrand, A.: Potassium movement in patients with familial periodic paralysis: Relationship to the defect in muscle function. Amer. J. Med., **23,** 356, 1957.
19. Zierler, K. L., and Andres, R.: Movement of potassium into skeletal muscle during spontaneous attack in family periodic paralysis. J. Clin. Invest., **36,** 730, 1957.
20. Shy, G. M., Wanko, T., Rowley, P. T., and Engel, A. G.: Studies in familial periodic paralysis. Exp. Neurol., **3,** 53, 1961.
21. Streeten, D. H. P.: Periodic Paralysis, in *The Metabolic Basis of Inherited Disease,* edited by J. B. Stanbury, J. B. Wyngaarden, and D. S. Fredrickson, 2nd ed. pp. 905–938. McGraw-Hill, New York, 1966.
22. Conn, J. W., Fajans, S. S., Louis, L. H., Streeten, D. H. P., and Johnson, R. D.: Intermittent aldosteronism in periodic paralysis: Dependence of attacks on retention of sodium, and failure to induce attacks by restriction of dietary sodium. Lancet, **1,** 802, 1957.
23. Rowley, P. T., and Kliman, B.: The effect of sodium loading and depletion on muscular strength and aldosterone excretion in familial periodic paralysis. Amer. J. Med., **28,** 376, 1960.
24. Vaughan Jones, R., McSwiney, R. R., and Brooks, R. V.: Periodic paralysis: Sodium metabolism and aldosterone output in two cases. Lancet, **1,** 177, 1959.
25. McArdle, B.: Familial periodic paralysis., Brit. Med. Bull., **12,** 226, 1956.
26. Satoyoshi, E., Suzuki, Y., and Abe, T.: Periodic paralysis: A study of carbohydrate and thiamine metabolism, Neurology (Minneap.), **13,** 24, 1963.
27. Olivarius, B. de F., and Christensen, E.: Histopathological muscular changes in familial periodic paralysis. Acta Neurol. Scand., **41,** 1, 1965.
28. Howes, E. L., Price, H. M., Pearson, C. M., and Blumberg, J. M.: Hypokalemic periodic paralysis. Electronmicroscopic changes in the sarcoplasm. Neurology (Minneap.), **16,** 242, 1966.
29. Engel, A. G.: Electron microscopic observations in primary hypokalemic and thyrotoxic periodic paralysis. Mayo Clinic Proc., **41,** 797, 1966.
30. Odor, D. L., Patel, A. N., and Pearce, L. A.: Familial hypokalemic periodic paralysis with permanent myopathy: A clinical and ultrastructural study. J. Neuropath. Exp. Neurol., **26,** 98, 1967.
31. Pratt, R. T. C.: *The Genetics of Neurological Disorders.* Oxford University Press, London, 1967.
32. MacLachlan, T. K.: Familial periodic paralysis: A description of six cases occurring in three generations of one family. Brain, **55,** 47, 1932.

33. Bickerstaff, E. R.: Periodic paralysis. J. Neurol. Neurosurg. Psychiat., **16,** 178, 1953.
34. Oliver, C. P., Ziegler, M., and McQuarrie, I.: Hereditary periodic paralysis in a family showing varied manifestations. Amer. J. Dis., Child., **68,** 308, 1944.
35. Helweg-Larsen, H. F., Hauge, M., and Sagild, U.: Hereditary transient muscular paralysis in Denmark: Genetic aspects of family periodic paralysis and family periodic adynamia. Acta. Genet. (Basel), **5,** 263, 1955.
36. Meyer, R. N.: Periodisk paralyse. Nord. Med., **48,** 1360–1365, 1952.
37. Gaupp, R. Jr.: Erblichkeitsuntersuchungen bei paroxysmaler Lähmung. Z. Ges. Neurol. Psychiat., **170,** 108, 1940.
38. Gaupp, R., and Kalden, O.: Erblichkeitsundersuchungen bei paroxysmaler Lahmung. Z. Ges. Neurol. Psychiat., **174,** 194, 1942.
39. Khan, M. Y.: Familial periodic paralysis. Indian Med. Gaz., **70,** 28, 1935.
40. McKusick, V. A.: *Mendelian Inheritance in Man,* Catalogue of: Johns Hopkins, Baltimore, 1966.
41. Sagild, U.: *Hereditary Transient Paralysis.* Munksgaard, Copenhagen, 1959.
42. Chen, K. M., et al.: Periodic paralysis in Taiwan: Clinical study of 28 cases. Arch. Neurol. (Chicago), **12,** 165–171, 1965.
43. Glynn, M. F., Talso, P. J., Oester, Y. T., and Fudema, J.: Studies in familial periodic paralysis. Clin. Res., **10,** 226, 1962.
44. Cusins, P. J., and Van Rooyen, R. J.: Familial periodic paralysis: Seven cases in a Durban family. S. Afr. Med. J., **37,** 1180, 1963.
45. Dalinghaus; E. A.: Die periodische oder paroxysmale Lahmung (Myoplegia paroxysmalis). Zbl. Ges. Neurol. Psychiat., **100,** 1, 1941.
46. McArdle, B.: Metabolic myopathies: The glycogenoses affecting muscle and hypo- and hyper-kalemic periodic paralysis. Amer. J. Med., **35,** 661, 1963.
47. Mankowsky, B. N.: Über die paroxysmale paralyse. Arch. Psychiat., **87,** 280, 1929.
48. Benedek, L., and Von Angyal, L.: Beitrage zue Pathogenese der paroxysmalen Lahmung (Myoplegia familaris). Z. Ges. Neurol. Psychiat., **174,** 213, 1942.
49. McArdle, B.: Metabolic and endocrine myopathies, in *Disorders of Voluntary Muscle,* edited by J. N. Walton, pp. 607-638. J. and A. Churchill Ltd., 1964.
50. Taylor, E. W.: Family periodic paralysis: With a report of cases hitherto unpublished. J. Nerv. Mental Dis., **25,** 637, 1898.
51. Zabriskie, E. G., and Frantz, A. M.: Familial periodic paralysis. Bull. Neurol. Inst., New York, **2,** 57, 1932.
52. Crafts, L. M.: A fifth case of family periodic paralysis. Amer. J. Med. Sci., **119,** 651, 1900.
53. Putnam, J. J.: A case of family periodic paralysis. Amer. J. Med. Sci., **119,** 160, 1900.
54. Gardner, H. W.: A case of periodic paralysis. Brain, **35,** 243, 1912–1913.
55. McArdle, B.: Le rôle du potassium dans la paralysié periodique familiale. Sem. Hop. Paris, **30,** 3724, 1954.
56. Conn, J. W., Louis, L. H., Fajans, S. S., Streeten, D. H. P., and Johnson, R. D.: Dependence of attacks of periodic paralysis upon retention of sodium and failure to induce either paralysis or sequestration of potassium when dietary sodium is restricted. Trans. Ass. Amer. Physicians, **70,** 167, 1957.
57. Stewart, H. J., Smith, J. J., and Milhorat, A. T.: Electrocardiographic and serum potassium changes in familial periodic paralysis, Amer. J. Med. Sci., **199,** 789, 1940.
58. Stoll, B., and Nisnewitz, S.: Electrocardiographic studies in a case of periodic paralysis. Arch. Intern. Med. (Chicago), **67,** 755, 1941.
59. Perelson, H. N., and Cosby, R. S.: The electrocardiogram in familial periodic paralysis. Amer. Heart J., **37,** 1126, 1949.
60. Klein, R., Ganelin, R., Marks, J. F., Usher, R., and Richards, C.: Periodic paralysis with cardiac arrhythmia. J. Pediat., **62,** 371–385, 1963.
61. Oppenheim, H.: Neue Mittheilungen uber den von Professor Westphal beschriebenen Fall von periodischer Lahmung aller vier Extremitaten. Charite-ann., **16,** 350, 1891.
62. Coppen, A. J., and Reynolds, E. H.: Electrolyte and water distribution in familial hypokalemic periodic paralysis. J. Neurol. Neurosurg. Psychiat., **29,** 107, 1966.
63. Pudenz, R. H., McIntosh, J. F., and McEachern, D.: The role of potassium in familial periodic paralysis. JAMA, **111,** 2253, 1938.
64. Gass, H., Cherkasky, M., and Savitsky, N.: Potassium and periodic paralysis: A metabolic study and physiological considerations. Medicine (Balt.), **27,** 105, 1948.
65. Eales, L., Linder, G. C., and Sakinofsky, I.: Sodium and potassium balance in relation to periodic paralysis and in a case of pyelonephritis with malignant hypertension. S. Afr. Med. J., **32,** 251, 1958.
66. Jung, R.: Physiologische untersuchungen beir der familiaren paroxysmalen Lahmung. *III. Congr. Neurol. Int.,* Copenhagen, 1939, p. 291.
67. Hammes, E. M.: Periodic paralysis: A report of three cases. JAMA, **146,** 1401, 1951.
68. Saunders, M. G.: Electroencephalograph findings in a case of familial periodic paralysis with hypopotassemia. Electroenceph. Clin. Neurophysiol., **6,** 499, 1954.
69. Fowler, W. M., and Pearson, C. M.: Diagnostic and prognostic significance of serum enzymes: II. Neurologic diseases other than muscular dystrophy. Arch. Phys. Med., **45,** 125, 1966.
70. Eichler, W., Jantz, H., and Jung, R.: Elektromyographische Untersuchungen uber die paroxysmale Lahmung. Z. Ges. Neurol. Psychiat., **170,** 531, 1940.
71. Satayoshi, E., et al.: Periodic paralysis in hyperthyroidism. Neurology (Minneap.), **13,** 746, 1963.
72. Resnick, J. S., and Engel, W. K.: Myotonic lid lag in hypokalemic periodic paralysis. J. Neurol. Neurosurg. Psychiat., **30,** 47, 1967.
73. Fudema, J. J., Oester, Y. T., Talso, P. J., and Glynn, M. F.: Electromyography and electrodiagnosis in familial periodic paralysis. Bull. Amer. Ass. Electromyog. Electrodiag., **9,** 7, 1962.
74. Engel, A. G., Lambert, E. H., Rosevear, J. W., and Newlon Tauxe, W.: Clinical and electromyographic studies in a patient with primary hypokalemic periodic paralysis. Amer. J. Med., **38,** 626, 1965.
75. Niall, J. F., and Pak Poy, R. K.: Studies in familial hypokalaemic periodic paralysis. Aust. Ann, Med., **15,** 352, 1966.
76. Danowski, T. S., Elkinton, J. R., Burrows, B. A., and Winkler, A.: Exchanges of sodium and potassium in familial periodic paralysis. J. Clin. Invest., **27,** 65, 1948.
77. McQuarrie, I., and Ziegler, M. R.: Hereditary periodic paralysis. II. Effects of fasting and of various types of diet on occurrence of paralytic attacks. Metabolism, **1,** 129, 1952.
78. Berliner, R. W.: The kidney. Ann. Rev. Physiol., **16,** 269, 1954.
79. Milne, M. D., Jones, N. C. H., and Evans, B. M.: Electrolyte excretion in states of potassium depletion in man, in *Ciba Foundation Symposium on the Kidney,* edited by A. A. G. Lewis, and G. E. W. Wolstenholme, pp. 212–223. Little, Brown, Boston, 1954.
80. Pullman, T. N., and McClure, W. W.: The effect of L-noradrenaline on electrolyte excretion in normal man. J. Lab. Clin. Med., **39,** 711, 1952.
81. Graeff, J. de, and Lameijer, L. D.: Periodic paralysis. Amer. J. Med., **39,** 70, 1965.
82. McArdle, B., and Merton, P. A.: The behavior of radio-potassium in man. J. Physiol. (London), **116,** 51, 1952.
83. Conn, J. W., and Streeten, D. H. P.: Periodic paralysis, in *The Metabolic Basis of Inherited Disease,* edited by J. B. Stanbury, J. B. Wyngaarden, and D. S. Fredrickson, 1st ed., p. 867. McGraw-Hill New York, 1960.
84. Talso, P. J., Glynn, M. F., Oester, Y. T., and Fudema, J.: Body composition in hypokalemic familial periodic paralysis. Ann. NY Acad. Sci., **110,** 993, 1963.
85. Kirk, E., and Moller, E.: Studies on a case of paroxysmal myoplegia. Acta Med. Scand., **80,** 64, 1933.
86. Cerny, A., and Katzenstein-Sutro, E.: Die paroxysmale Lahmung. Schweiz. Arch. Neurol. Neurochiv. Psychiat., **70,** 259, 1952.
87. Engel, A. G.: Thyroid function and periodic paralysis. Amer. J. Med., **30,** 327, 1961.
88. Jantz, H.: Stoff Wechseluntersuchungen bei paroxysmaler Lahmung. Nervenarzt, **18,** 360, 1947.

89. Vastola, E. F., and Bertrand, C. A.: Intracellular water and potassium in periodic paralysis. Neurology (Minneap.), **6**, 523, 1956.
90. Darrow, D. C., Schwartz, R., Iannucci, J. F., and Coville, R.: The relation of serum bicarbonate concentration to muscle composition. J. Clin. Invest., **27**, 198, 1948.
91. Hofmann, W. W., and Smith, R. A.: Hypokalemic periodic paralysis studied *in vitro*. Brain, **93**, 445, 1970.
92. Hazelwood, C. F., Nichols, B. L., and Chamberlin, N. F.: Evidence for the existence of a minimum of two phases of ordered water in skeletal muscle. Nature (London), **222**, 747, 1969.
93. Ling, G. N., and Cope, F. W.: Potassium ion: Is the bulk of intracellular K^+ adsorbed? Science, **163**, 1335, 1969.
94. Engel, A. G., Potter, C. S., and Rosevear, J. W.: Nucleotides and adenosine monophosphate deaminase activity of muscle in primary hypokalaemic periodic paralysis. Nature (London), **202**, 670, 1964.
95. Goldflam, S.: Dritte Mitteilung uber die paroxysmale, familiar Lahmung. Deutsch. Z. Nervenheilk., **11**, 242, 1897.
96. Holtzapple, G. E.: Periodic paralysis. JAMA, **45**, 1224, 1905.
97. Bekeny, G.: Uber irreversible Muskelveranderungen bei der paroxysmalen Lahmung auf Grund bioptischer Muskeluntersuchungen. Deutsch. Z. Nervenheilk., **182**, 119, 1961.
98. Bekeny, G., Haznos, T., and Solti, F.: Uber die hypokalamische form der paroxysmalen Lahmung Untersuchungen an einem Geschwisterpaar. Deutsch. Z. Nervenheilk., **182**, 69, 1961.
99. Bekeny, G., Hasznos, T., and Solti, F.: Uber die hyperkalamische Form der paroxysmalen Lahmung zur Frage der Adynamia episodica hereditaria. Deutsch. Z. Nervenheilk., **182**, 92, 1961.
100. Adams, R. D., Denny-Brown, D., and Pearson, C. M.: *Diseases of Muscle: A Study in Pathology,* 2d ed. Hoeber-Harper, New York, 1962.
101. Gruner, J. E., and Porte, A.: Les Lesions Musculaires de la paralysie Periodique Familiale. Rev. Neurol. (Paris), **101**, 501, 1959.
102. Humphreys, E. M., and Kato, K.: Glycogen storage disease: Thesaurismosis glycogenica (von Gierke). Amer. J. Path., **10**, 589, 1934.
103. Engel, A. G.: Electron microscopic observations in metabolic myopathies (three types of hypokalemic periodic paralysis, thyrotoxic myopathy and steroid induced myopathy). J. Neuropath. Exp. Neurol., **24**, 141, 1965.
104. MacDonald, R. D., Rewcastle, N. B., and Humphrey, J. G.: Myopathy of hypokalemic periodic paralysis. Arch. Neurol. (Chicago), **20**, 566, 1969.
105. Biczyskowa, W., Fidzianska, A., and Jedrzejowska, H.: Light and electron microscopic study of the muscles in hypokalemic periodic paralysis. Acta Neuropath. (Berlin), **12**, 329, 1969.
106. Engel, W. K.: Mitochondrial aggregates in muscle diseases. J. Histochem. Cytochem., **12**, 46, 1964.
107. Kuchel, O., Kandrae, J., and Charvat, J.: Einige probleme der pathogenese hypokalamischer muskelahmungen. Endokrinologie, **41**, 129, 1961.
108. Conn, J. W.: Presidential address. Part I. Painting background. Part II. Primary aldosteronism, a new clinical syndrome. J. Lab. Clin. Med., **45**, 3, 1955.
109. Giroire, H., Charbonnel, A., Vercelletto, P., and Delhumeaw: Une nouvelle observation de paralysies avec hypokaliemic par ingestion excessive d'extrait de reglisse. Rev. Neurol. (Paris), **104**, 539, 1961.
110. Gross, E. G., Dexter, J. D., and Roth, R. G.: Hypokalemic myopathy with myoglobinuria associated with licorice ingestion. New Eng. J. Med., **274**, 602, 1966.
111. Ferrebee, J. W., Parker, D., Carnes, W. H., Gerity, M. K., Atchley, D. W., and Loeb, R. W.: Certain effects of deoxycorticosterone: The development of "diabetes insipidus" and the replacement of muscle potassium by sodium in normal dogs. Amer. J. Physiol., **135**, 230, 1941.
112. Engel, A. G., Potter, C. S., and Rosevear, J. W.: Studies on carbohydrate metabolism and mitochondrial respiratory activities in primary hypokalemic periodic paralysis. Neurology (Minneap.), **17**, 329, 1967.
113. Johns, R. J.: The electrical and mechanical events of neuromuscular transmission. Amer. J. Med., **35**, 611, 1963.
114. Creutzfeldt, O., Abbott, B. C., Fowler, W. M., and Pearson, C. M.: Muscle membrane potentials in episodic adynamia. Electroenceph. Clin. Neurophysiol., **15**, 508, 1963.
115. Rieker, G., and Bolte, H. D.: Membranpotentiale einzelner Skeletmuskelzellen bei hypokaliamischer periodischer Muskelparalyse. Klin. Wschr., **44**, 804, 1966.
116. McComas, A. J., Mrozek, K., and Bradley, W. G.: The nature of the electrophysiological disorder in adynamia episodica. J. Neurol. Neurosurg. Psychiat., **31**, 48, 1968.
117. Adrian, R. H.: Movement of inorganic ions across the membrane of striated muscle. Circulation, **26**, 1214, 1962.
118. Skou, J. C.: Studies on the $Na^+ + K^+$ activated ATP hydrolyzing enzyme system: The role of SH groups. Biochem. Biophys. Res. Commun., **10**, 79, 1963.
119. Hokin, L. E., and Hokin, M. R.: Phosphatidic acid metabolism and active transport of sodium. Fed. Proc., **22**, 8, 1963.
120. Judah, J. D., Ahmed, K., and McLean, A. E. M.: Phosphoproteins and sodium transport. Nature (London), **196**, 484, 1962.
121. Adrian, R. H.: In *The Cellular Function of Membrane Transport,* edited by J. F. Hoffman, pp. 55–70. Prentice-Hall, Englewood Cliffs, N.J., 1964.
122. Hodgkin, A. L., and Horowicz, P.: The influence of potassium and chloride ions on the membrane potential of single muscle fibers. J. Physiol. (London), **148**, 127, 1959.
123. Engel, A. G., and Lambert, E. H.: Effects of calcium on isolated muscle fibers in hypokalemic periodic paralysis. Neurology (Minneap.), **18**, 275, 1968.
124. Solomon, S.: Theoretical diencephalic factors in periodic paralysis. Arch. Neurol. (Chicago), **9**, 55, 1963.
125. Grossman, C.: Periodic paralysis associated with obesity of hypothalamic origin: Observations in a case with changes in the electrocardiogram and serum potassium level. Arch. Neurol. Psychiat., **62**, 105, 1949.
126. Prader, A., and Zellweger, H.: Periodic hypopotassemic paralysis with hyperelectrolytemia in a case of dystrophia adiposogenitalia. Helv. Paediat. Acta, **7**, 42, 1952.
127. Kjerulf-Jensen, K., Krarup, N. B., and Warming-Larsen, A.: Persistent hypokalemia requiring constant potassium therapy. Lancet, **1**, 372, 1951.
128. Valso, R.: Periodic paralysis and the hypothalamus: A neurohumoral disorder. Nord. Med., **46**, 1134, 1951.
129. Poskanzer, D. C., and Kerr, D. N. S.: Periodic paralysis with response to spirinolactone. Lancet, **2**, 511, 1961.
130. Okinaka, S., Ohsawa, N., Shizume, K., Motohashi, K., Fujita, T., Murakawa, S., Matsuzake, F., Morii, H., and Uchikawa, T.: Effect of aldosterone antagonist (Sc 9420) on periodic paralysis. J. Clin. Endocr., **22**, 549, 1962.
131. Resnick, J. S., Engel, W. K., Griggs, R. C., and Stam, A. C.: Acetozolamide prophylaxis in hypokalemic periodic paralysis. New Eng. J. Med., **278**, 582–86, 1968.
132. Maas, O., and Paterson, A. S.: Myotonia congenita, dystrophia myotonia and paramyotonia: Reaffirmation of their identity. Brain, **73**, 318, 1950.
133. Tyler, F. H., Stephens, F. E., Gunn, F. D., and Perkoff, G. T.: Studies on disorders of muscle. VII. Clinical manifestations on inheritance of a type of periodic paralysis without hypopotassemia. J. Clin. Invest., **30**, 492, 1951.
134. Gamstorp, I.: Adynamia episodica hereditaria. Acta Paediat., **45**, (suppl. 108), 1, 1956.
135. Eulenberg, A.: Uber eine familiare, durch 6 Generationen urfolgbare Form congenitaler Paramyotonie. Neurol. Centralb., **5**, 265, 1886.
136. French, E. B., and Kilpatrick, R.: A variety of paramyotonia congenita. J. Neurol. Neurosurg. Psychiat., **20**, 40, 1957.
137. Bull, G. M., Carter, A. B., and Loure, K. G.: Hyperpotassemic paralysis. Lancet, **2**, 60, 1953.
138. Kaplan, M., et al.: L'Adynamie episodique hereditaire. Presse Med., **65**, 1305, 1957.
139. Egan, T. J., and Klein, R.: Hyperkalemic familial periodic paralysis. Pediatrics, **24**, 761, 1959.
140. Doak, P. B., and Eyre, K. E. D.: Adynamia episodica hereditaria or hyperkalemic periodic paralysis. New Zeal. Med. J., **60**, 19, 1961.
141. Van der Meulen, J. P., Gilbert, G. J., and Kane, C. A.: Familial hyperkalemic paralysis with myotonia. New Eng. J. Med., **26**, 1, 1961.
142. McArdle, B.: Adynamia episodica hereditaria and its treatment. Brain, **85**, 121, 1962.

143. Van't Hoff, W.: Familial myotonic periodic paralyses. Quart. J. Med., **31,** 385, 1962.
144. Armstrong, F. S.: Hyperkalemic familial periodic paralysis (adynamia episodica hereditaria). Ann. Intern. Med., **57,** 455, 1962.
145. Iverson, T. O.: Familial episodic adynamia. Acta Med. Scand., **171,** 737, 1962.
146. Gamstorp, I.: Adynamia episodica hereditaria and myotonia. Acta Neurol. Scand., **39,** 41, 1963.
147. Herman, R. H., and McDowell, M. K.: Hyperkalemic periodic paralysis (adynamia episodica hereditaria). Amer. J. Med., **35,** 749, 1963.
148. Allsop, J. L., et al.: Familial hyperkalaemic periodic paralysis. Aust. Ann. Med., **13,** 55, 1964.
149. Carson, M. J., and Pearson, C. M.: Familial hyperkalemic periodic paralysis with myotonic features. J. Pediat., **64,** 853, 1964.
150. Samaha, F. J.: Hyperkalemic periodic paralysis. Arch. Neurol. (Chicago), **12,** 145, 1965.
151. Layzer, R. B., Lovelace, R. E., and Rowland, L. P.: Hyperkalemic periodic paralysis. Arch. Neurol. (Chicago), **16,** 455, 1967.
152. Saunders, M., Ashworth, B., Emery, A. E. H., and Benedikz, J. E. G.: Familial myotonic periodic paralysis with muscle wasting. Brain, **91,** 295, 1968.
153. Bradley, W. G.: Adynamia episodica hereditaria. Clinical, pathological and electrophysiological studies in an affected family. Brain, **92,** 345, 1969.
154. Drager, G. A., Hammill, J. F., and Shy, G. M.: Paramyotonia congenita. Arch. Neurol. Psychiat., **80,** 1, 1958.
155. Dyken, M. L., and Timmons, G. D.: Hyperkalemic periodic paralysis with hypokalemic episodes. Arch. Neurol. (Chicago), **9,** 508, 1963.
156. Feneck, F., and Soler, N. G.: Hyperkalaemic periodic paralysis starting at age 48. Brit. Med. J., **2,** 2472, 1968.
157. Brooks, J. E.: Hyperkalemic periodic paralysis: Intracellular electromyographic studies. Arch. Neurol. (Chicago), **20,** 13, 1969.
158. Morrison, J. B.: The electromyographic changes in hyperkalemic familial periodic paralysis. Ann. Phys. Med., **5,** 153, 1960.
159. Klein, R., Egan, T., and Usher, P.: Changes in sodium, potassium and water in hyperkalemic familial periodic paralysis. Metabolism, **9,** 1005, 1960.
160. Hudson, A. J., Strickland, K. P., and Wilensky, A. J.: Serum enzyme studies in familial hyperkalemic periodic paralysis. Clin. Chim. Acta, **17,** 331, 1967.
161. Liljestrand, A.: A case of adynamia episodica hereditaria. Opusc. Med. (Stockh.), **2,** 183, 1957.
162. Krull, G. H., Leijnse, B., Vietor, W. P. J., Blieger, M., Ter Braak, J. W. G. and Gerbrandy, J.: Myotonia produced by an unknown humoral substance. Lancet, **2,** 668, 1966.
163. Jaffurs, W. J., Herman, R. H., McDowell, M. K., and Blumberg, J. E.: Hyperkalemic paralysis (adynamia episodica hereditaria): Ultrastructural studies of muscle in two cases. Metabolism, **12,** 740, 1963.
164. Bradley, W. G.: Ultrastructural changes in adynamia episodica hereditaria and normokalemic familial periodic paralysis. Brain, **92,** 379, 1969.
165. Caughey, J. E. and Myrianthopoulos, N. C.: *Dystrophia Myotonica and Related Disorders.* Thomas, Springfield, Illinois, 1963.
166. Magee, K. R.: A study of paramyotonia congenita. Arch. Neurol., **8,** 461, 1963.
167. Magee, K. R.: Paramyotonia congenita. Arch. Neurol., **14,** 590, 1966.
168. Gamstorp, I.: A study of transient muscular weakness. Acta Neurol. Scand., **38,** 3, 1962.
169. Merteus, H. G., et al.: Elektrolylund Aldosteronstoffwechsel bei der Adynamia episodica hereditaria, der hyperkaliamischen Form der periodischen Lahmung. Klin. Wschr., **42,** 65, 1964.
170. Bell, H., Hayes, W. L., and Vosburgh, J.: Hyperkalemic paralysis due to adrenal insufficiency. Arch. Int. Med., **115,** 418, 1965.
171. Buchthal, F., Engback, L., and Gamstorp, I.: Paresis and hyperexcitability in adynamia episodica hereditaria. Neurology, **7:** 347, 1958.
172. McFadzean, A. J. S., and Yeung, R.: Periodic paralysis complicating thyrotoxicosis in Chinese. Brit. Med. Journ. **1,** 451, 1967.
173. Chen, K. M., and Hung, T. P.: Periodic paralysis in Taiwan. Arch. Neurol., **12,** 165, 1965.
174. Norris, F. H., and Panner, B. J.: Thyrotoxic periodic paralysis. Arch. Neurol., **19,** 89, 1968.
175. Okihiro, M. M., and Beddow, R. M.: Thyrotoxic periodic paralysis in Hawaii. Neurology, **15,** 253, 1965.
176. Shizume, K., and Shishiba, Y.: Studies on electrolyte metabolism in idiopathic and thyrotoxic periodic paralysis. Metabolism, **15,** 138, 1966.
177. Shizume, K., et al.: Studies on electrolyte metabolism in idiopathic and thyrotoxic periodic paralysis. Metabolism, **15,** 145, 1966.
178. Shishiba, K., et al.: Studies on electrolyte metabolism in idiopathic and thyrotoxic periodic paralysis. Metabolism **15,** 153, 1966.
179. Schutta, H. S., and Armitage, J. L.: Thyrotoxic hypokalemic periodic paralysis. J. Neuropath. Exp. Neurol., **29,** 321, 1969.
180. Schutta, H. S., and Armitage, J. L.: The sarcoplasmic reticulum in thyrotoxic hypokalemic periodic paralysis. Metabolism **18,** (2), 81, 1969.
181. Engel, A. G.: Electron microscopic observations in primary hypokalemic and thyrotoxic periodic paralyses. Mayo Clin. Proc., **41,** 797, 1966.
182. Engel, A. G.: Evolution and content of vacuoles in primary hypokalemic periodic paralysis. Mayo Clinic Proc., **45,** 774, 1970.

CHAPTER FORTY-EIGHT
MUSCULAR DYSTROPHIES

Frank H. Tyler

Among the genetically determined disorders of man is a kind of abiotrophy of muscular tissue referred to as *muscular dystrophy.* This is not a single disease process but rather a category of disorders which are presently grouped together because of the histologic appearance of the damaged skeletal muscle and the absence of any primary neural lesion.

In the century since these disorders were differentiated from those with neural causes of muscular atrophy by the great European neurologists [1-3], many attempts have been made to explain their pathogenesis. It is now recognized that a number of clinically and genetically distinct disorders fall into this category. Unfortunately, many investigators in the past have failed to recognize this fact and thereby have compromised the usefulness of their data by pooling information from a variety of types of muscular dystrophy.

The prominent manifestation of muscular dystrophy is weakness and atrophy of skeletal muscle, but the disease process is not entirely limited to this structure. For example, there is evidence of myocardial involvement in most types of muscular dystrophy, and it is probable that smooth muscle is affected in at least the myotonic form. Involvement of nonmuscular tissue also occurs. The most striking example is myotonic dystrophy, in which baldness, lenticular cataracts, and testicular disease indicate effects of the abnormal gene on nonmuscular tissue.

A number of models of skeletal muscle disease have been developed in the experimental animal, and much information has been derived from study of several of these disorders. From the historical point of view the classic model has been that induced in many experimental animals by vitamin E deficiency. For a variety of reasons it now seems evident that this model is not closely related to the human disorders. In particular the very high rates of oxidation within the muscle and in the whole animal, as well as the marked regeneration of muscle tissue, are strikingly different. Somewhat similar muscular disorders can be induced in animals by glycine deficiency, potassium deficiency, and a number of other methods.

Most promising has been the discovery that genetically determined disorders of skeletal muscle occur spontaneously in a number of animal species. Extensive studies have been made of the Bar Harbor 129 dystrophic mouse [4], and preliminary investigations have been made of types of genetically determined muscle disease in chickens [5], hamsters [6], and sheep [7]. There is no certainty that any of these types of muscle disease is closely related to the human disorders in spite of histologic resemblance. Because of these difficulties no attempt will be made here to describe in detail the studies of these animal models except as they relate specifically to observations made in man.

The present discussion includes a description of the clinical manifestations of the commoner types of human muscular dystrophy. This is followed by an analysis of available information, from which a hypothesis is developed concerning the possible mechanisms which might result in the progressive muscular destruction that characterizes these disorders. The evidence has been derived primarily from histologic and histochemical studies of muscle structure, from studies of the biochemical constituents of the muscular tissue, and from abnormalities in the blood plasma which are apparently secondary to the process in the muscle itself. The possibility that the primary biochemical anomaly is not in muscle has been little pursued in recent times, but there is also evidence that certain abnormalities exist in the vascular system unrelated to myocardial disease per se, at least in some types of muscular dystrophy. And finally many therapeutic trials have been carried out over the years in an attempt to modify the clinical course of this distressingly disabling group of disorders; some information, at least of negative value, bearing on the pathogenesis of the disease may be derived from a brief discussion of these trials.

TYPES OF MUSCULAR DYSTROPHY

In recent years a clinical classification of the muscular dystrophies has been developed on which there is general agreement at the present time [8-10]. The more frequent types are usually called *Duchenne's, facioscapulohumeral, limb-girdle,* and *myotonic dystrophy.* A brief description of each of these and an attempt to evaluate their specificity and the clinical and genetic homogeneity of each will be helpful in demonstrating the complexities which limit any attempt to understand the pathogenesis of these disorders.

Duchenne's Muscular Dystrophy

Clinical Features

The Duchenne type [4, 11] of muscular dystrophy is primarily a disorder of boys. The onset of symptoms usually occurs between the ages of 2 and 6 years, and begins with weakness in the pelvic girdle musculature. In most patients the disorder runs an insidious but relatively rapid course. The progressive muscular disability extends rapidly to the pectoral girdle and trunk musculature and somewhat more slowly to the distal muscles of the extremities. The muscle atrophy is not a diffuse process at the beginning but rather affects individual muscles and even parts of proximal muscles selectively. For example, the sternal head of the pectoralis major is more affected than are the clavicular fibers of this muscle. This pattern of muscle atrophy is the best clinical sign in establishing the diagnosis of this and other dystrophies. The progression tends to be symmetric in its development.

Pseudohypertrophy

A peculiar and intriguing finding is the so-called pseudohypertrophy in some muscles in this disorder. The enlarging muscles are among the first clinical features of the disease, and they tend to maintain their abnormal size over a prolonged period of time. The rate of progression of muscular weakness is slower in these muscles than it is in other muscles in which the infiltration is less marked. Nearly all the patients show this phenomenon in the calf muscles, and some will show it in the deltoids and triceps as well. An occasional patient has pseudohypertrophy of many muscle groups. Clinically it consists of an enlarged but weakened muscle mass which has an inelastic and fibrous texture on palpation. Pathologically the muscle shows much increase in fat and fibrous tissue. This is only an exaggeration of the phenomena regularly present in all dystrophic muscle tissue. It is not specific for this particular kind of muscular dystrophy nor universal among the patients who in other respects fit into this group. In my series approximately 90 percent of the patients with childhood dystrophy have shown typical pseudohypertrophy, but it has also been present in a small percentage of each of the other major types of muscular dystrophy.

Other Features

The development of contractures of muscle and tendon limiting the extension or flexion of joints is also a typical feature. This is usually first apparent in the calf muscles and tendons, but also involves knees, hips, and elbows in the majority of patients as the disease progresses.

The progression of the disease results in muscular disability which may prevent the patient from walking because of weakness and contracture as early as at 8 years of age. The majority of patients become wheelchair or bed invalids before adolescence. In a small proportion of patients the disease progresses less rapidly in childhood and they enter adolescence with severe disability which nonetheless is compatible with ambulation or wheelchair existence. In these patients the disease appears to stabilize and progress at a much less rapid rate, if at all; a number of my patients have survived into early adult life.

Genetics

The inheritance of the disorder conforms to that of an X-linked recessive trait [12] (Fig. 48-1). Transmission in a pedigree occurs through the female line, and the disorder develops in 50 percent of the male offspring of known carrier females. Normal male children of carriers do not transmit the trait.

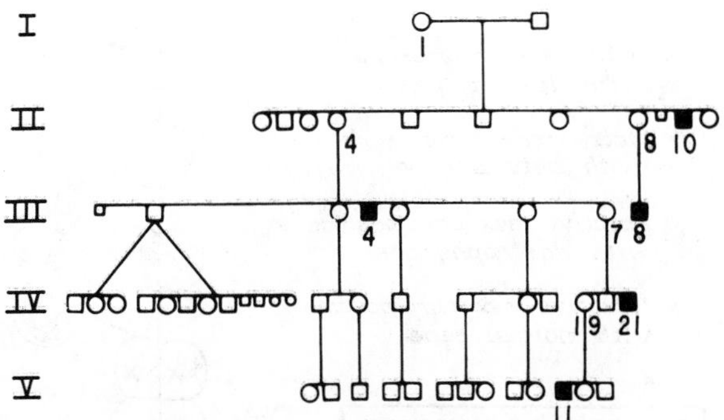

Figure 48-1. Pedigree of a family in which five patients with childhood muscular dystrophy are known. Note the transmission through certain females but not through unaffected males, and failure of patients with dystrophy to have children. This is typical X-linked recessive inheritance with failure of patients to reproduce.

An occasional pedigree has been reported in which sisters of patients with apparently typical Duchenne's dystrophy were affected with a similar kind of disorder. Interpretation of these cases is difficult. In many reports the disease has not been sufficiently clearly defined as typical Duchenne's muscular dystrophy, and it seems probable that infantile muscular atrophy and other diseases have been confused with this primary muscular disorder. On the other hand, some of these are typical and there has been good histologic evidence for the dystrophic muscular lesion. It may be that a clinically indistinguishable disease is transmitted in some families as an autosomal trait.

Pertinent to this consideration is the recent observation that many of the carrier females for this disorder can be identified by the presence of elevated aldolase or creatine phosphokinase levels in the plasma [13–15]. These are the muscle enzymes with the most strikingly elevated level in the serum of the affected subjects. A few such carrier females have had very high serum levels, and show some muscular weakness and a histologic lesion on biopsy consistent with muscular dystrophy [16].

The hypothesis (Lyon's, see Chap. 3) that only one X chromosome is active in each somatic cell can be invoked to explain these observations (Fig. 48-2). It is proposed that inactivation of one X chromosome occurs early in embryogenesis and that in subsequent generations of somatic cells the same X chromosome remains active as in the parent cell of that line. It thus is possible to have wide variations from the average situation in which half the cells have one X chromosome active and half have the other. One is tempted to speculate that the previously reported instances of affected female sibs represented the extreme degree of this manifestation in the heterozygous female. If indeed only a small part of the total body cells are important in the

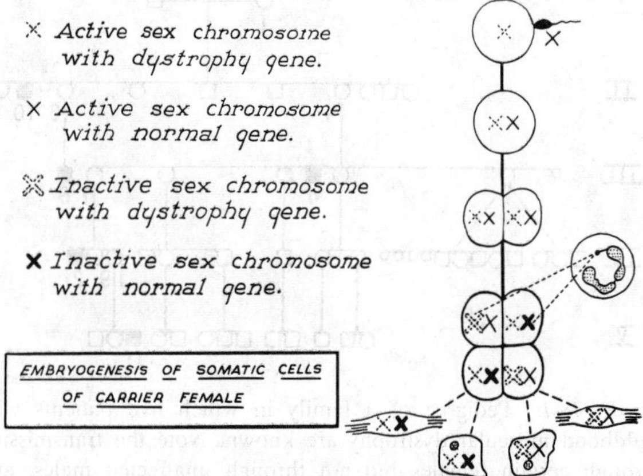

Figure 48-2. Diagrammatic representation of Lyon's hypothesis in the development of the heterozygous female zygote for childhood dystrophy. Differentiated cells on the right would be normal, and the cells on the left would be "dystrophic."

determination of the genetic anomaly, the extreme variability of plasma levels of creatine phosphokinase in the carrier female is satisfactorily explained.

In most series a third or more of cases appear to be sporadic in origin, and in many pedigrees it can be demonstrated conclusively from the statistical point of view that the trait was not transmitted in the female line antecedent to the involved male [12]. Most investigators have assumed that these sporadic cases represent new mutants of the same gene which causes the abnormality in the families in which the trait is obviously transmitted. This assumption requires a higher mutation rate than is usually seen in human genetic material, and in some series there are more apparently sporadic cases than would be accounted for by total failure of reproduction on the part of the involved males [17–19]. The reason for this excess of sporadic cases is not clear at the present time. In my studies [15] only an occasional mother of a patient with an apparently sporadic case has been found to have an increased plasma creatine phosphokinase level. One should find this in about half the mothers if the mutation occurs at the same rate in all X chromosomes and all the sporadic cases are the result of new mutations.

Two other explanations should not be neglected until the biochemical pathogenesis of this disorder is defined. The first is the possibility that more than one genic mutant is involved or that some anomaly occurs which makes the mutant appear initially in the male instead of the female [17]. Another possibility, which is equally probable in our present state of knowledge, is that some of these sporadic cases are caused by an acquired anomaly which simulates the genetic situation, i.e., that these are phenocopies of the genetic disease.

Becker's Dystrophy

Becker described a group of patients with a condition which has been referred to as benign Duchenne's dystrophy. It is more appropriately called Becker's type of dystrophy. These patients resemble those with Duchenne's dystrophy in X-linked inheritance and pseudohypertrophy of the calf muscles. They are different in that the first symptoms are extremely mild and frequently not noted until after 6 years of age. Significant disability may begin in adolescence, but many of these patients show real progression only in the fifth or sixth decade. Dystrophic myocardiopathy is common.

Facioscapulohumeral Progressive Muscular Dystrophy

The disorder first described by Landouzy and Déjèrine [20] has a classic clinical appearance easily recognized by an experienced observer. It is a relatively benign disease of adult life in the majority of patients, but definite abnormalities of muscular pattern and strength are present in all or nearly all individuals who carry the trait [21].

Clinical Features

Symptoms usually begin in adolescence, with weakness in the pectoral girdle and facial muscles. Atrophy progresses slowly and insidiously to a pattern similar to that in Duchenne's dystrophy except for the greater involvement of the pectoral than the pelvic girdle in most of the patients. Characteristic facial involvement and appearance develop which are rarely present in other dystrophies. This is a peculiar kind of focal atrophy resulting in inability to pucker the mouth and whistle normally, as well as in weakness of the orbicularis oculi and other facial muscles. Minimal manifestations can sometimes be observed as early as at age 6; essentially all the patients who carry the trait can be identified by age 12. Nevertheless, the total progression of the disease is extremely variable, and not infrequently patients in middle or late life fail to recognize their disability. Indeed, the benignity of the disorder in many patients has led one to suspect that its frequency is probably not very much different from that of Duchenne's dystrophy but that only an occasional patient is sufficiently disabled to seek medical attention. Its total incidence is unknown.

Genetics

The disorder is regularly inherited as an autosomal dominant trait. The disease in the homozygote is not clearly identified but may well be much more severe than in the heterozygote.

Limb-girdle Dystrophy

This term has been introduced [9] to identify a disorder that is different from either of the well-defined syndromes discussed above. It is uncertain whether it is a single clinical syndrome or simply a group of dystrophies without presently well-defined differentiating features. In general its manifestations are similar to those of Duchenne's and facioscapulohumeral dystrophy. In typical cases the disorder begins in preadolescence and progresses more rapidly than does facioscapulohumeral dystrophy. The face is usually spared. Many of the patients become disabled in late adolescence or early adult life so that they can no longer walk, but the course is variable. Usually the involvement is most severe in the pelvic girdle, but a number of patients are seen with initial symptoms at puberty in whom the disorder is first manifest in the pectoral girdle.

Genetics

Not infrequently two or more members of a sibship have similar manifestations, but pedigrees with multiple generations involved are unusual. Because of this it has been thought that this disorder is an autosomal recessive trait, but there is not sufficient evidence to establish this as the pattern of inheritance. The rather widely variable clinical manifestations, especially among different pedigrees, raise considerable doubt as to the specificity of this diagnosis from a clinical and genetic point of view. Nevertheless, it is a useful designation, because it covers most of the patients who have clinical dystrophy but do not have the clearly defined Duchenne's or facioscapulohumeral disease.

Rare Types

A number of other patients whose disorder fits the original definition of dystrophic muscle disease cannot easily be placed in the groups already described. The best defined of these is a distal disorder which is usually inherited as an autosomal dominant trait [22, 23]. It is slowly progressive, beginning in adolescence and producing only moderate disability.

A number of cases of extraocular muscle involvement have been seen which are referred to as the *ophthalmic type* [24]. The atrophy tends to remain restricted to the extraocular muscles. Most of the patients do not have affected relatives.

A number of other well-defined dystrophies have occurred in one or more families. A classic example is one described by Barnes [25] many years ago. These are obviously primary disorders of muscle which are closely related and not the same as the other dystrophies. Thus on the basis of clinical manifestations a variety of different disorders can be differentiated among the muscular dystrophies.

Myotonic Dystrophy

Myotonic dystrophy is one of the more common of the primary muscle diseases in which progressive atrophy occurs [26]. It differs considerably from the other types even though sharing with them a similar histologic pattern, lack of neural involvement, and obvious familial incidence.

Clinical Features

The disease begins in childhood with the appearance of myotonia. This frequently is mild and often is not recognized by the patient. During adolescence significant weakness, particularly in the dorsiflexors of the foot, tends to appear, and the patients begin to have significant difficulty with ambulation. In addition to focal involvement of proximal girdle muscles, there is involvement of peripheral musculature, with weakness in lower leg and foot, hand, and forearm. Progression is insidious and associated with loss of muscle mass and strength. The histologic picture is somewhat different from that in the other dystrophies, yet often it is not specific [27].

In addition to entailing muscle atrophy and weakness, myotonia can be demonstrated in well over 95 percent of patients at the time of first examination. Even in those in whom it is not present on grasp or percussion it can be identified electromyographically. In addition to this curious phenomenon, which is absent in the other types of dystrophy, baldness, lenticular cataracts, testicular atrophy, and rather characteristic and progressive emotional and intellectual changes are present.

Genetics

Occasionally an investigator has tried to classify each of the system involvements as a specific genetic trait, but this entire syndrome is the result of a single autosomal dominant trait (Fig. 48-3). It may well be that it is modified by environmental or other genetic factors which determine the severity of involvement not only of muscle but also of the extramuscular systems [28].

ANATOMIC CHANGES

The observation was made over 100 years ago that atrophy of the dystrophic muscle in the absence of a neural lesion is the means for differentiating between neural atrophy and dystrophic disease. The histologic lesion in the muscle itself is a random progressive destruction of individual muscle fibers and their replacement by fat and fibrous tissue. A characteristic lesion is a swollen fiber lacking its fibrillar structure, with the nuclei moved to the center. In biopsies taken very early in the course of Duchenne's dystrophy one also sees necrosis of fibers, macrophages, and occasionally even inflammatory cells. By the time the clinical disease is well established, these findings are uncommon, and most of the fibers are small and atrophic and show marked increase in sarcolemmal nuclei. These types of fibers are randomly mixed with fibers in the same fasciculus which appear normal.

Most observers have assumed that the increase in fibrous tissue within the muscle fasciculus is entirely secondary to the lesion of the muscle fiber itself, simply a scar replacing the normal fibers and fasciculi. Gollarz, Bourne, and

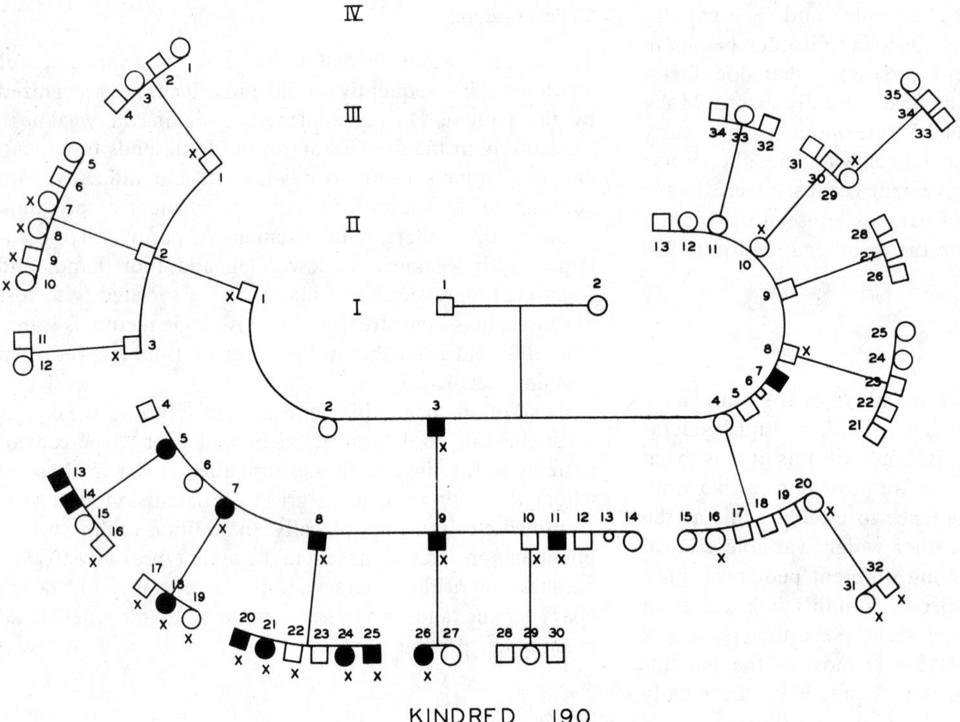

Figure 48-3. Pedigree of a family in which myotonic dystrophy occurs. Note the transmission by involved members to some of their children, without regard to sex, and failure of the disease to reappear in the descendants of nonaffected individuals. It is typical autosomal dominant inheritance.

Richardson [29] have made the interesting suggestion that the fibrous tissue may actually invade and destroy the normal muscle fibers. They have demonstrated that there is an increase in certain enzymes, particularly 5′-nucleotidase, relatively early in the course of the histologic change in the muscular tissue. This enzyme is a normal constituent of connective tissue, particularly of young and growing connective tissue. Thus the enzymatic changes are compatible with replacement fibrosis as well as with abnormal proliferation of connective tissue.

Another striking phenomenon in the muscular tissue is the presence of large amounts of fat within the fasciculi. This is uncommon both in neural and in inflammatory disease of muscle. Indeed pseudohypertrophy, a characteristic feature of Duchenne's dystrophy, is caused primarily by fatty and fibrous tissue within the muscle. The muscle fibers also are large and frequently show the round shape and hyaline change described above. Strength in the pseudohypertrophic muscle is relatively preserved but is not as great as would be predicted from the total muscle mass.

Fat infiltration also occurs in other muscles in which pseudohypertrophy is not present; it may reflect an important pathologic process in the development of the disease. Few studies have been carried out on the fatty tissue, and the specificity of the phenomenon is obscure. The fat of the pseudohypertrophic muscle appears to be relatively resistant to mobilization, since marked degrees of inanition may occur without loss of the typical lesion in the calf muscles.

When normal muscle is injured by such processes as polymyositis or acute crushing injury, rapid regeneration of muscle occurs. Regenerating muscle fibers are not prominent in the dystrophic muscle, and it has been proposed that an important defect in muscular dystrophy is the inability of the muscle to regenerate normally [30]. Regeneration is essentially normal after acute injury and can sometimes be found in association with active fiber destruction in the patient with incipient childhood dystrophy.

Vascular and Myocardial Abnormalities

The patient with Duchenne's dystrophy frequently has a number of clinical abnormalities of vasomotor control. The most striking are mottling and coldness of the extremities. These abnormalities become more prominent when the disease is advanced. A number of observations indicate that this is not part of the advancing muscular atrophy. The majority of these patients have a sinus tachycardia at rest with pulse rates above 100 per min. This tachycardia may be present early in the disease before there is extensive

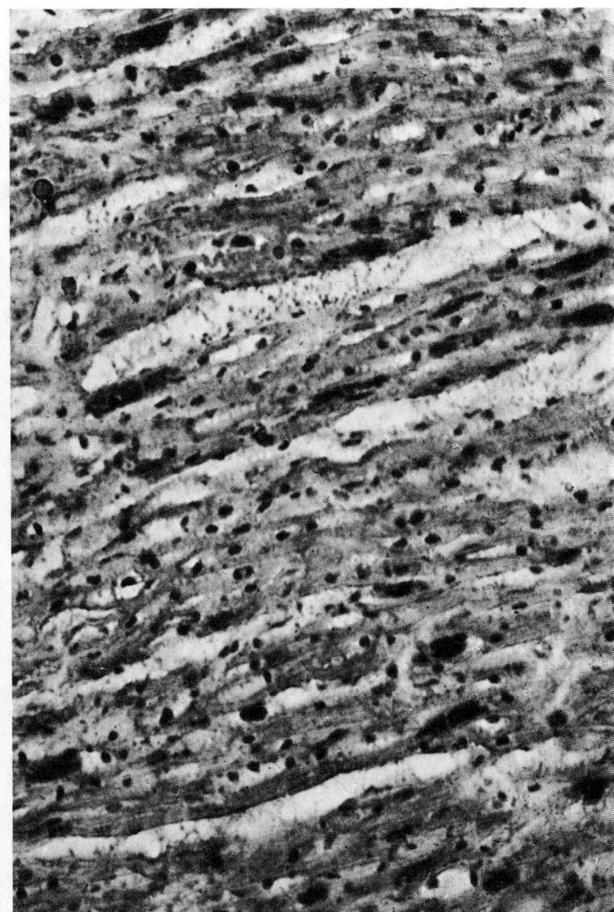

Figure 48-4. Myocardial fibrosis in childhood dystrophy. Note the diffuseness of the process, with normal vessels and adjacent normal-appearing myocardial fibers.

muscular atrophy, other evidence of myocardial involvement, or congestive heart failure.

Myocardial fibrosis may occur later in the course of this disease. The myocardial lesion is similar to that in the skeletal muscle. Characteristically it is a lacy fibrous tissue which seems to invade myocardial fibers directly. Indeed, histologically these lesions are more compatible with Bourne's hypothesis than is the lesion in the skeletal muscle itself (Fig. 48-4).

Additional evidence that the vascular phenomena are not entirely secondary to the skeletal muscle change has been presented by Demos and other investigators in Paris [13, 31]. Studying patients with Duchenne's dystrophy, they demonstrated that very early in the disease arm-to-arm circulation time was prolonged, but with advancing disease it became shorter than normal, and peripheral arteriovenous shunts developed. The histologic equivalent of this peripheral shunting is unclear, and it is difficult to correlate these observations with the progression of the disease. Oxygen consumption decreases as atrophy of muscles advances, and it certainly could be that anoxia contributes to the damage which the muscle fibers suffer. On the other hand, the random distribution of the damage within a microscopic fasciculus and the proximal occurrence of the initial muscle changes make it difficult to believe that this is the fundamental anomaly which leads to the damage. The decrease in oxygen consumption is more probably a consequence than a cause of the muscle atrophy.

Demos has observed that some of the female carriers of the gene for Duchenne's dystrophy show accelerated circulation times from arm to arm. It is unclear why these subjects without significant muscle disability should have the same circulatory disturbances which are found in their children only when the disease is advanced. In the carriers there was no correlation between increased serum aldolase levels and circulatory disturbance, as one might expect if indeed the latter were the cause of the progression of the muscle disease. It does appear that involvement of the vasculature is an important part of the dystrophic process and that it is probably independent of the skeletal muscle atrophy itself.

BIOCHEMICAL ABNORMALITIES IN MUSCULAR DYSTROPHY

The Creatine Anomaly

The first biochemical anomaly recognized in the dystrophic patient was creatinuria [32]. Creatine is normally formed in the liver by transmethylation of glycocyamine from methionine or other methyl donors (Fig. 48-5). Glycocyamine is formed from arginine and glycine by transamidinase. This enzyme is found in many tissues, particularly the kidney, pancreas, small intestinal mucosa, and probably in the liver. In man a large part of the glycocyamine is formed in the splanchnic circulation [33]. Creatine circulates in the plasma and is picked up and stored in the muscle largely as creatine phosphate. It forms a reserve energy pool for muscular activity.

In the muscle creatine is converted at an essentially constant rate of approximately 2 percent per day to creatinine, which diffuses back into the plasma and is excreted by the kidney (Fig. 48-6). As the body pool of creatine decreases, the creatinine excretion per unit time is decreased. Creatinine excretion is a useful index of body creatine stores and of the total muscle mass of the body. Thus the reduction in creatinine excretion which characterizes the dystrophic

$$\text{Arginine} + \text{Glycine} \xrightarrow{\text{TRANSAMINIDASE}} \text{Glycocyamine}$$

$$+ \text{Methionine} \xrightarrow{\text{TRANS-METHYLATION}} \text{Creatine} \xrightarrow{\text{CREATINE PHOSPHOKINASE}} \text{Creatine phosphate}$$

$$\rightarrow \text{Creatinine} \rightarrow \text{Excretion}$$

Figure 48-5. Synthesis of creatine: its metabolism and excretion.

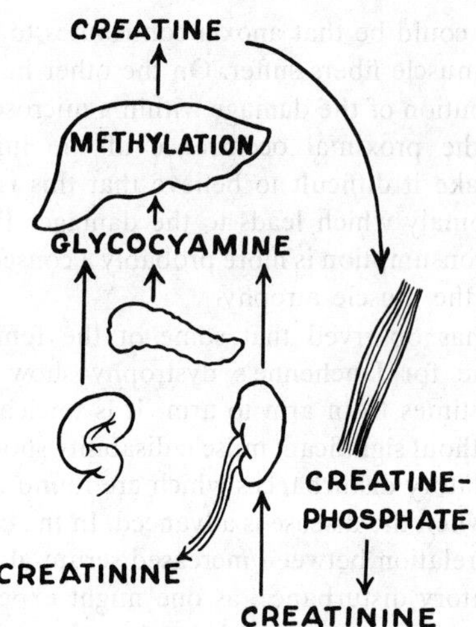

Figure 48-6. Formation, metabolism, and excretion of creatine and creatinine.

patient is simply a reflection of the loss of muscle from the dystrophic process.

It has been suggested that there might be abnormal renal handling of creatine which is responsible for the creatinuria [34]. Little evidence has been presented which supports such an abnormality. Creatinine clearance, as calculated from determinations done by the usual techniques (uncorrected Jaffé values), shows a marked decrease in the dystrophic patient as compared with normal individuals. Nonetheless, other tests of renal function including inulin and PAH clearance are normal (Table 48-1). The apparent abnormality of creatinine clearance is actually the result of an artifact related to the use of the alkaline picrate reaction for determination of creatinine. In normal plasma approximately 0.2 mg per 100 ml apparent creatinine is the result of the presence in plasma of other substances which give the reaction. These are not decreased in the dystrophic individual, but because actual creatinine is decreased, they represent an increasing fraction of the total Jaffé color which is obtained. Thus the creatinine clearance appears to be low. The same artifact is present in creatinine clearance in normal subjects but is largely compensated for by a small secretion of creatinine by the renal tubules. The two opposing factors result in values which roughly approximate inulin clearance in normal man.

Creatinuria is almost universal in patients with Duchenne's dystrophy and in most of the patients with limb-girdle dystrophy. It is quite irregular in patients with facioscapulohumeral dystrophy and myotonic dystrophy, and may be entirely absent even in advanced disease with extensive muscle atrophy and reduction in total muscle mass sufficient to lower creatinine excretion. Plasma levels of creatine are regularly increased in patients who have creatinuria.

The significance of creatinuria in patients with Duchenne's dystrophy is still unclear. In the normal subject administration of exogenous creatine suppresses creatine synthesis [35]. In the rat this operates by means of an enzyme-repression mechanism which reduces the concentration of transamidinase, the enzyme which makes glycocyamine [36]. The statement is frequently made that the creatinuria of dystrophy simply reflects an inability of the muscle to take up creatine in normal amounts [37, 38]. If this were true and the suppressive mechanism operated normally, the excess of creatine would suppress creatine synthesis rather than produce an overflow creatinuria. In patients who have muscle atrophy as the result of inanition or certain other processes, such as myotonic dystrophy, no creatinuria occurs. On the other hand, in patients with polymyositis and dermatomyositis, and to a lesser degree in patients with neural atrophy of muscle, creatinuria does occur and may be as severe as in Duchenne's dystrophy. It is clear that creatinuria is not specific to dystrophy, nor is it uniform in all the various kinds of dystrophy.

In the normal subject the creatine remains in the muscle after it has been removed from the plasma [35]. Unpublished studies of Tyler and those of Fitch and Sinton [39] with labeled creatine suggest that this is not true in the dystrophic muscle, but rather that the muscle creatine is exchanged with plasma creatine. This led Tyler to postulate that the abnormality in the skeletal muscle is one of membrane permeability, rather than a primary disorder in the regulation of creatine synthesis or renal handling of creatine. As we shall see, this concept of an abnormality in the permeability of the muscle membrane has much to recommend it as an explanation of certain other biochemical findings in studies of the muscle.

Enzymes of Muscle

Many studies have been made of the enzymes of muscle. One of the most difficult problems which has faced all investigators studying atrophic muscle has been the selection of a reference base. Because of the increase in fat and fibrous tissue, the use of wet or dry weight as a standard is obviously faulty. Various standards have been used, and none has been entirely satisfactory. At present the two most commonly used indices are noncollagen nitrogen and total nitrogen of the tissue. Noncollagen nitrogen, as suggested by Lilienthal [40], is that fraction of nitrogen of muscle which is soluble in dilute alkali and is presumably that primarily in the muscle cells themselves. Although not as sound theoretically, the determination of total tissue nitrogen correlates as well with intracellular constituents as do noncollagen nitrogen values. This is probably because the connective and fatty tissues contribute relatively little to the total amount of nitrogen. Other indices, such as creatine content and fat-free dry weight, have also been used; although they vary considerably in their relation to noncollagen nitrogen from muscle to muscle, even in biopsies from normal tissue, they give values that are just as satisfactory as are those of noncollagen nitrogen or total nitrogen.

Table 48-1. RENAL CLEARANCE AND OTHER TEST RESULTS IN PROGRESSIVE MUSCULAR DYSTROPHY

Patient	Age, yr	Severity	Type	*Clearance, ml/min*			Tubular resorption of creatine,* mg/min	Serum creatinine, mg/100 ml	Serum creatine,* mg/100 ml	*Corrected to 1.73 m³ surface area*			
										Clearance, ml/min			Tubular resorption of creatine,* mg/min
				Inulin	PAH	Creatinine				Inulin	PAH	Creatinine	
Endogenous creatine-creatinine:													
D.A.	8	++	Childhood	76	496	47	0.56	0.33	1.13	143	942	89	1.05
R.C.	9	++	Childhood	76	340	28	0.69	0.34	1.35	135	605	50	1.23
L.A.	11	+++	Childhood	96	489	44	0.90	0.33	1.45	154	792	71	1.44
L.C.	15	+++	Childhood	93	477	32	1.04	0.29	1.62	152	777	52	1.70
D.G.	18	++++	Childhood	108	573	32	1.25	0.39	1.79	143	770	42	1.65
J.S.	20	++++	Childhood	113	592	41	1.35	0.34	1.63	123	644	45	1.48
R.W.	21	++++	Childhood	67	357	33	1.28	0.41	2.14	87	465	42	1.62
L.L.	37	++	Facioscapulohumeral	114	570	75	1.34	0.69	1.37	124	620	82	1.46
C.C.	27	+	Facioscapulohumeral	121	. . .	110	1.52	0.77	1.51	117	. . .	106	1.47
Exogenous creatine-creatinine:†													
R.W.	21	++++	Childhood	64	. . .	58	1.26	1.08	5.80	83	. . .	75	1.64
C.C.	27	+	Facioscapulohumeral	113	. . .	145	1.68	1.26	8.00	109	. . .	140	1.62

* All creatine values are expressed as creatinine.
† Creatine and creatinine levels artificially increased by infusion of a solution kindly prepared by Armour Laboratories.

Glycolytic activity of muscle from Duchenne's muscular dystrophy is much reduced [41, 42]. Activities of the individual enzymes concerned in glycolysis show lowered levels, including α-glucan phosphorylase, aldolase, and phosphoglucomutase. On the other hand, Ronzoni et al. reported that hexokinase and lactic dehydrogenase are not decreased in relation to noncollagen nitrogen, and indeed there is some rise in lactic dehydrogenase levels [43].

A number of enzymes concerned in other metabolic processes have also been assayed. Creatine phosphokinase activity is strikingly reduced [42]. AMP (adenosine monophosphate) deaminase [44], present in high levels in normal muscle, is markedly decreased in muscle from dystrophic patients. In contrast, transaminases, aconitase, fumarase, cytochrome oxidase, and succinic dehydrogenase show no significant deviation from normal.

We have, then, a confusing array of information. Some enzyme activities are much decreased, and others are normal or slightly elevated. The large number of different biochemical processes carried out by enzymes whose activity is reduced suggests that these findings are relatively nonspecific. The enzymes which are most strikingly reduced are generally those which are primarily in the sarcoplasmic phase of the muscle and which might leak from the muscle if the membrane were abnormal. This explanation is not entirely adequate. It does not explain the rise in lactic dehydrogenase but fits well with changes in other glycolytic enzymes and in creatine phosphokinase.

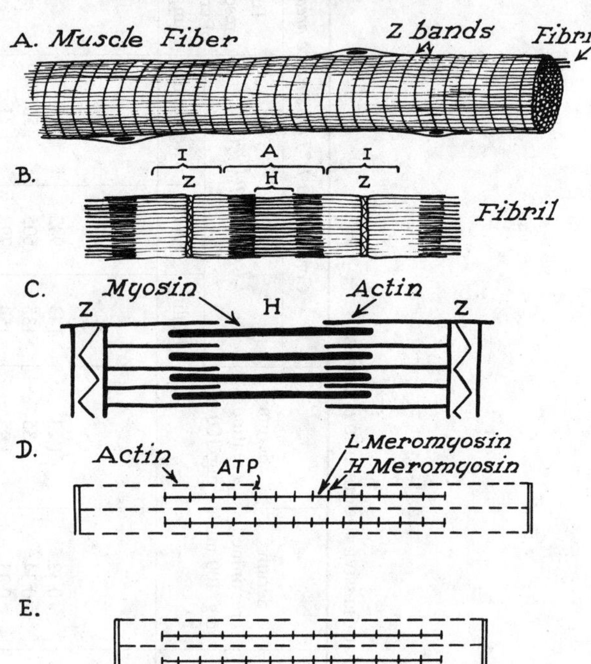

Figure 48-7. Schematic representation of a muscle fiber. The structure and contraction of actomyosin in muscle fibril is shown. The fibril shortens between the last two drawings as a result of movement of the myosin filaments along the actin filaments.

Actomyosin

Among the most interesting of the proteins in skeletal muscle are actin and myosin. They make up a large part of the total protein in striated muscle and account for the cross-striation, a characteristic feature of the tissue (Fig. 48-7). The ability of this pair of proteins to contract can be demonstrated both in vivo and in vitro.

The actin in the muscle fiber is present as a chain of protein molecules attached to a structural element which is the Z disk as seen microscopically (Fig. 48-7). The myosin is present as protein chains about which the actin chains are arranged hexagonally. The myosin chains themselves consist of two different peptide chains which are arranged systematically. The light meromyosin is continuous in the filament. The heavy meromyosins are attached to it and form cross links to the actin chains.

The two proteins form a complex in vitro called *actomyosin,* which is an active ATPase (adenosinetriphosphatase). Studies of separated fractions indicate that the activity is in the actin and heavy meromyosin molecules; the light meromyosin is inactive. It seems clear that during contraction, the heavy meromyosin bridges move along the actin chain to cause shortening of the muscle, and that the energy is derived from hydrolysis of ATP by the structural proteins. ATP is then regenerated by the glycolytic and Krebs cycles, or acutely from creatine phosphate by the mediation of creatine phosphokinase acting as a transfer enzyme for the high-energy phosphate.

One serious problem in understanding this model of the contraction of striated muscle has been that of the control of the enzymatic activity. Energy proportional to the work performed is released during contraction of muscle. Yet in vitro actomyosin fibers are in the contracted state in the presence of ATP, while in vivo relaxed muscle contains a large amount of ATP as well as the actin-heavy meromyosin bridges, which might be expected to hydrolyze the ATP and to contract. This paradox apparently relates to the dependence of the ATPase activity on a small but definite concentration of calcium ions. At rest the Ca^{++} is concentrated in specific areas of the endoplasmic reticulum. Electrical discharge of the fiber membrane effects release of Ca^{++} from these stores and thereby causes mechanical contraction. As the Ca^{++} is reaccumulated in the storage sites, relaxation occurs and ATP is regenerated.

Recently it has been suggested that the heavy meromyosin-actin bridges are not in contact with each other in the relaxed state. Ca^{++}, by means of its reaction with another structural protein called *troponin,* modifies the relationship of the other peptide chains in such a way that they are approximated and become enzymatically active. With reaccumulation of the Ca^{++} in the endoplasmic reticulum, the process is reversed.

The accumulation of Ca^{++} by the endoplasmic reticulum has been studied in detail in recent years [45, 46]. It is an active process dependent on an ATPase of the membrane. In the endoplasmic reticulum of the dystrophic mouse this process is clearly deficient, and recent data suggest that it is abnormal in Duchenne's dystrophy. In both situations it results in a small but significant delay in relaxation of the muscle.

Schapira et al. [41] have demonstrated that there is a marked reduction of the actomyosin concentrating in dystrophic muscle and a proportional drop in ATPase activity.

Several other structural proteins have been recognized more recently. All are reduced in concentration in dystrophic muscle.

Myoglobin

The myoglobin of normal and dystrophic human muscle has been studied in some detail in recent years. Interest was stimulated by two observations. The first was that the dystrophic muscle becomes pale very early in the disease process. Early German workers referred to it as "like fish flesh." This is particularly striking in Duchenne's muscular dystrophy but is also a feature of the adult forms of dystrophy. It was thought that the situation might be comparable to the now well-known anomalies of hemoglobin structure which result from mutation.

In normal human adult muscle approximately 80 percent of the myoglobin consists of a single molecular species. Confusion arose for a time from the fact that this fraction could be separated into two or three subfractions, but Perkoff et al. [47] demonstrated that these were artifacts introduced by modification of the state of the heme iron and were not caused by a change in the apomyoglobin structure. Indeed, the fractions can be easily interconverted in vitro.

Other iron-containing proteins in smaller amounts are also found which appear to be similar in general physical characteristics to adult myoglobin but can be separated from it on properly prepared fractionating columns. A small amount of the myoglobin of normal adult muscle is similar to the major component in the muscle of the fetus and has been generally referred to as fetal myoglobin. The other components which fractionate with the myoglobin are heterogeneous, and it is not certain at present that they are true myoglobins, although some of them contain a similar concentration of iron. A small fraction of myoglobin prepared from normal muscle has physical characteristics similar to those of myoglobin but does not contain heme iron. It has been suggested that this may be the apomyoglobin without its prosthetic group, but this has not been proved.

A number of changes have now been defined in autopsy material from patients with muscular dystrophy [48]. Muscle from all types of dystrophy shows a marked reduction in total concentration of myoglobin and myoglobin-like substances, even after correction for fat and fibrous tissue. The decrease is most striking in muscle from Duchenne's dystrophy. The small amounts of pure myoglobin which can be isolated contain proportions of adult and fetal myoglobin different from those observed in normal muscle. Only minimal quantities of normal adult myoglobin are found, and there is a relative but not absolute increase in the amount of "fetal" myoglobin and in the other minor fractions, including that which does not contain heme iron. Isolated "adult myoglobins" from skeletal muscle of facioscapulohumeral and myotonic dystrophy and from myocardium of Duchenne's dystrophy have the same spectral absorbency and electrophoretic and ultracentrifuge patterns and give the same peptides on trypsin hydrolysis as adult myoglobin from normal human muscle. Thus the abnormalities appear to be in the concentration and relative proportion of myoglobin, rather than in its qualitative characteristics.

The interpretation of these observations is difficult. The findings are consistent with the hypothesis that a change in membrane permeability has allowed the adult myoglobin to escape from the sarcoplasm. Under the stimulus of an attempt to form the protein at a greatly accelerated rate in Duchenne's dystrophy a greater proportion of "fetal" myoglobin is made.

Although the total concentration of myoglobin in muscle from patients with facioscapulohumeral and myotonic dystrophy is reduced, proportions of the various fractions are quite normal. Thus, evidence suggests that the various forms of dystrophy may not be closely related in their pathogenesis.

Creatine Phosphokinase (Creatine-ATP Transphosphorylase)

This enzyme has been of great interest because of the sarcoplasmic enzymes in plasma it has the most strikingly elevated level. Under ordinary circumstances it exists in the muscle as a dimer of two identical peptide chains. In nervous system tissue there is an enzyme with similar enzymatic activity. It also is a dimer of similar molecular weight but distinct peptide sequence. Isolation of the enzymes from dystrophic tissue by Kuby and associates [49] has demonstrated that most of the enzyme in the muscle from Duchenne's dystrophy is a hybrid of the two peptide chains. The significance of this observation is not clear. We may be observing once again a reversion to a more primitive state under the stress of continued loss of intracellular protein, just as has been suggested for myoglobin. On the other hand, a failure of normal maturation of the system controlling synthesis of creatine phosphokinase could be responsible for the enzymatic abnormality, and lack of normal enzyme activity might lead to muscle destruction.

High-energy Phosphate Compounds

Vignos and Warner [50] have evidence for an additional difference between the Duchenne type of dystrophy and the other dystrophies. It has been known for years that the total creatine and ATP content of muscle from patients with dystrophies and neurogenic atrophy is reduced even when corrected for noncollagen nitrogen. They found that the decrease is more marked in the muscle of patients with Duchenne's dystrophy. This may possibly be the result of an inability to retain creatine phosphate in the muscle.

Carbohydrate Metabolism

From time to time it has been reported that there is a characteristic abnormality of carbohydrate metabolism in some patients with muscular dystrophy, particularly myotonic dystrophy. Although an occasional patient has clearly had diabetes, no consistent abnormality has been observed in glucose tolerance. Studies of the fall in plasma phosphate concentration after glucose administration have shown that it may be impaired, as it is in the diabetic subject. Other subjects with severe muscle atrophy of other origins may show the same anomaly. It presumably is related to lack of skeletal muscle mass in which glycogen can be stored.

More recently measurements of plasma immunoreactive insulin levels after carbohydrate administration to patients with myotonic dystrophy have shown a striking overresponse of insulin [51, 52]. Levels after an overnight fast were also high. In spite of the high insulin level, the glucose tolerance curves were not clearly abnormal, although some showed a diminished peak at the usual 60-min sample. This is not infrequently found also in normal subjects. The insulin response to arginine and sulfonureas also was somewhat exaggerated in the patients with myotonic dystrophy. In spite of the excess insulin, no hypoglycemia was observed, but sensitivity to exogenous insulin was normal. The explanation of the paradox is not entirely clear. There is no evidence that the insulin is immunologically or functionally abnormal. In other types of dystrophy no similar abnormality of insulin response has been demonstrated.

Electrolyte and Other Abnormalities

The only electrolyte abnormality consistently found in studies of the muscle tissue is a decrease in intracellular potassium. In addition, the rate of exchange of intra- and extracellular potassium is accelerated. These changes are particularly striking in Duchenne's dystrophy but also appear in the more slowly progressive types [53, 54]. Zundel and Mays in our laboratories have studied the turnover of radioactive cesium and rubidium. Both are accelerated. All these effects may reflect altered membrane permeability.

Some investigators have also observed an increase in the relative concentration of intracellular sodium. Danowski and coworkers [55] reported a small but significant increase in serum phosphate and calcium in patients with Duchenne's dystrophy. This has not been found by other workers [56].

Small changes in the electrophoretic pattern of serum proteins have been observed. These consist primarily in a rise in α_2-globulin and a tendency toward a lower level of γ-globulin. The latter was found primarily in those patients with Duchenne's dystrophy [56] and may well be related to the relative isolation and freedom from infections of these patients. The change in α_2-globulin probably is a nonspecific response to injury. It is found commonly in many chronic diseases.

In myotonic dystrophy an acceleration of the turnover of the γ-globulin fraction IgG has been demonstrated [57]. The abnormality has not been found in the other dystrophies, and its significance is obscure.

A number of other changes have been reported but have not been found consistently. The most interesting of these is the report of moderate aminoaciduria [58], but the specificity of the finding is open to doubt [13].

Some years ago the claim was made that there is an excess of bound ribose in the urine of patients with muscular dystrophy which is not observed in patients with neural atrophy [59]. Other workers have been unable to confirm this observation as a specific and consistent abnormality [60].

Plasma Enzymes

One of the most striking and consistent observations of recent years is that certain enzymes which are normally present in muscle tissue also appear in excess amounts in the plasma in muscular dystrophy. The initial observation was made by Sibley and Lehninger, who found an elevation of serum aldolase [61]. Subsequent work has shown that concentration of a large number of enzymes is elevated. These include lactic dehydrogenase, glutamic oxaloacetic transaminase, α-glucan phosphorylase, phosphoglucomutase, glycerophosphate isomerase, and creatine phosphokinase [62]. The plasma activities are much lower than in muscle, but if plasma turnover is rapid, they probably could not result from destruction of muscle tissue alone. Enzyme levels are also elevated in the plasma in inflammatory and traumatic lesions of the muscle, but usually to a lesser degree and for a much shorter period of time. In Duchenne's dystrophy the serum enzyme levels tend to be highest early in the disease and the rise may be observed before any clinical manifestation of the disorder is present. In slowly progressive adult forms, such as facioscapulohumeral dystrophy, or in the advanced state of other types there may be no abnormality of the plasma enzymes. Among these enzymes the elevation of creatine phosphokinase is striking and relatively specific, and serves as a useful diagnostic tool. The abnormality of aldolase is next most marked. Determinations of lactic dehydrogenase or glutamic oxaloacetic transaminase are useful when the others are not available.

THEORY OF PATHOGENESIS

It seems obvious that an adequate theory of the pathogenesis of any of the genetic traits associated with progressive muscular dystrophy cannot be made at the present time. Any theory must account for the random and progressive destruction of muscle fibers over a very long period of time, the changes in the enzymes in the serum, and the changes in the constituents of the muscle tissue itself as the expression of a genetic mechanism.

It is tempting to consider that there is a primary defect in the permeability of the muscle membrane which allows the important intracellular constituents to diffuse abnormally into the extracellular fluid and that this results in inability of the muscle to maintain normal structure and function. Unfortunately there is at present little insight into the possible nature of such changes in permeability. Preliminary observations in Tyler's laboratory suggest that there may be a substance in the serum of patients with Duchenne's muscular dystrophy which changes the permeability of rat skeletal muscle in vitro [15]. This requires confirmation and further study.

THERAPY

Over the years a great many substances have been recommended as effective in preventing progression or causing regression of the muscular atrophy and weakness of muscular dystrophy. In our experience no regimen has yet proved to be effective.

Dowben [63] has claimed that a vigorous exercise program combined with administration of digitoxin and an anabolic steroid has resulted in stabilization of the course of muscular dystrophy, particularly adult dystrophy, and also has produced some delay in the progression of Duchenne's dystrophy. The therapeutic program is based on the hypothesis that digitalis glycosides change permeability in a nonspecific pharmacologic way and that anabolic steroid tends to promote accumulation of the lost protein constituents of the muscle. Further evaluation of this therapy has failed to confirm a long-term beneficial effect.

Two other groups of investigators have reported that administration of certain nucleotides retards progression of muscular dystrophy [64, 65]. Only limited information is available from either of these groups at the present time.

Evaluation of treatment has proved to be extremely difficult in these insidiously progressive disorders. Placebo effect is striking. Quantitative end points and double-blind design are essential but have not been employed until recently. Changes in creatinuria and plasma enzyme levels have been disappointing because of nonspecific effects of the agents employed. For example, hyperthyroidism will increase creatinuria and decrease plasma creatine phosphokinase in Duchenne's dystrophy but has similar effects in normal subjects.

SUMMARY

1 The term *muscular dystrophy* includes a group of disorders in which there is a common histologic appearance and progressive atrophy of skeletal muscle. The important types are Duchenne's, limb-girdle, facioscapulohumeral, and myotonic dystrophy. Most if not all of these disorders are genetically determined.

2 The histologic lesion is characterized by random progressive destruction of individual muscle fibers. Certain muscles are involved earlier and more severely than others. The myocardium is also frequently affected, and there is evidence of peripheral vascular abnormalities.

3 Creatinuria is characteristic of Duchenne's dystrophy and may occur in other diseases of muscle. Its significance and cause are not apparent at present.

4 Many glycolytic enzymes and certain other enzymes are reduced in concentration in the dystrophic muscle. Myoglobin concentration is reduced in muscle from all types of dystrophy, and the proportion of adult myoglobin is decreased in Duchenne's dystrophy. No qualitative abnormality has been identified.

5 Creatine phosphate and ATP are reduced in all types of dystrophy. Intracellular potassium is reduced in dystrophic muscle. Many enzymes of the sarcoplasm are increased in plasma in dystrophic patients.

6 Many of the biochemical abnormalities which have been identified in the atrophic muscle can be interpreted as a failure to retain soluble sarcoplasmic substances within the muscle fiber.

BIBLIOGRAPHY

1. Aran, F. A.: Recherches sur une maladie non encore décrite du système musculaire (atrophie musculaire progressive). Arch. Gen. Med., **24**, 5, 1850.
2. Meyron, E.: On granular or fatty degeneration of the voluntary muscles. Med.-chir. Trans., **35**, 72, 1852.
3. Oppenheimer, Z.: *Ueber progressive fettige Muskelentartung.* Heidelberg, 1855.
4. Michelson, A. M., Russell, E. S., and Pinckney, J. H.: Dystrophia muscularis: a hereditary primary myopathy in the house mouse. Proc. Nat. Acad. Sci. U.S.A., **41**, 1079, 1955.
5. Cornelius, C. E., Law, G. R. J., Julian, L. M., and Asmundson, V. S.: Plasma aldolase and glutamicoxaloacetic transaminase activities in inherited muscular dystrophy of domestic chickens. Proc. Soc. Exp. Biol. Med., **101**, 41, 1959.
6. Homburger, F., Baker, J. R., Nixon, C. W., and Wilgram, G.: New hereditary disease of Syrian hamsters. Arch. Intern. Med., **110**, 660, 1962.
7. Draper, G. J., and Parry, H. B.: Scrapie in sheep: the hereditary component in a high incidence environment. Nature (London), **195**, 670, 1962.

8. Tyler, F. H., and Wintrobe, M. M.: Studies in disorders of muscle. I. The problem of progressive muscular dystrophy. Ann. Intern. Med., **32,** 72, 1950.
9. Walton, J. N., and Natrass, F. J.: On the classification, natural history and treatment of the myopathies. Brain, **77,** 169, 1954.
10. Stevenson, A. C.: Muscular dystrophy in Northern Ireland. I. An account of the condition in fifty-one families. Ann. Eugen. **18,** 50, 1953.
11. Gowers, W.: *Pseudohypertrophic Muscular Paralysis.* J. & A. Churchill, Ltd., London, 1879.
12. Stephens, F. E., and Tyler, F. H.: Studies in disorders of muscle. V. The inheritance of childhood progressive muscular dystrophy in 33 kindreds. Amer. J. Hum. Genet., **3,** 111, 1951.
13. Dreyfus, J. C., and Schapira, G.: *Biochemistry of Hereditary Myopathies,* American Lecture Series, publ. 452. Charles C Thomas, Springfield, Ill., 1962.
14. Leyburn, P., Thomson, W. H. S., and Walton, J. N.: An investigation of the carrier state in the Duchenne type muscular dystrophy. Ann. Hum. Genet., **25,** 41, 1961.
15. Sugita, H., and Tyler, F. H.: Pathogenesis of muscular dystrophy. Trans. Ass. Amer. Physicians, **76,** 231, 1963.
16. Emery, A. E. H.: Clinical manifestation in two carriers of Duchenne muscular dystrophy. Lancet, **1,** 1126, 1963.
17. Haldane, J. B. S.: Mutation in the sex-linked recessive type of muscular dystrophy: a possible sex difference. Ann. Hum. Genet., **20,** 344, 1956.
18. Chung, C. A., and Morton, N. E.: Discrimination of genetic entities in muscular dystrophy. Ann. J. Hum. Genet., **11,** 339, 1959.
19. Cheeseman, E. A., Kilpatrick, S. J., Stevenson, A. C., and Smith, C. A. B.: The sex ratio of mutation rates of sex-linked recessive genes in man with particular reference to Duchenne type muscular dystrophy. Ann. Hum. Genet., **22,** 245, 1958.
20. Landouzy, L., and Déjèrine, J.: De la myopathie atrophique progressive. Rev. Med. Franc., **5,** 81, 1885; **5,** 253, 1885; **6,** 977, 1886.
21. Tyler, F. H., and Stephens, F. E.: Studies in disorders of muscle. II. Clinical manifestations and inheritance of facioscapulohumeral dystrophy in a large family. Ann. Intern. Med., **32,** 640, 1950.
22. Gowers, W. R.: A lecture on myopathy and a distal form. Brit. Med. J., **2,** 89, 1902.
23. Welander, L.: Myopathia distalis tarda hereditaria. Acta. Med. Scand., suppl. **265,** 1–124, 1951.
24. Kiloh, L. G., and Nevin, S.: Progressive dystrophy of external ocular muscles (ocular myopathy). Brain, **74,** 115, 1951.
25. Barnes, S.: A myopathic family; with hypertrophic, pseudohypertrophic, atrophic and terminal distal (in upper extremities) stages. Brain, **55,** 1, 1932.
26. Thomasen, E.: *Myotonia, Thompson's Disease, Paramyotonia and Dystrophia Myotonica: A Clinical and Heredobiologic Investigation.* Aarhus, Universitetsforlaget, Copenhagen, 1948.
27. Adams, R. D., Denny-Brown, D., and Pearson, C. M.: *Diseases of Muscle,* 2d ed. Hoeber-Harper, New York, 1962.
28. Penrose, L. S.: The problem of anticipation in pedigrees of dystrophia myotonica. Ann. Eugen. **14,** 125, 1948.
29. Gollarz, M. N., Bourne, G. H., and Richardson, H. D.: Histochemical studies on human muscular dystrophy, J. Histochem., **9,** 132, 1961.
30. Walton, J. N., and Adams, R. D.: The response of the normal, the denervated and the dystrophic muscle-cell to injury. J. Path. Bact., **72,** 273, 1956.
31. Demos, J.: Un nouveau problème posé par la myopathie humaine: les troubles des temps de circulation et leur liaison avec l'activité enzymatique sérique. Bull. Soc. Med. Hop. Paris, **77,** 636, 1961.
32. Milhorat, A. T.: Creatine and creatinine metabolism. Ass. Res. Nerv. Ment. Dis. Proc., **32,** 400, 1953.
33. Sandberg, A. A., Hecht, H. H., and Tyler, F. H.: Studies in disorders of muscle. X. The site of creatine synthesis in the human. Metabolism, **2,** 22, 1953.
34. Zierler, K. L., Folk, B. P., Magladery, J. W., and Lilienthal, J. L., Jr.: On creatinuria in man: the roles of the renal tubule and of the muscle mass. Johns Hopkins Hosp. Bull., **85,** 370, 1949.
35. Hoberman, H. D., Sims, E. A. H., and Peters, J. H.: Creatine and creatine metabolism in normal male adult studies with the aid of isotopic nitrogen. J. Biol. Chem., **172,** 45, 1948.
36. Walker, J. B.: Metabolic control of creatine biosynthesis. II. Restoration of transamidinase activity following creatine repression. J. Biol. Chem., **236,** 493, 1961.
37. Roche, M., Benedict, J. D., Yü, T. F., Bien, F. J., and Stetten, DeW., Jr.: Origin of urinary creatine in progressive muscular dystrophy. Metabolism, **1,** 13, 1952.
38. Benedict, J. D., Kalinsky, H. J., Scarrone, L. A., Wertheim, A. P., and Stetten, DeW., Jr.: The origin of urinary creatine in progressive muscular dystrophy. J. Clin. Invest., **34,** 141, 1955.
39. Fitch, C. C., and Sinton, D. W.: A study of creatine metabolism in diseases causing muscle wasting. J. Clin. Invest., **43,** 444, 1964.
40. Lilienthal, J. L., Jr., Zierler, K. L., Folk, B. P., Buka, R., and Riley, N. J.: A reference base and system for analysis of muscle constituents. J. Biol. Chem., **182,** 501, 1950.
41. Schapira, G., Dreyfus, J. C., Schapira, F., and Kruh, J.: Glycogenolytic enzymes in human progressive muscular dystrophy. Amer. J. Phys. Med., **34,** 313, 1955.
42. Vignos, P. J., Jr., and Keftowitz, M.: A biochemical study of certain skeletal muscle constituents in human progressive muscular dystrophy. J. Clin. Invest., **38,** 873, 1959.
43. Ronzoni, E., Berg, L., and Landau, W.: Enzyme studies in progressive muscular dystrophy. 38th Annual Meeting, ARNMD, New York. Ass. Res. Nerv. Ment. Dis., **38,** 721, 1960.
44. Pennington, R. J.: Muscular dystrophy in man: biochemical aspects. Proc. Nutr. Soc., **21,** 206, 1962.
45. Samaha, F. J., and Gergely, J.: Biochemical abnormalities of the sarcoplasmic reticulum in muscular dystrophy. New Eng. J. Med., **280,** 184, 1969.
46. Peter, J. B., and Worsfold, M: Muscular dystrophy and other myopathies: sarcotubular vesicles in early disease. Biochem. Med., **2,** 364, 1969.
47. Perkoff, G. T., Hill, R. L., Brown, D. M., and Tyler, F. H.: The characterization of adult human myoglobin. J. Biol. Chem., **237,** 2820, 1962.
48. Perkoff, G. T.: Studies of human myoglobin in several muscle diseases. New Eng. J. Med., **270,** 263, 1964.
49. Jacobs, H., Kabe, K. O., Yue, R., Keutel, H., Ziter, F., Palmieri, R., Tyler, F., and Kuby, S. A.: A comparison of normal human ATPase-creatine transphosphorylases with those from progressive muscular dystrophic tissues. Fed. Proc., **28,** 495, 1969.
50. Vignos, P. J., Jr., and Warner, J. L.: Glycogen, creatine and high energy phosphate in human muscle disease. J. Lab. Clin. Med., **62,** 579, 1963.
51. Huff, T. A., and Lebovitz, H. E.: Dynamics of insulin secretion in myotonic dystrophy. J. Clin. Endocr., **28,** 992, 1968.
52. Engel, W. K.: Studies of plasma insulin in myotonic dystrophy. J. Clin. Endocr., **29,** 684, 1969.
53. Horvath, B., and Proctor, J. B.: Muscular dystrophy: quantitative studies in the composition of dystrophic muscle. 38th Annual Meeting, ARNMD, New York. Ass. Res. Nerv. Ment. Dis., **38,** 740, 1960.
54. Williams, J. D., Ansell, B., Reiffel, L., Stone, C. A., and Kark, R. M.: Electrolyte levels in normal and dystrophic muscle determined by neutron activation. Lancet, **273,** 464, 1957.
55. Danowski, T. S., Wirth, P. M., Leinberger, M. H., Randall, L. A., and Peters, J. H.: Muscular dystrophy. III. Serum and blood solutes and other laboratory indices. A.M.A. J. Dis. Child., **91,** 346, 1956 (and following).
56. Tyler, F. H., and Perkoff, G. T.: Studies in disorders of muscle. VI. Is progressive muscular dystrophy an endocrine or metabolic disorder? A.M.A. Arch. Intern. Med., **88,** 175, 1951.
57. Engel, W. K., McFarlin, D. E., Drews, G. A., and Wochner, R. D.: Protein abnormalities in neuromuscular diseases. J.A.M.A., **195,** 754, 1966.
58. Ames, S., and Risley, H.: Amino aciduria in progressive muscular dystrophy. Proc. Soc. Exp. Biol. Med., **68,** 131, 1948.
59. Ronzoni, E., Wald, S., Lam, R. L., and Gildea, E. F.: Ribosuria in muscular dystrophy. Neurology, **5,** 412, 1955.
60. Walton, J. N., and Latner, A. L.: Ribosuria in muscular dystrophy. A.M.A. Arch. Neurol. Psychiat., **72,** 362, 1954.

61. Sibley, J. A., and Lehninger, A. L.: Aldolase in the serum and tissues of tumor-bearing animals. J. Nat. Cancer Inst., **9**, 303, 1949.
62. Ebashi, S., Toyokura, Y., Momoi, H., and Sugita, H.: High creatine phosphokinase activity of sera of progressive muscular dystrophy. J. Biochem. (Tokyo), **46**, 103, 1959.
63. Dowben, R. M.: Treatment of muscular dystrophy with steroids. New Eng. J. Med., **268**, 912, 1963.
64. Bourne, G. H., and Golarz, M. N.: Use of nucleotides in the treatment of muscular dystrophy. J.A.M.A., **180**, 761, 1962.
65. Thomson, W. H. S., and Guest, K. E.: A trial of therapy by nucleosides and nucleotides in muscular dystrophy. J. Neurol. Neurosurg. Psychiat., **26**, 111, 1963.

CHAPTER FORTY-NINE

THE MUCOPOLYSACCHARIDOSES *

Albert Dorfman and Reuben Matalon

The term *mucopolysaccharidosis,* originally introduced by Brante [1], is now widely used for a group of heritable diseases characterized by abnormal deposition in tissues and/or excretion in urine of acid mucopolysaccharides. It is difficult to delineate accurately this group of diseases since recent findings [2] indicate that abnormalities of mucopolysaccharide metabolism occur concomitantly with other metabolic aberrations in glycolipid storage diseases and cystic fibrosis. The basis of these metabolic interrelationships is not clear. This chapter will deal primarily with the group of diseases which show clear-cut abnormalities of the metabolism of mucopolysaccharides and will mention only briefly other related syndromes.

There exist a large number of heritable diseases of cartilage and bone which probably involve molecular abnormalities of connective tissue components, but no definitive information regarding their cause is now available. Included in this category are such syndromes as the *chondrodystrophies, achondroplasia, osteogenesis imperfecta, osteopetrosis, Ehlers-Danlos syndrome,* and numerous less well-defined entities. Some of these have been reviewed in detail in the excellent monograph by McKusick [3].

HISTORICAL ASPECTS

Space does not permit a detailed historical review of all of the mucopolysaccharidoses, but it is important to note the original descriptions which led to the recognition of this group of diseases. A much more detailed historical review has been given by McKusick [3].

Hurler's syndrome was first delineated, according to Henderson [4], by Dr. John Thompson at the Royal Infirmary, Edinburgh, in 1900. He named it *Johnny McL's disease.* Figure 49-1 is a photograph reproduced from Henderson's publication in 1940 of one of the three brothers studied by Thompson. Hunter [5] first described in 1917 two brothers whose features fit in most details our current conception of the X-linked form of the disease. The elder brother was not mentally retarded, but the younger brother was said to display evidence of impaired mentation.

In 1919, Gertrud Hurler [6], an assistant to Prof. Meinhard von Pfaundler of Munich, described two unrelated boys with findings which conformed entirely to the syndrome now associated with her name. In addition to the characteristics described by Hunter, she added corneal clouding, gibbus deformity, and severe mental retardation. Since these early publications, this syndrome has appeared in numerous reports under a variety of names, among which are *dysostosis multiplex, chondroosteodystrophy, polydystrophie, lipochondrodysplasia, dysostosis enchondralis dysostotische, idiotegargoylism, osteochondrodystrophie, osteoarthropathie, lipochondrodystrophy,* and *gargoylism.* The name *lipochondrodystrophy* was erroneously applied by Washington [7], in keeping with the earlier concept that this disease was due to lipid storage. The term *gargoylism* was introduced by Ellis et al. [8] because of a supposed resemblance of the patients to the gargoyles of certain cathedrals. Not only has this term a most unpleasant connotation for families, but it is etymologically incorrect since the term gargoyle refers to the original function of these structures in carrying rainwater away from columns rather than to the hideous chimeras which were portrayed.

It seems likely that the syndromes described by Hurler and Hunter were different and, as indicated below, the term Hunter's disease is now reserved for the X-linked recessive variant while Hurler's disease is used to indicate one of the autosomal variants. Earlier discussions of terminology are obsolete in that a number of different syndromes, phenotypically similar (although not identical), involve abnormalities of mucopolysaccharide metabolism. Attempts at rationalization of nomenclature are necessarily premature in view of the paucity of information regarding the basic defect (i.e., the nature of the mutant gene product responsible for the diseases). Nevertheless, for purposes of communication such classifications are necessary and will be detailed below.

CHEMISTRY OF MUCOPOLYSACCHARIDES

All multicellular organisms contain extracellular material which, in its simplest state, is similar to the jelly-like coat found about unicellular forms, while in more complex organisms this material becomes highly differentiated into the many specialized structures of the connective tissues. The chemical nature of intercellular substances is remarkably similar throughout the animal kingdom. Certain chemical analogies may be drawn between the ground substance of connective tissue and the capsules of bacteria.

For the purposes of this chapter, our interest will be confined to the connective tissue of higher organisms. Figure 49-2 is a sketch of an idealized connective tissue. Between the circulation and parenchymal cells is the connective tissue compartment. It is composed of fibers, specialized cells, and the amorphous ground substance. For simplicity, only two cell types, the fibroblast and the mast cell, are illustrated.

*Original investigations referred to in this manuscript were supported by grants from the following sources: USPHS No. AM-05996, USPHS No. HD-04583, USPHS No. RR-00305, the Chicago and Illinois Heart Association No. RN69-30, and the National Cystic Fibrosis Foundation.

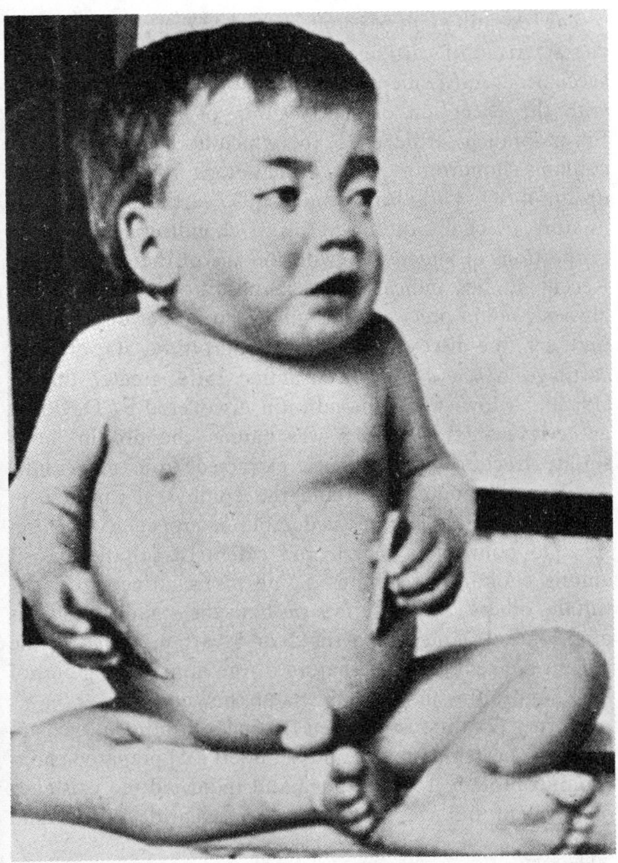

Figure 49-1. One of Thompson's original patients. (*Reproduced from Henderson* [4].)

These have a peculiar metabolic relationship to connective tissue. The fibroblasts, or specialized derivatives thereof, are responsible for the biosynthesis of both the acid mucopolysaccharides of connective tissue and the collagen fibers. The mast cells probably both synthesize and store heparin. Two chemically and morphologically distinct varieties of fibers, collagen and elastin, occur in connective tissues. The ground substance is a complex mixture which contains substances in transit between cells and circulation, as well as the special components peculiar to this compartment. Of the latter, the acid mucopolysaccharides have been most extensively studied and will be discussed in greatest detail in this chapter.

The idealized structure illustrated in Fig. 49-2 serves as a basis for understanding the more specialized types of connective tissue. Actually, connective tissue varies from the synovial fluid, which may be considered as a simplified ground substance, to the complex organization of bone in which an inorganic crystalline structure is superimposed on the fibers and ground substance.

The acid mucopolysaccharides are a group of closely related yet specific substances found singly in some tissues or in mixtures in others. Considerable confusion exists in the literature concerning the nomenclature of macromolecular carbohydrate compounds. Jeanloz [9] has suggested a new nomenclature which is being gradually adopted. For clarification, Table 49-1 lists that nomenclature with some modifications together with the older terminology. Since the term *acid mucopolysaccharide* is so widely accepted, it will be employed in this chapter. Table 49-2 lists certain structural features of the known acid mucopolysaccharides.

Hyaluronic acid is a polymer of N-acetylglucosamine and D-glucuronic acid whose molecular weight may be as high

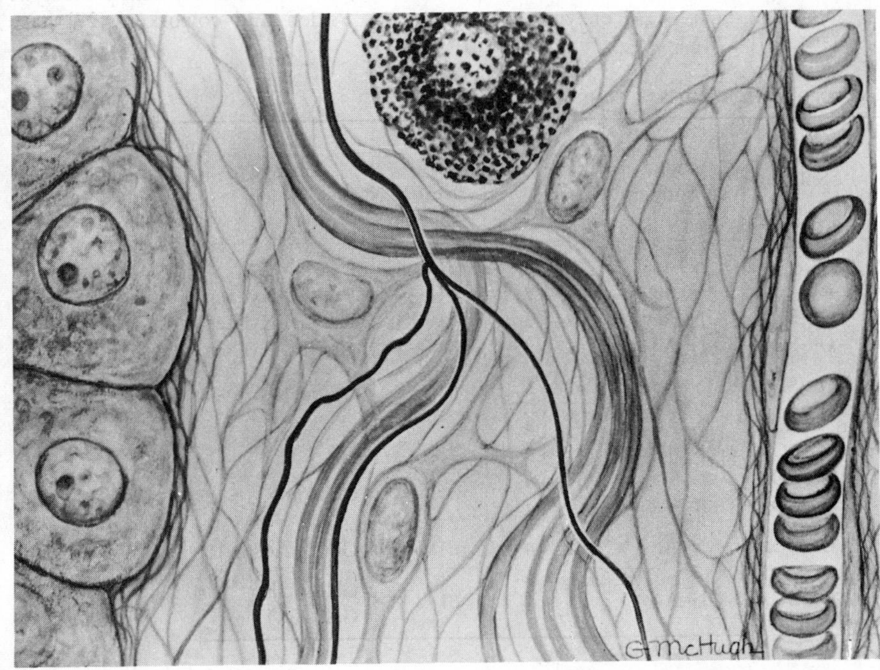

Figure 49-2. An idealized connective tissue between parenchymal cells and a capillary.

Table 49-1. NOMENCLATURE OF ACID MUCOPOLYSACCHARIDES

Old names	New names
Acid mucopolysaccharides	Glycosaminoglycuronoglycans*
Chondroitin Chondroitin sulfate A Chondroitin sulfate C	Chondroitin Chondroitin-4-sulfate Chondroitin-6-sulfate
Chondroitin sulfate B β-Heparin	Dermatan sulfate
Heparitin sulfate Heparin monosulfate	Heparan sulfate
Corneal keratosulfate Skeletal keratosulfate	Keratan sulfate I Keratan sulfate II
Chondromucoprotein Protein-polysaccharide complex	Proteoglycan

* Keratan sulfate would not qualify as a glycosaminoglycuronoglycan by the new nomenclature.

as 10^6 or as low as 8×10^4. Direct visualization of the molecule by electron microscopy [10] indicates that it is probably a linear molecule.

The linkage of hyaluronic acid to protein in mammalian tissues remains unsettled. Hamerman et al. [11] suggested that hyaluronic acid may be linked to protein through a glycopeptide containing glucose and galactose, while Wardi et al. [12] have claimed involvement of arabinose in the linkage to protein. Hyaluronic acid typically occurs in tissues of high water content such as vitreous humor, Wharton's jelly, synovial fluid, and the sex skin of certain primates [13], and is increased in myxedema [14]. In some tissues such as skin, it occurs in association with chondroitin-4/6-sulfate and dermatan sulfate.

The repeating unit of chondroitin-4-SO_4, a polysaccharide characteristic of cartilage, is shown in Fig. 49-3. This disaccharide unit is identical with that of chondroitin-6-SO_4, with the exception of the position of the ester sulfate. Elasmobranch cartilage [15, 16], which does not form bone, contains chondroitin-6-SO_4, while notochord contains chondroitin-4-SO_4 [17]. Embryonic chick cartilage contains a mixture of chondroitin-4-SO_4 and chondroitin-6-SO_4, the proportions of which vary with the age of the embryo [18]. Recent studies indicate that chondroitin sulfates do not always contain precisely one sulfate group per disaccharide unit, e.g., the discovery that the chondroitin-6-SO_4 of shark cartilage has a sulfate/hexosamine ratio greater than 1 [19, 20]. A low-sulfate chondroitin discovered by Davidson and Meyer [21] in cornea was named chondroitin. Low-sulfate fractions may also be extracted from the cranial cartilage of tadpoles [22] and the epiphyseal cartilage of embryonic chicks [18]. Considerable heterogeneity with respect to both chain length and extent of sulfation exists among chondroitin sulfates. Some disaccharide units lack sulfate, others contain sulfate on both the 4 and 6 positions of the hexosamine or on the 2 or 3 carbon atoms of the glucuronic acid [23]. The nature of the nonreducing end of the chondroitin sulfate chains is unknown.

Mörner [24] first recognized that chondroitin sulfates are linked to protein. Shatton and Schubert [25] prepared chondromucoprotein from cartilage and indicated the existence of covalent linkages between polysaccharide chains and protein.

The nature of the linkage between carbohydrate and protein was suggested by the finding of Muir [26] of a preponderance of serine residues in hydrolysates of chondroitin-4-SO_4 previously treated extensively with proteolytic enzymes. Subsequently, Rodén and coworkers [27] have

Table 49-2. MUCOPOLYSACCHARIDES OF CONNECTIVE TISSUE

Name	Amino sugar	Uronic acid	Sulfate	Amino substitution	*Linkage* Uronide	*Linkage* Hexos-aminidic	Linkage to protein
Hyaluronic acid	D-GlcN	D-GlcUA	......	N–Ac	$\beta 1 \rightarrow 3$	$\beta 1 \rightarrow 4$	?
Chondroitin	D-GalN	D-GlcUA	......	N–Ac	$\beta 1 \rightarrow 3$	$\beta 1 \rightarrow 4$	Gal-Gal-Xyl-Ser
Chondroitin-4-SO_4	D-GalN	D-GlcUA	O—SO_4	N–Ac	$\beta 1 \rightarrow 3$	$\beta 1 \rightarrow 4$	Gal-Gal-Xyl-Ser
Chondroitin-6-SO_4	D-GalN	D-GlcUA	O—SO_4	N–Ac	$\beta 1 \rightarrow 3$	$\beta 1 \rightarrow 4$	Gal-Gal-Xyl-Ser
Dermatan sulfate	D-GalN	L-IdUA D-GlcUA	O—SO_4	N–Ac	$\alpha 1 \rightarrow 3$	$\beta 1 \rightarrow 4$	Gal-Gal-Xyl-Ser
Heparan sulfate	D-GlcN	D-GlcUA L-IdUA	N—SO_4 O—SO_4	N–Ac N-SO_4	$\beta 1 \rightarrow 4$ $\alpha 1 \rightarrow 4$	$\alpha 1 \rightarrow 4$	Gal-Gal-Xyl-Ser
Heparin	D-GlcN	D-GlcUA L-IdUA	N—SO_4 O—SO_4	N-SO_4 (N-Ac)	$\beta 1 \rightarrow 4$ $\alpha 1 \rightarrow 4$	$\alpha 1 \rightarrow 4$	Gal-Gal-Xyl-Ser
Keratan sulfate I (cornea)	D-GlcN	Gal (mann)	O—SO_4	N–Ac	$\beta 1 \rightarrow 4$	$\beta 1 \rightarrow 3$	GlcNAc-AspNH$_2$
Keratan sulfate II (skeletal)	D-GlcN D-GalN	Gal (mann)	O—SO_4	N–Ac	$\beta 1 \rightarrow 4$	$\beta 1 \rightarrow 3$	GalNAc-Ser GalNAc-Thr

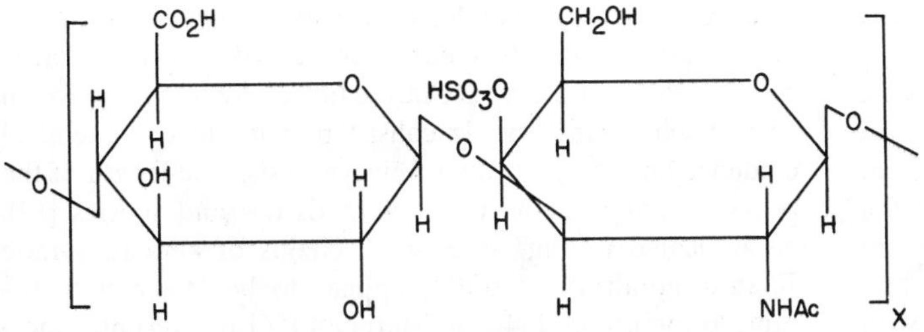

Figure 49-3. The disaccharide repeating unit of CS-4-SO_4.

determined the structure of the linkage region between several mucopolysaccharides and their respective proteins. Chondroitin-4-SO_4, chondroitin-6-SO_4, dermatan sulfate, heparan sulfate, and heparin polysaccharide chains are linked through the trisaccharide galactosylgalactosylxylose to the hydroxyl groups of serine residues. The details of this linkage region are illustrated in Fig. 49-4. Serine functions as the point at which the polysaccharide branches from the protein.

Dermatan sulfate differs from chondroitin-4- and chondroitin-6-sulfates in that its predominant uronic acid is L-iduronic acid although D-glucuronic acid [28, 29] is present in variable amounts. The glycosidic linkages are the same in position and configuration as in the chondroitin sulfates. (Since iduronic acid is L in configuration, the iduronosyl linkage is α.) In the dermatan sulfate of skin the sulfate group is in the 4 position, while in that of the umbilical cord it is in the 6 position [30]. Dermatan sulfates with sulfate/hexosamine ratios greater than 1 have been found both in normal tissues [23] and Hurler's tissues [31]. Sulfate may be linked to uronic acid [23] in addition to that linked to N-acetylgalactosamine.

The physiological functions of dermatan sulfate are poorly understood. In contrast to chondroitin-4- and chondroitin-6-sulfates, dermatan sulfate is antithrombic as is heparin, but in contrast to heparin it shows only minimal whole blood anticoagulant and blood lipid-clearing activities [32].

Perhaps even more than in the case of other mucopolysaccharides, keratan sulfate is characterized by considerable molecular heterogeneity. This polysaccharide is composed principally of a repeating disaccharide unit of N-acetylglucosamine and galactose with no uronic acid in the molecule. Sulfate content is variable, with ester sulfate present on carbon 6 of both the galactose and N-acetylglucosamine. At least two types of keratan sulfate, keratan sulfate I in cornea and keratan sulfate II in skeletal tissues, have been distinguished. In addition to the principal monosaccharides, mannose, fucose, sialic acid, and N-acetylgalactosamine have been found in keratan sulfates. The latter sugar appears to be characteristic only of keratan sulfate II. Keratan sulfate has been found in the urine of patients with Morquio's disease [33, 34] and, as described elsewhere in this volume, a keratan sulfate-like material has been found in the tissues and urine of patients with G_{M1} gangliosidosis [35–37]. The chemical structure of keratan sulfates from these sources has not yet been studied.

Linkage to protein in corneal keratan sulfate is between N-acetylglucosamine and asparagine to form the N-glycoside linkage typical of glycoproteins [38]. In contrast, at least a portion of the linkage to protein of skeletal keratan sulfate is by way of hydroxyl groups of serine and threonine. Details of this linkage region are not well understood, but galactosamine appears to be linked to the hydroxyamino acids [39].

Heparin differs from other acid mucopolysaccharides in a number of important respects. D-Glucuronic acid and D-glucosamine are the principal monosaccharides, but L-iduronic acid has been demonstrated in heparin in a number of laboratories [40–43]. The possibility that the finding of L-iduronic acid is an artifact of the isolation procedure has been raised but seems unlikely [44]. In contrast to mucopolysaccharides of ground substance, heparin contains α-glycosidic linkages. The sulfate content of heparin, although varying somewhat in different preparations, approaches 2.5 sulfate residues per disaccharide unit in preparations of highest biological activity. Almost all glucosamine residues are bound in sulfamide linkages, but a small number of glucosamine residues are N-acetylated in the region of the molecule proximal to linkage to protein [45, 46]. Sulfate groups are also linked to carbon-6 of glucosamine, and additional sulfate groups have been found on carbon-3 of the hexosamine and carbon-2 of the uronic acid.

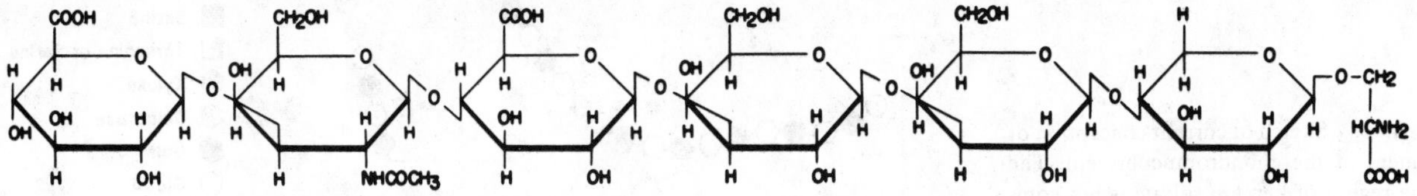

Figure 49-4. The linkage region of chondromucoprotein.

Recently Lindahl [47] has suggested that L-iduronic acid is the only uronic acid which is sulfated in heparin.

Unlike other acid mucopolysaccharides which occur in the extracellular ground substance, heparin appears to be an intracellular component of mast cells. The anticoagulant and lipid-clearing activities of heparin are well known, but the physiological role of this polysaccharide remains obscure since it has never been found in blood.

Heparan sulfate shares many structural features with heparin. These include the presence of D-glucosamine, D-glucuronic acid, and L-iduronic acid bound in α-glycoside linkages. Heparan sulfates appear to be a family of compounds with variable amounts of total sulfate and variable ratios of N-sulfated glucosamine to N-acetylated glucosamine [48]. In general the glucosamine residues proximal to the protein linkage are N-acetylated while the more distal residues are N-sulfated, although N-acetylated residues are present throughout the chain. As in the case of heparin, there remains a possibility that branch points may occur in the molecule. Heparan sulfate appears to be extracellular in distribution and has been isolated from blood vessel walls (primarily aorta) [49], amyloid [49], and brain [50]. Dorfman and Ho [51] have shown that heparan sulfate is formed in tissue culture by a strain of rat glial tumor cells.

Sulfated acid mucopolysaccharides are covalently bound to proteins. Although the nature of linkage to protein is known, other aspects of the macromolecular structure of the protein-polysaccharide are not yet fully understood. The basic concept of structure of chondromucoprotein was first proposed by Mathews and Lozaityte [52]. Figure 49-5 is a modification of this structure incorporating the additional information now available. This structure envisions a number of polysaccharide chains bound covalently to serine residues through the trisaccharide linkage region to a protein core. Such a structure is consistent with recent chemical evidence and the pathway of biosynthesis. The length of the polysaccharide chains varies with tissues and species [53]. As indicated in Fig. 49-5, some chains of keratan sulfate II and chondroitin-4/6-SO_4 appear to be attached to the same protein core [54, 55]. Mathews [56] has recently indicated that polysaccharide chains are spaced along the protein backbone in doublets; that is, two chains are separated by a relatively small number of amino acids while a larger number of amino acids separate such doublets. Doublets containing keratan sulfate and chondroitin sulfate have been isolated by Seno et al. [57], and a peptide containing both keratan sulfate and chondroitin sulfate was found in normal urine and in greatly increased amounts in the urine of patients with Morquio's disease by Kaplan et al. [58].

There remains considerable uncertainty regarding the nature of the protein of mucopolysaccharide-protein complexes. Chondromucoprotein preparations obtained by different investigators have exhibited a diversity of size, protein content, and amino acid composition. Evidence for multiple N-terminal amino acids has been presented. This lack of homogeneity may be derived from the association of chondromucoprotein with other proteins. Following treatment of chondromucoprotein preparations with 4*M* guanidinium chloride, Hascall and Sajdera [59, 60] isolated two components; one was designated a glycoprotein, and the other a chondroitin protein complex. Recombination of the two components produced aggregation which was de-

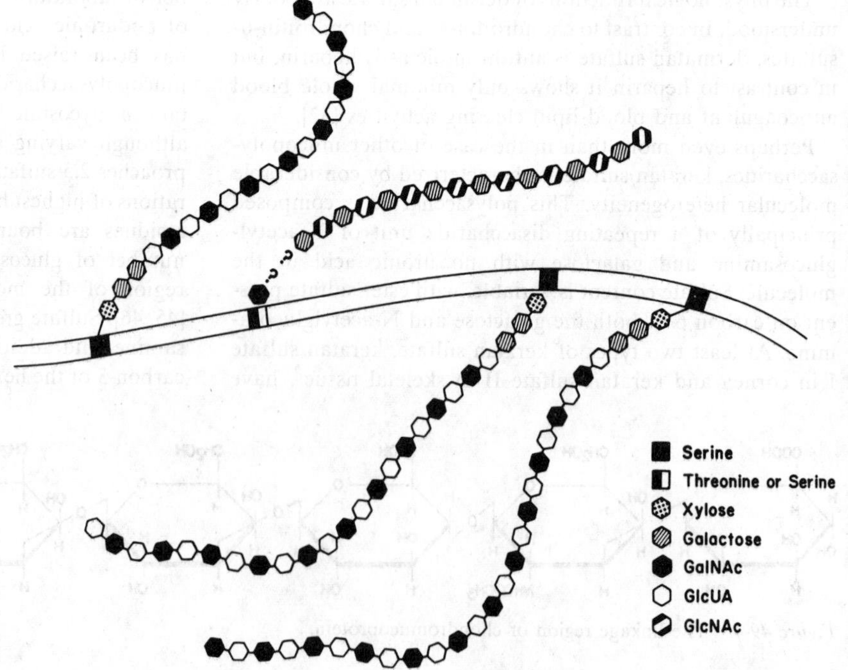

Figure 49-5. Sketch of current conception of a segment of the chondromucoprotein. The linkage region of keratan sulfate is not completely known. The carbohydrate chains are considerably longer than illustrated.

pendent on ionic strength and pH. Reduction and alkylation of cystine residues prevented reaggregation. The configuration of such aggregates is unknown.

Even less is known concerning the structure of protein complexes of mucopolysaccharides other than chondroitin sulfate. Toole and Lowther [61] have isolated a protein-polysaccharide complex of dermatan sulfate containing 50 percent protein. This complex appears to be firmly bound in tissues to collagen. The molecular weight of 100,000 to 200,000 is considerably less than that of the protein complexes of chondroitin sulfates.

The nature of the binding of heparin to protein has been a source of controversy which has not been resolved. Heparin preparations not treated with alkali were shown by Lindahl and Rodén [62] to contain serine and the galactosylgalactosylxylose linkage region. However, attempts to isolate protein-polysaccharide complexes from liver capsule or mast cell tumor granules have led to variable results [63, 64]. Lindahl [47] found that heparin prepared without alkali or proteolysis contained less than 1 mole of xylose and serine per polysaccharide chain. Interpretation of these findings is difficult but may be pertinent to some problems of the metabolism of mucopolysaccharides in the mucopolysaccharidoses. If it is assumed that the pathway of biosynthesis of heparin is similar to that of chondromucoprotein, it is to be expected that all heparin is initially synthesized as part of a protein complex. Since heparin normally remains within the cell (perhaps to be released only when mast cells are stimulated), intracellular heparin might be freed from the protein core by an endoglycosidase action which results in the release of free polysaccharide chains. The protein may be removed by proteolytic action either prior to or subsequent to such endoglycosidase action.

The binding of heparan sulfate to protein is even more poorly understood. There is, however, evidence that the heparan sulfate isolated from aorta or Hurler's urine or tissues contains serine, galactose, and xylose [65] in appropriate ratios, indicating the existence of a protein complex.

BIOSYNTHESIS OF MUCOPOLYSACCHARIDES

The widespread occurrence of heteropolysaccharides covalently linked to proteins and to lipids has enhanced interest in the study of the biosynthesis of this class of natural products. For the most part the pathways of biosynthesis of these materials are similar in a wide variety of cells. The mechanism of biosynthesis follows certain general principles.

1 The monosaccharide units are derived from glucose by a series of enzymic steps which alter steric configuration, state of oxidation, and length of carbon chain, and add amino groups.
2 Amino sugars are formed by the transfer of the amide group of glutamine to ketosugars.
3 The glycosyl residues are transferred to acceptors from precursor nucleotide diphosphate sugars or, in some cases, by way of lipid intermediates.
4 Unlike proteins and nucleic acids, the ordering of sugars is not specified by a template but rather by the specificity of the enzymes for both donor and acceptor groups. Genetic control is accordingly exerted by the specificity of the enzyme.
5 Carbohydrate chains are elongated in most cases from the nonreducing end of the chains by the transfer of glycosyl residues from nucleotide sugars. Exceptions are formation of the gram-negative lipopolysaccharides [66, 67] and bacterial cell walls [68], which involve a polyterpenoid lipid intermediate. A similar intermediate has been implicated in the transfer of mannose in both yeast and mammalian tissues [69, 70] and, more recently, perhaps in glycoprotein synthesis [71].
6 The glycosyl transferase enzymes appear to be membrane associated.

The interconversion of sugars and the formation of precursor nucleotides has been reviewed elsewhere [72].

The pathways for the formation of sugar nucleotides required for the synthesis of acid mucopolysaccharides are illustrated in Fig. 49-6. Mucopolysaccharide synthesis involving each of these nucleotides, with the exception of UDP-IdUA, has been directly demonstrated. It is assumed that UDP-IdUA is an intermediate in the formation of dermatan sulfate although in vitro biosynthesis of this polysaccharide has not yet been achieved. The epimerization of UDP-GlcUA to UDP-IdUA was discovered by Jacobson and Davidson [73] in rabbit skin and has more recently been found in intestinal mucosa by Fransson [74]. Of the precursors illustrated in Fig. 49-6, only UDP-IdUA and possibly UDP-xylose are uniquely associated with mucopolysaccharide syntheses. The remaining sugar nucleotides are intermediates for other cellular processes.

Inhibition of UDP-Glc dehydrogenase by UDP-xylose [75] and inhibition of fructose-6-PO_4 glutamine transamidase by UDP-GlcNAc [76] appear to be regulators of nucleotide levels.

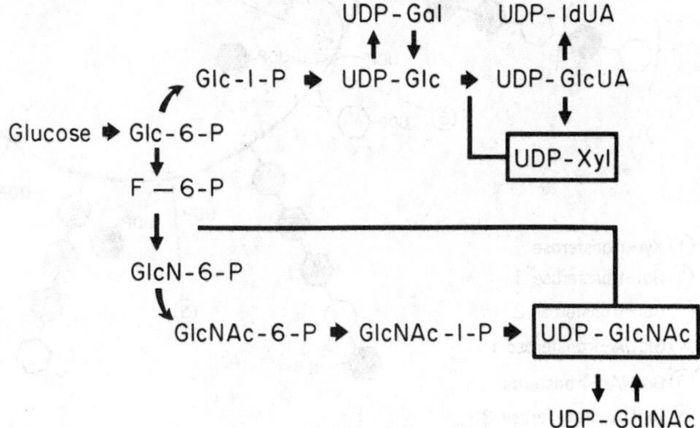

Figure 49-6. The pathway of formation of uridine nucleotide sugars involved in mucopolysaccharide biosynthesis.

Since the biosynthesis of the chondroitin sulfates is now most thoroughly understood, this pathway will be discussed as a prototype of mucopolysaccharide formation. The formation of macromolecules containing carbohydrate covalently bound to protein raises important questions of integration of synthesis of the two portions of the molecule. Three obvious possibilities exist: (1) independent synthesis of protein and polysaccharide followed by conjugation, (2) initial synthesis of protein followed by addition of carbohydrate, or (3) initial synthesis of polysaccharide followed by addition of protein. Studies utilizing puromycin and cycloheximide demonstrated that protein synthesis is required for the formation of the polysaccharide chain [77–79]. Similar results have been obtained in the study of various glycoproteins [80–83]. It may be concluded, therefore, that initially protein is synthesized, and carbohydrate is then added. Whether the initiation of polysaccharide chain growth precedes completion of the peptide chain and release from the ribosomes has not been definitively determined.

The pathway of formation of chondromucoprotein is illustrated in Fig. 49-7. Polysaccharide chains are initiated by the transfer of xylose from UDP-xylose to appropriate serine residues in the protein. Baker and Rodén [84] have demonstrated the transfer of xylose from UDP-xylose to a protein obtained by the Smith degradation of chondromucoprotein of the bovine nasal septum, and to a peptide mixture obtained by Smith degradation of a trypsin digest of chondromucoprotein, and to serylglycylglycine. The enzyme (enzyme 1) responsible for this transfer has been solubilized and purified from embryonic chick epiphyses by Horwitz et al. [85]. The exact sequence of amino acids in the region of attachment of polysaccharide chain has not yet been ascertained, although Katsura and Davidson [86] have indicated a sequence of glutamylglycylserylglycine in this region. More information is needed regarding the mechanism and determinants of specificity for the initiation of polysaccharide chain growth.

The details of further elongation of the polysaccharide chain have been immensely facilitated by the utilization of small molecular weight acceptors. Enzymes 2 and 3, which have been defined by Helting and Rodén [87], are responsible for the sequential addition of the two galactosyl residues to xylose to complete the linkage region. Although enzymes 2 and 3 have not yet been separated, competition experiments indicate that they are distinct and specific for appropriate acceptor groups. The configuration of the penultimate monosaccharide probably does not confer absolute specificity but may influence reaction rates [88].

Enzyme 4, also studied by Helting and Rodén [88], which is responsible for initiation of the mucopolysaccharide chain proper, transfers a uronsyl residue to a nonreducing galactose residue. As might be expected, inhibition experiments indicate that enzyme 4 is distinct from enzyme 6 which transfers uronosyl residues to N-acetylgalactosamine.

Enzyme 5 transfers N-acetylgalactosamine to uronic acid and, acting in concert with enzyme 6, results in alternation to produce the disaccharide units. Studies of the specificity of enzymes 5 and 6 indicate that glucuronic acid and

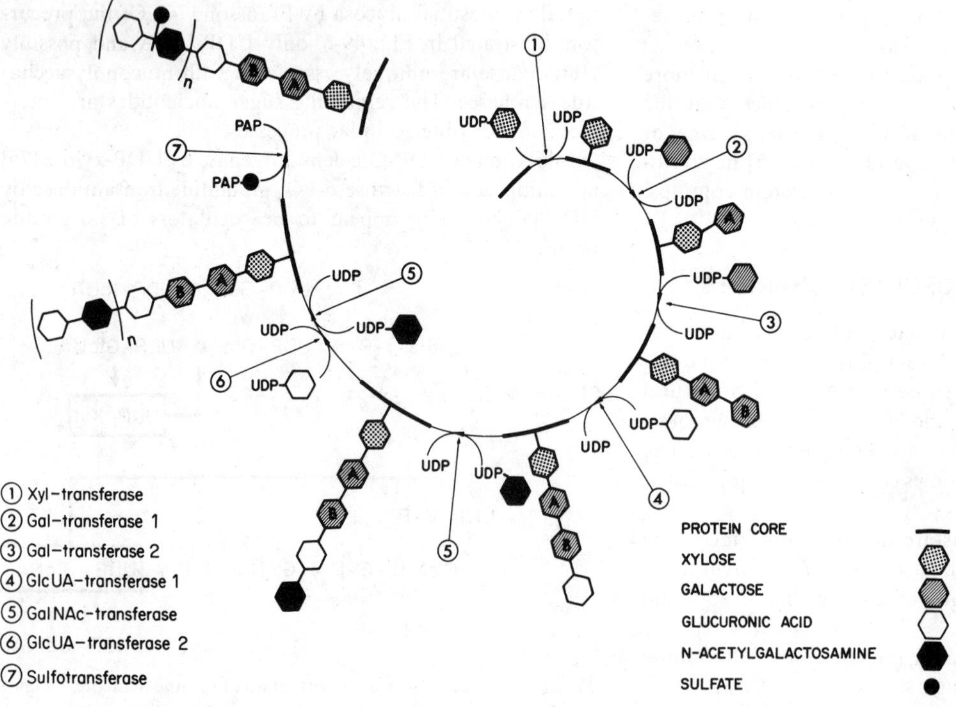

Figure 49-7. The pathway of biosynthesis of chondroitin-4-SO_4.

N-acetylgalactosamine are added to the nonreducing terminus of the polysaccharide chain without participation of an intermediate disaccharide. The enzymes are highly specific for alternation of glycosyl units, i.e., glucuronic acid is not added to an acceptor with a nonreducing glucuronic acid, and N-acetylgalactosamine is not transfered to an acceptor with a nonreducing N-acetylgalactosamine terminus. Enzyme 5 of cartilage does not transfer glucuronic acid to an acceptor with a nonreducing N-acetylglucosamine terminus; this indicates specificity for the configuration at C-4 of the hexosamine acceptor. A hybrid oligosaccharide was, however, formed by the transfer of N-acetylgalactosamine to a hexasaccharide prepared from hyaluronic acid. The enzyme, therefore, does not exhibit absolute specificity for the configuration of the penultimate monosaccharide. A sulfate group on position 4, but not on position 6, of the N-acetylgalactosamine nonreducing terminus prevented transfer of glucuronic acid. This phenomenon may have some pertinence to the mechanism of chain termination. If sulfation in position 4 of the nonreducing terminal N-acetylgalactosamine occurs, chain elongation may cease. Since such a mechanism would not account for chain termination of chondroitin-6-SO_4, it is likely that other mechanisms are involved. The polydispersity of chains indicates that relatively nonspecific factors may be operative. For example, if the K_m of the binding of the chondromucoprotein to the transferases decreases as the molecule increases in size, the product may be released as size increases, with consequent chain termination.

Robbins and Lipmann [90, 91] discovered that esterification of sulfate results from the transfer of sulfate from 3′-phosphoadenosine-5′-phosphosulfate (PAPS) to various acceptors. Since D'Abramo and Lipmann [92] showed that this mechanism was operative in the transfer of sulfate to chondroitin sulfate, numerous studies on the mechanism of sulfation of mucopolysaccharides have been reported [72]. Davidson and Meyer [21] proposed that chondroitin is an intermediate in chondroitin sulfate synthesis. However, the discovery of UDP-GalNAc-4-SO_4 in hen oviduct by Suzuki and Strominger [93] and its subsequent demonstration in cartilage by Picard and Gardais [94] raised the possibility that this compound may be an intermediate in mucopolysaccharide synthesis. No enzyme system has been discovered which utilizes UDP-GalNAc-4-SO_4 in mucopolysaccharide biosynthesis, while considerable evidence supports the concept that polymerization precedes sulfation. The function of UDP-GalNAc-4-SO_4 remains unknown.

Although the weight of evidence indicates that sulfation occurs at the macromolecular state, it is not yet clear whether the polysaccharide chain is completed before sulfation begins. The studies of Perlman and associates [95] indicate that polysaccharide chain formation occurs in the absence of sulfation, but the more recent studies of Silbert and DeLuca [96] suggest that sulfation proceeds as the polysaccharide chain grows.

Considerable confusion exists concerning the specificity of sulfotransferases. Since few studies have attempted purification of these enzymes, the apparent lack of specificity must be accepted with caution. Indeed when more detailed studies are undertaken, greater specificity becomes more evident. Details of the activity of sulfotransferases on various substrates have been reviewed by Stoolmiller and Dorfman [72] and Rodén [97].

Investigation of the biosynthesis of hyaluronic acid has been most extensive in group A streptococci [98–100]. As in the case of chondroitin sulfate, the polysaccharide chain is formed by the sequential addition of acetylated hexosamine and glucuronic acid units by transfer from the appropriate nucleotide sugars. The enzyme(s) in streptococci are bound to the protoplast membranes and, so far, have not been solubilized. In contrast to the chondroitin sulfate synthesizing system of cartilage, the use of small molecular weight acceptors has been unsuccessful, although single uronic acid residues may be added to nascent chains bound to the enzyme [100]. Treatment of streptococci with chloramphenicol or puromycin, under conditions which inhibit protein synthesis, does not prevent formation of hyaluronic acid. In contrast, both cycloheximide and puromycin partially inhibit hyaluronic acid synthesis in cultured human fibroblasts [79]. In view of the role of a lipid intermediate in the synthesis of the O antigen of *Salmonella,* the possibility of the participation of such an intermediate in hyaluronic acid has been examined by Stoolmiller and Dorfman [100]. No evidence for the involvement of such an intermediate was found. Preliminary studies by Stoolmiller and Dorfman [101] suggest that the reducing end of the streptococcal hyaluronic acid is N-acetylglucosamine. These studies, taken together with kinetic data, favor N-acetylglycosamine as the first sugar in the chain in hyaluronic acid formed by streptococci.

Understanding of the mechanism of hyaluronic acid formation in eucaryotic cells is more limited. Hyaluronic acid synthesis has been demonstrated in extracts of Rous sarcoma [102] and in Rous sarcoma-converted fibroblasts [103]. Schiller et al. [104] demonstrated hyaluronic acid synthesis in extracts of fetal rat skin, the enzymes for which were partially "solubilized" by mild papein treatment. Österlin and Jacobson [105, 106] found hyaluronic acid synthesizing activity in homogenates of the cortical layer of the vitreous body (presumably from the hyalocytes). Enzymic activity was found in both the supernatant solution and a sedimenting fraction.

Radioactive N-acetylglucosamine and glucuronic acid were transferred from the appropriate nucleotides to an endogenous acceptor as well as to an oligosaccharide mixture resulting from the digestion of hyaluronic acid by testicular hyaluronidase. Additionally, these investigators reported the formation of radioactive oligosaccharides on incubation of the enzyme with precursor nucleotides in the absence of added acceptors. Such a reaction requires that a nucleotide sugar (or some intermediate derived therefrom) act as an acceptor, with subsequent hydrolysis of the product to an oligosaccharide. Such a mechanism has not yet been reported, although nucleotide trisaccharides have been found [107]. Obviously many problems regarding the biosynthesis of hyaluronic acid remain to be elucidated, perhaps the most important of which is the resolution of the question of binding of hyaluronic acid to protein.

No cell-free system has been obtained which catalyzes the biosynthesis of dermatan sulfate. The study of the possible mechanisms of this biosynthesis raises two interesting problems not considered with respect to chondromucoprotein synthesis: (1) the origin of L-iduronic acid, and (2) the mechanism of hybrid polysaccharide formation. L-Iduronic acid residues probably derive from UDP-IdUA although more information is required regarding the UDP-GlcUA→UDP-IdUA epimerase. On the basis of available information concerning the specificity of glycosyl transferases, it is to be anticipated that cells which form dermatan sulfate should contain separate enzymes for the transfer of D-glucuronic acid and L-iduronic acid. The D-glucuronic acid transferase might be expected to be the same as that involved in chondroitin sulfate synthesis (enzyme 6, Fig. 49-7). This enzyme has been demonstrated in cultured skin fibroblasts which synthesize dermatan sulfate [108]. If the configuration of the penultimate group does not restrict the action of the enzyme, then this enzyme may participate in the formation of a hybrid polysaccharide, i.e., it could transfer D-glucuronic acid to an acceptor which contains L-iduronic acid in the penultimate position. It would be expected that two different N-acetylgalactosamine transferases are present, one to transfer N-acetylgalactosamine to L-iduronic acid nonreducing terminal acceptors and one to transfer N-acetylgalactosamine to D-glucuronic acid nonreducing terminal acceptors. The latter enzyme would be the same as that involved in chondroitin sulfate synthesis (enzyme 5, Fig. 49-7). If these speculations are correct, cells which synthesize dermatan sulfate should also contain the enzyme complement required for biosynthesis of chondroitin sulfate. A number of tissues which contain dermatan sulfate also contain chondroitin sulfate. The mechanisms responsible for the control of the relative amounts of the two polysaccharides or the extent of hybridization in dermatan sulfate are unknown. The possible role of the specific protein core remains to be elucidated. Preliminary studies by Stern and Rodén [109] indicate that the amino acid sequence in the region of polysaccharide attachment differs in the protein of skin dermatan sulfate from that of the chondromucoprotein of bovine nasal cartilage.

The pathway of sulfation of dermatan sulfate appears to follow that of other sulfated mucopolysaccharides. Since sulfate may occur in three different positions in dermatan sulfate, the 4 and 6 positions of N-acetylgalactosamine and on the uronic acid, as many as three different sulfotransferases may be required. That the sulfotransferases required for dermatan sulfate synthesis differ from those involved in chondroitin sulfate synthesis is indicated by studies of sulfotransferase of rabbit skin by Davidson and Riley [110] and of sulfotransferases of a leiomyosarcoma by Adams and Meaney [111].

Heparin and heparan sulfate biosynthesis presents problems which differ from those encountered in the study of the biosynthesis of other mucopolysaccharides. These include (1) the formation of α-glycoside linkages, (2) the formation of sulfamide linkages, and (3) the possible formation of branch points. The formation of α linkages from sugar nucleotides (which presumably are α linked) is not unique in that many such linkages occur in other polysaccharides. If transfer occurs by way of a two-step reaction, the α linkage will be maintained. Such a double displacement reaction might occur if the sugar is transferred through an additional intermediate or preliminary binding to the enzyme.

The formation of heparin in vitro has been studied in mast cell tumors primarily by Silbert [112–115]. A particulate enzyme preparation catalyzed the transfer of glucuronic acid and N-acetylglucosamine from the respective UDP derivatives to an endogenous acceptor to form a substance resistant to testicular hyaluronidase but not resistant to bacterial heparinase. Addition of 3′-phosphoadenyl-5′-phosphosulfate to the reaction mixture resulted in the appearance of both O and N sulfate esters and the concomitant loss of acetyl groups.

These observations indicate that heparin is formed by way of an N-acetylated glucosamine polysaccharide intermediate. A somewhat different pathway was suggested by Balasubramanian and coworkers [116], who isolated a soluble enzyme from a mast cell tumor which catalyzed the transfer of sulfate from 3′-phosphoadenyl-5′-phosphosulfate to N-desulfated heparan sulfate. Acetylation of the free amino groups decreased the efficiency of the acceptor. Addition of xylose to an endogenous acceptor in mast cell and chick oviduct preparations appears to follow the same pattern as occurs in chondromucoprotein synthesis [117,118].

The biosynthetic relationship of heparan sulfate to heparin is unknown. The presence of N-acetyl groups in heparin and the demonstration of an exchange of N-sulfate for N-acetyl groups suggest that the two compounds differ only with respect to the extent of replacement of N-acetyl groups by N-sulfate groups. The existence of a family of heparan sulfates containing various amounts of N-sulfate should be noted [48]. The fact that heparin is intracellular in mast cells and heparan sulfate appears to be extracellular may indicate both a metabolic and physiological distinction. Heparan sulfate has also been demonstrated in mast cell tumors [119].

It may be postulated that initial synthesis involves formation of an N-acetylated polysaccharide which may be partially N-sulfated and excreted from the cell as heparan sulfate. The same intermediate may be more thoroughly N-sulfated and O-sulfated and perhaps separated from the protein core (see above) while it is stored in the cell to give the granules of mast cells. The problems of introduction of L-iduronic and D-glucuronic acid residues are similar to those discussed for dermatan sulfate.

No cell-free system has yet been obtained for the in vitro biosynthesis of keratosulfate. This problem is considerably complicated by the many unknowns regarding the structure of both keratan sulfate I and keratan sulfate II. Sulfation of keratan sulfate has been reported in extracts of cornea by Wortman [120].

The Intracellular Localization of Polysaccharide Synthesis

A more complete understanding of the mechanism of intracellular synthesis of complex macromolecules destined for export requires not only an elucidation of the pathway of biosynthesis but an understanding of the integration of this process with respect to both cell function and structure. A number of pertinent questions must be considered: (1) What is the localization of synthesis of the core protein? (2) What is the site and time of addition of the initial carbohydrate unit? (3) What is the site of and spatial organization of the enzymes responsible for chain elongation and sulfation? (4) When and where do chain elongation and sulfation occur? (5) What mechanism is responsible for chain termination? (6) How is the completed product transported and released from the cell?

The cytoplasmic membrane system clearly plays a major role in polysaccharide synthesis [121]. It seems reasonable to assume that the core protein is synthesized at the ribosome by a conventional pattern of protein synthesis. Differentiated connective tissue cells engaged in matrix synthesis generally show an extensive rough endoplasmic reticulum [122]. Whether the first sugar unit is attached to the core protein before the peptide is completed is not clear.

Radioautographic studies have been carried out in attempts to locate the cellular sites of the synthesis of chondroitin sulfate [123, 124]. Goodman and Lane [124] found that, in minced tibiofemoral cartilage, sulfate is esterified within 3 min. Radioautography showed that only the vesicular component of the Golgi apparatus contains the radioactivity. It was postulated that the last step of biosynthesis occurs at this site. Neutra and Leblond [125], utilizing uptake of ^{3}H-glucose and ^{3}H-galactose in chondrocytes of tracheal and epiphyseal cartilage, observed by radioautography the accumulation of radioactivity in the region of the Golgi complex, beginning 15 to 20 min after the administration of labeled sugars. Numerous radioautographic studies suggested a major role for the Golgi complex in the synthesis and storage of mucopolysaccharides.

Roy and Ghadially [126] attempted to locate the site of hyaluronic acid synthesis in synovial membrane with combined histochemical and electron microscopic techniques utilizing colloidal iron staining. The localization of iron particles in small vesicles of the Golgi complex of the synovial cell suggested that this complex is involved in the secretion of hyaluronic acid. Barland and associates [127] studied intracellular hyaluronic acid synthesis by exposing cultured human synovial cells to ^{3}H-glucosamine. After 5 min of labeling, 47 percent of all grains were situated over the Golgi apparatus. The remaining grains were evenly distributed over the rest of the cytoplasmic organelles in proportion to the approximate areas occupied by these structures. When labeling was prolonged, the grains appeared to be predominantly associated with the Golgi apparatus.

These investigations were interpreted to indicate that the Golgi apparatus is the site of hyaluronic acid and chondroitin sulfate biosynthesis. Lack of resolution in thick sections with relatively high energy $^{35}SO_4$ and the absence of electronmicroscopic evidence in the tritiated galactose studies limit the validity of the conclusions. The appearance of most of the radioactivity in the Golgi apparatus may simply reflect a concentration of product in this area.

The role of the rough and smooth endoplasmic reticulum, including the Golgi complex, in the synthesis, transfer, and export of extracellular proteins has been investigated in such tissues as liver and pancreas [128–130]. Substances for export from the cell may be modified in various ways. The simplest form, perhaps, is aggregation and condensation to form secretory granules. Thus, for pancreatic enzymes, the zymogens are accumulated and condensed, and the vesicles are separated from the Golgi complex [129].

Liver glycoproteins are modified by the addition of short carbohydrate units. The hexosamine is believed to be added at least in part at the ribosomes [131] and perhaps additional sugars are added as the proteins traverse the cisternal spaces. Eylar [132] has proposed that interaction of the bound carbohydrate of a glycoprotein with the appropriate receptor in the cellular membrane permits transport of the macromolecule into the extracellular environment. Another interesting example of modification prior to export is that of protocollagen which must be hydroxylated before export [133].

Chondromucoprotein may be considered an extreme case of modification of a protein which involves the addition of extended polysaccharide chains. These chains are further modified by sulfation. Since chondromucoprotein biosynthesis proceeds by the stepwise addition of monosaccharide units to an acceptor protein, the actual subcellular distribution of enzymic activities involved in this biosynthetic sequence can be examined. In a preliminary communication, Suzuki et al. [134] examined xylose, galactose, glucuronic acid, galactosamine, and sulfate transferase activities in heavy and light particulate fractions obtained from a homogenate of chick embryo cartilage. Enzymic activities were demonstrable in both fractions with respect to the transfer of each sugar from the appropriate UDP derivative to endogenous acceptor. Horwitz and Dorfman [121] have studied in detail the localization of enzymic activities involved in chondroitin sulfate synthesis in preparations derived from embryonic chick chondroblasts which were fractionated by density gradient centrifugation. Both the total and specific activities for the enzymic transfer of xylose from UDP-Xyl to the hydroxyl groups of serine in the protein core are much higher in the rough endoplasmic reticulum than in the smooth. The distribution of the activity for transfer of galactose was similar. In these studies the measure of activity of xylosyl transferase and galactosyl transferase depended upon two variables: (1) the concentration of enzyme, and (2) the concentration of acceptor protein. More recent studies [135] utilizing artificial acceptors also showed that the total enzymic activity for addition of the linkage-region sugars, xylose and galactose, was greater in the rough than in the smooth microsomes.

The specific activity of the chondroitin sulfate polymerase enzymes (enzymes 5 and 6, Fig. 49-7) was approximately equal in the smooth and rough fractions. The incorporation of radioactivity from UDP-GalNAc^{3}H is stimulated by UDP-GlcUA in both the rough and smooth fractions, in accord with previous observations [95]. These findings indicate that chain elongation occurs when both nucleotides are present. As in the case of xylose and galactose incorporation, the polymerase assay utilizing both nucleotide sugars is dependent upon the concentration of endogenous acceptor as well as upon the concentration of polymerase. The measure of chondroitin sulfate polymerase activity using oligosaccharide acceptors obviates the problem of endogenous acceptors [121]. As in the case of polysaccharide synthesis, the specific activity was approximately the same in the smooth and rough fractions with hexasaccharide acceptors. For the pentasaccharide assay, the activity of the rough subfraction was somewhat higher.

The transfer of sulfate from 3′-phosphoadenyl-5′-phosphosulfate to chondroitin sulfate is also catalyzed by the microsomal fractions. When this enzyme was assayed with both endogenous and exogenous (chondroitin) acceptors, the specific activity of the smooth subfraction was four to five times that of the rough. The exact nature of the endogenous acceptor is unknown, but the smooth subfraction contained approximately four times as much endogenous acceptor as did the rough fraction. The sulfotransferase was readily solubilized.

On the basis of these studies and other information, the data were interpreted as follows: The synthesis of chondromucoprotein is initiated by formation of the core protein at the ribosome. The linkage-region sugars are added primarily at the rough endoplasmic reticulum, and the molecule is elongated and completed as it proceeds through the smooth endoplasmic reticulum and the Golgi apparatus.

Irrespective of the intracellular localization indicated by these studies, it is quite clear that the various enzymes are closely associated with membranes. The localization in membranes of enzymes involved in synthesis of complex macromolecules has been widely recognized. Although hypothetical, it is reasonable to assume that the specific spatial arrangement of enzymes active in a series of metabolic reactions may be highly advantageous from a kinetic point of view. If all reactions were to proceed randomly in free solution, each product would have to achieve relatively high concentrations before it could saturate the next enzyme in the biosynthetic pathway. If instead, as is apparently true, the enzymes are inserted into membranes, the progression of biosynthetic reactions may be promoted by the spatial relationships of the enzymes. Recent evidence suggests that at least some of the enzymes involved in chondromucoprotein synthesis are closely associated on multienzyme particles which in turn are attached to the membranes [136].

One may consider the intracellular synthesis of chondromucoproteins based on an assembly line of enzymes oriented in an orderly fashion on the cell membrane system. Along this path travels a product which is being fabricated by this enzymic machinery. The product travels with a half-life time probably of an order of magnitude of minutes. Whether the product is in solution in the cisternae of the endoplasmic reticulum or is attached to a membrane with a rapid transport is not clear.

Such a formulation raises interesting questions, many of which cannot yet be answered:

1 What fundamental control mechanisms determine the qualitative nature of the polysaccharides that are formed? It is clear that connective tissue cells in a number of locations possess the capacity for synthesis of mucopolysaccharides. Nevertheless, specific cells seem to become highly differentiated for the production of specific mucopolysaccharides. Chondrocytes appear to be limited to the formation of chondroitin-4- and chondroitin-6-sulfates and keratan sulfate II, while skin fibroblasts form a mixture of hyaluronic acid, dermatan sulfate, and chondroitin sulfates.

It is apparent from Fig. 49-6 that qualitative control of this differentiation is probably not dependent solely on synthesis of the nucleotide precursors since the requisite nucleotide sugars (with the possible exception of UDP-IdUA and UDP-xylose) are common to the formation of a large number of mucopolysaccharides, glycoproteins, and glycolipids. The synthesis of amino sugar precursors seems to be internally controlled. The studies of Kornfeld et al. [76] indicate that UDP-GlcNAc inhibits the fructose-6-PO_4 glutamine transamidase, thus serving as a feedback inhibitor of both UDP-GlcNAc and UDP-GalNAc. It seems more likely that the formation of specific glycosyl transferases or the specific acceptor proteins account for the qualitative specificity of connective tissue cells.

2 What factors control the rate of synthesis of mucopolysaccharides? Control of protein synthesis may affect mucopolysaccharide synthesis by virtue of control of both formation of acceptor proteins and formation of appropriate glycosyl transferases. Whether the synthesis of the protein acceptor is coordinated with the synthesis of the glycosyl transferases remains to be determined. A mechanism for the control of nucleotide interconversions by the level of acceptor protein is afforded by the observation of Neufeld and Hall [75] that UDP-xylose inhibits the conversion of UDP-Glc to UDP-GlcUA. In the absence of acceptor protein, formation of UDP-GlcUA would be inhibited.

Of great importance is further elucidation of the mechanisms controlling the flow of materials from the rough endoplasmic reticulum through the Golgi apparatus to the cell exterior. Jamieson and Palade [129, 137] proposed a scheme which involves two important locks. The first, which is dependent upon respiration, is between the rough endoplasmic reticulum and the Golgi apparatus, and the second involves the release of secretion vacuoles to the exterior and, apparently, also involves oxidative energy. Whether similar locks are involved in secretion of acid mucopolysaccharide production is not clear.

In the normal formation of extracellular matrix, it is probable that the amount of extracellular matrix influences the rate of formation of mucopolysaccharides. This type of control requires some communication from the extracellular material to the biosynthetic machinery of the cell. Although little is known regarding the nature of this communication, recent studies utilizing enzymes in organ culture indicate that depletion of matrix does indeed result in increase of intracellular synthetic rates [138].

Communication of extracellular matrix to biosynthetic machinery of the cell affords a possible mechanism for communication between cells.

A series of investigations concerned with factors that affect the metabolism of acid mucopolysaccharides of mammalian skin has been carried out by Schiller et al. [139–146]. It was found that hyaluronic acid of rat and rabbit skin is metabolically active, with a half-life varying from 2.5 to 4.0 days. The sulfated mucopolysaccharides turn over more slowly with a half-life of from 7 to 10 days. Similar half-life times were obtained whether the hexose moieties, the N-acetyl groups, or the sulfate groups were labeled.

Determination of these indices of normal metabolism facilitated studies of the influence of hormones on mucopolysaccharide metabolism [141, 142]. Administration of hydrocortisone resulted in a progressive decrease in the rate of turnover of both the hyaluronic acid and sulfated polysaccharide fractions. Induction of alloxan diabetes in rats caused a similar decrease in turnover rates of both fractions. The metabolic rates were restored to normal by the administration of insulin.

Studies of the effect of thyroxine and growth hormone on the metabolism of acid mucopolysaccharides of skin yielded discrepancies between uptake and decay measurements which suggested that rapid changes in pool size sufficient to invalidate the interpretation of turnover data may have occurred in hypophysectomized animals.

A fall in hyaluronic acid content with increasing age was found [143, 144]. The absolute amount of sulfated polysaccharide also decreases but less strikingly. Surprisingly, large amounts of heparin were found which had eluded detection by previous methods. The concentration of heparin decreases strikingly with age.

Following induction of hypothyroidism in rats fed propylthiouracil, there was a marked increase in the concentration of hyaluronic acid and a decrease in the concentration of sulfated mucopolysaccharides [14]. Treatment with thyroxine resulted in restoration toward normal. These changes did not follow the administration of thyrotropic hormone preparations, irrespective of whether or not they were contaminated with exophthalmic factor.

An impressive increase of hyaluronic acid concentration and a drop in sulfated polysaccharide content were observed following hypophysectomy [146]. Administration of growth hormone restored the sulfated fraction content toward normal, but the hyaluronic acid concentration was further increased. Administration of thyroxine to hypophysectomized animals resulted in a diminution of the hyaluronic acid concentration.

DEGRADATION OF MUCOPOLYSACCHARIDES

Discovery of lysosomes and recognition of the accumulation of partially degraded carbohydrate-containing macromolecules in a variety of storage diseases has focused attention on the physiological significance of glycosidases, many of which have been long known to be present in tissues. Studies in vivo had demonstrated that acid mucopolysaccharides turn over at a reasonably rapid rate in connective tissues. This implied the presence of enzymic pathways for the degradation of these compounds [13].

Since the original discovery by Meyer et al. [147] of an enzyme in pneumococci which degrades hyaluronic acid, an extensive literature has been concerned with enzymes which hydrolyze this polysaccharide [148]. The existence of hyaluronidase in mammalian tissues became clear when Chain and Duthie [149] demonstrated that the "spreading factor" of Duran-Reynals [150] was identical with this enzyme.

Mammalian hyaluronidases are endoglycosidases which hydrolyze endo-N-acetylglucosaminyl and endo-N-acetylgalactosaminyl-D-glucuronic acid bonds and catalyze transglycosylation. Testicular hyaluronidase hydrolyzes hyaluronic acid and chondroitin sulfates primarily to tetrasaccharides with the simultaneous production of disaccharides and hexasaccharides. In contrast, bacterial hyaluronidases split hyaluronic acid by an elimination reaction to produce disaccharides with 4, 5 unsaturation of the glucuronic acid moiety. Most bacterial enzymes do not act on sulfated polysaccharides; however, the enzymes isolated from *Proteus vulgaris* produce $\Delta^{4,5}$-disaccharides from chondroitin-4- and chondroitin-6-sulfates, as well as from dermatan sulfate [20]. Leech hyaluronidase hydrolyzes the endoglucosuronicyl$(1 \rightarrow 3)$ N-acetylglucosamine bond of hyaluronic acid [151].

Most studies on the purification and properties of hyaluronidase have concerned the enzyme extracted from mammalian testes. This enzyme is heat stable at acid pH and is optimally active in the region of pH 4.0. Speculation regarding the role of hyaluronidase of sperm in fertilization has not received firm experimental support.

The widespread occurrence of hyaluronidase as a lysosomal enzyme has recently become clear. Bollet and associates [152] demonstrated hyaluronidase in rat and guinea pig liver and kidney, rat spleen, human kidney, urine, plasma, synovial fluid, and synovial tissue. Hyaluronidase of lysosomes of liver, reported by Hutterer [153], has been purified by Aronson and Davidson [154] and found to have a pH optimum of 3.5 (lower than that of testicular hyaluronidase) and a molecular weight of 80,000. Other properties were similar to those of testicular hyaluronidase [155]. Like that enzyme, liver hyaluronidase acts on hyaluronic acid and chondroitin-4-SO_4 and chondroitin-6-SO_4 to produce oligosaccharides and is a transglycosidase. Hyaluronidase has also been found in the lysosomes of rat bone [156], kidney [157], canine submandibular gland [158], bovine aorta [159], rat skin [160], and tadpole tissues [161]. Cashman and coworkers [160] showed that skin hyaluronidase is polymorphic since it contains isozymes characterized by different isoelectric points, a variation apparently attributable to sialic acid content. Like the liver enzyme, the skin enzyme has a lower pH optimum and less affinity toward hexasaccharide than does the testicular enzyme. Bowness and Tan [162] have demonstrated that human serum hyaluronidase differs from bovine testis hyaluronidase in the elution pattern on chromatography and like lysosomal hyaluronidases shows a lower pH optimum.

Fransson and Rodén [28, 29] found that dermatan sulfate is a hybrid polysaccharide which contains both D-glucuronic acid and L-iduronic acid. Testicular hyaluronidase accordingly partially degrades this polysaccharide by hydrolysis of the interspersed endo-N-acetylgalactosaminyl-D-glucuronic acid linkages but not the endo-N-acetylgalactosaminyl-L-iduronic acid linkages.

Since hyaluronidase degrades hyaluronic acid and chondroitin-4- and chondroitin-6-SO_4 only to oligosaccharides, further degradation requires participation of other glycosidases. Oligosaccharides produced by mammalian hyaluronidases contain nonreducing terminal glucuronic acid residues linked in β linkage. β-Glucuronidase is a widely distributed enzyme which was demonstrated in lysosomes by deDuve et al. [163]. The ability of β-glucuronidase to remove uronic acid residues from hyaluronic acid oligosaccharides was demonstrated by Weissmann [164] and Linker et al. [165]. However, β-glucuronidase does not hydrolyze the disaccharide, hyalobiuronic acid.

Removal of glucuronic acid from higher oligosaccharides results in the exposure of nonreducing β-N-acetylglycosaminyl residues. β-N-Acetylhexosaminidases have been recently studied more intensively because of their possible role in the degradation of mucopolysaccharides, glycoproteins, and glycolipids. Weissmann and coworkers [166] showed that highly purified β-N-acetyl-D-glucosaminidase of beef liver removes the nonreducing N-acetylglucosamine residue from a trisaccharide prepared by β-glucuronidase digestion of a tetrasaccharide derived from hyaluronic acid. The ratio of activities toward the synthetic substrate, phenyl-β-N-acetylglucosaminide, and toward the trisaccharide derived from hyaluronic acid was the same for both the crude and purified enzyme. Activity of the purified enzyme toward phenyl β-D-N-acetylgalactosaminide was one-seventh of that observed toward the corresponding glucosamine derivative.

N-Acetylhexosaminidases have been studied extensively with respect to Tay-Sachs disease, a subject reviewed in detail elsewhere in this volume (Chap. 29). Robinson and Stirling [167] discovered two hexosaminidase components in human spleen homogenates which were separable chromatographically and electrophoretically. The more rapidly migrating activity was designated β-N-acetylhexosaminidase A, while the more slowly migrating activity was designated β-N-acetylhexosaminidase B. Both forms had identical K_m values, a pH optimum of 4.5, and the ratio of activity toward N-acetylglucosaminides and N-acetylgalactosaminides was found to be 8:1. Treatment of β-N-acetylglucosaminidase A with neuraminidase resulted in marked changes of electrophoretic mobility with the production of multiple forms. When the preparation was treated with sufficient neuraminidase for a longer period of time, all of the enzyme was converted to a material with an electrophoretic mobility of N-acetylhexosaminidase B.

The lack of specificity of the spleen enzyme toward the C-4 configuration of the amino sugars contrasts to the finding by Frohwein and Gatt [168] of hexosaminidases in calf brain with greater amino sugar specificity. However, Woollen et al. [169] found no difference between the relative N-acetyl-β-glucosaminidase and N-acetyl-β-galactosaminidase activities of a large number of β-N-acetylhexosaminidase preparations derived from mammalian, bacterial, and invertebrate sources. In all cases, N-acetylglucosaminides were better substrates. The two activities were never additive. Brain preparations were not studied.

The findings of Robinson and Stirling [167] have assumed added significance in view of the discovery by Okada and O'Brien [170], Sandhoff [171], and Hultberg [172] of the absence of a specific β-N-acetylhexosaminidase component in Tay-Sachs disease. Sandhoff et al. [173] discovered a complete absence of β-N-acetylhexosaminidase in a variant of Tay-Sachs disease characterized by the storage of globoside in the kidney. Okada and O'Brien [170] showed that in conventional Tay-Sachs disease only the A component of β-N-acetylhexosaminidase was absent in brain, liver, kidney, skin, cultured skin fibroblasts, blood plasma, and leukocytes. The level of β-N-acetylhexosaminidase B was markedly increased in Tay-Sachs brain tissue as compared with normal brain. Similarly, using an isoelectric focusing technique, Sandhoff [171] and Hultberg [172] found the absence of an enzyme component with an isoelectric point of pH 5.0 in all but one patient with conventional Tay-Sachs disease. This component is presumably identical with the β-N-acetylhexosaminidase A of Robinson and Stirling. A second component, presumably identical with β-N-acetylhexosaminidase B, isoelectric point 7.3, was found to be increased three- to fourfold in extracts of brains of conventional cases of Tay-Sachs disease. Dance et al. [174] found that urine and serum contain almost exclusively β-N-acetylhexosaminidase A. Following the suggestion of Robinson and Stirling that the A form of the enzyme is the transport form, Hultberg [172] suggested that Tay-Sachs disease results from the failure of the A form to come in contact with the stored G_{M2}.

The structural interrelationships of β-N-acetylhexosaminidase A and B are of considerable interest. The findings of Robinson and Stirling suggest that both forms may represent the same gene product which has been altered by the addition of sialic acid residues in the case of hexosaminidase B. If this be the case, the absence of only hexosaminidase A in Tay-Sachs disease might result from a failure of addition of sialic acid rather than from a structural gene mutation involving the hexosaminidase. Such a situation would introduce a new mechanism for the production of genetic disease, i.e., a mutation which affects the modification of an enzyme with respect to carbohydrate side chains rather than the amino acid sequence of the glycosidase.

Inadequate data are available concerning the role of the β-N-acetylhexosaminidases in mucopolysaccharide degradation. Aronson and de Duve [175] demonstrated that preparations of rat liver lysosomes degrade hyaluronic acid to a mixture of N-acetylglucosamine, glucuronic acid, and hyalobiuronic acid. The finding of hyalobiuronic acid suggested that β-glucuronidase does not hydrolyze the disaccharide, a fact already noted by Linker et al. [165]. Mahadevan and associates [157] reported the release of N-acetylhexosamine groups from chondroitin-4-sulfate as well as from hyaluronic acid by rat liver lysosome particles.

Buddecke and Werries [176, 177] have found that purified β-hexosaminidases from spleen and aorta are active on oligosaccharides derived from chondroitin-4-SO_4, chondroitin-6-SO_4, and hyaluronic acid. They were inhibited by hyaluronic acid, heparin, dermatan sulfate, chondroitin-4-sulfate, chondroitin-6-SO_4, and keratan sulfate.

In view of the complete absence of β-N-acetylhexosaminidase in the variant form of Tay-Sachs disease, mucopolysaccharides might be expected to accumulate in such patients. No report of such findings has appeared.

Indirect evidence for the existence of sulfatases active on chondroitin sulfate or its metabolic products was provided by Dohlman [178] and Dziewiatkowski [179] who found that subcutaneous administration of ^{35}S-chondroitin sulfate to rats resulted in the excretion of inorganic radioactive sulfate. Aronson and Davidson [180] studied the localization of ^{35}S-chondroitin-4- and ^{35}S-chondroitin-6-sulfate and ^{3}H-dermatan sulfate in rat liver lysosomes. Fifteen minutes after administration of the respective compounds, approximately 1 percent of the injected compounds was localized in lysosomes. Four days later the chondroitin-4- and chondroitin-6-sulfates had disappeared, while 40 percent of the dermatan sulfate remained. It is difficult to relate these results to the mechanisms of degradation of the respective polysaccharides since chondroitin-4- and chondroitin-6-sulfate metabolism was measured by the disappearance of $^{35}SO_4$, while dermatan sulfate metabolism was measured by the disappearance of ^{3}H attached to the carbon chain. The apparently more rapid disappearance of chondroitin sulfates than that of dermatan sulfate may have been due to the removal of sulfate rather than to the breakdown of the polysaccharide backbone. However, it is possible that the results validly reflected a slower metabolism of dermatan sulfate than chondroitin sulfates.

Kaplan and Meyer [181] found that chondroitin-4- and chondroitin-6-sulfates injected into dogs and humans disappeared from the blood in less than 4 hr. At low doses no polysaccharide appeared in the urine, but at higher doses a significant portion of the injected polysaccharide was excreted. Dermatan sulfate and heparan sulfate also disappeared from the blood relatively rapidly, but larger proportions of the injected dose than that of the chondroitin sulfates appeared in the urine.

Sulfatase in rat liver lysosomes active against oligosaccharides derived from chondroitin sulfate has been reported by Tudball and Davidson [182]. Sulfate groups were not removed from undegraded chondroitin-4-SO_4, oligosaccharides smaller than octasaccharides, or oligosaccharides which contain nonreducing terminal glucuronic acid groups. If this enzyme is concerned with the physiological degradation of chondroitin sulfates, its action would appear to be restricted to products first partially degraded by the action of hyaluronidase and β-glucuronidase.

In order to determine the site of degradation of mucopolysaccharide-protein complexes, Platt and Stein [183] surveyed the activities of five enzymes in human tissues. They considered it likely that mucopolysaccharide-protein complexes were degraded by the synergistic action of hyaluronidase, β-N-acetylhexosaminidase, β-glucuronidase, cathepsin D and "acid" carboxypeptidases. The highest activities for these enzymes were found in thymus, liver, spleen, and adrenals. Low activity was found in heart muscle and skin.

The extensive literature on aryl sulfatases is reviewed elsewhere in this book. Murphy et al. [184] found an absence of aryl sulfatases A, B, and C in a variant of metachromatic leukodystrophy characterized by the accumulation of acid mucopolysaccharides (see Chap. 32).

Sulfatase activity in cultured fibroblasts has been demonstrated indirectly by Matalon and Dorfman [185]. When dermatan sulfate, isolated from Hurler fibroblasts, was added to the medium of both normal and Hurler fibroblast cultures, approximately 20 percent of $^{35}SO_4$ was recovered as inorganic sulfate.

Beta-xylosidase was demonstrated by Fischer et al. [186] in rat liver and in pig kidney by Robinson and Abrahams [187]. Studies of the pig kidney enzyme by Robinson and Abrahams, the rat liver lysosomal enzyme by Patel and Tappel [188], and the rat liver lysosomal enzyme by Fisher and Kent [189] indicate that a single enzyme is responsible for β-D-xylosidase activity and β-D-glucosidase activity. In view of the presence of β-D-xylosylserine linkages in acid mucopolysaccharides, β-xylosidase might be expected to participate in the degradation of acid mucopolysaccharide–protein complexes. Aronson and de Duve [175] and Patel and Tappel [188] found no hydrolysis of xylosylserine by rat liver lysosomal enzyme preparations. The possibility exists that xylosylserine is hydrolyzed only if the serine is linked in a peptide. However, the xylosidase preparations of Fisher and Kent [189] did not hydrolyze the β-O-xylosides of glycylserine, serylglycine, and glycylserylglycine. That all of the xylosylserine linkages are not hydrolyzed in vivo is indicated by the finding of xylosylserine in urine by Tominga and associates [190].

The role of β-galactosidases in degradation of mucopolysaccharides is unclear. In mucopolysaccharides other than keratan sulfate, galactose is restricted to the linkage region. If β-galactosidase plays a significant role in the degradation of these polysaccharides, then it must act only on the linkage fragments which remain after chain degradation or as an endogalactosidase to separate polysaccharide chains from protein. This question will be discussed in greater detail in a subsequent section of this chapter.

That heparin is degraded in the body is known from the many years of experience with the therapeutic use of this compound. Following intravenous injection of heparin, the duration of physiological action is limited. A small portion of the injected heparin is taken up in tissues, principally in the liver and lung [191]. Most of the administered heparin is excreted in the urine in a partially desulfated form, probably the uroheparin of earlier literature [192–194]. The primary chemical change involved in the conversion of heparin to uroheparin appears to be the removal of N-sulfate groups, which accompanies the loss of physiological activity. This hydrolysis is perhaps due to heparinase, discovered by Cho and Jacques in liver [195], which brings about a decrease in metachromasia and physiological activity.

The possible pathway of dermatan sulfate, heparin, and heparan sulfate degradation has become more evident as a result of the recent discovery by Matalon et al. [474] of an enzyme in cultured fibroblasts and liver which releases L-iduronic acid from desulfated dermatan sulfate and heparan sulfate in the presence of β-glucuronidase and β-N-acetylhexosaminidase. Enzyme activity was also found in leukocytes and urine [475]. The activity of this enzyme was diminished in fibroblasts cultured from Hurler's patients.

Hutterer [153], in his study on the degradation of several mucopolysaccharides by the lysosomal enzymes of rat liver, found evidence of degradation of heparan sulfate but no cleavage of dermatan sulfate. The products of heparan sulfate cleavage were not identified, although the release of N-acetylhexosamine reducing groups was detected.

In view of the fact that heparin and heparan sulfate appear to have α-glycosaminidase linkages, α-N-acetylglucosaminidase in mammalian tissues may be important in their degradation [196]. This enzyme appears to be lysosomal [197–199] but, unlike the β-N-acetylhexosaminidases, it is specific for the configuration of the C-4 carbon atom since α-N-acetylgalactosaminidase appears to be distinct from α-N-acetylglucosaminidase.

Little work has yet appeared on the degradation of keratan sulfate. The accumulation of a keratan sulfate-like substance in the absence of β-galactosidase in G_{M1} gangliosidosis suggests that this glycosidase participates in the degradation of keratan sulfate. The demonstration by MacBrinn et al. [200] of the release of 38.9 percent of galactose from the keratan sulfate-like substance accumulated in generalized gangliosidosis by a liver lysosome preparation probably requires the simultaneous presence of β-N-acetylhexosaminidase acting in concert with the β-galactosidase.

As indicated above, with the possible exception of hyaluronic acid, acid mucopolysaccharides are synthesized in the cell as protein complexes in which the polysaccharide chains are joined to core protein by a linkage region consisting of galactosylgalactosylxylose. It remains to be determined whether degradation of the polysaccharide chain precedes or follows proteolytic digestion. Most studies of the proteolytic breakdown of protein-polysaccharide complexes have been concerned with cartilage. The striking effect of the intravenous injection of papain on the rabbit ear cartilage demonstrated by Thomas [201] drew attention to the role of the protein of chondromucoprotein in maintaining the physical integrity of cartilage. Subsequent inquiry into the effect of toxic doses of vitamin A on cartilage in organ cultures led to the development of the concept that release of proteolytic enzymes from lysosomes by various toxic agents may be responsible for the dissolution of cartilage matrix [202, 203]. This concept has been extended to the possible role of lysosomal proteases in the pathogenesis of acquired connective tissue disease [204]. Lysosomes contain an acid protease which acts like cathepsin D in the hydrolysis of chondromucoprotein [205]. The products of this degradation are chondroitin sulfate chains bound to small peptides or only to serine. The structure of the heparan sulfate fragments found by Knecht, et al. [65] in Hurler's tissues and urine is consistent with such a pathway of degradation.

Degradation of corneal keratan sulfate may occur by the splitting of the 1-aspartamido-β-N-acetylglucosamine bond by the action of the glycosidase, 1-aspartamino-β-N-acetylglucosamine hydrolyase, discovered by Makino and coworkers [206] and studied more recently in detail by Conchie and Strachan [207]. This enzyme apparently splits 1-L-aspartimido-β-N-acetylglucosamine to 1-amino-N-acetylglucosamine and aspartic acid. The former product decomposes spontaneously to N-acetylglucosamine and ammonia. Pollitt and associates [208] found an excretion of 300 mg per day of 1-aspartamido-β-N-acetylglucosamine in two mentally retarded patients presumably afflicted by a genetic defect of this enzyme. Widely distributed in mammalian tissues, this enzyme probably plays a major role in glycoprotein degradation. Conchie and Strachan [207] found a pH optimum of 7.0 for the enzyme in rat liver, but Makino et al. [206] observed a lower pH optimum for serum enzyme. Latency of this enzyme, demonstrated by Mahadevan and Tappel [209], suggests that it is lysosomal despite its high pH optimum.

The preceding review of enzymes possibly involved in the

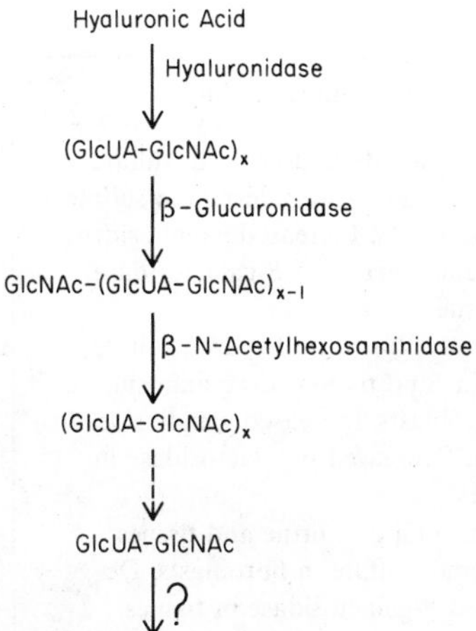

Figure 49-8. Possible pathway of degradation of hyaluronic acid.

degradation of the mucopolysaccharides indicates many gaps in our knowledge. In order to summarize some of the available information, Figs. 49-8 and 49-9 indicate possible pathways of hyaluronic acid and dermatan sulfate degradation. Figure 49-8 shows the probable pathway of hyaluronic acid degradation. Several uncertainties remain. Whether the β-N-acetylhexosaminidase involved in ganglioside metabolism is the same as that involved in hyaluronic acid degradation is unclear in view of the lack of accumulation of acid mucopolysaccharides in Tay-Sachs disease. The fate of hyalobiuronic acid is unknown.

More speculative is the pathway for degradation of the dermatan sulfate–protein complex indicated in Fig. 49-9. This pathway highlights the problems of understanding the mucopolysaccharidoses. Whether proteolysis precedes or follows polysaccharide degradation is not clear. Likewise,

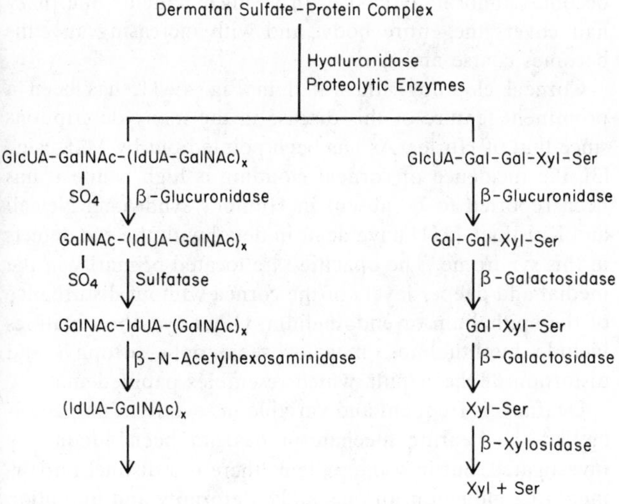

Figure 49-9. Possible pathway of degradation of dermatan sulfate–protein complex.

the number of proteolytic enzymes involved is unknown. Platt and Stein [183] suggested that cathepsin D and acid carboxypeptidase may play a major role in the degradation of the protein portion of the acid mucopolysaccharide–protein complex. Separation of the linkage region by the action of hyaluronidase seems reasonable on the basis of its known action on dermatan sulfate. The nature of the β-galactosidases involved in further degradation awaits study. β-Xylosidase splitting of xylosylserine seems logical, but so far has not been demonstrated. The finding of xylosylserine in urine suggests that this hydrolysis is incomplete.

The pathway of degradation of the polysaccharide chain must also be regarded as speculative. The existence of a sulfatase is clear; its indicated action is based on the limited evidence of Tudball and Davidson [182]. Whether the known β-N-acetylhexosaminidases account for removal of nonreducing N-acetylgalactosamine residues linked to L-iduronic acid is not known. Finally, the required α-L-iduronidase has now been found.

Similar pathways for heparin, heparan sulfate, and the keratan sulfates must, at present, be considered even more speculative. The postulated L-iduronase may also be concerned with the degradation of heparin and heparan sulfate.

CLINICAL ASPECTS OF MUCOPOLYSACCHARIDOSES

The discovery of acid mucopolysaccharides in tissues and urine in Hurler's disease and particularly the development of tissue culture techniques have led to an increasing number of descriptions of distinct acid mucopolysaccharidoses. Since detailed clinical description of each of these syndromes is prohibitive of space, an initial clinicopathological description of the prototype of the mucopolysaccharidoses, Hurler's disease, will be included followed by briefer descriptions of the reported variants.

Many investigators now follow the classification of McKusick [3, 210] whose scholarly work has contributed considerably to the recognition of the phenotypic and genotypic diversity of mucopolysaccharidoses. Table 49-3 includes McKusick's original classification to which have been added other syndromes which appear distinct.

The Hurler Syndrome—Mucopolysaccharidosis I

Clinical Manifestations

The most striking features are moderate dwarfism, grotesque facial appearance, protuberant abdomen, joint contractures, and mental retardation. Typical patients bear a striking resemblance to one another. The abnormal facies is illustrated in Fig. 49-10. The large head frequently shows a prominent ridge along the sagittal suture. Hypertelorism is evident even in mildly affected patients and in infants who

Table 49-3. THE MUCOPOLYSACCHARIDOSES AND RELATED DISORDERS

Disease	Clinical characteristics	Biochemical findings	Genetics
Hurler's syndrome—Mucopolysaccharidosis I	Severe mental retardation; skeletal deformities; marked corneal opacity, marked somatic changes	Dermatan sulfate and heparan sulfate in urine and tissues; dermatan sulfate in fibroblasts. Increased gangliosides in brain. Decreased β-galactosidase in tissues	Autosomal recessive
Hunter's syndrome—Mucopolysaccharidosis II	Moderate mental retardation; marked skeletal deformities; no corneal clouding; early deafness; marked somatic change	Dermatan sulfate and heparan sulfate in urine and tissues; dermatan sulfate in fibroblasts. Increased gangliosides in brain. Decreased β-galactosidase in tissues	X-linked recessive
Sanfilippo's syndrome—Mucopolysaccharidosis III (two types may exist)	Severe mental retardation; mild skeletal changes; corneal clouding questionable	Heparan sulfate in urine and tissues; dermatan sulfate in fibroblasts. Decreased β-galactosidase in tissues	Autosomal recessive
Morquio's syndrome—Mucopolysaccharidosis IV	Severe skeletal deformities; marked spondylepiphyseal dysplasia; no mental retardation; corneal opacities may occur	Keratan sulfate and chondroitin-%-sulfate in urine	Autosomal recessive
Scheie's syndrome—Mucopolysaccharidosis V	Mild skeletal changes; no mental retardation; severe corneal opacity	Dermatan sulfate in urine	Autosomal recessive
Maroteaux-Lamy syndrome—Mucopolysaccharidosis VI	Severe skeletal deformities; gross corneal opacity; no mental retardation	Dermatan sulfate in urine	Autosomal recessive
"I-cell" disease—Hurler variant	Severe mental retardation; skeletal deformities	Increased urinary mucopolysaccharides variable; dermatan sulfate in fibroblasts. Increased lipids in fibroblasts	Autosomal recessive
Lipomucopolysaccharidosis—Gal + disease	Severe mental retardation and skeletal deformities; corneal clouding	No increase in mucopolysaccharide in urine. Increased mucopolysaccharides and lipids in tissues (histochemical)	?
Mucopolysaccharidosis VII	Skeletal findings similar to Morquio's	Results not conclusive	?
G_{M1}-gangliosidosis—neurovisceral lipidosis	Severe early mental retardation (late form may occur); marked skeletal changes	Keratan sulfate-like material in tissues and urine. Very low β-galactosidase in tissues	Autosomal recessive

do not yet show the full-blown syndrome. The thick lips are usually separated to reveal a large tongue, widely spaced peg-like teeth, and hypertrophic gums. The bridge of the nose is depressed under a prominent forehead frequently covered by an abnormal amount of dark, coarse hair. The chest is usually enlarged with marked flaring of the lower ribs. Characteristic of a large percentage of patients is a prominent gibbus. The extremities are strikingly abnormal. The hands are usually broad, and the fingers short and stubby. The lower extremities similarly give the impression of heaviness. Contractures at the hips, knees, ankles, and elbows are common and usually involve the fingers. The spleen and liver are generally much enlarged, but in some patients splenic enlargement is absent. Diastasis of the recti and umbilical and inguinal hernias are common. Hernias appear early in life, and many of the patients seen by the authors had been subjected to herniorrhaphy before the diagnosis of the Hurler syndrome was established.

The skin is usually thick. In some cases elevated white nodules appear over the scapular region; these are more typical of the Hunter syndrome. Hirsutism is the rule, and as the patient becomes older, the hair of the body and head becomes abnormally coarse. In younger patients fine fuzzy hair covers the entire body, and with increasing age this becomes coarse and dark.

Corneal clouding, illustrated in Fig. 49-11, has been a prominent feature of this disease in the many descriptions since that of Hurler. As has been pointed out by McKusick [3], the incidence of corneal clouding is high, while it has been reported to be absent in Hunter's syndrome. Newell and Koistinen [211] have dealt in detail with the eye defects in this syndrome. The opacities are located primarily in the medial and deeper layers of the cornea without disturbance of the epithelium or endothelium. Other eye abnormalities include buphthalmos, megalocornea, optic atrophy, and distortion of the papilla which resembles papilledema.

Deafness is frequent and variable in severity. The pathology of the hearing mechanism has not been adequately investigated, but in some patients there is a distinct impairment of conduction. In one study, deformity and limitation of motion of the ossicles has been described [212].

The respiratory disease, so common in the more severely

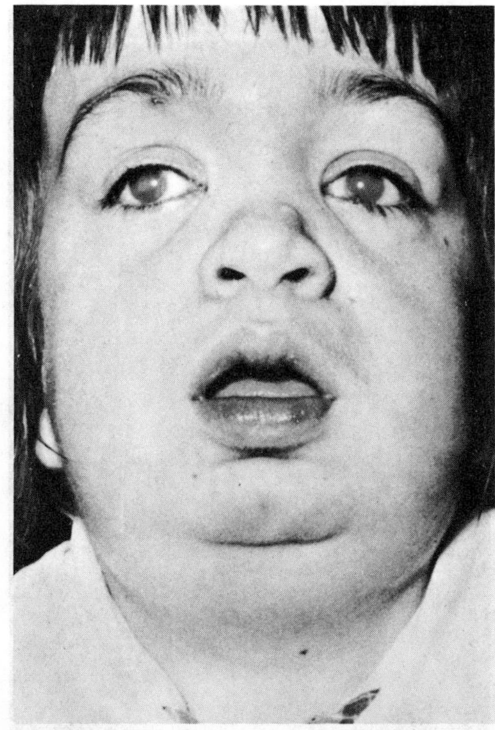

Figure 49-10. A severely affected patient.

affected individuals, undoubtedly results from the deformity of the nasal and facial bones.

Heart damage has been recognized as a part of the mucopolysaccharidoses since the original description by Hunter [5]. The earlier inadequate descriptions have now been replaced by more specific pathologic studies [213–215]. Berenson and Greer [216] have reported detailed findings in 21 cases and have confirmed the earlier claims of specific valvular lesions indicated by mitral and basal murmurs. Figure 49-11 illustrates the valvular lesion of Hurler's disease. McKusick [3] pointed out the similarity of the distribution of valvular lesions in the Hurler syndrome and in rheumatic heart disease. The order of frequency of involvement in both conditions is mitral, aortic, tricuspid, and pulmonary. This order corresponds to the peak pressures sustained by the four valves and suggests that hemodynamic factors may determine the localization of lesions which are based fundamentally on metabolic derangements.

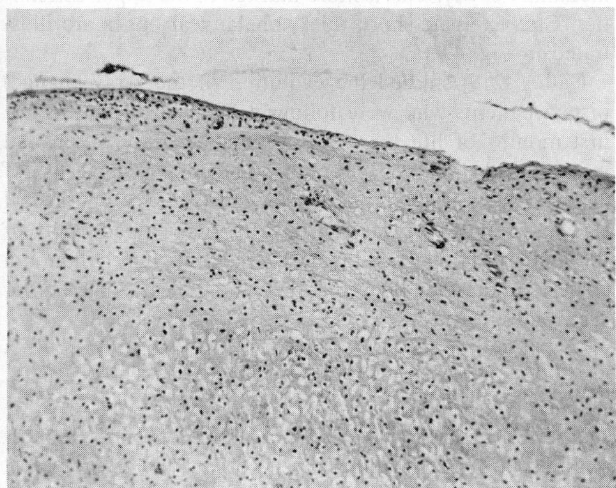

Figure 49-11. Cross section of the mitral valve in the Hurler syndrome.

Valvular disease is only one aspect of a widespread cardiopathy. Coronary artery disease and endocardial, pericardial, and myocardial disease also occur. Angina pectoris at age 4-$^3/_4$ years has been reported [217], and myocardial infarction at the age of 4 years has been observed by the authors. This undoubtedly results from the narrowing of the lumen by large numbers of "Hurler cells," as illustrated in the coronary artery shown in Fig. 49-12. Congestive failure is common in the Hurler syndrome, and death is frequently due to cardiac disease.

Neurologic findings are variable. Spasticity has been frequently reported, but it is difficult to differentiate from functional derangements secondary to connective tissue and skeletal deformities. Severe mental retardation is found in the vast majority of patients, and it has been questioned whether normal mental development is consistent with a diagnosis of the Hurler syndrome. This problem is complicated by inadequate psychologic testing in many of the reported cases and by the progressive nature of the disease itself. In some of the patients reported before 1957 as *forme*

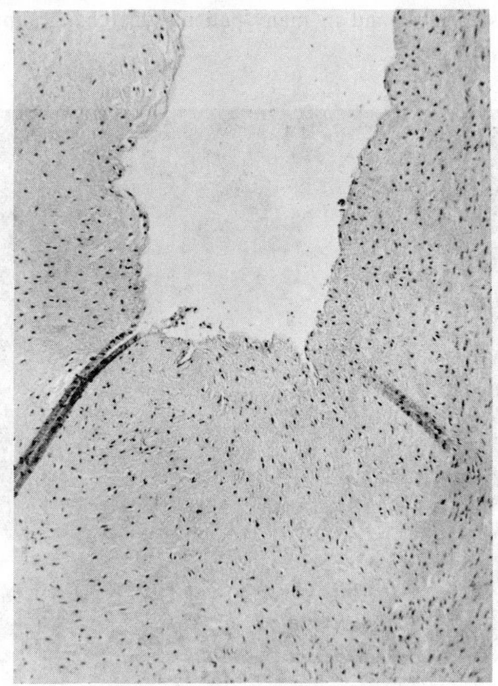

Figure 49-12. Coronary artery in the Hurler syndrome.

fruste of the Hurler syndrome, definitive conclusions cannot be reached, since no independent test for the existence of the disease was then available. It is the authors' experience, confirmed by many published reports, that early development may be reasonably normal and then followed by gradual deterioration.

Radiologic Findings

Roentgenographic changes in the Hurler syndrome are usually of considerable diagnostic help. Characteristic are the distortions of the skull, hyperostosis, and marked abnormality of the sella turcica. The unusually long sella with anterior pocketing has frequently been referred to as "boot-shaped" or "shoe-shaped". In some cases it appears to be unusually deep. The abnormalities of the sella (Fig. 49-13) are thought to arise primarily in bone rather than from changes in the pituitary. The understanding of the abnormal sella turcica in Hurler's syndrome has recently been furthered by the report of Neuhauser et al. [218] that sphenoidal erosions in Hurler's disease are associated with a high frequency of leptomeningeal cysts which cause erosion of the anterior clinoids. Abnormalities of the facial bones are also prominent.

The ribs assume an unusual flattened appearance which has been characterized as *spatulate.* The vertebral ends of ribs are unusually narrow. The gibbus formation is illustrated in Fig. 49-14. The bodies of certain vertebrae, particularly in the lower dorsal and upper lumbar regions, are wedge-shaped and have hooklike projections anteriorly, the so-called *beaked vertebrae.* The extent of vertebral deformities is variable and in many patients this change appears early in life.

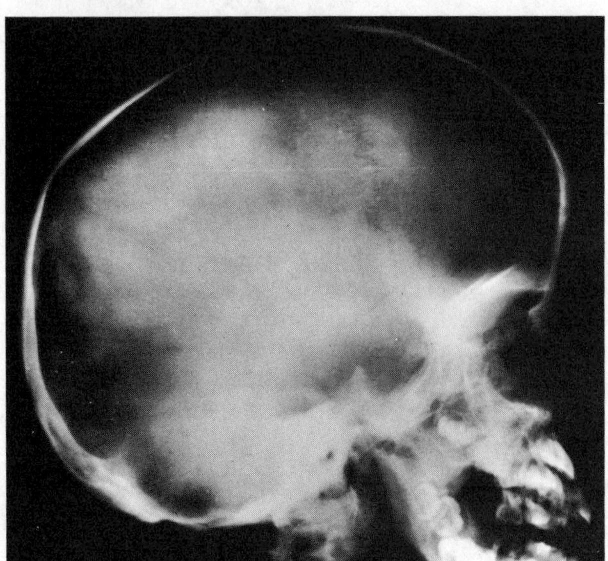

Figure 49-13. Lateral skull x-ray of patient with the Hurler syndrome. The marked deformity of the sella turcica is evident.

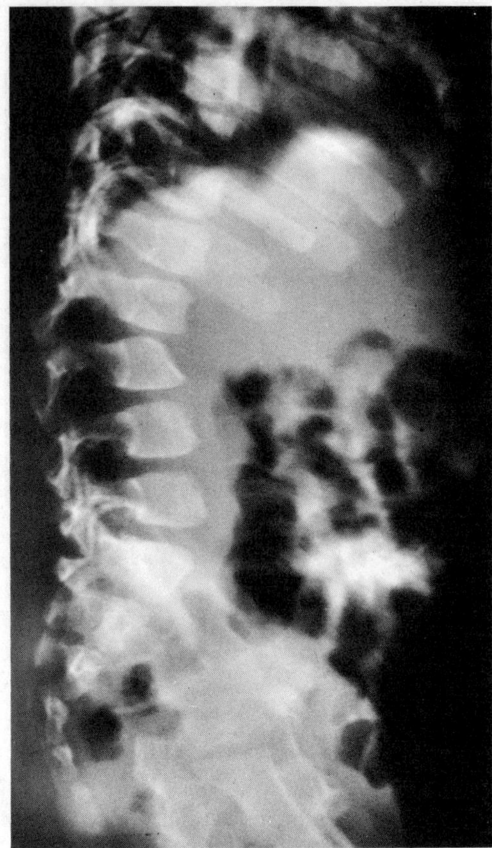

Figure 49-14. Lateral x-ray of the spine of a patient with the Hurler syndrome. The deformity of the vertebrae is evident. The spatulate ribs are easily noted.

Almost all bones of the extremities appear heavy or otherwise abnormal. The tubular bones show a swelling of the medullary cavity. This is more marked in the upper extremities. Characteristic short, thick, phalangeal bones are illustrated in Fig. 49-15.

Caffey [219] studied the evolution of the x-ray changes in two patients who were followed from birth. During the first months of life there was generalized rarefaction and metaphyseal spreading, cupping, and spurring, suggestive of active rickets or hyperparathyroidism. Extra subperiosteal sleeves of cortex of varying thickness enveloped many of the shafts and thickened them externally. By the sixth month changes in the long bones had become typical of the Hurler syndrome.

Pathology

In the Hurler syndrome gross examination shows abnormalities throughout almost every organ and tissue. Most involved are the brain, heart, liver, and spleen. In some instances there is a striking thickening of the dura which may achieve a width in excess of 1 cm. The weight of the

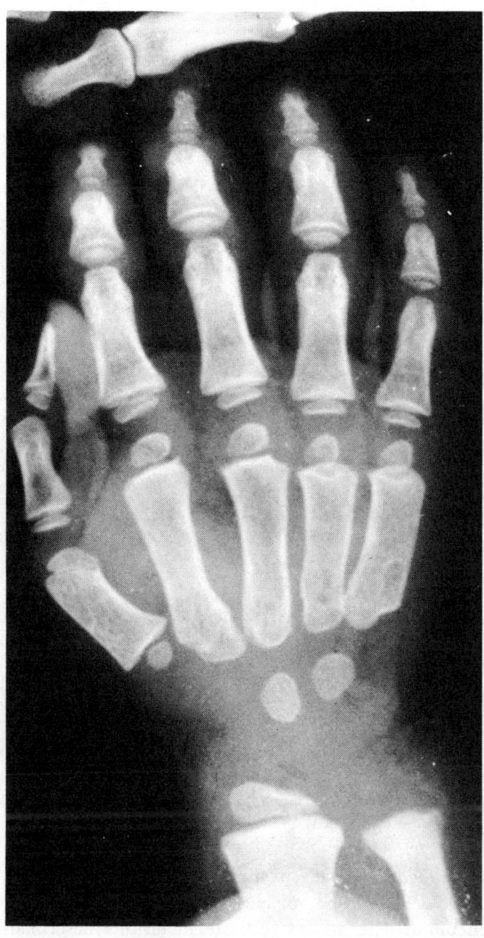

Figure 49-15. X-ray of the hand of a patient with typical Hurler syndrome.

brain has been variously reported as increased or decreased, and mild internal hydrocephalus has been observed. The principal cortical patterns may be normal, but atrophy of the convolutions has been observed [220].

There are striking changes in the valves, endocardium, myocardium, and coronary vessels [215, 216]. The heart may be grossly enlarged. The endocardium is thickened, sometimes nodular, particularly on the mitral valves and the chordae tendineae, as illustrated in Fig. 49-16. In addition to the thickening of the coronary arteries, changes may be observed in the aorta (Fig. 49-12). In some cases, the pericardium is thickened.

The liver and spleen are usually strikingly enlarged and have a peculiar hard consistency and grayish color. The kidneys are relatively normal in appearance, but histologic abnormalities have been reported [221].

Since the report of Tuthill in 1934 [222], who autopsied one of Hurler's original patients, there has been an appreciation of the presence of abnormal intracellular storage material. Tuthill, as did many of the early investigators, believed this to be lipid in nature, but even in this original report he noted that the storage material was soluble in formalin but not in alcohol. For the most part appropriate fixatives have not been used. Haust and Landing [223] have studied this problem in some detail, particularly with respect to the use of lead acetate for fixation.

Abnormalities based on the presence of large cells distended with storage material have been described in cartilage, fascia, tendons, periosteum, blood vessel walls, heart valves, meninges, and cornea. These cells, variously called *clear cells, gargoyle cells, Hurler's cells,* or *balloon cells,* characterize this disease. Lagunoff et al. [224] have given a description of these cells in a mitral leaflet especially prepared and examined by both light and electron micros-

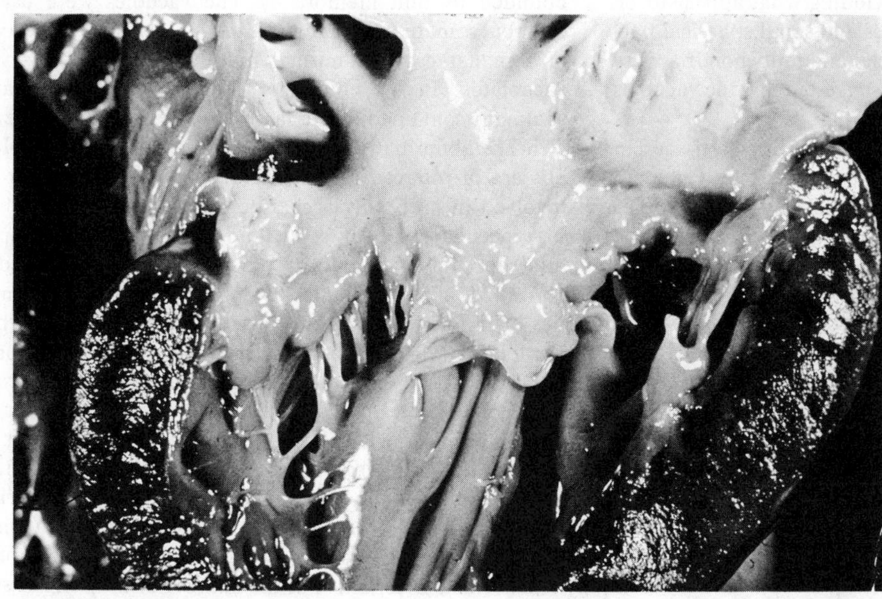

Figure 49-16. The heart of a patient with Hurler's syndrome. The nodular thickening of the mitral valve and chordae tendineae is evident.

copy. They describe them as large oval or polygonal cells, 20 microns in diameter, with a pale central nucleus. The cytoplasm was devoid of material stainable with hematoxylin and eosin or acidic toluidine blue. When frozen-dried sections were vapor-fixed in formaldehyde, deparaffined, dehydrated in 75 percent ethanol, and stained with toluidine blue, the cells were filled with intensely metachromatic granular material. No such material was observed extracellularly. Intracellular storage material was also retained when sections were stained in a 50 percent acidified ethanol solution of toluidine blue without removal of paraffin. The storage material was only weakly stained with the periodic acid-Schiff stain (PAS). On electron microscopic examination, the cytoplasm of the clear cells was found to be filled with large irregular clear vacuoles varying in size from 0.5 to 2.0 microns. The membranes of the vacuoles were often disrupted and the ruptured ends curled. Occasionally mitochondria and cisternae of endoplasmic reticulum were interspersed between the vacuoles. The mitochondria had irregular shapes and short cristae. Ribosomes were often missing from the endoplasmic reticulum.

Wolfe et al. [225] used a 10 percent solution of cetyltrimethylammonium bromide in the formalin fixative in order to preserve the very soluble acid mucopolysaccharides. They noted that polysaccharides accumulated in the form of fine cytoplasmic granules, not only in the obvious "gargoyle" cells, but also in the fibrocytes throughout the entire body. In addition to the polysaccharides, the authors noted accumulation of glycolipids in the brain and visceral organs of one of the two patients they studied.

On electron microscopy of liver biopsies, Van Hoof and Hers [226] found a large number of round or oval vacuoles surrounded by a unit membrane. These vacuoles contained a granular substance of low density. Figure 49-17 illustrates these vacuoles. Many contain polymorphous bodies, indicated by arrows in Fig. 49-17, including what appear to be rolled-up fragments of membranes and small spherical particles of variable density. The nuclei and mitochondria were quite normal. Van Hoof and Hers suggested that the vacuoles were derived from lysosomes.

Recently, studies of Hurler's and Sanfilippo's tissues in the electron microscope have been reviewed by Callahan and Lorincz [227] and Loeb et al. [228], who like other workers found in the Kupffer cells and hepatocytes a striking accumulation of single membrane-limited vacuoles which were nearly empty after lead staining. In one patient, typical rosettes indistinguishable from α-glycogen were observed in some vacuoles [229]. Lagunoff and Gritzka [230] found vacuoles in heart valves as well as in liver that showed the presence of acid phosphatase and were believed to be lysosomes.

The report of the structure of skin in Hurler's syndrome by DeCloux and Friederici [231] is of interest since it permits comparison of electron microscope studies of fibroblasts in vivo with cultured fibroblasts. Fibroblasts and macrophages were found to contain large numbers of cytoplasmic vacuoles

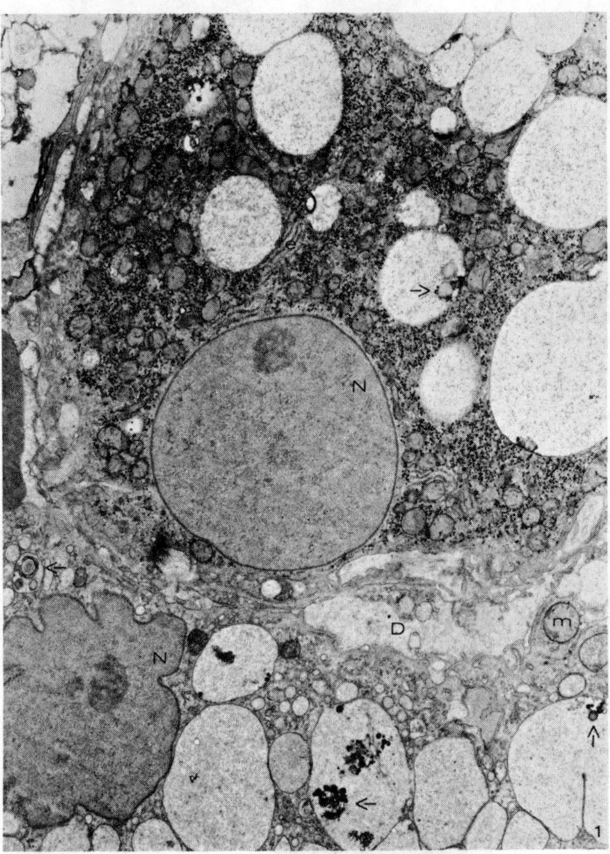

Figure 49-17. An electron photomicrograph of a liver biopsy specimen (×9,000). N, nucleus; M, mitochondria; re, endoplasmic reticulum. The arrows indicate inclusions described in the text. (*This photograph was kindly furnished by Dr. H. G. Hers.*)

bounded by unit membranes. The vacuoles were usually clear but sometimes contained lamellar inclusions. The axons of skin nerves were normal but the Schwann cells were vacuolated. In the epidermis, many cells of the stratum Malpighi contained single large vacuoles indenting the nuclei. The abnormalities in the Schwann cells and the epidermis are of interest in that these cells are not known to be involved in mucopolysaccharide metabolism.

A peculiar type of crystalloid structure in the hepatic mitochondria of Sanfilippo tissues has been described by Haust [232]. Berard-Badier et al. [233] found no abnormalities of mitochondria but confirmed the presence of typical vacuoles in cases of both Hurler and Hunter syndromes.

Bartman and Blanc [234] observed single membrane-bounded vacuoles in cultured fibroblasts in the Hurler and Hunter syndromes. Dilated cisternae were found in the rough endoplasmic reticulum. Ducket et al. [235] also noted abnormalities of the mitochondria. Conrad and associates [236] observed a strikingly increased quantity of single membrane-bound vacuoles in Hurler fibroblasts, compared with normals irrespective of the number of transfers or stage

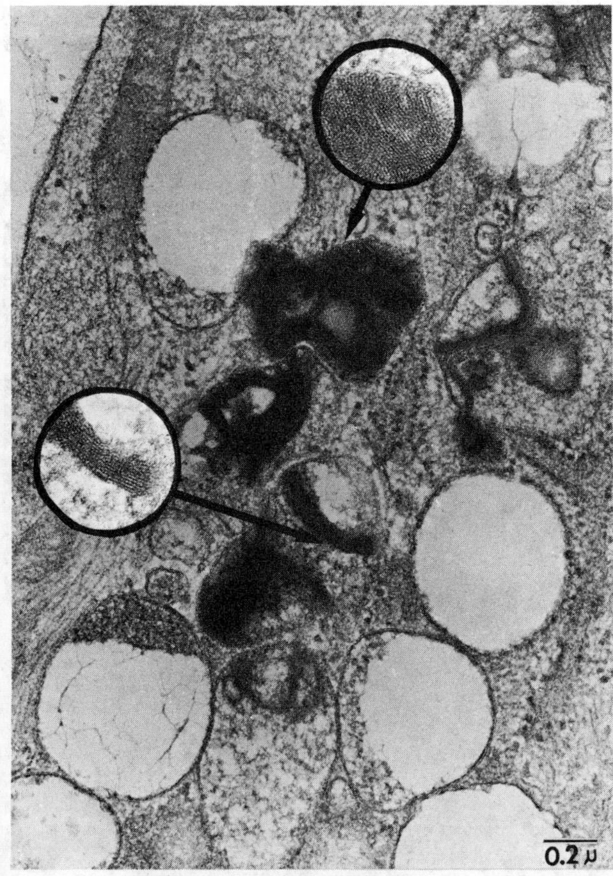

Figure 49-18. An electron micrograph of a cultured Hurler fibroblast (×59,250). Insert shows residual bodies (×150,000).

of the culture cycle. Such vacuoles were occasionally observed in small numbers in normal cells. Figure 49-18 illustrates a cultured fibroblast from a Hurler patient. In some vacuoles, lamellated bodies were present. No abnormalities of mitochondria were observed. The extent of dilatation of the rough endoplasmic reticulum did not exceed that observed in normal cells. However, strikingly dilated sacs were noted in the region of the Golgi apparatus. These are illustrated in Fig. 49-19. The material included in these sacs is considerably more electron dense than that in the vacuoles, which suggests the presence of a protein-polysaccharide complex. It was difficult to demonstrate acid phosphatase or aryl sulfatase in the large vacuoles. The vacuoles may contain material entering the cell by pinocytosis since colloidal gold added to the culture was demonstrated in these vacuoles.

Earlier attempts to identify the storage of the material in typical Hurler cells are only of historical interest. The storage material is predominantly acid mucopolysaccharide. Conclusions that this material is predominantly lipid are erroneous. The presence of some lipid deposits similar to those present in certain lipid storage diseases is evident.

Histologic changes in the brain have been described in considerable detail by various investigators. Among these is the excellent report by Jervis [220] who concluded that the most striking changes are in the gray matter. In preparations stained by the Nissl method, the body of the cell was swollen and distorted. The cytoplasm contained small vacuoles and few, if any, Nissl bodies. The nucleus was displaced toward the periphery of the cell and often showed degenerative changes. Special stains demonstrated disappearance of neurofibrils and the appearance of granular material. This material was best maintained in the tissues by the use of special methods of fixation. Jervis pointed out that the staining and solubility characteristics of the stored materials were not typical of lipid deposits. Characteristic changes were detected throughout the nervous system including neurons of plexuses. Changes found in glial cells were not as marked as those in neuronal cells. No abnormalities were observed in the white matter of the hemispheres. In some cases perivascular cells were found distended with fatty material, but unlike that found in the neuronal cells, this material stained typically for lipids and was readily soluble in fat solvents. On the basis of staining studies as well as chemical isolations Brante [1] concluded that there is indeed an increase in gangliosides in the central nervous system of afflicted patients. Lagunoff and coworkers [224] have described a second type of abnormal cell in the mitral leaflet which could not be identified in ordinary formalin-fixed paraffin-embedded tissues but was found with lipid stains in frozen-dried sections fixed in formaldehyde vapor. Characteristically, these structures appeared as elongated aggregations of lipid droplets pressed between collagen bundles. It was frequently difficult to identify these lipid-containing bodies as cells. When a nucleus was evident, it was located at one end of the cell but was not obviously different from a clear-cell nucleus. The lipid-containing cells were much less abundant than those containing metachromatic granules. In general, cells contained either metachromatic granules or lipids and only rarely were both types of inclusions seen in the same cell.

Several ultrastructural studies of the nervous system in mucopolysaccharidoses have now been reported [237–241]. One of the patients reported by Aleu and coworkers [238] was subsequently shown by Matalon et al. to be a Hurler variant. In all of these studies, including the more recent one by Loeb et al. [228], numerous lamellar bodies have been found in the cytoplasm of neurons. These resemble the membranous cytoplasmic bodies of Tay-Sachs disease. Both Loeb et al. [228] and Escourolle et al. [239] found inclusions in astrocytes, sometimes lamellar but usually clear and finely granular. In capillary pericytes, finely granular structures were found which resembled the inclusions of the hepatocytes.

Inclusion bodies in the polymorphonuclear leukocytes in Hurler's syndrome are of some theoretical as well as practical significance. These have been called *Alder* [242] or *Reilly bodies* [243]. The large granules take on a dark color with a Giemsa-Wright stain but are better differentiated by their

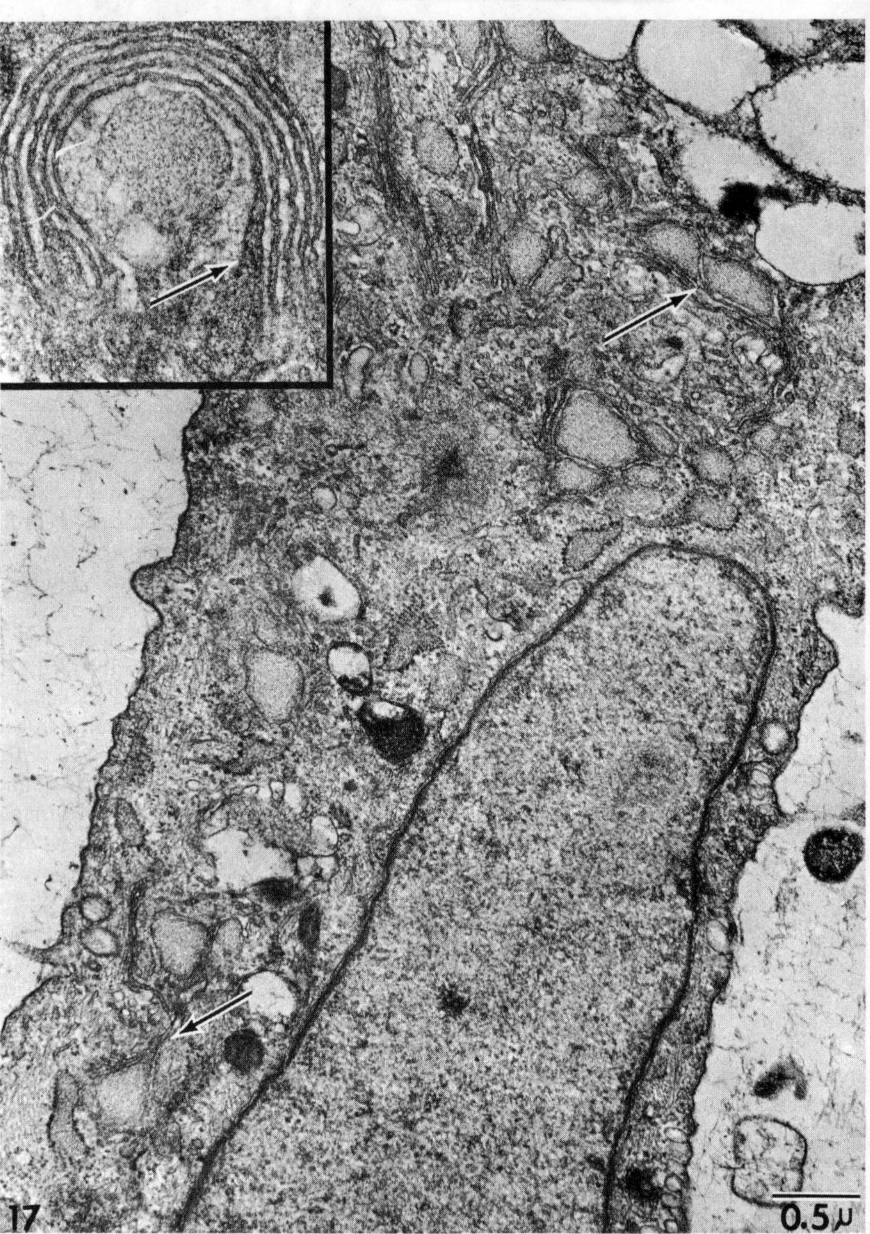

Figure 49-19. An electron micrograph of a cultured Hurler fibroblast (×28,500) showing dilated Golgi sacs. Insert, ×60,000. (See also Plate II-5.)

metachromatic staining with toluidine blue. Similar inclusions can be demonstrated with great regularity in bone marrow, particularly in the large histiocytes and in lymphocytes. These metachromatic inclusions persist in lymphocytes cultured from patients with the Hurler syndrome [244, 245]. Carlisle and Good [246] have shown that, following abrasion of the skin, cells which contain characteristic metachromatic granules appear in the exudate. Granules are more readily demonstrated in bone marrow than in peripheral blood cells [247].

Broad and hyalinized collagen bundles have been described in Hurler's disease by Lindsay et al. [248]. Lagunoff and associates [224] found a typical 700-Å spacing in collagen fibers by electron microscopy. Meyer and Hoffman [249] have commented on the association of broad collagen bundles with the presence of dermatan sulfate in tissues such as skin.

On the basis of cross-correction studies, Danes and Bearn [250] have suggested the existence of more than one genetic type of Hurler's disease.

The Hunter Syndrome—Mucopolysaccharidosis II

Patients with the Hunter syndrome have similar clinical features to those with Hurler's syndrome but are less severely affected. The gross facial appearance is similar and "gargoyle"-like; they suffer from dwarfism, "noisy" breathing, hepatosplenomegaly, inguinal hernias, skin changes, and stiffness of joints. Typical skin changes consisting of numerous nodules extending from the angle of the scapula toward the axillary line were described in a patient with Hunter's syndrome by Anderssen and Tandberg [251]. Mental retardation is less severe than in Hurler's syndrome. Such patients live longer and often survive to their twenties or thirties and occasionally beyond. Lumbar gibbus does not usually occur in the Hunter syndrome as it does in the Hurler's. Deafness is a more frequent feature of the Hunter syndrome. Cardiac involvement and death from congestive failure or coronary insufficiency often complicate the course of the disease. Hunter [5] noticed cardiomegaly and systolic and diastolic murmurs in one of his patients.

The pathological changes in the Hunter syndrome appear the same as those found in the Hurler patients. The radiological findings are also similar, with the exception of less vertebral involvement in the Hunter syndrome.

Although clinically and biochemically similar, the Hunter and Hurler syndromes are genetically distinct. The Hunter syndrome is X-linked [212, 252–261], while the Hurler syndrome is autosomal recessive. The Hunter syndrome is more frequent than the Hurler syndrome.

Although corneal clouding has been considered to be absent in Hunter's disease, exceptions have been reported by Van Pelt and Huizenga [261].

The Sanfilippo Syndrome—Mucopolysaccharidosis III

Lorincz [262], Harris [263], and, subsequently, Sanfilippo et al. [264] described patients who excreted heparan sulfate exclusively. The latter investigators pointed out that such patients show severe mental retardation in the absence of marked bone changes. Since that time a number of authors [3] have recognized this group of patients as differing in a variety of respects from those with typical Hurler's syndrome. Such patients now have been denoted after McKusick as *Sanfilippo syndrome* or *Mucopolysaccharidosis III*. Maroteaux and Lamy [265] have proposed the name *polydystrophic oligophrenia,* and Langer [266] has suggested the name *mucopolysaccharidosis H. S.* Figure 49-20 is a photograph of a patient with Sanfilippo's disease.

These patients show less craniofacial changes than the Hurler patients, but the overall appearance is abnormal. Dwarfism is not a prominent feature. The restriction of joint movements is more frequently associated with the prominence of neurological symptoms than the contractures which typically develop in Hurler disease. Corneal cloudiness and cardiac complications have not been described in this variant. Most striking is the early and progressive development of neurological symptoms with seizures, athetosis, and severe mental retardation. Death usually occurs by 10 to 14 years of age.

Although x-ray abnormalities are present, they are less severe than in the Hurler syndrome. Berggård and Bearn [267] noted minimum long bone involvement in patients who excreted exclusively heparan sulfate. Maroteaux and Lamy [265] have stressed the appearance and reduced height of the iliac wings with a decreased development of the heads of the femurs. Kyphosis does not occur, but an ovoid appearance of the vertebral bodies is frequently present.

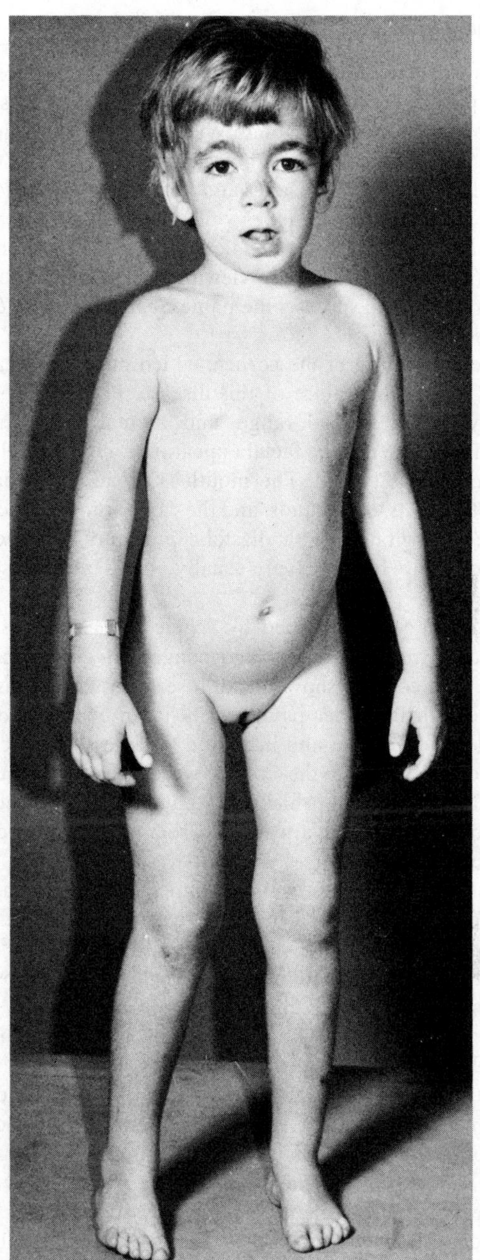

Figure 49-20. Photograph of patient with Sanfilippo's syndrome.

The Sanfilippo syndrome is an autosomal recessive disease. There is no accurate estimate of its frequency, but it appears to be less frequent than Hurler or Hunter variants. On the basis of fibroblast complementation studies, Wiesmann et al. [268] have suggested the existence of two distinct genetic forms of Sanfilippo's disease.

Scheie Syndrome—Mucopolysaccharidosis V

This syndrome, first described by Scheie et al. [269] and subsequently by McKusick et al. [210], is now considered to be a distinct entity, although Wiesmann and Neufeld [270] found no cross correction between Hurler's and Scheie's fibroblasts (see below). Danes and Bearn have suggested that there are two distinct types of Scheie's syndrome [250]. Rampini [271] has reviewed 14 cases from the literature and added an additional one. In view of the earlier descriptions of the disease, he suggests the name *Spate-Hurler* or *Ulrich-Scheie's disease.*

Severe clouding of the cornea, which may occur early in life, is a striking feature of this disease. Physical growth is usually in the normal range, and mental impairment is minimal or absent. The facial appearance, not gargoyle-like, is described as typical. The mouth is broad. Such patients have stiff joints, claw hands, and the carpal tunnel syndrome. Aortic regurgitation with diastolic murmurs has been described [210]. Hepatomegaly usually occurs without splenomegaly.

In the 10 cases described by Scheie and associates [269], familial corneal dystrophy and congenital glaucoma were noted. The corneas showed a diffuse haze which was most advanced in the older patients. Slit-lamp examination disclosed diffuse edema and increased thickness of the cornea. The central parts of the cornea were occasionally clearer than the periphery. A thickening and decrease in the elasticity of the conjunctiva was also observed. Hearing defects have been described.

Histological findings in the conjunctiva, cornea, and skin resemble those observed in Hurler's syndrome [269]. X-ray findings resemble those of Hurler's disease but are much less striking. Some spatulation of the ribs may be observed and changes in the vertebrae occur.

The original report of Scheie et al. [269] is somewhat difficult to interpret since there was a wide range in the severity of clinical manifestations. Kaplan [272] indicates that one of his patients was considered to have Scheie's syndrome at age 7 but Hurler's syndrome at age 9.

The frequency of Scheie's syndrome is not known, but it appears to be rarer than the mucopolysaccharidoses previously described. On the basis the series of Scheie et al. [269] and of McKusick et al. [210] inheritance appears to be autosomal recessive.

The Maroteaux-Lamy Syndrome—Mucopolysaccharidosis VI

This syndrome, sometimes designated *polydystrophic dwarfism,* was first delineated by Maroteaux et al. [273]. Skeletal changes and marked retardation of growth are striking features of this syndrome.

Additionally, lumbar kyphosis, protrusion of the sternum, and genu valgum were found. Abnormal facial appearance is not as striking as in Hurler's syndrome. Much different from Hurler's syndrome, this variant is characterized by lack of mental retardation. Hepatosplenomegaly and corneal opacities are usually present.

Patients with this mucopolysaccharidosis excrete large amounts of dermatan sulfate in the urine. X-ray changes are similar to those seen in Hurler's disease but without the anterior beaking of the vertebrae.

This disease is rare, and the gene frequency not known. In the cases described by Maroteaux et al. [273] and McKusick et al. [210] autosomal recessive mode of inheritance is suggested.

Morquio's Syndrome—Mucopolysaccharidosis IV

This syndrome, described independently by Morquio [274] and Brailsford [275], has become known as the *Morquio syndrome* or the *Morquio-Brailsford syndrome.* Attention has been primarily focused on the cartilaginous and bony structures primarily affected in this disease. Since the initial description, a number of cases, probably unrelated to this syndrome, were published under the name *Morquio's disease* [3]. A number of diseases exist which involve spondyloepiphyseal dysplasias, which may or may not have other manifestations of Morquio's syndrome.

Skeletal changes and linear growth are most strikingly affected. Patients with this disorder are dwarfed, have characteristically flat vertebrae, platyspondyly, knock knees, changes in the epiphyses, and generalized osteoporosis. The wrists are large but without the stiffness of joints typical of other mucopolysaccharidoses. The skeletal deformities of Morquio's syndrome are illustrated in Fig. 49-21, which shows the marked shortening of trunk with the relatively less shortening of the extremities. These two brothers have been reported by Zellweger et al. [276]. The changes in the acetabula and epiphyses result in marked deformities of the extremities and the chest. The spinal curvatures, together with rib deformities, result in a typical barrel chest with pigeon breast and short neck. The facial appearance is also characteristic, showing prominent maxilla, broad mouth, short nose, and widely spaced teeth with defective enamel. More recently, corneal opacities have been noted along with hepatosplenomegaly, deafness, and metachromatic granulation of leukocytes. Wiedemann [277] and Maroteaux and Lamy [278, 279] have pointed out the frequency of corneal opacities and used the term *Morquio-Ulrich's syndrome* to designate such patients as a distinct entity.

Neurological symptoms may result from the deformity of the spine. In contrast to Hurler's syndrome, intelligence is normal. Cardiac complications have been reported by McKusick et al. [210] but are probably secondary to the distortion of the chest.

The pathology of Morquio's disorder has not been adequately studied. Einhorn et al. [280, 281] described irregular growth of articular cartilage with focal aseptic necrosis of

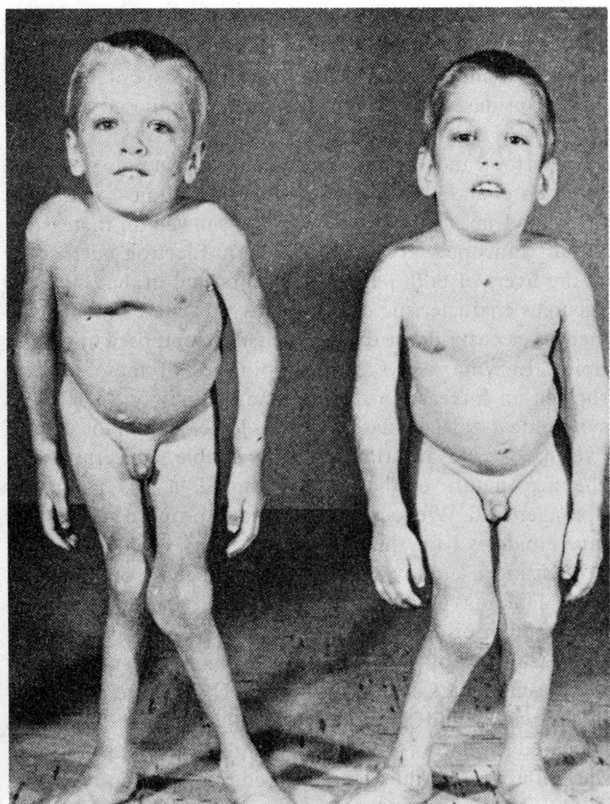

Figure 49-21. Brothers with Morquio-Ullrich disease. (*Reproduced with the kind permission of Dr. Hans Zellweger* [276].)

cartilage and bone. A more detailed pathological study by Schenk and Haggerty [282] indicates marked distortion of the cartilage matrix with striking change of cartilage architecture. The cells, recognizable as chondrocytes, were markedly enlarged. Additionally, large cells with foamy cytoplasm were thought on histochemical evidence to contain acid mucopolysaccharides. Hypertrophy and vacuolization of chondrocytes and Reilly bodies in granulocytes were reported in an iliac crest biopsy by Zellweger et al. [276]. Tondeur and Loeb [283] have examined liver biopsies of two patients, one with corneal opacities and the other with normal corneas. The Kupffer cells demonstrated large (0.3 to 4 microns) relatively electron-lucid inclusions, bound by unit membranes and containing a fine protein-like precipitate. The inclusions occasionally appeared as compact bodies, and membrane "myelin-like" round bodies were infrequently seen in the vacuoles. Hepatocytes were usually normal but occasionally contained structures resembling those found in the Kupffer cells. In general, the inclusions resembled those of Hurler's cells.

The fact that Morquio's syndrome is a mucopolysaccharidosis was clearly established by the discovery of keratan sulfate in the urine of patients with this disorder by Pedrini and coworkers [33].

It seems definite that there is at least one syndrome which is characterized by spondyloepiphyseal dysplasia, corneal opacity, and keratan sulfaturia for which the name *Morquio's syndrome* seems appropriate. Further studies will be required before the various types of epiphyseal dysplasias are unravelled. The complexity of the problem is illustrated by the report of Danes and Grossman [284] who attempted to separate these syndromes into spondyloepiphyseal dysplasias and epiphysiometaphyseal dysplasias.

The Morquio's syndrome is inherited as an autosomal recessive. The frequency is less than 1 in 40,000 births. Jacobsen [285] has suggested X linkage for Morquio's disease, but it is not clear whether he was studying the same disease.

G_{M1}-Gangliosidosis, Pseudo-Hurler's Disease

A group of patients described by Craig et al. [286] as *Hurler variants,* by Norman et al. [287] as *a Tay-Sachs variant,* and by Landing et al. [288] as *pseudo-Hurler's disease,* now appears to be *G_{M1}-gangliosidosis* or *generalized gangliosidosis* [36]. This syndrome, described in detail in Chap. 30, is characterized by the accumulation of G_{M1}-ganglioside and a "keratan sulfate-like" polysaccharide [35]. In the tissues of such patients, there is a lack of activity of the enzyme β-galactosidase [289]. Patients with this syndrome share the clinical features of both lipid and mucopolysaccharide storage diseases. A variant of G_{M1}-gangliosidosis showing keratan sulfate in the urine has been described by Pinsky, et al. [290]. Wolfe et al. [37] isolated from the urine of this patient a low-sulfate keratan sulfate-like compound which contained sialic acid.

Mucopolysaccharidosis VII

This syndrome was described by Dyggve et al. [291] in a family of Eskimo sibs in Greenland. The radiological findings of Morquio's diseases were present, together with corneal clouding and calcification of the ilium. One patient was mentally retarded. Chemical studies on the urine were inconclusive, though the authors suggest the presence of "altered" hyaluronic acid and dermatan sulfate. McKusick [3] has suggested that this might be a distinct syndrome justifying a designation as *Mucopolysaccharidosis VII.*

"I-cell" Disease

DeMars and LeRoy [292] have described a family with the clinical characteristics of Hurler's syndrome in which cultured fibroblasts, in phase microscopy, show a striking accumulation of inclusion bodies. The cells were not metachromatic. In a subsequent report, LeRoy and DeMars [293] added another patient, unrelated to the previous one, with a Hurler-like appearance and slight elevation of urinary mucopolysaccharides but no corneal clouding. The fibroblasts of both patients appeared similar under phase microscopy. The inclusions stained intensely for acid phosphatase which was present in much higher concentrations in the fibroblasts of these two patients than in the fibroblasts of patients with Hurler, Hunter, Sanfilippo, or Scheie syndromes, relatives of the patients, and unrelated controls. Beta-glucuronidase in fibroblasts was diminished as compared to other strains of fibroblasts. Cultured fibroblasts derived from the father and paternal uncle of one of the patients, but not from the mother, showed some cells which were similar to those of the patient.

The material accumulated in this disease has not been identified. The name *"I-cell" disease* was suggested because of the inclusions in the fibroblasts.

What may have been a similar syndrome has been studied in some detail by Matalon et al. [294]. A study of the brain biopsy of this patient was previously reported by Aleu and coworkers [238]. Limited joint mobility, hypertrophied gums, hepatomegaly, and inguinal hernias at the age of 2 months were also found in this patient. X-rays demonstrated small iliac bones, shallow acetabula and irregular ossification at the proximal ends of the femurs, and tapering metacarpals with a coarse trabecular pattern were present. The patient deteriorated neurologically by age 2-½ years, developed heart failure, and died at age 5 years, 3 months. There was slight kyphosis but no corneal clouding.

Fibroblast cultures were tinctorially strikingly different from Hurler fibroblasts. Toluidine blue staining revealed dark blue cytoplasm. Following the extraction of lipids with chloroform-methanol, metachromasia became apparent. Chemical study showed increased mucopolysaccharide content, primarily dermatan sulfate. Additionally, there was a marked increase in gangliosides, particularly G_{M3} and G_{D3}, phospholipids, and neutral lipids [295]. There was a marked decrease in a number of lysosomal enzymes, particularly β-N-acetylhexosaminidases and β-galactosidase [296]. Spranger and Wiedemann [476] have proposed the name mucolipidosis II for this disease.

Lipomucopolysaccharidosis; Mucolipidoses; Gal + Disease

Spranger et al. [297] reported two unrelated boys with features of Hurler's syndrome but with normal urinary mucopolysaccharide levels. Metachromatic granules were found in lymphocytes, liver cells, bone marrow, urinary sediment cells, and cultured fibroblasts. The urine was thought to have an abnormal amount of glycoprotein which was not characterized. On the basis of staining, increased amounts of lipids were thought to be present, but chemical characterization of neither the polysaccharide nor the lipids was performed. The term *lipomucopolysaccharidosis* was proposed. Originally it was thought that these cases were identical with the "I-cell" disease described by LeRoy and DeMars [293], but in a subsequent report [298] the authors indicated that these patients could be differentiated, on the basis of increased β-galactosidase activity in the liver. They proposed the name *mucolipidosis* for this disorder.

Van Hoof and Hers [299] studied two patients described by Loeb et al. [300] who displayed some clinical symptoms of gargoylism. One of these patients showed an increase in urinary mucopolysaccharide excretion. Electron microscopy of the livers of both patients were unusual in that the clear vacuoles characteristic of Hurler's syndrome contained numerous electron-dense droplets possibly composed of neutral lipids. Enzyme assays of liver biopsies of these patients showed an increase in β-galactosidase activity. In Hurler's syndrome β-galactosidase activity is lower than in the normal liver [299]. No information is available concerning the chemical nature of the material stored in this syndrome. Spranger and Wiedemann [476] have proposed the name mucolipidosis I for this disease.

Luchsinger et al. [301] have described a patient with clinical findings indicative of mucopolysaccharidosis but with no excretion or deposition in the liver of mucopolysaccharides. Cultures of fibroblasts showed luminescent granular cytoplasm on dark-field examination. Diminished β-galactosidase was found in the liver. Although the fibroblasts appeared similar to "I-cell" disease, the low β-galactosidase was different from the case described by LeRoy and DeMars [292].

The relationship of "I-cell" disease, the case described by Matalon et al., the cases described by Spranger et al., and the case of Luchsinger et al. remains unclear. Further chemical and enzymic studies are obviously required to delineate these mucopolysaccharide variants.

Mannosidosis

Öckerman [302] and Kjellman et al. [303] proposed the name *mannosidosis* for the disease of a single patient who died at age 4 with psychomotor retardation, gargoyle-like facies, increased stature, slight hepatosplenomegaly, muscular hypotonia, gibbus, abnormal bone structure, widely spaced teeth, cloudiness in the capsule of the lens, and hypogammaglobulinemia. Histological examination revealed markedly ballooned storage cells in the central nervous system. An increase in a mannose-containing substance and a decrease in α-mannosidase activity was found in the liver. Activities of other lysosomal enzymes such as β-galactosidase, β-glucuronidase, β-N-acetylglucosaminidase, α-fucosidase, and acid phosphatase were increased. The material isolated from the brain was heterogeneous and contained mannose and glucosamine. The molecular weight was less than 5,000. It was suggested that the accumulated material is an incompletely degraded product derived from glycoproteins.

Alpha-fucosidosis

Durand et al. [304, 305] described two sibs, male and female, born of a consanguine marriage, with severe progressive cerebral degeneration, increasing mental retardation, progressive dementia, gradual loss of muscle strength followed by intense spasticity, decerebrate rigidity, emaciation, thick skin, profuse sweating, cardiomegaly, and repeated respiratory infections. Increased sweat and saliva electrolytes combined with inability to concentrate dyes in the gall bladder were found. The patients died at 3-½ and 5-½ years of age. Histologic studies showed intracellular deposition of granular material which was weakly basophilic and sometimes stained with the periodic acid–Schiff reagent. Electron microscopy showed large clear vacuoles together with numerous lamellar structures. On the basis of solubility studies, the stored material was thought to be a mixture of carbohydrate, highly soluble in water, and a complex lipid. Durand et al. [306] found a ceramide tetra- and pentahexoside which exhibited H and h Lewis blood group activity in the liver and brain of these patients.

Dawson [477] found a large accumulation in the liver of the patient described by Freitag et al. [478] of a glycolipid containing fucose, galactose, glucose, and N-acetylglucosamine in a ratio of 1:2:1:1. It seems likely that this disease results from impaired degradation of glycoproteins and glycolipids containing α-fucose terminal groups. The non-reducing hexose of these glycolipids was found to be fucose. Van Hoof and Hers [307] discovered the absence of α-fucosidase activity in the liver of both of these patients, although other glycosidase activities were elevated. Loeb et al. [308] described a third patient with this disease who is possibly a distant cousin to the patients described by Durand et al. The name *α-fucosidosis* has been proposed for this disease. Van Hoof and Hers [299] found increased mucopolysaccharide levels in the livers of these patients and the presence of fucose in these fractions. Fucose has not been found previously in mucopolysaccharides other than keratan sulfate. Skin fibroblasts from the patient described by Loeb et al. [308] and studied by the authors showed no increase in mucopolysaccharide content and were ametachromatic.

Freitag et al. [478] in a detailed electron microscopic study of a liver, found large central deposits of reticulogranular material surrounded by a peripheral ring of electron-dense material deposited in membrane-invested storage elements. Other membrane-bound elements contained numerous lamellar structures with parallel or concentric orientation or both.

Metachromatic Leukodystrophy Variant

Szabo et al. [309] have described a patient with a gargoyle-like facies with an underdeveloped upper jaw, unusually long limbs, conduction deafness, cardiac abnormalities, and biconcave vertebral bodies with beak-like projections. Unusual was the finding of rounded, sharply outlined whitish changes scattered irregularly under the retinal veins. The urine contained large amounts of acid mucopolysaccharides, primarily dermatan sulfate and heparan sulfate. In the same paper, a 12-year-old girl is mentioned with severe bone deformities and idiocy and strikingly large amounts of dermatan sulfate in the urine. The fundus was reminiscent of Tay-Sachs disease, and metachromatic granules were present in a sural nerve biopsy. Bischel, Austin and Kemeny [310] have reported mucopolysaccharide abnormalities in the urine and tissues of two sibs with metachromatic leukodystrophy. The increase was in heparan sulfate. Dermatan sulfate was not excreted in abnormal quantities. Definition of these cases as distinct syndromes must await more detailed information. Murphy et al. [184] have made a detailed study of the tissues of such a patient and have found heparan sulfate and dermatan sulfate accumulated in the liver in quantities comparable to those found in mucopolysaccharidoses. No elevation of urinary mucopolysaccharides was present. Absence of arylsulfatases A, B, and C was demonstrated in the tissues of this patient. They accordingly suggest the possibility that these enzymes are involved in mucopolysaccharide degradation. Since arylsulfatase A is absent in the conventional form of metachromatic leukodystrophy, it is possible that aryl sulfatases B or C may be specifically related to desulfation of heparan and dermatan sulfates or oligosaccharide sulfates derived from these compounds.

Farber's Disease

Abul-Haj et al. [311] suggested that Farber's disease is a mucopolysaccharidosis. This syndrome is characterized by development early in infancy of irritability, a hoarse cry, swellings at many joints, and severe motor and mental retardation. In the reported cases, death always occurred by the age of 2 years. Characteristic granulomatous lesions containing cells distended by stored material were found throughout the body, particularly in all the regions of connective tissue and brain. No chemical studies have been reported regarding the nature of the stored material. Abul-Haj et al. [311] concluded that it was a mucopolysaccharide on the basis of histochemical studies and its widespread occurrence in connective tissue cells.

Chondroitin Sulfaturia

Philippart and Sugarman [312] have recently reported a patient with clinical and electron microscopic findings suggestive of Hurler's syndrome but with chondroitin-4-sulfate in the urine. The presence of an increased excretion of chondroitin sulfate in patients with symptoms resembling Morquio's disease has been previously reported by Kaplan et al. [58] and Dorfman and Ho [313].

Other Variants

Pincus and coworkers [314] described two sibs with a disorder characterized by progressive cerebral deterioration in the first decade associated with diffuse involvement of the reticuloendothelial system and infiltration of swollen histiocytes. One case developed corneal opacities 9 years after onset. Vertebral changes were similar to those of Hurler and Morquio's disease. The liver showed increased ganglioside content and on electron microscopy single membrane–limited vacuoles similar to those seen in Hurler's disease were observed. Acid mucopolysacchariduria (primarily chondroitin-4, 6-sulfate) occurred late in the course of the disease.

Winchester et al. [315] have described two sibs, products of a consanguine marriage, with a grotesque deforming disease of the limbs and trunk, characterized by severe progressive destruction of the large joints, accompanied by marked soft tissue swelling and later ankylosis and osteoporosis of the long bones. Kyphoscoliosis of the thoracolumbar spine was present. There were peripheral corneal opacities; however there was no increase in urinary acid mucopolysaccharide content. Skin fibroblasts showed metachromasia and increased intracellular uronic acid content.

Schimke and Horton [316] described two adolescent sibs who excreted both heparan sulfate and dermatan sulfate and had mild clinical symptoms of Hurler's disease, including corneal clouding, but no mental retardation. In contrast, Steinbach et al. [317] reported two patients with severe mental retardation, marked skeletal deformities, corneal clouding, and mucopolysacchariduria.

Langer and associates [318] described a case of a 61-year-old dwarfed man of presumed normal intelligence with many roentgen and clinical features which simulated Hunter's disease. No mucopolysaccharides were found in the urine, but an unidentified acid mucoid substance was said to be present in increased amounts.

Zugibe and associates [319] described a 52-year-old man with splenomegaly and limitation of motion of a left metatarsalphalangeal joint. On the basis of high urinary hexosamine and histochemical evidence, the storage material in the spleen was thought to be glycoprotein. The presence of excess urinary hexosamine in the father and in three sisters led to the suggestion of autosomal dominance. Berard-Badier et al. [233] have described a 15-year-old girl with hepatomegaly, osteochondrodystrophy, corneal clouding, cherry-red spots in both fundi, epileptic seizures, myoclonic jerks, and progressive psychomotor deficiency. Foamy cells were found in several tissues. Electron microscopy showed Kupffer cells containing vacuoles limited by single-unit membranes not unlike those seen in Hurler's disease. No increase in acid mucopolysaccharides was found in the urine. The nature of the storage material remains unknown.

CHEMISTRY OF MUCOPOLYSACCHARIDOSES

Early studies on the chemistry of the Hurler syndrome are largely of historical interest only and have been reviewed in great detail by Van Pelt [258]. The possibility that the storage material might be carbohydrate was initially proposed by deLange et al. [320] and Strauss [321] who considered that it might be glycogen. Lindsay et al. [248] suggested storage of a water-soluble substance, possibly a complex carbohydrate.

Modern knowledge concerning the biochemistry of this disease dates from Brante's report in 1952 [1] of the isolation from the livers of patients with the Hurler syndrome of a substance analytically similar to chondroitin sulfate. Uzman [322] proposed a genetic defect in the metabolism of a structural polysaccharide, although his data did not permit identification of the polysaccharide. Further indication of the chemical nature of the storage material was supplied by Stacey and Barker [323] in an addendum to a paper by Bishton et al. [324]. The liver of their patient contained a large amount of mucopolysaccharide which had a positive optical rotation and an infrared spectrum similar to heparin. The chemical nature of the polysaccharides involved in Hurler's syndrome and their excretion in the urine were reported in 1957 by Dorfman and Lorincz [325] who isolated 100 to 150 mg of acid mucopolysaccharides from the 24-hr urine of a 6-year-old girl with Hurler syndrome. The polysaccharide was identified as a mixture of dermatan sulfate and heparan sulfate. The relationship of the mucopolysaccharides in the urine to the storage material became clear when Brown [326] detected heparan sulfate in the liver of patients with the Hurler syndrome. The excretion of dermatan sulfate and heparan sulfate in urine was confirmed by Meyer et al. [327]. Chemical studies carried out by Meyer et al. [328] revealed these two polysaccharides in various organs of five autopsied cases. In four livers heparan sulfate was 90 percent of the total, while in one case equal amounts of the two polysaccharides were isolated from liver, kidney, spleen, and brain. The brain of a normal child did not yield any dermatan sulfate but did contain hyaluronic acid and heparan sulfate. Since these original observations, a large number of reports have confirmed the excretion of acid mucopolysaccharides as well as their deposition in tissues.

Methodology

Certain general principles are important for the isolation and determination of acid mucopolysaccharides. Since these macromolecules are polyanionic, their charge has been used for most separations. Three basic methods depending on charge have been employed: (1) precipitation by polycations such as cetylpyridinium chloride, cetyltrimethylammonium bromide, and 5-aminoacridine, (2) chromatography on ion-exchange resin columns such as Dowex-1 and Ecteola, and

(3) various types of electrophoresis. Additionally mucopolysaccharides may be separated by the differential alcohol solubility of their calcium salts. Scott [329] has studied in great detail the relationship of ionic strength and pH to the solubility of mucopolysaccharide-polycation complexes. The relative solubility of such complexes depends in general on the charge density of the mucopolysaccharides. Keratan sulfates behave anomalously. Hyaluronic acid–cetylpyridinium complex is soluble at lower salt concentrations than is the complex of chondroitin sulfates, which in turn is soluble at lower salt concentrations than the complex of heparin.

In applying purification methods to urine or tissue extracts it is important to recognize that whereas a given method may be successful in the separation and recovery of a mixture of pure polysaccharides, less reliable results are frequently obtained when a crude tissue extract is studied. Particularly anomalous results may be obtained with urine in view of the low molecular weight of dermatan sulfate and heparan sulfate fragments found in the mucopolysaccharidoses.

Analyses for mucopolysaccharides pose special problems. Hexosamine determinations can only be applied to highly purified preparations in view of the ubiquitous presence of hexosamines in glycoproteins and glycolipids. The available colorimetric methods for uronic acid analysis are not reliable when applied to crude tissue extracts of the various mucopolysaccharides. Heparin and heparan sulfate are most easily determined because of the specific reaction of N-sulfated groups with nitrous acid in the method of Lagunoff and Warren [330]. Keratan sulfate poses particular difficulties in that it behaves anomalously both on ion-exchange columns and on precipitation with cationic reagents. Since this mucopolysaccharide does not contain uronic acid, sugar analyses are limited to hexosamine and galactose, both of which are also present in glycoproteins. The problem is further complicated by the fact that according to Kaplan et al. [58] keratan sulfate and chondroitin sulfate may be attached to the same peptide in urine. Purification of keratan sulfate thus requires more specialized procedures [34].

Final identification of mucopolysaccharides requires isolation of highly purified compounds, complete chemical analyses, and characterization of physical properties. These procedures are not readily available in all laboratories and are not necessary for clinical use but are required for the confirmation of novel findings.

Table 49-4 presents commonly used properties for the identification of acid mucopolysaccharides. Partial identification of mucopolysaccharides may be achieved by a combination of enzymic and colorimetric methods as indicated in Table 49-4. The use of chondroitinase prepared from *P. vulgaris* permits more specific identification if the products are separated by chromatography [23].

The quantity of acid mucopolysaccharides excreted in the Hurler syndrome is sufficiently large so that many methods suffice for their demonstration, but the small increases reported in other diseases must be interpreted with care.

Several simplified screening methods have been reported for clinical purposes.

Acid Albumin Turbidity

This method is based on the fact that acid mucopolysaccharides at an acid pH react with albumin to form a precipitate. The method used in the authors' laboratory [331] is based on a previously published method for the assay of hyaluronidase [332]. Under appropriately controlled conditions of pH, ionic strength, temperature, and time, this method can be used for the semiquantitative estimation of acid mucopolysaccharides. The urine is centrifuged and dialyzed with external stirring against distilled water for at least 3 hr. Dialyzed urine, 1.5 ml, is mixed with 0.5 ml of a 0.3*M* phosphate-citrate buffer, pH 5.6, containing 0.45*M* NaCl. All reagents should be at room temperature. To this mixture

Table 49-4. CRITERIA FOR THE IDENTIFICATION OF THE ACID MUCOPOLYSACCHARIDES

Acid mucopolysaccharide	Susceptibility to: Testicular hyaluronidase	Streptococcal hyaluronidase	Proteus chondroitinases	Carbazole/ orcinol	Elution from Dowex-1, *M* NaCl
Hyaluronic acid	+	+	+	1.5–2.0(†)	0.5
Chondroitin	+	+	+	2.0	1.0
Chondroitin-4-sulfate	+	−	+	2.0	1.5
Chondroitin-6-sulfate	+	−	+	2.0	1.5
Dermatan sulfate	*	−	+	0.25–0.35	1.7
Heparan sulfate	−	−	−	3.0–4.0	1.3
Heparin	−	−	−	3.0–4.0	2.0
Keratan sulfate	−	−	−		3.0–4.0

* Dermatan sulfate is variably degraded by testicular hyaluronidase depending on the amount of glucuronic acid in the molecule.

† These are approximate values and may vary according to the course of material and its purity.

is added 10 ml of an acid albumin reagent. This reagent contains 0.1 percent of purified serum albumin in a 0.1*M* acetate buffer adjusted to pH 3.75. In the presence of acid mucopolysaccharides, a uniform turbidity develops which may be quantitated in a photoelectric colorimeter at 540 mμ. The optical density depends on the optical system employed. Controls should be carried out to correct for any urine color and to demonstrate that the reagents give appropriate turbidity with known chondroitin sulfate samples. With a light path of 1 cm optical densities above 0.050 have been found only in Hurler's or closely related syndromes. In the author's experience no well-authenticated patient with Hurler's syndrome has given a negative test by this method. Turbidities with an optical density of less than 0.050 have sometimes been found in young infants who are apparently normal.

Spot Test

A somewhat simpler test has been reported by Berry and Spinanger [333]. To perform the test 5, 10, and 25 μl urine are placed on a piece of Whatman No. 1 filter paper. A micropipette is used to spot 5 μl. Each application should dry thoroughly before the next one is made. The paper is dipped for about 1 min in an aqueous solution of 0.04 percent toluidine blue O, buffered at pH 2, drained, and rinsed in 95 percent ethyl alcohol. Urine from patients with the Hurler syndrome gives a purple spot against a blue background. When 260 samples from children with a variety of diseases were tested with amounts of urine of up to 5 to 10 times those which gave positive test results in patients with Hurler syndrome, faint positive spots were found in four specimens. Positive tests were found in normal specimens from newborns. When the method was applied to 2,200 specimens obtained by collecting infants' urine on filter paper, 0.02 percent positive test results were obtained.

Another spot test utilizing Alcian blue instead of toluidine blue has been described by Carson and Neill [334]. Turbidity tests using cetyltrimethylammonium bromide have been developed by Renuart [335] and using cetylpyridinium chloride by Manley and Hawksworth [336].

Steiness [337] evaluated the albumin turbidity test on urines of normal controls, families of patients with Hurler's disease, 13 patients with various other diseases, and on Hurler's disease patients. Only the urine of patients with Hurler's disease gave positive reactions. Carter et al. [338] evaluated the albumin turbidity test and the toluidine blue spot test on 800 mentally retarded control patients and 54 patients with the Hurler syndrome. The spot test was within the normal range for 98.5 percent of the control patients and 31.7 percent of the Hurler's patients. A gross acid albumin turbidimetric test (turbidity evaluated visually) was normal in 93.7 percent of normal urines and 9.3 percent of Hurler's urines. The quantitative acid albumin test was normal in 82.8 percent of the normals and 9.2 percent of Hurler's. The results obtained with different specimens of Hurler's urine showed some fluctuation with time. The cetyltrimethylammonium bromide turbidity test was found to be unreliable in the hands of Procopis et al. [339]. In contrast, Manley and Hawksworth found the cetylpyridinium chloride turbidity method quite reliable.

On evaluation of various screening tests, Pennock and coworkers [340] found no false positives but one false negative with acid albumin turbidity tests. Since they found the toluidine blue and Alcian blue spot tests unsatisfactory, they employed a cetylpyridinium chloride citrate test to screen 1,000 children. Thirty-six positive results were obtained, including four patients with mucopolysaccharidoses. The remaining patients comprised a wide variety of diagnoses, some of which were thought to excrete acid mucopolysaccharides. None of the screening tests described are adequate for the detection of keratan sulfate in Morquio's disease or G_{M1}-gangliosidosis.

Quantitative Methods

Several methods have been proposed which permit more adequate quantitative and qualitative determination of mucopolysaccharides and yet do not necessitate tedious purification. Manley and Hawksworth [336] have described an electrophoretic method on cellulose acetate strips with Alcian blue staining and densitometric measurement of the stained areas. Azure A staining was used to distinguish the metachromatically staining mucopolysaccharides from the orthochromatically staining mucoprotein.

Electrophoresis for the rapid identification of mucopolysaccharides is carried out in the author's laboratory on cellulose polyacetate strips (Sepraphore III) 2.5 × 15 cm. Samples of 5 μl containing 0.25 to 0.5 percent of mucopolysaccharide solution are applied with micropipettes and electrophoresed for 1 hr at 100 volts in a 0.1*M* pyridine–formic acid buffer, pH 3.0. Mucopolysaccharides are stained with 0.5 percent of acridine orange in water. Under these conditions good separations of hyaluronic acid, dermatan sulfate, chondroitin-4/6-SO_4, and heparan sulfate are obtained. Such studies are adequate for the preliminary identification of acid mucopolysaccharides in mixtures.

A relatively simple quantitative method for the further study of urine samples screened by the acid albumin turbidity method has been developed by Ho and Dorfman [341]. Between one-tenth and one-fifth of a 24-hr urine specimen is used for analysis, depending on urine volume. Samples are concentrated to approximately 5 ml, centrifuged, and after two washings of the sediment with water, the supernatant solutions and washings are combined and applied in a volume not exceeding 15 ml to a Sephadex G-25 column (superfine, 48 × 2.4 cm outside diameter). The column is packed and eluted with 0.05*M* sodium chloride. The mucopolysaccharide appears in the first 50 ml after the void volume. Urinary pigment and salts are retarded. The polysaccharide-containing fraction is concentrated to approximately 2 ml. Two 0.08 ml aliquots of this sample are chromatographed on duplicate Sephadex columns (G-25, superfine, 54 × 1.0 cm outside diameter) with 0.2*M* sodium chloride as eluent. The first 4 ml after the void volume contains the mucopolysaccharide fraction. The acid mucopolysaccharides are precipitated with 5 percent cetylpyridinium chloride added dropwise until no further precipitation occurs. After 1 hr at 38°C, the precipitate is collected by centrifugation and the supernatant solution is discarded. The polysaccharide–cetylpyridinium chloride complex is dissolved in 2*M* sodium chloride, 1 to 5 ml, depending on the amount of precipitate, and uronic acid is determined by the carbazole method [342]. The total mucopolysaccharide in a 24-hr urine specimen is expressed in terms of milligrams of uronic acid. If uronic acid is also determined by the orcinol method [343], the relative amounts of dermatan sulfate and heparan sulfate may be estimated. Hexosamine may be estimated by the modified method of Boas [344]. The presence of relatively large amounts of non-uronic acid–containing polysaccharides, such as keratan sulfate and glycoproteins in crude mixtures, may lead to low carbazole/hexosamine ratios. Precautions must be taken not to use excessive amounts of cetylpyridinium chloride, since keratan sulfate may be redissolved and appear in the supernatant fraction. Generally speaking, keratan sulfate is more difficult to isolate by this method, and chromatography on Dowex-1 is the preferable method. Keratan sulfate cannot, of course, be estimated by either the carbazole or orcinol methods.

By the use of Sephadex G-200, Constantopoulos [345] noted that urines which contain heparan sulfate show an elution peak with an average molecular weight of 2,300 while dermatan sulfate is found in a peak with an average molecular weight of 9,000 (some heparan sulfate is also found in this peak). He proposed that this method is valuable in giving a qualitative picture of the polysaccharide distribution in urine.

Most investigators have used some modification of the quantitative method originally described by DiFerrante and Rich [346]. This method depends upon the precipitation of mucopolysaccharide with cetyltrimethylammonium bromide, followed by determination of uronic acid in the redissolved precipitate. The variations of results obtained with this method led DiFerrante [347] to examine carefully the efficiency of precipitating agents. He concluded that under optimum conditions cetyltrimethylammonium bromide and cetylpyridinium chloride are superior to 5-aminoacridine as precipitants. Losses may occur due to dialysis or incomplete precipitation of low-molecular-weight compounds. However, Linker and associates [348] have demonstrated that failure to dialyze concentrated urine results in incomplete precipitation of urinary mucopolysaccharides by cationic reagents. For these reasons, concentration on Sephadex columns have considerable advantage.

Acid Mucopolysaccharides in Normal Urine

Since DiFerrante and Rich [346] demonstrated the presence of chondroitin sulfate in normal urine, a number of studies have been aimed at defining the qualitative and quantitative mucopolysaccharide content of normal urine. DiFerrante [349] found that normal urine contains chondroitin-4-sulfate and chondroitin-6-SO_4, some of which is incompletely sulfated. Additionally, smaller amounts of dermatan sulfate and possibly heparan sulfate were indicated. Linker and Terry [350] found that normal urine contains approximately 80 percent chondroitin sulfates and 20 percent of a mixture of approximately equal parts of dermatan sulfate and heparan sulfate. Berenson and Dalferes [351] found primarily chondroitin-4- and chondroitin-6-SO_4 and dermatan sulfate, with small amounts of chondroitin, heparan sulfate, and keratan sulfate in normal urine. Varadi and coworkers [352] characterized the mucopolysaccharide of a pool of normal male adult urine. The proportions found were chondroitin-6-SO_4, 34 percent; chondroitin-4-SO_4, 31 percent; chondroitin, 25 percent; heparan sulfate, 8 percent; dermatan sulfate, 1 percent; hyaluronic acid, 1 percent; keratan sulfate, 1 percent. The chondroitin sulfates were of low molecular weight, and some chains were bound to a peptide containing predominantly serine, glycine, and glutamic acids. Orii [353] also found low-sulfate chondroitin sulfate in urine, and Chakrapani and Bachhawat [354] found xylose and galactose in the chondroitin sulfate fraction of pooled normal urine and arabinose and glucose in a mixed fraction which contained hyaluronic acid. They observed somewhat higher levels of hyaluronic acid than reported by Varadi et al. Orii [355] found a distribution of polysaccharides in normal male children similar to that reported by Varadi et al., except for somewhat larger amounts of keratan sulfate.

These studies suggest that the chondroitin sulfates of urine represent fragments of chondromucoprotein which have undergone proteolysis, chain degradation, and desulfation.

The colorimetric determination of heparan sulfate by Lagunoff and associates [356] in normal urine indicated ratios of heparan sulfate to total mucopolysaccharides varying from 0 to 0.26 with a mean of 0.076. Teller [357] and Manley et al. [358] found a higher content of dermatan sulfate than did Varadi et al. Manley et al. noted that the proportion of chondroitin sulfates reached a peak in childhood while heparan sulfate content was increased in adults. A similar decrease in the proportion of chondroitin sulfates in the urine of adults has been noted by Mayes and Hansen [359] who also observed the presence of hyaluronic acid in the urine of infants.

Although some variation in proportions of mucopolysaccharides has been observed by different investigators, it is clear that low-molecular-weight chondroitin sulfates comprise the bulk of urinary mucopolysaccharides. Heparan sulfate is also present in significant quantities, together with smaller amounts of other acid mucopolysaccharides.

The reported normal levels of excretion of acid mucopolysaccharides are summarized in Table 49-5. Some variation in results is probably based on methodological differences. Difficulty is experienced in comparing various studies because of the differences in manner of expression of results. Spranger et al. [360] noted a wide daily variation in acid mucopolysaccharide excretion.

Several investigators have attempted to relate acid mucopolysaccharide excretion to urinary creatinine levels in order to obtain a more sensitive index for the comparison of normal to abnormal urinary mucopolysaccharide excretion and to obviate the necessity of 24-hr urine collections. Teller et al. [361] found a decrease in mucopolysaccharide/creatinine ratios in children between ages 0 to 14 years. Similar results were obtained by Mayes and Hansen [359], Manley et al. [358], and Spranger et al. [360]. The ratio becomes constant in adults, although the latter investigators found some increase in old age which was attributed to an artifact introduced by elevated glycoprotein content which interfered with their method.

The various studies seem reasonably consistent in indicating a peak of mucopolysaccharide excretion coincident with the major growth spurt.

Table 49-5. ACID MUCOPOLYSACCHARIDE EXCRETION IN NORMAL URINE

	Sex	Age, years	mg/24 hr
Kerby [392]	F	Adult	7.5
	M	Adult	12.2
DiFerrante and Rich [346]	F	Adult	9.4
	M	Adult	15.0
	F	7–8	14.0
	M	7–16	18.6
Rich et al. [393]	M	1 month	6.5
	M	13–15	18–23
Teller et al. [361]	..	4	8.9
		14	18.2
Muir et al. [394]		......	12–30
Lin [395]	..	Adult	4–9
Øhlenschaeger and Firman [389]	M	19–83	15.5
	F	19–78	11.2
DiFerrante [347]	M	Adult	13.3
	F	Adult	11.3
Ho and Dorfman [341]	..	0–1	3.8
		2–8	10.1
		9–12	15.6
	M	22–40	6.8
	F	22–40	4.8
		40–64	6.5
Thompson and Castor [384]	M	Adult	7.5
	F	Adult	6.8
Wessler [378]	M	21–57	11.9
	F	21–53	12.0

Abnormal Excretion of Mucopolysaccharides

A marked increase in excretion of acid mucopolysaccharides in various mucopolysaccharidoses has been so uniformly observed that detailed review of these data seems superfluous. Since the original report of Dorfman and Lorincz [325], it has been found that the augmented excretion is also characterized by a striking qualitative change in urinary mucopolysaccharide composition in Hurler and Hunter syndromes. Knecht and associates [65] compared the chemical structure of heparan sulfate isolated from the urine of a patient with Sanfilippo's syndrome with heparan sulfate isolated from normal human aorta. The urinary heparan sulfate was polydispersed with molecular weights ranging from 2,700 to 5,500. Resolution of the crude material yielded a fraction with a high N-sulfate content, which was almost completely devoid of amino acids and linkage sugars (xylose and galactose), and a second fraction containing more N-acetyl groups and serine, xylose, and galactose in molar proportions of 1:1:2. It was postulated that both fragments result from the degradation of a parent molecule similar to that of aorta heparan sulfate which showed a number average molecular weight of 24,000 to 29,000 and contained serine, xylose, and galactose in a molar ratio of 1:1:2. The fractions of high N-sulfate content presumably originate from parts of the heparan sulfate chains distal to the areas of protein binding. Kaplan [362] also isolated a heparan sulfate–serine compound from the urine of a patient with Sanfilippo's disease. Dermatan sulfate in the urine of Hurler's patients is also partially degraded [31]. As noted earlier, dermatan sulfate is a hybrid polymer containing both D-glucuronic acid and L-iduronic acid and is hydrolyzed at N-acetylgalactosaminyl-glucuronic acid linkages. The products found in urine behave as if they were derived from dermatan sulfate which had been cleaved by hyaluronidase. In addition to the large fragments of dermatan sulfate, Fransson and Dorfman [363] showed that Hurler's urine contains small oligosaccharides partially devoid of nonreducing D-glucuronic acid, indicating digestion by β-glucuronidase. Low molecular weights of urinary heparan sulfate and dermatan sulfate in urine have also been observed by Constantopoulos [345].

The occurrence of keratan sulfate in the urine of patients with Morquio's disease was first discovered by Pedrini and coworkers [33] and confirmed by Robins et al. [34]. Dorfman and associates [364] found an elevated concentration of chondroitin-4/6 SO_4 in a patient with Morquio's disease. The finding of both keratan sulfate and chondroitin sulfate in this syndrome is readily explained by the discovery of Kaplan et al. [58]. This discovery is consistent with the presence of both polysaccharides on a single peptide in cartilage described earlier in this chapter.

Linker et al. [479] have confirmed the presence of two to three times the normal amount of keratan sulfate in the urine of 12 patients with Morquio's disease. Although the increased proportion of keratan sulfate was maintained, the concentration of keratan sulfate in these patients declined with age.

As methodology has improved, attempts have been made to correlate the spectrum of urinary mucopolysaccharide excretion with the clinical classification of mucopolysaccharidoses. Following the description of Lorincz [262] and Harris [263] of patients who excreted only heparan sulfate, Sanfilippo et al. [264] suggested that the exclusive excretion of heparan sulfate is characteristic of a specific group of patients. Terry and Linker [365] suggested that the phenotype and genotype of mucopolysaccharidoses could be correlated with the pattern of mucopolysaccharide excretion. This question has now been studied in detail utilizing improved methodology by Kaplan [272] and Spranger [366]. In the urines of 46 patients with mucopolysaccharidoses, the following four discrete patterns were found: (1) solely excess heparan sulfate, (2) solely excess dermatan sulfate, (3) excess heparan sulfate and dermatan sulfate in approximately equal amounts, and (4) excess heparan sulfate and dermatan sulfate with a ratio of dermatan sulfate to heparan sulfate of 2 to 3 : 1. Kaplan proposed that mental retardation does not occur without the excretion of heparan sulfate and that the probability of mental retardation increased with an increasing concentration of heparan sulfate in urine. Similarly, it was suggested that no corneal opacity or aortic disease occurs in the absence of dermatan sulfate in the urine and that there is an increasing probability of the existence of these two abnormalities with an increasing concentration of dermatan sulfate. This correlation is of interest in view of the fact already mentioned that rat glial cell tumor and a human glial cell tumor produce heparan sulfate in tissue culture. The pure heparan sulfate excretors would appear to correspond to the generally accepted Sanfilippo's syndrome or Type III mucopolysaccharidosis, while pure dermatan sulfate excretors correspond to the Maroteaux-Lamy syndrome of Type VI mucopolysaccharidosis. The patients who showed approximately equal quantities of heparan sulfate and dermatan sulfate were all males and conform mostly to the clinical picture of Hunter's syndrome or Type II mucopolysaccharidosis. The patients who showed a predominance of dermatan sulfate include patients with clinical diagnoses of Hurler's syndrome, Hunter's syndrome, and Scheie's syndrome.

Spranger [366] studied the pattern of mucopolysaccharide excretion in 72 patients with a variety of mucopolysaccharidoses. Although the actual ratios found differed from those of Kaplan, trends were similar. Hurler's disease was characterized by excretion of both polysaccharides, but heparan sulfate predominated. Urine from patients with Sanfilippo's disease showed only heparan sulfate. Urine from patients with Morquio's disease showed keratan sulfate and chondroitin-$^4/_6$-sulfate. Urines of patients classified as Ullrich-Scheie's were inconstant, some showing only dermatan sulfate, while urines from others contained herparan sulfate as well. Maroteaux-Lamy patients showed only dermatan sulfate.

The confusion of the earlier literature seems to be disappearing, with improved methodology demonstrating increasingly clear-cut urine polysaccharide patterns. Patterns for mucopolysaccharidoses, I, II, III, IV, and VI seem reasonably clear, but more information regarding mucopolysaccharidosis V is required. One patient described by Spranger [366] excreted normal amounts of mucopolysaccharide, but with an increase in the proportion of dermatan sulfate.

The excretion of excess mucopolysaccharides in heterozygous individuals was reported by Teller, et al. [367] but denied by Terry and Linker [365] and Bergaard and Bearn [267]. Kaplan was likewise unable to find an elevation of polysaccharides in the urine of parents of some of his patients. A study carried out in the authors' laboratory similarly showed no striking difference between urine mucopolysaccharide levels in heterozygotes and normals. On a statistical basis there was a small increase in heterozygotes, but there was considerable overlap between the levels in normals and heterozygotes.

Teller et al. [368] found normal total levels of mucopolysaccharides in the parents of a patient with Sanfilippo's disease but an increase in the heparan sulfate fraction.

Studies on abnormalities of other urinary components in Hurler's syndrome have generally been negative, although Rennart and Dekaban [369] found an increase of serine in both plasma and urine and an increase of tryptophan in urine in Hurler's disease.

Relatively few studies have been reported on plasma mucopolysaccharide levels. In agreement with previous isolation studies [370], the bulk of polysaccharide in normal plasma was found by Calatroni and coworkers [371] to be chondroitin sulfate. A significantly larger concentration of acid mucopolysaccharide was found in the plasma of children than in that of adults. No difference was found between males and females. In three patients with Hurler's disease, the plasma level was higher than normal. A similar increase in serum mucopolysaccharide was found by Usui et al. [372].

Constantapoulos and Dekaban [373] found small quantities (0.010 mg per 100 ml) of mucopolysaccharides in the normal cerebrospinal fluid and considerably larger amounts (0.2 to 1.0 mg per ml) in Hurler's and Sanfilippo's syndrome. Carbazole/orcinol ratios indicated primarily heparan sulfate in Sanfilippo's syndrome and a mixture of heparan and dermatan sulfate in Hurler's syndrome. Both compounds were of low molecular weight.

The finding of increased mucopolysaccharide excretion in mucopolysaccharidoses has led to the study of polysaccharide excretion in other diseases. Berenson and Serra [374] and Berenson and Dalferes [351] found a two- to fourfold increase in the excretion of mucopolysaccharides in Marfan's syndrome, primarily due to an increased content of chondroitin-4- and chondroitin-6-sulfate. Earlier claims by Bacchus [375] of increased mucopolysaccharide in serum are open to question in view of the methods employed.

Lorincz [376] has reported an increased excretion of acid mucopolysaccharides in two families with hereditary deforming chondroplasia (diaphysial aclasis). This report was based only on the turbidity method. The quantities excreted were thought to be comparable to those obtained in the Hurler syndrome but consisted of chondroitin-4-SO_4 or chondroitin-6-SO_4, or both, and dialyzed slowly through a cellophane membrane. Lorincz [377] has also reported an increase in mucopolysaccharide excretion in six of eight children with arthrosteo-onychondysplasia (nail-patella syndrome). No increase was found in the urine of adults with the syndrome. Preliminary identification suggested that the polysaccharide in the urine resembled hyaluronic acid. These results could not be confirmed by Wessler [378].

Lorincz [379] indicated that "snorter cattle" have a disease akin to the Hurler syndrome on the basis of the excretion of excess mucopolysaccharide including dermatan sulfate. This claim has not been verified by Tyler et al. [380] and Mayer et al. [381].

DiFerrante [382] found an increase in urinary mucopolysaccharide excretion in rheumatoid arthritis which was suppressed by salicylate therapy. The extent of increase was small and qualitatively the material appeared to be primarily chondroitin sulfate. An increase of a similar order of magnitude was found by DiFerrante et al. [383] in lupus erythematosus. Thompson and Castor [384] found a similar increase in rheumatoid arthritis and other inflammatory connective tissue diseases, but they also found an increase in a variety of conditions not related to connective tissue disorders. Brunish and Sorensen [385] found a small increase in mucopolysaccharide excretion in nummular psoriasis and a more striking increase in psoriasis pustulosa and arthritic psoriasis.

Loewi [386] also found an increase in rheumatoid arthritis in adults but a decrease in children with this disease. No increase was found in dermatomyositis or rheumatic fever.

An increased excretion of hyaluronic acid and chondroitin sulfate in urticaria pigmentosa was reported by Asboe-Hansen and Clausen [387]. An increase in the excretion of polysaccharides in exophthalmos has been reported by Winand [388]. The observed increase was not correlated with hyperthyroidism. The qualitative distribution of polysaccharides was normal.

Øhlenschlaeger and Friman [389], in accordance with the findings of Thompson and Castor [384] and Wessler [378], discovered that urinary acid mucopolysaccharides were increased in active scleroderma but not during the inactive phase of the disease.

Hyaluronic acid has been detected in the serum and urine of a patient with neuroblastoma by Morse and Nussbaum [390] and chondroitin sulfate in the serum of three patients with myxomas of the heart by Matalon et al. [391].

Gangliosides in Hurler's Disease

Since the recognition of the role of mucopolysaccharides in the pathogenesis of Hurler's disease, relatively less attention has been given to the abnormal levels of the gangliosides in this syndrome. Jervis [396] first reported increased ganglioside levels in the brain. Similarly Brante [1,397] found an increase of gangliosides, diminished cerebrosides, and normal phospholipid and cholesterol levels. Subsequent studies by Taghavy and coworkers [398], Ledeen et al. [399], Gonatas and Gonatas [400], Suzuki [401], and Taketomi and Yamakawa [402] all indicated an increase in the gangliosides in the brain and an abnormal distribution but no evidence of the accumulation of a specific compound as is characteristic of the gangliosidoses. Increases were found in ceramide lactoside, G_{M2}, and G_{M1}, while the content of G_{T1a} was diminished. Taketomi and Yamakawa [402] noted particularly the increase in ceramide lactoside, and in two additional components of hematoside and two additional gangliosides which were not completely identified. The fatty acid composition of the ceramide lactoside was similar to hematoside. Both the hematoside and other gangliosides contained only C_{18}-sphingosine and a small amount of C_{18}-dehydrosphingosine.

Dawson [480] found a marked increase in ceramide mono-, di-, tri-, and tetrahexoside and in ganglioside G_{M3} in livers from patients with Hurler's disease but not in livers from patients with Sanfilippo's disease.

TISSUE CULTURE STUDIES

The application of tissue culture to the study of storage diseases was initiated by the discovery by Danes and Bearn [403] that fibroblasts cultured from patients with Hurler and Hunter syndromes contain metachromatic granules and the demonstration by Matalon and Dorfman [404] that metachromasia was due to the intracellular accumulation of large amounts of acid mucopolysaccharides. The striking presence of metachromatic granules in Hurler's fibroblasts is illustrated in Plate II–5. Fibroblasts cultured from patients with Hurler, Hunter, and Sanfilippo syndromes contain 5 to 10 times as much intracellular mucopolysaccharides as do normal fibroblasts. The major increase in mucopolysaccharides was accounted for by dermatan sulfate although levels of hyaluronic acid were greater than those in normal cells. Schafer et al. [405] demonstrated that the extent of the increase of dermatan sulfate was dependent on the presence of ascorbic acid in the growth medium.

The finding of increased concentration of dermatan sulfate in cells cultured from a patient with Sanfilippo's disease was surprising in view of the fact that the mucopolysaccharide found in the urine of the patient was almost exclusively heparan sulfate. In the many isolations of acid mucopolysaccharides from cultured human skin fibroblasts, a large increase of heparan sulfate has not been found in this laboratory.

Matalon and Dorfman [481] have more recently found small amounts of heparan sulfate in normal Hurler's and Sanfilippo's fibroblasts. A possible source of heparan sulfate in mucopolysaccharidoses has become apparent as a result

Table 49-6. METACHROMASIA OF CULTURED HUMAN FIBROBLASTS IN VARIOUS DISEASES

Diseases of connective tissue	Lipid storage diseases	Others
Hurler [424]	Fabry [411]	Cystic fibrosis [409]
Hunter [424]	Gaucher [430]	Juvenile amaurotic idiocy [431]
Sanfilippo [424]	Krabbe [432]	Myotonic muscular dystrophy [432]
Scheie [424]	Late infantile amaurotic idiocy [2]	
Morquio [423]	Hurler variant [294]	
Marfan [410]		
Pseudoxanthoma elasticum [429]		
Hurler variant [294]		

of the discovery by Dorfman and Ho [51] that a clone of glial cells cultured from a rat glial-cell tumor produces heparan sulfate in culture. Heparan sulfate is also produced in culture by a clone of human glial cells derived from a human glioma [406].

Upon studying fibroblasts from six families of patients with Hurler's syndrome, Danes and Bearn [407] found metachromatic cells not only in the cultures of the probands but also in those of both parents. The extent of metachromasia in the heterozygous carriers was comparable to that in the cells of the patients. In two of the families, abnormal genes were traced through two unaffected generations. In one family, both paternal grandfathers yielded metachromatic fibroblasts. The finding of metachromasia in the fibroblasts of both parents in two families of patients with Sanfilippo's disease indicated that this disease, like Hurler's, is an autosomal recessive disorder.

In three families of the X-linked disease (Hunter's), fibroblasts cultured from the skin of the fathers contained no metachromatic granules whereas those of the heterozygous mothers contained both metachromatic and ametachromatic cells. In one family, the skin fibroblasts of the maternal great-grandmother, maternal grandmother, maternal great-aunt, and the maternal half-aunt all contained positive cells. The abnormal gene was thus traced for three generations. Again the extent of cellular metachromasia could not be distinguished between the propositus and the heterozygous carriers. However, the cultures of the propositus showed an almost homogeneous population of metachromatic fibroblasts, whereas only approximately half of the cells of the heterozygous mothers contained metachromatic granules.

Further confirmation of the distinction between Hurler's and Hunter's diseases has been obtained by the use of cloning techniques [408]. All clones derived from patients and heterozygous carriers of the autosomal disease (Hurler's) showed marked metachromasia and increased intracellular uronic acid–containing macromolecules. Clones derived from affected subjects with the X-linked disease (Hunter's) also contained uniform metachromasia and increased uronic acid content. Clones obtained from fathers of patients with Hunter's disease showed neither metachromasia nor increased intracellular uronic acid. In contrast, two types of clones were derived from heterozygous mothers and sisters of patients. On the average, 72 percent of these clones were metachromatic and all showed increased uronic acid content, while 28 percent of the clones showed no metachromasia and a normal uronic acid content. These results provide further support for the Lyon hypothesis.

The discovery of metachromasia in fibroblasts of patients with mucopolysaccharidoses originally gave promise that this phenomenon might be diagnostic for this group of diseases. The situation became increasingly confusing with the appearance of metachromasia in a wide number of syndromes, including some not obviously related pathogenetically to Hurler's disease. This was particularly striking with the discovery by Danes and Bearn [409] that fibroblasts cultured from patients with cystic fibrosis demonstrate metachromasia.

Table 49-6 lists the diseases in which metachromasia of fibroblasts has been reported. Additionally, metachromasia has been found in our laboratory in fibroblast cultures of single patients with the following diseases: hyperlipemia, carotenemia, Jakob-Creutzfeldt disease, epidermolysis bullosa, mosaicism for multiple trisomies, scleroderma, unilateral nevus, and vitamin D–resistant rickets [2]. Since it is now known that metachromasia occurs in the unaffected heterozygotes of a number of diseases, it is not possible to draw final conclusions on individual patients in the absence of a study of multiple cases or of a study of families.

In order to establish more definitively the significance of metachromasia, the isolation and identification of mucopolysaccharides from cultured cells was undertaken [2]. Table 49-7 summarizes the results of a group of such experiments. In fibroblasts that show increased content of mucopolysaccharides, three different patterns emerged. A marked increase in dermatan sulfate occurs in Hurler's, Hunter's and Sanfilippo's diseases, a case of late infantile amaurotic idiocy, and a Hurler variant. In Marfan's disease the increase of total polysaccharide is primarily due to hyaluronic acid [410], whereas in Fabry's disease [411], Gaucher's disease, Krabbe's disease, cystic fibrosis, and Morquio's disease, although the quantity of polysaccharide is markedly in-

Table 49-7. INTRACELLULAR MUCOPOLYSACCHARIDES IN CULTURED HUMAN FIBROBLASTS

Diseases	Total acid mucopoly-saccharide, mg*	Hyaluronic acid, percent	Dermatan sulfate, percent	Chondroitin (4/6) sulfate, percent
Normal	0.6	68	16	16
Hurler	5.5	22	73	5
Hunter	6.5	23	67	10
Sanfilippo	3.3	45	48	7
Morquio	3.0	62	27	11
Marfan	4.8	92	2	6
Hurler variant	5.5	25	66	9
Cystic fibrosis	1.2	68	19	13
Cystic fibrosis	5.5	71	18	11
Cystic fibrosis (P. K.) one patient	0.6	22	65	13
Fabry	4.1	80	12	8
Gaucher	1.7	69	21	10
Late infantile amaurotic idiocy	3.8	40	51	9
Krabbe	4.8	84	10	6
Hurler heterozygote	4.2	45	43	12
Hunter heterozygote	2.0	51	35	14
Sanfilippo heterozygote	1.2	43	45	12
Hurler variant heterozygote	3.3	46	38	16
Cystic fibrosis heterozygote	2.2	70	18	12
Fabry heterozygote	2.9	72	18	10
Late infantile amaurotic idiocy heterozygote	2.5	55	34	11

* Results are based on isolation of polysaccharides from 10 Falcon tissue culture plates (100 mm) after 3 weeks growth. Each plate contained approximately 14×10^6 cells with a dry weight of 15 mg. The quantity of mucopolysaccharides is based on 33 percent hexosamine.

creased, the qualitative distribution is the same as in normal cells. The total amount of polysaccharide in the heterozygotes is, in general, less than in the corresponding homozygotes, but the qualitative pattern of the heterozygote is similar to the corresponding homozygotes.

Danes and associates [412] have developed a histochemical method for the study of cultured fibroblasts which involves the use of Alcian blue at various ionic strengths. Staining by Alcian blue in 0.3M $MgCl_2$ is restricted to fibroblasts from those diseases in which dermatan sulfate would be expected to accumulate, although failure to observe staining in Sanfilippo's disease is unexplained. Fibroblasts from a patient with the Maroteaux-Lamy syndrome were said to stain with Alcian blue but did not demonstrate toluidine blue metachromasia. The occasional fibroblasts of normal individuals as well as those of cystic fibrosis, Gaucher's disease, familial amaurotic idiocy, and pseudoxanthoma elasticum, which are metachromatic when stained with toluidine blue, did not stain with Alcian blue. The authors concluded that metachromasia in normal fibroblasts, "false positive," are genuine and due to some genetically determined cellular characteristic different from an increased mucopolysaccharide concentration.

These conclusions differ from those of Matalon and Dorfman [2] who have found metachromasia to correspond to increased intracellular mucopolysaccharide concentration. Again it is important to emphasize that metachromasia and increased intracellular mucopolysaccharide content in many diseases represents increased amounts of acid mucopolysaccharides in normal proportions rather than the specific pattern evident in mucopolysaccharidoses.

An unusual type of fibroblast reported by LeRoy and DeMars [293] in "I-cell" disease has already been discussed. What appeared to be an identical situation has been encountered by the authors in a case showing clinical manifestations of the Hurler syndrome (294]. It was proposed that this patient might be homozygous for Hurler's disease but might have an additional heterozygous genetic defect, perhaps related metabolically.

Foley and coworkers [413] have reported the use of white blood cell cultures for the study of metachromasia. Following the separation of leukocytes by the dextran procedure, metachromasia observed after 3 days in culture persisted for up to 14 days. The cells appeared to be pleomorphic. Metachromasia was found in the cultures derived from patients with Hurler's disease, heterozygous mothers and fathers, a patient with Sanfilippo's disease, patients with Hunter's disease, and in heterozygous mothers of patients with Hunter's disease but not in fathers of patients with Hunter's disease or controls. After 14 days in culture, metachromasia disappeared from cultures derived from heterozygotes but not from cultures derived from homozygotes. This phenomenon was interpreted as reflecting a difference in gene dosage in heterozygotes and homozygotes. Danes [414] has reported metachromasia in cultured leukocytes in the Scheie syndrome, generalized gangliosidosis, and cystic fibrosis. Metachromasia was not found in leukocytes cultured from patients with Gaucher's disease and Marfan's syndrome, although fibroblast cultures were positive.

Danes et al. [415] have applied leukocyte cultures to the study of the genetics of cystic fibrosis. Again, no metachromasia was observed in normal controls but, in cultures derived from 17 affected individuals, metachromasia developed on the fourth day in culture and reached a maximum within 7 to 10 days. In cultures derived from nine affected individuals, the metachromasia was vesicular, whereas the cells derived from eight other affected individuals showed diffuse metachromasia. After 10 days in culture the cytoplasmic metachromasia was significantly reduced, and in many cultures it had disappeared after 14 days. All cultures were ametachromatic by 29 days. Leukocyte cultures established from the heterozygous parents of all 17 affected patients showed the same class of metachromasia as observed in the cultures of their affected offspring. Cultures derived from three other affected individuals, as well as their parents, showed no metachromasia. On the basis of the three different kinds of cells observed in cultures, vesicular metachromasia, diffuse metachromasia, and no metachromasia, these authors propose the existence of three different, perhaps allelic, types of cystic fibrosis.

In another report, Danes and Bearn [416] have indicated a variation of metachromasia both qualitatively and quantitatively in fibroblast cultures. In the course of a study of 16 affected families, 2 were found whose fibroblasts showed vesicular metachromasia, but only a few vesicles per cell were found. These were designated as Class IA. Two other families were found with cells exhibiting many vesicles per cell and were designated as Class IB. By contrast, in 12 families more extensive vesicular granular cytoplasm was observed. This type was designated as Class II. Cultures derived from parents and other family members showed the same type of metachromasia as the respective probands. Fibroblasts derived from patients with the Class II disease showed a marked increase in intracellular acid mucopolysaccharide content. Incorporation of acetate-^{3}H and $^{35}SO_4$ into mucopolysaccharides was normal in the Class I disease but much elevated in the Class II disease. The mucopolysaccharides isolated were not identified, nor was their purity established.

Subsequently, Danes and Bearn [417] have reported that the major increase in mucopolysaccharides produced by fibroblasts derived from patients with cystic fibrosis (Class II) was due to an increase in the mucopolysaccharides in the medium, although the published data do show an increase in intracellular mucopolysaccharides. No attempt was made to identify the mucopolysaccharides chemically. The data in this paper are not entirely consistent with other publications from the same laboratory. Wiesmann and Neufeld [418] studied the metabolism of sulfated mucopolysaccharides in fibroblasts of cystic fibrosis patients, utilizing $^{35}SO_4$. They found only a small increase in intracellular accumulation or excretion of labeled polysaccharide. Matalon and Dorfman [419] were unable to detect the large increase in extracellular mucopolysaccharides reported by Danes and Bearn. The studies reported by Matalon and Dorfman [420] indicated that cystic fibrosis cells accumulated mucopolysaccharides which were similar in qualitative distribution to normal cells and consisted primarily of hyaluronic acid. Thus, the lack of marked changes in metabolism observed by Wiesmann and Neufeld is not surprising, since $^{35}SO_4$ was used in those studies. It is difficult at present to interpret the large increase in extracellular mucopolysaccharides reported by Danes and Bearn.

The significance of metachromasia in cultured fibroblasts has been questioned by Taysi et al. [421]. Fibroblast cultures from 91 patients were examined for metachromasia. As in previous reports, metachromasia was demonstrated in all homozygotes and heterozygotes of mucopolysaccharidoses and cystic fibrosis. In a control population consisting of hospitalized patients studied in a cytogenics laboratory for the presence of genetic metabolic defects or suspected chromosomal abnormalities, 27 percent of cultures exhibited metachromasia. The control group included patients with spondylepiphyseal dysplasia and idiopathic central nervous system degeneration. The high incidence of metachromasia in this group compared to the 6 to 8 percent found in normal controls by both Dorfman and Matalon and Danes and Bearn is difficult to explain [422]. It is not clear whether this discrepancy is due to technical difficulties or the rather selective population studied.

Considerable confusion exists in the literature concerning the extent of metachromasia in fibroblasts derived from patients with Morquio's syndrome. Following the original report by Fraccaro et al. [423], conflicting reports of findings have appeared. Most of these have centered on the clinical definition of this entity. Danes and Bearn [424] suggested that metachromasia occurs only in those patients with extraskeletal involvement, a criteria for diagnosis which has been challenged by Romano and Sietti [425] in view of the late appearance of extraskeletal findings in some patients. Durand and associates [426] reported the presence of metachromasia with the presumed accumulation of dermatan sulfate in a patient with Morquio's disease who excreted dermatan sulfate. This patient had many of the extraskeletal findings typical of Hurler's disease. As already indicated, Danes and Grossman [284] have attempted unsuccessfully to correlate the metachromasia and polysaccharide content of cultured fibroblasts with the x-ray appearance in a variety of patients with bone dysplasia.

It is apparent that there still exists confusion regarding

fibroblast abnormalities in the epiphyseal dysplasias. The finding of high hexose (presumably in macromolecules) by Danes and Grossman is of some interest and should point out a need for further identification of this material. As noted elsewhere in this chapter, keratan sulfate is excreted in the urine of patients with Morquio's disease, but this material has not been found in the fibroblasts of these patients by Matalon and Dorfman [2]. This is not remarkable, in view of the fact that keratan sulfate is probably synthesized by chondrocytes and corneal stromal cells rather than by skin fibroblasts.

In view of the diversity of results on metachromasia, some comment on the technique is indicated. Various investigators have employed different methods of growth, staining, and fixation. Plate II–5 illustrates normal and Hurler fibroblasts after 4 days of growth following five transfers. Cells for staining were grown on glass cover slips for 4 to 7 days. After removal from the medium the cover slips were rinsed in Earle's balanced salt solution, air-dried, and fixed in a tetrahydrofuran/acetone ratio of 1:1 for 5 min. The cover slips were then stained with 0.5 percent toluidine blue O (Fisher Scientific Co.) in 30 percent acetone. Staining varies from 30 to 60 sec, depending upon the density of cells on the cover slip. Following staining, the cover slips were dipped successively in 30 and 100 percent acetone and mounted with Permount.

In the course of our own studies, little difference was found in the metachromasia in early transfer or late transfer cells. This has been confirmed by electron microscope studies of such cells which show the marked accumulation of vacuoles in Hurler's fibroblasts irrespective of the number of transfers.

Danes and Bearn [407] noted that the culture of Hurler's fibroblasts in human serum prevented the appearance of metachromasia. Hors-Cayla et al. [427] showed that the addition of human serum to Hurler's cells previously cultured in fetal calf serum results in the disappearance of metachromasia. The disappearance of intracellular metachromasia was accompanied by an increase of mucopolysaccharide in the medium. This finding is of interest in view of the experiments of Neufeld and Fratantoni [428] described later. The discovery by these workers of the normalization of mucopolysaccharide metabolism in Hurler's fibroblasts by culture in the presence of other fibroblasts may explain the early observations of Danes and Bearn and Hors-Cayla et al.

The reports on tissue culture reviewed above indicate that the application of this technique has opened new vistas for the study of mucopolysaccharidoses, as well as for other genetic diseases.

GENETICS AND INCIDENCE

There are no adequate data for the determination of the frequency of the mucopolysaccharidoses. In 1957 Lamy et al. [433] collected 269 cases from the literature. Since the discovery of the role of acid mucopolysaccharides and the application of tissue culture techniques in these diseases, the number of reported cases has increased rapidly.

Hurler's disease is widely distributed in different racial groups, including American Negroes [434], Chinese [435], Oriental Indians [436], and Japanese [437]. Adequate data are not available for determining the relative racial frequency.

In 1942 Halpern and Curtis [438] examined the family history of 57 patients representing 40 sibships. They found 32 affected males and 25 affected females, a difference which they did not consider significant. They concluded that the Hurler syndrome is inherited as an autosomal recessive disease. A more complete survey was carried out by Jervis [396] in 1950 on 103 families. Eighty-four sibships were analyzed and corrected by the method of Lenz and Bernstein. The data were consistent with a single autosomal form of inheritance. No attempt was made to assess the possibility that the sample was not homogeneous. Jervis noted the high rate of consanguinity of his sample; the parents were cousins in at least 11 of the 103 families; histories were considered inadequate in 52 families. On the basis of Hogben's formula he estimated a gene frequency of 1:40,000, a figure derived from a 10 percent incidence of cousin marriages. Jervis commented upon the rarity of the disease in uncles and aunts, but more recent studies showed a significant incidence in uncles in X-linked groups of cases.

Better understanding of the genetics of this syndrome has come with the recognition of an X-linked form of the disease. Njå [252] described a family with five definitely affected individuals in two generations. All were males, and the genealogy was consistent with transmission through a female carrier. He observed that none of the affected males had corneal opacities and, accordingly, suggested the existence of a special genetic form of gargoylism linked to the X chromosome which occurs in males and is transmitted through females. Since this report, a number of other genealogies have been published which are consistent with this hypothesis. Beebe and Formel [255] have described nine cases in four generations of a family of Dutch extraction which has resided in the Catskill Mountains ouside Albany, New York, for about 250 years. Of 19 males, 9 were affected, while none of the 16 female sibs was affected. Figure 49-22 shows the genealogy of this family. Several members of this family have been studied by the author, and all the surviving affected males were found to excrete acid mucopolysaccharides.

Herndon et al., as quoted by Neel [439], have attempted to study the incidence of the two types of the disease and to correlate the phenotype with the mode of inheritance. In 246 cases from the literature, they found 167 males and 79 females. They confirmed Njå's impression that corneal clouding is characteristic of the autosomal recessive form and added the suggestion that deafness is more common in the X-linked form.

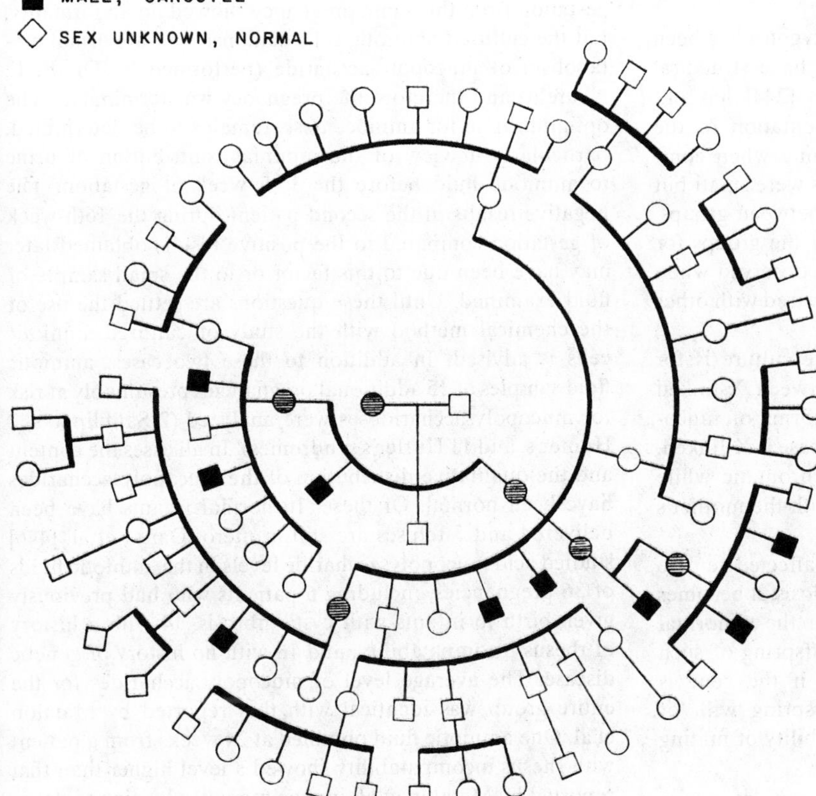

Figure 49-22. Genealogy of a family with the X-linked type of the Hurler syndrome. (*Taken from Beebe and Formel* [255].)

Lamy et al. [433] have made a most detailed and careful study of 269 cases. The first group of families consisted of those with at least one female case. In 47 families, 24 of which contained 1 or more affected individuals, other than the propositus, there were 119 children after elimination of the propositi. Of this group, 29 were affected (24.3 percent). In cases in which the sex of the sibships was completely known, 13 of 39 brothers and 9 of 27 sisters were affected. When one adds the families in which the sex in the sibship was not always known, the total number of affected males was 16 while the females numbered 13. Among the families which contained female patients, consanguinity was present in 16 of the 49 families in which adequate information was available.

It was concluded that the population of male patients could be divided into three groups, those belonging to: (1) sibships containing affected females, (2) families which contained no affected females but in which the type of inheritance could not be ascertained on the basis of the available information, and (3) families clearly displaying X linkage. When clinical symptoms in the two forms of the disease were analyzed, the autosomal recessive form was found to be characterized by greater frequency of corneal opacities, more severe dwarfing, and a more rapid evolution of the disease. In males with the X-linked form of the disease, corneal opacities were absent, but deafness was more common.

The study of Lamy et al. [433] considered the problem of the evolution of the disease in the two types. Adequate control analyses were included to show that the differences in manifestations were not due to differences in age of the two samples.

On the basis of the incidence of corneal opacities in the autosomal recessive type, the preponderance of males and the incidence of affected sisters of male cases, Lamy et al. [433] estimated that 31.4 $\pm$ 6.8 percent of male patients are of the X-linked type. Since this estimate appears high in view of the published genealogies, it was concluded that a significant number of patients of the X-linked type are new mutations.

McKusick [482] has recently indicated that the incidence of Hunter's disease is greater than that of Hurler's disease.

Berg et al. [440] found that the locus for Hunter's syndrome was close to the locus for $Xm_{(a)}$ serum antigen, with a recombination fraction of 0.09.

The Hurler syndrome has been described in identical twin

sisters [441] and in a twin brother and sister [217], while discordance has been described in twins who were presumably dizygotic [442]. The chromosome number and morphology have been described as normal by Gayler and Fried [443].

The problem of manifestations in heterozygotes has been examined by several investigators. In none have structural abnormalities been documented. Mittwoch [244] has observed increased polymorphonuclear segmentation in the parents of patients with the Hurler syndrome when compared to normal individuals. The differences were small but significant; however, there was an overlap between groups. No evidence is given for rigorous control of the groups for other variables. A similar difference was not observed when patients with the Hurler syndrome were compared with other mentally retarded children.

A particularly useful application of tissue culture is for genetic counseling when the distinction between X-linked Hunter's disease and autosomal recessive forms of mucopolysaccharidoses is necessary. When the disease is X-linked, some of the mother's fibroblasts are metachromatic while when it is an autosomal recessive disease, both the mother's and father's fibroblasts are metachromatic.

When metachromasia is present in a nonaffected female sib of a male patient with mucopolysaccharidosis, it becomes particularly important to determine whether the abnormal genes are X-linked. One half of the male offspring of such a carrier may be expected to be affected if the gene is X-linked, while if autosomal, affected offspring will, of course, be expected only in the remote possibility of mating with another carrier.

AMNIOCENTESIS

The development of the technique of amniocentesis has resulted in an interest in the prenatal diagnosis of mucopolysaccharidoses. Fratantoni et al. [444] reported the intrauterine diagnosis of a case of Hurler's disease and one of Hunter's disease. Diagnosis was accomplished on the basis of increased intracellular uptake of radioactive sulfate by cells cultured from the amniotic fluid. Matalon et al. [445] have reported the intrauterine diagnosis of a case of Hurler's disease by the direct determination of acid mucopolysaccharides in amniotic fluid obtained at the fourteenth week of pregnancy. The mucopolysaccharide content of fluid obtained from a pregnancy leading to the delivery of an afflicted infant contained approximately four times as much mucopolysaccharides as the average of normal fluids. More striking was the direct demonstration of the presence of heparan sulfate in the Hurler amniotic fluid in contrast to the complete absence of this mucopolysaccharide in normal fluids.

Another sample of amniotic fluid, obtained during abortion at 22 weeks of gestation, contained abnormal quantities of sulfated polysaccharides including dermatan and heparan sulfates [483]. In the liver of the aborted fetus large amounts of dermatan sulfate and heparan sulfate were found, in contrast to their absence in an unaffected fetus. A 2.0 ml sample of amniotic fluid obtained during the 16th week of gestation from this same pregnancy showed no abnormality, but the cultured amniotic cells demonstrated abnormal metabolism of mucopolysaccharide (performed by Dr. E. F. Neufeld) and therefore the pregnancy was terminated. The optimum time for amniocentesis remains to be determined, particularly in view of the minimal contribution of urine to amniotic fluid before the 16th week of gestation. The negative results in the second patient during the 16th week of gestation compared to the positive results obtained later may have been due to this factor or to the small sample of fluid examined. Until these questions are settled the use of the chemical method with the study of cultured amniotic cells is advised. In addition to these two cases, amniotic fluid samples of 15 additional pregnancies presumably at risk for mucopolysaccharidoses were analyzed (2 Sanfilippo's, 2 Hunter's, and 11 Hurler's syndromes). In all cases the content and the qualitative distribution of the mucopolysaccharides have been normal. Of these, 10 normal infants have been delivered and 5 fetuses are still in utero. Danes et al. [446] studied acid mucopolysaccharide levels in the amniotic fluids of 36 pregnancies, including 6 patients who had previously given birth to infants with cystic fibrosis, 14 with a history of rhesus incompatability, and 16 with no history of genetic disease. The average level of mucopolysaccharides for the entire group was identical with that reported by Matalon et al. One amniotic fluid obtained at 24 weeks from a patient with rhesus incompatability showed a level higher than that reported by Matalon et al. in the pregnancy leading to delivery of an infant with Hurler's disease. Danes et al [446] also showed that the level of acid mucopolysaccharides in amniotic fluid declined with progression of the pregnancy.

THE PATHOGENESIS OF THE MUCOPOLYSACCHARIDOSES

Understanding of the mucopolysaccharidoses requires, as in all genetic diseases, identification of the defective gene products. This has not yet been achieved for any of the mucopolysaccharidoses. Many important recent investigations suggest that this objective will soon be met.

Although many details of our understanding need further investigation, it is clear that the pathological features of these diseases stem from the intracellular deposition of mucopolysaccharides in a number of tissues of the body. An explanation of the pathogenesis must, therefore, cope with the fundamental cause of the intracellular accumulation of mucopolysaccharides. In considering this problem, one troublesome question which has been frequently disregarded needs to be emphasized. Pathological studies show the accumulation of mucopolysaccharides in cells which are not ordinarily involved in the synthesis of connective tissue matrix. To account for such widespread storage, one of the following mechanisms must obtain: (1) accumulation of mucopolysaccharides in certain tissues (e.g., liver, spleen) results from the ingestion by pinocytosis of polysaccharides produced elsewhere, (2) such cells synthesize acid mucopolysaccharides in abnormal amounts in these diseases, or (3) such cells manufacture acid mucopolysaccharides which are normally degraded. The finding by Olsson [447] of the synthesis by leukocytes of chondroitin sulfate and of the synthesis by glial cells of hyaluronic acid, chondroitin sulfate, and heparan sulfate [51] indicates that synthesis of acid mucopolysaccharide may not be confined to connective tissue cells as previously suspected.

The acid mucopolysaccharides stored in the liver and spleen and excreted in the urine in Hurler's and Sanfilippo's disease are partially degraded [65]. In the case of dermatan sulfate, the products isolated appear to result from degradation by the combined action of hyaluronidase, β-glucuronidase, and proteolytic enzymes. In contrast, the dermatan sulfate isolated from cultured fibroblasts appears to consist of intact polysaccharide chains. The extent of degradation of the protein core is not clear, but the studies of Fratantoni, Hall, and Neufeld [448] suggest that the molecular size of the material deposited intracellularly is smaller than that secreted by the fibroblasts.

Since cultured fibroblasts definitely demonstrate an abnormality in the metabolism of dermatan sulfate, metabolic studies on fibroblasts may most readily lead to elucidation of the pathogenesis.

Acid mucopolysaccharide–protein complexes are synthesized by a series of reactions which starts with the synthesis of the protein core at the rough endoplasmic reticulum and is followed by the stepwise addition of the appropriate sugars and sulfate groups. The molecule is probably completed in the smooth membranes of the Golgi apparatus. Following completion of the molecule, it seems likely that the product is "packaged" in excretion vacuoles which make their way to the cell surface for discharge of the protein–polysaccharide to the extracellular matrix. Matalon and Dorfman [404] showed that in Hurler's fibroblasts there was a marked accumulation of intracellular polysaccharide, even though the cells were secreting as much or more polysaccharide into the medium as normal fibroblasts. These studies were interpreted as indicating excessive synthesis or a defect in the secretion mechanism. This possibility contrasted with the suggesion by Van Hoof and Hers [226] that Hurler's disease is really a storage disease which results from the absence of a degradative enzyme. Their conclusions were based on the demonstration that mucopolysaccharides are stored in lysosomal structures. The earler suggestion by Dorfman [31] that Hurler's syndrome might result from the defective binding of polysaccharides to protein became untenable when Matalon and Dorfman [79] showed that mucopolysaccharide synthesis is inhibited by puromycin and cycloheximide in Hurler fibroblasts as in normal fibroblasts.

On the basis of kinetic studies, Fratantoni et al. [448] concluded that the accumulation of dermatan sulfate in Hurler and Hunter fibroblasts results from faulty degradation. In order to explain their observations, the existence of two pools of mucopolysaccharides in fibroblasts was suggested. The first pool turns over rapidly and represents about two-thirds of the mucopolysaccharide synthesized. This material is presumably a high-molecular-weight protein-polysaccharide complex secreted from the fibroblast to make an extracellular matrix. A second pool representing approximately one-third of the polysaccharide synthesized remains within the cell and is degraded. This may also contain material which is reingested from the medium. A defect in degradation of this pool was suggested by Fratantoni et al. as the cause of Hurler's and Hunter's disease. The data presented by these investigators indicate that intracellular mucopolysaccharide is degraded in a manner which releases dialyzable sulfate. Since the experiments were carried out with $^{35}SO_4$, it was not possible to determine whether the polysaccharide chain was degraded. The authors [296] showed that dermatan $^{35}SO_4$ was desulfated when exposed to either normal or Hurler fibroblast cultures.

Fratantoni et al. [448] showed a difference in the rate of the disappearance of radioactivity from intracellular $^{35}SO_4$-labeled polysaccharide among Hurler, Hunter, and normal cells. The differences are significant when plotted on the basis of the percentage of radioactivity disappearing from Hurler and Hunter cells. Assuming that the rate of degradation is dependent on pool size, Hurler and Hunter cells degrade polysaccharide less efficiently than do normal cells. No complete block in degradation exists since the absolute amounts of radioactivity which disappear are about the same for Hurler, Hunter, and normal cells.

Final acceptance of a defect of degradation has been hampered by the lack of definition of the missing or defective degradative enzyme, as well as by incomplete understanding of the pathways of degradation of the polysaccharides involved. Recently, attention has been focused on β-galactosidase. Öckerman [449] reported a decrease in β-galactosidase in the skin of patients with Hurler's disease while Gerich [450] found 25 and 33 percent of normal β-galactosidase activity in the skin homogenates of two sibs with Hunter's syndrome. The skin of the mother of one patient exhibited 54 percent of the normal value.

An attempt to study the kinetics of polysaccharide turnover in vivo has been made by Bartsocas and Moser [451]. After injection of $^{35}SO_4$, the ratio of disappearance of labeled polysaccharides from urine was much slower in Hurler's patients than in normals, but in twins with the Sanfilippo syndrome no such decrease in turnover rate was observed. In one patient with combined sulfatide and mucopolysaccharide storage, who showed a deficiency of arylsulfatases A, B, and C, the most prolonged excretion of radioactive mucopolysaccharides occurred.

Using 13 different substrates Van Hoof and Hers [299] have studied the hydrolase activities with tissue extracts of normal subjects and 32 different patients with Hurler's disease and related syndromes. In 14 patients thought to have Hurler's, Hunter's, or Sanfilippo's disease, a marked decrease in liver β-galactosidase measured at pH 3.6 was observed, whereas at a higher pH no difference in activity was found. Decreases of β-galactosidase activity were also observed in extracts of skin and brain but not in extracts of kidney, spleen, lung, and leukocytes of some patients. The livers of the same 14 patients showed a large increase in the activity of β-N-acetylglucosaminidase, β-N-acetylgalactosaminidase, α-fucosidase, and β-glucuronidase. The activities of α-glucosidase, cathepsin, and acid phosphatase were also above normal, whereas α-galactosidase, β-glucosidase, α-mannosidase, and β-xylosidase activities were normal.

Somewhat similar studies have been reported by Öckerman [452] who studied six hydrolases in the livers of six patients. Three of these patients were thought to be afflcted with Hurler's disease whereas two others were thought to represent Hunter's syndrome. Again, a marked decrease in acid β-galactosidase was observed, while β-glucuronidase, β-N-acetylglucosaminidase, acid phosphatase, and α-fucosidase were significantly increased in some of the specimens. The activity of α-mannosidase was not significantly different from that of normal specimens.

Austin et al. [453] have also studied hydrolases in autopsy material from two patients with Hurler's disease and urine from five other patients. In the liver, the mean arylsulfatase B activity was normal but was much elevated in white matter, cortex, and kidney. Activity of arylsulfatase A, acid phosphatase, and α-galactosidase were normal or in the low normal range in the tissues of the patients with Hurler's disease. Van Gemund et al. [454] similarly found a decrease in the β-galactosidase of seven patients with Hurler's and Hunter's disease. No abnormality of β-glucuronidase levels was found, but acid phosphatase was elevated.

Öckerman and associates [455] in a more detailed study of β-galactosidases, using 4-methylumbelliferyl substrates, found evidence in the liver of two β-galactosidases on gel filtration, an enzyme A with an apparent molecular weight of 85,000, and an enzyme B with an apparent molecular weight of 45,000. Enzyme A activity was decreased in liver, kidney, and spleen extracts of Hurler's and Hunter's patients, but the levels of enzyme A were normal or increased in urine and plasma.

MacBrinn et al [456] found a deficiency of β-galactosidase (pH 5.0) in extracts of autopsy samples of brain, liver, kidney, and spleen from 10 patients with Hurler's, Hunter's, and Sanfilippo's diseases. The diminished activity of the enzyme was demonstrated with nitrophenyl-β-galactosides, G_{M1}-ganglioside, and the keratan sulfate-like material of G_{M1}-gangliosidosis as substrates. Other lysosomal enzymes were normal or increased.

Thomas [457] found low levels of β-galactosidase in the urine of patients with mucopolysaccharidoses, but the activity was higher than that found in G_{M1}-gangliosidosis.

Upon more detailed comparison of the β-galactosidases of tissues from patients with Hurler's, Hunter's, and Sanfilippo's diseases with those from normal subjects, differences in temperature optima, pH optima, and heat stability were found by Ho and O'Brien [458]. Starch-gel electrophoresis revealed that control livers contained three separable β-galactosidase components with activity at pH 4 to 5. A marked deficiency of the slow-moving β-galactosidase components was observed in liver tissues from the three types of mucopolysaccharidoses. In normal kidney four β-galactosidase components were found, two of which were slow moving. In the patients with Hurler's disease both slow-moving components were markedly deficient, but the degree of deficiency was not as great as in the liver, except in the patient with Sanfilippo's disease.

The situation with regard to β-galactosidase is further complicated by the finding by Matalon and Dorfman [459] that although Hurler fibroblasts showed somewhat lower levels of β-galactosidase than normal fibroblasts, absence of a specific band on starch-gel electrophoresis was not apparent. Furthermore, the addition of heparan sulfate inhibits β-galactosidase, but this inhibition is prevented by the presence of chloride ion, which appears to prevent enzyme inactivation.

Benson et al. [484] found no qualitative or quantitative deficiency of β-galactosidase in cultured skin fibroblasts of patients with Hurler's or Sanfilippo's disease. Fluharty et al. [485] found a 50 percent increase in β-galactosidase levels in skin fibroblasts of Hurler's, Hunter's, and Sanfilippo's patients but could find no absence of any of the forms of β-galactosidase present in fibroblasts cultured from normal individuals. A study of β-galactosidase of leukocytes by Singer and Schafer [486] revealed no qualitative or quantitative differences between normal and Hurler's cells or cells derived from Hurler's heterozygotes. The expected low levels in leukocytes from patients with G_{M1} gangliosidosis were demonstrated. Gordon and Feleki [487] found that the level of serum β-galactosidase, β-glucuronidase, hyaluronidase, and arylsulfatase A decreases as the child's age increases, but that serum acid phosphatase increases with advancing age. Compared with age-matched controls there was no significant decrease in serum β-galactosidase activity in either Hurler's or Sanfilippo's disease. Although low β-galactosidase levels were found in liver of patients with Hurler's and Sanfilippo's disease, as compared to normal, the changes were not statistically significant. Patel et al. [488] found a decreased activity of hyaluronidase in livers of patients with Hurler's, Hunter's, and Sanfilippo's disease and a decrease in sulfatase activity measured at pH 5.6 in Hurler's disease.

That defective degradation underlies the pathogenesis of mucopolysaccharidoses has received further support from the studies on the interaction of cultured fibroblasts. Fratantoni and coworkers [460] observed that growth of Hunter or Hurler fibroblasts in the presence of normal fibroblasts results in the disappearance of metachromasia and the correction of the metabolic defect as measured by the uptake or disappearance of radioactive sulfate. Correction could also be achieved in mixed cultures of Hurler and Hunter syndromes [461]. Addition of the appropriate factor to either Hunter or Hurler cells results in the restoration of the kinetics of mucopolysaccharide turnover toward normal in both Hunter and Hurler fibroblasts. The disappearance of accumulated intracellular mucopolysaccharide resulting from treatment with the corrective factor is accompanied by a concomitant increase in extracellular dialyzable radioactivity. This finding suggests that the corrective factor promotes degradation. These observations have been confirmed in the authors' laboratory.

Neufeld and Cantz [462] found that certain patients with Sanfilippo's disease cross correct each other. The Sanfilippo's patients were found to fall into two groups, each presumably lacking a different factor required for normal mucopolysaccharide metabolism. In contrast Wiesmann and Neufeld [270] found no cross correction between Scheie's and Hurler's fibroblasts. In view of the clinical differences between these two syndromes, the finding indicating that they have the same biochemical defect is somewhat surprising. A possible explanation is that these two diseases involve different allelic mutations which would not be expected to produce cross correction.

Neufeld and Cantz [462] also indicated that correction of "I-cell" disease required both the Hurler and Hunter factors. Danes et al. [250] has recently indicated that the situation may be even more complex, since they have observed cross correction by the different groups of Hurler's patients and Hunter's patients. Thus each of these syndromes may be composed of several different variants. These studies were confined to observations of metachromasia.

The nature of the corrective factors is not yet determined. Neufeld and Cantz [462] found the factors in homogenates of newborn mouse skin and bovine sclera. Corrective factors for Hurler, Hunter, and Sanfilippo fibroblasts were found in normal human urine. The urine factors were phenotypically specific: a preparation from the urine of a 6-year-old Hunter patient corrected Hurler and Sanfilippo fibroblasts but contained only one-sixth the normal activity toward Hunter fibroblasts. In a second Hunter patient, the amount of Hunter factor was only 5 percent of that present in normal urine. In the case of one Hurler patient, much diminished activity (less than 25 percent) of the Hurler factor was found, while in the urine of a Sanfilippo patient, one of the two Sanfilippo factors was present but the other three factors were at the normal level.

Wiesmann and Neufeld [489] found that fibroblasts from Scheie's and Hurler's disease appear to require the same specific factor for their correction. These findings suggest that the two diseases may be allelic.

Using analytic polyacrylamide electrophoresis, Cantz et al. [463] have concluded that the Hunter factor is a protein of molecular weight 65,000. It is unstable above pH 8.0. It has been suggested that this factor is the "missing enzyme" although no enzymic activity has so far been demonstrated for any of the factors.

The recent discovery of L-iduronidase [474, 475] raises the possibility that absence or diminution of the activity of this enzyme may play an important role in the pathogenesis of the mucopolysaccharidoses. Whether the corrective factors demonstrate L-iduronidase activity remains to be determined.

TREATMENT

Methods of treatment suggested in the earlier literature are without theoretical justification or practical efficacy. The demonstration that large doses of adrenocortical hormones inhibit the synthesis of acid mucopolysaccharides [141] suggested that these compounds might be beneficial in the Hurler syndrome. A decrease in mucopolysaccharide excretion following such therapy was mentioned by Meyer et al. [328] while a claim of both decreased excretion and some clinical benefit has been made by Wolfson et al. [464]. Schuffler and Rosenthal [465] found an initial decrease after the institution of large doses of prednisone, following which there was an irregular decrease of mucopolysaccharide excretion. Similar results have been reported by Usui and associates [372]. They also observed a decrease in the ratio of dermatan sulfate to heparan sulfate with treatment of a patient with Hurler's syndrome. Renuart [466] treated one patient with high doses of steroids. Postmortem urine was said to have a low level of mucopolysaccharides but a large amount of lipids.

Nanivadekar and Nanivadekar [467] claimed clearing of corneal clouding in Hurler's syndrome following treatment with the anabolic steroid, nandrolone. Rennert and Dekaban [468] indicated a decreased excretion of acid mucopolysaccharides during treatment with glucosteroids but an increased excretion while receiving hydroxychloroquine. There were also indications of a change in dermatan sulfate/heparan sulfate ratios during the administration of thyroid and glucosteroids, but not with chloroquine, salicytes, or growth hormone.

Another approach to therapy stemmed from the observation of Danes and Bearn [469] that the addition of retinol (vitamin A alcohol) to cultures of Hurler's fibroblasts diminished metachromasia and decreased intracellular uronic acid content. The same investigators [470] reported an increase in urinary mucopolysaccharide excretion when 20 times the daily requirement of vitamin A was administered to seven patients with Hurler or Hunter syndromes [470]. No information was given regarding clinical changes in the patients.

Madsen and Linker [471] studied the effect of 4,000 units of vitamin A per kg per day on seven patients, comprising two with Hurler's disease, one with Hunter's disease, two with Sanfilippo's disease, and two with Morquio-Brailsford's disease. They concluded that (1) there are wide variations in the quantity of mucopolysaccharides excreted by individual patients, (2) the effect of vitamin A on mucopolysaccharide excretion is not uniform even among patients with the same syndrome, (3) vitamin A has no beneficial effect on the course of the clinical progression of these syndromes, and (4) vitamin A, in fact, may potentiate the effects of disordered mucopolysaccharide metabolism in these patients. A more limited experience in the authors' laboratory showed no beneficial effect from vitamin A therapy. No change in urinary mucopolysaccharides was found by Renuart [466] after treatment with large doses of vitamin A.

Gordon and Thursby-Pelham [472] report possible but not conclusive improvement of two patients with Sanfilippo's syndrome treated with large doses of vitamin A.

Schafer et al. [405] reported that the accumulation of dermatan sulfate in cultured Hurler's fibroblasts is dependent on the presence of ascorbic acid in the culture medium. On this basis, DeJong et al. [473] attempted to treat Hurler's disease with an ascorbic acid–free diet and concluded that patients with Hurler's disease were unusually resistant to the development of scurvy.

DiFerrante et al. [490] reported a decrease in excretion of large molecular weight glycosaminoglycans and an increased excretion of their degradative products following infusion of normal plasma. On treatment of two Hurler's and five Hunter's patients a marked decrease in hyperactive behavior was observed. It was claimed that the skin which was thick and cold before plasma infusion became soft and warm after the infusion. A dramatic improvement in the "claw hands" of the Hurler's patients was described. One month after treatment the patients' behavior returned abruptly to that observed before treatment.

SUMMARY

A simple summation of the available information regarding the pathogenesis of the mucopolysaccharidoses is difficult. Perhaps this can best be approached by the following listing of pertinent facts which require explanation in any final understanding of the problems of the mucopolysaccharidoses:

1 There are a number of heritable diseases which are characterized by the storage of dermatan sulfate and heparan sulfate. Available evidence indicates that at least Hurler's disease, Hunter's disease, Sanfilippo's disease, Scheie's disease, Maroteaux-Lamy disease, "I-cell" disease, and the lipomucopolysaccharidoses of Spranger and Weidemann (Gal + disease of Van Hoof and Hers) are all distinct syndromes. It has been proposed that there are two distinct Sanfilippo's genotypes, two distinct Hurler genotypes, and three distinct Hunter genotypes. It is possible that Scheie's disease and Hurler's disease are allelic.

Evidence for the existence of different corrective factors for Hurler's, Hunter's, and Sanfilippo's variants indicate that these are not allelic. That Hunter's disease is not allelic with any of the other diseases is clear from the chromosomal pattern: it is an X-linked disease while all of the others seem to be autosomal.

2 Morquio's disease appears to be phenotypically, genetically, and chemically distinct and probably involves a defect in the metabolism of the mucopolysaccharides of cartilage.

3 Marfan's syndrome is phenotypically, genetically, and chemically distinct. The relationship of the accumulation of hyaluronic acid in fibroblasts to the phenotypic expression of the disease is unclear.

4 The accumulation of mucopolysaccharides in fibroblast cultures in a variety of other syndromes, including lipid storage diseases and cystic fibrosis, does not seem to involve specific interference with the metabolism of dermatan sulfate and heparan sulfate. The mechanism or significance of this accumulation is unknown.

5 β-Galactosidase activity is decreased in the tissues of patients with Hurler, Hunter, and Sanfilippo diseases, and there is an absence of specific fractions of β-galactosidase in certain tissues. In cultured Hurler fibroblasts, although the level of β-galactosidase is depressed, the electrophoretic pattern is normal. Since β-galactoside linkages occur only internally in heparan sulfate and dermatan sulfate, β-galactosidase can only be expected to be involved in the degradation of these polysaccharides if it acts as an endogalactosidase or in the final degradation of the linkage region after removal of the distal portion of the polysaccharide chain. Furthermore, it seems unlikely that β-galactosidase (as measured with artificial substrates) is critical in dermatan sulfate and heparan sulfate accumulation, because these polysaccharides do not accumulate in G_{M1}-gangliosidosis (which is characterized by the complete absence of β-galactosidase).

6 Of the enzymes expected to participate in the degradation of mucopolysaccharides, hyaluronidase, β-glucuronidase, β-N-acetylhexosaminidase, and sulfatases appear to be present in the tissues of at least certain of the mucopolysaccharidoses. Whether the β-N-acetylhexosaminidase measured with artificial substrates and absent in one form of Tay-Sachs disease is critical in mucopolysaccharide degradation is indefinite in view of the lack of accumulation of mucopolysaccharides in either type of Tay-Sachs disease.

7 Dermatan sulfate and heparan sulfate both contain L-iduronic acid. An enzyme responsible for the hydrolysis of L-iduronosidic linkages which has recently been described might well be critical in the metabolism of these two polysaccharides. Since skin fibroblasts do not contain hyaluronidase, degradation of the dermatan sulfate molecule in the cells may require the alternate removal of N-acetylgalactosamine residues and L-iduronic acid residues. In the liver, which contains hyaluronidase, the dermatan sulfate would be degraded to oligosaccharides with further degradation impaired by the absence of L-iduronidase. This interpretation would account for the difference in the molecular size of dermatan sulfate found in the liver, spleen, and urine and that which accumulates in cultured fibroblasts of Hurler's patients.

8 An explanation is required for the accumulation of gangliosides in Hurler's syndrome. The simplest explanation would be the lack of an enzyme which acts on both mucopolysaccharides and the gangliosides. The observed low level of β-galactosidase might be of importance in this respect, but acceptance of this as the primary defect is difficult. It is possible that the accumulation of gangliosides is secondary to the inhibition of their degradation by mucopolysaccharides present in the tissues.

9 The available evidence suggests that faulty degradation is the most likely explanation of the mucopolysaccharidoses. It should be emphasized that many of the arguments would be equally valid if there were some error in the secretion process coupled with limited degradation of dermatan sulfate and heparan sulfate. A final decision can only be made when a specific enzyme defect is demonstrated.

10 No satisfactory treatment of the mucopolysaccharidoses has so far been discovered. The recent report of the beneficial effect of plasma infusion is of great interest.

BIBLIOGRAPHY

1. Brante, G.: Gargoylism: A mucopolysaccharidosis. Scand. J. Clin. Lab. Invest., **4,** 43, 1952.
2. Matalon, R., and Dorfman, A.: Acid mucopolysaccharides in cultured human fibroblasts. Lancet, **2,** 838, 1969.
3. McKusick, V. A.: *Heritable Disorders of Connective Tissue,* 3d ed. Mosby, St. Louis, 1966.
4. Henderson, J. L.: Gargoylism: Review of principal features with report of five cases. Arch. Dis. Child. **15,** 215, 1940.
5. Hunter, C.: A rare disease in two brothers. Proc. Roy. Soc. Med., **10,** 104, 1917.
6. Hurler, G.: Über eninen typ multipler abartungen, vorwiegend am skelettsystem. Z. Kinderheilk., **24,** 220, 1919.
7. Washington, J. A.: Lipochondrodystrophy, in *Practice of Pediatrics,* edited by J. Brenneman, vol. 4, suppl., 1939. W. F. Prior Co., Inc., Hagerstown, Md., 1937.
8. Ellis, R. W. B., Sheldon, W., and Capon, N. B.: Gargoylism (chondro-osteo-dystrophy, corneal opacities, hepatosplenomegaly and mental deficiency). Quart. J. Med., **5,** 119, 1936.
9. Jeanloz, R. W.: The nomenclature of acid mucopolysaccharides. Arthritis Rheum., **3,** 323, 1960.
10. Fessler, J. H., and Fessler, L. J.: Electron microscopic visualization of the polysaccharide hyaluronic acid. Proc. Nat. Acad. Sci. U.S.A., **56,** 141, 1966.
11. Hamerman, D., Rojkind, M., and Sandson, J.: Analyses of the protein moiety of hyaluronate. Fed. Proc., **25,** 790, 1966.
12. Wardi, A. H., Allen, W. S., Turner, D. L., and Stary, Z.: Hyaluronate-peptide linkage group. Biochim. Biophys. Acta, **192,** 151, 1969.
13. Dorfman, A., and Schiller, S.: Mucopolysaccharides of connective tissue, in *Biological Structure and Function,* edited by T. W. Goodwin and O. Lindberg, vol. 1, p. 327. Academic, New York, 1961.
14. Schiller, S., Slover, G., and Dorfman, A.: Effect of the thyroid gland on metabolism of acid mucopolysaccharides in skin. Biochim. Biophys. Acta, **58,** 27, 1962.
15. Nakanishi, K., Takahashi, N., and Egami, F.: Infra red spectra of charonin-sulfuric acid, chondroitin-sulfuric acid, and some related polysaccharides. Bull. Chem. Soc. Jap., **29,** 434, 1956.
16. Mathews, M. B.: Sodium chondroitin sulfate-protein complexes of cartilage. III. Preparation from shark. Biochim. Biophys. Acta, **58,** 92, 1962.
17. Mathews, M. B.: Comparative biochemistry of connective tissue ground substance. Biol. Bull., **119,** 283, 1960.
18. Robinson, H. C., and Dorfman, A.: The sulfation of chondroitin sulfate in embryonic chick cartilage epiphyses. J. Biol. Chem., **244,** 348, 1969.
19. Soda, T., Egami, F., and Horigome, T.: On chondroitin sulfuric acid: Preparation of chondroitin sulfuric acid by the use of trypaflavine. J. Chem. Soc. [Org.], **61,** 43, 1940.
20. Suzuki, S.: Isolation of novel disaccharides from chondroitin sulfates. J. Biol. Chem., **235,** 3580, 1960.
21. Davidson, E. A., and Meyer, K.: Chondroitin, a new mucopolysaccharide. J. Biol. Chem., **211,** 605, 1954.
22. Mathews, M. B., and Hinds, L.: Acid mucopolysaccharides and frog metamorphosis. Fed. Proc., **21,** 167, 1962.
23. Suzuki, S., Saito, H., Yamagata, T., Anno, K., Seno, N., Kawai, Y., and Furuhashi, T.: Formation of three types of disulfated disaccharides from chondroitin sulfates by chondroitinase digestion. J. Biol. Chem., **243,** 1543, 1968.
24. Mörner, C. T.: Chemische studien über den trachealknorpel. Skand. Arch. Physiol., **1,** 210, 1889.
25. Shatton, J., and Schubert, M.: Isolation of a mucoprotein from cartilage. J. Biol. Chem., **211,** 565, 1954.
26. Muir, H.: The nature of the link between protein and carbohydrate of a chondroitin sulfate complex from hyaline cartilage. Biochem. J., **69,** 195, 1958.
27. Rodén, L.: Cystic fibrosis, part II, in *Biochemistry of Glycoproteins and Related Substances,* edited by E. Rossi and E. Stobl, pp. 185–202. Karger, Basel, 1968.
28. Fransson, L.-Å., and Rodén, L.: Structure of dermatan sulfate. I. Degradation by testicular hyaluronidase. J. Biol. Chem., **242,** 4161, 1967.
29. Fransson, L.-Å., and Rodén, L.: Structure of dermatan sulfate. II. Characterization of products obtained by hyaluronidase digestion of dermatan sulfate. J. Biol. Chem., **242,** 4170, 1967.
30. Fransson, L.-Å.: Structure of dermatan sulfate. III. The hybrid structure of dermatan sulfate from umbilical cord. J. Biol. Chem., **243,** 1504, 1968.
31. Dorfman, A.: Metabolism of acid mucopolysaccharides. Biophys. J., **4,** 155, 1964.
32. Grossman, B. J., and Dorfman, A.: *In vitro* comparison of the antithrombic action of heparin and chondroitin-sulfuric acid-B. Pediatrics, **20,** 506, 1957.
33. Pedrini, V., Lennzi, L., and Zambotti, V.: Isolation and identification of keratosulphate in urine of patients affected by Morquio-Ullrich disease. Proc. Soc. Exp. Biol. Med., **110,** 847, 1962.
34. Robbins, M. M., Stevens, H. F., and Linker, A.: Morquio's disease: An abnormality of mucopolysaccharide metabolism. J. Pediat., **62,** 881, 1963.
35. Suzuki, K.: Cerebral GM_1 gangliosidosis: Chemical pathology of visceral organs. Science, **159,** 1471, 1968.
36. O'Brien, J.: Generalized gangliosidosis. J. Pediat., **75,** 167, 1969.
37. Wolfe, L. S., Callahan, J., Fawcett, J. S., Andermann, F., and Scriver, C. R.: G_{M1}-gangliosidosis without chondrodystrophy or visceromegaly: β-Galactosidase deficiency with gangliosidosis and the excessive excretion of a keratan sulfate. Neurology (Minneap.), **20,** 23, 1970.
38. Baker, J. R., Cifonelli, J. A., Mathews, M. B., and Rodén, L.: Mannose-containing glycopeptides from keratosulfate (KS). Fed. Proc., **28,** 605, 1969.
39. Bhavanandan, V. P., and Meyer, K.: Studies on keratosulfates (methylation, desulfation, and acid hydrolysis studies on old human rib cartilage keratosulfate). J. Biol. Chem., **243,** 1052, 1968.
40. Cifonelli, J. A., and Dorfman, A.: The uronic acid of heparin. Biochem. Biophys. Res. Commun., **7,** 41, 1962.
41. Radhakrishnamurthy, B., and Berenson, G. S.: Identification of uronic acids in mucopolysaccharides. Arch. Biochem., **101,** 360, 1963.
42. Wolfrom, M. L., Honda, S., and Wang, P. Y.: The isolation of L-iduronic acid from the crystalline barium acid salt of heparin. Carb. Res., **10,** 259, 1969.
43. Perlin, A. S., and Mazurek, M.: A proton magnetic resonance spectral study of heparin. Carb. Res., **7,** 369, 1968.
44. Yamauchi, F., Kosakai, M., and Yosizawa, Z.: Epimerization of D-glucuronic acid to L-iduronic acid by deaminization of heparins. Biochem. Biophys. Res. Commun., **33,** 721, 1968.

45. Lindahl, U.: The structures of xylosylserine and galactosylxylosyl serine from heparin. Biochim. Biophys. Acta, **130,** 361, 1966.
46. Cifonelli, J. A.: Reaction of heparitin sulfate with nitrous acid. Carb. Res., **8,** 233, 1968.
47. Lindahl, U.: Structure of heparin, heparan sulfate and their proteoglycans. In *NATO Advanced Study Institute on the Chemistry and Molecular Biology of the Intercellular Matrix,* edited by E. A. Balazs, vol. II, p. 943, Academic, London, 1970.
48. Cifonelli, J. A., and Dorfman, A.: Properties of heparin monosulfate (heparitin monosulfate). J. Biol. Chem., **235,** 3283, 1960.
49. Linker, A., Hoffman, P., Sampson, P., and Meyer, K.: Heparitin sulfate. Biochim. Biophys. Acta, **29,** 443, 1958.
50. Singh, M., and Bachhawat, B. K.: The distribution of variation with age of different uronic acid–containing mucopolysaccharides in brain. J. Neurochem., **12,** 519, 1965.
51. Dorfman, A., and Ho, P.-L.: Synthesis of acid mucopolysaccharides by glial tumor cells in tissue culture. Proc. Nat. Acad. Sci. U.S.A., **66,** 495, 1970.
52. Mathews, M. B., and Lozaityte, I.: Sodium chondroitin sulfate protein complexes of cartilage. I. Molecular weight and shape. Arch. Biochem., **74,** 158, 1957.
53. Mathews, M. B.: Macromolecular evolution of connective tissue. Biol. Rev., **42,** 499, 1967.
54. Tsiganos, C. P., and Muir, H.: Studies on protein-polysaccharide from pig laryngeal cartilage: Extraction and purification. Biochem. J., **113,** 879, 1969.
55. Rosenblum, E. L., and Cifonelli, J. A.: Linkage of chondroitin sulfate (CS) and keratan sulfate (KS) to a common protein. Fed. Proc., **26,** 282, 1967.
56. Mathews, M. B.: Sub-structure of cartilage chondroitin sulfate-proteins (CSP): Doublets. Fed. Proc., **27,** 529, 1968.
57. Seno, N., Meyer, K., Anderson, B., and Hoffman, P.: Variations in keratosulfates. J. Biol. Chem., **240,** 1005, 1965.
58. Kaplan, D., McKusick, V., Trebach, S., and Lazarus, B.: Keratosulfate–chondroitin sulfate peptide from normal urine and from urine of patients with Morquio syndrome (mucopolysaccharidosis IV). J. Lab. Clin. Med., **71,** 48, 1968.
59. Hascall, V. C., and Sajdera, S. W.: Proteinpolysaccharide complex from bovine nasal cartilage: The function of glycoprotein in the formation of aggregates. J. Biol. Chem., **244,** 2384, 1969.
60. Sajdera, S. W., and Hascall, V. C.: Protein polysaccharide complex from bovine nasal cartilage. (A comparison of low and high shear extraction procedures.) J. Biol. Chem., **244,** 77, 1969.
61. Toole, B. P., and Lowther, D. A.: Dermatan sulfate-protein: Isolation from and interaction with collagen. Arch. Biochem., **128,** 567, 1968.
62. Lindahl, U., and Rodén, L.: The role of galactose and xylose in the linkage of heparin to protein. J. Biol. Chem., **240,** 2821, 1965.
63. Lloyd, A. G., Bloom, G. D., and Balazs, E. A.: Evidence for the covalent association of heparin and protein in mast-cell granules. Biochem. J., **103,** 76P, 1967.
64. Serafini-Fracassini, A., and Durward, J. J.: Isolation of a heparin-protein complex from ox liver capsule. Biochem. J., **109,** 693, 1968.
65. Knecht, J., Cifonelli, J. A., and Dorfman, A.: Structural studies on heparitin sulfate of normal and Hurler tissues. J. Biol. Chem., **242,** 4652, 1967.
66. Dankert, M., Wright, A., Kelly, W. S., and Robbins, P. W.: Isolation, purification and properties of the lipid-linked intermediates of O-antigen biosynthesis. Arch. Biochem., **116,** 425, 1966.
67. Weiner, I. M., Higuchi, T., Rothfield, L., Saltmarsh-Andrew, M., Osborn, M. J., and Horecker, B. L.: Biosynthesis of bacterial lipopolysaccharide. V. Lipid-linked intermediates in the biosynthesis of the O-antigen groups of *Salmonella typhimurium.* Proc. Nat. Acad. Sci. U.S.A., **54,** 228, 1965.
68. Anderson, J. S., Matsuhashi, M., Haskin, M. A., and Strominger, J. L.: Lipid-phosphoacetylmuramyl-pentapeptide and lipid-phosphodisaccharide-pentopeptide: Presumed membrane transport intermediates in cell wall synthesis. Proc. Nat. Acad. Sci. U.S.A., **53,** 881, 1965.
69. Scher, M., Lennarz, W. J., and Sweeley, C. C.: The biosynthesis of mannosyl-l-phosphoryl-polyisoprenol in micrococcus lysodeikticus and its role in mannan synthesis. Proc. Nat. Acad. Sci. U.S.A., **59,** 1313, 1968.
70. Caccam, J. F., Jackson, J. J., and Eylar, E. H.: The biosynthesis of mannose-containing glycoproteins: A possible lipid intermediate. Biochem. Biophys. Res. Commun., **35,** 505, 1969.
71. Behrens, N. H., and Leloir, L. F.: Dolichol monophosphate glucose: An intermediate in glucose transfer in liver. Proc. Nat. Acad. Sci. U.S.A., **66,** 153, 1970.
72. Stoolmiller, A. C., and Dorfman, A.: The metabolism of glycosaminoglycans, in *Carbohydrate Metabolism,* edited by M. Florkin and E. Stotz, vol. 17, p. 241. Elsevier, Amsterdam, 1969.
73. Jacobson, B., and Davidson, E. A.: Biosynthesis of uronic acids by skin enzymes. II. Uridine diphosphate-D-glucuronic acid-5-epimerase. J. Biol. Chem., **237,** 638, 1962.
74. Fransson, L.-Å.: Structure and metabolism of the proteoglycans of dermatan sulfate. In *NATO Advanced Study Institute on the Chemistry and Molecular Biology of the Intercellular Matrix,* edited by E. A. Balazs, vol. II, p. 823, Academic, London, 1970.
75. Neufeld, E. F., and Hall, C. W.: Inhibition of UDP-D-glucose dehydrogenase by UDP-D-xylose: A possible regulatory mechanism. Biochem. Biophys. Res. Commun., **19,** 456, 1965.
76. Kornfeld, S., Kornfeld, R., Neufeld, E. F., and O'Brien, P. J.: The feedback control of sugar nucleotide biosynthesis in liver. Proc. Nat. Acad. Sci. U.S.A., **52,** 371, 1964.
77. Telser, A., Robinson, H. C., and Dorfman, A.: The biosynthesis of chondroitin-sulfate protein complex. Proc. Nat. Acad. Sci. U.S.A., **54,** 912, 1965.
78. De La Haba, G., and Holtzer, H.: Chondroitin sulfate: Inhibition of synthesis by puromycin. Science, **149,** 1263, 1965.
79. Matalon, R., and Dorfman, A.: The structure of acid mucopolysaccharides produced by Hurler fibroblasts in tissue culture. Proc. Nat. Acad. Sci. U.S.A., **60,** 179, 1968.
80. Molnar, J., Robinson, G. B., and Winzler, R. J.: Biosynthesis of glycoproteins. IV. The subcellular sites of incorporation of glucosamine-1-^{14}C into glycoprotein in rat liver. J. Biol. Chem., **240,** 1882, 1965.
81. Sarcione, E. J.: The initial subcellular site in incorporation of hexose into liver protein. J. Biol. Chem., **239,** 1686, 1964.
82. Spiro, R. G., and Spiro, M. J.: Glycoprotein biosynthesis: Studies on thyroglobulin. Characterization of a particular precursor and radioisotope incorporation by thyroid slices and particle systems. J. Biol. Chem., **241,** 1271, 1966.
83. Moroz, C., and Uhr, J. W.: A role of the carbohydrate moiety in the regulation of immunoglobulin synthesis and secretin. Fed. Proc., **27,** 735, 1968.
84. Baker, J. R., and Rodén, L.: Biosynthesis of chondroitin sulfate (CS): The xylosyltransferase reaction. Fed. Proc., **29,** 338, 1970.
85. Horwitz, A. L., Stoolmiller, A. C., and Dorfman, A.: Unpublished results.
86. Katsura, N., and Davidson, E. A.: Studies on porcine costal cartilage protein–polysaccharide complex. I. Enzymatic degradation. Biochim. Biophys. Acta, **121,** 120, 1966.
87. Helting, T., and Rodén, L.: Biosynthesis of chondroitin sulfate. I. Galactosyl transfer in the formation of the carbohydrate-protein linkage region. J. Biol. Chem., **244,** 2790, 1968.
88. Helting, T., and Rodén, L.: Biosynthesis of chondroitin sulfate. II. Glucuronosyl transfer in the formation of the carbohydrate-protein linkage region. J. Biol. Chem., **244,** 2799, 1969.
89. Telser, A., Robinson, H. C., and Dorfman, A.: The biosynthesis of chondroitin sulfate. Arch. Biochem., **116,** 458, 1966.
90. Robbins, P. W., and Lipmann, F.: Identification of enzymatically active sulfate as adenosine-3′-phosphate-5′-phosphosulfate. J. Amer. Chem. Soc., **78,** 6409, 1956.
91. Robbins, P. W., and Lipmann, F.: Isolation and identification of active sulfate. J. Biol. Chem., **229,** 837, 1957.
92. D'Abramo, F., and Lipmann, F.: The formation of adenosine-3′-phosphate-5′-phosphosulfate in extracts of chick embryo cartilage and its conversion into chondroitin sulfate. Biochim. Biophys. Acta, **25,** 211, 1957.
93. Suzuki, S., and Strominger, J. L.: Enzymatic sulfation of mucopoly-

saccharides in hen oviduct. I. Transfer of sulfate from 3′-phosphoadenosine 5′-phosphosulfate to mucopolysaccharides. J. Biol. Chem., **235,** 257, 1960.

94. Picard, J., and Gardais, A.: Structure and function of connective and skeletal tissue. *Pro. NATO Advanced Study Conference,* St. Andrews, 1964, p. 338. Butterworth, London, 1965.
95. Perlman, R. L., Telser, A., and Dorfman, A.: The biosynthesis of chondroitin sulfate by a cell-free preparation. J. Biol. Chem., **239,** 3623, 1964.
96. Silbert, J. E., and DeLuca, S.: Biosynthesis of chondroitin sulfate. III. Formation of a sulfated glycosaminoglycan with a microsomal preparation from chick embryo cartilage. J. Biol. Chem., **244,** 876, 1969.
97. Rodén, L.: Biosynthesis of acidic glycoaminoglycans (mucopolysaccharides), in *Metabolic Conjugation and Metabolic Hydrolysis,* vol. II. Academic, New York, 1970.
98. Markovitz, A., Cifonelli, J. A., and Dorfman, A.: The biosynthesis of hyaluronic acid by group A streptococcus. VI. Biosynthesis from uridine nucleotides in cell-free extracts. J. Biol. Chem., **234,** 2343, 1959.
99. Markovitz, A., and Dorfman, A.: Synthesis of capsular polysaccharide (hyaluronic acid) by protoplast membrane preparations of group A streptococcus. J. Biol. Chem., **237,** 273, 1962.
100. Stoolmiller, A. C., and Dorfman, A.: The biosynthesis of hyaluronic acid by streptococcus. J. Biol. Chem., **244,** 236, 1969.
101. Stoolmiller, A. C., and Dorfman, A.: Unpublished results.
102. Glaser, L., and Brown, D. H.: The enzymatic synthesis *in vitro* of hyaluronic acid chains. Proc. Nat. Acad. Sci. U.S.A., **41,** 253, 1955.
103. Ishimoto, N., Temin, H. M., and Strominger, J. L.: Studies of carcinogenesis by avian sarcoma viruses. II. Virus-induced increase in hyaluronic acid synthetase in chicken fibroblasts. J. Biol. Chem., **241,** 2052, 1966.
104. Schiller, S.: Synthesis of hyaluronic acid by a soluble enzyme system from mammalian tissue. Biochem. Biophys. Res. Commun., **15,** 250, 1964.
105. Osterlin, S. E., and Jacobson, B.: The synthesis of hyaluronic acid in vitreous. I. Soluble and particulate transferases in hyalocytes. Exp. Eye Res., **7,** 497, 1968.
106. Osterlin, S. E., and Jacobson, B.: The synthesis of hyaluronic acid in vitreous. II. The presence of soluble transferase and nucleotide sugar in the accellular vitreous gel. Exp. Eye Res., **7,** 511, 1968.
107. Kobata, A.: Isolation and identification of two novel uridine nucleotide oligosaccharides from human milk. Biochem. Biophys. Res. Commun., **7,** 346, 1962.
108. Dorfman, A.: Differential function of connective tissue cells, in *NATO Advanced Study Institute on the Chemistry and Molecular Biology of the Intercellular Matrix,* edited by E. A. Balazs. vol. III, p. 1421. Academic, London, 1970.
109. Stern, E. L., and Rodén, L.: Unpublished results.
110. Davidson, E. A., and Riley, J.: Enzymatic sulfation of chondroitin B. J. Biol. Chem., **235,** 3367, 1960.
111. Adams, J. B., and Meaney, M. F.: Specificity of sulfate transfer to chondroitin sulfate in human tumor extracts. Biochim. Biophys. Acta, **54,** 592, 1961.
112. Silbert, J. E.: Incorporation of ^{14}C and ^{3}H from nucleotide sugars into a polysaccharide in the presence of a cell-free preparation from mouse mast cell tumors. J. Biol. Chem., **238,** 3542, 1963.
113. Silbert, J. E.: Incorporation of $^{35}SO_4$ into endogenous heparin by a microsomal fraction from mast cell tumors. J. Biol. Chem., **242,** 2301, 1967.
114. Silbert, J. E.: Biosynthesis of heparin. III. Formation of a sulfated glycosaminoglycan with a microsomal preparation from mast cell tumors. J. Biol. Chem., **242,** 5146, 1967.
115. Silbert, J. E.: Biosynthesis of heparin. IV. N-Deacetylation of a precursor glycosaminoglycan. J. Biol. Chem., **242,** 5153, 1967.
116. Balasubramanian, A. S., Joun, N. S., and Marx, W.: Sulfation of N-desulfoheparin and heparan sulfate by a purified enzyme from mastocytoma. Arch. Biochem., **128,** 623, 1968.
117. Grebner, E. E., Hall, C. W., and Neufeld, E. F.: Glycosylation of serine residues by a uridine diphosphate-xylose: Protein xylosyltransferase from mouse mastocytoma. Arch. Biochem., **116,** 391, 1966.
118. Grebner, E. E., Hall, C. W., and Neufeld, E. F.: Incorporation of D-xylose-^{14}C into glycoprotein by particles from hen oviduct. Biochem. Biophys. Res. Commun., **22,** 672, 1966.
119. Rodén, L., and Dorfman, A.: The acid mucopolysaccharides of Furth's mastocytoma in the mouse. Acta Chem. Scand., **13,** 2121, 1960.
120. Wortman, B.: Enzymic sulfation of corneal mucopolysaccharides by beef corneal epithelial extract. J. Biol. Chem., **236,** 974, 1961.
121. Hortwitz, A. L., and Dorfman, A.: Subcellular sites for synthesis of chondromucoprotein of cartilage. J. Cell. Biol., **38,** 358, 1968.
122. Godman, G., and Porter, K. R.: Chondrogenesis, studied with the electron microscope. J. Biophys. Biochem. Cytol., **8,** 719, 1960.
123. Revel, J. P., and Hay, E. D.: An autoradiographic and electron microscopic study of collagen synthesis in differentiating cartilage. Z. Zellforsch., **61,** 110, 1963.
124. Godman, G., and Lane, N.: On the site of sulfation in the chondrocyte. J. Cell Biol., **21,** 353, 1964.
125. Neutra, M., and Leblond, C. P.: Radioautographic comparison of the uptake of galactose-H^3 and glucose-^3H in the Golgi region of various cells secreting glycoproteins or mucopolysaccharides. J. Cell Biol., **30,** 137, 1966.
126. Roy, S., and Ghadially, F. N.: Synthesis of hyaluronic acid by synovial cells. J. Bact., **93,** 555, 1967.
127. Barland, P., Smith, C., and Hamerman, D.: Localization of hyaluronic acid in synovial cells by radioautography. J. Cell. Biol., **37,** 13, 1968.
128. Redman, C. M., Siekevitz, P., and Palade, G. E.: Synthesis and transfer of amylase in pigeon pancreatic microsomes. J. Biol. Chem., **241,** 1150, 1966.
129. Jamieson, J. D., and Palade, G. E.: Intracellular transport of secretory proteins in the pancreatic exocrine cell. I. Role of the peripheral element of the Golgi complex. J. Cell Biol., **34,** 577, 1967.
130. Jamieson, J. D., and Palade, G. E.: Intracellular transport of secretory protein in the pancreatic exocrine cell. II. Transport to condensing vacuoles and zymogen granules. J. Cell Biol., **34,** 597–615, 1967.
131. Lawford, G. R., and Schacter, H.: Biosynthesis of glycoprotein by liver: The incorporation *in vivo* of ^{14}C-glucosamine into protein-bound hexosamine and sialic acid of rat liver subcellular fractions. J. Biol. Chem., **241,** 5408, 1968.
132. Eylar, E. H.: On the biological role of glycoproteins. J. Theor. Biol., **10,** 89, 1965.
133. Juva, K., Prockop, D. J., Cooper, G. W., and Lash, J. W.: Hydroxylation of proline and the intracellular accumulation of a polypeptide precursor of collagen. Science, **152,** 92, 1966.
134. Suzuki, S., Okayama, M., Kimata, K., Yamagata, T., Saito, H., Hoshino, M., and Suzuki, I.: Biosynthesis of chondromucoproteins. *7th Int. Congr. Biochem.,* Tokyo, 1967, vol. 4, p. 704.
135. Horwitz, A. L., and Dorfman, A.: Unpublished results.
136. Horwitz, A., Stoolmiller, A. C., and Dorfman, A.: Purification of the chondromucoprotein (CM-P) synthetase complex. Fed. Proc., **29,** 337, 1970.
137. Jamieson, J. D., and Palade, G. E.: Intracellular transport of secretory proteins in the pancreatic exocrine cell. IV. Metabolic requirements. J. Cell Biol., **39,** 589, 1968.
138. Bosmann, H. B.: Cellular control of macromolecular synthesis: Rates of synthetis of extracellular macromolecules during and after depletion by papain, Proc. Roy. Soc. London, [Biol.], **169,** 399, 1968.
139. Schiller, S., Mathews, M. B., Goldfaber, L., Ludowieg, J., and Dorfman, A.: The metabolism of mucopolysaccharides in animals. II. Studies in skin utilizing labeled acetate. J. Biol. Chem., **212,** 531, 1955.
140. Schiller, S., Mathews, M. B., Cifonelli, J. A., and Dorfman, A.: The metabolism of mucopolysaccharides in animals. III. Further studies on skin utilizing C^{14}-glucose, C^{11}-acetate, and S^{35}-sodium sulfate. J. Biol. Chem., **218,** 139, 1956.
141. Schiller, S., and Dorfman, A.: The metabolism of mucopolysaccharides in aminals: The effect of cortisone and hydrocortisone on rat skin. Endocrinology, **60,** 376, 1957.
142. Schiller, S., and Dorfman, A.: The metabolism of mucopolysaccharides in animals. IV. The influence of insulin. J. Biol. Chem., **227,** 625, 1957.
143. Schiller, S., Slover, G., and Dorfman, A.: A method for the separation

of acid mucopolysaccharides: Its application to the isolation of heparin from skin of rats. J. Biol. Chem., **236,** 983, 1961.
144. Schiller, S., and Dorfman, A.: Effect of age on the heparin content of rat skin. Nature (London), **185,** 111, 1960.
145. Schiller, S., and Dorfman, A.: The distribution of acid mucopolysaccharides in skin of diabetic rats. Biochim. Biophys. Acta, **78,** 371, 1963.
146. Schiller, S.: Mucopolysaccharides in relation to growth and thyroid hormones: J. Chronic Dis., **16,** 291, 1963.
147. Meyer, K., Dubos, R., and Smyth, E. M.: The hydrolysis of the polysaccharide acids of vitreous humor, of umbilical cord and of streptococcus by the autolytic enzyme of pneumococcus. J. Biol. Chem., **118,** 71, 1937.
148. Meyer, K., Hoffman, P., and Linker, A.: Hyaluronidases, in *The Enzymes* edited by P. D. Boyer, H. Lardy, and K. Myrbäck, 2 ed., vol. 4, p. 447. Academic, New York, 1960.
149. Chain, E., and Duthie, E. S.: Identity of hyaluronidase and spreading factor. Brit. J. Exp. Path., **21,** 324, 1940.
150. Duran-Reynals, F.: Exaltation de l'activite du virus vaccinal par les extraits des certaines organes. C. R. Soc. Biol. (Paris), **99,** 6, 1928.
151. Linker, A., Hoffman, P., and Meyer, K.: The hyaluronidase of the leech: An endoglucuronidase. Nature (London), **180,** 810, 1957.
152. Bollet, A. J., Bonner, W. M., and Nance, J. L.: The presence of hyaluronidase in various mammalian tissues. J. Biol. Chem., **238,** 3522, 1963.
153. Hutterer, F.: Degradation of mucopolysaccharides by hepatic lysosomes. Biochim. Biophys. Acta, **115,** 312, 1966.
154. Aronson, N. N., Jr., and Davidson, E. A.: Lysosomal hyaluronidase from rat liver. I. Preparation. J. Biol. Chem., **242,** 437, 1967.
155. Aronson, N. N., Jr., and Davidson, Eugene A.: Lysosomal hyaluronidase from rat liver. II. Properties. J. Biol. Chem., **242,** 441, 1967.
156. Vaes, G.: Hyaluronidase activity in lysosomes of bone tissue. Biochem. J., **103,** 802, 1967.
157. Mahadevan, S., Dillard, C. J., and Tappel, A. L.: Degradation of polysaccharides, mucopolysaccharides, and glycoproteins by lysosomal glycosidases. Arch. Biochem. Biophys., **129,** 525, 1969.
158. Tan, Y. H., and Bowness, J. J.: Canine submandibular-gland hyaluronidase: Purification and properties. Biochem. J., **110,** 9, 1968.
159. Buddecke, E., and Platt, D.: Untersuchungen zur chemie der arterienwand. 8. Nachweis, reinigung und eigenschaften der Hyaluronidase aus der Aorta des Rindes. Hoppe-Seyler's Z. Physiol. Chem., **343,** 61, 1965.
160. Cashman, D. C., Laryea, J. U., and Weissmann, B.: The hyaluronidase of rat skin. Arch. Biochem. Biophys., **135,** 387, 1969.
161. Silbert, J. E., Nagai, Y., and Gross, J.: Hyaluronidase from tadpole tissue. J. Biol. Chem., **240,** 1509, 1965.
162. Bowness, J. M., and Tan, Y. H.: Chromatographic distinction between hyaluronidases from human serum and ovine testes. Biochim. Biophys. Acta, **151,** 288, 1968.
163. de Duve, C., Pressman, B. C., Gianetto, R., Wattiaux, R., and Appelmans, F.: Tissue fractionation studies. 6. Intracellular distribution patterns of enzymes in rat liver tissue. Biochem. J., **60,** 604, 1955.
164. Weissmann, B.: The transglycosylative action of testicular hyaluronidase. J. Biol. Chem., **216,** 783, 1955.
165. Linker, A., Meyer, K., and Weissmann, B.: Enzymatic formation of monosaccharides from hyaluronate. J. Biol. Chem., **213,** 237, 1955.
166. Weissmann, B., Hadjiioannou, S., and Tornheim, J.: Oligosaccharase activity of β-N-acetyl-D-glucosaminidase of beef liver. J. Biol. Chem., **239,** 59, 1964.
167. Robinson, D., and Stirling, J. L.: N-acetyl-β-glucosaminidases in human spleen. Biochem. J., **107,** 321, 1968.
168. Frohwein, Y., and Gatt, S.: Separation of β-acetylglucosaminidase and β-N-acetylgalactosaminidase from calf brain cytoplasm. Biochim. Biophys. Acta, **128,** 216, 1966.
169. Woollen, J. W., Walker, P. G., and Heyworth, R.: Studies on glucosaminidase. 6. N-Acetyl-β-glucosaminidase and N-acetyl-β-galactosaminidase activities of a variety of enzyme preparations. Biochem. J., **79,** 294, 1961.
170. Okada, S., and O'Brien, J. S.: Tay-Sachs disease: Generalized absence of a beta-D-N-acetylhexosaminidase component. Science, **165,** 698, 1969.
171. Sandhoff, K.: Variation of β-N-acetylhexosaminidase-pattern in Tay-Sachs disease. FEBS Ltrs., **4,** 351, 1969.
172. Hultberg, B.: N-Acetylhexosaminidase activities in Tay-Sachs disease. Lancet, **2,** 1195, 1969.
173. Sandhoff, K., Andreae, U., and Jatzkewitz, H.: Deficient hexosaminidase activity in an exceptional case of Tay-Sachs disease with additional storage of kidney globoside in visceral organs. Life Sci., **7,** 283, 1968.
174. Dance, N., Price, R. G., Robinson, D., and Stirling, J. L.: Beta-galactosidase, beta-glucosidase and N-acetyl-beta-glucosaminidase in human kidney. Clin. Chim. Acta, **24,** 189, 1969.
175. Aronson, N. N., Jr., and de Duve, C.: Digestive activity of lysosomes. II. The digestion of macromolecule carbohydrates of extracts of rat liver lysosomes. J. Biol. Chem., **243,** 4564, 1968.
176. Buddecke, E., and Werries, E.: Reinigung und eigenschaften einer β-N-acetyl-D-hexosaminidase aus rindermilz. Z. Naturforsch. [B], **19B,** 798, 1964.
177. Buddecke, E., and Werries, E.: Untersuchungen zur chemie der arterienwand. VII. Reinigung und eigenschaften der β-acetyl-glucosaminidase aus der aorta des rindes. Hoppe-Seyler's Z. Physiol. Chem., **340,** 257, 1965.
178. Dohlman, C. -H.: The fate of the sulfate groups of chondroitin sulfate after administration to rats. Acta Physiol. Scand., **37,** 220, 1956.
179. Dziewiatkowski, D. D.: Some aspects of the metabolism of chondroitin sulfate-S^{35} in the rat. J. Biol. Chem., **223,** 239, 1956.
180. Aronson, N. N., Jr., and Davidson, E. A.: Catabolism of mucopolysaccharides by rat liver lysosomes *in vivo*. J. Biol. Chem., **243,** 4494, 1968.
181. Kaplan, D., and Meyer, K.: The fate of injected mucopolysaccharides. J. Clin. Invest., **41,** 743, 1962.
182. Tudball, N., and Davidson, E. A.: Isolation of a novel sulphatase from rat liver. Biochim. Biophys. Acta, **171,** 113, 1968.
183. Platt, D., and Stein, U.: Untersuchungen zum katabolen mucopolysaccharid-protein Stoffwechsel in menschlichen Organen. (Studies on the catabolic mucopolysaccharide-protein metabolism in human organs). Z. Klin. Chem., **7,** 374, 1969.
184. Murphy, J. V., Wolfe, H. J., Balazs, E. A., and Moser, H. W.: Personal communication.
185. Matalon, R., and Dorfman, A.: Unpublished results.
186. Fisher, D., Higham, M., Kent, P. W., and Pritchard, P.: β-Xylosidases of animal and other sources in relation to the degradation of chondroitin sulphate–peptide complexes. Biochem. J., **98,** 46P, 1966.
187. Robinson, D., and Abrahams, H. E.: β-D-Xylosidase in pig kidney. Biochim. Biophys. Acta, **132,** 214, 1967.
188. Patel, V., and Tappel, A. L.: Identity of β-glucosidase and β-xylosidase activities in rat liver lysosomes. Biochim. Biophys. Acta, **191,** 86, 1969.
189. Fisher, D., and Kent, P. W.: Rat liver β-xylosidase, a lysosomal membrane enzyme. Biochem. J., **115,** 50, 1969.
190. Tominaga, F., Oka, K., and Yoshida, H.: The isolation and identification of O-xylosyl-serine and S-methyl-cysteine sulfoxide from human urine. J. Biochem. (Tokyo), **57,** 717, 1965.
191. Eiber, H. B., and Borrelli, F. J.: Physiological disposition of heparin. Proc. Soc. Exp. Biol. Med., **98,** 672, 1958.
192. McAllister, B. M., and Demis, D. J.: Heparin metabolism: Isolation and characterization of uroheparin. Nature (London), **212,** 293, 1966.
193. Lloyd, A. G., Embery, G., Wusteman, F. S., and Dodgson, K. S.: The metabolic fate of ^{35}S-labelled heparin and related compounds. Biochem. J., **98,** 33P, 1966.
194. Lemaire, A., Picard, J., and Gardais, A.: Le catabolisme de l'heparine: Étude *in vivo* de la desulfatation de l'heparine chez le rat, par MM. C. R. Soc. Biol. (Paris), **264,** 949, 1967.
195. Cho, M. H., and Jaques, L. B.: Heparinase, III. Preparation and properties of the enzyme. Canad. J. Biochem., **34,** 799, 1956.
196. Roseman, S., and Dorfman, A.: α Glucosaminidase. J. Biol. Chem., **191,** 607, 1951.
197. Weissmann, B., Rowin, G., Marshall, J., and Friederici, D.: Mammalian α-acetylglucosaminidase: Enzymic properties, tissue distribution, and intracellular localization. Biochemistry (Wash.), **6,** 207, 1967.
198. Werries, E., Wollek, E., Gottschalk, A., and Buddecke, E.: Separation

of N-acetyl-α-glucosaminidase and N-acetyl-α-galactosaminidase from ox spleen: Cleavage of the O-glycosidic linkage between carbohydrate and polypeptide in ovine and bovine submaxillary glycoprotein by N-acetyl-α-galactosaminidase. Europ. J. Biochem., **10,** 445, 1969.

199. Weissmann, B., and Hinrichsen, D. F.: Mammalian α-acetylgalactosaminidase: Occurrence, partial purification, and action on linkages in submaxillary mucins. Biochemestry (Wash.), **8,** 2034, 1969.
200. MacBrinn, M. C., Okada, S., Ho, M. W., Hu, C. C., and O'Brien, J. S.: Generalized gangliosidosis: Impaired cleavage of galactose from a mucopolysaccharide and a glycoprotein. Science, **163,** 946, 1969.
201. Thomas, L.: Reversible collapse of rabbit ears after intravenous papain. and prevention of recovery by cortisone. J. Exp. Med., **104,** 245, 1956.
202. Lucy, J. A., Dingle, J. T., and Fell, H. B.: Studies on the mode of action of excess of vitamin A. I. A possible role of intracellular proteases in the degradation of cartilage matrix. Biochem. J., **79,** 500, 1961.
203. Weissman, G., and Thomas, L.: Studies on lysosomes. II. The effect of cortisone on the release of acid hydrolases from a large granule fraction of rabbit liver induced by an excess of vitamin A. J. Clin. Invest., **42,** 661, 1963.
204. Weissman, G., and Spilberg, I.: Breakdown of cartilage protein-polysaccharide by lysosomes. Arthritis Rheum., **11,** 162, 1968.
205. Ali, S. Y.: The degradation of cartilage matrix by an intracellular protease. Biochem. J., **87,** 403, 1963.
206. Makino, M., Kojima, T., and Yamashina, I.: Enzymatic cleavage of glycopeptides. Biochem, Biophys. Res. Commun., **24,** 961, 1966.
207. Conchie, J., and Strachan, I.: Distribution purification and properties of L-aspartamido-β-N-acetylglucosamine amidohydrolase. Biochem. J., **115,** 709, 1969.
208. Pollitt, R. J., Jenner, F. A., and Merskey, H.: Aspartylglucosaminuria: An inborn error of metabolism associated with mental defect. Lancet, **2,** 253, 1968.
209. Mahadevan, S., and Tappel, A. L.: Arylaminidases of rat liver and kidney. J. Biol. Chem., **242,** 2369, 1967.
210. McKusick, V. A., Kaplan, D., Wise, D., Hanley, W. B., Suddarth, S. B., Sevick, M. E., and Maumenee, A. E.: The genetic mucopolysaccharidoses. Medicine (Balt.), **44,** 445, 1965.
211. Newell, F. W., and Koistinen, A.: Lipochondrodystrophy (gargoylism), pathologic findings in five eyes of three patients. Arch. Opthal. (Chicago), **53,** 45, 1955.
212. Wolff, D.: Microscopic study of temporal bones in dysotosis multiplex (gargoylism). Laryngoscope, **52,** 218, 1942.
213. Lindsay, S.: The cardiovascular system in gargoylism. Brit. Heart J., **12,** 17, 1950.
214. Emanuel, R. W.: Gargoylism with cardiovascular involvement in two brothers. Brit. Heart J., **16,** 417, 1954.
215. Okada, R., Rosenthal, T. M., Scaravelli, G., and Lev, M.: A histopathologic study of the heart in gargoylism. Arch. Path. (Chicago), **84,** 20, 1967.
216. Berenson, G. S., and Greer, J. C.: Heart disease in the Hurler and Marfan syndromes. Arch. Intern. Med. (Chicago), **111,** 58, 1963.
217. Craig, W. S.: Gargoylism in a twin brother and sister. Arch. Dis. Child., **29,** 293, 1954.
218. Neuhauser, E. B. D., Griscom, N. T., Gilles, F. H., and Crocker, A. C.: Arachnoid cyst in the Hurler-Hunter syndrome. Ann. Radiol. (Paris), **11,** 1, 1968.
219. Caffey, J.: Gargoylism (Hunter-Hurler disease, dysostosis multiplex, lipochondrodystrophy): Prenatal and neonatal bone lesions and their early postnatal evaluation. Amer. J. Roentgen., **67,** 715, 1952.
220. Jervis, G. A.: Gargoylism: Study of 10 cases with emphasis on the *formes frustes.* Arch. Neurol. Psychiat., **63,** 681, 1950.
221. Kobayashi, N.: Acid mucopolysaccharide granules in the glomerular epithelium in gargoylism. Amer. J. Path., **35,** 591, 1959.
222. Tuthill, C. R.: Juvenile amaurotic idiocy, marked adventitial growth associated with skeletal malformations and tuberculomas. Arch. Neurol. Psychiat., **32,** 198, 1934.
223. Haust, M. D., and Landing, B. H.: Histochemical studies in Hurler's disease; a new method for localization of acid mucopolysaccharide, and analysis of lead acetate "fixation." J. Histochem. Cytochem., **9,** 79, 1961.
224. Lagunoff, D., Ross, R., and Benditt, E. P.: Histochemical and electron microscopic study in a case of Hurler's syndrome. Amer. J. Path., **41,** 273, 1962,
225. Wolfe, H. J., Blennerhasset, J. B., Young, G. F., and Cohen, R. F.: Hurler's syndrome: A histochemical study. New techniques for localization of very water-soluble acid mucopolysaccharides. Amer. J. Path., **45,** 1007, 1964.
226. Van Hoof, F., and Hers, H. G.: The ultrastructure of hepatic cells in Hurler's disease (gargoylism). C. R. Acad. Sci. [D] (Paris), **259,** 1281, 1964.
227. Callahan, W. P., and Lorincz, A. E.: Hepatic ultrastructures in the Hurler syndrome. Amer. J. Path., **48,** 277, 1966.
228. Loeb, H., Jonnieaux, G., Resibois, A., Cremer, N., Dodion, J., Tondeur, M., Gregoire, P. E., Richard, J., and Cieters, P.: Biochemical and ultrastructural studies in Hurler's syndrome. J. Pediat., **73,** 860, 1968.
229. Callahan, W. P., Hackett, R. L., and Lorincz, A. E.: New observations by light microscopy on liver histology in the Hurler's syndrome. Arch. Path. (Chicago), **83,** 507, 1967.
230. Lagunoff, D., and Gritzka, T. L.: The site of mucopolysaccharide accumulation in Hurler syndrome. Lab. Invest., **15,** 1578, 1966.
231. De Cloux, R. J., and Friederici, H. H. R.: Ultrastructural studies of the skin in Hurler's syndrome. Arch. Path. (Chicago), **88,** 350, 1969.
232. Haust, M. D.: Crystaloid structures of hepatic mitochondria in children with heparitin sulfate mucopolysaccharidosis (Sanfilippo type). Exp. Molec. Path., **8,** 123, 1968.
233. Berard-Badier, M., Adechy-Benkoel, L., Chamilian, A., Dubois-Gambarelli, D., Casanova, P., and Mariani, A.: Étude ultrastructurale du parenchyme hepatique dans les mucopolysaccharidoses. Path. Biol. (Paris), **18,** 117, 1970.
234. Bartman, J., and Blanc, W. A.: Fibroblast cultures in Hurler's and Hunter's syndromes. Arch. Path. (Chicago), **89,** 279, 1970.
235. Duckett, S., Christian, J. C., Thompson, J. N., and Drew, A. L.: The ultrastructure of metachromatic bodies in cultured fibroblasts in Hunter's syndrome. Develop. Med. Child. Neurol., **11,** 764, 1969.
236. Conrad, G., Sherman, D., and Dorfman, A.: Unpublished results.
237. Aleu, F. P., Terry, R. D., and Zellweger, H.: Electron microscopy of two cerebral biopsies in gargoylism. J. Neuropath. Exp. Neurol., **24,** 304, 1965.
238. Aleu, F. P., Suzuki, K., and Zellweger, H.: Ultrastructural and biochemical observations of three cerebral biopsies in gargoylism. *Proc. 5th Int. Congr. Neuropathology,* Zurich, Sept., 1965, vol. 100, 149.
239. Escourolle, R., Berger, B., and Poiries, J.: Biopsie cerebrele d'un cas de mucopolysaccharidose H. S. (oligophrenie polydystrophighe au maladie de Sanfilippo) étude histochemique et ultrastructurale. Presse Med., **74,** 2869, 1966.
240. Gonatas, N. K., and Gonatas, J.: Ultrastructural and biochemical observations on a case of infantile lipidosis and its relationship to Tay Sachs disease and gargoylism. J. Neuropath. Exp. Neurol., **24,** 318, 1965.
241. Wallace, B. J., Kaplan, H., Adachie, M., Schneck, L., and Volk, B. W.: Mucopolysaccharidosis Type III. Arch. Path. (Chicago), **82,** 462, 1966.
242. Alder, A. von: Konstitutionell bedingte granulationsveränderungen der leucocyten and knochenveränderungen. Schweiz. Med. Wschr., **80,** 1095, 1950.
243. Reilly, W. A.: The granules in the leucocytes in gargoylism. Amer. J. Dis. Child., **62,** 489, 1941.
244. Mittwoch, U.: Nuclear segmentation of the neutrophils in heterozygous carriers of gargoylism. Nature (London), **193,** 1209, 1962.
245. Bowman, J. E., Mittwoch, U., and Schneiderman, L. J.: Persistence of mucopolysaccharide inclusions in culture of lymphocytes from patients with gargoylism. Nature (London), **195,** 612, 1962.
246. Carlisle, J. W., and Good, R. A.: The inflammatory cycle. Amer. J. Dis. Child., **99,** 193, 1960.
247. Jermain, L. F., Rohn, R. J., and Bond, W. H.: Studies on the role of the reticuloendothelial system in Hurler's disease. Clin. Res., **7,** 216, 1959.
248. Lindsay, S., Reilly, W. A., Gotham, T. J., and Skahen, R.: Gargoylism. II. Study of pathologic lesions and clinical review of twelve cases. Amer. J. Dis. Child., **76,** 239, 1948.

249. Meyer, K., and Hoffman, P.: Hurler's syndrome. Arthritis Rheumat., **4**, 552, 1961.
250. Danes, B. S., and Bearn, A. G.: The correction of cellular metachromasia in cultured fibroblasts in several inherited mucopolysaccharidoses. Proc. Nat. Acad. Sci., U.S.A., **67**, 357, 1970.
251. Anderssen, B., and Tandberg, O.: Lipochondrodystrophy (gargoylism, Hurler syndrome) with specific cutaneous deposits. Acta Paediat. **41**, 162, 1952.
252. Njå, A.: A sex-linked type of gargoylism. Acta Paediat., **33**, 267, 1946.
253. Lundstrom, R.: Gargoylism; three cases. Nord. Med., **33**, 41, 1947.
254. Hooper, J. M. D.: Unusual case of gargoylism. Guy. Hosp. Rep., **101**, 222, 1952.
255. Beebe, R. T., and Formel, P. F.: Gargoylism: Sex linked transmissions in nine males. Trans. Amer. Clin. Climat. Ass., **66**, 199, 1954.
256. Millman, G., and Whittick, J. W.: A sex-linked variant of gargoylism. J. Neurol. Neurosurg. Psychiat., **15**, 253, 1952.
257. Cunningham, R. C.: A contribution to the genetics of gargoylism. J. Neurol. Neurosurg. Psychiat., **17**, 191, 1954.
258. Van Pelt, J. F.: Gargoylism. Thesis, Nijmegen University, 1960.
259. Campbell, T. N., and Fried, M.: Urinary mucopolysaccharide excretion in the sex-linked form of the Hurler syndrome. Proc. Soc. Exp. Biol. Med., **108**, 529, 1961.
260. Teller, W. M., Rosevear, J. W., and Burke, E. C.: Identification of heterozygous carriers of gargoylism. Proc. Soc. Exp. Biol. Med., **108**, 276, 1961.
261. Van Pelt, J. F., and Huizinga, J.: Some observations on the genetics of gargoylism. Acta Genet. (Basel), **12**, 1, 1962.
262. Lorincz, A. E.: Acid mucopolysaccharides in the Hurler syndrome. Fed. Proc., **17**, 266, 1958.
263. Harris, R. C.: Mucopolysaccharide disorder: A possible new genotype of Hurler's syndrome (abstract). Amer. J. Dis. Child. **102**. 741, 1961.
264. Sanfilippo, S. J., Podosin, R., Langer, L. O., Jr., and Good, R. A.: Mental retardation associated with acid mucopolysaccharides (heparitin sulfate type). J. Pediat., **63**, 837, 1963.
265. Maroteaux, P., and Lamy, M.: La pseudo-polydystrophie de Hurler. Presse Med., **74**, No. 55, 2889, 1966.
266. Langer, L. O.: The radiographic manifestations of the HS-mucopolysaccharidosis of Sanfilippo, with discussion of this condition in relation to the other mucopolysaccharidoses and a classification of these fundamentally similar entities. Ann. Radiol. (Paris), **7**, 315, 1964.
267. Berggård, I., and Bearn, A. G.: The Hurler syndrome: A biochemical and clinical study. Amer. J. Med., **39**, 221, 1965.
268. Kresse, H., Wiesmann, U., Cantz, M., Hall, C. W., and Neufeld, E. F.: Biochemical heterogeneity of the Sanfilippo syndrome: preliminary characterization of two deficient factors. Biochem. Biophys. Res. Commun., **42**, 892, 1971.
269. Scheie, H. G., Hambrick, G. W., Jr., and Barness, L. A.: A newly recognized *forme fruste* of Hurler's disease (gargoylism). Amer. J. Ophthal., **53**, 753, 1962.
270. Wiesmann, U., and Neufeld, E. F.: Scheie and Hurler syndromes: Apparent identity of the biochemical defect. Science, **169**, 72, 1970.
271. Rampini, S.: Der Spät-Hurler: Ullrich-Scheie Syndrome, mukopolysaccharodose V. Schweiz. Med. Wschr., **99**, 1769, 1969.
272. Kaplan, D.: Classification of the mucopolysaccharidoses based on the pattern of mucopolysacchariduria. Amer. J. Med., **47**, 721, 1969.
273. Maroteaux, P., Lévêque, B., Marie, J., and Lamy, M.: Une nouvelle dysostose avec elimination urinaire de chondroitine-sulfate B. Presse Med., **71**, 1849, 1963.
274. Morquio, L.: Sur une forme de dystrophie osseuses familiale,. Bull. Soc. Pediat., Paris, **27**, 536, 1929.
275. Brailsford, J. F.: Chondro-osteo-dystrophy: Roentgenographic and clinical features of child with dislocation of vertebrae. Amer. J. Surg., **7**, 404, 1929.
276. Zellweger, H., Ponseti, I. V. Pedrini, V., Stamler, F. S., and von Moorden, G. K.: Morquio-Ullrich's disease. J. Pediat., **59**, 549, 1961.
277. Wiedemann, H. R.: Ausgedehnte und allgemeine erblich bedingte Bildungs—und Wachstumsfehler des Knochengerustes. Mschr. Kinderheilk., **102**, 136. 1954.
278. Maroteaux, P., and Lamy, M.: Opacités cornéennes et trouble metabolique dans la maladie de Morquio. Rev. Franc. Étud. Clin. Biol., **6**, 481, 1961.
279. Maroteaux, P., and Lamy, M.: Hurler's disease, Morquio's disease and related mucopolysaccharidoses. J. Pediat., **67**, 312, 1965.
280. Einhorn, N. H., Moore, J. R., Ostrum, H. W., and Rountree, L. G.: Osteochondrodystrophia deformans (Morquio's disease): Report of three cases. Amer. J. Dis. Child. **61**, 776, 1941.
281. Einhorn, N. H., Moore, J. R., and Rountree, L. G.: Osteochondrodystrophia deformans (Morquio's disease): Observations at autopsy in one case. Amer. J. Dis. Child., **72**, 536, 1946.
282. Schenk, E. A., and Haggerty, J.: Morquio's disease, a radiologic and morphologic study. Pediatrics, **34**, 839, 1964.
283. Tondeur, M., and Loeb, H.: Étude ultrastructurelle du foie dans la maladie de Morquio. Pediat. Res., **3**, 19, 1969.
284. Danes, B. S., and Grossman, H.: Bone dysplasia including Morquio's syndrome, studied in skin fibroblast cultures. Amer. J. Med., **47**, 708, 1969.
285. Jacobsen, A. W.: Hereditary osteochondrodystrophia deformans: A family with twenty members affected in five generations. JAMA, **113**, 121, 1939.
286. Craig, J. M., Clarke, J. T., and Banker, B. Q.: Metabolic neurovisceral disorder with accumulation of an unidentified substance: Variant of Hurler's syndrome? Amer. J. Dis. Child., **98**, 577, 1959.
287. Norman, R. M., Tingey, A. H., Newman, C. G. H., and Ward, S. P.: Tay-Sachs disease with visceral involvement and its relation to gargoylism. Arch. Dis. Child. **39**, 634, 1964.
288. Landing, B. H., Silverman, F. N., Craig, J. M., Jacoby, M. D., Lahey, M. E., and Chadwick, D. L.: Familial neurovisceral lipidosis: An analysis of eight cases of a syndrome previously reported as "Hurler-variant," "Pseudo-Hurler disease," and "Tay-Sachs disease with visceral involvement." Am. J. Dis. Child., **108**, 503, 1964.
289. MacBrinn, M. C., Okada, S., Ho, M. W., Hu, C. C., and O'Brien, J. S.: Generalized gangliosidoses: Impaired cleavage of galactose from mucopolysaccharide and a glycoprotein. Science, **163**, 946, 1969.
290. Pinsky, L., Callahan, J. W., and Wolfe, L. S.: Fucosidosis? Lancet, **2**, 1080, 1968.
291. Dyggve, H. V., Melchior, J. C., and Clausen, J.: Morquio-Ulrich's disease: An inborn error of metabolism? Arch. Dis. Child. **37**, 525, 1962.
292. De Mars, R., and Leroy, J. G.: The remarkable cells cultured from a human with Hurler's syndrome: An approach to visual selection for *in vitro* genetic studies. In Vitro, **2**, 107, 1966.
293. Leroy, J. G., and DeMars, R.: Mutant enzymatic and cytological phenotypes in cultured human fibroblasts. Science, **157**, 804, 1967.
294. Matalon, R., Cifonelli, J. A., Zellweger, H., and Dorfman, A.: Lipid abnormalities in a variant of the Hurler syndrome. Proc. Nat. Acad. Sci., U.S.A., **59**, 1097, 1968.
295. Hof, L., Dawson, G., Matalon, R., and Dorfman, A.: Unpublished data.
296. Matalon, R., and Dorman, A.: Unpublished results.
297. Spranger, J. W., Wiedemann, H. R., Tolksdorf, M., Graucob, E., and Caesar, R.: Lipomucopolysaccharidose: Eine neue speicherkrankheit. Z. Kinderheilk., **103**, 285, 1968.
298. Spranger, J. W., and Wiedemann, H. R.: Lipomucopolysaccharidosis: A second look. Lancet, **2**, 270, 1969.
299. Van Hoof, F., and Hers, H. G.: The abnormalities of lysosomal enzymes in mucopolysaccharidosis. Europ. J. Biochem., **7**, 34, 1968.
300. Loeb, H., Tondeur, M., Toppet, M., and Cremer, M.: Clinical biochemical and ultrastructural studies of an atypical form of mucopolysaccharidosis. Acta Paediat. Scand., **58**, 220, 1969.
301. Luchsinger, U., Bühler, E. M., Méhes, K., and Kint, H. R.: I-cell disease. New Eng. J. Med., **282**, 1374, 1970.
302. Öckerman, P.-A.: A generalized storage disease resembling Hurler's syndrome. Lancet, **2**, 293. 1967.
303. Kjellman, B., Gamstrop, I., Brun, A., Öckerman, P.-A., and Palmgren, B.: Mannosidosis: A clinical and histopathologic study. J. Pediat., **75**, 366, 1969.
304. Durand, P., Phillipart, M., Barrone, C., Della Cella, G., and Bugiani, O.: Una nuova malattia da occumuola di glicolipidi. Minerva Pediat., **19**, 2187, 1967.

305. Durand, P., Barrone, C., and Della Cella, G.: Fucosidosis. J. Pediat., **75**, 665, 1969.
306. Durand, P., Barrone, C., Della Cella, G., and Philippart, M.: Fucosidosis. Lancet, **1**, 1198, 1968.
307. Van Hoof, F., and Hers, H. G.: Mucopolysaccharidosis by absence of α-fucosidase. Lancet, **1**, 1198, 1968.
308. Loeb, H., Tondeur, M., Jonniaux, G., Mockel-Pohl, S., and Vamos-Hurwitz, E.: Biochemical and ultracentrifugal studies in a case of mucopolysaccharidosis "F" (fucosidosis). Helv. Paediat. Acta, **24**, 519, 1969.
309. Szabo, L., Polgar, J., Vass, Z., and Jozsa, L: A Hurler's syndrome variant. Lancet, **2**, 1314, 1967.
310. Bischel, M. D., Austin, J. H., and Kemeny, M. D.: Metachromatic leukodystrophy. VII. Elevated sulfated acid polysaccharide levels in urine and post-mortem tissues. Arch. Neurol. (Chicago), **15**, 13, 1966.
311. Abul-Haj, S. K., Martz, D. G., Douglas, W. F., and Geppert, L. J.: Farber's disease: Report of a case with observations on its histogenesis and notes on the nature of the stored material. J. Pediat., **61**, 221, 1962.
312. Philippart, M., and Sugarman, G. I.: Chondroitin-4-sulfphate mucopolysaccharidosis—a new variant of Hurler's syndrome. Lancet, **2**, 854, 1969.
313. Dorfman, A., and Ho, P. L.: Unpublished results.
314. Pincus, J. H., Rossi, J. P., and Daroff, R. B.: Delayed development of disturbed mucopolysaccharide metabolism in a Hurler variant. Arch. Neurol. (Chicago), **16**, 244, 1967.
315. Winchester, P., Grossman, H., Lim, W. N., and Danes, B. S.: A new acid mucopolysaccharidosis with skeletal deformities stimulating rheumatoid arthritis. Amer. Roentgen., **106**, 121, 1969.
316. Schimke, R. N., and Horton, W. A.: A new mucopolysaccharidosis. Clin. Res., **17**, 530, 1969.
317. Steinback, H. L., Preger, L., Williams, H. E., and Cohen, P.: The Hurler syndrome without abnormal mucopolysacchariduria. Radiology, **90**, 472, 1968.
318. Langer, L. O., Jr., Kronenberg, R. S., and Gorlin, R. J.: A case simulating Hurler syndrome of unusual longevity, without abnormal mucopolysacchariduria. Amer. J. Med., **40**, 448, 1966.
319. Zugibe, F. T., Gilbert, E. F., and Gaziano, D.: Glycoprotein storage disease, a new entity. Amer. J. Med., **47**, 135, 1969.
320. de Lange, C., Gerlings, P. G., de Kleyn, A., and Lettinga, T. W.: Some remarks on gargoylism. Acta Paediat., **31**, 398, 1944.
321. Strauss, L.: The pathology of gargoylism: Report of a case and review of the literature. Amer. J. Path., **24**, 855, 1948.
322. Uzman, L. L.: Chemical nature of the storage substance in gargoylism. Arch. Path. (Chicago), **60**, 308, 1955.
323. Stacey, M., and Barker, S. A.: Chemical analysis of tissue polysaccharides. J. Clin. Path., **9**, 314, 1956.
324. Bishton, R. L., Norman, R. M., and Tingey, A.: The pathology and chemistry of a case of gargoylism. J. Clin. Path., **9**, 305, 1956.
325. Dorfman, A., and Lorincz, A. E.: Occurrence of urinary acid mucopolysaccharides in the Hurler syndrome. Proc. Nat. Acad. Sci., U.S.A., **43**, 443, 1957.
326. Brown, D. H.: Tissue storage of mucopolysaccharides in Hurler-Pfaundler's disease. Proc. Nat. Acad. Sci., U.S.A., **43**, 783, 1957.
327. Meyer, K., Grumbach, M. M., Linker, A., and Hoffman, P.: Excretion of sulfated mucopolysaccharides in gargoylism (Hurler's syndrome). Proc. Soc. Exp. Biol. Med., **97**, 275, 1958.
328. Meyer, K., Hoffman, P., Linker, A., Grumbach, M. M., and Sampson, P.: Sulfated mucopolysaccharides in urine and organs in gargoylism (Hurler's syndrome). II. Additional studies. Proc. Soc. Exp. Biol. Med., **102**, 587, 1959.
329. Scott, J. E.: Aliphatic ammonium salts in the assay of acidic polysaccharides from tissues, in *Methods of Biochemical Analyses,* edited by D. Glick, 2d printing, vol. 8, p. 145. Interscience, New York, 1960.
330. Lagunoff, D., and Warren, G.: Determination of 2-deoxy-D-sulfoaminohexose content of mucopolysaccharides. Arch. Biochem., **99**, 396, 1962.
331. Dorfman, A.: Studies on the biochemistry of connective tissue. Pediatrics, **22**, 576, 1958.
332. Dorfman, A., and Ott, M. L.: A turbidimetric method for the assay of hyaluronidase. J. Biol. Chem., **176**, 267, 1948.
333. Berry, H., and Spinanger, J.: Screening test for Hurler's syndrome. J. Lab. Clin. Med., **55**, 136, 1960.
334. Carson, N. A. J., and Neill, D. W.: Metabolic abnormalities detected in a survey of mentally backward individuals of Northern Ireland. Arch. Dis. Child., **37**, 505, 1962.
335. Renuart, A. W.: Screening of inborn errors of metabolism associated with mental deficiency or neurological disorders or both. New Eng. J. Med., **274**, 384, 1966.
336. Manley, G., and Hawksworth, J.: Diagnosis of Hurler's syndrome in the hospital laboratory and the determination of its genetic type. Arch. Dis. Child., **41**, 91, 1966.
337. Steiness, T. B.: Acid mucopolysaccharides in urine in gargoylism. Pediatrics, **27**, 112, 1961.
338. Carter, C. H., Wan, A. T., and Carpenter, D. G.: Commonly used tests in the detection of Hurler's syndrome. J. Pediat., **73**, 217, 1968.
339. Procopis, P. G., Turner, B., Ruxton, J. T., and Brown, D. A.: Screening tests for mucopolysaccharidoses. J. Ment. Defic. Res., **12**, 13, 1968.
340. Pennock, C. A., Mott, M. G., and Batstone, G. F.: Screening for mucopolysaccharidoses. Clin. Chim. Acta, **27**, 93, 1970.
341. Ho, P. L., and Dorfman, A.: Unpublished data.
342. Dische, Z.: A new specific color reaction of hexuronic acids. J. Biol. Chem., **167**, 189, 1947.
343. Brown, A. H.: Determination of pentose in the presence of large quantities of glucose. Arch. Biochem., **24**, 269, 1946.
344. Boas, N. F.: Method for determination of hexosamines in tissues. J. Biol. Chem., **204**, 553, 1953.
345. Constantopoulos, G.: Hurler-Hunter syndromes: Gel filtration and dialysis of urinary mucopolysaccharides. Nature (London), **220**, 583, 1968.
346. DiFerrante, N., and Rich, C.: The determination of aminopolysaccharides in urine. J. Lab. Clin. Med., **48**, 491, 1956.
347. DiFerrante, N.: The measurement of urinary mucopolysaccharides. Anal. Biochem., **21**, 98, 1967.
348. Linker, A., Evans, L. R., and Madsen, J. A.: Problems in the analysis of urinary mucopolysaccharide excretion. Biochem. Med., **2**, 448, 1969.
349. DiFerrante, N.: Acid mucopolysaccharides in normal human urine. J. Lab. Clin. Med., **61**, 633, 1963.
350. Linker, A., and Terry, K. D.: Urinary acid mucopolysaccharides in normal man and in Hurler's syndrome. Proc. Soc. Exp. Biol. Med., **113**, 743, 1963.
351. Berenson, G. S., and Dalferes, E. R., Jr.: Urinary excretion of mucopolysaccharide in normal individuals and in the Marfan syndrome. Biochim. Biophys. Acta, **101**, 183, 1968.
352. Varadi, D. P., Cifonelli, J. A., and Dorfman, A.: The acid mucopolysaccharides in normal urine. Biochim. Biophys. Acta, **141**, 103, 1967.
353. Orii, T.: Non-sulfated acid mucopolysaccharide excretion in normal male children and adults. Biochim. Biophys. Acta, **170**, 204, 1968.
354. Chakrapani, B., and Bachhawat, B. K.: Glycosaminoglycans of human urine. Part I. Protein-polysaccharide linkage region in the non-sulphated glycosaminoglycans of normal urine. Indian J. Biochem., **5**, 9, 1968.
355. Orii, T.: The urinary acid mucopolysaccharides in normal male children. Hoppe-Seyler's Z. Physiol. Chem., **349**, 816, 1968.
356. Lagunoff, D., Pritzl, P., and Scott, C. R.: Urinary N-sulfate glycosaminoglycan excretion in children: Normal and abnormal values. Proc. Soc. Exp. Biol. Med., **126**, 34, 1967.
357. Teller, W. M.: Urinary excretion patterns of individual acid mucopolysaccharides. Nature (London), **213**, 1132, 1967.
358. Manley, G., Severn, M., and Hawksworth, J.: Excretion patterns of glycosaminoglycans and glycoproteins in normal human urine. J. Clin. Path., **21**, 339, 1968.
359. Mayes, J. S., and Hansen, R. G.: Mucopolysaccharide excretion in patients with Hurler's syndrome, their families and normal man. Proc. Soc. Exp. Biol. Med., **122**, 927, 1966.
360. Spranger, J. W., Todt, H., and Wiedemann, H. R.: Untersuchungen zur zusammensetzung der urinmukopolysaccharide bei kindern und erwachsenen. Clin. Chim. Acta, **17**, 142, 1967.

361. Teller, W. M., Burke, E. C., Rosevear, J. W., and McKenzie, B. F.: Urinary excretion of acid mucopolysaccharides in normal children and patient with gargoylism. J. Lab. Clin. Med., **59,** 95, 1962.
362. Kaplan, D.: A heparitin serine compound from human urine. Biochim. Biophys. Acta, **136,** 394, 1967.
363. Fransson, L.-Å., and Dorfman, A.: Unpublished results.
364. Dorfman, A., Ho, P. L., and Warkany, J.: Unpublished data.
365. Terry, K., and Linker, A.: Distinction among four forms of Hurler's syndrome. Proc. Soc. Exp. Biol. Med., **115,** 394, 1964.
366. Spranger, J. W.: Biochemical definition of the mucopolysaccharidoses. Z. Kinderheilk, **108,** 17, 1970.
367. Teller, W. M., Rosevear, J. W., and Burke, E. C.: Identification of heterozygous carriers of gargoylism. Proc. Soc. Exp. Biol. Med., **108,** 276, 1961.
368. Teller, W. M., Bechtelsheimer, H., and Totovic, V.: Die heparitin-sulfat-mucopolysaccharidose (Sanfilippo) Klinsche, biochemische, genetische und morphologische untersuchen. Klin. Wschr., **45,** 497, 1967.
369. Rennert, O. M., and Dekaban, A. S.: Amino acid metabolism in patients with Hurler's syndrome. Metabolism, **15,** 429, 1966.
370. Schiller, S.: The isolation of chondroitin sulfuric acid from normal human plasma. Biochim. Biophys. Acta, **28,** 413, 1958.
371. Calatroni, A., Donnelly, P. V., and DiFerrante, N.: The glycosaminoglycans of human plasma J. Clin. Invest., **48,** 332, 1969.
372. Usui, T., Sano, T., and Matsuura, A.: Effect of prednisolone on serum and urinary mucopolysaccharides in Hurler's disease. Ann. Pediat. Japon., **14,** 213, 1968.
373. Constantopoulos, G., and Dekaban, A. S.: Acid mucopolysaccharides in cerebrospinal fluid of patients with Hunter-Hurler's syndrome. J. Neurochem., **17,** 117, 1970.
374. Berenson, G. S., and Serra, M. T.: Mucopolysaccharides in urine from patients with Marfan's syndrome. Fed. Proc., **18,** 749, 1959.
375. Bacchus, H.: Serum seromucoid and acid mucopolysaccharides in the Marfan syndrome. J. Lab. Clin. Med., **55,** 221, 1960.
376. Lorincz, A. E.: Urinary acid mucopolysaccharides in hereditary deforming chondrodysplasia (diphysical aclasis) Fed. Proc., **19,** 148, 1960.
377. Lorincz, A. E.: Mucopolysacchariduria in children with hereditary arthro-osteo-onychondysplasia. Fed. Proc., **21,** 173, 1962.
378. Wessler, E.: Determination of acidic glycosaminoglycans (mucopolysaccharides) in urine by an ion exchange method. Application to "collagenoses," gargoylism, the nail-patella syndrome and Farber's disease. Clin. Chim. Acta, **16,** 235, 1967.
379. Lorincz, A. E.: Hurler's syndrome in man and snorter dwarfism in cattle. Clin. Orthop., **33,** 104, 1964.
380. Tyler, W. S., Gregory, P. W., and Meyer, K.: Sulfated mucopolysaccharides of urine from brachycephalic bovine dwarfs. Amer. J. Vet. Res., **23,** 1109, 1962.
381. Mayer, J. S., Hansen, R. G., Gregory, P. W., and Tyler, W. S.: Mucopolysaccharide excretion in dwarf cattle. Fed. Proc., **22,** 412, 1963.
382. DiFerrante, N.: Urinary excretion of acid mucopolysaccharides by patients with rheumatoid arthritis. J. Lab. Clin. Med., **36,** 1516, 1957.
383. DiFerrante, N., Robbins, W. C., and Rich, C.: Urinary excretion of acid mucopolysaccharides by patients with lupus erythematosus. J. Lab. Clin. Med., **50,** 897, 1957.
384. Thompson, G. R., and Castor, C. W.: The excretion of nondialyzable urinary mucopolysaccharide in rheumatic and other systemic disease states. J. Lab. Clin. Med., **68,** 617, 1966.
385. Brunish, R., and Sorensen, B.: Urinary excretion of acid mucopolysaccharides and hydroxyproline in psoriasis. Dermatologica (Basel), **130,** 165, 1965.
386. Loewi, G.: Urinary excretion of acid polysaccharide in rheumatoid arthritis and other diseases. Ann. Rheum. Dis., **18,** 239, 1959.
387. Asboe-Hansen, G., and Clausen, J.: Mastocytosis (urticaria pigmentosa) with urinary excretion of hyaluronic acid and chondroitin sulfuric acid. Amer. J. Med., **36,** 144, 1964.
388. Winand, R. J.: Increased urinary excretion of acidic mucopolysaccharides in exophthalmos. J. Clin. Invest., **47,** 2563, 1968.
389. Øhlenschlaeger, K., and Friman, C.: A normal urinary excretion of acid mucopolysaccharides in generalized scleroderma. Scand. J. Clin. Lab. Invest., **21,** 364, 1968.
390. Morse, B. S., and Nussbaum, M.: The detection of hyaluronic acid in the serum and urine of a patient with nephroblastoma. Amer. J. Med., **42,** 996, 1967.
391. Matalon, R., Arcilla, R., Thilenius, O., and Replogle, R.: Unpublished data.
392. Kerby, G. P.: The excretion of glucuronic acid and of acid mucopolysaccharides in normal human urine. J. Clin. Invest., **33,** 1168, 1954.
393. Rich, C., DiFerrante, N., and Archibald, R. M.: Acid mucopolysaccharide excretion in the urine of children. J. Lab. Clin. Med., **50,** 686, 1957.
394. Muir, H., Mittwoch, U., and Bitter, T.: The diagnostic value of isolated urinary mucopolysaccharides and of lymphocytic inclusions in gargoylism. Arch. Dis. Child., **38,** 358, 1963.
395. Lin, M. C., Hall, W. K., Thevaos, T. G., and Coryell, M. B.: Mucopolysaccharide excretion in man. Fed. Proc., **23,** 483, 1964.
396. Jervis, G. A.: Familial mental deficiency akin to amaurotic idiocy and gargoylism: An apparently new type. Arch. Neurol. Psychiat., **47,** 943, 1942.
397. Brante, G.: Chemical pathology in gargoylism, in *Cerebral Lipidoses,* edited by J. M. Cumings and M. Lowenthal, p. 164. Blackwell, Oxford, 1957.
398. Taghavy, A., Salsman, K., and Ledeen, R.: An abnormal ganglioside pattern from a gargoyle brain. Fed. Proc., **23,** 128, 1964.
399. Ledeen, R., Salsman, K., Gonatas, J., and Taghavy, A.: Structure comparison of the major monosialogangliosides from brains of normal human, gargoylism, and late infantile systemic lipidosis. Part I. J. Neuropath. Exp. Neurol., **24,** 341, 1965.
400. Gonatas, N. K., and Gonatas, J.: Ultrastructural and biochemical observations on a case of systemic late infantile lipidosis and its relationship to Tay-Sachs disease and gargoylismus. J. Neuropath. Exp. Neurol., **24,** 318, 1965.
401. Suzuki, K.: Ganglioside patterns of normal and pathological brains, in *Sphingolipidoses,* edited by S. M. Aronson and B. W. Volk. 3rd Int. Symp. Sphingolipidoses, 1965, Pergamon, New York, 1966.
402. Taketomi, T., and Yamakawa, T.: Glycolipids of the brain in gargoylism. Jap. J. Exp. Med., **37,** 11, 1967.
403. Danes, B. S., and Bearn, A. G.: Hurler's syndrome: Demonstration of an inherited disorder of connective tissue in cell culture. Science, **149,** 989, 1965.
404. Matalon, R., and Dorfman, A.: Hurler's syndrome: Biosynthesis of acid mucopolysaccharides in tissue culture. Proc. Nat. Acad. Sci., USA, **56,** 1310, 1966.
405. Schafer, I. A., Sullivan, J. C., Svejcar, J., Kofoed, J., and Robertson, W. van B.: Vitamin C–induced increase of dermatan sulfate in cultured Hurler's fibroblasts. Science, **153,** 1008, 1966.
406. Dorfman, A., and Ho, P. L.: Unpublished data.
407. Danes, B. S., and Bearn, A. G.: Hurler's syndrome: A genetic study in cell culture. J. Exp. Med., **123,** 1, 1966.
408. Danes, B. S., and Bearn, A. G.: Hurler's syndrome: A genetic study of clones in cell cultures with particular reference to the Lyon hypothesis. J. Exp. Med., **126,** 509, 1967.
409. Danes, B. S., and Bearn, A. G.: A genetic cell marker in cystic fibrosis of the pancreas. Lancet, **1,** 1061, 1968.
410. Matalon, R., and Dorfman, A.: The accumulation of hyaluronic acid in cultured fibroblasts of the Marfan syndrome. Biochem. Biophys. Res. Commun., **32,** 150, 1968.
411. Matalon, R., Dorfman, A., Dawson, G., and Sweeley, C. C.: Glycolipid and mucopolysaccharide abnormality in fibroblasts of Fabry's disease. Science, **164,** 1522, 1969.
412. Danes, B. S., Scott, J. E., and Bearn, A. G.: Cell culture studies: Staining of glycosaminoglycans (mucopolysaccharides) by Alcian blue in salt solution. J. Exp. Med., **132,** 765, 1970.
413. Foley, K. M., Danes, B. S., and Bearn, A. G.: White blood cell cultures in genetic studies on the human mucopolysaccharidoses. Science, **164,** 424, 1969.
414. Danes, B. S.: The use of WBC cultures in the study of genetic metabolic diseases. Hosp. Practice, vol. 52, 1970.
415. Danes, B. S., Foley, K. M., Dillon, S. D., and Bearn, A. G.: Genetic study of cystic fibrosis of the pancreas using white blood cell cultures. Nature (London), **222,** 685, 1969.

416. Danes, B. S., and Bearn, A. G.: Cystic fibrosis of the pancreas. J. Exp. Med., **129,** 775, 1969.
417. Danes, B. S., and Bearn, A. G.: Cystic fibrosis: Distribution of mucopolysaccharides in fibroblast cultures. Biochem. Biophys. Res. Commun., **36,** 919, 1969.
418. Wiesmann, U., and Neufeld, E. F.: Metabolism of sulfated mucopolysaccharide in cultured fibroblasts from cystic fibrosis patients. J. Pediat., **77,** 685, 1970.
419. Matalon, R., and Dorfman, A.: Unpublished data.
420. Matalon, R., and Dorfman, A.: Acid mucopolysaccharides in cultured fibroblasts of cystic fibrosis of the pancreas. Biochem. Biophys. Res. Commun., **33,** 954, 1968.
421. Taysi, K., Kistenmacher, M. L., Punnett, H. H., and Mellman, W. J.: Limitations of metachromasia as a diagnostic aid in pediatrics. New Eng. J. Med., **281,** 1108, 1969.
422. Dorfman, A., and Matalon, R.: The Hurler and Hunter syndromes. Amer. J. Med., **47,** 691, 1969.
423. Fraccaro, M., Mannini, A., Lenzi, L., Magrini, U., Perona, P., and Sartori, E.: Morquio's disease: Metachromatic granules in cultured fibroblasts. Lancet, **1,** 508, 1967.
424. Danes, B. S., and Bearn, A. G.: Studying the mucopolysaccharidoses. Lancet, **1,** 793, 1967.
425. Romano, C., and Sietti, C.: Studying the mucopolysaccharidoses. Lancet, **2,** 210, 1967.
426. Durand, P., Borrone, C., and Della Cella, G.: Studying the mucopolysaccharidoses. Lancet, **1,** 1278, 1967.
427. Hors-Cayla, M.-C., Maroteaux, P., and deGrouchy, J.: Fibroblastes en culture au cours de mucopolysaccharidoses: Influence du serum sur la metachromasie. Ann. Genet. (Paris), **11,** 265, 1968.
428. Neufeld, E. F., and Fratantoni, J. C.: Inborn errors of mucopolysaccharide metabolism. Science, **169,** 141, 1970.
429. Cartwright, E., Danks, D. M., and Jack, I.: Metachromatic fibroblasts in pseudoxanthoma elasticum and Marfan's syndrome. Lancet, **1,** 533, 1969.
430. Danes, B. S., and Bearn, A. G.: Gaucher's disease: A genetic disease detected in skin fibroblast cultures. Science, **161,** 1347, 1968.
431. Danes, B. S., and Bearn, A. G.: Metachromasia and skin fibroblast cultures in juvenile familial amaurotic idiocy. Lancet, **2,** 855, 1968.
432. Swift, M. R., and Feingold, M. J.: Myotonic muscular dystrophy: Abnormalities in fibroblast cultures. Science, **165,** 294, 1969.
433. Lamy, M., Maroteaux, P., and Bader, J. P.: Étude génétique du gargoylisme. J. Genet. Hum. **6,** 156, 1957.
434. Aycock, E. K., and Paul, J. R., Jr.: Gargoylism: A report of two cases in Negroes. J. S. Carolina Med. Ass., **53,** 128, 1957.
435. Engle, D.: Dysostosis multiplex (Pfaundler-Hurler Syndrome): Two cases. Arch. Dis. Child., **14,** 217, 1939.
436. Griffiths, S. B., and Findlay, M.: Gargoylism: Clinical, radiological and haematological features in two siblings. Arch. Dis. Child., **32,** 229, 1958.
437. Kitagawa, M., Nishimura, H., and Makita, A.: Gargoylism and amaurotic family idiocy: Case report with histochemical and chemical survey. Acta Path. Jap., **12,** 129, 1962.
438. Halpern, S. L., and Curtis, G.: The genetics of gargoylism. Amer. J. Ment. Defic., **46,** 298, 1942.
439. Herndon, C. N., Goodman, H. O., and David, P. R. quoted by Neel, J. V.: On some pitfalls in developing an adequate genetic hypothesis. Amer. J. Hum. Genet., **7,** 1, 1955.
440. Berg, K., Danes, B. S., and Bearn, A. G.: The linkage relation of the loci for the *Xm* serum system and the X-linked form of Hurler's syndrome (Hunter's syndrome). Amer. J. Hum. Genet., **20,** 398, 1968.
441. Nonne, M.: Familiaries verkommen (3 geschwister) einer kombination von imperrfekter chondrodystrophie mit imperfekten myxoedema infantile. Z. Nervenheilk., **83,** 263, 1925.
442. Gasteiger, H., and Liebenam, L.: Beitrag zur dysostosis multiplex unter besonderer beruchsichtigung des augenbefundes. Klin. Mbl. Augenheilk., **99,** 333, 1937.
443. Gayler, B. W., and Fried, M.: Chromosome number and morphology in Hurler's syndrome. J. Clin, Path., **38,** 590, 1962.
444. Fratantoni, J. C., Neufeld, E. F., Uhlendorf, W., and Jacobson, C. B.: Intrauterine diagnosis of Hunter and Hurler syndromes. New Eng. J. Med., **280,** 686, 1969.
445. Matalon, R., Dorfman, A., Jacobson, C. B., and Nadler, H. L.: A chemical method for the antenatal diagnosis of mucopolysaccharidoses. Lancet, **1,** 85, 1970.
446. Danes, B. S., Queenan, J. T., Gadon, E., and Cederquist, L. L.: Antenatal diagnosis of mucopolysaccharidoses. Lancet, **1,** 946, 1970.
447. Olsson, T., Gardell, S., and Thunell, S.: Biosynthesis of glycosaminoglycans (mucopolysaccharides) in human leukocytes. Biochim. Biophys. Acta, **165,** 309, 1968.
448. Fratantoni, J. C., Hall, C. W., and Neufeld, E. F.: The defect in Hurler's and Hunter's syndromes: Faulty degradation of mucopolysaccharide. Proc. Nat. Acad. Sci., U.S.A., **60,** 699, 1968.
449. Öckerman, P. A.: Acid hydrolases in skin and plasma in gargoylism: Deficiency of β-galactosidase in skin. Clin. Chim. Acta, **20,** 1, 1968.
450. Gerich, J. E.: Hunter's syndrome: β-galactosidase deficiency in skin. New Eng. J. Med., **280,** 799, 1969.
451. Bartsocas, C. S., and Moser, H. W.: In vivo kinetics of polysaccharides in the Hurler and Sanfilippo syndromes. *Presented at Meetings of Amer. Pediat. Soc. Soc. Pediat. Res.,* Atlantic City, N. J., April 29, 1970 to May 2, 1970.
452. Öckerman, P. A.: Lysosomal acid hydrolases in the liver in gargoylism: Deficiency of 4-methyl umbelliferyl-β-galactosidase. Scand. J. Clin. Lab. Invest., **22,** 142, 1968.
453. Austin, J. H., McAfree, D., Armstrong, D., Rourke, M., Shearer, L., and Bachhawat, B. K.: Abnormal sulfatase activities in two human diseases (metachromatic leucodystrophy and gargoylism). Biochem. J., **93,** 15, 1964.
454. Van Gemund, J. J., Giesberts, M. A., Gorsira, M. C., and Willighagen, R. G.: Deficiency of 4-methyl umbelliferyl-β-galactosidase activity in the livers of seven patients with Hurler's disease. Maandschr. Kindergeneesk., **36,** 377, 1969.
455. Öckerman, P., Hultberg, B., and Erickson, O.: Enzyme patterns in tissues and body fluids in mucopolysaccharidoses. Clin. Chim. Acta, **25,** 97, 1969.
456. MacBrinn, M., Okada, S., Woolacott, M., Patel, V., Ho, M. W., Tappel, A. L., and O'Brien, J. S.: Beta galactosidase deficiency in the Hurler syndrome. New Eng. J. Med., **281,** 338, 1969.
457. Thomas, G.: β-D-Galactosidase in human urine: Deficiency in generalized gangliosidosis, J. Lab. Clin. Med., **74,** 725, 1969.
458. Ho, M. W., and O'Brien, J. S.: Hurler's syndrome: Deficiency of a specific beta galactosidase isoenzyme. Science, **165,** 611, 1969.
459. Matalon, R., and Dorfman, A.: Unpublished data.
460. Fratantoni, J. C., Hall, C. W., and Neufeld, E. F.: Hurler and Hunter syndromes. I. Mutual correction of the defect in cultured fibroblasts. Science, **162,** 570, 1968.
461. Fratantoni, J. C., Hall, C. W., and Neufeld, E. F.: The defect in Hurler and Hunter syndromes. II. Deficiency of specific factors involved in mucopolysaccharide degradation. Proc. Nat. Acad. Sci., U.S.A., **64,** 360, 1969.
462. Neufeld, E. F., and Cantz, M. J.: Corrective factors for inborn errors of mucopolysaccharide metabolism. Ann. NY Acad. Sci., in press.
463. Cantz, M., Chrambach, A., and Neufeld, E. F.: Characterization of the factor deficient in the Hunter syndrome by polyacrylamide gel electrophoresis. Biochem. Biophys. Res. Commun., **39,** 936, 1970.
464. Wolfson, S., Davidson, E. A., Harris, J., Kahana, L., and Lorincz, A. E.: Long-term corticosteroid therapy in Hurler syndrome. Amer. J. Dis. Child., **106,** 3, 1963.
465. Schuffler, M., and Rosenthal, I.: Personal communication.
466. Renuart, A. W.: Mucopolysaccharides in Hurler's syndrome. Lancet, **2,** 152, 1967.
467. Nanivadekar, S. A., and Nanivadekar, A. S., Quoted by Gordon, N., and Thursby-Pelham, D.: The Sanfilippo syndrome—an unusual disorder of mucopolysaccharide metabolism. Develop. Med. Child. Neurol., **11,** 485, 1969.
468. Rennert, M., and Dekaban, A.: Hurler-Hunter syndrome: Clinical and Biochemical study. Clin. Pharmacol. Ther., **7,** 283, 1966.
469. Danes, B. S., and Bearn, A. G.: Hurler's syndrome: Effect of retinol

(vitamin A alcohol) on cellular mucopolysaccharides in cultured human skin fibroblasts. J. Exp. Med., **124**, 1181, 1966.
470. Danes, B. S., and Bearn, A. G.: The effect of retinol (vitamin A alcohol) on urinary excretion of mucopolysaccharides in the Hurler syndrome. Lancet, **1**, 1029, 1967.
471. Madsen, J. A., and Linker, A.: Vitamin A and mucopolysaccharidosis: A clinical, biochemical evaluation. J. Pediat., **75**, 843, 1969.
472. Gordon, N., and Thursby-Pelham, D.: The Sanfilippo syndrome: An unusual disorder of mucopolysaccharide metabolism. Develop. Med. Child. Neurol., **11**, 485, 1969.
473. De Jong, B. P., Robertson, W. van B., and Schafer, I. A.: Failure to induce scurvy by ascorbic acid depletion in a patient with Hurler's syndrome. Pediatrics, **48**, 889, 1968.
474. Matalon, R., Cifonelli, J. A., and Dorfman, A.: L-iduronidase in cultured human fibroblasts and liver. Biochem. Biophys. Acta, **42**, 340, 1971.
475. Matalon, R., and Dorfman, A.: Unpublished results.
476. Spranger, J. W., and Wiedemann, H. R.: The genetic mucolipidoses, Humangenetik **9**, 113, 1970.
477. Dawson, G.: Unpublished results.
478. Freitag, F., Kücheman, K., Blümcke, S., and Spranger, J.: Hepatic ultrastructure in fucosidosis. Virchows Arch. Abt. B. Zellpath., **7**, 99, 1971.
479. Linker, A., Evans, L. R., and Langer, L. O.: Morquio's disease and mucopolysaccharide excretion. J. Pediat. **77**, 1039, 1970.
480. Dawson, G.: Unpublished results.
481. Matalon, R., and Dorfman, A.: Unpublished results.
482. McKusick, V. A.: The relative frequency of the Hurler and Hunter syndromes. New Eng. J. Med., **283**, 853, 1970.
483. Matalon, R., and Dorfman, A.: The antenatal diagnosis of mucopolysaccharidoses, in *Antenatal Diagnosis,* edited by A. Dorfman, University of Chicago, Chicago, 1971.
484. Benson, P. F., Browser-Riley, F., Gianelli, F.: β-Galactosidases in fibroblasts: Hurler and Sanfilippo syndromes. New Eng. J. Med., **283**, 999, 1970.
485. Fluharty, A. L., Porter, M. T., Lassila, E. L., Trammell, J., Currel, R. E., and Kihara, H.: Acid glycosidases in mucopolysaccharidoses' fibroblasts. Biochem. Med., **4**, 110, 1970.
486. Singer, H. S., and Schafer, I. A.: White-cell β-galactosidase activity. New Eng. J. Med., **282**, 571, 1970.
487. Gordon, B. A., and Feleki, V.: Acid hydrolases in the serum and liver in mucopolysaccharidoses types I and III. Clin. Biochem., **3**, 193, 1970.
488. Patel, V., Tappel, A. L., O'Brien, J. S.: Hyaluronidase and sulfatase deficiency in Hurler's syndrome. Biochem. Med., **3**, 447, 1970.
489. Wiesmann, U., and Neufeld, E. F.: Scheie and Hurler syndromes: apparent identity of the biochemical defect. Science, **169**, 72, 1970.
490. DiFerrante, N., Nichols, B. L., Donnelly, P. V., Neri, G., Hrgovcic, R., and Berglund, R. K.: Induced degradation of glycosaminoglycans in Hurler's and Hunter's syndromes by plasma infusion. Proc. Nat. Acad. Sci. USA, **68**, 303, 1971.
491. Dorfman, A., Matalon, R., Cifonelli, J. A., Thompson, J., and Dawson, G.: The degradation of acid mucopolysaccharides and the mucopolysaccharidoses, in *Sphingolipids, Sphingolipidoses and Allied Disorders,* edited by B. W. Volk and S. M. Aronson, p. 195, Plenum, New York, 1972.
492. Matalon, R., and Dorfman, A.: Hurler's syndrome: an α-L-iduronidase deficiency. Biochem. Biophys. Res. Commun., **47**, 959, 1972.
493. Bach, G., Friedman, R., Weissmann, B., and Neufeld, E. F.: The defect in the Hurler and Scheie syndromes: deficiency of α-L-iduronidase. Proc. Nat. Acad. Sci. U.S.A., in press.
494. Matalon, R., and Dorfman, A.: Unpublished data.
495. Barton, R. W., and Neufeld, E. F.: The Hurler corrective factor: purification and some properties. J. Biol. Chem., **246**, 7773, 1971.
496. Kresse, H., and Neufeld, E. F.: The Sanfilippo A corrective factor: purification and mode of action. J. Biol. Chem., **247**, 2164, 1972.
497. O'Brien, J. S.: Sanfilippo Syndrome: profound deficiency of alpha-acetylglucosaminidase activity in organs and skin fibroblasts from type B patients. Proc. Nat. Acad. Sci. U.S.A., in press.
498. Hall, C. W., Cantz, M., Neufeld, E. F., Sly, W. S., Quinton, B. A., McAlister, W. H., and Rimoin, D. L.: Personal communication.
499. Matalon, R., Dorfman, A., and Nadler, H. L.: A chemical method for the antenatal diagnosis of mucopolysaccharidoses. Lancet, **1**, 798, 1972.

ADDENDUM

Since this article was prepared rapid progress has been made in the identification of the enzymic defects of several of the mucopolysaccharidoses. The absent α-L-iduronidase activity in extracts of Hurler fibroblasts has now been confirmed using two natural substrates [474, 491] and one artificial substrate [492, 493]. Absence of α-L-iduronidase has also been demonstrated in Hurler liver, urine, and leukocytes. Normal levels of enzyme have been found in extracts of Hunter, Sanfilippo A and Sanfilippo B fibroblasts, and Sanfilippo A liver.

The Hurler factor, which has been partially purified by Barton and Neufeld [495], has been shown to demonstrate α-L-iduronidase activity [493]. An absence of α-L-iduronidase has also been demonstrated in extracts of Scheie fibroblasts [493, 494] confirming the previous impression that Scheie and Hurler disease are probably allelic mutations.

Kresse and Neufeld [496] have purified the Sanfilippo A factor and presented evidence that it is a sulfamidase which acts on heparan sulfate. An absence of α-N-acetylglucosaminidase in extracts of Sanfilippo B fibroblasts has been demonstrated by O'Brien [497] and confirmed by Matalon and Dorfman [494].

The absence of β-glucuronidase has been demonstrated by Hall et al. [498] in fibroblasts of a patient with symptoms and signs suggestive of a mucopolysaccharidosis. Further experience with mucopolysaccharide levels in amniotic fluid indicate that this method is not reliable for the prenatal diagnosis of mucopolysaccharidoses [499]. Since α-L-iduronidase has been demonstrated in fibroblasts cultured from normal amniotic fluid, it seems likely that antenatal diagnosis of Hurler disease can best be made by specific enzymic methods.

CHAPTER FIFTY

INHERITED SYSTEMIC AMYLOIDOSIS

Alan S. Cohen

Amyloidosis is a disorder characterized by the extracellular deposition of *amyloid,* a unique fibrous protein, in the connective tissue of the body. The deposit may be small and localized and have little apparent clinical effect on the individual; the amyloid may be widespread throughout the body with massive involvement of various organs and serious clinical consequences. The deposits may fall anywhere between these two extremes [1]. Little is known about the natural history of amyloidosis in man since the diagnosis is often not made until the disease is far advanced.

HISTORY

In 1842 Rokitansky [2] described in his "Treatise on abnormalities of the Liver" a disease in which the liver was enlarged, elastic, and waxy, and was occasionally accompanied by similar changes in the spleen. The description of firm, nonpainful enlargement of the liver in association with inflammatory disease exists as far back as Wainewright's paper of 1737 [3], but it remained for Virchow in 1854 [4, 5] to define and name the infiltrating substance. When he observed that the corpora amylacea of the nervous system stained blue with iodine and, subsequently, that the "sago spleen" after gentle application of iodine and sulfuric acid turned blue, he considered them as cellulose-like substances and named the material amyloid. This substance was studied for 60 years at the autopsy table or in experimental animals before direct biopsy procedures [6] and the Congo red test and stain were introduced in the 1920s [7, 8]. Since then a wide variety of studies both clinical and experimental have been carried out on what has often been considered an extremely rare "degenerative" condition. Recently, it has become apparent that amyloidosis is far more common than had been thought, that it is often of great clinical significance, that it is associated with an extraordinarily wide variety of diseases, and that there are a number of genetically determined amyloidoses.

CLASSIFICATION

While early studies showed that amyloid was often an accompaniment of chronic suppuration, it became apparent over 100 years ago that amyloidosis also occurs in the absence of predisposing disease [9, 10, 11]. This led to a variety of classifications of amyloid, starting with that of Lubarsch [12] (typical, common, or secondary variety versus atypical, uncommon, or primary variety) and leading to the popular classification proposed by Reimann et al. [13]:

1. Primary amyloidosis (no antecedent or coexisting disease, mesodermal tissue involvement, variability of staining, tendency to nodular deposits)
2. Secondary amyloidosis (chronic disease association, liver, spleen, kidney, adrenal involvement, constant staining properties)
3. Tumor forming (single or multiple masses of amyloid in eye, genitourinary, or respiratory tract)
4. Amyloidosis associated with multiple myeloma

Subsequently, King [14] commented on the overlap in organ involvement and staining properties and proposed that amyloid be called typical (parenchymal organ distribution), with or without associated disease. Dahlin [15] returned to the use of primary (systemic or focal), secondary (systemic or focal), and myeloma-related disease. Symmers [16] emphasized the overlap in the many parameters and suggested a scheme of generalized amyloidosis associated with a recognizable predisposing disease (generalized secondary amyloidosis), generalized amyloidosis in the absence of a recognized predisposing disease (generalized primary amyloidosis), and localized amyloidosis.

In recent years it has become apparent that the heredofamilial amyloidoses with their varying clinical manifestations are not accommodated in the above schemes. A new system of classification was devised based on the polarization optical properties of amyloid as defined by Missmahl and Hartwig [17]. These investigators, who had reaffirmed the green birefringence of amyloid after Congo red staining (see below), believe that amyloid is laid down either along reticulin fibers or collagen fibers. Accordingly, with Heller and associates [18], Missmahl classified the various amyloidoses as (1) perireticular, i.e., generalized vascular amyloid with the deposit starting in the basement membrane area and spreading outward to the tunica media, and (2) pericollagen, i.e., involving connective tissue of the tunica adventitia of the blood vessel and spreading inward to affect the media. The perireticulin class is said to include most secondary amyloidoses, several hereditary varieties (notably that associated with familial Mediterranean fever), and some cases of primary amyloid. Pericollagen distribution is found in several hereditary amyloidoses, as well as in association with multiple myeloma and several primary types.

This interesting scheme has been criticized for several reasons, which are discussed below, and appears to be rather empirical. Disorders have already been described by

Grants in support of studies mentioned in this chapter have been received from the Public Health Service, the National Institute of Arthritis and Metabolic Diseases (AM 5285 and AM 04599), the Arthritis Foundation, and University Hospital (Research Grant 827).

Missmahl in which both types of distribution are said to occur (i.e., systemic lupus erythematosus complicated by amyloid), and the classification has not been completely verified by other investigators although some cases seem to conform [20].

It would seem reasonable and clinically useful at present to classify amyloid in accordance with the presence or absence of other disease (secondary and primary amyloid) and the heredofamilial aspects. Undoubtedly as information accrues regarding the basic chemical and immunologic properties of amyloid, a more precise system may become available.

INCIDENCE

The incidence of amyloidosis in the population at large is not known. The only data available are those based on postmortem studies, which, for the most part, give a falsely low indication of the autopsy incidence since the special stains which are required to identify the presence of amyloid are not carried out routinely. There are a few studies on selected populations (patients with leprosy, chronic tuberculosis, etc.) where an exceedingly high incidence (up to 50 percent) of amyloid disease has been observed at postmortem examination. In the heredofamilial form of amyloid associated with familial Mediterranean fever, where clinical and postmortem data have been carefully assessed, evidence of amyloidosis has been obtained in 26.5 percent of 470 patients [21].

At a 1964 meeting, an attempt was made to draw together data on the geographic distribution of amyloid [22–24]. These studies were all based on routine postmortem data and reaffirmed that in many general hospitals the incidence of amyloid at postmortem was about 0.5 percent, that in Japan the incidence was low (about 0.1 percent), and that when special hospitals were included or countries where there existed a known genetic predisposition (Portugal and Israel) the overall incidence was significantly higher. There is general agreement that with antibiotics available for treating chronic infections such as tuberculosis and leprosy the incidence of secondary amyloidosis is decreasing. It would also appear that the increase in primary amyloid is disproportionately high, but whether this reflects an increased awareness and better diagnostic tools, or a true increased incidence is not clear. A high incidence of primary amyloid in Papua and New Guinea has been reported [25].

In a review of 400 consecutive necropsies, Ravid et al. [26] excluded 9 cases of generalized amyloid and still found focal small amyloid lesions in 18.4 percent of the remaining postmortem examinations. Cohen and Wills [27] recut and restained tissues from 100 consecutive autopsies and found 16 with amyloid. An even higher incidence of lesions in the aged population has been emphasized by Schwartz et al. [28]. Wright et al. [29] examined in detail a series of consecutive necropsies excluding those with diseases known to predispose to amyloid. They reported a striking incidence of 89 percent in those age 70 years and over and $37\frac{1}{2}$ percent in those age 30 to 70 years.

Thus small deposits of amyloid are almost the rule rather than the exception, and they are of unknown clinical significance.

PATHOLOGY

Gross Appearance

Amyloid is an amorphous, eosinophilic, glassy, hyalin extracellular substance which is ubiquitous in its distribution. Grossly, it may be identified by the classical iodine and dilute sulfuric acid stain first used by Virchow. When successful, this stain imparts a blue-purple color to the amyloid, but this is inconstant and primarily of historical interest. When small amounts of amyloid are present no gross organ abnormalities are demonstrable. With larger amounts the involved organs take on a firm rubbery consistency. They may have a waxy, pink, or gray appearance. Organ enlargement (especially liver, kidney, spleen, and heart) may be prominent when the deposits are large. In patients with long-standing renal involvement, the kidneys may become small and pale. The gastrointestinal tract may be locally or generally thickened, and gastric and intestinal ulcerations are not uncommon. The heart, in addition to being enlarged because of interstitial myocardial involvement, may have nodular elevations on its pericardial and endocardial surfaces, as well as lesions in the valves. Other gross findings are variable and dependent upon the presence or absence of local nodular deposits of amyloid.

Tinctorial Properties

Microscopically, amyloid is stained pink with the hematoxylin and eosin dyes and shows metachromasia with crystal violet or methyl violet, but it is othochromatic when stained with toluidine blue. The van Gieson stain for collagen stains the latter red and most of the background yellow, but imparts a khaki color to amyloid. The periodic acid–Schiff (PAS) stain gives amyloid a violaceous hue.

Congo red, introduced in 1922 [7], remains one of the most widely used stains. It is not completely specific, for it stains elastic tissue and unless carefully decolorized will stain dense bundles of collagen. When sections fixed in formalin and stained with Congo red are viewed in the polarizing microscope, a unique green birefringence is seen. This is the single most useful procedure for establishing the presence of amyloid. Recently, amyloid has been stained with fluorochromes to produce a secondary fluorescence. Thioflavine dyes in particular have been found to be sensitive indicators of amyloid [30]. The lack of specificity of these dyes makes it mandatory that they be employed primarily for screening and followed by more specific stains. Cotton dyes, especially Sirius red have also been found quite useful and specific [31]. A recent comparative evaluation of these stains has borne out the high degree of sensitivity and specificity of the green birefringence after Congo red or Sirius red staining [32].

Light Microscopic Appearance

In the light microscope, amyloid is almost invariably extracellular in the connective tissue. The deposits may be focal in almost any area of the body but most often the amyloid is perivascular. Amyloid may involve bone marrow, spleen capillaries, venules, veins, arterioles, or arteries. The heart may have focal or diffuse interstitial deposits in the myocardium, endocardium, or pericardium. In the kidney the glomerulus is primarily affected, but interstitial peritubular and vascular amyloid may be prominent. In early lesions small nodular or diffuse deposits appear near the basement membrane, and as the disease progresses the glomerulus may be so massively laden as to occlude the capillary bed (Fig. 50-1). Atrophic glomeruli laden with amyloid may show marked thickening in the area of Bowman's capsule and rarely the glomerulus may be almost replaced by connective tissue. Tubular dilatation, casts, and interstitial amyloid deposits may appear in the medulla.

In the gastrointestinal tract there may be perivascular deposits only, or irregular or diffuse deposits may occur in the submucosa, the muscularis mucosa, or subserosa. The

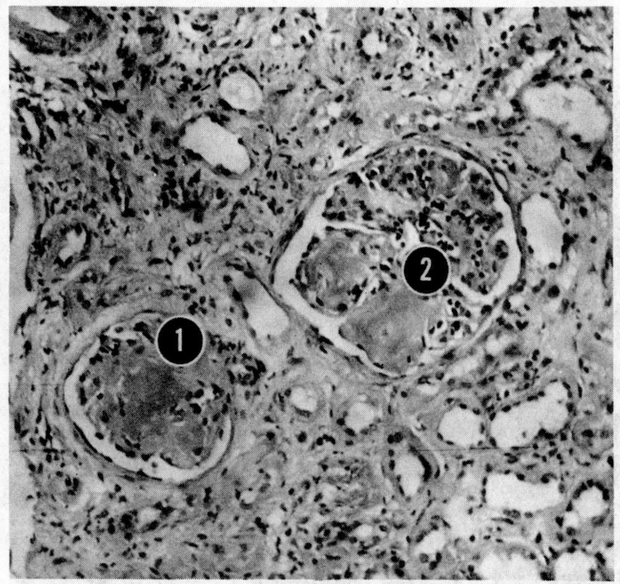

Figure 50-1. Light microscopic view of two glomeruli obtained from a patient with amyloidosis. Glomerulus 1 is almost totally obliterated by amyloid, while glomerulus 2 has total involvement of the glomerular loop in the lower left and diffuse subendothelial and mesangial amyloid. Congo red stain. ×120.

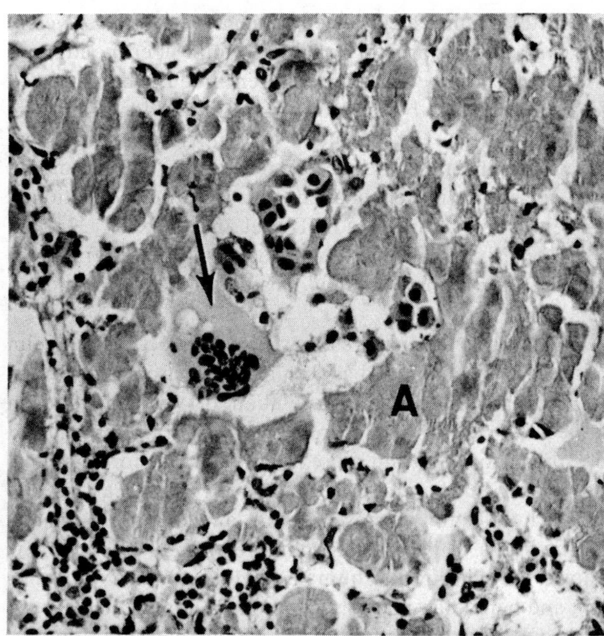

Figure 50-2. Light microscopic view of lung biopsy obtained from a patient with primary amyloidosis. Widespread amyloid (A) deposits are obvious, and a giant cell is indicated by the arrow. Congo red stain. ×175.

amyloid may appear in any level or appendage of the gastrointestinal tract, including the gallbladder and pancreas. Hepatic deposits may be perivascular only or, more frequently, diffuse amyloid is found between the Kupffer and parenchymal cells. In the nervous system, amyloid has been described along peripheral nerves, in autonomic ganglia, and in senile plaques and vessels of the central nervous system. It may be found in any part of the orbit including the vitreous humor and cornea.

The bronchopulmonary tract may be involved focally or extensively. The unique aspect of pulmonary or pleural involvement is that while amyloid in virtually all other locations of the body causes no resorption or foreign body reaction, pulmonary amyloid deposits may be accompanied by large numbers of macrophages about and within the lesions (Fig. 50-2). These deposits may also contain islets of cartilage and of ossification.

Thus, virtually no area of the body is spared. This ubiquitous distribution elicits a wide variety of clinical symptoms and signs [1].

Fine Structure of Amyloid

Divry and Florkin [33] in 1927 clearly observed the birefringence of amyloid when viewed in the polarizing microscope. This has been amply confirmed [34]. The extensive studies of Missmahl [17, 35] have demonstrated its positive form birefringence. He further concluded that there were areas where this could be converted to negative only by glycerol ("a characteristic property of the reticulin fiber") and areas where the positive form birefringence could be corrected to negative only by phenol ("properties identifying the collagen fiber"). He concluded that amyloid is laid down on preexisting reticulin or collagen fibers. This prompted the perireticulin-pericollagen classification mentioned earlier. The investigations of Diezel and Pfleiderer [36], on the other hand, led them to conclude that the birefringence is an intrinsic property of amyloid and is not dependent upon reticulin.

The latter conclusion is supported by the fact that reticulin has never been identified as such in the electron microscope. It probably represents a population of younger collagen molecules, perhaps with a greater carbohydrate content and possibly associated with more lipid to account for its optical properties. Furthermore, in 1959, Cohen and Calkins [37] found by electron microscopy that amyloid itself consists of fine fibrils. This has been confirmed [19, 38–40]. It is now known that all types of human amyloid—primary, secondary, and heredofamilial [41, 42]—consist of fine, nonbranching rigid fibrils, which in tissue sections measure approximately 100 Å in diameter (Fig. 50-3). They are usually arranged in random array when distant from the cell, but close to it they may be parallel or perpendicular to the plasmalemma, with which they occasionally appear to merge. Intracellular fibrils of dimensions comparable to those outside the cell are occasionally observed. Their precise nature has not been established.

The amyloid fibrils are usually seen in earliest and closest relationship to the mesangial cell in the kidney [43], although as deposits enlarge they appear in comparable relationship to the endothelial and finally epithelial cell. In the liver, they first border the Kupffer cell, but finally fill the space of Disse and abut the hepatic cell as well. In many other locations they are formed close to blood vessels, pericytes, and endothelial cells. Thus, while the cell synthesizing amyloid fibrils appears in many instances to be in the reticuloendothelial or macrophage family, it is possible that under some circumstances or in advanced disease the ability to produce these fibrils may be a more widespread phenomenon. The production of amyloid fibrils by reticuloendothelial cells in isolated spleen explants [44] and cultures [45] has been demonstrated by autoradiographic techniques at the light and electron microscopic levels.

PATHOGENESIS

The etiology of amyloidosis is not known. Throughout the years, amyloid has been regarded as (1) a disorder of serum proteins with associated hyperglobulinemia; (2) a disorder of protein metabolism; (3) related to an abnormality of the reticuloendothelial system; (4) the result of chronic immunologic stimulation leading to excessive antibody production and the deposition of antibody or antibody-antigen complexes as amyloid; (5) a disorder of delayed hypersensitivity; or (6) a combination of the aforementioned. These hypotheses are not mutually exclusive and since the etiology is unknown, when a specific abnormality is present it is difficult to be certain whether it is of primary significance or is a secondary phenomenon.

Amyloid occurs spontaneously throughout the animal kingdom and can readily be produced by a wide variety

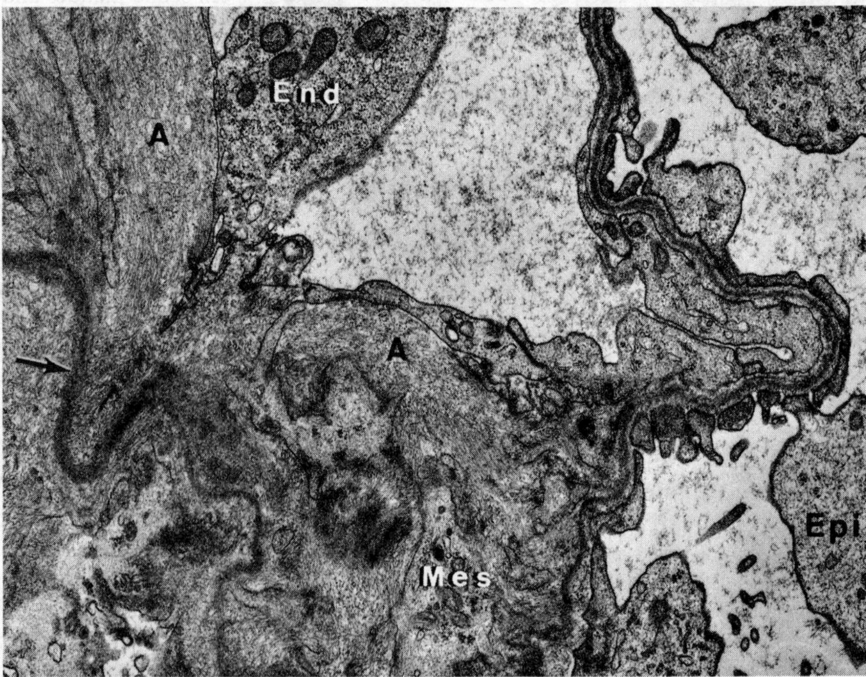

Figure 50-3. Electron micrograph of a kidney with diffuse amyloid (A) present in close approximation to the mesangial cell (Mes) and to the endothelial cell (End). The basement membrane (arrow) is intact, and only a small amount of amyloid approximates the epithelial cell (Epi) in the lower right. ×15,000.

of unrelated stimuli [19]. Most early data centered about its production by infectious agents, but as early as 1916 Bailey [46] found that it could be induced without suppuration by injections of broth cultures of the colon bacillus. Since then bacterial toxins, antitoxins, plasma proteins, casein, dietary manipulations, ribonucleic acid, methylcholanthrene, colloidal sulfur or selenium, cadmium, manganese chloride, thiouracil, mucopolysaccharides, endotoxin, parabiosis, sex-segregated grouping, and gamma irradiation have all been used to induce amyloid.

Plasma Proteins and Circulating Antibodies

It has become apparent that amyloid can occur without hyperglobulinemia; indeed it has been reported in patients with primary agammaglobulinemia [47]. The fact that amyloid in man and animals is often associated with chronic inflammatory or infectious diseases and that horses given repeated toxin injections for producing antitoxins developed amyloid has persuaded many that amyloid is the result of an antigen-antibody reaction. The concept that amyloid itself is or contains γ-globulin was furthered by fluorescent antibody studies demonstrating the presence of γ-globulin in the area of the amyloid deposit [48, 49]. Finally, because of the association of multiple myeloma and amyloid, it has been suggested that it might be the result of the plasma cell abnormality and that γ-globulin or its subunits (especially light chains) could in themselves constitute the amyloid [50]. The possible role of a circulating antibody was reviewed extensively by Schneider [51].

The results of other fluorescent antibody studies have varied, and one such investigation demonstrated γ-globulin on amyloid when hyperglobulinemia was present and fibrinogen when hyperfibrinogenemia was present [52]. Furthermore, plasmacytosis is not always present in amyloid disease and in fact is strikingly absent in the hereditary amyloidoses. Extensive studies of patients with primary amyloid for evidence of myeloma have shown only the occasional "M" spike and Bence-Jones proteinuria—without evidence of immature plasma cells in the marrow and without bone lesions. This has suggested that these are the occasional accompaniments of amyloidosis rather than its cause [53, 54].

More direct evidence bearing on the nature of amyloid has been obtained. Its fibrous ultrastructure is different from that of the immunoglobulins. The fibrils have been isolated in pure form and when studied by immune electron microscopy (incubation with ferritin-conjugated antihuman γ-globulin) no adherence of the ferritin conjugates to the amyloid was found [55]. Even a direct overlay of the conjugate onto the amyloid tissue demonstrated no specific γ-globulin localization. Furthermore, when intact lyophilized amyloid fibrils were tested against specific antisera to whole human γ-globulin and some of its components [56], no reaction was obtained. Others have also observed the lack of immunogenicity of whole amyloid fibrils [57, 58].

Extracts of amyloid fibrils have been prepared independently in a number of laboratories and have uniformly proved to be free of γ-globulin [59, 60, 61, 62]. Finally, immune tolerance to casein has been induced in mice soon after birth, and later it was found that tolerant and control mice given casein developed amyloid to the same degree. This observation indicated again the absence of a direct role for a circulating antibody in the genesis of amyloid [63]. Similar experiments in mice thymectomized at birth showed them to have as much amyloid as control groups when both were subsequently challenged with casein [64].

Delayed Hypersensitivity

The role of delayed hypersensitivity, lymphocytes, and the reticuloendothelial system (RES) in the genesis of amyloidosis is more difficult to assess. It was apparent as early as 1926 [65] that the RES probably plays a role in the production of amyloid. Teilum [66] in 1956 indicated that there are two phases in the genesis of amyloid and presented histologic data supporting this thesis. Carbon clearance studies have verified an early hyperactivity of the RES during casein induction of amyloid, and this is followed by a falloff in RES activity [67, 68]. The production of amyloid by RES cells or macrophages in a tissue explant system [44] and in tissue culture [45] has already been mentioned. Zschiesche and colleagues [69, 70] have related the known strain variation in susceptibility to amyloidosis to functional variations in RES activity in these species, while Ram et al. [71] observed histologically that the degree of lymphoreticular proliferation in a number of species does not relate to the amount of amyloid deposited.

Lymphocyte depletion is associated with the appearance of amyloid in experimental animals [72, 73, 74]. This phenomenon was emphasized by Druet and Janigan [75], who suggested that lymphocyte depletion might have a rate-limiting influence on the timing of the appearance of amyloidosis during experimental induction. In addition casein injections (which ultimately induce amyloid) initially suppress the immune response to other antigens (i.e., ferritin [76], SRBC [77]).

Impairment of the immune mechanism in amyloidosis was further demonstrated by Ranlov and Jensen [78]. They found prolonged homograft survival in amyloidotic mice. Impairment of cellular immune function by amyloidogenic agents has also been demonstrated by the response in vitro of mouse spleen cells to phytohemagglutinin [79] and by the migration inhibition technique using peritoneal cells of the guinea pig [80]. The latter investigation [196, 197] then demonstrated that the cellular unresponsiveness was specific to casein, while cellular immunity to other antigens remained the same. They suggested that in this model, amyloidosis might be a positive expression of tolerance.

A series of reports have now appeared on the isologous and homologous transfer of amyloidosis. It was shown that sensitized donor spleen cells—whether living or dead—could induce amyloid in recipient mice within 3 to 7 days following intravenous or intraperitoneal injection [81, 82, 83]. In addition, serum from sensitized isogenic donor mice was found to accelerate induction of amyloidosis in an x-irradiated recipient [84]. The latter studies were refined to demonstrate that ammonium sulfate fractions of donor spleens had amyloid enhancing factor activity and that a specific immune response to injected protein was not a necessary condition in the pathogenesis of amyloidosis [85]. Subsequently, it was found that human amyloid spleen homogenate, together with casein and without immunosuppression, caused amyloid in recipient mice within 5 days [86] and that there was strain dependence in recipients [87]. Several investigators have not been able to transfer passively the amyloid by means of thoracic duct cells [88, 89]. This further suggested that the amyloid-enhancing effect was not simple adoptive transfer. To date, therefore, it appears that an amyloid-enhancing or transfer factor exists in the tissues and serum of amyloidotic and preamyloidotic hosts. Studies of these factors may well shed further light on the cellular and immune mechanisms involved in the pathogenesis of amyloidosis.

ULTRASTRUCTURE OF ISOLATED COMPONENTS OF AMYLOID

After it was found that all human and animal amyloid has a fibrillar ultrastructure in tissue section, attempts were made to isolate the material [90–93].

Amyloid Fibrils

Using several different methods, one can obtain a preparation of fibrils of high purity which is positive to Congo red, shows crystal violet "metachromasia" and green birefringence in the polarizing microscope after Congo red staining, and (as will be subsequently discussed) can be made free of contaminating plasma proteins and the pentagonal unit (P component) as demonstrated by immunologic methods.

These fibrils constitute the starting material for the ultrastructural, biochemical, and x-ray diffraction studies to be described later and are thought to constitute the bulk of amyloid tissue deposits. Studies of high resolution ultrastructure have been carried out on fibrils shadowed with platinum-palladium and on fibrils negatively stained with phosphotungstic acid or uranyl acetate. The shadowed preparations clearly demonstrate long, thin, nonbranching fibrils, with a tendency toward lateral aggregation and a faint suggestion of periodicity (Fig. 50-4). More precise structural configuration can be displayed by negative staining [94]. The amyloid *fibril* is made up of laterally aggregated *filaments,* usually 1 to 4 in a group but occasionally more. This aggregate has a loose random twist. The center-to-center distance of the filaments is about 70 to 75 Å with no significant space between them. Filaments usually are equal in length and

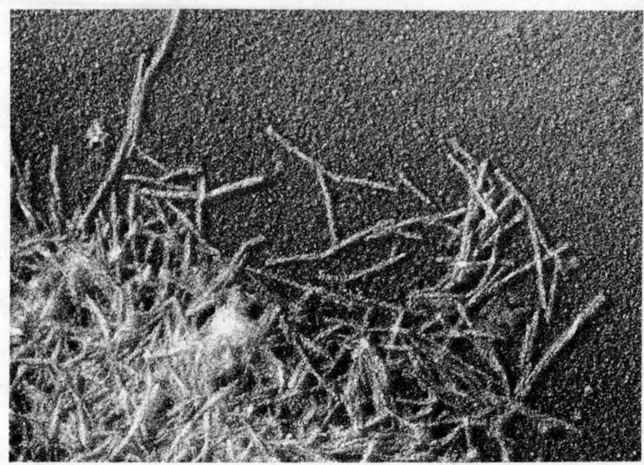

Figure 50-4. Electron micrograph of isolated and purified amyloid fibrils shadowed with platinum-palladium. ×60,000.

"break" cleanly. These fibrils are composed of subunits termed amyloid protofibrils (Fig. 50-5), which are 25 to 35 Å wide. Review of several thousand electron micrographs has led us to the interpretation that the filament is composed of five such protofibrils, arranged parallel to one another and longitudinally or slightly obliquely to the long axis of the filament. The protofibril itself is beaded and has a 35 to 50 Å repeat. Further resolution suggests that each protofibril is made up of two subprotofibril units, each 10 to 15 Å wide that form a helical structure. This model can explain the various types of fibril structure reported in the literature (see [94, figs. 28 and 29]).

While our interpretations of fibril structure, i.e., five units or protofibrils constituting the filament and two subprotofibrils in each protofibril, are still open to further investigation and verification, the 70 to 75 Å filament or fibril diameter in negatively stained preparations, and the presence of a 35 to 50 Å unit equivalent to the protofibril have been reported from several laboratories [95]. Other investigators have interpreted their data as indicating that two protofibrils constitute the 70 to 75 Å filament.

Pentagonal Unit (or P Component)

Bladen, et al. in 1966 [96] separated amyloid as described by Cohen and Calkins [37] but altered the procedure by collecting supernatants after the first several washes. These they sonicated and recentrifuged at high speed and obtained a pellet which was examined in the electron microscope after negative staining. The pellet, which originally was described as Congo red positive, was found to contain two types of particles. The first was a small pentagonal structure, 90 Å in diameter, made up of five 20 to 25 Å units about a central core. The second was a clear-cut 100 Å wide rod with a periodicity of about 40 Å. They suggested that the pentagonal structures were single units of the rods which were lying

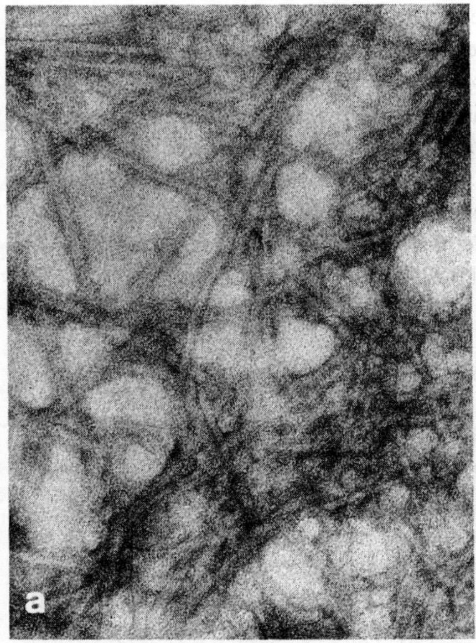

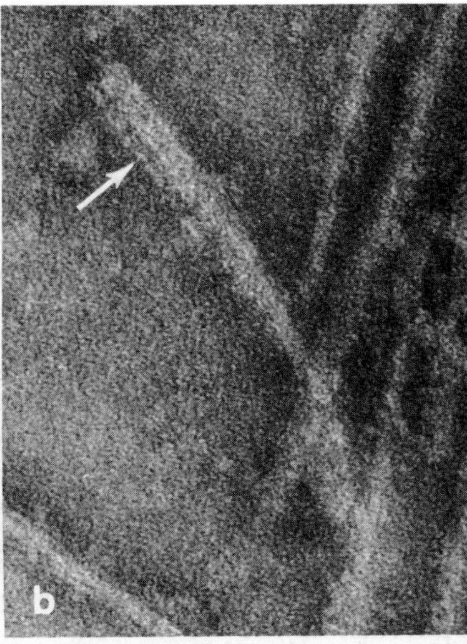

Figure 50-5. Electron micrograph of isolated purified amyloid fibrils negatively stained with 1% phosphotungstic acid. A. Each fibril (or filament) is about 75 Å in diameter. ×160,000. B. At higher magnification the protofibril (arrow) of about 35 Å diameter and with a 35 to 45 Å periodicity can be discerned. ×500,000.

on their flat side affording an end view of the amyloid rod. The authors first interpreted these findings as delineating the unit structure of amyloid.

It has become clear that these interesting observations, while valid new findings, were the first ultrastructural observations of a new component found in amyloid but *not* part of the fibril itself [97, 98]. The pentagonal unit when purified shows neither crystal violet metachromasia nor green birefringence on Congo red staining, unless contaminated by amyloid fibrils. It is a minor constituent of amyloid deposits, is not responsible for its characteristic staining properties, and is identical with a circulating α-globulin (see below). It can be isolated as originally described, or in simple saline washes or alkaline extracts of amyloid (Fig. 50-6).

BIOCHEMISTRY OF AMYLOID

Fibrils

Painstaking analyses of whole organs laden with amyloid have been done by many investigators in the past. While these studies anticipated in part some of the findings later made on purified preparations it is important at this time to define the precise components being analyzed and to separate clearly analyses of fibrils and those obtained from the P component (pentagonal unit). Whole tissue analyses have been reviewed in detail [19] and will not be discussed.

The purity of fibril preparations and their method of preparation are important and no standard procedures are yet available. We have used for separation at least the four methods referred to earlier and judge purity as follows:

1. Electron microscopically homogeneous preparation of characteristic fibrils with 70 to 75 Å diameter on negative staining without contaminating collagen fibrin or pentagonal units
2. Green birefringence after Congo red staining
3. Absence of plasma proteins determined immunologically
4. Absence of P component (pentagonal unit) determined immunologically
5. X-ray diffraction pattern characteristic of cross beta protein with a 4.6 Å meridional arc and a 9.8 Å equatorial arc

With these as initial criteria, one can perform analyses of amyloid derived from different tissues, different species, and different human varieties. There are variations in analyses which are sufficient to lead one to suspect that there

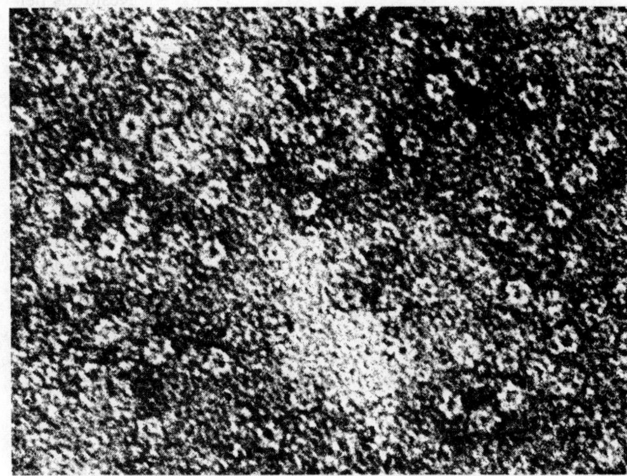

Figure 50-6. Electron micrograph of plasma component (P component; pentagonal unit) of amyloid, isolated from alkaline extracts and purified. The pentagonal nature of these units with a central core is apparent. ×400,000.

may be either other substances uniquely carried along in amyloid fibrils or subtle variations in the composition of different fibrils, even though they fulfill the above or other criteria of homogeneity and purity.

At any rate, amyloid is a protein with a nitrogen content of approximately 14.6 percent of the dry weight [91]. Hydroxylysine, hydroxyproline, desmosine, isodesmosine, and lysinonorlysine are absent. There is a predominance of acidic amino acid residues (glutamic acid and aspartic acid) and a small amount of tryptophan. A more recent amino acid analysis appears in Table 50-1. Similar analyses have been reported by others [93, 98], with some minor differences. Neutral sugars constitute less than 2 percent of the dry weight, and uronic acid and sialic acid less than 1 percent of the dry weight each [91, 93, 98]. The presence of neutral hexoses including glucose was recently reported in a glycopeptide fragment obtained after pronase treatment of amyloid fibrils [99]. Lipid is present only as a contaminant [92].

Whether or not mucopolysaccharide is part of the amyloid fibril molecule is not known. Increased amounts of heparin sulfate have been found in amyloid-laden organs [100]. In addition, isolated amyloid fibrils have been shown to contain more mucopolysaccharide than the comparable whole organ [101, 102]. Heparin sulfate was not the only mucopolysaccharide associated with the fibril. In one study, dermatan sulfate and chondroitin sulfate were also present [101]. One group has reported even greater amounts of mucopolysaccharide in amyloid-laden hearts, and has attributed this increase primarily to hyaluronic acid [103]. How any of these substances specifically relate to the structure of the amyloid fibril protein is not yet clear.

Table 50-1. AMINO ACID ANALYSIS OF AMYLOID FIBRILS ISOLATED FROM TISSUE OF A PATIENT WITH PRIMARY AMYLOIDOSIS*

	Residues per 1,000 residues
Aspartic acid	83.5
Threonine	68.4
Serine	85.4
Glutamic acid	117.8
Proline	72.1
Glycine	90.0
Alanine	79.2
Valine	52.2
Cystine (half)	30.6
Methionine	10.4
Isoleucine	35.9
Leucine	90.6
Tyrosine	43.4
Phenylalanine	37.8
Lysine	40.0
Histidine	14.1
Arginine	49.3
Tryptophan**	

* Tissue A.M. (AC 68–43)

** Not determined, but found in other preparations [91].

A major problem in analyzing amyloid fibrils has been their apparent insolubility and resistance to certain types of enzymatic digestion. While they are not digested by collagenase or hyaluronidase [90], the molecule can be partially hydrolyzed by pronase, Nagarse, trypsin, and papain [104].

Pras et al. [93] isolated amyloid in water and obtained a single homogeneous peak with an $s^{\circ}_{20}w$ of 45 to 50S. A comparable sedimentation coefficient was reported by Shirahama and Cohen [105] after an alkaline extraction of fibrils in a glycine buffer at pH 11.5. Subsequently, Pras et al. [106] found additional sedimentation coefficients in their water extracts of different amyloid fibril preparations and disparaties by polypeptide map analyses as well.

Skinner and Cohen [107] observed different amino terminal amino acids (i.e., glutamic acid, aspartic acid, or no amino terminal, along with small amounts of serine) among fibril preparations from tissues of patients with different clinical types of amyloid. No one amino terminal was identified with any one type of disease. The findings, plus the variations noted above [106] and the immunologic differences in degraded amyloid preparations reported by Franklin and Pras [58], suggest that continuing study will identify more precisely variations in the amyloid fibril protein. A recent publication has suggested (based on an amino-terminal amino acid sequence of seven amino acids) that amyloid protein is derived from the variable amino-terminal segment of immunoglobulin kappa chain [199]. This interesting work awaits verification but is consistent with the previously reported amino-terminal amino acids [107]. If verified, it will not negate the earlier mentioned facts concerning immunoglobulins and amyloid, but will require new interpretations of the data.

The configuration of the amyloid fibril protein as defined by x-ray diffraction studies has been reported independently from three laboratories. Virtually identical patterns and interpretations were obtained by two groups (sharp ring at 4.75 Å overlaying a diffuse halo at 4.3 Å and a less intense ring at 9.8 Å [108])(a sharp meridional arc at 4.68 Å and a more diffuse equatorial arc at 9.8 Å [109]. These patterns are most consistent with the pleated sheet pattern or cross-β configuration. The third group found reflections of (1) 9.4 Å, (2) 6.1 to 2.55 Å, and (3) 10 Å and 4.6 Å [110]. It seems probable that this last report differs from the other two because of the different method of preparation of the amyloid fibrils. It is our impression that the cross-β pattern holds for all amyloid fibril proteins studied up to the present. This finding affords another method of identifying "pure" fibril preparations and is not inconsistent with any of the ultrastructural analyses of amyloid mentioned earlier.

Pentagonal Unit (P Component)

When the amyloid fibrils were first isolated their solubility at various pH's was studied [111]. Material solubilized at pH 9.5 was injected into rabbits and antibody prepared. A series of studies demonstrated that the antigen (1) was an unusual α-globulin (referred to as a P component) which lacked identity with other known plasma proteins [112]; (2) was present in normal as well as amyloidotic and other pathologic sera; and (3) was present in variable amounts in amyloidotic tissue and absent from normal tissue. The material was purified, sprayed on a grid, and negatively stained [113]. A homogeneous preparation of pentagonal units was observed in the electron microscope. These were identical with those prepared by Bladen, Nylen, and Glenner [96] by other techniques. Thus, the unusual α-globulin identified and separated from amyloid fibrils was apparently not an intrinsic part of the fibril but corresponded to the pentagonal unit described earlier.

The pentagonal unit is distinguished from amyloid fibrils in its ultrastructure in its tinctorial properties (*no* crystal violet metachromasia, *no* green birefringence on polarization microscopy after Congo red staining) and in its immunologic properties. With regard to the last, whole amyloid fibrils are nonimmunogenic, while antibodies to the P component or pentagonal unit can easily be prepared [198].

Chemical studies on the pentagonal unit of amyloid are limited. It is a protein which according to Glenner and coworkers [98] is deficient in tryptophan and methionine. The total hexose content and N-acetylneuraminic acid content are said to be increased and the uronic acid content decreased, when compared to the fibril. On x-ray diffraction this component gives a diffuse pattern consistent with a globular protein.

CLINICAL FEATURES

Whether a patient has primary, secondary, or heredofamilial amyloidosis, the clinical manifestations depend upon the anatomic site of the deposit and the degree of interference with normal organ function. In the genetically determined forms, clinical patterns are usually recognizable and will be discussed in detail under these separate disorders. Renal involvement is potentially the most serious manifestation of the disease and the major cause of death in most series. Despite this, renal amyloid may be present and asymptomatic for many years and does not inevitably progress rapidly. Most patients will exhibit proteinuria which may at times be massive, and a classic nephrotic syndrome may be the presenting manifestation. Patients with renal amyloid may also have hematuria, but the presence of casts is unusual. Radiologically, the kidneys may be large, but with increased duration of the disease, small shrunken kidneys develop. Hypertension is rare early in the course, but as patients with renal amyloid survive longer the incidence of hypertension is increasing.

Cardiac amyloid when present may also be asymptomatic but on occasion may be severe enough to cause congestive heart failure. Electrocardiographic abnormalities include a wide variety of conduction abnormalities, especially heart block, with auricular flutter and fibrillation. Patients with cardiac amyloid may have arrhythmias precipitated by digitalis. This drug should be used with caution. The electrocardiogram in cardiac amyloidosis may indicate coronary artery disease in the absence of clinical symptoms. The reading is usually that of anterior or anteroseptal infarction.

Gastrointestinal symptoms in amyloidosis are common. They may result from direct involvement of the gastrointestinal tract at any level or from infiltration of the autonomic nervous system with amyloid. The symptoms include those of obstruction, ulceration, malabsorption, hemorrhage, protein loss, and diarrhea. While hepatic involvement is common, abnormalities of liver function are unusual and occur late in the disease. The two tests most useful in indicating hepatic amyloid are the bromsulfalein extraction and the serum level of alkaline phosphatase. Ascites and jaundice are rare. Since amyloidosis can involve any level of the respiratory tract, symptoms vary widely and include hoarseness, hemoptysis, epistaxis, and dysphagia. Neurologic symptoms are especially prominent in several of the heredofamilial amyloidoses. A patient may show an asymmetric or symmetric sensory neuropathy, severe autononic nervous symptoms, or even isolated cranial nerve lesions. Amyloid of the eye or orbit may cause proptosis, decreased visual acuity, muscle weakness, or ptosis.

Thus, virtually any organ of the body may be involved and the symptoms will depend upon the site of the deposit and its size.

Laboratory Findings

There are no laboratory abnormalities specific or unique for amyloid. Routine blood studies (hematocrit, white cell count, and differential count) are within normal limits unless blood loss or complicating disease is present. The sedimentation rate and other nonspecific indices of inflammation may or may not be elevated. Occasionally, the fibrinogen level is elevated nonspecifically (especially in familial Mediterranean fever [114]) but no uniform changes in serum complement have been found [115]. The bleeding which is occasionally reported is usually due to injury to blood vessels infiltrated with amyloid. In severe hepatic amyloid, the prothrombin time may be slightly elevated [116], and in a few patients with primary amyloid a selective deficiency of factor X (Stuart factor) has been found and attributed to an increased activation or consumption in vivo [117, 118, 119]. Other rare clotting abnormalities have also been reported [120, 121].

There are no specific changes in serum proteins. Patients may have hypogammaglobulinemia [47, 122] or macroglobulinemia [123] or increased IgA, IgG, or IgM at various times in the disease. No clear-cut sequential patterns of abnormality are known. Patients with multiple myeloma may have the usual monoclonal increases in IgG, IgA, IgD, kappa, or lambda chains in their serums, or monoclonal kappa or lambda chains in their urine. Plasmacytosis, while present in myeloma, is not necessarily found in patients with primary or secondary disease [53, 54, 124, 125]. A unique α-globulin

(P component or pentagonal unit) isolated from amyloid deposits has been found in the blood of patients with amyloidosis, but it also occurs in other disease states as well as in normal persons [112].

Urinary abnormalities include proteinuria, hematuria and occasionally casts. Liver function and electrocardiographic abnormalities have been mentioned earlier. Radiologic findings are protean and vary with the system involved.

Diagnosis

The diagnosis of amyloidosis rests first on clinical acumen, i.e., the recognition of a typical pattern of symptoms and signs attributable to a heredofamilial amyloid syndrome, or the recognition of a patient with a predisposing disorder such as rheumatoid arthritis when proteinuria and hepatomegaly develop. Inevitably the diagnosis depends upon biopsy (preferably rectal), use of the appropriate stain (Congo red), and observation of stained tissue in the polarizing microscope for the characteristic green birefringence (Fig. 50-7) [126].

The Congo red test introduced by Bennhold [8] is still of some use and may be interpreted as follows: with 20 percent or less serum retention (that is, 80 percent or more extraction), amyloid is almost certainly present; with 21 to 40 percent serum retention (that is, 60 to 79 percent extraction), amyloid is probably present; with 41 to 60 percent serum retention (40 to 59 percent extraction), the result is not diagnostic, and the test should be repeated in several months; and a serum retention of about 60 percent or more (less than 40 percent extraction) is negative for amyloid. A

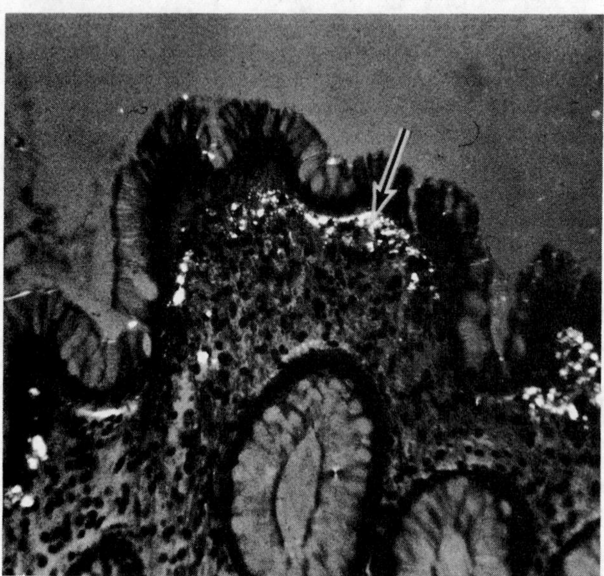

Figure 50-7. Light micrograph of a rectal biopsy demonstrating the green birefringence of amyloid in a patient with secondary disease. × 200. (See color plate II-2 opposite page 115).

negative test does not rule out the diagnosis of amyloid.

Biopsy is safe if an accessible site (gingiva, rectum) is utilized and simple precautions taken [127, 128, 129]. In general, to cope with potential bleeding, it is preferable to obtain the biopsy from sites that can be visualized directly. Amyloid lends tissue a certain rubbery rigidity which makes it apt to bleed. This is seen with the ecchymoses associated with amyloid of the skin, the hematuria seen in renal amyloid, and the startling gastrointestinal bleeding which may occur when amyloid is present in the intestinal tract. With appropriate precautions and with knowledge of the platelet count and the prothrombin, bleeding and clotting times, closed biopsies can be undertaken with relative impunity. Renal biopsy has been successfully performed in many patients with suspected or known amyloid of the kidney. Liver biopsy is usually safe, but the procedure should be approached cautiously in the patients with massive hepatomegaly. Peroral mucosal biopsy has been performed as well as splenic biopsy. In patients with respiratory-tract masses direct biopsy of laryngeal or bronchial lesions may enable one to establish the diagnosis. Bone-marrow biopsy has also been a useful method of establishing the diagnosis.

Treatment and Prognosis

There is no specific treatment for any type of amyloidosis. Eradication of the predisposing disease slows the progress of secondary amyloidosis, and in some organs serial biopsy suggests that reabsorption takes place. Cure of the underlying disease does not guarantee freedom from amyloid, for there are a number of recorded cases of its appearance many years after the cessation of activity of the primary disorder. In most of the reported cures of amyloid, direct biopsy proof is lacking, and the judgment is made on a basis of a clinical diagnosis (that is, hepatomegaly with subsequent improvement) or retention of Congo red dye and subsequent decreased retention. In some of these instances the circumstantial evidence for amyloid and its regression is quite strong. Among the agents which have been used or recommended are whole liver extract, adrenalcortical steroids, ascorbic acid, and immunosuppressive agents. None has caused clear-cut improvement. It is important to emphasize that with conservative supportive measures (e.g., treatment of complicating infections) the prognosis is far better than once had been thought [130]. We have followed patients with renal amyloid for over 12 years.

Two patients with renal amyloid who were severely azotemic and for whom no other form of treatment was available were recently given renal transplants [200]. One died of complicating infection 6 months after transplantation while the second is doing well 17 months posttransplant. The first showed no amyloid in the donor kidney at postmortem, and the second showed none in the donor kidney on biopsy 1 year later. This approach is limited and still should be considered in selected patients only.

HEREDOFAMILIAL AMYLOIDOSES

There is no generally accepted nosology for the increasing numbers of heredofamilial amyloid syndromes that have been described since Ostertag's early report on inherited renal amyloid [131]. The anatomic site of the early deposition of amyloid has been used by one group ("perireticulin-pericollagen classification") [18], some emphasize the site of predominant organ involvement (neuropathic versus nephropathic versus cardopathic amyloid), while others stress the genetic aspects. To date, virtually all analyses of pedigrees have shown that with one major exception the mode of inheritance is autosomal dominant. The exception, amyloidosis of familial Mediterranean fever, is inherited as an autosomal recessive disorder. Since there are no specific biochemical, hematologic, or immunologic tests that allow the differentiation of one type of amyloid from another, one must rely upon the specific and recognizable clinical patterns for classification. The classification utilized here is tentative and based largely on the major site of organ involvement, in addition to genetic data and ethnic background where available (Table 50-2).

Table 50-2. HEREDOFAMILIAL AMYLOIDOSES

Neuropathy
1. Lower limb (D)
   a. Portuguese
   b. Japanese
   c. Other (? U.S.A.—Greek variety)
2. Upper limb—carpal tunnel—vitreous opacities (D)
   a. Swiss (Indiana)
   b. German (Maryland)
3. Lower then upper limb plus nephropathy (D)
   a. English—Irish—Scottish (Iowa)

Nephropathy
1. With marked neuropathy [(3) above]
2. Familial Mediterranean fever (r)
   Non-Ashkenazi Jews; Armenians; Arabs; Turks
3. Fever and abdominal pain (D)
   Swedish
   Sicilian
4. Urticaria, deafness, and renal disease (D)
5. Renal failure and hypertension (D)

Cardiopathy
1. Progressive heart failure
   Danish (D)
2. Persistent atrial standstill

Miscellaneous
1. Medullary carcinoma of the thyroid
2. Lattice corneal dystrophy
3. Cutaneous

HEREDITARY AMYLOID NEUROPATHIES

Lower Limb Neuropathy

Portugal

In 1939, Andrade observed a peculiar type of lower limb neuropathy in a 37-year-old woman who lived in Povoa de Varzim, a fishing town in the Oporto region of Portugal. Since it was known that an unusual illness called *mal dos pesinhos* ("foot disease") existed in that area, further investigations were carried out. These revealed that the patient and others with "foot disease" had a familial type of generalized amyloidosis with major involvement of the nervous system. From the time of his original report [132] to the present, 249 affected individuals out of 623 persons distributed over 148 sibships have been identified for genetic analysis [133].

The disorder is inherited as an autosomal dominant with an equal sex ratio (Fig. 50-8). Sporadic cases of this disorder in individuals of Portuguese descent have been reported in Brazil, France, and Africa. In a study of one patient from the Ruhr region, an extra chromosome with a subterminal centromere in 10 percent of the bone marrow mitoses was found [134]. The age of onset is 25 to 35, with slow steady progression to cachexia and death in 10 to 12 years.

The beginnings of the disease are insidious, with hypesthesias and paresthesias in the lower limbs, followed by limb pain and difficulty in walking. Loss of heat, then pain, and touch and postural sensation take place. Trophic ulcers may appear. Autonomic involvement causes impotance and disturbances of gastrointestinal motility, such as severe constipation alternating with diarrhea. Cardiac involvement may

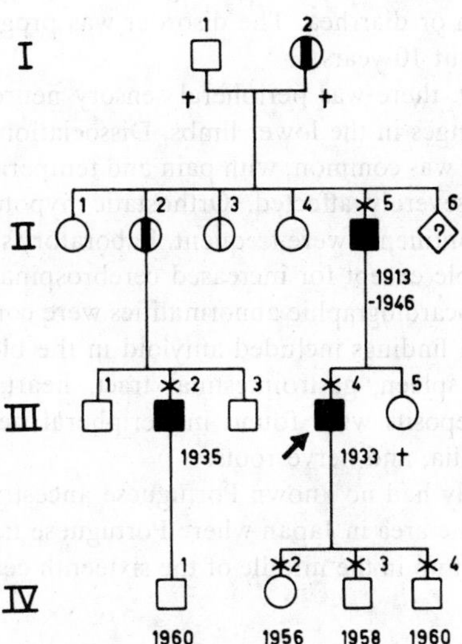

Figure 50-8. Dominant inheritance of hereditary amyloid neuropathy—Portuguese variety. Solid figures represent patients with amyloid and those with vertical bars are patients reliably reported as affected. Patients who are indicated with an asterisk were examined. (*From Andrade* [133], *with permission of the publisher.*)

be manifest by the electrocardiographic evidence of bundle branch block, left ventricular hypertrophy, atrioventricular dissociation, and signs of ischemia [135]. While not frequent, vitreous opacities may occur. Other eye signs include irregular and unequal pupil size. The carpal tunnel syndrome is not found. There are no data concerning clinical renal disease, but the kidneys are usually found involved at autopsy. Diagnosis is suggested by the typical clinical syndrome and confirmed by skin biopsy. No specific laboratory abnormalities have been detected. There is no known therapy.

Postmortem findings include classic amyloid in the peripheral nerves, autonomic nervous system, ganglia, and choroid plexus [136]. Blood vessels of all sizes are involved as is skin, smooth muscle, and occasionally striated muscle. Amyloid may be prominent in the heart as well as at various levels of the gastrointestinal system. The spleen in some cases is heavily involved, while the liver is usually spared except for its blood vessels. Pericollagen distribution of the amyloid has been reported, but not confirmed [18, 42]. Ultrastructural studies of the amyloid have demonstrated fibrils comparable to all other types of amyloid fibrils thus far described [42].

Japan

While amyloidosis was once considered rare in Japan [24], a number of families with this disease have recently been recognized. Araki and colleagues [137] in Arao City, Kyushu, studied four generations of 25 individuals in one family affected by amyloid peripheral neuropathy. The pattern was strikingly similar to the Portuguese polyneuropathy. The inheritance was as an autosomal dominant with high penetrance and equal sex ratio. Symptoms started between ages 30 to 47 with paresthesias in the legs, sexual impotence, and constipation or diarrhea. The disorder was progressive and fatal in about 10 years.

Clinically, there was peripheral sensory neuropathy and trophic changes in the lower limbs. Dissociation of sensory impairment was common, with pain and temperature sensation most severely affected. Orthostatic hypotension and urinary incontinence were frequent. Laboratory studies were unremarkable except for increased cerebrospinal fluid protein. Electrocardiographic abnormalities were common. The postmortem findings included amyloid in the blood vessels of kidney, spleen, gastrointestinal tract, heart, and skin. Amyloid deposits were found in peripheral nerves, autonomic ganglia, and nerve roots.

The family had no known Portuguese ancestry, although Kyushu is the area in Japan where Portuguese trading posts were first set up in the middle of the sixteenth century [138].

Other

Kantarjian and DeJorg in 1953 [139] reported a family in which three members had a similar syndrome consisting of severe peripheral neuropathy (especially of the lower limb), trophic lesions, gastrointestinal and sphincteric disturbances, vitreous opacities, and cardiac abnormalities. Autopsies of two members of the family showed generalized amyloidosis and no other associated disease.

Delank and coworkers in 1965 [140] described a familial amyloid neuropathy in two generations of a family residing in the Ruhr. The inheritance, sex ratio, age of onset, length of life, symptoms, and postmortem findings were almost identical with those described by Andrade. One of these patients had the chromosome abnormalities noted earlier [134]. In 1969, three persons of Greek origin in two kinships were reported to have an amyloid lower limb neuropathy with dissociated sensation and the other features characteristic of the Portuguese type of neuropathy [141]. Other reports in the literature are often not detailed enough to determine with certainty their relation to this particular type of neuropathy but it is likely that a family reported from Poland [142] and a kindred that has been the subject of scattered and multiple overlapping reports in the United States [143–148] suffered from a similar if not identical syndrome.

A Swedish family with hereditary (autosomal dominant) amyloid and lower limb neuropathy; gastrointestinal, autonomic nervous system, and cardiac abnormalities: and vitreous opacities has recently been reported [195].

Finally, a family originally described by Hicks in 1922 [149] with hereditary perforating ulcer of the foot, was subsequently reviewed by Denny-Brown [150] who observed hyalin bodies in ganglia and amyloid in the arterioles, but regarded these changes as secondary. It is not possible to be certain whether or not this family should be classified with the cases above.

Upper Limb Neuropathy with Carpal Tunnel Syndrome

Swiss Family (of Indiana)

Falls and coworkers in 1955 reported [151] a group of patients with ocular abnormalities believed to be associated with familial amyloidosis. One of the families presented with sheathlike semiopalescent hyaline vitreous opacities. The original two patients (cousins) had amyloid on gingival biopsy and ultimately extensive generalized amyloidosis at postmortem examination [152, 138].

This family has been described in detail by Rukavina et al. [152] and followed now for over 15 years by Jackson [138]. Examination of 156 members established the inheritance pattern as an autosomal dominant trait [153]. No chromosomal abnormalities have been observed. The disorder is characterized by a peripheral neuropathy of the upper limb, especially the hands. A carpal tunnel syndrome is frequent and sensory disturbances along the distribution of the median nerve have been documented. The age of onset is in the fourth or fifth decade and the progression is slow, with duration of life from the time of diagnosis varying from 16 to 35 years.

The symptoms consist of pain and numbness in the hands, especially at night. Symptomatic lower limb neuropathy or trophic ulcers are rare or absent. Visual symptoms include "specks" and "floaters". Blindness may ensue. Cardiovascular arrhythmias may appear. Gastrointestinal symptoms are not common. On clinical examination the hands are smooth and shiny and the wrists slightly thickened. There may be thenar atrophy and signs of sensory loss over the distribution of the median nerve. The eyes have vitreous opacities. Cardiomegaly with conduction disturbances may be present. Hepatomegaly has also been reported.

Routine hematologic and bone marrow studies in these patients are normal and no renal abnormalities have been reported. Alpha$_2$-globulin abnormalities are nonspecific [138, 152, 153]. Serum hexosamine levels, urinary mucopolysaccharide excretion [154], and blood amino acid levels are also normal. Pathologic studies have shown extensive amyloidosis of the heart and tongue, with involvement of larynx, liver, spleen, adrenal, pancreas, lungs, prostate, and kidneys. No amyloid was found in bone marrow or skin in one extensive postmortem [152]. The diagnosis is usually established by gingival or rectal biopsy. Skin biopsy is not as useful as in the Portuguese amyloid neuropathy.

No specific treatment for this slowly progressive disorder has been successful. Jackson has found excellent symptomatic relief of the carpal tunnel syndrome by decompressive surgery in four patients. In all of these the diagnosis of local amyloid in the carpal ligament, perineurium, and peritendinous structures was established [138]. Treatment of vitreous opacities in the past has not been successful but a new technical approach has allowed the successful treatment of one patient [138].

German Family (of Maryland)

In Washington County, Maryland, a common ancestry was recently described for 11 families of German origin, many of whom had an unusual neuropathy. Biopsies established that this was an amyloid polyneuropathy, while clinical and genetic analyses showed it to be almost identical with the disorder described in Indiana [155]. Fifty-three of fifty-nine affected living members were examined and a pattern of autosomal dominant inheritance was established. No chromosomal abnormalities were found. Slightly different clinical patterns predominated within each family.

The age of onset ranged from 15 to 66 years (mean 43 years) and the disorder ranged widely in duration but was present for at least 14 years in all. Men were more severely affected than women. The initial symptoms in most patients were consistent with a carpal tunnel syndrome, i.e., pain, paresthesias, or numbness (at night or after a day's work) in the median nerve distribution. Thenar wasting and loss of power followed. In some, these were the only symptoms for periods of up to 20 years. In others, similar discomfort in the feet followed in 8 to 10 years. Gastrointestinal, sphincteric, and bladder symptoms were rare. Blisters, burns, and ulcers were found occasionally in analgesic areas. Cardiovascular complaints were not marked.

Signs were those of median nerve compression and gradual development of more widespread sensory loss. Vitreous opacities, were found in only one patient. No specific laboratory abnormalities were detected in the blood chemistry, routine blood studies, or urinalyses. Sedimentation rates were, on occasion, slightly elevated. Serum immunoglobulins, cerebrospinal fluid, and liver function tests were normal. X-rays of the hands demonstrated small translucent areas of unknown significance in carpal, metacarpal, and phalangeal bones, respectively in three instances. Several patients had ECG evidence of myocardial disease, or arrythmias occurred attributable to amyloid. Electromyographic studies demonstrated prolonged latency of the median nerve in 33 of 39 tests.

Postmortem examinations have been performed of two patients from this family group. In one, almost all tissues were involved. The heart had extensive amyloid, and there were amyloid deposits in blood vessels of skin, skeletal muscle, nerves, lymph nodes, testis, prostate, lungs, intestine, adrenal, thyroid, parathyroid, pituitary, parasympathetic nerves, and ganglia. There was no amyloid in the spleen and only small amounts in vessels of the liver and kidneys. The second patient had deposits of amyloid in the heart, blood vessels, kidneys, and peripheral nerves, as well as some in the splenic and hepatic blood vessels [155]. Further pathologic material was obtained at the time of surgery for the carpal tunnel syndrome from 12 additional patients. Amyloid was found in the soft tissues of 8 of them [155]. Lambird and Hartmann [156] reported that 7 of 10 of these patients had amyloid in the flexor retinaculum. The ultrastructure of this material is the same as that of nonhereditofamilial amyloid, i.e., composed of fine rigid nonbranching fibrils, usually collected in discreet dense bundles among bundles of collagen.

Surgical decompression of the flexor retinaculum has given relief of the carpal tunnel syndrome in all but one or two patients [156]. Nerve conduction tests have shown improved function postoperatively and the symptomatic improvement has been striking.

A common ancestry could not be ascertained, even though both families have been traced back to the eighteenth century, yet the Swiss (Indiana) and German (Maryland) varieties of amyloid are virtually identical. Mahloudji and coworkers [155] determined that the familial peripheral neuropathy reported earlier by Schlesinger et al. [157] was one of the pedigrees which they had described. In that particular pedigree vitreous opacities, as well as the carpal tunnel syndrome, were present in the propositus.

Lower Then Upper Limb Neuropathy and Nephropathy

Amyloidosis in a family whose ancestors originated in Scotland, England, and Ireland was described by Van Allen and coworkers. They obtained pathologic verification of the diagnosis in eight members of two generations, including three father-son pairs [158]. The neuropathy differed from the preceding one in that both the upper and lower limbs were severely affected and there were no classical carpal tunnel syndromes. The disorder was inherited as an autosomal dominant. The average age of onset was 33 to 36 and the average life span was 17 years in the generation of the propositus [138].

The symptoms of neuropathy started in the lower limb with pain, dysesthesias, and weakness, followed by loss of pain sensation. The upper limbs were also frequently involved. The general course was progression of the neuropathy. Unlike the two preceding types of neuropathy this syndrome was accompanied by severe and progressive renal amyloid leading to death in uremia. Clinical nephrosis was not observed. Symptoms of peptic ulcer were clinically prominent (they appeared in six out of eight cases) and were often proved radiologically; however, the ulcer could not always be directly attributed to the amyloid. Cardiac symptoms were negligible except for hypertension associated with the progressive renal disease. Several patients had diminished hearing. In three persons cataracts occurred early in life. Neither vitreous opacities nor macroglossia was seen.

Routine laboratory studies showed only changes associated with the progressive renal disease. Cerebrospinal fluid protein was elevated (84 to 204 mg per 100 ml) in all patients subjected to lumbar puncture. At postmortem examination there was predominant involvement of liver, spleen, adrenal, kidney, testis, and nerve. Amyloid infiltration was found in sympathetic nerves and ganglia and in dorsal root ganglia, with crowding and destruction of cell bodies. In the kidney the deposition was largely arteriolar. Liver amyloid was present but with few clinical signs and symptoms. Similarly, marked adrenal amyloid occurred in four cases, without clinical signs of adrenal insufficiency. An ultrastructural analysis of the amyloid showed it to consist of 70 to 100 Å fibrils.

Thus, this unique syndrome, because of widespread neurologic involvement, severe renal amyloid, lack of vitreous amyloid, and lack of clear-cut carpal tunnel syndrome, appears to constitute a third variety of neuropathic amyloid.

NEPHROPATHY

With Marked Neuropathy (See Above)

The inadequacy of a clinical classification is obvious when one considers the severe renal lesion in the cases listed immediately above, for this family could equally well be classified as having a severe form of amyloid nephropathy—with associated neuropathy.

Familial Mediterranean Fever

In 1945, Siegal described 11 cases of benign paroxysmal peritonitis, a clinical entity characterized by recurrent attacks of peritoneal and pleural pain of unknown cause [159]. A myriad of names have been applied to this syndrome, depending upon which symptom or sign an author chose to emphasize. In 1955 and 1958 [160] Heller and associates, wishing to draw attention to the hereditary aspects of the disease, its prevalence amongst peoples of Mediterranean stock, and its striking febrile episodes, introduced the term familial Mediterranean fever (FMF). They also clearly indicated its strong association with amyloidosis and the relentless course of the renal amyloid disease. Previously, Cattan and Mamou had observed the disease, called *la maladie periodique,* in North Africa [161, 162], and it has been described in the United States as "familial recurring polyserositis" [163]. It is likely that some cases of "periodic disease" also fit within this descriptive framework [164].

The disorder is found largely in families of Mediterranean stock, especially non-Ashkenazi Jews (Sephardic primarily) and Armenians [165, 166]. It has been reported amongst Arabs [159] and it is probably not uncommon in individuals of Turkish origin [167]. It has been reported sporadically in individuals of other ethnic background but in many cases the clear-cut delineation of the clinical syndrome or the presence of amyloid has been lacking. The recent descriptions of a syndrome remarkably like FMF but of different inheritance and in other ethnic groups (Swedish [168] and Italian [169]) will be commented upon later.

Familial Mediterranean fever is inherited as an autosomal recessive trait. As such it is unique amongst the various forms of hereditary amyloidosis, for all others reported to date are autosomal dominant disorders. The most detailed genetic analyses were derived by Sohar and colleagues [165, 21] from a large population of Sephardic (North African) Jews. Analyses of 229 families suggested a homozygote incidence of 1:2,000 and a gene frequency of 1:45 or 0.022. Most pedigrees showed that the disease occurred amongst sibs and that first cousin marriages in this group were high. They observed that while amyloid was almost invariably associated with FMF, its occurrence did not seem to be secondary to the FMF nor related to its severity or frequency of attacks. Indeed amyloidosis as a sole manifestation of FMF was reported [170]. This strengthened the concept that two phenotypes exist: phenotype I in which clinical attacks precede amyloid, and phenotype II in which amyloid precedes the attacks.

Familial Mediterranean fever is characterized by attacks of fever which may be accompanied by pain in the abdomen, chest, or joints. These attacks usually occur in childhood, recur at irregular intervals, follow no predictable pattern, last 12 to 36 hours, and have no anatomic sequellae. The fever may be the sole manifestation. Abdominal pain is severe, gives a clinical picture of peritoneal inflammation, and has often led to fruitless surgical intervention. It was seen in 95 percent of Sohar and Gafni's patients [21] and was the presenting manifestation in 55 percent of these cases. Chest pain was typically pleuritic in nature, occurred in 40 percent of the patients, and was occasionally associated with a small pleural exudate. Joint pains which occurred in 75 percent of their patients were unique in that they tended to last longer (even up to 1 year), were associated with mild to severe inflammatory joint effusions, and usually were not associated with progressive bone or joint damage. An erysipelas-like erythema was another manifestation of acute FMF. It usually occurred on the lower leg and subsided spontaneously with remission of the attack.

Prior to the beginning of renal amyloidosis no specific laboratory abnormalities are detected. Plasma fibrinogen has been reported to be elevated [114]. No clear-cut clinical or electrocardiographic evidence of pericarditis has been found. The peripheral white cell count may be transiently elevated, but extensive search for infectious agents, pyrogenic steroids, and the like have not been fruitful. The cause of the attacks is completely unknown.

Amyloidosis is present in 27 percent of 316 FMF patients being followed by Gafni and coworkers [171]. They have found that the frequency of amyloid increased from 18 percent amongst patients born between 1955 and 1959 to 75 percent of those born before 1930, and believe that virtually all patients with FMF ultimately develop and die of amyloidosis. The amyloid usually manifests itself by proteinuria, and progresses to an amyloid nephrotic syndrome and ultimately to death from uremia. Renal failure was the cause of death in all patients except one who died of severe malabsorption due to gastrointestinal amyloid. In spite of widespread amyloid in other organs, clinical manifestations have been few. Splenomegaly is common while hepatomegaly is not. Adrenal insufficiency has not been seen. Macroglossia, carpal tunnel syndrome, severe neuropathy, and vitreous opacities are not found in this form of hereditary amyloid. The overall duration of life in 11 patients with clinically apparent renal amyloid ranged from $3\frac{1}{2}$ to 13 years, with an average of 7 years.

The diagnosis of amyloid can be made directly by renal biopsy but is most easily established by rectal biopsy, in spite of the paucity of gastrointestinal symptoms [172]. There is no specific treatment for the amyloid of familial Mediterranean fever, but supportive measures are usually helpful in prolonging life. It has been suggested that a low fat diet [173] will decrease the clinical attacks of FMF in patients of Armenian origin, but this has not been demonstrable in the group in Israel [174].

A wide variety of other agents including adrenal cortical steroids have no clear-cut effect either on the clinical attacks of FMF or on the amyloid disease.

At postmortem examination, extensive deposits of amyloid are found in the kidneys, especially the glomeruli, including the interstitial areas. Amyloid is widespread about blood vessels, especially the arterioles throughout the body. Splenic and adrenal amyloid is common and pulmonary deposits often occur adjacent to the pleura. Deposits are also found in the gastrointestinal tract, thyroid, and seminiferous tubules. Amyloid of the liver may be strikingly absent except for blood vessel involvement. Cardiac amyloid is minimal. The fine structure of the amyloid is comparable to that previously described [41].

Fever with Abdominal Pain

Several sporadic syndromes have been described that are characterized by recurrent attacks of abdominal pain. These have often been diagnosed as periodic disease when other causes have been eliminated. They have occasionally been found to be familial. One such family was described in Sweden in 1964 [175]. Subsequently, a member of the family succumbed to renal disease and was found to have renal amyloid [168]. Since he had recurrent attacks of abdominal pain with fever and died of renal amyloid he would seem to fit the syndrome of FMF. At postmortem examination widespread vascular as well as renal amyloid was found, including amyloid in the spleen and portal areas of the liver, much as in FMF amyloid.

Genetic analysis indicated that this syndrome was inherited as an autosomal dominant. Furthermore, the patients in this group had abdominal pain without any chest or joint pain and no skin rash. Their pain and fever lasted from days to weeks. Thus, while it is possibly a related syndrome, striking differences exist.

Another family was reported by Reich and Franklin [169]. The propositus, of Italian descent, had abdominal pain and was found to have amyloid in the gastrointestinal tract. Detailed family study revealed that his daughter and granddaughter had recurrent abdominal pain and fever suggestive of FMF. The dominant pattern of inheritance, the age of the propositus (80 years), and the lack of renal disease all suggest that this syndrome is not identical with FMF.

Thus while both the Swedish and Italian families bear a clinical similarity to FMF, the difference in the pattern of inheritance would necessitate separate classification at present. It should also be noted that etiocholanolone fever does not fit into any of these categories and in unequivocal FMF patients, abnormalities of etiocholanolone metabolism have not been identified [176].

Urticaria, Deafness, and Amyloid Renal Disease

A syndrome which begins with an urticarial rash, chills, and fever in adolescence, and is followed in a number of years by progressive perceptive deafness and eventually by nephropathy, was described by Muckle and Wells in 1962 [177]. They were able to demonstrate amyloid in two patients and suspected it in two others in their sibship of six. Family data were collected on 101 persons covering five generations in the area of Derbyshire, England. Nephritis, deafness, "aguey bouts," and urticarial rash were found in significant numbers. The authors thought that the symptom complex had an autosomal dominant inheritance.

No specific reason for the urticaria could be elicited. Three of the four patients whom the authors regarded as having amyloid (proved in two) were female. Other findings included loss of libido, skin thickening, glaucoma, pes cavus, and elevated sedimentation rates. Nonspecific serum protein changes were present, and one patient had hyperglycinuria. The amyloid deposits were extensive in the two who died of uremia. In the first patient the other organ involved was the adrenal gland, whereas in the second, amyloid of the spleen, liver, and testes occurred. The inner ear was examined in both cases, and in neither was amyloid demonstrable.

Subsequently, a solitary patient with amyloidosis associated with uriticaria, pes cavus, perceptive deafness, and renal disease was reported [178]. This patient reproduced in almost all respects the entire symptom complex reported in the sibship described above, and although no family relationship could be elicited, the patient was born on the outskirts of Derbyshire. It is possible that another family with comparable findings, first attributed to toxoplasmosis, truly represented another variant of this syndrome [179, 180]. An isolated case of deafness, urticaria, and amyloid was reported from Denmark in 1967 [181]. Detailed family examination was negative except for deafness in two members. Chromosome analysis of the propositus showed a small isochromatic gap in 20 percent of metaphases. This was difficult to interpret since the patient had been treated with cytotoxic agents.

Another family, possibly of Norwegian descent, was recently found to have a similar constellation, i.e., amyloidosis, deafness, urticaria, and limb pains [182]. Three generations were analyzed and amyloid proven in the propositus and a sib, both with the full syndrome. It was suspected in two other generations in which the full clinical syndrome was also present. Dominant inheritance was likely. Chromosome study was negative in the propositus.

It is also possible that this unusual group of findings was present in one of the earliest reports of familial amyloidosis [183]. Thirty years ago, three brothers (aged 42, 43, and 45) were reported to have died of renal amyloid. All three had had frequent attacks of chills and fever in childhood. Family follow-up in 1967 [155] indicated that the son of one had developed amyloidosis and that two of his five children had fevers, transient joint pains, and maculopapular rashes.

Renal Failure, Hypertension, and Amyloid

Although hypertension had long been considered a rare or late manifestation of renal amyloidosis, the earliest report of familial amyloid was that of Ostertag [131], who in 1932 and, subsequently, in 1950 [184] reported a family in which four members had hypertension, renal disease, and hepatosplenomegaly, and died at an early age. Autopsy examination of the propositus and one other member revealed amyloid in the kidney, liver, spleen, adrenals, and throughout the blood vessels. The syndrome was suspected in several others in the family and since it affected three consecutive generations, an autosomal dominant inheritance was proposed.

HEREDITARY CARDIAC AMYLOID

Progressive Heart Failure

In 1962, Frederiksen and his coworkers [185], in Denmark, described a sibship of 12 members, of whom 5 (3 females and 2 males) had proven amyloid, and in 2 of whom (1 female and 1 male) there was reason to suspect the same diagnosis. Of the remaining 5, 2 died in infancy, so that at least 5 and possibly 7 of the 10 adult sibs were severely affected by the disorder. The disease in these patients had its onset as dyspnea on exertion at 37 to 46 years of age. Three had had transient nonprogressive paresthesias in the hands. The dyspnea was rapidly progressive, and evidence of severe failure of the right side of the heart, leading to incapacity in a matter of months, was the usual course. The patients had neither macroglossia nor vitreous opacities. Renal, neurologic, and gastrointestinal manifestations were apparently not significant. The cardiac disease was similar in all patients studied. From the electrocardiographic tracings in five patients, the authors divided the myocardial amyloidosis into two types, the first with right bundle branch block with left-axis deviation and prolonged PR interval and the second with left ventricular hypertrophy and strain and with left-axis deviation or low voltage in the standard limb leads.

Hemodynamic studies of the five patients were uniform and showed elevated right atrial and pulmonary wedge pressures. The dip plateau configuration seen in diseases with impaired diastolic ventricular filling was present in all. The duration of illness from the beginning of symptoms to death was 2 or 3 years in three subjects, 6 years in one subject, and unknown in the two who had died (in their forties) before the study.

Laboratory assays in the patients showed no striking serum protein abnormalities, although a question arose of elevated α_1- and α_2-globulins in other members of the family. Clinical studies of first-degree and second-degree relatives gave no evidence of amyloidosis. Pathological studies showed extensive amyloid deposits in the myocardium and endocardium, and scattered small deposits in other organs. The spleen and kidney were spared in two and involved in one case. Only two patients had complete autopsies. Small vessels, adipose tissue, and skin were also generally involved.

Persistent Atrial Standstill

No other series of cases of hereditary amyloid with major involvement of the heart was reported until a recent family study of Allensworth and associates [186]. They reported three sibs who had slow heart rates, absent P waves on ECG, and apparent absence of atrial activity. A biopsy of the atrium of one patient demonstrated interstitial and perivascular amyloid.

The propositus was a Latin American woman who had pseudoxanthoma elasticum as well as the atrial standstill. Her brother, who presented with dyspnea and fever, was subjected to biopsy of the right atrial appendage and amyloid was demonstrated. Liver biopsies of both patients were negative. No direct evidence of more widespread amyloid was obtained. Their sister also was found to have atrial standstill, and a limited examination in a fourth sib revealed strong evidence of the identical abnormality. Data were not available on three other sibs (two living and one deceased). Chromosome studies were normal.

The clinical syndrome was characterized by slow pulse and cardiac enlargement with associated mild congestive heart failure. The latter responded to bed rest and salt restriction. The murmur of mitral regurgitation was present in two of the patients. At rest, heart rates were 35 to 50 per min, and increased after exercise or atropine. Electrocardiograms showed regular QRS complexes but no P waves. The absence of atrial activity was confirmed by intracardiac electrocardiograms. These patients differ from those of Frederiksen in the mildness of the congestive failure, and in the normal pressure measurements and cardiac outputs in two of the three patients. In addition, skin biopsies in the present series did not demonstrate amyloid. Their disease thus far has not been progressive.

MISCELLANEOUS HEREDITARY AMYLOIDOSES

Medullary Carcinoma of the Thyroid

In a study of pheochromocytoma and thyroid carcinoma, it was found that a mother and daughter in one of two families had amyloid-producing medullary thyroid carcinomas. The authors [187] reviewed several other reported kindreds of familial phenochromocytoma and medullary thyroid carcinoma. The latter often produced amyloid locally or in metastases. A single-gene autosomal-dominant inheritance pattern has been suggested for this unusual entity.

These associations had been known since the 1930s but it was Sipple in 1961 [188] who documented two cases of his own, reviewed the material of others, and brought the distinctive relationship to amyloid to the forefront. Of the multiple other family studies of this syndrome [187, 189] perhaps the most extensive is that of Steiner and coworkers [190], who studied a kindred of 186 patients and reviewed the literature in detail. They suggested that this entity be called multiple endocrine neoplasia, Type 2 (MEN-Type 2) to distinguish it from the entity involving tumors of the pituitary, parathyroids, and pancreatic islet cells (multiple endocrine neoplasia Type 1). They concluded that MEN-Type 2 is inherited as an autosomal dominant with high penetrance and variable expressivity.

Lattice Corneal Dystrophy

In addition to the generalized inherited amyloidoses, several forms of local amyloid have been described. One unusual corneal lesion, lattice dystrophy, was shown by several investigators to be comparable in all its histologic aspects to amyloid [191]. Klintworth [192] examined in detail five corneal buttons obtained from three sibs with this lesion. Histochemical stains and electron microscopic studies confirmed its similarity to amyloid of other varieties. The disorder is inherited as an autosomal dominant.

There have been no post-mortems on such patients, but limited biopsy data indicate that this curious lesion is a local form of inherited amyloid.

Cutaneous Amyloidosis

In 1950, localized amyloid deposits in the legs of two sibs, who also had psoriasis, were reported [193]. More recently [194] a local cutaneous amyloid was described in three members of different generations in the same family (a woman, her son, and his daughter). In all, the cutaneous lesion was a pigmented nonlichenified lesion (on the back), that absorbed Congo red on intradermal injection. Biopsies revealed papillary deposits that demonstrated methyl violet metachromasia. No evidence of diffuse involvement with amyloid was reported, and there was no evidence of similar lesions in other members of the family. One of the three affected also had psoriasis.

SUMMARY

1 Amyloid is a fibrous glycoprotein which accumulates extracellularly in the connective tissue, either appearing in association with another disease (often infectious or inflammatory) or appearing spontaneously for no apparent cause. In the former instance, the clinical condition is known as secondary amyloidosis, and in the latter, primary amyloidosis. It has been identified as a concomitant of aging. In recent years an increased number of heredofamilial amyloid syndromes have been recognized.

2 The extracellular substance amyloid, is eosinophilic, shows "crystal violet metachromasia," and most characteristically demonstrates green birefringence when viewed in the polarizing microscope after Congo red staining. By electron microscopy it has been discovered that tissue sections of all varieties of human and animal amyloid are made up of long, thin, rigid nonbranching fibrils, with an apparent diameter of about 100 Å. By use of negative staining techniques, further subunit structure and periodicity has been ascribed to the fibrils. X-ray diffraction studies have consistently demonstrated that the amyloid fibril has a cross-β pattern. Chemical analysis of the fibril has shown it to be a protein that contains a small amount (2 to 5 percent) of carbohydrate. It is distinct from collagen in the absence of hydroxyproline, hydroxylysine, and tryptophan and distinct from elastin in the absence of desmosine and isodesmosine. It is nonimmunogenic in native form and is not composed of antigen-antibody complexes, or whole immunoglobulin molecules.

3 A second component in amyloid is the plasma component (P component or pentagonal unit), which is also a glycoprotein, is immunogenic, has a sedimentation coefficient of about 10S, and a different ultrastructure. On x-ray diffraction it does not give a cross-β pattern; on isolation it does not stain with Congo red or crystal violet.

4 The pathogenesis of amyloidosis is not known. No abnormalities in circulating antibody have been identified but it is possible that alterations in delayed hypersensitivity exist.

5 Heredofamilial amyloidoses include a group primarily involving the nervous system. Among these a lower limb neuropathy, first described in Portugal, has a poor prognosis and is characterized by progressively severe neuropathy including marked autonomic nervous system involvement. This variety has been described in Japan and in a family of Greek origin in the United States. The second type of neuropathy has been found in families of Swiss origin in Indiana and in Maryland. It is a milder disease, and is often associated with a carpal tunnel syndrome and vitreous opacities. A more severe variety of generalized neuropathy and renal amyloid has been described in Iowa in a family of English-Irish-Scottish ancestry.

6 Several types of severe familial renal disease in association with amyloid have been described. Possibly the most remarkable is familial Mediterranean fever (FMF), a disorder subdivided into phenotype I with irregularly occurring fever and abdominal, chest, or joint pain, preceding or accompanying renal amyloid, and phenotype II in which amyloidosis is the first or only manifestation of the disease. All inherited amyloidoses thus far described, with the exception of FMF, are autosomal dominant diseases. FMF is an autosomal recessive. It is most commonly seen in Sephardic Jews, Armenians, Turks, and Arabs. Sporadically, other hereditary renal amyloids have been described, including the curious association of urticaria, deafness, and renal amyloid.

7 Severe familial amyloid heart disease has been described in a Danish family, and familial persistent atrial standstill in a family of Latin American origin.

8 Miscellaneous hereditary amyloid syndromes include those of hereditary multiple endocrine neoplasias—Type 2 (including medullary carcinoma of the thyroid with amyloid) and familial lattice corneal dystrophy.

9 While the etiology of amyloid is unknown, the course variable, and the prognosis uncertain, many patients do well and live many years. Studies are currently directed toward the further definition of the pathogenesis, the characterization of the fibril and pentagonal component, and ultimately toward rational treatment of this unusual disorder.

BIBLIOGRAPHY

1. Cohen, A. S.: Amyloidosis. New Eng. J. Med., **277**, 522–530, 574–583, 628–638, 1967.
2. Rokitansky, C.: *Handbuch der Pathologischen Anatomie,* vol. 3, p. 311. Braumuller and Seidel, Vienna, 1842.
3. Wainewright, J.: *A Treatise of the Liver* appended to *A Mechanical Account of the Non-Naturals,* 5th ed., 1737.
4. Virchow, R.: Weitere Mittheilungen uber des Vorkommen der pflanzlichen cellulose beim Menchen. Virchow. Arch. Path. Anat., **6**, 268–271, 1854*b*.
5. Virchow, R.: Zur Cellulose-Frage. Virchow. Arch. Path. Anat., **6**, 416–426, 1854*c*.
6. Waldenström, H.: On the formation and disappearance of amyloid in man. Acta Chir. Scand., **63**, 479–530, 1928.
7. Bennhold, H.: Eine spezifische Amyloidfärbung mit Kongorot. Munchen. Med. Wschr., **69**, 1537–1538, 1922.
8. Bennhold, H.: Üeber die Ausscheidung intravenös einverleibter Kongorotes bei den verschiedensten Erkrankungen insbesondere bei Amyloidosis. Deutsch. Arch. Klin. Med., **142**, 32–46, 1923.
9. Wilks, S.: Cases of lardaceous disease and some allied affections: With remarks. Guy. Hosp. Rep., **2**, 103–132, 1856.
10. Soyka, J.: Ueber amyloide degeneration. Prag. Med. Wschr., **1**, 165–171, 1876.
11. Wild, C.: Beitrag zur Kenntniss der amyloiden und der hyalinen Degeneration des bindegewebes. Beitr. Path. Anat., **1**, 175–200, 1886.
12. Lubarsch, O.: Zur Kenntnis ungewoehnlicher Amyloid Ablegerungen. Virchow. Arch. Path. Anat., **271**, 867–889, 1929.
13. Reimann, H. A., Koucky, R. F., and Eklumd, C. M.: Primary amyloidosis limited to tissue of mesenchymal origin. Amer. J. Pathol., **11**, 977–988, 1935.
14. King, L. S.: Atypical amyloid disease: With observations on a new silver stain for amyloid. Amer. J. Path., **24**, 1095–1116, 1948.
15. Dahlin, D. C.: Classification and general aspects of amyloidosis. Med. Clin. N. Amer., **34**, 1107–1111, 1950.
16. Symmers, W. St. C.: Primary amyloidosis: A review. J. Clin. Path., **9**, 187–211, 1956.
17. Missmahl, H. P., and Iartwig, M.: Polarisationsoptische untersuchungen an der amyloidsubstanz. Virchow. Arch. Path. Anat., **324**, 489–508, 1953.
18. Heller, H., Missmahl, H. P., Sohar, E., and Gafni, J.: Amyloidosis: Its differentiation into perireticulin and pericollagen types. J. Path. Bact., **88**, 15–34, 1964.
19. Cohen, A. S.: The constitution and genesis of amyloid, in *International Review of Experimental Pathology,* vol. IV, edited by G. W., Richter and M. A. Epstein. Academic, New York, 1965.
20. Hoedemaeker, P. H., Andrade, C., and Pick, A. I.: Discussion of "Reticulin and collagen as important factors for the localization of amyloid," in *Proceedings of the Symposium on Amyloidosis,* edited by E. Mandema, L. Ruinen, J. H. Scholten, and A. S. Cohen, pp. 29–33. Excerpta Medica, Amsterdam, 1968.
21. Sohar, E., Gafni, J., Pras, M., and Heller, H.: Familial Mediterranean fever. A survey of 470 cases and review of the literature. Amer. J. Med., **43**, 227–253, 1967.
22. Battaglia, S.: Results of a statistical investigation on amyloidosis. Path. Microbiol. (Basel), **27**, 792–808, 1964.

23. Edington, G. M., and Mainwaring, A. R.: Amyloidosis in Western Nigeria. Path. Microbiol. (Basel), **27,** 841–847, 1964.
24. Nakagawa, S., and Suzue, K.: Amyloidosis in Japan. Path. Microbiol. (Basel), **27,** 850–854, 1964.
25. Cooke, R. A., and Champness, L. T.: Amyloidosis in Papua and New Guinea—a preliminary communication. Papua and New Guinea Med. J., **10,** 43–46, 1967.
26. Ravid, M., Gafni, J., Sohar, E., and Missmahl, H. P.: Incidence and origin of nonsystemic microdeposits of amyloid. J. Clin. Path., **20,** 15–20, 1967.
27. Cohen, A. S., and Wills, A. A.: III. The incidence of amyloid deposits in 100 consecutive postmortem examinations, in *Proceedings of the Symposium on Amyloidosis,* edited by E. Mandema, L. Ruinen, J. H. Scholten, and A. S. Cohen, pp. 438–445. Excerpta Medica, Amsterdam, 1968.
28. Schwartz, P.: Senile cerebral pancreatic insular and cardiac amyloidosis. Trans. NY Acad. Sci., **27,** 393–413, 1965.
29. Wright, J. R., Calkins, E., Breen, W. J., Stolte, G., and Schultz, R. T.: Relationship of amyloid to aging. Medicine (Balt.), **48,** 39–60, 1969.
30. Vassar, P. S., and Culling, C. T. A.: Fluorescent stains with special reference to amyloid and connective tissues. Arch. Path. (Chicago), **68,** 487–498, 1959.
31. Sweat, F., and Puchtler, H.: Demonstration of amyloid with direct cotton dyes. Arch. Path. (Chicago), **80,** 613–620, 1965.
32. Cooper, J. H.: An evaluation of current methods for the diagnostic histochemistry of amyloid. J. Clin. Path., **22,** 410–413, 1969.
33. Divry, P., and Florkin, M.: Sur les proprietes optiques l'amyloide. C. R. Soc. Biol. (Paris), **97,** 1808–1810, 1927.
34. Ladewig, P.: Double-refringence of the amyloid-Congo red-complex in histological sections. Nature (London), **156,** 81–82, 1945.
35. Missmahl, H. P.: Polarisationsoptische beitrag zur Kongorotfarbung des amyloid. Zeit. Wiss. Mikr., **63,** 133–139, 1957.
36. Diezel, P. B. and Pfleiderer, A., Jr.: Histochemische und polarisationsoptische Untersuchungen am Amyloid. Virchow. Arch. Path. Anat., **332,** 552–567, 1959.
37. Cohen, A. S., and Calkins, E.: Electron microscopic observations on a fibrous component in amyloid of diverse origins. Nature (London), **183,** 1202–1203, 1959.
38. Caesar, R.: Elektronenmikroskopische Untersuchungen an menschlichem Amyloid bei verschiedenen Grundkrankheiten. Path. Microbiol. (Basel), **24,** 387–396, 1961.
39. Manitz, G., and Themann, H.: Elektronenmikroskopischer Beitrag zur Feinstruktur menschlichen leber amyloids. Beit. Path. Anat., **128,** 103–121, 1962.
40. Boere, H., Ruinen, L., and Scholten, J. H.: Electron microscopic studies on the fibrillar component of human splenic amyloid. J. Lab. Clin. Med., **66,** 943–951, 1965.
41. Cohen, A. S., Frensdorff, A., Lamprecht, M. A. and Calkins, E.: A study of the fine structure of the amyloid associated with familial Mediterranean fever. Amer. J. Path., **41,** 567–578, 1962.
42. Andrade, C.: Familial amyloidotic polyneuropathy, in *Proceedings of the Symposium on Amyloidosis,* edited by E. Mandema, L. Ruinen, J. H. Scholten, and A. S. Cohen. Excerpta Medica, Amsterdam, 1968.
43. Shirahama, T., and Cohen, A. S.: The fine structure of the glomerulus in human and experimental renal amyloidosis. Amer. J. Path., **51,** 869–911, 1967.
44. Cohen, A. S., Gross, E. and Shirahama, T.: The light and electron microscopic autoradiographic demonstration of local amyloid formation in spleen explants. Amer. J. Path., **47,** 1079–1111, 1965.
45. Bari, W. A., Pettengill, O. S. and Sorenson, G. D.: Electron microscopy and electron microscopic autoradiography of splenic cell cultures from mice with amyloidosis. Lab. Invest., **20,** 234–242, 1969.
46. Bailey, C. H.: The production of amyloid disease and chronic nephritis in rabbits by repeated intravenous injections of living colon bacilli. J. Exp. Med., **23,** 773–790, 1916.
47. Mawas, C., Sors, C. and Bernier, J.-J.: Amyloidosis associated with primary agammaglobulinemia, severe diarrhea and familial hypogammaglobulinemia. Amer. J. Med., **46,** 624–634, 1969.
48. Mellors, R. C. and Ortega, L. G.: Analytical pathology. III. New observations on the pathogenesis of glomerulonephritis, lipid nephrosis, periarteritis nodosa, and secondary amyloidosis in man. Amer. J. Path., **32,** 455–500, 1956.
49. Vasquez, J. J. and Dixon, F. J.: Immunohistochemical analysis of amyloid by the fluorescence technique. J. Exp. Med., **104,** 727–736, 1956.
50. Osserman, E. J., Takatsuki, K., and Talal, N.: Multiple myeloma. I. The pathogenesis of "Amyloidosis." Seminars Hema., **1,** 1–85, 1964.
51. Schneider, G.: Uber die Pathogenese der Amyloidose: Immunologische, histochemische und morphologische Untersuchungen. Ergebn. Allg. Path., **44,** 1–102, 1964.
52. Horowitz, R. E., Stuyvesant, V. W., Wigmore, W., and Tatter, D.: Fibrinogen as a component of amyloid. Arch. Path. (Chicago), **79,** 238–244, 1965.
53. Cathcart, E. S., Ritchie, R. F., Brandt, K., and Cohen, A. S.: Serologic and urinary studies in patients with amyloidosis, in *Proceedings of Symposium on Amyloidosis,* edited by E. Mandema, L. Ruinen, J. H. Scholten, and A. S. Cohen. Excerpta Medica, Amsterdam, 1968.
54. Barth, W. F., Willerson, J. T., Waldmann, T. A., and Decker, J. L.: Primary amyloidosis. Amer. J. Med., **47,** 259–273, 1969.
55. Paul, W. P., and Cohen, A. S.: Electron microscopic studies of amyloid fibrils with ferritin conjugated antibody. Amer. J. Path., **43,** 721–738, 1963.
56. Cathcart, E. S., and Cohen, A. S.: The relation between isolated human amyloid fibrils and human γ-globulin and its subunits. J. Immun. **96,** 239–244, 1966.
57. Ram, J. S., DeLellis, R. A., and Glenner, G. G.: Amyloid. IV. Is human amyloid immunogenic? Int. Arch. Alleg., **34,** 269–282, 1968.
58. Franklin, E. L. and Pras, M.: Immunologic studies of water-soluble human amyloid fibrils. J. Exp. Med., **130,** 797–808, 1969.
59. Benditt, E. P., Lagunoff, D., Eriksen, E., and Iseri, O. A.: Amyloid: Extraction and preliminary characterization of some proteins. Arch. Path. (Chicago), **74,** 323–330, 1962.
60. Cagli, V., Carbonara, A., and Mancini, G.: Le proprieta antigene della sostanza amiloide. Boll. Soc. Ital. Biol. Sper., **38,** 353–355, 1962.
61. Muckle, T. J.: Protein components of amyloid. Nature (London), **203,** 773–774, 1964.
62. Cathcart, E. S., Wollheim, F. A., and Cohen, A. S.: Plasma protein constituents of amyloid fibrils. J. Immun., **99,** 376–385, 1967.
63. Clerici, E., Pierpaoli, W., and Romussi, M.: Experimental amyloidosis in immunity. Path. Microbiol. (Basel), **28,** 806–815, 1965.
64. Rohde, R.: Über die experimentelle Amyloidose bei thymektomierten Maüsen. Z. Immunitsetsforsch, **129,** 268–277, 1965.
65. Smetana, H.: The relation of the reticuloendothelial system to the formation of amyloid. J. Exp. Med. **45,** 619–632, 1926.
66. Teilum, G.: Periodic acid-Schiff-positive reticuloendothelial cells producing glycoprotein: Functional significance during formation of amyloid. Amer. J. Path., **32,** 945–959, 1956.
67. Shearing, S. P., Comerford, F. R. and Cohen, A. S.: Effect of an amyloid inducing regimen on phagocytosis of carbon particles. Proc. Soc. Exp. Biol. Med., **119,** 673–676, 1965.
68. Ranlov, P.: Phagocytosis in experimental mouse amyloidosis. Acta Path. Microbiol. Scand., **68,** 19–28, 1966.
69. Zschiesche, W. and Ghatak, S.: Genetische Reaktionsunterschiede im Amyloidexperiment bei Maüsen. Verh. Deutsch. Ges. Path., **49,** 284–287, 1965.
70. Zschiesche, W., Heinecke, H. and Klaus, S.: Die phagocytoseaktivitat des reticulohistiocytaren systems und ihre Beziehungen zur experimentellen Amyloidose der Maus. Beitr. Path.Anat., **135,** 277–290, 1967.
71. Ram, S. J., DeLellis, R. A., and Glenner, G. G.: Amyloid. VIII. On strain variability in experimental murine amyloidosis. Proc. Soc. Exp. Biol. Med., **130,** 462–464, 1969.
72. Bradbury, S., and Micklem, H. S.: Amyloidosis and lymphoid aplasia in mouse radiation chimeras. Amer. J. Path., **46,** 263–277, 1965.
73. Kellum, M. J., Sutherland, D. E. R., Eckert, E., Peterson, R. D. A., and Good, R. A.: Wasting disease, Coombs-positivity, and amyloidosis in rabbits subjected to central lymphoid tissue extirpation and irradiation. Int. Arch. Allerg., **27,** 6–26, 1965.

74. Ranløv, P.: The role of the thymus in experimental mouse amyloidosis. Acta Path. Microbiol. Scand., **67,** 42–54, 1966.
75. Druet, R. L., and Janigan, D. T.: Experimental amyloidosis: Rates of induction, lymphocyte depletion and thymic atrophy. Amer. J. Path., **49,** 911–929, 1966.
76. Ranløv, P.: Humoral immunity during the induction of experimental amyloidosis. Acta Path. Microbiol. Scand., **69,** 375–383, 1967.
77. Rodey, G. E., Becker, G., and Pisciotta, A. V.: Casein-induced suppression of the immune response in mice. Fed. Proc., **27,** 307, 1968.
78. Ranløv, P., and Jensen, E.: Homograft reaction in amyloidotic mice. Acta Path. Microbiol. Scand., **67,** 161–164, 1966.
79. Rodey, G. E., and Good, R. A.: Modification of the in vitro response to phytohemagglutinin of mouse spleen cells by amyloidogenic agents. Proc. Soc. Exp. Biol. Med., **131,** 457–461, 1969.
80. Mullarkey, M., Cathcart, E. S., and Cohen, A. S.: Acquisition and loss of delayed hypersensitivity to casein. Fed. Proc., **29,** 306, 1970.
81. Werdelin, O., and Ranløv, P.: Amyloidosis in mice produced by transplantation of spleen cells from casein-treated mice. Acta Path. Microbiol. Scand., **68,** 1–18, 1966.
82. Hardt, F., and Ranløv, P.: Transfer amyloidosis. Acta Path. Microbiol. Scand., **73,** 549–558, 1968.
83. Ranløv, P. J.: Den eksperimentelle amyloidoses immunologi og patogenese. Thesis, Kobenhavn, 1968.
84. Hultgren, M. K., Druet, R. L., and Janigan, D. T.: Experimental amyloidosis in isogeneic x-irradiated recipients of sensitized spleen tissue. Amer. J. Path., **50,** 943–955, 1967.
85. Janigan, D. T.: Pathogenetic mechanisms in protein-induced amyloidosis. Amer. J. Path., **55,** 379–393, 1969.
86. Shirahama, T., Lawless, O. J., and Cohen, A. S.: Heterologous transfer of amyloid-human to mouse. Proc. Soc. Exp. Biol. Med., **130,** 516–519, 1969.
87. Willerson, J. T., Gordon, J. K., Talal, N., and Barth, W. F.: Murine amyloid. II. Transfer of an amyloid accelerating substance. Arthritis Rheum., **12,** 232–240, 1969.
88. Clerici, E., Mocarelli, P., de Ferari, F., and Villa, M. L.: Studies on the passive transfer of amyloidosis by cells. J. Lab. Clin. Med., **74,** 145–152, 1969.
89. Luders, K.: Leukozytentransfer und Amyloidose. Z. Immunitaetsforsch, **137,** 474–491, 1969.
90. Cohen, A. S., and Calkins, E.: The isolation of amyloid fibrils and a study of the effect of collagenase and hyaluronidase. J. Cell Biol., **21,** 481–486, 1964.
91. Cohen, A. S.: Preliminary chemical analysis of partially purified amyloid fibrils. Lab. Invest., **15,** 66–83, 1966.
92. Kim, I. C., Shirahama, T., and Cohen, A. S.: The lipid content of amyloid fibrils purified by a variety of methods. Amer. J. Path., **50,** 869–886, 1967.
93. Pras, M., Schubert, M., Zucker-Franklin, D., Rimon, A., and Franklin, E. C.: The characterization of soluble amyloid prepared in water. J. Clin. Invest., **47,** 924–933, 1968.
94. Shirahama, T., and Cohen, A. S.: High resolution electron microscopic analysis of the amyloid fibril. J. Cell Biol., **33,** 679–708, 1967.
95. Cohen, A. S., Gueft, B., Sorenson, G. D., Ruinen, L., Benditt, E. P., and Glenner, G. G.: Part IV. Electron microscopy of amyloid, in *Amyloidosis,* edited by E. Mandema, L. Ruinen, J. H., Scholten, and A. S. Cohen. Excerpta Medica, Amsterdam, 1968.
96. Bladen, H. A., Nylen, M. U., and Glenner, G. G.: The ultrastructure of human amyloid as revealed by the negative staining technique. J. Ultrastruct. Res., **14,** 449–459, 1966.
97. Cohen, A. S.: Aspects of the high resolution ultrastructure, immunology and biochemistry of amyloid, in *Amyloidosis,* edited by E. Mandema, L. Ruinen, J. H. Scholten, and A. S. Cohen. Excerpta Medica, Amsterdam, 1968.
98. Glenner, G. G., Keiser, H. R., Bladen, H. A., Cuatrecasas, P., Eanes, E. D., Ram, J. S., Kanfer, J. N., and DeLellis, R. A.: Amyloid VI: A comparison of two morphologic components of human amyloid deposits. J. Histochem. Cytochem., **16,** 633–644, 1968.
99. Nichols, R. B., and Clamp, J. R.: Investigation of glycoprotein material associated with hepatic amyloid. Clin. Chim. Acta, **17,** 415–421, 1967.
100. Bitter, T., and Muir, H.: Mucopolysaccharides of whole human spleens in generalized amyloidosis. J. Clin. Invest., **45,** 963–975, 1966.
101. Muir, H., and Cohen, A. S.: Mucopolysaccharides as components of amyloid, in *Amyloidosis,* edited by E. Mandema, L. Ruinen, J. H. Scholten, and A. S. Cohen. Excerpta Medica, Amsterdam, 1968.
102. Pennock, C. A.: Association of acid mucopolysaccharides with isolated amyloid fibrils. Nature (London), **217,** 753–754, 1968.
103. Berenson, G. S., Dalferes, E. R., Jr., Ruiz, H., and Radhakrishnamurthy, B.: Changes of acid mucopolysaccharides in the heart involved by amyloidosis. Amer. J. Cardiol., **24,** 358–364, 1969.
104. Kim, I. C., Franzblau, C., Shirahama, T., and Cohen, A. S.: The effect of papain, pronase, Nagarse and trypsin on isolated amyloid fibrils. Biochim. Biophys. Acta, **181,** 465–467, 1969.
105. Shirahama, T., and Cohen, A. S.: Reconstitution of amyloid fibrils from alkaline extracts. J. Cell Biol., **35,** 459–464, 1967.
106. Pras, M., Zucker-Franklin, D., Rimon, A., and Franklin, E. C.: Physical, chemical and ultrastructural studies of water-soluble human amyloid fibrils. J. Exp. Med., **130,** 777–795, 1969.
107. Skinner, M. M., and Cohen, A. S.: Chemical differences in the amyloid fibril protein demonstrated by amino-terminal amino acid analysis. Arthritis Rheum., **12,** 333, 1969.
108. Eanes, E. D., and Glenner, G. G.: X-ray diffraction studies on amyloid filaments. J. Histochem. Cytochem., **16,** 673–677, 1968.
109. Bonar, L., Cohen, A. S., and Skinner, M. M.: Characterization of the amyloid fibril as a cross-β protein. Proc. Soc. Exp. Biol. Med., **131,** 1373–1375, 1969.
110. Schmueli, U., Gafni, J., Sohar, E., and Ashkenazi, Y.: An x-ray study of amyloid. J. Molec. Biol., **41,** 309–311, 1969.
111. Newcombe, D. S., and Cohen, A. S.: Solubility characteristics of isolated amyloid fibrils. Biochim. Biophys. Acta., **104,** 480–486, 1965.
112. Cathcart, E. S., Comerford, F. R., and Cohen, A. S.: Immunologic studies on a protein extracted from human secondary amyloid. New Eng. J. Med., **273,** 143–146, 1965.
113. Cathcart, E. S., Shirahama, T., and Cohen, A. S.: Isolation and identification of a plasma component of amyloid. Biochim. Biophys. Acta, **147,** 392–393, 1967.
114. Frensdorff, A., Sohar, E., and Heller, H.: Plasma fibrinogen in familial Mediterranean fever. Ann. Intern. Med., **55,** 448–455, 1961.
115. Williams, R. C. Jr., and Law, D. H.: IV. Serum complement in amyloidosis. J. Lab. Clin. Med., **56,** 629–633, 1960.
116. Levine, R. A.: Amyloid disease of liver: Correlation of clinical, functional and morphologic features in 47 patients. Amer. J. Med., **33,** 349–357, 1962.
117. Korsan-Bengtsen, K., Hjort, P. F., and Ygge, J.: Acquired factor X deficiency in patient with amyloidosis. Thromb. Diath. Haemorrh., **7,** 558–566, 1962.
118. Howell, M.: Acquired factor X deficiency associated with systematized amyloidosis: Report of case. Blood, **21,** 739–744, 1963.
119. Pechet, L., and Kastrul, J. J.: Amyloidosis associated with factor X (Stuart) deficiency. Ann. Intern. Med., **61,** 315–318, 1964.
120. Pudlak, P., Vorlova, Z., and Stejskal, J.: Unusual haemorrhagic diathesis in atypical primary amyloidosis. Acta Haemat. (Basel), **25,** 321–334, 1961.
121. Redleaf, P. D., Davis, R. B., Kucinski, C., Hoilund, L., and Gans, H.: Amyloidosis with unusual bleeding diathesis: observations on use of epsilon amino acid. Ann. Intern. Med., **58,** 347–354, 1963.
122. Teilum, G.: Amyloidosis secondary to agammaglobulinemia. J. Path. Bact., **88,** 317–320, 1964.
123. Ranløv, P., and Nielsen, P. E.: Systemic (primary) amyloidosis associated with an IgM (B_2M) paraproteinemia. Acta Path. Microbiol. Scand., **66,** 154–168, 1966.
124. Aly, F. W., Braun, H. J., and Missmahl, H. P.: Dys und paraproteinamien bei Amyloidbefall. Klin. Wschr., **46,** 762–768, 1968.
125. Sellin, D., and Haferkamp, O.: Bence Jones protein und amyloid. Z. Ges. Exp. Med., **147,** 173–189, 1968.
126. Cohen, A. S.: Diagnosis of amyloidosis, in *Laboratory Diagnostic Methods in the Rheumatic Diseases,* edited by A. S. Cohen. Little, Brown, Boston, 1967.
127. Trieger, N., Cohen, A. S., Calkins, E.: Gingival biopsy as a diagnostic aid in amyloid disease. Arch. Oral Biol., **1,** 187–192, 1959.

128. Gafni, J., and Sohar, E.: Rectal biopsy for diagnosis of amyloidosis. Amer. J. Med. Sci., **240,** 332–336, 1960.
129. Kyle, R. A., Spencer, R. J., and Dahlin, D. C.: Value of rectal biopsy in the diagnosis of primary systemic amyloidosis. Amer. J. Med. Sci., **251,** 501–506, 1966.
130. Brandt, K., Cathcart, E. S., and Cohen, A. S.: A clinical analysis of the course and prognosis of 42 patients with amyloidosis. Amer. J. Med., **44,** 995–969, 1968.
131. Ostertang, B.: Demonstration einer eigenartigen familiaren "Paraamyloidose." Zbl. Allg. Path., **56,** 253–254, 1932.
132. Andrade, C.: A peculiar form of peripheral neuropathy. Brain, **75,** 408–427, 1952.
133. Andrade, C., Canijo, M., Klein, D. and Kaelin, A.: The genetic aspect of the familial amyloidotic polyneuropathy: Portuguese type of paramyloidosis. Humangenetik, **7,** 163–175, 1969.
134. Missmahl, H. P., and Siebner, H.: Chromosome studies in familial pericollagenous amyloidosis. German Med. Monthly, **10,** 374–378, 1965.
135. Coelho, E., and Pimentel, J. C.: Cardiac involvement in a peculiar form of paramyloidosis. Amer. J. Cardiol., **8,** 624, 1961.
136. Horta, J. S., Filipe, I., and Duarte, S.: Portuguese polyneuritic familial type of amyloidosis. Path. Microbiol. (Basel), **27,** 809–825, 1964.
137. Araki, S., Mawatari, S., Ohta, M., Nakajima, A., and Kuroiwa, Y.: Polyneuritic amyloidosis in a Japanese family. Arch. Neurol. (Chicago), **18,** 593–602, 1968.
138. Andrade, A., Araki, S., Block, W. D., Cohen, A. S., Jackson, C. E., Kuroiwa, Y., McKusick, V. A., Nissim, J., Sohar, E., and Van Allen, M. W.: Hereditary amyloidosis. Arthritis Rheum., **13,** 902, 1970.
139. Kantarjian, A. D., and DeJong, R. N.: Familial primary amyloidosis with nervous system involvement. Neurology (Minneap.), **3,** 399–409, 1953.
140. Delank, H. W., Koch, G., Könn, G., Missmahl, H. P., and Suwelack, K.: Familiäre amyloid-polyneuropathie typus Wohlwill-Corino Andrade. Arzneimittelforschung, **19,** 401–416, 1965.
141. Dyck, J. P., and Lambert, E. H.: Dissociated sensation in amyloidosis. Arch. Neurol. (Chicago), **20,** 490–507, 1969.
142. Kulisiewicz, T., Zielinski, J., and Kozlowska-Kowarska, A.: Przypadek neuropaltii obwodowej w pierwotnej amyloidozie rodzinnej. Neurol. Neurochir. Pol., **14,** 243–245, 1964.
143. Von Sallmann, L., Kaufman, H. E., Haase, G. R., Bartter, F. C., and Thomas, L. B.: Primary amyloidosis. Ann. Intern. Med., **52,** 668–681, 1960.
144. Kaufman, H. E., and Thomas, L. B.: Vitreous opacities diagnostic of familial amyloidosis. New Eng. J. Med., **261,** 1267–1271, 1959.
145. Duke, J. R., and Paton, D.: Primary familial amyloidosis: Occular manifestations with histopathologic observations. Trans. Amer. Ophthal. Soc., **63,** 146–167, 1965.
146. Paton, D., and Duke, J. R.: Primary familial amyloidosis. Amer. J. Opthal., **61,** 736–747, 1966.
147. Shulman, L. E., and Bartter, F. C.: Familial primary amyloidosis. Johns Hopkins Med. J., **98,** 238–239, 1956.
148. Kaufman, H. E.: Primary familial amyloidosis. Arch. Ophthal. (Chicago), **60,** 1036–1043, 1958.
149. Hicks, E. P.: Hereditary perforating ulcer of the foot. Lancet, **1,** 319–321, 1922.
150. Denny-Brown, D.: Hereditary sensory radicular neuropathy. J. Neurol. Neurosurg. Psychiat., **14,** 237–252, 1951.
151. Falls, H. F., Jackson, J. H., Carey, J. G., Rukavina, J. G., and Block, W. D.: Ocular manifestations of hereditary primary systemic amyloidosis. Arch. Opthal (Chicago), **54,** 660–664, 1955.
152. Rukavina, J. G., Block, W. D., Jackson, C. E., Falls, H. F., Carey, J. H., and Curtis, A. C.: Primary systemic amyloidosis: A review and an experimental, genetic, and clinical study of 29 cases with particular emphasis on the familial form. Medicine (Balt.), **35,** 239–334, 1956.
153. Jackson, C. E., Falls, H. F., Block, W. D., Rukavina, J. K., and Carey, J. H.: Inheritance of primary systemic amyloidosis. Amer. J. Hum. Genet., **12,** 434–439, 1960.
154. Jackson, C. E., Block, W. D., and Ratcliff, W. C.: Serum hexosamine content and urinary mucopolysaccharide excretion in hereditary primary amyloidosis. J. Lab. Clin. Med., **56,** 544–546, 1960.
155. Mahloudji, M., Teasdall, R. D., Adamkiewicz, J. J., Hartmann, W. H., Lambird, P. A., and McKusick, V. A.: The genetic amyloidosis: With particular reference to hereditary neuropathic amyloidosis, Type II (Indiana or Rukavina Type). Medicine (Balt.), **48,** 1–37, 1969.
156. Lambird, P. A., and Hartmann, W. H.: Hereditary amyloidosis, the flexor retinaculum, and the carpal tunnel syndrome. Amer. J. Clin. Path., **52,** 714–719, 1969.
157. Schlesinger, A. S., Duggins, V. A., and Masucci, E. I.: Peripheral neuropathy in familial primary amyloidosis. Brain, **85,** 357–370, 1962.
158. Van Allen, M. W., Frohlich, J. A., and Davis, J. R.: Inherited predisposition to generalized amyloidosis. Neurology (Minneap.), **19,** 10–25, 1969.
159. Siegal, S.: Benign paroxysmal peritonitis. Ann. Intern. Med., **23,** 1–21, 1945.
160. Heller, H., Sohar, E., and Sherf, L.: Familial Mediterranean fever. Arch. Intern. Med. (Chicago), **102,** 50–71, 1958.
161. Cattan, R., and Mamou, H.: 14 cas de maladie périodique dont 8 compliques de néphropathies. Bull. Soc. Med. Hop. Paris, **67,** 1104–1107, 1951.
162. Mamou, H.: Maladie périodique amylogène. Sem. Hop. Paris, **31,** 388–391, 1955.
163. Priest, R. J., and Nixon, R. K.: Familial recurring polyserositis: A disease entity. Ann. Intern. Med., **51,** 1253–1274, 1959.
164. Reimann, H. A.: Periodic disease. Medicine (Balt.), **30,** 219–245, 1951.
165. Sohar, E., Pras, M., Heller, J., and Heller, H.: Genetics of familial Mediterranean fever (FMF). Arch. Intern. Med. (Chicago), **107,** 529–538, 1961.
166. Kechejian, S. J.: Familial Mediterranean fever. Boston Med. Quart., **14,** 59–75, 1963.
167. Ozdemir, A. I., and Sokmen, C.: Familial Mediterranean fever among the Turkish people. Amer. J. Gastroent., **51,** 311–316, 1969.
168. Bergman, F., and Warmenius, S.: Familial perireticular amyloidosis in a Swedish family. Amer. J. Med., **45,** 601–606, 1968.
169. Reich, C. B., and Franklin, E. C.: Familial Mediterranean fever in an Italian family. Arch. Intern. Med. (Chicago), **125,** 337–340, 1970.
170. Blum, A., Gafni, J., Sohar, E., Shibolet, S., and Heller, H.: Amyloidosis as the sole manifestation of familial Mediterranean fever. Ann. Intern. Med., **57,** 795–799, 1962.
171. Gafni, J., Ravid, M., and Sohar, E.: The role of amyloidosis in familial Mediterranean fever. Israel J. Med. Sci., **4,** 995–999, 1968.
172. Gafni, J., and Sohar, E.: Rectal biopsy for the diagnosis of amyloidosis. Amer. J. Med. Sci., **240,** 332–336, 1960.
173. Mellinkoff, S. H., Snodgrass, R. W., Schwabe, A. D., Meade, J. F., Weimer, H. E., and Frankland, M.: Familial Mediterranean fever: Plasma protein abnormalities, low-fat diet and possible implications in pathogenesis. Ann. Intern. Med., **56,** 171–182, 1962.
174. Sohar, E., Gafni, J., Chaimow, M., Pras, M., and Heller, H.: Low-fat diet in familial Mediterranean fever. Arch. Intern. Med. (Chicago), **110,** 150–154, 1962.
175. Nilsson, S. E., and Floderus, S.: Nine cases of hereditary and nonhereditary periodic diseases. Acta Med. Scand., **175,** 341–346, 1964.
176. Bondy, P. K., Cohn, G. L., and Gregory, P. B.: Etiocholanolone fever. Medicine (Balt.), **44,** 249–262, 1965.
177. Muckle, T. J., and Wells, M.: Urticaria, deafness and amyloidosis: A new heredo-familial syndrome. Quart. J. Med., **31,** 235–248, 1962.
178. Kennedy, D. D., Rosenthal, F. D., and Sneddon, I. B.: Amyloidosis presenting as urticaria. Brit. Med. J., **1,** 31–32, 1966.
179. Campbell, A. M. G., and Clifton, I.: Adult toxoplasmosis in one family. Brain, **73,** 281–290, 1950.
180. Campbell, A. M. G.: The inherited amyloidoses. Lancet, **1,** 220, 1964.
181. Andersen, V., Buch, N. H., Jensen, M. K., and Killmann, S. A.: Deafness, urticaria and amyloidosis. Amer. J. Med., **42,** 449–456, 1967.
182. Black, J. T.: Amyloidosis, deafness, urticaria and limb pains: A hereditary syndrome. Ann. Intern. Med., **70,** 989–994, 1969.
183. Maxwell, E. S., and Kimbell, I.: Familial amyloidosis, with case reports. Med. Bull. Veterans Admin., **12,** 365–369, 1936.
184. Ostertag, B.: Familiare Amyloid-Erkrankung. Z. menschl. Vererb.-u. Konstit. lehre, **30,** 105–115, 1950.
185. Frederiksen, T., Gotzsche, H., Harboe, N., Kiaer, W., and Mellemgaard, K.: Primary familial amyloidosis with severe amyloid heart disease. Amer. J. Med., **33,** 328–348, 1962.

186. Allensworth, D. C., Rice, G. J., and Lowe, G. W.: Persistent atrial standstill in a family with myocardial disease. Amer. J. Med., **47**, 775–784, 1969.
187. Schimke, R. N., and Hartmann, W. H.: Familial amyloid-producing medullary thyroid carcinoma and pheochromocytoma: Distinct genetic entity. Ann. Intern. Med., **63**, 1027–1039, 1965.
188. Sipple, J. H.: The association of pheochromocytoma with carcinoma of the thyroid gland. Amer. J. Med., **31**, 163–166, 1961.
189. Sarosi, G., and Doe, P.: Familial occurrence of parathyroid adenomas, pheochromocytoma, and medullary carcinoma of the thyroid with amyloid stroma (Sipple's syndrome). Ann. Intern. Med., **68**, 1305–1309, 1968.
190. Steiner, L., Goodman, A. D., and Powers, R.: Study of a kindred with pheochromocytoma, medullary thyroid carcinoma, hyperparathyroidism and Cushing's disease: Multiple endocrine neoplasia, Type 2. Medicine (Balt.), **47**, 371–409, 1968.
191. Smith, M. E., and Zimmerman, L. E.: Amyloid in corneal dystophies. Arch. Ophthal. (Chicago), **79**, 407–412, 1968.
192. Klintworth, G. K.: Lattice corneal dystrophy: An inherited form of amyloidosis restricted to the cornea. Amer. J. Path., **50**, 371–400, 1967.
193. Isaak, L.: Localized amyloidosis cutis associated with psoriasis in siblings. Arch. Derm. Syphilol., **61**, 859–862, 1950.
194. Sagher, F., and Shanon, J.: Amyloidosis cutis: Familial occurrence in 3 generations. Arch. Derm. (Chicago), **87**, 171–175, 1963.
195. Andersson, R.: Hereditary amyloidosis with polyneuropathy. Acta Med. Scand., **188**, 85–94, 1970.
196. Cathcart, E. S., Mullarkey, M., and Cohen, A. S.: Amyloidosis: an expression of immunological tolerance? Lancet, **2**, 639–640, 1970.
197. Cathcart, E. S., Mullarkey, M., and Cohen, A. S.: Cellular immunity in casein-induced amyloidosis. Immunology, **20**, 1971 (in press).
198. Cohen, A. S.: Chemical and immunologic characterization of two components of amyloid, in *Chemistry and Molecular Biology of the Intercellular Matrix,* edited by E. A. Balacz, vol. 3, pp 1517–1536, Academic Press, New York, 1970.
199. Glenner, G. G., Harbaugh, J., Ohms, J. I., Harada, M., and Cuatrecasas, P.: An amyloid protein: the aminoterminal variable fragment of an immunoglobulin light chain. Biochem. Biophys. Res. Commun., **41**, 1287–1289, 1970.
200. Cohen, A. S., Bricetti, A., Harrington, J., and Mannick, J.: Renal transplantation in amyloid disease. (In preparation.)

CHAPTER FIFTY-ONE

HYPOPHOSPHATASIA

Frederic C. Bartter

Hypophosphatasia is a familial disease characterized by abnormalities of the skeleton, subnormal values of the serum alkaline phosphatase, and the presence of excessive quantities of phosphorylethanolamine in the plasma and urine. Hypercalcemia, renal damage, and occasionally premature synostosis of the cranial vault may also be found.

HISTORICAL ASPECTS

Although the disease was first given its present name by Rathbun [1] in 1948, there are scattered reports of what is undoubtedly the same entity going back 20 years before that time. The historical aspects are covered in detail in the reviews by Fraser [2], by Currarino and associates [3], and by Rasmussen [4]. The following reports are of especial interest in the development of currently accepted concepts of the disease: Huhne and Schonfeld [5] in 1929 described a patient with a syndrome clearly recognizable in retrospect as hypophosphatasia. Chown [6] in 1935 described two similar patients who at autopsy were also found to have had nephrocalcinosis. Kubatsch [7] in 1938 described a patient with "islands" of bone in the skull, whose father had evidence of premature synostosis. Alkaline phosphatase values were not reported in any of these cases. Anspach and Clifton [8] in 1939 noted hypercalcemia in a child with pathognomonic changes in the bones, including premature synostosis. Serum alkaline phosphatase concentrations in this child, determined on a number of occasions, were very low, except for one value in early infancy. Macey [9], in 1940, described two brothers (one 36 years of age) with hypophosphatasia who gave a history of severe rickets in childhood and of numerous fractures in adult life. Rathbun, in his classic description, reported that alkaline phosphatase activity was low in bone, intestinal mucosa, and kidney. Sobel and associates [10], in 1953, considerably advanced our knowledge of this syndrome. They noted for the first time premature loss of deciduous teeth as part of the syndrome and observed that the serum of their patient did not inhibit normal phosphatase activity. They found low alkaline phosphatase activity in bone, cartilage, liver, and a tooth; finally, they presented data strongly suggestive of hypersensitivity to vitamin D in their patient.

Fraser and associates [11] and McCance [12] discovered simultaneously, in 1954, that the excretion of phosphorylethanolamine (PEA) in the urine is an integral feature of the disease. They showed also that the parents of patients might have abnormally low serum alkaline phosphatase values. Fraser et al. [11] found that PEA might appear in the plasma of patients and in the urine of the otherwise normal parents of patients with hypophosphatasia. Fraser and Yendt [13] also showed that the cartilage of rachitic rats would calcify in the serum of patients with hypophosphatasia but that costochondral cartilage and osteoid from a patient would not calcify in the serum of normal people or in a synthetic medium containing appropriate concentrations of calcium and phosphate ions. Scaglione [14] reported in 1956 that a patient with abnormally low phosphatase activity in bone might nevertheless have normal phosphatase activity in the liver, duodenal juice, and, indeed, in osteoblasts in tissue culture. In 1958, Kretchmer and associates [15] reported alkaline phosphatase absent from the leukocytes of a patient and normal in the leukocytes of the mother (whose serum phosphatase concentration was low).

Pimstone et al. [16] showed that the serum alkaline phosphatase could be normal in patients known on genetic grounds to have hypophosphatasia—including even one patient with bone disease, excessive urinary PEA, and premature loss of deciduous teeth. In an adult patient with the full syndrome [17] they showed reciprocal fluctuations of serum alkaline phosphatase and urinary PEA over a 5-year period, though each was normal on several occasions. This patient also excreted phosphorylcholine in excessive amounts. The significance of serum alkaline phosphatase values in hypophosphatasia can be clarified only when the source of the phosphatase can be identified. Scriver and Cameron [18] reported that in a patient with normal total values the only significant abnormality appeared to be a decrease in affinity of the plasma phosphatase (isoenzyme) for PEA. Rasmussen [4] showed that the renal clearance of PEA varies directly with plasma PEA, approaching the creatinine clearance in homozygotes with the highest plasma values. His elegant chemical studies by refined techniques establish for the first time *normal* urinary, plasma, and clearance values for PEA.

CLINICAL FINDINGS

The clinical findings in hypophosphatasia are probably all attributable to the defect in formation of true bone, to premature synostosis of the skull, or to the hypercalcemia which is a frequent but not constant feature. Since the essential feature of the generalized bone disease is inadequacy of mature bone formation, the earlier the appearance of the disorder, the more severe the clinical manifestations. When the disease appears in utero, infants are often stillborn and lack adequate bony support for cranial and thoracic cavities. When it appears in adult life, patients may be asymptomatic or have only the symptoms attendant upon an occasional fracture. The disease of bone includes the gross changes of true rickets, with beading of costochondral junctions, bowing of the legs, and widening of the ends of the long bones. It may resemble the disorder *congenital bowing of the long bones,* in which the histologic and biochemical defects of hypophosphatasia are not found [19]. Genu valgum is commonly seen in hypophosphatasia. The ends of the long bones may assume a characteristic "notched" appearance by x-ray, which differs clearly from the smooth "cupping" of untreated rickets and resembles that of metaphyseal dysplasia. Figure 51-1 shows such lesions in a child of 39 months with hypophosphatasia.

Premature synostosis may be anticipated in infancy by the *absence* of radiologically demonstrable bone over large areas of skull, giving the appearance of wide sutures separating plaques of bone.

As in the syndrome of oxycephaly or acrocephalosyndactyly [20, 21], these areas represent in fact uncalcified osteoid without fibrous septums [22]. As they calcify, exophthalmos and an increase in intracranial pressure may appear. The skull may take on a "beaten silver" appearance by x-ray [23, 24]. Convulsions, serious brain damage, and death may ensue if surgical decompression is not performed. The late manifestations are those of oxycephaly. The sutures may show characteristic prominent bony ridges.

Subperiosteal new bone formation, not normally seen in rickets, has been reported in three cases [1, 2, 25]. Premature loss of the anterior deciduous teeth is frequently seen. Indeed, this valuable sign, which may appear without other evidence of bone disease [16], may provide a valuable genetic marker for cases with a minimal expression of the syndrome.

Hypercalcemia is common, especially in infants, and hypercalciuria results. The nausea and vomiting of some patients is clearly attributable to the hypercalcemia.

Eleven patients have come to medical attention for the first time as adults [9, 17, 24, 26, 27, 28, 29, 30, 32]. In many of these, rickets was said to have been present in childhood, followed by an interim period of apparently normal health for a number of years. They were later found in adulthood to have radiolucent bones and, in most instances, pseudofractures; roentgenologic evidence was obtained that one had had craniostenosis in childhood. In some, the rib cage still showed the classic deformities of infantile rickets [24]. One patient had "osteoporosis," hypophosphatasia, and phosphorylethanolaminuria, but no evidence of earlier disease. It thus appears that spontaneous, virtually complete remissions may occur and that new manifestations may not appear for a number of years.

LABORATORY DIAGNOSIS

Laboratory diagnosis consists of (1) demonstration of serum alkaline phosphatase values below normal for the patient's age, (2) histologic characterization of the bone lesions, and (3) demonstration of abnormal quantities of phosphorylethanolamine (PEA) in the urine and plasma. This compound has been found in small quantities in the urine and plasma of some normal subjects, and is identified as a small area of the ninhydrin-positive curve which comes off a Moore-Stein automatic column immediately before taurine [31, 33]. Rasmussen [4], by preliminary treatment with charcoal, followed by desalting on an anion exchange resin before chromatography on Dowex, provided the first quan-

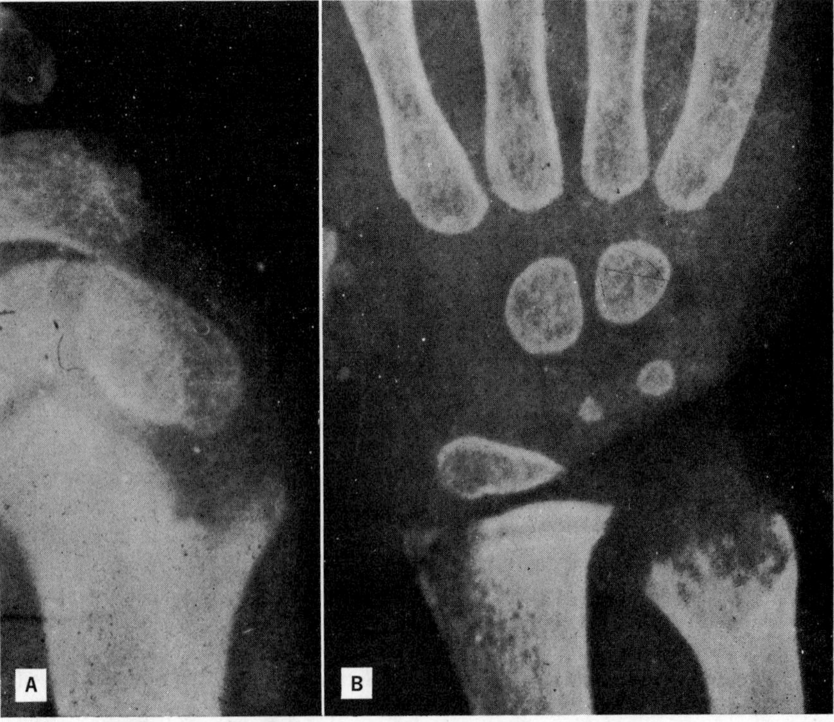

Figure 51-1. X-ray of the shoulder (A) and wrist (B) of a 39-year-old female with hypophosphatasia. Note defects in epiphyseal ossification. (*By permission of Dr. Edna Sobel.*)

titative values for urinary excretion, plasma concentration, and renal clearance of PEA in normal controls as well as in patients. The values so obtained for the normal controls were 17 to 99 μmoles per 24 hr, 0.21 to 0.33 μmoles per 100 ml, and 4 to 12 ml per min, respectively. Heterozygotes for hypophosphatasia (see below) showed urinary values three to eight times normal, plasma values about twice those of normal controls, and clearances about four times normal. Patients with hypophosphatasia showed urinary values from 10 to 50 times normal and plasma values about twice those of heterozygotes (0.75 to 0.85 μmoles per 100 ml). The renal clearance of PEA in these patients approached the creatinine clearance.

Rasmussen also studied the fate of "loads" of PEA in normal people, in heterozygous carriers of hypophosphatasia, and in patients with the full syndrome. Whereas the clearance data so obtained are difficult to interpret in view of the rapidly changing plasma values and the limitations of endogenous creatinine clearance as an estimate of glomerular filtration rate, all the results show an apparent "tubular maximum" for reabsorption of PEA of about 0.3 μmoles per min (Fig. 51-2). Accordingly, normal subjects, filtering only slightly more than this, excrete very little (about 7 percent of the "load"), whereas homozygotic patients, filtering only three to four times as much, reabsorb the same absolute amount and excrete about 90 percent of the load. Rasmussen's experiments showed also that patients, as compared to normal subjects, achieved higher plasma concentrations of PEA for a given load (e.g., 16 μmoles per 100 ml following a load of 21 μmoles per kg body weight in

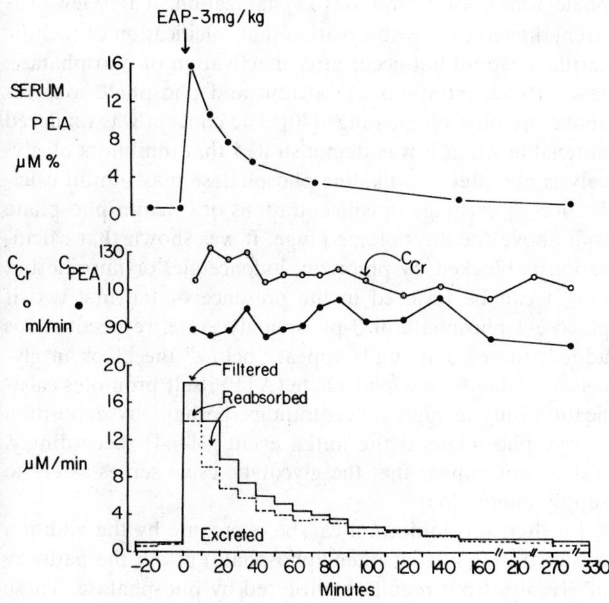

Figure 51-2. Clearance of phosphorylethanolamine (C_{PEA}) following intravenous infusion of a single dose given to a patient with homozygous hypophosphatasia. C_{cr} = creatinine clearance. Data plotted from Rasmussen [4].

patients, versus 10 μmoles per 100 ml in a normal control) and showed a lower rate of decline despite the higher renal clearance.

The higher plasma values (lower volume of distribution) suggested limited ability of PEA to enter cells in the patients; alternatively, their plasma "pool" may exchange with a saturated intracellular pool.

Hydroxyproline excretion, which serves as an index of collagen metabolism [34], may be extremely low in hypophosphatasia [35], whereas it is high in vitamin D–resistant rickets. This suggests that hydroxyproline excretion in hypophosphatasia reflects bone destruction (which is clearly decreased in the syndrome) rather than osteoid formation (which is clearly increased).

The histologic picture is generally indistinguishable from that of true rickets. The defect in ossification of cartilage appears, as in rickets, as a widening of the zones of provisional calcification, disruption of the normal columnar arrangement of cells, and failure of calcification of degenerating cartilage. Figure 51-3 shows a section from a costochondral junction of a child with the disorder [10]. The defect in appositional and subperiosteal bone formation appears as wide zones of uncalcified osteoid lined with osteoblasts. There is virtually no osteoclasis, nor is there fibrosis of the marrow or other evidence of bone destruction. As in osteomalacia, the total mass of bone plus matrix may appear greater than normal [22]. The defect in membranous bone, which may be so extensive as to leave only plaques of true bone in the skull [1], is histologically similar, showing wide areas of uncalcified osteoid. It has been observed in microradiologic studies that the true bone in this disease may have a relatively primitive structure for the patient's age, and that the collagen fibrils may be correspondingly poorly arranged [36]. Material from patients with true rickets of similar degree and severity is not available for comparison. It may be that the primitive structure results from the relative absence of remodeling of osteoid as compared with that in true bone. The first step in remodeling is, of course, bone destruction, which is indicated histologically by the presence of osteoclasts. Osteoclasts are extremely rare in bones with active rickets or osteomalacia.

THE CALCIFICATION PROCESS

It is not known how the biochemical defects (decreased serum alkaline phosphatase activity, elevated plasma and urinary phosphoethanolamine, and occasionally elevated serum and urinary calcium concentration) are interrelated. The disorder may be better understood in the light of current concepts of bone physiology.

Bone formation begins with the deposition of matrix in apposition to preexisting bone or calcified cartilage, or with its formation *de novo* in intramembranous sites. The osteoid is deposited by osteoblasts, which contain alkaline phosphatase. Some alkaline phosphatase from osteoblasts is liberated

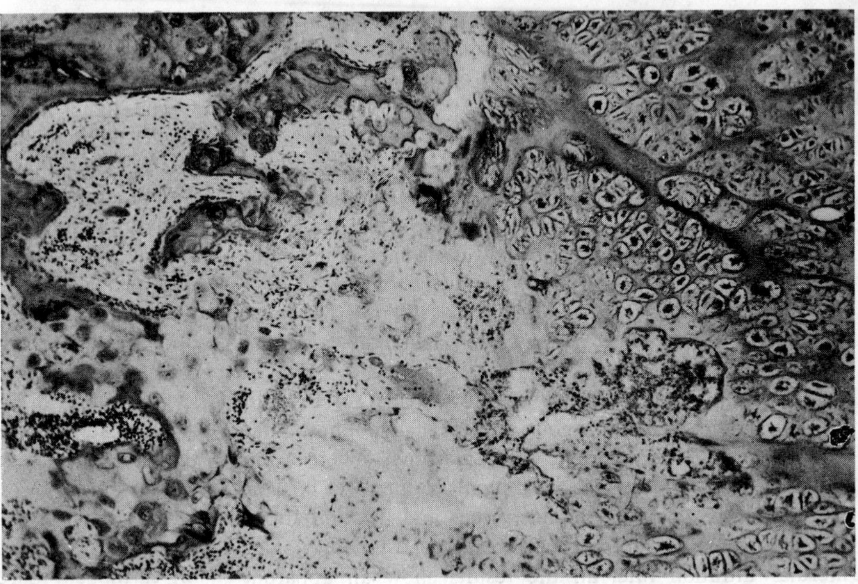

Figure 51-3. Costochondral junction of a rib of a 39-month-old girl with hypophosphatasia. Note the disorganization of cartilage and osteoid seams lined with osteoblasts. Undecalcified. (*By permission of Dr. Edna Sobel.*)

into the circulating fluids. In the absence of liver disease, the serum alkaline phosphatase concentration closely parallels, and serves as an index of, the number and activity of osteoblasts.

The earliest deposition of mineral in osteoid (nucleation) probably begins with the formation of an initial complex of calcium and phosphorus, which in all probability is $CaHPO_4$ [37]. The formation of this complex depends in part upon the activity product of $Ca^{++} \times HPO_4^{=}$ surrounding the osteoid. It has been suggested that the initial event is an ester linkage of phosphate (—O—P—) and that this is accomplished by phosphokinase and a suitable phosphate donor [38]. If such phosphate molecules are appropriately spaced and oriented and still possess free valence electrons, they can initiate nucleation by uniting electrostatically with calcium ions.

Once an initial complex is formed, it is spontaneously rearranged at physiologic pH to the hydroxyapatite structure of bone. Experimental evidence regarding the essential ion product has been derived largely from studies with rachitic cartilage. It has been assumed, without good evidence, that calcification of osteoid follows the same principles. Recent studies with reconstituted "native" collagen have largely supported the assumption. Calcification does not appear in rachitic cartilage incubated in solutions with a solubility product below a critical figure. The same applies, of course, to solutions of calcium phosphate alone. With rachitic cartilage (and with native collagen), however, the first precipitation occurs in spite of an activity product of $Ca^{++} \times HPO_4^{=}$ as little as one-third of that required for spontaneous precipitation. Hydroxyapatite, the mineral phase of formed bone, will remove calcium and phosphate from solutions with activity products of $Ca^{++} \times HPO_4^{=}$ below that of serum. The present problem concerns the failure of calcification *de novo* (nucleation) of newly formed osteoid or "calcifiable" cartilage.

A number of attempts have been made to explain the phenomenon of nucleation despite low solubility products. The first (which antedated accurate knowledge of the appropriate activity products) was that of Robison [39], who observed that alkaline phosphatase is present in all areas where calcification occurs. He suggested that phosphatase acts to liberate inorganic phosphate at the site of calcification and thus, by raising the activity product of calcium by phosphate ions locally, initiates crystallization. This view was strengthened by the observation that calcification of rachitic cartilage would not occur after inactivation of phosphatase, save at concentrations of calcium and phosphate ions far above the physiologic range [40]. The concept was rendered untenable when it was demonstrated that inhibitors of glycolysis not affecting alkaline phosphatase may inhibit calcification of cartilage in concentrations of calcium phosphate well above the physiologic range. It was shown that calcification is blocked by phlorizin, iodoacetate, or fluoride but that it can be restored in the presence of the first two if glucose-1-phosphate or 3-phosphoglycerate, respectively, is added; these compounds appear "below" the block in glycolysis. Adenosine triphosphate (ATP) itself promotes calcification only in high concentrations, perhaps by deposition of pyrophosphate as the initial event [41–44]. Accordingly, it does not appear that the glycolytic cycle serves solely to supply energy [45].

Further, this inhibition can be overcome by the addition of substrates (such as phenylphosphate) not in the pathway of glycolysis but readily hydrolyzed by phosphatase. These observations led Gutman and Yu to propose that phosphatase acts as a transferase of phosphate from organic phosphate esters to available sites on the matrix [45]. In this view, phosphatase assumes the role ascribed to phosphokinase in the initial transfer of phosphate to collagen discussed above.

Two other theories have been proposed to explain the place of phosphatase in bone formation: It has been suggested that it has no direct role in calcification but is associated with the formation of organic matrix. This view would find support if it could be regularly shown that nucleation occurs spontaneously in collagen reconstituted from solution at physiologic concentrations of calcium and phosphate [46], providing that the collagen had the structure of "native" cartilage (with 640 Å axial repeat). (This would, of course, pose again the question as to why all native cartilage does not calcify in vivo.) It has been suggested that traces of an essential mucopolysacharide are present even in these purified solutions [47]. It has been shown that beryllium, which inhibits alkaline phosphatase activity, inhibits calcification. This does not establish a role for phosphatase in the calcification process, since beryllium has this property in concentrations which do not affect the liberation of inorganic phosphate from β-glycerophosphate [48].

Finally, it has been suggested that phosphatase serves to destroy phosphate esters which inhibit calcification as crystal poisons [49]. In this view, the phosphate esters which are promoting calcification in slice experiments "protect" phosphate-containing sites from phosphatase leached from the slices [37]. A modified form of the last theory has been the suggestion that pyrophosphates or organic polyphosphates serve to inhibit calcification normally and that calcification can occur only when pyrophosphatase removes such an inhibitor. Since pyrophosphatase is present quite generally, this hypothesis requires a further explanation of the failure of most native collagen to calcify. It has been suggested that a form of bound pyrophosphate in native collagen which does not calcify is protected from the action of pyrophosphatase.

BIOCHEMICAL DEFECTS IN HYPOPHOSPHATASIA

Although rachitic cartilage (and probably the uncalcified osteoid in osteomalacia) normally calcifies readily in physiologic concentrations of calcium and phosphate ions, this does not occur in patients with hypophosphatasia. In this syndrome the serum phosphorus concentration is normal, and the serum calcium concentration is frequently elevated, in spite of the presence of histologic rickets. Furthermore, Fraser showed that rachitic cartilage will calcify in the serum of a patient with hypophosphatasia. This makes it unlikely that the defect in calcification results from too low an activity product of circulating calcium and phosphate ions. It also renders it unlikely that the calcium is present in a complexed, nonionized form. (This is suggested by the observation that vitamin D in average doses may rapidly elevate the serum calcium concentration of patients with hypophosphatasia [10]. Anning and associates [50] showed that vitamin D can increase significantly the concentration of diffusible, nonionized calcium.) On the other hand, if nucleation depends upon the activity of phosphate locally at osteoid sites and this is dependent upon phosphatase, the disorder may indeed involve a decrease of effective ion product.

The syndrome thus provides strong clinical evidence that alkaline phosphatase plays a role in the nucleation process. Since osteoid is present in abundance, it appears likely that phosphatase is not required for its formation. There remains the possibility that osteoid formed without alkaline phosphatase is abnormal. For example, it might lack a phosphorus-containing compound required for in vivo calcification, such as the mucopolysaccharide described by DiStefano and associates [51]. As noted above, the rachitic cartilage of a patient with hypophosphatasia did not calcify in normal serum [13]. Attempts to define further the relationship between the enzyme deficiency and the bone disease have proved unsuccessful.

An inhibitor of alkaline phosphatase could not be found in the serum of patients, although carefully sought for by four groups of investigators [10, 11, 22, 36]. There are no data available on the concentrations of circulating pyrophosphate or of tissue pyrophosphatase in hypophosphatasia.

PEA has been isolated from the urine and plasma of patients and of some parents of patients. Although alkaline phosphatase readily hydrolyzes this ester, there is no reasonable explanation for the association of the two biochemical defects in the disease. It has been suggested that PEA is the "true substrate" for bone alkaline phosphatase [27]. Thus, a hereditary defect resulting in a block in the reaction

$$NH_2CH_2CH_2{-}O{-}P(OH)_2{=}O + H_2O \xrightarrow[\text{phosphatase}]{\text{alkaline}} H_3PO_4 + NH_2CH_2CH_2OH$$

would lead to an excess of plasma and urinary phosphoethanolamine. A block in hydrolysis of the ester could lead to a defect in calcification whether the phosphatase acts as a liberator of inorganic phosphate, as a transferase, or to remove a "metabolic poison," as suggested by Neuman [49]. There is no evidence for or against such a hypothesis.

PEA is normally found in serum or urine [4]. It is a normal constituent of brain tissue. It may appear in excess in the urine of patients with liver disease [52], celiac disease, and erythroblastosis fetalis [53].

The known reactions involving PEA are shown diagramatically in Fig. 51-4. Because phosphorylcholine (PC) has been found in excess in the urine of a patient with hypophosphatasia [17] the figure includes the reactions involving PC as well.

PEA may be formed (1) by phosphorylation of ethanolamine, (2) by hydrolysis of phosphatidyl-ethanolamine, (3) by hydrolysis of an α-PEA-plasmalogen, and (4) by the aldolase cleavage of phosphoryl sphingosine. PC is formed by a series of reactions analogous to (1), (2), and (3).

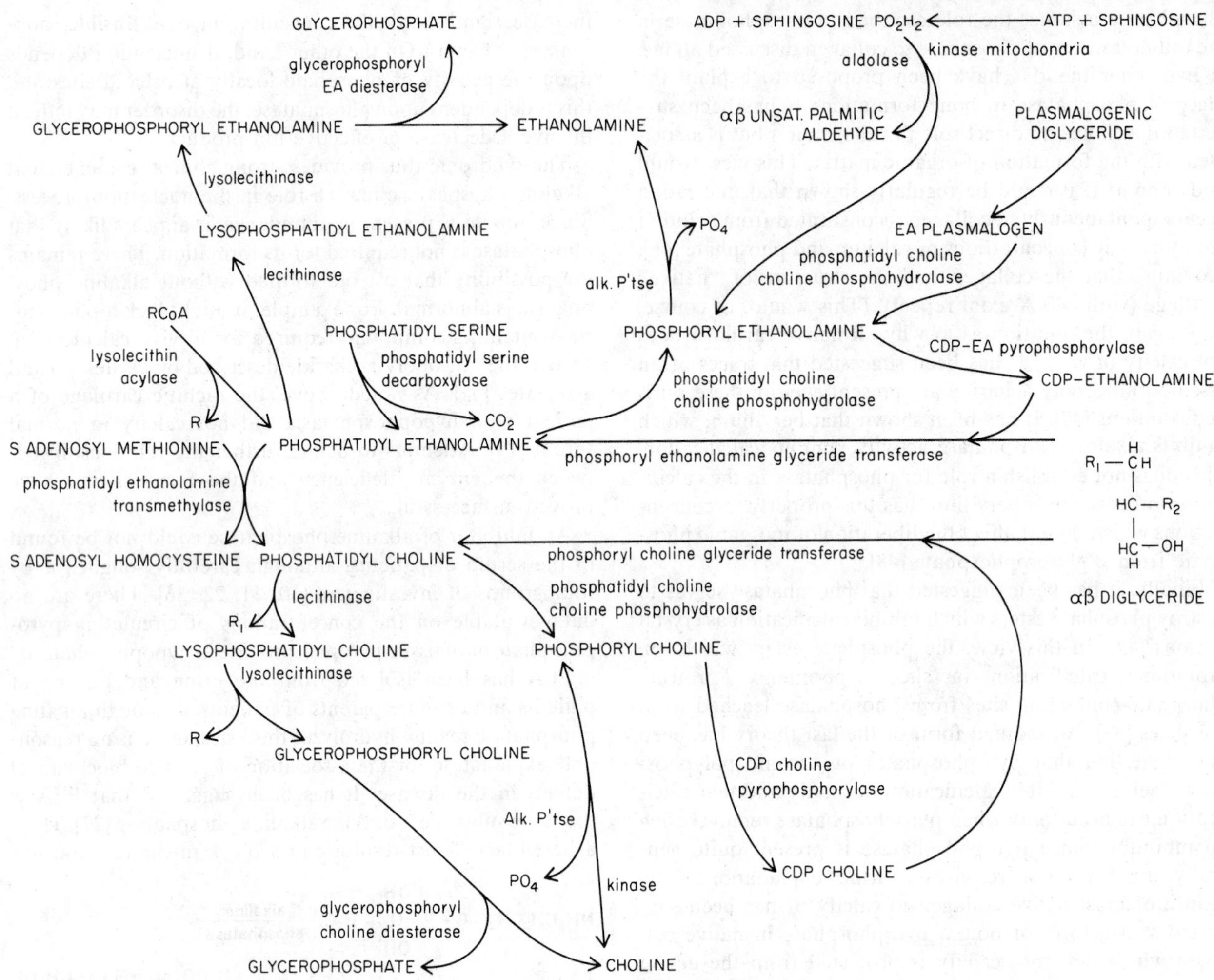

Figure 51-4. Metabolic pathways for phosphorylethanolamine and phosphorylcholine.

$$\textbf{Choline} \xrightarrow[\textbf{kinase}]{\textbf{choline}} \textbf{phosphorylcholine} \quad (1)$$

$$\alpha,\beta\textbf{-Diglyceride} + \textbf{CDP-choline} \xrightarrow[\textbf{glyceride transferase}]{\textbf{phosphorylcholine}} \textbf{phosphatidyl choline} \quad (2)$$

$$\textbf{Phosphatidyl choline} \xrightarrow[\textbf{choline phosphohydrolase}]{\textbf{phosphatidyl choline}} \textbf{phosphoryl choline}$$

$$\alpha\textbf{-Choline plasmalogen} \longrightarrow \textbf{phosphoryl choline} + \textbf{plasmalogen glyceride} \quad (3)$$

Indeed, phosphatidyl ethanolamine (itself readily converted to phosphatidyl choline) and phosphatidyl choline are converted to PEA and PC, respectively, by identical enzymes, i.e., lecithinase, lysolecithinase, and glycerophosphoryl choline diesterase, followed by choline kinase requiring ATP. Finally, both may lose the phosphate radical through the action of alkaline phosphatase. PEA may also be formed from phosphoryl sphingosine through the action of an aldolase (R. Brady, personal communication). Since the origin of the excessive PEA in hypophosphatasia is as obscure as its function, these observations do not even clarify the question of whether excessive production or decreased utilization (or degradation) of PEA is the ultimate defect. It is, of course, tempting to relate all aspects of the disorder to the deficiency of alkaline phosphatase and to attribute the excess of both PEA and CP (if it occurs regularly) to a failure of the hydrolysis of these compounds at the site (e.g., bone surface) at which they may function.

Hypercalcemia and hypercalciuria occur frequently but not constantly in hypophosphatasia. When they do occur, there may be nitrogen retention and nephrocalcinosis. A serum calcium concentration greater than 11 mg per 100 ml was noted on one or more occasions in 20 of the 31 patients for whom data were available [2].

The serum calcium may undergo wide fluctuations without

apparent cause and hypercalcemia may result from therapy with moderate doses of vitamin D. It may also occur in subjects who have never received supplemental vitamin D. Thus, one patient developed a serum calcium concentration of 17 mg per 100 ml after 10 days on 50,000 units a day [10]; another, who had a serum calcium concentration of 12 to 15 mg per 100 ml before therapy with the vitamin, showed a return of serum calcium to normal while receiving 50,000 units a day [25].

Inasmuch as the bones are surrounded with osteoid and little or no osteoclastic activity is seen histologically, it has been generally assumed that the hypercalcemia results from hyperabsorption of calcium. Even with normal calcium absorption hypercalcemia might indeed develop if the bone matrix were unable to deposit calcium (as is apparently the case in hypophosphatasia). The occurrence of all the other abnormalities of hypophosphatasia in many patients with normal serum calcium, who have not had supplemental vitamin D throughout their clinical course, eliminates the possibility that the alkaline phosphatase in this disease is depressed as a result of hypervitaminosis D and hypercalcemia [54, 55].

TREATMENT

There is no generally accepted therapy for hypophosphatasia. Vitamin D has been tried because the bone disease is like that found in rickets, with apparent improvement in one case [25]. This same patient and several others so treated [2, 10, 56] developed hypercalcemia and signs of vitamin D intoxication. There is no further evidence that vitamin D deficiency plays a part in the disease or that therapy with vitamin D is effective.

In a single patient, cortisone seemed to produce rapid improvement in the radiologic defects in the bones and to raise the serum alkaline phosphatase concentration to twice pretreatment values, but not to normal levels. Relapse occurred when cortisone was omitted, and there was a comparable response when it was reinstituted. On the other hand, five cases are said to have shown no response to cortisone [26, 57–59]. In three cases, osteotomy allowed healing of pseudofractures [9, 24, 26].

There is no record of the use of phosphate supplements to induce hyperphosphatemia as a therapeutic measure. It is possible that acalcification in hypophosphatasia results from a subnormal ion product at osteoid sites and that this is normally overcome through an action of phosphatase. Possibly the defect could be overcome by inducing an abnormally high solubility product in circulating fluids.

GENETICS

The reliability of a genetic analysis clearly depends upon the number of "markers" available, and the precision with which each can be analyzed: the less sensitive the chemical method, the poorer the "penetrance" will appear to be for the marker. In hypophosphatasia, for which the propositus always has bone disease, such markers include premature shedding of deciduous teeth, urinary and plasma PEA, and, of course, a low serum alkaline phosphatase. With the development of sensitive tests for urinary and plasma PEA [4], the detection of heterozygotes and the differentiation of hetero- from homozygotes is almost a quantitative procedure. As regards serum alkaline phosphatase, normal values are not infrequently found in subjects who are clearly affected [16]; indeed, in one patient, values fluctuated from normal to very low ones at different times [17] (with reciprocal variations in urinary PEA)! In very few cases has the source of the phosphatase been sought by modern means—thus, tests for the isozymes of phosphatase [60] might reveal that only one is consistently low in the syndrome. A single case of hypophosphatasia positive for *all* other markers, whose plasma was reported to contain normal quantities of intestinal *and bone* phosphatase isozymes [18] was thought to have as the sole defect an isozyme whose high K_m for EAP prevented hydrolysis of PEA at plasma concentrations. If further studies should show that urinary phosphoryl choline is another marker for hypophosphatasia [17], the genetic analysis should be greatly facilitated.

Published data are almost all consistent with the inheritance of hypophosphatasia as an autosomal recessive trait. This conclusion was reached on the basis of bone disease and alkaline phosphatase alone [61] on the assumption that all parents of cases must be heterozygotes. Since 70 percent of them showed low values, Steinberg used 70 percent as an estimate of "penetrance" of this trait.

Then, since two-thirds of all clinically normal sibs of patients should be heterozygotic, about 50 percent (0.70×0.66) should then have low serum phosphatase values. This compared well with an observed ratio of three affected in seven clinically healthy sibs tested. The high frequency of the disease in the last-born sib suggests that families with an affected child avoid future pregnancies or that medical reports have appeared before the families were complete.

When values for PEA are available for the detection of heterozygosity, especially now that a quantitative range for urinary PEA is established [4], the hereditary aspects of hypophosphatasia are considerably clarified. (Fraser noted that there is no good evidence that the defect of phosphatase and that of PEA metabolism are carried on the same gene and that there is suggestive evidence that they are not: relatives who excrete PEA tend to have higher serum phosphatase values than those who do not). In a study of 481 families of 16 patients with hypophosphatasia, Harris and Robson [62], using semiquantitative paper chromatography for PEA, concluded that only 58 percent of the presumed heterozygotes may be detected by this method.

A recent study in which all the indices for heterozygosity were used suggested a dominant mode of inheritance. Silver-

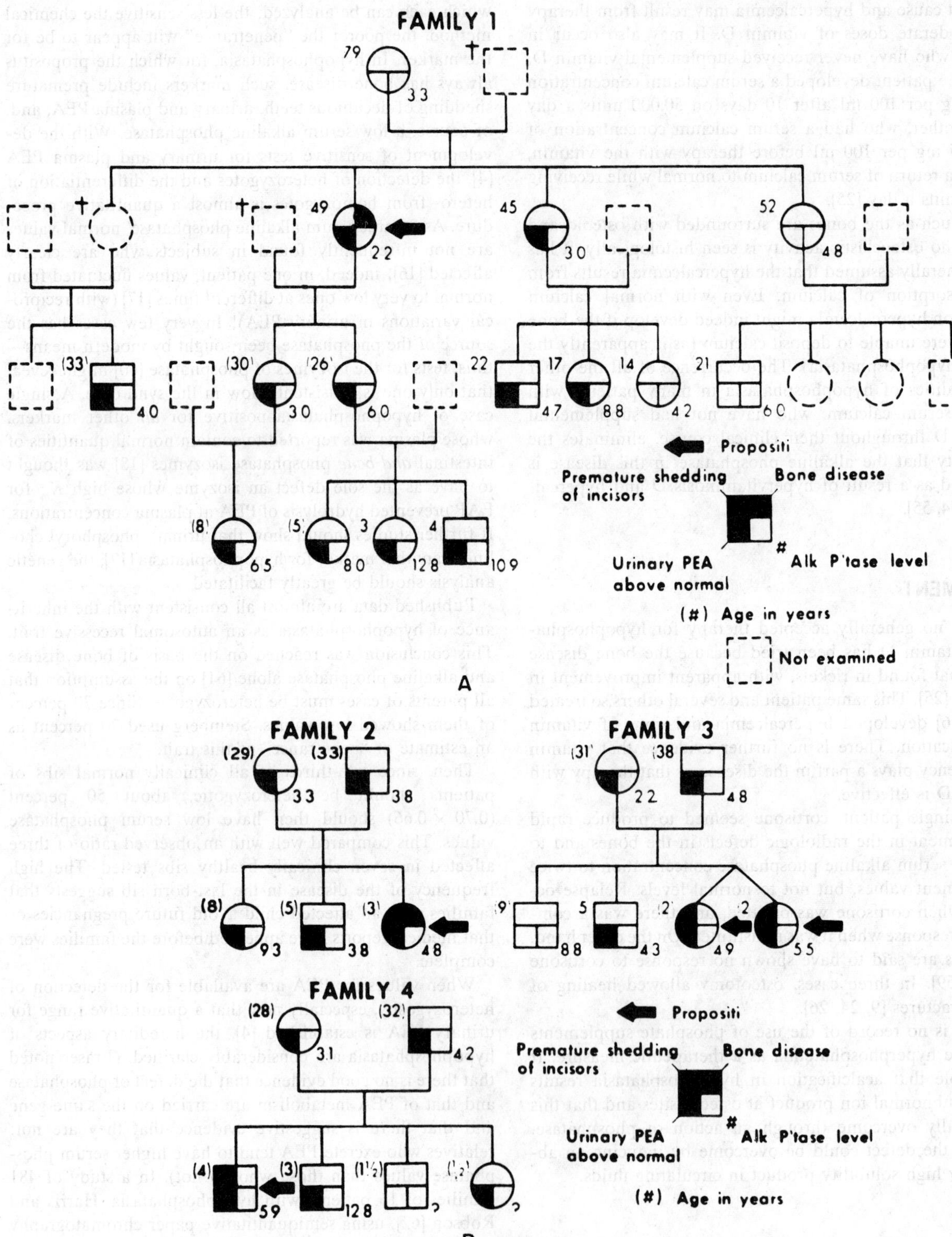

Figure 51-5. A. Pedigree of Patient L. B., adult patient with hypophosphatasia. B. Pedigrees of three patients with childhood form of hypophosphatasia. (*From Pimstone et al.* [16], *with permission.*)

man [23] found normal alkaline phosphatase values in the serum and no PEA in the urine of a mother and two of her children in a family in which the father and two other children had hypophosphatasia. According to accepted concepts, they should all have been heterozygotes for hypophosphatasia. It is possible that they were: as noted above, serum alkaline phosphatase may be normal in heterozygotes. On the other hand, the two affected sibs (Silverman's III 8 and III 9) were mild cases, with early loss of teeth and slight bone disease, whose PEA excretion was "good" (quantitative test not done) in one and "slightly increased" in the other. Thus, these two might be heterozygotes and the mother indeed normal.

In another study of four families, in which all markers were used [16], premature shedding of the deciduous teeth was the only overt sign of disease in two pedigrees. Of 24 family members presumed to be heterozygotes (on the basis of urinary PEA), none showed serum phosphatase values clearly *below* normal (Fig. 51-5).

In all these, inheritance is best explained on the basis of an autosomal recessive trait which must be present in homozygous form for severe bone disease.

SUMMARY

1 Hypophosphatasia is a familial disease in which severe skeletal defects result from a failure of deposition of apatite in osteoid and of normal ossification at epiphyseal plates. The serum alkaline phosphatase activity is below normal, and phosphorylethanolamine is found in excessive quantities in plasma and urine. There may be premature synostosis of the cranial vault, hypercalcemia, nephrocalcinosis, and premature loss of teeth.

2 The disease may be first detected in infancy or in adulthood. Diagnosis is based on the demonstration of radiologic and histologic changes in bone indistinguishable from those of rickets, a high concentration of phosphorylethanolamine in the plasma or urine, and serum alkaline phosphatase activity that is subnormal for the patient's age. Renal clearance of phosphorylethanolamine is high, since reabsorption does not increase with the filtered load.

3 The cardinal pathologic feature is inadequate calcification of bone matrix. The biochemical basis for this and its relation to the other biochemical defects are not known. It is possible that alkaline phosphatase is necessary for the formation of normal osteoid or that phosphorylethanolamine normally has an integral place in the calcification process.

4 The disease picture offers strong support for a role for alkaline phosphatase in normal calcification of bone.

5 There is no adequate therapy.

6 The disease appears to be inherited as an autosomal recessive trait. Heterozygotes may have low serum alkaline phosphatase concentrations, high urinary excretion of phosphorylethanolamine, or both, without bone disease.

BIBLIOGRAPHY

1. Rathbun, J. C.: Hypophosphatasia, a new developmental anomaly. Amer. J. Dis. Child., **75**, 822, 1948.
2. Fraser, D.: Hypophosphatasia. Amer. J. Med., **22**, 730, 1957.
3. Currarino, G., Neuhauser, E., Reyersback, G., and Sobel, E.: Hypophosphatasia. Amer. J. Roentgen., **78**, 392, 1957.
4. Rasmussen, K.: Phosphorylethanolamine and hypophosphatasia. Danish Med. Bull., **15**, 1, 1968.
5. Huhne, T., and Schonfeld, E.: Eine eigenartige Wachstumstorung in Kindesalter. Mschr. Kinderheilk., **42**, 267, 1929.
6. Chown, B.: Renal rickets and dwarfism: A pituitary disease. Brit. J. Surg., **23**, 552, 1935–1936.
7. Kubatsch, H.: Über eine seltene Knochenerkrankung. Mschr. Kinderheilk., **75**, 253, 1938.
8. Anspach, W. E., and Clifton, W. M.: Hyperparathyroidism in children. Amer. J. Dis. Child., **58**, 540, 1939.
9. Macey, H. B.: Multiple pseudofractures: Report of case. Proc. Staff Meet. Mayo Clin., **15**, 789, 1940.
10. Sobel, E. H., Clark, L. C., Fox, R. P., and Robinow, M.: Rickets, deficiency of "alkaline" phosphatase activity and premature loss of teeth in childhood. Pediatrics, **11**, 309, 1953.
11. Fraser, D., Yendt, E. R., and Christie, F. H.: Metabolic abnormalities in hypophosphatasia. Lancet, **1**, 286, 1955.
12. McCance, R. A.: The excretion of phosphoethanolamine and hypophosphatasia. Lancet, **1**, 131, 1955.
13. Fraser, D., and Yendt, E. R.: Metabolic abnormalities in hypophosphatasia. Amer. J. Dis. Child., **90**, 552, 1955.
14. Scaglione, P. R., and Lucey, J. F.: Further observations on hypophosphatasia. Amer. J. Dis. Child., **92**, 493, 1956.
15. Kretchmer, N., Stone, M., and Bauer, C.: Hereditary enzymatic effects as illustrated by hypophosphatasia. Ann. NY Acad. Sci., **75**, 279, 1958.
16. Pimstone, B., Eisenberg, E., and Silverman, S.: Hypophosphatasia: Genetic and dental studies. Ann. Intern. Med., **65**, 722, 1966.
17. Eisenberg, E., and Pimstone, B.: Hypophosphatasia in an adult. Clin. Orthop., **52**, 199, 1967.
18. Scriver, C. R., and Camerom, D.: Pseudohypophosphatasia. New Eng. J. Med., **281**, 604, 1969.
19. Kellsey, D. C.: Hypophosphatasia and congenital bowing of the long bones. JAMA, **179**, 187, 1962.
20. Park, E. A., and Powers, C. F.: Acrocephaly and scaphocephaly with symmetrically distributed malformation of the extremities. Amer. J. Dis. Child., **20**, 235, 1920.
21. Bartter, F. C.: Oxycephaly, in *Textbook of Medicine,* 11th ed., edited by P. B. Beeson and W. McDermott, p. 1517. Saunders, Philadelphia, 1963.
22. McCance, R. A., Fairweather, D. V. I., Barrett, A. M., and Morrison, A. B.: Genetic, clinical, biochemical and pathological features of hypophosphatasia. Quart. J. Med., n.s., **25**, 523, 1956.
23. Silverman, J. L.: Apparent dominant inheritance of hypophosphatasia. Arch. Intern. Med. (Chicago), **110**, 191, 1962.
24. Bethune, J., and Dent, C. E.: Hypophosphatasia in the adult. Amer. J. Med., **28**, 615, 1960.
25. Schlesinger, B., Luder, J., and Bodian, M.: Rickets with alkaline phosphatase deficiency: An osteoblastic dysplasia. Arch. Dis. Child, **30**, 265, 1955.
26. Henneman, P.: Personal communication.
27. Dent, C. E.: in *Bone Structure and Metabolism, CIBA Foundation Symposium,* p. 266. Churchill, London, 1956.
28. Owen, J. A., and Peskin, H.: Clinical study of an adult with hypophosphatasia. Clin. Res., **6**, 249, 1958.
29. Ryssing, E.: 2 tilfaelde of hypophosphatasia. Ugeskr. Laeg., **124**, 1997, 1962.
30. Beisel, W. R., Benjamin, N., and Austen, K. F.: Absence of leucocyte alkaline phosphatase activity in hypophosphatasia. Blood, **14**, 975, 1959.
31. Scriver, C. R., and Davies, E.: Endogenous renal clearance rates of free amino acids in pre-pubertal children. Pediatrics, **36**, 592, 1965.
32. Birtwell, V. M., Jr., Riggs, B. L., Peterson, L. F. A., and Jones, J. D.: Hypophosphatasia in an adult. Arch. Intern. Med. (Chicago), **120**, 90, 1967.

33. Goyer, R. A.: Ethanolamine phosphate excretion in a family with hypophosphatasia. Arch. Dis. Child, **38,** 205, 1963.
34. Keiser, H. R., Gill, J. R., Jr., Sjoerdsma, A., and Bartter, F. C.: Relation between urinary hydroxyproline and parathyroid function. J. Clin. Invest., **43,** 1073, 1964.
35. Teree, R. M., and Klein, L.: Hypophosphatasia: Clinical and metabolic studies. Pediatrics, **72,** 41, 1968.
36. Engfeldt, B., and Zetterstrom, R.: Osteodysmetamorphosis fetalis: Clinical pathological study of congenital skeletal disease with retarded growth, hypophosphatasemia and renal damage. J. Pediat., **45,** 125, 1954.
37. Neuman, W. F., and Neuman, M. W.: *The Chemical Dynamics of Bone Mineral.* The University of Chicago Press, Chicago, 1958.
38. Glimcher, M. J., and Krane, S. M.: Studies of the interactions of collagen and phosphate. I. The nature of inorganic orthophosphate binding, in *Radioisotopes and Bone,* edited by P. Lacraix and A. M. Budy, pp. 393–418. Blackwell Scientific Publications, Ltd., Oxford, 1962.
39. Robison, R.: Possible significance of hexosephosphoric esters in ossification. Biochem. J., **17,** 286, 1923.
40. Waldman, J.: Calcification of hypertrophic epiphyseal cartilage in vitro following inactivation of phosphatase and other enzymes. Proc. Soc. Exp. Biol. Med., **69,** 262, 1948.
41. Fleisch, H.: Role of nucleation and inhibition in calcification. Clin. Orthop., **32,** 170, 1964.
42. Cartier, P., and Picard, J.: La mineralisation du cartilage ossifiable: I. La mineralisation du cartilage in vitro. Bull. Soc. Chim. Biol. (Paris), **37,** 485, 1955.
43. Saito, S.: Studies on the mechanism of ossification in tissue culture: II Effects of adenosinetriphosphate and phosphocreatine on the growth of chick embryo femur. Jap. J. Exp. Med., **29,** 91, 1959.
44. Sobel, A. E., Burger, M., and Nobel, S.: Mechanisms of nuclei formation in mineralizing tissues. Clin. Orthop., **17,** 103, 1960.
45. Gutman, A. B., and Yu, T. F.: Concept of role of enzymes in endochondral calcification, in *Tr. Conf. Metabolic Interrelations,* vol. 2, p. 167. Josiah Macy, Jr. Foundation, New York, 1950.
46. Glimcher, M. J., Hodge, A. J., and Schmitt, F. O.: Macromolecular aggregation states in relation to mineralization: The collagen hydroxyapatite system as studied in vitro. Proc. Nat. Acad. Sci. USA, **43,** 860, 1957.
47. Kendrew, J. C.: in *The Proteins,* edited by H. Neurath and K. Bailey, vol. II, part B., chap. 23. Academic, New York, 1954.
48. Hiatt, H. H., and Shorr, E.: Inhibition of endochondral calcification in vitro by beryllium and L-histidine, in *Tr. Conf. Metabolic Interrelations,* vol. 3, p. 105. Josiah Macy, Jr. Foundation, New York, 1951.
49. Neuman, W. F., DiStefano, V., and Mulryan, B. J.: Surface chemistry of bone. III. Observations on role of phosphatase. J. Biol. Chem., **193,** 227, 1951.
50. Anning, S. T., Dawson, J., Dolby, D. E., and Ingram, J. T.: The toxic effects of calciferol. Quart. J. Med., **27,** 203, 1948.
51. DiStefano, V., Neuman, W. F., and Rouser, G.: The isolation of a phosphate ester from calcifiable cartilage. Arch. Biochem. **47,** 218, 1953.
52. Walshe, J. M.: Disturbances of amino acid metabolism following liver injury: A study by means of paper chromatography. Quart. J. Med., n.s., **22,** 483, 1953.
53. Fisher, O. D., and Neill, D. W.: Excretion of ethanolamine phosphoric acid in coeliac disease. Lancet, **1,** 334, 1955.
54. Nordin, B. E. C., and Fraser, R.: in *Bone Structure and Metabolism, CIBA Foundation Symposium,* p. 222. Churchill, London, 1956.
55. von Fanconi, G., and de Chastonay, E.: Die D-Hypervitaminose in Sauglingsalter. Helv. Paediat. Acta, **5,** 5, 1950.
56. Felder, J., and Schreirer, K.: Hypophosphatasie. Mschr. Kinderheilk., **103,** 437, 1955.
57. Lachsdal, O. E.: Quoted in Hypophosphatasia, by D. Fraser, Amer. J. Med., **22,** 730, 1957.
58. Schlesinger, B.: Quoted in Hypophosphatasia, by D. Fraser. Amer. J. Med., **22,** 730, 1957.
59. Dent, C. E.: Quoted in Hypophosphatasia, by D. Fraser. Amer. J. Med., **22,** 730, 1957.
60. Sussman, H. H., Small, P. A., Jr., and Cotlove, E.: Human alkaline phosphatase. J. Biol. Chem., **243,** 160, 1968.
61. Steinberg, A. G.: Quoted in Hypophosphatasia, by G. Currarino et al. Amer. J. Roentgen., **78,** 392, 1957.
62. Harris, H., and Robson, E. B.: A genetical study of ethanolamine phosphate excretion in hypophosphatasia, Hum. Gen., **23,** 421, 1958.

CHAPTER FIFTY-TWO

PSEUDOHYPOPARATHYROIDISM

John T. Potts, Jr.

Pseudohypoparathyroidism is a rare hereditary disorder characterized by symptoms and signs of hypoparathyroidism in association with distinctive skeletal and developmental defects. The hypoparathyroidism is due to deficient end-organ response to the endogenous hormone. Thus, the cause of the disease differs from that of true hypoparathyroidism; in the latter there is deficient parathyroid hormone production. In fact, pseudohypoparathyroidism is characterized by excessive secretion of parathyroid hormone and hyperplasia of the parathyroids, a response to the resistance to hormone action at the target tissues—the kidney and the bone. Satisfactory relief of the symptoms and complications of hypoparathyroidism can be achieved in these patients by treatment with a high intake of calcium and vitamin D.

Many aspects of pseudohypoparathyroidism remain unclarified, including the relation between the skeletal and developmental defects and the hypoparathyroidism. Relatives of patients with pseudohypoparathyroidism often have skeletal and developmental defects without any symptoms or chemical evidence of hypoparathyroidism. The term pseudo-pseudohypoparathyroidism has been applied to the distinctive developmental anomalies in these family members who lack evidence of hypoparathyroidism. Many details of the pathophysiology of pseudohypoparathyroidism remain uncertain, although recent studies have suggested the nature of the biochemical defect responsible for end-organ resistance to the parathyroid hormone. Similarly, many aspects of the genetics of this disorder are still under review, particularly the suggestion that a defective sex chromosome may be responsible for both the hypoparathyroidism and the growth and developmental defects.

HISTORY AND ETIOLOGY

The initial recognition of this syndrome in 1942 by Albright and his colleagues [1] resulted from a careful analysis of a patient with symptoms and signs of hypoparathyroidism but no metabolic response to the administration of parathyroid hormone. The latter was appreciated to be in sharp contrast to the exquisite sensitivity to parathyroid hormone of patients with true hypoparathyroidism and a deficiency of endogenous parathyroid hormone. Additional patients with this syndrome were recognized and in several parathyroid explorations revealed enlarged parathyroids [1].

Since there was evidence of increased endogenous parathyroid hormone production (the enlarged parathyroid glands) and a lack of response to the exogenous hormone, Albright et al. [*1a*] reasoned that in pseudohypoparathyroidism there must be a deficient end-organ response in kidney and bone. There has been general agreement that there was little to suggest a true deficiency of parathyroid hormone production. In recent years, however, as additional patients with this syndrome have been seen, other explanations for the disease have been considered [2]: (1) The parathyroid hormone made by these patients is biologically inactive and thereby interferes even with the effects of exogenous hormone; (2) there are circulating antibodies or other factors which inactivate parathyroid hormone; or (3) there is overproduction of a physiological antagonist to parathyroid hormone such as thyrocalcitonin [3].

Until the last several years it was impossible to test these various possibilities properly. A definitive explanation for the pathophysiology of the disorder required preparation of pure parathyroid hormone for study of hormone action, bioassays of sufficient sensitivity to test extracts of glands removed from patients with pseudohypoparathyroidism, and sensitive and specific immunological assays to measure the concentration of parathyroid hormone or to detect the presence of circulating antibodies. With the development of the necessary test procedures evidence for the existence of a discrete biochemical defect that explains end-organ resistance has been obtained, and the alternative hypotheses have been discarded. It has been shown that (1) there is an increased concentration of circulating parathyroid hormone in all subjects with pseudohypoparathyroidism (at least, if studied when they are hypocalcemic prior to the institution of vitamin D therapy) [1, 4]; (2) there is no evidence for circulating antibodies in any of these patients, although techniques have been developed which can reliably demonstrate such antibodies when present [5]; (3) there is evidence in support of the concept that the hormone made by these patients is biologically active [4]; and (4) there is normal production of calcitonin in pseudohypoparathyroidism. The last point is based on preliminary tests by bioassay which have indicated normal circulating concentrations of calcitonin [6] and the finding that thyroidectomy in a few patients has not resulted in the disappearance of hypocalcemia, in spite of the removal of the source of calcitonin production [3].

Direct evidence has been accumulated by Aurbach, Chase and their associates for a biochemical defect that would explain end-organ resistance [7–15]. The initial effect of parathyroid hormone on the kidney appears to be a stimulation of membrane bound adenyl cyclase, with a consequent rise in urinary 3′,5′ cyclic AMP [13]. Normal subjects and patients with true hypoparathyroidism have an increase of ten- to twentyfold in urinary cyclic AMP following administration of exogenous parathyroid hormone; patients with pseudohypoparathyroidism have essentially no response [7].

This test for urinary exretion of 3′,5′ cyclic AMP gives great promise of providing for the first time a definitive laboratory diagnosis of pseudohypoparathyroidism.

PATHOPHYSIOLOGY

The abnormalities in calcium metabolism and parathyroid function that are found in pseudohypoparathyroidism may be better understood by reviewing current information about the physiological actions of parathyroid hormone, the mediation of hormonal effects at the end organ by an increase of intracellular cyclic AMP, and the pattern of control of hormone secretion in secondary hypoparathyroidism.

Effects of Parathyroid Hormone

The physiological function of parathyroid hormone in man as well as in other mammalian species is to maintain extracellular fluid calcium concentration [1]. The hormone acts on bone, kidney, and intestine to increase serum calcium; in turn, parathyroid hormone production is closely regulated by serum calcium concentration [1]. This feedback system involving the parathyroids is one of the most important homeostatic mechanisms for the close regulation of extracellular fluid calcium concentration. Any tendency toward hypocalcemia, such as might be induced by prolonged starvation, is counteracted by an increased rate of secretion of parathyroid hormone. This in turn (1) acts to increase the rate of dissolution of bone mineral, thereby providing an increased flow of calcium from bone into blood, (2) reduces the renal clearance of calcium, returning more of the calcium filtered at the glomerulus into extracellular fluid, and (3) increases, perhaps by an indirect mechanism, the efficiency of calcium absorption in the intestine. The relative physiological importance of these three actions of parathyroid hormone, stimulation of calcium transport in bone, kidney, and intestine, has never been definitely resolved. It is technically difficult to characterize fully the action of parathyroid hormone on bone or to assess acute effects of the hormone on the intestine. Most workers have believed that the effect of the hormone on bone is the most important in maintaining calcium homeostasis. This is because evidence from metabolic balance and calcium kinetic studies indicates a transfer between extracellular fluid and bone of as much as 500 mg calcium daily (an amount large in relation to the total extracellular fluid calcium pool), and parathyroid hormone is known to influence this movement of calcium from bone into blood. It has become more apparent in the last several years that the action of parathyroid hormone on kidney to preserve calcium by increasing the percentage of filtered calcium that is reabsorbed is also important in the minute-to-minute regulation of blood calcium concentration [16].

Methods for assessing bone-blood mineral exchange in vivo are indirect. Studies of the effect of parathyroid hormone on bone in tissue culture and in bone perfusion systems, as well as cytologic studies of bone cells after long-term administration of parathyroid hormone to animals, have led to the concept of a dual action of parathyroid hormone on bone [1, 17]. These two effects have been termed the "calcium replacement" and the "bone remodeling" effects of parathyroid hormone [1]. It can be shown in vitro that there is an increased rate of release of calcium from bone into blood within minutes of the administration of parathyroid hormone [17]; this is consistent with the view that the major homeostatic mechanism for the prevention of hypocalcemia is a rapid mobilization of calcium from bone into extracellular fluid under the influence of parathyroid hormone. On the other hand, the more chronic effects of parathyroid hormone, mainly an increase in the number and activity of osteoclasts and a general increase in the remodeling of bone, appear only hours after the hormone is given. These actions, which involve increased protein synthesis, persist for hours after parathyroid hormone has been given. It is the latter effect, bone remodeling, which seems to be most closely related to the radiologic and histologic picture of the bone disease that results from long-standing excessive parathyroid action, osteitis fibrosa cystica [1].

It is not clear whether the two effects of parathyroid action on bone represent a continuous spectrum with a common initiating biochemical event, or whether the two effects of the hormone on bone are in some way separable. This uncertainty is further compounded by clinical findings. There are recent reports of osteitis fibrosa (excessive bone remodeling) in some patients with pseudohypoparathyroidism who are hypocalcemic (apparently deficient bone-blood mineral exchange). It has long been appreciated, but without apparent explanation, that osteitis fibrosa occurs infrequently in hyperparathyroidism in spite of the invariable presence of hypercalcemia [1]. These perplexing questions about the variable picture of bone disease in pseudohypoparathyroidism and hyperparathyroidism have been reviewed extensively elsewhere [1]. Much further information about fundamental processes of bone turnover and renewal will be required in order to clarify our understanding of the pathophysiology of bone disease in parathyroid disorders.

Role of Adenyl Cyclase

An important clue to the mode of action of parathyroid hormone at the biochemical level has been provided by investigations concerning the effects of parathyroid hormone on adenyl cyclase in the cells of the target tissue. The initial effect of parathyroid hormone on kidney cells both in vivo and in vitro [9, 10, 13, 14] and on bone cells in vitro [12] is a stimulation of adenyl cyclase. The cyclase enzyme is membrane bound. Stimulation of enzyme activity during specific hormone–target cell membrane interaction leads to an increase in intracellular 3′,5′ cyclic AMP. It has not yet been conclusively demonstrated that this rapidly effected rise in intracellular 3′,5′ cyclic AMP is the initial biochemical step in all of the physiological effects of parathyroid hormone, but there is considerable evidence in support of this thesis.

It has been shown that following the administration of parathyroid hormone there is, within minutes, a rise in urinary cyclic AMP that precedes in time any observable increase in phosphate excretion in the kidney [13] (the latter action of the hormone was previously the most rapidly detected hormonal effect [1].) Likewise, the effects on bone cell adenyl cyclase activity can be detected within 1 min of the addition of parathyroid hormone to a suspension of bone cells [12].

In addition, administration of dibutyryl cyclic AMP, which as a more soluble analogue of 3′,5′ cyclic AMP penetrates cells more effectively, simulating the actions of parathyroid hormone in parathyroidectomized animals [6, 19]. Dibutyryl cyclic AMP leads to a rise in serum calcium, a lowering of serum phosphate, and an increased excretion of calcium, phosphate, and hydroxyproline in urine [6, 19]. Other studies have indicated that the administration of drugs which influence the enzymes concerned with the destruction of intracellular 3′,5′ cyclic AMP have effects in vivo that are consistent with the mediation of parathyroid hormone action through an increased intracellular concentration of the cyclic nucleotide [6, 18]. Phosphodiesterase is one enzyme responsible for the degradation of intracellular cyclic AMP; the administration of theophylline, which inhibits phosphodiesterase, leads to an increase in serum calcium in parathyroidectomized rats, whereas the administration of imidazole, which stimulates phosphodiesterase, causes hypocalcemia or blocks the hypercalcemic effects of parathyroid hormone [18].

Important clinical confirmation of the significance of the cyclic AMP mechanism has come from the observations of Chase and associates already discussed above [7]. Patients with pseudohypoparathyroidism show a complete loss of the normal increase in urinary cyclic AMP following the administration of parathyroid hormone. This finding in patients with known end-organ resistance to parathyroid hormone supports the concept that stimulation of the membrane-bound adenyl cyclase must reflect the specific interaction between parathyroid hormone and the membrane of the target cell in kidney.

There have not yet been any definitive biochemical data that point to specific intracellular processes that are directly influenced by the increase in intracellular concentration of cyclic AMP. Essential to the hypothesis of a mediating role for cyclic AMP would be the demonstration that the cyclic nucleotide is responsible for stimulating one or more intracellular enzymic systems, the activity of which is ultimately responsible for the known physiological actions of the hormone on calcium and phosphate transport. It has now been shown that a stimulation of adenyl cyclase and an increased concentration of 3′,5′ cyclic AMP may be central in the mode of action of a variety of hormones including epinephrine, glucagon, corticotrophin, and thyrotropin [9]. A plausible link between the physiological actions of the hormone and the stimulation of a rate-limiting enzymic step has, so far, been demonstrated only with epinephrine and glucagon [20]. It has been shown that cyclic AMP is an essential cofactor or "allosteric inducer" of a series of linked phosphorylation reactions that ultimately result in the activation of phosphorylase and thereby in a stimulation of glycogenolysis [20]. With regard to parathyroid action, it has been proposed that cyclic AMP may increase cell membrane permeability and thereby cause a sudden influx of calcium into the cells. It has been further speculated that the increase in calcium or cyclic AMP then stimulates enzymic activity that ultimately leads to phosphaturia and hypercalcemia. Possible models of hormone action based on these effects have been proposed [21]. In order to validate any model of parathyroid hormone action it will be necessary to define more closely the events subsequent to hormone-membrane interaction in kidney and bone cells that would provide a link between cyclic AMP and hormone action.

Control of Parathyroid Hormone Secretion

The homeostatic role of parathyroid hormone in extracellular fluid calcium regulation has also been clarified from the opposite point of view, namely, the mode of control of hormone production in relation to physiological need [1]. Extensive studies, employing principally the immunoassay technique, have indicated that the secretion of the parathyroids is under the control of blood or extracellular fluid calcium concentration [1]. The precision of this regulation is remarkable. Under all types of experimental conditions in which blood calcium concentration is altered in animals or in man it has been shown that the parathyroid hormone secretory rate is under inverse proportional control by blood calcium concentration. Under normal conditions, hormone is continuously secreted. Hormone secretion is abolished only when blood calcium rises above 12 mg per 100 ml of blood. There is a continuous stepwise increase in the parathyroid hormone secretory rate as blood calcium concentration is lowered from 12 mg per 100 ml toward the lower limits of physiological tolerance, 4 to 5 mg per 100 ml [1].

There is an almost instantaneous modulation of the rate of hormone secretion in response to any change in blood calcium concentration. In addition, it has been shown that the hormone once secreted disappears rapidly from the circulation; effective systems for the destruction of the hormone located in one or more organs of the body (as yet not identified conclusively) remove or degrade the hormone with such rapidity that the half-time of the survival of the hormone in the circulation is of the order of 15 to 20 min [1, 22]. This system involving rapid modulation of the rate of secretion in response to hypocalcemia and a fixed and rapid rate of hormone destruction, provides for minute-to-minute regulation of the parathyroid hormone concentration in the blood in response to any change in serum calcium concentration. Since the effect of an increased concentration of hormone at the receptors is rapidly expressed, the parathyroids represent a most efficient homeostatic mechanism for regulation of extracellular fluid calcium concentration [1, 22].

Studies of the biosynthesis and secretion of parathyroid hormone show that the apparent concentration of preformed hormone in the gland is small in relation to the rate of hormone secretion. The fractional turnover of the hormone content of the gland per minute is high, even with basal rates of secretion. At maximal rates of hormone secretion (about fivefold above basal levels), the rate of new hormone biosynthesis appears to become almost rate limiting for secretion [1, 22]. The relative importance of hormone stores versus new hormone biosynthesis in the parathyroids is at variance with the situation found with many other peptide hormones. In the pituitary and the pancreas, stores of hormone are large in relation to rates of basal secretion [1, 22]. It seems likely that these findings explain the unusual adaptation that is found in secondary hyperparathyroidism, which develops whenever resistance to hormone action requires greater rates of hormone secretion than can be accomplished with maximal stimulation of the normal parathyroids. In animal models such as the parturient cow, which seem to reflect closely the conditions found in secondary hyperparathyroidism in man, the parathyroid glands become hyperplastic; the increase in the number or size of cells participating in hormone biosynthesis results in much greater rates of hormone secretion in response to any given change in blood calcium concentration [1, 22]. There is no change in the pattern of the control of hormone production by blood calcium. There is still a linear inverse proportional relationship between parathyroid secretory rate and blood calcium, but the slope of the line that describes the rate of hormone production as a function of blood calcium concentration is much steeper. This pattern is illustrated in Fig. 52-1.

The stimulus responsible for hyperplasia of the parathyroids has not been identified. It seems possible that in all of the conditions in which secondary hyperparathyroidism is found, resistance to hormone action accounts for persistent hypocalcemia in spite of increased hormone secretion. Chronic, even though partly compensated, hypocalcemia results in parathyroid hyperplasia [1].

In pseudohypoparathyroidism there is an inadequate flow of calcium into extracellular fluid because of the reduced effectiveness of parathyroid hormone in some or all of the target cells. This deficient action of the hormone on calcium transport leads to a serious reduction in extracellular fluid calcium concentration. In addition, due to the failure of the normal action of the parathyroid hormone to promote phosphate excretion in the kidney, hyperphosphatemia develops. There are several important physiological consequences of the hyperphosphatemia [1]. It is well known that a high

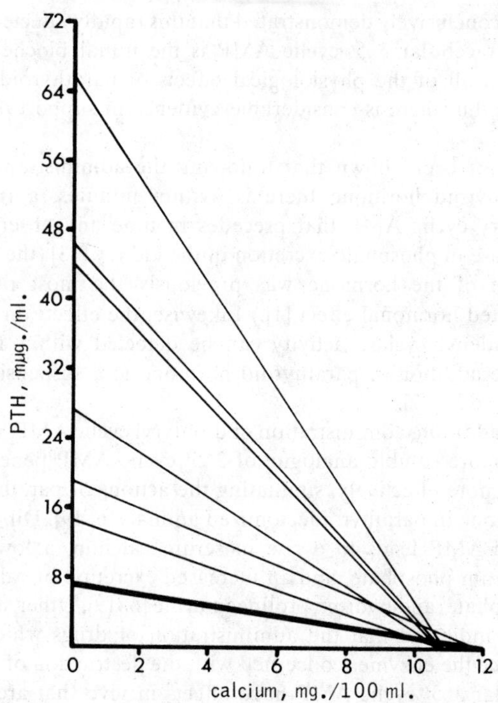

Figure 52-1. Comparison of the relationship between blood calcium concentration (independent variable) and parathyroid hormone concentration in a series of parturient cows with secondary hypoparathyroidism. The slope of the line relating hormone concentration as a function of blood calcium concentration is steeper in all animals with secondary hyperparathyroidism than in animals of normal size (heavy line—data taken from normal animals; extrapolation to zero calcium concentration).

blood phosphate concentration tends to lower blood calcium in many experimental situations or in disease states; the mechanism of the phosphate effect is still unclear. Present data indicate that an elevated blood phosphate concentration leads to an increased rate of deposition of calcium from extracellular fluid into bone and also into extraosseous tissues. In addition, there is evidence that a high blood phosphate concentration inhibits bone resorption.

The metabolic effects of hyperphosphatemia appear to act synergistically with deficient calcium transport to produce severe hypocalcemia. In response to the persistent hypocalcemia in untreated subjects with pseudohypoparathyroidism, secondary hyperparathyroidism develops. All patients who have been examined have markedly increased peripheral concentrations of hormone. In studies with our assay, three patients with pseudohypoparathyroidism had concentrations of 1.8, 3.0, and 3.1 ng per ml, values two-to fourfold above normal [1, 7]. As is consistent with secondary hyperparathyroidism, calcium infusion lowered hormone concentrations toward undetectable values. Hormone production was still under the control of blood calcium concentration. Increased concentrations of parathyroid hormone in several patients have also been reported from Tashjian's laboratory [4].

Peripheral Response to Parathyroid Hormone

Since all patients with the complete syndrome by definition are hypocalcemic and hyperphosphatemic, it has generally been believed that both bone and kidney are unresponsive. Some evidence is contradictory to this thesis. It was observed in the early studies of patients with the syndrome that some patients showed an essentially normal phosphaturia following the injection of parathyroid hormone [23]. There have also been reports that repeated intramuscular injections of parathyroid extract caused a slight rise in blood calcium. Four of the thirteen patients studied by Chase et al. showed a detectable, even though subnormal, increase in 3′,5′ AMP after parathyroid extract [7]. One patient had a completely normal rise in cyclic AMP after the administration of the hormone [7]. (Details of the latter patient's physical and laboratory data are not available.)

During the study of one patient with pseudohypoparathyroidism previously treated with vitamin D, Krane et al. in our clinic (unpublished) found that the removal of all four parathyroid glands was accomplished by a striking fall in serum calcium requiring a massive increase in vitamin D to restore serum calcium towards normal. These findings may mean that at least in some patients, perhaps when on chronic vitamin D treatment, there is a significant contribution to extracellular fluid calcium from parathyroid hormone-driven bone resorption when sufficient parathyroid hypersecretion has developed, despite osseous resistance to parathyroid action.

Additional support for the possibility that bone resistance may be only partial has come from case reports of unusual skeletal findings in some patients believed to have pseudohypoparathyroidism [24–30]. Reports have accumulated concerning approximately a dozen patients with hypocalcemia and hyperphosphatemia in whom evidence of osteitis fibrosa has been found by both x-ray and biopsy. This has led to the speculation that the renal end-organ defect may be the most severe if not the sole abnormality in some patients. Some have attributed the hypocalcemia solely to the hyperphosphatemia and have speculated that the skeleton is fully responsive; accordingly, it is believed that osteitis develops because of secondary hyperparathyroidism. On the other hand, detailed analysis of the clinical features of these dozen patients suggests that many may not be typical genetically or even match the physical findings of patients with true pseudohypoparathyroidism (see genetics, below). If this is true, then the findings in these patients are not relevant to the pathophysiology of pseudohypoparathyroidism.

Recently a report has appeared which carefully documents the restoration of a sensitivity to parathyroid hormone after vitamin D therapy in a patient with typical pseudohypoparathyroidism [3]. The patient had hypocalcemia and hyperphosphatemia prior to vitamin D therapy. There was no increase in serum calcium or urine phosphate nor a fall in serum phosphate, notwithstanding 10 days of parathyroid extract intramuscularly. (The preparation of hormone was shown to be active.) After treatment for many weeks with 100,000 units of vitamin D daily, serum calcium rose and serum phosphate fell into the normal range. A repeat trial of chronic intramuscular parathyroid extract (using the same batch of hormone) resulted in an apparently fully normal, acute, elevation in serum calcium to hypercalcemic levels, and brisk phosphaturia [3]. Subjects with pseudohypoparathyroidism, unlike patients with true hypoparathyroidism, do not excrete excessive quantities of calcium in urine when their blood calcium is made normal after vitamin D treatment [31]. This suggests that there is a normal renal end-organ response with regard to the action of the hormone to reduce renal calcium clearance.

These varied observations suggest that end-organ resistance may be less severe in some patients than in others or that vitamin D treatment alters end-organ sensitivity. In addition, it may be true that the bone is more responsive to hormone than the kidney in certain patients with pseudohypoparathyroidism. For clarification of these aspects of pathophysiology it would be essential to study directly the sensitivity of bone cell adenyl cyclase as well as kidney cyclase and to evaluate the urinary cyclic AMP response to administered hormone before and after vitamin D therapy. Such studies have not been reported. At least, the earlier view that a greater degree of bone versus renal abnormality could be explained by two different forms of parathyroid hormone, one effective on kidney the other on bone, has been largely disproved. During the course of our recent studies on the structure of parathyroid hormone, a peptide has been synthesized which corresponds to the amino terminal 34 amino acids of the major bovine parathyroid hormone. The synthetic peptide (Fig. 52-2) is highly active in vivo and in vitro on renal and skeletal tissue [32]. This indicates that a single short peptide sequence is indeed sufficient for expression of the action of the hormone on both physiological receptors, kidney and bone [32].

Thus, in spite of unresolved questions about variation or changes in end-organ sensitivity in some patients with pseudohypoparathyroidism, the overall evidence suggests that the disturbances in calcium and phosphorus metabolism in most patients with pseudohypoparathyroidism result from at least partial unresponsiveness of the receptors in both bone and kidney. It is difficult to attribute the severe hypocalcemia in these patients entirely to the renal end-organ defect with associated hyperphosphatemia. The concentration of circulating parathyroid hormone is in the same range as is found with severe hypercalcemia in primary hyperparathyroidism. Under these circumstances the severe hypocalcemia must be explained by at least a partial unresponsiveness in bone-blood calcium exchange.

Little can be said at the present time about the pathophysiology of the multiple skeletal and developmental effects in these patients. The genetics of the disorder are compatible with an abnormality in the X chromosome. Since identical short stature, abnormal metacarpals and metatarsals, and

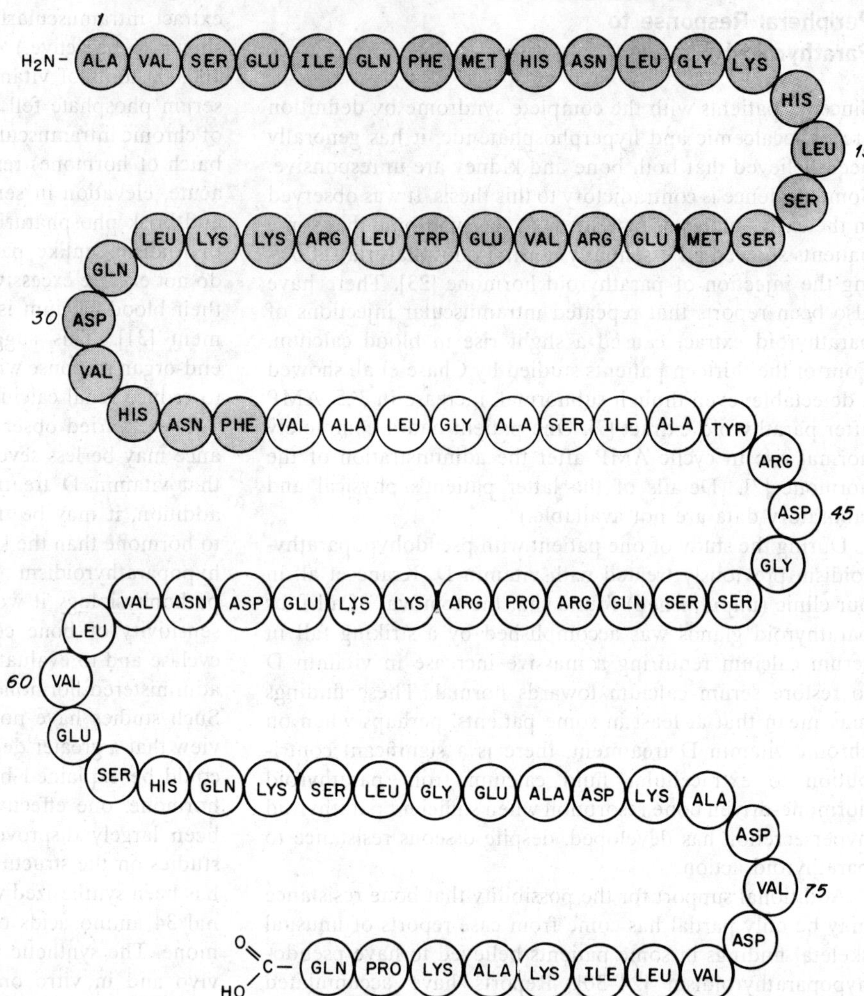

Figure 52-2. The amino acid sequence of bovine parathyroid hormone [60, 61]. The shaded residues represent the sequence of a biologically active fragment produced by peptide synthesis [32].

other physical features of the disease are found without hypocalcemia or hyperphosphatemia in patients with pseudopseudohypoparathyroidism (who have an apparently normal renal cell adenyl cyclase system), it seems likely that the skeletal and developmental defects are an independently inherited aspect of the illness reflecting X-chromosome deficits rather than a consequence of hypoparathyroidism per se.

CLINICAL FEATURES

Signs and Symptoms

Most of the symptoms of pseudohypoparathyroidism reflect increased neuromuscular irritability resulting from the abnormally low concentration of calcium in the blood and extracellular fluid. It has been established that it is the ionized fraction, constituting about 50 percent of the blood calcium (the remainder being bound to plasma proteins or present as chelates), that is the controlling factor in neuromuscular irritability and the numerous other biological functions in which calcium ion plays an important role [1]. It has been difficult to make precise correlations between the severity of symptoms and the degree of hypocalcemia in patients with pseudohypoparathyroidism. This difficulty may reflect the fact that most methods for the estimation of serum calcium provide only the total concentration of calcium, both ionized and protein bound.

The average age of onset of symptoms is about 8 years [33, 34]. Symptoms include tetany, convulsions, muscle cramps, and seizures. Episodes of laryngeal spasm are reported. Poor vision may occur as a result of cataracts.

Signs of the disease detected on physical and laboratory examination are referable either to the hypoparathyroidism or to the associated skeletal and developmental defects. Hypocalcemia and hyperphosphatemia are present in untreated pseudohypoparathyroidism as in hypoparathyroidism of any cause. Alkaline phosphatase is usually normal except for the small number of patients discussed above in whom there is evidence of osteitis fibrosa. A complication, particularly of the hyperphosphatemia, is the frequent occurrence of soft tissue calcifications. In pseudohypoparathyroidism the mineral deposits in ectopic sites may include the development of true bone. True bone formation in ectopic sites is never seen in idiopathic hypoparathyroidism [1]. Amorphous deposits of calcium and phosphate are also found in subcutaneous tissue and particularly in the basal ganglia. Calcification of the basal ganglia is noted in as many as 50 percent of the patients. The original patient reported with pseudopseudohypoparathyroidism had extensive ectopic calcification in spite of normal blood calcium and phosphate concentrations [35]. Most patients with pseudopseudohypoparathyroidism do not have ectopic calcium deposits.

The multiple skeletal and developmental abnormalities that are found in both pseudohypoparathyroidism and pseudopseudohypoparathyroidism include short stature, round face, short neck, thick, stocky body build and multiple discrete abnormalities in individual bones of the skeleton (Fig. 52-3) [1, 33, 34]. The latter abnormalities include shortness of the metacarpal and metatarsal bones and sometimes the phalanges. These defects seem to be due to premature closure of the epiphyses (Fig. 52-4). The most classic finding is an abnormally short fourth and fifth metacarpal or metatarsal. This defect may be unilateral. When only one digit is involved it is invariably the fourth; the least frequently involved is the second. When the hand is closed the knuckles on the affected fingers are replaced by dimples (Fig. 52-4). Exostoses are frequently reported. Usually there are only one or two detected, but occasionally multiple exostoses are found. Radius curvus may be present in some patients. There may be only a mild curvature or there may be extreme bowing with displacement of the epiphysis [36].

Although as mentioned elsewhere, a few patients with the syndrome that may not be genetically related to pseudohypoparathyroidism have shown evidence of osteitis fibrosa, the usual picture on x-ray examination in pseudohypoparathyroidism is a normal or even increased density, particularly in the skull [33, 34]. The calvarium may be thickened. In addition, multiple abnormalities are detected in tooth for-

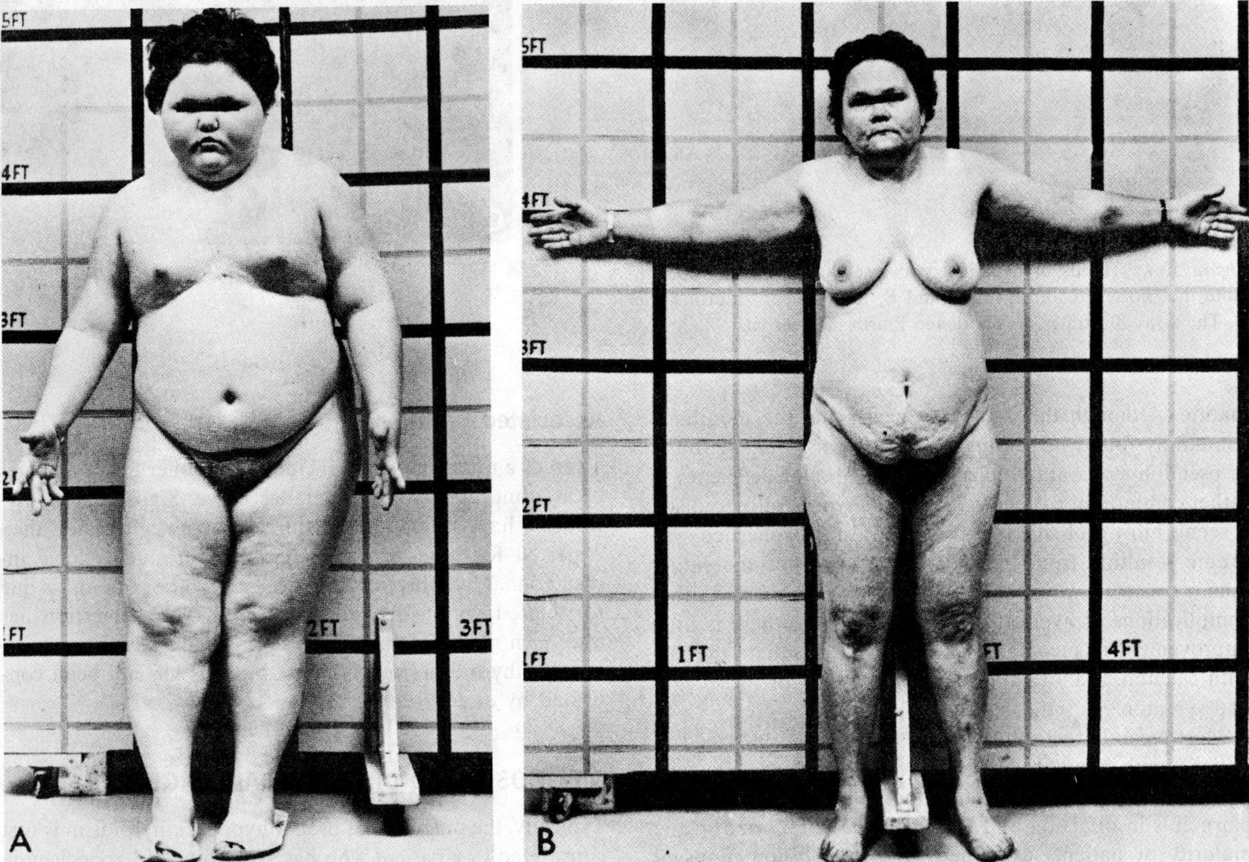

Figure 52-3. A. A young girl with pseudohypoparathyroidism. B. Her mother with pseudopseudohypoparathyroidism. Both exhibit short stature, obesity, rounded faces, and shortened metacarpals. Only the girl had the chemical abnormalities of hypoparathyroidism.

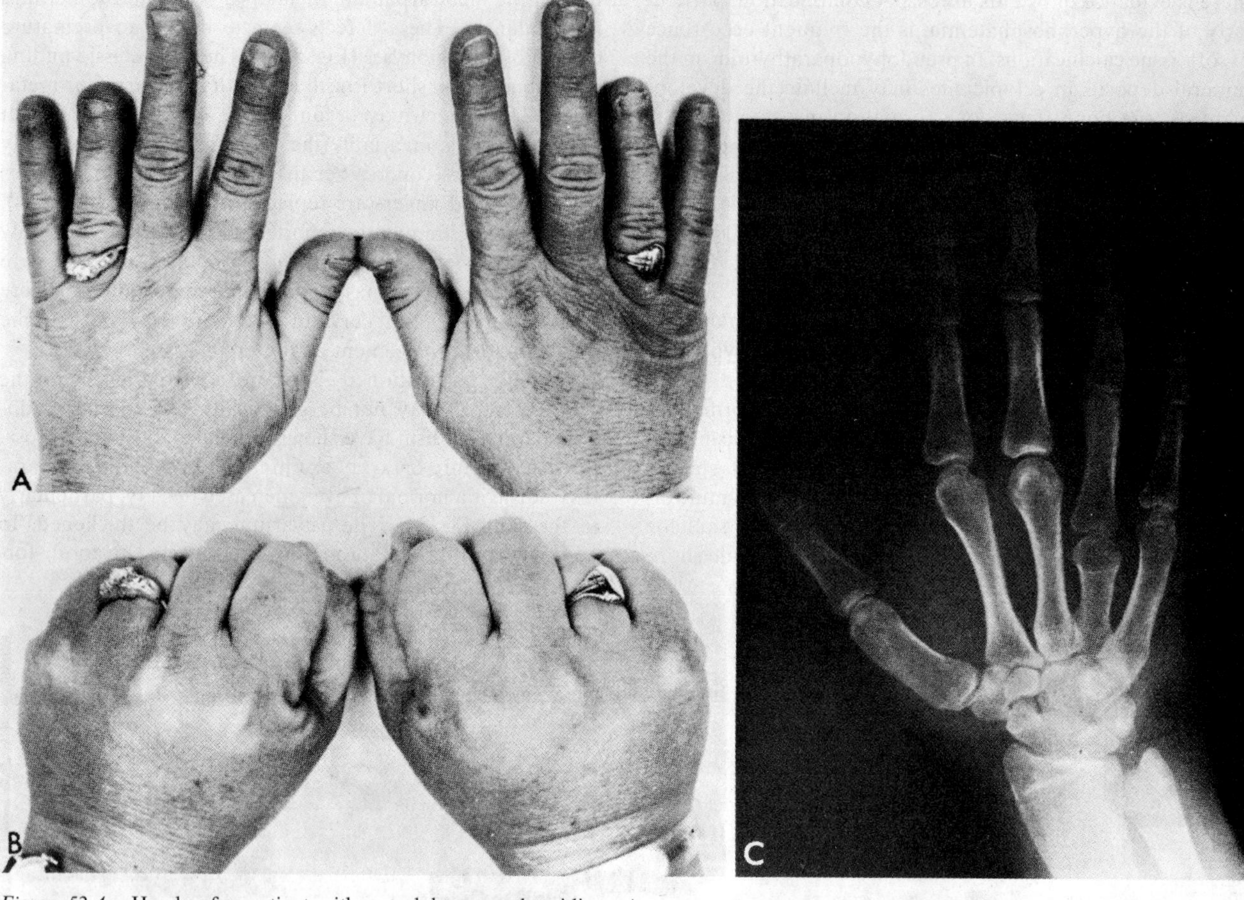

Figure 52-4. Hands of a patient with pseudohypoparathyroidism. A. Note the shortened fourth finger and B. the "absent" fourth knuckle. C. The x-ray illustrates the shortened fourth metacarpal.

mation. Although the nails may be fragile, the moniliasis commonly found in true hypoparathyroidism is not found in pseudohypoparathyroidism [33, 34]. Mental deficiency is rather common in patients with pseudohypoparathyroidism. It seems most probable that this is part of the inherited syndrome resulting from the deficient X chromosome rather than a consequence of basal ganglia calcification and other complications of hypocalcemia. In any event, there is little improvement in mental status even with adequate therapy with calcium and vitamin D. The frequency of these signs and symptoms is indicated in Table 52-1 [33, 34].

Most recently two other features have been described in patients with pseudohypoparathyroidism that appear to be part of the abnormal genetic inheritance. Distinctive impairments in olfaction and taste have been reported in the majority of patients examined [37]. In addition, unusual dermatoglyphic abnormalities have been detected by Forbes, including features such as frequent hypothenar patterns and distally located triradii [38].

Associated Features

There is a much increased incidence of either frank diabetes or an abnormal glucose tolerance curve. Signs of hypothyroidism have been noted with a frequency greater than expected for random occurrence. Recent studies have indicated that hypothyroidism, at least in some patients, is due to isolated thyrotropin deficiency [39]. The suggestion has also been made that in some patients there may be a resistance to thyroid hormone action, but this has not been confirmed by direct study.

DIAGNOSIS AND DIFFERENTIAL DIAGNOSIS

Typically, the diagnosis of pseudohypoparathyroidism is first considered in a patient who has symptoms of hypocalcemia and is found to have both hypocalcemia and hyperphosphatemia in the presence of normal renal function. Clinically, pseudohypoparathyroidism is more likely than true

Table 52-1. INCIDENCE OF SIGNS AND SYMPTOMS IN PSEUDOHYPOPARATHYROIDISM

	Percent
Signs	
Hypocalcemia	100
Soft tissue calcifications	
Subcutaneous	60
Cataracts	35
Basal ganglia	50
Skeletal abnormalities	
Increased density	15
Decreased density	15
Thickened calvarian	20
Developmental abnormalities	
Round face, short neck	75
Thick-set, stocky body build	50
Brachydactyly	
Metacarpals	70
Metatarsals	40
Symptoms	
Tetany	65
Convulsions	65
Muscle cramps	40
Laryngeal spasm	10
Parasthesias	10
Mental and personality changes	10
Parkinsonism	10

hypoparathyroidism if the unusual skeletal and developmental defects are detected or if there is a family history of other sibs with short stature and skeletal anomalies. A definitive diagnosis of pseudohypoparathyroidism must be established through application of specific laboratory tests. Previously these tests have centered around the demonstration of a lack of response to the administered parathyroid hormone (lack of phosphaturia or elevation of blood calcium), thus establishing end-organ resistance rather than deficiency of parathyroid hormone.

There have been many difficulties in performance and interpretation of these indirect tests of parathyroid hormone responsiveness in these patients. It is fortunate, therefore, that the development of newer test procedures offers great promise of providing a definitive diagnosis. Two principal tests should be employed, namely, the parathyroid hormone radioimmunoassay, and measurement of urinary cyclic AMP excretion following the administration of parathyroid hormone. Although not yet established, even in many referral centers, these tests are being performed by a sufficient number of investigators for access to the procedures to be now possible.

Diagnosis

Patients with symptomatic hypocalcemia, particularly if the history and physical examination suggest chronicity of the hypocalcemia (such as gradual onset of symptoms and evidence of ectopic calcification), would be expected to have secondary hyperparathyroidism if the parathyroid glands are functional. If no parathyroid hormone is detected by radioimmunoassay, notwithstanding the stimulus of marked hypocalcemia, then true hypoparathyroidism is the most likely diagnosis; if elevated concentrations of parathyroid hormone are found, then hypoparathyroidism on the basis of end-organ resistance is more likely [1]. If high circulating concentrations of hormone are found, the renal end-organ resistance to the parathyroid hormone can be demonstrated by measuring the urinary excretion of 3′,5′ cyclic AMP in response to the injection of a standard dose of parathyroid hormone. Typical responses in normal subjects, patients with idiopathic or postsurgical hypoparathyroidism, pseudohypoparathyroidism, and pseudopseudohypoparathyroidism are shown in Fig. 52-5. Chase, et al. found that there was a ten- to twentyfold increase in urinary cyclic AMP excretion in all groups, except those with pseudohypoparathyroidism, in whom very little, if any, response was noted [7].

As presently described, the latter test is performed over a several day period on hospitalized patients. All urine is collected at hourly intervals from 8:00 A.M. until noon on the control and test day. On the test day 300 U.S.P units of purified parathyroid hormone are infused at 9:00 A.M. over a 15-min period [7]. Urine is collected in two one-half hour aliquots between 9:00 and 10:00 A.M. The rise in cyclic AMP is usually maximal in the 30 min specimen. Results, expressed either as nanamoles of cyclic AMP per milligram of creatinine or as nanamoles per minute, normally show a ten- to twentyfold rise over basal values in either the 30- or 60-min urine collection after infusion except in those patients with pseudohypoparathyroidism. (In their initial studies Chase et al. [7] controlled the possibility that failure to detect an increased urinary excretion of 3′,5′ cyclic AMP in pseudohypoparathyroidism was due to excessive concentrations of endogenous hormone that interfered with normal responsiveness. Infusions of calcium, which suppressed endogenous parathyroid hormone as measured by radioimmunoassay, did not restore normal renal responsiveness after a second administration of parathyroid hormone. In addition, the patient discussed above, in whom all four parathyroid glands had been removed, also had a deficient response in urinary 3′,5′ cyclic AMP after the administration of parathyroid hormone.)

Prior to the availability of these newer techniques, the principal test for the evaluation of responsiveness to parathyroid hormone was the Ellsworth-Howard test. In this test measurements [36] of urinary phosphorus excretion are made following the administration of the hormone. Fasting patients have urine collected for a 3-hr period for measurement of phosphorus content. Then, 200 units of parathyroid hormone are given intravenously and urinary and serum phosphorus are measured for an additional period of 3 hr. In normal subjects there is usually an increase in urinary phos-

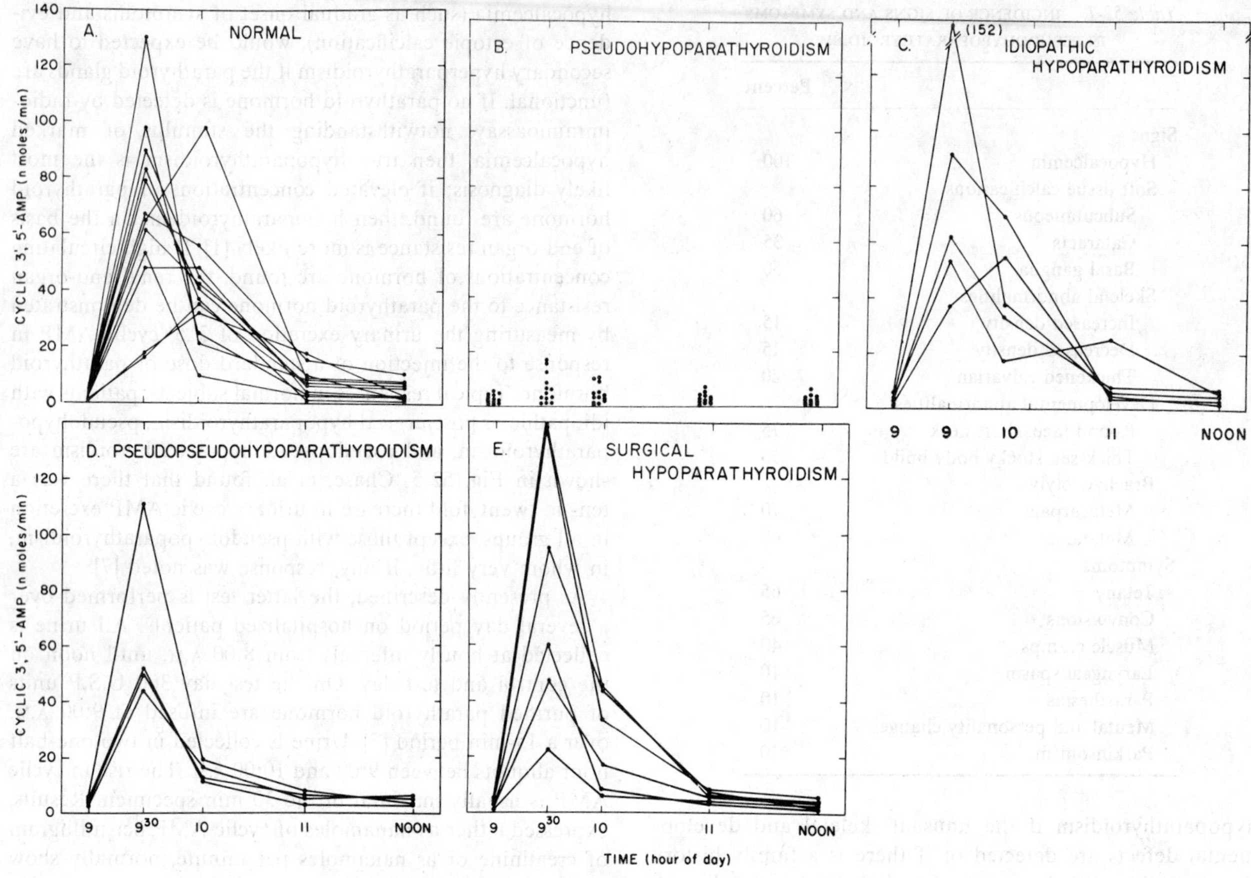

Figure 52-5. Cyclic AMP excretion in urine in response to the injection of parathyroid hormone (300 U.S.P units of parathyroid hormone given at 9 A.M.)

phorus of two to four times control values, and the serum phosphorus may fall as much as 1 mg per 100 ml [36]. Patients with hypoparathyroidism are more sensitive to the effects of administered hormone and they may show an increase in urinary phosphorus of 5 to 10 times the control value and a serum phosphorus fall of 1 to 2 mg per 100 ml. In patients with pseudohypoparathyroidism urinary phosphorus shows no change or less than a twofold rise. Unfortunately, there have been serious difficulties with these tests, including the difficulty of assessing the potency of the commercially available parathyroid hormone and the highly variable phosphaturic response even in normal subjects. The problems with these procedures have been reviewed by Bartter [36]. Aurbach et al. [40], have recently reemphasized the variable or misleading results that come from measurements of phosphate clearance in contrast to the clear-cut separation of patients with pseudohypoparathyroidism from normal subjects by the use of cyclic AMP measurements.

Another approach to a demonstration of parathyroid hormone unresponsiveness has been the administration of several hundred units of parathyroid extract daily for a week or more. Only a few patients with pseudohypoparathyroidism have been tested in this manner and there is not much experience with the response to such a test procedure in normal subjects. Even so, the lack of any rise in serum calcium in spite of the administration of parathormone for 7 to 10 days has occasionally been useful as a further indication of parathyroid hormone unresponsiveness.

Differential Diagnosis

The differential diagnosis of pseudohypoparathyroidism involves two principal categories of illness: (1) other causes of hypocalcemia, and (2) other unusual syndromes featuring skeletal and developmental anomalies that may simulate many of the constitutional features of pseudohypoparathyroidism.

Hypocalcemia may be encountered in true hypoparathyroidism (of which there are several variants), malabsorption, osteomalacia secondary to true vitamin D lack or vitamin D resistance, renal failure, hypoproteinemia, pancreatitis, and acute nutritional deficiency with associated hypomagnesemia [1]. Hypoparathyroidism in former years was most frequently the result of extensive thyroid surgery during which the parathyroids were inadvertently removed. A history of previous thyroid surgery, a lack of skeletal and developmental defects of the type commonly seen in pseudohypoparathyroidism, and, most definitively, lack of detectable circulating parathyroid hormone in conjunction with severe hypocalcemia are useful criteria for distinguishing postsurgical hypoparathyroidism from pseudohypoparathyroidism.

Idiopathic hypoparathyroidism is a relatively rare disease. A total lack of parathyroid function can be detected (1) as an isolated entity, idiopathic hypoparathyroidism; (2) in association with agenesis of the thymus (the DiGeorge syndrome) [41, 42], or (3) in association with a familial disorder in which there may be a deficiency of thyroid and adrenal function, pernicious anemia, and other defects [43]. In the last patients autoimmune mechanisms seem important, because in some patients antibodies have been detected that are directed against the various endocrine organs or the parietal cells of the stomach [43]. In any of these patients with a variant of parathyroid failure, the steps in the establishment of the correct diagnosis should include the clinical findings (together with the absence of the skeletal and developmental defects associated with pseudohypoparathyroidism), failure to detect parathyroid hormone by radioimmunoassay, and finally, if necessary, a demonstration of a normal rise in urinary cyclic AMP excretion after the administration of parathyroid hormone.

The DiGeorge syndrome is a rare disorder in which there is congenital absence of the thymus and the parathyroids, organs embryologically derived from the third and fourth branchial pouches [41, 42]. Patients with this syndrome usually die at 1 to 2 years of age of severe hypocalcemia or persistent infection, or both. The immune deficiency is of the fixed cellular type. Delayed hypersensitivity reactions are deficient and allograft rejections are absent. Humoral and circulating antibody mechanisms are intact [41, 42]. These striking features that result from the absence of the thymus make this unusual syndrome quite distinctive. There has been one attempt at parathyroid transplant. Although in theory this might have achieved a successful cure of the hypoparathyroidism, the transplant did not survive. A later thymic transplant was successful [41].

The familial syndrome of hypoparathyroidism is most unusual in several respects. Although an autoimmune basis for this disease has been suspected, it is often not possible to demonstrate antibodies against parathyroid, adrenal, thyroid, or stomach tissue [43]. These patients frequently have moniliasis, particularly in the fingernails. Recognition of the associated features is important because of the clinical problems encountered when adrenal failure or anemia develops. Careful and periodic evaluation of hematopoietic, adrenal, and thyroid status is important. In addition, other members of the kindreds should be carefully observed for the development of signs of hypoparathyroidism.

In patients with malabsorption, true vitamin D lack, vitamin D resistance, or renal failure, tests by the parathyroid radioimmunoassay have invariably shown an increased concentration of hormone in the plasma. Secondary hyperparathyroidism apparently results from the chronic hypocalcemia that accompanies these diseases [1]. The manifestations of renal failure, including phosphate retention, are usually obvious when hypocalcemia is found. Patients with osteomalacia usually show a low serum phosphorus, an apparent reflection of the persistence of the action of parathyroid hormone on renal phosphate excretion in spite of the deficiency of the vitamin D that interferes with the effective action of the hormone on bone.

Hypoproteinemia causes a reduction in total serum calcium because of the deficient binding of calcium. Subjects with this abnormality have a normal ionized serum calcium concentration and lack symptoms of hypocalcemia. Simple correction for the total calcium concentration based on the known binding of calcium by albumin and globulin can be made. Episodes of acute pancreatitis are associated with marked hypocalcemia, but this is present only during the acute phase of the illness. The explanation for this hypocalcemia, although much discussed, remains unknown [1].

There is an increasingly frequent recognition of the syndrome of hypocalcemia in patients with a recent history of a poor nutritional intake and hypomagnesemia. Estep et al. [44] have studied a group of alcoholics with severe hypomagnesemia. Hypocalcemia and refractoriness to exogenous parathyroid hormone were found, including a lack of the normal urinary cyclic AMP response. Other alcoholics with an apparently similar nutritional history who were not hypomagnesemic were normocalcemic and responsive to hormone. Parenteral correction of the hypomagnesemia over several days completely restored normal parathyroid responsiveness, including the urinary cyclic AMP response. It has been observed subsequently in similar patients that with a normal dietary intake in the hospital, serum magnesium rises with the improved diet and the hypocalcemia disappears within a week without specific treatment. Recognition of this syndrome is important in order to avoid an unnecessary diagnostic evaluation of these patients for some unusual cause of parathyroid failure. The implication is that it will also be important to measure serum magnesium levels in any patient suspected of pseudohypoparathyroidism prior to tests for parathyroid hormone responsiveness. Clinical observations in this group of patients have confirmed the long held suspicion that hypomagnesemia results in a blockade of parathyroid hormone action. It has been observed that magnesium may simulate calcium in its effects on parathyroid hormone secretion, i.e., hypomagnesemia leads to increased parathyroid secretion [45]. Severe hypomagnesemia, on the other hand, inhibits parathyroid hormone release from glands in vitro [45]. Correlations between parathyroid hormone concentrations and hypocalcemia in the hypomagnesemic syndromes prior to and after magnesium treatment would be important but have not yet been reported.

Patients with a variety of unusual skeletal and developmental defects, including the basal cell nevus syndrome [46–48], familial calcification of the cerebral basal ganglia [49–51], Gardner's syndrome [52, 53], vitamin D–resistant osteomalacia [1], and Turner's syndrome share certain features observed in pseudohypoparathyroidism. There have also been occasional reports that these patients are unresponsive to parathyroid hormone [52]. These findings have led some to suspect that these diseases are related to pseudohypoparathyroidism. All tests showing parathyroid responsiveness in these circumstances have been indirect, and most of these patients have not been reported to have any abnormalities in calcium and phosphorus metabolism. Because of the great interest in the genetics of these disorders, it is important to know whether any of these disease states is related to pseudohypoparathyroidism. Studies by Aurbach and associates [40] have established that these patients have a normal excretion of 3′,5′ cyclic AMP following the administration of parathyroid hormone. Only two patients with Turner's syndrome were tested. Also it was observed that patients with Gardner's syndrome, vitamin D–resistant rickets, and the basal ganglia calcification syndrome had higher baseline rates of excretion of cyclic AMP than normal subjects [40]. This has also been observed in primary hyperparathyroidism and in biochemically normal subjects with pseudopseudohypoparathyroidism. Although further study of these unusual syndromes will undoubtedly be required in order to understand fully many features of these diseases, it does not appear that they are genetically or biochemically related to true pseudohypoparathyroidism.

TREATMENT

Neuromuscular symptoms in pseudohypoparathyroidism can usually be controlled by restoring the blood calcium concentration toward normal with supplementary dietary calcium and vitamin D. The lenticular opacities may progress in spite of therapy [54]. The blood calcium concentration in hypoparathyroidism cannot be maintained without some preparation of vitamin D. The beneficial effects depend not only on enhanced efficiency of gastrointestinal absorption of calcium but also on increased resorption of bone (a direct action of the vitamin).

Unfortunately, vitamin D intoxication may develop without any apparent change in a dosage of vitamin D that has been optimal for several years. If hypercalcemia occurs, the long duration of the action of vitamin D may result in persistence of hypercalcemia for weeks or months after the vitamin D has been discontinued [1, 55]. Fortunately, vitamin D intoxication seems much less common in pseudohypoparathyroidism than in post-surgical or idiopathic hypoparathyroidism.

Recent developments in the pharmacology and biochemistry of vitamin D provide promise that the long-term management of patients with hypoparathyroidism may be considerably refined, if necessary, by newer forms of therapy [1]. Harrison et al. [55] have reinvestigated the relative pharmacological properties of dihydrotachysterol and vitamin D. Dihydrotachysterol is relatively more potent and more closely approximates the actions of parathyroid hormone in parathyroid-deficient animals or hypoparathyroid human subjects than either vitamin D_2 or D_3. It is essential to use pure crystalline dihydrotachysterol. Earlier commercial preparations contained multiple forms of the irradiated vitamin [1]. (The historical differences between AT-10, Hytakerol, and dihydrotachysterol are of interest in view of the older experience with AT-10 [1].)

Further improvements in the pharmacology of vitamin D are likely to result from the recent investigations of DeLuca and his associates of the biological properties of compounds such as 25-hydroxycholecalciferol, the apparent biologically active metabolite of vitamin D [56]. The 25-hydroxylated compounds may have more desirable properties with respect to duration and spectrum of action than vitamin D_2 or D_3. Less difficulty is encountered in the management of pseudohypoparathyroidism than true hypoparathyroidism, since only the latter patients have the additional problem of excessive urinary calcium excretion [31].

With the recognition of these several considerations, practical therapeutic programs can be recommended. Vitamin D is given, usually as ergocalciferol (D_2) at a dose of 50,000 to 100,000 units per day. Several grams of additional calcium as lactate or gluconate can be added as well but are often not required. Appropriate adjustments in dosage are made to achieve a blood calcium of 8.5 to 9.5 mg per 100 ml. It is important to appreciate that often weeks are required before the full effects of an increased dose of vitamin D are achieved. Patients should be seen at frequent intervals, particularly when dose schedules are initially established or readjusted. Blood and urine calcium estimations provide the early clues to excessive or inadequate dosages of vitamin D.

GENETICS

The hereditary aspects of pseudohypoparathyroidism have been well established [1, 34]. Pseudohypoparathyroidism is usually found within kindreds in which some other family members also have pseudohypoparathyroidism or the metabolically normal variant of the disorder, pseudopseudohypoparathyroidism. The variable expression of metabolic abnormalities in affected individuals is not understood.

In a detailed review of the hereditary aspects of pseudohypoparathyroidism made in 1962, Mann et al. [57] analyzed the incidence of the disorder in a total of 22 families. Sixty-nine cases of pseudohypoparathyroidism and thirty-eight cases of pseudopseudohypoparathyroidism were identified, mostly from published records, and accepted as clinically proven. It was concluded that the two disorders, pseudohypoparathyroidism and pseudopseudohypoparathyroidism, were genetically linked and were transmitted as sex-linked dominants. In support of this contention it was found that the sex incidence of affected females to males was 2 to 1. At present this view that pseudohypoparathyroidism is inherited as a sex-linked dominant cannot be unequivocally accepted. The disease is extremely rare, so that the total number of patients or of involved sibships is small for statistical analysis. Furthermore, acceptance of cases as authentic examples of the syndrome on the basis of literature reports is difficult, particularly with respect to the metabolically normal individuals, i.e., those with pseudopseudohypoparathyroidism. Certain of the developmental defects, such as short stature, short metacarpal or metatarsal bones, or even basal ganglia calcification are found in Turner's syndrome [58], Gardner's syndrome, basal cell nevus syndrome, or other hereditary disorders. These disorders are believed to be genetically distinct, since some of them are associated with chromosomal defects or appear to be autosomal dominant traits. These disorders also seem distinct from pseudohypoparathyroidism since they have apparently normal renal adenyl cyclase responses [40]. Hence, the finding of skeletal or developmental defects per se cannot be used as an absolute indication of pseudopseudohypoparathyroidism. Further, difficulties have been encountered even in interpretation of the diagnosis of pseudohypoparathyroidism. Most of the earlier reports used in analyses of hereditary patterns were based only on indirect tests of parathyroid function. These considerations about difficulties in interpreting published case reports help to explain the uncertainty about proposed genetic mechanisms. For example, four cases of apparent male-to-male transmission are recorded [57]. This mode of inheritance does not fit in with sex-linked dominance.

The possibility has not been excluded that the X chromosome is structurally deficient. In addition, even if the concept of simple sex-linked dominant inheritance is accepted, it is difficult to explain the occurrence of developmental defects in pseudopseudohypoparathyroidism without coexistent abnormality in renal adenyl cyclase responses or calcium or phosphate metabolism, if the genetic defect is identical in pseudohypoparathyroidism and pseudopseudohypoparathyroidism.

Aurbach [59] has proposed that this discrepancy might be explained, in females at least, by the Lyon hypothesis, i.e., one or the other of the X chromosomes might be inactivated to a relatively greater extent. Thus, if the abnormal X chromosome is inactivated the adenyl cyclase enzyme system would be competent, and pseudopseudohypoparathyroidism would be the result in the affected individual. If, on the other hand, the normal X chromosome is inactivated, then the adenyl cyclase system would be deficient and pseudohypoparathyroidism would be the clinical result. This explanation could not account for the occurrence of pseudopseudohypoparathyroidism in the male. Furthermore, the hypothesis would require that it be the normal X chromosome which is randomly inactivated in almost all cells in bone and particularly in kidney, since tests of adenyl cyclase response in kidney have revealed an almost total deficiency. Finally, it is not consistent with the concept of random inactivation of the X chromosome.

It is apparent that many aspects of the genetics remain unresolved. Two concepts may serve as useful models for further detailed clinical and biochemical study. These are (1) that the disorder is a sex-linked dominant (which serves to focus on deficiencies in the X chromosome system), and (2) that the variable expression of the disease might be explained in part by the Lyon hypothesis. It will be important to reevaluate hereditary patterns when patients have been studied by specific criteria such as urinary cyclic AMP responses after hormone administration. Detailed study of X-chromosome morphology might be revealing. Finally, observations of bone and kidney cells in vitro, particularly in tissue culture, might enable testing of the interesting hypothesis that the expression of the biochemical disorder is related to the suppression of the normal or the abnormal X chromosome.

SUMMARY

1 Pseudohypoparathyroidism is an inherited disorder characterized by skeletal and developmental defects, and signs and symptoms of hypoparathyroidism, the latter due to a deficient end-organ response to endogenous parathyroid hormone.

2 The disturbances in calcium and phosphate metabolism and in parathyroid function that are observed in these patients are attributable to partial or complete unresponsiveness of the receptors to parathyroid hormone in both bone and kidney. There is a failure of the receptors to respond to parathyroid hormone with a normal stimulation of membrane-bound adenyl cyclase. This deficient end-organ response results in deficiencies in calcium and phosphate transport. This in turn leads to secondary hyperparathyroidism; the concentration of parathyroid hormone in blood is increased in these patients.

3 Precise laboratory diagnosis can now be established in these patients by the demonstration of a failure of parathyroid hormone to cause the normal rise in cyclic AMP in urine. Little or no 3′,5′ cyclic adenosine monophosphate appears in the urine after the administration of parathyroid hormone to subjects with pseudohypoparathyroidism, whereas there is a ten- to twentyfold increase in normal subjects or those with true hypoparathyroidism. This test serves to differentiate pseudohypoparathyroidism from the apparently clinically related syndromes.

4 The neuromuscular symptoms of pseudohypoparathyroidism can usually be controlled by the judicious use of large doses of vitamin D. The occasional development of vitamin D intoxication requires careful control of medication in these patients.

5 Pseudohypoparathyroidism is clearly a hereditary disorder. Some individuals in affected sibships exhibit the skeletal and developmental defects without hypoparathyroidism; the latter defect is termed pseudopseudohypoparathyroidism. Analysis of such kindreds suggests that pseudohypoparathyroidism is inherited as a sex-linked dominant trait. Difficulties in definitive genetic analysis are encountered, however, due to the rarity of the disorder and the diagnostic difficulties encountered in the analysis of patients with pseudopseudohypoparathyroidism and other unusual syndromes that resemble pseudohypoparathyroidism.

BIBLIOGRAPHY

1. Potts, J. T., Jr., and Deftos, L. J.: Parathyroid hormone, thyrocalcitonin, vitamin D, bone and mineral metabolism, in *Duncan's Diseases of Metabolism,* edited by P. K. Bondy, 6th ed., p. 904. Saunders, Philadelphia, 1969.

1*a*. Albright, F., Burnett, C. H., Smith, P. H., and Parson, W.: Pseudohypoparathyroidism—an example of the "Seabright-Bantam syndrome." Endocrinology, **30,** 922, 1942.

2. Krane, S. M.: Selected features of the clinical course of hypoparathyroidism. JAMA. **178,** 472, 1961.

3. Se Mo Suh, Fraser, D., and Sang Whay Kooh: Pseudohypoparathyroidism: Responsiveness to parathyroid extract induced by vitamin D_2 therapy. J. Clin. Endocr., **30,** 609, 1970.

4. Tashjian, A. H., Jr., Frantz, A. G., and Lee, J. B.: Pseudohypoparathyroidism: Assays of parathyroid hormone and thyrocalcitonin. Proc. Nat. Acad. Sci. USA, **56,** 1138, 1966.

5. Melick, R. A., Gill, J. R., Berson, S. A., Yallow, R. S., Bartter, F. C., Potts, J. T., Jr., and Aurbach, G. D.: Antibodies and clinical resistance to parathyroid hormone. New Eng. J. Med., **276,** 144, 1967.

6. Gudmundsson, T. V., Galante, L., Horton, R., Matthews, E. W., Woodhouse, N. J. Y., and MacIntyre, I.: Human plasma calcitonin, in *Calcitonin, 1969,* p. 102. Proc. Second Internat. Symp., Heinemann, London, 1969.

7. Chase, L. R., Melson, G. L., and Aurbach, G. D.: Pseudohypoparathyroidism: Defective excretion of 3′,5′-AMP in response to parathyroid hormone. J. Clin. Invest., **48,** 1832, 1969.

8. Aurbach, G. D., and Houston, B. A.: Determination of 3′,5′-adenosine monophosphate with a method based on a radioactive phosphate exchange reaction. J. Biol. Chem., **22,** 5935, 1968.

9. Chase, L. R., and Aurbach, G. D.: Cyclic AMP and the mechanism of action of parathyroid hormone. *Proc. Third Parathyroid Conf., Parathyroid Hormone and Thyrocalcitonin* (*Calcitonin*). Excerpta Medica, October, 1967.

10. Melson, G. L., Chase, L. R., and Aurbach, G. D.: Parathyroid hormone-sensitive adenyl cyclase in isolated renal tubules. Endocrinology, **86,** 511, 1970.

11. Marcus, R., and Aurbach, G. D.: Bioassay of parathyroid hormone *in vitro* with a stable preparation of adenyl cyclase from rat kidney. Endocrinology, **85,** 801, 1969.

12. Chase, L. R., Fedak, S. A., and Aurbach, G. D.: Activation of skeletal adenyl cyclase by parathyroid hormone *in vitro.* Endocrinology, **84,** 761, 1969.

13. Chase, L. R., and Aurbach, G. D.: Parathyroid function and the renal excretion of 3′,5′-adenylic acid. Proc. Nat. Acad. Sci., USA, **58,** 518, 1967.

14. Chase, L. R., and Aurbach, G. D.: Renal adenyl cyclase: Anatomically separate sites for parathyroid hormone and vasopressin. Science, **159,** 545, 1968.

15. Chase, L. R., and Aurbach, G. D.: The effect of parathyroid hormone on the concentration of adenosine 3′,5′-monophosphate in skeletal tissue *in vitro.* J. Biol. Chem., **245,** 1520, 1970.

16. Nordin, B. E. C., and Peacock, M.: Role of kidney in regulation of plasma-calcium. Lancet, **2,** 1280, 1969.

17. Parsons, J. A., and Robinson, C. J.: A rapid indirect hypercalcemic action of parathyroid hormone demonstrated in isolated blood-perfused bone. Lancet, **2,** 329, 1969.

18. Wells, H., and Lloyd, W.: Hypercalcemic action of dibutyryl cyclic 3′,5′-adenosine monophosphate in rats after parathyroidectomy. Fed. Proc., **27,** 354, 1968.

19. Rasmussen, H., Pechet, M., and Fast, D.: Effect of dibutyryl cyclic adenosine 3′,5′-monophosphate, theophylline, and other nucleotides upon calcium and phosphate metabolism. J. Clin. Invest., **47,** 1843, 1968.

20. Walsh, D. A., Perkins, J. P., and Krebs, E. G.: An adenosine 3′,5′ monophosphate-dependent protein kinase from rabbit skeletal muscle. J. Biol. Chem., **243,** 3763, 1968.

21. Tenenhouse, A., Rasmussen, H., and Nagata, N.: Parathyroid hormone, 3′,5′-AMP and Ca^{++} in *Calcitonin, 1969,* p. 102. Proc. Second Internat. Symp., Heinemann, London, 1969.

22. Potts, J. T., Jr., Deftos, L. J., Buckle, R. M., Sherwood, L. M., and Aurbach, G. D.: Radioimmunoassay of parathyroid hormone: Studies of the control of secretion of the hormone and parathyroid function in clinical disorders, in *Radioisotopes in Medicine: In Vitro Studies* edited by R. L. Hayes, F. A. Goswitz, and B. E. P. Murphy, p. 207. U.S. Atomic Energy Commission, Oak Ridge, Tennessee, 1968.

23. Elrick, H., Albright, F., Bartter, F. C., Forbes, A. P., and Reeves, J.: Further studies on pseudo-hypoparathyroidism: Report of four new cases. Acta Endocr. (Copenhagen), **5,** 199, 1950.

24. Bell, N. H., Gerard, E. S., and Bartter, F. C.: Pseudohypoparathyroidism with osteitis fibrosa cystica and impaired absorption of calcium. J. Clin. Endocr., **23,** 759, 1963.

25. Kolb, F. O., and Steinbach, H. L.: Pseudohypoparathyroidism with secondary hyperparathyroidism and osteitis fibrosa. J. Clin. Endocr. **22,** 59, 1962.

26. Zampa, G. A., and Zucchelli, P. C.: Pseudohypoparathyroidism and bone demineralization: Case report and metabolic studies. J. Clin. Endocr., **25,** 1616, 1965.

27. Allen, E. H., Millard, F. J. C., and Nassim, J. R.: Hypo-hyperparathyroidism. Arch. Dis. Child., **43,** 295, 1968.

28. Singleton, E. B., and Teng, C. T.: Pseudohypoparathyroidism with bone changes simulating hyperparathyroidism (report of a case). Radiology, **78,** 388, 1962.

29. Costello, J. M., and Dent, C. E.: Hypo-hyperparathyroidism. Arch. Dis. Child., **38,** 397, 1963.

30. Cohen, R. D., and Vince, F. P.: Pseudohypoparathyroidism with raised plasma alkaline phosphatase. Arch. Dis. Child., **44,** 96, 1969.

31. Litvak, J., Moldawer, M. P., Forbes, A. P., and Henneman, P. H.: Hypocalcemic hypercalciuria during vitamin D and dihydrotachysterol therapy of hypoparathyroidism. J. Clin. Endocr., **18,** 246, 1958.

32. Potts, J. T., Jr., Tregear, G. W., Keutmann, H. T., Niall, H. D., Sauer, R., Deftos, L. J., Dawson, B. F., Hogan, M. L., and Aurbach, G. D.: Synthesis of a biologically active N-terminal tetratriacontapeptide of parathyroid hormone. Proc. Nat. Acad. Sci. USA, **68,** 63, 1971.

33. Bronsky, D., Kushner, D. S., Dubin, A., and Snapper, I.: Idiopathic hypoparathyroidism and pseudohypoparathyroidism: Case reports and review of the literature. Medicine (Balt.), **37,** 317, 1958.

34. Aurbach, G. D., and Potts, J. T., Jr.: The parathyroids, in *Advances in Metabolic Disorders* edited by R. Levine and R. Luft, vol. 1, p. 45. Academic, New York, 1964.

35. Albright, F., Forbes, A. P., and Henneman, P. H.: Pseudopseudohypoparathyroidism. Trans. Ass. Amer. Physicians, **65,** 337, 1952.

36. Bartter, F. C.: Pseudohypoparathyroidism and pseudopseudohypoparathyroidism, in *The Metabolic Basis of Inherited Disease* edited by J. B. Stanbury, J. B. Wyngaarden, and D. S. Fredrickson, p. 1024. McGraw-Hill, New York, 1966.

37. Henkin, R. I.: Impairment of olfaction and of the tastes of sour and bitter in pseudohyperparathyroidism. J. Clin. Endocr., **28,** 624, 1968.

38. Forbes, A. P.: Fingerprints and palm prints (dermatoglyphics) and Palmer-flexion creases in gonadal dysgenesis, pseudohypoparathyroidism and Klinefelter's syndrome. New Eng. J. Med., **270,** 1268, 1964.

39. Winnacker, J. L., Becker, K. L., and Moore, C. F.: Pseudohypoparathyroidism and selective deficiency of thyrotropin: An interesting association. Metabolism, **16,** 644, 1967.

40. Aurbach, G. D., Marcus, R., Winickoff, R. N., Epstein, E. H., and Nigra, T. P.: Urinary excretion of 3′,5′-AMP in syndromes considered refractory to parathyroid hormone. Metabolism, **19**, 799, 1970.
41. Cleveland, W. W., Fogel, B. J., Brown, W. T., and Kay, H. E. M.: Foetal thymic transplant in a case of DiGeorge's syndrome. Lancet, **2**, 1211, 1968.
42. Kretschmer, R., Say, B., Brown, D., and Rosen, F. S.: Congenital aplasia of the thymus gland (DiGeorge's syndrome). New Eng. J. Med., **279**, 1295, 1968.
43. Blizzard, R. M., Chee, D., and Davis, W.: The incidence of parathyroid and other antibodies in the sera of patients with idiopathic hypoparathyroidism. Clin. Exp. Immun., **1**, 119, 1966.
44. Estep, H. L., Martinez, G. R., and Jones, D.: Parathyroid hormone (PTH) unresponsiveness and 3′,5′-AMP excretion. Abstract #145, Endocrine Society Meeting, 1969.
45. Sherwood, L. M., Herrman, I., and Bassett, C. A.: Parathyroid hormone secretion *in vitro*: Regulation by calcium and magnesium ions. Nature (London), **225**, 1056, 1970.
46. Block, J. B., and Clendenning, W. E.: Parathyroid hormone hyporesponsiveness in patients with basal-cell nevi and bone defects. New Eng. J. Med., **262**, 908, 1960.
47. Gorlin, R. J., and Goltz, R. W.: Multiple nevoid basal-cell epithelioma, jaw cysts and bifid rib: a syndrome. New Eng. J. Med. **262**, 908, 1960. Med., **262**, 908, 1960.
48. Clendenning, W. E., Block, J. B., and Radde, I. G.: Basal cell nevus syndrome. Arch. Derm. (Chicago), **90**, 38, 1964.
49. Roberts, P. D.: Familial calcification of the cerebral basal ganglia and its relation to hypoparathyroidism. Brain, **82**, 599, 1959.
50. Matthews, W. B.: Familial calcification of the basal ganglia with response to parathormone. J. Neurol. Neurosurg. Psychiat., **20**, 172, 1957.
51. Roberts, P. D.: Familial calcification of the cerebral basal ganglia and its relation to hypoparathyroidism. Brain, **82**, 599, 1959.
52. Trygstad, C. W., Zisman, E., Witkip, C. J., and Bartter, F. C.: Resistance to parathyroid extract in Gardner's syndrome. J. Clin. Endocr., **28**, 1153, 1968.
53. Gardner, E. J.: Follow-up study of a family group exhibiting dominant inheritance for a syndrome including intestinal polyps, osteomas, fibromas and epidermal cysts. Am. J. Hum. Genet., **14**, 376, 1962.
54. Dimich, A., Bedrossian, P. B., and Wallach, S.: Hypoparathyroidism. Arch. Intern. Med. (Chicago), **120**, 449, 1967.
55. Harrison, H. E., Lifshitz, F., and Blizzard, R. M.: Comparison between crystalline dihydrotachysterol and calciferol in patients requiring pharmacologic vitamin D therapy. New Eng. J. Med., **276**, 894, 1967.
56. DeLuca, H. F.: Recent advances in the metabolism and function of vitamin D. Fed. Proc., **28**, 1678, 1969.
57. Mann, J. B., Alterman, S., and Hills, A. G.: Albright's hereditary osteodystrophy comprising pseudohypoparathyroidism and pseudo-pseudohypoparathyroidism: With a report of two cases representing the complete syndrome occurring in successive generations. Ann. Intern. Med., **56**, 315, 1962.
58. Van der Werff ten Bosch, J. J.: The syndrome of brachymetacarpal dwarfism ("pseudo-pseudohypoparathyroidism"). Lancet, **1**, 69, 1959.
59. Aurbach, G. D.: Parathyroids, in *Cecil and Loeb Textbook in Medicine,* edited by Beeson and McDermott, 13th ed. Saunders, Philadelphia, (in press).
60. Niall, H. D., Keutmann, H. T., Sauer, R., Hogan, M. L., Dawson, B. F., Aurbach, G. D., and Potts, J. T., Jr.: Hoppe Seyler Physiol. Chem., December, 1970.
61. Brewer, H. B., Jr., and Ronan, R.: Bovine parathyroid hormone: Amino acid sequence. Proc. Nat. Acad. Sci. (USA), **67**, 1862, 1970.

PART TEN

DISEASES MANIFEST PRIMARILY IN THE BLOOD AND BLOOD-FORMING TISSUES

CHAPTER FIFTY-THREE

HEREDITARY SPHEROCYTOSIS

James H. Jandl and Richard A. Cooper

In hereditary spherocytosis a hemolytic process is associated with an intrinsic ("intracorpuscular") defect in the red blood cell. The cardinal features of this disease are (1) increased rate of red blood cell destruction, (2) spherocytosis, (3) splenomegaly, (4) familial occurrence, and (5) almost invariable benefit from splenectomy. Among the many synonyms for this hemolytic disease, the most common are congenital hemolytic anemia and congenital hemolytic jaundice.

Although not restricted to any single race, hereditary spherocytosis is most frequent in people of European origin. Among those of Northern European descent it is the most prevalent of the hereditary hemolytic disorders. This disease affects the sexes equally and often is manifest in early infancy [1, 2].

CLINICAL FEATURES

There are three major clinical manifestations: anemia, jaundice, and splenomegaly. The severity of the anemia varies from time to time and from patient to patient. In most otherwise healthy patients the anemia is only moderate or mild and often is inappreciable. Whether or not frank anemia exists, the chronic hemolysis usually causes some degree of acholuric jaundice, although this may be variable or intermittent and tends to be less pronounced in early childhood [2]. Gallstones of the pigment type are common, even in childhood [3], and presumably are precipitated from bile containing high concentrations of bilirubin. The spleen is usually palpable, but the liver is usually normal in size. Although less frequent than in sickle-cell anemia, chronic leg ulcers occasionally develop, particularly in adulthood. These are usually bilateral, just above the malleoli, and ordinarily disappear after splenectomy. A wide assortment of skeletal abnormalities has been described in patients with hereditary spherocytosis. Some of these are presumably caused by the expanding force of the hyperplastic erythroid bone marrow during the formative years. Other apparently congenital abnormalities of the skeleton and eye [4, 5] have been encountered sporadically in association with hereditary spherocytosis [1, 2] and may be fortuitous associations from inbreeding rather than the result of a true "hemolytic constitution" [4].

PATHOLOGY

As in other chronic hemolytic disorders, there is compensatory normoblastic hyperplasia of the bone marrow with extension of the red marrow into the midshafts of the long bones. Occasionally extramedullary erythropoiesis may appear, often with formation of paravertebral masses; these may be mistaken for neoplasms, particularly when visible on chest x-ray. The spleen as observed at operation is darkly congested with blood and usually weighs from 500 to 2,000 gm. A precise weight is often difficult to establish because of a continuing leakage of blood. On section of the spleen, the sinuses are often observed to be dilated and empty, whereas the pulp cords are congested with red blood cells. By histologic criteria there is true hyperplasia of the splenic components, especially the perifollicular reticulum cells [6, 7]. Foci of hemopoiesis are often found [8], but as in most chronic hemolytic disorders, these usually are not striking.

LABORATORY FINDINGS

The laboratory findings are those common to all chronic hemolytic processes: anemia, an increased concentration of reticulocytes, a slight to moderate rise in indirect-reacting (nonglucuronide) bilirubin in the serum, and an elevated fecal excretion of urobilinogen. There is little or no hemoglobin in the plasma. The hemoglobin released from destroyed red blood cells is catabolized to bilirubin at the site of destruction (so-called "extravascular" hemolysis).

The severity of the manifestations of the disease depends upon the balance between the rate of red blood cell destruction, which may range from slightly to greatly increased, and the rate of compensatory red blood cell production by the marrow. The erythropoietic response to anemia in this disease is unusually brisk. Accordingly, the anemia may be minimal in spite of moderately rapid rates of red blood cell destruction, and in approximately 10 percent of patients, particularly young men, hemoglobin levels are perfectly normal. Patients having little or no anemia but with disproportionately severe icterus and reticulocytosis are said to have a "compensated form" of hemolytic anemia [4]. On the other hand, the equilibrium between the rates of red blood cell destruction and production may be dramatically upset by episodes of bone marrow failure ("aplastic crises"), during which erythroid hypoplasia and reticulocytopenia may ensue [9]. Most commonly such episodes are precipitated by infections. These infections may be otherwise mild but if highly communicable may cause an "epidemic" of aplastic crises in an afflicted family.

Aplastic crises of more gradual onset have been observed in patients with chronic hemolytic disorders on the basis of a "relative deficiency" of folic acid [10]. In these patients, folic acid utilization is evidently accelerated [11], presumably because of a net increase in the rate of deoxyribonucleic acid synthesis. Nutritional arrest in hereditary spherocytosis is particularly common in pregnancy [12, 13], during which time the marrow may become megaloblastic. Anemic crises due to a sharp acceleration of hemolysis ("hemolytic crises") are probably much less common than aplastic crises in hereditary spherocytosis. One identified cause of hemolytic crises is acute or subacute infection [14], at which time reticulocyte levels and osmotic fragility may be increased and splenomegaly enhanced.

The Spherocyte

The characteristic feature of this type of hereditary hemolytic anemia is the spherocyte (more accurately, a red blood cell more nearly spherical than normal). Similar cells may be observed in acquired hemolytic anemias caused by "autoantibodies" or by certain oxidant drugs. The spheroidal appearance on smear of red blood cells from patients with hereditary spherocytosis tends to be more uniform than is the case in acquired hemolytic anemias, where morphologic variation is usually pronounced. In hereditary spherocytosis the red blood cell mean corpuscular volume is usually in the normal or low-normal range, while the hemoglobin concentration (MCHC) tends to be above normal. The reverse is usually true of the red blood cells in acquired hemolytic anemia with spherocytosis. The red blood cell in hereditary spherocytosis is deficient in surface area [15].

Spherocytes are identified by microscopic examination of peripheral blood smears or suspensions. They appear as dark rounded cells lacking a central pale area and are smaller in diameter and greater in thickness than normal red blood cells. Spheroidicity may be measured quantitatively in terms of osmotic fragility. In the osmotic fragility test red blood cells are suspended in aqueous solutions containing various concentrations of sodium chloride. Since there is almost no exchange of cations during the relatively short duration of the test, osmotic equilibrium is achieved entirely by the rapid movement of water across the red blood cell membrane. In hypotonic solution the red blood cell swells until it approaches a sphere. Any further uptake of water renders the cell membrane porous and permits leakage of intracellular contents, of which hemoglobin is the most easily measured. Accordingly, assuming that the blood has a normal osmolarity, the pH is kept constant, and the duration of the test is sufficiently short to obviate significant transmembrane movement of cation, the osmotic fragility test is a precise measure of how nearly spherical a cell is at the time of exposure to the hypotonic medium [16]. The red blood cells, possibly including the newly formed reticulocytes [17], of patients with hereditary spherocytosis usually have an increase in osmotic fragility. Thus, spheroidicity is attained at higher concentrations of sodium chloride than is the case with normal red blood cells (Fig. 53-1). On microscopic examination spherocytes are usually detected even when in very small numbers. As ordinarily executed, the osmotic fragility test will not reveal spherocytes unless they constitute at least 1 or 2 percent of the total cell population. Thus it is not uncommon in mild forms of the disease to find some spherocytes on smear and yet a normal osmotic fragility. In such cases the incubation fragility (see section on The Hereditary Spherocytosis Red Blood Cell) is of particular diagnostic importance.

MECHANISM OF RED BLOOD CELL DESTRUCTION AND ROLE OF THE SPLEEN

Hereditary spherocytes have a diminished life-span in the patient or in the normal subject [2] when the spleen is present, but their survival is almost normal in patients or normal subjects after splenectomy [18, 19]. Normal red blood cells survive normally when transfused into patients with

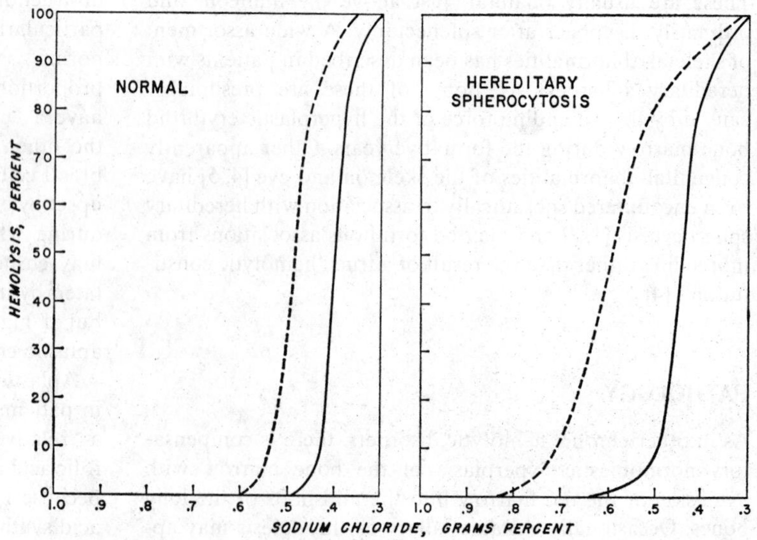

Figure 53.1. Comparison of osmotic fragility curves of normal red blood cells and of hereditary spherocytosis cells. These are summation curves depicting the portion of red blood cells hemolyzed at various concentrations of sodium chloride; they represent average values as determined by Emerson and his associates [28]. As indicated by the continuous lines, freshly drawn hereditary spherocytes are, on the average, slightly more susceptible to hypotonic lysis than normal red blood cells, and a small portion of these cells is striking in this respect, as indicated by a leftward tail in the osmotic fragility curve. After 24 hr of sterile incubation at 37°C (interrupted lines), hereditary spherocytes increase their thickness/diameter ratio more rapidly than do normal red blood cells, as indicated by the greater leftward shift in the osmotic fragility curve.

hereditary spherocytosis [20]. Thus, the red blood cell defect is intrinsic, is nontransferrable, and causes significant destruction of the cell only in the presence of the spleen.

Spherocytosis persists after splenectomy, but excessive destruction of the spherocyte ceases. The following observations have shown that the spleen is the principal site of abnormal red blood cell destruction and does not simply exert an intermediate influence: (1) The spleens of patients are characteristically engorged with blood, and the bilirubin content of splenic vein blood considerably exceeds that of the peripheral blood [21]. (2) Hereditary spherocytes labeled with ^{51}Cr and reinjected into patients or into normal subjects are sequestered in the spleen but not elsewhere [22, 23], and prior to actual sequestration their circulation time through the spleen is abnormally slow [24].

Direct observations of splenic blood in hereditary spherocytosis have shown that the red blood cells in the splenic pulp are more nearly spherical than those in the peripheral circulation [25–28] (Fig. 53-2). Spherocytes are selectively retained in the pulp of spleens, as determined after transfusion in vivo [25–29] and after splenic perfusion in vitro [27, 30]. Indeed, it has been shown [31] that spherocytes can be partially separated from normal red blood cells simply by passage through mechanical (Millipore) filters in vitro. The basis for such a physical selection of HS red blood cells may be either their plumper shape or greater intracellular viscosity (rigidity), or both, for in addition to being abnormally thick, HS cells are more rigid by virtue of their high hemoglobin concentration [32]. These observations support in all essential details the hypothesis of Ham and Castle [33, 34] that hereditary spherocytes are trapped in the spleen, where they are subject to hemoconcentration [35] and erythrostasis. There they undergo metabolic changes to which they are peculiarly susceptible and which lead to their destruction. In recent years efforts have been made to identify the biochemical lesion underlying the spherical shape and the abnormal susceptibility to injury by erythrostasis.

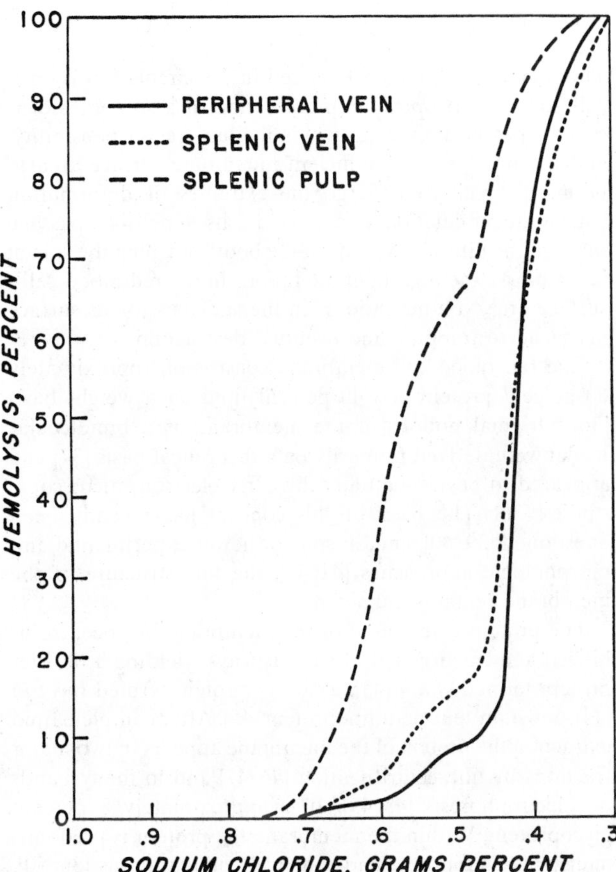

Figure 53.2. Influence of the spleen on the osmotic fragility of hereditary spherocytes. The majority of the red blood cells were only slightly more spherical than normal. However, 10 percent of the red blood cells in the peripheral blood (continuous line) represent an apparently separate population which distributes around a maximum increment of osmotic lysis at a sodium chloride concentration of between 0.55 and 0.60 gm per 100 ml. A similar but proportionately larger population of spherical cells was found simultaneously emerging from the splenic vein (dotted line). In the splenic pulp itself (interrupted line) the highly spherical population of red blood cells constituted a majority of those present. Observations such as this indicate that hereditary spherocytes trapped in the spleen undergo further spherical transformation much as they do on incubation in vitro (Fig. 53-1).

MAINTENANCE OF NORMAL RED BLOOD CELL INTEGRITY

Role of Red Blood Cell Metabolism

While the immature red blood cell is uniquely concerned with the synthesis of hemoglobin, it is otherwise comparable in its metabolic activity to many other tissue cells. When its maturation is complete, shortly after entering the circulation, the red blood cell functions primarily in transporting oxyhemoglobin. This task requires the preservation of (1) functional hemoglobin molecules, and (2) the structural integrity of the cell. The preservation of hemoglobin depends to a large extent upon intracellular reducing mechanisms and involves the adequate regeneration of NADPH and NADH. Normally NADPH is the preferred hydrogen donor in enzyme-linked reactions for reducing oxidized glutathione and presumably for other thiol compounds important in red blood cell integrity. Hereditary hemolytic disorders involving the metabolism of NADPH and of glutathione are dealt with in Chap. 55. Normally NADH is the preferred hydrogen donor in the enzymatic reduction of methemoglobin (Chap. 56). The metabolic activities necessary for the structural preservation of the cell are incompletely understood but are known to include the maintenance of electrolyte gradients across the cell membrane; this in turn depends upon the sustained generation of high-energy phosphate compounds. It is in this general respect that hereditary spherocytes appear to be defective.

Membrane Structure

The survival of the red blood cell in the circulation is critically dependent upon the preservation of a smooth biconcave shape, the maintenance of individual free suspensibility, and the possession of sufficient membrane surface area to permit the cell to undergo the extremes of deformation which the circulation demands. In its repetitive passage through the filtering systems of the body, of which the spleen is the most exacting, slight alterations in the red blood cell's surface area/volume ratio or in the stickiness of its surface may lead to trapping and eventual destruction.

The red blood cell membrane consists of approximately 60 percent protein and 40 percent lipid on a weight basis [36]. Original notions of the membrane as a bimolecular leaflet were derived primarily on a theoretical basis [37] and appeared to be substantiated by early electron microscopic studies [38]. The basis of this concept has recently been questioned [39, 40], and, in spite of newer experimental and morphologic approaches [41, 42], the fine structure of the membrane remains unknown.

The protein component of the membrane has been solubilized and fractionated in various ways, yielding a fibrillar protein termed *elinin* [43], a fibrous protein termed *spectrin* [44], and a protein-poor lipoprotein [45]. After complete lipid extraction the protein of the membrane appears in two major fractions by ultracentrifugation [46, 47] and in many bands on electrophoresis [48, 49]. It is approximately 8 percent glycoprotein. Within the membrane the protein is predominantly in random coil and α-helical configurations [36, 50]. Lipid forms the remainder of the membrane. The mature red blood cell appears unable to synthesize lipid [51], and all of its lipid is confined to the membrane [52]. Approximately 30 percent of the lipid is cholesterol, which is entirely free (nonesterified) and exchangeable with plasma-free cholesterol [52] through an equilibrium process not requiring energy [54]. It is uncertain how cholesterol is structurally incorporated, but recent studies [55, 56] suggest that the cholesterol of the membrane is important in determining the surface area and osmotic resistance of red blood cells. Most of the remaining red blood cell lipids are phospholipids, primarily lecithin, sphingomyelin, phosphatidyl serine, and phosphatidyl ethanolamine [57, 58]. One-fourth to one-half of the phospholipid in the membrane turns over slowly by exchange with serum phospholipids [59, 60]. The remainder is fixed and may play a more important functional or structural role. The fatty acid moieties of phospholipids exchange with plasma fatty acids independent of the exchange process involving the entire phospholipid molecule [61, 62]. The density and placement of the surface phospholipids may be critical to the permeability and "pore" structure of the red blood cell membrane. Glycolipids, free fatty acids, and triglycerides are all present within the membrane in small amounts. Although factors determining the overall lipid content of the membrane are incompletely understood, one significant factor is the equilibrium that exists between red blood cells and serum lipoproteins [63].

Ion Transport

The volume and thickness of red blood cells depend upon the control of ion transport across the cell membrane. The normal plasma anions, chloride and bicarbonate, permeate the red blood cell membrane almost as freely as does water. The cations, sodium and potassium, cross the normal membrane only at a relatively slow rate. In order to regulate volume and maintain osmotic balance [64], in the face of the osmotic pressure of its impermeant constituents (principally hemoglobin and the various glycolytic intermediates), the red blood cell must maintain active (energy-dependent) transport of cations. In man sodium enters the cell by passive transfer along an electrochemical gradient and is actively "pumped" out; potassium is actively transported into the cell against a gradient and diffuses out passively [65, 66]. Diffusion may, of course, be facilitated. Although the necessity for regulating the total cation content of the cell is understandable, the significance of the individual ion gradients is not clear, for the relative levels of sodium and potassium vary among, and even within, the various species. Presumably the high cell/plasma concentration ratio for potassium (approximately 25:1) and the correspondingly low ratio for sodium (approximately 1:12) provide a form of potential energy of importance to cellular metabolism.

The Na^+-K^+ exchange pump of human red blood cells extrudes 3 mEq of Na^+ for each 2 mEq of K^+ actively transported into the cell [69]. It is stimulated by a rise in intracellular Na^+ or extracellular K^+ [70, 71], and it is partially inhibited by cardiac glycosides [70–74] and ethacrynic acid [75]. Portions of this pump activity have been segregated from the total on the basis of their sensitivity to these ions and inhibitors. The ouabain-inhibitable portion, which accounts for 70 percent of the total activity in the steady state, increases in response to a rise in intercellular Na^+ [76]. Regulation appears to be achieved by the activation of adenosine triphosphatase (ATPase) activity [72, 73] in the membrane, which facilitates the hydrolysis of ATP and, thereby, the release of energy, either as work or heat. The ATP for this reaction is derived principally from the conversion of 1,3-diphosphoglycerate to 3-phosphoglycerate by the membrane-associated enzyme, phosphoglycerate kinase [77]. It is thought that cardiac glycosides inhibit the Na^+ efflux and glycolysis at this enzymatic site [77]. While ouabain affects the glycolytic rate of normal red blood cells only slightly [78], it appreciably decreases glycolysis in cells whose metabolism has been increased by Na^+ loading [76, 79]. The conversion of ATP energy to osmotic work may be accomplished by producing conformational changes in groups attached to the cell membrane lipoproteins [80–82]. Phosphatidic acids or phosphoproteins may function as carriers having cyclic and perhaps reciprocal changes in affinity for Na^+ and K^+. The mechanism outlined here for cation regulation obviously will break down if glycolysis is inhibited, if the formation or cleavage of high-energy phosphate bonds is suppressed, or if the rate of passive transfer accelerates beyond the capacity of active transport to offset it.

Glycolysis

Energy for the functions of the adult red blood cell is derived entirely from the metabolism of glucose. Unlike immature red blood cells, including reticulocytes [83], the mature red blood cell lacks cytochromes and many of the components of the tricarboxylic acid cycle. Since the red blood cell has a limited ability to utilize oxygen and cannot utilize pyruvate, glucose is mainly catabolized by the "anaerobic" (Embden-Meyerhof) pathway (Fig. 53-3), and lactic acid accumulates. In addition to this pathway, the mature red blood cell possesses an alternative, oxidative pathway, the hexose monophosphate shunt [85, 86] (pentose phosphate pathway; see also Chap. 55). This pathway cycles glucose-6-phosphate through several intermediate steps, the first two of which are oxidations in which NADP serves as a hydrogen acceptor. Reduced NADP is involved as a hydrogen donor in several enzyme-linked processes important to the red blood cell, particularly the reduction of oxidized glutathione. When this shunt is stimulated, for every three glucose molecules which take this pathway three molecules of fructose-6-phosphate and one molecule of triose phosphate are formed. Ordinarily, this pathway is relatively dormant, as indicated by the low rate of oxidation of glucose to carbon dioxide in vitro. When suspended in vitro red blood cells oxidize at most 11 percent [87], but usually 3 to 5 percent [88, 89], of glucose. The relative activity of the shunt is governed by the availability of NADP, and this in turn depends in large part upon the oxidation-reduction state of glutathione [88, 89]. When substances such as methylene blue and other permeant and reversibly reducible dyes are added, this oxidative shunt is activated to full capacity, and cellular respiration is increased dramatically [85, 86]. These substances substitute for the otherwise deficient mechanism for carrying electrons directly from NADPH to substrates and to oxygen. This "metabolic hiatus" between the high concentration of stored oxygen in red blood cells and the cellular constituents is an essential feature of the cell, for when it is breached by electron carriers, hemolysis ensues [90]. Except during an "oxidative stress," red blood cells normally depend relatively little upon the hexose monophosphate shunt in vivo, for in patients with only 15 to 20 percent of normal shunt activity (glucose-6-P-dehydrogenase deficiency; see Chap. 55) red blood cell life-span is only mildly curtailed [91]. Impairment of the anaerobic pathway (pyruvate kinase deficiency, Chap. 54) [92] severely restricts red blood cell survival.

Since the red blood cell normally is lacking in glycogen [93], except possibly during its early nucleated stages [94], and has no creatine [95], metabolic activity depends directly upon the availability of glucose in the surrounding medium. At physiologic plasma levels glucose can be rapidly transported across the cell membrane so as to maintain equal glucose levels in plasma water and cell water [96]. Glucose penetrates the cell by a process of facilitated diffusion [86] that does not require insulin [96]. The rate at which intracellular glucose is utilized is inversely proportional to the glucose-6-phosphate concentration [97], which in turn is a function of the rates of subsequent glycolytic steps (Fig. 53-3).

Phosphate Metabolism

Phosphate may enter the red blood cell by diffusion [98]; it is rapidly incorporated into organic esters [99–100]. The rate of phosphate uptake is dependent at least in part upon the rate of glycolysis. The first organic compound in which labeled phosphate can be found in large amounts is ATP [101], the terminal two phosphates of which turn over rapidly [102].

It is probable that phosphate is incorporated initially into glyceraldehyde-3-phosphate to form a diester through the action of glyceraldehyde-3-phosphate dehydrogenase [103], NAD acting as a hydrogen acceptor. The 1,3-diphosphoglycerate generated then donates the phosphate to ADP in the presence of phosphoglycerate kinase, to yield ATP and 3-phosphoglycerate (Fig. 53-3). Appropriately, the two enzymes required for incorporating plasma phosphate into cellular ATP are situated as a complex on the red blood cell membrane [104]. Fresh normal red blood cells contain very little [105] inorganic phosphate but have about 12 mmoles of water-soluble organic phosphate per liter of red blood cells. This is almost entirely in the form of glycolytic intermediates (Table 53-1). In contrast to previous studies [102, 107, 108], Minakami et al. [109] have found low levels of hexose diphosphate within the red blood cell.

The relatively stable diester, 2,3-diphosphoglycerate (2,3-DPG), has a conspicuously high concentration in the red blood cell. It serves as a phosphate depot, which is available for rephosphorylating ADP during metabolic deprivation [106]. The 2,3-DPG is partly depleted during brief incubations without glucose, and ATP levels are thereby maintained [106]. When incubation without added glucose is allowed to continue from 12 to 24 hr, 2,3-DPG is almost wholly consumed, and ATP levels decline [108, 110, 111]. When, on the other hand, the utilization of monophosphoglycerates [112] and of 2,3-DPG [108] is impaired, as by a deficiency of pyruvate kinase, very little is consumed during prolonged glucose deprivation [108]. The utilization of phosphate from 2,3-DPG is also blocked by fluoride, which is believed to suppress especially enolase [93]. Mature red blood cells appear to lack glycogen [93]. It is of interest that the red blood cells (contaminated with some white blood

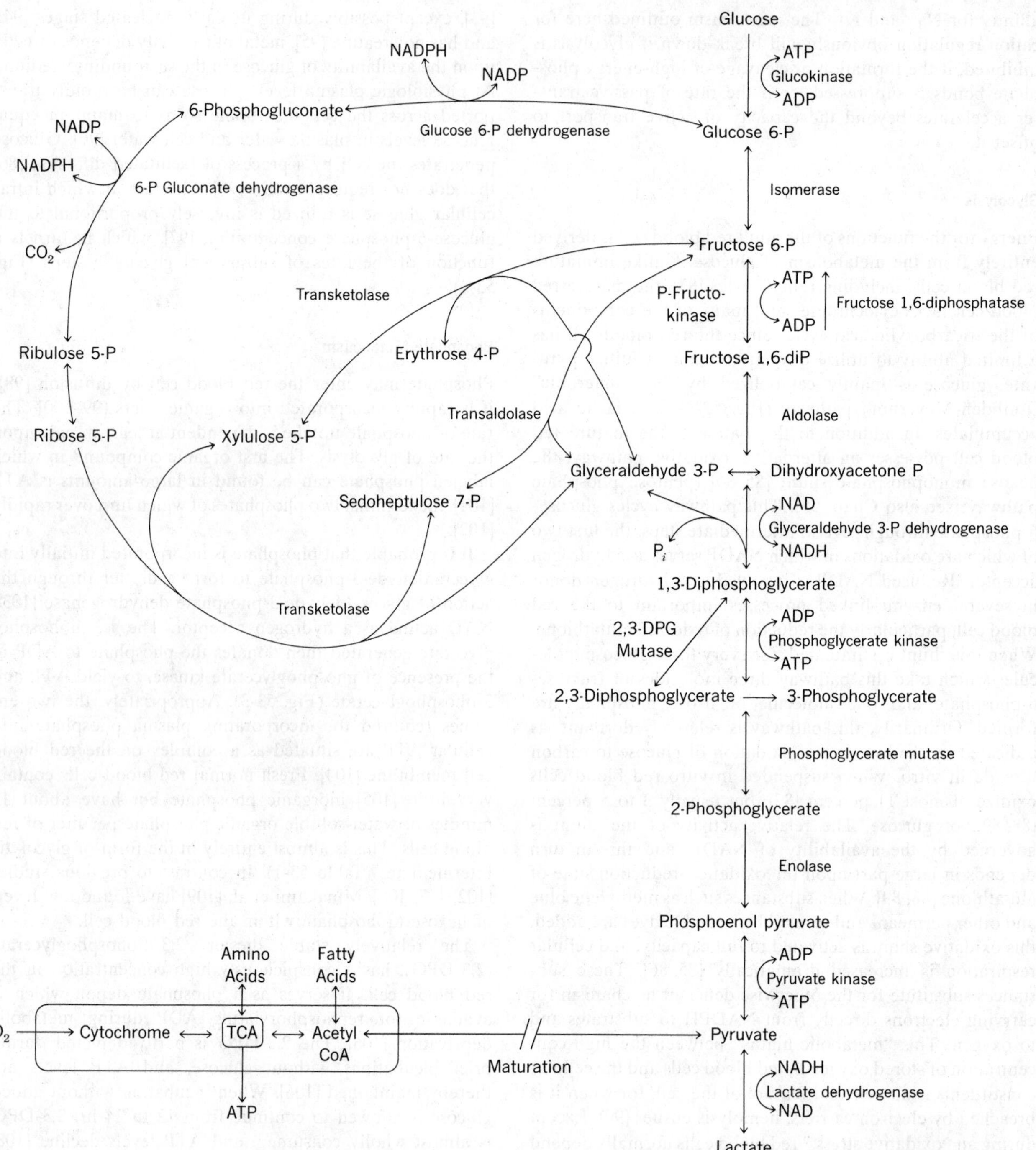

Figure 53-3. Metabolism of glucose by red blood cells. The main pathway in red blood cells is the anaerobic (Embden-Meyerhof) pathway portrayed vertically in this scheme. For every mole of glucose consumed in this chain of reactions, 2 moles of ATP and 2 moles of inorganic phosphate are utilized; in return 4 moles of ATP are generated and 2 moles of lactate are lost. The cyclic pathway at the upper left represents the hexose monophosphate shunt (pentose phosphate pathway) which serves the important function of generating NADPH. This pathway is solely responsible for the capacity of the red blood cell to generate carbon dioxide. The tricarboxylic acid (TCA) cycle portrayed in the lower left is present in reticulocytes but absent in mature red blood cells and can utilize substrates other than glucose [84].

Table 53-1. PHOSPHATE COMPOUNDS IN HUMAN RED BLOOD CELLS

	Bartlett [107] mmole/liter	Robinson et al. [108] mmole/liter	Gerlach et al. [102] mmole/kg	Minakami et al. [109] mmole/liter
Organic phosphate compounds:				
2,3-Diphosphoglycerate	3.60–5.10	3.10–4.53	3.07–4.30	4.00
Adenosine triphosphate	0.90–1.23	0.84–1.10	0.52–0.84	0.87–1.38
Hexose diphosphates	0.25–0.36	0.24–0.42	0.34–0.53	0.04–0.06
Adenosine diphosphate	0.19–0.25	0.08–0.15	0.24–0.40	0.10–0.15
Weak acid phosphates*	0.20–0.33	0.31–0.52	....	0.09
Inorganic phosphate	0.28–0.48	0.30–0.53	0.10–0.38	
Total phosphate	....	10.90–14.51	11.45–14.97	

* Adenosine monophosphate, glucose-6-phosphate, fructose-6-phosphate, ribose-5-phosphate, NADP.

cells) of patients with Type III (amylo-1,6-glucosidase deficiency) glycogen storage disease have been reported to have high levels of glycogen. This suggests that glycogen synthesis may occur normally in immature red blood cells [94].

Recently 2,3-DPG, which contains 75 to 80 percent of the organic phosphate of the cell, has been shown to be the principal modulator of oxygen binding by hemoglobin. In addition the option of switching glycolysis so as to generate (via a mutase) 2,3-DPG, a compound possessing only one high-energy phosphate, gives the red blood cell control of the net rate of synthesis of ATP, in amounts not exceeding energy requirements. This regulating mechanism is essentially an "uncoupling" of the rates of glycolysis and of ATP synthesis (see Chap. 54).

Effect of Erythrostasis

It is evident from the foregoing that the red blood cell is deficient in reserves of carbohydrate and other high-energy phosphate compounds. Degenerative changes commence shortly after the red blood cells are separated from its metabolites, namely glucose and inorganic phosphate. When normal red blood cells are incubated in vitro under sterile conditions, as in the autohemolysis test, they undergo progressive structural and chemical changes. A loss of volume control is one of the earliest. During the first 24 hr the cells swell and show an increase in osmotic fragility (Fig. 53-1) [25, 28, 33]. Swelling is accomplished by a net gain of sodium with net loss of potassium [113, 114]. The sodium flux is more rapid than that of potassium [113, 115]. As the active transport mechanisms fail, the sodium "leak" into the cells gradually exceeds the rate of active sodium extrusion. In addition there is an increase in cellular osmolarity as the various glycolytic intermediates are broken down. At this point the cells have begun to lose their viability, as judged by their inability to survive when reinjected into the circulation [116, 117]. Between 24 and 48 hr of erythrostasis the intracellular and extracellular concentrations of the cations approach equilibrium with the medium, and the red blood cells return to their original volume [114]. During this "shrinking" phase, potassium loss is prominent [114] and is accompanied by the loss of phosphate and of a number of glycolytic intermediates [108]. The loss of these osmotically active constituents probably accounts for the reduction in cell volume. Concomitantly, membrane lipids are lost [118, 119], decreasing the critical hemolytic volume of the cells [120]. After about 48 hr of incubation the cells become increasingly permeable to hemoglobin, and "autohemolysis" occurs visibly [114, 121].

These degenerative changes in red blood cells which occur when they are subjected to erythrostasis in vitro follow a depletion of glucose and an accumulation of lactic acid. Normal red blood cells consume from 1 to 2 μmoles of glucose (0.36 mg) per ml of cells per hr, and normal whole blood is depleted of glucose within 5 or 6 hr at 37°C. If the cells are washed free of glucose or are packed together, they lose their viability within a few hours. If glucose levels are maintained and the cells are kept in suspension, viability, structure, and metabolic integrity are preserved for over 24 hr [117, 119, 122]. Indeed, glycolysis will continue for at least 72 hr if glucose is available and the pH is kept constant [119, 122].

Within a few hours after glucose has been depleted, normal red blood cells at 37°C show a decline in 2,3-DPG and ATP levels and smaller rises in ADP and then AMP and a steady accumulation of inorganic phosphate [100, 108, 123]. If glucose is restored within a few hours, ATP and 2,3-DPG are regenerated and inorganic phosphate falls [123]. Similar but slower metabolic changes take place when red blood cells are stored for several weeks in the cold [124]. These changes and the loss of viability can be inhibited or partly reversed not only by glucose but also by purine nucleosides such as adenosine and inosine [125, 126]. This effect was originally attributed to ribose phosphate serving as an energy source [106, 125] through the action of purine nucleoside phosphorylase on inosine in the presence of phosphate [127, 129], but much of the beneficial effect may be from the condensation of adenine with phosphoribosylpyrophosphate to form AMP, which is then converted to ATP by mature red blood cells [130–132]. The addition of small amounts of adenine not only helps sustain cellular viability and ATP levels [131], but, when added with inosine, it also improves the morphologic appearance of stored red blood cells [133]. Although direct mechanisms for phosphorylating adenosine or for cleaving it to adenine and ribose have not been demonstrated in human red blood cells [129, 132, 134, 135], inosine and adenosine may contribute phosphorylated ribose for entrance into the hexose monophosphate shunt (Fig. 53-3). By entry into this pathway and conversion to triose phosphate, ribose from nucleosides can participate in the Embden-Meyerhof pathway. In this way ATP regeneration may be sustained in spite of a shortage of glucose or deficiencies in hexokinase (glucokinase) or hexose monophosphate isomerase. From the foregoing it is apparent that the maintenance of adequate levels of ATP is of critical importance in preserving the shape and function of the red blood cell membrane.

THE HEREDITARY SPHEROCYTOSIS RED BLOOD CELL

Susceptibility to Erythrostasis

The first and still the best evidence for an intrinsic defect in the metabolism of the red blood cells in hereditary spherocytosis (HS red blood cells) is the finding of Emerson et al. [25, 26, 28] that these cells undergo an abnormally rapid increase in osmotic fragility on sterile incubation (Fig. 53-1). The exaggerated increase in spheroidicity during erythrostasis in vitro is a constant feature of the red blood cells, even of patients whose peripheral red blood cells are not appreciably spheroidal when fresh. While it is the most dependable single test available for detecting hereditary spherocytosis [1, 2] the incubation fragility is also occasionally positive in acquired hemolytic anemia, especially that associated with myelofibrosis [121]. HS red blood cells undergo spontaneous autohemolysis to an abnormal extent [33, 34, 136], and this correlates with the rapidity of increase in osmotic fragility [114], but it is slower to evolve and usually becomes pronounced between 24 and 48 hr of incubation [1, 2, 121, 136]. Autohemolysis may be regarded as an extension of the same process as that measured in the osmotic fragility test, for both are prevented by oncotic or impermeant osmotic agents in the medium [117, 137].

The abnormally rapid autohemolysis and increase in osmotic fragility of HS red blood cells take place in saline as well as serum or plasma [2, 136]. These changes are suppressed in the cold and are much inhibited by periodic additions of fresh serum [34] and by supplements of glucose [114, 138, 139] or, to a lesser extent, of purine nucleosides [140, 141]. The protective effect of glucose is striking. It brings about a reduction in autohemolysis after 48 hr of incubation from 25 or 30 percent to about 5 percent [2, 113, 121, 137–139]. This effect is nullified by fluoride [142], to which HS red blood cells are abnormally susceptible [143].

Prior to splenectomy HS red cells are much less reliably protected by glucose, and occasionally glucose is ineffectual in inhibiting autohemolysis; in part, this may represent a "Crabtree effect" on the reticulocytes present in excess before splenectomy. After splenectomy, however, glucose invariably protects HS red cells subjected to prolonged incubation at 37°C.

Metabolic Abnormalities

The hypersusceptibility of HS red blood cells to erythrostasis in vitro and the protective effect of glucose has suggested that there is an intracorpuscular error in glycolysis. These cells show no overall deficiency in glycolysis in terms of glucose consumption [114] or phosphate exchange [140], but Prankerd et al. [140] found that when ^{32}P-labeled orthophosphate is added to the medium, it appears principally as an inorganic phosphate rather than in organic ester form. This low recovery of ^{32}P in organic form suggested to them that HS red blood cells are deficient in their ability to generate high-energy phosphate compounds essential to the preservation of the cell [140, 144]. Subsequent studies by others [145–150] have found no abnormality in the levels or relative distribution of phosphorylated intermediates. These seemingly discrepant observations are apparently attributable to the fact that the earlier studies were carried out over a period of hours rather than of minutes as were the later studies and may have largely reflected catabolic rather than anabolic events. This interpretation is supported by the findings of several workers [108, 123, 151] that within a few hours of standing in vitro HS red blood cells show a rapid and premature decline in ATP and 2,3-DPG, while ADP and inorganic phosphate increase. These degenerative changes are accompanied by abnormal increments in cell water and total cation [123] and later by an abnormal loss of stromal lipids [118, 119, 123]. The overall rate of glycolysis, as determined by glucose consumption and lactate formation, is actually higher in HS than normal, even in red blood cells from splenectomized patients [117, 151, 152]. This represents an acceleration of anaerobic glycolysis, as there is no acceleration in the oxidative (hexose monophosphate) pathway [117]. In another respect as well, HS red blood cells display an acceleration rather than a deceleration of metabolism: the active transport of sodium is increased [117, 153, 154] and this is associated with an increase in that portion of the membrane ATPase susceptible to inhibition by ouabain [155]. A relationship between these findings is revealed by the observation that cardiac glycosides largely suppress the excess glycolysis of HS red blood cells, whereas in fresh normal red blood cells glycolysis is less affected by the glycoside ATPase inhibitors [78, 117, 156]. The products of the accelerated breakdown of ATP in these cells are ADP and inorganic phosphate; both act as stimulants to glycolysis [117, 157] and presumably are directly responsible for the heightened rate of glycolysis. When ATP breakdown is inhibited by ouabain, HS red blood cells undergo even more striking autohemolysis in 48 hr, whereas normal red blood cells are affected little by ouabain [117, 151].

Nature of the Defect in Hereditary Spherocytosis

It has been concluded [117] from the information discussed above that (1) the membranes of HS red blood cells are inherently more permeable to sodium, (2) the resulting tendency for intracellular sodium levels to rise activates the sodium pump by activating ATPase, and (3) this in turn results in an accelerated breakdown of ATP into ADP and inorganic phosphate which act as stimulants to glycolysis. In support of this sequence, it was found that slowing sodium entry by suspending HS red blood cells in solutions containing impermeant osmotic agents such as sucrose, divalent cations, or ATP protects cellular viability during erythrostasis and prevents abnormal autohemolysis [117, 137]. Thus, it appears that the HS red blood cell depends for its preservation on a sustained and somewhat accelerated glycolysis to compensate for an inborn abnormality of the cell membrane.

The precise relation between the increased permeability of HS cells and their impaired survival is unclear. A quantitative correlation has not been found between sodium flux and survival in vivo [158]. Under homeostatic conditions compensation for the sodium leak usually is complete, protecting the cell from an accumulation of sodium [177]. Following splenectomy HS cell survival is either normal or near normal in spite of the persistence of a sodium leak [18, 19]. Patients without HS whose red blood cells have a much increased Na^+ flux do not necessarily have proportionately increased hemolysis [159]. Thus, factors in addition to an altered sodium flux appear important in HS cell survival. It seems probable that one factor is the spherocytic shape resulting from a decrease in membrane surface area. This predisposes the HS cell to "pooling" in the spleen, where the extreme conditions of erythrostasis interfere with its delicate metabolic compensation and destruction ensues. Increasing the surface area of the HS cell by the addition of membrane cholesterol, employing conditions favoring the membrane binding of cholesterol attached to lipoprotein, does not alter its sodium flux or glycolytic rate, but does increase the surface/volume ratio, "flattens" the red cell, and thereby improves cellular deformability. Inferentially, this permits the HS red cell to escape splenic entrapment and, thereby, to survive longer [160].

The molecular nature of the presumed membrane defect in hereditary spherocytosis is not yet defined. Because lipids determine many properties of the membrane, attention has been directed to the possibility that the primary defect is in stromal lipid metabolism. The total lipid content of HS cells prior to splenectomy is decreased [118, 161] in spite of the presence of a young cell population, which would tend to increase lipid values [162, 163]. After splenectomy, values are similar to those obtained from normal subjects with spleens [93, 118, 160]. That splenectomy in normal subjects results in an increase in membrane cholesterol and phospholipid [160] has been overlooked in most comparisons of lipid content. When HS red cells of splenectomized patients are compared with red blood cells from normal subjects who have all undergone splenectomy, a decreased lipid content of HS cells is readily apparent [160]. However, the surface area of HS cells is less than can be accounted for by a decreased membrane lipid content alone. The relative proportions of cholesterol and phospholipid and of the various phospholipids are normal in HS cells [118, 164–167], although earlier reports had indicated an abnormality in the relative concentrations of lysophosphatidyl ethanolamine and phosphatidyl ethanolamine [168, 169]. HS cells also incorporate oleic acid normally into lysophosphatides [170]. Conflicting data exist regarding the turnover rate of phospholipid phosphorus in HS cells [171, 172], a point of interest since certain phospholipids may function in cation transport [80–82]. Contrary to initial reports [173, 174], when glucose is not limited, the membrane lipids of HS cells have a stability equal to that of normal red blood cells [119, 160]. Instability is only evident under nonhomeostatic conditions, as when glucose is depleted the pH is low, etc. Clearly it follows that active transport of cations is not the cause of phospholipid instability, for the latter is elicited by conditions preventing active transport [118, 119]. There is inferential evidence that the basic inherited defect is one affecting a membrane protein, presumably one affecting sodium flux but not potassium flux. Whether this hypothetical abnormality directly involves a component protein of the system for transporting sodium or another protein that normally is involved in transport, per se, is unknown. By exposing normal red blood cells to small amounts of an impermeable sulfhydryl inhibitor, it is possible to create a cell defect closely resembling that of hereditary spherocytosis [175, 176]. Both in HS red blood cells and in sulfhydryl-inhibited cells erythrostasis causes a loss of cell surface area and a simultaneous gain in volume. As a consequence, the cell rapidly reaches its limiting ("hemolytic") volume.

Effect of Splenectomy

Within the microcirculation of the splenic red pulp, a portion of the red blood cells must traverse the screen-like basement membrane separating the cords and sinuses. The apertures in this discontinuous basement membrane are quite regular, measuring about 3 microns in diameter [177]. The decreased surface/volume ratio of HS cells, particularly at the lower pH of the spleen [178], decreases their ability to deform sufficiently to traverse these apertures. Consequently, the spleen subjects HS red blood cells to injurious erythrostasis, and, in addition, acts to filter out those cells most severely injured. The in vivo studies of Griggs et al. [179] demonstrated that HS red blood cells undergo several days of repetitious "conditioning" while circulating repetitively through the spleen before they acquire the "hyperspheroidal" shape that presages lysis. Thus a minor population of very spheroidal "conditioned" cells is generated that adds a tail to the osmotic fragility curve. This population continually gains newly conditioned cells and loses older cells. After splenectomy there may be a transient pile-up in the circulation of very spheroidal cells, but shortly thereafter this population disappears. Thereafter, the osmotic fragility curve indicates that the bimodal population of cells, characteristic of untreated hereditary spherocytosis, is replaced by a uniform population of cells of intermediate fragility [1, 18, 28].

While the exact nature of the biochemical defect in hereditary spherocytosis remains unknown, it is apparent that the defect is not merely a consequence of the metabolic change induced by the spleen. The increased osmotic fragility and membrane permeability for sodium of HS red cells persist after cure of the hemolytic process by splenectomy, and their metabolic lability during erythrostasis is still demonstrable [28, 121, 138]. Furthermore, these cells remain susceptible to splenic sequestration if transfused into normal subjects [2]. Thus the inherited defect remains after splenectomy but its clinical expression is prevented. So specific is the spleen in detecting and aggravating this red blood cell defect that splenectomy is invariably curative clinically. The rare relapses reported are attributable to postoperative growth of splenic autotransplants ("splenosis") [180] or to the hyperplasia of splenunculi that were overlooked during the operation [181].

GENETICS

The hereditary nature of what is now called hereditary spherocytosis has been known for many years [182], but a precise genetic characterization was hampered in some series by uncertain diagnostic criteria and by the variability with which the disease may be expressed. Nonetheless virtually all family studies of this disorder, even when rather insensitive methods have been used, have led to the conclusion that hereditary spherocytosis is inherited as a dominant character, i.e., that the disease is manifest in heterozygotes [183–190]. A slight deficiency of affected sibs was noted by Race [185] and by Young et al. [1, 187], and a number of cases have been reported in which neither parent had a demonstrable hematologic abnormality [187]. Some of these parents may be "carriers" whose disease is so mild as to escape ascertainment. Many patients without affected parents appear to be sporadic and are presumed to arise from mutation [190, 191]. If sporadic cases are excluded, and they may comprise one-quarter of all the patients, the incidence among sibs is close to 0.5 [190]. Careful studies in large families afflicted with hereditary spherocytosis have generally revealed a family incidence of about 0.5 [188]. In its inheritance, then, hereditary spherocytosis in man differs distinctly from a closely similar disease of the deer mouse [192], in which a homozygous (double-dose) inheritance is necessary to produce the disease. It has been suggested that the mutation for hereditary spherocytosis initially may have had the same "dominant" inheritance in the deer mouse as in man; later an accumulation of beneficial genetic modifiers gradually may have dampened the deleterious gene effect to the point where a double dose was required to produce manifest disease [192]. An alternative interpretation is that the human disease may be heterogeneous and that one form is manifest with dominant inheritance and another form, less common, is recessive and requires homozygous inheritance as in the deer mouse. Evidence for heterogeneity within the clinical entity of hereditary spherocytosis has been cited [187] but is inconclusive. Against the possibility of a recessive form of hereditary spherocytosis is the fact that the disorder has not been observed in the children of normal consanguineous parents [190].

The prevalence of hereditary spherocytosis in the United States and England is estimated to be about 220 per million [190] and is comparable to that of another dominant defect of red blood cells, hereditary elliptocytosis. Unlike one form of hereditary elliptocytosis having linkage to the Rh locus, the inheritance of hereditary spherocytosis is not linked to that of any of the blood groups or to other marker loci [185]. In its degree of severity, hereditary elliptocytosis is much more variable than is HS. In general it is far less likely to be severe or even manifest; most patients are entirely symptomless.

There is no certain example of hereditary spherocytosis in which the patients were homozygous for the trait, but it has been presumed in a family of 13 children, all with hereditary spherocytosis, and 9 of them with physical or mental retardation [189]. Race [185] reported a mating of first cousins, both of whom had hereditary spherocytosis. Three of the children were affected, one was normal, and there were two miscarriages.

SUMMARY

1 Hereditary spherocytosis is a congenital hemolytic anemia that is manifest in heterozygotes. It is caused by an intrinsic defect in the red blood cell.

2 The exact nature of this defect is unknown. It is characterized by red blood cells which are slightly deficient in surface and which tend to have a spherical rather than a normal discoidal form. These red blood cells characteristically undergo rapid degenerative changes in vitro when deprived of glucose or subjected to erythrostasis. These changes include an increase in osmotic fragility, disruption of cation gradients, loss of stromal lipids, breakdown of ATP, and finally autohemolysis. No deficiency in energy metabolism has been found. Glycolysis actually is increased. The most basic defect so far described is in the membrane, which is abnormally permeable to sodium. The increased leak rate for sodium is compensated for under optimal conditions by the activation of ATPase; this in turn accelerates the outward transport of sodium and increases the rate of glycolysis.

3 Unlike most body cells, red blood cells are limited in their ability to utilize oxygen and normally depend almost entirely upon anaerobic glycolysis for the generation of energy as ATP. There is rapid depletion of the energy sources necessary for ion transport and for maintenance of cell structure under erythrostatic conditions. Hereditary spherocytosis red blood cells are unusually vulnerable to metabolic inhibition and bear an increased metabolic burden caused by a defective membrane. In essence, hemolysis arises not from deficient energy but from excessive requirements.

4 Based on present knowledge, the following hypothesis is proposed:

a. There is an inherent abnormality of the membrane of hereditary spherocytosis red blood cells; these are characterized by decreased surface area, a selective increase in permeability to sodium, and structural instability on metabolic deprivation.

b. Under optimal metabolic conditions, as when freely suspended in plasma in the general circulation, the increased influx of sodium is compensated for by the activation of the ATPase system and increased glycolysis.

c. When, largely because of their decreased surface area, hereditary spherocytosis red blood cells are trapped and transiently separated from glucose-containing plasma in the spleen (erythrostasis), the compensation for their sodium permeability is prevented, leading to cell swelling. Later, prolonged or repetitious metabolic depletion causes a nonspecific permeability change of the cell membrane. This becomes reversible with the loss of cytoplasmic constituents, accompanied by loss of membrane lipids, and a diminished surface/volume ratio.

d. After repeated passage through the spleen these irreversibly damaged red blood cells are recognized as a minor population of very spheroidal and osmotically fragile cells in the peripheral blood.

e. Because of the thickness and rigidity of these "conditioned" red cells, the injured cell is slowed in its passage through the spleen by retention in the "cordal compartment" and is subjected to even more prolonged erythrostasis. This vicious cycle eventually traps the hereditary spherocytosis red blood cell in the spleen, wherein it undergoes hemolysis.

BIBLIOGRAPHY

1. Young, L. E., Izzo, M. J., and Platzer, R. F.: Hereditary spherocytosis. I. Clinical, hematologic and genetic features in 28 cases, with particular reference to the osmotic and mechanical fragility of incubated erythrocytes. Blood, **6**, 1073, 1951.
2. Dacie, J. V.: *The Haemolytic Anaemias, Congenital and Acquired.* Part I, *The Congenital Anaemias,* chap. 2. Grune & Stratton, New York, 1960.
3. Gairdner, D.: The association of gallstones with acholuric jaundice in children. Arch. Dis. Child, **14**, 109, 1939.
4. Gänsslen, M., Zipperlen, E., and Schüz, E.: Die hämolyische Konstitution. Arch. Klin. Med., **146**, 1, 1925.
5. Otto, J.: Seltene Augenhintergrundveränderung bei hämolytische Konstitution. Klin Mbl. Augenheilk, **126**, 327, 1955.
6. Von Haam, E., and Awny, A. J.: The pathology of hypersplenism. Amer. J. Clin. Path., **18**, 313, 1948.
7. Leffler, R. J.: The spleen in hypersplenism. Amer. J. Path., **28**, 303, 1952.
8. Wiland, O. K., and Smith, E. B.: The morphology of the spleen in congenital hemolytic anemia (hereditary spherocytosis). Amer. J. Clin. Path., **26**, 619, 1956.
9. Owren, P. A.: Congenital hemolytic jaundice: The pathogenesis of the "hemolytic crisis." Blood, **3**, 231, 1948.
10. Jandl, J. H., and Greenberg, M. S.: Bone-marrow failure due to relative nutritional deficiency in Cooley's hemolytic anemia: Painful "erythropoietic crises in response to folic acid." New Eng. J. Med., **260**, 461, 1959.
11. Chanarin, I., Dacie, J. V., and Mollin, D. L.: Folic-acid deficiency in haemolytic anaemia. Brit. J. Haemat., **5**, 245, 1959.
12. Delamore, I. W., Richmond, J., and Davies, S. H.: Megaloblastic anaemia in congenital spherocytosis. Brit. Med. J., **1**, 543, 1961.
13. Kohler, H. G., Meynell, M. J., and Cooke, W. T.: Spherocytic anaemia, complicated by megaloblastic anaemia of pregnancy. Brit. Med. J., **1**, 779, 1960.
14. Jandl, J. H., Jacob, H. S., and Daland, G. A.: Hypersplenism due to infection: A study of five cases manifesting hemolytic anemia. New Eng. J. Med., **264**, 1063, 1961.
15. Crosby, W. H.: The pathogenesis of spherocytes and leptocytes (target cells). Blood, **7**, 261, 1952.
16. Castle, W. B., and Daland, G. A.: Susceptibility of erythrocytes in hypotonic hemolysis as a function of discoidal form. Amer. J. Physiol., **120**, 371, 1937.
17. Paolino, W.: Variations of the mean diameter in the ripening of the erythrocyte. Acta Med. Scand., **136**, 141, 1949.
18. Emerson, C. P.: The influence of the spleen on the osmotic behavior and the longevity of red cells in hereditary spherocytosis (congenital hemolytic jaundice): A case study. Boston Med. Quart., **5**, 65, 1954.
19. Schrumph, A.: Duree de vie des globules rouges dans la sphérocytose héréditaire. Rev. Hemat., **11**, 140, 1956.
20. Dacie, J. V., and Mollison, P. L.: Survival of normal erythrocytes after transfusion to patients with familial haemolytic anaemia (alcholuric jaundice). Lancet, **1**, 550, 1943.
21. Gripwall, E.: Zur Klinik und Pathologie des hereditären häemolytischen Ikterus: Mit besonderer Berücksichtigung des Verhaltens der roten Blutörperchen. Acta Med. Scand., suppl. **96**, 1938.
22. Jandl, J. H., Greenberg, M. S., Yonemoto, R. H., and Castle, W. B.: Clinical determination of the sites of red cell sequestration in hemolytic anemias. J. Clin, Invest., **35**, 842, 1956.
23. Schlosser, L. L., Korst, D. R., Clatanoff, D. V., and Schilling, R. F.: Radioactivity over the spleen and liver following the transfusion of chromium ^{51}-labelled erythrocytes in hemolytic anemia. J. Clin. Invest., **36**, 1470, 1957.
24. Harris, I. M., McAlister, J. M., and Prankerd, T. A. J.: The relationship of abnormal red cells to the normal spleen. Clin. Sci., **16**, 223, 1957.
25. Emerson, C. P., Jr., Shen, S. C., and Castle, W. B.: The osmotic fragility of the red cells of the peripheral and splenic blood in patients with congenital hemolytic jaundice transfused with normal red cells. J. Clin. Invest., **25**, 922, 1946.
26. Emerson, C. P., Jr., Shen, S. C., Ham, T. H., and Castle, W. B.: The mechanism of blood destruction in congenital hemolytic jaundice. J. Clin. Invest., **26**, 1180, 1947.
27. Young, L. E., Platzer, R. F., Ervin, D. M., and Izzo, M. J.: Hereditary spherocytosis. II. Observations on the role of the spleen. Blood, **6**, 1099, 1951.
28. Emerson, C. P., Jr., Shen S. C., Ham, T. H., Fleming. E. M., and Castle. W. B.: Studies on the destruction of red blood cells. IX. Quantitative methods for determining the osmotic and mechanical fragility of red

cells in the peripheral blood and splenic pulp; the mechanism of increased hemolysis in hereditary spherocytosis (congenital hemolytic jaundice) as related to the functions of the spleen. Arch. Intern. Med. **97**, 38, 1956.
29. Weisman, R., Jr., Hurley, T. H., Harris, J. W., and Ham, T. H.: Studies of the function of the spleen in the hemolysis of red cells in hereditary spherocytosis and sickle cell disorders. J. Lab. Clin. Med., **42**, 965, 1953.
30. Dacie, J. V.: Familial haemolytic anaemia (acholuric jaundice), with particular reference to changes in fragility produced by splenectomy. Quart. J. Med., **12**, 101, 1943.
31. Jandl, J. H., Simmons, R. S., and Castle, W. B.: Red cell filtration and the pathogenesis of certain hemolytic anemias. Blood, **18**, 133, 1961.
32. Erslev, A. J., and Atwater, J.: Effect of mean corpuscular hemoglobin concentration on viscosity. J. Lab. Clin. Med., **62**, 401, 1963.
33. Ham, T. H., and Castle, W. B.: Relation of increased hypotonic fragility and of erythrostasis to the mechanism of hemolysis in certain anemias. Trans. Ass. Amer. Physicians, **55**, 127, 1940.
34. Ham, T. H., and Castle, W. B.: Studies on the destruction of red blood cells: Relation of increased hypotonic fragility and of erythrostasis to the mechanism of hemolysis in certain anemias. Proc. Amer. Phil. Soc., **82**, 411, 1940.
35. Barcroft, J., and Poole, L. T.: The blood in the spleen pulp. J. Physiol. (London), **64**, 23, 1927.
36. Maddy, A. H., and Malcolm, B. R.: Protein conformations in the plasma membrane. Science., **150**, 1616, 1965.
37. Danielli, J. F., and Davson, H.: A contribution to the theory of permeability of thin films. J. Cell. Physiol., **5**, 495, 1935.
38. Robertson, J. D.: Unit membranes: A review with recent new studies of experimental alterations and a new subunit structure in synaptic membranes, in *Cellular Membranes in Development*, edited by M. Locke. Academic New York, 1964.
39. Korn, E. D.: Structure of biological membranes. Science, **153**, 1491, 1966.
40. Korn, E. D.: Structure and function of the plasma membrane. J. Gen. Physiol., **52**, 257s, 1968.
41. Green, D. E., Allmann, D. W., Bachmann, E., Baum, H., Kopaczky, K., Korman, E. F., Lipton, S., MacLennon, D. H., McConnell, D. C., Perdue, J. F., Ruske, J. S., and Tzagoloff, A.: Formation of membranes by repeating units. Arch. Biophys., **119**, 312, 1967.
42. Weinstein, R. S., and Koo, V. M.: Penetration of red cell membranes by some membrane-associated particles. Proc. Soc. Exp. Biol. Med., **128**, 353, 1968.
43. Moskowitz, M., and Calvin, M.: On the components and structure of the human red cell membrane. Exp. Cell. Res., **3**, 33, 1952.
44. Marchesi, V. T., and Steers, E.: Selective solubilization of a protein component of the red cell membrane. Science, **159**, 203, 1968.
45. Morgan, T. E., and Hanahan, D. H.: Solubilization and characterization of a lipoprotein from erythrocyte stroma. Biochemistry (Wash.), **5**, 1050, 1966.
46. Rega, A. F., Weed, R. I., Reed, C. F., Berg, G. G., and Rothstein, A.: Changes in the properties of human erythrocyte membrane protein after solubilization by butanol extraction. Biochim. Biophys. Acta, **147**, 297, 1967.
47. Maddy, A. H.: The properties of the protein of the plasma membrane of ox erythrocytes. Biochim. Biophys. Acta, **117**, 193, 1966.
48. Lauf, P. K., and Poulik, M. D.: Solubilization and structural integrity of the human red cell membrane. Brit. J. Haemat., **15**, 191, 1968.
49. Rosenberg, S. A., and Guidotti, G.: The protein of human erythrocyte membranes. I. Preparation, solubilization, and partial characterization. J. Biol. Chem., **243**, 1985, 1968.
50. Wallach, D. F. H., and Gordon, A.: Lipid proten interactions in cellular membranes. Fed. Proc., **27**, 1263, 1968.
51. Marks, P. A., Bellhorn, A., and Kidson, C.: Lipid synthesis in human leukocytes, platelets and erythrocytes. J. Biol. Chem., **235**, 2579, 1960.
52. Dodge, J. T., Mitchell, C., Hanahan, D. J.: The preparation and characteristics of hemoglobin-free ghosts of human erythrocytes. Arch. Biochem., **180**, 119, 1963.
53. Hagerman, J. S., and Gould, R. G.: The in vitro interchange of cholesterol between plasma and red cells. Proc. Soc. Exp. Biol. Med., **78**, 329, 1951.
54. Murphy, J. R.: Erythrocyte metabolism. IV. Equilibration of cholesterol-4-C^{14} between erythrocytes and variously treated sera. J. Lab. Clin. Med., **60**, 571, 1962.
55. Murphy, J. R.: Erythrocyte metabolism. III. Relationship of energy, metabolism and serum factors to the osmotic fragility following incubation. J. Lab. Clin. Med., **60**, 86, 1962.
56. Cooper, R. A., and Jandl, J. H.: Bile salts and cholesterol in the pathogenesis of target cells in obstructive jaundice. J. Clin. Invest., **47**, 809, 1968.
57. Reed, C. F., Swisher, S. N., Marinetti, G. V., and Eden, E. G.: Studies of the lipids of the erythrocyte. I. Quantitative analysis of the lipids of normal human red blood cells. J. Lab. Clin. Med., **56**, 281, 1960.
58. Ways, P., Hanahan, D. H.: Characterization and quantification of red cell lipids in normal man. J. Lipid Res., **5**, 318, 1964.
59. Reed, C. F.: Phospholipid exchange between plasma and erythrocytes in man and the dog. J. Clin. Invest., **47**, 749, 1968.
60. Tarlov, A. R., and Mulder, E.: Phospholipid metabolism in rat erythrocytes: Quantitative studies of lecithin biosynthesis. Blood, **30**, 853, 1967. (Abstract.)
61. Farquhar, J. W., and Ahrens, E. H., Jr.: Effects of dietary fats on human erythrocyte fatty acid patterns. J. Clin. Invest., **42**, 617, 1963.
62. Shohet, S. B., Nathan, D. G., and Karnovsky, M. L.: Stages in the incorporation of fatty acids into red blood cells. J. Clin. Invest., **47**, 1096, 1968.
63. Cooper, R. A., and Jandl, J. H.: Red cell cholesterol content: A manifestation of the serum affinity for free cholesterol. Trans. Ass. Amer. Physicians, **82**, 324, 1969.
64. Williams, T. F., Fordham, C. C., III, Hollander, W., Jr., and Welt, L. G.: A study of the osmotic behavior of the human erythrocyte. J. Clin. Invest., **38**, 1587, 1959.
65. Maizels, M.: Cation transfer in human red cells, in *Membrane Transport and Metabolism*, edited by A. Kleinzeller and A. Kotyk. Academic, New York, 1961.
66. Hoffman, J. F.: Cation transport and the structure of the red cell plasma membrane. Circulation, **26**, 1201, 1962.
67. Czaczkes, J. W., Ullmann, T. D., Ullman, L., and Bar-Kochba, Z.: Determination of the red blood cell content of water, sodium, and potassium in normal subjects. J. Lab. Clin. Med., **61**, 873, 1963.
68. Valberg, L. S., Holt, J. M., Paulson, E., and Szivek, J.: Spectrochemical analysis of sodium, potassium, calcium, magnesium, copper, and zinc in normal human erythrocytes. J. Clin. Invest., **44**, 379, 1965.
69. Post, R. L., and Jolly, P. C.: The linkage of sodium, potassium and ammonium active transport across the human erythrocyte membrane. Biochim. Biophys. Acta, **25**, 118, 1957.
70. Whittam, R.: The asymmetrical stimulation of a membrane adenosine triphosphatase in relation to active cation transport. Biochem. J., **84**, 110, 1962.
71. Chan, P. C., Calabrese, V., and Theil, L. S.: Species differences in the effect of sodium and potassium ions on the ATPase of erythrocyte membranes. Biochim. Biophys. Acta, **79**, 424, 1964.
72. Post, R. L., Merritt, C. R., Kinsolving, C. R., and Albright, C. D.: Membrane adenosine triphosphatase as a participant in the active transport of sodium and potassium in the human erythrocyte. J. Biol. Chem., **235**, 1796, 1960.
73. Dunham, E. T., and Glynn, I. M.: Adenosine triphosphatase activity and the active movements of alkali metal ions. J. Physiol. (London), **156**, 274, 1961.
74. Charnock, J. S., and Post, R. L.: Evidence of the mechanism of ouabain inhibition of cation activated adenosine triphosphatase. Nature (London), **199**, 910, 1963.
75. Hoffman, J. F.: The red cell membrane and the transport of sodium and potassium. Amer. J. Med., **41**, 666, 1966.
76. Wallas, C. H., Parker, J. C., Gitelman, G. J. and Welt, L. G.: Relationships between erythrocyte active transport of sodium, lactate production, and erythrocyte sodium concentration. Clin. Res. **17**, 55, 1969.
77. Parker, J. C., and Hoffman, J. F.: The role of membrane phosphoglycerate kinase in the control of glycolytic rate by active cation transport in human red blood cells. J. Gen. Physiol., **50**, 893, 1967.
78. Minakami, S., and Yoshikawa, H.: Studies on erythrocyte glycolysis.

III. The effects of active cation transport, pH, and inorganic phosphate concentration on erythrocyte glycolysis. J. Biochem. (Tokyo), **59,** 145, 1966.
79. Whittam, R., and Ager, M. E.: The connection between active cation transport and metabolism in erythrocytes. Biochem. J., **97,** 214, 1965.
80. Hokin, L. E., and Hokin, M. R.: Phosphatidic acid metabolism and active transport of sodium. Fed. Proc., **22,** 8, 1963.
81. Hokin, L. E., and Hokin, M. R.: Diglyceride kinase and phosphatidic acid phosphatase in erythrocyte membranes. Nature (London), **189,** 836, 1961.
82. Ahmed, K., and Judah, J. D.: Role of phosphoproteins in ion transport in liver slices. Biochim. Biophys. Acta, **57,** 245, 1962.
83. Rapaport, S., and Hofmann, E. C. G.: Untersuchungen uber den Atmungsstoffwechsel von Reticulocyten. Biochem. Z., **326,** 493, 1955.
84. Schweiger, H. G., Rapaport, S., and Scholzel, E.: Der N-Stoffwechsel bei der erythrozyten reifung: Atmung und ammoniakbildung. Acta Biol. Med. German, **1,** 422, 1958.
85. Guzman Barron, E. S., and Hoffman, L. A.: The catalytic effect of dyes on the oxygen consumption of living cells. J. Gen. Physiol., **13,** 483, 1930.
86. Brin, M., and Yonemoto, R. H.: Stimulation of the glucose oxidative pathway in human erythrocytes by methylene blue. J. Biol. Chem., **230,** 307, 1958.
87. Murphy, J. R.: Erythrocyte metabolism. II. Glucose metabolism and pathways. J. Lab. Clin. Med., **55,** 286, 1960.
88. Carson, P. E., and Okita, G. T.: Metabolic patterns of hemolytic susceptibility, J. Clin. Invest., **42,** 922, 1963.
89. Jandl, J. H., and Jacob., H. S.: Unpublished observations.
90. Jandl, J. H., Engle, L. K., and Allen, D. W.: Oxidative hemolysis and precipitation of hemoglobin. I. Heinz body anemias as an acceleration of red cell aging. J. Clin. Invest., **39,** 1818, 1960.
91. Brewer, G. J., Tarlov, A. R., and Kellermeyer, R. W.: The hemolytic effect of primaquine. XII. Shortened erythrocyte life span in primaquine sensitive male Negroes in the absence of drug administration. J. Lab. Clin. Med., **58,** 217, 1961.
92. Tanaka, K. R., Valentine, W. N., and Miwa, S.: Pyruvate kinase (PK) deficiency hereditary nonspherocytic hemolytic anemia. Blood, **19,** 267, 1962.
93. Prankerd, T. A. J.: *The Red Cell.* Blackwell Scientific Publications, Ltd., Oxford, 1961.
94. Sidbury, J. B., Cornblath, M., Fisher, J., and House, E.: Glycogen in erythrocytes of patients with glycogen storage disease. Pediatrics, **27,** 103, 1961.
95. Eggleton, G. P., and Eggleton, P.: A method of estimating phosphagen and some other phosphorus compounds in muscle tissue. Brit. J. Physiol., **68,** 193, 1929.
96. Park, C. R., Post., R. L., Kalmen, C. F., Wright, J. H., Jr., Johnson, L. H., and Morgan, H. E.: The transport of glucose and other sugars across cell membranes and the effect of insulin in *Internal Secretions of the Pancreas,* vol. 9, p. 240. Ciba Found. Colloq. Endocrinol., 1956.
97. Rose, L. A., and O'Connell, E. L.: The role of glucose 6-phosphate in the regulation of glucose metabolism in human erythrocytes. J. Biol. Chem., **293,** 12, 1964.
98. Whittam, R.: *Transport and Diffusion in Red Blood Cells.* E. Arnold, London, 1964.
99. Gourley, D. R. H.: Glycolysis and phosphate turnover in the human erythrocyte. Arch. Biochem., **40,** 13, 1952.
100. Prankerd, T. A. J., and Altman, K. I.: A study of the metabolism of phosphorus in mammalian red cells. Biochem. J., **58,** 622, 1954.
101. Gourley, D. R. H.: The role of adenosine triphosphate in the transport of phosphate in the human erythrocyte. Arch. Biochem., **40,** 1, 1952.
102. Gerlach, E., Fleckenstein, A., and Gross, E.: Der intermediare Phosphat-stoffwechsel des Menschen-erythrocyten. Arch. Ges. Physiol., **266,** 528, 1958.
103. Bartlett, G. R.: Organization of red cell glycolytic enzymes: Cell coat phosphorus transfer. Ann. NY Acad. Sci., **75,** 110, 1958.
104. Schier, S. L.: Studies of the metabolism of human erythrocyte membranes. J. Clin. Invest., **42,** 756, 1963.
105. Skaug, O. E., and Natvig, R. A.: Inorganic phosphate in human erythrocytes. Scand. J. Clin. Lab. Invest., **9,** 39, 1957.
106. Prankerd, T. A. J.: The metabolism of the human erythrocyte: A review. Brit. J. Haemat., **I,** 131, 1955.
107. Bartlett, G. R.: Human red cell glycolytic intermediates. J. Biol. Chem., **234,** 449, 1959.
108. Robinson, M. A., Loder, P. B., and DeGruchy, G. C.: Red-cell metabolism in non-spherocytic congenital haemolytic anaemia. Brit. J. Haemat., **7,** 327, 1961.
109. Minakani, S. C., Suzuki, T. Soto, and Yoshikawa, H.: Studies on erythrocyte glycolysis. I. Determination of the glycolytic intermediates in human erythrocytes., J. Biochem. (Tokyo), **58,** 543, 1965.
110. Whittam, R.: Potassium movements and ATP in human red cells. J. Physiol. (London), **140,** 479, 1958.
111. Mills, G. C., and Summens, L. B.: The metabolism of nucleotides and other phosphate esters in erythrocytes during in vitro incubation at 37°. Arch. Biochem., **84,** 7, 1959.
112. Shafer, A. W.: Personal communication.
113. Maizels, M.: Cation control in human erythrocytes. J. Physiol. (London), **108,** 247, 1949.
114. Selwyn, J. G., and Dacie, J. V.: Autohemolysis and other changes resulting from the incubation in vitro of red cells from patients with congenital hemolytic anemia. Blood, **9,** 414, 1954.
115. Solomon, A. K.: The permeability of the human erythrocyte to sodium and potassium. J. Gen. Physiol., **36,** 57, 1952.
116. Jandl, J. H., and Tomlinson, A. S.: The destruction of red cells by antibodies in man. II. Pyrogenic, leukocytic and dermal responses to immune hemolysis. J. Clin. Invest., **37,** 1202, 1958.
117. Jacob, H. S., and Jandl, J. H.: Increased cell membrane permeability in the pathogenesis of hereditary spherocytosis. J. Clin. Invest., **43,** 1704, 1964.
118. Reed, C. F., and Swisher, S. N.: Erythrocyte lipid loss in hereditary spherocytosis. J. Clin. Invest., **45,** 777, 1966.
119. Cooper, R. A., and Jandl, J. H.: The selective and conjoint loss of red cell lipids. J. Clin. Invest., **48,** 906, 1969.
120. Weed, R. I., and Bowdler, A. J.: Metabolic dependence of critical hemolytic volume of human erythrocytes: Relationship to osmotic fragility and autohemolysis in hereditary spherocytosis and normal red cells. J. Clin. Invest., **45,** 1137, 1966.
121. Young, L. E., Izzo, M. J., Altman, K. I., and Swisher, S. N.: Studies on spontaneous in vitro autohemolysis in hemolytic disorders. Blood, **11,** 977, 1956.
122. Bishop, C.: Maintenance of ATP level of incubated human red cells by controlling the pH. Transfusion, **2,** 408, 1962.
123. Prankerd, T. A. J.: Studies on the pathogenesis of haemolysis in spherocytosis. Quart. J. Med., **24,** 1944, 1960.
124. Rapaport, S.: Dimensional, osmotic, and chemical changes of erythrocytes in stored blood. I. Blood preserved in sodium citrate, neutral, and acid-citrate-glucose (ACD) mixtures. J. Clin. Invest., **26,** 591, 1947.
125. Gabrio, B. W., Hennessey, M., Thomasson, J., and Finch, C. A.: Erythrocyte preservation. IV. In vitro reversibility of the storage lesion. J. Biol. Chem., **215,** 357, 1955.
126. Gabrio, B. W., Donohue, D. M., Huennekens, F. M., and Finch, C. A.: Erythrocyte preservation. VII. Acid-citrate-dextrose-inosine (ACDI) as a preservative for blood during storage at 4°C. J. Clin. Invest., **35,** 657, 1956.
127. Sandberg, A. A., Lee, G. R., Cartwright, G. E., and Wintrobe, M. M.: Purine nucleoside phosphorylase activity of blood. I. Erythrocytes. J. Clin. Invest., **34,** 1823, 1955.
128. Prankerd, T. A. J.: Cleavage of adenosine by human red cells. Brit. J. Haemat., **I,** 406, 1955.
129. Huennekens, F. M., Nurk, E., and Gabrio, B. W.: Erythrocyte metabolism. I. Purine nucleoside phosphorylase. J. Biol. Chem., **221,** 971, 1961.
130. Lowy, B. A., Ramot, B., and London, I. M.: Adenosine triphosphate metabolism in the rabbit erythrocyte in vivo and in vitro. Ann. NY Acad. Sci., **75,** 148, 1958.
131. Simon, E. R., Chapman, R. G., and Finch, C. A.: Adenine in red cell preservation. J. Clin. Invest., **41,** 351, 1962.
132. Lowy, B. A., Williams, M. K., and London, I. M.: The utilization of

purines and their ribosyl derivatives for the formation of adenosine triphosphate and guanosine triphosphate in the mature rabbit erythrocyte. J. Biol. Chem., **236,** 1439, 1961.
133. Nakao, M., Nakao, T., Tatibana, M., and Yoshikawa, H.: Phosphorus metabolism in human erythrocyte. III. Regeneration of adenosine triphosphate in long-stored erythrocytes by incubation with inosine and adenine. J. Biochem. (Tokyo), **47,** 661, 1960.
134. Schlenk, F.: Biosynthesis of nucleosides and nucleotides, in *The Nucleic Acids,* edited by E. Chargoff and J. N. Davidson, vol. 3, chap. 24, p. 309. Academic, New York, 1955.
135. Rubinstein, D., and Dentedt, O. F.: The metabolism of nucleosides by the erythrocyte. XIV. Metabolism of nucleosides by the erythrocyte. Canad. J. Biochem., **34,** 927, 1956.
136. Dacie, J. V.: Observations on autohaemolysis in familial acholuric jaundice. J. Path. Bact., **52,** 331, 1941.
137. Mohler, D. N.: Reduction of in vitro autohemolysis in hereditary spherocytosis in impermeant molecules. Blood, **30,** 449, 1967.
138. MacKinney, A. A., Jr., Morton, N. E., Kosower, N. S., and Schilling, R. F.: Ascertaining genetic carriers of hereditary spherocytosis by statistical analysis of multiple laboratory tests. J. Clin. Invest., **41,** 554, 1962.
139. Simon, E. R.: Expanded autohemolysis as an investigative and diagnostic tool in hemolytic disorders. Clin. Res. **11,** 200, 1963.
140. Prankerd, T. A. J., Altman, K. I., and Young, L. E.: Abnormalities of carbohydrate metabolism of red cells in hereditary spherocytosis. J. Clin. Invest., **34,** 1268, 1955.
141. Motulsky, A. G., Gabrio, B. W., Burkhardt, J., and Finch, C. A.: Erythrocyte carbohydrate metabolism in hereditary hemolytic anemias. Amer. J. Med., **19,** 291, 1955.
142. Altman, K. I., and Izzo, M. J., quoted in Young, L. E.: Hereditary spherocytosis. Amer. J. Med., **18,** 486, 1955.
143. Tabechian, H., Altman, K. I., and Young, L. E.: Inhibition of P^{32}-orthophosphate exchange by sodium fluoride in erythrocytes from patients with hereditary spherocytosis. Proc. Soc. Exp. Biol. Med., **92,** 712, 1956.
144. Prankerd, T. A. J.: Inborn errors of metabolism in red cells of congenital hemolytic anemias. Amer. J. Med., **22,** 724, 1957.
145. Weinstein, I. M., Dunn, I., Coe, E. L., and Ibsen, K. H.: Erythrocyte carbohydrate metabolism in hereditary spherocytosis. Clin. Res., **8,** 133, 1960.
146. Shafer, A. W.: Glycolytic intermediates of erythrocytes in hereditary spherocytosis. Clin. Res., **9,** 67, 1961.
147. Zipursky, A., Mayman, D., and Israels, L. G.: Phosphate metabolism in erythrocytes of normal humans and of patients with hereditary spherocytosis. Canad. J. Biochem., **40,** 95, 1962.
148. Tanaka, K. R., Valentine, W. N., and Miwa, S.: Studies on hereditary spherocytosis and other hemolytic anemias. Clin. Res., **10,** 109, 1962.
149. Shafer, A. W.: The phosphorylated carbohydrate intermediates from erythrocytes in hereditary spherocytosis. Blood, **23,** 417, 1964.
150. Dunn, I., Ibsen, K. H., Coe, E. L., Schneider, A. S., and Weinstein, I. M.: Erythrocyte carbohydrate metabolism in hereditary spherocytosis. J. Clin. Invest., **42,** 1535, 1963.
151. Mohler, D. N.: Adenosine triphosphate metabolism in hereditary spherocytosis J. Clin. Invest., **44,** 1417, 1965.
152. Reed, C. F. and Young, L. E.: Erythrocyte energy metabolism in hereditary spherocytosis. J. Clin. Invest., **46,** 1196, 1967.
153. Harris, E. J., and Prankerd, T. A. J.: The rate of sodium extrusion from human erythrocytes. J. Physiol. (London), **121,** 470, 1953.
154. Bertles, J. F.: Sodium transport across the surface membrane of red blood cells in hereditary spherocytosis. J. Clin. Invest., **36,** 816, 1957.
155. Nakao, K., Kurashina, S., and Nakao, M.: Adenosinetriphosphatase activity of erythrocyte membrane in hereditary spherocytosis. Life Sci., **6,** 595, 1967.
156. Konsek, J., and Bishop, C.: Relationship between adenosine triphosphate and cation transport in the human red cell. Proc. Soc. Exp. Biol. Med., **110,** 813, 1962.
157. Rose, I. A., Warms, J. V. B., and O'Connell, E. L.: Role of inorganic phosphate in stimulating the glucose utilization of human red cells. Biochem. Biophys. Res. Commun., **15,** 33, 1964.
158. Wiley, J. S.: Dominant inheritance of the sodium leak in hereditary spherocytic red cells and a comparison of sodium leak with red cell survival. Aust. Ann. Med., **17,** 177, 1968. (Abstract.)
159. Oski, F. A., Naiman, J. L., Blum, S. F., Zarkowsky, Whaun, J., Shohet, S. B., Green, A., and Nathan, D. G.: Congenital hemolytic anemia with high-sodium, low-potassium red cells. New Eng. J. Med., **280,** 909, 1969.
160. Cooper, R. A., and Jandl, J. H.: The role of membrane lipids in the survival of red cells in hereditary spherocytosis. J. Clin. Invest., **48,** 736, 1969.
161. Langley, G. R., and Felderhof, C. H.: Atypical autohemolysis in hereditary spherocytosis as a reflection of two cell populations: Relationship of cell lipids to conditioning by the spleen. Blood, **32,** 569, 1968.
162. Westerman, M. P., Pierce, L. E., and Jensen, W. N.: Erythrocyte lipids: A comparison of normal young and normal old populations. J. Lab. Clin. Med., **62,** 394, 1963.
163. van Gastel, C., van Den Berg, D., De Gier, J., van Deenen, L. L. M.: Some lipid characteristics of normal red blood cells of different age. Brit. J. Haemat., **11,** 193–199, 1965.
164. Phillips, G. B., and Roome, N. S.: Quantitative chromatographic analysis of the phospholipids of abnormal human red blood cells. Proc. Soc. Exp. Biol. Med., **109,** 360, 1962.
165. De Gier, J., van Deenen, L. L. M., Geerdink, R. A., Punt, K., and Verloop, M. C.: Phosphatide patterns of normal, spherocytic and elliptocytic red blood cells. Biochim. Biophys. Acta, **50,** 383–384, 1961.
166. De Gier. J., van Deenen, L. L. M., Verloop, M. C., and van Gastel, C.: Phospholipid and fatty acid characteristics of erythrocytes in some cases of anaemia. Brit. J. Haemat., **10,** 246, 1964.
167. Bradlow, B. A., Lee, J., and Rubenstein, R.: Erythrocyte phospholipids: Quantitative thin layer chromatography in paroxysmal nocturnal haemoglobinuria and hereditary spherocytosis. Brit. J. Haemat., **11,** 315, 1965.
168. Allison, A. C., Kates, M., and James, A. T.: An abnormality of blood lipids in hereditary spherocytosis. Brit. Med. J., **2,** 1766, 1960.
169. Kates, M., Allison, A. C., and James, A. T.: Phosphatides of human blood cells and their role in spherocytosis. Biochim. Biophys. Acta, **48,** 571, 1961.
170. Robertson, A. F., and Lands, W. E. M.: Metabolism of phospholipids in normal and spherocytic human erythrocytes. J. Lipid Res., **5,** 88, 1964.
171. Jacob, H. S., and Karnovsky, M. L.: Concomitant alterations of sodium flux and membrane phospholipid metabolism in red blood cells: Studies in hereditary spherocytosis. J. Clin. Invest., **46,** 173–185, 1967.
172. Reed, C. F.: Incorporation of orthophosphate-^{32}P into erythrocyte phospholipids in normal subjects and in patients with hereditary spherocytosis. J. Clin. Invest., **47,** 2630, 1968.
173. Jacob, H. S.: Membrane lipid depletion in hyperpermeable red blood cells: Its role in the genesis of spherocytes in hereditary spherocytosis. J. Clin. Invest., **46,** 2080, 1967.
174. Jacob, H. S.: Abnormalities in the physiology of the erythrocyte membrane in hereditary spherocytosis. Amer. J. Med., **41,** 734, 1966.
175. Jacob, H. S., and Jandl, J. H.: Effects of sulfhydryl inhibition on red blood cells. I. Mechanism of hemolysis. J. Clin. Invest., **41,** 779, 1962.
176. Jacob, H. S., and Jandl, J. H.: Effects of sulfhydryl inhibition on red blood cells. II. Studies in vivo. J. Clin. Invest., **41,** 1514, 1962.
177. Björkman, S. E.: The splenic circulation. Acta Med. Scand., suppl. 191, 1947.
178. Murphy, J. R.: The influence of pH and temperature on some physical properties of normal erythrocytes and erythrocytes from patients with hereditary spherocytosis. J. Lab. Clin. Med., **69,** 758–775, 1967.
179. Griggs, R. C., Weisman, R., Jr., and Harris, J. W.: Alterations in osmotic and mechanical fragility related to in vivo erythrocyte aging and splenic sequestration in hereditary spherocytosis. J. Clin. Invest., **39,** 89, 1960.
180. Stobie, G. H.: Splenosis. Canad. Med. Ass. J., **56,** 374, 1947.
181. Mackenzie, F. A. F., Elliot, D. H., Eastcott, H. G., II., Hughes-Jones, N. C., Barkhan, P., and Mollison, P. L.: Relapse in hereditary spherocytosis with proven splenunculus. Lancet, **I,** 1102, 1962.
182. Wilson, C.: Some cases showing hereditary enlargement of the spleen. Trans. Clin. Soc. London, **23,** 162, 1890.

183. Meulengracht, E.: Über die Erblichkeitsverhältnisse beim chronischen hereditären hämolyischen Ikterus. Deutsch. Arch. Klin. Med., **136,** 33, 1921.
184. Campbell, J. M. H., and Warner, E. C.: Heredity in acholuric jaundice. Quart. J. Med., **19,** 333, 1925–1926.
185. Race, R. R.: On the inheritance and linkage relations of acholuric jaundice. Ann. Eugenics, **11,** 365, 1942.
186. Abrams, M., and Battle, J. D., Jr.: A genetic study in hereditary spherocytosis. Amer. J. Hum. Genet., **4,** 350, 1952.
187. Young, L. E.: Observations on inheritance and heterogeneity of chronic spherocytosis. Trans. Ass. Amer. Physicians, **68,** 141, 1955.
188. Lawrence, J.: A genetic study of a family with hereditary spherocytosis (H.S.) and hyperuricemia. Clin. Res., **8,** 211, 1960.
189. Bernard, I., Boiron, M., and Estager, J.: Une grande famille hémolytique: Treize cas de maladie de Minkowski-Chaufford observés dans le méme patrie. Sem. Hop. Paris, **28,** 3741, 1952.
190. Morton, N. E., Mackinney, A. A., Kosower, N., Schiling, R. F., and Gray, M. P.: Genetics of spherocytosis. Amer. J. Hum. Genet., **14,** 170, 1962.
191. Neel, J. V.: Haemopoietic system. I. Inherited abnormalities of the cellular constituents of the blood, in *Clinical Genetics,* edited by A. Sorsby, p. 446. Mosby, St. Louis, 1953.
192. Anderson, R., Huetis, R. R., and Motulsky, A. G.: Hereditary spherocytosis in the deer mouse: Its similarity to the human disease. Blood, **15,** 491, 1960.
193. Morton, N. E.: The detection and estimation of linkage between the genes for elliptocytosis and Rh blood type. Amer. J. Hum. Genet., **8,** 80, 1956.
194. Crosby, W. H., and Conrad, M. E.: Hereditary spherocytosis: Observations on hemolytic mechanisms and iron metabolism. Blood, **15,** 662, 1960.

CHAPTER FIFTY-FOUR

PYRUVATE KINASE DEFICIENCY AND OTHER ENZYME-DEFICIENCY HEREDITARY HEMOLYTIC ANEMIAS*

William N. Valentine and Kouichi R. Tanaka

The hereditary hemolytic anemias of man are a heterogeneous group of diseases. In some an abnormal hemoglobin is present; in some, the thalassemic syndromes, there is an inability to synthesize quantitatively one or another of the peptide chains of globin; in some, which are the subject of this chapter, specific enzyme deficiencies appear to constitute the molecular basis of anemia. In still other instances, such as hereditary spherocytosis, the precise etiology remains obscure.

The emergence of hereditary hemolytic anemias associated with enzyme deficiency as clinical entities derived impetus from two main sources. The first was the definition of a specific deficiency of glucose-6-phosphate dehydrogenase (G-6-PD) [1] as the common denominator responsible for hemolytic episodes in persons receiving antimalarial agents such as primaquine and certain other drugs, or who were subject to favism [2]. The second was the studies of Dacie and his colleagues [3] of certain hereditary anemias which they described as "nonspherocytic," in contrast to the better known disorder of hereditary spherocytosis. These were clearly of heterogeneous etiology, but had in common the absence of detectable abnormal hemoglobin, a negative antiglobulin test, the absence of more than a rare spherocyte, a normal osmotic fragility when fresh red cells were tested, and only partial benefit from splenectomy. Selwyn and Dacie [4] categorized such cases as Type I or Type II on the basis of different behavior in an in vitro autohemolysis test. When sterile blood was incubated for 48 hr, the degree of hemolysis was comparable to or only slightly greater than that of normal blood in cases classified as Type I. Addition of glucose reduced the autohemolysis somewhat less than was true with normal cells. Type II erythrocytes generally showed marked autohemolysis not corrected by glucose; these red cells were found to have impaired conversion of glucose to lactate, and a defect in glycolysis was postulated. These findings were substantiated and extended by de Gruchy and his associates [5, 6] and Robinson et al. [7], who found abnormally low glucose utilization, reduced erythrocyte ATP, and an accumulation of certain phosphorylated intermediates. A defect in glycolysis beyond the point of 2,3-diphosphoglycerate (2,3-DPG) was suspected in Type II erythrocytes.

In 1961, Valentine, Tanaka, and Miwa [8] demonstrated a specific erythrocyte deficiency of the glycolytic enzyme, pyruvate kinase (PK), in three patients with congenital hemolytic anemia conforming to the Type II category. These findings and corollary studies were soon extended to additional patients [9] and similar cases have now been documented in many laboratories throughout the world [10–59]. Since 1961 a number of other hemolytic anemias associated with erythrocyte enzyme deficiencies due to inborn errors have been identified [60]. These may be categorized as (1) deficiencies in enzymes of the anaerobic, Embden-Meyerhof pathway; (2) deficiencies in the oxidative hexosemonophosphate (HMP) shunt pathway; and (3) deficiencies in certain nonglycolytic enzymes (Table 54-1).

In addition to pyruvate kinase deficiency, deficiencies of anaerobic glycolytic pathway enzymes associated with hereditary hemolytic disorders include those involving hexokinase (HK) [61–63], glucosephosphate isomerase (GPI) [64, 65], triosephosphate isomerase (TPI) [66–69], phosphoglycerate kinase (PGK) [70–72], and 2,3-diphosphoglyceromutase (2,3-DPGM) [16, 28, 73–75]. In addition, mild hemolytic disease has been reported in association with an inherited myopathy in which phosphofructokinase (PFK) activity is severely deficient in muscle and partially deficient in red cells [76–78]. Partial, and in one kindred, marked, deficiency of 6-phosphogluconate dehydrogenase (6-PGD), the second enzyme of the HMP shunt pathway, has been identified, but the clinical correlation with hemolytic anemia remains somewhat uncertain [79–85]. Among nonglycolytic enzyme deficiencies, that of glutathione reductase (GSSG-R) [86–93] is well documented as associated with a hereditary hemolytic syndrome. In a Dutch kindred a moderately severe hemolytic process has been observed in several members whose erythrocytes exhibit almost total lack of either oxidized or reduced glutathione [94–97]. The inborn error is thought to reside in the glutathione synthetase system [97, 98], with an inability to fully synthesize the tripeptide, glutathione (GSH). Possibly, but less certainly, related to chronic hemolysis are reported deficiencies in the enzymes ATPase [99] and glutathione peroxidase [100]. In addition, four different types of erythrocytes with high ATP content are known to occur [101]. In two, no hemolytic disorder has been found, while in the remaining two types hemolysis has been present [101–105].

NORMAL RED CELL METABOLISM

Erythrocyte metabolism is discussed in Chaps. 53, 55, and 56. The developing erythrocyte has the full metabolic machinery for replication, differentiation, and self-sustenance, and the reticulocyte (although nonnucleated) still has a

*Certain reported studies from the authors' laboratories were supported by Public Health Service Research Grants HE-1069 and HE-08757 from the National Heart Institute.

limited capacity for protein and lipid synthesis and the incorporation of iron into hemoglobin. Beyond the reticulocyte stage, the mature, nonnucleated red cell possesses no DNA, RNA, mitochondria or other intracellular organelles and only ineffectual vestiges of Kreb cycle metabolism. It can synthesize no new protein and hence no new enzymes. Its catalytic proteins, each with its own biologic half-life under any given set of conditions, decay at various rates as the cell ages. It is uniquely dependent essentially upon anaerobic and aerobic production of lactate from glucose to supply its small but definite energy requirements. The Embden-Meyerhof pathway of anaerobic glycolysis provides a mechanism for generating ATP and for cycling NAD to NADH and back again. The intact HMP pathway is associated with the conversion of NADP to NADPH, the latter serving primarily to maintain reduced glutathione since it is the cofactor necessary for glutathione reductase activity. No mechanism exists in the red cell for converting the energy of NADPH into high-energy phosphate bonds.

The concentration of two organic phosphate intermediates of glucose metabolism, 2,3-DPG and glucose-1,6-diphosphate, is uniquely high in human and certain mammalian erythrocytes [106, 107]. While the full metabolic significance of this is unknown, it is known that 2,3-DPG (formed from 1,3-DPG by the action of 2,3-DPGM) can be returned to the mainstream of glycolysis as 3-phosphomonoglycerate (3-PG) through the action of a phosphatase. This pathway (the Rapoport-Luebering shunt) [108, 109] bypasses one of the ATP-generating steps of the Embden-Meyerhof pathway—that mediated by phosphoglycerate kinase. About 90 percent of glucose metabolized normally traverses the anaerobic pathway [110], but HMP shunt pathway metabolism is greatly enhanced by any drug or agent capable of oxidizing GSH. Through the action of transketolase and transaldolase, intermediates of the HMP and Embden-Meyerhof pathway are interconvertible. Pentose phosphate generated in the former may thus be metabolized to lactate and result in production of ATP. In the simplest illustration, 1 mole of glucose progressing anaerobically to lactate is associated with a net gain of 2 moles of ATP. However, because variable amounts of glucose may be metabolized through the Rapoport-Luebering shunt, a net gain of between 0 and 2 moles of ATP actually results, depending on the fraction of glucose entering the 2,3-DPG pool. The adult red cell has small energy requirements, but it must maintain its shape, pump cations across its membrane against electrochemical gradients, protect itself against oxidative environmental stresses, and resist the conversion of its oxyhemoglobin to methemoglobin. Under normal circumstances, it is thought to approach ultimate destruction as a result of the slow denaturation of its irreplaceable metabolic machinery and is finally unable to maintain the energy requirements for survival [111–115]. Genetically imposed handicaps, further restricting its already limited resources, can be expected, when severe, to shorten survival in vivo and lead to hemolytic anemia.

PYRUVATE KINASE (PK) DEFICIENCY

Clinical Aspects

Incidence

Over 100 documented cases [9–59, 116–121] of pyruvate kinase deficiency hemolytic anemia have appeared in the world literature since the original description in 1961 [8]. A number of patients previously described as atypical or familial, or as having Dacie's Type II nonspherocytic hemolytic anemia, have been found deficient in this red cell enzyme when specifically assayed for pyruvate kinase [14, 17, 26, 46, 56]. It now appears that PK deficiency and G-6-PD deficiency are the most common of the known enzyme deficiency hereditary hemolytic anemias [42, 117, 122]. Other inborn errors of the Embden-Meyerhof pathway, which have been described subsequently and are discussed elsewhere in this chapter, are comparatively rare.

Patients with this disorder have been found primarily in the United States and Europe [117, 121], but also in Australia [14, 33], New Zealand [52], Canada [43, 51], and Japan [34]. The disease is most common in people of Northern European origin [8, 9, 117, 121] (Table 54-2), but it has been noted in Italians [10, 12, 13, 18, 23, 57], a girl of Syrian descent [56], a Spanish infant [59], a Mexican child [9], American Negroes [56, 123, 124], and in the Japanese [34]. A particularly high incidence of this disorder has been identified in the Mifflin County (Pennsylvania) Amish deme [32]. Both sexes are affected equally [9, 11, 30, 34, 116, 122].

Clinical Features

Patients with PK deficiency hemolytic anemia have no distinguishing or pathognomonic clinical features. They have the usual hallmarks of most chronic hemolytic processes, such as jaundice of varying degree, slight to moderate splenomegaly as a rule, and an increased incidence of gallstones [9, 11, 12, 15, 20–22, 27, 40, 42, 43, 48, 52, 116]. Considerable variation exists in the severity of the clinical disease [9]. The spectrum ranges from severe neonatal anemia requiring exchange or multiple transfusions, at one extreme [9, 11, 20, 21, 39, 41, 43, 52, 56–58], to a fully compensated hemolytic process in healthy adults at the other [9, 50, 52]. Transfusion requirements vary considerably [9]. The majority of patients have required transfusions but a significant number have maintained a comfortable hemoglobin level without them [9, 15, 34, 42, 50, 52]. A temporary exacerbation in the hemolytic process may occur in association with an intercurrent illness or surgical treatment [9, 24, 42]. On the whole, PK deficiency is a more severe disease than is hereditary spherocytosis [58].

In the majority of cases of PK deficiency, anemia or jaundice, or both, are noted in infancy or early childhood [9, 34, 58], but some patients apparently escape detection until adulthood [9, 15, 34, 40, 43, 50, 52, 58]. The deficiency

Table 54-1. HEREDITARY HEMOLYTIC ANEMIAS DUE TO ENZYME DEFICIENCIES

Enzyme deficiency	Frequency	RBC	WBC	Genetics	Comments
A. Embden-Meyerhof pathway					
1. Hexokinase (HK)	Rare	Deficient	Normal	Probably autosomal recessive	Utilization of glucose and fructose greatly reduced in comparison to nondeficient reticulocyte-rich blood.
2. Glucosephosphate isomerase (GPI)	Rare	Deficient	Deficient	Autosomal recessive	Starch-gel electrophoresis indicates genetic heterogeneity.
3. Phosphofructokinase (PFK)	Rare	About 50% deficient			Minimal, compensated hemolysis is clinically insignificant part of a severe muscle disorder (glycogen storage disease, Type VII).
4. Triosephosphate isomerase (TPI)	Rare	Deficient	Deficient	Autosomal recessive	Plasma, spinal fluid, skeletal muscle also very low in TPI. Homozygotes have severe neurologic syndrome and tendency to unexplained, sudden death. Nine homozygotes now recognized.
5. 2,3-Diphosphoglyceromutase (2,3-DPGM)	Rare	Deficient		Possibly autosomal recessive	Atypical features require further study in clearly defined cases. (See text.)
6. Phosphoglycerate kinase (PGK)	Rare	Deficient	Deficient	X-chromosome linked	So far rare. Neurologic and behavioral abnormalities are possibly associated with severe deficiency.
7. Pyruvate kinase (PK)	Most common next to G-6-PD	Deficient	Normal	Autosomal recessive	Predominantly Northern European ancestry reported. Wide clinical variability. Clear evidence of genetic heterogeneity.
B. Hexosemonophosphate (HMP) shunt pathway					
1. Glucose-6-phosphate dehydrogenase (G-6-PD)	Common	Deficient	Partially deficient —some types only	X-chromosome linked	See Chap. 55 for detailed discussion.
2. 6-Phosphogluconate dehydrogenase (6-PGD)	Rare	Partially deficient	Deficient in some variants only	Autosomal recessive	Relation of partial deficiency to hemolysis in few available reports not conclusive.
C. Nonglycolytic pathways					
1. Glutathione reductase (GSSG-R)	Uncertain	Usually partially deficient		?	Many syndromes including hemolytic anemia reported with partial to (rarely) severe deficiency. Clinical heterogeneity and role of riboflavin nutrition in coenzyme FAD availability often render interpretation uncertain. (See text.)

Table 54-1. (*Continued*)

Enzyme deficiency	Frequency	RBC	WBC	Genetics	Comments
2. Glutathione peroxidase (GSH-Px)	Rare	Deficient		?	RBC showed 25 to 30% normal activity of GSH-Px.
3. Glutathione synthetase Reaction II	Rare	Deficient		Autosomal recessive, presumably	GSH nearly totally absent in RBC. Primaquine sensitive. Chronic hemolytic anemia present in absence of drug administration. Defect is deficiency in enzyme-catalyzing γ-glutamyl cysteine + glycine $\xrightarrow[Mg^{++}]{ATP}$ GSH.
4. ATPase					Data too fragmentary to permit conclusions. A single report of partial deficiency in hemolytic anemia of undetermined cause.

has been recognized at birth [25], as well as in a woman of 65 years [45]. In spite of a moderately severe hemolytic anemia in most instances, survival to adulthood is common [9, 12, 15, 20, 23, 30, 34, 40, 42, 43, 46, 48, 50, 52, 56]. A particularly severe form found in the Amish kindreds is often fatal in early childhood unless splenectomy is performed [11, 32].

Splenomegaly of slight to moderate degree is the rule [9, 11, 12, 15, 20, 21, 34, 40, 43, 56] but is not invariable [34, 52]. Hepatomegaly is inconstant. Chronic leg ulcers may occur, though rarely [116]. Growth retardation and prominent frontal bosses may be observed in some of the severely affected children [9, 11, 20], but general development is usually normal. Women with PK deficiency seem to tolerate pregnancy with no unusual complications [34, 42, 43, 117].

Table 54-2. ANCESTRAL BACKGROUND OF PK-DEFICIENT PATIENTS

	No. of cases
"Northern European" origin	Predominant
United States, England, France, Germany, Canada, Australia, New Zealand, Netherlands, Denmark, Sweden, Switzerland	100+
Mediterranean area	
Italian	4
Syrian	1
Japanese	4
Negro	3
Mexican	1
Spanish	1

Hematologic Findings

The levels of hemoglobin and packed red cell volumes vary widely, but generally fall in the range of 6 to 12 gm per 100 ml and 17 to 37 ml per 100 ml blood, respectively [9, 12, 21, 30, 34, 40, 42, 43, 52]. A fairly uniform macrocytosis of slight to moderate degree is characteristic of adults [9, 12, 34, 42] and is probably related to the moderate to marked reticulocytosis which is usually present [9, 12, 30, 42]. Folic acid deficiency is not an etiologic factor [21]. Very high reticulocyte counts occur only after splenectomy [30, 42, 117]. The erythrocytes are normochromic with only slight anisocytosis and poikilocytosis [9, 12, 34, 40, 42]. Moderate polychromasia is present. Irregularly contracted red cells or cells with irregular borders, tailed poikilocytes, and elongated oval forms may be occasionally observed, as well as variable numbers of nucleated red cells [9, 12, 21, 24, 34, 42]. In infants or young children with severe anemia, greater degrees of morphologic change may occur. In a few cases, bizarre red cells resembling acanthocytes have been seen [24, 119]. Certain features such as Pappenheimer bodies, siderocytes, Howell-Jolly bodies, and target cells may appear following splenectomy [9, 21, 42], but are not specific for this disorder. The white blood count and platelet count are normal or slightly increased [9, 11, 21].

There is usually modest to moderate elevation of the serum bilirubin, which is mostly indirect reacting [9, 11, 21, 40, 43]. Plasma hemoglobin is not elevated [11], but serum haptoglobin may be decreased or absent [11, 21]. Fecal urobilinogen excretion is increased [9, 11, 34]. The serum iron is normal or slightly increased, and total iron binding capacity is normal [9, 42, 43]. The osmotic fragility of fresh red cells is normal, but the incubated fragility test may show varying degrees of abnormality [9, 11, 12, 21, 34, 40, 43, 52]. The autohemolysis test is described elsewhere in this chapter.

The Coombs' test and acid serum (Ham's) test are negative [9, 11, 12, 21, 40, 43, 52]. Donath-Landsteiner antibody and cold agglutinins are also absent [9, 11]. Hemoglobin is of the normal adult type (AA) [9, 11, 40]; fetal hemoglobin [9, 11, 15] and hemoglobin A_2 [11] are within normal limits. No Heinz bodies are observed by supravital staining [9, 42].

Other Laboratory Findings

Liver function tests are normal except for the bilirubinemia already mentioned. Routine urinalysis is normal, but urobilinogen may be increased [9]. Bone changes consistent with a hyperplastic marrow such as that seen in chronic hemolytic anemias may be observed in some of the severe cases during infancy or early childhood [11, 21].

Pathology

As expected, the bone marrow undergoes normoblastic hyperplasia [9–11, 24, 27, 40, 43, 52]. Hemosiderin is usually present in increased quantities. The spleen is moderately enlarged at the time of splenectomy and demonstrates no other remarkable gross features [9–11, 40, 41, 43]. Likewise, there are no specific histologic findings, but reticuloendothelial hyperplasia, variable degrees of congestion and deposits of hemosiderin, and erythrophagocytosis may be observed [9–11, 41, 46, 52]. Extramedullary hematopoiesis is usually not seen, but may occur. The liver is histologically normal [125]. As in any chronic hemolytic disease, cholelithiasis may appear at an early age.

Ferrokinetics and Red Cell Life Span Studies

Studies of ferrokinetics utilizing ^{59}Fe demonstrate a short plasma clearance time, before or after splenectomy [9]. A rapid maximal or near maximal appearance of radioiron in circulating erythrocytes is usually seen.

In most instances there is moderate to severe shortening of red cell life span as determined with the ^{51}Cr procedure for erythrocyte labeling [9, 11, 19, 24, 28, 34, 40, 41, 47, 48, 117]. Some splenic sequestration has been noted in a few patients [9, 11] but not in others [19, 20, 34, 43, 49]. Half-life times of 3.5, 4.3, and 5.7 days (normal = 27), with mean cell life estimated as 5.4, 6.7, and 9.3 days, respectively (normal = 110 to 120 days), were observed when red cells of three severely affected, splenectomized children were transfused into normal compatible recipients [11]. After autotransfusion of two of these splenectomized children, the red cell survival was greater than in the circulation of their corresponding normal recipients with intact spleens, as simultaneously determined. Similar findings are described by Oski, Nathan, and colleagues [24, 54]. In both autologous and isologous survival studies with PK-deficient erythrocytes from *splenectomized* patients, the ^{51}Cr survival curves are complex and suggest the destruction of variably affected red cells at different rates.

Contrary to the results seen when deficient erythrocytes from a *splenectomized* PK patient were studied as mentioned above, the autologous and isologous survival curves were virtually identical when PK-deficient red cells of a patient with an intact spleen were investigated [54]. Furthermore, no advantage is conferred on these cells when they circulate in splenectomized "normal" recipients. The spleen and liver scan patterns also differ somewhat from those observed during survival studies of red cells derived from splenectomized deficient subjects. In addition, by utilizing doubly labeled PK erythrocytes, Nathan and associates [54] have shown that a population of "young" PK cells contains more seriously damaged cells than a population of older cells, the latter surviving to an older age because of their improved initial outlook. These investigations also provide a reasonable explanation for the minimal or slight shortening of ^{51}Cr half-times reported in some patients with clinical and laboratory evidence of overt hemolysis [27, 43, 117].

Role of Spleen

The role of the spleen in the hemolytic anemia of PK deficiency is not clearly understood. As alluded to above, the ^{51}Cr data are conflicting in regard to splenic sequestration. There is increasing evidence that PK-deficient reticulocytes are selectively sequestered in the spleen [11, 42, 54]. On the basis of their extensive studies, Nathan and associates suggest that the spleen may "temper" the PK-deficient cell, and particularly the reticulocyte, so that its destruction in the liver is enhanced [54]. Splenectomy permits longer survival of newly formed cells, and hence the absolute reticulocyte count usually rises after removal of the spleen in this disease.

Clinical Effect of Splenectomy

Although initially it was thought that splenectomy is of little benefit in PK deficiency [9, 14, 26], there is now sufficient experience [11, 20, 21, 24, 40–43, 52, 54, 58] to indicate that some degree of improvement frequently occurs following removal of the spleen, especially in infants or young children with severe disease. The level of packed cell volume may increase significantly, transfusion requirements may decrease or be eliminated, growth and development in severely affected children may be accelerated, and osseous changes may revert toward normal. In the severe Amish cases it appears that splenectomy may be necessary for survival [11]. Nevertheless, in contrast to splenectomy in hereditary spherocytosis, the hemolytic process clearly persists in all cases.

Treatment

There is no specific therapy. The usual hematopoietic agents are not efficacious [9], although supplementary folic acid may be of value in some patients as in any chronic hemolytic process. Splenectomy is not curative, but often is of distinct value. It is indicated for those severely affected patients who need repeated blood transfusions or whose anemia is significantly symptomatic.

Biochemistry and Metabolism

Pyruvate Kinase Assay

Pyruvate kinase catalyzes the conversion of phosphoenolpyruvate to pyruvate with regeneration of ATP. The assay procedure employs phosphoenolpyruvate as substrate, buffer, ADP, KCl, $MgSO_4$, crystalline lactate dehydrogenase, NADH, and hemolysate, and is quantitated in terms of the linked reaction by which the pyruvate formed is transformed to lactate. The conversion of NADH to NAD is measured spectrophotometrically at 340 mμ (Fig. 54-1). Pyruvate kinase activity is defined in arbitrary units, as indicated in Table 54-3. The absolute activities observed in any laboratory, of course, may vary with the temperature at which the assay is performed as well as with the concentration of reactants. This procedure has been widely used and has proven to be a fairly reliable index for separating homozygous, heterozygous, and normal subjects [117, 120] (Table 54-3). Two screening methods [126, 127], as well as an automated assay system [128], have been described, but as yet have not been employed extensively.

Pyruvate Kinase Activity

A review of the clinical reports indicates that most PK-deficient patients have 5 to 25 percent of the normal (mean) red cell enzyme level and heterozygotes have about half the normal activity. Red cell PK values obtained by the spectrophotometric method, employing the assay conditions described previously [9], are shown in Table 54-3 for the initial nine PK patients examined in our laboratories. Although there is considerable variability in activity within the homozygous and heterozygous range, the values seldom overlap [117]. When clinically affected patients have PK values in the normal or heterozygous range, the possibility of a kinetically aberrant isozyme of pyruvate kinase should be considered [118]. Erythrocyte pyruvate kinase has not been found to be reduced markedly (in the homozygous range) in any other condition [9, 117, 120, 129] and is usually increased in other hemolytic disorders (Table 54-4), since reticulocytes and young red cells have greater activity than older cells [9, 130].

The fact that there is poor quantitative correlation between PK activity and clinical severity and that some asymptomatic heterozygotes have PK values within the homozygous range [9, 44, 56, 117] indicates that the assay, although useful, does not provide a precise quantitative measure of the metabolic derangement in the intact cell. It must be remembered that only metabolically affluent young cells, still capable of com-

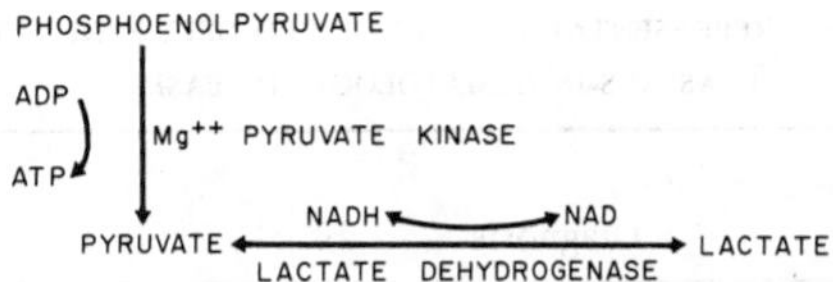

Figure 54-1. Schematic illustration of the glycolytic reaction catalyzed by pyruvate kinase and the subsequent conversion of pyruvate to lactate.

Table 54-3. PYRUVATE KINASE* ACTIVITY IN HEREDITARY HEMOLYTIC ANEMIA DUE TO PYRUVATE KINASE DEFICIENCY

		RBC			WBC		
Subject	No.	Mean	s.d.	Range	Mean	s.d.	Range
Normal	40	2.65	±0.34	2.00–3.40	850	±195	547–1,260
Presumed heterozygotes	47	1.20	±0.32	0.63–1.73†	1,018	±284	513–1,883
J.L.		0.00			729		
R.C.		0.18			697		
H.C.		0.14			627		
E.T.		0.30			1,144		
S.H.		0.00			670		
K.H.‡		0.81			621		
M.M.‡		0.83			638		
W.N.		0.29			664		
S.R.‡		0.71			810		

* One unit = that activity resulting in the conversion of 1 μmole NADH to NAD per min by 10^{10} RBC or WBC at 37°C under the assay conditions of these experiments.

† Except for single value of 0.35.

‡ Not entirely free of transfused cells when studied.

Table 54-4. REPRESENTATIVE DATA OF RED CELL PYRUVATE KINASE ASSAYS IN HEMATOLOGIC DISEASES

Diagnosis	PK activity*
Normal subjects (40) (mean and s.d.)	2.65 ± 0.34
Cord blood (mean of 7 samples)	4.71
Hereditary nonspherocytic hemolytic anemia, Type I	3.78
Hereditary Heinz body hemolytic anemia due to unstable hemoglobin	10.33
Nonspherocytic hemolytic anemia, unknown type	10.55
Nonspherocytic hemolytic anemia due to G-6-PD deficiency	6.19
Acquired hemolytic anemia (Coombs-negative)	8.25
Acquired hemolytic anemia (Coombs-positive)	5.00
Hereditary spherocytosis	4.14
Hereditary spherocytosis (postsplenectomy)	2.20
Hereditary elliptocytosis with anemia	4.44
Sickle-cell anemia (SS)	5.84
Sickle-cell hemoglobin C disease	3.26
Paroxysmal nocturnal hemoglobinuria	5.84
Thalassemia minor	4.50
Pernicious anemia in relapse	6.97
Polycythemia rubra vera	2.49
Myelofibrosis with myeloid metaplasia	3.67
Aplastic anemia	2.51
Iron deficiency anemia	4.25

* See Table 54-3 for definition of unit of pyruvate kinase activity.

pensating for their glycolytic deficiency, are available for assay. Furthermore, the PK assay measures the maximal enzyme activity under near optimal conditions, which do not necessarily obtain within the cell.

Autohemolysis

Most cases of pyruvate kinase deficiency demonstrate clearly increased hemolysis after 48 hr of sterile incubation that is not reduced by glucose (Type II as originally defined by Selwyn and Dacie [4]), but is largely or entirely correctable by ATP [9, 30]. While it appears that severe Type II autohemolysis correlates to a degree with clinical severity and reticulocyte count, it should be recognized that the autohemolysis pattern is quite variable. Autohemolysis may be only slightly increased and partially prevented by glucose (Type I) [19, 34, 39, 40, 43, 50] or essentially unchanged by glucose [22, 30, 43]. Indeed, in some instances glucose may accentuate hemolysis [9, 30, 42]. Keitt [42] has postulated that inhibition of reticulocyte respiration by glucose may account for this phenomenon. Rarely, the test may not be grossly abnormal in mildly affected individuals [9].

The increased autohemolysis of PK-deficient red cells is usually prevented by the addition of ATP. The mechanism of this effect is unclear. A variety of other compounds, such as AMP, ADP, NAD, and coenzyme A [9], as well as ATPase inhibitors (ethacrynic acid, ouabain, and *p*-chloromercuribenzoate [49]) may also reduce the degree of autohemolysis.

As Dacie [26] has reemphasized, the autohemolysis test, although retaining some usefulness in practice, is nonspecific. Any impairment of glycolysis, if sufficiently severe, is likely to result in increased hemolysis which is corrected only partially, if at all, by the addition of glucose.

Red Cell Metabolism in Pyruvate Kinase Deficiency

Enzymes

The specific deficiency of red cell pyruvate kinase occurs near the final step in the main pathway of glycolysis (Fig. 54-2). All other reactions of the Embden-Meyerhof and hexosemonophosphate shunt pathways, as well as a number of nonglycolytic reactions, are normally active [9–12, 15, 21, 33, 131]. Indeed, conforming to the pattern in erythrocyte populations of young mean cell age, many enzymatic activities are greater than normal. Unlike the erythrocytes with G-6-PD deficiency, PK-deficient red cells have a normal complement of reduced glutathione [12, 15, 19, 33, 132] and a normal glutathione stability test [11, 12, 15, 21, 42, 132].

Coenzymes

Pyruvate kinase catalyzes an important step in the regeneration of ATP from ADP and provides the pyruvate for the subsequent conversion to lactate. Therefore, PK-deficient erythrocytes would be expected to have difficulty in maintaining normal levels of ATP and NAD. Indeed, most patients with PK deficiency have low red cell ATP levels [12, 16, 17, 19, 21, 23, 30, 117, 131, 133], which may be unstable on incubation [14, 19, 21]. Occasionally, the concentration of ATP may be within the normal range [21, 42, 117, 120] or even increased [36, 43, 49, 117, 120]. The role which the residual mitochondrial oxidative phosphorylation plays in ATP generation in the reticulocyte in order to account for these findings remains unclear [42, 49]. Elevated levels of ATP have been observed in some cases in spite of increased ATP requirements because of increased ATPase activity [49]. The concentration of ADP is normal [12, 21, 30, 39] or increased [12, 15], while the content of AMP is variable [12, 15, 21, 30, 39]. Inorganic phosphate may be slightly greater in amount than in normal cells [30, 49]. The content of NAD and NADH determined together [30] or separately [19, 33] is reduced, and Oski and Diamond [21] have observed a marked fall in red cell NAD during an 8-hr incubation. The virtual disappearance of NAD under these circumstances is in keeping with the nature of the red cell defect of these patients.

Glycolytic Intermediates and Products

As would be expected with a metabolic defect late in the Embden-Meyerhof pathway, assay of glycolytic interme-

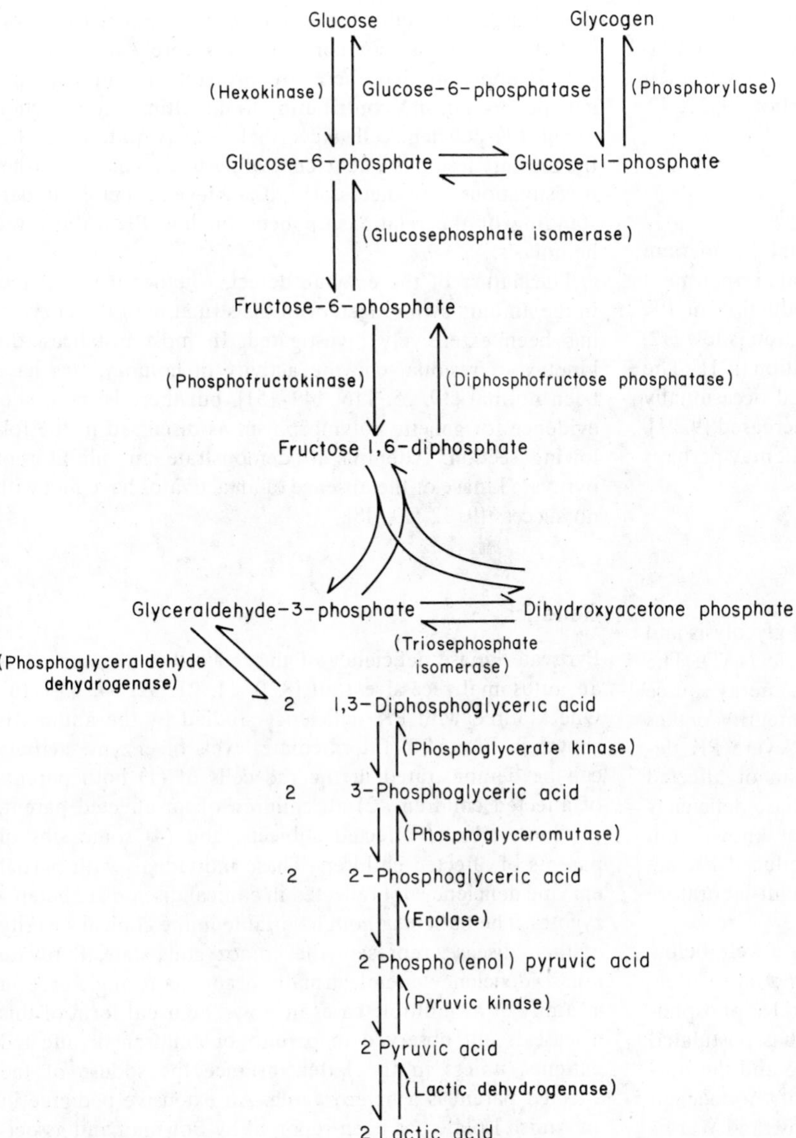

Figure 54-2. The principal metabolic pathways of glycolysis.

diates in PK-deficient red cells frequently reveals abnormal accumulations of phosphoenolpyruvate, 3-phosphoglycerate, and especially 2,3-diphosphoglycerate, whereas pyruvate and lactate levels are decreased or normal [15, 17, 19, 30, 31, 35, 133] (Fig. 54-2). Even glucose-6-phosphate, which is near the beginning of the glycolytic sequence, has been found increased to twice the normal level [134].

Although the high content and persistence on incubation of 2,3-DPG led Robinson and her associates [7] to predict an enzyme defect between 2,3-DPG and pyruvate in Type II nonspherocytic hemolytic anemias, and although this high level of 2,3-DPG has been called a metabolic hallmark of PK deficiency [42], this elevation is not specific for PK deficiency [135–138]. While the precise mechanism of the accumulation of 2,3-DPG has not been clarified [42], a reasonable explanation is that the increase in 3-PG proximal to the deficient PK enzyme favors the synthesis of 2,3-DPG while inhibiting its breakdown. Alternately, Zurcher et al. [139] and Loos [140] have suggested an increase in the turnover of the 2,3-DPG cycle, with a resultant decrease in the glycolytic yield of ATP. Of interest is the recent recognition that the high content of 2,3-DPG decreases the oxygen affinity of hemoglobin [141–146], thereby permitting a greater delivery of oxygen to tissues in PK deficiency [147] as well as in other states [135–137].

Glucose Utilization

Impairment of glucose utilization was observed initially in Type II nonspherocytic hemolytic anemia by Selwyn and

Dacie [4]. It has now been amply demonstrated that glucose utilization is defective in PK deficiency when account is taken of the increased percentage of reticulocytes with their extremely high capacity for glucose consumption [9, 30, 42, 117, 134].

Metabolism in Pyruvate Kinase Heterozygotes

Although the PK heterozygote has a normal hemogram, there is increasing evidence for some metabolic impairment in the red cells as a result of the partial reduction in PK activity. In some instances the ATP concentration is low [12, 34, 42, 117, 120] or unstable upon incubation [21]. The content of 2,3-DPG may be slightly increased occasionally [34, 39] and autohemolysis may be slightly increased [9, 21]. Red cell life span is usually normal [17, 24], but may perhaps be minimally decreased [34] in heterozygotes.

Pathogenesis of Hemolysis and the Nature of the Pyruvate Kinase Defect

Pyruvate kinase deficiency results in impaired glycolysis and impaired ability to generate ATP and to cycle NAD. The dependence of erythrocyes on glycolysis as an energy source necessary for the maintenance of cellular integrity makes it probable that the metabolic handicap of severe PK deficiency accounts for the diminished life span of affected erythrocytes. The critical level of pyruvate kinase deficiency which results in premature hemolysis is not known, but presumed heterozygotes with substantially reduced PK activity are asymptomatic [9], even though certain laboratory findings may be minimally abnormal.

Pyruvate kinase, which ordinarily operates well below substrate saturation in the cell [148], is rendered more effective by the greater availability of the substrate, phosphoenolypyruvate, in PK deficiency. Busch [19] has postulated that because of this accumulation of substrate and the normal excess of PK activity, the actual PK activity in deficient cells may not be rate limiting for glycolysis. Rose and Warms [148], on the basis of their studies utilizing whole glycolyzing cells, have suggested that at high glycolytic rates in normal and PK-deficient cells, glyceraldehyde phosphate dehydrogenase becomes rate limiting as a result of an increased ratio of NADH to NAD and an increased concentration of 1,3 diphosphoglyceric acid.

In some cases of PK deficiency the cells may have a severe membrane defect which results in cation leakage in addition to the profound block in glycolysis. Nathan and associates [134] have postulated that the combination of membrane injury and declining ATP produces spiculation of the cell surface, which leads in turn to trapping and destruction of the cells in the reticuloendothelial system, particularly in the spleen and liver. In further studies [54] they show that in PK deficiency the reticulocytes are variably damaged, and that this causes immediate destruction of some and better survival for others. Thus, the youngest population of the deficient cells contains the group with the poorest outlook, and an older population contains less severely affected cells.

It is apparent that there are probably multiple pathogenetic mechanisms contributing to the ultimate destruction of the PK-deficient cell. Nevertheless, it is quite clear that the primary lesion is a deficiency of pyruvate kinase. Further investigations, are necessary to achieve a better understanding of the relationship between low PK values and hemolysis.

The nature of the enzyme defect, whether it is a defect in the amount synthesized or in the structure of the enzyme, has been extensively investigated. In most instances, the kinetics of residual enzyme activity in homozygotes have been normal [19, 25, 116, 149–151], but there is increasing evidence for genetic polymorphism as discussed in the following section. Attempts to demonstrate an inhibitor of pyruvate kinase or the absence of an activator have met with no success [9, 12, 19, 48].

Genetics

Pyruvate kinase deficiency of the red cell is transmitted as an autosomal recessive trait [8, 9, 11, 21, 32, 34, 43, 116]. One kindred with PK deficiency studied by the authors is shown in Fig. 54-3. Intermediate levels of enzyme activity can be demonstrated in the red cells of (1) both parents of affected children, (2) all children of an affected parent, (3) some sibs of affected subjects, and (4) some sibs of parents of affected children. These individuals with partial enzyme deficiency not reflected in clinical disease are heterozygotes. The patients, though variable in the clinical severity of their disease, represent the homozygous state. Pyruvate kinase deficiency anemia usually occurs as a single case in a family or as multiple cases in sibs. The usual form of this disease is not observed in parents or children of affected patients, unless in the latter instance the spouse of the affected parent is a heterozygote. An extensive pedigree in an Amish isolate has been reported by Bowman and associates [32].

Leukocytes of patients with erythrocyte PK deficiency have normal enzyme activity [8, 9, 12]. This cellular difference in genetic control is also reflected in immunological and physiochemical [25, 152], as well as kinetic [149], differences between the PK of the human erythrocyte and leukocyte. Pyruvate kinase activity is also normal in plasma [22, 120]. The initial observations of normal activity in leukocytes [8, 9] and muscle [12], and reduced activity in liver [10], in PK deficiency are consistent with the subsequent demonstration by Bigley and associates [153] that three isozymes of pyruvate kinase occur in human tissues. Isozyme I is found in erythrocytes and liver, isozyme II in kidney, and isozyme III in liver, kidney, leukocytes, skeletal muscle, and cardiac muscle. Bigley and Koler [125] have further shown that liver from a patient with red cell PK deficiency has deficient PK I but normal PK III, thereby supporting

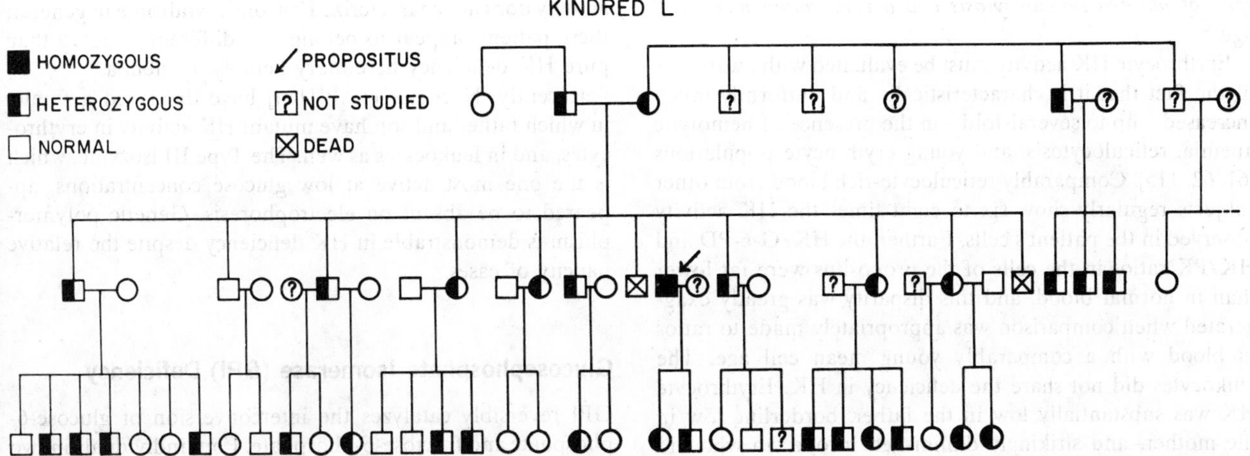

Figure 54-3. Pattern of inheritance of pyruvate kinase deficiency in Family L[8, 9]. An autosomal recessive mode of transmission is demonstrated. Squares designate males and circles females. The chart is constructed on the assumption that intermediate values for pyruvate kinase for a member of the kindred without the disease indicates the heterozygous state and that the disease indicates homozygosity.

the hypothesis of the identity of erythrocyte PK with one of the liver isozymes.

A review of the reported cases as well as our own observations indicate that pyruvate kinase deficiency hemolytic anemia is a heterogeneous disorder. There is marked variation in the clinical severity and poor correlation with PK assay values. Considerable variation is also present in PK values in apparent heterozygotes *among* families as well as *within* families [9].

It is becoming increasingly apparent, as in G-6-PD deficiency, that there is genetic polymorphism. In most cases residual enzyme activity in homozygotes has been normal [19, 25, 116, 149–151, 154], but may be increased [15, 154] or decreased [154–156]. In our laboratory Paglia and coworkers [118] have studied four patients in two unrelated families with clinical and biochemical features of erythrocyte PK deficiency, but with assay values in either the normal or high heterozygous range. In both families, the apparent dilemma was resolved by the finding that affected subjects had inherited from one side the "usual" gene resulting in PK deficiency, and from the other a gene resulting in a grossly abnormal pyruvate kinase with a K_m for PEP some 10 times greater than that of the normal enzyme. Differences in pH optimum, and heat and storage stability were also demonstrable. Cases with similar intermediate or normal PK assay values, and with the usual picture of homozygous deficiency have been noted by others [25, 31, 33, 39, 47, 117, 121, 157]. In some instances, the PK enzyme activity in this type of patient may be increased by fructose diphosphate [121, 122], whereas the usual PK-deficient enzyme is not activated. Hsu and associates [44] and subsequently Zuelzer and coworkers [56] have described extreme intrafamilial differences between PK-deficient phenotypes in respect to hemolysis, ATP stability, and glucose consumption. Their genetic analysis was consistent with heterozygosity for two distinct interacting mutants in minimally affected relatives of severely anemic homozygotes.

In addition, further genetic heterogeneity is suggested by the small group of patients who conform to the usual clinical picture of PK deficiency, but who may be heterozygous for the abnormal gene [23, 39, 50, 55, 57, 158]. In spite of the diverse observations, there is strong evidence that hereditary hemolytic anemia, conforming in virtually all respects to the PK-deficient type, may be associated with either a quantitative or a qualitative defect of the enzyme [182, 183].

No linkage of pyruvate kinase deficiency to ABO blood groups, Rh type, or haptoglobin types has been described [9, 11, 21, 48]. The accumulating reports on PK patients from various parts of the world suggest a rather wide geographic distribution of the gene, but more data are necessary to determine distribution as well as frequency of the mutant gene.

OTHER EMBDEN-MEYERHOF PATHWAY ENZYME DEFICIENCIES

Hexokinase (HK) Deficiency

In 1967 hereditary hemolytic anemia was observed in a child who had hematologic and clinical features similar to those described in PK deficiency. The erythrocytes exhibited a severe deficiency in hexokinase activity [61]. The erythrocytes possessed HK activity below the lower limits of normal *in spite of marked reticulocytosis and a very young mean cell age.*

Erythrocyte HK activity must be evaluated with awareness of the fact that it is characteristically and uniformly much increased—up to several-fold—in the presence of hemolytic anemia, reticulocytosis, and young erythrocyte populations [61, 62, 115]. Comparably reticulocyte-rich blood from other subjects regularly show six to eight times the HK activity observed in the patient's cells. Further, the HK/G-6-PD and HK/PK ratios in the cells of the propositus were far lower than in normal blood, and this disparity was greatly exaggerated when comparison was appropriately made to ratios in blood with a comparably young mean cell age. The leukocytes did not share the deficiency in HK. Erythrocyte HK was substantially low in the father, borderline low in the mother, and strikingly diminished in one sib who did not have hemolytic anemia. An autosomal recessive mode of transmission seemed probable.

Both glucose and fructose were consumed at rates below those of normal erythrocyte populations and far below those of comparably young, high-reticulocyte blood. The autohemolysis test resembled that categorized as Type I. Splenectomy, performed at age 5 months, ameliorated the hemolytic process, but it persisted with moderate, fluctuating anemia and reticulocytosis of 7 to 24 percent.

Hexokinase has been suspected to be a decisive link in determining the glycolytic rate of normal cells on the basis of its low in vitro activity, its strategic role as the first step in glycolysis, and on the basis of certain inferential evidence in various mammalian species [159–162]. In the HK deficient patient the reticulocytes and young erythrocytes have HK activity several-fold less than expected and appropriate to that present in normal blood. Measured on the HK scale of aging, even the reticulocytes are approaching physiological senility. Presumably such handicapped erythrocytes lack the capacity for normal survival.

Keitt [63] has recently studied two sisters with overt chronic hemolysis and deficient erythrocyte HK activity. Low red cell G-6-P, the product of the HK reaction, was observed in both patients, as well as in presumed heterozygous family members. HK activity in hemolysates derived from cells of the patients was low unless protected by glucose, mercaptoethanol, or EDTA. Further, the HK activity differed from that of normal cells in that glucose was not utilized efficiently at concentrations below 0.2 mM, whereas normal cells show linear glucose consumption down to at least 0.05 mM. It appeared that HK in the cells of the proposita was unstable and unusually susceptible to oxidation of its reactive sulfhydryl group.

In 1965, Löhr et al. [163] described diminished HK activity in all the blood elements—erythrocytes, leukocytes, and platelets—in three juvenile males with Fanconi's syndrome. These patients had absent or only low-grade reticulocytosis, panmyelopathy, multiple congenital abnormalities classically characteristic of the Fanconi syndrome, abnormal enzyme kinetics, and marked chromosomal aberrations. Low HK activity does not characterize Fanconi's syndrome in general; these patients appear to belong to a different category than pure HK deficiency hereditary hemolytic anemia.

Recently, Necheles et al. [184] have described a family in which father and son have mutant HK activity in erythrocytes, and in leukocytes as well. The Type III isozyme, which is the one most active at low glucose concentrations, appeared to be absent on electrophoresis. Genetic polymorphism is demonstrable in HK deficiency despite the relative paucity of cases.

Glucosephosphate Isomerase (GPI) Deficiency

GPI reversibly catalyzes the interconversion of glucose-6-phosphate and fructose-6-phosphate. Four individuals in two unrelated kindreds are known with severe erythrocyte GPI deficiency and severe, lifelong hereditary hemolytic anemia [64, 65]. Splenectomy partially ameliorated hemolysis in some of the affected children. Family studies demonstrated an autosomal mode of inheritance, the heterozygous parents and certain relatives being phenotypically normal but biochemically detectable in terms of partial GPI deficiency. The autohemolysis test has been variably positive and largely correctable by the addition of glucose or adenosine.

The leukocytes as well as the erythrocytes are deficient in GPI. Other body tissues may, therefore, be involved, but if so, no clinical evidence of deficient function has been detected. Production of $^{14}CO_2$ from carbon-2-labeled glucose in methylene-blue-stimulated cells reflects that fraction of glucose which traverses the HMP oxidative shunt. It reenters the Embden-Meyerhof pathway by way of F-6-P, is isomerized to G-6-P and then is recycled through the HMP shunt. In GPI-deficient cells this recycling was far below normal [64, 65]. Although homozygotes in the two known affected families cannot be distinguished by hematologic or clinical criteria nor by routine GPI assay techniques, a distinction between the two kindreds was readily apparent when starch-gel electrophoresis was performed [64, 65, 164]. In one kindred, the GPI electrophoretic patterns of both parents differed from normal and from each other. Their affected child appears to have inherited a different mutant enzyme from each parent. In this kindred, the zymogram of the propositus showed an increase in cathodal migration of GPI; neither major nor minor components corresponded to normal controls. In the second kindred, zymograms of the parents and of unaffected sibs were indistinguishable from normal, but the GPI of two severely affected children showed a significant decrease in cathodal migration of its major components and virtual absence of minor bands. Figure 54-4 shows the representative zymogram of one affected child in this kindred (Propositus B). Thus, in GPI deficiency genetic polymorphism has already been demonstrated. Similar hemolytic syndromes result from GPI deficiency, presumably because of more than one mutation at the GPI gene locus. In GPI deficiency, enzyme inhibitors

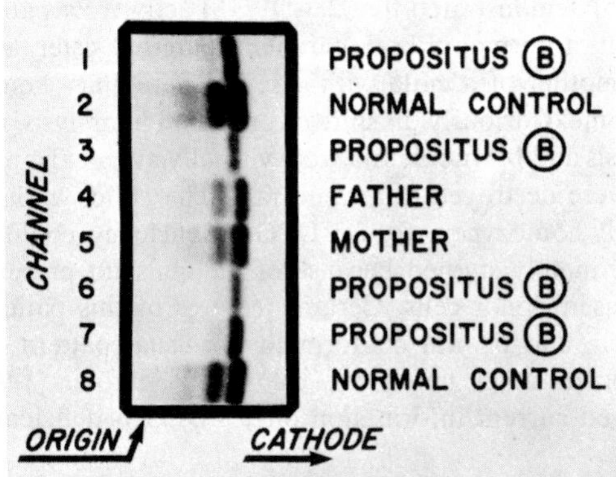

Figure 54-4. Starch-gel electrophoresis patterns of erythrocyte GPI from an affected child (here designated Propositus B), his parents, and a normal control. Propositus hemolysates in channels 1 and 7 were contaminated with white cells. Channels 3 and 6 contained erythrocyte preparations that were essentially devoid of leukocytes. (*Reproduced by courtesy of the New England Journal of Medicine.*)

have not been demonstrated and reaction kinetics are normal.

Since the description of the original two GPI deficient kindreds, additional cases have been added [185–189]. In at least two, the already documented genetic polymorphism has been augmented by the demonstration that leukocytes were unaffected or only slightly affected by the deficiency [185, 189]. In two others, G-6-PD deficiency and GPI deficiency have coexisted [187, 188].

Triosephosphate Isomerase (TPI) Deficiency

Severe hemolytic anemia has been demonstrated in certain highly consanguineous kindreds of French-Negro ancestry in association with a severe deficiency of TPI in both erythrocytes and leukocytes [66–69]. Similar findings are known in the United States in two unrelated persons [68, 165], both of English Caucasian derivation, and another has been found in England [166]. Patients with the severe disorder now are nine in number. Most affected children have died before the age of 5 years. The oldest known living patient with severe TPI deficiency has now survived to age 21 years. The disorder has an autosomal recessive inheritance pattern. Heterozygotes are clinically well and hematologically normal. In all homozygotes who have lived for as long as a few months there has been a severe and usually progressive atypical neurologic disorder [66, 67]. The patient who has now survived 21 years is severely handicapped by spasticity but the neurologic deficit appears to have stabilized [165]. Since the deficiency is known to involve leukocytes [66, 67] and skeletal muscle [68], in addition to erythrocytes, it is quite possible that concomitant neurologic disease may result from the same deficiency in nervous tissue. Interestingly, the spinal fluid TPI activity of affected subjects is far below that of normal persons. Three subjects have died suddenly from what appeared to be cardiac arrest or ventricular fibrillation. This raises the question of the involvement of cardiac muscle in TPI deficiency. Other tissues, with the exception of blood plasma where TPI activity is also low, have not been adequately studied. Thus, the present evidence strongly suggests a widespread tissue deficiency in TPI, with the hematologic and neurologic consequences dominating the clinical picture. TPI deficiency has been found to coexist in certain affected kindreds with G-6-PD deficiency and sickle-cell trait (Fig. 54-5) [67]. Two female subjects are known heterozygotes for both TPI and G-6-PD deficiencies and have no obvious clinical consequences, at least in the absence of drug challenge.

TPI catalyzes the interconversion of dihydroxyacetone phosphate (DHAP) and 3-phosphoglyceraldehyde (G-3-P). The equilibrium is far in the direction of DHAP, and DHAP accumulates intracellularly in the homozygous deficiency state [68]. The precise metabolic consequences of TPI deficiency, other than the accumulation of DHAP itself, are not well understood.

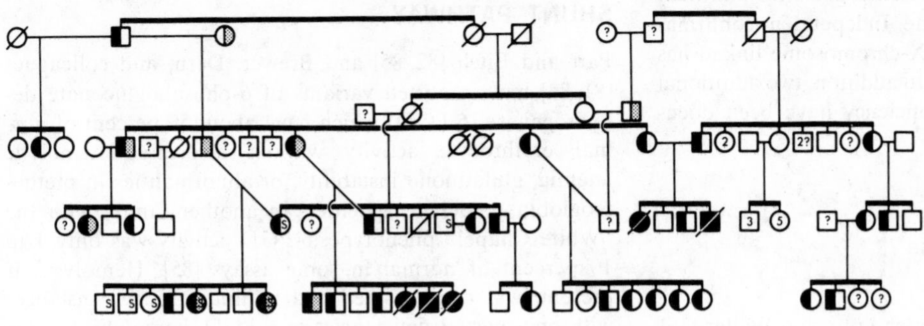

Figure 54-5. An unusual kindred in which TPI and G-6-PD deficiency and sickle-cell trait coexist.

Phosphoglycerate Kinase (PGK) Deficiency

PGK deficiency has been demonstrated in a single woman without known family [70] and in two male third cousins of a Chinese kindred [71, 72]. Both of the latter had severe hemolytic anemia which necessitated transfusions during periods of crisis often brought on by intercurrent infections. In one, splenectomy partially alleviated the severity of hemolysis, although reticulocytosis and moderate anemia persisted. Both children had mild mental retardation and behavioral aberrations which may or may not have been associated with the deficiency. Leukocytes as well as erythrocytes shared the deficiency [71, 72]. No information is available on other tissues.

The erythrocyte PGK deficiency was severe—less than 5 percent of normal. The fathers and all paternal relatives of both children were normal by all criteria including direct assay of erythrocytes. The mother and maternal grandmother of the propositus had a chronic, relatively mild, hemolytic process with mild PGK deficiency. The maternal second cousin and mother of a severely affected child, an obligate heterozygote, was normal by all criteria including assay. There was a highly suggestive family history of early deaths occurring in certain male members with unexplained anemia and sometimes neurological symptoms. The findings suggest that PGK deficiency, like G-6-PD deficiency, may be X-linked. The mild hemolytic process in the mother and maternal grandmother of the propositus suggests that they may be heterozygotes, and additional data [71, 72] suggesting mosaicism of their erythrocytes with respect to PGK activity lends inferential support to this hypothesis. Mosaicism is well demonstrated in G-6-PD deficiency [167–170]. The fact that the mother of a severely affected male child, the third cousin of the propositus, is apparently normal by all criteria is compatible with a similar, established situation occurring in X-linked G-6-PD deficiency, and is in accord with the Lyon hypothesis [171, 172]. The evidence based on this single kindred cannot be regarded as conclusive, but the inference is strong that the severely affected males may be hemizygotes and the mildly affected females heterozygotes for a mutant gene located on the X chromosome. Independent confirmation that PGK activity is indeed X-chromosome linked has recently been achieved [190, 191]. In addition, two additional instances of erythrocyte PGK deficiency have been documented [192, 193].

2,3-Diphosphoglycerate Mutase (2,3-DPGM) Deficiency

Bowdler and Prankerd [28] and later Löhr and Waller [16] have inferred a deficiency of 2,3-DPGM in certain subjects with hereditary hemolytic anemia. The indirect nature of the evidence demands some reservation as to the interpretation of the findings. Using direct methods, Schröter [74, 75] demonstrated that 2,3-DPGM activity was about 50 percent of normal in both parents, a paternal sister, and the grandmother of a child with a severe hereditary hemolytic syndrome. Curiously, in spite of profound hemolysis, reticulocytosis and bilirubinemia were virtually absent. Transfused cells were destroyed at a rapid rate. The child, while quite possibly homozygous for 2,3-DPGM deficiency, could never be adequately studied because of the constant presence of transfused donor cells. Certain features of this patient are puzzling and do not conform to the usual pattern of hemolysis in other hereditary disorders. Schröter [194] has reviewed current information on 2,3-DPGM deficiency.

Phosphofructokinase (PFK) Deficiency

Muscle PFK deficiency [76–78], a relatively recently defined inherited myopathy now designated as Type VII glycogen storage disease, is associated with almost total lack of PFK in muscle and about half the normal PFK activity in erythrocytes (cf. Chap. 7). Immunochemical studies have shown that erythrocyte PFK has two or more components and that about 50 percent of enzyme activity is attributable to "muscle type" PFK isozyme [78]. Although affected subjects have had neither anemia nor splenomegaly, a moderately reduced life span of ^{51}Cr-labeled erythrocytes, marrow erythroid hyperplasia, and reticulocytosis of the order of 3 to 7 percent have indicated a mild, compensated hemolytic process [78]. PFK phosphorylates F-6-P to F-1,6-diP. The reduction of erythrocyte PFK activity to 50 percent of normal may in this instance be the cause of the compensated hemolysis, but in most other situations enzyme deficiencies of this order of magnitude have not produced a detectable hemolytic disorder. Congenital hemolytic anemia associated with a 50 percent reduction in PFK activity of erythrocytes but unassociated with myopathy has likewise been reported [195].

DEFICIENCIES OF ENZYMES OF THE HMP SHUNT PATHWAY

Parr and Fitch [82, 85] and Brewer, Dern, and colleagues [81, 84] have reported variants of 6-phosphogluconate dehydrogenase (6-PGD) which have about 50 percent of normal erythrocyte activity without associated hemolytic anemia, glutathione instability, or abnormalities in methemoglobin reducing capacities. In another family with the "White Chapel" phenotype, 6-PGD activity was only 1 to 10 percent of normal in some assays [85]. Hemolysis, if present, was compensated and minimal. In two instances with only partial deficiencies in 6-PGD, hemolytic anemia has been present [79, 80], but in neither was it certain that the enzyme deficiency was the cause of the hemolysis. While severe 6-PGD deficiency might be expected to give a syndrome similar to G-6-PD deficiency, it is as yet uncertain that this is the case. Carson, studying the erythrocytes of one of Parr's 6-PGD-deficient subjects, found them indeed to be primaquine sensitive [173].

DEFICIENCIES OF THE NONGLYCOLYTIC ENZYMES

Glutathione Reductase (GSSG-R) Deficiency

The flavin enzyme, GSSG-R, reduces 1 mole of GSSG to 2 moles of GSH; NADPH is oxidized simultaneously to NADP. Carson and coworkers [87] have briefly reported susceptibility to primaquine, but not chronic hemolysis or anemia in a partially deficient subject. Löhr and Waller [86] and others [87–93] have observed partial GSSG-R deficiency in association with hereditary hemolytic anemia and sometimes with a panmyelopathy or with neurologic disturbances [92, 93]. The deficiency has been partial, GSH stability has been normal or nearly so, but the Heinz body formation test in the large series reported by Waller was always abnormal [93]. Kinetic and pH optima studies have suggested the production of an abnormal enzyme. Since in the largest available series, that reported by Waller [93], GSSG-R activities were only reduced to about one-half of normal, it is of interest that concomitant hematologic and neurologic findings were often severe. Because of this, Waller and colleagues [92, 93] have postulated a codominant autosomal mode of transmission of GSSG-R deficiency. The diversity of hematologic and other syndromes observed in association with only partial GSSG-R deficiency suggests that further study is necessary before the role of the deficiency in the syndromes can be fully assessed. Beutler [174, 175] has shown that GSSG-R activity as measured in hemolysates represents only a part of that available and that small amounts of flavin-adenine-dinucleotide (FAD) enhance the observed activity variably and, often, substantially. FAD is a coenzyme for GSSG-R. Beutler [175] further observed that even in normal subjects GSSG-R activity in hemolysates varies with the riboflavin content of the diet and is enhanced by riboflavin supplementation. It appears, then, that GSSG-R activity can be profoundly affected by riboflavin intake and metabolism. Clinical states associated with apparently partial deficiencies in GSSG-R may possibly have multiple bases, one of which may be abnormalities in riboflavin nutrition or in the synthesis of FAD from riboflavin.

Adenosine Triphosphatase (ATPase) Deficiency

Harvald and associates [99] have briefly reported three unrelated persons, two with chronic hemolytic anemia, in whom ATPase activities in the erythrocyte were about half of normal. While a relationship between ATPase deficiency and hemolysis was considered likely, it is not clear that this was necessarily the case, since it is well known that an Na^+-K^+-Mg^{++}-dependent ATPase hydrolyzes ATP and provides energy for the active transport of sodium and potassium across membranes. The data in Harvald's cases do not permit any conclusion as to whether transport ATPase or some other form of ATPase activity was involved. A single case of partial deficiency of erythrocyte ATPase has been reported from France [196]. It should be noted that Balfe and coworkers [197] have observed decreased ATPase activity and elevated red cell sodium concentration in a large number of members of a kindred in which no evidence of a hemolytic disorder existed.

Glutathione Peroxidase (GSH-Px) Deficiency

Necheles and his associates [100] have described a single Puerto Rican male whose erythrocytes possessed about one-fourth of the normal GSH-Px activity, while the red cells of his parents had about one-half of the normal activity. This patient had a hemolytic reaction following a blood transfusion, but after recovery a mild reticulocytosis suggested persistence of a compensated hemolytic process. GSH-Px catalyzes the detoxification of hydrogen peroxide and the simultaneous oxidation of GSH to GSSG [176–178]. It presumably protects against peroxidative injury and, since it plays a role in the production of GSSG, is indirectly linked to the HMP shunt pathway. It is of interest that while hydrogen peroxide decidedly stimulated HMP shunt pathway in normal erythrocytes, it failed to do so in the GSH-Px-deficient cells. A partial deficiency of GSH-Px has been observed in the neonatal period in conjunction with transient, mild hemolysis [179].

Boivin and associates [180] have recently described a 67-year-old male patient with chronic hemolytic anemia, methemoglobinemia, Heinz bodies, normal erythrocyte GSH, drug sensitivity, and a red cell GSH-Px activity which was only about 30 percent of that present in comparable reticulocyte-rich blood. Other erythrocytic oxido-reduction systems were normal and congenital deficiency of GSH-Px was postulated as the cause of the hemolytic process. The deficiency has been reviewed by Necheles and associates [198].

Glutathione (GSH) Deficiency

Moderately severe hereditary hemolytic anemia has been studied in a kindred in which red cells of certain members were almost totally lacking in oxidized or reduced glutathione [94–97]. In studies on two unrelated patients with the same findings, the second reaction of the GSH-synthetase system was found to be at fault [98, 181]. Deficient cells apparently are unable to convert γ-glutamyl cysteine to the full tripeptide. Unlike normal erythrocytes, the cells of patients with severe deficiency had an inherited inability to incorporate radioactive glycine into GSH. The cells of affected subjects are primaquine sensitive and also exquisitely sensitive to minute amounts of chromate. It is remarkable that so severe a deficiency of GSH should be compatible with survival, in view of the physiologic importance usually assigned to this tripeptide [199].

THE "HIGH-ATP" SYNDROMES

The erythrocytes of certain patients have been shown to contain ATP at levels up to twice normal. In one form of "high-ATP" cells no demonstrable abnormality has been found and hemolysis was not present [102–104]. In a second type there was likewise no hemolysis, but a marked increase in PK activity was consistently associated with and believed to be responsible for the high ATP [101]. High erythrocyte ATP has also been reported to coexist with a red cell 2,3-DPG phosphatase deficiency and a multiplicity of anomalies in two infants [105]. Finally, Busch has studied a patient with severe, hereditary nonspherocytic hemolytic anemia in which the only detectable abnormality was a marked elevation of red cell ATP. Disturbed regulation of *de novo* adenine nucleotide synthesis was assumed but not pinpointed [200, 201]. A similar case with substantial deficiency of erythrocyte ribosephosphate pyrophosphokinase (PRPP synthetase) is currently under study in the laboratory of one of the authors [202]. Hereditary nonspherocytic hemolytic anemia has likewise been observed as a dominantly transmitted syndrome associated with low erythrocyte ATP [203]. No associated enzyme deficiency has as yet been defined, but intensive studies have also thus far failed to yield a clue as to any other cause.

SUMMARY

1 Pyruvate kinase deficiency hemolytic anemia is the most common and best characterized of the hemolytic anemias resulting from a metabolic block in the Embden-Meyerhof pathway. The disorder occurs predominantly in patients of Northern European ancestry. It is characterized clinically by hemolytic anemia of variable but often severe degree, absence of spherocytosis, partial but frequently significant improvement after splenectomy in the severe cases, and usually by substantial autohemolysis.

Pyruvate kinase deficiency results in a diminished capacity to regenerate ATP and to cycle NAD in erythrocytes. Impairment of energy metabolism causes symptomatic hemolysis, but the precise mechanism of hemolysis remains to be clarified.

The disease is transmitted as an autosomal recessive trait. Leukocytes are not affected. Heterozygotes have about one-half the normal amount of PK activity in their erythrocytes; they usually have no clinically or hematologically detectable evidence of disease.

There is now ample evidence that genetic polymorphism exists in this disorder. PK deficiency usually appears to be a quantitative defect, but in some instances a qualitative defect in the enzyme has been detected.

2 Severe deficiencies of certain other enzymes of the Embden-Meyerhof pathway—hexokinase, glucosephosphate isomerase, triosephosphate isomerase, phosphoglycerate kinase, and 2,3-diphosphoglyceromutase—have also been detected in association with hereditary hemolytic anemias whose characteristics closely resemble those seen in pyruvate kinase deficiency. Thus far all appear to be much rarer than pyruvate kinase deficiency. Initial evidence suggests that phosphoglycerate kinase deficiency may be X-linked; in all others where data are satisfactory for analysis, the disorders are transmitted as autosomal recessive traits.

A mild compensated hemolytic process with partial red cell deficiency of phosphofructokinase is a concomitant of a severe muscle disorder due to a severe deficiency of the enzyme.

Triosephosphate isomerase deficiency is accompanied by a severe neurologic as well as hematologic syndrome, and probably by widespread deficiency of the enzyme in many tissues. Glucosephosphate isomerase and phosphoglycerate kinase deficiencies occur in leukocytes as well as erythrocytes.

3 Certain deficiencies of nonglycolytic enzymes have also been found in association with hereditary hemolytic anemias. In some, data are scanty as yet, and a cause and effect relationship is not entirely certain. The syndromes reported with partial erythrocyte glutathione reductase activity are difficult to evaluate since the enzyme has been shown to vary widely with nutritional status and with riboflavin metabolism. The coenzyme, flavin-adenine-dinucleotide, is strongly dependent on nutritional and perhaps metabolic factors.

4 Hereditary hemolytic anemia associated with a nearly total absence of oxidized or reduced glutathione in the red cell has been demonstrated. Inability to incorporate glycine into the tripeptide in the second reaction of the glutathione synthetase system presumably represents the hereditary defect.

5 Several "high-ATP" syndromes exist, but only two have been reported to be associated with chronic hemolysis.

BIBLIOGRAPHY

1. Carson, P. E., Flanagan, C. L., Ickes, C. E., and Alving, A. S.: Enzymatic deficiency in primaquine-sensitive erythrocytes. Science, **24,** 484, 1956.
2. Beutler, E.: Glucose-6-phosphate dehydrogenase activity. This volume, Chap. 55.
3. Dacie, J. V., Mollison, P. L., Richardson, N., Selwyn, J. G., and Shapiro, L.: Atypical congenital haemolytic anaemia. Quart. J. Med., **22,** 79, 1953.

4. Selwyn, J. G., and Dacie, J. V.: Autohemolysis and other changes resulting from the incubation in vitro of red cells from patients with congenital hemolytic anemia. Blood, **9,** 414, 1954.
5. de Gruchy, G. C., Santamaria, J. N., Parsons, I. C., and Crawford, H.: Nonspherocytic congenital hemolytic anemia. Blood, **16,** 1371, 1960.
6. de Gruchy, G. C., Crawford, H., and Morton, D.: Atypical (nonspherocytic) congenital haemolytic anaemia. *Proc. VII Congr. Internat. Soc. Hemat.,* Rome, 1958, **2,** part 1, 425. II Pensiero Scientifico, Rome.
7. Robinson, M. A., Loder, P. B., and de Gruchy, G. C.: Red-cell metabolism in nonspherocytic congenital haemolytic anaemia. Brit. J. Haemat., **7,** 327, 1961.
8. Valentine, W. N., Tanaka, K. R., and Miwa, S.: A specific erythrocyte glycolytic enzyme defect (pyruvate kinase) in three subjects with congenital non-spherocytic hemolytic anemia. Trans. Ass. Amer. Physicians, **74,** 100, 1961.
9. Tanaka, K. R., Valentine, W. N., and Miwa, S.: Pyruvate (PK) deficiency hereditary non-spherocytic hemolytic anemia. Blood, **18,** 784, 1961 (abstract); Blood, **19,** 267, 1962.
10. Brunetti, P., Puxeddu, A., and Nenci, G.: Anemia emolitica congenita non sferocitica de carenza di piruvico-chinasi (PK). Haematologica, **47,** 505, 1962.
11. Bowman, H. S., and Procopio, F.: Hereditary non-spherocytic hemolytic anemia of the pyruvate-kinase deficient type. Ann. Intern. Med., **58,** 567, 1963.
12. Brunetti, P., Puxeddu, A., Nenci, G., and Migliorini, E.: Congenital nonspherocytic haemolytic anaemia due to pyruvate-kinase deficiency. Acta Haemat. (Basel), **30,** 88, 1963.
13. Brunetti, P., Puxeddu, A., Nenci, G., and Migliorini, E.: Haemolytic anaemia due to pyruvate-kinase deficiency. Lancet, **2,** 169, 1963.
14. de Gruchy, G. C.: Red-cell metabolism in congenital haemolytic anaemias. Aust. Ann. Med., **12,** 6, 1963.
15. Waller, H. D., and Löhr, G. W.: Hereditary nonspherocytic enzymopenic hemolytic anemia with pyruvate kinase deficiency. *Proc. IX Congr. Internat. Soc. Hemat.,* Mexico City, 1962, **1,** 257. Universidad Nacional Autónoma de Mexico, Mexico, D. F., 1964.
16. Löhr, G. W., and Waller, H. D.: Zur biochemie einiger angeborener hämolytischer anämien. Folia Haemat. (Leipzig), **8,** 377, 1963.
17. Prankerd, T. A. J.: Inherited enzyme defects in congenital haemolytic anaemias. *Proc. IX Congr. Europ. Soc. Haemat.,* Lisbon, 1963, **2,** part 1, 735. S. Karger, Basel, 1963.
18. Larizza, P., Brunetti, P., and Grignani, F.: Biochemical and genetic aspects of erythrocyte pyruvate kinase deficiency. *Proc. IX Congr. Europ. Soc. Haemat.,* Lisbon, 1963, **2,** part 1, 745. S. Karger, Basel, 1963.
19. Busch, D.: Erythrocyte metabolism in three persons with hereditary nonspherocytic haemolytic anaemia, deficient in pyruvate-kinase. *Proc. IX Congr. Europ. Soc. Haemat.,* Lisbon, 1963, **2,** part 1, 783. S. Karger, Basel, 1963.
20. Mallarmé, J., and Boivin, P.: Nouvelles observations d'icteres hemolytique hereditaire nonspherocytaire avec deficit en pyruvate kinase. *Proc. IX Congr. Europ. Soc. Haemat.,* Lisbon, 1963, **2,** part 1, 789. S. Karger, Basel, 1963.
21. Oski, F. A., and Diamond, L. K.: Erythrocyte pyruvate kinase deficiency resulting in congenital nonspherocytic hemolytic anemia. New Eng. J. Med., **269,** 763, 1963.
22. Busch, D.: Congenitale nichtspharozytare hamolytische anamie mit mangel an erythrozytarer pyruvatkinase. Folia Haemat. (Leipzig), **9,** 89, 1964.
23. Bestetti, A., Rossi, U., Loos, J. A., and Prins, H. K.: A case of congenital atypical haemolytic anaemia with pyruvate kinase deficiency. Vox Sang., **9,** 492, 1964.
24. Oski, F. A., Nathan, D. G., Sidel, V. W., and Diamond, L. K.: Extreme hemolysis and red-cell distortion in erythrocyte pyruvate kinase deficiency. I. Morphology, erythrokinetics, and family enzyme studies. New Eng. J. Med., **270,** 1023, 1964.
25. Koler, R. D., Bigley, R. H., Jones, R. T., Rigas, D. A., VanBellinghen, P., and Thompson, P.: Pyruvate kinase: Molecular differences between human red cell and leukocyte enzyme. *Cold Spring Harbor Symposia Quant. Biol.,* **29,** 213, 1964.
26. Dacie, J. V.: The hereditary non-spherocytic haemolytic anaemias. Acta Haemat. (Basel), **31,** 177, 1964.
27. Mallarmé, J., Boivin, P., and Gerbeaux, J.: L'anemie hémolytique congénitale nonsphérocytaire par déficit en pyruvate-kinase. Bull. Soc. Med. Hop. Paris, **115,** 483, 1964.
28. Bowdler, A. J., and Prankerd, T. A. J.: Studies in congenital nonspherocytic haemolytic anaemias with specific enzyme defects. Acta Haemat. (Basel), 31, 65, 1964.
29. Kaars Sijpesteijn, J. A.: Een meisje met een congenitale nietsferocytaire hemolytische anemie (type Dacie II) en deficientie van het enzym pyruvaatkinase. Nederl. T. Geneesk., **108,** 440, 1964.
30. Grimes, A. J., Meisler, A., and Dacie, J. V.: Hereditary non-spherocytic haemolytic anaemia: A study of red-cell carbohydrate metabolism in twelve cases of pyruvatekinase deficiency. Brit. J. Haemat., **10,** 403, 1964.
31. Hjelm, M., and de Verdier, C.-H.: Non-spherocytic hemolytic anemia and changes in phosphoglycerate and phosphopyruvate metabolism of the red blood cell. *Abstr. Xth Congr. Int. Soc. Haemat.,* Stockholm, Sweden, 1964, p. K:41.
32. Bowman, H. S., McKusick, V. A., and Dronamraju, K. R.: Pyruvate kinase deficient hemolytic anemia in an Amish isolate. Amer. J. Hum. Genet., **17,** 1, 1965.
33. Loder, P. B., and de Gruchy, G. C.: Red-cell enzymes and co-enzymes in nonspherocytic congenital haemolytic anaemias. Brit. J. Haemat., **11,** 21, 1965.
34. Miwa, S., and Nagata, M.: Pyruvate kinase deficiency hereditary nonspherocytic hemolytic anemia: Report of two cases in a Japanese family and review of literature. Acta Haemat. Jap., **28,** 1, 1965.
35. Busch, D.: Probleme des erythrozytenstoffwechsels bei anamien mit pyruvatkinasemangel. Folia Haemat. (Leipzig), **83,** 395, 1965.
36. Jacobasch, G., Syllm-Rapoport, I., Scharfschwerdt, H., Otto, F. M. G., and Pester, H.: Pyruvatkinasemangel und einige probleme der glykolyseregulierung. Folia Haemat. (Leipzig), **83,** 407, 1965.
37. Hurez, A., Debray, H., Boivin, P., Brault, J., and d'Angély, Mlle.: Un cas d'anémie hémolytique par déficit en pyruvate-kinase. Arch. Franc. Pediat., **22,** 1219, 1965.
38. Verger, P., Bentégeat, J., Tönz, O., Guillard, J. M., and Boisseau, M.: A propos d'un cas de deficit en pyruvate-kinase: Etude clinique, investigations familiales et enzymologiques. *Xth Congr. Europ. Soc. Haemat.,* Strasbourg, 1965, p. 258. (Abstract.)
39. Busch, D., Witt, I., Berger, M., and Künzer, W.: Deficiency of pyruvate kinase in the erythrocytes of a child with hereditary non-spherocytic hemolytic anemia. Acta Paediat. Scand., **55,** 177, 1966.
40. Perry, L. V., and Alfrey, C. P., Jr.: Red cell pyruvate kinase deficiency in adults: A report of 2 cases. Med. Rec., **59,** 137, 1966.
41. Necheles, T. F., Finkel, H. E., Sheehan, R. G., and Allen, D. M.: Red cell pyruvate kinase deficiency: The effect of splenectomy. Arch. Intern. Med. (Chicago), **118,** 75, 1966.
42. Keitt, A. S.: Pyruvate kinase deficiency and related disorders of red cell glycolysis. Amer. J. Med., **41,** 762, 1966.
43. Collier, H. B., Ashford, D. R., and Bell, R. E.: Three cases of hemolytic anemia with erythrocyte pyruvate kinase deficiency in Alberta. Canad. Med. Ass. J., **95,** 1188, 1966.
44. Hsu, T. H. J., Robinson, A. R., and Zuelzer, W. W.: Genetic polymorphism of hemolytic anemias associated with erythrocyte pyruvic kinase deficiency. Blood, **28,** 977, 1966. (Abstract.)
45. Nathan, D. G., Oski, F. A., Sidel, V. W., Gardner, F. H., and Diamond, L. K.: Studies of erythrocyte spicule formation in haemolytic anaemia. Brit. J. Haemat., **12,** 385, 1966.
46. Gasser, C., and Marti, H. R.: Pyruvatkinasemangel bei hereditärer, nicht-sphärocytärer häemolytischer Anämie. Schweiz. Med. Wschr., **96,** 1264, 1966.
47. Fusco, F. A., Busch, D., Negrini, A. C., and Azzolini, A.: Anemia emolitica congentia non sferocitica da anomalie della piruvatochinasi. Haematologica, **51,** 836, 1966.
48. Hanel, H. K., Harvald, B., Mor, G., Christensen, N., and Deckert, T.: A case of haemolytic anaemia due to pyruvate kinase deficiency. Scand. J. Haemat., **4,** 53, 1967.
49. Twomey, J. J., O'Neal, F. B., Alfrey, C. P., and Moser, R. H.: ATP

metabolism in pyruvate kinase deficient erythrocytes. Blood, **30,** 576, 1967.

50. Roberts, P. D., and Leets, I.: Further observations on red cell pyruvate-kinase deficiency. *Proc. Xth Congr. Europ. Soc. Haemat.,* Strasbourg, 1965, part II, p. 306. S. Karger, Basel/New York, 1967.
51. Laurin, S., Letellier, G., Blais, M., and Marcil, G.: Anémie hémolytique nonspherocytaire par déficience en pyruvate-kinase. L. Union Med. Canada, **96,** 689, 1967.
52. Nixon, A. D., and Buchanan, J. G.: Haemolytic anaemia due to pyruvate kinase deficiency. New Zeal. Med. J., **66,** 859, 1967.
53. Boivin, P., and Galand, C.: Les anémies enzymopéniques, Un bilan. Path. Biol. (Paris), **15,** 1089, 1967.
54. Nathan, D. G., Oski, F. A., Miller, D. R., and Gardner, F. H.: Life-span and organ sequestration of the red cells in pyruvate kinase deficiency. New Eng. J. Med., **278,** 73, 1968.
55. Sachs, J. R., Wicker, D. J., Gilcher, R. O., Conrad, M. E., and Cohen, R. J.: Familial hemolytic anemia resulting from an abnormal red blood cell pyruvate kinase. J. Lab. Clin. Med., **72,** 359, 1968.
56. Zuelzer, W. W., Robinson, A. R., and Hsu, T. H. J.: Erythrocyte pyruvate kinase deficiency in non-spherocytic hemolytic anemia: A system of multiple genetic markers? Blood, **32,** 33, 1968.
57. Volpato, S., Vigi, V., and Cattarozzi, G.: Nonspherocytic haemolytic anaemia and severe jaundice in a newborn with partial pyruvate kinase deficiency. Acta Paediat. Scand., **57,** 59, 1968.
58. Dacie, J. V.: Recent advances in knowledge of the hereditary haemolytic anaemias. Schweiz. Med. Wschr., **98,** 1624, 1968.
59. Woessner, S., and Carbonell, M.: Hemolitica congenita no esferocitica por deficit de piruvatoquinasa: Presentacion de un caso clinico. Sangre (Barc.), **13,** 61, 1968.
60. Valentine, W. N.: Hereditary hemolytic anemias associated with specific erythrocyte enzymopathies. Calif. Med., **108,** 280, 1968.
61. Valentine, W. N., Oski, F. A., Paglia, D. E., Baughan, M. A., Schneider, A. S., and Naiman, J. L.: Hereditary hemolytic anemia with hexokinase deficiency: Role of hexokinase in erythrocyte aging. New Eng. J. Med., **276,** 1, 1967.
62. Valentine, W. N., Oski, F. A., Paglia, D. E., Baughan, M. A., Schneider, A. S., and Naiman, J. L.: Erythrocyte hexokinase and hereditary hemolytic anemia, in *Hereditary Disorders of Erythrocyte Metabolism,* edited by E. Beutler, p. 288. Grune & Stratton, New York, 1968.
63. Keitt, A. S.: Hemolytic anemia with impaired hexokinase activity. J. Clin. Invest., **48,** 1997, 1969.
64. Baughan, M. A., Valentine, W. N., Paglia, D. E., Ways, P. O., Simon, E. R., and DeMarsh, Q. B.: Hereditary hemolytic anemia associated with glucosephosphate isomerase (GPI) deficiency—a new enzyme defect of human erythrocytes. Blood, **32,** 236, 1968.
65. Paglia, D. E., Holland, P., Baughan, M. A., and Valentine, W. N.: Occurrence of defective hexosephosphate isomerization in human erythrocytes and leukocytes. New Eng. J. Med., **280,** 66, 1969.
66. Schneider, A. S., Valentine, W. N., Hattori, M., and Heins, H. L., Jr.: Hereditary hemolytic anemia with triosephosphate isomerase deficiency. New Eng. J. Med., **272,** 229, 1965.
67. Valentine, W. N., Schneider, A. S., Baughan, M. A., Paglia, D. E., and Heins, H. L., Jr.: Hereditary hemolytic anemia with triosephosphate isomerase deficiency: Studies in kindreds with co-existent sickle cell trait and erythrocyte glucose-6-phosphate dehydrogenase deficiency. Amer. J. Med., **41,** 27, 1966.
68. Schneider, A. S., Valentine, W. N., Baughan, M. A., Paglia, D. E., Shore, N. A., and Heins, H. L., Jr.: Triosephosphate isomerase deficiency. A. A multi-system inherited enzyme disorder: Clinical and genetic aspects, in *Hereditary Disorders of Erythrocyte Metabolism,* edited by E. Beutler, p. 265. Grune & Stratton, New York, 1968.
69. Schneider, A. S., Dunn, I., Ibsen, K. H., and Weinstein, I. M.: Triosephosphate isomerase deficiency. B. Inherited triosephosphate isomerase deficiency: Erythrocyte carbohydrate metabolism and preliminary studies of the erythrocyte enzyme. *Ibid,* p. 273.
70. Kraus, A. P., Langston, M. F., and Lynch, B. L.: Red cell phosphoglycerate kinase deficiency: A new cause of non-spherocytic hemolytic anemia. Biochem. Biophys. Res. Commun., **30,** 173, 1968.
71. Valentine, W. N., Hsieh, H., Paglia, D. E., Anderson, H. M., Baughan, M. A., Jaffé, E. R., and Garson, O. M.: Hereditary hemolytic anemia: Association with phosphoglycerate kinase deficiency in erythrocytes and leukocytes. Trans. Ass. Amer. Physicians, **81,** 49, 1968.
72. Valentine, W. N., Hsieh, H., Paglia, D. E., Anderson, H. M., Baughan, M. A., Jaffé, E. R., and Garson, O. M.: Hereditary hemolytic anemia associated with phosphoglycerate kinase deficiency in erythrocytes and leukocytes: A probable X-chromosome-linked syndrome. New Eng. J. Med., **280,** 528, 1969.
73. Alagille, D., Fleury, J., and Odièvre, M.: Déficit congénital en 2,3-diphosphoglycéromutase. Bull. Soc. Med. Hop., Paris, **115,** 493, 1964.
74. Schröter, W.: Kongenitale nichtsphärocytäre hämolytische anämie bei 2,3-diphosphoglyceratmutose-mangel der erythrocyten im frühen sauglingsalter. Klin. Wschr., **43,** 1147, 1965.
75. Schröter, W., and Heyden, H. V.: Kinetik des 2,3-diphosphoglyceratumsatzes in menschlichen erythrocyter. Biochem. Zeitsch., **341,** 387, 1965.
76. Tarui, S., Okuno, G., Ikura, Y., Tanaka, T., Suda, M., and Nishikawa, M.: Phosphofructokinase deficiency in skeletal muscle: A new type of glycogenosis. Biochem. Biophys. Res. Commun., **19,** 517, 1965.
77. Layzer, R. B., Rowland, L. P., and Ranney, H. M.: Muscle phosphofructokinase deficiency. Arch. Neurol. (Chicago), **17,** 512, 1967.
78. Tarui, S., Kono, N., Nasu, T., and Nishikawa, M.: Enzymatic basis for the coexistance of myopathy and hemolytic disease in inherited muscle phosphofructokinase deficiency. Biochem. Biophys. Res. Commun., **34,** 77, 1969.
79. Lausecker, C., Heidt, P., Fischer, D., Hartleyb, H., and Löhr, G. W.: Anémie hémolytique constitutionnelle avec deficit en 6-phosphogluconate-deshydrogenase Arch. Franc. Pediat., **22,** 789, 1965.
80. Scialom, C., Najean, Y., and Bernard, J.: Anémie hémolytique congénitale nonsphérocytaire avec déficit incomplet en 6-phosphogluconatedeshydrogenase. Nouv. Rev. Franc. Hemat., **6,** 452, 1966.
81. Brewer, G. J., and Dern, R. J.: A new inherited enzymatic deficiency of human erythrocytes: 6-phosphogluconate dehydrogenase deficiency. Amer. J. Hum. Genet., **16,** 472, 1964.
82. Parr, C. W., and Fitch, L. I.: Hereditary partial deficiency of human erythrocyte phosphogluconate dehydrogenase. Biochem. J., **93,** 28c, 1964.
83. Carter, N. D., Fildes, R. A., Fitch, L. I., and Parr, C. W.: Genetically determined electrophoretic variations of human phosphogluconate dehydrogenase. Acta Genet. (Basel), **18,** 109, 1968.
84. Dern, R. J., Brewer, G. J., Tashian, R. E., and Shows, T. B.: Hereditary variation of erythrocytic 6-phosphogluconate dehydrogenase. J. Lab. Clin. Med., **67,** 255, 1966.
85. Parr, C. W., and Fitch, L. I.: Inherited quantitative variations of human phosphogluconate dehydrogenase. Ann. Hum. Genet., **30,** 339, 1967.
86. Löhr, G. W., and Waller, H. D.: Eine neue enzymopenische hämolytische anämie mit glutathionreduktase-mangel. Med. Klin., **57,** 1521, 1962.
87. Carson, P. E., Brewer, G. J., and Ickes, C.: Decreased glutathione reductase with susceptibility to hemolysis. J. Lab. Clin. Med., **58,** 804, 1961. (Abstract.)
88. Blume, K. G., Gottwik, M., Löhr, G. W., and Rudiger, H. W.: Familienuntersuchungen zum glutathionreduktasemangel menschlicher erythrocyten. Humangenetik, **6,** 163, 1968.
89. Brittinger, G., Löffler, G., and König, E.: Angeborene nichtsphärocytäre hämolytische anämie bei familiärem mangel an DPNH- und TPNH-abhängiger glutathionreduktase der erythrocyten. I. Mitt. Klin. Wschr., **43,** 427, 1965.
90. Punt, K., Helleman, P. W., Staal, G., and Verloop, M. C.: A possible case of alpha-thalassemia (Hb.H-disease) in a Dutch family, associated with a deficiency of glutathione reductase in the erythrocytes. *Proc. Xth Congr. Europ. Soc. Haemat.,* Strasbourg, 1965, part II, p. 262. S. Karger, Basel/New York, 1967.
91. Fornaini, G., Bianchini, E., Leoncini, G., and Fantoni, A.: Metabolic aspects of red cells in congenital nonspherocytic haemolytic anaemia. Brit. J. Haemat., **10,** 23, 1964.
92. Waller, H. D., Löhr, G. W., Zysno, E., Gerok, W., Voss, D., and Strauss, G.: Glutathionreduktasemangel mit hämatologischen und neurologischen störungen (Autosomal dominant vererbliche bildung eines pathologischen enzyms). Klin. Wschr., **43,** 413, 1965.

93. Waller, H. D.: Glutathione reductase deficiency, in *Hereditary Disorders of Erythrocyte Metabolism,* edited by E. Beutler, p. 185. Grune & Stratton, New York, 1968.
94. Oort, M., Loos, J. A., and Prins, H. K.: Hereditary absence of reduced glutathione in the erythrocytes—a new clinical and biochemical entity. Vox Sang., **6,** 370, 1961.
95. Prins, H. K., Oort, M., Loos, J. A., Zürcher, C., and Beckers, T.: Congenital nonspherocytic hemolytic anemia, associated with glutathione deficiency of the erythrocytes: Hematologic, biochemical, and genetic studies. Blood, **27,** 145, 1966.
96. Prins, H. K., Oort, M., Loos, J. A., Zürcher, C., and Beckers, T.: Hereditary absence of glutathione in the erythrocytes: Biochemical, haematological, and genetical studies. *Proc. IX Congr. Europ. Soc. Haemat.,* Lisbon, 1963, p. 721. S. Karger, Basel, 1963.
97. Prins, H. K., Loos, J. A., and Zürcher, C.: Glutathione deficiency, in *Hereditary Disorders of Erythrocyte Metabolism,* edited by E. Beutler, p. 165. Grune & Stratton, New York, 1968.
98. Boivin, P., and Galand, C.: La synthèse du glutathion au cours de l'anémie hémolytique congénitale avec déficit en glutathion reduit. Nouv. Rev. Franc. Hemat., **5,** 707, 1965.
99. Harvald, B., Hanel, K. H., Squires, R., and Trap-Jensen, J.: Adenosine-triphosphatase deficiency in patients with nonspherocytic haemolytic anaemia. Lancet, **2,** 18, 1964.
100. Necheles, T. F., Maldonado, N., Barquet-Chediak, A., and Allen, D. M.: Homozygous erythrocyte glutathione-peroxidase deficiency: Clinical and biochemical studies. Blood, **33,** 164, 1969.
101. Loos, J. A., Prins, H. K., and Zürcher, C.: Elevated ATP levels in human erythrocytes, in *Hereditary Disorders of Erythrocyte Metabolism,* edited by E. Beutler, p. 280. Grune & Stratton, New York, 1968.
102. Brewer, G. J.: A new inherited metabolic abnormality of human erythrocytes characterized by elevated levels of adenosine triphosphate (ATP). J. Clin. Invest., **43,** 1287, 1964. (Abstract.)
103. Brewer, G. J.: A new inherited abnormality of human erythrocytes—elevated erythrocytic adenosine triphosphate. Biochem. Biophys. Res. Commun., **18,** 430, 1965.
104. Brewer, G. J., and Powell, R. D.: The adenosine triphosphate content of glucose-6-phosphate dehydrogenase-deficient and normal erythrocytes, including studies of a glucose-6-phosphate dehydrogenase-deficient man with "elevated erythrocytic ATP." J. Lab. Clin. Med., **67,** 726, 1966.
105. Jacobasch, G., Syllm-Rapoport, I., Roigas, H., and Rapoport, S.: 2,3-PGase-mangel als mögliche ursache erhöhten ATP-gehaltes. Clin. Chim. Acta, **10,** 477, 1964.
106. Bartlett, G. R.: Human red cell glycolytic intermediates. J. Biol. Chem., **234,** 449, 1959.
107. Bartlett, G. R.: Colorimetric assay methods for free and phosphorylated glyceric acids. J. Biol. Chem., **234,** 469, 1959.
108. Rapoport, S., and Luebering, J.: The formation of 2,3-diphosphoglycerate in rabbit erythrocytes: The existence of a diphosphoglycerate mutase. J. Biol. Chem., **183,** 507, 1950.
109. Rapoport, S., and Luebering, J.: An optical study of diphosphoglycerate mutase. J. Biol. Chem., **196,** 583, 1952.
110. Murphy, J. R.: Erythrocyte metabolism. II. Glucose metabolism and pathways. J. Lab. Clin. Med., **55,** 286, 1960.
111. Allison, A. C., and Burn, G. P.: Enzyme activity as a function of age in the human erythrocyte. Brit. J. Haemat., **1,** 291, 1955.
112. Marks, P. A., Johnson, A. B., Hirschberg, E., and Banks, J.: Studies on the mechanism of aging of human red blood cells. Ann. N.Y. Acad. Sci., **75,** 95, 1958.
113. Marks, P. A., Johnson, A. B., and Hirschberg, E.: Effect of age on enzyme activity in erythrocytes. Proc. Nat. Acad. Sci. USA, **44,** 529, 1958.
114. Sass, M. D., Vorsanger, E., and Spear, P. W.: Enzyme activity as an indicator of red cell age. Clin. Chim. Acta, **10,** 21, 1964.
115. Brok, F., Ramot, B., Zwang, E., and Danon, D.: Enzyme activities in human red blood cells of different age groups. Israel J. Med. Sci., **2,** 291, 1966.
116. Tanaka, K. R., Valentine, W. N., and Schneider, A. S.: Pyruvate kinase deficiency in hereditary nonspherocytic hemolytic anemia: An inborn error of metabolism. *Proc. IX Cong. Europ. Soc. Haemat.,* Lisbon, 1963, **2,** part 1, 739. S. Karger, Basel, 1963.
117. Tanaka, K. R., and Valentine, W. N.: Pyruvate kinase deficiency, in *Hereditary Disorders of Erythrocyte Metabolism,* edited by E. Beutler, p. 229. Grune & Stratton, New York, 1968.
118. Paglia, D. E., Valentine, W. N., Baughan, M. A., Miller, D. R., Reed, C. F., and McIntyre, O. R.: An inherited molecular lesion of erythrocyte pyruvate kinase: Identification of a kinetically aberrant isozyme associated with premature hemolysis. J. Clin. Invest., **47,** 1929, 1968.
119. Baughan, M. A., Paglia, D. E., Schneider, A. S., and Valentine, W. N.: An unusual hematological syndrome with pyruvate-kinase deficiency and Thalassemia minor in the kindreds. Acta Haemat. (Basel), **39,** 345, 1968.
120. Tanaka, K. R.: Pyruvate kinase, in *Biochemical Methods in Red Cell Genetics,* edited by J. J. Yunis, p. 167. Academic, New York, 1969.
121. Tanaka, K. R.: Pyruvate kinase deficiency hereditary hemolytic anemia. Jap. J. Hum. Genet., **44** (Supp.) 286, 1969.
122. Tanaka, K. R.: Unpublished data.
123. Brewer, G. J.: Personal communication, 1969.
124. Paglia, D. E., and Valentine, W. N.: Unpublished data.
125. Bigley, R. H., and Koler, R. D.: Liver pyruvate kinase (PK) isozymes in a PK-deficient patient. Ann. Hum. Genet., **31,** 383, 1968.
126. Brunetti, P., and Nenci, G.: A screening method for the detection of erythrocyte pyruvate kinase deficiency. Enzym. Biol. Clin. (Basel), **4,** 51, 1964.
127. Beutler, E.: A series of new screening procedures for pyruvate kinase deficiency, glucose-6-phosphate dehydrogenase deficiency, and glutathione reductase deficiency. Blood, **28,** 553, 1966.
128. Miwa, S., Kanai, M., and Nomoto, S.: Use of the AutoAnalyzer for determination of erythrocyte pyruvate kinase, glucose-6-phosphate dehydrogenase and cholinesterase. Brit. J. Haemat., **13** (Supp.) 54, 1967.
129. Miwa, S., Tanaka, K. R., and Valentine, W. N.: Erythrocytic and leukocytic glycolytic enzyme studies in hematologic and nonhematologic diseases. Acta Haemat. Jap., **25,** 12, 1962.
130. Powell, R. D., and DeGowin, R. L.: Relationship between activity of pyruvate kinase and age of the normal human erythrocyte. Nature (London), **205,** 507, 1965.
131. Löhr, G. W.: Hamatologische enzymologie. Helv. Med. Acta, **30,** 428, 1963.
132. Tanaka, K. R., and Valentine, W. N.: Unpublished data.
133. Shafer, A. W.: Glycolytic intermediates in erythrocytes in nonspherocytic hemolytic anemia with deficiency of glucose 6-phosphate dehydrogenase (G6-PD) or pyruvate kinase (PK). Clin. Res., **11,** 103, 1963. (Abstract.)
134. Nathan, D. G., Oski, F. A., Sidel, V. W., and Diamond, L. K.: Extreme hemolysis and red cell distortion in erythrocyte pyruvate kinase deficiency. II. Measurements of erythrocyte glucose consumption, potassium flux and adenosine triphosphate stability. New Eng. J. Med., **272,** 118, 1965.
135. Lenfant, C., Torrance, J., English, E., Finch, C. A., Reynafarje, C., Ramos, J., and Faura, J.: Effect of altitude on oxygen binding by hemoglobin and on organic phosphate levels. J. Clin. Invest., **47,** 2652, 1968.
136. Oski, F. A., Gottlieb, A. J., Delivoria-Papadopoulos, M., and Miller, W. W.: Red-cell 2,3-diphosphoglycerate levels in subjects with chronic hypoxemia. New Eng. J. Med., **280,** 1165, 1969.
137. Eaton, J. W., Brewer, G. J., and Grover, R. F.: Role of red cell 2,3-diphosphoglycerate in the adaptation of man to altitude. J. Lab. Clin. Med., **73,** 603, 1969.
138. Eaton, J. W., and Brewer, G. J.: The relationship between red cell 2,3-diphosphoglycerate and levels of hemoglobin in the human. Proc. Nat. Acad. Sci. USA, **61,** 756, 1968.
139. Zürcher, C., Loos, J. A., and Prins, H. K.: Hereditary high ATP content of human erythrocytes. Folia Haemat. (Leipzig), **83,** 366, 1965.
140. Loos, J. A.: Een vergelijkend biochemisch onderzoek bij normale en afwijkende menselijke erytrocyten. Doctoral Thesis, University of Amsterdam. Drukkerij "Aemstelstad," Amsterdam, 1965.
141. Benesch, R., and Benesch, R. E.: The effect of organic phosphates from

the human erythrocyte on the allosteric properties of hemoglobin. Biochem. Biophys. Res. Commun., **26**, 162, 1967.

142. Chanutin, A., and Curnish, R. R.: Effect of organic and inorganic phosphates on the oxygen equilibrium of human erythrocytes. Arch. Biochem. Biophys., **121**, 96, 1967.
143. Astrup, P., Garby, L., and de Verdier, C.-H.: Displacements of the oxyhemoglobin dissociation curve. Scand. J. Clin. Lab. Invest., **22**, 171, 1968.
144. Benesch, R., Benesch, R. E., and Yu, C. I.: Reciprocal binding of oxygen and diphosphoglycerate by human hemoglobin. Proc. Nat. Acad. Sci. USA, **59**, 526, 1968.
145. Benesch, R., and Benesch, R. E.: Intracellular organic phosphates as regulators of oxygen released by haemoglobin. Nature (London), **221**, 618, 1969.
146. de Verdier, C.-H., Garby, L., and Hjelm, M.: Regulation of oxygen transport. New Eng. J. Med., **280**, 1360, 1969.
147. Mourdjinis, A., Walters, C., Edwards, M. J., Koler, R. D., Vanderheiden, B., and Metcalfe, J.: Improved oxygen delivery in pyruvate kinase deficiency (PK-def). Clin. Res., **17**, 153, 1969. (Abstract.)
148. Rose, I. A., and Warms, J. V. B.: Control of glycolysis in the human red blood cell. J. Biol. Chem., **241**, 4848, 1966.
149. Campos, J. O., Koler, R. D., and Bigley, R. H.: Kinetic differences between human red cell and leucocyte pyruvate kinase. Nature (London), **208**, 194, 1965.
150. Wiesmann, U., and Tönz, O.: Investigations of the kinetics of red cell pyruvate kinase in normal individuals and in a patient with pyruvate kinase deficiency. Nature (London), **209**, 612, 1966.
151. Wiesmann, U., Tönz, O., Richterich, R., and Verger, P.: Die erythrocyten-pyruvat-kinase bei gesunden und bei nichtsphärocytärer, hämolytischer pyruvat-kinase-mangel-anämie. Klin. Wschr., **43**, 1311, 1965.
152. Koler, R. D., Bigley, R. H., and Stenzel, P.: Biochemical properties of human erythrocyte and leukocyte pyruvate kinase, in *Hereditary Disorders of Erythrocyte Metabolism,* edited by E. Beutler, p. 249. Grune & Stratton, New York, 1968.
153. Bigley, R. H., Stenzel, P., Jones, R. T., Campos, J. O., and Koler, R. D.: Tissue distribution of human pyruvate kinase isozymes. Enzym. Biol. Clin. (Basel), **9**, 10, 1968.
154. Boivin, P., and Galand, C.: Recherche d'une anomalie moléculaire lors des déficits en pyruvate kinase érythrocytaire. Nouv. Rev. Franc. Hemat., **8**, 201, 1968.
155. Boivin, P., and Galand, C.: Constante de Michaelis anormale pour le phosphoenol-pyruvate au cours d'un deficit en pyruvate-kinase erythrocytaire. Rev. Franc. Etud. Clin. Biol., **12**, 372, 1967.
156. Oski, F., and Bowman, H.: A low K_m phosphoenolpyruvate mutant in the Amish with red cell pyruvate kinase (PK) deficiency. Clin. Res., **16**, 540, 1968. (Abstract.)
157. Miwa, S., Nishina, T., Kakehashi, Y., Ohyama, H., and Moriguchi, O.: Kinetically abnormal erythrocyte pyruvate kinase (PK) associated with hereditary hemolytic anemia: a new variant? *Abstr. XIIIth Int. Congr. Hemat.,* Munich, Germany, 1970, p. 123.
158. Gross, R. T.: Clinical applications of some recent studies of erythrocyte enzymes. Bull. N.Y. Acad. Med., **39**, 90, 1963.
159. Grignani, F., and Löhr, G. W.: Uber die hexokinase in menschlichen blutzellen. Klin. Wschr., **38**, 796, 1960.
160. Hinterberger, U., Ockel, E., Gerischer-Mothes, W., and Rapoport, S.: Grofze und pH-abhängigkeit der anaeroben glykolyse und der hexokinäse aktivitat von erythrozyten und retikulozyten des kaninchens. Acta Biol. Med. German., **7**, 50, 1961.
161. Ockel, E., Rapoport, S., Hinterberger, U., and Gerischer-Mothes, W.: Die pH-abhängigkeit der anaeroben glykolyse und der hexokinäse. Folia Haemat. (Leipzig), **78**, 477, 1962.
162. Rapoport, S., Hinterberger, U., and Hofmann, E. C. G.: Die Begrenzende rolle der hexokinäse-reaktion für die anaerobe glykolyse der roten blutzellen. Naturwissenschaften, **48**, 501, 1961.
163. Löhr, G. W., Waller, H. D., Anschütz, F., and Knoop, A.: Biochemische defekte in den blutzellen bei familiärer panmyelopathie (Typ Fanconi). Humangenetik, **1**, 383, 1965.
164. Detter, J. C., Ways, P. O., Giblett, E. R., Baughan, M. A., Hopkinson, D. A., Povey, S., and Harris, H.: Inherited variations in human phosphohexose isomerase. Ann. Hum. Genet., **31**, 329, 1968.
165. Harris, S. R., Paglia, D. E., Jaffé, E. R., Valentine, W. N., and Klein, R. L.: Triosephosphate isomerase deficiency in an adult. Clin. Res., **18**, 529, 1970.
166. Angelman, H., Brain, M. L., and MacIver, J. E.: A case of triosephosphate isomerase deficiency with sudden death. *Abstr. XIIIth Int. Congr. Hemat.,* Munich, Germany, 1970, p. 122.
167. Davidson, R. G., Nitowsky, H. M., and Childs, B.: Demonstration of two populations of cells in the human female heterozygous for glucose-6-phosphate dehydrogenase variants. Proc. Nat. Acad. Sci. USA, **50**, 481, 1963.
168. Beutler, E., Yeh, M., and Fairbanks, V. F.: The normal human female as a mosaic of X-chromosome activity: Studies using the gene for G-6-PD deficiency as a marker. Proc. Nat. Acad. Sci. USA, **48**, 9, 1962.
169. Grumbach, M. M., Marks, P. A., and Morishima, A.: Erythrocyte glucose-6-phosphate dehydrogenase activity and X-chromosome polysomy. Lancet, **1**, 1330, 1962.
170. Tönz, O., and Rossi, E.: Morphological demonstration of two red cell populations in human females heterozygous for glucose-6-phosphate dehydrogenase deficiency. Nature (London), **202**, 606, 1964.
171. Lyon, M. F.: Gene action in the X-chromosomes of the mouse (*Mus musculus L.*): Nature (London), **190**, 372, 1961.
172. Lyon, M. F.: Sex chromatin and gene action in the mammalian X-chromosome. Amer. J. Hum. Genet., **14**, 135, 1962.
173. Carson, P. E., cited by Waller, H.D.: Discussion of glutathione reductase deficiency, in *Hereditary Disorders of Erythrocyte Metabolism,* edited by E. Beutler, p. 204. Grune & Stratton, New York, 1968.
174. Beutler, E.: The effect of flavin compounds on glutathione reductase activity: In vivo and in vitro studies. J. Clin. Invest., **48**, 1957, 1969.
175. Beutler, E.: Glutathione reductase stimulation in normal subjects by riboflavin supplementation. Science **165**, 613, 1969.
176. Mills, G. C.: Hemoglobin catabolism. I. Glutathione peroxidase, an erythrocyte enzyme which protects hemoglobin from oxidative breakdown. J. Biol. Chem., **229**, 189, 1957.
177. Mills, G. C., and Randall, H. P.: Hemoglobin catabolism. II. The protection of hemoglobin from oxidative breakdown in the intact erythrocyte. J. Biol. Chem., **232**, 589, 1958.
178. Paglia, D. E., and Valentine, W. N.: Studies on the quantitative and qualitative characterization of erythrocyte glutathione peroxidase. J. Lab. Clin. Med., **70**, 158, 1967.
179. Necheles, T. F., Boles, T. A., and Allen, D. M.: Erythrocyte glutathione-peroxidase deficiency and hemolytic disease of the newborn. J. Pediat., **72**, 319, 1968.
180. Boivin, P., Galand, C., Hakim, J., Rogé, J., and Guéroult, N.: Anémie hemolytique avec déficit en glutathione-peroxydase chez un adulte. Enzym. Biol. Clin. (Basel), **10**, 68, 1969.
181. Boivin, P., Galand, C., André, R., and Debray, J.: Anémies hémolytiques congénitales avec déficit isolé en glutathion réduit par déficit en glutathion synthétase. *Proc. Xth Congr. Europ. Soc. Haemat.,* Strasbourg, 1965, part II, p. 300. S. Karger, Basel/New York, 1967.
182. Tanaka, K. R., and Paglia, D. E.: Pyruvate kinase deficiency. Seminars in Hematology, **8**, 367, 1971.
183. Paglia, D. E., and Valentine, W. N.: Additional kinetic distinctions between normal pyruvate kinase and a mutant isozyme from human erythrocytes. Correction of the kinetic anomaly by fructose-1,6-diphosphate. Blood, **37**, 311, 1971.
184. Necheles, T. F., Rai, U. S., and Cameron, D.: Congenital nonspherocytic hemolytic anemia associated with an unusual hexokinase abnormality. J. Lab. Clin. Med., **76**, 593, 1970.
185. Arnold, H., Blume, K. G., Busch, D., Leikert, V., Löhr, G. W., and Lübs, E.: Klinische und biochemische Untersuchungen zur Glucosephosphatisomerase normaler menschlicher Erythrocyten und bei Glucose-phosphatisomerase-Mangel. Klin. Wschr. **48**, 1299, 1970.
186. Beutler, E.: Personal communication. 1971.
187. Schroeder, M., Foerster, J., and Beutler, E.: Personal communication. 1971.

188. Schröter, W., Brittinger, G., Zimmerschitt, E., and König, E.: A new haemolytic syndrome with glucose-phosphate isomerase (GPI) and glucose-6-phosphate dehydrogenase (G6PD) deficiency of the erythrocytes. Biochemical studies. Eur. J. Clin. Invest., **1**, 145, 1970, (Abstract).
189. Valentine, W. N., Paredes, R., Paglia, D. E., and Konrad, P. N.: Unpublished data.
190. Chen, S. H., Malcolm, L. A., Yoshida, A., and Giblett, E. R.: Phosphoglycerate kinase: an X-linked polymorphism in man. Amer. J. Hum. Genet., **23**, 87, 1971.
191. Meera Khan, P., Westerveld, A., Gryeschik, K.-H., Deys, B. F., Garson, O. M., and Siniscalio, M.: X-linkage of human phosphoglycerate kinase confirmed in man-mouse and man-Chinese hamster somatic cell hybrids. Am. J. Hum. Genet., **23**, 614, 1971.
192. Hjelm, M., and Wadman, B.: Nonspherocytic haemolytic anemia with phosphoglycerate kinase deficiency. *Abstr. XIIIth Int. Congr. Hemat.*, Munich, Germany, 1970, p. 121.
193. Mazza, U., Arese, P., Bosia, A., Gallo, E., and Pescarmona, G. P.: Red cell metabolism in a case of 3-phosphoglycerate kinase deficiency. *Abstr. XIIIth Int. Congr. Hemat.*, Munich, Germany, 1970, p. 121.
194. Schröter, W.: 2,3-Diphosphoglyceratstoffwechsel und 2,3-Diphosphoglyceratmutase-Mangel in Erythrocyten. Blut, **20**, 1, 1970.
195. Waterbury, L., and Frenkel, E. P.: Phosphofructokinase deficiency in congenital nonspherocytic hemolytic anemia. Clin. Res., **17**, 347, 1969.
196. Cotte, J., Kissin, C., Mathieu, M., Poncet, J., Monnet, P., Salle, B., and Germain, D.: Observation d'un cas de déficit partiel en ATPas intraérythrocytaire. Rev. Franc. Etud. Clin. Biol., **13**, 284, 1968.
197. Balfe, J. W., Cole, C., Smith, E. K. M., Graham, J. B., and Welt, L. G.: A hereditary sodium transport defect in the human red blood cell. J. Clin. Invest., **47**, 4a, 1968.
198. Necheles, T. F., Steinberg, M. H., and Cameron, D.: Erythrocyte glutathione-peroxidase deficiency. Brit. J. Haemat., **19**, 605, 1970.
199. Mohler, D. N., Majerus, P. W., Minnich, V., Hess, C. E., and Garrick, M. D.: Glutathione synthetase deficiency as a cause of hereditary hemolytic disease. New Eng. J. Med., **283**, 1253, 1970.
200. Busch, D.: Überhölter Erythrocyten-ATP-Spiegel-Merkmal einer hereditären nichtsphärocytären hämolytischen Anämie bei gestorter ATP-Utilisation und einer Stoffwechselunomalie roter Zellen ohne Krankheitswert. Klin. Wschr., **48**, 543, 1970.
201. Busch, D., and Heimpel, H.: Hereditäre nichtsphärocytäre hämolytische Anämie mit hohen Erythrocyten-ATP. Blut, **19**, 293, 1969.
202. Valentine, W. N., Anderson, H. M., Paglia, D. E., Jaffé, E. R., Konrad, P. N., and Harris, S. P.: Nonspherotytic hemolytic anemia, high red cell ATP and ribosephosphate pyrophosphokinase (RPK, E.C. 2.7.6.1) deficiency. Clin. Res., **19**, 567, 1971 (Abstract).
203. Paglia, D. E., Valentine, W. N., Tartaglia, A. P., and Konrad, P. N.: Adenine nucleotide reductions associated with a dominantly transmitted form of nonspherocytic hemolytic anemia. Blood, **36**, 837, 1970.

CHAPTER FIFTY-FIVE

GLUCOSE-6-PHOSPHATE DEHYDROGENASE DEFICIENCY*

Ernest Beutler

Over the years persons charged with the care of the sick have often been dismayed to find that a drug innocuous to many patients produced catastrophic results in a few. In 1953 it first became possible to study in detail one such drug-sensitivity reaction, the hemolytic effect of the 8-aminoquinoline antimalarial primaquine. These studies not only helped to clarify the mechanism of sensitivity to this drug but also led to the demonstration that a hereditary biochemical lesion of the erythrocyte, glucose-6-phosphate dehydrogenase (G-6-PD) deficiency, was responsible for many other drug-induced hemolytic anemias and for favism. Only the history of 8-aminoquinoline hemolytic anemia will be reviewed. That of related drug sensitivities is similar.

The history of the 8-aminoquinoline compounds resembles that of many drugs: the compound was hailed as harmless to the blood when it was first introduced in 1926; scarcely a year later severe, even fatal, hemolytic anemias were reported. The first of the 8-aminoquinolines in clinical medicine was plasmoquin (pamaquine), which was used by Mühlens [1] to treat syphilitics who had been inoculated with malaria.

Following the initial report of Cordes [2] on the hemolytic anemia associated with the administration of this drug, many similar reports appeared from all over the world [3–35]. Typically, the patient developed dark, often black, urine a few days after pamaquine therapy was begun. Jaundice appeared, and the red blood count and hemoglobin became much diminished. Usually the patient recovered, but sometimes he succumbed to massive destruction of red blood cells.

Attempts were made to implicate immune mechanisms in the etiology of hemolytic anemia due to pamaquine. A nonspecific hemagglutinin was described in the blood of one patient [21], but it was later demonstrated [33] that autoagglutinins could be found in the blood of patients receiving pamaquine who did not develop hemolytic anemia. Skin testing was attempted [27]. Fragility studies [11, 29, 33, 34] and Donath-Landsteiner tests [19, 25] were carried out. In addition, in vitro studies were made of hemolysis induced by pamaquine and related compounds, or by the plasma of patients who had recently received pamaquine [29, 36]. None of these studies solved the problem of why some persons developed acute hemolytic anemia when given pamaquine and others did not.

A few observations were made which, in retrospect, were much more significant. Heinz bodies in the red cells of a patient with mild hemolytic anemia occurring during pamaquine therapy were observed in 1928 [8]. Attention was called to the familial nature of pamaquine sensitivity, and analogies were drawn between this disorder and favism [31]. The difference in susceptibility of different races to hemolysis by pamaquine was recognized [18, 22, 25, 27, 29, 33].

It was not until after the introduction of primaquine, a therapeutically more effective 8-aminoquinoline [37], that it became possible to study intensively the hemolytic anemia induced by these compounds. The demonstration [38] that the sensitivity which induced the hemolytic anemia resided in the red blood cells made it possible to focus attention on the central problem, the abnormality of the erythrocyte.

Studies of the biochemistry of primaquine-sensitive cells suggested that their sensitivity to hemolysis was related in some way to their glutathione (GSH) content [39] and the stability of their GSH [40]. Examination of the pathways of GSH metabolism in drug-sensitive red cells [41] disclosed the probable primary defect, a deficiency of the enzyme glucose-6-phosphate dehydrogenase (G-6-PD). Subsequent observations established unequivocally that patients with favism [42–60], and a small group of subjects with nonspherocytic congenital hemolytic anemia [61–67], had many of the same biochemical abnormalities. It became apparent that there are many variants of G-6-PD deficiency which are distinguished from one another by certain clinical and biochemical differences [68, 69]. The most common types of deficiency in Western populations are the A− type, found chiefly in Negroes, and the Mediterranean type found most commonly in persons from the Mediterranean area. Other common types are A+, also found chiefly in Negroes, and the Canton type found among south Chinese. Since G-6-PD variants are being detected in many different laboratories and comparison with previously described variants is difficult when different methods of characterization have been employed, a series of standardized techniques for the characterization of variants has been proposed by a World Health Organization scientific group [70]. The recommendations of this group have been generally adopted, and are adhered to in this chapter. To aid further in the correlation of findings from many different laboratories, an international reference center for G-6-PD variants has been set up at the University of Washington, Seattle, Washington under the direction of Dr. Arno G. Motulsky. Regional centers have been established at Tel-Hashomer Government Hospital, Israel, under the direction of Dr. Bracha Ramot and at the University College Hospital, Ibadan, Nigeria under the direction of Dr. Lucio Luzzatto.

Recognition that this group of enzyme defects is inherited as an X-linked condition has made glucose-6-phosphate

*This work was supported in part by Public Health Service Grant No. HE 07449 from the National Heart Institute, National Institutes of Health.

dehydrogenase deficiency particularly important from a genetic point of view. It has made possible detailed mapping of the X chromosome, and indeed the genetics of the defect was one of the original observations which led to the X-inactivation hypothesis [71]. A number of reviews of G-6-PD deficiency have been published [70, 72–75].

CLINICAL ASPECTS

The A− Type of G-6-PD Deficiency

Negro subjects with the A− type of G-6-PD deficiency are essentially asymptomatic except under stress such as that imposed by drug administration and by infection. Although neonatal jaundice in a G-6-PD-deficient Negro infant has been reported [76–79], the bilirubin levels of G-6-PD-deficient Negro infants are, in general, normal [80] or only slightly increased [81].

The clinical course of primaquine-induced hemolysis has been studied under carefully controlled conditions [82]. When a G-6-PD-deficient Negro subject is given 30 mg primaquine daily, there is little or no evidence of hemolysis during the first 2 or 3 days. Then the urine begins to turn dark. In mild cases the patient often observes no other abnormality. In more severe cases, the patient complains of weakness and abdominal and back pain, and develops icterus and black urine. Heinz bodies appear in many of the red cells [83]; the hemoglobin, red blood cell, and hematocrit values fall rapidly, and the number of reticulocytes increases. This "acute hemolytic phase" ends spontaneously in about 1 week, even when drug administration is continued, and the "recovery phase" begins. The patient feels better, the color of the urine becomes normal, and the hemoglobin, red cell, and hematocrit values begin to rise. The reticulocyte count remains high at first and then declines. Throughout this time the Coombs' test result is negative, and red cell fragility remains unaltered. The only morphologic change in the blood is polychromasia and the appearance of Heinz bodies in the red cells during the first stages of hemolysis. Finally, the peripheral blood picture returns to normal, and the symptoms vanish, even though administration of the drug is continued in the same dosage that initially caused hemolysis. The refractory state which develops in G-6-PD deficiency is not due to altered metabolism of the drug after prolonged administration but rather to an alteration in reactivity of the red cell population [82].

Sensitivity to the hemolytic action of primaquine was found to be a function of red cell age [83]. There is a marked decrease in red cell G-6-PD activity with increasing cell age, even in normal red cells, and the decline in activity with aging is accelerated in red cells with the A− type of enzyme [73, 85, 86]. The relatively normal enzyme levels in younger cells of G-6-PD-deficient Negro subjects [73, 85, 86] provide some degree of protection against drug-induced hemolysis.

Acetanilid, sulfanilamide, diaphenylsulfon, and a number of other drugs [82, 87] were also given under controlled laboratory conditions to subjects known to be G-6-PD-deficient. In addition, there are many case reports of hemolytic anemia induced accidentally by naphthalene [52, 88–92], phenacetin [93], and nitrofurantoin (Furadantin) [94–97] in Negroes who are G-6-PD-deficient or who on clinical grounds may be presumed to have been enzyme deficient. The hemolytic anemia induced by acetanilid, sulfonamides, Furadantin, or naphthalene is similar to that induced by primaquine. Furadantin differs in not causing Heinz body formation [98]. Naphthalene-induced hemolytic anemia may at times be considerably more explosive than that observed with primaquine administration. Hemolysis induced by thiazolsulfone may vary greatly in intensity. Studies of the mechanism of this variability suggest that it is due to differences in absorption or metabolism of the drug [82]. Drugs known to cause hemolytic anemia in G-6-PD-deficient Negroes are listed in Table 55-1. Infections, too, appear to have the capacity to precipitate hemolytic reactions in those with the A− type of G-6-PD deficiency [120–122].

The Mediterranean Type of 6-P-PD Deficiency

Most patients with G-6-PD deficiency of the Mediterranean type also have no clinical signs or symptoms unless exposed to drugs. Under some conditions, contact with the fava bean [45, 46, 53, 56, 123, 124] and infections [47, 125] also appear to induce hemolytic crises. Jaundice is particularly severe when G-6-PD-deficient subjects contract hepatitis [126–128]. On occasion, hemolysis occurs even when there is no known inciting cause [129–132]. Hemolytic disease of the newborn may result from this enzyme deficiency. This has occurred among several Mediterranean and Oriental populations which have been studied [133–140], but not among Sephardic Jews in Israel [141], except in an instance when a triple dye was used to sterilize the umbilical stump [142].

In general, the clinical course of hemolysis is similar to that in subjects with the A− type deficiency, but it may be somewhat more severe [52, 115, 143, 144] in some cases, and in others it has not been self-limited [124, 146]. At least one drug, chloramphenicol, which failed to cause hemolysis in Negroes with G-6-PD deficiency [108, 109] has caused hemolysis in some Caucasians with G-6-PD deficiency [57, 113]. It may be, therefore, that the spectrum of drugs which may cause hemolysis in subjects with the Mediterranean type deficiency is wider than that in those with the A− type defect. Fava bean-induced hemolysis does not seem to occur with the A− type of defect, but may occur in Mediterranean subjects with G-6-PD deficiency within hours of contact with the fava beans and is often more severe than primaquine-induced hemolysis. Some factor other than red cell G-6-PD deficiency is required for the production of fava bean-induced hemolysis. In every case of favism in

Table 55-1. COMPOUNDS KNOWN TO HAVE INDUCED HEMOLYSIS OF GLUCOSE-6-PHOSPHATE DEHYDROGENASE–DEFICIENT RED CELLS

Analgesics:
- Acetanilid [99]
- Acetylsalicylic acid [100]*
- Acetophenetidin (phenacetin) [39, 99]*
- Antipyrine [100]
- Pyramidone [54]

Sulfonamides and sulfones:
- Sulfanilamide [99]
- Sulfapyridine [101, 102]
- Diaphenylsulfone [79, 87, 103]
- N_2-Acetylsulfanilamide [99]
- Sulfacetamide [99]
- Sulfisoxazole (Gantrisin) [102, 104]*
- Thiazolsulfone [99]
- Salicylazosulfapyridine (Azulfadine) [100]
- Sulfoxone [99]*
- Sulfamethoxypyridazine (Kynex) [100, 105, 106]

Antimalarials:
- Primaquine
- Pamaquine [107]
- Pentaquine [108, 109]
- Quinocide [104, 110]
- Quinacrine (Atabrine) [104]

Nonsulfonamide antibacterial agents:
- Furazolidone [100]
- Furmethonol [111]
- Nitrofurantoin (Furadantin) [94, 112]
- Nitrofurazone [97]
- Chloramphenicol [57, 113]‡
- Paraaminosalicylic acid [104]
- Neoarsphenamine [114]

Miscellaneous:
- Naphthalene [52, 88–90, 115]
- Trinitrotoluene [57]
- Methylene blue [116]*
- Nalidixic acid [117]
- Dimercaprol (BAL) [118]*
- Phenylhydrazine [99]
- Quinine [57, 102]†
- Quinidine [57]†
- Mestranol [119]

* Slightly hemolytic in Negroes, or only in very large doses.
† Hemolytic in Caucasians, but not in Negroes [109].
‡ Possibly hemolytic in Caucasians, but not in Negroes [109] or Orientals.

which the red cells have been studied the erythrocyte defect has been demonstrated, but subjects known to have G-6-PD deficiency have eaten fava beans with impunity [45, 147]. In addition, ^{51}Cr-labeled G-6-PD–deficient red cells are not necessarily destroyed in vivo when fava beans are eaten [56, 148, 149]. The possibility has been suggested that an additional genetic defect is required for sensitivity to the hemolytic effect of fava beans [150].

Congenital Nonspherocytic Hemolytic Anemia Associated with G-6-PD Deficiency

Unlike those with the more common forms of G-6-PD deficiency, some patients with rare and usually unstable variants of G-6-PD have a clinical syndrome of congenital nonspherocytic hemolytic anemia. These patients have varying degrees of anemia, even in the absence of drug administration. The anemia is usually mild and may appear in the neonatal period with jaundice. Increased hemolysis is commonly associated with drug administration and infections [60, 62–67, 131, 151–168]. The results of splenectomy are generally unsatisfactory.

GLUCOSE AND GSH METABOLISM IN THE NORMAL ERYTHROCYTE

Overall Metabolism of the Erythrocyte

Several reviews of the metabolism of the mature mammalian erythrocyte are available [169–171]. Although complex, it may be considered incomplete when compared with that of most other cells. For example, the mature red cell is unable to synthesize protein but does synthesize certain simpler compounds, such as GSH [172–176], nicotinamide mononucleotide, NAD [177–179], FAD [180], and ATP [181, 182]. While it was at one time believed that fat synthesis takes place in erythrocytes [183, 184], more recent studies indicate that lipid synthesis occurs only in reticulocytes and white cells [185, 186].

The red cell requires a source of energy for synthetic processes, for the maintenance of ion concentration gradients, and for the reduction of methemoglobin, which is continuously formed. The chief source of energy comes from the breakdown of glucose, but, in vitro, inosine, fructose, mannose, and galactose may be used as well (Fig. 55-1). Prior to further metabolism, glucose must be phosphorylated to glucose-6-phosphate. This is accomplished by the hexokinase reaction. In the erythrocyte, hexokinase activity is low compared to that of enzymes involved in the later stages of glucose metabolism, and hexokinase activity appears to be one of the rate-limiting steps in the utilization of glucose by the red cells [187, 188]. Subsequent to phosphorylation, glucose may be metabolized either anaerobically or aerobically. The relative rates of anaerobic glycolysis and aerobic metabolism of glucose can be influenced greatly by factors such as the pH of the suspending medium [189], the activity of G-6-PD [190, 191], and the rate of oxidation of GSH [192].

Anaerobic Metabolism

Under physiologic conditions glucose metabolism in the red cell is primarily anaerobic and yields lactic acid. The derived energy is stored in the form of high-energy phosphate bonds

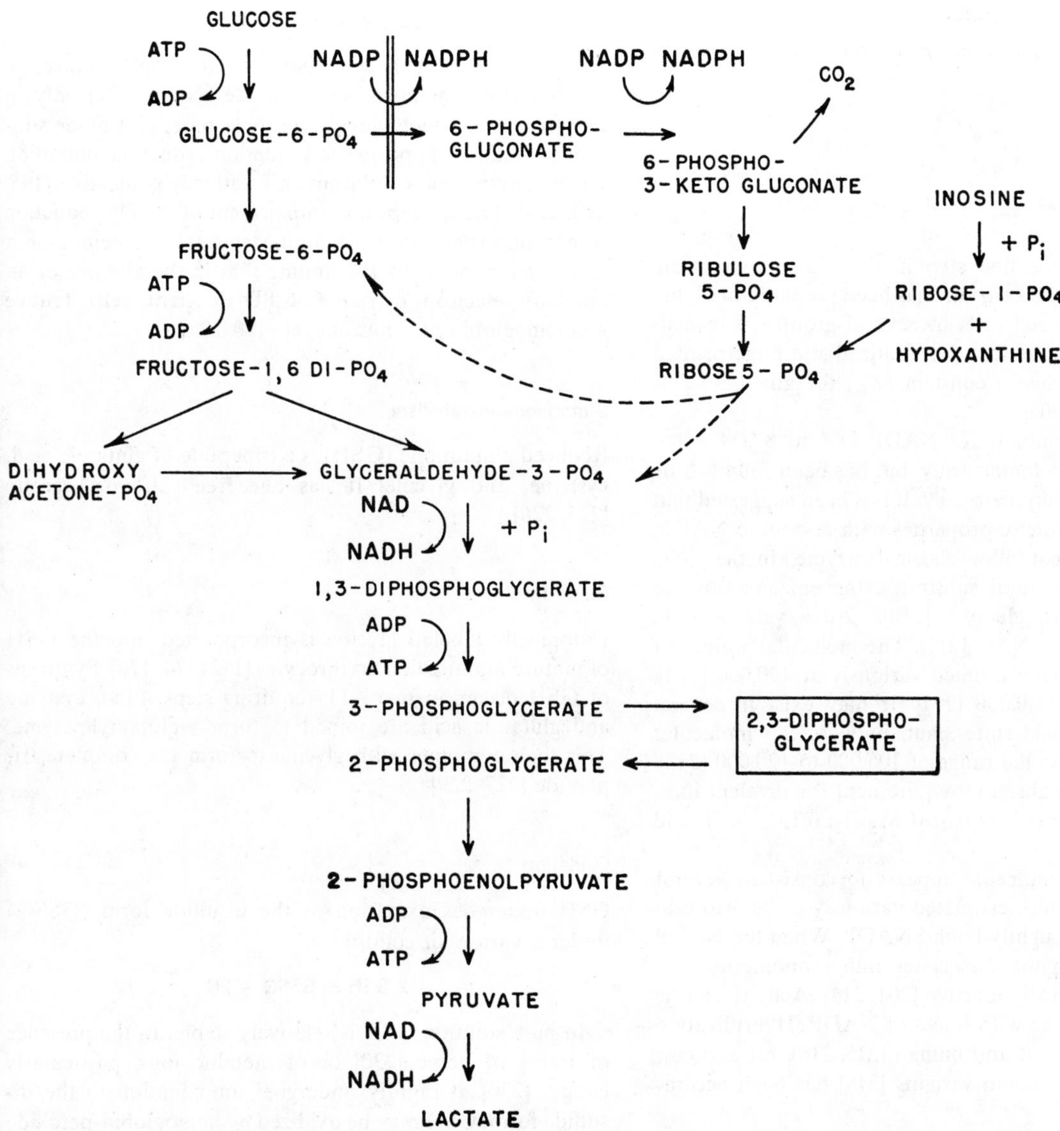

Figure 55-1. Glucose metabolism in the red blood cell. The site of the metabolic block in primaquine-sensitive erythrocytes is indicated by the double line between glucose-6-phosphate and 6-phosphogluconate.

by phosphorylation of ADP to ATP. During glycolysis, 1 mole of NAD is reduced in the oxidation of glyceraldehyde-3-phosphate to 1,3-diphosphoglyceric acid, and 1 mole of reduced NAD is oxidized in the reduction of pyruvic to lactic acid.

Oxidative Metabolism of Glucose

The direct oxidative pathway of glucose metabolism normally accounts for only a small proportion of the glucose utilized by the red blood cell [192, 189]. Methylene blue and certain other dyes [193–195], drugs such as acetylphenylhydrazine or primaquine, and certain physiologic substances such as cysteine and pyruvate [196] readily activate this route of metabolism by linking it to molecular oxygen, hydrogen peroxide, or methemoglobin. Glucose-6-P undergoes oxidation to 6-phosphogluconic acid through the action of G-6-PD. In this step, 1 mole of NADP is reduced. Phosphogluconic acid then undergoes oxidation to 6-phospho-3-keto gluconate and then to ribulose-5-P. Again, 1 mole of NADP is reduced. Various cleavages and condensations take place

[197, 198] which result ultimately in the formation of fructose-6-P and glyceraldehyde-3-P, normal intermediates in the anaerobic pathway.

G-6-PD

G-6-PD catalyzes the first step in the phosphogluconate oxidative pathway. This enzyme has been prepared in highly purified form from red cells by several groups of investigators [199–206] and has been crystallized and fingerprinted [207, 208]. The Michaelis constant (K_m) for glucose-6-P is 35 to 60 μM [199, 202].

The Michaelis constant for NADP is 4 to 8 μM when measured spectrophotometrically, but has been found to be 2 to 4 μM spectrofluorometrically. It has been suggested that the enzyme has allosteric properties with respect to NADP, and therefore does not follow classical enzyme kinetics [209]. In addition to its natural substrates, the enzyme can use analogues such as glucose [210], 2-deoxyglucose-6-P, deamino-NADP, and NAD [211]. The molecular weight of the enzyme has been estimated variously at 190,000 [202], 105,000 [201], and 240,000 [204]. It may exist in several different aggregational states, but, in vivo, the molecular weight is probably in the range of 105,000 to 120,000 [212]. It does not have an absolute requirement for divalent ions, but activity is increased by 0.01*M* $MgCl_2$, 0.1*M* NaCl, and 0.1*M* KCl [203].

The glucose-6-P molecule appears to consist of several identical [213] subunits, estimated variously to be 3 to 6 in number, containing tightly bound NADP. When the NADP is removed the enzyme dissociates into monomeric units which are enzymatically inactive [201, 214]. Activity can be restored by incubating with traces of NADP. Hybridization of the enzyme from rat and human [215, 216], rat and cow [217], and different human variants [218] has been accomplished.

Pathways of Oxidation of NADPH in the Erythrocyte

Several alternative routes of oxidation of NADPH are available in the red cell. Presumably these reflect some of the physiologic roles of NADPH and of the NADPH-generating system in the red cell.

Reduction of Oxidized Glutathione (GSSG)

NADPH is oxidized in the course of the enzymatic reduction of oxidized glutathione (GSSG) [219, 220].

$$\text{GSSG} + \text{NADPH} + \text{H}^+ \xrightarrow{\text{GSH reductase}} \text{2GSH} + \text{NADP}^+$$

The normal route of electron transfer from NADPH may involve the GSSG-GSH reaction [192, 221].

Reduction of Methemoglobin

NADPH is used for the reduction of methemoglobin through the NADP-methemoglobin reductase system [222] only in the presence of methylene blue, Nile blue, and other substances with an appropriate oxidation-reduction potential. Under physiologic conditions this pathway is inactive [195, 223, 224]. The concept that impairment of NADP reduction is not important in maintaining normal methemoglobin levels is supported by the finding that in the absence of an auxiliary electron carrier G-6-PD–deficient cells reduce methemoglobin at a normal rate [90, 223].

Glutathione Metabolism

Reduced glutathione (GSH) is a tripeptide of glutamic acid, cysteine, and glycine. It has one free sulfhydryl group [225, 226].

Biosynthesis

Isotopically labeled glycine is incorporated into the GSH of mature mammalian erythrocytes [172–174, 176]. Synthesis of GSH occurs in two ATP-requiring steps. First, cysteine and glutamic acid are joined to form γ-glutamylcysteine. This then combines with glycine to form the complete tripeptide [227–229].

Oxidation

GSH undergoes oxidation to the disulfide form (GSSG) under a variety of conditions.

$$2\ \text{GSH} \rightleftharpoons \text{GSSG} + 2\text{H}$$

In pure solution GSH is relatively stable. In the presence of traces of heme [230] or of metallic ions, particularly copper [230], it rapidly undergoes autoxidation to the disulfide form. GSH may be oxidized by hemoglobin-peroxide through the mediation of GSH peroxidase [231]. While it appears likely that it can serve as a hydrogen donor for the reduction of methemoglobin [231–233, 192], the rate of reaction is very slow or negligible under in vivo conditions [234]. It is oxidized rapidly when red cells are oxygenated in the absence of glucose [235–237], or are exposed to low levels of hydrogen peroxide by diffusion [231, 232, 238].

Reduction

Human red cells contain an enzyme, GSSG-reductase, which catalyzes the reduction of GSSG with NADPH serving as a hydrogen donor [220, 239].

Although NADH can also serve as a relatively inefficient hydrogen donor for GSSG reduction [220, 237, 239], physiologic reduction of GSSG appears to be accomplished solely through the NADPH route [240, 237]. The steady state concentration of GSSG is probably less than one-quarter of 1 percent of the total amount of glutathione in the cell [241].

Catabolism and Transport

In addition to the interconversion of GSH and GSSG, other pathways for the metabolism of red cell GSH exist. While biosynthesis of GSH proceeds in circulating red cells, it does not accumulate. Furthermore, when red cells are incubated with acetylphenylhydrazine in the absence of glucose there is a decrease not only of GSH, but also of total glutathione [242]. GSSG forms complexes with hemoglobin [243, 244], presumably through formation of a mixed disulfide with the cysteine residue in position 93 of the β chain [245]. This complex can apparently be split by the action of glutathione reductase and NADPH [577]. In addition, an active transport system extrudes GSSG from the erythrocyte [246, 247]. It has been suggested that a cysteinylglycine transpeptidase exists in red cells and that it can transfer γ-glutamate from glutathione to an amino acid receptor [229].

Function in the Economy of the Cell

A hereditary state has been discovered in which there is a virtual absence of red cell GSH, probably because of a failure in synthesis of the tripeptide [248]. GSH deficiency (with normal erythrocyte G-6-PD activity) results in a non-spherocytic congenital hemolytic anemia [249] associated with drug sensitivity [250]. These findings demonstrate unequivocally that GSH plays an important role in red cell metabolism. Complexing of most of red cell GSH with N-ethyl maleimide (NEM), on the other hand, has little effect on red cell survival [251]. This suggested that even small amounts of red cell GSH permit normal function, but our recent investigations infer that red cells can release GSH from the GSH-NEM complex [252]. GSH can prevent the accumulation of peroxide-hemoglobin complexes and thereby reduce the formation of choleglobin and methemoglobin in intact red cells which have been poisoned with azide [232]. Although the red cell is rich in catalase, the kinetic properties of this enzyme are such that it is relatively impotent in disposing of low levels of hydrogen peroxide. Thus, low levels of H_2O_2 can oxidize red cell GSH, even when catalase is not inhibited [238]. It may be, as suggested by Barron [253] for other tissues, that GSH helps to maintain-SH groups in the reduced state. G-6-PD [254] and GSH-reductase [255], both of which serve to keep GSH in the reduced state, are inhibited by sulfhydryl reagents. Accordingly, GSH and the glycolytic enzymes may be thought of as a "self-stabilizing chain" [256, 257]. In addition, oxidized glutathione may inhibit certain red cell enzymes, particularly hexokinase [258–260], but levels higher than may be encountered in vivo are required to produce inhibition [261].

BIOCHEMISTRY OF G-6-PD–DEFICIENT ERYTHROCYTES

Abnormalities Found Independently of Drug Administration

G-6-PD

The basic abnormality in G-6-PD deficiency is the formation of mature red cells which have diminished G-6-PD activity. It must be recognized that a deficiency of enzyme is only one of several abnormalities which affect this enzyme. Even those changes which do not result in clinically significant enzyme lack may be of considerable biochemical and genetic interest. Many variants of G-6-PD can be distinguished on the basis of enzyme activity found in the red cells, electrophoretic mobility of the enzyme, the Michaelis constant for its substrates, glucose-6-P and NADP, capacity to utilize 2-deoxyglucose-6-phosphate, galactose-6-phosphate, and deamino NADP, and NAD, heat stability, and pH optimum. In addition, certain variants can be distinguished by susceptibility to inhibition by sulfhydryl reagents [262], chromatographic mobility on ion exchange columns [263–265], transition temperatures [263], and heat sensitivity in tissue culture [266]. Table 55-2 lists those variants which have been characterized fairly completely in accordance with criteria set up by the WHO Scientific Group. In addition to these, other variants have been described but have been only incompletely characterized, among them "Madison" [300], "Tübingen" [166], "Berlin" [167], "Eyssen" [168], and "Hamburg" [160]. The purification of G-6-PD has been achieved [204–206]. The feat of fingerprinting highly purified G-6-PD (Type B+) from 20 units of normal blood has been accomplished and the fingerprints compared with those from 20 units of G-6-PD Type A+. A single amino acid substitution, a change from asparagine to aspartic acid, was found [207–208]. Similarly, the purified enzyme from G-6-PD Hektoen has been proved to have a single amino acid mutation, in this case histidine to tyrosine [575]. In addition, the recent development of a method for purifying G-6-PD 80,000-fold from a single unit of blood with a yield of 80 percent may make possible the molecular characterization of many other G-6-PD variants [206].

A deficiency of G-6-PD activity can occur because of decreased production of enzyme molecules, formation of enzyme molecules with decreased catalytic activity, or production of enzyme molecules with reduced stability. These mechanisms appear to be operative in various combinations. In the A− type of deficiency, electrophoretic studies on the purified enzyme [301], fluorescence studies on enzymes titrated with NADPH [301], and immunologic investigations [264, 265, 302, 303] have established that the number of enzyme molecules is decreased. Production of the enzyme appears to be normal, i.e., activity of the enzyme in bone marrow cells and reticulocytes is not appreciably diminished [86]. In the Mediterranean type of enzyme defect the amount

Table 55-2. G-6-PD VARIANTS

Variant	Population	RBC activity, percent of normal	Electrophoretic mobility, approx. percent of normal	K_m G-6-P, μM	K_m NADP, μM	2dG-6-P utilization, percent of G-6-P	Heat stability	pH optima	Population frequency
Normal B	Various	100	100	50–78	2.9–4.4	<4	Normal	Normal	Usual
Hektoen [267, 268]	U.S. White	400–500	100 129 (PO_4 – pH 6.7)	51	3.0	3	Normal	Normal	Rare
King County [269]	Negro	100	105	61	4	6	?	Normal	Rare
Ijebu-Ode [262, 270]	Negro	100	85	60	24	11 (14 mM)	Reduced	Biphasic	Rare
Ita-Bale [262, 270]	Negro	100	65	91	11	14 (14 mM)	Slightly reduced	Normal	Rare
Glendale [563]	Negro	100	94 (TEB) 95 (Tris) 82 (PO_4)	45	3.8	4	Normal	Normal	Rare
Inhambane [564]	Bantu	100	112 (TEB) 115 (PO_4)	38	4.7	<4	Normal	Slightly biphasic	Rare
Lourenzo Marques [564]	Bantu	100	106 (TEB) 106 (PO_4)	66	4.3	<4	Normal	Normal	Rare
Manjacaze [564]	Bantu	100	90 (TEB) 90 (PO_4)	141	3.8	<4	Normal	Normal	Rare
A+ [167, 271]	Negro	88	110	Normal	Normal	<4	Normal	Normal	Very common
Baltimore-Austin [272]	Negro	75	90	68	3.1	<4	Normal	Normal	Rare
Ibadan-Austin [272, 273]	Negro	72	80	62–72	3.3	<4	Normal	Normal	Rare
Minas Gerais [274]	Brazilian	<70	95	41	4	9	?	Normal	Rare
Madrona [275]	Negro	70–80	80	32	3.5	Normal	?	Normal	Rare
Barbieri [276]	Italian	40–60	135	Increased	Increased	?	Normal	?	Rare

Capetown [277]	Cape Colored Norwegian	53–80	55–65 (TEB) 76–88 (Tris) 35–48 (PO_4)	11–14	0.2–1	7–16	Normal	Biphasic	?
Kerala [278]	Asian SE Indian	50	75 (TEB) 90 (Tris)	23	1.5	7.4	Normal	Biphasic	Rare
Attica [279]	Greek	50	110	37–44	5	1.8	Normal	Normal	
Columbus [280]	Negro	35	100	Normal	Normal	Normal	?	?	Rare
Tripler [281]	U.S. White	35	97 (TEB) 97 (Tris) 90 (PO_4)	30		3.7	Markedly reduced	Slightly biphasic	
Tel-Hashomer [282]	Sephardic (Tunisian) Jew	25–40	60–70	30–40	?	Normal	Normal	Slightly biphasic	Rare
Kephalonia [279]	Greek	20	110	31–37	4	2	Normal	Normal	
Athens [283]	Greek	20	98	19	3	15	Slightly reduced	Slightly	
Chibuto [564]	Bantu	20	108 (TEB) 109 (PO_4)	30	8.2	<4	Slightly increased	Normal	Rare
Puerto Rico [284]	Puerto Rican	19	112	18.6		2.7	Slightly reduced	Slightly biphasic	
Washington [284]	Negro	16	95	57.4		1.6	Normal	Normal	
Constantine [567]	Arab	16	110 (PO_4)	19	1.9	4	Normal	Normal	Common
Markham [73]	New Guinea	15–10	105 108	4.4 6.3	?	162–222	? Reduced	Very biphasic	?
Kabyle [285]	Algerian	14–36	104 (TEB) 110 (PO_4)	68		10 (same as control)	Normal	Normal	
Freiburg [162, 286]	German	10–20	85 (TEB) 90 (PO_4)	87–118	4			Biphasic	
Carswell [568]	Irish	10	78 (TEB) 92 (Tris) 78 (PO_4)	44	6.4	3.5	Normal	Normal or slightly displaced	Rare
San Juan [569]	Puerto Rican	10	110 (Tris) 105 (PO_4)	16.2 ± 0.7		21.6	Markedly reduced	Biphasic 7.0 and 9.5	Rare

Table 55-2. (Continued)

Variant	Population	RBC activity, percent of normal	Electro-phoretic mobility, approx. percent of normal	K_m G-6-P, μM	K_m NADP, μM	2dG-6-P utilization, percent of G-6-P	Heat stability	pH optima	Population frequency
"El Morro" [569]	Puerto Rican	9	100 (Tris) 100 (PO_4)	35.6 ± 2.1		7.2	Moderately reduced	Biphasic 7.0 and 9.5	Rare
Johnstown* [565]	English American	8	110 (Tris)	62.0		2.5	Normal	Abnormally flat 7.5–8.5	Rare
Taipei Hakka [570]	Hakka Chinese	6–9	105 (Tris) 110 (PO_4)	27.7 – 43.4		3.3–5.4	Normal or slightly reduced	Normal	Rare
West Bengal [278]	Asian Indian	9	90 (TEB) 82 (Tris)	31	6.6	4	Normal	Normal	Rare
Chicago [157]	West European	9–26	100	58–76	3.1–3.7	<4	Markedly reduced	Normal	Rare
Seattle [279, 287, 288]	Welsh-Scottish	8–21	90	15–25	2.4–2.8	7–11	Normal	Slightly biphasic	Rare
Alhambra [289]	Finnish-Swedish	9–20	96 (TEB) 95 (Tris) 85 (PO_4)	55	2.6	2	Moderately reduced	Normal	Rare
A– [168, 271, 211]	Negro	8–20	110	Normal	Normal	<4	Normal	Normal	Common
Duarte* [290]	U.S.	8.5	100	58	5	5.4	Markedly reduced	7.0	Rare
Hong Kong [291]	Chinese	<8	100	Half normal	Normal	Sl.↑	Normal	Normal	?
Mediterranean [131, 276, 292, 293]	Asian Greek Sardinian Sephardic Jews N. W. Indian	0–7	100	19–26	1.2–1.6	23–27	Reduced	Biphasic	Common
Benevento [284]	Italian	7	93	4.6		245	Decreased	Biphasic	
Bangkok* [163]	Thai	5	100	60	5.3	8.4	Markedly reduced	8.0–8.5	

Panay [294]	Visayan Islands, Philippines	<5	96	30	4.7	Normal	Slightly increased	Biphasic	
Canton [295]	South Chinese	4–24	105	20–36	2.0–2.4	4–15	Slightly reduced	Biphasic	Common
Oklahoma* [296]	West European	4–10	100	127–200	20	<4	Low	Narrow peak	Rare
Paris [165]	French	4	?	280			Markedly reduced	High peak at 9.5	Rare
Union [297]	Philippino	<3	Fast	8–12	3.6–5.2	180	?	Biphasic	?
Ohio* [280]	Italian	2–16	Fast 110	Slightly increased	Slightly increased	Normal	Markedly reduced	?	Rare
Torrance* [164]	U.S.	2.4	103 (PO_4)	48 60	6	2.4	Markedly reduced	Normal	Rare
Clichy* [165]	Greek	2	100	178			?	Abnormal plateau 9–10	Rare
Albuquerque* [131]	U.S.	1	100	115	11	0	Markedly reduced	Peaked with optimum at 8.5	Rare
Ashdod* [298]	North African Jewish	0.5	92	100		40	Normal	Biphasic	Rare
Milwaukee* [299]	Puerto Rican White	0.5	92	224		3.7		8	Rare
Beaujon* [165]	French	0	Fast	182				Peak at 9.5	Rare
Ramat-Gan* [298]	Jewish Iraqui	0	92	35		40	Markedly reduced		Rare
Bat-Yam* [298]	Jewish Iraqui	0	100	27		45	Markedly reduced		Rare
Lifta [298]	Jewish Iraqui	0	90	25		60	Markedly reduced		Rare

Table 55-2. (Continued)

Variant	Population	RBC activity, percent of normal	Electro-phoretic mobility, approx. percent of normal	K_m G-6-P, μM	K_m NADP, μM	2dG-6-P utilization, percent of G-6-P	Heat stability	pH optima	Population frequency
Benevento [565]	Italian	7	95 (Tris)	4.6		245	Moderately reduced	Biphasic 5.5 and 7.5	Rare
Taiwan Hakka [570]	Hakka Chinese	2–9	105 (Tris) 110 (PO_4) pH 7.0	10.7 – 12.2		9.8 – 21.1	Normal or slightly reduced	Biphasic 7.0 and 9.5–10.0	Rare
Campbellpur [571]	Pakistani	2–7	100 (Tris)	11.4 – 13.9		5.6–16.4	Markedly reduced	Biphasic 7.5 and 9.5	Rare
"Zähringen" [572, 573]	German	1–4	104 (PO_4)	28	4.7	30	Reduced	7.5 and 8.5	Rare
Teheran [566]	Iran	<1	105 (Tris)	6.1		44	Moderately reduced	Biphasic 5.5 and 10.0	Rare

* Associated with nonspherocytic congenital hemolytic disease.
TEB = Tris-EDTA-borate buffer
Tris = Tris-HCl buffer
PO_4 = Phosphate buffer

of enzyme even in very young red cells is decreased [86]. In addition, each enzyme molecule has decreased catalytic activity [303].

Mixtures of normal and G-6-PD–deficient hemolysates reveal no evidence of enzyme inhibition [304]. At one time it was suggested that G-6-PD deficiency might be due to the absence of a normal stromal activator [305, 306], but it now seems probable that the phenomenon was a complex artifact [293].

Effects of G-6-PD Deficiency

GSH Deficiency

GSH deficiency was demonstrated originally in primaquine-sensitive subjects both by GSH assay with a nitroprusside method of relatively low specificity and by the use of the more specific alloxan "305" technique [39]. The deficiency of red cell GSH in G-6-PD–deficient persons is fairly consistent, especially if the determinations of several days are averaged [39], but individual values may be within normal limits [40]. Although at one time it was believed that the amount of GSSG in G-6-PD–deficient cells is also diminished [307, 308], new and improved techniques for estimation of GSSG [309] have shown that the GSSG content is actually three times normal [241]. Even so, the amount of GSSG in normal red cells is so small that the total glutathione (GSH + 2GSSG) is substantially diminished in these cells.

There is a rapid destruction of GSH [242] when red cells from a G-6-PD–deficient or normal subject are suspended in a saline-phosphate buffer and incubated with acetylphenylhydrazine. Concurrently, there is an increase in red cell GSSG. Subsequently, the GSSG falls slightly, so that a significant decline in total glutathione takes place during the course of the experiment [310]. The same effect can be demonstrated with other reducing agents, such as primaquine, phenylhydrazine, ascorbic acid [40, 311], Furadantin [94], α- and β-naphthoquinone [88], and certain vitamin K derivatives [88, 115]. If glucose or inosine is added to the system, normal red cells protect their GSH completely, but protection in enzyme-deficient red cells is incomplete [242, 311]. Substrates other than glucose and inosine, including ribose, lactate, pyruvate, malate, and fumarate, have little or no protective properties [242]. Recently methylphenylazoformate has proved to be especially useful in rapidly oxidizing GSH in red cells [312].

The mechanism by which acetylphenylhydrazine destroys GSH in red cells in vitro has been investigated in some detail. Oxygenation of the red cells is required for the destruction of GSH. A carbon dioxide–nitrogen mixture or carbon monoxide is extremely effective in protecting the GSH of deficient red cells from destruction [242]. Acetylphenylhydrazine modifies oxyhemoglobin in such a way that it rapidly oxidizes GSH [242]. The nature of the intermediate compound has not been determined. In addition, evidence has been presented that oxidation products of acetylphenylhydrazine may represent an important factor leading to the oxidation of red cell GSH [313, 314], and both modified hemoglobin and acetylphenylhydrazine oxidation products may play a role in the oxidation of GSH [315]. Once GSH has been oxidized, it can be reduced rapidly by normal red cells, which have the capacity of reducing NADP by the oxidation of glucose. Normal cells deprived of glucose and cells lacking G-6-PD do not reduce enough NADP to maintain GSH in the reduced state.

CO_2 Production and O_2 Consumption

Since the hexose monophosphate pathway is the only known pathway of oxygen consumption and CO_2 production in the red cell [194], any enzyme deficiency along this route should decrease O_2 consumption and CO_2 production. Red cells with the relatively mild A− type of defect are able to oxidize glucose at a normal rate when the demand for NADPH is normal, but when the rate of NADPH oxidation is hastened by the addition of agents such as methylene blue, the enzyme-deficient cells are unable to increase adequately the rate of glucose oxidation and carbon dioxide production [190, 316].

Methemoglobin Formation and Reduction

Reduction of methemoglobin in the presence of methylene blue, largely a NADPH-linked process, is diminished in G-6-PD–deficient red cells [90]. In the absence of an auxiliary dye such as methylene blue, the rate of methemoglobin reduction in deficient cells is normal [90, 223]. There is much less methemoglobin formation in G-6-PD–deficient red cells than in normal red cells when they are exposed to nitrosobenzol. Presumably, nitrosobenzol is reduced to phenylhydroxylamine by NADPH in order to form methemoglobin [317]. In the absence of NADPH phenylhydroxylamine is not formed and methemoglobin formation does not take place. Similarly, the inhibition of glutathione reductase by chromate, a process requiring NADPH [318, 319] presumably to change the configuration of the glutathione reductase molecule, occurs in normal, but not in G-6-PD–deficient cells.

NADP/NADPH Ratio

The ratio of NADP to NADPH is increased in enzyme-deficient cells [320–322], as might be predicted with a defect in the NADP-reducing system. A slight increase in the NAD/NADH ratio has also been described [317, 322]. However, recent studies suggest that the methods used for determining NADP/NADPH ratios are probably not reliable [576].

Other Biochemical Abnormalities

A number of other enzymatic changes have also been observed in G-6-PD–deficient red cells independently of drug administration. Increased activities of red cell GSH reductase [221], aldolase [53, 321, 323–325], glyceraldehyde phosphate dehydrogenase [53], hexokinase [326], and lactic dehydrogenase [53] have been reported. Activity of the last four enzymes has also been reported to be normal [191, 321, 327, 328]. Activities of phosphogluconate dehydrogenase [52], phosphohexose isomerase [52], purine nucleoside phosphorylase [52], triose isomerase [321], 3-phosphoglycerate kinase [321], pyruvate kinase [321], isocitric dehydrogenase [327], malic dehydrogenase [325], and glyoxylase [329] have also been measured in G-6-PD–deficient red cells and have been found normal. Enolase activity was normal in one subject but decreased in another [321].

The concentrations of at least three enzymes other than G-6-PD have been found diminished in enzyme-deficient red cells. These are NADPH diaphorase (NADP-linked methemoglobin reductase) [223, 330], acid phosphomonoesterase [330], (although not confirmed [332, 333]), and pyrophosphatase [334, 335]. Catalase activity has been reported normal in G-6-PD–deficient cells [46, 83]; a single report of diminished catalase activity [336] is not confirmed [337, 338]. It has been suggested that the decrease in catalase activity found G-6-PD–deficient subjects may have been due to the formation of complex II [339]. A patient with marked hypocatalasemia and G-6-PD deficiency apparently is a unique example of coincidence of two separate genetic abnormalities [340]. The author has found the activity of NADPH diaphorase diminished, not only in the Negro and non-Negro types of G-6-PD deficiency, but also in patients with nonspherocytic congenital hemolytic anemia associated with G-6-PD deficiency [341]. The reason for alterations in the activities of enzymes other than G-6-PD is not clear and deserves further study. The number of surface sulfhydryl groups of G-6-PD–deficient cells are normal but there is a slight decrease in protein sulfhydryl groups [342].

Chromatography of the amino acid residues of hydrolyzed hemoglobin from sensitive red cells has disclosed no abnormality [46], but a decrease in the quantity of Hb A_2 has been found [343]. It has been suggested that the intracellular K^+ of affected cells is significantly diminished [321]. No abnormality has been detected in stromal lipid fractions [321], but it has been reported that there is a small (5 percent) but statistically significant decrease in the total lipids of G-6-PD–deficient red cells [344].

Hematologic Properties of G-6-PD–deficient Erythrocytes

Although the structure of erythrocytes with G-6-PD deficiency is normal under light microscopy[83], abnormalities of the stroma resembling changes found in normal aging [345] have been detected by electron microscopy. G-6-PD–deficient erythrocytes are normal when examined by Coombs' antiglobulin technique [38, 83], the Ham acid hemolysis test [83], mechanical fragility tests [83], and sickle tests [83, 107, 346]. They contain no excess of methemoglobin [38, 83, 107], and the percentage of alkali-resistant hemoglobin and the electrophoretic mobility of the hemoglobin are normal [83]. In vitro hemolysis of G-6-PD–deficient cells by primaquine is normal [83], as is the prelytic loss of K^+ [347, 348]. Osmotic fragility is normal [83, 344]. The life span of the red cells with both the A– [349] and Mediterranean type [350] is slightly less than normal.

Changes Occurring in Erythrocytes during Drug Administration

G-6-PD

Only the older members of a red cell population are destroyed when primaquine is administered to a G-6-PD–deficient Negro patient [84]. Studies based on age-fractionated red cells show higher levels of G-6-PD in young cells than in old [73, 86, 351–353]. This disparity is accentuated in the A– type of deficiency [73, 85, 86, 191, 354]. Thus when primaquine is administered to subjects with the A– type deficiency, a slight rise in dehydrogenase activity is observed as the older, more enzyme-deficient, red cells are eliminated from the circulation [307].

Near-normal dehydrogenase levels have been found in persons with naphthalene-induced hemolytic anemia [90] and in subjects with favic crises [55, 355]. Since even young cells of patients with the Mediterranean type of deficiency have low levels of dehydrogenase, increases in enzyme activity may be minimal in subjects with this type of defect [356, 357].

GSH

The administration of primaquine to a G-6-PD–deficient subject results in a rapid fall in the average GSH level of the red cell. This precedes the major red cell destruction. There is then a return of average red cell GSH to the same level or a slightly higher level than that prior to taking the drug [307]. Similar observations have been made in patients with favism [47, 51, 53, 54] and sulfonamide-induced [47] hemolytic anemia. It has been suggested that initially GSH in the older red cells is almost completely destroyed and that GSH-depleted cells are then removed from the circulation [242].

The fate of GSH in sensitive red cells challenged in vivo by a drug requires further study. Early studies suggested that the loss of GSH was not accompanied by an increase in red cell GSSG [307]; however, the methods of analysis in those studies were inadequate [241, 309]. Some of the GSH which is lost from the red cells may form mixed disulfides with hemoglobin [244, 245], particularly with the exposed sulfhydryl group of the cysteine residue in the 93 position of the β chain. There is probably some loss of GSSG from the enzyme-deficient red cells by outward transport [246].

It has been reported that the results of the GSH stability test (see below) are not affected by primaquine administration [307], but transient GSH instability in the red cells of sensitive subjects has been reported following naphthalene- [90] and fava bean-induced hemolysis [47, 53, 355].

Methemoglobin Formation

The levels of methemoglobin found in the blood of deficient subjects given hemolytic drugs are not greater than those observed in normal subjects [33, 107] and may even be less [109]. When deficient subjects are given the nonhemolytic drug, sodium nitrite, higher levels of methemoglobin are found in their red cells than in the red cells of control subjects [358]. It is not known whether this is due to altered metabolism of sodium nitrite, greater susceptibility to methemoglobin formation, or faulty reduction of methemoglobin. The best available evidence [223] suggests that methemoglobin reduction in the absence of dye is normal in G-6-PD–deficient red cells. It has been suggested [358] that since older red cells have a diminished capacity to reduce methemoglobin [359–361], the preferential destruction of older cells [84] may account for the lower methemoglobin levels found in G-6-PD–deficient subjects. It may also be significant that at least one aromatic compound, nitrosobenzol, is a potent methemoglobin-forming agent in normal but not in enzyme-deficient cells [311].

MECHANISM OF RED CELL DESTRUCTION

Primaquine and related compounds do not lyse G-6-PD–deficient red cells more readily than normal red cells in vitro [83]. Hemolytic compounds probably cause changes in the erythrocytes which render them more susceptible to destruction by the reticuloendothelial system in vivo. Cells which have been damaged by a drug may have abnormal surface characteristics which are detected by the reticuloendothelial cells. Such changes might include the charge of the surface of the cell or alterations in its shape or plastic properties.

In 1931 Warburg et al. [362] pointed out that when red cells are treated with phenylhydrazine, hemoglobin is denatured. It was observed early in the studies of primaquine-induced hemolysis that formation of Heinz bodies and depletion of GSH precedes the destruction of G-6-PD–deficient erythrocytes [83, 307]. Heinz bodies appear to consist, at least in part, of hemoglobin denaturation products, including derivatives such as verdeglobin and choleglobin [363, 364]. Hemolytic drugs also promote the oxidation of GSH to GSSG, at least in the presence of hemoglobin. The mechanism of this effect is not entirely clear. Hemolytic drugs have the capacity to generate hydrogen peroxide when they react with hemoglobin [365]. Peroxide, itself, is a potent oxidant of hemoglobin and, through GSH peroxidase, of GSH. It has also been proposed that free radical intermediates of the drugs themselves may react with glutathione [314] to form free GS^- radicals or with the exposed sulfhydryl groups of hemoglobin.

The role of methemoglobin formation in the sequence of events leading to red cell destruction remains uncertain. Apparently, those drugs which have the capacity to oxidize hemoglobin irreversibly are also able to facilitate a shift of the equilibrium between oxyhemoglobin and methemoglobin toward methemoglobin [313, 315]; earlier observations indicating that phenylhydrazine treatment did not result in methemoglobin formation [109, 362, 366] were apparently in error. Methemoglobin formation per se does not hasten the rate of destruction of erythrocytes, since red cell survival after nitrite treatment or in congenital methemoglobinemia is normal. Because of the correlation between methemoglobin formation and drug-induced hemolysis, it has been suggested [313, 367, 368] that methemoglobin may be a precursor of degradation products such as choleglobin and verdeglobin. Furthermore, oxidation of hemoglobin to methemoglobin increases the tendency for heme to dissociate from globin [369]. Since heme-free globin is particularly unstable [370], loss of heme could lead to the formation of irreversibly denatured globin. No direct evidence for such a relationship has been presented. On the other hand, degradation of hemoglobin by "oxidant" hemolytic drugs and the rate of hemolysis in rats is uninfluenced by nitrite-induced methemoglobinemia [371–374], and Heinz bodies may be formed without perceptible methemoglobinemia [375, 376]. Whether or not methemoglobin plays an obligatory intermediate role in the degradation of hemoglobin during the course of drug-induced hemolysis, irreversibly denatured products of hemoglobin appear with eventual precipitation in the form of Heinz bodies [363, 364]. This may be associated with the formation of mixed disulfide with glutathione at the cysteine residue in position 93 of the β chain, and with the unfolding of the hemoglobin molecule and oxidation of its hidden sulfhydryl groups [245]. It has been suggested that the binding of Heinz bodies to the cell membrane involves formation of sulfhydryl bridges, and that fragments of the membrane are lost. Heinz bodies within the cell and possibly rigidity of the damaged membrane may make it difficult for G-6-PD–deficient cells to negotiate the splenic sinusoids and other small vessels in the body and these cells may be doomed to destruction [377].

Other biochemical alterations may also play a role in the death of the cell. The role of GSH in the economy of the erythrocyte, and the possible toxic effects of GSSG have already been described. Conceivably, hemolytic drugs may interfere with the metabolism of G-6-PD–deficient cells by oxidizing NADH or interfering in some way with glycolysis and ATP levels [317, 378]. The likelihood of inhibition of the enzyme directly by drugs has also received some attention [379].

The mechanism of hemolysis after exposure to fava beans,

in patients with infections, in the neonatal period, and in patients with nonspherocytic congenital hemolytic anemia is even more obscure than the mechanism of hemolysis induced by drugs. A fraction derived from fava beans has the capacity to destroy the GSH of deficient red cells [380, 381] and to damage deficient cells so that they are quickly destroyed in vivo [381]. It seems possible that substances derived from fava beans may act in some individuals like oxidant drugs such as primaquine. Influenza A virus preferentially lyses G-6-PD–deficient red cells [382]. It is conceivable that similar effects occur in vivo. Levels of certain red cell enzymes, particularly NADH-diaphorase [383], glutathione peroxidase [384], and catalase [385] are decreased in the newborn. The relative lack of these may make the cell more vulnerable to the destructive influence of low levels of peroxide which may develop in vivo without drug administration. Similarly, red cells with severe deficits of G-6-PD, as in patients with nonspherocytic congenital hemolytic anemia, may be destroyed even at naturally occurring levels of peroxide.

GENETICS OF G-6-PD DEFICIENCY

The biochemical and clinical stigmata of G-6-PD deficiency are most commonly found among males [52, 53, 147, 386, 387]. Intermediate degrees of enzyme deficiency or glutathione stability appears in females [52, 115, 147, 386–388]. Pedigrees of G-6-PD–deficient subjects almost invariably show that the mother of affected males carries the disorder, if it is demonstrable in either parent [45, 52, 147, 386, 387]. Further evidence for the sex linkage of G-6-PD deficiency has come from observations of the linkage of this defect with color-blindness [389–391].

The recombination fraction between the gene for G-6-PD and deuteranopia has been estimated at 5 percent [392]. In a study from Sardinia the two genes were most frequently in the coupling phase [389], while in a study from Israel [390] the repulsion phase was significantly more frequent. It has been suggested that the genes for deuteranopia and proteranopia may lie relatively far apart on the X chromosome and that the gene for G-6-PD lies between their loci [393]. No linkage has been found between the Xg^a locus and the locus for G-6-PD [394–396]. The linkage data have recently been discussed in some detail [397, 398].

While a large proportion of females heterozygous for G-6-PD deficiency have intermediate levels of enzyme activity, numerous exceptions are found. For example, as indicated in Fig. 55–2, affected subjects have been found in whom the defect could be demonstrated in neither parent when the criterion for classification was the GSH stability test (cf. Family 12, LA: III-7,8 produced IV-12). The fact that neither parent of some propositi has a demonstrable defect indicates that the gene can be carried without causing a detectable disorder of the red cell. Conversely, some females with marked GSH instability and G-6-PD deficiency are heterozygous, because they have borne boys who are not affected [cf. Fig. 55–2, Family K: II-A.K. and E.K. have produced four negative sons (III-J.K., P.K., Go.K., and G.K.)]. In one such case it has been shown that the heterozygote had a normal female chromosomal complement [399]. Females, who possess two X chromosomes, have no more G-6-PD activity [85, 400] or only slightly more [401] than males possessing only one X chromosome. Also persons with more than two X chromosomes do not have greater than normal red cell G-6-PD activity [400]. These findings, as well as the markedly variable expression of G-6-PD activity in heterozygotes could be explained by the "inactive X" hypothesis [71, 402–404]. If one of the two X chromosomes of females is genetically inactive, then the heterozygote with intermediate enzyme activity should have two red cell populations, red cells with normal activity and red cells that are grossly deficient in G-6-PD activity. It has been shown that the curve of reduction of methemoglobin in the presence of Nile blue sulfate has two components when red cells of heterozygotes for G-6-PD deficiency are studied [71, 405]. These curves resemble exactly those obtained from artificial mixtures of cells obtained from normal subjects and from hemizygotes for G-6-PD deficiency. Similarly, the disappearance of GSH from the red cells of heterozygotes when challenged in vitro with acetylphenylhydrazine, or the regeneration of GSH in azoester treated cells, takes place in two components just as in artificial mixtures from normal subjects and hemizygotes [71, 312].

The separation of enzyme-deficient cells from the blood of heterozygous subjects has been accomplished [406]. This was done by studying subjects heterozygous for both G-6-PD deficiency and sickle-cell trait. After 3 hr of methemoglobin reduction, cell suspensions were deoxygenated. This permitted cells containing hemoglobin to sickle, while methemoglobin-containing cells remained unsickled. The unsickled forms were separated by millipore filtration and were found to contain as little enzyme and as much methemoglobin as red cells from hemizygous males [406]. The bimodality of red cell populations with respect to G-6-PD deficiency has been confirmed by the microspectrophotometric measurement of individual red cell methemoglobin levels [407]. Red cell survival studies have also indicated the presence of two populations [408]. Several investigators have employed histochemical methods for the detection of methemoglobin in demonstrating mosaicism in heterozygotes for G-6-PD deficiency [409–414]. Since it is possible to produce mosaicism or pseudomosaicism in preparations made from normal cells or from cells of males hemizygous for mild G-6-PD deficiency, only limited weight can be given to these findings [415–417]. Even so, these procedures when carefully standardized may be useful in detection of heterozygotes (see below).

The fact that only one gene for G-6-PD is active in each somatic cell has been confirmed by cloning studies [418] and in naturally occurring clones, i.e., tumors [419–422].

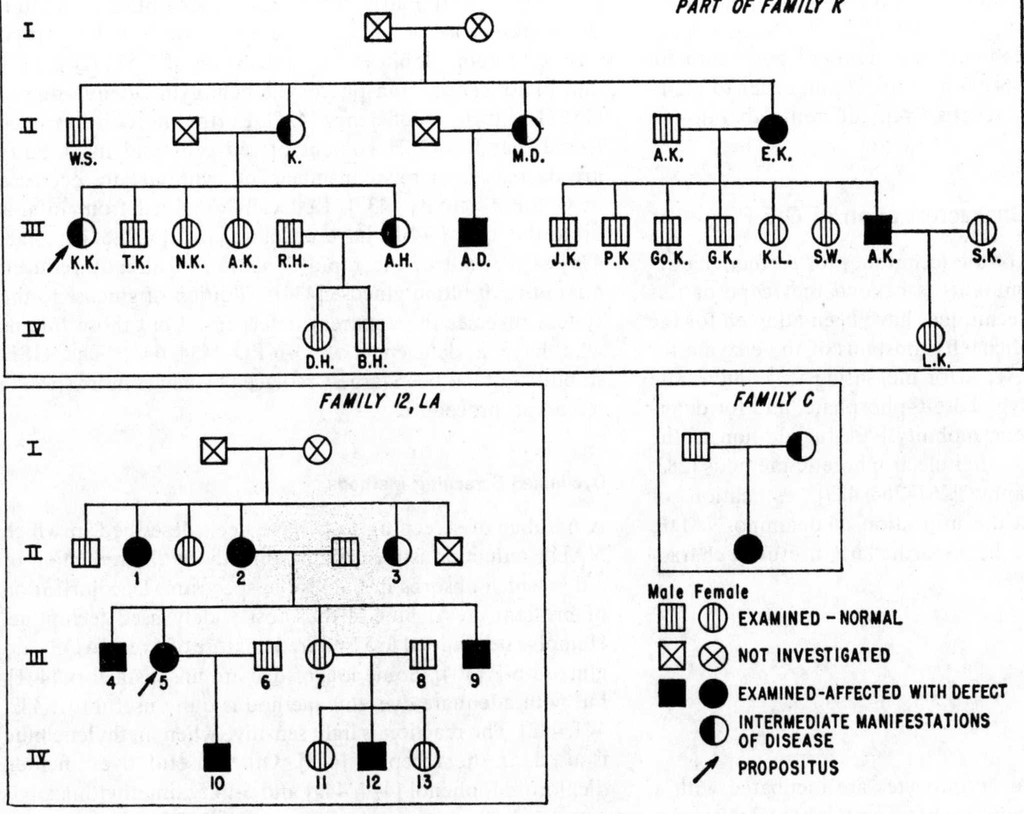

Figure 55-2. Some revealing pedigrees of families with primaquine sensitivity. The K family, only a part of which is presented, and the C family were studies by Gross et al. [52] using an assay for glucose-6-phosphate dehydrogenase as the criterion for designation of subjects. LA in Family 12 was studied by Childs et al. [386], using the GSH stability test as a criterion of sensitivity. Open symbols indicate subjects who had normal glucose-6-phosphate dehydrogenase activity or GSH stability tests. Solid symbols indicate a well-marked deficiency of glucose-6-phosphate dehydrogenase or marked GSH instability. Half-shaded symbols indicate intermediate manifestations of the defect. Symbols with a cross indicate that the subject was not examined.

METHODS OF DETECTION OF G-6-PD DEFICIENCY

Many methods for distinguishing the apparently normal red cells of G-6-PD–deficient subjects from those of normal persons are now available.

Quantitative Enzyme Assays

Quantitative assay for G-6-PD is carried out by measuring the rate of NADP reduction in the presence of glucose-6-phosphate. This may be measured by the increase in optical density at 340 mμ, or by the fluorescence of the reduced pyridine nucleotide. It is important to recognize that the 6-phosphogluconic acid which is formed in the G-6-PD reaction will be partially oxidized in the phosphogluconic dehydrogenase reaction, yielding additional NADPH. Thus, the simple one-step assay does not measure G-6-PD activity alone. This difficulty may be overcome by determining the phosphogluconic dehydrogenase activity in a cuvette containing no glucose-6-phosphate, but containing a saturating quantity of 6-phosphogluconic acid. Subtraction of the phosphogluconate dehydrogenase activity from the system in which both activities are being measured gives an accurate appraisal of the G-6-PD activity [254]. This technique is not suitable when G-6-PD activity is very low, since it is then necessary to subtract a large value from a value which is only slightly greater. Alternatively, purified phosphogluconate dehydrogenase may be added to the system to make certain that the second reaction proceeds at maximum velocity [254].

There has been agreement on a standard procedure for the measurement of G-6-PD activity [70], in order to facilitate the comparison of results from different laboratories.

Further Qualitative Characterization of G-6-PD

Detailed consideration of the techniques for further characterization of G-6-PD mutants is beyond the scope of this chapter. Standardized techniques have been adopted for the determination of the Michaelis constants of the enzyme for glucose-6-P and for NADP, for measuring its relative rate of utilization of 2-deoxyglucose-6-phosphate, and for determining its electrophoretic mobility [70]. In addition to the standard systems, many other electrophoretic methods [283, 423–428], chromatography [262–264, 429], estimation of pH-activity curves, and the utilization of deamino-NADP, NAD, and glucose have been particularly useful in characterizing new variants.

Screening Tests

Heinz Body Formation

When G-6-PD–deficient erythrocytes are incubated with a variety of reducing agents such as acetylphenylhydrazine, phenylhydrazine, primaquine, or ascorbic acid, a different pattern of Heinz body formation is observed from that which occurs when normal cells are incubated under identical conditions [430]. This forms the basis of the first in vitro method by which a fairly reliable differentiation of drug-sensitive from nonsensitive subjects can be made [53, 94, 115, 355, 440]. Disadvantages include the sensitivity of the test to changes in oxygen tension and to changes in the hematocrit [430]. This procedure has now been superceded by more specific screening methods.

GSH Stability Test

The incubation of red cells with acetylphenylhydrazine and the measurement of GSH stability is a useful method for the detection of the red cell defect of drug sensitivity [40, 311]. This test is somewhat more time-consuming than the Heinz body method but can be performed relatively simply and rapidly, especially with newer techniques of GSH estimation [431]. It is considerably less sensitive to changes in oxygen tension and hematocrit than is the Heinz body procedure. It gives clear separation of enzyme-deficient from normal males but is less reliable for the detection of heterozygotes. Correlation between G-6-PD assays and GSH stability tests has been good in the hands of most investigators [49, 52, 53, 355, 432, 433], but occasional discrepancies between GSH stability tests and enzyme assays are observed [48, 53, 432–434]. False positive results are obtained in Hb E thalassemia disease [435], probably because of the participation of hemoglobin in the destruction of GSH [242, 315], and in congenital nonspherocytic hemolytic anemia due to GSSG-reductase deficiency [436]. Furthermore, it has been found that the GSH content of red cells and its stability are decreased in renal insufficiency, without any decrease in G-6-PD activity [437]. Red cells obtained from infants up to the age of 74 hr have unstable GSH [52, 88, 434, 438, 439] as a result of the rapid depletion of already reduced quantities of blood glucose [434]. Addition of glucose to the system reverses the apparent defect in all but those infants who have a deficiency of G-6-PD [434, 440]. The GSH stability test has been largely replaced by newer more specific screening procedures.

Dye-linked Screening Methods

A number of screening tests have been described in which NADP reduction is measured indirectly by the reduction of a dye which absorbs in the visible spectrum. Decolorization of brilliant cresyl blue is the most widely used technique. Hemolysate is added to a buffered mixture of dye, NADP, and glucose-6-P [304]. Some lots of dye are unsatisfactory [441], but with adequate dye, this method is quite useful [91, 432, 441, 442]. The reaction is light sensitive when methylene blue is used as the receptor [443]. Other useful dyes include dichloroindophenol [444, 445] and 3-(4,5-dimethylthiazolyl-1-2)-2,5-diphenyltetrazolium bromide (MTT) [446].

The Methemoglobin Reduction Test

This test [447] takes advantage of the fact that methemoglobin reduction in the presence of methylene blue proceeds largely through the hexose monophosphate shunt pathway. When G-6-PD activity is impaired, the rate of methemoglobin reduction is diminished. The test is relatively simple and requires no expensive reagents. The blood must be fresh. Abnormal results may be obtained when the blood of patients with NADPH-diaphorase deficiency [448] is examined.

Methylene Blue Absorption Test

There is a tendency for leukomethylene blue to become tightly bound to red cells. The absorption of methylene blue by erythrocytes has formed the basis of two tests. Relatively fresh blood must be used [449, 450].

The Ascorbate Cyanide Test

This test [451, 452] depends on the fact that incubation with ascorbate results in denaturation of the hemoglobin in G-6-PD–deficient cells when catalase is inhibited by cyanide. The test is simple and requires no expensive reagents. The results can be interpreted visually. Two milliliters of fresh blood are required. There are many conditions other than

G-6-PD deficiency which give a positive test. These include glutathione deficiency [453], glutathione reductase deficiency, hemoglobinopathies with unstable hemoglobins, and pyruvate kinase deficiency [454].

The Fluorescent Spot Test

This test is highly specific, is exceedingly simple to perform, requires only a small volume of blood, and is not costly. It is based upon the fact that reduced pyridine nucleotides fluoresce, while oxidized pyridine nucleotides do not. Five to ten minutes incubation of a blood sample which may be several weeks old suffices. The blood may even be dried on filter paper. A screening reagent containing glucose-6-phosphate, NADP, buffer, and saponin are required to carry out this test [455]. The mixture is spotted on filter paper and inspected under long-wave ultraviolet light. If the spot fluoresces, G-6-PD deficiency is not present. The incorporation of GSSG into the test reagent makes it sufficiently sensitive to detect mild G-6-PD deficiency by reoxidation, through the glutathione reductase reaction, of the small amounts of NADP which may have been reduced to NADPH [456].

Heterozygote Detection

The detection of heterozygotes poses serious problems which have been described in considerable detail elsewhere [454, 457]. Since the red cells of the heterozygote are a mixture of normal and enzyme-deficient red cells, a cell lysate may not reveal the fact that it was prepared from a heterozygous individual if the proportion of enzyme-deficient cells is relatively small. Methods which depend upon the activity of individual red cells, such as the methemoglobin elution test [411], the tetrazolium-linked cytochemical method [458], or the ascorbate cyanide test, have proved to be more sensitive in the detection of small populations of G-6-PD–deficient cells than a quantitative enzyme assay.

G-6-PD ACTIVITY IN CELLS OTHER THAN ERYTHROCYTES

Because G-6-PD deficiency is genetically determined, it would appear reasonable to suppose that the synthesis of this enzyme might also be impaired in tissues other than the red blood cells.

Leukocyte G-6-PD is normal in subjects with the A− type of deficiency [459] but is decreased in leukocytes from deficient Mediterranean [460] and Chinese [461] subjects. Inconsistent abnormalities of leukocyte G-6-PD, not well correlated with red cell activities, have also been reported [462], and although it has been claimed that the leukocyte enzyme differs from the red cell enzyme [463] the consensus appears to be that the leukocyte enzyme and the red cell enzyme are genetically and structurally identical [464, 465].

Another form of G-6-PD (hexose-6-PD) has been found in mammalian liver [466]. This enzyme is inherited through an autosomal gene [466] and has broad substrate specificity [467, 468]. It is found in many tissues, including kidney, heart, lung, testis, and adrenal, but not in erythrocytes, leukocytes, brain, or breast [469]. This enzyme appears to be identical to an enzyme formerly known as glucose-dehydrogenase [468] and should not be confused with the sex-linked form of G-6-PD. In G-6-PD deficiency a decrease in enzyme activity has also been described in lens tissue [470, 471], kidney [461], adrenal [461], platelets [461, 472], skin culture [461, 473], saliva [474], breast milk [475], and liver [135, 461, 476, 477]. The magnitude of decrease is generally less in other tissues, particularly those with nucleated cells, than in erythrocytes. It may be that lack of protein-synthesizing ability and relatively long life span allow the defect to reach its maximum extent in the red cell.

There is some evidence to suggest that G-6-PD deficiency may have effects in tissues other than the erythrocyte. Several patients with G-6-PD deficiency and cataracts have been reported [167, 299]. Following intravenous injection of either glucose-1-^{14}C or glucose-6-^{14}C, the percentage of expired labeled CO_2 was found to be abnormally low [478]. An alteration in glucose tolerance curves has been reported [479], but not confirmed [480]. It has also been shown that the metabolism of intravenously infused cortisol and the excretion of 6-β-hydroxycortisol are abnormal in G-6-PD–deficient subjects. This suggests an inability to reduce the A ring [481]. A decline in serum cholesterol upon primaquine administration in G-6-PD–deficient but not in normal subjects has also been reported [482]. While the overall incidence of G-6-PD deficiency is approximately normal in schizophrenic patients, those subjects with a diagnosis of catatonic schizophrenia have a much higher than normal incidence of the deficiency, and those with paranoid schizophrenia a greatly decreased incidence [483]. This was not confirmed in another study [484].

THE INCIDENCE AND DISTRIBUTION OF G-6-PD DEFICIENCY

G-6-PD deficiency is widely distributed. It is found in virtually all racial groups [304, 70]. The A− type is found chiefly in Africa and in areas to which African Negroes have migrated [79, 97, 102, 304, 397, 486–498]. The gene frequency is approximately 11 percent among American Negroes. Other surveys have revealed an appreciable incidence of the deficiency around the Mediterranean basin [57, 134, 145, 499, 147, 304, 500–517] and in East Indians [304, 434, 492, 518–523], Orientals [304, 447, 518, 524–537], Oceanians [538–543], Philippinos [294, 537, 544, 545], and some American Indians [304, 546–548]. Occasional cases have been reported from various parts of Europe [58, 517, 549–558].

The geographic distribution has led to the suggestion that the gene may confer some protection against falciparum malaria [304, 485, 516, 559, 560]. It was pointed out that malarial parasites require the oxidative shunt and GSH for optimal growth. The similarity between the distribution of falciparum malaria and the gene for G-6-PD deficiency has been confirmed in a number of studies [489, 504, 505], but lack of correlation has been observed in New Guinea and New Britain [543]. Conflicting data have been presented for parasite counts in children with enzyme deficiency [304, 489, 493, 561]. Parasite counts on the blood of heterozygotes for G-6-PD deficiency indicate that deficient cells are less frequently parasitized in the same individual than cells with normal enzyme activity [562]. Most of the available data seem to suggest that malarial infection may be less severe in small children with G-6-PD deficiency. It is possible that other factors may also play a role in favoring the survival of individuals with G-6-PD deficiency. This remains a problem for the future.

SUMMARY

1 When certain ordinarily harmless drugs are administered to susceptible patients, an acute hemolytic anemia results. Among these drugs are the 8-aminoquinoline antimalarials, such as primaquine, certain sulfonamides, acetanilid, phenacetin, Furadantin, and many others.

2 Susceptibility to drug-induced hemolytic disease may be due to a deficiency of glucose-6-phosphate dehydrogenase (G-6-PD) activity in the erythrocyte. This enzyme normally catalyzes the oxidation of glucose-6-phosphate, which is coupled to the reduction of NADP. NADPH in turn, maintains glutathione in its reduced form (GSH).

3 Many mutant forms of G-6-PD are known and are distinguished by their biochemical characteristics. Two mutants have been fingerprinted and found to be due to single amino acid substitutions.

4 G-6-PD deficiency can be detected by an NADP-linked assay in which the rate of reduction of NADP is measured spectrophotometrically. A number of screening methods are also available.

5 G-6-PD deficiency is inherited as a sex-linked trait. Female heterozygotes have two populations of red cells, those with normal enzyme activity and those with deficient enzyme activity.

6 G-6-PD deficiency is widely distributed in the populations of the world. One of the factors which may cause the high incidence of this abnormality to be maintained in some populations is its possible protective ability against falciparum malaria, due to the specific enzyme deficiency of the erythrocytes.

BIBLIOGRAPHY

1. Mühlens, P.: Die Behandlung der naturlichen menschlichen Malariainfektion mit Plasmochin. Naturwissenschaften, **14**, 1162, 1926.
2. Cordes, W.: Experiences with plasmochin in malaria: Preliminary reports. *15th Annual Report, United Fruit Co. (Med. Dept.)*, p. 66, 1926.
3. Cordes, W.: Observations on the toxic effect of plasmochin. *16th Annual Report, United Fruit Co. (Med. Dept.)*, p. 62, 1927.
4. Eiselberg, K. P.: Poisoning (plasmochin): 2 cases. Wien. Klin. Wschr., **40**, 525, 1927.
5. Brosius, O. T.: Plasmochin in malaria. *16th Annual Report, United Fruit Co. (Med. Dept.)*, p. 26, 1927.
6. Brosius, O. T.: Plasmochin in malaria. *17th Annual Report, United Fruit Co. (Med. Dept.)*, p. 51, 1928.
7. Cordes, W.: Zwischenfalle bei der Plasmochinbehandlung. Arch. Schiffs- u. Tropenhyg., **32**, 143, 1928.
8. Palma, M. D.: Plasmochin therapy in malaria. Riforma Med., **44**, 753, 1928.
9. Namikawa, H.: Symptoms of poisoning in the treatment of malaria. Taiwan Igakkai Zasshi, **284**, 1298, 1928.
10. Menk, W.: Combined quinine and plasmochin treatment for malaria in Haitian Negroes. *16th Annual Report, United Fruit Co. (Med. Dept.)*, p. 78, 1928.
11. Roskott, E. R., and Seno, R.: Experience of plasmochin. Genesk. tijdschr. Nederl. Indie, **68**, 80, 1928.
12. Kligler, I. F., and Reitler, R.: Studies in malaria. IV. Prophylactic use of plasmochin in a Bedouin population. Riv. Malar., **8**, 28, 1929.
13. Manai, A.: Ittero da plasmochina. Policlinico [Prat.], **36**, 1215, 1929.
14. Baermann, G., and Smits, E.: Über Plasmochin. II. Mitteilung. Arch. Schiffs- u. Tropenhyg., **33**, 24, 1929.
15. Freiman, M.: Plasmoquine and plasmoquine compound in the treatment of malaria. J. Trop. Med., **32**, 165, 1929.
16. Manifold, J. A.: Report on a trial of plasmoquine and quinine in the treatment of benign tertian malaria. J. Roy. Army Med. Corps., **56**, 321, 1931.
17. Missiroli, A., and Marino, P.: Anwendung des Chinoplasmin zur Malariasanierung. Arch. Schiffs- u. Tropenhyg., **38**, 1, 1934.
18. Amy, A. C.: Hemoglobinuria: A new problem on the Indian frontier. J. Roy. Army Med. Corps., **62**, 178, 269, 318, 1934.
19. Ficacci, L.: Emoglobinuria da plasmochina. Policlinico [Prat.], **42**, 136, 1935.
20. Sein, M.: Case of hemoglobinuria caused by plasmochin, taken as prophylactic against malaria. Indian Med. Gaz., **72**, 86, 1937.
21. Mann, W. N.: Haemoglobinuria following the administration of plasmoquine. Trans. Roy. Soc. Trop. Med. Hyg., **37**, 151, 1943.
22. Smith, S.: Note regarding hemoglobinuria following the administration of plasmochin. Trans. Roy. Soc. Trop. Med. Hyg., **37**, 151, 1943.
23. Braun, K., and de Vries, A.: Plasmochin and quinine as the cause of acute haemolytic anemia. Harefuah, **27**, 219, 1944.
24. West, J. B., and Henderson, A. B.: Plasmochin intoxication. Bull. U.S. Army Med. Dept., **82**, 87, 1944.
25. Swantz, H. E., and Bayliss, M.: Hemoglobinuria: Report of ten cases of its occurrence in Negroes during convalescence from malaria. War Med., **7**, 104, 1945.
26. Hardgrove, M., and Applebaum, I. L.: Plasmochin toxicity: Analysis of 258 cases. Ann. Intern. Med., **25**, 103, 1946.
27. Dimson, S. B., and McMartin, R. B.: Pamaquine haemoglobinuria. Quart. J. Med., **15**, 25, 1946.
28. Loeb, R. F.: Activity of a new antimalarial agent, pentaquine (SN-13, 276): Statement approved by the Board for Coordination of Malarial Studies. J.A.M.A., **132**, 321, 1946.
29. Feldman, A., II., Packer, H., Murphy, F. D., and Watson, R. B.: Pamaquine naphthoate as a prophylactic for malarial infections. J. Clin. Invest., **26**, 77, 1947.
30. Atchley, J. A., Yount, E. H., Husted, J. R., Pullman, T. N., Alving, A. S., and Eichelberger, L.: Reactions observed during treatment with pentaquine, administered with quinacrine (Atabrine) metachloridine (SN-11, 437) and with sulfadiazine. J. Nat. Malaria Soc., **7**, 118, 1948.
31. Turchetti, A.: Forme poco frequenti di emoglobinuria da farmaci in corso di infezione malarica. Riforma Med., **62**, 325, 1948.
32. Keng, K. L.: Een geval van zwartwaterkoorts met cyanose (methaemoglobinaemia), waarschijnlijk door plasmochine. Med. Maandbl., **1**, 342, 1948.

33. Earle, D. P., Jr., Bigelow, F. S., Zubrod, C. G., and Kane, C. A.: Studies on the chemotherapy of the human malarias. IX. Effect of pamaquine on the blood cells of man. J. Clin. Invest., **27**, 121, suppl., 1948.
34. Mer, G., Birnbaum, D., and Kligler, I. J.: Lysis of blood of malaria patients by bile or bile salts. Trans Roy. Soc. Trop. Med. Hyg., **34**, 373, 1940–1941.
35. Coatney, G. R., Cooper, W. G., Eyles, D. E., Culwell, W. B., White, W. C., and Lints, H. A.: Studies in human malaria. XXVII. Observations on the use of pentaquine in the prevention and treatment of Chesson strain vivax malaria. J. Nat. Malaria Soc., **9**, 222, 1950.
36. Zylmann, G.: In vitro und in vivo Versuche über die haemolytischen Eigenschaften der synthetischen Malariamittel. Deutsch. Tropenmed. Z., **48**, 7, 1944.
37. Edgcomb, J. H., Arnold, J., Yount, E. H., Alving, A. S., and Eichelberger, L.: Primaquine (SN-13, 272), a new curative agent in vivax malaria: A preliminary report., J. Nat. Malaria Soc., **9**, 284, 1950.
38. Dern, R. J., Weinstein, I. M., LeRoy, G. V., Talmage, D. W., and Alving, A. S.: The hemolytic effect of primaquine. I. The localization of the drug-induced hemolytic defect in primaquine-sensitive individuals. J. Lab. Clin. Med., **43**, 303, 1954.
39. Beutler, E., Dern, R. J., Flanagan, C. L., and Alving, A. S.: The hemolytic effect of primaquine. VII. Biochemical studies of drug-sensitive erythrocytes. J. Lab. Clin. Med., **45**, 286, 1955.
40. Beutler, E.: The glutathione instability of drug-sensitive red cells: A new method for the in vitro detection of drug sensitivity. J. Lab. Clin. Med., **49**, 84, 1957.
41. Carson, P. E., Flanagan, C. L., Ickes, C. E., and Alving, A. S.: Enzymatic deficiency in primaquine-sensitive erythrocytes. Science, **124**, 484, 1956.
42. Sansone, G., and Segni, G.: Prime determinazioni del glutathione (GSH) ematico nel favismo. Boll. Soc. Ital. Biol. Sper., **32**, 456, 1956.
43. Sansone, G., and Segni, G.: L'instabilita del glutathione ematico (GSH) nel favismo: Utilizzasione di un test selettivo: Introduzione al problema genetico. Boll. Soc. Ital. Biol. Sper., **33**, 1057, 1957.
44. Sansone, G., and Segni, G.: Nuovi aspetti dell'alterato biochimismo degli eritrociti de favici: Assenza pressoché completa della glucoso-6-p deidrogenasi. Boll. Soc. Ital. Biol. Sper., **34**, 327, 1958.
45. Sansone, G., Piga, A. M., and Segni, G.: Il favisimo. Edizioni Minerva Medica, Torino, 1958.
46. Szeinberg, A., Sheba, C., Hirshorn, N., and Bodonyi, E.: Studies on erythrocytes in cases with past history of favism and drug-induced acute hemolytic anemia. Blood, **12**, 603, 1957.
47. Szeinberg, A., Asher, Y., and Sheba, C.: Studies on glutathione stability in erythrocytes of cases with past history of favism or sulfa-drug-induced hemolysis. Blood, **13**, 348, 1958.
48. Szeinberg, A., Sheba, C., and Adam, A.: Enzymatic abnormality in erythrocytes of a population sensitive to Vicia fava or drug-induced hemolytic anemia. Nature (London). **181**, 1256, 1958.
49. Zinkham, W. H., Lenhard, R. E., Jr., and Childs, E.: A deficiency of glucose-6-phosphate dehydrogenase activity in erythrocytes from patients with favism. Bull. Johns Hopkins Hosp., **102**, 169, 1958.
50. Panizon, F.: Sul comportamento delle emazie dei fabici di fronte all'idrossilamina in vitro. Studi sassaresi, **35**, 164, 1957.
51. Panizon, F., and Pujatti, G.: Studio sul fluctuatione eritrocitario nel favismo. Acta Paediat. Latina (Parma), **11**, 71, 1958.
52. Gross, R. T., Hurwitz, R. E., and Marks, P. A.: An hereditary enzymatic defect in erythrocyte metabolism: Glucose-6-phosphate dehydrogenase deficiency. J. Clin. Invest., **37**, 1176, 1958.
53. Larizza, P., Brunetti, P., Grignani, F., and Ventura, S.: L'individualita bioqnzimatica dell'eritrocite "fabico" sopra alcune anomalie biochemiche ed enzimatiche delle emazie nei pazienti affetti da favismo e nei loro familiari. Haematologica, **43**, 205, 1958.
54. Sartori, E., and Panizon, F.: Nuove prospettive nelle studio del favismo. Studi Sassaresi, **35**, 363, 1957.
55. Grignani, F., and Brunetti, P.: Carenza di glucosio-6-fosfato deidrogenasi nelle emazie dei fabici nel crisi emolitica ed a distanza dalla stessa. Rass. Med. Sard, **60**, 399, 1958.
56. Davies, P.: Favism: A family study. Quart. J. Med., **31**, 157, 1962.
57. Larizza, P., Brunetti, P., and Grignani, F.: Anemie emolitiche enzimopeniche. Haematologica, **45**, 1, 129, 1960.
58. Brodribb, H. S., and Worssam, A. R.: Favism in an Englishwoman. Brit. Med. J., **1**, 1367, 1961.
59. Vullo, C., and Panizon, F.: The mechanism of haemolysis in favism. Acta Haemat. (Basel), **22**, 146, 1959.
60. Kattamis, C. A., Kyriazakou, M., and Chaidas, S.: Favism. Clinical and biochemical data. J. Med. Genet., **6**, 34, 1969.
61. Newton, W. A., Jr., and Bass, J. C.: Glutathione sensitive chronic non-spherocytic hemolytic anemia. A.M.A. J. Dis. Child., **96**, 501, 1958.
62. Zinkham, W. H., and Lenhard, R. E.: Metabolic abnormalities of erythrocytes from patients with congenital non-spherocytic hemolytic anemia. J. Pediat., **55**, 319, 1959.
63. Shahidi, N. T., and Diamond, L. K.: Enzyme deficiency in erythrocytes in congenital nonspherocytic hemolytic anemia. Pediatrics, **24**, 245, 1959.
64. Zinkham, W. H., and Lenhard, R. E., Jr.: Observations on the significance of primaquine sensitive erythrocytes in patients with congenital nonspherocytic hemolytic anemia. A.M.A.J. Dis. Child., **98**, 443, 1959.
65. Furunhjelm, U., and Vuopio, P.: Glucose-6-phosphate-dehydrogenase deficiency. Lancet, **2**, 1366, 1961.
66. Tada, K.: Enzymatic anomaly of erythrocytes in congenital nonspherocytic hemolytic anemia. Tohoku J. Exp. Med., **75**, 263, 1961.
67. Kirkman, H. N., and Riley, H. D., Jr.: Congenital nonspherocytic hemolytic anemia. Amer. J. Dis. Child., **102**, 313, 1961.
68. Kirkman, H. N.: Genetic control of human enzymes. Pediat. Clin. N. Amer., **10**, 299, 1963.
69. Kirkman, H. N., Brinson, G. A., and Pickard, B. M.: New variants of glucose-6-phosphate dehydrogenase in Caucasian males. *Proc. IX Cong. Europ. Soc. Haemat.*, Lisbon, 1963, part II, p. 685. S. Karger, Basel.
70. WHO Technical Report: Standardization of procedures for the study of glucose-6-phosphate dehydrogenase. WHO Techn. Rep. Ser., No. 366, 1967.
71. Beutler, E., Yeh, M., and Fairbanks, V. F.: The normal human female as a mosaic of X-chromosome activity: Studies using the gene for g-6-pd deficiency as a marker. Proc. Nat. Acad. Sci. U.S.A., **48**, 9, 1962.
72. Motulsky, A. G.: Theoretical and clinical problems of glucose-6-phosphate dehydrogenase deficiency: Its occurrence in Africans and its combination with hemoglobinopathy, in *Abnormal Haemoglobins in Africa,* p. 143. Blackwell, Oxford, 1965.
73. Kirkman, H. N., Kidson, C., and Kennedy, M.: Variants of human glucose-6-phosphate dehydrogenase: Studies of samples from New Guinea, in *Hereditary Disorders of Erythrocyte Metabolism,* edited by E. Beutler, p. 126. Grune & Stratton, New York, 1968.
74. Beutler, E.: Drug-induced hemolytic anemia. Pharmacol. Rev., **21**, 73, 1969.
75. Boivin, P., Piguet, H., and Galand, C.: Anomalies des enzymes de la dégradation du glucose érythrocytaire. Nouv. Rev. Franc. Hemat., **6**, 769, 1966.
76. Eshaghpour, E., Oski, F. A., and Williams, M.: The relationship of erythrocyte glucose-6-phosphate dehydrogenase deficiency to hyperbilirubinemia in Negro premature infants. J. Pediat., **70**, 595, 1967.
77. Ifekwunigwe, A. E., and Luzzatto, L.: Kernicterus in G.-6-P.D.-deficiency. Lancet, **1**, 677, 1966.
78. Hendrickse, R. G., discussion of paper by Motulsky, A.: Theoretical and clinical problems of glucose-6-phosphate dehydrogenase deficiency: Its occurrence in Africans and its combination with hemoglobinopathy, in *Abnormal Haemoglobins in Africa,* p. 208. Blackwell, Oxford, 1965.
79. Gilles, H. M., and Taylor, B. G.: The existence of the glucose-6-phosphate dehydrogenase deficiency trait in Nigeria and its clinical implications. Ann. Trop. Med., **55**, 64, 1961.
80. O'Flynn, M. E. D., and Hsia, D. Y.: Serum bilirubin levels and glucose-6-phosphate dehydrogenase deficiency in newborn American Negroes. J. Pediat., **63**, 160, 1963.
81. Zinkham, W. G.: Peripheral blood and bilirubin values in normal full-term primaquine-sensitive Negro infants: Effect of vitamin K. Pediatrics, **31**, 983, 1963.
82. Dern, R. J., Beutler, E., and Alving, A. S.: The hemolytic effect of primaquine. II. The natural course of the hemolytic anemia and the mechanism of its self-limited character. J. Lab. Clin. Med., **44**, 171, 1954.
83. Beutler, E., Dern, R. J., and Alving, A. S.: The hemolytic effect of

primaquine. III. A study of primaquine-sensitive erythrocytes. J. Lab. Clin. Med., **44,** 177, 1954.

84. Beutler, E., Dern, R. J., and Alving, A. S.: The hemolytic effect of primaquine. IV. The relationship of cell age to hemolysis. J. Lab. Clin. Med., **44,** 439, 1954.
85. Marks, P. A., and Gross, R. T.: Erythrocyte glucose-6-phosphate dehydrogenase deficiency: Evidence of differences between Negroes and Caucasians with respect to this genetically determined trait. J. Clin. Invest., **38,** 2253, 1959.
86. Piomelli, S., Corash, L. M., Davenport, D. D., Miraglia, J., and Amorosi, E. L.: In vivo lability of glucose-6-phosphate dehydrogenase in GD^{A-} and $Gd^{Mediterranean}$ deficiency. J. Clin. Invest., **47,** 940, 1968.
87. Degowin, R. L., Eppes, R. B., Powell, R. D., and Carson, P. E.: The haemolytic effects of diaphenylsulfone (DDS) in normal subjects and in those with glucose-6-phosphate dehydrogenase deficiency. WHO Bull., **35,** 165–179, 1966.
88. Zinkham, W. H., and Childs, B.: A defect in GSH metabolism in erythrocytes from patients with a naphthalene-induced hemolytic anemia. Pediatrics, **22,** 461, 1958.
89. McGovern, J. J., Isselbacher, K., Rose, P. J., and Grossman. M. S.: Observations on the glutathione (GSH) stability of red blood cells. A.M.A. J. Dis. Child., **96,** 502, 1958.
90. Dawson, J. P., Thayer, W. W., and Desforges, J. F.: Acute hemolytic anemia in the newborn infant due to naphthalene poisoning; report of two cases with investigations into the mechanism of the disease. Blood, **13,** 1113, 1958.
91. Gilles, H. M., and Ikeme, A. C.: Hemoglobinuria among adult Nigerians due to glucose-6-phosphate dehydrogenase deficiency with drug sensitivity. Lancet, **2,** 889, 1960.
92. Zuelzer, W. W., and Apt, L.: Acute hemolytic anemia due to naphthalene poisoning. J.A.M.A., **141,** 185, 1949.
93. Houston, I. B., and Barlow, A. M.: Acute haemolytic anaemia and methemoglobinuria produced by phenacetin. Lancet, **2,** 1062, 1959.
94. Kimbro, E. I., Jr., Sachs, M. V., and Torbert, J. V.: Mechanism of the hemolytic anemia induced by nitrofurantoin (Furadantin). Bull. Johns Hopkins Hosp., **101,** 245, 1957.
95. West, M., and Zimmerman, H. J.: Hemolytic anemia in patient receiving nitrofurantoin (Furadantin). J.A.M.A., **162,** 637, 1956.
96. Sonnet, J., Vandepitte, J., and Haumont, A.: Anaemie hemolytique par la nitrofurazone revelatrice d'une deficience globulair en glucose-6-phosphate dehydrogenase. Ann. Soc. Belg. Med. Trop., **39,** 691, 1959.
97. Robertson, D. H. H.: Nitrofurazone-induced haemolytic anaemia in a refractory case of Trypanosoma rhodesiense sleeping sickness: The haemolytic trait and self-limiting haemolytic anaemia. Ann. Trop. Med., **55,** 49, 1961.
98. Szeinberg, A., Adam, A., and Sheba, C.: Effect of nitrofurantoin in erythrocyte viability. Proc. Tel-Hashomer Hosp., **1,** 49, 1962.
99. Dern, R. J., Beutler, E., and Alving, A. S.: The hemolytic effect of primaquine. V. Primaquine sensitivity as a manifestation of a multiple drug sensitivity. J. Lab. Clin. Med., **45,** 30, 1955.
100. Kellermeyer, R. W., Tarlov, A. K., Schrier, S. L., and Alving, A. S.: Hemolytic effect of commonly used drugs on erythrocytes deficient in glucose-6-phosphate dehydrogenase. J. Lab. Clin. Med., **52,** 827, 1958 (abstract).
101. Szeinberg, A., Sheba, C., Ramot, B., and Adam, A.: Differences in hemolytic susceptibility among subjects with glucose-6-phosphate dehydrogenase. Clin. Res., **8,** 18, 1960 (abstract).
102. Zail, S. S., Charlton, R. W., and Bothwell, T. H.: The haemolytic effect of certain drugs in Bantu subjects with a deficiency of glucose-6-phosphate dehydrogenase. S. Afr. J. Med. Sci., **27,** 95, 1962.
103. Chernof, D.: Dapsone-induced hemolysis in G-6-PD deficiency. J.A.M.A., **201,** 554, 1967.
104. Kellermeyer, R. W., Tarlov, A. R., Brewer, G. J., Carson, P. E., and Alving, A. S.: Hemolytic effect of therapeutic drugs: Clinical considerations of the primaquine-type hemolysis. J.A.M.A., **180,** 388, 1962.
105. Brown, A., and Cevik, N.: Hemolysis and jaundice in the newborn following maternal treatment with sulfamethoxypyridazine (kynex). Pediatrics, **36,** 742, 1965.
106. Premuzić-Lampić, M., and Prica, M.: The hemolytic effect of sulamin (sulfamethoxypyridazine) on erythrocytes with glucose-6-phosphate dehydrogenase deficiency. Blood Transf. Bull., **21,** 61, 1967.
107. Hockwald, R. S., Arnold, J., Clayman, C. B., and Alving, A. S.: Status of primaquine. IV. Toxicity of primaquine in Negroes. J.A.M.A., **149,** 1568, 1952.
108. Beutler, E., Dern, R. J., and Alving, A. S.: Studies of the hemolytic anemia induced by primaquine and related compounds. Unpublished.
109. Beutler, E.: The hemolytic effect of primaquine and related compounds: A review. Blood, **14,** 103, 1959.
110. Alving, A. S., Johnson, C. F., Tarlov, A. R., Brewer, G. J., Kellermeyer, R. W., and Carson, P. E.: Mitigation of the haemolytic effect of primaquine and enhancement of its action against exoerythrocytic forms of the Chesson strain of plasmodium vivax by intermittent regimens of drug administration. WHO Bull., **22,** 621, 1960.
111. Brewer, G. J., Tarlov, A. R., and Alving, A. S.: Cited in Standardization of procedures for the study of glucose-6-phosphate dehydrogenase. WHO Techn. Rep. Ser., No. 366, pp. 27, 1967.
112. Jeannet, M., Perrier, C. V., and Tönz, O.: Anémie hémolytique aigüe par la nitrofurantoïne chez une Iranienne présentant un déficit en glucose-6-phosphate-déhydrogénase érythrocytaire. Schweiz. Med. Wschr., **94,** 939, 1964.
113. Chatterjea. S. C., and Das, P. K.: Chloramphenicol induced haemolytic anaemia due to enzymatic deficiency of erythrocytes. J. Indian Med. Ass., **40,** 172, 1963.
114. Michot, F., Rastetter, J., and Gronauer, H.: Durch neosalvarsan ausgelöste hämolyse bei glukose-6-phosphat-dehydrogenase-mangel, kombiniert mit hepatischem icterus. Schweiz. Med. Wschr., **96,** 985, 1966.
115. Sansone, G., and Segni, G.: Difetto biochimico eritrocitario: a carattere genetico, in un bambino con anemia emolitica acuta da naftalina. Boll. Soc. Ital. Biol. Sper., **34,** 615, 1958.
116. Brewer, G. J., and Tarlov, A. R.: Studies on the mechanism of primaquine-type hemolysis: The effect of methylene blue. Clin. Res., **9,** 65, 1961 (abstract).
117. Belton, E. M., and Jones, R. V.: Haemolytic anaemia due to Nalidixic acid. Lancet, **2,** 691, 1965.
118. Tarlov, A. R.: Unpublished, cited in Tarlov et al. ref. 344.
119. Westring, D. W., and Calas, C.: Hemolytic effect of estrogen on G-6-PD deficient erythrocytes. Clin. Res., **16,** 544, 1968 (abstract).
120. Burka, E. R., Weaver, Z., III, and Marks, P. A.: Clinical spectrum of hemolytic anemia associated with G-6-PD deficiency. Ann. Intern. Med., **64,** 817, 1966.
121. Mengel, C. E., Metz, E., and Yancey, W. S.: Anemia during acute infections: Role of glucose-6-phosphate dehydrogenase deficiency in Negroes. Arch. Intern. Med. (Chicago), **119,** 187, 1967.
122. Berry, D. H., and Vietti, T. J.: Clinical manifestations of primaquine-sensitive anemia. Amer. J. Dis. Child., **110,** 166, 1965.
123. Kattamis, C. A., Kyriazukou, M., and Chaidas, S.: Favism. J. Med. Genet., **6,** 34, 1969.
124. George J. N., Sears, D. A., McCurdy, P., and Conrad, M. E.: Primaquine sensitivity in caucasians: Hemolytic reactions induced by primaquine in G-6-PD deficient subjects. J. Lab. Clin. Med., **70,** 80, 1967.
125. Hersko, C., and Vardy, P. A.: Haemolysis in typhoid fever in children with G-6-PD deficiency. Brit. Med. J., **1,** 214, 1967.
126. Choremis, C., Kattamis, Ch. A., Kyriazakou, M., and Gavriilidou, E.: Viral hepatitis in G-6-PD deficiency: Lancet, **1,** 269, 1966.
127. Boon, W. H.: Viral hepatitis in G-6-PD deficiency. Lancet, **1,** 882, 1966.
128. Sutton, R. N. P.: Viral hepatitis in G-6-PD deficiency. Lancet, **1,** 550, 1966.
129. Lisker, R., Loria, A., and Strygler, I.: Hemolytic anemia associated with instability of the reduced glutathione of the erythrocyte: Family affected with this defect. Prensa Med. Mex., **25,** 2, 1960.
130. Ben-Ishay, D., and Izak, G.: Chronic hemolysis associated with glucose-6-phosphate deficiency. J. Lab. Clin. Med., **63,** 1002, 1964.
131. Beutler, E., Mathai, C. K., and Smith, J. E.: Biochemical variants of glucose-6-phosphate dehydrogenase giving rise to congenital nonspherocytic hemolytic disease. Blood, **31,** 131, 1968.
132. Schettini, F., and Meloni, T.: Characterization of glucose-6-phosphate dehydrogenase in Sardinian children with congenital nonspherocytic haemolytic anaemia. Acta Haemat., **37,** 198, 1967.

133. Schärer, K., Herzka, H., and Marti, H. R.: Kernicterus bei Mangel an Glukose-6-phosphat Dehydrogenase der Erythrocyten. Helv. Paediat. Acta, **2**, 148, 1963.
134. Doxiadis, S. A., Fessas, Ph., Valaes, T., and Mastrokalos, W.: Glucose-6-phosphate dehydrogenase deficiency. Lancet, **1**, 297, 1961.
135. Panizon, F.: Dimonstrazione della anomalia enzimatica nel fegato di soggetti con difetto eritrocitario di glucose-6-fosfato deidrogenasi. Boll. Soc. Ital. Biol. Sper., **36**, 106, 1960.
136. Doxiadis, S. A., Fessas, Ph., and Valaes, T.: Erythrocyte enzyme deficiency in unexplained kernicterus. Lancet, **2**, 44, 1960.
137. Smith, G., and Vella, F.: Erythrocyte enzyme deficiency in unexplained kernicterus. Lancet, **1**, 1133, 1960.
138. Weatherall, D. J.: Enzyme deficiency in haemolytic disease of the newborn. Lancet, **2**, 835, 1960.
139. Panizon, F.: L'ictère grave du nouveau-né associé à une défivience en glucose-6-phosphate déhydrogenase. Biol. Neonat., **2**, 167, 1960.
140. Lu, T. C., Wei, H., and Blackwell, R. Q.: Increased incidence of severe hyperbilirubinemia among newborn Chinese infants with G-6-PD deficiency. Pediatrics, **37**, 994, 1966.
141. Szeinberg, A., Oliver, M., Schmidt, R., Adam, A., and Sheba, C.: Glucose-6-phosphate dehydrogenase deficiency and haemolytic disease of the newborn in Israel. Arch. Dis. Child., **38**, 23, 1963.
142. Freier, S., Mayer, K., Abrahamov, A., and Levene, C. Neonatal jaundice in infants with enzymatic defect of the red blood cell. Israel J. Med. Sci., **1**, 844, 1965.
143. Szeinberg, A., Pras, M., Sheba, C., Adam. A., and Ramot, B.: The hemolytic effect of various sulfonamides on subjects with a deficiency of glucose-6-phosphate dehydrogenase of erythrocytes. Israel M. I., **18**, 176, 1959.
144. Bernard, J., and Dreyfus, J. C.: Hémolyse aiguë familiale et déficit de la glucose-6-phosphate déhydrogenase des érythrocytes. Nouv. Rev. Franc. Hemat., **2**, 135, 1962.
145. Salvidio, E., Pannacciulli, I., and Tizianello, A.: G-6-pd deficient states in Sardinians. *Proc. IX Cong. Europ. Soc. Haemat.*, Lisbon, 1963, part II/1, p. 707. S. Karger, Basel.
146. Larizza, P., Brunetti, P., Grignani, F., and Ventura, S.: I fabici sono sensibili alla primachina. Minerva Med., **49**, 3769, 1958.
147. Szeinberg, A., Sheba, C., and Adam, A.: Selective occurrence of glutathione instability in red blood corpuscles of the various Jewish tribes. Blood, **13**, 1043, 1959.
148. Greenberg, M. S., and Wong, H.: Studies on the destruction of glutathione-unstable red blood cells: The influence of fava beans and primaquine upon such cells in vivo. J. Lab. Clin. Med., **57**, 733, 1961.
149. Panizon, F., and Vullo, C.: The mechanism of haemolysis in favism. Acta Haemat., **26**, 337, 1961.
150. Stamatoyannopoulos, G., Fraser, G. R., Motulsky, A. G., Fessas, P. H., Akrivakis, A., and Papayannopoulou, T.: On the familial predisposition to favism. Amer. J. Hum. Genet., **18**, 253, 1966.
151. Bowdler, A. J., and Prankerd, T. A. J.: Studies in congenital nonsperocytic haemolytic anaemias with specific enzyme defects. Acta Haemat., **31**, 65, 1964.
152. Cloutier, M. D., Burgert, E. O.: Congenital nonspherocytic hemolytic disease secondary to G-6-PD deficiency: Report of 3 cases. Mayo Clin. Proc., **41**, 316, 1966.
153. Escobar, M. A., Heller, P., and Trobaugh, F. E., Jr.: "Complete" erythrocyte glucose-6-phosphate dehydrogenase deficiency. Arch. Intern. Med. (Chicago), **113**, 428, 1964.
154. Fornaini, G., Bianchini, E., Leoncini, G., and Fantoni, A.: Metabolic aspects of red cells in congenital nonspherocytic hemolytic anaemia. Brit. J. Haemat., **10**, 23, 1964.
155. Greenberg, L. H., and Tanaka, K. R.: Hereditary hemolytic anemia due to glucose-6-phosphate dehydrogenase deficiency. Amer. J. Dis. Child., **110**, 206, 1965.
156. Grossman, A., Ramanathan, K., Justice, P., Gordon, J., Shahidi, N. T., and Hsia, D.: Congenital nonspherocytic hemolytic anemia associated with erythrocyte G-6-PD deficiency in a Negro family. Pediatrics, **37**, 624, 1966.
157. Kirkman, H. N., Rosenthal, I. M., Simon, E. R., Carson, P. E., and Brinson, A. G.: "Chicago I" variant of glucose-6-phosphate dehydrogenase in congenital hemolytic disease. J. Lab. Clin. Med., **63**, 715, 1964.
158. Kühböck, V. J., Pietschmann, H., and Rothenbuchner, G.: Enzymopenische hämolytische Anämie bei einer österreichischen Familie. Wien. Klin. Wschr., **81**, 135, 1969.
159. Messerschmitt, J., Suaudeau, C., Benallegue, V. R., Fabre, S., Bon, J., Andre, L., Khati, B., Dubois, M., Benabdallan, S., and Kotchoyan, P.: Defaut en G-6-PD et anemies hemolytiques en Algerie. Nouv. Rev. Franc. Hemat., **7**, 827, 1967.
160. Schröter, W., Drescher, J., and Fischer, K.: Uber eine seltene form des glucose-6-phosphatdehydrogenase-Mangels mit kongenitaler nichtsphärocytärer hämolytischer anämie. Klin. Wschr., **45**, 355, 1967.
161. Puxeddu, A., Santeusanio, F., Migliorini, E., Siracusa, A., and Merlitti, A.: Studio di un Gruppo Familiare Umbro-Marchigiano con Anemia Emolitica Congenita Non Sferocitica da Carenza di Glucosio-t-Fosfato-Deidrogenase (G6PD). Haemat. Arch., **53**, 30, 1968.
162. Weinreich, J., Busch, D., Gottstein, U., Schaefer, J., and Rohr, J.: Über zwei neue Fälle von hereditärer nichtsphärocytärer hämolytischer anämie bei glucose-6-phosphat-dehydrogenase-defekt in einer nord Deutschen familie. Klin. Wschr., **46**, 146, 1968.
163. Talalak, P., and Beutler, E.: G-6-PD Bangkok: A new variant found in congenital nonspherocytic hemolytic disease (CNHD). Blood, **33**, 772, 1969.
164. Tanaka, K. R., and Beutler, E.: Hereditary hemolytic anemia due to glucose-6-phosphate dehydrogenase Torrance: A new variant. J. Lab. Clin. Med., **73**, 657, 1969.
165. Boivin, P., and Galand, C.: Nouvelles variantes de la glucose-6-phosphate dehydrogenase erythrocytaire. Rev. Franc. Etud. Clin. Biol., **13**, 30, 1968.
166. Waller, H. D., Löhr, G. W., and Gayer, J.: Hereditäre Nichtsphärocytäre Hämolytische Anämie Durch Glucose-6-Phosphatdehydrogenase-Mangel. (Bildung Eines Enzymproteins mit Veränderten Eigenschaften in den Blutzellen Einer Deutschen Familie). Klin. Wschr., **44**, 122, 1966.
167. Helge, H., and Börner, K.: Kongenitale nichtsphärozytäre hämolytische Anämie, Katarakt und Glucose-6-phosphat-Dehydrogenase-Mangel. Deutsch. Med. Wschr., **91**, 1584, 1966.
168. Boyer, S. H., Porter, I. H., and Weilbacher, R. G.: Electrophoretic heterogeneity of glucose-6-phosphate dehydrogenase and its relationship to enzyme deficiency in man. Proc. Nat. Acad. Sci. U.S.A. **48**, 1868, 1962.
168*a*. Abe, T., Takafuji, H., and Yamamoto, M.: Congenital nonspherocytic hemolytic anemia due to a deficiency of glucose-6-phosphate dehydrogenase in the red blood cells in a Japanese family. Blut, **17**, 143, 1968.
169. Bishop, C.: Overall red cell metabolism, in *The Red Blood Cell*, edited by C. Bishop and D. M. Surgenor, p. 147. Academic, New York, 1964.
170. Valentine, W. N.: Hereditary hemolytic anemias associated with specific erythrocyte enzymopathies. Calif. Med., **108**, 280, 1968.
171. Beutler, E.: Genetic disorders of red cell metabolism. Med. Clin. N. Amer., **53**, 813, 1969.
172. Prins, H. K., Oort, M., Loos, J. A., Zürcher, C., and Beckers, T.: Hereditary absence of glutathione in erythrocytes: Biochemical, haematological and genetical. *Proc. IX Cong. Europ. Soc. Haemat.*, Lisbon, 1963, part II/1, p. 721. S. Karger, Basel.
173. Dimant, E., Landberg, E., and London, I. M.: The metabolic behavior of reduced glutathione in human and avian erythrocytes. J. Biol. Chem., **213**, 769, 1955.
174. Elder, H. A., and Mortensen, R. A.: The incorporation of labeled glycine into erythrocyte glutathione. J. Biol. Chem., **218**, 261, 1956.
175. Mortensen, R. A., Haley, M. I., and Elder, H. A.: The turnover of erythrocyte glutathione in the rat. J. Biol. Chem., **218**, 269, 1956.
176. Szeinberg, A., Adam, A., Ramot, B., Sheba, C., and Meyers, F.: The incorporation of isotopically labelled glycine into the glutathione of erythrocytes with glucose-6-phosphate dehydrogenase deficiency. Biochim. Biophys. Acta, **36**, 65, 1959.
177. Leder, I. G., and Handler, P.: Synthesis of nicotinamide mononucleotide by human erythrocytes *in vitro*. J. Biol. Chem., **189**, 889, 1951.
178. Tulpule, P. G.: Species difference in pyridine nucleotide synthesis by erythrocytes. Nature (London), **181**, 1804, 1958.
179. Jaffé, E. R., and Gordon, E. W.: The incorporation of nicotinic acid

and of nicotinamide into the pyridine nucleotides of erythrocytes and reticulocytes of rabbits in vitro. J. Clin. Invest., **42,** 1017, 1963.

180. Mandula, B. and Beutler, E.: Synthesis of riboflavin nucleotides by mature human erythrocytes. Blood, **36,** 491, 1970.
181. Lowy, B. A., Ramot, B., and London, I. M.: The biosynthesis of adenosine triphosphate and guanosine triphosphate in the rabbit erythrocyte *in vivo* and *in vitro.* J. Biol. Chem., **235,** 1920, 1960.
182. Lowy, B. A., Williams, M. K., and London, I. M.: The utilization of purines and their ribosyl derivatives for the formation of adenosine triphosphate and guanosine triphosphate in the mature rabbit erythrocyte. J. Biol. Chem., **236,** 1439, 1961.
183. Altman, K. I.: The *in vitro* incorporation of a C-14 acetate into the stroma of erythrocytes. Arch. Biochem., **42,** 478, 1953.
184. James, A. T., Lovelock, J. E., and Webb, J.: The biosynthesis of fatty acids by human red blood cells. Biochemistry (Wash.), **66,** 60, 1957.
185. O'Donnell, V. J., Ottolenghi, P., Malkin, A., Denstedt, O. F., and Heard, R. D. H.: The biosynthesis from acetate-1-C^{14} of fatty acids and cholesterol in formed blood elements. Canad. J. Biochem. Physiol., **36,** 1125, 1958.
186. Marks, P. A., and Gellhorn, A.: Lipid synthesis in human leucocytes and erythrocytes *in vitro.* Fed. Proc., **18,** 281, 1959.
187. Chapman, R. G., Hennessey, M. A., Waltersdorph, A. M., Huennekens, F. M., and Gabrio, B. W.: Erythrocyte metabolism. V. Levels of glycolytic enzymes and regulation of glycolysis. J. Clin. Invest., **41,** 1249, 1962.
188. Ockel, E., Rapoport, S., Hinterberger, U., and Gerischer-Mothes, W.: Die pH-abhängigkeit der anaeroben Glykolyse und der Hexokinase. Folia Haemat. (Leipzig), **78,** 477, 1962.
189. Murphy, J. R.: Erythrocyte metabolism. II. Glucose metabolism and pathways. J. Lab. Clin. Med., **55,** 286, 1960.
190. Kellermeyer, R. W., Carson, P. E., Schrier, S. L., Tarlov, A. R., and Alving, A. S.: The hemolytic effect of primaquine. XIV. Pentose metabolism in primiquine-sensitive erythrocytes. J. Lab. Clin. Med., **58,** 715, 1961.
191. Johnson, A. B., and Marks, P. A.: Glucose metabolism and oxygen consumption in normal and glucose-6-phosphate dehydrogenase deficient human erythrocytes. Clin. Res., **6,** 187, 1958 (abstract).
192. Jacob, H. S., and Jandl, J. H.: Effects of sulfhydryl inhibition on red blood cells. III. Glutathione in the regulation of the hexose monophosphate pathway. J. Biol. Chem., **241,** 4243, 1966.
193. Harrop, G. A., Jr., and Barron, E. S. G.: Studies on blood cell metabolism: Effect of methylene blue and other dyes upon the oxygen consumption of mammalian and avian erythrocytes. J. Exp. Med., **48,** 207, 1928.
194. Brin, M., and Yonemoto, R. H.: Stimulation of the glucose oxidative pathway in human erythrocytes by methylene blue. J. Biol. Chem., **230,** 307, 1958.
195. Gibson, Q. H.: The reduction of methemoglobin in red blood cells and studies on the cause of idiopathic methemoglobinemia. Biochem. J., **42,** 13, 1948.
196. Szeinberg, A., and Marks, P. A.: Substances stimulating glucose catabolism by the oxidative reactions of the pentose phosphate pathway in human erythrocytes. J. Clin. Invest., **40,** 914, 1961.
197. Beutler, E.: Abnormalities of glycolysis (HMP shunt). Bibl. Haemat., **29,** 146, 1968.
198. Dische, Z.: The pentose phosphate metabolism in red cells, in *The Red Blood Cell,* C. Bishop and D. M. Surgenor, p. 189. Academic, New York, 1964.
199. Marks, P. A., Szeinberg, A., and Banks, J.: Erythrocyte glucose-6-phosphate dehydrogenase of normal and mutant human subjects: Properties of the purified enzyme. J. Biol. Chem., **236,** 10, 1961.
200. Kirkman, H. N.: Glucose 6-phosphate dehydrogenase from human erythrocytes. I. Further purification and characterization. J. Biol. Chem., **237,** 2364, 1962.
201. Kirkman, H. N., and Hendrickson, E. M.: Glucose-6-phosphate dehydrogenase from human erythrocytes. II. Subactive states of the enzyme from normal persons. J. Biol. Chem., **237,** 2371, 1962.
202. Chung, A. E., and Langdon, R. G.: Human erythrocyte glucose-6-phosphate dehydrogenase. I. Isolation and properties of the enzyme. J. Biol. Chem., **238,** 2309, 1963.
203. Balinsky, D., and Bernstein, R. E.: The purification and properties of glucose-6-phosphate dehydrogenase from human erythrocytes. Biochim. Biophys. Acta, **67,** 313, 1963.
204. Yoshida, A.: Glucose-6-phosphate dehydrogenase of human erythrocytes. I. Purification and characterization of normal (B+) enzyme. J. Biol. Chem., **241,** 4966, 1966.
205. Soldin, S. J., and Balinsky, D.: The kinetic properties of human erythrocyte glucose-6-phosphate dehydrogenase. Biochemistry, **7,** 1077, 1968.
206. Rattazzi, M. C.: Isolation and purification of human erythrocyte glucose-6-phosphate dehydrogenase from small amounts of blood. Biochim. Biophys. Acta, **181,** 1, 1969.
207. Yoshida, A.: A single amino acid substitution (asparagine to aspartic acid) between normal (B+) and the common Negro variant (A+) of human glucose-6-phosphate dehydrogenase. Proc. Nat. Acad. Sci. U.S.A., **57,** 835, 1967.
208. Yoshida, A.: Human glucose-6-phosphate dehydrogenase: Purification and characterization of Negro type variant (A+) and comparison with normal enzyme (B+). Biochem. Genet., **1,** 81, 1967.
209. Luzzatto, L.: Regulation of the activity of glucose-6-phosphate dehydrogenase by $NADP^+$ and NADPH. Biochim. Biophys. Acta, **146,** 18, 1967.
210. Kissin, C., and Beutler, E.: The utilization of glucose by normal glucose-6-phosphate dehydrogenase and by glucose-6-phosphate dehydrogenase Mediterranean. Proc. Soc. Exp. Biol. Med., **128,** 595, 1968.
211. Kirkman, H. N., McCurdy, P. R., and Naiman, J. L.: Functionally abnormal glucose-6-phosphate dehydrogenases. *Cold Spring Harbor Symposia on Quantitative Biology,* vol. *29,* p. 391, 1964.
212. Rattazzi, M. C.: Glucose-6-phosphate dehydrogenase from human erythrocytes: Molecular weight determination by gel filtration. Biochem. Biophys. Res. Commun., **31,** 16, 1968.
213. Yoshida, A.: Subunit structure of human glucose-6-phosphate dehydrogenase and its genetic implication. Biochem. Genet., **2,** 237, 1968.
214. Chung, A. E., and Langdon, R. G.: Human erythrocyte glucose-6-phosphate dehydrogenase. II. Enzyme-coenzyme interrelationship. J. Biol. Chem., **238,** 2317, 1963.
215. Beutler, E., and Collins, Z.: Hybridization studies in the further characterization of erythrocyte G-6-PD. Experientia, **22,** 827, 1966.
216. Rosa, R., and Dreyfus, J. C.: Hybridation de la glucose-6-phosphate deshydrogenase des globules rouges et des globules blancs. Clin. Chim. Acta, **24,** 199, 1969.
217. Beutler, E., and Collins, Z.: Hybridization of glucose-6-phosphate dehydrogenase from rat and human erythrocytes. Science, **150,** 1306, 1965.
218. Yoshida, A., Steinmann, L., and Harbert, P.: In vitro hybridization of normal and variant human glucose-6-phosphate dehydrogenase. Nature (London), **216,** 175, 1967.
219. Rall, T. W., and Lehninger, A. L.: Glutathione reductase of animal tissues. J. Biol. Chem., **194,** 119, 1952.
220. Francoeur, M., and Denstedt, O. F.: Metabolism of mammalian erythrocytes. VII. The glutathione reductase of the mammalian erythrocyte. Canad. J. Biochem., **32,** 663, 1954.
221. Schrier, S. L., Kellermeyer, R. W., Carson, P. E., Ickes, C. E., and Alving, A. S.: The hemolytic effect of primaquine. IX. Enzymatic abnormalities in primaquine-sensitive erythrocytes. J. Lab. Clin. Med., **52,** 109, 1958.
222. Huennekens, F. M., Caffrey, R. W., Basford, R. E., and Gabrio, B. W.: Erythrocyte metabolism. IV. Isolation and properties of methemoglobin reductase. J. Biol. Chem., **227,** 261, 1957.
223. Jaffé, E.: The reduction of methemoglobin in erythrocytes of a patient with congenital methemoglobinemia, subjects with erythrocyte glucose-6-phosphate dehydrogenase deficiency, and normal individuals. Blood, **21,** 561, 1963.
224. Strömme, J. H., and Eldjarn, L.: The role of the pentose phosphate pathway in the reduction of methaemoglobin in human erythrocytes. Biochem. J., **84,** 406, 1962.
225. Wieland, T.: Chemistry and properties of glutathione. *Glutathione Proc. Symp.,* Ridgefield, Conn., 1953, p. 45. Academic, New York, 1953.
226. Calvin, M.: Mercaptans and disulfides: Some physics, chemistry, and

speculation. *Glutathione Proc. Symp.* Ridgefield, Conn., 1953, p. 3. Academic, New York, 1953.
227. Boivin, P., Galand, C., André, R., and Debray, J.: Anémies hémolytiques congénitales avec déficit isolé en glutathion réduit par déficit en glutathion synthétase. Nouv. Rev. Franc. Hemat., **6,** 859, 1966.
228. Sass, D.: Glutathione synthesis in cell-free preparations from erythrocytes of different ages. Clin. Chim. Acta, **22,** 207, 1968.
229. Jackson, R. C.: Studies in the enzymology of glutathione metabolism in human erythrocytes. Biochem. J., **111,** 309, 1969.
230. Lyman, C. M., and Barron, E. S. G.: Studies on biological oxidations. VIII. The oxidation of glutathione with copper and hemochromogens as catalysts. J. Biol. Chem., **121,** 275, 1937.
231. Mills, G. C.: Hemoglobin catabolism. I. Glutathione peroxidase, an erythrocyte enzyme which protects hemoglobin from oxidative breakdown. J. Biol. Chem., **229,** 189, 1957.
232. Mills, G. C., and Randall, H. P.: Hemoglobin catabolism. II. The protection of hemoglobin from oxidative breakdown in the intact erythrocyte. J. Biol. Chem., **232,** 589, 1958.
233. Eggleton, P., and Fegler, G.: Reduced glutathione and spontaneous methaemoglobin formation in haemolysates. Quart. J. Physiol., **37,** 163, 1952.
234. Beutler, E., and Kelly, B. M.: The effect of sodium nitrite on red cell GSH. Experientia, **19,** 96, 1963.
235. Fegler, G.: Relationship between reduced glutathione content and spontaneous haemolysis in shed blood. Nature (London), **170,** 624, 1952.
236. Klebanoff, S. J.: Glutathione metabolism. II. The oxidation and reduction of glutathione in intact erythrocytes. Biochem. J., **65,** 423, 1957.
237. Beutler, E., and Yeh, M. K. Y.: Erythrocyte glutathione reductase. Blood, **21,** 573, 1963.
238. Cohen, G., and Hochstein, P.: Glucose-6-phosphate dehydrogenase and detoxification of hydrogen peroxide in human erythrocytes. Science, **134,** 1756, 1961.
239. Carson, P., Schrier, S., and Flanagan, C. L.: Use of DPNH as coenzyme for glutathione reductase of hemolysates. Fed. Proc., **16,** 19, 1957 (abstract).
240. Rieber, E. E., Kosower, N. S., and Jaffe, E. R.: Reduced nicotinamide adenine dinucleotide and the reduction of oxidized glutathione in human erythrocytes. J. Clin. Invest., **47,** 66, 1968.
241. Srivastava, S. K., and Beutler, E.: Oxidized glutathione levels in erythrocytes of glucose-6-phosphate dehydrogenase deficient subjects. Lancet, **11,** 23, 1968.
242. Beutler, E., Robson, M., and Buttenwieser, E.: The mechanism of glutathione destruction and protection in drug-sensitive and non-sensitive erythrocytes: *In vitro* studies, J. Clin. Invest., **36,** 617, 1957.
243. Huisman, T. H. J., and Dozy, A. M.: Studies on the heterogeneity of hemoglobin. V. Binding of hemoglobin with oxidized glutathione. J. Lab. Clin. Med., **60,** 302, 1962.
244. Allen, D. W., and Jandl, J. H.: Oxidative hemolysis and precipitation of hemoglobin. II. Role of thiols in oxidant drug action. J. Clin. Invest., **40,** 454, 1961.
245. Jacob, H. S., Brain, M. C., Dacie, J. V., Carrell, R. W., and Lehmann, H.: Abnormal haem binding and globin SH group blockade in unstable haemoglobins. Nature (London), **218,** 1214, 1968.
246. Srivastava, S. K., and Beutler, E.: The transport of oxidized glutathione from human erythrocytes. J. Biol. Chem., **244,** 9, 1969.
247. Beutler, E., and Srivastava, S. K.: The efflux of GSSG from human erythrocytes. Metabolism and Membrane Permeability of Erythrocytes and Thrombocytes, 1st Int. Symp., Vienna, 1968, p. 91. Thieme, Stuttgart.
248. Boivin, P., and Galand, C.: La synthese du glutathion au cours de l'anemie hemolytique congenitale avec deficit en glutathion reduit. Deficit congenital en glutathionsynthetase erythrocytaire? Nouv. Rev. Franc. Hemat., **5,** 606, 1965.
249. Oort, M., Loos, J. A., and Prins, H. K.: Hereditary absence of reduced glutathione in the erythrocytes—a new clinical and biochemical entity? Vox Sang., **6,** 370, 1961.
250. Prins, H. K., Oort, M., Loos, J. A., Zürcher, C., and Beckers, T: Congenital nonspherocytic hemolytic anemia, associated with glutathione deficiency of the erythrocytes. Blood, **27,** 145, 1966.
251. Jacob, H. S., and Jandl, J. H.: Effects of sulfhydryl inhibition on red blood cells. II. Studies *in vivo.* J. Clin. Invest., **41,** 1514, 1962.
252. Beutler, E., Srivastava, S. K., and West, C.: The reversibility of N-ethylmaleimide (NEM) alkylation of red cell glutathione. Biochem. Biophys. Res. Comm., **38,** 341, 1970.
253. Barron, E. S. G., and Singer, T. P.: Enzyme systems containing active sulfhydryl groups: The role of glutathione. Science, **97,** 356, 1943.
254. Glock, G. E., and McLean, P.: Further studies on the properties and assay of glucose-6-phosphate dehydrogenase and 6-phosphogluconate dehydrogenase of rat liver. Biochem. J., **55,** 400, 1953.
255. Langdon, R. G.: Properties and mechanism of action of purified glutathione reductase. Biochim. Biophys. Acta, **30,** 432, 1958.
256. Rapoport, S., and Scheuch, D.: Glutathione stability and pyrophosphatase activity in reticulocytes: Direct evidence for the importance of glutathione for the enzyme status in intact cells. Nature (London), **186,** 967, 1960.
257. Scheuch, D., Kahrig, C., Ockel, E., Wagenknecht, C., and Rapoport, S. M.: Role of glutathione and of a self-stabilizing chain of SH-enzymes and substrates in the metabolic regulation of erythrocytes. Nature (London), **190,** 631, 1961.
258. Rapoport, S. M.: Mechanisms of maintenance and inactivation of SH-enzymes. *Proc. IX Cong. Europ. Soc. Haemat.,* Lisbon, 1963, p. 648.
259. Eldjarn, L., and Bremer, J.: The inhibitory effect at the hexokinase level of disulphides on glucose metabolism in human erythrocytes. Biochem. J., **84,** 286, 1962.
260. Mager, J., Razin, A., Hershko, A., and Izak, G.: The mechanism of red-cell hexokinase inhibition induced by oxidation of intracellular glutathione and its relation to drug sensitivity. Biochem. Biophys. Res. Commun. **17,** 703, 1964.
261. Beutler, E., and Teeple, L.: The effect of oxidized glutathione (GSSG) on human erythrocyte hexokinase activity. Acta Biol. Med. German, **22,** 707, 1969.
262. Luzzatto, L., and Afolayan, A.: Enzymic properties of different types of human erythrocyte glucose-6-phosphate dehydrogenase, with characterization of two new genetic variants. J. Clin. Invest., **47,** 1833, 1968.
263. Luzzatto, L., and Allan, N. C.: Different properties of glucose-6-phosphate dehydrogenase from human erythrocytes with normal and abnormal enzyme levels. Biochem. Biophys. Res. Commun., **21,** 547, 1965.
264. Yoshida, A.: The structure of normal and variant human glucose-6-phosphate dehydrogenase, in *Genetically Determined Abnormalities of Red Cell Metabolism.* City of Hope Symp. Ser., vol. I, p. 126, Grune & Stratton, New York, 1967.
265. Yoshida, A., Stamatoyannopoulos, G. and Motulsky, A.: Negro variant of glucose-6-phosphate dehydrogenase deficiency (A−) in man. Science. **155,** 97, 1967.
266. DeMars, R.: A temperature-sensitive glucose-6-phosphate dehydrogenase in mutant cultured human cells. Proc. Nat. Acad. Sci. U.S.A., **61,** 562, 1968.
267. Dern, R. J.: A new hereditary quantitative variant of G-6-PD characterized by a marked increase in enzyme activity, J. Lab. Clin. Med., **68,** 560, 1966.
268. Dern, R. J., McCurdy, P. R., and Yoshida, A.: A new structural variant of glucose-6-phosphate dehydrogenase with a high production rate (G6PD Hektoen). J. Lab. Clin. Med., **73,** 283, 1969.
269. Yoshida, A., Baur, E., and Motulsky, A. G.: To be published.
270. Luzzatto, L. Personal communication.
271. Kirkman, H. N., and Hendrickson, E. M.: Sex-linked electrophoretic difference in glucose-6-phosphate dehydrogenase. Amer. J. Hum. Genet., **15,** 241, 1963.
272. Long, W. K., Kirkman, H. N., and Sutton, H. E.: Electrophoretically slow variants of glucose-6-phosphate dehydrogenase from red cells of Negroes. J. Lab. Clin. Med., **65,** 81, 1965.
273. Porter, I. H., Boyer, S. H., Watson-Williams, E. J., Adam, A., and Siniscalco, M.: Variation of glucose-6-phosphate dehydrogenase in different populations. Lancet, **1,** 895, 1964.
274. Azevado, E., and Yoshida, A.: Minas Gerais—another variant of glucose-6-phosphate dehydrogenase in man, in press.

275. Hook, E. B., Stamatoyannopoulos, G., Yoshida, A., and Motulsky, A. G.: Glucose-6-phosphate dehydrogenase Madrona: A slow electrophoretic glucose-6-phosphate dehydrogenase variant with kinetic characteristics similar to those of normal type. J. Lab. Clin. Med., **72**, 404, 1968.
276. Marks, P. A., Banks, J., and Gross, R. T.: Genetic heterogeneity of glucose-6-phosphate dehydrogenase deficiency. Nature (London), **194**, 454, 1962.
277. Botha, M. C., Dern, R. J., Mitchell, M., West, C., and Beutler, E.: G6PD Capetown, a variant of glucose-6-phosphate dehydrogenase. Am. J. Human Genet., **21**, 547, 1969.
278. Azevado, E., Kirkman, H. N., Morrow, A. C., and Motulsky, A. G.: Variants of red cell glucose-6-phosphate dehydrogenase among Asiatic Indians. Ann. Hum. Genet., **31**, 373, 1968.
279. Rattazzi, M. C., Lenzerini, L., Khan, P. M., and Luzzatto, L.: Characterization of glucose-6-phosphate dehydrogenase variants. II. G6PD Kephalonia, G6PD Attica, and G6PD "Seattle-like" found in Greece.: Amer. J. Hum. Genet., **21**, 154, 1969.
280. Pinto, P. V. C., Newton, W. A., Jr., and Richardson, D. E.: Evidence for four types of erythrocyte glucose-6-phosphate dehydrogenase from G-6-PD deficient human subjects. J. Clin. Invest., **45**, 823, 1966.
281. Engstrom, P. F., and Beutler, E.: G-6-PD Tripler: A unique variant associated with chronic hemolytic disease. Blood, **36**, 10, 1970.
282. Ramot, B., and Brok, F.: A new glucose-6-phosphate dehydrogenase mutant (Tel-Hashomer mutant). Ann. Hum. Genet., **28**, 167, 1964.
283. Stamatoyannopoulos, G., Yoshida, A., Bacopoulos, C., and Motulsky, A. G.: Athens variant of glucose-6-phosphate dehydrogenase. Science, **157**, 831, 1967.
284. McCurdy, P. R.: Personal communication, 1968.
285. Kaplan, J. C., Rosa, R., Seringe, P., and Hoeffel, J. C.: Le polymorphisme génétique de la glucose-6-phosphate déshydrogénase erythrocytaire chez l'homme. II. Etude d'une nouvelle variété a activite diminuée: le type "kabyle." Enzym. Biol. Clin., (Basel), **8**, 332, 1967.
286. Busch, D., and Boie, K.: Glucose-6-Phosphat-Dehydrogenase-Defekt in Deutschland II. Eigenschaften des Enzyms (Typ, Freiburg). Klin. Wschr. **48**, 74, 1970.
287. Kirkman, H. N., Simon, E. R., and Pickard, B. M.: Seattle variant of glucose-6-phosphate dehydrogenase. J. Lab. Clin. Med., **66**, 834, 1965.
288. Shows, T. B., Jr., Tashian, R. E., Brewer, G. J., and Dern, R. J.: Erythrocyte glucose-6-phosphate dehydrogenase in Caucasians: New inherited variant. Science, **145**, 1056, 1964.
289. Beutler, E., and Rosen, R.: Nonspherocytic congenital hemolytic anemia due to a new G-6-PD variant: G-6-PD Alhambra. Pediatrics, **45**, 230, 1970.
290. Beutler, E.: The Duarte variant, in *Galactosemia,* edited by D. Y. Y. Hsia. Charles C Thomas, Springfield, Ill., in press.
291. Wong, P. W. K., Shih, L-Y., and Hsia, D. Y. Y.: Characterization of glucose-6-phosphate dehydrogenase among Chinese. Nature (London), **208**, 1323, 1965.
292. Kirkman, H. N., Schettini, F., and Pickard, B. M.: Mediterranean variant of glucose-6-phosphate dehydrogenase. J. Lab. Clin. Med., **63**, 726, 1964.
293. Ramot, B., Bauminger, S., Brok, F., Gafni, D., and Schwartz, J.: Characterization of glucose-6-phosphate dehydrogenase in Jewish mutants. J. Lab. Clin. Med., **64**, 895, 1964.
294. Fernandez, M. N., and Fairbanks, V. F.: Glucose-6-phosphate dehydrogenase deficiency in the Philippines: Report of a new variant-G6PD Panay. Mayo Clin. Proc., **43**, 645, 1968.
295. McCurdy, P. R., Kirkman, H. N., Naiman, J. L., Jim, R. T. S., and Pickard, B. M.: A Chinese variant of glucose-6-phosphate dehydrogenase. J. Lab. Clin. Med., **67**, 374, 1966.
296. Kirkman, H. N., and Riley, H. D., Jr.: Congenital nonspherocytic hemolytic anemia. Amer. J. Dis. Child., **102**, 313, 1961.
297. Yoshida, A., Baur, E. W., and Motulsky, A. G.: A Philippino glucose-6-phosphate dehydrogenase variant (G6PD union) with enzyme deficiency and altered substrate specificity. Blood, **35**, 506, 1970.
298. Ramot, B., Ben-Bassat, I., and Shchory, M.: New glucose-6-phosphate dehydrogenase variants observed in Israel. Association with congenital non-spherocytic hemolytic disease. J. Lab. Clin. Med., **74**, 895, 1969.
299. Westring, D. W., and Pisciotta, A. V.: Anemia, cataracts, and seizures in patient with glucose-6-phosphate dehydrogenase deficiency. Arch. Intern. Med. (Chicago), **118**, 385, 1966.
300. Nance, W. E., and Uchida, I.: Turner's syndrome, twinning, and an unusual variant of glucose-6-phosphate dehydrogenase. Amer. J. Hum. Genet., **16**, 380, 1964.
301. Kirkman, H. N., and Crowell, B. B.: Molecular deficiency of glucose-6-phosphate dehydrogenase in primaquine sensitivity. Nature (London), **197**, 286, 1963.
302. Marks, P.: G6PD deficiency in different population groups, in *The Genetics of Migrant and Isolate Populations,* edited by E. Goldschmidt, p. 75. Williams & Wilkins, Baltimore, 1963.
303. Marks, P. A., and Tsutsui, E. A.: Human glucose-6-P dehydrogenase: Studies on the relation between antigenicity and catalytic activity—the role of TPN. Ann. N.Y. Acad. Sci, **103**, 903, 1963.
304. Motulsky, A. G., and Campbell-Kraut, J. M.: Population genetics of glucose-6-phosphate dehydrogenase deficiency of the red cell. *Proc. Conf. Genetic Polymorphisms and Geographic Variations in Diseases.* p. 159. Grune & Stratton, New York, 1961.
305. Rimon, A., Askenazi, I., Ramot, B., and Sheba, C.: Activation of glucose-6-phosphate dehydrogenase of enzyme deficient subjects: I. Activation by stroma of normal erythrocytes. Biochem. Biophys. Res. Commun. **2**, 138, 1960.
306. Ramot, B., Ashkenazi, I., Rimon, A., Adam, A., and Sheba, C.: Activation of glucose-6-phosphate dehydrogenase of enzyme-deficient subjects. II. Properties of the activator and the activation reaction. J. Clin. Invest., **40**, 611, 1961.
307. Flanagan, C. L., Schrier, S. L., Carson, P. E., and Alving, A. S.: The hemolytic effect of primaquine. VIII. The effect of drug administration on parameters of primaquine sensitivity. J. Lab. Clin. Med., **51**, 600, 1958.
308. Szeinberg, A., and Chari-Bitron, A.: Blood glutathione concentration after haemolytic anemia due to *Vicia faba* or sulphonamides. Acta Haemat. (Basel), **18**, 229, 1957.
309. Srivastava, S. K., and Beutler, E.: Accurate measurements of oxidized glutathione content of human, rabbit, and rat red blood cells and tissues. Anal. Biochem., **25**, 70, 1968.
310. Beutler, E.: Unpublished observations.
311. Beutler, E.: In vitro studies of the stability of red cell glutathione: A new test for drug sensitivity. J. Clin. Invest., **35**, 690, 1956 (abstract).
312. Kosower, N. S., Vanderhoff, G. A., and London, I. M.: The regeneration of reduced glutathione in normal and glucose-6-phosphate dehydrogenase deficient human red blood cells. Blood, **29**, 313, 1967.
313. Jandl, J. H., Engle, L. K., and Allen, D. W.: Oxidative hemolysis and precipitation of hemoglobin. I. Heinz body anemias as an acceleration of red cell aging. J. Clin. Invest., **39**, 1818, 1960.
314. Kosower, N. D.: Discussion of Glutathione Deficiency by H. K. Prins, J. A. Loos, and C. Zürcher, in *Hereditary Disorders of Erythrocyte Metabolism,* edited by E. Beutler. City of Hope Symp. Ser., vol. 1, p. 176, Grune & Stratton, New York, 1968.
315. Balinsky, D., and Bernstein, R. E.: Oxidation of reduced glutathione by acetylphenylhydrazine, haemoglobin and erythrocytes. Nature (London), **199**, 187, 1963.
316. Davidson, W. D., and Tanaka, K. R.: Continuous measurement of pentose phosphate pathway activity in erythrocytes: An ionization chamber method. J. Lab. Clin. Med., **73**, 173, 1969.
317. Löhr, G. S., and Waller, H. D.: Biochemie und Pathogenese der enzymopenischen hämolytischen Anämien. Deutsch. Med. Wschr., **86**, 27, 1961.
318. Koutras, G. A., Hattori, M., Schneider. A. S., Ebaugh, F. G., Jr., and Valentine, W. N.: Studies on chromated erythrocytes: Effect of sodium chromate on erythrocyte glutathione reductase. J. Clin. Invest., **43**, 323, 1964.
319. Koutras, G. A., Schneider, A. S., Hattori, M., and Valentine, W. N.: Studies on chromated erythrocytes: Mechanisms of chromate inhibition of glutathione reductase. Brit. J. Haemat., **11**, 360, 1965.
320. Waller, H. D., Löhr, G. W., and Tabatabai, M.: Hämolyse und Fehlen von Glucose-6-phosphatdehydrogenase in roten Blutzellen (eine Fermenanomalie der Erythrocyten). Klin. Wschr., **35**, 1022, 1957.

321. Löhr, G. W., and Waller, H. D.: Hämolytische Erythrocytopathie durch Fehlen von Glucose-6-phosphatdehydrogenase in roten Blutzellen als Dominant verebliche Krankheit. Klin. Wschr., **36**, 865, 1958.
322. Schrier, S., Kellermeyer, R., and Alving, A. S.: Coenzyme studies in primaquine-sensitive erythrocytes. Proc. Soc. Exp. Biol. Med., **99**, 354, 1958.
323. Bonsignore, A., Fornaini, G., Segni, G., and Seitun, A.: Transketolase and transaldolase reactions in the erythrocytes of human subjects with favism history. Biochem. Biophys. Res. Commun., **4**, 147, 1961.
324. Bonsignore, A., Fornaini, G., Fantoni, A., Segni, P., Spanu, G., and Fancello, F.: Attivitá enzimatiche dell'eritrocita favico nel perido emolitico. Boll. Soc. Ital. Biol. Sper., **38**, 1127, 1962.
325. Schrier, S. L., Kellermeyer, R. W., Carson, P. E., Ickes, C. E., and Alving, A. S.: The hemolytic effect of primaquine. X. Aldolase and glyceraldehyde-3-phosphate dehydrogenase activity in primaquine-sensitive erythrocytes. J. Lab. Clin. Med., **54**, 232, 1959.
326. Brewer, G. J., Powell, R. D., Swanson, S. H., and Alving, A. S.: Hemolytic effect of primaquine. XVII. Hexokinase activity of glucose-6-phosphate dehydrogenase-deficient and normal erythrocytes. J. Lab. Clin. Med., **64**, 601, 1964.
327. Heller, P., and Weinstein, H. G.: Aldolase, isocitric dehydrogenase and malic dehydrogenase in glucose-6-phosphate dehydrogenase deficient erythrocytes. J. Lab. Clin. Med., **54**, 824, 1959.
328. Löhr, G., and Waller, H.: Erythrozytenfermente. (Blutbildung und Blutumsatz bie Feten und Neugeborenen). Z. Geburtsh. Gynaek., **159**, suppl., 120, 1962.
329. Brewer, G. J., Powell, R. D., Tarlov, A. R., and Alving, A. S.: Hemolytic effect of primaquine. XVI. Glyoxalase activity of primaquine-sensitive and normal erythrocytes. J. Lab. Clin. Med., **63**, 106, 1964.
330. Bonsignore, A., Fornaini, G., Segni, G., and Fantoni, F.: Glutathione-reductase and methaemoglobin-reductase in erythrocytes of human subjects with a case history of favism. Ital. J. Biochem., **9**, 345, 1960.
331. Oski, F. A., Shahidi, N. T., and Diamond, L. K.: Erythrocyte acid phosphomonoesterase and glucose-6-phosphate dehydrogenase deficiency in Caucasians. Science, **139**, 409, 1963.
332. Schettini, F., Meloni, T., Mela, C., and Fanciulli, G.: Red cell acid phosphatase in normal and glucose-6-phosphatase deficiency Sardinian subjects. Acta Haemat. (Basel), **33**, 230, 1965.
333. Lu, T. C., and Wei, H.: Erythrocyte acid phosphomonoesterase activity in newly born Chinese deficient in glucose-6-phosphate dehydrogenase. Nature (London), **213**, 707, 1967.
334. Brunetti, P., Grignani, F., and Ernisli, G.: Behaviour of the erythrocyte pyrophosphatase activity in the enzyme-deficiency haemolytic anaemias. II. A new test for the detection of the enzyme defect. Acta Haemat. (Basel), **27**, 246, 1962.
335. Brunetti, P., Grignani, F., and Ernisli, G.: Behaviour of the erythrocyte pyrophosphatase activity in the enzyme-deficiency haemolytic anaemias. I. Quantitative modifications of the enzyme. Acta Haemat. (Basel), **27**, 146, 1962.
336. Tarlov, A., and Kellermeyer, R. W.: The hemolytic effect of primaquine. XI. Decreased catalase activity in primaquine-sensitive erythrocytes. J. Lab. Clin. Med., **58**, 204, 1961.
337. Ezra, R., Szeinberg, A., and Sheba, Ch.: Catalase activity in normal and glucose-6-phosphate dehydrogenase deficient red cells. Israel J. Med. Sci., **I**, 847, 1965.
338. Haut, A., and Taylor, E. H.: Catalase function in glucose-6-phosphate dehydrogenase deficiency. J. Clin. Invest., **46**, 1068, 1967 (abstract).
339. Liebowitz, J., and Cohen, G.: Increased hydrogen peroxide levels in glucose-6-phosphate dehydrogenase deficient erythrocytes exposed to acetylphenylhydrazine. Biochem. Pharmacol., **17**, 983, 1968.
340. Pinkhas, J., Djaldetti, M., Joshua, H., Resnick, C., and DeVries, A.: Sulfhemoglobinemia and acute hemolytic anemia with Heinz bodies following contact with a fungicide—zinc ethylene bisidithiocarbamate—in a subject with glucose-6-phosphate dehydrogenase deficiency and hypocatalasemia. Blood, **21**, 484, 1963.
341. Beutler, E., and Collins, Z.: Unpublished observations.
342. Szeinberg, A., and Clejan, L.: Sulfhydryl groups in the red cells of normal and glucose-6-phosphate dehydrogenase-deficient subjects. Biochim. Biophysica Acta, **93**, 564, 1964.
343. Zaidman, J.: On the heterogeneity of hemoglobin from normal and glucose-6-phosphate dehydrogenase-deficient individuals. Clin. Chim. Acta, **23**, 67, 1969.
344. Tarlov, A. R., Brewer, G. J., Carson, P. E., and Alving, A. S.: Primaquine sensitivity: Glucose-6-phosphate dehydrogenase deficiency; an inborn error of metabolism of medical and biological significance. Arch. Intern. Med. (Chicago), **109**, 209, 1962.
345. Danon, D., Sheba, C., and Ramot, B.: The morphology of glucose-6-phosphate dehydrogenase deficient erythrocytes: Electronmicroscopic studies. Blood, **17**, 229, 1961.
346. Jones, R., Jr., Jackson, L. S., DiLorenzo, A., Marx, R. L., Levy, B. L., Kenny, E. C., Gilbert, M., Johnson, M. N., and Alving, A. S.: Korean vivax malaria. III. Curative effect and toxicity of primaquine in doses from 10–30 mg daily. Amer. J. Trop. Med., **2**, 977, 1953.
347. Weed, R., Eber, J., and Rothstein, A.: Effects of primaquine and other related compounds on the red blood cell membrane. I. Na^+ and K^+ permeability in normal human cells. J. Clin. Invest., **40**, 130, 1961.
348. Weed, R.: Effects of primaquine on the red blood cell membrane. II. K^+ permeability in glucose-6-phosphate dehydrogenase deficient erythrocytes. J. Clin. Invest., **40**, 140, 1961.
349. Brewer, G. J., Tarlov, A. R., and Kellermeyer, R. W.: The hemolytic effect of primaquine. XII. Shortened erythrocyte life span in primaquine-sensitive male Negroes in the absence of drug administration. J. Lab. Clin. Med., **58**, 217, 1961.
350. Bernini, L., Latte, B., Siniscalco, M., Piomelli, S., Spada, U., Adinolfi, M., and Mollison, P. L.: Survival of ^{51}Cr-labelled red cells in subjects with thalassaemia-trait or g6pd deficiency or both abnormalities. Brit. J. Haemat., **10**, 171, 1964.
351. Rubinstein, D., Ottolenghi, P., and Denstedt, O. F.: The metabolism of the erythrocyte. XIII. Enzyme activity in the reticulocyte. Canad. J. Biochem. Physiol., **34**, 222, 1956.
352. Marks, P. A., Johnson, A. B., and Hirschberg, E.: Effect of age on the enzyme activity in erythrocytes. Proc. Nat. Acad. Sci. U.S.A., **44**, 529, 1958.
353. Löhr, G. W., Waller, H. D., Karges, O., Schlegel, B., and Müller, A. A.: Zur Biochemie der Alterung menschlicher Erythrocyten. Klin. Wschr., **36**, 1008, 1958.
354. Marks, P. A., and Gross, R. T.: Drug-induced hemolytic anemias and congenital galactosemia. Bull. N.Y. Acad. Med., **35**, 433, 1959.
355. Sansone, G., Borrone, C., and Robei, S.: Suscettibilita degli eritrociti a formare corpi di Heinz in vitro in condizioni normali (neonati e lattanti) e pathologiche (favismo e talessemia). Boll. Soc. Ital. Biol. Sper., **34**, 1561, 1958.
356. Bonsignore, A., Fornaini, G., Fantoni, A., Leoncini, G., and Segni, P.: Relationship between age and enzymatic activities in human erythrocytes from normal and fava-bean-sensitive subjects. J. Clin. Invest., **43**, 834, 1964.
357. Salvidio, E., Pannacciulli, I., Tizianello, A., and Ajmar, F.: Nature of hemolytic crises and the fate of G6PD deficient, drug-damaged erythrocytes in Sardinians. New Eng. J. Med., **276**, 1339, 1967.
358. Brewer, G. J., Tarlov, A. R., Kellermeyer, R. W., and Alving, A. S.: The hemolytic effect of primaquine. XV. Role of methemoglobin. J. Lab. Clin. Med., **59**, 905, 1962.
359. Jalavisto, E.: Bleeding anemia and methemoglobin reduction in dog erythrocytes. Acta Physiol. Scand., **46**, 252, 1959.
360. Jung, F.: The relation of age, hemolytic resistance and methemoglobin content of erythrocytes. Deutsch. Arch. Klin. Med., **195**, 454, 1949.
361. Waller, H. D., Schlegel, B., Müller, A. A., and Löhr, G. W.: Der Hemoglobingehalt in alternden Erythrocyten. Klin. Wschr., **37**, 898, 1959.
362. Warburg, C., Kubowitz, F., and Christian, W.: Ueber die Wirkung von Phenylhydrazine und Phenylhydroxlamin auf den Stoffwechsel der roten Blutzellen (Methode zur Messung des Stoffwechsels roter Blutzellen). Biochem. Z., **242**, 170, 1931.
363. Webster, S. H.: Heinz body phenomenon in erythrocytes: A review. Blood, **4**, 479, 1949.
364. Fertman, M. H., and Fertman, M. D.: Toxic anemias and Heinz bodies. Medicine (Balt.), **34**, 131, 1955.
365. Cohen, G., and Hochstein, P.: Generation of hydrogen peroxide in erythrocytes by hemolytic agents. Biochemistry (Wash.), **3**, 895, 1964.

366. Finch, C. A.: Methemoglobinemia and sulfhemoglobinemia. New Eng. J. Med., **239,** 470, 1948.
367. Harley, J. D., and Mauer. A. M.: Studies on the formation of Heinz bodies. I. Methemoglobin production and oxyhemoglobin destruction. Blood, **16,** 1722, 1960.
368. Jandl, J. H.: The Heinz body hemolytic anemias. Ann. Intern. Med., **58,** 702, 1963.
369. Bunn, H. F., and Jandl, J. H.: Exchange of heme among hemoglobins and between hemoglobin and albumin. J. Biol. Chem., **243,** 465, 1968.
370. Rossi-Fanelli, A., Antonini, E., and Caputo, A.: Studies on the structure of human hemoglobin. I. Physicochemical properties of human globin. Biochim. Biophys. Acta, **30,** 608, 1958.
371. Beutler, E., and Baluda, M. C.: The role of methemoglobin in oxidative degradation of hemoglobin. Acta Haemat. (Basel), **27,** 321, 1962.
372. Magos, L.: Effect of the methemoglobinemia on Heinz body formation. Experientia, **15,** 197, 1960.
373. Beutler, E.: Drug-induced haemolytic anaemias and the mechanism and significance of Heinz body formation in red blood cells. Nature (London), **196,** 1095, 1962.
374. Beutler, E., Baluda, M. C., and Kelly, B. M.: The role of methemoglobin in the mechanism of drug-induced hemolytic anemia. *Proc. IX Cong. Internat. Soc. Hemat.,* Mexico City, 1962, p. 233. Grune & Stratton, New York, 1964.
375. Rentsch, G.: Genesis of Heinz bodies and methemoglobin formation. Biochem. Pharmacol., **17,** 423, 1967.
376. Martin, H., Wörner, W., and Rittmeister, B.: Hämolytische Anämie Durch Inhalation von Hydroxylaminen. Klin. Wschr., **42,** 725, 1964.
377. Rifkind, R. A.: Destruction of injured red cells *in vivo.* Amer. J. Med., **41,** 711, 1966.
378. Mohler, D. N., and Williams, W. J.: The effect of phenylhydrazine on the adenosine triphosphate content of normal and glucose-6-phosphate dehydrogenase-deficient human blood. J. Clin. Invest., **40,** 1735, 1961.
379. Desforges, J. F., Kalaw, E., and Gilchrist, P.: Inhibition of glucose-6-phosphate dehydrogenase by hemolysis inducing drugs. J. Lab. Clin. Med., **55,** 757, 1960.
380. Mager, J., Glaser, G., Razin, A., Izak, G., Bien, S., and Noam, M.: Metabolic effects of pyrimidines derived from fava bean glycosides on human erythrocytes deficient in glucose-6-phosphate dehydrogenase.: Biochem. Biophys. Res. Commun. **20,** 235, 1965.
381. Panizon, F., and Zacchelo, F.: The mechanism of haemolysis in favism. Acta Haemat. (Basel), **33,** 129, 1965.
382. Necheles, T. F., and Gorshein, D.: Virus-induced hemolysis in erythrocytes deficient in glucose-6-phosphate dehydrogenase. Science, **160,** 535, 1968.
383. Ross, J. D.: Deficient activity of DPNH-dependent methemoglobin diaphorase in cord blood erythrocytes. Blood, **21,** 51, 1963.
384. Necheles, T. F., Boles, T. A., and Allen, D. M.: Erythrocyte glutathione-peroxidase deficiency and hemolytic disease of the newborn infant. J. Pediat., **72,** 319, 1968.
385. Jones, P. E. H., and McCance, R. A.: Enzyme activities in the blood of infants and adults. Biochem. J., **45,** 464, 1949.
386. Childs, B., Zinkham, W., Browne, E. A., Kimbro, E. L., and Torbert, J. V.: A genetic study of a defect in glutathione metabolism of the erythrocyte. Bull. Johns Hopkins Hosp., **102,** 21, 1958.
387. Browne, E. A.: The inheritance of an intrinsic abnormality of the red blood cell predisposing to drug-induced hemolytic anemia. Bull. Johns Hopkins Hosp., **101,** 115, 1957.
388. Sansone, G., and Segni, G.: Sensitivity to broad beans. Lancet, **2,** 295, 1957.
389. Siniscalco, M., Motulsky, A. G., Latte, B., Bernini, L., and Montalenti, G.: Indagnini genetiche sulla predisposizione al favismo. II. Dati familiari: associazoine genica con il daltonismo. Accad. naz. dei lincei, ser. VIII, 28, 1960.
390. Adam, A.: Linkage between deficiency of glucose-6-phosphate dehydrogenase and colour-blindness. Nature (London), **189,** 686, 1961.
391. Siniscalco, M., and Filippi, G.: Recombination between protan and deutan genes: Data on their relative positions in respect of the G6PD locus. Nature (London), **204,** 1064, 1964.
392. Porter, I. H., Schulze, J., and McKusick, V. A.: Genetical-linkage between the loci for glucose-6-phosphate dehydrogenase deficiency and colour-blindness in American Negroes. Ann. Hum. Genet., **26,** 107, 1962.
393. Kalmus, H.: Distance and sequence of the loci for protan and deutan defects and for glucose-6-phosphate dehydrogenase deficiency. Nature (London), **194,** 214, 1962.
394. Adam, A., Sheba, Ch., Sanger, R., and Race, R. R.: The linkage relation of G6PD to Xg (letter to the editor). Amer. J. Hum. Genet., **18,** 110, 1966.
395. Bowman, J. E., Carson, P. E., and Frischer, H.: The segregation in one family of three alleles at the glucose-6-phosphate dehydrogenase locus. Hum. Heredity, **19,** 25, 1969.
396. Siniscalco, M., Filippi, G., Latte, B., Piomelli, S., Rattazzi, M., Gavin. J., Sanger, R., and Race, R. R.: Failure to detect linkage between Xg and other X-borne loci in Sardinians. Ann. Hum. Genet., **29,** 231, 1966.
397. Motulsky, A. G.: Theoretical and clinical problems of glucose-6-phosphate dehydrogenase deficiency: Its occurrence in Africans and its combination with hemoglobinopathy. *Proc. 2nd Symp. on Abnormal Haemoglobins,* sponsored by C.I.O.M.S., Ibadan, Nigeria, 1963.
398. Motulsky, A. G.: Contributions of hereditary disorders of red cell metabolism to human genetics, in *Genetically Determined Abnormalities of Red Cell Metabolism,* edited by E. Beutler. City of Hope Symp. Ser., vol. 1, p. 303, Grune & Stratton, New York, 1968.
399. Trujillo, J., Fairbanks, V., Ohno, S., and Beutler, E.: Chromosomal constitution in glucose-6-phosphate-dehydrogenase deficiency. Lancet, **2,** 1454, 1961.
400. Grumbach, M. M., Marks, P. A., and Morishima, A.: Erythrocyte glucose-6-phosphate dehydrogenase activity and X-chromosome polysomy. Lancet, **1,** 1330, 1962.
401. Davidson, R. G., Migeon, B. R., Borden, M., and Childs, B.: Dosage compensation in the regulation of erythrocyte glucose-6-phosphate dehydrogenase activity. Bull. Johns Hopkins Hosp., **112,** 318, 1963.
402. Lyon, M. F.: Gene action in the x-chromosome of the mouse (*Mus musculus L.*). Nature (London), **190,** 372, 1961.
403. Beutler, E.: Biochemical abnormalities associated with hemolytic states, in *Mechanisms of Anemia,* edited by I. M. Weinstein and E. Beutler, p. 195. McGraw-Hill, New York, 1962.
404. Lyon, M. F.: Sex chromatin and gene action in the mammalian X-chromatin. Amer. J. Hum. Genet., **14,** 135, 1962.
405. Beutler, E., and Fairbanks, V. F.: The normal human female as a mosaic of X-chromosome activity: Studies using glucose-6-phosphate dehydrogenase as a genetic marker. *Proc. IX Cong. Internat. Soc. Hemat.,* Mexico City, 1962, p. 43. Grune & Stratton, New York, 1964.
406. Beutler, E., and Baluda, M. C.: The separation of glucose-6-phosphate deficient erythrocytes from the blood of heterozygotes for g-6-pd deficiency. Lancet, **1,** 189, 1964.
407. Kaplan, J. C., Dreyfus, J. C., and Bessis, M.: La structure en mosaique du chromosome X chez la femme. Nouv. Rev. Franc. Hemat., **5,** 835, 1965.
408. Sartori, E., Panizon, F., and Zacchello, F.: Bimodal distribution of erythrocytes in heterozygotes for strong Mediterranean glucose-6-phosphate dehydrogenase deficiency. J. Med. Genet., **3,** 42, 1966.
409. Sansone, G., Rasore-Quartino, A., and Veneziano, G.: Two red-cell populations in the human female heterozygous for g-6-pd deficiency. Lancet. **1,** 329, 1964.
410. Tönz, O., and Rossi, E.: Morphological demonstration of two red cell populations in human females heterozygous for glucose-6-phosphate dehydrogenase deficiency. Nature (London), **202,** 606, 1964.
411. Gall, J. C., Jr., Brewer, G. J., and Dern, R. J.: Studies of glucose-6-phosphate dehydrogenase activity of individual erythrocytes: The methemoglobin-elution test for identification of females heterozygous for G6PD deficiency. Amer. J. Hum. Genet., **17,** 359, 1965.
412. Tönz, O.: The problem of defining the heterozygous carrier in glucose-6-phosphate dehydrogenase deficiency. Ann. Paediat., **204,** 24, 1965.
413. Kattamis, C. A.: Glucose-6-phosphate dehydrogenase deficiency in female heterozygotes and the X-inactivation hypothesis. Acta Paediat. Scand., suppl. **172,** 103, 1967.
414. Stamatoyannopoulos, G., Papayannopoulou, Th., Bakopoulos, Chr., and

Motulsky, A. G.: Detection of glucose-6-phosphate dehydrogenase deficient heterozygotes. Blood, **29**, 87, 1967.

415. Beutler, E., and Collins, Z.: Pseudo-mosaicism in males with mild glucose-6-phosphate-dehydrogenase deficiency. Lancet, **1**, 552, 1965.

416. Papayannopoulou, T., and Stamatoyannopoulos, G.: Pseudomosaicism in males with mild glucose-6-phosphate dehydrogenase deficiency. Lancet, **2**, 1215, 1964.

417. Betke, K., Kleihauer, E., and Knotek, Z.: Zytologische untersuchungen zur frage des zellmosaiks bei heterozygoten frauen mit glukose-6-phosphatdehydrogenase Mangel. Acta Paediat. Scand., suppl. **172**, 30, 1967.

418. Davidson, R. G., Nitowsky, H. M., and Childs, B.: Demonstration of two populations of cells in the human female heterozygous for glucose-6-phosphate dehydrogenase variants. Proc. Nat. Acad. Sci. U.S.A., **50**, 481, 1963.

419. Linder, D., and Gartler, S. M.: Glucose-6-phosphate dehydrogenase mosaicism: Utilization as a cell marker in the study of leiomyomas. Science, **150**, 67, 1965.

420. Gartler, S. M., Ziprkowski, L., Krakowski, A., Ezra, R., Szeinberg, A., and Adam, A.: G-6-PD mosaicism as a tracer in the study of hereditary multiple trichoepithelioma. Amer. J. Hum. Genet., **18**, 282, 1966.

421. Beutler, E., Collins, Z., and Irwin, L.: Value of genetic variants of glucose-6-phosphate dehydrogenase in tracing the origin of malignant tumors. New Eng. J. Med., **276**, 389, 1967.

422. Fialkow, P. J., Gartler, S. M., and Yoshida, A.: Clonal origin of chronic myelocytic leukemia in man. Proc. Nat. Acad. Sci. U.S.A., **58**, 1468, 1967.

423. Rattazzi, M. C., Bernini, L. F., Fiorelli, G., and Mannucci, P. M.: Electrophoresis of glucose-6-phosphate dehydrogenase: A new technique. Nature (London), **213**, 79, 1967.

424. Haywood, B., Starkweather, W., Spencer, H., and Zarafonetis, C.: Electrophoretic separation of glucose-6-phosphate dehydrogenase from human erythrocytes with agar gels. J. Lab. Clin. Med., **71**, 324, 1968.

425. Peterson, W. D., Jr., Stulberg, C. S., Swanborg, N. K., and Robinson, A. R.: Glucose-6-phosphate dehydrogenase isoenzymes in human cell cultures determined by sucrose-agar gel and cellulose acetate zymograms. Proc. Soc. Exp. Biol. Med., **128**, 772, 1968.

426. Sparkes, R. S., Baluda, M. C., and Townsend, D. E.: Cellulose acetate electrophoresis of human glucose-6-phosphate dehydrogenase. J. Lab. Clin. Med., **73**, 531, 1969.

427. Louderback, A., Beutler, E., Natland, M., and Temianka, D.: Agar gel electrophoresis of G-6-PD isoenzymes. Clin. Res., **17**, 149, 1969 (abstract).

428. Mathai, C. K., Ohno, S., and Beutler, E.: Sex-linkage of the glucose-6-phosphate dehydrogenase gene in the family *Equidae.* Nature (London), **210**, 115, 1966.

429. Luzzatto, L., and Okoye, V. C. N.: Resolution of genetic variants of human erythrocyte glucose-6-phosphate dehydrogenase by thin layer chromatography. Biochem. Biophys. Res. Commun., **29**, 705, 1967.

430. Beutler, E., Dern, R. J., and Alving, A. S.: The hemolytic effect of primaquine. VI. An in vitro test for sensitivity of erythrocytes to primaquine. J. Lab. Clin. Med., **45**, 40, 1955.

431. Beutler, E., Duron, O., and Kelly, B. M.: Improved method for the determination of blood glutathione. J. Lab. Clin. Med., **61**, 882, 1963.

432. Kraus, A. P., Neely, C. L., Carey, F. T., and Kraus, L. M.: Detection of deficient erythrocyte regeneration of reduced triphosphopyridine nucleotide from glucose-6-phosphate: Evaluation of a rapid screening test. Ann. Intern. Med., **55**, 765, 1962.

433. Salvidio, E., Pannacciulli, I., and Tizianello, A.: Evaluation experimentale de quelques méthodes biochimiques permettant de déceler la susceptibilité à l'hémolyse due aux médicaments. Nouv. Rev. Franc. Hemat., **3**, 233, 1963.

434. Zinkham, W. H.: An *in vitro* abnormality of glutathione metabolism in erythrocytes from normal newborns: Mechanism and clinical significance. Pediatrics, **23**, 18, 1959.

435. Swarup, S., Ghosh, S. K., and Chatterjea, J. B.: Glutathione stability test in haemoglobin E-thalassemia disease. Nature (London), **188**, 153, 1960.

436. Löhr, G. W., and Waller, H. D.: Eine neue enzymopenische hämolytische Anämie mit Glutathionreduktase-mangel. Med. Klin., **57**, 1521, 1962.

437. Theil, G. E., Brodine, C. E., and Doolan, P. D.: Red cell glutathione content and stability in renal sufficiency. J. Lab. Clin. Med. **58**, 736, 1961.

438. Szeinberg, A., Ramot, B., Adam, A., and Sheba, C.: Glutathione metabolism in cord blood and in the newborn infant. A.M.A.J. Dis. Child. **96**, 542, 1958.

439. Gross, R. T., and Hurwitz, R. E.: The pentose phosphate pathway in human erythrocytes, relationship between age of the subject and enzyme activity. Pediatrics, **22**, 453, 1958.

440. Szeinberg, A., Ramot, B., Sheba, C., Adam, A., Halbrecht, I., Rikover, M., Wishnievsky, S., and Rabau, E.: Glutathione metabolism in cord and newborn infant blood. J. Clin. Invest., **37**, 1436, 1958.

441. Bernstein, R. E.: Brilliant cresyl blue screening test for demonstrating glucose-6-phosphate dehydrogenase deficiency in red cells. Clin. Chim. Acta, **8**, 158, 1963.

442. Lee, T. C., Shih, L. Y., Huang, P. C., Lin, C. C., Blackwell, B. N., Blackwell, R. Q., and Hsia, D. Y.: Glucose-6-phosphate dehydrogenase deficiency in Taiwan. Amer. J. Hum. Genet., **15**, 126, 1963.

443. Tönz, O., and Betke, K.: Einfacher Farbtest zur Bestimmung der Glucose-6-phosphatdehydrogenase in menschlichen Erythrocyten. Klin. Wschr., **40**, 1962.

444. Ells, H. A., and Kirkman, H. N.: A colorimetric method for assay of erythrocytic glucose-6-phosphate dehydrogenase. Proc. Soc. Exp. Biol. Med., **106**, 607, 1961.

445. Bernstein, R. E.: A rapid screening dye test for the detection of glucose-6-phosphate dehydrogenase deficiency in red cells. Nature (London), **194**, 192, 1962.

446. Fairbanks, V. F., and Beutler, E.: A simple method for detection of erythrocyte glucose-6-phosphate dehydrogenase (G-6-PD spot test). Blood, **20**, 591, 1962.

447. Brewer, G. J., Tarlov, A. R., and Alving, A. S.: The methemoglobin reduction test for primaquine-type sensitivity of erythrocytes. J.A.M.A., **180**, 386, 1962.

448. Sass, M. D., Caruso, C. J., and Farhangi, M.: TPNH-methemoglobin reductase deficiency: A new red-cell enzyme defect. J. Lab. Clin. Med., **70**, 760, 1967.

449. Oski, F. A., and Growney, P. M.: A simple micromethod for the detection of erythrocyte glucose-6-phosphate dehydrogenase deficiency. J. Pediat., **66**, 90, 1965.

450. Sass, M. D., Caruso, C. J., and Axelrod, D. R.: Rapid screening for D-glucose-6-phosphate: NADP oxidoreductase deficiency with methylene blue. J. Lab. Clin. Med., **68**, 156, 1966.

451. Rakitzis, E. T.: Test for glucose-6-phosphate dehydrogenase deficiency. Lancet, **2**, 1182, 1964.

452. Jacob, H. S., and Jandl, J. H.: A simple visual screening test for G-6-PD deficiency employing ascorbate and cyanide. New Eng. J. Med., **274**, 1162, 1966.

453. Prins, H. K., Loos, J. A., and Zurcher, C.: Glutathione deficiency, in *Hereditary Disorders of Erythrocyte Metabolism,* edited by E. Beutler. City of Hope Symp. Ser., vol. 1, p. 165, Grune & Stratton, New York, 1968.

454. Fairbanks, V. F., and Fernandez, M. N.: The identification of metabolic errors associated with hemolytic anemia. J.A.M.A., **208**, 316, 1969.

455. Beutler, E.: A series of new screening procedures for pyruvate kinase deficiency, glucose-6-phosphate dehydrogenase deficiency, and glutathione reductase deficiency. Blood, **28**, 553, 1966.

456. Beutler, E. and Mitchell, M.: Special modifications of the fluorescent screening method for glucose-6-phosphate dehydrogenase deficiency. Blood, **32**, 816, 1968.

457. Beutler, E.: G-6-PD activity of individual erythrocytes and X-chromosomal inactivation, in *Biochemical Methods in Red Cell Genetics,* edited by J. J. Yunis, p. 95. Academic, New York, 1969.

458. Fairbanks, V. F., and Lampe, L. T.: A tetrazolium-linked cytochemical method for estimation of glucose-6-phosphate dehydrogenase activity in individual erythrocytes: Applications in the study of heterozygotes for glucose-6-phosphate dehydrogenase deficiency. Blood, **31**, 589, 1968.

459. Marks, P. A., Gross, R. T., and Hurwitz, R. E.: Gene action in erythrocyte

deficiency of glucose-6-phosphate dehydrogenase: Tissue enzyme levels. Nature (London), **183,** 1266, 1959.

460. Ramot, B., Fisher, S., Szeinberg, A., Adam, A., Sheba, C., and Gafni, D.: A study of subjects with erythrocyte glucose-6-phosphate dehydrogenase deficiency. II. Investigation of leukocyte enzymes. J. Clin. Invest., **38,** 2234, 1959.
461. Chan, T. K., Todd, D., and Wong, C. C.: Tissue enzyme levels in erythrocyte glucose-6-phosphate dehydrogenase deficiency. J. Lab. Clin. Med., **56,** 937, 1965.
462. Sabine, J. C., Jung, E. D., Fish, M. B., Pestaner, L. C., and Rankin, R. E.: Observations on the inheritance of glucose-6-phosphate dehydrogenase deficiency in erythrocytes and in leucocytes. Brit. J. Haemat., **9,** 164, 1963.
463. Bonsignore, A., Fornaini, G., Leoncini, G., Fantoni, A., and Segni, P.: Characterization of leukocyte glucose-6-phosphate dehydrogenase in Sardinian mutants. J. Clin. Invest., **45,** 1865, 1966.
464. Justice, P., Shih, L. Y., Gordon, J., Grossman, A., and Hsia, D.: Characterization of leukocyte glucose-6-phosphate dehydrogenase in normal and mutant human subjects. J. Lab. Clin. Med., **68,** 552, 1966.
465. Yoshida, A., Stamatoyannopoulos, G., and Motulsky, A. G.: Biochemical genetics of glucose-6-phosphate dehydrogenase variation. Ann. N.Y. Acad. Sci., **155,** 868, 1968.
466. Shaw, C. R., and Barto, E.: Autosomally determined polymorphism of glucose-6-phosphate dehydrogenase in peromyscus. Science, **148,** 1099, 1965.
467. Ohno, S., Morrison, M., and Beutler, E.: Hexose-6-phosphate dehydrogenase found in human liver. Science, **153,** 1015, 1966.
468. Beutler, E., and Morrison, M.: Localization and characteristics of hexose-6-phosphate dehydrogenase (glucose dehydrogenase). J. Biol. Chem., **242,** 5289, 1967.
469. Mandula, B., Srivastava, S. K., and Beutler, E.: Hexose-6-phosphate dehydrogenase: Distribution in rat tissues and effect of diet, age and steroids. Arch. Biochem. Biophys., **141,** 155, 1970.
470. Zinkham, W. H.: Enzyme studies on lenses from persons with primaquine-sensitive erythrocytes. A.M.A.J. Dis. Child., **100,** 525, 1960.
471. Zinkham, W. H.: A deficiency of glucose-6-phosphate dehydrogenase activity in lens from individuals with primaquinesensitive erythrocytes. Bull. Johns Hopkins Hosp., **109,** 306, 1961.
472. Ramot, B., Szeinberg, A., Adam, A., Sheba, C., and Gafni, D.: A study of subjects with erythrocyte glucose-6-phosphate dehydrogenase deficiency. I. Investigation of platelet enzymes. J. Clin. Invest., **38,** 1659, 1959.
473. Gartler, S. M., Gandini, E., and Ceppellini, R.: Glucose-6-phosphate dehydrogenase deficient mutant in human cell culture. Nature (London), **193,** 602, 1962.
474. Ramot, B., Sheba, C., Adam, A., and Ashkenasi, I.: Erythrocyte glucose-6-phosphate dehydrogenase deficient subjects: Enzyme-level in saliva. Nature (London), **185,** 931, 1960.
475. Sklavunu-Zurukzoglu, S., Mameletzis, C., and Katriu, D. Observations on the glucose-6-phosphate dehydrogenase of the breast milk. Helv. Paediat. Acta, **20,** 193, 1965.
476. Panizon, F.: Erythrocyte enzyme deficiency in unexplained kernicterus. Lancet, **2,** 1093, 1960.
477. Brunetti, P., Rossetti, R., and Broccia, G.: New findings on the bio-enzymology of icteric-hemoglobinuric favism. III. The activity of glucose-6-phosphate-dehydrogenase in the liver parenchyma. Rass. Fisiopat. Clin., **32,** 338, 1960.
478. Carson, P. E., and Okita, G. T.: Metabolic patterns of hemolytic susceptibility. J. Clin. Invest., **42,** 922, 1963 (abstract).
479. Chanmugam, D., and Frumin, A. M.: Abnormal oral glucose tolerance response in erythrocyte glucose-6-phosphate dehydrogenase deficiency. New Eng. J. Med., **271,** 1202, 1964.
480. Eppes, R., Brewer, G., DeGowin, R., McNamara, J., Flanagan, C., Schrier, S., Tarlov, A., Powell, R., and Carson, P.: Oral glucose tolerance in Negro men deficient in G-6-PD. New Eng. J. Med., **275,** 855, 1966.
481. Borkowski, A. J., Marks, P. A., Katz, F. H., Lipman, M. M., and Christy, N. P.: An abnormal pathway of steroid metabolism in patients with glucose-6-phosphate dehydrogenase deficiency. J. Clin. Invest., **41,** 1346, 1962 (abstract).
482. Tarlov, A. R., Brewer, G. J., and Swanson, S. H.: The effect of primaquine administration on the serum cholesterol of drug-sensitive American Negroes. Clin. Res., **9,** 190, 1961.
483. Dern, R. J., Glynn, M. F., and Brewer, G. J.: Studies on the correlation of the genetically determined trait, glucose-6-phosphate dehydrogenase deficiency, with behavioral manifestations in schizophrenia. J. Lab. Clin. Med., **62,** 319, 1963.
484. Bowman, J. E., Brewer, G. J., Frischer, H., Carter, J. L., Eisenstein, R. B., and Bayrakci, C.: A re-evaluation of the relationship between glucose-6-phosphate dehydrogenase deficiency and the behavioral manifestations of schizophrenia. J. Lab. Clin. Med., **65,** 222, 1965.
485. Motulsky, A. G.: Metabolic metamorphisms and the role of infectious diseases in human evolution. Hum. Biol., **32,** 28, 1960.
486. Sonnet, J., and Michaux, J. L.: Glucose-6-phosphate dehydrogenase deficiency, haptoglobin groups, blood groups and sickle-cell trait in the Bantus of West Belgian Congo. Nature (London), **188,** 504, 1960.
487. Allison, A. C.: Glucose-6-phosphate dehydrogenase deficiency in red blood cells of East Africans. Nature (London), **186,** 531, 1960.
488. Charles, L. J.: Observations of the haemolytic effect of primaquine in 100 Ghanaian children. Ann. Trop. Med., **54,** 460, 1960.
489. Allison, A. C., and Clyde, D. F.: Malaria in African children with deficient erythrocyte glucose-6-phosphate dehydrogenase. Brit. Med. J., **1,** 1346, 1961.
490. Allison, A. C., Charles, L. J., and McGregor, I. A.: Erythrocyte glucose-6-phosphate dehydrogenase deficiency in West Africa. Nature (London), **190,** 1198, 1961.
491. Charlton, R. W., and Bothwell, T., II.: Primaquine-sensitivity of red cells in various races in southern Africa. Brit. Med. J., **1,** 194, 1961.
492. Sutton, R. N. P.: Erythrocyte glucose-6-phosphate-dehydrogenase deficiency in Trinidad. Lancet, **1,** 855, 1963.
493. Harris, R., and Gilles, H. M.: Glucose-6-phosphate dehydrogenase deficiency in the peoples of the Niger Delta. Ann. Hum. Genet., **25,** 199, 1961.
494. Van Der Sar, A., Schouten, H., and Struyker Boudier, A. M.: Glucose-6-phosphate dehydrogenase deficiency in red cells: Incidence in the Curacao population, its clinical and genetic aspects. Enzymologia, **27,** 289, 1964.
495. Levin, S. E., Charlton, R. W., and Freiman, I.: Glucose-6-phosphate dehydrogenase deficiency and neonatal jaundice in South African Bantu infants. J. Pediat., **65,** 757, 1964.
496. Lewis, R. A., and Hathorn, M.: Correlation of S hemoglobin with glucose-6-phosphate dehydrogenase deficiency and its significance. Blood, **26,** 176, 1965.
497. Marti, H. R., Schoepf, K., and Gsell, O. R.: Frequency of haemoglobin S and glucose-6-phosphate dehydrogenase deficiency in Southern Tanzania. Brit. Med. J. **1,** 1476, 1965.
498. Lothe, F.: Erythrocyte glucose-6-phosphate dehydrogenase deficiency in Uganda. Nature (London), **215,** 299, 1967.
499. Szeinberg, A.: G6PD deficiency among Jews—genetic and anthropological considerations, in *The Genetics of Migrant and Isolate Populations,* edited by E. Goldschmidt, p. 69. Williams & Wilkins, Baltimore, 1963.
500. Sansone, G., Segni, G., and de Cecco, C.: Il difetto biochimico critrocitario predisponente all'emolisi favica: Prime ricerche sulla popolazione ligure e su quella sarda. Boll. Soc. Ital. Biol. Sper., **34,** 1558, 1958.
501. Walker, D. G., and Bowman, J. E.: Glutathione stability of the erythrocytes in Iranians. Nature (London), **184,** 1325, 1959.
502. Bowman, J. E., and Walker, D. G.: Virtual absence of glutathione instability of the erythrocytes among Armenians in Iran. Nature (London), **191,** 221, 1961.
503. Lenzerini, L., and Contu, L.: Instability of erythrocytic, reduced glutathione (GSH) in the pathogenesis of icterichemoglobinuric favism. Rass. Fisiopat. Clin., **32,** 312, 1960.
504. Siniscalco, M., Bernini, L., Latte, B., and Motulsky, A. G.: Favism and thalassemia in Sardinia and their relationship to malaria. Nature (London), **190,** 1179, 1961.
505. Choremis, C., Zannos-Mariolea, L., and Kattamis, M. D. C.: Frequency

of glucose-6-phosphate-dehydrogenase deficiency in certain highly malarious areas of Greece. Lancet, **1,** 17, 1962.

506. Salvioli, G. P., Jr., and Babini, B.: La fréquence de la déficience congénitale en glucose-6-phosphate-deshydrogenase chez les nouveau-néz de la ville de Bologne. Arch. Franc. Pediat., **20,** 459, 1963.

507. Stamatoyannopoulos, G., Panayotopoulos, A., and Papayannopoulou, T.: Mild glucose-6-phosphate dehydrogenase deficiency in Greek males. Lancet, **2,** 932, 1964.

508. Plato, C. C., Rucknagel, D. L., and Gershowitz, H.: Studies on the distribution of glucose-6-phosphate dehydrogenase deficiency, thalassemia, and other genetic traits in the coastal and mountain village of Cyprus. Amer. J. Hum. Genet., **16,** 267, 1964.

509. Taleb, N., Loiselet, J., Ghorra, F., and Sfeir, H.: Sur la déficience en glucose-6-phosphate-deshydrogénase dans les populations autochtones du Linan. C. R. Acad. Sci. [D] (Paris), **258,** 5749, 1964.

510. Ruffié, J., and Taleb, N.: Étude hémotypologique des ethnies libanaises. Monograph, Hermann, Paris, 1965.

511. Say, B., Ozand, P., Berkel, I., and Cevik, N.: Erythrocyte glucose-6-phosphate dehydrogenase deficiency in Turkey. Acta Paediat. Scand., **54,** 319, 1965.

512. Ragab, A. H., El-Alfi, O. S., and Abboud, M. A.: Incidence of glucose-6-phosphate dehydrogenase deficiency in Egypt. Amer. J. Hum. Genet., **18,** 21, 1966.

513. Stamatoyannopoulos, G., Panayotopoulos, A., and Motulsky, A. G.: The distribution of G-6-PD deficiency in Greece. Amer. J. Hum. Genet., **18,** 296, 1966.

514. Gelpi, A. P.: Glucose-6-phosphate dehydrogenase deficiency, the sickling trait, and malaria in Saudi Arab children. Trop. Pediat., **71,** 138, 1967.

515. Stamatoyannopoulos, G., and Fessas, Ph.: Thalassemia, glucose-6-phosphate dehydrogenase deficiency, sickling, and malarial endemicity in Greece: A study of five areas. Brit. Med. J., **1,** 875, 1964.

516. Siniscalco, M., Bernini, L., Filippi, G., Latte, B., Meera Khan, P., Piomelli, S., and Rattazzi, M.: Population genetics of haemoglobin variants, thalassaemia and G-6-pd deficiency, with particular reference to the malaria hypothesis. Bull. WHO, **34,** 379, 1966.

517. Dreyfus, J. C., Maleknia, N., and Kaplan, J. C.: Recherches sur de déficit en glucose-6-phosphate deshydrogenase en France: A propos de 200 dosages. Nouv. Rev. Franc. Hemat., **4,** 791, 1964.

518. Vella, F.: Favism in Asia. Med. J. Aust., **2,** 196, 1959.

519. Baxi, A. J., Balakrishnan, V., and Sanghvi, L. D.: Deficiency of glucose-6-phosphate dehydrogenase: Observations on a sample from Bombay. Curr. Sci., **30,** 16, 1961.

520. Baxi, A. J., Balakrishnan, V., Undevia, J. V., and Sanghvi, L. D.: Glucose-6-phosphate dehydrogenase deficiency in the Parsee community, Bombay. Indian J. Med. Sci., **17,** 493, 1963.

521. Kahn, P. M.: Glucose-6-phosphate dehydrogenase deficiency in an Indian rural area. J. Genet. **59,** 14, 1964.

522. Chatterjea, J. B.: Haemoglobinopathies, glucose-6-phosphate dehydrogenase deficiency and allied problems in the Indian subcontinent. Bull. WHO, **35,** 837, 1966.

523. Deshmukh, V. V., and Sharma, K. D.: Deficiency of erythrocyte glucose-6-phosphate dehydrogenase and sickle cell trait: A survey of Mahar students at Aurangabad, Maharashtra. Indian Med. Res., **56,** 821, 1968.

524. Jim, R. T. S., and Chu, F. K.: Hyperbilirubinemia due to glucose-6-phosphate dehydrogenase deficiency in a newborn Chinese infant. Pediatrics, **31,** 1046, 1963.

525. Chan, T. K., Todd, D., and Wong, C. C.: Erythrocyte glucose-6-phosphate dehydrogenase deficiency in Chinese. Brit. Med. J., **2,** 102, 1964.

526. Eng, L. L., and Chin, J.: Abnormal haemoglobin and glucose-6-phosphate dehydrogenase deficiency in Malayan aborigines. Nature (London), **204,** 291, 1964.

527. Eng, L. L., and Ti, T. S.: Glucose-6-phosphate dehydrogenase deficiency in Malayans. Trans. Royal Soc. Trop. Med. Hyg., **58,** 500, 1964.

528. Eng, L. L., and Giok, P. H.: Glucose-6-phosphate dehydrogenase deficiency in Indonesia. Nature (London), **204,** 88, 1964.

529. Flatz, G., Thanangkul, O., Simarak, S., and Manmontri, M.: Glucose-6-phosphate dehydrogenase deficiency and jaundice in new born infants in Northern Thailand. Ann. Paediat., **203,** 39, 1964.

530. Miwa, S., Teramura, K., Irisawa, K., and Oyama, H.: Glucose-6-phosphate dehydrogenase (G-6-PD) deficiency. II. Incidence of G-6-PD deficiency in Japanese. Acta Haemat. Jap., **28,** 590, 1965.

531. Wasi, P., Na-Nakorn, S., and Suingdumrong, A.: Studies of the distribution of haemoglobin E: Thalassemias and glucose-6-phosphate dehydrogenase deficiency in North-eastern Thailand. Nature (London), **214,** 501, 1967.

532. Tuchinda, S., Rucknagel, D. L., Na-Nakorn, S., and Wasi, P.: The Thai variant and the distribution of alleles of 6-phosphogluconate dehydrogenase and the distribution of glucose-6-phosphate dehydrogenase deficiency in Thailand. Biochem. Genet., **2,** 253, 1968.

533. Blackwell, R. Q., Ro, I. H., and Yen, L.: Low incidence of erythrocyte G-6-PD deficiency in Koreans. Vox Sang., **14,** 299, 1968.

534. Lai, H. C., Lai, M. P. Y., and Leung, K. S. N.: Glucose-6-phosphate dehydrogenase deficiency in Chinese. J. Clin. Path., **21,** 44, 1968.

535. Motulsky, A. G., Lee, T. C., and Fraser, G. R.: Glucose-6-phosphate dehydrogenase (G6PD) deficiency, thalassaemia, and abnormal haemoglobins in Taiwan. J. Med. Genet, **2,** 18, 1965.

536. Yue, P. C. K., and Strickland, M.: Glucose-6-phosphate dehydrogenase deficiency and neonatal jaundice in Chinese male infants in Hong Kong. Lancet, **1,** 350, 1965.

537. Jim, R. T. S.: Survey for erythrocyte glucose-6-phosphate de-hydrogenase deficiency in Hawaii. Acta Haemat. (Basel), **37,** 94, 1967.

538. Ryan, B. P. D., and Parsons, I. C.: Glucose-6-phosphate dehydrogenase activity in Papuans. Nature (London), **192,** 4801, 1961.

539. Kidson, C., and Gorman, J. G.: Contribution of red cell enzyme deficiency trait to an understanding of genetic relationships between Melanesian and other populations. Amer. J. Phys. Anthrop., **20,** 357, 1962.

540. Kidson, C., and Gajdusek, D. C.: Glucose-6-phosphate dehydrogenase deficiency in Micronesian peoples. Aust. J. Sci., **25,** 61, 1962.

541. Gorman, J. G., and Kidson, C.: Distribution pattern of an inherited trait, red cell enzyme deficiency, in New Guinea and New Britain. Amer. J. Phys. Anthrop., **20,** 347, 1962.

542. Ryan, B. P. K., and Parsons, I. C.: Glucose-6-phosphate dehydrogenase activity in anaemic Papuans. Blood, **19,** 258, 1962.

543. Kidson, C., and Gorman, J. G.: A challenge to the concept of selection by malaria in glucose-6-phosphate dehydrogenase deficiency. Nature, (London), **196,** 49, 1962.

544. Nitowsky, H. M., Soderman, D. D., and Herz, F.: Glucose-6-phosphate dehydrogenase deficiency in Filipinos. Lancet, **1,** 917, 1965.

545. Motulsky, A. G., Stransky, E., and Fraser, G. R.: Glucose-6-phosphate dehydrogenase (G6PD) deficiency, thalassaemia, and abnormal haemoglobins in the Philippines. J. Med. Genet., **1,** 102, 1964.

546. Best, W. R.: Absence of erythrocyte glucose-6-phosphate dehydrogenase deficiency in certain Peruvian Indians. J. Lab. Clin. Med., **54,** 791, 1959.

547. Lisker, R., Loria, A., and Cordova, M. S.: Studies on several genetic hematological traits of the Mexican population. VIII. Hemoglobin S, glucose-6-phosphate dehydrogenase deficiency, and other characteristics in a malarial region. Amer. J., Hum. Genet., **17,** 179, 1965.

548. Vergnes, H., and Larrouy, G.: Les déficits en G6PD dans les populations des Andes boliviennes. Soc. Franc. Hemat., **7,** 124, 1967.

549. Erdohazi, M., and Highman, W. J.: Glucose-6-phosphate dehydrogenase deficiency in Britain. Lancet, **2,** 1274, 1962.

550. Holt, J. M., and Sladden, R. A.: Favism in England—two more cases. Arch. Dis. Child., **40,** 271, 1965.

551. Chan, T. K.: G-6-PD in West Scotland. Lancet, **2,** 752, 1966.

552. Fraser, G. R., Grunwald, P., and Stamatoyannopoulos, G.: Glucose-6-phosphate dehydrogenase (G6PD) deficiency, abnormal haemoglobins, and thalassaemia in Yugoslavia. J. Med. Genet., **3,** 35, 1966.

553. Flatz, G., and Düren, R.: Glucose-6-phosphate dehydrogenase deficiency in Spain. Humangenetik, **4,** 81, 1967.

554. Rosta, J., Makói, Z., and Reif, M.: Investigations regarding glucose-6-phosphate dehydrogenase deficiency in Hungary. Acta Paediat. Acad. Sci. Hung., **8,** 41, 1967.

555. Schneer, J. H.: A Survey for erythrocyte glucose-6-phosphate dehydrogenase deficiency in Rumania. Acta Haemat. (Basel), **40,** 44, 1968.

556. Johannsen, L. P., Witt, I., and Künzer, W.: Favismus bei einer deutschen Familie. Deutsch. Med. Wschr., **93,** 2463, 1968.
557. Obbink, H. J. K.: Glucose-6-phosphate dehydrogenase deficiency in a Dutch family. Acta Genet. (Basel), **15,** 21, 1965.
558. Schmidt, P. M.: Syndrome hémolytique par déficit en glucose-6-phosphate-déhydrogénase chez un Autrichien. Schweiz. Med. Wschr., **86,** 1262, 1966.
559. Motulsky, A., Kraut, J. M., Thiems, W. T., and Musto, D. F.: Biochemical genetics of glucose-6-phosphate dehydrogenase deficiency. Clin. Res., **7,** 78, 1959 (abstract).
560. Motulsky, A. G.: Glucose-6-phosphate dehydrogenase deficiency, haemolytic disease of the newborn, and malaria. Lancet, **1,** 1168, 1961.
561. Krautrachue, M., Na-Nakorn, S., Charoeniarp, P., and Suwanakul, L.: Haemoglobin E and malaria in South-East Thailand. Ann. Trop. Med., **55,** 468, 1961.
562. Luzzatto, L., Usanga, E. A., and Reddy, S.: Glucose 6-phosphate dehydrogenase deficient red cells: Resistance to infection by malarial parasites. Science, **164,** 839, 1969.
563. Beutler, E., Louderback, A., and Natland, M.: Unpublished.
564. Reys, L., Manso, C., and Stamatoyannopoulos, G.: Genetic studies on Southeastern Bantu of Mozambique. I. Variants of glucose-6-phosphate dehydrogenase. Amer. J. Hum. Genet., **22,** 203–215, 1970.
565. McCurdy, P. R., Dillon, D., and Conrad, M.: Personal communication.
566. McCurdy, P. R.: Personal communication.
567. Kissin, C., and Cotte, J.: Etude d'un variant de glucose-6-phosphate deshydrogenase: Le type Constantine. Enzym. Biol. Clin. (Basel), **11,** 277–284, 1970.
568. Siegel, N. H., and Beutler, E.: Unpublished observation.
569. McCurdy, P. R., and Maldonado, N.: Personal communication.
570. McCurdy, P. R., Blackwell, R. Q., Todd, D., Tso, S. C., and Tuchinda. S.: Further studies on G-6-PD deficiency in Chinese subjects. J. Lab. Clin. Med., **75,** 788–797, 1970.
571. McCurdy, P. R., and Mahmood, L.: Personal communication.
572. Johannsen, L. P., Witt, I., and Künzer, W.: Favismus bei einer deutschen Familie. Deutsch. Med. Wschr., **93,** 2463–2470, 1968.
573. Witt, I., and Joshioka, S.: Personal communication.
574. Chan, T. K., Chesterman, C. N., McFadzean, A. J. S., and Todd, D.: The survival of glucose-6-phosphate dehydrogenase-deficient erythrocytes in patients with typhoid fever on chloramphenicol therapy. J. Lab. Clin. Med., **77,** 177, 1971.
575. Yoshida, A.: Amino acid substitution (histidine to tyrosine) in a glucose-6-phosphate dehydrogenase variant (G6PD Hektoen) associated with over-production. J. Mol. Biol., **52,** 483, 1970.
576. Burch, H. B., Bradley, M. E., and Lowry, O. H.: The measurement of triphosphopyridine nucleotide and reduced triphosphopyridine nucleotide and the role of hemoglobin in producing erroneous triphosphopyridine nucleotide values. J. Biol. Chem., **242,** 4546, 1967.
577. Srivastava, S. K., and Beutler, E.: Glutathione metabolism of the erythrocyte. The enzymic cleavage of glutathione-haemoglobin preparations by glutathione reductase. Biochem. J., **119,** 353, 1970.

CHAPTER FIFTY-SIX

HEREDITARY METHEMOGLOBINEMIA WITH DEFICIENCY OF NADH-METHEMOGLOBIN REDUCTASE *

Alan S. Keitt

With certain rare and incompletely characterized exceptions, congenital methemoglobinemia in man occurs either in association with an inherited deficiency in the NADH-methemoglobin reductase activity of erythrocytes, or in the presence of one of the hemoglobins M.† Whereas the enzyme deficiency limits the capacity for reduction of normal methemoglobin, the mutant M hemoglobins, once oxidized, are resistant to normal cellular reducing mechanisms. The methemoglobinemia associated with defective reducing enzyme activity is recessively inherited and responds to therapy with methylene blue (MB) with the prompt disappearance of cyanosis. By contrast, the hemoglobin M disorders are dominant traits which are resistant to therapy with methylene blue.

Many insights into the mechanisms by which erythrocytes reduce methemoglobin have been derived from investigations of the interrelationships between glycolysis and methemoglobin reduction in cells with various inherited metabolic disorders. These studies have established the primacy of an NADH-linked pathway for methemoglobin reduction in normal cells and furnish strong evidence that a defect in NADH-methemoglobin reductase activity underlies the methemoglobinemia of those patients who have only normal hemoglobin A. Attempts to purify and characterize this enzyme have yielded conflicting results in regard to pyridine nucleotide specificity and electron transport mechanism. The metabolic and clinical aspects of congenital methemoglobinemia have been reviewed in a series of comprehensive papers by Jaffé(1–3).

HISTORY

Methemoglobinemia in man was first recognized in individuals who were exposed to certain chemicals that are capable of increasing the rate of oxidation of hemoglobin. Patients with methemoglobinemia without known exposure to such agents were presumed to absorb or produce toxic compounds in their gastrointestinal tract [4, 5]. This colorful concept of "autotoxic enterogenous cyanosis" has not withstood subsequent careful scrutiny. The familial nature of the disease was not established until the report of Hitzenberger in 1932 [5]. Only in 1945 in the reports of Barcroft et al. [6] and Sievers and Ryon [7] did it become apparent that impaired reduction of methemoglobin rather than increased oxidation of hemoglobin was the primary defect in most cases of congenital methemoglobinemia. Virtually all of the subsequent developments in the field were anticipated by Gibson in his classic paper of 1948 [8]. Hemoglobin M, the first abnormal hemoglobin to be described, was reported in the same year by Horlein and Weber in a German family with dominant transmission of congenital methemoglobinemia [9].

METHEMOGLOBIN METABOLISM

Properties of Methemoglobin

Methemoglobin (ferrihemoglobin, hemiglobin) is a trivial name for hemoglobin in which ferrohemes are oxidized to ferrihemes and are thus unable to bind oxygen reversibly. In partially oxidized hemoglobin solutions, methemoglobin presumably represents a mixture of hemoglobin species with different ratios of ferri- to ferroheme. In this state the affinity of the ferrohemes for oxygen is increased.

The spontaneous oxidation of normal hemoglobin by oxygen is slow. This is in part a result of the intensely hydrophobic nature of the heme "pocket" within the globin moiety [10]. Alterations in this nonpolar milieu in certain mutant hemoglobins result in a marked increase in their rate of spontaneous oxidation to methemoglobin. Various substances can greatly increase the rate of oxidation of methemoglobin by direct oxidation (e.g., ferricyanide), by cyclic oxidation (e.g., methylene blue), or by the formation of labile complexes (e.g., nitrite). Methemoglobin forms complexes with several ions which affect its properties. Reaction with cyanide stabilizes the molecule and obliterates its characteristic absorption peak at 632 mμ. Nitrite forms a complex with methemoglobin which also alters its spectral properties

* Personal investigations cited were supported by grants T1-AM-5391 and HE-07652 from the National Institutes of Health.

† Confusing terminology has plagued students of methemoglobin metabolism and its disorders, in part because of the incomplete characterization and apparent nonspecifity of the enzymes involved in methemoglobin reduction. NADH-methemoglobin reductase is frequently termed *diaphorase* because it is customarily assayed with a dye rather than methemoglobin as a terminal electron acceptor. It is more properly called *NADH-ferrihemoglobin oxidoreductase,* and has been variously termed *DPNH-dehydrogenase I, coenzyme factor I, ferrihemoglobin reductase,* etc. In this chapter, *NADPH-dehydrogenase* is used rather than *NADPH-methemoglobin reductase* in view of the lack of evidence that NADPH and methemoglobin react directly in the presence of the enzyme. It has been variously designated *TPNH-dehydrogenase, Hämiglobinreduktase, coenzyme factor II,* etc.

[11]. Ferrocyanide, in direct contrast to cyanide, greatly enhances both enzymatic and nonenzymatic reduction of methemoglobin [12, 13].

Regulation of Methemoglobin Levels in Red Cells

The maintenance of the methemoglobin level at less than ½ of a percent [14] of the total hemoglobin in the normal red cell reflects a balance between the slow formation of methemoglobin and the rate of its reduction. For purposes of methemoglobin reduction, the glycolytic apparatus of the red cell may be considered to consist of two distinct pathways which differ in their coenzyme linkages. The anaerobic glycolytic pathway (or Embden-Meyerhof pathway) contains two NADH-linked dehydrogenases, glyceraldehyde-3-phosphate dehydrogenase (G-3-PD) and lactic dehydrogenase (LDH). The reactions governed by these enzymes normally proceed in opposite directions in regard to NADH, that is, during normal steady state glycolysis these reactions are coupled so that there is no net production of NADH. The oxidative glycolytic pathway (hexose monophosphate, or HMP shunt), on the other hand, contains two NADPH-linked dehydrogenases, glucose-6-phosphate dehydrogenase (G-6-PD) and 6-phosphogluconate dehydrogenase (6-PGD) which are set in tandem and are capable of the rapid production of NADPH. Both glycolytic pathways may participate in methemoglobin reduction but do so under differing conditions. The relative rates of reduction by the respective pathways depend in part on the arrangement of these dehydrogenases which determines their potential for the generation of reduced pyridine nucleotides.

Interactions between Methemoglobin Reduction and Red Cell Glycolysis

The NADH-linked Pathway

When normal red cells are incubated with glucose after exposure to nitrite, reduction of methemoglobin occurs at a linear rate of approximately 1 μmole heme per ml cells per hr [8, 15, 16]. The reduction occurs almost entirely by an NADH-linked pathway and results in the accumulation of a stoichiometric amount of pyruvate [8].* The latter serves as an indicator of a decrease in the level of intracellular NADH. With glucose as the substrate, NADH is generated by the G-3-PD reaction. The linkage between G-3-PD and methemoglobin reduction is not a direct one, since any reaction leading to the generation of NADH can result in the reduction of methemoglobin. Thus, lactate, fumarate, malate, formaldehyde, and xylitol [17] are all efficient substrates for reduction without passing through G-3-PD [2].

The rate of methemoglobin reduction is determined by the availability of NADH rather than by the rate of glycolysis per se. Thus, stimulation of lactate formation by phosphate results in a minimal increase in reduction rate [18], whereas preincubation of cells with nicotinic acid in order to increase their level of NAD (and presumably NADH) causes a significant increase in rate [19]. Further evidence that the rate of reduction is limited by the concentration of NADH is provided by the effects of sodium fluoride on the rate of methemoglobin reduction. Since fluoride inhibits glycolysis beyond the G-3-PD reaction, it does not inhibit methemoglobin reduction [8]. Under these conditions there is a marked increase in the level of red cell 2,3-diphosphoglycerate (2,3-DPG). A reexamination of the effect of fluoride revealed that, in fact, the rate of methemoglobin reduction was stimulated (Fig. 56-1). The most plausible explanation is that by diverting glycolysis toward 2,3-DPG and away from pyruvate, NADH utilization by the LDH reaction is decreased and, consequently, more NADH is available for methemoglobin reduction. Similar conclusions were reached by Schröter [20], who found that 2,3-DPG formation was increased in hemolysates during methemoglobin reduction and suggested that the NADH sparing effect would benefit reduction of methemoglobin.The stimulatory effect of fluoride occurred at concentrations which completely inhibit glucose consumption and even occurred when glucose was absent from the incubation medium. This effect was not observed in a patient with NADH-methemoglobin reductase deficiency [18]. It is apparent, therefore, that there is a significant amount of endogenous substrate, probably including ribose from catabolism of adenine nucleotides, for reducing methemoglobin by way of the NADH-linked pathway.

The NADPH-linked Pathway

The remarkable catalytic effect of methylene blue (MB) on oxygen consumption and methemoglobin reduction in red

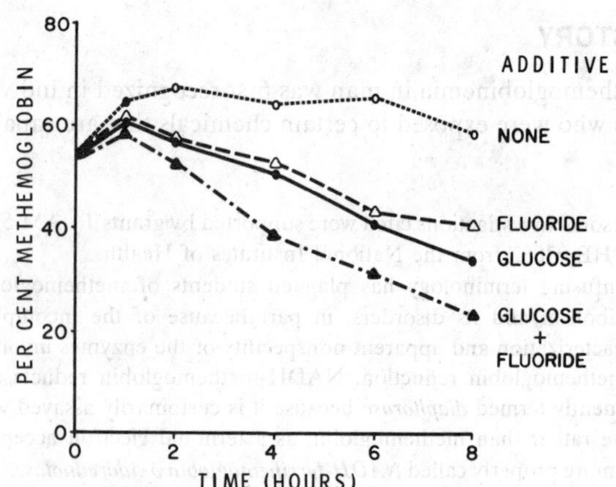

Figure 56-1. Effect of fluoride on methemoglobin reduction rate. Incubations were performed according to previously published methods [16]. Final concentration of fluoride 24 mM.

*One mole of NADH will reduce two moles of ferriheme.

cells has been recognized for over 30 years [21, 22]. MB shuttles electrons between oxygen or methemoglobin and NADPH. The initial electron transfer from NADPH to MB may occur spontaneously, a process which is activated by light [23], or it may be mediated by a red cell enzyme which is loosely called NADPH-dehydrogenase. Leukomethylene blue (LMB), a product of this reaction, may spontaneously reduce oxygen or methemoglobin, with regeneration of MB [24]. The full catalytic effect of MB depends upon the rapid regeneration of NADPH by the dehydrogenases of the HMP shunt [25]. Accordingly, patients who are deficient in red cell G-6-PD fail to show the normal stimulation of methemoglobin reduction in the presence of MB [26], a test which has served as a useful screening procedure for the detection of this metabolic defect. The overall series of reactions can be represented as follows:

$$\text{MB} + \text{NADPH} \xrightarrow{\text{NADPH-dehydrogenase (light)}} \text{LMB} + \text{NADP} \quad (1)$$

$$\text{LMB} + O_2 \longrightarrow \text{MB} + H_2O \quad (2a)$$

$$\text{LMB} + \text{ferriheme} \longrightarrow \text{MB} + \text{ferroheme} \quad (2b)$$

$$\text{NADP} + \text{HMP} \xrightarrow{\text{G-6-PD, 6-PGD}} \text{NADPH} + \text{ribose phosphate} + CO_2 \quad (3)$$

In contrast to the readily observable alterations in the NADH-linked glycolytic sequence during methemoglobin reduction, evidence for interaction between NADPH and methemoglobin in intact cells in the absence of MB is tenuous. Any participation of an NADPH-linked mechanism in normal reduction of methemoglobin should be accompanied by an increased regeneration of NADPH through the HMP shunt, and this would be indicated by an increase in evolution of labeled CO_2 from radioactive glucose. A measure of the contribution of the NADPH-linked pathway to normal reduction of methemoglobin might be provided by the assay of a decrease in HMP shunt activity induced by cyanide, since an excess of cyanide quantitatively removes methemoglobin by formation of inert cyanmethemoglobin.

Nitrite increases the oxygen consumption of red cells, and this is blocked by cyanide [27]. Although this increase has been interpreted as a stimulation of the HMP shunt by methemoglobin, the continuing presence of nitrite and the possible uptake of oxygen by deoxyhemoglobin as methemoglobin is reduced permits alternative explanations. When nitrite is removed from the cells by careful washing, a slight increase in evolution of labeled CO_2 can be detected during incubation with ^{14}C-labeled glucose [28], and this can be abolished by adding an excess of cyanide [18]. This has been attributed to nonenzymatic reduction of methemoglobin by glutathione, and regeneration of reduced glutathione by NADPH-linked glutathione reductase [28]. It was found that, during anaerobic incubations, reduced glutathione decreased in the presence of methemoglobin (but not with deoxyhemoglobin) by an amount which was roughly equivalent to the methemoglobin which became reduced.

An alternative or contributory explanation for the slight stimulation of HMP shunt activity during methemoglobin reduction derives from the observation that pyruvate may increase shunt metabolism to a similar extent [29]. Since pyruvate accumulates during the reduction of methemoglobin in normal cells, it is difficult to rule out an effect of this pyruvate on activity of the shunt. Studies in patients with congenital methemoglobinemia are perhaps informative in this regard since exposure to nitrite is not needed and there is no accumulation of pyruvate during incubation. The presence of methemoglobin in these cells is not associated with an increase in the HMP shunt and no significant change is induced by complexing methemoglobin with cyanide (Table 56-1). Since the NADPH-linked pathway is preserved in these cells, as indicated by their normal reduction with methylene blue [8, 16], it is apparent that there must be little, if any, interaction between methemoglobin and NADPH in the absence of an artificial electron carrier.

Enzymatic Mediators of Methemoglobin Reduction

While the initial steps of the reaction sequences leading to methemoglobin reduction through the generation of reduced

Table 56-1. EFFECT OF METHEMOGLOBIN, WITH AND WITHOUT ADDED CYANIDE, ON THE RATE OF UTILIZATION OF GLUCOSE BY THE HMP SHUNT PATHWAY [16]

Red cells	Cyanide added	Glucose consumed, μmoles/ml cells/hr	Glucose via HMP shunt		Methemoglobin, percent
			μmoles/ml cells/hr	Percent of glucose consumed	
Patient	0	1.81	0.091	5.0	19.2
	+	1.49	0.084	5.6	0.0
Normal	0	1.53	0.086	5.6	<1.0
subject 1	+	1.39	0.080	5.8	0.0
Normal	0	1.88	0.105	5.6	<1.0
subject 2	+	1.71	0.087	5.1	0.0
Normal	0	1.70	0.089	5.2	<1.0
subject 3	+	1.62	0.083	5.1	0.0

pyridine nucleotides are clearly separable, the mechanisms of the terminal steps linking NADH and NADPH to methemoglobin remain controversial. It has generally been assumed from the findings of Gibson [8] and Scott [30] that there are two or more distinct methemoglobin reducing enzymes with differing coenzyme requirements in normal red cells. An alternative suggestion has been made by Huennekens and coworkers [31] that a single protein (or group of proteins) mediates reduction with either NADH or NADPH. At present no satisfactory resolution of the problem is available. Nevertheless, there are compelling reasons, based on studies of the methemoglobin reducing pathways in red cells from patients with discrete genetic defects, for retaining the concept that NADH- and NADPH-linked reducing activities reside in separate and distinct enzymes.

As a group, the enzymes which are methemoglobin reductases require an artificial activator for full activity and are nonspecific in their requirements for a terminal electron acceptor. The activities reside in multiple fractions, each with differing properties. Because of differences in isolation procedures and choice of activators, direct comparison between the various fractions isolated by different investigators is exceedingly difficult.

Kiese first attempted to purify a methemoglobin reducing enzyme, which he called Hämiglobinreduktase [32]. This enzyme required NADPH and methylene blue in order to reduce methemoglobin. It contained flavin which was thought to be the prosthetic group.

Scott [30] has isolated four proteins from red cells which have reduced pyridine nucleotide dehydrogenase activity in the presence of a redox dye, dichlorophenolindophenol (DCIP). The major fraction, called NADH-dehydrogenase I, had a ratio of activity with NADH to that with NADPH of 100:1.5. It contained flavin and reduced methemoglobin at a rate sufficient to account for most of the reduction observed in intact cells. Its primary role in methemoglobin reduction in vivo has been deduced from its absence from the red cells of Eskimo patients with congenital methemoglobinemia [33]. Two other proteins with relative NADPH specificity do not contain flavin and are weak methemoglobin reductases. They may account for only 5 percent of the reducing capacity of intact cells. Scott has estimated that at least 95 percent of methemoglobin reduction in vivo is accomplished by "DPNH-dehydrogenase I" [34].

Huennekens and his colleagues have reported that there are three separate protein fractions capable of reducing methemoglobin in red cells [31]. All lack flavin, have an absolute requirement for a redox catalyst such as methylene blue, and have a ratio of activity with NADH and NADPH of approximately 4:1. The suggestion was made that an unidentified mediator is present in red cells which is lost during purification and which takes the place of methylene blue in vivo. The Michaelis constant (K_m) of the fractions for NADPH is an order of magnitude below that for NADH. They further suggest that the normal preponderance of NADH-linked methemoglobin reduction would arise from the approximately tenfold greater production of NADH by anaerobic glycolysis than of NADPH by the HMP shunt during steady state glycolysis.

Hegesh and Avron have recently made the important observation that ferrocyanide greatly enhances the rate of reduction of methemoglobin in hemolysates fortified with NADH [12]. Convincing evidence has been presented that ferrocyanide acts by forming a complex with methemoglobin rather than as an electron transporting intermediary. The binding site for ferrocyanide is unknown, but optimal activation is achieved at a molar ratio of ferrocyanide to methemoglobin of 4:1. These workers have purified a "ferrihemoglobin reductase" which is specific for NADH when the methemoglobin ferrocyanide complex is used as an electron acceptor [35]. When redox dyes such as methylene blue are used as activators rather than ferrocyanide, the NADH specificity is not absolute. This may explain the cross reactivity of the Huennekens enzyme preparation. The elution behavior of the enzyme was similar to that of Scott's "DPNH-dehydrogenase 1" but the enzyme was virtually devoid of flavin. The authors postulate that the ferrocyanide binding alters the conformation of methemoglobin and allows the NADH-linked reductase closer access to the heme groups.

In a fortuitous observation which may have a bearing on this controversy, Sass described a patient with a deficiency in erythrocyte NADPH-dehydrogenase [36]. These red cells do not show the customary stimulation of methemoglobin reduction with methylene blue, but they have normal G-6-PD activity, normal methemoglobin content and NADH-methemoglobin reductase activity, and a normal capacity for methemoglobin reduction in the absence of methylene blue. This enzyme is apparently required for the rapid oxidation of NADPH by methylene blue, since stimulation of the HMP shunt by methylene blue is much impaired in its absence [37]. The activity of this NADPH-dehydrogenase has been separated electrophoretically from the NADH-linked enzyme [38, 39] and is selectively lacking in hemolysate from the deficient patient [39]. The activity of this enzyme is presumably normal in patients with congenital methemoglobinemia due to deficient NADH-methemoglobin reductase activity whose erythrocytes reduce methemoglobin rapidly in the presence of methylene blue [8].

The independent genetic transmission of these two rare inborn errors of metabolism seems incompatible with the formulation of Huennekens and his coworkers that the NADH and NADPH methemoglobin reducing activities are present on a single enzyme. The suggestion that red cells contain an endogenous mediator which is capable of transporting electrons between NADPH and methemoglobin also is difficult to accept in view of the insignificant stimulation of the HMP shunt by methemoglobin. If such an intermediary exists one would predict from the kinetics of the Huennekens enzymes that NADPH-linked methemoglobin reduction would predominate, since the affinity of the enzyme for NADPH is greater than its affinity for NADH by a factor of 10, whereas the concentrations of these nucleotides are of the same order of magnitude in normal cells. Why then does the HMP shunt not respond to methemoglobin? One might speculate that the dye-dependent pyridine nucleotide dehydrogenases are vestigial red cell enzymes whose naturally occurring cofactor has been lost, not during purification but by mutation. A genetic event of this kind might confer an evolutionary advantage on the red cell by fostering a relative insulation between reduced pyridine nucleotides and potential intracellular oxidants, including methemoglobin [40].

RED CELL METABOLISM IN FAMILIAL METHEMOGLOBINEMIA

When red cells from patients with deficient NADH-methemoglobin reductase activity are exposed to moderate amounts of nitrite and subsequently incubated with glucose, the slow reduction of methemoglobin proceeds at one-third to one-quarter of the normal rate [16, 30] and pyruvate does not accumulate [8]. Nevertheless, as previously noted, rapid methemoglobin reduction occurs in the presence of methylene blue. The failure of pyruvate accumulation led Gibson to conclude that these patients lack a previously unsuspected NADH-linked enzyme which is the preferred route for methemoglobin reduction, and that methylene blue opens a separate NADPH-linked pathway which is normally dormant [8]. No other consistent metabolic abnormality has been detected in methemoglobinemic cells. The overall conversion of glucose to lactate, the individual enzyme activities of the Embden-Meyerhof pathway, and the concentration and generation of pyridine and adenine nucleotides have all been found normal [3]. The HMP shunt proceeds at a rate which is identical to that of normal cells [16] and is fully responsive to the catalytic effects of methylene blue [18]. The enzyme defect seems limited to red cells, since leukocyte [41] and muscle [42] soluble NADH-diaphorase activity is normal and no increase in muscle metmyoglobin is detectable [42].

The extent to which the residual reducing capacity in methemoglobinemic cells can be attributed to persistent NADH-methemoglobin reductase activity or to the contribution of ancillary pathways is unclear. Enzyme activity measured by the assay method of Scott [33] has ranged from 0 to 50 percent of normal. Because of the use of DCIP as an intermediary in this assay and the considerable blank activity, it is difficult to extrapolate from hemolysate activity to reducing capacity in intact cells. Recently Hegesh [43] has developed an assay using ferrocyanide and methemoglobin as the terminal electron acceptor. It has a distinctly lower blank and faster rate and is therefore probably more accurate at low levels of activity. Using this method, low but measurable activity has been detected in all homozygotes studied by Hsieh and Jaffé [44].

This residual NADH-methemoglobin reductase activity probably accounts for the small but finite reducing capacity which can be observed in deficient cells with lactate as the substrate [16, 45]. When glucose is substituted for lactate a small but potentially critical increment in reduction rate can be observed in relatively young but not in older cells [16]. Histochemical techniques have demonstrated that methemoglobin is heterogenously distributed within the red cell population [16] (Fig. 56-2). Those cells containing the most methemoglobin are found in the older fraction as obtained by differential centrifugation [16]. It is probable that a decline in reducing capacity, perhaps involving the regeneration of reduced glutathione, occurs in older cells and accounts for the age-dependent accumulation of methemoglobin. The failure of the HMP shunt to respond to the presumed increase in oxidation of GSH remains unexplained. It should also be noted that because of genetic heterogeneity in the methemoglobin reductases, studies conducted on the red cells of individual patients may not necessarily apply to all patients with this disease. Nevertheless, some of the common clinical features can be explained in part by segregation of methemoglobin into a minor cell fraction.

Clinical Features

The effects of the accumulation of methemoglobin in the blood of patients with deficient NADH-methemoglobin reductase activity are mild and differ little from those observed in chronic anemia with an equivalent reduction in oxygen carrying capacity. The cyanosis, which may vary from being barely detectable to profound, is usually observed at birth* and is often attributed to cardiac or pulmonary anomalies with venous shunting. The degree of methemoglobinemia is variable among patients but usually reaches a plateau between 15 and 30 percent, although it may occasionally reach 45 percent. Patients generally complain only of mild fatigue and dyspnea on exertion and it is often surprising how little these symptoms are affected by treatment which markedly decreases the level of circulating methemoglobin.

There is a distinct increase in the incidence of severe mental retardation associated with deficiency of NADH-methemoglobin reductase activity [41, 47]. The retardation, which is often associated with severe developmental anomalies, is not invariably transmitted with the methemoglobinemia in members of the same family [41]. Nonetheless, most patients are normal mentally. The α-chain variants of the hemoglobin M group are not associated with an increased incidence of mental retardation, in spite of a comparable degree of methemoglobinemia in utero.

Little information is available concerning the magnitude

*This may help in distinguishing this disease from the hemoglobin M diseases with β-chain anomalies in which cyanosis occurs only after fetal hemoglobin decreases.

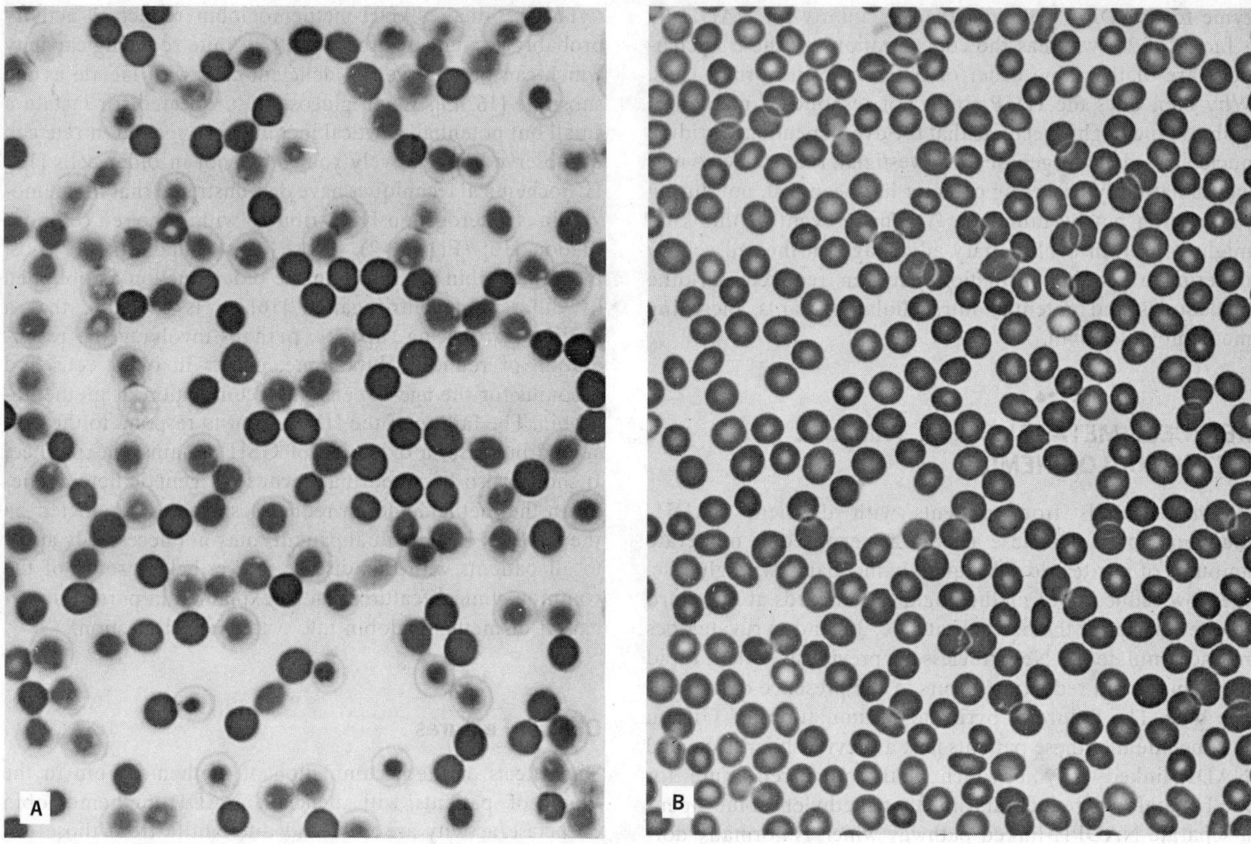

Figure 56-2. Heterogeneous distribution of methemoglobin in untreated cells from a patient with deficient NADH-methemoglobin reductase activity (A) compared with a normal control (B). The staining procedure is that of Kleihauer and Betke [46] in which cells containing methemoglobin become decolorized while normal cells stain darkly. (*Reprinted from New Eng. J. Med.* [16].)

and nature of the physiologic compensatory mechanisms in this disease. Occasional patients have moderate polycythemia, but both the frequency and adequacy of bone marrow compensation falls short of what would be predicted from the loss in oxygen carrying capacity. Since red cell survival is normal, it appears that the erythropoietin mechanism fails to detect or the marrow is unable to respond to the loss in oxygen carrying capacity in many cases.

Conflicting evidence has been reported concerning hemoglobin-oxygen dissociation curves in patients with congenital methemoglobinemia. In some studies a shift of the curve to the left indicated an increased affinity of hemoglobin for oxygen, while an equal number of investigators have reported no change in the character of the dissociation curve [3]. The molecular conformation of methemoglobin resembles that of oxyhemoglobin. Thus, partial oxidation of heme in a hemoglobin tetramer results in an increased affinity for oxygen by the remaining ferrohemes. A shift to the left has been found in methemoglobinemia induced by nitrite treatment of normal red cells [48]. Failure to find a comparable shift in the blood of methemoglobinemic patients stems in part from the segregation of methemoglobin within a discrete population of older cells. This would decrease the total intramolecular interaction between ferri- and ferrohemes [16, 49].

Both methylene blue (1 to 3 mg per kg) and ascorbic acid (500 mg per day) are effective in lowering the methemoglobin levels in patients with deficient NADH-methemoglobin reductase activity. Ascorbic acid apparently reduces methemoglobin directly and may be regenerated by reduced glutathione [13]. The finding of low serum ascorbate levels in several patients with congenital methemoglobinemia [50, 51] suggests that it, like glutathione, may contribute to methemoglobin reduction in some cases. Following therapy with methylene blue, methemoglobin reaccumulates at a fairly constant rate of about 2 to 3 percent per day before leveling off at pretreatment levels in 10 to 14 days [16, 50]. This observation furnishes additional strong evidence that methemoglobin reducing capacity is critically impaired in only a minority of cells. If the predominance of methemoglobin in the older cells occurred as a result of a slow, continuous accumulation of methemoglobin throughout the life span of the cells, it would take several months to reach equilibrium after cessation of therapy. The ability of the younger cells to withstand the metabolic defect presumably accounts for the self-limited nature of the disease.

Diagnosis

This disorder must be distinguished from cyanosis associated with congenital heart disease or an abnormal hemoglobin with decreased oxygen affinity (e.g., hemoglobin Kansas). The presence of methemoglobin may be suspected by the persistence of the chocolate brown color of shed blood after thorough oxygenation and can be confirmed spectroscopically by the method of Evelyn and Malloy [52]. Differentiation from hemoglobin M disease can usually be suspected clinically (see above) and can be simply tested by adding methylene blue to whole blood and observing whether visible reduction (brown to red) takes place. Definite diagnosis rests on the assay methods of Scott [33] or Hegesh [43].

Genetics

Family studies have indicated that this disease is transmitted as an autosomal recessive trait in virtually all instances [3]. Parents of affected children and children of affected parents have intermediate levels of activity of the diaphorase by the assay of Scott, and similar intermediate levels are found by the assay method of Hegesh. Methemoglobin content in the heterozygote is nearly normal, but the rate of reduction of methemoglobin in intact cells is distinctly decreased [47, 53]. This impairment in reducing capacity may become clinically apparent during exposure to drugs which form methemoglobin. Primaquine, chloroquine, and diaminodiphenylsulfone may cause methemoglobinemia in heterozygotes [53].

Genetic Variation in NADH-Methemoglobin Reductase

Successful application of electrophoretic techniques to the study of methemoglobin reductase has resulted in the detection of several genetic variants of the NADH-linked enzyme in patients with congenital methemoglobinemia. Kaplan and Beutler [38] and West et al. [54] have independently reported abnormalities in the electrophoretic mobility of NADH-methemoglobin reductase in patients with methemoglobinemia. The abnormal bands were probably distinct from one another but technical differences do not permit direct comparison. The fast-migrating band of Kaplan and Beutler was termed the *California* variant. Several patients with methemoglobinemia showed either faint bands with normal mobility or total absence of activity. Bloom and Zarkowsky [39] obtained similar results in five additional patients, one of whom showed a band with decreased mobility. NADPH-linked dye reduction was distinct from that with NADH and had normal mobility and staining intensity in all of the patients with abnormal NADH patterns.

Recently Hsieh and Jaffé [44] have studied some of these patients again and several more of their own, including a number of heterozygous persons. By concentrating the enzyme approximately thirtyfold prior to electrophoresis, bands of NADH-methemoglobin reductase activity were obtained in all the homozygotes. Six abnormal bands were identified on the basis of differing mobilities on starch gel (Table 56-2). Heterozygotes displayed a normal band and a weak additional band which corresponded to that found in related homozygotes. It is of interest that the same mutations tended to occur in individuals of similar ethnic background. This suggests that they may have stemmed from a common source.

Several recent studies have demonstrated additional electrophoretic variation in NADH-methemoglobin reductase among individuals with normal methemoglobin concentrations and normal reducing capacity [55, 56].

The foregoing studies indicate that there are several alleles for the enzyme, which when present are expressed as methemoglobinemia with a decrease in NADH-methemoglobin reductase activity. At present only variations in electrophoretic mobility have been detected; more precise characterization of the mutant enzymes awaits further study.

SUMMARY

1 Red cells normally maintain a low concentration of methemoglobin because of the considerable excess of methemoglobin reducing capacity relative to the rate of hemoglobin oxidation. Most of the reduction of methemoglobin is accomplished by the enzyme NADH-methemoglobin reductase. An auxiliary reduction pathway in normal cells requires the generation of NADPH, an NADPH dehy-

Table 56-2. VARIANTS OF NADH-METHEMOGLOBIN REDUCTASE*

Origin	Preliminary designation	Ethnic group	Electrophoretic mobility†, percent of normal
California	California	Unknown	133
Boston	Boston Fast	Italian	127
New York area	Puerto Rico	Puerto Rican	117–120
Princeton	Princeton	Anglo-Saxon	113
California	Duarte	English/Polish	108
Boston	Boston Slow	Irish	90

* Data of H. S. Hsieh, and E. R. Jaffe, [44].
† Method of Kaplan and Beutler [38].

drogenase, and an autoxidizable dye such as methylene blue. Glutathione and ascorbic acid may also reduce methemoglobin directly, although at a slow rate.

2 Both inherited or acquired deficiencies in each of these reduction mechanisms have been observed, but methemoglobinemia occurs only with a deficiency in the activity of NADH-methemoglobin reductase. This results in a benign lifelong cyanosis which can be corrected with methylene blue or ascorbic acid.

3 The genetic basis for this disease in most cases involves inheritance of an altered enzyme with decreased activity and abnormal electrophoretic migration. The diversity of mutants that has been detected indicates that the disease derives from a set of allelic genes which have a reasonably uniform clinical expression. Discrepancies in severity and associated metabolic abnormalities may at least in part be attributed to varying properties of the enzymes corresponding to the different allelic genes.

BIBLIOGRAPHY

1. Jaffé, E. R., and Heller, P.: Methemoglobinemia in man, in *Progress in Hematology,* edited by C. V. Moore and E. B. Brown, vol. IV. Grune & Stratton, New York, 1964.
2. Jaffé, E. R.: Metabolic processes involved in the formation and reduction of methemoglobin in human erythrocytes, in *The Red Blood Cell,* edited by C. Bishop and D. M. Surgenor. Academic, New York, 1964.
3. Jaffé, E. R.: Hereditary methemoglobinemias associated with abnormalities in the metabolism of erythrocytes. Amer. J. Med., **41,** 786, 1966.
4. Stokvis, B. J.: Zur Casuistic der autotoxischen enterogenen Cyanosen. (Met-Haemoglobinaemia et enteritis parasitaria). Internat. Beitr. Inn. Med., **1,** 597, 1902.
5. Hitzenberger, K.: Autotoxische Zyanose (Intraglobulaire Methamoglobinamie.) Wien. Arch. Inn. Med. **23,** 85, 1932.
6. Barcroft, H., Gibson, Q. H., Harrison, D. C., and McMurray, J.: Familial idiopathic methaemoglobinaemia and its treatment with ascorbic acid. Clin. Sci., **5,** 145, 1945.
7. Sievers, R. F., and Ryon, J. B.: Congenital idiopathic methemoglobinemia: Favorable response to ascorbic acid therapy. Arch. Intern. Med. (Chicago), **76,** 299, 1945.
8. Gibson, Q. H.: The reduction of methaemoglobin in red blood cells and studies on the cause of idiopathic methaemoglobinaemia. Biochem. J., **42,** 13, 1948.
9. Horlein, H., and Weber, G.: Uber chronische familiare Methamoglobinamie und eine neue Modifikation des Methamoglobins. Deutsch. Med. Wschr., **73,** 476, 1948.
10. Carrell, R. W., and Lehmann, H.: The unstable haemoglobin haemolytic anaemias. Seminars Hemat., **6,** 116, 1969.
11. Smith, R. P.: The nitrite-methemoglobin complex—its significance in methemoglobin analyses and its possible role in methemoglobinemia. Biochem. Pharmacol., **16,** 1655, 1967.
12. Hegesh, E., and Avron, M.: The enzymatic reduction of ferrihemoglobin. I. The reduction of ferrihemoglobin in red blood cells and hemolysates. Biochim. Biophys. Acta., **146,** 91, 1967.
13. Gibson, Q. H.: The reduction of methaemoglobin by ascorbic acid. Biochem. J., **37,** 615, 1943.
14. Van Slyke, D. D., Hiller, A., Weisiger, J. R., and Cruz, W. O.: Determination of carbon monoxide in blood and of total and active hemoglobin by carbon monoxide capacity: Inactive hemoglobin and methemoglobin contents of normal blood. J. Biol. Chem., **166,** 121–148, 1946.
15. Jaffé, E. R.: The reduction of methemoglobin in human erythrocytes incubated with purine nucleotides. J. Clin. Invest., **38,** 1555, 1959.
16. Keitt, A. S., Smith, T. W., and Jandl, J. H.: Red cell "pseudomosaicism" in congenital methemoglobinemia. New Eng. J. Med., **275,** 398, 1966.
17. Asakura, T., Adachi, K., Minakami, S., and Yoshikawa, H.: Non-glycolytic sugar metabolism in human erythrocytes. I. Xylitol metabolism. J. Biochem. (Tokyo), **62,** 184, 1967.
18. Keitt, A. S.: Unpublished observations.
19. Jaffé, E. R., and Neumann, G.: Hereditary methemoglobinemia, toxic methemoglobinemia and the reduction of methemoglobin. Ann. NY Acad. Sci., **151,** 795, 1968.
20. Schröter, W., and Winter, P.: Zur Bedeutung des 2,3-Diphosphoglycerat-Zyklus in Erythrozyten: Beziehungen zwischen Methamoglobin-und 2,3-Dichlorophenolindophenol-Reduktion, Glykolyse, und 2,3-Diphosphoglyceratbildung. Blut, **14,** 1, 1966.
21. Barron, E. S. G., and Harrop, G. A.: Studies on blood cell metabolism. II. The effect of glycolysis and lactic acid formation of mammalian and avian erythrocytes. J. Biol. Chem., **79,** 65, 1928.
22. Warburg, O. F., Kubowitz, F., and Christian, W.: Uber die katalytische Wirkung von Methylenblau in lebenden Zellen. Biochem. Z., **227,** 254, 1930.
23. Tonz, O.: *The Congenital Methemoglobinemias.* S. Karger, Basel, 1968. (Bibliotheca Haematologica No. 28.)
24. Beutler, E., and Baluda, M. C.: Methemoglobin reduction: Studies of interaction between cell populations and the role of methylene blue. Blood, **22,** 323, 1963.
25. Brin, M., and Yonemoto, R. H.: Stimulation of the glucose oxidative pathway in human erythrocytes by methylene blue. J. Biol. Chem., **230,** 307, 1958.
26. Dawson, J. P., Thayer, W. W., and Desforges, J. F.: Acute hemolytic anemia in the newborn infant due to naphthalene poisoning: Report of two cases with investigations into the mechanisms of the disease. Blood, **13,** 1113, 1958.
27. DeLoecker, W. C. J., and Prankerd, T. A. J.: Factors influencing the hexose monophosphate shunt in red cells. Clin. Chim. Acta, **6,** 641, 1961.
28. Stromme, J. H., and Eldjarn, L.: The role of the pentose phosphate pathway in the reduction of methaemoglobin in human erythrocytes. Biochem. J., **84,** 406, 1962.
29. Szeinberg, A., and Marks, P. A.: Substances stimulating glucose catabolism by the oxidative reactions of the pentose phosphate pathway in human erythrocytes. J. Clin. Invest., **40,** 914, 1961.
30. Scott, E. M., Duncan, I. W., and Ekstrand, V.: The reduced pyridine nucleotide dehydrogenases of human erythrocytes. J. Biol. Chem., **240,** 481, 1965.
31. Kajita, A., Kerwar, G. W., and Huennekens, F. M.: Multiple forms of methemoglobin reductase. Arch. Biochim. Biophys., **130,** 662, 1969.
32. Kiese, M., Schneider, C., and Waller, H. D.: Hämiglobinreduktase Naunyn-Schmiedebergs. Arch. Exp. Path., **231,** 158, 1957.
33. Scott, E. M.: The relation of diaphorase of human erythrocytes to inheritance of methemoglobinemia. J. Clin. Invest., **39,** 1176, 1960.
34. Scott, E. M.: Congenital methemoglobinemia due to DPNH-diaphorase deficiency, in *Hereditary Disorders of Erythrocyte Metabolism,* edited by E. Beutler. Grune & Stratton, New York, 1968.
35. Hegesh, E., and Avron, M.: The enzymatic reduction of ferrihemoglobin. II. Purification of a ferrihemoglobin reductase from human erythrocytes. Biochim. Biophys. Acta., **146,** 397, 1967.
36. Sass, M. D., Caruso, C. J., Farhangi, M.: TPNH-methemoglobin reductase deficiency: A new red-cell enzyme defect. J. Lab. Clin. Med., **70,** 760, 1967.
37. Sass, M. D.: Observations on the role of TPNH dehydrogenase in human red cells. Clin. Chim. Acta, **21,** 101, 1968.
38. Kaplan, J. C., and Beutler, E.: Electrophoresis of red cell NADH and NADPH-diaphorases in normal subjects and patients with congenital methemoglobinemia. Biochem. Biophys. Res. Commun., **29,** 605, 1967.
39. Bloom, G., and Zarkowsky, H.: Heterogeneity of the enzymatic defect in congenital methemoglobinemia. New Eng. J. Med., **281,** 919, 1969.
40. Jandl, J. H.: The Heinz body hemolytic anemias. Ann. Intern. Med., **58,** 702, 1963.
41. Fialkow, P. J., Browder, J. A., Sparkes, R. S., and Motulsky, A. G.: Mental retardation in methemoglobinemia due to diaphorase deficiency. New Eng. J. Med., **273,** 840, 1965.

42. Smith, R. F., and Graybiel, A.: Personal communication.
43. Hegesh, E., Calmanovici, N., and Avron, M.: New method for determining ferrihemoglobin reductase (NADH methemoglobin reductase) in erythrocytes. J. Lab. Clin. Med., **72**, 339, 1968.
44. Hsieh, H., and Jaffé, E. R.: Electrophoretic and functional variants of NADH-methemoglobin reductase in hereditary methemoglobinemia. J. Clin. Invest., **50**, 196, 1971.
45. Jaffé, E. R.: The methemoglobin reductase systems of human erythrocytes, in *Metabolism and Membrane Permeability of Erythrocytes and Thrombocytes,* edited by E. Deutsch, E. Gerlach, and K. Moser. Thieme, Stuttgart, 1968.
46. Kleihauer, E., and Betke, K.: Elution procedure for demonstration of methaemoglobin in red cells of human blood smears. Nature (London), **199**, 1196, 1963.
47. Jaffé, E. R., Neumann, G., Rothberg, H., Wilson, F. T., Webster, R. M., and Wolff, J. A.: Hereditary methemoglobinemia with and without mental retardation: A study of three families. Amer. J. Med., **41**, 42, 1966.
48. Darling, R. C., and Roughton, F. J. W.: The effect of methemoglobin on the equilibrium between oxygen and hemoglobin. Amer. J. Physiol., **137**, 56, 1942.
49. Gibson, Q. H.: Methaemoglobin and sulfhaemoglobin, in *The Chemical Pathology of Animal Pigments,* edited by R. T. Williams. Biochemical Society Symposia (No. 12), Cambridge, New York, 1954.
50. Eder, H. A., Finch, C., and McKee, R. W.: Congenital methemoglobinemia: A clinical and biochemical study of a case. J. Clin. Invest., **28**, 269, 1949.
51. Scott, E. M., and Hoskins, D. D.: Hereditary methemoglobinemia in Alaskan Eskimos and Indians. Blood, **13**, 795, 1958.
52. Evelyn, K., and Malloy, H.: Microdetermination of oxyhemoglobin, methemoglobin and sulfhemoglobin in a single sample of blood. J. Biol. Chem., **126**, 655, 1938.
53. Cohen, R. J., Sachs, J. R., Wicher, D. J., and Conrad, M.: Methemoglobinemia provoked by malarial chemoprophyllaxis in Vietnam. New Eng. J. Med., **279**, 1127, 1968.
54. West, C. A., Gomperts, B. D., Huehns, E. R., Kessell, E., and Ashby, J. R.: Demonstration of an enzyme variant in a case of congenital methaemoglobinemia. Brit. Med. J., **4**, 212, 1967.
55. Detter, J. C., Anderson, J. E., and Giblett, E. R.: NADH diaphorase: An inherited variant associated with normal methemoglobin reduction. Amer. J. Hum. Genet., **22**, 100, 1970.
56. Hopkinson, D. A., Corney, G., Cook, P. J. L., Robson, E. B., and Harris, H.: Genetically determined electrophoretic variants of human red cell NADH diaphorase. Ann. Hum. Genet., **34**, 1, 1970.

CHAPTER FIFTY-SEVEN

THE HEMOGLOBINOPATHIES

Hermann Lehmann and R. G. Huntsman

The observations of Pauling and his collaborators on the electrophoretic characteristics of human hemoglobins, first published in 1949, form a landmark in biochemical genetics. Their observations, and many that have followed, have firmly established the existence of various species of human hemoglobin and have shown that a subject may have various combinations of these species circulating in his blood at the same time. The inheritance of the hemoglobins follows strict genetic patterns, and certain dyscrasias of the blood may quite precisely reflect the genetic pattern of the constituent hemoglobins.

This chapter will include a review of present information on the chemical nature of the hemoglobins and the genetics of their inheritance, and will attempt to classify the variant hemoglobins. In addition, the diseases deriving from an endowment of abnormal hemoglobin will be described and interpreted.

HUMAN HEMOGLOBIN

Hemoglobin is the principal protein of man concerned with oxygen transport. Each molecule of hemoglobin consists of one molecule of globin to which are attached four molecules of ferroprotoporphyrin IX (Fig. 57-1). The heme does not lie flat on the surface but is embedded in the protein part of the molecule and has been likened to a half-dollar piece pushed into a doughnut (or a penny into a bun—J. C. Kendrew). This prosthetic group is common to groups of compounds concerned in redox processes in both the plant and animal kingdoms, from the peroxidase of horse radish to the cytochromes of man. The protein part of the hemoglobin molecule shows a wide variation of molecular weight in the lower animals, but in the vertebrates the molecular weight is relatively constant at about 68,000 (66,700 for man).

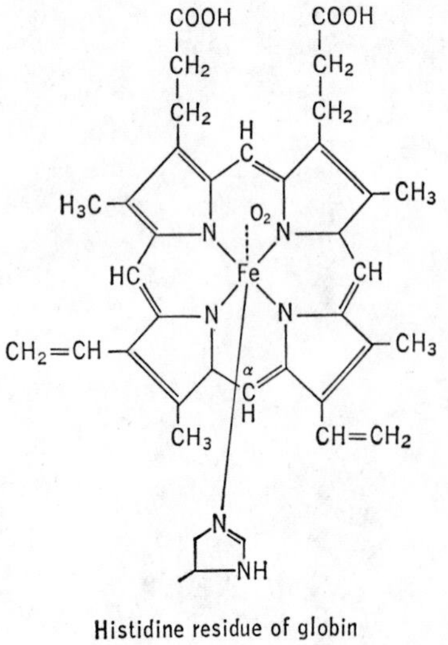

Histidine residue of globin

Figure 57-1. Heme, one of the four identical prosthetic groups attached to one molecule of globin.

Adult and Fetal Hemoglobin

About one hundred years ago von Körber [1] noticed that the blood of the adult is more easily denatured by alkali than that from the placenta. He concluded that there are two human hemoglobins, adult and fetal. These are now designated A and F. Hemoglobin F is present in infants at birth, when it varies in concentration from approximately 60 to 90 percent. It then gradually disappears from the circulation, and by the age of 4 months only traces persist. Several observers have noted that Hb F persists for more than 4 months in normal Negro childern.

Jonxis [2] has pointed out that with a red cell life of only 120 days the presence of Hb F in the blood of normal children over 3 months old may be explained only by the synthesis of this pigment after birth. Formation of Hb F may persist in pathologic states which begin at an age when Hb F is still being produced, and if the cause of the infantile disorder, usually an anemia, is not removed, Hb F may still be found in adult life. This was first observed in thalassemia [3–6] but was later also found in sickle-cell anemia [7] and other hemoglobinopathies. The phenomenon is not specifically associated with this group of disorders but can be observed in many other syndromes, such as spherocytic jaundice, leukemia, and nutritional anemias.

The numerous physical differences between adult and fetal hemoglobins have been summarized by White and Beaven [8], Betke [9], and Bertles [10]. These include differences in solubility and ultraviolet spectrum, and resistance to alkali denaturation. There may be differences also for oxygen affinity and in antigenic activity. Hemoglobin F is inherited independently of all the adult hemoglobin variants. These and other properties listed below divide it sharply from Hb A and its variants.

Alkali denaturation: At pH 12.8 (0.04*N* alkali) and at room temperature, the half reaction time of denaturation (t ½) for Hb A is 10 sec, and for Hb F is 1,000 sec.

Ultraviolet spectrum: The tryptophan fine-spectrum band for Hb A is 291.0 mμ, and for Hb F is 289.8 mμ.

Electrophoresis: The isoelectric point of Hb A is 6.87 and of Hb F is 6.98. On open boundary electrophoresis at pH 6.5, A and F separate. On paper electrophoresis at pH 8.6, A and F do not separate, but when present in a mixture, F causes slowing of the A band. Upon starch-gel electrophoresis at pH 8.6, Hb F separates as a distinct

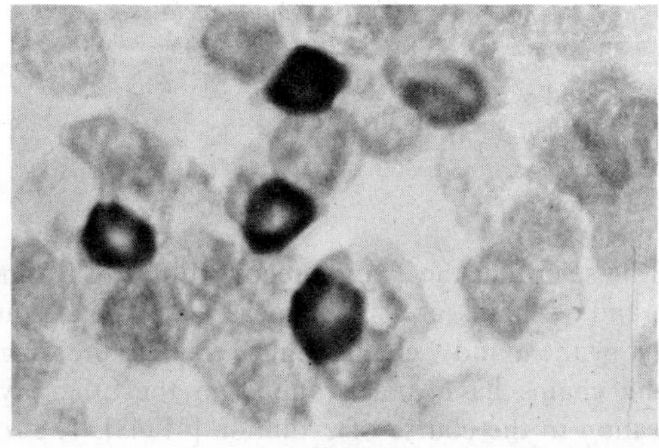

Figure 57-2. Cells of an adult and of a newborn infant stained after Kleihauer and Betke [11]. The adult cells appear as ghosts, and the newborn cells are fully stained.

band behind Hb A. With agar "electrochromatography" at pH 6.2, Hb F separates as a distinct band in front of Hb A.

Chromatography: Hemoglobin F separates as a distinct band in front of Hb A on Amberlite IRC 50 at pH 6 or on carboxymethylcellulose.

Solubility: Hb A is soluble at pH 3.2; Hb F is not. This can be used to identify cells containing Hb F. Slides are immersed in a citrate buffer, pH 3.2. On subsequent staining Hb A cells will appear as ghosts, and Hb F cells will be fully stained (Fig. 57-2).

Immunology: Antiserums have been prepared from chickens, rabbits, and other species which precipitate specifically Hb A and F, respectively. Agglutinating serums have been prepared from rabbits which act on the red cells of the newborn but not on those of the adult, except when the adult blood contains Hb F.

Oxygen dissociation: The oxygen affinity of cord blood is greater than that of adult blood and yet, after dialysis, fetal hemoglobin is less avid for oxygen than adult hemoglobin [12]. It is now known that the avidity of hemoglobin for molecular oxygen is dependent upon the concentration within the red cell of a normal cellular metabolite 2,3-diphosphoglycerate. Hemoglobin "stripped" of 2,3-diphosphoglycerate by dialysis becomes extremely avid for oxygen [13, 14]. The hemoglobin in the red cell of a patient with sickle-cell anemia is less avid for oxygen and this helps to compensate the patient for the anemia from which he suffers [15]. The altered oxygen affinity of the other abnormal hemoglobins is considered later in the section on unstable hemoglobins.

Hemoglobin A_2 and Other Minor Fractions

Hemoglobin A is not a homogeneous protein. Derrien [16] has summarized his own experiences and that of other workers with fractional "salting out" of Hb A. He found six different components. Itano [17] considers these results due to the transition of soluble protein into the solid phase, where the crystal forms differ at different salt concentrations. There can be no doubt that adult hemoglobin consists of at least two fractions, which can easily be separated by electrophoresis: a major component, Hb A_1, and a minor component amounting to about 2 percent, Hb A_2 [18].

Hemoglobin A_2 is an adult hemoglobin in its own right and is inherited independently from Hb A_1. Like fetal hemoglobin, hemoglobin A_2 has its own variants. Hemoglobin A_2 is found in the absence of Hb A_1 in sickle-cell homozygotes. Also, like Hb F it is increased in thalassemia, in which the Hb A_1 formation is decreased. Other minor fractions undoubtedly exist [19] (Fig. 57-3). Hb A_3 may be a combination of Hb A_1 with glutathione [20]. In the case of hemoglobin F a minor fraction has been isolated by chromatography and has been found to be an acetylated derivative [21]. It has been suggested that some of the minor components seen after the electrophoresis of myoglobin may be due to partial unfolding of the polypeptide chain [22], and the same may also be true for hemoglobin.

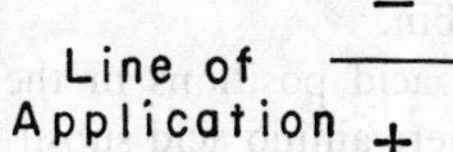

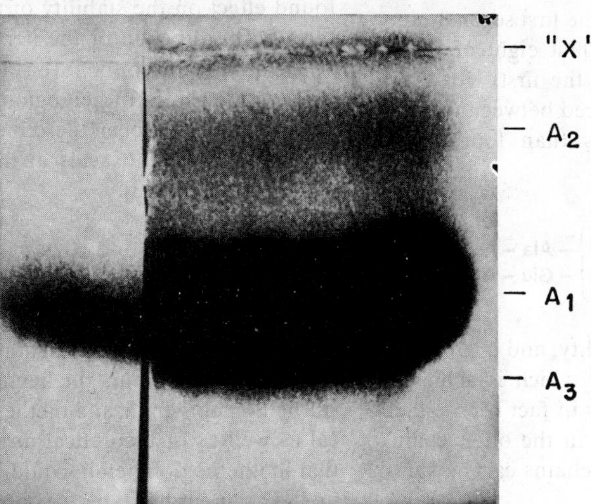

Figure 57-3. The heterogeneity of hemoglobin. When normal adult hemoglobin is examined by paper electrophoresis at pH 8.6, a single fraction is observed (see left, unstained strip). On staining, several additional minor fractions appear. These are Hb A_2 and A_3, and a nonhemoglobin component X.

The Polypeptide Chains of the Different Human Hemoglobins

Human hemoglobin has a molecular weight of 66,700. X-ray studies of horse hemoglobin have shown that this molecule is composed of two equal halves which together form an ellipsoid of the dimensions 55 × 55 × 70 Å [23]. In human hemoglobin each molecule contains four polypeptide chains of which two named α are common to Hb A, F, and A_2. The second pair consists of either β, γ, or δ chains, and differs in each of these three hemoglobins [24–31].

$$\text{Hb A} = \alpha_2\beta_2$$
$$\text{Hb F} = \alpha_2\gamma_2$$
$$\text{Hb A}_2 = \alpha_2\delta_2$$

There are two types of embryonic hemoglobin:

$$\text{Gower I} = \epsilon_4$$
$$\text{Gower II} = \alpha_2\epsilon_2$$

The last two have disappeared by the time the embryo is 10 cm crown-rump length [32–33]. They are considered in a later subsection (Prefetal Hemoglobin) of this chapter. Yet another physiological polypeptide chain called the Portland chain has been described [34, 35].

The α chain has 141 amino acid residues, and the others are composed of 146 each [36–39]. A comparison of the amino acid sequence shows the great similarity of the four chains. The resemblance can be made to appear even greater if the α and β chains are laid side by side and the α-chain residues are realigned over the β-chain residues by introducing occasional "gaps" [40].

	1	2	3	4	5	6	7	8
α chain—	Val	– Leu	– Ser	– Pro	– Ala	– Asp	– Lys –	
β chain—	Val	– His	– Leu	– Thr	– Pro	– Glu	– Glu	– Lys

Note: Val = valyl, Leu = leucyl, Ser = seryl, Pro = prolyl, Ala = alanyl, Asp = aspartyl, Lys = lysyl, His = histidyl, Thr = threonyl, Glu = glutamyl.

Thus if one compares, as shown above, the first seven amino acid residues of the α chain with the first eight of the β chain, agreement can be seen only for the first. However, if a Braunitzer *Lücke* ("gap") is introduced between the first two residues of the α chain, no less than four correspondences will appear.

α chain—	Val	–	–	Leu	– Ser –	Pro	– Ala	– Asp –	Lys
β chain—	Val	– His	–	Leu	– Thr –	Pro	– Glu	– Glu –	Lys

This gap does not, of course, exist in reality, and one cannot say whether the increased resemblance which is achieved by introducing it indicates that there has in fact been either a deletion in one chain or an insertion in the other chain. The correspondences between the four chains can be summarized as follows and as in Fig. 57-4.

Chains	*Identical amino acid sequences, percent*
α and γ	39
α and β	42
β and γ	71
β and δ	96

It will be seen that the β and δ chains differ little, and that the β and γ chains are much more alike than either the α and β or the α and γ chains. This has led to the suggestion that the chains have arisen one from the other by gene duplication in the course of evolution [41–43]. The α chain may be considered to be the oldest. By gene duplication a second α-chain gene would have arisen, and these two would have evolved independently, so that eventually there would be two different genes, one for the α chain and one perhaps for the γ chain. It is reasonable to assume that the γ chain which occurs in Hb F is the oldest of the non-α chains, and indeed it is the one which differs most from the α chain. By the same principle the β chain would have arisen from the γ chain, and finally the δ chain gene would have split away from the gene for the β chain. Zuckerkandl and Pauling [44] have attempted to estimate the time of derivation of different hemoglobin polypeptide chains in the course of evolution. They arrive at a figure of 11 to 18 million years per amino acid substitution in a chain of about 150 amino acids, with a median figure of 14.5 million years. These calculations assume that the play of mutagenic forces has been fairly evenly distributed over the last 600 million years (Table 57-1)!

It is now appreciated that the human γ chain may possess either an alanyl or a glycyl residue at position 136. This suggests that there are multiple structural genes for the γ chain of human fetal hemoglobin [45]. It is possible that the human α chain gene is also duplicated [46, 47].

Perhaps the two most important residues in each chain are the histidines in α 58 and α 87, and β 63 and β 92, because the heme radical is "suspended" between these residues. Any mutational changes in this area have a profound effect on the stability of the ferrous atom and therefore on the function of the hemoglobin.

There are now only seven amino acid positions in the polypeptide chains of hemoglobin where amino acid substitutions have not been described in either man or other animals. The amino acids at these sites are called the invariant residues [48].

The Abnormal Hemoglobins

Until 15 years ago interest in adult hemoglobin was centered on its prosthetic group, the heme. Carboxyhemoglobinemia, sulfhemoglobinemia, and methemoglobinemia were of clinical as well as of theoretical importance, and it was known that methemoglobinemia could be either acquired or inherited. The inherited type was attributed to abnormalities in

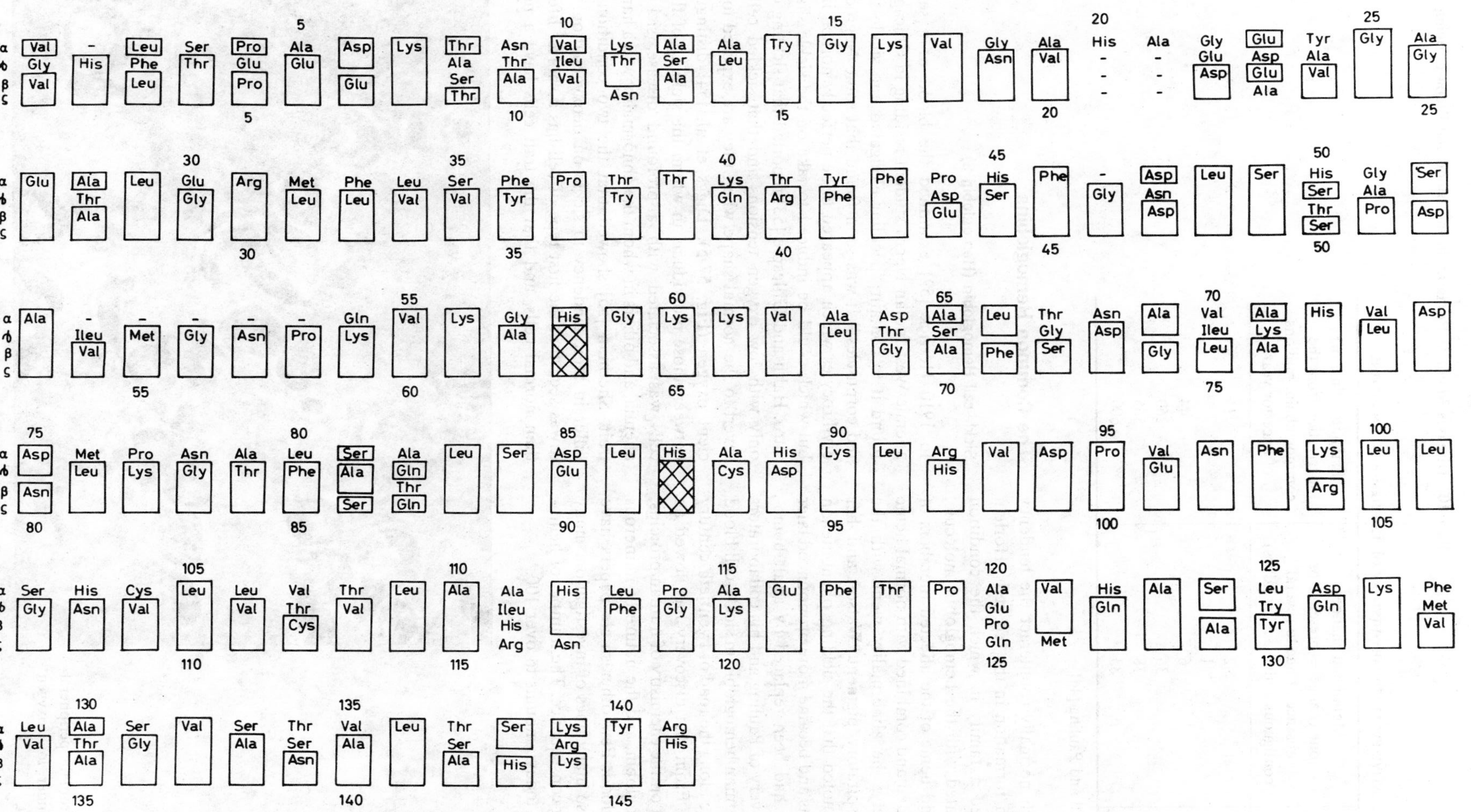

Figure 57-4. The α, γ, β, and δ chains of human hemoglobin. Similar residues are boxed (after Ingram). The areas where similarity of the chains is most evident may represent vital areas where mutation would be lethal. Alternatively, they may represent stable areas compared with the "hot spots" where mutations are more likely to occur. γ^{136} can be either Gly or Ala.

Table 57-1. SPECULATIVE EVOLUTIONARY HISTORY OF THE HEMOGLOBIN CHAINS

Chains being compared	Mutational changes (one change = presence or absence of one to several contiguous amino acid residues)	Estimated time of derivation from the common chain, millions of ancestor years
Gorilla α and human α	2	11
Gorilla β and human β	1	
Human β and δ	6	44
Human β and γ	36	260
Human α and β	78	565
Human α and γ	83	600

Source: After Zuckerkandl and Pauling [44].

reducing systems which normally counteract the tendency toward methemoglobin formation in the red cells. Hörlein and Weber [49] studied a family in which the condition appeared to be associated with the hemoglobin molecule, for when the globin and heme of the affected members of this family were separated and combined with normal heme and globin, respectively, the abnormality went with the globin part of the respiratory pigment. Watson and her collaborators [50] had noted that the sickling phenomenon was only slight in infants and became more pronounced later when the fetal variant had been replaced by adult hemoglobin. It was the discovery of Pauling and his collaborators [51] of a second adult human hemoglobin in sickle-cell blood that became a milestone along the road of twentieth-century investigative medicine. From that discovery has flowed an abundance of new light on the chemistry of human proteins, the physiology of hemoglobin, and the nature of numerous disease states of the blood. Few other single papers have been the beginning of so many lines of investigation, many of them of far-reaching consequence. The number of hemoglobin variants known today amounts to over 100.

The Common Hemoglobins

Sickle-cell Hemoglobin (Hemoglobin S)

In 1910 Herrick [52] examined the blood of a severely anemic West Indian Negro student residing in Chicago and found it to contain "peculiar elongated and sickle-shaped red corpuscles." It was soon found that some Negroes had erythrocytes which appeared to be perfectly normal in vivo but which could be induced to take on the sickle shape in vitro. Hahn and Gillespie [53] reported that sickling occurs only with low oxygen tensions and that sickled cells can revert to the normal shape when they are exposed to sufficient oxygen (Fig. 57-5). Diggs et al. [54] distinguished between those individuals in whom the sickling of the red cells was associated with a profound disease, sickle-cell anemia, and others in whom the abnormality was a harmless trait. Sherman [55] showed that the two conditions also differ in their tendency to sickle on deoxygenation. Later it was seen that the first type of cell has a shorter life span than normal cells, and that the trait cells have a normal

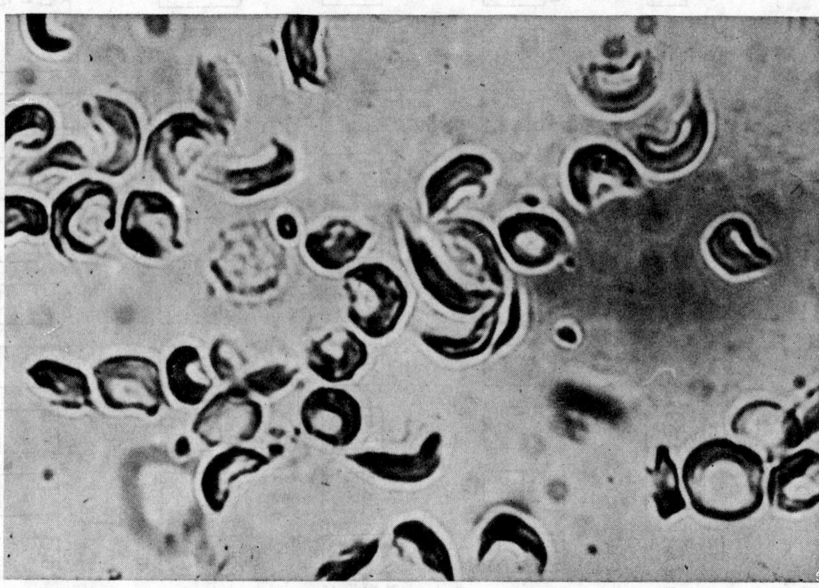

Figure 57-5. Sickle cells from the peripheral blood as they appear under low oxygen tension, in the sickling test.

survival time even when transfused into patients with sickle-cell anemia [56, 57].

The sickling phenomenon is familial, and the mode of inheritance is that of a single Mendelian dominant [58, 59]. At first it was generally assumed that the same gene produces in some persons an asymptomatic condition, the sickling trait, and in others is responsible for the severe form with anemia and other changes. Neel suggested in 1947 [60] that there might be an alternative hypothesis similar to that which had differentiated between severe and mild thalassemia in terms of their being homozygous and heterozygous states. In 1949 the same theory together with supporting evidence was put forward by Beet [61], and Neel presented conclusive proof based on numerous family studies [62].

The discovery of the sickle-cell hemoglobin correlated all the data that had been accumulating. Sickling was due to an abnormal hemoglobin, and whereas in the heterozygous carriers of the sickle-cell trait both Hb A and Hb S were found, no A was present in patients with sickle-cell anemia who were homozygous for the abnormal gene. Thus the gene for Hb A found expression in the phenotype in the presence of another for Hb S (Fig. 57-6). Another hemoglobin besides S was found in small amounts in the blood of patients homozygous for sickling, but this was not Hb A. It was later shown to be Hb F persisting in these patients beyond the age of infancy [7].

Almost all the findings in sickle-cell disease can be explained by the physical properties of reduced Hb S and particularly by its low solubility at low oxygen tension. Harris [63] found that the deoxygenation of concentrated solutions of Hb S results in a semisolid gel. Under the microscope, tactoids 1 to 15 microns long may be observed which are remarkably similar in shape to sickled cells. On reoxygenation the tactoids disappear, but they form again when the oxygen is removed. Perutz and his collaborators [64, 65] reported that reduced Hb S is much less soluble than reduced Hb A. Oxygenated Hb A and Hb S have the same solubility, but upon deoxygenation the solubility of Hb A falls by one-half, whereas that of the sickle-cell hemoglobin becomes 50 times less. Sickling may therefore be understood as the outcome of intracellular tactoid formation in reduced sickle cells. The greater the concentration of the reduced Hb S, the more it is likely to form tactoids, and accordingly the tendency to sickle is more pronounced in sickle-cell anemia than in sickle trait. The gelling of hemoglobin inside the cells, resulting in a deformity of the red cells, increases blood viscosity. Indeed virtually all of the features of the disease can be related directly or indirectly to the increase in blood viscosity which accompanies deoxygenation [66, 67]. The slower the blood flow, the greater will be the deoxygenation, and the more intense will be the transformation of the discoid red cell into the spiked sickled cell. These abnormally shaped cells will be phagocytized by reticuloendothelial cells; this may explain why sickle cells have a shorter life span. Sickle-cell anemia is by far the most severe of the hemolytic anemias arising from variants of Hb A. In addition to the common hemolytic element the in vivo sickling of red cells adds further to the destruction. Should the viscous bizarre-shaped cells cause blockage of small vessels, a vicious circle is set up. Deoxygenation becomes more intense, and the cell shape becomes more and more abnormal.

The time factor is important in the development of sickling [68]. With a normal circulation time, sickle cells remain in the deoxygenated state less than the 15 sec required for sickling to begin, but if for any reason they are held up in organs with a low oxygen tension there will be time for sickling. A few sickled cells are invariably found in the

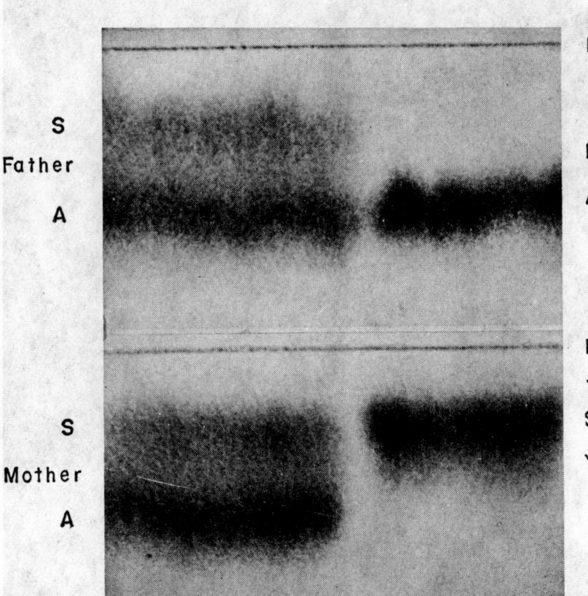

Figure 57-6. The paper electrophoretic pattern (barbiturate buffer, pH 8.6) of a sample of blood obtained from two children of parents, each of whom was a sickle-cell trait carrier. On the left, above, a sample from the father; below, one from the mother. On the right above is a sample from the elder child, who is normal; the younger child (below) has sickle-cell anemia.

circulating blood in sickle-cell anemia. These irreversibly sickled cells have undergone some structural damage to the cell membrane. They do not revert to normal shape even when fully oxygenated and their number gives some indication of the severity of the hemolytic process [69].

The clogging of small blood vessels is responsible for the "crises" of sickle-cell anemia. Infarctions, which can occur in any part of the body, may appear as acute abdominal emergencies, pneumonia, priapism, heart disease, or hematuria. Necrotic areas in the long bones arising from the closure of nutrient vessels tend to become infected, and osteomyelitis is a frequent complication. A *Salmonella* osteomyelitis is almost pathognomonic of sickle-cell disease, [70]. The curious x-ray appearance of the skull sometimes seen in sickle-cell anemia is a manifestation of the erythroid hyperplasia found in any severe chronic hemolytic process. A calcified cerebral infarct is also shown in Fig. 57-7. In contrast, sickle cells are not present in the circulating blood of the sickle-cell trait carrier.

On the whole, and for practical purposes, one can assume that the sickle-cell trait is harmless. For example African athletes with the sickle-cell trait, undergoing extreme stress at high altitude in the Mexican Olympic Games, did not experience any ill effects [71]. On the other hand sudden death has recently been reported in four young males, heterozygous for Hb S, while undergoing vigorous physical exercise at an altitude of 4,060 ft [72].

The red cells of the sickle-cell trait carrier have on average about 20 to 40 percent of sickle hemoglobin and they will sickle only when the oxygen tension is reduced to below about 10 mm Hg [73]. Undue deoxygenation should therefore be avoided during the administration of an anesthetic and it should be remembered that this may well occur during the relatively unsupervised "recovery period" [74]. Severe, otherwise unexplained hematuria, presumably by a renal sickling lesion, has been recorded in patients whose only abnormality was found to be a sickle-cell trait [75, 76]. Splenic infarction can occur when sickle-cell trait carriers fly at high altitude in unpressurized aircraft [77] or possibly even on very rare occasions, in pressurized aircraft. It should be remembered that even an adequately pressurized plane flies at an equivalent of 5,000 ft and this not uncommonly has proved a dangerous experience for a patient with sickle-cell anemia or sickle-cell-Hb C disease [78]. It appears reasonable that the sickle-cell trait carrier, although fit, should be protected from unphysiological anoxic stresses and would be probably ill-advised to take a responsible job, such as mine rescue or aircrew work, which might involve accidental deoxygenation.

When genes for Hb A and Hb S are inherited together, both hemoglobins are incorporated into the same cells. This can be concluded because in sickle-cell preparations from trait carriers almost all cells take on the abnormal shape. However, the proportion of the two hemoglobins is unequal; only 20 to 40 percent is Hb S. There are two possible explanations for the higher proportion of Hb A in the hetero-

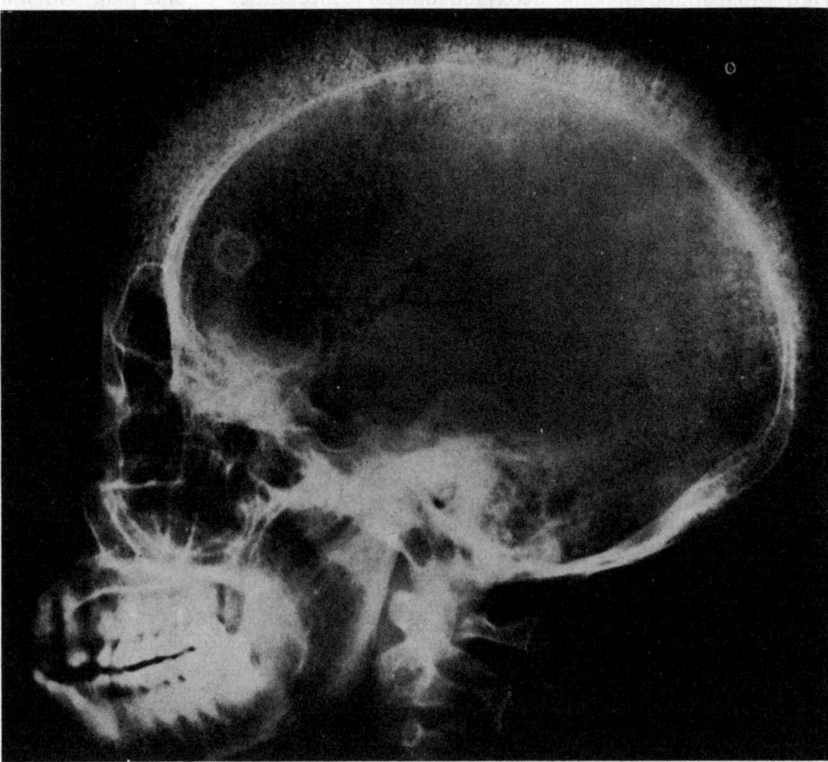

Figure 57-7. X-ray appearance of the skull of an adolescent patient with sickle-cell anemia. The thickened diploë with the absence of an outer table results in a "hair on end" appearance. This severe degree of "hair on end" appearance (representing erythroid marrow hyperplasia) is characteristic of β thalassemia major rather than sickle-cell anemia. There appears to be a ring infarct in the frontal region. (*By permission of Dr. W. P. Cockshutt, University College Hospital, Ibadan, Nigeria.*)

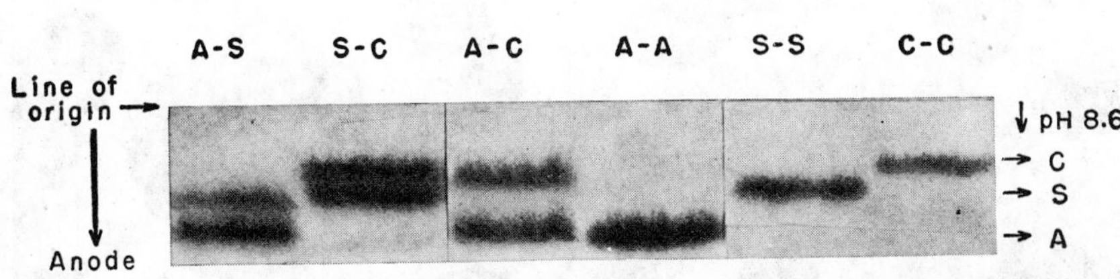

Figure 57-8. The identification of different hemoglobins by filter paper electrophoresis. In an alkaline buffer, hemoglobin will travel toward the positive pole. The speed of migration differs; adult hemoglobin (A) is faster than sickle hemoglobin (S), and S is faster than hemoglobin C. Hemoglobin D travels at the same speed as S, but it can be differentiated by its inability to form a gel in the reduced state. (*By permission of G. M. Edington and H. Lehmann* [85].)

zygote. One is that Hb A is produced at a greater rate [79]. It is also possible that the heterozygote produces a series of cells with varying proportions of A and S [80] and that those containing more S are preferentially destroyed. In either case, in any one moment circulating blood would show more Hb A than Hb S.

Almost every cell from a sickle-cell trait carrier can be made to sickle on extreme deoxygenation in vitro—such as occurs in the sickling test. The sickling test is, therefore, positive in both the patient with sickle-cell anemia and the fit sickle-cell trait carrier. This widely used test merely detects the presence of sickle hemoglobin and does not distinguish between their two very different genetic (and clinical) states.

The recognition of Hb S, the studies of its biochemical and physical properties, and the examination of individual patients and their families went far to support the genetic theory that sickle-cell anemia is a disease of the homozygote. Contradictions to this hypothesis led to the discovery of two other abnormal hemoglobins.

Hemoglobin C

The observation of atypical cases of sickle-cell disease with failure to find sickling in one of the two parents led to the discovery by Neel and his colleagues of a new second abnormal hemoglobin in the nonsickling parent and to the demonstration of the same pigment in the children with the intermediate type of sickle-cell disease called Hemoglobin S C disease (or sickle-cell–Hb C disease) [81, 82]. In these patients, who are doubly abnormal heterozygotes, the S gene is inherited from one parent and the C gene from the other. In this condition hemoglobin S amounts to more than half the total hemoglobin; the consequence is that heterozygotes for these two abnormal hemoglobin genes suffer from sickle-cell disease. The clinical disability is less severe than sickle-cell anemia because the total amount of Hb S in the cells is still less than that formed in the homozygous sickling condition [81–83].

Hemoglobin C was shown to produce a symptomless trait in heterozygotes, and its proportion in the trait-carrying parents was less than that in the children with Hb S and C. The homozygous state for Hb C was not encountered by Neel et al. [81] but they predicted it, and it was found shortly afterward by several other workers. Ranney and her colleagues [84] were able to show that the genes for Hb A, S, and C were allelic; i.e., the β-chain chromosome could have a locus only for the A, S, or C gene. Electrophoretic patterns of hemoglobin samples for several combinations of these hemoglobins appear in Fig. 57-8.

Although the Hb C trait is completely harmless, the homozygous state for Hb C is definitely a disease. Under favorable conditions the hemoglobinopathy is latent, but the decreased life span of the erythrocytes will exacerbate any additional stress. It is of clinical importance that sickle-cell–Hb C disease is usually and Hb C disease is always associated with splenomegaly, whereas in adults with sickle-cell anemia the spleen can only very rarely be felt. In sickle-cell anemia numerous splenic infarcts eventually lead to autosplenectomy. The cells of the Hb C disease are thin, and numerous "target cells" can be seen (Fig. 57-9). The amino acid substitution in Hb C is that of lysine for glutamic acid in the 6th position of the β chain [86].

Hemoglobin D

Hemoglobin D was first found in a patient with atypical hemolytic anemia. Electrophoresis revealed a single hemoglobin migrating in the position of Hb S [87, 88]. One of the parents failed to show sickle cells on repeated tests, but on electrophoresis a sickle-cell trait pattern was found. It was then discovered that a hemoglobin with the electrophoretic properties of Hb S but without its abnormally low solubility in the reduced state was responsible for the conflicting observations. The propositus was in fact suffering not from sickle-cell anemia but from "sickle-cell–Hb D" disease. The parent was a Hb D trait carrier. At one time thought to be a rare hemoglobin, D is now known to occur in 2 percent of Punjabis and in 1 percent of Gujarati-speaking Lohana in Southern India [89]. This common variant was originally described in Los Angeles but it is also known as D_{Punjab}. The term *Hb D* is used for any hemoglobin variant which travels on starch gel or paper at alkaline pH in an electrophoretic position identical with sickle hemoglobin and yet is normally soluble in the reduced state and therefore gives a negative sickling test [87]. A number of such variants having different amino acid substitutions are now known [90], but of these D_{Punjab} is by far the commonest.

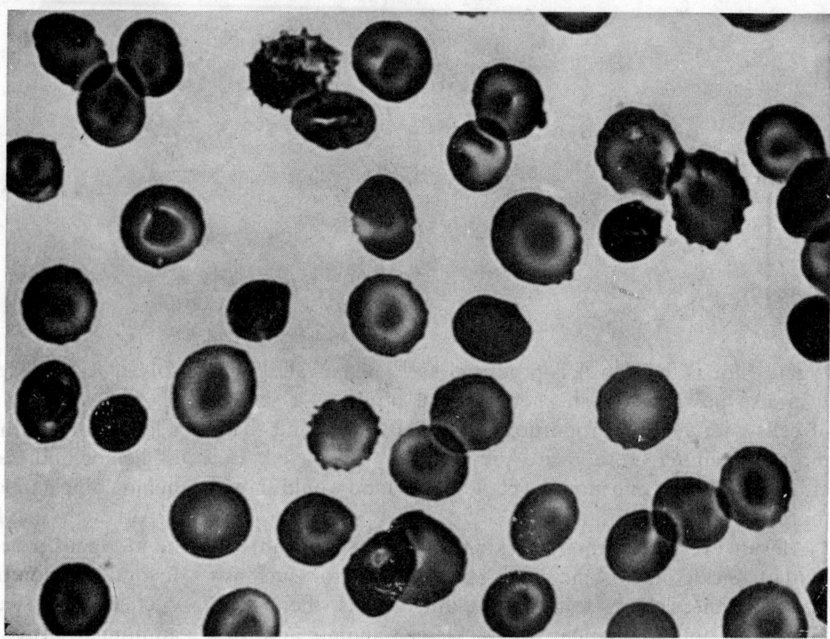

Figure 57-9. The red cells of the Hb C disease as they appear in the peripheral blood.

Hemoglobin E

Hemoglobin E was discovered in a family in California [91] and independently in Thailand [92, 93]. The observations in Thailand provided the first evidence that abnormal hemoglobins other than Hb S exist at high frequency in non-Negroids. On electrophoresis at alkaline pH, Hb E is very similar to Hb C (Fig. 57-10). This is not surprising because both these variants are glutamic acid → lysine mutations. In the case of Hb C this has occurred in the 6th position [86] and in Hb E the 26th position of the β chain [94].

As noted above, Hb S and C are allelic characters [84]. The first record of a family in which Hb S and Hb E occurred together made it likely, though not certain, that Hb S and Hb E were also allelic [95]. The son of a woman with Hb S and E presented the same hemoglobin combination (Fig. 57-11). If the son had inherited both hemoglobins from the mother, this observation would exclude the possibility that S and E could be alleles. However, the son could have inherited one of the two hemoglobins from his father, and one-fifth of the population to which the father belonged carried the sickle-cell trait. The father had died. Thus the observations on mother and son would exclude the possibility that the genes for Hb S and E are alleles only *if* the father had been proved not to carry the sickle-cell trait. On the other hand, in the next generation four children of the man with the two abnormal hemoglobins and of his normal wife had only one abnormal hemoglobin each. Thus on the whole the evidence favors allelism or close linkage of the genes for Hb E and S.

Further observations in sickle-cell–Hb E disease added to the evidence in favor of allelism of the two hemoglobin genes [97], but the best evidence came from the analysis of the chemical change in the hemoglobin molecule when

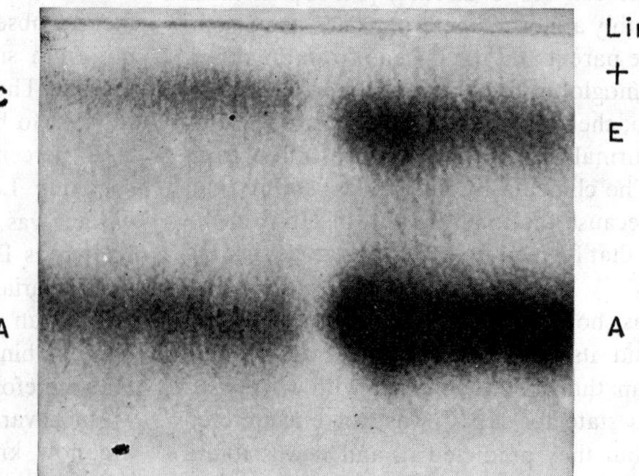

Figure 57-10. A comparison of Hb C and Hb E traits. Hb E moves slightly faster than Hb C. (Paper electrophoresis at pH 8.6 barbiturate buffer.)

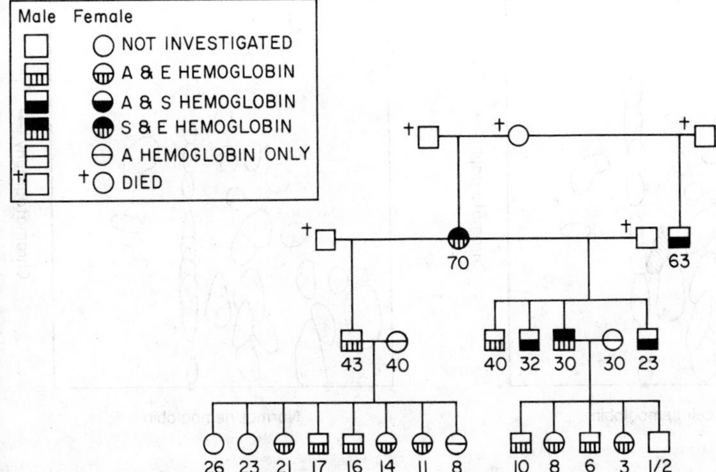

Figure 57-11. The inheritance pattern in a family with Hb A, S, and E. For further discussion see text. (*By permission of Aksoy et al.* [96].)

it was found that this occurred in the same (the β) peptide chain in Hb S, Hb C, and Hb E [98]. Hemoglobins S, C, E and one of the D variants are the common abnormal variants occurring in millions of men in Africa and Asia; following their characterization other human hemoglobins have been described, many of them rare. Their classification will be discussed later, but it may be appropriate at this stage to describe the molecular changes which underlie the variations in the globin molecule.

The Chemistry of the Hemoglobin Variants

Ingram's finding that the difference between Hb A and Hb S is in the amino acid sequence of the polypeptide chains forming the globin molecule resulted in an entirely new insight into the nature of protein polymorphism. At that time it was equally possible that the explanation might lie in a physical difference, for example in a difference in "folding" of the polypeptide chains such as has been suggested recently to account for minor myoglobin components [22]. It was not realized then that the shape of a polypeptide chain and its amino acid sequence were dependent on each other [48, 99] and that one might one day deduce the tertiary structure of a protein from its amino acid composition and arrangement, just as one might one day conclude from the shape of a polypeptide chain the nature of some of the amino acid sequences.

Indications of a difference in the free carboxylic residues such as aspartyl or glutamyl along the polypeptide chains had come from an ingenious differential titration by means of paper electrophoresis [100, 101]. It had been calculated from the differences in isoelectric points that Hb S differs from Hb A by possessing two to four more net positive charges per molecule [51]. Scheinberg et al. [100, 101] brought forward evidence that the difference is due to a smaller free carboxylic group content in Hb S. On electrophoresis at pH 11.7, the two pigments differ in their mobility, and since lysine and arginine would lose their electric charge at pH 11.7, the difference cannot be due to one of the free amino groups. On the other hand, at pH 4 and below, free carboxylic groups would lose their charge; at this pH, Hb A and S fail to differ on electrophoresis. From this it could be concluded that Hb S carries a smaller number of aspartic or glutamic acid residues, or both. Such a difference of overall charge could have been due to an arrangement by which the globins were chemically identical but differed in the arrangements of the polypeptide chains, so that fewer free carboxylic groups could influence the overall charge in Hb S. Or it could have been due to a difference in chemical nature, Hb S possessing a lesser number of free carboxylic groups. Since one molecule consists of 574 amino acids, such a small difference in amino acid composition might well have been thought impossible to establish. As the hemoglobin molecule consists of two identical halves, it would not have been necessary to look for a difference in all 574 amino acids, but only in 287 of them, but that is still a formidable number. In spite of this there was an indication that valine was involved, although at the time this result was thought possibly to be artifactual [102]. Ingram therefore decided to break down the molecule by tryptic digestion and to examine the smaller components separately [103, 104]. Trypsin hydrolysis breaks peptide chains where the amino acids lysine and arginine occur, but nowhere else. Since there are 27 molecules of lysine and arginine in each half molecule of globin, the digested protein resolves into 28 short amino acid chains (Fig. 57-12). These peptides were separated in one direction by electrophoresis and in another by chromatography on the same large sheet of paper [105]. These maps, or "fingerprints," of the hemoglobin molecule split into small peptide components permitted detection of small differences between specific peptide fragments of Hb A and Hb S. Of the 28 peptide spots, all but one were identical in the two fingerprints. Hunt and Ingram found that this peptide contained eight amino acids. Seven of these were identical in both peptides, but one, the sixth, was glutamic acid in Hb

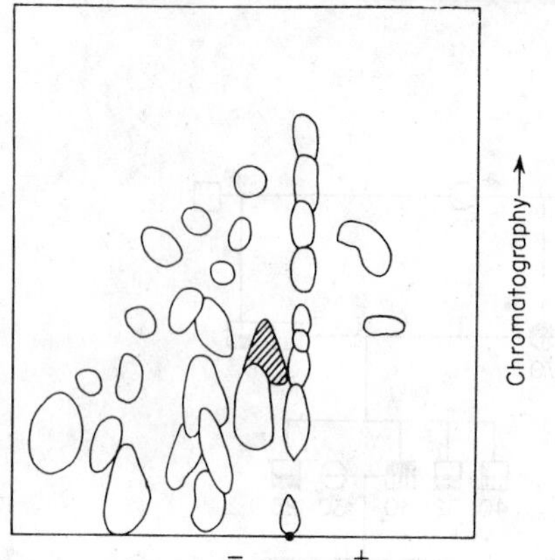

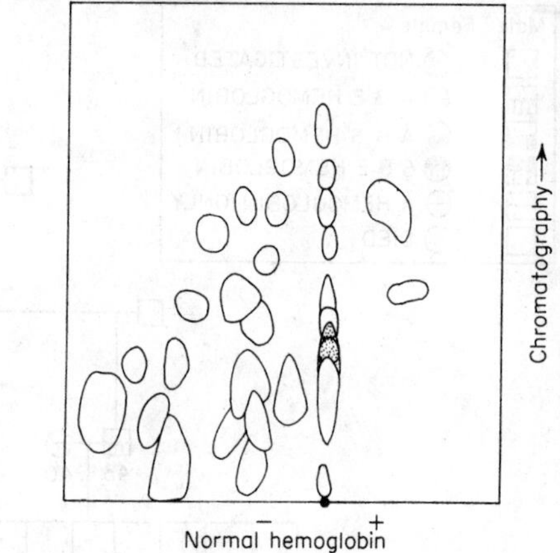

Figure 57-12. A fingerprint of the polypeptides from Hb A (*right*) and from Hb S (*left*). Electrophoresis was performed from left to right, and chromatography vertically. Note that the peptides all correspond, except for one indicated by the shaded area. (*By permission of V. M. Ingram* [103].)

A and valine in Hb S [101]. This observation confirmed independently and indeed brilliantly the earlier predictions of Pauling et al. [51] and Scheinberg et al. [100, 101] that the charge difference between the two proteins could be due to a loss of two carboxylic residues in Hb S, and showed that this variation was of a chemical rather than a positional character. The low solubility of Hb S in its reduced state was not explained by Ingram, but he pointed out that the solubility of a protein depends upon the distribution of positive and negative charges upon its surface. Amino acids with uncharged nonpolar hydrophobic side chains are found in the center of the globin. In contrast, hydrophilic amino acids with either charged or polar side chains aggregate on the exterior surface [48]. Because the charged and polar groups attract the surrounding water molecules, the hemeglobin unit is normally extremely soluble. A change in surface charge pattern through the removal of a charged glutamic acid and its replacement with a hydrophobic valine could result in aggregation of the hemoglobin molecules together and precipitation out of solution [51, 107, 108].

Ingram's clarification of the chemical difference between the two hemoglobins also indicated for the first time just how a gene might act in the synthesis of polymorphic proteins, for the only alteration caused by the Hb S mutation was the substitution of one in 287 amino acids.

When Hb C was examined by the same methods [109], it was seen that again the same peptide was affected. In this case two others had taken its place. This indicated that Hb C possesses an arginine or lysine where Hb A and S have no bond that can be attacked by trypsin. It was then found that the glutamic acid of Hb A and the valine of Hb S are replaced by lysine in Hb C. Thus a negative charge lost in Hb S is replaced by a positive charge in Hb C. This difference explains the electrophoretic behavior of Hb C, which on electrophoresis at alkaline pH (8.6) migrates behind Hb A toward the positive pole about twice as slowly as Hb S. A change from glutamic acid to lysine involves a difference of two units of electric charge. Furthermore, these findings reinforce the genetic evidence that the two mutations occur in the same place on the gene, since they affect the same amino acid. These findings are summarized in Table 57-2. An investigation of three samples of hemoglobin D already referred to [90] demonstrated the fallacy of identifying a hemoglobin on the basis of its electrophoretic properties alone. With the exception of glutamic acid → lysine and lysine → glutamic acid mutations (see Figs. 57-13 and 57-19, Table 57-3, and page 1420), the electrophoretic position does not pinpoint which of the many amino acids may be involved. The electrophoretic position is merely an indication of the charge change resulting from the amino acid substitution. For example, it has already been mentioned that the position occupied by Hb S and the many Hb D's after paper or starch-gel electrophoresis are identical [87, 88]. This is not surprising because this position (Fig 57-13) merely indicates that there has been an amino acid substitution which has given a single increased unit of positivity. In the case of Hb S, a negatively charged glutamic acid has been replaced by a neutral valine [106]. In the case of D_{Punjab}, a negatively charged glutamic acid has been replaced by a neutral glutamine [110]. In the case of D_{Ibadan}, a neutral threonine has been replaced by a positively charged lysine [111]. A fifth amino acid, histidine, carries only a *weak* positive charge (which is suppressed at alkaline pH) and plays an important part in the function of the hemoglobin molecule as a buffer. Since electrophoresis merely detects a charge change in a polypeptide chain it follows that a hemoglobin variant, detectable on electrophoresis at alkaline

Table 57-2. AMINO ACID SEQUENCE IN PEPTIDE NO. 1

Hemoglobin	*β* chain
A	Val-His-Leu-Thr-Pro-Glu^--Glu-Lys
S	Val-His-Leu-Thr-Pro-Val-Glu-Lys
C	Val-His-Leu-Thr-Pro-Lys^+-Glu-Lys

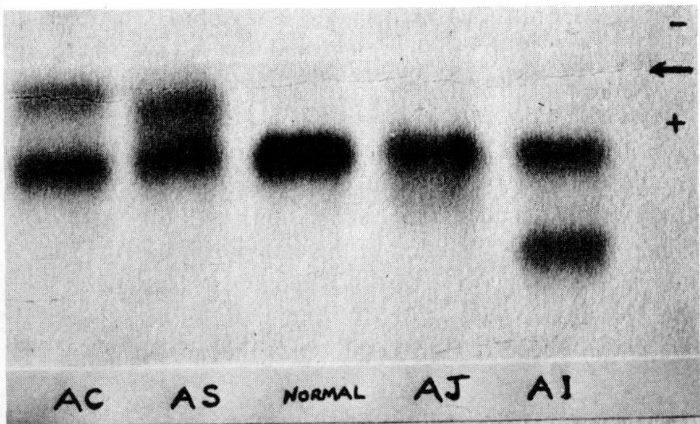

Figure 57-13. Paper electrophoresis (tris buffer) of a variety of hemoglobins selected because of the varied charge differences resulting from the specific amino acid substitutions involved.

pH, must have an amino acid substitution involving one of the four strongly charged amino acids (see Fig. 57-13). Hemoglobin Köln (see section on Unstable Hemoglobins) is detectable on electrophoresis because of an altered polypeptide chain configuration.

Of the 20 amino acids occuring in the hemoglobin polypeptide chains, only 4 carry *strong* charges on their side chains throughout a wide range of pH:

Lysine, Arginine } positive charge Glutamic acid, Aspartic acid } negative charge

Ingram and his collaborators now went further and determined in which of the two polypeptide chains, α or β, the amino acid sequence was altered [106, 112]. The results made it clear that the peptides with the alterations for S, C, D_{Punjab}, and E are parts of the β chain (Fig. 57-14). Thus, the α chains of Hb A, S, C, D_{Punjab}, and E are all identical and normal. In contrast the peptide which carries the differences found in the original Hb I belongs to the α chain [114]. It therefore follows that the β chains of Hb A and this are identical and normal.

Table 57-3. CHARGE CHANGES ACCOMPANYING CERTAIN AMINO ACID SUBSTITUTIONS

Hemoglobin	Amino acid substitution		Position	Charge change
C	Glu (−)	Lys (+)	β 6	2+
S	Glu (−)	Val (0)	β 6	+
J	Gly (0)	Asp (−)	α 15	−
I	Lys (+)	Glu (−)	α 59	2−

Note: (1) Amino acid substitutions involving 2+ and 1+ changes (i.e., C and S) are poorly distinguished on the tris buffer paper electrophoretic system used. (2) All D hemoglobins (e.g., D_{Punjab} β 121, Glu → Gln) have an amino acid substitution resulting in a gain of one unit of positivity and occupy on paper and starch-gel electrophoresis an identical position to Hb S. They can easily be distinguished on agar-gel electrophoresis (see Fig. 57-15*B*). (3) All hemoglobin variants which have a 2+ or 2− charge change must be due to Lys ⇌ Glu substitutions. The genetic code (Fig. 57-19 and text) does not allow Lys ⇌ Asp, Arg ⇌ Glu, Arg ⇌ Asp substitutions with only one change of DNA base.

This work found full confirmation from some ingenious "hybridization" experiments carried out by Itano and Schroeder, and their respective collaborators. Singer and Itano [115] had observed that human hemoglobin dissociates at pH 4.3 into two unequal halves. One might have expected to find the two symmetrical half molecules which had been recognized in x-ray studies, each consisting of one α and one β chain: $\alpha\beta$ and $\alpha\beta$. However, at acid pH the two halves which were obtained were asymmetrical and consisted of the two α chains and the two β chains, respectively: α_2 and β_2. The dissociation of the hemoglobin molecule has been intensively studied [116], and it appears that this could well occur in two stages: $\alpha_2\beta_2 \rightarrow \alpha\beta + \alpha\beta \rightarrow \alpha_2 + \beta_2$. When mixtures of Hb A and Hb S [115, 117] were submitted to this dissociation of the chains and when these were then recombined by changing the pH from acid to alkaline, the subunits of the globin molecule combined indiscriminately. The α chains from Hb A ($\alpha_2{}^A$) combined both with the β chains from Hb A ($\beta_2{}^A$) and from Hb S ($\beta_2{}^S$), and vice versa. Of the four possible combinations, only those with the β chains of Hb S had the properties of sickle-cell hemoglobin, regardless of whether the α chains were derived from Hb A or Hb S. Thus both from Ingram's direct analysis and from the hybridization studies, it may be concluded that the α chains of Hb A and Hb S are interchangeable. A logical next step was to attempt hybridization of an abnormal α chain with an abnormal β chain, in order to see whether this would result in a new and hitherto unobserved hemoglobin. Itano succeeded in preparing such pigments by dissociating and recombining mixtures of Hb I, S, and C [118], and was even able to combine the asymmetrical subunits of human and canine hemoglobin molecules, producing thereby two new hemoglobins [119].

Independent Genetic Control of α and β Chains

At that time Smith and Torbert [120] published a family tree in which both Hb S with its abnormality in the β chain and a new Hb (Hopkins II) with its abnormality in the α chain were found to segregate. In one individual, three hemoglobins were found: Hb A, Hb S, and Hb Hopkins II. From this they concluded that Hb S and Hb Hopkins II could not be alleles and that there were at least two independent genes controlling the production of adult hemoglobin. Ingram suggested that the two hemoglobin genes might correspond to the two peptide chains of human globin, one determining the α chain, and the other the β chain.

Itano and Robinson [119] found by dissociation and recombination that the individual with Hb A, S, and Hopkins

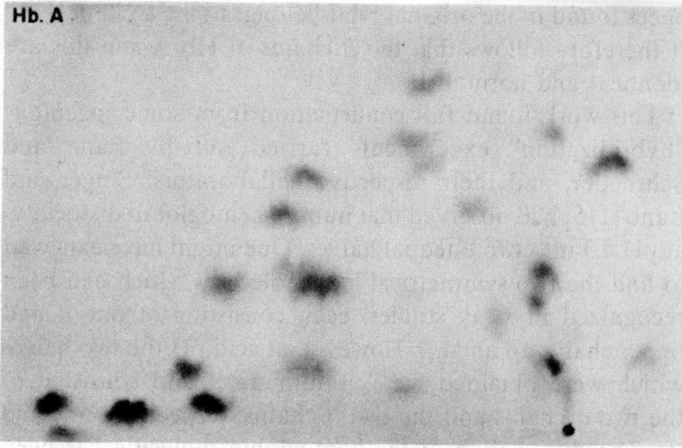

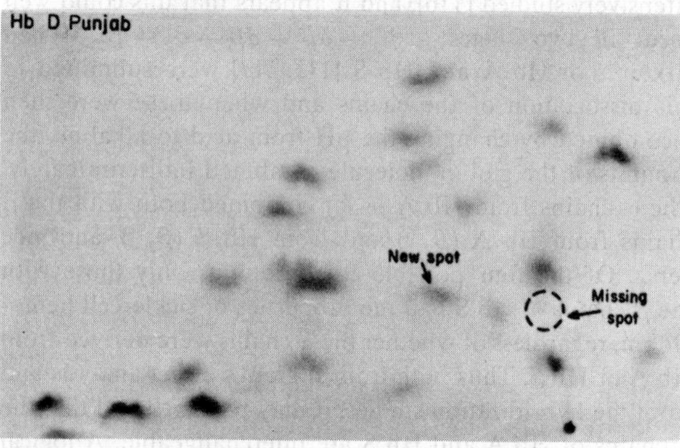

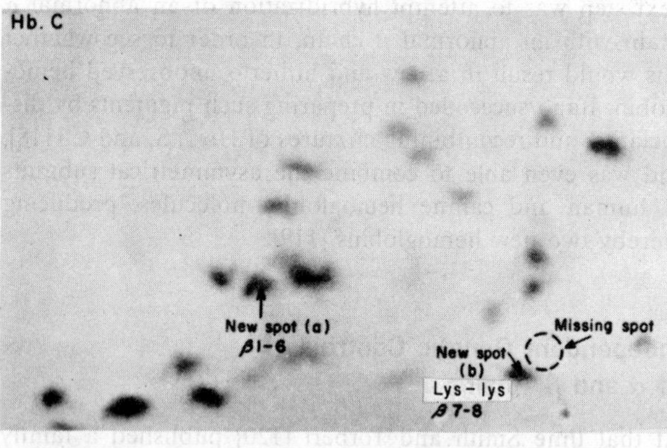

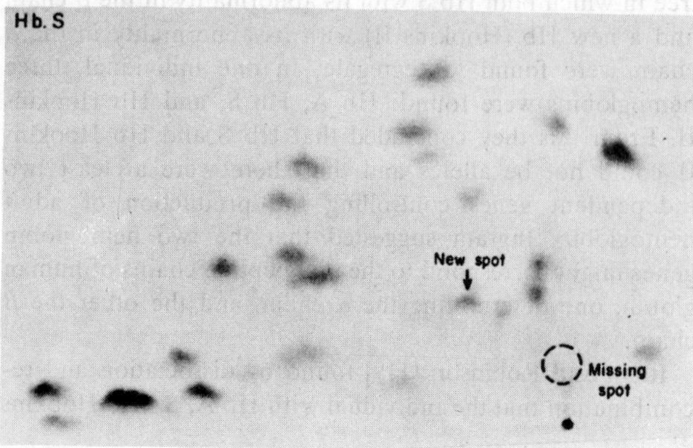

II possessed in fact a fourth hemoglobin. Hemoglobin Hopkins II was an α-chain abnormal variant, and the fourth hemoglobin was a mixture of the abnormal α chains of Hb Hopkins II and the β chain of Hb S. Hemoglobin Hopkins II is as fast on electrophoresis at pH 8.6 as Hb S is slow, compared with Hb A. The doubly abnormal hybrid, Hb Hopkins II-S, had therefore the same mobility as Hb A. When the "Hb A" fraction of this individual was dissociated and recombined, some of the β^S chains formed Hb S with the normal α chains of Hb A, and some of the $\alpha^{\text{Hopkins II}}$ chains formed Hb Hopkins II with the normal β chains.

Normal α-chain gene + normal β-chain gene = Hb A
Abnormal α-chain gene + normal β-chain gene = Hb Hopkins II
Normal α-chain gene + abnormal β-chain gene = Hb S
Abnormal α-chain gene + abnormal β-chain gene = Hb Hopkins II-S (doubly abnormal hybrid)

Four different hemoglobins in one individual could be easily demonstrated by electrophoresis when both the abnormal α and β chains were slow moving. Their combination into a doubly abnormal hybrid resulted in doubly slow-moving hemoglobin which could be demonstrated without difficulty. The two slow-moving hemoglobins were Hb $G_{\text{Philadelphia}}$ ($\alpha_2{}^G\beta_2$) and Hb C ($\alpha_2\beta_2{}^C$), and this situation was found independently in a United States Negro and a West Indian family, respectively. The four hemoglobins found were hemoglobin G ($\alpha_2{}^G\beta_2$), hemoglobin C ($\alpha_2\beta_2{}^C$), normal adult hemoglobin ($\alpha_2\beta_2$), and a doubly abnormal hybrid ($\alpha_2{}^G\beta_2{}^C$) [121–123].

All these findings fully supported Ingram's new genetic interpretation of two independent genes controlling the α chain and β chain, respectively [112]. On the basis of this theory it should be comparatively easy to determine the genotype of the carrier of an abnormal hemoglobin. A fingerprint would show whether the alteration occurs in a peptide belonging to the α or to the β chain. Further, hybridization with Hb S or C (β-chain mutation) would result in a new abnormal hybrid if the hemoglobin under test were the outcome of an α-chain mutation. Hybridization with Hb I or $G_{\text{Philadelphia}}$ (α-chain mutations) similarly would give a new abnormal hemoglobin hybrid if the tested pigment were the result of a β-chain mutation. By this method a considerable number of variants could be classified [124]. The situation as explained at the commencement of this chapter is likely to be more complex, with the probable duplication of the α-chain gene [47].

Figure 57-14. Peptide analysis of Hb A, C, D_{Punjab}, and S. The alterations are in the β chain. The top figure is a fingerprint of Hb A. Note the missing spots and the new spots in the other hemoglobins. The interpretation of fingerprints is discussed in Lehmann and Huntsman [113].

The Rare Hemoglobins

Following the discovery of Hb S, Hb C, Hb D, and Hb E, less common hemoglobin variants were described. At first they were classified according to their electrophoretic mobility.

In 1953 Chernoff and his colleagues [125] proposed that for mnemonic reasons the following letters be assigned to hemoglobins known at the time:

F, fetal hemoglobin
A, normal adult hemoglobin
S, sickle-cell hemoglobin

Later Singer [126] proposed that the letter M should be used for the abnormal methemoglobin of Hörlein and Weber [51]. All other hemoglobins which might be discovered later were to be known by letters of the alphabet in the order of their discovery beginning with the letter C (b or B had at one time been used for the sickle-cell hemoglobin). Difficulties arose when different hemoglobins were given the same letter by their discoverers, or when two or more designations were suggested for the same hemoglobin.

In 1956 Robinson et al. [127] suggested a way out of this dilemma by naming two hemoglobins "Liberian I" and "Liberian II," after the place where they had been discovered.

It was finally decided to discontinue naming new variants by letters, and at present only the letters A to Q and the letter S, with the exception of B, are in use. All other hemoglobins are given names of the hospital, area, or country where they were discovered; family names and names of communities have also been used.

These hemoglobins, with the exception of the Hb M's and the unstable hemoglobins (see later) have been discovered because they showed electrophoretic properties different from hemoglobin A. For every amino acid substitution resulting in an electrophoretically demonstrable charge (e.g., Glu $\rightarrow$ Val in Hb S) there would be many more in which one neutral amino acid in the peptide chain is substituted by another neutral amino acid. Such a substitution would not be demonstrable by electrophoresis, because there has been no alteration of electrical charge.

That hemoglobins with identical electrophoretic properties need not have identical amino acid substitutions has already been discussed [90]. Once this was appreciated, attempts were made to differentiate hemoglobins by means other than electrophoresis on paper or starch gel at alkaline pH. Electrophoresis at varying pH and chromatography on Amberlite IRC 50 were found to be useful [128] in differentiating hemoglobins which have closely similar electrophoretic properties at alkaline pH. At the present time only agar-gel electrophoresis at pH 6 [129] is widely used to differentiate hemoglobins which occupy similar positions on paper or starch-gel electrophoresis at alkaline pH (Fig. 57-15 A and B).

Facilities for peptide analysis of "fingerprinting" are now much more readily available. As a result, the exact amino acid substitution is now usually ascertained prior to the publication of a new variant. Hemoglobin variants are now tabulated according to the position in a particular polypeptide chain, where the amino acid substitution has occurred. Sickle hemoglobin would then become $\alpha_2\beta_2^{6\,\mathrm{Glu}\rightarrow\mathrm{Val}}$ or $\alpha_2\beta_2^{6\,\mathrm{Val}}$, i.e., a valine has been substituted for glutamic acid in the 6th position of the β chain.

Thus there are at present two types of nomenclature for hemoglobin variants. The more important is the chemical nomenclature which can be applied when the mutational change in a variant has been defined chemically [130, 131]. This step has by now been taken for about 100 hemoglobin variants (Table 57-4).

The great majority of variants have been found in the α or β chains of adult hemoglobin. This only represents the ease of surveying and detecting such variants. Adult blood samples are easy to obtain and the detection of variants requires no expert technical skills. In contrast, γ-chain variants have to be found in the blood of neonates (commonly blood "milked" from the umbilical cord) and δ-chain variants are found at levels of only about 1 percent of the total hemoglobin present, their detection therefore requiring some expertise. Schroeder [248] has repeatedly warned that the mere search for an abnormal peptide and the finding of one difference in its amino acid sequence do not represent the complete examination of a hemoglobin. Such an investigation requires the determination of all amino acid sequences, step by step, of both the α and the β chains.

Table 57-4 lists the variants known at present which have been defined according to the position of their mutation change in the α, β, γ, or δ polypeptide chains. An examination of Fig. 57-4 demonstrates that it is possible to equate one amino acid position with another. In this figure homologous amino acids are boxed together. It is apparent that, because of the Braunitzer gaps, such amino acids may have a different number if their position is enumerated by counting from the amino terminal end of the polypeptide chain. For example the two histidines, between which the heme group is slung (crosshatched in Fig. 57-4), are residues 58 and 87 in the α chain and residues 63 and 92 in the β, γ, and δ chains. In order to overcome this difficulty, it is more logical to enumerate an amino acid according to the position it occupies in the helical or nonhelical parts of the molecule (see Fig. 57-16) [48, 249]. The helical segments are labeled A, B, C, etc. The nonhelical segment is given the letter of the preceding and following helix, e.g., the nonhelical segment between helix A and helix B is labeled AB. The few nonhelical amino acids at the commencement and termination of the polypeptide chain are referred to as NA and HC, respectively. If one examines Table 57-4 it will be seen that, with this nomenclature, the two histidine residues mentioned above would be labeled E7 and F8 (i.e., they are the 7th residue in the E helix and the 8th residue in the F helix), irrespective of whether they occur in the α, β, γ, or δ chain of hemoglobin or even in myoglobin.

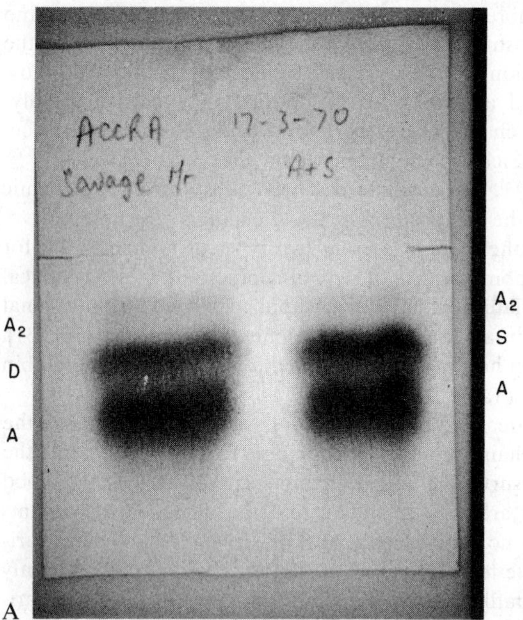

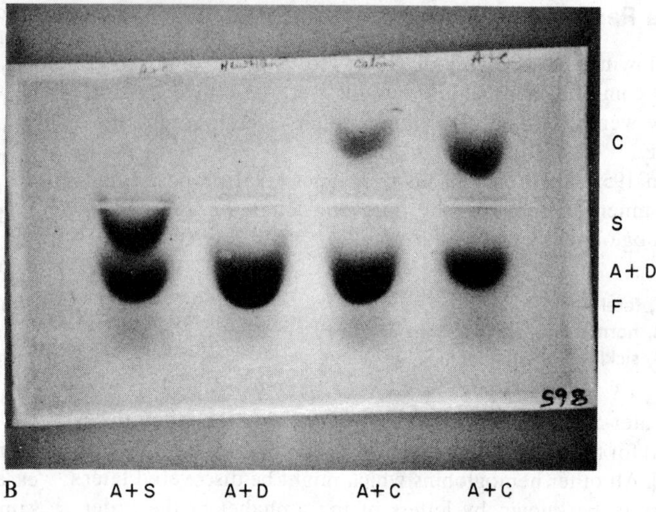

Figure 57-15. A. Paper electrophoresis (tris buffer, alkaline pH) of (*left*) blood from a heterozygote of Hb A and Hb D_{Punjab} and (*right*) blood from a heterozygote of Hb A and Hb S. As hemoglobins D and S occupy similar positions, they cannot be distinguished by this technique. B. Agar-gel electrophoresis (pH 6) of (*left to right*) heterozygotes of hemoglobins A and S, A and D_{Punjab}, and A and C (two). As hemoglobins A and D do not separate on this electrophoretic system, heterozygotes of hemoglobins A and D are easily distinguished from those of A and S. If agar gel were used as the initial electrophoretic screening system, D_{Punjab} would not be detected.

Since all three hemoglobins A, A_2, and F contain α chains, an α-chain abnormality will be reflected in all three, and heterozygotes with a normal and an abnormal α-chain hemoglobin, $\alpha_2{}^x\beta_2$, will possess two hemoglobins A_2, one $\alpha_2\delta_2$, and one $\alpha_2{}^x\delta_2$. This was shown for Hb $G_{Philadelphia}$, and Hb Norfolk [150, 249*a*]. At birth they will possess two fetal hemoglobins: $\alpha_2\gamma_2$ and $\alpha_2{}^x\gamma_2$ [249*b*].

In addition to the hemoglobins listed in Table 57-4, there are others known which have been identified only by their electrophoretic properties or in which the abnormal peptide chain has been identified by hybridization experiments but not yet by its exact amino acid substitution.

THE M HEMOGLOBINS

Oxyhemoglobin donates O_2 to the tissues and thereby becomes deoxyhemoglobin when the oxygen pressure in the blood falls. Methemoglobin cannot give up O_2 in this manner, and however low the blood oxygen pressure, methemoglobin remains in the oxidized state with its heme iron in the trivalent (ferric) form. It was thought that methemoglobin represented the "oxidized" form of hemoglobin while oxyhemoglobin was merely "oxygenated," a reduced hemoglobin with the iron in the ferrous state but differing from deoxyhemoglobin by having an oxygen molecule attached to its divalent (ferrous) heme iron. It is now known from studies on myoglobin [250] that in oxyhemoglobin an electron is transferred from the divalent iron to the oxygen molecule, and that in oxyhemoglobin the iron atom is therefore trivalent. One can assume that the same occurs in hemoglobin, and that as in oxymyoglobin, so in oxyhemoglobin the electron is transferred back to the heme iron when the oxygen leaves the hemoglobin to enter the tissue, so that in deoxyhemoglobin the iron is again in the ferrous state.

Oxyhemoglobin and methemoglobin differ in their ability to become deoxyhemoglobin, because water is present in the heme pocket of methemoglobin and absent in that of the oxyhemoglobin [251, 252]. The water permits the iron atom to become stabilized in the ferric form, and only a chemical reaction can reduce the ferric heme to ferrous heme. In oxyhemoglobin the oxygen can be removed by the physical process of lowering the oxygen pressure.

The hereditary methemoglobinemias can be divided into two major groups. In one the methemoglobin is normal, but there is a genetically determined deficiency of the enzymes

Table 57-4. LIST OF KNOWN HEMOGLOBIN SUBSTITUTIONS AND DELETIONS

Reference number	Amino acid position	Substitution	Name	Helical number	Reference number	Amino acid position	Substitution	Name
		α-chain variants					*β-chain variants*	
[132]	5	Ala → Asp	$\text{J}_{\text{Toronto}}$	NA2	[174]	2	His → Tyr	Tokuchi
				A3	[175]	6	Glu → Val	S
				A3	[86]	6	Glu → Lys	C
				A3 or A4	[176]	6 or 7	Glu → (deleted)	Leiden
				A4	[177]	7	Glu → Gly	$\text{G}_{\text{San Jose}}$
				A4	[178]	7	Glu → Lys	Siriraj
				A6	[179]	9	Ser → Cys	Porto Alegre
[133]	12	Ala → Asp	J_{Paris}	A10				
				A11	[180]	14	Leu → Arg	Sogn
[134]	15	Gly → Asp	J_{Oxford}	A13	[181]	16	Gly → Asp	$\text{J}_{\text{Baltimore}}$
				A13	[182]	16	Gly → Arg	$\text{D}_{\text{Bushman}}$
[135]	16	Lys → Glu	I	A14				
				A15	[183]	17	Lys → Glu	Nagasaki
[136]	22	Gly → Asp	$\text{J}_{\text{Medellin}}$	B3				
[137]	23	Glu → Gln	Memphis	B4	[184, 185]	22	Glu → Ala	$\text{G}_{\text{Coushatta}}$
[138]	23	Glu → Val	$\text{G}_{\text{Audhali}}$	B4	[186]	22	Glu → Lys	$\text{E}_{\text{Saskatoon}}$
[139]	23	Glu → Lys	Chad	B4	[187]	22	Glu → Gly	Taipei
				B5	[188]	23	Val → (deleted)	$\text{M}_{\text{Freiburg}}$
				B6	[189]	24	Gly → Arg	Riverdale-Bronx
				B7	[190]	25	Gly → Arg	$\text{G}_{\text{Taiwan-Ami}}$
				B8	[94]	26	Glu → Lys	E
				B10	[191]	28	Leu → Pro	Genova
[140]	30	Glu → Gln	$\text{G}_{\text{Chinese}}$ (Honolulu)	B11				
				B12	[192]	30	Arg → Ser	Tacoma
				C1	[193]	35	Tyr → Phe	Philly
				C3	[194]	37	Tyr → Ser	Hirose
[141]	43	Phe → Val	Torino	CD1	[195]	42	Phe → Ser	Hammersmith
				CD2	[196]	43	Glu → Ala	$\text{G}_{\text{Galveston}}$
[142]	47	Asp → Gly	$\text{L}_{\text{Ferrara}}$	CD5	[197]	46	Gly → Glu	K_{Ibadan}
[143]	47	Asp → His	Hasharon	CD5				
				CD6	[198]	47	Asp → Asn	$\text{G}_{\text{Copenhagen}}$
[144]	50	His → Asp	$\text{J}_{\text{Sardegna}}$	CD8				
[145]	51	Gly → Arg	Russ	CD9				
[146]	51	Gly → Asp	$\text{J}_{\text{Abidjan}}$	CD9				
				D3	[199]	52	Asp → Asn	Osu Christiansborg
				D7	[165]	56	Gly → Asp	$\text{J}_{\text{Bangkok}}$
				E2	[198a]	58	Pro → Arg	Dhofar
[147]	54	Gln → Arg	Shimonoseki	E3	[199a]	59	Lys → Glu	1-High Wycombe
[148]	54	Gln → Glu	Mexico	E3				
				E5	[200]	61	Lys → Glu	$\text{N}_{\text{Seattle}}$
				E5	[201]	61	Lys → Asn	Hikari
[149]	57	Gly → Arg	$\text{L}_{\text{Persian Gulf}}$	E6				

Table 57-4. *(Continued)*

Reference number	Amino acid position	Substitution	Name	Helical number	Reference number	Amino acid position	Substitution	Name
		α-chain variants					*β-chain variants*	
[150]	57	Gly → Asp	Norfolk	E6				
[151]	58	His → Tyr	M_{Boston}	E7	[151]	63	His → Tyr	$M_{Saskatoon}$
				E7	[202]	63	His → Arg	Zurich
[152]	60	Lys → Asn	Zambia	E9				
				E10	[203]	66	Lys → Glu	$I_{Toulouse}$
				E11	[151]	67	Val → Glu	$M_{Milwaukee}$
				E11	[204]	67	Val → Ala	Sydney
				E11	[205]	67	Val → Asp	Bristol
				E13	[198]	69	Gly → Asp	$J_{Cambridge}$
[153]	68	Asn → Lys	$G_{Philadelphia}$	E17	[206]	73	Asp → Asn	Korle Bu
[154]	68	Asn → Asp	Ube II	E17				
				A3		6	Glu → Val	C_{Harlem}
				E17	[207]	73	Asp → Asn	
				E18	[208]	74	Gly → Asp	Shepherds Bush
				E20	[209]	76	Ala → Glu	Seattle
				EF1	[210]	77	His → Asp	J_{Iran}
[155]	74	Asp → His	$Q_{(S.E. Asia)}$	EF3				
[156]	75	Asp → His	$Q_{(Iran)}$	EF4	[211]	80	Asn → Lys	G_{Szuhu}
[157]	78	Asn → Lys	Stanleyville II	EF7				
[158]	80	Leu → Arg	Ann Arbor	F1				
				F3	[111]	87	Thr → Lys	D_{Ibadan}
				F4	[212]	88	Leu → Pro	Santa Ana
				F4	[213]	88	Leu → Arg	Boras
[159]	84	Ser → Arg	Etobicoke	F5				
[160]	85	Asp → Asn	$G_{Norfolk}$	F6	[214]	90	Glu → Lys	Agenogi
[161]	85	Asp → Tyr	Atago	F6				
				F7	[215]	91	Leu → Pro	Sabine
[162]	87	His → Tyr	M_{Iwate}	F8	[216]	92	His → Tyr	$M_{Hyde Park}$
				FG1	[217]	94	Asp → Asn	Oak Ridge
[163]	90	Lys → Asn	Broussais	FG2	[218]	95	Lys → Glu	W
				F7-FG2 or F8-FG3 or F9-FG4	[219]	91–95 or 92–96 or 93–97	Deleted	Gun Hill
[164]	92	Arg → Gln	$J_{Capetown}$	FG4				
[165]	92	Arg → Leu	Chesapeake	FG4	[220]	97	His → Gln	Malmo
				FG5	[221]	98	Val → Met	Köln
				G1	[222]	99	Asp → His	Yakima
				G1	[223]	99	Asp → Asn	Kempsey
[166]	95	Pro → Leu	$G_{Georgia}$	G2	[224]	102	Asn → Thr	Kansas

Reference number	Amino acid position	Substitution	Name	Helical number	Reference number	Amino acid position	Substitution	Name
		α-chain variants					*β-chain variants*	
				G4	[225]	102	Asn → Lys	Richmond
[167]	102	Ser → Arg	Manitoba	G9	[226]	108	Asn → Asp	Yoshizuka
				G10	[227]	113	Val → Glu	New York
				G15	[228]	117	His → Arg	P
				G16				
[168]	112	His → Gln	Dakar	G19		120	Lys → Glu	Hijiyama
[148]	114	Pro → Arg	Chiapas	GH2	[229]			
[169]	115	Ala → Asp	$J_{Tongariki}$	GH3				
[170]	116	Glu → Lys	$O_{Indonesia}$	GH4	[170]	121	Glu → Lys	O_{Arab}
				GH4	[110]	121	Glu → Gln	O_{Punjab}
				H2	[172]	124	Pro → Arg	Khartoum
				H4	[230]	126	Val → Glu	Hofu
				H7	[231]	129	Ala → Asp	$J_{Taichung}$
				H8	[232]	130	Tyr → Asp	Wien
				H10	[197]	132	Lys → Gln	$K_{Woolwich}$
				H14	[233]	136	Gly → Asp	Hope
[171]	136	Leu → Pro	Bibba	H19	[220]	141	Leu → Arg	Olmsted
				H21	[235]	145	Tyr → His	Rainier
				HC2	[234]	146	His → Asp	Hiroshima
[172]	141	Arg → Pro	Singapore	HC3				
[173]	141	Arg split off on hemolysis in plasma	Koellicker	HC3				
				HC4-HC13	[236]	Additional residues at C terminal		Tak
		γ-chain variants					*δ-chain variants*	
				NA2	[243]	2	His → Arg	$A_{2\ Sphakia}$
[237]	5	Glu → Lys	$F_{Texas\ I}$	A2				
[238]	6	Glu → Lys	$F_{Texas\ II}$	A3				
[239]	12	Thr → Lys	$F_{Alexandra}$	A9	[244]	12	Asn → Lys	N.Y.U.
				A13	[245]	16	Gly → Arg	A_2'
				B4	[246]	22	Ala → Glu	$A_{2\ Flatbush}$
[240]	61	Lys → Glu	$F_{Jamaica}$ (136 Ala)	E5				
[241]	117	His → Arg	F_{Malta} (136 Gly)	G19				
[242]	121	Glu → Lys	F_{Hull}	GH4				
				H14	[247]	136	Gly → Asp	$A_{2\ Babinga}$

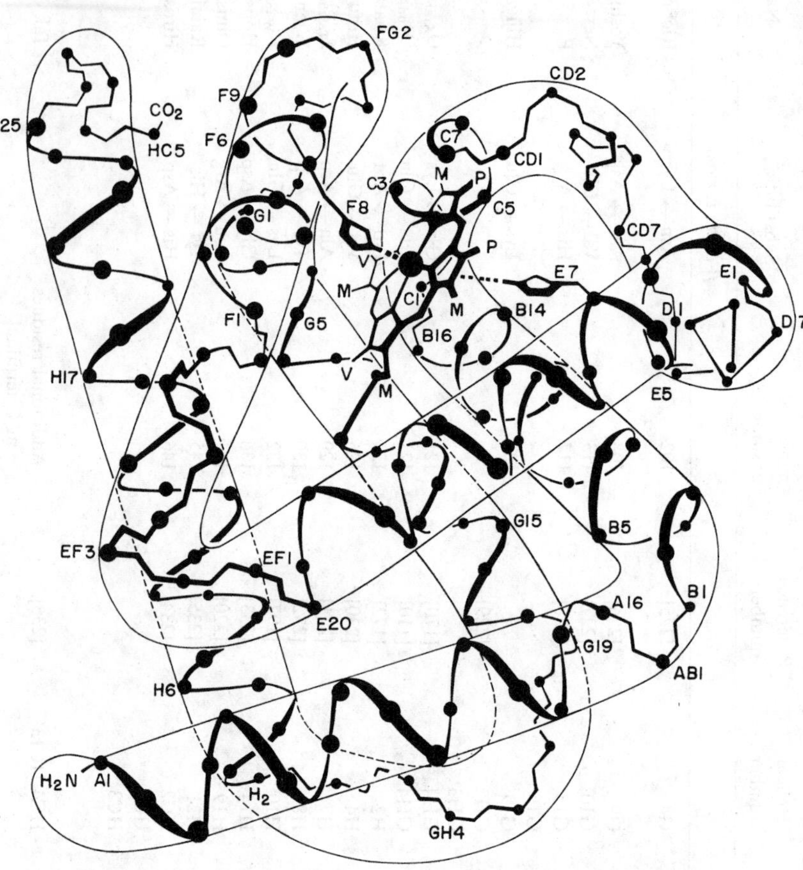

Figure 57-16. About 80 percent of amino acids in the polypeptide chains of myoglobin and hemoglobin are in a helical structure. Note the heme group between the two histidyls E7 and F8. (*By courtesy of Dr. R. E. Dickerson, published in The Proteins, Academic Press. The H helix in the original figure has been renumbered.*)

that normally reduce the traces of the methemoglobin which are constantly produced. In the other group of methemoglobinemias there is no enzymopenia but the heme is in the ferric form because the globin is abnormal and does not provide the tight hydrophobic heme pocket that protects the heme iron against stabilization in the trivalent (ferric) state. Singer [126] proposed in 1955 that the letter M should be used to denote a methemoglobin with an abnormal globin, described in 1948 by Hörlein and Weber [49].

We have already referred to the two important histidines in the α and β chains (α 58 and 87, and β 63 and 92) or, as they can be described in the helical notation, α and β E7 and α and β F8. Alpha 58 (E7) histidine and β63 (E7) histidine lie opposite the heme iron in the heme pocket but are not linked to it chemically, and accordingly are called the two distal histidines. F8 α 87 and β 92 are the positions of the two proximal histidines, so named because they are chemically linked to the heme iron. In all four positions substitutions of tyrosine for histidine can occur (Table 57-5). They all result in M hemoglobins because the phenol group

Table 57-5. THE M HEMOGLOBINS

Hemoglobin	Substitution	Position	Position to heme	Reference
Amino acid substitutions involving proximal or distal histidine				
M_{Boston}	His → Tyr	α 58 (E7)	Distal	[151]
M_{Iwate}	His → Tyr	α 87 (F8)	Proximal	[162]
$M_{Saskatoon}$	His → Tyr	β 63 (E7)	Distal	[151]
$M_{Hyde\ Park}$	His → Tyr	β 92 (F8)	Proximal	[216]
Amino acid substitutions not *involving proximal or distal histidines*				
$M_{Freiburg}$	Val → (deleted)	β 23 (B5)		[188]
$M_{Milwaukee}$	Val → Glu	β 67 (E11)		[151]

of tyrosine forms an ionic link with the iron atom and thereby stabilizes it in the ferric state [253].

A fifth Hb M is the outcome of a substitution of β 67 (Ell) valine by glutamic acid—Hb $M_{Milwaukee}$ [151]. The residue in this position points toward the heme, and a glutamic acid side chain would push the side chain of β 63 (E7) histidine out of the heme pocket and form a salt bridge with the iron atom. As in the other M hemoglobins the result would be that the iron atom becomes stabilized in the ferric form [249, 253, 254].

The four M hemoglobins in which tyrosine is substituted for histidine have different properties, not according to whether the distal or the proximal histidine is substituted, but according to whether they occur in the α or the β chain. The two β chain variants, Hb $M_{Saskatoon}$ and Hb $M_{Hyde\ Park}$, have an oxygen affinity comparable to that of Hb A, and exhibit a Bohr effect, whereas both the α-chain mutants M_{Boston} and M_{Iwate} have an abnormally low oxygen affinity and show a similarly decreased Bohr effect [255].

The M hemoglobins differ in their rate of oxidation by potassium ferricyanide or hydrogen peroxide. These properties have been reviewed by Tönz [256]: for example, the hemolysate from heterozygotes containing Hb A and Hb M_{Iwate} shows a normal rate of oxidation with potassium ferricyanide, and this can be related to the fact that in this case a prior reduction of the M fraction by sodium dithionite had not been possible, so that only the reaction of the normal Hb A was measured. Hb M_{Boston} reacts slowly with dithionite and $M_{Saskatoon}$ almost normally. Hb $M_{Hyde\ Park}$ is difficult to study in this respect because of its instability.

The hemolysates of the various heterozygotes differ in their spectroscopic properties. The usual method for estimating methemoglobin spectroscopically is that by Evelyn and Malloy [257]. The methemoglobin is treated with potassium ferricyanide to form cyanoferric hemoglobin and the change in absorption at 632 mμ is measured. Since some M hemoglobins do not react with cyanide, although the color of the blood clearly indicates the presence of methemoglobin, the method of Evelyn and Malloy will produce a negative result. To demonstrate a Hb M by spectroscopy the whole range of the spectrum has to be measured. Figure 57-17 shows the methemoglobin spectrum of Hb A and Hb M_{Boston}, Hb $M_{Saskatoon}$, and Hb Milwaukee I. Whereas in normal methemoglobin A absorbance is decreased at 600 mμ (compared with 632 mμ), no decrease is seen in Hb M_{Boston} and Hb $M_{Saskatoon}$. Since these hemolysates come from heterozygotes, and the spectra are each the outcome of mixtures of Hb A and Hb M, the abnormal M hemoglobins by themselves differ even more from methemoglobin A in their absorption at 600 mμ.

UNSTABLE HEMOGLOBINS

The stability of the hemoglobin molecule depends to a large degree on the close fit around the heme of a heme pocket lined with hydrophobic amino acid side chains. These side chains form van der Waals bonds with the heme and this bonding increases the helical contact of the molecule, and confers on it a general stability which includes heat stability [258]. Thus, whereas the heme-free globin is thermolabile and readily precipitates at 50°C, hemoglobin is quite stable at this temperature [259, 260].

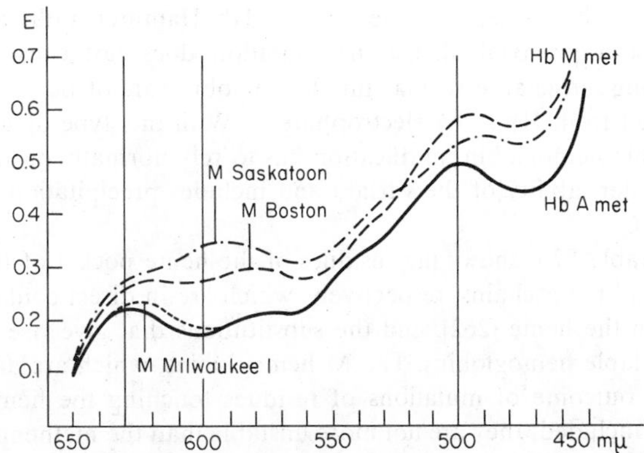

Figure 57-17. Methemoglobin spectrum in hemolysate of patients with various hemoglobin M types. (*By permission of Tönz* [256].)

Any interference with the nature of the heme pocket which results in its being less tightly fitting than in normal hemoglobin, or a substitution of nonpolar by polar residues, will allow access of water to the heme. This will result in methemoglobin formation. Methemoglobin loses its heme much more easily than oxy and deoxy hemoglobin, and as already stated, free globin is much less stable than hemoglobin. Without the heme it tends to form mixed disulfide proteins by linking β 93 cysteine with sulfhydryl groups, particularly of the cell membranes, when it then precipitates. These inclusion bodies, also called Heinz bodies, are removed by the spleen, which at the same time causes some damage to the cell membrane and thereby a reduction of the red cell life span [261].

The great majority of the unstable hemoglobins arise from mutations in the heme pocket. The first to be described was Hb Zürich β 63 (E7) histidine → arginine. Other examples are Hb Köln β 98 (FG5) valine → methionine [221] and Hb Hammersmith β 42 (CD1) phenylalanine → serine [195]. It will be noted that the histidine → arginine mutation in Hb Zürich confers an increase in positive charge. In particular, on electrophoresis at pH 8.9 arginine side chains will be positively charged, while the histidine side chain does not carry a charge at that pH. Hb Köln and Hb Hammersmith are the outcome of neutral mutations. Nevertheless, the first can be separated from Hb A by simple electrophoresis, but Hb Hammersmith cannot be so isolated. In Hb Köln the replacement of the β 98 (FG5) valine by the larger molecule methionine alters the configuration so that the molecule is more positively charged. A tendency to methemoglobin formation and heme loss also will increase the positive charge, because the acidic side chains of the heme will no longer be present. In the case of Hb Hammersmith, the neutral phenylalanine-serine mutation does not cause a change in charge so that this hemoglobin cannot be separated from Hb A by electrophoresis. With this type of unstable hemoglobin, purification has to rely normally on the greater lability of the variant and includes precipitation at 50°C.

Table 57-6 shows the residues of the heme pocket of the α and the β chains, respectively, which are in direct contact with the heme [262], and the substitutions that give rise to unstable hemoglobins. The M hemoglobins, which are also the outcome of mutations of residues touching the heme, are included; they are not more unstable than the methemoglobin of Hb A.

While the mutations of residues touching the heme are the most frequent causes of hemoglobin instability, there are also other such mutations occurring within the heme pocket, for example β 74 (E18) glycine $\rightarrow$ aspartic acid (Hb Shepherds Bush) [208], or introducing charges which alter internal arrangements, for example β 130 tyrosine $\rightarrow$ aspartic acid (Hb Wien) [232].

Deletion of amino acids distorts the conformation of the whole molecule, and as a consequence of such deletions Hb Freiburg [188], Hb Gun Hill [219], and Hb Leiden [176] are unstable.

Although the polypeptide chain may be normal, for the stability of the human hemoglobin molecule the interaction of two α and two non-α chains is necessary. Free α chains are notoriously unstable and it is thought that they precipitate in the erythrocytes of patients with β thalassemia, thereby causing a shortened life-span of these cells in the same manner as Hb Köln or Hb Hammersmith cause hemolytic anemia [263]. In α thalassemia this role is undertaken by the unstable β and γ tetramers, Hb H and Hb Bart's. The tetramers $\alpha_2\beta_2$ and the $\alpha\beta$ dimers are in equilibrium with each other (Fig. 57-18). The $\alpha_1\beta_1$ and $\alpha_2\beta_2$ contacts are "gluing" contacts, forming the $\alpha\beta$ dimer. The $\alpha_1\beta_2$ and $\alpha_2\beta_1$ contacts grip the two dimers and form a tetramer. These latter contacts undergo considerable structural alteration in the change from oxy to deoxy hemoglobin and vice versa [262]. Changes at the $\alpha_1\beta_1$ contacts may therefore lead to increased dissociation to the monomer and to precipitation.

Table 57-6. RESIDUES TOUCHING THE HEME AND THEIR SUBSTITUTIONS

Helical Number	Sequential number and residue in Hb A		Substitution		Reference number
	α	β			
B13	32 Met	31 Leu			
C4	39 Thr	38 Thr			
C7	42 Tyr	41 Phe			
CD1	43 Phe	42 Phe	α Val Torino	unstable	[141]
			β Ser Hammersmith	unstable	[195]
CD3	45 His	44 Ser			
CD4	46 Phe	45 Phe			
E7	58 His	63 His	α Tyr Boston	Hb M	[151]
			β Tyr Saskatoon	Hb M	[151]
			β Arg Zürich	unstable	[202]
E10	....	66 Lys	β Glu Toulouse		[203]
E11	62 Val	67 Val	β Tyr Milwaukee	Hb M	[151]
			β Ala Sidney	unstable	[204]
			β Asp Bristol	unstable	[205]
E14	....	70 Ser			
E15	....	71 Phe	β Ser Christchurch		[225]
F4	83 Leu	88 Leu	β Pro Santa Ana	unstable	[212]
			β Arg Borås	unstable	[213]
F7	86 Leu	91 Leu	β Pro Sabine	unstable	[215]
F8	87 His	92 His	α Tyr Iwate	Hb M	[162]
			β Tyr Hyde Park	Hb M	[216]
FG3	91 Leu	96 Leu			
FG5	93 Val	98 Val	β Met Köln	unstable	[221]
G4	97 Asn	102 Asn	β Thr Kansas	unstable	[224]
G5	98 Phe	103 Phe			
G8	101 Leu	106 Leu			
H15	132 Val	137 Val			
H19	136 Leu	141 Leu	α Pro Bibba	unstable	[171]
			β Arg Olmsted	unstable	[220]

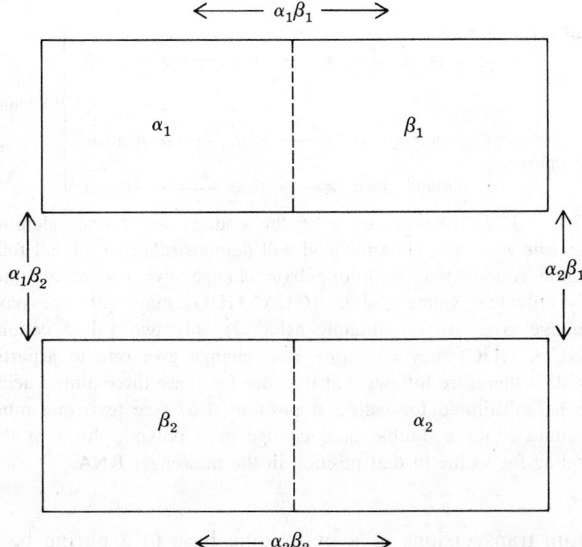

Figure 57-18. One α and one β polypeptide chain are joined together by an $\alpha_1\beta_1$ contact to form a dimer. The $\alpha_1\beta_1$ and $\alpha_2\beta_2$ dimers are joined together by an $\alpha_1\beta_2$ contact to form a tetramer. *Note:* (1) The $\alpha_1\beta_1$ and $\alpha_2\beta_2$ contact are identical. (2) The $\alpha_1\beta_2$ and $\alpha_2\beta_1$ contact are identical. (3) The expression $\alpha_2\beta_2$ normally refers to the complete tetramer containing two α and two β chains. It can refer also to the specific $\alpha_2\beta_2$ dimer as in the above figure.

This is the case in Hb Philly [193] where the $\alpha_1\beta_1$ contact is weakened by a mutation of β 35 (Cl) tyrosine → phenylalanine. The diminished affinity of the normal α chains for the β chains of Hb E [β 26 (B9) glutamic acid → lysine] [193], which has been shown to cause the low levels of Hb E in Hb AE heterozygotes with α thalassemia [264], can be related to the effect of this mutation on the $\alpha_1\beta_1$ contact at β 30 (B12) [253].

Changes in Hemoglobin Structures Affecting Oxygen Affinity

The subunits of the hemoglobin molecule move on deoxygenation, with both the α and β chains rotating, the former more than the latter [265]. Mutations at contacts between the subunits $\alpha_1\beta_2$ can be expected to affect the oxygen affinity, the Bohr effect, and the heme-heme interaction. It is not possible to draw a strict dividing line between the "unstable hemoglobins" and the hemoglobins with altered oxygen affinity, because many mutations have secondary effects in the overall structure of the tetramer. Most of the unstable hemoglobins, notably Hb Köln [221], have an increased oxygen affinity. Hb Hammersmith [195] and Hb Kansas [224], on the other hand, have a decreased oxygen affinity, and, because of cyanosis, carriers of these hemoglobins have on several occasions been provisionally designated as patients with methemoglobinemia.

As a rule all hemoglobins with alterations in or near the $\alpha_1\beta_2$ contacts—the contacts that determine the stability of the tetramer—show an increased oxygen affinity. Examples are Hb Malmö, Hb Chesapeake [166], Hb Cape Town [104], Hb Yakima [222], and Hb Kempsey [223].

A complete system to explain oxygen transport has been developed by Perutz [330]. It involves the N terminals of the α and the C terminals of the β chains. Mutations in these should alter the oxygen transport, including heme-heme interaction and the Bohr effect.

Abnormal Hemoglobins and the Genetic Code

The amino acid sequence of a polypeptide chain depends on the nucleotide sequence of the RNA along which the amino acids are assembled on the ribosomes. The code according to which a certain nucleotide sequence predetermines which amino acid is incorporated (Fig. 57-19) has been determined in virus and bacterial protein synthesis. There are four possible nucleotides in RNA: uridylic (U), guanylic (G), cytidylic (C), and adenylic (A). For example, an RNA consisting entirely of uridylic nucleotide residues results in a protein consisting entirely of phenylalanine residues. Assuming that the nucleotide code consists of three

-U-		-C-		-A-		-G-	
UUU	Phe	UCU	Ser	UAU	Tyr	UGU	Cys
UUC		UCC		UAC		UGC	
UUA	Leu	UCA	Ser	UAA	Ochre	UGA	Nonsense
UUG		UCG		UAG	Amber	UGG	Trp
CUU	Leu	CCU	Pro	CAU	His	CGU	Arg
CUC		CCC		CAC		CGC	
CUA	Leu	CCA	Pro	CAA	Gln	CGA	Arg
CUG		CCG		CAG		CGG	
AUU	Ile	ACU	Thr	AAU	Asn	AGU	Ser
AUC		ACC		AAC		AGC	
AUA	Ile	ACA	Thr	AAA	Lys	AGA	Arg
AUG	Met	ACG		AAG		AGG	
GUU	Val	GCU	Ala	GAU	Asp	GGU	Gly
GUC		GCC		GAC		GGC	
GUA	Val	GCA	Ala	GAA	Glu	GGA	Gly
GUG		GCG		GAG		GGG	

Figure 57-19. The genetic code. The code is degenerate, i.e., more than one base triplet may code for one amino acid. The Ochre and Amber triplets UAA and UAG probably terminate the polypeptide chain. The present information as regards polypeptide chain initiation and termination is nearly complete, and the genetic code has been established for eukaryotic as well as for viral and bacterial systems.

letters, the coding for phenylalanine would then be UUU (uridylic-uridylic-uridylic).

Although the genetic code was primarily derived from studies of bacterial and virus RNA, its application to man was demonstrated by its use in predicting permissible amino acid replacements in human hemoglobin [135]. It was shown that amino acid substitutions in human hemoglobin variants could all be explained on the basis of point mutations. This confinement to a single base change allows, for instance, the substitution

Lysine ⟷	glutamic acid
A A A	G A A
A A G	G A G

in which there has been an interchange of adenine and guanine. However, the substitution

Lysine ⟷	aspartic acid
A A A	G A C
A A G	G A U

is not found, since this involves a double base change. Study of the genetic code (Fig. 57-19) will demonstrate that arginine ↔ glutamic acid and arginine ↔ aspartic acid again involves a double base change. The only interchange between a positively and a negatively charged amino acid with one base change is the Lys ↔ Glu substitution (see Fig. 57-13).

No exception to the rule that variants arise from single point mutations has yet been found. Nevertheless, there may be polymorphism for the codons responsible for the same amino acid; i.e., various persons may have different codons at a certain base triplet position in the messenger RNA, and yet these codons will code for the same amino acid and there will be no alteration in the polypeptide chain constructed. For example CUA, which codes for leucine, can undergo nine point mutations involving any one of the three bases, and four of the resulting triplets will still code for leucine. The same valine residue in the chain is replaced by alanine in Hb Sydney [204], glutamic acid in Hb Milwaukee [151], and aspartic acid in Hb Bristol [205]. For these three substitutions to be point mutations, one has to assume a polymorphism for the valine at position β 67 (see Fig. 57-20). Of the four DNA bases, two, adenine and guanine, are purine bases and two, thymine (or uracil in RNA) and cytosine, are pyrimidine bases. A substitution of one purine for another (A ⇌ G) or a pyrimidine for a pyrimidine (T ⇌ C) is called *transition.* A substitution of a purine for a pyrimidine (A → C, A → T, G → C, and G → T) and a pyrimidine for a purine (T → A, T → G, C → A, and C → G) is called *transversion.*

It is of interest to compare the number of variants arising from transversions in the DNA with those caused by transitions. In terms of messenger RNA, which has a uracil in place of the thymine of DNA, each base can undergo two transversions (A ⇌ C, A ⇌ U, G ⇌ C, G ⇌ U) but only one transition (A ⇌ G, U ⇌ C). The number of variants, arising

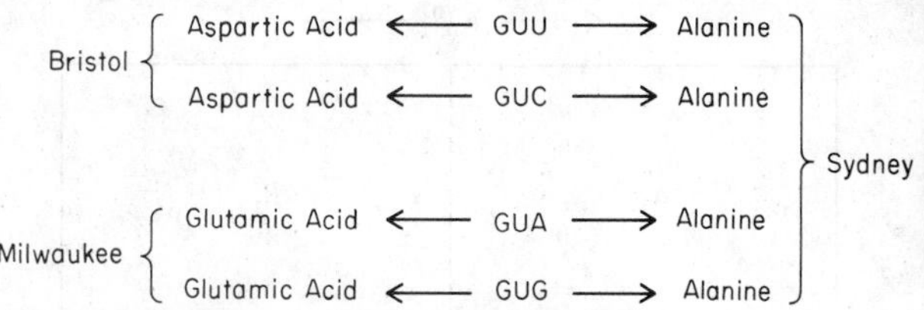

Figure 57-20. Examination of the codons for valine, alanine, aspartic acid, and glutamic acid will demonstrate that, (1) all four valine codons may with one base change give rise to alanine, (2) only two valine codons (GUA, GUG) may with one base change give rise to glutamic acid, (3) only two valine codons (GUU, GUC) may with one base change give one to aspartic acid. It therefore follows that in order for these three amino acids to be substituted for valine at position β 67 (see text) one must assume either a double base change or a polymorphism in the coding for valine in that position in the messenger RNA.

from transversions of a pyrimidine base to a purine base and vice versa, is not twice that of those caused by the transitions from one purine to the other and one pyrimidine to the other, respectively. In fact the number of transversions and transitions are more or less equal, indicating that the more radical transversion is less frequent than one would expect from purely random change. Of the transitions the G → A change in the messenger RNA, or A → G change in DNA, accounts for a considerably larger number of variants than any other mutation [266, 267]. These considerations apply to the hemoglobin molecule as a whole. Further analysis shows that for substitutions on the outside of the globin molecule the number of mutations due to transversions to that due to transitions approaches the expected 2:1 ratio, but that transversions are rare in the interior of the molecule [266].

Two hemoglobins have been described which have elongated polypeptide chains. Hb Constant Spring [326] has about 30 residues attached to the α chain, the first of which is a glutamine. A possible explanation is that a stop codon has undergone a single point mutation to one for glutamine. In Hb Tak [327] eight residues are attached, and the first is a threonine. As this cannot have arisen from a single point mutation in a stop codon or an insertion or deletion, it is suggested that the nascent chains may be longer normally and be shortened by hydrolysis after synthesis. It is known that nascent rabbit hemoglobin has an additional residue of methionine at the N terminal which is cleaved off during the later stages of biosynthesis [328, 329].

Prefetal Hemoglobin

Just as Hb F precedes Hb A in human development, so another more primitive hemoglobin precedes Hb F in the fetus. There is no evidence that Hb F precedes the adult pigment in the true sense of the word, for although the proportion of Hb F is higher in the embryo than at birth, Hb A has been found in the youngest embryos examined.

There has been evidence both in favor of and against the existence of a "prefetal primitive" hemoglobin. Allison's primitive "hemoglobin P" [268] was not a human hemoglobin but was found in rat embryos. In man, investigation is difficult because of the small amount of blood which can be obtained from embryos when they become available. Halbrecht, Klibanski, and Bar Ilan [269, 270] found in embryos an alkali-resistant hemoglobin with a lower mobility on paper electrophoresis at pH 8.6 than that of either Hb F or A. Drescher and Künzer [271–273] also found a primitive alkali-resistant hemoglobin with an ultraviolet spectrum of the Hb F type.

In 1961 Huehns and his collaborators [274] described two hemoglobin fractions Gower I and Gower II, in a very young human embryo. Recent work has indicated that these two fractions represent a primitive "embryonic" hemoglobin and possibly a fourth physiologic human hemoglobin, $\alpha_2\epsilon_2$. The faster moving fraction (Hb Gower I) might consist of ϵ chains only [32, 33].

The structure of the ϵ chain has not yet been completely determined [275]. It has already been mentioned [34, 35] that there is yet another physiological hemoglobin polypeptide, the Portland chain consisting of ζ and γ chains.

The γ Chain of Hb F

The change from fetal to adult hemoglobin in early infancy must be envisaged as a closing down of γ-chain production in favor of β-chain formation; $\alpha_2\gamma_2$ is replaced by $\alpha_2\beta_2$. When infants suffer from anemias of any kind, inherited or acquired, Hb F continues to remain present, and thus several percent of Hb F is a regular feature of sickle-cell anemia or spherocytosis as well as of early nutritional anemia. Staining of blood smears for Hb F [11] demonstrates that this is not equally distributed but that it is carried in relatively few cells. There is, however, a condition when fetal hemoglobin is found in later life, not as a consequence of the survival of a few Hb F producing clones, but as a feature of all cells.

This condition was first seen in Ghana [276] and in Liberia [277], and then in East Africa [278], and was named *hereditary persistence of high fetal hemoglobin*. It has since been seen in many places and has been extensively studied in American Negroes [279, 280]. There are no clinical or hematologic abnormalities associated with this condition; Hb F simply replaces Hb A in the phenotype. For example, in the person with both the sickle-cell trait and hereditary persistence of high fetal hemoglobin there is about 70 percent Hb S, no Hb A, and 30 percent Hb F. A homozygote for the persistent high-fetal-hemoglobin gene was seen to have 100 percent Hb F in his cells. It was particularly notable that Hb A_2 was completely absent [281]. This homozygote had thus not only failed completely to "switch" on his β-chain production but also had been unable to produce the δ chains for Hb A_2. From this it was concluded that an operator gene for the β-chain gene also controlled the gene for the δ chain [282, 283]. This led to the conclusion that the two loci must be on the same chromosome, and probably next to each other [284, 285].

The δ Chain of Hb A_2

The position of Hb A_2 as a pigment under independent genetic control from Hb A and Hb F found its support in chemical investigations [286–288]. Its close linkage to Hb A had been concluded from the findings in carriers of the gene for persistent high fetal hemoglobin. This close linkage became more apparent when Hb Lepore was also examined chemically [289] (see below).

The Lepore hemoglobin (named after the family in which it was discovered [290]) was found during family studies of patients with thalassemia major. Both parents were of Italian extraction. The propositus, an infant apparently suffering from thalassemia major, was found to possess, in addition to Hb A, 74 percent Hb F, 1.2 percent Hb A_2, and 5 percent Hb Lepore. Since the mother possessed 11 percent of Hb Lepore and the father had thalassemia minor with an Hb A_2 concentration of 5.5 percent, it was concluded that the child suffered from a combination of the two abnormalities. Four other members of the family showed the Lepore hemoglobin, in combination with Hb A and a slightly raised level of Hb F (2.3 to 2.6 percent); they were considered to be heterozygotes.

On the basis of peptide analysis Gerald and his colleagues [291] suggested that the mutation responsible for Hb Lepore involved more than one gene. Homozygotes were seen to have a suppression of both Hb A and Hb A_2 formation, which indicated an involvement of both the loci for the genes responsible for the β chain and the δ chain [292, 293]. The peptide analysis of the non-α chains showed indeed some of the features of the β chain and some of the δ chain [294]. Baglioni [295] showed then that the non-α chain of the Lepore hemoglobin was in its N-terminal part δ chain, and in its C-terminal part β chain. Baglioni suggested that this type of chain would arise if the δ and the β genes were next to each other on the chromosome and if a nonhomologous crossing took place between the two genes. It is of interest that one Hb Lepore from an Italian family [295] had a longer δ section than another from New Guinea [296].

Hemoglobin Lepore (Fig. 57-21) is the outcome of an unequal crossover between two chromosomes following nonhomologous pairing. The deficiency fusion product would then be the only adult non-α-chain gene on one chromosome, whereas the other fusion product would be present together with genes for the normal δ and β chains [296–297]. The fact that Hb Lepore ($\delta\beta$) indeed occurs without Hb A and A_2 in the homozygote confirms this concept. The other fusion product ($\beta\delta$) has now also been described: Hb Miyada [298] differs from a second such $\beta\delta$ product by having a shorter β section. The latter is Hb P (Congo type) which has actually been found in several individuals together with Hb A and Hb S [299, 300]. Since

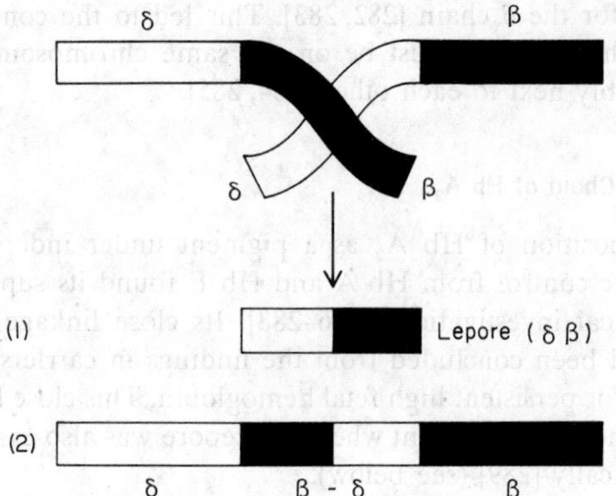

Figure 57-21. Unequal crossing over of two normal chromosomes each containing one δ and one β gene. The product of such an unequal crossing over is (1) a chromosome with only one δβ gene and (2) a chromosome with three genes, δ, βδ, and β.

β^A and β^S are alleles it would not be possible for the third hemoglobin also to be a β-chain variant. For this reason it was at one time thought that Hb P Congo was an α-chain abnormal hemoglobin. It has now been demonstrated to have the chemical features of a βδ fusion product [301].

Dintzis [302, 303] and Naughton and Dintzis [304] incubated reticulocytes with labeled leucine. In these cells hemoglobin is still synthesized, and it could be demonstrated that the growth of the peptide chains proceeds by a steady sequential addition of amino acids to the growing chain. Furthermore, it was possible to show that the growth proceeds from the free amino group end of the chains toward the COOH-terminus. Thus the numbering of the amino acid residues corresponds to the sequential incorporation into the peptide chains. The sequence of the amino acids is now known, in phage at least, to be collinear with the genes on the chromosome [305]. One can therefore picture the position of the loci for the δ and the β genes as neighbors on the chromosome, the δ locus being above the β locus.

World Distribution of Abnormal Hemoglobins

Anthropologists are particularly interested in human characters which are not so rare as to be of no general importance nor so widespread that they lose their value in distinguishing among different human populations. For anthropologic purposes perhaps the ideal characters among the abnormal hemoglobins are Hb C and Hb E. Both pigments are present in millions of human beings, but at the same time they are peculiarly associated only with certain well-circumscribed groups of people [306, 307]. Hemoglobin C, discovered in American Negroes, could be expected to have come with their ancestors from West Africa, but it was surprising to find that hemoglobin C, which is not frequent in American Negroes, should turn up in 10 percent of the inhabitants of Accra in Ghana. On the other hand, no Hb C is seen in East Africa, nor is it found in the Belgian Congo. Occasionally examples have been seen in South Africa, or in Central Africa, but there is always a readily traced connection with West Africa. Within that part of the continent, again fairly sharp geographic demarcations are noted. Westward from Ghana the incidence falls until it becomes very low in Liberia, and there is a similar decline eastward; in the Yoruba in Western Nigeria the incidence is only about half that found in the coastal region of Ghana. This is even more impressive when it is seen that within Nigeria the Niger River forms a barrier to the spread of Hb C; westward, in the Yoruba, Hb C is found in 5 to 6 percent of the population; east of the river in the Ibo, the incidence amounts to only a fraction of 1 percent. In Ghana itself the frequency of the Hb C gene increases toward the north; in the northernmost territories of Ghana and in the neighboring high Volta territory, one-fifth of the population possesses Hb C in its red cells. There is, therefore, a center of high frequency somewhere in the north of Ghana, with a fall in frequency to the south, east, and west. Neel once stated that "never in the history of genetics, with the possible exception of Ford's melanism story in the moth, have geneticists and those with kindred interests been quite so close to having a ringside seat at the origin and dissemination of a 'new gene'" (Fig. 57-22). Alternatively Hb C may occur in an older population later displaced.

Hemoglobin E presents a similar situation. Again a very high frequency is found in the Burmese and their immediate neighbors, but not in the Indians in nearby Bengal, the Tibetans, or the Indonesians. There are small foci with a high incidence in the Indonesian archipelago, but such a local increase would be expected for any gene in small islands with an inbreeding population. Of particular interest is that Hb E is found in the Indo-Chinese but not in the

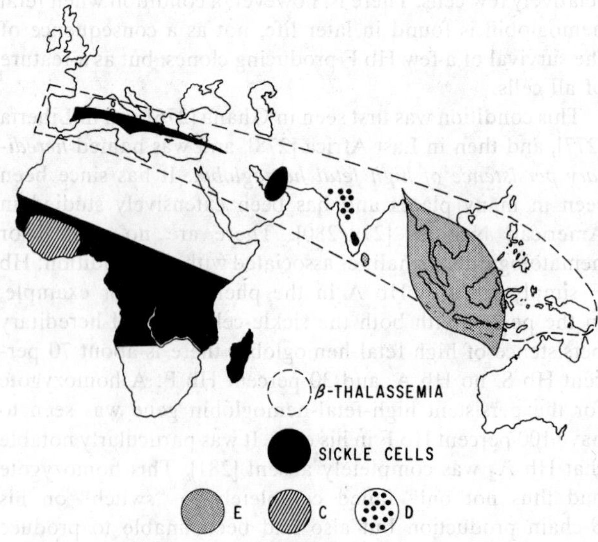

Figure 57-22. World distribution of major hemoglobin abnormalities.

Chinese, and that it is therefore linked with the earlier Mongolian populations of Southeast Asia. In Malaya there is a higher incidence in the north. Less hemoglobin E appears in the south, where immigration from Indonesia has been of greater importance. Of the primitive populations, the Vedda of Ceylon have a high Hb E frequency, which links them with the proto-Malays rather than with the "Veddoids" of Southern India, in whom sickling but no Hb E is found. This throws an entirely new light on the racial affinities of these Veddas, which is actually borne out by their physical appearance. Of the few proto-Malayan Pygmies examined, several were Hb E trait carriers but no Hb E was discovered in the Negritos of the nearby Andaman Islands.

Hemoglobin S is more widely spread [308]. It is found in tropical Africa, in the west as well as in the east. In the east there are striking differences between the Hamitic tribes, with few if any sickle cells, and the Bantus and Nilotes, with high sickling rates. There is evidence for a westward spread of the sickling gene, and in Liberia sickling is less frequent in the older and longer-established populations. Hemoglobin S is also found in India, but predominantly in primitive tribes which are the least likely to have been in contact with Africa. It has been proposed that the African continent and India inherited the sickling gene independently but from a common source in the Middle East. This would well agree with what is known of population movements from the Middle East toward the southeast into India.

Hemoglobin D_{Punjab} is found in 2 percent of Punjabis, in 1 percent in the Gujarati-speaking Lohanas south of them, and in 1 percent of Iranians. This hemoglobin also occurs sporadically in Caucasians, and has been found in Turks, Britishers, and Portuguese, and has been seen in American Indians. It is identical with the first Hb D discovered in Los Angeles and strictly speaking should now be called Hb $D_{Los\ Angeles}$.

The distribution of the rarer variants may be of anthropological interest. The recent finding of Hb $G_{Coushatta}$ in American Indians [184] and a single finding of it in Southeast Asia [185] may be an indication of a link between Asia and the North American continent.

POPULATION DYNAMICS OF THE ABNORMAL HEMOGLOBINS

It is tragic that in Africa very few homozygotes for the sickling gene reach adult life. Many surveys, particularly in East, West, and Central Africa, have either failed to find sickle-cell homozygotes in the adult population or have discovered them only exceptionally. It is therefore surprising that the gene is present at a high frequency in many parts of that continent [309]. The steady drain caused by the early death of homozygotes would be expected to cause a fall in the incidence of Hb S. Frequencies of 40 percent and more of the sickle-cell trait can be understood only if there exists a special compensating mechanism which replenishes the Hb S pool in every generation. Neel [310] in 1953 discussed the implications of a situation in which the sickling gene was constantly eliminated by early death of homozygotes but in which a high frequency was nevertheless maintained. One possibility is that a high mutation rate for the sickling gene is a peculiar characteristic of these populations and replaces the genes lost in every generation by sickle-cell anemia. Such an explanation would require a mutation rate about 3,000 times greater than those hitherto calculated for man [311] and in a search for evidence to put this theory to the test in tropical Africa no support could be found for it in an extensive survey [312]. The other possibility suggested by Neel is that a balanced polymorphism exists by which the A + S heterozygote enjoys advantages not shared by either homozygote. Allison [311] found evidence that sickle-cell trait carriers enjoy an immunity against malaria which is not shared by the normal homozygote.

Several investigators have shared in developing the concept of balanced polymorphism as the genetic mechanism supporting the persistence of the sickling gene at high frequency. Early observations were made in Rhodesia [313, 314]. It is of the greatest importance that two points be kept in mind: It is necessary to single out for investigation the effect of *Plasmodium falciparum* and to separate it from the part played by other parasites, because only *P. falciparum* causes malignant malaria which kills children in infancy. In these children it is necessary to consider only the age at which immunity against the parasite had not yet been acquired. Immunity is acquired very early in hyperendemic areas, and studies of adults or even of children above the age of 2 include many individuals with partial protection against *P. falciparum,* some of whom would be sickle-cell trait carriers and normal homozygotes [315]. The protection against malaria afforded to sickling infants could by itself fully explain the high sickling rate in some African populations. The mechanism of protection might be a failure of *P. falciparum* to thrive on sickle-cell hemoglobin, or it might be related to the fact that cells infected with this parasite tend to adhere to the vessel wall, where they would become deoxygenated. This would cause them to alter their shape, and the sickled cells would then be phagocytosed [316]. The latter is the more probable explanation, because cells containing Hb S do not differ from normal cells when they are used for the culture of *P. falciparum* in vitro [317]. Survival of homozygotes plays little part in maintaining the sickling gene, at least in some parts of Africa [318, 319]. The protection in infancy of the heterozygotes against malignant malaria is not only the first but also the most striking example of balanced polymorphism acting in the natural selection of the human race. It is noteworthy that no case of cerebral malaria resulting in death has as yet been seen in a sickle-cell trait child.

There is a remarkable correlation between a high sickling rate and a low social status [320]. The lower the social level of a human group, usually the greater is its isolation, and inbreeding populations are notoriously likely to accumulate specific characters at a higher frequency than societies with a larger gene pool. There is yet another factor which would tend to raise the sickling frequency in the more primitive tribes in the less accessible parts of Africa. Although the malarial pressure may not be greater, the malarial death rate will be increased with unfavorable living conditions [321]. This would explain why the sickling rate is higher in some areas of Africa where the intensity of malarial infection is less than in others with a greater incidence of the sickle-cell trait. With an overall increase in the death rate, any differences due to protection against malaria will become more significant. This suggests that the improvement of living conditions, as well as the eradication of malaria, will cause a fall in the sickling incidence in future generations.

In marked contrast to the severe course of sickle-cell anemia in Africa, the apparently similar disease in the West Indies runs a benign course [322].

The position of Hb C and Hb E in relation to malaria is still controversial. It has been suggested that Hb F might be responsible in part for the "inborn" protection of infants against malaria; as for Hb E and Hb D, it has been pointed out that homozygotes who would on the whole be viable and are known to produce children would be protected against thalassemia [323]. Thalassemia acts by interference with the production of Hb A and should therefore have no effect on homozygotes for Hb E or D. In heterozygotes the only conditions which could arise would be Hb E thalassemia and Hb D thalassemia, respectively. These hemoglobinopathies are much less severe than thalassemia major. It is noteworthy that both Hb E and Hb D are found in parts of the world where it is now known that the incidence of thalassemia is high and where thalassemia major is the only hemoglobin disease which will cause the death of the affected persons with near certainty before they are able to produce children. Other advantages of Hb E and Hb D might be related to the red cell morphology of the homozygous conditions. The blood picture resembles that of patients with a compensated iron deficiency. There is a polycythemia without a rise in total red cell volume, and perhaps such individuals can adapt themselves more easily to an iron-deficient diet or to secondary iron deficiency in hookworm disease [324].

SUMMARY

1 The hemoglobins of man are a group of pigments, each of which is composed of four molecules of ferroprotoporphyrin IX attached to one molecule of globin. The hemoglobins differ in the properties of the globin moiety.

2 At birth, fetal hemoglobin, Hb F, predominates. In normal man this is rapidly replaced by the normal adult pigment, Hb A. Hemoglobin A consists of at least two components, a major one, Hb A_1, and a minor component, Hb A_2.

3 The globin molecule consists of two identical half molecules, each of which contains two different long peptide chains. In Hb A these are the α and β chains, in Hb F, the α and the γ chains, and in Hb A_2, the α and δ chains. The variant hemoglobins contain either altered combinations of the four chains or altered amino acid sequence within the chains. Each type of chain is thought to correspond to one gene, and the inheritance of the polypeptide chains is codominant.

4 Abnormal hemoglobins were principally identified by their electrophoretic properties but are now characterized by the mutational change in their amino acid sequence. The most important abnormal hemoglobin is sickle-cell hemoglobin, Hb S, which is responsible for the sickling phenomenon in sickle-cell disease. Reduced solubility of Hb S under reduced oxygen tension is responsible for the various clinical and laboratory phenomena of the disease. Heterozygotes for Hb S and Hb A are not anemic, but heterozygotes for Hb S and for other abnormal hemoglobins or for thalassemia may be anemic if Hb S becomes the predominant hemoglobin.

5 The world distribution of the variant hemoglobins has provided important anthropologic data and has contributed to the study of population dynamics. In the case of Hb S, the high frequency of trait carriers is thought to derive from a selective advantage of Hb AS heterozygotes in areas with high mortality from *P. falciparum.*

BIBLIOGRAPHY

1. von Körber, E.: Über Differenzen des Blutfarbstoffes. (Dissertation), Dorpat, 1886 Zentralbl. med. Wissensch., **177**, 1867.
2. Jonxis, J. H. P.: Foetal haemoglobin in children, in *Abnormal Haemoglobins,* p. 114. Blackwell, Oxford, 1959.
3. Bianco, I.: La resistenza emoglobinica nei portatori di microcithemia e di falcemia. Policlinico [prat], **55,** 103, 1948.
4. Putignano, T., and Fiore-Donati, L.: La resistenza emoglobinica nel M. di Cooley (del bambino e dell'adulto) e forme affini. Bull. Soc. ital. biol. sper., **24,** 277, 1948.
5. Vecchio, F.: Sulla resistenza dell'emoglobinica alla denaturazione alcalina negli ammalati di anemia di Cooley e nei loro familiari. Prog. med. Napoli, **4,** 201, 1948.
6. Liquori, A. M.: Presence of foetal haemoglobin in Cooley's anaemia. Nature (London), **167,** 950, 1951.
7. Singer, K., Chernoff, A. I., and Singer, L.: Studies on abnormal hemoglobins. Blood, **6,** 413, 1951.
8. White, J. C., and Beaven, G. H.: Review of varieties of human haemoglobin in health and disease. J. Clin. Path., **7,** 175, 1954.
9. Betke, K.: Der menschliche Blutfarbstoff bei Fetus und reifem Organismus. Springer, Berlin, 1954.
10. Bertles, J. F.: The occurrence and significance of fetal hemoglobins, in *Regulation of Hematopoiesis,* edited by A. S. Gordon. Appleton-Century-Crofts, New York, 1969.
11. Kleihauer, E., and Betke, K.: Praktische Anwendung des Nachweises von Hb F haltigen zellen in fixierten Blut-ausstrichen. Internist, **1,** 292, 1960.
12. Allen, D. W., Wyman, J., Jr., and Smith, C. A.: The oxygen equilibrium of fetal and adult human hemoglobin. J. Biol. Chem., **203,** 81, 1953.
13. Beutler, E.: "A shift to the left" or "a shift to the right" in the regulation of erythropoiesis. Blood, **33,** 496, 1969.

14. Benesch, R., and Benesch, R. E.: Intracellular organic phosphates as regulators of oxygen release by haemoglobin. Nature (London), **221,** 618, 1969.
15. Bellingham, A. J., and Huehns, E. R.: Compensation in haemolytic anaemias caused by abnormal haemoglobins. Nature (London), **218,** 924, 1968.
16. Derrien, Y.: On the heterogeneity of normal human haemoglobins, in *Abnormal Haemoglobins,* p. 63. Blackwell, Oxford, 1959.
17. Itano, H. A.: Solubilities of naturally occurring mixtures of human hemoglobin. Arch. Biochem., **47,** 148, 1953.
18. Kunkel, H. G., and Wallenius, G.: New hemoglobin in normal adult blood. Science, **122,** 288, 1955.
19. Schroeder, W. A., and Holmquist, W. R.: A function for hemoglobin A_{1c} in *Structural Chemistry and Molecular Biology,* edited by A. Rich and N. Davidson. Freeman, San Francisco, 1968.
20. Muller, C. J.: A comparative study on the structure of mammalian and avian haemoglobins (Ph.D. thesis). Van Gorcum & Co., Assen, Netherlands, 1961.
21. Schroeder, W. A.: Hemoglobin F_1 and a few remarks on γ-F chain sequence. Conference on Hemoglobin, Columbia University. New York, 1962.
22. Epstein, C. J., and Schechter, A. N.: An approach to the problems of conformation of isoenzymes. Ann. NY Acad. Sci., **151,** 85, 1968.
23. Perutz, M. F., Muirhead, H., Cox, J. M., Goaman, L. C. G., Mathews, F. S., McGandy, E. L., and Webb, L. E.: Three-dimensional Fourier synthesis of horse oxyhaemoglobin at 2.8 Å resolution. Nature (London), **219,** 28, 1968.
24. Rhinesmith, H. S., Schroeder, W. A., and Pauling, L.: The N-terminal amino acid residues of normal adult hemoglobin: A quantitative study of certain aspects of Sanger's DNP-method. J. Am. Chem. Soc., **79,** 609, 1957.
25. Rhinesmith, H. S., Schroeder, W. A., and Martin, N.: The N-terminal sequence of the β chains of normal adult human hemoglobin. J. Am. Chem. Soc., **80,** 3358, 1958.
26. Schroeder, W. A., and Matsuda, G.: N-terminal residues of human fetal hemoglobin. J. Amer. Chem. Soc., **80,** 1521, 1958.
27. Hunt, J. A.: Identity of the α-chains of adult and foetal human haemoglobins. Nature (London), **183,** 1373, 1959.
28. Katz, A. M., and Chernoff, A. I.: Structural similarities between hemoglobins A and J. Science, **130,** 1574, 1959.
29. Stretton, A. O. W., and Ingram, V. M.: An amino acid difference between human hemoglobins A and A_2. Fed. Proc., **19,** 343, part 1, 1960.
30. Muller, C. J., and Jonxis, H. J. P.: Identity of Haemoglobin A_2. Nature, London, **188,** 949, 1960.
31. Huehns, E. R., and Shooter, E. M.: The molecular composition of haemoglobins A_2 and G_2. Biochem. J., **78,** 13*P,* 1961.
32. Huehns, E. R., Dance, N., Beaven, G. H., Keil, J. V., Hecht, F., and Motulsky, A. G.: Human embryonic haemoglobins. Nature (London), **201,** 1095, 1964.
33. Huehns, E. R., and Shooter, E. M.: Human haemoglobins. J. Med. Genet., **2,** 48, 1965.
34. Weatherall, D. J., Clegg, J. B., and Cauchi, M. N.: The haemoglobin constitution of infants with the haemoglobin Bart's hydrops foetalis syndrome. Brit. J. Haemat., **18,** 349, 1970.
35. Capp, G. O., Rigas, D. A., and Jones, R. T.: Hemoglobin Portland 1: A new human hemoglobin unique in structure. Science, **157,** 65, 1967.
36. Braunitzer, G., Gehring-Müller, R., Hilschmann, N., Hilse, K., Hobom, G., Rudloff, V., and Wittmann-Liebold, B.: Die Konstitution des normalen adulten Humenhämoglobins. Z. Physiol. Chem., **325,** 283, 1961.
37. Schroeder, W. A., Shelton, J. R., Shelton, J. B., and Cormick, J.: Further sequences in the γ-chain of human fetal hemoglobin. Proc. Nat. Acad. Sci. USA, **48,** 284, 1962.
38. Konigsberg, W., and Hill, R. J.: The structure of human hemoglobin. III. The sequence of amino-acids in the tryptic peptides of the α-chain. J. Biol. Chem., **237,** 2547, 1962.
39. Braunitzer, G., Hilse, K., Rudloff, V., and Hilschmann. N.: *The Hemoglobins: Advances in Protein Chemistry,* vol. 19, p. 1. Academic, New York, 1964.
40. Braunitzer, F.: Das normale adulte Humanhämoglobin, in *Haemoglobin Colloquium,* edited by H. Lehmann and K. Betke, p. 15. Thieme, Stuttgart, 1962.
41. Ingram, V. M.: Gene evolution and the haemoglobins. Nature (London), **189,** 704, 1961.
42. Ingram, V. M.: *The Hemoglobins in Genetics and Evolution,* Columbia, New York, 1963.
43. Zuckerkandl, E.: Hemoglobins, Haeckels "biogenetic law," and molecular aspects of development, in *Structural Chemistry and Molecular Biology,* edited by A. Rich and N. Davidson. Freeman, San Francisco, 1968.
44. Zuckerkandl, E., and Pauling, L.: Molecular disease, evolution, and genic heterogeneity, in *Horizons in Biochemistry,* edited by M. Kasha and B. Pullman, p. 189. Academic, New York, 1962.
45. Schroeder, W. A., Huisman, T. H. J., Shelton, J. R., Shelton, J. B., Kleihauer, E. F., Dozy, A. M., and Robberson, B.: Evidence for multiple structural genes for the γ chain of human fetal hemoglobin. Proc. Nat. Acad. Sci. USA, **60,** 537, 1968.
46. Lehmann, H., and Carrell, R. W.: Differences between the α and β chain mutants of human haemoglobin and between α and β thalassaemia: Possible duplication of the α chain gene. Brit. Med. J., **4,** 748, 1968.
47. Brimhall, B., Hollan, S., Jones, R. T., Koler, R. D., Stocklen, Z., and Szelenyi, J. G.: Multiple alpha-chain loci for human hemoglobin. Clin. Res. **18,** 184, 1970.
48. Perutz, M. F.: The haemoglobin molecule. Proc. Roy. Soc. [Biol], **173,** 113, 1969.
49. Hörlein, H., and Weber, G.: Uber chronische familiäre Methämoglobinämie und eine neue Modifikation des Methämoglobins, Deutsch. Med. Wschr., **73,** 476, 1948.
50. Watson, J.: The significance of the paucity of sickle cells in newborn Negro infants. Amer. J. Med. Sci., **215,** 419, 1948.
51. Pauling, L., Itano, H. A., Singer, S. J., and Wells, I. C.: Sickle cell anemia, a molecular disease. Science, **110,** 543, 1949.
52. Herrick, J. B.: Peculiar elongated and sickle-shaped red blood corpuscles in a case of severe anemia. Arch. Intern. Med. (Chicago), **6,** 517, 1910.
53. Hahn, E. V., and Gillespie, E. B.: Sickle cell anemia. Arch. Intern. Med. (Chicago), **39,** 233, 1927.
54. Diggs, L. W., Ahmann, C. F., and Bibb, J.: The incidence and significance of the sickle cell trait. Ann. Intern. Med., **7,** 769, 1933.
55. Sherman, I. J.: The sickling phenomenon, with special reference to the differentiation of sickle cell anemia from the sickle cell trait. Bull. Johns Hopkins Hosp., **67,** 309, 1940.
56. Singer, K., Robin, S., King, J. C., and Jefferson, R. N.: The life span of the sickle cell and the pathogenesis of sickle cell anemia. J. Lab. Clin. Med., **33,** 975, 1948.
57. Callender, S. T. E., Nickel, J. F., Moore, C. V., and Powell, E. O.: Sickle cell disease: Studied by measuring the survival of transfused red blood cells. J. Lab. Clin. Med., **34,** 90, 1949.
58. Emmel, V. E.: A study of the erythrocytes in a case of severe anemia with elongated and sickle-shaped red blood corpuscles. Arch. Intern. Med. (Chicago), **20,** 586, 1917.
59. Taliaferro, W. H., and Huck, J. G.: The inheritance of sickle-cell anemia in man. Genetics, **8,** 594, 1923.
60. Neel, J. V.: The clinical detection of genetic carriers of inherited disease. Medicine (Balt.), **26,** 115, 1947.
61. Beet, E. A.: Genetics of sickle-cell trait in a Bantu tribe. Ann. Eugenics, **14,** 279, 1949.
62. Neel, J. V.: The inheritance of sickle cell anemia. Science, **110,** 64, 1949.
63. Harris, J. W.: Studies on the destruction of red blood cells. VIII. Molecular orientation in sickle cell hemoglobin solutions. Proc. Soc. Exp. Biol. Med., **75,** 197, 1950.
64. Perutz, M. F., and Mitchison, J. M.: State of haemoglobin in sickle-cell anemia. Nature (London), **166,** 677, 1950.
65. Perutz, M. F., and Liquori, A. M.: X-ray and solubility studies of the

haemoglobins of sickle-cell anemia patients. Nature (London), **167**, 929, 1951.

66. Greenberg, M. S., Kass, E. H., and Castle, W. B.: Studies on the destruction of red blood cells. XII. Factors influencing the role of hemoglobin in the pathologic physiology of sickle cell anemia and related disorders. J. Clin. Invest., **36**, 833, 1957.
67. Harris, J. W., Brewster, H. H., Ham, T. H., and Castle, W. B.: Studies on destruction of red blood cells: biophysics and biology of sickle-cell disease. AMA Arch. Intern. Med., **97**, 145, 1956.
68. Allison, A. C.: Observations on the sickling phenomenon and on the distribution of different haemoglobin types in erythrocyte populations. Clin. Sci., **15**, 497, 1956.
69. Serjeant, G. R., Serjeant, B. E., and Milner, P. F.: The irreversibly sickled cell: A determinant of haemolysis in sickle cell anaemia. Brit. J. Haemat., **17**, 527, 1969.
70. Roberts, A. R., and Hilburg, L. E.: Sickle cell disease with salmonella osteomyelitis. J. Pediat., **52**, 170, 1958.
71. Romero-Herrera, A. E., Personal communication.
72. Jones, S. R., Binder, R. A., and Donowho, E. M.: Sudden death in sickle-cell trait. New Eng. J. Med., **282**, 232, 1970.
73. Griggs, R. L., and Harris, J. W.: The biophysics of the variants of sickle-cell disease. AMA Arch. Intern. Med., **97**, 315, 1956.
74. Konotey-Ahulu, F. I. D.: Anaesthetic deaths and the sickle-cell trait. Lancet, **1**, 267, 1969.
75. Goodwin, W. E., Alston, E. F., and Semans, J. H.: Hematuria and sickle cell disease: Unexplained, gross, unilateral, renal hematuria in Negroes, coincident with the blood sickling trait. J. Urol., 63, 79, 1950.
76. Chernoff, A. I.: The human hemoglobins in health and disease. New Eng. J. Med., **253**, 322, 365, 416, 1955.
77. Cooley, J. C., Peterson, W. L., Engel, C. E., and Jemigan, J. P.: Clinical trait of massive splenic infarction, sicklemia trait and high altitude flying. JAMA, **154**, 111, 1954.
78. Smith, E. W., and Conley, C. L.: Sicklemia and infarction of the spleen during aerial flight. Bull. Johns Hopkins Hosp., **96**, 35, 1955.
79. Itano, H. A.: The human hemoglobins: Their properties and genetic control. Advances Protein Chem., **12**, 215, 1957.
80. Levere, R. D., Lichtman, H. C., and Levine, J.: Effect of iron deficiency anaemia on the metabolism of the heterogenic haemoglobins in sickle-cell trait. Nature (London), **202**, 499, 1964.
81. Neel, J. V., Kaplan, E., Zuelzer, W. W.: Further studies on hemoglobin C. I. A description of 3 additional families segregating for hemoglobin C and sickle cell hemoglobin. Blood, **8**, 724, 1953.
82. Itano, H. A., and Neel, J. V.: A new inherited abnormality of human hemoglobin. Proc. Nat. Acad. Sci. USA, **36**, 613, 1950.
83. River, G. L., Robbins, A. B., and Schwartz, S. O.: S-C hemoglobin: A clinical study. Blood, **18**, 385, 1961.
84. Ranney, H. M., Larson, D. L., and McCormack, G. H., Jr.: Some clinical, biochemical, and genetic observations on hemoglobin C. J. Clin, Invest., **32**, 1277, 1953.
85. Edington, G. M., and Lehmann, H.: A case of sickle-cell haemoglobin C disease and a survey of haemoglobin C incidence in West Africa. Trans. Roy. Soc. Trop. Med. Hyg., **48**, 332, 1954.
86. Hunt, J. A., and Ingram, V. M.: Abnormal human haemoglobins. IV. The chemical difference between normal haemoglobin and haemoglobin C. Biochim. Biophys. Acta, **42**, 409, 1960.
87. Itano, H. A.: A third abnormal hemoglobin associated with hereditary hemolytic anemia. Proc. Nat. Acad. Sci. USA, **37**, 775, 1951.
88. Sturgeon, P., Itano, H. A., and Bergren, W. R.: Clinical manifestations of inherited abnormal hemoglobins. I. The interaction of hemoglobin-S with hemoglobin-D. Blood, **10**, 389, 1955.
89. Lehmann, H.: Distribution of abnormal haemoglobins. J. Clin. Path., **9**, 180, 1956.
90. Benzer, S., Ingram, V. M., and Lehmann, H.: Three varieties of human haemoglobin D. Nature (London), **182**, 853, 1958.
91. Itano, H. A., Bergren, W. R., and Sturgeon, P.: Identification of a fourth abnormal human hemoglobin. J. Amer. Chem. Soc., **76**, 2278, 1954.
92. Minnich, V., Na-Nakorn, S., Chongchareonsuk, S., and Kochaseni, S.: Mediterranean anemia: A study of thirty-two cases in Thailand. Blood, **9**, 1, 1954.
93. Chernoff, A. I., Minnich, V., and Chongchareonsuk, S.: Hemoglobin E, a hereditary abnormality of human hemoglobin. Science, **120**, 605, 1954.
94. Hunt, J. A., and Ingram, V. M.: Abnormal human haemoglobins. VI. The chemical difference between haemoglobins A and E. Biochim. Biophys. Acta, **49**, 520, 1961.
95. Aksoy, M., and Lehmann, H.: The first observation of sickle-cell haemoglobin E disease. Nature (London), **179**, 1248, 1957.
96. Aksoy, M., Ikin, E. W., Mourant, A. E., and Lehmann, H.: Blood groups, haemoglobins and thalassaemia in Turks in Southern Turkey and Eti-Turks. Brit. Med. J., **2**, 937, 1958.
97. Aksoy, M.: Hemoglobin E syndromes. II. Sickle-cell hemoglobin E disease. Blood, **15**, 610, 1960.
98. Hunt, J. A., and Ingram, V. M.: Human haemoglobin E: The chemical effect of gene mutation. Nature (London), **184**, 870, 1959.
99. Perutz, M. F., Kendrew, J. C., and Watson, H. C.: Structure and function of haemoglobins. II. Some relations between polypeptide chain configuration and amino acid sequence. J. Molec. Biol., **13**, 669, 1965.
100. Scheinberg, I. H., Harris, R. S., and Spitzer, J. L.: Differential titration by means of paper electrophoresis and the structure of human hemoglobins. Proc. Nat. Acad. Sci. USA, **40**, 777, 1954.
101. Scheinberg, I. H.: The structural basis of differences in electrophoretic behavior of human hemoglobins, in *Conference on Hemoglobin,* p. 227. National Academy of Sciences, National Research Council Publication 557, Washington, 1958.
102. Havinga, E.: Comparison of the phosphorus content, optical rotation, separation of hemes and globin, and terminal amino acid residues of normal adult human hemoglobin and sickle cell hemoglobin. Proc. Nat. Acad. Sci. USA, **39**, 59, 1953.
103. Ingram, V. M.: A specific chemical difference between globins of normal human and sickle-cell anaemia haemoglobin. Nature (London), **178**, 792, 1956.
104. Ingram, V. M.: Gene mutations in human haemoglobin: The chemical difference between normal and sickle cell haemoglobin. Nature (London), **180**, 326, 1957.
105. Ingram, V. M.: Abnormal human haemoglobins. I. The comparison of normal human and sickle-cell haemoglobins by "fingerprinting." Biochim. Biophys. Acta, **28**, 539, 1958.
106. Hunt, J. A., and Ingram, V. M.: A terminal peptide sequence of human haemoglobin. Nature (London), **184**, 640, 1959.
107. Murayama, M.: Molecular mechanism of red cell "sickling." Science, **153**, 145, 1966.
108. Perutz, M. F., and Lehmann, H.: Molecular pathology of human haemoglobins. Nature (London), **219**, 902, 1968.
109. Hunt, J. A., and Ingram, V. M.: Allelomorphism and the chemical differences of the human haemoglobins A, S, and C. Nature (London), **184**, 1062, 1958.
110. Baglioni, C., and Punjab, D.: Abnormal human haemoglobins. VIII. Chemical studies on haemoglobin D. Biochim. Biophys. Acta, **59**, 437, 1962.
111. Watson-Williams, E. J., Beale, D., Irvine, D., and Lehmann, H.: A new haemoglobin D Ibadan (β-87 threonine-lysine) producing no sickle-cell haemoglobin D disease with haemoglobin S. Nature (London), **205**, 1273, 1965.
112. Ingram, V. M.: Chemistry of the abnormal human haemoglobins. Brit. Med. Bull., **15**, 27, 1959.
113. Lehmann, H., and Huntsman, R. G.: *Man's Haemoglobins,* North Holland Publishing Co., Amsterdam, 1966.
114. Murayama, M., and Ingram, V. M.: Comparison of normal adult human haemoglobin with haemoglobin I by "fingerprinting." Nature (London), **183**, 1798, 1958.
115. Singer, S. J., and Itano, H. A.: On the asymmetrical dissociation of human hemoglobin. Proc. Nat. Acad. Sci. USA, **45**, 174, 1959.
116. Rosemeyer, M. A., and Huehns, E. R.: On the mechanism of the dissociation of haemoglobin. J. Molec. Biol., **25**, 253, 1967.
117. Vinograd, J. R., Hutchison, W. D., and Schroeder, W. A.: C^{14}-hybrids of human hemoglobins. II. The identification of the aberrant chain in human hemoglobin S. J. Amer. Chem. Soc., **81**, 3168, 1959.
118. Itano, H. A., and Robinson, E.: Formation of normal and doubly

abnormal haemoglobins by recombination of haemoglobin I with S and C. Nature (London), **183,** 1799, 1959.

119. Itano, H. A., and Robinson, E.: Properties and inheritance of hemoglobin by asymmetric recombination. Nature (London), **184,** 1468, 1959.
120. Smith, E. W., and Torbert, J. V.: Study of two abnormal hemoglobins with evidence for a new genetic locus for hemoglobin formation. Bull. Johns Hopkins Hosp., **102,** 38, 1958.
121. Atwater, J., Schwartz, I. R., and Tocantins, L. M.: A variety of human hemoglobin with 4 distinct electrophoretic components. Blood, **15,** 901, 1960.
122. Raper, A. B., Gammack, D. B., Huehns, E. R., and Shooter, E. M.: Four hemoglobins in one individual: A study of the genetic interaction of Hb-G and Hb-C. Brit. Med. J., **2,** 1257, 1960.
123. Baglioni, C., and Ingram, V. M.: Four adult hemoglobin types in one person. Nature (London), **189,** 465, 1961.
124. Gammack, D. B., Huehns, E. R., Lehmann, H., and Shooter, E. M.: The abnormal polypeptide chains in a number of haemoglobin variants. Acta Genet. (Basel), **11,** 1, 1961.
125. Chernoff, A. I., Fisher, B., Harris, J. W., Itano, H. A., Kaplan, E., Singer, K., and Neel, J. V.: A system of nomenclature for the varieties of human hemoglobin. Science, **118,** 116, 1953.
126. Singer, K.: Hereditary hemolytic disorders associated with abnormal hemoglobins. Amer. J. Med., **18,** 633, 1955.
127. Robinson, A. R., Zuelzer, W. W., Neel, J. V., Livingstone, F. B., and Miller, M.: Two "fast" hemoglobin components in Liberian blood samples. Blood, **11,** 902, 1956.
128. Huisman, T. H., and Prins, H. K.: The chromatographic behaviour of different abnormal human haemoglobins on the cation exchanger amberlite IRC 50. Clin. Chim. Acta, **2,** 307, 1957.
129. Robinson, R., Robson, M., Harrison, A. P., and Zuelzer, W. W.: A new technique for differentiation of hemoglobin. J. Lab. Clin. Med., **50,** 745, 1957.
130. Gerald, P. S., and Ingram, V. M.: Recommendation for the nomenclature of hemoglobins. J. Biol. Chem., **236,** 2155, 1961.
131. Recommendations of the International Society of Haematology on the nomenclature of abnormal haemoglobins. Brit. J. Haemat., **II,** 121, 1965.
132. Crookston, J. H., Beale, D., Irvine, D., and Lehmann, H.: A new haemoglobin, J Toronto (α_5 alanine-aspartic acid). Nature (London), **208,** 1059, 1965.
133. Rosa, J., Maleknia, N., Vergos, D., and Dunet, R.: Une nouvelle hemoglobine anormale; l'hemoglobine. J α Paris. 12 Ala-Asp. Nouv. Rev. Franc. Hemat., **6,** 423, 1966.
134. Liddell, J., Brown, D., Beale, D., Lehmann, H., and Huntsman, R. G.: A new haemoglobin J α Oxford found during a survey of an English population. Nature (London), **204,** 269, 1964.
135. Schneider, R. G., Alperin, J. B., Beale, D., and Lehmann, H.: Hemoglobin I in an American Negro family: Structural and hematologic studies. J. Lab. Clin. Med., **68,** 940, 1966.
136. Gottlieb, A. J., Restrepo, A., and Itano, H. A.: Hb J Medellin: Chemical and genetic study. Fed. Proc. Amer. Soc. Exp. Biol., **23,** 172, 1964.
137. Kraus, A. P., Miyaji, T., Iuchi, I., and Kraus, L. M.: Memphis: A new variety of sickle cell anemia with clinically mild symptoms due to an α-chain variant of hemoglobin ($\alpha_{23}{}^{\mathrm{GluNH_2}}$). J. Lab. Clin. Med., **66,** 886, 1965.
138. Marengo-Rowe, A. J., Beale, D., and Lehmann, H.: A new haemoglobin variant from Southern Arabia: G-Audhali [α23 (B4) glutamic acid-valine] and the variability of B4 in human haemoglobin. Nature (London), **219,** 1164, 1968.
139. Boyer, S. H., Crosby, E. F., Fuller, G. F., Ulenurn, L., and Buck, A. A.: A survey of hemoglobins in the Republic of Chad and characterization of hemoglobin Chad: $\alpha_2{}^{23\,\mathrm{Glu\text{-}Lys}}\beta_2$. Amer. J. Hum. Genet., **20,** 570, 1969.
140. Swenson, R. T., Hill, R. L., Lehmann, H., and Jim, R. T. S.: A chemical abnormality in hemoglobin G from Chinese individuals. J. Biol. Chem., **237,** 1517, 1962.
141. Beretta, A., Prato, V., Gallo, E., and Lehmann, H.: Haemoglobin Torino α43 (CDl) phenylalanine-valine. Nature (London), **217,** 1016, 1968.
142. Bianco, J., Modiano, G., Bottini, E., and Lucci, R.: Alteration in the α-chain of haemoglobin L Ferrara. Nature (London), **198,** 395, 1963.
143. Halbrecht, I., Isaacs, W. A., Lehmann, H., and Ben-Porat, F.: Hemoglobin Hasharon (α47 aspartic acid-histidine). Israel J. Med. Sci., **3,** 827, 1967.
144. Tangheroni, W., Zorcolo, G., Gallo, E., and Lehmann, H.: Haemoglobin J Sardegna: α50 D6 histidine-aspartic acid. Nature (London), **218,** 470, 1968.
145. Reynolds, C. A., and Huisman, T. H. J.: Hemoglobin Russ or $\alpha_2{}^{51\,\mathrm{Arg}}\beta_2$. Biochim. Biophys. Acta, **130,** 541, 1966.
146. Cabannes, R., Price, B., and Lehmann, H.: To be published.
147. Miyaji, T., Iuchi, I., Takeda, I., and Shibata, S.: Hemoglobin Shimonoseki ($\alpha_2{}^{54\,\mathrm{Arg}}\beta_2{}^{A}$), a slow moving hemoglobin found in a Japanese family, with special reference to its chemistry. Acta. Haemat. Jap., **26,** 531, 1963.
148. Jones, R. T., Brimhill, B., and Lisker, R.: Chemical characterisation of hemoglobin Mexico and hemoglobin Chiapas. Biochim. Biophys. Acta, **154,** 488, 1968.
149. Rahbar, S., Kinderlerer, Judith L., and Lehmann, H.: Haemoglobin L Persian Gulf: α57 (E6) glycine$\rightarrow$arginine, Acta. Haemat., **42,** 169, 1969.
150. Baglioni, C.: A chemical study of hemoglobin Norfolk. J. Biol. Chem., **237,** 69, 1962.
151. Gerald, P. S., and Efron, M. L.: Haemoglobin Boston: Chemical studies of several varieties of Hb M. Proc. Nat. Acad. Sci. USA, **47,** 1758, 1961.
152. Barclay, G. P. T., Charlesworth, Deborah, and Lehmann, H.: Abnormal haemoglobins in Zambia: A new haemoglobin Zambia α60 (E9) lysine-asparagine. Brit. Med. J., **4,** 595, 1969.
153. Baglioni, C., and Ingram, V. M.: G Philadelphia: Abnormal human haemoglobins. V. Clinical investigation of haemoglobins, A.G.C.X. from one individual. Biochim. Biophys. Acta, **48,** 253, 1961.
154. Miyaji, T., Iuchi, I., Yamamoto, K., Ohba, Y., and Shibata, S.: Amino acid substitution of hemoglobin Ube II ($\alpha_2{}^{68\,\mathrm{Asp}}\beta_2$): An example of successful application of partial hydrolysis of peptide with 5% acetic acid. Clin. Chim. Acta., **16,** 347, 1967.
155. Blackwell, R. Q., and Lin, C-S.: Hemoglobin G Taichung: α74 Asp$\rightarrow$His. Biochim. Biophys. Acta, **200,** 70, 1970.
156. Lorkin, P. A., Charlesworth, D., Lehmann, H., Rahbah, S., Tuchinda, S., and Lie, Injo Luan Eng. Two haemoglobins Q, α74 (EF3) and α75 (EF4) aspartic acid$\rightarrow$histidine. Brit. J. Haemat., **19,** 17, 1970.
157. Van Ros, G., Beale, D., and Lehmann, H. Haemoglobin Stanleyville II (α78 asparagine-lysine). Brit. Med. J., **4,** 92, 1968.
158. Rucknagel, D. L.: Personal communication.
159. Crookston, J. H., Farquharson, Helen A., Beale, D., and Lehmann, H.: Haemoglobin Etobicoke: α84 (F5) serine-arginine. Canad. J. Biochem., **47,** 143, 1969.
160. Huntsman, R. G., Lorkin, P. A., and Lehmann, H.: Unpublished observations.
161. Matsuda, G.: Personal communication.
162. Miyaji, T., Iuchi, I., Shibata, S., Takeda, I., and Tamura, A.: Possible amino acid substitution in the α-chain (α87 Tyr) of Hb M Iwate. Acta Haemat. Jap., **26,** 538, 1963.
163. De Traverse, P. M., Lehmann, H., Coquelet, M. L., Beale, D., and Isaacs, W. A.: Etude d'une hemoglobine Jα nom encore decrite, dans une famille francais. C. R. Soc. Biol. (Paris), **160,** 2270, 1966.
164. Botha, M. C., Beale, D., Isaacs, W. A., and Lehmann, H.: Haemoglobin J Capetown α_2 92 arginine-glutamine β_2. Nature, **212,** 792, 1966.
165. Clegg, J. B., Naughton, M. A., and Weatherall, D. J.: Abnormal human haemoglobin: Separation and characterisation of the α and β chains by chromatography and the determination of two new variants Hb Chesapeake and Hb J (Bangkok). J. Molec. Biol., **19,** 91, 1966.
166. Huisman, T. H. J., Adams, H. R., Wilson, J. B., Efremou, G. D., Reynolds, Cecelia A., and Wrightstone, Ruth N.: Haemoglobin G Georgia or $\alpha_2{}^{95\mathrm{Leu}(G\text{-}2)}\beta_2$. Biochim. Biophys. Acta, **200,** 578–80, 1970.
167. Crookston, J. H., Farquharson, H., Kinderlerer, J., and Lehmann, H.: Hemoglobin Manitoba: α102 (G9) serine replaced by arginine. Canad. J. Biochem, **48,** 911, 1970.
168. Rosa, J., Oudart, J. L., Pagnier, J., Belkhodja, O., Boigne, J. M., and Labie, D.: Abs. papers 12th. Congress Int. Soc. Haemat., New York, p. 73, 1968.
169. Gajdusek, D. C., Guiart, J., Kirk, R. L., Carrell, R. W., Irvine, D., Kynoch, P. A. M., and Lehmann, H.: Haemoglobin J. Tongariki (α115

alanine-aspartic acid) the first new haemoglobin variant found in a Pacific (Melanesian) population. J. Med. Genet., **4,** 1, 1967.

170. Baglioni, C., and Lehmann, H.: Haemoglobin O Indonesia: Chemical heterogeneity of haemoglobin O. Nature (London), **196,** 229, 1962.
171. Kleihauer, E. F., Reynolds, C. A., Dozy, A. M., Wilson, J. B., Moores, R. R., Berenson, M. P., Wright, C. S., and Huisman, T. H. J.: Hemoglobin Bibba or $\alpha_2^{136Pro}\beta_2$ an unstable α-chain abnormal hemoglobin. Biochim. Biophys. Acta, **154,** 220, 1968.
172. Clegg, J. B., Weatherall, D. J., and Wong, Hock Boon: Haemoglobin Singapore: Two new human haemoglobin variants involving proline substitutions. Nature (London), **222,** 379, 1969.
173. Marti, H. R., Beale, D., and Lehmann, H.: Haemoglobin Koellicker: A new acquired haemoglobin appearing after severe haemolysis = α_2 minus 141 Arg β_2. Acta Haemat. (Basel), **37,** 174, 1967.
174. Miyaji, T., Takeda, I., and Shibata, S.: A new hemoglobin, Hb. Tokuchi ($\alpha_2{}^A\beta_2{}^{2Tyr}$), discovered in Hofu City. Acta Haemat. Jap., **26,** (I) suppl. 45, 1963.
175. Ingram, V. M.: Haemoglobin S: Abnormal human haemoglobins. III. The chemical difference between normal and sickle cell haemoglobins. Biochim. Biophys. Acta, **36,** 402, 1969.
176. de Jong, W. W. W., Went, L. N., and Bernini, L. F.: Haemoglobin Leiden: Deletion of β6 or 7 glutamic acid. Nature (London), **220,** 788, 1968.
177. Hill, R. I., Swenson, R. T., and Schwartz, H. C.: G San Jose: Characterization of a chemical abnormality in hemoglobin G. J. Biol. Chem., **235,** 3182, 1960.
178. Tuchinda, S., Beale, D., and Lehmann, H.: A new haemoglobin in a Thai family: A case of haemoglobin Siriraj-β Thalassaemia. Brit. Med. J., **1,** 1583, 1965.
179. Bonaventura, J., and Riggs, A.: Haemoglobin Port Alegre: Polymerisation of hemoglobin of mouse and man. Structural basis. Science, **158,** 800, 1967.
180. Monn, D., Gaffney, P. J., and Lehmann, H.: Haemoglobin Sogn: A new haemoglobin variant β14 leucine-arginine. Scand. J. Haemat., **5,** 353, 1968.
181. Baglioni, C., and Weatherall, D. J.: Abnormal hemoglobin IX: Chemistry of hemoglobin J Baltimore. Biochim. Biophys. Acta, **78,** 637, 1963.
182. Wade, Patricia T., Jenkins, T., and Huehns, E. R.: Haemoglobin variant in a Bushman: Haemoglobin D β Bushman $\alpha_2\beta_2{}^{16Gly\text{-}Arg}$. Nature (London), **216,** 688, 1967.
183. Mackawa, M., Mackawa, T., Fujiwara, N., Tabara, K., and Matsuda, G.: Hemoglobin Nagasaki ($\alpha_2{}^A\beta_2{}^{17Glu}$): A new abnormal human hemoglobin found in a family in Nagasaki. Personal communication.
184. Bowman, B. H., Barnett, D. R., and Hite, R.: Hemoglobin G Coushatta: A beta variant with a delta-like substitution. Biochem. Biophys. Res. Commun., **26,** 466, 1967.
185. Blackwell, R. Q., Chen-Sheng, Liu, Hung-fu, Yang, Cheng-Chang, Wang, and Tung-Hsiang, Huang J.: Hemoglobin variant common to Chinese and North American Indians: $\alpha_2\beta_2{}^{22Glu\rightarrow Ala}$. Science, **161,** 381, 1968.
186. Vella, F., Lorkin, P. A., Carrell, R. W., and Lehmann, H.: A new haemoglobin variant resembling haemoglobin E, haemoglobin E Saskatoon β22 Glu-Lys. Canad. J. Biochem., **45,** 1385, 1967.
187. Blackwell, R. Q., Yang, H. J., and Wang, C. C.: Hemoglobin G Taipei: $\alpha_2\beta_2{}^{22Glu\rightarrow Gly}$. Biochim. Biophys. Acta, **175,** 237, 1969.
188. Jones, R. T., Brimhall, B., Huisman, T. H. J., Kleihauer, E., and Betke, K.: Hemoglobin Freiburg: Abnormal hemoglobin due to deletion of a single amino acid residue. Science, **154,** 1024. 1966.
189. Ranney, H. M., Jacobs, A. S., Udem, L., and Zalusky, R.: Hemoglobin Riverdale-Bronx, an unstable hemoglobin resulting from the substitution of arginine for glycine at helical residue B6 of the β polypeptide chain. Biochem. Biophys. Res. Commun., **33,** 1004, 1968.
190. Blackwell, R. Q., and Lin, C. S.: Haemoglobin G Taiwan-Ami $\alpha_2\beta_2{}^{25Gly\text{-}Arg}$. Biochem. Biophys. Res. Commun., **30,** 690, 1968.
191. Sansone, G., Carrell, R. W., and Lehmann, H.: Haemoglobin Genova: β28 (B10) leucine-proline. Nature (London), **214,** 877, 1967.
192. Baur, E. W., and Motulski, A. G.: Hemoglobin Tacoma: A β-chain variant associated with increased A_2. Humangenetik, **1,** 621, 1965.
193. Rieder, R. F., Oski, F. A., and Clegg, J. B.: Personal communication.
194. Yanase, T., Hanada., M., Seita, M., Ohya, I., Ohta, Y., Imamura, T., and Fijimura, T.: Molecular basis of morbidity: From a series of studies of hemoglobinopathy in west Japan. Jap. J. Hum. Genet., **13,** 40, 1968.
195. Dacie, J. V., Shinton, N. J., Gaffney, P. J., Jr., Carrell, R. W., and Lehmann, H.: Haemoglobin Hammersmith [β42 (CDI) Phe-Ser]. Nature (London), **216,** 663, 1967.
196. Bowman, B. H., Oliver, C. P., Barnett, D. R., Cunningham, J. E., and Schneider, R. G.: G Galveston: Chemical characterization of three hemoglobins G. Blood, **23,** 193, 1964.
197. Allen, N., Beale, D., Irvine, D., and Lehmann, H.: Three haemoglobins K: Woolwich an abnormal, Cameroon and Ibadan, two unusual variants of human haemoglobin A. Nature (London), **208,** 658, 1965.
198. Sick, K., Beale, D., Irvine, D., Lehmann, H., Goodall, P. T., and Macdougall, Sheona: Haemoglobin G Copenhagen and haemoglobin J Cambridge: Two new β-chain variants of haemoglobin A. Biochim. Biophys. Acta, **140,** 231, 1967.
198*a*. Marengo-Rowe, A. J., Lorkin, P. A., Gallo, E., and Lehmann, H.: Haemoglobin Dhofar—a new variant from Southern Arabia. Biochim. Biophys. Acta, **168,** 58, 1968.
199. Konotey-Ahula, F. I. D., Kinderlerer, Judith L., Lehmann, H., and Rinngelhann, B.: Unpublished observations.
199*a*. Boulton, F. E., Huntsman, R. G., Lehmann, H., Lorkin, P. A., and Romero, Herrera A. E.: Myoglobin variants. Proc. Brit. Soc. Haemat., April, 1970.
200. Jones, R. T., Brimhall, Bernadine, Huehns, E. R., and Motulsky, A. G.: Structural characterization of hemoglobin N Seattle $\alpha_2\beta_2{}^{61Lys\text{-}Glu}$. Biochim. Biophys. Acta, **154,** 278, 1968.
201. Shibata, S., Miyaji, T., Iuchi, I., Ueda, S., and Takeda, I.: Hemoglobin Hikari ($\alpha_2\beta_2{}^{61Asp\,NH_2}$). A fast moving hemoglobin found in two unrelated Japanese families. Clin. Chim. Acta, **10,** 101, 1964.
202. Muller, C. J., and Kingma, S.: Haemoglobin Zurich $\alpha_2{}^A\beta_2{}^{63Arg}$. Biochim. Biophys. Acta, **50,** 595, 1961.
203. Rosa, J., Labie, D., Wajcman, H., Boigne, J. M. Cabannes, R., Bierme, R., and Ruffie, J.: Haemoglobin I Toulouse: β66 (E10) Lys-Glu: A new abnormal haemoglobin with a mutation localized on the E10 porphyrin surrounding zone. Nature (London), **223,** 190, 1969.
204. Carrell, R. W., Lehmann, H., Lorkin, P. A., Raik, Eva, and Hunter, Elizabeth: Haemoglobin Sydney: β67 (E11) valine-alanine: An emerging pattern of unstable haemoglobins. Nature (London), **215,** 626, 1967.
205. Steadman, J. H., Yates, A., and Huehns, E. R. Idiopathic Heinz body anaemia: Hb-Bristol β67 (E11) Val→ Asp. Brit. J. Haemat., **18,** 435, 1970.
206. Konotey-Ahulu, F. I. D., Gallo, E., Lehmann, H., and Ringelhann, B.: Haemoglobin Korle-Bu (β73 aspartic acid-asparagine) showing one of the two amino acid substitutions of haemoglobin C Harlem. J. Med. Genet., **5,** 107, 1968.
207. Bookchin, R. M., Nagel, R. L., Ranney, H. M., and Jacob, A. S.: Hemoglobin C Harlem: A sickling variant containing amino acid substitutions in two residues of the β-polypeptide chain. Biochem. Biophys. Res. Commun., **23,** 122, 1966.
208. White, J. M., Brain, M. C., Lorkin, P. A., Lehmann, H., and Smith, M.: Mild "unstable haemoglobin haemolytic anaemia" caused by haemoglobin Shepherds Bush [β74 (E18) Gly→ Asp], Nature (London), **225,** 939, 1970.
209. Motulsky, A. G.: Personal communication.
210. Rahbar, S., Beale, D., Isaacs, W. A., and Lehmann, H.: Abnormal haemoglobins in Iran: Observations of a new variant—haemoglobin J Iran ($\alpha_2\beta_2{}^{77His\text{-}Asp}$). Brit. Med. J., **1,** 674, 1967.
211. Blackwell, R. Q., Yang, H. Y., and Wang, C. C.: Hemoglobin G Szuhu: β80 Asn-Lys. Biochim. Biophys. Acta, **188,** 59, 1969.
212. Opfell, R. W., Lorkin, P. A., and Lehmann, H.: Hereditary nonspherocytic haemolytic anaemia with post-splenectomy inclusion bodies and pigmenturia caused by an unstable haemoglobin Santa Ana β88 (F4) leucine-proline. J. Med. Genet., **5,** 292, 1968.
213. Hollender, A., Lorkin, P. A., Lehmann, H., and Svensson, B.: New unstable haemoglobin Borås: β88 (F4) leucine-arginine. Nature (London), **222,** 953, 1969.
214. Miyaji, T., Suzuki, H., Ohba, Y., and Shibata, S.: Hemoglobin Agenogi ($\alpha_2\beta_2{}^{90Lys}$). A slow moving hemoglobin of a Japanese family resembling Hb-E. Clin. Chim. Acta, **14,** 624, 1966.
215. Schneider, R. G., Satoshi, U., Alperin, J. B., Brimhill, B., and Jones,

R. T.: Hemoglobin Sabone beta 91 (F7) Leu-Pro. An unstable variant causing severe anemia with inclusion bodies. New Eng. J. Med., **280,** 739, 1969.

216. Heller, P., Coleman, R. D., and Yakulis, V.: Hemoglobin M Hyde Park: A new variant of abnormal methemoglobin. J. Clin. Invest., **45,** 1021, 1966.
217. Kraus, L.: Personal communication.
218. Clegg, J. B., Naughton, M. A., and Weatherall, D. J.: An improved method for characterization of human haemoglobin mutants: identification of $\alpha_2\beta_2$ 95 Glu, haemoglobin N (Baltimore), Nature (London), **207,** 945, 1965.
219. Bradley, T. B., Wohl, R. C., and Rieder, R. F.: Hemoglobin Gun Hill: Deletion of five amino acid residues and impaired heme-globin binding. Science, **157,** 1581, 1967.
220. Lorkin, P. A., Lehmann, H., Fairbanks, V. F., Berglund, G., and Leonhardt, T.: Two new pathological haemoglobins Olmsted β141 (H19) Leu$\rightarrow$ Arg and Malmo β97 (FG4) His$\rightarrow$ Glu. Proc. Biochem. Soc., July, 1970.
221. Carrell, R. W., Lehmann, H., and Hutchinson, H. E.: Haemoglobin Köln (β98 valine-methionine): An unstable protein causing inclusion-body anaemia. Nature (London), **210,** 915, 1966.
222. Jones, R. T., Osgood, E. E., Brimhall, B., and Koler, R. D.: Hemoglobin Yakima: 1. Clinical and biochemical studies. J. Clin. Invest., **46,** 1840, 1967.
223. Reed, C. S., Hampson, R., Gordon, S., Jones, R. T., Novy, M. J., Brimhall, B., Edwards, M. J., and Koler, R. D.: Erythrocytosis secondary to increased oxygen affinity of a mutant hemoglobin, hemoglobin Kempsey. Blood, **31,** 623, 1968.
224. Bonaventura, J., and Riggs, A.: Hemoglobin Kansas, a human hemoglobin with a neutral amino acid substitution and an abnormal oxygen equilibrium. J. Biol. Chem., **243,** 980, 1968.
225. Efremon, G. D., Huisman, T. H. J., Smith, Linda L., Wilson, J. B., Kitchens, Janice L., Wrightstone, Ruth N., and Adams, H. R.: Hemoglobin Richmond, a human hemoglobin which forms asymmetric hybrids with other hemoglobins. J. Biol. Chem., **244,** 6105, 1969.
226. Imamura, T., Fujita, S., Ohta, Y., Hanada, M., and Yanase, T.: Hemoglobin Yoshizuka [G 10 (108) β asparagine$\rightarrow$ aspartic acid]: A new variant with a reduced oxygen affinity from a Japanese family. J. Clin. Invest., **48,** 2341, 1969.
227. Ranney, H. M., Jacobs, A. S., and Nagel, R. L.: Haemoglobin New York. Nature (London), **213,** 876, 1967.
228. Schneider, R. G., Alperin, J. B., Brimhall, B., and Jones, R. T.: Hemoglobin P ($\alpha_2\beta_2{}^{117\,Arg}$): Structure and properties. J. Lab. Clin. Med., **73,** 616, 1969.
229. Miyaji, T., Ohba, Y., Yamamoto, K., Shibata, S., Iuchi, I., and Hamilton, H. B.: Hemoglobin Hijiyama: A new fast-moving hemoglobin in a Japanese family. Science, **159,** 204, 1968.
230. Miyaji, T., Ohba, Y., Yamamoto, K., Shibata, S., Iuchi, I., and Takenaka, H.: Japanese haemoglobin variant (Hb Hofu $\alpha_2\beta_2{}^{126\,Glu}$). Nature (London), **217,** 89, 1968.
231. Blackwell, R. Q., Yang, H. J., and Wang, C. C.: Hemoglobin J Taichung: β129 Ala-Asp. Biochim. Biophys. Acta, **194,** 1, 1969.
232. Pietschmann, H., Lorkin, P. A., Lehmann, H., and Braunsteiner, H.: Unpublished observations.
233. Minnich, V., Hill, R. J., Khuri, P. D., and Anderson, M. E. Hemoglobin Hope: a beta chain variant. Blood, **25,** 830, 1965.
234. Hamilton, H. B., Iuchi, I., Miyaji, T., and Shibata, S.: Hemoglobin Hiroshima (β^{143} histidine-aspartic acid): A newly identified fast moving beta chain variant associated with increased oxygen affinity and compensatory erythremia. J. Clin. Invest., **48,** 525, 1969, and personal communication.
235. Stammatoyannopoulos, G., Adamson, J., Yoshida, A., and Heienberg, S.: Hemoglobin Rainier: An adult alkali resistant hemoglobin associated with erythrocytosis. Blood, **30,** 879, 1967.
236. Lehmann, H.: Unpublished observations.
237. Jenkins, G. C., Beale, D., Black, A. J., Huntsman, R. G., and Lehmann, H.: Haemoglobin F Texas I ($\alpha_2\gamma_2{}^{5\,Glu\text{-}Lys}$): A variant of haemoglobin F. Brit. J. Haemat., **13,** 252, 1967.
238. Larkin, I. L. M., Baker, T., Lorkin, P. A., Lehmann, H., Black, A. J., and Huntsman, R. G.: Haemoglobin F Texas II ($\alpha_2\gamma_2{}^{6\,Glu\text{-}Lys}$), the second of the haemoglobin F Texas variants. Brit. J. Haemat., **14,** 233, 1968.
239. Loukopoulos, D., Kaltsoya, A., and Fessas, P.: On the chemical abnormality of the Hb "Alexandria," a fetal hemoglobin variant. Blood, **33,** 114, 1969.
240. Ahern, E. J., Jones, R. T., Brimhall, B., and Gray, R. H.: Haemoglobin F Jamaica ($\alpha_2\gamma_2$ 61 Lys$\rightarrow$ Glu: 136 Ala). Brit. J. Haemat., **18,** 369, 1970.
241. Cauchi, M. N., Clegg, J. B., and Weatherall, D. J.: Haemoglobin F (Malta): A new foetal haemoglobin variant with a high incidence in Maltese infants. Nature (London), **223,** 311, 1969.
242. Sacker, L. S., Beale, D., Black, A. J., Huntsman, R. G., Lehmann, H., and Lorkin, P. A.: Haemoglobin F Hull (γ121 glutamic acid-lysine) Homologous with haemoglobins O Arab and O Indonesia. Brit. Med. J., **3,** 531, 1967.
243. Jones, R. T., Brimhall, B., Huehns, E. R., and Barnicot, N. A.: Hemoglobin Sphakia: A Delta-Chain Variant of Hemoglobin A_2 from Crete. Science, **151,** 1406, 1966.
244. Ranney, H. M. Personal communication.
245. Ball, E. W., Maynell, M. J., Beale, D., Kynoch, Pamela, Lehmann, H., and Stretton, A. O. W. Haemoglobin A_2' $\alpha_2\delta_2{}^{16\,Gly\text{-}Arg}$. Nature (London), **209,** 1217, 1966.
246. Jones, R. T., Brimhall, B., and Huisman, T. H. J.: Chemical studies of hemoglobin A_2 δ Flatbush. $\alpha_2\delta_2{}^{22\,Glu}$. Clin. Res., **14,** 168, 1966.
247. de Jong, W. W. W., and Bernini, L. F.: Haemoglobin Babinga (δ136 glycine-aspartic acid): A new delta chain variant. Nature (London), **219,** 1360, 1968.
248. Schroeder, W. A.: The hemoglobins. Ann. Rev. Biochem., **32,** 301, 1963.
249. Watson, H. C., and Kendrew, J. C.: Comparison between the amino-acid sequences of sperm whale myoglobin and of human haemoglobin. Nature (London), **190,** 670, 1961.
249*a*. Huehns, E. R., and Shooter, E. M.: The polypeptide chains of Hb-A_2 and Hb-G_2. J. Molec. Biol., **3,** 257, 1961.
249*b*. Minnich, V., Cordonnier, J. K., Williams, W. J., and Moore, C. V.: Alpha, beta, and gamma hemoglobin polypeptide chains during the neonatal period with description of a fetal form of Hb-D_{alpha} St. Louis. Blood, **19,** 137, 1962.
250. Nobbs, C. L., Watson, H. C., and Kendrew, J. C.: Structure of deoxyhaemoglobin: A crystallographic study. Nature (London), **209,** 339, 1966.
251. Weiss, J. J.: Nature of the iron-oxygen bond in oxyhaemoglobin. Nature (London), **202,** 83, 1964.
252. Weiss, J. J.: Nature of the iron-oxygen bond in oxyhaemoglobin. Nature (London), **203,** 182, 1964.
253. Perutz, M. F., and Lehmann, H.: Molecular pathology of human haemoglobins. Nature (London), **219,** 902, 1968.
254. Hayashi, A., Suzuki, T., Imai, K., Morimoto, H., and Watari, H. L.: Properties of hemoglobin M Milwaukee-1 variant and its unique characteristic. Biochim. Biophys. Acta, **194,** 6, 1969.
255. Ranney, H. M., Nagel, R. L., Heller, P., and Idem, L.: Oxygen equilibrium of hemoglobin M Hyde Park. Biochim. Biophys. Acta, **160,** 112, 1968.
256. Tönz, O.: The congenital methemoglobinemias: *Physiology and Pathophysiology of Hemoglobin Metabolism.* Karger, Basel, 1968.
257. Evelyn, K., and Malloy, H.: Microdetermination of oxyhemoglobin, methemoglobin, and sulfhemoglobin in a single sample of blood. J. Biol. Chem., **126,** 655, 1938.
258. Watson, H. C.: in *Hemes and Hemoproteins,* edited by B. Chance, R. W. Estabrook, and I. Yonetani, p. 63. Academic, New York, 1966.
259. Fanelli, A. R., Antonini, E., and Caputo, A.: Studies on the structure of hemoglobin. 1. Physicochemical properties of human globin. Biochim. Biophys. Acta, **30,** 608, 1958; **35,** 93, 1958.
260. Hrkal, Z., and Vodrazka, Z.: A study of the conformation of human globin in solution by optical methods. Biochim. Biophys. Acta, **133,** 527, 1967.
261. Jacob, H. S., Brain, M. C., Dacie, J. V., Carrell, R. W., and Lehmann, H.: Abnormal haem binding and globin SH group blockade in unstable haemoglobins. Nature (London), **218,** 1214, 1966.
262. Perutz, M. F., Muirhead, H., Cox, J. M., and Goaman, L. C. G.: Three-dimensional Fourier synthesis of horse oxyhaemoglobin at 2.8 Å resolution. II. The atomic model. Nature (London), **219,** 131, 1968.

263. Fessas, P., Loukopoulas, D., and Kaltsoya, A.: Peptide analysis of the inclusions of erythroid cells in β-thalassaemia. Biochim. Biophys. Acta, **124**, 430, 1966.
264. Tuchinda, S., Beale, D., and Lehmann, H.: The suppression of haemoglobin E synthesis where haemoglobin H disease and haemoglobin E occur together. Humangenetik, **3**, 312, 1967.
265. Muirhead, H., Cox, J. M., Mazzarella, L., and Perutz, M. F.: Structure and function of haemoglobin. III. A three-dimensional Fourier synthesis of human deoxyhaemoglobin at 5.5 Å resolution. J. Molec. Biol., **28**, 117, 1967.
266. Lehmann, H., and Carrell, R. W.: Variations in the structure of human haemoglobins. Brit. Med. Bull., **25**, 14, 1969.
267. Vogel, F.: Point mutations and human hemoglobin variants. Humangenetik, **8**, 1, 1969.
268. Allison, A. C.: Notation for hemoglobin types and genes controlling their synthesis. Science, **122**, 640, 1955.
269. Halbrecht, I., and Klibanski, C.: Identification of a new normal embryonic haemoglobin. Nature (London), **178**, 794, 1956.
270. Halbrecht, I., Klibanski, C., and Bar Ilan, F.: Coexistence of the embryonic (third normal) haemoglobin fraction with erythroblastosis in the blood of two full-term new-born babies with multiple malformations. Nature (London), **183**, 327, 1959.
271. Drescher, H., and Künzer, W.: Der Blutfarbstoff des menschlichen Feten. Klin. Wschr., **32**, 92, 1954.
272. Künzer, W., and Drescher, H.: Spektrophotometrische Untersuchungen am Blutfarbstoff menschlicher Feten. Klin. Wschr., **34**, 918, 1956.
273. Künzer, W.: Human embryo haemoglobins. Nature, **179**, 477, 1957.
274. Huehns, E. R., Flynn, F. V., Butler, E. A., and Beaven, G. H.: Two new haemoglobin variants in a very young human embryo. Nature (London), **189**, 496, 1961.
275. Szelényi, J. G., and Hollan, S. R.: Studies on the structure of human embryonic haemoglobin. Acta Biochim. Biophys. Acad. Sci. Hung., **4**, 47–55, 1969.
276. Edington, G. M., and Lehmann, H.: Expression of the sickle-cell gene in Africa. Brit. Med. J., **1**, 1308; **2**, 1328, 1955.
277. Neel, J. V., Hiernaux, J., Linhard, J., Robinson, A., Zuelzer, W. W., and Livingstone, F. R.: Data on occurrence of hemoglobin C and other abnormal hemoglobins in some African populations. Amer. J. Hum. Genet., **8**, 138, 1956.
278. Jacob, G. F., and Raper, A. B.: Hereditary persistence of foetal haemoglobin production, and its interaction with the sickle-cell trait. Brit. J. Haemat., **4**, 138, 1958.
279. Herman, E. C., and Conley, C. L.: Hereditary persistence of fetal hemoglobin: A family study. Amer. J. Med., **29**, 9, 1960.
280. Conley, C. L., Weatherall, D. J., Richardson, S. N., Shephard, M. K., and Charache, S.: Hereditary persistence of fetal hemoglobin: A study of 79 affected persons in 15 Negro families in Baltimore. Blood, **21**, 261, 1963.
281. Wheeler, J. T., and Krevans, J. R.: The homozygous state of persistent fetal hemoglobin and the interaction of persistent fetal hemoglobin with thalassemia. Bull. Johns Hopkins Hosp., **109**, 215, 1961.
282. Motulsky, A. G.: Controller genes in synthesis of human haemoglobin. Nature (London), **194**, 607, 1962.
283. Neel, J. V.: The hemoglobin genes: A remarkable example of the clustering of related genetic functions on a single mammalian chromosome. Blood, **18**, 769, 1961.
284. Boyer, S. H., Rucknagel, D. L., Weatherall, D. J., and Watson-Williams, E. J.: Further evidence for linkage between the β and δ loci governing human hemoglobin and the population dynamics of linked genes. Amer. J. Hum. Genet., **15**, 438, 1963.
285. Horton, B. F., and Huisman, T. H. J.: Linkage of the β-chain and the δ-chain structural genes of human hemoglobins. Amer. J. Hum. Genet., **15**, 394, 1963.
286. Ingram, V. M., and Stretton, A. O. W.: Human haemoglobin A_2: Chemistry, genetics, and evolution. Nature (London), **190**, 1079, 1961.
287. Muller, C. J., and Jonxis, J. H. P.: Identity of haemoglobin A_2. Nature (London), **188**, 949, 1960.
288. Gammack, D. B., Huehns, E. R., Shooter, E. M., and Gerald, P. A.: Identification of the abnormal peptide chain in haemoglobin G_{Ibadan}. J. Molec. Biol., **2**, 372, 1960.
289. Labie, D., Schroeder, W. A., and Huisman, T. H. J.: The amino acid sequence of the δ-β chains of haemoglobin Lepore Augusta and Lepore Washington. Biochim. Biophys. Acta, **127**, 428, 1966.
290. Gerald, P. S., and Diamond, L. K.: A new hereditary hemoglobinopathy (the Lepore trait) and its interaction with thalassemia trait. Blood, **13**, 835, 1958.
291. Gerald, P. S., Efron, M. L., and Diamond, L. K.: A human mutation (the Lepore hemoglobinopathy) possibly involving two "cistrons." Amer. J. Dis. Child., **102**, 514, 1961.
292. Neeb, H., Beiboer, J. L., Jonxis, J. H. P., Kaars-Sijpestejn, J. A., and Muller, C. J.: Homozygous Lepore haemoglobin disease appearing as thalassemia major in two Papuan siblings. Trop. Geogr. Med., **13**, 207, 1961.
293. Fessas, P., Stomatoyannopoulos, G., and Karaklis, A.: Hemoglobin "Pylos": Study of hemoglobinopathy resembling thalassemia in the heterozygous, homozygous, and double heterozygous state. Blood, **19**, 1, 1962.
294. Barnabas, J., and Muller, C. J.: Haemoglobin Lepore hollandi. Nature (London), **194**, 931, 1962.
295. Baglioni, C.: The fusion of two peptide chains in hemoglobin Lepore and its interpretation as a genetic deletion. Proc. Nat. Acad. Sci. USA, **48**, 1880, 1962.
296. Smithies, O.: Chromosomal rearrangements and protein structure. Cold Spring Harbor Symposia on Quantitative Biology, **19**, 309–319, 1964.
297. Harris, H.: *The Principles of Human Biochemical Genetics.* North Holland Publishing Co., Amsterdam, 1970.
298. Yanase, T., Handa, M., Seita, H., Ohya, I., Ohta, Y., Imamura, T., Fujimura, T., Kawasaki, K., and Yamaoka, K.: Molecular basis of morbidity from a series of studies of hemoglobinopathies in Western Japan. Jap. J. Hum. Genet., **13**, 40, 1968.
299. Dherte, P., Lehmann, H., and Vandepitte, J.: Haemoglobin P in a family in the Belgian Congo. Nature (London), **184**, 1133, 1959.
300. Lambotte-Legrand, J., Lambotte-Legrand, C., Ager, J. A. M., and Lehmann, H.: L'hémoglobinose P: à propos d'un cas d'association des hémoglobines P et S. Rev. hémat., **15**, 10, 1960.
301. Lehmann, H., and Charlesworth, Deborah.: Observations on haemoglobin P (Congo type). Proc. Biochem. Soc., July, 1970.
302. Dintzis, H. M.: Assembly of the peptide chains of hemoglobin. Proc. Nat. Acad. Sci. USA, **47**, 247, 1961.
303. Dintzis, H. M.: Biosynthesis of hemoglobin. Conference on Hemoglobin, Columbia University, New York, 1962.
304. Naughton, M. A., and Dintzis, H. M.: Sequential biosynthesis of the peptide chains of hemoglobin. Proc. Nat. Acad. Sci. USA, **48**, 1822, 1962.
305. Sarabhai, A. S., Stretton, A. O. W., Brenner, S., and Bolle, A.: Colinearity of the gene with the polypeptide chain. Nature (London), **201**, 13, 1964.
306. Lehmann, H.: Distributions of variations in human haemoglobin synthesis, in *Abnormal Haemoglobins,* p. 202. Blackwell, Oxford, 1959.
307. Rucknagel, D. L., and Neel, J. V.: The hemoglobinopathies, in *Progress in Medical Genetics,* edited by A. G. Steinberg, vol. 1, p. 158. Grune & Stratton, New York, 1961.
308. Livingstone, F. B.: *Abnormal Hemoglobins in Human Populations,* Aldine, Chicago, 1967.
309. Lehmann, H.: The maintenance of the haemoglobinopathies at high frequency: A consideration of the relation between sickling and malaria and of allied problems, in *Abnormal Haemoglobins,* p. 307. Blackwell, Oxford, 1959.
310. Neel, J. V.: Data pertaining to population dynamics of sickle cell disease. J. Hum. Genet., **5**, 154, 1953.
311. Allison, A. C.: Protection afforded by sickle-cell trait against subtertian malarial infection. Brit. Med. J., **1**, 290, 1954.
312. Vandepitte, J. M., Zuelzer, W. W., Neel, J. V., and Colaert, J.: Evidence concerning the inadequacy of mutation as an explanation of the frequency of the sickle cell gene in the Belgian Congo. Blood, **10**, 341, 1955.
313. Beet, E. A.: Sickle cell disease in the Balovale district of Northern Rhodesia. E. Afr. Med. J., **23**, 75, 1956.

314. Brain, P.: Sickle cell trait: Its clinical significance. S. Afr. Med. J., **26**, 925, 1952.
315. Raper, A. B.: Malaria and the sickling trait. Brit. Med. J., **1**, 1186, 1955.
316. Miller, M. J., Neel, J. V., and Livingstone, F. B.: Distribution of parasites in the red cells of sickle-cell trait carriers infected with *Plasmodium falciparum,* Trans. Roy. Soc. Trop. Med. Hyg., **50**, 924, 1956.
317. Raper, A. B.: Further observations on sickling and malaria. Trans. Roy. Soc. Trop. Med. Hyg., **53**, 110, 1959.
318. Lehmann, H., and Raper, A. B.: Maintenance of high sickling rate in an African community. Brit. Med. J., **2**, 333, 1956.
319. Allison, A. C.: Sickle cell and haemoglobin C genes in some African populations. Ann. Hum. Genet., **21**, 67, 1956.
320. Lehmann, H.: Distribution of the sickle cell gene: A new light on the origin of the East Africans. Eugenics Rev., **46**, 101, 1954.
321. Lehmann, H., and Raper, A. B.: The maintenance of different sickling rates in similar populations. J. Physiol., **133**, 15*P*, 1956.
322. Serjeant, G. R., Richards, R., Barbor, P. R. H., and Milner, P. F.: Relatively benign sickle cell anaemia in 60 patients aged over 30 in the West Indies. Brit. Med. J., **3**, 86, 1968.
323. Lehmann, H.: Variations in human haemoglobin synthesis and factors governing their inheritance. Brit. Med. Bull., **15**, 40, 1959.
324. Haldane, J. B. S.: Disease and evolution. Ric. Sci., **19**, suppl. 68, 1949.
325. Carrell, R. W.: Personal communication.
326. Milner, P. F., Clegg, J. B., and Weatherall, D. J.: Haemoglobin-H disease due to a unique haemoglobin variant with an elongated α-chain. Lancet, **1**, 729, 1971.
327. Flatz, G., Kinderlerer, J. L., Kilmartin, J. V., and Lehmann, H.: Haemoglobin Tak: a variant with additional residues at the end of the β-chains. Lancet, **1**, 732, 1971.
328. Jackson, R., and Hunter, T.: Role of methionine in the initiation of haemoglobin synthesis. Nature, **227**, 672, 1970.
329. Wilson, D. B., and Dintzis, H. M.: Protein chain initiation in rabbit reticulocytes. Proc. Nat. Acad. Sci. USA, **66**, 1282, 1970.
330. Perutz, M. F.: Stereochemistry of cooperative effects in haemoglobin. Nature, **228**, 726, 1970.

CHAPTER FIFTY-EIGHT

THE THALASSEMIAS

D. J. Weatherall

A form of severe anemia, occurring early in life and associated with splenomegaly and bone changes, was first described by Cooley and Lee in 1925 [1]. The condition was later named *thalassemia* from θαλασσα "the sea," since early cases were all of Mediterranean background. It was only in the period after 1940 that the true genetic character of this disorder was fully appreciated. It became clear that the disease described by Cooley was the homozygous state for a partially dominant autosomal gene, while the heterozygous state was associated with much milder hematological changes. The severely affected homozygous condition became known as *thalassemia major*, while the heterozygous states, according to their severity, were designated *thalassemia minor* or *minima*. Several extensive reviews have dealt with the historical aspects of thalassemia in detail [2, 3].

Since 1950 it has been established that *thalassemia* is not a single disease entity but a group of disorders which result from an inherited abnormality of globin production and are therefore classifiable as *hemoglobinopathies* [4]. It is now clear that inherited hemoglobinopathies are of two types. First there are those, like sickle-cell anemia, which result from an inherited structural abnormality in one of the constituent globin chains. Although these abnormal hemoglobins may be synthesized at a slower rate or broken down more rapidly than normal adult hemoglobin, the associated clinical abnormalities result from the physical properties of the abnormal hemoglobin. The second major group of inherited abnormalities of hemoglobin synthesis, the thalassemias, result from inherited defects in the *rate* of synthesis of *normal* hemoglobin. In this group of disorders the clinical abnormalities are the result of a deficient overall rate of production of normal hemoglobin, combined with the deleterious results of imbalanced globin chain synthesis [4, 5, 6, 7].

Since the structural hemoglobin variants and the thalassemias occur frequently in the same population groups it is not surprising that the two genetic defects frequently occur together in the same individual. The different genetic types of thalassemia and their combinations with the genes for abnormal hemoglobins produce a complex series of disorders known collectively as the thalassemia syndromes. Before considering each of these disorders in detail, it will be necessary to review briefly the genetic control of hemoglobin structure and the mechanisms which govern its rate of synthesis. These subjects have been extensively reviewed [6, 8, 9, 10], and only those aspects with particular relevance to the thalassemia problem will be discussed.

THE GENETIC CONTROL OF HEMOGLOBIN SYNTHESIS

Genetic Control

The structure of hemoglobin has been fully reviewed in the previous chapter and will only be briefly mentioned here. Human adult hemoglobin is a heterogeneous mixture of proteins, consisting of a major component, hemoglobin A, and a minor fraction constituting 2.5 percent of the total, hemoglobin A_2. In intrauterine life, the main hemoglobin pigment is hemoglobin F. The structure of these hemoglobins is basically similar, each consisting of two separate pairs of like globin chains. All the normal human hemoglobins have one pair of chains in common, the α-chains; in hemoglobin A these are combined with β-chains ($\alpha_2\beta_2$), in hemoglobin A_2 with δ-chains ($\alpha_2\delta_2$), and in hemoglobin F with γ-chains ($\alpha_2\gamma_2$).

Critical family studies have provided clear evidence regarding the organization of the genetic control of hemoglobin structure (Fig. 58-1). The same locus (or loci) controls the synthesis of α-chains in fetal and adult life. In intrauterine life α-chains combine with γ-chains to produce hemoglobin F, and hemoglobin A forms only a minor part of the total pigment. At birth the β- and δ-loci are fully activated and the γ-locus is "switched off." Alpha chains now combine with β-chains and δ-chains to produce hemoglobins A and A_2. This switchover is extremely smooth, there being only a slight excess of γ- or β-chains produced in the neonatal period during the switchover from γ- to β- and δ-chain synthesis.

The scheme outlined above for the genetic control of hemoglobin synthesis is rather oversimplified and recent work has indicated that there may be multiple structural loci controlling both α- and γ-chain synthesis. It has been shown that human fetal hemoglobin is a mixture of molecules with the following formulae: $\alpha_2\gamma_2^{136\text{Gly}}$, $\alpha_2\gamma_2^{136\text{Ala}}$ [78]. There is very good evidence that the synthesis of these γ-chains is directed by distinct structural genes [78, 79]. The precise number of these structural loci and their relationship to each other have not yet been worked out. There is also recent evidence that at least in some populations there may be more than one structural gene controlling α-chain synthesis in normal adult hemoglobin. Furthermore one family study [80] suggests that these α-loci are not linked and indeed may be on different chromosomes. These recent discoveries make the genetic definition of some of the thalassemia

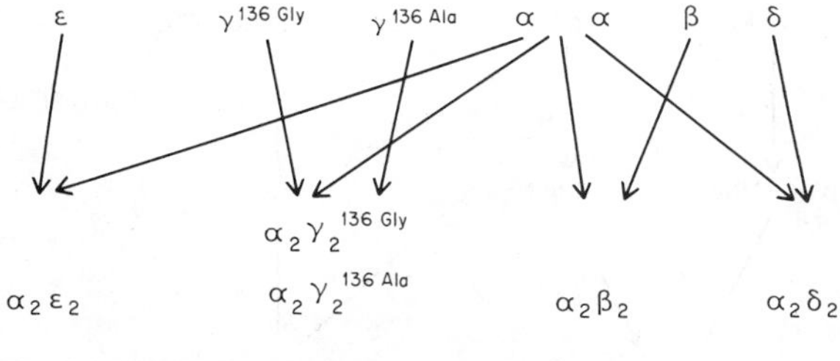

Figure 58-1. Genetic control of hemoglobin synthesis. At least two structural genes on each chromosome direct the synthesis of the γ chains of fetal hemoglobin. In addition, it now seems likely that, in some individuals, there are at least two α-chain genes on each chromosome.

disorders, particularly the α-thalassemias, extremely complex.

Little is known about the chromosomal location of the hemoglobin genes except that the δ- and β-chain genes are closely linked [11], whereas the genes for the α and β chains are either some distance apart on the same chromosome or possibly on different chromosomes [12]. The location of the γ-chain locus is still uncertain.

Synthesis of Hemoglobin

The mechanisms involved in the control of this genetic system are poorly understood, and this is probably why the basic biosynthetic defect in thalassemia awaits elucidation. Current knowledge about this important topic has been fully reviewed elsewhere [9].

The genetic information which determines the structure of the globin chains is contained in the sequences of the base pairs of their constituent genes. A 9S fraction with the labeling and functional properties of messenger RNA has now been obtained from mouse, rabbit, and human reticulocytes. The 9S material from human reticulocytes appears to be genuine messenger RNA since it can direct the synthesis of human α- and β-chains in a rabbit cell free system [13,87].

There is now good evidence from work in both rabbit and human reticulocytes that α-chains are released into a small pool before combining with β-chains [20, 21]. It has been suggested that α-chains from this pool combine with partially completed β-chains on the ribosomes and that α-chains are required for the removal of β-chains from the ribosomes. While this is an attractive mechanism for synchronizing the production of both α- and β-chains it does not fit in with the findings in certain forms of thalassemia. It appears that α- and β-chains first combine as the $\alpha\beta$ unit; heme is then inserted and the two $\alpha\beta$ units combine to form a stable tetramer. There is increasing evidence that the incorporation of heme occurs after the release of the globin chain from the ribosome [22].

Clearly this complex series of synthetic steps requires control and coordination. Control can occur at the transcriptional level. Since no RNA is synthesized beyond the orthochromatic normoblast stage, this form of control can only be applicable to early red cell precursors. Control can also be exerted at the level of translation. This could occur in the reticulocyte.

There is good evidence that the β- and δ-loci are linked and that the C-terminal end of the δ-chain lies close to the N-terminal end of the β-chain [23]. These observations have resulted in much speculation about the possibility of a $\delta\beta$-operon. Such a unit would be under the control of a hypothetical operator gene, thus providing a mechanism for activation of the δ- and β-loci in the neonatal period and for control of specific messenger RNA production in adult life. These speculations have followed from the findings in patients with hereditary persistence of fetal hemoglobin [24]. There is no other evidence for the existence of such a coordinated unit of genetic expression. Arguments against this general concept have been fully reviewed elsewhere [9].

There are several mechanisms which might control the rate of globin chain synthesis during its assembly on the polysomes. The overall rate of chain synthesis could be modified by the rate of binding of individual amino acyl transfer RNAs and their combination in peptide linkage; the rate of chain initiation, termination, and release; the rate of folding to a tertiary configuration; the availability of heme; and the rate of association with other chains to form a stable hemoglobin molecule. In addition, since the genetic code is degenerate, availability of different transfer RNAs may be rate limiting in chain assembly [6]. Any of these mechanisms could be abnormal in the various types of thalassemia.

There is fairly strong evidence that heme and globin production are coordinated [25]. The complex series of steps in which heme is synthesized from glycine and active succinate have been fully worked out [26] and the rate limiting step in this pathway is known. Thus it appears that the step in which glycine and succinate combine to produce δ-amino levulinic acid, which is catalyzed by δ-amino-levulinic acid synthetase, is inhibited as heme accumulates in the red cell [26]. The relationships between heme and globin synthesis and the control of heme synthesis are summarized in Fig. 58-2.

THE DIFFERENT FORMS OF THALASSEMIA

Just as there are abnormal hemoglobins resulting from structural changes in either the α- or β-chains, so there are two main types of thalassemia, α and β, depending upon whether the rate of α-chain or β-chain synthesis is retarded [7].

The β-thalassemias are usually characterized by persistent

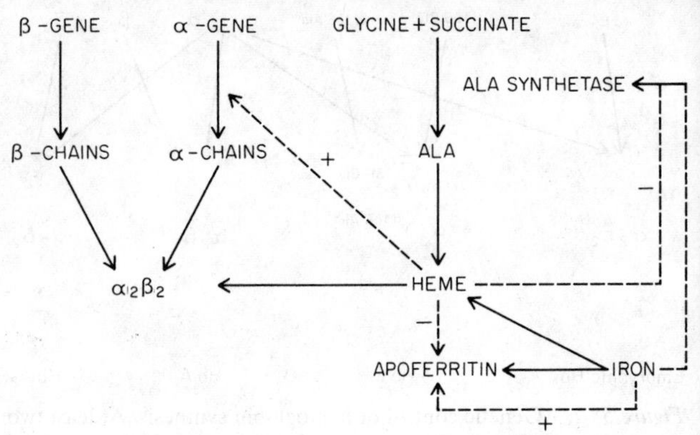

Figure 58-2. Control of hemoglobin production. Heme inhibits its own rate of synthesis by "negative feedback." It also stimulates the synthesis of globin chains. Iron also stimulates heme synthesis directly and excess iron may inhibit the early stages of heme synthesis. Iron stimulates apoferritin synthesis in the red cell precursor, while heme has the opposite effect. This diagram underlines the central place of heme in the control of both hemoglobin and iron metabolism.

Table 58-1. THE GENOTYPE, CLINICAL FINDINGS, AND HEMOGLOBIN PATTERN IN DIFFERENT FORMS OF β-THALASSEMIA

Genotype	Clinical features	Hemoglobin pattern
$\delta\beta\,\delta\beta$	Normal.	Normal
1. $\delta\beta^{\text{thal}+}\,\delta\beta^{\text{thal}+}$	Cooley's anemia.	20 to 80% hemoglobin F. Variable hemoglobin A_2. Free α chain present.
2. $\delta\beta\,\delta\beta^{\text{thal}+}$	Thalassemia minor. Variable anemia.	3.5 to 7.5% hemoglobin A_2. Slight elevation in hemoglobin F in 50% of the cases.
3. $\delta\beta^{\text{thal o}}\,\delta\beta^{\text{thal o}}$	Cooley's anemia.	Hemoglobin entirely fetal except for a small amount of hemoglobin A_2. Free α chain present.
4. $\delta\beta\,\delta\beta^{\text{thal o}}$	Thalassemia minor.	As for (2).
5. $(\delta\beta)^{\text{thal o}}\,(\delta\beta)^{\text{thal o}}$	Cooley's anemia but milder than above.	Hemoglobin entirely of fetal type.
6. $\delta\beta\,(\delta\beta)^{\text{thal o}}$	Thalassemia minor.	Hemoglobin F in 5 to 20% range. Hemoglobin A_2 normal.
7. $\delta\beta^{\text{thal o}}\,(\delta\beta)^{\text{thal o}}$	Mild Cooley's anemia.	Hemoglobin F makes up total hemoglobin except for a trace of hemoglobin A_2 in 1% range.
8. $\delta\beta^{\text{thal ?}}\,\delta\beta$	Nil.	Normal. Silent β-thalassemia gene.
9. $\delta\beta^{\text{S}}\,\delta\beta^{\text{thal o}}$	Similar to sickle-cell anemia.	Hemoglobin consists mainly of hemoglobin S with increased levels of hemoglobin A_2 and F. No hemoglobin A.
10. $\delta\beta^{\text{S}}\,\delta\beta^{\text{thal}+}$	As above but usually milder.	Hemoglobin S makes up about 70% of total hemoglobin. Hemoglobin A present at about 20% with increased hemoglobins A_2 and F.
11. $\delta\beta^{\text{S}}\,(\delta\beta)^{\text{thal o}}$	As above.	Hemoglobin made up of hemoglobin S with hemoglobin F and A_2. No hemoglobin A.
12. $(\delta\beta)^{\text{Lepore}}\,(\delta\beta)^{\text{Lepore}}$	Cooley's anemia.	Hemoglobin consists of F and Lepore. No A or A_2.
13. $(\delta\beta)^{\text{Lepore}}\,\delta\beta$	Thalassemia minor.	Hemoglobin consists of A with about 8% Lepore, increased hemoglobin F and low hemoglobin A_2.

Note: The δ and β loci which are normal are written $\delta\beta$. The α and γ loci are normal and are not shown. Several conditions have been left out of this table, for example, hemoglobin C and hemoglobin E thalassemia. Both of these occur with β-thalassemia^{o} and β-thalassemia^{+} as shown for sickle-cell thalassemia. It is also possible that $\delta\beta$-thalassemia exists in a form with some β- and δ-chain synthesis.

synthesis of fetal hemoglobin beyond the neonatal period. Thus, in an absence of sufficient β-chains, γ-chains are synthesized, but at a rate which is insufficient to compensate for the deficiency of β-chains. As will be seen later, there are several different types of β-thalassemia depending upon whether there is a total or partial deficiency of β-chains and whether the synthesis of δ-chains of hemoglobin A_2 is normal or defective. Furthermore, there are several disorders resulting from the combination of β-thalassemia with β-structural hemoglobin variants (Table 58-1).

Since α-chains are shared by fetal and adult hemoglobins a deficiency of α-chain production might be expected to affect hemoglobin synthesis in fetal as well as in adult life. A reduced rate of α-chain synthesis in fetal life results [27] in an excess of γ-chains, which form γ_4 tetramers or hemoglobin Bart's. In adult life a deficiency of α-chains also results in an excess of β-chains which form β_4 tetramers or hemoglobin H [28, 29]. Several disorders result from the interactions of the α-thalassemia genes, either with other α-thalassemia genes or with the α- or β-chain structural hemoglobin variants (Table 58-2).

There are other thalassemia-like disorders resulting from a series of unequal genetic crossovers at the $\delta\beta$-gene complex. This type of mechanism results in a composite $\delta\beta$-chain and $\beta\delta$-chain which are synthesized at a reduced rate (see previous chapter).

Table 58-2. THE GENOTYPE, CLINICAL FINDINGS, AND HEMOGLOBIN PATTERN IN DIFFERENT FORMS OF α-THALASSEMIA

Genotype	Clinical findings	Hemoglobin pattern
$\alpha\ \alpha$ / $\beta\ \beta$	Normal	Normal
1. $\alpha^{thal\ 1}\ \alpha^{thal\ 1}$ / $\beta\ \beta$	Hydrops fetalis	80 to 90% hemoglobin Bart's. The remainder is hemoglobins H and Portland.
2. $\alpha^{thal\ 1}\ \alpha$ / $\beta\ \beta$	Mild thalassemic picture	Normal in adult life. 5 to 10% hemoglobin Bart's in infants.
3. $\alpha^{thal\ 2}\ \alpha$ / $\beta\ \beta$	Normal	Normal in adult life. 1 to 2% hemoglobin Bart's in infancy.
4. $\alpha^{thal\ 1}\ \alpha^{thal\ 2}$ / $\beta\ \beta$	Moderate hemolytic anemia	Hemoglobin H makes up 5 to 30% of the hemoglobin with small amount of hemoglobin Bart's.
5. $\alpha^{thal\ 1}\ \alpha^{Q}$ / $\beta\ \beta$	Moderate hemolytic anemia	Hemoglobin consists of Q, Q_2, H, and Bart's.
6. $\alpha^{thal\ 1}\ \alpha$ / $\beta\ \beta^{E}$	Moderate hemolytic anemia	Hemoglobin consists of E, A, and Bart's.
7. $\alpha^{thal\ 1}\ \alpha$ / $\beta^{E}\ \beta^{E}$	Picture similar to Cooley's anemia	Hemoglobin consists of E, Bart's, and H.
8. $\alpha^{thal\ 1}\ \alpha^{thal\ 2}$ / $\beta^{S}\ \beta^{S}$	Moderate hemolytic anemia	Hemoglobin consists of S, A_2, and 20% Bart's.

Note: The genotype is derived from studies of the level of hemoglobin Bart's in infancy. For simplicity, only a single α-chain gene on each chromosome has been shown. It is possible that the α-thalassemia 1 and α-thalassemia 2 genes represent specific mutations at different α-chain loci on the same chromosome or on different chromosomes. All possible combinations of α-thalassemia with β chain variants have not been included. Other interpretations of these findings are discussed in the text.

Finally there are some poorly defined conditions which may arise from defective δ- or γ-chain synthesis. Each of these types of thalassemia will be considered in detail in the following sections.

THE β-THALASSEMIAS

The β-thalassemias are summarized in Table 58-1. The group is comprised of two main varieties, β-thalassemia$^+$ and β-thalassemia^o in which there is a partial or total deficiency of β-chain synthesis, respectively. In addition there are several disorders resulting from defective δ- and β-chain production, the $\delta\beta$-thalassemias. Finally, there are the conditions arising from heterozygosity for one of these forms of β-thalassemia and α- or β-chain structural hemoglobin variants.

True β-Thalassemia

Clinical Features

The homozygous state for this form of thalassemia produces the clinical picture first described by Thomas Cooley in 1925. Affected children are well at birth. Anemia is usually noticed during the first few months of life and becomes progressively severe. The victim fails to thrive. As he grows older the typical appearances of Cooley's anemia develop. There is stunting of growth, bossing of the skull, and overgrowth of the maxillary region, the whole face gradually assuming a "mongoloid" appearance. These changes are associated with characteristic radiological appearances of the long bones. The liver and spleen are invariably enlarged. There is increasing pigmentation of the skin.

The clinical course is one of severe anemia during childhood and frequent complications. These children are particularly prone to infection and this is a common cause of death. Because of the overactivity of the bone marrow, folic acid deficiency frequently occurs. Spontaneous fractures occur commonly as a result of the expansion of the marrow cavities, with thinning of the long bones and skull. Maxillary deformities often lead to dental problems from malocclusion. The formation of massive deposits of extramedullary hemopoietic tissue may cause pressure symptoms such as spinal compression or may be mistaken for a pulmonary neoplasm on chest x-ray. With the gross splenomegaly which may occur a secondary thrombocytopenia and leukopenia frequently develop, leading to a further tendency to infection and bleeding. Many of these children have a bleeding tendency in the absence of thrombocytopenia. Epistaxis is particularly common. This has been associated with poor liver function in some cases.

If these patients can be tided over the first years of life with repeated blood transfusions they nearly all develop hemochromatosis as they grow older and many of them die in the second and third decades of cardiac failure because of siderosis of the myocardium. Puberty is invariably delayed and other endocrine disturbances such as diabetes mellitus are not uncommon and are probably associated with hemochromatosis.

Hemoglobin levels may be in the 2 to 3 gm per 100 ml range. The blood film shows gross aniso-poikilocytosis with hypochromia, target cell formation, and a variable degree of basophilic stippling of the red cells. The appearance of the blood film varies somewhat depending on whether the spleen is intact or not [5]. In nonsplenectomized patients, large poikilocytes are common, whereas after splenectomy large flat macrocytes and small deformed microcytes are frequently seen. The reticulocyte count is moderately elevated and there are nearly always nucleated red cells in the peripheral blood. The white cell and platelet counts are slightly raised unless there is secondary hypersplenism. Staining of the peripheral blood with methyl violet, particularly in splenectomized subjects, reveals stippling or ragged inclusion bodies in the red cells [30]. These inclusions can nearly always be found in the red cell precursors in the bone marrow. The marrow usually shows erythroid hyperplasia with morphological abnormalities of the erythroblasts associated with striking basophilic stippling and increased iron deposition. In some cases there may be an increase in ringed sideroblasts, but these changes are not as marked as in the primary sideroblastic anemias.

Hemoglobin Pattern

The hemoglobin pattern is characterized by an increased level of fetal hemoglobin, ranging from less than 10 percent to over 90 percent. In some instances there may be a total deficiency of hemoglobin A synthesis. This represents a specific type of β-thalassemia (β-thalassemia^o), since other affected family members also show a similar absence of hemoglobin A. This type of β-thalassemia occurs in specific areas such as Northern Italy and Southeast Asia [31, 32].

The acid elution test shows that the fetal hemoglobin is quite heterogeneously distributed among the red cells. Hemoglobin A_2 levels in homozygous β-thalassemia are highly variable, giving either a low, normal, or high result. If expressed as a proportion of hemoglobin A, however, the hemoglobin A_2 level is almost invariably elevated. On an alkaline starch-gel electrophoresis of hemolysates which have been prepared by high-speed centrifugation, traces of free α chain remaining in the region of the origin can be found in some instances [33].

Heterozygous β-Thalassemia

Clinical findings in heterozygous β-thalassemia are variable. In some the disorder is completely silent while in other patients the clinical findings may be almost as severe as in the homozygous form of the disorder. The names *thalassemia intermedia, thalassemia minor,* and *thalassemia minima* have been used to describe these various clinical degrees of heterozygous β-thalassemia. Genetic studies have shown a marked heterogeneity of the disorders designated *thalassemia intermedia* [34].

Most patients with heterozygous β-thalassemia have a mild degree of anemia and a peripheral blood film characterized by a variable degree of aniso-poikilocytosis and hypochromia of the red cells. The reticulocyte count is rarely elevated. Often there is a moderate degree of erythrocytosis. The anemia may worsen during periods of stress, particularly during pregnancy, and affected women often present with refractory anemia during the second or third trimesters. Clinical examination is usually normal, but occasionally the spleen may be enlarged.

The hemoglobin pattern in β-thalassemia minor is characterized by an increase of hemoglobin A_2 into the 3.5 to 8 percent range. Fetal hemoglobin is elevated in about half of the patients, is usually in the range of 1 to 3 percent, and is rarely more than 5 percent. The hemoglobin A_2 value may be artificially depressed in patients with β-thalassemia who have coexistent iron deficiency, and it may rise to the β-thalassemia range with the institution of iron therapy [35].

$\delta\beta$-Thalassemia (F Thalassemia)

The homozygous state for $\delta\beta$-thalassemia has been observed in only a few patients [36, 37]. It is characterized clinically as milder than Cooley's anemia. The hemoglobin pattern consists entirely of hemoglobin F; hemoglobins A and A_2 are absent.

The heterozygous state for $\delta\beta$-thalassemia is characterized by a hematological disorder similar to that of β-thalassemia minor. The hemoglobin pattern is different in that the fetal hemoglobin level is higher, being in the 5 to 20 percent range, and the hemoglobin A_2 value is normal or slightly reduced. As in β-thalassemia the fetal hemoglobin is quite heterogeneously distributed among the red cells, thus distinguishing this disorder from hereditary persistence of fetal hemoglobin.

There is now a well-documented condition resulting from heterozygosity for both β-thalassemia and $\delta\beta$-thalassemia. The clinical pattern is similar but slightly milder than that of classical Cooley's anemia; the hemoglobin consists almost entirely of hemoglobin F with a small amount of hemoglobin A_2.

$\delta\beta$-thalassemia has also been observed in individuals heterozygous for hemoglobin S [38]. Hemoglobin A was not present in these patients. Thus the finding of no hemoglobins A or A_2 in the homozygous state and no hemoglobin A in a patient heterozygous for $\delta\beta$-thalassemia and hemoglobin S provides clear genetic proof that $\delta\beta$-thalassemia is characterized by a total deficit of β- and δ-chain synthesis on the affected chromosomes. It is possible that a form of this disorder also occurs in which only a partial deficit of δ- and β-chain production is present [34].

Other Forms of $\delta\beta$-Thalassemia

The Hemoglobin Lepore Syndromes

In 1958 Gerald and Diamond [49] noted that, in one parent of a child with clinical Cooley's anemia, instead of the usual pattern of heterozygous β-thalassemia the hematological picture of thalassemia was associated with the presence of a hemoglobin variant which migrated in the position of hemoglobin S. This variant, which comprised about 8 percent of the total hemoglobin, was named Lepore after the family name of the patient. With the finding of other Lepore hemoglobins this variant was subsequently named hemoglobin Lepore (Washington). Similar hemoglobin variants associated with thalassemia have been found in Indonesia, [hemoglobin Lepore (Hollandia)] [50], Greece (hemoglobin Pylos) [51], and sporadically in many other racial groups.

The hemoglobin Lepore disorder has been described in the homozygous state, heterozygous state, and heterozygous state in association with thalassemia or hemoglobin S. In the homozygous state, the hemoglobin consists of Lepore and fetal hemoglobin only and the clinical picture is that of severe Cooley's anemia. Hemoglobins A and A_2 are not synthesized. In the heterozygous state, the findings are those of β-thalassemia minor, the hemoglobin consisting of about 8 percent hemoglobin Lepore, a low level of hemoglobin A_2, and an increased fetal hemoglobin.

Hemoglobin Lepore has been analyzed chemically [52] and found to have normal α-chains combined with a pair of chains consisting of the N-terminal residues of the δ-chain fused to the C-terminal end of the β-chain. The point of fusion is variable. In hemoglobin Lepore (Washington) it lies between the 85th and 120th residues, whereas in hemoglobin Lepore (Hollandia) it is much nearer the N-terminal end of the δ-chain.

The composite $\delta\beta$ chain of the Lepore hemoglobin is thought to have arisen after chromosomal misalignment and unequal crossing-over at the $\beta\delta$ gene complex, resulting in a composite $\delta\beta$ chain. This type of unequal crossing-over is also thought to be the basis for the structure of the α chain of human haptoglobin and has been frequently observed in *Drosophila* genetics.

Nearly all of the Lepore hemoglobins analyzed to date seem to be identical to hemoglobin Lepore (Washington). This has certainly been true for the hemoglobins Pylos and Lepore (Nicoscia), and a hemoglobin Lepore recently found in the Negro population in Jamaica. It seems likely that there will be other Lepore-like hemoglobins, and it is possible that some of them may have a charge similar to hemoglobins A or A_2 and accordingly not be detectable by standard electrophoretic techniques. This mechanism would produce clinical thalassemia without an apparent alteration in the hemoglobin pattern. Thus there may be several forms of $\delta\beta$-thalassemia which await recognition [4].

The clinical consequences of the Lepore abnormality presumably follow the reduced rate of synthesis of the composite $\delta\beta$ chain. This in turn produces a poorly hemoglobinized red cell and clinical thalassemia.

β-Thalassemia with Normal Levels of Hemoglobins A_2 and F: The "Silent" Gene

In some families with children who have typical Cooley's anemia one parent has been found to be normal [4, 53a]. Recently, biosynthetic studies on such an individual indicated that there was an inequality of globin chain production [53], and it was suggested that this is yet another form of β-thalassemia. While this is certainly possible it should be remembered that several other conditions such as iron deficiency and other defects of heme synthesis may alter the normal α/β ratio. Further studies of this group are needed.

Hereditary Persistence of Fetal Hemoglobin (HPFH)

This condition resembles $\delta\beta$-thalassemia in that there is a total deficiency of β- and δ-chain synthesis in the cis position. Synthesis of γ-chains remains active and there is no overall chain imbalance and thus no hematological abnormality.

The various combinations of HPFH have been fully reviewed elsewhere [4]. The heterozygous state can be differentiated from $\delta\beta$-thalassemia by determining the distribution of hemoglobin F in individual red cells by the acid elution technique. In $\delta\beta$-thalassemia the fetal hemoglobin

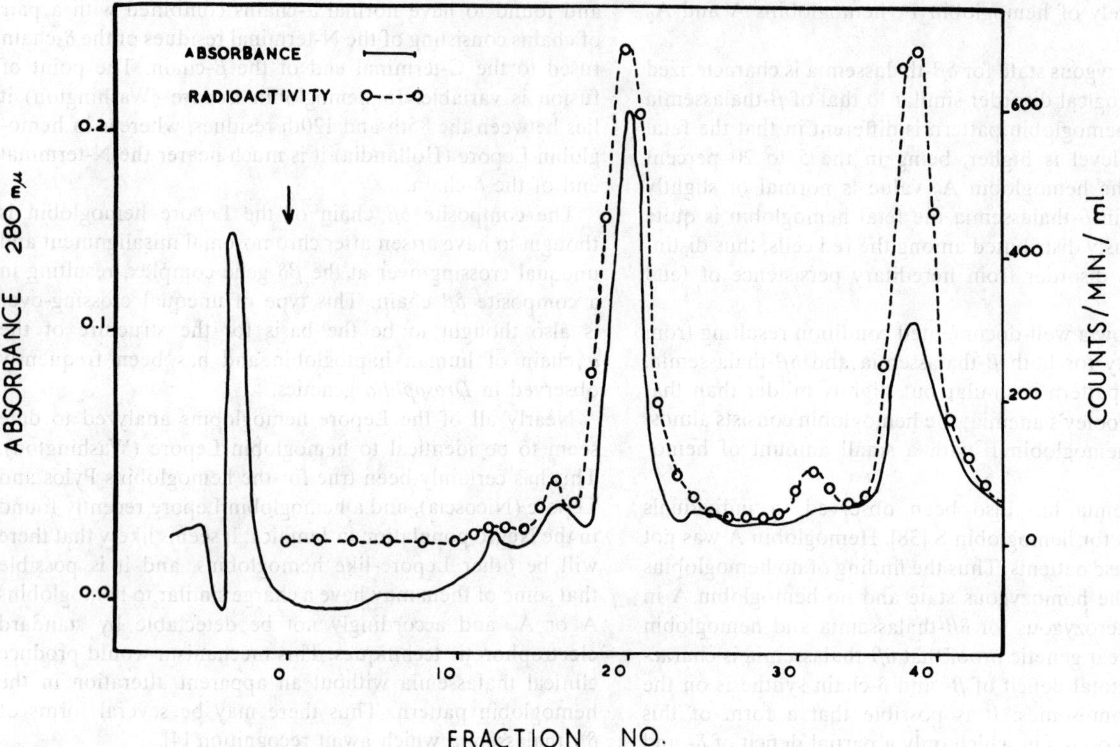

Figure 58-3. The incorporation of radioactivity into the α- and β-chains of nonthalassemic reticulocytes. Reticulocytes were incubated with ^{14}C-leucine and the globin precipitated after 1 hr. The chains were separated on urea columns. The first main peak is β-chain and the second peak α-chain. It will be seen that the amount of radioactive label incorporated into each chain is similar.

is unevenly distributed, while in HPFH each red cell contains similar amounts of acid resistant hemoglobin.

β-Thalassemia Associated with β-Structural Hemoglobin Variants

The β-thalassemia–β-structural hemoglobin variant combinations of most clinical importance are sickle-cell thalassemia, hemoglobin C thalassemia, and hemoglobin E thalassemia.

Sickle-cell thalassemia occurs in parts of Africa and in the Mediterranean population, particularly in Greece and Italy. The clinical results of carrying one gene for hemoglobin S and the corresponding gene for β-thalassemia depend mainly on the type of β-thalassemia gene. Where no normal β chain is synthesized, the hemoglobin pattern consists wholly of hemoglobin S with an increase in hemoglobins F and A_2. The associated clinical events are similar to sickle-cell anemia, with severe anemia and recurrent sickling crises. Where the β-thalassemia gene only partly depresses β-chain production, the adult hemoglobin consists of about 70 percent hemoglobin S and about 25 percent hemoglobin A. The associated clinical findings tend to be less severe than sickle-cell disease, with mild anemia and few sickling crises. The relation between the hemoglobin pattern and the clinical findings in sickle-cell thalassemia is not invariable and some patients with hemoglobin A–producing type of sickle-cell thalassemia (β-thalassemia$^+$) have had a severe clinical course.

Hemoglobin C thalassemia is characterized by a mild hemolytic disorder associated with splenomegaly. The hemoglobin pattern is variable depending upon whether the thalassemia gene is of the hemoglobin A or "non-hemoglobin A–producing" type. In the latter instance, the hemoglobin consists of hemoglobin C only and the clinical impact tends to be more severe. This disorder has been recorded mainly in North Africa, but a recent patient has been described in the American Negro population. Where some hemoglobin A is produced, the hemolytic disorder is extremely mild and may be present only during pregnancy as a refractory anemia or with folic acid deficiency.

Hemoglobin E thalassemia is a severe public health problem in Southeast Asia. The β-thalassemia gene in that area is mainly of the "non-hemoglobin A–producing" or β-thalassemia^0 type. The hemoglobin pattern in this disorder, therefore, consists of hemoglobins E, F, and A_2, with no hemoglobin A. The clinical picture is similar to that of homozygous β-thalassemia.

The Pathophysiology of the Anemia of the β-Thalassemias

In the last few years in vitro studies of globin chain synthesis in β-thalassemia have provided evidence regarding the mechanism of the anemia of this disorder [21, 39, 40, 41, 42]. Globin synthesis has been studied by measuring the rate of incorporation of radioactive amino acids into the globin chains of hemoglobins A and F in short-term experiments using reticulocytes from patients with various forms of β-thalassemia. In all patients studied, α-chain synthesis has exceeded that of the combined synthesis of β- and δ-chains by several-fold (Figs. 58-3 and 58-4). This suggests that an excess of free chains is released into the red cells of patients with β-thalassemia. In some experiments, β-chain synthesis appears to be completely deficient, only hemoglobins F and A_2, and free α chain being synthesized [31]. Similar studies on the cells of patients with hemoglobin E thalassemia and sickle-cell thalassemia [21] confirm that these disorders are of two types, i.e., those in which hemoglobin A is produced and those in which there is a total deficiency of β chains. These correspond to β-thalassemia$^+$ and β-thalassemia^o, respectively.

Free α-chains can be isolated from the cells of patients with β-thalassemia by electrophoresis on starch gel or, following incubation with radioactive amino acids, by gel filtration on Sephadex [21, 42] or by DEAE chromatography [21]. This pool of α-chains is unstable and rapidly becomes associated with the red cell stroma [44]. It is almost certain that this excess of unstable α-chains forms the inclusion bodies found in the red cell precursors in this disorder.

Thalassemic erythrocytes have been shown to have several well defined metabolic abnormalities. Thus the membrane is more permeable to potassium and there is a reduced ability to regenerate ATP [5]. This "leakiness" of the red cell membrane has also been found in patients with various unstable hemoglobin disorders such as hemoglobin Köln. It seems probable that the inclusion bodies resulting from the precipitated α chain are in some way responsible for this change in membrane physiology. Possibly damage results from mechanical trauma as the inclusion bodies are

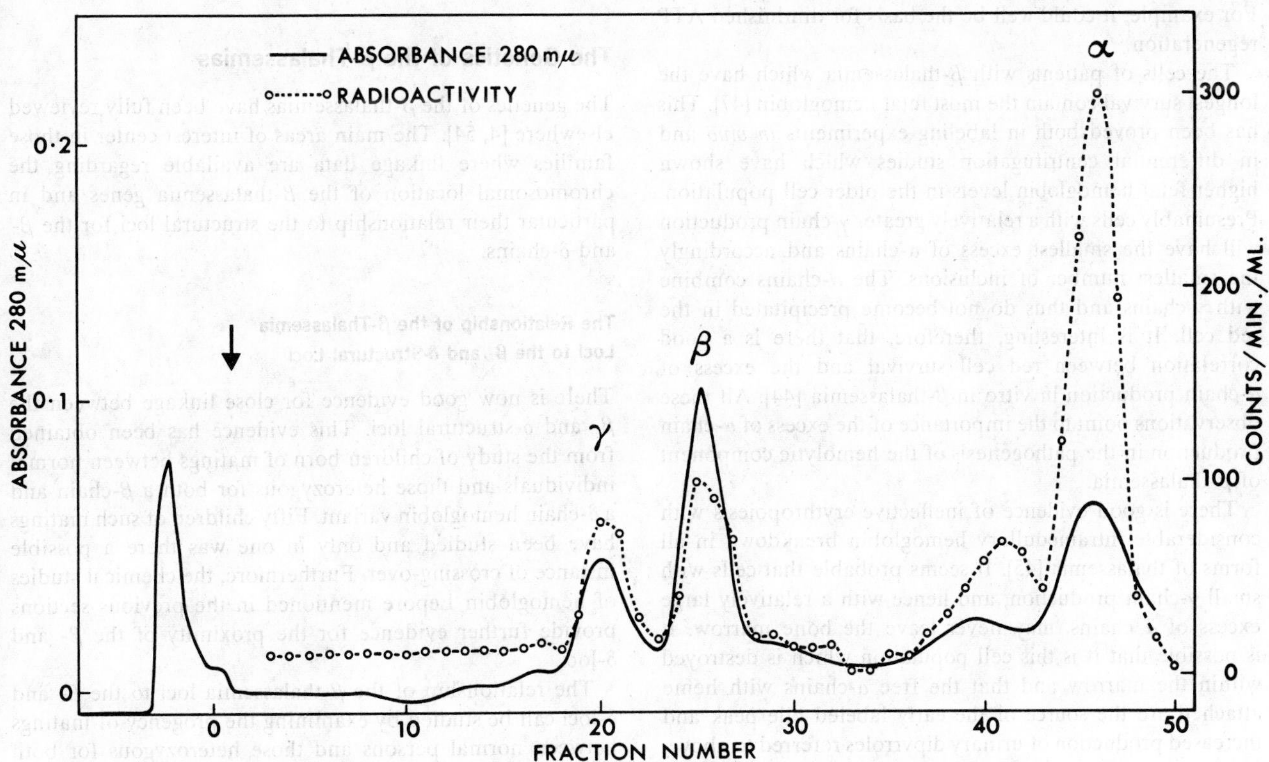

Figure 58-4. The incorporation of ^{14}C-leucine into the globin chains of a child with homozygous β-thalassemia. The experimental conditions are exactly the same as in Fig. 58-3. It will be seen that there is a large excess of α-chain radioactivity, indicating imbalance of globin chain synthesis and the liberation of free α-chains into the cell.

"pitted out" of the red cells during passage through the splenic sinusoids. Membrane damage might also follow the binding of membrane sulfhydryl groups by precipitating α chains.

Defective heme synthesis has been clearly demonstrated in β-thalassemia [2]. Heme inhibits ALA-synthetase which is responsible for heme synthesis, and thus controls its rate of synthesis by "feedback" inhibition. It seems probable, therefore, that the defect in heme production is the result of a "pile up" of heme due to defective globin chain synthesis. Some of this heme will be combined with free α chain and be degraded in the red cell precursor. It seems probable that it is this material which is responsible for the large "early labeled bile" peak found in kinetic studies in vivo of the red cells of patients with homozygous β-thalassemia [45] and also for the increase in the urinary dipyrroles described in this disorder [46].

In addition to the pile-up of heme because of defective globin chain synthesis, there appears to be an accumulation of iron within the red cell precursors. This iron is distributed throughout the cytoplasm and also in the perinuclear region, although ringed sideroblasts are not as commonly seen in thalassemia as in the sideroblastic anemias. The excess iron in the mitochondrial region is probably the cause of at least some of the metabolic changes in the red cell precursors. For example, it could well be the basis for diminished ATP regeneration.

The cells of patients with β-thalassemia which have the longest survival contain the most fetal hemoglobin [47]. This has been proved both in labeling experiments *in vivo* and in differential centrifugation studies which have shown higher fetal hemoglobin levels in the older cell population. Presumably cells with a relatively greater γ-chain production will have the smallest excess of α-chains and accordingly the smallest number of inclusions. The α-chains combine with γ-chains and thus do not become precipitated in the red cell. It is interesting, therefore, that there is a good correlation between red cell survival and the excess of α-chain production in vitro in β-thalassemia [44]. All these observations point to the importance of the excess of α-chain production in the pathogenesis of the hemolytic component of β-thalassemia.

There is good evidence of ineffective erythropoiesis with considerable intramedullary hemoglobin breakdown in all forms of thalassemia [45]. It seems probable that cells with small γ-chain production, and hence with a relatively large excess of α chains, may never leave the bone marrow. It is possible that it is this cell population which is destroyed within the marrow and that the free α-chains with heme attached are the source of the early labeled bile peak and increased production of urinary dipyrroles referred to above. Similar metabolic changes have been observed in patients with various unstable hemoglobin disorders [48]. Thus a rather similar pattern is emerging in the thalassemias and in all conditions associated with intracellular precipitation of either whole hemoglobin molecules or an excess of single globin chains. These relationships are summarized in Fig. 58-5.

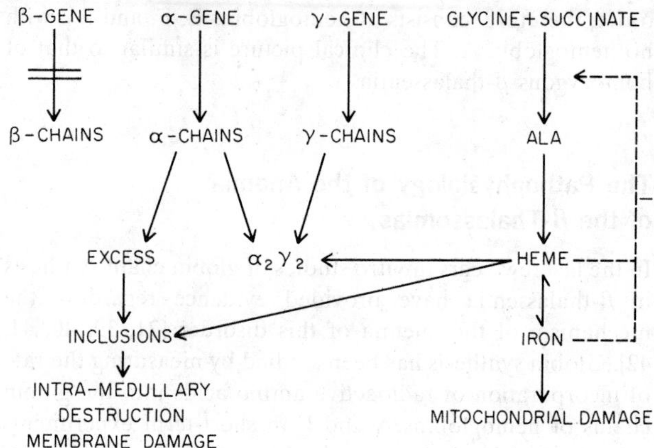

Figure 58-5. The breakdown of intracellular control in β-thalassemia. In the absence of β-chains there is an excess of α-chain production with inclusion body formation and red cell membrane damage. Some of the α-chains and heme form hemoglobin F but there is an overall excess of heme production with a secondary feedback inhibition.

The Genetics of the β-Thalassemias

The genetics of the β-thalassemias have been fully reviewed elsewhere [4, 54]. The main areas of interest center in those families where linkage data are available regarding the chromosomal location of the β-thalassemia genes and in particular their relationship to the structural loci for the β- and δ-chains.

The Relationship of the β-Thalassemia Loci to the β- and δ-Structural Loci

There is now good evidence for close linkage between the β- and δ-structural loci. This evidence has been obtained from the study of children born of matings between normal individuals and those heterozygous for both a β-chain and a δ-chain hemoglobin variant. Fifty children of such matings have been studied and only in one was there a possible instance of crossing-over. Furthermore, the chemical studies of hemoglobin Lepore mentioned in the previous sections provide further evidence for the proximity of the β- and δ-loci.

The relationship of the β-thalassemia loci to the β- and δ-loci can be studied by examining the progency of matings between normal persons and those heterozygous for both β-thalassemia and either a β- or a δ-chain hemoglobin variant. Such matings have recently been summarized [4, 54]. There have been 71 reported instances of children born of matings between individuals heterozygous for both sickle-cell and thalassemia genes and normal persons. In two instances, the thalassemia was of the noninteracting type, while in two other families no electrophoretic studies were reported. Exclusion of these families leaves one doubtful crossover. The findings in 46 individuals born of persons with hemoglobin C thalassemia have also been summarized and there are 3 possible but not definite instances of crossing-over between the β-thalassemia and β-structural loci. Unfortunately, categorical blood group data were not provided and so these reports must be regarded with caution. The β-thalassemia and β-structural variant genes have only been seen together in the repulsion phase. It is probable that if they occurred together on the same chromosome the abnormal β chains would either not be produced at all or would be produced in very small quantities. In the former instance the pattern would be that of thalassemia trait, while the latter would resemble "noninteracting" sickle-cell thalassemia.

Four families have been reported in which individuals heterozygous for both hemoglobin A_2' (also called B_2) and β-thalassemia have had one or more children from a mating with a normal person. In one family a crossover could not be ruled out. Two further families have been described in which the genes were clearly shown to be in the repulsion phase, i.e., the abnormal genes on opposite chromosomes. In one family eleven children were studied and one was a possible example of crossing-over, while in the other family among seven children one possible crossover was found. Thus in 31 possible chances for crossing-over between β-thalassemia and δ-structural loci there have been 2 probable examples of crossing-over. Adequate blood group data are available with each of these studies.

It is difficult to interpret this type of linkage data in man, particularly since adequate blood group data and information on other genetic markers have not always been given. It appears that the β-structural and δ-structural loci are closely linked and that the β-structural and β-thalassemia loci are alleles or very closely linked. Probably, the β-thalassemia and δ-structural loci are not so close together as are the β-structural and δ-structural loci.

α-THALASSEMIA

The α-thalassemias have been much harder to define because defective α-chain synthesis affects hemoglobins A, F, and A_2, and therefore alterations in relative amounts of hemoglobins A_2 and F would not be expected in this disorder. Furthermore, it appears that compensation for a total deficiency of α-chain synthesis on one chromosome can be accomplished with much greater facility than a similar deficiency of β-chain production. Thus, the heterozygous states for α-thalassemia are extremely difficult to identify in adult life.

During the switch from fetal to adult hemoglobin synthesis there is a period when both γ- and β-chains are competing for the available α-chains. During this time a slight imbalance of chain production occurs even in normal infants and a small excess of γ-chains is produced, forming traces of hemoglobin Bart's [55]. The level of hemoglobin Bart's in normal infants never exceeds 1 percent of the total hemoglobin. When there is a slight deficiency of α-chains as compared with γ- and β-chains, hemoglobin A is produced rather than hemoglobin F because of the greater affinity of α-chains for β-chains than for γ-chains. Thus the level of hemoglobin Bart's in the neonatal period offers a general guide to the presence of the α-thalassemia gene.

A series of different forms of α-thalassemia can be described, depending on the level of hemoglobin Bart's in infancy [55, 56]. Infants with 5 to 15 percent hemoglobin Bart's show a mild thalassemic blood pattern, the hemoglobin Bart's disappearing as they grow older. This condition has been called α-thalassemia 1, and can be recognized as a mild thalassemia-like state in adult life. Some infants are born with 1 to 2 percent hemoglobin Bart's and a completely normal blood picture. This milder form of α-thalassemia has been called α-thalassemia 2, the expression of a "silent" α-thalassemia gene. The α-thalassemia syndromes result from the interactions of these thalassemia genes both with themselves and with α-chain or β-chain structural hemoglobin variants. These complex disorders are summarized in Table 58-2.

Homozygous α-Thalassemia 1 Disease: The Hemoglobin Bart's Hydrops Fetalis Syndrome

This disorder is a frequent cause of stillbirth in Southeast Asia [57, 58]. Infants are stillborn between 34 and 40 weeks with severe hydrops fetalis. Occasionally they survive delivery but die within a short time. There is pallor, edema, and hepatosplenomegaly. Autopsy discloses massive extramedullary hematopoiesis. The blood film is that of a severe thalassemia with many nucleated red cells.

The hemoglobin in this disorder is comprised mainly of hemoglobin Bart's with small amounts of a slower component which has been identified as hemoglobin Portland, a normal minor component of cord blood [59]. A complete absence of hemoglobins A and F suggests a total deficiency of α-chain synthesis in these babies [59]. In some, a faint trace of hemoglobin A has been found on starch-gel electrophoresis but it is not absolutely certain whether this might have come from contamination with maternal blood.

Examination of parents of these infants shows a mild thalassemia-like disorder, with normal levels of hemoglobins F and A_2. In some patients an occasional cell containing inclusion bodies may be demonstrated after the incubation of blood samples with brilliant cresyl blue. Isotope incorporation studies in vitro may disclose a deficiency of α-chain synthesis in these presumed α-thalassemia 1 carriers [60]. These findings and family studies have led to the hypothesis that the hemoglobin Bart's hydrops syndrome results from homozygosity for the α-thalassemia 1 gene.

Hemoglobin H Disease (α-Thalassemia 1–α-Thalassemia 2 Disease)

Hemoglobin H disease was described independently in the United States and Greece in 1955 [28, 29]. The clinical findings are variable, the worst affected patients being similar to those homozygous for β-thalassemia, while many have a much milder course. There is a variable degree of anemia with hypochromia and aniso-poikilocytosis of the red cells. The reticulocyte count is usually in the 5 percent range. Incubation of the red cells with brilliant cresyl blue discloses ragged inclusion bodies in practically all of the cells. After splenectomy large single Heinz bodies are observed in some cells. These are thought to be formed by the precipitation of the unstable hemoglobin H molecule *in vivo.* These are seen only after splenectomy. The inclusions which form on incubation with brilliant cresyl blue are due to precipitation of hemoglobin H *in vitro* as a result of interaction of the dye and the hemoglobin.

The hemoglobin pattern in hemoglobin H disease is somewhat variable. Hemoglobin A always constitutes the major component, while the level of hemoglobin H varies from 5 to 30 percent. In addition there is nearly always a small amount of hemoglobin Bart's and a component consisting entirely of the δ chains of hemoglobin A_2. Hemoglobins H and Bart's are unique among the hemoglobin variants in that they migrate anodally at pH 6.5 to 7.0 and therefore are easily identified.

The physical properties of hemoglobin H are unusual. The oxygen association curve is shifted to the left and virtually no oxygen is given up at physiological tensions [61]. Furthermore, it exhibits no Bohr effect. Thus, hemoglobin H is useless as a physiological oxygen carrier, a fact which must be important for patients with high levels of this hemoglobin.

The inheritance of hemoglobin H disease is not entirely established. One of the parents of one affected patient usually shows a mild thalassemia with normal levels of hemoglobins A_2 and F, while the other parent is normal. Children born of matings between patients with hemoglobin H disease and apparently normal persons may be normal, may have a mild thalassemia-like disorder, or may have hemoglobin H disease. From extensive studies in Thailand it has been suggested that hemoglobin H disease results from the inheritance of both the α-thalassemia 1 and the α-thalassemia 2 genes [56]. If this is the case, infants born of parents with hemoglobin H disease should show either 5 to 15 percent hemoglobin Bart's (α-thalassemia 1) or 1 to 2 percent hemoglobin Bart's (α-thalassemia 2), and indeed this appears to be the case [62]. If the two genes are alleles, transmission of the hemoglobin H disease from parent to child must result from a mating with a carrier of either the α-thalassemia 1 or α-thalassemia 2 traits. This is a distinct possibility in populations such as Thailand where both genes appear to occur with a high frequency. It is interesting that no example of transmission of hemoglobin H disease from one generation to the next has been recorded in areas where the disease seems to be rare, e.g., the Northern European population.

An imbalance of globin chain production accompanied by the formation of hemoglobin H has also been reported in a small number of elderly patients with erythro-leukemia. The genetic basis for this finding is unknown.

α-Thalassemia 1 and α-Thalassemia 2 Traits

Alpha-thalassemia 1 carriers appear to have a mild thalassemia-like disorder which can be recognized only with difficulty in adult life. In the neonatal period hemoglobin Bart's is increased to the 5 to 10 percent range. In adult life the blood shows only slight changes, but incubation of red cells with brilliant cresyl blue may reveal a rare cell with hemoglobin H inclusion bodies. Hemoglobin electrophoresis is usually normal, but on starch-gel electrophoreses in phosphate buffer pH 7.0 it is occasionally possible to demonstrate traces of hemoglobins H or Bart's. Furthermore, chromatography on Amberlite IRC 50 may demonstrate small amounts of Bart's in some of these subjects. It is not possible to make a diagnosis of the α-thalassemia carrier state in adult life with any real certainty. Claims that this can be achieved by measuring the rate of globin chain synthesis [60] await confirmation.

Alpha-thalassemia 2 appears to be a completely silent gene in adult life and is characterized by a slight elevation of hemoglobin Bart's in the neonatal period. This condition has only been delineated with any certainty in Thailand, and population studies to determine the significance of small elevations of hemoglobin Bart's in other racial groups remain to be done.

Although population surveys and studies of hemoglobin Bart's levels in the neonatal period have provided strong evidence for the existence of α-thalassemia 1 and 2 genes, the genetic transmission of these disorders remains uncertain. The genetic transmission of the α-thalassemias in Thailand has recently been extensively studied and an attempt has been made to correlate the findings with recent evidence that there are multiple structural genes controlling α-chain synthesis in some populations [80, 82, 83].

Most of the data from Thailand would suggest that the α-thalassemia 1 and 2 genes are alleles or are at very closely linked loci on the same chromosome. However this material has recently been completely restudied [84] and apparently it is consistent with there being two different α-thalassemia genes at independent α loci. Clearly much more work is required before it is possible to give a dogmatic answer about the genetic transmission of α-thalassemia.

α-Thalassemia Associated with α-Chain Hemoglobin Variants

α-Thalassemia has been found in association with several α-chain hemoglobin variants, notably hemoglobins Q and I. In hemoglobin Q α-thalassemia [63] which has been found in Orientals, the clinical findings are similar to those of hemoglobin H disease. The hemoglobin pattern consists of hemoglobins H, Bart's, Q, and Q_2 ($\alpha_2{}^Q\delta_2$). It appears that in these patients the α-thalassemia gene causes complete suppression of α-chain synthesis on the affected chromosome, hemoglobins Q and Q_2 having been synthesized under the direction of the homologous chromosome. In hemoglobin I α-thalassemia, found in a Negro woman [64], the pigment consisted of hemoglobin I ($\alpha_2{}^I\beta_2$) which made up about 70 percent of the hemoglobin, the rest being hemoglobin A. Clearly, in this instance, production of α-chains was not completely suppressed.

These observations suggest that, like β-thalassemia, the α-thalassemias are heterogeneous; in some cases the gene results in a total deficiency of α-chain production while in others there is only partial suppression of synthesis.

Recently another α-chain variant has been found in association with α-thalassemia. This hemoglobin, designated hemoglobin Constant Spring, has been found to interact with α-thalassemia 1 to produce a severe type of haemoglobin H disease [83]. It is unique in that in addition to the usual 141 amino acid residues it has approximately 31 extra residues attached to the C-terminal end of the α-chain. It is synthesized at a slow rate and for this reason interacts with the severe α-thalassemia gene to produce hemoglobin H disease. Structural analysis of the additional piece on the end of the α-chain of hemoglobin Constant Spring is compatible with this variant having arisen by mutation of the terminating codon [88]. Recent studies in southeast Asia and Greece indicate that this variant is an extremely common cause of hemoglobin H disease and in Thailand and Malaya may be responsible for over 50 percent of cases of this disorder [89].

α-Thalassemia Associated with β-Chain Hemoglobin Variants

It has become clear that in populations in which both α-thalassemia and β-chain hemoglobin variants occur frequently there are thalassemia-like disorders which arise from combinations of these genetic abnormalities. The best characterized of these complex syndromes is that of α-thalassemia 1–α-thalassemia 2 hemoglobin E disease [65]. This genetic combination results clinically in thalassemia intermedia, with moderate anemia and hepatosplenomegaly. The blood pigment consists of hemoglobins A, E, and Bart's, and sometimes hemoglobin H. The presence of the α-thalassemia gene appears to reduce the level of hemoglobin E below that usually found in individuals heterozygous for the hemoglobin E gene alone.

Another combination of α-thalassemia and a β-chain hemoglobin variant has recently been identified in Saudi Arabia [66]. This combination consists of homozygous sickle-cell anemia with α-thalassemias 1 and 2. This combination resulted in chronic anemia and the appearance of hemoglobins S and F, and 20 percent hemoglobin Bart's. The molecule $\beta_4{}^S$ was not identified in this particular child. This suggests that, if it exists, it must be extremely unstable. The high levels of hemoglobins F and Bart's appeared to provide protection from the deleterious effects of the sickle-cell gene, since there were no sickling crises and the associated anemia was far less than that usually seen in homozygous sickle-cell anemia.

The α-thalassemia gene modifies the levels of hemoglobins in patients also heterozygous for a β-hemoglobin variant. For example the α-thalassemia gene reduces the amount of hemoglobin S and hemoglobin E in carriers of the hemoglobin S or E traits. The reason for this is that, if α chains are in limited supply, they will combine with normal β chains in preference to β^E or β^S chains. The reduction in the amount of β-chain hemoglobin variants in heterozygotes offers a possible method for recognition of the α-thalassemia gene in adult life.

Several families have now been reported in which patients with the clinical picture of thalassemia have received an α-thalassemia gene from one parent and a β-thalassemia gene from the other [85]. These individuals have marked hypochromia and variation in shape and size of their red cells, but there is no increase in hemoglobin F and usually the hemoglobin A_2 value is only marginally elevated. Biosynthetic studies have shown that the α/β production ratio in these patients is almost unity and their red cell survival is normal, indicating that the shortened red cell survival in thalassemia is due to chain imbalance with the formation of insoluble precipitates within the red cell.

Hemoglobin Synthesis in α-Thalassemia

It has recently been possible to study hemoglobin synthesis in vitro in infants with the hemoglobin Bart's hydrops fetalis syndrome [59]. Complete deficiency of α-chain synthesis has been confirmed. If reticulocytes from patients with hemoglobin H disease are incubated with radioactive amino acids and the globin chains separated it can be demonstrated that the rate of β-chain synthesis exceeds that of α-chain synthesis by two or three times [67]. Most of the β chains are freely released into the cell and form hemoglobin H. A small fraction exists as a pool capable of combining with newly made α chains as they are released. Free intracellular exchange of subunits between hemoglobin A and hemoglobin H has been demonstrated.

From studies of the specific activities of hemoglobins A and H after both in vitro and in vivo labeling experiments, it is clear that hemoglobin H is preferentially destroyed in the circulation. Since differential centrifugation studies have shown clear evidence that the amount of hemoglobin H is reduced in the older cell population [68], it appears that it is precipitated and removed from erythrocytes as they age. Presumably it precipitates in the form of Heinz bodies which are removed in the spleen. These can, in fact, be seen in the peripheral blood only after splenectomy.

Metabolic studies on the cells of patients with hemoglobin H disease have shown the same abnormalities as occur in β-thalassemia [5], i.e., increased membrane permeability and reduced ability to regenerate ATP. It seems probable therefore that the same mechanisms of red cell destruction occur in both conditions. The kinetic studies mentioned above suggest that these membrane changes are the result of precipitating globin chains, in this case the excess of β-chains. The difference in clinical severity between the two conditions may, at least in part, be due to the relatively greater stability of hemoglobin H as compared with the free α chains that occur in β-thalassemia.

Studies of hemoglobin synthesis have also been performed in α-thalassemia carrier states and it has been claimed that the presence of both α-thalassemias 1 and 2 can be detected by in vitro studies of globin chain synthesis [60]. This important observation awaits confirmation.

THE POPULATION GENETICS OF THALASSEMIA

The thalassemias have been observed in most racial groups. It is clear that there is a particularly high incidence in the Mediterranean region, the Middle East, and the Orient, although few large-scale surveys using a wide variety of screening techniques have been reported.

Surveys in Italy based on an osmotic fragility screening procedure have given an incidence of 7 to 15 percent in the Po delta region and Sicily [69]. Although this method includes individuals with iron deficiency and does not distinguish between different types of thalassemia, it is probable that a large proportion of the samples associated with reduced osmotic fragility represented different forms of β-thalassemia. In a survey of 1,600 Greek males using starch-gel and starch-block electrophoresis, with full hematological studies, 85 were found to have increased levels of hemoglobin A_2 and there was associated hematological evidence of thalassemia in all but 1 [70]. There is probably a high incidence of β-thalassemia in India, the Sudan, Turkey, and parts of Israel. Recent surveys of Thailand have demonstrated a remarkable prevalence of all the thalassemia genes (Table 58-3), and the incidence rate in Malaya and Indonesia is probably also high. The high A_2 β-thalassemia gene was thought to be rare in Africa, but the incidence in American Negroes has been estimated at 0.8 percent. Surveys using quantitative hemoglobin A_2 estimations in Nigeria have given low incidence figures but the gene occurs more commonly in Ghana [71, 72]. Sporadic reports of high A_2 β-thalassemia have appeared from practically every racial group.

Far less information regarding the incidence of $\delta\beta$-thalassemia is available. This condition is readily recognized on starch-gel electrophoresis and, in a survey of 1,500 adult Negroes in the United States, two instances were found [4]. It was found in 11 of 1,600 Greek males [70], and once in a survey of 2,790 individuals in Thailand [73]. It also occurs in Italy but its incidence is unknown.

The incidence of α-thalassemia is even more difficult to assess because of the difficulty in recognizing the carrier state in adult life. In a survey in Greece using red cell inclusion bodies and starch-gel electrophoresis as an indicator of the presence of hemoglobin H, an incidence of 0.6 percent carriers was found [70]. In Thailand, approximately 25 percent of newborns have increased levels of hemoglobin Bart's. This indicates a high incidence of α-thalassemia [32].

Since the homozygous states for the thalassemias are not usually compatible with survival into reproductive age, high gene frequencies can only be maintained if the heterozygotes have an advantage. Presumably the thalassemias have arisen in different areas by mutation and reached a high frequency where advantage exists. The selective factors in this balanced polymorphism have not yet been worked out.

Thalassemia carriers may be more resistant to malaria than normal persons. Certainly the high-frequency areas are those where malaria was common. In Sardinia, a much higher incidence of thalassemia was detected in the low-lying, marshy areas where malaria was frequent, than in the mountainous regions [15]. Similar findings have been reported from New Guinea and North Borneo. The relationship of the frequency of the sickle-cell trait and glucose-6-phosphate dehydrogenase deficiency to malaria is now well established, but studies in Greece have revealed a nonparallel distribution between enzyme deficiency and thalassemia in the Arta region. Similar results have been obtained from surveys in Thailand.

It has also been suggested that increased iron absorption in thalassemia might be an advantage in periods of iron depletion such as pregnancy. In fact, heterozygotes for thalassemia do not have an increased absorption of iron, or if iron absorption is increased total body iron levels are

Table 58-3. MAJOR HEMOGLOBIN TYPES IN THE MORE COMMON THALASSEMIC DISEASES SEEN IN THAILAND [32]

Diseases	Major hemoglobin types	Estimated number of patients*
β-thalassemia homozygosity	F or F + A	18,750
β-thalassemia/Hb E	E + F	48,750
Hb H	A + H	151,986
Hb H/Hb E	A + E + Bart's	22,709
Hb Bart's hydrops fetalis	Bart's	80,790
		322,790

* Estimated for the population of 30 million.

not elevated above normal. Whether the higher mean fetal hemoglobin levels found in thalassemics between the ages of 6 months and 1 year have any protective value has not yet been determined. Preliminary studies in Thailand suggest that this is not the case (personal communication from Dr. M. Kruatrachue).

Clearly the factors which maintain the high thalassemia gene frequencies are not fully understood. One complicating factor is the tendency for the β-thalassemia gene frequency to be depressed in areas where there is a high frequency of β-chain hemoglobin variants, because of the severe clinical sequelae of the interaction of the two genes. This mechanism is more important in Thailand, which has a high incidence of hemoglobin E, than in Greece. It appears that malaria is a more important selective agent for maintaining the high frequency of sickle-cell and G-6-PD deficiency genes than thalassemia. Whether the proposed tendency for gene reduplication and nonhomologous crossing at the βδ-gene complex is an important factor in maintaining the high frequency of thalassemia is uncertain, but even if this is true strong selective environmental forces would still be required.

THE CLINICAL MANAGEMENT OF THALASSEMIA

There is no definitive treatment for any of the thalassemia syndromes. Therapy is entirely supportive. Blood transfusion is the only useful form of treatment in homozygous β-thalassemia. It has been suggested that thalassemic children develop better if their hemoglobin is maintained at a normal level [75], but this necessitates frequent blood transfusions, and it is still not certain whether children treated in this way develop hemosiderosis and hemochromatosis earlier [76]. At present it seems wiser to maintain the hemoglobin at about 10 to 12 gm per 100 ml.

These children are prone to transfusion reactions. Hyperpyrexial episodes may be due to white cell antibodies or sensitivity to plasma components. The use of washed cells or white cell filters is helpful and some of these children respond fairly well to transfusion while receiving an adrenal steroid. Recent reports indicate that the use of frozen cell transfusions is particularly valuable to patients with thalassemia because the cells are washed free of most of the plasma before freezing. Thus it would be valuable to start thalassemic babies on a regime of frozen cell transfusion at the beginning of their treatment.

Since thalassemics have increased folic acid requirements they should be kept on regular supplements. Other hematinics, particularly iron, are contraindicated. The main complication of early infancy is that of infection. All infections should be treated early with antibiotics and a careful watch kept on the hemoglobin level since the anemia is always made worse by infection.

The role of splenectomy in β-thalassemia is clear. While it does not improve the basic defect in hemoglobin production, it corrects the secondary hypersplenism characterized by leukopenia and thrombocytopenia with a worsening of the anemia. Hemodynamic studies show evidence of splenic pooling in some patients. The development of this complication is the only real indication for splenectomy unless the enlargement of the spleen is causing pressure symptoms. There is a high risk of infection after splenectomy, particularly in early childhood, and accordingly it is best to postpone the operation until age 5 years or more.

If anemia and infection in early childhood can be adequately managed the main danger is that of iron overload. Many patients die in the second or third decade of generalized hemosiderosis and hemochromatosis. The main cause of death is hemochromatosis of the myocardium with cardiac failure, but there is also a high incidence of endocrine deficiency and liver damage. There appears to be no adequate method of preventing iron overload, since none of the chelating agents is effective in preventing iron absorption from the gastrointestinal tract. Furthermore they are unable to remove iron until the body stores are much increased. It is important, therefore, that thalassemic children do not receive oral iron therapy. Once the iron stores are increased, the most active agents are desferrioxamine and DTPA (diethylene triamine penta-acetate). The parents can be taught to use desferrioxamine as an intramuscular injection two or three times a week, and DTPA can be put into each transfusion bottle in doses ranging from 2 to 6 gm. In this way it is sometimes possible to remove almost as much iron as is being given during a year's transfusional program. Since iron is not easily removed until the child is already overloaded, these chelating agents do not really solve the problem of iron overload.

Certain other thalassemia syndromes offer particular clinical problems. Heterozygous β-thalassemia is not usually associated with any clinical problems except during periods of stress such as pregnancy. It is most important to see that these patients receive adequate folic acid supplements at this time. Patients heterozygous for β-thalassemia and the sickle-cell gene have a variable clinical course but the more severely affected have a course similar to homozygous sickle-cell anemia. Their management should be similar to that for sickle-cell anemia. Hemoglobin H disease should be managed as β-thalassemia. Since the hemoglobin H inclusion bodies are removed in the spleen, splenectomy might seem to be indicated early in this disorder, but in fact the results are not uniformly good. Because there is evidence that hemoglobin H tends to precipitate in the presence of various oxidant drugs such as sulfonamides they are better avoided.

Certain problems are common to all the thalassemia syndromes. Dental disorders deriving from maxillary deformity are particularly frequent. Recurrent fractures are also troublesome and it is probably better to transfuse to a high level if this becomes a major difficulty. Bleeding, particularly from the nose, is also a frequent feature and may be associated with liver disease. Attacks of chest pain associated with pericarditis occur and should be treated symptomatically.

More definitive therapy such as bone marrow transplantation is under study at several centers but at the moment has no place in thalassemia. When contemplating experimental approaches of this kind it should be remembered that these children, if treated carefully, have a reasonable future for at least 10 to 15 years, and this must be compared with the possible dangerous side effects of bone marrow transplantation. It should be explained that this technique is entirely experimental at present.

THE MOLECULAR DEFECT IN THALASSEMIA

From the evidence which has been reviewed in the sections on hemoglobin synthesis in both β- and α-thalassemia, it is clear that both disorders result from an imbalance of globin chain synthesis. In some cases there is a total absence of globin synthesis, while in others the production of globin chains is grossly retarded. Practically all the clinical and hematological findings in these syndromes can be explained on the basis of this imbalance.

There are two main levels at which the basic genetic defect might be operative (Fig. 58-6). First, there might be a reduction in the amount of messenger RNA for the affected globin chain, the structure of any messenger RNA being normal. Second, the messenger RNA might be structurally abnormal so that polypeptide chain initiation, assembly, or termination might be abnormal. It is not possible at present to study the rate of messenger RNA synthesis since functional messenger RNA has not yet been isolated from the mammalian cells, but it is possible to measure the assembly time of globin chains and thus indirectly the processes of chain initiation, assembly, and termination in reticulocytes. This type of experiment has been performed in reticulocytes from nonthalassemic individuals and from patients with β-thalassemia, and no differences in the assembly times between normal and β-thalassemic reticulocytes have been found [77]. This observation provides strong evidence that the processes of chain assembly and termination are normal in β-thalassemia. It does not rule out a defect in the initiating step. Thus, unless initiation is abnormal the basic defect in the forms of β-thalassemia studied in this way appears to be a deficiency in the amount of messenger RNA for that particular chain. No evidence for the presence of fragments of chains has been found.

Recent studies on the effect of initiation factors obtained from rabbit reticulocytes on hemoglobin synthesis in thalassemic reticulocytes indicate that the latter respond normally to rabbit initiation factors and the resultant hemoglobin synthesis still shows an imbalance of chain production with a defect in β-chain synthesis [86]. These results suggest that a mutation involving initiation factors is not responsible for the defective β-chain production in this disorder.

There are many ways in which such a deficiency of messenger RNA might come about. In those cases where no hemoglobin chains are produced there might be a total deletion of the gene involved. Where some globin chain is synthesized it is necessary to invoke some form of defective

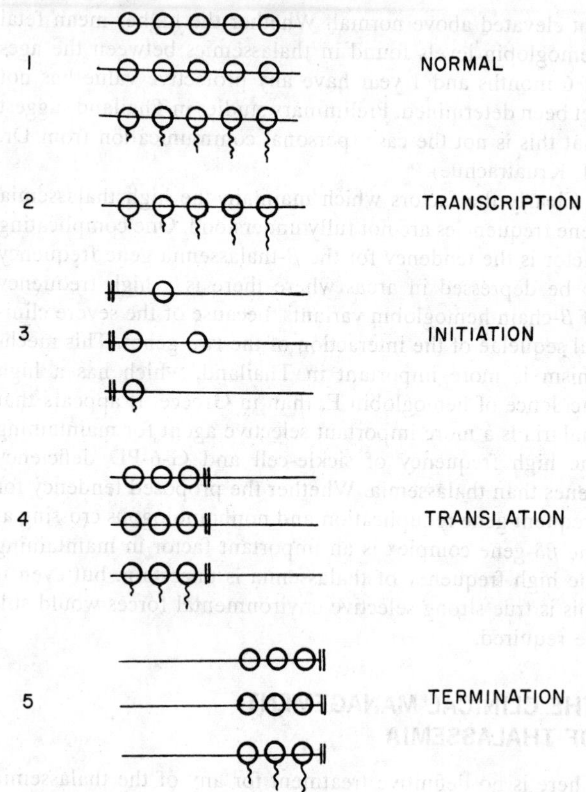

Figure 58-6. Models of the defect in thalassemia. In model 2 there is a deficiency of messenger RNA but the process of globin chain assembly is normal. In model 3 there is an abnormality of chain initiation but the assembly time of globin chains is also normal. In models 4 and 5 the assembly time of the globin chain would be delayed. Current experimental evidence suggests that the defect in some forms of thalassemia is that shown by model 2 or 3.

control of globin chain production. Many models of this type have been constructed, but at the moment there is no convincing evidence to support any of them. As pointed out earlier, there is a small amount of evidence suggesting that the β-thalassemia and β-structural loci can be separated by linkage studies. If this proves true, and the β-thalassemia mutation appears to be some distance from the β-structural loci, then the whole controller gene hypothesis would be much more attractive.

The recent observation [78] that human fetal hemoglobin is a mixture of molecules, some having the formula $\alpha_2\gamma_2{}^{136\ \mathrm{Gly}}$ and others $\alpha_2\gamma_2{}^{136\ \mathrm{Ala}}$, is of particular relevance to thalassemia. It is now clear that these γ chains are the products of different structural loci [78, 79]. If it is shown that the γ- and β-loci are linked, and if the hemoglobin F in thalassemia is found to have different ratios of $\gamma^{136\ \mathrm{Gly}}/\gamma^{136\ \mathrm{Ala}}$ chains, then it may be possible to delineate a series of deletions on the chromosome loci coding for hemoglobin as the molecular basis for thalassemia.

Another recent advance in the field of hemoglobin genetics

which has implications for thalassemia is the observation that, at least in some populations, there are multiple structural loci directing the synthesis of α chains [80]. Although this work awaits confirmation, it has particular relevance to the α-thalassemia problem. A speculative interpretation of some of the observations described in the section on α-thalassemia has recently been put forward based on this new knowledge about the α-loci [81].

It has been suggested that there are four possible α-thalassemia mutations in any one person, each involving one structural locus. If all four genes are inactive, the hemoglobin Bart's hydrops syndrome will result. If three genes are inactive, hemoglobin H disease results. While if one or two loci are inactive, the various forms of heterozygous α-thalassemia are found. Since hemoglobin Q α-thalassemia is always found in association with a total absence of hemoglobin A it follows that this α-chain variant must always be linked to an α-thalassemia gene. Evidence for this has been accumulated from the study of several persons heterozygous for hemoglobin Q.

SUMMARY

1 The thalassemias are a group of genetic disorders of hemoglobin synthesis which result from a defective rate of synthesis of one or more of the globin chains.

2 There are two main groups of thalassemias, the α-thalassemias and the β-thalassemias characterized by a deficiency of α- or β-chain synthesis, respectively. Each of these main groups consists of several genetically distinct disorders which can be recognized by the associated hematological and hemoglobin electrophoretic characteristics.

3 The clinical pictures in the thalassemia syndromes are the result of both the nonproduction of hemoglobin and imbalanced globin chain synthesis, with the formation of unstable aggregates of precipitated globin. This material results in damage to the red cell membrane and shortened red cell survival.

4 The basic molecular defect in the different forms of thalassemia is still unknown, but there is increasing evidence that at least some forms of the disorder result from a deficiency of messenger RNA for the affected chain.

5 The treatment of the thalassemia syndromes is unsatisfactory and mainly symptomatic.

BIBLIOGRAPHY

1. Cooley, T. B., and Lee, P.: A series of cases of splenomegaly in children with anemia and peculiar bone changes. Trans. Amer. Pediat. Soc., **37**, 29, 1925.
2. Bannerman, R. M.: *Thalassemia: A survey of some aspects.* Grune & Stratton, New York and London, 1961.
3. Chernoff, A. I.: The distribution of the thalassemia gene: A historical review. Blood, **14**, 899, 1959.
4. Weatherall, D. J.: *The Thalassemia Syndromes,* Blackwell Scientific Publications, Oxford, 1965.
5. Nathan, D. G., and Gunn, R. B.: Thalassemia: The consequences of unbalanced hemoglobin synthesis. Amer. J. Med., **41**, 815, 1966.
6. Itano, H. A.: The synthesis and structure of normal and abnormal hemoglobins, in *Abnormal Haemoglobins in Africa,* edited by J. H. P. Jonxis. C.I.O.M.S. Symp., Blackwell Scientific Publications, Oxford, 1965.
7. Ingram, V. M., and Stretton, A. O. W.: Genetic basis of the thalassaemia diseases. Nature (London), **184**, 1903, 1959.
8. Huehns, E. R., and Shooter, E. M. Review Article: Human haemoglobins. J. Med. Genet., **2**, 1, 1965.
9. Weatherall, D. J., and Clegg, J. B.: The control of human hemoglobin synthesis and function in health and disease, in *Progress in Hematology,* edited by E. Brown, C. V. Morre, vol. 6, p. 261. Grune & Stratton, New York, 1969.
10. Lehmann, H., and Carrell, R. W.: Variations in the structure of human hemoglobin with particular reference to the unstable haemoglobins. Brit. Med. Bull., **25**, 14, 1969.
11. Boyer, S. H., Rucknagel, D. L., Weatherall, D. J., and Watson-Williams, E. J.: Further evidence for linkage between the β- and δ-loci governing human hemoglobin and the population dynamics of linked genes, Amer. J. Hum. Genet., **15**, 438, 1963.
12. Bradley, T. B., Boyer, S. H., and Allen, F. H.: Hopkins-2-hemoglobin: A revised pedigree with data on blood and serum groups. Bull. Johns Hopkins Hosp., **108**, 75, 1961.
13. Labrie, F.: Isolation of an RNA with the properties of haemoglobin messenger. Nature (London), **221**, 1217, 1969.
14. Weisblum, R., Benzer, S., and Holley, R. W.: A physical basis for degeneracy in the amino acid code. Proc. Nat. Acad. Sci., USA, **48**, 1449, 1962.
15. Smith A. E., and Marcker, K. A.: Cytoplasmic methionine transfer RNA's from eukaryotes, Nature (London), **226**, 607, 1970.
16. Clark, B. F. C., and Marcker, K. A.: The role of N-formyl-methionyl-sRNA in protein synthesis. J. Molec. Biol., **17**, 394, 1966.
17. Dintzis, H. M.: Assembly of the peptide chains of hemoglobin. Proc. Nat. Acad. Sci. USA, **47**, 247, 1961.
20. Baglioni, C., and Campana, T.: Alpha chain and globin: Intermediates in the synthesis of rabbit hemoglobin. Europ. J. Biochem., **2**, 480, 1967.
21. Weatherall, D. J., Clegg, J. B., Na-Nakorn, S., and Wasi, P.: The pattern of disordered haemoglobin synthesis in homozygous and heterozygous β-thalassaemia. Brit. J. Haemat., **16**, 251, 1969.
22. Felicetti, L., Colombo, B., and Baglioni, C.: Assembly of hemoglobin. Biochim. Biophys. Acta, **380**, 129, 1966.
23. Baglioni, C.: The chemical structure of hemoglobin Lepore and its interpretation as the result of non-homologous crossing-over: Genetics today. *Proc. XI Internat. Cong. Genetics,* The Hague, vol. 1, p. 294. Macmillan, New York, 1963.
24. Neel, J. V.: The haemoglobin genes; a remarkable example of the clustering of related genetic functions on a single mammalian chromosome. Blood, **18**, 769, 1961.
25. London, I. M., Bruns, G. P., and Karibian, O.: The regulation of hemoglobin synthesis and the pathogenesis of some hypochromic anaemias. Medicine (Balt.), **43**, 789, 1964.
26. Granick, S., and Levere, R. D.: Controls of hemoglobin synthesis. Plenary Session Papers of XII Cong. Int. Soc. Haematol., p. 247, 1968.
27. Ager, J. A. M., and Lehmann, H.: Observations on some "fast" haemoglobins: K, J, N, and 'Bart's.' Brit. Med. J., **1**, 929, 1958.
28. Rigas, D. A., Koler, R. D., and Osgood, E. E.: New hemoglobin possessing a higher electrophoretic mobility than normal adult hemoglobin. Science, **121**, 372, 1955.
29. Gouttas, A., Fessas, P., Tsevrenis, H., and Xefteri, E.: Description d'une nouvelle variete d'anemie hemolytique congenitale. (Etude hematologique, electrophoretique et genetique). Sang., **26**, 911, 1955.
30. Fessas, P.: Inclusions of hemoglobin in erythroblasts and erythrocytes of thalassemia. Blood, **21**, 21, 1963.
31. Bargellesi, A., Pontremoli, S., and Conconi, F.: Absence of beta-globin synthesis and excess of alpha-globin synthesis in homozygous beta-thalassemia. Europ. J. Biochem., **1**, 73, 1967.

32. Wasi, P., Na-Nakorn, S., Pootrakul, S., Sookanck, M., Pornputkul, M., and Panich, V.: Alpha and beta-thalassemia in Thailand. Ann. NY Acad. Sci., **165**, 60, 1969.
33. Fessas, P., and Loukopoulos, D.: Alpha-chain of human hemoglobin: Occurrence *in vivo.* Science, **143**, 590, 1964.
34. Pearson, H. A.: Thalassemia intermedia: Genetic and biochemical considerations. Ann. NY Acad. Sci., **119**, 390, 1964.
35. Wasi, P., Disthasongchan, P., and Na-Nakorn, S.: The effect of iron deficiency on the levels of hemoglobins A_2 and E. J. Lab. Clin. Med., **71**, (1), 85, 1968.
36. Brancati, C., and Baglioni, C.: Homozygous β-δ-thalassaemia ($\beta\delta$ microcythaemia). Nature (London), **212**, 262, 1966.
37. Ramot, B., Ben-Bassat, I., Gafni, D., and Zaanoon, R.: A family with three $\beta\delta$-thalassemia homozygotes. Blood, **35**, 158, 1970.
38. Stamatoyannopoulos, G., Papayannopoulou, T., Fessas, P., and Motulsky, A. G.: The beta-delta thalassemias. Ann. NY Acad. Sci., **165**, 25, 1969.
39. Weatherall, D. J., Clegg, J. B., and Naughton, M. A.: Globin synthesis in thalassaemia: An in vitro study. Nature (London), **208**, 1061, 1965.
40. Heywood, J. D., Karon, M., and Weissman, S.: Asymmetrical incorporation of amino acids into the alpha and beta chains of hemoglobin synthesised in thalassemic reticulocytes. J. Lab. Clin. Med., **66**, 476, 1965.
41. Bank, A., and Marks, P.: Excess alpha chain synthesis relative to beta chain synthesis in thalassemia major and minor. Nature (London), **212**, 1198, 1966.
42. Huehns, E. R., and Modell, C. B.: Haemoglobin synthesis in thalassaemia. Trans. Roy. Soc. Trop. Med. Hyg., **61**, 157, 1967.
43. Bank, A., Braverman, S., O'Donnell, J. V., and Marks, P. A.: Absolute rates of globin chain synthesis in thalassemia. Blood, **31**, 226, 1968.
44. Bargellesi, A., Pontremoli, S., Menini, C., and Conconi, F.: Excess of alpha globin synthesis in homozygous beta-thalassemia and its removal from the red blood cell cytoplasm. Europ. J. Biochem., **3**, 364, 1968.
45. Sturgeon, P., and Finch, C. A.: Erythrokinetics in Cooley's anemia. Blood, **12**, 64, 1957.
46. Kreimer-Birnbaum, M., Pinkerton, P. H., Bannerman, R. M., and Hutchison, H. E.: Urinary "dipyrroles"; their occurrence and significance in thalassemia and other disorders. Blood **28**, 993, 1966.
47. Gabuzda, T. G., Nathan, D. G., and Gardner, F. H.: The turnover of hemoglobins A, F, and A_2 in the peripheral blood of three patients with thalassemia. J. Clin. Invest., **42**, 1678, 1963.
48. Carrell, R. W., and Lehmann, H.: The unstable haemoglobin haemolytic anaemias. Seminars Hemat., **6**, 116, 1969.
49. Gerald, P. S., and Diamond, L. K.: The diagnosis of thalassemia trait by starch block electrophoresis of the hemoglobin. Blood, **13**, 61, 1958.
50. Neeb, H., Beiboer, J. L., Jonxis, J. H. P., Sijpesteijn, J. A. K., and Müller, C. J.: Homozygous Lepore haemoglobin disease appearing as thalassaemia major in two Papuan siblings. Trop. Geogr. Med., **13**, 207, 1961.
51. Fessas, P., Stamatoyannopoulos, G., and Karaklis, A.: Hemoglobin "Pylos": Study of a hemoglobinopathy resembling thalassemia in the heterozygous, homozygous, and double heterozygous state. Blood, **19**, 1, 1962.
52. Baglioni, C.: The fusion of two peptide chains in hemoglobin Lepore and its interpretation as a genetic deletion. Proc. Nat. Acad. Sci. USA, **48**, 1880, 1962.
53. Schwartz, E.: The silent carrier of beta-thalassemia. New Eng. J. Med., **81**, 1327, 1969.
53a. Marti, H. R., and Grieder, H. R.: Heterozygote β-thalassemie ohne vermehrung von haemoglobin A_2. Schweiz. Med. Wschr., **100**, 663, 1970.
54. Weatherall, D. J.: The thalassemias, in *Progress in Medical Genetics,* edited by A. G. Steinberg and A. G. Bearn, vol. V, p. 8. Grune & Stratton, New York, 1966.
55. Weatherall, D. J.: Abnormal haemoglobins in the neonatal period and their relationship to thalassaemia. Brit. J. Haemat., **9**, 265, 1963.
56. Wasi, P., Na-Nakorn, S., Pootrakul, S., Pornpatkul, M., and Suingdumrong, A.: Haemoglobin H—an α-thalassaemia$_1$/α-thalassaemia$_2$ disease. *XII Cong. Internat. Soc. Haemat,* New York, p. 59, 1968. Abstracts of simultaneous sessions.
57. Lie, Injo Luan Eng: Alpha-chain thalassemia and hydrops fetalis in Malaya: Report of five cases. Blood, **20**, 581, 1962.
58. Lie, Injo Luan Eng, and Lie, Hong Gie: Abnormal haemoglobin production as a probable cause of erythroblastosis and hydrops foetalis in uniovular twins. Acta Haemat. (Basel), **25**, 192, 1961.
59. Weatherall, D. J., Clegg, J. B., and Wong, H. B.: The haemoglobin constitution of infants with the haemoglobin Bart's hydrops foetalis syndrome. Brit. J. Haemat., **18**, 357, 1970.
60. Schwartz, E., Kan, Y. W., and Nathan, D. G.: Unbalanced globin chain synthesis in alpha-thalassemia heterozygotes. Ann. NY Acad. Sci., **165**, 288, 1969.
61. Benesch, R. E., Ranney, H. M., Benesch, R., and Smith, G. M.: The chemistry of the Bohr effect. II. Some properties of hemoglobin H. J. Biol. Chem., **236**, 2926, 1961.
62. Na-Nakorn, S., Wasi, P., Pornpatkul, M., and Pootrakul, S.: Further evidence for a genetic basis for haemoglobin H disease from newborn offspring of patients. Nature (London), **223**, 59, 1969.
63. Dormandy, K. M., Lock, S. P., and Lehmann, H.: Haemoglobin Q-alpha-thalassaemia, Brit. Med. J., **1**, 1582, 1961.
64. Atwater, J., Schwartz, I. R., Erslev, A. J., Montgomery, T. D., and Tocantins, L. M.: Sickling of erythrocytes in a patient with thalassemia-hemoglobin I disease. New Eng. J. Med., **263**, 1215, 1960.
65. Wasi, P., Sookanek, M., Pootrakul, S., Na-Nakorn, S., and Suingdumrong, A.: Haemoglobin E and alpha thalassaemia. Brit. Med. J., **4**, 29, 1967.
66. Weatherall, D. J., Clegg, J. B., Blankson, J., and McNiel, J. R.: A new sickling disorder resulting from interaction of the genes for haemoglobin S and α-thalassaemia. Brit. J. Haemat., **17**, 517, 1969.
67. Clegg, J. B., and Weatherall, D. J.: Haemoglobin synthesis in alpha-thalassaemia (Haemoglobin H disease). Nature (London), **215**, 1241, 1967.
68. Rigas, D. A., and Koler, R. D.: Decreased erythrocyte survival in hemoglobin H disease as a result of the abnormal properties of hemoglobin H: The benefit of splenectomy. Blood, **18**, 1, 1961.
69. Silvestroni, E., and Bianco, I.: The distribution of the microcythaemias (or thalassaemias) in Italy: Some aspects of the haematological and haemoglobinic picture in these haemopathies, in *Abnormal Haemoglobins—A symposium,* edited by J. H. P. Jonxis and J. F. Delafresnaye, p. 242. Blackwell Scientific Publications, Oxford, 1959.
70. Malamos, B., Fessas, P., Stamatoyannopoulos, G.: Types of thalassaemia-trait carriers as revealed by a study of their incidence in Greece. Brit. J. Haemat., **8**, 5, 1962.
71. Ringelhann, B., Dodu, S. R. A., Konotey-Ahulu, F. I. D., Lehmann, H.: 1. A survey for haemoglobin variants, thalassaemia and glucose-6-phosphate dehydrogenase deficiency in Northern Ghana. Ghana Med. J., **7**, 120, 1968.
72. Weatherall, D. J., Gilles, H. M., Mustafa, D., Blankson, J., and Clegg, J. B.: Thalassaemia in some African populations: preliminary surveys. In preparation.
73. Flatz, G., Pik, C., and Sringam, S.: Haemoglobinopathies in Thailand. II. Incidence and distribution of elevations of haemoglobin A_2 and haemoglobin F, a survey of 2790 people. Brit. J. Haemat., **11**, 227, 1965.
74. Carcassi, V., Ceppellini, R., and Siniscalco, M.: Il tracciato elettroforetico dell'emoglobina per una migliore discriminazione della talassemie. Haematologica, **42**, 1635, 1957.
75. Wolman, I. J.: Transfusion therapy in Cooley's anemia: Growth and health as related to long-range hemoglobin levels, a progress report. Problems of Cooley's anemia. Ann. NY Acad. Sci., **119**, 736, 1964.
76. Wolman, I. J., and Ortolani, M.: Some clinical features of Cooley's anemia patients as related to transfusion schedules. Ann. NY Acad. Sci., **165**, 407, 1969.
77. Clegg, J. B., Weatherall, D. J., Na-Nakorn, S., and Wasi, P.: Haemoglobin synthesis in β-thalassaemia. Nature (London), **220**, 664, 1968.
78. Schroeder, W. A., Huismann, T. J. H., Shelton, J. R., Shelton, J. B., Kleihauer, E. F., Dozy, A. M., and Robberson, B.: Evidence for multiple structural genes for the γ-chain of human fetal hemoglobin. Proc. Nat. Acad. Sci. USA, **60**, 537, 1968.
79. Cauchi, M. N., Clegg, J. B., and Weatherall, D. J. Haemoglobin F (Malta): A new foetal haemoglobin variant with a high incidence in Maltese infants. Nature (London), **223**, 311, 1969.
80. Brimhall, B., Hollán, S., Jones, R. T., Koler, R. D., Stocklen, Z., and Szelenyi, J. G.: Abst. Clin Res., **18**, 184, 1970.

81. Lehman, H.: Differences between α- and β-chain mutants of human haemoglobin and between α-and β-thalasseamia: Possible duplication of the α-chain gene. Brit. Med. J., **4,** 748, 1968.
82. Wasi, P.: The alpha thalassemic genes. J. Med. Assoc. Thailand, **53,** 677, 1970.
83. Milner, P. F., Clegg, J. B., and Weatherall, D. J.: Haemoglobin H disease due to a unique haemoglobin variant with an elongated α-chain. Lancet, **1,** 729, 1971.
84. Koler, R. D., Jones, R. T., Wasi, P., and Pootrakul, S.: Genetics of hemoglobin H and α-thalassemia. Am. J. Hum. Genet., 1971 (in press).
85. Kan, Y. W., and Nathan, D. G.: Mild thalassemia: the result of interactions of alpha and beta thalassemia genes. J. Clin. Invest., **49,** 635, 1970.
86. Gilbert, J. M., Thornton, A. G., Nienhuis, A. W., and Anderson, W. F.: Cell-free hemoglobin synthesis in beta-thalassemia. Proc. Nat. Acad. Sci., **67,** 1854, 1970.
87. Nienuis, A. W., Laycock, D. G., and Anderson, W. F.: Translation of rabbit haemoglobin messenger RNA by thalassaemic and non-thalassaemic ribosomes. Nature (London), **231,** 205, 1971.
88. Clegg, J. B., Weatherall, D. J., and Milner, P. F.: Haemoglobin Constant Spring—a chain termination mutant? Nature (London), **234,** 337, 1971.
89. Fessas, P., Lio-Injo Luan Eng, Na-Nakorn, S., Todd, D., Clegg, J. B., and Weatherall, D. J.: The identification of the slow moving haemoglobin components found in patients with haemoglobin H disease from different racial groups. Submitted for publication.

PART ELEVEN

DISEASES MANIFEST PRIMARILY AS TRANSPORT DISORDERS

CHAPTER FIFTY-NINE

INTESTINAL DISACCHARIDASE DEFICIENCIES AND GLUCOSE-GALACTOSE MALABSORPTION*

Gary M. Gray†

Intolerance to the dietary disaccharides, sucrose and lactose, and to the hydrolytic products of starch (maltose, maltotriose, and the α-dextrins), results from a deficiency of one or more of the specific intestinal mucosal enzymes responsible for their hydrolysis. Rarely is a patient seen who cannot tolerate any dietary carbohydrate because of an inability to absorb the final hydrolytic products, glucose and galactose. Symptoms of carbohydrate maldigestion or malabsorption include abdominal bloating and distention, nausea, cramping pain, and diarrhea. A secondary malabsorption of other nutrients may develop. It is particularly important to distinguish these syndromes from "irritable" colon or "spastic" colitis since treatment of disaccharidase deficiency is quite different and highly successful.

For many years European physicians [1, 2] have observed that certain children develop abdominal distention and diarrhea after ingestion of milk or sugar, but the clinical syndrome lacked a biochemical explanation until methods became available for obtaining [3, 4] and assaying [5] peroral biopsies of the small intestine. An important reason for the slow development of these methods was a general acceptance of the erroneous concept that digestive enzymes are secreted from the intestinal wall into the lumen. Intestinal disaccharidases were clearly demonstrated to be most active at the luminal pole of the intestinal cell in the limiting brush border membrane less than 10 years ago [6]. Studies in man then demonstrated that disaccharides are hydrolyzed by mucosal-bound enzymes [7, 8]. Analysis of small intestinal biopsies for these enzymes has now become a useful technique for estimating the digestion and absorption of carbohydrates.

*Supported in part by Grant No. AM-11270 from the National Institute of Arthritis and Metabolic Diseases, National Institutes of Health.

†Recipient of a Career Development Award (IK4-Am47443) from the N.I.A.M.D.

DIGESTION AND ABSORPTION OF CARBOHYDRATES

The Sites of Hydrolysis and Transport

A brief consideration of intestinal handling of carbohydrates will facilitate an understanding of enzymatic and transport defects. Much confusion about the hydrolysis and absorption of carbohydrates has been erased in the last few years [6-10].

Starch constitutes 60 percent of the carbohydrate ingested daily. Both the branched form (amylopectin) and straight chain form (amylose) of this glucose polymer are hydrolyzed extremely rapidly by salivary and pancreatic α-amylase within the duodenal luminal contents. The extent of the hydrolysis of amylopectin is diagramed in Fig. 59-1. α-Amylase attacks at the interior 1, 4α-glucose-glucose links to yield maltose, maltotriose, and the α-dextrins (branched oligosaccharides averaging six glucose units) [9, 10].

Figure 59-2 is a diagram of the overall process of digestion and absorption, with emphasis on the intestinal phase where the final steps of breakdown and transport occur. The oligosaccharides released from starch as well as the disaccharides sucrose and lactose can be hydrolyzed only by specific enzymes which are an integral part of the mucosal surface. After hydrolysis by the appropriate mucosal enzyme, the released monosaccharides, glucose, galactose, and fructose, are then absorbed into the epithelial cell by two specific mechanisms. Glucose and galactose, which have almost identical chemical structure, are transported against their

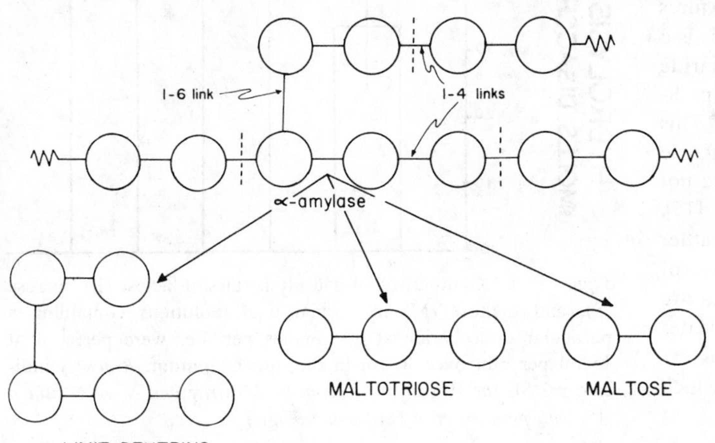

Figure 59-1. Final products of amylopectin hydrolysis by α-amylase. A segment of the amylopectin is shown, with each circle representing a glucose unit. The sites of amylase action are indicated by the dotted lines. (*Reproduced from G. M. Gray* [10] *with permission of Fed. Proc.*)

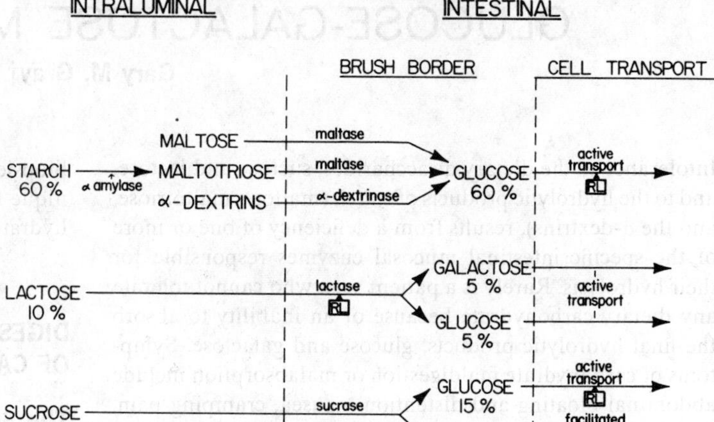

Figure 59-2. Outline of carbohydrate digestion and absorption in man. Percentages refer to fraction of total carbohydrate in the diet. RL indicates the rate-limiting step in the overall digestive-absorptive process for each carbohydrate ingested. (*Reproduced from G. M. Gray* [93] *with permission of Gastroenterology.*)

own concentration gradients by an active process requiring energy and Na^+ [11, 12]. The kinetics of this process suggest that there is a binding-and-release phenomenon similar to that which exists between enzyme and substrate. This concept has been made more plausible by the recent demonstration that there is a glucose-binding protein in microorganisms that transport this monosaccharide [13]. Fructose utilizes a separate mechanism for transport across the cell. It is absorbed more slowly and moves down a concentration gradient [14]. Unlike many other small molecules, such as mannitol, that are excluded from entry into the intestinal cell, fructose utilizes a specific mechanism which allows efficient absorption.

Rate-limiting Steps in Carbohydrate Hydrolysis and Absorption

By intestinal perfusion studies with disaccharides and perfusion with equivalent amounts of monosaccharide mixtures in man [8, 15], it has been demonstrated that hydrolysis is a rapid process which can release sufficient monosaccharide to saturate the glucose-galactose and fructose transport pathways. The sole exception is the hydrolysis of lactose. This proceeds in vivo at only about half the rate of sucrose (Fig. 59-3), and the glucose and galactose released are not sufficient to give maximal rates of active transport [15]. Hence, unlike other disaccharides, lactose hydrolysis rather than transport is rate limiting in the overall process of hydrolysis and transport [15] (Fig. 59-2). This unique feature of lactose digestion and absorption in normal man indicates a relative lack of reserve of lactase activity and helps explain the peculiar vulnerability of lactose digestion which will be considered in detail below.

CARBOHYDRATE MALDIGESTION AND MALABSORPTION

Pathogenesis

Carbohydrates are digested and absorbed in a specific steplike fashion under normal conditions. A defect at any level will permit free carbohydrate to remain within the intestinal lumen. Because of the small molecular size of these sugars, they have a relatively large osmotic activity per gram and attract much water from the extracellular space into the intestinal cavity. Patients with carbohydrate malabsorption complain of abdominal fullness, bloating, and cramping pain

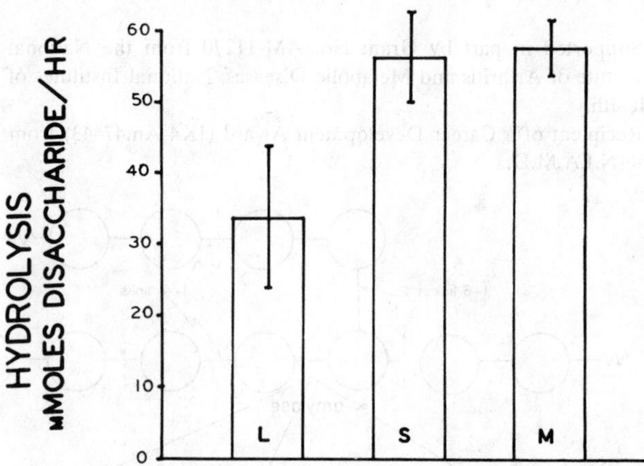

Figure 59-3. Comparison of hydrolysis rates of lactose (L), sucrose (S), and maltose (M) in normal man. Solutions containing a particular disaccharide at 80 mmoles per liter were perfused at 15 ml per min over 30 cm in the upper jejunum. *Brackets* indicate ±2 SE for 10 subjects. (*From G. M. Gray and N. A. Santiago* [15] *with permission of Gastroenterology.*)

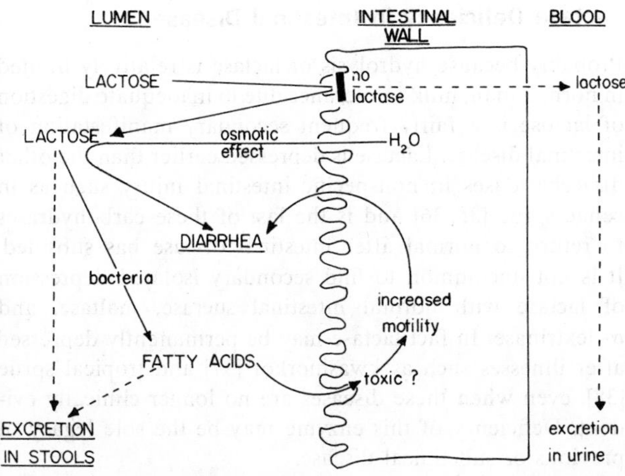

Figure 59-4. Diagrammatic representation of the pathogenesis of the disaccharidase deficiency syndrome. See text for elaboration.

within 5 to 30 min after ingesting the offending carbohydrate. Since the unabsorbed sugar continues to exert its osmotic action in the colon, watery diarrhea containing carbohydrate often occurs from within a few minutes to as much as 5 hr after ingestion of the offending sugar. Bacteria in the lower ileum and colon metabolize the carbohydrate to fatty acids [16]. These fatty acids cause a low pH (<6) of the stool in children, but lowering of pH is not consistently found in adults with the syndrome. The increased fluid in the intestinal lumen and the acid environment stimulate intestinal motility and accelerate intestinal transit time. The mechanisms responsible for the diarrhea of patients with lactase deficiency are shown in Fig. 59-4.

Disacchariduria

An increase in the excretion of intact disaccharide in the urine may occur in some patients with disaccharidase deficiency. Under normal conditions the intestine is almost impermeable to disaccharides, but trace amounts may be absorbed without hydrolysis. There is little if any metabolism of disaccharides after absorption, and only 50 mg or less of any particular disaccharide is customarily excreted in 24 hr in normal man [17]. This may increase to 300 mg or more in patients with intestinal damage [e.g., celiac sprue [18]] or in those who have a high intraluminal concentration of disaccharide, as may be the case in the disaccharidase deficiencies [19]. Disacchariduria is a nonspecific finding which never accounts for more than 1 percent of the ingested carbohydrate and does not serve as a test for disaccharidase deficiency. In fact there appears to be little reason for undertaking the cumbersome analysis for carbohydrate in the urine in patients suspected of having malabsorption of carbohydrate.

TYPES OF LACTOSE INTOLERANCE

Idiopathic Lactase Deficiency in Adolescents and Adults

Most of the patients with lactase deficiency belong to this category. There is a wide variation in prevalence among different racial groups (Table 59-1). While the white population has a relatively low prevalence rate, a remarkably high proportion of American Negroes (70 percent), Orientals (100 percent), and African Bantus (50 percent) have been found with an isolated deficiency of this one disaccharidase.

Typically an adolescent or young adult reports a dislike for milk. This symptom often is ill-defined since the symptoms of intolerance are no longer recalled because the patient had long ago eliminated milk from his diet. The patients usually learn to avoid milk and have no further symptoms. Occasionally they may recall that intolerance began with fever and infection or gastroenteritis, but most cannot relate the onset to a particular illness.

Nearly all lactase-deficient patients in racial groups of high risk for this disorder give a history of appreciable milk ingestion without symptoms as infants and children. They become intolerant as adolescents or young adults [26]. Because of this delayed development of lactase deficiency and the high prevalence of the malady in many racial groups, it has been suggested that man possesses a neonatal lactase which is replaced later by an adult enzyme [27, 28]. This is improbable in view of the recent studies on human intestinal lactases which have disclosed that young children have an enzymatic complement of β-galactosidases that is identical to that of adults [29].

Lactase Deficiency in Infants and Young Children

Oral lactose tolerance tests show that children have full capacity to digest lactose at birth even if they are members

Table 59-1. PREVALENCE OF LACTASE DEFICIENCY IN HEALTHY POPULATION GROUPS

Group	Number tested	Location	Percent lactase deficient	Reference
White	18	Baltimore	5	[20]
	14	San Juan, P. R.	14	[15]
	100	Rochester, Minn.	10	[21]
	93	Chicago	19	[22]
	700	Copenhagen	3	[23]
American Negro	20	Baltimore	70	[20]
	24	Chicago	75	[22]
African Bantu	40	Uganda	50	[24]
Puerto Rican	28	San Juan, P. R.	21	[15]
Oriental	11	Rochester, Minn.	100	[25]

of population groups with a high prevalence of adult lactase deficiency [26, 30]. While manifest deficiency of intestinal lactase in infants and young children is relatively rare, definite cases have been recorded in the first few months of life, and some children with the syndrome eventually develop normal lactase activity within from several months to a year or two after the deficiency is first discovered [31, 32]. Possibly fleeting intestinal injury or the delayed acquisition of lactase may account for these instances. It is important to distinguish this form of lactase deficiency in infants from the peculiar toxic response to lactose without enzyme deficiency which is described next.

Lactose Intolerance in Children without Lactase Deficiency

Occasionally an infant develops overwhelming symptoms of inanition, severe dehydration, and cachexia, sometimes culminating in death, after the ingestion of milk or lactose [2]. In these children the sugar can be digested and absorbed normally, at least as estimated from the blood sugar rise after lactose ingestion. Instead, the response to lactose suggests a direct toxic effect on the intestine, and the immediate withdrawal of milk may be lifesaving. Lactosuria is usually a prominent feature. Thus the intestine may be so damaged that it becomes permeable to the disaccharide. Although there appear to be several authenticated cases of this entity [1, 2, 33, 34], little has been published in the last several years.

Many pediatricians with whom I have discussed this syndrome say that they have observed an occasional patient who fits the description. Comparative features of lactase deficiency and lactose intolerance without the enzyme deficiency are given in Table 59-2. Until further experimental data are available, pediatricians should carefully attempt to categorize cases of milk intolerance according to clinical criteria, with verification by disaccharidase assay. Only in this way will it be possible to ascertain whether indeed there is any toxic response to lactose in the presence of normal intestinal lactase.

Table 59-2. LACTOSE INTOLERANCE IN INFANCY

Lactase deficiency	Intolerance without lactase deficiency
Failure to gain weight; no severe reaction	Diarrhea, vomiting, toxic state after lactose
Flat lactose tolerance test and lactase deficiency	Normal lactose tolerance or only transient lactase deficiency
Lactosuria (variable)	Lactosuria (characteristic)
Normal absorption other nutrients	Decreased xylose absorption
	Amino aciduria, renal acidosis (common)

Lactase Deficiency in Intestinal Disease

Probably because hydrolysis of lactase is relatively limited in normal man, milk intolerance due to inadequate digestion of lactose is a fairly frequent secondary manifestation of intestinal disease. Lactase is depressed earlier than the other disaccharidases in nonspecific intestinal injury such as in celiac sprue [35, 36] and is the last of these carbohydrases to return to normal after intestinal disease has subsided. It is not uncommon to find secondary isolated depression of lactase with normal intestinal sucrase, maltase, and α-dextrinase. In fact lactase may be permanently depressed after illnesses such as kwashiorkor [37] and tropical sprue [38], even when these diseases are no longer clinically evident. Deficiency of this enzyme may be the sole legacy of previous or subclinical disease.

Diseases involving the small intestine that are frequently associated with lactase deficiency and other disaccharidase deficiencies appear in Table 59-3. In general, patients with surface cell abnormalities of the intestine due to these diseases will have lactase deficiency, and 60 to 70 percent of them will also have sucrase and maltase deficiency. This enzyme deficiency state is especially found after gastrectomy, because patients with a normal concentration of lactase may have so rapid a rate of delivery of ingested lactose that the capacity of the small intestine to hydrolyze it is exceeded. After small bowel resections it is said that the total remaining lactase activity may be insufficient to digest completely the lactose of the diet, but few reports actually confirm this [46, 47].

Lactase Deficiency in Diseases Other Than of the Small Intestine

At one time or another claims have been made for an association between lactase deficiency and a variety of diseases in which the small intestine is not directly involved. Ulcerative colitis [48, 49], duodenal ulcer [50], and osteoporosis [51] are but a few of these. In general the associations were made before it was appreciated that there is a high prevalence of lactase deficiency in many racial groups. Further studies are required before a relationship between lactase deficiency and these diseases can be established.

Clinical Diagnosis of Lactase Deficiency

Patients with symptoms of abdominal fullness, nausea, and diarrhea after ingestion of 1 to 3 glasses of milk may be evaluated by analysis of a 3 to 10 mg biopsy of the small intestine. The remainder of the biopsy may be used for conventional histology. The assay has been standardized [5] in international enzyme units (U) per gram protein or per gram wet weight, based on specific measurements of glucose released from the disaccharide substrate. Results have been

Table 59-3. DISACCHARIDASE DEFICIENCY IN GASTROINTESTINAL DISORDERS*

Diagnosis	Number of patients	Percent lactase deficient	Percent sucrase or maltase deficient	References
Celiac sprue				
Untreated	51	100	76	[18, 35, 36, 39, 40, 41]
Treated	14	64	50	[41]
Tropical sprue				
Untreated	46	100	72	[38, 39]
Treated	48	63	0	[38]
Kwashiorkor				
Treated	17	100	0	[37]
"Irritable" colon	71	38	0	[42, 43]
Infant diarrhea	10	40	30	[31]
Postgastrectomy	42	36	0	[44, 45]

* Most patients were white with a presumed prevalence of lactase deficiency in the healthy control group of 5 to 19 percent (see Table 59-1).

reproducible the world over as long as the biopsy is obtained at the ligament of Treitz or up to 30 cm beyond. The typical range of normal values is shown in Table 59-4. It is of interest that lactase activity, in agreement with in vivo studies, is appreciably lower than activity of the other disaccharidases. Activities below those given are usually associated with symptoms of enzyme deficiency. Jejunal assay for these enzymes is critical for diagnosis.

Oral lactose tolerance tests with analyses of blood sugar at 15, 30, 60, 90, and 120 min have been advocated as being highly reliable in ascertaining lactase deficiency [52, 53], but 30 percent of patients with normal lactase activity by assay of intestinal biopsy have flat responses (less than 20 mg per 100 ml rise in blood sugar concentration) when venous blood is analyzed [54]. Use of capillary blood eliminates these falsely flat tests but apparently produces a falsely normal increase in blood sugar in 40 percent of lactase deficient patients [54, 55]. More recent studies of a large group of patients by Welch and his colleagues [56] suggest that the capillary lactose tolerance test after the ingestion of 1 gm of the sugar per kilogram body weight may be associated with few false positive or negative results. A mixture of glucose and galactose causes a greater rise in blood sugar than does the equivalent amount of lactose in normal man. This supports the view that lactose is not well handled even under ideal circumstances. Because hydrolysis of lactose is normally the slowest of all carbohydrate digestive and absorptive processes [15], oral tolerance tests with this sugar probably cannot be expected to separate reliably normal patients from those with lactase deficiency. The assay of peroral biopsies is quite simple and is the procedure of choice, except in small children in whom intestinal biopsy may be hazardous [57].

Symptoms produced by ingestion of lactose usually reflect the fate of the sugar in the intestine. Patients with lactase deficiency develop typical symptoms of the clinical syndrome when undergoing a lactose tolerance test. We have uniformly found lactose, glucose, and galactose in the stools of these patients [58]. Unfortunately, some patients who digest lactose normally also show symptoms after ingestion of the sugar for reasons which are unknown.

Final confirmation of a diagnosis of lactase deficiency is the dramatic response usually seen when the sugar is completely eliminated from the diet. If there is still doubt about the diagnosis, symptoms should return upon resumption of milk or lactose intake.

Treatment of Lactase Deficiency

Elimination of lactose from the diet is the only practical way to eliminate symptoms, and it is very successful. Addi-

Table 59-4. NORMAL VALUES OF INTESTINAL DISACCHARIDASES*

	Lactase	Sucrase	Isomaltase†	Maltase	Sucrase/ lactase
U per gm protein	45 (15–95)	93 (40–165)	99 (50–160)	262 (128–461)	2.1 (1.0–4.5)
U per gm wet weight	3.5 (1.0–6.5)	8.1 (3.5–14)	8.3 (3.8–14)	20 (10–36)	2.3 (1.0–4.5)

* From combined data on 50 patients from Puerto Rico and the United States. U = μmoles per min. Mean values with range in parentheses.

† α-Dextrinase is a more proper name for this enzyme, but the term isomaltase is commonly used.

Table 59-5. FOODS CONTAINING LACTOSE*

Food	Source of lactose
Milk (including nonfat, dried, condensed)	Natural
Processed meat (cold cuts, sausage, wieners)	Milk added in processing
Potatoes (French fried or instant)	Lactose filler added in processing
Prepared mixes (muffins, biscuits, cakes, cookies, pancakes, waffles, dry cereals)	Milk added in manufacture
Prepared soups	Lactose added in processing
Canned and frozen fruits	Lactose added in processing
Salad dressings	Lactose added in processing
Instant coffee	Lactose added in processing
Portagen (medium chain triglyceride preparation)	Lactose added as calorie source

* Summarized from Koch et al. [59] and a Mead Johnson Co. brochure on Portagen [60].

tion of crude lactase preparations to food without avoidance of lactose-containing foods also is effective but is an unwieldy and more expensive method than simple substitution of other sources of calories. Patients with underlying intestinal disease must, of course, receive appropriate therapy for the primary illness.

Total elimination of lactose is not always necessary since many patients can tolerate one or even two glasses of milk without symptoms. A minority of patients cannot tolerate a single 8-oz glass of milk (12 gm lactose) and may require strict elimination of all sources of lactose. Table 59-5 lists some dietary sources of lactose that are not usually considered. Prepackaged and ready-to-eat foods are particularly suspect since lactose is often added as a filler. Individual foods may not contain a large amount of lactose, but, as the list indicates, the varied sources may allow a substantial total intake. It is important that the patient read the statement of contents on the labels of suspect foods. Interestingly enough, Portagen (Mead Johnson Co.), a popular medium chain triglyceride preparation, contains 37 gm lactose per 8 oz. Since it is frequently used as a source of readily absorbable fat in patients with malabsorption who may also have lactase deficiency, care must be taken when giving it to patients with a history suggestive of milk intolerance.

Causes of Lactase Deficiency: Genetic and Environmental Considerations

Most mammals other than man have abundant intestinal lactase at birth which wanes within days to months with weaning [61]. It has been suggested that loss of lactase occurs with maturation and is probably the normal condition for man [27, 62]. If so, white persons of European origin must have somehow acquired a mutant lactase which persists in the adult. Possibly an inability to digest lactose was at one time so deleterious for European adults that there was a selective advantage for those who could continue digestion of lactose throughout life. Much more study is needed of the milk-drinking patterns of earlier generations [63], there being no evidence that milk has been an absolute requirement for the survival of a population.

The frequency of lactase deficiency in healthy adult members of several racial groups (Table 59-1) has prompted the belief that the enzyme deficiency is an inherited disorder. There is no doubt that at least half the members of non-European population groups have milk intolerance and lactose intolerance as adolescents or young adults. Furthermore, probability analysis of the American Negro and white groups is compatible with autosomal recessive inheritance for isolated lactase deficiency [64]. Unfortunately, only preliminary (two-generation) family studies have been carried out [65, 66] and data, while compatible with recessive inheritance, are insufficient to exclude a dominant pattern. Furthermore, adult lactase deficiency cannot be established as an inherited trait as long as other factors contributing to the deficiency state have not been adequately controlled. Among these are the peculiar sensitivity of intestinal lactase to intestinal injury, persistence of the isolated deficiency state long after any underlying intestinal disease has become quiescent [37, 38], dietary influences, and the unknown residue of subclinical intestinal disease in a given population. Hopefully, the critical family studies of multiple generations will soon be available.

In general it has been assumed in population studies (Table 59-1) that environmental factors do not play a role in lactase deficiency and that the variable to consider is the gene. In this regard it is interesting that Australian aboriginal [67] and Baganda children [68] have a sudden decline in rate of growth at about 12 months of age that is presumably the result of a high incidence of gastrointestinal and respiratory diseases [67] and suboptimal nutrition [68]. These same children begin to have flat lactose tolerance tests at the same age, and nearly all are lactose intolerant by age 4 years [30, 67]. It may be possible that these children develop transitory malnutrition or temporary subclinical disease which leaves them with permanent lactase deficiency.

While lactase deficiency in infancy is quite rare, it has

occurred in sibs [34] and is probably inherited as an autosomal recessive gene. Diarrhea of any origin is often associated with transient lactase deficiency [31]. More thorough family studies are needed but there is more security in attributing the infant type than the adult type to a genetic cause.

SUCRASE-α-DEXTRINASE DEFICIENCY

Reports of intolerance to sucrose in the diet have come from many areas of the world. There are probably 65 to 75 known instances of sucrase deficiency [69, 70]. The malady appears to be inherited as an autosomal recessive gene. All patients have had low activity not only of sucrase but also of α-dextrinase (isomaltase) in the mucosa of the small intestine. Symptoms occur in early childhood when the offending sugar is ingested and are indistinguishable from those of lactase deficiency, except that they are evoked by table sugar rather than by milk. Starch is usually well tolerated because the undigestible α-dextrins have a high molecular weight (1,500 average). They provide only 10 to 20 percent of the osmotic activity per gram of sucrose and attract correspondingly less water into the intestinal lumen. Patients nearly always discover the inability to tolerate sweets and modify their diet to avoid symptoms. Tolerance to sucrose tends to increase with age, so that several grams may be taken without ill effect by the young adult. Deletion of sucrose from the diet eliminates the symptoms but may encroach upon the obligate source of calories in some areas of the world. As noted above for lactase deficiency, determination of enzyme activity in a small intestinal biopsy specimen is required to establish the diagnosis.

Identification of the Intestinal Oligosaccharidases and Disaccharidases

These enzymes have been very difficult to separate and characterize because they are an integral part of the brush border membrane and are similar to each other in biochemical behavior. Early studies, based on partial separation by gel filtration chromatography [71] and heat inactivation of the disaccharidase peaks [72, 73], suggested that there are two β-galactosidases with a specificity for lactose and cellobiose and five α-glucosidases, two with sucrase activity, one with isomaltase activity, and two with only maltase activity.

There has been little advancement in our knowledge of the α-glucosidases in the last few years, but recently it has been possible to separate three human intestinal β-galactosidases [29] by density gradient centrifugation, as outlined in Fig. 59-5. As shown in Fig. 59-6, patients with lactase deficiency uniformly lack one of the two lactases (enzyme I) [74]. Enzyme II is presumably too deep within the intestinal cell to be effective against dietary lactose. In addition, the nonspecific β-galactosidase (enzyme III), which is incapable of splitting lactase, is also absent in some lactase deficient patients. This suggests that enzymes I and III may be related. It is possible that enzyme III is a precursor of the specific lactase. If this is true then a failure of synthesis of enzyme III would be a type of defect in which both enzymes would be absent, and a block of the conversion of III to I would explain the defect in those patients who retain enzyme III at normal levels.

Table 59-6 lists the properties of the oligo- and disaccharidases currently known in the normal human intestine, along with the biochemical techniques used for their identi-

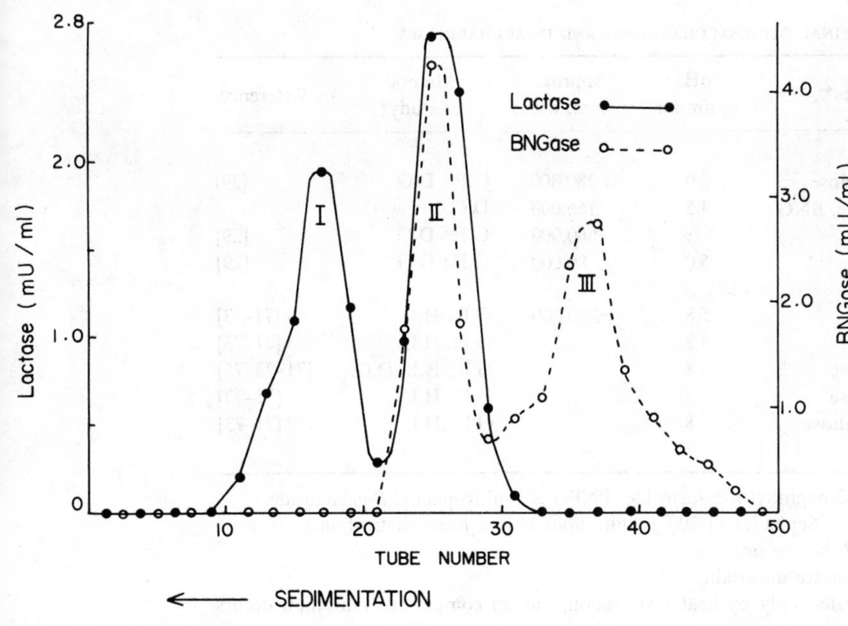

Figure 59-5. Separation of human intestinal β-galactosidases by density gradient ultracentrifugation on 5 to 20% NaCl for 9 hr in the SW50L rotor. 0.1 ml intestinal supernatant was layered on the 5 ml gradient. BNGase = 6-bromo-2-naphthyl-β-galactosidase; U = μmoles per min of substrate split. (*Reproduced from G. M. Gray and N. A. Santiago* [29], *with permission of J. Clin. Invest.*)

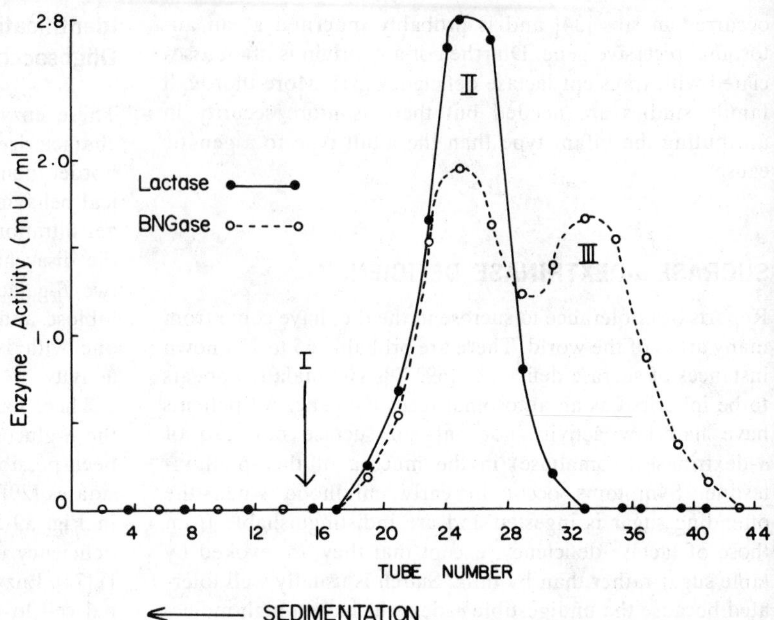

Figure 59-6. Density gradient centrifugation of intestinal preparation from a patient with lactose intolerance and lactase deficiency. Conditions are the same as in Fig. 59-5. Note that enzyme I is undetectable. (*Reproduced from G. M. Gray et al.* [74], *with permission of J. Clin. Invest.*)

fication. Further study of these enzymes should yield a better understanding of their hydrolytic roles in health and disease.

Interrelations of Sucrase and α-Dextrinase

The activities of sucrase are essentially equal to those of α-dextrinase (isomaltase), and patients with hereditary sucrase deficiency have always been found lacking in α-dextrinase as well, although the depression of the latter enzyme is usually less [76]. This has prompted the suggestion that sucrase and α-dextrinase either are under the same biosynthetic control, an analogy to the regulator gene concept for bacterial systems [77], or else the two enzyme activities are on the same protein molecule, as in the "two-headed" enzyme which has both transferase and glucosidase activities against glycogen phosphorylase limit dextrin [78]. It has not been possible to separate human sucrase and α-dextrinase into separate protein species, but these enzymes do appear to occupy separate active sites, because there is no competitive inhibition between their appropriate substrates, and heat inactivation of each activity occurs at different rates

Table 59-6. HUMAN INTESTINAL OLIGOSACCHARIDASES AND DISACCHARIDASES

Class (Trivial name)	Number	Substrates*	pH optimum	Approx. mol. wt	Method of study†	Reference
β-Galactosidases						
Lactase	I	*Lactose,* cellobiose	6.0	280,000	G.F.; D.G.	[29]
	II‡	*PNPG,* Lactose, BNG	4.5	156,000	D.G.	
				660,000	G.F.; D.G.	[29]
	III	*BNG, PNPG*	6.0	80,000	G.F.; D.G.	[29]
α-Glucosidases						
	I§	*Maltose*	5.8	>200,000	G.F., H.I.	[71–73]
	II§	*Maltose*	5.8	....	G.F., H.I.	[71–73]
Sucrase 1	III	*Sucrose,* maltose	5.8	....	G.F., H.I., D.G.	[71–73, 75]
Sucrase 2¶	IV	*Sucrose,* maltose	5.8	....	G.F., H.I.	[71–73]
α-Dextrinase¶	V	*α-Dextrins,* maltose isomaltose	5.8	....	G.F., H.I.	[71–73]

* Principal substrate in *italics.* BNG = 6-bromo-2-naphthyl-β-galactoside; PNPG = ρ-nitro-phenyl-β-galactoside.
†D.G. = density gradient centrifugation; G.F. = Sephadex G-200 gel filtration; H.I. = heat inactivation.
‡Ineffective in vivo against lactose; not a brush border enzyme.
§Location in intestinal cell and role in digestion are uncertain.
¶Sucrase 2 and α-dextranase have been separated only by heat inactivation, but no competitive inhibition occurs between their principal substrates.

[73, 75]. Perhaps the reason why these two enzymes share the same protein molecule is that they work in concert to hydrolyze the α-1-4 (maltose) links and the adjacent α-1-6 (isomaltose) branching points of the α-dextrins.

Elucidation of the interaction of sucrase and α-dextrinase is critical for understanding the mechanism of the terminal digestion of starch in the normal and diseased intestine.

Development and Control of Disaccharidases in Man

Sucrase, maltase, and α-dextrinase activities are acquired by the eleventh week of gestation, but lactase activity remains low until at least 28 weeks of gestation [79]. Lactase is high in newborn infants. Presumably, it reaches its maximum concentration shortly before term.

Little is known about induction or repression of these enzymes by food and drugs. Feeding of sucrose or fructose increases intestinal sucrase in man after 2 to 5 days [80]; approximately the same time is required for turnover of the intestinal digestive-absorptive cell. Lactase deficient patients fed lactose for 6 to 12 months do not increase their intestinal lactase [81, 82], and patients with galactosemia who are kept on a lactose-free diet from birth maintain their lactase activity at normal levels [83]. Thus in man there is no evidence that lactose has any influence whatsoever on lactase activity.

Cortisone promotes precocious acquisition of disaccharidases in the developing rat intestine [61] but has no effect on sucrase or maltase in the adult rat. The effect of corticosteroids on man has not been studied.

GLUCOSE-GALACTOSE MALABSORPTION

There have been at least 20 patients reported with malabsorption of glucose and galactose [84–87]. Children with this abnormality have diarrhea, dehydration, and sugar in the stools after ingestion of almost any dietary carbohydrate, because they contain at least one of these hexoses. All patients who have been carefully tested have had an associated mild defect in renal tubular reabsorption of glucose. Customarily, they excrete 250 to 1,000 mg glucose per 100 ml in the urine. If the disorder is not recognized, the child may die of dehydration and malnutrition. Elimination of all dietary carbohydrate is required, and fructose, with a transport system that is not affected, is substituted as the source of carbohydrate calories (cf. Fig. 59-2). Some patients tolerate sucrose better than other disaccharides because one of its monosaccharide components is the readily absorbed fructose.

The diagnosis should be suspected in a child who tolerates all dietary carbohydrate poorly and who has little or no rise in blood sugar after a meal. Stools are acid and contain glucose and galactose. Perfusion of the intestine with a solution containing glucose and fructose demonstrates the paradoxical finding of more rapid disappearance (absorption) of the passively transported fructose than of the glucose [88]. In vitro study of a small intestinal biopsy demonstrates loss of normal accumulation of glucose beyond the concentration in the medium [89]. Indeed, tissue concentrations always are less than in the incubation medium. This rare malady may be distinguished from disaccharidase deficiencies because there is no significant rise in blood sugar concentration in the course of a glucose-galactose oral tolerance test.

As shown in Fig. 59-7, glucose and Na^+ are currently thought to be bound to a carrier and then released after entry into the intestinal cell to go their separate ways [90]. Na^+ is pumped out of the base and sides of the cell and may provide the driving force for active glucose transport. Glucose transport is facilitated by entry of K^+ which hastens its metabolism to glycogen and lactic acid [91]. Patients with glucose-galactose malabsorption probably have a defect at the carrier-mediated entry step, rather than a defect of K^+ facilitation, or at the Na^+ pump site, since they do not accumulate glucose within the intestinal cells and yet are capable of absorbing Na^+. Exact definition of the defect will not be possible until the molecular basis for active glucose transport is completely understood.

Genetic Aspects

A study of relatives of an intermarried Swedish family going back 10 generations to the eighteenth century has shown that the defect probably has an autosomal recessive mode of inheritance [92]. As there have only been a few patients reported since the first description of the malady in 1962 [85, 86], the frequency of the gene in the world population is probably low. All patients reported have either been

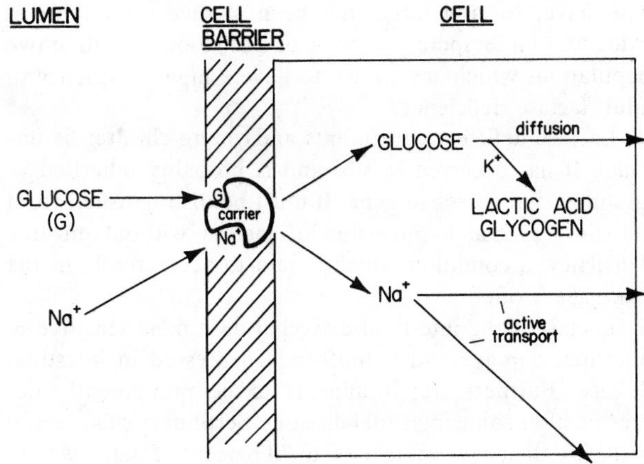

Figure 59-7. Schematic diagram of active glucose transport by the intestinal cell. The sugar accumulates in the cell by virtue of active Na^+ transport and then moves out of the cell with facilitation provided by K^+-stimulated conversion to metabolic products. (*Modified from Crane* [90] *and Csáky and Ho* [91]. *Reproduced from G. M. Gray* [93], *with permission of Gastroenterology.*)

white or their racial origin has not been mentioned. One patient had a Chinese mother and a white father, so it would appear that the gene is not confined to a single population group, unless that patient was a new mutant.

SUMMARY

1 The breakdown products of dietary starch (maltose, maltotriose, and α-dextrins), as well as sucrose and lactose, are hydrolyzed by their specific carbohydrases localized at the luminal pole of the small intestinal mucosal cell. After hydrolysis the released monosaccharides are transported by specific mechanisms. Glucose and galactose share an active Na^+-requiring process that accumulates these monosaccharides in the cell against a concentration gradient. Fructose, the other monosaccharide produced by hydrolysis, is absorbed by facilitated passive diffusion.

2 Clinically, a deficiency of a particular disaccharidase is accompanied by abdominal fullness and bloating, cramping pain, and diarrhea. The unhydrolyzed disaccharide, which is initially unabsorbed, remains free in the intestinal lumen where it exerts an osmotic effect. Bacteria in the lower ileum and colon metabolize the undigested sugar to monosaccharides and fatty acids. These are poorly absorbed in the more distal intestine and further aggravate the osmotic diarrhea.

3 Intestinal lactase deficiency occurs in 3 to 19 percent of healthy white people of European origin, 70 percent of American Negroes, 50 percent of African Bantus, and in virtually all Orientals that have been tested. These patients appear to become intolerant of lactose in adolescence or as young adults, and claims have been made that the deficiency is inherited as an autosomal recessive characteristic. Environmental factors of diet and subclinical intestinal disease have, by and large, not been studied, and there is evidence of a temporary slowing of childhood growth in two populations which are known to have a high prevalence of adult lactase deficiency.

4 Lactase deficiency in infants and young children is unusual. It has occurred in sibs and is probably inherited as an autosomal recessive gene. It must be distinguished from a toxic response to ingestion of lactose without enzyme deficiency, a condition which is said to occur rarely in the same age group.

5 Lactase is the intestinal disaccharidase most sensitive to intestinal damage and is uniformly depressed in intestinal disease. Furthermore, it appears to be permanently depressed after some intestinal diseases. Secondary sucrase and maltase deficiency occurs in 60 to 70 percent of patients with malabsorptive disease of the small intestine, but both return to normal when the disease undergoes remission.

6 Sucrase-α-dextrinase deficiency is a rare malady inherited as an autosomal recessive gene. Intolerance to sugar is discovered in childhood, and the patient and his family usually learn to eliminate sucrose from the diet. The α-dextrins, being of larger molecular size, have little osmotic effect, and accordingly starch is usually well tolerated. Many older children eventually are able to tolerate moderate amounts of sucrose.

7 Assay of enzyme activity in a small intestinal biopsy is critical for the diagnosis of disaccharidase deficiency. Oral sugar tolerance tests serve as helpful screening procedures. The dramatic amelioration of symptoms upon withdrawal of the offending sugar from the diet confirms the diagnosis.

8 Glucose-galactase malabsorption is a rare defect in the transport of these sugars. The clinical syndrome is indistinguishable from disaccharidase deficiency, except that there is intolerance to almost all dietary sugars because most of them contain at least one of these monosaccharides. In contrast to disaccharidase deficiency, the glucose tolerance test produces little or no rise in blood sugar, and intestinal mucosal biopsies do not accumulate glucose against a concentration gradient. Replacement of all dietary carbohydrate with fructose is successful, since this monosaccharide is absorbed by a different mechanism than glucose or galactose. As estimated from an extensive family study, this malady is a genetic defect with an autosomal recessive pattern of inheritance.

BIBLIOGRAPHY

1. Durand, P.: Lattosuria idiopatica in una paziente con diarrea cronica ed acidosi. Minerva Pediat., **10,** 706, 1958.
2. Holzel, A., Mereu, T., and Thomson, M. L.: Severe lactose intolerance in infancy. Lancet, **2,** 1346, 1962.
3. Crosby, W. H., and Kugler, H. W.: Intraluminal biopsy of the small intestine. Amer. J. Dig. Dis., **2,** 236, 1957.
4. Brandborg, L. L., Rubin, C. E., and Quinton, W. E.: A multipurpose instrument for suction biopsy of the esophagus, stomach, small bowel and colon. Gastroenterology, **37,** 1, 1959.
5. Dahlquist, A.: Method for assay of intestinal disaccharidases. Anal. Biochem., **7,** 18, 1964.
6. Miller, D., and Crane, R. K.: The digestive function of the epithelium of the small intestine. II. Localization of disaccharide hydrolysis in the isolated brush border portion of intestinal epithelial cells. Biochim. Biophys. Acta, **52,** 293, 1961.
7. Dahlqvist, A., and Borgström, B.: Digestion and absorption of disaccharides in man. Biochem. J., **81,** 411, 1961.
8. Gray, G. M., and Ingelfinger, F. J.: Intestinal absorption of sucrose in man: The site of hydrolysis and absorption. J. Clin. Invest., **44,** 390, 1965.
9. Roberts, P. J. P., and Whelan, W. J.: The mechanism of carbohydrase action. 5. Action of human salivary α-amylase on amylopectin and glycogen. Biochem. J., **76,** 246, 1960.
10. Gray, G. M.: Malabsorption of carbohydrate. Fed. Proc., **26,** 1415, 1967.
11. Barnett, J. E. G., Jarvis, W. T. S., and Munday, K. A.: Structural requirements for active intestinal sugar transport. The involvement of hydrogen bonds at C-1 and C-6 of the sugar. Biochem. J., **109,** 61, 1968.
12. Riklis, E., and Quastel, J. H.: Effects of cations on sugar absorption by isolated surviving guinea pig intestine. Canad. J. Biochem. Physiol., **36,** 347, 1958.
13. Anraku, Y.: Transport of sugars and amino acids in bacteria. I. Purification and specificity of the galactose—and leucine—binding proteins. J. Biol. Chem., **243,** 3116, 1968.
14. Fridhandler, L., and Quastel, J. H.: Absorption of sugars from isolated surviving intestine. Arch. Biochem. Biophys., **56,** 412, 1955.
15. Gray, G. M., and Santiago, N. S.: Disaccharide absorption in normal and diseased human intestine. Gastroenterology, **51,** 489, 1966.

16. Christopher, N. L., and Bayless, T. M.: Role of small bowel and colon in lactose-induced diarrhea. Gastroenterology, **56,** 1250, 1969. (Abstract.)
17. Bickel, H.: Mellituria: paper chromatographic study. J. Pediat., **59,** 641, 1961.
18. Weser, E., and Sleisenger, M. H.: Lactosuria and lactase deficiency in adult celiac disease. Gastroenterology, **48,** 571, 1965.
19. Durand, P.: Lactose intolerance, in *Disorders Due to Intestinal Defective Carbohydrate Digestion and Absorption,* p. 105, edited by P. Durand. "Il Pensiero Scientifico" Publisher, Rome, 1964.
20. Bayless, T. M., and Rosensweig, N. S.: A racial difference in incidence of lactase deficiency. JAMA, **197,** 968, 1966.
21. Newcomer, A. D., and McGill, D. B.: Disaccharidase activity in the small intestine: Prevalence of lactase deficiency in 100 healthy subjects. Gastroenterology, **53,** 881, 1967.
22. Littman, A., Cady, A. B., and Rhodes, J.: Lactase and other disaccharidase deficiencies in the hospital population. Israel J. Med. Sci., **4,** 110, 1968.
23. Gudmand-Höyer, E., Dahlqvist, A., and Jarnum, S.: Specific small-intestinal lactase deficiency in adults. Scand. J. Gastroent., **4,** 377, 1969.
24. Cook, G. C., and Kajubi, S. K.: Tribal incidence of lactase deficiency in Uganda. Lancet, **1,** 725, 1966.
25. Chung, M. H., and McGill, D. B.: Lactase deficiency in Orientals. Gastroenterology, **54,** 225, 1968.
26. Huang, Shi-Shung, and Bayless, T. M.: Lactose intolerance in healthy children. New Eng. J. Med., **276,** 1283, 1967.
27. Ferguson, A., and Maxwell, J. D.: Genetic aetiology of lactose intolerance. Lancet, **2,** 188, 1967.
28. Huang, Shi-Shung, and Bayless, T. M.: Milk and lactose intolerance in healthy Orientals. Science, **160,** 83, 1968.
29. Gray, G. M., and Santiago, N. A.: Intestinal β-galactosidases. I. Separation and characterization of three enzymes in normal human intestine. J. Clin. Invest., **48,** 716, 1969.
30. Cook, G. C.: Lactase activity in newborn and infant Baganda. Brit. Med. J., **1,** 527, 1967.
31. Burke, V., Kerry, K. R., and Anderson, C. M.: The relationship of dietary lactose to refractory diarrhoea in infancy. Aust. Paed. J., **1,** 147, 1965.
32. Sunshine, P., and Kretchmer, N.: Studies of small intestine during development. III. Infantile diarrhea associated with intolerance to disaccharides. Pediatrics, **34,** 38, 1964.
33. Darling, S., Mortensen, O., and Søndergaard, G.: Lactosuria and aminoaciduria in infancy: A new inborn error of metabolism. Acta Paediat. (Uppsala), **49,** 281, 1960.
34. Holzel, A.: Sugar malabsorption and sugar intolerance in childhood. Proc. Roy. Soc. Med., **61,** 1095, 1968.
35. Plotkin, G. R., and Isselbacher, K. J.: Secondary disaccharidase deficiency in adult celiac disease (non-tropical sprue) and other malabsorption states. New Eng. J. Med., **271,** 1033, 1964.
36. Shmerling, D. H., Auricchio, S., Rubino, A., Hadorn, B., and Prader, A.: Der sekundäre Mangel an intestinaler Disaccharidaseaktivität bei der Cöliake: Quantitative Bestimmung der Enzymaktivität and Klinische Beurteilung. Helv. Paediat. Acta, **19,** 507, 1964.
37. Cook, G. C., and Lee, F. D.: The jejunum after kwashiorkor. Lancet, **2,** 1263, 1966.
38. Gray, G. M., Walter, W. M., Jr., and Colver, E. H.: Persistent deficiency of intestinal lactase in apparently cured tropical sprue. Gastroenterology, **54,** 552, 1968.
39. Sheehy, T. W., and Anderson, P. R.: Disaccharidase activity in normal and diseased small bowel. Lancet, **2,** 1, 1965.
40. Welsh, J. D., Rohrer, V. G., Drewry, R., May, J. C., and Walker, A.: Human intestinal disaccharidase activity. II. Diseases of the small intestine and deficiency states. Arch. Intern. Med. (Chicago), **117,** 495, 1966.
41. Welsh, J. D., Zschiesche, O. M., Anderson, J., and Walker, A.: Intestinal disaccharidase activity in celiac sprue (gluten-sensitive enteropathy). Arch. Intern. Med. (Chicago), **123,** 33, 1969.
42. McMichael, H. B., Webb, J., and Dawson, A. M.: Lactase deficiency in adults: A cause of "functional" diarrhoea. Lancet, **1,** 717, 1965.
43. Weser, E., Rubin, W., Ross, L., and Sleisenger, M. H.: Lactase deficiency in patients with the "irritable-colon syndrome." New Eng. J. Med., **273,** 1070, 1965.
44. Kojecký, Z., and Matlocha, Z.: Quantitative differences of intestinal disaccharidase activity following the resection of stomach. Gastroenterologia (Basel), **104,** 343, 1965.
45. Welsh, J. D., Shaw, R. W., and Walker, A.: Isolated lactase deficiency producing postgastrectomy milk intolerance. Ann. Intern. Med., **64,** 1252, 1966.
46. Weijers, H. A., and Van de Kamer, J. H.: Diarrhoea caused by deficiency of sugar splitting enzymes. II. Acta Paediat., **51,** 371, 1962.
47. Kern, F., Struthers, J. E., and Attwood, W. L.: Lactose intolerance as a cause of steatorrhea in an adult. Gastroenterology, **45,** 477, 1963.
48. Cady, A. B., Rhodes, J. B., Littman, A., and Crane, R. K.: Significance of lactase deficit in ulcerative colitis. J. Lab. Clin. Med., **70,** 279, 1967.
49. Newcomer, A. D., and McGill, D. B.: Incidence of lactase deficiency in ulcerative colitis. Gastroenterology, **53,** 890, 1967.
50. Auricchio, S., Rubino, A., Landolt, M., Semenza, G., and Prader, A.: Isolated intestinal lactase deficiency in the adult. Lancet, **2,** 324, 1963.
51. Birge, S. J., Jr., Keutmann, H. T., Cuatrecasas, P., and Whedon, G. D.: Osteoporosis, intestinal lactase deficiency and low dietary calcium intake. New Eng. J. Med., **276,** 445, 1967.
52. Peternel, W. W.: Lactose tolerance in relation to intestinal lactase activity. Gastroenterology, **48,** 299, 1965.
53. Littman, A., and Hammond, J. B.: Diarrhea in adults caused by deficiency in intestinal disaccharidases, Gastroenterology, **48,** 237, 1965.
54. McGill, D. B., and Newcomer, A. D.: Comparison of venous and capillary blood samples in lactose tolerance testing. Gastroenterology, **53,** 371, 1967.
55. Gray, G. M.: Problems with lactose tolerance tests. Gastroenterology, **53,** 496, 1967.
56. Welsh, J. D.: Isolated lactase deficiency in humans. Report on 100 patients. Medicine, **40,** 257, 1970.
57. Partin, J. C., and Schubert, W. K.: Precautionary note on the use of the intestinal-biopsy capsule in infants and emaciated children. New Eng. J. Med., **274,** 94, 1966.
58. Rosenquist, C. J., Heaton, J. W., Friedland, G. W., Gray, G. M., and Zboralske, F. F.: Assessment of a radiographic method for diagnosis of intestinal lactase deficiency: a prospective study. Invest. Rad., **6,** 40, 1971.
59. Koch, R., Acosta, P., Ragsdale, N., and Donnell, G. N.: Nutrition in the treatment of galactosemia. J. Amer. Dietetic Assoc., **43,** 216, 1963.
60. Physicians Handbook: Portagen. Mead Johnson and Co., 1967, p. 13.
61. Doell, R. G., and Kretchmer, N.: Studies of small intestine during development. I. Distribution and activity of β-galactosidase. Biochim. Biophys. Acta, **62,** 353, 1962.
62. Cook, G. C.: Some observations on racial lactase deficiency. Proc. Roy. Soc. Med., **61,** 1102, 1968.
63. Simoons, F.: The non-milking area of Africa. Anthropos, **49,** 58, 1954.
64. Bayless, T. M., Christopher, N. L., and Boyer, S. H.: Autosomal recessive inheritance of intestinal lactase deficiency: Evidence from ethnic differences. J. Clin. Invest., **48,** 6a, 1969 (abstract).
65. Welsh, J. D., Zschiesche, O. M., Willits, V. L., Jr., and Russell, L.: Studies of lactose intolerance in families. Arch. Intern. Med. (Chicago), **122,** 315, 1968.
66. Neale, G.: The diagnosis, incidence and significance of disaccharidase deficiency in adults. Proc. Roy. Soc. Med., **61,** 1099, 1968.
67. Elliott, R. B., and Maxwell, G. M.: Lactose maldigestion in Australian aboriginal children. Med. J. Aust., **1,** 46, 1967.
68. Rutishauser, I. H. E.: Heights and weights of middle class Baganda children. Lancet, **2,** 565, 1965.
69. Burgess, E. A., Levin, B., Mahalanabis, D., and Tonge, R. E.: Hereditary sucrose intolerance: Levels of sucrase activity in jejunal mucosa. Arch. Dis. Child., **39,** 431, 1964.
70. Prader, A., and Auricchio, S.: Defects of intestinal disaccharide absorption. Ann. Rev. Med., **16,** 345, 1965.
71. Semenza, G., Auricchio, S., and Rubino, A.: Multiplicity of human intestinal disaccharidases. I. Chromatographic separation of maltases and two lactases. Biochim. Biophys. Acta, **96,** 487, 1965.
72. Dahlquist, A.: Specificity of the human intestinal disaccharidases and implications for hereditary disaccharide intolerance. J. Clin. Invest., **41,** 463, 1962.
73. Auricchio, S., Semenza, G., and Rubino, A.: Multiplicity of human

intestinal disaccharidases. II. Characterization of the individual maltases. Biochim. Biophys. Acta, **96,** 498, 1965.
74. Gray, G. M., Santiago, N. A., Colver, E. H., and Genel, M.: Intestinal β-galactosidases. II. Biochemical alteration in human lactase deficiency. J. Clin. Invest., **48,** 729, 1969.
75. Eggermont, E.: The biochemical defects in sucrose intolerance and in glucose-galactose malabsorption. Thesis. Faculté de Médecine, Université Catholique de Louvain, 1968.
76. Auricchio, S., Rubino, A., Prader, A., Rey, J., Jos, J., Frezal, J., and Davidson, M.: Intestinal glycosidase activities in congenital malabsorption of disaccharides. J. Pediat., **66,** 555, 1965.
77. Jacob, F., and Monod, J.: Genetic regulatory mechanisms in the synthesis of proteins. J. Molec. Biol., **3,** 318, 1961.
78. Nelson, T. E., Kolb, E., and Larner, J.: Purification and properties of rabbit muscle amylo-1,6-glucosidase-oligo-1,4→1,4-transferase. Biochemistry (U.S.A.), **8,** 1419, 1969.
79. Dahlqvist, A., and Lindberg, T.: Development of the intestinal disaccharidase and alkaline phosphatase activities in the human foetus. Clin. Sci., **30,** 517, 1966.
80. Rosensweig, N. S., and Herman, R. H.: Time response of jejunal sucrase and maltase activity to a high sucrose diet in normal man. Gastroenterology, **56,** 500, 1969.
81. Cuatrecasas, P., Lockwood, D. H., and Caldwell, J. R.: Lactase deficiency in the adult: A common occurrence, Lancet, **1,** 14, 1965.
82. Gray, G. M.: Unpublished observations.
83. Kogut, M. D., Donnell, G. N., and Shaw, K. N. F.: Studies of lactose absorption in patients with galactosemia. J. Pediat., **71,** 75, 1967.
84. Lindquist, B., and Meeuwisse, G. W.: Chronic diarrhoea caused by monosaccharide malabsorption. Acta Paediat. Scand., **51,** 674, 1962.
85. Laplane, R., Polonovski, C., Etienne, M., Debray, P., Lods, J.-C., and Pissarro, B.: L'intolérance aux sucres á transfert intestinal actif: Ses rapports avec l'intolérance au lactose et le syndrome coeliaque. Arch. Franc. Pediat., **19,** 895, 1962.
86. Schneider, A. J., Kinter, W. B., and Stirling, C. E.: Glucose-galactose malabsorption. New Eng. J. Med., **274,** 305, 1966.
87. Meeuwisse, G. W., and Dahlqvist, A.: Glucose-galactose malabsorption. Acta Paediat, Scand., **57,** 273, 1968.
88. Meeuwisse, G., and Melin, K.: Glucose-galactose malabsorption. Acta Paediat. Scand., suppl., **188,** 3, 1969.
89. Eggermont, E., and Loeb, H.: Glucose-galactose intolerance. Lancet, **2,** 343, 1966.
90. Crane, R. K.: Hypothesis for mechanism of intestinal active transport of sugars. Fed. Proc., **21,** 891, 1962.
91. Csáky, T. Z., and Ho, P. M.: The effect of potassium on the intestinal transport of glucose. J. Gen. Physiol., **50,** 113, 1966.
92. Melin, K., and Meeuwisse, G. W.: Glucose-galactose malabsorption: A genetic study. Acta Paediat. Scand., suppl., **188,** 19, 1969.
93. Gray, G. M.: Progress in gastroenterology: Carbohydrate digestion and absorption. Gastroenterology, **58,** 906, 1970.

CHAPTER SIXTY

FAMILIAL (HEREDITARY) VITAMIN D-RESISTANT RICKETS WITH HYPOPHOSPHATEMIA

T. Franklin Williams and Robert W. Winters

Familial (hereditary) vitamin D-resistant rickets with hypophosphatemia is a specific disorder characterized by (1) familial occurrence, the inheritance of the abnormality being, with possible rare exceptions, a single-dose effect of an X-linked gene ("X-linked dominant"); (2) hypophosphatemia associated with decreased renal tubular reabsorption of inorganic phosphate as the consistent inherited abnormality; (3) rickets or osteomalacia in some but not all affected persons, not responsive to physiological amounts of vitamin D; (4) diminished gastrointestinal absorption of calcium, demonstrable in affected children with rickets; and (5) an abnormality in the metabolism of vitamin D.

Identification of this disorder by these characteristics sets it apart from other conditions that may share some of the same features but not the clear-cut genetic pattern, such as vitamin D-resistant rickets associated with normal or high serum concentration of inorganic phosphate and patients with multiple abnormalities of renal tubular function (Fanconi syndrome, renal tubular acidosis). By limiting this discussion to the genetically distinct disorder, we can have some confidence that we are dealing with a disease affecting a substantial number of persons in the same fundamental ways.

HISTORICAL DEVELOPMENT

The growth of the understanding of this disorder has proceeded along clinical, physiologic, and genetic pathways. Rickets which failed to respond to the usual doses of vitamin D was recognized only after vitamin D-deficiency rickets had been largely eliminated by prophylaxis. In such a patient, Albright et al. [1] in 1937 first showed that very large doses of vitamin D would bring about healing of the rickets. That hypophosphatemia was due either primarily or secondarily to decreased renal tubular reabsorption of phosphate was first recognized by Robertson et al. [2] in 1942.

The first description of familial occurrence of vitamin D-resistant rickets with hypophosphatemia was in 1941 by Christensen [3], who reported a mother and her son and daughter with typical features of the disease. Earlier instances of familial occurrence are probable [4]. On the basis of skeletal manifestations several workers proposed an autosomal dominant mode of inheritance with variable degrees of manifestation of recognizable bone disease [5, 6]. However, Winters and his collaborators [7, 8] and Graham et al. [9] were able to show that the occurrence of hypophosphatemia in involved families follows an X-linked mode of inheritance, with virtually complete generation-to-generation manifestations of the biochemical abnormality.

More recently, as a part of the rapid advancements being made in understanding vitamin D, an abnormality in the conversion of vitamin D to its biologically active metabolite has been demonstrated in affected family members [10, 11]. This points to the possibility of a single genetic locus for the expression of the disorder.

These advances still leave unanswered a number of important questions: the cause of the phosphaturia, i.e., whether it is an intrinsic renal tubular defect, or due to secondary hyperparathyroidism, or the result of the abnormality in metabolism in vitamin D; a full explanation of the failure of growth in affected children; and the cause of bony overgrowth which appears at tendinous attachments in affected adults and can be a source of morbidity.

CLINICAL AND RADIOLOGIC FINDINGS

The mildest abnormality is purely biochemical. This is hypophosphatemia (see below, under Hypophosphatemia, for criteria for hypophosphatemia) without clinical manifestations other than a slight decrease in height, when compared with normophosphatemic sibs. This is a common finding in kindreds with the disorder [7–9, 12].

In hypophosphatemic adults the varying degrees of deformities due to rickets in childhood include bowing of the legs and shortening of stature, usually without evidence of continuing active bone disease. A few affected adults have evidence of active osteomalacia, as judged by the presence of pseudofractures and an elevated serum alkaline phosphatase level. These changes revert toward normal with treatment with large doses of vitamin D.

In clinically affected adults, bony overgrowth at the site of major muscular attachments and around joints may cause significant limitation of motion, particularly in elbows, shoulders, and hips [8, 13, 14]. Such overgrowth within the spinal canal has produced symptomatic cord compression requiring surgical intervention [15–17].

In affected children with rickets the disease is usually first recognized when the child begins to walk, but the history or x-ray examination often reveals abnormalities dating to the first year of life, including growth failure, deformities of the skull, late dentition and "sitting" deformities of the legs. Spine and pelvis do not show active rickets, in contrast to vitamin D-deficiency rickets [18]. These children have usually received prophylactic doses of vitamin D or have failed to respond to what was initially diagnosed as vitamin D-deficiency rickets. Healing of the active rickets occurs upon treatment with large doses of vitamin D, or vitamin D plus oral phosphate preparations, or 25-hydroxycholecalciferol (see Treatment, below). Permanent deformities and shortened stature usually persist. In adults and children the use of the massive doses of vitamin D required for healing frequently results in vitamin D intoxication with hypercalcemia. Upon discontinuance of the vitamin the rickets usually becomes active again. Thus vitamin D-resistant rickets differs clinically from vitamin D-deficiency rickets both in the 100-fold greater dose required to induce healing and in the fact that a permanent "cure" is rarely achieved until growth is completed.

Among family members with hypophosphatemia, females have a lower incidence of bone disease than males [8, 12], but when present it may be of the same severity [18]. Few patients have the muscular weakness and atony that are such prominent and frequent features of vitamin D-deficiency rickets. Active rickets of the spine or pelvis is not found [19]. There has been no steatorrhea, liver disease, or renal disease other than the specific abnormality in tubular reabsorption of phosphate. Craniostenosis and convulsions in infancy have been described in association with this disorder.

The primary, diagnostic radiologic findings in this syndrome are the same as those seen in rickets and osteomalacia from other causes. In children with rickets, the typical changes in the epiphyseal regions of the long bones are the most common characteristic findings (Figs. 60-1, 60-2).

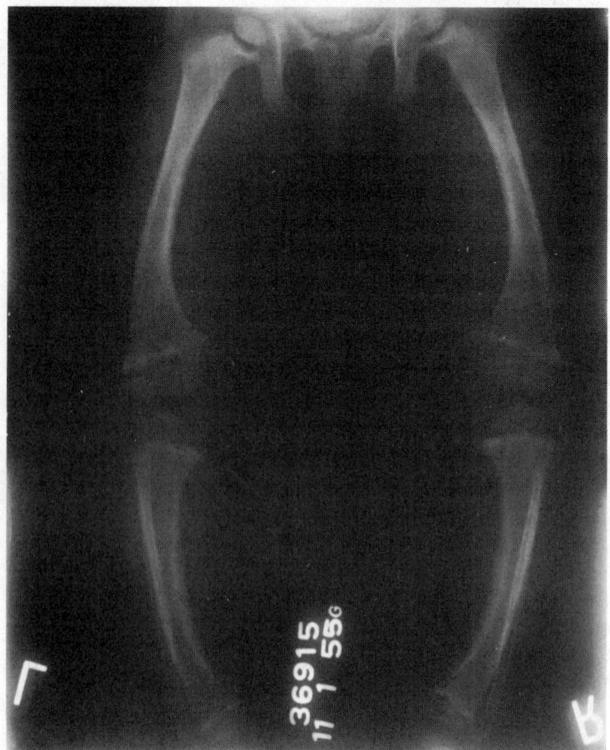

Figure 60-1. Anteroposterior view of the knees of a 4-year-old boy (VI-9 of E kindred of Winters et al. [8]), showing marked rachitic changes, with early healing, and lateral curvature of femora and tibiae.

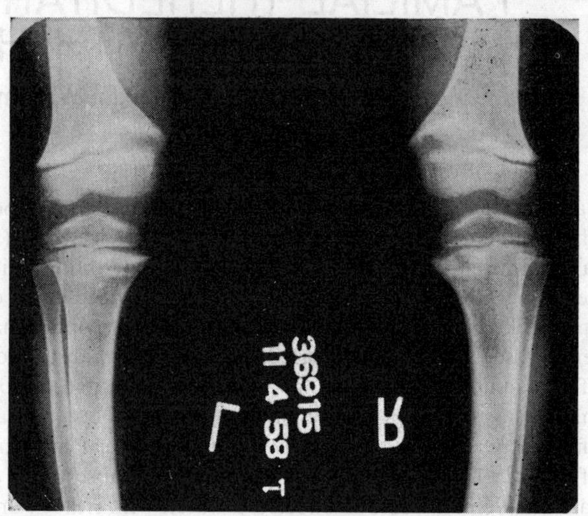

Figure 60-2. View of the knees of same patient as that in Fig. 60-1 after 3 years of treatment with large doses of vitamin D. Healing is still not complete.

Fractures, pseudofractures, and deformities of the skull, thorax, and long bones are also seen. Additional changes which are occasionally present in children and adults are similar to those seen in certain osteochondrodystrophies, including coarsened trabecular patterns in long bones, cystic-appearing areas in metaphyses and epiphyses, and shortening and broadening of the long bones. In adults, in addition to postrachitic deformities, pseudofractures may be seen (Fig. 60-3), as well as the abnormal bony protuberances already referred to (Fig. 60-4).

Table 60-1 summarizes the principal clinical findings of this disorder. Original reports of familial instances may be consulted for additional details [3, 5-9, 12, 13, 19-40].

A few cases of resistant rickets have had additional findings of hypocalcemia, tetany, and usually amino aciduria, with excellent clinical response to large doses of vitamin D [12, 20, 41-44]. These cases show evidence of transmission by an autosomal gene, which may be recessive, and probably represent a different entity; it has been called pseudovitamin D-deficiency rickets.

HYPOPHOSPHATEMIA—THE MAJOR CHEMICAL ABNORMALITY IN THE BLOOD

The significant place that a low serum or plasma concentration of inorganic phosphate* occupies in this disease is highlighted by two lines of evidence: (1) almost all patients who would be designated as having resistant rickets on other grounds have also had hypophosphatemia (the normal values for serum phosphorus reported by Linnerloth et al.

*Subsequently in this chapter the expression *serum phosphorus* will be used to designate serum or plasma concentrations of inorganic phosphate.

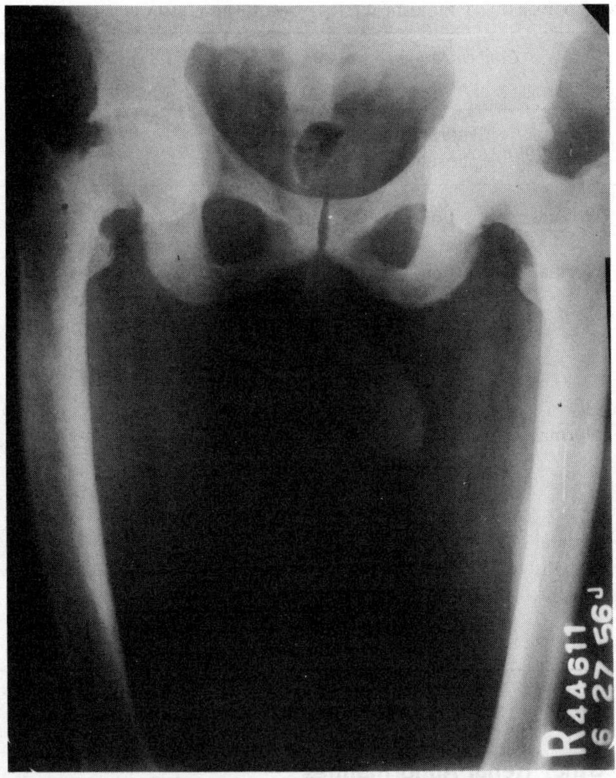

Figure 60-3. Anteroposterior view of femur of a 41-year-old man (V-12 of E kindred of Winters et al. [8]). Note coxa vara, lateral curvature of femur, and pseudofracture of the femoral neck.

[32] and Christiansson [23] may represent a different entity); and (2) the mode of inheritance has been best revealed by using hypophosphatemia as the discriminant.

In designating a person as hypophosphatemic, allowance must be made for the normal changes in serum phosphorus with age and for differences between the sexes. Greenberg and coworkers [45], using a large number of observations on normal persons, have expressed mathematically and graphically, with limits of statistical confidence, the relationship between serum phosphorus and age for each sex.

The age at which hypophosphatemia first appears seems to be variable. Thus Harrison et al. [46] have reported normophosphatemia from birth up to the age of 6 months or later in children who then developed hypophosphatemia, growth retardation, and rickets; our experience is similar, Harrison et al. suggested that the relatively low glomerular filtration rate which is characteristic of the first few months of life may result in normal serum phosphorus, even though a tubular defect in phosphate reabsorption may already be present. On the other hand, Stickler et al. [47] have found consistently low serum phosphorus values from birth. Variability also exists in reported sex differences: Winters et al. [8] found that hypophosphatemic females in affected families had slightly higher values for serum phosphorus than males in the same family, whereas McNair et al. [18] found no sex differences, but their studies did not include individuals who had hypophosphatemia without rickets.

The serum alkaline phosphatase level is elevated in affected persons with active rickets and osteomalacia. Treatment with sufficient vitamin D to produce healing of the rickets is accompanied by a return of the alkaline phosphatase to or toward normal, although initially a transient increase may occur. In some instances the serum phosphorus has risen with treatment, but healing has often been observed with no significant rise in phosphorus.

Other related serum chemical determinations are usually normal. The calcium concentration is normal or, rarely, slightly low. Total protein, albumin, globulins, urea nitrogen, amino acids, sodium, potassium, chloride, carbon dioxide content, and pH are uniformly normal. Hypomagnesemia has been reported in one patient [48] but has been found normal in others (unpublished observation of the authors).

RENAL FINDINGS

The Renal Abnormality in Phosphate Excretion

In every instance in which it has been studied the hypophosphatemia of this disorder has been associated with

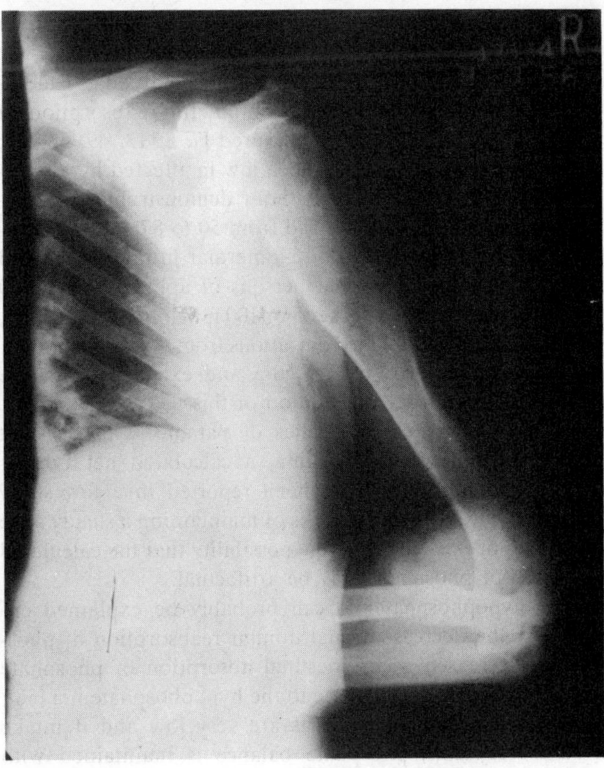

Figure 60-4. Anteroposterior view of the humerus of a 58-year-old man (IV-5 of the E kindred of Winters et al. [8]), showing coarse trabeculation and a bony protuberance at the site of insertion of the deltoid muscle.

Table 60-1. SUMMARY OF FINDINGS IN FAMILIAL VITAMIN D–RESISTANT RICKETS WITH HYPOPHOSPHATEMIA

Type of hypophosphatemia	Age at onset, years	Clinical and radiologic abnormalities	*Concentration in serum or plasma*			Other observations
			Calcium	Inorganic phosphate	Alkaline phosphatase	
1. Asymptomatic hypophosphatemia	Under 1	Slightly shortened stature	Normal	Low	Normal	No other abnormalities
2. Hypophosphatemia in adults with inactive postrachitic deformities	Under 1	Lateral (and usually anteroposterior) bowing of legs; shortened stature; occasionally coarsened trabeculation, rarefied areas, bony overgrowth	Normal	Low	Normal or slightly high	More frequent among hypophosphatemic males
3. Hypophosphatemia in adults with deformities and active osteomalacia	Under 1	Same as for (2) plus pseudofractures	Normal	Low	Slightly high	
4. Hypophosphatemia with resistant rickets in childhood	Under 1	Active rickets; occasionally coarsened trabeculation; shortened stature	Normal or slightly low	Low	High	More severe in affected males; craniostenosis and convulsions in a few instances

increased renal excretion and decreased net renal tubular reabsorption of phosphate [2, 3, 5, 27, 31, 38, 39, 49–53]. The most quantitative data have been obtained in studies in which the renal tubular maximum for reabsorption of phosphate (Tm_P) has been measured [7, 8, 13, 49, 53–55]; in all instances the Tm_P has been low in affected hypophosphatemic persons, with or without demonstrable bone involvement. Values have ranged from 50 to 87 μmoles phosphate reabsorbed per 100 ml glomerular filtrate, compared to a mean value in normal persons of approximately 130 μmoles phosphate reabsorbed per 100 ml glomerular filtrate, with limits of two standard deviations from 90 to 150 μmoles. Typical data appear in Fig. 60-5 and extensive data are tabulated in the previous edition of this text [53].

On rare occasions in studies of patients with resistant rickets with phosphate loading, a calculated net tubular secretion of phosphate has been reported in a few study periods [56, 57]. The difficulties of maintaining a steady state in studies of this type raise the possibility that the calculated secretion of phosphate may be artifactual.

The hypophosphatemia can probably be explained entirely by the decreased renal tubular reabsorption of phosphate. Decreased gastrointestinal absorption of phosphate probably does not contribute to the hypophosphatemia [58]; if levels of serum phosphorus are very low and if intake is also very low, phosphate balance is maintained with minimal phosphate excretion [59].

Possible pathogenetic explanations for the decreased renal tubular reabsorption of phosphate are discussed below.

Other Renal Abnormalities

Except for the low tubular reabsorption of phosphate, renal function is normal as far as can be determined from the available data. The glomerular filtration rate has been nor-

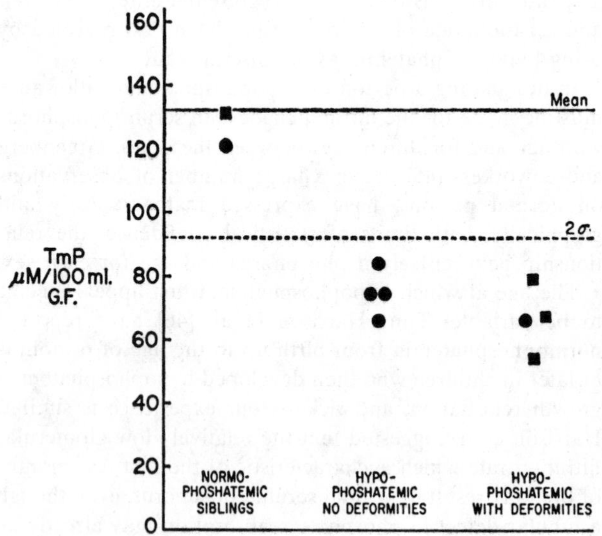

Figure 60-5. Values for maximal tubular reabsorption of phosphate (Tm_P, μmoles per 100 ml glomerular filtrate) on 10 members of the E kindred of Winters et al. ■ = male, ● = female. The mean and 2 s.d. (2σ) for the values of Tm_P of 26 normal subjects [185, 186, and unpublished observations of the authors] are represented by the lines.

mal in the affected persons in whom it has been measured [53, 55, 60, 61], and clearance and tubular maximum for the excretion of para-aminohippurate are reported normal [55, 61]. The carbon dioxide content of the blood is normal with rare exceptions, which are probably atypical cases [27, 39], and the ability to acidify the urine is normal [19, 31, 55, 59, 61, 62]. Concentration and dilution tests are normal [27, 31, 55].

Amino acid excretion in familial instances of the disorder has been normal [8, 19, 23, 31, 38, 39, 55] with rare exceptions [12, 63, 64], one of which may represent more than simple vitamin D–resistant rickets [27, 39]. Mild glycinuria has been observed in a few families with typical vitamin D–resistant rickets [12]. Observations in patients without a family history have been more varied: some have had no abnormal amino aciduria [38, 39, 65], while others have had abnormally high excretions of various amino acids and a decrease upon the administration of large doses of vitamin D [31, 33, 42, 44, 66], a response similar to that of the amino aciduria of vitamin D–deficiency rickets to smaller doses [66, 67]. The excretory patterns of amino acids after loading with histidine and arginine [66] or methionine [68] are probably abnormal in patients with vitamin D–resistant rickets, but more detailed information is needed, including comparable studies of normal persons.

Mild renal glycosuria has been rarely reported in association with vitamin D–resistant rickets in familial cases [12, 27, 39, 50, 55] and in nonfamilial instances [60, 69]. The large body of negative evidence suggests that an abnormality in glucose reabsorption does not participate in the production of increased phosphate excretion. Furthermore, in two affected members of one family (one of whom had renal glycosuria and a low glucose *Tm*), glucose loading to levels saturating glucose reabsorption produced no change in the already elevated phosphate clearance [55]. On the other hand, evidence has been presented in abstract form, from two affected persons (one with a family history), that infusion of 10 percent glucose led to complete suppression of tubular reabsorption of phosphate [70].

Histologic and histochemical information is limited largely to renal biopsies performed after prolonged therapy with vitamin D. The kidney tissue has varied from appearing completely normal [71] to showing varying degrees of nephrocalcinosis [71–75], probably related to the degree of hypercalcemia the patient had experienced during treatment. The single autopsy report, that of a 45-year-old man with a typical family history and prolonged treatment with vitamin D who died of acute alcoholism, revealed no gross, microscopic, or histochemical abnormalities, and no abnormalities on microdissection of nephrons [64, 73]. In renal biopsy material, a decrease in NAD-diaphorase and alkaline phosphatase [72] and acid phosphatase [56] has been reported, but the use of qualitative histochemical techniques for drawing quantitative conclusions has been questioned [76].

Effects of Vitamin D on Renal Function in Vitamin D-resistant Rickets

The renal effects of vitamin D in this disorder have been incompletely studied. Typically, treatment with large doses of vitamin D produces little or no change in the serum phosphorus or the phosphaturia [1, 2, 5, 19, 27, 59, 62, 77, 78], unless vitamin D overdosage, with hypercalcemia, has led to impaired glomerular function accompanied by a rise in serum phosphorus [46]. Measurements of Tm_P both soon after beginning vitamin D therapy and after prolonged therapy have shown variable and inconsistent changes [49, 53, 61, 77, 79, 80].

The glomerular filtration rate has also been reported variably to rise [81], fall [79], or remain unchanged [5, 53, 77, 78], with vitamin D therapy short of intoxication.

Occasional observations of a decreased tubular reabsorption of phosphate with vitamin D therapy may fit into pathogenetic speculations (see below). Zetterström and Winberg [82] reported a fall in serum phosphorus without a change in absorption or excretion as the initial response to treatment with 100,000 to 200,000 I.U. per day orally. If the glomerular filtration rate did not change (and this was not measured), then tubular reabsorption must have decreased. Magid et al. [55] reported a lower Tm_P in one patient after treatment with 600,000 units vitamin D for 3 months.

INTESTINAL ABSORPTION OF CALCIUM AND PHOSPHATE

Normal Features and the Role of Vitamin D and Its Metabolites

Beginning almost 50 years ago, studies which have become classics established our basic knowledge about the importance of vitamin D in calcium absorption. Normal children and adults, supplied with physiologic amounts of vitamin D and dietary calcium above a minimum level (0.45 to 1.0 gm per day) [83–85], absorb enough calcium to remain in calcium balance. Children achieve enough positive balance for normal growth of bone. A deficiency of vitamin D intake uniformly leads to progressively lowered absorption of calcium until fecal excretion of calcium equals intake. The resulting deficiency in calcium is the major cause of the development of rickets, i.e., uncalcified osteoid, in growing bone (although the direct effects of vitamin D or its metabolites on bone also appear to play a role; see below). The administration of vitamin D to vitamin D–deficient subjects leads to a striking increase in calcium absorption [86–88]. This action of vitamin D is the most clearly established role of the vitamin in maintaining the normal metabolism of calcium.

Within the past decade, major advances have been made

in our understanding of the conversion of vitamin D to more active metabolites and the probable mechanisms of action of the metabolites in promoting intestinal calcium absorption. Through the development of preparations of tritium-labeled vitamin D with high specific activity, and of methods for the separation of the products of its metabolism, DeLuca and his associates have been able to trace the path of vitamin D through the animal organism, to identify and subsequently synthesize the major active metabolites of vitamin D, and to localize their cellular sites and probable mechanisms of action. This and other simultaneous work have established the following features:

1 Vitamin D is rapidly absorbed from the jejunum and ileum, requires bile for the absorption, first enters lymphatic channels predominately, and circulates bound primarily to α_2-globulin, with some binding also to albumin and α_1-globulin (see Avioli [89] for review).

2 Circulating vitamin D is rapidly taken up by the liver—within the first 2 hr—and there is converted to one or more biologically active metabolites [90]. For vitamin D_3, cholecalciferol, the quantitatively most important metabolite is 25-hydroxycholecalciferol (25-HCC) (Fig. 60-6) [91, 92]. This product has 1.4 to 1.5 times the biologic potency of vitamin D_3. Vitamin D_2 is similarly converted largely to 25-hydroxyergocalciferol [93] (Fig. 60-6). This active metabolite rapidly enters the circulation from the liver, reaches a near-maximum concentration within 4 hr (in studies in rats), and again circulates bound largely to α_2-globulin. The liver appears to be the only organ capable of converting cholecalciferol to 25-HCC, and a hydroxylating enzyme system has been demonstrated in liver preparations [94].

3 In the intestine 25-HCC has the direct and almost immediate effect of increasing calcium absorption. This has been most clearly demonstrated in isolated, perfused intestines from vitamin D–deficient rats, preparations in which large doses of vitamin D itself have no direct effect [95, 96]. Other support for the role of 25-HCC as the biologically active form of vitamin D appears in studies of vitamin D action on calcium absorption in vivo. There is a lag of 6 to 8 hr after administration, compared to a response to 25-HCC within 2 hr, as is consistent with the time required for conversion of vitamin D to 25-HCC [96, 97].

4 Vitamin D (in vivo) stimulates at least two intestinal cellular systems involved in the absorption and transport of

OH CH₂ HO A — OH CH₂ HO B

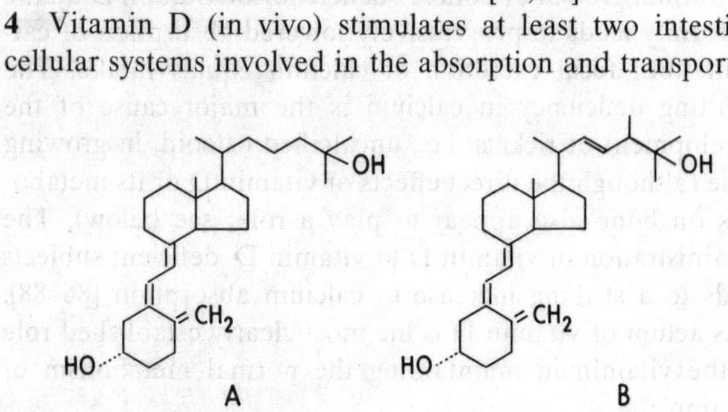

Figure 60-6. Chemical configurations of 25-hydroxycholecalciferol (*A*) and 25-hydroxyergocalciferol (*B*).

calcium: there is an increase in amount of a calcium-dependent ATPase located in the brush border of the mucosal surface, accompanied by an increase in calcium uptake across the mucosa [96, 98, 99]. Also, there is an increase in a calcium-binding protein which exists in the supernatant fraction of intestinal cells and is involved in calcium transport across the cell [100–102].

5 Within the intestinal cell, labeled 25-HCC becomes located primarily on the nuclear membrane [96, 103, 104] (with some evidence also for localization on chromatin [105, 106], a finding disputed by DeLuca). Agents which block RNA synthesis such as actinomycin D, block the physiological action of vitamin D or 25-HCC, and experiments with pulse labeling of nuclear RNA show increases after the administration of vitamin preparations to vitamin D–deficient animals (maximum effect in 5 hr after intravenous administration of vitamin D_3, and within 30 min after administration of 25-HCC) [96]. Furthermore, increased template activity of DNA chromatin for production of RNA-polymerase has been shown [96]. From these data DeLuca concludes that 25-HCC, acting at the nuclear membrane, is "unmasking" a specific set of genes which code for the synthesis of proteins involved in calcium transport, i.e., mucosal ATPase or calcium-binding protein. Thus, understanding of the metabolism and action of vitamin D at the cellular and genetic level is rapidly developing and will undoubtedly serve as the basis for unravelling the genetic defect(s) in vitamin D–resistant rickets.

It has also been shown that vitamin D is necessary for the enhancement of intestinal calcium absorption which can be produced by dibutyryl cyclic adenylic acid [107], an observation which is consistent with the evidence that parathyroid hormone, presumably through activation of adenyl cyclase, increases intestinal calcium absorption when vitamin D is present. Thus, the effects of vitamin D are required for another system involved in calcium absorption, although the nature of the vitamin D requirement has not yet been determined.

Most vitamin D–mediated calcium absorption occurs in the duodenum [108–110]. Phosphate absorption is probably not fully dependent upon vitamin D. It is strongly influenced by the presence of unabsorbed calcium in the intestinal lumen, which presumably sequesters the phosphate as calcium phosphate [111, 112]. Recent work also indicates a selective action of vitamin D on phosphate absorption, primarily in the jejunum [113].

Abnormalities in Absorption of Calcium and Phosphate in Familial Vitamin D–resistant Rickets

Before treatment with massive doses of vitamin D, children with familial vitamin D–resistant rickets excrete virtually all their ingested calcium in the feces. Urinary calcium excretion is low. These subjects have slightly positive or slightly negative balances for calcium, but they lack the degree of positive balance which is characteristic of the normal growing child. Total phosphate balance is comparable to the calcium balance, but a larger proportion of the ingested phosphate is absorbed and excreted in the urine. Data from the literature which illustrate the differences between normal subjects and persons with vitamin D–resistant rickets are summarized by Stickler [114]; typical data can also be found elsewhere [3, 5, 19, 27, 115, 116]. There is recent evidence from two affected half brothers, based on combined balance and radiokinetic calcium studies, that increased fecal endogenous calcium excretion was a significant component of the calcium balance in the absence of large amounts of vitamin D [117].

In affected adults receiving adequate calcium but only the usual dietary amounts of vitamin D, the calcium and phosphate balance is usually as positive as in normal persons [14, 52, 116, 118, 119].

In vitamin D–resistant rickets large doses of vitamin D (2.5 to 37.5 mg or 100,000 to 1,500,000 I.U. per day) uniformly increase the absorption of calcium, while urinary excretion remains low. Simultaneously, the phosphate balance becomes positive, primarily because of increased absorption. This response to very large doses of vitamin D is the same as the response of patients with vitamin D–deficiency rickets to small doses. Dihydrotachysterol in doses in the same range as vitamin D (1.25 to 12.5 mg per day) produces similar changes in calcium absorption in vitamin D–resistant rickets [114, 115, 120–122] and probably, at this dosage, in vitamin D–deficiency rickets [123, 124]. Normal persons and patients with primary hypoparathyroidism also respond similarly to large doses [86, 120, 125].

The effects of various doses of 25-hydroxycholecalciferol (25-HCC), the major biologically active metabolite of vitamin D_3 (see above), on calcium absorption in persons with familial vitamin D–resistant rickets are not yet clear. Presumably, if this disorder were due primarily to decreased conversion of vitamin D to the active metabolite (the evidence for which is discussed below), then supplying 25-HCC in the usual physiological amounts should lead to improved calcium absorption and healing of rickets. However, in a study of five patients treated with 2,500 I.U. of 25-HCC daily for 3 weeks, there was a positive effect on calcium balance in only one patient. This suggested that any defect in conversion of vitamin D to 25-HCC could not be the only cause of this disorder [126]. One feature of that study which limits its interpretability is the fact that previous large doses of vitamin D had been discontinued only 4 weeks prior to the evaluation of the effects of the 25-HCC. Such a time interval may have been so short that continuing effects of the vitamin D could have masked any effects of the 25-HCC. Other preliminary reports indicate a healing action (and thus presumably increased calcium absorption) of 25-HCC on resistant rickets in daily doses of 4,800 I.U. or higher, doses which are considerably lower than the effective doses of vitamin D [127].

Further evidence that poor absorption of calcium, arising from a lack of vitamin D effect, is not the only defect in vitamin D–resistant rickets is furnished by several studies, in which the administration of large amounts of phosphate, orally or intravenously, has produced increased calcium absorption, a positive balance of calcium and phosphate, and the healing of rickets [56, 115, 128, 129]. Healing cannot be continued by use of added phosphate alone [12, 130].

METABOLISM OF BONE

Role of Vitamin D in Normal Bone Physiology

As already indicated, the primary action of vitamin D and its metabolites in preventing or healing rickets is by way of promoting increased intestinal calcium absorption. This action, plus the secondary effect of the increased calcium absorption on diminishing parathyroid hormone activity (and the possible promotion of increased calcitonin activity), serves to provide extracellular concentrations of calcium and phosphate which are favorable for the calcification of osteoid. Whether a direct action of vitamin D (or its metabolites) on osteoid is also a necessary component of normal bone formation has not been established.

Vitamin D, through a role in bone *resorption,* may contribute to providing calcium and phosphate for the calcification of new osteoid. Vitamin D in physiological amounts in vitamin D–deficient rats probably causes increased bone resorption in some regions [131, 132], and very small amounts of 25-HCC will stimulate the release of previously incorporated ^{45}Ca from fetal rat bone in vitro, an effect that vitamin D itself does not produce even in large doses [133]. The bone-resorptive effects of vitamin D in vivo are dependent upon the presence of parathyroid hormone and are opposed by calcitonin [63, 134–137].

In rats [86, 138] and dogs [139] an abnormal trabecular appearance and increase in noncalcium content of the shaft of the long bones is a distinctive feature of vitamin D deficiency and is not directly related to absorption of calcium and phosphate; this evidence also suggests that vitamin D has a direct function in normal bone formation.

Toxic doses of vitamin D in vivo clearly produce abnormal amounts of bone resorption [86].

Abnormalities in Bone Metabolism in Familial Vitamin D–resistant Rickets with Hypophosphatemia

It is noteworthy first of all that this inherited disorder can be expressed by hypophosphatemia and diminished renal tubular reabsorption of phosphate alone, with *no apparent bone disease.* The only clinically discernible abnormality may be a stature slightly shorter than that of normophosphatemic sibs [8, 12]. There are no radiologic abnormalities. This virtual lack of bone disease in spite of hypophosphatemia indicates that factors other than simply a low serum phosphorus are participating in those affected persons who develop bone disease.

Two different types of bony abnormalities have been described in patients with vitamin D–resistant rickets. First, the characteristic finding which gives the disease its name is the rachitic appearance of the epiphyseal region. There is a markedly expanded zone of proliferating cartilage, with increased osteoid tissue and invasion by wide, tortuous blood vessels [1, 26, 38, 59, 140, 141]. These changes are present in patients with and without family histories. The radiologic changes in the epiphyseal area are entirely characteristic of vitamin D–deficiency rickets.

The epiphyseal lesion heals in most instances when the patients are treated with large doses of vitamin D. Healing can also be initiated by supplying large amounts of phosphate, as already noted, and is accelerated by immobilization of patients at the time of osteotomy [31, 36, 39, 62]. Symptomatic improvement has been reported in association with an increased positive balance of calcium and phosphate produced by a large calcium intake [118]. This lack of need for vitamin D itself in order to heal the epiphyseal lesion is also characteristic of vitamin D–deficiency rickets [128].

It is also noteworthy that the healing of the epiphyseal lesion which occurs upon therapy with large doses of vitamin D usually proceeds without any significant rise in serum phosphorus.

The second type of bony abnormality in familial vitamin D–resistant rickets consists of a distortion of the compact bone of the metaphyses of long bones. Biopsy material (taken before as well as after vitamin D therapy) has shown an abnormal irregular mosaic formation of the Haversian system and trabeculae, and probably an increase in osteoblastic borders and areas of active resorption [3, 26, 39]. Other biopsy studies, using fresh, undecalcified sections, have shown perilacunar "halos" of low-density bone and slow bone turnover [142–144]. Abnormal metabolism of chondroitin sulfate and alkaline phosphatase has also been described [145]. The bone may appear unusually dense radiologically [58, 118, 119, 146]. The histologic pattern has some features suggestive of Paget's disease or of experimental hyperparathyroidism [147]. In some patients, bone from the metaphysis has been almost normal [27, 39].

This distortion of trabecular structure may simply be another manifestation of rickets, slow to develop and slow to heal, and accordingly more evident in vitamin D–resistant than in vitamin D–deficiency rickets. Reference has already been made to abnormal trabecular patterns in experimental vitamin D deficiency. It may also be related in some way to the defect in metabolism of vitamin D, discussed below. On the other hand, the similarity of these changes with those seen on osteochondrodystrophy raises the possibility that this bony abnormality is another congenital, presumably inherited, defect in these patients.

Studies of bone turnover rates in vitamin D–resistant rickets, before and after treatment with vitamin D, with or without added phosphate, have produced variable results. Bauer et al. [21] found such an increased accretion of phosphate into bone with vitamin D therapy that some of it could only have come from other bone. Hall et al. [117], on the other hand, found increased bone turnover rates after previous vitamin D therapy was discontinued. Other normal [129] and high [119, 148] turnover rates have been reported. Smith and Dick [149] have reported increased hydroxyproline excretion, presumably arising in bone, when vitamin D or dihydrotachysterol was administered together with oral phosphate, but not when the vitamin preparations were given alone, in one subject with vitamin D–resistant rickets. They suggest that the phosphate itself may have a direct action on mobilizing bone collagen. Variable degrees of retention (presumably by bone) of acute intravenous loads of calcium have been reported in patients with resistant rickets [78, 150, 151].

POSSIBLE MECHANISMS OF PATHOGENESIS AND QUESTIONS STILL UNANSWERED

Any discussion of the pathogenesis of familial vitamin D–resistant rickets with hypophosphatemia must take into consideration the following characteristic features: (1) hypophosphatemia and decreased renal tubular reabsorption of phosphate, the one (and often only) abnormality present in all genetically affected persons; (2) decreased intestinal absorption of calcium, present to varying degrees; (3) bony abnormalities, consisting not only of rickets or osteomalacia but also of other histological changes and bony overgrowth, and not fully accounted for simply by hypophosphatemia; and (4) the response of intestinal calcium absorption and rickets, but not the phosphaturia, to large doses of vitamin D.

Until recently, the predominant debate about pathogenesis has concerned the question whether the hypophosphatemia is due to a primary intrinsic renal tubular defect in phosphate reabsorption, or whether it is due to secondary hyperparathyroidism arising as a result of decreased calcium absorption in the intestine. The new finding that persons with familial hypophosphatemia have an abnormality in metabolism of vitamin D has now become a logical starting point in the effort to provide a unified pathogenetic picture. As will be seen, no present approach fully accounts for all of the above characteristics.

An Abnormality in Metabolism of Vitamin D

For some time, a defect in the metabolism of vitamin D has been suggested [152, 153] as an explanation for the apparent "resistance" to the action of vitamin D despite demonstrably elevated blood levels [35, 150, 153, 154] during the treatment of affected persons. In 1965 and 1967, utilizing tritium-labeled vitamin D_3 orally [155] or intravenously [10], a delayed disappearance of tritium-labeled vitamin D_3 from the plasma of persons with vitamin D–resistant rickets was recorded, and abnormally low levels of lipid-soluble plasma radioactivity were found. Those studies were followed by a more definitive evaluation of the metabolism of tritiated vitamin D (D_3-^3H) in this disorder by Avioli and associates [11]. Four children with familial vitamin D–resistant rickets (one on treatment with vitamin D, the others untreated) and four adult family members with persistent hypophosphatemia were compared with seven normal subjects in terms of the metabolic fate of plasma D_3-^3H following an intravenous injection of 5 to 8 microcuries. Urinary and fecal excretory products were measured. The distribution of radioactivity between aqueous and chloroform-extractable (lipid-soluble) phases, and the distribution of the lipid-soluble phase on silicic acid column chromatography were determined.

Delayed disappearance of plasma radioactivity was again demonstrated, with mean plasma half-times of 39 ± 4, 25 ± 2, and 22 ± 1 hr for children with resistant rickets, adults with familial hypophosphatemia, and normal subjects, respectively. Furthermore, there was a marked diminution in lipid-soluble plasma radioactivity (the component containing unchanged vitamin D and its biologically active metabolites) and corresponding increases in polar, water-soluble metabolites. As shown in Table 60-2, *A*, these changes were greatest in the children with resistant rickets and intermediate in the adults with hypophosphatemia without active bone disease.

In other studies on normal subjects and animals, separation of the lipid-soluble phase on silicic acid column chromatography has previously yielded several peaks, the largest

Table 60-2.

A. Distribution of plasma radioactivity between the aqueous phase and the chloroform phase 24 hr after intravenous vitamin D_3-^3H

	Aqueous	*Chloroform*
	Percent total plasma radioactivity*	
Vitamin D-resistant rickets (4 affected children)	28.5 ± 5.4	71.5 ± 5.4
Familial hypophosphatemia (4 adults)	13.3 ± 5.4	86.7 ± 5.4
Normals (7, spanning the ages of the above)	1.9 ± 0.7	98.1 ± 0.7

B. Distribution of plasma chloroform extracts during silicic acid column chromatography at 24 hr

	Peak 3	*Peak 4*
	Percent total radioactivity*	
Vitamin D–resistant rickets	88 ± 4	8 ± 4
Familial hypophosphatemia	79 ± 5	19 ± 5
Normal	61 ± 3	35 ± 3

* Values are means ± SEM.
Source: Avioli et al. [11].

of which were Peak 3, identified as unaltered vitamin D, and Peak 4, identified as 25-hydroxycholecalciferol (25-HCC), the major biologically active metabolite of vitamin D_3 (see earlier discussion) [91, 96, 156]. Table 60-2, *B* shows that in subjects with resistant rickets there is a major reduction in conversion of vitamin D to Peak 4 (25-HCC), and again those with hypophosphatemia but no active bone disease occupy an intermediate place.

Total urinary excretion of radioactivity was approximately the same in the three groups, but the percent that was water soluble (and probably biologically inactive) was higher in the affected persons: 92.4 ± 1.7, 86.9 ± 1.3, and 85.5 ± 0.8 percent for those with resistant rickets, those with hypophosphatemia, and normal subjects, respectively. Fecal analyses showed increases in lipid-soluble radioactivity and in the Peak 3 (unaltered vitamin D) component in the affected persons [11].

Thus, persons with familial vitamin D–resistant rickets and hypophosphatemia show an abnormality in metabolism of vitamin D, which is characterized by a decrease in conversion of the vitamin to its biologically active product, 25-HCC, an increase in plasma and urinary water-soluble metabolites which are probably biologically inactive, and an increase in fecal excretion of unchanged vitamin D. Such an abnormality in vitamin D metabolism could well be the result of a genetic defect and offers the first clue to localizing and identifying the specific mechanism for genetic determination of this disorder. Further elucidation awaits future work.

Possible Consequences of Abnormal Vitamin D Metabolism

Some of the cardinal manifestations of this syndrome can be readily accounted for by the abnormalities in vitamin D metabolism, whereas the explanation of others becomes conjectural.

First, a decrease in production of 25-HCC might explain the decreased intestinal absorption of calcium in this disorder. As already discussed (see above, Intestinal Absorption of Calcium and Phosphate), it now appears that 25-HCC is the principal form in which vitamin D exerts its effects on intestinal cells to promote calcium absorption. It remains to be established whether the defect in conversion of vitamin D to 25-HCC can account quantitatively for the deficient calcium absorption. One study [126] raises doubt that this is the complete explanation: treatment with 2,500 units 25-HCC, an amount which should have been more than physiological replacement for any defect in conversion, did not produce any significant changes in balance of calcium or phosphate, or in serum calcium, phosphate, or alkaline phosphatase. It is possible that the continuing effects of previous vitamin D therapy masked any effects of 25-HCC in that study.

Deficient intestinal absorption of calcium could in turn lead to rickets or osteomalacia, secondary hyperparathyroidism with phosphaturia, and hypophosphatemia. For the reasons discussed in detail below, it seems unlikely that the hypophosphatemia and phosphaturia can be explained solely by secondary hyperparathyroidism.

Second, the phosphaturia and hypophosphatemia could conceivably be produced by a direct action on the renal tubules of one or more of the water-soluble metabolites of vitamin D which appear in plasma and urine in excessive amounts in this disorder [11, 157]. In support of such a view is the fact that other steroid compounds (cortisone, hydrocortisone, diethylstilbesterol) have been found to decrease net renal tubular phosphate reabsorption [158–160]. Also consistent with such a mechanism is the lack of a decrease, or an actual increase, in phosphaturia with large doses of vitamin D [55, 82]; presumably, large doses would lead to large amounts of the water-soluble metabolites. No direct observations on the possible effects of these metabolites of vitamin D on renal handling of phosphate have been reported.

Third, it is possible that the various bony abnormalities seen in this disorder could be attributed directly to the deficient production of 25-HCC. This compound has been shown to localize in bone as well as in intestine and to promote bone resorption (see above, Metabolism of Bone). It may be that the distorted bone formation of resistant rickets is a result of inadequate 25-HCC action on bone. Such a suggestion can only be conjectural at this time, especially in view of the lack of consistency in studies of these bony abnormalities. As noted earlier, somewhat similar if less marked bony changes have been described in vitamin D–deficiency rickets.

Thus the abnormalities in vitamin D metabolism observed in this disorder could explain its major clinical and physiologic manifestations. Even so, a number of essential elements in this explanation await factual confirmation or rejection.

Possible Abnormalities in Vitamin D Absorption or Binding

It is unlikely that there is an abnormality in the absorption of vitamin D in vitamin D–resistant rickets. The blood level of the vitamin as measured by the bioassay technique of Warkany is normal or only slightly low prior to oral treatment with massive doses and is markedly elevated afterward [35, 150, 153, 154]. In addition, the bone disease is not prevented or cured by parenterally administered, conventional doses of vitamin D [1, 22, 30, 34, 38, 39]; nor is ultraviolet light effective in curing rickets of the resistant type [1, 20, 31, 153, 161, 162].

Scott et al. [155] found a decrease in lipid-soluble plasma radioactivity in patients with resistant rickets compared to normals after an oral dose of tritiated vitamin D, which they attributed to decreased intestinal absorption. Subsequent work with D_3-^3H, already discussed, indicates that their observation is related to the abnormal metabolism of vitamin D which leads to decreased lipid-soluble plasma radioactivity [10, 11].

Vitamin D or its biologically active metabolites might be abnormally bound to the globulin with which it circulates. One preliminary report described a longer than normal circulation of such a metabolite, bound on an α-globulin, in one patient with resistant rickets [163]. Another study reported no evidence for abnormal binding of vitamin D in two affected patients [164]. Clearly more data are needed.

The Possible Role of Secondary Hyperparathyroidism

On the basis of their studies on the first patient for whom the diagnosis of vitamin D–resistant rickets was made, Albright and his colleagues [1, 111] proposed that the primary event is decreased intestinal absorption of calcium due to "resistance" to vitamin D. This leads to a low serum calcium concentration, which in turn stimulates parathyroid secretion. Increased parathyroid hormone activity causes decreased tubular reabsorption of phosphate and hypophosphatemia, as well as returning the serum calcium concentration toward normal. If the compensatory overactivity of the parathyroid glands should be just sufficient, the final results of this sequence could be normal serum calcium, low serum phosphorus, and diminished renal tubular reabsorption of phosphate, which are the findings in patients with vitamin D–resistant rickets. The recently discovered defect in the metabolism of vitamin D is consistent with this sequence. Here we consider the evidence on the degree to which secondary hyperparathyroidism may account for the phosphaturia and hypophosphatemia.

It is well established that excessive parathyroid hormone can decrease the net renal tubular reabsorption of phosphate to the range seen in vitamin D–resistant rickets. For example, Hiatt and Thompson [165] showed that parathyroid extract, given intramuscularly for 3 to 5 days to normal humans, lowered the Tm_P to 31 to 91 μmoles per 100 ml glomerular filtrate (mean = 68) (compare with Fig. 60-5).

If secondary hyperparathyroidism is present in this disorder, one would expect histologic evidence of parathyroid hyperplasia and bony changes characteristic of hyperparathyroidism. Parathyroid glands biopsied or removed from affected persons have been variously reported: Albright et al. [1], White et al. [64], and Frame and Smith [166] described hyperplastic glands, whereas Wilson et al. [56], Frame et al. [143], and Howard [167] have reported normal glands. The only radiologic changes in bone suggesting hyperparathyroidism have been absence of lamina dura in several patients [29], which may be nonspecific [120]. Assay of serum for parathyroid activity, reported high in one patient with probable resistant rickets [168], has not been extensively applied.

The response of the phosphaturia to intravenous calcium infusion has been used as indirect evidence about the state of parathyroid activity and its contribution to the hypophosphatemia. If the phosphaturia is due to secondary hyperparathyroidism, then raising the serum calcium concentration should suppress parathyroid secretion and phosphaturia. In most patients with resistant rickets studied in this manner, a calcium infusion for 3 to 24 hr has resulted in a significant decrease in phosphate excretion [8, 13, 14, 31, 54, 55, 56, 61, 72, 78, 119, 150, 169–171]. Falls et al. [13] found that a 6 to 8 hr calcium infusion suppressed phosphaturia whereas a 4-hr infusion with a lesser load did not, and suggested that with a chronic state of secondary hyperparathyroidism more prolonged hypercalcemia is necessary to achieve suppression. Serum phosphorus remained below normal in most of these studies. Thus the amount of phosphate actually being reabsorbed remained low and one cannot state whether the tubular capacity for reabsorbing phosphate was normal or not. The calculated tubular reabsorption of phosphate rose into the normal range in one case reported by Fraser et al. [170], in four of five cases reported by Lafferty et al. [119], and in one of three cases reported by Vaandrager [78].

In instances in which Tm_P has been measured before and after calcium infusion, the Tm_P has remained below normal. Thus Blackard et al. [14] found only a small rise, from 41 to 74 μmoles per 100 ml glomerular filtrate, and Magid et al. [55] in two patients and the present authors in one patient found no change from previously low values [53].

Marked suppression of phosphate excretion has also been observed following calcium infusion in some patients with various diseases thought to have unequivocal renal tubular defects, e.g., cystinosis, Fanconi syndrome, and renal tubular acidosis [72, 173]. Thus, response to calcium infusion does not exclude intrinsic tubular disease directly contributing to phosphaturia.

The responsiveness of the kidneys in persons with resistant rickets to changes in parathyroid activity has also been studied by administering parathyroid extract and by following the diurnal variation in phosphaturia. Parathyroid extract administered intramuscularly or subcutaneously [1, 169, 170] has produced increased phosphaturia. Other studies with intravenous parathyroid extract are difficult to interpret because of the variable effects on the glomerular filtration rate [165]. In three patients, Wilson et al. [56] reported a spontaneous loss of diurnal variation in serum phosphorus but normal diurnal changes in urinary phosphorus, which are the opposite of changes found in primary hyperparathyroidism.

On the basis of observed versus expected proportions of calcium proteinate in the total serum calcium, Rose [174] found no evidence for secondary hyperparathyroidism in seven patients with various forms of resistant rickets.

In summary, the renal tubular mechanism for reabsorption of phosphate in persons with resistant rickets appears to be responsive to changes in parathyroid hormone activity. There is evidence, particularly from biopsy of parathyroid glands, for a variable degree of secondary hyperparathyroidism. This is an expected feature of active rickets of any type. There is no conclusive evidence that secondary hyperparathyroidism accounts fully for the phosphaturia and hypophosphatemia, and a number of the above findings suggest that there is a tubular abnormality in handling phosphate, in addition to the effect of excessive parathyroid hormone. Finally, in family members with hypophosphatemia without bone disease, and in those with active bone disease in whom treatment with vitamin D has produced healing (and even hypercalcemia) but in whom hypophosphatemia persists, it seems improbable that secondary hyperparathyroidism is present.

The Possible Role of an Intrinsic Renal Tubular Defect in Reabsorption of Phosphate

It has frequently been suggested, as an alternative to the original Albright hypothesis, that the primary abnormality in familial vitamin D–resistant rickets and hypophosphatemia is a specific, genetically determined defect in the renal tubular mechanism for transport of phosphate [2, 27, 37, 51, 166, 175–178]. This is the simplest explanation to account for the genetic pattern which is so clearly related to the hypophosphatemia itself, with or without bone disease.

It seems clear that such a tubular defect resulting in hypophosphatemia could only account in part for the other characteristics of this disorder. With regard to the deficient intestinal calcium absorption and development of rickets, it has been suggested that these are secondary to decreased deposition of bone salts as a direct result of the hypophosphatemia [176], and it has been shown that added phosphate (orally or intravenously) will increase calcium absorption and initiate the healing of rickets [47, 56, 115, 128, 143]. It has generally proved impossible to sustain the healing or positive calcium balance through use of added phosphate alone or with added calcium [12, 130, 178, 179].

A primary renal tubular defect would not explain the distorted bony structure and bony overgrowth which are common features of this disorder; nor would it account for the observed abnormality in metabolism of vitamin D, although an abnormal amount of a metabolite of vitamin D might itself cause the decreased renal tubular reabsorption of phosphate.

Summary of Possible Mechanisms of Pathogenesis

In spite of extensive efforts to establish a unified explanation for the various abnormalities which characterize familial hypophosphatemia and vitamin D–resistant rickets, there remain inadequacies in each proposal. The renal tubular defect in reabsorption of phosphate and the impaired intestinal absorption of calcium appear to be at least partly independent of each other. The various bony abnormalities other than the rickets, probably including shortened stature as well, do not have a satisfactory explanation. It is possible that the abnormality in the metabolism of vitamin D which has been demonstrated in affected families will, through the effects of different metabolic products on different end organs, ultimately account for the full constellation of derangements.

GENETIC ASPECTS

In familial vitamin D–resistant rickets with hypophosphatemia, it has been clearly demonstrated that the inherited trait may vary in the degree of manifestation from individuals who have severe to mild bone disease and hypophosphatemia to those in whom only hypophosphatemia can be demonstrated. In this latter group it has not been possible clearly to establish any evidence of active or former rickets. In each of 21 affected families studied by the authors and their colleagues [8, 9, 12, 180], if hypophosphatemia is used as the discriminant, transmission can best be explained by the presence of a single abnormal gene on an X chromosome. Further, the gene has a single-dose effect, or is dominant, in that it is transmitted from generation to generation without interruption. The segregation ratios in the progeny of affected parents were, with some exceptions discussed below, those to be anticipated with such a gene.

These points are illustrated in Fig. 60-7 which is a part of the original large North Carolina kindred reported by Winters et al. [8]. If individuals were classified as affected solely on the basis of active rickets or postrachitic deformities, there was no clear-cut pattern of inheritance, and several instances of "skipping" of a generation would have occurred. On the other hand, if the presence of hypophosphatemia was used as the criterion for the presence of the trait, a clear generation-to-generation transmission emerged.

Studies in 20 additional families in North Carolina and Great Britain are in essential agreement with the original report. These results are summarized in Tables 60-3 and 60-4 and permit the following conclusions: (1) All 97 subjects with active rickets or postrachitic deformities were hypophosphatemic. (2) An additional 49 (47 females and 2 males) were hypophosphatemic with no evidence of active or previous rickets. (3) Included in these 49 were all 13 instances of proved or probable "skipping" when skeletal disease was used as the sole criterion for classification. (4) In 88 of 92 instances, where the requisite data were available, hypophosphatemia was inherited in a predictable fashion in that all hypophosphatemic progeny had one hypophosphatemic parent. A possible explanation of the four exceptions is discussed below. (5) No hypophosphatemic child had more than one hypophosphatemic parent in numerous matings where both parents were examined. (6) Among the progeny of all hypophosphatemic parents, including both normal and affected persons, the total number of brothers was approximately equal to the total number of sisters (86 males and 92 females, Table 60-3). (7) The total number of *affected* male children was half that of *affected* females (31:61) (Table 60-3). A similar ratio for all affected individuals was (46:100, Table 60-4).

These results strongly suggest that hypophosphatemia is almost uniformly inherited in this disorder, whereas overt bone disease varies considerably. In some families it is expressed in those inheriting the trait to a greater degree than in others. Hypophosphatemia, then, is an important but not the sole determinant of bone disease, and to date provides the best discriminant for identifying the presence of the trait. It should be emphasized that, from the experience of the authors and their colleagues, repeated sampling

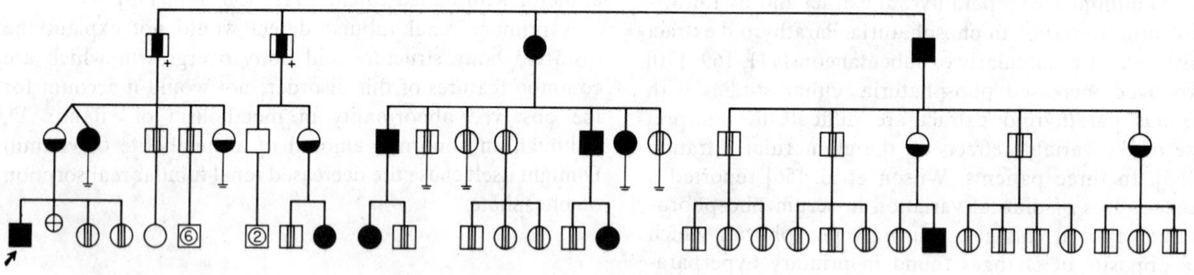

Figure 60-7. Portion of original (E) pedigree [8]. Note (1) regularity of generation-to-generation transmission, if hypophosphatemia without evidence of skeletal disease is used as a criterion for the presence of the inherited abnormality, and (2) no affected sons but uniformly affected daughters of affected fathers.

Table 60-3. DATA ON 178 CLASSIFIED PROGENY OF HYPOPHOSPHATEMIC PARENTS IN 21 PEDIGREES

Pedigree		No. of parents	*Classified progeny*				
			Male		Female		Total
Origin	Total		Affected*	Normal	Affected*	Normal	
Hypophosphatemic fathers							
North Carolina	5	16	0	19	24	0	43
Great Britain	6	6	0	9	7	0	16
Total	11	22	0	28	31	0	59
Hypophosphatemic mothers							
North Carolina	4	29	21	22	14	27	84
Great Britain	14	16	10	5	16	4	35
Total	18	45	31	27	30	31	119
Grand total	29	67	31	55	61	31	178

* Affected signifies hypophosphatemia with or without skeletal disease.
Source: From [8, 9, 12, 180].

may be necessary to establish the presence of hypophosphatemia. In several instances involving individuals known from previous observations to have been hypophosphatemic, an initial resurvey did not reestablish this biochemical abnormality, but additional multiple sampling did. Provided the samples were drawn more than 2 hr after eating, the frequency of demonstration of a low serum or plasma phosphorus was as great as in those in whom early morning fasting samples were obtained [12]. The reverse problem of false positives, i.e., a single low serum phosphorus with subsequent normal ones, was encountered much less frequently if the 99 percent confidence limit was observed [45].

These results also indicate that transmission is due to an abnormal gene on an X chromosome. In Table 60-3, in the classified progeny of 22 affected fathers all 28 males were normal, while all 31 females were affected. The chance of this distribution occurring on the basis of an autosomal gene is virtually nil.

With an abnormal gene residing on an X chromosome, an affected female is therefore heterozygous (X^-X), whereas an affected male lacking the normal allele is hemizygous (X^-Y). Since the male progeny of an affected male receive the Y chromosome from their fathers, they would all be normal. On the other hand, the female progeny of an affected male receive the single X^- chromosome of the father and are, therefore, all affected. This hypothesis also predicts that half the progeny of an affected female should be normal and half affected without regard to sex. Data on this point are also shown in Table 60-3. While the pooled data from the North Carolina and British studies meet the expected ratios with a high degree of significance, they do so because of opposite discrepancies in the two series, especially in respect to the female progeny of affected mothers. Thus, in the former (and larger) series there were almost twice as many normal as compared to affected daughters, whereas only 4 of 20 comparable daughters in Great Britain were normal. There is no satisfactory explanation for these discrepancies.

Thirty-three females from the four families reported by Graham et al. [9] were resurveyed in 1963 and 1964 by

Table 60-4. SUMMARY CLASSIFICATION OF ALL AFFECTED AND CHEMICALLY CLASSIFIED SUBJECTS WITH FAMILIAL VITAMIN D–RESISTANT RICKETS AND HYPOPHOSPHATEMIA

Pedigree		*Hypophosphatemic males*			*Hypophosphatemic females*			
Origin	Total	Bone disease	No bone disease	Total	Bone disease	No bone disease	Total	Grand total
North Carolina	5	30	2	32	19	44	63	95
Great Britain	16	14	0	14	34	3	37	51
Total	21	44	2	46	53	47	100	146

Source: From [8, 9, 12, 180].

reexamination and by repeating the serum phosphorus 4 to 7 years after their first classification. In 10 of these, originally normal, there was no change in classification. One child classified questionably as normal at ages 2 and 3 was found to have hypophosphatemia without evidence of bone disease at age 6 (H-V-7). Of 22 hypophosphatemic females without evidence of bone disease, 21 remained hypophosphatemic. The exception was a female classified as hypophosphatemic at age 9 months who was normophosphatemic and clinically normal at age 6 years. It should be noted, in addition, that had single specimens drawn in the field been accepted, 7 of the 22 might have been classified as normal during the resurvey utilizing the curves of Greenberg et al. [45] for separating normals from abnormals. Multiple sampling re-established the presence of hypophosphatemia.

The hypothesis that this trait is transmitted as a single-dose effect by a gene on an X chromosome offers the best explanation of the great majority of the data in other published reports [3, 5, 6, 13, 14, 22–25, 29, 30, 33–39]. The clearest rejection of an X-linked gene would be a documented instance of male-to-male transmission. A few such instances have been described [20, 41, 56, 181], which may represent a different disorder.

In the first kindred studied by Winters et al. [7, 8] a marked difference was observed between heterozygotes and hemizygotes with respect to the severity of bone disease. Hypophosphatemic males nearly always had obvious rickets or postrachitic deformities, while hypophosphatemic females tended to have much less skeletal involvement. In general this difference has been confirmed in the pedigrees subsequently studied [9, 12, 180]. Only two males had no demonstrable bone disease. McNair et al. [18] have reported no sex difference in severity but their data do not include information about family members with hypophosphatemia alone.

The relative immunity of the female from severe skeletal disease has at least three possible explanations: (1) The normal allele may modify the action of the abnormal gene so that the female escapes severe bone disease because of heterozygosity. (2) The relative immunity of the female is a factor independent of gene dosage. Since there is no proved instance of a homozygous female, this problem remains unresolved. (3) If one of the X chromosomes becomes inactivated, mosaicism and variation in degree of manifestation could result [182].

Not all cases of vitamin D–resistant rickets are clearly inherited. Sporadic cases could be due to phenocopy, a recessive trait, or new mutations. We have encountered one such female in North Carolina [183]. In the British study of Burnett et al. [12] there were five females and three males in regard to whom the evidence from a fairly extensive study of relatives and sibs indicated that they were the only affected members in their respective kindred. In this same study an additional four affected mothers, who had borne severely affected children, had apparently normal parents. In two of these, repeated examination of the parents and

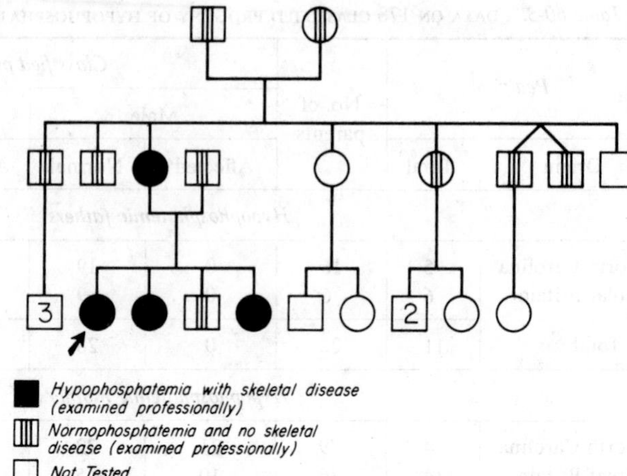

Figure 60-8. Portion of kindred 11. S. E. [12]. Note affected mother with three affected children. Spouse of affected mother, her parents, and five of seven sibs had no clinical evidence of former rickets and were normophosphatemic on several occasions including under fasting conditions. The two chemically unclassified sibs were reported to be normal.

sibs of the affected mother was not possible, and in each of these two there was a possibility that complicating renal disease rendered the normal plasma phosphorus suspect in the parents. In the two others, a fairly complete survey with resampling of plasma phosphorus was possible. One such kindred is shown in Fig. 60-8 and suggests that the mother represented a new mutation.

On the assumption that the last two affected mothers with affected progeny and the eight sporadic cases in the British series were new mutations, rough estimates of mutation rates are possible. For an X-linked gene, the mutation rates per gene per generation were 6.4×10^{-6} and 5.3×10^{-6} for males and females, respectively [12]. These rough estimates are sufficiently similar to those better established in other hereditary diseases to warrant further attempts to ascertain what proportion of sporadic cases represent new mutations.

Normal karyotypes have been reported in two affected family members [55].

DIFFERENTIAL DIAGNOSIS

The problem of differential diagnosis usually arises in a patient with clinical and chemical evidence of rickets or osteomalacia. Rarely, an unexpected finding of asymptomatic hypophosphatemia may be the clue to identifying a new family with this disorder, a step which may have considerable preventive value to potentially affected children.

In general, the diagnosis of familial vitamin D–resistant rickets is arrived at by (1) excluding other causes, and (2) establishing the presence of hypophosphatemia with or without bone disease in other family members. Among other causes of rickets or osteomalacia one should consider principally diseases of intestinal malabsorption, renal tubular disease (renal tubular acidosis; Fanconi's syndrome), and uremic renal disease in which vitamin D–resistant osteomalacia or rickets may be a significant component of the renal osteodystrophy. Deficiency of vitamin D intake remains an unusual cause of rickets.

A newly recognized entity is hypophosphatemic osteomalacia associated with hemangiomas and giant cell granulomas, in which removal of the tumor has been associated with a disappearance of phosphaturia, hypophosphatemia, and osteomalacia [184]. The possibility that such a tumor may be producing a hormone which directly affects the kidney (and perhaps bone and intestine), or antagonizes the action of vitamin D, also gives promise that this disease may shed some light on the pathogenetic mechanisms in familial vitamin D–resistant rickets.

A detailed discussion of differential diagnosis is contained in a recent review by Arnstein et al. [178].

In searching for other hypophosphatemic family members, it is important to obtain several determinations in equivocal situations, on blood samples obtained in the fasting state or 2 hr or more after a meal.

TREATMENT

The treatment of vitamin D–resistant rickets must be highly individualized; it is based on recognition not only of the age and growth potential of the patient and the severity of his skeletal disease but also of the real risks of hypervitaminosis D.

In general, treatment should be undertaken in children with active rickets and in adults with active osteomalacia. Cautious treatment should also be considered in genetically affected infants (i.e., with hypophosphatemia) who, on careful and frequent observation, are having a decline in growth rate, in particular if this is associated with rising serum alkaline phosphatase or bowing of the legs.

Treatment with Vitamin D, with or without Oral Phosphate

Until there is further availability of and experience with 25-hydroxycholecalciferol, vitamin D in pharmacologic doses remains the cornerstone of effective treatment. Oral phosphate may be added to the program with the aim of keeping the effective dose of vitamin D as low as possible.

It has been shown that the ingestion of 1 to 3 gm phosphorus per day (as a neutral phosphate solution) may alone initiate and for a time sustain healing [115, 128, 129, 179]. In more prolonged observations with phosphate alone, or alternating with calcium supplements, it has been found that healing does not continue or may regress [12, 130, 179]. The combined use of oral phosphate and vitamin D in a daily dosage of 25,000 to 50,000 I.U. has produced satisfactory healing in a number of patients [56, 187] without evidence of toxicity. Similar unpublished experience in a number of centers has also been favorable. At times diarrhea produced by the phosphate solution may limit its usefulness.

A typical starting regimen consists of a neutral phosphate solution providing 250 to 500 mg phosphorus four times a day (such solutions are commercially available or may be prepared by a pharmacist from mixtures of sodium or potassium mono- and dihydrogen phosphate in 4:1 molar ratio, to give a pH of approximately 7.4). The starting dose of vitamin D should be 10,000 to 25,000 I.U. per day. The patient is seen at intervals of 4 to 6 weeks and the vitamin D increased in increments of 10,000 to 25,000 I.U. per day, as needed to achieve evidence of healing, i.e., a falling serum level of alkaline phosphatase and radiographic improvement.

At the same time the patient must be carefully followed for evidence of hypervitaminosis D, for often the effective therapeutic dose lies in the toxic range. In order to avoid serious degrees of hypercalcemia, continuous medical supervision is required and should include a search for signs and symptoms of hypercalcemia, serial measurements of serum calcium, and frequent urinalyses and estimations of blood urea nitrogen or serum creatinine concentration. Mild but significant hypercalcemia is often unaccompanied by objective signs and clear-cut symptoms. The Sulkowitch test for calcium in the urine is not of great value in the early recognition of vitamin D poisoning, but it may be helpful to have the parents perform the test regularly to focus their attention on this ever-present problem.

Careful quantitative measurements of urinary calcium excretion (e.g., on a 24-hr collection made just before each visit to the physician) may be an additional helpful guide to vitamin D therapy [58, 188, 189]. Calcium excretion may rise from very low to normal levels just before the serum calcium rises detectably [78].

During healing the phosphate and calcium balances become positive, but serum phosphorus usually does not rise to normal values unless renal insufficiency has supervened as a result of vitamin D intoxication [46, 122, 191]. At first glance, healing in the face of hypophosphatemia may seem to contradict the view that hypophosphatemia is a principal determinant of the rickets. The experiments of Yendt and Howard [190] provide an explanation. They found that transient increases in the level of phosphate in rachitic rats may be sufficient to initiate calcification, which continues even though ambient concentration of phosphate is again reduced to levels associated with rickets. This has also been suggested by clinical data [129].

Healing of the rickets is often associated with some improvement in the severity of deformities [188, and personal experience]. The use of braces during prepubertal years may help [191, 192]. For serious and persistent deformity, subsequent osteotomy is often indicated. Surgical correction should be undertaken only after the active process is fully controlled. Before and during the period of immobilization the dose of vitamin D must be greatly reduced or eliminated and then reinstituted with mobilization.

Treatment should be continued at least until all epiphyses are closed. Usually thereafter there is no evidence of active bone disease. Recurrences do occasionally appear, especially in the age range of 40 to 50 years, and accordingly a person with this disorder needs continued periodic reevaluation.

The potentiality for permanent renal damage is the greatest hazard of overtreatment with vitamin D, and concern has been expressed that this may develop with prolonged therapy even when there has been no other evidence of vitamin D poisoning. Renal biopsies after treatment have shown both normal tissue [56, 64, 71, 73] and varying degrees of glomerular sclerosis, intratubular and interstitial calcium deposits, and fibrosis and atrophy [19, 72–75]; the more severe examples have occurred in association with unequivocal hypercalcemia and were accompanied by deteriorated renal function. With discontinuance of vitamin D after an episode of intoxication, the degree and speed of recovery of renal function are quite variable.

Oral phosphate therapy may also involve some hazards to renal function [193], and patients so treated must be followed closely for this possibility. In one adult with the familial disease and a pseudofracture of the hip (Fig. 60-3) the addition of oral phosphate therapy to a regimen of 300,000 I.U. vitamin D per day (a dose found necessary to produce any evidence of healing) was followed by a gradual rise in blood pressure from 130/80 to 160/100, appearance of trace to 1+ albuminuria, and rise in BUN from 12 to 25 mg per 100 ml, all without any change in his normal serum calcium and low serum phosphorus. Discontinuance of the added phosphate with continuance of the vitamin D at the same dose was followed by a reversal of all abnormalities.

The Problem of Growth Retardation

A problem of continuing concern is the fact that most children with resistant rickets never achieve normal height. Several factors contribute to this problem.

First, the diagnosis may not be made and effective treatment begun until deformities and growth retardation have already developed. Whether growth retardation is or can be reversed by treatment is discussed below.

Second, it is notoriously difficult to maintain adequate treatment, and yet avoid hypervitaminosis D, throughout the growing years. As is true with most chronic illnesses requiring continuous treatment, patients with this disorder, their parents, and their physicians frequently let therapy lapse. Or an episode of vitamin D intoxication may require discontinuance of therapy, which is usually not reinstituted until evidence of active rickets has reappeared. Thus any possible beneficial effect of continuous treatment on growth itself is lost. Stickler et al. [19], for example, recorded at least one episode of hypercalcemia among 23 of 43 treated patients. Others have also documented the difficulties in achieving continuing effective therapy [188, 191, 192].

Third, the persistence of leg deformities contributes to shortened stature, and in fact in already-deformed long bones an improvement in longitudinal growth of bone as a result of treatment adds more to the deformity than to the total height [194].

Finally, there may be an abnormality in growth of the legs of affected persons which is distinct from active rickets and not corrected by present modes of treatment. In an extensive retrospective evaluation of this problem, McNair and Stickler [18] found that upper-segment growth was not significantly different from normal, but lower segments averaged 15 percent below normal. Height was not correlated with extent of recorded treatment nor could short stature be accounted for solely by residual deformity.

It has been pointed out that in virtually all of the patients described above treatment was not started before significant growth retardation had probably already occurred [195]. Furthermore, Schoen has reported a patient in whom treatment was begun at age 5 months, and who maintained normal growth [194, 196]. Also, Bourgeois and Bierich [197] have reported a sharp acceleration in growth *rate* to above normal and increases in height relative to age, with adequate treatment.

It has been suggested that growth deficiency is another result of refractory hypophosphatemia per se. In support of this view is the fact that serum phosphorus and growth are often normal for the first 5 to 12 months after birth [46, 47, 181, 188, 194]. The appearance of hypophosphatemia at that time is associated with the appearance of both a declining growth rate and active rickets [46, 181]. Also, Harrison et al. [46], in a review of experience with 20 patients, found only 1 in whom normal growth rate was achieved. This occurred in association with a rise in serum phosphorus to normal as a result of renal insufficiency from an episode of hypervitaminosis D. Others have reported low serum phosphorus as early as the second day after birth [47], and either no correlation or only a poor correlation between serum phosphorus and degree of shortening [19, 198].

Mandibular growth, dental eruption, and dental age have been reported normal in affected children [199]. Administration of human growth hormone along with vitamin D in two children failed to improve growth [200].

Thus the cause and degree of preventibility of growth retardation in resistant rickets is not clear. At this time the most reasonable approach seems to be to follow closely the rate of growth and other parameters related to the diagnosis of rickets in potentially affected infants throughout the first months of life, to initiate treatment with vitamin D and phosphate as early as possible once unequivocal evidence of rickets has appeared, and to consider using oral phosphate alone for growth retardation without active rickets.

Other Therapeutic Agents

Dihydrotachysterol has been effective in the treatment of resistant rickets, including patients who seemed not to respond to large doses of vitamin D [162, 181] (see also earlier section on abnormalities in absorption of calcium and phosphate). It has the potential advantages of a quicker onset of action and shorter duration.

Of most interest at present is the potential use of 25-hydroxycholecalciferol (25-HCC) (Fig. 60-6). Doses as low as 4,800 I.U. per day are effective in promoting healing of familial vitamin D–resistant rickets [127], a dose far lower than minimal effective doses of vitamin D but still higher than one would expect to be required if a defect in conversion of vitamin D to its active metabolite were the only abnormality in this disorder [126; see earlier discussion]. Another preliminary report describes the effective treatment of an adult with late-onset resistant osteomalacia with 2,000 I.U. 25-HCC or less per day [201]. It may be expected that more definitive data on the role of 25-HCC in the treatment of resistant rickets will soon be available.

PREVENTIVE MEASURES

Once the mode of inheritance of the trait has been determined in a particular family (and this will be X-linked dominant in almost all instances), the affected individuals and their spouses should be fully informed of the nature of the transmission of the gene as well as the chances and probable consequences of having a child with the disease. Potentially affected progeny of such a mating should then be studied as early as practicable in order to establish the genotype, with the aim of as early an institution of therapy as necessary to prevent serious degrees of deformity. As already noted, the detection of hypophosphatemia is difficult in the young infant. The diagnosis can be made or excluded with confidence only by obtaining multiple determinations throughout at least the first year of life.

SUMMARY

1 Familial (hereditary) vitamin D–resistant rickets with hypophosphatemia is a disorder in which (*a*) the rickets or osteomalacia which may develop is not responsive to physiological amounts of vitamin D; (*b*) the most distinctive feature is hypophosphatemia associated with diminished renal tubular reabsorption of phosphate; (*c*) the inheritance pattern, best seen in terms of hypophosphatemia, is a single-dose effect on the X chromosome ("X-linked dominance"); (*d*) decreased intestinal absorption of calcium of varying degrees and distinctive bony changes in addition to rickets occur; and (*e*) an abnormality in metabolism of vitamin D exists.

2 The genetically related abnormal vitamin D metabolism, consisting of decreased conversion of vitamin D to its biologically active metabolite, 25-hydroxycholecalciferol, and increased conversion to water-soluble, nonactive metabolites, could account for the decreased intestinal calcium absorption.

3 Secondary hyperparathyroidism, developing as a result of the diminished calcium absorption, appears to be present in many patients and probably accounts in part for the phosphaturia and hypophosphatemia. However, this seems an unlikely explanation for the occurence of hypophosphatemia without rickets or the persistence of hypophosphatemia and phosphaturia in the face of adequate treatment. It is conjectured that the increased water-soluble steroidal metabolites may have a renal phosphaturic action, analogous to certain other steroids, or that there is a primary renal tubular defect in phosphate reabsorption.

4 There is as yet no satisfactory explanation for the various bony abnormalities other than the rickets, including distortion of trabeculae, overgrowth at tendinous attachments, and possibly shortened stature.

5 From genetic considerations, it is possible to predict individuals likely to develop the disorder and to take the necessary steps for early detection and prevention of the deforming features.

6 Treatment consists of the cautious use of increasing doses of vitamin D or dihydrotachysterol with or without oral phosphate; with further availability of and experience with 25-hydroxycholecalciferol, it is probable that this or a similar active form of the vitamin will become the treatment of choice.

BIBLIOGRAPHY

1. Albright, F., Butler, A. M., and Bloomberg, E.: Rickets resistant to vitamin D therapy. Amer. J. Dis. Child., **54**, 529, 1937.
2. Robertson, B. R., Harris, R. C., and McCune, D. J.: Refractory rickets: Mechanism of therapeutic action of calciferol. Amer. J. Dis. Child., **64**, 948, 1942.
3. Christensen, J. F.: Three familial cases of atypical late rickets. Acta Paediat. Scand., **28**, 247, 1940–41.
4. Baagoe, K.: Rachitis tarda. Ugeskr. Laeg., **86**, 175, 1924.
5. Dent, C. E., and Harris, H. Hereditary forms of rickets and osteomalacia. J. Bone Joint Surg. [Amer.], **38-B**, 204, 1956.
6. Mitchell, F. N., and Mitchell, J. E.: Vitamin-D–resistant rickets. A.M.A. J. Dis. Child., **93**, 385, 1957.
7. Winters, R. W., Graham, J. B., Williams, T. F., McFalls, V. W., and Burnett, C. H.: A genetic study of familial hypophosphatemia and vitamin D resistant rickets. Trans. Ass. Amer. Physicians, **70**, 234, 1957.
8. Winters, R. W., Graham, J. B., Williams, T. F., McFalls, V. W., and Burnett, C. H.: A genetic study of familial hypophosphatemia and vitamin D resistant rickets with a review of the literature. Medicine (Balt.), **37**, 97, 1958.
9. Graham, J. B., McFalls, V. W., and Winters, R. W.: Familial hypophosphatemia with vitamin D-resistant rickets. II. Three additional kindreds of the sex-linked dominant type with a genetic analysis of four such families. Amer. J. Hum. Genet., **11**, 311, 1959.

10. DeLuca, H. F., Lund, J., Rosenbloom, A., and Lobeck, C. C.: Metabolism of tritiated vitamin D_3 in familial vitamin D-resistant rickets with hypophosphatemia. J. Pediat., **70,** 828, 1967.
11. Avioli, L. V., Williams, T. F., Lund, J., and DeLuca, H. F.: Metabolism of vitamin D_3-^3H in vitamin D-resistant rickets and familial hypophosphatemia. J. Clin. Invest., **46,** 1907, 1967.
12. Burnett, C. H., Dent, C. E., Harper, C., and Warland, B. J.: Vitamin D-resistant rickets: Analysis of twenty-four pedigrees with hereditary and sporadic cases. Amer. J. Med., **36,** 222, 1964.
13. Falls, W. F., Jr., Carter, N. W., Rector, F. W., Jr., and Seldin, D. W.: Familial vitamin D-resistant rickets: Study of six cases with evaluation of the pathogenetic role of secondary hyperparathyroidism. Ann. Intern. Med., **68,** 553, 1968.
14. Blackard, W. G., Robinson, R. R., and White, J. E.: Familial hypophosphatemia: Report of a case, with observations regarding pathogenesis. New Eng. J. Med., **266,** 899, 1962.
15. Johnston, C. C., Jr., Kurlander, G. J., Smith, D. M., Goodman, J. M., and Campbell, R. L.: Familial vitamin D resistant rickets in untreated adult. Arch. Intern. Med. (Chicago), **117,** 141, 1966.
16. Dugger, G. S., and Vandiver, R. W.: Spinal cord compression caused by vitamin D resistant rickets. J. Neurosurg., **25,** 300, 1966.
17. Yoshikawa, S., Shiba, M., and Suzuki, A.: Spinal-cord compression in untreated adult cases of vitamin-D resistant rickets. J. Bone Joint Surg. [Amer.], **50-A,** 743, 1968.
18. McNair, S. L., and Stickler, G. B.: Growth in familial hypophosphatemic vitamin-D-resistant rickets. New Eng. J. Med., **281,** 511, 1969.
19. Stickler, G. B., Beabout, J. W., and Riggs, B. L.: Vitamin D-resistant rickets: Clinical experience with 41 typical familial hypophosphatemic patients and 2 atypical nonfamilial cases. Mayo Clin. Proc., **45,** 197, 1970.
20. Liebe, S.: Über night heilbare Rachitis. Mschr. Kinderheilk., **78,** 221, 1939.
21. Bauer, G. O. H., Carlsson, A., and Lundquist, B.: Bone salt metabolism in human rickets studied with radioactive phosphorus. Metabolism, **5,** 573, 1956.
22. Carlgren, L.-E.: A case of vitamin D resistant rickets treated with massive doses of vitamin D_2. Acta Paediat., **35,** 367, 1948.
23. Christiansson, G.: Emergence of primary vitamin D resistant rickets at puberty: Genetic study of primary rickets with familial disposition. Acta Paediat., **47,** 288, 1958.
24. Coleman, E. N., and Foote, J. B.: Craniostenosis with familial vitamin-D-resistant rickets. Brit. Med. J., **1,** 561, 1954.
25. Daeschner, C. W., Jr.: Vitamin D resistant rickets: Diagnosis and management. Texas J. Med., **53,** 324, 1957.
26. Engfeldt, B., Zetterström, R., and Winberg, J.: Primary vitamin-D resistant rickets. III. Biophysical studies of skeletal tissue. J. Bone Joint Surg. [Amer.], **38-A,** 1323, 1956.
27. Fanconi, G., and Girardet, P.: Familiärer persistierended Phosphatdiabetes mit D-vitamin resistenter Rachitis. Helv. Paediat. Acta, **7,** 14, 1952.
28. Gardner, L. I.: Vitamin D-refractory rickets, in *Textbook of Pediatrics,* edited by W. E. Nelson, 6th ed. Saunders, Philadelphia, 1954.
29. Holt, J. F.: Vitamin D resistant rickets (refractory rickets). Amer. J. Roentgen., **64,** 590, 1950.
30. Imerslund, O.: Craniostenosis and vitamin D resistant rickets. Acta Paediat., **40,** 449, 1951.
31. Lamy, M., Royer, P., Frézal, J., and Lestradet, H.: Le rachitisme vitamino-résistant familial hypophosphatémique primitif. Arch. Franc. Pédiat., **15,** 1, 1958.
32. Linnerloth, K., Hallgren, B., Palmén, K., and Zetterström, R.: Primary (genuine) vitamin D resistant rickets. IV. A clinical and genetic study. Acta Paediat., **47,** 568, 1958.
33. Litman, N. N., Ulstrom, R. A., and Westin, W. W.: Vitamin D resistant rickets. Calif. Med., **86,** 248, 1957.
34. MacKay, H., and May, Q. I.: Rickets resistant to vitamin D: Healing with very heavy dosage of vitamin D, fluctuations in vitamin D requirement, development of hypercalcemia. Proc. Roy. Soc. Med., **38,** 565, 1944–1945.
35. McCune, D. J.: Refractory rickets in identical twins. Amer. J. Dis. Child., **63,** 1008, 1942.
36. Pedersen, H. E., and McCarroll, H. R.: Vitamin-resistant rickets. J. Bone Joint Surg. [Amer.], **33-A,** 203, 1951.
37. Peterson, R. E.: Hypophosphatemic rickets: Description and case reports of renal tubular form of this deficiency disease. J. Kansas Med. Soc., **57,** 582, 1956.
38. Swoboda, W.: Die genuine vitamin D-resistente Rachitis. Wien. Beitr. Kinderheilk., **6,** 1, 1956.
39. Tobler, R., Prader, A., and Taillard, W.: Die familiäre primäre vitamin-D-resistent Rachitis (Phosphatdiabetes). Helv. Paediat. Acta, **11,** 209, 1956.
40. Hsia, D.Y.-Y., Kraus, M., and Samuels, J.: Genetic studies on vitamin D resistant rickets (familial hypophosphatemia). Amer. J. Hum. Genet., **11,** 156, 1959.
41. Prader, A., Illig, R., and Heierli, E.: Eine besondere Form der Primären vitamin-D-resistenten Rachitis mit Hypocalcämie und autosomal-dominanten Erbgang: Die Hereditäre Pseudomangelrachitis. Helv. Paediat. Acta, **16,** 452, 1961.
42. Stoop, J. W., Schragen, M. J. C., and Tiddens, H. A. W. M.: Pseudo vitamin D deficiency rickets: Report of four new cases. Acta Paediat., **56,** 607, 1967.
43. Dent, C. E., Friedman, M., and Watson, L.: Hereditary pseudo-vitamin D deficiency rickets ("Hereditäre Pseudo-mangelrachitis"). J. Bone Joint Surg. [Amer.], **50-B,** 708, 1968.
44. Suster, P., and Paala, J. V.: Pseudovitamin D-deficiency rickets. J. Pediat., **76,** 937, 1970.
45. Greenberg, B. G., Winters, R. W., and Graham, J. B.: The normal range of serum inorganic phosphorus and its utility as a discriminant in the diagnosis of congenital hypophosphatemia. J. Clin. Endocr., **20,** 364, 1960.
46. Harrison, H. E., Harrison, H. C., Lifshitz, F., and Johnson, A. D.: Growth disturbance in hereditary hypophosphatemia. Amer. J. Dis. Child., **112,** 290, 1966.
47. Stickler, G. B.: Familial hypophosphatemic vitamin D resistant rickets. Acta Paediat., **58,** 213, 1969.
48. Prasad, A. S., Flink, E. B., and McCollister, R.: Ultrafiltration studies on serum magnesium in normal and diseased states. J. Lab. Clin. Med., **58,** 531, 1961.
49. Rupp, W., and Swoboda, W.: Untersuchungen des PO_4-stoffwechsels bei vitamin-D-resistenter Rachitis ("Phosphat-diabetes"). I. Mittelung. Helv. Paediat. Acta, **9,** 249, 1054; II. Mittelung. Helv. Paediat. Acta, **10,** 135, 1955.
50. Dent, C. E.: Rickets and osteomalacia from renal tubular defects. J. Bone Joint Surg. [Brit.], **34-B,** 266, 1952.
51. McCance, R. A.: Osteomalacia with Looser's nodes (Milkman's syndrome) due to a raised resistance to vitamin D acquired about the age of 15 years. Quart. J. Med., N.S., **16,** 33, 1947.
52. Rupp, W., and Swoboda, W.: Clearance-untersuchungen bei vitamin D-resistenter Rachitis. Mschr. Kinderheilk., **102,** 173, 1954.
53. Williams, T. F., Winters, R. W., and Burnett, C. H.: Familial (hereditary) vitamin D-resistant rickets with hypophosphatemia, in *The Metabolic Basis of Inherited Disease,* edited by J. B. Stanbury et al., 2nd ed., pp. 1183–1184. McGraw-Hill, New York 1966.
54. Jackson, W. P. U., Dowdle, E., and Linder, G. C.: Vitamin-D-resistant osteomalacia. Brit. Med. J., **1,** 1269, 1958.
55. Magid, G. J., Maloney, J. R., Sirota, J. H., and Schwab, E. A.: Familial hypophosphatemia: Studies on its pathogenesis in an affected mother and son. Ann. Intern. Med., **64,** 1009, 1966.
56. Wilson, D. R., York, S. E., Jaworski, Z. F., and Yendt, E. R.: Studies in hypophosphatemic vitamin D-refractory osteomalacia in adults: Oral phosphate supplements as an adjunct to therapy. Medicine (Balt.), **44,** 99, 1965.
57. Ryan, W. G., Nibbe, A. F., and Schwartz, T. B.: Fibrous dysplasia of bone with vitamin D resistant rickets: A case study. Metabolism, **17,** 988, 1968.
58. Steendijk, R.: On the pathogenesis of vitamin D deficient rickets and primary vitamin D resistant rickets. Helv. Pediat. Acta, **17,** 65, 1962.

59. Winberg, J., Bergstrand, C. G., Engfeldt, B., and Zetterström, R.: Primary vitamin D refractory rickets. I. Report of two cases treated with high doses of vitamin D. Acta Paediat., **43,** 347, 1954.
60. Freeman, S., and Dunsky, I.: Resistant rickets. Amer. J. Dis. Child, **79,** 409, 1950.
61. Dodge, W. F., Travis, L. B., and Daeschner, C. W.: Vitamin-D resistant rickets: Studies of renal tubular function. *Proc. Southern Soc. Pediat. Res.,* Memphis, Tenn., Nov. 8–9, 1963.
62. Kajdi, L.: Comparison of the effect of vitamin D and citrates on mineral metabolism in late rickets. Amer. J. Dis. Child., **68,** 352, 1944.
63. Jonxis, J. H. P.: Some investigations on rickets. J. Pediat., **59,** 607, 1961.
64. White, J. E., Binford, C. C., Robinson, R. R., and Blackard, W. G.: Familial hypophosphatemia: Clinical course and necropsy. Arch. Intern. Med. (Chicago), **111,** 460, 1963.
65. Bickel, H.: Discussion of Jonxis, ref. 66. Helv. Paediat. Acta, **10,** 257, 1955.
66. Jonxis, J. H. P.: Amino-aciduria and rickets. Helv. Paediat. Acta, **10,** 245, 1955.
67. Jonxis, J. H. P., Smith, P. A., and Huisman, T. H. J.: Rickets and aminoaciduria. Lancet, **2,** 1015, 1952.
68. Fishman, W. H.: Methionine-induced aminoaciduria in vitamin D resistant rickets. Metabolism, **4,** 107, 1955.
69. Milkman, L. A.: Multiple spontaneous idiopathic symmetrical fractures. Amer. J. Roentgen., **32,** 622, 1934.
70. Barbour, B. H., Kronfield, S. J., and Pawlicki, A.: On the mechanism of tubular reabsorption of phosphorus in vitamin D resistant rickets. Clin. Res., **12,** 247, 1964 (abstract).
71. Paunier, L., Conen, P. E., Gibson, A. A. M., and Fraser, D.: Renal function and histology after long-term vitamin D therapy of vitamin D refractory rickets. J. Pediat., **73,** 833, 1968.
72. Nigrin, G., Cochrane, W. A., Jannigan, D., and Ernst, A.: Results of calcium infusion and renal biopsy studies in refractory rickets. Amer. J. Dis. Child., **104,** 478, 1962 (abstract).
73. Darmady, E. M., and Robinson, R. R.: Personal communication.
74. Darmady, E. M., and Stranack, F.: Microdissection of the nephron in disease. Brit. Med. Bull., **13,** 21, 1957.
75. Montcriff, M. W., and Chance, G. W.: Nephrotoxic effect of vitamin D therapy in vitamin D refractory rickets. Arch. Dis. Child., **44,** 571, 1969.
76. Reiner, C.: Discussion of Nigrin et al., ref. 72.
77. Dancaster, C. P., and Jackson, W. P. U.: Familial vitamin D–resistant rickets. Arch. Dis. Child., **34,** 383, 1959.
78. Vaandrager, G. J.: Primaire vitamin D–refractaire rachitis: Criteria voor diagnose en therapie. Thesis, Utrecht, 1960.
79. Robinson, H. W., and Nelson, W. E.: Phosphorus clearance in children with vitamin D resistant rickets. Amer. J. Dis. Child., **69,** 323, 1945.
80. Dent, C. E., Anderson, J., and Senior, B.: Effect of vitamin D on renal reabsorption of phosphorus. J. Bone Joint Surg. [Brit.], **37-B,** 171, 1955 (abstract).
81. Klein, R., and Gow, R. C.: Interaction of parathyroid hormone and vitamin D on the renal excretion of phosphate. J. Clin. Endocr., **13,** 271, 1953.
82. Zetterström, R., and Winberg, J.: Primary vitamin D refractory rickets. II. Metabolic studies during treatment with massive doses of vitamin D. Acta Paediat., **44,** 45, 1955.
83. Bauer, W., Albright, F., and Aub, J. C.: Studies of calcium and phosphorus metabolism. II. The calcium excretion of normal individuals on a low calcium diet, also data on a case of pregnancy. J. Clin. Invest., **7,** 75, 1929.
84. Sherman, H. C., and Hawley, E.: Calcium and phosphorus metabolism in childhood. J. Biol. Chem., **53,** 375, 1922.
85. Stearns, G., Oelke, M. J., and Boyd, J. D.: Mineral metabolism in late rickets. Amer. J. Dis. Child., **42,** 88, 1931.
86. Nicolaysen, R., and Eeg-Larsen, N.: The biochemistry and physiology of vitamin D. Vitamins Hormones (NY), **11,** 29, 1953.
87. Orr, W. J., Holt, L. E., Jr., Wilkins, L., and Boone, F. H.: The calcium and phosphorus metabolism in rickets with special reference to ultraviolet ray therapy. Amer. J. Dis. Child., **26,** 362, 1923.
88. Telfer, S. V.: Studies in calcium and phosphorus metabolism. V. Infantile rickets: The excretion and absorption of the mineral elements and the influence of fats in the diet on mineral absorption. Quart. J. Med., **20,** 7, 1926–1927.
89. Avioli, L. V.: Absorption and metabolism of vitamin D_3 in man. Amer. J. Clin. Nutr., **22,** 437, 1969.
90. Ponchon, G., and DeLuca, H. F.: The role of the liver in the metabolism of vitamin D. J. Clin. Invest., **48,** 1273, 1969.
91. Blunt, J. W., DeLuca, H. F., and Schnoes, H. K.: 25-Hydroxycholecalciferol: A biologically active metabolite of vitamin D_3. Biochemistry (Wash.), **7,** 3317, 1968.
92. Blunt, J. W., and DeLuca, H. F.: The synthesis of 25-hydroxycholecalciferol: A biologically active metabolite of vitamin D_3. Biochemistry (Wash.), **8,** 671, 1969.
93. Suda, T., DeLuca, H. F., Schnoes, H., and Blunt, J. W.: 25-Hydroxyergocalciferol: A biologically active metabolite of vitamin D_2. Biochem. Biophys. Res. Commun., **35,** 182, 1969.
94. Horsting, M., and DeLuca, H. F.: Enzymatic conversion of cholecalciferol to 25-hydroxycholecalciferol. Fed. Proc., **28,** 351, 1969 (abstract).
95. Olson, E. B., and DeLuca, H. F.: 25-Hydroxycholecalciferol: Direct effect on calcium transport. Science, **165,** 405, 1969.
96. DeLuca, H. F.: Recent advances in the metabolism and function of vitamin D. Fed. Proc., **28,** 1678, 1969.
97. Blunt, J. W., and DeLuca, H. F.: The biological activity of 25-hydroxycholecalciferol, a metabolite of vitamin D_3. Proc. Nat. Acad. Sci. USA, **61,** 1503, 1968.
98. Martin, D. L., Melancon, M. J., and DeLuca, H. F.: Vitamin D stimulated, calcium-dependent adenosine triphosphatase from brush borders of rat small intestine. Biochem. Biophys. Res. Commun., **35,** 819, 1969.
99. Melancon, M. J., and DeLuca, H. F.: Vitamin D stimulation of calcium-dependent adenosine triphosphatase in chick intestinal brush borders. Biochemistry (Wash.), **9,** 1658, 1970.
100. Wasserman, R. H., Corradino, R. A., and Taylor, A. N.: Vitamin D–dependent calcium-binding protein: Purification and some properties. J. Biol. Chem., **243,** 3978, 1968.
101. Wasserman, R. H., and Taylor, A. N.: Vitamin D–dependent calcium-binding protein: Response to some physiological and nutritional variables. J. Biol. Chem., **243,** 3987, 1968.
102. Taylor, A. N., and Wasserman, R. H.: Correlations between the vitamin D–induced calcium binding protein and intestinal absorption of calcium. Fed. Proc., **28,** 1834, 1969.
103. Stohs, S. J., and DeLuca, H. F.: Subcellular location of vitamin D and its metabolites in intestinal mucosa after a 10-IU dose. Biochemistry (Wash.), **6,** 3338, 1967.
104. Cousins, R. J., DeLuca, H. F., Suda, T., Chen, T., and Tanaka, Y.: Metabolism and subcellular location of 25-hydroxycholecalciferol in intestinal mucosa. Biochemistry (Wash.), **9,** 1453, 1970.
105. Haussler, M. R., Myrtle, J. F., and Norman, A. W.: The association of a metabolite of vitamin D_3 with intestinal mucosal chromatin in vivo. J. Biol. Chem., **243,** 4055, 1968.
106. Haussler, M. R., and Norman, A. W.: Chromosomal receptor for a vitamin D metabolite. Proc. Nat. Acad. Sci. USA, **62,** 155, 1969.
107. Harrison, H. C., and Harrison, H. E.: Dibutyryl cyclic AMP, vitamin D and intestinal permeability to calcium. Endocrinology, **86,** 756, 1970.
108. Harrison, H. E., and Harrison, H. C.: Transfer of Ca^{45} across intestinal wall in vitro in relation to action of vitamin D and cortisol. Amer. J. Physiol., **199,** 265, 1960.
109. Harrison, H. E.: Vitamin D and calcium and phosphate transport. Pediatrics, **28,** 531, 1961.
110. Urban, E., and Schedl, H. P.: Comparison of in vivo and in vitro effects of vitamin D on calcium transport in the rat. Amer. J. Physiol., **217,** 126, 1969.
111. Albright, F., and Sulkowitch, H. W.: The effect of vitamin D on calcium and phosphorus metabolism; studies on four patients. J. Clin. Invest., **17,** 305, 1938.
112. Nicolaysen, R.: XV. Studies upon the mode of action of vitamin D. III. The influence of vitamin D on the absorption of calcium and phosphorus in the rat. Biochem. J., **31,** 122, 1937.

113. Kowarski, S., and Schachter, D.: Effects of vitamin D on phosphate transport and incorporation into mucosal constituents of rat intestinal mucosa. J. Biol. Chem., **244,** 211, 1969.
114. Stickler, G. B.: External calcium and phosphorus balances in vitamin D-resistant rickets. J. Pediat., **63,** 942, 1963.
115. Saville, P. D., Nassim, J. R., Stevenson, F. H., Mulligan, L., and Carey, M.: The effect of A.T.10 on calcium and phosphorus metabolism in resistant rickets. Clin. Sci., **14,** 489, 1955.
116. Williams, T. F., Winters, R. W., and Burnett, C. H.: Familial (hereditary) vitamin D-resistant rickets with hypophosphatemia, in *The Metabolic Basis of Inherited Disease,* edited by J. B. Stanbury, et al., 2nd ed., p. 1187.
117. Hall, B. D., MacMillan, D. R., and Bronner, F.: Vitamin D-resistant rickets and high fecal endogenous calcium output: A report of two cases. Amer. J. Clin. Nutr., **22,** 448, 1969.
118. Stanbury, S. W.: Osteomalacia. Schweiz. Med. Wschr., **92,** 883, 1962.
119. Lafferty, F. W., Herndon, C. H., and Pearson, O. H.: Pathogenesis of vitamin D-resistant rickets and the response to high calcium intake. J. Clin. Endocr., **23,** 903, 1963.
120. Albright, F., Burnett, C. H., Parson, W., Reifenstein, E. C., Jr., and Roos, A.: Osteomalacia and late rickets: The various etiologies met in the United States, with emphasis on that resulting from a specific form of renal acidosis, the therapeutic indications for each etiological subgroup, and the relationship between osteomalacia and Milkman's syndrome. Medicine (Balt.), **25,** 399, 1946.
121. Albright, F., Sulkowitch, H. W., and Bloomberg, E.: A comparison of the effects of vitamin D, dihydrotachysterol (A.T.10), and parathyroid extract on the disordered metabolism of rickets. J. Clin. Invest., **18,** 165, 1939.
122. Harrison, H. E.: The varieties of rickets and osteomalacia associated with hypophosphatemia. Clin. Orthop., **9,** 61, 1957.
123. Swoboda, W.: Die Wirksamkeit von Dihydrotachysterin bei vitamin-D-resistenter Rachitis und Mangelrachitis. Helv. Paediat. Acta, **14,** 472, 1959.
124. Illig, R., Antener, I., and Prader, A.: Die Wirkung von Dihydrotachysterin$_2$ (DHT) bei Mangelrachitis und die antirachitische Aktivität des Serums nach Verabreichung von DHT and Vitamin D. Helv. Paediat. Acta, **16,** 469, 1961.
125. Bauer, W., Marble, A., and Claflin, D.: Studies on the mode of action of irradiated ergosterol. I. Its effect on the calcium, phosphorus and nitrogen metabolism of normal individuals. J. Clin. Invest., **11,** 1, 1932.
126. Earp, H. S., Ney, R. L., Gitelman, H. J., Richman, R., and DeLuca, H. F.: Effects of 25-hydroxycholecalciferol in patients with familial hypophosphatemia and vitamin-D-resistant rickets. New Eng. J. Med., **283,** 627, 1970.
127. Seely, J. R., Coussons, H., Smith, J. D., and DeLuca, H. F.: Effective treatment of hypophosphatemic vitamin D resistant rickets (VDRR) with 25-hydroxycholecalciferol (25-HCC), *Amer. Pediat. Soc.,* Atlantic City, N.J., April 29-May 2, 1970, p. 48 Abstracts.
128. Fraser, D., Geiger, D. W., Munn, J. D., Slater, P. E., Jahn, R., and Liu, E.: Calcification studies in clinical vitamin D deficiency and in hypophosphatemic vitamin D-refractory rickets: The induction of calcium deposition in rachitic cartilage without the administration of vitamin D. A.M.A. J. Dis. Child., **96,** 460, 1958.
129. Nagant de Deuxchaisnes, C., and Krane, S. M.: The treatment of adult phosphate diabetes and Fanconi syndrome with neutral sodium phosphate. Amer. J. Med., **43,** 508, 1967.
130. Frame, B., Smith, R. W., Jr., Fleming, J. L., and Manson, G.: Oral phosphates in vitamin-D-refractory rickets and osteomalacia. Amer. J. Dis. Child., **106,** 147, 1963.
131. Carlsson, A.: Tracer experiments on the effect of vitamin D on the skeletal metabolism of calcium and phosphorus. Acta Physiol. Scand., **26,** 212, 1952.
132. Nicolaysen, R., and Eeg-Larsen, N.: The mode of action of vitamin D, in *Bone Structure and Metabolism,* edited by G. E. W. Wolstenholme and C. M. O'Connor, p. 175. Ciba Found. Symp., Little, Brown, Boston, 1956.
133. Trummel, C. L., Raisz, L. G., Blunt, J. W., and DeLuca, H. F.: 25-Hydroxycholecalciferol: Stimulation of bone resorption in tissue culture. Science, **163,** 1450, 1969.
134. Rasmussen, H., DeLuca, H., Arnaud, C., Hawker, C., and Von Stedingk, M.: The relationship between vitamin D and parathyroid hormone. J. Clin. Invest., **42,** 1940, 1963.
135. Harrison, H. C., Harrison, H. E., and Park, E. A.: Vitamin D and citrate metabolism: Effect of vitamin D in rats fed diets adequate in both calcium and phosphorus. Amer. J. Physiol., **192,** 432, 1958.
136. Pechet, M. M., Bobadilla, E., Carroll, E. L., and Hesse, R. H.: Regulation of bone resorption and formation: Influence of thyrocalcitonin, parathyroid hormone, neutral phosphate and vitamin D$_3$. Amer. J. Med., **43,** 696, 1967.
137. Melancon, M. J., and DeLuca, H. F.: Interrelationships between thyrocalcitonin, parathyroid hormone and vitamin D: Control of serum calcium in hypervitaminosis D. Endocrinology, **85,** 704, 1969.
138. Nicolaysen, R., and Jansen, J.: Vitamin D and bone formation in rats. Acta Pediat., **23,** 405, 1939.
139. Mellanby, E.: The rickets-producing and anticalcifying action of phytate. J. Physiol. (London), **109,** 488, 1949.
140. Gregersen, E.: Primary vitamin-resistant rickets. Acta Pediat., **44,** 491, 1955.
141. Lüssy, M.: Über sogenannte vitamin-resistente Rachitis. Ann. Pediat. (Paris), **166,** 11, 1946.
142. Frost, H. M.: A unique histological feature of vitamin D resistant rickets observed in four cases. Acta Ortho. Scand., **33,** 220, 1963.
143. Frame, B., Arnstein, A. R., Frost, H. M., and Smith, R. W.: Resistant osteomalacia: Studies with tetracycline bone labeling and metabolic balance. Amer. J. Med., **38,** 134, 1965.
144. Villaneuva, A. R., Ilnicki, L., Frost, L. N., and Arnstein, R.: Measurement of the bone formation in a case of familial hypophosphatemic vitamin D-resistant rickets. J. Lab. Clin. Med., **67,** 973, 1966.
145. Kuhlman, R. E., and Stamp, W. G.: Biochemical biopsy evaluation of the epiphyseal mechanism in a patient with vitamin D-resistant rickets. J. Lab. Clin. Med., **64,** 14, 1964.
146. Silverman, F. N., and Currarino, G.: Roentgen manifestations of hereditary metabolic diseases in childhood. Metabolism, **9,** 248, 1960.
147. Engfeldt, B., and Zetterström, R.: Biophysical and chemical investigation on bone tissue in experimental hyperparathyroidism. Endocrinology, **54,** 506, 1954.
148. Ray, R. D., Mueller, K. H., Sankaran, B., Mensen, E. D., and Schwartz, T. B.: Metabolic disease of bone: Kinetic studies. Med. Clin. N. Amer., **49,** 241, 1965.
149. Smith, R., and Dick, M.: The effect of vitamin D and phosphate on urinary total hydroxyproline excretion in adult-presenting "vitamin D resistant" type I renal tubular osteomalacia. Clin. Sci., **35,** 575, 1968.
150. Ko, K. W., and Fellers, F. X.: On the mechanisms of simple familial hypophosphatemic rickets. Amer. J. Dis. Child., **102,** 437, 1961 (abstract).
151. Haas, H. G., Canary, J. J., Kyle, L. H., Meyer, R. J., and Schaaf, M.: Skeletal calcium retention in osteoporosis and in osteomalacia. J. Clin. Endocr., **23,** 605, 1963.
152. Beumer, H.: Zur Frage der D-vitamin resistenz und der Rachitisprophylaxe mit reinen D-vitaminpräparaten. Z. Kinderheilk., **63,** 744, 1942-43.
153. Bakwin, H., Bodansky, O., and Schorr, R.: Refractory rickets. Amer. J. Dis. Child., **59,** 560, 1940.
154. Eliot, M. M., and Park, E. A.: Rickets, in *Brennemann's Practice of Pediatrics,* edited by I. McQuarrie, vol. I, chap. 36. W. F. Prior Co, Hagerstown, Md., 1938.
155. Scott, K. G., Smyth, F. S., Peng, C. T., Reilly, W. A., Stevenson, E. A., and Castle, J. N.: Measurements of the plasma levels of tritiated labelled vitamin D$_3$ in control and rachitic, cirrhotic and osteoporotic patients. Strahlentherapie, suppl. **60,** 317, 1965.
156. Avioli, L. V., McDonald, J. E., Lund, J., and DeLuca, H. F.: Metabolism of vitamin D$_3$-^{3}H in human subjects: Distribution in blood, bile, feces and urine. J. Clin. Invest., **46,** 983, 1967.
157. Williams, T. F.: Pathogenesis of familial vitamin D-resistant rickets (editorial). Ann. Intern. Med., **68,** 706, 1968.
158. Roberts, K. E., and Pitts, R. F.: The effects of cortisone and desoxycorti-

costerone on the renal tubular reabsorption of phosphate and the excretion of titratable acid and potassium in dogs. Endocrinology, **52,** 324, 1953.

159. Mills, J. N., and Thomas, S.: The acute effects of cortisone and cortisol upon renal function in man. J. Endocr., **17,** 41, 1958.
160. Nassim, J. R., Saville, P. D., and Mulligan, L.: The effect of stilboestrol on urinary phosphate excretion. Clin. Sci., **15,** 367, 1956.
161. Gunther, L., Cohn, E. T., Cohn, W. E., and Greenberg, D. M.: Metabolism of bone salts in resistant rickets: Report of a case, with balance and radioactive tracer studies. Amer. J. Dis. Child., **66,** 517, 1943.
162. Bessau, G., and Löhr, H.: Über eine Heilungsmöglichkeit gewisser vitamin D-resistenter Rachitisformen. Mschr. Kinderheilk., **90,** 1, 1942.
163. Rikkers, H., and DeLuca, H.: Metabolism and serum protein binding of ^{3}H-vitamin D_4 in vitamin D-resistant rickets. J. Pediat., **74,** 828, 1969 (abstract and discussion).
164. Jacobs, R. L., and Day, R. D.: Studies of vitamin D binding in normal and rachitic serum. Clin. Orthop., **56,** 275, 1968.
165. Hiatt, H. H., and Thompson, D. D.: The effects of parathyroid extract on renal function in man. J. Clin. Invest., **36,** 557, 1957.
166. Frame, B., and Smith, R. W., Jr.: Phosphate diabetes. Amer. J. Med., **25,** 771, 1958.
167. Howard, J. E.: In case records of Massachusetts General Hospital. New Eng. J. Med., **273,** 494, 1965.
168. Highman, W. J., and Hamilton, B.: Calcium and phosphorus metabolism in a case of intractable rickets. J. Pediat., **9,** 56, 1936.
169. Fraser, D., Leeming, J. M., Cerwenka, E. A., and Keneres, K.: Studies of the pathogenesis of the high renal clearance of phosphate in hypophosphatemic vitamin D-refractory rickets of the simple type. A.M.A. J. Dis. Child., **98,** 586, 1959.
170. Fraser, D., Leeming, J. M., and Cerwenka, E. A.: Über die Handhabung von Phosphat dürch die Nieren bei hypophosphatämischer vitamin-D-resistenter Rachitis der einfachen Art und bei Cystinspeicher-krankheit. Helv. Paediat. Acta, **14,** 497, 1959.
171. Field, M. H., and Reiss, E.: Vitamin-D-resistant rickets: The effect of calcium infusion on phosphate reabsorption. J. Clin. Invest., **39,** 1807, 1960.
172. (Omitted.)
173. Haquani, A. H., and Ram, M. M.: Renal tubular insufficiency. J. Pediat., **61,** 242, 1962.
174. Rose, G. A.: Parathyroid gland function as assessed from the plasma ionized and protein-bound calcium fractions. Mem. Soc. Endocr., **9,** 148, 1960.
175. Fanconi, G.: Tubular insufficiency and renal dwarfism. Arch. Dis. Child., **29,** 1, 1954.
176. Fanconi, G.: Variations in sensitivity to vitamin D: From vitamin D-resistant rickets, vitamin D avitaminotic rickets and hypervitaminosis D to idiopathic hypercalcemia, in *Bone Structure and Metabolism,* edited by G. E. W. Wolstenholme and C. M. O'Connor, p. 187. Ciba Found. Symp., Little, Brown, Boston, 1956.
177. Winters, R. W., and Graham, J. B.: Multiple genetic mechanisms in vitamin D-resistant rickets. Pediatrics, **25,** 932, 1960.
178. Arnstein, A. R., Frame, B., and Frost, H. M.: Recent progress in osteomalacia and rickets. Ann. Intern. Med., **67,** 1296, 1967.
179. Stickler, G. B., Hayles, A. B., and Rosevear, J. W.: Familial hypophosphatemic vitamin D resistant rickets: Effect of increased oral calcium and phosphorus intake without high doses of vitamin D. Amer. J. Dis. Child., **110,** 664, 1965.
180. Williams, T. F., and Arnold, M. B.: Unpublished observations.
181. Harrison, H. E., and Harrison, H. C.: Hereditary metabolic bone diseases. Clin. Orthop., **33,** 147, 1964.
182. Lyon, M. F.: Sex chromatin and gene action in the mammalian X-chromosome. Amer. J. Hum. Genet., **14,** 135, 1962.
183. Winters, R. W., McFalls, V. W., and Graham, J. B.: "Sporadic" hypophosphatemia and vitamin D-resistant rickets. Pediatrics, **25,** 959, 1960.
184. Salassa, R. M., Jowsey, J., and Arnaud, C. D.: Hypophosphatemic osteomalacia associated with "nonendocrine" tumors. New Eng. J. Med., **283,** 65, 1970.
185. Anderson, J.: A method for estimating *Tm* for phosphate in man. J. Physiol. (London), **130,** 268, 1955.
186. Longson, D., Mills, J. N., Thomas, S., and Yates, P. A.: Handling of phosphate by the human kidney at high plasma concentrations. J. Physiol., **131,** 555, 1956.
187. West, C. D., Blanton, J. D., Silverman, F. N., and Holland, N. H.: Use of phosphate salts as an adjunct to vitamin D in the treatment of hypophosphatemic vitamin D refractory rickets. J. Pediat., **64,** 469, 1964.
188. Tapia, J., Stearns, G., and Ponseti, I. V.: Vitamin-D resistant rickets: A long-term clinical study of eleven patients. J. Bone Joint Surg. [Amer.], **46-A,** 935, 1964.
189. Stearns, G.: A guide to adequacy of therapy in resistant rickets due to familial or essential hypophosphatemia. J. Bone Joint Surg. [Amer.], **46-A,** 959, 1964.
190. Yendt, E. R., and Howard, J. E.: Studies on the mode of action of citrate therapy in rickets. Bull. Johns Hopkins Hosp., **96,** 101, 1955.
191. Stamp, W. G., Whitesides, T. E., Field, M. H., and Scheer, G. E.: Treatment of vitamin-D resistant rickets: A long-term evaluation of its effectiveness. J. Bone Joint Surg. [Amer.], **46-A,** 965, 1964.
192. Pierce, D. S., Wallace, W. M., and Herndon, C. H.: Long-term treatment of vitamin-D resistant rickets. J. Bone Joint Surg. [Amer.], **46-A,** 978, 1964.
193. Fraser, D.: Personal communication.
194. Schoen, E. J. The question of normal height in patients with vitamin D-resistant rickets. JAMA, **195,** 524, 1966.
195. Schoen, E. J.: Letter to editor. New Eng. J. Med., **281,** 1195, 1969.
196. Schoen, E. J.: Hereditary hypophosphatemia (letter). Amer. J. Dis. Child., **114,** 214, 1967.
197. Bourgeois, M., and Bierich, J. R.: Die genuine Vitamin-D resistente Rachitis und ihre Behandlung mit höhen Vigantoldosen. Mschr. Kinderheilk., **114,** 472, 1966.
198. Steendijk, R.: Growth in vitamin D-resistant rickets. Calcif. Tissue Res., **2,** suppl., 60, 1968.
199. Tracy, W. E., and Campbell, R. A.: Dentofacial development in children with vitamin D-resistant rickets. J. Amer. Dent. Ass., **76,** 1026, 1968.
200. Gershberg, H., Neumann, L. L., and Mari, J.: Studies on vitamin D-resistant rickets; effects of human growth hormone. Metabolism, **13,** 636, 1964.
201. Pak, C. Y. C., DeLuca, H. F., Chavez de los Riva, J. R., and Suda, T.: Treatment of vitamin D resistant rickets with 25-hydroxycholecalciferol. Clin. Res., **17,** 291, 1969 (abstract).

CHAPTER SIXTY-ONE

HARTNUP DISEASE

John B. Jepson

Hartnup disease is a rare familial condition in which the one constant feature is a specific hyperaminoaciduria. This is due to a diminished capacity for renal reabsorption of a group of monoamino-monocarboxylic acids which share a common, and in this case defective, transport system. The publication which first fully reported the existence of this disease [1] bore the title "Hereditary Pellagra-like Skin Rash with Temporary Cerebellar Ataxia, Constant Renal Amino Aciduria, and Other Bizarre Biochemical Features." As a description of the main aspects of the disease this title cannot be bettered. The family in which the condition was first found consented to the use of their surname, *Hartnup*, as an appropriate appellation. The original report [1] referred only obliquely to the name Hartnup and used the term *H disease*; occasional reference had earlier been made to *Hart's syndrome*. Hartnup *disorder* would be more appropriate than *disease*. The disorder has a physiological interest out of all proportion to its rare clinical occurrence ("a unique experiment of Nature which cannot be simulated experimentally" [30]). Its study has already shed light on general problems of renal absorption, amino acid transport, protein digestion, nicotinamide metabolism, and intestinal bacterial reactions. Because further developments can confidently be expected, interest has not slackened since the previous edition of this book [31], and work with new and old cases is such that Hartnup disease now rates a subject heading in *Index Medicus*.

HISTORY

In 1951, a boy, aged 12, E. Hartnup, was admitted to the Middlesex Hospital, London, England, with mild cerebellar ataxia and a red, scaly rash on the exposed areas of his body. His mother avowed that he had pellagra, for her eldest daughter (P.H.), with identical symptoms, had been treated at the hospital in 1937 for that disease. Although the rash in E.H. was quite consistent with pellagra, other findings were not, and a diagnosis of pellagra as a *dietary* deficiency disease was untenable.

Apart from variable cerebellar signs and retarded mental development, the only abnormality detected at that time was in the urinary excretion of free amino acids. Paper chromatography of the urine disclosed an excretion pattern of amino acids quite unlike that seen in any other disease.

At about the same time, P.H., then aged 19, had a recurrence of ataxia without a rash similar to that which she had had in childhood when the pellagra-like rash was most severe. The excretion pattern of amino acids in her urine was identical with that of her brother E.H.

It was then clear that these two sibs were affected by the same disease. An inherited condition seemed probable when it was learned that the parents were first cousins.

The Hartnup Family

Neither parent and none of their six other children gave a clinical history to suggest that they were similarly affected, although one girl (M.H.) was mentally retarded. However, two younger sibs of E.H., Jh.H. and H.H., also had gross aminoaciduria with the characteristic chromatographic pattern. No abnormality was detected in the urine of the other four siblings or in either parent. In the affected children, the amino acid excretion has persisted unchanged in pattern and amount up to the present. The skin and neurologic disturbances have gradually lessened in P.H. and E.H. but have made a fleeting appearance in the younger boys. The mental defect in M.H. does not seem related to the main abnormality.

The pedigree of the Hartnup family (as of 1953), with a diagrammatic representation of the chromatographic findings, is given in Fig. 61-1. No other relatives of the Hartnup parents show the abnormality.

Other Cases

In the definitive report on the Hartnup family [1] two other cases of "pellagra" in English children, reported earlier by Hickish [2] and Hersov [3], were reexamined. Chromatography of the urines [1] indicated that these two patients were not true dietary pellagrins but had Hartnup disease.

Thirty-seven other cases have since been discovered, bringing the total to forty-three. Details are given in Table 61-1, which includes the forty-one documented cases and two cases as yet unpublished (as of March 1971). Those cases printed below the horizontal line have been reported since the previous list was published in 1966 [31]; they include the youngest known patient, the oldest known case, the first cases with children, and the first patients from the American continent.

CLINICAL ASPECTS

The clinical manifestations of Hartnup disease are intermittent and variable. Although the biochemical lesion as represented by aminoaciduria is always present, clinically recognizable "attacks" may occur only rarely and in widely different forms, and grow milder with increasing age. Indeed,

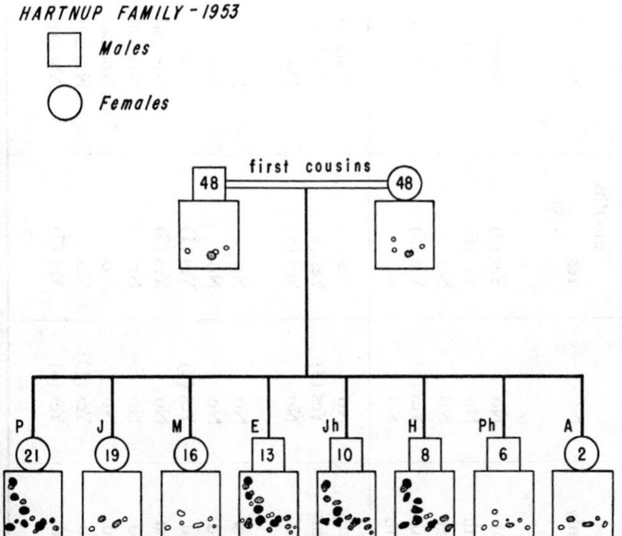

Figure 61-1. The genealogy of Hartnup disease as illustrated in the Hartnup family. The parents were first cousins. The age of the subject in 1953 is indicated by the numbers; in the squares are the chromatography patterns of urine samples in two-dimensional chromatograms stained for amino acids.

several of the recently described cases have only come to light through routine screening [21, 23, 29]—"disorder" without "disease."

Skin Lesions

In the original Hartnup cases, and in most of those found subsequently, the primary cause of referral to hospital has been a red, scaly rash, sometimes dry, sometimes raw and blistered. The rash appears intermittently, usually in summertime, with a distribution on exposed parts of the face, neck, hands, and legs, suggesting photosensitivity [1, 6, 9]. Hartnup patients learn to avoid exposure to direct light [23], but photosensitivity has not been convincingly demonstrated by experiment. The appearance and distribution of the dermatitis closely resemble that seen in dietary pellagra. Two cases [14, 20] had the condition diagnosed as hydroa vacciniforme (vesiculobullous photodermatosis leaving residual scarring).

Neurologic Manifestations

Several of the patients with Hartnup disease have developed a severe but fully reversible cerebellar ataxia. These neurologic crises seem to be precipitated at those times when the skin rash is most severe, but occasionally they may follow infectious disease without rash [1, 6, 7]. During attacks the patient has an unsteady gait and walks with a wide base. Arm movements are jerky, and there is an intention tremor. Nystagmus and double vision are present. No sensory abnormalities are found. The ataxia develops suddenly and rapidly reaches a peak. The manifestations may vary from day to day. Gradual improvement follows over a period of weeks, and complete recovery is the rule.

Some patients have never shown severe ataxia but have experienced a period of "collapsing" or fainting attacks without warning [5, 18]. Stubborn headache is common and may be the only sign of cerebral involvement [8]. Intermittent muscle pains and weaknesses occur [9, 10]. EEG examinations [1, 5, 9, 10] show considerable, but variable, dysrhythmia which has defied interpretation.

Psychologic Changes

Psychiatric features have ranged from mild emotional instability to complete delirium, a range similar to that of the psychiatric disturbances of classic pellagra. They were the cause for referral to hospital in only two cases—bizarre delusions and vivid hallucinations in one [3] and depersonalization in the other (Patient E) [5]. Nine of the known Hartnup patients are mentally retarded (IQ 60 to 90). This suggests some relationship between the genetically determined lesion and mental development or capacity, but several of the older patients have high intelligence and ability (one is president of a bank!) and the original suggestion [1] of a progressive mental deterioration is no longer tenable. Indeed, increasing age seems to bring a general improvement in attitude and attainment, if not in IQ.

Precipitating Factors

Attacks have been precipitated by exposure to sunlight, fever [1], sulfonamides [6], and psychologic stress [5], coupled in every instance with an inadequate or irregular diet. For example, one patient had lived for months on corn flakes [6]; another provoked her first rash by changing to a maize-containing African diet [26]. It seems that clinical signs seldom appear except under the provocation of rather poor nutrition [25]. The clinical deterioration during childhood, followed by improvement in adult life, also points to some nutrient being in limited supply because of a biochemical abnormality; growth, stress, or poor diet exacerbate the situation. There is general agreement that this nutrient is nicotinamide, for the following reasons:

1 Dietary pellagra (nicotinamide deficiency) is characterized by dermatitis and dementia. The rash of Hartnup disease is similar in all respects to that of pellagra. The neuropsychiatric effects are rather less severe.
2 Hartnup patients show marked clinical improvement following oral nicotinamide therapy (page 1498).
3 The abnormal amino acid transport mechanisms which characterize Hartnup disease result in a diversion of trypto-

Table 61-1. THE KNOWN CASES OF HARTNUP DISEASE

Clinical investigators	Relationship of parents	No. of children	Designation of patient	Sex	Year of birth	Position in family	Clinical symptoms (and age when first noticed)		Intelligence and psychological status
							Ataxia	Rash	
[1]	First cousins (Hartnup family)	8	P.H.	F	1932	1st	Yes (5)	Yes (3)	Retarded
			E.H.	M	1939	4th	Yes (12)	Yes (9)	Retarded
			Jh.H.	M	1943	5th	Yes (11)	Yes (8)	Fair
			H.H.	M	1945	6th	No	No	High
[1, 2]	Not reported	1	Not reported (initials T.S.)	F	1949	Only	No	Yes (4)	Normal
[3, 4, 5]	Unrelated	4	M.H.	M	1942	4th	Slight	Yes (10)	Fair
[6]	Unrelated	2	Angela P.	F	1947	2d	Yes (5)	Yes (5)	Normal
[7]	Second cousins	9	D	F	1948	7th	Yes	Yes (3)	Low
			Sister of D	F	1954	9th	Yes	Yes (3)	Normal
[7]	Related but relationship not specified	3	C	F	1947	1st	Yes (5)	Yes (6)	Below normal
[5]	Unrelated	3	J	F	1931	1st	Yes (18)	Yes (9)	High
			E	F	1932	2d	Yes (17)	Yes (8)	Normal
[8]	Unrelated	2	Gudrun B.	F	1947	1st	No	Yes (7)	Normal
[9]	Unrelated	4	N.A.	F	1947	1st	Yes (12)	Yes (1)	Retarded
			E.A.	M	1951	3d	No	Yes (5)	Normal
[10]	Not reported	3	H.H.	F	1954	1st	Yes (1)	Yes (1)	Retarded
[11]	Unrelated	5	Hans B.D.	M	1960	5th	No	Yes 3 months	Normal
[11]	Not reported	1	Bart N. (nephew of Hans B.D.)	M	1954	Only	No	Yes	Normal
[12]	Unrelated	5 (1 dead)	E.P.	F	1945 (died 1959)	2d	No	Yes (9)	Normal
			S.P.	F	1948	4th	No	Yes (6)	Normal
[13]	First cousins	4 (1 dead)	R.	F	1951	1st	No	No	Normal
			Y.	M	1956	3d	Yes (5)	Yes (5)	Normal
			Sister of Y.	F	1961	4th	No	No	Normal
[14]	Unrelated	1	Angelika H	F	1954	Only	No	Yes (2)	Normal
[15]	Not reported	1	M.L.	M	1955	Only	Yes (8)	Yes (8)	Normal
[16]	Unrelated	6	Monika G	F	1951 (died 1962)	1st	No	Yes (5)	Disturbed
[17]	Unrelated	3	H.P.	F	1949	1st	No	No	Normal
			K.P.	F	1960	2d	No	No	Normal
			T.P.	F	1963	3d	Yes (2)	Yes (1)	Normal
[18, 19, 20]	Unrelated	2	Case 1 (S.R.)	M	1960	1st	No	Yes (3)	Normal
[18, 19]	Unrelated	2	Case 2	M	1965	2d	No	No	Normal
[21]	Unrelated	2	Christopher S	M	1964	2d	No	No	Normal
[22]	Second cousins	5 (eldest dead)	K.M.	M	1946	2d	Yes (13)	Yes	Normal
			A.M.	F	1948	3d	Yes (6)	Yes (7)	Abnormal

Table 61-1. THE KNOWN CASES OF HARTNUP DISEASE (CONT'D)

Clinical investigators	Relationship of parents	No. of children	Designation of patient	Sex	Year of birth	Position in family	Clinical symptoms (and age when first noticed)		Intelligence and psychological status
							Ataxia	Rash	
[23]	Unrelated	6	III 4	F	1913	3d	No	No	Deaf mute and defective
		(2 dead)	III 6	F	1924	5th	No	No	High
			III 7	M	1928	6th	No	No	High
[24]	Uncle—niece	1	Not reported	M	1966 ?	. . .	No	Yes (1)	
[25]	Second cousins	10	H.R.R.	M	1954	1st	Yes (6)	Yes (1)	Retarded
		(3 dead— 2 of these probably affected)	M.E.R.R.	M	1962	7th	Yes (5)	Yes (1)	Normal
[26, 27]	Unrelated	2	Not reported (initials J.S.)	F	1945	2d	Yes	Yes	Normal (except on maize diet)
[28]	Unrelated	2	S.H.	F	1968	2d	No	No	
[29]	Unrelated	2	L	M	1949	1st	No	Yes	Retarded

phan dissimilation, which lessens the normal metabolic conversion of tryptophan to nicotinamide. The usual supplementation of dietary nicotinamide from "internal" sources is thereby diminished.

Much emphasis has accordingly been placed on the deranged tryptophan metabolism of Hartnup disease, perhaps to the intellectual exclusion of some other amino acid whose abnormal fate or unavailability may also be important, although less easily studied.

METABOLISM OF TRYPTOPHAN

Tryptophan is not synthesized by man and is, therefore, an essential dietary constituent. It is released from its combination in proteins by hydrolysis in the intestine. It is possible that some absorption can occur as small peptides.

Absorption

It is only within the last decade that information has been collected on the site and mechanisms for the intestinal absorption of amino acids, including tryptophan. This development has been partly under the stimulus of the discovery of "diseases" of cellular transport, such as Hartnup disease. It is now clear that the principal site for absorption by diffusion and active transport is the columnar epithelial cells of the jejunum.

Several types of transport "system" are involved, at least some being against a concentration gradient (i.e., "active") [32, 33]. For active intestinal absorption (and in kidney), protein amino acids fall into four groups, each with its own high-capacity system: the glycine-proline-hydroxyproline group; the dicarboxylic group; the dibasic-cystine group; and the monoamino-monocarboxylic group, which includes tryptophan. No details are known of the mechanisms involved, but any theory will have to accommodate the fact that specific impairments can be genetically determined. In addition, there are independent transport systems of lower capacity, probably specific for individual amino acids and under independent genetic control (see Chaps. 62, 63, 64).

Degradation

The degradation of tryptophan is of particular interest because of its partial conversion to the physiologically important compounds nicotinic acid and serotonin. Figure 61-2 shows some of the many pathways along which tryptophan catabolism can proceed. Only those transformations which at present seem relevant to Hartnup disease are discussed below. (For more detailed consideration, see Refs. 31, 34.)

Metabolism to Kynurenine

Tryptophan is first converted to formylkynurenine by the liver enzyme tryptophan pyrrolase; increased activity of this enzyme is readily brought about by tryptophan administration or by corticoids [35, 35*a*]. Formylkynurenine is hydrolyzed to kynurenine by the liver enzyme, formylase. A unique case of congenital tryptophanuria with dwarfism and pellagra-like rash has been reported by Tada [36]. The patient could absorb tryptophan but could not convert it to kynurenine. The significance of this for the understanding of Hartnup disease is discussed on page 1497.

Kynurenine to Nicotinamide

Liver and kidney mitochondria cause hydroxylation of kynurenine to 3-hydroxykynurenine, which can be cleaved by the pyridoxal-requiring enzyme, kynureninase, to alanine and 3-hydroxyanthranilic acid. This product is oxidized to a labile ring-opened aldehyde intermediate, as shown in Fig. 61-2. Ring closure and decarboxylation then occur simultaneously, with the formation of either nicotinic acid or picolinic acid, each by its specific enzyme.

From a quantitative point of view, little tryptophan appears to be converted to nicotinic acid under normal conditions. The dietary equivalent of 1 mg nicotinamide is approximately 60 mg tryptophan [37]. Nevertheless, it may well be that some specialized or localized requirement for nicotinamide can only be met by production *in situ*.

Derivatives

Another pathway of tryptophan metabolism is conversion to indolic acids. Armstrong et al. have shown that normal urine contains a large number of indolic acids, the main ones of which are indoleacetic acid, indolelactic acid, 5-hydroxyindoleacetic acid, and indoleacetylglutamine [38]. Studies by Weissbach et al. [39] have indicated that the urinary indoleacetic acid excreted is a product of the metabolism of both intestinal microorganisms and mammalian tissues. This conversion occurs mainly by transamination of tryptophan to indolepyruvic acid, with subsequent decarboxylation to indoleacetic acid. Small amounts of tryptophan are also converted to indoleacetic acid by way of tryptamine. The normal tryptamine excretion by man is very low but can be raised manyfold by the administration of monamine oxidase inhibitors [40].

If intestinal absorption of tryptophan is delayed for some reason (see below), colonic bacteria can transform tryptophan into indolylpropionic acid (indolyl—$CH_2 \cdot CH_2 \cdot COOH$). This is absorbed from the intestine and converted by tissues into indolylacrylic acid (indolyl—$CH{=}CH \cdot COOH$), which is finally excreted as the urinary conjugate, indolylacryloylglycine [41, 42]. Apparently mammalian tissue produces neither indolylpropionic nor indolylacrylic acids directly from tryptophan.

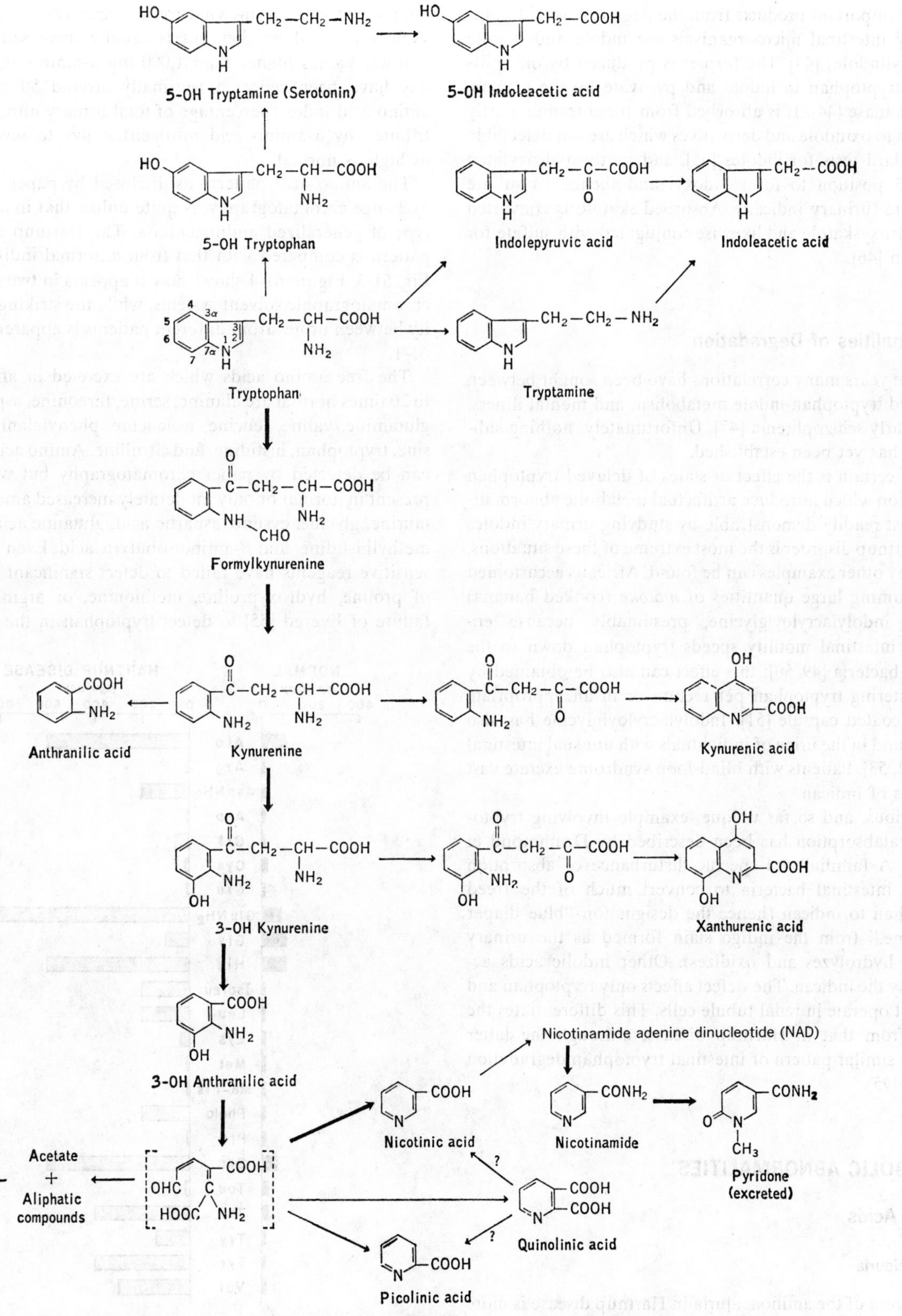

5-OH Tryptamine (Serotonin)

5-OH Indoleacetic acid

5-OH Tryptophan

Indolepyruvic acid

Indoleacetic acid

Tryptophan

Tryptamine

Formylkynurenine

Anthranilic acid

Kynurenine

Kynurenic acid

3-OH Kynurenine

Xanthurenic acid

3-OH Anthranilic acid

Nicotinamide adenine dinucleotide (NAD)

Nicotinic acid

Nicotinamide

Pyridone (excreted)

CO_2 ← Acetate + Aliphatic compounds

Quinolinic acid

Picolinic acid

Figure 61-2. Metabolic pathways which are open to tryptophan. Main pathways are shown in bold arrows.

Other important products from the degradation of tryptophan by intestinal microorganisms are indole and skatole (3-methylindole) [43]. The former is produced by the splitting of tryptophan to indole and pyruvate by the enzyme tryptophanase [44]. It is absorbed from the intestine, partly oxidized to oxindole and derivatives which are not detectable by standard tests for indoles [45], and partly hydroxylated in the 3 position to form indoxyl and thence its sulfate conjugate (urinary indican). Absorbed skatole is converted to 6-hydroxyskatole and likewise conjugated with sulfate for excretion [46].

Abnormalities of Degradation

Over the years many correlations have been sought between deranged tryptophan-indole metabolism and mental illness, particularly schizophrenia [47]. Unfortunately, nothing substantial has yet been established.

More certain is the effect of states of delayed tryptophan absorption which introduce artifactual metabolic abnormalities, most readily demonstrable by studying urinary indoles [48]. Hartnup disorder is the most extreme of these situations, but many other examples can be found. Africans accustomed to consuming large quantities of *matoke* (cooked banana) excrete indolylacryloylglycine, presumably because enhanced intestinal motility speeds tryptophan down to the colonic bacteria [49, 50]; this effect can also be obtained by administering tryptophan per rectum or in an appropriate enteric coated capsule [51]. Indolylacryloylglycine has also been found in the urine of individuals with unusual intestinal flora [52, 53]. Patients with blind-loop syndrome excrete vast amounts of indican.

A serious, and so far unique, example involving tryptophan malabsorption has been described by Drummond et al. [54]. A familial and specific disturbance of absorption permits intestinal bacteria to convert much of the freed tryptophan to indican (hence the designation "blue diaper syndrome," from the indigo stain formed as the urinary indican hydrolyzes and oxidizes). Other indolic acids accompany the indican. The defect affects only tryptophan and does not operate in renal tubule cells. This differentiates the lesion from that in Hartnup disease, although the latter shows a similar pattern of intestinal tryptophan degradation (page 1495).

METABOLIC ABNORMALITIES

Amino Acids

Aminoaciduria

The *pattern* of the aminoaciduria in Hartnup disease is more significant than the total amount of amino acids excreted, so that chromatography must be used in the diagnosis. Total amino acid varies somewhat from case to case and may be slightly affected by diet but is usually increased at least tenfold. Values higher than 1,000 mg α-amino acid-N per day have been reported (normally around 50 mg). The amino acid index (percentage of total urinary nitrogen contributed by α-amino acid nitrogen) is five to seven times as high as normal.

The amino acid pattern, as disclosed by paper and ion-exchange chromatography, is quite unlike that in any other type of generalized aminoaciduria. The Hartnup excretion pattern is compared with that from a normal individual in Fig. 61-3. Figure 61-4 shows how it appears in two different chromatographic solvent systems, while the striking similarity between urines from different patients is apparent in Fig. 61-1.

The free amino acids which are excreted in amounts 5 to 20 times normal are alanine, serine, threonine, asparagine, glutamine, valine, leucine, isoleucine, phenylalanine, tyrosine, tryptophan, histidine, and citrulline. Amino acids which can be detected by paper chromatography but which are present in normal or only moderately increased amounts are taurine, glycine, cystine, aspartic acid, glutamic acid, lysine, methylhistidine, and β-aminoisobutyric acid. Even the most sensitive reagents have failed to detect significant amounts of proline, hydroxyproline, methionine, or arginine. The failure of Evered [55] to detect tryptophan in the urine of

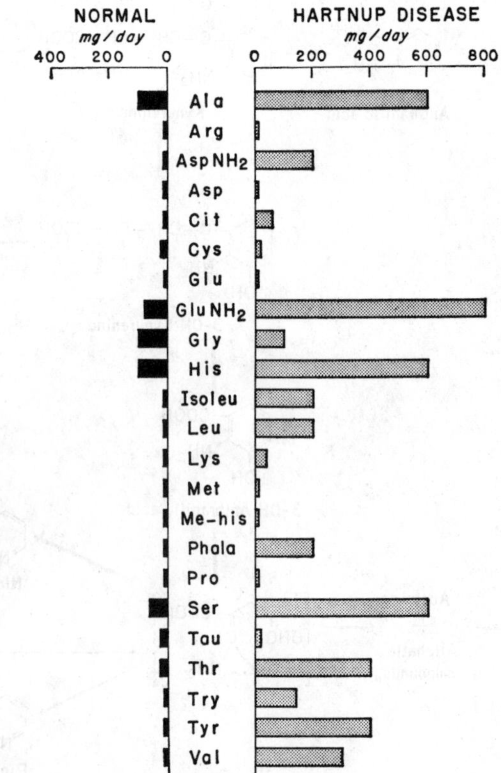

Figure 61-3. The excretion of free amino acids in the urine of normal subjects and patients with Hartnup disease.

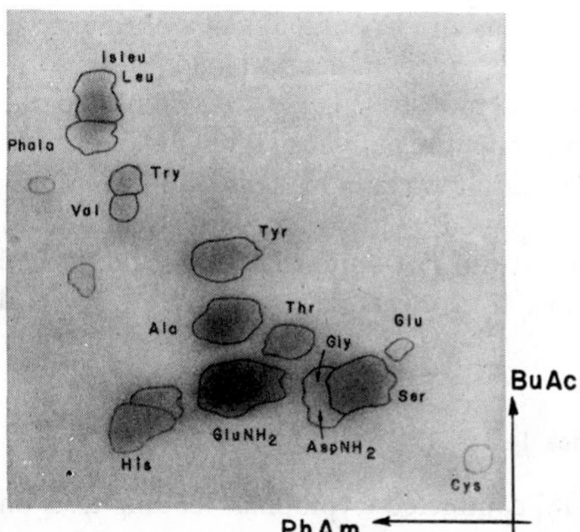

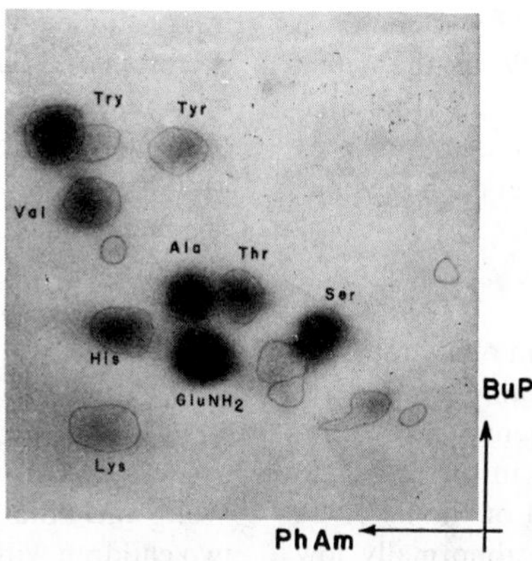

Figure 61-4. Chromatogram of a urine sample from a patient with Hartnup disease in two different solvent systems. On the left the first chromatographic system was butanol–acetic acid–water, and on the right the first system was a butanol–pyridine–water system. In each case the second chromatographic solvent system was phenol–ammonia. The urine was desalted electrolytically.

patients with Hartnup disease was due to the destruction of this amino acid on cation-exchange resins [56], and others have had this difficulty. The excretion of free glutamic acid and aspartic acid is low (as in normal urine), but that of the respective amides is very high. If the urine is left at room temperature for a few hours, the level of free glutamic acid rises at the expense of glutamine, but specimens can be kept deep-frozen for years without deterioration. The free amino acids are all of the L- configuration [57].

Acid hydrolysis of the urine releases no new amino acids and *relatively* little additional amino acid nitrogen, although increased excretion of certain conjugates (e.g., indolylacetylglutamine) undoubtedly occurs.

The aminoaciduria is of *renal* origin, not an "overflow" phenomenon. The renal clearance of total amino acid nitrogen, both in the fasting state [56] and following an oral load of casein [58], is very much higher than normal. Similarly, the renal clearances of those individual amino acids which are excreted in excess are grossly elevated above normal, although the clearances of the amino acids which are not excreted in excess are but little elevated.

Table 61-2 gives some examples from the work of Dent

Table 61-2. RENAL CLEARANCE OF AMINO ACIDS IN HARTNUP DISEASE

Amino acid	Excretion in Hartnup disease	Clearance, ml per min	
		Hartnup	Normal
Total amino acid-N			
Fasting	High	6–22	1.5
Maximum on oral protein load	Very high	25–50	3.0
Threonine	High	70	1.0
Tyrosine	High	66	1.5
Histidine	High	122	6.0
Taurine	Low	1.9	5.0
Proline	Low	0.3	0.1
Cystine	Low	0.4	0.5
Lysine	Low	3.0	0.4

[58], Evered [55], Tada [59], and Halvorsen [60]. Clearances of up to 140 ml per min for histidine [7] approximate the normal glomerular filtration rate, and indeed one patient [60] excreted 17 percent of an intravenous load of L-histidine unchanged within 4 hr (a control yielded only 0.3 percent). For the other amino acids excreted by Hartnup patients, the tubular *reabsorption* of the filtered load at physiological concentrations is calculated to be 50 to 80 percent, as compared to about 98 percent for normal subjects. Either the lesion is far from complete, or, more probably, it only blocks one of several transport mechanisms applicable to each amino acid [33, 61].

These excretion studies indicate a specific disturbance in the renal tubular reabsorption of a certain group of amino acids, namely, those of the monoamino-monocarboxylic group, which are known to share a common system for renal membrane transport. The quartet of amino acids excreted in cystinuria (cystine, lysine, arginine, and ornithine; see Chap. 62) share another transport system, and this is obviously intact in Hartnup patients, as is the third distinct transport system, for the glycine-imino acid group, the system which is defective in certain types of glycinuria (Chap. 63). This concept, that Hartnup disease is one of a trio of genetic errors each involving only one of the systems for amino acid transport, was first suggested by Milne et al. [62] and extended by them to apply to the absorptive systems of the intestine as well as of the renal tubule.

The amino acid excretion pattern is remarkably constant, and is usually unchanged by nicotinamide or other vitamins, drugs, or antibiotics. Isolated reports to the contrary [15, 63] are generally discounted, but there remains the possibility that some variant of the condition is involved.

All other tests of tubular function and renal clearance have given normal results. No urinary reducing sugars are found. The mother of the Hartnup family showed no evidence of an abnormal amino acid clearance, even in response to an oral casein load. In one patient with Hartnup disease to come to autopsy [12], microdissection of kidney nephrons [64] showed that the descending limb of the loop of Henle was completely missing. This severely affected patient had certain unusual features, such as hypoproteinemia and hepatic insufficiency; no equivalent renal abnormality was found in the patients studied by Dauth et al. [16]. While the defect will surely be found at the enzymic, rather than the anatomic, level, in vitro experiments on amino acid uptake by renal cells from Hartnup patients have not yet been possible.

Amino Acid Absorption

It is less easy to demonstrate that the defect in renal transport applies also to absorption in the small intestine, but several studies have shown that: (1) Hartnup patients excrete elevated amounts of the affected amino acids in the feces; (2) the rise in plasma concentration of several of the involved amino acids following an oral loading is abnormally low or delayed, although normal concentrations are found after intravenous administration; and (3) bacterial degradation products from unabsorbed amino acids are found in excess in urine. This has been especially investigated for tryptophan.

Fecal Amino Acids

Fecal amino acid excretion has been studied by two-dimensional paper electrophoresis/chromatography of appropriate fecal extracts [65, 66]. Strong support for the specific lesion of intestinal absorption was provided by the findings of Scriver [65] that the total amount of free amino acids in the feces of a Hartnup patient (on a controlled diet low in plant materials) was manyfold that in normal feces, and that the Hartnup fecal excretion pattern of amino acids closely mirrored the typical Hartnup urinary pattern. When L-tryptophan is given orally, its fecal excretion increases severalfold in patients, but not at all in normal subjects [18]. In Hartnup disease it seems that virtually no D-tryptophan is absorbed, and large amounts of it appear in feces after oral DL-tryptophan [67]. On the other hand, the symptomless infant studied by Seakins and Ersser [66] had a normal fecal excretion of amino acids except under oral load. Malabsorption of tyrosine was demonstrated, and this inhibited the absorption of the other neutral amino acids but not of proline. Malabsorption of histidine was not evident from examining the feces; this also applied to the adult patient studied by Halvorsen [60], and it did not seem that the histidine had been completely lost by conversion to histamine by fecal bacteria.

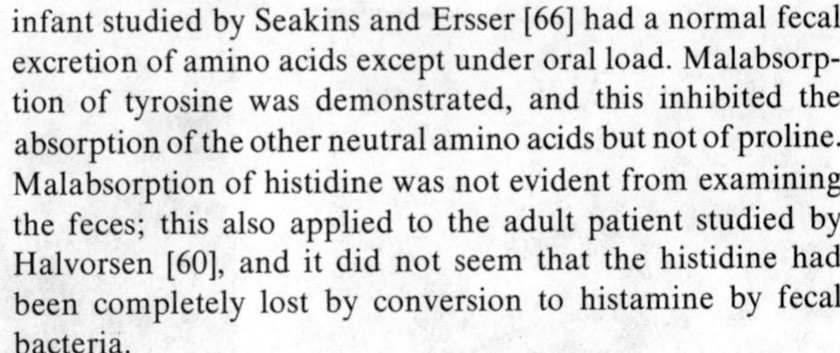

Amino Acid Tolerance Tests

Wong and Pillai [18] conducted tryptophan loading tests on two children with Hartnup disease maintained on a constant protein diet, with 100 mg per kg L-tryptophan added either orally or intravenously. The plasma tryptophan levels were measured at 2-hr intervals. The results (Fig. 61-5) show that intestinal absorption of free tryptophan is delayed and incomplete. In another patient [23], similar studies with single amino acids showed a severely defective intestinal absorption of phenylalanine. Methionine and leucine had delayed absorption; the absorption of proline was normal.

Administration of oral L-histidine gave flat tolerance curves extending over 6 hr, while normal subjects under the same conditions showed a high peak in plasma concentration within 1 hr [60]. The low plasma concentration was interpreted as being due more to the rapid kidney clearance of histidine than to defective absorption. Doubt is cast on this interpretation by recent work of Milne et al. [27*a*]: a *normal* peaked curve for free histidine in plasma is found when this amino acid is given to a Hartnup subject in the form of oral carnosine (β-alanyl-L-histidine); presumably the dipeptide is absorbed normally and then hydrolyzed, in which case the urinary loss of histidine should produce a flat histidine curve if this was the cause of the low plasma concentration found after free histidine. This Hartnup sub-

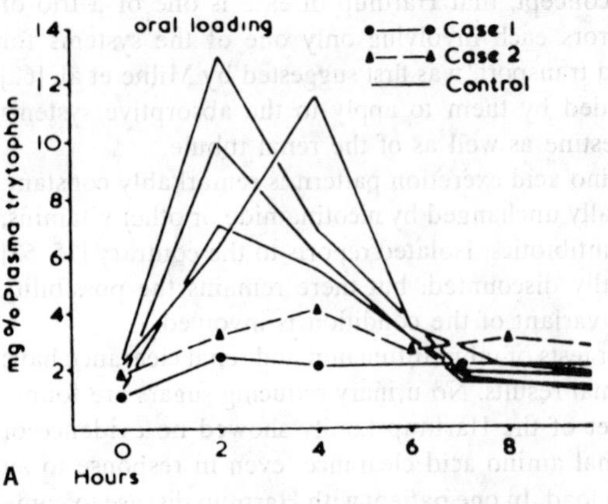

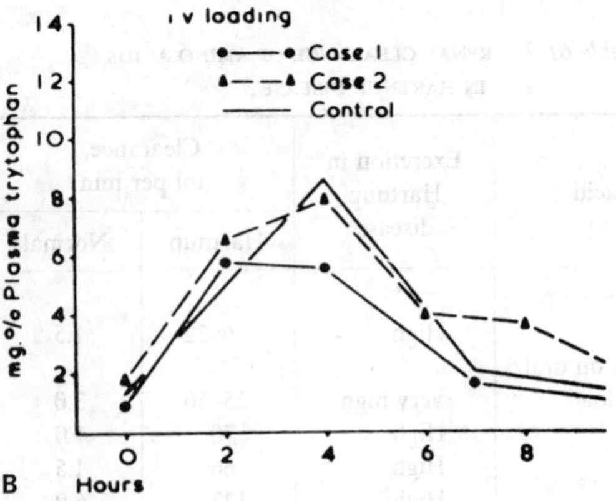

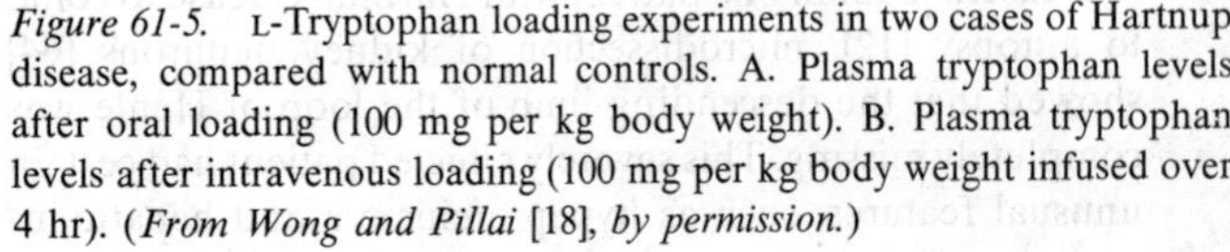

Figure 61-5. L-Tryptophan loading experiments in two cases of Hartnup disease, compared with normal controls. A. Plasma tryptophan levels after oral loading (100 mg per kg body weight). B. Plasma tryptophan levels after intravenous loading (100 mg per kg body weight infused over 4 hr). (*From Wong and Pillai* [18], *by permission.*)

ject also absorbed phenylalanine and tryptophan better when they were in dipeptide form than as the corresponding mixed free amino acids, while the reverse is true in normal subjects. This suggests that amino acid nutrition in Hartnup disease (and possibly in analogous situations) is maintained more by absorption of small peptides than by essential amino acids in free form.

In the two patients who died [16, 64], the intestinal mucosa was not histologically unusual, but study at the electron microscope level is obviously needed. Experiments in vitro on amino acid uptake by intestinal tissue from patients have not been attempted.

Plasma Amino Acids

Many measurements [e.g., 55, 59, 60] have shown that the plasma concentrations of the affected amino acids under standardized conditions are on the low side of normal, down to about 30 percent lower. This could be anticipated from the diminished absorption and increased excretion.

Other Transport Systems for Amino Acids

Sweat and saliva from Hartnup patients have a normal amino acid composition [1]. In vitro, leucocytes from a Hartnup patient concentrated tryptophan and proline against a concentration gradient, but in neither was the uptake significantly different from normal values [68]. A technique for studying amino acid transport in cell cultures of human fibroblasts [69] has been applied to skin cultures from three Hartnup patients. There are strong indications that the rate of uptake of tryptophan by these cells is lower than with normal controls [70].

All these observations emphasize that many biochemically independent transport mechanisms must exist in man, and that Hartnup disease affects only one (or a few) of the different types, and only in specific tissues.

Metabolites of Tryptophan and Indole

Early in the investigations of the Hartnup family [1], a high but variable urinary excretion of indigogenic material (indican) was apparent. This led to a more complete investigation of urinary indoles by paper chromatography. A raised excretion of the indolic acids derived from tryptophan was thus revealed, but this has not proved to be so constant a feature of the disease as was first thought.

Indicanuria

All individuals with "Hartnup" aminoaciduria can also excrete large but variable amounts of indican, almost entirely as indoxyl sulfate. But a small amount of indoxyl-β-glucuronide can accompany it.

Patients of Rodnight and McIlwain and of Hersov and Rodnight [4, 5] excreted up to 400 mg per day compared with the less than 100 mg excreted by normal subjects of the same age. As with normal subjects, indican excretion fell rapidly during a course of oral chlortetracycline. After only 4 days on the antibiotic, indican was barely detectable, even when L-tryptophan was fed in addition [1]. A similar result was obtained using neomycin [11, 71], but succinylsulfathiazole for 7 days had no effect [4]. Antibiotics did not alter the urinary amino acid excretion, and the indicanuria returned to its high level a few days after the cessation of treatment.

Even in Hartnup patients showing a reasonably normal indican excretion, this could be raised dramatically by oral administration of L-tryptophan [1]. The process can be followed by measurements on serial urine samples [18, 67]. In normal subjects there was a slight, variable rise in indican, followed by a fall to normal within 12 hr, representing a tryptophan-to-indican conversion of less than 1.5 percent. By contrast, in Hartnup disease there was a greatly raised excretion, which reached a maximum after 12 hr and persisted for more than 24 hr, with a conversion of 7 to 13 percent.

A patient investigated by Srikantia et al. [13] was exceptional in showing a fivefold rise in indican excretion rate within 1 hr of a tryptophan load. This returned to normal within 3 hr, with a further peak after 3 hr more. It has been suggested that this patient represents a variant of Hartnup disease, with the absorption defect applying only in the kidney tubule. This is discussed later.

The urinary indoxyl derivatives are final excretion products, which are formed in the liver from indole absorbed from the colon. Here it must arise from the action of intestinal microorganisms on the tryptophan which was not absorbed from the jejunum because of the transport defect. Studies of the indole-producing bacteria from the feces of Hartnup patients [72] have failed to show that chronic exposure to tryptophan has altered the colonic flora in type or amount from that normally found. On the other hand, there is little or no excretion of 6-hydroxyskatole sulfate, the final product of intestinal skatole formation characteristic of malabsorption syndromes.

The intestinal indole does not appear to have any direct effect on the amino acid transport, but De Laey et al. [63] have suggested an indirect effect by way of nicotinamide formation. This will be discussed later. Certainly patients with blindloop syndrome excrete vast amounts of indican without the development of amino aciduria.

Indolylacetic Acid and Its Congeners

Paper chromatographic studies [73] revealed that E.H., the first of the Hartnup family investigated, excreted indolylacetic acid (IAA) at a considerably higher level than normal [1]. This was particularly true during his acute bouts of ataxia and rash, but even after clinical recovery the urinary abnormality was generally present. The IAA was always ac-

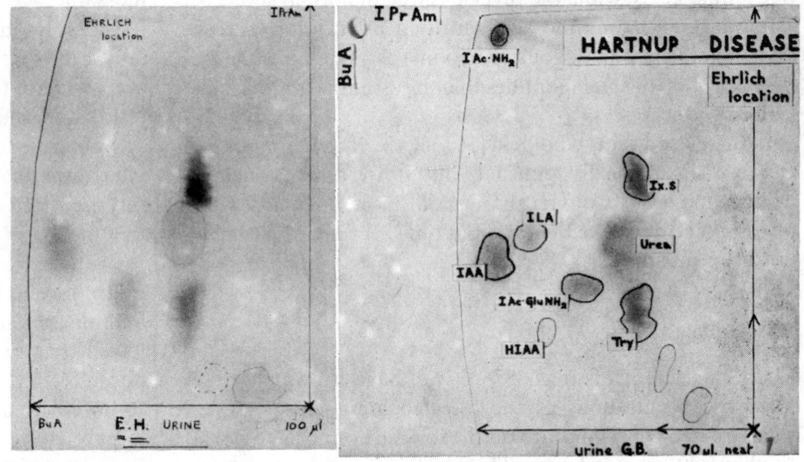

Figure 61-6. Urinary indole patterns in Hartnup disease. *Left:* Paper chromatogram of urine from patient E.H. [1]. 100 μl urine was chromatographed with ascending solvents: isopropanol-ammonia, first and up; butanol-acetic acid, second, right to left. Compounds were located with *p*-dimethylaminobenzaldehyde (Ehrlich's reagent). The key is found in the right-hand photograph. Note the central urea spot (normally yellow), the indican spot (*Ix.S*) (brown), and the triad of spots due to indolylacetic acid (IAA), indolylacetylglutamine, and tryptophan. This pattern is typical of Hartnup disease, although the relative intensity of spots is variable. *Right:* Paper chromatogram of urine from patient G.B. [8]. This chromatogram shows an additional spot due to indolyllactic acid (ILA) not found in other cases of Hartnup disease. (*By permission of Baron et al.* [1]; *Weyers and Bickel* [8].)

companied by a conjugation product, indolylacetyl-L-glutamine. This conjugation product is the one expected from the liver "detoxication" of IAA in man. The other possible conjugate, indolylacetylglucuronide, has been present occasionally but only in moderate amount [8].

These indoles, after two-dimensional paper chromatography and location with Ehrlich's reagent, showed a distribution pattern quite as characteristic as the amino acid pattern (Fig. 61-6). Similar indolic patterns were found with urine from the other affected members of the Hartnup family; the unaffected members had normal (barely detectable) excretion of indolic acid (less than 10 mg per day). During one period of hospitalization, the free IAA excretion in E.H. varied from 50 to 200 mg per day on a normal varied diet. Five years later his IAA excretion was normal, although that of a younger brother was 70 mg per day (35 percent in the conjugated form). Almost all the known cases of Hartnup disease have shown a higher-than-normal excretion of indolic acids on some occasion. Exact comparisons are not possible because IAA is excreted by man through a diffusion mechanism involving increase of clearance with rise of urinary pH [74] and few of the measurements have been made under conditions of pH control. It is under the stimulus of an oral tryptophan load that indolic acid production becomes an obvious and invariant feature of Hartnup disease.

Effect of Tryptophan Loading

The oral administration of L-tryptophan to normal subjects in quantities of about 70 mg per kg body weight causes a sharp sixfold rise in free and conjugated urinary IAA [67]. The peak is reached at 2 hr, and the excretion is back to its normal low level in 8 hr. The total conversion of such a load to urinary indolic acids is about 0.2 percent. In Hartnup disease, the rise is several times larger still, does not reach its peak until the eighth to tenth hour, and persists at a high level for at least 24 hr (Fig. 61-7). The total conversion can be as high as 2 percent, not allowing for unchanged tryptophan still found in the feces.

Hartnup patients on oral tryptophan loading also excrete large quantities of indolylacryloylglycine (I-Acr-Gly), with the same 8-hr lag period that applies to IAA production [71, 75]; they may even excrete small amounts of I-Acr-Gly on a normal diet. In contrast, normal subjects never produce I-Acr-Gly unless free tryptophan is forced into contact with the colonic bacteria (see Abnormalities of Degradation, above); even a large oral load will not do this provided the usual absorption mechanisms are operative.

The direct or indirect source of these indolic acids is the bacterial metabolism of tryptophan. It is therefore obvious that, in Hartnup disease, tryptophan taken orally, or released from protein *in situ,* may be in prolonged contact with the flora of the lower reaches of the intestine, resulting in the production of abnormally large amounts of decomposition products. Some of these are absorbed, and finally excreted in the urine.

Full support for this explanation comes from the effect of intestinal antibiotics in Hartnup patients. Neomycin (with nystatin) not only lowers the excretion of all the indolic acids to somewhat below the "normal" level but virtually abolishes any rise after oral tryptophan loading [9, 63, 71]. It is possible that the neomycin slightly inhibits tryptophan or IAA absorption from the intestine [76], but this could not account for more than a small part of the dramatic effect.

Crawford [50] has applied the term *pseudo Hartnup* to conditions where a florid urinary indolic excretion is produced by dietary measures. This terminology is to be deprecated, because the situation lacks the only constant characteristic of Hartnup disorder, namely the specific hyperamino aciduria.

There is no difference between normal and Hartnup subjects in the output of indican and indolic acids after intravenous tryptophan [18].

If DL-tryptophan is fed to normal subjects, indolyllactic acid (ILA) appears in the urine in large quantities, and is presumably formed from indolylpyruvic acid produced by the action of D-amino acid oxidase. Hartnup patients react quite differently. There is little excretion of ILA, and most of the D-tryptophan is recovered from the feces, presumably because the absorption block for the D-isomer is virtually complete [67]. It is remarkable, therefore, that in one case of Hartnup disease, but one only, ILA was a constant urinary component [8] (Fig. 61-6). This lack of ILA indicates that most of the urinary IAA is derived from tryptophan through bacterially produced tryptamine and not through indolylpyruvic acid.

Other Urinary Indoles

Chromatographic methods have failed to disclose indolylpyruvic acid or its decomposition products in the urine of Hartnup patients [77]. Oral indolylpyruvic acid is treated identically by normal subjects and Hartnup patients, except that the latter show an increased tryptophan output [71]. This suggests that the amino acid transport defect does not extend to the corresponding oxo-acids.

The urinary excretion of tryptamine is within normal limits in Hartnup patients [5, 51]. This may only be tryptamine produced locally in the kidney and does not indicate the possible rate of tryptamine formation in other tissues or in the intestine [72]. Tryptamine is metabolized to IAA by way of the corresponding aldehyde. Experiments to see if this oxidative pathway could be diverted through a reductive pathway by the administration of ethanol [78] were unsuccessful; no urinary tryptophol or its conjugates were detectable in Hartnup or control subjects, before or after the consumption of large quantities of alcohol [51].

Indolic Acids in the Blood

The whole blood and plasma indolic acids have been studied chromatographically in some patients with Hartnup disease [5]. Apart from a slightly elevated concentration of indoxyl sulfate, patients and normal subjects were indistinguishable. The renal clearance values for indolic acids are normally very high [79]. The clearance of indolylacetylglutamine is at least 150 ml per min, and it may be synthesized, at least in part, from IAA in the kidney.

The whole blood and serum levels for serotonin (5-hydroxytryptamine) were on the low side of the normal range, in parallel with the low urinary 5-HT and 5-HIAA excretions [5, 18]. This may represent a slight diversion of tryptophan from serotonin formation.

Nicotinic Acid Intermediates

Because of the pellagra-like symptoms of Hartnup disease, a possible enzymic block in the usual tryptophan-kynurenine-nicotinic acid pathway (Fig. 61-2) was early suspected [1]. In one patient on a normal diet the urinary excretion of nicotinic acid and its derivatives was on the low side of normal and was surprisingly little elevated by the oral administration of tryptophan [1].

Although complicated by the possibility that the amino acid kynurenine is one of those affected by the Hartnup transport defect, later work has corroborated the earlier findings. Normal subjects converted 3 to 7 percent of oral L-tryptophan to urinary kynurenine, with the peak excretion rate (about 80 mg per hr) after 2 to 4 hr. Hartnup patients converted only 0.5 to 1.5 percent to kynurenine, with a maximum excretion rate of 10 mg per hr although still after 2 to 4 hr [18, 67].

This is shown in Fig. 61-7, which makes it clear that kynurenine is only formed from absorbed tryptophan and is therefore liable to be in short supply in Hartnup disease. Following the oral tryptophan load in affected subjects, there was no accumulation of formylkynurenine, the intermediate before kynurenine [67], or increase in products after kynurenine, such as xanthurenic acid [71], N-methylnicotinamide [68], or N-methylpyridone carboxamide [10]. Administered nicotinamide was handled normally, as judged by urinary products [10].

All of this strongly supports the original suggestion [1] that there is diminished operation of the tryptophan-kynurenine-nicotinamide metabolic pathway in Hartnup patients, but whether this is solely due to the diminished availability of tryptophan, or is also due to some noxious

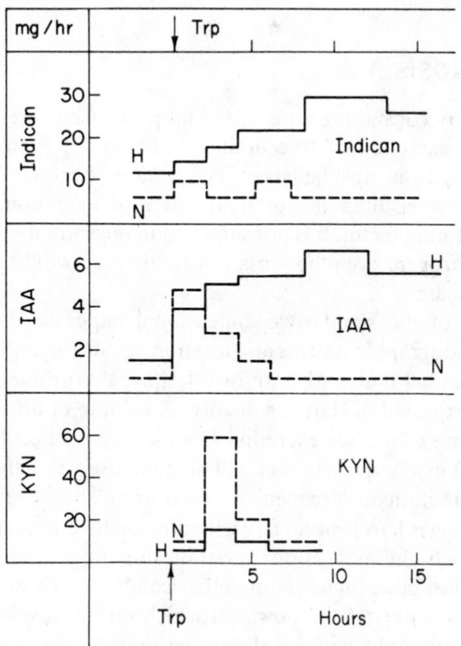

Figure 61-7. Urinary excretion (mg per hr) of tryptophan derivatives following oral L-tryptophan (about 70 mg per kg body weight) administered to normal subjects (N – – –) and to Hartnup patients (H ——). These are idealized responses, averaged from the results of several investigators.

factor, or to some enzymic abnormality, remains an open question.

De Laey and his group [63] claimed that, in rats, the uptake and metabolism of tryptophan were enhanced by nicotinamide and depressed by indole. If this applies to man, then the biochemical abnormalities of Hartnup disease would represent a vicious circle which could be broken by massive nicotinamide therapy. Although there is general agreement that the dermatitis and neuropsychiatric symptoms are improved by nicotinamide (as with pellagra), only De Laey [63] and Fois [15] have ever claimed that the hyperamino aciduria or the amino acid uptake were measurably affected by nicotinamide (see [19] and [21] for contrary observations).

Other Biochemical Investigations

Considering the ominous nature of the Hartnup amino acid lesion, it is remarkable how normal the other biochemical and physiologic processes appear to remain.

It might be expected that tryptophan would not be the only poorly absorbed amino acid to undergo intestinal decomposition, yet Hartnup patients have a normal excretion pattern of urinary phenolic acids, even after an oral load of tyrosine [21, 51].

Studies of urinary and fecal porphyrins [1, 20] have failed to show anything that could cause or exacerbate the photosensitivity.

DIAGNOSIS

The only constant feature of Hartnup disease is the characteristic excretion of free amino acids, and it is upon this that diagnosis must be based. The *pattern* of excreted amino acids, rather than the total amino acid excretion, is the determining factor. It is not sufficient to measure total amino acid nitrogen, even though a low total value would exclude the disease.

Any of the simple two-dimensional paper or thin-layer chromatographic systems and location agents for amino acids will serve. Figures 61-3 and 61-4 show the urinary amino acids expected in Hartnup disease. A volume of urine corresponding to a 2-sec excretion from a 24-hr collection on a normal or low-protein diet will give intensely reacting spots with the ninhydrin reagent. Normal urine shows very little. Desalting is hardly necessary with this small volume. Patients show only the most minor variation in pattern, and nothing like it has been found in any other condition. Those screening procedures of the newborn which do not involve *urine* chromatography will not detect the defect.

The only alternative diagnosis for Hartnup disease would be pellagra, and in the few cases of true dietary pellagra examined [1] the amino acid excretion was low or normal.

The indolic excretion is not constant enough to be the basis of a diagnostic test, but the abnormal response to oral L-tryptophan loading (70 mg per kg) accompanied by chromatography of serial samples might be used. Hartnup disease would be associated with a greater-than-normal excretion of indolylacetic acid, indolylacryloylglycine, and indican, persisting for 24 hr at least.

Hartnup disease is not excluded by a normal indole excretion, but all patients with a high indican or high IAA excretion should be further examined for the Hartnup amino acid excretion pattern.

Hartnup disease should be suspected in patients with the following signs: pellagra not due to gross dietary deficiency; photosensitive rash, especially if accompanied by neurologic changes; reversible ataxia, especially when siblings are affected similarly; high excretion of indican or indolylacetic acid. The disorder is so rare that every case should be reported in the medical literature without delay; otherwise, it may never be possible to find those minor variants in the condition which will ultimately enable the lesion to be located at a molecular level.

TREATMENT

The paucity of cases and their variability have not made it easy to evaluate possible courses of treatment. Similarity of the symptoms to those of pellagra has led in many instances to oral nicotinamide therapy (40 to 200 mg amide or acid per day). Marked improvement in the dermatitis and neurologic picture has usually followed [9, 19, 26], but improvement may occur without treatment. In view of the high urinary loss of amino acids, a high-protein diet or supplement has been prescribed and seems beneficial. Oral neomycin would seem worth trying during an acute attack. Barrier creams have not usually improved the skin sensitivity [14, 20]. Monoamine oxidase inhibitors are contraindicated.

The ultimate prognosis seems good. Amelioration comes with adulthood. Two symptomless Hartnup subjects have children, all in excellent health [23].

GENETICS

The 43 proved cases (18 males, 25 females) are distributed among 28 families with a total of 99 children (Table 61-1). Sibs are affected in 10 families. In at least seven families, the parents are consanguine, although two families [8, 23] know of no blood relationship as far back as 1416 and 1630, respectively! Ten of the families come from England, ten from continental Europe, two from Scandinavia, two from the United States, and one each from South America, India, Japan, and Australia.

The consanguinity rate and the segregation ratios are not significantly different from those expected if Hartnup disease is the homozygous (double dose) manifestation of a non-X-linked rare allele (not necessarily the same allele in every case).

This conclusion must be considered in the light of the biochemical pedigree of the Japanese family extensively studied by Oyanagi et al. [22]. Two of the four living children from a second-cousin marriage had the biochemical and clinical characteristics of Hartnup disease. The other two children (symptomless) were described as also showing the characteristic chromatographic patterns of urinary amino acids and indoles, and the same was claimed for the healthy paternal and maternal grandfathers (first cousins), and for two healthy first cousins of the parents on the maternal side. Oyanagi did not count these six individuals as cases of Hartnup disease because they were clinically healthy, and they are not therefore included in Table 61-1 or the totals given above, although they should be by the criteria generally applied. These subjects were considered to be "carrier members of Hartnup disease." On the basis of autosomal recessive transmission, this conclusion fits the pedigree perfectly were it not for the fact that no other obligate heterozygote shows the slightest defect in renal amino acid reabsorption. Admittedly the two obvious patients were severely affected, and the allele concerned may be a vicious variant that even shows in single dose.

Heterozygosity

Both parents of each fully affected (homozygous) individual would be heterozygous carriers of the offending allele, and might be expected to show a mild form of the defect. All the parents and most of the near relatives of Hartnup cases have been examined for the characteristic amino aciduria; all were uniformly normal, with the exception discussed above [22]. The mother of the Hartnup children has a normal amino acid clearance, even in response to a casein load [58]. The progeny of an individual with Hartnup disorder have a normal amino acid excretion [23].

There are several indications that a heterozygote can often be distinguished from a normal subject by the response to tryptophan. The parents of two Hartnup patients [18] had a delayed peak for plasma tryptophan following an oral load. Similarly challenged, all the children from the Hartnup patients excreted abnormally large amounts of indican, IAA, and I-Acr-Gly [23]. One of these obligate heterozygotes also has a skin reaction to sunlight, in line with other observations [8, 9] of a high incidence of photosensitivity in apparently nonaffected kindred. The patient erroneously diagnosed as having Hartnup disease solely on the basis of a rash and an indolic excretion [80] might therefore be a heterozygote for the disorder. It is strange that some heterozygotes should appear to be almost as sensitive as are homozygotes to tryptophan-nicotinamide insufficiency.

In complex organs like intestine or kidney, the total transport difference between the heterozygote and the normal homozygote could be small indeed. Confirmation of the mode of genetic transmission of the disorder may require the discovery of a simpler in vitro system possessing only the "group" transport mechanisms for amino acids—perhaps cells cultured from intestine or kidney with the more specific transport mechanisms chemically suppressed.

ATTEMPTED RATIONALIZATION OF CLINICAL MANIFESTATIONS AND BIOCHEMICAL DISORDERS

It has already been hinted that even the small number of Hartnup subjects so far uncovered may include several variants of the condition. Any present attempt to relate the total clinical manifestations to the total biochemical findings may be doomed to failure from the start. Nevertheless, a tolerably satisfying picture is beginning to emerge, at least on the nutritional side. The renal defect does not seem important (contrast cystinuria). Even the urinary loss of amino acid is quantitatively small compared to variations of dietary intake. It is the intestinal defect which is the key, not only to the obvious consequences of the disorder but also to why the consequences are not more striking than they are.

Nicotinamide Deficiency

Hartnup subjects lose much of their dietary tryptophan by fecal and urinary excretion of the free amino acid and by its bacterial decomposition to nutritionally useless indolic acids. There is no reason to doubt that the pellagrinous rash is due to inefficient tryptophan utilization and metabolism, which contributes to mild nicotinamide insufficiency, possibly in those tissues which prefer that this factor be formed *in situ*. In other words, the threshold below which diets become inadequate for requirements of nicotinamide has been raised. In the rat, all the enzymes needed for the biosynthesis of nicotinamide from tryptophan are detectable in liver but not in brain [81]. Thus it is reasonable to suppose that one tissue has priority over another for the available dietary nicotinamide. Any situation which diminishes the tryptophan-nicotinamide conversion could be expected to have similar results. One such patient, a Japanese girl from a first-cousin marriage, has been described. The defect was termed *tryptophanuria with dwarfism* [36] and was associated not with impaired tryptophan transport, for the blood tryptophan level was high, but with an enzymic inability to effect an adequate conversion of tryptophan to kynurenine. The similarity of this clinical condition to Hartnup disease strongly supports the belief that, in the latter too, it is a deficiency of endogenous nicotinamide formed from intracellular tryptophan by way of kynurenine that is responsible for the photosensitive rash, and possibly the ataxia. On the other hand, why is the pellagrinous rash not characteristic of the "blue diaper syndrome" [54], in which tryptophan malabsorption also occurs? The diminished production of nicotinamide in Hartnup subjects could stem from causes other than the lessened amount of available tryptophan. For example, it could arise through a partial failure in the stabilization of tryptophan pyrrolase because of lack of tryptophan substrate [35, 35*a*] or because the transport lesion prevents tryptophan from gaining access to a special nicotinamide-synthesizing "compartment."

Toxic Episodes

The causes of the short-lived neurological and psychotic disturbances are less clear. They could be equivalent to the dementia of dietary pellagra (presumably due to nicotinamide deficiency in the nervous system), a possibility supported by their appearance only during periods of intense rash or obviously inadequate nutrition. Alternatively, they could represent the toxic effect on the nervous system of metabolites produced by the intestinal flora from unabsorbed amino acids. Milne originally cast indolic acids in this role [67], but IAA can be consumed and absorbed in vast quantities without ill effects [82]. Tryptamine has also been indicted as the culprit [83], but attempts to detect an elevated turnover of tissue tryptamine in Hartnup patients have been unsuccessful (p. 1497). Non-Hartnup patients on monoamine oxidase blockade, or with tryptamine-producing tumors [84], show no ataxia, rash, or amino aciduria. Indolylacrylic acid could be expected to have unfortunate effects when absorbed. It can inhibit liver tryptophan pyrrolase in vitro [85] and could thereby diminish still further an already strained conversion of tryptophan to nicotinamide. It has been claimed to cause photosensitivity in animals [14].

Persistent neonatal diarrhea has been a feature of some clinical cases [9]; indeed, one infant was originally thought to have disaccharidase deficiency [28]. The cause could be acidic products from the bacterial fermentation of free amino acids remaining unabsorbed in the intestine.

Alternative Absorption Systems

Hartnup disease causes some minor generalized nutritional defects, not unexpectedly in view of the poor absorption and accelerated loss of many of the essential amino acids. From childhood, almost all Hartnup patients are short in stature, with a mean height about 5 cm below the normal mean of adult males [86]. What *is* surprising is the mildness of the manifestations of a disorder that might be imagined to be equivalent to gross protein malnutrition. For example, in a healthy adult with the disorder, the absorption of L-phenylalanine from an oral dose of the free amino acid was only 25 percent of the average normal absorption [27]. This degree of impaired absorption for this essential amino acid would rapidly cause a negative nitrogen balance, which was certainly not the case. The *normal* intestinal absorption of amino acids fed in dipeptide form suggests that amino acid nutrition in Hartnup disorder is maintained more by the unaffected transport of small peptides derived from the partial hydrolysis of protein than by the impaired transport of the free amino acids.

This intestinal system for peptide absorption is an additional complication to add to the multitude of alternative transport systems already postulated to apply to amino acids. In "true" Hartnup disease, the defect applies to the high-capacity system for the monoamino-monocarboxylic acids in intestine and in renal tubule. Such a system probably operates under conditions of amino acid abundance, to conserve these desirable materials against less fortunate times to come [32]. It is unlikely that group transport systems could be used to control the amino acid milieu of internal cells, so the Hartnup transport defect probably does not apply at many sites other than intestine and kidney. There is no reason why the genetically determined defect *must* apply to both tissues. If the lesion affects a factor common to the intestinal and the renal mechanisms then both will be affected, as in true Hartnup disease. But if the defect disturbed a component unique to the renal mechanism, then the typical hyperaminoaciduria could be present without intestinal disturbances. Such variants have been suggested [13, 87].

On the other hand, even if the characteristic defect is present in intestine and kidney, the intestinal defect could be overwhelmed by simultaneous hyperactivity of the alternative absorption systems; almost nothing is known about the genetic variability of these latter.

Individual Amino Acids

Hartnup disease is considered to affect the group transport of the monoamino-monocarboxylic acids. It might be expected that this group would include *methionine,* but it does not. This could mean the operation of an independent system for methionine transport, a possibility strengthened by the existence of the *methionine malabsorption syndrome* [88], which is probably identical with "oasthouse disease" [89]. In this familial condition there is defective transport which largely affects methionine, with some diminished absorption of aromatic and branched-chain amino acids as well. Intestine and kidney are both affected, and methionine appears in the urine, especially after an oral load. Some of the unabsorbed methionine is covered by colonic bacteria to α-hydroxybutyric acid (the "oasthouse" smell); this acid may be responsible for the severe neurological abnormalities, because a low-methionine diet rapidly ameliorates the clinical picture [87].

There is no doubt that, in Hartnup disease, the renal clearance of *lysine* is raised manyfold, and elevated urinary excretion of lysine has been reported, especially by Seakins and Ersser [21]. Lysine is one of the dibasic transport group, and again this is out of line. Of course, there is no reason why the transport groups should not overlap a little, and the continued study of patients with Hartnup disorder and its variants may be the best way of finding out if they do.

SUMMARY

1 Hartnup disease is characterized by an intermittent red, scaly, pellagra-like rash appearing after exposure to sunlight, by attacks of cerebellar ataxia, and occasionally by psychiatric changes ranging from emotional instability to delirium. A considerable proportion of patients are of somewhat lowered intelligence, but this is not a necessary accompaniment.

2 The disease was originally observed in four out of eight offspring of a first-cousin marriage. Other patients, including 9 more sets of sibs, have brought the total of known cases to 43. Present information is consistent with the disease being the homozygous manifestation of a rare autosomal allele, but no test for the heterozygous state is known.

3 The single recognized constant feature of the disease is a massive amino aciduria involving only that group of monoamino-monocarboxylic acids known to share a common renal reabsorption mechanism. This provides the only certain diagnostic test.

4 The amino aciduria arises because patients with the disease have a diminished power for the tubular reabsorption of these particular amino acids. The specific defect also applies to intestinal absorption from the jejunum, so that patients retain these specific amino acids in the intestine for abnormally long periods. This allows intestinal bacteria to convert them into decomposition products, some of which are absorbed.

5 The effect of intestinal decomposition is particularly noticeable in the case of tryptophan: often on a normal diet and always after an oral tryptophan load, patients excrete large quantities of indoxyl sulfate (indican), indolylacetic acid, and indolylacryloylglycine, all of which can be shown by intestinal sterilization to be products of bacterial action.

6 Patients have a lowered ability to convert tryptophan to kynurenine and nicotinamide. This is attributed to the deviation of tryptophan from its normal metabolic route because of the absorption defect, but other reasons cannot be excluded.

7 In general patients have responded satisfactorily to prolonged oral administration of nicotinamide.

8 Unlike the related condition of cystinuria, the pathologic significance of Hartnup disease does not seem to lie in the amino aciduria which provides its diagnosis. It is suggested that it is the accompanying absorption defect in intestine or other nonrenal sites, which:

(*a*) Allows formation of decomposition products which are toxic to the central nervous system but the nature of which is still conjectural.

(*b*) Diminishes the amount of nicotinamide synthesized from tryptophan, thus causing "pellagra" at times of metabolic strain.

(*c*) Diminishes somewhat the availability of essential amino acids, with consequent general or specific malnutrition. Alternative intestinal mechanisms must be responsible for much compensatory absorption.

9 The importance of Hartnup disease lies in the clue it has already provided to the existence of general absorption defects in other diseases. It may yet help to elucidate the mechanism by which a genetic defect can specifically diminish the absorption of certain amino acids across particular types of cell membranes.

BIBLIOGRAPHY

1. Baron, D. N., Dent, C. E., Harris, H., Hart, E. W., and Jepson, J. B.: Hereditary pellagra-like skin rash with temporary cerebellar ataxia, constant renal amino aciduria, and other bizarre biochemical features. Lancet, **2**, 421, 1956.
2. Hickish, G. W.: Pellagra in an English child. Arch. Dis. Child., **30**, 195, 1955.
3. Hersov, L. A.: A case of childhood pellagra with psychosis. J. Ment. Sci., **101**, 878, 1955.
4. Rodnight, R., and McIlwain, H.: Indicanuria and the psychosis of a pellagrin. J. Ment. Sci., **101**, 884, 1955.
5. Hersov, L. A., and Rodnight, R.: Hartnup disease in psychiatric practice; clinical and biochemical features of three cases. J. Neurol. Neurosurg. Psychiat., **23**, 40, 1960.
6. Henderson, W.: A case of Hartnup disease. Arch. Dis. Child., **33**, 114, 1958.
7. Jonxis, J. H.: Oligophrenia phenylpyruvica en de Hartnupziekte. Nederl. T. Geneesk., **101**, 569, 1957.
8. Weyers, H., and Bickel, H.: Photodermatose mit Aminoacidurie, Indolaceturie, und cerebralen Manifestationen (Hartnup-Syndrom). Klin. Wschr., **36**, 893, 1958.
9. Halvorsen, K., and Halvorsen, S.: Hartnup disease. Pediatrics, **31**, 29, 1963.
10. Albers, F. H., and Wadman, S. K.: Een patiënte met H-ziekte. Maandschr. Kindergeneesk., **29**, 102, 1961.
11. Hooft, C., De Laey, P., Timmermans, J., and Snoeck, J.: La maladie de Hartnup. Acta Paediat. Belg., **16**, 281, 1962 [in French]; De Hartnupziekte. Maandschr. Kindergeneesk., **31**, 75, 1963 [in Flemish]. (See also ref. 63.)
12. Visakorpi, J. K., Hjelt, L., Lahikainen, T., and Ohman, S.: Hartnup disease in two siblings. Ann. Paediat. Fenn., **10**, 42, 1964.
13. Srikantia, S. G., Venkatachalam, P. S., and Reddy, V.: Clinical and biochemical features of a case of Hartnup disease. Brit. Med. J., **1**, 282, 1964.
14. Kimmig, J.: Hartnup-syndrom. Arch. Klin. Exp. Derm., **219**, 753, 1964.
15. Fois, A., and Lecchini, L.: Acute cerebellar ataxia associated with some features of the Hartnup syndrome. Helv. Paediat. Acta, **19**, 42, 1964.
16. Dauth, K. H., Dietel, K., and Erbert, W.: Das Hartnupsyndrom. Bericht über einen tödlichen Krankheitsverlauf. Z. Kinderheilk., **95**, 103, 1966.
17. Nielsen, E. G., Vedso, S., and Zimmerman-Nielsen, C.: Hartnup disease in three siblings. Danish Med. Bull., **13**, 155, 1966.
18. Wong, P. W. K., and Pillai, P. M.: Clinical and biochemical observations in two cases of Hartnup disease. Arch. Dis. Child., **41**, 383, 1966.
19. Wong, P. W. K., Lambert, A. M., Pillai, P. M., and Jones, P. M.: Observations on nicotinic acid therapy in Hartnup disease. Arch. Dis. Child., **42**, 642, 1967.
20. Ashurst, P. J.: Hydroa vacciniforme occurring in association with Hartnup disease. Brit. J. Derm., **81**, 486, 1969.
21. Seakins, J. W. T., and Ersser, R. S.: Effects of amino acid loads on a healthy infant with the biochemical features of Hartnup disease. Arch. Dis. Child., **42**, 682, 1967.
22. Oyanagi, K., Takagi, N., Kitabatake, M., and Nakao, T.: Hartnup disease. Tohoku J. Exp. Med., **91**, 383, 1967.
23. Pomeroy, J., Efron, M. L., Dayman, J., and Hoefnagel, D.: Hartnup disorder in a New England family. New Eng. J. Med., **278**, 1214, 1968.
24. Boat, T., and Yarbro, M.: Hartnup's disease in an infant. *Abstracts Soc. Pediat. Res.*, 38th annual meeting, May 1968, p. 159.

25. Lopez, F., Velez, H., and Toro, G.: Hartnup disease in two Colombian siblings. Neurology (Minneap.), **19,** 71, 1969.
26. Milne, M. D.: Hartnup disease. Biochem. J., **111,** 3P, 1969.
27. Asatoor, A. M., and Navab, F.: Studies on intestinal absorption of amino acids and a dipeptide in a case of Hartnup disease. Gut, **11,** 373, 1970.
27a. Asatoor, A. M., Cheng, B., Edwards, K. D. G., Lant, A. F., Matthews, D. M., Milne, M. D., Navab, F., and Richards, A. J.: Intestinal absorption of two dipeptides in Hartnup disease. Gut, **11,** 380, 1970.
28. Raine, D. N. [Birmingham, England]: Unpublished observations.
29. Stevens, B. J., and Pitt, D. [Melbourne, Australia]: Unpublished observations.
30. Milne, M. D.: Disorders of aminoacid metabolism. Scientific Basis of Medicine, Annual Reviews, p. 149, 1961.
31. Jepson, J. B.: Hartnup disease, in *The Metabolic Basis of Inherited Disease,* edited by J. B. Stanbury, J. B. Wyngaarden, and D. S. Fredrickson, 2d ed., chap. 57, New York, 1966.
32. Scriver, C. R.: Inborn errors of aminoacid metabolism. Brit. Med. Bull., **25,** 35, 1969.
33. Scriver, C. R.: The human biochemical genetics of aminoacid transport. Pediatrics, **44,** 348, 1969.
34. Meister, A.: *Biochemistry of the Amino Acids,* 2d ed., Academic, New York, 1965.
35. Feigelson, P., Feigelson, M., and Greengard, O.: Comparison of the mechanisms of hormonal and substrate induction of rat liver tryptophan pyrrolase. Recent Progr. Hormone Res., **18,** 491, 1962.
35a. Schimke, R. T., Sweeney, E. W., and Berlin, C. M.: The roles of synthesis and degradation in the control of rat liver tryptophan pyrrolase. J. Biol. Chem., **240,** 322, 1965.
36. Tada, K., Ito, H., Wada, Y., and Arakawa, T.: Congenital tryptophanuria with dwarfism. Tohoku J. Exp. Med., **80,** 118, 1963.
37. Goldsmith, G. A.: Niacin-tryptophan relationships in man and niacin requirement. Amer. J. Clin. Nutr., **6,** 479, 1958.
38. Armstrong, M. D., Shaw, K. N. F., Gortatowski, M. J., and Singer, H.: The indole acids of human urine. J. Biol. Chem., **232,** 17, 1958.
39. Weissbach, H., King, W., Sjoerdsma, A., and Udenfriend, S.: Formation of indole-3-acetic acid and tryptamine in animals. J. Biol. Chem., **234,** 81, 1959.
40. Sjoerdsma, A., Oates, J. A., Zaltzman, P., and Udenfriend, S.: Identification and assay of urinary tryptamine. J. Pharmacol. Exp. Ther., **126,** 217, 1959.
41. Smith, Heather G., Smith, W. R. D., and Jepson, J. B.: Interconversions of indolic acids by bacteria and rat tissue—possible relevance to Hartnup disorder. Clin. Sci., **34,** 333, 1968.
42. Smith, Heather G., Smith W. R. D., Jepson, J. B., and Sorensen, K.: The metabolism and excretion of indolylacrylic acid in the rat. Biochem. Pharmacol., **19,** 1689, 1970.
43. Fordtran, J. S., Scroggie, W. B., and Polter, D. E.: Colonic absorption of tryptophan metabolites in man. J. Lab. Clin. Med., **64,** 125, 1964.
44. Happold, F. C.: Tryptophanase-tryptophan reaction. Advances enzym., **10,** 51, 1950.
45. King, L. J., Parke, D. V., and Williams, R. T.: Metabolism of indole-2-^{14}C. Biochem. J., **88,** 66P, 1963.
46. Nakao, A., and Ball, M.: The appearance of a skatole derivative in the urine of schizophrenics. J. Nerv. Ment. Dis., **130,** 417, 1960.
47. Sprince, H.: Indole metabolism in mental illness. Clin. Chem., **7,** 203, 1961.
48. Scriver, C. R.: Abnormalities of tryptophan metabolism in a patient with malabsorption syndrome. J. Lab. Clin. Med., **58,** 908, 1961.
49. Crawford, M. A.: Degradation of aminoacids in the large gut of East Africans and its possible significance. E. Afr. Med. J., **41,** 228, 1964.
50. Crawford, M. A.: Discussion of indole metabolism in Hartnup disease. Advances Pharmacol., **6B,** 176, 1968.
51. Dayman, J., and Jepson, J. B.: Unpublished observations.
52. Mellman, W. U., Barness, L. A., Tedesco, T. A., and Besselman, D.: Indolylacryloyl-glycine excretion in a family with mental retardation. Clin. Chim. Acta, **8,** 843, 1963.
53. Szeinberg, A., Bar-Or, R., Pollak, S., Cohen, B. E., and Jepson, J. B.: Observations on urinary excretion of indolylacryloyl-glycine. Clin. Chim. Acta, **11,** 506, 1965.
54. Drummond, K. N., Michael, A. F., Ulstrom, R. A., and Good, R. A.: The blue diaper syndrome: Familial hypercalcemia with nephrocalcinosis and indicanuria. Amer. J. Med., **37,** 928, 1964.
55. Evered, D. F.: The excretion of aminoacids by the human: A quantitative study with ion-exchange chromatography. Biochem. J., **62,** 416, 1956.
56. Cusworth, D. C., and Dent, C. E.: Renal clearances of aminoacids in normal adults and in patients with aminoaciduria. Biochem. J., **74,** 551, 1960.
57. Bonetti, E., and Dent, C. E.: The determination of optical configuration of naturally occurring amino acids using specific enzymes and paper chromatography. Biochem. J., **57,** 77, 1954.
58. Dent, C. E.: The renal aminoacidurias. Exp. Med. Surg., **12,** 229, 1954.
59. Tada, K., Hirono, H., and Arakawa, T.: Endogenous renal clearance rates of free aminoacids in prolinuric and Hartnup patients. Tohoku J. Exp. Med., **93,** 57, 1967.
60. Halvorsen, S., Hygstedt, O., Jagenburg, R., and Sjaasted, O.: Cellular transport of L-histidine in Hartnup disease. J. Clin. Invest., **48,** 1552, 1969.
61. Scriver, C. R.: In *Aminoacid Metabolism and Genetic Variation,* edited by W. L. Nyhan, chap. 22, p. 327. McGraw-Hill, New York, 1967.
62. Milne, M. D., Asatoor, A., and Loughridge, L.: Hartnup disease and cystinuria. Lancet, **1,** 51, 1961.
63. De Laey, P., Hooft, C., Timmermans, J., and Snoeck, J.: Biochemical aspects of the Hartnup disease. Ann. Paediat., **202,** 145, 253, 1964.
64. Hjelt, L., Paatela, M., and Visakorpi, J. K.: Autopsy findings in Hartnup disease. *Proc. 13th Northern Pediat. Cong.,* Copenhagen, 1961.
65. Scriver, C. R.: Hartnup disease. New Eng. J. Med., **273,** 530, 1965.
66. Seakins, J. W. T., and Ersser, R. S.: Effects of aminoacid loads on a healthy infant with the biochemical features of Hartnup disease. Arch. Dis. Child., **42,** 682, 1967.
67. Milne, M. D., Crawford, M. A., Girao, C. B., and Loughridge, L. W.: The metabolic disorder in Hartnup disease. Quart. J. Med., **29,** 407, 1960.
68. Tada, K., Morikawa, T., and Arakawa, T.: Tryptophan load and uptake of tryptophan by leukocytes in Hartnup disease. Tohoku J. Exp. Med., **90,** 337, 1966.
69. Platter, H., and Martin, G. M.: Tryptophan transport in cultures of human fibroblasts. Proc. Soc. Exp. Biol. Med., **123,** 140, 1966.
70. Martin, G. M. [Seattle, Washington, U.S.A.]: Unpublished observations.
71. Shaw, K. N. F., Redlich, D., Wright, S. W., and Jepson, J. B.: Dependence of urinary indole excretion in Hartnup disease upon gut flora. Fed.Proc., **19,** 194, 1960.
72. Asatoor, A. M., Craske, J., London, D. R., and Milne, M. D.: Indole production in Hartnup disease. Lancet, **1,** 126, 1963.
73. Jepson, J. B.: In *Chromatographic and Electrophoretic Techniques,* edited by I. Smith, 3rd ed., vol. 1, chap. 9. Heinemann, London, 1969.
74. Milne, M. D., Crawford, M. A., Girao, C. B., and Loughridge, L. W.: The excretion of indolylacetic acid and related indolic acids in man and the rat. Clin. Sci., **19,** 165, 1960.
75. Jepson, J. B.: Indole metabolism in Hartnup disease. Advances Pharmacol., **6B,** 171, 1968.
76. Hvidt, S., and Kjeldsen, K.: Malabsorption induced by small doses of neomycin sulphate. Acta Med. Scand., **173,** 699, 1963.
77. Jepson, J. B.: Indolylacetamide, a chromatographic artifact from the natural indoles indolylacetylglucosiduronic acid and indolylpyruvic acid. Biochem. J., **69,** 22 P, 1958.
78. Davis, V. E., Brown, H., Huff, J. A., and Cashaw, J. L.: Alteration of serotonin metabolism to 5-hydroxytryptophol by ethanol ingestion in man. J. Lab. Clin. Med., **69,** 132, 1967.
79. Despopoulos, A., and Weissbach, H.: Renal metabolism of 5-hydroxyindoleacetic acid. Amer. J. Physiol., **189,** 548, 1957.
80. Borrie, P. F., and Lewis, C. A.: Hartnup disease. Proc. Roy. Soc. Med., **55,** 231, 1962.
81. Ikeda, M., Tsiyi, H., Nakamura, S., Ichiyama, A., Nishizuka, Y., and Hayaishi, O.: Studies on the biosynthesis of nicotinamide adenine dinucleotide. J. Biol. Chem., **240,** 1395, 1965.
82. Mirsky, J. A.: Insulinase, insulinase inhibitors and diabetes mellitus. Recent Progr. Hormone Res., **13,** 429, 1957.
83. Milne, M. D.: Disorders of aminoacid transport. Brit. Med. J., **1,** 327, 1964.

84. Crawford, T. B. B., Ashcroft, M. B., Eccleston, D., and Smith, A. N.: Some observations on the metabolism of indoles in two patients with carcinoid syndrome. Gastroenterology, **48**, 745, 1965.
85. Frieden, E., Westmark, G. W., and Schor, J. M.: Inhibition of tryptophan pyrrolase by serotonin, epinephrine and tryptophan analogues. Arch. Biochem. Biophys., **92**, 176, 1961.
86. Colliss, Jane E., Levi, A. J., and Milne, M. D.: Stature and nutrition in cystinuria and Hartnup disease. Brit. Med. J., **1**, 590, 1963.
87. Efron, M. L., and Ampola, M. G.: The aminoacidurias. Pediat. Clin. N. Amer., **14**, 881, 1967.
88. Hooft, C., Timmermans, J., Snoeck, J., Antener, T., Oyaert, W., and van den Hende, C.: Methionine malabsorption syndrome. Ann. Paediat., **205**, 73, 1965.
89. Jepson, J. B., Smith, A. J., and Strang, L. B.: An inborn error of metabolism with urinary excretion of hydroxyacids, ketoacids and aminoacids. Lancet, **2**, 1334, 1958.

CHAPTER SIXTY-TWO

CYSTINURIA*

Samuel O. Thier and Stanton Segal

Cystinuria is an inheritable disorder of amino acid transport affecting the epithelial cells of the renal tubules and gastrointestinal tract. The disease is expressed clinically by the formation of calculi in the urinary tract, with the potential for obstruction, infection, and ultimately renal insufficiency. The disease is characterized primarily by the precipitation of cystine, the least soluble of the naturally occurring amino acids; lysine, arginine, ornithine, and cysteine-homocysteine mixed disulfide are also present in excess in the urine. Since this aminoaciduria occurs with a normal or reduced filtered load of cystine and the dibasic amino acids, it was postulated earlier that cystinuria is a disorder of tubular transport in the kidney. The subsequent demonstration of comparably defective transport in the intestine established the present view of this disorder as an inherited defect in a specific transepithelial transport mechanism, which is expressed in two areas, the kidney and the intestine.

HISTORY

The historical development of a theory of the pathogenesis of cystinuria was anything but orderly. Although the data suggesting renal and intestinal lesions appeared in random order, it is easier to trace the history of the renal lesion before that of the intestinal defect.

In 1810 Wollaston analyzed two stones recovered from urinary bladders and discerned that they differed from all previously described calculi. Because of their bladder origin and supposed chemical nature, they were named cystic oxide stones [1]. In 1824 Stromeyer noted hexagonal platelike crystals in the urine of patients with cystinuria [2]. The finding of cystine crystals served for many years as the chief means of diagnosing the disease and remains helpful even today.

In 1833 Berzelius, recognizing that the compound was not an oxide, renamed the substance "cystine," perpetuating the fallacy that it originated in the bladder [3]. Although improved descriptions of the chemistry of cystine were developed over the next 70 years, it was not until 1902 that Friedman defined the chemical structure of cystine [4]. In his 1908 Croonian lectures, Garrod discussed cystinuria among the inborn errors of metabolism and postulated that a defect in the metabolism of cystine was responsible for the disorder [5]. During the next 40 years, in spite of the reports of increased lysine in the urine of cystinuric subjects, there was little advance in our understanding of the disease. The present concepts of cystinuria emerged after the advent of paper chromatography and development of polarographic and microbiologic assays. With these methods, Yeh et al. demonstrated in 1947 that lysinuria and argininuria also occur in cystinuria [6], and Stein found that a large quantity of ornithine was also present [7]. Subsequently, Dent et al. [8] and Arrow and Westall [9] noted that plasma levels of cystine and of dibasic amino acids were normal or low. Dent and Rose observed that cystine and the dibasic amino acids had structural similarities, i.e., two amino groups separated by 4 to 6 chemical bonds. They postulated that there was a single renal transport mechanism shared by these amino acids, and proposed that this mechanism was defective or absent in cystinuria [10] (Fig. 62-1). This formulation remains the best explanation of the renal defect in cystinuria.

The intestinal defect was not recognized as promptly. Von Udranszky and Baumann in 1889 observed that cadaverine and putrescine, decarboxylation products of lysine and arginine, were present in large amounts in urine of cystinuric subjects [11]. These findings were confirmed by Loewy and Neuberg [12]. Subsequently an increase of urinary cystine excretion was reported in cystinuria in response to protein feeding, but feeding of cystine itself was not observed to increase either serum or urine cystine [13, 14]. After half a century these data were finally interpreted by Milne, who had already recognized the intestinal transport defect associated with the renal aminoaciduria in Hartnup's disease [15]. Milne performed experiments which demonstrated reduced intestinal absorption of the dibasic amino acids in patients with cystinuria [16, 17]. His findings have subsequently been confirmed in vitro by studies of transport in jejunal biopsies [18–20].

CLINICAL ASPECTS

Cystinuria is a rare disease, with a complex recessive mode of inheritance. The incidence is difficult to estimate. Figures range from 1 per 200 to 250 individuals excreting excess cystine in the urine to 1/100,000 homozygous for the trait. Crawhall et al. estimated the incidence on the basis of urine nitroprusside tests. On the assumption that there are twice as many individuals with truly recessive cystinuria as individuals with the incompletely recessive trait, they estimated that 1 per 20,000 persons are homozygous for cystinuria [21, 22]. The disease occurs equally in both sexes, but males are more severely affected and have a higher mortality rate. The greater severity of the disease in males may be related to urinary tract anatomy, with a greater likelihood of urethral obstruction in males. Although clinical expression of the disease may occur in the first year of life or as late as the ninth decade, the second and third decades appear to be the peak times for expression of cystinuria. Colic, the most common presentation, may be associated with obstruction

*Supported by Grant AM 10894 from the National Institutes of Health.

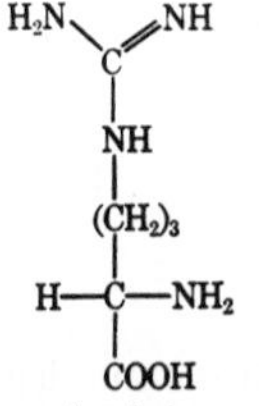

$S{-}S$; CH_2 CH_2; $H{-}C{-}NH_2$ $H{-}C{-}NH_2$; $COOH$ $COOH$
Cystine

NH_2; $(CH_2)_4$; $H{-}C{-}NH_2$; $COOH$
Lysine

H; $H{-}C{-}NH_2$; $(CH_2)_2$; $H{-}C{-}NH_2$; $COOH$
Ornithine

$H_2N{-}C({=}NH)$; NH; $(CH_2)_3$; $H{-}C{-}NH_2$; $COOH$
Arginine

Figure 62-1. Chemical structures of the amino acids excreted in excessive amounts in the urine in cystinuria.

of the urinary tract, subsequent infection, and eventual loss of function. Infection, hypertension, and renal failure may occur occasionally and cause the patient first to seek medical attention.

Cystine Stones

Both cystine stones and uric acid stones form readily in acid urine, and the two are frequently confused. However, the cystine stone, with its yellow-brown color and maple sugar crystal surface, is much firmer than uric acid and is radiopaque [23, 24]. The radiopacity of cystine is due to the density of the sulfur molecules. On roentgenograms cystine stones appear smooth and are less dense than calcium stones. Cystine calculi tend to occur as staghorn or multiple recurrent stones, frequently necessitating surgery (Fig. 62-2). Calcium stones may also be formed as a result of infection secondary to cystine calculi.

DIAGNOSIS

The diagnosis of cystinuria should be entertained in every patient with urinary calculi or with urinary tract symptoms suggestive of calculi. The simplest diagnostic procedure is the miscroscopic examination of urinary sediment, preferably in the first voiding in the morning or other concentrated urine, for typical cystine crystals (Fig. 62-3).

The cyanide-nitroprusside test has been widely applied as a chemical screening procedure [25, 26]. It is important that the color obtained be compared with that of a specimen of normal urine to which cystine has been added. Since the lower limit of sensitivity of the reaction is about 75 to 125 mg per gm creatinine, the reaction permits easy detection of homozygous stone formers, who usually excrete more than 250 mg per gm creatinine [27, 28]. Some but not all of those heterozygotes with increased urinary cystine may also be detected by this procedure. A positive nitroprusside test may be seen in homocystinuria as well as in patients with acetonuria. Patients with crystalluria or a positive cyanide-nitroprusside test should be further studied for identification of urinary amino acids by such methods as thin-layer chromatography [29] or high-voltage electrophoresis [30]. Quantitation of cystine may be made easily following its electrolytic reduction to the thiol, which can be colorimetrically determined [29]. Quantitative ion-exchange chromatography is the most sophisticated procedure and should be performed whenever possible [31, 32]. By this method the upper limits of normal values for cystine, lysine, arginine, and ornithine in the adult are 18, 130, 16, and 22 mg per gm creatinine, respectively [22].

Cystinuria has been associated with hyperuricemia [33], hemophilia [34], retinitis pigmentosa [35], muscular dystrophy [36], muscular hypotonia [37], mongolism [38], and hereditary pancreatitis [39], and it occurs as an isolated aminoaciduria with hypocalcemic tetany [40]. As a group, cystinuric subjects are believed to be shorter than the general

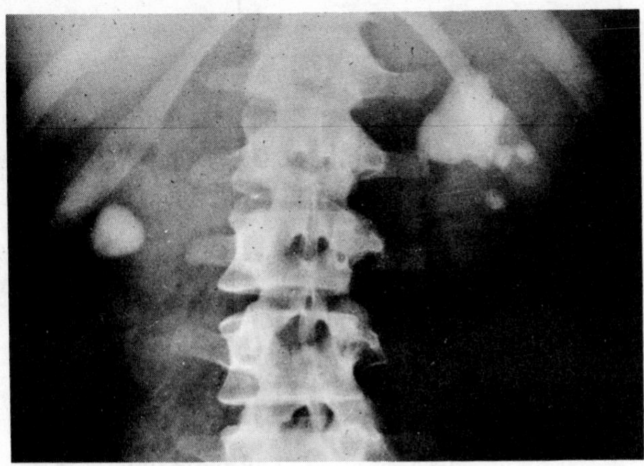

Figure 62-2. Roentgenogram of the abdomen of a cystinuric patient showing bilateral radiopaque calculi.

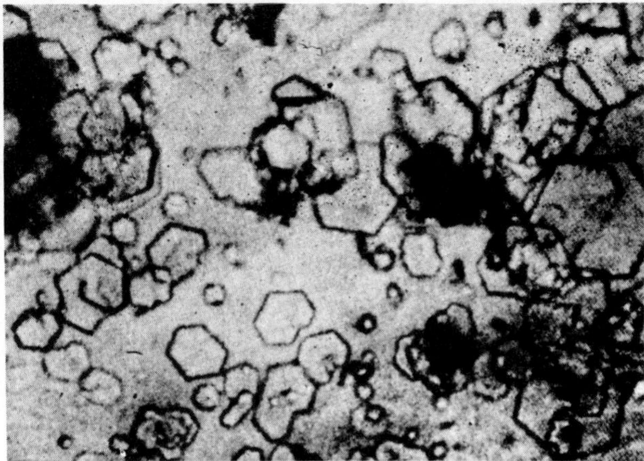

Figure 62-3. Cystine crystals as they appear in the urinary sediment in cystinuria.

population, perhaps because of malabsorption of essential amino acids [41].

BIOCHEMISTRY OF CYSTINURIA

Consideration of cystinuria as an inborn error of metabolism by Garrod [5] was based on the assumption that an enzyme responsible for cystine catabolism was missing or defective. Although Garrod's concept of a missing enzyme in a metabolic pathway has been substantiated for the other diseases upon which his theory was based, this has not been done for cystinuria. Garrod was not truly incorrect about cystinuria, since the modern view that the disease is an inherited disorder of membrane transport supposes the genetic loss of a mechanism located in the membrane which is responsible for movement of extracellular cystine into the confines of the cell. The concept of a membrane transport mechanism involving an amino acid–binding site and genetic control is consistent with the function of a "carrier" protein. An abnormality of the function of this first step in metabolism, involving transport of the substrate into the cell, is certainly consistent with Garrod's original view. What Garrod did not anticipate was the membrane nature of the disorder and the primary involvement of the kidney and intestine.

Garrod's concept stimulated the elucidation of the transsulfuration metabolic pathway shown in Fig. 62-4. The feeding experiments of Brand and his colleagues demonstrated that methionine [13] and proteins high in methionine [42] resulted in higher cystine excretion, since methionine is converted to cysteine and then to cystine. Feeding of cystine itself did not give rise to increased amounts of urinary cystine, but giving cysteine did [14]. This can now be interpreted on the basis of an intestinal defect in cystine absorption which does not involve cysteine (see later). The role of cystathionine as an intermediate was shown in du Vigneaud's laboratory when that compound gave rise to cystine [43]. Most recent observations have been concerned with the enzymes of the pathway in relation to homocystinuria [44] and cystathioninuria [45]. The observation that the body can

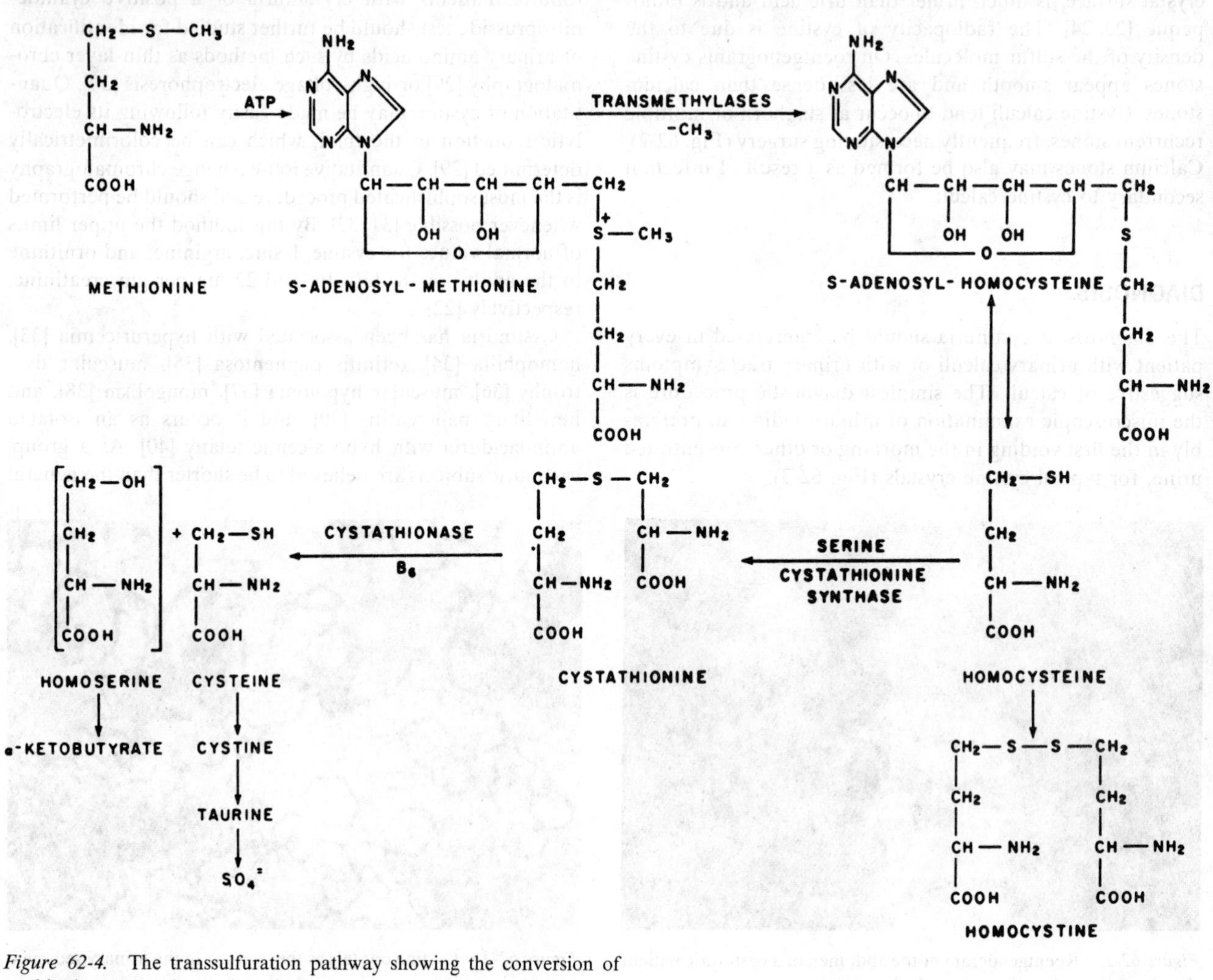

Figure 62-4. The transsulfuration pathway showing the conversion of methionine to cysteine and cystine.

Table 62-1. INTRACELLULAR FORMS OF ^{35}S AFTER INCUBATION OF RAT KIDNEY CORTEX SLICES WITH LABELED L-CYSTINE AND L-CYSTEINE [52]

Age of animal	Transported substrate	Concentration, mM	*Intracellular form of ^{35}S as percent of intracellular ^{35}S*			
			Cystine	Reduced glutathione	Cysteine	Other
5 days	Cystine	0.07	0	25	62	13
5 days	Cysteine	0.07	6	24	62	8
Adult	Cystine	0.07	0	12	68	20
Adult	Cysteine	0.07	14	20	64	8

convert methionine or homocystine to cystine by way of the transsulfuration pathway has relegated cystine to the position of a nonessential amino acid, but the demonstration that cystathionase is not active in fetal tissues implies that cystine may be an essential amino acid in fetal development [46].

Relatively less seems to be known of the catabolism of cystine or cysteine to sulfate. Oxidation to cysteinsulfonate, taurine, cysteic acid, and sulfite appears to be involved [47, 48]. Increased urinary sulfate excretion in cystinuric patients fed cystine may involve the oxidation of unabsorbed cystine in the gastrointestinal tract and subsequent absorption of the inorganic ion [49].

These aspects of cystine catabolism may be more appropriately considered with regard to the human cystine storage disease, cystinosis [50], which should not be confused with cystinuria. Although a generalized aminoaciduria is present with cystinosis, the large amounts of cystine or dibasic amino acids found with cystinuria are not found. Cystine storage disease is associated with deposition of cystine in various tissues; in cystinuria there is no tissue deposition, only urinary loss.

Of importance to a basic understanding of both human diseases involving cystine is the fact that the intracellular form of the amino acid is not the disulfide but the free thiol, cysteine [51, 52]. If cystine-^{35}S is incubated with kidney cortex slices or other tissues, the ^{35}S within the cell is mainly in cysteine or glutathione, little or none being maintained as cystine [52] (Table 62-1). Reduction of cystine to cysteine is believed to take place within the cell by a mechanism mediated by glutathione-cysteine transhydrogenase [53].

RENAL TRANSPORT DEFECTS

Cystinuria is a classic example of a disorder of renal tubular function. In discussing aminoaciduria it should be kept clearly in mind that most aminoacidurias are not disorders of tubular function. Normally amino acids are filtered and are almost entirely reabsorbed in the proximal nephron. There is a maximal capacity to the reabsorptive mechanism which is exceeded in certain disorders. In most cases of aminoaciduria an extrarenal metabolic defect leads to the accumulation of an amino acid in the plasma, which is then filtered in amounts exceeding the normal capacity of the nephron for reabsorption. These are not disorders of tubular function. With normal or low plasma levels and diminished filtered loads of amino acid, if excessive loss still occurs in the urine, then the reabsorptive capacity of the tubule is said to be below normal and tubular dysfunction exists. The latter situation obtains in cystinuria. Excessive urinary losses of cystine and dibasic amino acids occur with normal or less than normal plasma levels of the affected amino acids [8, 9].

Of all amino acids studied, only cystine and the dibasic amino acids are involved in cystinuria. On the basis of this information Dent and Rose postulated a single transport mechanism shared by cystine and the dibasic amino acids which is defective in cystinuria [10]. This postulate predicted that increasing the filtered load of one amino acid in the group should reduce the reabsorption of the others. Robson and Rose [54] demonstrated that this was indeed true in normal man, and similar data were derived from animal studies by Webber, Brown, and Pitts [55]. Since infusion of lysine did not increase cystine excretion in cystinuria, it was proposed that the transport mechanism for these amino acids was absent; therefore, the normal functional interactions could not be demonstrated.

Cystine and Dibasic Amino Acid Transport

The concept of cystinuria developed by Dent and Rose remains the most useful theory of this disease, but it will have to be extended to explain several recent observations. In the first place there are discrepancies between observations in vivo and results in vitro. Studies in vitro in slices of rat and human renal cortex have demonstrated that the dibasic amino acids, lysine, arginine, and ornithine, do indeed share a common transport mechanism which is defective in cystinuria [56, 57], but cystine does not compete for this mechanism, and the cystine transport mechanism is not itself affected by the dibasic amino acids. Lysine participates in exchange diffusion with the other dibasic amino acids but not with cystine [58]. Furthermore, kidney slices from cystinuric and normal subjects concentrate cystine equally well [57].

Numerous experiments have been performed, using kidney slice transport techniques in vitro which clearly demonstrate that the transport systems for lysine and cystine in rat kidney cortex are not the same [59, 60] (Table 62-2). In addition to the lack of mutual inhibition between these two amino acids and their nonparticipation in heteroexchange diffusion mentioned above, certain biochemical differences exist in their transport characteristics. Lysine transport is only partially dependent on the presence of sodium ion and aerobic conditions, and over a pH range of 6 to 8.5 shows little change of influx rate [59]. Cystine transport, on the other hand, is completely dependent on sodium and oxygen and shows marked differences in influx pH, with an optimum of about pH 7.4 [60].

Perhaps the best evidence for the distinction between dibasic amino acid and cystine transport systems is based on differences in ontogeny [61]. In newborn rat kidney cortex the lysine transport system is fully operative, whereas the cystine transport mechanism is impaired and does not reach the normal adult level until 15 days of age. It is difficult to conceive of a single carrier mechanism that behaves differently toward both substrates. Support for the separate nature of the lysine and cystine transport systems is offered also by the recent discovery of clinical disorders in which cystine and dibasic aminoacidurias occurred independently. Brodehl [40] has found isolated cystinuria without dibasic aminoaciduria. Also, many dogs with cystinuria have no lysinuria [62]. Conversely, dibasic aminoaciduria (lysinuria) without cystinuria has also been reported [63, 64].

Cystine and Cysteine Transport

The reduced form of cystine, cysteine, may play an important role in the underlying abnormality. Plasma cysteine in cystinuric patients is decreased proportionally more than cystine or the dibasic amino acids, but little cysteine appears in urine, and no increased conversion of cysteine to cystine has yet been demonstrated [65, 66]. Frimpter [67], having found an arteriovenous difference for cysteine but not for cystine across the kidney of a single patient, postulated that urinary cystine may be derived from plasma cysteine. Rosenberg et al. [68], however, found no increase in cysteine extraction in two patients when compared with controls. An increase in cysteine clearance by the kidney would seem an unlikely source of urinary cystine. The plasma level of cysteine is only about 25 percent of that of cystine, too low to explain the large amounts of urinary cystine on the basis of a total loss of filtered cysteine.

Measurement in vitro of cysteine uptake by renal cortex obtained at surgery from cystinuric patients has failed to show any difference from control tissue [69]. Similar normal results have been seen in experiments employing intestinal mucosa from cystinuric subjects, although, as pointed out below, there is a defect in cystine uptake by the mucosa [70]. Further kinetic studies in rat kidney cortex slices have furnished evidence, based on response to alteration of pH, temperature changes, oxygen lack, and sodium deprivation, that the kidney cystine and cysteine transport systems are different [60]. Confirmation of this supposition has come from ontogenetic studies which show a separate developmental time pattern for cystine and cysteine transport in rat kidney cortex [52].

An examination of the transport interaction of cysteine with dibasic amino acids in vitro showed no mutual inhibition of uptake, a result also obtained for cystine and lysine [71]. Even so, incubation of cysteine with lysine causes an enhanced accumulation of the sulfur amino acid by kidney cortex [58, 71]. Schwartzman, Blair, and Segal [71] have explained the lysine-enhanced accumulation of cystine by showing that the dibasic amino acids inhibit the efflux of intracellular cysteine into the incubation fluid. This is the first demonstration in vitro of an interaction between the sulfur amino acids and the dibasic amino acids, and it may have physiologic importance since the natural intracellular form is cysteine even if cystine is the compound being transported [51, 52].

Renal Extractions

Examination of the extraction of cystine from blood flowing through the kidneys of cystinuric patients has revealed

Table 62-2. CHARACTERISTICS OF CYSTINE AND LYSINE TRANSPORT IN MAMMALIAN KIDNEY CORTEX SLICES [58–61]

Experimental parameter	Cystine	Lysine
1. Oxygen dependence	Complete	Partial
2. Sodium dependence	Complete	Partial
3. pH dependence	Marked	Little
4. Inhibition by arginine and ornithine	None	Present, competitive
5. Auto-exchange diffusion	None	Present
6. Hetero-exchange diffusion with arginine and ornithine	None	Present
7. Developmental pattern	Decreased at birth	Normal at birth

minimal arteriovenous differences [67, 68] and no alteration from the normal. Assuming that total failure of tubular reabsorption of cystine accounts for cystinuria, a large arteriovenous difference for cystine should be discernible. The inability to demonstrate this has raised the possibility of cystine synthesis *de novo* or kidney protein catabolism to account for the presence of urinary cystine in the face of normal plasma extraction. Frimpter [66] has attempted to answer this by comparing the specific activity of plasma and urinary cystine after infusing cystine-^{35}S. The fact that these activities were the same argues against an endogenous kidney production of cystine, but it is possible that the long infusion period may have labeled the kidney pools of cystine so that the sought-for specific activity differences would not be detected. The picture is complicated further by the evidence that certain patients with cystinuria have a cystine clearance greater than the glomerular filtration rate, with a ratio of $C_{cystine}$ to C_{inulin} ranging between 1 and 2 [72, 73]. From a physiologic viewpoint this is consistent with cystine secretion and raises the question of bidirectional cystine transport.

Transport in Vivo and in Vitro

Thus, there appears to be no discrepancy between renal clearance data upon which the Dent and Rose hypothesis is based and observations in vitro of dibasic amino acid transport in kidney cortex slices. The renal clearance data for cystine and the observations in vitro regarding cystine and cysteine transport are the most difficult to reconcile. It appears that the hypothesis of Dent and Rose is only a partial explanation. Thus far the basis of hyperexcretion of cystine by cystinuric patients is enigmatic. Schwartzman, Blair, and Segal [71] have observed that lysine inhibits cysteine efflux from renal tubule cells, and have postulated that an efflux system shared by lysine and cysteine may be defective in cystinuria. The fact that the sulfur amino acid within the cell is cysteine gives special significance to the interaction of cysteine and dibasic amino acids during efflux, an interaction not shown by cystine and lysine for the entry process. The theory proposes that if cysteine movement out of cells into the peritubular capillary is defective, an elevation of intracellular cysteine would occur which could affect cystine entry at the brush border. Such an elevation of kidney intracellular cysteine (which remains to be demonstrated) could prevent reduction of the incoming disulfide amino acid and thereby slow influx. The predicted alteration of cystine or cysteine accumulation in vitro by kidney cortex from cystinuric patients has not been observed, but this may be because of the disruption of the normal transtubular direction of cysteine fluxes by the slice technique.

The possibility of multiple transport cellular systems with overlapping affinities may provide alternate explanations. Studies with human kidney slices indicate that there are perhaps two distinct influx systems for lysine [74], one for cystine [74], and two for cysteine [69]. Though there is some evidence to suggest a loss of shared systems [74, 75], the possibility of bidirectional amino acid transport remains unsupported and unrefuted.

URINARY EXCRETION OF OTHER AMINO ACIDS IN CYSTINURIA

Although hyperexcretion of lysine, arginine, ornithine, and cystine in the urine is the hallmark of cystinuria, other amino acids have been found in higher than normal amounts in the urine of some patients. These include glycine [72], methionine [76], cystathionine [77], and homocystine-cysteine disulfide [78] (Fig. 62-5). The latter is most consistently present in variable amounts up to 224 mg per 24 hr [67], the amount being related directly to the amount of cystine excreted [79]. This mixed disulfide has also been found in the urine of patients with Fanconi's syndrome on the basis of Wilson's disease, as well as in dogs with cystinuria [67]. Subsequently, the mixed disulfide was demonstrated in normal plasma and in increased amount in the plasma of a patient with homocystinuria [80]. Although it was thought at first to be uniquely associated with cystinuria, homocysteine-cysteine mixed disulfide probably is a normal plasma constituent which is overexcreted because it participates in the renal tubular defect responsible for the loss of cystine.

INTESTINAL TRANSPORT DEFECTS

When an amino acid is fed absorption occurs, and the unabsorbed amino acid will be used by the intestinal flora. The less an amino acid is absorbed, the lower the blood levels will be after feeding, and the greater will be the levels of bacterial breakdown products in the stool and perhaps also in plasma and urine. If bacterial flora are suppressed, the nonabsorbed amino acid should be demonstrable in the stool. Lysine, arginine, and ornithine are decarboxylated by bacteria in the intestine to the diamines cadaverine, agma-

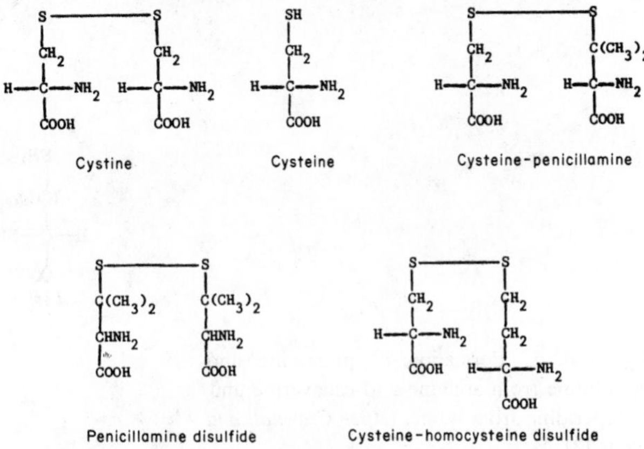

Figure 62-5. The structure of cystine and related compounds.

tine, and putrescine. Piperidine is formed from lysine breakdown, and pyrrolidine from arginine and ornithine metabolism (Fig. 62-6). These heterocyclic amines are formed from the diamines. As mentioned earlier, the data suggesting an intestinal transport defect in cystinuric patients were available by the late nineteenth century, when diamines were detected in the urine of these patients [11, 12]. It was only after Milne and coworkers demonstrated defective tryptophan absorption from the intestine of patients with the neutral aminoaciduria, Hartnup's disease, in 1960, that the data on cystinuria were finally brought into focus [15]. Milne et al. observed increased putrescine and pyrrolidine in the urine after feeding arginine, and increased cadaverine, piperidine, and pyrrolidine after feeding lysine. Since the pyrrolidine could not have been derived from lysine, it was concluded that lysine was competitively inhibiting arginine transport in the intestine. The role of bacterial degradation in this process was proved in patients treated with oral neomycin; pyrrolidine and putrescine decreased in stool and urine, while lysine, arginine, and ornithine increased in the stool of patients so treated [16, 17]. Evidence for a failure of cystine absorption was presented by Brand, Cahill, and Harris [13], by Dent et al. [8], and more recently by London and Foley [49] and Rosenberg et al. [68], using ion-exchange chromatography to measure plasma cystine concentration after oral loading. In all these studies cysteine absorption by cystinuric patients was not impaired [81].

The concept of impaired intestinal amino acid transport derived from feeding experiments received direct confirmation by the demonstration in vitro of defective amino acid accumulation in specimens of jejunal mucosa obtained by peroral biopsy [18–20]. The results of further studies showed that there were some patients who had total impairment of cystine, lysine, and arginine accumulation, others who had small but detectable cystine transport but no dibasic amino acid transport, and still a third group who had normal or only slightly impaired cystine uptake and demonstrable but diminished lysine and arginine accumulation [82] (Fig. 62-7). Later experiments showed that intestinal mucosa from the different types of cystinuria had no impairment of cysteine accumulation in vitro [70]. This finding not only established the independence of the cystine and cysteine transport mechanism but with the results of studies of cystine uptake in vitro explained the many oral feeding experiments previously performed which showed a rise in plasma and urinary cystine after cysteine feeding but not after cystine feeding [49, 81]. The contrasts between findings of intestine and kidney in vitro are striking. The impaired cystine transport in the mucosa of most cystinuric patients [82] differs markedly from the normal transport of cystine observed in kidney slices from the same patients [57]. Furthermore, while active transport of lysine is absent in mucosa of the patients [82], it is only reduced by about one-half in kidney slices [57]. Finally, mutual competitive inhibition of lysine and

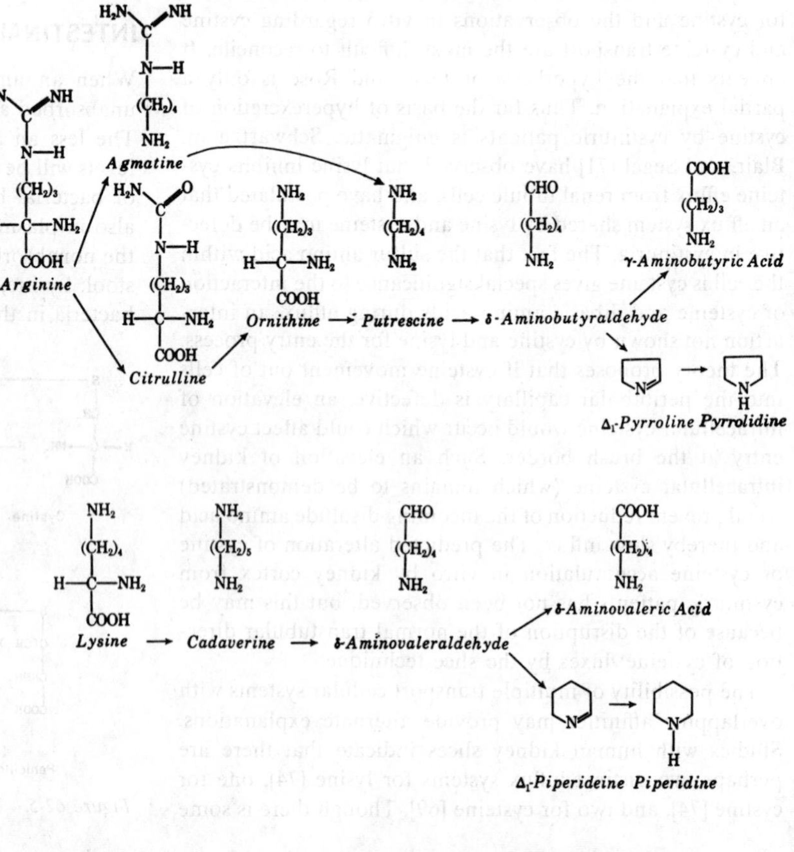

Figure 62-6. Formation of putrescine and pyrrolidine from arginine and cadaverine and of piperidine from lysine. (*After Crawhall and Watts* [21].)

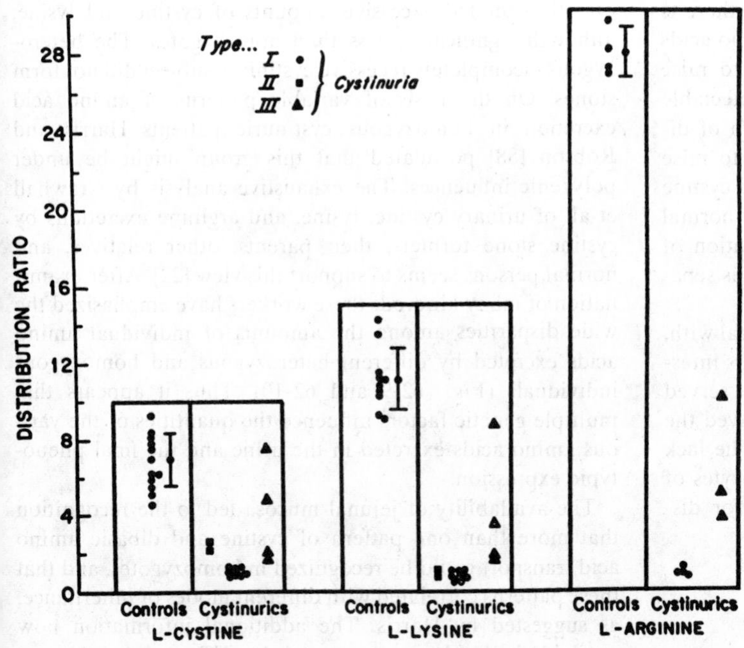

Figure 62-7. Uptake of cystine, lysine, and arginine by jejunal mucosa from control and cystinuric subjects expressed as the distribution ratio, i.e., the ratio of radioactive amino acid inside the cell to that in the medium, after a 45-min incubation [82].

cystine is demonstrable in intestinal mucosa but not in kidney slices. The results of the intestinal transport studies in vitro thus fit the postulates of Dent and Rose made from the urinary findings that cystine and the basic amino acids share a common transport system.

Differences between the characteristics of intestinal and renal transport of lysine in vitro have been clearly demonstrated in the rat. Lysine uptake by intestinal mucosa is sodium- and oxygen-dependent and sensitive to pH changes; that by the kidney is only minimally affected by changes in sodium, oxygen, or pH [83]. These findings, along with the evidence for separate lysine and cystine transport mechanisms in kidney [59–61], prompted Segal [84] to propose a model of a membrane carrier system that could explain cystine and lysine transport in the intestine and kidney of cystinuric patients.

Family studies of cystine excretion alone allowed differentiation of phenotypically identical cystinuric subjects into two genetically different groups [27, 85, 86]. Additional consideration of the intestinal mucosal transport patterns for the dibasic amino acids allows homozygous cystinuric subjects to be differentiated into three groups [82] (Table 62-3).

Table 62-3. CLASSIFICATION OF CASES OF CYSTINURIA

Experimental observations	Type I	Type II	Type III
Intestine:			
In vitro transport	No transport of cystine, lysine, or arginine; normal cysteine transport	No transport of lysine; markedly reduced cystine transport	Transport of cystine reduced but may be normal; lysine variably reduced
Oral cystine administration	No plasma cystine elevation	No plasma cystine elevation	Slow increase in plasma cystine to normal elevation
Kidney:			
In vitro transport	Normal cystine, cysteine; reduced lysine transport	....	Normal cystine; reduced lysine transport
Urinary amino acid excretion	Increased cystine, lysine, arginine, ornithine	Increased cystine, lysine, arginine, ornithine excretion	Increased cystine, lysine, arginine, ornithine excretion
Urinary amino acid excretion in heterozygotes	Normal	Cystine and lysine above normal	Cystine and lysine above normal

In Type I, which includes the majority of patients, there is no accumulation of either cystine or the dibasic amino acids against a gradient, and oral cystine loading fails to raise serum cystine levels (Fig. 62-8). In Type II there is detectable active accumulation of cystine but no accumulation of dibasic amino acids; as in Type I oral loading fails to raise serum cystine levels. In Type III accumulation of cystine and dibasic amino acids does occur but not to the normal extent; oral cystine loading results in normal elevation of plasma cystine levels. The family studies based on this separation will be discussed under "Genetics."

Thus, an intestinal defect similar to, but not identical with, the renal lesion is inherited in cystinuria. Though this intestinal defect may be of little clinical importance, it has served as an extremely sensitive genetic marker and has paved the way for a new genetic classification of cystinuria. The lack of amino acid transport defects in circulating leukocytes of cystinuric patients has precluded their usefulness for discerning genetic aspects of the disease [87].

GENETICS

The genetics of cystinuria has been a field of expanding knowledge in recent years. An understanding of the genetics of this disorder depends on a clear definition of the phenotypically homozygous state. This state is suggested by (1) the excretion of over 250 mg cystine per gm creatinine, often with formation of urinary calculi, and (2) the presence of an intestinal absorptive defect for cystine and the dibasic amino acids. In the first large-scale genetic studies, Harris and coworkers divided cystinuria into two groups in which phenotypically homozygous subjects were indistinguishable [86]. In one group the disease was transmitted as a true recessive trait; no family members other than the homozygous individual had aminoaciduria. The second group was designated as incompletely recessive; family members frequently excreted excessive amounts of cystine and lysine, although significantly less than homozygotes. The heterozygous incompletely recessive cystinuric subject did not form stones. On the basis of variable patterns of amino acid excretion in homozygous cystinuric patients Harris and Robson [88] postulated that this group might be under polygenic influences. The exhaustive analysis by Crawhall et al. of urinary cystine, lysine, and arginine excretions by cystine stone formers, their parents, other relatives, and normal persons seems to support this view [22]. After examination of many kindreds these workers have emphasized the wide disparities among the amounts of individual amino acids excreted by different heterozygous and homozygous individuals (Figs. 62-9 and 62-10). Thus it appears that multiple genetic factors influence the quantities of the various amino acids excreted in the urine and the final phenotypic expression.

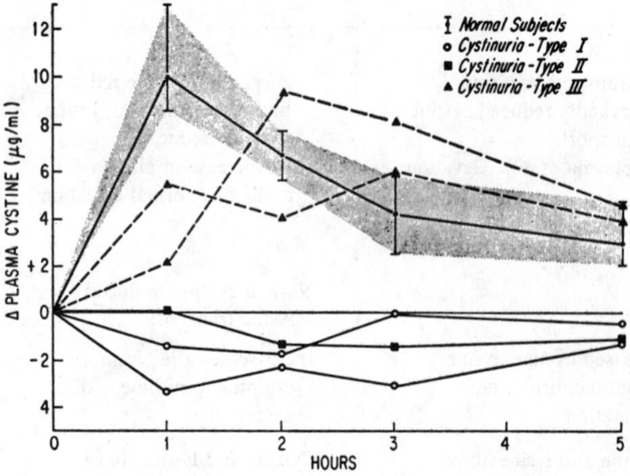

Figure 62-8. The change of plasma cystine levels after oral cystine administration of 0.05 micromole per kg [82].

The availability of jejunal mucosa led to the recognition that more than one pattern of cystine and dibasic amino acid transport could be recognized in homozygotes, and that these patterns correlated with different modes of inheritance, as suggested by Harris. The additional information now available is that homozygotes can be differentiated without recourse to family studies. The pattern of jejunal mucosal transport discussed above under "Intestinal Transport Defects" is summarized in Table 62-3. Note that three classes of cystinuria may now be developed and that the last two were combined in the incompletely recessive group II of Harris.

With the ability to separate homozygous cystinuric subjects into distinct groups based on intestinal transport, Rosenberg restudied the families of these individuals and found distinctive urinary amino acid patterns [89]. Families of Type I patients had no abnormal urinary amino acid excretion. Type II and Type III heterozygous individuals excreted excessive amounts of cystine and the dibasic amino acids in their urine. The quantities excreted were consistently higher in the Type II heterozygotes.

The presence of at least three distinct genetic types raised the question of whether cystinuria represented a group of diseases with defects in separate steps of amino acid transport, or different defects in the same genetically controlled step; i.e., were the different types the result of nonallelic or allelic mutations? The results of matings between Type I and Type II or III heterozygous individuals could provide an answer. If the defects were allelic, a fully expressed homozygous state (a better term is "compound heterozygous state") might appear in the offspring. If the defects were in separate genes, then only the expressed heterozygous state should appear in the offspring, i.e., Type II or III. The fact that "homozygous" children were found suggested that the defects were allelic [90, 91]. Although studies in vitro of intestinal transport have defined what seem to be three phenotypes [82], it should be pointed out that within the third type the cystine uptake by mucosal biopsies ranges from normal to an impairment almost as severe as in the

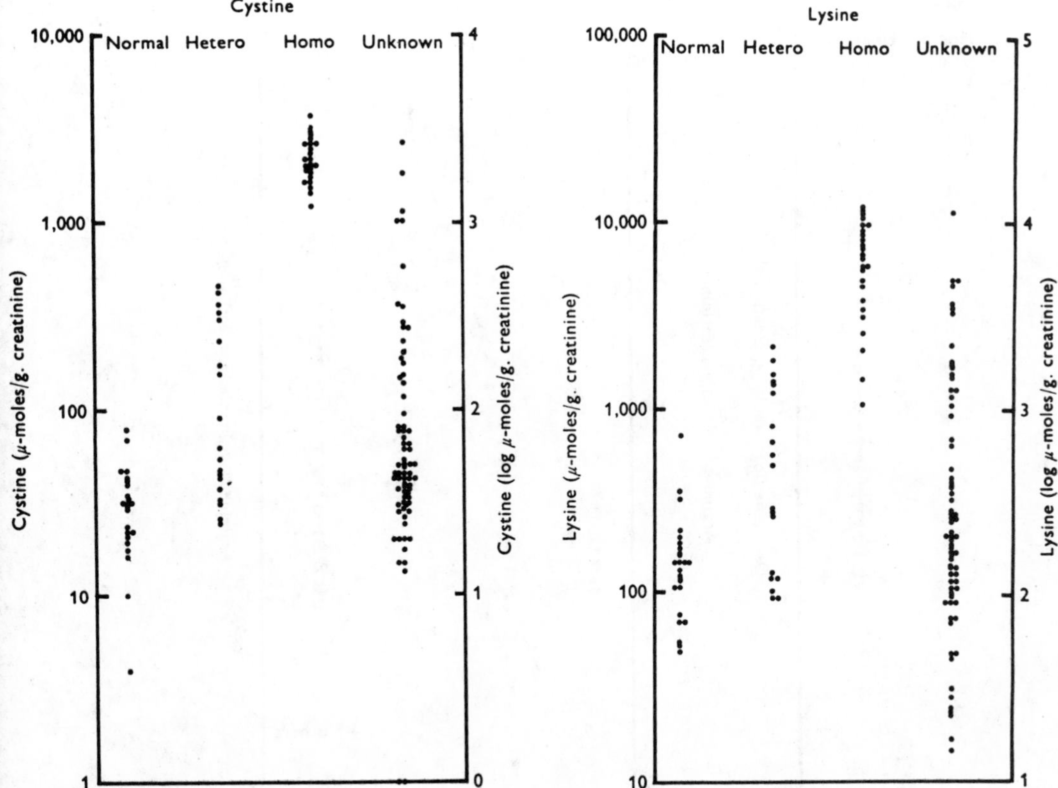

Figure 62-9. The excretion of cystine and lysine by normal subjects, patients with cystinuria, heterozygotes for cystinuria, and relatives of cystinuric patients [22].

first type (Fig. 62-7). The third type may be an expression of an even greater multiplicity of genetic factors involved in the intestinal transport phenotype.

Thus cystinuria is defined as a genetic disorder with a complex recessive mode of inheritance resulting from allelic mutations. At least some of the mutations may be expressed in the heterozygous state. The most sensitive means for differentiating the three types of homozygous cystinuric subjects is the study of the intestinal transport of cystine and the dibasic amino acids in vitro. Similar differentiation can be attempted from studies of urinary amino acid excretion in families of cystinuric subjects. This approach is neither as sensitive nor as direct as the study of transport in vitro.

TREATMENT

Were it not for the insolubility of cystine, cystinuria would be a metabolic oddity of no clinical significance except under conditions of critical limitation of protein intake. Therefore treatment is designed to reduce excretion and increase the solubility of cystine. Therapeutic approaches may be divided into three categories: (1) dietary restriction aimed at reducing cystine production and excretion; (2) attempts to increase cystine solubility by physical means; (3) attempts to convert cystine to a more soluble compound.

Dietary Therapy

The production of cystine from the essential amino acid methionine by a series of defined metabolic events is outlined in Fig. 62-4. Numerous attempts have been made to design diets low in methionine, yet adequate for nutritional purposes. The results of use of such diets are extremely variable. Disappearance of cystinuria while the patient was on one of these diets has been reported by some investigators, whereas others have been unable to demonstrate any significant reduction in urinary cystine with careful methionine restriction [92, 93]. It is probably reasonable to avoid excessive methionine intake, but it is clear that discomforting diets are not indicated.

Physical Factors

At urinary pH values below 7.5 about 300 mg cystine per liter of urine will be in solution. Increasing urine volume

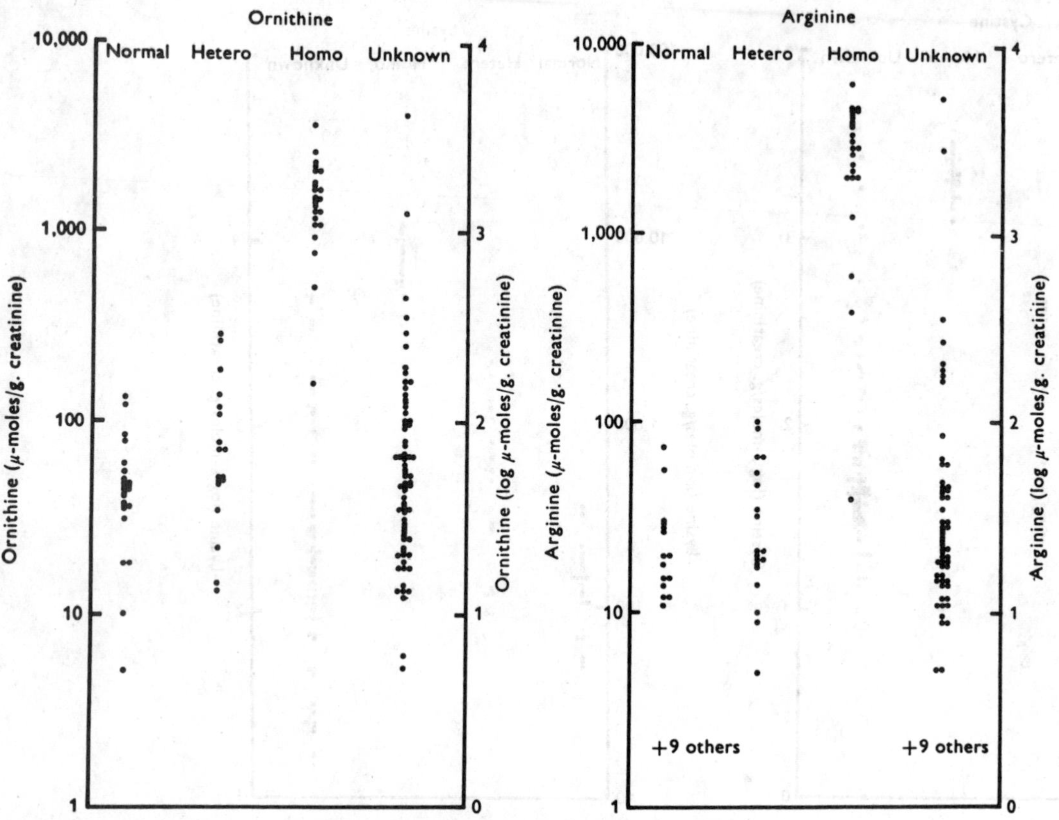

Figure 62-10. The excretion of arginine and ornithine by normal subjects, cystinuric patients, heterozygotes for cystinuria, and relatives of cystinuric patients [22].

provides a progressive reduction in urinary cystine concentration and reduces the likelihood of precipitation. Some reports of stone dissolution on high fluid intake programs have appeared [94]. Many cystinuric subjects excrete in the range of 1 gm cystine per day and will require a fluid intake of 4 or more liters per day. Cystine solubility can also be enhanced by providing an alkaline pH, but the solubility does not increase significantly until the pH is above 7.5 (Fig. 62-11). Since the maximum urine pH which can be achieved is about 8, there is little leeway in the alkalinizing program. Administration of bicarbonate, citrate, and carbonic anhydrase inhibitors has been advocated for improving solubility, but while theoretically reasonable it is not clear that much practical benefit occurs. Since varying physical factors, high fluid intake, and alkalinization are logical and simple, they should be included in the first therapeutic program in all cystinuric subjects. In considering high fluid intake therapy, Dent and Senior [95] pointed out the importance of preventing supersaturation of urine with cystine at night when urine flow is low. The intake of two glasses of water at bedtime repeated at 2 or 3 A.M. is recommended. Dent et al. [94] found hydration therapy to be successful in preventing stone formation in about two-thirds of patients who adhered to it, during a 10-year study. Their therapeutic hydration regimen is well outlined in their paper.

Penicillamine

In spite of the best and most controlled therapeutic efforts, some patients with cystinuria will repeatedly form and pass stones, and a significant number will require surgery for

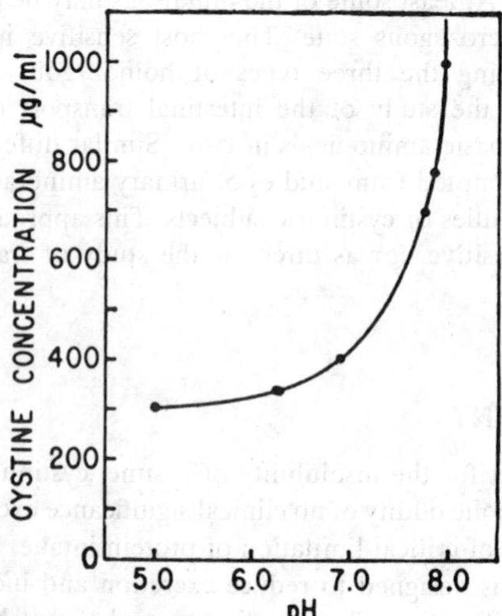

Figure 62-11. The solubility of cystine in relation to urinary pH. (*From Dent and Senior* [95].)

relief of urinary tract obstruction. For those who were apparently not helped by diet, fluid, and alkalinization, there was little to be done until Crawhall, Scowen, and Watts introduced the use of D-penicillamine ($\beta\beta$-dimethyl-cysteine). Through a disulfide exchange reaction, this drug can produce the mixed disulfide of cysteine-penicillamine, which is significantly more soluble than cystine [96, 97] (Fig. 62-5). On adequate penicillamine therapy, usually 1 to 2 gm per 24 hr, cystine excretion may be kept below 200 mg per gm creatinine, a level at which stone formation is minimal. The reduction of urinary cystine does not appear to be balanced by the amount of cysteine which is combined with penicillamine into the cysteine-penicillamine mixed disulfide. The total molar amount of half-cystine excreted on penicillamine therapy, i.e., the sum of cystine plus the cysteine moiety of the mixed disulfide, is much less than prior to drug treatment. This plus the reduction of plasma cystine levels by the drug suggests another biochemical effect of penicillamine besides disulfide exchange [98, 99]. In contrast to the results on cystinuric subjects, the total molar amount of half-cystine in urine of normal individuals given penicillamine is greatly increased [98]. This finding has not been satisfactorily explained.

Although strikingly effective, penicillamine has certain undesirable side effects. As high as 50 percent of patients receiving the drug will develop allergic reactions, usually fever and rash; rarely arthralgias appear [98]. More severe reactions include development of a nephrotic syndrome [103–105] and of pancytopenia [106]. Epidermolysis [107–109], thrombocytosis [110], and loss of taste have also been reported [111]. In addition, a possible problem resulting from inhibition of pyridoxine should be recognized and treated with supplemental pyridoxine phosphate. The possible reaction of penicillamine with pyridoxine to form a thiazolidine led to studies demonstrating reduced pyridoxal effect in patients on penicillamine therapy (increased kynurenic acid excretion) [112]. The chelating properties of penicillamine are responsible for increased copper and zinc excretion in the urine and less significant effects on calcium, mercury, and iron excretion [113–115]. There is evidence to suggest that at least part of the increase in copper excretion is independent of chelation [115] and is as yet unexplained. No interference with growth is seen in children, and pregnancies have been successfully completed on the drug [102, 116].

In view of the drawbacks of D-penicillamine therapy, its use should be restricted to patients in whom more conservative therapy has failed or who have lost one kidney from cystine stone disease. Therapy should be started in the hospital in order to monitor reactions of hypersensitivity. In those patients initially sensitive to the drug, adequate results have been obtained by readministering the medication in gradually increasing doses over a period of 1 to 2 months. A related compound, N-acetyl-D-penicillamine, has been developed which is effective in disulfide formation and thus in reducing cystine content; this compound appears to have fewer side effects, perhaps because of the unavailability of an amino group for chemical reaction [22, 117]. Cross sensitivity between penicillamine and penicillin has not been a problem.

The apparent reduction in cystine crystalluria in patients receiving diazepoxide remains unexplained but bears further investigation [118].

ANIMAL MODELS OF CYSTINURIA

Three animal models have been suggested for the study of cystinuria. As a result of studies of amino acid excretion patterns of animals in the London Zoo, Harris thought that the blotched genet excreted very large amounts of cystine [119]. The genet appeared to be unique in that "cystine" was excreted without the dibasic amino acids, and was excreted in concentrations far greater than would ordinarily remain in solution. The latter observation led to postulation of substances in genet urine which would enhance cystine solubility. Recently Crawhall and Segal have demonstrated that the genet excretes not cystine, but the far more soluble sulfur amino acid, S-sulfo-L-cysteine [120]. There is in fact no abnormality of cystine transport in the genet, and this apparent animal model must be discarded.

In 1956 a male mink with large numbers of apparently pure cystine stones was reported. This was a ranch mink on a higher than usual protein intake but otherwise unremarkable [121]. The presence of cystinuria in an animal group already carefully bred and therefore easily studied bears further investigation, but at present little further information is available.

Canine cystinuria represents potentially the most useful model for study. Although cystine stones in dogs were described as early as 1823, it was not until Brand and Cahill bred a group of Irish terriers with cystinuria that any systematic observations were made [122–126]. The expression of cystinuria corresponded to a sex-linked inheritance pattern. As in man, their animals responded with rises in cystine excretion after methionine feeding, and had no change after cystine feeding. Most, if not all, canine cystinuria has appeared in males. Though this may be due to the narrow urethra of male dogs, which brings stone production to clinical attention, amino acid chromatography has not revealed the disease in females to date.

The exact amino acid excretion pattern in canine cystinuria is not clear. Isolated cystinuria, cystinuria plus lysinuria, and the full pattern of cystine and all dibasic amino acids appearing in excess in the urine have been reported [62, 127–130]. An intestinal defect in amino acid transport has been postulated [131].

Recent application of transport techniques in vitro to both intestinal and kidney biopsies of cystine stone–forming dogs has disclosed a defect neither in cystine nor in lysine accumulation by either tissue [62]. The absence of a demonstrable lysine transport defect in these dog tissues is unlike the findings in human biopsies, while the absence of a cystine transport defect is consistent with findings in man. It would appear that canine cystinuria is a heterogeneous entity. The presence of large amounts of cystine in the urine of these dogs makes this strain an excellent model for evaluating the nature of hyperexcretion of cystine and assessment of therapeutic approaches for decreasing the amounts of urinary cystine in man. To date, fluid intake, alkalinization, and D-penicillamine have all been observed to alter the clinical course favorably [132].

One human experimental model has been described by Brown [133]. He produced increased urinary excretion of several amino acids (principally cystine, lysine, ornithine, and arginine) in amounts similar to homozygous cystinuria in patients fed the nonmetabolizable amino acid, cycloleucine. The rat also shows this response to cycloleucine administration [134]. Holtzapple et al. [135] have shown that cycloleucine is a competitive inhibitor of the transport of both neutral and dibasic amino acid by slices of human kidney cortex.

SUMMARY

1 Cystinuria is a disorder of amino acid transport affecting the epithelial cells of the renal tubule and the gastrointestinal tract. The defective transport of cystine, lysine, arginine, and ornithine is transmitted as an autosomal recessive trait. The heterozygous state may reflect true recessive or incompletely recessive inheritance. In the latter state the affected amino acids are excreted in urine in quantities greater than normal but less than in the homozygous state. By use of the intestinal transport system as a sensitive genetic marker, three types of cystinuric homozygotes can be defined, and the evidence is that these types result from allelic mutations.

2 The intestinal transport defect can be demonstrated in vivo by oral loading studies. The involved amino acids are fed, and blood and stool levels of the amino acids and their breakdown products are measured. Complementary data supporting the studies in vivo have been derived from studies in vitro of intestinal mucosal transport.

3 The renal lesions demonstrable for all four amino acids and the mixed disulfide of cysteine-homocysteine can be demonstrated by clearance studies. Studies in vitro of amino acid transport by renal cortical slices demonstrate a defect for dibasic amino acids but not for cystine. In fact, no interaction of cystine and dibasic amino acid is demonstrable in vitro. Cysteine, the precursor and intracellular form of cystine, can be shown to share a cellular efflux system with the dibasic amino acids. The discrepancy between results of studies in the kidney in vivo and in vitro remains to be explained.

4 Cystinuria is expressed clinically as urinary tract calculus disease. Radiopaque cystine stones are formed, and hexagonal cystine crystals appear in the urine. Diagnosis may be pursued by testing urine with nitroprusside, high-voltage electrophoresis, or column amino acid analysis. Stones generally form at cystine excretion rates of greater than 300 mg cystine per gm creatinine in acid urine. Cystinuric patients are susceptible to all complications of stone disease. Treatment is directed at reducing the concentration of cystine in urine by increasing urine volume, increasing cystine solubility by alkalinizing the urine, and reducing cystine excretion by use of D-penicillamine. D-penicillamine, although extremely effective, is not without risk and should be reserved for patients who fail to respond to conservative therapy.

5 Models of human cystinuria have been described in animals. Studies of these models may help clarify the cellular defect in cystinuria and may provide a system for testing new drug therapy.

BIBLIOGRAPHY

1. Wollaston, W. H.: On cystic oxide: a new species of urinary calculus. Trans. Roy. Soc. London, **100,** 223, 1810.
2. Noehden, G. H.: Scientific notices—chemistry, cystic oxide—communicated in a letter from Dr. Noehden to Mr. Children. Ann. Philos., **7,** 146, 1824.
3. Berzelius, J. J.: Calculus urinaires. Traite Chem., **7,** 424, 1833.
4. Friedman, E.: Der Kreislauf des Schwefels in der organischen Natur. Ergebn. Physiol., **1,** 15, 1902.
5. Garrod, A. E.: Inborn errors of metabolism. Lancet, **2,** 1908. (Lecture I, p. 1; Lecture II, p 73; Lecture III, p. 142; Lecture IV, p. 214.)
6. Yeh, H. L., Frankl, W., Dunn, M. S., Parker, P., Hugher, B., and Gyorgy, P.: The urinary excretion of amino acids by a cystinuric subject. Amer. J. Med. Sci., **214,** 507, 1947.
7. Stein, W. H.: Excretion of amino acids in cystinuria. Proc. Soc. Exp. Biol. Med., **78,** 705, 1951.
8. Dent, C. E., Senior, B., and Walshe, J. M.: The pathogenesis of cystinuria. II. Polarographic studies of the metabolism of sulphur-containing amino-acids. J. Clin. Invest., **33,** 1216, 1954.
9. Arrow, V. K., and Westall, R. G.: Amino acid clearances in cystinuria. J. Physiol., **142,** 141, 1958.
10. Dent, C. E., and Rose, G. A.: Amino acid metabolism in cystinuria. Quart. J. Med., **20,** 205, 1951.
11. von Udranszky, L., and Baumann, E.: Ueber das Vorkommen von Diaminen, sogenannten Ptomainen, bei Cystinurie. Z. Physiol. Chem., **13,** 562, 1889.
12. Loewy, A., and Neuberg, C.: Über Cystinurie. S. Physiol. Chem., **43,** 338, 1904.
13. Brand, E., Cahill, G. F., and Harris, M. M.: Cystinuria. II. The metabolism of cysteine, methionine and glutathione. J. Biol. Chem., **109,** 69, 1935.
14. Brand, E., and Cahill, G. F.: Further studies on metabolism of sulfur compounds in cystinuria. Proc. Soc. Exp. Biol. Med., **31,** 1247, 1934.
15. Milne, M. D., et al.: The metabolic disorder in Hartnup disease. Quart. J. Med., **29,** 407, 1960.
16. Milne, M. D., Asatoor, A. M., Edwards, K. D. G., and Loughridge, L. W.: The intestinal absorption defect in cystinuria. Gut, **2,** 323, 1961.
17. Asatoor, A. M., Lacey, B. W., London, D. R., and Milne, M. D.: Amino acid metabolism in cystinuria. Clin. Sci., **23,** 285, 1962.
18. Thier, S., Fox, M., Segal, S., and Rosenberg, L. E.: Cystinuria: in vitro demonstration of an intestinal transport defect. Science, **143,** 482, 1964.
19. McCarthy, C. F., Borland, J. L., Lynch, H. J., Owen, E. E., and Tyor, M. P.: Defective uptake of basic amino acids and L-cystine by intestinal mucosa of patients with cystinuria. J. Clin. Invest., **43,** 1518, 1964.
20. Thier, S., Segal, S., Fox, M., Blair, A., and Rosenberg, L. E.: Cystinuria: defective intestinal transport of dibasic amino acids and cystine. J. Clin. Invest., **44,** 442, 1965.
21. Crawhall, J. C., and Watts, R. W. E.: Cystinuria. Amer. J. Med., **45,** 736, 1968.

22. Crawhall, J. C., Purkiss, P., Watts, R. W. E., and Young, E. P.: The excretion of amino acids by cystinuric patients and their relatives. Ann. Hum. Genet., **33**, 149, 1969.
23. Renander, A.: The roentgen density of the cystine calculus. Acta Radiol., suppl. **41**, 1941.
24. Hambraeus, L., and Lagergren, C.: Cystinuria in Sweden. VI, Biophysical and roentgenological studies of urinary calculi from cystinurics. J. Urol., **88**, 826, 1962.
25. Brand, E., Harris, M. M., and Biloon, S.: Cystinuria: excretion of a cystine complex which decomposes in the urine with the liberation of free cystine. J. Biol. Chem., **86**, 315, 1930.
26. Lewis, H. B.: Cystinuria: a review of some recent investigations. Yale J. Biol. Med., **4**, 437, 1932.
27. Harris, H., Mittwoch, U., Robson, E. B., and Warren, F. L.: Pattern of amino acid excretion in cystinuria. Ann. Hum. Genet., **19**, 196, 1955.
28. Hambraeus, L.: Comparative studies of the value of two cyanide-nitroprusside methods in the diagnosis of cystinuria. Scand. J. Lab. Clin. Invest., **15**, 657, 1963.
29. Crawhall, J. C., Saunders, E. P., and Thompson, C. J.: Heterozygotes for cystinuria. Ann. Hum. Genet., **29**, 257, 1966.
30. Sackett, D. L.: Adaptation of monodirectional high voltage electrophoresis on long papers to the rapid qualitative identification of urinary amino acids. J. Lab. Clin. Med., **63**, 306, 1964.
31. Stein, W. H.: A chromatographic investigation of the amino acid constituents of normal urine. J. Biol. Chem., **201**, 45, 1953.
32. Soupart, P.: Free amino acids of blood and urine in the human, in *Amino Acid Pools,* edited by J. T. Holden, p. 220. Elsevier, Amsterdam, 1962.
33. Meloni, C. R., and Canary, J. J.: Cystinuria with hyperuricemia. J.A.M.A., **200**, 169, 1967.
34. Dent, C. E., and Harris, H.: The genetics of cystinuria. Ann. Hum. Genet., **16**, 60, 1951.
35. Brooks, W. D. W., Heasman, M. A., and Lovell, R. R. H.: Retinitis pigmentosa associated with cystinuria; 2 uncommon inherited conditions occurring in family. Lancet, **1**, 1096, 1949.
36. Hurwitz, L. J., Carson, N. A. J., Allen, I. V., Fannin, T. F., Lyttle, J. A., and Neill, D. W.: Clinical, biochemical and histopathological findings in a family with muscular dystrophy. Brain, **90**, 799, 1967.
37. Clara, R., and Lowenthal, A.: Familial and congenital lysine-cystinuria with benign myopathy and dwarfism. J. Neurol. Sci., **3**, 434, 1966.
38. Tanguay, R. B., and Galindo, J.: Cystinuria associated with mongolism and identification of an abnormal pyrrolidine compound in urine. Amer. J. Clin. Path., **46**, 442, 1966.
39. Gross, J. B., Ulrich, J. A., and Jones, J. D.: Urinary excretion of amino acids in a kindred with hereditary pancreatitis and aminoaciduria. Gastroenterology, **47**, 41, 1964.
40. Brodehl, J., Gallissen, K., and Kowalewski, S.: Isolated cystinuria (without lysine-ornithine-argininuria) in a family with hypocalcemic tetany. Klin. Wschr., **45**, 38, 1967.
41. Collis, J. E., Levi, A. J., and Milne, M. D.: Stature and nutrition in cystinuria and Hartnup disease. Brit. Med. J., **1**, 590, 1963.
42. Brand, E., Block, R. J., Kassell, B., and Cahill, G. F.: Cystinuria. V. The metabolism of casein and lactalbumin. J. Biol. Chem., **119**, 669, 1937.
43. Rachele, J. R., Reed, L. J., Kidwai, A. R., Ferger, M. F., and du Vigneaud, V.: Conversion of cystathionine labeled with S^{35} to cystine *in vivo.* J. Biol. Chem., **185**, 817, 1950.
44. Schimke, R. N., McKusick, V. A., and Weilbaecher, R. G.: Homocystinuria, in *Amino Acid Metabolism and Genetic Variation,* edited by W. L. Nyhan, pp. 297–313. McGraw-Hill, New York, 1967.
45. Frimpter, G. W.: Cystathionuria, in *Amino Acid Metabolism and Genetic Variation,* edited by W. L. Nyhan, pp. 315–523. McGraw-Hill, New York, 1967.
46. Sturman, J. A., Gaull, G., and Raihs, N. C. R.: Absence of cystathionase in human fetal liver: Is cystine essential? Science, **169**, 74, 1970.
47. Gaitonde, M. K., and Gaull, G.: A procedure for the quantitative analysis of the sulphur amino acids of rat tissues. Biochem. J., **102**, 959, 1967.
48. Wheldrake, J. F., and Pasternak, C. A.: The oxidation of cystine by mast-cell tumor, p. 815 in Culture. Biochem. J., **106**, 437, 1968.
49. London, D. R., and Foley, T. H.: Cystine metabolism in cystinuria. Clin. Sci., **29**, 133, 1965.
50. Crawhall, J. C., Lietman, P. S., Schneider, J. A., and Seegmiller, J. E.: Cystinosis: plasma cystine and cysteine concentrations and effect of D-penicillamine and dietary treatment. Amer. J. Med., **44**, 330, 1968.
51. Crawhall, J. C., and Segal, S.: The intracellular ratio of cysteine and cystine in various tissues. Biochem. J., **105**, 891, 1967.
52. Segal, S., and Smith, I.: Delineation of cystine and cysteine transport systems in rat kidney cortex by developmental patterns. Proc. Nat. Acad. Sci., U.S.A., **63**, 926, 1969.
53. States, B., and Segal, S.: Distribution of glutathione-cystine transhydrogenase activity in subcellular fractions of rat intestinal mucosa. Biochem. J., **113**, 443, 1969.
54. Robson, E. B., and Rose, G. A.: The effect of intravenous lysine on the renal clearances of cystine, arginine and ornithine in normal subjects, in patients with cystinuria and Fanconi syndrome and their relatives. Clin. Sci., **16**, 75, 1957.
55. Webber, W. A., Brown, J. L., and Pitts, R. F.: Interactions of amino acids in renal tubular transport. Amer. J. Physiol., **200**, 380, 1961.
56. Rosenberg, L. E., Downing, S. J., and Segal, S.: Competitive inhibition of dibasic amino acid transport in rat kidney. J. Biol. Chem., **237**, 2265, 1962.
57. Fox, M., Thier, S., Rosenberg, L. E., Kiser, W., and Segal, S.: Evidence against a single renal transport defect in cystinuria. New Eng. J. Med., **270**, 556, 1964.
58. Schwartzman, L., Blair, A., and Segal, S.: Exchange diffusion of dibasic amino acids in rat-kidney cortex slices. Biochim. Biophys. Acta, **135**, 120, 1967.
59. Segal, S., Schwartzman, L., Blair, A., and Bertoli, D.: Dibasic amino acid transport in rat kidney cortex slices. Biochim. Biophys. Acta, **135**, 127, 1967.
60. Segal, S., and Crawhall, J. C.: Characteristics of cystine and cysteine transport in rat kidney cortex slices. Proc. Nat. Acad. Sci. U.S.A., **59**, 231, 1968.
61. Segal, S., and Smith, I.: Delineation of separate transport systems in rat-kidney cortex for L-lysine and L-cystine by developmental patterns. Biochem. Biophys. Res. Commun., **35**, 771, 1969.
62. Holtzapple, P. G., Bovee, K., Rea, C. F., and Segal, S.: Amino acid uptake by kidney and jejunal tissue from dogs with cystine stones. Science, **166**, 1525, 1969.
63. Whelan, D. T., and Scriver, C. R.: Hyperdibasicaminoaciduria: an inherited disorder of amino acid transport. Pediat. Res., **2**, 525, 1968.
64. Oyanagi, K., Miura, R., and Yamanouchi, T.: Congenital lysinuria: a new inherited transport disorder of dibasic amino acids. J. Pediat., **77**, 259, 1970.
65. Stein, W. H., and Moore, S.: The free amino acids of human blood plasma. J. Biol. Chem., **211**, 915, 1954.
66. Frimpter, G. W.: Cystinuria: intravenous administration of S^{35} cystine and S^{35} cysteine. Clin. Sci., **31**, 207, 1966.
67. Frimpter, G. W.: Cystinuria: metabolism of the disulfide of cysteine and homocysteine. J. Clin. Invest., **42**, 1956, 1963.
68. Rosenberg, L. E., Durant, J. L., and Holland, J. M.: Intestinal absorption and renal extraction of cystine and cysteine in cystinuria. New Eng. J. Med., **273**, 1239, 1965.
69. Segal, S., and Crawhall, J. C.: Transport of cysteine by human kidney cortex. Biochem. Med., **1**, 141, 1967.
70. Rosenberg, L. E., Crawhall, J. C., and Segal, S.: Intestinal transport of cystine and cysteine in man: evidence for separate mechanisms. J. Clin. Invest., **46**, 30, 1967.
71. Schwartzman, L., Blair, A., and Segal, S.: A common renal transport system for lysine, ornithine, arginine and cysteine. Biochem. Biophys. Res. Commun., **23**, 220, 1966.
72. Frimpter, G. W., Horwith, M., Furth, E., Fellows, R. E., and Thompson, D. D.: Inulin and endogenous amino acid renal clearances in cystinuria: evidence for tubular secretion. J. Clin. Invest., **41**, 281, 1962.
73. Crawhall, J. C., Scowen, E. F., Thompson, C. J., and Watts, R. W. E.:

The renal clearance of amino acids in cystinuria. J. Clin. Invest., **46,** 1162, 1967.

74. Rosenberg, L. E., Albrecht, I., and Segal, S.: Lysine transport in human kidney: evidence for two systems. Science, **155,** 1426, 1967.
75. Scriver, S. R., and Wilson, O. H.: Amino acid transport: evidence for genetic control of two types in human kidney. Science, **155,** 1428, 1967.
76. King, J. S., Jr., and Wainer A.: Cystinuria with hyperuricemia and methioninuria: biochemical study of a case. Amer. J. Med., **43,** 125, 1967.
77. Frimpter, G. W.: Cystathioninuria in a patient with cystinuria. Amer. J. Med., **46,** 832, 1969.
78. Frimpter, G. W.: The disulfide of L-cysteine and L-homocysteine in urine of patients with cystinuria. J. Biol. Chem., **236,** 651, 1961.
79. Hambraeus, L.: Cystinuria in Sweden: quantitative studies of urinary amino acid excretion in cystinurics. Acta Soc. Med Upsal., **6,** 1, 1964.
80. Schneider, J. A., Bradley, K. H., and Seegmiller, J. E.: Identification and measurement of cysteine-homocysteine mixed disulfide in plasma. J. Lab. Clin. Med., **71,** 122, 1968.
81. Foley, T. H., and London, D. R.: Cysteine metabolism in cystinuria. Clin. Sci., **29,** 549, 1965.
82. Rosenberg, L. E., Downing, S., Durant, J. L., and Segal, S.: Cystinuria: biochemical evidence for three genetically distinct diseases. J. Clin. Invest., **45,** 365, 1966.
83. Segal, S., Lowenstein, L. M., and Wallace, A.: Comparison of the transport characteristics by rat intestine and kidney cortex. Gastroenterology, **55,** 386, 1968.
84. Segal, S.: Tissue transport defects of dibasic amino acids, in Symposium on Intestinal Absorption and Malabsorption. Mod. Probl. Pediat., **11,** 56, 1968.
85. Harris, H., and Warren, F. L.: Quantitative studies on the urinary cystine in patients with cystine stone formation and their relatives. Ann. Eugen., **18,** 125, 1953.
86. Harris, H., Mittwoch, U., Robson, E. B., and Warren, F. L.: Phenotypes and genotypes in cystinuria. Ann. Hum. Genet., **20,** 57, 1955.
87. Rosenberg, L. E., and Downing, S.: Transport of neutral and dibasic amino acids by human leucocytes: Absence of a defect in cystinuria. J. Clin. Invest., **44,** 1382, 1965.
88. Harris, H., and Robson, E. B.: Variation in homozygous cystinuria. Acta Genet. (Basel), **5,** 581, 1955.
89. Rosenberg, L. E., Durant, J. L., and Albrecht, I.: Genetic heterogeneity in cystinuria: evidence for allelism. Trans. Ass. Amer. Physicians, **79,** 284, 1966.
90. Rosenberg, L. E.: Genetic heterogeneity in cystinuria, in *Amino Acid Metabolism and Genetic Variation,* edited by W. L. Nyhan, p. 341. McGraw-Hill, New York, 1967.
91. Hershko, C., Ben-Ami, E., Paciorkovski, J., and Levin, N.: Alleomorphism in cystinuria. Proc. Tel-Hashomer Hosp., **4,** 21, 1965.
92. Kolb, F. O., Earll, J. M., and Harris, H. A.: Disappearance of cystinuria in a patient treated with prolonged low methionine diet. Metabolism, **16,** 378, 1967.
93. Zinneman, H. H., and Jones, J. E.: Dietary methionine and its influence on cystine excretion in cystinuric patients. Metabolism, **15,** 915, 1966.
94. Dent, C. E., Friedmann, M., Green, H., and Watson, L. C. A.: Treatment of cystinuria. Brit. Med. J., **1,** 403, 1965.
95. Dent, C. E., and Senior, B.: Studies on the treatment of cystinuria. Brit. J. Urol., **27,** 317, 1955.
96. Crawhall, J. C., Scowen, E. F., and Watts, R. W. E.: Effect of penicillamine on cystinuria. Brit. Med. J., **1,** 585, 1963.
97. Crawhall, J. C., Scowen, E. F., and Watts, R. W. E.: Further observations on use of D-penicillamine in cystinuria. Brit. Med. J., **1,** 1411, 1964.
98. Bartter, F. C., Lotz, M., Thier, S., Rosenberg, L. E., and Potts, J. T.: Cystinuria: combined clinical staff conference at the National Institutes of Health. Ann. Intern. Med., **62,** 796, 1965.
99. Crawhall, J. C., and Thompson, C. J.: Cystinuria: effect of D-penicillamine on plasma and urinary cystine concentrations. Science, **147,** 1459, 1965.
100. Lotz, M., and Potts, J. T.: Quantitation of the effects of penicillamine therapy in cystinuria. J. Clin. Invest., **43,** 1293, 1964.
101. McDonald, J. E., and Henneman, P. H.: Stone dissolution in vivo and control of cystinuria with D-penicillamine. New Eng. J. Med., **273,** 578, 1965.
102. Crawhall, J. C., Scowen, E. F., Thompson, C. J., and Watts, R. W. E.: Dissolution of cystine stones during D-penicillamine treatment of a pregnant patient with cystinuria. Brit. Med. J., **1,** 216, 1967.
103. Fellers, F. X., and Shahidi, N. T.: The nephrotic syndrome induced by penicillamine therapy. Amer. J. Dis. Child., **98,** 669, 1959.
104. Adams, D. A., Goldman, R., Maxwell, M. H., and Latta, H.: Nephrotic syndrome associated with penicillamine therapy of Wilson's disease. Amer. J. Med., **36,** 330, 1964.
105. Rosenberg, L. E., and Hayslett, J. P.: Nephrotoxic effects of penicillamine in cystinuria. J.A.M.A., **201,** 698, 1967.
106. Corcos, J. M., Soler-Bechera, J., Mayer, K., Freyberg, R. H., Goldstein, R., and Jaffé, I.: Neutrophilic agranulocytosis during administration of penicillamine. J.A.M.A., **189,** 265, 1964.
107. Beer, W. E., and Cooke, K. B.: Epidermolysis bullosa induced by penicillamine. Brit. J. Derm., **79,** 123, 1967.
108. Katz, R.: Penicillamine-induced skin lesions, a possible example of human lathyrism. Arch. Derm. Syph., **95,** 196, 1967.
109. Harris, E. D., and Sjoerdsma, A.: Effect of penicillamine on human collagen and its possible application to treatment of scleroderma. Lancet, **1,** 996, 1966.
110. Fawcett, N. P., Nyhan, W. L., and Anderson, W. W.: Thrombocytosis during treatment of cystinuria with penicillamine. J. Pediat., **69,** 976, 1966.
111. Keiser, H. R., Henkin, R. I., Bartter, F. C., and Sjoerdsma, A.: Loss of taste during therapy with penicillamine. J.A.M.A., **203,** 381, 1968.
112. Jaffe, I. A., Altman, K., and Merryman, P.: The antipyridoxine effect of penicillamine in man. J. Clin. Invest., **43,** 1969, 1964.
113. Walsh, J. M., and Patston, V.: Effect of penicillamine on serum iron. Arch. Dis. Child., **40,** 651, 1965.
114. Bostrom, H., and Wester, P. O.: Excretion of trace elements in two penicillamine-treated cases of cystinuria. Acta Med. Scand., **181,** 475, 1967.
115. McCall, J. T., Goldstein, N. P., Randall, R. V., and Gross, J. B.: Comparative metabolism of copper and zinc in patients with Wilson's disease (hepatolenticular degeneration). Amer. J. Med. Sci., **254,** 35, 1967.
116. Pruzanski, W.: Cystinuria and cystine urolithiasis in childhood. Acta Paediat. Scand., **55,** 97, 1966.
117. Stokes, G. S., Potts, J. T., Lotz, M., and Bartter, F.: A new agent in the treatment of cystinuria: N-acetyl-D-penicillamine. Brit. Med. J., **1,** 284, 1968.
118. Fariss, B. L., and Kolb, F. O.: Preliminary communication: factors involved in crystal formation in cystinuria. J.A.M.A., **205,** 138, 1968.
119. Datta, S. P., and Harris, H.: Urinary amino acid patterns of some mammals. Ann. Eugen., **18,** 107, 1953.
120. Crawhall, J. C., and Segal, S.: Sulphocysteine in the urine of the blotched Kenya genet. Nature (London), **208,** 1320, 1965.
121. Oldfield, J. E., Allen, P. H., and Adair, J.: Identification of cystine calculi in mink. Proc. Soc. Exp. Biol. Med., **91,** 560, 1956.
122. Lassaigne, J. L.: Observation sur l'existence de l'oxide cystique dans un calcul vésical du chien, et essai analytique sur la composition élémentaire de cette substance particuliere. Ann. Chim. Phys., 2d ser., **23,** 328, 1823.
123. Morris, M. L., Green, D. F., Dinkel, J. H., and Brand, E.: Canine cystinuria. North Amer. Vet., **16,** 16, 1935.
124. Brand, E., and Cahill, G. F.: Canine cystinuria. III. J. Biol. Chem., **114,** XV, 1936.
125. Brand, E., Cahill, G. F., and Kassell, B.: Canine cystinuria. V. Family history of two cystinuric Irish terriers and cystine determinations in dog urine. J. Biol. Chem., **133,** 431, 1940.
126. Green, D. F., Morris, M. L., Cahill, G. F., and Brand, E.: Canine cystinuria. II. Analysis of cystine calculi and sulfur distribution in the urine. J. Biol. Chem., **114,** 91, 1936.
127. Crane, C. W., and Turner, A. W.: Amino acid patterns of urine and blood plasma in a cystinuric Labrador dog. Nature (London), **177,** 237, 1956.

128. Treacher, R. J.: Amino acid excretion in canine cystine-stone disease. Vet. Rec., **74,** 503, 1962.
129. Cornelius, C. E., Bishop, J. A., and Schaffer, M. H.: A quantitative study of amino aciduria in dachshunds with a history of cystine urolithiasis. Cornell Vet., **177,** April, 1967.
130. Goulden, B. E., and Leaver, J. L.: Low voltage paper electrophoresis as a screening test for the diagnosis of canine cystinuria. Vet. Rec., **80,** 244, 1967.
131. Treacher, R. J.: Intestinal absorption of lysine in cystinuric dogs. J. Comp. Path., **75,** 309, 1965.
132. Frimpter, G. W., Thouin, P., and Ewalds, B. H.: Penicillamine in canine cystinuria. J. Amer. Vet. Med. Ass., **151,** 1084, 1967.
133. Brown, R. R.: Aminoaciduria resulting from cycloleucine administration in man. Science, **157,** 432, 1967.
134. Goyer, R. A., Reynolds, J. O., Jr., and Elston, R. C.: Characteristics of the aminoaciduria resulting from cycloleucine administration in pair fed rats. Proc. Soc. Exp. Biol. Med., **130,** 860, 1969.
135. Holtzapple, P., Rea, C., Genel, M., and Segal, S.: Cycloleucine inhibition of amino acid transport in human and rat kidney cortex. J. Lab. Clin. Med., **75,** 818, 1970.

CHAPTER SIXTY-THREE

FAMILIAL IMINOGLYCINURIA*

Charles R. Scriver

Familial iminoglycinuria is an inborn error of membrane transport characterized by exaggerated renal clearance of free proline, hydroxyproline, and glycine[1] in the presence of normal plasma concentrations of all three compounds; the renal clearance of other amino acids is normal. The trait has been discovered in patients with a variety of illnesses and also in healthy subjects; familial iminoglycinuria is probably a harmless condition.

The iminoglycinuric phenotype constitutes the homozygous form of the trait; the heterozygote has no iminoaciduria but may or may not show hyperglycinuria. Heterogeneity of the heterozygous phenotype may be an indication that more than one mutant allele occurs at the gene locus controlling the relevant membrane transport protein. The urinary phenotype of homozygotes born to parents of similar phenotype is identical to that of iminoglycinuric subjects born to parents of dissimilar phenotypes. Genetic heterogeneity at the relevant locus is also suggested by the segregation of homozygotes with an associated intestinal transport defect from those without this finding.

Mutant homozygotes, regardless of their postulated genotype, retain considerable tubular absorptive function under the normal endogenous plasma load; this probably reflects the presence of more than one mode of membrane transport available to the imino acids and glycine. A transport site shared by the three compounds and with large capacity is believed to be deleted or inactivated by the iminoglycinuria mutation, while other membrane systems with different specificity and smaller capacity for imino acids and glycine remain active.

DISCOVERY OF FAMILIAL IMINOGLYCINURIA

Chromatographic techniques provide the clinician with a means for evaluating the distribution of amino acids in body fluids. The initial application by Dent [1] of chromatographic methods to medical investigation fostered an exponential increase in the number of diseases of amino acid metabolism that were discovered between 1948 and the present time [2]. Chromatographic interest at first focused primarily on variations in the excretion of the amino acids in the urine [3]. It was soon recognized that urine of young infants normally contains a large quantity of the two imino acids[2], proline and hydroxyproline, and of the amino acid, glycine. Imino aciduria of the newborn disappears as the infant reaches about 6 months of age, and thereafter urine normally does not contain detectable amounts of proline or hydroxyproline; the intensity of glycinuria also diminishes at this time.

Several investigators over the years have studied the origin of hyperiminoglycinuria in the human infant [7–10]. Their data indicate that net tubular absorption of several amino acids, including the imino acids and glycine, is impaired in the newborn by comparison with the older subject (Fig. 63-1). The subsequent suppression of iminoglycinuria during the later infantile period is associated with enhanced net tubular absorption of the three solutes. It appears then that a particular transport function in the renal tubule undergoes maturation postnatally. This function may be the membrane transport system preferentially shared by the imino acids and glycine [11].

Persistence of iminoglycinuria beyond early infancy constitutes an abnormality of amino acid metabolism. It occurs under three different circumstances:

1. As a complex "combined" aminoaciduria in the presence of hyperprolinemia or hyperhydroxyprolinemia (see Chap. 16 on these diseases)
2. As a specific inborn error of membrane transport of amino acids now usually known as *familial* (*renal*) *iminoglycinuria* (the subject of this chapter)
3. As a component of a generalized disturbance of membrane transport, e.g., in Fanconi's syndrome

It is the second form of iminoglycinuria which concerns us here (Table 63-1). Joseph and colleagues [12] described familial iminoglycinuria for the first time in 1958 and attributed it to an abnormality of renal tubular transport. Because the trait was associated with a familial convulsive disorder, and because the relation of the one to the other was poorly understood, it was temporarily given the eponym, "Joseph's syndrome" [13]. Shortly thereafter, Jonxis in Holland observed another family with a convulsive disorder in which some members had an iminoglycinuria of renal origin [14]. The second published report appeared in 1965 from Japan [15]. Tada and colleagues [15] described "proli-

*This work was supported in part by an associateship of the Medical Research Council of Canada.

[1] These compounds are also excreted in bound form as oligopeptides (see Chap. 16, Disorders of Proline and Hydroxyproline Metabolism). Familial iminoglycinuria is a trait affecting only the free forms of proline, hydroxyproline, and glycine.

[2] "Imino acid" is a popular term used to distinguish the configuration of the secondary amine group (RC—NHCH—COOH) of the heterocyclic amino acids from the usual primary amine group (NH_2—CHR—COOH) of other amino acids. The term "imino acid" is freely used in standard texts on the biochemistry and metabolism of amino acids [4, 5], but reservations have been expressed about the accuracy of its use in this way [6].

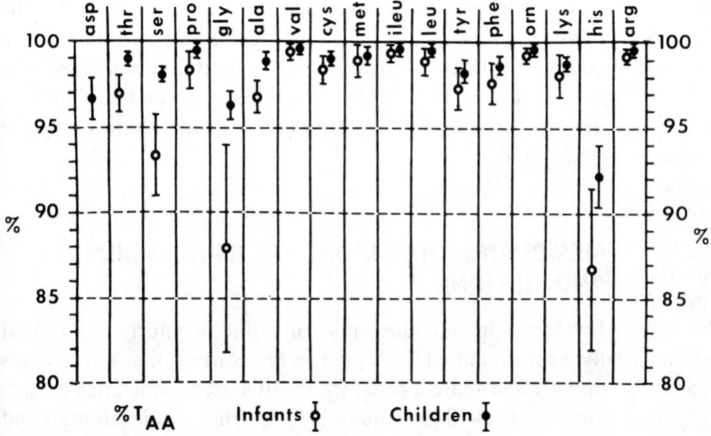

Figure 63-1. Net tubular absorption of amino acids (expressed as percent of filtered load) is less efficient in the newborn human subject when compared with older subjects. Glycine absorption is particularly impaired, and the presence of imino acids in the urine of the neonate and young infant is noteworthy. (*Redrawn from Brodehl and Gellissen* [10]. *Reproduced from Pediatrics with permission.*)

nuria: a new renal tubular defect in transport of proline and glycine," in two unrelated probands. Both patients were mentally retarded, and consanguinity was present in one of the families. A year later Morikawa et al. [16] reported a third Japanese patient with iminoglycinuria and mental retardation. They described a new feature, an associated intestinal transport defect, which also involved the imino acids and glycine. Familial iminoglycinuria was first reported from North America after its discovery in an Ashkenazic Jewish pedigree [17]. The proband was a healthy adult male in whom the trait was found incidentally during investigation of the family for the cause of liver cirrhosis in a relative

Table 63-1. SUMMARY OF CLINICAL FEATURES IN FAMILIES WITH RENAL IMINOGLYCINURIA

Pedigree	Source of data	Age of homozygote at diagnosis, yr	Sex	Reason for medical attention	Hyperglycinuria in obligate heterozygote	Intestinal transport defect	Special features
A	Joseph et al. (1958) [12]	$1\frac{9}{12}$	M	Seizures	No	Not studied	Proband and 2 sibs died with seizures
B	Tada et al. (1965) [15]	$\frac{9}{12}$	F	Mental retardation with cortical atrophy	No	No	
C	Tada et al. (1965) [15]	$\frac{4}{12}$*	M	Mental retardation with cortical atrophy	No	Not studied	Parental consanguinity
D	Morikawa et al. (1966) [16]	$1\frac{5}{12}$	F	Mental retardation and hypsarrhythmia	No‡	Yes	
E	Scriver & Wilson (1967) [17, 21]	42	M	None†	Yes	No	Pedigree contains compound heterozygote
F	Goodman et al. (1967) [19]	18	F	Mental retardation after encephalitis	Yes/No§	Yes	
G	Hoefnagel & Pomeroy (1968) [24]	11	F	Hypophosphatemic rickets and mild mental retardation	Yes/No§	Not studied	
H	Scriver (1968) [21]	29	F	None†	Yes	No	Cystinosis also present in pedigree
I	Whelan & Scriver (1968) [21, 22]	21	F	None†	Yes	Not studied	Cystathioninuria also present in pedigree
J	Rosenberg et al. (1968) [23]	6	M	Deafness	Yes	No	
K	Fraser et al. (1968) [25]	16	M	Deafness and Leber's optic atrophy	No (only mother tested)	Not studied	Parental consanguinity suspected

* Iminoglycinuria was still present at 12 months of age.
† Discovered during investigation of another trait in the pedigree.
‡ Personal communication from Dr. Keiya Tada (1969).
§ One parent is hyperglycinuric, the other is not; therefore, the child is probably a compound heterozygote (see Fig. 63-9).

[18]. Other cases of familial iminoglycinuria were then recognized in the United States and in Canada [19–24], and recently in Great Britain [25]. Thus, the trait appears to be widely distibuted.

In every reported instance iminoglycinuria has been discovered during investigations carried out for other purposes. In the majority of the pedigrees, the proband with iminoglycinuria was initially investigated for a serious medical problem (Table 63-1).[3] However, the diversity of the clinical abnormalities in probands with familial iminoglycinuria suggests that there is little or no direct relationship between the inherited disorder of membrane transport and the accompanying illness. Several investigators have proposed that familial iminoglycinuria is indeed a benign inborn error of membrane transport [22, 23, 25], a conclusion which is borne out by the occurrence of nine healthy iminoglycinuric subjects in Pedigrees E, H, and I (Table 63-1) (see also Fig. 63-9).

LABORATORY METHODS FOR DETECTION AND INVESTIGATION

Iminoglycinuria can be easily detected by chromatographic and electrophoretic methods applied to urine. The presence of even small amounts of proline and hydroxyproline in the urine of older infants, children, and adults is abnormal. Case finding is enhanced if methods are used which effectively demonstrate the imino acids. Two-dimensional partition methods are usually more sensitive than one-dimensional separations. The analytic systems described by Dent [27] and by Smith in his text on chromatographic and electrophoretic methods [28] include a variety of techniques for separating amino acids on filter paper. Proline, hydroxyproline, and glycine produce distinctive colors in clearly defined positions on the chromatogram if it is stained with the appropriate reagents [28]. We have found that the phenol-lutidine partition system of Dent [27] will produce a filter-paper chromatogram which can be stained with a mixture of ninhydrin (0.25 percent w/v) and isatin (0.01 percent w/v) in acetone, containing 1 percent lutidine to give characteristic colors for proline (yellow-pink), hydroxyproline (mauve), and glycine (brown-orange) after heating for 10 min at 80°C. Ehrlich's reagent [28] applied over the ninhydrin-isatin stain will erase most ninhydrin-positive spots, while staining hydroxyproline purple.

Accurate quantitative analysis can be performed by elution chromatography on ion-exchange resin columns. Several semiautomated instruments will perform accurate analyses using the recommended procedures for operation. Modified procedures have been devised for rapid analysis of the neutral amino acids in physiologic fluids on short resin columns with the Technicon instrument [29] and the Beckman analyzer [30]. These methods can facilitate investigation, particularly if loading and infusion studies must be performed.

[3] The interesting pedigree described by deVries et al. [26] is omitted from Table 63-1. These authors described several female members with nephrolithiasis and dominantly inherited hyperglycinuria in three generations of Ashkenazic Jews living in Israel. This pedigree probably reflects the heterozygous phenotype of the iminoglycinuric trait (see "Genetics," below).

MEMBRANE TRANSPORT OF IMINO ACIDS AND GLYCINE

Investigation into the cause of iminoglycinuria in familial hyperprolinemia [31, 32] led to the concept that imino acids and glycine share a renal transport system which has preference for these three solutes [11]. Further studies in man and other mammals, both in vivo and in vitro, have revealed that membrane transport of proline, hydroxyproline, and glycine is a complex process, apparently involving several reactive membrane sites which are under the control of several genes.

Studies in Vivo

Titration studies performed on human subjects by the methods of Smith and coworkers [33] show that net tubular absorption of L-proline in man undergoes saturation as the plasma concentration is increased [32]. A maximum rate for net tubular absorption of proline (T_m proline) has been determined [32]. Renal tubular transport of hydroxy-L-proline has also been studied in man by similar titration techniques, and transport of this imino acid can also be saturated [34].

The capacity of the normal renal tubule to transport proline and hydroxyproline is shown in Table 63-2 and in Fig. 63-6. Although studies of glycine transport have not yet been performed in man, data from the dog [35] imply that its uptake is saturated in vivo at concentrations considerably in excess of those which are required of the imino acids to saturate their membrane transport systems. Thus, it can be said that the amount of membrane available for the transport of imino acids and glycine into tubular cells is finite. The restrictive nature of membrane transport under these conditions indicates that uptake is mediated by membrane functions which control solute migration.

The role of membrane sites or permeases or mediators [36, 37], as they have been variously named, which mediate solute migration is further delineated in the particular interactions which occur between amino acids during tubular absorption. Infusion of one imino acid increases urinary excretion of the other and of glycine in man [32, 34], yet there is little or no effect on the excretion of other amino acids. The same selective interaction between imino acids and glycine is also observed in vivo in the rat [38], and to some extent in the dog [39], although in the dog the interaction is much less selective. Patients with familial hyper-

Table 63-2. RENAL CLEARANCE, NET TUBULAR ABSORPTION, AND T_m OF IMINO ACIDS AND GLYCINE IN FAMILIAL IMINOGLYCINURIA

Phenotype	*Proline*			*Hydroxyproline*			*Glycine*	
	Endog. Clear., ml/min/1.73 m²	Reabsorbed, %	T_m, μmoles/min/1.73 m²	Endog. Clear., ml/min/1.73 m²	Reabsorbed, %	T_m μmoles/min/1.73 m²	Endog. Clear., ml/min/1.73 m²	Reabsorbed, %
Normal*	0–0.03	>99.8	180–300	0	100	60–135	1.2–8.6	93–99
Homozygous†								
Mean	6.7	....	....	13	...	......	27	
Range	0.5–19.6	77–99.5	10–18	1–33.6	65–99	6	17.0–41.6	61–77
Heterozygous‡ ("hyperglycinuric")	0	100	35–117	0	100	50	14.3 8.6–26.2	82–95
Heterozygous§ ("silent")	0	100	?	0	100	?	3.1–6.7	>93

* From Rosenberg and Scriver [53]. T_m data from Scriver [21].

† Compiled from Goodman et al. [19], Scriver [21], Rosenberg et al. [23], Hoefnagel and Pomeroy [24], and Tada et al. [51].

‡ Compiled from Goodman et al. [19], Scriver [21], Rosenberg et al. [23], and Hoefnagel and Pomeroy [24].

§ Compiled from Goodman [20], Scriver [21], and Hoefnagel and Pomeroy [24].

prolinemia have iminoglycinuria [31, 32] which is directly proportional to the concentration of proline in their plasma when the concentration of proline exceeds 1 mM; this is the level at which proline itself begins to saturate its own transport system and appears in the urine [32].

Thus, data on imino acid and glycine transport from normal human subjects and from patients with disordered imino acid catabolism complement each other and suggest that the renal tubule has a membrane transport system which is selective in its preference for proline, hydroxyproline, and glycine, and which is finite in its capacity.

Studies in Vitro

The rat kidney cortex slice method of Rosenberg and colleagues [44] has been used to study membrane transport of imino acids and glycine. These solutes are accumulated by a mechanism which can be saturated [38, 45] and which follows Michaelis-Menten kinetics. There are selective competitive interactions between these substrates [45] in accord with sharing of reactive sites. Nevertheless an intensive kinetic analysis of the competitive interactions by methods which test for homogeneity in so-called "common" transport sites used by several substrates [45, 46] has indicated that it is not possible to attribute all the uptake of imino acids and glycine to a single membrane system [38, 45]. Extensive studies of L-proline and glycine uptake by kidney cortex slices [47], and of glycine [48*a*] and L-proline [48*b*] by isolated tubules, have shown that both substrates are transported by more than one system (Fig. 63-2).

In addition to the differences in transport kinetics which distinguish one system from another, a number of qualitative characteristics, such as the response to competitive and noncompetitive inhibitors, were used in these investigations for delineating the heterogeneity of sites available to each substrate. As a result of these studies and of many others addressed to the same problem (cited in [37] and [49]), it is now generally assumed that membrane transport sites exhibit two types of specificity toward their substrates (Fig. 63-3): one type distinguishes between substrates of different chemical composition; the other type determines the manner in which a single substrate is taken up over a broad concentration range. This heterogeneity of renal uptake is not confined to the imino acids and glycine. It has been clearly described for the metabolically inert amino acid, α-amino isobutyric acid (AIB) [50], for the essential amino acid lysine [50*a*], and also for monosaccharides [50*b*]. Diversity of trans-

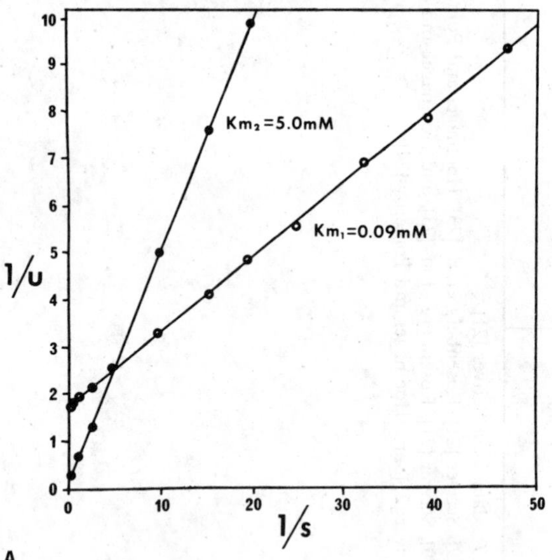

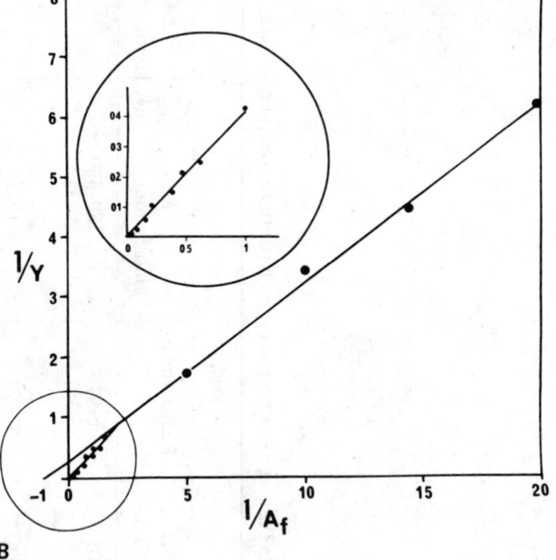

Figure 63-2. Evidence for more than one mode of uptake for L-proline and for glycine in mammalian kidney. *A.* Lineweaver-Burk plot of L-proline uptake at low and high concentrations by rat kidney cortex slice. The contributions to total uptake from each of two systems have been specifically calculated, and the K_m value shown is the actual value for each system. (*From* [47], *with permission of the American Journal of Physiology.*) *B.* Lineweaver-Burk plot of glycine uptake by isolated rabbit kidney tubules indicates the presence of more than one system. The actual uptake contributed by the individual systems has not been determined; thus the K_m values are only first approximations. (*Redrawn from* [48*a*], *with permission of the Journal of Biological Chemistry.*)

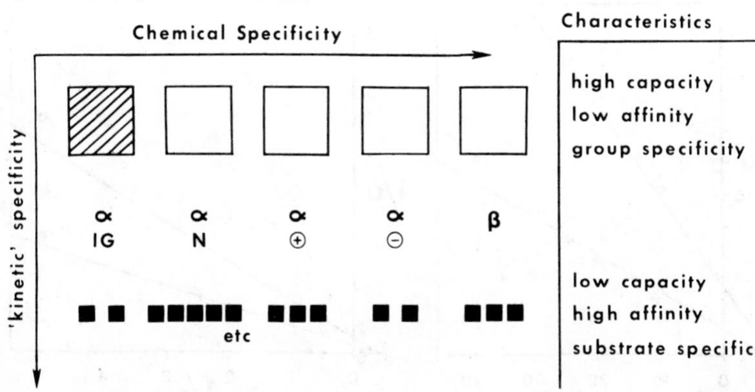

Figure 63-3. A model showing two species of "reactive sites" ("transport proteins" or "permeases") in kidney. *Upper series:* five types of sites, each of which shares a family of substrates, and whose respective preferences for substrates are (*left to right*) α-amino acids—imino acids and glycine (IG), neutral amino acid (N), cationic (+), and anionic (−) α-amino acids; and β-amino acids (β). These sites have characteristics which distinguish them from a second species (*lower series*), which have greater substrate specificity. Familial iminoglycinuria is believed to be an inborn error of membrane transport in which the membrane protein serving shared transport of imino acids and glycine is deleted (hatched symbol).

port processes is clearly evident in kidney, and it seems to be one explanation for the phenomenon of *residual transport* in mutant homozygotes who have an inborn error of transport. Nonetheless heterogeneity is not necessarily expressed equivalently in all tissues of a metazoan organism such as man, and this could account for the inconsistent expression of a mutant transport phenotype in various organs.

Efflux of solute from mammalian cells is also accomplished by mediated processes which are not necessarily identical to those serving influx. Oxender and Christensen [50*c*] discerned that reactive sites for efflux transport are less specific than those mediating influx.

Development of Renal Transport

It has long been known that excretion of imino acids and glycine in the urine is particularly prominent relative to the general hyperaminoaciduria which persists for several months after birth [3, 7–10]. Excessive iminoglycinuria in the early postnatal period of life also is seen in the rat [40, 41], and in the mouse, guinea pig, and kitten [41]. Investigation of this phenomenon in man [7–10] and in the rat [40, 41] has shown that it is directly related to reduced net tubular reabsorption (Fig. 63-1). The age-dependent change in efficiency of tubular conservation, with particular reference to the imino acids and glycine, suggests that the activity of the transport system(s) used by these compounds increases with age. It has been shown that the relative activities of membrane transport systems with different substrate preferences change at different rates in the intestine during development [42]. Accordingly it seems reasonable that differential rates of maturation of renal transport systems account for the distinctive character of postnatal aminoaciduria [43].

Recent studies [41] have defined the ontogeny of the transport systems for imino acids and glycine in Long-Evans rat kidney. Iminoaciduria disappears about 1 week after birth; glycinuria diminishes to adult levels at about 3 weeks of age. Studies in vitro reveal the emergence of a low-K_m system for L-proline at about 10 days in kidney; a low-K_m system for glycine appears in the third week after birth. Until the appearance of these two systems, transport occurs on a high-K_m, high-capacity system with two characteristics of the "common" system found in mature kidney. The developing kidney thus expresses differential gene activity reflected in the changing specific activity of various transport systems. It was also noted that efflux systems for imino acids and glycine in kidney behaved independently of the influx systems.

The findings in rat kidney are probably informative about the events which take place during human renal ontogeny. It has now been shown (K. Baerlocher, C. Clow, S. Mackenzie, and C. R. Scriver; unpublished) that renal imino aciduria persists for about 3 months after full-term birth whereas hyperglycinuria persists about 6 months. Phased changes in the specific activity of tubular transport systems in the human infant seem evident from these findings.

METABOLISM AND TRANSPORT

The influence of the catabolism of L-proline on its own transport has been assessed in vitro. L-Proline is normally converted to several derivatives, notably glutamic acid, glutamine, and ornithine. It is also oxidized with evolution of CO_2. In experiments concerned with transport and metabolism of L-proline [47] it was found that the rate of metabolism of proline did not change the affinity of the substrate for its own transport system (Fig. 63-4). On the other hand, the observed rate of transport of proline was dependent both on the external concentration of substrate available for transport and the amount determined to have reached the intracellular space. When these events are considered, there is still evidence for two different systems of proline transport, one at high and one at low external concentrations. It follows that predictions concerning the nature of the membrane sites at which transport occurs are not likely to be affected by intracellular metabolism. These considerations are relevant to the interpretation of the mutant transport phenotypes described below.

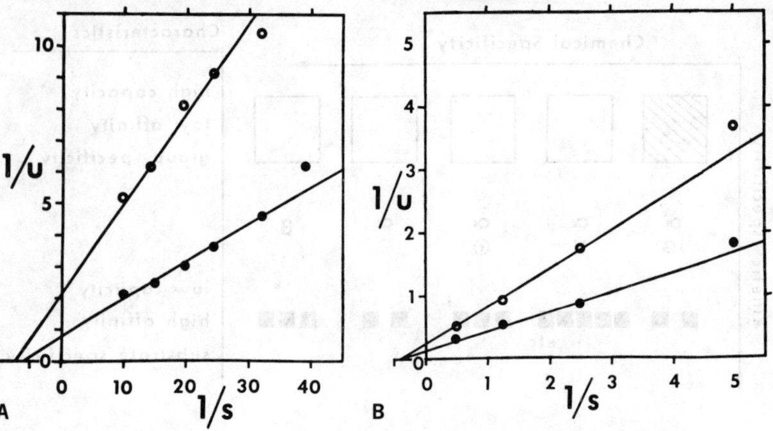

Figure 63-4. Effect of metabolism on uptake of L-proline. Lineweaver-Burk plots show that the V_{max} (intercept on ordinate), but not K_m (intercept on abscissa), is altered when the amount of proline which is oxidized to $^{14}CO_2$ after uptake of L-proline-U-^{14}C is included (closed circles), or ignored (open circles) in the calculations of the kinetic constants for L-proline transport at low (*A*) and high (*B*) external concentrations. Thus, catabolism of substrate following its own uptake, in this case, does not affect the affinity of the substrate for its own transport protein. (*From* [47] *with permission of the American Journal of Physiology.*)

Nature of Membrane Transport Sites for Imino Acids and Glycine

The foregoing reveals that the migration and concentration of imino acids and glycine across the renal tubular cell membrane are mediated by processes which can be saturated, which have specificity, and which are constitutive in the sense that intracellular metabolism of the solute after its uptake does not modulate the actual process of uptake. Christensen defined the modality serving transport of a solute as a "reactive site" [36], and Pardee [50*d*] has recently reviewed the evidence for the protein nature of such sites.

Membrane transport proteins or permeases comprise a means whereby the cell can achieve specificity in the uptake of metabolites; it then follows that mutation in the gene which controls a transport protein will modify a specific membrane function; this will be reflected by a phenotype which could be called an inborn error of transport. Familial iminoglycinuria is one of 30 such traits now known in man [49]. Mutations which affect the transport of proline or of glycine independently have been identified in bacteria (cited in [49]), and since both substrates are not necessarily affected together, it may be assumed that uptake of imino acids and glycine in microorganisms is achieved, at least in part, by more than one site.

MECHANISM OF FAMILIAL IMINOGLYCINURIA

Probands with familial iminoglycinuria are discovered because their urine contains excessive amounts of proline, hydroxyproline, and glycine. The excretion of other amino acids is normal, and the concentration of all the amino acids in the plasma of these subjects is normal. The endogenous renal clearance rates of amino acids and their net tubular absorption rates have been calculated in a number of subjects [19, 21, 23, 24, 51]; only the imino acids and glycine have elevated clearance rates and impaired net absorption rates (Table 63-2). Familial iminoglycinuria is, therefore, the reflection of impaired function of a specific renal tubular transport system. Two related and important observations emerge from these relatively simple studies:

1 Net tubular absorption of imino acids and glycine is not completely eliminated in homozygotes.
2 The abnormal prolinuria may disappear at low plasma proline concentrations in homozygotes (Fig. 63-5), even though the venous plasma "threshold" for prolinuria is very low in homozygotes (about 0.1 mM) compared to normal subjects (about 0.8 mM).

The ability of the homozygote to retain a considerable fraction of his specific tubular absorptive function is a feature shared by homozygotes with other inborn errors of membrane transport [42]. For example, the homozygote with

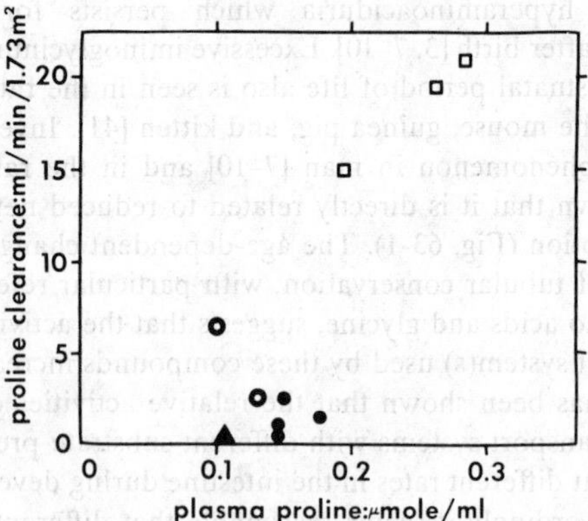

Figure 63-5. Endogenous renal clearance of L-proline related to its concentration in plasma in homozygotes with familial iminoglycinuria. The "venous plasma threshold concentration" at which prolinuria appears is about 0.1 mM; the normal value is about 0.8 mM [21]. Abnormal prolinuria disappears in mutant homozygotes at low plasma proline concentrations, indicating the existence of a small but efficient tubular capacity to transport proline. (*Redrawn from* [21] *with permission of the Journal of Clinical Investigation, with data, symbol O, added from* [23] and other data, symbol ▲, added from [51].)

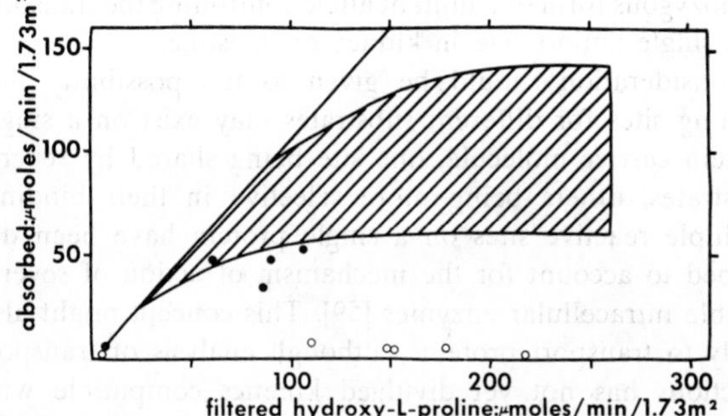

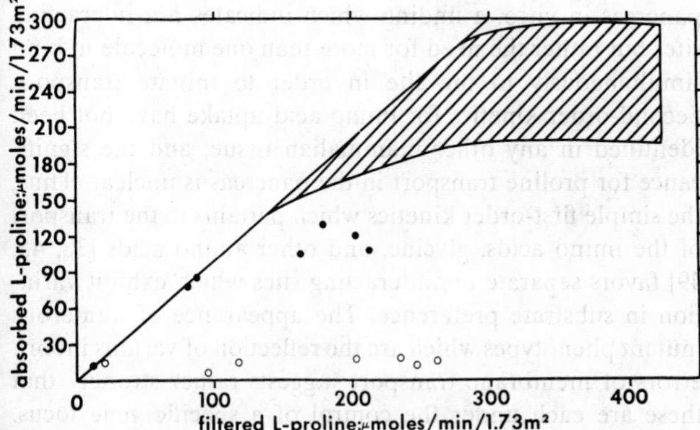

Figure 63-6. Maximum rates of tubular absorption (T_m) of L-proline and hydroxy-L-proline in normal subjects (hatched), heterozygotes (solid circles), and mutant homozygotes with iminoglycinuria. (*Reprinted from* [21] *with permission of the Journal of Clinical Investigation.*)

classical cystinuria, or with the hypercystinuric trait, or with Hartnup's disease, usually retains some capacity to transport the relevant amino acids. A similar characteristic is also observed for hexose transport in glucose-galactose malabsorption in regard to renal tubular absorption of glucose [50*b*]. An interpretation of this phenomenon is that more than one type of transport site serves the migration of a substrate across the cell membrane. The studies of iminoglycine transport in mammalian kidney in vitro support this interpretation.

Transport Saturation in the Mutant Phenotype

Mutant homozygotes and obligate heterozygotes have been infused with L-proline and hydroxy-L-proline in order to determine the equivalent T_m values [17, 21, 23]. These investigations disclosed that imino acid transport is saturated in the mutant homozygote at normal plasma concentration of proline and hydroxyproline (Fig. 63-6). The heterozygote has a T_m which is intermediate between normal and abnormal values (Fig. 63-6); in these subjects imino acid absorption is normal at concentrations below the T_m. This suggests that the affinity of the available imino acid transport sites in the heterozygote is normal. Taken together, these findings indicate that the mutation causes deletion of a transport system which has a capacity well above the normal plasma concentration of imino acids. Another modality of uptake with a small but recognizable capacity is retained.

Interaction between Imino Acids and Glycine in the Mutant Phenotype

Imino acids and glycine normally interact competitively during uptake by the kidney both in vivo and in vitro. These interactions have been studied in subjects with the iminoglycinuric trait, and they are distinctly different from the normal. Though proline or hydroxyproline progressively inhibits tubular absorption of glycine in normal subjects as the concentration in the tubular fluid is increased (Fig. 63-7), neither imino acid inhibits glycine uptake in the mutant homozygote. This can be explained if it is assumed that the persistent glycine transport in the mutant homozygote occurs at a tubular site which is not inhibited by either imino acid [17, 21]. Imino acids are partially effective as competitive inhibitors of glycine transport in heterozygotes (Fig. 63-7), but there is a limit to which glycine transport can be inhibited. Between 8 and 16 μmoles per min per 1.73 m² cannot be inhibited in either the normal or the mutant

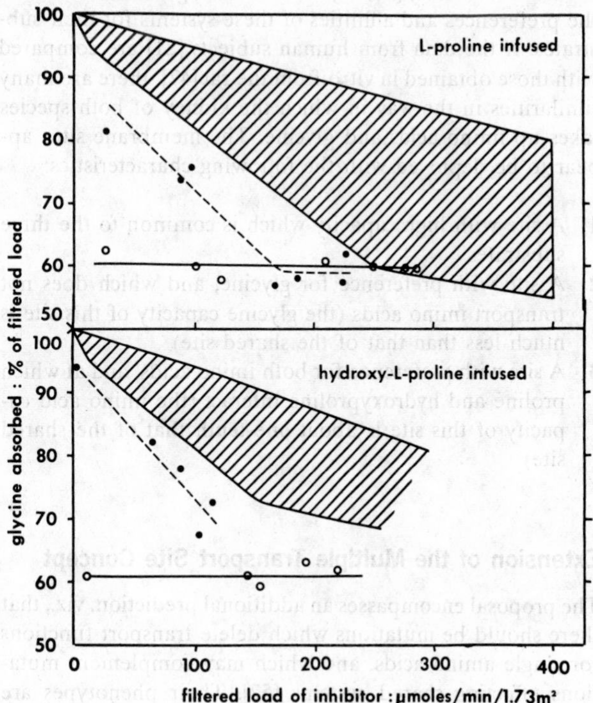

Figure 63-7. Effect of L-proline and hydroxy-L-proline on net tubular absorption of glycine in normal subjects (hatched), heterozygotes (solid circles), and mutant homozygotes with iminoglycinuria. (*Reprinted from* [21] *with permission of the Journal of Clinical Investigation.*)

phenotypes. This presumably represents the noninhibitable portion of glycine transport which is not affected by the mutation.

Imino acids also interact competitively with each other during absorption by the normal tubule [31, 34]. Some degree of interaction is also found in mutant homozygotes [21]. This suggests that the alternate site at which imino acids are transported in the mutant homozygote is shared by these two substrates. It is noteworthy in this context that a specific separate site for hydroxyproline transport has not been identified either in *Escherichia coli* [54], where proline and glycine transport sites have been clearly delineated, or in bone cells [55], where hydroxyproline is an important constituent of collagen. There is apparently no advantage to be gained from a separate membrane transport site for hydroxyproline, since hydroxyproline is synthesized in peptide linkage from proline after the latter has been incorporated into a precollagen polypeptide.

THE APPARENT DEPLOYMENT OF MEMBRANE TRANSPORT SITES FOR UPTAKE OF IMINO ACIDS AND GLYCINE

Calculations have been made of the relative capacities of the systems for transport of imino acids and glycine in mammalian kidney [21, 47], and something can be said about the preferences and affinities of these systems for their substrates. If the data from human subjects [21] are compared with those obtained in vitro from the rat [47], there are many similarities in the way in which the kidney of both species takes up imino acids and glycine. The membrane sites appear to be deployed with the following characteristics:

1 A site with high capacity which is common to the three substrates
2 A site with preference for glycine, and which does not transport imino acids (the glycine capacity of this site is much less than that of the shared site)
3 A site with preference for both imino acids, and at which proline and hydroxyproline interact (the imino acid capacity of this site is about one-tenth that of the shared site)

Extension of the Multiple Transport Site Concept

The proposal encompasses an additional prediction, viz., that there should be mutations which delete transport functions for single amino acids, and which may complement mutations affecting shared systems [52]. Their phenotypes are apparently found in the diseases such as isolated cystinuria [56], which has been seen in a family with idiopathic hyperparathyroidism, methionine malabsorption [57], and tryptophan malabsorption [58], each of which seems to be the homozygous form of a mutant allele controlling the transport of a single amino acid in kidney or intestine.

Consideration should be given to the possibility that binding sites for different substrates may exist on a single protein carrier molecule, one site being shared by several substrates, others being more selective in their binding. Multiple reactive sites on a single protein have been described to account for the mechanism of action of several soluble intracellular enzymes [59]. This concept might also apply to transport proteins, although analysis of transport functions has not yet divulged kinetics compatible with multiple interacting sites [59]. Bégin and Scholefield [60] observed second-order kinetics for proline uptake by mouse pancreas in vitro, a finding which indicates not interacting sites but rather the need for more than one molecule to bind simultaneously to the site in order to initiate transport. Second-order kinetics for imino acid uptake have not been identified in any other mammalian tissue, and the significance for proline transport in the pancreas is unclear. Thus, the simple first-order kinetics which pertains to the transport of the imino acids, glycine, and other amino acids [38, 45, 49] favors separate noninteracting sites which exhibit variation in substrate preference. The appearance of numerous mutant phenotypes which are the reflection of various inborn errors of membrane transport suggests rather strongly that these are each under the control of a specific gene locus.

EXPRESSION OF THE PHENOTYPE IN NONRENAL TISSUES

Intestine

Intestinal transport of imino acids and glycine has been examined in vivo in several homozygotes [15, 16, 19, 21, 23] and in intestinal biopsy material in one subject [23]. Two phenotypes have been identified in vivo in terms of proline absorption (Fig. 63-8). Some homozygotes have normal intestinal transport of L-proline [15, 21, 23], while others have a delayed and depressed uptake of this imino acid into plasma [16, 19]. The association of different intestinal phenotypes with a single renal phenotype suggests that more than one mutant allele is responsible for the iminoglycinuric trait.

Fecal excretion of amino acids has also been examined in homozygotes. In patients with a normal plasma response to oral proline loading [21, 23], the fecal excretion of amino acids is normal. On the other hand, homozygotes with impaired plasma response curves have an elevated concentration of proline in the feces [16, 19]. Morikawa et al. [16] also found a modest excess of glycine in the feces before and after an oral glycine load, even though the plasma glycine response curve was normal after an oral load. It is of interest that the plasma response to glycine loading by mouth is normal in patients with and without any demonstrable impairment of proline absorption [16, 19, 23]. This

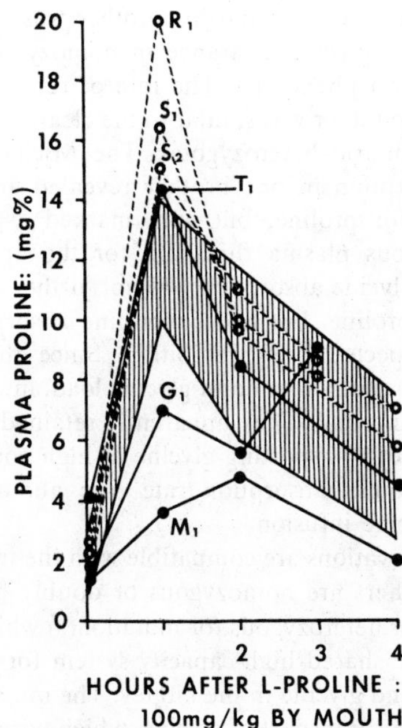

Figure 63-8. Postabsorptive concentration of proline in plasma after an oral load of L-proline (100 mg per kg) in normal subjects (hatched area), and in mutant homozygotes with familial iminoglycinuria. Two types of plasma response are seen in the latter; an increase indicating normal intestinal absorption in subjects S_1 and S_2 [21], R_1 [23], and T_1 [15]; a flattened response indicating impaired absorption in subjects M_1 [16] and G_1 [19].

may indicate that the imino-glycine transport systems of the intestine are qualitatively different from those in the kidney.

Leukocytes

Tada and colleagues [61] examined the accumulation of proline in peripheral leukocytes obtained from a mutant homozygote with impaired intestinal and renal transport. The ability of the leukocytes to accumulate proline was normal. Tada [61] proposed that leukocytes do not express the mutant transport allele for the high-capacity transport system. These leukocyte studies were done at low substrate concentrations (about 0.006 mM), low enough, in fact, that uptake could have occurred almost exclusively on the low-capacity system (Fig. 63-2), which is apparently retained in the mutant trait. Thus, the experiment and its interpretations must be considered inconclusive.

Skin Fibroblasts

Tada and his colleagues [61] also studied the incorporation of L-proline into the collagen of fibroblasts from a skin biopsy during incubation for 2 hr. The rate of incorporation was not different from the rate obtained with normal skin. The same reservation expressed about the leukocyte studies applies also to this experiment. The substrate concentration was only 0.05 mM, and proline uptake could have been achieved by the low-capacity system, the activity of which would not have been affected in the iminoglycinuric phenotype.

DIAGNOSIS

Criteria for Abnormal Iminoglycinuria

Any degree of *iminoaciduria* after 6 months of age may be considered abnormal. Hyperglycinuria may be recognized on partition chromatograms when the glycine spot is disproportionately intense in comparison with other amino acids. The quantitative criteria for *hyperglycinuria* are: urinary excretion exceeding 160 μmoles per gm total nitrogen [21], or 150 mg per 24 hr [62], or an endogenous clearance rate exceeding 8.6 ml per min per 1.73 m^2 [63].

Physiologic Considerations

There are three mechanisms by which abnormal iminoglycinuria can occur:

COMBINED MECHANISM. One substrate is present in high concentration. If it shares a transport site with other molecules it will displace the cosubstrates competitively. Thus, although only one substrate is present in excess in plasma, several may appear in increased amounts in the urine.

MODIFIED REACTIVE SITE (SPECIFIC, RENAL MECHANISM). The substrate concentration in plasma is normal, but the transport site is modified, and access of the substrate is impaired.

MODIFIED TRANSFER OF SUBSTRATE (GENERALIZED OR SPECIFIC RENAL MECHANISM). The substrate combines adequately with the reactive site, but either the number of sites is limited, or migration of substrate after it combines with the site is impaired.

Differential Diagnosis

HYPERPROLINEMIA AND HYDROXYPROLINEMIA. Iminoglycinuria occurs by a "combined" mechanism when there is hyperprolinemia in excess of about 0.8 mM [32]. Hyperprolinemia, Type I or Type II (see Chap. 16), is usually accompanied by iminoglycinuria. Though the single patient with hydroxyprolinemia [64] did not exhibit iminoglycinuria, the concentration of hydroxyproline in the plasma was no greater than 0.4 mM; hydroxyproline must be present in plasma at this concentration at least in order to inhibit tubular absorption of proline and glycine competitively [34]. Hyperprolinemia and hydroxyprolinemia can be ruled out as a cause of iminoglycinuria if the concentration of both imino acids in plasma is normal in subjects with iminoglycinuria.

FANCONI'S SYNDROME. Iminoglycinuria occurs in this syndrome as part of a generalized inhibition of tubular transport. Thus, a generalized hyperaminoaciduria occurs in Fanconi's syndrome in contrast to the selective nature of the hyperaminoaciduria in familial iminoglycinuria. Maleic acid, which produces Fanconi's syndrome in vivo, inhibits transport noncompetitively in vitro [65].

NEONATAL IMINOGLYCINURIA. The human infant normally has some degree of renal iminoglycinuria until about the third month of postnatal life.

RENAL GLYCINURIA. There have been numerous reports of hyperglycinuria without iminoaciduria. Since this phenotype may represent one form of the heterozygote with the iminoglycinuria mutation, it merits special attention.

The pedigree with dominantly inherited renal hyperglycinuria and nephrolithiasis, reported by deVries et al. [26], has already been mentioned and will be discussed below.

Käser and colleagues [66] described autosomal dominant glucoglycinuria. The 9-year-old male proband was thought to have cystic fibrosis as well as glucoglycinuria. Glucosuria occurred by the Type B mechanism of Reubi (see Chap. 64), i.e., the renal threshold for glucosuria was low (79 mg per 100 ml), but the T_{mG} was normal (386 mg per min per 1.73 m^2). Thirteen healthy relatives of the forty-four who were examined also had glucoglycinuria; no subjects with glucosuria or glycinuria alone were found. Glycinuria apparently occurred through a mechanism similar to that responsible for glucosuria.

Scriver et al. [67] reported a 16-year-old male with hypophosphatemic rickets. Glucoglycinuria was also present. The glucosuria accorded with the Reubi Type A mechanism (low T_m). The impairment of glycine transport was apparently a fault of transport, not of binding of glycine to its site. Thus the glucoglycinuria occurred through a mechanism different from that described by Käser et al. [66]. Since the phosphaturia also involved impaired net uptake in this patient, it seems that there was an inhibition of transport analogous to that which is believed to occur in Fanconi's syndrome; but only three metabolites, instead of a great many, were significantly affected. Dent and Harris [68] described other patients in whom hypophosphatemic rickets and glycinuria occurred, and further examples are cited in the paper by Scriver et al. [67].

A particularly interesting form of hyperglycinuria without endogenous iminoaciduria has been discovered in two brothers and their father [69]. The renal clearance of glycine in the healthy proband and his brother was equivalent to the values for glycine clearance in homozygotes with the iminoglycinuria phenotype. The rate of renal clearance of glycine by the father was similar to the clearance rate found in iminoglycinuric heterozygotes. The Michaelis plot for proline absorption in one brother revealed an apparently normal T_m for proline, but with marked "splay" and a reduced venous plasma threshold for the appearance of prolinuria. Glycine absorption was not further depressed by infusion of proline, but hydroxyproline absorption underwent the expected brisk inhibition. Since these patients responded normally to an oral glycine load, intestinal transport seemed normal. They apparently retained a renal system capable of transporting glycine at high concentrations, since the tubular absorption rate rose about twentyfold during a glycine infusion.

These observations are compatible with the interpretation that the brothers are homozygous or doubly heterozygous and the father heterozygous for mutation(s) which affect the affinity of the shared high-capacity system for transport of imino acids and glycine in the kidney. The mutation is most unfavorable for transport of glycine, which normally has the lowest affinity for the system [38], whereas imino acids gain efficient access to the system at normal plasma concentrations.

The mother of the patients had no hyperglycinuria. She may carry a mutation which is different from that of her husband, or the mutant allele may be variably expressed. In any event, this pedigree illustrates the existence of several mutant alleles at the gene locus controlling the iminoglycinuric system.

These examples indicate that a number of mutant alleles (or, in some cases, perhaps acquired abnormalities) may affect glycine transport in the kidney. All these traits should be distinguished from the "prerenal" form of hyperglycinuria which is found in hyperglycinemia [70].

GENETICS

Familial renal iminoglycinuria evidently occurs when two mutant autosomal alleles occur at the locus which controls the shared imino-glycine transport site. Close consanguinity in the parents of iminoglycinuric children in two of the eleven pedigrees [15, 25] supports the belief that the trait is recessively inherited. There is no evidence that it is X-linked (see Fig. 63-9).

Obligate heterozygotes for the familial iminoglycinuric trait have had hyperglycinuria in some pedigrees (Pedigrees E, H, and I, Fig. 63-9). Hyperglycinuria, therefore, might appear as a dominant trait if iminoglycinuric subjects were not also present in the same pedigree. Dominantly inherited hyperglycinuria was, in fact, described in an Ashkenazic Jewish pedigree by deVries and associates [26], and this pedigree has been classified in the second edition of the present book as a particular form of "hyperglycinuria." It

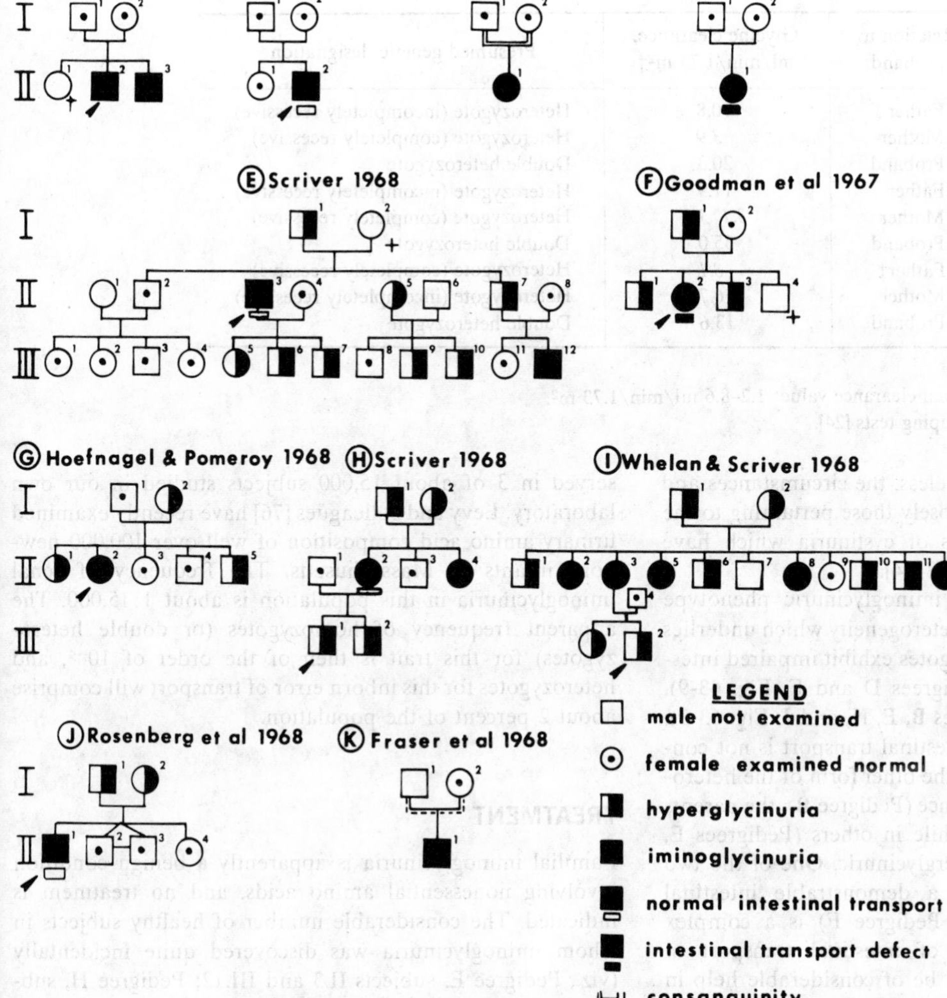

Figure 63-9. Pedigrees of patients with familial iminoglycinuria. Additional information received by personal communication to the author [20, 75] updates the published reports on heterozygous phenotypes in Pedigrees D and F.

is more likely that deVries and colleagues described the heterozygous phenotype of familial iminoglycinuria but did not recognize this because no subject with iminoglycinuria was found in the pedigree. The heterozygous form of iminoglycinuria should be considered in the differential diagnosis of any patient who shows hyperglycinuria.

Obligate heterozygotes for the iminoglycinuric trait do not always exhibit hyperglycinuria. Four pedigrees are known (A, B, C, and D, Fig. 63-9) in which neither parent of the iminoglycinuric proband has hyperglycinuria. The presence of two types of heterozygotes for the iminoglycinuric trait suggest that the mutant allele occurs in more than one form. When the mutant allele is expressed (as hyperglycinuria) in the heterozygote, the situation is analogous to the "incompletely recessive" form of cystinuria [71]; when the mutant allele is silent in the heterozygote, the situation is analogous to the "completely recessive" form of cystinuria.

It would be important to know whether both mutations occur at the same gene locus. There are three pedigrees (E, F, and G, Fig. 63-9) in which one parent of an iminoglycinuric member is hyperglycinuric and the other parent is not (Table 63-3). Nonetheless, the renal phenotype of the presumably doubly heterozygous child born to these matings is indistinguishable from that of homozygotes with two hyperglycinuric parents, or with two "silent" parents. Thus, it is likely that the complex heterozygote is heteroallelic for two different mutant alleles which occur at the same gene locus. Further proof is needed to secure this conclusion and

Table 63-3. EVIDENCE FOR MORE THAN ONE ALLELIC MUTATION FOR THE FAMILIAL IMINOGLYCINURIC TRAIT: PHENOTYPIC HETEROGENEITY IN HETEROZYGOTES

Pedigree	Subject*	Relation to proband	Glycine clearance, ml/min/1.73 m²†	Presumed genetic designation
E[21]	II.7	Father	10.8	Heterozygote (incompletely recessive)
	II.8	Mother	*3.9*	Heterozygote (completely recessive)
	III.12	Proband	20.3	Double heterozygote
F[19, 20]	I.1	Father	11.9	Heterozygote (incompletely recessive)
	I.2	Mother	*3.1, 3.2*	Heterozygote (completely recessive)
	II.2	Proband	35.0	Double heterozygote
G[24]	I.1	Father‡	*8.1*	Heterozygote (completely recessive)
	I.2	Mother	6.7	Heterozygote (incompletely recessive)
	II.2	Proband	13.6	Double heterozygote

* Designations refer to Fig. 63-9.
† Italicized values are normal. Normal clearance value: 1.2–8.6 ml/min/1.73 m².
‡ Paternity confirmed by blood grouping tests [24].

to rule out nonallelism; nonetheless, the circumstances and their interpretation resemble closely those pertaining to the presumably heteroallelic forms of cystinuria which have been described by Rosenberg [72–74].

Yet another feature of the iminoglycinuric phenotype indicates the apparent genetic heterogeneity which underlies this trait. Some mutant homozygotes exhibit impaired intestinal transport of proline (Pedigrees D and F, Fig. 63-9), whereas others do not (Pedigrees B, E, H, and J, Fig. 63-9). The phenotype with normal intestinal transport is not consistently associated with one or the other form of the heterozygous phenotypes. In one instance (Pedigree B), the parents are of the silent phenotype, while in others (Pedigrees E, H, and J), the parents are hyperglycinuric. One of the two iminoglycinuric subjects with a demonstrable intestinal transport defect (Subject II.2, Pedigree F) is a complex heterozygote. Further studies of intestinal transport in homozygotes of this type could be of considerable help in correlating phenotype with genotype (Table 63-4), as Rosenberg has done for cystinuria [74].

The prevalence of familial iminoglycinuria in the population is unknown. The disorder was detected once in 19,000 individuals in Woolf's laboratory [25], and it has been observed in 3 of about 15,000 subjects studied in our own laboratory. Levy and colleagues [76] have recently examined urinary amino acid composition of well over 100,000 newborn infants in Massachusetts. The frequency of renal iminoglycinuria in this population is about 1:15,000. The apparent frequency of homozygotes (or double heterozygotes) for this trait is then of the order of 10^{-4}, and heterozygotes for this inborn error of transport will comprise about 2 percent of the population.

TREATMENT

Familial iminoglycinuria is apparently a benign condition involving nonessential amino acids, and no treatment is indicated. The considerable number of healthy subjects in whom iminoglycinuria was discovered quite incidentally (viz., Pedigree E, subjects II.3 and III.12; Pedigree H, subjects II.2 and II.4; and all homozygous members of Pedigree I) support this interpretation. The various illnesses which have been associated with the iminoglycinuric trait apparently served only to bring the transport mutation to attention.

Table 63-4. EVIDENCE FOR SEVERAL GENETICALLY DISTINCT TYPES OF FAMILIAL IMINOGLYCINURIA

Allele	Renal trait (homozygotes)	Plasma proline response after oral proline load (homozygotes)	Renal trait (heterozygotes)	Ref.
Normal	Normal	Increase	Normal	
Mutant:				
Type I	IG	Impaired	Normal	[16, 75]
Type II	IG	Normal increase	Normal	[15]
Type III	IG	Normal increase	G	[21, 23]

Note: IG = iminoglycinuria; G = hyperglycinuria.

NEW DEVELOPMENTS

Another pedigree (L, in the present listing) of familial iminoglycinuria has been reported [77]. The 12 year-old female proband was identified in a screening of a school for the blind (see also pedigree K [22]); achromatopsia and iminoglycinuria were found. Investigation of the proband and her large family revealed absence of an intestinal transport defect and hyperglycinuria in both parents. Thus, the patient is apparently homozygous for the type III allele characterized in Table 63-4. The iminoglycinuria allele was considered benign by the authors and seemed to segregate independently of the achromatopsia allele.

SUMMARY

1 Familial iminoglycinuria is an inborn error of membrane transport in which apparently there is deletion or inactivation of the membrane transport protein of the renal tubule which selectively binds L-proline, hydroxy-L-proline, and glycine during cellular uptake. The iminoglycinuria phenotype is autosomal recessive.
2 There is no consistent or typical illness associated with the abnormality, and many who have it are entirely healthy.
3 Homozygotes retain significant tubular absorption of the imino acids and glycine. The residual transport system is saturated at endogenous concentrations of substrate, and the normal competitive interactions between the imino acids and glycine during tubular uptake are not observed. These seemingly paradoxical observations can be explained if several species of membrane transport proteins participate in the migration of the imino acids and glycine. Loss of a carrier which is shared by the imino acids and glycine, and retention of other more selective carriers which bind either glycine or imino acids, but not both simultaneously, would account for the homozygous iminoglycinuric phenotype.
4 Impaired intestinal transport of L-proline has been demonstrated in some homozygotes. A transport defect has not been demonstrated in the leukocytes or skin fibroblasts of these subjects.
5 Obligate heterozygotes may be "hyperglycinuric" (incompletely recessive) or "silent" (completely recessive) with regard to their phenotypic expression of the mutant allele. Some homozygotes have impaired intestinal absorption of the imino acids and glycine. Thus there is genetic heterogeneity.
6 The different mutations appear to be allelic. Homozygotes with two "silent" mutant alleles, or with two "hyperglycinuric" alleles, or double heterozygotes with two mutant alleles of different types, are all of the same renal phenotype.
7 The differential diagnosis of familial iminoglycinuria includes the iminoacidopathies; hyperprolinemia and hydroxyprolinemia, in which iminoglycinuria occurs by a combined saturation-inhibition mechanism; Fanconi's syndrome, in which iminoglycinuria occurs as part of a generalized disturbance of transport; and the newborn, who may have iminoglycinuria as part of the normal hyperaminoaciduria in the first 3 months of life.
8 Several different forms of renal hyperglycinuria are known. These must be distinguished from the hyperglycinuric phenotype of the heterozygote with renal iminoglycinuria.

BIBLIOGRAPHY

1. Dent, C. E.: Detection of amino acids in urine and other fluids. Lancet, **2,** 637, 1946.
2. Scriver, C. R.: Inborn errors of amino acid metabolism. Brit. Med. Bull., **25,** 35, 1969.
3. Scriver, C. R.: Hereditary aminoaciduria, in *Progress in Medical Genetics,* edited by A. Bearn and A. G. Steinberg, vol. 2, p. 83. Grune & Stratton, New York, 1962.
4. Greenstein, J. P., and Winitz, M.: *Chemistry of the Amino Acids,* 3 vols. Wiley, New York, 1961.
5. Meister, A.: *Biochemistry of the Amino Acids,* 2d ed., 2 vols., 1084 pp. Academic, New York, 1965.
6. McMillan, D. E.: Letter to the Editor. New Eng. J. Med., **273,** 771, 1965.
7. Sereni, F., McNamara, H., Shibuya, M., Kretchmer, N., and Barnett, H. L.: Concentration in plasma and rate of urinary excretion of amino acids in premature infants. Pediatrics, **15,** 575, 1955.
8. Woolf, L. I., and Norman, A. P.: The urinary excretion of amino acids and sugars in early infancy. J. Pediat., **50,** 271, 1957.
9. O'Brien, D., and Butterfield, L. J.: Further studies on renal tubular conservation of free amino acids in early infancy. Arch. Dis. Child., **38,** 437, 1963.
10. Brodehl, J., and Gellissen, K.: Endogenous renal transport of free amino acids in infancy and childhood. Pediatrics, **42,** 395, 1968.
11. Scriver, C. R., Schafer, I. A. and Efron, M. L.: New renal tubular amino acid transport system and a new hereditary disorder of amino acid metabolism. Nature (London), **192,** 672, 1961.
12. Joseph, R., Ribierre, M., Job, J-C., and Girault, M.: Maladie familiale associante des convulsions a début très precoce, une hyperalbuminorachie et une hyperaminoacidurie. Arch. Franc. Pediat., **15,** 374, 1958.
13. Paine, R. S.: Evaluation of familial biochemically determined mental retardation in children, with special reference to aminoaciduria. New Eng. J. Med., **262,** 658, 1966.
14. Jonxis, J. H. P.: Personal communications, 1962 (cited in [18]) and 1969.
15. Tada, K., Morikawa, T., Ando, T., Yoshida, T. and Miragawa, A.: Prolinuria: a new renal tubular defect in transport of proline and glycine. Tohoku J. Exp. Med., **87,** 133, 1965.
16. Morikawa, T., Tada, K., Ando, T., Yoshida, T., Yokoyama, Y., and Arakawa, T.: Prolinuria: defect in intestinal absorption of imino acids and glycine. Tohoku J. Exp. Med., **90,** 105, 1966.
17. Scriver, C. R., and Wilson, O. H.: Amino acid transport in human kidney: evidence for genetic control of two types. Science, **155,** 1428, 1967.
18. Miller, M.: Familial cirrhosis with hepatoma. Amer. J. Dig. Dis., **12,** 633, 1967.
19. Goodman, S. I., McIntyre, C. A., and O'Brien, D.: Impaired intestinal transport of proline in a patient with familial iminoaciduria. J. Pediat., **71,** 246, 1967.
20. Goodman, S. I.: Personal communication, 1969.
21. Scriver, C. R.: Renal tubular transport of proline, hydroxyproline and glycine. III. Genetic basis for more than one mode of transport in human kidney. J. Clin. Invest., **47,** 823, 1968.
22. Whelan, D. T., and Scriver, C. R.: Cystathioninuria and renal iminoglycinuria in a pedigree: a perspective on counseling. New Eng. J. Med., **278,** 924, 1968.
23. Rosenberg, L. E., Durant, J. L., and Elsas, II, L. J.: Familial imino-

glycinuria: an inborn error of renal tubular transport. New Eng. J. Med., **278,** 1407, 1968.

24. Hoefnagel, D., and Pomeroy, J.: Personal communication of unpublished data, 1968 and 1969.
25. Fraser, G. R., Friedmann, A. I., Patton, V. M., Wade, D. N., and Woolf, L. I.: Iminoglycinuria—a "harmless" inborn error of metabolism? Humangenetik, **6,** 362, 1968.
26. DeVries, A., Kochwa, S., Lazebnik, J., Frank, M., and Djaldetti, M.: Glycinuria, a hereditary disorder associated with nephrolithiasis. Amer. J. Med., **23,** 408, 1957.
27. Dent, C. E.: A study of the behaviour of some sixty amino acids and other ninhydrin reacting substances on phenol-"collidine" filter paper chromatograms with notes as to the occurrence of some of them in biological fluids. Biochem. J., **43,** 169, 1948.
28. Smith, I. (ed.): *Chromatographic and Electrophoretic Techniques,* 2 vols. Interscience, New York, 1960 and 1968.
29. Shih, V., Efron, M. L., and Mechanic, G. L.: Rapid short column chromatography of amino acids: a method for blood and urine specimens in the diagnosis and treatment of metabolic diseases. Anal. Biochem., **20,** 299, 1967.
30. Scriver, C. R., Davies, E., and Lamm, P.: Accelerated selective short column chromatography of neutral and acidic amino acids on a Beckman-Spinco analyzer, modified for simultaneous analysis of two samples. Clin. Biochem., **1,** 179, 1968.
31. Schafer, I. A., Scriver, C. R., and Efron, M. L.: Familial hyperprolinemia, cerebral dysfunction and renal anomalies occurring in a family with hereditary nephritis and deafness. New Eng. J. Med., **267,** 51, 1962.
32. Scriver, C. R., Efron, M. L., and Schafer, I. A.: Renal tubular transport of proline, hydroxyproline and glycine in health and in familial hyperprolinemia. J. Clin. Invest., **43,** 374, 1964.
33. Smith, H. W., Goldring, W., Chasis, H., Ranges, H. A., and Bradley, S. E.: The application of saturation methods to the study of glomerular and tubular function in the human kidney. J. Mount Sinai Hosp. N.Y., **10,** 59, 1943.
34. Scriver, C. R., and Goldman, H.: Renal tubular transport of proline, hydroxyproline and glycine. II. Hydroxy-L-proline as substrate and as inhibitor in-vivo. J. Clin. Invest., **45,** 1357, 1966.
35. Pitts, R. F.: A renal reabsorptive mechanism in the dog common to glycine and creatine. Amer. J. Physiol., **140,** 156, 1943.
36. Christensen, H. N.: Reactive sites and biological transport. Advances Protein Chem., **15,** 239, 1960.
37. Christensen, H. N.: Some transport lessons taught by the organic solute. Perspect. Biol. Med., **10,** 471, 1967.
38. Wilson, O. H., and Scriver, C. R.: Specificity of transport of neutral and basic amino acids in rat kidney. Amer. J. Physiol., **213,** 185, 1967.
39. Webber, W. A.: Interactions of neutral and acidic amino acids in renal tubular transport. Amer. J. Physiol., **202,** 577, 1962.
40. Webber, W. A.: Amino acid excretion patterns in developing rats. Canad. J. Physiol. Pharmacol., **45,** 867, 1967.
41. Baerlocher, K., Scriver, C. R., and Mohyuddin, F.: Ontogeny of iminoglycine transport in mammalian kidney. Proc. Nat. Acad. Sci., **65,** 1009, 1970.
42. Deren, J. J., Strauss, E. W., and Wilson, T. H.: The development of structure and transport systems of the fetal rabbit intestine. Develop. Biol., **12,** 467, 1965.
43. Webber, W. A., and Cairns, J. A.: A comparison of the amino acid concentrating ability of the kidney cortex of newborn and mature rats. Canad. J. Physiol. Pharmacol., **46,** 165, 1968.
44. Rosenberg, L. E., Blair, A., and Segal, S.: Transport of amino acids by slices of rat-kidney cortex. Biochim. Biophys. Acta, **54,** 479, 1961.
45. Scriver, C. R., and Wilson, O. H.: Possible location for a common gene product in membrane transport of imino acids and glycine. Nature (London), **202,** 92, 1964.
46. Ahmed, K., and Scholefield, P. G.: Biochemical studies of 1-aminocyclopentane carboxylic acid. Canad. J. Biochem. Physiol., **40,** 1101, 1962.
47. Mohyuddin, F., and Scriver, C. R.: Amino acid transport in mammalian kidney. Identification and analysis of multiple systems for iminoacids and glycine in rat kidney. Amer. J. Physiol., **219,** 1, 1970.

48*a*. Hillman, R. E., Albrecht, I., and Rosenberg, L. E.: Identification and analysis of multiple glycine transport systems in isolated mammalian renal tubules. J. Biol. Chem., **243,** 5566, 1968.

48*b*. Hillman, R. E., and Rosenberg, L. E.: Amino acid transport by isolated mammalian renal tubules. II. Transport systems for L-proline. J. Biol. Chem., **244,** 4494, 1969.

49. Scriver, C. R., and Hechtman, P.: Human genetics of membrane transport with emphasis on amino acids. Advances in Human Genetics, **1,** 211, 1970.
50. Scriver, C. R., and Mohyuddin, F.: Amino acid transport in kidney: heterogeneity of AIB uptake. J. Biol. Chem., **243,** 3207, 1968.

50*a*. Rosenberg, L. E., Albrecht, I., and Segal, S.: Lysine transport in human kidney: evidence for two systems. Science, **155,** 1426, 1967.

50*b*. Elsas, L. J., Hillman, R. E., Patterson, J. H., and Rosenberg, L. E.: Renal and intestinal hexose transport in familial glucose-galactose malabsorption. J. Clin. Invest., **49,** 576, 1970.

50*c*. Oxender, D. L., and Christensen, H. N.: Distinct mediating systems for the transport of neutral amino acids by the Ehrlich cell. J. Biol. Chem., **238,** 3686, 1963.

50*d*. Pardee, A. B.: Membrane transport proteins. Science, **162,** 632, 1968.

51. Tada, K., Hirono, H., and Arakawa, T.: Endogenous renal clearance rates of free amino acids in prolinuric and Hartnup patients. Tohoku J. Exp. Med., **93,** 57, 1967.
52. Scriver, C. R.: Amino acid transport in mammalian kidney, in *Amino Acid Metabolism and Genetic Variation,* edited by W. L. Nyhan, p. 327. McGraw-Hill, New York, 1967.
53. Rosenberg, L. E., and Scriver, C. R.: Amino acid metabolism. In *Duncan's Diseases of Metabolism,* 6th ed., edited by P. K. Bondy, p. 366. Saunders, Philadelphia, 1969.
54. Wilson, O. H.: Amino acid transport in proline auxotrophs of *E. coli.* Ph. D. Thesis, McGill University, Montreal, 1966.
55. Finerman, G. A. M., and Rosenberg, L. E.: Amino acid transport in bone: evidence for separate transport systems for neutral amino and imino acids. J. Biol. Chem., **241,** 1487, 1966.
56. Brodehl, J., Gellisen, K., and Kowalewski, S.: Isolierter Defekt der tubulären Cystin-rück Resorption in einer Familie mit idiopathischem Hypoparathyroidismus. Klin. Wschr., **45,** 38, 1967.
57. Hooft, C., Carton, D., Snoeck, J., Timmermans, J., Antener, I., van den Hende, C., and Oyaert, W.: Further investigations in the methionine malabsorption syndrome. Helv. Paediat. Acta, **23,** 334, 1968.
58. Drummond, K. N., Michael, A. F., Ulstrom, R. A., and Good, R. A.: Blue diaper syndrome: familial hypercalcemia with nephrocalcinosis and indicanuria. Amer. J. Med., **37,** 928, 1964.
59. La Du, B. N.: Genetic variation in metabolic disorders, in *Amino Acid Metabolism and Genetic Variation,* edited by W. L. Nyhan, p. 121. McGraw-Hill, 1967.
60. Bégin, N., and Scholefield, P. G.: The uptake of amino acids by mouse pancreas in-vitro. III. The kinetic characteristics of the transport of L-proline. Biochim. Biophys. Acta, **104,** 566, 1965.
61. Tada, K., Morikawa, T., and Arakawa, T.: Prolinuria: transport of proline by leukocytes. Tohoku J. Exp. Med., **90,** 189, 1966.
62. Carver, M. J., and Paska, R.: Ion-exchange chromatography of urinary amino acids. I. Normal children. Clin. Chim. Acta, **6,** 721, 1961.
63. Scriver, C. R., and Davies, E.: Endogenous renal clearance rates of free amino acids in pre-pubertal children. Pediatrics, **36,** 592, 1965.
64. Efron, M. L., Bixby, E. M., Palattao, L. G., and Pryles, C. V.: Hydroxyprolinemia associated with mental deficiency. New Eng. J. Med., **267,** 1193, 1962.
65. Rosenberg, L. E., and Segal, S.: Maleic acid-induced inhibition of amino acid transport in rat kidney. Biochem. J., **92,** 345, 1964.
66. Käser, H., Cottier, P., and Antener, I.: Glucoglycinuria, a new familial syndrome. J. Pediat., **61,** 386, 1962.
67. Scriver, C. R., Goldbloom, R. B., and Roy, C. C.: Hypophosphatemic rickets with renal hyperglycinuria, renal glucosuria and glycylprolinuria: a syndrome with evidence for renal tubular secretion of phosphorus. Pediatrics, **34,** 357, 1964.
68. Dent, C. E., and Harris, H.: Hereditary forms of rickets and osteomalacia. J. Bone Joint Surg., **38B,** 204, 1956.

69. Greene, M. L., Lietman, P. S., Rosenberg, L. E., and Seegmiller, J. E.: Familial hyperglycinuria (in press), 1971.
70. Nyhan, W. L., Ando, T., and Gerritsen, T.: Hyperglycinemia, in *Amino Acid Metabolism and Genetic Variation,* edited by W. L. Nyhan, p. 255. McGraw-Hill, New York.
71. Harris, H., Mittwoch, U., Robson, E. B., and Warren, F. L.: Pattern of amino acid excretion in cystinuria. Ann. Hum. Genet., **19,** 195, 1955.
72. Rosenberg, L. E.: Cystinuria: genetic heterogeneity and allelism. Science, **154,** 1341, 1966.
73. Rosenberg, L. E., Durant, J. L., and Albrecht, I.: Genetic heterogeneity in cystinuria: evidence for allelism. Trans. Ass. Amer. Physicians, **79,** 284, 1966.
74. Rosenberg, L. E.: Genetic heterogeneity in cystinuria, in *Amino Acid Metabolism and Genetic Variation,* edited by W. L. Nyhan, p. 341. McGraw-Hill, New York, 1967.
75. Tada, K.: Personal communication, 1969.
76. Levy, H. L.: Personal communication, 1970.
77. Tancredi, F., Guazzi, G., and Aurichio, S.: Renal iminoglycinuria without intestinal malabsorption of glycine and iminoacids. J. Pediat., **76,** 386, 1970.

CHAPTER SIXTY-FOUR

RENAL GLYCOSURIA

Stephen M. Krane

Renal glycosuria denotes the renal tubular abnormality in individuals who excrete a variable amount of glucose in the urine at normal levels of blood glucose. For purposes of this discussion, attention will be limited to those subjects in whom the abnormality in glucose excretion is the only apparent tubular defect, although the same considerations are applicable to the glycosuria occurring in more widespread disorders of the renal tubule, such as Fanconi's syndrome.

DEFINITION AND CLINICAL DESCRIPTION

In the past, there has been considerable confusion as to whether different types of renal glycosuria exist. On the basis of more recent data, it appears probable that the phenotypic expression of the defect in different individuals with familial renal glycosuria is the result of a number of different mutations. The use of more refined techniques has made it possible to distinguish these variations, rather than base a classification on such criteria as severity of the glycosuria, relationship to carbohydrate intake, or the degree of lowering of the threshold for glucose excretion in the urine [1, 2].

The criteria proposed by Marble for "true" renal glycosuria seem most reasonable if one is to avoid "an unwieldy hodgepodge of cases difficult to study and follow over a period of years" [1, 3]. They are as follows:

1 Glycosuria is present without hyperglycemia. The amount of glucose excreted may vary from less than 10 gm to more than 100 gm per 24 hr.
2 The degree of glycosuria is largely independent of diet but may fluctuate somewhat according to the amount of carbohydrate ingested. In general, all specimens of urine examined, including those after an overnight fast, should contain sugar.
3 Levels of blood glucose are influenced only slightly by dietary carbohydrate. The oral glucose tolerance curve is normal or slightly "flat."
4 The type of sugar excreted is glucose by chemical test. Other meliturias are excluded (pentosuria, fructosuria, galactosuria, sucrosuria, maltosuria, mannoheptulosuria) [4]. Simple and specific methods, employing glucose oxidase for the identification of glucose, are now readily available.
5 Subjects with the disorder are able to store and utilize carbohydrate normally.

If the above criteria are rigidly adhered to, the condition is not common. Only 94 cases have been observed among 50,000 cases of melituria seen at the Joslin Clinic [1]. On the other hand, Lawrence proposes that renal glycosuria is proved whenever glycosuria occurs with a normal glucose tolerance test, whether or not the urine contains sugar at the beginning of the test [2]. On the basis of this more liberal definition, he found that 65 percent of 800 selectees with glycosuria fell into this category.

All authors agree that the condition is benign and symptomless except during pregnancy or starvation, when dehydration and ketosis may develop. There is still considerable disagreement as to whether these patients ever develop true diabetes mellitus. On the basis of his experience Marble does not believe they do, although diabetes mellitus was present in the families of 15 of the 22 patients that he originally discussed. A convincing report of diabetes mellitus developing in a 19-year-old male with renal glycosuria documented since the age of 8 years suggests that these conditions may rarely be associated [5]. Ackerman et al., using Lawrence's criteria for the diagnosis of renal glycosuria, found that of 27 patients in whom the diagnosis had originally been made, 17 (63 percent) were found to be diabetic when retested 3 months to 13 years later [6]. Until the defect in renal glycosuria is more clearly defined in terms of its fundamental mechanism, it cannot be stated whether or not those patients who clearly fall into Marble's classification represent a different entity from those patients observed by Ackerman et al. It would appear from the findings of Ackerman et al. that the patients diagnosed by Lawrence's criteria should be followed for possible development of diabetes mellitus.

The age at which the disorder is first detected varies, but in the majority of patients it is in the second decade. One case was discovered when the patient was only 4 weeks old [7]. Another patient, followed for 64 years with invariable glycosuria, at times excreted as much as 5 percent glucose in the urine [1]. The abnormality in glucose transfer thus appears to persist throughout life.

NATURE OF THE MECHANISM OF GLUCOSE TRANSPORT

In considering renal glycosuria as an inborn error of metabolism, it should be stressed that the fundamental mechanism for the active transport of glucose in the renal tubules has not been defined. The "error" cannot, therefore, be localized biochemically as it has in some other disorders. Indeed, the existence of a chemical reaction involving the transported substance, glucose, has not been demonstrated. Nevertheless, it is possible to describe certain characteristics of tubular transport of glucose. This subject has been reviewed by Taggart [8].

The application of micropuncture techniques has demonstrated in various amphibians and mammals that glucose is present in the glomerular filtrate in the same concentration as in the plasma water [9, 10]. In the proximal convoluted tubule sugar is reabsorbed against an increasing concentration gradient, so that by the midpoint of this tubule little glucose remains in the lumen. The reabsorptive process, which is blocked by the glycoside phlorizin, is not restricted to any particular segment of the proximal tubule, but it is not demonstrable in the distal tubule. In the presence of phlorizin the concentration of reducing substance in the tubular urine may increase to as high as three times that of plasma as water is reabsorbed. In phlorizinized *Necturus* glucose can diffuse back toward the plasma if the concentration in the tubular lumen is much greater than in plasma.

It has been shown in the dog by Shannon and Fisher [11] and in man by Smith [12, 13] that as the concentration of glucose in the blood is progressively increased, the amount reabsorbed (T) by the tubules approaches a maximum (T_m) (curve 1, Fig. 64-1). Shannon assumed that as the load of glucose presented to the tubules increases, progressive saturation of the reabsorptive mechanism occurs until a maximum level is reached and the excess is excreted in the urine. He postulated that the sequence of reactions in glucose transfer involves (1) a reversible combination of the solute with a hypothetical cellular element present in constant but limiting amounts and (2) decomposition of this complex by a reaction which is first-order in type and rate-limiting for the whole process.

Although Shannon's data fitted well with this hypothesis, clearance data obtained in man show variable deviations, or "splay," from the ideal curve [13] (curve 2, Fig. 64-1). The explanation has been offered that even in the normal kidney with loads less than the maximal average, the transport in some individual nephrons will be less than in others [14]. Since the capacity of some tubules for reabsorption will be exceeded at relatively low levels, glucose would be excreted from these nephrons before the average maximal load is reached. It has been further assumed that the titration curves for both kidneys would deviate from the "theoretical" in proportion to the degree of heterogeneity in the nephron population.

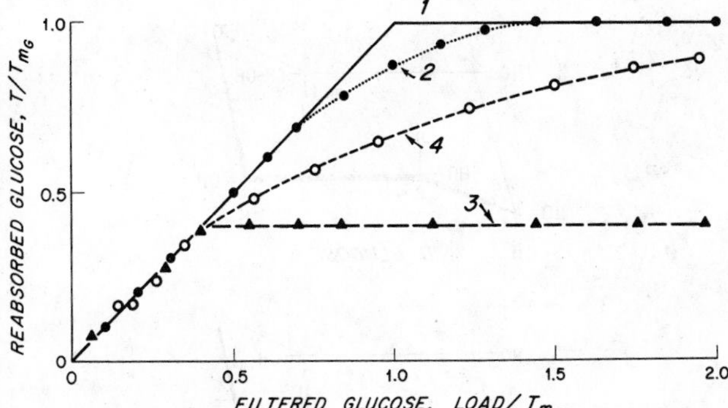

Figure 64-1. Renal tubular glucose reabsorption as a function of load presented to the tubule. Curve 1 is theoretical and based on the assumptions of Shannon and Fisher [11]. Curve 2 is seen in normal man, showing the slight splay from the theoretical. Curve 3 is seen in patients with low T_m. Curve 4 is seen in a patient with renal glycosuria showing an exaggerated splay.

Support for this hypothesis has been obtained in dogs by correlation of the anatomic heterogeneity of nephrons determined by microdissection with the functional heterogeneity determined by glucose titrations prior to sacrifice [15, 16]. The data are consistent with the idea that the glomerular filtration rate is determined by the area of the external surface of the capillary tuft and that the maximum glucose reabsorptive capacity depends on the mass of proximal convoluted tubule cells. The curves for T/T_m versus load/T_m closely fitted the curves for "glucose titration" obtained from the anatomic data.

It has, however, been pointed out by Mudge [14] and Berliner [17] that the assumptions on which this explanation is based can be only an approximation, i.e., that each nephron excretes no glucose until completely saturated. There are no experimental data which conclusively prove this. Mudge [14] stated that if Michaelis-Menten kinetics are applicable to the process of glucose transport across a tubule cell, it is apparent that maximal rates would not be attained until concentration of the substrate reached levels severalfold greater than the concentration in glomerular filtrate at T_m. The splay in the glucose titration curve for the whole kidney as well as for the individual nephron could be explained on this basis. Calculation of the rate constant for the glucose transport system, assuming Michaelis-Menten kinetics, revealed a K_m for glucose of less than $2.5 \times 10^{-4}M$ [18]. It was therefore concluded that the departure of the observed data from the theoretical curves could be attributed not to an unsaturated transport system but rather to a dispersal of reabsorptive capacity in a log-normal distribution.

However, hexose transport, when studied in vitro in tissues in which a concentrative mechanism exists, such as intestinal mucosa as well as renal cortex, does appear to follow Michaelis-Menten kinetics as usually applied to enzymatic reactions. The saturation of renal tubular glucose reabsorption as observed in vivo using titration techniques has been considered to be a process similar to saturation of an enzyme with substrate [19]. As the filtered load[1] of glucose (substrate, S) increases, the amount of glucose reabsorbed (T) increases

[1]The amount of glucose reabsorbed per minute (T) is calculated by subtracting the amount appearing in the urine per minute from the filtered load (plasma concentration $\times$ glomerular filtration rate in milliliters per minute). Apparently T glucose represents a mean rate of tubular reabsorption, since the amount reabsorbed decreases progressively along the proximal convoluted tubule. Furthermore, as glucose is reabsorbed, its concentration becomes lowest near the walls and highest in the center of the tubular lumen [20]. As water is reabsorbed, the concentration difference would be reversed. Until the maximal rate of reabsorption (T_m) is reached, it is usually considered that T is a function of load. However, since the glomerular filtration rate does not change significantly in any one study as plasma glucose concentration is increased, T may be considered a function of plasma glucose concentration. Although T does not represent true initial velocity for the reabsorption process, if the system follows Michaelis-Menten kinetics, then an approximate apparent K_m would be the concentration of plasma glucose when $T/T_m = 0.5$ ($v/V_{max} = 0.5$).

(velocity, v) until a maximum velocity of reabsorption, T_m, is reached (analogous to maximal velocity of the enzymatic reaction, or V). If the initial step in transport of glucose (G) requires coupling with an hypothetical carrier (C) to form a glucose-carrier complex (GC), then the equation for the interaction may be written:

$$[G] + [C] \rightleftharpoons [GC] \tag{1}$$

and

$$K = \frac{[G][C]}{[GC]} \tag{2}$$

This expression implies that there will always be unbound glucose and unbound carrier, the amount depending on the magnitude of K. If K is large, the affinity of glucose for the carrier would be low and more glucose would appear in the urine at low loads (concentration) [19]. Woolf, Goodwin, and Phelps [20] have derived expressions and plotted curves for glucose reabsorption in a model nephron using such calculations. When a normal amount of carrier per unit area of tubular wall is assumed, with abnormal affinity (K_m) of carrier for glucose, the calculated curves resemble those obtained with normal renal glucose titration data.

Active Transport

Most of the information pertaining to the mechanism of active transport of sugars has been obtained through studies of the small intestine [27, 28], where the situation is presumed to be analogous, although obviously not identical, to that in the renal tubule. As will be discussed subsequently in detail, in human disease defects in renal tubular transport of glucose have been accompanied in some instances by a similar defect in intestinal transport, whereas in other instances, possibly the majority, intestinal transport has not been impaired. Nevertheless, enough similarities have been described in renal and intestinal transport to warrant detailed consideration of the findings in the intestine, as they may reflect the situation in the renal tubule.

With several different in vitro systems, including isolated loops [29], everted sacs [30–32], or isolated rings [33], it has been possible to show transport of certain sugars and accumulation within the tissue against a concentration gradient. The cells involved in active transport of these sugars, present in proximal convoluted tubules as well as in the small intestine, have projections on the luminal brush border known as microvilli [34–37]. When the concentrations of the actively transported sugar, D-galactose, were measured in various parts of hamster intestine, the relationships of these concentrations indicated that the active transport is mediated by a process which lies in or near the brush border end of the epithelial cells [38]. Further data obtained using galactose-^{14}C and radioautographic techniques [39] showed the earliest concentration of label at the brush border pole of the intestinal cells and support the concept that entry and accumulation of hexoses are located near the brush border.

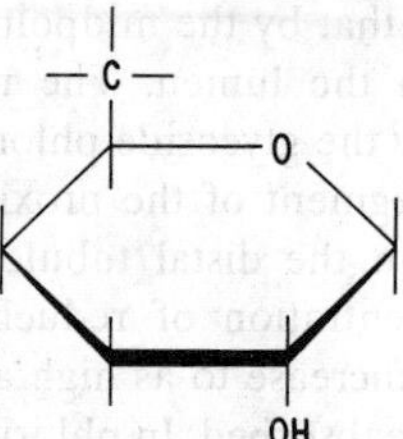

Figure 64-2. Structural features common to sugars actively transported by the intestine [27].

The process of active transport of sugars by the intestine exhibits apparent stereochemical and configurational specificity. Although the structural requirements for transport are not absolute and are dependent on the method used to measure active transport, there are structural features that are common to those compounds that are actively absorbed [27]. The common structure of such sugars may be described as a D-pyranose ring, a methyl or hydroxymethyl group at carbon-5, and a hydroxyl group in the glucose configuration at carbon-2 (Fig. 64-2). This may be an oversimplification, since, for example, it has been shown more recently that L-glucose is actively transported by hamster intestine and interacts specifically with the sugar transport system shared by D-glucose [40]. D- and L-glucose can both present the same conformation of the underlying tetrahydropyranose structure as illustrated in Fig. 64-3. Whatever substrate specificity the structure shown in Fig. 64-2 has, it differs distinctly from that of mammalian hexokinase; several hexoses actively transported by the intestine are not phosphorylated by intestinal homogenates, and this is further evidence against the phosphorylation-dephosphorylation hypothesis discussed previously [41].

As mentioned earlier, the kinetics of interaction of glucose and analogues possessing the minimal structural requirements resemble the kinetics of enzymes. Mutual competitive inhibition between pairs of sugars actively transported by

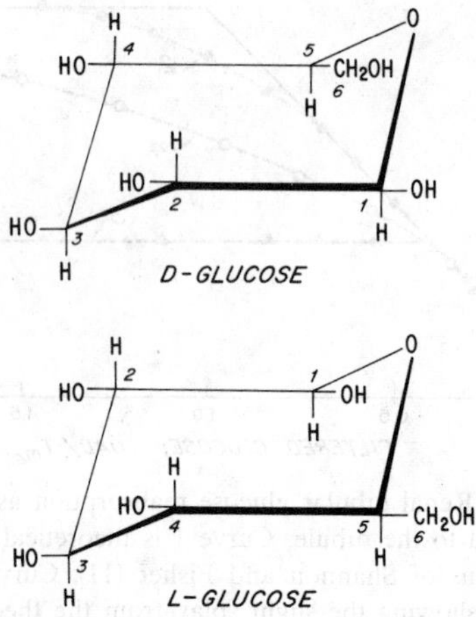

Figure 64-3. Conformational and configurational relationships of D- and L-glucose [28].

the intestine of small animals has been shown, and the data indicate that these substances share a single common pathway [27, 42]. Kinetics of a similar type have now been described for human specimens of jejunal mucosa obtained by biopsy [19, 43] with an apparent K_m for glucose of 4.2 mM, somewhat higher than that calculated for hamster jejunum (1.5 mM [42]). Values for K_m calculated from in vivo studies in man are even higher, an observation so far unexplained [28].

In animal intestine glucose is transported without breakdown and resynthesis of the six-carbon chain [44]. Reactions which involve removal or transfer of oxygen at carbon-2 of the sugar molecule or which require the presence of carbon-bound hydrogen at the same position have been excluded as reactions essential for the transport of the sugar [45].

Active transport is an energy-requiring process. Absence of air (oxygen) or inhibition of reactions yielding energy results in inhibition of accumulation of sugars against a concentration difference, using preparations of small intestine [29, 30]. The phenomenon of transport is not itself a part of intracellular metabolism [28]. There are no known chemical reactions in which the transported sugars participate in the process of transport. Data have now been accumulated by many investigators working with different animal species indicating that the presence of Na^+ is essential for the active transport process [46–49]. Cardiac glycosides such as strophanthidin and ouabain, which are inhibitors of active ion transport, also inhibit active sugar transport in vitro [50]. Furthermore, it has recently been shown in isolated rabbit ileum that the addition of an actively transported sugar, whether metabolizable or not, results in an increase in the transmural electrical potential (serosa positive), whereas sugars which are not actively transported, even if metabolized, do not produce such increases [51]. Present evidence suggests that active transport of sugars consists of two processes [52, 53]: (1) *penetration* into the cell at the brush border by a process which has an absolute dependence on Na^+ but is independent of oxygen and (2) *accumulation* within the cell, which not only requires Na^+ but also requires oxygen for energy-yielding reactions.

The Cellular Carrier

The nature of the hypothetical cellular carrier, if indeed one exists, has not been elucidated. It has been postulated that the initial step in transport is phosphorylation of glucose mediated by hexokinase and adenosine triphosphate, with subsequent dephosphorylation through the action of a phosphatase [21, 22]. The glucose-6-phosphate formed in the first reaction is assumed not to diffuse out of the cell, and the removal of *free* glucose by phosphorylation would then favor the inward movement of glucose in the direction of the concentration gradient. Hexokinase, nonspecific alkaline phosphatase, and the specific glucose-6-phosphatase are found in proximal tubular cells. Nonetheless, the weight of evidence is heavily against a phosphorylated sugar as an intermediate in the transport process [8]. When phlorizin was administered to animals to produce almost complete block of glucose reabsorption, no inhibition of alkaline phosphatase in the proximal convoluted tubules could be demonstrated histochemically [23]. Phlorizin, in doses which produced profound glycosuria, did not alter the time curve of disappearance of injected ^{32}P-labeled inorganic phosphate from the plasma of cats [24]. These data of Dratz and Handler [24] indicated that in the presence of phlorizin, normal or even accelerated synthesis of glucose esters is seen. The authors concluded that if a highly active fraction of either glucose-1-phosphate or glucose-6-phosphate mediates renal tubular transport of glucose, then this must be present in amounts too minute to be detected by their technique. In addition, there are two clinical observations which fail to support the unique role of either alkaline or glucose-6-phosphatase in the transport reactions. Cori noted the absence of glycosuria in patients with glycogen storage disease in whom the specific glucose-6-phosphatase was lacking [25]. Similarly normal carbohydrate metabolism has been observed in subjects with hypophosphatasia in whom alkaline phosphatase activity is decreased or absent [26].

One interpretation of the data involves a model such as that illustrated in Fig. 64-4, in which there are two binding sites on the same mobile carrier, one of them specific for Na^+ and the other for the sugar [54, 28]. In this model, binding of Na^+ is assumed to activate the movement of a restricted group of sugars across the mucosal membrane. A Na^+ gradient, operating synergistically with an opposing K^+ gradient, is presumed to be the driving force for active sugar transport. In addition, another asymmetry in the system results from the fact that the affinity between a sugar and the carrier is inversely related to the Na^+ concentration [55]. Furthermore the presence of K^+ decreases the affinity beyond that caused only by the lack of Na^+.

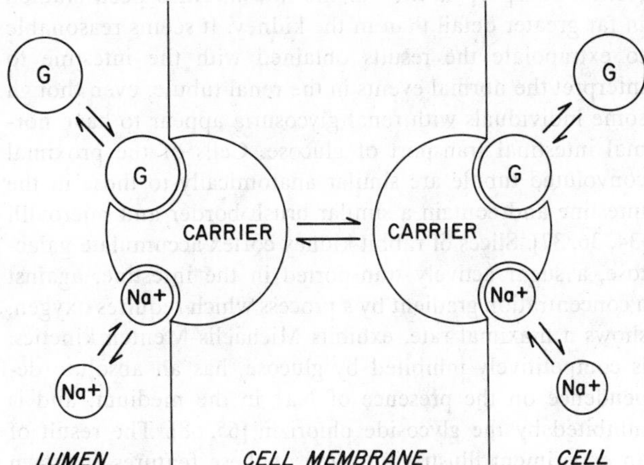

Figure 64-4. Model for a mobile carrier located at the brush border end of the epithelial cell, showing separate binding sites for glucose (*G*) and Na^+ on the carrier. (*Adapted from Crane* [28].)

Some comment concerning the inhibitory effect on sugar transport of the glycoside phlorizin is pertinent, since many of the hypotheses discussed above assume that the action of this compound is highly specific. Phlorizin inhibits several enzyme systems that require or are stimulated by adenine nucleotides. These include inhibition of phosphorylase [56], Ehrlich ascites tumor hexokinase [27], and aerobic phosphorylation by homogenates of guinea pig kidney cortex [57]. Phlorizin also induces adenosine triphosphate—reversible swelling of mitochondria [58] and inhibits the enzyme mutarotase [59–61] postulated to be involved in sugar transport. These inhibitions occur at concentrations of phlorizin considerably higher than those required to inhibit active sugar transport in vivo. Phlorizin also inhibits entrance of sugar into erythrocytes [62], Ehrlich ascites tumor cells [63], and isolated perfused heart [64]. The glycoside, at low concentrations, inhibits the entry of galactose into slices of rabbit kidney cortex, not only under conditions where accumulation against a concentration difference occurs, but also when the latter is prevented by the addition of a metabolic inhibitor [65]. It appears likely that the action of phlorizin in inhibiting active transport of sugars occurs at the first, or penetration step, which involves a competition between phlorizin and the sugars for a specific site on a "carrier" in the brush border membrane [66–67].

It should be noted that most of the features that characterize glucose absorption in small-animal intestine are also observed in transport by human intestine. In addition to the similar value for K_m of glucose transport noted earlier, glucose transport in human jejunum is against a concentration gradient, is inhibited by low temperature, metabolic poisons, absence of Na^+, or presence of ouabain, and exhibits competitive inhibition by sugars such as galactose but not by fructose or xylose [43].

Transport by the Kidney

Active transport in vitro in the intestine has been studied in far greater detail than in the kidney. It seems reasonable to extrapolate the results obtained with the intestine to interpret the normal events in the renal tubule, even though some individuals with renal glycosuria appear to have normal intestinal transport of glucose. Cells of the proximal convoluted tubule are similar anatomically to those in the intestine and contain a similar brush border and microvilli [34, 36, 37]. Slices of rabbit kidney cortex accumulate galactose, a sugar actively transported in the intestine, against a concentration gradient by a process which requires oxygen, shows a maximal rate, exhibits Michaelis-Menten kinetics, is competitively inhibited by glucose, has an absolute dependence on the presence of Na^+ in the medium, and is inhibited by the glycoside phlorizin [65, 68]. The result of an experiment illustrating some of these features is shown in Fig. 64-5. The apparent K_m for galactose transport [65] was 2 mM, a value similar to that calculated for hamster intestine [42], and that for glucose was about 10 mM.

A hypothesis originally advanced to account for glucose transport by the kidney involved enzyme-catalyzed mutarotation as the fundamental event [59–61, 69]. Mutarotases are enzymes that possess catalytic activity against free sugars and are relatively abundant in kidney, liver, and intestine. The specificity of animal mutarotases for substrates and inhibitors resembles that of the transport process. On the other hand the fact that sugars lacking a hydroxyl function at carbon-1 can be actively transported but cannot mutarotate is strong evidence against the role of mutarotase in transport. Other arguments against this hypothesis are equally compelling [28].

In summary, glucose of the glomerular filtrate which is present in concentration equal to that in the plasma water is reabsorbed in the proximal convoluted tubules against an ever-increasing concentration gradient. Reabsorption of the sugar is mediated by energy-requiring processes analogous to those involved in active transport by the small intestine, has a restricted specificity, requires the presence of Na^+, and is susceptible to inhibition by phlorizin. A maximal rate of transport is observed both in vitro and in vivo. The transport mechanism, located at the luminal or brush border end of the cell, is intimately linked to ion transport. No chemical reaction involving the transported sugar has been demonstrated; the six-carbon chain is transported intact without breakdown and resynthesis [70].

Recently a number of studies have suggested that there may be some interaction of the transport systems for sugars and amino acids in both intestine [74–73] and kidney [74, 75]. Glucose, galactose, and fructose all inhibit the intracellular accumulation of certain neutral amino acids by slices of renal cortex, by a mechanism which is noncompetitive in type [74]. In dogs, on the other hand, glycine and alanine inhibit maximal tubular reabsorption of glucose, whereas leucine does not [75].

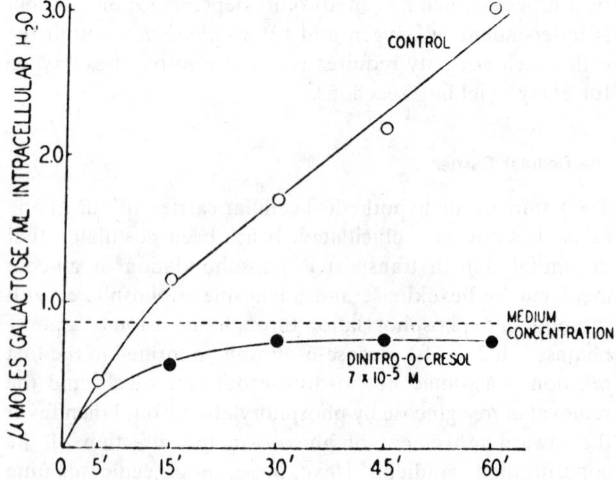

Figure 64-5. Time-course of accumulation of ^{14}C-galactose by rabbit kidney cortex slices. (*From Krane and Crane* [65].)

NATURE OF THE TUBULAR ABNORMALITY IN RENAL GLYCOSURIA

Patients with true renal glycosuria usually lead a normal life, and it has not been possible to obtain samples of renal cortex for adequate study in order to characterize the defect in hexose transport. In those instances in which tissue has been obtained, it has been examined using only morphologic techniques. The latter will be considered subsequently. The data on which interpretation of the tubular abnormality is based have been derived from studies of patients with renal glycosuria using clearance techniques [19, 36, 37, 76–83]. The diagnosis in most of these patients was made using the criteria developed by Marble [1, 3]. The amount of glucose excreted was variable but easily detectable by screening techniques, and usually well in excess of 1 gm per 24 hr. Normal individuals on a diet containing 30 cal per kg and 50 percent of calories as carbohydrate excrete less than 325 mg per 24 hr [19].

The glomerular filtration rate [76–80], secretion of *p*-aminohippuric acid [78], and reabsorption of phosphate [83] and amino acids [14] have been reported to be normal in these patients. There is no evidence of generalized progressive renal failure. High urinary lactate clearance in patients with renal glycosuria has been noted [84]. It was suggested that some patients with renal glycosuria have a tubular defect which affects lactate as well as glucose.

It was originally proposed by Reubi [78] and Bradley et al. [80] that patients with renal glycosuria seemed to fall within two separate groups, those with normal glucose T_m and those with low glucose T_m. Reubi concluded that in those patients with low glucose T_m a familial tendency was evident. Bradley thought the reverse was true. Taggart [85], in reviewing the available literature, including the data collected by Bradley, Reubi, and Lambert, concluded that the cases did not appear to fall into two distinct categories according to the glucose T_m but were evenly distributed from the lowest to the highest values. The data for glucose T_m in reported cases of renal glycosuria compared to normal subjects are shown in Fig. 64-6. The distribution does not appear to suggest two distinct groups, although the techniques might not be sensitive and reproducible enough to detect such a distinction.

Data obtained with the titration method of Smith [12, 13] are of considerable interest. Use of this technique in the patients with low glucose T_m (curve 3, Fig. 64-1), so called Type A renal glycosuria, led to the conclusion that the defect in glucose reabsorption is diffuse, involving most, if not all, nephrons. In the other individuals with renal glycosuria (Type B) in whom the glucose T_m was within the normal range (Type B), both Reubi [78] and Bradley et al. [80] commented on the exaggerated splay in the titration curves (curve 4, Fig. 64-1). They attributed this to a heterogeneity among nephrons, whether on a functional or anatomic basis. Reubi further suggested that in these individuals there were actually two distinct groups of nephrons. As previously mentioned, configuration of the titration curve may be a function of the kinetics of the tubular transfer reactions, rather than an expression of heterogeneity among nephrons. For example, a decrease in the affinity of the substrate (glucose) for the transfer system could result in a shift of the curve to the right without altering T_m. Thus the point at which the ratio T/T_m reaches 0.5 would occur at higher plasma concentrations of glucose.

The data in Fig. 64-6 have been obtained in many different laboratories, where variations in technique or variations in the population studied may influence the results. An attempt to obtain more accurate data in a normal population of young men has been published [108]. The glucose T_m was 325 ± 36 mg per min per 1.73 m^2 in 16 healthy men ranging in age from 17 to 28. The splay in these normal subjects was considerably less than that reported by others. Young men with renal glycosuria were all found to have increased splay, although those with consistent as opposed to intermittent glycosuria tended in addition to have low values for glucose T_m. It was suggested that the degree of splay determines the threshold for appearance of recognizable glycosuria, whereas the T_m is the major determinant of the magnitude of measured glycosuria.

The calculations of Woolf, Goodwin, and Phelps [20], previously discussed, reveal that if it is assumed that the number of carrier units is reduced (decreased C in Eqs. 1 and 2), the theoretical titration curve is characteristic of patients with Type A renal glycosuria (curve 3, Fig. 64-1). Altering K_m (increase K of Eq. 2), so that the affinity of glucose (G) for the carrier (C) decreases, produces a curve with exaggerated splay characteristic of the patient with Type B renal glycosuria. Decrease in functional carrier units could theoretically be spotty as well as diffuse. Decrease in affinity of glucose for the carrier could theoretically result not only

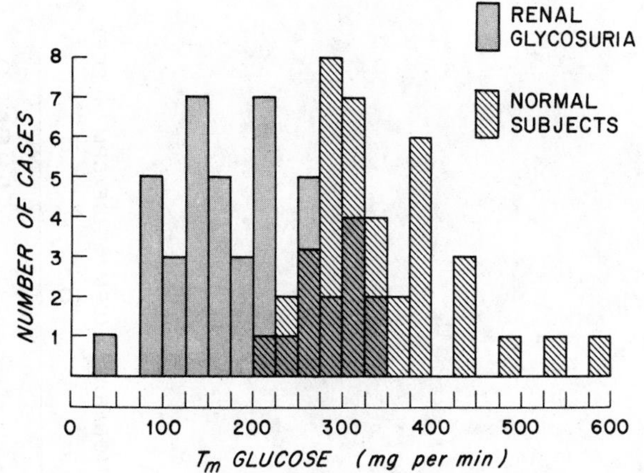

Figure 64-6. Distribution of values for glucose T_m among reported patients with renal glycosuria versus normal subjects. The values for renal glycosuric subjects are obtained from the reports of several authors [36, 37, 76–82, 105]. The normal values corrected to 1.73 m^2 body surface are taken from Smith *et al.* [107] and Elsas and Rosenberg [19].

from mutations involving the glucose-binding site on the carrier but also from other mutations such as might involve the Na^+-binding site which would allosterically alter glucose binding. Changes in the permeability characteristics of the tubular membrane toward the entry of glucose into the tubular cell could also result in a change in the shape of the titration curve.

One report describes a 9-year-old boy with cystic fibrosis of the pancreas and renal glycosuria (identified as glucose) with a normal glucose T_m (386 mg per min per 1.73 m²), but with increased splay of the curve [86]. This boy also demonstrated hyperglycinuria and a normal serum glycine level but no other aminoaciduria or other urinary abnormality. Study of 45 members of the family of the propositus revealed 13 asymptomatic subjects with glycosuria and hyperglycinuria. Inheritance of these abnormalities, thought to represent a new syndrome ("glucoglycinuria"), was that of an autosomal dominant trait.

In 1962, patients were reported with an abnormality in glucose transport in both the kidney and intestine [87], an intriguing observation especially in view of the similarities in renal and intestinal transport previously discussed. Three children and one adult all had diarrhea which appeared shortly after birth, was worse after meals, and resulted in profound weight loss and severe malnutrition [87]. Elimination of lactose from the diet produced no improvement. No disaccharides were found in the stools, and the only monosaccharides which were identified were glucose and galactose. Loading with these sugars produced flat blood curves. All the patients showed "slight renal glycosuria." Fructose, on the other hand, was rapidly absorbed, and when this was the only dietary carbohydrate, clinical improvement resulted. Fructose, which does not have the structure shown in Fig. 64-2, is not actively transported by intestine in vitro and does not inhibit glucose and galactose accumulation. In addition, the absorption of D-xylose, another sugar which does not have the structure in Fig. 64-2, is also normal [43]. A total of 14 cases have now been reported [87–98], all with similar findings, including several other cases with glycosuria [43, 96, 98]. Intestinal biopsies studied in vitro revealed no concentration of glucose against a gradient, whereas transport of alanine was normal [98]. Although phlorizin markedly inhibited glucose accumulation by control tissue, there was no effect on that from the patient.

Further studies of the transport of sugars by samples of jejunum obtained by Rubin tube biopsy from a patient, her parents, and her sibs are the subject of the most recent report [43]. As mentioned previously, normal jejunum can transport glucose actively to establish a large concentration difference by a process which exhibits Michaelis-Menten kinetics and is inhibited by metabolic poisons or the absence of Na^+ in the medium. In contrast, jejunum from the patient with glucose-galactose malabsorption was unable to accumulate glucose, although uptake of fructose was indistinguishable from that of normal subjects [43, 98].

These observations confirm the earlier study of Schneider et al. [91], who noted failure of uptake of ^{14}C-labeled galactose at the brush border of jejunal epithelium incubated in vitro. Both parents had rates of glucose transport which fell between those of the patient and normal controls (Fig. 64-7). The pattern of inheritance based on these studies, as well as those in other reported cases, is thus consistent with that of an autosomal recessive trait, with evidence for the presence of the mutant gene in the heterozygote. Since there is no detectable glucose accumulation by the homozygote, the possible mechanism (decreased carrier units versus decreased affinity of carrier for substrate) cannot be tested. The results in the heterozygote suggest that K_m is not different from controls, although the velocity V of transport is decreased. The proband in this report also showed a defect

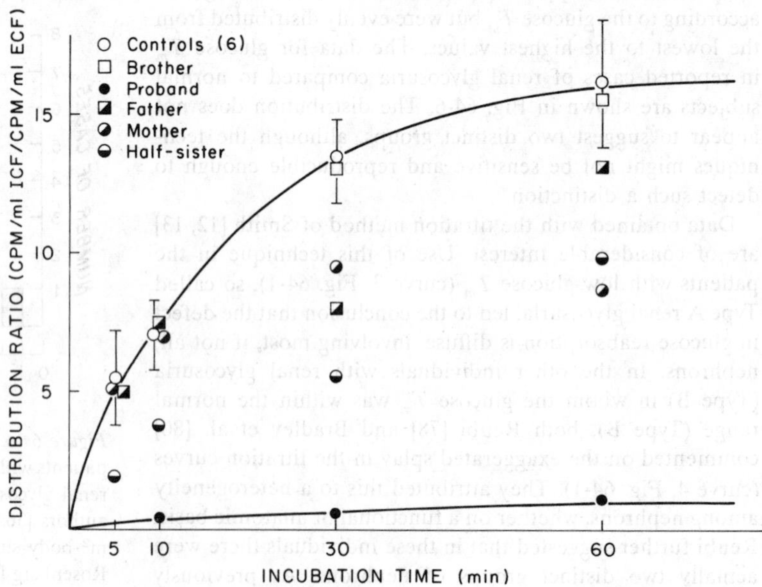

Figure 64-7. Transport of D-glucose-^{14}C by biopsy samples of jejunal mucosa in a family with intestinal glucose-galactose malabsorption. (*From Elsas et al.* [43].)

in renal transport of glucose, and although the renal phase of the study was inconclusive, it is suggested that glucose T_m is not reduced. It is, therefore, possible that the kidney may have glucose transport systems in addition to those in the intestine. The observations that other patients with true renal glycosuria have normal intestinal transport of glucose, measured by studies in vitro of jejunal biopsy specimen, are consistent with this idea [19]. It should be noted that correlation between abnormalities in renal and intestinal absorption of substances other than glucose have been recognized previously in cystinuria, Hartnup disease, and prolinuria [43].

Structural Abnormalities in Renal Glycosuria

There were two early reports of histologic examination of renal tissue from patients with renal glycosuria. Marble [4] has pointed out that in the earlier publication of Grote and Heilmann [99] the patient probably had true diabetes mellitus. The other case, reported by Monasterio [100], was evidently one of true renal glycosuria, with a similar disease in a sibling and diabetes mellitus in one parent. Histologic examination of a biopsy specimen of one kidney showed in many places marked flattening of tubular epithelium; this was occasionally so striking that the epithelium resembled endothelium. The author was careful to note that the relationship of this change to the functional abnormality was not certain.

Leonardi et al. studied needle biopsies from five members of two different families [76]. The glucose T_m was low in the two individuals in whom it was measured. In these subjects as well as the others, renal function was normal. Results of routine histologic examination and of histochemical estimation of alkaline phosphatase activity in the brush borders of the proximal convoluted tubules were within normal limits. Electron microscopic examination of two of the biopsies revealed no significant changes "which would be considered typical for renal glycosuria." In another report the electron microscopic appearance in biopsies from five patients with renal glycosuria and low glucose T_m revealed no abnormalities in two and slight thickening of the basement membrane in the remainder [77]. Such changes were considered to be nonspecific. Thus no anatomic defect in renal glycosuria has been demonstrated. The presence of normal alkaline phosphatase in the one report provides further evidence against a role of this enzyme in glucose transport.

Monasterio et al. were able to follow 15 patients with renal glycosuria, in 9 of whom measurements of glucose T_m were performed [36]. Needle biopsy specimens of the kidney in three of these revealed findings that were similar, although less marked than those in the earlier report [100]. Subsequently, Monasterio et al. reported the findings in a large sample of renal tissue from two patients with renal glycosuria obtained at surgery and fixed immediately in appropriate media [37]. Both patients were males and had "flat" glucose tolerance curves. One had a low glucose T_m (180 mg per min) and excreted between 27 and 100 gm glucose for 24 hr; the other had a normal glucose T_m (338 mg per min) and excreted between 6 and 51 gm glucose per 24 hr. Glomerular filtration rates were normal in each (150 and 130 ml per min, respectively). Routine histologic examination, microdissection of nephrons, and electron microscopy were performed on each sample of kidney. From the measurements of 50 complete nephrons in each instance, it was concluded that there was no significant difference in the ratio of glomerular surface to the proximal volume of the nephrons and, therefore, no significant difference between the dimensions of the portions of the nephrons concerned with the handling of glucose in these two patients with renal glycosuria and in normal subjects. Thus there was no *anatomic* basis for "glomerular tubular imbalance," proposed by some to account for the glycosuria [78, 80]. What was observed were lesions of the proximal convolutions of the nephron characterized by cellular changes including vacuolization, accumulation of abnormal PAS-positive material, and dissolution of elements of the brush border at the luminal surface and of the mitochondria. They assumed that these lesions must be reversible, although the evidence was indirect, and that lesions were not specific for renal glycosuria. Monasterio et al. indicated that about 35 percent of the proximal tubules showed easily recognizable lesions in the patient with the most severe disorder, and about 13 percent in the patient with the milder functional impairment. They attributed the failure of others to recognize structural abnormalities to the inadequate sampling inherent in the needle biopsy method.

Although a spotty disruption of the integrity of epithelial cells in portions of the proximal convoluted tubule might account for the functional abnormality in glucose transport, it is obvious that a minor alteration in the primary structure of the carrier protein could markedly alter the functional capacity of the carrier or its affinity for substrate and not be observable with the most sophisticated of available morphologic techniques. As an example, the extraordinary functional impairment of jejunal epithelium in glucosegalactose malabsorption [43, 98] is not accompanied by detectable morphologic abnormality [98].

GENETICS

It is apparent from the preceding discussion that there is probably no single defect that characterizes all subjects with renal glycosuria. Although there is no clear-cut separation of groups of patients on the basis of glucose T_m alone, it is likely that the different patterns obtained by the glucose titration method (low T_m with "normal" shape and near-normal T_m with increased splay) represent different abnormalities. The recognition of the defect in renal tubular transport of glucose in intestinal glucose-galactose malabsorption indicates yet another distinct abnormality. In many of the reports describing families with renal glycosuria, information is incomplete or the techniques for detection insensitive or inaccurate. Even with the use of titration methods, as noted previously, different observers reached opposite conclusions about possible patterns of inheritance [78, 80].

The most complete study of the heredity of renal glycosuria was published in 1927 [101]. Hjärne was able to obtain information on 141 out of 199 individuals, in three generations, who had common ancestors in the eighteenth century. Glycosuria with normal blood sugar levels was found in 18 on unlimited carbohydrate intake, and an additional 6 persons had glycosuria during the course of a glucose tolerance test only. Hjärne concluded that the defect was inherited as an autosomal dominant characteristic in view of the following:

1 Glycosuria occurred in male as well as female members of the family.
2 Where neither parent had glycosuria, none of the offspring had the abnormality.
3 Where either of the parents had glycosuria, some of the children generally had it.

Although true diabetes mellitus was present in seven members of the family studied by Hjärne, the mode of inheritance of this defect was not similar to that of renal glycosuria. Similar conclusions regarding inheritance of renal glycosuria were reached by Schnell [102] and supported by the report of Brown and Poleshuck [103] and by that of Houston and Merrivale [104].

These conclusions have been questioned by Elsas and Rosenberg [19], who pointed out that the affected members of those pedigrees demonstrating a dominant pattern of inheritance might actually represent heterozygotes and homozygotes for different mutations in the glucose transport process. The variation in severity of the abnormality had previously led Froesch et al. [105] to conclude that the defect may be expressed in the heterozygote but more distinctly in the homozygote. Khachadurian and Khachadurian [106] observed different patterns of inheritance in different pedigrees. They concluded that continuous heavy glucosuria did not occur in successive generations and that the parents of patients with marked glucosuria usually had mild intermittent glucosuria or none at all. Elsas and Rosenberg [19] interpreted these observations as indicating that the offspring were homozygotes for the mutant gene, whereas the parents were heterozygotes, a pattern more consistent with an autosomal recessive mode of inheritance.

In their own detailed studies of two pedigrees, Elsas and Rosenberg [19] observed a brother and sister with mild intermittent glycosuria who excreted 1,040 and 811 mg glucose per 25 hr (Fig. 64-8, Pedigree Cov) respectively. The patients showed mild decrease in glucose T_m, with a normal shape of the titration curve. Both parents were normal. They interpreted these findings as indicating a Type A renal glycosuria inherited as an autosomal recessive trait. The situation in the second pedigree was more complicated (Fig. 64-8, Pedigree Hol). In this family two brothers had severe Type A renal glycosuria and the fourth brother was considered to have mild Type B glycosuria. This pattern could be interpreted as the variable expression of an autosomal dominant mutation. Alternatively, it was suggested that the so-called Type A renal glycosuria is a mutation reflecting decreased capacity of the transport system, and that Type B is a mutation representing decreased affinity of the transport system for its substrate glucose, as discussed earlier. Therefore, the two severely affected brothers might be doubly heterozygous for two mutant genes.

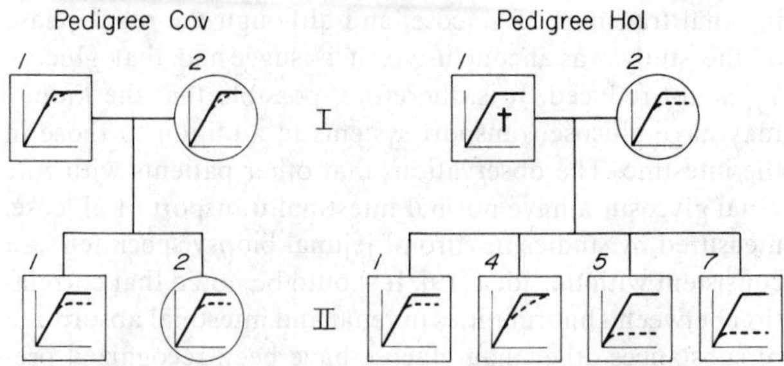

Figure 64-8. Differences in pattern of inheritance in two families with renal glycosuria. The normal pattern is illustrated in Cov, I, *1*; increased splay, in Hol, II, *4*; and low T_m, in Hol, II, *5*. (*From Elsas and Rosenberg* [19].)

The pattern of inheritance of intestinal glucose-galactose malabsorption is more clearly autosomal recessive [43]. In this disorder, the data from the intestine suggest that the mutation is reflected in decreased *capacity* of the transport system.

SUMMARY

1 Renal glycosuria is an abnormality in which glucose is excreted in the urine at normal concentrations of blood glucose. In spite of the urinary excretion of large amounts of glucose in some patients, the condition is clinically benign and usually symptomless.

2 It is probable that several different abnormalities are included under the term renal glycosuria. The majority of patients show a decrease in glucose T_m and a variable degree of splay of the titration curve. It is possible that those with low glucose T_m have a decreased functional capacity of the glucose carrier and those with increased splay have decreased affinity of carrier for glucose, analogies based on models employing Michaelis-Menten kinetics. Some patients may have mixtures of abnormalities. Others have defects in intestinal transport of hexoses that are associated with the renal defect, although in so-called intestinal glucose-galactose malabsorption the intestinal defect is severe and the renal abnormality mild.

3 In a few patients careful study has shown structural defects in the renal proximal convoluted tubules; in others no such abnormalities have been detected.

4 Although the pattern of inheritance in some pedigrees is interpreted as autosomal dominant, the pattern in other families is most consistent with that of an autosomal recessive trait.

5 The mechanism of renal tubular transport of glucose is probably similar to that of the intestine in that it is concentrative and characterized by stereospecific structural requirements, mutual competitive inhibitors of transported sugars, saturation kinetics, dependency on aerobic energy generation, and a dependency on Na^+ concentration.

6 In the light of present knowledge of the mechanism of the renal tubular transport of glucose the excretion of excessive amounts of glucose in the urine at normal levels of blood glucose could result from any of the following: (*a*) decrease in the anatomic mass of the proximal convoluted tubule relative to the glomerular surface, (*b*) decrease in the functional capacity of the system responsible for accumulation of glucose against a concentration difference within the tubule cell, (*c*) abnormal distribution of the transport system relative to glomerular filtration whether on an anatomic or functional basis, (*d*) reduction in the permeability toward glucose of the luminal membrane of the cell, (*e*) decrease in the affinity for glucose of the hypothetical membrane carrier.

BIBLIOGRAPHY

1. Marble, A.: Non-diabetic melituria, in E. P. Joslin, H. F. Root, P. White, and A. Marble (editors). *The Treatment of Diabetes Mellitus.* Lea & Febiger, Philadelphia, 1959.
2. Lawrence, R. D.: Symptomless glycosurias: differentiation by sugar tolerance tests. Med. Clin. N. Amer., **31**, 289, 1947.
3. Marble, A.: Renal glycosuria. Amer. J. Med. Sci., **183**, 811, 1932.
4. Marble, A.: The diagnosis of the less common meliturias including pentosuria and fructosuria. Med. Clin. N. Amer., **31**, 313, 1947.
5. Drucker, W. D., Fitch, R. F., and Gaston, J. H.: Diabetes mellitus and preexisting renal glycosuria. Arch. Intern. Med., **110**, 199, 1962.
6. Ackerman, I. P., Fajans, S. S., and Conn, J. W.: The development of diabetes mellitus in patients with nondiabetic glycosuria. Clin. Res. Proc., **6**, 251, 1958.
7. Horowitz, L., and Schwarzer, S.: Renal glycosuria: occurrence in two siblings and a review of the literature. J. Pediat., **47**, 639, 1955.
8. Taggart, J. V.: Mechanisms of renal tubular transport. Amer. J. Med., **24**, 774, 1958.
9. Walker, A. M., and Hudson, C. L.: The reabsorption of glucose from the renal tubules in amphibia and the action of phlorizin upon it. Amer. J. Physiol., **118**, 130, 1937.
10. Walker, A. M., Bott, P. A., Oliver, J., and MacDowell, M. C.: The collection and analysis of fluid from single nephrons of the mammalian kidney. Amer. J. Physiol., **134**, 580, 1941.
11. Shannon, J. A., and Fisher, S.: The renal tubular reabsorption of glucose in the normal dog. Amer. J. Physiol., **122**, 765, 1938.
12. Smith, H. W.: *Lectures on the Kidney.* University of Kansas, Lawrence, 1943.
13. Smith, H. W.: *The Kidney: Structure and Function in Health and Disease,* Oxford University Press, Fair Lawn, N.J., 1951.
14. Mudge, G. H.: Clinical patterns of tubular dysfunction. Amer. J. Med., **24**, 785, 1958.
15. Oliver, J.: The antithesis of structure and function in renal activity: the problem of its correlation in the nephrons and the kidney and an approach towards its resolution by structural-functional equivalents. Bull. N.Y. Acad. Med., **37**, 81, 1961.
16. Bradley, S., Laragh, J., Wheeler, H., MacDowell, M., and Oliver, J.: Correlation of structure and function in the handling of glucose by the nephrons of the canine kidney. J. Clin. Invest., **40**, 1113, 1961.
17. Berliner, R.: Discussion of Reubi in [78].
18. Burgen, A. S. V.: A theoretical treatment of glucose reabsorption in the kidney. Canad. J. Biochem. Physiol., **34**, 466, 1956.
19. Elsas, L. J., and Rosenberg, L. E.: Familial renal glycosuria: a genetic reappraisal of hexose transport by kidney and intestine. J. Clin. Invest., **48**, 1845, 1969.
20. Woolf, L. I., Goodwin, B. L., and Phelps, C. E.: T_m-limited renal tubular reabsorption and the genetics of renal glycosuria. J. Theor. Biol., **11**, 10, 1966.
21. Lundsgaard, E.: Die Wirkung von Phlorrhizin auf die Glucoseresorption. Biochem. Z., **264**, 221, 1933.
22. Kalckar, H.: Phosphorylation in kidney tissue. Enzymologia, **2**, 47, 1937.
23. Kritzler, R. A., and Gutman, A. B.: Alkaline phosphatase activity of the proximal convoluted tubules and the mechanism of phlorizin glycosuria. Amer. J. Physiol., **134**, 94, 1941.
24. Dratz, A. F., and Handler, P.: Renal phosphate and carbohydrate metabolism studied with the aid of radiophosphorus. J. Biol. Chem., **197**, 419, 1952.
25. Cori, G. T.: Glycogen structure and enzyme deficiencies in glycogen storage disease. Harvey Lect., **48**, 145, 1954.
26. Frazer, D.: Hypophosphatasia. Amer. J. Med., **22**, 730, 1957.
27. Crane, R. K.: Intestinal absorption of sugars. Physiol. Rev., **40**, 789, 1960.
28. Crane, R. K.: Absorption of sugars, in *Handbook of Physiology,* sec. 6, Alimentary Canal, vol. III, Intestinal Absorption, chap. 69, pp. 1323–1351. American Physiological Society, Washington, 1968.
29. Darlington, W. A., and Quastel, J. H.: Absorption of sugars from isolated surviving intestine. Arch. Biochem., **43**, 194, 1953.
30. Wilson, T. H., and Vincent, T. N.: Absorption of sugars in vitro by the intestine of the golden hamster. J. Biol. Chem., **216**, 851, 1955.
31. Crane, R. K., and Krane, S. M.: On the mechanism of the intestinal absorption of sugars. Biochim. Biophys. Acta, **20**, 568, 1956.
32. Wilson, T. H., and Crane, R. K.: The specificity of sugar transport by the hamster intestine. Biochim. Biophys. Acta, **29**, 30, 1958.
33. Crane, R. K., and Mandelstam, P.: The active transport of sugars by various preparations of hamster intestine. Biochim. Biophys. Acta, **45**, 460, 1960.
34. Rhodin, J.: Electron microscopy of the kidney. Amer. J. Med., **24**, 661, 1958.
35. Clark, S. L.: Ingestion of proteins and colloidal materials by columnar absorptive cells of the small intestine in suckling rats and mice. J. Biophys. Biochem. Cytol., **5**, 41, 1959.
36. Monasterio, G., Muiesan, G., Pardelli, G., Marinozzi, V., and Bosman, C.: Diabete renale o tubulo-displasia glicosurica. Minerva Nefrol., **10**, 42, 1963.
37. Monasterio, G., Oliver, J., Muiesan, G., Pardelli, G., Marinozzi, V., and MacDowell, M.: Renal diabetes as a congenital tubular dysplasia. Amer. J. Med., **37**, 44, 1964.
38. McDougal, D. B., Jr., Little, K. D., and Crane, R. K.: Studies on the mechanism of intestinal absorption of sugars. IV. Localization of galactose concentrations within the intestinal wall during active transport *in vitro.* Biochim. Biophys. Acta, **45**, 483, 1960.
39. Kinter, W. B., and Wilson, T. H.: Autoradiographic study of sugar and amino acid absorption by everted sacs of hamster intestine. J. Cell Biol., **25**, 19, 1965.
40. Caspary, W. F., and Crane, R. K.: Inclusion of L-glucose within the specificity limits of the active sugar transport of hamster small intestine. Biochim. Biophys. Acta, **163**, 395, 1968.
41. Sols, A.: The hexokinase activity of the intestinal mucosa. Biochim. Biophys. Acta, **19**, 144, 1956.
42. Crane, R. K.: Studies on the mechanism of the intestinal absorption

of sugars. III. Mutual inhibition, *in vitro,* between some actively transported sugars. Biochim. Biophys. Acta, **45,** 477, 1960.

43. Elsas, L. J., Hillman, R. E., Patterson, J. H., and Rosenberg, L. E.: Renal and intestinal hexose transport in familial glucose-galactose malabsorption. J. Clin. Invest., **49,** 576, 1970.
44. Taylor, W. R., and Langdon, R. G.: Intestinal absorption of glucose in the rat. Biochim. Biophys. Acta, **12,** 384, 1956.
45. Crane, R. K., and Krane, S. M.: Studies on the mechanism of the intestinal active transport of sugars. Biochim. Biophys. Acta, **31,** 397, 1959.
46. Riklis, E., and Quastel, J. H.: Effects of cations on sugar absorption by isolated surviving guinea pig intestine. Canad. J. Biochem. Physiol., **36,** 347, 1958.
47. Csaky, T. Z., and Thale, M.: Effect of ionic environment on the intestinal sugar transport. J. Physiol., **151,** 59, 1960.
48. Csaky, T. Z., and Zollicoffer, L.: Ionic effect on intestinal transport of glucose in the rat. Amer. J. Physiol., **198,** 1056, 1960.
49. Bihler, I., and Crane, R. K.: Studies on the mechanism of intestinal absorption of sugars. V. The influence of several cations and anions on the active transport of sugars, *in vitro,* by various preparations of hamster small intestine. Biochim. Biophys. Acta, **59,** 78, 1962.
50. Crane, R. K., Miller, D., and Bihler, I.: The restrictions on possible mechanisms of intestinal active transport of sugars, in *Membrane Transport and Metabolism,* edited by A. Kleinzeller and A. Kotyk. Academic, New York, 1961.
51. Schultz, S. G., and Zalusky, R.: The interaction between active sodium transport and active sugar transport in the isolated rabbit ileum. Biochim. Biophys. Acta, **71,** 503, 1963.
52. Crane, R. K.: Hypothesis for mechanism of intestinal active transport of sugars. Fed. Proc., **21,** 891, 1962.
53. Faust, R. G.: The effect of anoxia and lithium ions on the absorption of D-glucose by the rat jejunum, in vitro. Biochim. Biophys. Acta, **60,** 604, 1962.
54. Crane, R. K.: Na^+ dependent transport in the intestine and other animal tissues. Fed. Proc., **24,** 1000, 1965.
55. Crane, R. K., Forstner, G., and Eichholz, A.: Studies on the mechanism of the intestinal absorption of sugars. X. An effect of Na^+ concentration on the apparent Michaelis constants for intestinal sugar transport, *in vitro.* Biochim. Biophys. Acta, **109,** 467, 1965.
56. Cori, C. F., Cori, G. T., and Green, A. A.: Crystalline muscle phosphorylase. III. Kinetics. J. Biol. Chem., **151,** 39, 1943.
57. Lotspeich, W. D., and Keller, D. M.: A study of some effects of phlorizin on the metabolism of kidney tissue in vitro. J. Biol. Chem., **222,** 843, 1956.
58. Keller, D. M., and Lotspeich, W. D.: Effect of phlorizin on the osmotic behavior of mitochondria in isotonic sucrose. J. Biol. Chem., **234,** 991, 1959.
59. Keston, A. S.: Occurrence of mutarotase in animals: its proposed relationship to transport and reabsorption of sugars and insulin. Science, **120,** 355, 1954.
60. Keston, A. S.: Purification of kidney mutarotase: evidence for proposed unitary sugar transport theory. Fed. Proc., **14,** 234, 1955.
61. Keston, A. S.: Mutarotase inhibition by 1-deoxyglucose. Science, **143,** 698, 1964.
62. LeFevre, P. G.: Evidence of active transfer of certain non-electrolytes across human red cell membrane. J. Gen. Physiol., **31,** 505, 1948.
63. Crane, R. K., Field, R. A., and Cori, C. F.: Studies of tissue permeability. I. The penetration of sugars into the Ehrlich ascites tumor cells. J. Biol. Chem., **224,** 649, 1957.
64. Park, C. R., Reinwein, D., Henderson, M. J., Cadenas, E., and Morgan, H. E.: Action of insulin on the transport of glucose through the cell membrane. Amer. J. Med., **26,** 674, 1959.
65. Krane, S. M., and Crane, R. K.: The accumulation of D-galactose against a concentration gradient by slices of rabbit kidney cortex. J. Biol. Chem., **234,** 211, 1959.
66. Lotspeich, W. D.: Phlorizin and the cellular transport of glucose. Harvey Lect., **56,** 63, 1961.
67. Alvarado, F., and Crane, R. K.: Phlorizin as a competitive inhibitor of the active transport of sugars by hamster small intestine, *in vitro.* Biochim. Biophys. Acta, **56,** 170, 1962.
68. Kleinzeller, A., and Kotyk, A.: Cations and transport of galactose in kidney-cortex slices. Biochim. Biophys. Acta, **54,** 367, 1961.
69. Keston, A. S.: Kinetics and distribution of mutarotases and their relation to sugar transport. J. Biol. Chem., **239,** 3241, 1964.
70. Chinard, F. P., Taylor, W. R., Nolan, L. F., and Enns, T.: Renal handling of glucose in dogs. Amer. J. Physiol., **196,** 535, 1959.
71. Dewey, H., and Smyth, D. H.: Effect of sugar on intestinal transfer of amino acids. Nature (London), **202,** 400, 1964.
72. Saunders, S. J., and Isselbacher, K. J.: Inhibition of intestinal amino acids transport by hexoses. Biochim. Biophys. Acta, **102,** 397, 1965.
73. Alvarado, F.: Transport of sugars and amino acids in the intestine: evidence for a common carrier. Science, **151,** 1010, 1966.
74. Thier, S., Fox, M., Rosenberg, L., and Segal, S.: Hexose inhibition of amino acid uptakes in rat kidney cortex slices. Biochim. Biophys. Acta, **93,** 106, 1964.
75. Webber, W. A., and Campbell, J. L.: Effects of amino acids on renal glucose reabsorption in dogs. Canad. J. Physiol. Pharmacol., **43,** 915, 1965.
76. Leonardi, P., Ruol, A., and Munari, R.: Morphologic aspects of renal glycosuria. Amer. J. Med. Sci., **239,** 721, 1960.
77. Freeman, J. A., and Roberts, K. E.: A fine structural study of renal glycosuria. Exp. Molec. Path., **2,** 83, 1963.
78. Reubi, F. C.: Glucose titration in renal glycosuria, in *Ciba Foundation Symposium on the Kidney.* Little, Brown, Boston, 1954.
79. Lambert, P. P.: A study of the mechanism by which toxic tubular damage changes the renal threshold, in *The Kidney,* Ciba Foundation Symposium. Little, Brown, Boston, 1954.
80. Bradley, S. E., Bradley, G. P., Tyson, C. J., Curry, J. J., and Blake, W. C.: Renal function in renal diseases. Amer. J. Med., **9,** 766, 1950.
81. Robertson, J. A., and Gray, C. H.: Renal-function rests in renal glycosuria including observations during pregnancy. Lancet, **2,** 15, 1950.
82. Nielsen, A. L.: On the mechanism of glycosuria. Acta Med. Scand., **130,** 219, 1948.
83. Govaerts, P., and Lambert, P. P.: Pathogénie du diabèt renal. Acta Clin. Belg., **4,** 1, 1949.
84. Anderson, J., and Mazza, R.: Pyruvate and lactate excretion in patients with diabetes mellitus and benign glycosuria. Lancet, **2,** 270, 1963.
85. Taggart, J. V.: in Combined clinics on disorders of renal tubular function. Amer. J. Med., **20,** 448, 1956.
86. Käser, H., Cottier, P., and Antener, I.: Glucoglycinuria, a new familial syndrome. J. Pediat., **61,** 386, 1962.
87. Lindquist, B., Meeuwisse, G., and Melin, K.: Glucose-galactose malabsorption. Lancet, **2,** 666, 1962.
88. Laplane, R., Polonovski, C., Etienne, M., Debray, P., Lods, J.-C., and Pissarro, B.: L'intolérance aux sucres a transfert intestinal actif: ses rapports avec intolérance au lactose et le syndrome coeliaque. Arch. Franc. Pediat., **19,** 895, 1962.
89. Anderson, C. H., Kerry, K. R., and Townley, R. W.: An inborn defect of intestinal absorption of certain monosaccharides. Arch. Dis. Child., **40,** 1, 1965.
90. Linneweh, F., Schaumloffel, E., and Barthelmai, W.: Angeborene Glucose- und Galaktose-malabsorption. Klin. Wschr., **43,** 405, 1965.
91. Schneider, A. J., Kinter, W. B., and Stirling, C. E.: Glucose-galactose malabsorption: report of a case with autoradiographic studies of a mucosal biopsy. New Eng. J. Med., **274,** 305, 1966.
92. Marks, J. F., Norton, J. B., and Fordtran, J. S.: Glucose-galactose malabsorption. J. Pediat., **69,** 225, 1966.
93. Eggermont, E., and Loeb, H.: Glucose-galactose intolerance. Lancet, **2,** 343, 1966.
94. Dubois, R., Loeb, H., Eggermont, E., and Mainguet, P.: Étude clinique et biochimique d'un cas de malabsorption congénitale du glucose et du galactose. Helv. Paediat. Acta, **21,** 577, 1966.
95. Nusslé, D., and Gautier, E.: Malabsorption congenitale du glucose et du galactose. Assemblée Ann. Soc. Suisse Pediatric, Lugano.
96. Liu, H., Anderson, G. J., Tsao, M. U., Moore, B., and Diday, Z.: T_m

glucose in a case of congenital intestinal and renal malabsorption of monosaccharides. Pediat. Res., **1,** 386, 1967.

97. Pruitt, A. W., Achord, J. L., Fales, F. W., and Patterson, J. H.: Glucose-galactose malabsorption complicated by monilial arthritis. Pediatrics, **43,** 106, 1969.
98. Meeuwisse, G. W., and Dahlquist, A.: Glucose-galactose malabsorption: a study with biopsy of the small intestinal mucosa. Acta Paediat. Scand., **57,** 273, 1968.
99. Grote, L. R., and Heilmann, P.: Ein anatomischer Befund bei renalem Diabetes. Zbl. Allg. Path., **64,** 65, 1935.
100. Monasterio, G.: Histologischer und physio-pathologischer Beitrag zur Pathogenese des Diabetes renalis. Klin. Wschr., **18,** 538, 1939.
101. Hjärne, V. A.: A study of orthoglycaemic glycosuria with particular reference to its hereditability. Acta Med. Scand., **67,** 422, 1927.
102. Schnell, A.: Das Wesen der essentiellen renal Glykosurie und ihre beziehung zum Diabetes mellitus, unter besonderer Berucksichtigung der Erhlichkeitsfrange. Acta Med. Scand., **92,** 153, 1937.
103. Brown, M. S., and Poleshuck, R.: Familial renal glycosuria. J. Lab. Clin. Med., **20,** 605, 1935.
104. Houston, J. C., and Merrivale, W. H. H.: Renal glycosuria in a family. Guy. Hosp. Rep., **98,** 233, 1949.
105. Froesch, E. R., Winegrad, A. I., and Renold, A. E.: Die tubuläre Nierenfunktion bei verscheidenen Formen des renalen Diabetes mellitus. Helv. Med. Acta, **24,** 548, 1957.
106. Khachadurian, A. K., and Khachadurian, L. A.: The inheritance of renal glycosuria. Amer. J. Hum. Genet., **16,** 189, 1964.
107. Smith, H. W., Goldring, W., Chasis, H., Ranges, H. A., and Bradley, S. E.: The application of saturation methods to the study of glomerular and tubular function in the human kidney. J. Mount Sinai Hosp., **10,** 59, 1943.
108. McPhaul, J. J., Jr., and Simonaitis, J. J.: Observations on the mechanisms of glycosuria during glucose loads in normal and diabetic subjects. J. Clin. Invest., **47,** 702, 1968.

CHAPTER SIXTY-FIVE

RENAL TUBULAR ACIDOSIS

Donald W. Seldin and Jean D. Wilson

Renal tubular acidosis is a clinical syndrome with the outstanding feature of a sustained metabolic acidosis, characterized by a low concentration of serum bicarbonate and an approximately commensurate elevation in serum chloride level. The disorder was first described by Lightwood [1] and Butler et al. [2], and then extensively delineated by Albright and his associates [3]. In addition to hyperchloremic acidosis, there is, in many patients, a variety of associated disturbances in electrolyte metabolism. Hypokalemia, with weakness or paralysis, may result from excessive potassium losses. Osteomalacia, nephrocalcinosis, and renal stones may be caused, at least in part, by hypercalciuria and hyperphosphaturia. Polyuria and impaired concentrating ability may be the consequence of nephrocalcinosis, potassium deficiency, or both.

Since the administration of sodium bicarbonate tends to correct not only hyperchloremic acidosis but the excessive urinary losses of potassium, calcium, and phosphorus, as well, it is tempting to regard the entire syndrome as the consequence of a single defect—the inability to excrete normal amounts of acid into the urine. Such a defect should be able to explain the cause not only of the acidosis but also of the associated electrolyte derangements.

Two types of defective urinary acidification have been identified among patients with hyperchloremic renal tubular acidosis. Some patients develop acidosis without any detectable depression in their capacity to reabsorb filtered bicarbonate; the hallmark of their deranged renal acidification appears to be an inability to lower the urine pH, no matter how severe the systemic acidosis, below the relatively high value of 6. Because this type of the disorder has been studied longest and most intensively, it is often called *classical* renal tubular acidosis. The present report will be concerned with an analysis of the pathogenesis, treatment, and genetic background of this syndrome. The second type of disturbance responsible for renal tubular acidosis is a defective capacity to reabsorb filtered bicarbonate. This derangement was explored in detail in Chap. 52 on Fanconi's syndrome in the second edition of this book, and will be examined here only to distinguish its pathogenesis and treatment from those of the classical form.

REGULATION OF ACID-BASE BALANCE

The pH of the plasma is given by the ratio of bicarbonate to dissolved CO_2, as formulated in the Henderson-Hasselbalch equation,

$$pH = 6.1 + \log \frac{[HCO_3^-]}{[CO_2]}$$

Under normal conditions the lungs and kidneys stabilize the pH at a value close to 7.4 by the regulated excretion of the acid end products of metabolism. The denominator of the Henderson-Hasselbalch equation, the plasma CO_2 tension, is maintained within very narrow limits by the excretion of CO_2 by the lungs. The kidneys are concerned with the stabilization of the numerator, the concentration of sodium bicarbonate in plasma. This is accomplished by two processes: (1) virtually complete reabsorption of filtered bicarbonate, and (2) regeneration of the sodium bicarbonate which has been decomposed by the invasion of strong acids into the plasma, a process which is dependent on the formation of titratable acid and the excretion of ammonia.

These processes appear to be mediated by a single mechanism, located in the proximal and distal nephrons, involving the reabsorption of sodium ions of the tubular urine in exchange for hydrogen ions of the tubular cell, the hydrogen ions being generated by the hydration of CO_2 under the catalytic influence of the enzyme carbonic anhydrase.

Reabsorption of Bicarbonate

Hydrogen Secretion

Four lines of evidence strongly support the hypothesis that the reabsorption of filtered sodium bicarbonate is mediated by hydrogen secretion. (1) Pitts and Lotspeich [4] demonstrated that alkaline urines contain CO_2 at very high tensions, an observation which was interpreted to mean that sodium bicarbonate is reabsorbed in the distal tubule by the exchange of tubular sodium for cellular hydrogen, thereby forming carbonic acid, which slowly dehydrates and therefore appears in the bladder urine as increased CO_2 tension. (2) Berliner [5] assumed, from the very high rates of sodium bicarbonate excretion following the administration of acetazoleamide, that hydrogen secretion and, therefore, sodium bicarbonate reabsorption are blocked in the proximal tubule as well. (3) The maximum reabsorptive capacity for sodium bicarbonate was demonstrated to vary with the CO_2 tension of the plasma, presumably because this influences the pH of the renal tubular cell [6–8]. Indeed, the reabsorption of bicarbonate appeared to be entirely dependent on the plasma CO_2 tension and an intact carbonic anhydrase enzyme system [9]. (4) Finally, micropuncture studies in rats during sodium bicarbonate diuresis furnished direct evidence for hydrogen secretion [10]. In the proximal tubule an excessive accumulation of carbonic acid could be demonstrated after carbonic anhydrase was inhibited. This was interpreted to mean that hydrogen secretion mediated bicarbonate reabsorption but that carbonic acid would not accumulate in the proximal tubular urine under normal circumstances because of the location of carbonic anhydrase on the luminal surface. In the distal tubule it was possible to demonstrate excess carbonic acid without inhibition of carbonic anhydrase. This indicated that bicarbonate reabsorption is mediated by hydrogen secretion and that carbonic acid can accumulate in the tubular urine because there is no luminal carbonic anhydrase in this segment of the nephron. These studies clearly establish that the bulk of bicarbonate reabsorption is mediated by hydrogen secretion. They do not exclude the possibility, however, that a small portion of the filtered bicarbonate may be reabsorbed directly, perhaps by a process of passive diffusion along favorable electrochemical gradients.

The pattern of proximal and distal bicarbonate reabsorption has been characterized by micropuncture studies in several species. In the nonacidotic rat, Gottschalk et at. [11] and Rector [12] have demonstrated that at the end of the accessible portion of the proximal tubule the tubular fluid pH falls to about 6.7 and the concentration of bicarbonate to about 7 mEq per liter. This means that about 85 to 90 percent of the filtered bicarbonate is normally reabsorbed in the rat proximal tubule. The remaining bicarbonate is reabsorbed in the distal tubule and the collecting duct. During metabolic acidosis in the rat the proximal tubule can acidify the tubular urine to a much greater extent, so that the bicarbonate concentration at the end of the accessible portion can be depressed to levels as low as 1 to 2 mEq per liter [11]. In the nonacidotic dog, the concentration of bicarbonate at the end of the accessible portion of the proximal tubule falls only slightly, from about 22 to 17 mEq per liter, leaving about 25 percent of the filtered bicarbonate unreabsorbed [13]. During metabolic acidosis, however, proximal tubular bicarbonate concentration falls in this species as well [14]. The pattern of proximal tubular bicarbonate concentration in man is unknown, but it is likely, from these studies, that the bulk of filtered bicarbonate is reabsorbed in the proximal tubule, that the distal nephron is fully capable of reabsorbing the 10 to 25 percent of filtered bicarbonate that escapes proximal reabsorption, and that during metabolic acidosis the amount of bicarbonate escaping proximal reabsorption is very small. No data available to date indicate that all filtered bicarbonate can be reabsorbed in the proximal tubule, even during severe metabolic acidosis.

At least five factors have been identified which influence the capacity to reabsorb bicarbonate: (1) plasma CO_2 tension, (2) carbonic anhydrase activity, (3) potassium, (4) effective arterial blood volume, (5) mineralocorticoids.

The overall pattern of bicarbonate reabsorption has been delineated by Pitts and his associates [4]. The reabsorptive capacity of the tubules, for unknown reasons, varies with the glomerular filtration rate. Consequently, rises and falls in filtration rate, although increasing or decreasing the filtered load of bicarbonate, do not influence bicarbonate excretion, since such changes seem precisely balanced by commensurate changes in tubular reabsorption. Bicarbonate excretion is much more critically related to the concentration of plasma bicarbonate. During metabolic acidosis, all filtered bicarbonate is reabsorbed and the urine is acid. As the plasma bicarbonate is increased, bicarbonate reabsorption is still complete until the plasma concentration reaches about 25 mEq per liter, when bicarbonate excretion commences. At 27 to 28 mEq per liter, the maximum reabsorptive capacity is attained, and further increases in bicarbonate concentration elicit no further rise in bicarbonate reabsorption. The excretion of bicarbonate at plasma concentrations below that at which the bicarbonate T_m is attained has been termed a *bicarbonate leak* [9].

Plasma CO_2 Tension

The capacity to reabsorb bicarbonate is increased by respiratory acidosis and diminished by respiratory alkalosis. These effects are due to changes in the plasma CO_2 tension per se, not to changes in plasma pH, since a high plasma CO_2 tension can be balanced by raising the plasma bicarbonate so that the pH is normal without influencing bicarbonate reabsorption [6–8]. The effect of plasma CO_2 tension is presumed to be mediated by its influence on the pH of the renal tubular cell. With chronic respiratory acidosis, there is a further increase in bicarbonate reabsorptive capacity beyond what is achieved at the same plasma CO_2 tensions during acute respiratory acidosis [15]. The nature of this adaptive response is unknown. Although changes in plasma CO_2 tension influence the maximum reabsorptive capacity, they have no effect on the bicarbonate leak. Thus when about 75 percent of the reabsorptive capacity is utilized, a similar bicarbonate leak commences in both respiratory alkalosis and acidosis [9].

Renal Carbonic Anhydrase Activity

The activity of carbonic anhydrase also influences bicarbonate reabsorption. Inhibition of this enzyme by acetazoleamide has two effects: the bicarbonate T_m is sharply reduced, and the bicarbonate leak is greatly augmented, so that a maximally acid urine cannot be elaborated even in metabolic acidosis [9]. As a result of these effects, bicarbonate is lost into the urine, and this results in a metabolic acidosis. The concentration of plasma bicarbonate stabilizes at a level where the uncatalyzed hydration of CO_2 in the renal tubular cell can generate sufficient hydrogen to reabsorb the reduced filtered load. Carbonic anhydrase activity has been demonstrated in both the proximal and distal nephron [10]. In both segments the enzyme appears to be located in the renal tubular cell, where it catalyzes the hydration of CO_2 to carbonic acid, thereby furnishing a plentiful supply of hydrogen for bicarbonate reabsorption. In addition, it appears to be present in the luminal membrane of the proximal tubular cells, where it can catalyze the decomposition of carbonic acid formed in the proximal tubular urine as a result of hydrogen secretion. This prevents the accumulation of carbonic acid, an excess of which would lower tubular fluid pH and prevent further hydrogen secretion.

Potassium

Potassium deficiency can augment the capacity to reabsorb bicarbonate. Evidence has been advanced, on the basis of micropuncture studies, suggesting that this effect is in the proximal tubules. Since the proximal tubule is a site for potassium reabsorption, not potassium secretion, enhanced bicarbonate reabsorption cannot readily be attributed to decreased competitive inhibition at a common potassium-hydrogen secretory pathway. It was suggested, therefore, that intracellular acidosis in the proximal tubular cell, as a result of potassium deficiency, stimulates increased hydrogen secretion [16, 17].

Effective Arterial Blood Volume

Schwartz and his associates [18–20] have developed a variety of experimental models in which metabolic alkalosis is sustained in spite of a normal plasma CO_2 tension, intact carbonic anhydrase activity, and the absence of potassium deficiency. The alkalosis is uniformly relieved by the administration of chloride. Sodium chloride relieves the alkalosis by inducing bicarbonate excretion. Hydrochloric acid relieves the alkalosis without appreciably altering urine pH. All the procedures used to produce alkalosis—sodium nitrate diuresis, the posthypercapneic state, aspiration of gastric juice—are associated with a contraction of extracellular volume, because of dietary salt restriction, urinary losses, or intracellular shifts. It is likely that a reduced extracellular volume stimulates overall reabsorption of sodium salts, so that virtually all the filtered anions are reabsorbed, even though the filtered bicarbonate is high. Administration of sodium chloride can alleviate alkalosis by expanding extracellular volume and relieving the stimulus to sodium retention; the normal discrimination between chloride and bicarbonate can then be made, and sodium bicarbonate excretion will correct the alkalosis. Hydrochloric acid administration leaves the stimulus for sodium retention unchanged. In consequence, no sodium bicarbonate excretion ensues, but the alkalosis is corrected because of the altered composition of the glomerular filtrate [17].

Mineralocorticoids

Salt-retaining mineralocorticoids, such as aldosterone and deoxycorticosterone, frequently are associated with the development and maintenance of metabolic alkalosis in man and animals [21, 22]. Part of this effect of mineralocorticoids may be the consequence of their capacity, in the presence of sodium salts, to accelerate potassium excretion by augmenting distal tubular potassium secretion. This would have the dual effect of promoting alkalosis because of a movement of hydrogen into cells as potassium deficiency develops, and maintaining the alkalosis because of enhanced bicarbonate reabsorptive capacity in the proximal tubule associated with potassium depletion. In addition, however, it is very likely that mineralocorticoids, by augmenting the reabsorption of sodium salts in the distal tubule, may directly enhance $NaHCO_3$ reabsorption in this segment.

Regeneration of Bicarbonate

By far the largest proportion of secreted hydrogen ion is concerned with the reabsorption of filtered bicarbonate. At normal plasma concentrations of about 25 mEq per liter, about 3,500 mEq hydrogen ion must be secreted daily to salvage the filtered bicarbonate. In addition from 50 to 100 mmoles of strong acids is discharged into the extracellular fluid daily as a result of metabolic processes. Under normal circumstances these acids consist principally of sulfuric and phosphoric acid, derived from the metabolism of protein and phospholipids from the diet and cellular breakdown. These acids (HA) invade the blood, where they are neutralized by the buffers, and appear in the glomerular filtrate as sodium salts (NaA). Since the principal buffer of plasma is sodium bicarbonate, the reaction may be written schematically thus:

$$\begin{array}{l} HA + NaHCO_3 \longrightarrow NaA + H_2CO_3 \\ \qquad\qquad\qquad\qquad\qquad\quad \Updownarrow \\ \qquad\qquad\qquad\qquad\qquad CO_2 + H_2O \end{array}$$

Even if all the filtered bicarbonate were reclaimed, metabolic acidosis would ensue if the sodium bicarbonate, decomposed in the body by the strong acids, were not regenerated in the kidney. The regeneration of sodium bicarbonate is accomplished by the formation of titratable acid and the secretion of ammonia.

The term titratable acid denotes the amount of alkali required to titrate an acid urine back to the pH of plasma. The magnitude of titratable acid excretion is a rough approximation of the amount of $NaHCO_3$ regenerated as a result of a reduction in urine pH below that of plasma. For any given reduction in urine pH, far more titratable acid will be present if the urine is heavily buffered than if it contains little buffer. This stems from the fact that in acid urines (i.e., urine pH below the pK of the buffer) the weak acid is present principally in an un-ionized form. Buffers thus permit a greater degree of sodium for hydrogen exchange for any given urine pH. Were it not for the presence of buffers, the reabsorption of sodium for hydrogen would quickly lower the urine pH to the limiting value of 4, at which point further hydrogen secretion would stop. The principal buffer in the glomerular filtrate is Na_2HPO_4. In acid urines the secondary sodium can be exchanged for hydrogen of the tubular cell; in consequence, $NaHCO_3$ is returned to the blood, while NaH_2PO_4 is excreted in the urine. At a normal plasma pH, phosphate is present as a mixture of Na_2HPO_4 and NaH_2PO_4, in a ratio of 4:1. Therefore, the excretion into the urine of 1 mmole of phosphate as NaH_2PO_4 is associated with the regeneration of 0.8 mmole of $NaHCO_3$, which is returned to the blood. Inasmuch as the proximal tubular fluid can be acidified, especially in metabolic acidosis [11, 12, 14], titratable acid can be formed in this segment. In the acidotic rat given phosphate, about 60 percent of the titratable acid is formed in the proximal tubule, about 35 percent is formed in the distal tubule, and about 5 percent is formed in the collecting duct [12]. Normally, titratable acid excretion is small, because only a small amount of buffer is excreted into the urine. When buffer is augmented by phosphate infusions, titratable acid excretion is greatly accelerated. Should the urine pH be acid and fixed, titratable acid excretion becomes a linear function of buffer excretion.

Ammonia excretion represents the second mechanism whereby bicarbonate can be regenerated. For each millimole of ammonia excreted into the urine, a millimole of bicarbonate is returned to the blood. Like the formation of titratable acid, the principal function of ammonia secretion is to prevent a fall in urinary pH to a limiting value, thereby facilitating the continued secretion of hydrogen in exchange for sodium [23]. Recent studies in dogs [24] and man [25] of renal arteriovenous differences of amino acids during normal circumstances and metabolic acidosis indicate that the principal precursor of ammonia is glutamine, which is actively transported into the renal tubular cell and deamidated by the enzyme glutaminase; in addition, glutamic acid, arising from glutamine deamidation, may also serve as a substrate for ammonia production.

Ammonia, thus produced, enters the urine by a process of diffusion-trapping, regulated by the pH of the tubular urine. As hydrogen-ion concentration in luminal fluid increases, ammonia, which is highly soluble in lipid membranes, diffuses out of the tubular cell and is converted to ammonium ion, to which the tubular membrane is thought to be virtually impermeable. This is why the excretion of ammonia varies inversely with urine pH. Although micropuncture studies disclose that ammonia is present in both the proximal and distal tubule of the rat [26, 27] and dog [14], it is not clear that it is produced in both these sites. Ammonia diffuses rapidly and attains diffusion equilibrium throughout all phases of the kidney [28]. It could conceivably be produced in the distal nephron, from which it might diffuse into the proximal nephron.

When the urine is in the acid range, ammonia excretion varies inversely with urine pH and is uninfluenced by urine flow. In more alkaline urines, beginning at a pH of about 6.2, urine flow exerts a considerable effect on ammonia excretion. This suggests that diffusion of ammonia between tubular cells and urine approaches equilibrium [23].

During chronic metabolic acidosis [29] and potassium deficiency [30] more ammonia is produced at any given urine pH than during acute metabolic acidosis. The mechanism of this adaptive response is unknown. In the rat it is correlated with an increase in the activity of the glutaminase enzyme system; in the dog, which exhibits similar adaptation, no increase in enzymatic activity has been demonstrated [31].

Hydrogen Secretory Capacity and Net Acidification

Figure 65-1 is a schematic diagram of the processes by which the kidney maintains a constant concentration of serum bicarbonate in the face of an acid load of about 100 mmoles per day. The filtered bicarbonate is reabsorbed in the proximal and distal nephron as a result of the reabsorption of sodium in exchange for hydrogen, a process which consumes about 3,500 mEq hydrogen daily. In addition, the bicarbonate decomposed by the invasion of acids into the blood is regenerated and returned to the body; this is "new" bicarbonate, or regenerated bicarbonate, and is associated with the excretion of an equivalent amount of ammonia plus titratable acid into the urine.

It is apparent that the vast bulk of the secretory capacity is involved in reclaiming filtered bicarbonate. Nevertheless, this process is associated with sufficient reduction of urine pH, certainly in the distal nephron and probably in the proximal nephron as well, so that titratable acid and ammonia excretion can proceed actively and regenerate the small amount of bicarbonate that has been decomposed.

The total hydrogen secretory capacity is given by the expression, bicarbonate T_m + titratable acid + ammonia. It can be tested during severe metabolic alkalosis. The filtered bicarbonate is far in excess of the hydrogen secretory capacity. Bicarbonate escapes into the urine, rendering it alkaline, and ammonia excretion and titratable acid formation are negligible. Even though the urine is alkaline, the secretion of hydrogen is at a maximum. Bicarbonate infusions, therefore, permit the assessment of hydrogen secretory capacity, but they mask entirely the ability of the kidney to regenerate bicarbonate.

During metabolic acidosis, hydrogen secretory capacity is in excess of the filtered load of bicarbonate. Filtered bicarbonate is completely reclaimed from the tubular urine, and the ability of the kidney to regenerate bicarbonate can be examined. The excretion of ammonia plus titratable acid minus bicarbonate—*net effective acidification*—expresses the capacity to regenerate bicarbonate. When net acidification equals acid production, the subject is in acid-base balance. If net acidification is less than acid production, metabolic acidosis results. A defect in net acidification can be the result either of deficient hydrogen secretory capacity or of a disturbance in the process of bicarbonate regeneration. Assuming that acid production is kept constant, therefore, the capacity of the kidneys to *reclaim* and *regenerate* bicarbonate must both be examined before the cause of a metabolic acidosis can be ascertained.

Since ammonia and titratable acid excretion are both

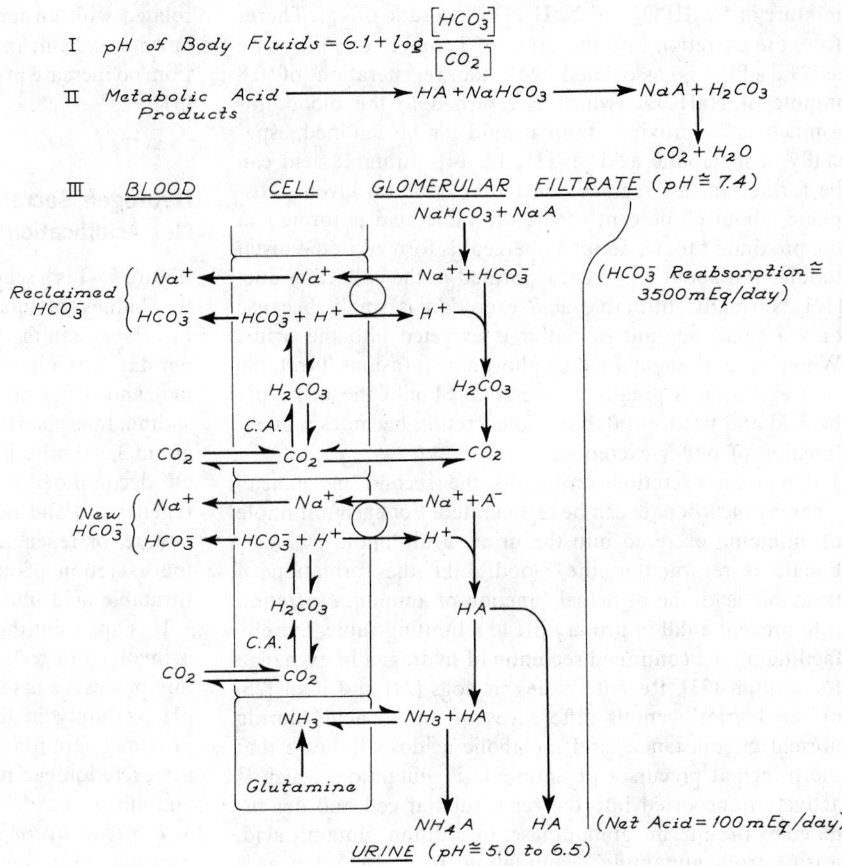

Figure 65-1. The role of the kidney in regulation of acid-base balance.

augmented as urine pH falls, a critical determinant of net acidification is the ability to lower urine pH to the limiting value of 4. The requirements for the generation of high pH gradients between urine and plasma are the following: (1) the hydrogen secretory capacity must be considerably in excess of the bicarbonate load, so that bicarbonate can be removed from the urine relatively early, thereby permitting the secretion of hydrogen into a bicarbonate-free distal tubular fluid. This is the circumstance in metabolic acidosis. (2) Sodium salts, particularly those with an impermeant anion, must reach the distal nephron and be reabsorbed there. The administration of sodium sulfate to subjects given a salt-retaining steroid or placed on a salt-free diet (to promote sodium retention) fulfills these requirements [32]. Hydrogen secretion in the distal nephron is stimulated by the reabsorption of sodium, while the presence of an impermeant anion, by promoting an increase in distal transtubular potential difference, facilitates the trapping of secreted hydrogen [33]. (3) Significant osmotic diuresis and buffer loads must not be present. Osmotic diuresis prevents maximum lowering of urine pH by depressing proximal reabsorption and sweeping sodium bicarbonate to the distal nephron. Buffer loads soak up secreted hydrogen; therefore, the collecting duct, which can generate very steep pH gradients but has a small capacity, cannot accomplish the final reduction in urine pH [12].

THE NATURE OF THE DISTURBANCE IN CLASSICAL RENAL TUBULAR ACIDOSIS: EVIDENCE FOR A GRADIENT DEFECT

On the basis of the foregoing analysis, the possible causes of the acidosis of classical renal tubular acidosis are listed in Table 65-1.

Bicarbonate titration studies disclose no evidence of a reduction in bicarbonate T_m [34, 35]. This is illustrated in a representative study from the laboratory of Seldin and Wilson [36]. (Fig. 65-2). The relation of plasma bicarbonate to bicarbonate reabsorption is plotted as plasma bicarbonate and is raised from 13 to 43 mEq per liter by an infusion of sodium bicarbonate. The bicarbonate T_m is, if anything, slightly high but certainly not depressed. Since virtually all bicarbonate reabsorption is mediated by hydrogen secretion (save, perhaps, a small amount of bicarbonate, the passive

Table 65-1. THEORETICAL CAUSES OF HYPERCHLOREMIC RENAL TUBULAR ACIDOSIS (GRADIENT DEFECT)

1. Impaired bicarbonate reabsorption
   a. Reduced bicarbonate T_m
   b. Excessive bicarbonate spillage below T_m
2. Impaired acid production
3. Impaired NH_3 production
4. Inability to elaborate acid urine

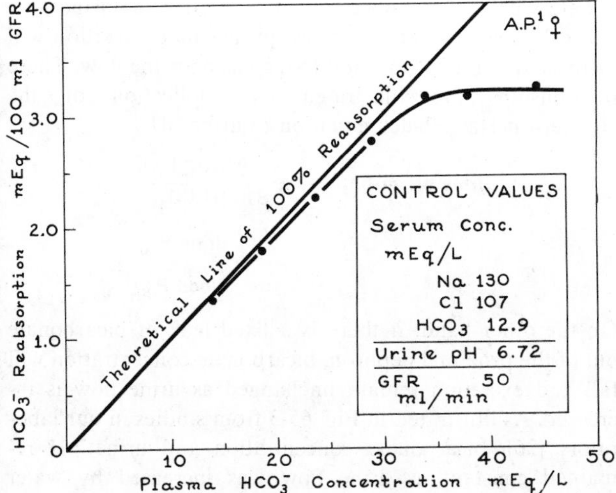

Figure 65-2. The relationship between bicarbonate reabsorption and plasma bicarbonate concentration in renal tubular acidosis—gradient defect.

reabsorption of which may be driven by favorable electrochemical gradients), it may be concluded that the total hydrogen secretory capacity is intact.

A similar inference can be drawn from the rise in titratable acid excretion, as neutral phosphate is infused, in direct proportion to the magnitude of phosphaturia [34, 35, 37]. Since in these studies [34, 35, 37], urine pH did not fall significantly with phosphate loads, the low titratable acid excretion usually noted in these patients must be due to the relatively high fixed urine pH, not to any deficiency in the total capacity to secrete hydrogen in exchange for sodium.

Different results were obtained by Latner and Burnard [38], who demonstrated a definite fall in urine pH and a rise in ammonia excretion with neutral phosphate infusions. They proposed that there was a defect in proximal tubular bicarbonate reabsorption which resulted in increased delivery to the distal nephron, thereby alkalinizing the urine and depressing ammonia and titratable acid formation. If this were so, the defect should be exaggerated when the plasma bicarbonate is elevated and should be detectable by a depressed bicarbonate T_m. Unfortunately, bicarbonate titration studies were not performed. Moreover, the studies cited above indicate that, in adults at least, phosphate infusion does not appreciably lower urine pH. It is possible that the patients studied by Latner and Burnard [38] did not have classical renal tubular acidosis, but developed hyperchloremic acidosis on the basis of bicarbonate wastage, a syndrome to be discussed subsequently.

A second possible explanation for the acidosis is that there is a slight bicarbonate leak before the T_m is reached, and this may accumulate over a period of days to significant bicarbonate wastage. In Fig. 65-2, it should be noted that there is a deviation of points from the theoretical line of 100 percent reabsorption to a greater extent than is noted in normal subjects. This should not necessarily be interpreted as an excessive leak of sodium bicarbonate into the urine. This small bicarbonate excretion, as well as the constant excretion of small amounts of bicarbonate even during severe acidosis, probably represents ammonium bicarbonate excretion, a process which has no influence on systemic acid-base balance. In favor of this explanation is the commensurate rise in ammonia and bicarbonate excretion as urine flow is increased from 0.5 to 4 ml per min by water diuresis (Fig. 65-3). Moreover, in the two patients studied by Schwartz and his associates [39], the increase in bicarbonate excretion, as the plasma bicarbonate was raised to normal, was small when compared with uremic subjects with bicarbonate wastage.

The third disturbance attributing acidosis to failure to reclaim filtered bicarbonate involves the assumption that the enzyme carbonic anhydrase is deficient. Although chronic inhibition of carbonic anhydrase in normal subjects by acetazoleamide can produce hyperchloremic acidosis, the mechanism is entirely different. Carbonic anhydrase inhibition produces a definite depression in the bicarbonate T_m, with a marked bicarbonate leak [9]. A pronounced sodium bicarbonate diuresis results. In renal tubular acidosis, the bicarbonate T_m is normal, and the bicarbonate leak is trivial; bicarbonate excretion is small and consists principally of ammonium bicarbonate, not sodium bicarbonate. A variety of studies have indicated a reduced response to acetazoleamide [35, 40, 41]. This is not surprising in view of the impaired glomerular filtration rate and the systemic acidosis—disturbances which will reduce the response to acetazoleamide in the absence of renal tubular acidosis. In Table 65-2 are summarized two of our studies [36] in which a brisk bicarbonate diuresis could be elicited by acetazoleamide when the serum bicarbonate was partially restored to normal by sodium bicarbonate administration. In addition, carbonic anhydrase activity was normal in renal tissue obtained by biopsy from a child with renal tubular acidosis [42].

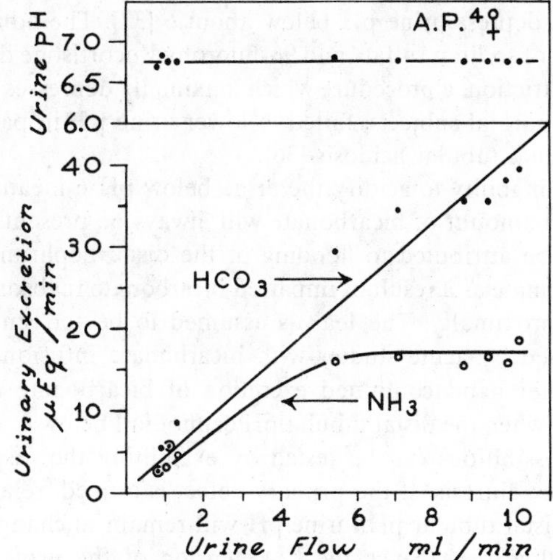

Figure 65-3. The effect of water diuresis on bicarbonate and ammonia excretion in renal tubular acidosis (gradient defect).

Table 65-2. EFFECT OF ACETAZOLEAMIDE ON HCO_3 EXCRETION IN RENAL TUBULAR ACIDOSIS (GRADIENT DEFECT)

		Mean values		
Subject	Condition	$[HCO_3^-]_S$, mEq/l	GFR, ml/min	ΔHCO_3^- excretion, μEq/min
A. P.	Acidosis	11.5	50	20
	Normal plasma pH	20	50	170
S. H.	Acidosis	16	40	0
	Normal plasma pH	24	40	120

From these studies, it may be concluded that total hydrogen secretory capacity is intact and that the acidosis does not result from an inability to reclaim filtered bicarbonate.

Albright and his associates originally attributed the acidosis to a defect in ammonia production [3]. It is true that ammonia excretion is usually reduced, but it has subsequently been demonstrated that ammonia excretion is normal or high for the urine pH, if correction is also made for the low glomerular filtration rate [37]. In addition, a recent study indicates that renal glutaminase activity is not depressed [42]. It may therefore be concluded that the reduced excretion of ammonia does not represent a primary disturbance in ammonia production or transport but rather is the passive consequence of a relatively high urine pH and a reduced glomerular filtration rate.

With the single exception of Latner and Burnard [38], all studies have revealed an inability of patients with this disorder to acidify the urine in spite of severe systemic acidosis. It has therefore been proposed by Reynolds [35] and others [34, 37] that the basic defect in renal tubular acidosis is an inability to establish high pH gradients between urine and plasma. Measures which usually depress urine pH well into the acid range have little effect. Ammonium chloride loads do not depress urine pH below about 6 [37]. The administration of sodium sulfate and 9α-fluorohydrocortisone during salt restriction, a procedure which maximally depresses urine pH in normal subjects, failed to lower urine pH in patients with renal tubular acidosis [36].

The inability to acidify the urine below pH 6 means that a small amount of bicarbonate will always be present. This might be attributed to flooding of the distal nephron with bicarbonate as a result of impaired bicarbonate reabsorption more proximally. The leak is assumed to be too small to be tested by acute studies with bicarbonate infusions. On the other hand continued excretion of bicarbonate is expected when the distal tubular pH cannot fall below 6. These two possibilities can be tested by examining the response to water diuresis. If the primary defect is a fixed, relatively high distal tubular pH, urine pH will remain unchanged as urine flow rises. Since the CO_2 tension of the urine is in equilibrium with that of blood, the concentration of bicarbonate will also remain constant. Therefore, as urine flow is accelerated by water diuresis, bicarbonate excretion will increase in direct proportion to increasing urine flow. These relationships are illustrated by application of the Henderson-Hasselbalch equation to urine pH:

$$\text{Urine pH} = pK' + \log \frac{[HCO_3^-]}{810\,[H_2CO_3]}$$

$$\Updownarrow$$
$$\text{urine } P_{CO_2}$$
$$\Updownarrow$$
$$\text{blood } P_{CO_2}$$

On the other hand, if there is a fixed leak of bicarbonate out of the proximal nephron, bicarbonate concentration will fall and excretion remain unchanged as urine flow is increased. As illustrated in Fig. 65-3 from studies in our laboratory [36], bicarbonate concentration and urine pH remained constant as urine flow was increased by water diuresis; therefore bicarbonate excretion rose in direct proportion to increasing urine flow. This constitutes strong evidence that the constant excretion of bicarbonate is due not to a leak out of the proximal tubule but rather to an inability to lower urine pH in the distal nephron.

It is also apparent from Fig. 65-3 that ammonia excretion is partially flow-dependent up to urine flows of about 5 ml per min, doubtless because ammonia diffusion approaches equilibrium between tubular cell and urine at about pH 6.2 [23]. Since the excretion of ammonium bicarbonate does not influence systemic acid-base balance, it may be concluded that bicarbonate wastage is not an important factor in the cause of the acidosis.

The explanation for the inability sharply to lower urine pH is unknown. It is possible that the hydrogen secretory system in the distal nephron is unable to perform the work required to establish high pH gradients. The fact, however, that bulk hydrogen secretion, as reflected in the bicarbonate T_m, is normal suggests that hydrogen secretion may not be disturbed. Instead, the defect might be due to excessive back-diffusion of secreted hydrogen as a result of increased permeability of the distal tubule. This type of disorder would be expected to become manifest only when buffer and bicarbonate were present in the urine in very small amounts and would be compatible with the finding of normal hydrogen secretory capacity and a defective ability to generate sharp pH gradients between urine and plasma.

The manner in which a relatively high, fixed urine pH can produce hyperchloremic acidosis was studied by the author [36] in patients placed on a low-salt diet (Fig. 65-4). After a control period of 5 days during which plasma composition was kept normal by Shohl's solution and sodium chloride, both were withdrawn from the diet. A mild acidosis and a minimal rise in serum chloride supervened. Extracellular volume shrank 2 to 3 liters, as reflected by a fall in body weight and radiosulfate space, and the urine remained alkaline and contained small amounts of ammonia, titratable acid, and bicarbonate. The administration of dietary salt markedly worsened the hyperchloremia and

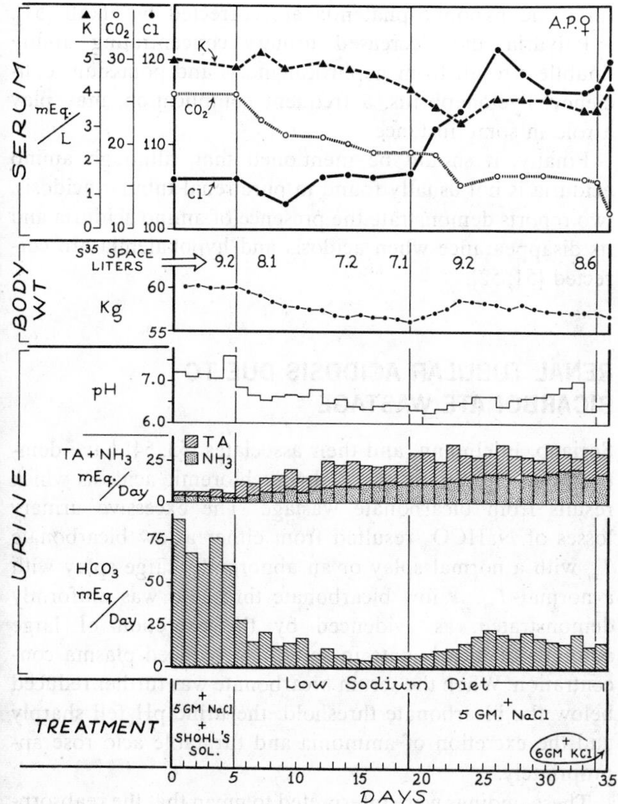

Figure 65-4. Metabolic balance study of a patient with renal tubular acidosis (gradient defect) while on a low-salt diet. *TA*, titratable acidity.

acidosis without significantly changing the external balance of acid. Finally, correction of the potassium deficit with potassium chloride aggravated the hyperchloremic acidosis.

From these studies a tentative reconstruction of the pathogenesis of classical hyperchloremic renal tubular acidosis may be ventured (Fig. 65-5). Metabolic acids (HA) enter the blood and decompose bicarbonate to NaA, which is filtered into the tubular urine. However, the exchange of tubular sodium for cellular hydrogen is diminished, since the formation of HA would reduce urine pH to its limiting value. In consequence, NaA is excreted into the urine. The reduced sodium-for-hydrogen exchange may be associated with increased sodium-for-potassium exchange, resulting in accelerated losses of KA. The loss of sodium bicarbonate as NaA or KA causes systemic acidosis, while the shrinkage of extracellular volume by the loss of bicarbonate without commensurate losses of chloride leads to mild hyperchloremia. Retention of dietary sodium chloride will reexpand extracellular volume and aggravate the acidosis by diluting plasma bicarbonate. Since the ratio of sodium to chloride in plasma is about 1.4:1, reexpansion of extracellular volume by sodium chloride will also increase the hyperchloremia. Loss of potassium mitigates the acidosis, probably because some of the potassium loss is associated with entrance of hydrogen into tissue cells.

Potassium Deficiency

Excessive potassium excretion with severe hypokalemia (notwithstanding the presence of marked systemic acidosis) is common in these patients. The most probable explanation

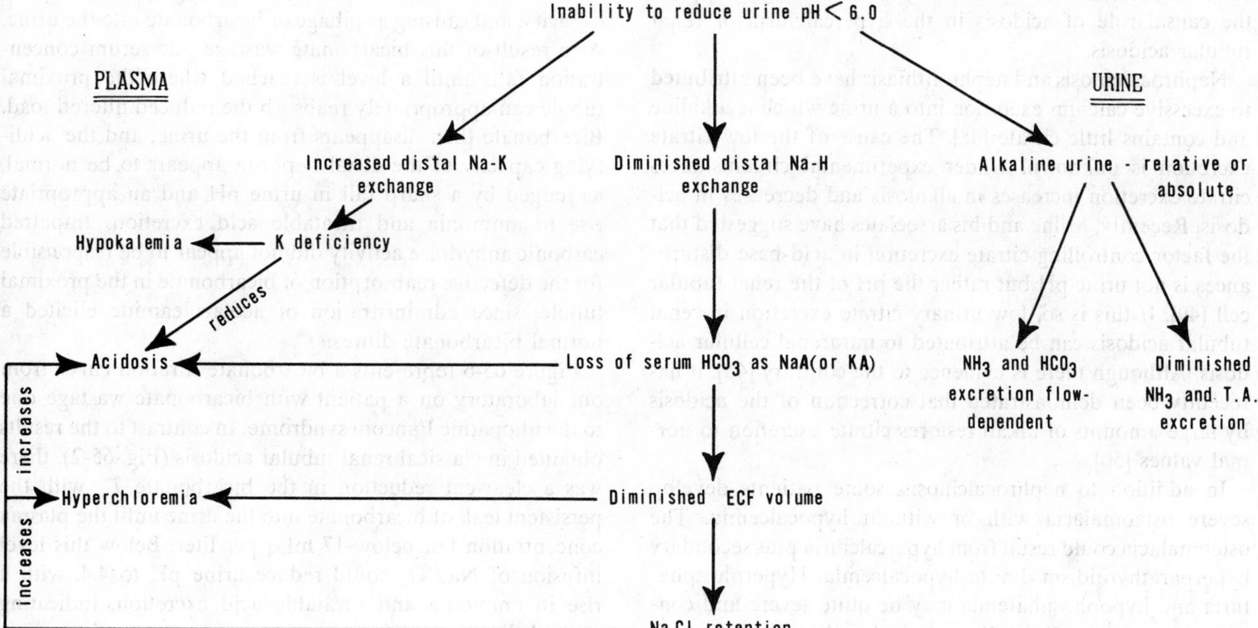

Figure 65-5. Pathogenesis of hyperchloremic renal tubular acidosis—gradient defect.

is that, as a result of diminished sodium-for-hydrogen exchange, increased amounts of NaR are present in the distal nephron, thereby stimulating sodium-for-potassium exchange (Fig. 65-5). The best evidence for this is the correction of potassium wastage when enough sodium bicarbonate is given to facilitate hydrogen secretion in the distal nephron [43]. In addition, secondary aldosteronism, resulting from salt depletion, may accentuate potassium loss [43].

Calcium and Phosphorus

Hypercalciuria, hypocalcemia, osteomalacia, nephrocalcinosis, and nephrolithiasis accompany renal tubular acidosis and probably are related, directly or indirectly, to the basic defect in urinary acidification.

Hypercalciuria has been attributed by Albright and Reifenstein to the effects of chronic acidosis [3], in analogy to the increased calcium excretion in normal subjects given ammonium chloride loads [3, 44]. Since metabolic acidosis will induce hypercalciuria in the parathyroidectomized animal, the effect cannot be attributed to enhanced parathormone secretion alone [45]. The recent studies of Goodman and his associates [46] and Lemann et al. [47] demonstrate that during a steady state of ammonium chloride acidosis in normal subjects as well as in a steady state of uremic acidosis, net acidification (the excretion of ammonia + titratable acid–bicarbonate) is considerably less than metabolic acid production, even though the serum bicarbonate remains constant. This suggests that acid is being neutralized somewhere in the body, presumably in part at least in bone. This, as well as the fall in calcium excretion following correction of acidosis by alkali, strongly supports the causal role of acidosis in the hypercalciuria of renal tubular acidosis.

Nephrocalcinosis and nephrolithiasis have been attributed to excessive calcium excretion into a urine which is alkaline and contains little citrate [48]. The cause of the low citrate excretion is unknown. Under experimental circumstances citrate excretion increases in alkalosis and decreases in acidosis. Recently, Milne and his associates have suggested that the factor controlling citrate excretion in acid-base disturbances is not urine pH but rather the pH of the renal tubular cell [49]. If this is so, low urinary citrate excretion in renal tubular acidosis can be attributed to intrarenal cellular acidosis. Although there is evidence to the contrary [48], it has recently been demonstrated that correction of the acidosis by large amounts of alkali restores citrate excretion to normal values [50].

In addition to nephrocalcinosis, some patients develop severe osteomalacia with or without hypocalcemia. The osteomalacia could result from hypercalciuria plus secondary hyperparathyroidism due to hypocalcemia. Hyperphosphaturia and hypophosphatemia may be quite severe and contribute to osteomalacia. Increased phosphate excretion, in the pure forms of the disease, seems to be a secondary phenomenon, related to the acidosis, since hyperphosphaturia and hypophosphatemia are corrected by alkali [51].

Polyuria and decreased urinary concentrating ability doubtless result from nephrocalcinosis and potassium deficiency. Pyelonephritis, a frequent complication, may play a role in some instances.

Finally, it should be mentioned that, although amino aciduria is not usually found in pure renal tubular acidosis, two reports demonstrate the presence of amino aciduria and its disappearance when acidosis and hypokalemia are corrected [51, 52].

RENAL TUBULAR ACIDOSIS DUE TO BICARBONATE WASTAGE

Soriano, Edelmann, and their associates [53, 54] have demonstrated a different type of hyperchloremic acidosis which results from bicarbonate wastage. The excessive urinary losses of $NaHCO_3$ resulted from either a low bicarbonate T_m with a normal splay or an abnormally large splay with a normal T_m. A low bicarbonate threshold was uniformly demonstrated, as evidenced by the excretion of large amounts of bicarbonate in spite of a reduced plasma concentration. When the serum bicarbonate was further reduced below the bicarbonate threshold, the urine pH fell sharply and the excretion of ammonia and titratable acid rose appropriately.

These findings were interpreted to mean that the reabsorption of bicarbonate in the proximal tubule was depressed, resulting in a reduced bicarbonate T_M or an increased splay. In consequence, increased amounts of bicarbonate are delivered to the distal nephron, exceeding its reabsorptive capacity, and causing a spillage of bicarbonate into the urine. As a result of this bicarbonate wastage, the serum concentration falls until a level is reached where the proximal tubule can appropriately reabsorb the reduced filtered load. Bicarbonate then disappears from the urine, and the acidifying capacity of the distal nephron appears to be normal, as judged by a sharp fall in urine pH and an appropriate rise in ammonia and titratable acid excretion. Impaired carbonic anhydrase activity did not appear to be responsible for the defective reabsorption of bicarbonate in the proximal tubule, since administration of acetazoleamide elicited a normal bicarbonate diuresis.

Figure 65-6 represents a bicarbonate titration curve from our laboratory on a patient with bicarbonate wastage due to the idiopathic Fanconi syndrome. In contrast to the results obtained in classical renal tubular acidosis (Fig. 65-2), there was a clear-cut reduction in the bicarbonate T_m with the persistent leak of bicarbonate into the urine until the plasma concentration fell below 17 mEq per liter. Below this level infusion of Na_2SO_4 could reduce urine pH to 4.4, with a rise in ammonia and titratable acid excretion, indicating normal distal acidifying capacity.

The studies of Soriano and Edelmann [53, 54], as well as the data cited here, constitute strong evidence that bicar-

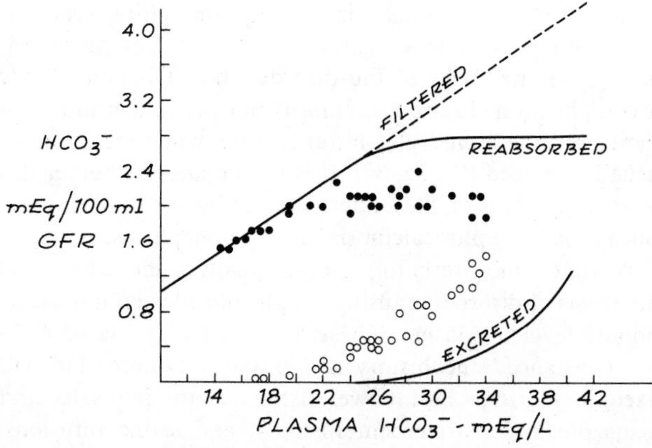

Figure 65-6. The relationship between bicarbonate reabsorption and plasma bicarbonate concentration in renal tubular acidosis of the bicarbonate wastage type. The closed circles represent the reabsorbed bicarbonate, and the open circles represent the excreted bicarbonate observed in the patient. Normal values are demonstrated by the lines labeled "reabsorbed" and "excreted."

bonate wastage is a result of a disturbance in the proximal tubule. No evidence of impaired distal acidification can be elicited when the plasma bicarbonate concentration has been reduced sufficiently to permit appropriate proximal reabsorption. It is possible, however, that some patients with classical renal tubular acidosis of the gradient type have a slight defect in proximal bicarbonate reabsorption in addition. Sebastian, McSherry, and Morris [55] reported studies in which some patients with classical renal tubular acidosis, given water loads when the plasma bicarbonate was moderately reduced, displayed a striking reduction in urine pH and bicarbonate concentration as urine flow increased. This was taken as evidence that the high urine pH was the consequence, not merely of the inability of the distal nephron to establish steep pH gradients, but also of a proximal bicarbonate leak. An alternative explanation would attribute the very alkaline urines at low urine flows to the accumulation of carbonic acid which reduces distal pH, thereby depressing hydrogen secretion and bicarbonate reabsorption [10, 56]. The lower urine pH and bicarbonate concentration at high urine flows could result from the fact that increased urine flow will decrease the concentration of carbonic acid in the distal nephron, thereby permitting further hydrogen secretion and bicarbonate reabsorption. Bicarbonate titration curves in such patients might clarify the issue.

CLINICAL FEATURES OF CLASSICAL RENAL TUBULAR ACIDOSIS

Renal tubular acidosis may occur in a pure form or as a feature of some more inclusive disease state. Hugh, Webster, and Elkinton [57] have suggested that the term, *primary renal tubular acidosis,* be applied to those cases in which there is no related antecedent disease and which are not part of another disease state. *Secondary renal tubular acidosis* refers to cases with antecedent or associated diseases. Primary renal tubular acidosis, in turn, may be subdivided into two forms: an infantile type and an adult type [57]. Lightwood and Butler [58] have pointed out that the "infantile" type may sometimes become manifest after the first year of life; the adult type has, on rare occasions, appeared within the first year. Since the distinguishing feature of cases beginning in infancy is the fact that the disease almost invariably disappears if the patient is treated while the adult form tends to be permanent, they have proposed that the primary cases be classified as transient or persistent.

Transient Primary Renal Tubular Acidosis

The disorder usually begins within the first year of life and is characterized by anorexia, vomiting, failure to thrive, apathy, wasting, weakness, and polyuria [59]. Carré and his associates [60] reported 5 of 17 cases with hypercalcemia. Nephrocalcinosis, detectable by x-ray, is rare. About 70 percent of the cases are in males [57]. If treatment is adequate, recovery is complete and without residua.

Persistent Primary Renal Tubular Acidosis

This disorder occurs predominately in females (about 70 percent of the cases) and tends to appear after the age of 2 years, although several cases clearly began within the first year. The majority of cases are sporadic, but the familial occurrence of the disorder is being increasingly reported.

The symptoms of the disorder are attributable to the electrolyte disturbances and their consequences, and are summarized in Table 65-3. Chronic acidosis may be responsible for anorexia, lethargy, and dyspnea on exertion, and may contribute to the failure of normal growth [61]. Osteomalacia, with bone pain and pathologic fractures, may result

Table 65-3. DERANGEMENTS IN HYPERCHLOREMIC RENAL TUBULAR ACIDOSIS (GRADIENT DEFECT)

Tendency toward disturbance		
Plasma	Urine	Systemic
Acidosis Hyperchloremia Hyponatremia Hypokalemia Hypocalcemia Hypophosphatemia Elevated alkaline phosphatase	Polyuria and isosthenuria Alkaline or relatively alkaline Decreased NH_3 and titratable acid Hyperkaliuria Hypercalciuria Hyperphosphaturia	Nephrocalcinosis and nephrolithiasis Osteomalacia and bone pain Weakness Periodic attacks of weakness or paralysis Familial or acquired

from hypercalciuria and hyperphosphaturia, and may be associated with a normal or reduced serum calcium and phosphorus levels and an elevated alkaline phosphatase concentration. Nephrocalcinosis and nephrolithiasis occur in 73 percent of the cases [37]. Ureteral colic results from renal stones, while nephrolithiasis gives rise to a striking roentgenogram of medullary calcification (Fig. 65-7) and is responsible, in part at least, for polyuria and impaired concentrating power of the kidney. Potassium loss may result in severe hypokalemia and is responsible for the frequent presenting picture of flaccid paralysis, sometimes including the respiratory muscles [62]. Cardiac arrhythmias may result from hypokalemia. Some patients come to the physician in a crisis, which may be precipitated by starvation and vomiting. Profound weakness or frank flaccid paralysis may be associated with either deep, powerful respiratory excursions or feeble and ineffectual respiratory motions, depending, no doubt, on the balance between the central drive to respiration caused by metabolic acidosis and the weakness of the respiratory muscles caused by hypokalemia. These features may be associated with drowsiness or coma and mild fever, and often simulate a central nervous system disorder. We have observed several patients in such a crisis whose spinal fluid protein level was elevated. Salt depletion, often associated with hyponatremia [63], may develop, especially in

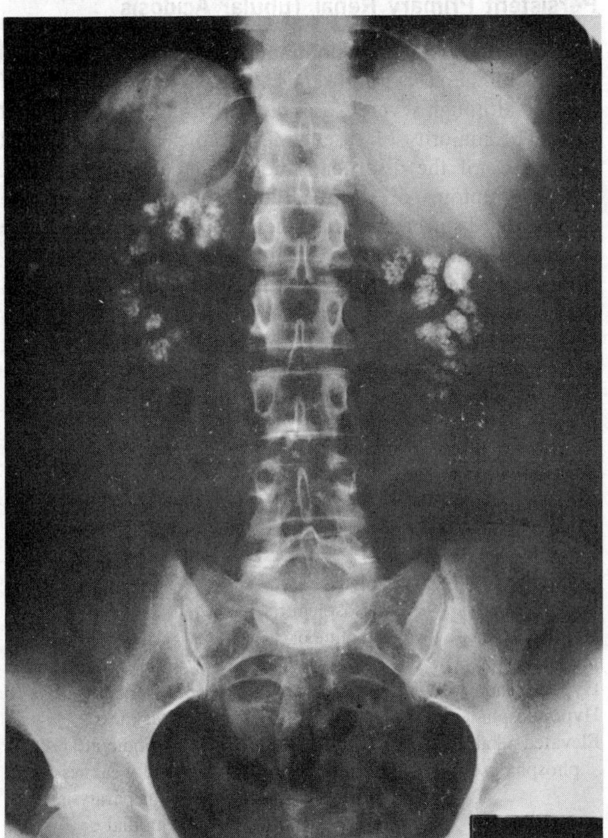

Figure 65-7. Renal stones in a patient with renal tubular acidosis (gradient defect).

patients whose salt intake is low. Pyelonephritis, which is frequently present, was regarded by Albright and his associates [3] as the cause of the disorder, but it is more likely a complication. Frank azotemia is not present in most patients, but the glomerular filtration rate, when measured, is usually reduced [63, 35, 37]. It is not apparent whether this is an expression of the underlying disease or of such complications as nephrocalcinosis and pyelonephritis.

At times, the presenting picture involves the differential diagnosis of disorders causing a high chloride and low bicarbonate level in plasma. These are listed in Table 65-4. In most instances, the history and physical examination will exclude diarrhea and bowel fistula, acidifying salts and acetazoleamide, ureteroenterostomy, and saline infusions. Nephrocalcinosis, if present, will favor classical renal tubular acidosis.

To distinguish renal tubular acidosis due to a gradient defect from that due to bicarbonate wastage may be difficult. The differences between the two disorders are summarized in Table 65-5. Both disorders present with hyperchloremic acidosis and hypokalemia. Four features are especially helpful for differential diagnosis: (1) bicarbonate reabsorption, as disclosed by a bicarbonate titration curve, is grossly impaired if bicarbonate wastage is present, but not with the gradient defect. (2) The urine pH is always relatively high in the gradient defect, no matter how severe the systemic acidosis. A low urine pH, therefore, excludes the gradient defect. (3) Patients with bicarbonate wastage tend to be relatively resistant to bicarbonate therapy, since the administered bicarbonate, by raising the plasma concentration, tends to be spilled promptly into the urine. By contrast, patients with the gradient defect are bicarbonate-sensitive, and their condition can be readily controlled by oral bicarbonate administration. (4) Such features of Fanconi's syndrome as glucosuria and amino aciduria are exceedingly rare in the gradient defect, while nephrocalcinosis, which occurs in about 73 percent of these patients, is very rarely associated with bicarbonate wastage. Bicarbonate wastage can occur as a primary disorder, either as an isolated renal tubular defect [53, 54] or as part of an idiopathic Fanconi syndrome. Bicarbonate wastage may also occur in a secondary form in association with heavy metals, such as cadmium [64] and mercury [65]; drugs, such as outdated tetracycline [66]; dysproteinemic states, such as multiple myeloma [67, 68] and Sjögren's syndrome [69]; during a rejection reaction following transplantation [70]; and in genetic diseases, such as Wilson's disease [71], Lowe's syndrome [72], galactosemia [73], and hereditary fructose intolerance [74, 75]. Osserman and his associates [76] and Morris [77] have emphasized that the common quality of many of these seemingly diverse disorders—heavy metal poisoning, dysproteinemic states, rejection reaction, hereditary fructose intolerance—is the presence of lysozymuria, derived either because of systemic overproduction or from a toxic, inflammatory, or metabolic injury of the kidney. Lysozyme is an extremely basic, low-molecular-weight protein, avidly bound in the proximal tubule, and could conceivably be the common causal factor

Table 65-4 CAUSES OF HIGH CHLORIDE AND LOW BICARBONATE CONCENTRATIONS IN PLASMA

Clinical disorder			Serum		
Classification	Physiologic disturbance	Clinical derangement	HCO_3^-	Cl^-	pH
Metabolic acidosis (primary alkali deficit)	Alkali loss or acid retention	1. Diarrhea and bowel fistula 2. NH_4Cl, organic acidifying salts (e.g., arginine hydrochloride), cation exchange resins 3. Acetazoleamide 4. Ureteroenterostomy 5. Hyperchloremic renal tubular acidosis—*gradient defect:* *a.* Primary *b.* Secondary 6. Hyperchloremic renal tubular acidosis—*bicarbonate wastage:* *a.* Primary *b.* Secondary 7. Renal insufficiency	Low	High	Low
	Dilution	Rapid saline infusions	Low	High	Low
Respiratory alkalosis (primary CO_2 deficit)	Alveolar over-ventilation	Stimulation of respiratory center by: 1. Chemical changes (salicylates, anoxia) 2. Reflexes (chest pain, diminished pulmonary compliance) 3. Central stimulation (psychic, CNS disease)	Low	High	High

in the proximal tubular lesion responsible for many of the secondary forms of Fanconi's syndrome and bicarbonate wastage.

The acidosis of chronic renal failure may sometimes appear as hyperchloremic acidosis. This disorder most commonly arises during the course of azotemic renal failure due to pyelonephritis. Azotemia is moderate, and hyperchloremic acidosis is associated with little or no rise in undetermined acids. The serum potassium level of these patients tends to be high, not low, and the patients, when acidotic, can elaborate a urine of maximum acidity [78].

Finally, severe respiratory alkalosis can reduce serum bicarbonate concentration, elevate serum chloride level, and result in the formation of an alkaline urine. At times profound hypokalemia may develop, owing to alkalinization of renal tubular cells with excessive exchange of sodium for potassium. In complicated instances a blood pH can establish the proper diagnosis.

Persistent Primary Renal Tubular Acidosis—Incomplete Type

Wrong and Davies [37] report three cases of nephrocalcinosis without hypercalciuria and without hyperchloremic acidosis. These patients were unable to excrete a highly acid urine, even after challenge with ammonium chloride (0.1 gm per kg body weight by mouth). The absence of hyperchloremic acidosis is demonstrated by the ability of the patients to excrete large amounts of ammonia.

Table 65-5 CHARACTERISTIC FEATURES OF THE TWO TYPES OF RENAL TUBULAR ACIDOSIS

Feature	Gradient defect	Bicarbonate wastage
Site of defect	Presumably distal tubule	Presumably proximal tubule
Renal amino aciduria and glucosuria	Rare	Common
Nephrocalcinosis	Common	Rare
NH_3 excretion (corrected for GFR* and urine pH)	Normal	Normal
Maximal reduction in urine pH:		
1. When ser $HCO_3^- > 18$ mEq/l	>6.0	>6.0
2. When ser $HCO_3^- < 13$ mEq/l	>6.0	<5.4
Response to alkali	Sensitive	Resistant

* Glomerular filtration rate.

Secondary Renal Tubular Acidosis

Classical renal tubular acidosis is termed secondary when it appears as an expression of an identifiable systemic disease. By far the most important identifiable disorders are various dysproteinemic states. Cohen and Way [79] reported two cases in young women with hyperglobulinemic purpura. Morris and Fudenberg [80] reviewed a variety of isolated reports and studied 22 patients with hypergammaglobulinemia. Of the 22 patients, 12 displayed defective urinary acidification, while 5 had overt hyperchloremic acidosis. Most of the patients displayed a broad-based elevation in 7S γ-globulin in association with such diseases as idiopathic hypergammaglobulinemia, lupoid hepatitis, and coccidioidomycosis. In 4 patients, the dysproteinemia was due, not to a rise in 7S γ-globulin, but to macroglobulinemia (Waldenström's). In addition to 7S γ-globulin and macroglobulin, cryoglobulin has been associated with classical renal tubular acidosis. LoSpalluto and his associates [81] demonstrated the presence of a peculiar cryoglobulin (which consisted of equal quantities of 7S and 19S γ-globulins) in a woman whose classical renal tubular acidosis antedated the onset of detectable dysproteinemia.

It is not clear how these dysproteinemic states produce the renal disorder. In contrast to the finding of lysozymuria in diverse types of Fanconi's syndrome and bicarbonate wastage [76, 77], Morris could find no detectable lysozymuria in 6 patients with classical renal tubular acidosis [77]. It would appear that in bicarbonate wastage, despite the various abnormalities in serum proteins, it is the lysozymuria which may be responsible for the proximal tubular lesion. In classical renal tubular acidosis, since there is no lysozymuria, the elevations in 7S γ-globulin, macroglobulin, or cryoglobulin may be responsible for the disorder.

It does not seem likely that the abnormal proteins cause a direct injury to tubular cells, since immunofluorescent antibody studies disclose no demonstrable immunoglobulin deposition in the tubules [82, 83]. An alternative hypothesis attributes the disorder to disturbed viscosity caused by the abnormal proteins in small medullary blood vessels [84]. This also seems unlikely, since, as Huth has pointed out [85], there is no demonstrable correlation between impaired urinary acidification and the magnitude and type of dysproteinemia.

In addition to dysproteinemic states, classical renal tubular acidosis has been reported secondary to hypercalcemia of vitamin D intoxication [86], hyperthyroidism [87, 88], and amphotericin B intoxication [89].

TREATMENT

Acidosis can be treated by the administration of Shohl's solution [90]: 140 gm citric acid and 98 gm hydrated crystalline salt of sodium citrate are dissolved in water to a final volume of 1 liter. Citric acid is included in the mixture to provide an acid buffer in the intestine to enhance calcium absorption. In the body citric acid is dissipated as CO_2 and water, while sodium citrate is converted to sodium bicarbonate. Shohl's solution contains 1 mEq sodium per milliliter of solution. About 50 to 100 ml is given daily in three divided doses. The solution is made more palatable by diluting it with ginger ale and chilling it. Shohl's solution is usually more satisfactory than sodium bicarbonate because it does not produce abdominal bloating or belching. If supplemental potassium is required, 50 gm sodium citrate and 50 gm potassium citrate can be mixed with 140 gm citric acid. The serum bicarbonate and potassium should be checked periodically to ascertain if alkalosis or hyperkalemia has developed. If edema appears, the patient should be placed on a diet low in sodium chloride; Shohl's solution can be continued, because the administration of sodium citrate will not usually lead to unrelenting sodium retention. If sodium chloride is restricted from the diet, potassium must be given as potassium chloride in order to replenish a potassium deficiency [91, 92]. Supplemental calcium salts and vitamin D are not required by most patients. Correction of acidosis stops hypercalciuria and facilitates remineralization of the skeleton. If severe symptomatic osteomalacia is present, calcium lactate and vitamin D can be given. The serum calcium should be checked to make certain hypercalcemia is not induced. Hypercalciuria should also be avoided by checking the urine for calcium by Sulkowitch's test. When remineralization is complete, calcium salts and vitamin D should be stopped.

In the fulminant crisis of renal tubular acidosis, with severe hypokalemia, infusions of sodium bicarbonate and potassium chloride must be given. The infusion of isotonic sodium bicarbonate should be given with care: too much sodium bicarbonate may lead to metabolic alkalosis; too rapid infusion can cause respiratory alkalosis, even when the serum bicarbonate level is not elevated above normal (owing to the persistent acidosis of the respiratory center which drives respiration). Both forms of alkalosis can precipitate tetany, especially in the presence of hypocalcemia. Tetany has also been precipitated by the correction of hypokalemia in the presence of marked hypocalcemia [62].

GENETICS

Most published cases of renal tubular acidosis appear to be sporadic in nature, 56 of the 60 cases reviewed by Piel [93] in 1957 having had negative family histories. A familial incidence of this disease has been described with greater frequency during the past few years, and 17 different families involving 72 affected individuals have now been reported with some combination of the constellation of inability to acidify the urine, persistent hyperchloremic acidosis, nephrocalcinosis, and nephrolithiasis. The family histories are summarized in Fig. 65-8. Although many of these family studies are so small as to be inadequate for analysis of the mode of inheritance, one of the reported families involves trans-

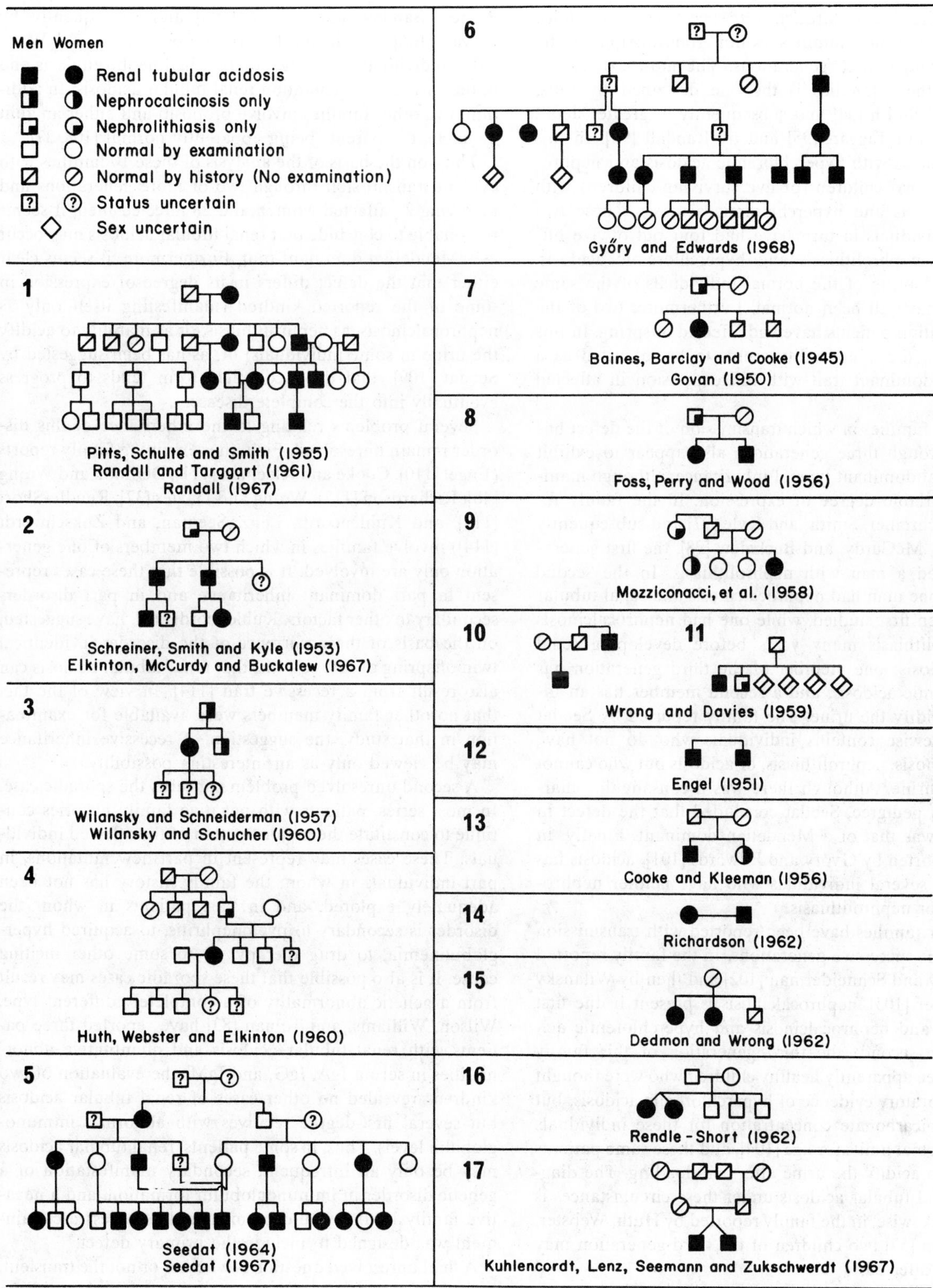

Figure 65-8. Genetic charts of 17 families with renal tubular acidosis (gradient defect).

mission of the disease through four successive generations, and three additional families exhibit transmission of the disorder through three generations. The most extensively studied of these families is the one described by Pitts, Schulte, and Smith [94] and subsequently in greater detail by Randall and Taggart [95] and by Randall [96]. In this family a woman with hyperchloremic acidosis and nephrolithiasis had two children (of five surviving children) with nephrocalcinosis and hyperchloremic acidosis. These two affected individuals in turn have had four out of five offspring with nephrolithiasis and hyperchloremic acidosis, while the offspring of the normal individuals of the same generation have all been normal. Furthermore, two of the third-generation patients have had affected offspring. In this family, then, the abnormality seems to be inherited as a Mendelian dominant trait with full expression in affected individuals.

The three families in which transmission of the defect has occurred through three generations also appear to exhibit an autosomal dominant type of inheritance, although manifesting a variable degree of expression. In the family reported by Schreiner, Smith, and Kyle [97] and subsequently by Elkinton, McCurdy, and Buckalew [98], the first generation included a man with nephrolithiasis. In the second generation one man had nephrocalcinosis and renal tubular acidosis when first studied, while one had nephrocalcinosis and nephrolithiasis many years before developing renal tubular acidosis; one member of the third generation has hyperchloremic acidosis, and a second member has an inability to acidify the urine. The family reported by Seedat [99, 100] likewise contains individuals who do not have nephrocalcinosis, nephrolithiasis, or acidosis but who cannot acidify the urine. Although there was a consanguine marriage in this pedigree, Seedat concluded that the defect in this family was that of a Mendelian dominant. Finally, in a family reported by Győry and Edwards [101], acidosis has occurred in several individuals who have neither nephrocalcinosis nor nephrolithiasis.

Two other families have been reported with transmission through three successive generations. In the family reported by Wilansky and Schneiderman [102] and then by Wilansky and Schucher [103], nephrocalcinosis is present in the first generation, and nephrocalcinosis and hyperchloremic acidosis in the second; the third generation of this family includes three apparently healthy children who were thought to have laboratory evidence of hyperchloremic acidosis, but the serum bicarbonate concentration for these individuals is within normal limits for age [104], and these same patients were able to acidify the urine after acid loading. The diagnosis of renal tubular acidosis under these circumstances is doubtful. Likewise, in the family reported by Huth, Webster, and Elkinton [57] two children of the third generation may possibly be affected.

Two other family trees involving two successive generations fit well with the possibility of a dominant defect with variable degrees of manifestation. In the family reported by Baines, Barclay, and Cooke [105] and subsequently by Govan [106], and in the family of Foss, Perry, and Wood [107], individuals in one generation had nephrolithiasis and in the succeeding generation renal tubular acidosis. In addition, two other families involve propositi and either an aunt or uncle, the parents being apparently normal [108, 37].

Thus, on the basis of the analysis of these 10 families with evident transmission through two or more generations and involving 27 affected women and 28 affected men, it seems reasonable to conclude that renal tubular acidosis may occur as a Mendelian dominant trait. Furthermore, it seems clear either that the defect differs in its degree of expression in some of the reported kindred (manifesting itself only as nephrocalcinosis, as nephrolithiasis, or as inability to acidify the urine in some individuals) or, as has been suggested by Seedat [109], that the incomplete form tends to progress eventually into the complete disease.

Several problems relating to the inheritance of this disorder remain unresolved. First, the remaining family reports (Engel [110], Cooke and Kleeman [111], Dedmon and Wrong [48], Richardson [112], Wrong and Davies [37], Rendle-Short [113], and Kuhlencordt, Lenz, Seeman, and Zukschwerdt [114]) involve families in which two members of one generation only are involved. It is possible that these cases represent in part dominant inheritance and in part disorders secondary to other factors. Kuhlencordt et al. have suggested, on the basis of the occurrence of the disorder in identical twin offspring of first cousins, that renal tubular acidosis can also result from a recessive trait [114]. In view of the fact that no other family members were available for examination in that study, the suggestion of recessive inheritance may be viewed only as an interesting possibility.

A second unresolved problem concerns the sporadic case. In most series, patients with negative family histories continue to constitute the major fraction of the affected individuals. These cases may represent in part new mutations, in part individuals in whom the family history has not been adequately explored, and in part patients in whom the disorder is secondary to pyelonephritis, to acquired hyperglobulinemia, to drug therapy, or to some other inciting cause. It is also possible that these sporadic cases may result from a genetic abnormality of a completely different type. Wilson, Williams, and Tobian [83] have reported three patients with renal tubular acidosis and quantitative abnormalities in serum IgA, IgG, and IgM; the evaluation of two kindreds revealed no other cases of renal tubular acidosis but several first-degree relatives with abnormal immunoglobulin levels. Thus, in some patients, renal tubular acidosis may be only an infrequent, secondary manifestation of a genetic disorder in immunoglobulin formation, and a negative family history would be meaningless unless ascertainment was designed to include the primary defect.

A final unresolved question is whether or not the transient, infantile form of the disease represents a variant of the persistent late childhood and adult form of renal tubular acidosis, or is a separate entity. Abundant evidence is available that the persistent disease may begin early in life. Thus, in one of the familial cases reported by Engel [110] there were nephrocalcinosis and nephrolithiasis by the age of 4 months, and in the case reported by Mozziconacci et al. [108] there was nephrocalcinosis at the age of 3 months. Indeed, the possibility seems attractive that the infantile form may be a variant of the adult form; those infants in whom the disease is mild, the diagnosis is made early, and treatment is begun before nephrocalcinosis ensues, may recover, while patients with severe cases or in whom therapy is begun late may suffer more severe consequences of the defect. In support of this view are 7 cases reported by Doxiadis [115] and 13 reported by Carré, Wood, and Smallwood [60] of infants who recovered from the infantile form of the disease and who had no radiologic evidence of nephrocalcinosis; the 3 babies who died in these two series all had nephrocalcinosis.

Against this unitary concept has been assembled a convincing argument. As has been pointed out by several investigators, the transient infantile form of renal tubular acidosis is striking for the negativity of the family histories [59, 60, 114]. Indeed, only one involved family has been reported in which an affected individual recovered. Of the twin sisters reported by Rendle-Short [112], one infant (with nephrocalcinosis) died of citrate intoxication, while the other apparently recovered completely following a course of citrate therapy. Of the other families with manifestation of the illness in infancy, no recoveries have been noted. Because of the striking negativity of the family histories and because of a preponderance of males in these cases, Huth, Webster, and Elkinton [57] have argued that the transient form of the disease is a separate entity, representing a delay of maturation of renal function due to a recessive trait or to some nongenetic cause. The report of Lightwood and Butler [58] lends support to the suggestion that an environmental factor may be responsible for the transient form of the disease. They noted an abrupt decrease in the incidence of the disorder in England after 1954. Although they considered the decrease in the administration of vitamin D, mercury, and sulfonamides as possible factors, none of these seemed to explain the sudden decline in the frequency of infantile renal tubular acidosis.

SUMMARY

1 Two types of defective urinary acidification have been identified among patients with hyperchloremic renal tubular acidosis. Some patients develop acidosis without any detectable depression in their capacity to reabsorb filtered bicarbonate; the hallmark of their deranged renal acidification appears to be an inability to lower the urine pH, no matter how severe the systemic acidosis, below the relatively high value of 6. This type of disorder has been termed classical renal tubular acidosis or renal tubular acidosis due to a gradient defect. The second type of disturbance responsible for renal tubular acidosis is a defective capacity to reabsorb filtered bicarbonate. This form of the disorder is termed bicarbonate wastage.

2 Classical renal tubular acidosis is characterized, in addition to the defect in distal acidification, by a variable constellation of features, consisting of hyperchloremic acidosis; hypokalemia, with weakness and paralysis owing to hyperkaluria; osteomalacia, nephrocalcinosis, and renal stones, caused, at least in part, by hypercalciuria and hypophosphaturia; and polyuria and impaired concentrating ability as a consequence of potassium deficiency, nephrocalcinosis, or both.

All the derangements can be traced to a single primary defect in the mechanism of urinary acidification. Intact reclamation of filtered bicarbonate indicates that total hydrogen secretory capacity is normal. No leak of bicarbonate out of the proximal tubule can be demonstrated. Ammonia excretion is not impaired if the excretory rate is corrected for urine pH and glomerular filtration rate. The defect thus appears to be an inability of the distal tubule to generate steep pH gradients between blood and tubular urine. The most plausible explanation of the defect is excessive back-diffusion of secreted hydrogen from tubular urine to blood, presumably because of increased permeability to hydrogen of the distal tubular cells.

Treatment with alkali is effective in correcting all the electrolyte disturbances (save, of course, those due to irreversible renal damage).

3 Bicarbonate wastage as a cause for renal tubular acidosis appears to be a defect in bicarbonate reclamation in the proximal tubule and is characterized by a low bicarbonate T_m or an increased splay or both. When the serum bicarbonate is reduced below the threshold value, the urine becomes very acid, and ammonia and titratable secretable acid rise normally. This disorder occurs in a primary form, either as an isolated defect or as part of Fanconi's syndrome. It may also appear as a secondary disturbance in a variety of disease states, such as heavy metal poisoning, dysproteinemic states, rejection reaction to a renal transplant, and hereditary fructose intolerance. The common property of these seemingly diverse disorders is the presence of lysozymuria, derived either from systemic overproduction or from a toxic, inflammatory, or metabolic injury of the kidney. Lysozyme appears to be avidly bound in the proximal tubule and could conceivably be the causal factor responsible for impaired proximal bicarbonate reabsorption.

4 Classical renal tubular acidosis may occur in a pure primary form, either as a transient disease in infancy or as a persistent disease with an onset usually in late childhood or adult life. The transient disease is very rarely familial, but the persistent disease, although more commonly sporadic, exhibits an appreciable familial incidence. Secondary causes of classical renal tubular acidosis include hypercalcemic states, various hyperglobulinemic disorders, and certain poisonings (amphotericin B).

5 Dominant transmission has been described in several families with the primary persistent form of the classical disease. In some families full expression has always occurred, whereas in others expression has been variable. The transient infantile form may not have a genetic basis, or if it does, it may have a different mode of inheritance.

BIBLIOGRAPHY

1. Lightwood, R.: Communication to British Pediatric Association. Arch. Dis. Child., **10**, 205, 1935.
2. Butler, A. M., Wilson, J. L., and Farber, S.: Dehydration and acidosis with calcification of renal tubules. J. Pediat., **8**, 489, 1936.
3. Albright, F., and Reifenstein, E. C., Jr.: *Parathyroid Glands and Metabolic Bone Disease.* Williams & Wilkins, Baltimore, 1948.
4. Pitts, R. F., and Lotspeich, W. D.: Bicarbonate and the renal regulation of acid-base balance. Amer. J. Physiol., **147**, 138, 1946.
5. Berliner, R. W.: Renal secretion of potassium and hydrogen ions. Fed. Proc., **11**, 695, 1952.
6. Brazeau, P., and Gilman, A.: Effect of plasma CO_2 tension on renal tubular reabsorption of bicarbonate. Amer. J. Physiol., **175**, 33, 1953.
7. Relman, A. S., Etsten, B., and Schwartz, W. B.: The regulation of renal bicarbonate reabsorption by plasma carbon dioxide tension. J. Clin. Invest., **32**, 972, 1953.
8. Dorman, P. J., Sullivan, W. J., and Pitts, R. F.: The renal response to acute respiratory acidosis. J. Clin. Invest., **33**, 82, 1954.
9. Rector, F. C., Jr., Seldin, D. W., Roberts, A. D., Jr., and Smith, J. S.: The role of plasma CO_2 tension and carbonic anhydrase activity in the renal reabsorption of bicarbonate. J. Clin. Invest., **39**, 1706, 1960.
10. Rector, F. C., Jr., Carter, N. W., and Seldin, D. W.: The mechanism of bicarbonate reabsorption in the proximal and distal tubules of the kidney. J. Clin. Invest., **44**, 278, 1965.
11. Gottschalk, C. W., Lassiter, W. E., and Mylle, M.: Localization of urine acidification in the mammalian kidney. Amer. J. Physiol., **198**, 581, 1960.
12. Rector, F. C., Jr.: Micropuncture studies on the mechanism of urinary acidification, in *Renal Metabolism and Epidemiology of Some Renal Diseases,* p. 9. National Kidney Foundation, New York, 1964.
13. Clapp, J. R., Watson, J. F., and Berliner, R. W.: Osmolality, bicarbonate concentration, and water reabsorption in proximal tubule of the dog nephron. Amer. J. Physiol., **205**, 273, 1963.
14. Clapp, J. R., Owen, E. E., and Robinson, R. R.: Contribution of the proximal tubule to urinary ammonia excretion by the dog. Amer. J. Physiol., **209**, 269, 1965.
15. Sullivan, W. J., and Dorman, P. J.: The renal response to chronic respiratory acidosis. J. Clin. Invest., **34**, 268, 1955.
16. Rector, F. C., Jr., Bloomer, H. A., and Seldin, D. W.: Effect of potassium deficiency on the reabsorption of bicarbonate in the proximal convolution of the rat kidney. J. Clin. Invest., **43**, 1976, 1964.
17. Kunau, R. T., Jr., Frick, A., Rector, F. C., Jr., and Seldin, D. W.: Micropuncture study of the proximal tubular factors responsible for the maintenance of alkalosis during potassium deficiency in the rat. Clin. Sci., **34**, 223, 1968.
18. Gulyassy, P. F., van Ypersele de Strihou, C., and Schwartz, W. B.: On the mechanism of nitrate-induced alkalosis: the possible role of selective chloride depletion in acid-base regulation. J. Clin. Invest., **41**, 1850, 1962.
19. Schwartz, W. B., Hays, R. M., Polak, A., and Haynie, G. D.: Effects of chronic hypercapnia on electrolyte and acid-base equilibrium. II. Recovery, with special reference to the influence of chloride intake. J. Clin. Invest., **40**, 1238, 1961.
20. Needle, M. A., Kaloyanides, G. J., and Schwartz, W. F.: The effects of selective depletion of hydrochloric acid on acid-base and electrolyte equilibrium. J. Clin. Invest., **43**, 1836, 1964.
21. Seldin, D. W., Welt, L. G., and Cort, J. H.: The role of sodium salts and adrenal steroids in the production of hypokalemic alkalosis. Yale J. Biol. Med., **29**, 229, 1956.
22. Luke, R. G., and Levitin, H.: Impaired renal conservation of chloride and acid-base changes associated with potassium depletion. Clin. Sci., **32**, 511, 1967.
23. Orloff, J., and Berliner, R. W.: The mechanism of the excretion of ammonia in the dog. J. Clin. Invest., **35**, 223, 1956.
24. Pitts, R. F., de Haas, J., and Klein, J.: Relation of renal anions and amide nitrogen extraction to ammonia production. Amer. J. Physiol., **204**, 187, 1963.
25. Owen, E. E., and Robinson, R. R.: Amino acid extraction and ammonia metabolism by the human kidney during prolonged administration of ammonium chloride. J. Clin. Invest., **42**, 263, 1963.
26. Glabman, S., Klose, R. M., and Giebisch, G.: Micropuncture study of ammonia excretion in the rat. Amer. J. Physiol., **205**, 127, 1963.
27. Hayes, C. P., Jr., Mayson, J. S., Owen, E. E., and Robinson, R. R.: A micropuncture evaluation of renal ammonia excretion in the rat. Amer. J. Physiol., **207**, 77, 1964.
28. Stone, W. J., Balagura, S., and Pitts, R. F.: Diffusion equilibrium for ammonia in the kidney of the acidotic dog. J. Clin. Invest., **46**, 1603, 1967.
29. Pitts, R. F.: Renal excretion of acid. Fed. Proc., **7**, 418, 1948.
30. Seldin, D. W., Rector, F. C., Jr., Carter, N., and Copenhaver, J.: The relation of hypokalemic alkalosis induced by adrenal steroids to renal acid secretion. J. Clin. Invest., **33**, 965, 1954.
31. Rector, F. C., Jr., and Orloff, J.: The effect of the administration of sodium bicarbonate and ammonium chloride on the excretion and production of ammonia: the absence of alterations in the activity of renal ammonia-producing enzymes in the dog. J. Clin. Invest., **38**, 366, 1959.
32. Schwartz, W. B., Jenson, R. L., and Relman, A. S.: Acidification of the urine and increased ammonium excretion without change in acid-base equilibrium: sodium reabsorption as a stimulus to the acidifying process. J. Clin. Invest., **34**, 673, 1955.
33. Clapp, J. R., Rector, F. C., Jr., and Seldin, D. W.: Effect of unreabsorbed anions on proximal and distal transtubular potentials in rats. Amer. J. Physiol., **202**, 781, 1962.
34. Smith, L. H., Jr., and Schreiner, G. E.: Studies on renal hyperchloremic acidosis. J. Lab. Clin, Med., **43**, 347, 1954.
35. Reynolds, T. B.: Observations on the pathogenesis of renal tubular acidosis. Amer. J. Med., **25**, 503, 1958.
36. Seldin, D. W., Rector, F. C., Jr., Portwood, R., and Carter, N.: Pathogenesis of hyperchloremic acidosis in renal tubular acidosis, in *Proceedings of the First International Congress on Nephrology,* p. 725. Karger, Basel, 1961.
37. Wrong, O., and Davies, H. E. F.: The excretion of acid in renal disease. Quart. J. Med., n.s., **28**, 259, 1959.
38. Latner, A. L., and Burnard, E. D.: Idiopathic hyperchloremic renal acidosis of infants: observations on the site and nature of the lesion. Quart. J. Med., n.s., **19**, 285, 1950.
39. Schwartz, W. B., Hall, P. W., Hays, R. M., and Relman, A. S.: On the mechanism of acidosis in chronic renal disease. J. Clin. Invest., **38**, 39, 1959.
40. Kaye, M.: The effect of a single oral dose of the carbonic anhydrase inhibitor, acetazoleamide, in renal disease. J. Clin. Invest., **34**, 277, 1955.
41. Webster, G. D., Jr., Huth, E. J., Elkinton, J. R., and McCance, R.: The renal excretion of hydrogen ion in renal tubular disease. II. Quantitative response to the carbonic anhydrase inhibitor, acetazolamide. Amer. J. Med., **29**, 576, 1960.
42. Yaffe, S. J., Craig, J. M., and Fellers, F. X.: Studies on renal enzymes in a patient with renal tubular acidosis. Amer. J. Med., **29**, 1968, 1960.
43. Gill, J. R., Jr., Bell, N. H., and Bartter, F. C.: Correction of renal sodium loss and secondary aldosteronism in renal tubular acidosis with bicarbonate loading. Clin. Res., **9**, 201, 1961.
44. Sartorius, O. W., Roemmelt, J. C., and Pitts, R. F.: The renal regulation of acid-base balance in man. IV. The nature of the renal compensations in ammonium chloride acidosis. J. Clin. Invest., **28**, 423, 1949.
45. Silberg, B., Calder, D., Carter, N., and Seldin, D. W.: Urinary calcium excretion in parathyroidectomized rats during metabolic and respiratory acidosis. Clin. Res., **12**, 50, 1964.
46. Goodman, A. D., Lemann, J., Jr., Lennon, E. J., and Relman, A. S.: Production, excretion, and net balance of fixed acid in patients with renal acidosis. J. Clin. Invest., **44**, 495, 1965.

47. Lemann, J., Jr., Lennon, E. J., Goodman, A. D., Litzow, J. R., and Relman, A. S.: The net balance of acid in subjects given large loads of acid or alkali. J. Clin. Invest., **44,** 507, 1965.
48. Dedmon, R. E., and Wrong, O.: The excretion of organic anion in renal tubular acidosis with particular reference to citrate. Clin. Sci., **22,** 19, 1962.
49. Evans, B. M., MacIntyre, I., MacPherson, C. R., and Milne, M. S.: Alkalosis in sodium and potassium depletion (with special reference to organic acid excretion). Clin. Sci., **16,** 53, 1957.
50. Morrissey, J. F., Ochoa, M., Jr., Lotspeich, W. D., and Waterhouse, C.: Citrate excretion in renal tubular acidosis. Ann. Intern. Med., **58,** 159, 1963.
51. Harrison, H. E., Chisolm, J. J., Jr., and Harrison, H. C.: Congenital renal tubular acidosis. A.M.A. J. Dis. Child., **96,** 588, 1958.
52. Denton, D. A., Wynn, V., McDonald, I. R., and Simon, S.: Renal regulation of the extracellular fluid. II. Renal physiology in electrolyte subtraction. Acta Med. Scand., suppl. **261,** 1, 1951.
53. Soriano, J. R., Boichis, H., Stark, H., and Edelmann, C. M., Jr.: Proximal renal tubular acidosis: a defect in bicarbonate reabsorption with normal urinary acidification. Pediat. Res., **1,** 81, 1967.
54. Soriano, J. R., Boichis, H., and Edelmann, C. M., Jr.: Bicarbonate reabsorption and hydrogen ion excretion in children with renal tubular acidosis. J. Pediat. **71,** 802, 1967.
55. Sebastian, A., McSherry, E., and Morris, R. C., Jr.: On the mechanism of the inappropriately high urinary pH in classic renal tubular acidosis, in *Abstracts of American Society of Nephrology,* p. 59, 1969.
56. Reid, E. L., and Hills, A. G.: The effect of delayed dehydration of carbonic acid in renal bicarbonate clearance, and its significance for acid-base balance. Clin. Sci., **37,** 381, 1969.
57. Huth, E., J., Webster, G. D., Jr., and Elkinton, J. R.: The renal excretion of hydrogen ion in renal tubular acidosis. III. An attempt to detect latent cases in a family: comments on nosology, genetics and etiology of the primary disease. Amer. J. Med., **29,** 586, 1960.
58. Lightwood, R., and Butler, N.: Decline in primary infantile renal acidosis; aetiological implications. Brit. Med. J., **1,** 855, 1963.
59. Lightwood, R., Payne, W. W., and Black, J. A.: Infantile renal acidosis. Pediatrics, **12,** 628, 1953.
60. Carré, I. J., Wood, B. S. B., and Smallwood, W. C.: Idiopathic renal acidosis in infancy. Arch. Dis. Child., **29,** 326, 1954.
61. Cooke, R. E., Boyden, D. G., and Haller, E.: The relationship of acidosis and growth retardation. J. Pediat., **57,** 326, 1960.
62. Owen, E. E., and Verner, J. V., and Jr.: Renal tubular disease with muscle paralysis and hypokalemia. Amer. J. Med., **28,** 8, 1960.
63. Pines, K. L., and Mudge, G. H.: Renal tubular acidosis with osteomalacia: report of three cases. Amer. J. Med., **11,** 302, 1951.
64. Kazantzis, G., Flynn, F. V., Spowage, J. S., and Trott, D. G.: Renal tubular malfunction and pulmonary emphysema in cadmium pigment workers. Quart. J. Med., n.s., **32,** 165, 1963.
65. MacGregor, M. E., and Rayner, P. H. W.: Pink disease and primary renal tubular acidosis. Lancet, **2,** 1083, 1964.
66. Frimpter, G. W., Timpanelli, A. E., Eisenmenger, W. J., Stein, H. S., and Ehrlich, L. I.: Reversible "Fanconi syndrome" caused by degraded tetracycline. J.A.M.A., **184,** 111, 1963.
67. Engle, R. L., and Wallis, L. A.: Multiple myelomatosis and the adult Fanconi syndrome. Amer. J. Med., **22,** 5, 1957.
68. Sanchez, L. M., and Domz, C. A.: Renal patterns in myeloma. Ann. Intern. Med., **52,** 44, 1960.
69. Talal, N., Zisman, E., and Schur, P. H.: Renal tubular acidosis, glomerulonephritis, and immunologic factors in Sjögren's syndrome. Arthritis and Rheum., **11,** 774, 1968.
70. Mookerjee, B., Gault, M. H., and Dossetor, J. B.: Hyperchloremic acidosis in early diagnosis of renal allograft rejection. Ann. Intern. Med., **71,** 47, 1969.
71. Morgan, H. G., Stewart, W. K., Lowe, K. G., Stowers, J. M., and Johnstone, J. H.: Wilson's disease and the Fanconi syndrome. Quart. J. Med., n.s., **31,** 361, 1962.
72. Schoen, E. J.: Lowe's syndrome: abnormalities in renal tubular function in combination with other congenital defects. Amer. J. Med., **27,** 781, 1959.
73. Bickel, H., and Thursby-Pelham, D. C.: Hyperaminoaciduria in Lignac-Fanconi disease, in galactosaemia and in an obscure syndrome. Arch. Dis. Child., **29,** 224, 1954.
74. Morris, R. C., Jr.: An experimental acidification defect in patients with hereditary fructose intolerance. I. Its resemblance to renal tubular acidosis. J. Clin. Invest., **47,** 1389, 1968.
75. Morris, R. C., Jr.: An experimental renal acidification defect in patients with hereditary fructose intolerance. II. Its distinction from classic renal tubular acidosis; its resemblance to the renal acidification defect associated with the Fanconi syndrome of children with cystinosis. J. Clin. Invest., **47,** 1648, 1968.
76. Muggia, F. M., Heinemann, H. O., Farbongi, M., and Osserman, E. F.: Lysozymuria and renal tubular dysfunction in monocytic and myelomonocytic leukemia. Amer. J. Med., **47,** 351, 1969.
77. Morris, R. C., Jr.: The clinical spectrum of Fanconi's syndrome. Calif. Med., **108,** 225, 1968.
78. Lathem, W.: Hyperchloremic acidosis in chronic pyelonephritis. New Eng. J. Med., **258,** 1031, 1958.
79. Cohen, A., and Way, B. J.: The association of renal tubular acidosis with hyperglobulinaemic purpura. Aust. Ann. Med., **11,** 189, 1962.
80. Morris, R. C., Jr., and Fudenberg, H. H.: Impaired renal acidification in patients with hypergammaglobulinemia. Medicine, **46,** 57, 1967.
81. LoSpalluto, J., Dorward, B., Miller, W. J., and Ziff, M.: Cryoglobulinemia based on interaction between a gamma macroglobulin and 7S gamma globulin. Amer. J. Med., **32,** 142, 1962.
82. McCurdy, D. K., Cornell, G. G., III, and DePratti, V. J.: Hyperglobulinemic renal tubular acidosis: report of two cases. Ann. Intern. Med., **67,** 110, 1967.
83. Wilson, I. D., Williams, R. C., Jr., and Tobian, L. J.: Renal tubular acidosis: three cases with immunoglobulin abnormalities in the patients and their kindreds. Amer. J. Med., **43,** 356, 1967.
84. Bennett, W. M., Hempel, K. H., Berland, J. E., and Porter, G. A.: Renal tubular acidosis. Arch. Intern. Med., **121,** 81, 1968.
85. Huth, E. J.: Renal tubular syndromes, immunologic disorders, and cancer. Ann. Intern. Med., **67,** 213, 1967.
86. Ferris, T., Kashgarian, M., Levitin, H., Braudt, I., and Epstein, F. H.: Renal tubular acidosis and renal potassium wasting acquired as a result of hypercalcemic nephropathy. New Eng. J. Med., **265,** 924, 1961.
87. Huth, E. J., Mayock, R. L., and Kerr, R. M.: Hyperthyroidism associated with renal tubular acidosis. Amer. J. Med., **26,** 818, 1959.
88. Zisman, E., Buccino, R. A., Gordon, P., and Bartter, F. C.: Hyperthyroidism and renal tubular acidosis. Arch. Intern. Med., **121,** 118, 1968.
89. McCurdy, D. K., Frederic, M., and Elkinton, J. R.: Renal tubular acidosis due to amphotericin B. New Eng. J. Med., **278,** 124, 1968.
90. Shohl, A. T.: The effect of the acid-base content of the diet upon the production and cure of rickets with special reference to citrates. J. Nutr., **14,** 69, 1937.
91. deGraeff, J., Struyvenberg, A., and Lameijer, L. D. F.: The role of chloride in hypokalemic alkalosis: balance studies in man. Amer. J. Med., **37,** 778, 1964.
92. Kassirer, J. P., Berkman, P. M., Lawrenz, D. R., and Schwartz, W. B.: The critical role of chloride in the correction of hypokalemic alkalosis in man. Amer. J. Med., **38,** 172, 1965.
93. Piel, C. F.: Disease of the renal tubules in childhood. Pediatrics, **20,** 337, 1957.
94. Pitts, H. H., Schulte, J. W., and Smith, D. R.: Nephrocalcinosis in a father and three children. J. Urol., **73,** 208, 1955.
95. Randall, R. E., and Targgart, W. H.: Familial renal tubular acidosis. Ann. Intern. Med., **54,** 1108, 1961.
96. Randall, R. E., Jr.: Familial renal tubular acidosis revisited. Ann. Intern. Med., **66,** 1024, 1967.
97. Schreiner, G. E., Smith, L. H., and Kyle, L. H.: Renal hyperchloremic acidosis. Amer. J. Med., **15,** 122, 1953.
98. Elkinton, J. R., McCurdy, D. K., and Buckalew, V. M., Jr.: Hydrogen ion and the kidney, in *Renal Disease,* p. 110. F. A. Davis Company, Philadelphia, 1967.
99. Seedat, Y. K.: Some observations of renal tubular acidosis—a family study. S. Afr. Med. J., **38,** 606, 1964.

100. Seedat, Y. K.: Renal tubular acidosis. S. Afr. Med. J., **41,** 1007, 1967.
101. Gyory, A. Z., and Edwards, K. D. G.: Renal tubular acidosis: A family with an autosomal dominant genetic defect in renal hydrogen ion transport, with proximal tubular and collecting duct dysfunction and increased metabolism of citrate and ammonia. Amer. J. Med., **45,** 43, 1968.
102. Wilansky, D. L., and Schneiderman, C.: Renal tubular acidosis with recurrent nephrolithiasis and nephrocalcinosis. New England J. Med., **257,** 399, 1957.
103. Wilansky, D. L., and Schucher, R.: Familial acidosis of renal tubular origin. Canad. Med. Ass. J., **83,** 308, 1960.
104. Elkinton, J. R., and Danowski, T. S.: *The Body Fluids,* p. 123. The Williams and Wilkins Co., Baltimore, 1955.
105. Baines, G. H., Barclay, J. A., and Cooke, W. T.: Nephrocalcinosis associated with hyperchloraemia and low plasma-bicarbonate. Quart. J. Med. (n.s.), **14,** 113, 1945.
106. Govan, A. D. T.: Nephrocalcinosis associated with hyperchloraemia and low plasma bicarbonate. Quart. J. Med. (n.s.), **19,** 277, 1950.
107. Foss, G. L., Perry, C. B., and Wood, F. J. Y.: Renal tubular acidosis. Quart. J. Med. (n.s.), **25,** 185, 1956.
108. Mozziconacci, P., Lestradet, H., Attal, C., Girard, F., and Pham-Huu-Trung: Acidose renale hyperchloremique avec nephrocalcinose familiale, retinite albescente et hypocalciurie. Semaine des Hopitaux, **2,** 3167, 1958.
109. Seedat, Y. K.: Letter and comments: Familial renal tubular acidosis. Ann. Intern. Med., **69,** 1329, 1968.
110. Engel, W. J.: Nephrocalcinosis. J.A.M.A., **145,** 288, 1951.
111. Cooke, R. E., and Kleeman, C. R.: Distal tubular function with renal calcification. Yale J. Biol. Med., **23,** 199, 1950.
112. Richardson, R. E.: Nephrocalcinosis with special reference to its occurrence in renal tubular acidosis. Clin. Radiol., **13,** 224, 1962.
113. Doxiadis, S. A.: Idiopathic renal acidosis in infancy. Arch. Dis. Child., **27,** 409, 1952.
114. Kuhlencordt, F., Lenz, W., Seemann, N., and Zukschwerdt, L.: Renal tubular acidosis and bilateral nephrocalcinosis in uniovular twins. German Med. Monthly, **11,** 565, 1967.

CHAPTER SIXTY-SIX

VASOPRESSIN-RESISTANT DIABETES INSIPIDUS

Jack Orloff and Maurice B. Burg

Vasopressin-resistant diabetes insipidus is a rare congenital and familial disease characterized by failure of the kidneys to respond to antidiuretic hormone. The essential features of the disorder are polyuria, polydipsia, and the excretion of persistently hypotonic urine. The disease was first described by Forssman [1] and Waring et al. [2], who, recognizing the inefficacy of vasopressin in promoting the excretion of hypertonic urine, distinguished it from diabetes insipidus due to insufficiency of neurohypophyseal hormone. Later, Williams and Henry [3] introduced the name *nephrogenic diabetes insipidus* in order to emphasize that insensitivity of the renal tubule cells to antidiuretic hormone is responsible for all the clinical findings in the disease.

PHYSIOLOGY OF WATER BALANCE

In normal man the osmotic pressure of plasma, in essence a reflection of the ratio of water to solute in the body, is virtually constant (285 to 295 mOsm per kg H_2O), despite wide variations in the intake of solute and water. Regulation is achieved by varying both the volume flow of urine and its osmotic pressure in response to changes in plasma osmolality. A fall in plasma osmolality, indicative of relative water excess, is normally attended by the excretion of large volumes of urine less concentrated than plasma. This loss of water without its equivalent content of solute (285 μOsm for every milliliter of water) restores plasma osmolality to normal. Conversely, hyperosmolality, whether due to water loss or retention of solute in excess of water, is corrected by the excretion of urine more concentrated than plasma.

The precise adjustment of urine flow and osmolality is in large part due to the remarkable efficiency of the pituitary-renal system. The kidney is capable of varying urine flow under physiologic conditions in the adult from less than 1 to more than 20 ml per min and urine concentration from a maximum of 1,400 to a minimum of 30 to 40 mOsm per kg H_2O. These changes are effected to a considerable degree by variations in the tubular reabsorption of water, largely determined by the action of the neurohypophyseal hormone, vasopressin.

Role of the Neurohypophysis in Water Balance

Vasopressin, an octapeptide [4], is elaborated in the supraoptic and paraventricular nuclei of the hypothalamus [7]. The hormone is thought to be stored in the posterior portion of the pituitary body, from which it is secreted into the blood in response to nervous stimuli originating in cells (*osmoreceptors*) in the anterior hypothalamus and transmitted to the pituitary along the supraopticohypophyseal tracts [8]. The hormone isolated from ox pituitary by du Vigneaud and his associates is a cyclic octapeptide with the following structure [4]:

Cys·Tyr·Phe·Glu(NH$_2$)·Asp(NH$_2$)·Cys·Pro·Arg·Gly(NH$_2$)

Hog vasopressin and that from certain other members of this suborder (Suina) contain lysine in the penultimate position. All other mammals studied, including man [5], are thought to secrete the arginine form shown above [6].

On the basis of Verney's [8] classic demonstrations, it has been concluded that shrinkage of the osmoreceptors, due to an elevation in the effective osmotic pressure[1] of plasma, effects the release of antidiuretic hormone (vasopressin) into the circulating blood. The resultant increase in urine osmolality restores plasma osmolality to normal, thereby diminishing the rate of secretion of hormone. Conversely, a reduction in effective osmotic pressure by virtue of swelling of the osmoreceptors leads to inhibition of antidiuretic hormone release and permits the excretion of large volumes of dilute urine. It is important to recognize that graded release of hormone is essential in order to afford the continuous regulation of urine flow and concentration necessary to minimize deviations in plasma osmolality. Although the renal regulation of water balance is inadequate in the absence of a properly functioning hypothalamicohypophyseal system or when the kidney is insensitive to the effect of antidiuretic hormone, as in the disease under discussion, the patient with either form of diabetes insipidus is capable of maintaining plasma osmolality within the normal range merely by adjusting fluid intake. As long as the volume of water ingested exceeds that excreted in the urine by an amount equivalent to that dissipated in the form of insensible loss and perspiration, excessive concentration of body fluids will not occur. In this situation, thirst, rather than variable reabsorption of water, assumes a regulatory role.

Renal Regulation of Water Balance

Although the antidiuretic effect of vasopressin and the physiologic factors involved in its release from the hypophysis

[1]Effective osmotic pressure is that exerted by solutes that do not penetrate cell membranes rapidly. Sodium and attendant anions represent the major osmotically effective constituents of the extracellular space. Urea, on the other hand, although it contributes to the total osmotic pressure, does not appreciably affect the distribution of water between cells and surrounding extracellular fluids, since it penetrates cells relatively freely and its concentration is approximately equal in the two phases.

have been recognized for many years, the intrarenal events which transpire in the elaboration of hypotonic or hypertonic urine are not yet completely understood. Sufficient data derived from a variety of sources are available to justify a tentative description of the process [9–19].

In order to account for the normal variations in urine flow and concentration the plasma ultrafiltrate formed at the glomerulus must be modified as it courses down the tubule. Two fundamental processes are involved: the selective abstraction of solute and the tubular reabsorption of water. Water reabsorption in the tubule is divided into at least three, and possibly four, functionally and anatomically distinct phases. It is believed that water flows passively out of the proximal segment, the descending limb of Henle's loop, the distal convoluted tubule, and the collecting duct into the surrounding renal tissue, along osmotic gradients established by prior solute removal. The proximal segment and descending limb of Henle's loop are considered to be freely permeable to water under all circumstances; the distal convolution and collecting duct are freely permeable only in the presence of antidiuretic hormone. Consequently variations in the permeability of the membrane to water in the latter segments impose restrictions on outward flow and permit the elaboration of urine of varying tonicity and volume. Furthermore, it has been established [21] that there is a progressive increase in the osmotic pressure of the renal interstitial fluid from cortex to papilla (Fig. 66-1), the medulla and papilla being hyperosmotic to plasma under all circumstances, whereas the cortex is isosmotic.

Normally, 20 percent of the plasma perfusing the kidney is filtered at the glomerulus. Of the ultrafiltrate, 80 to 85 percent is reabsorbed in the proximal segment essentially as an isosmotic solution [9, 10, 14, 22]. As noted above, the luminal membrane in this area is freely permeable to water under all circumstances. Sodium and attendant anion are reabsorbed by a process involving active sodium transport (i.e., transport against an electrochemical gradient); water then flows passively out of the tubule along the resultant osmotic gradient. The reduced volume of isosmotic fluid is then delivered to the loop of Henle, where, as Wirz and his associates [13, 21] originally suggested, the urine is progressively concentrated as it flows downward in the descending limb and is then diluted in the upward ascent in the ascending limb. In support of this are the observations (1) that urine at the tip of Henle's loop is hypertonic to plasma [14, 16], (2) that urine in the ascending limb is less concentrated than that in the adjacent descending limb at the same level in the medulla [20], and (3) that urine in the first portion of the distal convolution is hypotonic to plasma irrespective of the final urine concentration [14, 16,

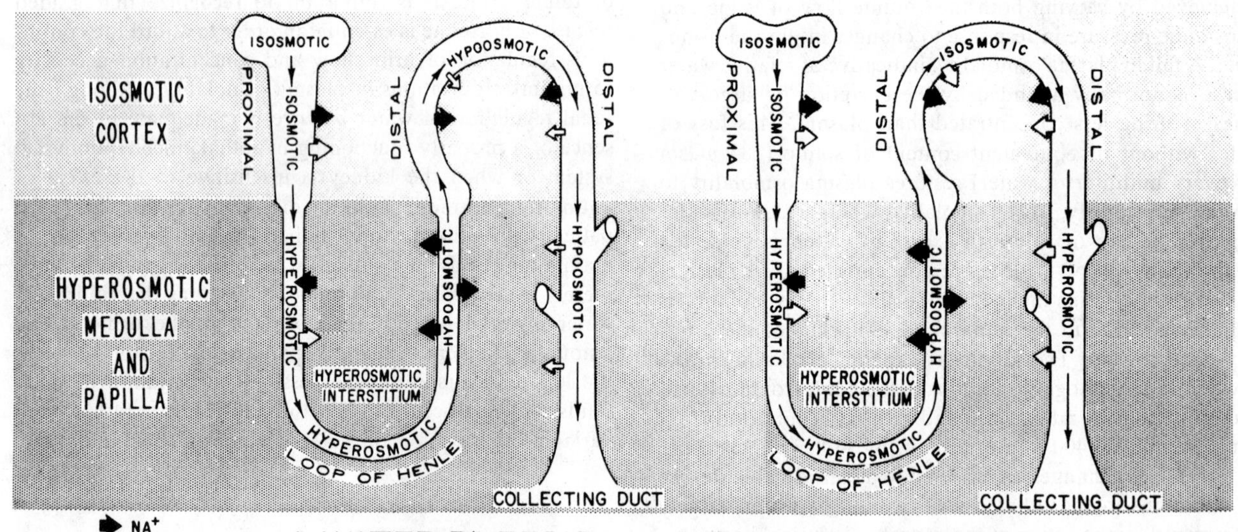

Figure 66-1. The nephron during water diuresis (A) and antidiuresis (B). The diagram is described in detail in the text, under "The Countercurrent Theory." Although not indicated in the figure, the longitudinal interstitial osmotic gradient increases progressively from corticomedullary junction to papilla. The size of the arrows representing H_2O and NaCl reabsorption indicates the relative extent of these processes. Although hyperosmolarity in the descending limb is probably the result of water abstraction, the movement of NaCl and other solutes from the interstitial space into the lumen also may be an important factor [23]. The role of urea in the concentrating and diluting processes discussed in the text has been omitted from the figure.

22]. In view of this it is reasonable to assume that the descending limb is freely permeable to water under all circumstances, hypertonicity being effected by loss of water without solute into the surrounding hypertonic interstitium, whereas the ascending limb is impermeable to water, dilution being achieved by the active extrusion of sodium chloride without water. It is essential to recognize that the processes described thus far are uninfluenced by vasopressin and occur as described whether or not the final urine is concentrated or dilute. Were no other factors involved, one could visualize the situation in vasopressin-resistant diabetes insipidus (and in water diuresis in general) as the excretion of most of the residual hypotonic urine leaving the loop of Henle. That this is an oversimplification is attested to by arguments to be presented subsequently.

The sequence of events in the distal convolution and collecting duct, unlike that in the proximal portions of the nephron, differs considerably in water diuresis and antidiuresis. In the absence of vasopressin and when a dilute urine is to be excreted, the luminal membrane in the distal nephron is thought to be relatively impermeable to water. Dilute urine which leaves Henle's loop is rendered more hypotonic by the continued abstraction of solute without water in the distal convolution and perhaps even in the collecting duct [24]. Consequently urine less concentrated than plasma is excreted into the bladder. Although some loss of water along its osmotic gradient takes place in the distal nephron even in the absence of vasopressin, it is generally insufficient to effect the excretion of either an isotonic or hypertonic urine.

In marked contrast, when vasopressin is present, hypertonic urine is elaborated. Antidiuretic hormone increases the permeability of the distal convolution [25], collecting tubule [26], and collecting duct [16, 27, 28] to water, so that these areas of the tubule function as does the proximal segment. Although electrolyte is still abstracted from hypotonic fluid entering the distal convolution as in water diuresis, in the presence of ADH, the excess water flows freely out of the tubule into the cortical interstitium until osmotic equilibrium is achieved. This has been established both by Wirz [22] and by Gottschalk and Mylle [14, 16], who observed that urine in the distal convolution, which remains hypotonic when ADH secretion is in abeyance, becomes isosmotic in antidiuresis. The residual isosmotic urine is then delivered to the collecting duct, where water in excess of solute is lost by osmotic flow into the hypertonic interstitium of the medullopapillary region, and the resultant hypertonic urine is excreted.

Cellular Mode of Action of Antidiuretic Hormone

The view that ADH increases the permeability of the tubule epithelium to water was initially deduced from studies in other tissues. Koefoed-Johnsen and Ussing [29] observed a marked increase in net water movement along an osmotic gradient across isolated frog skin under the influence of neurohypophyseal extract. Similar results have been obtained utilizing the urinary bladder of the toad [30, 31]. More recently a direct effect of vasopressin on osmotic flow has been demonstrated in the isolated perfused collecting tubule of the rabbit [26]. The addition of vasopressin to the inner, or blood, surface of these tissues results in an acceleration of osmotic flow of water greater than that predicted on the basis of diffusion alone [26, 29, 30]. Because of the disproportionate increase in water movement as well as other evidence, Koefoed-Johnsen and Ussing concluded that the hormone induces its permeability effect by increasing the size or number of aqueous channels or pores within the epithelial membrane through which water may flow. The rate-limiting barrier for water, the permeability of which is altered by vasopressin, is at the luminal surface of the epithelial cell in the pertinent portions of the nephron [32].

Although the molecular basis of the action of ADH is as yet unknown, some of the current views are discussed below. The first step in the action of the hormone must be attachment and interaction with specific receptor sites near the blood surface of the epithelial cell. This presumably initiates a series of events, biochemical or physical, which ultimately results in a change in the permeability of the luminal membrane to water. Fong and coworkers [33] initially concluded that the reaction between the disulfide bridge of vasopressin and sulfhydryl groups in the membrane was involved, not only in the primary attachment of the hormone to the receptor tissue, but also in the mechanical triggering of the alteration in water permeability. This is no longer a tenable hypothesis, particularly since non-disulfide-containing analogues of vasopressin still elicit a physiologic effect [34]. Ginetzinsky and Ivanova [35, 36] suggested that vasopressin induces the secretion by collecting duct cells of hyaluronidase into the urine. Subsequent depolymerization of intercellular and basement membrane hyaluronic acid by the enzyme is thought to be responsible for the increase in the permeability of the tubule membrane to water. Dicker and Eggleton [37] have adopted this thesis and have implicated the hyaluronidase system in the pathogenesis of nephrogenic diabetes insipidus [38]. Their findings and those of Ginetzinsky have not been confirmed by others, and both the interpretation and methods have been severely criticized [39–42]. Furthermore, the addition of hyaluronidase to those epithelial membranes which do respond to antidiuretic hormone in a characteristic fashion results in no change in water permeability [43, 44].

More recently Orloff and Handler [45–47] have proposed that vasopressin stimulates the production of an intracellular intermediate, cyclic adenosine-3′,5′monophosphate (3′,5′-AMP), which is responsible for the changes in permeability induced by vasopressin. The role of the cyclic nucleotide in the action of many other hormones in their respective receptor tissues was first suggested by Sutherland and Rall [48]. Orloff and Handler subsequently observed that cyclic 3′,5′-AMP effectively mimics vasopressin in toad bladder in

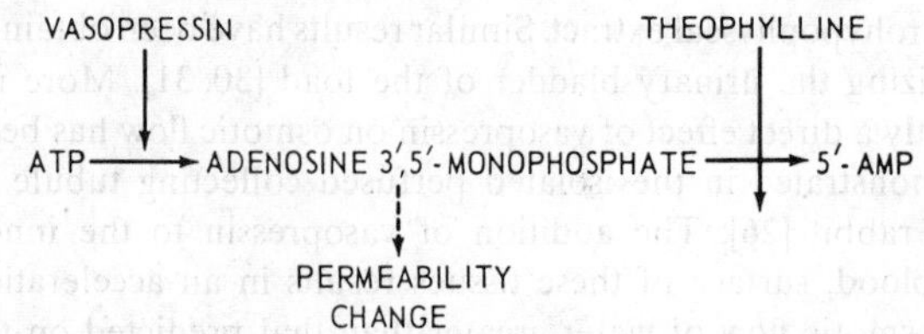

Figure 66-2. The role of adenosine-3',5'-monophosphate in the action of vasopressin and the effect of theophylline on this mechanism. (See text for details.)

that it induces a similar increase in osmotic flow of water [45]. An analogous effect of cyclic-AMP has been demonstrated in the collecting tubule as well [26]. The hypothesis is illustrated in Fig. 66-2. The conversion of ATP to cyclic AMP is accelerated by antidiuretic hormone in both toad bladder and kidney [49–51]. Furthermore, methyl xanthines, such as theophylline, which increase the concentration of cyclic AMP in toad bladder [50] and other tissues [48] by interfering with the degradation of cyclic AMP, accelerate the osmotic flow of water across toad bladder and collecting tubule as do vasopressin and the nucleotide [45, 52]. Although this thesis does not afford an explanation of the pertinent physical and chemical changes in the membrane which must occur in order to account for the increase in permeability, it does implicate a metabolic process in the action of the hormone.

The Countercurrent Theory

The view that water movement in all segments of the nephron, including that in the collecting duct, is passive has only recently been proposed. The terminal process which results in the elaboration of urine more concentrated than plasma had been assumed to be an active process, since it apparently required "uphill" transport of water, i.e., movement of water from a solution in which the activity of water is less than that of the surrounding interstitium. The argument was based on the belief that the osmotic pressure of the renal interstitial space approximated that of all other tissues of the body and was 290 mOsm per kg H_2O. Wirz et al. [21] resolved this problem and provided a rational basis for considering that water movement out of the tubule lumen is passive (along its activity gradient) even when urine is markedly hypertonic. Wirz observed, by direct cryoscopic analysis, that the solute concentration of kidney water increases progressively from cortex to papilla and that both the inner medulla and papilla are markedly hypertonic to peripheral plasma. He concluded that the hypertonic environment surrounding the collecting duct provides the osmotic force necessary for passive movement of water out of this segment. He was the first to suggest that the achievement of diffusion equilibrium when the membrane is made freely permeable to water by vasopressin results in the elaboration of hypertonic urine. It is a testimony to Wirz's ingenuity to recall that hypertonicity of the medulla had been noted earlier [53], only to be ignored by most renal physiologists.

Wirz [22] considered the hypertonicity of the medulla and papilla (the longitudinal concentration gradient) to be due to deposition of sodium chloride transported out of the ascending limb of Henle's loop into the surrounding interstitium. Although not explicitly stated as such in his original description, it is likely, as noted above, that loss of water without solute in the descending limb raises the concentration of the urine in this segment above that of plasma. This process, concomitant concentration and dilution of urine in opposing segments of a looplike structure in which the flow of urine in one segment is counter to that of the other, has a particular physiologic advantage. Since the NaCl concentration of ascending-limb urine is from the beginning approximately equal to that of the environment, the transport of sodium salts out of this segment is nowhere against a steep concentration gradient. This minimizes any energetic difficulties which might arise were sodium salts transported from hypotonic urine to a markedly hypertonic environment, as has been suggested by Berliner et al. [15].

Both the anatomic arrangement of the loop and the processes described have all the features of a hairpin countercurrent multiplier system. The principle of the multiplier has been described in detail by Hargitay and Kuhn [54] and was originally applied in a somewhat modified fashion to the kidney by these workers and Wirz et al. [21]. It is evident that deposition of NaCl in excess of water in the interstitial space of the medulla and papilla will raise the osmotic pressure of this area above that of the cortex. Progressive multiplication of this longitudinal gradient to the extent observed experimentally is visualized in the following manner: In a hypothetical first circulation through the loop, the intraluminal fluid has the same concentration throughout, equal to that of the cortex. Active transport of NaCl from the water-impermeable ascending limb lowers the concentration of ascending-limb contents and raises that of the interstitial fluid and descending limb (see above). The slightly hypertonic descending-limb fluid moves around through the hairpin bend in the loop into the ascending limb, temporarily abolishing the concentration gradient between the opposing segments. However, continuing transport of NaCl from the ascending limb, now containing fluid more concentrated than in the previous circulation, raises the osmotic pressure of the interstitial and descending-limb fluids once again. Descending-limb fluid more concentrated than previously moves into the ascending limb, and the process continues until in the steady state the longitudinal gradient is multiplied manyfold, whereas the small transverse gradient between loop contents and interstitium is at each point in the renal medulla equal and unchanged. In other terms, the hairpin countercurrent multiplier system, by permitting transport against a minimal gradient, provides the basis for multiplying the small gradient between loop contents and interstitium manyfold in the longitudinal axis.

Whether or not urinary dilution in the ascending section

of the loop and concentration of the interstitial spaces occurs as described and is accomplished by a hairpin countercurrent multiplier device, sequestration of trapping of NaCl in the interstitial space in order to maintain the concentration gradient cannot be explained simply on the basis of this hypothesis. Since blood courses through this area, one would expect the excess solute to be dissipated and the solute concentration never to exceed appreciably that of the inflowing blood. This aspect, discussed by Wirz [55], has been emphasized and developed in detail by Berliner et al. [15]. Noting that the postglomerular capillaries in this area do not course directly through the kidney but also bend back upon each other in the shape of loops, they suggested that the capillaries may act as countercurrent exchangers. This is illustrated in Fig. 66-3. Free diffusion of solute from the outflowing to the inflowing limb of the capillary loop permits recirculation of solute in the medulla, minimizing the loss of excess NaCl and other solutes (notably urea) from the area. The concentration gradient is thereby maintained and not dissipated as it would be were blood flowing through in one direction only. The capillary countercurrent exchanger not only maintains the interstitial NaCl concentration, indirectly providing the osmotic force necessary for the terminal concentrating process, but also serves to trap any urea which diffuses into the interstitial space from the collecting duct [56]. The concentration of urea in medullary water approaches that of collecting-duct contents, being approximately equal in antidiuresis. In view of this, Berliner et al. [15] have pointed out that insofar as collecting-duct urea is osmotically balanced by urea in the surrounding interstitial fluid, it will increase the osmotic pressure of urine beyond that attained by simple equilibration of collecting-duct contents with interstitial NaCl. In other terms, the urine urea does not need to be balanced by an equivalent concentration of NaCl in the interstitial fluid, as do the other solutes. Consequently, final urine osmolality will be greater or lesser depending on the urea load presented to the collecting duct, even though no change in interstitial NaCl content occurs. The clinical significance of this is considerable. Inadequacy of urea load may limit the apparent concentrating ability of the kidney, though no defect in either the permeability of the membrane to water or in the so-called sodium "pump" may be present [56, 57].

Figure 66-1 is a schematic drawing of the nephron. The cortex containing the glomerulus and the proximal and distal convolutions is represented as being isosmotic with peripheral plasma. The medulla and papilla, in which the loops of Henle, the collecting duct, and the deeper portions of the capillary loops are embedded, are represented as being hyperosmotic to plasma. Vasopressin affects only the distal convolution and collecting system. In diabetes insipidus or whenever vasopressin is either ineffective or not secreted, urine made dilute by transport of electrolyte out of both Henle's loop and the distal convolution loses only a small fraction of its water as it passes through the distal portions of the nephron and is excreted as such in the bladder. In the presence of vasopressin, free permeability of the distal-convolution and collecting-duct membrane to water permits osmotic flow of water out of the lumen. Consequently the osmolality of urine in each segment approximates that of the tubular environment, becoming isosmotic to plasma in the distal convolution and hyperosmotic in the collecting duct. It is important to recognize that the major effect of vasopressin insofar as water balance is concerned is in the distal convolution. The promotion of osmotic equilibrium in this area and the formation of isosmotic urine results in the restoration of as much as ±15 percent of the filtered water to the body, whereas the reduction in volume in the collecting duct, though resulting in urine hypertonicity, restores considerably less (±5 percent).

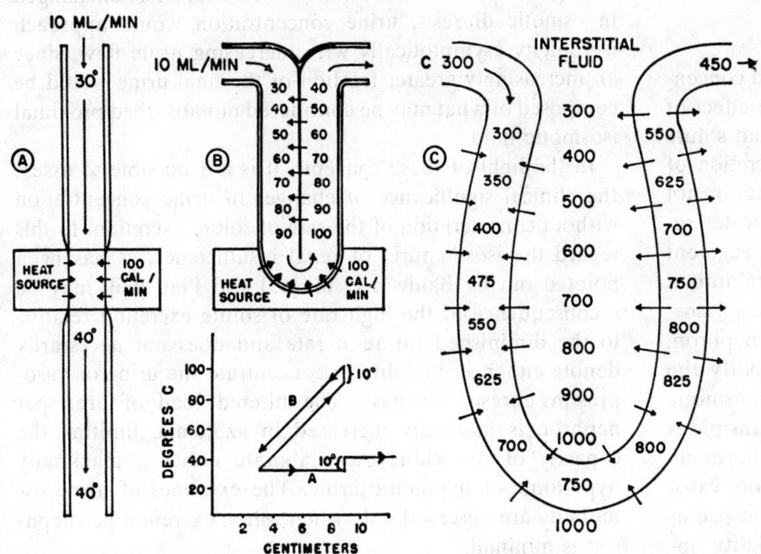

Figure 66-3. Principle of the countercurrent exchanger. A and B. The effect of heating water flowing at the rate of 10 ml per min through a pipe. The addition of 100 cal per min raises the temperature 10° in both A (straight flow) and B (countercurrent flow). However, since the incoming water is heated by the outgoing water in B, the maximum temperature attained in the countercurrent system is considerably higher than with straight flow. The graph compares the temperature along the flow tubes in each system. C. Countercurrent flow as applied to the capillary loop, showing that it is not necessary for the limbs of the loop to be in direct contact. In the hypothetical illustration given, both limbs are in contact with the same interstitial fluid, of progressively increasing concentration. Sodium salts (arrows) at first enter the capillary blood, later partly return to the interstitial fluid. Note the analogy between B, in which heat is recirculated, and C, in which sodium salts are similarly retained in an area. (*Reproduced from Berliner et al. [15], with permission of the author and publishers.*)

Factors Other than Vasopressin

Effects of Filtration Rate

In order properly to evaluate the significance of changes in urine flow and osmolality in patients suspected of having vasopressin-resistant diabetes insipidus, it is essential to recognize the influence of at least two other factors, filtration rate and solute excretion, on the concentrating process. Berliner and Davidson [58] have demonstrated that a reduction in filtration rate may, even in the absence of vasopressin (or at least when its secretion is minimal and constant), promote the excretion of hypertonic urine. Presumably volume flow of hypotonic urine to the collecting duct is significantly diminished by this procedure. Consequently although outward movement of water in the terminal segment is minimal under these circumstances, it may be sufficient to concentrate the small volume of urine delivered to the collecting duct. An additional factor may be a reduction in medullary blood flow, which would increase the efficiency of the countercurrent exchanger and elevate the interstitial osmolality. In view of this observation, minor increases in urine osmolality in diabetes insipidus following dehydration need not necessarily signify residual antidiuretic hormone activity. On the other hand, it is not at all certain that the elaboration of hypertonic urine in patients with the pituitary disorder following protracted dehydration of manipulations designed to reduce filtration rate can uniformly be ascribed to the fall in filtration rate itself. Residual antidiuretic hormone activity can never be completely excluded except in patients with the severe form of vasopressin-resistant diabetes insipidus. In one such patient, although urine osmolality rose during dehydration in association with a fall in filtration rate, it never exceeded that of plasma [59]. Similarly, in another patient in whom filtration rate was experimentally decreased by orthostatic hypotension, urine osmolality rose but did not exceed that in plasma [60].

Effects of Solute Excretion

The influence of solute excretion on urine flow and concentration is clinically of greater significance than the effect of filtration rate. Osmotic diuretics diminish water and solute reabsorption in the nephron and result in the excretion of large volumes of essentially isosmotic urine, whether or not vasopressin is acting. Both sodium transport and water reabsorption are interfered with in the proximal segment because of the osmotic restraint of nonabsorbed intraluminal solute. Consequently a larger than normal volume of isosmotic urine enters the more distal portions of the nephron, overwhelming the capacity of the segment to modify the concentration of the urine. Urine osmolality rises in osmotic diuresis both in patients with nephrogenic diabetes insipidus [61] and in normal persons [62] during antidiuretic hormone suppression, whereas in hydropenic subjects in whom vasopressin is acting, the converse, a progressive fall in osmolality, occurs [63]. In both instances, urine osmolality approaches that of unmodified glomerular filtrate as the fraction of proximal urine delivered to the distal segment increases.

It is important to emphasize that no fundamental processes other than proximal reabsorption need be disturbed during osmotic diuresis to account for the observations. It is probable that in the presence of vasopressin more water is actually removed in the collecting duct during solute diuresis than at low rates of solute excretion [64]. That this does not result in the achievement of maximal hypertonicity is due in part at least to the resultant dilution of the medullary interstitial space. Even were osmotic equilibrium to obtain in this segment, which is unlikely during the rapid flow of solute diuresis, the maximal osmotic pressure which could be obtained would be considerably less than normal.

The effects of osmotic diuresis are more easily visualized if one considers, as do Wesson and Anslow [12], that hypotonic urine is made up of two hypothetical moieties: (1) an isosmotic portion (referred to as the "osmolar clearance") equal in volume to the number of milliliters of fluid containing all the urine solute at the concentration of plasma, and (2) an additional amount of distilled water (referred to as solute-free water) equal in volume to that which would have to be added to the isosmotic moiety to reduce its concentration to that observed. Hypertonic urine, on the other hand, is depicted as being made up of an isosmotic portion less that amount of solute-free water which would have to be abstracted from it to produce the observed hypertonicity (referred to as negative solute-free water). In this view, the removal of solute from isosmotic filtrate (the process of urinary dilution) results in the elaboration of solute-free water, and conversely the abstraction of solute-free water from isosmotic filtrate results in the addition of negative-free water to the interstitium and the production of hypertonic urine. Clearly, even were the amount of solute-free water formed in water diuresis or the amount of negative-free water abstracted in antidiuresis unchanged in osmotic diuresis, urine concentration would approach isotonicity asymptotically with increasing urine flow, since an increasingly greater fraction of the final urine would be composed of what may be considered nonabsorbed proximal isosmotic fluid.

In the light of these concepts, it is not possible to assess the clinical significance of changes in urine concentration without consideration of the rate of solute excretion. In this regard the isosthenuria of renal insufficiency, as has been pointed out by Baldwin et al. [65] and Platt [66], may be a consequence of the high rate of solute excretion relative to the diminished filtration rate and does not necessarily denote either an inability to concentrate the urine or vasopressin unresponsiveness. The filtered load of urea per nephron is markedly increased in azotemia, limiting the capacity of the kidney to elaborate either a maximally hypertonic or hypotonic urine. The extremes of urine osmolality are observed only when solute excretion per nephron is minimal.

Even in the absence of antidiuretic hormone, as noted above, water may flow out of the relatively impermeable distal segment and collecting duct, although at a considerably lesser rate than when vasopressin is present [61, 67]. In the course of solute diuresis in vasopressin-resistant diabetes insipidus, Orloff and Walser [61] noted (Fig. 66-4) not only a progressive rise in urine osmolality but also an increasingly greater rate of solute-free water excretion. They concluded that this phenomenon is in part due to a progressive decline in the rate of outward movement of water initially freed in Henle's loop and the distal convolution as a consequence of the osmotic restraint of intraluminal solute. Thus the presence of solute in tubule urine increases the intraluminal osmolality and thereby decreases the rate of outward flow of water in both the distal convoluted tubule and collecting duct. Even in the presence of vasopressin, massive solute diuresis may so limit outward movement of water as to result in the excretion of hypotonic urine. Results of this nature have been observed during vasopressin administration in patients with pituitary diabetes insipidus [68] and in dogs undergoing combined water and solute diuresis [67]. This is not a reflection of insensitivity to vasopressin but indicates that despite relatively free permeability to water in the distal nephron, the reduction in both the transit time and the osmotic gradient limits the loss of free water in this segment. In addition the delivery of more sodium to the diluting segment in osmotic diuresis may result in an increased rate of sodium reabsorption and thereby greater free-water generation.

In view of these observations it is important to determine the normal relationship between urine osmolality and solute excretion before ascribing isosthenuria (see above) or even hyposthenuria[2] to true vasopressin insensitivity.

[2] The excretion of urine less concentrated than plasma.

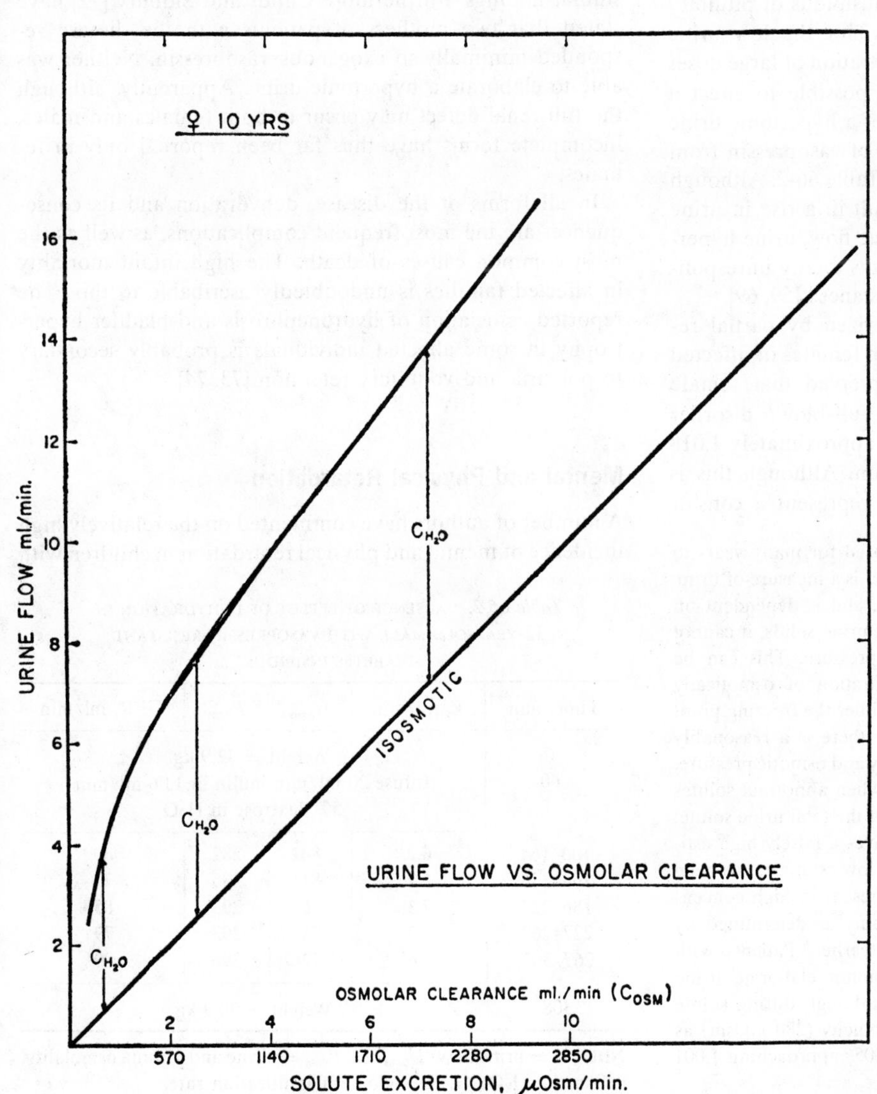

Figure 66-4. The relationship between urine flow and solute excretion in a 10-year-old girl with vasopressin-resistant diabetes insipidus. The diagonal line represents the excretion of isosmotic urine, the curvilinear line that observed experimentally. The difference between the hypothetical and observed lines represents solute-free water excretion (CH_2O), which rose progressively throughout the study.

CLINICAL ASPECTS

Vasopressin-resistant diabetes insipidus manifests itself soon after birth, but since polyuria in infancy is rarely considered a symptom of disease even in the first-born of the most apprehensive parent, it is frequently undiagnosed in early life. Furthermore the presenting signs, which in fact may be alarming, are often nonspecific, being those associated with severe dehydration: fever, convulsions in infants, vomiting, constipation, and hyperosmolality. The characteristic syndrome—polydipsia, polyuria, and persistent hyposthenuria (specific gravity generally less than 1.005*)—diagnostic in offspring of affected families, is noted only when hydration is adequate. Under these circumstances, other causes of dehydration can generally be excluded.

Response to Vasopressin

In contrast to what occurs in diabetes insipidus of pituitary origin, neither the copious urine flow nor the low urine concentration is affected by the administration of large doses of vasopressin (Table 66-1). Nor is it possible to effect a diminution in flow or the elaboration of a hypertonic urine by stimuli known to enhance secretion of vasopressin from the pituitary body. This is illustrated in Table 66-2. Although severe dehydration may ultimately result in a rise in urine osmolality and an associated fall in urine flow, urine hypertonicity has not been observed in patients totally unresponsive to vasopressin under these circumstances [59, 69].

Mild forms of the disease, characterized by partial responsiveness to vasopressin, may exist in females of affected families. Carter and Simpkiss [71] observed that female sibs and relatives of patients with the full-blown disorder were able to concentrate their urine to approximately 1.018 to 1.019 following 12 hr of dehydration. Although this is significantly less than normal, it does represent a considerable degree of responsiveness. Forssman [1] has reported similar findings. Furthermore Childs and Sidbury [72] have stated that two mothers of patients with the disease responded minimally to exogenous vasopressin. Neither was able to elaborate a hypertonic urine. Apparently, although the full renal defect may occur in both females and males, incomplete forms have thus far been reported only in females.

In all forms of the disease, dehydration and its consequences are the most frequent complications, as well as the most common causes of death. The high infant mortality in affected families is undoubtedly ascribable to this. The reported association of hydronephrosis and bladder hypertrophy in some affected individuals is probably secondary to polyuria and voluntary retention [73, 74].

*Specific gravity measurements have been used for many years to estimate urine concentration. Since the former is a measure of urine density, rather than of solute concentration, and is dependent on both the weight and volume displacement of urine solids, it cannot be used as a precise estimate of osmotic pressure. This can be determined only by measuring the concentration of osmotically active constituents in urine, by determining either the freezing point or vapor pressure of the urine. Despite this there is a reasonably good correlation between urine specific gravity and osmotic pressure. Significant discrepancies are observed only when abnormal solutes (glucose, protein) constitute a large fraction of the total urine solute. Under these circumstances specific gravity gives a falsely high estimate of urine concentration. The converse, a low estimate, has been reported by Miles et al. [70] when urea is present in high concentration in urine. The limits of urine osmolality as determined by cryoscopic analysis have been referred to earlier. Patients with nephrogenic diabetes insipidus generally cannot elaborate urine more concentrated than 50 to 100 mOsm, although during solute diuresis urine osmolality may approach isotonicity (280 mOsm) as a limit. Urine specific gravity is less than 1.005, approaching 1.001 during osmotic diuresis.

Table 66-1. LACK OF EFFECT OF PURIFIED VASOPRESSIN IN A 12-YEAR-OLD MALE WITH VASOPRESSIN-RESISTANT DIABETES INSIPIDUS

Time, min	V, ml/min	U_{osm}	P_{osm}	GFR, ml/min
0	Infuse 10 mg/min inulin in 6.1 ml/min 5% dextrose			
50–70	10.2	44	293	83
70–90	10.8	48	293	87
130	Infuse 50 mU/min vasopressin			
130–150	11.1	44	290	87
150–170	10.7	48	287	89

Note: V = urine flow; U_{osm} and P_{osm} = urine and plasma osmolality, mOsm/kg H_2O; GFR = glomerular filtration rate.

Mental and Physical Retardation

A number of authors have commented on the relatively high incidence of mental and physical retardation in children with

Table 66-2. ABSENCE OF EFFECT OF DEHYDRATION IN 12-YEAR-OLD MALE WITH VASOPRESSIN-RESISTANT DIABETES INSIPIDUS

Time, min	V, ml/min	U_{osm}	P_{osm}	GFR, ml/min
0	Weight = 32.9 kg			
60	Infuse 20 ml/min inulin in 1.06 ml/min 5% dextrose in H_2O			
100–164	6.2	84	282	69
164–186	5.7	81	285	71
186–227	7.3	76	293	85
227–267	7.7	72	293	79
267–307	7.6	72	296	80
308	Weight = 30.9 kg			

Note: V = urine flow; U_{osm} and P_{osm} = urine and plasma osmolality, mOsm/kg H_2O; GFR = glomerular filtration rate.

this disorder [3, 75–81]. It is not at all clear that these are primary accompaniments of the renal defect. More likely, structural brain damage, if present, is secondary to repeated episodes of severe dehydration [75, 77, 78] and to the altered growth pattern occasioned by inadequate food intake because of the exhausting influence of uncontrolled polydipsia. Hillman et al. [81] observed that an infant suffering from the disease became so exhausted from polydipsia when subsisting on a regular diet that he was unable to eat and play normally. Mental performance and nutritional status were improved by altering the protein and salt content of the diet so as to decrease obligatory solute and water loss. The reduction in polyuria diminished the time required for drinking and enabled the child to play, eat, and sleep adequately.

Renal Function

The only physiologic abnormality present in the disease is defective water reabsorption. In all other respects renal function may be considered to be normal. Changes in glomerular filtration rate, renal blood flow, and discrete tubular processes which have been reported are probably ascribable to dehydration or hydronephrosis, both of which are common complications of the disease, or associated but unrelated structural disease of the kidney. In the absence of these conditions blood flow, filtration rate, glucose, phosphate, and amino acid transport, etc., are unaffected [2, 3, 61, 76, 80, 82]. Abnormalities of acid-base balance and electrolyte metabolism are excluded by the normal plasma electrolyte patterns observed when hydration is adequate.

PATHOGENESIS

The disease is clearly of renal origin. The neurohypophyseal system is intact, as shown by absence of anatomic abnormalities and the presence of antidiuretic substance in blood and urine of patients under appropriate conditions [79, 80, 83–87]. Chemical characterization of the antidiuretic substance in blood and urine has not been accomplished. It is unlikely that an abnormal hormone is produced to which the kidney is unresponsive [88, 89]. Nor is rapid inactivation of hormone likely as the basis for the disease, since administration of large doses of vasopressin results in abdominal pain and blanching, known side effects of the hormone, even though there is no effect on urine flow and concentration [80, 85, 90, 91]. Other preparations of vasopressin, the synthetic arginine and lysine forms, are also ineffective [91].

On the basis of all the studies it is assumed that end-organ unresponsiveness in the distal convolution and collecting system is responsible for the inefficacy of the hormone in this disorder. The current view of the cellular mode of action of antidiuretic hormone discussed above provides possible explanations for the defect in nephrogenic diabetes insipidus. Thus it is conceivable that the hypothetical receptor is defective in the tissue and thereby prevents hormone binding and interaction. Alternatively the adenyl cyclase system may be absent from the tubule cells involved in water movement in patients with nephrogenic diabetes insipidus. Either suggestion would account for the clinical findings of unremitting water diuresis in these patients. Neither is based on fact.

Although gross and microscopic examination of renal tissue by conventional techniques has not revealed any abnormality [2, 76, 79, 80, 92], MacDonald [80] has reported some shortening of the proximal segment in a microdissected specimen from one child. This has been confirmed by Darmady et al. [92]. These authors proposed that an associated reduction in proximal reabsorption and resultant increased delivery of hypotonic fluid from the ascending limb of the loop of Henle to the distal portion of the nephron is responsible for the concentrating defect in this disorder, rather than unresponsiveness to vasopressin. Their thesis, somewhat analogous to that proposed to account for isosthenuria in renal insufficiency and in solute diuresis, cannot account for the observed excretion of persistently dilute urine of low osmolality in patients with nephrogenic diabetes insipidus. Furthermore, although patients with cystinosis also may have shortened proximal tubules [92], any defect in concentrating ability which they may have is considerably less than that in patients with nephrogenic diabetes insipidus.

DIAGNOSIS

The diagnosis is established without difficulty in the adequately hydrated subject in whom no response to vasopressin is observed. Persistent hypotonicity of the urine is the only specific laboratory finding in this disease. Abnormalities in urine and plasma composition when observed are consequent to severe dehydration or associated disorders.

Other causes of isosthenuria or hyposthenuria may be mistaken for the incompletely expressed form of the disease. However, the characteristic findings of the underlying disorder should preclude errors in diagnosis. Diminished ability to concentrate urine maximally has been observed in a large variety of conditions. These include hypokalemic nephropathy [93], hypercalcemia [94], sickle-cell disease [95], so-called water-losing nephritis [96], juvenile nephronophthisis [97], postobstructive uropathy [98, 99], azotemia [66], medullary cystic disease [99], cystic disease of the kidney [99], and amyloid disease of the kidney [96]. In all but a few of these, although the urine may be hypertonic to plasma following vasopressin, it is not maximally concentrated.

Isosthenuria in renal insufficiency is due in large part to solute diuresis (see above) and is generally not attended by true unresponsiveness to vasopressin. Although it is possible that some patients may have structural disease with resultant insensitivity to vasopressin, this has not been established. Whether the reports of decreased concentrating ability in tubular acidosis [100] and in congenital tubular defects associated with aminoaciduria [101] are indicative of true unresponsiveness to vasopressin cannot be established on the basis of the available evidence.

Psychogenic polydipsia may be associated with diminished responsiveness to vasopressin [102]. DeWardener and Herxheimer [103] observed a reversible limitation in concentrating ability in these and in normal subjects following prolonged chronic and excessive water ingestion. DeWardener [102] has also stated that patients with pituitary diabetes insipidus may demonstrate this on occasion. The cause of the temporary alteration in tubule permeability is unknown. Prolonged administration of vasopressin and water in both man and dog may also be associated with an apparent diminution in responsiveness to the hormone [104–106]. Hays and Leaf [107] contend that a reversible decrease in the permeability of the membrane to water may be produced by the chronic depression of the osmolality of the fluid bathing the blood border of the tubule cell. Harrington and Valtin [108], on the other hand, believe that membrane permeability is normal but that a persistently subnormal osmolality of the renal papilla is responsible for the concentrating defect.

Hereditary Pituitary Diabetes Insipidus

Although the distinction between pituitary diabetes insipidus and the renal form generally is not difficult, mild cases of vasopressin-resistant diabetes insipidus have been confused with hereditary pituitary diabetes insipidus [1]. The latter disorder is familial and also appears in early infancy. However, it is a less severe disease than the fully expressed form of vasopressin-resistant diabetes insipidus. Consequently dehydration and retarded development are uncommon. Nonspecific atrophy of the posterior lobe of the pituitary and hypoplasia of the paraventricular and supraoptic nuclei have been observed at autopsy. According to Forssman [1], two forms of this disease exist, one transmitted as a sex-linked recessive, the other as an autosomal dominant trait.

GENETICS

The renal form of diabetes insipidus is an inherited disease which appears with greater frequency in male members of affected families than in females. It was originally considered by Forssman [1] and Williams and Henry [3] to be transmitted as a sex-linked recessive characteristic. All 17 patients examined by these authors were males whose parents and female sibs were thought to be unaffected. Furthermore the female sibs repeatedly passed the trait on to their male offspring. No example of male-to-male transmission was observed. It has since been established that the disease may be incompletely manifest in female heterozygotes [71, 109]. Although all the males thus far reported exhibit complete unresponsiveness to vasopressin, mild forms of the disease have been observed in female sibs and relatives of affected males [1, 71, 109]. In addition, in families in which there is no evidence that the fathers were affected, several females have been reported in whom the disease is fully as severe as in males [61, 85, 110, 111]. On the basis of these observations it appears that nephrogenic diabetes insipidus is an X-linked disorder with variable degrees of manifestation in heterozygous females. If this is so, mothers and half the sisters of affected males should either be carriers of the defect or exhibit some form of the disease. More careful studies in the future may establish this. In the only affected families studied with this in mind, 14 of 20 females examined were unable to concentrate their urine normally following dehydration [71, 109].

Bode and Crawford [112] have suggested that most North American cases of the disease are descended from immigrants of the "Ulster Scot" clan who reached Nova Scotia in 1761 on the ship Hopewell. Among these people there is a long tradition and legendary origin of "water drinkers," precisely conforming to inheritance of a sex-linked recessive pattern.

Childs and Sidbury [72], although conceding that the disease is most reasonably viewed as due to a gene occupying the X chromosome, have suggested an alternative hypothesis, i.e., autosomal inheritance with some degree of sex limitation. The latter view of the mode of inheritance has been emphasized by Cannon [110] and others [113]. Cannon described a large pedigree in which 5 of 55 affected males were reported to have affected sons. Cannon explained this pedigree by assuming that in some kindreds, at least, the disease is autosomal with a low degree of manifestation in females. G. Allen (personal communication) has pointed out that Cannon's pedigree conforms closely to X-linked inheritance with the exception of the four cases of male-to-male transmission. If inheritance were autosomal, half the male offspring of affected males should have the disease, and only half the female offspring of such males should be carriers. According to Cannon's pedigree chart, only 6 of the 44 male children were affected, and of 19 females who had children 16 were affected or had affected children. Either of these discrepancies, alone, is sufficient to preclude an autosomal theory of inheritance in this family.

TREATMENT

There is no specific therapy for the disease. Adequate hydration, easily achieved in the adult by allowing free access to water, is essential to prevent the deteriorating effect of repeated episodes of dehydration. Although polyuria may be minimized by reducing solute intake, this is rarely necessary except in infants.

On the other hand, the introduction of chlorothiazide and its congeners as a therapeutic agent in the disease has proved useful. Crawford and Kennedy [111] first noted that chronic administration of these derivatives to patients with diabetes insipidus resulted in a marked reduction in urine flow and a moderate increase in urine concentration. The effect of the thiazide diuretics may be enhanced to a considerable degree if the patients are also maintained on a low sodium intake. The observed increase in urine concentration provided by chlorothiazide is in accord with its effect in normal animals and man during water diuresis [114, 115]. In these, the drug interferes with sodium chloride reabsorption in the distal portions of the nephron, thereby reducing the formation of solute-free water. However, this effect alone cannot account for the reduction in urine flow. The latter is undoubtedly attributable to a decrease in the fraction of glomerular filtrate escaping reabsorption in the proximal segment. The diminution in flow of tubule fluid to the distal nephron provides the basis for the reduction in urine volume observed following administration of the chlorothiazide derivatives and contributes to some extent to the observed rise in urine osmolality. Earley and Orloff have presented evidence consistent with the view that the enhanced reabsorption of isosmotic fluid in the proximal nephron may be related to the mild degree of sodium depletion induced by the drug [116]. They have shown that once a sodium deficiency is achieved by the diuretic agent, antidiuresis persists without further drug administration as long as the sodium deficiency is maintained by salt restriction. When salt losses are restored, polyuria rapidly returns. Their observations and conclusions are similar to those of Havard and Wood [117] and of Cutler et al. [60].

Although chlorothiazide is a useful therapeutic agent in this disorder, particularly since it limits nocturia in children, it is notable that administration is not necessarily without hazard. The drug must be given in association with a low-sodium diet in order to exert its maximal antidiuretic effect, and potassium must be added to the diet in order to prevent the development of hypokalemia.

Other diuretics, insofar as they induce some degree of salt depletion, have an effect similar to that of chlorothiazide [116, 118–121]. The proposal that the various diuretics may interfere with aldosterone activity [122] is not supported by the data of other investigators [116].

The benzene sulfonylurea compound, chlorpropamide, which is purported to be an effective antidiuretic agent in patients with pituitary diabetes insipidus, does not reduce urine flow in those afflicted with nephrogenic diabetes insipidus, or for that matter in normal individuals undergoing water diuresis [123].

The therapy of the acute episode of dehydration may differ from that in other situations. If sufficient water can be administered orally, hyperosmolality of body fluids is easily overcome. On the other hand, if parenteral therapy is necessary, 5 percent dextrose in water, although the fluid of choice in other instances of dehydration, may aggravate the hypertonicity. Orloff and Walser [91] observed that the rapid infusion of isosmotic dextrose in water in nephrogenic diabetes insipidus, insofar as it produces solute diuresis (glycosuria), will so increase solute-free water excretion as to promote the development of hyperosmolality and cellular dehydration. The dextrose is not metabolized with sufficient speed to "release" solute-free water in excess of that excreted in the urine. It is virtually impossible to maintain positive water balance if 5 percent dextrose is administered to patients with this disorder. Hyperosmolality may be successfully corrected by administering 2½ to 3 percent dextrose in water,[3] since under these circumstances it is possible to limit the extent of the urinary solute and water loss. It is advisable to administer water without solute orally as soon as is clinically feasible.

SUMMARY

1 Vasopressin-resistant diabetes insipidus is a renal disorder characterized by polydipsia, polyuria, and the excretion of persistently hypotonic urine. It is distinguished from diabetes insipidus due to insufficiency of antidiuretic hormone by a lack of response to exogenous vasopressin.

2 All males thus far reported are completely unresponsive to antidiuretic hormone. Mild forms of the disease, in which a limited response to vasopressin occurs, are observed in some female members of affected families.

3 The only known defect present in the disease is insensitivity of the renal tubule cells to vasopressin. No anatomic or biochemical basis for the end-organ unresponsiveness has been determined. The hormone normally accelerates the passive reabsorption of water in the distal nephron, ultimately resulting in a reduction in urine flow and a rise in urine osmolality. In its absence, or when the pertinent tubule cells are insensitive to its effect, water diuresis is continuous.

4 Maintenance of water balance by ingestion of adequate amounts of water is sufficient treatment. When the amount of water required is inconveniently large, this can be reduced by restriction of solute intake and by the administration of chlorothiazide or its congeners. Life expectancy is normal if episodes of dehydration are prevented.

5 The genetic pattern of the disorder is consistent with transmission as an X-linked characteristic with variable degrees of manifestation in females. The suggestion that an autosomal form of inheritance may be present in some families is not fully supported by the available data.

BIBLIOGRAPHY

1. Forssman, H.: On hereditary diabetes insipidus: with special reference to a sex-linked form. Acta Med. Scand., **121**, suppl. 159, 1, 1956.
2. Waring, A. J., Laslo, K., and Tappan, V.: A congenital defect of water metabolism. Amer. J. Dis. Child., **69**, 323, 1945.
3. Williams, R. H., and Henry, C.: Nephrogenic diabetes insipidus: transmitted by females and appearing during infancy in males. Ann. Intern. Med., **27**, 84, 1957.

[3]Intravascular hemolysis is not observed if 2½ to 3 percent dextrose in water is administered parenterally. Less concentrated solutions may be hazardous.

4. du Vigneaud, V., Lawler, H. C., and Popenoe, E. A.: Enzymatic cleavage of glycinamide from vasopressin and a proposed structure for this pressor-antidiuretic hormone of the posterior pituitary. J. Amer. Chem. Soc., **75**, 4880, 1953.
5. Light, A., and du Vigneaud, V.: On the nature of oxytocin and vasopressin from human pituitary. Proc. Soc. Exp. Biol. Med., **98**, 692, 1958.
6. Sawyer, W. H.: Evolution of antidiuretic hormones and their functions. Amer. J. Med., **42**, 678, 1967.
7. Scharrer, E., and Scharrer, B.: Hormones produced by neurosecretory cells. Recent Progr. Hormone Res., **10**, 183, 1954.
8. Verney, E. B.: Renal excretion of water and salt. Lancet, **2**, 1237, 1295, 1957.
9. Richards, A. N.: The Croonian Lecture. Processes of urine formation. Proc. Roy. Soc. London S. B., **126**, 398, 1938.
10. Walker, A. M., Bott, P. A., Oliver, J., and MacDowell, M. C.: The collection and analysis of fluid from single nephrons of the mammalian kidney. Amer. J. Physiol., **134**, 580, 1941.
11. Smith, H. W.: *The Kidney: Structure and Function in Health and Disease.* Oxford University Press, Fair Lawn, N.J., 1951.
12. Wesson, L. G., Jr., and Anslow, W. P.: Effect of osmotic and mercurial diuresis on simultaneous water diuresis. Amer. J. Physiol., **170**, 255, 1952.
13. Wirz, H.: The localization of antidiuretic action in the mammalian kidney, in *The Neurohypophysis,* edited by H. Heller, p. 157. Academic, New York, 1957.
14. Gottschalk, C. W., and Mylle, M.: Micropuncture study of the mammalian urinary concentrating mechanism: evidence for the countercurrent hypothesis. Amer. J. Physiol., **196**, 927, 1959.
15. Berliner, R. W., Levinsky, N. G., Davidson, D. G., and Eden, M.: Dilution and concentration of the urine and the action of antidiuretic hormone. Amer. J. Med., **24**, 730, 1958.
16. Gottschalk, C. W.: Micropuncture studies of tubular function in the mammalian kidney. Physiologist, **4**, 35, 1961.
17. Ullrich, K. J., Kramer, K., and Boylan, J. W.: Present knowledge of the countercurrent system in the mammalian kidney. Progr. Cardiovasc. Dis., **3**, 395, 1961.
18. Gottschalk, C. W.: Osmotic concentration and dilution of the urine. Amer. J. Med., **36**, 670, 1964.
19. Berliner, R. W., and Bennett, C. M.: Concentration of urine in the mammalian kidney. Amer. J. Med., **42**, 777, 1967.
20. Jamison, R. L., Bennett, C. M., and Berliner, R. W.: Countercurrent multiplication by the thin loops of Henle. Amer. J. Physiol., **212**, 357, 1967.
21. Wirz, H., Hargitay, B., and Kuhn, W.: Lokalisation des Konzentrierungsprozesses in der Niere durch direkte Kryoskopie. Helv. Physiol. Pharmacol. Acta, **9**, 196, 1951.
22. Wirz, H.: Der osmotische Druck in den corticalen Tubuli der Rattenniere. Helv. Physiol. Pharmacol. Acta, **14**, 353, 1956.
23. de Rouffignac, C., and Morel, F.: Micropuncture study of water, electrolytes, and urea movements along the loops of Henle in *Psammomys.* J. Clin. Invest., **48**, 474, 1969.
24. Hilger, H. H., Klümper, J. D., and Ullrich, K. J.: Reabsorption of water and ion transport by the cells of the collecting ducts of the mammalian kidney (microanalytical studies). Arch. Ges. Physiol., **267**, 218, 1958.
25. Ullrich, K. J., Rumrich, G., and Fuchs, G.: Wasserpermeabilität und transtubulärer Wasserfluss corticaler Nephronabschnitte bei verschiedenen Diuresezuständen. Arch. Ges. Physiol., **280**, 99, 1964.
26. Grantham, J. J., and Burg, M. B.: Effect of vasopressin and cyclic AMP on permeability of isolated collecting tubules. Amer. J. Physiol., **211**, 255, 1966.
27. Jaenike, J. R.: The influence of vasopressin on the permeability of the mammalian collecting duct to urea. J. Clin. Invest., **40**, 144, 1961.
28. Morgan, T., Sakai, F., and Berliner, R. W.: In vitro permeability of medullary collecting ducts to water and urea. Amer. J. Physiol., **214**, 574, 1968.
29. Koefoed-Johnsen, V., and Ussing, H. H.: The contributions of diffusion and flow to the passage of H_2O through living membranes: effect of neurohypophyseal hormone on isolated Anuran skin. Acta Physiol. Scand., **28**, 60, 1953.
30. Leaf, A.: Action of neurohypophyseal hormones on the toad bladder. Gen. Comp. Endocr., **2**, 148, 1962.
31. Bentley, P. J.: The effects of neurohypophysial extracts on water transfer across the wall of the isolated urinary bladder of the toad *Bufo marinus.* J. Endocr., **17**, 201, 1958.
32. Ganote, C. W., Grantham, J. J., Moses, H. L., Burg, M. B. and Orloff, J.: Ultrastructural studies of vasopressin effect on isolated perfused renal collecting tubules of the rabbit. J. Cell Biol., **36**, 355, 1968.
33. Fong, C. T. O., Silver, L., Christman, D. R., and Schwartz, I. L.: On the mechanism of action of the antidiuretic hormone (vasopressin). Proc. Nat. Acad. Sci. U.S.A., **46**, 1273, 1960.
34. Schwartz, I. L., Rasmussen, H., and Rudinger, J.: Activity of neurohypophysial hormone analogues lacking a disulfide bridge. Proc. Nat. Acad. Sci. U.S.A., **52**, 1044, 1964.
35. Ginetzinsky, A. G.: Role of hyaluronidase in the reabsorption of water in renal tubules: the mechanism of action of the antidiuretic hormone. Nature (London), **182**, 1218, 1958.
36. Ginetzinsky, A. G., and Ivanova, L. N.: Role of the hyaluronic acid-hyaluronidase system in the process of water reabsorption in the renal tubules. Dokl. Akad. Nauk S.S.S.R., **119**, 1048, 1958.
37. Dicker, S. E., and Eggleton, M. G.: Renal excretion of hyaluronidase and calcium in man during the antidiuretic action of vasopressins and some analogues. J. Physiol., **157**, 351, 1961.
38. Dicker, S. E., and Eggleton, M. G.: Nephrogenic diabetes insipidus. Clin. Sci., **24**, 81, 1963.
39. Berlyne, G. M.: Urinary hyaluronidase. Nature (London), **185**, 389, 1960.
40. Knudsen, P. J., and Koefoed, J.: Urinary inhibitors of hyaluronidase. Nature (London), **191**, 1306, 1961.
41. Breddy, P., Cooper, G. F., and Boss, J. M. N.: Antidiuretic hormone and renal collecting tubules. Nature (London), **192**, 76, 1961.
42. Berlyne, G. M.: Urinary hyaluronidase: a method of assay and investigation of its relationship to the urine concentrating mechanism. Clin. Sci., **19**, 619, 1960.
43. Bentley, P. J.: Hyaluronidase, corticosteroids and the action of neurohypophysial hormone on the urinary bladder of the frog. J. Endocr., **24**, 407, 1962.
44. Leaf, A.: Some actions of neurohypophyseal hormones on a living membrane. J. Gen. Physiol., **43**, 175, 1960.
45. Orloff, J., and Handler, J. S.: The similarity of effects of vasopressin, adenosine-3′,5′-phosphate (cyclic AMP) and theophylline on the toad bladder. J. Clin. Invest., **41**, 702, 1962.
46. Orloff, J., and Handler, J. S.: The cellular mode of action of antidiuretic hormone. Amer. J. Med., **36**, 686, 1964.
47. Orloff, J., and Handler, J. S.: The role of adenosine 3′,5′-phosphate in the action of antidiuretic hormone. Amer. J. Med., **42**, 757, 1967.
48. Sutherland, E. W., and Rall, T. W.: The relation of adenosine 3′,5′-phosphate and phosphorylase to the actions of catecholamines and other hormones. Pharmacol. Rev., **12**, 265, 1960.
49. Brown, E., Clarke, D. L., Roux, V., and Sherman, G. H.: The stimulation of adenosine 3′,5′-monophosphate production by antidiuretic factors. J. Biol. Chem., **238**, 852, 1963.
50. Handler, J. S., Butcher, R. W., Sutherland, E. W., and Orloff, J.: Unpublished observations.
51. Chase, L., and Aurbach, G.: Renal adenyl cyclase: anatomically separate site for parathyroid hormone and vasopressin. Science, **159**, 545, 1968.
52. Grantham, J. J., and Orloff, J.: Effect of prostaglandin E_1 on the permeability response of the isolated collecting tubule to vasopressin, adenosine 3′,5′-monophosphate and theophylline. J. Clin. Invest., **47**, 1154, 1968.
53. Ljungberg, E.: On the reabsorption of chlorides in the kidney of the rabbit. Acta Med. Scand., suppl., **127**, 186, 1, 1947.
54. Hargitay, B., and Kuhn, W.: Das Multiplikationsprinzik als Grundlage der Harnkonzentrierung in der Niere. Z. Elektrochem., **55**, 539, 1951.
55. Wirz, H.: Der osmotische Druck des Blutes in der nieren Papille. Helv. Physiol. Pharmacol. Acta, **11**, 20, 1953.
56. Levinsky, N. G., and Berliner, R. W.: The role of urea in the urine concentrating mechanism. J. Clin. Invest., **38**, 741, 1959.
57. Epstein, F. H., Kleeman, C. R., Pursel, S., and Hendrikx, A.: The effect

of feeding protein and urea on the renal concentrating process. J. Clin. Invest., **36,** 635, 1957.
58. Berliner, R. W., and Davidson, D. G.: Production of hypertonic urine in the absence of pituitary antidiuretic hormone. J. Clin. Invest., **36,** 1416, 1957.
59. Keitel, H. G., Walser, M., and Orloff, J.: Unpublished data.
60. Cutler, R. E., Kleeman, C. R., Maxwell, M. H., and Dowling, T. J.: Physiological studies in nephrogenic diabetes insipidus. J. Clin. Endocr., **22,** 827, 1962.
61. Orloff, J., and Walser, M.: Water and solute excretion in pitressin-resistant diabetes insipidus. Clin. Res. Proc., **4,** 136, 1956.
62. Kleeman, C. R., Epstein, F. H., and White, C.: The effect of variations in solute excretion and glomerular filtration on water diuresis. J. Clin. Invest., **35,** 749, 1956.
63. McCance, R. A.: The excretion of urea, salts and water during periods of hydropenia in man. J. Physiol., **104,** 196, 1945.
64. Page, L. B., and Reem, G. H.: Urinary concentrating mechanism in the dog. Amer. J. Physiol., **171,** 572, 1952.
65. Baldwin, D. S., Berman, H. J., Heinemann, H. O., and Smith, H. W.: The elaboration of osmotically concentrated urine in renal disease. J. Clin. Invest., **34,** 800, 1955.
66. Platt, R.: Renal failure. Lancet, **1,** 1239, 1951.
67. Orloff, J., Wagner, H. N., and Davidson, D. G.: The effect of variations in solute excretion and vasopressin dosage on the excretion of water in the dog. J. Clin. Invest., **37,** 458, 1958.
68. de Wardener, H. E., and del Greco, F.: The influence of solute excretion rate on the production of a hypotonic urine in man. Clin. Sci., **14,** 715, 1955.
69. Childs, B.: Personal communication.
70. Miles, B. E., Paton, A., and de Wardener, H. E.: Maximum urine concentration. Brit. Med. J., **2,** 901, 1954.
71. Carter, C., and Simpkiss, M.: The "carrier" state in nephrogenic diabetes insipidus. Lancet, **2,** 1069, 1956.
72. Childs, B., and Sidbury, J. B.: A survey of genetics as it applies to problems in medicine. Pediatrics, **20,** 177, 1957.
73. Chung, R. C. H., and Mantell, L. K.: Urographic changes in diabetes insipidus. J.A.M.A., **150,** 1307, 1952.
74. Silverstein, E., and Tobian, L.: Pitressin-resistant diabetes insipidus with massive hydronephrosis. Amer. J. Med., **27,** 819, 1961.
75. Ruess, A. L., and Rosenthal, I. M.: Intelligence in nephrogenic diabetes insipidus, Amer. J. Dis. Child., **105,** 358, 1963.
76. Kirman, B. H., Black, J. A., Wilkinson, R. H., and Evans, P. R.: Familial pitressin-resistant diabetes insipidus with mental defect. Arch. Dis. Child., **31,** 59, 1956.
77. Ellborg, A., and Forssman, H.: Nephrogenic diabetes insipidus in children. Acta Paediat., **44,** 209, 1955.
78. Gautier, E., and Simpkiss, M.: The management of nephrogenic diabetes insipidus in early life. Acta Paediat., **46,** 354, 1957.
79. Wattiez, P. R., Loeb, H., Bellens, R., and van Geffel, R.: Diabète-insipide pitressino-résistant. Helv. Paediat. Acta, **12,** 643, 1957.
80. MacDonald, W. B.: Congenital pitressin resistant diabetes insipidus of renal origin. Pediatrics, **15,** 298, 1955.
81. Hillman, D. A., Olcay, N., Porter, P., Cushman, A., and Talbot, N. B: Renal (vasopressin-resistant) diabetes insipidus: definition of the effects of a homeostatic limitation in capacity to conserve water on the physical, intellectual, and emotional development of a child. Pediatrics, **21,** 430, 1958.
82. Schoen, E. J.: Renal diabetes insipidus. Pediatrics, **26,** 808, 1960.
83. Linneweh, F., Buchborn, E., and Dellbrück, B.: Familiärer renaler Diabetes insipidus. Klin. Wschr., **35,** 22, 1957.
84. Holliday, M. A., Burstin, C., and Hurrah, J.: Evidence that the antidiuretic substance in the plasma of children with nephrogenic diabetes insipidus is ADH. Pediatrics, **32,** 384, 1963.
85. Dancis, J., Birmingham, J. R., and Leslie, S. H.: Congenital diabetes insipidus resistant to treatment with pitressin. Amer. J. Dis. Child., **75,** 316, 1948.
86. Luder, J., and Burnett, D.: A congenital renal tubular defect. Arch. Dis. Child., **29,** 44, 1954.
87. Baratz, R. A., Doig, A., and Adatto, I. J.: Plasma antidiuretic activity and free water clearance following osmoreceptor and neurohypophyseal stimulation in human subjects. J. Clin. Invest., **39,** 1539, 1960.
88. Dicker, S. E., and Eggleton, M. G.: Nephrogenic diabetes insipidus. Clin. Sci., **24,** 81, 1963.
89. Holliday, M., Burstin, C., and Hurrah, J.: Evidence that the antidiuretic substance in the plasma of children with nephrogenic diabetes insipidus is antidiuretic hormone. Pediatrics, **32,** 384, 1963.
90. Kao, M. Y. C., and Steiner, M. M.: Diabetes insipidus in infancy resistant to pitressin. Pediatrics, **12,** 400, 1958.
91. Orloff, J., and Walser, M.: Unpublished observations.
92. Darmady, E., Prince, J., and Stranack, F.: The proximal convoluted tubule in the renal handling of water. Lancet, **2,** p. 1254, 1964.
93. Relman, A. S., and Schwartz, W. B.: The kidney in potassium depletion. Amer. J. Med., **24,** 764, 1958.
94. Cohen, S. I., Fitzgerald, M. G., Fourman, P., Griffeths, W. J., and de Wardener, H. E.: Polyuria in hyperparathyroidism. Quart. J. Med., **26,** 423, 1957.
95. Keitel, H. G., Thompson, D., and Itano, H. A.: Hyposthenuria in sickle cell anemia: a reversible renal defect. J. Clin. Invest., **35,** 998, 1956.
96. Roussak, N. J., and Oleesky, S.: Water losing nephritis: a syndrome simulating diabetes insipidus. Quart. J. Med., **23,** 147, 1954.
97. Broberger, O., Winberg, J., and Zetterstrom, R.: Juvenile nephronophthisis. Part I. A genetically determined nephropathy with hypotonic polyuria and azotemia. Acta Paediat. Scand., **49,** 470, 1960.
98. Earley, L. E.: Extreme polyuria in obstructive uropathy: report of a case of "water-losing nephritis" in an infant, with a discussion of polyuria. New Eng. J. Med., **255,** 600, 1956.
99. Holliday, M., Eagan, T., Morris, C., Janah, A., and Hurrah, J.: Pitressin-resistant hyposthenuria in chronic renal disease. Amer. J. Med., **42,** 378, 1967.
100. Cooke, R. E., and Kleeman, C. R.: Distal tubular dysfunction with renal calcification. Yale J. Biol. Med., **23,** 199, 1950.
101. Bickel, H., Baar, H. S., Astley, R., Douglas, A. A., Finch, E., Harris, H., Harvey, C. C., Hickmans, E. M., Philpott, M. G., Smallwood, W. C., Smellie, J. M., and Teall, C. G.: Cystine storage disease with aminoaciduria and dwarfism (Lignac-Fanconi disease). Acta Paediat. Scand., **42,** suppl. 90, 1, 1952.
102. de Wardener, H. E.: *The Kidney.* Little, Brown, Boston, 1958.
103. de Wardener, H. E., and Herxheimer, A.: The effect of a high water intake on the kidney's ability to concentrate the urine in man. J. Physiol., **139,** 42, 1957.
104. Jaenike, J. R., and Waterhouse, C.: The effects of sustained vasopressin administration in man. Clin. Res. Proc., **7,** 272, 1959.
105. Davis, J. O., Howell, D. S., and Hyatt, R. E.: Effect of chronic pitressin administration on electrolyte excretion in normal dogs and in dogs with experimental ascites. Endocrinology, **55,** 409, 1954.
106. Levinsky, N. G., Davidson, D. G., and Berliner, R. W.: Changes in urine concentration during prolonged administration of vasopressin and water. Amer. J. Physiol., **196,** 451, 1959.
107. Hays, R. M., and Leaf, A.: The problem of clinical vasopressin resistance: in vitro studies. Ann. Intern. Med., **54,** 700, 1961.
108. Harrington, A., and Valtin, H.: Impaired urinary concentration after vasopressin and its gradual correction in hypothalmic diabetes insipidus. J. Clin. Invest., **47,** 502, 1968.
109. Schoen, E. J.: Renal diabetes insipidus. Pediatrics, **26,** 808, 1960.
110. Cannon, J. F.: Diabetes insipidus: clinical and experimental studies with consideration of genetic relationships. A.M.A. Arch. Intern. Med., **96,** 215, 1955.
111. Crawford, J. D., and Kennedy, G. C.: Chlorothiazide in diabetes insipidus. Nature (London), **183,** 891, 1959.
112. Bode, H. H., and Crawford, J. D.: Nephrogenic diabetes insipidus in North America—the Hopewell Hypothesis. New Eng. J. Med., **208,** 750, 1969.
113. Robinson, M. G., and Kaplan, S. A.: Inheritance of vasopressin-resistant ("nephrogenic") diabetes insipidus. A.M.A. J. Dis. Child., **99,** 164, 1960.
114. Earley, L. E., Kahn, M., and Orloff, J.: The effects of infusions of

chlorothiazide on urinary dilution and concentration in the dog, J. Clin. Invest., **40,** 857, 1961.

115. Heinemann, H. O., Demartini, F. E., and Laragh, J. H.: The effect of chlorothiazide on renal excretion of electrolytes and free water, Amer. J. Med., **26,** 853, 1959.
116. Earley, L. E., and Orloff, J.: The mechanism of antidiuresis associated with the administration of hydrochlorothiazide to patients with vasopressin-resistant diabetes insipidus. J. Clin. Invest., **41,** 1988, 1962.
117. Havard, C. W. H., and Wood, P. H. N.: Antidiuretic properties of hydrochlorothiazide in diabetes insipidus. Brit. Med. J., **1,** 1306, 1960.
118. Brown, D., Reynolds, J., Michael, A., and Ulstrom, R.: The use and mode of action of ethacrynic acid in nephrogenic diabetes insipidus. Pediatrics, **37,** 447, 1966.
119. Kowarski, A., Berant, M., Grossman, M., and Migeon, C.: Antidiuretic properties of aldactone (spironolactone) in diabetes insipidus: studies on the mechanism of antidiuresis. Johns Hopkins Hosp. Bull. **119,** 413, 1966.
120. Ramos, G., Rivera, A., Pena, J., and Dies, F.: Mechanism of the antidiuretic effect of soluretic drugs. Clin. Pharmacol. Therap., **8,** 557, 1967.
121. Skadhauge, E.: Studies of the antidiuresis induced by natrichloriuretic drugs in rats with diabetes insipidus. Quart. J. Exp. Physiol., **51,** 297, 1966.
122. Kennedy, G. C., and Crawford, J. D.: A comparison of the effects of adrenalectomy and of chlorothiazide in experimental diabetes insipidus. J. Endocr., **22,** 77, 1961.
123. Arduino, F., Ferraz, F. P. J., and Rodriguez, J.: Antidiuretic action of chlorpropamide in idiopathic diabetes insipidus. J. Clin. Endocr., **26,** 1325, 1966.

CHAPTER SIXTY-SEVEN

CYSTINOSIS AND THE FANCONI SYNDROME

J. A. Schneider and J. E. Seegmiller

Cystinosis is a recessively inherited metabolic disorder characterized biochemically by a high intracellular content of cystine localized in a subcellular compartment of phagocytic cells, which results in crystal deposition in the cornea, conjunctiva, bone marrow, lymph nodes, leukocytes, and internal organs. The primary abnormal gene product leading to cystine accumulation remains to be identified.

Clinical expression ranges widely from one family to another. Symptoms of its most severe form, nephropathic cystinosis, result from an impairment of both tubular and glomerular functions and consist primarily of renal abnormalities of the Fanconi syndrome, with the usual deficiency in tubular reabsorption of water, phosphate, sodium, potassium, bicarbonate, glucose, amino acids, and other organic acids. The defect in water reabsorption usually accounts for the presenting symptoms of the disease, which are polyuria, polydipsia, and recurrent unexplained fevers, probably the result of dehydration. Symptoms usually appear within the first year of life. The renal loss of phosphate accounts for the subsequent development of hypophosphatemic rickets resistant to the usual antirachitic doses of vitamin D. The loss of potassium and bicarbonate results in hypokalemia and chronic acidosis. In addition, affected children show severe growth retardation and progressive glomerular damage which usually progresses to death from uremia within the first decade of life. In other families, attenuated clinical expression permits survival of patients into the second or third decade. In still other families with a somewhat lower intracellular concentration of cystine, the kidney is spared, and the disorder is benign.

Genetic heterogeneity of this disease is suggested by the variations in severity between families and the similar degrees of severity of clinical expression of the disease within a given family. Several reviews of cystinosis and the Fanconi syndrome have appeared over the years and reflect the changing concepts of the disease [1–11].

Although the essential elements of the Fanconi syndrome appear in a variety of other primary hereditary and acquired disorders (Table 67-1), cystinosis is the most common cause of the Fanconi syndrome in children.

HISTORICAL RESUMÉ

Recognition of the various clinical and pathologic features of cystinosis and the Fanconi syndrome was fragmented in time and confounded by chance association with other disorders. This confusion began with the first recognition of the disease by Abderhalden in 1903, who described cystine crystals in the liver and spleen at autopsy of a 21-month-old infant who died of "inanition" [12]. Two additional sibs had died previously of a similar illness. Since the urine of the child's father, paternal grandfather, and two sibs contained excessive quantities of cystine, he called the condition a "familial cystine diathesis." This led to an early and unwarranted view that cystinosis was a more severe expression of cystinuria.

Lignac's report in 1924 of cystine deposits in each of three infants with rickets, dwarfism, renal disease, and wasting had provided some delineation of the clinical expression of cystinosis [13, 14]. The finding of ureteral cystine stones in one of these children further compounded the confusion with cystinuria. Subsequent reports of other cases of cystine storage without evidence of cystinuria by Russell and Barrie in 1936 [15] and Beumer in 1937 [16] further delineated the multisystem syndrome of "cystine storage disease." The distinction between cystinosis and cystinuria first suspected on clinical grounds was clearly established with the subsequent demonstration by Dent and Harris that patients with cystinuria excreted other dibasic amino acids, lysine, arginine, and ornithine, in addition to cystine [17].

Additional aspects of the clinical expression of this disease emerged from the association of rickets and stunted growth in a child with glycosuria and albuminuria found by Fanconi in 1931 [18]. Vitamin D-resistant rickets with spontaneous fractures was described in 1933 by deToni in a dwarfed child who also showed a low concentration of phosphorus in the serum, acidosis, albuminuria, and glycosuria [19]. A report of a similar child by Debré in 1934 [20] led Fanconi in 1936 to propose a syndrome of "nephrotic-glycosuric dwarfism with hypophosphatemic rickets" [21, 22].

The possibility that the Fanconi syndrome and cystinosis were but two aspects of the same entity, proposed by Beumer

Table 67-1 CAUSES OF THE RENAL FANCONI SYNDROME

I. Metabolic defect with Fanconi syndrome as a major finding
   - *A.* Cystinosis
   - *B.* Idiopathic [2, 25, 184]
   - *C.* Lowe's syndrome [170, 185]
   - *D.* Tyrosinemia [165, 186]

II. Metabolic defect with Fanconi syndrome not a major finding
   - *A.* Galactosemia [187, 188, 189]
   - *B.* Glycogen storage disease (glucose-6-phosphatase deficiency) [24, 190, 208]
   - *C.* Hereditary fructose intolerance [191]
   - *D.* Wilson's disease [159–161]

III. Other conditions
   - *A.* Human kidney transplantation [192, 193]
   - *B.* Multiple myeloma [40, 171–173]

IV. Exogenous toxins
   - *A.* Heavy metals [155–158]
   - *B.* Lysol (cresol) burn [168]
   - *C.* Maleic acid (in rats) [162]
   - *D.* Methyl-3-chromone [163]
   - *E.* Degraded tetracycline [164, 194–198]

and Wepler in 1937 [23], was supported by the demonstration of cystine crystals in the tissues at necropsy of one of Fanconi's original patients [24]. The detailed study by Bickel in 1952 in a larger series of patients [1] provided further evidence of the association of cystinosis with the Fanconi syndrome and progressive glomerular damage.

The delay in making this association was undoubtedly due in part to the solubility of cystine in formalin or aqueous solutions used in the routine fixation and staining of autopsy tissues. Not all cases of the Fanconi syndrome show evidence of crystalline cystine deposits, particularly those with onset in adult life [25]. Conversely, not all individuals with cystine deposits show the Fanconi syndrome and progressive renal damage as demonstrated by the benign form of cystinosis in adults [26–29].

The finding of an intracellular concentration of cystine 80 to 100 times normal in leukocytes [30] or in fibroblasts [31] cultured in vitro from skin biopsies of patients with cystinosis has extended the biochemical understanding of this disease. It has led to the chemical identification of heterozygotes for this disorder who tend to show moderately elevated intracellular concentrations of cystine [30, 31]. In addition a retinal lesion consisting of a patchy depigmentation has been found in patients with nephropathic but not in those with benign cystinosis [32].

CLINICAL FEATURES

Nephropathic Cystinosis

The major clinical symptomatology of nephropathic cystinosis can, for the most part, be related to the progressive impairment of initially tubular, then glomerular function to produce an unremitting course and fatal outcome. Other aspects of the disease, such as the growth retardation and fair complexion, are less readily explained. A tendency to photophobia can be related either to the corneal deposits of crystals or to the retinopathy (see below).

Early Symptoms

Clinical Course

Children with nephropathic cystinosis appear normal at birth and during their first 6 months or so of life. The first overt signs of the disease are usually produced by the renal tubular defect in water reabsorption. The resulting polyuria and polydipsia make affected children especially vulnerable to dehydration, and this leads to recurrent fever as one of the most common presenting symptoms. In addition, by 1 year of age they usually show growth retardation, rickets, acidosis, and other chemical evidence of renal tubular abnormalities, such as increased renal excretion of glucose, amino acids, phosphate, and potassium. There usually is some evidence of glomerular damage as well, and the subsequent course is determined by the rate at which glomerular insufficiency progresses. Less overt clinical and biochemical evidence of the disease has been found at a much earlier age by careful examination of children known to be at risk because of an older affected sib [33, 34]. Some but not all patients show recurrent episodes of acute prostration, weakness, and cardiovascular collapse, which can lead to early and sudden death. This has been observed during intravenous infusion of glucose but can also occur without known precipitating cause. This disturbance is associated with gross changes in serum electrolytes, and most of the symptomatology is thought to be related to profound hypokalemia.

Failure to thrive is one of the more prominent features of the disease. Affected children show growth failure within the first year or so of life and remain below the 3rd percentile in both height and weight throughout life. Mental development is normal.

Rickets develops at an early age in most patients even on the usual preventive doses of vitamin D. Frontal bossing, genu valgum, thickening of the wrists and ankles, rachitic rosary, and Harrison's groove are frequently seen. X-rays of the long bones show the broadened and frayed epiphyses characteristic of rickets. The glomerular damage progresses in a sporadic but unremitting manner. Careful study of affected patients shows that glomerular dysfunction may remain constant for many months or even years, followed by periods of fairly rapid deterioration that seem to be unrelated to any environmental or biochemical factor yet detected. The possibility has been suggested that excessive quantities of vitamin D used to control the rickets may contribute to progressive renal dysfunction [4]. Nevertheless, advanced renal dysfunction has been found in patients first diagnosed at 2 years of age or older who have never been treated with vitamin D in large amounts [35].

In addition to the glomerular damage, these children show a number of other clinical features not obviously related to the renal abnormalities. The majority have blond hair and a fair complexion, often having substantially less pigmentation than their parents (Fig. 67-1). Exposure to sunlight produces skin tanning with far less tendency to sunburn than would be expected from the lack of skin pigment. In addition, they tolerate infections well and show no unusual susceptibility to intercurrent illness.

Severe photophobia develops in most affected children within the first few years of life. Characteristic changes in the eye provide some of the most consistent features of the disease, and a detailed ophthalmologic examination often establishes the clinical diagnosis. The first ophthalmic manifestations were described by Burki in 1941 [36]. Slit-lamp examination discloses homogeneously dispersed tinsellike refractile opacities in the cornea and the conjunctiva. Crystalline cystine has been identified by x-ray diffraction in the conjunctival but not in the corneal deposits [37]. The crys-

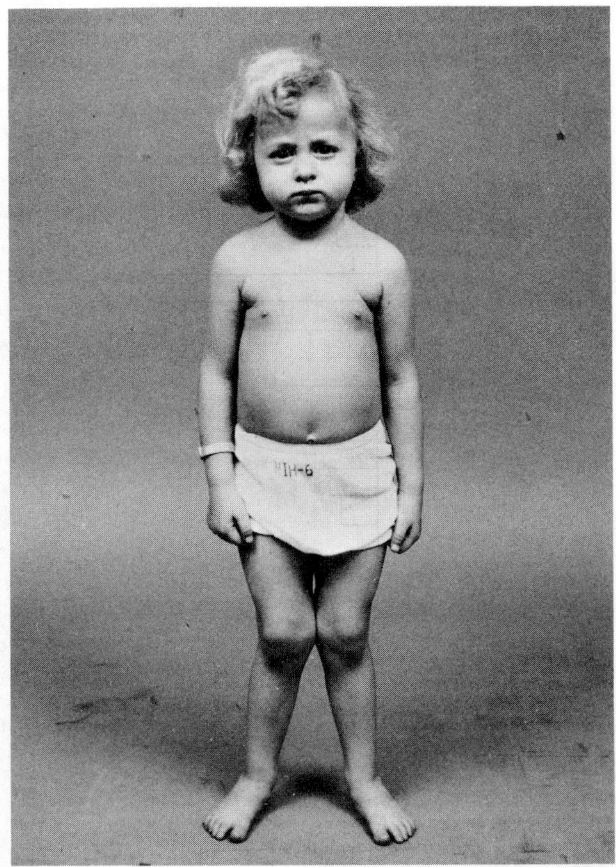

Figure 67-1. Child with cystinosis showing decreased pigmentation and genu valgum from rickets.

talline opacities in the periphery of the cornea occupy the entire corneal thickness, while in the central region of the cornea only the anterior one-third to two-thirds is affected. These iridescent crystalline particles are so typical as to be diagnostic of all forms of cystinosis and appear before the full clinical manifestations of nephropathic cystinosis are expressed. However, other disorders are known in which corneal deposits are found [38].

In addition to the corneal and conjunctival changes, a peripheral retinopathy has recently been found [32] which is characteristic only of the nephropathic form of cystinosis. The pathologic change consists of a generalized pigment disturbance that often assumes a depigmented patchy pattern with superimposed pigment clumps of regular distribution, varying in size from about one-tenth disc diameter to a fine pepperlike stippling. These changes affect the temporal side more extensively than the nasal side and are marked in the peripheral regions of the retina whereas the central regions are generally devoid of abnormal pigmentation. This retinopathy has permitted a diagnosis of cystinosis to be made with accuracy in a child as young as 5 weeks of age, even though only a rare crystal was present in the iris at that age [34]. Evidently, the retinal changes precede those in the cornea.

Early Laboratory Findings

The development of clinical symptoms of the Fanconi syndrome is paralleled by the appearance of laboratory evidence of renal tubular dysfunction. This includes glycosuria, with excretion of from traces to 4 to 5 gm glucose per 100 ml urine [33, 39], organic aciduria, and amino aciduria. Excessive quantities of 10 or more amino acids appear in the urine (Fig. 67-2) and generally account for about 80 percent of the organic acids. Cystine excretion is generally increased in the same proportion as other amino acids. Renal calculi composed of cystine have been reported in only one patient [14, 15]. An increased phosphate excretion is usually found [3], and a decreased intestinal absorption of phosphate has also been reported [7]. Proteinuria is often present and consists of the so-called tubular protein associated with the Fanconi syndrome. This includes around 200 times the normal excretion of the light chain of gamma-globulin [40]. The significance of this characteristic finding remains to be determined. In spite of systemic acidosis the urine tends to be alkaline and contains increased amounts of ammonium ion. In addition, microscopic examination reveals many granular casts and occasional erythrocytes as glomerular damage progresses.

The blood sugar concentration is normal. Metabolic acidosis with diminished plasma carbon dioxide reflects the renal loss of bicarbonate. Hypophosphatemia is related to the appearance of rickets, the activity of which is reflected in an increased serum concentration of alkaline phosphatase. An increased blood pyruvate concentration has been found in some but not all patients and presumably results from an effect of the cystine on SH enzymes [35, 41]. There is a tendency to severe hypokalemia. BUN and serum creatinine are usually in the normal range early in the disease, even though creatinine and urea clearance are substantially diminished. The erythrocyte sedimentation rate is always elevated. The exact reason for this finding is not known.

Late Symptoms and Findings

The clinical course of the disease is one of periodic but unremitting progression of glomerular damage, leading eventually to death in uremia before puberty. As in other forms of renal dysfunction, children are able to maintain relatively normal degrees of activity until the renal insufficiency becomes advanced, so that only in the last 6 months to 1 year of life are the children seriously incapacitated.

In some patients advanced renal disease with elevated BUN and creatinine is found as early as 2 years of age. In these patients the amino aciduria is often masked by the severely diminished glomerular filtration rate, so that the total amino acid excretion is in the normal range. Other aspects

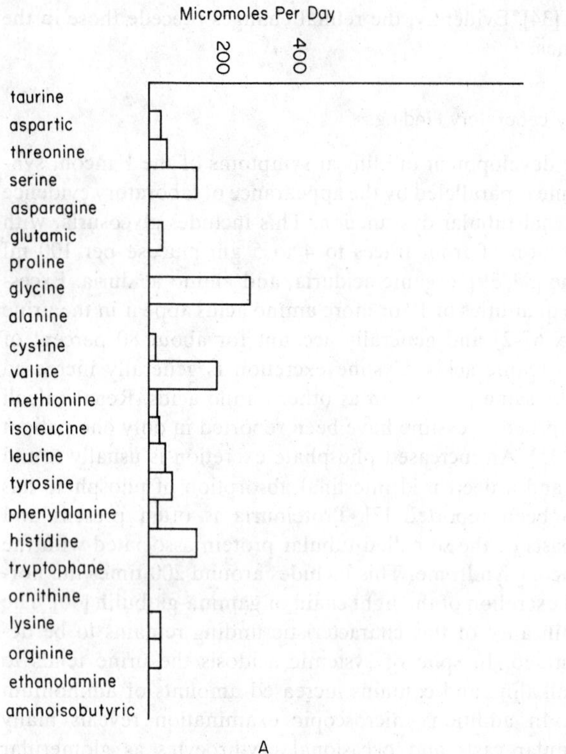

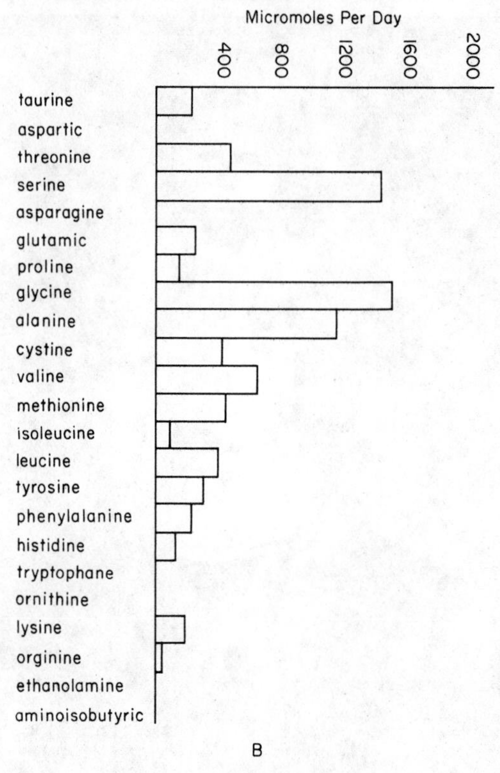

Figure 67-2. Comparison of 24-hr amino acid excretion in a normal (*A*) and cystinotic (*B*) child. *A*, data of Jonxis [199], recalculated and *B*, data of Harrison and Harrison [137]. (*Reproduced with permission of J.A.M.A.*)

of the Fanconi syndrome may also be obscured in some patients by advanced glomerular damage [35]. In the same manner the hypophosphatemia and hypokalemia are corrected as renal deterioration progresses and are eventually replaced by hyperphosphatemia, hyperkalemia, and a secondary hypocalcemia. The acidosis may then become even more marked. Correction of the acidosis by administration of alkali salts can then result in tetany. Growth failure, progressive renal dysfunction, and acidosis can also ameliorate the clinical symptoms of rickets in occasional patients. Polyuria and polydipsia also diminish as glomerular insufficiency supervenes. The clinical symptomatology then becomes primarily that associated with severe renal failure and uremia. Weakness and lethargy with edema and congestive cardiac failure result from salt retention and from the profound anemia of renal failure.

The children remain dwarfed throughout life. In only one patient has a spontaneous remission been noted. The patient presented with grave manifestations in infancy, but by age 8 years had spontaneously showed considerable clinical improvement, and at age 28 years showed only short stature, mild renal insufficiency, hypercalciuria, hypercalcemia, and amino aciduria. Cystine crystals were not found in the cornea upon examination at age 28 and were not mentioned at earlier examinations [42].

Intermediate Forms

Patients with cystinosis have been described who appear to have an attenuated form of the disease which permits them to survive well into the second [15] or even third decade of life [43]. In addition patients are reported who failed to show abnormalities of renal tubular function [7, 44]. In general, affected members of a given family tend to have a similar clinical course. This suggests a genetic basis. Patients in three separate families have all had less severe elevations of intracellular free-cystine than observed in the usual patients with nephropathic cystinosis [65, 200–202].

Benign Cystinosis

What appears to be a completely benign variant of cystinosis has been identified in nine patients [26–29, 45]. Brief reference has been made to additional children who may belong in this category [7, 44]. The primary clinical distinction between the benign and the nephropathic form of the disease is failure of these patients to show either retinopathy or renal dysfunction. Nevertheless, they show crystalline deposits in the cornea, bone marrow, and leukocytes, but this causes no disability. These patients live to adult life, and their cystinosis is usually identified only incidentally during a routine ophthalmologic examination with a slit lamp. This benign variant of the disease appears to represent one end of the spectrum of clinical expression. These patients tend to show somewhat lower concentration of intracellular cystine [45] than do patients with nephropathic cystinosis.

Genetics

Both the nephrophatic and benign forms of cystinosis show an autosomal recessive pattern of inheritance. As a result the disease appears in greater frequency in consanguineous matings such as that shown in Fig. 67-3. The frequency of the disease in the general population has not been assessed. Genetic heterogeneity is suggested by the differences in clinical expression of the disease in different families. An even greater range of both genetic and environmental factors undoubtedly underlie the renal tubular abnormalities of other forms of the Fanconi syndrome.

Pathology

The pathologic changes observed at autopsy in patients dying of nephropathic cystinosis can be related to two different processes, the terminal uremia and the primary pathologic changes of cystinosis.

Cystine Crystals

The specific and characteristic pathologic lesion of cystinosis is a deposition of cystine crystals primarily in reticuloendothelial cells of the bone marrow, liver, spleen, and lymphatic system. Different patients show considerable variation in the extent of crystal deposition. Crystals are also found within

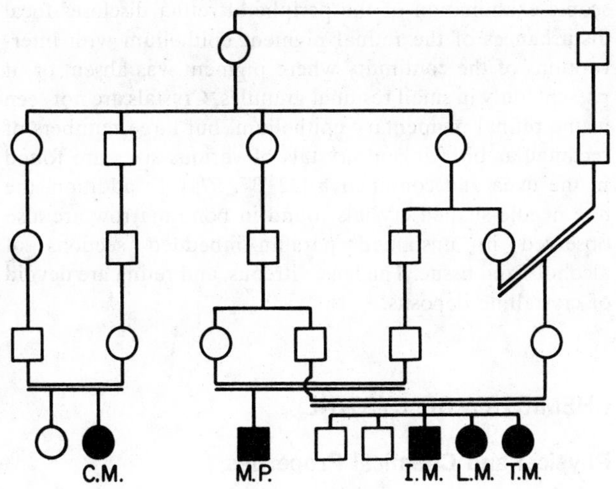

Figure 67-3. Pedigree showing consanguinity of a family with cystinosis.

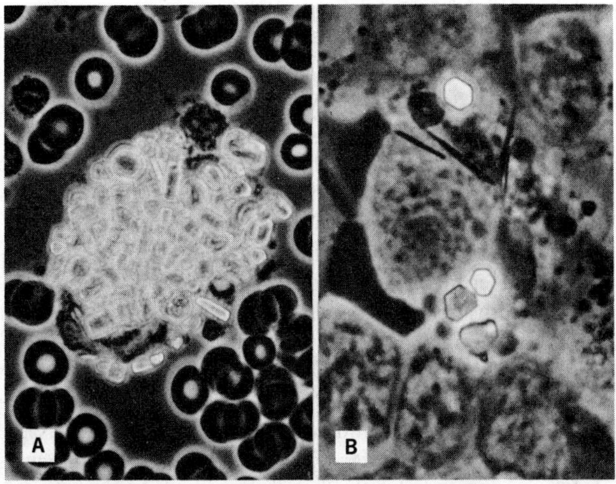

Figure 67-4. Cystine crystals in bone marrow showing (A) rectangular forms (B) hexagonal plates and unidentified needle-shaped crystals.

the kidney and are more numerous in the medulla than in the cortex. Occasionally a few crystals are seen in the mesangium of a glomerulus. At times crystals may be seen in the lumen of a tubule forming a minute calculus. Cells with a foamy cytoplasm are also frequently found in the kidneys and other tissues and are thought to represent cells from which cystine crystals have been removed during preparation of the histologic section.

The solubility of cystine in acid solutions and formalin commonly used as fixatives undoubtedly contributes to the wide variation in the amount of crystal formation observed in histologic preparations. Even in tissues fixed in absolute alcohol or frozen, instances are known in which essentially all crystals were lost during the final exposure to the aqueous solutions used in staining. The cystine crystals are, therefore, best observed in their natural state in frozen or alcohol-fixed tissues before staining, using cross-polarizing filters and phase microscopy. Treatment with organic solvents will remove birefringent lipid materials. The cystine crystals show several different forms including, most frequently, clusters of brick-shaped birefringent crystals, shown in Fig. 67-4A and less commonly, the typical nonbirefringent hexagonal plates shown in Fig. 67-4B. In addition, needle-shaped crystals are also observed (Fig. 67-4B) in some preparations, but their composition remains to be determined. The medium in which the crystallization occurs can affect the crystal form [1]. The autolysis and resulting acid production accompanying post-mortem changes could also contribute to dissolution of crystals.

Kidneys

Detailed descriptions of the pathologic changes in a large number of patients have appeared in the literature. The major changes are found in the kidneys, which are characteristically pale and shrunken, weighing as little as one-quarter of the normal. The capsule is adherent and practically no normal markings are discernible at the corticomedullary junction. Minute white granules can be seen with a magnifying glass on the cut surface.

The precise location of the crystals is often difficult to ascertain. Barr and Bickel concluded that they were primarily intracellular and within reticuloendothelial cells [1, 46]. They found no deposits within lymphocytes, but in severe cases some crystals were scattered throughout almost every organ. Microscopically, there is complete disorganization of the renal parenchyma and a marked but irregularly distributed increase in the amount of connective tissue in both the medulla and the cortex. The degree of fibrosis is more severe the longer the child has survived. In some areas the interstitial tissue is cellular with predominantly lymphocytes and large mononuclear cells, whereas in other areas it is fibrous with few cells. In the far-advanced case the glomeruli are virtually bloodless and contain no patent capillaries. A patchy necrosis of the glomerular tuft is found in many areas. These glomeruli also show a hyaline thickening of the basement membrane of the parietal layer of Bowman's capsule. Glomerular fibrosis appears to be preceded by a periglomerular fibrosis.

Renal Tubules

The renal tubules show replacement of their normal epithelial lining by a cuboidal epithelium, making differentiation of the various segments of the tubule difficult. Two characteristic features emerge upon microdissection of the nephron. Many nephrons are hypotrophic, particularly in the proximal convoluted tubules, with narrowing in the first part of the tubule forming the "swan neck" lesion described by Clay and colleagues [47]. These lesions are more commonly seen in the more advanced cases than in patients dying early in the course of the disease. The second feature is a marked shortening of the proximal convoluted tubules. These abnormalities are difficult to see in ordinary histologic sections because of the problem of obtaining the glomerulus and proximal convoluted tubule in one plane.

Although these swan neck lesions were originally regarded as congenital tubular malformations, more recent studies by Darmady and associates show that they are not specific for cystinosis. They are also found occasionally in microcystic disease [48], renal homotransplants [49, 50], hepatolenticular degeneration, and possibly in chronic Bright's disease [51]. The fact that children with cystinosis who survive longer are more severely affected than those dying early in infancy suggests that the renal malformation may be a secondary manifestation of the disease process. The mechanism for the formation of the swan neck deformity proposed by Darmady is an initial necrosis of the proximal tubular epithelium as a result of high cystine concentrations within the cell, followed by a downgrowth of the cells lining the glomerulus to form the swan neck lesion. This mechanism also accounts for the failure of the renal tubular defects to be apparent during the first few months of life. Nephrotoxicity has been observed in experimental animals given a diet rich in cystine [52–54] (see below).

Histologic examination also shows gross disorganization and atrophy of the proximal convoluted tubular epithelium. Many of the glomeruli show fibrotic obliteration. The interstitial fibrosis is the most striking pathologic feature. Local areas show round-cell infiltration and occasional pyroninophilic macrophages. Secondary pyelonephritis occasionally occurs.

Electron Microscopy

Precise intracellular location of the cystine crystals has been achieved by examination with the electron microscope. The profiles of the intracellular cystine crystals are shown surrounded by a membrane. Studies of a lymph node [55] shown in Fig. 67-5 as well as those of macrophages within conjunctival biopsy specimens [56] suggest that lysosomes are the subcellular structures containing cystine crystals. Incubation of tissues with ferritin granules results in ferritin accumulation within the same compartment containing the cystine crystals [56]. Hummeler et al. have demonstrated inclusions of amorphous material in lysosomes from rectal mucosa, leukocytes, and fibroblasts of patients with nephropathic cystinosis [144]. The lysosomes of rectal mucosa also contained crystals. Even noncrystalline cystine within peripheral leukocytes of cystinotic patients shows sedimentation in a density gradient in the same fractions containing enzymes characteristic of lysosomes [57].

Ocular Pathology

Pathologic examination of the eyes discloses the same patchy depigmentation of the peripheral areas of the retina that was observed on funduscopic examination in vivo. Microscopic examination of the peripheral retina discloses focal disturbances of the retinal pigment epithelium with interruptions of the continuity where pigment was absent or, if present, only in small residual granules. Crystals are not seen in the retinal pigmentary epithelium, but large numbers of rectangular birefringent crystals of various sizes are found in the uvea and conjunctiva [32, 37, 57a]. In addition, the fine needle-shaped crystals found in bone marrow are also observed in unstained paraffin-imbedded sections of alcohol-fixed tissue. The lens, vitreous, and retina are devoid of crystalline deposits.

CHEMISTRY OF CYSTINE

Physical and Chemical Properties

L-cystine crystallizes from water in hexagonal plates that show no birefringence in polarized light. Although hexago-

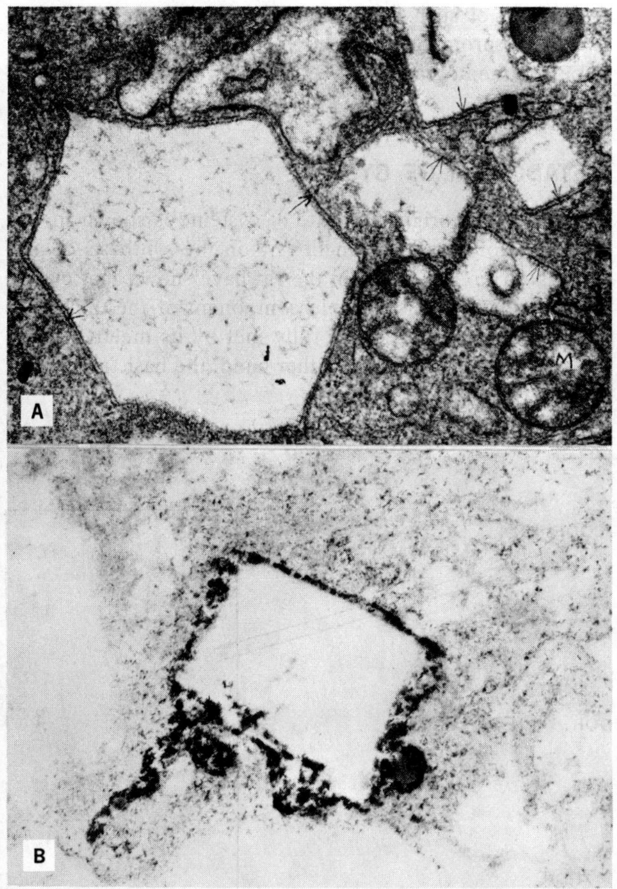

Figure 67-5. Electron photomicrographs of a lymph node biopsy of a patient with cystinosis showing (A) profiles of intracellular cystine crystals within intact limiting membrane as revealed by uranyl acetate stain, and (B) location of acid phosphatase activity at the periphery of a cystine crystal profile as shown by lead deposition after incubation with glycerophosphate. Scale mark is 1 μ in each photo. (*Reproduced from Patrick & Lake* [55] *with permission of J. Clin. Path.*)

nal plates are also found occasionally in bone marrow and other tissues, the most common form is a birefringent rectangular block that is often brick-shaped. The crystalline form varies with the solvent. The rectangular birefringent crystals most frequently found in vivo probably represent side views of short hexagonal prisms with two underdeveloped faces [1]. Hydrochlorides of either D- or L-cystine crystallize in large prismatic needles. Cystine decomposes in a sealed tube at 260 to 261°C and in aqueous solution shows dissociation constants of $pK_{a_1} = 8.00$; $pK_{a_2} = 10.25$; $pK_{b_1} = 11.95$; $pK_{b_2} = 12.96$.

Solubility

At 25°C water can carry in solution 112 mg L-cystine per liter, 239 mg at 50°C, 523 mg at 75°C, and 1.142 gm at 100°C. The solubility is greatly increased by either lowering or raising the pH [58, 59]. Human plasma at 37°C and pH 7.4 can carry around 380 mg cystine per liter (320 μmoles half-cystine/100 ml) [11, 30]. Cystine is insoluble in alcohol.

Redox Potential

The interconversion of cystine and cysteine constitutes a reversible oxidation-reduction system. Values reported for the absolute redox potential range from −0.21 and −0.23 ev [60, 61] to −0.34 and −0.39 ev [62, 63]. Much of the difficulty in this measurement arises from the chemical reaction of the sulfhydryl groups with the metal electrodes commonly employed. The same difficulties hold for the analogous determination of the redox potential of glutathione (GSH). Indirect comparative methods have therefore been used, and they agree that the redox potential for cysteine/cystine relative to GSH/GSSG is +0.017 to 0.018 ev. The disulfide bond of cystine therefore readily reacts with sulfhydryl groups (SH) of glutathione and a large number of other compounds to form cysteine and mixed disulfide of the original SH compound. This kind of interaction constitutes the rationale behind the successful clinical use of penicillamine in treatment of cystinuria [64]. Similar reasoning has suggested its use for treatment of cystinosis, but this has proved unsuccessful [11]. Dithiothreitol is an effective reducing agent for disulfide groups. It diminishes the intracellular cystine content of cultured cystinotic fibroblasts [65].

Reactivity of Sulfhydryl Groups

The disulfide-sulfhydryl interconversion makes cystine capable of interacting with a large number of compounds, including heavy metals, proteins, and a wide variety of chemical groups, particularly in the presence of a substance with an appropriate redox potential. Sulfhydryl groups have been implicated in formation of a large number of pigments, presumably through interaction with phenolic groups.

Determination of Cystine and Cysteine

The quantitative determination of cystine and cysteine-containing compounds can be performed by a variety of procedures. Cysteine (or cystine after reduction to cysteine) gives a red color in alkaline solution with sodium 1,2-naphthoquinone-4-sulfonate in the presence of the strong reducing agent, sodium thiosulfate ($Na_2S_2O_4$) [66]. Another reaction commonly employed is a nonspecific test in which the sulfhydryl group of cysteine reduces the disulfide group of 5-5 dithiobis-2-nitrobenzoic acid (Ellman's reagent) to produce a compound with a more intense yellow color [67].

The ninhydrin reaction of amino acids, although nonspecific, permits the specific determination of cysteine or cystine after separation from other amino acids by ion-exchange chromatography [68, 69]. A highly specific colorimetric determination of cysteine is based on its reaction with noradrenachrome to form a yellow complex having an absorption maximum of 414 mμ [70, 71]. A recurring problem in any biochemical study of sulfur amino acid metabolism is the tendency of sulfhydryl groups to undergo spontaneous oxidation to disulfide groups or sulfonic acids upon exposure to the oxygen of air. This problem is especially difficult when a determination of the sulfhydryl and disulfide forms of the same compound (cysteine and cystine) is required. The identity of the sulfhydryl group can be maintained by treatment with a reagent that forms a stable compound with sulfhydryl groups, such as iodoacetamide or N-ethylmaleimide. The sulfhydryl derivative can then be separated from the disulfide compound and determined with ninhydrin. Separation of such compounds can be achieved with ion-exchange chromatography, high-voltage electrophoresis, or paper chromatography [72, 73].

METABOLISM OF CYSTINE

The metabolic origin and fate of cysteine is shown in Fig. 67-6. One of its major functions is in the synthesis of proteins. Nutritional studies in the rat have shown that cystine (or cysteine) is a dispensable component of the diet, since the need for cystine can be fully met by its metabolic precursor, methionine. On the other hand, the basic nutritional

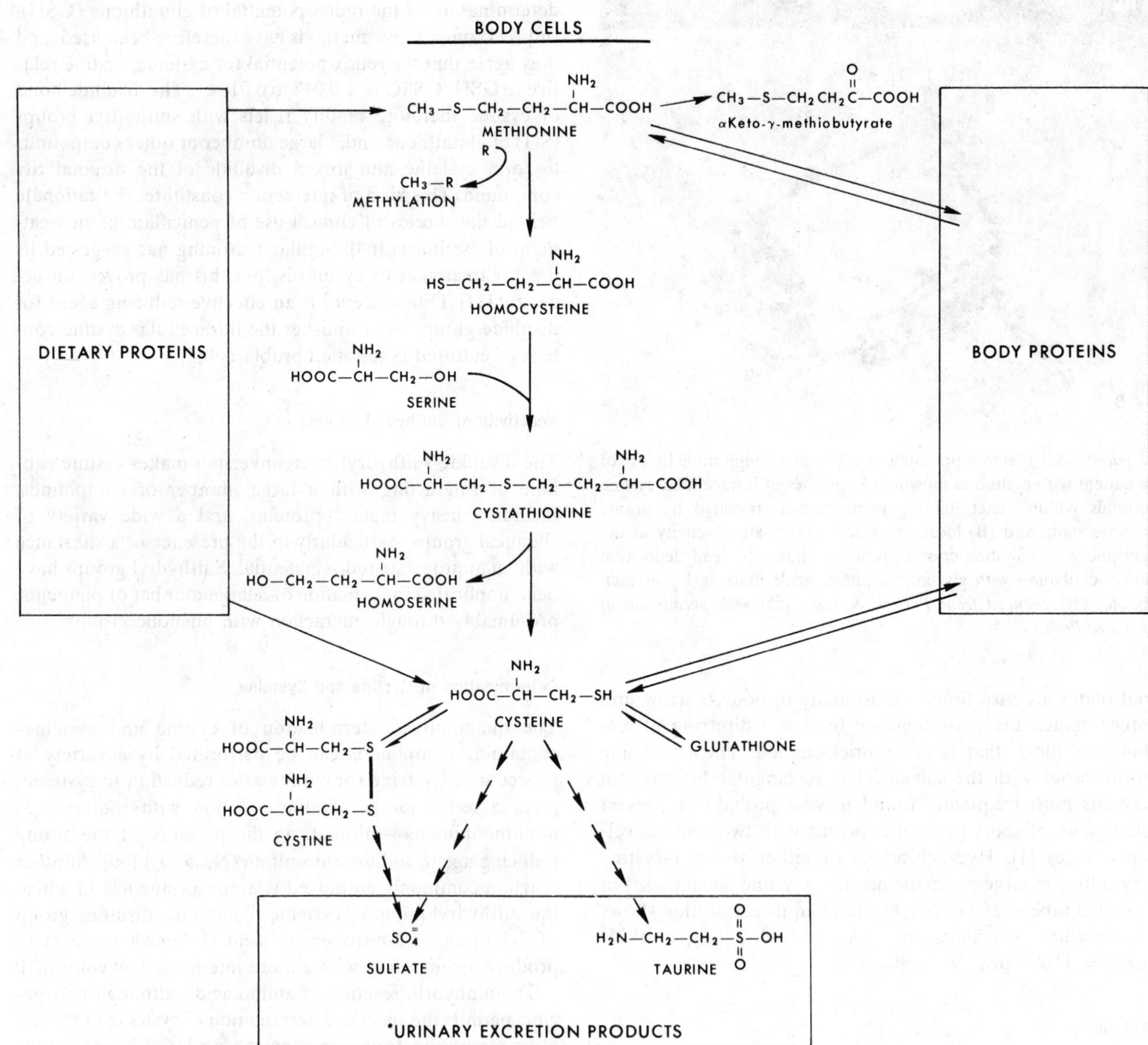

Figure 67-6. Metabolic origin and fate of cysteine in mammals. (*Reproduced from Seegmiller et al.* [11] *with permission of Ann. Intern. Med.*)

requirement for methionine can be met only incompletely by cystine in the diet. Cystine is, therefore, classed as a nonessential amino acid. Evidence that a similar interconversion occurs in the human being has come from the increased excretion of cystine observed after administration of methionine to patients with cystinuria [74]. Furthermore, when methionine-^{35}S was administered to a cystinuric patient, the isotope was found in urinary cystine [75]. The origin of the carbon and nitrogen skeleton of cystine from serine was first shown by the recovery of ^{15}N in cystine when ^{15}N-labeled serine was administered to rats [76]. The increased cystine formed by a patient with cystinuria upon administration of homocysteine [77] suggested the intermediate formation of cystathionine [78]. This was further supported by the demonstration that L-cystathionine is capable of supporting the growth of rats in place of cysteine [79]. Homoserine, formed by cystathionine cleavage, is deaminated to ketobutyric acid, which can then be reaminated to aminobutyric acid. This pathway accounts for the increased amounts of aminobutyric acid found in the urine of human subjects who have ingested methionine [80, 81]. L-Cystathionine has been isolated from human brain, where it is present in concentrations of 22.5 to 56.6 mg per 100 gm wet weight of the tissue [82]. Although cystine is required for optimal growth of human cell lines in tissue culture, such cells are capable of converting methionine sulfur to cysteine [83, 84]. Pyridoxal phosphate is a cofactor for the enzymes that both form and cleave cystathionine, shown in Fig. 67-6. The same enzyme from rat liver that catalyzes cystathionine cleavage also deaminates homoserine [85, 86]. Crystalline cystathionase also cleaves the carbon-sulfur bond in djenkolic acid, lanthionine, and L-cysteine. The latter compounds are converted to a keto acid and hydrogen sulfide (see also Chaps. 19 and 20).

The formation of homocysteine from methionine involves the transfer of an intact methyl group [87]. This reversible reaction requires the intermediate formation of S-adenosylmethionine as the active methyl donor [88–90].

In addition to the pathway for cystine biosynthesis through transulfuration from homocysteine to serine described above, inorganic sulfide can be utilized directly for cystine formation from serine in lower forms of life by the enzyme serine sulfhydrase. This enzyme has been extensively studied in yeast [91, 92]. It has been purified from *S. typhimurium*, and the mechanism responsible for regulation of the activity of this enzyme has been studied in detail by Becker, Kredich and Tomkins, [93]. A similar reaction has also been found in liver of rat and chicken [94], and in the allantoic sac and liver of the chick embryo [95].

Oxidation and Reduction of Cysteine and Cystine

As shown in Figure 67-7, cysteine has a variety of possible metabolic fates. It undergoes a facile oxidation of the sulfhydryl groups to form the disulfide molecule, cystine. Enzymatic reactions catalyze both the oxidation of cysteine to cystine and the reduction of cystine to cysteine, even though both reactions occur nonenzymatically at a significant rate. Cytochrome c and cytochrome oxidase catalyze the oxidation [96], while the reduction of cystine to cysteine is catalyzed by a NADH-requiring reaction in yeast and higher plants [97, 98] and mammalian systems [99]. Transhydrogenation between cystine and reduced glutathione is a more active system for achieving this reduction in most mammalian tissues [100–102]. The resulting oxidized glutathione is in turn reduced to the sulfhydryl form by an enzyme requiring NADPH, glutathione reductase (Fig. 67-8). In addition, an active system in plasma for oxidation of cysteine to cystine has been observed [103]. Recently, a NADPH-requiring disulfide reductase has been demonstrated in rat liver [203, 204].

The desulfuration of cysteine to form pyruvate, hydrogen sulfide, and ammonia was first observed in 1933 [104] and was later shown to occur in preparations of mammalian liver, kidney, and pancreas, as well as in certain microorganisms [105–107]. Enzyme preparations that catalyze this reaction also catalyze the incorporation of ^{35}S-sulfide into cysteine. This suggests that this reaction is to some extent reversible [108, 109]. Several different enzymatic mechanisms evidently lead to this desulfuration. One of these is catalyzed by cystathionase, while several reactions are involved in another mechanism, which includes desulfuration of β-mercaptopyruvate. The latter substance is formed by transamination of cysteine with a keto acid [110]. The subsequent desulfuration produces pyruvate and inorganic sulfur, which can be further reduced to hydrogen sulfide in the presence of excess cysteine, glutathione, or other strong reducing agent. A close association of cysteine desulfhydrase and cystathionase activity has been noted [111, 112].

Within the cell most of the cysteine is maintained in the reduced form. The most active system for maintaining this reducing potential is the cysteine-glutathione transhydrogenase system, which in turn is linked to oxidation of glucose-6-phosphate by NADP, as shown in Figure 67-8. The glutathione reductase from a variety of sources contains flavine adenine dinucleotide and is extremely sensitive to sulfhydryl inhibitors [102]. The mechanism of action of glutathione reductase proposed by Mize et al. [100, 101], is as follows:

$$\text{Enzyme-SH} + \text{GSSG} \longrightarrow \text{Enzyme-SSG} + \text{GSH}$$
$$\text{Enzyme-SSG} + \text{NADPH} + \text{H}^+ \longrightarrow \text{Enzyme-SH} + \text{GSH} + \text{NADP}$$

Oxidation of Cysteine

The stepwise oxidation of the sulfur group of cysteine (Fig. 67-7) to cysteine sulfenic acid, cysteine sulfinic acid, and cysteic acid is apparently an irreversible reaction sequence [113], since cysteine sulfinic acid does not replace dietary cysteine in supporting growth [114]. A transamination of cysteine sulfinic acid with α-ketoglutarate or oxaloacetate

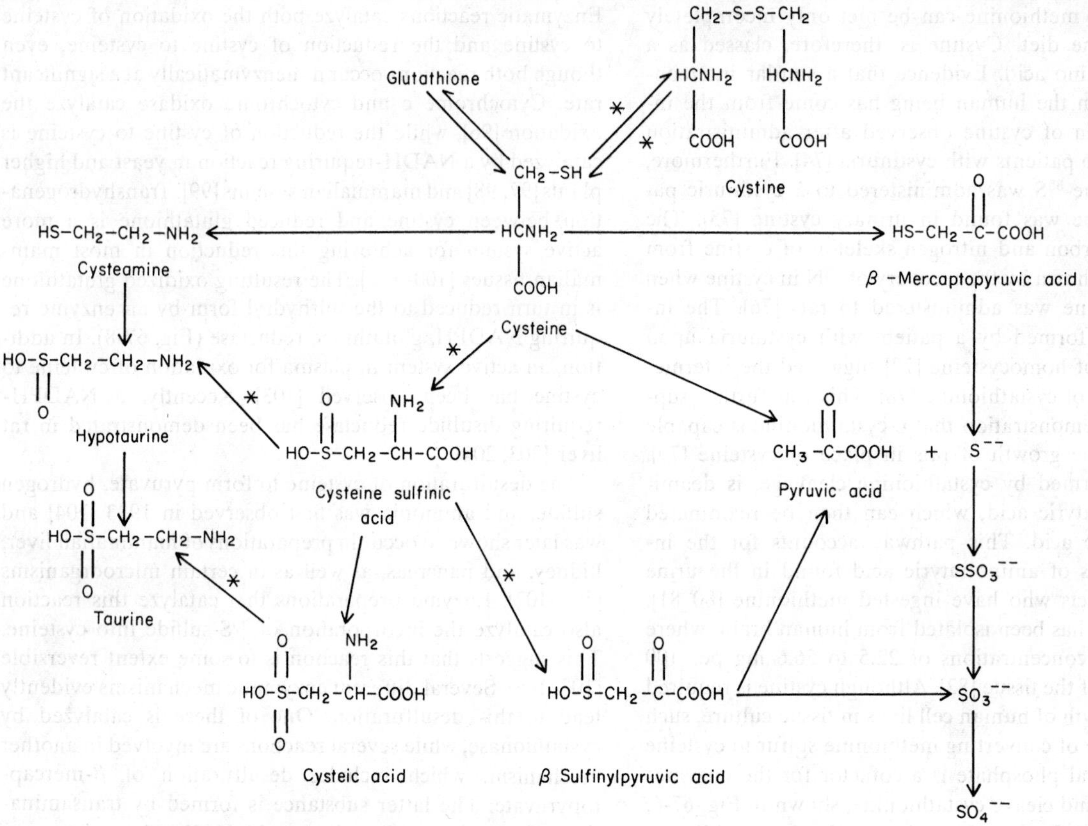

Figure 67-7. Metabolic pathways for degradation of cysteine. Asterisk indicates enzymes found by Patrick [135] to have normal activity in cystinotic tissue.

results in formation of inorganic sulfite and pyruvate. The intermediate produced, sulfinyl pyruvic acid, has never been isolated and is presumably extremely unstable. This transamination is catalyzed by purified preparations of glutamic-aspartic transaminase, which is thought to be responsible for conversion of cysteine sulfinic acid to sulfite [115]. In addition, an oxidative deamination reaction catalyzed by rat liver mitochondria also results in the oxidation of cysteine sulfinic acid to pyruvate, sulfate, and ammonia in the presence of diphosphopyridine nucleotide [116]. Direct desulfuration of cysteine sulfinic acid by the cross-reaction of aspartate-decarboxylase of bacterial origin has been demonstrated [117]. Whether or not the mammalian enzyme also participates in such a direct "desulfinase" reaction is not yet known. A hemoprotein with an absorption spectrum resembling that of cytochrome b_5 has been identified as the enzyme catalyzing the oxidation of sulfite to sulfate (205–207). This enzyme, sulfite oxidase, was deficient in a patient with severe retardation who excreted in the urine S-sulfo-L-cysteine, sulfite and thiosulfate [118]. As seen in Fig. 67-7, there are at least two pathways of taurine formation, involving either cysteic acid or hypotaurine as intermediates [118a].

Physiologic Significance of Disulfide Bonds

The intracellular and extracellular milieu show marked differences in content of disulfide compounds. The high intracellular concentration of glutathione tends to maintain sulfhydryl groups of amino acids and proteins in the reduced SH form, while an active system found in plasma oxidizes many sulfhydryl compounds to their disulfide form [103]. A cyclic change in SH groups in the fertilized sea urchin egg during the cell division cycle is associated with a fibrous protein substance precipitated by saturated ammonium sulfate but not by trichloracetic acid [119]. A possible role for this protein in cell division has been proposed [120]. Ability of these threadlike structures to contract is related apparently to the SH content of the thread. Contraction is presumably the result of formation of SS bonds [121, 122]. Masia has reviewed work on the possible involvement of SH and SS bonds in the cell division process [123]. He suggests that the meiotic apparatus of the sea urchin egg may be a "disulfide-bonded structure" on the basis of its stabilization by the disulfide form of mercaptoethanol and its loss of structure in the presence of SH substances.

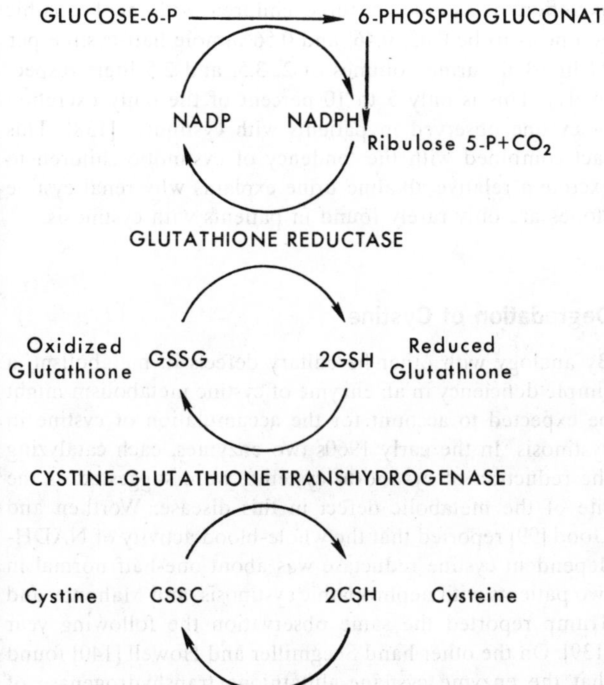

Figure 67-8. Diagram of cystine glutathione reductase link to carbohydrate metabolism.

Renal Tubular Transport

The possibility that a decrease in SH groups in kidney tubules may be associated with physiologic and pathologic variations in tubular function is suggested by recent studies. Pitressin reduces the quantity of histochemically detectable SH groups in kidney tubules [124]. The possibility that a thiol group may be involved in the antidiuretic action of this hormone was further supported by the finding that tritium-labeled rat vasopressin is bound to rat kidney tissue through an S—S (i.e., thio-cleavable) bond. By contrast, muscle tissue, which does not respond to this hormone, showed no such binding [125, 126]. Further correlations between membrane permeability and formation of S—S bonds between the hormone and receptor sites were found in studies of the toad bladder [127, 128]. Correlation was found between the capacity of the membrane to allow a passive non-energy-dependent transfer of water between regions of different osmotic pressure and its capacity to form an S—S bond between the hormone and receptor sites under various conditions of inhibition, of oxygen or glucose deprivation. Both processes were inhibited by SH group reagents such as N-ethylmaleimide, which at low concentrations mimicked the physiologic action of the hormone and at high concentrations interfered with its action, presumably through binding SH receptor sites.

Production of the Fanconi syndrome in both the rat and man by administration of a wide variety of compounds that have in common the ability to bind sulfhydryl groups suggest that binding of the sulfhydryl groups of renal tubules may mediate this action.

CYSTINE METABOLISM IN CYSTINOSIS

The precise abnormality in gene product responsible for the development of cystinosis continues to be elusive, but substantial progress has been made. Many hypotheses have been proposed only to be discarded by lack of support by subsequent investigations. Only with a systematic approach have answers to fundamental questions on the pathogenesis of the disease been obtained. The application of the amino acid analyzer to the problem has greatly facilitated investigations of this problem. The underlying cause of the accumulation of excessive quantities of cystine remains to be identified, but the site of crystal formation has been established as intracellular and has been further localized to a subcellular organelle, probably a lysosome, as already noted.

In the course of systematic investigations the handling of cystine by man has been examined at several levels of organization.

Intestinal Absorption of Cystine and Cysteine

The intestinal absorption of excessive quantities of cystine could theoretically provide a simple explanation of this disease providing the absorption was incomplete in normal subjects. Although cells of the gastrointestinal tract contain crystalline deposits of cystine in nephropathic cystinosis [129–131] intestinal absorption of both cystine and cysteine is unimpaired in this disease. Fasting cystine and cysteine tolerance tests were performed in three children, aged 5 to 7 years, with nephropathic cystinosis [132]. Following the ingestion of 0.5 mmole cystine per kg body weight, the plasma cyst(e)ine concentration increased approximately twofold in 1 to 2 hr and returned to normal or near-normal levels by 5 hr. A load of 0.5 mmole cysteine hydrochloride per kg body weight caused a three- to fourfold increase in plasma cyst(e)ine concentration and a seven- to tenfold increase in plasma cysteine concentration (as measured using iodoacetic acid [133]) in 1 to 2 hr, with a return to normal concentrations by 5 hr. Both results agree closely with published values for normal *adults* given the same or comparable oral loads on a body weight basis [134, 135]. Comparable data on normal children are not available.

Plasma Cystine and Cysteine Concentrations

Cystine exists primarily in its oxidized form in the plasma and in the extracellular compartment. In the earliest measurements of fasting plasma cystine and cysteine concentrations, Brigham, Stein, and Moore [133] studied two children with nephropathic cystinosis and found the cysteine concentration to be normal but the cystine concentration to be slightly elevated. Crawhall et al. have reported normal fasting plasma cystine and cysteine concentrations in six children with this disease [35], and Schneider et al. could find no consistent abnormality in the fasting plasma cyst(e)ine concentration in patients with either nephropathic or benign cystinosis [45] (Table 67-2).

Solubility of Cystine in Plasma

Although cystine has a limited solubility, the concentrations normally found in human plasma are far below saturation. The concentration of cystine found in solution in normal plasma of 4 to 10 μmoles of half-cystine per 100 ml [133] was increased around fiftyfold to 303 μmoles half-cystine per 100 ml of normal plasma upon incubation at 37° C, pH 7.3, with excess cystine. Plasma from a child with cystinosis when similarly treated showed a concentration of 341 μmoles half-cystine per 100 ml of plasma [11, 30]. Thus, cystine solubility in cystinotic plasma is around fifty times greater than the fasting plasma cystine concentration in patients with cystinosis and at least fourteen times greater than the peak plasma cyst(e)ine concentration observed following the ingestion of 0.5 mmole cystine or cysteine hydrochloride per kg body weight by children with nephropathic cystinosis [136]. These facts appear to preclude the extracellular crystallization of cystine in this disease and have focused attention on the cystine content of the intracellular compartments.

Urinary Excretion of Cystine

All patients with nephropathic cystinosis have a generalized amino aciduria, but increased excretion of cystine is in the same relative proportion as the increased excretion of many other amino acids [1, 137]. Crawhall et al. [35] reported the

Table 67-2. FASTING PLASMA CYSTINE CONCENTRATIONS

Subjects	μmole half-cystine/100ml
Adults with benign cystinosis:	
N.T.	12.4
H.S.	9.2
J.B.	9.0
Adult Controls:	
J.E.S.	9.8
F.R.	9.1
J.S.	9.0
9 Children with nephropathic cystinosis	6.8 ± 1.2*
11 Control children	7.2 ± 1.4

* Mean ± 1 s.d.

Source: Reproduced from Schneider et al. [45] with permission of New Eng. J. Med.

excretion of cystine in three children with nephropathic cystinosis to be 0.45, 0.46, and 0.56 mmole half-cystine per 24 hr (daily urine volumes of 2, 3.5, and 2.5 liters respectively). This is only 5 to 10 percent of the daily excretion of cystine observed in patients with cystinuria [138]. This fact combined with the tendency of cystinotic children to excrete a relative alkaline urine explains why renal cystine stones are only rarely found in patients with cystinosis.

Degradation of Cystine

By analogy with other hereditary defects in metabolism, a simple deficiency in an enzyme of cystine metabolism might be expected to account for the accumulation of cystine in cystinosis. In the early 1960s two enzymes, each catalyzing the reduction of cystine to cysteine, were suggested as the site of the metabolic defect in this disease. Worthen and Good [99] reported that the whole-blood activity of NADH-dependent cystine reductase was about one-half normal in two patients with nephropathic cystinosis, and Mahoney and Trump reported the same observation the following year [139]. On the other hand Seegmiller and Howell [140] found that the enzyme cysteine-glutathione transhydrogenase of erythrocytes was much more active than cystine reductase in reducing cystine. Furthermore they found that it was present in liver tissue from two children with cystinosis.

Patrick reported an extensive study of the activity of a large number of enzymes concerned with the degradation of cysteine and cystine in post-mortem liver from children with nephropathic cystinosis and found no metabolic block [141]. The enzymes he studied (Fig. 67-7) included those responsible for the decarboxylation of cysteine sulfinic acid and cysteic acid, the oxidation of cystine and cysteine to inorganic sulfate, and the transamination of cysteine sulfinic acid with α-ketoglutarate, which yields β-sulfinylpyruvic acid which is then "desulfinated" to pyruvic acid and sulfate. All these enzyme systems showed a normal activity in cystinotic liver.

In subsequent studies he was able to show a grossly deficient activity in several enzymes that require reduced sulfhydryl groups for activity (see below) [142].

Intracellular Concentration of Free Cystine

Since histologic examination of cystinotic tissue shows cystine crystals primarily in reticuloendothelial cells, the simplest explanation is that the crystals are first formed extracellularly and are then phagocytized. On the other hand, almost 20 years ago Barr concluded on histologic grounds that the crystals form inside these cells and are not trapped by phagocytosis [46]. This question could be answered definitively by studying the intracellular cystine content of crystal-free cells from patients with cystinosis. Increased intracellular cystine content could lead to crystal formation.

Earlier measurements of cystine content in cystinotic tissue have merely reflected the presence of cystine crystals [1].

Leukocyte Content of Cystine

Mixed populations of peripheral leukocytes from patients with cystinosis were found to contain much more free cystine than normal cells, and thus, they provided the first meaningful biochemical measurement of cystine accumulation in this disease [30]. Cells containing crystals did not withstand the brief exposure to hypotonic solutions used to lyse erythrocytes during the preparation procedure and were, therefore, never observed in the final leukocyte preparations. Furthermore subsequent studies of such leukocyte preparations by electron microscopy have revealed no intracellular crystals [143, 144]. The mean free-cystine (i.e., nonprotein cystine) content of white cells from nine children with nephropathic cystinosis was, nevertheless, 80 times normal and from three patients with benign cystinosis, 30 times normal [30, 45] (Fig. 67-9). Subsequent studies have demonstrated that cystine stores are in the polymorphonuclear leukocytes and macrophages, but not in lymphocytes [145].

In many studies, the leukocyte preparation has been lysed in the presence of an excess of N-ethylmaleimide (NEM) so that both the reduced form, cysteine, as its NEM adduct, as well as cystine might be measured separately. Although a system of analysis that could detect as little as 1 mμmole of the cysteine-NEM derivative was used [69] none was identified in 100 mg (wet weight) of normal or heterozygote cells or in 25 mg of homozygous cells [30]. This was unexpected because cystine transported into other mammalian

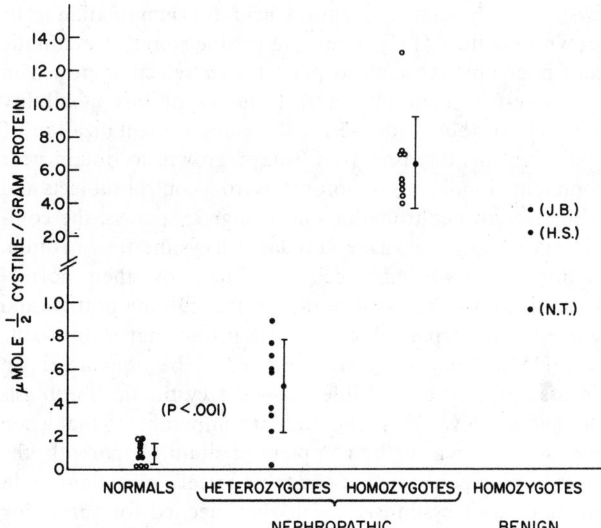

Figure 67-9. Free cystine content of leukocytes in children (o o) and adults (• •) with nephropathic and benign cystinosis. Note the scale change on the ordinate. The brackets indicate ±1 s.d. from the mean. (*Reproduced from Schneider et al.* [45] *with permission of New Eng. J. Med.*)

tissue is found intracellularly primarily in the reduced form [146, 147]. The possibility that the intracellular cysteine may have been leached out of the leukocytes during preparation has not been eliminated. The content of another reduced sulfhydryl compound of larger molecular weight, glutathione, is normal in leukocytes from patients with cystinosis [132].

Transport of Cystine-^{35}S and Cysteine-^{35}S by Leukocytes

Studies of the intracellular transport of cystine-^{35}S and cysteine-^{35}S have shown important differences in normal and cystinotic cells [72]. Cystine-^{35}S was transported into this cell relatively ineffectively by either cystinotic or control leukocytes, but cysteine-^{35}S was well incorporated by both cell populations. The cysteine was kept in its reduced state in the extracellular medium by the use of thiolated Sephadex [148] and was the form actually transported. Under steady state conditions, leukocytes from nine patients with nephropathic cystinosis established a distribution ratio (counts per unit volume intracellular/counts per unit volume extracellular) for ^{35}S of 34 ± 7.7 compared to 21 ± 8.3 in leukocytes from nine age-matched controls ($p < 0.01$). When the intracellular ^{35}S was identified, approximately 30 percent was found in glutathione in both cystinotic and control cells. Whereas only 2 percent of the ^{35}S was found in the oxidized form, cystine, in normal leukocytes, 40 percent was found as cystine in cystinotic cells. When the distribution ratio was recalculated to represent only cysteine-^{35}S, the values were 10 ± 3.2 in cystinotic cells compared to 13 ± 6.9 in normal cells ($p > 0.2$). The large amount of ^{35}S found as cystine-^{35}S in cystinotic cells could have resulted from an inability of these cells to maintain the cysteine ^{35}S in its reduced state, an exchange of half-cystine moieties with the preexisting cystine pool, or a combination of both. Although these data show an enhanced total uptake of cysteine-^{35}S by these cystinotic cells they did not permit a definite conclusion as to whether or not a primary defect in cysteine transport exists in this disease.

Cystine Content of Fibroblasts

Fibroblasts cultured in vitro from skin biopsies of patients with cystinosis and maintained in culture through several generations also contain greatly increased amounts of free cystine [31]. Fibroblasts from patients with either nephropathic or benign cystinosis grow normally and appear normal except that fibroblasts from two of six children with nephropathic cystinosis appeared somewhat larger than normal. Cystine crystals have not been seen in these fibroblasts by either phase or electron microscopy [143]. Yet, fibroblasts from patients with nephropathic cystinosis contain over 100 times the normal content of free cystine, and from patients with benign cystinosis about 50 times the normal free cystine content [31, 45] (Fig. 67-10). These findings suggest that a quantitative biochemical difference underlies the differences in clinical expression of these two variants of cystinosis.

Detection of the Heterozygote

The free-cystine content of peripheral leukocytes and of skin fibroblasts cultured from parents of cystinotic children has provided the first biochemical identification of the heterozygote in this disorder [30, 31]. As shown in Figs. 67-9 and 67-10, the mean intracellular content of free cystine in leukocytes and fibroblasts from obligate heterozygotes for nephropathic cystinosis is five to six times greater than the mean normal value. Although there is occasional overlap between control and heterozygote values, the differences between these groups is statistically significant ($p < 0.001$ for leukocyte values and about 0.01 for fibroblasts values). The fact that the cystine content of heterozygote tissues is substantially less than half that observed in tissues from homozygous patients means that the cystine content is not directly proportional to gene dosage in this recessively inherited disease.

Intracellular Location of Cystine

Cystinotic cells contain large amounts of free cystine in spite of normal activities of the soluble enzyme systems which reduce and further metabolize this amino acid [141]. One explanation for this paradox would be an intracellular compartmentalization of cystine in a location where it is not available to the reductive enzymes. This concept was first

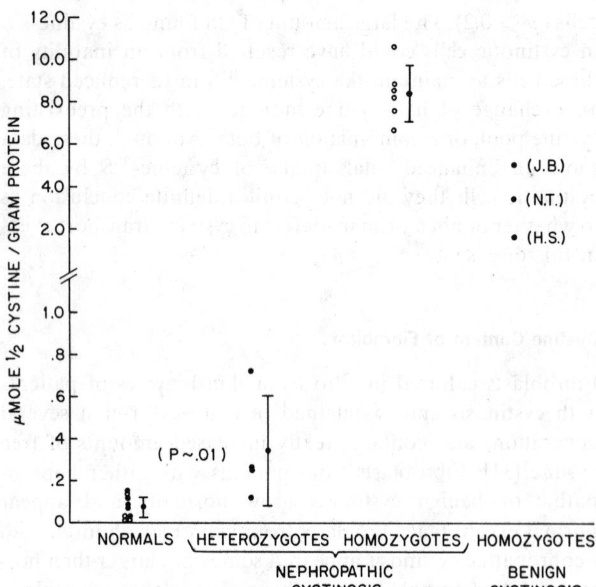

Figure 67-10. Free cystine content of fibroblasts cultured from children (o o) and adults (● ●) with nephropathic and benign cystinosis. Note the scale change on the ordinate. The brackets indicate ±1 s.d. from the mean. (*Reproduced from Schneider et al.* [45] *with permission of New Eng. J. Med.*)

advocated in glycogen storage disease, type II, where no defect in glycogen metabolism was found in studies of whole cell homogenates, but the enzyme defect was demonstrated when isolated lysosomes were studied [149].

To test this hypothesis, lysates of cystinotic leukocytes were separated into nuclear, granular (acid-phosphatase-rich), and soluble fractions, and each fraction was then assayed for cystine (Table 67-3). In white cells from four children with nephropathic cystinosis, 76.7 ± 4.5 percent (mean ± 1 s.d.) of the total free cystine was found in the granular fraction [30]. Similar results were obtained with lysates of cultured skin fibroblasts [31], and in both leukocytes and fibroblasts from patients with benign cystinosis [45]. In fact, these same tissues from parents (obligate heterozygotes) of children with nephropathic cystinosis show similar findings [150]. These studies are difficult to perform in normal tissues because of the extremely small amount of cystine present, but in one experiment 60 percent of the cystine was found in the granular fraction [30].

If the granular fraction of cystinotic leukocytes is treated with a detergent (Triton X-100) before acid precipitation of protein prior to amino acid analysis, the recovery of cystine increases almost twofold [30]. Studies using NEM showed that the new cystine uncovered is all in the oxidized state. Cystine is released from the granular fraction of cystinotic fibroblasts following treatment with Triton X-100, sodium deoxycholate, or hypotonic solution [31]. Thus, in cystinotic cells the cystine appears to be separated from the bulk of the cytoplasm by a lipid-containing membrane.

Further Evidence of the Compartmentalization of Cystine in Cystinosis

Cystine is an essential amino acid for mammalian cells grown in culture [151]. Thus, the cystine stores of cystinotic cells might be expected to permit their selective growth in a cystine-free medium. In fact studies of this possibility provided further evidence for the compartmentalization of cystine in this disease. After 3-days' growth to obtain near confluent monolayers of fibroblasts from control subjects and patients with nephropathic and benign cystinosis, the complete growth media was replaced with a cystine-free medium. Within 24 hr all three cell types had lost their normal attachment to the glass walls of the culture bottles and stained with trypan blue, a dye that does not stain viable cells [152]. Thus, the cells appeared to be nonviable; yet on assay for cystine (Table 67-4) the cystinotic fibroblasts still had an elevated cystine content comparable to that when they were grown in the complete medium. Apparently the large cystine pool was not available to cells of patients with either type of cystinosis, even when needed for sustaining normal metabolism [45].

None of these studies [30, 31, 45] identified the exact site of cystine storage. Although, the fact that cystine was found in the fraction containing acid phosphatase suggested that the cystine is present in lysosomes, this fraction undoubtedly

Table 67-3. SUBCELLULAR FRACTIONATION OF CYSTINOTIC LEUKOCYTES

Fraction	Nephropathic cystinosis				Benign cystinosis			
	Acid phosphatase		*Cystine*		*Acid phosphatase*		*Cystine*	
	μmole ρNP*/ 30 min/ mg prot.	Percent total	μmole half-cystine/ gm prot.	Percent total	μmole ρNP*/ 30 min/ mg prot.	Percent total	μmole half-cystine/ gm prot.	Percent total
Nuclear, 1,000 × g	1.8	0.9	31.8	4.8	11.6	4.3	3.2	9.7
Granular, 27,000 × g	12.5	53.5	59.0	78.8	7.8	40.2	10.2	78.7
Supernatant	2.9	45.6	3.3	16.4	2.3	55.5	0.26	11.6

* ρNP = para-nitrophenylphosphate.
Source: Reproduced in part from Schneider et al. [30] with permission of Science and from Schneider et al. [45] with permission of New Eng. J. Med.

contained mitochondria and other particles as well as lysosomes. In another experiment hypotonicity caused a greater release of cystine than of acid phosphatase from the granular fraction of fibroblasts [31]. This suggested a mitochondrial site for the cystine, since they are more sensitive than lysosomes to such treatment [153]. More recently, careful sucrose-gradient centrifugation studies of cystinotic leukocytes by Schulman et al. showed the cystine to be localized in a fraction rich in lysosomal enzymes and completely separate from the mitochondrial fraction [57]. They also found that there are two lysosomal fractions in leukocytes, a dense one containing the cystine, and a lighter fraction containing most of the acid phosphatase. If there are also two populations of lysosomes in fibroblasts this might explain the results of the hypotonic treatment described above (i.e., the dense lysosomes might be more sensitive to hypotonicity).

Electron Microscopic Studies

Further definition of the subcellular compartment containing cystine has come from electron photomicrographs. In 1962, Jackson, et al. [154], reported electron microscopic studies of kidney tissue from patients with nephropathic cystinosis. They observed cystine crystals in interstitial cells and tubular epithelial cells and described mitochondria which had lost their rodlike form and appeared as swollen, round or oval structures. In addition, they saw vacuolization or swelling of the endoplasmic reticulum and numerous granular cytoplasmic bodies. In 1968, Morecki, et al. [130] reported an electron microscopic study of intestinal mucosa from a child with nephropathic cystinosis. These investigators interpreted their micrographs as showing cystine crystals deposited in altered mitochondria in reticuloendothelial cells of the lamina propria.

In the same year Patrick presented compelling evidence in electron photomicrographs for the presence of cystine crystals within lysosomes [55]. He studied a lymph node from a patient with nephropathic cystinosis and demonstrated intracellular cystine crystals which were enclosed by intact membranes. Using a technique which combined lead deposition with the hydrolysis of the substrate, β-glycerophosphate, he showed the localization of acid phosphatase activity at the periphery of a cystine crystal profile (Fig. 67-5).

Since then, electron microscopic studies of conjunctival mononuclear cells [56, 57, 57a] and rectal mucosal lamina propria [144] have been interpreted as showing microcrystals of cystine in lysosomes. Schulman et al. have incubated conjunctival biopsies with ferritin crystals and electron micrographs have shown that the ingested ferritin particles are

Table 67-4. FREE CYSTINE CONTENT OF FIBROBLASTS WITH AND WITHOUT CYSTINE IN THE GROWTH MEDIUM

Type of cells	Complete medium, μmole half-cystine/ gm protein	Cystine-free medium, μmole half-cystine/ gm protein
Control:		
E.H. (9-year-old girl)	0.07	0.28
Patient with nephropathic cystinosis:		
S.R. (6-year-old girl)	7.5	9.0
Patients with benign cystinosis:		
N.T.	0.96	0.97
J.B.	3.6	4.0

Source: Reproduced from Schneider et al. [45] with permission of the New Eng. J. Med.

localized at the periphery of the cystine crystal profile [56]. The high cystine content of conjunctival biopsy specimens has been used to diagnose cystinosis [154*a*].

Finding a crystal in a particular location does not prove that it crystallized there. Thus, the exact site of cystine accumulation will not be definitely known until the exact biochemical defect, and its intracellular location are known.

Biochemical Interactions of Cystine

As a result of the facile sulfhydryl-disulfide interaction occurring between cystine and sulfhydryl groups, cystine can inhibit many sulfhydryl-dependent enzyme systems. This has several implications in the understanding of this disease. The renal tubular defect in cystinosis could very well result from an inhibition of sulfhydryl-dependent enzyme systems presumably involved in tubular reabsorptive processes. This will be discussed in greater detail below.

The sulfhydryl-disulfide interaction provides an indirect argument for compartmentalization of the cystine pool in cystinotic cells so that it is not in physical contact with cytoplasmic enzymes. Otherwise the 100-fold increase in cystine concentration, with its consequent inhibition of so many enzymes, would probably be incompatible with life. Such considerations also argue against the mitochondria as the site of cystine storage, since many vital mitochondrial enzymes are inhibited by the oxidized form of this amino acid. Finally, one must evaluate the primary enzyme defect in cystinosis with circumspection and be able to prove that a missing enzyme activity is a cause and not a result of the cystine accumulation.

Patrick has reported deficient activities of several sulfhydryl-dependent enzymes in post-mortem liver and kidney tissue from patients with nephropathic cystinosis (Fig. 67-7) [142]. These enzymes included glucose-6-phosphate dehydrogenase, 6-phosphogluconate dehydrogenase, hexokinase, succinate dehydrogenase, alcohol dehydrogenase, and δ-aminolevulinate dehydrase. Other enzymes not dependent on sulfhydryl groups for activity showed either normal activity in the cystinotic tissue or activities in the range found in other tissues subject to chronic inflammation from other causes.

Patrick was able to reproduce these decreases in activity of sulfhydryl-requiring enzymes in control tissues by the addition of cystine, but these changes were quickly corrected by the addition of cysteine. The decreased enzyme activities in cystinotic tissue were in general only partially restored following the addition of cysteine. It is difficult to evaluate fully the possible significance of such findings, especially since the measurements were made in post-mortem tissue that had been chronically involved in the disease process. Activities of glucose-6-phosphate dehydrogenase and 6-phosphogluconate dehydrogenase were virtually absent in leukocyte lysates from patients with nephropathic cystinosis, but both activities were restored to normal following dialysis in a solution of cysteine [136]. Presumably these enzymes have normal activities in the intact cell, but are inhibited by cystine following lysis of the cells and partial release of the compartmentalized cystine.

CLINICAL AND BIOCHEMICAL CORRELATIONS

Other Causes of the Fanconi Syndrome

The multiple causes of the renal Fanconi syndrome (Table 67-1) have encouraged investigators to seek a unifying concept to explain the tubular dysfunction which occurs [3–5, 7, 8, 11]. Many of the agents which cause the renal Fanconi syndrome are known inhibitors of sulfhydryl-requiring enzymes. This is true of the heavy metals, cadmium [155], lead [156–158], uranium [157], mercury [157], copper in Wilson's disease [159–161], maleic acid [162], and cystine [52–54]. Stave and Schlaak produced a generalized amino aciduria and glucosuria in rabbits by feeding them large amounts of cystine [52, 53], and Schwartz-Tiene et al. produced the full triad of amino aciduria, glucosuria, and phosphaturia in rats fed large amounts of cystine [54].

Renal tubular dysfunction has also resulted from apparent intoxication by the aromatic compounds shown in Fig. 67-11. Otten and Vis have recently reported a case of Fanconi syndrome due to methyl-3-chromone, and have drawn attention to the similarity of this compound to tetracycline [163]. Benitz and Diermeier have shown that anhydro-4-epi-tetracycline is the degradation product of tetracycline which is toxic to the renal tubules [164]. In tyrosinemia, *p*-hydroxyphenyllactic acid and *p*-hydroxyphenylpyruvic acid accumulate [165] and are the likely causes of tubular damage. These same compounds accumulate in scurvy since ascorbic acid is required by the enzyme which is lacking in tyrosinemia, *p*-hydroxyphenyl-pyruvic acid oxidase (see Chap. 12). Amino aciduria, but not the full Fanconi syndrome, has been reported in scurvy [166, 167]. This syndrome has also been reported following a "Lysol" burn [a mixture of meta, ortho, and para cresol) [168].

To our knowledge, none of these aromatic compounds is an inhibitor of sulfhydryl enzymes, but they all have some similarity in structure to *p*-benzoquinone (also illustrated in Fig. 67-11), and the quinones are well-known inhibitors of sulfhydryl-requiring enzymes [169].

In galactosemia (see Chap. 8), glycogen storage disease (see Chap. 7), and hereditary fructose intolerance (see Chap. 6) the accumulated (and presumably toxic) product is known but the mechanism by which these products cause tubular damage is not. In Lowe's syndrome [170] and in idiopathic Fanconi syndrome the nature of a toxic substance (if any) is also, of course, unknown. In the human kidney allograft the tubular damage may be related to the rejection phenomenon [192, 193]. Renal tubular damage is a known consequence of multiple myeloma, and so it is not surprising

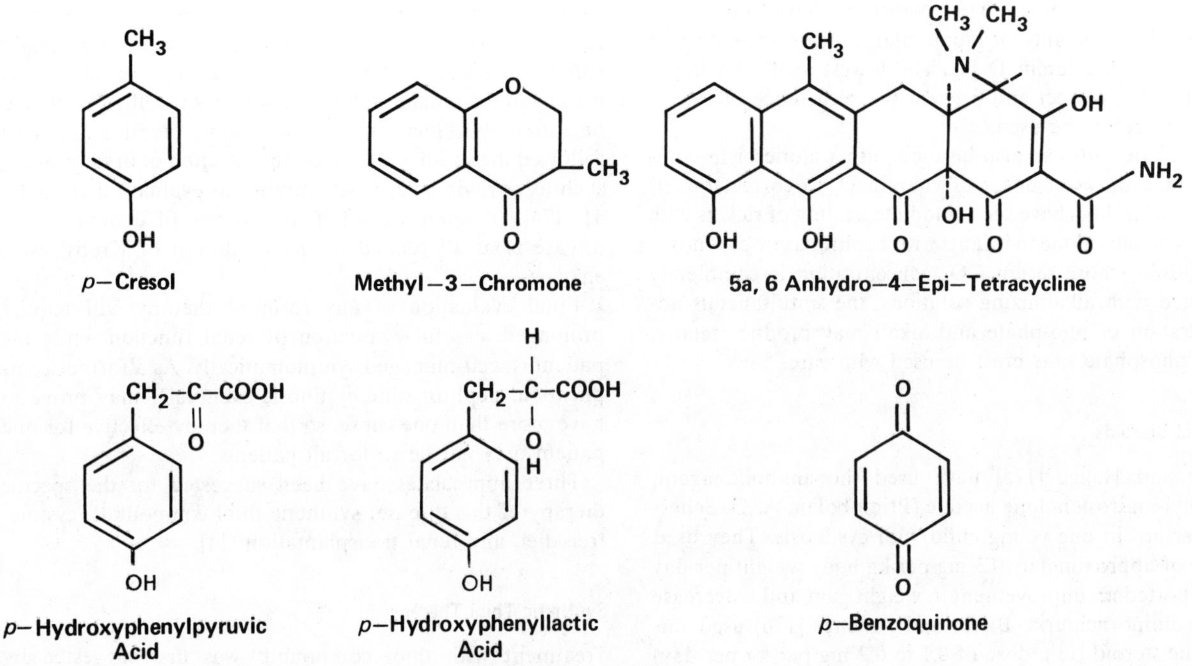

Figure 67-11. Aromatic compounds which may produce the renal Fanconi syndrome.

that occasional patients with this disease demonstrate the Fanconi syndrome [171–173]. Since all patients with the renal Fanconi syndrome excrete excessive amounts of L chains from immunoglobulins [40], care must be taken in establishing the diagnosis of multiple myeloma in an adult patient who presents with the Fanconi syndrome.

The occasional finding of an elevation of the blood pyruvate concentration in cystinosis [35, 41] could be the result of several different types of metabolic abnormalities. The fair complexion and hair of children with nephropathic cystinosis probably results from an inhibition of melanin production by cystine, but no direct biochemical evidence of such an interference is available. The organic aciduria which occurs in nephropathic cystinosis, in addition to the amino aciduria, may result from a combination of elevated blood concentrations and defective renal tubular reabsorption of these acids. Schärer and Antener have recently reviewed the possible causes of organic aciduria in this disorder [9].

TREATMENT

Symptomatic Treatment

The symptomatic treatment of nephropathic cystinosis consists of providing an adequate fluid intake, correcting the metabolic acidosis and potassium deficit, and healing the rickets. In most patients this is readily accomplished and results in a salutary improvement in the child's personality, eating, activity, and "general well-being." When under proper therapy, these children tolerate the usual infectious diseases of childhood very well.

Patients with benign cystinosis, of course, require no therapy.

Correction of the Metabolic Acidosis and Hypokalemia

The acidosis and hypokalemia are most easily corrected by the use of a potassium-containing alkalinizing mixture such as a solution of sodium and potassium citrate [3]. The authors have used the commercially available preparation Polycitra (Willen Drug Company, Baltimore) which contains 2.0 gm citric acid, 3.0 gm sodium citrate, and 3.3 gm potassium citrate per 30 ml. This preparation is well tolerated and provides 1 mEq sodium and 1 mEq potassium per ml. The average dosage is 45 ml to 60 ml per day. In some patients, as in the two cases reported by Worthen and Good [4], the serum concentration of bicarbonate cannot be raised above 20 mEq per liter regardless of the amount of alkalinizing solution used, but in other patients the serum bicarbonate concentration can be completely corrected. On this therapy the serum potassium concentration usually remains at a low normal level or slightly less, but no signs of hypokalemia, such as ECG changes, are present.

Correction of Rickets

In most patients the skeletal changes are readily corrected with doses of 10,000 to 15,000 units per day of vitamin D (ergocalciferol, vitamin D_2). Worthen and Good have stressed the possibility of glomerular damage secondary to large doses of vitamin D [4]. The lowest dose of vitamin D which will correct and prevent the recurrence of rickets should therefore be used.

Phosphate salts can also be used, either alone or in combination with lower doses of vitamin D, to correct rickets [174]. The authors have seen complete healing of rickets with phosphate salts alone in infants with nephropathic cystinosis. In children whose serum CO_2 concentration is completely corrected with alkalinizing solutions, the simultaneous administration of phosphate and alkali may produce tetany. Thus, phosphate salts must be used with care.

Anabolic Steroids

Weber and Hagge [175] have used the anabolic agent, 1-methyl-androstenolone acetate (Primobolan, A. G. Schering, Berlin), in one young child with cystinosis. They used a dose of approximately 0.3 mg per kg body weight per day and reported an improvement in weight gain and a decrease in the amino aciduria. Bauer and Antener [176] used this anabolic steroid (in a dose of 0.1 to 0.2 mg per kg per day) in a patient who seemed to do well while on a low-cystine diet. This treatment is claimed to improve the appetite and strength of the children. We have had no experience with these steroids and are of the opinion that patients whose electrolyte imbalance is well controlled do well without additional agents.

Specific Therapy

Attempts at specific therapy for nephropathic cystinosis have been difficult to evaluate for three reasons. First, there has not been a specific, objective parameter in evaluating therapy. Next, these children often show much improvement including improved glomerular function [136] with only symptomatic therapy. Finally, the natural course of the disease is not uniform, and some patients may go several years without a further decrease in glomerular function in the absence of any specific therapy.

Ideally, a successful therapeutic regimen would rid these children of their cystine stores. The recent findings of increased amounts of free cystine in tissue containing no cystine crystals should provide the best measurement of cystine accumulation and be helpful in evaluating therapy. Lacking an actual decrease in cystine storage, therapy might still be effective if it protected the actual site of cystine toxicity in the renal tubular and glomerular cells. This would be extremely difficult to evaluate. Some investigators have followed the serum and urine concentration of organic acids, such as pyruvic acid, in attempting to evaluate therapy [9, 41, 176]. It is not known if the toxicity of cystine in this disease is at all related to the inhibition of Krebs' cycle enzymes.

Final evaluation of any form of therapy will require prolonged, careful evaluation of renal function while the patient is well-managed symptomatically. As a further complication, nephropathic cystinosis eventually may prove to have more than one cause, so that therapy effective for one patient may not be so for all patients.

Three approaches have been suggested for the specific therapy of this disease: synthetic thiol compounds, cystine-free diet, and renal transplantation [11].

Synthetic Thiol Therapy

Treatment with thiol compounds was first suggested by Clayton and Patrick [41], who tried both dimercaprol (BAL) and penicillamine (β,β-dimethyl cysteine) in the hope of reactivating or maintaining thiol-dependent enzyme systems. They found that both drugs lowered the blood pyruvate concentration and each of their three patients showed an improvement in general well-being and one began to gain weight coincident with therapy. Since then most investigators have used D-penicillamine, which is less toxic than its L isomer. Schärer and Antener [9] found that penicillamine decreased the urinary pyruvate excretion to near-normal levels in this disease, but Bauer and Antener [176] reported that the pyruvate excretion increased when penicillamine was given. Crawhall et al. [35] treated four patients with high doses of D-penicillamine (200 to 400 mg per day) for 9 months to 3½ years. None showed any clinical improvement. Only one of the four children had an elevated blood pyruvate concentration. Although this child's blood pyruvate concentration decreased to normal, renal glomerular function worsened and she died after approximately 2 years' treatment with D-penicillamine. This drug reduced the fasting plasma concentration of free cystine by about one-half (Table 67-5), but did not lower the leukocyte content of free cystine [11]. Although both penicillamine and its mixed

Table 67-5. EFFECT OF THERAPY ON FASTING PLASMA CYSTINE CONCENTRATION IN NEPHROPATHIC CYSTINOSIS

	No. of patients	Before, μmole half-cystine/100 ml plasma ± 1 s.d.	After, μmole half-cystine/100 ml plasma ± 1 s.d.
D-penicillamine, 200–400 mg/day	3	7.46 ± 1.64	3.77 ± 0.77 ($p < 0.05$)
Cystine-free diet	4	6.78 ± 1.09	2.61 ± 1.03 ($p < 0.01$)

disulfide with cysteine are easily identified in the ion-exchange chromatographic technique used for measurement of cystine [69, 146] neither compound was ever detected in the leukocytes from patients treated with this drug. Thus, we are not certain that D-penicillamine even enters the body cells. Hambraeus and Broberger [177] were also unable to demonstrate clinical improvement with this drug.

A promising new approach to treatment has been suggested by the observation of Goldman et al. that dithiothreitol is an effective drug for the lowering of intracellular cystine in fibroblasts cultured from a patient with cystinosis [65]. The full clinical assessment of its efficacy remains to be determined.

Dietary Therapy

Treatment with a cystine-free diet was first suggested by Linneweh [6] and Schärer and Antener [9]. The latter investigators used lentils as the protein source and were able to provide a diet containing 20 mg methionine and 10 mg cystine per kg body weight per day for their 2-year-old patient. Evaluation of their study is complicated by their use of an anabolic steroid (1-methyl-androstenolone acetate, 0.1 to 0.2 mg per kg body weight per day). The clinical condition improved, and the child grew 8 cm in length and gained 2.5 kg during the 9 months of therapy. The endogenous creatinine clearance rose from 20 to 33 ml per min per 1.73 m^2. Meanwhile the corneal crystal deposits also appeared to regress. This is difficult to understand since the corneal crystals in this disease may not be cystine crystals [37]. Recently, Seip et al. [178] have treated two brothers with the same diet and reported an improvement in well-being after 8 months of treatment.

A completely synthetic diet given to four children with nephropathic cystinosis at age 3, 4, 10, and 21 months, contained a mixture of L-amino acids and no protein [11]. It supplied no cystine and 44 mg methionine per kg body weight per day, which is the minimum requirement for infants [179]. Although this diet reduced the fasting plasma concentration of free cystine (Table 67-5) it effected no clinical improvement and did not decrease the leukocyte content of free cystine.

Renal Transplantation

Since the primary abnormality leading to renal failure in cystinosis appears to be a genetically determined defect of the intracellular environment, most likely involving lysosomes, cells without this genetic defect transplanted into a cystinotic patient should not accumulate cystine. Therefore, a cystinotic child should be as good a candidate for renal transplantation as any other child with chronic renal disease.

To our knowledge, three medical centers have now accumulated extensive experience on kidney transplantation in patients with nephropathic cystinosis [180–182]. Six patients have been followed for 8 to 32 months after transplantation. The authors know of two other cases in which the recipient died within a few months after transplantation from causes unrelated to cystinosis. None of the six children developed recurrence of the complete Fanconi syndrome and all have benefited from the procedure. Although these children had been in terminal renal failure at the time of transplantation, two now have endogenous creatinine clearances of 30 to 40, one of 66, and three of over 100 ml per min per 1.73 m^2. Two of the patients have had an accelerated rejection phenomenon. One of these has mild proteinuria and amino aciduria, and both have mild hypertension which was not present before transplantation [182]. Both had parent (obligate heterozygote) donors. Three of the other four children also had parent donors, but did not have unusual rejection problems. Two of the six patients had growth spurts after transplantation [180, 183], but this is difficult to evaluate since all six were kept on immunosuppressive regimens which might be expected to prevent growth.

Surprisingly, cystine appears to accumulate in donor kidneys. Serial renal biopsies of the donor kidneys have demonstrated the gradual appearance of cystine crystals in the interstitial regions of the kidney, but not in tubular epithelial cells, and only in one instance in glomerular cells [180, 182]. This accumulation of cystine crystals is also demonstrated by an increase in the free cystine content of donor kidney [180, 181]. In the one child who received a kidney from an unrelated donor, the free cystine content of the donor kidney was 10 times normal in a biopsy obtained 5 months after transplantation. It is possible that the crystal-containing cells are of host origin and migrated into the donor kidney as part of the mononuclear cell infiltration frequently observed in allografts.

At present, renal transplantation for patients in the terminal stages of nephropathic cystinosis appears to be a justifiable therapeutic procedure. The long-term follow-up of such patients promises to provide useful information which should aid in the eventual complete understanding of cystinosis.

SUMMARY

1 Cystinosis is a recessively inherited metabolic disorder characterized biochemically by an abnormally high intracellular content of free cystine which results in cystine crystal deposition in the conjunctiva, bone marrow, lymph nodes, leukocytes, and internal organs. There are at least three forms of this disease. The nephropathic form has been the most thoroughly studied. Children with this form of cystinosis present in the first year of life with the renal tubular defects characteristic of the Fanconi syndrome, and also have progressive renal glomerular damage which leads to death in uremia before ten years of age. Other patients have a completely benign form of cystinosis, and are only discovered when an ophthalmological examination is done for another reason and reveals characteristic crystalline opacities in the cornea and conjunctiva. Finally, some patients have an intermediate type of cystinosis characterized by less severe renal disease than occurs in the nephropathic variety.

2 A characteristic lesion in the peripheral retina, a patchy depigmentation, is found consistently in the nephropathic form, but never in the benign form. It has been found in some, but not all, patients with the intermediate form of cystinosis. This lesion was detectable in a 5-week-old infant with nephropathic cystinosis.

3 The renal defects in nephropathic cystinosis are probably caused by the large intracellular accumulation of free cystine. Cystine is known to inhibit many sulfhydryl-requiring enzymes, but the cystinotic cell has some protection because this amino acid is compartmentalized in these cells, and thus separated from other cellular enzymes. Both electron microscopic studies and sucrose gradient centrifugation studies of cystinotic tissues have identified the intracellular site of cystine storage as the lysosome. The exact mechanism leading to this storage, and the identity of the abnormal gene product, are not known.

4 The symptomatic management of patients with nephropathic cystinosis is usually uncomplicated, but attempts at specific therapy have been unsuccessful. Renal transplantation has been life-saving in several children, but must still be considered an experimental procedure.

BIBLIOGRAPHY

1. Bickel, H., Baar, H. S., Astley, R., Douglas, A. A., Finch, E., Harris, H., Harvey, C. C., Hickmans, E. M., Philpott, M. G., Smallwood, W. C., Smellie, J. M., and Teall, C. G.: Cystine storage disease with aminoaciduria and dwarfism (Lignac-Fanconi Disease). Acta Paediat., **42(suppl. 90),** 1, 1952.
2. Dent, C. E., and Harris, H.: Hereditary forms of rickets and osteomalacia. J. Bone Joint Surgery, **38B,** 204, 1956.
3. Harrison, H. E.: The Fanconi Syndrome. J. Chronic Dis., **7,** 346, 1958.
4. Worthen, H. G., and Good, R. A.: The de Toni-Fanconi Syndrome with cystinosis. A.M.A. J. Dis. Child., **95,** 653, 1958.
5. Mudge, G. H.: Clinical patterns of tubular dysfunction. Amer. J. Med., **24,** 785, 1958.
6. Linneweh, F.: Storüngen des Aminosauren-Stoffwechsels, in *Erbliche Stoffwechselkrankheiten,* edited by F. Linneweh, p. 141, Urban and Schwarzenberg, Munich, 1962.
7. Bickel, H.: Proximal tubular defects, in *Renal Disease,* edited by D. A. K. Black, p. 347, Blackwell, Oxford, 1962 or F. A. Davis Co., Philadelphia, 1964.
8. Milne, M. D.: Renal tubular dysfunction, in *Diseases of the Kidney,* edited by M. B. Strauss & L. G. Welt, p. 786, Little, Brown, Boston, 1963.
9. Schärer, K., and Antener, I.: Zur Biochemie und Therapie der Cystinose. Ann. Paediat., **203 (suppl. 1),** 1, 1964.
10. Leaf, A.: The syndrome of osteomalacia, renal glycosuria, aminoaciduria, and increased phosphorus clearance (The Fanconi Syndrome), in *Metabolic Basis of Inherited Disease,* edited by J. B. Stanbury, J. B. Wyngaarden, and D. S. Fredrickson, 2nd ed., p. 1205, McGraw-Hill, New York, 1966.
11. Seegmiller, J. E., Friedmann, T., Harrison, H. E., Wong, V., and Schneider, J. A.: Cystinosis, Combined Clinical Staff Conference at the National Institutes of Health, Ann. Intern. Med., **68,** 883, 1968.
12. Abderhalden, F.: Familiare Cystindiathese. Z. Physiol. Chem., **38,** 557, 1903.
13. Lignac, G. O. E.: Stooris der cystine-stofwisseling byj Kinderen. Nederl. T. Geneesk., **68,** 2987, 1924.
14. Lignac, G. O. E.: Uber Storung des Cystinstoffwechsels bei Kindern. Deutsch. Arch. Klin. Med., **145,** 139, 1924.
15. Russell, D. S., and Barrie, H. J.: Storage of cystine in the reticuloendothelial system and its association with chronic nephritis and renal rickets. Lancet, **2,** 899, 1936.
16. Beumer, H.: Über die Cystinkrankheit. Mschr. Kinderheilk., **68,** 251, 1937.
17. Dent, C. E., and Harris, H.: The Genetics of 'Cystinuria'. Ann. Eugenics, **16,** 60, 1951.
18. Fanconi, G.: Die nicht diabetischen Glykosurien und Hyperglykämien des ältern Kindes: Jahrb. Kinderh., **133,** 257, 1931.
19. deToni, G.: Remarks on the relations between renal rickets (renal dwarfism) and renal diabetes. Acta Paediat., **16,** 479, 1933.
20. Debré, R., Marie, J., Clétet, F., and Messimy, R.: Rachitisme tardif coexistent avec une néphrite chronique et une glycosurie. Arch. Méd. Enf., **37,** 597, 1934.
21. Fanconi, G.: Der nephrotisch-glykosurische Zwergwuchs mit hypophosphatämischer Rachitis. Deutsch Med. Wschr., **62,** 1169, 1936.
22. Fanconi, G.: Der fruhinfantile nephrotisch-glykosurische Zwergwuchsmit hypophosphatämischer Rachitis. Jahrb. Kinderh., **147,** 299, 1936.
23. Beumer, H., and Wepler, W.: Über die Cystinkrankheit der Ersten Lebenszeit. Klin. Wschr., **16,** 8, 1937.
24. Fanconi, G., and Bickel, H.: Die chronische Aminoacidurie (Aminosäurediabetes oder nephrotisch-glukosurischer Zwergwuchs) bei der Glykogenose und der Cystinkrankheit. Helv. Paediat. Acta., **4,** 359, 1949.
25. Wallis, L. A., and Engle, R. L., Jr.: The adult Fanconi syndrome. II. Review of eighteen cases. Amer. J. Med., **22,** 13, 1957.
26. Cogan, D. G., Kuwabara, T., Hurlbut, C. S., Jr., and McMurray, V.: Further observations on cystinosis in the adult. J.A.M.A., **166,** 1725, 1958.
27. Cogan, D. G., Kuwabara, T., Kinoshita, J., Sheehan, L., and Merola, L.: Cystinosis in an adult. J.A.M.A., **164,** 394, 1957.
28. Lietman, P. S., Frazier, P. D., Wong, V. G., Shotton, D., and Seegmiller, J. E.: Adult cystinosis—a benign disorder. Amer. J. Med., **40,** 511, 1966.
29. Brubaker, R. F., Wong, V. G., Schulman, J. D., Seegmiller, J. E., and Kuwabara, T.: Benign cystinosis: the clinical, biochemical and morphologic findings in a family with two affected siblings. Amer. J. Med. **49,** 546, 1970.
30. Schneider, J. A., Bradley, K., and Seegmiller, J. E.: Increased cystine in leukocytes from individuals homozygous and heterozygous for cystinosis. Science, **157,** 1321, 1967.
31. Schneider, J. A., Rosenbloom, F. M., Bradley, K. H., and Seegmiller, J. E.: Increased free-cystine content of fibroblasts cultured from patients with cystinosis. Biochem. Biophys. Res. Commun., **29,** 527, 1967.
32. Wong, V. G., Lietman, P. S., and Seegmiller, J. E.: Alterations of pigment epithelium in cystinosis. Arch. Ophthal; **77,** 361, 1967.
33. Bickel, H.: Die Entwicklung der biochemischen Läsion bei der Lignac-Fanconischen Krankheit. Helv. Paediat. Acta, **10,** 259, 1955.
34. Schneider, J. A., Wong, V., and Seegmiller, J. E.: The early diagnosis of cystinosis. J. Pediat., **74,** 114, 1969.
35. Crawhall, J. C., Lietman, P. S., Schneider, J. A., and Seegmiller, J. E.: Cystinosis: plasma cystine and cysteine concentrations and the effect of D-penicillamine and dietary treatment. Amer. J. Med., **44,** 330, 1968.
36. Burki, V. E.: Über die Cystinkrankheit im Klienkindesalter unter besonderer Berücksichtigung des Augenbefundes. Ophthalmologica, **101,** 257, 1941.
37. Frazier, P. D., and Wong, V. G.: Cystinosis: histologic and crystallographic examination of crystals in eye tissues. Arch. Ophthal. (Chicago), **80,** 87, 1968.
38. Burki, V. E.: Über Hornhautveranderungen bei einem Fall von multiplem Myelom (Plasmocytom). Ophthalmologica (Basel), **135,** 565, 1958.
39. McCune, D. J., Mason, H. H., and Clarke, H. T.: Intractable hypophosphatemic rickets with renal glycosuria and acidosis (the Fanconi syndrome). Amer. J. Dis. Child., **65,** 81, 1943.
40. Waldmann, T. A., and Strober, W.: Metabolism of immunoglobulins. Progr. Allergy **13,** 89, 1969.

41. Clayton, B. E., and Patrick, A. D.: Use of dimercaprol or penicillamine in the treatment of cystinosis. Lancet, **2,** 909, 1961.
42. deToni, G., and Durand, P.: Guarigione clinica del drabete renale e del rachitismo renale in un grave caso di sindrome di Toni-Debré Fanconi giunto all'eta'adulta con persistenza del nanismo e della iper-aminoaciduria. Minerva Pediat., **7,** 1053, 1955.
43. Linder, G. C., Bull. G. M., and Grayce, I.: Hypophosphatemic glycosuric rickets (Fanconi syndrome). 1. A study of the acid-base balance and amino acid excretion. Report of a case with retinitis pigmentosa. Clinical Proc. J. Cape Town Post-Grad Med. Assn., **8,** 1, 1949.
44. Weber, V. H.: Beitrag zur Frage der Nierenfunktionsstörung bei Cystinosis. Helv. Paediat. Acta, **8,** 348, 1953.
45. Schneider, J. A., Wong, V., Bradley, K. H., and Seegmiller, J. E.: Biochemical comparisons of the adult and childhood forms of cystinosis. New Eng. J. Med., **279,** 1253, 1968.
46. Barr, H. S.: Pathologie des Aminosäuren-Diabetes. Mschr. Kinderheilk., **99,** 35, 1951.
47. Clay, R. D., Darmady, E. M., and Hawkins, M.: The nature of the renal lesion in Fanconi syndrome. J. Path. Bact., **65,** 551, 1953.
48. Giles, H. McC., Pugh, R. C. B., Darmady, E. M., Stranack, F., and Woolf, L. I.: The nephrotic syndrome in early infancy: A report of three cases. Arch. Dis. Child., **32,** 167, 1957.
49. Darmady, E. M., Offer, J. M., and Stranack, F.: Study of renal vessels by microdissection in human transplantation. Brit. Med. J., **2,** 976, 1964.
50. Darmady, E. M., Dempster, W. J., and Stranack, F.: The evolution of interstitial and tubular changes in homotransplanted kidneys. J. Path. Bact., **70,** 225, 1955.
51. Darmady, E. M.: The renal changes in some metabolic diseases in *The Kidney,* p. 253, edited by F. K. Mostofi and D. E. Smith. Williams & Wilkins, Baltimore, 1966.
52. Stave, U.: Aminosäuren-Verfütterung and Tubulusschaden. II. Mitteilung. Die tubuläre Funktion nach Cystine-Verfütterung bei Kaninchen. Z. Kinderheilk., **78,** 275, 1956.
53. Stave, U., and Schlaak, E.: Aminosäuren-Verfütterung und Tubulusschaden. I. Mitteilung. Aminoacidurie nach Cystine-Verfütterung bei Kaninchen. Z. Kinderheilk., **78,** 261, 1956.
54. Schwarz-Tiene, E., Careddu, P., and Cabassa, N.: Alterazioni funzionali e anatomiche renali nella intossicazione sperimentale da cistina. Minerva Pediat., **9,** 239, 1957.
55. Patrick, A. D., and Lake, B. D.: Cystinosis: Electron microscopic evidence of lysosomal storage of cystine in lymph node. J. Clin. Path., **21,** 571, 1968.
56. Schulman, J. D., Wong, V., Olson, W. H., and Seegmiller, J. E.: Lysosomal site of crystalline deposits in cystinosis as shown by ferritin uptake. Arch. Path., **90,** 259, 1970.
57. Schulman, J. D., Bradley, K. H., and Seegmiller, J. E.: Cystine: Compartmentalization within lysosomes in cystinotic leukocytes. Science, **166,** 1152, 1969.
57a. Wong, V. G., Kuwabara, T., Brubaker, R., Olson, W., Schulman, J., and Seegmiller, J. E.: Intralysosomal cystine crytals in cystinosis. Invest. Ophthal., **9,** 83, 1970.
58. Sano, K.: Solubility of amino acids with changes of pH. Biochem. Z., **168,** 14, 1926.
59. Smith, D. R., Kolb, F. O., and Harper, H. A.: Management of cystinuria and cystine-stone disease. J. Urol. **81,** 61, 1959.
60. Eldjarn, L., and Pihl, A.: Equilibrium constants and oxidation—reduction potentials of some thiol-disulfide systems. J. Amer. Chem. Soc., **79,** 4589, 1957.
61. Jocelyn, P. C.: The standard redox potential of cysteine—cystine from the thioldisulphide exchange reaction with glutathione and lipoic acid. Europ. J. Biochem., **2,** 327, 1967.
62. Clark, W. M.: *Oxidation-reduction Potentials of Organic Systems.* p. 471, Williams & Wilkins, Baltimore, 1960.
63. Gorin, G., and Doughty, G.: Equilibrium constants for the reaction of glutathione with cystine and their relative oxidation-reduction potentials. Arch. Biochem. Biophys., **126,** 547, 1968.
64. Crawhall, J. C., Scowen, E. F., and Watts, R. W. E.: Effect of penicillamine on cystinuria. Brit. Med. J., **1,** 588, 1963.
65. Goldman, H., Scriver, C. R., Aaron, K., and Pinsky, L.: Use of dithiothreitol to correct cystine storage in cultured cystinotic fibroblasts. Lancet, **1,** 811, 1970.
66. Sullivan, M. X., and Hess, W. C.: The determination of cystine in urine. J. Biol. Chem., **116,** 221, 1936.
67. Ellman, G. L.: Tissue sulfhydryl groups. Arch. Biochem. Biophys., **82,** 70, 1959.
68. Moore, S., Spackman, D. H., and Stein, W. H.: Chromatography of amino acids on sulfonated polystyrene resins; an improved system. Anal. Chem., **30,** 1185, 1958.
69. Crawhill, J. C., Thompson, C. J., and Bradley, K. H.: Separation of cystine, penicillamine disulphide and cysteine-penicillamine mixed disulphide by automatic amino acid analysis. Anal. Biochem., **14,** 405, 1966.
70. Roston, S.: Determination of cysteine. Anal. Biochem., **6,** 486, 1963.
71. Schneider, J. A., Bradley, K. H., and Seegmiller, J. E.: Colorimetric assay of cystine using noradrenochrome. Anal. Biochem., **23,** 129, 1968.
72. Schneider, J. A., Bradley, K. H., and Seegmiller, J. E.: Transport and intracellular fate of cysteine-^{35}S in leukocytes from normal subjects and patients with cystinosis. Pediat. Res., **2,** 441, 1968.
73. Smith, I., Ed.: *Chromatographic and Electrophoretic Techniques,* 2 vol., Interscience publishers, New York, 1960.
74. Brand, E., Cahill, G. F., and Harris, M. M.: Cystinuria, II. The metabolism of cystine, cysteine, methionine and glutathione. J. Biol. Chem., **109,** 69, 1935.
75. Reed, L. J., Cavallini, D., Plum, F., Rachele, J. R., and du Vigneaud. V.: The conversion of methionine to cystine in a human cystinuric. J. Biol. Chem., **180,** 783, 1949.
76. Stetten, De W. Jr.: The fate of dietary serine in the body of the rat. J. Biol. Chem., **144,** 501, 1942.
77. Brand, E., Cahill, G. F., and Block, R. J.: Cystinuria, IV. The metabolism of homocysteine and homocystine. J. Biol. Chem., **110,** 399, 1935.
78. Brand, E., Block, R. J., Kassell, B., and Cahill, G. F.: Carboxymethylcystine metabolism, its implications on therapy in cystinuria and on methionine-cysteine relationship. Proc. Soc. Exp. Biol. Med., **35,** 501, 1936.
79. Anslow, W. P., Jr., Simmonds, S., and du Vigneaud, V.: The synthesis of the isomers of cystathionine and a study of their availability in sulfur metabolism. J. Biol. Chem., **166,** 35, 1946.
80. Dent, C. E.: Partition chromatography on paper as applied to investigation of amino acids and peptides in normal and pathological urines. Biochem. J., **40** (4), XLIV, 1946.
81. Dent, C. E.: Methionine metabolism and α-aminobutyric acid. Science. **105,** 335, 1947.
82. Tallan, H. H., Moore, S., and Stein, W. H.: L-cystathionine in human brain. J. Biol. Chem., **230,** 707, 1958.
83. Eagle, H., Piez, K. A., and Oyama, V. I.: The biosynthesis of cystine in human cell cultures. J. Biol. Chem., **236,** 1425, 1961.
84. Uhlendorf, B. W., and Mudd, S. H.: Cystathionine synthase in tissue culture derived from human skin. Enzyme defect in homocystinuria. Science, **160,** 1007, 1968.
85. Matsuo Y., and Greenberg, D. M.: A crystalline enzyme that cleaves homoserine and cystathione, I. Isolation procedure and some physiochemical properties. J. Biol. Chem., **230,** 545, 1958.
86, Matsuo, Y., and Greenberg, D. M.: A crystalline enzyme that cleaves homoserine and cystathionine, Ill. Coenzyme resolution, activators, and inhibitors. J. Biol. Chem., **234,** 507, 1959.
87. Keller, E. B., Rachele, J. R., and du Vigneaud, V.: A study of transmethylation with methionine containing deuterium and ^{14}C in the methyl group. J. Biol. Chem., **177,** 733, 1949.
88. Cantoni, G. L.: *Phosphorous Metabolism,* edited by W. D. McElroy, and B. Glass, vol. I, p. 641, Johns Hopkins, Baltimore, 1951.
89. Cantoni, G. L.: Activation of methionine for transmethylation. J. Biol. Chem. **189,** 745, 1951.
90. Cantoni, G. L.: Methylation of nicotinamide with a soluble enzyme system from rat liver. J. Biol. Chem., **189,** 203, 1951.
91. Schlossmann, K., Brüggemann, J., and Lynen, F.: Biosynthese des Cysteins, I. Nachweis and Isolierung der Serinsulfhydrase aus Bächerhefe. Biochem. Z., **336,** 258, 1962.

92. Schlossmann, K., and Lynen, F.: Biosynthese des Cysteins aus Serin und Schwefelwasserstoff. Biochem. Z. **328,** 591, 1957.
93. Becker, M. A., Kredich, N. M., and Tomkins, G. M.: The purification and characterization of O-acetylserine sulfhydrase-A from salmonella typhimurium. J. Biol. Chem., **244,** 2418, 1969.
94. Sentenae, A., and Fromageot, P.: La Sérinehydrolyase de L'oiseau mise, an évidence dans l'embryon et Mécanisme d'action. Biochim. Biophys., Acta, **81,** 289, 1964.
95. Brüggemann, J., Schlossman, K., Merkenschlager, M., and Waldschmidt, M.: Zur Frage des Vorkommens der Serinsulfhydrase. Biochem. Z., **335,** 392, 1962.
96. Keilin, D.: Cytochrome and intracellular oxidase. Proc. Roy. Soc. [Biol.],
97. Nickerson, W. J., and Romano, A. H.: Enzymatic reduction of cystine by coenzyme I (DPNH). Science, **115,** 676, 1952.
98. Romano, A. H., and Nickerson, W. J.: Cystine reductase of pea seeds and yeasts. J. Biol. Chem., **208,** 409, 1954.
99. Worthen, H. G., and Good, R. A.: The pathogenesis of cystinosis. Amer. J. Dis. Child., **102,** 494, 1961.
100. Mize, C. E., and Langdon, R. G.: Hepatic glutathione reductase: I Purification and general kinetic properties. J. Biol. Chem., **237,** 1589, 1962.
101. Mize, C. E., Thompson, T. E., and Langdon, R. G.: Hepatic glutathione reductase: II. Physical properties and mechanism of action. J. Biol. Chem. **237,** 1596, 1962.
102. Black, S.: The biochemistry of sulfur containing compounds. Ann. Rev. Biochem., **32,** 399, 1963.
103. Seegmiller, J. E.: Unpublished observations.
104. Tarr, H. L. A.: The enzymic formation of hydrogen sulfide by certain heterotrophic bacteria. Biochem. J., **27,** 1869, 1933.
105. Fromageot, C., Wookey, E., and Chaix, P.: Sur la dégradation anaérobie de la cystéine par la désulfurase du foie. Enzymologia, **9,** 198, 1940.
106. Fromageot, C.: Oxidation of organic sulfur in animals. Advances Enzym., **7,** 369, 1947.
107. Fromageot, C.: *The Enzymes;* edited by J. B. Sumner, and K. Myrbäck, Vol. 2, p. 248, Academic, New York, 1951.
108. Smythe, C. V.: Some enzyme reactions of S compounds and their possible interrelationships. Ann. N.Y. Acad. Sci., **45,** 425, 1944.
109. Smythe, C. V., and Halliday, D.: An enzymatic conversion of radioactive sulfide sulfur to cysteine sulfur. J. Biol. Chem., **144,** 237, 1942.
110. Meister, A., Fraser, P. E., and Tice, S. V.: Enzymatic desulfuration of B-mercaptopyruvate to pyruvate. J. Biol. Chem., **206,** 561, 1954.
111. Binkley, F.: Synthesis of cystathionine by preparations from rat liver. J. Biol. Chem., **191,** 531, 1951.
112. Flavin, M.: Microbial transsulfuration: The mechanism of an enzymatic disulfide elimination reaction. J. Biol. Chem., **237,** 768, 1962.
113. Meister, A.: *Biochemistry of the Amino Acids,* 2d ed. Academic, New York, 1965.
114. Bennett, M. A.: Metabolism of sulfur. V. The replaceability of *l*-cystine in the diets of rats with some partially oxidized derivatives. Biochem. J., **31,** 962, 1937.
115. Singer, T. P., and Kearney, E. B.: Enzymatic pathways in the degradation of sulfur-containing amino acids. In *Amino Acid Mėtabolism,* edited by W. D. McElroy and H. B. Glass, p. 558, Johns Hopkins, Baltimore, 1955.
116. Kearney, E. B., and Singer, T. P.: Enzymic transformations of L-cysteine sulfinic acid. Biochim. Biophys. Acta, **11,** 276, 1953.
117. Soda, K., Novogrodsky, A., and Meister, A.: Enzymatic desulfination of cysteine sulfinic acid. Biochemistry, **3,** 1450, 1964.
118. Laster, L., Irreverre, F., Mudd, S. H., and Heizer, W. D.: A previously unrecognized disorder of metabolism of sulfur-containing compounds-abnormal urinary excretion of S-sulfo-l-cysteine sulfite and thiosulfate in a severely retarded child with ectopia lentis. J. Clin. Invest., **46,** 1082, 1967.
118a. Jacobsen, J. G., and Smith, L. H.: Biochemistry and physiology of taurine and taurine derivatives. Physiol. Rev. **48,** 424, 1968.
119. Sakai, H., and Dan, K.: Studies on sulfhydryl groups during cell division of sea urchin egg. Exp. Cell Res., **16,** 24, 1959.
120. Kane, R. E., and Hersh, R. T.: The isolation and preliminary characterization of a major soluble protein of the sea urchin egg. Exp. Cell Res., **16,** 59, 1959.
121. Sakai, H.: Studies on sulfhydryl groups during cell division of sea urchin egg. IV. Contractile properties of the thread model of KCl-soluble protein from the sea urchin egg. J. Gen. Physiol., **45,** 411, 1962.
122. Sakai, H.: Studies on sulfhydryl groups during cell division of sea urchin egg. V. Change in contractility of the thread model in relation to cell division. J. Gen. Physiol., **45,** 427, 1962.
123. Mazia, D.: The Role of Thiol Groups in the Structure and Function of the Mitotic Apparatus in *Sulfur in Proteins,* edited by R. Benesch, I. M. Klotz, W. R. Middlebrook, P. D. Boyer, A. G. Szent Gyorgi, and D. R. Schwarz, p. 367. Academic, New York, 1959.
124. Cafruny, E. J., Carhart, E., and Farah, A.: Effects of hypophysectomy and hormones on sulfhydryl concentrations in rat kidney cells. Endrocrinology, **61,** 143, 1957.
125. Fong, C. T. O., Schwartz, I. L., Popenoe, E. A., Silver, L., and Schoessler, M. A.: On the molecular binding of lysine vasopressin at its renal receptor site. J. Amer. Chem., Soc. **81,** 2592, 1959.
126. Fong, C. T. O., Silver, L., Christman, D. R., and Schwartz, I. L.: On the mechanism of action of the antidiuretic hormone (vasopressin). Proc. Nat. Acad. Sci. USA, **46,** 1273, 1960.
127. Rasmussen, H., Schwartz, I. L., Schoessler, M. A., and Hochster, G.: Studies on the mechanism of action of vasopressin. Proc. Nat. Acad. Sci. USA, **46,** 1278, 1960.
128. Schwartz, I. L., Rasmussen, H., Schlossler, M. A., Silver, L., and Fong, C. T. O.: Relation of chemical attachment to physiological action of vasopressin. Proc. Nat. Acad. Sci. USA, **46,** 1288, 1960.
129. Schneider, J. A., Nolan, S. P., and Seegmiller, J. E.: Appendicitis in a child with cystinosis. Arch. Surg., **97,** 565, 1968.
130. Morecki, R., Paunier, L., Hamilton, J. R.: Intestinal mucosa in cystinosis: A fine structure study. Arch. Pathol., **86,** 297, 1968.
131. Holtzapple, P. G., Genel, M., Yakovac, W. C., Hummeler, K., and Segal, S.: The diagnosis of cystinosis by rectal biopsy. New Eng. J. Med., **281,** 143, 1969.
132. Schneider, J. A.: Unpublished observation.
133. Brigham, M. P., Stein, W. H., and Moore, S.: The concentrations of cysteine and cystine in human blood plasma. J. Clin. Invest., **39,** 1633, 1960.
134. Rosenberg, L. E., Durant, J. L., and Holland, J. M.: Intestinal absorption and renal extraction of cystine and cysteine in cystinuria. New Eng. J. Med., **273,** 1239, 1965.
135. London, D. R., and Foley, T. H.: Cystine metabolism in cystinuria. Clin. Sci., **29,** 129, 1965.
136. Schneider, J. A., and Seegmiller, J. E.: Unpublished observation.
137. Harrison, H. E., and Harrison, H. C.: Aminoaciduria in relation to deficiency diseases and kidney function. J.A.M.A., **164,** 1571, 1957.
138. Dent, C. E., and Senior, B.: Studies on the treatment of cystinuria. Brit. J. Urol., **27,** 317, 1955.
139. Mahoney, C. P., and Trump, B. F.: Studies in cystinosis. Amer. J. Dis. Child. **104,** 563, 1962.
140. Seegmiller, J. E., and Howell, R. R.: Cystine metabolism in deToni-Fanconi syndrome with cystinosis. Clin. Res., **9,** 189, 1961.
141. Patrick, A. D.: The degradative metabolism of L-cysteine and L-cystine *in vitro* by liver in cystinosis. Biochem. J., **83,** 248, 1962.
142. Patrick, A. D.: Deficiencies of SH-dependent enzymes in cystinosis. Clin. Sci., **28,** 427, 1965.
143. Schulman, J. D.: Unpublished observation.
144. Hummeler, K., Zajac, B. A., Genel, M., Holtzapple, P. G., and Segal, S.: Human cystinosis: Intracellular deposition of cystine. Science, **168,** 859, 1970.
145. Schulman, J. D., Wong, V. G., Kuwabara, T., Bradley, K. H., and Seegmiller, J. E.: Intracellular cystine content of leukocyte populations in cystinosis. Arch. Intern. Med., **125,** 660, 1970.
146. Crawhall, J. C., and Segal, S.: The intracellular cysteine/cystine ratio in kidney cortex. Biochem. J., **99,** 19c, 1966.
147. Rosenberg, L. E., Crawhall, J. C., and Segal, S.: Intestinal transport of cystine and cysteine in man: Evidence for separate mechanisms. J. Clin. Invest., **46,** 30, 1967.

148. Jellum, E.: The prevention of thiol autoxidation in biological systems by means of thiolated sephadex. Acta Chem. Scand., **18**, 1887, 1964.
149. Hers, M. G.: In *Advances in Metabolic Disorders,* edited by R. Levine and R. Luft. p. 1, Academic, New York, 1969.
150. Schulman, J. D., Schneider, J. A., Bradley, K. H., and Seegmiller, J. E.: Heterozygote studies in cystinosis. Clin. Chim. Acta, **29**, 73, 1970.
151. Eagle, H.: Amino acid metabolism in mammalian cell cultures. Science, **130**, 432, 1959.
152. Pappenheimer, A. M.: Experimental studies upon lymphocytes. 1. Reactions of lymphocytes under various experimental conditions. J. Exp. Med., **25**, 633, 1917.
153. Novikoff, A.: In *Lysosomes* (Ciba Foundation Symposium), edited by de Reuck. p. 402, Churchill, London, 1963.
154. Jackson, J. D., Smith, F. G., Litman, N. N., Yuile, C. L., and Latta, H.: The Fanconi syndrome with cystinosis. Electron microscopy of renal biopsy specimens from five patients. Amer. J. Med., **33**, 893, 1962.
154a. Schulman, J. D., Wong, V. G., Bradley, K. H., and Seegmiller, J. E.: A simple technique for the biochemical diagnosis of cystinosis. J. Pediat. **76**, 289, 1970.
155. Nicaud, P., Lafitte, A., Gros. A., and Guatier, J. P.: Les Lésions osseuses de l'intoxication chronique par le cadmium. Aspects radiologique à type de syndrome de Milkman. Efficacité du traitement calcique et vitaminique (Vitamine D). Bull. Mém. Soc. Med. Hop., Paris, **18**, 204, 1942.
156. Wilson, V. K., Thomson, M. L., and Dent, C. E.: Amino-aciduria in lead poisoning: a case in childhood. Lancet, **2**, 66, 1953.
157. Clarkson, T. W., and Kench, J. E.: Urinary excretion of amino acids by men absorbing heavy metals. Biochem. J., **62**, 361, 1956.
158. Chisolm, J. J.: Aminoaciduria as a manifestation of renal tubular injury in lead intoxication and a comparison with patterns of aminoaciduria seen in other diseases. J. Pediat., **60**, 1, 1962.
159. Uzman, L., and Denny-Brown, D.: Amino-aciduria in hepatolenticular degeneration (Wilson's disease). Amer. J. Med. Sci., **215**, 599, 1948.
160. Cooper, A. M., Eckhardt, R. D., Faloon, W. W., and Davidson, C. S.: Investigation of the aminoaciduria in Wilson's disease (hepatolenticular degeneration): demonstration of a defect in renal function. J. Clin. Invest, **29**, 265, 1950.
161. Bearn, A. G., Yü, T. F., and Gutman, A. B.: Renal function in Wilson's disease. J. Clin. Invest., **36**, 1107, 1957.
162. Harrison, H. E., and Harrison, H. C.: Experimental production of renal glycosuria, phosphaturia and aminoaciduria by injection of maleic acid. Science, **120**, 606, 1954.
163. Otten, J., and Vis, H. L.: Acute reversible renal tubular dysfunction following intoxication with methyl-3-chromone. J. Pediat., **73**, 422, 1968.
164. Benitz, K. F., and Diermeier, H. F.: Renal toxicity of tetracycline degradation products. Proc. Soc. Exp. Biol. Med., **115**, 930, 1964.
165. Gentz, J., Jagenburg, R., and Zetterstrom, R.: Tyrosinemia. An inborn error of tyrosine metabolism with cirrhosis of the liver and multiple renal tubular defects (de Toni-Debré-Fanconi syndrome). J. Pediat., **66**, 670, 1965.
166. Harrison, H. E.: Personal communication.
167. Jonxis, J. H. P., and Huisman, T. H. J.: Aminoaciduria and ascorbic acid deficiency. Pediatrics, **14**, 238, 1954.
168. Spencer, A. G., and Franglen, G. T.: Gross aminoaciduria following a lysol burn. Lancet, **1**, 190, 1952.
169. Webb, J. L.: *Enzyme and Metabolic Inhibitors.* Vol. III, p. 421, Academic, New York, 1966.
170. Lowe, C. U., Terrey, M., and MacLachlan, E. A.: Organic-aciduria, decreased renal ammonia production, hydrophthalmos, and mental retardation; clinical entity. Amer. J. Dis. Child., **83**, 164, 1952.
171. Sirota, J. H., and Hamerman, D.: Renal function studies in an adult subject with the Fanconi syndrome. Amer. J. Med., **16**, 138, 1954.
172. Dragsted, P. J., and Hjorth, N.: The association of the Fanconi syndrome with malignant disease. Danish Med. Bull., **3**, 177, 1956.
173. Engle, R. L. Jr., and Wallis, L. A.: Multiple myeloma and the adult Fanconi syndrome. 1. Report of a case with crystal-like deposits in the tumor cells and in the epithelial cells of the kidney. Amer. J. Med., **22**, 5, 1957.
174. West, C. D., Blanton, J. C., Silverman, F. N., and Holland, N. H.: Use of phosphate salts as an adjunct to vitamin D in the treatment of hypophosphatemic vitamin D refractory rickets. J. Pediat., **64**, 469, 1964.
175. Weber, V. H., and Hagge, W.: Über die erfolgreiche Behandlung der Zystinose mit einem Anabolicum. Arch. Kinderheilk., **168**, 110, 1963.
176. Bauer, B., and Antener, I.: Eine wirksame diätetische und medikamentöse Cystinose-behandlung. Helv. Paediat. Acta, **21**, 19, 1966.
177. Hambraeus, L., and Broberger, O.: Penicillamine treatment of cystinosis. Acta Paediat. Scand., **56**, 243, 1967.
178. Seip, M., Steen-Johnsen, J. Vellan, J. E., and Gjessing, L. R.: Dietary treatment of cystinosis. Acta Paediat. Scand. **57**, 409, 1968.
179. Snyderman, S. E., Boyer, A., Norton, P. M., Roitman, E., and Holt, L. E., Jr.: The essential amino acid requirements of infants. X. Methionine. Amer. J. Clin. Nutr., **15**, 322, 1964.
180. Mahoney, C. P., Striker, G. E., Hickman, R. O., Manning, G. B., and Marchioro, T. L.: Renal transplantation for childhood cystinosis. New Eng. J. Med., **283**, 397, 1970.
181. Hambidge, K. M., Goodman, S. I., Walravens, P. A., Mauer, S. M., Brettschneider, L., Penn, I., and Starzl, T. E.: Accumulation of cystine following renal homotransplantation for cystinosis. Pediat. Res., **3**, 364, 1969.
182. Lucas, Z. J., Kempson, R. L., Palmer, J., Korn, D., and Cohn, R. B.: Renal allotransplantation in man: II. Transplantation in cystinosis, a metabolic disease. Amer. J. Surg., **118**, 158, 1969.
183. Goodman, S. I.: Personal communication.
184. Hunt, D. D., Stearns, G., McKinley, J. B., Froning, E., Hicks, P., and Bonfiglio, M.: Long-term study of family with Fanconi syndrome without cystinosis (deToni-Debré-Fanconi syndrome). Amer. J. Med., **40**, 492, 1966.
185. Debré, R., Royer, P., Lestradet, H., and Straub, W.: L'insuffisance tubulaire congénitale avec arriération mentale, cataracte et glaucome (syndrome de Lowe). Arch. Franc. Pediat., **12**, 337, 1955.
186. Halvorsen, S., and Gjessing, L. R.: Studies on tyrosinosis: I. Effect of low-tyrosine and low-phenylalanine diet. Brit. Med. J., **2**, 1171, 1964.
187. Holzel, A., Komrower, G. M., and Wilson, V. K.: Amino-aciduria in galactosaemia. Brit. Med. J., **1**, 194, 1952.
188. Hsia, D., Y-Y., Hsia, H.-H., Green, S., Kay, M., and Gellis, S. S.: Amino aciduria in galactosaemia. A.M.A. J. Dis. Child., **88**, 458, 1954.
189. Cusworth, D. C., Dent, C. E., and Flynn, F. V.: The aminoaciduria in galactosaemia. Arch. Dis. Child., **30**, 150, 1955.
190. Lampert, F., and Mayer, H.: Glykogenose der Leber mit Galaktoseverwertungsstörung und schwerem Fanconi-Syndrom. Z. kinderheilk., **98**, 133, 1967.
191. Morris, R. C., Ueki, L., Loh, D., Eanes, R. Z., and McLin, P.: Absence of renal fructose-1-phosphate aldolase activity in hereditary fructose intolerance. Nature, **214**, 920, 1967.
192. Massry, S. G., Preuss, H. G., Maher, J. F., and Schreiner, G. E.: Renal tubular acidosis after cadaver kidney homotransplantation. Studies on mechanism. Amer. J. Med., **42**, 284, 1967.
193. Gyory, A. Z., Stewart, J. H., George, C. R. P., Tiller, D. J., and Edwards, K. D. G.: Renal tubular acidosis, acidosis due to hyperkalaemia, hypercalcaemia, disordered citrate metabolism and other tubular dysfunctions following human renal transplantation. Quart. J. Med., **38**, 231, 1969.
194. Frimpter, G. W., Timpanelli, A. E., Eisenmenger, W. J., Stein, H. S., and Ehrlich, L. I.: Reversible "Fanconi syndrome" caused by degraded tetracycline. J.A.M.A., **184**, 111, 1963.
195. Gross, J. M.: Fanconi syndrome (adult type) developing secondary to the ingestion of outdated tetracycline. Ann. Intern. Med., **58**, 523, 1963.
196. Cleveland, W. W., Adams, W. C., Mann, J. B., and Nyhan, W. L.: Acquired Fanconi syndrome following degraded tetracycline. J. Pediat., **66**, 333, 1965.
197. Fulop, M., and Drapkin, A.: Potassium-depletion syndrome secondary to nephropathy apparently caused by "outdated tetracycline". New Eng. J. Med., **272**, 986, 1965.
198. Brodehl, J., Gellissen, K., Hagge, W., and Schumacher, H.: Reversible renales Fanconi-syndrome durch toxisches Abbawprodukt des Tetrazyklins. Helv. Paediat. Acta, **23**, 373, 1968.
199. Jonxis, J. H. P.: Aminoaciduria and rickets. Helv. Paediat. Acta **10**, 245, 1955.

200. Pittman, G., Deodhar, S., Schulman, J. D., and Lando, J. B.: Nephropathic cystinosis in a young adult. Presented at the Annual Meeting of the International Academy of Pathology, March 10, 1971, Montreal.
201. Aaron, K. Goldman, H., and Scriver, C. R.: Adolescent Cystinosis. A "new" phenotype. A possible role for dithiotreitol (DTT) in treatment. In *Hereditary Disorders of Sulphur Metabolism.* Eighth annual conference of the Society for the Study of Inborn Errors of Metabolism. Belfast, 1970.
202. Van Hooft, C., Carton, D., and DeSchrijver, F.: Juvenile cystinosis in two siblings. In *Hereditary Disorders of Sulphur Metabolism.* Eighth annual conference of the Society of Inborn Errors of Metabolism. Belfast, 1970.
203. Tietze, F.: Disulfide reduction in rat liver. I. Evidence for the presence of nonspecific nucleotide-dependent disulfide reductase and GSH-disulfide transhydrogenase activities in the high-speed supernatant fraction. Arch. Biochem. Biophys., **138**, 177, 1970.
204. Tietze, F.: Disulfide reduction in rat liver. II. Chromatographic separation of nucleotide-dependent disulfide reductase and GSH-disulfide transhydrogenase activities of the high-speed supernatant fraction. Biochem. Biophys. Acta, **220**, 449, 1970.
205. Cohen, H. J., and Fridovich, I.: Hepatic sulfite oxidase. Purification and properties. J. Biol. Chem., **246**, 359, 1971.
206. Cohen H. J., and Fridovich, I.: Hepatic sulfite oxidase. The nature and function of the heme prosthetic groups. J. Biol. Chem., **246**, 367, 1971.
207. Cohen, H. J., and Fridovich, I.: Hepatic sulfite oxidase. A functional role for molybdenum. J. Biol. Chem., **246**, 374, 1971.
208. Hers, G.: Glycogen storage disease, in *Carbohydrate Metabolism and its Disorders,* edited by F. Dickens, P. J. Randle, and W. J. Whelan, vol. II, Academic, New York, 1968.

CHAPTER SIXTY-EIGHT

CYSTIC FIBROSIS*

Charles C. Lobeck

Cystic fibrosis is a common disease of children and young adults in countries with large Caucasian populations. If it is assumed that the incidence is 1 in 2,000 Caucasian live births, about 1,500 Caucasian infants were born in the United States with the disease in 1966. It is clearly an inherited disorder, but its molecular basis is unknown. The classic features are chronic bronchiolar obstruction and infection of the lungs, steatorrhea and azotorrhea, increase in the salinity of sweat, malnutrition, and growth failure. Clinical manifestations vary, even in the same sibship.

Fanconi first related congenital cystic pancreatic fibrosis and bronchiectasis in 1936 [1]. Many other reports describing the pathology of the pancreas, meconium ileus, and various clinical manifestations of the disease had been published, beginning with Landsteiner in 1905 [2]. As early as 1912, Garrod [3], ascribed Mendelian recessive inheritance to familial congenital steatorrhea, which was probably cystic fibrosis. The pathologic lesion of the pancreas was differentiated from vitamin A deficiency by Blackfan and Wolbach in 1933 [4] and reported as a separate entity by Blackfan and May [5], and Harper [6], in 1938. Andersen [7] used the term *cystic fibrosis of the pancreas* in 1938, when she reviewed the literature and described the disease as a distinct entity. Twenty years later, Andersen [8] listed 13 names that had been given to the disease. The most popular of these, *mucoviscidosis,* was proposed by Farber in 1945 [9] to describe the increased viscosity of mucous secretions and is still commonly used in continental Europe. Since the discovery by di Sant'Agnese [10], in 1953, that the salinity of sweat is increased and that the disease is a generalized exocrinopathy with various abnormalities of exocrine secretion, a shortened form of the original name, *cystic fibrosis,* has become most common.

CLINICAL FEATURES

Gestation for infants with cystic fibrosis is uneventful and of normal duration. The average birth weight is less than that of healthy controls [11, 12].

Gastrointestinal

The disease may make its initial appearance at birth as intestinal obstruction characterized by dilatation of the small intestine proximal to a terminal ileum filled with thickened meconium. The colon is narrowed but returns to a normal caliber after relief of the obstruction. This condition is called *meconium ileus* and is virtually pathognomonic of cystic fibrosis. Volvulus and ileal atresias are commonly associated with meconium ileus, but congenital malformations of other organ systems are rare. Hydramnios is sometimes present, and prenatal perforation of the bowel with aseptic peritonitis may be a complication [13–15]. The incidence of meconium ileus in 106 patients in the author's clinic was 16 percent, approximately the same as that reported by others [15, 16]. Intestinal obstruction from fecal plugs, intussusception, and volvulus occasionally occurs in older children and adults with cystic fibrosis [17, 18].

During the first year of life most patients have frequent, large, foul stools, increase in appetite, poor weight gain, and abdominal distension. Steathorrhea may be severe. Twelve of the author's patients, ranging in age from 4 to 9 years, excreted an average of 41 gm fat per day during a 4-day stool collection while off all treatment. Control subjects excreted less than 7 gm per day.

Hypoproteinemia and edema may occur in infants with cystic fibrosis fed human milk or soybean preparations [19]. The poor assimilation of soybean protein [20] and the lower protein content of human milk are probably etiologic factors. Hypoalbuminemia may occur in older patients, associated with increased plasma volume and cor pulmonale [21]. Older children with pulmonary disease may have slight polycythemia with increased intestinal absorption of iron and moderate hypoferremia [22, 23].

Intermittent abdominal cramps and pain are among the most troublesome complaints for patients with the disease. A relation of these to duodenal ulceration, steatorrhea, pancreatitis, and fecal impaction has not been proven [13]. Rectal prolapse, uncommon in other children, has occurred in 19 percent of the author's patients in the first 3 years of life, and the same incidence has been observed by others [24].

Before the general use of vitamin preparations, symptoms of vitamin A deficiency, such as xerophthalmia and corneal ulceration, were frequently described in association with steatorrhea in cystic fibrosis [25, 26]. Rickets is rare [27], but deposition of ceroid pigment in the smooth muscle of the gastrointestinal tract [28], eosinophilic masses in nerve axons [29], and decreased concentration of plasma tocopherol suggesting vitamin E deficiency have been observed [30]. Vitamin K deficiency with decreased prothrombin and bleeding occasionally occurs [31, 32]. The disease may present as a hemorrhagic diathesis from this cause [33]. Disaccharide intolerance [34] and deficiency of intestinal lactase [35, 36] have been observed in some patients (see Chap. 59).

Pulmonary involvement

The first signs of pulmonary involvement appear at any time after birth but most frequently before the age of 1 year [37].

*Supported by Grant AM06365 from the National Institutes of Health and by the National Cystic Fibrosis Research Foundation, New York. The author recognizes the contribution of his associates, John A. Mangos and Nona R. McSherry to this work.

They have not appeared until the second decade in some of the author's patients. Cough, wheezing, and stertorous breathing in the infant are the cardinal symptoms. Repeated bouts of pneumonia may ensue but need not be frequent. Viral infections affecting the lungs often develop into bacterial pneumonias. A most important bacterial invader is *Staphylococcus aureus,* which is present in the respiratory tract from very early in life [38]. No single phage type is prevalent [39]. *Pseudomonas aeruginosa* is also frequently present [38, 40]. Evidence that this organism is atypical [40] has not been confirmed [41].

Pulmonary involvement later in childhood may be suggested by increased chest diameter and clubbing of the fingers and toes. Decreased exercise tolerance, chronic productive cough, tachypnea, and chronic cor pulmonale may become increasingly severe. Characteristic radiographic findings are flattening of the diaphragmatic leaves, an increased anteroposterior diameter of the chest, a small heart shadow, and a "honeycomb" appearance of the lung parenchyma. Atelactasis and pneumothorax may occur. Death most frequently is the result of pneumonia, anoxia, and exhaustion after a long period of respiratory insufficiency.

Other systems

Shock from sodium depletion may occur during sweating [42]. The danger is greatest in infants and very ill, debilitated patients who cannot express their craving for salt.

Signs of portal hypertension including enlargement of the spleen, leukopenia, thrombocytopenia, and hematemesis have occurred in 3 percent of the patients in the author's clinic. This syndrome was due to hepatic cirrhosis, termed *multilobular biliary cirrhosis with concretions,* in the patients observed by di Sant'Agnese [43]. Although it must be generalized to produce symptoms, most patients are found to have focal areas of biliary cirrhosis at autopsy [43].

Duodenal ulcer has been reported [44–46]. Andersen saw a high incidence at autopsy in older children [47]. It has been found in two of the author's patients, both males older than 16 years.

The incidence of diabetes mellitus is higher than in the general population [48]. A report of a higher incidence of diabetes mellitus in the families of affected children [49] was not confirmed [50]. Abnormal oral glucose tolerance was found by Handwerger [51] in 36 percent of 31 patients with cystic fibrosis. The rise in plasma insulin following oral glucose was prompt but subnormal in all patients with cystic fibrosis who were tested. Intravenous glucose administration was followed by glucose and insulin responses which were much less impaired. The response to oral tolbutamide was a rise in plasma insulin in all cases. Human growth hormone responses to hypoglycemia may be deficient in cystic fibrosis patients with growth retardation and malnutrition [52]. The diabetes of cystic fibrosis is usually mild, rarely ketotic, and sometimes responsive to tolbutamide, unlike classical juvenile diabetes mellitus.

Children with cystic fibrosis do not suffer from clinical disorders of the nervous system. The median IQ of 21 patients in the author's clinic selected at random was 118. Edema of the optic disks and retrobulbar neuritis associated with severe pulmonary insufficiency [53] is probably an effect of long-term chloramphenicol administration [54]. A report [55] of a high incidence of abnormal electroencephalograms has not been confirmed [56].

Increased acuity of the senses of taste and smell, similar to that of adrenal insufficiency, has been observed [57]. Hydrocortisone did not alter the threshold for perception in cystic fibrosis. Salt taste thresholds are normal [58], but the ratio of tasters to nontasters of phenylthiocarbamide is lower in patients with cystic fibrosis than in unaffected members of the family or the normal population [59].

Growth

Rates of linear growth and osseous maturation are frequently depressed [60]. Body weight is usually below that expected for height. Accordingly, these children may be short and appear emaciated (Fig. 68-1). The buttocks are small, the abdomen distended, and the extremities thin. In some, if therapy has been vigorous, growth may be normal.

As the children grow older, sinusitis [61] and nasal polyposis [62] become frequent and troublesome. The submaxillary glands may become palpably enlarged [63], and frequently chest deformity and clubbing of the extremities become more severe. Puberty is frequently delayed, but the disease may progress more slowly during adolescence [64].

In recent years many children with cystic fibrosis have grown to adulthood. There is a preponderance of male survivors. Shwachman [65] reported 65 percent of 65 patients over 17 years of age were male. Final height attainment may be normal in the adult [66]. Women with cystic fibrosis have reproduced [67], although the risk of pregnancy to maternal and fetal health may be great. Men with cystic fibrosis have aspermia and are sterile [68, 69]. Survival beyond the fourth decade is rare.

The prognosis of cystic fibrosis has improved dramatically with adequate treatment. In a recent national study, Warwick [70] showed that the median age at death before treatment became available was 8 months. With modern treatment, in 1964, the median age at death was 12 years, and in one clinic where intensive prophylactic treatment is used the median age at death is 21 years.

PATHOGENESIS

The clinical features of cystic fibrosis could only be the result of a widespread disorder. Strong evidence indicates that the disorder is chiefly of exocrine glands. Analysis of exocrine secretory fluids has not led to detection of an isolated specific abnormality of one biochemical system which could become a single focus for metabolic investigation. Instead, varying

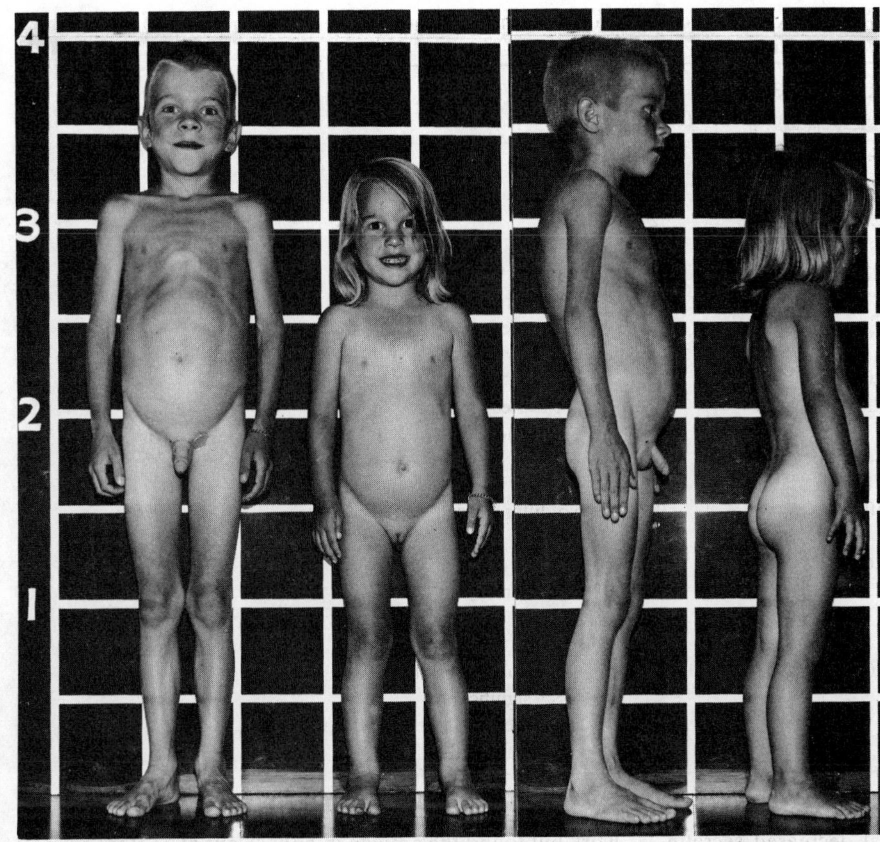

Figure 68-1. Sibs with cystic fibrosis. The boy, photographed at age 7 years 9 months, the average height of a 6-year-old and weight of a 5-year-old, died at age 9 of progressive pulmonary failure. He had a history of steatorrhea and severe pulmonary disease. The girl at age 3 years 11 months when photographed had steatorrhea and mild pulmonary disease until age 5 when she developed a series of respiratory infections and died at age 5½ years with respiratory and cardiac failure. Two other sibs are healthy, and a third died with meconium ileus.

abnormal properties and compositions have been found in fluids from different exocrine tissues. These abnormal fluids are responsible for the pathology of the disease.

Gastrointestinal Tract

Pancreas

Pathologic changes in the pancreas may be observed during fetal life. At first, small casts of eosinophilic material may be found in the acini. The acini then become irregular with cellular proliferation, and casts appear in the ducts. The ducts become distended and occluded by fibrous tissue. Cyst formation and acinar atrophy are followed by infiltration with adipose tissue. After 2 years of age the pancreas may be unrecognizable except as islets clustered in fibrous or adipose tissue (71, 72). The process occurs at varying speeds, and approximately 15 percent of patients do not develop signs of pancreatic disease.

The steatorrhea and azotorrhea of cystic fibrosis are due to the deficiency of pancreatic lipase, trypsin, chymotrypsin, and carboxypeptidase. Malabsorption of fatty acids which do not require digestion with pancreatic enzymes has been reported [73], but patients can absorb fatty acids of low molecular weight [74]. In some instances when an enzyme was found to be absent from duodenal fluid in the fasting state, its presence could be detected after instillation of olive oil into the duodenum [75]. Deficiencies of chymotrypsin and trypsin have also been detected in the stool [76, 77]. Repeated duodenal intubation has revealed the postnatal development of pancreatic insufficiency in some patients [75]. We have not observed the development of clinical signs of pancreatic insufficiency if it was not present in the first few years of life. Abnormalities of the electrolyte concentration of duodenal fluid have not been detected (Table 68-1) [78], but the pH is depressed. Increased viscosity is a more prominent feature than decreased enzyme activity.

Hadorn and his associates [79, 80] have studied pancreatic function in patients with cystic fibrosis who do not have steatorrhea. Enzyme secretion in response to pancreozymin was almost normal, but secretin response was much decreased. In contrast [81], children with pancreatic insufficiency without cystic fibrosis had a more normal secretin response but deficient enzyme secretion. In 8 of 10 patients with cystic fibrosis the viscosity of the duodenal juice was increased after secretin stimulation. The bicarbonate concentration did not rise, and chloride concentration remained high as the rate of flow increased. The same findings have been reported by Rick [82] in an adult with cystic fibrosis, and a qualitative difference of the effect of secretin on the rectal mucosa has been observed without the presence of

Table 68-1. REPRESENTATIVE AVERAGE OF THE ELECTROLYTE COMPOSITION OF VARIOUS SECRETIONS IN CYSTIC FIBROSIS

Secretion	Na^+ (mEq/l)	K^+ (mEq/l)	Ca^{++} (mEq/l)	Cl^- (mEq/l)	Comment
Mixed saliva [78]					
Control	16	20		16	Na^+ and Cl^- elevated
Cystic fibrosis	27	21		24	
Parotid saliva [111]					
Control	24	22	2	19	Na^+, Ca^{++}, Cl^- and rate of secretion slightly elevated
Cystic fibrosis	31	23	3	24	
Submaxillary saliva [116]					
Control	30	20	3.6	17	Na^+, Ca^{++}, and Cl^- elevated; rate of secretion normal
Cystic fibrosis	46	23	6.1	25	
Duodenal fluid [78]					
Control	107	11		94	
Cystic fibrosis	125	10		90	No differences
Tears [218]					
Control	140	26		134	
Cystic fibrosis	137	23		133	No differences
Sweat [165]					
Control	25	11	2–4 [167]	20	Na^+, Cl^- above range of controls in childhood; K^+ significantly elevated in large series; Ca^{++} normal
Cystic fibrosis	110	16	2–4	117	

steatorrhea [83]. Hadorn concludes that decreased secretin response may contribute to the obstructive pathology in the pancreas and also may indicate a primary abnormality of the duct cells.

Glycoproteins of the Intestinal Tract

Di Sant'Agnese and his colleagues [84] have observed an increased susceptibility to denaturation of a fraction of the glycoprotein of duodenal fluid after treatment with organic solvents. This abnormality was found in some patients in whom a deficiency of pancreatic enzymes could not be detected. Further study [85] demonstrated differences in the composition of the carbohydrate moiety of this denatured glycoprotein. Most characteristic was a decreased sialic acid and an increased fucose content when compared to glycoproteins from control subjects. The total amount of glycoprotein was normal. Roelfs found an increased fucose content and fucose to sialic acid ratio in rectal mucus [86]. It has been postulated that the ratio of fucose to sialic acid may determine glycoprotein solubility and thus be a factor in the pathogenesis of cystic fibrosis.

Lowe and his colleagues [87] observed an antigenically distinct glycoprotein in the stool of patients with cystic fibrosis. This was also found by immunofluorescence in the cytoplasm of epithelial cells of colonic and pulmonary glands. Broglio [88] and his group were able to repeat this work but found the antigen in only 26 out of 71 stool extracts from patients with cystic fibrosis. They also found the antigen in 14 of 54 stool extracts from normal patients.

Serum Proteins in the Intestinal Tract

Several investigators [89–92] have found serum albumin and globulins in duodenal fluid and meconium from patients with cystic fibrosis in excess of that found in controls. Green reported [93] that a simple immunologic and chemical test detected serum protein in 9 subjects with meconium ileus and 36 of 40 other patients with cystic fibrosis. He also found positive tests in 30 percent of healthy sibs and only 4 weakly positive results in 1,200 randomly collected meconium specimens from normal infants. These results suggested that the presence of serum in meconium may be characteristic of heterozygotes as well as homozygotes.

Intestinal Mucous Glands

Goblet cell hyperplasia has been observed in the epithelium lining the tracheobronchial tree, intestines, and pancreatic ducts near the ampulla [94]. An increase in sulfomucins and in the intensity of PAS staining was found in these epithelial mucins by histochemical staining. The latter corresponds to the increase in fucose observed chemically. On the other hand, peroral intestinal biopsies reported by Freye et al. [95]

were normal except for an abnormally thick fibrillar mucinous covering of the epithelial cells. Goblet cells were normal. Andersen [47] observed that the intestinal glands and appendix are variably occluded by inspissated material. The rectal glands [96] are also frequently distended with secretions.

Meconium Ileus

Meconium ileus has been observed in patients with minimal microscopic alterations of the pancreas [97] and is related more to abnormalities of the intestinal glands than to pancreatic insufficiency [98]. Analyses of meconium from patients with meconium ileus have disclosed the presence of serum proteins and decreased amounts of ash and mucopolysaccharide [99] when compared to meconium from healthy infants.

Liver and Gallbladder

The pathogenesis of the hepatic cirrhosis is obscure but may be the inspissation of bile in the liver [47, 100]. Hemosiderosis, seen microscopically in untreated patients, is probably due to increased absorption of iron.

Submucosal cysts and thick colorless mucus were found in 23 percent of gallbladders from patients with cystic fibrosis at the Johns Hopkins Hospital [101]. A histochemical study of cystic fibrosis gallbaldders revealed increased sulfomucins and engorgement of epithelial cells with mucins [102]. Symptoms of gallbladder disease do not usually occur.

Salivary Glands

The concentration of electrolytes in mixed saliva is abnormal (Table 68-1) [78, 103–105]. Sodium and chloride concentrations are elevated. The major contributors to the mixed saliva are the parotid and submaxillary glands. The first, a serous gland, is not histologically abnormal, but the second, with a secretion rich in glycoprotein, frequently shows partial destruction.

The parotid saliva of the rat, a hypotonic fluid, varies in composition with the rate of secretion per unit mass of the gland [106]. The interpretation of electrolyte concentrations in parotid saliva from human subjects is complicated by the inability to measure the mass of the gland. Since the gland could be enlarged in cystic fibrosis, differences between cystic fibrosis and normal are difficult to determine. Some investigators have observed increased concentrations of sodium [105, 107], chloride, and iodide [108] in parotid saliva (Table 68-1). Lawson [109] found that the sodium concentration normally decreased during the first 3 to 4 months of life, and at that time the levels in cystic fibrosis saliva were distinctly higher and did not overlap with controls. There are conflicting reports on the rate of parotid salivary secretion. It has been recorded as elevated [78, 105, 110] and normal [111, 112]. In healthy subjects the sodium concentration of parotid saliva increases and approaches a maximum as the rate of secretion increases [113]. This is also true for patients with cystic fibrosis but higher values are attained [114]. There are conflicting reports of differences in calcium and phosphorous excretion [111, 115]. Assays for amylase in parotid saliva have not revealed significant differences from healthy controls [116].

The rate of secretion of the submaxillary gland is not increased [116, 117] but the sodium, chloride, calcium, and phosphorous concentrations in the secretion are elevated (Table 68-1) [116, 41]. Electrolyte concentrations of submaxillary saliva are also dependent upon rate of flow [118]. Since the gland is frequently palpably enlarged and partially destroyed, the same caution of interpretation applies to data from this gland as from the parotid. The concentrations of the organic components in submaxillary saliva, including amylase and glycoproteins are elevated [116, 119]. The fucose to sialic acid ratio of the glycoproteins is increased [116]. Reflex stimulation of the submaxillary gland produces a saliva which is turbid and contains higher concentrations of calcium and nitrogen than controls [117]. Chernick and Barbero [120] found that the intravenous administration of guanethidine to patients with cystic fibrosis was followed by a rapid clearing of the submaxillary saliva and drop in the nitrogen content. The amylase and sialic acid concentrations also decreased toward normal, but calcium concentration did not change. This effect was specific for guanethidine and could not be reproduced by vasodilators or other agents causing adrenergic blockade. Gugler and his associates [121] found that chelation of calcium from reflexly produced submaxillary saliva in cystic fibrosis caused clearing of the saliva and conversely the addition of calcium to normal saliva increased the turbidity. They did not find abnormal glycoproteins using polyacrylamide gel electrophoresis, but the intensity of the bands in cystic fibrosis could be simulated by the addition of calcium to normal saliva. Thus the turbidity of submaxillary saliva from patients with cystic fibrosis can be reversed toward normal by either reduction of the concentration of protein or of calcium.

When the submaxillary gland of the dog is stimulated with increasing doses of pilocarpine, the ratio of fucose to sialic acid in the carbohydrate fraction in the saliva increases [122]. This finding suggests [123] that the abnormal fucose to sialic ratio of glycoproteins in cystic fibrosis may be a result of increased intensity of physiologic stimulation.

The levels of 11S IgA in submaxillary saliva have been reported as elevated [124] but normal in parotid saliva [125]. Serum 7S IgA and IgG are elevated [124–126] in cystic fibrosis, as is IgM with severe pulmonary disease.

Warwick [127] observed increased eosinophilic material in the acini and ducts of the labial salivary gland in children with cystic fibrosis. This was also found in normal adults [128] but was more frequent and severe in heterozygous adults [129]. The cellular morphology of these salivary glands is normal [128] except for the abundance of lysosomes in acinar cells [130]. The output of the glands is more viscid and scantier than normal [131].

Mangos [103] has observed that following retrograde injection, the mixed saliva from patients with untreated cystic fibrosis causes inhibition of sodium reabsorption (Fig. 68-2) in the rat parotid gland similar to that achieved with ouabain. On the other hand, cystic fibrosis saliva did not reduce the ATPase activity of heavy membranes or microsomes from beef parotid glands. Similar inhibition of sodium reabsorption could be achieved by the retrograde injection of various polycations [132]. Heparin, a negatively charged protein, reversed the effect of cystic fibrosis saliva and the polycations when mixed with them prior to retrograde injection. Further, it has been observed [133] that after 3 weeks of daily injections of isoproterenol, rats develop marked enlargement of the parotid and submaxillary glands, increased sodium and protein concentrations in parotid saliva at all flow rates, and the appearance of a factor in the serum which caused ciliary dyskinesis of rabbit respiratory epithelium in culture.

The feeding of pancreatin, raw pancreas, and proteolytic enzymes to rats causes enlargement of the parotid and submaxillary glands [134] with an increased salivary flow rate

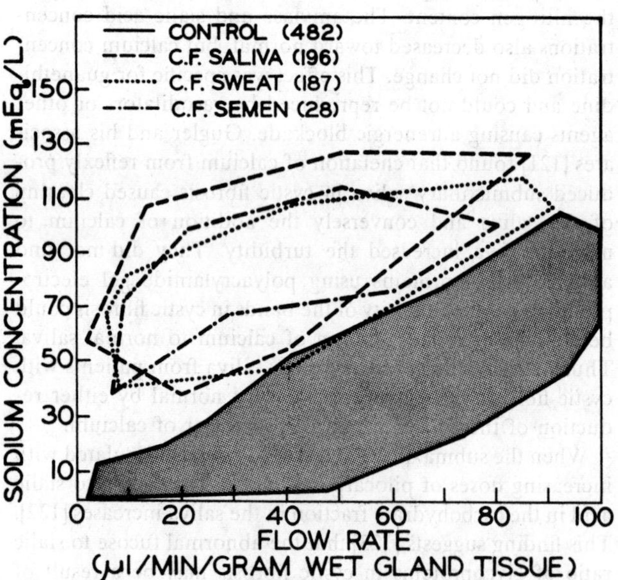

Figure 68-2. The relationship of sodium concentration to flow rate in rat parotid saliva following retrograde perfusion of the duct system of the gland with mixed saliva (– – –), sweat (. . . . .), and semen (– · – · –) from patients with cystic fibrosis. The shaded area enclosed by the solid line is the range of measurement obtained after retrograde perfusion of the duct system with isotonic saline and saliva, sweat and semen from control individuals matching the patients for age and sex. The parotid glands of the rats were stimulated with pilocarpine (0.05 to 0.1 mg per 100 gm body weight) injected intravenously. The numbers in parentheses indicate the number of individual measurements. For details see references.

of parotid saliva but a decreased flow rate from the submaxillary gland [135]. After this treatment elevated sodium concentrations were found in parotid saliva and elevated calcium and protein concentrations in submaxillary saliva. Since patients with cystic fibrosis are frequently fed pancreatic enzymes, the effect of this treatment may alter or accentuate some of the pathologic findings mentioned in this section.

Lungs

Clinically, the lungs may not be affected until far into the first or even second decade of life. Pathologically the earliest changes are distension of the mucous glands of the tracheobronchial tree and upper respiratory tract [47]. Without treatment the pattern of ventilatory dysfunction which develops is characteristic of obstructive pulmonary disease [136]. Vital capacity, as percent of the predicted value, decreases steadily with increasing age. Expressed in the same way, functional residual capacity, and to a greater degree, the ratio of residual volume to total lung capacity remains constantly elevated [137]. The maximum midexpiratory flow rate is greatly reduced, and there is an early uneven distribution of intrapulmonary gas distribution [138]. There is uneven ventilation and overinflation of the lung. Mucoid impaction of the large bronchi may be associated with the latter [139]. Zelkowitz and Giammona [140] have observed an abnormal diffusion capacity after exercise in children with cystic fibrosis who have normal lung volumes, mechanics of breathing, and gas mixing. Right ventricular hypertrophy, pulmonary hypertension, and cor pulmonale are frequent complications [141–143].

Uncontaminated mucus has not been obtained for analysis. Material obtained by bronchoscopy or coughing is always contaminated with bacteria, elements of blood, and exudates. There is an increased content of organic material and decreased content of sodium, chloride, and total ash in secretions from patients with cystic fibrosis compared to those from patients with laryngectomy. The fact that secretions from patients with bronchiectasis have intermediate values of these constituents indicates that infection plays a major role in determining the chemical composition of pulmonary secretions [144]. The increased bacterial DNA content of material from the bronchial tree in cystic fibrosis may increase the viscosity of the secretions [145]. The carbohydrates present in the glycoproteins, such as fucose and hexosamine, are decreased, while sialic acid is increased [146]. The relationship of sialic acid to fucose is opposite to that observed by Dische et al. [85] in duodenal fluid.

Immunofluorescent staining for immune globulins has revealed an increase in IgA-producing plasma cells in the bronchial mucosa and an increase in IgG-producing cells in the bronchial lymph nodes [147]. Findings such as these were not present in a patient without severe pulmonary disease.

Reproductive System

The glands of the uterine cervix are frequently distended with mucus in newly born females with meconium ileus [72]. The same is true of the penile and urethral glands of Littré and Cowper from older boys with cystic fibrosis. Blanc [148] found an increased incidence of periurethral and prostatic concretions in older children with cystic fibrosis but normal testicular histology. In 1968, Denning [68] demonstrated aspermia in the ejaculate from men with cystic fibrosis and found that seminal fluid viscosity was normal, turbidity increased, but volume was reduced. She also found normal testicular histology but observed many abnormal spermatocytes and spermatids. Kaplan [69] confirmed these findings but added the important observation that the vas deferens was atresic in all patients examined and the epididymis incompletely developed in most. This was observed as early as 38 days of age and confirmed by another group at 15 months of age [149]. Kaplan also observed a decrease in fructose and increase in citric acid and acid phosphatase concentrations in seminal fluid. This suggested that most of the semen originated in the prostate, with a decreased or abnormal contribution from the seminal vesicles. More recently, Rule [150] compared 18 patients with cystic fibrosis to 3 adults with ligated vas deferentia and found the fructose concentration depressed and the glucose elevated but no differences in fucose or sialic acid-fucose ratios. She suggested a primary abnormality of the seminal vesicle in addition to atresia of the vas deferens. Mangos (Fig. 68-2) [151] has found that the ejaculate from patients with cystic fibrosis inhibits sodium reabsorption in the rat parotid gland, whereas that of healthy controls does not.

The question remains unanswered as to whether there is a developmental anomaly of the mesonephric ducts causing atresia of the vas deferens in cystic fibrosis, or, as has been pointed out by di Sant'Agnese [152], whether the atresia is caused by an abnormality of the secretory process analogous to the ileal atresia, gall bladder atrophy, or disappearance of the pancreatic duct often found in cystic fibrosis.

Eccrine Sweat

The increased sodium and chloride concentrations of eccrine sweat are the most constant and clearly defined abnormality that has been detected in cystic fibrosis (Table 68-1). We have not observed a patient with the other clinical features of the disease who did not also have increased concentrations of sodium and chloride in sweat. This characteristic finding is present at birth in those infants from whom adequate volumes of sweat can be obtained for analysis [153].

The potassium concentration is also increased, but there is considerable overlap with controls. It is decreased to normal by the parenteral administration of acetazoleamide [154]. The sodium and chloride concentrations are unaffected by this drug.

Healthy subjects reduce the salinity of sweat in response to salt restriction or increased environmental temperature and physical exercise [155]. Failure of acclimatization in cystic fibrosis was first detected by Kessler and Andersen [42] at the Babies Hospital in New York City, when they observed that five of ten children suffering acute circulatory collapse in the hot summer of 1948 were children with this disease. This led in turn to the important discovery of the abnormal composition of sweat by di Sant'Agnese and his colleagues first reported in 1953 [10]. Vascular collapse is still a threat to the child with cystic fibrosis when he sweats excessively, but the use of salt replacement has lessened this danger.

In spite of failure of acclimatization in cystic fibrosis, the elevated sodium and chloride concentrations of sweat are variably reduced to levels which are still above those of acclimatized control subjects by dietary salt deprivation or the intramuscular administration of aldosterone [156–160]. The potassium concentration rises in the sweat, and there is a significant decrease in the sodium to potassium ratio. This effect is not immediate but occurs maximally on the fifth day after the beginning of the stimulus [157]. The administration of aldosterone, desoxycorticosterone, or 9-alpha-fluorohydrocortisone or dietary salt deprivation are therefore not clinically useful as tests for cystic fibrosis, since there is a response to these agents, and the test is expensive, must be extended over a long period, and has potential dangers. Even in adults the persistence of elevated sodium or chloride levels in sweat associated with the clinical history and signs of the disease are the best criteria for diagnosis.

In healthy subjects the sodium concentration in sweat rises with increase in the rate of sweating when consecutive collections are made on a single subject from the same area of the skin [161]. Since the number of active sweat glands per unit surface area decreases [162] and their length and diameter increases with aging [163], differences in sweating rate between different individuals do not necessarily reflect different rates of flow through the duct of the gland. Fortunately the sweat gland is of normal size in cystic fibrosis [164]. Even so, rates of sweating compared in age-matched subjects do not reflect absolute rates of flow through the duct because the output of large numbers of glands are sampled and their absolute size is unknown. When rates of sweating are compared, no differences are found between control and cystic fibrosis patients, but the sodium and chloride concentrations are extremely variable and always higher in cystic fibrosis [165]. During sleep the spontaneous sweating of patients is increased over that of healthy children [166], so that in a normal environment over a 24-hr period, rate of sweating may be increased.

Emrich and his colleagues [167] collected sweat droplets from only 60 to 250 glands and stimulated flow with various agents. They found that the average sweat output per gland was within the normal range in cystic fibrosis. Lobeck and McSherry [168] confirmed this using another technique. In the study of Emrich sodium and chloride concentrations rose with increasing output, but the lowest values in cystic fibrosis were considerably above those of the controls. Calcium and potassium concentrations decreased as output increased. Potassium concentrations were clearly elevated, but calcium was normal. Lactic acid and urea also decreased hyperbolically with increasing outputs and were slightly lower in cystic fibrosis. The sweat urea concentration is always above that of plasma and has been used as a means of identifying water reabsorption in the sweat gland [169]. Since Brusilow [170] has observed that there are nonplasma sources of urea in sweat, this method is questionable. Emrich also observed that sweat creatinine concentration was higher than that of plasma in patients with cystic fibrosis and controls but decreased with increasing output to less than plasma levels. Glucose concentrations were independent of sweat output and not elevated in cystic fibrosis. As expected from the changes in other constituents, osmolality was initially high, decreased, and then rose again at high outputs per gland. The pH of cystic fibrosis sweat and control sweat was acid (3.5 to 6.0) at low outputs and slightly alkaline at high outputs (7.0 to 8.5). The viscosity of cystic fibrosis sweat was higher than control sweat but this could be explained by the higher salt content. Other investigators have found that other organic constituents such as amino acids [171, 172] do not differ in cystic fibrosis from those found in controls. Glycoproteins have been isolated from sweat and an increased ratio of fucose to sialic acid found in the carbohydrate fraction in cystic fibrosis [173].

By use of the consecutive measurement of sweating rate and the rate of sweat sodium excretion in children with cystic fibrosis, Cage and his colleague [174], using the method of Schwartz [161], have calculated that the duct of the sweat gland in cystic fibrosis has a greatly reduced capacity to reabsorb sodium. Emrich [167] and Slegers [160] have reached similar conclusions, as have Schulz and her colleagues using direct micropuncture measurements [175, 176]. Mangos and McSherry [177] have demonstrated that sweat from patients with cystic fibrosis contains a heat-labile, nondialyzable factor which inhibits sodium reabsorption in the duct of the parotid gland of the rat (Fig. 68-2). This has been confirmed by Kaiser [334] by retrograde injection of cystic fibrosis sweat into normal sweat glands.

Whether the fluid secreted in the coil of the sweat gland is slightly hypertonic [176, 178, 179] or isotonic [161, 167, 174] is not settled. Few direct measurements have been made and, in those few, no abnormality was found in cystic fibrosis [175]. Thus, the cause of the increased sweat salinity in cystic fibrosis appears to be a decrease of sodium reabsorption in the duct of the gland.

Analysis of sweat collected from a small area of the skin surface after pilocarpine iontophoresis is used for clinical diagnosis [180]. This technique, although it may cause minor burning [181], is simple, safe, and accurate enough for this purpose. Increased sweat salinity can also be detected in cystic fibrosis by application to the skin of electrodes sensitive to sodium [182] and chloride [183, 184] or measurement of sweat electrical conductivity [185] and skin electrical resistance [186]. These techniques have not yet gained clinical acceptance.

The wide use of sweat analysis has led to discovery of some of the causes of variability in sweat composition of healthy Caucasian subjects of European origin (Fig. 68-3). Sweat sodium concentrations are higher and more variable in adults than in children when local sweating is produced with parasympathomimetic agents [165, 187]. This is correlated with a higher output of sweat per gland in adults, which is more marked in men [168]. During the first month of life, at the time of initiation of spontaneous sweating, sodium and chloride concentrations are at the adult level but are lower in the remainder of the first year of life [153]. Sex differences are not apparent until maturity. Women produce less sweat of lower sodium concentration than men, and the potassium concentration is the same in children and women but is significantly lower and approaches the concentration of potassium in extracellular fluid in men. In the Bantus of Uganda, McCance [188], using the same technique, found that Negro children produced less sweat than Caucasians (Indians and Europeans) [189] living in the same area and that adult Negro men do not produce more sweat than women or children of the same race. Sweat sodium concentration also did not rise with increasing age in Negroes but was slightly higher in adult men than women. Europeans living in Uganda exhibited the same dependence of sweat rate and sodium concentration upon age and sex as those living in Wisconsin, but sodium concentrations were much lower, probably due to acclimatization.

The sweat chloride concentration in healthy subjects averages 20 mEq per liter less than the sum of the sodium and potassium concentrations and is usually significantly lower

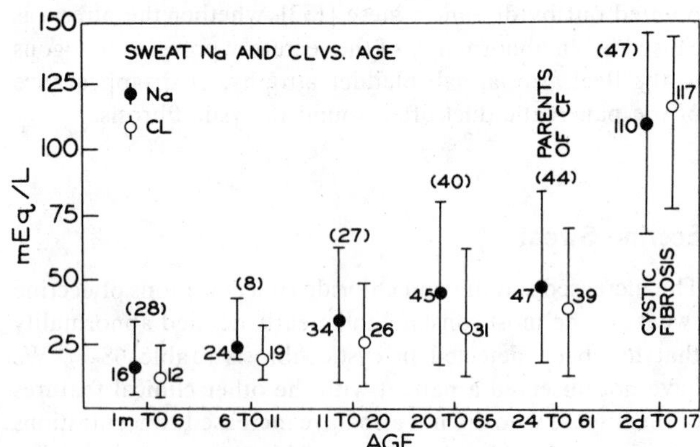

Figure 68-3. Variation of sweat sodium and chloride concentrations with age. Numbers and circles represent mean concentrations and range. Numbers in parentheses are numbers of subjects. Average concentrations of sodium and chloride are seen to increase with aging. In healthy subjects, chloride concentration is less than sodium; in cystic fibrosis the reverse is true. There is overlap of sodium concentration between adults and patients with cystic fibrosis. There is no overlap of chloride.

than that of sodium (Fig. 68-3). In the author's experience the chloride and sodium concentrations in cystic fibrosis may be almost equal because of the higher potassium concentration in these patients. Thus the chloride concentration in cystic fibrosis is less likely to overlap the values of control subjects and is more useful in diagnosis than is the sodium concentration (Fig. 68-3). In the adult there is overlap of sweat sodium and, to a lesser degree, chloride concentration with values from patients with cystic fibrosis, and clear abnormalities in some instances may be difficult to ascertain.

Other diseases may be associated with elevation of the sodium and chloride concentrations of the sweat, but these are not difficult to differentiate clinically (Table 68-2). It has been known for some time that Addison's disease is associated with elevated sweat sodium and chloride concentrations and that these can be decreased by treatment with mineralocorticoids (Table 68-2) [190]. Elevated sweat sodium or chloride concentrations have been reported in a sibship with hypoparathyroidism and signs of ectodermal dysplasia [191] and in another family with ectodermal dysplasia associated with sensorineural deafness and other anomalies (Table 68-2) [192]. A patient with autonomic dysfunction and segmental hypohidrosis, also probably related to ectodermal dysplasia, had elevated sweat sodium and chloride concentrations (Table 68-2) [193]. Patients with hereditary nephrogenic diabetes insipidus may have transient elevations of sweat sodium, potassium, and chloride concentrations (Table 68-2) [194], but with a single exception [195], these patients have only been those with relatively decreased thirst. This finding has been used successfully in our clinic as an aid to diagnosis of this disease in infancy, when excessive thirst and polyuria are absent. Some years ago Moseley [196] observed high sweat sodium concentrations in the sweat of patients with hypothyroidism and low sweat sodium concentrations in thyrotoxicosis. More recently Grand [197] and his colleagues, and Madoff (Table 68-2) [198] have observed the same findings in hypothyroidism. Sweat salinity can be reduced by treatment of the hypothyroidism. The unconfirmed observation (Table 68-2) [199] has been made that males with glucose-6-phosphatase deficiency (hepatorenal glycogen storage disease, Chap. 7) have sweat sodium and chloride concentrations comparable to those in cystic fibrosis. Unlike the response in cystic fibrosis, these were reduced to normal levels by decrease in sodium intake.

McCance [188] has found a slight depression of sweat rate in Bantu children with kwashiorkor and marasmus but no increase in sweat sodium concentration. The author has observed anhidrosis and sweat sodium concentrations in the 40 to 70 mEq per liter range upon resumption of sweating in malnourished Caucasian children. The rate of sweating of these children increased, and sodium concentrations returned to normal levels with restoration of good nutrition.

Several series of patients [200–213] with various forms of chronic pulmonary disease particularly chronic bronchitis have been reported with elevated average sweat sodium or chloride concentrations. In all these reports there has been considerable overlap of the values with those of controls. The significance of these observations is difficult to judge because the adequacy of controls for age, sex, diet, season of the year, physical activity, or indications of the state of acclimatization are frequently not reported. In many the number of patients is small. The report [214] of increased sweat salinity in patients with asthma has not been confirmed by others [215–217].

Table 68-2. REPORTED CONDITIONS OTHER THAN CYSTIC FIBROSIS WITH ELEVATED CONCENTRATION OF SODIUM AND CHLORIDE IN SWEAT

Disease	*Sweat electrolytes (mEq/l)*		Comment
	Na^+	Cl^-	
Addison's disease [190]	90–110	80–125	Decreased by treatment with mineralocorticoids
Familial hypoparathyroidism with anodontia [191]	178	127	Apparently unassociated with adrenal insufficiency
Familial hidrotic ectodermal dysplasia with sensorineural deafness [192]	74	53	Adults have higher values
Pupillotonia, hyporeflexia, and segmental hypohidrosis with autonomic dysfunction [193]	30–128	30–120	
Hereditary nephrogenic diabetes insipidus [194]	60–70	50–60	In infancy, without thirst
Hypothyroidism [198]		63–90	
Glucose-6-phosphatase deficiency [199]	73	71	Decreased by treatment of hypothyroidism Males, unconfirmed

Tears

In 1958 di Sant'Agnese et al. [78] reported a slight increase in the sodium chloride concentration of tears from patients with cystic fibrosis, but Khaw and Shwachman [218] did not confirm this finding (Table 68-1). Normally tears are isotonic or slightly hypertonic and have a sodium concentration which is similar to that of extracellular fluid, but the potassium concentration is considerably higher.

Hair and Nails

Hair and nails from children with cystic fibrosis have a higher content of sodium and potassium than normal [219–221]. This probably results from absorption of electrolytes by these tissues from sweat [41, 222]. In the case of hair the sodium content varies throughout its length, but in nails it is uniform. Neutron activation analysis of nails has been used for mass screening for cystic fibrosis with some success [222, 223]. The hair and nails of patients with cystic fibrosis appear to have a normal growth rate, appearance, and color.

Urine

Patients with cystic fibrosis can reduce urine sodium excretion after dietary salt deprivation to the same degree as controls [157]. Robson et al. [224] have reported that inulin clearance and fractional excretion of sodium are not abnormal, but in four of eight subjects with cystic fibrosis free water clearance was much reduced. This suggests impairment of sodium transport in the ascending loop of Henle.

Maxfield and Wolins [225] reported that the Tamm-Horsfall protein of urine has abnormal physical properties in cystic fibrosis. Extensive study of this finding has not led to the detection of differences in composition or physical behavior of this glycoprotein in controls and patients with cystic fibrosis [226–229].

Blood

Erythrocytes

The sodium and potassium concentration [230–231] and the morphology of erythrocytes are normal in cystic fibrosis. In studies of the sodium efflux from these cells, Balfe et al. [231] found a decrease in the ouabain-inhibited sodium transport and a marked decrease in the ethacrynic acid–sensitive transport of sodium. Ouabain-sensitive ATPase activity was decreased in ghosts but the ouabain-insensitive ATPase activity was normal. Parents of patients with cystic fibrosis were found to have a decreased ethacrynic acid–sensitive sodium transport. Since the erythrocytes have a normal composition in cystic fibrosis, they postulate that the rate of diffusion of sodium into the cells is slow, and balances the low transport rate out of the cell. Lobeck [230] and Mangos [232] have not been able to confirm these observations.

Leukocytes

Metachromasia is not demonstrable in leukocytes from fresh peripheral blood of patients with cystic fibrosis but develops in cultured leukocytes stained with toluidine blue about 4 days after the beginning of the culture [233]. Control leukocytes in these studies were ametachromatic. The metachromasia was not present in all patients with the disease. Human serum in the culture medium did not suppress the development of metachromasia. Leukocytes are not known to function abnormally in the disease.

Plasma and Serum

There is a substance in serum from patients with cystic fibrosis which causes disorganization of the ciliary beat of explants of rabbit trachea [234] and cessation of the beat of oyster cilia [235]. This substance is nondialyzable and heat labile, properties it shares with the substance found by Mangos in the sweat [177] and saliva [103] of patients with cystic fibrosis. Cessation of the beat of oyster cilia also followed application of parotid saliva from patients with cystic fibrosis and the polycations, polylysine and polyornithine. Mangos [132] has observed that these substances also inhibit sodium transport in the rat parotid gland.

The intestinal malabsorption of cystic fibrosis is associated with a decrease in lipoprotein lipase [236] and an electrophoretically slow-moving form of alkaline phosphatase in serum [237]. Relative increases in certain nonessential fatty acids particularly palmitoleic and oleic [238, 239], and depression of linoleic and arachidonic acids in plasma are probably also related to malabsorption. The slightly elevated tyrosine levels in plasma [240, 241] and urinary excretion of *p*-hydroxyphenylacetic acid [242, 243] are probably related to absorption of fecal tyrosine and tyramine found in increased amounts in cystic fibrosis [243].

Similarly, the pulmonary disease of cystic fibrosis is associated with high levels of precipitating antibodies in serum to *H. influenza, Pseudomonas aeruginosa* and *Staphylococcus aureus* [244], *Aspergillus fumigatus* [245, 246], and to lung tissue itself [247].

In the well-controlled patient the electrolyte concentrations in plasma are normal.

GENETICS

Cystic fibrosis is an inherited disease expressed only in the homozygous state without X linkage (autosomal recessive). Some of or all the stigmata are present from birth. The chromosomes are normal in number [248] and appearance [249]. At birth, both sexes are affected with equal frequency [153] even though later males may predominate [65, 250, 251] as a result of a higher mortality in females. Parents are unaffected. As expected, when mothers with cystic fibrosis have reproduced, their children have not had the disease [67, 252]. Discordance for cystic fibrosis has not been reported in monozygotic twins. No characteristic environmental insult to mothers has been demonstrated. The disease occurs without regard to maternal age or birth order [250, 253] or season of the year [254]. The high incidence of cystic fibrosis has only been found in Caucasians of European origin. The disease does occur in American Negroes [255, 256], American Indians [256, 257], and Orientals [258]. Reports of its occurrence in other Caucasian groups [259, 260], African Negroes [261], and Japanese [262–264] are frequently based on post-mortem findings or not substantiated by sweat analysis and classical clinical features. Records are sometimes not made of racial origin in these reports. Wright and Morton [265] in a study of cystic fibrosis in Hawaii from 1950 to 1965, estimated the gene frequency as fivefold higher in Caucasians than in non-Caucasians. Parental consanguinity in Caucasians has not been observed by us and has been so only rarely by others [253, 266, 267]. As expected, stepchildren in a sibship are rarely affected, but the incidence in first cousins is higher than in the general population [253, 268].

The disease has a high incidence in sibs (Fig. 68-4). Crow [269] estimated the segregation frequency as 0.267 with a s.d. of 0.033; Danks [250] estimated 0.243 with an s.d. of 0.016; and Wright and Morton [265] estimated 0.2599 with an s.d. of 0.0168. These estimates, arrived at by a maximum likelihood method, are not significantly different from 0.25 expected for a gene expressed only in the homozygous state (autosomal recessive). No evidence for a large fraction of sporadic cases (due to mutation, phenocopies, and other causes) was found in these data.

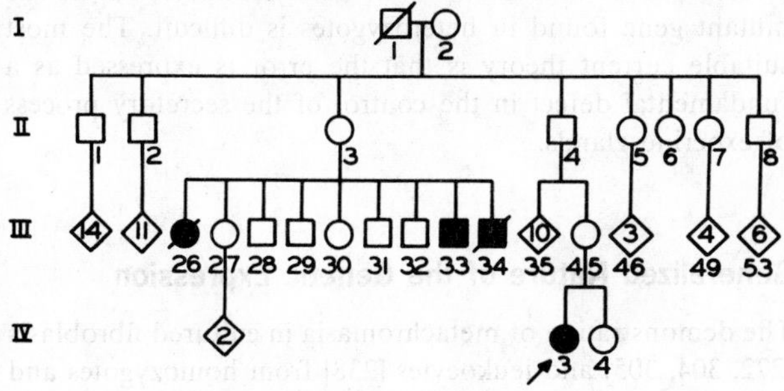

Figure 68-4. Pedigree of a kindred with cystic fibrosis. Propositus is Patient IV-3, with surgically corrected meconium ileus. Probands III-26 and III-34 died of meconium ileus shortly after birth. Proband III-33 has mild pulmonary and gastrointestinal disease at age 13. Parent I-1 died at age 65 of cancer; I-2 is living at age 80. Recessive inheritance is strongly suggested by lack of affected individuals in generations I and II and sibship III-35-45.

Heterozygotes

Presumed heterozygotes for cystic fibrosis (parents and sibs) may have higher average sweat sodium [270] and chloride [271] concentrations than controls, higher sodium content of nails [221], more frequent presence of serum protein in meconium [93], and a decrease in ethacrynic acid–sensitive sodium transport in erythrocytes [231]. These reports either show a great overlap of values for cystic fibrosis with controls or are as yet unconfirmed. The presence in heterozygotes of a factor in serum which causes disruption of ciliary activity [234] has been confirmed [235]. The very low prevalence of this factor in control subjects is compatible with the prevalence of the gene in the general population. The observation of metachromasia in cultured fibroblasts [272, 273] or leukocytes [233] from heterozygotes by Danes and Bearn has not yet been confirmed in other laboratories. It is also now a nonspecific marker for many diseases. On the other hand, the uniformity of the observation in the kindreds studied [273] leaves little doubt that metachromasia can occur in heterozygotes. The similarity of the appearance of metachromasia in some families to that seen in the mucopolysaccharidoses or other diseases detected by this technique makes certain heterozygote identification impossible. It is not known whether the sodium transport inhibitory substance found by Mangos is present in the sweat or saliva of heterozygotes.

These observations are strong evidence that cystic fibrosis is a genetic disease observed only in the homozygous state. The possibility of causation by multiple alleles or alleles at different loci cannot be excluded. The agreement between the expected and observed incidence of the disease in cousins of index cases and the low rate of parental consanguinity in Caucasians suggests that few loci are involved. On the other hand, Danes and Bearn [273] have detected several different types of metachromasia in cultured fibroblasts from heterozygotes and affected subjects. In each kindred only one type was found. Although this might suggest the action of genes at several loci, it could also be the result of multiple (noncomplementary) alleles for different types of metachromasia, all of which produce the cystic fibrosis phenotype, or could simply be an artifact of the culture system.

Linkage with blood group loci was not found in an analysis by Steinberg et al. [274], and the proportion of children with cystic fibrosis who are secretors of ABO blood group antigens is the same as in controls [275].

Associated Disorders

Isolated association of cystic fibrosis with Wiskott-Aldrich [276], Kartagener's [277], Down's [278], and *cri du chat* syndromes [279] have been described. In the last patient, the serum factor causing ciliary dyskinesis was present in the patient and her father, but not her mother. Based on this fact, the suggestion was made that the patient might be hemizygous for the cystic fibrosis gene on the intact short arm of chromosome 5. Later vesicular metachromasia was found in both parents and the patient [280]. Dallaire [281] studied a family with one child with cystic fibrosis and another with *cri du chat* syndrome. The latter child did not have any sign of cystic fibrosis, but a fibroblast culture exhibited metachromasia and his serum produced ciliary dyskinesis. Therefore he was probably heterozygous but not hemizygous, although it is possible that the deletion was not large enough to unmask the mutant gene. The author has not observed cystic fibrosis among patients with *cri du chat* syndrome or vice versa. In summary, these observations seem to shed doubt on the hypothesis that the cystic fibrosis gene is located on the short arm of chromosome 5.

Incidence

Many estimates have been made of the incidence of cystic fibrosis in the United States [265, 267, 282–286], Australia [250], and Europe [253, 287–289]. The most recent of these, based on population surveys, range from 1 in 2,000 to 1 in 4,000 live births, except for a Swedish estimate [287] of 1 in 7,700 live births. Thus, the incidence of heterozygotes in the Caucasian population is approximately 4 percent, but in Sweden may be only 2 percent. In order that this high incidence be maintained by mutation alone, a mutation rate would be required of an order of magnitude higher than has been observed for most other recessive conditions [290]. For this reason many have postulated that there must be a reproductive or survival advantage for heterozygotes. An advantage of only 1.6 percent is needed to maintain an incidence of 1 in 3,700 live births. Epidemiologic studies are not likely to detect an advantage of this small magnitude. Baumann [291] found that in Switzerland the sibships of index cases included an average of 4.27 children, whereas control families had only 2.48. Danks [250], and Knudson [292] studied the average family size of grandparental matings, since one of the grandparents must have been heterozygous: it was significantly larger than that of control families. The advantage implied by these studies is far in excess of that required and could lead to a rising incidence of the disease in Caucasian populations. Perhaps the composition of the mucus of the uterine cervix in heterozygous women [293] or the composition of seminal fluid in heterozygous men confers increased fertility.

In their study of cystic fibrosis in Hawaii, Wright and Morton [265] suggested that the differences between the incidence in Caucasians and non-Caucasians may be related to the presence of different alleles in the two groups, a selection differential or genetic drift. They conclude that heterozygous advantage in Caucasians might be limited to this race. They could not exclude genetic drift as the cause of the difference between the frequency in Caucasians and non-Caucasians.

Heterozygotes for cystic fibrosis do not have clinical findings of cystic fibrosis. Parents do not have an increased incidence of chronic pulmonary or gastrointestinal disease [294, 295, 50, 296]. Ascertainment of adult heterozygotes as patients with "adult mucoviscidosis," expressed as pulmonary disease [200–213], gastrointestinal ulcers [297], diabetes mellitus [298, 299], and immune deficiency disease [300] associated with slightly elevated levels of sodium or chloride in sweat is not good enough to be acceptable in the light of present methods of heterozygote detection. It is also contrary to the expectation of a heterozygote advantage in Caucasians. In addition, the extreme variability of sweat electrolyte concentrations makes the use of sweat analysis for this purpose questionable. Although it is true that the ascertainment of heterozygotes as the parents of probands excludes most of the heterozygotes in the population, it is unlikely that the latter group would differ significantly from parents. Chronic bronchitis may be associated with a tendency to higher sweat sodium and chloride concentrations. It would certainly seem more fruitful to investigate physiologic or biochemical reasons for this association than to implicate these syndromes as the heterozygous state of cystic fibrosis.

HYPOTHESES REGARDING THE FUNDAMENTAL DEFECT

Hypotheses regarding the fundamental defect in cystic fibrosis have evolved as knowledge of the pathophysiology and genetics has increased and modern techniques of study have been applied. Vitamin A deficiency was suggested [25], since this was a common accompaniment of the early cases, but the pathologic findings of vitamin A deficiency have become much less frequent and are now known to have been superimposed on the basic disease process [301]. Similarly the theory of Baggenstoss et al. [302] that secretin deficiency underlies the pancreatic changes had to be rejected when it was found that the amount of the hormone in intestinal tissue was normal [303].

Formation of a hypothesis that includes new knowledge of the secretory process and the various expressions of the mutant gene found in heterozygotes is difficult. The most suitable current theory is that the error is expressed as a fundamental defect in the control of the secretory process of exocrine glands.

Generalized Nature of the Genetic Expression

The demonstration of metachromasia in cultured fibroblasts [272, 304, 305] and leukocytes [238] from homozygotes and heterozygotes with cystic fibrosis indicates that the mutant gene can express itself in cells other than those of exocrine glands. Metachromatic granules and vesicles are not present in skin [273] or leukocytes [233] before culture. Two different laboratories [273, 304] have demonstrated that, in some cases, the metachromasia is associated with increase in the cellular content of mucopolysaccharides. Matalon and Dorfman

[304] compared the mucopolysaccharide composition of fibroblasts from patients with cystic fibrosis with those cultured from patients with a number of the diseases associated with metachromasia. Unlike some of these, the total amount of acid mucopolysaccharides was variably increased, and specific acid mucopolysaccharides were present in normal proportion. This does not mean that cystic fibrosis is a mucopolysaccharidosis but rather that under certain special environmental conditions, the mutant gene may be expressed as an abnormality in the metabolism of these substances. The defect may be in systems that control mucopolysaccharide synthesis, degradation and release under tissue culture conditions and be quite distinct from direct involvement in mucopolysaccharide metabolism in the intact host. Nevertheless the search for a molecular abnormality in cultured cells could be rewarding as it has been in other diseases.

The Process of Secretion

All evidence suggests that cystic fibrosis is primarily a disease of exocrine glands. It appears that in the most constantly involved gland, the eccrine sweat gland, the major cause of increased sweat sodium and chloride concentrations is reduction in sodium reabsorption in the duct of the gland. On the basis of many assumptions Slegers [160] postulated that reabsorption of sodium occurs in two stages in the duct of the eccrine sweat gland. Sodium, accompanied by chloride, is reabsorbed proximally in the duct, and distally it is reabsorbed by an ion exchange mechanism for potassium or hydrogen ion. The latter mechanism is thought to be intact in cystic fibrosis because of the high potassium excretion of cystic fibrosis sweat, its inverse relationship to ammonia excretion as an indicator of hydrogen ion production, and the response of cystic fibrosis sweat glands to aldosterone. Sodium reabsorption in the proximal duct is postulated to be defective, but the primary secretory fluid is normal. Gordon and Cage [306] did not agree that the high potassium concentration in the sweat is due solely to sodium exchange and suggested that the potassium concentration of the precursor fluid is elevated and that in cystic fibrosis there is an increased resistance to passive diffusion of sodium into the secretory fluid as well as out of the lumen of the duct. Their theory is based on the hypothesis that the primary event in sweat secretion is the release of lactate from anaerobic glycolysis in the secretory coil since lactate is found in high concentration in sweat.

The observation that there may be deficient pancreatic response to secretin in patients with cystic fibrosis who still retain pancreatic function stimulated Johansen, Anderson, and Hadorn [307] to suggest that there is an inhibition of fluid movement from the extracellular space into secretory cells throughout the body. They suggested that water reabsorption out of the duct lumen of eccrine glands may be reduced because of decreased sodium reabsorption, and since the output of sweat by the glands is normal in cystic fibrosis, the rate of secretion must be reduced. Thus, the increased viscosity of mucus and increased solute concentration of secretory fluids from exocrine glands in cystic fibrosis would be due to the relative paucity of water and electrolytes accompanying the secretion of macromolecules.

The observation by Mangos of a substance present in sweat [177] and saliva [103] in cystic fibrosis which inhibits sodium reabsorption in the duct of the rat parotid gland suggests that the primary defect could be in the secretory process. The presence of an abnormal molecule or a normal molecule in larger than usual amounts in these secretory fluids suggests a defect in the control or function of the exocrine cell. Support for this hypothesis is gained from the observation that long-term isoproterenol administration to rats [133] can induce the appearance of the ciliary dyskinetic factor in the serum and sodium transport inhibition in the parotid gland of the rat, just as in cystic fibrosis. The effect of guanethidine, a repressor of exocrine activity, in reducing the protein content and turbidity of submaxillary saliva in cystic fibrosis also suggests a similar defect.

These recently advanced hypotheses suggest that the pathology of cystic fibrosis has its origin in an abnormality in the secretory process of exocrine cells. Since there has been no clear abnormality demonstrated in the structure of the glycoproteins of exocrine secretions, the observations of Gugler et al. [121] suggest that alterations in the ionic composition of secretory fluids, particularly in the concentration of calcium, could account for hypothetical changes in the physical properties of glycoproteins. This hypothesis, as well as the suggestion of Chernick and Barbero [120] that increased secretion of these proteins by secretory cells is the cause of the high protein concentration of submaxillary saliva, are not incompatible with the hypothesis that the exocrine cell is the site of the defect. Further knowledge of the process of exocrine secretion may eventually lead to the understanding of pathogenesis of cystic fibrosis.

Origin of Serum Factors

The presence of a substance or substances in the serum which can cause ciliary dyskinesis [234] or cessation of beat [235] brings into focus the question of their relationship to abnormal exocrine gland function. Two possible sources of these factors can be mentioned. Either they originate in exocrine glands and are released into the circulation as a result of abnormal function of the gland or there is production of the factors in other tissues. In the latter event, they may cause a defect in the process of secretion and be primary in the production of the disease. At present there is no direct evidence for either of these possibilities. There is ample precedent for release of the products of secretion by exocrine glands, particularly the pancreas, into the circulation. The similarity between the sodium transport–inhibiting factor and ciliary dyskinesis factor, the presence of ciliary dyskinesis factor in the saliva of patients with cystic fibrosis [235], and the results of the isoproterenol experiments in rats [133] suggest that this may be the case. On the other hand the presence of these factors in the plasma of heterozygotes in the absence of any abnormality of exocrine gland function suggests that they may be primary effectors of the abnormality of exocrine secretion.

The question of the origin and relationship of serum factors to exocrine function cannot be answered without further knowledge of the mechanism of exocrine gland function and its relation to substances in plasma and secretions.

Defect in the Control of Secretion

There is a possibility that cystic fibrosis is due to a defect in the control of exocrine secretion rather than in the synthesis of a molecule secreted by exocrine glands. The abnormality could be in the autonomic nervous system or in the response of the exocrine tissue to stimulation.

Clinical evidence of a generalized disturbance of any segment of the autonomic nervous system is lacking. Heart rate is normal, tearing is not excessive, and intestinal motility and vasomotor responses are normal. The observation by Rubin et al. [308] that the rate of pupillary dilatation in response to darkness was distinctly slowed in cystic fibrosis did not suggest a generalized defect in the autonomic nervous system but rather a deficiency of an adrenergic mediator. Adrenergic sweating is present in cystic fibrosis [309], and other functions controlled by adrenergic nerves do not seem impaired.

Many observations suggest that the exocrine glands are hyperfunctioning in cystic fibrosis. Hypertrophy of rat parotid glands with findings simulating cystic fibrosis can be produced by isoproterenol injection [133]. Decreased rate of sweating and increased concentration of electrolytes following prolonged diaphoresis [310, 311] occurs more rapidly in patients with cystic fibrosis than in controls [312]. The increased fucose-sialic acid ratio in the glycoproteins may reflect increased intensity of secretory stimulation [122]. The turbidity, nitrogen, and calcium content and ratio of fucose to sialic acid of submaxillary saliva when reflexly stimulated in cystic fibrosis is similar to that obtained from control children after more vigorous stimulation with pharmacologic amounts of parasympathomimetic drugs [117]. The histologic appearance of the tracheobronchial and intestinal glands suggest hypersecretion [47].

Since increased production and release or decreased destruction of acetylcholine [313, 314] does not seem to be the cause of this hypersecretion [315–317], it is possible that the defect of exocrine gland function lies within the exocrine cell. The adenyl cyclase, cyclic adenosine-3'-5' monophosphate (cylic AMP) system can control protein synthesis or membrane permeability of a variety of cells [318]. It is active in the control of the secretory cells of the rat parotid [319, 320]. This system or another, controlling the translation of neurogenic stimulation into secretion within the cell, could be at fault in cystic fibrosis.

TREATMENT

The prognosis of cystic fibrosis depends upon the treatment. The extent to which surgical skill and facilities are available for the infant with meconium ileus and the intensity of the management of the progressive pulmonary involvement are major determinants of mortality. To prevent morbidity, the patient with cystic fibrosis requires continuing optimistic management. The greatest success in reduction of morbidity and mortality have come in those centers in which intensive management is provided [70].

Since pulmonary involvement is the most common cause of death and chronic disability, the principal effort of treatment has been to alleviate obstruction of airflow and reduce infection. The most useful measures have been water aerosol therapy in a mist tent or by mask, antibiotics, and physical therapy including postural drainage, chest vibration, clapping and compression and breathing exercises. The availability of large number of agents has made tests of the efficacy of any one of them difficult. Mist therapy is most widely used and is of benefit [321]. Some use it prophylactically before the onset of clinical pulmonary disease [322]. Recently the physiologic basis of the benefit from mist tent therapy has been questioned [323].

Particularly effective as antibiotics for treatment of acute infections are chloramphenicol and semisynthetic penicillins. Bone marrow depression from use of the former has been reported rarely, although there can be toxicity to the central nervous system [54]. An effective means of treating *Pseudomonas* infection has not been developed, but carbenicillin and gentomycin show some promise [324]. Continuous antibiotic therapy is occasionally used in management but is of unknown effectiveness. Low-dose prophylactic antibiotic therapy should be avoided. Mucolytic agents such as hypertonic salt solutions and *n*-acetyl cysteine inhaled as aerosols have been of value in occasional patients. Bronchodilators such as isoproterenol administered by aerosol are also used. Bronchial lavage with saline or mucolytic agents has not proved to be of long-term value and can be lethal [325, 326].

Meconium ileus is treated with immediate surgical exploration. Recently a gentle gastrografin enema has been found effective in relieving the obstruction without surgery [327]. This may be particularly effective in the treatment of intestinal obstruction in later childhood but can be dangerous. The Bishop-Koop procedure, resection of the enlarged intestine and end-to-side ileoileostomy, has been the most successful surgical operation for meconium ileus [13].

Treatment of gastrointestinal malabsorption is directed at improving nutrition and relieving abdominal cramps and foul diarrhea. The diet should be individualized because of variation in the degree of malabsorption [328]. Medium-chain triglyceride feeding may improve nutrition [329, 330].

When administered orally, various extracts of animal pancreas sometimes give subjective relief from diarrhea and cramps, and may decrease steatorrhea to a variable degree. Supplementary vitamins A and D should be added to the diet in water-miscible form. Vitamin E is frequently administered but has no proven clinical value. Vitamin K should be given to infants before surgical treatment or during treatment with broad-spectrum antibiotics.

Growth, development, and physical strength may be enhanced by the administration of anabolic steroids [331–333]. These are most useful in patients with severe pulmonary disease, particularly preadolescent girls.

Other complications such as portal hypertension and cirrhosis, rectal prolapse, pneumothroax, atelectasis, nasal polyposis, and duodenal ulcer are treated in the conventional ways.

SUMMARY

1 Cystic fibrosis (mucoviscidosis) of the pancreas is a relatively common inherited disease of childhood and early adulthood in Caucasians of European origin. The clinical features of the disease stem from an unknown defect in exocrine gland function. Both serous and mucous glands are known to be affected.

2 Exocrine glands which are known to have reabsorbing surfaces (eccrine sweat gland, parotid and submaxillary gland) have increased concentrations of sodium and chloride in their final secretory product. The lacrimal apparatus without reabsorbing surfaces produce tears of normal composition. The increased salinity of eccrine sweat is the most useful diagnostic test for the disease.

3 Exocrine glands with secretions of high protein content show the greatest histologic abnormality. Mucous secretions are tenacious and thick. The pancreas frequently does not function at birth and, when functioning, has a deficient response to secretin. Increased viscosity of mucus is a major cause of the obstructive pulmonary disease which is life-threatening.

4 Women with cystic fibrosis have reproduced, but men are sterile. Atresia of the vas deferentia and abnormality of the exocrine glands of the male reproductive system are responsible for the sterility in spite of the occurrence of spermatogenesis.

5 The major clinical manifestations of cystic fibrosis are pulmonary and gastrointestinal. Frequent findings are progressive bronchiolar obstruction with complicating pulmonary infection, hyperaeration, and cor pulmonale. Meconium ileus is pathognomonic, and generalized cirrhosis of the liver occurs occasionally. Steatorrhea and azotorrhea with malnutrition and growth retardation are common consequences of pancreatic insufficiency. Sweating can lead to sodium and chloride depletion. Without treatment the prognosis is grave.

6 There are reports of abnormalities in sites other than the exocrine glands. Erythrocyte sodium transport or permeability may be abnormal, and there is a substance in plasma which causes ciliary dyskinesia in explants of rabbit cilia and cessation of beat of oyster cilia. The central and autonomic nervous system do not appear to be affected.

7 The fundamental defect is unknown but is most probably in the process or control of secretion by the exocrine gland. Increased sodium and chloride concentrations in secretory products are best explained by the presence of a substance or substances in secretory fluids which inhibit reabsorption. No abnormality of the glycoprotein composition of secretory fluids, other than increased concentration and increased fucose/sialic acid ratio has been found. An abnormality of exocrine cell function seems more likely than synthesis of an abnormal molecule as the cause of the disease.

8 Cystic fibrosis is manifest clinically only in the homozygous state. Probably only one genetic locus is involved. Reproductive advantage for heterozygous individuals is presumably responsible for the high incidence of the disease in Causcasians of European origin. Heterozygotes have the ciliary dyskinesis factor in their serum. The mutant gene may also express itself as metachromasia in fibroblasts and leukocytes in tissue culture. Metachromasia occurs in both heterozygotes and homozygotes with equal intensity. This is associated in some with an increase in mucopolysaccharide content.

9 Treatment lengthens survival and is directed mainly at preventing chronic disability from progression of pulmonary involvement, malnutrition, and steatorrhea. Meconium ileus is treated surgically.

BIBLIOGRAPHY

1. Fanconi, G., Uehlinger, E., and Knauer, C.: Das Coeliaksyndrom bei angeborener zystischer Pankreasfibromatose und Bronchiektasien. Wien. Med. Wschr., **86**, 753, 1936.
2. Landsteiner, K.: Darmverschluss durch eingedicktes Meconium Pancreatitis. Zbl. Allg. Path., **16**, 903, 1905.
3. Garrod, A. E., Hurtley, W. H.: Congenital family steathorrhea. Quart. J. Med., **6**, 242, 1912.
4. Blackfan, K. D., and Wolbach, S. B.: Vitamin A deficiency in infants: a clinical and pathological study. J. Pediat., **3**, 679, 1933.
5. Blackfan, K. D., and May, C. D.: Inspissation of secretions, dilation of the ducts and acini, atrophy and fibrosis of the pancreas in infants. J. Pediat., **13**, 627, 1938.
6. Harper, M. H.: Congenital steatorrhoea due to pancreatic defect. Arch. Dis. Child., **13**, 45, 1938.
7. Andersen, D. H.: Cystic fibrosis of the pancreas and its relation to celiac disease. Amer. J. Dis. Child., **56**, 344, 1938.
8. Andersen, D. H.: Cystic fibrosis of the pancreas. J. Chronic Dis., **7**, 58, 1959.
9. Farber, S.: Some organic digestive disturbances in early life. J. Mich. Med. Soc., **44**, 587, 1945.
10. di Sant'Agnese, P. A., Darling, R. C., Perera, G. A., and Shea, E.: Abnormal electrolyte composition of sweat in cystic fibrosis of the pancreas. Pediatrics, **12**, 549, 1953.
11. Boyer, P. H.: Low birth weight in fibrocystic disease of the pancreas. Pediatrics, **16**, 778, 1955.
12. Hsia, D. Y. Y.: Birth weight in cystic fibrosis of the pancreas. Ann. Hum. Genet., **23**, 289, 1959.

13. Holsclaw, D. S., Eckstein, H. B., and Nixon, H. H.: Meconium ileus. Amer. J. Dis. Child., **109**, 101, 1965.
14. Oppenheimer, E. H., and Esterly, J. R.: Observations in cystic fibrosis of the pancreas. II. Neonatal intestinal obstruction. Bull. Johns Hopkins Hosp., **111**, 1, 1962.
15. Donnison, A. B., Schwachman, H., and Gross, R. E.: A review of 164 children with meconium ileus seen at the Children's Hospital Medical Center, Boston. Pediatrics, **37**, 833, 1966.
16. May, C. G., and Lowe, C. U.: Fibrosis of pancreas in infants and children. J. Pediat., **34**, 663, 1949.
17. Mullins, F., Talamo, R., and di Sant'Agnese, P. A.: Late intestinal complications of cystic fibrosis. J.A.M.A., **192**, 741, 1965.
18. Hunton, D. B., Long, W. K., and Tsumagari, H. Y.: Meconium ileus equivalent: an adult complication of fibrocystic disease. Gastroenterology, **50**, 99, 1966.
19. Fleisher, D. S., Di George, A. M., Barness, L. A., and Cornfeld, D.: Hypoproteinemia and edema in infants with cystic fibrosis of the pancreas. J. Pediat., **64**, 341, 1964.
20. Fleisher, D. S., Di George, A. M., Auerbach, V. H., Huang, N. N., and Barness, L. A.: Protein metabolism in cystic fibrosis of the pancreas. J. Pediat., **64**, 349, 1964.
21. Strober, W., Peter, G., and Schwartz, R. H.: Albumin metabolism in cystic fibrosis. Pediatrics, **43**, 416, 1969.
22. Caplan, A., and Gross, S.: Hematologic and serologic studies in cystic fibrosis. J. Pediat., **73**, 540, 1968.
23. Tönz, O., and Rossi, E.: Iron absorption in cystic fibrosis, in *4th International Conference on Cystic Fibrosis of the Pancreas* (mucoviscidosis), Mod. Prob. Pediat., **10**, 259, 1967.
24. Kulczycki, L. L., and Shwachman, H.: Studies in cystic fibrosis of the pancreas: occurrence of rectal prolapse. New Eng. J. Med., **259**, 409, 1958.
25. Andersen, D. H.: Cystic fibrosis, vitamin A deficiency and bronchiectasis. J. Pediat., **15**, 763, 1939.
26. Zuelzer, W. W., and Newton, W. A., Jr.: The pathogenesis of fibrocystic disease of the pancreas. Pediatrics, **4**, 53, 1949.
27. Bodian, M. (ed.): *Fibrocystic Disease of the Pancreas: A Congenital Disorder of Mucus Production-Mucosis,* p. 143. Heinemann, London, 1952.
28. Blanc, W. A., Reid, J. D., and Andersen, D. H.: Avitaminosis E in cystic fibrosis of the pancreas. Pediatrics, **22**, 494, 1958.
29. Sung, J. H.: Neuroaxonal dystrophy in mucoviscidosis. J. Neuropath. Exp. Neurol., **23**, 567, 1964.
30. Gordon, H. H., and Nitowsky, H. M.: Some studies of tocopherol in infants and children. Amer. J. Clin. Nutrition, **4**, 391, 1956.
31. di Sant'Agnese, P. A.: Cystic fibrosis of the pancreas. J.A.M.A., **172**, 135, 1960.
32. Shwachman, H.: Therapy of cystic fibrosis of the pancreas. Pediatrics, **25**, 155, 1960.
33. Torstenson, O. L., Humphrey, G. B., Edson, J. R., and Warwick, W. J.: Cystic fibrosis presenting with severe hemorrhage due to vitamin K malabsorption: a report of 3 cases. Pediatrics, **45**, 857, 1970.
34. Gibbons, I. S. E.: Disaccharides and cystic fibrosis of the pancreas. Arch. Dis. Child., **44**, 63, 1969.
35. Antonowicz, I., Reddy, V., Khaw, K. T., and Shwachman, H.: Lactase deficiency in patients with cystic fibrosis. Pediatrics, **42**, 492, 1968.
36. Cozetto, F. J.: Intestinal lactase deficiency in a patient with cystic fibrosis. Pediatrics, **32**, 228, 1963.
37. Royce, S. W.: Cardiac and pulmonary complications in fibrocystic disease of the pancreas, in *Fibrocystic Disease of the Pancreas: Report 18th Ross Pediat. Res. Conf.* Ross Lab., Columbus, Ohio, 1956.
38. Iacocca, V. F., Sibinga, M. S., and Barbero, G. J.: Respiratory tract bacteriology in cystic fibrosis. Amer. J. Dis. Child., **106**, 315, 1963.
39. Pittman, F. E., Calderon, H., Goode, L., and di Sant'Agnese, P. A.: Phage groups and antibiotic sensitivity of staphylococcus aureus associated with cystic fibrosis of the pancreas. Pediatrics, **24**, 40, 1959.
40. Doggett, R. G., Harrison, G. M., Stillwell, R. N., and Wallis, E. S.: An atypical *pseudomonas aeruginosa* associated with cystic fibrosis of the pancreas. J. Pediat., **68**, 215, 1966.
41. di Sant'Agnese, P. A., and Talamo, R. C.: Pathogenesis and physiopathology of cystic fibrosis of the pancreas, fibrocystic disease of the pancreas (mucoviscidosis). New Eng. J. Med., **277**, 1287, 1343, 1399, 1967.
42. Kessler, W. R., and Andersen, D. H.: Heat prostration in fibrocystic disease of pancreas and other conditions. Pediatrics, **8**, 648, 1951.
43. di Sant'Agnese, P. A., and Blanc, W. A.: A distinctive type of biliary cirrhosis of the liver associated with fibrocystic disease of the pancreas, recognition through signs of portal hypertension. Pediatrics, **18**, 387, 1956.
44. Aterman, K.: Duodenal ulceration and fibrocystic pancreas disease. Amer. J. Dis. Child., **101**, 210, 1961.
45. Wurm, H.: Ulcus duodeni mit Pankreasentwicklungsstorüng bei einem 7 Wochen alter Säugling. Z. Kinderheilk, **43**, 286, 1927.
46. Markel, I. J.: Fibrocystic disease of the pancreas with an unusual lesion. J. Indiana Med. Ass., **37**, 674, 1944.
47. Andersen, D. H.: Pathology of cystic fibrosis. Ann. N. Y. Acad. Sci., **93**, 500, 1962.
48. Rosan, R. C., Shwachman, H., and Kulczycki, L. L.: Diabetes mellitus and cystic fibrosis of the pancreas. Amer. J. Dis. Child., **104**, 625, 1962.
49. Charles, R. N., and Kelley, M. L.: Occurrence of diabetes mellitus in families of patients with cystic fibrosis of the pancreas. J. Chron. Dis., **14**, 381, 1961.
50. Orzales, M. M., Kohner, D., Cook, C. D., and Shwachman, H.: Anamnesis, sweat electrolyte and pulmonary function studies in parents of patients with cystic fibrosis of the pancreas. Acta Paediat. Scand., **52**, 267, 1963.
51. Handwerger, S., Roth, J., Gorden, P., di Sant'Agnese, P., Carpenter, D. F., and Peter, G.: Glucose intolerance in cystic fibrosis. New Eng. J. Med., **281**, 451, 1969.
52. Green, O. C., Fefferman, R., and Nair, S.: Plasma growth hormone levels in children with cystic fibrosis and short stature. Unresponsiveness to hypoglycemia. J. Clin. Endocr., **27**, 1059, 1967.
53. Bruce, G. M., Denning, C. R., and Spalter, H. F.: Ocular findings in cystic fibrosis of the pancreas. Arch. Ophthal., **63**, 391, 1960.
54. Huang, N. N., Harley, R. D., Promadhattavedi, V., and Sproul, A.: Visual disturbances in cystic fibrosis following chloramphenicol administration. J. Pediat., **68**, 32, 1966.
55. Greutzner, A., and Geletneky, C. L.: E.E.G.—Befunde bei Erwachsenen Mucoviscidosis. Zbl. Neuro. Psychiat., **161**, 6, 1960.
56. Spock, A., and Wilson, W. P.: Electroencephalograms of patients with cystic fibrosis. Amer. J. Dis. Child., **108**, 144, 1964.
57. Henkin, R. I., and Powell, G. F.: Increased sensitivity of taste and smell in cystic fibrosis. Science, **138**, 1107, 1962.
58. Wotman, S., Mandel, I. D., Khotim, S., Thompson, R. H., Jr., Kutscher, A. H., Zegarelli, E. V., and Denning, C. R.: Salt taste thresholds in cystic fibrosis. Amer. J. Dis. Child., **108**, 372, 1964.
59. Manalapas, F. C., Stein, A. A., Pagliara, A. S., Apicelli, A. A., Porter, I. H., and Patterson, P. R.: Phenylthiocarbamide taste sensitivity in cystic fibrosis. J. Pediat., **66**, 8, 1965.
60. Sproul, A., and Huang, N.: Growth patterns in children with cystic fibrosis. J. Pediat., **65**, 664, 1964.
61. Gharib, R., Allen, R. P., Joos, H. A., and Bravo, L. R.: Paranasal sinuses in cystic fibrosis. Amer. J. Dis. Child., **108**, 499, 1964.
62. Shwachman, H., Kulczycki, L. L., Mueller, H. L., and Flake, C. G.: Nasal polyposis in patients with cystic fibrosis. Pediatrics, **30**, 389, 1962.
63. Barbero, G. J., and Sibinga, M. S.: Enlargement of the submaxillary salivary glands in cystic fibrosis. Pediatrics, **29**, 788, 1962.
64. McIntosh, R.: Cystic fibrosis of the pancreas in patients over 10 years of age. Acta Paediat. Scand., Suppl., 100, **43**, 469, 1954.
65. Shwachman, H., Kulczycki, L. L., and Khaw, K.: Studies in cystic fibrosis: a report on sixty-five patients over 17 years of age. Pediatrics, **36**, 689, 1965.
66. di Sant'Agnese, P. A.: Cystic fibrosis in adolescents and young adults, in *4th International Conference on Cystic Fibrosis of the Pancreas* (mucoviscidosis), Mod. Prob. Pediat., **10**, 135, 1967.
67. Grand, R. J., Talamo, R. C., di Sant'Agnese, P. A., and Schwartz, R. H.: Pregnancy in cystic fibrosis of the pancreas. J.A.M.A., **195**, 993, 1966.

68. Denning, C. R., Sommers, S. C., and Quigley, H. J.: Infertility in male patients with cystic fibrosis. Pediatrics, **41,** 7, 1968.
69. Kaplan, E., Shwachman, H., Perlmutter, A. D., Rule, A., Khaw, K. T., and Holsclaw, D. S.: Reproductive failure in males with cystic fibrosis. New Eng. J. Med., **279,** 65, 1968.
70. Warwick, W. J., and Pogue, R. E.: The prognosis for children with cystic fibrosis based on reasoned approaches to therapy: past, present, and future. J. Asthma Res., **5,** 277, 1968.
71. Andersen, P. H.: Pathology of cystic fibrosis. Ann. N.Y. Acad. Sci., **93,** 500, 1962.
72. Bodian, M. (ed.): *Fibrocystic Disease of the Pancreas: A Congenital Disorder of Mucus Production-Mucosis,* pp. 86–104. Heinemann, London, 1952.
73. Reemtsma, K., di Sant'Agnese, P. A., Malm, J. R., and Barker, H. G.: Cystic fibrosis of pancreas. Intestinal absorption of fat and fatty acid labeled with I^{131}. Pediatrics, **22,** 525, 1958.
74. Kuo, P. T., and Huang, N. N.: The effect of medium chain triglyceride upon fat absorption and plasma lipid and depot fat of children with cystic fibrosis of the pancreas. J. Clin. Invest., **44,** 1924, 1965.
75. Shwachman, H., and Leubner, H.: Mucoviscidosis. Advan. Pediat., **7,** 249, 1955.
76. Dyck, W. P.: Titrimetric measurements of fecal trypsin and chymotrypsin in cystic fibrosis with pancreatic exocrine insufficiency. Am. J. Dig. Dis., New Series, **12,** 310, 1967.
77. Barbero, G. J., Sibinga, M. S., Marino, J. M., and Seibel, R.: Stool trypsin and chymotrypsin. Am. J. Dis. Child., **112,** 536, 1966.
78. di Sant'Agnese, P. A., Grossman, H., Darling, R. C., and Denning, C. R.: Saliva, tears and duodenal contents in cystic fibrosis of the pancreas. Pediatrics, **22,** 507, 1958.
79. Hadorn, B., Johansen, P. G., and Anderson, C. M.: Pancreozymin secretin test of exocrine pancreatic function in cystic fibrosis and the significance of the result for the pathogenesis of the disease. Canad. Med. Ass. J., **98,** 377, 1968.
80. Hadorn, B., Johansen, P. G., and Anderson, C. M.: Pancreozymin secretin tests of exocrine pancreatic function in cystic fibrosis and the significance of the results for the pathogenesis of the disease. Aust. Pediat. J., **4,** 8, 1968.
81. Hadorn, B., Zoppi, G., Shmerling, D. H., Prader, A., McIntyre, I., and Anderson, C. M.: Quantitative assessment of exocrine pancreatic function in infants and children. J. Pediat., **73,** 39, 1968.
82. Rick, W.: Untersuchung zur exokrinen Funktion des Pankreas bei Zystischer Pankreasfibrose. Med. Welt, **42,** 2158, 1963.
83. Johansen, P. G., Hadorn, B., and Anderson, C. M.: The effect of secretin on human rectal mucosa *in vivo.* Nature (London), **217,** 468, 1968.
84. di Sant'Agnese, P. A., Dische, Z., and Danilchenko, A.: Physicochemical differences of mucoproteins in duodenal fluid of patients with cystic fibrosis of the pancreas and controls: clinical aspects. Pediatrics, **19,** 252, 1957.
85. Dische, Z., di Sant'Agnese, P. A., Pallavicini, C., and Youlos, J.: Composition of mucoprotein fractions from duodenal fluid of patients with cystic fibrosis of the pancreas and from controls. Pediatrics, **24,** 74, 1959.
86. Roelfs, R. E., Gibbs, G. E., and Griffin, G. D.: The composition of rectal mucus in cystic fibrosis. Amer. J. Dis. Child., **113,** 419, 1967.
87. Lowe, C. V., Adler, W., Broberger, O., Walsh, J., and Neter, E.: Mucopolysaccharide from patients with cystic fibrosis of the pancreas. Science, **153,** 1124, 1966.
88. Broglio, A. L., Saari, T. N., Blackwell, C., Carlson, D. M., and Matthews, L. W.: Comparison of stool antigens from normal and cystic fibrosis children. Cystic Fibrosis Club Abstracts., p. 15, April 26, 1967.
89. Chodos, D. D. I., Ely, R. S., and Kelly, V. C.: Paper electrophoresis of duodenal fluid from patients with cystic fibrosis. Proc. Soc. Exp. Biol. Med., **99,** 775, 1958.
90. Wiser, W. C. and Beier, F. R.: Albumin in the meconium of infants with cystic fibrosis: a preliminary report. Pediatrics, **33,** 115, 1964.
91. Schacter, H., and Dixon, G. H.: A comparative study of the proteins in normal meconium and in meconium ileus patients. Canad. J. Biochem., **43,** 381, 1965.
92. Knauff, R. E., and Adams, J. A.: Proteins and mucoproteins in the duodenal fluids of cystic fibrosis and control subjects. Clin. Chem. Acta, **19,** 245, 1968.
93. Green, M. N., and Shwachman, H.: Presumptive tests for cystic fibrosis based on serum protein in meconium. Pediatrics, **41,** 989, 1968.
94. Lev. R., and Spicer, S. S.: Histochemical comparison of human epithelial mucins in normal and in hypersecretory states including pancreatic cystic fibrosis. Amer. J. Path., **46,** 23, 1965.
95. Freye, H. B., Kurtz, S. M., Spock, A., and Capp, P. M.: Light and electron microscopic examination of the small bowel of children with cystic fibrosis. J. Pediat., **64,** 575, 1964.
96. Parkins, R. A., Rubin, C. E., Eidelman, S., Dobins, W. O., III, and Phelps, P. C.: The diagnosis of cystic fibrosis by rectal suction biopsy. Lancet, **2,** 851, 1963.
97. Fanconi, G.: Fünf Fälle von angeborenem Darmörschluss. Arch. path. Anat., **229,** 207, 1921.
98. Thomaidis, T. S., and Arey, J. B.: The intestinal lesions in cystic fibrosis of the pancreas. J. Pediat., **63,** 44, 1963.
99. Buchanan, D. J., and Rapaport, S.: Chemical comparison of normal meconium and meconium from a patient with meconium ileus. Pediatrics, **9,** 304, 1952.
100. Porta, E. A., Stein, A. A., and Patterson, P.: Ultra-structural changes of pancreas and liver in cystic fibrosis. Amer. J. Clin. Path., **42,** 451, 1964.
101. Esterly, J. R., and Oppenheimer, E. H.: Observations in cystic fibrosis of the pancreas. I. The gallbladder. Bull. Johns Hopkins Hosp., **110,** 247, 1962.
102. Esterly, J. R., and Spicer, S. S.: Mucin histochemistry of human gallbladder: changes in adenocarcinoma, cystic fibrosis, and cholecystitis. J. Nat. Cancer Inst., **40,** 1, 1968.
103. Mangos, J. A., McSherry, N. R., and Benke, P. J.: A sodium transport inhibitory factor in the saliva of patients with cystic fibrosis of the pancreas. Pediat. Res., **1,** 436, 1967.
104. Prader, A., and Gautier, E.: Die Na und K-konzentration in gemischten Speichel: II. Erhöhte Werte bei der Pankreasfibrose. Helv. Paediat. Acta, **10,** 56, 1955.
105. Barbero, G. J., and Chernick, W.: Function of the salivary glands in cystic fibrosis of the pancreas. Pediatrics, **22,** 945, 1958.
106. Mangos, J. A., and Braun-Schubert, G.: Micropuncture study of the rat parotid gland. *4th International Conference on Cystic Fibrosis of the Pancreas* (mucoviscidosis). Mod. Prob. Pediat., **10,** 107, 1967.
107. Johnston, W. H.: Salivary electrolytes in fibrocytic disease of the pancreas. Arch. Dis. Child., **31,** 477, 1956.
108. Bessman, S. P.: Comment, in *Fibrocystic Disease of the Pancreas: Report 18th Ross Pediat. Res. Conf.,* p. 22. Ross Lab., Columbus, Ohio, 1956.
109. Lawson, D., Saggers, B. A., and Chapman, M. J.: Screening for cystic fibrosis by measurement of unstimulated parotid saliva sodium levels. Arch. Dis. Child., **42,** 689, 1967.
110. di Sant'Agnese, P. A.: Studies of sweat in fibrocystic disease of the pancreas, in *Fibrocystic Disease of the Pancreas: Report 18th Ross Pediat. Res. Conf.,* p. 47. Ross Lab., Columbus, Ohio, 1956.
111. Chauncey, H. H., Levine, D. M., Kass, G., Shwachman, H., Henriques, B. L., and Kulczyiki, L. L.: Composition of human saliva; parotid gland secretory rate and electrolyte concentration in children with cystic fibrosis. Arch. Oral Biol., **7,** 707, 1962.
112. Kutscher, A. H., Mandel, I. D., Thompson, R. H., Wotman, S., Zegarelli, E. V., Fahn, B. S., Denning, C. R., Goldstein, J. A., Taubman, M., and Khotim, S.: Parotid saliva in cystic fibrosis. I. Flow rate. Amer. J. Dis. Child., **110,** 643, 1965.
113. Thaysen, J. H., Thorn, N. A., and Schwartz, I. L.: Excretion of sodium, potassium, chloride and carbon dioxide in human parotid saliva. Amer. J. Physiol., **178,** 155, 1954.
114. Sibinga, M. S., Marmar, J., and Barbero, G. J.: Excretion of sodium in parotid saliva in cystic fibrosis. Cystic Fibrosis Club Abstracts, 4th Annual Meeting, Atlantic City, N.J., April 30, 1963.
115. Mandel, I. D., Thompson, R. H., Wotman, S., Taubman, M., Kutscher, A. H., Zegarelli, E. V., Denning, C. R., Botwick, J. T., and Fahn, B. S.: Parotid saliva in cystic fibrosis. II. Electrolytes and protein-bound carbohydrates. Amer. J. Dis. Child., **110,** 646, 1965.

116. Mandel, I. D., Kutscher, A., Denning, C. R., Thompson, R. H., Jr., and Zegarelli, E. V.: Salivary studies in cystic fibrosis. Amer. J. Dis. Child., **113**, 431, 1967.
117. Chernick, W. S., Barbero, G. J., and Parkins, F. H.: Studies on submaxillary saliva in cystic fibrosis. J. Pediat., **59**, 890, 1961.
118. Wiesmann, V., Pallavicini, J. C., Swerdlow, H., and di Sant'Agnese, P. A.: Effect of rate on electrolytes and carbohydrates in normal submaxillary saliva. Fed. Proc., **27**, 676, 1968.
119. Chernick, W. S., Eichel, H. J., and Barbero, G. J.: Submaxillary salivary enzymes as a measure of glandular activity in cystic fibrosis. J. Pediat., **65**, 694, 1964.
120. Chernick, W. S., and Barbero, G. J.: Reversal of submaxillary salivary alterations in cystic fibrosis by guanethidine. *4th International Conference on Cystic Fibrosis of the Pancreas* (mucoviscidosis). Mod. Prob. Pediat., **10**, 125, 1967.
121. Gugler, E., Pallavicini, J. C., Swerdlow, H., and di Sant'Agnese, P. A.: Role of calcium in submaxillary saliva of patients with cystic fibrosis. J. Pediat., **71**, 585, 1967.
122. Dische, Z., Pallavicini, C., Cizek, L. H., and Chien, S.: Changes in the control of the secretion of mucus glycoproteins as possible pathogenic factor in cystic fibrosis of the pancreas. Ann. N.Y. Acad. Sci., **93**, 526, 1962.
123. Chernick, W. S., and Barbero, G. J.: Studies on human trachiobronchial and submaxillary secretions in normal and pathophysiological conditions. Ann. N.Y. Acad. Sci., **106**, 698, 1963.
124. Gugler, E., Pallavicini, J. C., Swerdlow, H., Zipkin, I. and di Sant'Agnese, P. A.: Immunological studies of submaxillary saliva from patients with cystic fibrosis and from normal children. J. Pediat., **73**, 548, 1968.
125. South, M. A., Warwick, W. J., Wollheim, F. A. and Good, R. A.: The IgA system. III. IgA levels in the serum and saliva of pediatric patients—evidence for a local immunological system. J. Pediat., **71**, 645, 1967.
126. Schwartz, R. H.: Serum immunoglobulin levels in cystic fibrosis. Amer. J. Dis. Child., **111**, 408, 1966.
127. Warwick, W. J., Bernard, B., and Meskin, L. H.: The involvement of the labial mucous salivary gland in patients with cystic fibrosis. Pediatrics, **34**, 621, 1964.
128. Sweney, L., and Warwick, W. J.: Involvement of the labial salivary gland in patients with cystic fibrosis. III. Ultrastructural changes. Arch. Path. **86**, 413, 1968.
129. Sweney, L. R., Hedrick, M. C., Meskin, L. H. and Warwick, W. J.: The involvement of the labial mucous salivary gland in patients with cystic fibrosis. II. The heterozygote state. Pediatrics, **40**, 421, 1967.
130. Tandler, B., Denning, C. R., Mandel, I. D., and Kutscher, A. H.: Comparative ultrastructure of labial salivary glands in normal and cystic fibrosis subjects. Cystic Fibrosis Club Abstracts., p. 11, April 26, 1967.
131. Kutscher, A. H., Denning, C. R., Zegarelli, E. V., Kessler, W., Eriv, A., Mandel. I. D., Ruiz, L., Mehrhof, A., Phelan, J., and Ellegood, K.: Capillary tube test for minor salivary gland secretion in cystic fibrosis of the pancreas. N.Y. J. Med., **68**, 2812, 1968.
132. Mangos, J. A., and McSherry, N. R.: Studies on the mechanism of inhibition of sodium transport in cystic fibrosis of the pancreas. Pediat. Res., **2**, 378, 1968.
133. Mangos, J. A., McSherry, N. R., Benke, P. J., and Spock, A.: Studies on the pathogenesis of cystic fibrosis: the isoproterenol treated rat as an experimental model. In *Proceedings of the 5th International Cystic Fibrosis Conference,* edited by D. Lawson, p. 25, Cystic Fibrosis Research Trust, London, 1969.
134. Wells, H., Peronace, A. A. V., and Stark, L. W.: Taste receptors and sialadenotrophic action of proteolytic enzymes in rats. Amer. J. Physiol. **208**, 877, 1965.
135. Mangos, J. A., Benke, P. J., and McSherry, N. R.: Salivary gland enlargement and functional changes during feeding of pancreatin to rats (possible relationship to pathophysiology of cystic fibrosis). (Abstract) J. Pediat., **74**, 823, 1969.
136. Beier, F. R., Renzetti, A. D., Jr., Mitchell, M., and Watanabe, S.: Pulmonary pathophysiology in cystic fibrosis. Amer. Rev. Resp. Dis., **94**, 430, 1966.
137. Zelkowitz, P. S., and Giammona, S. T.: Cystic fibrosis pulmonary studies in children, adolescents, and young adults. Amer. J. Dis. Child., **117**, 543, 1969.
138. DeMuth, G. R., Howatt, W. F., and Talner, N. S.: Intrapulmonary gas distribution in cystic fibrosis. Amer. J. Dis. Child., **103**, 129, 1962.
139. Waring, W. W., Brunt, C. H., and Hilman, B. C.: Mucoid impaction of bronchi in cystic fibrosis. Pediatrics, **39**, 166, 1967.
140. Zelkowitz, P. S. and Giammona, S. T.: Effects of gravity and exercise on the pulmonary diffusing capacity in children with cystic fibrosis. J. Pediat., **74**, 393, 1969.
141. Goldring, R. M.: Pulmonary hypertension and cor pulmonale in cystic fibrosis of the pancreas. J. Pediat., **65**, 501, 1964.
142. Bowden, D. H., Fischer, V. W. and Wyatt, J. P.: Cor pulmonale in cystic fibrosis: a morphometric analysis. Amer. J. Med., **38**, 226, 1965.
143. Moss, A. J., Harper, W. H., Dooley, R. R., Murray, J. F., and Mack, J. F.: Cor pulmonale in cystic fibrosis of the pancreas. J. Pediat., **67**, 797, 1965.
144. Potter, J. L., Matthews, L. W., Spector, S., and Lemm, J.: Studies on pulmonary secretions. II. Osmolarity and the ionic environment of pulmonary secretions from patients with cystic fibrosis, bronchiectosis, and laryngectomy. Amer. Rev. Resp. Dis., **96**, 83, 1967.
145. Lieberman, J., and Kurnick, N. B.: Proteolytic enzyme activity and the role of desoxyribose nucleic acid (DNA) in cystic fibrosis sputum. Pediatrics, **31**, 1028, 1963.
146. Potter, J. L., Matthews, L. W., Lemm, J., and Spector, S.: Human pulmonary secretions in health and disease. Ann. N.Y. Acad. Sci., **106**, 692, 1963.
147. Martinez-Tello, F. J., Braun, D. G., and Blanc, W. A.: Immunoglobulin production in bronchial mucosa and bronchial lymph nodes, particularly in cystic fibrosis of the pancreas. J. Immunol., **101**, 989, 1968.
148. Blanc, W. A., Franciosi, R., and Wigger, H. J.: Pathology of the organs of reproduction in cystic fibrosis. I. Testis and prostate in prepuberal and early puberal cases. Cystic Fibrosis Club Abstracts, p. 13, May 3, 1965.
149. Valman, H. B., and France, N. E.: The vas deferens in cystic fibrosis. Lancet, **2**, 566, 1969.
150. Rule, A. H., Kopito, L., and Shwachman, H.: Chemical analyses of ejaculates from patients with cystic fibrosis compared with ligated and normal controls. Cystic Fibrosis Club Abstracts. p. 13, April 29, 1969.
151. Mangos, J. A.: Personal Communication.
152. di Sant'Agnese, P. A.: Guest Editorial—Fertility and the young adult with cystic fibrosis. New Eng. J. Med., **279**, 103, 1968.
153. Shwachman, H., and Mahmoodian, A.: Pilocarpine iontophoresis sweat testing results of seven years' experience. *4th International Conference on Cystic Fibrosis of the Pancreas* (mucoviscidosis). Mod. Prob. Pediat., **10**, 158, 1967.
154. Richterich, R., and Friolet, B.: The effect of acetazolamide on sweat electrolytes in mucoviscidosis. Metabolism, **12**, 1112, 1963.
155. Conn, J. W.: Aldosteronism in man: some clinical and climatological aspects. Part I. J.A.M.A., **183**, 775, 1963.
156. Grand, R. J., di Sant'Agnese, P. A., Talamo, R. C., and Pallavicini, J. C.: The effects of exogenous aldosterone on sweat electrolytes. I. normal subjects. J. Pediat., **70**, 346, 1967.
157. Grand, R. J., di Sant'Agnese, P. A., Talamo, R. C. and Pallavicini, J. C.: The effects of exogenous aldosterone on sweat electrolytes. II. Patients with cystic fibrosis of the pancreas. J. Pediat., **70**, 357, 1967.
158. DeHaller, R., Siegenthaler, P., and Muller, A. F.: Influence de l'aldostérone sur la concentration du sodium et du chlore sudoral dans la mucoviscidose et chez le sujet normal. Helv. Med. Acta., **30**, 534, 1963.
159. Emrich, H. M., Stoll, E., Friolet, B., Colombo, J. P., Rossi, E. and Richterich, R.: Excretion of different substances in the sweat of children with cystic fibrosis and controls. *4th International Conference on Cystic Fibrosis of the Pancreas* (mucoviscidosis). Mod. Prob. Pediat., **10**, 58, 1967.
160. Slegers, J. F. G.: *The Secretion and Reabsorption of Salt and Water in the Sweat Gland.* Drukkerij Gebr. Janssen N.J., Nijmegen, 1966.
161. Schwartz, I. L., and Thaysen, J. H.: Excretion of sodium and potassium in human sweat. J. Clin. Invest., **35**, 114, 1956.
162. Huebner, D. E., Lobeck, C. C., and McSherry, N. R.: Density and

secretory activity of eccrine sweat glands in patients with cystic fibrosis and in healthy controls. Pediatrics, **38,** 613, 1966.

163. Landing, B. H., Wells, T. R., and Williamson, M. L.: Studies on growth of eccrine sweat glands, in *Human Growth, Body Composition, Cell Growth, Energy and Intelligence,* edited by D. B. Cheek, p. 382–395. Lea & Febiger, Philadelphia, 1968.
164. Bartman, J., and Landing, B. H.: Morphology of the sweat apparatus in cystic fibrosis. Amer. J. Clin. Path., **45,** 455, 1966.
165. Lobeck, C. C., and Huebner, D.: Effect of age, sex, and cystic fibrosis on the sodium and potassium content of human sweat. Pediatrics, **30,** 172, 1962.
166. Sibinga, M. S., and Barbero, G. J.: Studies in the physiology of sweating in cystic fibrosis. Arch. Dis. Child., **36,** 537, 1961.
167. Emrich, H. M., Stoll, E., Friolet, B., Colombo, J. P., Richterich, R., and Rossi, E.: Sweat composition in relation to rate of sweating in patients with cystic fibrosis of the pancreas. Pediat. Res., **2,** 464, 1968.
168. Lobeck, C. C., and McSherry, N. R.: The ionic composition of pilocarpine induced sweat in relation to gland output during aging and in cystic fibrosis. *4th International Conference on Cystic Fibrosis of the Pancreas* (mucoviscidosis). Mod. Prob. Pediat., **10,** 41, 1967.
169. Schwartz, I. L., Thaysen, J. H., and Dole, V. P.: Urea excretion in human sweat as a tracer for movement of water within the gland. J. Exp. Med., **97,** 429, 1953.
170. Brusilow, S. W.: Evidence for a non-plasma source of urea in sweat. Nature (London), **214,** 506, 1967.
171. Ghadimi, H., Stern, M., and Shwachman, H.: Study of free amino acids in sweat from patients with cystic fibrosis. Amer. J. Dis. Child., **99,** 333, 1960.
172. Clarke, J. T., Elian, E., and Shwachman, H.: Components of sweat. Amer. J. Dis. Child., **101,** 490, 1961.
173. Pallavicini, J. C., Gabriel, O., di Sant'Agnese, P. A., and Buskirk, E. R.: Isolation and characterization of carbohydrate-protein complexes from human sweat. Ann. N.Y. Acad. Sci., **106,** 330, 1963.
174. Cage, G. W., Dobson, R. L., and Waller, R.: Sweat gland function in cystic fibrosis. J. Clin. Invest., **45,** 1373, 1966.
175. Schulz, I. J.: Micropuncture studies of the sweat formation in cystic fibrosis patients. J. Clin. Invest., **48,** 1470, 1969.
176. Schulz, I., Ullrich, K. J., Frömter, E., Holzgreve, H., Frick, A., and Hegel, J.: Mikropunktion und elektrische Potentialmessung an Schweissdrüsen des Menschen. Pflüger Arch., **284,** 360, 1965.
177. Mangos, J. A., and McSherry, N. R.: Sodium transport: inhibitory factor in sweat of patients with cystic fibrosis. Science, **158,** 135, 1967.
178. Gibson, L. E., and di Sant'Agnese, P. A.: Studies of salt excretion in sweat. J. Pediat., **62,** 855, 1963.
179. Brusilow, S. W., and Gordes, E. H.: Solute and water secretion in sweat. J. Clin. Invest., **43,** 477, 1964.
180. Gibson, L. E., and Cooke, R. E.: A test for concentration of electrolytes in sweat in cystic fibrosis of the pancreas utilizing pilocarpine by iontophoresis. Pediatrics, **23,** 545, 1959.
181. Schwarz, V., Sutcliffe, C. H., and Style, P. P.: Some hazards of the sweat test. Arch. Dis. Child., **43,** 695, 1968.
182. Goldbloom, R. B., and Sekelj, P.: Cystic fibrosis of the pancreas: diagnosis by application of a sodium electrode to the skin. New Eng. J. Med., **269,** 1349, 1963.
183. Warwick, W. J., and Hansen, L.: The silver electrode method for rapid analysis of sweat chloride. Pediatrics, **36,** 261, 1965.
184. Kopito, L., and Shwachman, H.: Studies in cystic fibrosis: determination of sweat electrolytes in situ with direct reading electrodes. Pediatrics, **43,** 794, 1969.
185. Licht, T. S., Stern, M., and Shwachman, H.: Measurement of electrical conductivity of sweat: its application to study of cystic fibrosis of the pancreas. Clin. Chem., **3,** 37, 1957.
186. Batson, R., Young, W. C., and Shepard, F. M.: Observations on skin resistance to electricity and sweat chloride content: preliminary report. J. Pediat., **60,** 716, 1962.
187. Anderson, C. M., and Freeman, M.: 'Sweat test' results in normal persons of different ages compared with families with fibrocystic disease of the pancreas. Arch. Dis. Child., **35,** 581, 1960.
188. McCance, R. A., Rutishauser, I. H. E., and Knight, H. C.: Response of sweat glands to pilocarpine in the Bantu of Uganda. Lancet, **1,** 663, 1968.
189. McCance, R. A., and Purottit, G.: Ethnic differences in the response of sweat glands to pilocarpine. Nature (London), **221,** 378, 1969.
190. Conn, J. W.: Electrolyte composition of sweat. A.M.A. Arch. Intern. Med., **83,** 416, 1949.
191. Morse, W. I., Cochrane, W. A., and Landrigan, P. L.: Familial hypoparathyroidism with pernicious anemia, steatorrhea and adrenocortical insufficiency: a variant of mucoviscidosis. New Eng. J. Med., **264,** 1021, 1961.
192. Robinson, G. C., Miller, J. R., and Bensimon, J. R.: Familial ectodermal dysplasia with sensorineural deafness and other anomalies. Pediatrics, **30,** 797, 1962.
193. Esterly, N. B., Cantolino, S. J., Alter, B. P., and Brusilow, S. W.: Pupillatonia, hyporeflexia, and segmental hypohidrosis: autonomic dysfunction in a child. J. Pediat., **73,** 852, 1968.
194. Lobeck, C. C., Barta, R. A., and Mangos, J. A.: Study of sweat in pitressin-resistant diabetes insipidus. J. Pediat., **62,** 868, 1963.
195. Weber, J. W., and Gautier, E.: Pitressin resistenter Diabetes insipidus: Therapie mit Salidiuretica. Helv. Paediat. Acta, **16,** 565, 1961.
196. Moseley, A. J., Fitzhugh, F. W., Jr., Hughes, D. J. and Merrill, A. J.: Adrenal activity in thyroid dysfunction (Abstract). Amer. J. Med., **9,** 259, 1950.
197. Grand, R. J., Rosen, S. W., di Sant'Agnese, P. A., and Kirkham, W. R.: Unusual case of XXY Klinefelter's syndrome with pancreatic insufficiency, hypothyroidism, deafness, chronic lung disease, dwarfism and microcephaly. Amer. J. Med., **41,** 478, 1966.
198. Madoff, L.: Elevated sweat chlorides and hypothyroidism. J. Pediat., **73,** 244, 1968.
199. Harris, R. C., and Cohen, H. I.: Sweat electrolytes in glycogen storage disease, type I. Pediatrics, **31,** 1044, 1963.
200. Toivonen, S.: Studies of the function of the sweat gland, parotid gland, and pancreas in chronic bronchitis and heterozygous mucoviscidosis or cystic fibrosis. Ann. Med. Intern. Fenn., **56,** Suppl. 50, 1967.
201. Coates, E. O., and Brinkman, G. L.: Sweat chloride in patients with chronic bronchial disease and its relation to mucoviscidosis (cystic fibrosis). Amer. Rev. Resp. Dis., **87,** 673, 1963.
202. Karlish, A. J.: *Mucoviscidosis in Adults, Further Studies in Chronic Lung Disease in Mucoviscidosis,* edited by E. Koch & F. Bohn, p. 121 Schattaververlag, Stuttgart., 1964.
203. Cabanel, G., Voog, R., and Rambaud, P.: Systematic research of the taint of mucoviscidosis in chronic bronchitis in adults. *4th International Conference on Cystic Fibrosis of the Pancreas* (mucoviscidosis). Mod. Prob. Pediat., **10,** 284, 1967.
204. Bernard, E., Israel, L., and Debris, M. D.: Chronic bronchitis and mucoviscidosis. Amer. Rev. Resp. Dis., **85,** 22, 1962.
205. Bernard, E., Israel, L. and Debris, M. D.: Sur 155 cas de broncho-emphysème de l'adulte étudiés avec le test de la sueur: du role étiologique de la mucoviscidose. Bull. Soc. Méd. Hôp. Paris, **113,** 394, 1962.
206. Bernard, E., Israel, L., and Debris, M. D.: Etudie sur le role de la mucoviscidose comme facteur étiologique dans les bronchites chronique de l'adulte. J. Franc. Méd. Chir. Thorac., **15,** 447, 1961.
207. Boucher, H., Sauquet, R., Roumagoux, J., Mergier, P., and Royer, G.: di Sant'Agnese's sweat test in pneumology: a critical study of 98 cases. Presse Méd., **69,** 57, 1961.
208. Bernard, E., Israel, L., and Debris, M. D.: Le rôle de la mucoviscidose dans la pathogénie de l'association emphysème-ulcère digestif. Presse Méd. **70,** 861, 1962.
209. Zeilhofer, R.: *Zur Interpretation des Schweisstestes am Beispiel der Chronischen Bronchitis in Mucoviscidosis.* Symposium am 20, Sept., 1962 in Giessen, edited by E. Koch, H. Bohn, and Fr. Koch, p. 97, Schattauer, Stuttgart, 1964.
210. Karlish, A. J., and Tárnoky, A. L.: Mucoviscidosis and chronic lung disease. Proc. Roy. Soc. Med., **54,** 980, 1963.
211. Toigo, A., Dietz, A. A., Crane, J. B., and Reisner, D.: Sweat electrolytes in chronic pulmonary disease. Ann. Intern. Med., **58,** 961, 1963.
212. Peterson, E. M.: Consideration of cystic fibrosis in adults with a study of sweat electrolyte values. J.A.M.A., **171,** 1, 1959.

213. Catta, J., and Belliard, P.: Résultant du test de la sueur effectué chez 55 malades. Concours Méd., **84,** 5493, 1962.
214. Hsia, D. Y. Y., Driscoll, S. G., Greenberg, D., Lee, T. D., and Lanoff. G.: Abnormal sweat electrolytes in patients with allergies. Am. J. Dis. Child., **96,** 685, 1958.
215. Perry, E. F., and Scott, R. B.: Sweat electrolytes in allergic children. J. Allerg., **32,** 528, 1961.
216. Van Metre, T. E., Cooke, R. E., Gibson, L. E., and Winkenwerder, W. L.: Evidence of allergy in patients with cystic fibrosis of the pancreas. J. Allerg., **31,** 141, 1960.
217. Andrews, B. F., Bruton, O. C., and Knoblock, E. C.: Sweat chloride concentration in children with allergy and with cystic fibrosis of the pancreas. Pediatrics, **29,** 204, 1962.
218. Shwachman, H., and Antoniwicz, I.: Observations by K. T. Khaw, in the sweat test in cystic fibrosis. Ann. N.Y. Acad. Sci., **93,** 603, 1962.
219. Kopito, L., and Shwachman, H.: Spectroscopic analysis of tissues from patients with cystic fibrosis and controls. Nature (London), **202,** 501, 1964.
220. Grosse, K. P., Stephan, U., and Sitzmann, F. C.: Untersuchungen über den Natrium und Kalium gehalt in Finger-und Zehennägeln. Z. Kinderheilk., **100,** 87, 1967.
221. Kopito, L., Mohmoodian, A., Townley, R. R. W., Khaw, K. T., and Shwachman, H.: Studies in cystic fibrosis: analysis of nail clippings for sodium and potassium. New Eng. J. Med., **272,** 504, 1965.
222. Stamm, S. J., Woodruff, G. L., and Babb, A. L.: Cystic fibrosis mass screening by neutron activation analysis. Cystic Fibrosis Club Abstracts, p. 22, April 29, 1969.
223. Harrison, G. M., Bickers, G., Dogget, R., Fite, L. E., Wainerdi, R. E. and Yule, H. P.: Automated neutron activation analysis of trace elements in tissue (nail clippings) of patients with cystic fibrosis. Cystic Fibrosis Club Abstracts. p. 38, April 29, 1969.
224. Robson, A. M., Tateishi, S., Strominger, D. B., and Klahr, S.: An abnormality in renal function in patients with cystic fibrosis. Abstracts. The Society for Pediatric Research. p. 119, May 2–3, 1969.
225. Maxfield, M., and Wolins, W.: A molecular abnormality of urinary mucoprotein in cystic fibrosis of the pancreas. J. Clin. Invest., **41,** 455, 1962.
226. Friedmann, T., and Johnson, P.: Structure of Tamm-Hansfall mucoproteins in fibrocystic disease. J. Lab. Clin. Med., **70,** 404, 1967.
227. Schwartz, R. H., and Pallavicini, J. C.: Immunological and chemical studies of cystic fibrosis and normal urinary glycoprotein of Tamm and Horsfall. J. Lab. Clin. Med., **70,** 725, 1967.
228. Talamo, R. C., Raunio, V., Gabriel, O., Pallavicini, J. C., Halbert, S., and di Sant'Agnese, P. A.: Immunologic and biochemical comparison of urinary glycoproteins in patients with cystic fibrosis of the pancreas and normal controls. J. Pediat., **65,** 480, 1964.
229. Stevenson, F. K.: The viscosity of Tamm-Horsfall mucoprotein and its relation to cystic fibrosis. Clin. Chem. Acta., **23,** 441, 1969.
230. Lobeck, C. C.: *Discussion in Research on Pathogenesis of Cystic Fibrosis,* edited by P. A. di Sant'Agnese, pp. 107–110, Wickersham Printing Co. Lancaster, Pa. 1966.
231. Balfe, J. W., Cole, C. and Welt, L. G.: Red-cell transport defect in patients with cystic fibrosis and in their parents. Science, **162,** 689, 1968.
232. Mangos, J. A. and McSherry, N. R.: Unpublished observations.
233. Danes, B. S., Foley, K. M., Dillon, S. D., and Bearn, A. G.: Genetic study of cystic fibrosis of the pancreas using white blood cell cultures. Nature (London), **222,** 685, 1969.
234. Spock, A., Heick, H. M. C., Cress, H., and Logan, W. S.: Abnormal serum factor in patients with cystic fibrosis of the pancreas. Pediat. Res., **1,** 173, 1967.
235. Bowman, B. H., Lockhart, L. H., and McCombs, M. L.: Oyster ciliary inhibition by cystic fibrosis factor. Science, **164,** 325, 1969.
236. Jakovcic, S., and Hsia, D. Y. Y.: Studies on mechanism for decreased lipoprotein lipase in cystic fibrosis of the pancreas. J. Pediat., **62,** 25, 1963.
237. Hsia, D. Y. Y., Shih, L. Y., Justice, P., O'Flynn, M. E.: Serum alkaline phosphatase in cystic fibrosis of the pancreas. Lancet, **1,** 106, 1969.
238. Kuo, P. T., Huang, N. N., and Bassett, D. R.: The fatty acid composition of the serum chylomicrons and adipose tissue of children with cystic fibrosis of the pancreas. J. Pediat., **60,** 394, 1962.
239. Caren, R., and Corbo, L.: Plasma fatty acids in pancreatic cystic fibrosis and liver disease. J. Clin. Endocr., **26,** 470, 1966.
240. Bonham, T. J., Robinson, R., and Macmahon, A. M. H.: Tyrosine in fibrocystic disease. Lancet, **2,** 1188, 1965.
241. Zack, P., Ross, P., Applegarth, D. A., and Israels, S.: Tyrosine in fibrocystic disease. J. Pediat., **72,** 692, 1968.
242. Robinson, R.: Tyrosine metabolism in cystic fibrosis. Clinica Chim. Acta. **14,** 166, 1966.
243. Gibbons, I. S. E., Seakins, J. W. T., and Ersser, R. S.: Tyrosine metabolism and faecal amino acids in cystic fibrosis of the pancreas. Lancet, **1,** 877, 1967.
244. Burns, M. W., and May, J. R.: Bacterial precipitins in serum of patients with cystic fibrosis. Lancet, **1,** 270, 1968.
245. Mearns, M., Longbottom, J., and Batten, J.: Precipitating antibodies to aspergillus fumigatus in cystic fibrosis. Lancet, **1,** 538, 1967.
246. Schwartz, R. H., Johnstone, D. E., Holsclaw, D. S., and Dooley, R. R.: Serum precipitins to *Aspergillus fumigatus.* Cystic Fibrosis Club Abstracts, p. 48, April 29, 1969.
247. Stein, A. A., Manlapas, F. C., Soike, K. F., and Patterson, P. R.: Specific isoantibodies in cystic fibrosis, a study of serum and bronchial mucus. J. Pediat., **65,** 495, 1964.
248. Peter, G., and Whang-Peng, J.: Chromosomes in cystic fibrosis. Lancet, **1,** 978, 1968.
249. Blanc, W. A., McGiluray, E. R. T., and Miller, O. J.: Chromosomes in cystic fibrosis. Lancet, **1,** 1152, 1968.
250. Danks, D. M., Allan, J., and Anderson, C. M.: A genetic study of fibrocystic disease of the pancreas. Ann. Hum. Genet., **28,** 323, 1965.
251. Martel, L., and Robert, J. M.: Remarques concernant le taux de masculineté dans les fratries attientes de mucoviscidose. Pediatrie, **17,** 409, 1962.
252. Rosenow, E. C., and Lee, R. A.: Cystic fibrosis and pregnancy. J.A.M.A., **203,** 227, 1968.
253. Carter, C. O.: in *Fibrocystic Disease of the Pancreas,* edited by M. Bodian, p. 50. Grune & Stratton, New York, 1953.
254. Lowe, C. U., May, C. D., and Reed, S. C.: Fibrosis of the pancreas in infants and children. Amer. J. Dis. Child., **78,** 349, 1949.
255. Kulczycki, L. L., Guin, G. H., and Mann, N.: Cystic fibrosis in Negro children: results of a search. Clin. Pediat., **3,** 692, 1964.
256. Oppenheimer, E. H., and Esterly, J. R.: Cystic fibrosis in non-Caucasian patients. Pediatrics, **42,** 547, 1968.
257. Harris, R. L., and Riley, H. D., Jr.: Cystic fibrosis in the American Indian. Pediatrics, **41,** 733, 1968.
258. Wang, C. I., Sumi, W. T., Stanton, R., Kwok, S., and Yamazaki, J. N.: Cystic fibrosis in an Oriental child. New Eng. J. Med., **279,** 1216, 1968.
259. Ahari, H., and Pakdaman, P.: Cystic fibrosis of the pancreas in Iran. J. Trop. Pediat., **11,** 14, 1965.
260. Bhakoo, O. N., Kumar, R., and Walia, B. N. S.: Mucoviscidosis of the lung. Indian J. Pediat., **35,** 183, 1968.
261. MacDougall, L. G.: Fibrocystic disease of the pancreas in African children. Lancet, **2,** 409, 1962.
262. Hamamoto, E., Otahara, S., and Iizuka, K.: A case report of fibrocystic disease of the pancreas. Acta Paediat. Jap., **65,** 502, 1961.
263. Kobayashi, Y., Tomisawa, T., Takai, Y., Izumi, R., and Hatakeyama, M.: An autopsied case of fibrocystic disease of the pancreas. Acta Paediat. Jap., **65,** 597, 1961.
264. Ikai, K., Sugie, I., Sugino, I., Nitta, H., Iida, T., Ogawa, J., and Suchi, T.: Cystic fibrosis cases found by re-examination of histology of pancreas and post mortem protocol in Japanese children and sweat test on the siblings. Acta Paediat. Jap., **7,** 23, 1965.
265. Wright, S. W., and Morton, N. E.: Genetic studies on cystic fibrosis in Hawaii. Amer. J. Hum. Genet., **20,** 157, 1968.
266. Carter, C. O.: Fibrocystic disease of the pancreas, in *Clinical Genetics,* edited by A. Sorsby, p. 413. Butterworth, London, 1953.
267. Goodman, H. O., and Reed, S. C.: Heredity of fibrosis of the pancreas: possible mutation rate of the gene. Am. J. Hum. Genet., **4,** 59, 1952.
268. Steinberg, A. G.: Dependence of the phenotype on environment and

heredity, in *The Genetics of Migrant and Isolate Populations,* edited by E. Goldschmidt, p. 139. Williams & Wilkins, Baltimore, 1963.
269. Crow, J. F.: Problems of ascertainment in the analysis of family data, in *Genetics and the Epidemiology of Chronic Diseases,* edited by J. V. Neel, M. W. Shaw, and W. J. Schull, Chap. 2. U.S. Dept. of Health, Education, and Welfare, P.H.S. Publication #1163, February, 1965.
270. di Sant'Agnese, P. A., and Powell, G. F.: The eccrine sweat defect in cystic fibrosis of the pancreas (mucoviscidosis). Ann. N.Y. Acad. Sci., **93,** 555, 1962.
271. Sproul, A., and Huang, N.: Diagnosis of heterozygosity for cystic fibrosis by discriminatory analysis of sweat chloride distribution. J. Pediat. **69,** 759, 1966.
272. Danes, B. S., and Bearn, A. G.: A genetic cell marker in cystic fibrosis of the pancreas. Lancet, **1,** 1061, 1968.
273. Danes, B. S., and Bearn, A. G.: Cystic fibrosis of the pancreas, a study in cell culture. J. Exp. Med., **129,** 775, 1969.
274. Steinberg, A. G., Shwachman, H., Allen, F. H., Jr., and Dooley, R. R.: Linkage studies with cystic fibrosis of the pancreas. Amer. J. Hum. Genet., **8,** 162, 1956.
275. Virtanen, S.: Salivary secretion of ABO blood group substances in cystic fibrosis of the pancreas. J. Pediat., **68,** 139, 1966.
276. Bitar, J., and Lightwood, R.: The Wiskott-Aldrich syndrome associated with mucoviscidosis in the same patient. J. Pediat., **71,** 123, 1967.
277. Brown, N. M., and Smith, A. N.: Kartagener's syndrome with fibrocystic disease. Brit. Med. J., **2,** 725, 1959.
278. Milunsky, A.: Cystic fibrosis and Down's syndrome. Pediatrics, **42,** 501, 1968.
279. Smith, D. W., Docter, J. M., Ferrier, P. E., Frias, J. L., and Spock, A.: Possible localization of the gene for cystic fibrosis of the pancreas to the short arm of chromosome 5. Lancet, **2,** 309, 1968.
280. Danes, B. S., and Bearn, A. G.: Localization of the cystic fibrosis gene. Lancet, **2,** 1303, 1968.
281. Dallaire, L., Destiné, M. L.: Localization of the cystic fibrosis gene. Lancet, **1,** 419, 1969.
282. Merritt, A. D., Hanna, B. L., Todd, C. W., Jr., and Myers, T. L.: Incidence and mode of inheritance of cystic fibrosis. J. Lab. Clin. Med., **60,** 998, 1962.
283. Steinberg, A. G., and Brown, D. C.: On the incidence of cystic fibrosis of the pancreas. Amer. J. Human Genet., **12,** 416, 1960.
284. Kulczycki, L. L., MacLeod, K. I. E., and Shwachman, H.: A survey of school children for cystic fibrosis. Amer. J. Dis. Child., **100,** 174, 1960.
285. Andersen, D. H., and Hodges, R. G.: Celiac syndrome. V. Genetics of cystic fibrosis of the pancreas with a consideration of etiology. Amer. J. Dis. Child., **72,** 62, 1946.
286. Kramm, E. R., Crane, M. M., Sirken, M. G., and Brown, M. L.: A cystic fibrosis pilot survey in three New England states. Amer. J. Public Health., **52,** 2041, 1962.
287. Selander, P.: The frequency of cystic fibrosis of the pancreas in Sweden. Acta Paediat., **51,** 65, 1962.
288. Pugh, R. J., and Pickup, J. D.: Cystic fibrosis in the Leeds Region: Incidence and life expectancy. Arch. Dis. Child., **42,** 544, 1967.
289. Houstek, J., and Vávrová, V.: Incidence of cystic fibrosis of pancreas in Czechoslovakia. Cesk. Pediat., **17,** 445, 1962.
290. Crow, J. F.: Mutation in man. Prog. M. Genet., **I,** 1, 1961.
291. Baumann, T.: Die Mucoviscidosis als rezessives und irregulär dominantes Erbleiden: eine klinische und genetische Studie. Helvet. paediat. acta, **13,** Suppl. 8, 4, 102, 1958.
292. Knudson, A. G., Wayne, L., and Hallett, W. Y.: On the selective advantage of cystic fibrosis heterozygotes. Amer. J. Hum. Genet., **19,** 388, 1967.
293. Anderson, C. M., Allan, J., and Johansen, P. G.: Comments on the possible existence and nature of a heterozygote advantage in cystic fibrosis. *4th International Conference on Cystic Fibrosis of the Pancreas* (mucoviscidosis) Mod. Prob. Pediat., **10,** 381, 1967.
294. Batten, J., Muir, D., Simon, G., Carter, C.: The prevalence of respiratory disease in heterozygotes for the gene for fibrocystic disease of the pancreas. Lancet, **1,** 1348, 1963.
295. Anderson, C. M., Freeman, M., Allan, J., and Hubbard, L.: Observations on (i) sweat sodium levels in relation to chronic respiratory disease in adults and (ii) the incidence of respiratory and other disease in parents and siblings of patients with fibrocystic disease of the pancreas. Med. J. Austr., **1,** 965, 1962.
296. Hallet, W. Y., Knudson, A. G., Jr., and Massey, F. J., Jr.: Absence of detrimental effect of the carrier state for the cystic fibrosis gene. Amer. Rev. Resp. Dis., **92,** 714, 1965.
297. Bohn, H.: Über die Erwachsenenmucoviscidosis, in. Mucoviscidosis (Zystische Parkreas fibrose), edited by E. Koch, H. Bohn, and Fr. Koch, p. 65, Schattauerverlag, Stuttgart, 1964.
298. Israel, L., Chimenes, H., Debris, M. D., and Klotz, H. P.: The incidence and aetiological role of mucoviscidosis in diabetes in adults: preliminary note. Presse Méd. **69,** 176, 1961.
299. Uhry, P., and Swynghedavw, B.: Mucoviscidose et diabēte sucre de l'adulte. Clin. Paris, **56,** 461, 1961.
300. Hanicki, Z., Hawiger, J., and Struzik, T.: Das Antikörpermangelsyndrom und die Mucoviscidosis. Wien. Klin. Wschr., **75,** 862, 1963.
301. Farber, S.: Pancreatic function and disease in early life. A.M.A. Arch. Path., **37,** 238, 1944.
302. Baggenstoss, A. H., Power, M. H., Grindlay, J. H.: The relationship of fibrocystic disease of the pancreas to a deficiency of secretin. Pediatrics, **2,** 435, 1948.
303. Gibbs, G. E., and Gershbein, L. L.: Presence of secretin in cystic fibrosis of the pancreas. Proc. Soc. Exp. Biol. Med., **74,** 336, 1950.
304. Matalon, R., and Dorfman, A.: Acid mucopolysaccharides in cultured human fibroblasts. Lancet, **2,** 838, 1969.
305. Punnett, H. H., Kistenmacher, M. L., and Niederer, B. S.: Metachromasia in fibroblasts. Lancet, **1,** 1433, 1968.
306. Gordon, R. H., and Cage, G. W.: Hypothesis, Mechanism of water and electrolyte excretion by the eccrine sweat gland. Lancet, **1,** 1246, 1966.
307. Johansen, P. G., Anderson, C. M., and Hadorn, B.: Cystic fibrosis of the pancreas: a generalized disturbance of water and electrolyte movement in exocrine tissues. Lancet, **1,** 455, 1968.
308. Rubin, L. S., Barbero, G. J., Chernick, W. S., and Sibinga, M. S.: Pupillary reactivity as a measure of autonomic balance in cystic fibrosis. J. Pediat., **63,** 1120, 1963.
309. Gibson, L. E.: The effect of adrenergic stimulation upon sweating in normal children and cystic fibrosis patients. Pediatrics, **42,** 458, 1968.
310. Hancock, W., Whitehouse, A. G. R., and Haldane, J. S.: The loss of water and salts through the skin, and corresponding physiological adjustments. Proc. Roy. Soc. [Biol.], **105,** 43, 1929.
311. Thaysen, J. H., and Schwartz, I. L.: Fatigue of the sweat glands. J. Clin. Invest., **34,** 1719, 1955.
312. Sibinga, M. S., and Barbero, G. J.: Studies in the physiology of sweating in cystic fibrosis. Pediatrics, **27,** 912, 1961.
313. Roberts, G. B. S.: Fundamental defect in fibrocystic disease of the pancreas. Lancet, **2,** 964, 1959.
314. Eyerman, E. L., Hurley, R. J., and Irwin, R. L.: Acetylcholine in sweat in fibrocystic disease of the pancreas. Nature, **192,** 77, 1961.
315. Gibbs, G. E.: Changes in sweat in research on cystic fibrosis: Transactions. Edited by R. McIntosh; pp. 145–174, French-Bray, Baltimore, 1960.
316. Hokin, L. E., Hokin, M. R., and Lobeck, C. C.: Effects of acetylcholine on the incorporation of P^{32} into the phospholipids in slices of skin from children with and without cystic fibrosis of the pancreas. J. Clin. Invest., **42,** 1232, 1963.
317. Holzel, A., Schwarz, V., Torkington, P., and Greville-Williams, G. E.: Mucoviscidosis and the autonomic nervous system. Lancet, **1,** 822, 1962.
318. Robinson, G. A., Butcher, R. W., and Sutherland, E. W.: Cyclic AMP in *Annual Review of Physiology,* edited by V. E. Hall, p. 149. Palo Alto, Calif., 1968.
319. Mangos, J. A., and McSherry, N. R.: Secretory function of isolated parotid acinar cells (abstract), p. 111, Society for Pediatric Research, 1971.
320. Grand, R. J.: Control of protein synthesis in rat parotid gland. Fed. Proc. **28,** 273, 1969.
321. Matthews, L. W., Doershuk, C. F., and Spector, S.: Mist tent therapy of the obstructive pulmonary lesion of cystic fibrosis. Pediatrics, **39,** 176, 1967.

322. Doershuk, C. F., Matthews, L. W., Tucker, A. S. and Spector, S.: Evaluation of a prophylactic and chiropeutic program for patients with cystic fibrosis. Pediatrics, **36,** 675, 1965.
323. Wolfsdorf, J., Swift, D. L., and Avery, M. E.: Mist therapy reconsidered; an evaluation of the respiratory deposition of labelled water aerosols produced by jet and ultrasonic nebulizers. Pediatrics, **43,** 799, 1969.
324. Boxerbaum, B., Doershuk, C. F., Pittman, S., and Matthews, L. W.: The efficacy and tolerance of carbenicillin in patients with cystic fibrosis. Cystic Fibrosis Club Abstracts. p. 19, April 29, 1969.
325. Cezeaux, G., Jr., Telford, J., Harrison, G. M., and Keats, A.: Bronchial lavage in cystic fibrosis. J.A.M.A., **199,** 15, 1967.
326. Khaw, K. T., Rowe, A. A., and Shwachman, H.: A controlled study of pulmonary lavage in patients with cystic fibrosis. Cystic Fibrosis Club Abstracts. p. 17, May 3, 1965.
327. Noblett, H. R.: Treatment of uncomplicated meconium ileus by gastrografin enema: a preliminary report. J. Pediat. Surg., **4,** 190, 1969.
328. Weihofen, D. M., and Pringle, D. J.: Dietary intake and food tolerances of children with cystic fibrosis. J. Amer. Diet. Ass., **54,** 206, 1969.
329. Kuo, P. T., and Huang, N. N.: The effect of medium chain triglyceride upon fat absorption and plasma lipid and depot fat of children with cystic fibrosis of the pancreas. J. Clin. Invest., **44,** 1924, 1965.
330. Anderson, C. M., and Burke, V.: Medium chain triglyceride feeding in cystic fibrosis. *4th International Conference on Cystic Fibrosis of the Pancreas* (mucoviscidosis). Mod. Prob. Pediat., **10,** 326, 1967.
331. Good, T. A., and Bessman, S. P.: Anabolic steroids in cystic fibrosis of the pancreas. Amer. J. Dis. Child., **111,** 272, 1966.
332. Dennis, J. L. and Panos. T. C.: Growth and bone-age retardation in cystic fibrosis. Response to anabolic steroid. J.A.M.A., **194,** 855, 1965.
333. Dooley, R. R., Moss, A. J., Wright, P. M., and Hassakis, P. C.: Norethandrolone in cystic fibrosis of the pancreas. J. Pediat., **74,** 95, 1969.
334. Kaiser, D., Drack, E., and Rossi, E.: Effect of cystic fibrosis sweat on sodium reabsorption by the normal sweat gland. Lancet, **1,** 1003, 1970.

PART TWELVE

DEFICIENCIES OF CIRCULATING ENZYMES AND PLASMA PROTEINS

CHAPTER SIXTY-NINE
GENETIC VARIATIONS OF PLASMA PROTEINS

Alexander G. Bearn and Hartwig Cleve

The synthesis of all proteins, including those in the blood plasma, is under genetic control. Although the variations which have been detected in health and disease are usually quantitative in character, a certain number are qualitative and represent structural variants. Many of the structural variants are not associated with clinical disease and represent part of the genetic diversity that exists in all populations. In this chapter, a selected number of serum proteins which show marked genetic variations will be discussed. The list is not comprehensive, and the reader is referred to the monograph of Schultze and Heremans [1] on "Molecular Biology of Human Proteins" for additional information and to the monograph by Giblett [2] entitled "Genetic Markers in Human Blood" for more extensive genetic discussions.

PLASMA ALBUMIN

Albumin constitutes approximately one-half of the total plasma proteins. The high concentration of albumin in plasma permitted isolation of highly purified preparations of this protein more than 2 decades ago. Albumin has thus served as a model for the development and refinement of physiochemical techniques for the investigation of proteins. For an extensive review of the voluminous literature on the methods of preparation, size, shape, chemical composition, and behavior of albumin in solution, the reader is referred to the standard works on plasma proteins [1, 3].

Properties of Albumin

Albumin appears to be composed exclusively of amino acids. There is no evidence for a carbohydrate prosthetic group, and although it is difficult to prepare albumin free of fatty acids and heavy metal ions, it seems that these substances represent contaminants tightly bound to the protein, rather than true constituents of the albumin molecule. The apparent heterogeneity of serum albumin observed by various electrophoretic, ultracentrifugal, and chromatographic procedures is probably due to the presence of albumin monomers and dimers. Albumin has a molecular weight of 65,000 to 70,000. The molecule consists of a single polypeptide chain which is folded by 17 disulfide bridges into four globular regions. Although these globular domains are connected by peptide linkages, the molecule can be regarded in a sense as consisting of subunits [4]. Because of its relatively small size and the high concentration in plasma, albumin contributes 75 to 80 percent of the colloid osmotic pressure of plasma. Therefore it plays a major role in the regulation of the intravascular volume. The data available on the shape of the albumin molecule suggest that it can be regarded as an elongated ellipsoid which can undergo extensive reversible configurational alterations. The high affinity of albumin for ions, especially anions, and its capacity to bind nonionic substances has been attributed to this "configurational adaptability." Albumin thus serves an important function as a transport protein. Albumin has no known enzymatic or hormonal activity.

Analbuminemia

Analbuminemia, the absence of albumin in serum, was observed first by Bennhold et al. [5] in two sibs from Germany. Additional cases have been reported in the United States, one of whom was a Negro, and in Switzerland [6]. Consanguinity was found in the ancestry of two families from Germany and Switzerland with this abnormality. Analbuminemia may, therefore, be inherited as an autosomal recessive trait. Although the albumin fraction is by examination with electrophoretic methods virtually absent, the defect is not complete. Examination of sera from patients with this condition using sensitive immunologic methods has revealed the presence of small quantities of albumin (1.6 to 24 mg per 100 ml), which was immunologically indistinguishable from albumin obtained from normal individuals. The concentration of albumin in the serum of presumed heterozygotes is normal.

In spite of the many functions commonly ascribed to albumin, the symptoms of analbuminemia are remarkably mild. Two of the females with analbuminemia consulted a physician for fatigue and slight pretibial edema, whereas the males in these families were virtually unaffected by their protein anomaly; they were detected only during the investigation of the family. Two patients with analbuminemia had mild anemia, and in two patients the condition was associated with mild diarrhea. The affected persons had no proteinuria, and the liver functions were normal. Analbuminemia causes a reduction of the colloid pressure to one-third or one-half the normal value. The increase of various plasma globulins, a slight decrease in blood pressure, and a marked decrease of the capillary pressure found in some patients have been interpreted as compensatory phenomena. A disorder of the transport function is indicated by an increase in the elimination rate of intravenously injected Congo red and Evans blue. A decreased blood calcium is occasionally observed. Most patients have elevated serum cholesterol and phospholipids, whereas serum triglyceride concentrations are normal.

The half-life of intravenously injected labeled albumin is prolonged in these patients. This is in agreement with the view that analbuminemia is caused by a decreased rate of albumin synthesis [7]. The lack of allergic reactions to repeated intravenous injections of human albumin has been ascribed to the presence of traces of normal albumin.

Serum Albumin Variants

Genetic variants of albumin are known to occur in two distinct forms that are both disclosed by electrophoretic procedures. One form is characterized by the presence of a variant albumin with a difference in electric charge; the second form is characterized by the occurrence of albumin dimers.

The electrophoretic albumin variants occur only infrequently in most populations. Most subjects in whom this anomaly is observed are, therefore, heterozygous for the albumin variant. Examination of serum by free, paper, or gel electrophoresis at the conventional slightly alkaline pH reveals in these persons two distinct albumin fractions. The term *bisalbuminemia,* therefore, has been proposed for this condition [8]. Since the first report by Knedel [9], albumin variants have been observed in more than twenty Caucasian families, and polymorphic albumin variation has been discovered in certain North American Indian tribes [10, 11]. Comparative analysis by starch gel electrophoresis with the use of different buffer systems has revealed the existence of at least eleven different genetic albumin variants. Five albumin variants migrate more rapidly than normal albumin, and six variants have a slower electrophoretic mobility than normal albumin [10, 12]. The albumin variants "fast," "very fast," "slow," and "very slow" have been observed in Caucasian families [10]. The albumin variant "faster" is also called *albumin Naskapi*. Albumin Naskapi has been observed in members of seven different tribes of North American Indians [11]. *Albumin Maku* was observed first in a woman from the South American Indian tribe Maku in Southern Venezuela. Albumin Maku migrates more rapidly than the "faster" variant at pH 6.9, but more slowly than this variant at pH 5.0 [12]. The slowly migrating variant, called *albumin Mexico,* was found in two Mexican Indians [13]. Another slow-moving variant, *albumin Gainesville,* was observed in a family of Irish descent [14]. *Albumin Cayemite* is a slow variant observed in Negroes [15]. *Albumin Uinba* is found in New Guinea indigenes in whom also a further faster-moving variant has been recognized [16].

These variants occur, apart from albumin Naskapi, at low frequency. Albumin Naskapi, however, is quite frequent in some Indian tribes, particularly in the Naskapi and Montagnais from Canada, the frequencies for the mutant gene being 0.13 and 0.08, respectively. In these tribes, also, persons homozygous for the albumin mutant were discovered [11]. Family data including observations on three generations within a family indicate that these albumin variants are inherited as autosomal codominant traits. Both the heterozygous carriers and the persons homozygous for an albumin variant are apparently healthy and not affected by their protein anomaly. Of interest is the observation that the structural loci for albumin and the group-specific component (Gc) are genetically linked [17].

The electrophoretic albumin variants are presumably caused by point mutations and arise from single amino acid substitutions in the primary sequence of the albumin polypeptide chain. Proof of this interpretation is lacking. The only data available were provided by Gitlin et al. [18] who compared the tryptic peptides of normal albumin and the "very slow" variant by fingerprint mapping. A substitution of a lysine residue for an acidic amino acid was assumed.

The second form of inherited albumin variation was observed first in a Welsh family [19]. This variation was subsequently found also in an American Negro family [20, 21] and several Swedish families [22]. It is first disclosed by electrophoretic examination of serum on starch or polyacrylamide gels. An additional albumin band in the post-albumin region is observed in the sera of the affected persons. But in contrast to the electrophoretic variants described in the preceding section, in which the normal and mutant albumin are present in approximately equal amounts, the additional albumin component in these persons represents only 10 to 15 percent of the total albumin. The abnormal albumin is immunologically indistinguishable from normal albumin. The variant has been characterized as an albumin dimer [21]. The dimer formation may involve both disulfide and noncovalent bonds. This type of albumin variant is inherited as an autosomal codominant trait [19, 21, 22].

HAPTOGLOBIN

In 1938 Polonovski and Jayle described a protein in human serum which had the unique property of binding hemoglobin [23]. This α_2-globulin was named *haptoglobin* and was extensively investigated by the French workers [24]. By 1946 it was apparent that there were two types of haptoglobin which varied in their precipitability toward ammonium sulfate. It was not until 1955, as a result of the introduction of the starch-gel technique, that it became possible to establish that haptoglobins are inherited as an autosomal system without dominance [25, 26].

The Common Haptoglobin Types

The two alleles, designated Hp^1 and Hp^2, determine the three common haptoglobin phenotypes Hp 1-1, Hp 2-1, and Hp 2-2. The haptoglobin of individuals homozygous for the Hp^1 allele migrates as a single component in the starch-gel system. Individuals homozygous for the Hp^2 alleles synthesize multiple haptoglobin components which form a series of stable polymers of increasing molecular weight and decreasing electrophoretic mobility in the gel system. Heterozygous individuals also synthesize a series of components whose mobilities differ from those of the Hp 2-2 polymers (Fig. 69-1). Cleavage of disulfide bridges in purified haptoglobins by reducing agents like β-mercaptoethanol produces

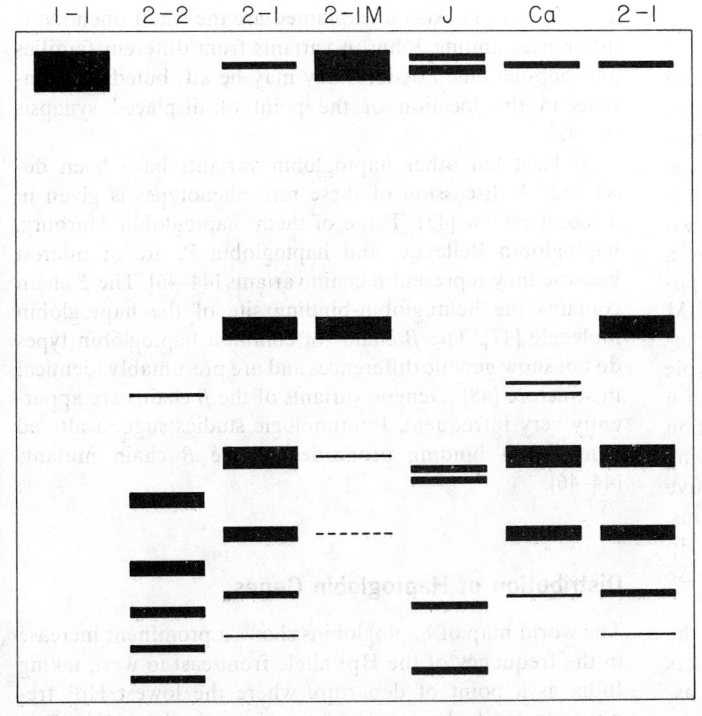

Figure 69-1. The various phenotypes of the haptoglobin system as disclosed by benzidine staining after starch-gel electrophoresis: Hp 2-1M (2-1 modified), Hp^J (Johnson), Hp^{Ca} (Carlsberg). Details of Hp 2-1M and Hp^J phenotypes found in text. Hp^{Ca} type is very rare.

two different types of molecular subunits, called α and β chains [27]. By starch-gel electrophoresis in acidic buffer systems and in the presence of 8*M* urea, these can be separated into the slower-migrating β- and the faster-migrating α-polypeptide chains. By this technique it can be shown that the haptoglobin polymorphism is associated with the α chains. This procedure permitted further division of the gene products of the Hp^1 allele into fast- and slow-migrating α^1 chains. Thus, three autosomal alleles, Hp α^{1F}, Hp α^{1S}, and Hp α^2, determine six common haptoglobin types, called Hp α1F-1F, Hp α1F-1S, Hp α1S-1S, Hp α2-1F, Hp α2-1S, and Hp α2-2.

Smithies and coworkers submitted the three different α chains to comparative analysis of their chymotryptic peptides, their terminal amino acids, and their molecular weights [28, 29]. From their studies it could be concluded that the two α^1 chains differ by a single amino acid residue. A lysine residue in the α^{1F} chain is replaced by a glutamic acid residue in the α^{1S} chain. The α^2 chain is almost twice as long as the α^1 chains and appears to result from the fusion of an α^{1F} chain with an α^{1S} chain with the deletion of segments of sequence from the C-terminal end of one chain and the N-terminal end of the other. As mechanism for the origin of the Hp α^2 gene, Smithies et al. proposed gene duplication of the Hp α^{1F} and Hp α^{1S} alleles by unequal nonhomologous crossing-over [29]. This concept was confirmed by Dixon and coworkers [30, 31], who determined the complete amino acid sequences of the three common α chains and found complete agreement with the results obtained by peptide analysis.

Haptoglobin 1-1 is a singular molecular species with a molecular weight of approximately 100,000. It is composed of two α^1 chains of 9,000 molecular weight each and a pair of β chains of 40,000 molecular weight each. The chains are linked by disulfide bonds, presumably three or four. The molecular model for haptoglobin 1-1 which has been deduced from this information has an apparent similarity to the molecular models proposed for the immunoglobulin IgG [32]. This analogy may be more than coincidental, since the amino acid sequence of the haptoglobin α chains has portions with homologies to the invariant part of a series of kappa and lambda Bence Jones proteins [31]. Also, examination of the secondary structure by optical rotatory dispersion and circular dichroism has shown similarities between haptoglobin 1-1 and IgG [33, 34]. The data on both proteins are compatible with the interpretation that both contain no α-helical structures—or only very small portions of them—and that both contain, in addition to random coil structures, portions with β structures. The structural and functional similarities between haptoglobin and immunoglobin IgG may reflect a common evolutionary origin. The Hp α genes may be related to the postulated precursor genes for L chains [31].

Hp 2-1 and Hp 2-2 are characterized by a series of polymers. Several plausible models for their composition have been proposed. In the most favored hypothesis the constitution of the Hp 2-2 polymers is in accord with the formula $(\alpha^2\beta)_4$ $(\alpha^2\beta)_6$ $(\alpha^2\beta)_8$ . . . , thus representing dimers, trimers, tetramers, etc. [35]. The Hp 2-1 components may be constituted as $(\alpha^1\beta)_2$, $(\alpha^1\beta)_2(\alpha^2\beta)_2$, $(\alpha^1\beta)_2(\alpha^2\beta)_4$, $(\alpha^1\beta)_2(\alpha^2\beta)_6$ . . . [35].

Genetic Variants of Haptoglobin

In addition to the common haptoglobin types, several variant phenotypes have been recognized (Fig. 69-1). The most frequent occurs in about 10 percent of Negroes. This phenotype is superficially very similar to the normal Hp 2-1 type and called, therefore, *Hp 2-1 modified,* or *Hp 2-1M* [36]. It is characterized by an increased proportion of the two faster-moving haptoglobin components accompanied by a greatly decreased concentration of the slow-moving components. Examination of several individuals of the Hp 2-1M phenotype shows that the slower-moving haptoglobin components may vary in staining intensity. The phenotypic appearance ranges from a normal Hp 2-1 phenotype to a Hp 2-1M type with a strong band in the Hp 1-1 position and a faint trace band in the position of the first slow-moving component [37]. The subtyping pattern after reductive cleavage reveals the presence of normal α^1 and α^2 chains, but there is a consistent distortion of their proportions: Hp 2-1M shows a relative increase of α^1 and a relative decrease of α^2 chains [38].

An additional phenotype Hp0 is characterized by the absence of haptoglobin. In cases where hemolytic disorders can be excluded, the absence of haptoglobin has been assigned a genetic basis. Distinction of these cases from persons with extreme hypohaptoglobinemia can be achieved by reexamination after concentration of their serum proteins. Individuals of the Hp0 phenotypes are also frequent among African or American Negroes and occur often in those families in which the variant Hp 2-1M is also observed [39].

The genetic control of the Hp 2-1M and Hp0 phenotypes is not completely understood. Giblett and Steinberg have postulated that the two variants are determined by an additional allele Hp^{2M} at the haptoglobin locus with variable phenotypic expression [39]. An alternate hypothesis ascribes these types to the action of genes which control the amount of haptoglobin synthesized. Thus, the Hp 2-1M phenotype represents reduced synthesis of Hp^2 gene product, and Hp0 is the manifestation of complete repression of haptoglobin synthesis [40]. These controller genes are presumably closely linked to the structural Hp α gene. The very rare type Hp Carlsberg (Fig. 69-1) is characterized also by distortion of the amount of α chains synthesized by the two haptoglobin alleles. Subtyping in these cases reveals an excess of α^2 chains over α^1 chains (38).

Haptoglobin Johnson (Fig. 69-1) is another variant which occurs only infrequently. It has been observed in widely different parts of the world and in different ethnic groups [38]. The subtype pattern shows a slowly migrating α chain, which has a molecular size corresponding to a tripling of an α^1 chain. Smithies et al. [29] have suggested that the Hp αJ-chain is the product of a gene Hp^J which is derived from a partial triplication of the original Hp α^1 gene by unequal homologous crossing-over in individuals homozygous for Hp^2. This attractive hypothesis does not conform to the double-band pattern observed in several Hp Johnson variants (Fig. 69-1). Also unexplained are the small phenotypic differences among Johnson variants from different families and populations. Possibly they may be attributed to variations in the location of the point of displaced synapsis [41, 42].

At least ten other haptoglobin variants have been described. A discussion of these rare phenotypes is given in a recent review [43]. Three of them, haptoglobin Marburg, haptoglobin Bellevue, and haptoglobin P, are of interest because they represent β chain variants [44–46]. The β chain contains the hemoglobin-binding site of the haptoglobin molecule [47]. The β chains of common haptoglobin types do not show genetic differences and are presumably identical in structure [48]. Genetic variants of the β chains are apparently very infrequent. Immunologic studies suggest altered hemoglobin binding properties of the β chain mutants [44–46].

Distribution of Haptoglobin Genes

The world map of haptoglobins shows a prominent increase in the frequency of the Hp^1 allele from east to west, taking India as a point of departure where the lowest Hp^1 frequencies are to be found (data summarized in [43]). The Hp^1 frequencies range from slightly less than 0.10 in Tamil and Irula populations from Southeast Asia to 0.80 in South American Indians and African Negroes. Information on the distribution of the two Hp^1 alleles is still limited. In Caucasians Hp^{1S} is more frequent than Hp^{1F}, and in Negroes Hp^{1S} and Hp^{1F} have approximately equal frequencies. In Oriental populations the allele Hp^{1F} is extremely rare [49, 50].

The selective factors which may be responsible for these variations in Hp gene frequencies are unknown. The biologic function of haptoglobin is probably directly related to its capacity to bind hemoglobin. The haptoglobin-hemoglobin complex is rapidly removed from the circulating blood, chiefly presumably by the liver [51, 52, 53]. Earlier interpretations emphasized the possible role this mechanism may play for the determination of the renal threshold for hemoglobin [51, 54]. In a study of patients with hemolytic anemias who were ahaptoglobinemic Whitten failed to demonstrate a significant increase in the urinary excretion of hemoglobin [55]. Nakajima and coworkers suggested a relationship between the formation of the haptoglobin-hemoglobin complex and the metabolic degradation of hemoglobin in the liver [56]. They suggested that an enzyme heme-α-methenyl-oxygenase catalyzes the oxidative cleavage of heme to produce a precursor of biliverdin. Using animal liver homogenates, they found that the heme in free hemoglobin is resistant to the action of this enzyme but is rapidly degraded after combination of hemoglobin with haptoglobin. In this function Hp 2-2 appears to be significantly more efficient than either Hp 2-1 or Hp 1-1. Smithies has suggested that this difference could be the basis for a selective advantage of the Hp^2 gene [57]. The existence of the enzyme heme-α-methenyl-oxygenase has been questioned, since its postulated activity can be attributed as well to a nonenzymatic, low-molecular-weight substance present in liver, conceivably ascorbic acid [58, 59]. Thus the exact biologic function of haptoglobin, as well as the significance of its genetic polymorphism, remains to be established.

Recent studies on haptoglobins have focused on the nature and mechanism of the binding of hemoglobin [154, 155], the subunit structure of the haptoglobin molecule [156], and the primary structure of its constituent β-chain [157]. An association of structural variations of chromosome 16 with the haptoglobin α chain variations permits the assignment of the Hp α locus to this chromosome with a high degree (0.97) of probability [158].

THE GROUP-SPECIFIC COMPONENT (Gc)

The α_2-globulin fraction of human serum is a complex mixture of proteins with similar electrophoretic mobilities. In addition to the major α_2-globulins comprising haptoglobin, α_2-macroglobulin, and ceruloplasmin, several other proteins in small amounts have been recognized. Some of these have been isolated and their physiochemical and chemical characteristics determined. Although many biologic activities have been assigned to the α_2-globulin fraction as a whole, only in a few instances can a specific function be allotted to a particular protein within the group. At present the biologic significance of most of the minor proteins has not been elucidated, but in one instance a complex genetic polymorphism has been revealed.

During immunoelectrophoretic analysis of human sera Hirschfeld observed variation in the electrophoretic mobility of a certain α_2-globulin which he called the group-specific component (Gc) [60]. He was able to classify normal human sera into three groups according to differences in the electrophoretic position of the precipitin arc of this protein (Fig. 69-2). The three common Gc types are designated Gc 1-1, Gc 2-1, and Gc 2-2. They are determined by a pair of autosomal alleles, called Gc^1 and Gc^2 [61]. Classification of Gc types can be performed by electrophoresis on starch or polyacrylamide gels [62, 63] as well as by the original immunoelectrophoretic procedure.

Extensive population surveys for this genetic marker have revealed a worldwide distribution of the two alleles Gc^1 and Gc^2 [64, 65]. In most populations, Gc^1 is more common than Gc^2. The frequency of the latter varies from 0.011 in an Australian Aborigine tribe from Cundeelee in the Western Desert [66], to 0.385 in a population of Finns from the island of Kokar [67]. In several South American Indian tribes Gc^2 is more common than Gc^1 [68]. Most Caucasian and Mongoloid populations have Gc^2 frequencies between 0.20 and 0.30. Negro populations have Gc^2 frequencies between 0.03 and 0.11. The mechanisms responsible for these distribution differences are not known.

A number of rare genetic variants in the Gc system have been discovered which include the faster migrating Gc Aborigine [69] and Gc Darmstadt [70], the slower migrating Gc Bangkok [71] and Gc Z [72], and the variants Gc Chippewa [69] and Gc Norway [73]. The structural loci for Gc and albumin are genetically linked [17].

The various genetic types of the group-specific components have a molecular weight of 50,000 and a sedimentation constant of 4.1S [74]. Gc contains 3.3 percent carbohydrates and is devoid of neuraminic acid and lipids. It is composed of structural subunits. The constituent polypeptide chains have a molecular weight of 25,000 [75, 76]. Gel electrophoresis, as well as immunoelectrophoresis with prolonged separation times, reveals that the group-specific components of the homozygous Gc types are electrophoretically hetero-

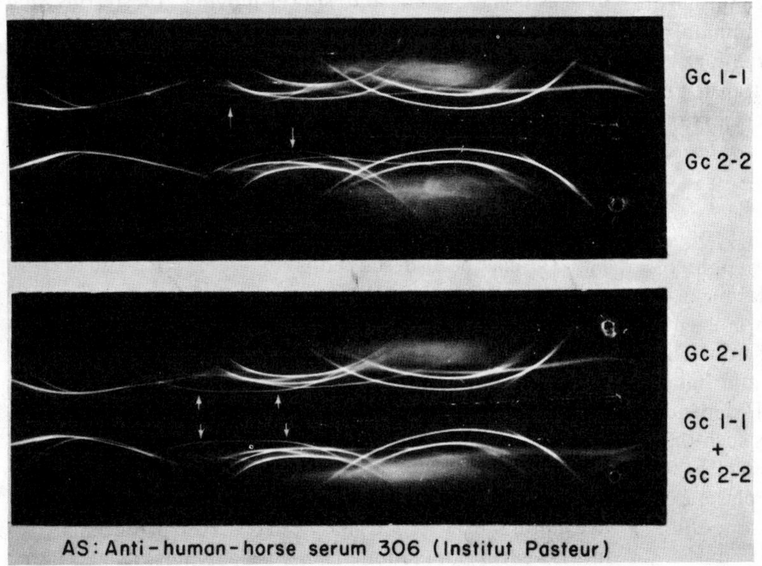

Figure 69-2. Comparative immunoelectrophoretic analysis of three normal human serums demonstrating the three common phenotypes of the group-specific component. The immunoelectrophoretic pattern of a mixture of equal amounts of Gc 1-1- and Gc 2-2-type serums is also illustrated. The Gc is indicated by arrows. The separation has been carried out from right (cathode) to left (anode).

geneous [77, 78]. Both Gc 1-1 and Gc 2-2 have a fast- and slow-migrating component, and Gc 2-1 has a three-band pattern. The Gc 1-1 fast, 1-1 slow, and 2-2 slow components have been isolated and analyzed [76]. The Gc molecule is probably composed of chains with very similar structures, but the structural differences among the various genetic types have not been identified. These may reside in single amino acid substitutions, as suggested by the available peptide map data [75, 79]. The subunit structure of the group-specific component has recently been further elucidated; it is probable that the Gc molecule is composed of three different types of polypeptide chains. They are under the control of three different structural gene loci, one of which reveals polymorphic genetic variations [159].

The biologic function of the group-specific component is unknown. The serum concentration of Gc in healthy individuals is approximately 40 mg per 100 ml [80]. There are slight but significant differences in the concentrations between the genetic types: persons with Gc 1-1 have on the average higher levels than those with Gc 2-1, and persons with Gc 2-1 have higher concentrations than subjects with Gc 2-2 [80]. Gc is increased in the sera of pregnant women. Since the group-specific component is synthesized in the liver [81], patients with severe liver diseases tend to have low Gc serum levels [80]. The application of the Gc system is presently restricted to its use as an additional marker in population studies, twin diagnosis, and in disputed paternity.

TRANSFERRIN

Iron in serum is bound to a serum protein called *transferrin.* Since the normal metabolism of iron requires a daily turnover of 10 times the amount of serum iron, it is clear that transferrin serves a transport function. The role of transferrin in iron metabolism has been reviewed by Laurell [82], Bowman [83], and by Giblett [2]. Jandl and Katz [84] have observed a specific attachment of transferrin to immature red cells. The affinity of iron-saturated transferrin for the cells is approximately fivefold that of iron-free transferrin and is considerably greater than that for synthetic chelating agents.

Properties of Transferrin

Transferrin is a glycoprotein with a molecular weight of approximately 90,000. It is present in normal plasma in a concentration of 250 to 300 mg per 100 ml. Each molecule of transferrin is capable of binding two atoms of iron. The bond is ionic, involves ferric, not ferrous, iron, and has a weak interaction between the binding sites. The pH dependence of the dissociation of iron from transferrin is such that dissociation is detected at approximately pH 7 and is 50 percent complete at approximately pH 6. In the plasma of normal individuals the circulating transferrin is one-third saturated with iron.

There are 10 groups in the pH 5.5 to 12 region that titrate in iron-free transferrin but do not titrate in iron-saturated transferrin. These are thought to indicate 3-tyrosine and 2-histidine groups at each iron-binding site. Although the nature of the site may be different for conalbumin, the iron-binding protein of egg white, Malmström et al. [85] have reported that the electron spin resonance spectrums of the iron complexes of the two proteins are very similar. The precise molecular weight of transferrin is probably somewhat lower than the commonly accepted value of 90,000. Charlwood [86] and Roberts and coworkers [87] have suggested the molecular weight of transferrin is approximately 75,000. Recent evidence clearly indicates that the protein, which is synthesized in the liver, is composed of a single polypeptide chain [88].

Genetics of Transferrin

Interest in the genetic aspects of transferrin began in 1957, when Smithies demonstrated by starch-gel electrophoresis the occurrence of two β-globulins in the serum of some individuals [89]. The β-globulin found in the serum of most people was named Type C; the faster-moving variant, which was observed in Caucasians, was named Type B, and the slower variant, observed in Negroes, was named Type D. Each of the variants was found to segregate in pedigrees, and an autosomal allelic system without dominance was postulated. Two years later Giblett [90] identified these β-globulins as transferrins by means of autoradiography. As subsequent genetically determined variants were described, a nomenclature was adopted in which subscripts were selected to distinguish the transferrins within the fast and slow B and D categories. There are now, in addition to the common transferrin C, eight transferrins in the B group and ten in the D group [2, 91]. The discovery by Harris et al. [92] of additional faster- and slower-moving transferrins that did not coincide with the B and D of Smithies led to the adoption of subscripts in order of decreasing mobility to differentiate variants within the fast- and slow-moving groups. Nineteen different molecular species of transferrin have been identified [2]. These encompass a wide range of electrophoretic mobility and cover the α-β region in the starch-gel pattern from the haptoglobin-2 position to ceruloplasmin (Fig. 69-3). Recently a further variant, transferrin $B_{Lambert}$, has been described [160].

Because of the low frequency of transferrin variants, the precise mode of inheritance of transferrin has not yet been established, but the data strongly support an autosomal allelic system without dominance. Partial evidence for this pattern of inheritance has been presented for most of the variants. Family studies have not been reported for many of the rarer transferrins, but it seems likely that a similar pattern of inheritance will be found. A particularly informative mating ($B_2D_1 \times CC$) has been observed by Beckman [93] in a Swedish population. The two daughters of the mating

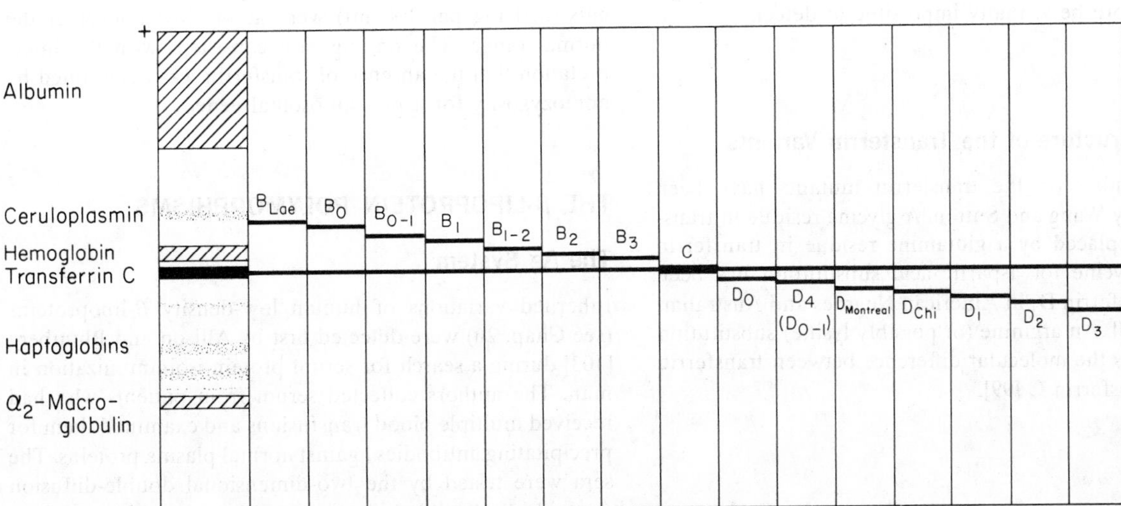

Figure 69-3. The inherited variations in the human transferrins.

were of transferrin phenotypes B_2C and CD_1, respectively; thus, three transferrin types are segregating in this family. A second family reported by Robinson and coworkers demonstrates segregation between transferrins $B_{1\text{-}2}$ and B_2 [94].

Polymorphism of Human Transferrin

The elaborate polymorphism of 19 different molecular species of transferrin can be distinguished by their mobilities in starch-gel electrophoresis. Transferrin C is by far the most frequent in all population studies; transferrins B_{Lae}, B_0, B_1, $B_{Atalanti}$, $B_{1\text{-}2}$, B_3, D_0, D_{Wigan}, $D_{Adelaide}$, $D_{0\text{-}1}$, $D_{Montreal}$, $D_{Finland}$, D_2, and D_3 have been reported only in isolated cases [95, 96]. Transferrin variants observed in measurable frequencies are the B_2 of Caucasian populations, the $B_{0\text{-}1}$ of Navaho Indians, the D_1 of Negroes, and the D_{Chi} of Chinese. The calculated gene frequency values for these populations are 0.005, 0.04, 0.06, and 0.03, respectively [95, 96]. The last three values are each higher than the generally accepted cutoff level of 1 percent, above which the frequency of a particular allele is unlikely to be maintained by mutation alone. The frequencies of individuals heterozygous for each variant are given in Table 69-1.

An interesting feature of the transferrin variations is the occurrence of a unique transferrin in a particular population. It appears that the transferrin gene locus is capable of numerous viable mutations and that in different populations a particular transferrin variant has been selected to accord with the adaptive situation in their local environments. Thus, random mutations to the transferrin variants $B_{0\text{-}1}$, D_{Chi}, and D_1 were apparently of selective advantage in the early North American, Oriental, and African environments where they originated.

The Caucasian, Navaho, Chinese, and Negro populations, with their relatively higher frequencies of unusual transferrins, may represent states of balanced polymorphism. The main function of transferrin is the transport of iron in the body. Since the principal genetic variations in transferrin appear to be expressed in terms of charge, it is possible that the equilibrium for the transport of iron may be altered by the charge differences which exist among the various transferrins. According to the equilibrium postulated by Laurell, the slower-moving, more positively charged transferrins should favor the formation of the Fe-Tf complex and hence the removal of iron from tissues, whereas the faster-moving, more negatively charged transferrins should favor dissociation of the iron complex and storage of iron. Thus far studies have detected no significant difference in the rate of disappearance of iron from the serum of transferrins B_0, B_1, C, and D_3 from serum or in utilization of iron for hemoglobin synthesis. If the frequencies of the unusual transferrin alleles are stable, the similar incidence of $B_{0\text{-}1}$ in Navaho Indians, D_{Chi} in Chinese, and D_1 in Negroes suggests that selective factors of approximately equivalent intensity may be operating in these three populations. If a balanced polymorphism is the correct explanation of the transferrin heterogeneity, the selective factors responsible for maintaining the

Table 69-1. PERCENT FREQUENCY OF INDIVIDUALS HETEROZYGOUS FOR TRANSFERRIN VARIANTS

Population	B_2	$B_{0\text{-}1}$	D_1	D_{Chi}
Caucasian	1	0	0	0
Navaho Indian	0	8	0	0
Negro	0	0	12	0
Chinese	0	0	0	6

observed gene frequencies need only be extremely small and would therefore be virtually impossible to detect.

Chemical Structure of the Transferrin Variants

Structural studies on the transferrin mutants have been undertaken by Wang and Sutton. A glycine residue in transferrin C is replaced by a glutamine residue in transferrin B_2 [97]; a glycine for aspartic acid substitution has been found in transferrin D_1 in American Negroes and Australian aborigines [98]. An arginine (or possibly lysine) substitution for histidine is the molecular difference between transferrin D_{Chi} and transferrin C [99].

Hereditary Absence of Transferrin

Only three patients have been reported with absent serum transferrin. The first two of these probably had an acquired deficiency of the protein. Riegel and Thomas [100] described an 85-year-old woman whose plasma, 2 days before death, showed an extreme diminution or absence of the β-globulin fraction by paper electrophoresis. Hitzig et al. [101] described a child of 2 years and 9 months with erythroleukemia with symptoms for 3 months. Transferrin could not be detected by immunoelectrophoresis of serum drawn 4 days before death. One month before death the serum showed a normal transferrin precipitin arc by immunoelectrophoresis.

The third case is that of Heilmeyer et al. [102]. A 7-year-old girl had a severe hypochromic anemia first diagnosed at age 3½ months. The mother had two miscarriages before the birth of the child, and a subsequent child died immediately after birth. Treatment with iron, cortisone, and vitamin B_{12} was ineffective, and transfusions were required at 3-month intervals. The child suffered from recurrent infections, had retarded growth, and was hospitalized 17 times in the course of treatment. Clinical findings revealed a low hemoglobin concentration (9.1 gm per 100 ml), normal levels of hemoglobin F and A_2 and of serum copper, and a decreased serum iron concentration (9 to 14 μg per 100 ml), total iron-binding capacity (33 μg per 100 ml), and unsaturated iron-binding capacity (19 μg per 100 ml). Normal levels for the latter three iron values are 150, 450, and 300 μg per 100 ml, respectively. The half-time for clearance from the plasma of injected radioactive iron (^{59}Fe) was 5 min, as compared to normal values of 70 to 140 min; the iron was localized in the liver, spleen, and bone marrow after clearance. After oral administration of ^{59}Fe, 70 percent of the dose was recovered in the feces, as compared to normal recovery of 80 to 90 percent. A slight decrease in erythrocyte survival time was observed.

The transferrin concentrations determined for both parents (220 mg per 100 ml) were at the lower level of the normal range. The findings are consistent with the interpretation that the absence of transferrin was determined by homozygosity for a rare autosomal gene.

THE β-LIPOPROTEIN POLYMORPHISMS

The Ag System

Inherited variations of human low-density β-lipoproteins (see Chap. 26) were detected first by Allison and Blumberg [103] during a search for serum protein isoimmunization in man. The authors collected serum from patients who had received multiple blood transfusions and examined them for precipitating antibodies against normal plasma proteins. The sera were tested by the two-dimensional double-diffusion method in agar gel against a panel of normal human sera. In the serum of one patient (C.deB.) a substance was found which behaved as a precipitating antibody against the β-lipoprotein of some normal sera but not of others [104]. The ability of normal sera to react or not to react with the serum of the patients was attributed to the presence or absence of a single antigen named Ag(a) which was supposedly controlled by a single gene Ag^A [103–105]. It is now known that this original serum contained three antibodies with different specificities, which have been named anti-Ag(x), anti-Ag(a_1), and anti-Ag(z) [106, 107]. In addition, two further antibody specificities have been found, which were labeled anti-Ag(y) and anti-Ag(t) [108, 109]. Corresponding to these five antibody specificities, five antigens or antigenic determinants called Ag(x), Ag(a_1), Ag(z), Ag(y), and Ag(t) are assumed to exist. Family studies have shown that Ag(x) and Ag(y) apparently behave like the gene products of antithetical alleles. Ag(a_1), Ag(z), and Ag(t) are also inherited as autosomal dominant traits [110, 111]. The five antigens are associated with each other.

Hirschfeld has developed two alternate models for the genetic control of the Ag antigens which are comparable to the two Rh models of Fisher-Race and Wiener. In the linkage model three closely linked loci with eight different Ag genes are assumed. In the single locus model the five Ag antigens are supposedly determined by a series of alleles [110]. The family data available at present can be reconciled with both models. In addition, nonprecipitating Ag antibodies with different specificities, named anti-Ag(c) and anti-Ag(e), have been described recently [112, 113].

The Lp System

Berg has demonstrated genetic polymorphism of human β-lipoproteins by the use of antisera obtained by heteroimmunization [114]. Purified β-lipoprotein fractions or whole human sera were used for immunization of rabbits. The antisera were absorbed with various individual normal sera, and the absorbed antisera were subsequently tested with the agar-gel diffusion technique against a panel of normal human sera. The system of genetic variants revealed by these antisera was named the Lp-system, and the first specificity defined in this system was labeled Lp(a). The system of Ag antigens and the Lp(a)-system are supposedly not genetically linked [115, 116, 117]. The Lp(a) antigen is inherited as an autosomal dominant trait. An electrophoretically homogeneous lipoprotein fraction of density $1.050 < \rho < 1.125$ gm per ml (corresponding to the HDL_1 class, see Chap. 26) has recently been isolated with Lp(a) specificity [118, 119]. It was shown that the Lp(a) reactivity was retained after removal of the lipid from the lipoprotein. This Lp(a)+ lipoprotein fraction appears to be absent in Lp(a)− sera [118, 119].

Double β-lipoprotein

An electrophoretic variant of β-lipoprotein, called *double beta-lipoprotein,* was observed by Seegers et al. [120]. The variant lipoprotein migrated faster than normal β-lipoprotein on paper and starch-block electrophoresis. On starch-gel electrophoresis the variant moved slower than normal β-lipoprotein. The variant was inherited as an autosomal codominant trait. No clinical condition was associated with this anomaly.

α_1-ANTITRYPSIN

In normal man the serum protein designated α_1-antitrypsin accounts for approximately 90 percent of the total trypsin inhibitory capacity of normal serum [121]. Although the most purified protein which is presently available is unstable and may be heterogeneous, a number of physical constants have been determined. Alpha$_1$-antitrypsin is a glycoprotein of 40,000 to 60,000 molecular weight [122, 123]. It has a carbohydrate content of approximately 12 percent and contains no cystine residues [124]. Alpha$_1$-antitrypsin comprises the major component of the α_1 region in the electropherogram of normal serum. Thus a deficiency of the protein may be suspected by inspection of routine serum electrophoretic patterns.

Confirmation of a suspected deficiency of α_1-antitrypsin requires additional immunologic, electrophoretic, or enzymatic measurements. Quantitative estimations of the protein using the Maneini technique show that the level of α_1-antitrypsin in normal serum is approximately 200 mg per 100 ml [125]. Alpha$_1$-antitrypsin can also be measured enzymatically using the synthetic substrate benzoyl-arginine-*p*-nitroanilide. The serum level is substantially increased in acute and chronic infections, in neoplasia, and in pregnancy [125]. An increased concentration also occurs in women taking contraceptive pills.

Interest in the serum α_1-antitrypsin greatly increased following the observation by Laurell and Eriksson in 1963 of an association between a deficiency of α_1-antitrypsin and chronic obstructive pulmonary disease [126]. This association was quickly confirmed in several laboratories in different countries [127–129]. In most instances the emphysema is characterized by early onset, a relative tendency to occur more frequently in females, and absence of a history of chronic bronchitis. In the few instances in which autopsy reports are available, the panacinar [130, 131] form of emphysema is uniformly present. Hyperinflation of the lower lobes is stressed by some authors [130]. It should be emphasized that homozygous α_1-antitrypsin deficiency occurs in probably no more than 2 percent of all patients with severe emphysema, although it may be more frequent in patients with emphysema under the age of 40 years. Moreover, not all subjects with homozygous antitrypsin deficiency are abnormal when they are found and studied. Two out of seven clinically asymptomatic homozygous subjects with a deficiency of α_1-antitrypsin had a low diffusion capacity and abnormal pulmonary perfusion [131]. In a series of 70 subjects with homozygous α_1-antitrypsin deficiency three over the age of 60 showed no clinical evidence of emphysema [125]. Whether individuals heterozygous for α_1-antitrypsin deficiency are more prone than normal subjects to develop emphysema is not yet resolved.

Recently, certain patients with recessively inherited infantile liver cirrhosis associated with α_1-antitrypsin deficiency have been recognized [146]. Electrophoretic classification of the deficiency state for α_1-antitrypsin revealed the Pi ZZ phenotype [147]. In several instances progressive cirrhosis developed from neonatal or infantile hepatitis. The role of the serum protease inhibitor defect in the pathogenesis of the disease remains to be established.

Some progress has been made in elucidating the pathogenetic role of the α_1-antitrypsin deficiency for chronic obstructive pulmonary disease (COPD). In an analysis of seven homozygous deficient individuals, four had mildly impaired air flow rates, hypoxemia, increased alveolar-arterial oxygen gradients, and decreased carbon monoxide diffusing capacity [148]. Studies using xenon-133 indicated an altered distribution of pulmonary capillary perfusion with loss of the normally occurring perfusion gradient from base to apex. This finding was also made in a 14-year-old subject with homozygous deficiency who was clinically and physiologically normal. Thus, an altered pulmonary blood flow pattern may be an early manifestation of α_1-antitrypsin deficiency. In another study [149] it was shown that α_1-antitrypsin acts as an inhibitor of leukocyte proteases in purulent sputum. A deficiency of α_1-antitrypsin may, therefore, be associated with a decreased resistance of pulmonary tissue to proteolytic digestion during the inflammatory response.

Several investigations have been devoted to the question

of whether in addition to homozygous deficient subjects, individuals who are heterozygous for α_1-antitrypsin deficiency and persons with certain rare Pi (protease inhibitor) mutants, are relatively more susceptible to the development of chronic obstructive pulmonary disease [125, 150–153]. A definitive conclusion cannot as yet be drawn from the data available. In the original material of Eriksson [136] the clinical evaluation of family members who were obligatory heterozygotes for α_1-antitrypsin deficiency did not provide evidence for a predisposition for emphysema in this group. Lieberman, however, in an analysis of 28 relatives of homozygous affected individuals [150] found 4 out of 19 heterozygotes with COPD. Electrophoretic and enzymatic assay of the trypsin inhibitor capacity of serum in 66 patients with emphysema revealed seven who were classified as homozygous and 10 as heterozygous deficient. Kueppers et al. [151] reported 98 patients with COPD, of whom 25 (25.5 percent) appeared to be heterozygous for the α_1-antitrypsin deficiency gene. In two control groups the heterozygous frequency was significantly lower, 14 percent and 9 percent, respectively. Electrophoretic classification by acid starch-gel electrophoresis and subsequent antigen-antibody crossed electrophoresis [152] permits a more accurate identification of the heterozygous state and was employed by these authors. These studies strongly suggest that heterozygous carriers of the α_1-antitrypsin deficiency gene are particularly liable to develop emphysema. The frequency of the heterozygous and homozgous states for α_1-antitrypsin deficiency, Pi MZ and Pi ZZ, and the frequency of other Pi mutants, especially Pi SS, Pi MS, and Pi SZ, have to be assessed with greater accuracy in the general population and in groups of patients with COPD. Prospective studies in those Pi types with supposedly increased risk will be needed to assess the pattern of development of emphysema and the influence of preventive measures.

Pathogenesis of Emphysema

Although the association between a deficiency of α_1-antitrypsin and emphysema is widely claimed, the cause of this association remains obscure. Gross and coworkers [132] were able to induce emphysema in rats by the intratracheal instillation of papain, and a similar observation has been made in the Syrian hamster by Goldring and coworkers following the administration of a papain aerosol [133]. It is well established that α_1-antitrypsin will inhibit the intracellular proteolytic enzymes of leukocytes and that it also has antielastase activity [134]. It seems plausible, therefore, that the association of emphysema with a deficiency of α_1-antitrypsin is due to the absence of effective antiprotease activity against intracellular leukocyte proteases which are liberated when the cell disintegrates. Further studies will be required before the precise mechanism responsible for the association of α_1-antitrypsin deficiency and emphysema is delineated [134, 135].

Genetics

The synthesis of α_1-antitrypsin is controlled by an autosomal allelic system [126, 136–140]. In persons homozygous for the most frequent deficiency gene, the serum α_1-antitrypsin is reduced to 10 to 15 percent of normal values; in individuals heterozygous for this gene the protein is decreased to approximately 60 percent of the normal concentration [125]. In American and Swedish populations the frequency of heterozygotes for the deficiency gene is approximately 2 to 4 percent. Some geographic variation has been observed. The deficiency is rare in Finnish populations.

Recent development in electrophoretic techniques have revealed a number of mutants at the α_1-antitrypsin locus collectively known as the *Pi* (protease inhibitor) *mutants* [139–141]. The common form of α_1-antitrypsin is controlled by a gene designated Pi^M; the deficiency allele is designated Pi^Z. Other variants include Pi^S, Pi^F, Pi^I, Pi^V, and Pi^W. Alleles Pi^Z and Pi^F occur relatively frequently in Caucasian populations. Reliable estimates for the serum α_1-antitrypsin concentration cannot be obtained unless the Pi type of α_1-antitrypsin is known. Thus Pi phenotypes SS, MS, and MZ have 63 percent, 83 percent, and 61 percent of the activity found for the normal Pi type MM [125]. These genetic refinements should not obscure the primary observation that most patients with the α_1-antitrypsin deficiency are homozygous ZZ. Of 16,190 healthy individuals, 13 (approximately 0.8 per 1000) from Norway and Sweden were found to have the ZZ phenotype [125]. Detailed studies on pulmonary function were not reported.

FURTHER GENETIC VARIATIONS OF SERUM PROTEINS

Ceruloplasmin variants are rare among Caucasians. In Negroes a genetic polymorphism has been recognized recently [142]. Three distinct electrophoretic forms exist, called CpA, CpB, and CpC. CpB is the common ceruloplasmin, CpA represents a faster-migrating, and CpC a slower-migrating variant.

Alpha$_2$-macroglobulin supposedly displays variations of its antigenic determinants. With an antiserum prepared in a rabbit by immunizing with whole serum from a female donor, inherited variations have been disclosed which were attributed to α_2-macroglobulin [143]. This trait, called Xm(a), appears to be inherited as an X-linked character. This marker is potentially useful for linkage studies. Unfortunately, the original reagent is depleted and attempts to obtain antisera with the same specificity have been unsuccessful.

Beta$_2$-glycoprotein I concentration in human serum appears to be under genetic control. Individuals with serum levels reduced to approximately half the normal serum concentration are relatively frequent. They are presumably heterozygous for a deficiency gene Bg^D [144].

Alpha$_1$-acid glycoprotein also has inherited electrophoretic variants [145].

SUMMARY

1 Several mutations have been recognized which influence the synthesis of serum albumin. Analbuminemia, the almost complete absence of albumin in serum, is extremely rare. The condition appears to be inherited as an autosomal recessive trait. Affected individuals are only mildly incapacitated. Fatigue, pretibial edema, mild anemia, or mild diarrhea are in some cases associated with the protein deficiency. Bisalbuminemia, the presence of two electrophoretically distinct albumins in serum, has been observed in several families from different populations. At least 11 different electrophoretic variants have been identified, 5 of them migrating faster and 6 of them migrating slower than normal albumin. These variants are inherited as autosomal codominant traits. They are infrequent in most populations. Inherited albumin dimer formation is another type of genetic albumin variation. It has been found in several families and is also inherited as an autosomal codominant trait. Bisalbuminemia and albumin dimer variants are not associated with clinical disease.

2 Haptoglobin is an α_2-globulin in human serum which binds hemoglobin. Three common phenotypes, called Hp 1-1, Hp 2-1, and Hp 2-2, can be distinguished by gel electrophoresis. After breakdown of the haptoglobin molecules into their constituent polypeptide chains through reductive cleavage of disulfide bonds it is possible to discriminate six common phenotypes. Subdivision of the Hp^1 gene product into fast- and slow-moving α chains accounts for this "hidden" variability. Thus, a total of six haptoglobin subtypes is determined by three common alleles, Hp^{1F}, Hp^{1S}, and Hp^2. Complete amino acid sequence data indicate as evolutionary origin of the Hp^2 gene partial gene duplication by fusion of parts of two Hp^1 genes. Several other genetic variants have been observed. Absence of haptoglobin, ahaptoglobinemia, may be genetically determined but is more frequently caused by in vivo hemolysis and subsequent removal of the formed haptoglobin-hemoglobin complex from the circulating blood.

3 The group-specific component (Gc) is an α_2-globulin of serum of unknown biologic function. Three common genetic types, Gc 1-1, Gc 2-1, and Gc 2-2, are determined by two autosomal alleles. They can be classified by gel or immunoelectrophoresis. Several additional genetic variants have been found.

4 Transferrin is the carrier protein for iron in the blood. Most persons are homozygous for the common transferrin, called transferrin C. A total of 18 genetic transferrin variants has been discovered. The faster-migrating variants are called B transferrins, and the slower-migrating variants D transferrins. Most of these variants are rare, but some occur at higher frequencies in certain populations. Their biologic significance in relation to iron metabolism is not clearly understood. Hereditary absence of transferrin, atransferrinemia, has been reported in a child with severe hypochromic anemia and generalized hemosiderosis.

5 Inherited variations of low-density β-lipoproteins have been discovered by immunologic methods. Certain patients who have received multiple blood transfusions develop precipitating antibodies which can discriminate the β-lipoproteins of some persons and not of others. With the use of these isoimmune sera a complex system of inherited β-lipoprotein variants, the Ag-system, has been established. A different approach, the use of antisera from rabbits immunized with β-lipoprotein fractions from individual blood donors, has led to the discovery of an additional genetic polymorphism of the β-lipoproteins, the Lp-system.

6 Genetic variants of ceruloplasmin and of acid-α_1-glycoprotein have been distinguished electrophoretically. Alpha$_2$-macroglobulin appears to display inherited variations of its antigenic determinants. Variations of serum concentrations of β_2-glycoprotein I are genetically controlled.

7 Approximately 90 percent of the total serum trypsin inhibitory activity resides in a protein, of 40,000 to 60,000 molecular weight, and a carbohydrate content of 12 percent, called serum α_1-antitrypsin. Low levels of this protein are characteristically associated with chronic obstructive pulmonary disease with emphysema. No more than 2 percent of patients with this disease have a deficiency of the protein. Clinical disease only occurs in homozygotes for the abnormal gene. The synthesis of the protein is controlled by a series of codominant alleles at a single locus. The frequency of the heterozygous trait in most populations is approximately 2 to 4 percent.

BIBLIOGRAPHY

1. Schultze, H. E., and Heremans, J. F.: Molecular Biology of Human Proteins: With Special Reference to Plasma Proteins. vol. 1, Elsevier, Amsterdam, 1966.
2. Giblett, E. R.: Genetic Markers in Human Blood. Blackwell Oxford, 1969.
3. Putnam, F. W. (Ed.): The Plasma Proteins. Academic, New York, 1960.
4. Pederson, D. M., and Foster, J. F.: Subtilisin cleavage of bovine plasma albumin. Reversible association of the two primary fragments and their relation to the structure of the parent protein. Biochemistry, **8**, 2357, 1969.
5. Bennhold, H., Peters, H., and Roth, E.: Über einen Fall von kompletter Analbuminaemie ohne wesentliche klinische Krankheitszeichen. Verh. Deutsch. Ges. Inn. Med. **60**, 630, 1954.
6. Waldmann, T. A., Gordon, R. S. Jr., and Rosse, W.: Studies on the metabolism of the serum proteins and lipids in a patient with analbuminemia. Amer. J. Med., **37**, 960, 1964.
7. Bennhold, H., and Kallee, E.: Comparative studies on the half-life of I^{131} labeled albumins and non-radioactive human serum albumin in a case of analbuminemia. J. Clin. Invest., **38**, 863, 1959.
8. Franglen, G., Martin, N. H., Hargreaves, I., Smith, M. J. H., and Williams, D. I.: Bisalbuminaemia: a hereditary albumin abnormality. Lancet, **1**, 307, 1960.
9. Knedel, M.: Die Doppel-albuminämie, eine neue erbliche Proteinanomalie. Blut, **3**, 129, 1957.

10. Weitkamp, L. R., Shreffler, D. C., Robbins, J. L., Drachmann, O., Adner, P. L., Wieme, R. J., Simon, N. M., Cooke, K. B., Sandor, G., Wuhrmann, F., Braend, M., and Tarnoky, A. L.: An electrophoretic comparison of serum albumin variants from nineteen unrelated families. Acta Genet. (Basel), **17**, 399, 1967.
11. Melartin, L., and Blumberg, B. S.: Albumin Naskapi: A new variant of serum albumin. Science, **153**, 1664, 1966.
12. Weitkamp, L. R., and Chagnon, N. A.: Albumin Maku: a new variant of serum albumin. Nature, **217**, 759, 1968.
13. Melartin, L., and Blumberg, B. S.: Inherited variants of human serum albumin. Clin. Res., **14**, 482, 1966.
14. Lau, T., Sunderman, F. W. Jr., Agarwal, S. S., Sutnick, A. I., and Blumberg, B. S.: Genetics of albumin Gainesville, a new variant of human serum albumin. Nature, **221**, 66, 1969.
15. Weitkamp, L. R., Basu, A., Gall, J. C., and Brown, W.: Albumin Cayemite: A Negro plasma albumin variant. Humangenetik, **7**, 180, 1969.
16. Weitkamp, L. R., Shreffler, D. C., and Saave, J. J.: Serum albumin variants in New Guinea indigenes. Vox Sang., **17**, 237, 1969.
17. Weitkamp, L. R., Rucknagel, D. L., and Gershowitz, H.: Genetic linkage between structural loci for albumin and group specific component (Gc). Amer. J. Hum. Genet., **18**, 559, 1966.
18. Gitlin, D., Schmid, K., Earle, D. P., and Givelber, H.: Observations on double albumin. II. A peptide difference between two genetically determined serum albumins. J. Clin. Invest., **40**, 820, 1961.
19. Fraser, G. R., Harris, H., and Robson, E. B.: A new genetically determined plasma protein in man. Lancet, **1**, 1023, 1959.
20. Jamieson, G. A., and Rohde, V. C.: Genetically determined albumin dimer in a normal blood donor. Proc. 11th Congr. Int. Soc. Blood Transf., Sydney, 1966. Bibl. Haemat., No. 29, Part I, Karger, Basel/New York, 1968, p. 415.
21. Jamieson, G. A., and Ganguly, P.: Studies on a genetically determined albumin dimer. Biochem. Genet., **3**, 403, 1969.
22. Laurell, C. B., and Nilehn, J. E.: A new type of inherited serum albumin anomaly. J. Clin. Invest., **45**, 1935, 1966.
23. Polonovski, M. and Jayle, M. F.: Existence dans le plasma sanguin d'une substance activant l'action peroxydasique de l'hémoglobine. C. R. Soc. Biol. (Paris) **129**, 457, 1938.
24. Jayle, M. F., and Moretti, J.: Haptoglobin: Biochemical, genetic and physiological aspects. Progr. Hemat., **3**, 342, 1962.
25. Smithies, O.: Zone electrophoresis in starch gels: group variations in the serum proteins of normal human adults. Biochem. J., **61**, 629, 1955.
26. Smithies, O., and Walker, N. F.: Notation for serum protein groups and the genes controlling their inheritance. Nature, **178**, 694, 1956.
27. Smithies, O., Connell, G. E., and Dixon, G. H.: Inheritance of haptoglobin subtypes. Amer. J. Hum. Genet., **14**, 14, 1962.
28. Connell, G. E., Dixon, G. H., and Smithies, O.: Subdivision of the three common haptoglobin types based on "hidden" differences. Nature, **193**, 505, 1962.
29. Smithies, O., Connell, G. E., and Dixon, G. H.: Chromosomal rearrangements and the evolution of haptoglobin genes. Nature, **196**, 232, 1962.
30. Dixon, G. H.: Mechanisms of protein evolution. In *Essays in Biochemistry,* vol. 2, p. 147/edited by P. N. Campbell and G. D. Greville, Academic, London, New York, 1966.
31. Black, J. A., and Dixon, G. H.: Amino-acid sequence of alpha chains of human haptoglobins. Nature, **218**, 736, 1968.
32. Shim, B.-S., and Bearn, A. G.: Immunological and biochemical studies on serum haptoglobin. J. Exp. Med., **120**, 611, 1964.
33. Waks, M. and Alfsen, A.: Structural studies of haptoglobins. I. Hydrogen in equilibria and optical rotatory dispersion of Hp 1-1 and Hp 2-2. Arch. Biochim. Biophys., **113**, 304, 1966.
34. Hamaguchi, H.: Purification and some properties of the three common genetic types of haptoglobins and the hemoglobin—haptoglobin complexes. Amer. J. Hum. Genet., **21**, 440, 1969.
35. Shim, B.-S., Lee, T.-H., and Kang, Y.-S.: Immunological and biochemical investigations of human serum haptoglobin: composition of haptoglobin-haemoglobin intermediates, haemoglobin binding sites and presence of additional alleles for the β-chain. Nature, **207**, 1264, 1965.
36. Giblett, E. R.: Haptoglobin types in American Negroes. Nature, **183**, 192, 1959.
37. Sutton, H. E., and Karp, G. W.: Variations in heterozygous expression at the haptoglobin locus. Amer. J. Hum. Genet., **16**, 419, 1964.
38. Giblett, E. R.: Variant haptoglobin phenotypes. Cold Spring Harbor Symp. Quant. Biol., **29**, 321, 1964.
39. Giblett, E. R. and Steinberg, A. G.: The inheritance of the serum haptoglobin types in American Negroes: evidence for a third allele Hp^{2M}. Amer. J. Hum. Genet., **12**, 160, 1960.
40. Parker, W. C. and Bearn, A. G.: Control gene mutations as a possible explanation of certain haptoglobin phenotypes. Amer. J. Hum. Genet., **15**, 159, 1963.
41. Giblett, E. R.: The haptoglobin system. Series Haematol., **1**, 3, 1968.
42. Cleve, H. and Herzog, P.: Phenotypic variations of haptoglobin Johnson types. Humangenetik, **7**, 218, 1969.
43. Kirk, R. L.: The haptoglobin groups in man. Monographs in *Human Genetics,* vol. 4, edited by L. Beckman and M. Hauge, S. Karger, New York, 1968.
44. Cleve, H., and Deicher, H.: Haptoglobin "Marburg": Untersuchungen über eine seltene erbliche Haptoglobinvariante mit zwei verschiedenen Phänotypen innerhalb einer Familie. Humangenetik, **1**, 537, 1965.
45. Javid, J.: Haptoglobin 2-1 Bellevue, a haptoglobin β-chain mutant. Proc. Nat. Acad. Sci., **57**, 920, 1967.
46. Choi, Y.-M., and Shim, B.-S.: Immunochemical characterization of haptoglobin P variants. Thesis of Catholic Med. Coll., Seoul, Korea, **13**, 277, 1967.
47. Gordon, S., and Bearn, A. G.: Hemoglobin binding capacity of isolated haptoglobin polypeptide chains. Proc. Soc. Exp. Biol. Med., **121**, 846, 1966.
48. Cleve, H., Gordon, S., Bowman, B. H., and Bearn, A. G.: Comparison of the tryptic peptides and amino acid composition of the beta polypeptide chains of the three common haptoglobin phenotypes. Amer. J. Hum. Genet., **19**, 713, 1967.
49. Giblett, E. R., and Brooks, L. E.: Haptoglobin sub-types in three racial groups. Nature, **197**, 576, 1963.
50. Shim, B.-S., and Bearn, A. G.: The distribution of haptoglobin subtypes in various populations, including subtype patterns in some non-human primates. Amer. J. Hum. Genet., **16**, 477, 1964.
51. Laurell, C. B., and Nyman, M.: Studies on serum haptoglobin level in haemoglobinaemia and its influence on renal excretion of haemoglobin. Blood, **12**, 493, 1957.
52. Murray, R. F., Connell, G. E., and Pert, J. H.: Role of haptoglobin in clearance and distribution of extracorpuscular haemoglobin. Blood, **17**, 45, 1961.
53. Keene, W. R., and Jandl, J. H.: The sites of haemoglobin catabolism. Blood, **26**, 705, 1965.
54. Allison, A. C., and Ap Rees, W.: The binding of haemoglobin by plasma proteins (haptoglobins). Brit. Med. J., **2**, 1137, 1957.
55. Whitten, C. F.: Studies on serum haptoglobin—a functional inquiry. New Eng. J. Med., **266**, 529, 1962.
56. Nakajima, H., Takemura, T., Nakajima, O., and Yamaoka, K.: Studies on heme α-methenyl oxygenase. J. Biol. Chem., **238**, 3784, 1963.
57. Smithies, O.: Chromosomal rearrangements and protein structure. Cold Spring Harbor Symp. Quant. Biol., **29**, 309, 1964.
58. Murphy, R. F., O'h Eocha, C., and O'Carra, P.: The formation of verdohaemochrome from pyridine protohaemechrome by extracts of red algae and of liver. Biochem. J., **104**, 6 C, 1967.
59. Levin, E. Y.: Conversion of protohemochrome to verdohemochrome with liver homogenates. Biochim. Biophys. Acta. **136**, 155, 1967.
60. Hirschfeld, J.: Immune-electrophoretic demonstration of qualitative differences in human sera and their relation to the haptoglobins. Acta Path. Microbiol. Scand., **47**, 160, 1959.
61. Hirschfeld, J., Jonsson, B., and Rasmuson, M.: Inheritance of a new group-specific system demonstrated in normal human sera by means of an immunoelectrophoretic technique. Nature, **185**, 931, 1960.
62. Parker, W. C., Cleve, H., and Bearn, A. G.: Determination of phenotypes in the human group-specific component (Gc) system by starch gel electrophoresis. Amer. J. Hum. Genet., **15**, 353, 1963.

63. Kitchin, F. D.: Demonstration of the inherited serum group-specific protein by acrylamide electrophoresis. Proc. Soc. Exp. Biol. Med. **119,** 1153, 1965.
64. Cleve, H., and Bearn, A. G.: The group-specific component of serum; genetic and chemical considerations. Progr. Med. Genet. **2,** 64, 1962.
65. Cleve, H., Kirk, R. L., Gajdusek, D. C., and Guiart, J.: On the distribution of the Gc variant Gc Aborigine in Melanesian populations; determination of Gc-types in sera from Tongariki Island, New Hebrides. Acta Genet. (Basel), **17,** 511, 1967.
66. Kirk, R. L., Cleve, H., and Bearn, A. G.: The distribution of the Gc-types in sera from Australian aborigines. Amer. J. Phys. Anthrop., **21,** 215, 1963.
67. Hirschfeld, J., Seppälä, M., Erikkson, A. W., and Forsius, H.: Distribution of the group-specific components (Gc) in Finland. Ann. Med. Exp. Biol. Fenniae (Helsinki), **41,** 382, 1963.
68. Neel, J. V., Salzano, F. M., Junqueira, P. C., Keiter, F., and Maybury-Lewis, D.: Studies on the Xavante Indians of the Brazilian Mato Grosso. Amer. J. Hum. Genet., **16,** 52, 1964.
69. Cleve, H., Kirk, R. L., Parker, W. C., Bearn, A. G., Schacht, L. E., Kleinman, H., and Horsfall, W. R.: Two genetic variants of the group-specific component of human serum: Gc Chippewa and Gc Aborigine. Amer. J. Hum. Genet., **15,** 368, 1963.
70. Cleve, H., Kitchin, F. D., Kirchberg, G., and Wendt, G. G.: A faster migrating Gc-variant: Gc Darmstadt. Humangenetik, **9,** 26, 1970.
71. Rucknagel, D. L., Shreffler, D. C., and Halstead, S. B.: The Bangkok variant of the serum group-specific component (Gc) and the frequency of the Gc alleles in Thailand. Amer. J. Hum. Genet., **20,** 478, 1968.
72. Hennig, W. and Hoppe, H. H.: A new allele in the Gc-system: Gc^Z. Vox Sang., **10,** 214, 1965.
73. Reinskou, T.: A new variant in the Gc system. Acta Genet. (Basel), **15,** 248, 1965.
74. Cleve, H., Prunier, J. H., and Bearn, A. G.: Isolation and partial characterization of the two principal inherited group-specific components of human serum. J. Exp. Med., **118,** 711, 1963.
75. Bowman, B. H., and Bearn, A. G.: The presence of subunits in the inherited group-specific component of human serum. Proc. Nat. Acad. Sci. (USA), **53,** 722, 1965.
76. Simons, K. and Bearn, A. G.: The use of preparative polyacrylamide-column electrophoresis in isolation of electrophoretically distinguishable components of the serum group-specific protein. Biochim. Biophys. Acta, **133,** 499, 1967.
77. Bearn, A. G., Kitchin, F. D., and Bowman, B. H.: Heterogeneity of the inherited group-specific component of human serum. J. Exp. Med., **120,** 83, 1964.
78. Reinskou, T.: A heterogeneity of the fast moving component of the Gc system. Acta Path. Microbiol. Scand., **59,** 526, 1963.
79. Ruoslahti, E.: Studies on the molecular basis of Gc polymorphism. Ann. Med. Exp. Biol. Fenn., **45,** 1, 1967.
80. Cleve, H. and Dencker, H.: Quantitative variations of the group-specific component (Gc) and the Barium-α_2-glycoprotein of human serum in health and disease. Edited by H. Peeters, p. 379, Proc. XIVth Coll. Prot. Biol. Fluids, Bruges, Elsevier, Amsterdam, 1966.
81. Prunier, J. H., Bearn, A. G., and Cleve, H.: Site of formation of the group-specific component and certain other serum proteins. Proc. Soc. Exp. Biol. Med., **115,** 1005, 1964.
82. Laurell, C. B.: Plasma iron and the transport of iron in the organism. Pharmacol. Rev., **4,** 371, 1952.
83. Bowman, B. H.: Serum transferrin. Series Haematologica I, **1,** 97, 1968.
84. Jandl, J. H., and Katz, J. H.: The plasma-to-cell cycle of transferrin. J. Clin. Invest., **42,** 314, 1963.
85. Malmström, B., Vanngard, T., Aasa, R., and Saltman, P.: On the nature of the metal-binding sites in transferrin and conalbumin. Fed. Proc., **22,** 595, 1963.
86. Charlwood, P. A.: Ultracentrifugal characteristics of human, monkey and rat transferrins. Biochemistry J., **88,** 394, 1963.
87. Roberts, R. C., Makey, D. G., and Seal, U. S.: Human transferrins; molecular weight and sedimentation properties. J. Biol. Chem., **241,** 4907, 1966.
88. Greene, F. C., and Feeney, R. E.: Physical evidence for transferrins as single polypeptide chains. Biochemistry, **7,** 1366, 1968.
89. Smithies, O.: Variations in human serum β-globulins. Nature, **180,** 1482, 1957.
90. Giblett, E. R., Hickman, C. G., and Smithies, O.: Serum transferrins, Nature (London), **183,** 1589, 1959.
91. Parker, W. C., and Bearn, A. G.: Additional genetic variation of human serum transferrin, Science, **137,** 854, 1962.
92. Harris, H., Robson, E. B., and Siniscalco, M.: β-globulin variants in man. Nature (London), **182,** 452, 1958.
93. Beckman, L.: Slow and fast transferrin variants in the same pedigree. Nature (London), **194,** 796, 1962.
94. Robinson, J. C., Blumberg, B. S., Pierce, J. E., Cooper, A. J., and Hanes, C. G.: Studies on the inherited variants of blood proteins. II. Familiar segregation of transferrins B, $B_{1\text{-}2}$, B_2. J. Lab. Clin. Med., **62,** 762, 1963.
95. Bearn, A. G., Parker, W. C., and Cleve, H.: Genetic variations in the serum proteins: studies on transferrin and the group-specific components. 2d Int. Conf. Congenital Malformations, New York, July, 1963, pp. 125–134.
96. Parker, W. C., and Bearn, A. G.: Haptoglobin and transferrin variation in humans and primates: two new transferrins in Chinese and Japanese populations. Ann. Hum. Genet., **25,** 227, 1961.
97. Wang, A. C., Sutton, H. E., and Riggs, A.: A chemical difference between human transferrins B_2 and C. Amer. J. Hum. Genet. **18,** 454, 1966.
98. Wang, A. C., Sutton, H. E., and Scott, I. D.: Transferrin D_1: Identity in Australian aboriginies and American Negroes, Science, **156,** 936, 1967.
99. Wang, A. C., Sutton, H. E., and Howard, P. N.: Human transferrins C and D_{Chi}: An amino acid difference, Biochem. Genet., **1,** 55, 1967.
100. Riegel, C., and Thomas, D.: Absence of beta-globulin fraction in the serum protein of a patient with unexplained anemia. New Eng. J. Med., **255,** 434, 1956.
101. Hitzig, W. H., Schmid, M., Betke, K., and Rothschild, M.: Erythroleukamie mit Hamoglobinpathie und Eisenstoffwechelstörung. Helvet. Paediat. Acta, **15,** 203, 1960.
102. Heilmeyer, L., Keller, W., Vivell, O., Keiderling, W., Betke, K., Wohler, F., and Schultze, H. E.: Kongenitale Atransferrinämie bei einem sieben Jahre alten Kind. Deutsch. Med. Wschr., **86,** 1745, 1961.
103. Allison, A. C., and Blumberg, B. S.: An isoprecipitation reaction distinguishing human serum protein types. Lancet, **1,** 634, 1961.
104. Blumberg, B. S., Dray, S., and Robinson, J. C.: Antigen polymorphism of a low density beta lipoprotein. Nature, **194,** 656, 1962.
105. Blumberg, B. S., Bernanke, D., and Allison, A. C.: A human lipoprotein polymorphism. J. Clin. Invest., **41,** 1936, 1962.
106. Hirschfeld, J.: Investigations of a new anti-Ag antiserum with particular reference to the reliability of Ag-typing by microimmunodiffusion tests in agar gel. Science Tools, **10,** 45, 1963.
107. Hirschfeld, J., Blumberg, B. S., and Allison, A. C.: Relationship of human anti-lipoprotein allotypic sera. Nature, **202,** 706, 1964.
108. Hirschfeld, J., Contu, L., and Blumberg, B. S.: Antilipoprotein neuroserum (C. P.) and its relation to sera C. de B. and L. L. Nature, **214,** 495, 1967.
109. Hirschfeld, J., Unger, P., and Ramgren, O.: A new anti-Ag serum (serum B. N.) Nature, **212,** 206, 1966.
110. Hirschfeld, J., and Rittner, C.: Inheritance of the Ag(x), Ag(y), (a_1) and Ag(z) antigens. Vox Sang., **16,** 146, 1969.
111. Morganti, G., Beolchini, P. E., Bütler, R., and Vierucci, A.: Contribution to the genetics of serum β-lipoproteins in man. II. Frequency, transmission and penetrance of the Ag(a_1) factor and its linkeage with the Ag(x) and Ag(y) factors. Humangenetik, **5,** 98, 1968.
112. Bütler, R., and Brunner, E.: A non-precipitating anti-Ag antibody. Vox Sang., **13,** 508, 1967.
113. Bütler, R., and Brunner, E.: A second example of a non-precipitating anti-Ag antibody. Vox Sang., **14,** 230, 1968.
114. Berg, K.: A new serum type system in man—the Lp system. Acta Path. Microbiol. Scand., **59,** 369, 1963.
115. Berg, K.: Comparative studies on the Lp and Ag serum type systems. Acta Path. Microbiol. Scand., **62,** 276, 1964.

116. Berg, K.: Lack of linkage between the Lp and Ag serum systems. Vox Sang., **12,** 71, 1967.
117. Rittner, C.: Bestehen Beziehungen zwischen dem Ag-und dem Lp-system? Z. Immunitätsforsch, **130,** 229, 1966.
118. Wiegandt, H., Lipp, K., and Wendt, G. G.: Identifizierung eines Lipoproteins mit Antigenwirksamkeit im Lp-System. Hoppe-Seyler's Z. Physiol. Chem., **349,** 489, 1968.
119. Schultz, J. S., Shreffler, D. C., and Harvie, N. R.: Genetic and antigenic studies and partial purification of a human serum lipoprotein carrying the Lp antigenic determinant. Proc. Nat. Acad. Sci., **61,** 963, 1968.
120. Seegers, W., Hirschhorn, K., Burnett, L., Robson, E. B., and Harris, H.: Double beta-lipoprotein: a new genetic variant in man. Science, **149,** 303, 1965.
121. Jacobsson, K.: Studies on the trypsin and plasmin inhibitors in human serum. Scand. J. Clin. Lab. Invest., Suppl. 14, 1955.
122. Rimon, A., Shamash, Y., and Shapiro, B.: The plasmin inhibitor of human plasma. J. Biol. Chem., **241,** 5102, 1966.
123. Schultze, H. E., Heide, K., and Haupt, H.: Alpha$_1$-antitrypsin aus Humanserum. Klin. Wschr., **40,** 427, 1962.
124. Shamash, Y., and Rimon, A.: The plasmin inhibitors of human plasma. Biochim. Biophys. Acta, **121,** 35, 1966.
125. Fagerhol, M. K., and Laurell, C. B.: The Pi system—Inherited variants of serum alpha$_1$-antitrypsin, in Progress in Medical Genetics, edited by A. G. Steinberg and A. G. Bearn, vol. 7. Grune & Stratton, New York. p. 96, 1970.
126. Laurell, C. B., and Eriksson, S.: The electrophoretic alpha$_1$-globulin pattern of serum in alpha$_1$-antitrypsin deficiency. Scand. J. Clin. Lab. Invest., **15,** 132, 1963.
127. Kueppers, F., and Bearn, A. G.: Inherited variations of human serum alpha$_1$-antitrypsin. Science, **154,** 407, 1966.
128. Mazodier, P.: Le deficit constitutionnel en alpha$_1$-antitrypsine, six rapports avec les maladies broncho-pulmonaires chronique et type obstructif. J. Franç. Med. Chir. Thorac., **20,** 247, 1966.
129. Meiers, H. G., Beizenherz, D., Bruster, H., Strassburger, D., and Grenel, H.: Alpha$_1$-antitrypsin-Defekt und Lungenemphysem. Deutsch. Med. Wschr., **93,** 1633, 1968.
130. Briscoe, W. A., Kueppers, F., Davis, A. L., and Bearn, A. G.: A case of inherited deficiency of serum alpha$_1$-antitrypsin associated with pulmonary emphysema. Amer. Rev. Resp. Dis., **94,** 529, 1966.
131. Guenter, C. A., Welch, M. H., Russel, T. R., Hyde, R. M., and Hammarsten, J. F.: The pattern of lung disease associated with alpha$_1$-antitrypsin deficiency. Arch. Intern. Med., **122,** 254, 1968.
132. Gross, P., Pfitzer, E. A., Tolker, E., Babyerk, M. A., and Kaschak, M.: Experimental emphysema. Arch. Env. Health, **11,** 50, 1965.
133. Goldring, I. P., Greenburg, L., and Ratner, I. M.: On the production of emphysema in Syrian hamster by aerosol inhalation of papain. Arch. Env. Health, **16,** 59, 1968.
134. Kueppers, F. and Bearn, A. G.: A possible experimental approach to the association of hereditary alpha$_1$-antitrypsin deficiency and pulmonary emphysema. Proc. Soc. Exp. Biol. Med., **121,** 1207, 1966.
135. Tarkoff, M. P., Kueppers, F., and Miller, W.: Pulmonary emphysema and alpha$_1$-antitrypsin deficiency. Amer. J. Med., **45,** 220, 1968.
136. Eriksson, S.: Studies in alpha$_1$-antitrypsin deficiency. Acta Med. Scand., **177,** Suppl. 175, 1965.
137. Talamo, R. C., Allen, J. D., Kahan, M. G., and Austen, K. F.: Hereditary alpha$_1$-antitrypsin deficiency. New Eng. J. Med., **278,** 345, 1968.
138. Talamo, R. C., Blennerhassett, J. B., and Austen, K. F.: Familial emphysema and alpha$_1$-antitrypsin deficiency. New Eng. J. Med., **275,** 1301, 1966.
139. Fagerhol, M. K.: Serum Pi types in Norwegians. Acta Path. Microbiol. Scand., **70,** 421, 1967.
140. Fagerhol, M. K., and Tenfjord, O. W.: Serum Pi types in some European, American, Asian and African populations. Acta Path. Microbiol. Scand., **72,** 601, 1968.
141. Fagerhol, M. K., and Hauge, H. E.: The Pi phenotype MP. Vox Sang., **15,** 396, 1968.
142. Shreffler, D. C., Brewer, G. J., Gall, J. C. and Honeyman, M. S.: Electrophoretic variation in human serum ceruloplasmin: a new genetic polymorphism. Biochem. Genet., **1,** 101, 1967.
143. Berg, K. and Bearn, A. G.: An inherited X-linked serum system in man—the X_m system. J. Exp. Med., **123,** 379, 1966.
144. Cleve, H.: Genetic studies on the deficiency of β_2-glycoprotein I of human serum. Humangenetik, **5,** 294, 1968.
145. Tokita, K. and Schmid, K. : The genetically determined α_1-acid glycoprotein variants. Genetics Today. Proc XIth Int. Congr. Genet., The Hague, 1963, vol. 1, p. 296.
146. Sharp, H. L., Bridges, R. A., Krivit, W., and Freier, E. F.: Cirrhosis associated with alpha$_1$-antitrypsin deficiency: A previously unrecognized inherited disorder. J. Lab. Clin. Med., **73,** 934, 1969.
147. Johnson, A. M., and Alper, C. A.: Deficiency of alpha$_1$-antitrypsin in childhood liver disease. Pediatrics, **46,** 921, 1970.
148. Levine, B. W., Talamo, R. C., Shannon, D. C., and Kazemi, H.: Alteration in distribution of pulmonary blood flow, an early manifestation of alpha$_1$-antitrypsin deficiency. Ann. Int. Med., **73,** 397, 1970.
149. Lieberman, J., Mohamed, M., and Mittmann, C.: Inhibition of leukocytic proteases in purulent sputum by alpha$_1$-antitrypsin. J. Clin. Invest., **49,** 58a, 1970 (Abstr.).
150. Lieberman, J.: Heterozygous and homozygous alpha$_1$-antitrypsin deficiency in patients with pulmonary emphysema. New Engl. J. Med., **281,** 279, 1969.
151. Kueppers, F., Fallat, R., and Larson, R. K.: Obstructive lung disease and α_1-antitrypsin deficiency gene heterozygosity. Science, **165,** 899, 1969.
152. Kueppers, F.: Identification of the heterozygous state for the α_1-antitrypsin deficiency gene in man. Biochem. Genet., **3,** 283, 1969.
153. Welch, M., Reinecke, M., Hammerstein, J., and Guenter, C.: Antitrypsin deficiency in pulmonary disease: The significance of intermediate levels. Ann. Int. Med., **73,** 533, 1969.
154. Chiancone, E., Alfsen, A., Ioppolo, C., Vecchini, P., Finazzi Agro, A., Wyman, J., and Antonini, E.: Studies on the reaction of haptoglobin with haemoglobin and haemoglobin chains. I. Stoichiometry and affinity. J. Mol. Biol., **34,** 347, 1968.
155. Alfsen, A., Chiancone, E., Antonini, E., Waks, M., and Wyman, J.: Studies on the reaction of haptoglobin with hemoglobin and hemoglobin chains. III. Observations on the kinetics of the reaction of the haptoglobin-hemoglobin complexes with carbon monoxide. Biochim. Biophys. Acta, **207,** 395, 1970.
156. Bernini, L. F., and Borri-Voltattorni, C.: Studies on the structure of human haptoglobins. I. Spontaneous refolding after extensive reduction and dissociation. Biochim. Biophys. Acta, **200,** 203, 1970.
157. Barnett, D. R., Lee, T.-H., and Bowman, B. H.: Amino-acid sequence of the carboxyl terminal octapeptide of human haptoglobin beta chain. Nature, **225,** 938, 1970.
158. Robson, E. B., Polani, P. E., Dart, S. J., Jacobs, P. A., and Renwick, J. H.: Probable assignment of the alpha locus of haptoglobin to chromosome 16 in man. Nature, **233,** 1163, 1969.
159. Bowman, B. H.: Composition and subunit structure of the inherited group-specific protein of human serum. Biochemistry, **11,** 4327, 1969.
160. Barnett, D. R., and Bowman, B. H.: A transferrin variant, $B_{Lambert}$. Acta Genet. (Basel), **18,** 573, 1968.

CHAPTER SEVENTY

GENETIC DEFECTS IN GAMMA-GLOBULIN SYNTHESIS*

Fred S. Rosen and Ezio Merler

In 1936 Tiselius first designated the γ-globulins as a distinct group of serum proteins which migrate most slowly toward the anode in an electrophoretic field [1]. In the following year, Tiselius and Kabat [2] showed that the antibodies in serum are associated with the γ-globulin fraction. Although it became known during the next 2 decades that immunization resulted in a heterogeneous antibody response in that γ-globulins of various molecular weights and "fast" or "slow" mobilities could be elicited, it was not appreciated until the late 1950s that the γ-globulins could be subdivided into various classes. At the present time, five classes of γ-globulins are recognized: IgG or γG; IgA or γA; IgM or γM; IgD or γD; and IgE or γE. The designations "Ig" or "γ" can and will be used interchangeably. These classes of immunoglobulins are related to one another in that they share a basic structural plan of four polypeptide chains that are symmetrical about the long axis of the molecule; two of the four polypeptide chains are common in all classes of immunoglobulins. An understanding of the structural relationships among the γ-globulin classes was made possible by the studies of Porter in 1959 on enzymatic cleavage of γ-globulin. These led to a hypothetical molecular model which has withstood the tests of many experimental verifications and direct visualization by electron microscopy.

STRUCTURE OF γ-GLOBULIN

In 1959 Porter reported that rabbit γ-globulin could be split into three fragments by the enzyme papain, in the presence of cysteine. Two of these are identical and contain the combining site for antigen, and a third can be crystallized and does not bind antigen [3]. The two identical fragments are designated Fab (for antigen binding) and the third Fc (for crystallizable). Fc fragments have a molecular weight of 48,000, and Fab fragments, 52,000. Thus, a mole of γ-globulin, upon papain digestion, yields 1 mole of Fc fragments and 2 moles of Fab fragments. The molecular weight of the intact molecule is estimated to be of the order of 150,000.

In 1961, Edelman and Poulik reduced γ-globulin with mercaptoethanol in the presence of urea. By subsequent gel filtration in acid solution, two types of polypeptide chains could be separated [4]. Heavy chains, designated H chains, have a molecular weight of 53,000, and light chains, or L chains, have a molecular weight of 22,000. It was discerned that Fab fragments are composed of L chains and portions of H chains and that Fc fragments are composed only of parts of H chains (Fig. 70-1).

In contrast to the plant enzyme papain, animal proteases, such as trypsin, chymotrypsin, and pepsin, digest the Fc fragment into small peptides while the two Fab fragments remain joined together and retain bivalent antibody activity in a molecule of 100,000 molecular weight. This type of altered molecule is designated $F(ab')_2$ [5].

L chains, with a single minor exception, are covalently linked by a disulfide bond to H chains through the ultimate or penultimate amino acid residue at the carboxy terminal end of the L chains, which is a cysteine residue. Variable numbers of disulfide bonds link the H chains together (see Table 70-1); depending on the class or subclass of immunoglobulin, there may be two to five inter-H-chain disulfides [6].

The Bence-Jones protein found in the urine of patients with multiple myeloma is composed of L chains or dimers of L chains [7]. When rabbits are immunized with individual Bence-Jones proteins, two types of antisera to L chains can be obtained. The two types of L chains recognized by such antisera are designated κ and λ L chains. All immunoglobulin molecules, regardless of class or subclass, contain L chains of the κ or λ type. No individual molecule contains a mixture of the two, so that each immunoglobulin molecule or molecular subunit contains either two κ chains or two λ chains [8].

The amino acid sequences of a number of Bence-Jones L chains of both κ and λ type have been worked out [9]. From these sequence data analogies between the C-terminal halves (residues 106 to 212) of the L chains are quite apparent, whereas the N-terminal halves (residues 1 to 105) exhibit considerable variability. The adjacent N-terminal portions of H chains also are highly variable in their amino acid

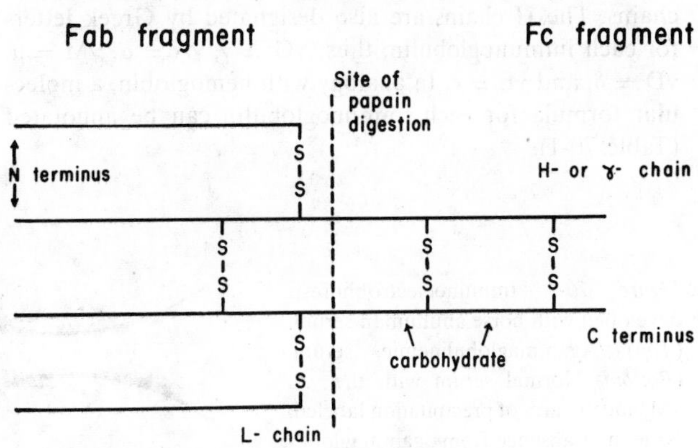

Figure 70-1. A schematic representation of the γ-globulin molecule by R. R. Porter.

*Supported by Public Health Service grants AI-05877 and K-3-AM 19,650 (FSR).

Table 70-1. PHYSICOCHEMICAL PROPERTIES OF THE IMMUNOGLOBULINS

Immuno-globulin	Sedimentation coefficients (S)	Approx. mol. wt. × 10^3	Carbohydrate content, %	Heavy chains	Total S—S interchain bonds	Molecular formulas
γG	6.6	150	2.8	γ1	4	$\gamma 1_2\kappa_2$; $\gamma 1_2\lambda_2$
				γ2	6	$\gamma 2_2\kappa_2$; $\gamma 2_2\lambda_2$
				γ3	7	$\gamma 3_2\kappa_2$; $\gamma 3_2\lambda_2$
				γ4	4	$\gamma 4_2\kappa_2$; $\gamma 4_2\lambda_2$
γA	7, 9, 11	$(170)_n$	6.4	α1	?3	$(\alpha 1_2\kappa_2)_n$; $(\alpha 1_2\lambda_2)_n$
				α2	?2	$(\alpha 2_2\kappa_2)_n$; $(\alpha 2_2\lambda_2)_n$
γM	18.6	900	10.2	μ	20	$(\mu_2\kappa_2)_5$; $(\mu_2\lambda_2)_5$
γD	7	160	?	δ	?	$\delta_2\lambda_2$; $\delta_2\kappa_2$
γE	7.9	190	11	ε	3	$\epsilon_2\lambda_2$; $\epsilon_2\kappa_2$

sequences, whereas the remainder of the H chains of various subclasses have constant homologies. The specific activity of the antibody molecule, that is, its ability to combine with an antigen, presumably resides in this variable portion of the Fab fragment. Although no more than 5 percent of the entire molecule is occupied by the combining site, at the present time the precise amino acid sequence is not known for any combining site. It is also not certain how the antigen dictates this structural alteration to render γ-globulin molecules into specific antibodies. Elaborations of the theories of antibody formation can be found in several reviews [10–12].

Before it was learned that there are two types of L chains, different classes of immunoglobulins were recognized by virtue of certain antigenic differences. It was first shown that the serum of boys with X-linked agammaglobulinemia lacked three classes of globulins, γG, γA, and γM, when the serum was examined with horse antiserum to human serum [13], and that the myeloma globulins and macroglobulins of Waldenström's disease were related to one or another of these three classes of globulins [14] (Fig. 70-2). Subsequently, a fourth class, γD, was found in certain myeloma patients whose M component was unrelated to the then-known three [15]. And, lastly, a fifth class, γE, has been identified with reaginic activity in man [16]. The differences among classes of the immunoglobulins reside in their H chains. The H chains are also designated by Greek letters for each immunoglobulin, thus: γG = γ, γA = α, γM = μ, γD = δ, and γE = ε. In analogy with hemoglobin, a molecular formula for each immunoglobulin can be annotated (Table 70-1).

CLASSES AND SUBCLASSES OF IMMUNOGLOBULINS

Pertinent physicochemical data for immunoglobulins are given in Table 70-1. Table 70-2 contains quantitative and metabolic information on each of the immunoglobulin classes [17].

Gamma-G-Globulin

Seventy-five to eighty-five percent of the serum antibodies are contained in the γG class. Antibodies to the pyogenic bacteria and viruses, and antitoxins are principally in the γG fraction.

Gamma-G-globulin contains 2.8 percent carbohydrate by weight. This is contained in two symmetrically arranged units attached to an asparagine residue of the H chain at amino acid residue 297 from the N terminus [18].

The human placenta efficiently transports γG from the maternal to fetal circulation, whereas the other immunoglobulins are almost completely excluded from the fetus. The mechanism for this active transport involves recognition of the Fc fragment [19].

Four subclasses of γG-globulin have been recognized by means of antigenic differences in individual γG myeloma proteins. They are designated γG1, γG2, γG3, and γG4. The frequency distribution of these subclasses in normal serum is 70:18:8:4 [20]. The ability of γG-globulin to fix complement is shared by γG1, γG2, and γG3, but not by γG4. The property of γG-globulin to fix to skin receptors, as measured by passive cutaneous anaphylaxis, is contained in

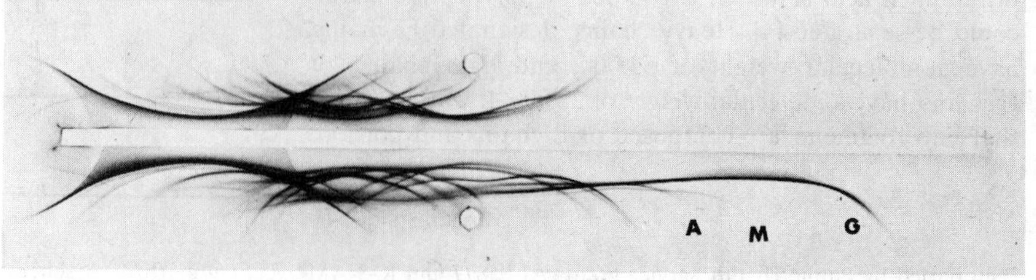

Figure 70-2. Immunoelectrophoresis developed with horse antihuman serum. (*Top*) Agammaglobulinemic serum. (*Bottom*) Normal serum with the γA, γM, and γG arcs of precipitation labeled. Note their absence from agammaglobulinemic serum.

Table 70-2. QUANTITATION AND METABOLISM OF IMMUNOGLOBULINS IN MAN [17]

Immuno-globulin	Serum concentration, mg/100 ml	% Total body pool in plasma	*t* ½ days	% Plasma pool catabolized/day	Synthetic rate, mg/kg/day
γG	600–1500	45	23	6.7	33
γA	200–300	42	5.8	25	24
γM	75–150	76	5.1	18	6.7
γD	0–3	75	2.8	37	0.4
γE	~0.05	51	2.5	89	0.016

the γG1, γG3, and γG4, but not γG2 molecules. All subclasses cross the placenta. Although the precise chemical localization of these functions is not yet known, chemical and genetic differences between the subclasses have been established.

Certain antibodies have been restricted to specific subclasses. For instance, antidextran antibodies are in the γG2 subclass; anti-Rh, in γG1 and γG3; anti-A substance, in γG1; and anti-factor VIII, principally in γG4. These restricted specificities may not bear up under further examination of individual sera.

Gamma-A-Globulins

The γA-globulins constitute about 15 percent of the antibodies of human serum. A large spectrum of specificities has been associated with γA globulins. These globulins have a tendency to polymerize, and about 5 to 10 percent of serum γA is found as a 9S dimer of the 7S form. Larger aggregates of 11S, 13S, and 15S are also found in serum in smaller amounts. The carbohydrate content of γA globulin is 6.4 percent. The sugar is linked to two asparagine residues of the H or α chain. N-acetylgalactosamine is linked to one serine residue of the α chain [21].

Gamma-A-globulins are encountered in relatively larger quantities in saliva, tears, colostrum, succus entericus, and nasal and bronchial secretions. Normal saliva contains 28 mg per 100 ml; colostrum, 151 mg per 100 ml; and tears, 7 mg per 100 ml [22]. Most of the γA in secretions is 11S globulin, along with lesser amounts of 15S and 7S forms. An additional structural unit is appended to γA in secretions; it has a molecular weight of approximately 50,000 and has been designated T chain because of a presumptive function in transporting γA-globulins across mucosal surfaces [23]. This "transport piece" is found only in mucosal cells and not in cells which synthesize γA-globulins. Critical evidence for a transport function for this transport piece is lacking at present.

Two classes of γA-globulin are known. Not only do the α chains of both subclasses differ, but the less common of the two also appears to have no inter L-H chain disulfide bonds. Hydrogen bonding and other tertiary forces hold L chains of the molecules of this subclass to the H chains [24].

Gamma-A-globulins do not fix complement, nor do they cross the placenta. They neutralize viruses. Local immunization of the nasal mucosa or gastrointestinal tract has been successfully effected with local production of γA viral-neutralizing globulins. Although newborn infants can synthesize γA-globulins at birth or in utero if the fetus is stimulated by infection, the serum γA-globulin level rises slowly throughout childhood and does not reach adult levels until the end of the first decade of life.

Gamma-M-Globulin

Between 5 and 10 percent of serum antibody is encountered in a class of immunoglobulins of large molecular size, the macroglobulins. They have a sedimentation coefficient of 19S and a molecular weight of 900,000. In 1957 Deutsch and Morton dissociated γM-globulins with mercaptoethanol into subunits of 6.5S [25]. The subunits, which have a molecular weight of 180,000, are designated γMs. The intact molecule is composed of five subunits, but each subunit is composed of two L chains and two μ chains and has two combining sites, so that the intact molecule has ten such combining sites [26]. From electron micrographs it appears that the subunits are arranged in a radial fashion and that the μ chains of the subunits are linked to adjacent subunits by disulfide bonds. The molecule contains 10.2 percent carbohydrate, all attached to the μ chains.

A large number of antibody specificities have been associated with γM. For example, antibodies to the large lipopolysaccharide antigens, such as the Wasserman, Forssman, blood group, and endotoxin antibodies, are principally γM-globulins. The γMs subunits may cross the placenta if they are present as free subunits in maternal serum. Little intact γM-globulin crosses the placental barrier. The fetus, if infected after the twentieth week of gestation, may synthesize considerable amounts of γM-globulins. Ordinarily they become detectable in the first week of extrauterine life and rise rapidly to achieve adult levels of serum concentration by the age of 6 months.

Approximately half of the γM-globulins fix complement. In most detection systems about 1,000-fold fewer γM molecules can be measured than other immunoglobulins. This ease of detectability had led to the assumption that γM antibodies are formed first following an antigenic stimulus, whereas this may in truth be an artifact of the detection system employed.

Gamma-D- and Gamma-E-Globulins

The Ishizakas have demonstrated that reaginic antibody in the serum of ragweed-sensitive people can be purified and identified with a unique class of immunoglobulins which are designated γE [27, 28]. These immunoglobulins exhibit all the properties of reaginic antibody in the classic Prausnitz-Küstner test in that they fix to human and monkey skin, are heat labile, are neutralized by allergens, and mediate histamine release. The discovery of two γE myelomas has facilitated structural studies of this immunoglobulin class, which is ordinarily present in only trace amounts [29, 30]. A large number of methionine and cysteine residues are present in the ε chain, as well as 11 percent by weight of carbohydrate. Elevated serum levels of γE globulin have been found in patients with extrinsic asthma, worm infestation, and various allergies [31, 32].

No antibody activity has been associated with γD-globulins. Over 20 patients with γD myeloma have been reported, but the physiologic significance of this class of globulins is not known.

Genetic Determinants of γ-Globulins

As previously intimated, allotypic differences which are genetically determined can be found on κ chains and on γ chains of γG1, γG2, and γG3 globulins. None has as yet been detected on α-, μ-, δ-, or ε chains or on λ chains. Several good reviews of this subject are available [33–35]. The detection system is complex, as are most inhibition methods. One is represented schematically in Fig. 70-3. An Rh positive red cell, coated with a maternal isoantibody of known genetic specificity, is agglutinated by an antibody of such restricted specificity that it recognizes minor antigenic differences expressed as genetic determinants in the Rh isoantibody. Such a source of agglutinating antibody has been found on occasion in normal serum or following multiple transfusions and in patients with rheumatoid arthritis (rheumatoid factor). At any rate, the specificity of γ-globulin in a serum sample can be ascertained by its ability to inhibit the agglutination reaction between an agglutinator and coated Rh positive cells, where the specificity of the coat and the agglutinator are known.

With such a cumbersome system it has been determined that there are three alleles at the Inv locus of the κ chains and nearly thirty alleles at the Gm locus of the γ chains. Although a system of numerical designation for the alleles at both loci has been devised, it is not yet widely used, and the original letter designations remain tenaciously in the literature.

The γ chains of γG1 contain the Gm (a), (x), (z), (y), and (f) factors, while γG3 contains the Gm (g) and all the (b) group of alleles. Only a single allele, Gm (n), can be discerned at present in γG2. The frequency distribution of the alleles is not random and has been ascertained in some detail for various racial and ethnic groups [20]. The frequency of alleles in the Caucasian population is shown in Table 70-3. Thus, γG1 molecules contain Gm (a) and Gm (z) or Gm (y) and Gm (f) but almost never another combination. Likewise, γG3 molecules have either Gm (b) or Gm (g) but not both. Thus there are six possible genes which can be hypothesized; Gm^{za}, Gm^{fy}, Gm^{b}, Gm^{g}, Gm^{n}, and Gm^{n-}, and three possible cistrons. They appear to be very closely linked. The finding of rare Gm complexes has given preliminary evidence for recombination of genes in kindred with offspring whose γ-globulins contain rare gene complexes. It appears that the order of the cistrons may be γG4—γG2—γG3—γG1 [20].

The amino acid differences among several alleles are known and are given in various reviews. The extensive homologies in amino acid sequences between the constant portions of the various immunoglobulins have given credence to the hypothesis that this complex system of immunoglobulins has arisen from gene duplications of a single primordial cistron.

In view of the expanding knowledge of the genes which control γ-globulin synthesis, it is somewhat disappointing that only a few patients have been identified in whom there is evidence for nonexpression of an allele governing immunoglobulin synthesis. On the other hand, a spectrum of genetic defects in γ-globulin synthesis results from a failure of development or maturation of cell populations which are involved in the synthesis of immunoglobulins.

X-LINKED AGAMMAGLOBULINEMIA

Historical Aspects

In 1952 Bruton reported the remarkable finding of the absence of γ-globulin from the serum of an 8-year-old boy who had been well up to the age of 4 years, when septic arthritis of the left knee developed. During the next 4 years the boy had 19 episodes of pneumococcal sepsis, repeated attacks of otitis media, and 2 bouts of pneumococcal pneumonia. Although these illnesses were successfully treated with antibiotics, immunization with polyvalent pneumococcal vaccines did not protect him or result in the appearance of serum antibodies. Further investigation demonstrated that he was unable to produce antibodies after typhoid vaccination, and a Schick test remained positive after attempted diphtheria immunization. Free electrophoresis of the serum revealed normal albumin and α- and β-globulins, but the γ fraction was undetectable. After adequate intramuscular injection of γ-globulin, the patient remained well [36].

These observations of susceptibility to bacterial infection accompanied by absence of γ-globulin and antibodies from

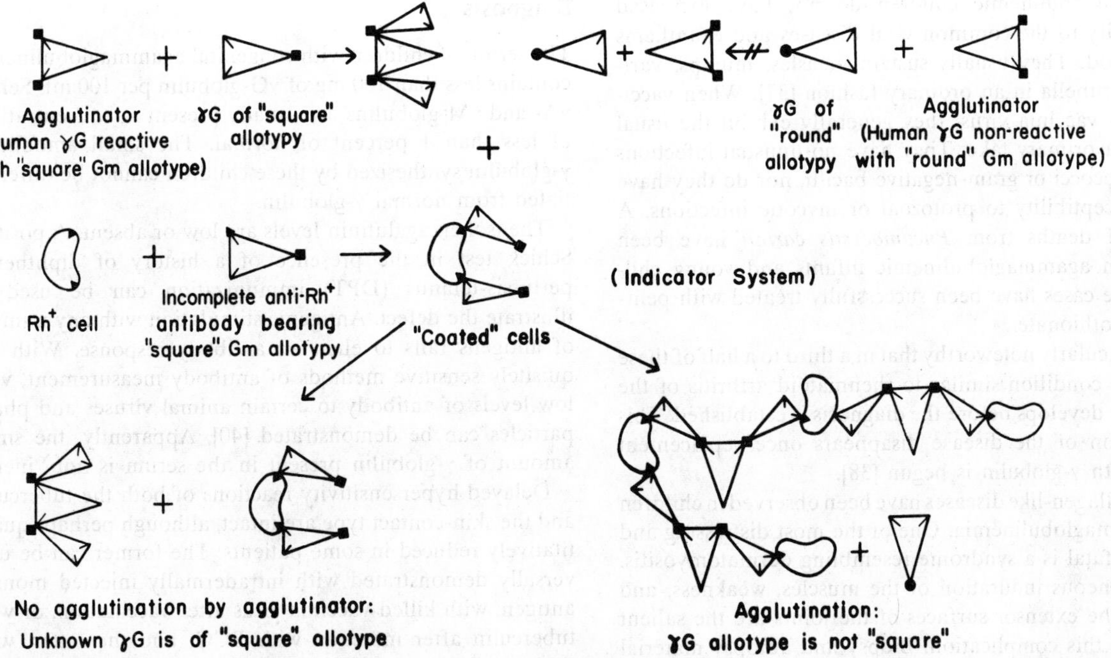

Figure 70-3. A schematic representation of the system for detecting genetic markers on γ-globulin by its ability or failure to inhibit agglutination of coated Rh^+ red cells by an agglutinator where the genetic specificity of the coat and the agglutinator are known.

the serum, as well as inability to synthesize antibody following appropriate antigenic stimulation, were confirmed in other patients by other observers within a short time. Over 200 cases of the disease have now been studied.

Clinical Features

Male infants with X-linked agammaglobulinemia usually remain well during the first 9 months of life, probably because of the passive protection afforded by the maternal γ-globulin. Undue susceptibility to infection becomes evident during the second year of life. Depending on the environment of the child, the presence of older sibs, and other circumstances, the onset of frequent infections may be even further delayed. Almost invariably these children contract infections from the pyogenic organisms, principally staphylococci, pneumococci, streptococci, and *Hemophilus influenzae.* The infections can usually be readily controlled with antimicrobial chemotherapy. Purulent sinusitis, pneumonia, sepsis, meningitis, and furunculosis are the most common types. These infections may be persistently recurrent until proper prophylactic therapy is undertaken. Untreated, many of these children develop chronic progressive bronchiectasis and ultimately die of the pulmonary complications if they survive the innumerable infections.

Table 70-3. CHARACTERISTICS OF γG-GLOBULIN SUBCLASSES [20]

Caucasoid gene complexes					Complement fixation	Transplacental passage	Fixation to skin	Frequency distribution
		x						
γG1	a	a	y	y	+	+	+	70
	z	z	f	f				
γG2	n-	n-	n	n-	+	+	0	18
γG3	g	g	b	b	+	+	+	8
γG4					0	+	+	4
Frequency of allelic complexes:	0.20	0.10	0.52	0.17				

Agammaglobulinemic children do not have increased susceptibility to the common viral diseases and exanthems of childhood. They usually sustain measles, mumps, varicella, and rubella in an ordinary fashion [37]. When vaccinated with vaccinia virus, they generally exhibit the usual course of a primary take. They have no unusual infections with enterococci or gram-negative bacilli, nor do they have undue susceptibility to protozoal or mycotic infections. A number of deaths from *Pneumocystis carinii* have been reported in agammaglobulinemic infants and young children. Some cases have been successfully treated with pentamidine isothionate.

It is particularly noteworthy that in a third to a half of these children, a condition similar to rheumatoid arthritis of the large joints develops before the diagnosis is established. This complication of the disease disappears once replacement therapy with γ-globulin is begun [38].

Other collagen-like diseases have been observed in children with agammaglobulinemia. One of the most distressing and uniformly fatal is a syndrome resembling dermatomyositis. Edema, ligneous induration of the muscles, weakness, and rash over the extensor surfaces of the joints are the salient features of this complication. Biopsy and autopsy material show lymphorrhages around the small blood vessels. Similar involvement of the central nervous system has been observed with progressive, ultimately fatal, neurologic disease. Although the distribution of the lymphocytic infiltrates is characteristic of neoplasia, the individual cells of the infiltrate appear to be normal. Neither steroids nor antimetabolites have prevented a fatal outcome. The possibility of a viral etiology for this syndrome has not been excluded. Adenovirus type 12 and echovirus type 9 were cultured from several organs at the time of death from two patients.

Hemolytic anemia, drug eruptions, atopic eczema, poison ivy, allergic rhinitis, and asthma have been observed in agammaglobulinemic patients with high frequency. Wheal and flare reactions cannot be elicited.

Genetics

The study of a large number of kindreds with multiple occurrences of agammaglobulinemia has disclosed an X-linked pattern of inheritance. Besides the occurrence of the disease in brothers, the diagnosis has been established in boys with sisters who subsequently had male children with the disease.

It has not been possible to do extensive linkage studies of the gene. The X-linked blood group Xg(a) is at least three crossover units distant from the agammaglobulinemia gene [39]. The position of the gene in relation to other X-linked traits is not known. The heterozygous female carrier of the gene cannot be detected by presently available methods. The incidence of the defect is not known. No ethnic group has an unusually high incidence of the defect.

Diagnosis

The serum of children with congenital agammaglobulinemia contains less than 100 mg of γG-globulin per 100 ml. Serum γA- and γM-globulins are usually present in concentrations of less than 1 percent of normal. The small amount of γ-globulin synthesized by these children cannot be differentiated from normal γ-globulin.

The isohemagglutinin levels are low or absent. A positive Schick test in the presence of a history of diphtheria-pertussis-tetanus (DPT) immunization can be used to illustrate the defect. Antigenic stimulation with any number of antigens fails to elicit an antibody response. With exquisitely sensitive methods of antibody measurement, very low levels of antibody to certain animal viruses and phage particles can be demonstrated [40]. Apparently, the small amount of γ-globulin present in the serum is not "inert."

Delayed hypersensitivity reactions of both the tuberculin and the skin-contact type are intact, although perhaps quantitatively reduced in some patients. The former can be universally demonstrated with intradermally injected monilia antigen, with killed vaccinia virus after vaccination, or with tuberculin after infection with BCG, and the latter, with dinitrochlorobenzene (DNCB) applied to the skin as a patch test after suitable provocation with a vesicant dose of DNCB [41].

Other serum constituents involved in resistance to infection are normal. Serum complement, lysozyme and properdin levels, phagocytosis, and interferon synthesis are within normal limits.

The *sine qua non* of the diagnosis of X-linked agammaglobulinemia is the demonstration of an absence of plasma cells in lymph nodes stimulated with antigen. The basic defect in the disease is, in fact, the absence of plasma cells from the lymph nodes, spleen, intestine, and bone marrow [42]. In addition to the absence of plasma cells from the usual sites, there is no normal follicular organization of lymphocytes. The thymus gland is normal.

Peripheral blood lymphocytes of agammaglobulinemic children appear to respond normally to phytohemagglutinin and to antigenic and allogeneic stimuli [43]. Homograft rejection is intact in a few agammaglobulinemic patients who have been studied. Several cases of delayed rejection have been recorded, although normal second-set rejection has been observed.

Treatment

The injection of γ-globulin has proved to be an effective means of preventing the severe, recurrent, pyogenic infections sustained by these patients. Patients with congenital agammaglobulinemia have received repeated injections at monthly intervals for as long as 16 years without any ill effect or untoward reaction. It was indeed fortuitous and unforeseen that this antigenic material would not produce isosensitization of these immunologically handicapped children.

The dose of γ-globulin that provides effective prophylaxis was found empirically [44]. If the serum level is raised by approximately 200 mg per 100 ml, invasive bacterial infections can be prevented. To achieve the desired level, a newly diagnosed patient is given 1.8 ml, or 300 mg, of γ-globulin per kg body weight, usually in three divided doses of 0.6 ml (100 mg) per kg. This raises the serum concentration by about 300 mg per 100 ml. Since the half-life of the γ-globulin injected is 30 days or more in these patients, they must receive a monthly injection of 0.6 ml (100 mg) per kg to maintain the desired level of approximately 200 mg per 100 ml. Smaller doses are ineffective.

PRIMARY ACQUIRED AGAMMAGLOBULINEMIA (LATE ONSET AGAMMAGLOBULINEMIA)

Shortly after the initial description of congenital agammaglobulinemia, an acquired form of the disease was described in adults [45, 46]. The acquisition of agammaglobulinemia has now been documented in several patients, but close observation has not revealed the cause for this sudden depression of γ-globulin synthesis [47, 48].

Primary acquired agammaglobulinemia has been found equally in males and females. Although there is no clear-cut genetic influence on the occurrence of primary acquired agammaglobulinemia, multiple cases in a single kindred have been reported [49]. Cruchaud et al., on the other hand, have reported acquired agammaglobulinemia in one of two identical twins [51]. There has been a high incidence of other immunologic abnormalities in relatives of patients with acquired agammaglobulinemia, such as lupus, hemolytic anemia, positive rheumatoid factor tests, and thrombocytopenic purpura [50].

Undue susceptibility to pyogenic infection, particularly recurrent sinusitis and pneumonia, is a prominent clinical feature of acquired agammaglobulinemia. Patients with chronic progressive bronchiectasis should be prime suspects for the diagnosis of acquired agammaglobulinemia.

A prominent and frequent complication of acquired agammaglobulinemia, which is almost never seen in the congenital disease, is a sprue-like syndrome. Diarrhea, steatorrhea, at times protein-losing enteropathy, and a whole range of malabsorption difficulties afflict more than half of all adults with acquired agammaglobulinemia. An intestinal biopsy is rarely rewarding, for, more often than not the characteristic flattening of the villi seen in nontropical sprue is absent, and the biopsy material appears to be perfectly normal. In some instances nodular lymphoid hyperplasia has been reported [52]. No explanation for this gastrointestinal complication has been forthcoming. Bacterial counts of succus entericus are not consistently different from normal. Some of these patients have improved on a gluten-free diet, and others upon elimination of milk from the diet. The most helpful therapy is found only by trial and error. The arthritis so frequently seen in the congenital form of the disease is rarer in the acquired disease.

Another distinguishing feature of the acquired form of the disease is the frequent occurrence of noncaseating granulomas. The lungs, spleen, skin, and liver are most frequently involved. No microorganisms have been found consistently in these lesions. Steroid therapy has been helpful. A number of patients with acquired agammaglobulinemia have splenomegaly, or hepatosplenomegaly, and lymphadenopathy. The complications of hypersplenism have developed in some of these patients. This syndrome has affected multiple members of at least one kindred [53]. Early onset of this syndrome has been recorded in young girls [54, 55].

Quantitation of immunoglobulins in the serums of patients with acquired agammaglobulinemia usually reveals levels of γG below 500 mg per 100 ml—higher than those encountered in the serums of children with congenital disease. Gamma-A and gamma-M may also be detected in significant quantity in the serums of these patients. The γG-globulin may show restricted heterogeneity [56].

Lymph nodes lack plasma cells, but in place of the absent follicles of congenital agammaglobulinemia, abiotrophy of the follicles or striking follicular hyperplasia may be found. Cultures of lymphocytes from patients with primary acquired agammaglobulinemia show decreased RNA and DNA synthesis when stimulated [57]. Lymph node transplants have survived and functioned for a time in these patients [58]. From in vitro and in vivo studies, it does not appear that there is any inhibitory factor causing this disease.

Patients with primary acquired agammaglobulinemia have an unusually high incidence of "autoimmune" disease, such as pernicious anemia, hemolytic anemia, and so on [59]. Although patients with lymphoma or chronic lymphocytic leukemia may present with or develop hypogammaglobulinemia, the progression of primary acquired agammaglobulinemia to lymphoreticular malignancy has only rarely been documented. There is a frequent association between thymoma and acquired agammaglobulinemia [60]. Patients with thymoma and agammaglobulinemia may show progressive deterioration of cellular immunity and aregenerative anemia.

THE DYSGAMMAGLOBULINEMIAS

The advent of immunoelectrophoretic techniques led to a more precise definition of immunoglobulin defects in a number of situations in which the hypogammaglobulinemia involved one or two of the immunoglobulin groups, whereas the others were normal or elevated. Six combinations of the deficits of the three major immunoglobulins are obviously possible, although only two of these have been extensively reported. There have been many attempts to classify these abnormalities, but it is presently more confusing and less helpful to abide by one or another system of designations than to describe the immunoelectrophoretic stigmata of the defect under discussion. It has been estimated that about 1 in 200 random hospital admissions have some form of dysgammaglobulinemia [61].

Absence of γA, γG, Normal or Elevated γM

One of the common partial immunoglobulin defects is characterized by a deficiency of γA- and γG-globulins and increased amounts of γM-globulin in the serum [62]. Gamma-M-globulin levels range from 150 to 1,000 mg per 100 ml in these patients. In spite of the enormous elevations of the γM-globulin levels, the γM-globulin does not form an M component. The γM-appears to be composed of normally distributed molecules with antibody activity, particularly those usually associated with the macroglobulins, and to have a normal distribution of κ and λ chains. Several, but not all, of these patients have an elevation of the serum γD-globulins and γMs subunits [63]. Both hereditary and acquired forms of this defect have been observed [64]. In addition to their undue susceptibility to infection, many of these patients acquire thrombocytopenia, neutropenia, renal lesions, and aplastic or hemolytic anemia, presumably manifestations of "autoimmune" processes. In one patient this was shown to involve the N antigen of the red cell [65]. Administration of exogenous γG-globulin has not generally decreased the γM-globulin levels, although Hitzig has reported that it did ameliorate the severe neutropenia in a boy whom he observed [66] and in a recent report the γM level was reduced by exogenous γG-globulin [67].

The defect can apparently be inherited as an X-linked phenomenon. In one instance four boys of one kindred and two boys of another were reported to have this defect, and identical male twins are known to be affected [68]. A number of the patients have been adult females and older girls, in whom the defect appears to be a primary acquired one [69].

The histopathology is interesting in that it provides a unique opportunity to study the γM-synthesizing cells. In the acquired form of this type of dysgammaglobulinemia, well-defined follicles are present, and in the periphery abundant cells virtually indistinguishable from plasma cells are found, except that they stain with PAS because of the high carbohydrate content of the γM-globulins, which can be identified with fluorescein-labeled anti-γM-globulin. In the hereditary disease follicle formation does not occur. In the spleen and other lymphoid tissues the lymphocytoid or plasmacytoid cells, similar to cells which are characteristic of Waldenström's disease, stain with PAS and fluorescein-labeled anti-γM-globulin. One of our patients died of a diffuse infiltrative process in which plasmacytoid cells proliferated diffusely in the intestine, gall bladder, liver, and other viscera. In another of our children with this defect, an enormous unilateral hypertrophy of the tonsil developed, necessitating removal. It was found to be diffusely infiltrated with plasmacytoid cells.

Absence of γA, Normal γG, and γM

The isolated absence of γA-globulin from the serum occurs in a significant but small proportion of the normal population [70]. Two healthy researchers have found their own serums to lack γA-globulin [71]. Gamma-A deficiency has been associated with steatorrhea and nontypical sprue [72]. These patients lack γA-producing cells in the lamina propria of the intestinal tract where γA-producing cells are found in greatest abundance. Other patients with connective tissue disease and about 80 percent of patients with ataxia telangiectasia lack serum and secretory γA [73].

Although familial lack of γA is well documented, the mode of inheritance of the defect is not clearly established [74]. Several patients with absent γA have circulating anti-γA antibodies. This may result in rapid catabolism of γA [75] or in plasma transfusion reactions [76, 77]. Gamma A deficiency has been associated with partial deletions of the long arm of chromosome 18, but this is not a regular finding in patients with this chromosomal abnormality.

Severe Combined Immunodeficiency

Historical Aspects

In 1950 Glanzmann and Riniker described two unrelated infants who succumbed to overwhelming infection during the second year of life after a lifelong succession of serious infections, including intractable diarrhea, thrush, and a persistent morbilliform rash [78]. They recorded persistent and profound lymphopenia in these two infants, and called the disorder "essential lymphocytophthisis." Over 100 cases of this disease have now been well described [79]. It has been variously designated as alymphocytosis, the Swiss type of agammaglobulinemia, thymic alymphoplasia, thymic dysplasia, lymphopenic agammaglobulinemia, and so on. At least part of this confusion in terminology results from the fact that two different modes of inheritance are fairly clearly established. In the early European descriptions it appeared that the disease was transmitted as an autosomal recessive; there was consanguinity among approximately one-third of parents of affected children [80]. Further studies of affected families in America and Europe strongly suggested an X-linked mode of transmission. This supposition was based on (1) the documentation of affected males in three generations, and (2) the appearance of the disease in sons of a single mother with differing paternities [81, 82]. The fact that the phenocopy can arise from two different modes of inheritance probably accounts for the 3:1 ratio of males/females observed in the reported cases.

Clinical Aspects

For purposes of clinical description it is probably easiest to lump the two genetic types because there is no discernible difference in their clinical course, nor, for that matter, in the morbid anatomy of the disease. In any case, infections start early, between 3 and 6 months of age, and a rapid succession of debilitating infections brings about an early demise. Death within the first 2 years of life is the rule. Almost all infants with this disease develop loose, watery, chronic diarrhea. Frequently, stool cultures grow out *Salmonella* or enteropathic *Escherichia coli* strains. Pulmonary infection is also almost universal. Abscess of the lung containing *Pseudomonas aeruginosa* is a common cause of death, as is pneumonitis due to *Pneumocystis carinii*. Extensive moniliasis of the mouth or diaper area persists beyond the neonatal period and is often a first sign of the disease. Thrush is usually present even before any antibiotic therapy. These infants are incapable of limiting and terminating the most benign viral infections. Death has resulted from generalized chickenpox, measles with Hecht's giant-cell pneumonia, and in a few instances from cytomegalovirus and adenovirus infection. Vaccination results in progressive, ultimately fatal, vaccinia infection. BCG inoculation has also resulted in progressive BCG infection. These infants fail to thrive. Lack of weight gain gives the appearance of "runting," which may be aggravated by protein-losing enteropathy.

Diagnosis

In 1958 the Swiss workers pointed out that agammaglobulinemia is a prominent feature of this disease entity [83, 84]. Serum concentrations of immunoglobulins are very low, and the γG may exhibit restricted heterogenity. No antibody synthesis can be detected.

Leukopenia is usually encountered because of the low lymphocyte counts, usually less than 2,000 per mm^3. The lymphocyte count may be variable and decline from initial normal neonatal levels ($>$3,000 per mm^3) to profoundly lymphopenic levels. A single lymphocyte count is, nonetheless, not a reliable index of the disease, since normal counts can be observed occasionally. Electron microscopy reveals that these blood lymphocytes are mostly immature forms resembling lymphoblasts. Granulocytes and platelets are normal, but leukocytosis may not occur in the presence of overt infection. Eosinophilia is common, and abnormal granulation of the eosinophils has been reported.

The bone marrow is uniformly deficient in plasma cells, lymphocytes, and lymphoblasts. Bone marrow of normal infants contains up to 20 percent of cells in the lymphocytic series. This deficiency may well be the primary defect in this disease, i.e., failure of formation of an immunopotential cell which originates from the marrow. Lymph node biopsy, when feasible, exhibits a complete lack of germinal elements, plasma cells, and lymphocytes. Only the stroma of the node is seen to contain occasional mast cells and eosinophils or, rarely, small collections of lymphoid cells without any apparent organization.

No indicators of delayed sensitivity can be elicited in these infants [85]. They are unresponsive to monilia antigen in the presence of overt, chronic monilia infection. They cannot be sensitized to DNFB. The peripheral blood lymphocytes are completely unresponsive to phytohemagglutinin or allogeneic stimulation [85]. Skin grafts are accepted with no microscopic or macroscopic signs of rejection. At autopsy lymphoid tissue is absent from the spleen, tonsils, appendix, and intestines. The thymus gland is found with difficulty in the neck and has usually failed to descend in the normal manner into the anterior mediastinum. It weighs less than a gram and is composed of primordial, spindle-shaped cells, occasionally forming swirls or rosettes. No Hassall's corpuscles and few, if any, lymphocytes are found. The dysplasia of the thymus gland is a uniformly characteristic feature of this disease.

Therapy

Gamma-globulin therapy is of no avail in steming the inexorably fatal progress of the defect. Attempts to restore immunologic competence with thymus grafts, fetal hematopoietic cells, and bone marrow transplants have, in the past, uniformly failed to achieve this end. Although transitory beneficial effects have been achieved, development of graft versus host disease has resulted in several fatalities. This complication has arisen following bone marrow or whole blood transfusion [86]. In one instance persistence of transplacentally acquired maternal lymphoid cells was recorded [87].

A characteristic maculopapular rash starting on the face heralds the onset of graft versus host disease about 7 days after the administration of histoincompatible immunocompetent cells. The rash spreads rapidly to involve ultimately all skin surfaces, including the palms and soles. Thrombocytopenia, leukopenia, jaundice, and anasarca follow in quick succession, and bone marrow aplasia leads to death from massive hemorrhage by the twelfth to fourteenth day. On the basis of experimental observations it has been reasoned that transplants of bone marrow cells as a source of immunopotential stem cells would restore immunologic competence to these infants. It is apparent from these misadventures that it would be necessary to circumvent the graft versus host disease by administering completely histocompatible bone marrow cells. A histocompatibility difference at only one allele of the HL-A locus has resulted in explosive graft versus host reactions [88]. A few cases of the X-linked type of hereditary thymic dysplasia have been immunologically restored with bone marrow cells from normal sibs who were histocompatible by direct leukocyte typing and by mixed leukocyte culture; thus, the patient's leukocytes did not provoke uptake of tritiated thymidine by the donor cells in vitro. In one attempted therapeutic transplant the donor and recipient were ABO incompatible, and the recipient developed an aplastic crisis which was treated with a second bone marrow transplant. This produced complete erythrocyte and leukocyte chimerism in the recipient. The patient had a minor and transient graft versus host reaction following the first marrow transplant [89]. This complication was presumably circumvented in the second case by eliminating antigen-sensitive cells from the transplant by albumin density gradient centrifugation [90]. A third patient (of the autosomal recessive type) treated with similarly prepared marrow cells died of intercurrent causes 3 weeks after the transplant. In this patient few if any of the stigmata of graft versus host disease were present at the time of autopsy. At the moment this therapeutic approach appears promising, not only in terms of restoring health, but also in the elucidating the ontogeny of immunologic competence in man.

In the preceding section it has been pointed out that hereditary thymic dysplasia may be inherited by one or another of two alternative mechanisms and that patients with this disease may exhibit varying degrees of circulating lymphopenia and of lymphoid tissue depletion. The constant pathologic hallmark of the disease resides in the dysplasia of the thymus gland, although this is most probably not the basic defect in the disease. The immunologic defect appears rather to result from the maturation failure of immunopotential cells in the bone marrow. Perhaps the abnormal embryogenesis of the thymus in these infants is a result of the absence of an inducer or organizer from lymphocytic cells which affects the thymic epithelial primordium. Such a construction remains at the present time entirely hypothetical but nonetheless useful in unifying the variations on the basic pattern. The most devastating of these variant forms is so-called *reticular dysgenesia* [91]. The few infants with this disease have died within the first week of life from overwhelming staphylococcal sepsis. In addition to the characteristic thymic dysplasia, lymphopenia, and lymphoid depletion, there is severe neutropenia and depletion of myeloid precursors from the marrow. If the myeloid and lymphoid cell lines stem from a common precursor element, one might assume a failure of formation of the common precursor cell in reticular dysgenesia.

At the opposite end of this spectrum are those infants with normal immunoglobulins associated with lymphopenia, lymphoid tissue depletion, and absent cellular immunity [92]. This form of lymphopenia with normal immunoglobulins has often been designated as *Nezelof's syndrome.* Nezelof termed the defect *aplasie lymphocytaire normoplasmocytaire et normoglobulinemique.* Indeed, abundant numbers of plasma cells are found in the spleen, intestine, and elsewhere at autopsy, along with the thymic dysplasia and lymphocyte depletion. The clinical course of these infants may be slightly less malignant, but death by the third or fourth year of life has been the rule. A high incidence of Coombs'-positive hemolytic anemia has been encountered in these infants, together with other "autoimmune" phenomena [93, 94]. Antigenic stimulation with phage particles, bacterial toxins, etc., does not result in a normal or even detectable antibody rise, and only one of these infants had a decent antibody response to poliovirus. At present it appears that the immune response of these infants is grossly abnormal in spite of normal immunoglobulin levels. All the reported kindreds thus far are consistent with autosomal recessive inheritance.

A number of infants with thymic dysplasia have also been reported with only γM, or γG and γA in their serums [95]. It may be spurious to classify all these variations by the presence of one or another immunoglobulin in the serum, since variations in immunoglobulin pattern have been observed in sibs of an affected kindred.

SUMMARY

1 The immunoglobulins of human serum can be subdivided into five major classes, γG, γA, γM, γD, and γE. Four subclasses of γG and two subclasses of γA have been identified. Chemical, genetic, and metabolic differences between the various classes and subclasses have been found. Twelve to fifteen closely linked cistrons may control the synthesis of the immunoglobulins, but only three of them have been identified thus far with any degree of certainty.

2 An X-linked disease, agammaglobulinemia, is characterized by recurrent pyogenic infections, failure to synthesize antibodies, and absence from the serum of all immunoglobulins. In affected males, plasma cells, which synthesize the immunoglobulins, are found to be absent from lymphoid tissue, bone marrow, spleen, and intestine. A form of the disease in which the onset of agammaglobulinemia is late, occurs in family clusters, but the genetic transmission of the defect is not clarified. Partial defects in immunoglobulin synthesis have been described. Gamma globulin replacement therapy offers adequate prophylaxis against recurrent infection in this group of syndromes.

3 A second large group of agammaglobulinemias is accompanied by lymphopenia, failure of normal thymic embryogenesis, an absence of cellular immunity, usually fatal, and susceptibility to bacterial fungal and viral infections. This defect may be transmitted as an X-linked or as an autosomal recessive phenomenon. A number of variants of lymphopenic agammaglobulinemia have been described. Normal immunologic reactivity has been established in affected infants by transplants of histocompatible bone marrow.

BIBLIOGRAPHY

1. Tiselius, A.: Electrophoresis of serum globulin. II. Electrophoretic analysis of normal and immune serum. Biochem. J., **31,** 1464, 1937.
2. Tiselius, A., and Kabat, E. A.: Electrophoresis of immune serum. Science, **87,** 416, 1938.
3. Porter, R. R.: Hydrolysis of rabbit γ-globulin and antibodies with crystalline papain. Biochem. J., **73,** 119, 1959.

4. Edelman, G. M., and Poulik, M. D.: Studies on structural units of the γ-globulins. J. Exp. Med., **113,** 861, 1961.
5. Nisonoff, A., Wissler, F. C., and Lipman, L. N.: Properties of a major component of peptic digest of rabbit antibody. Science, **132,** 1770, 1960.
6. Frangione, B., Milstein, C., and Pink, J. R. L.: Structural studies of immunoglobulin G. Nature, **221,** 145, 1969.
7. Edelman, G. M., and Gally, J. A.: Nature of Bence Jones proteins: Chemical similarities to polypeptide chains of myeloma globulins and normal γ-globulins. J. Exp. Med., **116,** 207, 1962.
8. Bernier, G. M., and Cebra, J. J.: Frequency distribution of α, γ, κ, and λ polypeptide chains in human lymphoid tissues. J. Immunol., **95,** 246, 1965.
9. Hilschmann, N., and Craig, L. C.: Amino acid sequence studies with Bence Jones proteins. Proc. Nat. Acad. Sci., **53,** 1403, 1965.
10. Smithies, O.: Gamma-globulin variability: genetic hypothesis. Nature **199,** 1231, 1963.
11. Haurowitz, F.: Antibody formation and coding problems. Nature, **205,** 847, 1965.
12. Burnet, M.: *Self and Not-self.* Cambridge, London, 1969.
13. Gitlin, D., Hitzig, W. H., and Janeway, C. A.: Multiple serum protein deficiencies in congenital and acquired agammaglobulinemia. J. Clin. Invest., **35,** 1199, 1956.
14. Heremans, J. F.: Immunochemical studies on protein pathology: immunoglobulin concept. Clin. Chim. Acta, **4,** 639, 1959.
15. Rowe, D. S., and Fahey, J. L.: New class of human immunoglobulins. I. Unique myeloma protein. J. Exp. Med., **121,** 171, 1965.
16. Ishizaka, K., and Ishizaka, T.: Physicochemical properties of reaginic antibody. I. Association of reaginic activity with immunoglobulin other than γA or γG globulin. J. Allerg. **37,** 169, 1966.
17. Waldmann, T. A.: Disorders of immunoglobulin metabolism. New Eng. J. Med., **281,** 1170, 1969.
18. Edelman, G. M., Cunningham, B. A., Gall, W. E., Gottlieb, P. D., Rutishauser, U., and Waxdal, M. J.: The covalent structure of an entire γG immunoglobulin molecule. Proc. Nat. Acad. Sci., **63,** 78, 1969.
19. Gitlin, D., Kumate, J., Urrusti, J., and Morales, C.: Selectivity of human placenta in the transfer of plasma proteins from mother to fetus. J. Clin. Invest., **43,** 1938, 1964.
20. Natvig, J. B., Kunkel, H. G., and Gedde-Dahl, T., Jr.: Genetic studies of the heavy chain subgroups of γG globulin. p. 313 in IIIrd Nobel Symposium, Gamma Globulins, edited by J. Killander. Almquist & Wiskell, Stockholm, 1967.
21. Dawson, G., and Clamp, J. R.: Investigations on the oligosaccharide units of an A myeloma globulin. Biochem. J., **107,** 341, 1968.
22. Chodirker, W. B., and Tomasi, T. B., Jr.: Gamma globulins: quantitative relationships in human serum and nonvascular fluids. Science **142,** 1080, 1963.
23. Cebra, J. J., and Small, P. A., Jr.: Polypeptide chain structure of rabbit immunoglobulins. II. Secretory γA globulin from colostrum. Biochem., **6,** 503, 1967.
24. Grey, H. M., Abel, C. A., Yount, W. J., and Kunkel, H. G.: A subclass of human γA-globulins (γA_2) which lacks the disulfide bonds linking heavy and light chains. J. Exp. Med., **128,** 1223, 1968.
25. Deutsch, H. F., and Morton, J. I.: Dissociation of human serum macroglobulins. Science, **125,** 600, 1957.
26. Merler, E., Matsumoto, S., and Karlin, L. I.: The valency of human γM immunoglobulin antibody. J. Biol. Chem., **243,** 386, 1968.
27. Ishizaka, K., Ishizaka, T., and Hornbrook, M. M.: Physicochemical properties of reaginic antibody. V. Correlation of reaginic activity with gamma-E-globulin antibody. J. Immun., **97,** 840, 1961.
28. Ishizaka, K., and Ishizaka, T.: Identification of gamma E-antibodies as a carrier of reaginic activity. J. Immun., **97,** 840, 1966.
29. Ogawa, M., Kochwa, S., Smith, C., Ishizaka, K., and McIntyre, O. R.: Clinical aspects of IgE myeloma. New Eng. J. Med., **281,** 1217, 1969.
30. Johansson, S. G. O., and Bennich, H.: Immunological studies of an atypical (myeloma) immunoglobulin. Immunology, **13,** 381, 1967.
31. Johansson, S. G. O.: Raised levels of a new immunoglobulin class in asthma. Lancet, **2,** 951, 1967.
32. Coombs, R. R. A., Hunter, A., Jonas, W. E., Bennich, H., Johansson, S. G. O., and Panzani, R.: Detection of IgE specific antibody (probably reagin) to castor-bean allergen by the red-cell-linked antigen-antiglobulin reaction. Lancet, **1,** 1115, 1968.
33. Franklin, E. C., and Fudenberg, H. H.: Genetic polymorphism of human γ-globulins. Rheumatology, **2,** 62, 1969.
34. Natvig, J. B., and Kunkel, H. G.: Genetic markers of human immunoglobulins. Series Haematologica, **1,** 66, 1968.
35. Steinberg, A. G.: Progress in the study of genetically determined human gamma globulin types (Gm and Inv groups). Prog. Med. Genet., **2,** 1, 1963.
36. Bruton, O. C.: Agammaglobulinemia. Pediatrics, **9,** 722, 1952.
37. Gitlin, D., Janeway, C. A., Apt, L., and Craig, J. M.: Agammaglobulinemia, in *Cellular and Humoral Aspects of Hypersensitivity States: Symposium,* edited by H. S. Lawrence. Hoeber-Harper, pp. 375–441, New York, 1959.
38. Janeway, C. A., Gitlin, D., Craig, J. M., and Grice, D. S.: Collagen disease in patients with congenital agammaglobulinemia. Trans. Ass. Amer. Physicians, **69,** 93, 1956.
39. Rosen, F. S., Hutchison, G. B., and Allen, F. H., Jr.: Xg blood groups and congenital hypogammaglobulinemia. Vox. Sanguin., **10,** 729, 1965.
40. Bacon, S., et al.: Antibody production by hypogammaglobulinemic patients. J. Immun., **88,** 443, 1962.
41. Porter, H. M.: Immunologic studies in congenital agammaglobulinemia with emphasis on delayed hypersensitivity. Pediatrics, **20,** 958, 1957.
42. Craig, J., Gitlin, D., and Jewett, T.: Response of lymph nodes of normal and congenital agammaglobulinemic children to antigenic stimulation. Amer. J. Dis. Child., **88,** 626, 1954.
43. Cooperband, S. R., Rosen, F. S., and Kibrick, S.: Studies on the *in vitro* behavior of agammaglobulinemic lymphocytes. J. Clin. Invest., **47,** 836–847, 1968.
44. Janeway, C. A., and Rosen, F. S.: The gamma globulins. IV. Therapeutic uses of gamma globulin. New Eng. J. Med., **275,** 826, 1966.
45. Prasad, A. S., and Koza, D. W.: Agammaglobulinemia. Ann. Intern. Med., **41,** 629, 1954.
46. Grant, G. H., and Wallace, W. D.: Agammaglobulinaemia. Lancet, **2,** 671, 1954.
47. Charache, P., Rosen, F. S., Janeway, C. A., Craig, J. M., and Rosenberg, H. A.: Acquired agammaglobulinaemia in siblings, Lancet **1,** 234, 1965.
48. Robbins, J. B., Eitzman, D. V., and Ellis, E. F.: Immunochemical evidence for development of "acquired" hypogammaglobulinemic state. New Eng. J. Med., **274,** 607, 1966.
49. Wolf, J. K.: Primary acquired agammaglobulinemia with family history of collagen disease and hematologic disorders. New Eng. J. Med., **266,** 473, 1962.
50. Fudenberg, H., German, J. L., III, and Kunkel, H. G.: Occurrence of rheumatoid factor and other abnormalities in families of patients with agammaglobulinemia. Arthritis Rheum., **5,** 565, 1962.
51. Cruchaud, A., Laperrouza, C., Dumitan, S. H., and Ferrier, P. E.: Agammaglobulinemia in one of two identical twins. Amer. J. Med., **40,** 127, 1966.
52. Hermans, P. E., Huizenga, K. A., Hoffman, H. N., II, Brown, A. L., Jr., and Markowitz, H.: Dysgammaglobulinemia associated with nodular lymphoid hyperplasia of small intestine. Amer. J. Med., **40,** 78, 1966.
53. Prasad, A. S., Reiner, E., and Watson, C. J.: Syndrome of hypogammaglobulinemia, splenomegaly and hypersplenism. Blood, **12,** 926, 1957.
54. Pearce, K. M., and Perinpanayagam, M. S.: Congenital idiopathic hypogammaglobulinaemia. Arch. Dis. Childhood, **32,** 422, 1957.
55. Traggis, D. G., Ruthig, D., Smith, G., and Cleveland, W.: Hypogammaglobulinemia in young girl: case report with clinical, immunological, and pathological data. Amer. J. Dis. Child., **102,** 8, 1961.
56. Hong, R., and Good, R. A.: Limited heterogeneity of gamma globulin in hypogammaglobulinemia. Science, **156,** 1102, 1967.
57. Tormey, D. C., Kamin, R., and Fudenberg, H. H.: Quantitative studies of phytohemagglutinin-induced DNA and RNA synthesis in normal and agammaglobulinemic leukocytes. J. Exp. Med., **125,** 863, 1967.
58. Martin, C. M., Waite, J. B., and McCullough, N. B.: Antibody protein

synthesis by lymph nodes homotransplanted to hypogammaglobulinemic adult. J. Clin. Invest., **36**, 405, 1957.

59. Fudenberg, H. H., and Solomon, A.: Acquired agammaglobulinemia with autoimmune hemolytic disease. Vox Sang., **6**, 68, 1961.
60. MacLean, L. D., Zak, S. J., Varco, R. L., and Good, R. A.: Thymic tumor and acquired agammaglobulinemia: clinical and experimental study of immune response. Surgery, **40**, 1010, 1956.
61. Hobbs, J. R.: Immune imbalance in dysgammaglobulinemia type IV. Lancet, **1**, 110, 1968.
62. Rosen, F. S., Kevy, S., Merler, E., Janeway, C. A., and Gitlin, D.: Recurrent bacterial infections and dysgammaglobulinemia, deficiency of 7S gamma-globulins in presence of elevated 19S gamma globulin: report of two cases. Pediatrics, **28**, 182, 1961.
63. Gleich, G. J., Uhr, J. W., and Vaughan, J. H.: Antibody formation in dysgammaglobulinemia. J. Clin. Invest., **45**, 1334, 1966.
64. Rosen, F. S., and Bougas, J. A.: Acquired dysgammaglobulinemia: elevation of 19S gamma globulin and deficiency of 7S globulin in woman with chronic progressive bronchiectasis. New Eng. J. Med., **269**, 1336, 1963.
65. Hinz, C. F., Jr., and Boyer, J. T.: Dysgammaglobulinemia in adult manifested as autoimmune hemolytic anemia: serologic and immunochemical characterization of antibody of unusual specificity. New Eng. J. Med., **269**, 1329, 1963.
66. Hitzig, W. H., and Schlapfer, A.: Chronic neutropenia and dysgammaglobulinemia: possible interrelations. In International Society of Haematology. Abstracts of the 10th Congress. Stockholm: Munksgaard, 1964. D:23.
67. Stiehm, E. R., and Fudenberg, H. H.: Clinical and immunologic features of dysgammaglobulinemia type I: report of case diagnosed in first year of life. Amer. J. Med., **40**, 805, 1966.
68. Jamieson, W. M., and Kerr, M. R.: Family with several cases of hypogammaglobulinaemia. Arch. Dis. Child., **37**, 330, 1962.
69. Barth, W. F., Asofsky, R., Liddy, F. J., Tanaka, Y., Rowe, D. S., and Fahey, J. L.: Antibody deficiency syndrome: selective immunoglobulin deficiency with reduced synthesis of gamma and alpha immunoglobulin polypeptide chains. Amer. J. Med., **39**, 319, 1965.
70. Bachmann, R.: Studies on serum γA-globulin level. III. Frequency of A-γA-globulinemia. J. Clin. Lab. Invest., **17**, 316–320, 1965.
71. Rockey, J. H., Hanson, L. A., Heremans, J. F., and Kunkel, H. G.: Beta-2A aglobulinemia in two healthy men. J. Lab. Clin. Med., **63**, 205, 1964.
72. Crabbe, P. A., and Heremans, J. F.: Selective IgA deficiency with steatorrhea. Amer. J. Med., **42**, 319, 1967.
73. Young R. R., Austen, K. F., and Moser, H. W.: Abnormalities of serum gamma-1-A globulin and ataxia telangiectasia. Medicine, **43**, 423, 1964.
74. Stocker, F., Ammann, P., and Rossi, E.: Selective γ-A-globulin deficiency with dominant autosomal inheritance in a Swiss family. Arch. Dis. Child., **43**, 585, 1968.
75. Strober, W., Wochner, R. D., Barlow, M. H., McFarlin, D. E., and Waldmann, T. A.: Immunoglobulin metabolism in ataxia telangiectasia. J. Clin. Invest., **47**, 1905, 1968.
76. Vyas, G. N., Perkins, H. A., and Fudenberg, H. H.: Anaphylactoid transfusion reactions associated with anti-IgA. Lancet, **2**, 312, 1968.
77. Schmidt, A. P., Taswell, H. F., and Gleich, G. J.: Anaphylactic transfusion reactions associated with anti-IgA antibody. New Eng. J. Med. **280**, 188, 1969.
78. Glanzmann, E., and Riniker, P.: Essentielle Lymphocytophthise: Ein neues Krankheitsbild aus der Säuglingspathologie. Ann. Paediat., **175**, 1, 1950.
79. Hitzig, W. H., Barandun, S., and Cottier, H.: Die schweizerische Form der Agammaglobulinämie. Ergebn. Inn. Med. Kinderheilk., **27**, 79, 1968.
80. Hitzig, W. H., and Willi, H.: Hereditäre lymphoplasmocytäre Dysgenesie. Schweiz. Med. Wchschr., **91**, 1625, 1961.
81. Gitlin, D., and Craig, J. M.: The thymus and other lymphoid tissues in congenital agammaglobulinemia. I. Thymic alymphoplasia and lymphocytic hypoplasia and their relation to infection. Pediatrics, **32**, 517, 1963.
82. Miller, M. E.: Thymic dysplasia ("Swiss agammaglobulinemia"). I. Graft versus host reaction following bone-marrow transfusion. J. Pediat., **70**, 730, 1967.
83. Tobler, R., and Cottier, H.: Familiäre Lymphopenie mit Agammaglobulinämie und schwerer Moniliasis: die "essentielle Agammaglobulinämie. Helv. Paediat. Acta, **13**, 313, 1958.
84. Hitzig, W. H., Biro, Z., Bosch, H., and Huser, H. J.: Agammaglobulinämie und Alymphocytose mit Schwund des lymphatischen Gewebes. Helv. Paediat. Acta, **13**, 551, 1958.
85. Rosen, F. S., and Janeway, C. A.: The gamma globulins, III. The antibody deficiency syndromes. New Eng. J. Med., **275**, 709, 1966.
86. Hathaway, W. E., Githens, J. H., Blackburn, W. R., Fulginiti, V., and Kempe, C. H.: Aplastic anemia, histiocytosis, and erythrodermia in immunologically deficient children—probably human runt disease. New Eng. J. Med., **273**, 953, 1965.
87. Kadowaki, J., Thompson, R. I., Zuelzer, W. W., Woolley, P. V., Brough, A. J., and Gruber, D.: XX/XY lymphoid chimaerism in congenital immunological deficiency syndrome with thymic alymphopenia. Lancet, **2**, 1152, 1965.
88. Kretschmer, R., Jeannet, M., Mereu, T. R., Kretschmer, K., Winn, H., and Rosen, F. S.: Hereditary thymic dysplasia: a graft-versus-host reaction induced by bone marrow cells with a partial 4a series histoincompatibility. Pediat. Res., **3**, 37, 1969.
89. Gatti, R. A., Meuwissen, H. J., Allen, H. D., Hong, R., and Good, R. A.: Immunologic reconstitution of sex-linked lymphopenic immunologic deficiency. Lancet, **2**, 1366, 1968.
90. DeKoning, J., van Bekkum, D. W., Dicke, K. A., Dooren, L. J., von Rood, J. J., and Radl, J.: Transplantation of bone-marrow cells and fetal thymus in an infant with lymphopenic immunological deficiency. Lancet, **1**, 1223, 1969.
91. DeVaal, O. M., and Seynhaeve, V.: Reticular dysgenesia. Lancet, **2**, 1123, 1959.
92. Nezelof, C., Jammet, M. L., Lortholary, P., Labrune, B., and Lamy, M.: L'hypoplasie héréditaire du thymus: sa place et sa responsabilité dans une observation d'aplasie lymphocytaire, normoplasmocytaire et normoglobulinémique du nourrisson. Arch. Franc. Pediat., **21**, 897, 1964.
93. Schaller, J., Ching, Y., Williams, C. P. S., Davis, S. D., Lagunoff, D., and Wedgewood, R. J.: Hypergammaglobulinaemia, antibody deficiency, autoimmune haemolytic anemia, and nephritis in an infant with a familial lymphopenic immune defect. Lancet, **2**, 825, 1966.
94. Goldman, A. S., Haggard, M. E., McFedden, J., Ritzman, S., Houston, E. W., Bratcher, R. L., Weiss, K. G., Box, E. M., and Szekrenyes, J. W.: Thymic alymphoplasia, lymphoma and dysglobulinemia. Hyper-γ-A, normo-γ-M, hypo-γ-G, a-γ-D, and γ-E-globulinemia, plasmacytosis, normal delayed hypersensitivity, severe allergic reactions, and Coombs positive anemia. Pediatrics, **39**, 348, 1967.
95. Sacrez, R., Willard, D., Levy, M., Moyer, S., and Bigel, P.: Lymphocytophthisie d'evolution atypique. Arch. Franc. Pediat., **22**, 975, 1965.

CHAPTER SEVENTY-ONE

INHERITED ABNORMALITIES OF THE COMPLEMENT SYSTEM IN MAN

Shaun Ruddy and K. Frank Austen

The complement system consists of a group of serum proteins which interact sequentially to mediate certain of the effects of antigen-antibody reactions. The series of complement reactions is initiated by the union of an appropriate antibody either with soluble antigen or with an antigen located on the surface of such target cells as erythrocytes, tumor cells, bacteria, or protozoa. The effects of this activation of the complement system are increased vascular permeability; attraction of polymorphonuclear leukocytes; adherence of the antigen-antibody complexes or target cells to erythrocytes, polymorphonuclear leukocytes, or platelets; increased phagocytosis by polymorphonuclear leukocytes; and finally, the production of a defect in the target cell membrane which leads to osmotic lysis and cell death.

Several inherited abnormalities in the structure or function of complement components or of inhibitors of the complement system have been observed in human serum. Three of these represent genetically controlled deficiency states: inherited absence of the activity of the normal serum inhibitor of the first component, which is associated with the disease hereditary angioedema [1]; deficiency of the second component [2]; and partial deficiency of the third component [3]. Inherited structural polymorphism has been described for the third [4] and fourth [5] components of complement. Abnormalities of the first [6, 7] and fifth [8, 9] components have been associated with defects in host resistance, but the mechanisms or genetic controls of these abnormalities, if any, are less well understood.

THE COMPLEMENT SYSTEM

Nomenclature

Rapid advances in the knowledge of the complement reactions, made by a number of different groups of workers, have resulted in a profusion of symbols for designating the ingredients of these reactions. Table 71-1 contains the nomenclature agreed upon at a series of discussions arranged by the World Health Organization [10] and the previous designations for these same materials. Most of the available information about the nature of the complement system has come from studies of the lysis of sheep erythrocytes (E) treated with rabbit antibody (A) by the complement (C) contained in fresh normal serum [11, 12, 13], and the nomenclature is therefore based primarily on this immune hemolytic sequence. Long-standing usage has resulted in the designation of the first three components in the reaction sequence as C1, C4, and C2 instead of the more logical ascending numerical order; but the terminal six components, which have only been fully appreciated during the past decade, are numbered sequentially. The first component comprises three distinct protein subcomponents, to which the names C1q, C1r, and C1s have been given. The terms β_{1E}, β_{1C}, and β_{1F}, which formerly designated C4, C3, and C5 respectively, are still prevalent in the literature.

Erythrocyte-antibody complexes which have interacted with certain of the complement components are named according to the reaction steps which they have completed, e.g., EAC$\overline{1}$, EAC$\overline{14}$, EAC$\overline{142}$. The bar over the component numbers on the complexes implies that the component is in the activated state. Both activated components and inactive products, which are designated by the suffix "i," e.g., C4i, C3i, can occur in the fluid phase of complement reactions. Fragments which result from the cleavage of complement components during the course of their reactions are suffixed sequentially, as, for example, C3a, C3b, C3c, and C3d.

Chemical Nature of Complement Proteins

Table 71-2 gives the electrophoretic mobilities, approximate molecular weights, sedimentation coefficients, and approximate serum concentrations of the components of human complement and of the three inhibitors or inactivators which interact with these components. C1 normally exists in serum as a single molecular species with an approximate molecular weight of 900,000. Calcium ions are required for the maintenance of the integrity of this molecule: when treated with chelating agents such as ethylenediaminetetraacetate (EDTA), it dissociates into three subunits, C1q, C1r, and C1s [14]. Data for each of these three subunits are given separately. The normal serum inhibitor of activated C1, C$\overline{1}$ INH, has been demonstrated to be immunochemically identical to the α_2-neuraminoglycoprotein [15]; it contains 12 percent hexose and 17 percent N-acetyl neuraminic acid. The fourth component, which occurs in relatively high concentrations in serum, contains 14 percent carbohydrate, consisting of hexose, hexosamine, and neuraminic acid [13]. The second component, C2, has an approximate molecular weight of 120,000 and is present in human serum in a concentration of 10 ± 2 μg per ml.

In human serum the concentration of the third component ranges from 900 to 1,500 μg per ml. Because of this high concentration, most antisera to whole human serum contain antibody directed against C3, making this component readily visible on routine immunoelectrophoretic analysis of human serum. On agarose electrophoresis of whole serum, C3 is visible as a discrete band in the β region. The precise

Table 71-1. COMPLEMENT NOMENCLATURE

Preferred Symbol	Interpretation	Synonyms
C	Complement	C′
E	Erythrocyte	
A	Antibody	amboceptor
C1	First	
C1q	component	C′0, 11-S component
C1r	and its	
C1s	subunits	C′1 esterase (in activated form)
C4	Fourth component	β_{1E}-globulin
C2	Second component	
C3	Third component	β_{1C}-globulin, C′3c, C′3a
C5	Fifth component	β_{1F}-globulin, C′3b
C6	Sixth component	C′3e, C′3a
C7	Seventh component	C′3f, C′3β
C8	Eighth component	C′3a, C′3c
C9	Ninth component	C′3d
C$\bar{1}$ INH*	Inhibitor of first component	EI, C′1 esterase inhibitor, C′1 INA
C3 INA*	Inactivator of cell-bound C3	KAF, conglutinogen activating factor
C6 INA*	Inactivator of cell-bound C6	
EAC1–*n*, e.g., EAC1–7	Intermediate complex formed by the reaction of the first "*n*" components	EAC1, 4, 2, 3, 5, 6, 7
Bar above number, e.g., C$\bar{1}$	Activated state of component	C′1a
Suffix "i," e.g., C3i	Component which has lost activity	
Suffix "a," "b," "c," e.g., C3a	Individual fragments of components produced during reaction	F(a)C′3

* These symbols were not generally agreed upon at the WHO discussions.

mobility of C3 observed with these techniques depends on the handling of the serum. When human serum is stored at temperatures above $-70°$C, C3 spontaneously converts to an electrophoretically faster material, which has been called β_{1A}-globulin [13]. This process of conversion is associated with a change in sedimentation coefficient to 6.9S [13], and the appearance of a separate, antigenically distinct fragment in the α_2 region on electrophoresis, called α_{2D}, which can be detected by certain antisera [16].

C3 inactivator has been partially purified from whole human serum [17]. It is a β_1-globulin with an approximate molecular weight of 100,000. The carbohydrate moiety of

Table 71-2. PROPERTIES OF HUMAN COMPLEMENT PROTEINS

	C1q	C1r	C1s	C1 INH	C4	C2	C3	C3 INA	C5	C6	C6 INA	C7	C8	C9
Electrophoretic mobility	γ_2	β	α_2	α_2	β_1	β_2	β_1	β_1	β_1	β_2	β_2	β_2	γ_1	α_2
Approx. molecular weight	400,000	....	110,000	90,000	230,000	117,000	185,000	100,000	....	....	....	....	....	75,000
S_w 20	11S	7S	4S	4S	10S	5.2S	9S	5S	8.7S	6.6S	6.6S	5.6S	8.5S	4.5S
Serum concentration (μg/ml)	100–200	....	24–46	130–210	200–600	8–12	900–1500	....	51–99	....	....	....	....	1–2

C3 INA appears to be required for its activity, since treatment with metaperiodate results in loss of activity [13]. C5 exists in serum in concentrations ranging from 50 to 100 μg per ml. This component also contains a high proportion (19 percent) of carbohydrate, chiefly in the form of hexose and hexosamine with very little neuraminic acid [13].

Little is known about the chemistry of C6 INA, C6, C7, C8, or C9. The last two components, which apparently exist in trace concentrations in serum, have been purified and antibody has been prepared against them [13]. Human C8 is said to be inactivated by treatment with the chelating agent EDTA [18]. The carbohydrate content of C9 is apparently required for activity, since treatment with periodate results in loss of activity [13].

The Complement Reaction Sequence (Fig. 1)

Fixation and Activation of C1

The sequence of complement reactions is initiated by IgG or IgM antibodies which have been altered as a result of union with their corresponding antigens or by IgG immunoglobulin which has been altered by heat aggregation [19]. In immune hemolysis, the fixation and activation of C1 usually requires either a doublet of IgG molecules in close proximity or a single IgM molecule [20]. The C1q portion of the C1 molecule bears the binding site of C1 for the immunoglobulin [14], and through it this subunit undergoes reversible binding, generating the complex EAC1. The combination of C1 with EA is followed by a temperature-dependent activation step in which the inactive precursor form, C1, is converted to an active esterase [21], $C\bar{1}$. This is the form of the component which reacts with the next two components in the sequence. Activation of C1 can also be accomplished by treatment with trypsin or plasmin [22]. The esteratic site on the C1 molecule resides on the C1s subunit, and active $C\bar{1}$ can be obtained either by direct purification [23], or by elution from $EAC\bar{1}$ by treatment with EDTA [21].

Action of $C\bar{1}$

$C\bar{1}$ splits C4 into at least two pieces [24]. C4a, a fragment of C4 with a molecular weight of approximately 7,400, appears free in the fluid phase. It is unclear whether or not biologic activity is associated with C4a. About 5 to 10 percent of the C4b fragments are bound to the cell membrane, forming the stable complex $EAC\overline{14}$, and the balance remains free in the fluid phase as the hemolytically inactive product, C4i [25].

The interaction of native C4 or C4i with $C\bar{1}$ markedly enhances the activity of the C1 enzyme on its other natural substrate, C2 [26]. In a fashion analogous to the reaction of C1 with C4, the C2 molecule is also split. The major fragment is bound to the cell surface, generating the cellular intermediate $EAC\overline{142}$ [27]. This intermediate is unstable and decays rapidly to the state $EAC\overline{14}$, liberating the hemolytically inactive product $C\bar{2}^d$, into the fluid phase. A smaller fragment of C2 produced by the action of $C\bar{1}$, which has a molecular weight of approximately 40,000 and appears directly in the fluid phase, has been demonstrated for guinea pig C2 [28], but not thus far for human C2. The possibility that the action of $C\bar{1}$ on C2 may liberate an additional fragment with kinin-like activities, which may be responsible for the lesions of hereditary angioedema, will be discussed below.

The C3 Step

The action of $C\bar{1}$ on C4 and C2 generates from these components a new enzymatic activity, C3 convertase [29]. This enzyme, which requires magnesium ions for its formation, can be produced in the fluid phase, but is more efficiently assembled on the cell surface, in the form of the $EAC\overline{142}$ cell. Through the action of C3 convertase a small fragment of the C3 molecule, C3a, is released into the fluid phase. This fragment is anaphylatoxin [30], and is a permeability factor. Anaphylatoxin causes a local wheal when injected intracutaneously into man. It releases histamine in vitro from rat peritoneal mast cells and causes the isolated guinea pig ileum to contract, with tachyphylaxis [30]. It seems likely that this fragment of C3 produces changes in permeability by releasing histamine from cells.

C3b, the major fragment of C3, is either bound to the cellular intermediate $EAC\overline{1423}$, or remains free in the fluid phase as the inactive product, C3i. The presence of C3b on the cell surface confers upon it the ability to participate in the immune adherence phenomenon, a reaction in which the C3b-coated cell binds to a specific receptor site on erythrocytes, polymorphonuclear leukocytes, or platelets [31]. This phenomenon is thought to enhance phagocytosis by polymorphonuclear leukocytes.

In an important control mechanism the C3 inactivator (C3 INA) acts on cell-bound C3b. It blocks all the biologic activities of this fragment, namely, induction of immune adherence, enhancement of phagocytosis, and reactivity with the subsequent components leading to immune hemolysis. C3 INA appears to function as an enzyme since it is not consumed during the course of its time- and temperature-dependent reaction with cell-bound C3b [17]. The C3 inactivator appears to be identical to the conglutinogen activating factor (KAF), a material in normal serum which confers upon $EAC\overline{1423}$ prepared with purified components the ability to react with conglutinin, a substance in bovine serum which agglutinates particles coated with KAF-treated C3 [32].

Reactions with C5, C6, and C7: Generation of Chemotactic Factors

The presence of C3b on the surface of the $EAC\overline{1423}$ intermediate permits its reaction with the next component in the sequence, C5. The binding and activation of C5 also appear to require the presence of C2 on the cell. Biologic activities have been observed for C5. A low-molecular-weight fragment with anaphylatoxin activity is liberated during the course of its reaction with EAC$\overline{1423}$ [33], and production of a material with chemotactic activity for polymorphonuclear leukocytes has also been described [34]. It seems likely that these anaphylatoxic and chemotactic activities reside in the same fragment.

The reaction mechanisms for C6 and C7 have been less well studied than those of the preceding components. Both of these components are physically bound to the cell surface and generate the stable intermediate EAC$\overline{1423567}$. An inactivator of C6 [35] functions at the C6 step and blocks the hemolytic activity of cell-bound C6. In the course of the formation of EAC$\overline{1\text{–}7}$ a chemotactic factor for polymorphonuclear leukocytes is generated [36]. This activity appears to reside in a high-molecular-weight complex formed by the interaction of C5, 6, and 7 and is distinct from the low-molecular-weight chemotactic factor generated from C5.

Cells coated with antibody achieve the "1–7" state by progressive binding and activation of the first seven complement components as diagramed in Fig. 71-1. In addition, it has recently been appreciated that cells *not* coated with antibody can be brought to an analogous state, in the sense of reactivity with C8 and C9, by entirely fluid phase activation of the complement system [37]. Erythrocytes present in reaction mixtures containing fluid phase C3 convertase, C3, and C5–7 progress to a state of susceptibility to C8 and C9. When added to whole serum, a factor from cobra venom appears to induce a similar state in nonsensitized erythrocytes [38]. So far, only sheep erythrocytes have been used in these lytic reactions induced by fluid phase interactions of complement components. If the capacity to participate in such reactions is a more universal property of cell membranes, the lysis of such "innocent bystander" nonsensitized cells by activation of the complement system might be an important mechanism of cell damage.

The Terminal Steps of Immune Hemolysis

The union of C8 and the EAC$\overline{1\text{–}7}$ cell initiates membrane damage: EAC$\overline{1\text{–}8}$ cells tend to lyse gradually upon incubation at 37°C [39]. The addition of C9 markedly increases the rate of lysis, although there is a distinct lag between the combination of EAC$\overline{1\text{–}8}$ and C9 and the appearance of hemoglobin in the supernatant fluid. Membrane damage by human complement is associated with the appearance of a characteristic 103-Å discontinuity which has been observed by electron microscopic studies of negatively stained membranes from lysed erythrocytes and other target cells [40]. These complement-induced "holes" appear to represent bubbles corresponding to micelle formation in the membrane, the tops of which have burst as a result of the negative stain [41]. The nature of the chemical change which corresponds to this lesion is not precisely known [42].

Methods of Measuring Complement Components

Radial Immunodiffusion

Techniques for quantitative immunochemical determinations of C1q [7], C$\overline{1}$ INH [43], C4 [44], C3 [45], and C5 [46] have

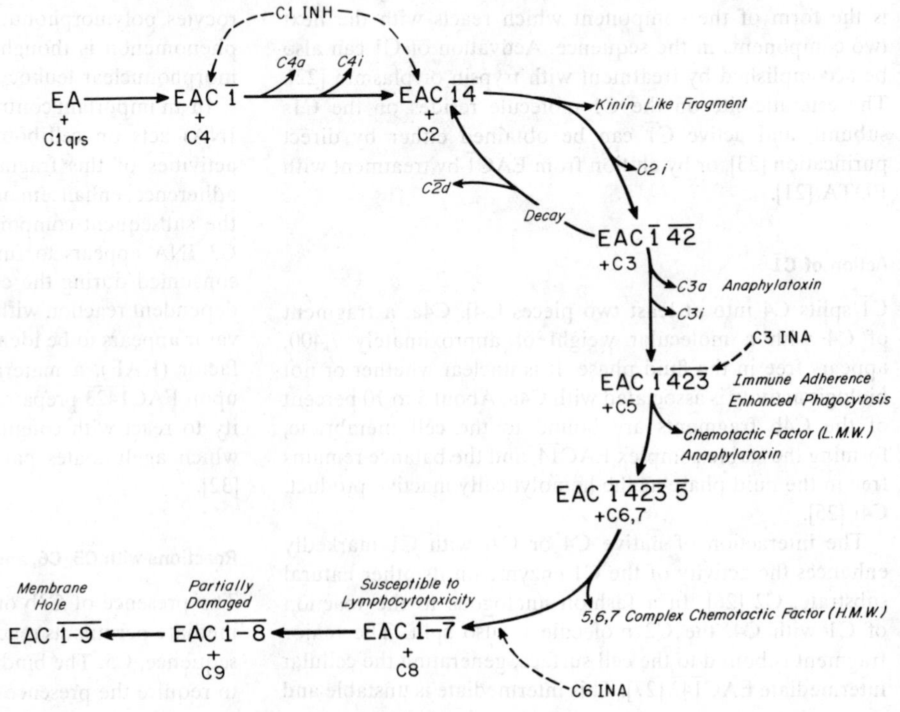

Figure 71-1. Reaction mechanisms and biologic results of the complement system.

been reported. Each of these depends on the ability of monospecific antisera directed against the component proteins to precipitate them as antigens. Modifications of the radial immunodiffusion technique of Mancini [47] are usually used: monospecific antibody is incorporated into buffered agarose gel, holes are punched in the gel, and the serum samples placed in these holes. After diffusion for a predetermined period of time, the size of the precipitin rings surrounding the holes is measured and compared with the size of rings produced in the same gel by known quantities of the component being measured. The concentration of the component can be expressed directly in terms of weight of complement protein per milliliter. The experimental error of such procedures is usually about 10 percent. Because immunochemical measurements depend on the antigenic integrity of the component protein, they have the advantage that special processing of serum samples is not usually required. Such determinations yield no information about the functional integrity of the component being measured.

Hemolytic Activity Measurements

The whole hemolytic complement activity, or CH50 [48], measures the resultant of the interaction of all nine components and three inactivators and is the procedure most often available to assess the functional state of the complement system. This test is useful for screening in suspected abnormalities of the complement system: it is always low in homozygous C2 deficiency, and may be reduced in hereditary angioedema. A normal CH50 does not, however, exclude partial deficiency states or hereditary angioedema.

As a result of the elaboration of the one-hit theory of immune hemolysis [11] and the availability of stable intermediates of the hemolytic system, effective molecular titrations of individual components are now possible. These functional assays require that the test serum supply the component being measured in a hemolytic system in which all other components are present in excess. For example, in the titration of serum C4 activity [49], the intermediate cells $EAC\overline{1}$, carrying an excess of $C\overline{1}$ sites, are incubated with the test serum diluted sufficiently to supply a limiting amount of C4. The extent of conversion of the $EAC\overline{1}$ to $EAC\overline{14}$ by the test serum is determined by first treating the cells with an excess of functionally pure C2 to convert all $EAC\overline{14}$ to $EAC\overline{142}$, and then lysing these cells by supplying excesses of C3, 5, 6, 7, 8, and 9. By an application of the Poisson distribution, the theoretical dose in terms of numbers of damaged sites per erythrocyte (Z) corresponding to the observed response in terms of percent lysis can be calculated. Arithmetic plots of Z versus the input of either test serum or purified C4 are linear over a wide range of C4 concentrations. The titer of the test serum is defined as the reciprocal of the dilution required to generate an average of 1.0 sites per cell. Stoichiometric hemolytic titrations have been described for C1 [50], $C\overline{1}$ INH [51], C4 [49], C2 [52], and C3 [17] in whole human serum. The day-to-day experimental error of these techniques is about 10 percent, and measurements performed on the same day with the same batch of cells vary by less than 5 percent.

$C\overline{1}$ INHIBITOR DEFICIENCY: HEREDITARY ANGIOEDEMA

History

Although the morphology of angioedema had been described several years earlier, it was William Osler who, in 1888, distinguished a hereditary form of this disease [53]. His summary of angioedema occurring in five generations of the same family called attention to most of the important clinical features of hereditary angioedema, including the prominence of gastrointestinal disturbances and the propensity for sudden death caused by upper respiratory obstruction. The autosomal dominant mode of inheritance was well documented by Crowder and Crowder [54], who described a kindred of 64 individuals, with 28 patients with angioedema, of whom 15 had died from the acute complications of the disease.

The biochemical defect in hereditary angioedema was first described by Donaldson and Evans in 1963 [1]. Rosen and his associates called attention to the "genetic variant" form of the disease, in which nonfunctional but antigenically intact inhibitor protein is present in the sera of affected individuals [43]. Donaldson and Rosen have reviewed their clinical experience with the disease [55].

Clinical Aspects

Subcutaneous Edema

Recurrent bouts of acute, circumscribed and transient edema of the skin are usually the chief complaint of patients with hereditary angioedema. The skin of any part of the body can be involved, but the most common site is either an area of the face or an extremity. Attacks may rarely be heralded by transient erythema or mottling of the skin, but characteristically no changes in the hue or temperature of the involved area are detectable. Patients sometimes experience subjective symptoms of vague discomfort in an area which subsequently swells. The edema usually spreads concentrically from a single site on the body, and the simultaneous appearance of multiple discrete areas of swelling during a single attack is distinctly unusual. The lesion ranges in size from an area a few centimeters in diameter to involvement of most of an extremity. The localized edema does not itch and cannot be pitted. The swelling may progress for up to 24 or 48 hr and then usually subsides over the next 2 or 3 days.

Gastrointestinal Edema

A clinical feature which is highly characteristic of hereditary angioedema is involvement of the gastrointestinal tract.

Edema of the wall of the gut, which has been observed both by x-ray [56] and at laparotomy [57], may lead to severe abdominal pain and profuse vomiting, resembling acute obstruction of the bowel. Cramping abdominal pain and watery diarrhea may also result. The symptoms may be sufficiently severe to lead to surgical intervention: healed laparotomy scars are a frequent physical finding among patients with hereditary angioedema. Clinical signs of peritonitis, fever, and marked leukocytosis do not occur. Improvement usually occurs within 48 hr, so that supportive therapy is all that is required.

Gastrointestinal attacks may accompany episodes of subcutaneous edema or may occur independently of them. In one family, abdominal complaints were the most prominent feature of the disease, and the occasional attacks of subcutaneous edema which all of the affected members also experienced were viewed as a minor unrelated nuisance [58]. A history of severe, self-limited attacks of abdominal pain, accompanied by vomiting or diarrhea or both is so characteristic of hereditary angioedema that its presence in any patient with angioedema should alert the physician to the possibility of this diagnosis.

Edema of the Upper Respiratory Tract

Another common feature of hereditary angioedema is submucosal edema of the upper respiratory tract, which may progress to laryngeal edema with death by asphyxiation. Although this problem may occur in other, nonfamilial forms of angioedema, it seems to be more frequent in patients with hereditary angioedema. A tracheostomy scar is another common physical finding in this disease. Among affected members of large kindreds mortality rates due to respiratory obstruction have ranged from as low as 6 percent [59] to as high as 54 percent [54]. Attacks may begin on the face or buccal mucosa and progress to involve the glottis and larynx within a few hours. The frequency of this life-threatening complication makes it important to distinguish hereditary angioedema from other more common nonfamilial forms.

Frequency of Attacks and Precipitating Factors

Ordinarily there is no periodicity to the attacks of hereditary angioedema. Some patients have episodes of swelling on an average of once weekly, and others report only a few attacks during their entire lifetime. Although attacks of angioedema may occur during early childhood, most members of previously undiagnosed kindreds come to the physician's attention at about the age of puberty. Not infrequently children who can be demonstrated to have the biochemical lesion of hereditary angioedema will experience an increasing frequency of attacks at this age. Bouts of edema appear to be most frequent during the reproductive years and occur less often during later life. Exceptions to this are not rare, and the onset of attacks at age 58 in a woman documented to have the biochemical lesion of hereditary angioedema has been reported [57].

When queried, most patients will cite local trauma as a definite factor which commonly precipitates attacks of angioedema. The extent of trauma may be so minor as to be forgotten until swelling ensues. Dental extractions are particularly dangerous: severe edema of the oropharynx and glottis may occur, and at least one such patient has died [55].

Although many patients assert that exposure to one or another food or other allergen is associated with attacks of angioedema, these impressions are difficult to substantiate. Skin testing with the suspected allergen is often negative, and reexposure to the suspected food often does not precipitate an attack.

Emotional trauma is cited second most commonly as a precipitating factor by patients with hereditary angioedema [55]. The original descriptions of "hereditary angio*neurotic*" edema underscores the importance which has been attributed to emotional factors in this disease. It is not surprising that a lifetime of recurrent swellings, some of which may be potentially asphyxiating, and of unexplained recurrent abdominal pain and gastrointestinal upset, should be accompanied by anxiety and frustration. Because there is little objective evidence to suggest that emotional factors have a primary role in the pathogenesis of this disease, the authors prefer the term *hereditary angioedema* to the older name.

Family History

The absence of a family history of cutaneous angioedema does not exclude the diagnosis of hereditary angioedema. Relevant history may include young relatives who have died suddenly of obscure causes or familial complaints related to the gastrointestinal tract. A sizable proportion of patients will report no knowledge of any familial abnormalities. Occasional cases may represent spontaneous mutations to the genetic defect associated with this disease [60].

Although hereditary angioedema was formerly considered to be a rare entity, during the past 5 years the authors have confirmed the diagnosis in over 100 patients, occurring among 29 kindreds. Other workers in the field have had similar experiences [55]. Any patient with angioedema, even those with negative family histories, therefore, should be evaluated for the "hereditary" form of the disease.

Pathology

The pathologic alterations occurring in hereditary angioedema have been observed in tissues obtained by skin and peroral jejunal biopsy, laparotomy, and at post-mortem examination [61]. Skin changes consisted of subcutaneous edema; leakage from the postcapillary venules was apparent on electron microscopic examination. Upper respiratory tract involvement always revealed laryngeal edema. Spongiosis of the mucosal epithelial cells with cytoplasmic vacuole formation was prominent. Marked submucosal edema with masking of the submucosal fibrous structures was also demonstrable, but there was little inflammatory response and no tissue eosinophilia. Diffuse edema and hemorrhage of the lungs presumably occurred secondary to asphyxiation. Jejunal tissue showed edema of the *lamina propria,* particularly of the superficial portion of the villi, giving a club-shaped appearance. Submucosal edema was present. The mucocutaneous and visceral tissue findings in hereditary angioedema can be distinguished from those of fatal systemic anaphylaxis, wherein the involved organs contain an inflammatory infiltrate, frequently with prominence of eosinophils.

Treatment

No specific therapy is presently available for hereditary angioedema. A variety of symptomatic remedies have been tried, mostly without success. In particular, salicylates, antihistamines, and adrenal cortical steroids are ineffective either in preventing the onset of an attack or in aborting an attack already under way. Local applications of cold or heat are similarly without benefit. Subcutaneous administration of aqueous epinephrine is a common practice, but its usefulness has never clearly been documented. Plasma transfusions have been reported to arrest an attack already in progress [62], although there are theoretical reasons why such therapy might be hazardous [63]. In patients with progressive oropharyngeal or laryngeal edema, tracheostomy can be lifesaving.

Epsilon-aminocaproic acid has been reported to decrease the frequency of attacks in two cases [64, 65]. Maintenance androgen therapy has been thought to decrease the frequency of attacks, although the rationale for the use of this hormone is unclear [66, 55, 58].

Pathogenesis of Edema

Role of Activated C1

The evidence for the involvement of the complement system in hereditary angioedema is abundant, and the mechanism for the edema has been partially elucidated. Patients with this disease have an inherited deficiency of the function of the inhibitor of $C\bar{1}$ ($C\bar{1}$ INH) [1]. There are three lines of evidence that the uninhibited activated $C\bar{1}$ is central to the pathogenesis of the edema. Clinical attacks are associated with the appearance of plasma esterase activity against N-acetyl-L-tyrosine ethyl ester [67], a synthetic amino acid ester substrate of $C\bar{1}$. C4 and C2, the natural substrates of $C\bar{1}$ [44], are reduced in activity in the sera of affected individuals, even during asymptomatic intervals, and further reductions occur during clinical attacks [60]. Metabolic studies with purified and radiolabeled C4 have demonstrated that this component is catabolized three to five times as rapidly in patients with hereditary angioedema as in normal control subjects [68].

When purified $C\overline{1s}$ is injected into the skin of normal volunteers, an intense wheal develops. Intradermal injection of the same material into patients with hereditary angioedema precipitates a full-blown local attack of angioedema. Similar injections into individuals homozygous for C2 deficiency disclose an inablility to respond even at a dose 10 times that which elicits a permeability change in normal subjects. It can be inferred from these studies [69] that the $C\bar{1}$ INH limits the capacity of $C\bar{1}$ to induce permeability changes and that C2 is an essential substrate.

The mechanism by which $C\bar{1}$ becomes activated and an attack of edema is precipitated in hereditary angioedema remains unclear. The finding [70] that soybean trypsin inhibitor interferes with the generation of a permeability factor from hereditary angioedema plasma implicates a serum protease such as kallikrein or plasmin. The capacity of both of these enzymes to activate C1 has been demonstrated [22]. The fact that $C\bar{1}$ INH is not only effective against C1 but also against kallikrein and plasmin [71] suggests that the inborn error may be responsible for both the episodic activation of C1 and its subsequent action in generating the pathogenetic permeability factor.

Chemical Mediator of the Edema

The precise chemical nature of the material which mediates the permeability change in hereditary angioedema remains unknown. When incubated at 37°C, plasma from patients with this disease develops the capacity to increase vascular permeability and to contract the isolated estrous rat uterus [70]. These activities apparently reside in a heat-stable polypeptide. Although this material resembles bradykinin in certain of its properties, it differs from the known kinins in being susceptible to degradation by trypsin and in producing a pressor effect in the rat. A preliminary report [72] has been made about the generation of a similar vasoactive factor following the in vitro combination of $C\bar{1}$, C4, and C2 purified from human serum. This material may represent an as yet uncharacterized split product of the second component of complement.

Other mediators of vascular permeability have also been implicated in hereditary angioedema. Urinary histamine levels are increased during attacks of angioedema [73]. This may reflect the release of anaphylatoxin by C3 convertase generated from the fluid phase action of $C\bar{1}$ on C4 and C2. The moderate hypercatabolism of C3 observed in turnover studies of this component in hereditary angioedema patients [68] supports the contention that some C3 convertase is formed. Histamine release due to anaphylatoxin does not appear to have a central role in the pathogenesis of the edema, since patients with acquired C3 deficiency show a normal cutaneous permeability response on $C\bar{1}$ injection [69] and antihistaminics do not affect the clinical course of hereditary angioedema.

Deficiency of a normal serum inhibitor of plasma kallikrein, the enzyme which generates bradykinin from kininogen, was described [74] in patients with hereditary angioedema before the complement abnormality was appreciated. It has subsequently been demonstrated that purified C$\bar{1}$ INH blocks kallikrein [72] through the formation of an inactive stoichiometric complex [75]. The extent of the contribution of bradykinin to the lesion of hereditary angioedema is as yet unclear.

In summary, current evidence indicates that the change in vascular permeability which occurs in hereditary angioedema is mediated by a polypeptide with kininlike activities but which is distinct from bradykinin. This polypeptide may be released from C2 by the action of C$\bar{1}$ in the presence of C4; components reacting beyond the C2 step do not appear to be involved in the clinical problem. Kallikrein or plasmin may be responsible for the activation of C1 to C$\bar{1}$.

Laboratory Diagnosis

Deficiency of the function of C$\bar{1}$ INH can be demonstrated either by direct measurements of the inhibitor, or by measuring the consequences of its absence, i.e., reductions in the serum levels of C4 and C2. Of these, the C4 protein determination is the simplest screening test available [76]. Less than 1 percent of individuals affected with hereditary angioedema have C4 protein levels within the normal range. Although a normal C4 protein level virtually excludes the diagnosis of hereditary angioedema, reduced levels are not

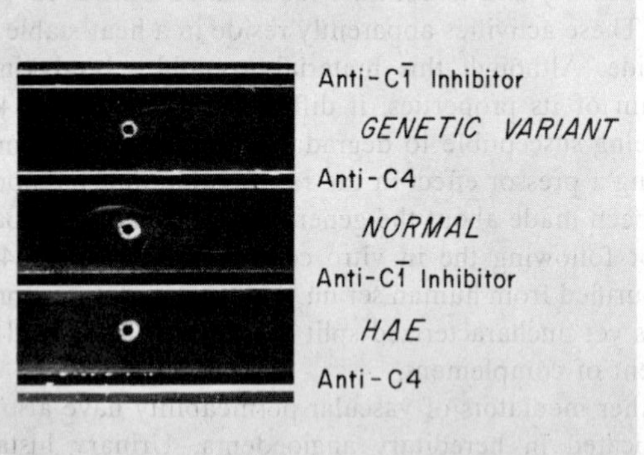

Figure 71-2. Immunoelectrophoresis of sera from a normal individual and two patients with hereditary angioedema, one with the "common" and the other with the "genetic variant" form of the disease. Precipitin arcs corresponding to C4 and C$\bar{1}$ INH are visible with the normal serum. Both are absent with the serum from the common form of hereditary angioedema. Only the arc corresponding to C$\bar{1}$ INH is present with the genetic variant serum. By hemolytic assay, the genetic variant serum contained $<$100 units C$\bar{1}$ INH per ml. (Normal, 38,000 $\pm$ 18,000 units/ml.) A slight shift in the mobility of the nonfunctional inhibitor protein present in the genetic variant serum is apparent.

specifically diagnostic of this disease. Low serum C4 levels are also found in such diseases as systemic lupus erythematosus, acute glomerulonephritis, and certain forms of cryoglobulinemia [77, 78].

A specific test for the absence of C$\bar{1}$ INH is therefore required to confirm the diagnosis. Because of its simplicity, radial immunodiffusion for C$\bar{1}$ INH protein is usually performed on the sera of hereditary angioedema suspects with low C4 protein [76]. A serum C$\bar{1}$ INH protein level of less than 100 μg per ml is diagnostic of hereditary angioedema, but a normal immunodiffusion result for C$\bar{1}$ INH does not exclude the diagnosis. Approximately 10 percent of kindreds will have a "genetic variant" form of the disease, in which normal serum concentrations of antigenically intact, but functionless, C$\bar{1}$ INH protein are present [43] (Fig. 71-2). In these cases, only a functional measurement of C$\bar{1}$ INH activity will be diagnostic. The hemolytic assay for C$\bar{1}$ INH determines the ability of the serum to inhibit a known amount of purified C$\bar{1}$ in immune hemolysis [51]. A less sensitive enzymatic assay measures the ability of the test serum to block the activity of a known amount of C$\overline{1s}$ on a synthetic amino acid ester substrate [79].

Genetics

Mode of Inheritance

Over 60 kindreds with hereditary angioedema have been reported in the literature. The disease has occurred in American Negroes, Irish, English, Scotch-Irish, Swedish, Italian, Dutch, French, Sephardic and Ashkenazi Jews and Turkish Armenians. Hereditary angioedema appears to be transmitted as an autosomal dominant trait, and affected individuals are heterozygous for the trait. Although there is usually good correspondence between the presence of the biochemical defect and symptoms of angioedema, occasional individuals who have no symptoms will have reduced C$\bar{1}$ INH levels [60]. The biochemical defect has been shown to occur in three successive generations in eight kindreds [55, 60]. One instance of hereditary angioedema occurring *de novo* in an individual whose parents had normal serum levels of C$\bar{1}$ INH has been reported [60]: one of four of the progeny of this subject was affected. The pedigree in this case was not verified with other independent tests such as blood groups analysis.

Serum Concentrations of C$\bar{1}$ Inhibitor in "Conventional" Hereditary Angioedema

Although individuals affected by hereditary angioedema appear to be heterozygous, only small amounts of C$\bar{1}$ INH are found in their sera. Serum levels are relatively constant for any given affected individual over periods of up to 2 years. When it has been determined, the C$\bar{1}$ INH in the sera of hereditary angioedema patients is as active on a weight basis in the inhibition of the hemolytic activity of $C\bar{1}$ as is that of normal serum [51].

Impaired synthesis of $C\bar{1}$ INH has been inferred from the reduced serum levels in the conventional form of hereditary angioedema. Immunofluorescent studies with antibody directed against $C\bar{1}$ INH also support this view: specific fluorescence has been observed in 5–10 percent of the hepatic parenchymal cells of normal individuals, but no fluorescent cells were found in the liver biopsy specimens obtained from two patients with hereditary angioedema [99]. Catabolic rates, measured with purified and radiolabeled $C\bar{1}$ INH, were similar in normals and in patients with hereditary angioedema, so that synthetic rates, calculated from serum levels and catabolic rates, were depressed in hereditary angioedema [100]. The autosomal dominant mode of inheritance of this synthetic defect suggests an abnormality of a regulator gene.

Genetic Variant Form: Polymorphism of $C\bar{1}$ INH

In certain kindreds with hereditary angioedema, the sera of affected individuals contain normal quantities of an antigenically intact but nonfunctional inhibitor protein [43]. Kindreds with this form breed true, and the mode of inheritance is similar to the more common form of the disease. "Genetic variant" hereditary angioedema almost certainly represents a structural mutation in inhibitor synthesis. On immunoelectrophoretic analysis, the nonfunctional inhibitor protein has an appearance which differs very slightly but distinctly from normal (Fig. 71-2). When analyzed by thin layer agarose electrophoresis, the difference in mobility is more apparent. Analyses of $C\bar{1}$ INH protein from five kindreds with genetic variant hereditary angioedema have demonstrated unique mobilities for each family which are constant for all affected members of the kindred [80]. Variant protein present in the sera of one kindred has also been found to vary in the extent to which it inhibits the activity of a highly purified plasma kallikrein [75].

C2 DEFICIENCY

History

The first observation of an isolated deficiency of the second component of complement was made by Woodworth in 1958 [81]. He found that serum from a single healthy donor would not promote the immune adherence of rice starch to human erythrocytes and that, furthermore, this serum was inactive in immune hemolysis. Using combinations of sera made partially deficient in one or more of the four "components" of complement known to exist at the time ("R reagents"), the defect was traced to the second component, but no family studies were done. A second individual with C2 deficiency was reported by Silverstein in 1960 [82]. No evidence for genetic transmission was obtained when the sera of two sibs and two children of the patient were studied with R reagents.

The inheritable aspect of C2 deficiency was documented by Klemperer and coworkers, who studied the C2-deficient patient described by Woodworth, and 31 members of the kindred (Family W.) [2]. When the activity of C2 was measured by a stoichiometric titration, and the other components detected with R reagents, an inherited deficiency for C2 was demonstrated. A similar inherited defect was established by more extensive examination of the kindred (Family P.) reported by Silverstein [83].

Specificity of the Defect for C2

Hemolytic Measurements

The validity of the observations reported by Klemperer et al. [2] has been established by reexamination of sera from homozygous and heterozygous deficient members of Families W. and P. Stoichiometric titrations of C1, C4, and C2, and specific assays for C3, 5, 6, 7, 8, and 9 performed with purified components have demonstrated that the deficiency is limited to C2 [84]. The possibility that deficient sera contained an inhibitor or inactivator of normal C2 was excluded by demonstrating that the activity of purified guinea pig C2 was uninfluenced by the presence of deficient serum [2]. Kinetic experiments excluded the possibility that deficient sera contained an unstable form of C2 which decayed more rapidly from the $\overline{142}$ sites than did normal C2 [2]. The specificity of the deficiency for C2 was confirmed by restoring the overall hemolytic activity of a deficient serum by the addition of purified human C2 [2].

Immunodiffusion Measurements

Radial immunodiffusion assays for C4, C3, and $C\bar{1}$ INH protein have all yielded normal results in C2 deficiency. Antibody prepared against human C2 has been used to measure the levels of C2 protein in normal and in C2 deficient sera [85]. The normal serum concentration of C2 is 10 ± 2 μg per ml [85]. No precipitation was observed with the sera of C2-deficient individuals [85, 86].

Biologic Implications

Consideration of the complement sequence suggests that individuals lacking C2 might also be deficient in the host defenses promoted by immune adherence, enhanced phagocytosis, anaphylatoxin release, leukochemotaxis, and immune cytolysis. None of the C2 deficient subjects has experienced any unusual susceptibility to infection. Either these complement-dependent reactions are not important in host resistance or they are not impaired in vivo in C2-deficient individuals to the extent suggested by in vitro determinations of immune hemolytic activity. The latter appears to be correct.

Immune Adherence Activity in C2 Deficiency

The immune adherence activities of C2-deficient sera were found to range from one-fortieth to one-ninth of normal using sensitized *Brucella abortus* as the test antigen [2, 83]. When sensitized erythrocytes were used, immune adherence activities were found to be normal [87, 88]. The discrepancies between these observations may relate to the concentrations of the test antigens in the system (10^{11} *B. abortus* per ml versus 10^7 sheep erythrocytes per ml), or to the efficiency with which the two test complexes bind C3b. The explanation for the observations that immune adherence is not impaired in C2 deficiency to the same extent as immune hemolysis lies in the differential requirements of the two systems for active C2. Immune adherence requires that the immune complex has reacted with the first four components so as to be coated with C3b. Cells from which C2 has decayed, resulting in the $\overline{143}$ state, are fully reactive. In order for the immune hemolytic reaction to proceed, the continued presence of active C2 on the site is required. It seems probable that C2 deficient serum contains sufficient C2 to generate some $\overline{1423}$ sites which, after decay to the $\overline{143}$ state, are fully reactive in immune adherence but will not interact with the remaining components so as to permit lysis. Since phagocytosis enhancement requires the same components as immune adherence, presumably this activity in C2-deficient serum would not be impaired to the same extent as immune hemolysis.

Bactericidal Activity of C2-deficient Serum

The results of bactericidal activity measurements of C2-deficient sera depend on how the tests are performed. Using organisms sensitized with an exogenous source of antibody, a system analogous to the immune hemolysis of optimally sensitized sheep erythrocytes, the bactericidal activity of C2-deficient sera is markedly reduced [2]. If unsensitized organisms are used, the test serum serving both as the source of natural antibody to the organisms and of complement, no difference is detectable between normal and C2-deficient sera [87]. It appears that the small quantities of C2 contained in deficient sera are adequate to convert all the $\overline{14}$ sites generated by the limited quantities of natural antibody present. Since the system using unsensitized organisms is more analogous to the conditions prevailing in vivo, the overall bactericidal activity of C2-deficient homozygotes may not be significantly impaired.

In summary, C2-deficient *sera* exhibit impaired performance in in vitro tests of host defense functions which tend to emphasize the complement requirement. C2-deficient *individuals,* on the other hand, exhibit no impairments of the host defenses associated with these functions, probably because the small quantities of circulating C2 present in their sera are adequate for their performance in vivo.

Genetics

Mode of Inheritance

In Families W. and P. pedigree studies demonstrated that C2 deficiency was transmitted as an autosomal trait, heterozygotes having approximately half-normal serum C2 levels and homozygotes having less than 5 percent of the normal activity [2, 83]. A third kindred (Family D.) was initially thought to represent a different form of inheritance because all affected individuals were males, and heterozygotes could not be detected [89]. Since the original report a C2-deficient female has been born. In addition more specific techniques for the measurement of C2 have demonstrated heterozygous members of this kindred [90]. A fourth kindred (Family C.) with a pattern of inheritance which is probably similar to the first three has also been reported [88].

Mechanism of Reduced C2 Levels

The defect in C2 deficiency is presumably one of synthesis, not increased catabolism. Serum C2 activities in hetero-

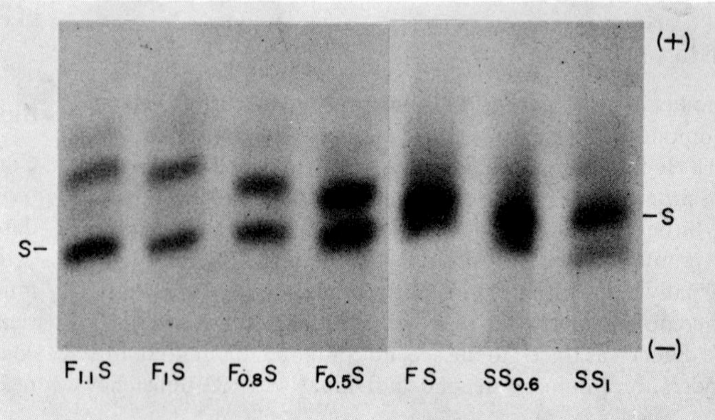

Figure 71-3. Appearance of the eight known allotypes of C3 following prolonged agarose electrophoresis (*Courtesy of Dr. C. Alper.*)

zygotes range from approximately 40 to 70 percent of the normal mean. Levels in homozygotes are less than 5 percent but are not zero. The small amounts of C2 present in the serum of homozygous deficient individuals have been measured by their ability to promote the binding of radiolabeled C3 to EAC$\overline{14}$ cells. By this technique C2 activities in homozygous deficient sera ranged from 2 to 4 percent of normal [88].

C2 protein determinations on heterozygous C2 deficient sera yield values which range from 30 to 60 percent of the normal mean [85]. On a weight basis, the C2 contained in the serum of heterozygous C2 deficient individuals is as active as normal C2 [90]. The C2 contained in the heterozygous deficient sera from all four kindreds is antigenically identical to normal C2 when analyzed with antibody prepared against the normal material [90]. Since this C2 is presumably the product of the normal, not the mutant, gene, no conclusion can be made about the product, if any, of the mutant gene. No antigenic analysis of the small quantity of C2 present in the serum of homozygotes has yet been reported. The evidence, therefore, does not permit a distinction between a regulatory and a structural defect of synthesis.

POLYMORPHISM OF COMPLEMENT COMPONENTS

Inherited Variations in C3 Mobility

History

Because of its high concentration in normal serum, C3 is readily visible as a dense band in the slow β region on agarose electrophoresis in calcium-containing buffer. Inherited variations in the mobility of C3 were observed simultaneously and independently by Alper and Propp [4] and by Wieme et al. [91]. Initially, only rare variants with unusually fast or slow mobilities were described, but techniques with higher resolving power demonstrated the electrophoretic heterogeneity of "normal" C3 [4]. Using starch gel electrophoresis, Azen and Smithies also observed the common polymorphism of C3 [92].

Further studies by Alper et al. [3] have demonstrated inheritance of a partial deficiency of C3, which results from nonexpression of one of the two C3 alleles. In addition, a variant with reduced synthesis is characterized by diminished, but not absent, amounts of the C3 corresponding to this allele [93].

Allotypes of C3

Figure 71-3 shows the eight known variations in the mobility of C3 for human serum. The nomenclature designated by subscripts is based on the relative mobilities of variants with respect to the common allotypes F and S. The distances between the mobility of F and S and the mobilities of the original fastest and slowest variants have been arbitrarily designated as 1.0. Thus, the $S_{0.6}$ variant migrates about 60 percent of the distance between S and $S_{1.0}$. The discovery of an allotype which migrates faster than $F_{1.0}$ has resulted in the designation $F_{1.1}$.

A variant of C3F with reduced synthesis has also been described [93]. Individuals with this allele have a 40/60 distribution of F and S protein, as opposed to the usual 50/50 distribution. Measurements of catabolic rates of C3F and C3S in these subjects yield normal values, implying decreased synthesis of C3F.

The identity of the bands observed on electrophoresis with C3 has been demonstrated by analysis with antigen-antibody crossed electrophoresis [94] against monospecific anti-C3. Furthermore, following purification, radiolabeling, and addition to whole serum, the mobilities of the isolated C3 allotypes were preserved. A similar persistence in the differences in mobilities has been observed following "conversion" of the C3 to the "β_{1A}" form. No differences in antigenicity were observed among the C3 allotypes when analyzed with antisera prepared against FS or $F_{1.0}$ F C3. Sedimentation of $F_{1.0}$S, $FS_{1.0}$, and $F_{1.0}$F types of C3 in sucrose density gradients has not shown any differences in size among these variants [4].

Clinical Implications

Few data are available concerning possible alterations in function corresponding to the differences in net charge of the C3 allotypes. Although the probands of several of the kindreds were originally studied because of such diseases as chronic idiopathic thrombocytopenic purpura and aplastic anemia, phenotypically identical members of the same kindreds are in excellent health. No differences in total hemolytic complement activity or in immune adherence activity are apparent among sera containing variant C3 protein. Sera containing different allotypes appear to be equal with respect to their ability to reconstitute the total hemolytic activity of a serum from a patient with an acquired deficiency of C3 [4].

Genetics

Inheritance of the known allotypes of C3 is consistent with autosomal codominance [4]. The concentrations of the two gene products in serum from heterozygotes are approximately equal. The S and F allotypes are relatively common, and all others are rare. Analyses of 152 sera from Caucasian, Negro, and Oriental subjects have permitted the calculation of F and S gene frequencies for each of these three groups. For Caucasians, the S/F distribution was 0.75/0.25; for Negroes, 0.90/0.10; and for Orientals, 0.98/0.02 [4].

Partial C3 Deficiency

A single kindred containing seven individuals with approximately half-normal serum concentrations of C3 has been described [3]. Analysis of the electrophoretic mobilities of the C3 in the sera of the partially deficient individuals revealed that they all had only a single allotype, either F or S. Analysis of the pedigree of this kindred suggested that an additional allele exists at the C3 locus. No gene product corresponding to this allele appears in the serum to cause an inherited deficiency of C3. Thus far only heterozygous individuals have been observed.

Synthesis of C3

Information about the site of synthesis of C3 has been obtained from studies of allotypes in donor and recipient of a hepatic allograft [95]. The recipient type was $FS_{0.6}$, and the donor SS. Following orthotopic transplantation of the liver, the recipient's type changed to that of the donor, and this type persisted until the recipient died of pulmonary sepsis 6 weeks postoperatively. These observations indicate that the liver is the primary, if not the sole, site of C3 synthesis in man. Allotypic differences in C3 observed between mothers and their newborns demonstrates that this component of complement is synthesized by the human fetus [96]. No evidence of transplacental passage has been observed. The finding that individuals with partial deficiency have approximately 50 percent of the normal concentration of this protein suggests that synthesis of C3 is probably independent of plasma concentration.

Polymorphism of C4

Because the concentration of the fourth component of complement is too low to permit direct visualization as a distinct protein band in agarose electrophoresis, plasma samples were examined [5] by antigen-antibody crossed electrophoresis. Heterogeneity of C4 mobility was shown by the repeated occurrence of seven different precipitin patterns. The patterns were formed by varying combinations of 3 subtypes of C4, which differed in electrophoretic mobility. These subtypes were designated C, A, and A_1, in order of increasing mobility toward the anode.

C4 of a given subtype retained its characteristic mobility after purification, when run alone or mixed with plasma containing C4 of other subtypes. The subtypes A_1 and C could be separated chromatographically as well as electrophoretically. The characteristic relative mobilities of different C4 subtypes, both in plasma or after purification, were retained even after conversion of C4 to C4i. Mixtures of plasmas containing only subtypes A alone or C alone were used to reproduce patterns composed of both of these subtypes in varying proportions [101]. Analysis of the precipitin patterns obtained with these mixtures of plasma agreed closely with their predicted content of subtypes A and C. Although there is evidence that the C4 subtypes are heritable characteristics, the mode of inheritance and the quantitative aspects of this inheritance remain unclear. The data that are available are consistent with the interpretation that subtypes A and A_1 are controlled by allelic genes, and that these genes are not allelic with that controlling subtype C.

The ratio of C4 hemolytic activity to protein concentration varied according to the subtype composition of individual samples. Highest ratios occurred with patterns composed of subtype C alone, intermediate values with patterns consisting of A and C, and the lowest values with patterns containing subtype A alone [5]. Analysis of C4 polymorphism in paired samples of maternal and fetal plasma has provided evidence for fetal synthesis of C4 and for the absence of transplacental passage of this component [101].

DEFICIENCIES OF COMPLEMENT COMPONENTS ASSOCIATED WITH DEFECTS IN HOST RESISTANCE

Possible Familial Deficiency in C5 Function

A familial defect in the capacity of plasma to enhance the phagocytosis of certain particles by polymorphonuclear leukocytes has been described by Miller et al. [8]. The proband was an 18-month infant with recurrent gram negative bacterial infections, who improved dramatically with plasma transfusion therapy. Plasma from this infant failed to enhance the phagocytosis of yeast, rice-starch, or *Staphylococcus aureus* to the same extent as did normal plasma. A similar deficiency of opsonization was found in plasma from the patient's mother and several other relatives. Inheritance of this abnormality followed an autosomal pattern, but the available data did not permit distinction between a dominant or recessive mode of transmission.

The defect has been tentatively attributed to an abnormality of C5 [9]. Normal mouse serum partially restored the ability of the plasma of the proband to enhance phagocytosis, but serum from mice congenitally deficient in C5 was inactive in this regard. Highly purified human C5 also partially reconstituted the plasma defect. The C5 contained in the serum of the proband was normal on immunoelectrophoresis when analyzed with specific antibody prepared against normal human C5. Antigenic analysis gave a reaction of identity between the patient's C5 and normal human C5 using the same antiserum. Precise measurements of the hemolytic activity of the C5 of the patient are not yet available. The quantity of active C5 in the serum was sufficient to produce a normal result for the measurement of total hemolytic complement. C5 hemolytic activity also appeared to be normal when measured by the ability of the serum to restore the hemolytic activity of normal serum which had been treated with KCNS to destroy C3, C4, and C5, and then supplemented with purified C3 and C4.

A defect of C5 which impairs its ability to enhance the phagocytosis of certain antigens, but not of others, and leaves intact its antigenicity and its function in immune hemolysis has been postulated [9]. Additional studies will be required to determine the precise nature of this defect and to confirm the role of C5 in the enhancement of phagocytosis of certain antigens which has been postulated on the basis of this familial abnormality.

Deficiency of C1q Associated with Impaired Immunoglobulin Synthesis

In their original description of the serum protein C1q, Müller-Eberhard and Kunkel [97] observed reduced levels of this component in the sera of three patients with sex-linked agammaglobulinemia. More recently, O'Connell et al. [6] have described an infant with Swiss-type agammaglobulinemia who died at age 7 weeks and had no detectable hemolytic complement activity. Component analysis revealed absent C1 hemolytic activity, and radial immunodiffusion indicated that the serum was markedly deficient in C1q; C1r and C1s were not measured. Subsequently, moderate reductions in serum concentrations of C1q have been described in a variety of hypogammaglobulinemic states, including the congenital sex-linked, Swiss-type, and acquired forms [98]. A direct correlation between serum IgG levels and serum C1q has been observed [7].

These reductions in serum C1q levels may reflect impaired synthesis of this complement protein associated with impaired synthesis of immunoglobulins, or they may be secondary in some way to the reduced serum levels of IgG. Measurements of the catabolic and synthetic rates of C1q will be required before the relationships between agammaglobulinemic states and reduced serum levels of this component are clarified.

SUMMARY

1 Knowledge of the chemical nature and the reaction mechanisms of the nine serum proteins which constitute the complement system has led to the recognition of genetically controlled abnormalities of the structure or function of these proteins.

2 A deficiency of the inhibitor of the first component of complement, inherited as an autosomal dominant trait, is associated with hereditary angioedema. This disease is marked by recurrent attacks of subepithelial edema of the skin and gastrointestinal and upper respiratory tracts. Striking clinical features of angioedema of the hereditary type are repeated crampy abdominal pains and a high frequency of laryngeal edema. Biochemically, the disease is characterized by markedly reduced or absent activity of the normal α_2-globulin inhibitor of the first component of complement. About 10 percent of kindreds have a genetic variant form of the deficiency in which an antigenically intact but nonfunctional inhibitor protein is synthesized. The pathogenesis of the edema appears to involve a vasoactive peptide which is released from the second (C2) component of complement by uninhibited first component acting in the presence of the fourth (C4) component.

3 Deficiency of the second component of complement has been described in four kindreds. The sera of homozygous deficient individuals contain approximately 4 percent of the normal serum C2 activity; the sera of heterozygous deficient individuals contain approximately one-half the normal amounts. Correlation of C2 activity measurements with immunochemical determinations of C2 protein indicates that the C2 present in the sera of deficient individuals functions normally. Although the deficiency state is readily demonstrable in vitro, the small amounts of C2 present in the sera are apparently adequate to mediate the effects of natural antibody, and affected individuals manifest no apparent defects in host resistance.

4 Inherited structural polymorphisms of the third (C3) and fourth (C4) components of complement have been demonstrated. The electrophoretic mobility of C3 has been shown to be controlled by a single set of alleles, inherited as autosomal codominants. Two of the allotypes of C3 are common, and the other six are rare. A ninth allele, which is not expressed and results in half-normal serum C3 levels, has also been described. Applications of C3 allotyping have provided evidence that the liver is the primary, if not sole, site of synthesis of human C3. Inherited variations in the electrophoretic mobility of C4 have also been described. The seven distinct patterns of C4 mobility which have been observed appear to result from variations in the amounts of three electrophoretic subtypes, of which two are allelic. Differences in mobility have been associated with variations in the functional efficiency of the C4 molecule.

5 Defects in host resistance have been tentatively associated with abnormalities of two other components; the genetic bases for these abnormalities remain to be established. Absent or reduced serum levels of C1q, the binding subunit of C1, have been described in hypogammaglobulinemic states. A defect of plasma-mediated phagocytosis enhancement has been associated with impaired function of the fifth component.

BIBLIOGRAPHY

1. Donaldson, V. H., and Evans, R. R.: A biochemical abnormality in hereditary angioneurotic edema. Amer. J. Med., **35,** 37, 1963.
2. Klemperer, M. R., Woodworth, H. C., Rosen, F. S., and Austen, K. F.: Hereditary deficiency of the second component of complement (C'2) in man. J. Clin. Invest., **45,** 880, 1966.
3. Alper, C. A., Propp, R. P., Klemperer, M. R., and Rosen, F. S.: Inherited deficiency of the third component of human complement (C'3). J. Clin. Invest., **48,** 553, 1969.
4. Alper, C. A., and Propp, R. P.: Genetic polymorphism of the third component of human complement (C'3). J. Clin. Invest., **47,** 2181, 1968.
5. Rosenfeld, S. I., Ruddy, S., and Austen, K. F.: Structural polymorphism of the fourth component of human complement. J. Clin. Invest., **48,** 2283, 1969.
6. O'Connell, E. J., Enriques, P., Linman, J. W., Gleich, G. J., and McDuffie, F. C.: Swiss type agammaglobulinemia associated with an abnormality of the inflammatory response (abstr.). J. Pediat., **69,** 981, 1966.

7. Kohler, P. F., and Müller-Eberhard, H. J.: Complement-immunoglobulin relation: Deficiency of C1q associated with impaired immunoglobulin G synthesis. Science, **163,** 474, 1969.
8. Miller, M. E., Seals, J., Kaye, R., and Lentsky, L.: A familial plasma-associated defect of phagocytosis. Lancet, **2,** 60, 1968.
9. Nilsson, U. R., and Heym, G.: Studies on the chemical nature of the fifth component of human complement (C5) (abstr.). Fed. Proc., **28,** 818, 1969.
10. World Health Organization: Nomenclature of complement. Bull. W.H.O., **39,** 935, 1968.
11. Mayer, M. M.: Mechanism of hemolysis by complement, in *Ciba Foundation Symposium on Complement,* edited by G. E. W. Wolstenholm and J. Knight, p. 4. Churchill, London, 1965.
12. Nelson, R. A.: The role of complement in immune phenomena, in *The Inflammatory Process,* edited by B. W. Zweifach, L. H. Grant, and R. T. McCluskey, p. 819. Academic, New York, 1965.
13. Müller-Eberhard, H. J.: Chemistry and reaction mechanisms of the complement system. Advances Immun., **8,** 1, 1968.
14. Lepow, I. H., Naff, G. B., Todd, E. W., Pensky, J., and Hinz, C. F.: Chromatographic resolution of the first component of human complement into three activities. J. Exp. Med., **117,** 983, 1961.
15. Pensky, J., and Schwick, H. G.: Human serum inhibitor of C′1 esterase. Identity with α2-neuraminoglycoprotein. Science, **163,** 698, 1969.
16. West, C. D., Davis, N. C., Forristal, J., Herbst, J., and Spitzer, R.: Antigenic determinants of human β1C and β1G globulins. J. Immun., **96,** 650, 1966.
17. Ruddy, S., and Austen, K. F.: C3 inactivator of man. I. Hemolytic measurement by the inactivation of cell-bound C3. J. Immun., **102,** 533, 1969.
18. Shultz, D. R., and Zarco, R. A.: Inhibition of the eighth component of complement (C8) by chelating agents. Fed. Proc., **28,** 818, 1969.
19. Christian, C. L.: Studies of aggregated γ globulin. J. Immun., **84,** 112, 1960.
20. Borsos, T., and Rapp, H. J.: Hemolysin titration based on fixation of the activated first component of complement. Evidence that one molecule of hemolysin suffices to sensitize an erythrocyte. J. Immun., **95,** 559, 1965.
21. Becker, E. L.: Concerning the mechanism of complement action. IV. The properties of activated first component of guinea pig complement. J. Immun., **82,** 43, 1958.
22. Ratnoff, O. D., and Naff, G. B.: The conversion of C′1s to C′1 esterase by plasmin and trypsin. J. Exp. Med., **125,** 337, 1967.
23. Lepow, I. H., Ratnoff, O. D., Rosen, F. S., and Pillemer, L.: Observations on a proesterase associated with partially purified first component of human complement (C′1). Proc. Soc. Exp. Biol. Med., **92,** 32, 1956.
24. Patrick, R. A., and Lepow, I. H.: Fragmentation of the fourth component of human complement by C1s (abstr.). Fed. Proc., **28,** 817, 1969.
25. Müller-Eberhard, H. J., and Biro, C. F.: Isolation and description of the fourth component of human complement. J. Exp. Med., **118,** 447, 1963.
26. Gigli, I., and Austen, K. F.: Fluid phase destruction of $C2^{hu}$ by $C1^{hu}$. I. Its enhancement and inhibition by homologous and heterologous C4. J. Exp. Med., **129,** 679, 1969.
27. Sitomer, G., Stroud, R. M., and Mayer, M. M.: Reversible adsorption of C2 by EAC′4: Role of Mg^{2+}, enumeration of competent SAC′4: two-step nature of C′2a fixation and estimation of its efficiency. Immunochem., **3,** 57, 1966.
28. Stroud, R. M., Mayer, M. M., Miller, J. A., and McKenzie, A. T.: $C'2a^{d}$, an inactive derivative of C′2 released during decay of EAC′4, 2a. Immunochem., **3,** 163, 1966.
29. Müller-Eberhard, H. J., Polley, M. J., and Calcott, M. A.: Formation and functional significance of a molecular complex derived from the second and the fourth components of human complement. J. Exp. Med., **125,** 359, 1967.
30. Dias da Silva, W., and Lepow, I. H.: Complement as a mediator of inflammation. II. Biological properties of anaphylatoxin prepared with purified components of human complement. J. Exp. Med., **125,** 921, 1967.
31. Gigli, I., and Nelson, R. A.: Complement dependent immune phagocytosis. Exp. Cell Res., **51,** 45, 1968.
32. Lachmann, P. J., and Müller-Eberhard, H. J.: The demonstration in human serum of "conglutinogen-activating factor" and its effect on the third component of complement. J. Immun., **100,** 691, 1968.
33. Cochrane, C. G., and Müller-Eberhard, H. J.: The derivation of two distinct anaphylatoxin activities from the third and fifth components of human complement. J. Exp. Med., **122,** 99, 1968.
34. Ward, P. A., and Newman, L. J.: A neutrophil chemotactic factor from human C5. J. Immun., **102,** 93, 1969.
35. Tamura, N., and Nelson, R. A.: Three naturally occurring inhibitors of components of complement in guinea pig and rabbit serum. J. Immun., **94,** 582, 1967.
36. Ward, P. A., Cochrane, C. G., and Müller-Eberhard, H. J.: Further studies on the chemotactic factor of complement and its formation *in vivo.* Immunology, **11,** 141, 1966.
37. Götze, O., and Müller-Eberhard, H. J.: Lysis of erythrocytes by complement in the absence of antibody. J. Exp. Med., **132** (5), 898, 1970.
38. Pickering, R. J., Wolfson, M. R., Good, R. A., and Gewurz, H.: Hemolysis induced by cobra venom factor activation of terminal complement components in guinea pig serum. Fed. Proc., **28,** 818, 1969.
39. Stolfi, R.: Immune lytic transformation. A state of irreversible damage generated as a result of the reaction of the eighth component of the guinea pig complement system. J. Immun., **100,** 46, 1968.
40. Rosse, W. F., Dourmashkin, R. R., and Humphrey, J. H.: Immune lysis of normal human and paroxysmal nocturnal hemoglobinuria (PNH) red blood cells. III. The membrane defects caused by complement lysis. J. Exp. Med., **123,** 969, 1966.
41. Borsos, T., Dourmashkin, R. R., and Humphrey, J. H.: Lesions in erythrocyte membranes caused by immune hemolysis. Nature (London), **202,** 251, 1964.
42. Smith, J. K., and Becker, E. L.: Serum complement and the enzymatic degradation of erythrocyte phospholipid. J. Immun., **100,** 459, 1968.
43. Rosen, F. S., Charache, P., Pensky, J., and Donaldson, V.: Hereditary angioneurotic edema: Two genetic variants. Science, **148,** 957, 1965.
44. Ruddy, S., Carpenter, C. B., Austen, K. F., and Müller-Eberhard, H. J.: Complement component levels in hereditary angioedema and isolated C2 deficiency in man, in *Mechanisms of Inflammation Induced by Immune Reactions,* 5th International Immunopathology Symposium, edited by P. A. Miescher and P. Grabar, p. 231. Schwabe & Co., Basel, 1968.
45. West, C. D., Northway, J. D., and Davis, N. C.: Serum levels of β1C globulin, a complement component, in the nephritides, lipoid nephrosis, and other conditions. J. Clin. Invest., **43,** 1507, 1964.
46. Kohler, P. F., and Müller-Eberhard, H. J.: Immunochemical quantitation of the third, fourth and fifth components of human complement: Concentrations in the serum of healthy adults. J. Immun., **99,** 1211, 1967.
47. Mancini, G., Vaerman, J. P., Carbonara, A. O., and Heremans, J. F.: Single radio-diffusion method for immunological quantitation of proteins, in *Colloquium on the Protides of Biological Fluids.* Proc. 10th/11th Colloqu., edited by H. Peeters, p. 370. Elsevier, Amsterdam, 1963.
48. Mayer, M. M.: Complement and complement fixation, in *Experimental Immunochemistry,* edited by E. A. Kabat and M. M. Mayer, p. 135. Charles C Thomas, Springfield, Ill., 1961.
49. Ruddy, S., and Austen, K. F.: Stoichiometric measurement of the activity of the fourth component of complement (C′4) in whole human serum. J. Immun., **99,** 1162, 1967.
50. Borsos, T., and Rapp, H. J.: Chromatographic separation of the first component of complement and its assay on a molecular basis. J. Immun., **91,** 851, 1963.
51. Gigli, I., Ruddy, S., and Austen, K. F.: The stoichiometric measurement of the serum inhibitor of the first component of complement by the inhibition of immune hemolysis. J. Immun., **100,** 1154, 1968.
52. Borsos, T., and Rapp, H. J.: Immune hemolysis. A simplified method for the preparation of EAC′4 with guinea pig or human complement. J. Immun., **99,** 263, 1967.
53. Osler, W.: Hereditary angio-neurotic edema. Amer. J. Med. Sci., **95,** 362, 1888.
54. Crowder, J. R., and Crowder, T. R.: Five generations of angioneurotic edema. Arch. Intern. Med., **20,** 840, 1917.
55. Donaldson, V. H., and Rosen, F. S.: Hereditary angioneurotic edema: A clinical survey. Pediatrics, **37,** 1017, 1966.

56. Landerman, N. S.: Hereditary angioneurotic edema. I. Case reports and review of the literature. J. Allerg., **33**, 316, 1962.
57. Thorvaldsson, S. E., Sedlack, R. E., Gleich, G. J., and Ruddy, S.: Angioneurotic edema and deficiency of C′1 esterase inhibitor in a 61 year old woman. Ann. Int. Med. **71**, 353, 1969.
58. Sheffer, A. L.: Personal communication.
59. Spaulding, W. B.: Hereditary angioneurotic edema in two families. Canad. Med. Ass. J., **73**, 181, 1955.
60. Austen, K. F., and Sheffer, A. L.: Detection of hereditary angioneurotic edema by demonstration of a reduction in the second component of human complement. New Eng. J. Med., **272**, 649, 1965.
61. Sheffer, A. L., Craig, J. M., Wilms-Kretschmer, K., Austen, K. F., and Rosen, F. S.: Histopathological and ultrastructural observations on tissues from patients with hereditary angioneurotic edema. J. Allerg., (in press).
62. Pickering, R. J., Kelly, J. R., Good, R. A., and Gewurz, H.: Replacement therapy in hereditary angioedema: Successful treatment of two patients with fresh frozen plasma. Lancet, **1**, 326, 1969.
63. Rosen, F. S., and Austen, K. F.: The "Neurotic Edema" (Hereditary Angioedema). (Editorial). New Eng. J. Med., **280**, 1356, 1969.
64. Nilsson, I. M., Andersson, L., and Bjorkman, S. E.: Epsilonaminocaproic acid (E-ACA) as a therapeutic agent. Based on 5 years' clinical experience. Acta Med. Scand. Suppl., **448**, 21, 1966.
65. Lundh, B., Laurell, A. B., Wetterquist, H., White, T., and Granerus, G.: A case of hereditary angioneurotic edema treated with E-aminocaproic acid. Clin. Exp. Immun., **3**, 733, 1968.
66. Spaulding, W. B.: Methyl testosterone therapy for hereditary episodic edema (hereditary angioneurotic edema). Ann. Intern. Med., **53**, 739, 1960.
67. Donaldson, V. H., and Rosen, F. S.: Action of complement in hereditary angioneurotic edema: Role of C′1 esterase. J. Clin. Invest., **43**, 2204, 1964.
68. Carpenter, C. B., Ruddy, S., Shehadeh, I. H., Müller-Eberhard, H. J., Merrill, J. P., and Austen, K. F.: Complement metabolism in man: Hypercatabolism of the fourth (C′4) and third (C′3) components in patients with renal allograft rejection and hereditary angioedema. J. Clin. Invest., **48**, 1495, 1969.
69. Klemperer, M. R., Donaldson, V. H., and Rosen, F. S.: Effect of C1 esterase on vascular permeability in man: Studies in normal and complement-deficient individuals and in patients with hereditary angioneurotic edema. J. Clin. Invest., **47**, 604, 1968.
70. Donaldson, V. H., Ratnoff, O. D., Dias da Silva, W., and Rosen, F. S.: Permeability-increasing activity in hereditary angioneurotic edema plasma. II. Mechanism of formation and partial characterization. J. Clin. Invest., **48**, 642, 1969.
71. Naff, G. B., and Ratnoff, O. D.: The enzymatic nature of C′1r: Conversion of C′1s to C′1 esterase and digestion of amino acid esters by C′1r. J. Exp. Med., **128**, 571, 1968.
72. Donaldson, V. H., Ratnoff, O. D., Klemperer, M. R., and Rosen, F. S.: Studies on a peptide from hereditary angioneurotic edema plasma with permeability factor and kinin activity (abstr.). J. Immun., **101**, 818, 1968.
73. Hallberg, G. G., Laurell, A. B., and Wetterquist, H.: Studies on the histamine metabolism and the complement system in hereditary angioneurotic edema. Acta Med. Scand., **182**, 11, 1967.
74. Landerman, N. S., Webster, M. E., Becker, E. L., and Ratcliffe, H. E.: Hereditary angioneurotic edema. II. Deficiency of inhibitor for serum globulin permeability factor and/or plasma kallikrein. J. Allerg., **33**, 330, 1962.
75. Gigli, I., Mason, J. W., Colman, R. W., and Austen, K. F.: Interaction of plasma kallikrein with the C′1 inhibitor (C′1a INH) J. Immun., **104**, 574, 1970.
76. Ruddy, S., Gigli, I., Sheffer, A. L., and Austen, K. F.: The laboratory diagnosis of hereditary angioedema, in *Allergology Proceedings of the Sixth Congress of the International Association of Allergology*, edited by B. Rose, M. Richter, A. Sehon and A. W. Frankland, Excerpta Medica Foundation, Amsterdam, 1968.
77. Schur, P. H., and Austen, K. F.: Complement in human disease. Ann. Rev. Med., **19**, 1, 1968.
78. Kohler, P. F., and tenBensel, R.: Serial complement component alterations in acute glomerulonephritis and systemic lupus erythematosus. Clin. Exp. Immun., **4**, 191, 1969.
79. Levy, L. R., and Lepow, I. H.: Assay and properties of a serum inhibitor of C1 esterase. Proc. Soc. Exp. Biol., **101**, 608, 1959.
80. Rosen, F. S.: Personal communication.
81. Woodworth, H. C.: Unpublished observations. 1958.
82. Silverstein, A. M.: Essential hypocomplementemia: Report of a case. Blood, **16**, 1338, 1960.
83. Klemperer, M. R., and Austen, K. F., and Rosen, F. S.: Hereditary deficiency of the second component of complement (C′2) in man: Further observations on a second kindred. J. Immun., **98**, 72, 1967.
84. Ruddy, S., and Austen, K. F.: Disease and non-disease associated with inherited disorders of the complement system in man, in *Protides of the Biological Fluids, 15th Colloquium*, edited by H. Peeters, p. 401. Elsevier, Amsterdam, 1968.
85. Klemperer, M. R.: Hereditary deficiency of the second component of complement in man: An immunochemical study. J. Immun., **102**, 168, 1969.
86. Polley, M. J.: Inherited C2 deficiency in man: Lack of immunochemically detectable C2 protein in serum from deficient individuals. Science, **161**, 1149, 1968.
87. Gewurz, H., Pickering, R. J., Muschel, L. H., Mergenhagen, S. E., and Good, R. A.: Complement dependent biological functions in complement deficiency in man. Lancet, **2**, 356, 1966.
88. Cooper, N. R., tenBensel, R., and Kohler, P. F.: Studies of an additional kindred with hereditary deficiency of the second component of human complement (C2) and description of a new method for the quantitation of C2. J. Immun., **101**, 1176, 1968.
89. Kumate, J.: Meningitis repetidas asocidas con hipocomplementemia. Presented at the 15th Meeting of the Associacion de Investigacion Pediatrica, Mexico D.F., 1962.
90. Ruddy, S., Klemperer, M. R., Rosen, F. S., Austen, K. F., and Kumate, J.: Hereditary deficiency of the second component of complement in man: Correlation of C2 hemolytic activity with immunochemical measurements of C2 protein. Immunology, **18**, 943, 1970.
91. Wieme, R. J., Demeulenaere, L., and Segers, J.: Familial occurrence of electrophoretic C′3 variant in man, in *Protides of the Biological Fluids, 15th Colloquium*, edited by H. Peeters, p. 499. Elsevier, Amsterdam, 1968.
92. Azen, E. A., and Smithies, O.: Genetic polymorphism of C′3 (β1C-globulin) in human serum. Science, **162**, 905, 1968.
93. Alper, C. A., and Rosen, F. S.: Studies of a hypomorphic variant of human C3, J. Clin. Invest., **50**, 324, 1971.
94. Laurell, C. B.: Antigen-antibody crossed electrophoresis. Anal. Biochem., **10**, 358, 1965.
95. Alper, C. A., Johnson, M. A., Birtch, A. G., and Moore, F. D.: Human C′3: Evidence for the liver as the primary site of synthesis. Science, **163**, 286, 1969.
96. Propp, R. P., and Alper, C. A.: C′3 synthesis in human fetus and lack of transplacental passage. Science, **162**, 672, 1968.
97. Müller-Eberhard, H. J., and Kunkel, H. G.: Isolation of a thermolabile serum protein which precipitates γglobulin aggregates and participates in immune hemolysis. Proc. Soc. Exp. Biol. Med., **106**, 291, 1961.
98. Gewurz, H., Pickering, R. J., Christian, R., Snyderman, R., Mergenhagen, S. E., and Good, R. A.: Decreased C1q protein concentration and agglutinating activity in agammaglobulinemia syndromes. An inborn error reflected in the complement system. Clin. Exp. Immun., **3**, 437, 1968.
99. Johnson, A. M., Alper, C. A., Rosen, F. S., and Craig, J. M.: $C\bar{1}$ inhibitor: Evidence for decreased hepatic synthesis in hereditary angioneurotic edema. (Submitted for publication.)
100. Rosen, F. S., Alper, C. A., Pensky, J., Klemperer, M. R., and Donaldson, V. H.: The genetic determinants of heterogeneity of the C1 esterase inhibitor in patients with hereditary angioneurotic edema. (Submitted for publication.)
101. Bach, S., Ruddy, S., MacLaren, J. A., and Austen, K. F.: Electrophoretic polymorphism of the fourth component of human complement (C4) in paired maternal and fetal plasmas. Immunology (in press).

CHAPTER SEVENTY-TWO

HEREDITARY DISORDERS OF HEMOSTASIS*

Oscar D. Ratnoff

In few areas of medicine has an understanding of hereditary pathologic states and of normal physiologic and biochemical processes been so mutually interdependent as in the study of hemostasis. Fortunately, the last few years have allowed us to see blood clotting as the product of a series of enzymatic reactions which do not differ essentially from other biochemical processes. The common assumption that knowledge about blood coagulation and its abnormalities is in a chaotic state has little justification. To some extent, this view arises from the confusing terminology which plagues this field. A glossary of the nomenclature used in this chapter is provided in Table 72-1.

PHYSIOLOGY OF HEMOSTASIS

Fibrinogen

In mammalian plasma, clotting results from the conversion of soluble *fibrinogen* into insoluble *fibrin* through the action of an enzyme, thrombin (Fig. 72-1). Fibrinogen is a protein, synthesized in the liver, as demonstrated in perfused organ [1–3] and tissue slice [4] preparations. It is the only clotting factor which can be assayed chemically or gravimetrically. In normal human plasma it has an average concentration of about 300 mg per 100 ml [5, 6]. Highly purified preparations of human fibrinogen can be made by alcohol [7, 8] or ether fractionation of plasma [9].

Fibrinogen of human or bovine origin has a molecular weight of about 340,000, a sedimentation coefficient of 7.6 to 7.9, and a molecular length variously estimated as 240 to 600 Å, depending on the technique used and the pH at which the measurement is made [9–14]. The suggestion has been offered that fibrinogen consists of a heterogeneous group of proteins [15, 16]. The molecule is long and thin. Its greatest width is 50 to 65 Å, and under the electron microscope it appears to consist of three small nodules held together by a thin thread [13]. Each molecule is composed of three pairs of polypeptide chains, α(A), β(B), and γ respectively, held together by sulfhydryl bonds [17, 18].

The long-suspected proteolytic nature of the action of thrombin on fibrinogen was established independently by Bettelheim and Bailey [19] and Lóránd and Middlebrook [20]. Thrombin probably splits arginylglycine bonds in fibrinogen molecules. This releases several small polypeptide fragments and decreases its molecular weight by about 3 percent [21, 22]. Two polypeptides are removed from the α(A) chains and two others from the β(B) chains; the polypeptides are probably split from the terminal nodules of the fibrinogen molecule [12, 23]. Fibrinopeptide B may have a physiologic function in hemostatis, since it possesses the capacity to potentiate the contraction of smooth muscle by bradykinin [24].

The monomers of fibrin polymerize to form strands in which each end of a molecule attaches to the opposite end of another, probably through hydrogen bonds [25], although the possibility that the linkage is through readily dissoluble covalent bonds has been suggested [26]. The strands also grow in thickness to as much as 0.1 micron in diameter, presumably by the formation of side-to-side linkages [23]. Under the electron microscope the fibers are seen to have cross striations, which perhaps reflect the submolecular nodules [13, 27]. These various reactions lead to the formation of macroscopic fibrin strands.

The coagulant properties of fibrinogen are linked in an unexplained way to its content of carbohydrate, some of which may be released during the cross-bonding of fibrinogen molecules brought about by fibrin stabilizing factor (*see below*) [25]. Carbohydrate accounts for 3 to 4 percent of the molecular weight [12, 28]. Fibrinogen also contains small amounts of phosphorus, a significant part of which is lost during clotting [29]. Coagulation is accelerated by the presence of calcium ions at physiologic concentrations [30–32] and by a heat-labile accelerator in normal plasma [33–35]. Calcium ions probably speed the polymerization of fibrin monomers, but the site of action of the plasma accelerator is not yet known.

Fibrin prepared by incubating purified fibrinogen and thrombin has low tensile strength [36] and is soluble in 30 percent urea [37, 38]. In contrast, fibrin formed in plasma has high tensile strength and is insoluble in urea. The differences in the properties of these fibrins are due to the presence in plasma of a specific globulin, *fibrin-stabilizing factor* [38, 39] (fibrinase [40], factor XIII). Fibrin-stabilizing factor is a relatively labile substance [37] with a molecular weight of about 300,000 [40]. Its effect upon fibrin depends upon its activation by thrombin [42], its content of sulfhydryl groups [43], and the presence of calcium ions in the milieu of the reaction [36]. Loewy et al. [44] envision that fibrin-stabilizing factor catalyzes formation of links between amide groups and amino groups on adjacent fibrin molecules, a process described as transamidation. This involves amides of γ-carboxyl glutamine and probably β-carboxyl asparagine residues of one fibrin monomer and the epsilon-amino groups of lysyl residues on adjacent fibrin monomers [41, 45], with the release of ammonia. Recognition of the transamidation function of fibrin-stabilizing factor has led to its

*Included in this chapter are the results of unpublished studies supported in part by Research Grant HE 01661 from the National Heart Institute of the National Institutes of Health, Public Health Service, and in part by a grant from the American Heart Association.

Table 72-1. GLOSSARY

Terms used in this chapter	Synonyms
Fibrinogen	Factor I
Thrombin	Biothrombin
Prothrombin	Factor II, prethrombin (?)
Tissue thromboplastin	Factor III, thrombokinase
Calcium	Factor IV
Accelerin	Thrombin-activated proaccelerin
Proaccelerin	Factor V, labile factor, plasma accelerator globulin, plasma Ac globulin
Stuart factor	Factor X, Stuart-Prower factor, autoprothrombin III
Activated Stuart factor	Autoprothrombin C, plasma thrombokinase
Factor VII	Pro-SPCA, precursor of serum prothrombin conversion accelerator, autoprothrombin I
Proconvertin	Usually applied collectively for Stuart factor and factor VII, but sometimes to factor VII alone; stable factor
Antihemophilic factor	Factor VIII, antihemophilic globulin, antihemophilic factor A, platelet cofactor I
Christmas factor	Factor IX, plasma thromboplastin component (PTC), autoprothrombin II, antihemophilic factor B
Plasma thromboplastin antecedent (PTA)	Factor XI, antihemophilic factor C
Hageman factor	Factor XII
Fibrin-stabilizing factor	Factor XIII, fibrinase
Prothrombin-converting principle	Prothrombinase

in vitro assay by measurement of incorporation of ^{14}C-glycine ethyl ester into casein or fibrin [41] or of monodansyl cadaverine into casein [46]. The carbohydrate moiety of fibrinogen is also intimately related to the functioning of fibrin-stabilizing factor [47]. An additional biologic function of this factor has been suggested by studies in which the growth of human fibroblasts in tissue culture was enhanced by its presence [48]. Platelets, as well as plasma, possess fibrin-stabilizing factor activity. Evidence has accrued that this activity arises within the megakaryocytes and is not adsorbed from plasma [49].

Thrombin

Thrombin evolves during clotting from a precursor, prothrombin. Its sedimentation constant and molecular weight are disputed [50–53], but the latter is probably 13,000 to 14,000 [54, 55]. Preparations with higher molecular weights may contain dimeric forms. The hydrolytic nature of thrombin has been inferred not only from its effect upon fibrinogen but also from its ability to digest synthetic substrates hydrolyzed by other proteases, for example, *p*-toluene sulfonyl-L-arginine methyl ester (TAMe) [56], various *p*-nitrophenylesters [57, 58], α-N-toluene-*p*-sulfonyl-L-lysine methyl ester [59], L-histidine methyl ester [60], and benzoyl arginyl *p*-nitroanilide (BAPA) [61]. Moreover, thrombin is said to digest other proteins such as the oxidized β chain of insulin [62] and albumin [63]. Like certain other hydrolytic enzymes, it is inactivated by diisopropylphosphofluoridate (DFP), which reacts with serine residues [22, 64, 65]. This observation has led to elucidation of the sequence of amino acids at the active site of thrombin, namely, glycyl-aspartyl-seryl-glycyl-glutamyl-alanine [66]. This arrangement is similar to trypsin, chymotrypsin, and elastase. Consonant with these observations is the finding that TAMe [56] and *p*-toluenesulfonylarginylglycine [67] inhibit fibrin formation, presumably in a competitive manner.

The best-known function of thrombin is conversion of fibrinogen to fibrin monomer by splitting off fibrinopeptides A and B. Additionally, its activates fibrin-stabilizing factor and alters antihemophilic factor (factor VIII) and proaccelerin (factor V) so as to potentiate their clot-promoting properties. Thrombin is also important for the hemostatic behavior of platelets, in that it participates in reactions leading to their aggregation and viscous metamorphosis and to the phenomenon of clot retraction.

The thrombin which forms during clotting disappears rapidly. In part this is due to its adsorption to the fibrin clot [68]. In addition plasma has potent thrombin-inhibitory activity [69], a property residing in the α-globulin fraction (see below). Heparin also exerts a powerful antithrombic effect but probably does not exist in normal blood. Teleologically, these thrombin-inactivating mechanisms are appealing, for they provide ways through which clot formation within the body may be self-limiting.

Prothrombin

Prothrombin, the precursor of thrombin, is a globulin with a sedimentation constant probably of 4.6 [70] and a molecu-

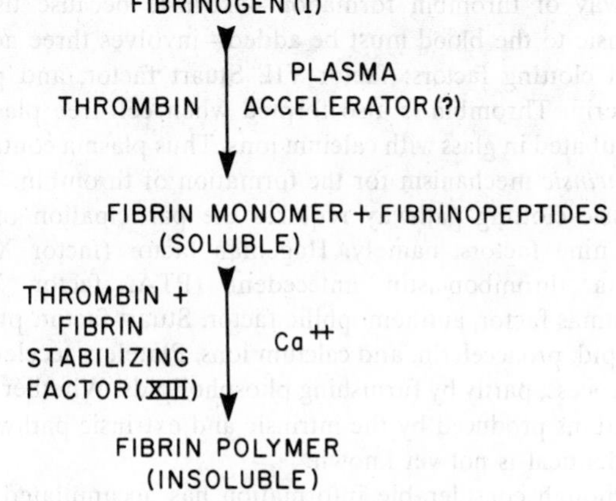

Figure 72-1. Steps in the formation of fibrin.

lar weight of 68,000. The molecule dissociates to a molecular weight of 34,000 on dilution [51, 71]. Studies of human prothrombin indicate that at most about 80 mg and probably much less are present per liter of plasma [72]. Human prothrombin migrates with the α_2-globulins on paper electrophoresis [73] and with the α_1-globulins upon curtain electrophoresis of plasma [74]. It is precipitated in fraction III-2 by Cohn's method [75]. Preparations of prothrombin contain carbohydrate [76, 77]. Prothrombin is synthesized in the liver [78–80], apparently by the parenchymal cells [81]. The synthesis takes place only when adequate supplies of vitamin K are available [82–84]. This important property is shared with Stuart factor (factor X), factor VII (the precursor of serum prothrombin conversion accelerator: pro-SPCA), and Christmas factor (factor IX, plasma thromboplastin component) (see below).

The purification of prothrombin has been difficult. Like the other vitamin K-dependent clotting factors, it is readily adsorbed onto certain insoluble alkaline earth compounds, such as barium sulfate, calcium phosphate, and aluminum or magnesium hydroxide, and can then be eluted with sodium citrate solution. Much of the controversy concerning the change of prothrombin to thrombin has arisen from problems of separation of prothrombin from other clotting factors [85]. In most procedures further purification has been achieved by column chromatography on calcium phosphate gel, diethylaminoethyl cellulose, or Amberlite IRC 50 [86–88]. The technique of Malhotra and Carter [89], in which bovine plasma is first adsorbed with barium sulfate under conditions which leave most of the prothrombin in solution, avoids the use of cellulose columns and still provides a prothrombin of high purity; this overcomes some of the theoretical objections raised by chromatographic procedures.

Most of the research in blood coagulation during the last 80 years has been stimulated by the effort to understand how prothrombin changes to thrombin. In general, two pathways have been delineated through which thrombin may evolve under physiologic conditions. When particles of tissue—*tissue thromboplastin*—are mixed with plasma and calcium ions, thrombin is rapidly generated. This *extrinsic* pathway of thrombin formation—extrinsic because tissue extrinsic to the blood must be added—involves three additional clotting factors: factor VII, Stuart factor, and proaccelerin. Thrombin is also formed when cell-free plasma is incubated in glass with calcium ions. Thus plasma contains an *intrinsic* mechanism for the formation of thrombin. The intrinsic clotting pathway requires the participation of at least nine factors, namely, Hageman factor (factor XII), plasma thromboplastin antecedent (PTA, factor XI), Christmas factor, antihemophilic factor, Stuart factor, phospholipid, proaccelerin, and calcium ions. Platelets accelerate the process, partly by furnishing phospholipids. Whether the thrombins produced by the intrinsic and extrinsic pathways are identical is not yet known.

Although considerable information has accumulated regarding the nature of the various clotting factors, an intimate knowledge of their mode of action is lacking. The sequence of events shown in Figs. 72-2 and 72-3 is one among several possible formulations and should be viewed critically. Clotting can be visualized as the end result of a series of enzymatic steps. Some of the clotting factors appear to be proenzymes, and the clotting process seems to be related to the activation of these substances.

Hageman Factor

The first identified reaction leading to thrombin formation in the intrinsic clotting pathway is the activation of Hageman factor by glass or similar surfaces [90–92]. Hageman factor is a protein found in plasma and serum in most mammalian species but lacking in the plasma of dolphins, killer whales [93], and fowl [92]. Its site of synthesis is unknown. Tentatively, a gene locus responsible for synthesis has been identified on the short arm of chromosome 6 [94].

Hageman factor is precipitated from human plasma maximally in Cohn fractions III and IV [95]. Hageman factor migrates in the area between β- and γ-globulins during paper electrophoresis of plasma, but with curtain electrophoresis activity attributed to this factor migrates over a wide range, encompassing α-, β-, and γ-globulins [74]. Hageman factor has been purified 3,000- to 5,000-fold [96, 97]; when separated from human plasma, preparations invariably contain a fraction in the activated form. The sedimentation constant of Hageman factor is about 5, and it has an apparent molecular weight of approximately 80,000 [98]. The effect of glass and similar surfaces in activating Hageman factor is not understood, but it can be duplicated by certain soluble substances, notably ellagic acid (4,4′,5,5′,6,6′-hexahydroxydiphenic acid-2,6,2′,6′-dilactone), an oxidation product of gallic acid [99]. The activated form of Hageman factor behaves as if

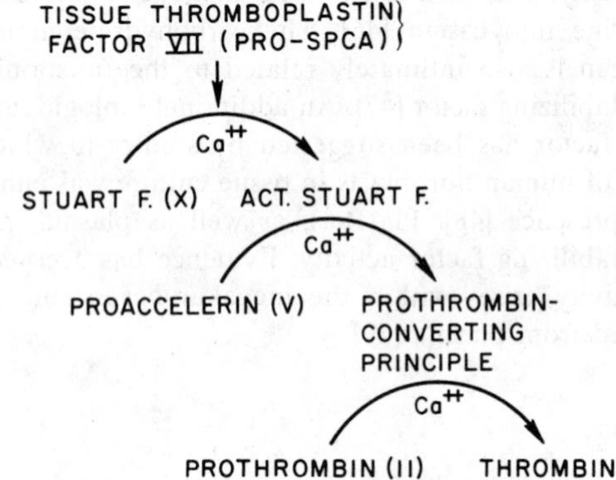

Figure 72-2. Extrinsic clotting pathway for the formation of thrombin. Omitted from the diagram are inhibitors of various steps and the alteration induced by thrombin in proaccelerin. The phospholipid portion of tissue thromboplastin may function in the formation and action of the prothrombin-converting principle. (*From Prentice and Ratnoff* [274].)

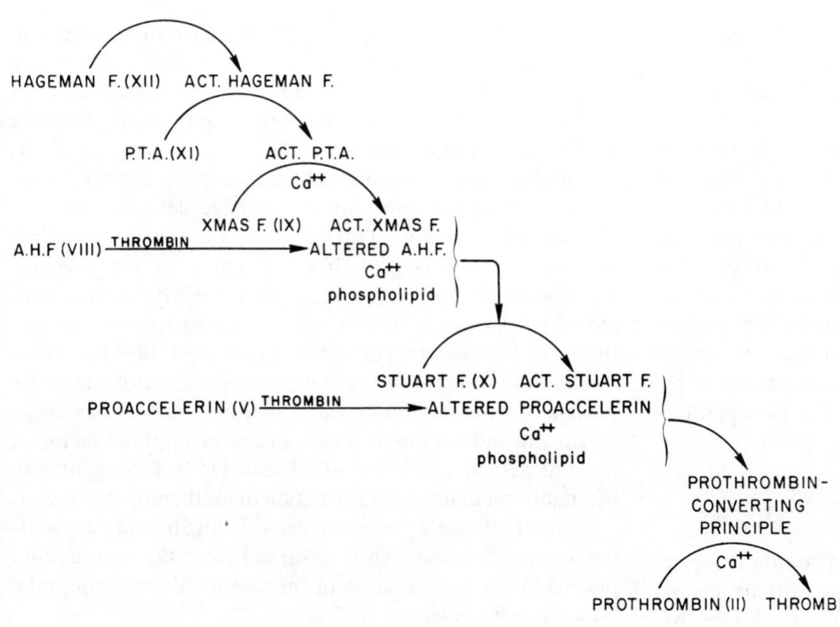

Figure 72-3. The intrinsic pathway of thrombin formation. (PTA = plasma thromboplastin antecedent; Xmas F = Christmas factor; AHF = antihemophilic factor.)

it were much less soluble in aqueous media than its precursor or as if polymerized [98].

What normally activates Hageman factor in vivo is not known. Contact with skin seems to induce activation, an effect attributed to sebum [100]. Further, collagen appears to activate Hageman factor, an action dependent upon the presence of free carboxyl groups on the collagen molecule [101, 102]. The asymptomatic nature of Hageman trait, the hereditary deficiency of plasma Hageman factor, may diminish the physiologic importance of these observations.

Activated Hageman factor acts like an enzyme but lacks the esterolytic activity of some proteases [103]. Hageman factor may also act directly on platelets to release a clot-promoting agent [104]. Its role in clotting is the activation of PTA [105–109]. Activated Hageman factor also participates in the activation of factors in plasma which increase vascular permeability [110, 111], dilate blood vessels [112], contract smooth muscle [113], provoke pain [114], promote white blood cell migration through small blood vessels [115], induce fibrinolysis[116–118], and convert the first component of complement to C′1 esterase [119].

Plasma Thromboplastin Antecedent (PTA)

Virtually nothing is known about the properties of PTA except that it is a protein which is found both in plasma and serum. Plasma adsorbed with aluminum hydroxide gel loses an appreciable fraction of PTA activity. Its tissue of origin is unknown. Purification of PTA has not been achieved, but trace amounts, lacking other clotting factors, have been prepared [105, 120]. Both on paper and on curtain electrophoresis, PTA migrates in the region of the β- and γ-globulins [74, 121]. When PTA is incubated with activated Hageman factor, clot-promoting properties rapidly appear which are attributable to *activated* PTA. Whatever the change which occurs during activation, no gross alteration occurs in the sedimentation constant, which is approximately 5 to 6, as determined by sucrose gradient ultracentrifugation [98]. Activated PTA has been highly purified [118, 122], but our best preparations are still contaminated with two other substrates of Hageman factor, plasma kallikrein, an agent participating in experimental inflammation, and Hageman factor-cofactor, which changes plasminogen to plasmin, a plasma proteolytic enzyme. Activated PTA is probably a hydrolytic enzyme since it can be inhibited by DFP [105, 122]; its molecular weight is approximately 165,000 [118]. Studies with radioactive DFP indicate that, like certain other hydrolytic enzymes, the active site of enzyme action contains serine [122]. Preparations free of kallikrein can be prepared by chromatography on hydroxyl apatite [61].

Hageman trait, the hereditary absence of Hageman factor, is not usually associated with a bleeding tendency. It is therefore of interest that crude preparations of PTA lacking detectable Hageman factor slowly form activated PTA [105]. This process is accelerated by the sodium soaps of saturated long-chain fatty acids [123]. Perhaps, then, mechanisms exist for initiating the clotting process independent of Hageman factor.

Christmas Factor

The next step in the intrinsic clotting process is the activation of Christmas factor by activated PTA [108, 121, 124–126]. This process requires calcium ions [124, 126] and is probably inhibited by small amounts of heparin [126]. Christmas factor is probably synthesized in the liver, and vitamin K is needed. Christmas factor has been only partially purified. Concentrates are readily made by taking advantage of its adsorption by the salts of alkaline earths, but attempts to separate it from the other vitamin K–dependent clotting factors only lead to deterioration. Christmas factor is a protein which migrates as a β_2-globulin on paper electrophoresis of plasma [127] but with the α-globulins and albumin upon curtain electrophoresis [74]. A sedimentation constant of 3.8 [128] and a molecular weight of 110,000 [129] have been reported. The chemical change induced in Christmas factor by activated PTA is not known, but probably the modification of the molecule is minor. Activated Christmas factor cannot be separated from its precursor by column chromatography [126], although it may be separated by starch-block electrophoresis [130].

Antihemophilic Factor

Activated Christmas factor reacts with antihemophilic factor to form an agent which, in turn, activates Stuart factor [126, 131]. The nature of this agent is not yet known. At one time it was thought that activated Christmas factor converted antihemophilic factor to an activated form. At present the source of the clot-promoting property which evolves in mixtures of activated Christmas factor and antihemophilic factor is not clear. Both calcium ions and phospholipid are needed for generation of clot-promoting activity [132], and the antihemophilic factor must first be altered by thrombin to function optimally [133]. Prepared from human plasma, the clot-promoting activity is unstable, lasting no more than 8 to 10 min [132]; a similar product isolated from bovine material is more stable.

The chemical nature of antihemophilic factor has been elusive because of its lability. Antihemophilic factor is present in fresh human plasma, but the titer decreases during the storage of blood or plasma at 4°C. The bulk of the antihemophilic activity of human plasma is contained in Cohn fraction 1 [75]. Fractions of human or animal plasma, rich in antihemophilic activity and suitable for clinical use, have been separated by many techniques [75, 134–142]. Preparations purified as much as 10,000-fold have been separated experimentally, but these are not yet practical for therapeutic use [143, 144].

Antihemophilic factor presumably is a protein, for it is destroyed by the plasma protease plasmin [145] and by highly purified thrombin [146]. These enzymes do not account for the instability of antihemophilic factor during storage of plasma [147]. In human plasma no more than 7 mg is present per liter [143]. Human antihemophilic factor has a sedimentation constant of approximately 40 and behaves like a glycoprotein with a minimal molecular weight of about 2,000,000 [144, 148]. The suggestion has been made that it contains phospholipid necessary for its activity [149], but this has not been true of our preparations. In the laboratory the macromolecule can be dissociated by succinic anhydride; one product of succinylation, with a molecular weight of 25,000, has rich activity [150]. Electrophoretic data are confused by adsorption of antihemophilic factor to paper and by interaction with other proteins; on curtain electrophoresis it migrates in a band spreading from the albumin to the α_2 fraction of plasma [74].

The site of formation of antihemophilic factor is unknown, but severe experimental hepatic damage decreases its concentration in the blood [151]. Although the data are controversial, synthesis is probably a function of the reticuloendothelial system and takes place largely in the liver [151–154]. Evidence that the spleen is a unique site of synthesis is less secure [153–155]. Studies of bleeders have disclosed two stages in the synthesis of the factor, since the plasma of patients with classic hemophilia contains an agent which can induce the synthesis of antihemophilic factor in patients with von Willebrand's disease [157]. This agent may be an intermediate in the formation of antihemophilic factor.

Normal platelets have an activity attributable to antihemophilic factor which is adsorbed from the surrounding plasma [158]. The function of this adsorbed antihemophilic factor is not evident.

Stuart Factor

Stuart factor, the substrate for the product formed by the interaction of activated Christmas factor and antihemophilic factor, is a protein which is synthesized in the liver when vitamin K is available [159]. Its properties are similar in many respects to those of prothrombin. In its native state in plasma it migrates on paper electrophoresis as an α-globulin [160]. Highly purified preparations have been separated from bovine plasma and serum by Esnouf and Williams [161]. In their hands Stuart factor prepared from plasma had a molecular weight of 87,000, but that prepared from serum, only 36,000. The factor can also be activated by Russell's viper venom [161–163], trypsin [164], papain [164], 25% sodium citrate [165], and, as will be noted shortly, the product of the interaction of tissue thromboplastin and Factor VII. Activation by Russell's viper venom occurs only if calcium ions are present. The molecule is split by the venom. A second component appears upon electrophoresis, and the N-terminal amino acids are changed. Activated Stuart factor may be a hydrolytic enzyme, for it is said to digest TAMe [161, 166], and this substrate inhibits its clot-promoting ability [167]. Moreover, soybean trypsin inhibitor blocks both the esterolytic [161, 166] and coagulant [168] properties. Activated Stuart factor may be identical with the clot-promoting activities designated as *intermediate product 1* by Bergsagel and Hougie [169, 170] *plasma thrombokinase* by Milstone [171] and *autoprothrombin C* by Seegers [172].

Stuart factor, activated by the intrinsic clotting system or by Russell's viper venom, participates with phospholipid and proaccelerin to form an agent which converts prothrombin to thrombin. In the coagulation of cell-free plasma by way of the intrinsic pathway, the plasma itself probably furnishes the necessary phospholipid, whereas in whole blood platelets may serve this function. The most effective plasma phospholipid is phosphatidyl ethanolamine [173], although two phospholipids derived from platelets, phosphatidyl ethanolamine and phosphatidyl serine, both have clot-promoting properties [174, 175]. The importance of the fatty acid composition of the phosphatides is not yet delineated. More than half of the fatty acid component of the clot-promoting phosphatides is arachidonic acid, and the rest is largely stearic and oleic acids [176].

Factor VII

The action of factor VII is probably limited to the extrinsic pathway. Vitamin K is required for its synthesis, and this probably takes place within the liver [80]. No more than 50 mg is present in a liter of plasma [177]. On paper electrophoresis it migrates between the α- and β-globulins. Like the other vitamin K–dependent factors, it is readily adsorbed by such compounds as barium sulfate and calcium phosphate and is easily eluted from these, but separation from other eluted factors is difficult. The molecular weight has been tentatively estimated as 63,000 [178]; the molecule contains about 50 percent hexose [178]. Preparations, free of other clotting factors, can be made from human plasma by chromatography [178].

Tissue Thromboplastin

The extrinsic pathway of clotting is initiated by contact of blood with tissues. The active agents of tissue are known generically as *tissue thromboplastin.* The thromboplastic activity of tissues has been related to the microsomes [179, 180]. Their clot-promoting effect resides in a heat-stable lipid fraction and a heat-labile protein fraction, possibly combined as a lipoprotein [181–183]. When tissue thromboplastin, factor VII, and calcium ions are incubated together, a product forms which can activate Stuart factor [184]. This reaction requires the presence of phospholipid, principally phosphatidyl ethanolamine and phosphatidyl choline, and if the tissues are freed of lipids, they lose their clot-promoting properties unless phospholipids are restored [183, 185]. Whether tissue thromboplastin itself behaves enzymatically is not clear [179, 186].

Proaccelerin and Formation of the Prothrombin-converting Principle

Activated Stuart factor, evolved either through the extrinsic or intrinsic pathways, reacts with proaccelerin in the presence of phospholipid to produce an agent which can change prothrombin to thrombin. Human proaccelerin is a labile plasma protein, readily destroyed by gentle heating, storage, trypsin, or plasmin [187, 188]. Activity attributable to proaccelerin is destroyed or consumed during clotting, so that serum is ordinarily devoid of this factor. Bovine serum is an exception.

The results of many attempts to purify human proaccelerin have been disappointing. Little is known about its chemical nature other than that it migrates with the albumin fraction on curtain electrophoresis [74] and in the area between the β- and γ-globulins on paper [73]. Purification of bovine proaccelerin, a much more stable substance, has been more successful; its molecular weight is about 300,000 [189, 190]. The observation that its concentration in plasma is decreased in patients or animals with hepatic damage suggests that the liver may be the site of synthesis [191]. A rare hereditary disorder characterized by deficiencies of both antihemophilic factor and proaccelerin suggests that the synthesis of these two factors may involve a common step (see page 1693).

Proaccelerin is adsorbed from the plasma by platelets and is tightly bound to their surfaces [192, 193]. Of interest in this regard is that asolectin, a mixture of phosphatides, readily removes proaccelerin from plasma [194]. The proaccelerin on platelets may contribute to their clot-promoting properties.

Still unsettled is whether activated Stuart factor converts proaccelerin into the agent which changes prothrombin into thrombin or vice versa. Currently, the most attractive hypothesis is that proaccelerin is first altered by thrombin (or some other protease) [195–198]. In the process, the molecular weight of proaccelerin is decreased from about 300,000 to about 200,000 [189]. The thrombin-altered proaccelerin, i.e., accelerin, then participates with activated Stuart factor in the generation of a *prothrombin-converting principle,* which splits prothrombin enzymatically [199] to form two immunologically distinct parts, thrombin and a second fragment [200]. The formation and action of the prothrombin converting principle require the presence of calcium ions and probably take place upon the surface of phospholipid micelles [197, 199, 201, 202]. The agent effecting the transformation of prothrombin to thrombin is probably activated Stuart factor itself [201–204].

Besides the intrinsic and extrinsic pathways of clotting, other mechanisms may play a role in the activation of prothrombin. Seegers [205] demonstrated that his preparations of prothrombin slowly formed thrombin in 25% sodium citrate solution. This activation may well be dependent upon the presence of contaminating substances, since more highly purified preparations of prothrombin do not undergo this activation [86, 206]. Spaet and Cintron [165] suggest that the effect of 25% sodium citrate is to activate Stuart factor.

Plasma Inhibitors Of Blood Clotting

Not unexpectedly, human plasma can limit the blood clotting process by inhibiting activated clotting factors. Of several mechanisms which have been delineated, those involving thrombin and the activated states of Hageman factor, PTA, and Stuart factors are best known. Activated Hageman factor and activated PTA deteriorate rapidly in plasma [92, 207]. The property of plasma responsible for these actions has been localized to a fraction soluble in half-saturated ammonium sulfate [92, 208]; studies of Niemetz and Nossel [209] suggest that the two clotting factors are inhibited by separate agents. Recently, the plasma inhibitor of C′1 esterase, an agent identical with α_2-neuraminoglycoprotein, has been found to inhibit both activated Hageman factor and activated PTA [210], but whether this substance is identical with the inhibitors described earlier is not yet known.

Normal plasma also inactivates activated Stuart factor [211] and neutralizes the clot-promoting properties of tissue thromboplastin [212]. The effects of thrombin are neutralized in several ways. Plasma contains an α-globulin, designated as *antithrombin III,* which gradually inactivates any thrombin which may form [213]. This antithrombin is probably identical with the agent in plasma which potentiates the antithrombic effect of heparin, earlier designated as *antithrombin II* and with the inhibitor of Stuart factor [614]. A second fraction of plasma, α_2-macroglobulin, also slowly inhibits thrombin [214]. Once clotting takes place, thrombin is also inactivated by adsorption onto fibrin. Besides these and possibly other circulating inhibitors, other devices are available to counter the consequences of inadvertent intravascular clotting, such as the rapid removal of procoagulant substances by the liver and reticuloendothelial system.

Platelets

This review of the steps leading to the formation of a fibrin clot seems to slight the important role which *platelets* play in hemostasis [215, 216]. For many years it was thought that platelets, disrupted by contact with a foreign surface, release a thromboplastin similar to that furnished by injured tissue. In point of fact, platelets are a poor source of thromboplastin, although Biggs et al. [104] have recently revived interest in this possibility, since a clot-promoting agent can be released from platelets by activated Hageman factor. Nonetheless, platelets serve several different functions in coagulation. Mention has already been made that platelets furnish phospholipids which accelerate the formation of the prothrombin-converting principle. The phospholipids, known generically as platelet factor 3, are present both in the cytoplasmic granules and the membrane of the platelets [217, 218]. Marcus [219] has suggested that the platelet phospholipid used in the intrinsic pathway of coagulation is derived from the membrane rather than from the platelet granules. PTA, antihemophilic factor, and proaccelerin, adsorbed to the platelet surface, may have a significant function in clotting. Evidence also exists that extracts of platelets may accelerate the formation of fibrin by thrombin [220]. Whether the fibrin-stabilizing factor found in platelets plays a significant role in hemostasis is not clear [221].

An important function of platelets is related to hemostasis after injury to the smallest blood vessels. Platelets accumulate at the site of vascular injury within a few seconds. They stick to the exposed subendothelial tissues. The presumption has been made that they adhere to collagen-like protein, since in vitro collagen brings about aggregation of platelets, a process mediated by the release of adenosine diphosphate (ADP) by these cells [216, 222]. As the platelets pile up, they release ADP, enhancing the adhesion of platelets to each other [223, 224]. Perhaps ADP is also liberated by the injured endothelial cells. Soon a sufficient mass of platelets forms to seal the wound. The platelets gradually lose their identity and undergo a process awkwardly called *viscous metamorphosis* in which one cell seems to fuse with another.

Present evidence links viscous metamorphosis to the phenomenon of *clot retraction,* in which the clot shrinks and its serum is expressed. These two processes appear to depend upon the action of thrombin, for, as it evolves during clotting, thrombin induces an agglutination of platelets [225, 226], in part mediated by release of ADP [216]. This aggregation occurs only in the presence of divalent cations [227] and may precede the appearance of macroscopic fibrin strands. At the same time the platelets undergo striking morphologic changes. They seem to swell, and the cytoplasmic granules form clumps. On a surface the platelets spread out, and cytoplasmic pseudopods appear which join those of other nearby platelets to form a network [227–229]. They discharge their granules and mitochondria into the surrounding medium [227, 230, 231]. The platelet network seems to act as a nidus toward which the developing fibrin strands are oriented [232]. When clot retraction occurs, bridges of fibrin can be seen between the enlarging platelet clumps. Clot retraction, contrary to earlier views, is primarily a platelet function in which these cells appear to contract; shrinking of the fibrin strands themselves cannot be demonstrated [216, 232, 233].

The forces which result in viscous metamorphosis and clot retraction have been investigated at length. Initiation of the two processes by thrombin is thought to be related to the presence of fibrinogen on the surface of the platelet [234] and within its cytoplasmic granules [235]. Perhaps the interaction of thrombin and platelet fibrinogen changes platelet permeability [236]. The viscous metamorphosis and clot retraction which follow are dependent upon adenosine triphosphate (ATP) in the platelets, which is probably synthesized by way of an intrinsic glycolytic system [237, 238]. The two processes are also linked to a protein in the platelets called *thrombosthenin,* similar to muscle actomyosin, which also contracts in the presence of ATP and divalent cations [239]. Thrombosthenin is an adenosine triphosphatase (ATPase) [240], and platelet ATP falls rapidly during clotting [240, 241]. The fibrin-stabilizing factor in platelets may also participate in these several reactions [242].

The morphologic changes of viscous metamorphosis observed in vitro may also be seen in the aggregates of platelets which accumulate at the site of experimental vascular injury [243, 244]. The significance of clot retraction for hemostasis has not been clarified. Still, when this function is impaired, either because of thrombocytopenia or because the platelets are qualitatively defective, a bleeding tendency ensues.

THE LABORATORY INVESTIGATION OF HEMORRHAGIC STATES

The differential diagnosis of the hereditary hemorrhagic disorders is, for the most part, a laboratory exercise, since the symptomatology of one is much the same as another. Many excellent summaries of laboratory techniques are available [245–250]. Only the principles underlying certain screening tests will be considered here. The typical findings in certain hereditary bleeding syndromes are summarized in Table 72-2.

Tests of Clotting Time

The *clotting time of whole blood* is an overall measure of the intrinsic blood clotting mechanism and as such depends upon the presence of all the clotting factors *except factor VII.* It is most accurately performed upon venous blood drawn with care to minimize the admixture of tissue. Methods employing capillary blood are relatively insensitive. Measured in glass tubes, the clotting time seldom helps to uncover minor defects where no history of significant hemorrhagic symptoms is obtained; a deficiency of Hageman factor, which is usually asymptomatic, is the exception. The clotting time of whole blood is usually normal in thrombocytopenia or in mild cases of hemophilia, Christmas disease, or PTA deficiency. Clotting in glass tubes is probably initiated partly by the surface activation of Hageman factor and partly by the effect of surfaces upon the blood cells, particularly the platelets. The use of polystyrene or silicone-coated tubes lengthens the clotting time of normal blood, since these surfaces are less efficient activators of clotting. By exaggerating minor differences, the clotting time under these conditions may be long if the blood contains defective platelets or is thrombocytopenic. Such tubes make the test more sensitive to minor coagulative abnormalities.

The *clotting time of recalcified plasma,* measured in glass tubes, is also insensitive, for it is abnormally long only if severe deficiencies of the clotting factors are present. Again, this test is not responsive to deficiencies of platelets or factor VII. The test is more sensitive to minor abnormalities if crude phospholipid mixtures of plant or animal origin are added, a procedure described as measurement of the *partial thromboplastin time* [252]. In a variant of this test, kaolin or celite, activators of Hageman factor, is added to the mixture to standardize the surface to which plasma is exposed. The *partial thromboplastin time* is useful in detecting coagulative defects, although it sometimes gives erratic and inexplicable results and must be interpreted with caution. In patients with mild hemophilia or Christmas disease, the partial thromboplastin time may be normal.

Several screening tests are available for locating in a general way the stage of clotting at which an abnormality resides. The *thrombin time,* the clotting time of a mixture of plasma and bovine thrombin, is abnormally long in hypofibrinogenemia or in the presence of anticoagulants which inhibit fibrin formation such as heparin or the digestion products of fibrinogen or fibrin. It may also be long if the fibrinogen is qualitatively abnormal or if the property of plasma which accelerates fibrin formation is deficient

Table 72-2. DIFFERENTIATION OF SOME HEMORRHAGIC DISORDERS (TYPICAL FINDINGS)

Disorder	Clotting time	Partial thromboplastin time	Bleeding time	Thrombin time	Prothrombin time	Serum prothrombic activity	Special tests
Classic hemophilia	Normal to long	Long	Normal	Normal	Normal	Normal to high	Corrected by fresh adsorbed plasma*
Christmas disease	Normal to long	Long	Normal	Normal	Normal	Normal to high	Corrected by serum
PTA deficiency	Normal to long	Long	Variable	Normal	Normal	Normal to high	Corrected by serum or adsorbed plasma†
Hageman trait	Long	Long	Normal	Normal	Normal	High	Corrected by serum or adsorbed plasma†
Factor VII deficiency	Normal	Normal	Normal	Normal	Long	Normal	Corrected by Russell's viper venom
Stuart factor deficiency	Normal to long	Long	Normal	Normal	Long	High	Corrected by serum, not by Russell's viper venom
Parahemophilia	Long	Long	Normal	Normal	Long	High	Corrected by fresh adsorbed plasma
Hypoprothrombinemia	Normal to long	Variable	Normal	Normal	Long	Normal	Corrected by aged plasma
Afibrinogenemia	Infinite	Infinite	Variable	Infinite	Infinite	Normal	Not corrected by thrombin
Fibrin-stabilizing factor deficiency	Normal	Normal	Normal	Normal	Normal	Normal	Clot dissolves in 1% monochloroacetic acid
Thrombocytopenia	Normal	Normal	Long	Normal	Normal	High	Platelet count <120,000; impaired clot retraction
Thrombopathic purpura	Normal	Normal	Long	Normal	Normal	Variable	ADP aggregation poor, clot-promoting function of platelets impaired
Glanzmann's disease	Normal	Normal	Long	Normal	Normal	Normal	ADP aggregation poor; impaired clot retraction
Thrombocythemia	Normal	Normal	Variable	Normal	Normal	Normal	Platelet count >800,000
von Willebrand's disease	Variable	Variable	Long	Normal	Normal	Normal to high	Antihemophilic factor titer may be low

* Plasma adsorbed with aluminum hydroxide, barium sulfate, etc.
† Distinguished by crossmatching plasmas with known defective plasmas.
Source: Ratnoff [251]. By permission of Harper and Row, New York.

[33, 34]. The thrombin time is not affected by a deficiency of fibrin-stabilizing factor.

Prothrombin Time

Abnormalities of the extrinsic clotting pathway are detected by measuring the *one-stage prothrombin time* of Quick et al. [253]. In this procedure the clotting time of recalcified plasma is tested in the presence of tissue thromboplastin. Abnormally long prothrombin times reflect deficiencies in prothrombin itself, factor VII, Stuart factor, proaccelerin, or fibrinogen. Moreover, the one-stage prothrombin time may be prolonged by anticoagulants, notably heparin and a circulating anticoagulant found in the plasma of some patients with systemic lupus erythematosus. The specific cause of a prolonged prothrombin time can be uncovered by suitable tests.

Serum Prothrombic Activity

If the thrombin time and prothrombin time are normal but a defect in coagulation is suspected, attention may be turned toward an abnormality in the early stages of the intrinsic clotting pathway. Measurement of *prothrombin "consumption,"* or *serum prothrombic activity,* may confirm this suspicion [254, 255]. Normally, when blood clots in a glass tube, the conversion of prothrombin to thrombin is gradual. Clotting occurs whenever sufficient thrombin has formed, but long after clotting is completed some prothrombin still remains. An estimate of the prothrombic activity remaining in the serum at a fixed time interval after blood is drawn is an excellent test of clotting function. The conversion of prothrombin to thrombin in venous blood is impeded by deficiencies of platelets or of any clotting factor except factor VII, prothrombin, or fibrinogen. When the formation of thrombin is retarded, the prothrombin content of serum is abnormally high, that is, prothrombin consumption is poor. Used for detecting the presence of a hemostatic defect, measurement of serum prothrombic activity is a helpful technique. On the other hand a variation of the method in which the ability of various normal or abnormal plasmas, serums, or fractions thereof to correct abnormal prothrombin consumption is measured, is less satisfactory. In the author's hands the results of these tests have often been misleading, and other procedures are of more value.

Thromboplastin Generation Test

Another screening technique of great importance is the *thromboplastin generation test* of Biggs and Douglas [256]. This test is designed to measure the evolution of prothrombin-converting activity, utilizing a system deficient in prothrombin. Serum, citrated plasma, and platelets are prepared from the blood of the patient and from a normal subject. The plasma is adsorbed with aluminum hydroxide to remove prothrombin, Christmas factor, factor VII, and Stuart factor. In the first step of the test a mixture of diluted serum, diluted adsorbed plasma, platelets, and calcium is prepared. This "incubation mixture," containing all recognized clotting factors except prothrombin, is incubated in a glass tube at 37°C. Samples are removed at intervals and added to normal platelet-deficient plasma ("substrate"). Biggs and Douglas postulated that "thromboplastic activity," evolved in the incubation mixture, could be quantified by measuring its effect upon the clotting of the substrate plasma. Thus:

Step 1: Serum (containing Hageman factor, PTA, Christmas factor, and Stuart factor) + adsorbed plasma (containing Hageman factor, PTA, antihemophilic factor, proaccelerin, and fibrinogen) + platelets + calcium → "thromboplastin" (that is, prothrombin-converting activity).
Step 2: "Thromboplastin" + platelet-deficient plasma (containing prothrombin, fibrinogen, and other clotting factors) + Ca^{++} → thrombin and the formation of a clot [257].

By testing successive samples of the incubation mixture, the rate of evolution of clot-promoting activity and its intensity can be measured. A deficiency of any clotting factor except factor VII causes impaired "thromboplastin generation" in the first step and is reflected by a long clotting time in the second step.

The thromboplastin generation test is a moderately sensitive indicator of impaired clotting, but it will give normal results in mild hemophilia or Christmas disease [245]. When abnormal, the test lends itself to a further analysis of clotting defect through substitution of normal reagents for those of the patient, one at a time [Table 72-3].

The theoretical basis of the thromboplastin generation test is less secure than this summary indicates. Normally, a clot always appears in the initial generating mixture when clot-promoting activity is maximal. Presumably thrombin has been generated in the supposedly prothrombin deficient mixture. The source of the thrombin is usually the normal serum reagent, for it is virtually impossible to free serum of prothrombin without special manipulations. Nevertheless, the thromboplastin generation test serves a useful diagnostic purpose, particularly when plasmas with known deficiencies are not available.

Assays for Specific Clotting Factors

The *concentration of each individual clotting factor* may be determined by measuring the effect of a small amount of plasma upon a mixture containing all known activities except the specific one to be tested. An exception is fibrinogen, which can be converted into fibrin and then assayed by conventional chemical techniques. The actual method of assay varies widely, depending upon the factor to be tested and the prejudices of the investigator. In general, variations

Table 72-3. USUAL RESULTS OF THROMBOPLASTIN GENERATION TEST IN SOME COAGULATIVE ABNORMALITIES

Source of $Al(OH)_3$-adsorbed plasma	Source of serum	Source of platelets or phospholipid	*Results*							
			Classic hemophilia	Christmas disease	PTA deficiency	Hageman trait	Parahemophilia	Factor VII deficiency	Stuart factor deficiency	Thrombopathic purpura
Normal	Patient	Normal	Normal	Abnormal	Normal	Normal	Normal	Normal	Abnormal	Normal
Patient	Normal	Normal	Abnormal	Normal	Normal	Normal	Abnormal	Normal	Normal	Normal
Patient	Patient	Normal	Abnormal	Abnormal	Abnormal	Abnormal	Abnormal	Normal	Abnormal	Normal
Normal	Normal	Patient	Normal	Normal	Normal	Normal	Normal	Normal	Normal	Abnormal

Source: Adapted from R. Biggs and L. W. Gaston: The blood-clotting factors in *The Metabolic Basis of Inherited Disease,* 1st ed., edited by J. B. Stanbury, J. B. Wyngaarden, and D. S. Fredrickson. McGraw-Hill, New York, 1960.

of the one-stage prothrombin time are used to test those factors required in the extrinsic clotting pathway, and variations of the thromboplastin generation test or partial thromboplastin time test are employed for testing for the other factors, that is, antihemophilic factor, Christmas factor, Hageman factor, and PTA. An excellent way to assay these last four factors is to perform the partial thromboplastin time test in the presence of kaolin. This ensures maximal activation of Hageman factor and PTA [258–260]. The presence of fibrin-stabilizing factor is usually measured qualitatively by determining whether a recalcified plasma clot is soluble in 5*M* urea or 1% monochloroacetic acid.

One must always be wary of two major pitfalls in the assay of clotting factors. The presence of a clotting factor in its *activated* form precludes the measurement of factors participating at an earlier step of clotting. For example, Hageman factor cannot be measured in the presence of activated PTA, and none of the clotting factors can be measured if thrombin is present. The second source of error is the presence of a circulating anticoagulant which may inhibit clotting and give the erroneous impression that the plasma is deficient in one or more clotting factors. Special techniques are needed for assaying clotting factors under these circumstances.

Tests of Platelet Function

In normal individuals the platelet count varies from about 150,000 to 350,000 per mm^3. When there are fewer than 100,000 platelets per mm^3, clot retraction may be impaired, the bleeding time may be prolonged, and serum prothrombic activity may be abnormally high. Qualitative defects in platelets may be assessed by measuring their coagulant function in the thromboplastin generation test or recalcified plasma clotting time; their adhesion to glass [261]; their aggregation by collagen, ADP, epinephrine, or thrombin; and their capacity to induce clot retraction. The bleeding time is long in most individuals whose platelets are qualitatively defective. The many variations of the tests available testify to the technical difficulties which accompany their use.

CLINICAL DISORDERS

Classic Hemophilia

The earliest record of a familial disorder of hemostasis is to be found in the Tract Yebamoth of the Babylonian Talmud, written before the sixth century A.D. Rabbi Simeon Ben Gamilieal exempted from circumcision a boy whose brothers had bled following this rite [262]. Six centuries later an Arabian physician, Khalaf Abul Kasim el Zahrewi, otherwise known as Alsaharavi or Albucasis, wrote about the men in a certain village who bled uncontrollably after injury [263]. Thereafter, virtually nothing was said about hereditary hemorrhagic conditions until 1803, when Otto described the "hemorrhagic disposition" which a "woman by the name of Smith, settled in the vicinity of Plymouth, New Hampshire" transmitted to her descendents. "It is a surprising circumstance," he noted, "that the males only are subject to this strange affliction, and that all of them are not liable to it. Although females are exempt, they are still capable of transmitting it to their male children" [264]. For whatever philosophic inferences one may wish to draw, Otto had not actually seen a bleeder when he wrote his article.

During the nineteenth century the chief concern among people interested in bleeders was to unravel the strange hereditary pattern. Not unexpectedly, rules were hard to deduce, for only in the last few years has it been clear that the syndrome which Schönlein named *hemophilia* may result from a dozen or more separable defects. The confusion was lessened by the coincidence that classic hemophilia and Christmas disease, the two commonest familial bleeding diseases, are inherited in the same way. In fact, no new principle was deduced beyond Otto's observations until Legg [265] reported that the daughter of a hemophiliac could pass the defect to her sons, a point not previously clear.

An appreciation that hemophilia might be related to a defect in blood coagulation was reached only in 1893, when Wright [266] observed the delay in clotting characteristic of the disease. His writings display his bewilderment concerning this discovery. As late as 1878, Immerman [263] could assert, "The hypothesis that the bleeding disease is dependent upon a congenital imperfection of the blood will have to be abandoned." Considerable attention was paid to the "remarkably thin and sometimes actually transparent" nature of the intima of the arteries in some cases. Nevertheless, ". . . very generally, the intima of both the large and the small arteries was distinctly seen to have undergone a partial fatty degeneration, . . ." an observation important because it was unconfused by the effects of blood transfusion. Indeed, the vascular lesion seemed so striking that it was thought "to constitute the anatomical substratum" of the disease [263]. Hemorrhages were thought to be due to a congenital disproportion between the volume of blood and the capacity of the vascular apparatus and to an abnormal increase in the lateral pressure within the vessels.

Our present-day concept of the nature of hemophilia was foreshadowed by Addis [267], who found that the formation of thrombin was abnormally slow in hemophilic blood and that a fraction of normal plasma shortened the abnormally long clotting time. Attention was directed away from the plasma as the site of the defect by Minot and Lee [268], who attributed hemophilia to an abnormality in the platelets. Frank and Hartmann [269], Govaerts and Gratia [270], Bendien and van Creveld [271], and Patek and Stetson [272] all clearly demonstrated that the defect in hemophilic blood was localized to the plasma. Some years later this simple concept was confounded by Pavlovsky's [273] report that a mixture of the blood of two "hemophiliacs" clotted more rapidly than either alone. This startling observation soon led to the division of cases into those with "classic hemophilia," with blood deficient in antihemophilia factor, and those with Christmas disease, with blood lacking Christmas factor, a chemically distinct protein. With the development of modern techniques, other hemophilia-like syndromes have been delineated, and many of the anomalies in the earlier literature have been resolved.

Clinical Findings

Classic hemophilia is the hereditary deficiency of antihemophilic factor. The disorder probably exists in about 1 of every 10,000 males in the United States and Europe, but is said to be uncommon in Bantu and in Japanese [274]. The clinical severity of the disorder varies from family to family and parallels in general the degree of deficiency of antihemophilic factor. In severe cases virtually no antihemophilic factor is detectable in the plasma, while in mild hemophilia the concentration of this substance may be as high as 20 percent of the average normal. Among the various affected members of a family the severity of the disease is approximately the same [245].

The person severely affected with hemophilia may bleed after neonatal circumcision. The newborn infant with hemophilia has no antihemophilic factor in the cord blood [275, 276]. More usually, the first evidence of a bleeding tendency, ecchymoses and subcutaneous and intramuscular hematomas, appears when the child begins to crawl and walk and, as a consequence, to fall. Bleeding into the joints is common, and after repeated hemorrhages permanent and crippling deformities may ensue. Bleeding may take place virtually anywhere. Hematuria, bleeding into the gastrointestinal tract, epistaxis, and gingival bleeding are frequent. Bleeding into the central nervous system is less common but may cause permanent or even lethal damage. Still more rarely, the person with hemophilia may bleed into the soft tissues of the neck, a crisis which may lead to asphyxia [277]. Even trivial injury and any dental extraction or surgical procedure may initiate persistent hemorrhage. Often bleeding seems to start spontaneously, the patient being unaware of any injury.

In at least half of cases, the bleeding tendency is milder than has just been described [278]. Spontaneous bleeding and hemarthroses may be unusual. Indeed, in some patients, hemorrhage may be induced only by injury or surgical procedures. There seems to be an almost continuous spectrum of severity, ranging from those cases in which the disorder is very mild to those in which the patient seems to spend as much time in the hospital as out of it.

Patients with hemophilia contend that their episodes of bleeding occur in bouts, and clinical observation seems to confirm this [246]. Not uncommonly, for example, a patient under treatment for hemarthrosis may have hematuria. The biologic basis for this hemostatic breakdown is unknown. In mild hemophilia, exercise [279] or the injection of epinephrine [280] may cause a transient increase in the concentration of antihemophilic factor in plasma, but this does not seem to happen in severely affected patients. Adults with hemophilia sometimes relate that their symptoms are milder than in childhood and that episodes of severe bleeding are less frequent. They often believe that the amelioration of their disability coincided with the emotional changes of adolescence, when they rejected the overprotection which their parents provided [281]. Whether their interpretation is correct, whether some subtle physiologic change takes place at adolescence, or indeed, whether they have just learned to avoid injury and to ignore minor episodes of bleeding, is uncertain. Whatever the mechanism, no evidence exists that the concentration of antihemophilic factor increases at the same time as the supposed amelioration.

Laboratory Studies

The fundamental defect in classic hemophilia appears to be a failure to synthesize normally functional antihemophilic factor. Among normal individuals the concentration of this clotting protein varies widely. Published values range from 50 to 200 percent of that of an average normal adult [282–284]. The author's data show a variation from 40 to 400 percent of a mean value [285]. Among normal sibs the variation in antihemophilic factor concentration is less than among individuals in different families, and statistically, a child's titer is determined by that of his parents [286]. These observations have been interpreted to mean that the concentration of this substance is controlled in part by autosomal genes.

The concentration of antihemophilic factor is relatively higher in the plasma of Australian aborigines [287] and Bantu [288] than in whites, but this may reflect a pathologic rather than a normal difference, since hypergammaglobulinemia, common in the aborigines, may be associated with elevated levels of antihemophilic factor [287]. Nonetheless, the concentration of antihemophilic factor is significantly higher in normal American Negroes compared to American whites [285]. No difference has been noted between normal males and females [285, 289].

Under basal conditions the concentration of antihemophilic factor in normal individuals is relatively constant from day to day. There is a gradual increase in titer with age [282], although this has been questioned [290]. The factors affecting variation in the concentration of antihemophilic factor from time to time are not clear, but a striking increase in titer follows exercise [274] or the intravenous injection of epinephrine [280]. Increases in the concentration of antihemophilic factor have also been reported during pregnancy [291] or the administration of oral contraceptives [292]; after surgical treatment [293], fever [294], or x-irradiation [295]; and in hyperthyroid states [296], atherosclerosis [297], and diabetes [298].

In the test tube, the deficiency of antihemophilic factor in the plasma of patients with hemophilia impairs clotting because it retards the development of the substance active in the conversion of prothrombin to thrombin [267, 299]. Presumably in these patients the same delay in thrombin formation impairs hemostasis following injury. Interestingly, the person with hemophilia does not ordinarily bleed excessively from minor wounds. Possibly clotting in such wounds is initiated by tissue thromboplastin originating in the injured tissue, or hemostasis is provided through other mechanisms. An explanation is lacking for the peculiar susceptibility of hemophilic joints to hemorrhage. Synovial fluid is a poor source of thromboplastin and thus may not support hemostasis by way of the extrinsic pathway [300].

The diagnosis of severe hemophilia is relatively simple. The clotting time of whole blood or plasma, measured in glass tubes, is prolonged. The defect is localized to the intrinsic clotting mechanism by demonstrating a normal one-stage prothrombin time [253]. Abnormally high serum prothrombic activity (poor prothrombin consumption), a long partial thromboplastin time, and impaired thromboplastin generation by the Biggs-Douglas test indicate that the development of the prothrombin-converting principle is impeded. The abnormality in the thromboplastin generation test is corrected by substitution of normal adsorbed plasma for that of the patient but is unaltered by the substitution of normal serum. The platelets, too, are defective in that they lack the antihemophilic factor normally adsorbed to their surface [158, 301].

The diagnosis of classic hemophilia is established by demonstrating that the plasma contains little or no antihemophilic factor. For this purpose the most accurate assays are those in which the plasma is tested for its capacity to correct the coagulative abnormality of known hemophilic plasma. If hemophilic plasma is not available, a presumptive diagnosis can be made by demonstrating that a crude antihemophilic fraction of normal plasma can correct the defect in the plasma of the patient. A similarly prepared fraction of the patient's plasma should lack this corrective effect.

In mildly or moderately affected patients, a diagnosis of hemophilia is more difficult. The clotting time of whole blood or plasma may be normal when measured in glass tubes, but in silicone-coated or polystyrene tubes the clotting time of whole blood is usually abnormally long. The measurement of prothrombin consumption, partial thromboplastin time, and thromboplastin generation may provide normal or only equivocally abnormal results. The diagnosis can only be established by quantitative estimation of the concentration of antihemophilic factor.

In classic hemophilia the tourniquet test of capillary "fragility" and the bleeding time, that is, the length of time elapsing until bleeding from a small stab wound stops, are normal. These findings coincide with the clinical observation that bleeding from minor injuries may be minimal. The normal bleeding time is in contradistinction to the abnormally long value often seen in von Willebrand's disease (see later), another disorder in which the concentration of antihemophilic factor may be depressed. Since the measurement of the bleeding time is difficult and the results variable, too much reliance should not be placed upon any single determination in the differential diagnosis of classic hemophilia and von Willebrand's disease.

Therapy

The principal therapeutic measure available for the treatment of bleeding in hemophilia is the temporary correction of the coagulative defect by the transfusion of plasma or fractions of plasma rich in antihemophilic factor. Whole blood is of value in sustaining the blood volume after major hemorrhage. Usually it cannot be used to raise the level of antihemophilic factor significantly, since the amount needed may increase the blood volume dangerously. To control bleeding from accidental or surgical wounds, the level of antihemophilic factor must be raised to 30 or 40 percent of normal or more and sustained for many hours or days. A lesser level, perhaps 10 or 20 percent of normal, is usually adequate to control bleeding into the soft tissues or joints, but even these levels cannot be achieved with whole blood. The use of plasma or antihemophilic factor–rich fractions of plasma avoids this difficulty. Until recently the treatment of choice was the administration of freshly frozen plasma at a dosage of approximately 15 ml per kg body weight, given over a period of 30 to 60 min [302]. Once transfused, the antihemophilic factor is quickly dissipated. In patients who are not bleeding, one-half of a single transfusion of this agent disappears from the circulation within 10 to 12 hr [303]. The fall may be even more precipitous if the patient is bleeding [304]. Thus additional plasma must be injected repeatedly. Our practice has been to transfuse 1.5 ml plasma per kg every 3 or 4 hr until symptoms have subsided. If the patient has suffered severe injury or is to undergo surgery, this regimen is usually inadequate to control bleeding, and larger volumes provide undue risk of hypervolemia.

Fortunately, the last few years have seen the development of several concentrates of antihemophilic factor. Of these, the most useful are frozen cryoprecipitates of antihemophilic factor and lyophilized antihemophilic factor-rich plasma fractions. The cryoprecipitated fraction is prepared by freezing freshly separated plasma and then allowing it to thaw at 4°C [142]. The small precipitate which remains, containing about half of the antihemophilic activity of the original plasma, is separated by centrifugation. The supernatant plasma is decanted and recombined with the blood cells; it can be used for routine blood transfusion in nonhemophilic individuals. A typical course of therapy consists of an initial transfusion of one bag of cryoprecipitate (about 100 units of antihemophilic activity, one unit being that in 1 ml of an average normal plasma) for each 6 kg body weight, followed by one bag for each 12 kg every 12 hr. Cryoprecipitates are routinely separated from blood donated to the Cuyahoga County Red Cross. Under such conditions, the amount of antihemophilic factor in each bag is only about 70 units and for this reason we now use one bag for every 4 kg of body weight initially and one bag for every 8 kg every 12 hr thereafter. The lyophilized preparations available commercially or through the American Red Cross have the advantages of accessibility in areas where cryoprecipitates are not readily obtained and of the possibility of using exceptionally high doses without expanding the plasma volume unduly. All forms of antihemophilic factor have the disadvantage that they may contain hepatitis virus. The details of therapy with plasma or its fractions have been the subject of a recent review [302].

In addition to the administration of plasma or its fractions to correct the specific defect of classic hemophilia, other measures may be helpful in the control of bleeding. Gentle pressure to accessible wounds, possibly combined with the local application of bovine thrombin or Russell's viper venom, may promote hemostasis. The affected part should be immobilized and cooled with ice bags. Rarely, bleeding into a closed space may threaten major nerves or blood vessels, or tissues may be so distended that necrosis seems imminent. Special attention must be paid to the care of hemarthroses in order to prevent permanent damage [305]. The availability of concentrated antihemophilic factor has made it possible to perform many types of surgical procedures, including those designed to restore the function of joints [303, 306–308].

Perhaps because gingival hemorrhages are so frequent in hemophilia, dental hygiene is poor and dental extractions are frequently necessary. These procedures should be performed only under the joint supervision of an oral surgeon and hematologist, both familiar with the problems of bleeders. In severe hemophilia transfusions are usually required before, and for several days after, extraction, but in milder cases transfusions may not be needed [309, 310].

An important aspect in the care of congenital bleeders of whatever type is the encouragement of normal emotional and intellectual development. The constant physical threat to their child and their own sense of guilt make the parents of bleeders characteristically overprotective. As a result, the bleeder is often emotionally immature. Moreover, schooling may be sporadic, and the bleeder often reaches adult life unprepared to make a living. The physician should take an active role in guiding the parents to allow the child as much freedom as possible and to encourage acquiring as much education as he is fitted for. The goal is a self-sufficient adult [257, 311–313].

Aspirin, because it interferes with the hemostatic function of platelets, is contraindicated in patients with hemophilia and other bleeding disorders. Patients should be instructed to read the labels of commercially available analgesic preparations and to avoid any containing this drug.

Genetics

Classic hemophilia is an example par excellence of a disorder inherited as an X-linked recessive trait [314]. The locus is close to those determining deutan color blindness [315] and glucose-6-phosphate dehydrogenase synthesis [316]. With few exceptions, hemophilia is limited to males whose sons are normal and cannot carry the trait to their children and whose daughters are invariably carriers. In turn, these carriers transmit the disorder to half their sons and the carrier state to half their daughters (Fig. 72-4). The abnormality in hemophilia is due to the presence on the X chromosome of a mutant allele for a gene controlling the synthesis of antihemophilic factor. Presumably the aberrant allele is inadequate to support the synthesis of normal antihemophilic factor. Two forms of hemophilia have been distinguished. In all patients tested, antigen related to antihemophilic factor can be detected in normal amounts, using heterologous specific antiserum [603]. A smaller group of patients can be identified in whom nonfunctional antihemophilic factor can be identified additionally by tests employing homologous circulating anticoagulants directed against this factor [317, 318]. These findings are not yet reconciled with the observations of Barrow and Graham [150] who treated fractions prepared from the plasma of patients with classic hemophilia or von Willebrand's disease with succinic anhydride and released molecular fragments with antihemophilic activity.

The synthesis of antihemophilic factor appears to be under the control of additional genes besides those on the X chromosome. A deficiency of antihemophilic factor is found in von Willebrand's disease, inherited as an autosomal recessive

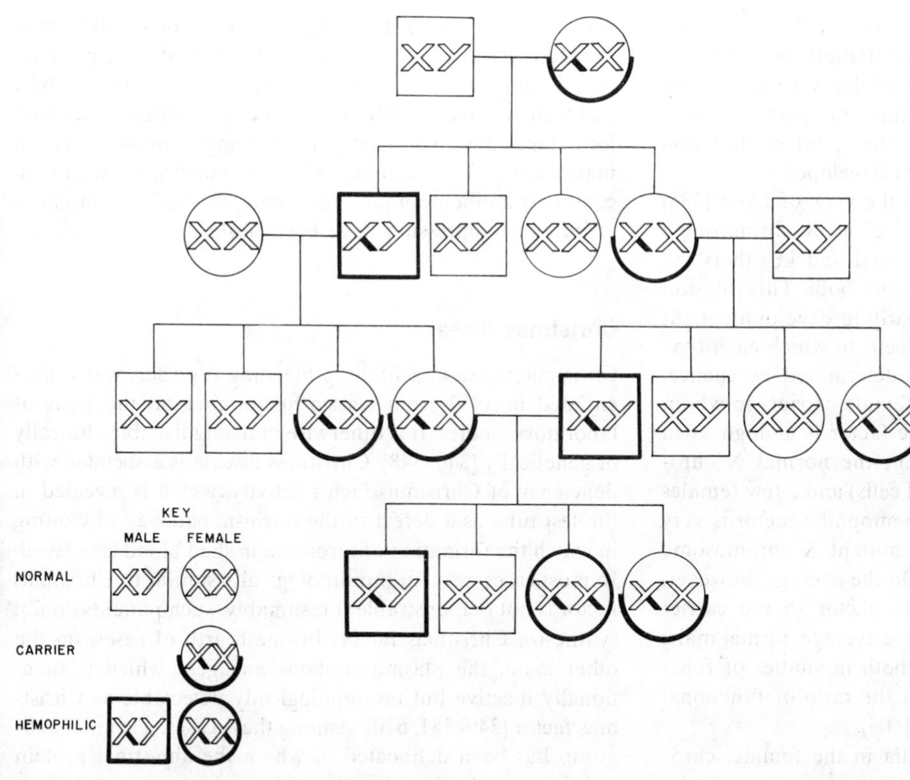

Figure 72-4. The pattern of inheritance in hemophilia and Christmas disease. The so-called sex chromosomes are represented as X and Y in accordance with convention. (*Reprinted from* [276] *by permission of the Year Book Medical Publishers, Chicago.*)

disorder. Hensen [319] described a family in which classic hemophilia was transmitted from father to son in an autosomal dominant way. How these various genes interact is not understood.

A few instances have been reported of true hemophilia in females. As one would expect, these bleeders are homozygous for the mutant allele and are the offspring of a hemophilic father and a carrier mother [320–322]. The same X-linked pattern of inheritance is found in canine hemophilia, a disorder indistinguishable in its clinical and laboratory features from the human disease [323]. Equine hemophilia has also been described [324].

In about one-third of cases the patient with hemophilia is unaware of a family history of bleeding [245, 275, 291]. In some instances this may be due to mutation of the antihemophilic gene on the X chromosome of the ovum from which he or his mother developed. More often, one suspects that a negative family history reflects the chance distribution of the mutant gene in earlier generations or merely an ignorance concerning the illnesses of the forebears. Sometimes a positive family history is concealed by the guilt-ridden parents. Strauss [325] has proposed that a negative family history is relatively commoner in patients with severe hemophilia; our own experience is in accord with this view.

In the cells of female carriers one of the pair of X chromosomes bears the normal gene and the other the mutant allele for the synthesis of antihemophilic factor. The female carriers are nearly always asymptomatic [326]. In a few, minor symptoms suggesting a bleeding tendency may be present, but these are difficult to evaluate because an awareness of hemorrhagic phenomena pervades a bleeder's family [327].

The concentration of antihemophilic factor varies widely from one carrier to the next. The average of many is 50 to 70 percent of normal [328, 329]. The genetic meaning of this depression in the *average* titer is not entirely clear. Studies on proved carriers demonstrate abnormally low titers in one-third or more of cases, depending upon the sensitivity of the method used. The carrier state seems more readily detected in the female relatives of persons with mild rather than severe hemophilia [326, 328, 330]. Rarely the titer of antihemophilic factor may be 5 percent of normal or less; these carriers may have symptoms suggestive of hemophilia [331–334]. Little information is available concerning the normal sons of carriers, who inherit the X chromosome bearing the normal maternal allele, but what there is suggests that they have a normal amount of antihemophilic factor in the plasma [289]. Recently, an improved method for the detection of carriers has been devised which takes advantage of the observation that hemophiliacs synthesize normal amounts of functionally defective antihemophilic factor [604]. In accordance with this, carriers often synthesize disproportionately more *antigenic* antihemophilic factor than *functional* antihemophilic factor. By measuring both antigen and functional antihemophilic factor one can identify at least 90 percent of carriers. Moreover, 4 of 10 mothers of patients who had no family history of hemophilia were normal by these criteria. Presumably some of these mothers may have been normal, the illness arising as the result of mutation in the ovum from which the patient developed.

All these data are consistent with the view of Lyon [335] that in some of the cells of a female the X chromosome inherited from the mother is functional and in others the X chromosome from her father, but not both. This division of cells, it is hypothesized, occurs early in development. At this critical stage the proportion of cells in which each type of X chromosome predominates is determined by chance. As a result, one should find a few female carriers in whom the concentration of antihemophilic factor is as high as in any male (that is, carriers in whom the normal X chromosome is functional in virtually all cells) and a few females in whom the concentration of antihemophilic factor is very low (that is, carriers in whom the mutant X chromosome is functional in virtually all cells). On the average, however, the concentration of antihemophilic factor in the carrier female should be about half that of the average normal male. Such indeed seems to be the case both in studies of functional antihemophilic factor and of the ratio of functional to antigenic antihemophilic factor [604].

In at least one case of hemophilia in the female, chromosomal studies revealed that the patient was genetically male [336]. In another, XX/XO mosaicism was found in a female whose maternal grandfather and brother had hemophilia [337]. Rare instances of seemingly true hemophilia in females with negative family histories have also been recorded; the genetic meaning of these cases remains a mystery [338, 339]. Confusion of sporadic hemophilia in the female with von Willebrand's disease (see later) is one of several explanations.

Occasionally hemophilia may be complicated by the presence in the plasma of an agent capable of inactivating or destroying antihemophilic factor [340]. This agent, called a *circulating anticoagulant,* may make the patient refractory to the beneficial effects of transfusion of normal plasma or its fractions. In the author's experience one-fifth of patients may have this complication [341], but circulating anticoagulants are less frequent in other series [245]. In such patients, plasma nonetheless contains normal amounts of antigen related to antihemophilic factor [603].

The origin of the circulating anticoagulant directed against antihemophilic factor is perplexing. Nearly always the patients have had transfusions of blood or plasma some time before its appearance, but this is equally true of other patients with hemophilia who do not develop the factor. The anticoagulant seems to be an antibody directed against antihemophilic factor. The antibody is of the IgG type [342–344]. The great majority are said to be monoclonal, with kappa light chains, although this view has been challenged on the basis of studies of idiopathic anti-antihemophilic factor anticoagulants [345]. The anticoagulant often disappears within months or a few years, only to reappear almost immediately after the patient is retransfused. The presence of an anticoagulant makes therapy with antihemophilic factor ineffective, and hemorrhage can be treated only with local measures, blood or plasma being valuable only for maintaining blood volume. Massive transfusions with concentrated antihemophilic factor may be tried, but attempts at immunosuppression have been futile.

Christmas disease

Christmas disease, a lifelong bleeding disorder, was differentiated in 1952 from classic hemophilia on the basis of laboratory studies. It is otherwise indistinguishable clinically or genetically [346–348]. Christmas disease is associated with deficiency of Christmas factor activity, which is revealed in the test tube as a defect in the intrinsic pathway of clotting in which the formation of thrombin in shed blood is delayed. In most cases, protein immunologically similar to Christmas factor is not demonstrable. Presumably, such patients do not synthesize Christmas factor. In one-fourth of cases, on the other hand, the plasma contains an agent which is functionally inactive but immunologically detectable as Christmas factor [349–351, 610]. Among these cases, a smaller subgroup has been delineated in whom the abnormal protein interferes with the clot-promoting properties of bovine thromboplastin [350].

Christmas disease occurs about one-tenth to one-fifth as often as classic hemophilia. The relative frequency varies from place to place [352–354]. It is particularly frequent among the Amish in Ohio [355], and it is relatively uncommon in Japan [356]. A similar disorder has been described in dogs [357].

Like classic hemophilia, Christmas disease varies in the severity of its symptoms, and this correlates with the degree of the deficiency measured in the laboratory. Christmas disease is more frequently mild than classic hemophilia [245, 358].

The concentration of Christmas factor in normal plasma varies widely. In one study the titer of Christmas factor ranged from 37 to 170 percent of the normal mean value [359], and from 50 to 180 percent in another [360]. No significant difference exists between the titer of Christmas factor in normal males and that in nonpregnant females, but the concentration rises dramatically during pregnancy [361]. A change in the concentration of Christmas factor with age [359] has been disputed [362].

Little or no Christmas factor activity may be detectable in the plasma of patients with severe Christmas disease. Titers of less than 5 percent of normal are usual [360, 363]. In contrast, in mildly affected patients the concentration of this substance may be 30 percent of normal or higher, values which inexplicably overlap the normal ranges [360]. Within a given family both the severity of symptoms and the titer of Christmas factor are approximately the same in affected persons. Some evidence exists that in patients with Christmas disease the titer of Christmas factor gradually rises with age [359].

Genetics

Christmas disease is inherited in the same way as classic hemophilia. It is an X-linked recessive which is virtually limited to males (Fig. 72-4). The locus for Christmas factor on the X chromosome is apparently far distant from that for antihemophilic factor [364] and for deutan color blindness [362], but it is close to that for serum protein Xm [364]. In approximately two-thirds of cases, a family history of bleeding can be obtained [275, 352]. Occasionally, as in two females studied in the author's laboratory, heterozygotes have symptoms suggestive of Christmas disease, but usually they are asymptomatic [365–367]. The titer of Christmas factor in the plasma of carriers is on the average only 45 to 65 percent of normal [359, 360, 368, 369]. The titer among carriers varies widely but nearly always overlaps the normal range. Thus diagnosis of the carrier state is difficult. The average titer in heterozygous females is about half that of normal individuals. This has been interpreted as meaning that in the cells of the female one of a pair of X chromosomes is genetically inactive [368], in accordance with Lyon's hypothesis [335]. Thus, in some cells of heterozygotes the X chromosome carrying the normal allele for the production of Christmas factor is functional, whereas in others only the mutant allele is active. The proportion of cells in which one or the other X chromosome is functional varies from individual to individual. This explains the extremely low titers of Christmas factor that may be encountered in some carriers, such as a young girl whose plasma contained only 2 percent Christmas factor; this child had a severe bleeding diathesis [370]. Karyotypic analysis has been used to confirm the sex in several such female patients [371, 372].

The great overlap in concentration of Christmas factor between normal individuals and proved carriers sharply limits the utility of assays for this factor in detecting the heterozygous state. An unsolved puzzle is why female carriers of Christmas disease may be asymptomatic and yet have titers of Christmas factor which are appreciably less than those of some affected males with clinical disease.

Laboratory Studies

Depending upon the severity of the defect, the clotting time in glass tubes of venous blood or plasma, the partial thromboplastin time, and prothrombin consumption may or may not be abnormal, but the clotting time of whole blood is usually prolonged in polystyrene or silicone-coated tubes. The bleeding time and the tourniquet test are normal. The one-stage prothrombin time is also ordinarily normal, but in several patients in whom nonfunctional material, antigenically related to Christmas factor, was found in plasma, this test gave abnormal results when ox brain thromboplastin was used [350, 372]. The prolonged prothrombin time was apparently due to inhibition of the reaction between thromboplastin and factor VII by the aberrent Christmas factor [373]. Usually, the results of the thromboplastin generation test are abnormal, but they may be normal in mild cases. The defect in this test is corrected by substituting normal serum for that of the patient, but not by substituting normal aluminum hydroxide-adsorbed plasma, which lacks Christmas factor. The diagnosis of Christmas disease depends upon the demonstration by a specific assay that the titer of Christmas factor is depressed. In mild Christmas disease the results of routine testing may be misleadingly normal. When there is a reasonable clinical suspicion that Christmas disease may be present, specific assays must be performed.

Therapy

The principles of therapy in Christmas disease do not differ from those of classic hemophilia. Fortunately Christmas factor is more stable both in vitro and in vivo. Ordinary bank blood retains essentially all its Christmas factor activity. Plasma prepared from bank blood and stored at $-20°C$ may be used for several months [374]. For adequate hemostasis the concentration of Christmas factor in the circulating plasma must be raised to 25 percent of normal or higher [375, 376]. Once the plasma level has been raised by transfusion, 20 to 40 hr elapse before the concentration has fallen by half. This is a significantly longer period than in classic hemophilia [376–378]. Nevertheless, as much plasma or more is needed to promote hemostasis in patients with Christmas disease as in those with classic hemophilia [245, 379]. Perhaps this is because the transfused Christmas factor must be distributed through a large extravascular pool, possibly as large as one-tenth of body weight, so that more plasma is needed to raise the concentration of this factor to a desired level [303, 376]. Because relatively large amounts of plasma are needed to treat patients with Christmas disease, a concentrate of Christmas factor would be of value. Several such preparations have been used effectively and are now commercially available [377, 380–384].

An unsupported impression exists that the prognosis of Christmas disease is better than that of hemophilia. In about one-eighth of cases the disorder has been complicated by the presence of a circulating anticoagulant directed against Christmas factor, so that transfusion therapy is ineffective [341, 351, 358]. The presence of a circulating anticoagulant probably does not influence prognosis [385].

Hageman trait

Hageman trait is the hereditary absence of detectable Hageman factor in the plasma [386]. With minor exceptions this abnormality is unassociated with clinical evidence of a bleeding tendency. Nor is there evidence of abnormalities in inflammatory response despite the participation of Hageman factor in experimental inflammation. The index cases have been found by chance. In the laboratory the clotting time of whole blood or recalcified plasma or both is greatly prolonged, and serum prothrombic activity is abnormally high. The thromboplastin generation test also gives abnormal values, and substitution of either normal serum or normal adsorbed plasma will correct this. The bleeding time is normal, and the tourniquet test usually gives normal results. The diagnosis is made by testing the effect of plasma on the clotting of plasma known to be deficient in Hageman factor. A tentative diagnosis of Hageman trait is possible if clot-promoting activity does not appear when plasma is exposed to glass or kaolin [258], but accurate diagnosis requires a direct comparison with a plasma known to possess this specific defect.

There is considerable variation in the normal concentration of Hageman factor. In a group of normal males varying in age from 19 to 40 the concentration varied from 35 to 185 percent of the mean, half of the values falling between 75 and 125 percent [61]. No information is available concerning the influence of various physiologic changes on its concentration.

Hageman trait is inherited as an autosomal recessive character [387, 388]. Severe deficiencies have been detected in neither the parents nor offspring of affected individuals, and consanguinity has been found in 8 of 85 families. In one apparent exception to this rule consanguineous unions during successive generations may have occurred [389]. Partial deficiencies of Hageman factor can be demonstrated in many heterozygotes. In some, the concentration of Hageman factor is about half of normal, and in others the concentration is much lower. This bimodal distribution was interpreted by Veltkamp [389, 390] to mean that at least two normally occurring alleles are needed for the synthesis of this factor.

The suggestion has been made that patients with Hageman trait synthesize a form of Hageman factor lacking procoagulant activity [391]. But antigenic material related to Hageman factor was not demonstrable in plasma in a large series of patients with Hageman trait. This suggests that a true deficiency exists [392]. Suitable tests demonstrate traces of Hageman factor in the plasma [61]. Significantly, the plasma of persons with Hageman trait inhibits the clot-promoting effect which glass has upon normal plasma [92, 393]. In at least one patient defective aggregation of platelets by ADP, epinephrine, and thrombin has been described [394]; this has not been true in our experience.

Interest in Hageman trait rests in the paradox implicit in its asymptomatic character in spite of laboratory abnormalities as marked as those in severe hemophilia or Christmas disease. No satisfactory explanation of this puzzle has been forthcoming, although it is notable that one substrate of activated Hageman factor, PTA, may be activated in the laboratory in its virtual absence [105, 123]. Surprisingly, Mr. Hageman, the index patient, died of pulmonary embolism after pelvic fracture. No significant abnormalities were found at autopsy [395].

No therapy is indicated for persons with Hageman trait, but prudence suggests that blood or plasma be readily available if surgical intervention is undertaken [374]. When normal plasma is transfused into someone with Hageman trait, half of the Hageman factor activity is dissipated within 40 to 50 hr [396, 397].

PTA deficiency

In 1953 Rosenthal et al. [398] studied three members of a family with a mild bleeding tendency "marked chiefly by bleeding after tooth extractions." The abnormality was clearly separable from hemophilia and Christmas disease, and appeared to result from deficiency of a new clotting factor, designated plasma thromboplastic antecedent, or PTA, since it seemed to function early during the clotting process. PTA deficiency is apparently a failure to synthesize normal amounts of the functionally deficient clotting factor; the deficiency can be demonstrated by immunologic techniques [605].

More than 200 similar cases have now been described [399, 400]. PTA deficiency occurs in both sexes and has been recognized somewhat more often in females. Spontaneous bleeding is unusual. The patients come to attention because of bleeding after dental extraction, tonsillectomy, other surgical procedures, or injuries. Curiously, surgical treatment or childbirth need not be accompanied by bleeding [401]. Epistaxes are relatively common, but menorrhagia or bleeding into the central nervous system are unusual. Hemarthroses and hematuria rarely if ever occur [400]. PTA deficiency has been detected in two Holstein cows, half-sisters, one of which had evidence of hemarthrosis [402].

Nothing is known concerning the influence of various physiologic conditions on the concentration of PTA in normal plasma. In two series normal individuals varied from 63 to 136 percent [403] and from 55 to 185 percent of the mean value [61].

The way in which PTA deficiency is inherited has been clarified by Rapaport and his associates [403]. They distinguish two groups of patients, those with "major" and those with "minor" deficiencies of PTA. In those with major deficiencies the concentration of PTA is 20 percent or less of average normal values. Probably none has an absolute deficiency of the factor. These patients usually have a bleeding tendency, although rarely they may be asymptomatic [404]. Patients with minor deficiencies of PTA have trivial symptoms or none, and their concentration of PTA ranges from 30 to 60 percent of the average normal. The difference between major and minor PTA deficiencies can be explained by the assumption that the allele responsible for the defect is incompletely dominant. Individuals homozygous for the mutant allele have major PTA deficiencies, while heterozygotes have minor deficiencies. Although other interpretations have been suggested, most of the published data are in accordance with this view [400, 405]. The majority of patients have been Jewish [363, 400, 403].

The recognition of PTA deficiency is difficult. The clotting time of whole blood is either normal or only slightly prolonged. Prothrombin consumption is often abnormal. This defect can be corrected by the addition of small amounts of the plasma or serum of normal persons or patients with other hemorrhagic disorders, but this is a technically difficult procedure. An important exception is that the plasma of patients with Hageman trait may be less effective than normal plasma [406]. In severe cases the thromboplastin generation test also gives abnormal results. The defect can be corrected by the substitution of either aluminum hydroxide-adsorbed normal plasma or normal serum. This distinguishes the abnormality from hemophilia or Christmas disease but not from Hageman trait. In a few patients the bleeding time has been prolonged [407].

The diagnosis of PTA deficiency can be made with certainty only by demonstrating that the abnormality in the plasma is not corrected by the plasma of a patient known to have PTA deficiency. Unfortunately, the defect seems to disappear when the plasma is stored for several days in a refrigerator or freezer, unless it is prepared in silicone-coated tubes and the platelets removed by high-speed centrifugation. Because of these technical problems, some of the published cases of PTA deficiency may not be genuine. An excellent specific assay for PTA has been described [259].

Information concerning the treatment of bleeding in PTA deficiency is meager. The use of stored blood or plasma has been suggested [408]. After transfusion, half of the administered PTA is no longer detectable after 60 hr [409]. In at least one patient resistance to the corrective effect of normal plasma was related to the presence of a circulating anticoagulant directed against PTA [410].

Deficiencies of Prothrombin, Factor VII, and Stuart Factor

Deficiencies of prothrombin, factor VII, and Stuart factor may be advantageously considered together, since these substances, with Christmas factor, compose a group of proteins with many common features. Chemically they are remarkably similar, and separation and purification have been difficult. The difficulties in separating one from another may be related to similarities in amino acid composition. The amino acids of three of the factors, prothrombin, Christmas factor, and Stuart factor, have been compared and are virtually the same except for a relatively high proportion of cystine in Stuart factor [56, 172]. The four factors are probably all proenzymes. Like some other proteolytic enzymes, thrombin and activated Stuart factor, the active forms of prothrombin and Stuart factor digest synthetic amino acid esters [56, 161].

The same four clotting factors have many biologic properties in common. They are synthesized only if vitamin K is available, and anything compromising its supply may induce simultaneous deficiencies of all four factors. Vitamin K is probably a coenzyme, participating in electron transport and coupled oxidative phosphorylation [411–414], but this hardly explains its role. These observations cannot be applied to the synthesis of proteins [612]. Why the action of vitamin K seems limited to the synthesis of these four proteins is an intriguing puzzle. Experiments of Olson [415], Suttie [416], Hemker [417], and Josso [418] indicate that the synthesis of the four factors proceeds in two stages. The first, the synthesis of polypeptides, does not require vitamin K. The second step, in which the completed protein is released from the ribosomes, takes place only if the vitamin is available. In its absence, the incomplete protein may enter the bloodstream where it acts as a competitive inhibitor of the vitamin K–dependent factors [417]. Hemker [417] has suggested that the function of vitamin K is to facilitate addition of carbohydrate to the structure.

The bulk of the vitamin K absorbed by the body is synthesized by the bacterial flora of the gastrointestinal tract. Before bacterial growth begins, the newborn infant is dependent upon supplies of vitamin K obtained prenatally from its mother or supplied by her milk. These exogenous supplies are marginal. The normal infant is deficient in each of the vitamin K–dependent clotting factors at birth, a deficiency which progresses for 2 to 5 days and then gradually disappears. A deficiency of vitamin K may result from inhibition of intestinal bacterial growth by orally administered antibiotics or from impairment of absorption of the vitamin because of intrinsic intestinal dysfunction or because bile salts, which are needed to emulsify the lipid-soluble vitamin, are excluded from the intestine by intra- or extrahepatic biliary obstruction. Once absorbed, vitamin K is utilized in the liver. Synthesis of the vitamin K–dependent clotting factors is impaired in patients with hepatic disease and in those to whom vitamin K antagonists such as coumarin or the phenindione compounds have been administered. Pregnancy and various stresses may be associated with elevated concentrations of the vitamin K–dependent clotting factors [361, 419].

No satisfactory hypothesis explains the similarities among the vitamin K-dependent clotting factors. Seegers' view [420] is attractive in many ways. He suggests that prothrombin is a complex molecule consisting of prothrombin (the immediate precursor of thrombin), autoprothrombin III (the precursor of autoprothrombin C, that is, activated Stuart factor), and a third, an inhibitory component. Autoprothrombin I (i.e., factor VII) and autoprothrombin II (i.e., Christmas factor) are also derived from the prothrombin molecule. Malhotra's [89] procedure for purification, however, seems to separate prothrombin from the other vitamin K-dependent factors by relatively atraumatic means, and thus contradicts Seegers' appealing hypothesis. Another major stumbling block to this idea is that the four recognized factors may be involved in separate hereditary deficiencies. Whether this apparently insurmountable obstacle is real is yet to be determined.

Hereditary deficiencies of the vitamin K–dependent clotting factors must be distinguished from the effects of self-administered coumarin-like drugs. Nearly always the latter disorder is a deliberate attempt to deceive the unwary physician, but in two of our patients bleeding followed the dispensing of Dicumarol in error. The diagnosis is readily made by demonstrating the presence of deficiencies of all four vitamin K–dependent clotting factors and of the offending drug in the plasma. Nearly all cases have been in persons who have ready access to drugs [421, 422].

Hereditary Deficiency of Prothrombin

Christmas disease, the hereditary deficiency of Christmas factor, has already been discussed. Only a handful of cases of the hereditary deficiency of prothrombin have been described. The hemorrhagic tendency in these cases is clinically similar to that in hemophilia. The patients bleed from the umbilicus at birth and later into the skin, muscle, and joints. Epistaxes, gingival bleeding, hematuria, and menorrhagia may be troublesome, and the patients may bleed after dental extraction, tonsillectomy, and other surgical procedures. The diagnosis is suggested by an abnormally long one-stage prothrombin time which is uncorrected either by normal serum or by normal plasma from which the vitamin K–dependent clotting factors have been adsorbed. The degree of the deficiency of prothrombin can be estimated by specific assays for this factor [423]. In normal, nonpregnant individuals the concentration of prothrombin varies from 65 to 150 percent of the mean value [61, 423, 424]. In most of the reported cases, in contrast, the concentration of prothrombin was about 10 percent of normal, and in at least two [425, 426] still less was present. To a degree the severity of bleeding reflects the severity of the defect noted in the laboratory. One patient, in whom the concentration of prothrombin was 10 to 13 percent of normal, had no symptoms until his thirteenth year [427]. In some patients the clotting and bleeding times have been prolonged, but the results of the prothrombin consumption and thromboplastin generation tests have been normal.

Hereditary deficiencies of prothrombin are inherited as autosomal traits which are almost completely recessive. Both sexes are affected with equal frequency. In three of eight families the parents were first cousins [427, 428]. In some cases the asymptomatic carriers may be identified by a slight prolongation of the one-stage prothrombin time [425, 426]. In two patients slight deficiencies of factor VII or Stuart factor, or of both, were also found [426, 429]. In one case the electrophoretic band corresponding to prothrombin was lacking in the plasma [427]. Some patients with congenital hypoprothrombinemia may be unable to synthesize protein recognizable immunologically as prothrombin [611]. In one family, on the other hand, although affected individuals had a partial functional deficiency of prothrombin, this protein appeared to be present in normal concentration, as if the patients synthesized an abnormal form of the molecule [430].

The transfusion of plasma may be used to control hemorrhage, although the amount required is not certain. The newly available concentrates of the vitamin K–dependent clotting factors, when prepared from plasma rather than serum, may be efficacious. The biologic half-life of prothrombin has been estimated at 3 to 5 days [427, 428], but in a patient with prothrombin deficiency treated with plasma, half of the transfused factor disappeared within 9 hr [431]. In one case transfused prothrombin was probably destroyed at an accelerated rate, but no anticoagulant substance could be demonstrated [245]. Vitamin K is without value in therapy.

Hereditary Deficiency of Factor VII

Hereditary deficiency of factor VII is probably rare. About 50 cases have been reported [432, 433]. It is probably a true deficiency, since the plasma of affected individuals does not contain antigen reacting with specific anti-factor VII antiserum [434, 435]. The clinical pattern is similar to what is seen in moderately severe hemophilia. Bleeding into the subcutaneous tissues, muscles, and joints is common. Other types of hemorrhage, gastrointestinal or central nervous system bleeding, hematuria, epistaxes, gingival bleeding, and menorrhagia, have been observed. Bleeding after surgical treatment or dental extraction is frequent but not invariable. Sometimes a bleeding tendency is recognized shortly after birth because of hemorrhage from the umbilicus [432]. In other cases the patients have been free from bleeding in spite of severe laboratory abnormalities [276, 436]. Indeed, two asymptomatic patients actually suffered pulmonary embolism [437, 438].

In normal adults the concentration of factor VII varies widely. In one series of 40 males values ranged between 55 and 185 percent of the mean [61]. Excessively high values have been described in association with pregnancy, surgical stress, and acute myocardial infarction [177]. A bleeding tendency may appear when the concentration of factor VII falls below 10 percent [177, 419].

The diagnosis of factor VII deficiency presents no difficulties. The prothrombin time is usually greatly prolonged, and this is corrected by addition of serum [432]. This test does not distinguish a deficiency of factor VII from that of Stuart factor, but unlike Stuart factor deficiency, the clotting time of recalcified plasma is normal in the presence of Russell's viper venom, an agent which promotes clotting by activating Stuart factor [159]. In cases of factor VII deficiency the clotting time of whole blood and prothrombin consumption are usually normal, and no defect can be demonstrated in the thromboplastin generation test, but these criteria are not absolute [257]. The bleeding time may be abnormally long [177]. A definitive diagnosis is best made by comparing the plasma of the suspected patient with that of a patient known to have factor VII deficiency.

Hereditary deficiency of factor VII may occur in either sex and appears to be the homozygous condition for an autosomal gene which in the heterozygous state causes a partial deficiency of this factor [276, 439]. A similar pattern of inheritance has been observed in a family of beagles with factor VII deficiency [440]. Unexplained is a preponderance of female patients [433, 439]. Not enough data are available concerning the sibs of probands to interpret this observation. In several instances the patients had parents who were related [439, 441, 442]. The concentration of factor VII in presumed homozygotes for the mutant allele has been 10 percent or less [177]; three of the author's patients have had virtually none. Heterozygous relatives have 25 to 75 percent of normal factor VII activity, a deficiency reflected in slight prolongation of the prothrombin time [439, 442]. The heterozygous state is usually not associated with significant bleeding. In two sibs under our care, the apparent concentration of factor VII has risen with adolescence, although it is still far below normal.

Bleeding due to factor VII deficiency can be life-threatening. Deaths have been described from bleeding into the central nervous system [443] and from menorrhagia [442]. No specific therapy is available. Transfusions of plasma may help to control hemorrhage. Since factor VII is stable during the usual period of storage, bank blood or plasma derived from bank blood may be used. The volume required can only be determined empirically. An initial dose of a liter of plasma to an adult continued at the rate of 100 ml every 3 or 4 hr is probably adequate. Concentrates of the vitamin K-dependent clotting factors should prove useful. The time which elapses until half of the transfused factor VII disappears from the circulating plasma is only 1 or 2 hr [444]. Hormonal suppression of menstrual bleeding may help in the treatment of menorrhagia.

Chevalier [445] observed that the plasma of one of his patients inactivated factor VII of normal plasma, but other cases complicated by circulating anticoagulants have not been described.

Stuart Factor Deficiency

Stuart factor deficiency is not distinguishable clinically from factor VII deficiency [159, 456, 457]. Immunologic studies suggest that in some cases the disorder is a true deficiency state [274, 434], while in others, material immunologically similar to Stuart factor is present in plasma [613]. Moreover, functional studies suggest that the defect varies from family to family [613]. The prothrombin time is prolonged, and this is corrected by the addition of normal serum. In contrast to factor VII deficiency, the clotting time of recalcified plasma is abnormally long in the presence of Russell's viper venom [159]. The clotting time of venous blood and partial thromboplastin time are also long, and the prothrombin consumption and thromboplastin generation test give abnormal results. In order to establish the diagnosis, the plasma of the patient should be compared directly with that of a patient with known Stuart factor deficiency.

Stuart factor deficiency has been reported somewhat less frequently than factor VII deficiency [274]. It is a penetrant, partially dominant autosomal trait [448]. The heterozygotes have little or no bleeding tendency, but slight prolongation of the prothrombin time and minor abnormalities in the thromboplastin generation test may be detected. The concentration of Stuart factor in the plasma of heterozygotes ranges from 20 to 52 percent of normal [448], whereas in normal persons the titer of this substance varied from 65 to 185 percent and from 72 to 115 percent of the mean in two studies [61, 449]. The concentration of Stuart factor in the plasma of homozygous patients is less than 10 percent of normal [450] and usually much lower. The parents of some homozygotes have been consanguineous [448, 451]. In one family moderate deficiency of Stuart factor was sometimes associated with a mild deficiency of factor VII [449]. Familial deficiency of Stuart factor must be distinguished from the acquired condition, as described in association with amyloidosis [452].

The treatment of bleeding in Stuart factor deficiency is similar to that in factor VII deficiency, but the transfusion of plasma may be more effective, since it takes 2 to 3 days for half of a given amount of Stuart factor to disappear from the plasma [453]. Again, vitamin K is not of value.

Congenital Combined Deficiency of the Vitamin K-dependent Clotting Factors

Although a combined deficiency of the four clotting factors which require vitamin K for synthesis has been reported several times, in nearly every instance the patient had access to coumarin-like drugs, suggesting that the disorder was surreptitiously induced. A true instance of concomitant deficiency of prothrombin, Stuart factor, factor VII, and Christmas factor has been described in an infant girl who had had bleeding from the first week of life [606]. No evidence of hepatic damage or of malabsorption was found, but the patient responded to the administration of vitamin K. Studies of both parents gave normal results. The pathogenesis of the deficiency state was not clarified further, and whether the patient's defect was inherited is not certain.

Hereditary Resistance to Coumarin-like Drugs

O'Reilly and his associates [454] recently described a kindred in which 7 individuals were unusually resistant to the effects of warfarin, bishydroxycoumarin, and phenindione. The abnormality was probably inherited in an autosomal dominant manner. The propositus required 20 times the usual dose of warfarin to obtain a therapeutic effect. The mechanism underlying the disorder is not yet elucidated, but plasma binding of warfarin was normal and the urine contained normal amounts of a warfarin metabolite. Affected individuals were unusually sensitive to the corrective effects of orally ingested vitamin K when they had been treated with warfarin. It seems possible either that the patients had an abnormal enzyme or receptor site with a decreased affinity for coumarin drugs or an increased affinity for vitamin K. A similar defect has been observed in wild rats, in which transmission as an autosomal dominant trait has been demonstrated [455]. Since warfarin inhibited the synthesis of factor VII in rat liver slices as readily in affected as in normal animals, the hypothesis has been proposed that the site of resistance is somewhere between the point of transfer from the binding site for the drug on plasma albumin and that part of the liver parenchymal cell which responds to warfarin in the in vitro system; this view remains unsubstantiated.

Parahemophilia

Parahemophilia is a familial disorder in which the concentration of proaccelerin in plasma is abnormally low [187]. More than 30 families with this disorder have been found. The symptoms resemble those of classic hemophilia, although hemarthroses are unusual [257, 456]. Menorrhagia is a serious problem which may cause death from exsanguination [457], and parturition may be followed after some days by severe hemorrhage [458].

Parahemophilia occurs in both sexes. It is apparently the homozygous state of a partially dominant trait. Affected individuals have virtually no proaccelerin in the plasma, and their heterozygous relatives may have partial deficiencies and sometimes such minor evidence of a bleeding tendency as epistaxes [192, 459]. The severity of bleeding varies from patient to patient. It is not clear whether different persons within a single family are affected to the same degree.

The concentration of proaccelerin in normal human plasma varies widely. In 40 normal males between the ages of 19 and 40, the concentration varied from 45 to 165 percent of the mean value, and 27 of the values were between 75 and 125 percent [61]. Dicumarol therapy is without effect. A moderate rise in the concentration of proaccelerin has been reported in patients with diabetes [298] and 2 to 4 days after the induction of fever by the intramuscular injection of milk [294].

The diagnosis of parahemophilia is easily established in the laboratory. The prothrombin time is abnormally long and is corrected by the addition of fresh normal plasma from which the vitamin K–dependent clotting factors have been removed but not by human serum or stored oxalated plasma, both of which are deficient in proaccelerin. Results of other clotting tests may be abnormal. The clotting time of whole blood or plasma and the partial thromboplastin time may be prolonged, and serum prothrombic activity is usually abnormally high. The results of the thromboplastin generation test are abnormal. This is most clearly demonstrated when the incubation mixture includes the patient's own platelets or crude "cephalin" instead of normal platelets. This observation reflects the fact that the platelets, unlike normal platelets, lack proaccelerin-like activity [192, 193]. This defect of platelets can be corrected by incubating them in normal plasma. The defect in the thromboplastin generation test is more readily discernible if the patient's own plasma is used as the substrate [301]. Rarely the bleeding time may be prolonged [460].

The prognosis of parahemophilia is usually good, but deaths have been reported. The treatment of bleeding is similar to that of classic hemophilia. Blood or plasma stored at 4°C is unreliable as a source of proaccelerin, but freshly frozen plasma retains its activity for several months [461]. Concentrates of antihemophilic factor are without benefit. How long the effects of transfusion last is uncertain; in different studies the time elapsing until half of an amount of transfused proaccelerin had disappeared was 12 to 36 hr [462–464]. The concentration of proaccelerin needed for hemostasis is not clear. Values between 10 and 25 percent of normal have been suggested as necessary to prevent bleeding even after surgical procedures [462, 464]. No information is available concerning the use of fractions of plasma rich in proaccelerin. Circulating anticoagulants inactivating proaccelerin have been described in a few patients. Under these circumstances, transfusions are effective only in maintaining the blood volume [465, 466].

Congenital Afibrinogenemia

Congenital afibrinogenemia is a rare disease in which little or no detectable fibrinogen is present in the plasma [467]. Notwithstanding the absence of a mechanism for the formation of clots, this disorder is compatible with life. Persons with congenital afibrinogenemia bleed severely after injury or surgery. Bleeding from the umbilicus within a few days of birth, after circumcision or dental extractions, or even from diaper rash is common. There may be repeated episodes of ecchymoses, epistaxes, hematomas, hemoptyses, or bleeding into the gastrointestinal or genitourinary tracts or the central nervous system. Hemarthroses are relatively rare. Permanent damage to tissues is distinctly unusual, perhaps because no fibrin forms at the site of the injury [245]. Pseudocysts of bone such as are seen in hemophilia occur [468]. The most striking characteristic of congenital afibrinogenemia is that the patients have long periods of freedom from bleeding. Curiously, girls who reach the menarche may have nearly normal menses [469, 470], although this is not always true. These observations underline the importance for hemostasis of other mechanisms besides clotting.

The hereditary nature of congenital afibrinogenemia was recognized soon after the first case was described. Consanguinity has been reported in 22 of 32 families for whom data are available. The patients have always appeared in the same generation. Among 65 sibs of probands 31 percent also had the disorder. The disease occurs in both sexes but is said to be more frequent in males. In a tabulation of 70 published cases 43 were males. This sex difference may not be genuine, since among the sibs of probands, 11 males and 10 females had the disorder. These various observations suggest that congenital afibrinogenemia is an autosomal recessive trait. The heterozygous carriers are usually asymptomatic and have normal plasma concentrations of fibrinogen. In occasional instances slight hypofibrinogenemia has been described in heterozygotes.

The clotting time of whole blood or plasma and the prothrombin time are, of course, infinite, and blood fails to clot upon the addition of thrombin. Assays for all other clotting factors have usually given normal results, except that in a few instances transient thrombocytopenia and slight depression of proaccelerin have been described. The bleeding time is usually prolonged, and when normal, bleeding may start afresh if the finger is flexed shortly after the test [471]. Results of the tourniquet test are usually normal. Needless to say, the erythrocyte sedimentation rate is virtually zero, the red cells remaining suspended even after 24 hr [233].

Whether a total deficiency of fibrinogen ever occurs is not clear. No band is detectable upon electrophoresis of plasma, nor can fibrinogen be precipitated by heating or "salting out." Nonetheless, in a few patients immunologic methods have demonstrated traces of fibrogen in the plasma [472, 473]. Only traces of fibrinogen-like material can be detected in platelet cytoplasmic granules [222]. The low concentration of fibrinogen in plasma may be responsible for defective adhesion of platelets to glass and for their poor aggregation by epinephrine or small amounts of ADP [474, 475]. Platelet aggregation by collagen or by larger amounts of ADP is normal. Although thrombin brings about aggregation of platelets at a nearly normal rate, the cells do not then undergo the usual sequential changes of viscous metamorphosis in a normal manner. Aggregates of platelets, formed in recalcified plasma, break up abnormally readily [476]. These observations suggest that the bleeding tendency of patients with afibrinogenemia is due not only to their inability to form a fibrin clot but also to deficiencies in the hemostatic behavior of their platelets.

The concentration of fibrinogen in normal plasma ranges from about 170 to 400 mg per 100 ml and averages approximately 300 mg [5, 6]. The concentration of fibrinogen is increased during pregnancy and in inflammatory states. ACTH [477] and pituitary growth hormone [478] increase its concentration, yet normal values are obtained in patients who have undergone hypophysectomy [479]. The level of fibrinogen is influenced by diet. Ingestion of large amounts of cooked pig stomach increases its concentration [480, 481]. These various observations fail to give a clear picture of the factors influencing the metabolism of this protein.

The basic defect in afibrinogenemia apparently is a failure of synthesis. Intravenously injected fibrinogen remains in the blood as long as in normal subjects. One-half to three-quarters of transfused fibrinogen disappears within the first 48 hr, but thereafter only 15 percent of what remains disappears each day [470, 472, 482]; some give a somewhat higher figure [470].

Bleeding in congenital afibrinogenemia is treated by the intravenous injection of concentrated human fibrinogen, usually in the form of Cohn fraction I [75]. A dose of 4 gm is sufficient to provide hemostasis in an adult. This raises the concentration to about 100 mg per 100 ml plasma, or about one-third of normal. Repeated injections may be needed. Such treatment is all too often complicated by homologous serum jaundice, the virus of which often contaminates fraction I, since this is made from pooled plasma. To some extent, this risk may be obviated by using cryoprecipitated antihemophilic factor as a source of fibrinogen; one bag of cryoprecipitate is given for each 2 kg body weight as an initial dose; thereafter, one bag for each 15 kg is sufficient [303]. Rarely, anticoagulant substances appear in the plasma of patients who have been transfused with fibrinogen and preclude further therapy [468, 484]. A number of patients have reached adult life, but the prognosis is generally poor. Usually death results from blood loss or bleeding into a vital area. Unbelievably, three patients have died of pulmonary embolism; the emboli were made up of masses of platelets, and in two cases these appeared to arise from lesions in the veins of the legs [484, 485]. The dangers of homologous serum jaundice or of acquiring circulating anticoagulants make it unwise to attempt prophylaxis by repeated injections of fibrinogen.

In addition to those patients in whom fibrinogen can be detected only by immunologic methods, there are a few in whom small but significant amounts are present. For example, 20 mg per 100 ml plasma has been reported [486]. This hypofibrinogenemic state is not distinguishable from afibrinogenemia in its mode of inheritance, but clinically the course of the disorder seems more benign.

Congenital Dysfibrinogenemia

In congenital afibrinogenemia, affected individuals seem incapable of synthesizing fibrinogen. In contrast, in at least eight families, individuals have been found who synthesize a functionally abnormal fibrinogen, detectable immunologically but from which fibrin is not formed at a normal rate [487–490]. The abnormality has been discovered because the thrombin time, that is, the clotting time of plasma upon the addition of thrombin, has been abnormally long. As a consequence, in most patients, the prothrombin time has also been above normal, the finding which brings the disorder to the physician's attention. The concentration of fibrinogen in plasma, measured in terms of the amount of fibrin which can be formed, has been normal or slightly depressed in most instances, but in one case none was detectable [489]. Functional and immunologic criteria suggest that the defect differs from family to family, but in nearly all it has been inherited in an autosomal dominant pattern. In most cases, the functional abnormality has been a failure of dissolved fibrin monomers or polymers to aggregate in a normal manner but in at least one, the rate at which thrombin changes fibrinogen to fibrin monomer has been below normal [607]. In one instance analysis demonstrated that an arginine residue in the N-terminal part of the α (A) chain of fibrinogen was replaced by a neutral amino acid, most likely serine [491]. This abnormal protein, designated as *fibrinogen Detroit,* contained less carbohydrate than normal fibrinogen [489].

Only a few patients with congenital dysfibrinogenemia have had a bleeding tendency, and that has usually been mild. Inexplicably, several have suffered thrombotic episodes. In at least two families some affected individuals have experienced dehiscence of operative wounds [488, 490]. One of our patients whose blood contained fibrinogen Cleveland, died recently and at autopsy had fibrinous pleurisy and pericarditis, probably infectious in origin. Experience in one patient with a bleeding tendency suggests that the transfusion of fibrinogen may have been beneficial [489].

What may be a variant of dysfibrinogenemia has been described in a patient whose fibrinogen clotted more rapidly than normally upon the addition of thrombin [492]. The defect was associated with a high incidence of thromboembolic phenomena. In another family, an abnormal fibrinogen manifested defective cross-linking between fibrin strands once clotting had occurred [608].

Deficiency of Fibrin-stabilizing Factor

At least 43 patients with congenital deficiency of fibrin-stabilizing factor activity have been detected since this disorder was first described by Duckert [493, 494]. The defect is more frequent in males than in females. The patients have had repeated episodes of serious bleeding after injury. Almost all bled from the umbilicus shortly after birth. In some patients the illness has been characterized by protracted bleeding lasting many weeks after an injury. Wounds may heal slowly or may break down repeatedly. Hematomas, hemarthroses, hematuria, and habitual abortion associated with uterine bleeding have been described. Intracranial bleeding, often lethal, is frequent.

All routine tests for hemostatic function have been normal, but fibrin prepared from the plasma of the patient, unlike normal plasma, is soluble in 5*M* urea or 1% monochloroacetic acid. The diagnosis of fibrin-stabilizing factor deficiency is firmly established by demonstrating deficient incorporation of C^{14}-glycine ethyl ester into fibrin or casein [495] or of monodansyl cadaverine into casein [46]. The transfusion of small amounts of plasma—fresh, stored, or frozen—readily controls bleeding and has been used prophylactically [493, 496, 497]. The half-life of fibrin-stabilizing factor after the transfusion of plasma has been estimated as 3 to 5 days [496, 498]. The patients may become refractory to transfusion as antibodies appear to the administered fibrin-stabilizing factor [46].

In a study of 10 families protein immunologically similar to fibrin-stabilizing factor was demonstrable in all affected individuals tested [499]. Thus, the patients are not deficient in the factor, but synthesize an inert form of the molecule. The method of inheritance of the disease is not clear. A review of the known cases suggested that in different families inheritance was through either autosomal recessive or sex-linked recessive genes. This would explain the preponderance of affected males [494]. Cases published subsequent to this report are in agreement with this interpretation. Carriers may have a diminished plasma concentration of functional fibrin-stabilizing factor [46].

Von Willebrand's Disease

Von Willebrand [500] described an unusual bleeding syndrome among the inhabitants of the Åland Islands in the Baltic Sea in 1926. Among those affected the severity of the clinical manifestations varies widely, but in general the symptoms resemble those of mild hemophilia. Both sexes are susceptible. Unlike hemophilia, cutaneous and mucosal petechiae may occur [501]. Menorrhagia, bleeding at childbirth and bleeding from the gastrointestinal tract may be troublesome and even fatal [501]. A long-recognized hemorrhagic disease of swine now seems to be strikingly similar to von Willebrand's disease [502, 503].

Von Willebrand found that the bleeding time in his patient was prolonged. He attributed the defect to a qualitative abnormality of the platelets. Borchgrevink [504] proposed that in von Willebrand's disease the adhesiveness of platelets to an injured vessel wall was impaired, a view which has been disputed [505]. Similarly, Salzman [506] and Zucker [507] reported that the adhesion of platelets to glass beads was reduced in this disorder. Although this is true in many instances normal adhesiveness to glass is observed with blood from typical von Willebrand's disease. In any event, there is no clear-cut evidence that any intrinsic abnormality of platelets exists.

A more satisfying explanation of the pathogenesis of bleeding in the Åland Islanders has emerged in a roundabout way. In 1953 three groups of investigators described patients with a lifelong bleeding tendency in whom the bleeding time was long and the concentration of antihemophilic factor in the plasma was reduced [508–510]. The long bleeding time and the fact that five of the seven patients were females made the diagnosis of classic hemophilia untenable. These observations were soon confirmed. Consistent with the deficiency of antihemophilic factor, the clotting time was sometimes prolonged, serum prothrombin consumption was often poor, and the thromboplastin generation test gave abnormal results. In this last test the alteration detected was indistinguishable from that observed in classic hemophilia.

Since these patients resembled those described by von

Willebrand, Jürgens [511] and Nilsson [512] and their associates reinvestigated the Åland Island bleeders. They found that these patients had the same combination of defects, i.e., a prolonged bleeding time and a deficiency of antihemophilic factor. For this reason, the syndrome is usually called *von Willebrand's disease.* The term *vascular hemophilia,* suggested by Schulman et al. [346], seems preferable and avoids confusion with *von Willebrand-Jürgen's thrombopathy,* a misnomer applied to one of the qualitative abnormalities of platelets, but this name has not gained acceptance.

The prolonged bleeding time of patients with von Willebrand's disease was soon found to be related to the absence of a plasma factor. Schulman et al. [513] observed that the bleeding time was shortened by the administration of plasma. The corrective effect is due to the presence of an agent which is concentrated in partially purified antihemophilic factor prepared by the method of Nilsson et al. [156], but it differs from this substance. This agent seems to increase the adhesion of platelets to an incised wound, a function possibly impaired in patients with von Willebrand's disease [154]. The correction of the bleeding time following transfusion is more certain if the blood or plasma is administered within a few hours after it is drawn [157, 515]. The effect of transfusion is transient, and within 8 hr the bleeding time is once more prolonged [515].

The transfusion of blood, plasma, cryoprecipitates of plasma, or serum also corrects the deficiency of antihemophilic factor [151, 513, 515, 516]. Unexpectedly the titer of antihemophilic factor in the recipient's plasma rises for 4 to 8 hr after transfusion and then decreases at a much slower rate than in true hemophilia [514, 517]. Equally unexpectedly, the same rise in the titer of antihemophilic factor occurs if the patient is transfused with the plasma of a patient with classic hemophilia [156, 157]. One can only conclude that both normal and hemophilic plasma contain an agent which induces the generation of antihemophilic factor in patients with von Willebrand's disease. Whether this means, as has been suggested, that this agent is an intermediate in the synthesis of antihemophilic factor remains unproved. Studies by Nilsson et al. [156] suggest that the factor inducing the synthesis of antihemophilic factor is distinct from that which shortens the bleeding time, but this also is not universally accepted [518, 519]. The deficiency of antihemophilic factor measured in clotting tests parallels a deficiency in antigens related to this clotting factor, measured immunologically, in contrast to the situation in classic hemophilia [603]. As in normal individuals, exercise sharply increases the concentration of antihemophilic factor in the plasma of patients with von Willebrand's disease. This occurs without a latent period [520].

The pattern of inheritance of von Willebrand's disease has been puzzling. In contradistinction to classic hemophilia, the severity of symptoms varies from patient to patient within a single family. Moreover, clinical severity does not correlate well with the magnitude of the two defects measurable in the laboratory, the bleeding time and the concentration of antihemophilic factor. Within the same family different individuals may have an abnormal bleeding time, a deficiency of antihemophilic factor, or both, and the intensity of these defects varies from person to person. Both sexes are affected, and there are instances in which the sons of affected males have von Willebrand's disease [521] while their daughters may be unaffected [61]. These data are consistent with transmission by an autosomal dominant gene of variable expressivity. What is unexplained is the consistent observation that the incidence of clinically apparent von Willebrand's disease is significantly greater in females than in males. Thus among 378 cases tabulated from published data, 247 were females. Perhaps this distribution reflects the common occurrence of unexplained menorrhagia as a presenting symptom [522]. We have studied 14 males and 15 females, but many of the males were asymptomatic and were investigated only because they had affected female relatives. Also unexplained is the coexistence of two abnormalities, clearly separable in the laboratory and often dissociated in different affected individuals. This confusion can be dissipated by invoking two separate genetic defects [523], but this is unconvincing.

In most instances patients with von Willebrand's disease are heterozygotes. In one interesting study two apparently homozygous individuals were severely affected, and the transfusion of plasma induced only a trivial increase in plasma antihemophilic activity beyond that which could be accounted for by the infusion itself [525]. Whether this resistance to transfusion is inherent in the homozygous state or reflects the effects of earlier transfusions in these severely affected individuals is not certain. A similar phenomenon was noted in one of our patients who is probably a heterozygote.

The treatment of von Willebrand's disease is similar to that of classic hemophilia. Individual episodes of bleeding may be treated by the transfusion of fresh plasma, freshly frozen plasma, or cryoprecipitates of plasma. After repeated transfusions patients may become refractory to stimulation of their own mechanisms for the synthesis of antihemophilic factor, so that the benefit of plasma is limited to its content of antihemophilic factor and any corrective effect it might have upon the bleeding time [524]. Menorrhagia may present a difficult therapeutic problem. Hormonal therapy to suppress menstruation should be tried. Pregnancy induces temporary remission in some cases and is demonstrated in the laboratory as a shortening of the bleeding time and an increase in antihemophilic factor activity [526, 527]. The possibility that clinical remission and an elevation of plasma antihemophilic activity may be induced in female patients by oral contraceptive therapy has been raised [528].

Combined Deficiency of Antihemophilic Factor and Proaccelerin

The coexistence of deficiencies of antihemophilic factor and proaccelerin has been described in 15 bleeders in 10 families [301, 529–532]. This extraordinary combination appears in both sexes. Although genetic data are scant, the frequency of consanguinity suggests that the defect is inherited as an autosomal recessive trait. One of the author's patients has two sons and a daughter whose plasmas contain normal amounts of antihemophilic factor and proaccelerin [61], but in other patients the plasma of the mother was partially deficient in proaccelerin [533]. Of many proposed explanations for the simultaneous deficiencies of these two factors, two seem most attractive. A single gene may control synthesis of a precursor common to both antihemophilic factor and proaccelerin. Alternatively a single gene may regulate the blood level of these two substances. There are no data to support these hypotheses. Whatever the genetic defect, it seems unrelated to that of von Willebrand's disease, since the transfusion of normal plasma does not lead to a delayed rise in antihemophilic factor [531, 532]. A recent report of Ménaché [534] questions this. In one patient physical exertion caused a remarkable increase in the concentrations of proaccelerin and antihemophilic factor, and in another, of antihemophilic factor alone [532]. In our patient, plasma contained normal amounts of antigen related to antihemophilic factor, as if he synthesized a nonfunctional type of this clotting factor [603].

Qualitative Abnormalities of Platelets

Among the most interesting of the hereditary hemorrhagic disorders are those in which platelets are qualitatively abnormal. The generic names *thromboasthenia* or *thrombocytopathic purpura* have been used for this group. As techniques have developed for the study of platelet behavior a bewildering number of syndromes have been described. In all likelihood many of these are the same disorder studied by different means. Three main groups can be discerned, those in which clot retraction is impaired (thromboasthenia, or Glanzmann's disease), those in which the primary defect is thought to be in the clot-promoting function of platelets (von Willebrand-Jürgen's syndrome, or thrombopathic purpura), and those in which aggregation of platelets by collagen or thrombin is impaired (sometimes called *thrombopathia,* a name used for other disorders as well).

Glanzmann's Disease

Glanzmann's disease is a lifelong disorder of both sexes clinically resembling mild thrombocytopenic purpura. The patients have ecchymoses and petechiae, bleeding from the gingiva, nosebleeds, gastrointestinal bleeding, menorrhagia or metrorrhagia, and excessive bleeding after surgical procedures. The bleeding time is prolonged, often to a remarkable degree, and capillary fragility as measured by the tourniquet test is increased. Although the platelet count is usually normal, mild thrombocytopenia may be present [535, 536]. The platelets often seem abnormally large and bizarre [537] and are usually isolated rather than clumped [538]. As clotting begins, pseudopods do not form as they normally would, and the fibrin strands do not orient to the platelets [537]. Electron microscopy demonstrates that the platelets are structurally abnormal [535] and do not spread out in a thin film in a normal manner [539, 540].

The platelet abnormalities in Glanzmann's disease are doubtless causally related to the impairment in clot retraction. The usual tests for the coagulant function of platelets give normal results [541]. The clotting time of whole blood and prothrombin consumption are normal (although two of our patients may be an exception, having a borderline defect in the latter test), while the platelets behave normally in the thromboplastin generation test [542]. Aggregation of platelets by ADP and thrombin is impaired in all cases [532, 535, 543] and platelets may not adhere to glass [61].

At least five different genotypic changes have been distinguished which lead to the phenotype. In one group, the concentration of ATP in the platelet is abnormally low and glycolysis is defective [238, 543, 544]. The concentrations of pyruvate kinase and phosphoglyceraldehyde dehydrogenase in the platelets are low. In a second variety, the concentration of ATP within the platelets has been low, but no enzyme defect has been discovered [545]. In other cases, ATPase seems deficient [546]. In some instances, which may belong to this same group, the concentration of ADP may be diminished [543]. In still another, platelets are deficient in glutathione reductase [547], and in still others, the platelet surface and cytoplasmic granules appear to lack the fibrinogen-like protein found normally [235, 548]. Thus, some patients seem unable to synthesize ATP and others to utilize it [543, 544]. In some, the addition of ATP and magnesium ions to the medium permits normal clot retraction. Patients with Glanzmann's disease, then, seem to lack the normal mechanisms required for viscous metamorphosis and clot retraction. Currently available data are so contradictory that no faith need be placed in this classification.

The limited data available are in agreement with the view that the several varieties of Glanzmann's disease are inherited as autosomal recessive traits [535, 540]. No specific form of therapy is available, but temporary correction of the defective clot retraction may follow the transfusion of fresh blood [535, 538]. The prognosis must be guarded because death from hemorrhage may occur [544]. The severity of bleeding may diminish as the patients grow older [544].

Thrombopathic Purpura

In a second type of hereditary qualitative platelet disorder, *thrombopathic purpura* (sometimes called *von Willebrand-Jürgen's syndrome*), the platelets lack normal clot-promoting activity. The clinical picture in affected individuals is not different from that of Glanzmann's disease, and both sexes are equally affected. The disorder is usually inherited as an autosomal recessive trait. The platelets are often large and bizarre in appearance [537, 549] and may be unclumped on a blood smear [550]. Impaired adhesiveness of the platelets to a glass surface may be demonstrated [551]. At least in some cases the defect seems to arise from failure of the platelets to release their phospholipid-rich granules into the plasma [552]. The defect may reside in the platelet membrane. These cells seem to be abnormally resistant to lysis by hypotonic solutions [552]. Once lysed by distilled water they discharge their granules, and normal clot-promoting activity results. As in Glanzmann's disease, aggregation of platelets by ADP and thrombin is impaired [553], but no intracellular enzymatic defect has been described, and the concentration of ATP in the platelet is normal [546].

The bleeding in patients with thrombopathic purpura is prolonged, and capillary fragility may be abnormal. The clotting time may be slightly prolonged. Prothrombin consumption is poor, and the platelets do not support thromboplastin generation in the Biggs-Douglas test. No specific therapy is available, but blood transfusion may shorten the bleeding time for several hours [554].

Occasionally, thrombocytopenia may occur in patients whose platelets seem to lack normal clot-promoting activity [555]. In one well-studied family the platelets were abnormally large, failed to adhere to glass, and were removed from the circulation abnormally rapidly [556]. The thrombocytopenic defect has been said to be transmitted as autosomal dominant [555], autosomal recessive [556], and X-linked [557] traits in other families. In one patient the platelet count rose to normal levels after splenectomy, but the hemorrhagic syndrome continued [537]. In another, platelet aggregation by ADP was normal and electron microscopy of the platelets in two affected relatives revealed a deficiency of α-granules. Linkage of the defect with blood group O was suggested [558].

Several patients have been reported in whom a combination of platelet abnormalities coexisted. In these, the platelets were defective both in clot retraction and in clot-promoting functions. Transfusion of normal blood corrected both abnormalities briefly [535, 559].

Thrombopathia

A third group of cases, not yet well defined, has been described under a variety of names, of which *thrombopathia* [560] is perhaps the simplest. Whether these are all representative of a single disease or, as is more likely, have features in common but are not identical, is not yet clear. Different investigators have used different techniques for study, so that variations in laboratory findings are difficult to interpret. In general the patients have had a mild bleeding disorder characterized by spontaneous bruising [561]. The existence of a hemostatic defect is demonstrated by a prolonged bleeding time. Aggregation of platelets by connective tissue is impaired in spite of normal release of ADP and ATP in the process [562, 563]. Impaired adhesion of platelets to glass and impaired aggregation by epinephrine, glass beads, and low concentrations of ADP have been observed in some cases. The aggregates formed by ADP may break up prematurely. In contrast, aggregation by larger amounts of ADP is normal [563]. Clot retraction and the release of clot-promoting phospholipids are normal. A similar disorder has been related to *albinism* [564]. Thrombopathia is probably the same as *essential athrombia,* in which the patients have had a long bleeding time and have had platelets which do not agglutinate yet seem to undergo viscous metamorphosis and to support clot retraction and coagulation [565]. Hopefully, the confusion posed by these cases will be ended as better methods for their study emerge. Since the ingestion of aspirin and certain other drugs impedes aggregation of platelets by collagen, it is important that tests be performed no sooner than a week after medication has been discontinued.

Other Disorders of Hemostasis

Many other factors concerned with clotting and inherited deficiencies of clotting have been described. Not all have survived scrutiny. Among those still to be established are Nishimine factor, Tatsumi factor, Fletcher factor, Dynia factor, and Flood factor. *Nishimine factor* is believed to be a substance in barium sulfate–adsorbed normal plasma, which is needed for the generation of thromboplastic activity but which is separable from antihemophilic factor and other recognized clot-promoting agents. It was recognized by its absence in a 3-year-old Japanese boy who died of uncontrollable epistaxis. His platelets seemed to share the defect, and his bleeding time was prolonged [566].

Tatsumi factor is said to be similar in its properties to Christmas factor but distinguishable from it by appropriate tests. A deficiency was found in two consanguineous families. The disorder occurred in both sexes and was manifested by hemorrhagic symptoms [567]. In these patients the clotting time was slightly prolonged, prothrombin consumption and thromboplastin generation were abnormal, and the bleeding time was long. The suggestion has been made that Tatsumi factor is needed for activation of Christmas factor by activated PTA [568].

Fletcher factor, deficient in the plasma of two boys and two girls, children of a consanguineous marriage, appears to participate in some unknown way in the early stages of the intrinsic pathway of thrombin formation. The affected individuals were asymptomatic [569]. Several additional cases have been described [615, 616].

Dynia factor was thought to be deficient in the plasma of a young boy with mild bleeding problems and in several asymptomatic relatives; its proposed site of action is related to the functioning of antihemophilic factor [570].

Flood factor is defined as an agent in plasma which shortens the slightly long prothrombin time of several asymptomatic individuals in the Flood family studied by Quick and Hussey [425]. Its properties are said to resemble those of factor VII, from which it was distinguishable.

Other hereditary disorders of hemostasis are associated

with thrombocytopenia, but their metabolic basis is uncertain. Schulman and his associates [571] have carried out intensive studies of a young girl with severe thrombocytopenia who did not respond to corticosteroid therapy or splenectomy but had a partial remission after the transfusion of plasma. The patient has been treated by repeated transfusions of normal plasma, which appears to contain a thrombopoetic factor lacking in the patient [572]. Whether her disorder is hereditary in nature is not yet known.

Congenital thrombocytopenia with eczema and repeated infections, described by Wiskott [573] and Aldrich et al. [574], is a sex-linked recessive trait occurring in male infants which is almost invariably fatal within a few years. The thrombocytopenia is probably due to failure of production of platelets [575]. The patients are said to have a peculiar propensity for severe infections with herpes simplex virus [576]. In patients studied by Krivit and Good [577] and Kildeberg [578] an almost total deficiency of natural isoagglutinins raised the possibility that the syndrome reflects a disordered immune mechanism. In two patients, besides the virtual absence of serum isoagglutinins, there was a striking elevation of the β_{2A}-globulin level [579]. Lymphopenia is commonplace. The possibility has been postulated that cellular mechanisms responsible for delayed hypersensitivity, related to the recognition of antigens by the host, are impaired [576, 580]. Malignant diseases of the reticuloendothelial system have been reported as complications of the syndrome [581, 582].

Familial thrombocytopenia has also been described in association with *aplastic anemia of infants* [583]. In *Fanconi's disease,* the aplastic anemia may occur in combination with multiple congenital anomalies of the genitourinary tract, dwarfism, microcephaly, deafness, or congenital heart disease [584]. This disorder appears to be a recessive trait, occurring in both sexes and usually fatal in the midteens. Acute leukemia occurs in some patients. A similar familial disorder in which skeletal abnormalities, cardiac anomalies, and thrombocytopenia coexist has also been delineated [585]. In these patients, the red and white blood cells are normal. The prognosis is poor. A more benign *familial thrombocytopenia,* unassociated with infections, aplastic anemia, or congenital anomalies, has been described [586]. In two carefully studied families, individuals of several generations were affected, the males more often than the females [587, 588]. In Bithell's [588] family, hypersegmentation of neutrophils and eosinophilia were present in thrombocytopenic individuals. Splenectomy was without benefit. *May-Hegglin anomaly* is an asymptomatic disorder in which basophilic bodies, apparently collections of ribonucleic acid, are found in the cytoplasm of granulocytes. The platelets are often of giant size, are poorly granulated, and have a shortened life-span, sometimes resulting in thrombocytopenia [589, 590]. Other familial thrombocytopenias are reviewed by Kurstjens [558].

A familial clotting disorder observed in a family of Mohawk Indians has been ascribed to the presence in the plasma of a substance which inactivated the thrombin which evolves during coagulation [591]. Affected subjects had a mild bleeding tendency, and clotting times were long. The antithrombin could not be identified with the known antithrombin substances in blood. The mode of inheritance of the disorder was not clear. In another family, in which a mild hemorrhagic tendency was present in four successive generations, an *inhibitor of activated Stuart factor,* resembling that commonly observed in systemic lupus erythematosus, was detected in affected individuals [211]. A similar agent was found in normal plasma but in much smaller amounts. Other truly hereditary disorders due to anticoagulant substances have not been defined, but individual instances of lifelong bleeding ascribed to *hyperheparinemia* have been reported [592]. A recurrent view that classic hemophilia is due to the presence in plasma of anticoagulant substances is unsupportable at this time. Patients with hereditary angioneurotic edema have a partial deficiency of plasma inhibitory activity against activated PTA [609]. No symptoms referable to this anomaly have been recognized.

Hemorrhagic symptoms may also complicate various connective tissue disorders, such as *Meekrin-Ehlers-Danlos syndrome, osteogenesis imperfecta,* and *pseudoxanthoma elasticum* [257]. The pathogenesis of the bleeding in these states is obscure. Perhaps the blood vessels lack adequate support. Several different hemostatic anomalies have been described in some patients with Meekrin-Ehlers-Danlos syndrome and osteogenesis imperfecta, but their genesis and indeed their relationship to the bleeding tendency is uncertain [593]. Physiologic and anatomic abnormalities have been observed in platelets in some instances of Meekrin-Ehlers-Danlos syndrome [594] and osteogenesis imperfecta [595].

Equally obscure in its pathogenesis is *hereditary hemorrhagic telangiectasis* (Osler-Rendu-Weber syndrome), an autosomal dominant trait in which bleeding occurs from the skin or mucosal membranes [596]. In many of these patients, the disorder is complicated by pulmonary arteriovenous fistulas [597]. The essence of the disorder seems to be the development of vascular telangiectatic lesions in which the endothelium is unsupported by muscular or elastic tissues [598]. Impaired adhesion of platelets to injured blood vessels has been reported [599]. Persistent nosebleeds, a cardinal symptom, sometimes remit during estrogen therapy [583]. Although the patients may survive to old age, chronic iron deficiency anemia may be troublesome. Death may occur prematurely from hemorrhage or from cerebral abscesses in patients with pulmonary arteriovenous fistulas.

Mention should be made of *pseudohemophilia,* a familial hemorrhagic disorder in which the bleeding time is long but no other abnormality can be demonstrated [257, 601]. Whether pseudohemophilia is a real entity or whether cases so diagnosed are really instances of such other disorders as von Willebrand's disease or qualitative disorders of platelets is not clear. The author has not resorted to this diagnosis in the last decade. The study of patients in whom this diagnosis has been made may be rewarding.

Finally, the converse of a hemorrhagic disorder has been

described. Egeberg [602] has observed a Norwegian family in which many individuals of both sexes suffered thrombosis. He correlated this tendency with a partial deficiency in plasma of an inhibitor of thrombin designated as antithrombin III. Presumably, in such persons the inadvertant intravascular formation of thrombin might not be checked in normal fashion.

SUMMARY

1 Blood coagulation can be visualized as the end result of a series of enzymatic reactions. Clotting follows the action of an enzyme, thrombin, upon fibrinogen. The tensile strength of the fibrin which forms is enhanced by the action of another enzyme, fibrin-stabilizing factor. Thrombin is derived from prothrombin by several pathways. In cell-free plasma, prothrombin formation takes place through the *intrinsic clotting pathway,* which involves the successive participation of Hageman factor, plasma thromboplastin antecedent, Christmas factor, antihemophilic factor, Stuart factor, phospholipid, and proaccelerin. Calcium ions are also required. When tissue thromboplastin is added to plasma, thrombin also forms through the *extrinsic clotting pathway.* This route requires factor VII, Stuart factor, proaccelerin, and calcium ions. Platelets participate in hemostasis by furnishing phospholipids for coagulation and by adhering to the walls of damaged blood vessels. Hereditary disorders have been described in which the plasma is deficient in one or more of each of the factors involved in hemostasis, excepting only calcium ions and phospholipids.

2 Screening tests, such as measurement of the clotting time, partial thromboplastin time, serum prothrombic activity, and thromboplastin generation, are useful in the recognition of abnormalities but are often insufficiently sensitive to detect minor changes. Currently the most useful tests for this purpose are those designed to quantify the concentration of individual clotting factors.

3 The clinical picture of the various hereditary hemorrhagic disorders is stereotyped, except that patients with purely coagulative defects seldom have petechiae. Differential diagnosis is based almost entirely upon family history and laboratory studies. Classic hemophilia and Christmas disease are inherited as X-linked recessive traits, and deficiencies of other clotting factors are either partially dominant or recessive autosomal traits. Unexplained is the discordance between the degree of the coagulative defect, as measured in the laboratory, and the severity of symptoms. Hageman trait, for example, is usually asymptomatic, while classic hemophilia may be associated with severe bleeding, yet the abnormality measured in the laboratory is of about the same magnitude in the two diseases.

4 Although hemorrhagic disorders have usually been thought to reflect deficient synthesis of clotting factors, more recent evidence suggests that in many instances the patients synthesize a nonfunctional variant of the supposedly missing substance. Classic hemophilia is one important example of this phenomenon.

5 The study of hemorrhagic disorders has been crucial to an understanding of hemostatic processes. The utility of these studies can be demonstrated by recent observations of von Willebrand's disease. In this disorder the bleeding time is prolonged, and the concentration of antihemophilic factor in plasma is abnormally low. The titer of antihemophilic factor rises to normal levels after the transfusion of plasma obtained from patients with severe classic hemophilia. This observation implies that the synthesis of antihemophilic factor proceeds in two steps, one of which is abnormal in classic hemophilia and the other in von Willebrand's disease. Thus, experience nourishes our expectation that close examination of the many still unexplained bleeding syndromes will continue to be helpful in elucidating normal mechanisms.

BIBLIOGRAPHY

1. Miller, L., and Bale, W. F.: Synthesis of all plasma protein fractions except gamma globulins by the liver; the use of zone electrophoresis and lysine-ε-C^{14} to define the plasma proteins synthesized by the isolated perfused liver. J. Exp. Med., **99,** 125, 1954.
2. Miller, L. L., Bly, C. F., Watson, M. L., and Bale, W. F.: The dominant role of the liver in plasma protein synthesis: a direct study of the isolated perfused rat liver with the aid of lysine-ε-C^{14}. J. Exp. Med., **94,** 431, 1951.
3. Goldsworthy, P. D., Peppers J., and Volwiler, W.: Pacific Slope Biochem. Conf., Abstr., p. 6, 1963.
4. Straub, P. W.: A study of fibrinogen production by human liver slices *in vitro* by an immunoprecipitin method. J. Clin. Invest., **42,** 130, 1963.
5. Gram, H. C.: The results of a new method for determining the fibrin percentage in blood and plasma. Acta Med. Scand., **56,** 107, 1922.
6. Ratnoff, O. D., and Menzie, C.: A new method for determining the fibrinogen in small samples of plasma. J. Lab. Clin. Med., **37,** 316, 1951.
7. Cohn, E. J., Strong, L. E., Hughes, W. L., Jr., Mulford, D. J., Ashworth, J. N., Melin, M., and Taylor, H. L.: Preparation and properties of serum and plasma proteins. IV. A system for the separation into fractions of the protein and lipoprotein components of biological tissues and fluids. J. Amer. Chem. Soc., **68,** 459, 1951.
8. Blombäck, B., and Blombäck, M.: Purification of human and bovine fibrinogen. Arkiv. Kemi, **10,** 415, 1956.
9. Caspary, E. A., and Kekwick, R. A.: Some physiocochemical properties of human fibrinogen. Biochem. J., **67,** 41, 1957.
10. Shulman, S.: The size and shape of bovine fibrinogen. Studies of sedimentation, diffusion and viscosity. J. Amer. Chem. Soc., **75,** 5846, 1953.
11. Fantl, P., and Ward, H. A.: Molecular weight of human fibrinogen derived from phosphorus determinations. Biochem. J., **96,** 886, 1965.
12. Scheraga, H. A., and Laskowski, M., Jr.: The fibrinogen fibrin conversion. Advances Protein Chem., **12,** 1, 1957.
13. Hall, C. E., and Slayter, H. S.: The fibrinogen molecule: its size, shape and mode of polymerization. Biophys. Biochem. Cytol., **5,** 11, 1959.
14. Hall, C. E., and Slayter, H. S.: Molecular features of fibrinogen and fibrin. *Proc. 5th Internat. Cong. Electron Microscopy,* edited by S. S. Breese, Jr., vol. 2, pp. 1–3. Academic, New York, 1962.
15. Finlayson, J. S., and Mosesson, M. W.: Heterogeneity of human fibrinogen. Biochemistry, **2,** 42, 1963.
16. Finlayson, J. S.: Chromatographic purification of fibrinogen, in *Fibrinogen,* edited by K. Laki, p. 39. Marcel Dekker, New York, 1968.
17. Mihalyi, E.: Structural aspects of fibrinogen, in *Fibrinogen,* edited by K. Laki, p. 61. Marcel Dekker, New York, 1968.

18. Blombäck, B., Blombäck, M., Henschen, A., Hessel, B., Iwanaga, S. and Woods, K. R.: N-terminal disulphide knot of human fibrinogen. Nature, **218**, 130, 1968.
19. Bettelheim, F. R., and Bailey, K.: The products of the action of thrombin on fibrinogen. Biochim. Biophys. Acta, **9**, 578, 1952.
20. Lóránd, L., and Middlebrook, W. R.: The action of thrombin on fibrinogen. Biochem. J., **52**, 196, 1952.
21. Lóránd, L.: Fibrino-peptide. Biochem. J., **52**, 200, 1952.
22. Bailey, K., and Bettelheim, F. R.: The clotting of fibrinogen. I. The liberation of peptide material. Biochim. Biophys. Acta, **18**, 405, 1955.
23. Laki, K., Gladner, J. A., and Folk, J. E.: Some aspects of the fibrinogen-fibrin transition. Nature (London), **187**, 758, 1960.
24. Osbahr, A. J., Jr., Gladner, J. A., and Laki, K.: The action of human thrombin on human fibrinogen. Biochem. Biophys. Res. Commun., **13**, 462, 1963.
25. Laki, K.: Introduction and summary, in *Fibrinogen,* edited by K. Laki, p. 1, Marcel Dekker, New York, 1968.
26. Endres, G. F., Ehrenpreis, S., and Scheraga, H. A.: Covalent bonding in the reversible polymerization of fibrin monomer. Biochem. Biophys. Acta., **104**, 620, 1965.
27. Hawn, C. V., and Porter, K. R.: The fine structure of clots formed from purified bovine fibrinogen and thrombin: a study with the electron microscope. J. Exp. Med., **82**, 285, 1947.
28. Laki, L., and Mester, L.: The role of the carbohydrate moiety in bovine fibrinogen. Biochim. Biophys. Acta, **57**, 152, 1962.
29. Fantl, P., and Ward, H. A.: Phosphorus content of fibrinogen and fibrin. Biochim. Biophys. Acta, **64**, 568, 1962.
30. Seegers, W. H., and Smith, H. P.: Factors which influence the activity of purified thrombin. Amer. J. Physiol., **137**, 348, 1942.
31. Rosenfeld, G., and Jánszky, B.: The accelerating effect of calcium on the fibrinogen-fibrin transformation. Science, **116**, 36, 1952.
32. Ratnoff, O. D., and Potts, A. M.: The accelerating effect of calcium and other cations on the conversion of fibrinogen to fibrin. J. Clin. Invest., **33**, 206, 1954.
33. Ratnoff, O. D.: An accelerating property of plasma for the coagulation of fibrinogen by thrombin. J. Clin. Invest., **33**, 1175, 1954.
34. Jim, R. T. S.: A study of the plasma thrombin time. J. Lab. Clin. Med., **50**, 451, 1957.
35. Triantaphyllopoulos, D. C.: Blood globulins reducing the anticoagulant activity of heparin. Canad. J. Biochem. Physiol., **34**, 939, 1956.
36. Ferry, J. D., Miller, M., and Shulman, S.: The conversion of fibrinogen to fibrin. VII. Rigidity and stress relaxation of fibrin clots: effect of calcium. Arch. Biochem., **34**, 424, 1951.
37. Lóránd, L.: Fibrin clots. Nature (London), **166**, 694, 1950.
38. Laki, K., and Lóránd, L.: On the solubility of fibrin clots. Science, **108**, 280, 1948.
39. Lóránd, L., and Jacobsen, A.: Studies on the polymerization of fibrin. The role of the globulin: fibrin-stabilizing factor. J. Biol. Chem., **230**, 421, 1958.
40. Loewy, A. G., Dunathan, K., Kriel, R., and Wolfinger, H. L., Jr.: Fibrinase. I: Purification of substrate and enzyme. J. Biol. Chem., **236**, 2625, 1961.
41. Loewy, A. G.: Enzymatic control of insoluble-fibrin formation, in *Fibrinogen,* edited by K. Laki, p. 185. Marcel Dekker, New York, 1968.
42. Lóránd, L., and Konishi, K.: Activation of fibrin stabilizing factor by thrombin. Fed. Proc., **21**, 62, 1962.
43. Lóránd, L., Chen, C. H., Fuchs, L. E., Jacobsen, A., and Lóránd, J. B.: A plasma globulin as a partner of fibrin in clot formation. *Proc. 4th Internat. Cong. Biochem.,* Vienna, 1958, **10**, 228. Pergamon, New York, 1959–1960.
44. Loewy, A. G., Dahlberg, J. E., Dorwart, W. V., Jr., Weber, M. J., and Eisele, J.: A transamidase mechanism for insoluble fibrin formation. Biochem. Biophys. Res. Commun., **15**, 177, 1964.
45. Pisano, J. J., Finlayson, J. S., and Peyton, M. P.: Cross-link in fibrin polymerized by factor XIII: Epsilon-(gamma-glutamyl) lysine. Science, **160**, 892, 1968.
46. Lóránd, L., Uragama, T., deKiewiet, J. W. C., and Nossel, H. L.: Diagnostic and genetic studies on fibrin-stabilizing factor with a new assay based on amine incorporation. J. Clin. Invest., **48**, 1054, 1969.
47. Mester, L.: Structure and possible role of the carbohydrate moiety in fibrinogen, in *Fibrinogen,* edited by K. Laki, p. 165. Marcel Dekker, New York, 1968.
48. Beck, E., Duckert, F., and Ernst, M.: The influence of fibrin stabilizing factor on the growth of fibroblasts in vitro and wound healing. Thromb. Diath. Haemorrh., **6**, 485, 1961.
49. Kiesselbach, T. H., and Wagner, R. H.: Origin of platelet factor XIII (Fibrin stabilizing factor) Fed. Proc., **28**, 745, 1969.
50. Scheraga, H. A.: Purification of clotting factors from a physico-chemical viewpoint. Thromb. Diath. Haemorrh., **7**, Suppl. 1, 186, 1962.
51. Seegers, W. H.: *Prothrombin.* Harvard, Cambridge, Mass., 1962.
52. Baughman, D. J., and Waugh, D. E.: Bovine thrombin. Purification and certain properties. J. Biol. Chem., **242**, 525, 1962.
53. Seegers, W. H., McCoy, L., Kipfer, R. K., and Murano, G.: Preparation and properties of thrombin. Arch. Biochem. Biophys., **128**, 194, 1968.
54. Gladner, J. A., Laki, K., and Stohlman, F.: Labeled DIP-thrombin. Biochim. Biophys. Acta, **27**, 218, 1958.
55. Berg, W., Korsan-Bergston, K., and Ygge, J.: Human and bovine plasminogen-free thrombin purified by means of gel filtration and ion exchange chromatography. Throm. Diath. Haemorrh., **15**, 501, 1966.
56. Sherry, S., and Troll, W.: Action of thrombin on synthetic substrates. J. Biol. Chem., **208**, 95, 1954.
57. Martin, C. J., Golubow, J., and Axelrod, A. E.: The hydrolysis of carbobenzoxy-l-tyrosine *p*-nitrophenyl ester by various enzymes. J. Biol. Chem., **234**, 1718, 1959.
58. Lóránd, L., Brannen, W. T., Jr., and Rule, N. G.: Thrombin-catalyzed hydrolysis of *p*-nitrophenyl esters. Arch. Biochem., **96**, 147, 1962.
59. Elmore, D. T., and Curragh, E.: Kinetic studies on the mechanism of thrombin-catalyzed reactions. Biochem. J., **86**, 9P, 1963.
60. Cole, E. R.: Hydrolysis of L-histidine methyl ester. I. The action of thrombin. Thromb. Diath. Haemorr., **19**, 321, 1968.
61. Ratnoff, O. D.: Unpublished observations.
62. Scherga, H. A.: Thrombin and its interaction with fibrinogen. Ann. N.Y. Acad. Sci., **75**, 189, 1958.
63. Thelin, G. M., and Wagner, R. H.: The action of thrombin on serum albumin. Biochem. Biophys. Res. Commun., **1**, 219, 1959.
64. Gladner, J. A., and Laki, K.: The inhibition of thrombin by diisopropyl phosphofluoridate. Arch. Biochem., **62**, 501, 1956.
65. Miller, K. D., and Van Vunakis, H.: The effect of diisopropyl fluorophosphate on the proteinase and esterase activities of thrombin and of prothrombin and its activators. J. Biol. Chem., **223**, 227, 1956.
66. Gladner, J. A., and Laki, K.: The active site of thrombin. J. Amer. Chem. Soc., **80**, 1263, 1958.
67. Lóránd, L., and Yudkin, E. P.: The effect of arginylpeptides on the clotting of fibrinogen with thrombin. Biochim. Biophys. Acta, **25**, 437, 1957.
68. Quick, A. J., and Favre-Gilly, J. E.: Fibrin: a factor influencing the consumption of prothrombin in coagulation. Amer. J. Physiol., **158**, 387, 1949.
69. Astrup, T., and Darling, S.: Measurement and properties of antithrombin. Acta Physiol. Scand., **4**, 203, 1942.
70. Alexander, B.: Some biochemical, physicochemical and immunochemical studies of prothrombin and proconvertin (factor VII): their biochemical significance. *Proc. 4th Internat. Cong. Biochem.,* Vienna, 1958, **10**, 37, Pergamon, New York, 1959–1960.
71. Lamy, F., and Waugh, D. F.: The physical changes of prothrombin under various experimental conditions. Thromb. Diath. Haemorrh., **2**, 188, 1958.
72. Lanchantin, G., and Friedmann, J. A.: Biochemical studies of human plasma prothrombin. Thromb. Diath. Haemorrh., **9**, 223, 1963.
73. Owen, C. A., Jr., and McKenzie, B. F.: Application of paper electrophoresis to separation of blood clotting factors. J. Appl. Physiol., **6**, 696, 1954.
74. Lewis, J. H., Walters, D., Didisheim, P., and Merchant, W. R.: Application of continuous flow electrophoresis to the study of the blood coagulation proteins and the fibrinolytic enzyme system. I. Normal human materials. J. Clin. Invest., **37**, 1323, 1958.
75. Cohn, E. J., Oncley, J. L., Strong, L. E., Hughes, W. L., Jr., and

Armstrong, S. H., Jr.: Chemical, clinical and immunological studies on the products of human plasma fractionation. I. The characterization of the protein fractions of human plasma. J. Clin. Invest., **23**, 417, 1944.

76. Miller, K. D., and Seegers, W. H.: The preparation of a carbohydrate fraction from prothrombin and its chemical nature. Arch. Biochem., **60**, 398, 1956.
77. Lóránd, L., Alkjaersig, N., and Seegers, W. H.: Carbohydrate and nitrogen distribution during the activation of purified prothrombin in sodium citrate solution. Arch. Biochem., **45**, 312, 1953.
78. Warner, E. D., Brinkhous, K. M., and Smith, H. P.: A quantitative study of blood clotting: prothrombin fluctuations under experimental conditions. Amer. J. Physiol., **114**, 667, 1936.
79. Smith, H. P., Warner, E. D., and Brinkhous, K. M.: Prothrombin deficiency and the bleeding tendency in liver injury (chloroform intoxication). J. Exp. Med., **66**, 801, 1937.
80. Pool, J., and Robinson, J.: *In vitro* synthesis of coagulation factors by rat liver slices. Amer. J. Physiol., **196**, 423, 1959.
81. Barnhart, M. I.: Cellular site for prothrombin synthesis. Amer. J. Physiol., **199**, 360, 1960.
82. Dam, H.: Hemorrhages in chicks reared on artificial diets: a new deficiency disease. Nature (London), **133**, 909, 1934.
83. Schönheyder, F.: The antihaemorrhagic vitamin of the chick: measurement and biological action, Nature (London), **135**, 652, 1935.
84. Quick, A. J.: The coagulation defect in sweet clover disease and in hemorrhagic chick disease of dietary origin. Amer. J. Physiol., **118**, 260, 1937.
85. Goldstein, R., Le Bolloc'h, A., Alexander, B., and Zonderman, E.: Preparation and properties of prothrombin. J. Biol. Chem., **234**, 2857, 1959.
86. Seegers, W. H., and Landaburu, R. H.: Purification of prothrombin and thrombin by chromatography on cellulose. Canad. J. Biochem. Physiol., **38**, 1405, 1960.
87. Miller, K. D.: Chromatographic isolation of plasma prothrombin and trans-γ-glucosylase. J. Biol. Chem., **231**, 987, 1958.
88. Shapiro, S. S., and Waugh, D. F.: The purification of human prothrombin. Thromb. Diath. Haemorrh., **16**, 469, 1966.
89. Malhotra, O. P., and Carter, J. R.: Modified method for the preparation of purified bovine prothrombin of high specific activity. Thromb. Diath. Haemorrh., **19**, 178, 1968.
90. Shafrir, E., and de Vries, A.: Studies on the clot-promoting activity of glass. J. Clin. Invest., **35**, 1183, 1956.
91. Margolis, J.: Glass surface and blood coagulation. Nature (London), **178**, 805, 1956.
92. Ratnoff, O. D., and Rosenblum, J. M.: Role of Hageman factor in the initiation of clotting by glass: evidence that glass frees Hageman factor from inhibition. Amer. J. Med., **25**, 160, 1958.
93. Robinson, J. A., and Aggeler, P. M.: To be published.
94. DeGrouchy, J., Veslot, J., Bonnette, J., and Roidot, M.: Case of ?6p-chromosomal aberration. Amer. J. Dis. Child., **115**, 93, 1968.
95. Jim, R. T. S., and Goldfein, S.: Hageman trait (Hageman factor deficiency). Amer. J. Med., **23**, 824, 1957.
96. Ratnoff, O. D., and Davie, E. W.: The purification of activated Hageman factor (Activated XII). Biochemistry, **1**, 967, 1962.
97. Schoenmakers, J. G., Kurstjens, R. M., Haanen, C. A., and Zilliken, F.: Purification of activated bovine Hageman factor. Fed. Proc., **22**, 163, 1963.
98. Donaldson, V. H., and Ratnoff, O. D.: Hageman factor: alterations in physical properties during activation. Science, **150**, 754, 1965.
99. Ratnoff, O. D., and Crum, J. D.: Activation of Hageman factor by solutions of ellagic acid. J. Lab. Clin. Med., **62**, 1006, 1963.
100. Ogston, D., Ogston, C. M., and Ratnoff, O. D.: Studies on the clot-promoting effect of skin. J. Lab. Clin. Med., **73**, 70, 1969.
101. Niewiarowski, S., Bankowski, E., and Rogowicka, I.: Studies on adsorption and activation of Hageman factor (Factor XIII) by collagen and elastin. Thromb. Diath. Haemorrh., **14**, 387, 1965.
102. Wilner, G. D., Nossel, H. L., and LeRoy, E. C.: Activation of Hageman factor by collagen. J. Clin. Invest., **47**, 2608, 1968.
103. Ratnoff, O. D., Davie, E. W., and Mallett, D. L.: The current status of knowledge about Hageman factor. Thromb. Diath. Haemorrh., **6**, Suppl. 1, 364, 1962.
104. Biggs, R., Denson, K. W. E., Risenberg, D., and McIntyre, C.: Coagulant activity of platelets. Brit. J. Haemat., **15**, 283, 1968.
105. Ratnoff, O. D., Davie, E. W., and Mallett, D. L.: Studies on the action of Hageman factor: evidence that activated Hageman factor in turn activates plasma thromboplastin antecedent. J. Clin. Invest., **40**, 803, 1961.
106. Waaler, B. A.: Contact activation in the intrinsic blood clotting system: studies on a plasma product formed on contact with glass and similar surfaces. Scandinav. J. Clin. Lab. Invest., **11**, Suppl. 37, 1, 1959.
107. Hardisty, R. M., and Margolis, J.: The role of Hageman factor in the initiation of blood coagulation. Brit. J. Haemat., **5**, 203, 1959.
108. Soulier, J. P., Wartelle, O., and Ménaché, D.: Differential characteristics of Hageman and PTA factors: role of contact in the initial phase of coagulation. Rev. Franc. Étud. Clin. Biol, **3**, 263, 1958.
109. Ratnoff, O. D.: Hageman trait. Thromb. Diath. Haemorrh., **4**, Suppl. 1, 116, 1960.
110. Margolis, J.: Activation of a permeability factor in plasma by contact with glass. Nature (London), **181**, 635, 1958.
111. Ratnoff, O. D., and Miles, A. A.: The induction of permeability-increasing activity in human plasma by activated Hageman factor. Brit. J. Exp. Path., **45**, 328, 1964.
112. Webster, M. D., and Ratnoff, O. D.: Role of Hageman factor in the activation of vasodilator activity in human plasma. Nature (London), **192**, 180, 1961.
113. Margolis, J.: Activation of plasma by contact with glass: evidence for a common reaction which releases plasma kinin and initiates coagulation. J. Physiol., **144**, 1, 1958.
114. Keele, C. A., and Armstrong, D.: *Substances Producing Pain and Itch.* Williams and Wilkins, Baltimore, 1964.
115. Graham, R. C., Jr., Ebert, R. H., Ratnoff, O. D., and Moses, J. H.: Pathogenesis of inflammation. II. *In vivo* observations of the inflammatory effects of activated Hageman factor and bradykinin. J. Exp. Med., **121**, 807, 1965.
116. Niewiarowski, S., and Prou-Wartelle, O.: Role du facteur contact (facteur Hageman) dans la fibrinolyse. Thromb. Diath. Haemorrh. **3**, 593, 1959.
117. Iatridis, S. G., and Ferguson, J. H.: Effect of surface and Hageman factor on the endogenous or spontaneous activation of the fibrinolytic system. Thromb. Diath. Haemorrh., **6**, 411, 1961.
118. Ogston, D., Ogston, C. M., Ratnoff, O. D., and Forbes, C. D.: Studies on a complex mechanism for the activation of plasminogen by kaolin and by chloroform: the participation of Hageman factor and additional factors. J. Clin. Invest., **48**, 1786, 1969.
119. Donaldson, V. H.: Mechanisms of activation of C'l esterase in hereditary angioneurotic edema plasma *in vitro*. The role of Hageman factor a clot-promoting agent. J. Exp. Med., **127**, 411, 1968.
120. Schiffman, S., Rapaport, S. I., Ware, A. G. and Mehl, J. W.: Separation of plasma thromboplastin antecedent (PTA) and Hageman factor (HF) from human plasma. Proc. Soc. Exp. Biol. Med. **105**, 453, 1960.
121. Bachmann, F., Duckert, F., Fisch, U., Streuli, F., Gerber, D., and Koller, F.: Der Gerinnungsdefekt beim kongenitalen PTA-mangel. Schweiz. Med. Wschr., **88**, 1037, 1958.
122. Kingdon, H. S., Davie, E. W., and Ratnoff, O. D.: The reaction between activated plasma thromboplastin antecedent and diisopropyl-phosphofluoridate. Biochemistry, **3**, 166, 1964.
123. Botti, R. E., and Ratnoff, O. D.: The clot-promoting effect of soaps of long chain saturated fatty acids. J. Clin. Invest., **42**, 1569, 1963.
124. Egli, H., and Buscha, H.: Zur Differenzierung und Kalzium-abhangigkeit von Kontaktwirkungen benetzbarer Oberflachen: ihr Einfluss auf die Bluthrombokinasebildung. Thromb. Diath. Haemorrh., **3**, 604, 1959.
125. Biggs, R., and Bidwell, E.: The kinetics of blood thromboplastin formation. *Proc. 4th Internat. Cong. Biochem.*, Vienna, 1958, vol. 10, p. 172. Pergamon, New York, 1959–1960.
126. Ratnoff, O. D., and Davie, E. W.: The activation of Christmas factor (Factor IX) by activated plasma thromboplastin antecedent (Factor XI). Biochemistry, **1**, 677, 1962.
127. Aggeler, P. M., Spaet, T. H., and Emery, B. E.: Purification of plasma

thromboplastin factor B (plasma thromboplastin component) and its identification as a beta$_2$ globulin. Science, **119**, 806, 1954.

128. Mammen, E.: Activation of bovine prothrombin to autoprothrombin II. Thromb. Diath. Haemorrh., **7**, Suppl. 1, 264, 1962.
129. Aronson, D. L., Preiss, J. W., and Mosesson, M. W.: Molecular weights of Factor VIII (AHF) and Factor IX (PTC) by electron irradiation. Thromb. Diath. Haemorrh., **8**, 270, 1962.
130. Schiffman, S., Rapaport, S. I., and Patch, M. J.: Starch block electrophoresis of clotting factors. Clin. Res., **12**, 110, 1964.
131. Macfarlane, R. G.: Purification of Factor X: its activation by Russell's viper venom and also by physiological factors. Thromb. Diath. Haemorrh., **7**, Suppl. 1, 222, 1962.
132. Lundblad, R. L., and Davie, E. W.: The activation of antihemophilic factor (Factor VIII) by activated Christmas factor (activated Factor IX)., **3**, 1720, 1964.
133. Rapaport, S. I., Schiffman, S., Patch, M. J., and Ames, S. B.: The importance of activation of antihemophilic globulin and proaccelerin by traces of thrombin in the generation of intrinsic prothrombinase activity. Blood, **21**, 221, 1963.
134. Kekwick, R. A., and Wolf, P.: A concentrate of human antihemophilic factor: its use in six cases of hemophilia. Lancet, **1**, 647, 1957.
135. Bidwell, E.: The purification of bovine antihaemophilic globulin. Brit. J. Haemat., **1**, 35, 1955.
136. Nilsson, I. M., Blombäck, M., Blombäck, B., and Ramgren, O.: The use of human AHF (Fraction I-O) in hemophilia A. Blut, **8**, 92, 1962.
137. van Creveld, S., Pascha, C. N., and Veder, H. A.: The separation of AHF from fibrinogen. III. Thromb. Diath. Haemorrh., **6**, 282, 1961.
138. Pavlovsky, A., Simonetti, C., Casillas, G., Bergna, L. J., Andino, A., and Bachman, A. E.: The use of Factor VIII freed from fibrinogen in the treatment of hemophilic patients. Brit. J. Haemat., **7**, 365, 1961.
139. Soulier, J. P., Blatrix, C., and Steinbuch, M.: Fractionation of the clotting factors in human blood. Vox Sang., **6**, 220, 1961.
140. Langdell, R. D.: Purification of Factor VIII. Thromb. Diath. Haemorrh., **7**, Suppl. 1, 192, 1962.
141. Pavlovsky, A., Peterson, H., Casillas, G., Simonetti, C., and Canaveri, A. M.: Purification of Factor VIII. Thromb. Diath. Haemorrh., **7**, Suppl. 1, 197, 1962.
142. Pool, J. G., and Shannon, A. E.: Production of high potency concentrates of antihemophilic globulin in a closed-bag system. New Eng. J. Med., **273**, 1443, 1965.
143. Johnson, A. J., Newman, J., Howell, M. B., and Puszkin, S.: Purification of antihemophilic factor (AHF) for clinical and experimental use. Thromb. Diath. Haemorrh., Suppl. **26**, 379, 1967.
144. Ratnoff, O. D., Kass, L., and Lang, P. D.: Studies on the purification of antihemophilic factor (Factor VIII). II. Separation of partially purified antihemophilic factor by gel filtration of plasma. J. Clin. Invest., **48**, 975, 1969.
145. Wagner, R. H., Pate, D., and Brinkhous, K. M.: Further purification of antihemophilic factor (AHF) from dog plasma. Fed. Proc., **13**, 445, 1954.
146. Penick, G. D.: Some factors that influence utilization of antihemophilic activity during clotting. Proc. Soc. Exp. Biol. Med., **96**, 277, 1957.
147. Kekwick, R. A., and Walton, P. L.: Conditions influencing the stability of human antihaemophilic factor. Nature (London), **194**, 878, 1962.
148. Kass, L., Ratnoff, O. D., and Leon, M. A.: Studies on the purification of antihemophilic factor (Factor VIII). I. Precipitation of antihemophilic factor by concanavalin A. J. Clin. Invest., **48**, 351, 1969.
149. Hershgold, E. J., Davidson, A. M., and Janszen, M. E.: Human factor VIII (AHG), a lipoprotein: activation and inactivation by phospholipases. Fed. Proc., **28**, 639, 1969.
150. Barrow, E. M., and Graham, J. B.: The dissociation of plasma antihemophilic factor. Fed. Proc., **28**, 746, 1969.
151. Penick, G. D., Roberts, H. R., Webster, W. P., and Brinkhous, K. M.: Hemorrhagic states secondary to intravascular clotting: an experimental study of their evolution and prevention. A.M.A. Arch. Path., **66**, 708, 1958.
152. Webster, W. P., Reddick, R. L., Roberts, H. R., and Penick, G. D.: Release of factor VIII (antihaemophilic factor) from perfused organs and tissues. Nature, **213**, 1146, 1967.
153. Dodds, W. J.: Storage, release and synthesis of coagulation factor in isolated perfused organs. Amer. J. Physiol., **217**, 879, 1969.
154. Marchioro, T. L., Hougie, C., Ragde, J., Epstein, R. B., and Thomas, E. D.: Hemophilia: role of organ homografts. Science, **163**, 188, 1969.
155. Norman, J. C., Lambilliotte, J. P., Kojima, Y., and Sise, H. S.: Antihemophilic factor release by perfused liver and spleen: relationship to hemophilia. Science, **158**, 1060, 1967.
156. Nilsson, I. M., Blombäck, M., and Francken, I. von: On an inherited autosomal hemorrhagic diathesis with antihemophilic globulin (AHG) deficiency and prolonged bleeding time. Acta Med. Scand., **159**, 35, 1957.
157. Nilsson, I. M., Blombäck, M., and Blombäck, B.: v. Willebrand's disease in Sweden: its pathogenesis and treatment. Acta Med. Scand., **164**, 263, 1959.
158. Mann, F. D.: Reactivity of hemophilic plasma to platelet thromboplastin. J. Lab. Clin. Med., **48**, 51, 1956.
159. Hougie, G., Barrow, E. M., and Graham, J. B.: Stuart clotting defect. I. Segregation of an hereditary hemorrhagic state from the heterozygous group heretofore called "stable factor." J. Clin. Invest., **36**, 485, 1957.
160. Fisch, U.: Über einen neuen Accelerator der Blutthrombokinasebildung. Thromb. Diath. Haemorrh., **2**, 60, 1958.
161. Esnouf, M. P., and Williams, W. J.: The isolation and purification of a bovine-plasma protein which is a substrate for the coagulant fraction of Russell's viper venom. Biochem. J., **84**, 62, 1962.
162. Macfarlane, R. G.: The coagulant action of Russell's viper venom: the use of antivenom in defining its reaction with a serum factor. Brit. J. Haemat., **7**, 496, 1961.
163. Macfarlane, R. G.: Progress in coagulation: perspectives. Thromb. Diath. Haemorrh., **7**, Suppl. 1, 17, 1962.
164. Alexander, B., Pechet, L., and Kliman, A.: Proteolysis, fibrinolysis and coagulation: significance in thrombolytic therapy. Circulation, **26**, 596, 1962.
165. Spaet, T. H., and Cintron, J.: Pathways to blood coagulation: Product I formation. Blood, **21**, 745, 1963.
166. Milstone, J. H.: Thrombokinase of the blood as trypsin-like enzyme. J. Gen. Physiol., **45**, 103, 1962.
167. Marciniak, E., and Seegers, W. H.: Autoprothrombin C: a second enzyme from prothrombin. Canad. J. Biochem. Physiol. **40**, 597, 1962.
168. Breckenridge, R. T., and Ratnoff, O. D.: The role of proaccelerin in human blood coagulation. J. Clin. Invest., **44**, 302, 1965.
169. Bergsagel, D. E., and Hougie, C.: Intermediate stages in the formation of blood thromboplastin. Brit. J. Haemat., **2**, 113, 1956.
170. Hougie, C.: The role of Factor V in the formation of blood thromboplastin. J. Lab. Clin. Med., **50**, 61, 1957.
171. Milstone, J. H.: On the evolution of blood clotting theory. Medicine, **31**, 411, 1952.
172. Seegers, W. H., Cole, E. R., Harmison, C. R., and Marciniak, E.: Purification and some properties of autoprothrombin C. Canad. J. Biochem. Physiol. **41**, 1047, 1963.
173. Rouser, G., White, S. G., and Schloredt, D.: Phospholipid structure and thromboplastic activity. I. The phosphatide fraction active in recalcified normal human plasma. Biochim. Biophys. Acta, **28**, 71, 1958.
174. Troup, S. B., Reed, C. F., Marinetti, G. W., and Swisher, S. N.: Thromboplastic factors in platelets and red blood cells: observations on their chemical nature and function in *in vitro* coagulation. J. Clin. Invest., **39**, 342, 1960.
175. Marcus, A. J., Ullman, H. L., Safier, L. B., and Ballard, H. S.: Platelet phosphatides: their fatty acid and aldehyde composition and activity in different clotting systems. J. Clin. Invest., **41**, 2198, 1962.
176. Marcus, A. J., Ullman, H. L., and Ballard, H. S.: Fatty acids of human platelet phosphatides. Proc. Soc. Exp. Biol. Med., **107**, 483, 1961.
177. Alexander, B.: Factor VII (proconvertin). Thromb. Diath. Haemorrh., **6**, Suppl. 1, 392, 1962.
178. Prydz, H.: Studies on proconvertin (factor VII). Some characteristics of purified factor VII preparations. Scand. J. Clin. Lab. Invest., **17**, Suppl. **84**, 78, 1965.
179. Williams, W. J.: The activity of lung microsomes in blood coagulation. J. Biol. Chem., **239**, 933, 1964.
180. Williams, W. J.: The activity of human placenta microsomes and brain particles in blood coagulation. J. Biol. Chem., **241**, 1840, 1966.

181. Howell, W. H.: The nature and action of the thromboplastic (zymoplastic) substance of the tissues. Amer. J. Physiol., **31**, 1, 1912.
182. Quick, A. J.: Biochemistry of clotting factors in tissues and erythrocytes. *Proc. 4th Internat. Cong. Biochem.,* Vienna, 1958, vol. 10, p. 123. Pergamon, New York, 1959–1960.
183. Nemerson, Y.: Characteristics and lipid requirement of coagulant proteins extracted from lung and brain: The specificity of the protein component of tissue factor. J. Clin. Invest., **48**, 322, 1969.
184. Nemerson, Y.: The reaction between bovine brain tissue factor and factors VII and X. Biochemistry, **5**, 601, 1966.
185. Nemerson, Y.: The phospholipid requirement of tissue factor in blood coagulation. J. Clin. Invest., **47**, 72, 1968.
186. Nemerson, Y., and Spaet, T. H.: The activation of factor X by extracts of rabbit brain. Blood, **23**, 657, 1964.
187. Owren, P. A.: The coagulation of blood: investigations of a new clotting factor. Acta Med. Scand., **128**, Suppl. 194, 1, 1947.
188. Lewis, J. H., Howe, A. C., and Ferguson, J. H.: Thrombin formation: effects of lysin (fibrinolysin, plasmin) on prothrombin, Ac globulin and tissue thromboplastin. J. Clin. Invest., **28**, 1507, 1949.
189. Papahadjopoulos, D., Hougie, C., and Hanahan, D. J.: Purification and properties of bovine factor V: a change in molecular size during blood coagulation. Biochemistry, **3**, 264, 1964.
190. Esnouf, M. P., and Jobin, F.: The isolation of factor V from bovine plasma. Biochem. J., **102**, 660, 1967.
191. Sykes, E. M., Jr., Seegers, W. H., and Ware, A. G.: Effect of acute liver damage on Ac-globulin activity of plasma. Proc. Soc. Exp. Biol. Med., **67**, 506, 1948.
192. Lewis, J. H., and Ferguson, J. H.: Hypoproaccelerinemia. Blood, **10**, 351, 1955.
193. Hjort, P., Rapaport, S. I., and Owren, P. A.: Evidence that platelet accelerator (platelet factor I) is adsorbed plasma proaccelerin. Blood, **10**, 1139, 1955.
194. Seamen, A. J., and Owren, P. A.: An asolectin adsorbed substrate for proaccelerin assay. J. Clin. Invest., **35**, 145, 1956.
195. Ware, A. G., Murphy, R. C., and Seegers, W. H.: The function of Ac-globulin in blood clotting. Science, **106**, 618, 1947.
196. Owren, P. A.: Prothrombin and accessory factors: clinical significance. Amer. J. Med., **14**, 201, 1953.
197. Prentice, C. R. M., Ratnoff, O. D., and Breckenridge, R. T.: Experiments on the nature of the prothrombin-converting principle: alteration of proaccelerin by thrombin. Brit. J. Haemat., **13**, 898, 1967.
198. Prentice, C. R. M., and Ratnoff, O. D.: The action of Russell's Viper Venom on factor V and the prothrombin converting principle. Brit. J. Haemat., **16**, 291, 1969.
199. Prentice, C. R. M., Breckenridge, R. T., and Ratnoff, O. D.: Studies on the conversion of prothrombin to thrombin: with notes on the cation requirements for this reaction. J. Lab. Clin. Med., **69**, 229, 1967.
200. Shapiro, S. S.: Human prothrombin activation: immunochemical study. Science, **162**, 127, 1968.
201. Esnouf, M. P., and Jobin, F.: Lipids in prothrombin conversion. Thromb. Diath. Haemorrh., **13**, Suppl., 103, 1965.
202. Hemker, H. C., Esnouf, M. P., Hemker, P. W., Swart, A. C. W., and Macfarlane, R. G.: Formation of prothrombin converting activity. Nature, **215**, 248, 1967.
203. Milstone, J. H.: Thrombokinase as prime activator of prothrombin: historic perspectives and present status. Fed. Proc., **23**, 742, 1964.
204. Prentice, C. R. M., and Ratnoff, O. D.: The action of Russell's viper venom on Factor V and the prothrombin-converting principle. Brit. J. Haemat., **16**, 291, 1969.
205. Seegers, W. H.: Activation of purified prothrombin. Proc. Soc. Exp. Biol. Med., **72**, 677, 1949.
206. Goldstein, R., and Alexander, B.: Further studies on proconvertin deficiency and the role of proconvertin, in *Hemophilia and Hemophilioid Diseases,* edited by K. M. Brinkhous, p. 93. University of North Carolina Press, Chapel Hill, N.C., 1957.
207. Margolis, J.: Initiation of blood coagulation by glass and related substances. J. Physiol., **137**, 95, 1957.
208. Nossel, H. L., and Niemetz, J.: A normal inhibitor of the blood contact reaction product. Blood, **25**, 712, 1065.
209. Niemetz, J., and Nossel, H.: Method of purification and properties of anti-XIa (inhibitor of the contact product). Thromb. Diath. Haemorrh., **17**, 335, 1967.
210. Forbes, C. D., Pensky, J., and Ratnoff, O. D.: Inhibition of activated Hageman factor and plasma thromboplastin antecedent by purified serum C1 inactivator. J. Lab. Clin. Med., **76**, 809, 1970.
211. Robinson, A. J., Aggeler, P. M., McNicol, G. P., and Douglas, A. S.: An atypical genetic hemorrhagic disease with increased concentration of a natural inhibitor of prothrombin consumption. Brit. J. Haemat., **13**, 510, 1967.
212. Thomas, L.: Studies on the intravascular thromboplastic effect of tissue suspensions in mice. II. A factor in normal rabbit serum which inhibits the thromboplastic effect of the sedimentable tissue component. Bull. Johns Hopkins Hosp., **81**, 26, 1947.
213. Astrup, T., and Darling, S.: The measurement and properties of antithrombin. Acta Physiol. Scand., **4**, 293, 1942.
214. Lanchantin, G. F., Plesset, M. L., Friedmann, J. A., and Hart, D. W.: Dissociation of esterolytic and clotting activities of thrombin by trypsin-binding macroglobulin. Proc. Soc. Exp. Biol. Med., **121**, 449, 1966.
215. Marcus, A. J., and Zucker, M. B.: *The Physiology of Blood Platelets.* Grune & Stratton, New York, 1964.
216. Davey, M. J., and Lüscher, E. F.: Biochemical aspects of platelet function and hemostasis. Seminars Hemat., **5**, 5, 1968.
217. Schulz, H., and Hiepler, E.: Über die Lokalisierung von gerinnungsphysiologischen Aktivitaten in submikroskopischen Strukturen der Thrombocytes. Klin. Wschr., **37**, 273, 1959.
218. Johnson, S. A., Sturrock, R. M., and Rebuck, J. W.: Morphological location of platelet factor 3 activity in normal platelets. *Proc. 4th Internat. Cong. Biochem.,* Vienna, 1958, vol. 10, p. 105. Pergamon, New York, 1959–1960.
219. Marcus, A. J., and Zucker-Franklin, D.: Studies on subcellular platelet particles. Blood, **23**, 389, 1964.
220. Ware, A. G., Fahey, J. L., and Seegers, W. H.: Platelet extracts, fibrin formation and interaction of purified prothrombin and thromboplastin. Amer. J. Physiol., **154**, 40, 1948.
221. McDonagh, J., McDonagh, R. P., Jr., Delâge, J.-M., and Wagner, R. H.: Factor XIII in human plasma and platelets. J. Clin. Invest., **48**, 940, 1969.
222. Spaet, T. H., and Zucker, M. B.: Mechanism of platelet plug formation and the role of adenosine diphosphate. Amer. J. Physiol., **206**, 1267, 1964.
223. Gaarder, A., Jonsen, J., Laland, S., Hellem, A., and Owren, P. A.: Adenosine diphosphate in red cells as a factor in the adhesiveness of human blood platelets. Nature (London), **192**, 531, 1961.
224. Kaser-Glanzmann, R., and Lüscher, E. F.: The mechanism of platelet aggregation in relation to hemostasis. Thromb. Diath. Haemorrh., 7, 480, 1962.
225. Fonio, A.: Neuere untersuchungen über Blutgerinnung, Schweiz. Med. Wschr., **4**, 36, 60, 1923.
226. Quick, A. J., and Hussey, C. V.: The mechanism of clot retraction. Science, **112**, 558, 1950.
227. Zucker, M. B., and Borrelli, J.: Viscous metamorphosis, clot retraction and other morphologic alterations of blood platelets. J. Appl. Physiol., **14**, 575, 1959.
228. Conley, C. L.: Platelets in clot retraction, in *Blood Platelets,* edited by S. A. Johnson, R. W. Monto, J. W. Rebuck, and R. C. Horn, p. 437, Little, Brown, Boston, 1961.
229. Gaintner, J. R., Jackson, D. P., and Conley, C. L.: Morphologic studies of clot retraction. Bull. Johns Hopkins Hosp., **111**, 266, 1962.
230. Hovig, T.: The ultrastructure of rabbit blood platelet aggregates. Thromb. Diath. Haemorrh., **8**, 455, 1962.
231. Parmeggiani, A.: Elektronenoptische Beobachtungen an menschlichen Blutplättchen während der viskösen Metemorphase. Thromb. Diath. Haemorrh., **6**, 517, 1961.
232. Tocantins, L. M.: Platelets and the structure and physical properties of blood clots. Amer. J. Physiol., **114**, 709, 1936.
233. Pinniger, J. L., and Prunty, F. T. S.: Some observations on the blood clotting mechanism: the role of fibrinogen and platelets with reference to a case of congenital afibrinogenemia. Brit. J. Exp. Path., **27**, 200, 1946.

234. Schmid, H. J., Jackson, D. P., and Conley, C. L.: Mechanism of action of thrombin on platelets. J. Clin. Invest., **41**, 543, 1962.
235. Nachman, R. L., Marcus, A. J., and Zucker-Franklin, D.: Immunologic studies of proteins associated with subcellular fractions of normal human platelets. J. Lab. Clin. Med., **69**, 651, 1967.
236. Hartmann, R. C., Auditore, J. V., and Jackson, D. P.: Studies on thrombocytosis. I. Hyperkalemia due to release of potassium from platelets during coagulation. J. Clin. Invest., **37**, 699, 1958.
237. Lüscher, E. F.: Retraction activity of the platelets: biochemical background and physiologic significance, in *Blood Platelets,* edited by S. A. Johnson, R. W. Monto, J. W. Rebuck, and R. C. Horn, p. 445. Little, Brown, Boston, 1961.
238. Gross, R.: Metabolic aspects of normal and pathological platelets, in *Blood Platelets,* edited by S. A. Johnson, R. W. Monto, J. W. Rebuck, and R. C. Horn, p. 407. Little, Brown, Boston, 1961.
239. Bettex-Galland, M., and Lüscher, E. F.: Extraction of actomyosin-like protein from human thrombocytes, Nature (London), **184**, 276, 1959.
240. Bettex-Galland, M., and Lüscher, E. F.: Thrombosthenin, a contractile protein from thrombocytes: its extraction from human blood platelets and some of its properties. Biochim. Biophys. Acta, **49**, 536, 1961.
241. Born, G. V. R.: The break-down of adenosine triphosphate in blood platelets during clotting. J. Physiol., **133**, 61–2P, 1956.
242. Kiesselbach, T. H., and Wagner, R. H.: Fibrin-stabilizing factor: a thrombin-labile platelet protein. Amer. J. Physiol., **211**, 1472, 1966.
243. Hughes, J.: Agglutination précose des plaquettes au cours de la formation du clou hémostatique. Thromb. Diath. Haemorrh., **3**, 177, 1959.
244. Kjaerheim, A., and Hovig, T.: The ultrastructure of haemostatic blood platelet plugs in rabbit mesenterium. Thromb. Diath. Haemorrh., **7**, 1, 1962.
245. Biggs, R., and MacFarlane, R. G.: *Human Blood Coagulation and Its Disorders,* 3d ed. Davis, Philadelphia, 1962.
246. Stefanini, M., and Dameshek, W.: *The Hemorrhagic Disorders: A Clinical and Therapeutic Approach,* 2d ed., Grune & Stratton, New York, 1962.
247. Douglas, A. S.: *Anticoagulant Therapy.* Blackwell, Oxford, 1962.
248. Quick, A. J.: *Hemorrhagic Diseases and Thrombosis,* 3d ed., Lea & Febiger, Philadelphia, 1966.
249. Hardisty, R. M., and Ingram, G. I. C. *Bleeding Disorders. Investigation and Management.* Davis, Philadelphia, 1965.
250. Tocantins, L. M., and Kazan, L. A. (edit.): *Blood Coagulation, Hemorrhage and Thrombosis, Methods of Study.* Grune & Stratton, New York, 1964.
251. Ratnoff, O. D.: An approach to the diagnosis of disorders of hemostasis. In *Treatment of Hemorrhagic Disorders,* edited by O. D. Ratnoff, p. 11, Harper and Row, New York, 1968.
252. Rodman, N. F., Jr., Barrow, E. M., and Graham, J. B.: Diagnosis and control of the hemophilioid states with partial thromboplastin time (PTT) test. Amer. J. Clin. Path., **29**, 525, 1958.
253. Quick, A. J., Stanley-Brown, M., and Bancroft, F. W.: A study of the coagulation defect in hemophilia and jaundice. Amer. J. Med. Sci., **190**, 501, 1935.
254. Alexander, B., and Landwehr, G.: Prothrombin consumption, serum prothrombic activity and prothrombin conversion accelerator in hemophilia and thrombocytopenia. J. Clin. Invest., **28**, 1511, 1949.
255. Quick, A. J., and Favre-Gilly, J. E.: The prothrombin consumption test: its clinical and theoretic implications. Blood, **4**, 1281, 1949.
256. Biggs, R., and Douglas, A. S.: The thromboplastin generation test. J. Clin. Path., **6**, 23, 1953.
257. Ratnoff, O. D.: *Bleeding Syndromes.* American Lecture Series. Charles C Thomas, Springfield, Ill., 1960.
258. Margolis, J.: The kaolin clotting time: a rapid one-stage method for diagnosis of coagulation defects. J. Clin. Path., **11**, 406, 1958.
259. Rapaport, S. I., Schiffman, S., Patch, M. J., and Ware, A. G.: A simple, specific one-stage assay for plasma thromboplastin antecedent (PTA) activity. J. Lab. Clin. Med., **57**, 771, 1961.
260. Hardisty, R. M., and Macpherson, J. C.: A one-stage Factor VIII (antihemophilic globulin) assay and its use on venous and capillary plasma. Thromb. Diath. Haemorrh., **7**, 215, 1962.
261. Hartmann, R. C.: Tests of platelet adhesiveness and their clinical significance. Seminars Hemat., **5**, 60, 1968.
262. *The Babylonian Talmud,* edited by I. Epstein. Yebamoth sect. 64B, vol. 1, p. 431. Soncino Press, London, 1936.
263. Immerman, N. H.: Haemophilia, scurvy and morbus maculosus, in *Cyclopedia of the Practice of Medicine,* edited by H. von Ziemssen, American ed. vol. 17, p. 1, Wood, Baltimore, 1878.
264. Otto, J. C.: An account of an hemorrhagic disposition existing in certain families. M. Repository, **6**, 1, 1803.
265. Legg, J. W.: Report on haemophilia with a note on the hereditary descent of colour-blindness. St. Bart. Hosp. Rep., **17**, 303, 1881.
266. Wright, A. E.: On a method of determining the condition of blood coagulability for clinical and experimental purposes, and on the effect of the administration of calcium salts in haemophilia and actual or threatened haemorrhage. Brit. Med. J., **2**, 334, 1893.
267. Addis, T.: The pathogenesis of hereditary haemophilia. J. Path. Bact., **15**, 427, 1911.
268. Minot, G. R., and Lee, R. I.: The blood platelets in hemophilia. Arch. Intern. Med., **18**, 474, 1916.
269. Frank, E., and Hartmann, E.: Über das Wesen und die therapeutische Korrektur der hämophilen Gerinnungstorung. Klin. Wschr., **6**, 435, 1927.
270. Govaerts, P., and Gratia, A.: Contribution à l'étude de l'hémophilie. Rev. Belg. Sci. Méd., **3**, 689, 1931.
271. Bendien, W. M., and van Creveld, S.: Investigation on haemophilia. Acta Brev. Nederl., **5**, 135, 1935.
272. Patek, A. J., Jr., and Stetson, R. J.: Hemophilia: abnormal coagulation of blood and its relation to blood platelets. J. Clin. Invest., **15**, 531, 1936.
273. Pavlovsky, A.: Contribution to the pathogenesis of hemophilia. Blood, **2**, 185, 1947.
274. Prentice, C. R. M., and Ratnoff, O. D.: Genetic disorders of blood coagulation. Seminars Hemat., **4**, 93, 1967.
275. Hartmann, J. R., and Diamond, L. K.: Natural history of seventy-three patients with hemophilia and related hemorrhagic diseases. A.M.A. J. Dis. Child., **90**, 594, 1955.
276. Ratnoff, O. D.: Hereditary defects in clotting mechanisms. Advances Intern. Med., **9**, 107, 1958.
277. Leatherdale, R. A. L.: Respiratory obstruction in haemophilic patients. Brit. Med. J., **1**, 1316, 1960.
278. Graham, J. B., McLendon, W., and Brinkhous, K. M.: Mild hemophilia: an allelic form of the disease. Amer. J. Med. Sci., **225**, 46, 1953.
279. Rizza, C. R.: The effect of exercise on the level of antihemophilic globulin in human blood. J. Physiol., **156**, 128, 1961.
280. Ingram, G. I. C.: Increase in antihemophilic globulin activity following infusion of adrenaline. J. Physiol., **156**, 217, 1961.
281. Agle, D.: Psychiatric studies of patients with hemophilia and related states. Arch. Intern. Med., **114**, 76, 1964.
282. Cooperberg, A. A., and Teitelbaum, J.: The concentration antihaemophilia globulin (AHG) related to age. Brit. J. Haemat., **6**, 281, 1960.
283. Hawkey, C. M., Anstall, H. B., and Grove-Rasmussen, M.: A study of comparative antihemophilic factor levels in fresh frozen plasma *in vitro* and *in vivo.* Transfusion, **2**, 94, 1962.
284. Pool, J. G., and Robinson, J.: Assay of plasma antihaemophilic globulin (AHF). Brit. J. Haemat., **5**, 17, 1959.
285. Ratnoff, O. D., Botti, R. E., Breckenridge, R. T., and Littell, A. S.: Some problems in the measurement of antihemophilic activity, in *The Hemophilias,* edited by K. M. Brinkhous. p. 3, University of North Carolina Press, Chapel Hill, 1964.
286. Pitney, W. R., Kirk, R. L., Arnold, B. J., and Stenhouse, N. S.: Plasma antihaemophilic factor (Factor VIII) concentrations in normal families. Brit. J. Haemat., **8**, 421, 1962.
287. Pitney, W. R., and Elliott, M. H.: Plasma antihaemophilic factor concentrations in the Australian aborigine and in conditions associated with hypergammaglobulinemia, Nature (London), **185**, 397, 1960.
288. Merskey, C., Gordon, H., Lackner, H., Schrire, V., Kaplan, B. J., Sougin-Mibashan, R., Nossel, H. L., and Moodie, A.: Blood coagulation and fibrinolysis in relation to coronary heart disease: a comparative study of normal white men, white men with overt coronary heart disease, and normal Bantu men. Brit. Med. J., **1**, 219, 1960.

289. Pitney, W. R., and Arnold, B. J.: Plasma antihaemophilic factor (AHF) concentrations in families of patients with haemorrhagic states. Brit. J. Haemat., **5,** 184, 1959.
290. Preston, A. E., and Barr, A.: The plasma concentration of factor VIII in the normal population. II. The effects of age, sex and blood group. Brit. J. Haemat., **10,** 238, 1964.
291. Jorpes, E., and Ramgren, O.: The haemophilia situation in Sweden. Acta Med. Scand., **171,** Suppl. 379, 23, 1962.
292. Egeberg, O., and Owren, P. A.: Oral contraceptives and blood coagulation. Brit. Med. J., **1,** 220, 1963.
293. Amundsen, M. A., Spittell, J. A., Jr., Thompson, J. H., Jr., and Owen, C. A., Jr.: Hypercoagulability associated with malignant disease and with the postoperative state: evidence for elevated levels of antihemophilic globulin. Ann. Intern. Med., **58,** 608, 1963.
294. Egeberg, O.: The effect of unspecific fever induction on the blood clotting system. Scand. J. Clin. Lab. Invest., **14,** 471, 1962.
295. Sise, H. S., Gauthier, J., Becker, R., and Bolger, J.: Blood coagulation factors in total body irritation. Blood, **18,** 702, 1961.
296. Egeberg, O.: Influence of thyroid function in the blood clotting system. Scand. J. Clin. Lab. Invest., **15,** 1, 1963.
297. Cooperberg, A. A., and Teitelbaum, J. I.: The concentration of antihemophilic globulin (AHG) in patients with coronary artery disease. Ann. Intern. Med., **54,** 899, 1961.
298. Egeberg, O.: The blood coagulability in diabetic patients. Scand. J. Clin. Lab. Invest., **15,** 533, 1963.
299. Brinkhous, K. M.: A study of the clotting defect in hemophilia: the delayed formation of thrombin. Amer. J. Med. Sci., **198,** 509, 1939.
300. Cho, M. H., and Neuhaus, O. W.: Absence of blood clotting substances from synovial fluid. Thromb. Diath. Haemorrh., **5,** 108, 1961.
301. Seibert, R. H., Margolius, A., Jr., and Ratnoff, O. D.: Observations on hemophilia, parahemophilia and coexistent hemophilia and parahemophilia. J. Lab. Clin. Med., **52,** 449, 1958.
302. Breckenridge, R. T., and Ratnoff, O. D.: Therapy of hereditary disorders of blood coagulation, in *Treatment of Hemorrhagic Disorders.* edited by O. D. Ratnoff. p. 39, Harper and Row, New York, 1968.
303. Shulman, N. R.: Surgical care of patients with hereditary disorders of blood coagulation, in *Treatment of Hemorrhagic Disorders,* edited by O. D. Ratnoff. p. 61, Harper and Row, New York, 1968.
304. van Creveld, S., and Mochtar, I. A.: Management of hemophilia, in *Hemophilia and Other Hemorrhagic States,* edited by K. M. Brinkhous, p. 27. The University of North Carolina Press, Chapel Hill, N. C., 1959.
305. Curtiss, P. H., Jr.: Orthopedic management of patients with hereditary disorders of blood coagulation, in *Treatment of Hemorrhagic Disorders,* edited by O. D. Ratnoff, p. 84, Harper and Row, New York, 1968.
306. Biggs, R.: Major surgery in haemophilic patients, in *Treatment of Haemophilia and other Coagulation Disorders,* edited by R. Biggs and R. G. Macfarlane, p. 166, Davis, Philadelphia, 1966.
307. Ingram, G. I. C.: Major surgery in hemophilia: use of animal antihemophilic factor in Britain. Transfusion, **2,** 88, 1962.
308. Tarnay, T. J.: *Surgery in the Hemophiliac.* Charles C Thomas, Springfield, Ill., 1968.
309. Webster, W. P., Roberts, H. R., and Penick, G. D.: Dental care of patients with hereditary disorders of blood coagulation, in *Treatment of Hemorrhagic Disorders,* edited by O. D. Ratnoff, p. 93, Harper and Row, New York, 1968.
310. Biggs, R., and Matthews, J. M.: The general treatment of haemophilic patients after dental extraction, in *Treatment of Haemophilia and Other Coagulation Disorders,* edited by R. Biggs and R. G. Macfarlane, p. 144, Davis, Philadelphia, 1966.
311. Alby, J. M., Alby, N., and Caen, J.: Problèmes psychologiques de l'hémophile. Nouv, Rev. franç Hemat., **2,** 119, 1962.
312. Soulier, J. P., and Josso, F. (edit.).: *Current studies in hemophilia.* Bibl. Haemat., **26,** 121, 1966.
313. Agle, D. P., and Mattson, Å.: Psychiatric and social care of patients with hereditary hemorrhagic disease, *in Treatment of Hemorrhagic Disorders,* edited by O. D. Ratnoff, p. 111, Harper and Row, New York, 1968.
314. Kerr, C. B.: Genetic counselling in hereditary disorders of blood coagulation, in *Treatment of Hemorrhagic Disorders,* edited by O. D. Ratnoff, p. 125, Harper and Row, New York, 1968.
315. Whittaker, D. L., Copeland, D. L., and Graham, J. B.: Linkage of color blindness to hemophilias A and B. Amer. J. Hum. Genet., **14,** 492, 1962.
316. McKusick, V. A.: On the X chromosome of man. Quart. Rev. Biol. **37,** 69, 1962.
317. Hoyer, L. W., and Breckenridge, R. T.: Immunologic studies of antihemophilic factor (AHF, factor VIII): Cross-reacting material in a genetic variant of hemophilia A. Blood, **32,** 962, 1969.
318. Feinstein, D., Chong, M. N. Y., Kaster, C. K., and Rapaport, S. I.: Hemophilia A: Polymorphism detectable by a factor VIII antibody. Science, **163,** 1072, 1969.
319. Hensen, A., Mattern, M. J., and Loeliger, E. A.: Haemophilia A with apparent autosomal dominant inheritance. Evidence for a second autosomal locus involved in factor VIII production. Thromb. Diath. Haemorrh., **14,** 341, 1965.
320. Merskey, C.: The occurrence of haemophilia in the human female. Quart. J. Med., N. S., **20,** 299, 1951.
321. Israels, M. C. G., Lempert, H., and Gilbertson, E.: Haemophilia in the female. Lancet, **1,** 1375, 1951.
322. Stefanovic, S., Rolovig, Z., and Zujevic, J.: Hémophilie A chez une fillette, Sang, **30,** 858, 1959.
323. Brinkhous, K. M., and Graham, J. B.: Hemophilia in the female dog. Science, **111,** 723, 1950.
324. Nossel, H. L., Archer, R. K., and Macfarlane, R. G.: Equine haemophilia: report of a case and its response to multiple infusions of heterospecific AHG. Brit. J. Haemat., **8,** 335, 1962.
325. Strauss, H. S.: The perpetuation of hemophilia by mutation. Pediatrics, **39,** 186, 1967.
326. Margolius, A., Jr., and Ratnoff, O. D.: A laboratory study of the carrier state in classic hemophilia. J. Clin. Invest., **35,** 1316, 1956.
327. Merskey, C., and Macfarlane, R. G.: Female carrier of haemophilia: clinical and laboratory study. Lancet, **1,** 487, 1951.
328. Rapaport, S. I., Patch, M. J., and Moore, F. J.: Anti-hemophilic globulin levels in carriers of hemophilia A. J. Clin. Invest., **39,** 1619, 1960.
329. Didisheim, P., Ferguson, J. H., and Lewis, J. H.: Hemostatic data in relatives of hemophiliacs A and B. A.M.A. Arch. Intern. Med., **101,** 347, 1958.
330. Douglas, A. S., and Cook, I. A.: Deficiency of antihaemophilic globulin in heterozygous haemophilic females. Lancet, **2,** 616, 1957.
331. McGovern, J. J., and Steinberg, A. G.: Antihemophilic factor deficiency in the female, J. Lab. Clin. Med., **51,** 386, 1958.
332. de la Chapelle, A., Ikkala, E., and Nevanlinna, H. R.: Haemophilia A in a girl; a probable exception from sex-linked recessive inheritance. Lancet, **2,** 578, 1961.
333. Taylor, K., and Biggs, R.: A mildly affected female haemophiliac. Brit. Med. J., **1,** 1494, 1957.
334. Mellman, W. J., Wolman, I. J., Wurzel, H. A., Moorehead, P. S., and Qualls, D. H.: A chromosomal female with hemophilia A. Blood, **17,** 719, 1961.
335. Lyon, M. F.: Gene action in the X-chromosome of the mouse (Mus musculus L.). Nature (London), **190,** 372, 1961.
336. Nilsson, I. M., Bergman, S., Reitalu, J., and Waldenström, J.: Haemophilia A in a "girl" with male sex-chromatin pattern. Lancet, **2,** 264, 1959.
337. Gilchrest, G. S., Hammond, D., and Melnyk, J.: Hemophilia A in a phenotypically normal female with XX/XO mosaicism. New Eng. J. Med., **273,** 1402, 1965.
338. Quick, A. J., and Hussey, C. V.: Haemophilia-like states in girls. Lancet, **1,** 1294, 1958.
339. Braun, E. H., and Stollar, D. B.: Spontaneous haemophilia in a female. Thromb. Diath. Haemorrh., **4,** 369, 1960.
340. Lawrence, J. S., and Johnson, J. B.: The presence of a circulating anticoagulant in a male member of a hemophiliac family. Trans. Amer. Clin. Climat. Ass., **57,** 223, 1942.
341. Margolius, A., Jr., Jackson, D. P., and Ratnoff, O. D.: Circulating

anticoagulants: a study of 40 cases and a review of the literature. Medicine, **40,** 145, 1961.

342. Leitner, A., Bidwell, E., and Dike, G. W. R.: An antihaemophilic globulin (Factor VIII) inhibitor: purification, characterization and reaction kinetics. Brit. J. Haemat., **9,** 245, 1963.
343. Shulman, N. R., Marder, V. J., and Leitner, A.: Inactivation of Factor VIII (AHF) by a gamma globulin anticoagulant. J. Clin. Invest., **42,** 970, 1963 (abstr.).
344. Shapiro, S. S.: Immunologic character of acquired inhibitors of antihemophilic globulin (factor VIII) and the kinetics of their interaction with factor VIII. J. Clin. Invest., **46,** 147, 1967.
345. Shulman, N. R., and Hirschman, R. J.: Acquired hemophilia. Clin. Res., **17,** 466, 1969.
346. Schulman, I., Smith, C. H.: Hemorrhagic disease in infant due to deficiency of a previously undescribed clotting factor. Blood, **7,** 794, 1952.
347. Biggs, R., Douglas, A. S., Macfarlane, R. G., Dacie, J. V., Pitney, W. R., Merskey, C., and O'Brien, J. R.: Christmas disease: a condition previously mistaken for haemophilia. Brit. Med. J., **2,** 1378, 1952.
348. Aggeler, P. M., White, S. G., Glendenning, M. B., Page, E. W., Leake, T. B., and Bates, G.: Plasma thromboplastin component (PTC) deficiency: a new disease resembling hemophilia, Proc. Soc. Exp. Biol. Med., **79,** 692, 1952.
349. Fantl., P., Sawers, R. J., and Mart, A. G.: Investigation of a haemorrhagic disease due to beta-prothromboplastin deficiency complicated by a specific inhibitor of thromboplastin formation. Aust. Ann. Med., **5,** 163, 1956.
350. Hougie, C., and Twomey, J. J.: Hemophilia B_M: a new type of Factor IX deficiency. Lancet, **1,** 698, 1967.
351. Roberts, H. R., Grizzle, J. E., McLester, W. D., and Penick, G. D.: Genetic variants of hemophilia B: detection by means of a specific PTC inhibitor. J. Clin. Invest., **47,** 360, 1968.
352. Macfarlane, R. G.: Factor IX (Christmas factor, PTC). Thromb. Diath. Haemorrh., **6,** Suppl. 1, 408, 1962.
353. Jung, E. G.: The relative frequency of haemophilia A and B. Thromb. Diath. Haemorrh., **4,** 331, 1960.
354. Ratnoff, O. D., and Margolius, A., Jr.: On the epidemiology of hemophilia and Christmas disease. New Eng. J. Med., **256,** 845, 1957.
355. Wall, R. L., McConnell, J. L., and Moore, D.: Christmas disease, deutan color blindness and the Xg^a blood group in the Amish. J. Lab. Clin. Med., **64,** 1015, 1964.
356. Yoshida, K.: Hemophilia and related diseases. Acta Haemat. Jap., **24,** 109, 1961.
357. Mustard, J. F., Rowsell, H. C., Robinson, T. D., Hoeksema, T. D., and Downie, H. G.: Canine haemophilia B (Christmas disease). Brit. J. Haemat., **6,** 259, 1960.
358. Burgensis-Desgaultieres, H.: *L'Hémophilie B, à propos de 50 observations. Thesis, Institut Pasteur de Lyon, 1962.*
359. Simpson, N. E., and Biggs, R.: The inheritance of Christmas factor. Brit. J. Haemat., **8,** 191, 1962.
360. Barrow, E. M., Bullock, W. R., and Graham, J. B.: A study of the carrier state for plasma thromboplastin component (PTC, Christmas factor) deficiency, utilizing a new assay procedure. J. Lab. Clin. Med., **55,** 936, 1960.
361. Ratnoff, O. D. and Holland, T. R.: Coagulation components in normal and abnormal pregnancies. Ann. N.Y. Acad. Sci., **75,** 626, 1959.
362. Wall, R. L., McConnell, J., Moore, D., Macpherson, C. R., and Marson, A.: Christmas disease, color-blindness and blood group Xg^a. Amer. J. Med., **43,** 214, 1967.
363. Biggs, R., and Macfarlane, R. G.: Haemophilia and related conditions: a survey of 187 cases. Brit. J. Haemat., **4,** 1, 1958.
364. Berg, K., and Bearn, A.: Common X-linked serum marker and its relation to other loci on the X chromosome. Trans. Ass. Amer. Physicians, **79,** 165, 1966.
365. Hardisty, R. M.: Christmas disease in a woman. Brit. Med. J., **1,** 1039, 1957.
366. Moor-Jankowski, J. K., Huser, H. F., Rosin, S., Troug, G., Schneeberger, M., and Geiger, M.: *Hemophilia B: Genetics, Hematology and Clinical Aspects.* S. Karger Basel, 1958.
367. Cook, I. A., and Douglas, A. S.: Demonstrable deficiency of Christmas factor in two sisters. Brit. Med. J., **1,** 479, 1960.
368. Frota-Pessoa, O., Gomes, E. L., and Calicchio, T. R.: Christmas factor: dosage compensation and the production of blood coagulation factor IX. Science, **139,** 348, 1963.
369. Bolton, F. G., and Clarke, J. E.: A method of assaying Christmas factor: its application to the study of Christmas disease (Factor IX deficiency). Brit. J. Haemat., **5,** 396, 1959.
370. Niléhn, J., and Nilsson, I. M.: Haemophilia B in a girl. Thromb. Diath. Haemorrh., **7,** 553, 1962.
371. Rozman, C., Castillo, R., Ribas-Mundó, M., and Surós, J.: Christmas disease in a girl with female karyotype. Acta Haemat., **37,** 217, 1967.
372. Kidd, P., Denson, K. W. E., and Biggs, R.: The thrombotest reagent and Christmas disease. Lancet, **2,** 522, 1963.
373. Twomey, J. J., Corless, J., Thornton, L. and Hougie, C.: Studies on the inheritance and nature of hemophilia B_M. Amer. J. Med., **46,** 372, 1969.
374. Geratz, J. D., and Graham, J. B.: Plasma thromboplastin component (Christmas factor, Factor IX) levels in stored human blood and plasma. Thromb. Diath. Haemorrh., **4,** 376, 1960.
375. Carter, S. H., Gougie, C., and Menk, K.: Fatal case of congenital plasma thromboplastin component deficiency: failure of response to therapy in Christmas disease. J.A.M.A., **173,** 631, 1960.
376. Loeliger, E. A., and Hensen, A.: Substitution therapy in haemophilia B. Thromb. Diath. Haemorrh., **6,** 391, 1961.
377. Biggs, R., Bidwell, E., Handley, D. A., Macfarlane, R. G., Trueta, J., Elliot-Smith, A., Dike, G. W. R., and Ash, B. J.: The preparation and assay of a Christmas factor (Factor IX) concentrate and its use in the treatment of two patients. Brit. J. Haemat., **7,** 349, 1961.
378. Adelson, E., Rheingold, J. J., Parker, O., Steiner, M., and Kirby, J. C.: Survival of plasma thromboplastin component and antihemophilic globulin in normal humans. Clin. Res., **8,** 369, 1960.
379. Ratnoff, O. D.: The therapy of hereditary disorders of blood coagulation. Arch. Intern. Med., **112,** 92, 1963.
380. Soulier, J. P., Blatrix, C., Prou-Wartelle, O., and Vignal, A.: Préparation d'une fraction sérique riche en convertine (VII), factor Stuart (X) et facteur antihémophilique B (IX). Nouv. Rev. Franç. Hemat., **2,** 27, 1962.
381. Birk, G.: Zur Therapie der Hämophile B. Klin. Wschr., **36,** 240, 1958.
382. Didisheim, P., Loeb, J., Blatrix, C., and Soulier, J. P.: Preparation of a human plasma fraction rich in prothrombin, proconvertin, Stuart factor, and PTC and a study of its activity and toxicity in rabbits and man. J. Lab. Clin. Med., **53,** 322, 1959.
383. Gilchrest, G. S., Ekert, J., Shanbroom, E., and Hammond, D.: Evaluation of a new concentrate for the treatment of factor IX deficiency. New Eng. J. Med., **280,** 291, 1969.
384. Hoag, M. D., Johnson, F. F., Robinson, J. A., and Aggeler, P. M.: Treatment of hemophilia B with a new clotting-factor concentrate. New Eng. J. Med., **280,** 581, 1969.
385. Hardisty, R. M.: A naturally occurring inhibitor of Christmas factor (Factor IX). Thromb. Diath. Haemorrh., **8,** 67, 1962.
386. Ratnoff, O. D., and Colopy, J. E.: A familial hemorrhagic trait associated with a deficiency of a clot-promoting fraction of plasma. J. Clin. Invest., **34,** 602, 1955.
387. Margolis, A., Jr., and Ratnoff, O. D.: Observations on the hereditary nature of Hageman trait. Blood, **11,** 565, 1956.
388. Ratnoff, O. D., and Steinberg, A. G.: Further studies on the inheritance of Hageman trait. J. Lab. Clin. Med., **59,** 980, 1962.
389. Veltkamp, J. J., Drion, E. F., and Loeliger, E. A.: Detection of the carrier state in hereditary coagulation disorders. II. Thromb. Diath. Haemorrh., **19,** 403, 1968.
390. Veltkamp, J. J., Hemker, H. C., and Loeliger, E. A.: Detection of heterozygotes for factors VIII, IX and XII deficiency. Thromb. Diath. Haemorrh., **12,** Suppl. 17, 181, 1965.
391. Loeliger, E. A., and Hansen, A.: Coagulation studies in a case of Hageman trait. Thromb. Diath. Haemorrh., **5,** 187, 1961.
392. Smink, M. McL., Daniel, T. M., Ratnoff, O. D., and Stavitsky, A. B.: Immunological demonstration of a deficiency of Hageman factor-like material in Hageman trait. J. Lab. Clin. Med., **69,** 819, 1967.
393. Soulier, J. P., Prou-Wartelle, O., and Ménaché, D.: Hageman trait and

PTA deficiency: the role of contact of blood with glass. Brit. J. Haemat., **5,** 121, 1959.

394. Post, R. M., Sise, H. S., and Okonkwo, P.: Platelet aggregation and factor XII. Fed. Proc., **28,** 509, 1969.
395. Ratnoff, O. D., Busse, R. J., Jr., and Sheon, R. P.: The demise of John Hageman. New Eng., J. Med., **279,** 760, 1968.
396. Fantl, P.: Discussion of Ratnoff, et al., [103].
397. Josso, F., Prou-Wartelle, O., and Charlas, J.: Durée de vie du Facteur Hageman (Facteur XII). Nouv. Rev. Franç. Hemat., **4,** 454, 1964.
398. Rosenthal, R. L., Dreskin, O. H., and Rosenthal, N.: New hemophilia-like disease caused by deficiency of a third plasma thromboplastin factor. Proc. Soc. Exp. Biol. Med., **82,** 171, 1953.
399. Kurtides, E. S.: Plasma thromboplastin antecedent: report of a case and review of literature. Quart Bull. Northwestern Univ. Med. School, **36,** 329, 1962.
400. Rosenthal, R. L.: Plasma thromboplastin antecedent (PTA) activity. Thromb. Diath. Haemorrh., **6,** Suppl. 1, 379, 1962.
401. Phillips, L. Discussion of Rosenthal, ref. 400.
402. Kociba, G. J., Ratnoff, O. D., Loeb, W. F., Wall, R. L., and Heider, L. E.: Bovine plasma thromboplastin antecedent (Factor IX) deficiency. J. Lab. Clin. Med., **74,** 37, 1969.
403. Rapaport, S. I., Proctor, R. P., Patch, M. J., and Yettra, M.: The mode of inheritance of PTA deficiency: evidence for the existence of major PTA deficiency. Blood, **18,** 149, 1961.
404. Todd, M. E., Panter, G., and Wright, I. S.: Deficiency of one or more factors of unusual interest. Thromb. Diath. Haemorrh., **4,** Suppl., 151, 1960.
405. Cavins, J. A., and Wall, R. L.: Clinical and laboratory studies of plasma thromboplastin antecedent deficiency (PTA). Amer. J. Med., **29,** 444, 1960.
406. Frick, P. G., and Hagen, P. S.: Severe coagulation defect without hemorrhagic symptoms caused by a deficiency of the fifth plasma thromboplastin precursor. J. Lab. Clin. Med., **47,** 592, 1956.
407. Ramot, B., and Fisher, S.: Plasma thromboplastin antecedent deficiency and its association with pseudohemophilia: a report of 2 cases. Israel Med. J., **19,** 85, 1960.
408. Rosenthal, R. L., Dreskin, O. H., and Rosenthal, N.: Plasma thromboplastin antecedent (PTA) deficiency: clinical, coagulation, therapeutic and hereditary aspects of a new hemophilia-like disease. Blood, **10,** 120, 1955.
409. Nossel, H. L., Niemetz, J., and Sawitsky, A.: Blood PTA (factor XI) levels following plasma infusion. Proc. Soc. Biol. Med., **115,** 896, 1964.
410. Josephson, A. M., and Lisker, R.: Demonstration of a circulating anticoagulant in plasma thromboplastin antecedent deficiency. J. Clin. Invest., **37,** 148, 1958.
411. Martius, C., and Nitz-Litzow, D.: Oxydative Phosphorylierung und Vitamin K Mangel. Biochim. Biophys. Acta, **13,** 152, 1954.
412. Beyer, R. E.: Vitamin K_1, a component of the mitochondrial oxidative phosphorylation system. Biochim. Biophys. Acta, **28,** 663, 1958.
413. Dallam, R. D.: Vitamin K and oxidative phosphorylation. Biochim. Biophys. Acta, **25,** 439, 1957.
414. Beyer, R. E.: The effect of ultraviolet light on mitochondria. II. Restoration of oxidative phosphorylation with vitamin K_1 after near-ultraviolet treatment. J. Biol. Chem., **234,** 688, 1959.
415. Olson, J. P., Miller, L. L., and Troup, S. B.: Synthesis of clotting factors by the isolated perfused liver. J. Clin. Invest., **45,** 690, 1966.
416. Suttie, J. W.: Control of prothrombin and factor VII biosynthesis by vitamin K. Arch. Biochem. Biophys., **118,** 166, 1967.
417. Hemker, H. C., Veltkamp, J. J., and Loeliger, E. A.: Kinetic aspects of the interaction of blood clotting enzymes. III. Demonstration of an inhibitor of prothrombin conversion in vitamin K deficiency. Thromb. Diath. Haemorrh., **19,** 346, 1968.
418. Josso, F., Lavergne, J. M., Gouault, M., Prou-Wartelle, O., and Soulier, J. P.: Différents états moléculaires du facteur II (prothrombine). Leur étude à l'aide de la staphylocagulase et d'anticorps anti-facteur II. I. Le facteur II chez les sujets traité par les antagoniste de la vitamine K. Thromb. Diath. Haemorrh., **20,** 88, 1968.
419. Alexander, B., Meyers, L., Kenny, J., Goldstein, R., Gurewich, V., and Grinspoon, L.: Blood coagulation in pregnancy: proconvertin and prothrombin, and the hypercoagulable state. New Eng. J. Med., **254,** 358, 1956.
420. Seegers, W. H.: Uses and regulation of blood clotting mechanisms. In *Blood Clotting Enzymology,* edited by W. H. Seegers, p. 1, Academic, New York, 1967.
421. O'Reilly, R. A., Aggeler, P. M., and Gibbs, J. O.: Hemorrhagic state due to surreptitious ingestion of bishydroxy coumarin (dicumarol). New Eng. J. Med., **267,** 19, 1962.
422. Bowie, E. J. W., Todd, M., Thompson, J. H. Jr., Owen, C. A. Jr., and Wright, I. S.: Anticoagulant malingerers (The "dicumarol-eaters"). Amer. J. Med., **39,** 855, 1965.
423. Alexander, B.: Estimation of plasma prothrombin by the one-stage method, in *The Coagulation of Blood: Methods of Study,* edited by L. M. Tocantins, p. 89. Grune & Stratton, New York, 1955.
424. Lewis, J. H., Ferguson, J. H., and Fresh, J. W.: Primary hemorrhagic diseases. J. Lab. Clin. Med., **49,** 211, 1957.
425. Quick, A. J., and Hussey, C. V.: Hereditary hypoprothrombinaemias. Lancet, **1,** 173, 1962.
426. Pool, J. G., Desai, R., and Kropatkin, M.: Severe congenital hypoprothrombinemia in a Negro boy. Thromb. Diath. Haemorrh., **8,** 235, 1962.
427. Josso, F., Prou-Wartelle, O., and Soulier, J. P.: Étude d'un cas d'hypoprothrombinémie congénitale. Nouv. Rev. Franç. Hémat., **2,** 647, 1962.
428. Borchgrevinck, C. F., Egeberg, O., Pool, J. G., Skulason, T., Stormorken, H., and Waaler, B.: A study of a case of congenital hypoprothrombinaemia. Brit. J. Haemat., **5,** 294, 1959.
429. van Creveld, S.: Congenital idiopathic hypoprothrombinemia. Acta Paediat., **43,** Suppl. 100, 245, 1954.
430. Shapiro, S., and Martinez, J.: Congenital dysprothrombinemia: an inherited structural disorder of human prothrombin. J. Clin. Invest. **48,** 2251, 1969.
431. Soulier, J. P., Prou-Wartelle, O., and Josso, F.: Demi-vie de la prothrombine vraie (Facteur II). Nouv. Rev. Franç. Hemat., **2,** 673, 1962.
432. Alexander, B., Goldstein, R., Landwehr, G., and Cook, C. D.: Congenital SPCA deficiency: a hitherto unrecognized coagulation defect with hemorrhage rectified by serum and serum factors. J. Clin. Invest., **30,** 596, 1951.
433. Owen, C. A., Amundsen, M. A., Thompson, J. H., Jr., Spitell, J. A., Bowie, E. J. W., Stilwell, J. G., Hewlett, J. S. Mills, S. D., Sauer, W. G., and Gage, R. P.: Congenital deficiency of factor VII (hypoconvertinemia). Amer. J. Med., **37,** 71, 1964.
434. Lewis, J. H.: Formation of heterologous antibodies to certain coagulation factors. *Proc. VIIth Intern. Conf. Int. Soc. Hemat.,* **2,** Sect. 1, 708, 1958.
435. Prydz, H.: Studies on proconvertin (factor VII). VI. The production in rabbits of an antiserum against factor VII. Scand. J. Clin. Lab. Invest., **17,** 66, 1965.
436. Glueck, H. I., and Sutherland, J. M.: Inherited Factor-VII defect in a Negro family. Pediatrics, **27,** 204, 1961.
437. Godal, H. C., Madsen, K., and Meyer, R. N.: Thrombo-embolism in patients with total proconvertin (Factor VII) deficiency: a report of two cases. Acta Med. Scand., **171,** 325, 1962.
438. Hall, C. A., Rapaport, S. I., Ames, S. B., and DeGroot, J. A.: A clinical and family study of hereditary proconvertin (factor VII) deficiency. Amer. J. Med., **37,** 172, 1964.
439. Dische, F. E., and Benfield, V.: Congenital Factor VII deficiency: haematological and genetic aspects. Acta Haemat., **21,** 257, 1959.
440. Mustard, J. F., Secord, D., Hoeksema, T. D., Downie, H. G., and Rowsell, H. C.: Canine Factor-VII deficiency. Brit. J. Haemat., **8,** 43, 1962.
441. Rabiner, S. F., Winick, M., and Smith, C. H.: Congenital deficiency of Factor VII complicated by coagulation defect of the newborn. A.M.A. J. Dis. Child., **98,** 501, 1959 (abstr.).
442. Cleton, F. J., and Loeliger, E. A.: Two typical hereditary charts of congenital Factor VII deficiency. Thromb. Diath. Haemorrh., **5,** 87, 1961.
443. van Creveld, S., Veder, H. A., and Blans, M. M.: Congenital hypoproconvertinemia. Ann. Paediat., **187,** 373, 1956.
444. Hoag, M. S., Aggeler, P. M., and Fowell, A. H.: Disappearance rate

of concentrated proconvertin extracts in congenital and acquired hypoproconvertinemia. J. Clin. Invest., **39**, 554, 1960.

445. Chevallier, P., Bernard, J., Fiehrer, A., Bilski-Pasquier, G., Samama, M., and Cerf. M.: Deux cas d'hypoconvertinémie familiale. Sang, **26**, 650, 1955.
446. Graham, J. B., and Hougie, C.: Factor X (Stuart-Prower factor). Thromb. Diath. Haemorrh., **6**, Suppl. 1, 416, 1962.
447. Telfer, T. P., Denson, K. W., and Wright, D. R.: A new coagulation defect. Brit. J. Haemat., **2**, 308, 1956.
448. Graham, J. B., Barrow, E. M., and Hougie, C.: Stuart factor defect. II. Genetic aspects of a "new" hemorrhagic state. J. Clin. Invest. **36**, 497, 1957.
449. Kroll, A. J., Alexander, B., Cochios, F., and Pechet, L.: Hereditary deficiencies of clotting factors VII and X associated with carotid-body tumors. New Eng. J. Med., **270**, 6, 1964.
450. Rabiner, S. F., and Kretchmer, N.: The Stuart-Prower factor: utilization of clotting factors obtained by starch-block electrophoresis for genetic evaluation. Brit. J. Haemat., **7**, 99, 1961.
451. Roos, J., van Arkel, C., Verloop, M. C., and Jordan, F. L. J.: A "new" family with Stuart-Prower deficiency. Thromb. Diath. Haemorrh., **3**, 59, 1959.
452. Graham, J. B., Barrow, E. M., and Wynne, T. R.: Stuart clotting defect. III. An acquired case with complete recovery, in *Hemophilia and Other Hemorrhagic States,* edited by K. M. Brinkhous, p. 158. The University of North Carolina Press, Chapel Hill, N.C., 1959.
453. Graham, J. B.: Stuart clotting defect and Stuart factor. Thromb. Diath. Haemorrh., Suppl. **4**, 22, 1960.
454. O'Reilly, R. A., Aggeler, P. M., Hoag, M. S., Leong, L. S., and Kropatkin, M. L.: Hereditary transmission of exceptional resistance to coumarin anticoagulant drugs. The first reported kindred. New Eng. J. Med., **271**, 809, 1964.
455. Pool, J. G., O'Reilly, R. A., Schneiderman, L. J., and Alexander, M.: Warfarin resistance in the rat. Amer. J. Physiol., **215**, 627, 1968.
456. Gobbi, F., Ascari, E., and Barbieri, U.: Congenital deficiency of proaccelerin (Owren's parahemophilia): clinical and physiopathological observations. Minerva Med., **51**, 78, 1960.
457. Brink, A. J., and Kingsley, C. S.: Familial disorder of blood coagulation due to deficiency of labile factor. Quart. J. Med., **21**, 19, 1952.
458. Fajardo, L. F., and Silvert, D.: Pregnancy and Ac-globulin deficiency. Amer. J. Obster. Gynec., **74**, 909, 1957.
459. Friedman, I. A., Quick, A. J., Higgins, F., Hussey, C. V., and Hickey, M. E.: Hereditary labile factor (Factor V) deficiency. J.A.M.A., **175**, 370, 1961.
460. Soulier, J. P., and Larrieu, M. J.: Deficit en 3 ème facteur prothromboplastique plasmatique: rapports entre le PTA et le facteur Hageman. Thromb. Diath. Haemorrh., **2**, 1, 1958.
461. Owren, P. A.: Factor V (proaccelerin). Thromb. Diath. Haemorrh., **6**, Suppl. 1, 387, 1962.
462. Webster, W. P., and Penick, G. D.: Hemostasis in congenital factor V deficiency. Fed. Proc., **22**, 328, 1963.
463. Alexander, B., and Goldstein, R.: Parahemophilia in 3 siblings (Owren's disease) with studies on certain plasma components affecting prothrombin conversion. Amer. J. Med., **13**, 255, 1952.
464. Borchgrevink, C. F., and Owren, P. A.: Surgery in a patient with Factor V (Proaccelerin) deficiency. Acta Med. Scand., **170**, 743, 1961.
465. Ferguson, J. H., Johnston, C. L., Jr., and Howell, D. A.: A circulating inhibitor (Anti-AcG) specific for the labile Factor-V of the blood-clotting mechanism. Blood, **13**, 382, 1958.
466. Hörder, M. H.: Isolierter Faktor V-mangel bedingt durch einen spezifischen Hemmkörper, Acta Haemat., **12**, 1, 1954.
467. Rabe, F., and Salomon, E.: Ueber Faserstoffmangel im Blut bei einem Falle von Hämophilie. Deutsch. Arch. Klin. Med., **132**, 240, 1920.
468. Brönnimann, R.: Kongenital afibrinogenämie. Acta Haemat., **11**, 41, 1954.
469. Lawson, H. A.: Congenital afibrinogenemia: report of case, New Eng. J. Med., **248**, 552, 1953.
470. Ingram, G. I. C., Pinniger, J. L., and Vallet, L.: Survival in an afibrinogenaemic subject of fibrinogen prepared from "time-expired" blood. Lancet, **1**, 135, 1960.
471. Opitz, H., and Frei, M.: Über eien neue Form der Pseudohämophile, Jahrb. Kinderh., **94**, 374, 1921.
472. Rausen, A. R., Cruchaud, A., McMillan, C. W., and Gitlin, D.: A study of fibrinogen turnover in classical hemophilia and congenital afibrinogenemia. Blood, **18**, 710, 1961.
473. Niewiarowski, S., Kozlawska, J., Gulmantowicz, A., and Pelczarska-Kasperka, E.: Congenital afibrinogenemia: biological study of 2 cases. Hemostase, **2**, 191, 1962.
474. Gugler, E., and Lüscher, E.: Die kongenitale Afibrinogenämie. Ann. Paediat., **200**, 125, 1963.
475. Inceman, S., Caen, J., and Bernard, J.: Aggregation, adhesion, and viscous metamorphosis of platelets in congenital fibrinogen deficiencies. J. Lab. Clin. Med., **68**, 21, 1966.
476. Rodman, N. F.: Sequential changes in platelet ultrastructure in a white thrombus model. In *Physiology of Hemostasis and Thrombosis,* edited by S. A. Johnson and W. H. Seegers, p. 266. Charles C Thomas, Springfield, Ill., 1967.
477. Atencio, A. C., Chao, P.-Y., Chen, A. Y., and Reeve, E. B.: Fibrinogen response to corticotropin preparations in rabbits. Amer. J. Physiol., **216**, 773, 1969.
478. Campbell, J., Hausler, H. R., Munroe, J. S., and Davidson, I. W. F.: Effects of growth hormone in dogs. Endocrinology, **53**, 134, 1953.
479. Pearson, O. H., and Ratnoff, O. D.: Unpublished observations.
480. Foster, D. P., and Whipple, G. H.: Blood fibrin studies. II. Normal fibrin values and the influence of diet. Amer. J. Physiol., **58**, 379, 1921.
481. Ham, T. H., and Curtis, F. C.: Plasma fibrinogen response in man: influence of the nutritional state, induced hyperpyrexia, infectious disease and liver damage. Medicine, **17**, 413, 1938.
482. Hammond, J. D., and Verel, D.: Observations on the distribution and biological half-life of human fibrinogen. Brit. J. Haemat., **5**, 431, 1959.
483. Adelson, E.: Fibrinogen metabolism. In *Fibrinogen,* edited by K. Laki. p. 225. Marcel Dekker, New York, 1968.
484. de vries, A., Rosenberg, T., Kochwa, S., and Boss, J. H.: Precipitating antifibrinogen antibody appearing after fibrinogen infusions in a patient with congenital afibrinogenemia. Amer. J. Med., **30**, 486, 1961.
485. Ingram, G. I. C., McBrien, D. J., and Spencer, H.: Fatal pulmonary embolus in congenital fibrinopenia. Report of two cases. Acta Haemat., **35**, 56, 1966.
486. Pavlovsky, A., and Berg, A. L. J.: Congenital fibrinopenia: comments on the evolution of a case followed for 20 years. Hemostase, **2**, 239, 1962.
487. Beck, E. A.: Congenital variants of human fibrinogen, in *Fibrinogen,* edited by K. Laki. p. 269, Marcel Dekker, New York, 1968.
488. Forman, W. B., Ratnoff, O. D., and Boyer, M. H.: An inherited qualitative abnormality in plasma fibrinogen: fibrinogen Cleveland. J. Lab. Clin. Med., **72**, 455, 1968.
489. Mammen, E. F., Prasad, A. S., Barnhart, M. I., and Au, C. C.: Congenital dysfibrinogenemia: fibrinogen Detroit. J. Clin. Invest., **48**, 235, 1969.
490. Ménaché, D.: Constitutional and familial abnormal fibrinogen. Thromb. Diath. Haemorrh., Suppl. **13**, 173, 1964.
491. Blombäck, M., Blombäck, B., Mammen, E. F., and Prasad, A. S.: Fibrinogen Detroit-a molecular defect in the N-terminal disulphide knot of human fibrinogen. Nature, **218**, 134, 1968.
492. Egeberg, O.: Inherited fibrinogen abnormality causing thrombophilia. Thromb. Diath. Haemorrh., **17**, 176, 1967.
493. Duckert, F., Jung, E., and Shmerling, D. H.: A hitherto undescribed congenital haemorrhagic diathesis probably due to fibrin stabilizing factor deficiency. Thromb Diath. Haemorrh., **5**, 179, 1961.
494. Ratnoff, O. D., and Steinberg, A. G.: Inheritance of fibrin-stabilising factor deficiency. Lancet, **1**, 25, 1968.
495. Britten, A. F. H.: Congenital deficiency of factor XIII (fibrin-stabilizing factor). Report of a case and review of the literature. Amer. J. Med., **43**, 751, 1967.
496. Amris, C. J., and Ranek, L.: A case of fibrin-stabilizing factor (FSF) deficiency. Thromb. Diath. Haemorrh., **14**, 332, 1965.
497. Barry, A., and Delâge, J. M.: Congenital deficiency of fibrin-stabilizing factor. New Eng. J. Med., **272**, 943, 1965.
498. Duckert, F.: Fibrin stabilizing factor (Factor XIII): consequence of its deficiency. Thromb. Diath. Haemorrh., Suppl. **13**, 115, 1963.

499. Duckert, F.: Le facteur XIII et la proteine XIII. Nouv. Rev. Franç. Hemat., **10**, 685, 1970.
500. von Willebrand, E. A.: Über hereditare Pseudohämophilie, Acta Med. Scand., **76**, 521, 1931.
501. Jürgens, R., and Ferlin, A.: Ueber den sog. Prothrombinkonsumptiontest bei Hämophilie (Hämophil Kondukortorinnen) und bei konstitutioneller Thrombopathie (v. Willebrand-Jürgens). Schweiz. Med. Wschr., **80**, 1098, 1950.
502. Cornell, C. M., and Muhrer, M. E.: Coagulation factors in normal and hemophiliac-type swine. Amer. J. Physiol., **206**, 926, 1964.
503. Chan, J. Y. S., Owen, C. A., Jr., Bowie, E. J. W., Didisheim, P., Thompson, J. H., Jr., Muhrer, M. E., and Zollman, P. E.: Von Willebrand's disease "stimulating factor" in porcine plasma. Amer. J. Physiol., **214**, 1219, 1968.
504. Borchgrevink, C. F.: Platelet adhesion in vivo in patients with bleeding disorders. Acta Med. Scand., **170**, 231, 1961.
505. Cronberg, S., Nilsson, I. M., and Silver, J.: Studies on the platelet adhesiveness in von Willebrand's disease. Acta Med. Scand., **180**, 43, 1966.
506. Salzman, E. W.: Measurement of platelet adhesiveness. J. Lab. Clin. Med., **62**, 724, 1963.
507. Zucker, M.: In vitro abnormality of the blood in von Willebrand's disease correctable by normal plasma. Nature, **197**, 601, 1963.
508. Alexander, B., and Goldstein, R.: Dual hemostatic defect in pseudo-hemophilia. J. Clin. Invest., **32**, 551, 1953.
509. Larrieu, M. J., and Soulier, J. P.: Déficit en facteur antihémophilique A chez une fille associé à un trouble de saignment. Rev. Hémat., **8**, 361, 1953.
510. Quick, A. J., and Hussey, C. V.: Hemophilic condition in the female. J. Lab. Clin. Med., **42**, 929, 1953.
511. Jürgens, R., Lehmann, W., Wegelius, O., Eriksson, A. W., and Heipler, E.: Mitteilung über den Mangel an antihamophilem Globulin (Faktor VIII) bei der aalandischen Thrombopathie (v. Willebrand-Jürgens). Thromb. Diath. Haemorrh., **1**, 257, 1957.
512. Nilsson, I. M., Blombäck, M., Jorpes, E., Blombäck, B., and Johansson, S.: v. Willebrand's disease and its correction with human plasma fraction 1-0. Acta Med. Scand., **159**, 179, 1957.
513. Schulman, I., Smith, C. H., Erlandson, M., and Fort, E.: Vascular hemophilia: a familial hemorrhagic disease in males and females characterized by combined antihemophilic globulin deficiency and vascular abnormalities. A.M.A. J. Dis. Child., **90**, 526, 1955.
514. Cornu, P., Larrieu, M. J., Caen, J., and Bernard, J.: Transfusion studies in von Willebrand's disease: effect on bleeding time and Factor VIII. Brit. J. Haemat., **9**, 189, 1963.
515. Cornu, P., Larrieu, M. J., Caen, J., and Bernard, J.: Données nouvelles concernant la maladie de Willebrand (angiohémophilia) Rev. Franç. Étud. Clin. Biol., **5**, 614, 1960.
516. Bennett, E., and Dormandy, K.: Pool's cryoprecipitate and exhausted plasma in the treatment of von Willebrand's disease and factor XI deficiency. Lancet, **2**, 731, 1966.
517. Biggs, R., and Matthews, J. M.: The treatment of haemorrhage in von Willebrand's disease and the blood level of Factor VIII (AHG). Brit. J. Haemat., **9**, 203, 1963.
518. Blomback, M., and Blomback, B.: Response to fractions in von Willebrand's disease, in *The Hemophilias*, edited by K. M. Brinkhous, p. 286, University of North Carolina Press, Chapel Hill, 1964.
519. Caen, J.: Effect of normal and hemophilic plasma on AHG activity and long bleeding time in von Willebrand's disease, in *The Hemophilias*, edited by K. M. Brinkhous. p. 276, University of North Carolina Press, Chapel Hill, 1964.
520. Egeberg, O.: The effect of exercise on the blood clotting system. Scand. J. Clin. Lab. Invest., **15**, 13, 1963.
521. Cornu, P., Larrieu, M. J., Caen, J., and Bernard, J.: Maladie de Willebrand étude clinique, génetique et biologique (a propos de 22 observations). Nouv. Rev. Franç. Hemat., **1**, 231, 1961.
522. Horowitz, H. I., and O'Leary, D.: Von Willebrand's disease. A critical evaluation of diagnostic criteria. N.Y. J. Med., **65**, 2236, 1965.
523. Graham, J.: The inheritance of "vascular hemophilia": a new and interesting problem in human genetics. J. Med. Educ., **34**, 385, 1959.
524. Winckelmann, G., Groh, R., Schneider, J., and Huber, P.: Pregnancy and childbirth in von Willebrand's disease. Factor VIII levels. Germ. Med. Monthly, **12**, 208, 1967.
525. Barrow, E. M., Heindel, C. C., Roberts, H. R., and Graham, J. B.: Heterozygosity and homozygosity in von Willebrand's disease. Proc. Soc. Exp. Biol. Med., **118**, 684, 1965.
526. Strauss, H. S., and Diamond, L. K.: Elevation of Factor VIII (anti-hemophilic factor) during pregnancy in normal persons and in a patient with von Willebrand's disease. New Eng. J. Med., **269**, 1251, 1963.
527. van Creveld, S., Kloosterman, G. J., Mochtar, I. A., and Koppe, J. G.: Interchange between blood of mother and fetus in vascular hemophilia. Biol. Neonat., **4**, 379, 1962.
528. Glueck, H. I., and Flessa, H.: The control of hemorrhage with a combination of norethynodrel-mestranol. J. Lab. Clin. Med., **70**, 877, 1967.
529. Oeri, J., Matter, M., Isenschmid, H., Hauser, F., and Koller, F.: Angeborener Mangel an Factor V (Parahaemophilie) verbunden mit echter Haemophilie A bei zwei Brüdern. Mod. Probl. Paediat., **1**, 575, 1954: Ann. Paediat., Suppl. **58.**
530. Iversen, T., and Bastrup-Madsen, P.: Congenital familial deficiency of Factor V (parahemophilia) combined with deficiency of antihemophilic globulin. Brit. J. Haemat., **2**, 265, 1956.
531. Jones, J. H., Rizza, C. R., Hardisty, R. M., Dormandy, K. M., and Macpherson, J. C.: Combined deficiency of Factor V and Factor VIII (antihaemophilic globulin): a report of 3 cases. Brit. J. Haemat., **8**, 120, 1962.
532. Seligsohn, U., and Ramot, B.: Combined factor-V and factor-VIII deficiency: report of 4 cases. Brit. J. Haemat., **16**, 475, 1969.
533. Gobbi, F.: Hereditary combined deficiency of AHG and proaccelerin. Scand. J. Haemat., **3**, 222, 1966.
534. Ménaché, D.: A new case of combined deficiency of factor V and factor VIII. *Proc. XII Congress Int. Soc. Hematology*, New York, **178**, 1968.
535. Caen, J. P., Castaldi, P. A., Leclerc, J. C., Inceman, S., Larrieu, M. J., Probst, M., and Bernard, J.: Congenital bleeding disorders with long bleeding time and normal platelet count. Amer. J. Med., **41**, 4, 1966.
536. Zucker, M. B., Pert, J. H., and Hilgartner, M. W.: Platelet function in a patient with thrombasthenia. Blood, **28**, 524, 1966.
537. Jackson, D. P., Hartmann, R. C., and Conley, C. L.: Clot retraction as measure of platelet function; clinical disorders associated with qualitative platelet defects (thrombocytopathic purpura). Bull. Johns Hopkins Hosp., **93**, 370, 1953.
538. de Vries, A., Shafrir, E., Efrati, P., and Shamir, Z.: Thrombocytopathic purpura with normal prothrombin consumption: hemorrhagic diathesis due to partial platelet dysfunction. Blood, **8**, 1000, 1953.
539. Braunsteiner, H., and Pakesch, F.: Thrombocytoasthenia and thrombocytopathia: old names and new diseases. Blood, **11**, 965, 1956.
540. Friedman, L., Bowie, E. J. W., Thompson, J. H., Jr., Brown, A. L., Jr., and Owen, C. A., Jr.: Familial Glanzmann's thrombasthenia. Proc. Staff Mayo Clinic, **39**, 908, 1964.
541. Weiss, H. J., and Kochwa, S.: Studies of platelet function and proteins in 3 patients with Glanzmann's thrombasthenia. J. Lab. Clin. Med., **71**, 153, 1968.
542. Hardisty, R. M., Dormandy, K. M., and Hutton, R. A.: Thromasthenia. Study of 3 cases. Brit. J. Haemat., **10**, 371, 1964.
543. Caen, J., and Cousin, C.: Le trouble d'adhésivité in vivo des plaquettes dans la maladie de Willebrand et les thrombasthénies de Glanzmann. Nouv. Rev. Franç. Hemat., **2**, 685, 1962.
544. Larrieu, M. J., Caen, J., Lelong, J. C., and Bernard, J.: Maladie de Glanzmann: Étude clinique, biologique et pathogénique à propos de cinq observations. Nouv. Rev. Franç. Hemat., **1**, 662, 1961.
545. Schettini, F., Berni Canani, M., DiFrancesco, L., and Rea, F.: Studies on the enzymes of blood platelets from healthy and thrombopathic children. Acta Haemat., **27**, 237, 1962.
546. Gross, R.: Biochemie normale und pathologischer Blutplättchen. *Proc. VIII Cong. Europ. Soc. Haemat.*, Vienna, 1961, vol. 16, S. Karger, Basel, 1962.
547. Moser, K., Lechner, K., and Vinazzer, H.: A hitherto not described enzyme defect in thrombasthenia: glutathione reductase deficiency. Thromb. Diath. Haemorrh., **19**, 46, 1968.
548. Jackson, D. P., Morse, E. E., Zieve, P. D., and Conley, C. L.: Thrombo-

cytopathic purpura associated with defective clot retraction and absence of platelet fibrinogen. Blood, **22**, 827, 1963.

549. Bernard, J., and Soulier, J. P.: Sur une nouvelle varieté de dystrophie thrombocytaire hémorragipare congénitale. Sem. Hop. Paris, **24**, 3217, 1948.
550. Soulier, J. P., Larrieu, M. J., and Wartelle, O.: La thromboplastinoformation dans les affections plaquettaires. Acta Haemat., **14**, 160, 1955.
551. Inceman, S., Ucar, S., and Ulutin, O. N.: Athrombia thrombocytopathia. Thromb. Diath. Haemorrh., **4**, 234, 1960.
552. Ulutin, O. N., and Karaca, M.: A study on the pathogenesis of thrombopathia using the platelet osmotic-resistance test. Brit. J. Haemat., **5**, 302, 1959.
553. Caen, J.: Adhésion des plaquettes aux lévres de la plaie vasculaire et aggrégation entre elles. *Proc. XXII Cong., Internat. Union Physiol. Soc.,* p. 248. Leiden, 1962.
554. Bernard, J., Caen, J., and Maroteau, P.: La dystrophie thrombocytaire hemorragipare congénitale. Rev. Haemat., **12**, 222, 1957.
555. Quick, A. J., and Hussey, C. V.: Hereditary thrombopathic thrombocytopenia. Amer. J. Med. Sci., **245**, 643, 1963.
556. Cullum, K., Cooney, D. P., and Schreier, S. L.: Familial thrombocytopenic thrombocytopathy. Brit. J. Haemat., **13**, 147, 1967.
557. Quick, A. J.: Hereditary thrombopathic thrombocytopenia: sex-linked inheritance pattern. Amer. J. Med. Sci., **250**, 527, 1965.
558. Kurstjens, R., Bolt, C., Vossen, M., and Haanen, C.: Familial thrombopathic thrombocytopenia. Brit. J. Haemat., **15**, 305, 1968.
559. van Creveld, S., and Veder, H. A.: Differentiation of Factor 3 and Factor 4 of the platelets in a patient with a haemorrhagic diathesis. Ann. Paediat., **185**, 236, 1955.
560. Weiss, H. J.: Platelet aggregation, adhesion and adenosine diphosphate release in thrombopathia (platelet factor 3 deficiency): comparison with Glanzmann's thrombasthenia and von Willebrand's disease. Amer. J. Med., **43**, 570, 1967.
561. Marcus, A. J.: Platelet function. New Eng. J. Med., **280**, 1213, 1278, 1330, 1969.
562. Hirsh, J., Castelan, D. J., and Loder, P. B.: Spontaneous bruising associated with a defect in the interaction of platelets with connective tissue. Lancet, **2**, 18, 1967.
563. Sahud, M. A., and Aggeler, P. M.: Platelet dysfunction-differentation of a newly recognized primary type from that produced by aspirin. New Eng. J. Med., **280**, 453, 1969.
564. Hardisty, R. M., and Hutton, R. A.: Bleeding tendency associated with a "new" abnormality of platelet behaviour. Lancet, **1**, 983, 1967.
565. Inceman, S., Unugur, A., and Aran, M.: Essential athrombia. Thromb. Diath. Haemorrh., **8**, 502, 1962.
566. Yoshida, K.: Haemorrhagic diathesia due to deficiency of an AHF-like factor (Nishimine factor) associated with a qualitative platelet dysfunction. *Proc. VI Cong. Europ. Soc. Haemat.,* 1957, p. 167, S. Karger, Copenhagen.
567. Yoshida, K., Umegaki, K., Yoshioka, K., Fukui, H., Majima, T., and Tagawa, N.: Hemorrhagic diathesis with prolonged bleeding time, serum defect and qualitative platelet dysfunction. *Proc. VIII Internat. Cong. Hemat.,* p. 1556. Tokyo Pan Pacific Press, 1960.
568. Kosaki, G., Tanaka, K., Inoshita, K., and Nagao, M.: A role of TF (Tatsumi-factor) on activation of factor IX, 2nd report. *Proc. XII Congress, Internat. Soc. Hematology,* p. 176. New York, 1968.
569. Hathaway, W. E., Behlasen, L. P., and Hathaway, H. S.: Evidence for a new plasma thromboplastin factor. I. Case report, coagulation studies and physiochemical properties. Blood, **26**, 521, 1965.
570. Pechet, L., Cochios, F., and Deykin, D.: Further studies on the "Dynia" clotting abnormality. Thromb. Diath. Haemorrh., **17**, 365, 1967.
571. Schulman, I., Pierce, M., Lukens, A., and Currimbhoy, Z.: Studies on thrombopoesis. I. A factor in normal human plasma required for platelet production; chronic thrombocytopenia due to its deficiency. Blood, **16**, 943, 1960.
572. Abilgaard, C. F., and Simone, J. V.: Thrombopoesis. Seminars Hemat., **4**, 424, 1967.
573. Wiskott, A.: Familiärer, angeborener Morbus Werlhofii? Mschr. Kinderheilk., **68**, 212, 1937.
574. Aldrich, R. A., Steinberg, A. G., and Campbell, D. C.: Pedigree demonstrating a sex-linked recessive condition characterized by draining ears, eczematoid dermatitis and bloody diarrhea. Pediatrics, **13**, 133, 1954.
575. Krivit, W., Yunis, E., and White, J. G.: Platelet survival studies in Aldrich syndrome. Pediatrics, **37**, 339, 1966.
576. St. Geme, J. W., Jr., Prince, J. T., Burke, B. A., Good, R. A., and Krivit, W.: Impaired cellular resistance to herpes-simplex virus in Wiskott-Aldrich syndrome. New Eng. J. Med., **273**, 229, 1965.
577. Krivit, W., and Good, R. A.: Aldrich's syndrome: thrombocytopenia, eczema and infection in infants. A.M.A. J. Dis. Child., **97**, 137, 1959.
578. Kildeberg, P.: The Aldrich syndrome. Pediatrics, **27**, 362, 1961.
579. West, C. D., Hong, R., and Holland, N. H.: Immunoglobin levels from the newborn period to adulthood and in immunoglobulin deficiency states. J. Clin. Invest., **41**, 2054, 1962.
580. Blaese, R. M., Strober, W., Brown, R. S., and Walkmann, T. A.: The Wiskott-Aldrich syndrome. A disorder with a possible defect in antigen processing or recognition. Lancet, **1**, 1056, 1968.
581. Sherry, S., and others: Rademacher's disease. Amer. J. Med., **32**, 80, 1962.
582. Ten Bensel, R. W., Stadlan, E. M., and Krivit, W.: The development of malignancy in the course of Aldrich syndrome. J. Pediat., **68**, 761, 1966.
583. Roberts, M. H., and Smith, M. H.: Thrombopenic purpura: report of four cases in one family. A.M.A. J. Dis. Child, **79**, 820, 1950.
584. Dawson, J. P.: Congenital pancytopenia associated with multiple congenital anomalies (Fanconi type): review of the literature and report of a 20-year-old female with a 10-year follow-up and apparently good response to splenectomy. Pediatrics, **15**, 325, 1955.
585. Hauser, F.: Über hereditäre und symptomatische congenitale Thrombopenie. Ann. Paediat., **171**, 86, 1948.
586. Wooley, E. J. S.: Familial idiopathic thrombocytopenic purpura. Brit. Med. J., **1**, 440, 1956.
587. Ata, M., Fisher, O. D., and Holman, C. A.: Inherited thrombocytopenia. Lancet, **1**, 119, 1965.
588. Bithell, T. C., Didisheim, P., Cartwright, G. E., and Wintrobe, M. M.: Thrombocytopenia inherited as an autosomal dominant trait. Blood, **25**, 231, 1965.
589. Wassmuth, D. R., Hamilton, H. E., and Sheets, R. F.: May-Hegglin anomaly. Hereditary affection of granulocytes and platelets. J. Amer. Med. Ass., **183**, 737, 1963.
590. Davis, J. W., and Wilson, S. J.: Platelet survival in the May-Hegglin anomaly. Brit. J. Haemat., **12**, 61, 1966.
591. Brown, G. M., Diamant, N. E., Galbraith, P. R., and Wilson, W. E. C.: A familial hemorrhagic diathesis due to an antithrombin. Blood, **21**, 298, 1963.
592. Quick, A. J., and Hussey, C. V.: Hyperheparinemia: clinical picture and treatment. J. Lab. Clin. Med., **48**, 932, 1956.
593. Estes, J. W.: Platelet size and function in the heritable disorders of connective tissue. Ann. Intern. Med., **68**, 1237, 1968.
594. Kasjiwagi, H., Riddle, J. M., Abraham, J. P., and Frame, B.: Function and ultrastructural abnormalities of platelets in the Ehlers-Danlos syndrome. Ann. Intern. Med., **63**, 249, 1965.
595. Riddle, J. M., quoted by Mammen, E. F.: Irregular blood coagulation. In *Blood Clotting Enzymology,* edited by W. H. Seegers, p. 421, Academic, New York, 1967.
596. Osler, W.: On multiple hereditary telangiectases with recurring haemorrhages. Quart. J. Med., **1**, 53, 1907.
597. Rodes, C. B.: Cavernous hemangiomas of the lung with secondary polycythemia. J.A.M.A., **110**, 1914, 1938.
598. Hanes, F. M.: Multiple hereditary hemorrhagic telangiectasia causing hemorrhage (hereditary hemorrhagic telangiectasia). Bull. Johns Hopkins Hosp., **20**, 63, 1909.
599. Muckle, T. J.: Low in-vivo adhesive-platelet count in hereditary haemorrhagic telangiectasia. Lancet, **2**, 880, 1964.
600. Harrison, D. F. N.: Familial hemorrhagic telangiectasia: 20 cases treated with systemic oestrogen. Quart. J. Med., **33**, N.S., 25, 1964.
601. Blackburn, E. K., Primary capillary hemorrhage. Brit. J. Haemat., **7**, 239, 1961.

602. Egeberg, O.: Thrombophilia caused by inheritable deficiency of blood antithrombin. Scand. J. Clin. Lab. Invest., **17,** 92, 1965.
603. Zimmerman, T. S., Ratnoff, O. D., and Powell, A. E.: Immunologic differentiation of classic hemophilia (Factor VIII deficiency) and von Willebrand's disease, with observations on combined deficiencies of antihemophilic factor and proaccelerin (Factor V) and on an acquired circulating anticoagulant against antihemophilic factor. J. Clin. Invest., **50,** 244, 1971.
604. Zimmerman, T. S., Ratnoff, O. D. and Littell, A. S.: Detection of carriers of classic hemophilia using an immunologic assay for antihemophilic factor (Factor VIII). J. Clin. Invest., **50,** 255, 1971.
605. Forbes, C. D. and Ratnoff, O. D. To be published.
606. McMillan, C. W. and Roberts, H. R.: Congenital combined deficiency of coagulation Factors II, VII, IX and X. New Engl. J. Med., **274,** 1313, 1966.
607. Gralnick, H. R., Givelber, H. and Finlayson, J. S.: A familial bleeding disorder associated with dysfibrinogenemia. Clin. Res., **18,** 405, 1970.
608. Hampton, J. W.: Qualitative fibrinogen defect associated with abnormal fibrin stabilization. J. Lab. Clin. Med., **72,** 882, 1968.
609. Forbes, C. D., Ratnoff, O. D. and Donaldson, V. H.: Unpublished observations.
610. Brown, P. E., Hougie, C. and Roberts, H. R.: The genetic heterogeneity of hemophilia B. New Engl. J. Med., **283,** 61, 1970.
611. Kattlove, H. E., Shapiro, S. S. and Spivak, M.: Hereditary prothrombin deficiency. New Engl. J. Med., **282,** 57, 1970.
612. Olson, R. E.: The mode of action of vitamin K. Nutrition Reviews, **28,** 171, 1970.
613. Denson, K. W. E., Lurie, A., DeCataldo, F. and Mannucci, P. M.: The Factor-X defect: recognition of abnormal forms of Factor X. Brit. J. Haemat., **18,** 317, 1970.
614. Yin, E. T., Wessler, S. and Stoll, P. J. To be published.
615. Hathaway, W. E. and Alsever, J.: The relation of 'Fletcher Factor' to Factors XI and XII. Brit. J. Haemat., **18,** 161, 1970.
616. Hattersley, P. G. and Hayse, D.: Fletcher factor deficiency: a report of three unrelated cases. Brit. J. Haemat., **18,** 411, 1970.
617. Robinson, A. J., Kropatkin, M. and Aggeler, P. M.: Hageman factor (Factor XII) deficiency in marine mammals. Science, **166,** 1420, 1969.
618. Lewis, J. H., Bayer, W. L. and Szeto, I. L. F.: Coagulation Factor XII deficiency in the porpoise, *Tursiops truncatus.* Comp. Biochem. Physiol. **31,** 667, 1969.

CHAPTER SEVENTY-THREE

ACATALASEMIA*

Hugo Aebi and Hedi Suter

DISTRIBUTION AND DEFINITION

Acatalasemia, a deficiency of the enzyme *catalase* inherited as an autosomal recessive trait, is a rare condition, first recognized in 1946 by Takahara among the Japanese [1–5]. Before 1962 all known patients homozygous for acatalasemia were located in Japan and Korea [6, 7]. More recently, the disorder has been detected in western countries, such as Switzerland [8, 9], Israel [10–12], and Germany [13]. Observations from Sweden [14–16] and the United States [17, 18] offer strong evidence that at least heterozygotes also do exist in these countries. Therefore the gene (or genes) for acatalasemia may have a worldwide distribution.

Several terms are synonymous with *acatalasemia.* Since the deficiency is not restricted to blood, but also involves other tissues, such as mucous membrane, tonsils, skin, liver, muscle, placenta, and bone marrow, the more general term *acatalasia* has been recommended [9]. Alternatives are *anenzymia catalasea* or *the acatalatic condition* [19, 20]. None of the proposed terms is strictly correct because traces of catalase can be detected in blood and in tissues of homozygous subjects. Nevertheless, the term *hypocatalasemia* should be reserved for those members of families with acatalasemia who are presumed heterozygous carriers of the acatalasemia gene. Since the mode of gene action as well as the level of residual activity may vary from family to family, in some instances the enzyme activity level in the blood of heterozygotes may be within the normal range.

Acatalasemia is not a single entity. It must be considered as a *group of mutations* which lead to a change in the activity level or other properties of the normal enzyme. Among other changes, the variations in the level of activity in blood and tissues of homozygotes and heterozygotes provide a rational base for the classification of the different subspecies of acatalasemia. Since acatalasemia is both rare and often without symptoms, the anomaly is of no particular clinical importance. There is much controversy about the biologic significance of catalase in the mammalian organism, and this enzyme deficiency is of special interest to the biochemist.

PROPERTIES AND FUNCTION OF CATALASE

History

Thénard [21] observed in 1818 that both plant and animal tissues degrade hydrogen peroxide, a substance which he himself had discovered some years earlier. In 1901 Loew [22] gave the name *catalase* to the substance responsible for this degradation. In 1923 Warburg [23] suggested that catalase is an iron-containing enzyme because it is inhibited by cyanide; evidence that its prosthetic group is hematin was offered in 1930 by Zeile and Hellström [24]. The enzyme was first crystallized from beef liver in 1937 by Sumner and Dounce [25]. Catalase activity is widely distributed in mammalian tissues but is most abundant in liver, kidney, and erythrocytes [26, 27]. It has been crystallized from these three tissues of a number of species, including man [27–31], as well as from bacteria [32].

Structure of Catalase

Animal catalase (E.C. 1.11.1.6; H_2O_2-H_2O_2 oxidoreductase) is a protein (molecular weight, 240,000) which contains four ferriprotoporphyrin (hematin) groups: 1.1 percent protohemin, 0.09 percent iron, and 16.8 percent nitrogen. The *primary structure* of the human erythrocyte catalase protein is not known. The complete sequence of the monomer of bovine liver catalase consisting of 505 amino acid residues was established in 1969 by Schroeder et al., [33]. The active enzyme is composed of four subunits. For some time there was a controversy regarding the number and type of subunits in the active catalase molecule, and alternatives between two and six were offered by various authors [34–36]. By applying drastic procedures, such as performic acid oxidation, even smaller degradation products, with a molecular weight of 25,000 to 29,000 (possibly "half-subunits") can be obtained [37]. The concept that catalase, like other hemin compounds, is a tetramer, is based not only on Schroeder's analytical data but also on dissociation experiments on the succinylated derivative, which yields a product with a molecular weight of about 65,000 [38], and on electron microscopic studies. Kiselev et al., [39, 40] found that red cell catalase can be crystallized in tubes, with monomolecular layer walls and the molecules formed in a helical arrangement. In the electron micrographs the catalase molecule is seen to be composed of two identical parts consistent with a structure built of four subunits arranged with 222 point-group symmetry.

Catalase preparations obtained from various species and organs can be differentiated by immunologic [41] and chromatographic [42, 43] methods. Variation in heat stability may serve the same purpose [44]. Furthermore, there is evidence that mammalian catalase exists in multiple or alternative molecular forms. Heterogeneity of liver catalase and of erythrocyte catalase [48] has been demonstrated by chromatographic separation procedures [45–47]. Three fractions (A, B, and C) can be obtained from human red cells [49], but they are unstable and can be interconverted. These forms probably represent different conformational states (conformers) of the same molecular species [48].

Catalase has characteristic spectroscopic and magnetic

*Supported by grants from the Swiss National Science Foundation.

properties. In the visible range it has absorption bands at 405, 505, 535, 538, and 623 mμ [50]. Extinction is highest at the Soret band (405 mμ), the wavelength that is commonly used for direct measurement of catalase concentration. The millimolar extinction coefficient at 405 mμ is 380 to 400 per mole enzyme or about 100 per hematin group. In human erythrocyte catalase, just as in beef liver catalase, the porphyrin nucleus is the ferric complex of protoporphyrin IX (corresponding to etioporphyrin isomer Type III, protohemin) [51]. It is identical with that found in horseradish peroxidase, methemoglobin, and metmyoglobin, and is similar to that of ferricytochrome C.

The catabolism of the hemin of catalase is apparently identical with that of hemoglobin and ultimately yields bilirubin [52]. The ferriprotoporphyrin of catalase is easily removed from the apoenzyme by acid-acetone. Recombination has not yet been achieved [53].

Separation of catalase from hemoglobin in a hemolysate can be accomplished by (1) gel filtration on Sephadex G-100 [54]; (2) adsorption of catalase on DEAE-cellulose [49]; or (3) differential destruction of hemoglobin in organic solvents such as ethanol and chloroform in which catalase is more stable [55]. Isolation procedures have been described by Bonnichsen et al., [56], by Herbert and Pinsent [31], and by Deutsch [57].

Reaction Mechanism

Catalase is one of the most active catalysts produced by nature. It decomposes hydrogen peroxide at an extremely rapid rate, corresponding to a catalytic center activity of about 10^7 min $^{-1}$. One molecule of catalase is capable of splitting up to 42,000 molecules of H_2O_2 per second at O °C, depending upon the concentration of H_2O_2. If the steady state concentration of H_2O_2 in the system is high, catalase acts mainly as an H_2O_2-decomposing catalyst. At low H_2O_2 concentration ($<10^{-6}M$) and in the presence of a suitable hydrogen donor, it acts mainly as a peroxidase. In 1936 Keilin and Hartree [58] demonstrated coupled oxidation of ethanol in the presence of a peroxide-generating system (xanthine oxidase and hypoxanthine) and catalase. It is now well established that with a high substrate concentration of methanol, ethanol, or formic acid, and at low concentrations of peroxide, catalase exhibits peroxidatic activity [59, 60].

The mechanism of catalase action is atypical. The main route consists of several sequential steps: The reaction is initiated by combination of one molecule of catalase with one of H_2O_2 to form the primary enzyme-substrate complex (= compound I)

$$\text{Catalase} + H_2O_2 \longrightarrow \text{catalase} - H_2O_2 \text{ (compound I)}$$

Compound I then reacts further by combining with a suitable hydrogen donor to form a ternary complex. Its dual function as a catalatic or as a peroxidatic catalyst is due to competition among several H-donors, including H_2O_2 itself for compound I. The alternatives using formate as an example of a typical hydrogen donor are

$$\text{(1) Catalase} - H_2O_2 + HCOOH \longrightarrow \text{catalase} + CO_2 + 2H_2O$$
(compound I)

$$\text{(2) Catalase} - H_2O_2 + H_2O_2 \longrightarrow \text{catalase} + O_2 + 2H_2O$$
(compound I)

The switch between the catalatic and peroxidatic actions of catalase is due to the fact that H_2O_2 may react with the free enzyme as well as with compound I. At low concentrations H_2O_2 is used exclusively for the formation of compound I; at high H_2O_2 concentrations it acts as a substrate and as a hydrogen donor as well. Within the whole experimental range the initial rate of H_2O_2 decomposition increases with rising H_2O_2 concentration. In the steady state there is an equilibrium between compound I and its alternative counterparts, compound II and compound III, which are practically inactive. Accordingly catalase is rapidly inactivated at higher H_2O_2 concentrations while compound I is being converted to compound II and III. As a result in an assay for catalase activity the initial hydrogen peroxide concentration and the duration of the incubation period are of crucial importance. The kinetics of catalatic and peroxidatic activity have been investigated in detail by Chance et al. [61]. More recently the kinetic properties of red cell catalase in solution as well as *in situ* have been studied by Nicholls [62]. Reference is also made to several reviews published in recent years [34, 50, 63–66].

Catalase Assay

Catalase activity in hemolysate or other biologic material can be determined (1) indirectly by following H_2O_2 decomposition or O_2 production under specified assay conditions, (2) directly by a quantitative immunoassay technique [41], or (3) by measuring the peroxidatic oxidation of a suitable hydrogen donor such as formate-^{14}C, $^{14}CO_2$ production being taken as an index [67].

For routine measurements indirect techniques are used exclusively. In principle, all methods for the detection of H_2O_2 may be used for measuring catalase activity [65, 68]. Decomposition of H_2O_2 can be measured by titrimetric, ultraviolet spectrophotometric (ΔE 240), photometric, or fluorimetric methods. Alternatively, O_2 production can be followed either manometrically or by means of the oxygen electrode. A number of methods which can be recommended for assay or detection of catalase in blood and tissues have been reviewed recently [65].

Distribution

Catalase is widely distributed in nature. The fact that it is missing in most anaerobic microorganisms but occurs abundantly in radioresistant species (e.g., *Micrococcus radiodurans;* Laser [69]) has considerably stimulated speculations about its physiologic role. In mammalian tissues the enzyme concentration is highest in liver and lowest in connective tissue. There is a great deal of variation among species, with activity in the liver being highest in herbivores, such as cow, horse, and guinea pig. Catalase activity can be detected in human liver at an early stage of embryonic development (about the sixth week) [70]. The level of catalase in liver depends on genetic and environmental factors [71]. The depressing action of certain malignant tumors on liver catalase in man and the rat is of particular interest [72–74].

In the liver cell catalase is mainly localized in peroxisomes [75–77] and in mitochondria [78]. Peroxisomes, formerly called *microbodies,* are particularly rich in catalase. So far this specialized organelle has been isolated from mammalian liver and kidney as well as from single-cell organisms (*Tetrahymena pyriformis*). In addition to organelle-bound catalase, there is also a small fraction in the cell sap. Whether this fraction is merely the enzyme in transit from the site of synthesis to the organelles or is due to a (reversible?) release of particle-bound catalase is not established [79, 80]. Catalase in the mature red cell is essentially free. Only traces are bound to stromal proteins [81]. There is considerable variation too in the catalase activity of erythrocytes. Normal human red cells are relatively rich in catalase, but duck erythrocytes contain almost none [19]. There is no correlation between catalase activity in tissues and in blood when different species are compared [67]. During the life-span of normal human erythrocytes there is only a moderate decrease, if any, in catalase activity [49, 82, 83].

Turnover

Theorell and associates [84] have shown that the red cell and the liver enzymes turn over at different rates. They investigated the origin of liver and blood catalase in guinea pigs using ^{59}Fe and ^{55}Fe. The specific activity in liver ferritin initially exceeded that in liver catalase, but equal labeling was approached at about 10 days and thereafter the specific activities declined in parallel. By contrast, blood catalase showed a slower increase that ran parallel to the hemoglobin iron activity. It was concluded that identical enzymes were being formed in different organs at different rates.

Additional evidence for independent origins of the heme of liver and erythrocyte catalase is provided by studies of Schmid et al. [85]. Administration of allylisopropylacetamide (AIA) to rabbits and rats causes a marked and rapid fall in liver catalase activity, a great increase in liver porphyrin concentration, and porphyrinuria. No significant change occurs in erythrocyte catalase activity, in hemoglobin concentration, or in activity of liver cytochrome oxidase or succinic dehydrogenase.

The turnover of catalase in rat liver has been studied in detail by Rechcigl and Price [86]. They have shown that 3-amino-1,2,4-triazole (AT) destroys catalase irreversibly without interfering with its resynthesis, whereas AIA blocks the synthesis of catalase without affecting its destruction. Based on these findings methods were devised for measuring the rate of synthesis and destruction of catalase in vivo. The rate of synthesis of catalase in the rat liver proved to be four times that of the kidney, and the rate constants of destruction were identical. The average half-life of rat liver catalase is about 3 days, which is obviously much less than the corresponding figure for red cell catalase [87, 88].

Physiologic Role of Catalase

General Considerations

It was originally thought that catalase serves as a physiologic safeguard for decomposing H_2O_2 which might otherwise accumulate within the cell [89, 90]. As early as 1933 Bingold [89] suggested that the role of erythrocyte catalase is to protect hemoglobin from oxidation by H_2O_2. It was shown that inhibition of catalase by hydroxylamine permitted rapid oxidation of hemoglobin to methemoglobin when peroxide was added. Even today the physiologic role of catalase is not at all clear. Most likely it may act either way, i.e., as a regulator of hydrogen peroxide concentration; small amounts of peroxide will saturate the peroxidatic function; larger amounts will be decomposed in the catalase reaction. The peroxidatic action of catalase requires only very low concentrations of peroxide, about $10^{-9}M$. Thus at a steady state concentration of $10^{-8}M$, as in *M. lysodeikticus* [91, 92], catalase is probably acting by a combination of catalatic and peroxidatic pathways.

Tissue Catalase

The role of catalase in tissues is strictly peroxidatic, at least insofar as the fraction in peroxisomes is concerned. This organelle, first observed by Rouiller and Bernhard [93] and studied in detail by de Duve and Baudhuin [75], contains H_2O_2-producing enzymes (e.g., uricase, D-amino acid oxidase, and monoamine oxidase) and catalase in high concentration. The peroxisomes may be regarded as specialized organelles well equipped to perform coupled oxidation reactions. They are constructed in such a way as to act as a trap for the hydrogen peroxide produced by the oxidases. According to Poole [77], it may well be that the reactions catalyzed by these oxidases are more important in cellular metabolism than is immediately apparent.

Little is known about the role of mitochondrial catalase. In their studies on the reversal of mitochondrial swelling caused by reduced glutathione, Neubert et al. [78] and Lehninger and Beck [94] identified the contraction factors I and II as glutathione peroxidase and catalase. Heppel and Porterfield [95] first showed that coupled peroxidatic reactions are of physiologic significance. They found that enough hydrogen peroxide is produced in rat liver homogenates to promote a readily measurable oxidation of nitrite to nitrate by catalase. Aebi and associates have investigated formate and methanol oxidation in vivo and in vitro using ^{14}C-labeled substrates [67, 96]. Comparing various species and different tissues, they found that there is a relatively close correlation between the level of catalase activity and the maximal oxidation rate. The overall capacity of rat liver for producing H_2O_2 as measured in a homogenate preparation by saturating all enzymes generating peroxide with substrate is about 10 μmoles per hr per gm wet weight.

Aerobic dehydrogenases also occur in bacteria. Production of H_2O_2 has been detected in several aerobic organisms which contain no catalase, such as pneumococci, *Bacillus acidophilus,* and certain streptococci. H_2O_2 presumably occurs also in other aerobic or facultative anaerobic organisms, but may escape accumulation because of the catalase, which is known to occur in *Escherichia coli, Bacillus subtilis, Staphylococcus aureus, Pseudomonas aeruginosa,* and others.

Erythrocyte Catalase

Protective Action

Red blood cell catalase is one of the enzyme systems capable of protecting hemoglobin and other cell components against oxidizing agents, such as reagent H_2O_2, ascorbate, peroxide-producing drugs, or radicals generated by x-rays [97, 98]. The relative contribution of catalase to protection of the red cell is still uncertain. Cohen and associates [99–101] have studied the competition between erythrocyte catalase and glutathione peroxidase for the common substrate, H_2O_2. Both normal erythrocytes and catalase-deficient erythrocytes (duck cells and azide-treated human cells) were protected against the toxic effects of low H_2O_2 concentrations by sustained glutathione peroxidase activity. At an extracellular H_2O_2 concentration of $10^{-7}M$ oxidation of glutathione accounted for the destruction of a major fraction of H_2O_2 added to these cells. In all types of erythrocytes oxidation of hemoglobin by H_2O_2 occurred only after intracellular glutathione was oxidized. They concluded that under physiologic conditions catalase plays no role in this respect [99–101]. Others consider it to be the main protecting enzyme [97]. Nicholls has studied the function of catalase in the intact red cell. His data led him to the conclusion that the interior of the red cell is shielded against exogenous peroxide by a permeability barrier, presumably the red cell membrane. In the intact red cell, catalase is fully active and is capable of destroying 99.0 to 99.9 percent of H_2O_2 entering the cell [62].

Competition for H_2O_2

It is reasonable to assume that all mechanisms operating in the red cell compete for the removal of H_2O_2 or other oxidizing species, such as OH-radicals [98]. The extent of the contribution of catalase and glutathione peroxidase to the removal probably depends on the rate of formation of peroxide and the experimental conditions (Fig. 73-1). The rate of generation of H_2O_2 in the erythrocyte is presumably low. It is assumed that three processes contribute to it: (1) the activity of yellow enzymes, (2) oxidation of thiol compounds (G—SH), and (3) autoxidation of hemoglobin [81]. Under physiologic conditions the ability of the red cells to protect hemoglobin from oxidation depends largely on the presence or absence of glucose. Glutathione peroxidase is of major importance in this scheme. If additional sources of peroxide formation are present, such as drugs or ionizing radiation, catalase concentration in the red cell becomes important. Under these conditions methemoglobin formation clearly depends on catalase concentration: the higher the catalase activity, the more resistant the cell [97, 98, 102].

There are three different ways by which the role of catalase in the red cell can be studied:

1 In normal human erythrocytes catalase can be blocked by inhibitors such as azide or hydroxylamine. Cells treated in this way react as if they contained almost no catalase.
2 Red cell catalase activity from different species varies within a wide range. The comparison between normal human red cells and those of the duck is particularly striking, with the former having about 500 times more activity than

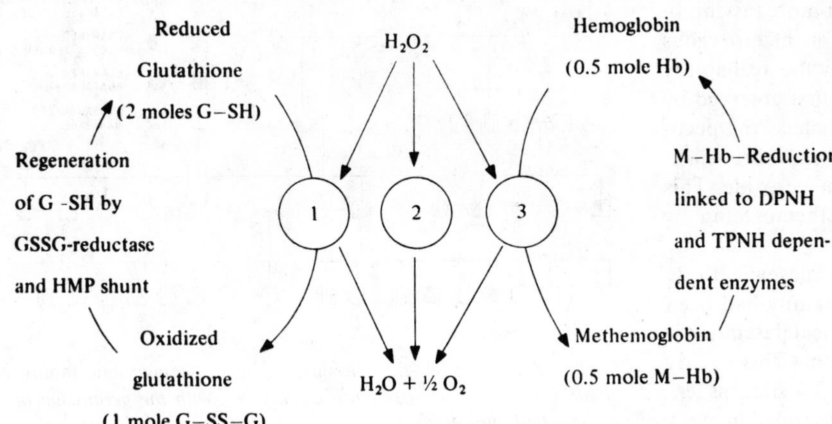

Figure 73-1. Competition for H_2O_2 in the erythrocyte: (1) glutathione peroxidase; (2) catalase; (3) nonenzymic oxidation. Tentative sequence of priority, $1 \rightarrow 2 \rightarrow 3$ [65].

the latter. Cells with differing activity may throw light on the role of catalase.

3 Individuals with practically no catalase activity in blood, and presumably also in tissues, represent a most suitable tool for the study of the physiologic function of catalase.

CLINICAL OBSERVATIONS

Acatalasemia in Japan

Discovery

The discovery of acatalasemia was a model of clinical investigation [1]. In 1946, Takahara, professor of otorhinolaryngology at Okayama Medical School operated upon an 11-year-old girl with a foul, friable, granulating tumor in the right nasal cavity and maxillary sinus. Following radical excision of the tumor, hydrogen peroxide was applied to the operative site. To his surprise the maxillary cavity and surface blood immediately turned brownish-black, and the usual bubbles did not appear. Takahara supposed silver nitrate had been applied by mistake. He promptly washed the wound with saline solution and applied hydrogen peroxide from a new bottle, only to observe a repetition of the color changes. Takahara then speculated that blood and tissues of the patient might be deficient in the enzyme catalase, which normally degrades hydrogen peroxide. Investigation revealed absence of catalase activity in the patient's erythrocytes and oral mucosa. Three of five sibs also lacked catalase activity in the blood. The parents were cousins.

Soon more instances of "Takahara's disease" were detected in Japan. In 1952, when nine cases in three families were known, Dr. Takahara modestly wrote that "the condition is probably inherited" [5]. Further investigation was undertaken in cooperation with several biochemists. One of them, Kaziro of Tokyo, found that lack of catalase was not limited to blood and oral mucosa, but also occurred in tissues such as liver, bone marrow, and muscle [19]. The majority of cases have been discovered at the time of operative treatment or during other prophylactic measures such as extraction of teeth or tonsillectomy. The search for more (asymptomatic) patients with acatalasemia and for heterozygous carriers (hypocatalasemia) was facilitated by the availability of rapid and simple screening methods. As first observed by Takahara the blood of homozygous patients has "the peculiar and striking property to change its color into brownish-black instantly upon contact with hydrogen peroxide. This blackening is due to the formation of methemoglobin by H_2O_2 in the absence of catalase" [1].

By the fall of 1967, 77 instances of acatalasemia in 39 Japanese families and 3 in a pure Korean family had been detected in Japan. [103, 104]. Most of the acatalasemic patients are children of consanguine marriages. This clearly favors homozygosity for a rare allele. In 17 sibships examined, consanguinity of some degree was recorded in every instance but one. Of the 17 marriages, 10 involved first cousins, and 2 involved not only first cousins but additional degrees of relationship [105]. A typical example is given in Fig. 73-2.

Gene Frequency and Geographic Distribution

In order to estimate the frequency of the gene(s) responsible for acatalasemia, a considerable number of screenings for homozygous and heterozygous cases have been performed in various regions of the Far East [107]. For this purpose Hamilton et al. [108] devised a method which identifies all samples exerting an activity below a preset level (e.g., more than three standard deviations below the mean catalase activity of a control population). As will be shown later, most hypocatalasemic individuals in Japan have catalase in their blood, the amount corresponding to about half that in the blood of a normal person. Takahara [103] in collaboration with the Atomic Bomb Casualty Commission [108] has investigated the frequency of hypocatalasemia in approximately 83,000 Asian subjects including Japanese and Koreans residing in Japan, residents of the Ryukyu Islands, and Chinese living in Taiwan. The distribution and frequency of the heterozygous carrier state in the population of these countries is summarized in Table 73-1. The frequency is highest among Koreans, followed by the Chinese of northern China, central China, southern China, and those Chinese in Taiwan residing there for many generations. The lowest rate is found in Okinawa, where only 1 hypocatalasemic individual was detected among 13,380 persons examined. Even within the Japanese population there is considerable variation. The gene frequency in the Japanese is assumed to be approximately 0.0025. With a population of almost 100 million, approximately 1,800 cases of acatalasemia and about 500,000 persons with hypocatalasemia would be anticipated [105]. Hamilton et al. [108] found that the frequence of hypocatalasemia was 0.0009 in Japanese residing in Hiroshima and 0.0003 (1 out of 2,968) in Japanese

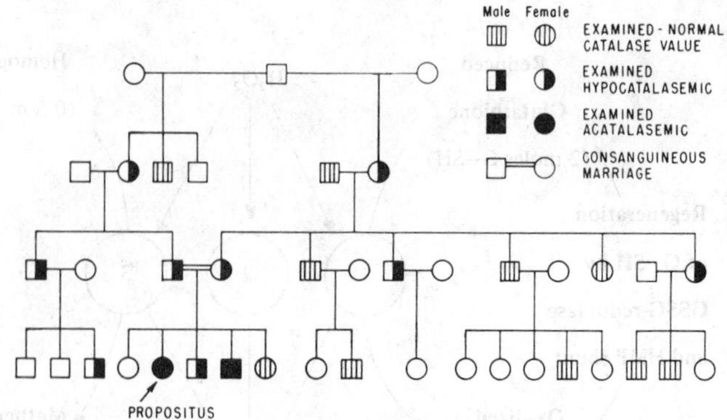

Figure 73-2. Genealogic relationships in an acatalasemic family. (*Redrawn from E. T. Nishimura et al.* [106], *with the permission of authors and publisher.*)

Table 73-1. FREQUENCY OF HYPOCATALASEMIA; RESULTS OF SCREENINGS AMONG FAR EASTERN POPULATIONS [103]

Race	Number of examinations	Number of hypocatalasemia cases	Frequency, %
Japanese	46,878	116	0.25
Ryukyuans			
in Miyako	10,083	1	0.01 } 0.007
in Okinawa	3,297	0	0
Koreans	922	11	1.29
Chinese	20,644	66	0.32
Aborigines in Taiwan	1,145	1	0.09
Total	82,969	195	0.235

in Nagasaki, whereas in Nagano a frequency of 0.012 (38 out of 3,296) was observed.

Although some of these differences appear large, calculations based on all the data available concerning consanguinity in the parents of affected individuals gave a range of carrier frequency (±1 s.d.) of 0 to 0.0121 [108]. The data at hand were derived from a study of 17 sibships. It was estimated that at least 100 additional sibships in which acatalasemia was segregating would be necessary to refine the gene frequency estimates to the point where comparisons between observation and expectation would become meaningful. This uneven distribution of the acatalasemia gene among the population of a single nation makes comparisons very difficult and favors the concept of pockets in which certain rare recessive genes are represented in unusually high frequencies [109].

It has been suggested that Japan may have received the gene from Korea a long time ago and that, in view of its widespread distribution throughout Japan, the gene must be of considerable antiquity [107, 108]. Speculations based on the observation that there is a frequency gradient on the mainland from the northern to the southern regions and to the islands of the Far East must be considered with caution, even if they seem to fit the concept of the migration of Mongolian races.

Takahara's Disease

Only about half of the individuals homozygous for acatalasemia have clinical manifestations. These patients are mostly under the age of 10 years, and some are in their infancy. Apparently the characteristic gangrene seldom occurs after puberty [1].

Symptoms

The clinical manifestations usually begin as a small painful ulcer in the crevices around the neck of a tooth or sometimes in the tonsillar lacunas. The disease appears in mild, moderate, and severe forms [104, 105]. In the mild type, ulcers appear in the dental alveoli. In the moderate type, alveolar gangrene and atrophy develop, and recession of alveolar bone exposes the necks of the teeth, causing them to loosen and fall out. Severe cases present widespread destruction. Inflammation develops into a far-advanced gangrene of the maxillas and the soft oral tissues, similar to the so-called Noma. After healing, there is a remarkable recession of the gum, which is characteristic of this disease, or there may be scarring which causes difficulty in opening the mouth.

Pathogenesis

This type of oral ulceration is attributed mainly to the lack of catalase in blood and probably in tissues. Bacteria in the crevices of the tooth or tonsillar lacunas produce hydrogen peroxide during metabolic proliferation. The most common organisms, hemolytic streptococci and pneumococci Type I, are producers of hydrogen peroxide and lack catalase. Since there is no catalase in the tissues to decompose the H_2O_2 produced by these bacteria, the hemoglobin is oxidized by the H_2O_2. This deprives the infected area of oxygen and causes ulceration, necrosis, and decay of the oral mucosa and other tissues [104].

Therapy

Treatment of the oral lesions has been highly successful in controlling the progression of the necrotic changes. Surgical excision of granulating tumors, curettage, drainage and irrigation of septic areas, extraction of teeth, and antibiotic therapy have been employed. Reconstructive surgical procedures and bone grafts may be required. According to Takahara, there is no difference in the healing rate of the wound between acatalasemic and normal individuals. Use of crystalline catalase suspensions has been suggested for the local treatment of ulcerations in acatalasemic patients [110]. Transfusion of normal whole blood should be an effective means for raising the catalase concentration in the mucosa above the critical level.

The Erratic Occurrence of Symptoms

It is not known why symptoms do not occur in all cases. They preferentially affect children only of certain acatalasemic families. By comparing catalase activity of fibroblast cultures grown from skin biopsy specimens of Swiss and Japanese patients, Krooth [111] has shown that there is a significant difference in the level of residual catalase activity. The former contained about one-twentieth the activity of fibroblasts of normal subjects, whereas in the Japanese no activity could be detected at all. These findings favor the assumption that at a low level of residual catalase activity the actual enzyme concentration may become critical: in certain cases it seems to be above, and in others below, this limit. In fact, Ogata et al. [112] have reported that the level of residual catalase activity is lower in patients affected with Takahara's disease than in asymptomatic subjects. It is also possible that the nutritional state or the immunologic state of the affected individuals or the composition of their oral flora may play a determining role. The observation that in Japan oral gangrene is only rarely seen today may be considered as evidence for the participation of environmental factors.

Acatalasemia in European Countries

In western countries the first patients homozygous for acatalasemia were detected during screening of essentially all male Swiss persons reaching the age of 19 in 1961 and in 1965. Out of 73,661 individuals tested in collaboration with the Swiss Red Cross Transfusion Service, 3 were acatalasemic [8, 113]. Thus the frequency of homozygotes is about 0.04 per 1,000. If it is assumed that all mutations are due to a change at the same locus and that this study is a valid representation, an average gene frequency of 0.012 can be calculated. Even if a large error may attend this estimate, it is an indication that acatalasemia is probably about as frequent in Europe as in Japan.

Examination of all members of the families of propositi has led to the detection of eight more cases [9, 114]. Thus a total of 11 (6 females and 5 males) individuals homozygous for acatalasemia and a considerable number of subjects with partially reduced blood catalase activity, presumably heterozygotes, have been detected. None of these has, or apparently ever had, severe gangrenous oral infections. Up to 1969 all the acatalesemic individuals detected in Switzerland are in good health, with good dental status.

Considerable screening has been done in East Germany, but apparently without success. A typical patient has been observed in Leipzig [13]. The case history, published in 1968, was of a male brought to the hospital 3 weeks after birth because of multiple infections of the skin, of the face and neck, and of the oral mucosa. From the beginning of the first dentition there was continuous inflammation of the gums and loosening of the teeth. Following a minor accident, when the child fell and hit his face, he lost eight teeth within a few weeks. The laboratory data are all normal except for a slightly elevated antistreptolysin titer (100 ASE per ml). Although length and weight correspond to age, bone development as shown by x-ray examination is retarded by at least 2 years. Bacteriologic examinations of the oral cavity were positive for hemolytic streptococci throughout the medical examination period. No exact information about the therapy and the sibship of this patient has been obtained.

Diagnosis in this instance has been made after a considerable lag of time. Takahara [115] made a "plea to the public" that every patient with oral ulcerations or intermittent inflammation of the oral mucosa should be considered suspicious for acatalasemia.

Acatalasemia in Israel

In 1963 Szeinberg and associates [10–12] reported a dual hereditary red cell defect with a deficiency both of glucose-6-phosphate dehydrogenase and of catalase. The propositus, an Iranian Jew, developed a severe hemolytic anemia with sulfhemoglobinemia following contact with a fungicide, zinc ethylene bisdithiocarbamate. Examination of red blood cells demonstrated a fully expressed deficiency of glucose-6-phosphate dehydrogenase combined with a severe deficiency of catalase. The activity of the latter was approximately 8 percent of the mean normal activity. Investigation of members of three generations of the family suggested that the two enzymatic defects were transmitted independently [12]. The heterozygous state was characterized by intermediate hypocatalasemia (50 to 65 percent of mean normal catalase activity). Similarly intermediate hypocatalasemia was detected in all the children of the propositus as well as in several other members of the family, both in those normal for glucose-6-phosphate dehydrogenase and those with glucose-6-phosphate dehydrogenase deficiency [116]. No difference in the degree of "intermediate hypocatalasemia" was observed between these two groups of subjects heterozygous for catalase deficiency. There was no suggestion of interaction between these mutants. Thus, in this family there is a unique, purely accidental combination of two enzymatic defects.

CLINICAL INVESTIGATIONS

Blood Catalase

For the determination of catalase in blood several rapid and accurate techniques are available [65]. In earlier studies titrimetric or spectrophotometric methods were principally used. In future screenings the automated procedure, as devised by Leighton et al. [76] and Lamy et al. [117] will probably be the method of choice.

Normal Level

In the standard assay for blood catalase activity as employed in the Japanese studies [105], whole blood is diluted approximately 1,000-fold to a final hemoglobin concentration of 0.14 gm per liter. Aliquots are then added immediately to a buffered solution of H_2O_2. Residual peroxide is determined by permanganate titration. At successive 15-sec intervals incubation is stopped by addition of H_2SO_4. Under these conditions the disappearance of peroxide follows first-order kinetics, and the velocity constant K_{cat} is used as a measure of catalase activity. The mean and standard deviation for one series of observations on 259 normal individuals was 5.38 ± 0.73 units [105], with a range of 3.90 to 7.47 units. A slightly lower mean value is obtained if blood is allowed to stand 1 day or more before analysis. This observation may become important whenever specimens obtained in field studies must be sent to a distant laboratory. As shown by Hübl and Bretschneider [118], the mode of predilution of the hemolysate is critical. After final dilution of the hemolysate, catalase is unstable. Furthermore, gross alterations in hemoglobin content have to be taken into account, since in normal individuals there is a linear relationship between catalase activity and hemoglobin concentration [105, 119, 120].

Hypocatalasemia

Using the technique described above, catalase assays were done on the blood of 175 members of 13 families by Nishimura and associates [106]. The distribution of catalase activity values was trimodal (Fig. 73-3), corresponding to the three phenotypes termed *acatalasemic, hypocatalasemic,* and *normal.* The sex distribution was equal among all phenotypes. In this study all persons who should have been genetic carriers were hypocatalasemic. As shown in Fig. 73-3 there was no overlap between the three groups. Thus, a clear distinction emerges between (1) normocatalasemic individuals, or nonaffected homozygotes; (2) hypocatalasemic subjects, or presumed heterozygous carriers; and (3) acatalasemic subjects, or affected homozygotes [105, 106]. In 37 hypocatalasemic individuals the mean value was 2.51 ± 0.27, with a range of 1.94 to 2.98 units, corresponding to 36 to 55 percent of the normal mean [105].

On the basis of the blood-catalase data of five sibships containing 13 cases of acatalasemia, Takahara et al. [2] postulated that acatalasemia is transmitted by "incompletely recessive monogenetic inheritance." Subsequent family studies have amply confirmed this "recessive" inheritance pattern in all known pedigrees. In a review of 17 segregating sibships

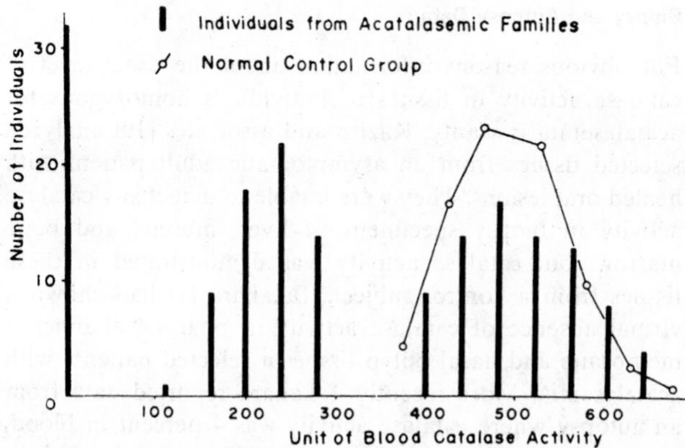

Figure 73-3. Distribution of catalase values for 175 members of 13 acatalasemic families and comparison with a percentage distribution curve of enzyme activity of 273 normal subjects. The column on the left represents acatalasemic subjects, the five columns in the center hypocatalasemic subjects, and those on the right, normal individuals in these families. (*By permission of S. Takahara and the publisher* [104].)

reported up to 1960, the ratio of acatalasemic to normal members was 36 : 57, with males and females affected in equal numbers [4, 5, 105]. If a correction for the 17 probands is made, on the assumption of ascertainment through a single affected individual for each segregating sibship, the numbers of affected and normal become 19 and 57 [105]. These correspond perfectly to the expectation of a 25 percent incidence of homozygosity for a recessive trait. A detailed consideration of pedigrees brought out a number of genetically significant facts: (1) hypocatalasemic values were found in every instance in which it was possible to study one or both parents of an acatalasemic individual; (2) the children of one acatalasemic and one normal parent were hypocatalasemic; (3) sibs of parents of affected subjects were either normal or hypocatalasemic; (4) the sex distribution among hypocatalasemic patients was 17 males and 13 females. All these findings indicate that hypocatalasemia is the heterozygous carrier state for the gene which, when homozygous, is responsible for acatalasemia.

Families Exerting an Atypical Mode of Inheritance

Further studies have revealed that there are at least two more forms of acatalasemia in Japan [105, 109]. First, in a large kindred (designated OH) of 116 members, in which two sibships are segregating for acatalasemia, carrier values overlap with normal. Here, in contrast to the classical nonoverlapping trimodal distribution, there is a broad continuum (3 homozygotes aside), ranging from 2.98 to 6.73, with a distinct frequency maximum at 5.40 to 5.59. This peak corresponds fairly well to the previously established mean of 5.38. The lowest K_{cat} values observed in this kindred (except the 3 acatalasemic patients) are at the upper limit of values reported previously for "regular" hypocatalasemic patients. Hamilton and associates [108, 109] are of the opinion that these findings are best explained by a previously undescribed gene, which may or may not be allelic to the mutant responsible for the "regular" type of acatalasemia. An investigation covering some 50 members of the Swiss acatalasemic sibships has led to the same result [9, 121]. Here again the normal range and that of the presumed heterozygotes merge considerably. As in the Family OH, all cases (but one) of the latter group show an activity level of 60 to 80 percent of normal.

Takahara et al. [105] have reported still another atypical instance (Family 13 MI), and suggested that there may be a third genetic type of acatalasemia among Japanese. A single male acatalasemic patient was found whose three children had catalase values well within the normal range (mean 4.95 K_{cat} units). This would be consistent with completely recessive inheritance.

Residual Catalase in Homozygotes

In his early papers Takahara [1] stated that acatalasemic blood has one-four-hundred-and-fiftieth to one-nine-hundredth of normal activity, but there was considerable scattering at these low levels. The values in blood vary between 0 and 3.2 percent. For the homozygous acatalasemic patients in Switzerland the range is 0.1 to 1.3 percent of normal. Feinstein's perborate method [122] has proved to be sensitive and particularly useful for the determination of residual enzyme activity. For an Iranian-born Jew considered to be a homozygote of another type of acatalasemia, Szeinberg et al. [10] reported a catalase activity level in blood of 8 percent. Thus, in the acatalasemic condition there is a situation similar to which developed in galactosemia after the discovery of the Duarte variant (cf. Chap. 8).

Cellular Distribution of Catalase in Blood

Heterozygotes

Heterozygous individuals in families with acatalasemia have intermediate catalase activity in red cells and other tissues which may be either due to the presence of two cell populations, one being virtually free of catalase, or to a single cell population of intermediate enzyme activity. In order to decide between these possibilities, two methods applicable to blood smears have been used:

1 A chemical procedure is based on the fact that the sensitivity of the erythrocyte towards H_2O_2 depends largely on its catalase content and that oxyhemoglobin, but not cyanmethemoglobin, is active as a peroxidase. This technique, devised by Aebi et al. [123, 124] is an extension of the differential staining method of Kleihauer and Betke [125].

2 The fluorescent antibody technique, as used by Hosoi et al. [126, 127], requires antihuman red cell catalase tagged with a fluorescent label as a reagent.

The former test is simpler, but shows a threshold phenomenon. Both methods have led to the same results. Heterozygotes of various Swiss and Japanese families have been analyzed, but no mosaicism or other evidence for two cell populations has been obtained. Additional evidence for even distribution of catalase in blood of heterozygotes was obtained by chemical estimation of methemoglobin formation in vitro at various rates of H_2O_2 generation [98].

Homozygotes

A pseudomosaicism may be seen in the blood of Swiss individuals homozygous for acatalasemia. Out of 100 to 150 red cells, 1 behaves chemically as if it contained approximately the same amount of catalase as a normal red cell [124]. Using the immunologic procedure, it becomes evident that the catalase-positive cells do not represent a uniform entity but seem to be composed of various stages of intermediate fluorescence intensity [127]. In whole blood the number of fluorescent (that is, catalase-positive) cells varies between 1 and 2 percent, a figure which is slightly higher than that obtained by using the Betke staining technique (0.5 to 1.0 percent). Fractionation experiments have revealed that the number of catalase-positive cells, as visualized by fluorescent anticatalase, steadily decreases from the top to the bottom fraction (Fig. 73-4). There is a direct proportionality between the fluorescent cell count and the number of reticulocytes. Catalase activity in reticulocytes and mature erythrocytes, as calculated by extrapolation, may differ by a ratio of up to to 300 to 1 [124]. When normal blood is analyzed in the same manner, the fractions have a similar distribution pattern with respect to the reticulocytes, but there is no significant difference in catalase activity. Study of homozygous acatalasemic subjects in a number of Japanese families [129] and of the Israeli case [116] have led to a different result. Here, a fractionation of the red cells according to density (and age) revealed no difference in catalase activity. The drastic decrease in catalase activity during the life-span of acatalasemic red cells of certain homozygotes can be explained in various ways. It is most probably due to the presence of an enzyme variant of reduced stability. Additional evidence for this assumption was obtained from incubation experiments with fractions enriched in reticulocytes [81] and from heat stability tests performed with the purified enzyme [113]. If there are no signs of an unequal distribution, the enzyme deficiency may be due to the synthesis of an enzyme variant of reduced specific activity. The data suggest that the Swiss cases represent the former and the Japanese—at least those investigated—as well as the Israeli, the latter type.

Catalase Activity in Tissues

Biopsy and Autopsy Data

For obvious reasons information about the exact level of catalase activity in tissues of individuals homozygous for acatalasemia is scanty. Kaziro and associates [19] analyzed selected tissues from an asymptomatic adult patient with healed oral lesions. They were unable to detect any catalase activity in biopsy specimens of liver, muscle, and bone marrow, but catalase activity was demonstrated in these tissues from a control subject. Takahara [1] had shown a virtual absence of catalase activity in pharyngeal mucous membrane and nasal polyp tissue in selected patients with acatalasemia. More recently Takahara reported data from an autopsy where catalase activity was 4 percent in blood, 40 percent in liver and spleen, and 50 percent in kidney as compared to the average found in normal man [104]. These figures are definitely higher than those reported earlier. On the other hand Aebi and associates [114] detected residual catalase activity in the palatine tonsils, liver, placenta, and skin biopsies from the patient. The level was relatively low in tissues with a high normal catalase activity

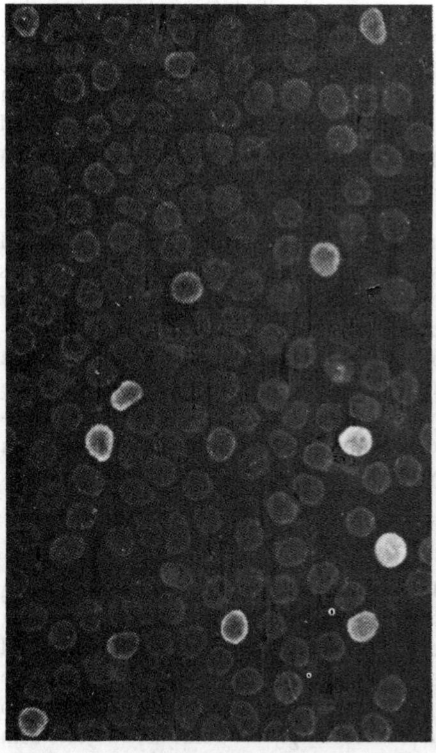

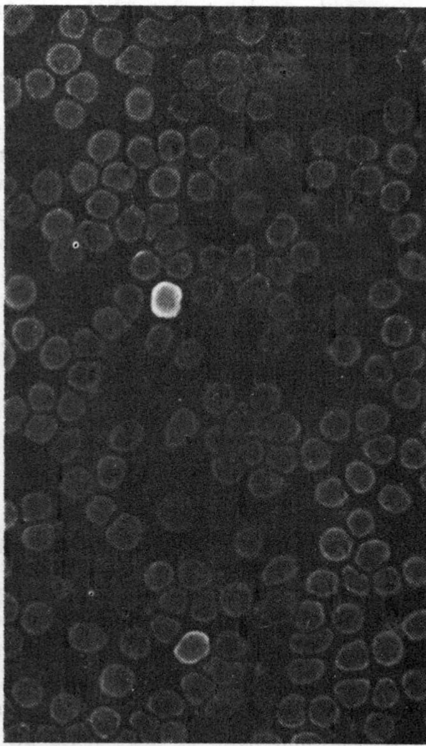

Figure 73-4. Blood smears treated with fluorescent anti-human erythrocyte catalase. Blood of a subject homozygous for Type III acatalasemia. Analysis of blood fractions obtained by centrifugation in 20 percent albumin solution according to Sass et al. [128]. (*Left*) Top fraction containing fluorescent (=catalase-positive) cells in high proportion (6.5 percent), the intensity varying considerably. (*Right*) Bottom fraction, fluorescent cells are seen only exceptionally (0.3 percent) (*By permission of authors and Experientia* [127].)

(e.g., liver <1 percent) and vice versa (e.g., fibroblasts cultivated in vitro from skin biopsy ~ 15 percent). Thus there are patients justifying the term *acatalasemia* and others to whom the more general term *acatalasia* applies.

Tissue Culture Studies

Experiments in several laboratories have shown that catalase-deficient cells retain their enzymatic abnormalities in culture [114, 130–132]. This was first demonstrated by Krooth et al. [130], who developed cell lines from skin biopsies on an acatalasemic patient, one with hypocatalasemia, and eight control subjects. They demonstrated that the three presumed genotypes retained the characteristic levels of catalase activity for up to a year in culture. Another enzyme, lactate dehydrogenase, was normal in all cell lines. Mixtures of sonicates of acatalasemic cells and normal cells, in varying proportions, showed the predicted levels of catalase activity. These experiments exclude the presence of a potent catalase inhibitor and also probably exclude the lack of a required catalase activator in the acatalasemic tissue. Further experiments have disclosed that fibroblasts do not differ significantly in respect to their sensitivity toward x-irradiation [114, 132].

The catalase activity of fibroblast cultures from Japanese was from 2 to 4 percent [132], and those from the Swiss patients were approximately 15 percent of the activity found in a normal strain. This difference was confirmed by Krooth [111], who investigated strains from both types under identical condition. Whereas the cells of the Japanese strain failed to develop measurable catalase throughout the growth of the culture, the Swiss-type cells, like normal cells, developed progressively higher specific catalase activity, but throughout growth they had much lower specific activities than normal cells. Sadamoto [132] found that the growth rates of normal and acatalasemic cell lines were similar in their propagating period (tenth–thirtieth generation). Subsequently they both proliferated again up to about the sixtieth generation and then gradually slowed. Acatalasemic cells were considerably more sensitive towards reagent H_2O_2 ($10^{-4}M$) than normal cells; their growth rate was reduced to less than a third as compared to that of normal cells equally treated with hydrogen peroxide. The activity of respiratory enzymes, such as succinic dehydrogenase or cytochrome oxidase was diminished by $10^{-4}M$ H_2O_2 to a greater extent in acatalasemic fibroblasts (−70 percent, −40 percent) than in normal fibroblasts (−20 percent, 0 percent). Full protection was obtained in either case by adding a small amount of pure catalase to the medium. This may be taken as an indication that the resistance of acatalasemic cells in vitro (and presumably also in the mucosa and connective tissue) to extrinsic peroxide is low. From these observations the author concludes that when acatalasemic cells are exposed to extrinsic hydrogen peroxide, as in the case of bacterial proliferation, the traces of residual catalase are not sufficient to accomplish a rapid decomposition of the peroxide. As a consequence of enzyme inactivation, cell death and tissue necrosis may occur. It must be kept in mind that a fibroblast culture is a system which is virtually free of hemoglobin and other blood components. In this context it is interesting to note, that Doi [133] was able to produce oral gangrene in ducks (which are physiologically acatalasemic) by submucous injection of hydrogen peroxide.

Fibroblasts from skin biopsy specimens have been used for a morphologic study of the chromosomes. A comparison of fibroblasts from hypocatalasemic and acatalasemic individuals as well as of their leukocytes with those of normal subjects disclosed no alterations [134, 135].

Metabolic Data Other Than on Catalase

Analysis of Enzymes in Blood

In Swiss cases enzyme activities in serum, white cells, and red cells have been measured [9]. Serum of individuals with acatalasemia are normal for amylase, cholinesterase, transaminase, and phosphatase activity as well as for ceruloplasmin. The same is true for glucose utilization, lactate production, and porphobilinogen synthesis in white cells. Glucose-6-phosphate dehydrogenase, glutamate dehydrogenase, transaminases, and peroxidase activities are slightly decreased. A considerable number of enzymes and metabolic activities have been measured in red cells of normal, hypocatalasemic, and acatalasemic members of families with acatalasemia. The data fall within the normal range, with the exception of glutathione reductase and glutathione peroxidase activities in erythrocytes. These are slightly elevated above the normal range in homozygotes, and to a smaller extent, in the other members of the Swiss acatalasemic families [81]. In this connection the finding of Jacob et al. [136] is of particular interest. Using glucose-1-^{14}C, they have found that human acatalasemic red cells, when incubated in vitro, produce $^{14}CO_2$ about three times faster than normal cells. If ascorbate (5 mmolar) is added as a hydrogen peroxide generator, glucose metabolism through the hexose monophosphate shunt is increased about twelve fold. In spite of this drastic enhancement of shunt activity, formation of lactate by these cells is unaltered. Since NADPH regeneration is required for several protective mechanisms in the red cell, this increase may be regarded as evidence for a compensatory stimulation of the hexose monophosphate shunt. If this assumption is correct, it would mean that lack of catalase in erythrocytes can be sufficiently compensated by an increased activity of the glutathione-regenerating mechanism.

Hemoglobin and Its Metabolites

Hemoglobin concentration is normal in patients with acatalasemia, except in patients with oral gangrene, in whom mild anemia occurs [1]. Although acatalasemic red cells are sensitive to oxidizing agents, no significant quantities of methemoglobin could be detected in circulating erythrocytes. None was detectable in fresh ACD blood samples. After storage at 4°C for 9 days the methemoglobin content varied between 0.2 and 1.1 percent. The rate of Heinz body formation tested with acetylphenylhydrazine was the same in blood from patients with acatalasemia as in normal blood samples. Methemoglobin reductase activity is normal at least in type III acatalasemia red cells. In one family (V) there are several subjects with a significant increase in hemoglobin F. This elevated Hb F content does not coincide with homozygosity for the enzyme deficiency [9].

The amounts of coproporphyrin and bilirubin in the urine are said to be up to five times as high as normal in the usual Japanese type of acatalasemia [137]. So far, no additional evidence for a derangement of homeostatic regulation of either heme synthesis or degradation has been obtained.

Formate Metabolism

Among the hydrogen donors specific for demonstrating peroxidatic catalase activity ethanol and methanol cannot be used, ethanol because of alternative pathways, and methanol because of toxicity. Formate has the advantage not only of being nontoxic, but also of being converted to CO_2 in a single step. Accordingly the ability of subjects with acatalasemia to perform coupled oxidation of formate by peroxidatic catalase activity was investigated. Loading tests with sodium formate were carried out in normal subjects and patients with acatalasemia. After a single oral dose of 5 gm only 2.4 to 4.4 percent of the formate was excreted in the urine of both groups. Similar loading tests in germ-free rats, performed with ^{14}C-formate disclosed a significant difference in comparison with controls. The data led Baggiolini et al. [138] to conclude that the intestinal flora may contribute significantly to the formate-oxidizing capacity of the intact rat (up to 25 percent of the total capacity). Experiments of this type have not been made in man, but experiments with intact red cells and hemolysates have been done. Whereas normal red cells use H_2O_2 generated by thiol oxidation for coupled oxidation of ^{14}C-formate, acatalasemic cells are almost completely unable to perform this peroxidatic reaction [114]. Clearly, it would be highly desirable to carry out incubation experiments with tissue specimens of individuals with acatalasemia.

CHEMICAL NATURE OF RESIDUAL CATALASE

Immunologic Studies

A particular effort has been made by the Japanese and the Swiss groups to elucidate the chemical nature of residual catalase activity in blood of subjects homozygous for acatalasemia [54, 139–143]. Initially Takahara et al. [139] attempted to determine by immunologic techniques whether catalase protein exists in the blood of subjects with acatalasemia. Their experiments with partially purified blood catalase (Herbert-Pinsent method stage 2 or 3) led them to state that "the catalase molecule is either absent or synthesized only in negligible amounts or altered to such an extent that it is no longer immunologically reactive." This conclusion was based on the observation that purified fractions from acatalasemic blood do not give a precipitin ring test with rabbit antiserum against a highly purified preparation (Kat.f. 60,000) of normal human erythrocyte catalase. In a later study the proportions of the quantities of immunologically detectable catalase protein in normal, hypocatalasemic, and acatalasemic hemolysates were 1.0:0.5:0.07. Nearly the same figures (1.0:0.5:0) were obtained by measuring catalase activity. Other investigators also have searched for catalase-like protein by immunologic techniques [144–147] but have failed, presumably because the material was not purified enough or a rough isolation procedure was used.

Catalase-active material from acatalasemic subjects was obtained by gel filtration with Sephadex (G-100) in sufficient quantity to compare its properties with those of the enzyme from normal human red cells. Preparations from Swiss patients with acatalasemia precipitated with anticatalase in Ouchterlony double diffusion plates [114, 143]. Semiquantitative evaluation of the results obtained with the Ouchterlony method indicated that the concentration of antigenic protein differed from normal by a factor of 100 to 200. This is of the same order of magnitude as the difference in catalase activity in acatalasemic and normal red cells and indicates that the residual activity in the Swiss-type acatalasemic hemolysates is ascribable to a protein similar to, or identical with, the enzyme of normal individuals.

The purified protein obtained from hemolysate of Japanese-type acatalasemic cells reacts with anticatalase, but it is not identical with purified catalase from normal individuals, nor does it show any enzyme activity. This material, identical with the "minor inactive component" also found in normal blood, has a molecular weight of 40,000 to 60,000 (i.e., about one-sixth of the fully constituted active catalase) and has no Soret absorption. Shibata et al. [148] consider it to be a subunit or precursor of catalase, or both. Nishimura et al. [149] have confirmed and extended this study, inasmuch as C-reactive protein, which is present in normal and acatalasemic hemolysates, is antigenically similar to erythrocyte catalase. This is in agreement with the finding of Hokama et al. [150] that an antiserum preparation reacting specifically against C-reactive protein (CRPA) can absorb the catalatic activity of purified erythrocyte catalase up to 54 percent. There is further evidence for a metabolic interrelationship between C-reactive protein and liver catalase. After a single injection of 3-amino-1,2,4-triazole in rabbits there is rapid depletion of hepatic catalase accompanied by a rise in C-reactive protein in the serum. Conversely, the restoration of catalatic activity is accompanied by a disappearance of C-reactive protein from the serum. There is also a striking chemical similarity between C-reactive protein and human hepatic catalase with respect to their tryptic peptide maps [151].

Physicochemical Approach

Attempts to demonstrate residual catalase spectrophotometrically [141] or electrophoretically [140] in preparations stage 2 and 3 of the Herbert-Pinsent procedure have failed, but active catalase material has been obtained in appreciable quantity from "acatalasemic" blood by applying the technique of gel filtration [54, 148, 152]. Its properties were compared with those of the enzyme from normal human red cells and were identical in respect to (1) mobility on a Sephadex G-100 (or G-200) column; (2) electrophoretic mobility on starch gel; and (3) sensitivity toward azide ($I_{50} \sim 10^{-6}M$). This procedure was used to demonstrate residual catalase in blood from Japanese and Swiss patients with acatalasemia. Residual (or "minimal") catalase activity can be separated into two peaks (Fig. 73-5) [104, 112]. The first contains a catalase-like component, which is heat labile and can be inhibited by $10^{-4}M$ Na-azide; the activity in the second peak is thermostable and is probably due to a methemoglobin-H_2O_2 complex derived from hemoglobin in the presence of hydrogen peroxide. The activity in the first peak has a higher degree of variation than that in the second peak. The first peak contains a catalase-like protein and represents about 25 to 50 percent of the total catalatic activity in acatalasemic blood. Preparations obtained from various Japanese patients show no difference between normal and acatalasemic blood with respect to (1) heat stability, (2) sensitivity towards azide and aminotriazole, and (3) reactivity against purified anti-human-blood-catalase [104].

Chromatographic methods have been devised for a separation of residual catalase from hemoglobin and other red cell constituents on a larger scale. Two fractions of red cell catalase are obtained by column chromatography on a calcium phosphate-DEAE-cellulose complex gel [153, 154]. Analysis by electrophoresis on a mixture of starch-agar-polyacrylamide gel has shown that both purified fractions of normal and acatalasemic red cell catalase have identical properties, but the two fractions from blood of heterozygotes are heterogenous, one fraction migrating as normal catalase, the other as catalase from a patient homozygous for acatalasemia. Thus, according to current terminology of isoenzymes, the formula of catalase in blood of normal, hypocatalasemic, and acatalasemic human beings may be expressed as I-I, I-II, and II-II respectively. Heat stability tests performed at 55°C [113] suggest that the material obtained from Swiss patients (in contrast to that from the Japanese) is considerably more labile at elevated temperature than is the normal enzyme.

Heterogeneity of erythrocyte catalase has also been inves-

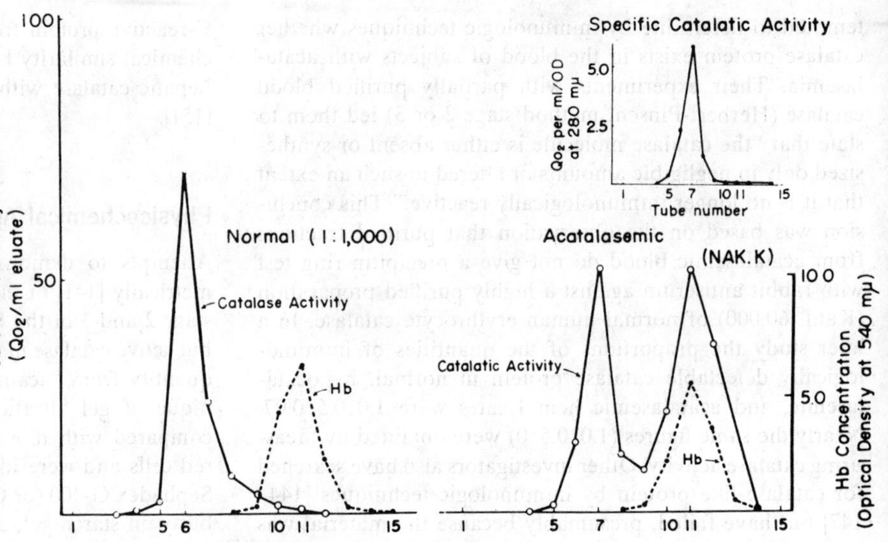

Figure 73-5. Separation of "minimal catalatic substance" in an acatalasemic hemolysate by Sephadex G-100 gel filtration according to Aebi et al. [54]. (*Right*) Blood of a Japanese subject homozygous for Type I acatalasemia. (*Left*) Normal blood, the scale for catalase activity reduced 1:1,000. The dotted lines represent hemoglobin concentration (OD 540 mμ). (*By permission of S. Takahara and publisher* [104].)

tigated by a fractionation technique as described by Thorup et al. [49]. Whole blood as well as reticulocyte-enriched preparations were used. Catalase-active material was separated into three different fractions, A, B, and C, both from normal blood and from blood from patients with hypocatalasemia and acatalasemia [104, 121]. Neither the Japanese nor the Swiss cases showed any gross differences in the elution patterns of red cell catalase. This heterogeneity is attributed to alternative molecular forms (conformers) of normal, as well as of variant erythrocyte catalase [48, 155].

GENETICS

Catalase Variants

There is growing evidence that catalase-active material obtained from subjects with acatalasemia may differ from the normal enzyme in physicochemical properties, although there is enzymatic and antigenic identity. If the acatalasemic condition is really due to a structural gene mutation, it would explain why in certain individuals an unstable enzyme variant or a variant of low specific activity is formed. Allocatalasia, a catalase anomaly observed in 1963 by Baur [17], may be another catalase variant. Six members of a family of Scandinavian-British extraction have a red cell catalase with atypical electrophoretic mobility. There is normal red cell catalase activity, and the patients have no symptoms or physical findings. There are reports from Sweden [14–16] as well as from the United States [18] of individuals who have lowered blood catalase activity. Whether they are heterozygotes for acatalasemia or homozygotes for another trait has not been ascertained. It should be emphasized that loss of enzyme activity permits no conclusions regarding the source of the findings. It may either be because of a mutation within the regulator gene system or an alteration in the primary structure and catalytic activity or stability of the enzyme molecule.

Heterogeneity in Acatalasemia

The present state of knowledge on acatalasemia is typical of the situation in many other inborn errors of metabolism. What once was considered as a single entity has turned out to be a group of anomalies. In the 17 sibships reported in 1960 by Takahara et al. [105] there was one which was anomalous. In this family there was a male with acatalasemia with three children who had normal values of blood catalase activity. Thus, in these obligate heterozygotes the trait was completely recessive.

Another Japanese kindred in which two sibships segregate for acatalasemia has been extensively studied by Hamilton and Neel [109]. Catalase activity values of carriers overlapped with the normal range. The Swiss families described by Aebi and associates [9] resemble the third Japanese variant more than either of the other two. The values are from 60 to 85 percent of the mean normal (with one exception of 15 percent). Swiss acatalasemia may thus be another genetic variant. The Israeli patient, in whom low catalase activity is combined with a deficiency of glucose-6-phosphate dehydrogenase, does not fit any of these categories. This is also true for the family in the State of Washington showing the phenomenon of allocatalasia. Accordingly an extension of the original classification is necessary. The classification as outlined in Table 73-2 is based on a number of clinical and biochemical observations:

I. Level of residual catalase activity in blood and tissues of homozygotes
II. Cellular distribution of residual catalase in blood as shown by a pseudomosaicism

III. Properties of the material responsible for residual (minimal) catalase activity, mainly heat stability and electrophoretic mobility
IV. Level of catalase activity in blood of heterozygotes
V. Clinical symptoms (Takahara's disease)

Types I to V differ in several respects. Type I acatalasemia shows a proportional gene dosage, with heterozygotes having half of the normal activity. This is evidently not true of types II and III because in all heterozygotes catalase activity is higher than 56 percent of normal, or even overlaps with the normal range. In the Israeli, type IV, residual catalase is high in the homozygote (8 percent of normal). This deficiency is accidentally combined with a lack of G6PD. By fractionating the red cell population, it has been shown that the level of residual catalase activity in juvenile and mature red cells is about the same in types I and IV acatalasemia [116, 129]. Contrariwise there is a considerable difference in catalase activity between juvenile and mature red cells in blood of three homozygotes of the Swiss-type acatalasemia [121, 124]. An analogous difference was observed in the heat stability test. Consequently, catalase activity of an unstable variant seems to fade off rapidly during red cell maturation. Takahara's disease has been observed in individuals homozygous for the "regular" Japanese form (type I) only. Although the information on the German case is incomplete, it is reasonable to assume that it is closely related to type I, because it shares most of the features shown by the Japanese patients.

CATALASE DEFICIENCY IN ANIMALS

There are several species of animals in which there is an abnormal level of catalase in blood or tissues. Since the situation is similar to acatalasemia in man, these animals may serve as valuable tools for study of the metabolic implications of this deficiency. Three types of anomalies may be distinguished:

Table 73-2. TENTATIVE CLASSIFICATION OF ACATALASEMIA CASES AND RELATED ANOMALIES REPORTED IN LITERATURE UNTIL 1969

Type (year of detection)	Origin (no. of families)	Number of homozygotes (Hom.) & heterozygotes (Het.)	Relative catalase activity (normal = 100%)	Remarks
I (1946)	Japan (37)	Hom: 73 Het: >100	Hom: 0–3.2% Het: 37–56%	Incomplete autosomal recessive inheritance: oral gangrene (e.g., Takahara's disease) in 50% of homozygotes. Activity: trimodal distribution curve; no overlap. Homogeneous distribution of residual catalase activity in red cell population [1, 6, !3]
(1959)	Korea (1)	Hom: 3 Het: ?		
(1967)	Germany (1)	Hom: 1 Het: ?		
II (1959)	Japan (1) Family 13 MI	Hom: 1 Het: ?	Hom: 3.2% Het: ∼100%	Complete autosomal recessive inheritance (involvement of modifier or suppressor genes?) [105]
IIIa (1962)	Japan (1) kindred 29 OHH	Hom: 3 Het: 17	Hom: 0 (?) Het: >56%	Overlap between heterozygous carrier and normals (dual allelic control?) [109]
IIIb (1961)	Switzerland (3) Families V., B., and G.	Hom: 11 Het: ∼30	Hom: 0.1–1.3% Het: 60–85% (1 case 15%)	Synthesis of two different types of catalase in heterozygotes (normal catalase plus unstable variant), all homozygotes in good state of health; pseudomosaicism in red cells of homozygotes [121]
IV (1963)	Israel (1) (Iranian born)	Hom: 1 Het: 15	Hom: 8% Het: 49–67%	Combination with deficiency of G-6-PD: intolerance to fungicide; homogeneous distribution of residual catalase activity in blood [10, 11, 18]
(1967)	United States (1)	Hom: — Het: 1	Hom: — Het: 50%	
V (1963)	United States (1) (Scandinavian and British extraction) Family B.	Hom: 0 Het: 6	All 100%	Allocatalasia: synthesis of a variant catalase; activity and stability as normal catalase [17]

1. Species which are physiologically acatalasemic (e.g., duck)
2. Species showing a polymorphism in the level of catalase activity (e.g., dog, guinea pig)
3. Species with acatalasemic mutants (e.g., mouse, guinea pig)

Catalase Level in Blood of Various Species

Comparative studies among a considerable number of species have been made [20, 44, 156–160]. Use of different methods and units makes a comparison of results difficult, and also factors of age, sex, nutritional status, and strain have often not been considered. All studies have confirmed the observation of Kaziro et al. [19] that catalase is by far lowest in ducks. Duck blood contains about 500 times less catalase than does human blood (5 versus 2,500 perborate units per ml). Catalase is also relatively low in fowl and some other birds, whereas in monkey, rabbit, and cat it is almost as high as in man. Because it is physiologically acatalasemic, the blood of ducks has often been used for the study of the role of catalase in protecting hemoglobin, structural proteins, and red cell enzymes against oxidizing agents and x-irradiation. Duck erythrocytes are far more radiation-sensitive than those of any other species, if methemoglobin formation is taken as an indicator. Analogous investigations have been made by applying vapors of H_2O_2 *in a two-compartment system or by generating* H_2O_2 enzymatically. Obviously, oxidizable chemicals yielding peroxide such as ascorbate, methylhydrazine, phenylhydrazine, menadione, and several 8-aminoquinoline antimalarials (e.g., primaquine, pamaquine) may also serve this purpose [9, 97–102, 162, 163]. Since the level of residual catalase in duck blood is even lower than in some of the patients with acatalasemia, the effects observed in duck blood may exceed those seen in homozygous persons.

Any comparison between the various species should take account of the fact that not only catalase but also other enzymes may display considerable variation. For example, the red cell of the duck, in addition to its low catalase, has a sixfold higher activity of glutathione peroxidase and a threefold higher reduced glutathione than that of man [34].

Catalase Polymorphisms

A nonunimodal distribution of red cell catalase activity has been observed in dogs, in guinea pigs, and in mice. Allison et al. [164] observed variations in erythrocyte catalase activity in a large group of dogs of various breeds. In some dogs activity values were quite low. Controlled breeding of these animals disclosed a simple mode of recessive inheritance, for which a single pair of alleles was proposed. Feinstein et al. [161] also observed a wide range of variation in a beagle colony. Among 83 animals blood catalase varied between 0 and 43 perborate units per ml. A clear-cut trimodal distribution was not seen. Radev [165] obtained similar results in a study of guinea pigs with normal and low blood catalase values. Animals with low blood values were also found to have low catalase activity in their livers. Whereas it was reduced about 20 times in blood, catalase activity in liver and spleen was reduced to about a fifth of normal. No signs of ill health were noted in either guinea pigs or dogs with low catalase activities. Studies on blood catalase in large populations of guinea pigs of diverse origin have revealed that there is also a wide range of variation with a trimodal but overlapping distribution. A uniform activity level was observed in liver [166].

Polymorphism of catalase activity in blood and tissues has been investigated most thoroughly in mice. Greenstein and Andervont [167] observed that inbred strains of mice may vary with respect to liver catalase activity. The fact that catalase activity in livers of mice of strain C57 BL is approximately half that of other strains was investigated in more detail by Heston et al. [168]. It was shown that this is due to a single major gene with low level of activity dominant to the high activity gene. This gene (C_e) controlling liver catalase has no apparent influence on blood or kidney catalase activity. Further studies disclosed that the differences in liver catalase of the substrains C57 BL/6 and C57 BL/He are due to different rates of degradation of the enzyme, whereas the rates of synthesis are identical in the two strains. This anomaly is probably specific for catalase, because it is not seen in a series of other liver enzymes, notably those localized in the same organelle, such as urate oxidase [169]. Ganschow and Schimke [88] have isolated liver catalase from both strains and have shown that they are identical. Findings with this mutant may be considered as a direct demonstration of genetic control of the amount of a specific protein in a mammalian organism. In discussing the nature of the mutation altering the rate of turnover of liver catalase, the authors offer two alternatives: (1) properties of the protein as a substrate for degradation may be changed, or, (2) the activity of the degradative system may be altered. In another mutant strain a marked difference in specific activity of the purified enzymes was observed; however, there were no differences in electrophoretic mobility, sedimentation constant, pH-optimum, hematin content, or stability to heat and proteolytic inactivation. Since the mutations affecting specific activity and the rate of degradation are not closely linked, all combinations can be observed among hybrid progeny. If this situation turns out to be typical rather than exceptional for any other species, it would explain the wide range of variation observed in dogs and, to a lesser extent, in man.

Hypocatalasemic and Acatalasemic Mutants in Mice

Feinstein et al. have investigated blood catalase in mice [170–172]. The approach and the result of this study are most relevant for any type of inborn error. After determination of the normal range (149 ± 14 perborate units per ml; $n = 110$) a total of 12,306 mice were screened semiquantitatively for subnormal blood catalase activity. Fifty-six prospective heterozygotes with an activity level below 112 perborate units per ml were found. By mating and backcrossing with the parents, five animals were clearly established as genetic heterozygotes. One of the mutants appears to be comparable to human acatalasemia, the heterozygote showing approximately 50 percent and the homozygote about 1 percent of normal catalase. The other four established mutant lines have no exact human counterpart. In heterozygotes catalase level is approximately 65 percent, and in homozygotes, about 20 percent, as compared to normal. From a comparison with regard to sensitivity to heat, pH extremes, ionizing radiation, and a variety of inhibitors (e.g., azide, aminotriazole, etc.) it is concluded that the catalase of the normal strain differs qualitatively from all the mutants. The catalase variants of the five mutants also differ among themselves [172]. The variant enzyme in blood and tissues of the mutant C_5b shows an unusual heat lability. It undergoes rapid inactivation when assayed at 37°C. If analyzed under appropriate conditions (15 sec, 20°C), the level in blood is 2 percent, and in liver, 85 percent as compared to normal mice [173].

An immunologic study has disclosed that in blood of the acatalasemic strain (as well as in the four hypocatalasemic strains) immunologically identical catalase protein is present in large amounts. Thus, the mutations most probably modify in the neighborhood of the active site without affecting the antigenic determinants [174]. The autosomal mutant causing acatalasemia in mice (C_5b has been analyzed for its linkage-relationship with other mutants and found to be located on linkage group V between the Danforth shorttail and agouti loci [175]. The mice of the mutant strain C_5b are extremely sensitive to intraperitoneally injected hydrogen peroxide, but exogenous catalase may protect the mice from otherwise lethal doses of H_2O_2 [176]. No difference in sensitivity to whole-body irradiation or hyperbaric oxygen was observed between normal and acatalasemic mice [177]. The existence of animal mutants with catalase variants of different specific activity and reduced stability or with difference in the rate of degradation may be taken as an indication of the complexity and the heterogeneity of this condition in man.

SUMMARY

1 Acatalasemia is a rare hereditary deficiency of erythrocyte catalase. In most but not all instances it is combined with a lack of tissue catalase. This justifies the more general term *acatalasia.*

2 Acatalasemia, transmitted as an autosomal recessive trait, has been found in Japanese, Korean, Swiss, German, and Israeli people. By 1968, 93 individuals homozygous for this trait among 45 families had been identified.

3 The disorder was discovered by Takahara in 1946 in a patient with ulcerating gangrenous lesions of the oral cavity. Addition of hydrogen peroxide to the operative site resulted in no foaming and caused the tissues to turn black. Takahara's disease, formerly observed in about 50 percent of the children has become considerably less frequent in recent years. Affected persons whose teeth are removed and whose lesions have been healed may remain entirely well thereafter.

4 Most individuals homozygous for acatalas(em)ia are asymptomatic. They were detected by screening tests for blood catalase activity. The detection of hypocatalasemia, the heterozygous carrier state, can be accomplished by screening as well, because most of these subjects show about half of normal activity. The gene frequency varies considerably (0.05 to 1.4 percent), but the genes for acatalasemia apparently have a worldwide distribution.

5 There is genetic heterogeneity inasmuch as at least five subspecies can be distinguished. These variant types differ in respect to the level of residual catalase activity in red cells (0 to 8 percent) and tissues of homozygotes. In most families blood catalase values show a trimodal distribution with no overlap between groups. In others, the ranges of normal and that of heterozygotes merge.

6 Analogous disorders of catalase synthesis (or degradation) with similar genetic characteristics have been observed in dogs, guinea pigs, and mice. In each of these species the level of blood catalase has a wide range of variation. This is due in part to polymorphism and in part to the existence of acatalasemic alleles. By systematic inbreeding of mice with subnormal catalase levels five different mutant strains were obtained.

7 The presence of small amounts of catalase activity in blood of individuals with acatalasemia as well as of mice is due to the synthesis of an enzyme variant of poor stability or of low specific activity. Evidence for both alternatives was obtained by means of heat stability tests, in vitro analysis of the cellular distribution of residual catalase in blood fractions, and by a study of the enzyme turnover in various organs.

BIBLIOGRAPHY

1. Takahara, S.: Progressive oral gangrene probably due to lack of catalase in the blood (acatalasemia). Lancet, **2,** 1101, 1952.
2. Takahara, S., Sato, H., Doi, M., and Mihara, S.: Acatalasemia. III. On the heredity of acatalasemia. Proc. Jap. Acad., **28,** 585, 1952.
3. Takahara, S.: Progressive oral gangrene due to acatalasemia. Laryngoscope, **64,** 685, 1954.
4. Takahara, S., and Doi, K.: Statistical observation on 35 cases of acatalasemia appearing in literature. Jap. J. Otol., **61,** 1727, 1958.
5. Takahara, S., and Doi, K.: Statistical study of acatalasemia (a review of thirty-eight cases appearing in the literature). Acta Med. Okayama, **13,** No. 1, 1959.
6. Yata, H.: A case of acatalasemia. Nihou Shika Hyoron, **204,** 7, 1959.
7. Takahara, S.: Acatalasemia (in Japanese). Naika Hokan, **7,** 488, 1961.
8. Aebi, H., Heiniger, J. P., Bütler, R., and Hässig, A.: Two cases of acatalasia in Switzerland. Experientia, **17,** 466, 1961.

9. Aebi, H., Jeunet, F., Richterich, R., Suter, H., Bütler, R., Frei, J., and Marti, H. R.: Observations in two Swiss families with acatalasia. Enzym. Biol. Clin. (Basel), **2,** 1, 1962/63.
10. Szeinberg, A., de Vries, A., Pinkhas, J., Djaldetti, M., and Ezra, R.: A dual hereditary red blood cell defect in one family: Hypocatalasemia and glucose-6-phosphate dehydrogenase deficiency. Acta Genet. Med. (Roma), **12,** 247, 1963.
11. Szeinberg, A., de Vries, A., Pinkhas, J., Djaldetti, M., and Ezra, R.: A dual hereditary red cell defect in one family: hypocatalasemia and glucose-6-phosphate dehydrogenase deficiency. Communication of the XI Int. Congress of Genetics, The Hague 1963, Abstract 15.60.
12. Pinkhas, J., Djaldetti, M., Joshua, H., Resnick, Ch., and de Vries, A.: Sulfhemoglobinemia and acute hemolytic anemia with Heinz bodies following contact with a fungicide—zinc ethylene bisdithiocarbamate-in a subject with glucose-6-phosphate dehydrogenase deficiency and hypocatalasemia. Blood, **21,** 484, 1963.
13. Polster, H., Beyreiss, K., and Nostitz, H.-J.: Akatalasie bei einem vierjährigen Jungen. Kinderärztl. Praxis, **8,** 367, 1968.
14. Paul, K. G., and Engstedt, L. M.: Normal and abnormal blood catalase activity in adults. Scand. J. Clin. Lab. Invest., **10,** 26, 1958.
15. Engstedt, L., and Paul, K. G.: Inter-individual variations in blood catalase activity. Scand. J. Clin. Lab. Invest., **12,** 502, 1960.
16. Engstedt, L., and Paul, K. G.: Non-hereditary hypocatalasia. Scand. J. Clin. Lab. Invest., **17,** 295, 1965.
17. Baur, E. W.: Catalase abnormality in a Caucasian family in the United States. Science, **140,** 816, 1963.
18. Taylor, E. H., and Haut, A.: Hypocatalasia in two American men. Clin. Res., **15,** 289, 1967.
19. Kaziro, K., Kikuchi, G., Nakamura, H., and Yoshiya, M.: Die Frage nach der physiologischen Funktion der Katalase im menschlichen Organismus: Notiz über die Entdeckung einer Konstitutionsanomalie "Anenzymia catalasea". Chem. Ber., **85,** 886, 1952.
20. Nakamura, H., Yoshiya, M., Kaziro, K., and Kikuchi, G.: On "Anenzymia catalasea" a new type of constitutional abnormality. Proc. Japan Acad., **28,** 59, 1952.
21. Thénard, L. J.: L'académie des sciences, Paris, 1818, cited in Theorell, ref. 84.
22. Loew, O.: Catalase, new enzyme of general occurrence, with special reference to the tobacco plant. U.S. Dept. Agriculture Report 68, p. 47, 1901.
23. Warburg. O.: Ueber die antikatalytische Wirkung der Blausäure. Biochem. Z., **136,** 266, 1923.
24. Zeile, K., and Hellström, H.: Ueber die aktive Gruppe der Leberkatalase. Z. Physiol. Chem., **192,** 171, 1930.
25. Sumner, J. B., and Dounce, A. L.: Crystalline catalase. J. Biol. Chem., **121,** 417, 1937.
26. Greenstein, J. B., and Thompson, J. W.: Range in activity of several enzymes in normal and neoplastic tissues of mice. J. Nat. Cancer Inst., **4,** 275, 1943–44.
27. Sumner, J. B., and Somers, G. F.: *Chemistry and Methods of Enzymes,* p. 216. Academic, New York, 1953.
28. Dixon, M., and Webb, E. C.: *Enzymes.* Academic, New York, 1958.
29. Bonnichsen, R. K.: Catalase from horse kidney and human liver. Acta Chem. Scand., **1,** 114, 1947.
30. Bonnichsen, R. K.: On the hematin and bile pigments in catalase. Acta Chem. Scand., **2,** 561, 1948.
31. Herbert, D., and Pinsent, J.: Crystalline human erythrocyte catalase. Biochem. J., **43,** 203, 1948.
32. Herbert, D., and Pinsent, J.: Crystalline bacterial catalase. Biochem. J., **43,** 193, 1948.
33. Schroeder, W. A., Shelton, J. R., Shelton, J. B., Robertson, B., and Apell, G.: The amino acid sequence of bovine liver catalase. A preliminary report. Arch. Biochem. Biophys., **131,** 653, 1969.
34. Aebi, H.: La catalase erythrocytaire, in *Exposés Annuels de Biochimie Médicale,* p. 139, 29ième serie Masson et Cie, Paris, 1969.
35. Samejima, T., and Shibata, K.: Denaturation of catalase by formamide and urea related to the subunit make-up of the molecule. Arch. Biochem. Biophys., **93,** 407, 1961.
36. Samejima, T., and Yang, J. T.: Reconstitution of acid-denatured catalase. J. Biol. Chem., **238,** 3256, 1963.
37. Hiraga, M., Abe, K., and Anan, F. K.: The subunit structure of catalase: estimation of molecular weight of performic acid-oxidized catalase. Bull. Tokyo Med. Dent. Univ., **14,** 293, 1967.
38. Weber, K., and Sund, H.: Zur Quartärstruktur der Katalase aus Rinderleber. Angew. Chem., **77,** 621, 1965.
39. Kiselev, N. A., Shpitzberg, C. L., and Vainshtein, B. K.: Crystallization of catalase in the form of tubes with monomolecular walls. J. Molec. Biol., **25,** 433, 1967.
40. Kiselev, N. A., de Rosier, D. J., and Klug, A.: Structure of the tubes of catalase: Analysis of electron micrographs by optical filtering. J. Molec. Biol., **35,** 561, 1968.
41. Higashi, T., Yagi, M., and Hirai, H.: Immunochemical studies on catalase. J. Biochem. (Tokyo), **49,** 707, 1961.
42. Schroeder, W. A., Saha, A., Fenninger, W. D., and Cua, J. T.: Preliminary chemical investigation of the structures of beef-liver and horse-liver catalases. Biochim. Biophys. Acta, **58,** 611, 1962.
43. Schroeder, W. A., Shelton, J. R., Shelton, J. B., and Olson, B. M.: Some amino acid sequences in bovine-liver catalase. Biochim. Biophys. Acta, **89,** 47, 1969.
44. Feinstein, R. N., Sacher, G. A., Howard, J. B., and Braun, J. T.: Comparative heat stability of blood catalase. Arch. Biochem. Biophys., **22,** 338, 1967.
45. Higashi, T., and Shibata, Y.: Studies on rat liver catalase. IV. Heterogeneity of mitochondrial and supernatant catalase. J. Biochem., **58,** 530, 1965.
46. Holmes, R. S., and Masters, C. J.: Catalase heterogeneity. Arch. Biochem. Biophys., **109,** 196, 1965.
47. Heidrich, H.-G.: New aspects of heterogeneity of beef liver catalase. Hoppe-Seyler Z. Physiol. Chem., **349,** 873, 1968.
48. Cantz, M., Mörikofer-Zwez, St., Bossi, E., Kaufmann, H., von Wartburg, J. P., and Aebi, H.: Alternative molecular forms of erythrocyte catalase. Experientia, **24,** 119, 1968.
49. Thorup, O. A. Jr., Carpenter, J. T., and Howard, P.: Human erythrocyte catalase: Demonstration of heterogeneity and relationship to erythrocyte ageing in vivo. Brit. J. Haemat., **10,** 542, 1964.
50. Nicholls, P., and Schonbaum, G. R.: Catalases, in *The Enzymes,* edited by P. D. Boyer, H. Lardy, and K. Myrbäck, vol. 8 pp. 147–225, Academic, New York, 1963.
51. Stern, K. G.: The constitution of the prosthetic group of catalase. J. Biol. Chem., **112,** 661, 1936.
52. Lemberg, R., Norris, M., and Legge, J. W.: Catalase. Nature (London), **144,** 551, 1939.
53. Sumner, J. B., and Dounce, A. L.: Catalase II. J. Biol. Chem., **127,** 439, 1939.
54. Aebi, H., Schneider, C. H., Gang, H., and Wiesmann, U.: Separation of catalase and other red cell enzymes from hemoglobin by gel filtration. Experientia, **20,** 103, 1964.
55. Tsuchihashi, M.: Zur Kenntnis der Blutkatalase. Biochem. Z., **140,** 63, 1923.
56. Bonnichsen, R. K., Chance, B., and Theorell, H.: Catalase activity. Acta Chem. Scand., **1,** 685, 1947.
57. Deutsch, H. F.: Properties of various crystalline horse erythrocyte catalase preparations. Acta Chem. Scand., **6,** 1516, 1952.
58. Keilin, D., and Hartree, E. F.: Coupled oxidation of alcohol. Proc. Roy. Soc. [Biol.], **119,** 141, 1936.
59. Frei, E., and Aebi, H.: Isotopie-Effekte bei der peroxydatischen Formiatoxydation durch Leberkatalase. Helv. Chim. Acta, **41,** 241, 1958.
60. Aebi, H., and Frei, E.: Gekoppelte Oxydation von Formiat und Thiolverbindungen durch Katalase. Helv. Chim. Acta, **41,** 361, 1958.
61. Chance, B., Greenstein, D. S., and Roughton, F. J. W.: The mechanism of catalase action. I. The steady-state analysis. Arch. Biochem. Biophys., **37,** 301, 1952.
62. Nicholls, P.: Activity of catalase in the red cell. Biochim. Biophys. Acta, **99,** 286, 1965.
63. Maehly, A. C., and Chance, B.: The assay of catalase and peroxidases,

in *Methods of Biochemical Analysis,* edited by D. Glick, vol. I, p. 357. Interscience, New York, 1954.

64. Colowick, S. P., and Kaplan, N. O. (eds.,): *Methods in Enzymology,* vol. II. pp. 764–791. Academic, New York, 1955.
65. Aebi, H., and Suter, H.: Catalase, in *Biochemical Methods in Red Cell Genetics,* edited by J. J. Yunis, p. 255. Academic, New York, 1969.

65*a*. Haining, J. L., and Legan, J. S.: Improved assay for catalase based upon steady-state substrate concentration. Anal. Biochemistry, **45,** 469, 1972.

66. Aebi, H.: Katalase, in *Die Methoden der enzymatischen Analysen.* edited by H. U. Bergmeyer, 2d ed., p. 636, Verlag Chemie GmbH, Weinheim, 1969.
67. Aebi, H., Frei, E., Knab, R., and Siegenthaler, P.: Untersuchungen über die Formiatoxydation in der Leber. Helv. Physiol. Pharmacol. Acta, **15,** 150, 1957.
68. Aebi, H.: Detection and fixation of radiation-produced peroxide by enzymes. Radiation Res., Suppl. **3,** 130, 1963.
69. Laser, H.: Micrococcus radiodurans. Meeting Europ. Soc. for Radiation Biology, Utrecht, N.L., 1965.
70. Orita, Y., Komiya, S., Konishi, N., and Ohkura, K.: Biochemical study of human embryo, with special reference to development of catalase. Jap. J. Hum. Genet., **8,** 141, 1963.
71. Aebi, H.: Mécanisme et rôle biologique de l'action peroxydatique de la catalase. Bull. Soc. Chim. Biol., **42,** 187, 1960.
72. Matuo, Y., Nishikawa, K., Horio, T., and Okunuki, K.: Effect of growth of rhodamine sarcoma in rat on some liver enzyme activities. Gann, **59,** 299, 1968.
73. Nakamura, T., Matuo, Y., Nishikawa, K., Horio, T., and Okunuki, K.: Effects on various types of liver catalase by growth of rhodamine sarcoma and by administration of in vivo catalase-depressing substance prepared from the tumor. Gann, **59,** 317, 1968.
74. Matuo, Y.: In vivo liver catalase-depressing substance from rhodamine sarcoma. Gann, **59,** 405, 1968.
75. De Duve, Ch., and Baudhuin, P.: Peroxisomes (Microbodies and related particles). Physiol. Rev., **46,** 323, 1966.
76. Leighton, F., Poole, B., Beaufay, H., Baudhuin, P., Coffey, J. W., Fowler. S., and de Duve, Ch.: The large-scale separation of peroxisomes, mitochondria, and lysosomes from the livers of rats injected with Triton WR-1339. J. Cell Biol., **37,** 482, 1968.
77. Poole, B., Leighton, F., and de Duve, Ch.: Synthesis and turnover of rat liver peroxisomes. 2. Turnover of peroxisome proteins. J. Cell Biol., **41,** 536, 1969.
78. Neubert, D., Wojtczak, A. B., and Lehninger, A. L.: Purification and identification of mitochondrial contraction factors. Proc. Nat. Acad. Sci. U.S.A., **48,** 1651, 1962.
79. Higashi, T., and Peters, T., Jr.: Studies on rat liver catalase. II. Incorporation of ^{14}C-leucine into catalase of liver cell fractions in vivo. J. Biol. Chem., **238,** 3952, 1963.
80. Adams, D. H., and Burgess, E. A.: The intracellular redistribution of catalase during the incubation of mouse-liver slices. Biochem. J., **71,** 340, 1959.
81. Aebi, H., Bossi, E., Cantz, M., Matsubara, S., and Suter, H.: Auswirkung von Enzymdefekten auf den Erythrocytenstoffwechsel (erläutert am Beispiel der Akatalasie). Folia Haemat. (Leipzig), **91,** 5, 1969.
82. Allison, A. C., and Burn, G. P.: Enzyme activity as a function of age in the human erythrocyte. Brit. J. Haemat., **1,** 291, 1955.
83. Sass, M. D.: Catalase activity in young red cells. Nature (London), **197,** 503, 1963.
84. Theorell, H., Beznak, H., Bonnichsen, R., Paul, K. G., and Akeson, A.: On the distribution of radioactive iron in guinea pigs and its rate of appearance in some hemoproteins and ferritins. Acta Chem. Scand., **5,** 445, 1951.
85. Schmid, R., Figen, J. F., and Schwartz, S.: Experimental porphyria. IV. Studies of liver catalase and other heme enzymes in Sedormid porphyria. J. Biol. Chem., **217,** 263, 1955.
86. Rechcigl, Jr. M., and Price, V. E.: Studies on the turnover of catalase in vivo. Prog. Exp. Tumor Res., **10,** 112, 1968.
87. Schimke, R. T.: Protein turnover and the regulation of enzyme levels in rat liver. International Symposium on Enzymatic Aspects of Metabolic Regulation, Mexico City, 1966.
88. Ganschow, R., and Schimke, R. T.: Genetic control of catalase in inbred mice, in *Some Aspects of the Control of Protein Synthesis in Animal Tissues.* Academic, New York, 1968.

88*a*. Ganschow, R. E. and Schimke, R. T.: Murine catalase phenotypes. Biochem. Genetics, **4,** 157, 1970.

89. Bingold, K.: Die Niere als blutzerstörendes Organ. Klin. Wschr., **12,** 1201, 1933.
90. Keilin, D., and Hartree, E. F.: Properties of catalase: Catalysis of coupled oxidation of alcohols. Biochem. J., **39,** 293, 1945.
91. Chance, B.: Enzyme-substrate compounds. Advances Enzym., **12,** 153, 1951.
92. Chance, B.: The state of catalase in the respiring bacterial cell. Science, **116,** 202, 1952.
93. Rouiller, C., and Bernhard, W.: "Microbodies" and the problem of mitochondrial regeneration in liver cells. J. Biophys. Biochem. Cytol., Suppl. **2,** 355, 1956.
94. Lehninger, A. L., and Beck, D. P.: The catalase requirement in the reversal and mitochondrial swelling caused by reduced glutathione and by trace metals. J. Biol. Chem., **242,** 2098, 1967.
95. Heppel, L. A., and Porterfield, V. T.: Metabolism of inorganic nitrite and nitrate esters. I. The coupled oxidation of nitrite by peroxide-forming systems and catalase. J. Biol. Chem., **178,** 549, 1949.
96. Aebi, H., Koblet, H., and von Wartburg, J. P.: Ueber den Mechanismus der biologischen Methanoloxydation. Helv. Physiol. Acta, **15,** 384, 1957.
97. Warburg, O., Schröder, W., and Gattung, H. W.: Ueber die Wirkung von Röntgenstrahlen auf Hämoglobin. Z. Naturforsch. [B], **15,** 163, 1960.
98. Aebi, H., and Suter, H.: Ueber die Peroxidempfindlichkeit von Akatalasie-Erythrocyten. Humangenetik, **2,** 328, 1966.
99. Cohen, G., and Hochstein, P.: Glutathione peroxidase: the primary agent for the elimination of hydrogen peroxide in erythrocytes. Biochemistry, **2,** 1420, 1963.
100. Cohen, G., and Hochstein, P.: Generation of hydrogen peroxide in erythrocytes by hemolytic agents. Biochemistry, **3,** 895, 1964.
101. Liebowitz, J., and Cohen, G.: Increased hydrogen peroxide levels in glucose-6-phosphate dehydrogenase deficient erythrocytes exposed to acetylphenylhydrazine. Biochem. Pharmacol., **17,** 983, 1968.
102. Aebi, H., Heiniger, J.-P., and Lauber, E.: Methämoglobinbildung in Erythrocyten durch Peroxydeinwirkung. Versuche zur Beurteilung der Schutzfunktion von Katalase und Glutathionperoxidase. Helv. Chim. Acta, **47,** 1428, 1964.
103. Takahara, S.: Acatalasemia. Asian Med. J., **10,** 46, 1967.
104. Takahara, S.: Acatalasemia in Japan, in *Hereditary Disorders of Erythrocyte Metabolism,* edited by E. Beutler, vol. I. p. 21. Grune & Stratton, New York, 1968.
105. Takahara, S., Hamilton, H. B., Neel, J. V., Kobara, T. Y., Ogura, Y., and Nishimura, E. T.: Hypocatalasemia: a new genetic carrier state. J. Clin. Invest., **39,** 610, 1960.
106. Nishimura, E. T., Hamilton, H. B., Kobara, T. Y., Takahara, S., Ogura, Y., and Doi, K.: Carrier state in human acatalasemia. Science, **130,** 333, 1959.
107. Ohkura, K., Ogura, Y., and Takahara, S.: Population studies of acatalasemia and hypocatalasemia in Japan, Ryukyu, and Taiwan. Communication to the 3d Int. Congress of Human Genetics, Chicago, 1966.
108. Hamilton, H. B., Neel, J. V., Kobara, T. Y., and Ozaki, K.: The frequency in Japan of carriers of the rare "recessive" gene causing acatalasemia. J. Clin. Invest., **40,** 2199, 1961.
109. Hamilton, H. B., and Neel, J. V.: Genetic heterogeneity in human acatalasia. Amer. J. Human Genet., **15,** 408, 1963.
110. "Annotations", Blood catalase and oral ulceration. Lancet, **2,** 1121, 1952.
111. Krooth, R. S.: Some properties of diploid cell strains developed from the tissues of patients with inherited biochemical disorders. In Vitro, **2,** 82, 1967.
112. Ogata, M., Sadamoto, M., and Takahara, S.: On minimal catalatic activity in Japanese acatalasemic blood. Proc. Jap. Acad., **42,** 828, 1966.

112*a*. Chang, T. M. S.: Effects of local applications of microencapsulated catalase on the response of oral lesions to hydrogen peroxide in acatalasemia. J. Dent. Res. Suppl., **51**, 319, 1972.
113. Aebi, H.: The investigation of inherited enzyme deficiencies with special reference to acatalasia. Proc. 3rd Int. Congress of Human Genetics, Chicago 1966, edited by J. F. Crow and J. V. Neel, p. 189, Johns Hopkins, Baltimore, 1967.
114. Aebi, H., Baggiolini, M., Dewald, B., Lauber, E., Suter, H., Micheli, A., and Frei, J.: Observations in two Swiss families with acatalasia II. Enzymol. Biol. Clin., **4**, 121, 1964.
115. Takahara, S., Ogura, Y., and Doi, K.: Statistical study of acatalasemia, a review of thirty-eight cases appearing in the literature. Acta Med. Okayama, **13**, 209, 1959.
116. Szeinberg, A., and Sosnowsky, A.: Personal communication 1967.
117. Lamy, J. N., Lamy-Provansal, J., de Russe, J., and Weill, J. D.: Dosage automatique de l'eau oxygénée et application à l'étude cinétique de la catalase. Bull. Soc. Chim. Biol., **49**, 1167, 1967.
118. Hübl, P., and Bretschneider, R.: Die Titanylsulfatmethode zur Bestimmung der Katalase im Blut, Serum und Harn. Hoppe-Seyler Z. Physiol., Chem., **335**, 146, 1964.
119. Funaki, H.: Thermal analysis of blood catalase reaction. Jap. J. Physiol., **5**, 183, 1955.
120. Miller, H.: The relationship between catalase and haemoglobin in human blood. Biochem. J., **68**, 275, 1958.
121. Aebi, H., Bossi, E., Cantz, M., Matsubara, S., and Suter, H.: Acatalasemia in Switzerland, in *Hereditary Disorders of Erythrocyte Metabolism,* edited by E. Beutler, vol. I. p. 41. Grune and Stratton, New York, 1968.
122. Feinstein, R. N.: Perborate as substrate in a new assay of catalase. J. Biol. Chem., **180**, 1197, 1949.
123. Aebi, H., Cantz, M., and Suter, H.: Cellular distribution of catalase activity in red cells of homozygous and heterozygous cases of acatalasia. Experientia, **21**, 713, 1965.
124. Aebi, H., and Cantz, M.: Ueber die celluläre Verteilung der Katalase im Blut homozygoter und heterozygoter Defektträger (Akatalasie). Humangenetik, **3**, 50, 1966.
125. Kleihauer, E., and Betke, K.: Elution procedure for the demonstration of methemoglobin in red cells of human blood smears. Nature (London), **199**, 1196, 1963.
126. Hosoi, T.: Fluorescent antibody technique utilized for studies on cellular distribution of erythrocytic antigens. Acta Haemat. Jap., **31**, 138, 1968.
127. Hosoi, T., Suter, H., Yahara, S., and Aebi, H.: Pseudomosaicism in acatalasemic red cells visualized by fluorescent antibody technique. Experientia, **25**, 313, 1969.
128. Sass, M. D., Caruso, C. J., and O'Connell D. J.: Decreased glutathione in ageing red cells. Clin. Chim. Acta, **11**, 334, 1965.
129. Ogata, M., and Takahara, S.: On minimal catalatic activity of Japanese acatalasemia and acatalasemic mice. Proc. XII. Int. Congress of Genetics, The Science Council of Japan, Tokyo 1968. Abstr. 7.5.8.
130. Krooth, R. S., Howell, R. R., and Hamilton, H. B.: Properties of acatalasic cells growing in vitro. J. Exp. Med., **115**, 313, 1962.
131. Kitamura, I., Ogata, M., and Takahara, S.: Tissue culture of skin in acatalasemia and hypocatalasemia. Proc. Jap. Acad., **38**, 365, 1962.
132. Sadamoto, M.: Nature of cultured cells of the skin from acatalasemic individuals with Takahara's disease. Acta Med. Okayama, **20**, 193, 1966.
133. Doi, K.: Experimental study on the oral gangrene appearing in acatalasemia. Okayama Igakkai Zasshi, **71**, 1125, 1959.
134. Ohkura, K., Nakagawa, H., Kosaka, N., Sadamoto, M., and Takahara, S.: Chromosome study of acatalasemia. Proc. Jap. Acad., **40**, 52, 1964.
135. Klinger, H.: Unpublished observations, 1964.
136. Jacob, H. S., Ingbar, S. H., and Jandl, J. H.: Oxidative hemolysis and erythrocyte metabolism in hereditary acatalasia. J. Clin. Invest., **44**, 1187, 1965.
137. Takahara, S.: Acatalasemia. Proc. 2nd Int. Congress Human Genet., Rome 1961, vol. 1, p. 539.
138. Baggiolini, M., Aebi, H., Sacquet, E., and Charlier, H.: Beteiligung der Darmflora an peroxydatischen Umsetzungen (Formiatoxydation) bei der Ratte. Helv. Physiol. Pharmacol. Acta, **22**, 53, 1964.
139. Takahara, S., Ogata, M., Kobara, T. Y., Nishimura, E. T., and Brown, W. J.: The "catalase protein" of acatalasemic red blood cells. Lab. Invest., **11**, 782, 1962.
140. Ogata, M., and Takahara, S.: Paper electrophoretic studies on the catalase protein in acatalasemic blood extract (stage 3 by Herbert-Pinsent). Proc. Jap. Acad., **38**, 361, 1962.
141. Takahara, S., and Ogata, M.: Spectrometric studies on the catalase in acatalasemic red blood cell extracts, stage 2 and 3 by Herbert-Pinsent. Proc. Jap. Acad., **38**, 779, 1962.
142. Ogata, M., and Takahara, S.: Quantitative precipitin studies on catalase protein in hemolysate and acetone extract from acatalasemia and hypocatalasemia. Proc. Jap. Acad., **39**, 783, 1963.
143. Micheli, A., and Aebi, H.: Recherche immunochimique de la catalase érythrocytaire dans l'hemolysat acatalasique. Rev. Franç. Etud. Clin. Biol., **10**, 431, 1965.
144. Kajiro, K.: Immunological study of acatalasemia, in "Study of Acatalesemia", a report compiled by the Education University of the Japanese Government. Cited in Hamilton and Neel [109].
145. Otani, A.: Immunological investigation of acatalasia. Jap. J. Biochem., **32**, 216, 1960.
146. Nishimura, E. T., Kobara, T. Y., Takahara, S., Hamilton, H. B., and Madden, S. C.: Immunologic evidence of catalase deficiency in human hereditary acatalasemia. Lab. Invest., **10**, 333, 1961.
147. Micheli, A.: Etude immunochimique d'hémolysats acatalasiques. Experientia, **19**, 138, 1963.
148. Shibata, Y., Higashi, T., Hirai, H., and Hamilton, H. B.: Immunochemical studies on catalase II. An anticatalase reacting component in normal, hypocatalasic, and acatalasic human erythrocytes. Arch. Biochem. Biophys., **118**, 200, 1967.
148*a*. Higashi, T., Kudo, H., and Kashiwagi, K.: Specific precipitation of catalase-synthesizing ribosomes by anti-catalase antiserum. J. Biochem., **71**, 463, 1972.
148*b*. Kashiwagi, K., Tobe, T., Higashi, T., and Warabioka, K.: Impaired synthesis of liver catalase in tumor-bearing rats. Gann, **63**, 57, 1972.
149. Nishimura, E. T., Takahara, S., and Hokama, Y.: Interrelationship of catalase and C-reactive protein in acatalasemic erythrocytes. Arch. Biochem. Biophys., **126**, 121, 1968.
150. Hokama, Y., Croxatto, H. D., Yamada, K., and Nishimura, E. T.: The occurrence of immunologically common antigenic components in C-reactive protein and human hepatic and erythrocyte catalases. Cancer Res., **27**, 2300, 1967.
151. Hokama, Y., Yamada, K., Moikeha, S. N., and Nishimura, E. T.: The metabolic interrelationship and physicochemical analysis of C-reative protein and hepatic catalase. Cancer Res., **29**, 542, 1969.
152. Andrews, P.: Estimation of the molecular weights of proteins by Sephadex gel-filtration. Biochem. J., **91**, 222, 1964.
153. Matsubara, S., Suter, H., and Aebi, H.: Heterogeneity of catalase in blood of heterozygous cases of acatalasia. Experientia, **22**, 428, 1966.
154. Matsubara, S., Suter, H., and Aebi, H.: Fractionation of erythrocyte catalase from normal, hypocatalatic, and acatalatic humans. Humangenetik, **4**, 29, 1967.
155. Mörikofer-Zwez, St., Cantz, M., Kaufmann, H., von Wartburg, J. P., and Aebi, H.: Heterogeneity of erythrocyte catalase: Correlations between sulfhydryl group content, chromatographic and electrophoretic properties. Europ. J. Biochem., **11**, 49, 1969.
156. Takahara, S., Mihara, S., Tsugawa, K., and Doi, M.: Acatalasemia II. Contents of catalase in blood and tissues of men and animals. Proc. Jap. Acad., **28**, 383, 1952.
157. Richardson, M., Huddleson, I. F., and Bethea, R.: Study of catalase in erythrocytes and bacteria. I. Procedure for the determination of the catalase activity of erythrocytes. Arch. Biochem. Biophys., **42**, 114, 1953.
158. Richardson, M., Huddleson, I. F., Bethea, R., and Trustdorf, M.: Study of catalase in erythrocytes and bacteria. II. Catalase activity of erythrocytes from different species of normal animals and from normal humans. Arch. Biochem. Biophys., **42**, 124, 1953.
159. Knab, R.: Vergleichende Biochemie der Leberkatalase. Inaugural Dissertation der Med. Fakultät der Universität Bern, 1960.

160. Paniker, N. V., and Iyer, G. Y. N.: Erythrocyte catalase and detoxication of hydrogen peroxide. Canad. J. Biochem., **43,** 1029, 1965.

160*a*. Butenandt, O.: Glutathion, Glutathionperoxydase, Glutathionreduktase, Glucose-6-Phosphatdehydrogenase, Lactatdehydrogenase und Katalase in Erythrocyten von Neugeborenen, Säuglingen und Kindern und ihre Beziehung zur Heinzkörperbildung. Z. Kinderheilk. **111,** 149–161, 1971.

161. Feinstein, R. N., Faulhaber, J. T., and Howard, J. B.: Acatalasemia and hypocatalasemia in the dog and the duck. Proc. Soc. Exp. Biol. Med., **127,** 1051, 1968.

162. Aebi, H., and Suter, H.: Wirkung peroxydbildender Cytostatica auf Methämoglobin und Glutathiongehalt normaler und akatalatischer Erythrocyten. Helv. Physiol. Acta, **23,** C9, 1965.

163. Aebi, H., Dewald, B., and Suter, H.: Peroxidbildung bei der Autoxidation N^2-substituierter Methylhydrazine. Helv. Chim. Acta, **48,** 1380, 1965.

164. Allison, A. C., Rees, W., and Burn, G. P.: Genetically controlled differences in catalase activity of dog erythrocytes. Nature (London), **180,** 649, 1957.

165. Radev. T.: Inheritance of hypocatalasemia in guinea pigs. J. Genet., **57,** 169, 1960.

166. Moosbrugger, G. A., Spuhler, V., and Meyer, K.: Katalasebestimmungen beim Meerschweinchen. Schweiz. Z. Path. Bakt., **19,** 781, 1956.

167. Greenstein, J. P., and Andervont, H. B.: The liver catalase activity of tumor bearing mice and the effect of spontaneous regression and of removal of certain tumors. J. Nat. Cancer Inst., **2,** 345, 1942.

168. Heston, W. E., Hoffman, H. A., and Rechcigle, M.: Genetic analysis of liver catalase activity in two substrains of C57BL mice. Genet. Res., **6,** 387, 1965.

169. Li, J. B.: Specificity of catalase degradation in C57BL mice: Comparison with other liver enzymes. Enzym. Biol. Clin., **9,** 161, 1968.

170. Feinstein, R. N., Seaholm, J. E., Howard, J. B., and Russell, W. L.: Acatalasemic mice. Proc. Nat. Acad. Sci. U.S.A., **52,** 661, 1964.

171. Feinstein, R. N., Howard, J. B., Braun, J. T., and Seaholm, J. E.: Acatalasemic and hypocatalasemic mouse mutants. Genetics, **53,** 925, 1966.

172. Feinstein, R. N., Braun, J. T., and Howard, J. B.: Acatalasemic and hypocatalasemic mouse mutants: II. Mutational variations in blood and solid tissue catalases. Arch. Biochem. Biophys., **120,** 165, 1967.

172*a*. Feinstein, R. N.: Acatalasemia in the mouse and other species. Biochem. Genetics, **4,** 135, 1970.

172*b*. Feinstein, R. N., Howard, J. B., and Savol, R.: Heat and urea stability of blood catalase of catalase-mutant mouse strains. Experientia, **27,** 1152, 1971.

172*c*. Feinstein, R. N., Savol, R., and Howard, J. B.: Conversion of catalatic to peroxidatic activity in livers of normal and acatalasemic mice. Enzymologia, **41,** 345, 1971.

172*d*. Feinstein, R. N., and Nelson, D. M.: Effects of supralethal gamma ray doses on survival time and certain blood parameters of normal, acatalasemic, and aminotriazole-treated mice. Kerntechnik, **13.** Jg. Heft 9, 400, 1971.

173. Aebi, H., Suter, H., and Feinstein, R. N.: Activity and stability of catalase in blood and tissues of normal and acatalasemic mice. Biochem. Genet., **2,** 245, 1968.

174. Feinstein, R. N., Suter, H., and Jaroslow, B. N.: Blood catalase polymorphism: Some immunological aspects. Science, **159,** 638, 1968.

175. Dickerman, R. C., Feinstein, R. N., and Grahn, D.: Position of the acatalasemia gene in linkage group V of the mouse. J. Hered., **59,** 177, 1968.

176. Feinstein, R. N., Braun, J. T., and Howard, J. B.: Reversal of H_2O_2 toxicity in the acatalasemic mouse by catalase administration: Suggested model for possible replacement therapy of inborn errors of metabolism. J. Lab. Clin. Med., **68,** 952, 1966.

177. Feinstein, R. N., Faulhaber, J. T., and Howard, J. B.: Sensitivity of acatalasemic mice to acute and chronic irradiation and related conditions. Rad. Res., **35,** 341, 1968.

CHAPTER SEVENTY-FOUR

THE CHOLINESTERASE VARIANTS

Hermann Lehmann and James Liddell

The cholinesterase variants may be considered as examples of pharmacogenetics. This term was introduced by Vogel in 1959 to describe those genetically determined disorders which are usually revealed by an altered response to specific drugs [1]. The term is not precise and its limits are arbitrary. A classic and typical example is drug-induced hemolytic anemia described in Chap. 55 on glucose-6-phosphate dehydrogenase deficiency.

Cholinesterase deficiency is usually symptomless, but the patient has a profound sensitivity to the muscle relaxant suxamethonium. Anesthetists have used this drug extensively for the last 20 years as a drug of choice because the muscular paralysis conveniently lasts for only 3 or 4 min after the usual dose of 20 to 100 mg. The short action is due to hydrolysis by cholinesterase.

Suxamethonium is the dicholine ester of succinic acid and can be regarded as two acetylcholine molecules joined by their acetate groups:

$$CH_3—COO—CH_2—CH_2—N^+(CH_3)_3$$

Acetylcholine

$$\begin{array}{l} CH_2—COO—CH_2—CH_2—N^+(CH_3)_3 \\ | \\ CH_2—COO—CH_2—CH_2—N^+(CH_3)_3 \end{array}$$

Suxamethonium

THE CHOLINESTERASES

The nomenclature of the cholinesterases has been set by the Report of the Commission on Enzymes of the International Union of Biochemistry [2]. Each enzyme has been given a trivial and a systematic name and a classifying number. Two cholinesterases are known: acetylcholinesterase and cholinesterase.

Acetylcholinesterase (acetylcholine acetyl-hydrolase 3.1.1.7). Because of its great physiologic importance, this enzyme was formerly known as *true cholinesterase.* It is a relatively specific enzyme which hydrolyzes acetylcholine faster than other choline esters. It is found in many tissues including the human red cell and nervous tissues and is responsible for inactivating acetylcholine produced at the neuromuscular junction during neurotransmission. This enzyme does not hydrolyze suxamethonium; indeed, it is inhibited by the drug.

Cholinesterase (acylcholine acyl-hydrolase, 3.1.1.8). This enzyme has previously been called *pseudocholinesterase.* Other names were *butyryl cholinesterase* and *nonspecific cholinesterase.* It hydrolyzes many cholinesters including suxamethonium. In man it is found in most tissues including the plasma but not the red cells. The plasma enzyme is synthesized in the liver. The physiologic function of the enzyme is unknown, but it has been plausibly suggested that the main role may be the hydrolysis of those cholinesters which inhibit acetylcholinesterase. These include substances such as propionylcholine and butyrylcholine which can be formed in vitro by the enzyme systems responsible for synthesis of acetylcholine and which may also be produced by bacterial action in the gut.

Mechanism of Action

The mechanism of action of both acetylcholinesterase and cholinesterase is partly understood. Each substrate molecule appears to combine with the enzyme at two different sites. The first of these, the anionic site, is a negatively charged region of the enzyme surface which combines with the positively charged quaternary nitrogen atom. Many inhibitors contain a similar radical and are thought to interfere with enzyme activity by combining reversibly with this site. The second, or esteratic, site appears to combine with the carbonyl group of the ester linkage and to be responsible for the actual hydrolysis. Other inhibitors act at this second site, particularly the organophosphorus compounds which combine irreversibly with the enzyme. The work on the mechanism of the active enzyme has been performed primarily with acetylcholinesterase. It is uncertain whether cholinesterase has two active sites, but this would be compatible with the biochemical behavior of the cholinesterase variants.

Properties of Normal Plasma Cholinesterase

Many methods of assay of cholinesterase are available. That of Kalow and Lindsay [3] has been used for most investigations on the cholinesterase variants: The specific substrate benzoylcholine absorbs ultraviolet light at a wavelength of 240 mμ, and hydrolysis can be followed spectrophotometrically. More recently thiocholine esters have been used [4, 5]. These techniques are more sensitive and can also be used to study the cholinesterase variants.

Plasma cholinesterase can be fractionated by gel electrophoresis, the exact number of bands obtained depending on the technique. Harris et al. [6] found four bands (C_1–C_4) by using two-dimensional electrophoresis on paper and starch gel with naphthyl acetate as substrate. The slowest band (C_4) contained 90 percent of the activity. Juul [7] detected 12 isoenzymes using polyacrylamide disk electrophoresis and butyrylthiocholine as substrate. The molecular weight of the major isoenzyme component is approximately 360,000 [5], but the results of gel filtration indicate that the minor components have a lower molecular weight [8].

Cholinesterase contains several molecules of sialic acid [9]. These can be removed by neuraminidase, with alteration of electrophoretic mobility.

THE CHOLINESTERASE VARIANTS

The Atypical Enzyme

Soon after suxamethonium was introduced a number of patients with sensitivity to the drug were described in whom the plasma cholinesterase level was low [10, 11]. These low cholinesterase levels were usually inherited and not due to acquired abnormalities such as liver disease [12, 13]. The evidence suggested that patients sensitive to suxamethonium were homozygous for an abnormal gene. Apparent heterozygotes had cholinesterase levels which overlapped both the lower limit of the normal range and the value found in sensitive subjects [14, 15]. Using the benzoylcholine assay [3], Kalow and his colleagues greatly improved the understanding of this genetic variant. They compared the kinetics of the cholinesterase found in a suxamethonium-sensitive subject with those from a normal person and found that the two differed in the following ways:

1. The normal enzyme had a higher affinity (i.e., lower Michaelis constant) for all substrates than the enzyme from the sensitive individual [16]. Figure 74-1 shows the results obtained with suxamethonium as a substrate. It can be seen that this experiment also shows that the plasma from a suxamethonium-sensitive individual has no detectable activity against this substrate when it is present in therapeutic concentrations.
2. The cholinesterase activity of a normal plasma was inhibited much more strongly by many, but not all, cholinesterase inhibitors [17].

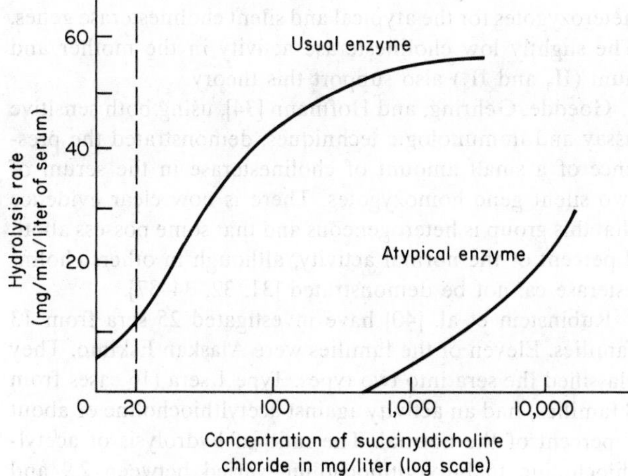

Figure 74-1. The rate of hydrolysis produced by the usual and atypical cholinesterase on varying concentrations of suxamethonium (succinyldicholine); the dotted line indicates the therapeutic plasma level. (*After Kalow* [39].)

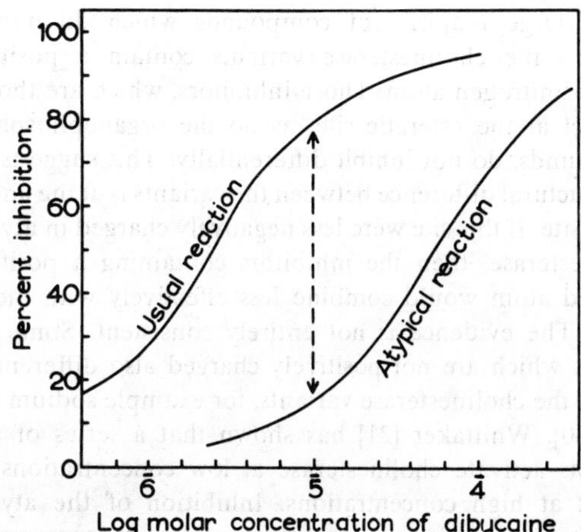

Figure 74-2. The percentage inhibition produced by varying concentrations of dibucaine on usual and atypical cholinesterase. (*After Kalow and Genest* [18].)

These two differences were strong evidence that the cholinesterase found in persons sensitive to suxamethonium was a different molecular species from the normal. It suggested that these patients were homozygotes possessing two mutant genes which determined the production of a cholinesterase molecule with an altered amino acid sequence. Kalow and Genest [18] suggested the term *atypical cholinesterase* for the unusual variant. One inhibitor produced a differential inhibition. This was the local anesthetic dibucaine (cinchocaine, Nupercaine). The degree of inhibition caused by varying concentrations of this substance on the normal and atypical enzyme is shown in Fig. 74-2. The maximal difference in inhibition is given by a $10^{-5}M$ concentration. Kalow and Genest [18] suggested the use of this concentration to identify the genotype of a subject. They called the percentage inhibition produced *the dibucaine number*, or DN. The dibucaine number clearly differentiates three types of persons: the normal homozygote with a dibucaine number of about 80; the atypical homozygote with a value below 30; and the heterozygote with a value between 45 and 69. This technique, unlike the estimation of cholinesterase activity, clearly identifies the heterozygote. It has therefore become a standard technique in the investigation of families and in population surveys.

Another inhibitor which distinguishes even more clearly between the genotypes is another positively charged substance, the dimethyl carbamate of (2-hydroxy-5-phenylbenzyl) trimethyl ammonium bromide, usually known by the manufacturer's (Hoffman-La Roche) code name of RO2-0683. At $10^{-8}M$ this substance will inhibit the normal enzyme by over 90 percent, the atypical variant by less than 10 percent, and the heterozygote by between 58 and 70 percent [19].

The large majority of compounds which differentiate between the cholinesterase variants contain a positively charged nitrogen atom. Those inhibitors, which are thought to react at the esteratic site, as do the organophosphorus compounds, do not inhibit differentially. This suggests that the structural difference between the variants is at the anionic active site. If this site were less negatively charged in atypical cholinesterase, then the inhibitors containing a positively charged atom would combine less effectively with the enzyme. The evidence is not entirely consistent. Some substances which are not positively charged also differentially inhibit the cholinesterase variants, for example sodium fluoride [20]. Whittaker [21] has shown that a series of alkyl alcohols activate cholinesterase at low concentrations and inhibit at high concentrations. Inhibition of the atypical variant occurs at lower concentrations and is more marked than with the usual enzyme. This is the reverse of the situation with dibucaine, where it is the usual enzyme which is strongly inhibited. It has been shown that 1 percent *n*-butanol activates normal cholinesterase by between 156 and 189 percent and inhibits atypical cholinesterase by between 36 and 61 percent [22]. Further evidence that the two cholinesterase variants are separate enzymes is provided by the fact that they can be separated by cation exchange chromatography using diethyl aminoethyl cellulose (DEAE) columns or by electrophoresis at high pH [23]. These techniques also show that both enzymes are present in the plasma of the heterozygote. The variant also appears in tissues other than plasma in an affected individual [24].

The Fluoride-resistant Enzyme

Harris and Whittaker [20] found that sodium fluoride is a differential inhibitor of the usual and atypical enzyme in a manner similar to dibucaine. They defined the percentage

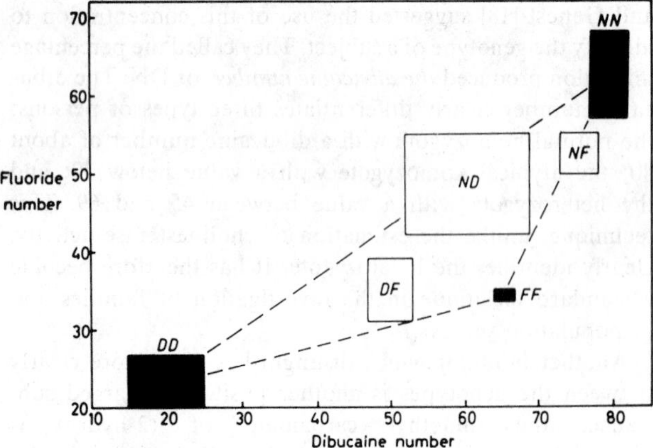

Figure 74-3. The relationship between the dibucaine and fluoride numbers of the cholinesterase variants determined by the three alleles for (1) the normal enzyme (N); (2) the atypical (dibucaine-resistant) enzyme (D); (3) the fluoride-resistant enzyme (F). The values found in the three homozygotes lie within the black rectangles and those for the heterozygotes, within the white rectangles. (*After Liddell, Lehmann, and Davies* [19].)

inhibition produced by $5 \times 10^{-2} M$ fluoride as *the flouride number.* They used both dibucaine and fluoride numbers in an investigation of number of families of suxamethonium-sensitive patients. It might be expected that the three groups of subjects corresponding to the two homozygotes and the heterozygotes would result. Surprisingly an additional two subgroups were detected with slightly lower dibucaine numbers and definitely lower fluoride numbers. Further work has shown that this increased resistance to fluoride is also inherited. It is due to the presence of a further cholinesterase gene, an allele of the others [25, 26]. The relationship of this new variant to the others is shown in Fig. 74-3. The heterozygote for the genes determining both fluoride and dibucaine resistance is sensitive to suxamethonium [27]. The homozygote with fluoride-resistant cholinesterase is also moderately sensitive, and three cases have been described [19, 28, 29].

The Silent Gene

In 1962 Liddell, Lehmann, and Silk found one patient with a marked sensitivity to suxamethonium who had no detectable cholinesterase activity [30]. The family data showed that this was inherited and that the person with no cholinesterase activity was homozygous for another cholinesterase gene. A total of 64 similar patients have now been reported, 48 in a population of 5,000 Alaskan Eskimo [31, 32]. The silent gene is an allele of those for the atypical and fluoride-resistant enzymes [33].

The existence of this gene can explain some family studies which do not fit the expected pattern. Such a family is shown in Fig. 74-4. It can be seen that the mother (II_3) of the two apparently abnormal homozygotes (III_1 and III_2) appears to possess only the normal enzyme. These results would be explained if the mother were a heterozygote for the normal and the silent genes. The two children would then be heterozygotes for the atypical and silent cholinesterase genes. The slightly low cholinesterase activity in the mother and aunt (II_3 and II_4) also support this theory.

Goedde, Gehring, and Hofmann [34], using both sensitive assay and immunologic techniques, demonstrated the presence of a small amount of cholinesterase in the serum of two silent gene homozygotes. There is now clear evidence that this group is heterogeneous and that some possess about 2 percent of the normal activity, although in others cholinesterase cannot be demonstrated [31, 32, 34–37].

Rubinstein et al. [40] have investigated 25 sera from 13 families. Eleven of the families were Alaskan Eskimo. They classified the sera into two types. Type 1 sera (16 cases from 8 families) had an activity against acetylthiocholine of about 1 percent of the normal. The ratio of hydrolysis of acetylthiocholine to butyrylthiocholine varied between 2.9 and 10.3. The average inhibition produced by dibucaine was 5 percent, by quinidine, 51 percent, and by Mytelase, 67 percent. The sera did not react with a cholinesterase antiserum. These properties were similar to those of acetylcholinesterase obtained from red cell stroma. Type 2 sera (8 cases from

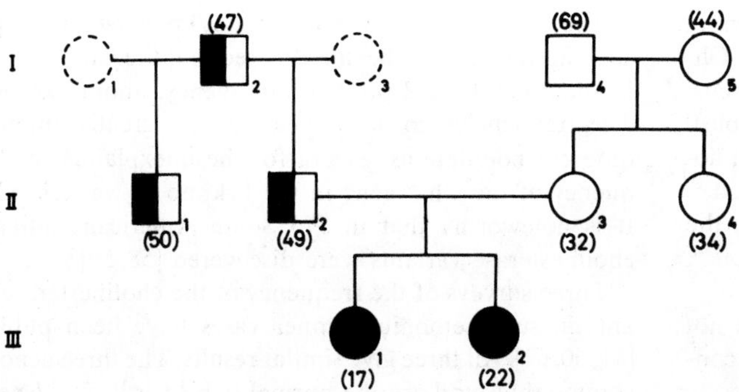

● Abnormal dibucaine number (presumed abnormal homozygote)

◐ Intermediate dibucaine number (presumed heterozygote)

○ Normal dibucaine number (presumed normal homozygote)

◌ Not tested

Figures in brackets show enzyme level

Figure 74-4. One family with an anomalous inheritance (see text). (*After Liddell, Lehmann, and Silk* [30].)

5 families) had an acetylthiocholine hydrolyzing activity of about 2 percent of normal, while the ratio of acetyl to butyrylthiocholine activity was less than 1. Dibucaine inhibited by 68 percent, quinidine, by 83 percent, and Mytelase, by 26 percent. The sera reacted with cholinesterase antisera. These results are similar to those seen with normal cholinesterase. One serum had properties intermediate between the two types. Rubinstein and his colleagues therefore suggested that type 1 sera were due to a truly "silent gene," with the residual cholinesterase activity probably coming from the red cell ghosts, whereas type 2 sera were due to a variant producing small amounts of normal enzyme. Scott [32], using different techniques from Rubinstein and his colleagues, studied 48 Alaskan Eskimo with cholinesterase deficiency. Thirty persons from fourteen families were completely deficient (Rubinstein et al., type 1), and fifteen persons from twelve families had a trace amount of enzyme (Rubinstein et al., type 2).

It is difficult to identify the heterozygote for the normal and silent genes. A review of the literature has shown that the serum cholinesterase level in this genotype varies between 28 percent and 114 percent of the normal mean, while 69 percent of patients had values within the normal range [41].

Two cases of suxamethonium apnea have been reported in heterozygotes for the silent gene and for fluoride resistance [42, 43].

The C_5 Variant

Harris, Hopkinson, and Robson [6] separated four cholinesterase isoenzymes by gel electrophoresis of normal serum. The slowest moving, C_4, contained about 90 percent of the activity. In about 10 percent of the British population a still slower-moving C_5 band is found. This is genetically determined [44, 45]. Penetrance is incomplete, and the affected individuals appear to be heterozygous or homozygous for another cholinesterase gene. These C_5^+ people are not sensitive to suxamethonium, and their mean activity is about 30 percent higher than normal.

This variant is not an allele of the others [4–6], which suggests that there are two genes responsible for cholinesterase synthesis. An alternative explanation might be that C_5^+ individuals possess in their sera another genetically determined protein of unknown function which can polymerize with cholinesterase. Gallango and Arends [47] found an increased incidence of C_5 and also another cholinesterase isoenzyme in patients with myelomatosis. This could be due to formation of a complex between cholinesterase and an abnormal protein produced by the disease process. The polymerization theory does not explain the increased enzyme level in C_5^+ individuals. The correct genetic interpretation of this variant is still uncertain.

OTHER CHOLINESTERASE VARIANTS

A few family studies have been reported which cannot be explained by the above classification [48–51]. It appears probable from genetic studies of other proteins that many more rare cholinesterase variants exist.

Nomenclature and Recognition of the Variants

Two different nomenclatures have been proposed for the five well-established cholinesterase genes. The first is that proposed by Motulsky [52] using the symbol E for esterase, the second proposed by Goedde and Baitsch [53] uses the symbol Ch. There are two cholinesterase loci, E_1 and E_2, or Ch_1 and Ch_2. There are four known variants at the first locus: the usual gene $E_1{}^u$, or $Ch_1{}^U$, the gene for the atypical dibucaine-resistant enzyme $E_1{}^a$, or $Ch_1{}^D$; the gene for fluoride resistance $E_1{}^f$, or $Ch_1{}^F$, and the silent gene, $E_1{}^s$, or $Ch_1{}^S$. There are only two known variants at the second locus: the usual enzyme $E_2{}^-$, or $Ch_2{}^-$ and the C_5 variant $E_2{}^+$, or $Ch_2{}^+$. The two systems are listed in Table 74-1.

The relationship and function of the two genes is not known. It is at least possible that the Ch_2 locus is not concerned with cholinesterase synthesis. The Ch_1 locus is closely linked with the transferrin locus [54].

The usual technique for phenotype identification uses the benzoylcholine assay with dibucaine [18] and fluoride [21]. Inhibition with butanol also gives good differentition of this variant [22], but it is difficult to distinguish $Ch_1{}^UCh_1{}^F$ individuals from $Ch_1{}^UCh_1{}^U$ and $Ch_1{}^UCh_1{}^D$, while $Ch_1{}^F$ homozygotes may be confused with the $Ch_1{}^UCh_1{}^D$ heterozygotes (see Table 74-1).

Das and Liddell [55] have proposed using the butyrylthiocholine assay and measuring RO2-0683 inhibition and activity remaining after 15-min incubation with 6 percent butanol (see Table 74-1). This improves the identification of some genotypes.

Suxamethonium Sensitivity

The frequency of the $Ch_1{}^D$ gene is about 0.019 in Western Europe and Canada [56, 57].

This figure has been derived from population surveys identifying the heterozygote. The $Ch_1{}^DCh_1{}^D$ homozygote should therefore occur with a frequency of 1 in 2,800, and this accords reasonably well with the occurrence of suxamethonium apnea in this genotype.

The other gene frequencies are not known with any precision, although it has been estimated that the $Ch_1{}^F$ frequency is about 0.0018 and the $Ch_1{}^S$ frequency, about 0.0029 [41]. The frequencies do not appear to vary greatly among the different populations, except for the unexplained high frequency of the $Ch_1{}^S$ gene in the Eskimo of western Alaska. It is noteworthy that in 576 South American Indians no cholinesterase variants were discovered [58, 59].

Three surveys of the frequency of the cholinesterase variants in suxamethonium apnea cases have been published [41, 60, 61]. All three give similar results. The three genotypes commonly found are the normal ($Ch_1{}^DCh_1{}^D$) in 37 percent of cases, the atypical homozygote ($Ch_1{}^DCh_1{}^D$), in 44 percent, and the atypical heterozygote ($Ch_1{}^UCh_1{}^D$), in 10 percent. The other genotypes are uncommon. The cause of suxamethonium apnea in patients with an apparently normal cholinesterase genotype is not known. It seems likely to be a number of unrelated causes, e.g., anoxia, although some cases might be due to a variant which present techniques cannot detect. We have seen at least one case where family studies showed that one sensitive individual was a $Ch_1{}^UCh_1{}^S$ heterozygote.

The $Ch_1{}^DCh_1{}^D$, $Ch_1{}^DCh_1{}^F$, $Ch_1{}^DCh_1{}^S$ and $Ch_1{}^SCh_1{}^S$ subjects usually have apnea lasting 2 or 3 hr, while the apnea in other sensitive genotypes is considerably shorter. In some genotypes only a proportion show suxamethonium sensitivity. Thus only about 1 in 500 of the atypical heterozygotes ($Ch_1{}^UCh_1{}^D$) appears to develop a prolonged apnea. These findings are summarized in the table.

SUMMARY

1 A number of cholinesterase variants are determined by two genetic loci (Ch_1 and Ch_2). The variants at the Ch_1 locus are recognized by an altered sensitivity of the enzyme to

Table 74-1. THE NOMENCLATURE, BIOCHEMICAL CHARACTERISTICS, FREQUENCY AND SUXAMETHONIUM SENSITIVITY OF THE CHOLINESTERASE GENOTYPES AT THE Ch_1 (E_1) LOCUS

Nomenclature		*Benzoylcholine assay*		*Butyrylthiocholine assay*				
Goedde and Baitsch (1964)	Motulsky (1964)	Dibucaine number	Fluoride number	R02-0683 inhibition	R02-0683 inhibition	Activity with 6% butanol	Frequency	Suxamethonium Sensitivity
Homozygotes								
$Ch_1{}^U\ Ch_1{}^U$	$E_1{}^u\ E_1{}^u$	80	62	95	97	100	Normal population	? 1 in 3,200 moderately sensitive
$Ch_1{}^D\ Ch_1{}^D$	$E_1{}^a\ E_1{}^a$	20	22	10	7	3	1 in 2,800	All markedly sensitive
$Ch_1{}^F\ Ch_1{}^F$	$E_1{}^f\ E_1{}^f$	65	35	80	73	3	? 1 in 300,000	? All moderately sensitive
$Ch_1{}^S\ Ch_1{}^S$	$E_1{}^s\ E_1{}^s$	....	....	....	....	....	? 1 in 140,000	All markedly sensitive
Heterozygotes								
$Ch_1{}^U\ Ch_1{}^D$	$E_1{}^u\ E_1{}^a$	60	50	65	70	74	1 in 26	? 1 in 500 moderately sensitive
$Ch_1{}^U\ Ch_1{}^F$	$E_1{}^u\ E_1{}^f$	75	52	90	87	74	? 1 in 280	? 1 in 200 moderately sensitive
$Ch_1{}^U\ Ch_1{}^S$	$E_1{}^u\ E_1{}^s$	80	62	95	97	100	? 1 in 190	Not known; probably similar to $Ch_1{}^U\ Ch_1{}^D$
$Ch_1{}^D\ Ch_1{}^F$	$E_1{}^a\ E_1{}^f$	50	35	55	63	11	? 1 in 29,000	? All markedly sensitive
$Ch_1{}^D\ Ch_1{}^S$	$E_1{}^a\ E_1{}^s$	20	22	10	7	3	? 1 in 20,000	All markedly sensitive
$Ch_1{}^F\ Ch_1{}^S$	$E_1{}^f\ E_1{}^s$	65	35	80	73	3	? 1 in 200,000	? All moderately sensitive

inhibitors such as dibucaine, RO2-0683, flouride, and butanol. The one unusual variant at the Ch_2 locus (Ch_2^+) produces an extra cholinesterase band on gel electrophoresis.
2 The most frequent variant at the Ch_1 locus is the atypical (Ch_1^D) gene. The homozygote for this trait is highly sensitive to the muscle relaxant suxamethonium, and a small proportion of heterozygotes are slightly sensitive.
3 Two further rare alleles have been found at the Ch_1 locus. The Ch_1^F gene directs synthesis of an enzyme recognized by an altered response to inhibition by sodium fluoride. The Ch_1^S (silent) gene appears to consist of at least two types. Type 1 determines a complete absence of cholinesterase activity. Type 2 produces an activity of about 2 percent of the normal level. Homozygotes for the Ch_1^F and Ch_1^S genes are also sensitive to suxamethonium.

BIBLIOGRAPHY

1. Vogel, F.: Moderne probleme der Humangenetik. Ergebn. Inn. Med. Kinderheilk., **12,** 52, 1959.
2. *Report of the Commission on Enzymes of the International Union of Biochemistry.* Pergamon, New York, 1961.
3. Kalow, W., and Lindsay, H. A.: A comparison of optical and manometric methods for the assay of human serum cholinesterase. Canad. J. Biochem. Physiol., **33,** 568, 1955.
4. Ellman, G. L., Courtney, K. D., Andres, V., and Featherstone, R. M.: A new and rapid colorimetric determination of acetylcholinesterase activity. Biochem. Pharm., **7,** 88, 1961.
5. Das, P. K., and Liddell, J.: Purification and properties of human serum cholinesterase. Biochem. J., **116,** 875, 1970.
6. Harris, H., Hopkinson, D. A., and Robson, E. B.: Two dimensional electrophoresis of pseudocholinesterase components in human serum. Nature (London), **196,** 1296, 1962.
7. Juul, P.: Human plasma cholinesterase isoenzymes. Clin. Chim. Acta, **19,** 205, 1968.
8. Harris, H., and Robson, E. B.: Fractionation of human serum cholinesterase components by gel filtration. Biochem. Biophys. Acta, **73,** 649, 1963.
9. Svensmark, O.: Human serum cholinesterase as a sialo-protein. Acta Physiol. Scand., **52,** 267, 1961.
10. Evans, F. T., Gray, P. W. S., Lehmann, H., and Silk, E.: Sensitivity to succinylcholine in relation to serum-cholinesterase. Lancet, **1,** 1229, 1952.
11. Bourne, J. G., Collier, H. O., and Somers, G. F.: Succinylcholine (succinoylcholine): muscle relaxant of short action. Lancet, **1,** 1225, 1952.
12. Forbat, A., Lehmann, H., and Silk, E.: Prolonged apnoea following injection of succinyldicholine. Lancet, **2,** 1067, 1953.
13. Lehmann, H., and Ryan, E.: The familial incidence of low pseudocholinesterase level. Lancet, **2,** 124, 1956.
14. Lehmann, H., Patston, V., and Ryan, E.: The inheritance of an idiopathic low plasma pseudocholinesterase level. J. Clin. Path., **11,** 554, 1958.
15. Lehmann, H., Silk, E, and Liddell, J.: Pseudocholinesterase. Brit. Med. Bull., **17,** 230, 1961.
16. Davies, R. O., Marton, A. V., and Kalow, W.: The action of normal and atypical cholinesterase of human serum upon a series of esters of choline. Canad. J. Biochem. Physiol., **38,** 545, 1960.
17. Kalow, W., and Davies, R. O.: The activity of various esterase inhibitors towards atypical human serum cholinesterase. Biochem. Pharmacol., **1,** 183, 1958.
18. Kalow, W., and Genest, K.: A method for the detection of atypical forms of human cholinesterase: determination of dibucaine numbers. Canad. J. Biochem. Physiol., **35,** 339. 1957.
19. Liddell, J., Lehmann, H., and Davies, D.: Harris and Whittakers pseudocholinesterase variant with increased resistance to fluoride: a study of four families and identification of the homozygote. Acta Genet., **13,** 95, 1963.
20. Harris, H., and Whittaker, M.: Differential inhibition of human serum cholinesterase with fluoride: recognition of two phenotypes. Nature (London), **191,** 496, 1961.
21. Whittaker, M.: The pseudocholinesterase variants: differentiation by means of alkyl alcohols. Acta Genet., **18,** 325, 1968.
22. Whittaker, M.: Differential inhibition of human serum cholinesterase with *n*-butyl alcohol: recognition of new phenotypes. Acta Genet., **18,** 335, 1968.
23. Liddell, J., Lehmann, H., Davies, D., and Sharih, A.: Physical separation of pseudocholinesterase variants in human serum. Lancet, **1,** 643, 1962.
24. Liddell, J., Newman, G. E., and Brown, D. F.: A pseudocholinesterase variant in human tissues. Nature (London), **198,** 1090, 1963.
25. Harris, H., and Whittaker, M.: The serum cholinesterase variants: a study of twenty-two families selected via the intermediate phenotype. Ann. Hum. Genet., **26,** 59, 1962.
26. Harris, H., and Whittaker. M.: Differential inhibition of "usual" and "atypical" serum cholinesterase by sodium chloride and sodium fluoride. Ann. Hum. Genet., **27,** 53, 1963.
27. Lehmann, H., Liddell, J., Blackwell, B., O'Connor, D. C., and Daws, Ann V.: Two further serum pseudocholinesterase phenotypes as causes of suxamethonium apnoea. Brit. Med. J., **1,** 1116, 1963.
28. Whittaker, M.: The pseudocholinesterase variants: esterase levels and increased resistance to fluoride. Acta Genet., **14,** 281, 1964.
29. Griffiths, P. D., Davies, D., and Lehmann, H.: A second family demonstrating the homozygote for the fluoride-resistant pseudocholinesterase variant. Brit. Med. J., **2,** 215, 1966.
30. Liddell, J., Lehmann, H., and Silk, E.: A "silent" pseudocholinesterase gene. Nature. (London), **193,** 1561, 1962.
31. Gutsche, B. B., Scott, E. M., and Wright, R. C.: Hereditary deficiency of pseudocholinesterase in Eskimos. Nature (London), **215,** 322, 1967.
32. Scott, E. M.: Properties of the trace enzyme in human serum cholinesterase deficiency. Biochem. Biophys. Res. Commun., **38,** 902, 1970.
33. Simpson, N. E. and Kalow, W.: The "silent" gene for serum cholinesterase. Amer. J. Hum. Genet., **18,** 243, 1964.
34. Goedde, H. W., Gehring, D., and Hofmann, R. A.: On the problem of a "silent gene" in pseudocholinesterase polymorphism. Biochim. Biophys. Acta, **107,** 391, 1965.
35. Hodgkin, W. E., Giblett, E. R., Levine, H., Bauer, E. W., and Motulsky, A. G.: Complete pseudocholinesterase deficiency: genetic and immunologic characterisation. J. Clin. Invest., **44,** 486, 1965.
36. Goedde, H. W., and Altand, K.: Evidence for different "silent genes" in the human serum pseudocholinesterase polymorphism. Ann. N.Y. Acad. Sci., **151,** 540, 1968.
37. Das, P. K.: Studies on human serum cholinesterase. Ph.D. Thesis, London University, 1969.
38. Gaffney, P. J., and Lehmann, H.: Residual enzyme activity in the serum of a homozygote for the silent pseudocholinesterase gene. Hum. Hered. **19,** 234, 1969.
39. Kalow, W.: Cholinesterase types; in Ciba Foundation, *Symposium on Biochemistry of Human Genetics,* edited by G. E. W. Wolstenholme, and C. M. O'Connor, Churchill, London, 1960.
40. Rubinstein, H. M., Dietz, A. A., Hodges, L. K., Lubrano, T., and Czebotar, V.: Silent cholinesterase gene: Variations in the properties of serum enzyme in apparent homozygotes. J. Clin. Invest., **49,** 479, 1970.
41. Lehmann, H., and Liddell, J.: Human cholinesterase (pseudocholinesterase) Genetic variants and their recognition. Brit. J. Anaesth., **41,** 235, 1969.
42. Whittaker, M.: The pseudocholinesterase variants: a study of fourteen families selected via the fluoride resistant phenotype. Acta Genet., **17,** 1, 1967.
43. Simpson, N. E.: A second heterozygote for "silent" and "fluoride resistant" genes for serum cholinesterase. J. Med. Genet., **4,** 264, 1967.
44. Harris, H., Hopkinson, D. A., Robson, E. B., and Whittaker, M.: Genetical studies on a new variant of serum cholinesterase detected by electrophoresis. Ann. Hum. Genet., **26,** 359, 1963.
45. Robson, E. B., and Harris, H.: Further data on the incidence and genetics

of the serum cholinesterase phenotype C_5^+. Ann. Hum. Genet., **29**, 403, 1966.

46. Harris, H., Robson, E. B., Glen-Blott, A. M., and Thornton, J. A.: Evidence for non-allelism between genes affecting human serum cholinesterase. Nature (London), **200**, 1185, 1963.
47. Gallango, M. L., and Arends, T.: Phenotypical variants of pseudocholinesterase in myeloma patients. Humangenetik. **7**, 104, 1969.
48. Lehmann, H., Silk, E., Harris, H., and Whittaker, M.: A new pseudocholinesterase phenotype? Acta Genet., **10**, 241, 1960.
49. Neitlich, H. W.: Increased plasma cholinesterase activity and succinylcholine resistance: a genetic variant. J. Clin. Invest., **45**, 380, 1966.
50. Whittaker, M.: An additional pseudocholinesterase phenotype occuring in suxamethonium apnoea. Brit. J. Anaesth., **40**, 579, 1968.
51. Yoshida, A., and Motulsky, A. G.: A pseudocholinesterase variant (E Cynthiana) associated with elevated plasma enzyme activity. Amer. J. Hum. Genet. **21**, 486, 1969.
52. Motulsky, A. G.: Pharmacogenetics, in *Progress in Medical Genetics,* vol. III, edited by A. G. Steinburg, and A. G. Bearn. Grune and Stratton, New York 1964.
53. Goedde, H. W., and Baitsch, H.: Nomenclature of pseudocholinesterase polymorphism. Brit. Med. J., **2**, 310, 1964.
54. Robson, E. B., Sutherland, O., and Harris, H.: Evidence for linkage between the transferrin locus (Tf) and the serum cholinesterase locus (E) in man. Ann. Hum. Genet., **29**, 325, 1966.
55. Das, P. K. and Liddell, J.: The diagnosis of the cholinesterase variants using butyrylthiocholine. J. Med. Genetics. In press.
56. Kalow, W., and Gunn, D. R.: Some statistical data on atypical cholinesterase of human serum. Ann. Hum. Genet., **23**, 239, 1958.
57. Kattamis, C., Zannos-Manolea, L., Franco, A. P., Liddell, J., Lehmann, H., and Davies, D.: Frequency of atypical pseudocholinesterase in British and Mediterranean populations. Nature (London), **196**, 599, 1962.
58. Arends, T., Davies, D. A. and Lehmann, H.: Absence of variants of usual pseudocholinesterase (acylcholine acyl hydrolase) in South American Indians. Acta Genet. (Basel), **17**, 13, 1967.
59. Tashian, R. E., Brewer, G. J., Lehmann, H., Davies, D. A. and Rucknagel, D. L.: Further studies on the Xavante Indians. Amer. J. Hum. Genet., **19**, 524, 1967.
60. Kalow, W.: Contribution of hereditary factors to the response drugs. Fed. Proc., **24**, 1259, 1965.
61. Thompson, J. C. and Whittaker, M.: A study of the pseudocholinesterase in 78 cases of apnoea following suxamethonium. Acta Genet., **16**, 209, 1966.

INDEX